Expert | CONSULT

Activate your access at expertconsult.com

1 REGISTER

- Visit **expertconsult.com.**
- Click **"Register Now."**
- Fill in your **user information.**
- Click **"Create Account."**

2 ACTIVATE YOUR BOOK

- Scratch off your **Activation Code** below and enter it into the **"Add a title"** box.
- **You're done!** Click on the book's title under **"My Titles."**

For technical assistance, email **online.help@elsevier.com** or call **800-401-9962** (inside the US) or **+1-314-995-3200** (outside the US).

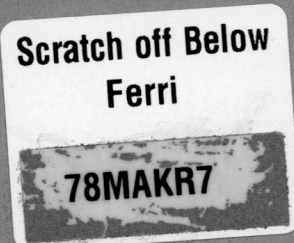

Scratch off Below
Ferri

78MAKR7

Activation Code

2012

Ferri's CLINICAL ADVISOR

5 Books in 1

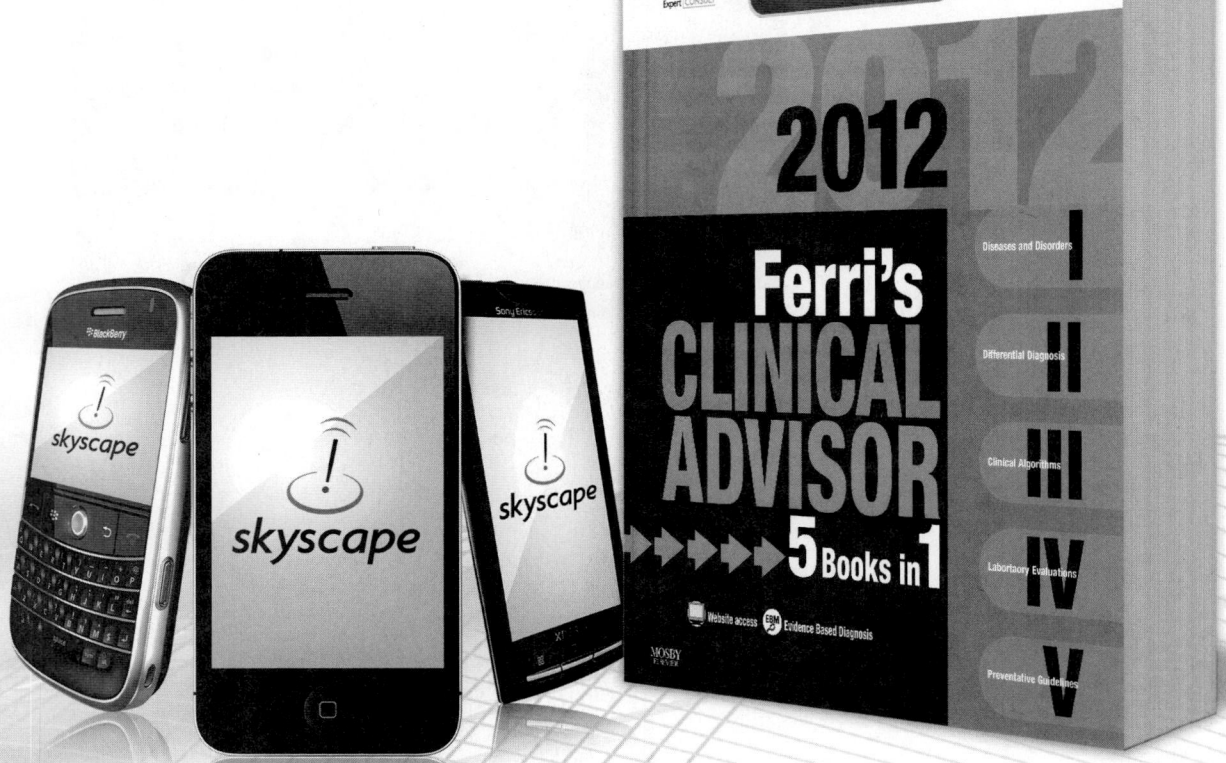

2012

Ferri's CLINICAL ADVISOR

5 Books in 1

FRED F. FERRI, M.D., F.A.C.P.
Clinical Professor
Alpert Medical School
Brown University
Providence, Rhode Island

ELSEVIER
MOSBY

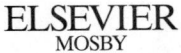

1600 John F. Kennedy Blvd.
Ste 1800
Philadelphia, PA 19103-2899

FERRI'S CLINICAL ADVISOR 2012: 5 BOOKS IN 1

ISBN: 978-0-323-05611-3
ISSN: 1541-4515

Copyright © 2012, 2011, 2010, 2009, 2008, 2007, 2006, 2005, 2004, 2003, 2002, 2001, 2000, 1999 by Mosby, Inc., an affiliate of Elsevier Inc.

Notices

Knowledge and best practice in this field are constantly changing. As new research and experience broaden our understanding, changes in research methods, professional practices, or medical treatment may become necessary.

Practitioners and researchers must always rely on their own experience and knowledge in evaluating and using any information, methods, compounds, or experiments described herein. In using such information or methods they should be mindful of their own safety and the safety of others, including parties for whom they have a professional responsibility.

With respect to any drug or pharmaceutical products identified, readers are advised to check the most current information provided (i) on procedures featured or (ii) by the manufacturer of each product to be administered, to verify the recommended dose or formula, the method and duration of administration, and contraindications. It is the responsibility of practitioners, relying on their own experience and knowledge of their patients, to make diagnoses, to determine dosages and the best treatment for each individual patient, and to take all appropriate safety precautions.

To the fullest extent of the law, neither the Publisher nor the authors, contributors, or editors, assume any liability for any injury and/or damage to persons or property as a matter of products liability, negligence or otherwise, or from any use or operation of any methods, products, instructions, or ideas contained in the material herein.

ISBN: 978-0-323-05611-3
ISSN: 1541-4515

Acquisitions Editor: Kate Dimock
Developmental Editor: Virginia Wilson
Editorial Assistant: Kate Crowley
Publishing Services Manager: Pat Joiner-Myers
Senior Project Manager: Joy Moore
Designer: Steven Stave
Marketing Manager: Tracie Pasker

Printed in the United States of America

Last digit is the print number: 9 8 7 6 5 4 3 2 1

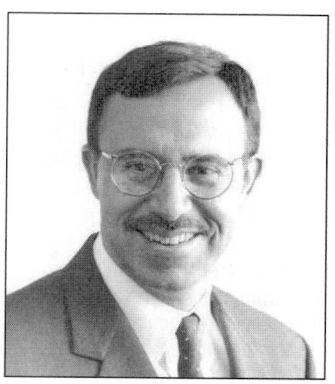

RUBEN ALVERO, M.D.
Director
Assisted Reproductive Technologies
Residency Program Director
Vice Chairman for Education
Department of Obstetrics and
    Gynecology
University of Colorado Denver
Aurora, Colorado
SECTION I

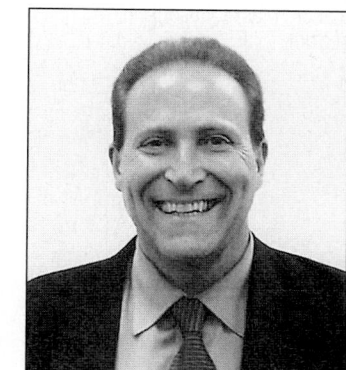

**FRED F. FERRI,
M.D., F.A.C.P.**
Clinical Professor
Alpert Medical School
Brown University
Providence, Rhode Island
SECTIONS I-V

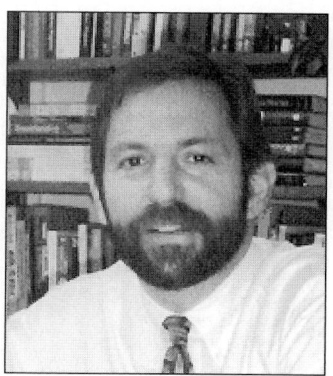

**JEFFREY M. BORKAN,
M.D., PH.D.**
Professor and Chair
Department of Family Medicine
Memorial Hospital of Rhode Island
Pawtucket, Rhode Island
Alpert Medical School
Brown University
Providence, Rhode Island
SECTION I

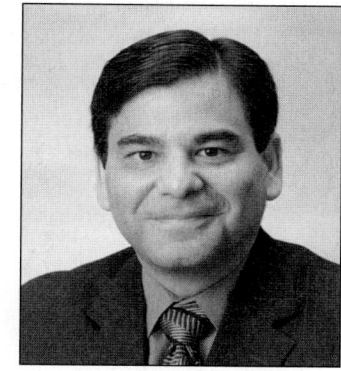

**GLENN G. FORT, M.D.,
M.P.H., F.A.C.P., F.I.D.S.A.**
Clinical Associate Professor of
    Medicine
Alpert Medical School
Brown University
Providence, Rhode Island
Chief
Infectious Diseases
Our Lady of Fatima Hospital
North Providence, Rhode Island
SECTION I

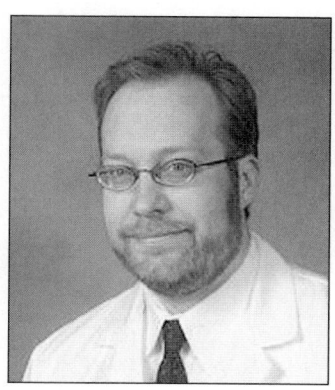

MICHAEL R. DOBBS, M.D.
Associate Professor and Vice-Chair
Assistant Professor
Neurology and Preventative
    Medicine
Neurology Residency Program
    Director
Medical Director
Stroke Care
Chandler Medical Center
University of Kentucky
Lexington, Kentucky
SECTION I

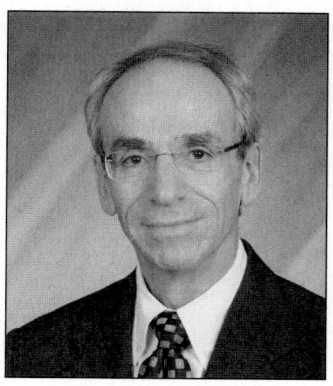

**RICHARD J. GOLDBERG,
M.D., M.S.**
Psychiatrist-in-Chief
Rhode Island Hospital and the
    Miriam Hospital
Professor
Department of Psychiatry and
    Human Behavior
Alpert Medical School
Brown University
Providence, Rhode Island
SECTION I

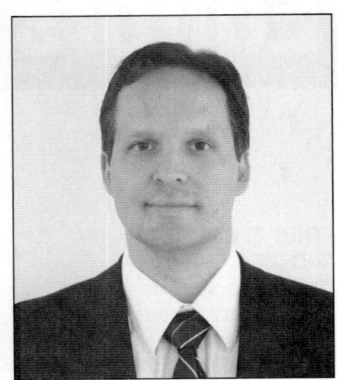

HARALD ALEXANDER HALL, M.D.
Director
Rheumatology Fellowship Program
Roger Williams Medical Center
Assistant Professor of Medicine
Boston University School of
   Medicine
Boston, Massachusetts
SECTION I

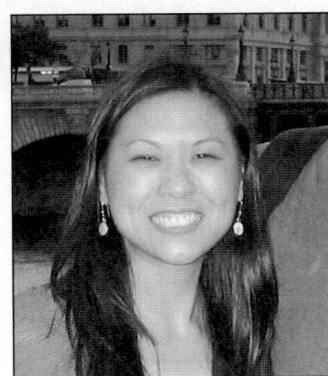

IRIS TONG, M.D.
Assistant Professor
Department of Medicine
Alpert Medical School
Brown University
Providence, Rhode Island
SECTION I

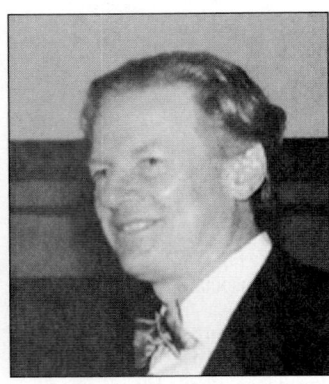

DENNIS J. MIKOLICH, M.D., F.A.C.P., F.C.C.P.
Chief
Division of Infectious Diseases
VA Medical Center
Clinical Associate Professor of
   Medicine
Brown Medical School
Providence, Rhode Island
SECTION I

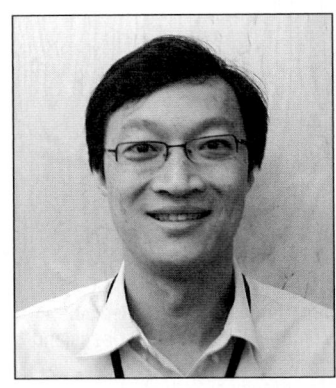

WEN-CHIH WU, M.D.
Staff Cardiologist
Providence VA Medical Center
Associate Professor of Medicine
Alpert Medical School
Brown University
Providence, Rhode Island
SECTION I

SONYA S. ABDEL-RAZEQ, M.D.
Clinical Assistant Instructor
Department of Obstetrics and Gynecology/Resident Education
State University of New York at Buffalo
Women's and Children's Hospital
Buffalo, New York

ABDULRAHMAN ABDULBAKI, M.D.
Cardiology Fellow
Louisiana State University and Health Science Center
Shreveport, Louisiana

MONZR M. AL MALKI, M.D.
Biotherapeutics Development Laboratory
Division of Surgical Research
Boston University School of Medicine
Roger Williams Medical Center
Providence, Rhode Island

TANYA ALI, M.D.
Clinical Assistant Professor of Medicine
Department of Medicine
Alpert Medical School
Brown University
Providence, Rhode Island

PHILIP J. ALIOTTA, M.D., M.S.H.A., F.A.C.S.
Clinical Instructor
Department of Urology
School of Medicine and Biomedical Sciences
State University of New York at Buffalo
Buffalo, New York
Medical Director
Center for Urologic Research of Western New York
Williamsville, New York

RUBEN ALVERO, M.D.
Director, Assisted Reproductive Technologies
Residency Program Director
Vice Chairman for Education
Department of Obstetrics and Gynecology
University of Colorado Denver
Aurora, Colorado

SRIVIDYA ANANDAN, M.D.
Attending Physician
Internal Medicine
Harvard Vanguard Medical Associates
Quincy, Massachusetts

GOWRI ANANDARAJAH, M.D.
Professor of Family Medicine (Clinical)
Clinical Associate Professor
Department of Family Medicine
Alpert Medical School
Brown University
Providence, Rhode Island

MEL L. ANDERSON, M.D., F.A.C.P.
Assistant Professor of Medicine
University of Colorado School of Medicine
Denver Veterans Affairs Medical Center
Denver, Colorado

MICHELLE STOZEK ANVAR, M.D.
Clinical Instructor
Division of General Internal Medicine
Rhode Island Hospital
Clinical Instructor
Alpert Medical School
Brown University
Providence, Rhode Island

ETSUKO AOKI, M.D., PH.D.
Attending Physician
Department of Hematology
Nagoya Medical Center
Nagoya, Japan

NICOLE APPELLE, M.D.
Assistant Professor of Internal Medicine
University of California, San Francisco
San Francisco, California

WISSAM S.Z. ASFAHANI, M.D.
Department of Neurosurgery
University of Kentucky
Lexington, Kentucky

SUDEEP KAUR AULAKH, M.D., C.M., F.R.C.P.C.
Director of Ambulatory Education
High Street Health Center Assistant
Professor of Medicine
Tufts University School of Medicine Baystate
Medical Center
Springfield, Massachusetts

CRISOSTOMO R. BALIOG, Jr., M.D.
Rheumatology Fellow
Division of Rheumatology
Roger Williams Hospital
Boston University School of Medicine
Providence, Rhode Island

PRIYA BANSAL, M.D., M.P.H.
Physician
Internal Medicine
Miriam Hospital/Rhode Island Hospital
Providence, Rhode Island

ROWLAND P. BARRETT, PH.D.
Associate Professor of Psychiatry & Human Behavior
Alpert Medical School
Brown University
Providence, Rhode Island

VIKRAM BEHERA, M.D.
Clinical Instructor of Medicine
Brown Medical School
Providence, Rhode Island

OMRI BERGER, M.D.
Fellow
Psychiatry and the Law Program
Department of Psychiatry
University of California, San Francisco
San Francisco, California

SETH A. BERKOWITZ, M.D.
Department of Medicine
University of California, San Francisco
San Francisco, California

MICHAEL BLUNDIN, M.D.
Pulmonary and Critical Care
Rhode Island Hospital
Providence, Rhode Island

SHEENAGH M. BODKIN, M.D.
Woman and Infants Hospital
Alpert Medical School
Brown University
Providence, Rhode Island

NIRALI BORA, M.D.
Assistant Clinical Instructor of Family Medicine
Alpert Medical School
Brown University
Providence, Rhode Island
Memorial Hospital of Rhode Island
Pawtucket, Rhode Island

JEFFREY M. BORKAN, M.D., PH.D.
Professor and Chair
Department of Family Medicine
Memorial Hospital of Rhode Island
Pawtucket, Rhode Island
Alpert Medical School
Brown University
Providence, Rhode Island

ALEXANDRA BOSKE, M.D.
Resident
Department of Neurology
University of Kentucky
Lexington, Kentucky

LYNN BOWLBY, M.D., F.A.C.P.
Medical Director
Duke Outpatient Clinic (DOC)
Duke Internal Medicine Residency Program
Durham, North Carolina

MARK F. BRADY, M.D., M.P.H., M.M.S.
Department of Emergency Medicine
Yale-New Haven Hospital
New Haven, Connecticut

MANDEEP K. BRAR, M.D.
Clinical Assistant Professor
Department of Obstetrics and Gynecology
State University of New York at Buffalo
Buffalo, New York

ELIZABETH BROWN, M.D.
Assistant Clinical Instructor of Family Medicine
Memorial Hospital of Rhode Island
Alpert Medical School
Brown University
Pawtucket, Rhode Island

GAVIN BROWN, M.D.
Neuromuscular Fellow
Emory University
Atlanta, Georgia

JENNIFER BUCKLEY, M.D.
Assistant Clinical Instructor of Family Medicine
Memorial Hospital of Rhode Island
Alpert Medical School
Brown University
Providence, Rhode Island

JONATHAN BURNS, M.A., M.D.
Assistant Clinical Instructor of Family Medicine
Alpert Medical School
Brown University
Providence, Rhode Island

D. BRANDON BURTIS, D.O.
Behavioral Neurology Fellow
Department of Neurology
College of Medicine
University of Florida
Gainesville, Florida

DOUGLAS BURTT, M.D.
Clinical Assistant Professor of Medicine
Division of Cardiology
Alpert Medical School
Brown University
Providence, Rhode Island

STEVEN BUSSELEN, M.D.
Medical Director
Tri-Town Health Center
Johnston, Rhode Island

CLAUDIA RODRIGUEZ CABRERA, M.D.
Internal Medicine Residency Program Director
Hospital Regional Universitario de Jose Maria
Cabral y Baez
Santiago, Dominican Republic

NIDA CHAUDHARY, M.D.
House Officer
Internal Medicine Residency Program
Alpert Medical School
Brown University
Providence, Rhode Island

GAURAV CHOUDHARY, M.D.
Assistant Professor of Medicine
Alpert Medical School
Brown University
Providence, Rhode Island

STEPHANIE W. CHOW, M.D.
Assistant Clinical Instructor of Family Medicine
Alpert Medical School
Brown University
Providence, Rhode Island

SCOTT COHEN, M.D.
Fellow in Cardiology
Alpert Medical School
Brown University
Providence, Rhode Island

KAILA COMPTON, M.D., Ph.D.
Department of Psychiatry
Residency Training Program
University of California, San Francisco
San Francisco, California

MARIA A. CORIGLIANO, M.D., F.A.C.O.G.
Clinical Assistant Professor
Department of Obstetrics and Gynecology
State University of New York at Buffalo
Buffalo, New York

BRIAN J. COWLES, PHARM.D.
Assistant Professor of Pharmacy
Department of Pharmacy Practice
Albany College of Pharmacy and Health Sciences, Vermont Campus
Colchester, Vermont

PATRICIA CRISTOFARO, M.D.
Assistant Professor of Medicine
Alpert Medical School
Brown University
Physician
Veterans' Hospital
Providence, Rhode Island

ALICIA J. CURTIN, Ph.D., G.N.P.
Assistant Professor
Division of Geriatrics
Alpert Medical School
Brown University
Providence, Rhode Island

KRISTY L. DALRYMPLE, Ph.D.
Assistant Professor (Research)
Department of Psychiatry and Human Behavior
Alpert Medical School
Brown University
Staff Psychologist
Department of Psychiatry
Rhode Island Hospital
Providence, Rhode Island

GEORGE T. DANAKAS, M.D., F.A.C.O.G.
Clinical Assistant Professor
Department of Obstetrics and Gynecology
State University of New York at Buffalo
Buffalo, New York

ALEXANDRA DEGENHARDT, M.D.
Director
Multiple Sclerosis Center
New York Methodist Hospital
Brooklyn, New York

GABRIEL A. DELGADO, M.D.
Fellow
Cardiology
Alpert Medical School
Brown University
Providence, Rhode Island

JOSEPH A. DIAZ, M.D.
Assistant Professor of Medicine
Division of General Internal Medicine
Memorial Hospital of Rhode Island
Alpert Medical School
Brown University
Providence, Rhode Island

MICHAEL R. DOBBS, M.D.
Associate Professor and Vice-Chair
Neurology and Preventative Medicine
Neurology Residency Program Director
Medical Director
Stroke Care
Chandler Medical Center
University of Kentucky
Lexington, Kentucky

AMANDA M. DONOHUE, D.O.
Fellow
Cardiovascular Medicine
University of California, Irvine
Irvine, California

WILLIAM F. DOTSON II, M.D.
Department of Neurology
Medical Center
University of Kentucky
Lexington, Kentucky

ANDREW DUKER, M.D.
Assistant Professor of Neurology
James J. and Joan A. Gardner Family Center for Parkinson's Disease
    and Movement Disorders
University of Cincinnati
Cincinnati, Ohio

THOMAS J. EARL, M.D.
Fellow
Cardiovascular Disease
Division of Cardiology
Department of Medicine
Alpert Medical School
Brown University
Providence, Rhode Island

AHMAD EDRIS, M.D.
Fellow
Cardiovascular Medicine
University of California, Irvine
Irvine, California

STUART J. EISENDRATH, M.D.
Professor of Clinical Psychiatry
Director of the UCSF Depression Center
Director of Clinical Services
Langley Porter Psychiatric Hospital and Clinics
University of California, San Francisco
San Francisco, California

CHRISTINE EISENHOWER, PHARM.D.
Doctor of Pharmacy Candidate
University of Rhode Island
Kingston, Rhode Island

PAMELA ELLSWORTH, M.D.
Associate Professor of Urology
Brown University
Providence, Rhode Island

HODA ELTOMI, M.D.
Assistant Clinical Instructor of Family Medicine
Memorial Hospital of Rhode Island
Pawtucket, Rhode Island
Alpert Medical School
Brown University
Providence, Rhode Island

GREGORY J. ESPER, M.D.
Director
General Neurology
Emory University
Atlanta, Georgia

PATRICIO SEBASTIAN ESPINOSA, M.D., M.P.H.
Adjunct Professor of Neurology and Pediatric Neurology
College of Health Sciences
Universidad San Francisco de Quito (USFQ)
Medical Staff
Hospital de los Valles
Cumbayá, Quito, Ecuador
Chairman
International Center of Neurosciences
Quito, Ecuador/New Orleans, Louisiana

VALERIA FABRE, M.D.
Resident
Internal Medicine
Memorial Hospital of Rhode Island
Pawtucket, Rhode Island
Alpert Medical School
Brown University
Providence, Rhode Island

MARK J. FAGAN, M.D.
Director
Medical Primary Care Unit
Rhode Island Hospital
Associate Professor of Medicine
Alpert Medical School
Brown University
Providence, Rhode Island

GIL M. FARKASH, M.D.
Assistant Clinical Professor
School of Medicine
State University of New York at Buffalo
Buffalo, New York

MITCHELL D. FELDMAN, M.D., M.PHIL.
Professor of Medicine
Director of Faculty Mentoring
Division of General Internal Medicine
University of California, San Francisco
San Francisco, California

FRED F. FERRI, M.D., F.A.C.P.
Clinical Professor
Alpert Medical School
Brown University
Providence, Rhode Island

GLEN FINNEY, M.D.
Assistant Professor
Department of Neurology
College of Medicine
University of Florida
Gainesville, Florida

STACI A. FISCHER, M.D., F.A.C.P., F.I.D.S.A.
Associate Professor of Medicine
Assistant Professor
Division of Infectious Diseases
Alpert Medical School
Brown University
Director
Graduate Medical Education Lifespan
Director
Transplant Infectious Diseases
Rhode Island Hospital
Providence, Rhode Island

MARLENE FISHMAN, M.P.H., C.I.C.
Director
Nosocomial Infection
St. Joseph Health Services of Rhode Island
North Providence, Rhode Island

ILJIE KIM FITZGERALD, M.D., M.S.
Department of Psychiatry
University of California, San Francisco
San Francisco, California
VA Greater Los Angeles Healthcare System
Los Angeles, California

TAMARA G. FONG, M.D., Ph.D.
Instructor in Neurology
Beth Israel Deaconess Medical Center
Harvard Medical School
Boston, Massachusetts

FRANK G. FORT, M.D., F.A.C.S.
Medical Director
Capital Region Vein Centre
Schenectady, New York

GLENN G. FORT, M.D., M.P.H., F.A.C.P., F.I.D.S.A.
Clinical Associate Professor of Medicine
Alpert Medical School
Brown University
Providence, Rhode Island
Chief
Infectious Diseases
Our Lady of Fatima Hospital
North Providence, Rhode Island

DAVID J. FORTUNATO, M.D., F.A.C.C.
Clinical Associate Professor of Medicine
Alpert Medical School
Brown University
Cardiology Section
VA Medical Center
Providence, Rhode Island

GREGORY K. FRITZ, M.D.
Professor and Director
Division of Child and Adolescent Psychiatry
Interim Vice Chair
Department of Psychiatry and Human Behavior
Alpert Medical School
Brown University
Academic Director
E.P. Bradley Hospital
Associate Chief and Director Child Psychiatry
Rhode Island Hospital
Hasbro Children's Hospital
Providence, Rhode Island

GENNA GEKHT, M.D.
Chief Resident in Neurology
Department of Neurology
Emory University
Atlanta, Georgia

ANTHONY S. GEMINIAGNI, M.D.
Fellow
Cardiology
Alpert Medical School
Brown University
Providence, Rhode Island

PAUL F. GEORGE, M.D.
Assistant Professor of Family Medicine
Memorial Hospital of Rhode Island
Alpert Medical School
Brown University
Providence, Rhode Island

ANNGENE A. GIUSTOZZI, M.D., M.P.H., F.A.A.F.P.
Assistant Professor
Department of Family Medicine
Alpert Medical School
Brown University
Providence, Rhode Island

CINDY GLEIT, M.D.
Assistant Clinical Instructor
Department of Family Medicine
Alpert Medical School
Brown University
Providence, Rhode Island

RICHARD J. GOLDBERG, M.D., M.S.
Psychiatrist-in-Chief
Rhode Island Hospital and The Miriam Hospital
Professor
Department of Psychiatry and Human Behavior
Alpert Medical School
Brown University
Providence, Rhode Island

GEETHA GOPALAKRISHNAN, M.D.
Assistant Professor of Medicine
Alpert Medical School
Brown University
Providence, Rhode Island

PAUL GORDON, M.D.
Clinical Assistant Professor of Medicine
Division of Cardiology
Alpert Medical School
Brown University
Providence, Rhode Island

NANCY R. GRAFF, M.D.
Associate Clinical Professor
Department of Pediatrics
University of California, San Diego
San Diego, California

JOHN A. GRAY, M.D., Ph.D.
Postdoctoral Fellow
Department of Cellular and Molecular Pharmacology
University of California, San Francisco
San Francisco, California

ALLISON D. GRAZIADEI, M.D.
Endocrinology Fellow
Division of Endocrinology
Alpert Medical School
Brown University
Providence, Rhode Island

PRIYA SARIN GUPTA, M.D.
Assistant Clinical Instructor of Family Medicine
Alpert School of Medicine
Brown University
Providence, Rhode Island

NAWAZ HACK, M.D.
Department of Neurology
Chandler Medical Center
University of Kentucky
Lexington, Kentucky

WILLIAM O. HAHN, M.D.
Brown Internal Medicine Residency Program
Providence, Rhode Island

HARALD ALEXANDER HALL, M.D.
Rheumatology Fellowship Program Director
Roger Williams Medical Center
Assistant Professor of Medicine
Boston University School of Medicine
Boston, Massachusetts

SAJEEV HANDA, M.D.
Director
Division of Hospitalist Medicine
Rhode Island Hospital
Clinical Instructor of Medicine
Alpert Medical School
Brown University
Providence, Rhode Island

TAYLOR HARRISON, M.D.
Assistant Professor of Neurology
Department of Neurology
Emory University
Atlanta, Georgia

DON HAYES, Jr., M.D.
Assistant Professor of Pediatrics and Internal Medicine
University of Kentucky College of Medicine
Director
University of Kentucky Pediatric Sleep Program
Kentucky Children's Hospital
Associate Director
University of Kentucky Healthcare Sleep Disorders Center
Lexington, Kentucky

CHRISTINE HEALY, D.O.
Assistant Clinical Instructor
Department of Family Medicine
Alpert Medical School
Brown University
Providence, Rhode Island

N. WILSON HOLLAND, M.D., F.A.C.P.
Assistant Professor of Medicine
Fellowship Director
Department of Medicine
Division of Geriatrics and Gerontology
Emory University School of Medicine
Atlanta Veterans Administration Medical Center
Atlanta, Georgia

SUSIE L. HU, M.D.
Assistant Professor of Medicine
Alpert Medical School
Brown University
Division of Kidney Disease and Hypertension
Rhode Island Hospital
Providence, Rhode Island

ANNE L. HUME, PHARM.D.
Professor of Pharmacy
Department of Pharmacy Practice
University of Rhode Island
Kingston, Rhode Island
Adjunct Professor of Family Medicine
Memorial Hospital of Rhode Island
Pawtucket, Rhode Island

RICHARD S. ISAACSON, M.D.
Resident in Neurology
Beth Israel Deaconess Medical Center
Harvard Medical School
Boston, Massachusetts

AHMAD M. ISMAIL, M.D.
Academic Hospitalist
Memorial Hospital of Rhode Island
Pawtucket, Rhode Island
Assistant Program Director
Internal Medicine Residency Program
Alpert Medical School
Brown University
Providence, Rhode Island

JENNIFER JEREMIAH, M.D.
Clinical Associate Professor of Medicine
Alpert Medical School
Brown University
Providence, Rhode Island

MICHAEL P. JOHNSON, M.D.
Staff Physician
Division of General Internal Medicine
Rhode Island Hospital
Assistant Professor of Medicine
Alpert Medical School
Brown University
Providence, Rhode Island

BREE JOHNSTON, M.D., M.P.H.
Associate Professor of Medicine
Division of Geriatrics
Department of Medicine
Veterans Affairs Medical Center
University of California, San Diego
San Diego, California

KIMBERLY JONES, M.D.
Resident Physician
Department of Child Neurology
University of Kentucky
Lexington, Kentucky

KOHAR JONES, M.D.
Clinical Assistant Professor
Department of Family Medicine
University of Chicago
Family Physician Chicago Family Health Center
Chicago, Illinois

LUCY KALANITHI, M.D.
Internal Medicine
Kaiser Permanente Medical Center
Oakland, California

MAHIM KAPOOR, M.D.
Resident in Internal Medicine
Alpert Medical School
Brown University
Providence, Rhode Island

EMILY R. KATZ, M.D.
Director
Child & Adolescent Psychiatry Consultation-Liaison Service
Hasbro Children's Hospital
Rhode Island Hospital
Assistant Professor (Clinical) of Psychiatry and Human Behavior
Alpert Medical School
Brown University
Providence, Rhode Island

ALI KAZIM, M.D.
Director
Psychiatry Emergency Service & Correctional Psychiatry
Rhode Island Hospital
Clinical Associate Professor
Department of Psychiatry and Human Behavior and Emergency Medicine
Alpert Medical School
Brown University
Providence, Rhode Island

BROOKE E. KEELEY, D.P.M.
Doctor of Podiatric Medicine
Roger Williams Medical Center
Department of Podiatric Surgery
Boston University School of Medicine
Boston, Massachusetts

KARA A. KENNEDY, D.O.
KY Clinic L-445
Department of Neurology
University of Kentucky
Lexington, Kentucky

BEVIN KENNEY, M.D.
Instructor in Medicine
Harvard University
Cambridge, Massachusetts
Primary Care Internist
Brookside Community Health Center
Jamaica Plain, Massachusetts

LARA KFOURY, M.D.
Renal Fellow
Division of Kidney Disease and Hypertension
Alpert Medical School
Brown University
Rhode Island Hospital
Providence, Rhode Island

WAN J. KIM, M.D.
Clinical Instructor
Department of Obstetrics and Gynecology
State University of New York at Buffalo
Buffalo, New York

ROBERT M. KIRCHNER, M.D.
Cardiology Fellow
Division of Cardiology
Alpert Medical School
Brown University
Providence, Rhode Island

MICHAEL KLEIN, M.D.
Clinical Assistant Professor
Department of Family Medicine
Alpert Medical School
Brown University
Providence, Rhode Island

MELVYN KOBY, M.D.
Associate Clinical Professor of Medicine
Department of Ophthalmology
University of Louisville School of Medicine
Louisville, Kentucky

ROBERT KOHN, M.D.
Professor
Department of Psychiatry and Human Behavior
Director
Geriatric Psychiatry Fellowship Training Program
Brown University
Providence, Rhode Island

KENNETH KORR, M.D.
Associate Professor of Medicine
Division of Cardiology
Alpert Medical School
Brown University
Providence, Rhode Island

KRISTINA KRAMER, M.D.
Medical Director
Intensive Care Unit
John Muir Medical Center
Walnut Creek, California

DAVID I. KURSS, M.D., F.A.C.O.G.
Clinical Assistant Professor
Department of Obstetrics and Gynecology
State University of New York at Buffalo
Buffalo, New York

CINDY LAI, M.D.
Associate Professor of Clinical Medicine
Intersessions Course Director
Site Director
Medicine Clerkships
University of California, San Francisco
San Francisco, California

EDWARD V. LALLY, M.D.
Director
Division of Rheumatology
Rhode Island Hospital
Professor of Medicine
Alpert School of Medicine
Brown University
Providence, Rhode Island

QUANG P. LE, M.D., M.P.H.
Assistant Instructor
Department of Family Medicine
Memorial Hospital of Rhode Island
Alpert Medical School
Brown University
Providence, Rhode Island

KACHIU LEE, B.A.
Medical Student
Department of Dermatology
Feinberg School of Medicine
Northwestern University
Chicago, Illinois

PHILIP LEE, M.D.
Cardiology Fellow
Department of Cardiology
Alpert Medicine School
Brown University
Providence, Rhode Island

MARGARET LEKANDER, M.D.
Assistant Instructor
Department of Family
Memorial Hospital of Rhode Island
Alpert Medical School
Brown University
Pawtucket, Rhode Island

DONITA DILLON LIGHTNER, M.D.
Pediatric Neurology
Department of Neurology
University of Kentucky
Lexington, Kentucky

CHUN LIM, M.D., Ph.D.
Department of Neurology
Beth Israel Deaconess Medical Center
Boston, Massachusetts

CUI LI LIN, M.D.
Gastroenterology Fellow
Division of Gastroenterology
Alpert Medical School
Brown University
Providence, Rhode Island

JEANNETTE P. LIN, M.D.
Fellow
Cardiovascular Medicine
University of California, Irvine
Irvine, California

RICHARD LONG, M.D.
Adjunct Clinical Associate Professor
Department of Family Medicine
Alpert Medical School
Brown University
Providence, Rhode Island
Clinical Associate Professor of Family Medicine
Department of Family Medicine
Boston University School of Medicine
Boston, Massachusetts

SUSANNA R. MAGEE, M.D., M.P.H.
Assistant Professor of Family Medicine
Department of Family Medicine
Alpert Medical School
Brown University
Providence, Rhode Island
Director of Maternal and Child Health
Memorial Hospital of Rhode Island
Pawtucket, Rhode Island

ACHRAF A. MAKKI, M.D., M.SC.
Resident
Department of Neurology
Emory University
Atlanta, Georgia

DOUGLAS W. MARTIN, M.D.
Fellow
Pulmonary Diseases and Critical Care
Alpert Medical School
Brown University
Providence, Rhode Island

ELISABETH B. MATSON, D.O.
Rheumatology Fellow
Rhode Island Hospital
Alpert School of Medicine
Brown University
Providence, Rhode Island

DANIEL T. MATTSON, M.D., M.SC. (MED.)
St. Louis Neurological Institute
St. Louis, Missouri

KATE MAVRICH, M.D.
Medical Resident
Alpert Medical School
Brown University
Providence, Rhode Island

ALISON MAY, M.D.
Department of Psychiatry
VA Medical Center
University of California, San Francisco
Clinical Instructor
Lyon-Martin Health Services
San Francisco, California

MAITREYI MAZUMDAR, M.D., M.P.H.
Instructor in Neurology
Harvard Medical School
Children's Hospital Boston
Department of Neurology
Boston, Massachusetts

JEFFREY C. McCLEAN II, M.D.
Chief of Electrodiagnostic Medicine
Department of Neurology
San Antonio Military Medical Center
San Antonio, Texas

KELLY A. McGARRY, M.D.
Program Director
General Internal Medicine Residency Program
Rhode Island Hospital
Assistant Professor of Medicine
Alpert Medical School
Brown University
Providence, Rhode Island

LYNN McNICOLL, M.D.
Assistant Professor of Medicine
Alpert Medical School
Brown University
Geriatrician
Division of Geriatrics
Rhode Island Hospital
Providence, Rhode Island

LAURA H. McPEAKE, M.D.
Assistant Professor of Emergency Medicine
Brown University Attending Physician of Emergency Medicine
Rhode Island Hospital/Miriam Hospital
Providence, Rhode Island

AKANKSHA MEHTA, M.D.
Surgical Resident
Department of Urology
Brown University
Providence, Rhode Island

DANIEL E. MENDEZ-ALLWOOD, M.D.
Rheumatology Fellow
Roger Williams Medical Center
Boston University School of Medicine
Boston, Massachusetts

LONNIE R. MERCIER, M.D.
Clinical Instructor
Department of Orthopedic Surgery
Creighton University School of Medicine
Omaha, Nebraska

DENNIS J. MIKOLICH, M.D., F.A.C.P., F.C.C.P.
Chief
Division of Infectious Diseases
VA Medical Center
Clinical Associate Professor of Medicine
Alpert Medical School
Brown University
Providence, Rhode Island

JENNIFER MIRANDA, M.D.
Endocrinology Fellow
Rhode Island Hospital
Alpert Medical School
Brown University
Providence, Rhode Island

NADIA MUJAHID, M.D.
Fellow
Department of Geriatrics
Rhode Island Hospital
Alpert Medical School
Brown University
Providence, Rhode Island

VINCENT A. MUKKADA, M.D.
Assistant Professor (Clinical) of Pediatrics
Alpert Medical School
Brown University
Pediatric Gastroenterologist
Hasbro Children's Hospital
Rhode Island Hospital
Providence, Rhode Island

BILAL H. NAQVI, M.D.
Hematologist/Oncologist
Marshfield Clinic Regional Cancer Center
Eau Claire, Wisconsin

JACK H. NASSAU, Ph.D.
Clinical Assistant Professor of Psychiatry and Human Behavior
Alpert Medical School
Brown University
Pediatric Psychologist
Rhode Island Hospital
Hasbro Children's Hospital
Providence, Rhode Island

TAKUMA NEMOTO, M.D.
Research Associate Professor of Surgery
State University of New York at Buffalo
Buffalo, New York

JAMES J. NG, M.D.
Staff Physician
The Vancouver Clinic
Vancouver, Washington

MELISSA NOTHNAGLE, M.D.
Assistant Professor of Family Medicine
Alpert Medical School
Brown University
Providence, Rhode Island

BETH NOWAK, M.D.
Fellow
Geriatric Medicine
Boston Medical Center
Boston, Massachusetts

JUDITH NUDELMAN, M.D.
Clinical Assistant Professor
Department of Family Medicine
Alpert Medical School
Brown University
Providence, Rhode Island

GAIL M. O'BRIEN, M.D.
Medical Director
Adult Ambulatory Services
Rhode Island Hospital
Clinical Associate Professor of Medicine
Alpert Medical School
Brown University
Providence, Rhode Island

CAROLYN J. O'CONNOR, M.D.
Assistant Clinical Professor
School of Medicine
Yale University
Department of Medicine
St. Mary's Hospital
Waterbury, Connecticut

ALEXANDER B. OLAWAIYE, M.D.
Fellow
Division of Gynecologic Oncology
Vincent Department of Obstetrics
Gynecology and Reproductive Biology
Massachusetts General Hospital
Harvard Medical School
Boston, Massachusetts

MICHAEL K. ONG, M.D., Ph.D.
Assistant Professor
UCLA Division of General Internal Medicine/Health Services Research
School of Medicine
University of California, Los Angeles
Los Angeles, California

STEVEN M. OPAL, M.D.
Professor of Medicine
Infectious Disease Division
Alpert Medical School
Brown University
Providence, Rhode Island

JOSEPH R. OWENS, M.D.
KY Clinic L-445
Department of Neurology
University of Kentucky
Lexington, Kentucky

CHRISTINA ANTONIO PACHECO, M.D.
Clinical Assistant Professor
Department of Family Medicine
Alpert Medical School
Brown University
Providence, Rhode Island

ROBERTO PACHECO, M.D.
Fellow
Interventional Cardiology
Alpert Medical School
Brown University
Providence, Rhode Island

JANICE PATACSIL-TRULL, M.D.
Family Practitioner
Family Medicine Associates of South Attleboro
South Attleboro, Massachusetts

BIRJU B. PATEL, M.D., F.A.C.P.
Assistant Professor of Medicine
Department of Medicine
Division of Geriatrics and Gerontology
Emory University School of Medicine
Atlanta Veterans Administration Medical Center
Atlanta, Georgia

PRANAV M. PATEL, M.D., F.A.C.C., F.S.C.A.I.
Assistant Professor of Medicine
Director
Cardiac Catheterization Laboratory
University of California, Irvine
Irvine, California

ELENI PATROZOU, M.D.
Clinical Instructor in Medicine
Alpert Medical School
Brown University
Providence, Rhode Island
Internist-Infectious Diseases Consultant
Hygeia Hospital Greece
Athens, Greece

STEVEN PELIGIAN, D.O.
Medical Director
CODAC Behavioral Healthcare
Providence, Rhode Island

HEIDI H. PETERSON, M.D.
Clinical Assistant Professor
Department of Family Medicine
Alpert Medical School
Brown University
Providence, Rhode Island
Memorial Hospital of Rhode Island
Pawtucket, Rhode Island

KATHARINE A. PHILLIPS, M.D.
Director
Body Dysmorphic Disorder Program
Director
Research for Adult Psychiatry
Rhode Island Hospital
Professor of Psychiatry and Human Behavior
Alpert Medical School
Brown University
Providence, Rhode Island

PAUL A. PIRRAGLIA, M.D., M.P.H.
Assistant Professor of Medicine
Alpert Medical School
Brown University
Rhode Island Hospital
Providence, Rhode Island

WENDY A. PLANTE, PH.D.
Clinical Assistant Professor of Psychiatry and Human Behavior
Alpert Medical School
Brown University
Pediatric Psychologist
Rhode Island Hospital
Hasbro Children's Hospital
Providence, Rhode Island

ANGELA PLETTE, M.D.
Assistant Professor of Medicine
Assistant Program Director
Hematology/Oncology Fellowship
Department of Medicine
Alpert Medical School
Brown University
Providence, Rhode Island

SHARON S. HARTMAN POLENSEK, M.D., PH.D.
Clinical Associate
Department of Neurology
Emory University
Atlanta, Georgia

DONN POSNER, PH.D., C.B.S.M.
Director, Clinical Behavioral Medicine
Behavioral Sleep Medicine
Sleep Disorders Center of Lifespan Hospitals
Clinical Associate Professor
Alpert Medical School
Brown University
Providence, Rhode Island

ARUNDATHI G. PRASAD, M.D.
Clinical Instructor
Department of Obstetrics and Gynecology/Resident Education
State University of New York at Buffalo
Women's and Children's Hospital
Buffalo, New York

KITTICHAI PROMRAT, M.D.
Assistant Professor
Division of Gastroenterology
Department of Medicine
Alpert Medical School
Brown University
Chief
Gastroenterology Section
Providence Veterans Affairs Medical Center
Providence, Rhode Island

SHAHNAZ PUNJANI, M.D.
Fellow
Preventive Cardiology
Providence VA Medical Center
Alpert Medical School
Brown University
Providence, Rhode Island

JOHN RAGSDALE, M.D.
Clinical Assistant Professor of Family Medicine
Duke University Medical Center
Department of Community and Family Medicine
Durham, North Carolina

RADHIKA A. RAMANAN, M.D., M.P.H.
Assistant Professor of Medicine
University of California, San Francisco
San Francisco, California

CHRISTIAN N. RAMSEY III, M.D.
Assistant Professor
Department of Neurosurgery
University of Kentucky
Lexington, Kentucky

WASIM RASHID, M.D.
Director
Geriatric Psychiatry
Rhode Island Hospital
Providence, Rhode Island

RICHARD REGNANTE, M.D.
Fellow in Cardiovascular Disease
Division of Cardiovascular Medicine
Alpert Medical School
Brown University
Providence, Rhode Island

VICTOR I. REUS, M.D.
Professor
Department of Psychiatry
School of Medicine
Langley Porter Psychiatric Institute
University of California, San Francisco
San Francisco, California

HARLAN G. RICH, M.D.
Director of Endoscopy
Rhode Island Hospital
Associate Professor of Medicine
Alpert Medical School
Brown University
Providence, Rhode Island

JESSICA RISSER, M.D., M.P.H.
Third Year Dermatology Resident
Department of Dermatology
Alpert Medical School
Brown University
Providence, Rhode Island

LUTHER K. ROBINSON, M.D.
Associate Professor of Pediatrics
Director
Dysmorphology and Clinical Genetics
State University of New York at Buffalo
Buffalo, New York

ANISHKA ROLLE, M.D.
Rheumatology Fellow
Roger Williams Medical Center
Boston University School of Medicine
Boston, Massachusetts

LAUREN ROTH, M.D.
Fellow
Reproductive Endocrinology and Infertility
Department of Obstetrics and Gynecology
University of Colorado
Aurora, Colorado

AMITY RUBEOR, D.O.
Assistant Professor (Clinical)
Department of Family Medicine
Alpert Medical
School Brown University
Providence, Rhode Island

IMMAD SADIQ, M.D.
Clinical Assistant Professor of Medicine
Division of Cardiology
Alpert Medical School
Brown University
Providence, Rhode Island

NUHA R. SAID, M.D.
Rheumatologist
Department of Rheumatology
Roger Williams Medical Center
Providence, Rhode Island

HEMANT K. SATPATHY, M.D.
Fellow
Division of Maternal Fetal Medicine
Department of Obstetrics and Gynecology
Emory University
Atlanta, Georgia

RUBY SATPATHY, M.D.
Fellow
Cardiology
Department of Internal Medicine
Creighton University
Omaha, Nebraska

JASON M. SATTERFIELD, Ph.D.
Director
Behavioral Medicine
Associate Professor of Clinical Medicine
University of California, San Francisco
San Francisco, California

SEAN I. SAVITZ, M.D.
Assistant Professor of Neurology
University of Texas
Houston, Texas

SYEDA M. SAYEED, M.D.
Internal Medicine Department
Memorial Hospital of Rhode Island
Alpert Medical School
Brown University
Providence, Rhode Island

MICHAEL SCHAEFER, M.D.
Endocrinology Fellow
Rhode Island Hospital
Alpert Medical School
Brown University
Providence, Rhode Island

PETER J. SELL, D. O.
Assistant Professor
Department of Pediatrics
University of Massachusetts Medical School
Worcester, Massachusetts

CATHERINE SHAFTS, D.O.
Assistant Clinical Instructor
Alpert Medical School
Brown University
Providence, Rhode Island

MADHAVI SHAH, M.D.
Assistant Clinical Instructor
Department of Family Medicine
Alpert Medical School
Brown University
Providence, Rhode Island

GRACE SHIH, M.D.
Assistant Clinical Instructor
Department of Family Medicine
Alpert Medical School
Brown University
Providence, Rhode Island

ASHA SHRESTHA, M.D.
Medical Resident
Memorial Hospital of Rhode Island
Alpert School of Medicine
Brown University
Providence, Rhode Island

NAUMAN SIDDIQI, M.D.
Fellow
Cardiovascular Medicine
University of California, Irvine
Irvine, California

MARK SIGMAN, M.D.
Associate Professor of Surgery (Urology)
Division of Urology
Alpert Medical School
Brown University
Providence, Rhode Island

JOSHUA R. SILVERSTEIN, M.D.
Cardiology Fellow
Alpert Medical School
Brown University
Providence, Rhode Island

JOANNE M. SILVIA, M.D.
Clinical Assistant Professor
Assistant Professor
Department of Family Medicine
Memorial Hospital of Rhode Island
Alpert Medical School
Brown University
Providence, Rhode Island

DIVYA SINGHAL, M.D.
Department of Neurology
University of Kentucky
Lexington, Kentucky

JOHN SLADKY, M.D.
Staff Neurologist
Associate Program Director
Wilford Hall Medical Center
San Antonio, Texas

U. SHIVRAJ SOHUR, M.D., Ph.D.
Assistant Professor of Neurology
Harvard Medical School
Boston, Massachusetts

DIVJOT SOOCH, M.D.
Department of Family Medicine
Memorial Hospital of Rhode Island
Pawtucket, Rhode Island

MARY BETH SUTTER, M.D.
Assistant Instructor of Family Medicine
Alpert Medical School
Brown University
Providence, Rhode Island

JULIE ANNE SZUMIGALA, M.D.
Clinical Instructor
Department of Obstetrics and Gynecology
State University of New York at Buffalo
Buffalo, New York

DOMINICK TAMMARO, M.D.
Associate Director
Categorical Internal Medicine Residency
Co-Director
Medicine-Pediatrics Residency
Division of General Internal Medicine
Rhode Island Hospital
Associate Professor of Medicine
Alpert Medical School
Brown University
Providence, Rhode Island

SARAH TAPYRIK, M.D.
Pulmonary Fellow
NYU Department of Pulmonary and Critical Care
New York, New York

GLADYS TELANG, M.D.
Associate Professor of Dermatology
Memorial Hospital of Rhode Island
Pawtucket, Rhode Island
Alpert Medical School
Brown University
Providence, Rhode Island

IRIS L. TONG, M.D.
Assistant Professor
Department of Medicine
Alpert Medical School
Brown University
Providence, Rhode Island

FREDERICK D. TRONCALES, M.D.
Fellow
Pulmonary Diseases and Critical Care
Alpert Medical School
Brown University
Providence, Rhode Island

ALEXANDER G. TRUESDELL, M.D.
Fellow
Cardiology
Alpert Medical School
Brown University
Providence, Rhode Island

MARGARET TRYFOROS, M.D.
Clinical Assistant Professor
Department of Family Medicine
Alpert Medical School
Brown University
Providence, Rhode Island
Memorial Hospital of Rhode Island
Pawtucket, Rhode Island

JOSEPH RALPH TUCCI M.D., F.A.C.P., F.A.C.E.
Professor of Medicine
Boston University School of Medicine
Boston, Massachusetts
Adjunct Professor of Medicine
Alpert Medical School
Brown University
Interim Chairman Department of Medicine
Director
Division of Endocrinology and Metabolism
Roger Williams Medical Center
Providence, Rhode Island

EROBOGHENE E. UBOGU, M.D.
Assistant Professor of Neurology
Director
Neuromuscular Immunopathology Research Laboratory
Department of Neurology
Baylor College of Medicine
Houston, Texas

SEAN H. UITERWYK, M.D.
Clinical Assistant Professor
Department of Family Medicine
Alpert Medical School
Brown University
Providence, Rhode Island

NICOLE J. ULLRICH, M.D., Ph.D.
Assistant Professor
Harvard Medical School
Department of Neurology
Children's Hospital Boston
Boston, Massachusetts

MARISA E. VAN POZNAK, M.D.
Attending Physician
Internal Medicine
Women and Infants Hospital
Alpert Medical School
Brown University
Providence, Rhode Island

JORGE A. VILLAFUERTE, M.D.
Attending Orthopedic Surgeon
VA Medical Center
West Roxbury, Massachusetts

HANNAH VU, D.O.
Assistant Clinical Instructor
Department of Family Medicine
Alpert Medical School
Brown University
Providence, Rhode Island

TARA M. WAYT, D.O.
Emergency Department Resident
Hartford Hospital
University of Connecticut School of Medicine
Hartford, Connecticut

DENNIS M. WEPPNER, M.D., F.A.C.O.G.
Associate Professor of Clinical Gynecology/Obstetrics
State University of New York at Buffalo
Clinical Chief
Department of Gynecology/Obstetrics
Millard Fillmore Hospital
Buffalo, New York

JORDAN WHITE, M.D.
Assistant Instructor
Department of Family Medicine
Alpert Medical School
Brown University
Memorial Hospital of Rhode Island
Pawtucket, Rhode Island

LAUREL M. WHITE, M.D.
Clinical Assistant Professor
Department of Obstetrics and Gynecology
Division of Maternal Fetal Medicine
State University of New York at Buffalo
Buffalo, New York

MATTHEW P. WICKLUND, M.D., F.A.A.N.
Professor of Neurology
Department of Neurology
Penn State College of Medicine
Hershey, Pennsylvania

CHARLES WOLFF, M.D.
Board Certified Family Medicine
Board Certified Hospice and Palliative Care Medicine
Interim Chief of Geriatrics and Assistant Professor of Clinical Medicine
Department of Family Medicine
Memorial Hospital of Rhode Island
Pawtucket, Rhode Island
Alpert Medical School
Brown University
Providence, Rhode Island

MARIE ELIZABETH WONG, M.D.
Physician
Family Medicine
Baystate Brightwood Health Center
Springfield, Massachusetts

WEN-CHIH WU, M.D.
Staff Cardiologist
Providence VA Medical Center
Associate Professor of Medicine
Alpert Medical School
Brown University
Providence, Rhode Island

BETH J. WUTZ, M.D.
Clinical Assistant Professor of Medicine
Division of Internal Medicine/Pediatrics
Kajeida Health–Buffalo General Hospital
State University of New York at Buffalo
Buffalo, New York

SARAH L. XAVIER, D.O.
Director of Psychiatric Services
Rhode Island Training School
Director
Child & Adolescent Forensic Psychiatry
Rhode Island Hospital
Clinical Assistant Professor of Psychiatry and Human Behavior
Alpert Medical School
Brown University
Providence, Rhode Island

AUGUSTIN G. YIP, M.D., Ph.D.
Butler Hospital
Department of Psychiatry and Human Behavior
Brown University
Providence, Rhode Island

JOHN Q. YOUNG, M.D., M.P.P.
Assistant Professor
Department of Psychiatry
School of Medicine
University of California, San Francisco
San Francisco, California

CANDICE YUVIENCO, M.D.
Rheumatology Fellow
Rhode Island Hospital
Alpert School of Medicine
Brown University
Providence, Rhode Island

CINDY ZADIKOFF, M.D., F.R.C.P.C.
Assistant Professor of Neurology
Parkinson's Disease and Movement Disorders Center
Feinberg School of Medicine
Northwestern University
Chicago, Illinois

FARIHA ZAHEER, M.D.
Department of Neurology
University of Kentucky
Lexington, Kentucky

MARK ZIMMERMAN, M.D.
Director
Outpatient Psychiatry
Rhode Island Hospital/The Miriam Hospital
Associate Professor
Department of Psychiatry
Alpert Medical School
Brown University
Providence, Rhode Island

BERNARD ZIMMERMANN, M.D.
Director
Division of Rheumatology
Roger Williams Medical Center
Associate Professor of Medicine
Boston University School of Medicine
Providence, Rhode Island

SCOTT J. ZUCCALA, D.O., F.A.C.O.G.
Staff Physician
Mercy Hospital of Buffalo
Buffalo, New York

RYAN W. ZUZEK, M.D.
Clinical Cardiology Fellow
Division of Cardiology
Alpert Medical School
Brown University
Providence, Rhode Island

To our families.
Their constant support and encouragement made this book a reality.

This book is intended to be a clear and concise reference for physicians and allied health professionals. Its user-friendly format was designed to provide a fast and efficient way to identify important clinical information and to offer practical guidance in patient management. The book is divided into five sections and an appendix, each with emphasis on clinical information.

The tremendous success of the previous editions and the enthusiastic comments from numerous colleagues have brought about several positive changes. Each section has been significantly expanded from prior editions, bringing the total number of medical topics covered in this book to more than 1000. Illustrations have been added to several topics to enhance recollection of clinically important facts. The use of ICD-9CM codes in all the topics will expedite claims submission and reimbursement.

Section I describes in detail more than 700 medical disorders. A total of 20 new topics, 75 new tables, and 60 new illustrations have been added to the 2012 edition. Each medical topic in this section is arranged alphabetically, and the material in each topic is presented in outline format for ease of retrieval. Topics with an accompanying algorithm in Section III are identified with an algorithm symbol (ALG). Similarly, if topics also have a Patient Teaching Guide (PTG) available online, this has been noted. More than 100 PTGs have been added to the 2012 edition. Throughout the text, key, quick-access information is consistently highlighted; clinical photographs are used to further illustrate selected medical conditions; and relevant ICD-9CM codes are listed. Most references focus on current peer-reviewed journal articles rather than outdated textbooks and old review articles. Evidence-based medicine data have been added to relevant topics.

Topics in this section use the following structured approach:
1. Basic Information (Definition, Synonyms, ICD-9CM Codes, Epidemiology & Demographics, Physical Findings & Clinical Presentation, Etiology)
2. Diagnosis (Differential Diagnosis, Workup, Laboratory Tests, Imaging Studies)
3. Treatment (Nonpharmacologic Therapy, Acute General Rx, Chronic Rx, Disposition, Referral)
4. Pearls & Considerations (Comments, Suggested Readings)
5. Evidence-Based Data and References

Section II includes the differential diagnosis, etiology, and classification of signs and symptoms. This section has been significantly expanded for the 2012 edition with the addition of 97 new topics. It is a practical section that allows the user investigating a physical complaint or abnormal laboratory value to follow a "workup" leading to a diagnosis. The physician can then easily look up the presumptive diagnosis in Section I for the information specific to that illness.

Section III includes clinical algorithms to guide and expedite the patient's workup and therapy. Many physicians describe this section as particularly valuable in today's managed-care environment.

Section IV includes normal laboratory values and interpretation of results of commonly ordered laboratory tests. By providing interpretation of abnormal results, this section facilitates the diagnosis of medical disorders and further adds to the comprehensive, "one-stop" nature of our text. This section has also expanded for the 2012 edition with the addition of several new lab tests.

Section V focuses on preventive medicine and offers essential guidelines from the U.S. Preventive Services Task Force. Information in this section includes recommendations for the periodic health examination, screening for major diseases and disorders, patient counseling, and immunization and chemoprophylaxis recommendations. A portion of this section has been moved to the electronic-only format to limit the total page count for the 2012 edition.

The **Appendix** has been divided into two major sections. Section I contains extensive information on complementary and alternative medicine (CAM). With the material in this appendix, we hope to lessen the current scarcity of exposure of allopathic and osteopathic physicians to the diversity of CAM therapies. Section II of the Appendix, available online, contains an extensive section on primary care procedures.

As clinicians, we all realize the importance of patient education and the need for clear communication with our patients. Toward that end, practical patient instruction sheets, organized alphabetically and covering the majority of the topics in this book, are available online and can be easily customized and printed from any computer. All of them have been updated, and more than 100 new ones have been added to the 2012 edition. They represent a valuable addition to patient care and are useful for improving physician–patient communication, patient satisfaction, and quality of care.

I believe that we have produced a state-of-the-art information system with significant differences from existing texts. It contains five sections and patient education guides that could be sold separately based on their content, yet are available under a single cover, offering the reader a tremendous value. I hope that the *Clinical Advisor*'s user-friendly approach, numerous unique features, and yearly updates will make this book a valuable medical reference, not only to primary care physicians but also to physicians in other specialties, medical students, and allied health professionals.

Fred F. Ferri, M.D., F.A.C.P.

Note: Comments from readers are always appreciated and can be forwarded directly to Dr. Ferri at fred_ferri@brown.edu.

EVALUATION OF EVIDENCE

Ferri's Clinical Advisor evaluates all evidence based on a rating system published by the American Academy of Family Physicians. In order to indicate the strength of the supporting evidence, each summary statement is accorded one of three levels:

LEVEL A
- Systematic reviews of randomized controlled trials, including meta-analyses
- Good-quality randomized controlled trials

LEVEL B
- Good-quality nonrandomized clinical trials
- Systematic reviews not in Level A
- Lower-quality randomized controlled trials not in Level A
- Other types of study: case-control studies, clinical cohort studies, cross-sectional studies, retrospective studies, and uncontrolled studies

LEVEL C
- Evidence-based consensus statements and expert guidelines

SOURCES OF EVIDENCE

Evidence is summarized principally from three critically evaluated, very highly regarded sources:

- **Cochrane Systematic Reviews** are respected throughout the world as one of the most rigorous searches of medical journals for randomized controlled trials. They provide highly structured systematic reviews, with evidence included or excluded on the basis of explicit quality-related criteria, and they often use meta-analyses to increase the power of the findings of numerous studies.
- *Clinical Evidence* is produced by the BMJ Publishing Group. It provides synopses of the best currently available evidence on the treatment and prevention of many clinical conditions, based on searches and appraisals of the available literature.
- **The National Guideline Clearinghouse™** is a comprehensive database of evidence-based clinical practice guidelines and related documents produced by the Agency for Healthcare Research and Quality in partnership with the American Medical Association and the American Association of Health Plans.

In addition, where evidence exists that has not yet been critically reviewed in one of the three sites above, the evidence is summarized briefly, categorized, and fully referenced. Guidelines are also sourced from government and professional bodies.

SECTION I Diseases and Disorders

PTG indicates that a Patient Teaching Guide is
available at www.expertconsult.com.

SECTION II Differential Diagnosis

SECTION III Clinical Algorithms

SECTION IV Laboratory Tests and Interpretation of Results

SECTION V Clinical Practice Guidelines

APPENDIX I Complementary and Alternative Medicine

APPENDIX II Primary Care Procedures, available at www.expertconsult.com

Additional *PTGs* Available at www.expertconsult.com
Not Linked to Topics in Section I

Additional Algorithms Available at www.expertconsult.com

Diseases and Disorders

BASIC INFORMATION

DEFINITION

Abruptio placentae is the separation of placenta from the uterine wall before delivery of the fetus. There are three classes of abruption based on maternal and fetal status, including an assessment of uterine contractions, quantity of bleeding, fetal heart rate monitoring, and abnormal coagulation studies (fibrinogen, prothrombin time, partial thromboplastin time).

- Grade I: mild vaginal bleeding, uterine irritability, stable vital signs, reassuring fetal heart rate, normal coagulation profile (fibrinogen 450 mg%)
- Grade II: moderate vaginal bleeding, hypertonic uterine contractions, orthostatic blood pressure measurements, unfavorable fetal status, fibrinogen 150 to 250 mg%
- Grade III: severe bleeding (may be concealed), hypertonic uterine contractions, overt signs of hypovolemic shock, fetal death, thrombocytopenia, fibrinogen <150 mg%

SYNONYMS

Premature separation of placenta

ICD-9CM CODES
641.2 Premature separation of placenta

EPIDEMIOLOGY & DEMOGRAPHICS

INCIDENCE (IN U.S.): One in 86 to 206 births; incidence by grade: I = 40%, II = 45%, III = 15%; 80% occur before the onset of labor
RISK FACTORS: Hypertension (greatest association), trauma, polyhydramnios, multifetal gestation, smoking, use of crack cocaine, chorioamnionitis, preterm premature rupture of membranes
RECURRENCE RATE: 5% to 17%; with two prior episodes, 25%

PHYSICAL FINDINGS & CLINICAL PRESENTATION

- Triad of uterine bleeding (concealed or per vagina), hypertonic uterine contractions or signs of preterm labor, and evidence of fetal compromise exists.
- More than 80% of cases have external bleeding; 20% of cases have no bleeding but have indirect evidence of abruption, such as failed tocolysis for preterm labor.
- Tetanic uterine contractions are found in only 17% of cases unless grade II or III abruption.

ETIOLOGY

- Primary etiology: unknown
- Hypertension: found in 40% to 50% of grade III abruptions
- Rapid decompression of uterine cavity, as can occur in polyhydramnios or multifetal gestation
- Blunt external trauma (motor vehicle accident, spousal abuse)

DIAGNOSIS

DIFFERENTIAL DIAGNOSIS

- Placenta previa
- Cervical or vaginal trauma
- Labor
- Cervical cancer
- Rupture of membranes
- The differential diagnosis of vaginal bleeding in pregnancy is described in Section II

WORKUP

- Initial assessment should evaluate for the source of bleeding, ruling out placenta previa that may contraindicate any type of vaginal examination (e.g., pelvic speculum examination).
- Continuous fetal heart monitoring is indicated for all viable gestations (60% incidence of fetal distress in labor); may show early signs of maternal hypovolemia (late decelerations or fetal tachycardia) before overt maternal vital sign changes.
- Actual amount of blood loss is often greater than initially perceived because of the possibility of concealed retroplacental bleeding and apparent "normal" vital signs. The relative hypervolemia of pregnancy initially protects the patient until late in the course of bleeding, when abrupt and sudden cardiovascular collapse can occur.

LABORATORY TESTS

- Baseline hemoglobin and hematocrit help quantify blood loss and establish baseline values for serial comparisons during expectant management.
- Coagulation profile: platelets, fibrinogen, prothrombin, and partial thromboplastin time. Diffuse intravascular coagulation can develop with severe abruption. If fibrinogen is <150 mg%, estimated blood loss is approximately 2000 ml; if fibrinogen is <100 mg%, consider fresh frozen plasma to prevent further bleeding.
- Type and antibody screen is important to identify Rh-negative patients who may need Rh immune globulin.

IMAGING STUDIES

Ultrasound should include fetal presentation and status, amniotic fluid volume, placental location, as well as any evidence of hematoma (retroplacental, subchorionic, or preplacental).

TREATMENT

ACUTE GENERAL Rx

- Stabilization of the mother is the first priority.
- Treatment depends on gestational age of the fetus, severity of the abruption, and maternal status.
- Initial assessment for signs of maternal hemodynamic compromise or hemorrhagic shock; large-bore intravenous access, with crystalloid fluid resuscitation using a replacement of 3 ml lactated Ringer's solution for every 1 ml estimated blood loss.
- Indwelling Foley catheter to monitor urine output and maternal volume status, with a goal of 30 ml/hr urine output.
- Assess fetal status and gestational age by sonogram and continuous fetal heart rate monitoring.
- Because of the unpredictable nature of abruptions, cross-matched blood should be made available during the initial resuscitation period.

CHRONIC Rx

- In the term fetus or when lung maturity has been documented, delivery is indicated.
- In the preterm fetus or a fetus with an immature lung profile, consider betamethasone 12.5 mg IM q24h for two doses and then delivery, depending on the severity of the abruption and the likelihood of fetal complications from preterm birth.
- Cesarean section should be reserved for cases of fetal distress or for standard obstetric indications.
- In select cases, such as severe prematurity with a stable mother and mild contractions, magnesium sulfate can be used for tocolysis, 6 g IV loading dose then 3 g/hr maintenance, to allow for course of steroids.

DISPOSITION

Because of the unpredictable nature of abruptions, expectant management should occur only under controlled circumstances and is rarely practiced.

REFERRAL

Abruptio placentae places mother and fetus in a high-risk situation and should be managed by a qualified obstetrician in a facility with capability for neonatal and maternal resuscitation and ability to perform emergency cesarean sections.

AUTHORS: **SCOTT J. ZUCCALA, D.O.,** and **RUBEN ALVERO, M.D.**

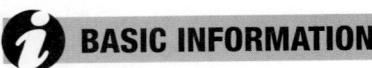

BASIC INFORMATION

DEFINITION

A brain abscess is a focal, intracerebral infection that begins as a localized area of cerebritis and develops into a collection of pus surrounded by a well-vascularized capsule.

ICD-9CM CODES
324.0 Brain abscess

EPIDEMIOLOGY & DEMOGRAPHICS

INCIDENCE: Quite uncommon (occurs about 2% as commonly as brain tumors)
PEAK INCIDENCE: Preadolescence and middle age
PREDOMINANT AGE: Occurs at any age
PREDOMINANT SEX:
- Men affected more than women
- Most common source of underlying infection: contiguous spread from the paranasal sinuses, middle ear, or teeth

PHYSICAL FINDINGS & CLINICAL PRESENTATION

- Classic triad: fever, headache, and focal neurologic deficit are present in 50% of cases.
- Fever is present in only 50% of patients.
- Headache is usually localized to the side of the abscess; onset can be gradual or severe; present in 70% of cases.
- Focal neurologic findings (e.g., seizures, hemiparesis, aphasia, ataxia) depend on the location of the abscess and are seen in 30% to 50% of cases.
- Papilledema is present in 25% of cases.
- Presence of adjacent infections (dental abscess, otitis media, and sinusitis) may be a clue to the underlying diagnosis and should be sought in any suspected case.
- Time course from symptom onset to presentation ranges from hours in fulminant cases to more than 1 mo; 75% present in the first 2 wk.
- The nonspecific presentation of a brain abscess warrants that clinicians maintain a high index of suspicion.

ETIOLOGY

- Brain abscesses arise from:
  Contiguous infection
  Hematogenous spread from a remote site
- They are classified based on the likely portal of entry.
Likely source of abscess:
A. Contiguous focus or primary infection (55% of all brain abscesses):
  1. Paranasal sinus: occur in frontal lobe; streptococci, *Bacteroides, Haemophilus,* and *Fusobacterium* spp.
  2. Otitis media/mastoiditis: occur in temporal lobe and cerebellum; streptococci, Enterobacteriaceae, *Bacteroides,* and *Pseudomonas* spp.
  3. Dental sepsis: occur in frontal lobe; mixed *Fusobacterium, Bacteroides,* and *Streptococcus* spp.

  4. Penetrating head injury: site of abscess depends on site of wound; *Staphylococcus aureus, Clostridium* spp., Enterobacteriaceae
  5. Postoperative: *Staphylococcus epidermidis* and *S. aureus,* Enterobacteriaceae, and Pseudomonadaceae
B. Hematogenous spread/distant site of infection (25% of all brain abscesses): abscesses most commonly multiple, especially in middle cerebral artery distribution; infecting organisms depend on source.
  1. Congenital heart disease: streptococci, *Haemophilus* spp.
  2. Endocarditis: *S. aureus,* viridans streptococci
  3. Urinary tract: Enterobacteriaceae, Pseudomonadaceae
  4. Intraabdominal: streptococci, Enterobacteriaceae, anaerobes
  5. Lung: streptococci, *Actinomyces* species, *Fusobacterium* spp.
  6. Immunocompromised host: *Toxoplasma* species, fungi, Enterobacteriaceae, *Nocardia* spp., tuberculosis, listeriosis
C. Cryptogenic (unknown source): 20% of all brain abscesses

DIAGNOSIS

DIFFERENTIAL DIAGNOSIS

- Other parameningeal infections: subdural empyema, epidural abscess, thrombophlebitis of the major dural venous sinuses and cortical veins
- Embolic strokes in patients with bacterial endocarditis
- Mycotic aneurysms with leakage
- Viral encephalitis (usually resulting from herpes simplex)
- Acute hemorrhagic leukoencephalitis
- Parasitic infections: toxoplasmosis, echinococcosis, cysticercosis
- Metastatic or primary brain tumors
- Cerebral infarction
- CNS vasculitis
- Chronic subdural hematoma

WORKUP

Physical examination, laboratory tests, and imaging studies

LABORATORY TESTS

- White blood cell counts are elevated in 60% of patients.
- Erythrocyte sedimentation rate is usually elevated but may be normal.
- Blood cultures are most often negative (10% positive).
- Lumbar puncture is contraindicated in patients with suspected abscess (20% die or experience neurologic decline).
- The yield of Gram stain and culture of material aspirated at time of surgical drainage approaches 100%.

IMAGING STUDIES

- MRI with and without gadolinium is the diagnostic procedure of choice; provides superior detail compared with CT scan (higher sensitivity and specificity than CT scan, but not always immediately available).
- CT scan (Fig. 1-1) with intravenous contrast is still an excellent test (sensitivity 95%-99%).
- Serial CT or MRI scanning is recommended to follow the response to therapy.

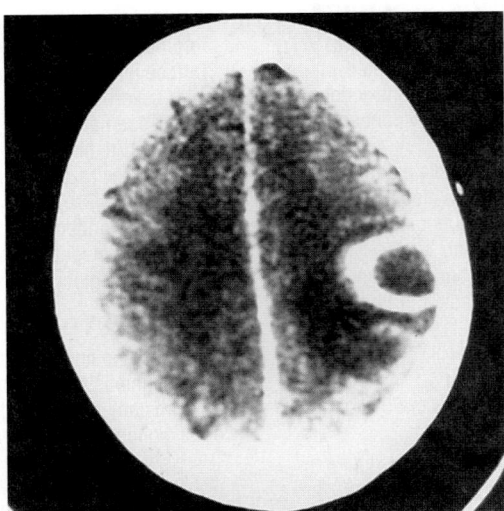

FIGURE 1-1 Computed tomographic (CT) scan showing a brain abscess. A woman presented to physicians after a focal seizure followed by headache and weakness of the arm. Dental work had been performed several weeks before. CT scan revealed a contrast-enhanced, ringlike mass surrounded by edema. It is not possible on this scan to differentiate tumor from abscess. At surgery a well-encapsulated abscess was encountered. (From Andreoli TE [ed]: *Cecil essentials of medicine,* ed 8, Philadelphia, 2010, WB Saunders.)

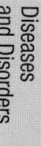

Rx TREATMENT

ACUTE GENERAL Rx

- Effective treatment involves a combination of empiric antibiotic therapy and timely excision or aspiration of the abscess.
- If evidence of edema or mass effect, treatment of elevated intracranial pressure is paramount.
  - Hyperventilation of mechanically ventilated patient.
  - Dexamethasone initially in a dosage of 10 mg IV followed by 4 mg IV q6h until symptoms of cerebral edema subside. Dosage may be reduced after 2 to 4 days and gradually discontinued over a period of 5 to 7 days.
  - Mannitol 0.25 to 1 g/kg IV over 20 to 30 min q6 to 8h; maximum of 6 g/kg in 24 hr.
- Medical therapy is never a substitute for surgical intervention to relieve increased intracranial pressure. Neurologic deterioration usually mandates surgery.
- Steroids should be limited to patients with severe cerebral edema or midline shift.

MEDICAL Rx

If abscess <2.5 cm and patient is neurologically stable and conscious, may start antibiotics and observe. Empiric antibiotic therapy guided by:
- Abscess location
- Suspicion of primary source
- Presence of single or multiple abscesses
- Patient's underlying medical conditions (e.g., HIV, immunocompromised)

Selection of empiric antibiotic therapy:
- Primary infection or contiguous source:
  1. Otitis media/mastoiditis, sinusitis, dental infection: third-generation cephalosporin (cefotaxime 2 g q6h IV or ceftriaxone 2 g q12h IV) plus metronidazole 15 mg/kg IV as a loading dose, then 7.5 mg/kg q6h IV or 15 mg/kg q12h IV

  2. Dental infection: penicillin G 6 million units q6h plus metronidazole 15 mg/kg IV as a loading dose, then 7.5 mg/kg IV q6h or 15 mg/kg IV q12h
  3. Head trauma: third-generation cephalosporin (cefotaxime 2 g IV q6h or ceftriaxone 2 g IV q12h) plus nafcillin 2 g IV q4h or vancomycin (30 mg/kg IV in two divided doses adjusted for renal function)
  4. Postoperative neurosurgery: vancomycin (dose as above) plus ceftazidime (2 g IV q8h)
- Hematogenous spread (congenital heart disease, endocarditis, urinary tract, lung, intraabdominal): nafcillin or vancomycin plus metronidazole plus third-generation cephalosporin (cefotaxime 2 g IV q6h or ceftriaxone 2 g IV q12h)

Duration of antibiotic therapy is unclear. Most recommend parenteral treatment for 4 to 8 wk, with repeated neuroimaging to ensure adequate treatment. (Imaging suggested every week for first 2 wk of therapy, then every 2 wk until antibiotics finished, and then every 2 to 4 mo for 1 yr to monitor for disease recurrence.)

SURGICAL Rx

- Two indications for surgical intervention:
  1. Collect specimens for culture and sensitivity
  2. Reduce mass effect
- Stereotactic biopsy or aspirate of the abscess if surgically feasible
- Essential to selection of targeted antimicrobial coverage
- Timing and choice of surgery depends on:
  - Primary infection source
  - Number and location of the abscesses
  - Whether the procedure is diagnostic or therapeutic
  - Neurologic status of the patient

DISPOSITION

- Prompt diagnostic consideration, early institution of appropriate antimicrobial therapy, and advanced neuroradiologic imaging have

reduced the mortality rate from brain abscesses from 40% to 80% in the preantibiotic era to 10% to 20% at present.
- Morbidity is usually manifest as persistent neurologic sequelae (seizures, intellectual or behavioral impairment, motor deficits) seen in 20% to 60% of patients.

REFERRAL

Consultation with a neurosurgeon is mandatory.

! PEARLS & CONSIDERATIONS

COMMENTS

- It is important to maintain a high index of suspicion because a brain abscess often presents with nonspecific symptoms.
- Rapid imaging and early institution of appropriate antimicrobial therapy improve patient morbidity and mortality.
- Neurosurgical consultation is mandatory.

PREVENTION

Because brain abscesses arise from either contiguous infections or hematogenously from a remote site, early and appropriate treatment of inciting infections is paramount to prevent brain abscess.

EBM EVIDENCE

available at www.expertconsult.com

SUGGESTED READINGS
available at www.expertconsult.com

AUTHOR: **KELLY A. MCGARRY, M.D.**

BASIC INFORMATION

DEFINITION

Breast abscess is an acute inflammatory process resulting in the formation of a collection of purulent material. Typically there is painful erythematous mass formation in the breast, occasionally draining through the overlying skin or nipple duct.

SYNONYMS

Subareolar abscess
Lactational or puerperal abscess

ICD-9CM CODES
6.110 Abscess of the breast
675.0 Abscess of the nipple related to childbirth
675.1 Abscess of the breast related to childbirth

EPIDEMIOLOGY & DEMOGRAPHICS

INCIDENCE: 10% to 30% of all breast abscesses are lactational; acute mastitis occurs in 2.5% of nursing mothers, with one in 15 of these women developing abscess.

PHYSICAL FINDINGS & CLINICAL PRESENTATION

Painful erythematous induration involving breast and leading to fluctuant abscess

ETIOLOGY

- Lactational abscess: milk stasis and bacterial infection leading to mastitis and then abscess, with *Staphylococcus aureus* the most common causative agent
- Subareolar abscess:
  1. Central ducts involved, with obstructive nipple duct changes leading to bacterial infection
  2. Cultured organisms mixed, including anaerobes, staphylococci, streptococci, and others

DIAGNOSIS

DIFFERENTIAL DIAGNOSIS

- Inflammatory carcinoma
- Advanced carcinoma with erythema, edema, and/or ulceration
- Tuberculous abscess (rare in the United States)
- Hydradenitis of breast skin
- Sebaceous cyst with infection

WORKUP

- Clinical examination sufficient
- If abscess suspected, referral to surgeon for incision, drainage, and biopsy
- If possible abscess or advanced carcinoma, referral for workup required

LABORATORY TESTS

- Perform culture and sensitivity test of abscess contents.
- If mammogram or ultrasound is required but prevented by discomfort, perform after treatment and subsequent resolution of abscess.

TREATMENT

NONPHARMACOLOGIC THERAPY

- Established abscess: incision and drainage
- Biopsy of abscess cavity wall to exclude carcinoma

ACUTE GENERAL Rx

- Antibiotics: generally staphylococci in lactational abscess. Recommended initial antibiotic therapy is nafcillin or oxacillin 2 g q4h IV or cefazolin 1 g q8h IV for 10 to 14 days. Alternative includes vancomycin 1 g IV q12h.
- If acute mastitis is identified and treated early without the development of an abscess, resolution without drainage is possible.
- Subareolar abscess: broad-spectrum antibiotic treatment (e.g., cephalexin 500 mg PO qid or cefazolin 1 g q8h IV for 10 to 14 days for more severe infection) and drainage are needed to control acute phase.

CHRONIC Rx

Further surgical treatment for recurrences or fistula

DISPOSITION

- Lactational abscess: possible to continue breastfeeding without risk of infection to the infant
- Subareolar abscess:
  1. High risk for recurrence or complication of fistula formation
  2. Patient informed and referred to General Surgery for evaluation and treatment

REFERRAL

- If abscess drainage required
- For surgical consultation if subareolar abscess involved

SUGGESTED READINGS
available at www.expertconsult.com

AUTHORS: **TAKUMA NEMOTO, M.D.,** and **RUBEN ALVERO, M.D.**

BASIC INFORMATION

DEFINITION

Liver abscess is a necrotic infection of the liver usually classified as pyogenic or amebic.

SYNONYMS

Pyogenic hepatic abscess
Amebic hepatic abscess

ICD-9CM CODES
572.0 Abscess of liver

EPIDEMIOLOGY & DEMOGRAPHICS

INCIDENCE: Incidence of pyogenic liver abscess is 2.3 cases per 100,000 population.
PREVALANCE (WORLDWIDE): Amebic liver abscess is more common than pyogenic liver abscess.
PREVALENCE (IN U.S.): Pyogenic liver abscess is more common than amebic liver abscess.
PREDOMINANT SEX AND AGE: More common in men than women; male/female ratio of 2:1; most common in fourth to sixth decades of life.

PHYSICAL FINDINGS & CLINICAL PRESENTATION

- Fever, chills, and sweats
- Weakness/malaise
- Anorexia with weight loss
- Nausea, vomiting, and diarrhea
- Cough with pleuritic chest pain
- Right upper quadrant abdominal pain
- Hepatomegaly
- Splenomegaly
- Jaundice
- Pleural effusions, rales, and friction rubs may be present
- Most abscesses occur on the right lobe of the liver

ETIOLOGY

- Pyogenic liver abscess is usually polymicrobial (*Klebsiella pneumoniae* [43%], *Escherichia coli* [33%], *Streptococcus* spp. [37%], *Pseudomonas aeruginosa*, *Proteus* spp., *Bacteroides* spp. [24%], *Fusobacterium* spp., *Actinomyces* spp., gram-positive anaerobes, and *Staphylococcus aureus*).
- Pyogenic liver abscess occurs from:
  1. Biliary disease with cholangitis (accounts for approximately 40% to 60%).
  2. Gallbladder disease with contiguous spread to the liver.
  3. Diverticulitis or appendicitis with spread via the portal circulation.
  4. Hematogenous spread via the hepatic artery, though uncommon; if a solitary organism is isolated, a distant source of hematogenous seeding should be sought.
  5. Penetrating wounds.
  6. Cryptogenic.
  7. Infection by way of portal system (portal pyemia).
  8. No causes found in approximately half of cases.
  9. Incidence increased in patients with diabetes and metastatic cancer.
- Amebic hepatic abscess is caused by the parasite *Entamoeba histolytica*. Amebiasis is usually due to fecal-oral contamination and invades the intestinal mucosa, gaining entry into the portal system to reach the liver.

DIAGNOSIS

The diagnosis of liver abscess requires a high index of suspicion after a detailed history and physical examination. Imaging studies and microbiologic, serologic, and percutaneous techniques (e.g., aspiration) confirm the presence of a liver abscess.

DIFFERENTIAL DIAGNOSIS

- Cholangitis
- Cholecystitis
- Diverticulitis
- Appendicitis
- Perforated viscus
- Mesentery ischemia
- Pulmonary embolism
- Pancreatitis

WORKUP

- The workup of a liver abscess should focus on differentiating between amebic and pyogenic causes.
- Features suggesting an amebic cause include travel to an endemic area, single abscess rather than multiple abscesses, subacute onset of symptoms, and absence of conditions predisposing to pyogenic liver abscess, as highlighted under "Etiology."
- Laboratory studies are not specific but are useful as adjunctive tests.
- Imaging studies cannot differentiate between the two, and bacteriologic cultures may be sterile in 50% of the cases.

LABORATORY TESTS

- Complete blood count: leukocytosis
- Liver function tests: alkaline phosphatase is most commonly elevated (95% to 100%); aspartate transaminase (AST) and alanine transaminase (ALT) elevated in 50% of cases; elevated bilirubin (28% to 30%); decreased albumin
- Prothrombin time (INR): prolonged (70%)
- Blood cultures: positive in 50% of cases
- Aspiration (50% sterile)
- Stool samples for *E. histolytica* trophozoites (positive in 10% to 15% of amebic liver abscess cases)
- Serologic testing for *E. histolytica* does not differentiate acute from old infections

IMAGING STUDIES

- Ultrasound (80% to 100% sensitivity in detecting abscesses) shows round or oval hypoechogenic mass.
- CT scan is more sensitive in detecting hepatic abscesses and contiguous organ extension and is the imaging study of choice (Fig. 1-2).
- Chest x-ray: abnormal in 50% of the cases, may reveal elevated right hemidiaphragm, subdiaphragmatic air-fluid levels, pleural effusions, and consolidating infiltrates.
- Most liver abscesses are single; however, multiple liver abscesses can occur with systemic bacteremia.

TREATMENT

NONPHARMACOLOGIC THERAPY

- The management of pyogenic liver abscess differs from that of amebic liver abscess.
- Medical management is the cornerstone of therapy in amebic liver abscess, whereas early intervention in the form of surgical therapy or catheter drainage and parenteral

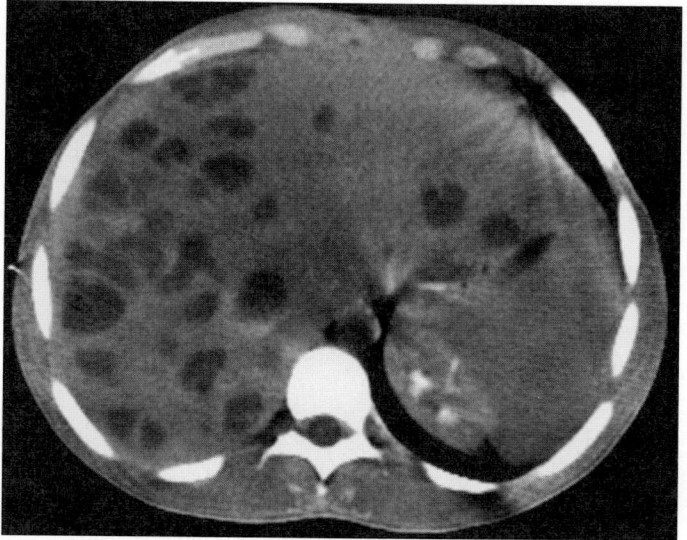

FIGURE 1-2 CT scan demonstrating multiple pyogenic liver abscesses in a 25-year-old man. (From Goldman L, Bennett JC [ed]: *Cecil textbook of medicine*, ed 22, Philadelphia, 2004, WB Saunders.)

antibiotics is the rule in pyogenic liver abscess.

ACUTE GENERAL Rx

- Percutaneous drainage under CT or ultrasound guidance is essential in the treatment of pyogenic liver abscesses.
- Aspiration of hepatic amebic abscesses is not required unless there is no response to treatment or a pyogenic cause is being considered.
- Empiric broad-spectrum antibiotics are recommended initially until culture results are available. Common choices include:
  1. Metronidazole (500 mg IV q8h) plus a fluoroquinolone (ciprofloxacin 400 mg IV q12h or levofloxacin 500 mg IV daily).
  2. Monotherapy with a beta-lactam/beta-lactamase inhibitor, such as piperacillin/tazobactam (4.5 g q6h), ticarcillin-clavulanate (3.1 g q4h), or ampicillin-sulbactam (3 g q6h).
  3. Monotherapy with a carbapenem, such as imipenem (500 mg IV q6h), meropenem (1 g q8h), or ertapenem (1 g daily).
  4. In patients with penicillin allergy, clindamycin 600 to 900 mg IV q8h with an aminoglycoside can be considered.
  5. Duration of antibiotic treatment is usually 4 to 6 wk with IV antibiotics used for the first 1 to 2 wk or until a favorable clinical response, followed thereafter with oral antibiotics (e.g., metronidazole 500 mg PO q8h plus ciprofloxacin 500 mg PO q12h).
  6. Third-generation cephalosporins should not be used for empiric therapy because of risk of the emergence of beta-lactamase-producing bacteria.

- Antibiotic coverage for amebic liver abscesses includes:
  1. Tissue agent: metronidazole 750 mg PO tid for 10 days
  2. Luminal agent: after therapy with tissue agent treatment with any luminal agent is required even if the stool is negative, such as paromomycin for 10 days or diiodohydroxyquin for 20 days.

CHRONIC Rx

- If fever persists for 2 wk despite percutaneous drainage and antibiotic therapy as outlined under "Acute General Rx," or if there is failure of aspiration or failure of percutaneous drainage, surgery is indicated.
- In patients not responding to intravenous antibiotics and percutaneous drainage, hepatic artery antibiotic infusion can be considered.
- In patients with evidence of metastatic disease that is causing biliary obstruction, a gastroenterology consultation for endoscopic retrograde cholangiopancreatography and stenting should be considered.

DISPOSITION

- Most patients with pyogenic liver abscesses defervesce within 2 wk of treatment with antibiotics and drainage.
- No randomized controlled studies have evaluated the optimal duration of antibiotic therapy for pyogenic liver abscess. Typical duration of antibiotic therapy is at least 4 to 6 wk.
- Pyogenic liver abscess cure rates using percutaneous drainage and antibiotics have been reported to be between 88% and 100%.

- Mortality rate of untreated pyogenic liver abscess is nearly 100%.
- Most patients with amebic liver abscesses defervesce within 4 to 5 days of treatment.
- Amebic liver abscess mortality rate is <1% unless complications occur (see "Comments").
- Follow-up imaging should be used to monitor response to therapy; continue treatment until CT scan shows complete or near complete resolution of cavity.

REFERRAL

Infectious disease, gastroenterology, interventional radiology, and general surgical consultations are recommended in any patient with hepatic abscess.

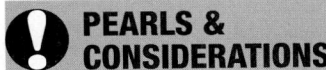

PEARLS & CONSIDERATIONS

COMMENTS

- Complications of pyogenic and amebic liver abscesses include:
  1. Pleuropulmonary extension, resulting in empyema, abscess, and fistula formation
  2. Peritonitis
  3. Purulent pericarditis
  4. Sepsis
- Amebic liver abscesses complicate amebic colitis in nearly 10% of cases.

SUGGESTED READINGS
available at www.expertconsult.com

AUTHOR: **TANYA ALI, M.D.**

❗ BASIC INFORMATION

DEFINITION

A lung abscess is an infection of the lung parenchyma resulting in a necrotic cavity containing pus.

SYNONYMS

Pulmonary abscess

ICD-9CM CODES
513.0 Abscess of lung

EPIDEMIOLOGY & DEMOGRAPHICS

INCIDENCE: Has decreased over the last 30 years as a result of antibiotic therapy.
- Lung abscess in patients age 50 and over is associated with primary lung neoplasia in 30% of the cases.
- Lung abscesses commonly coexist with empyemas.

RISK FACTORS (see Table 1-1):
1. Alcohol-related problems
2. Seizure disorders
3. Cerebrovascular disorders with dysphagia
4. Drug abuse
5. Esophageal disorders (e.g., scleroderma, esophageal carcinoma, etc.)
6. Poor oral hygiene
7. Obstructive malignant lung disease
8. Bronchiectasis

PHYSICAL FINDINGS & CLINICAL PRESENTATION

- Symptoms are generally insidious and prolonged, occurring for weeks to months
- Fever, chills, and sweats
- Cough
- Sputum production (purulent with foul odor)
- Pleuritic chest pain
- Hemoptysis
- Dyspnea
- Malaise, fatigue, and weakness
- Tachycardia and tachypnea
- Dullness to percussion, whispered pectoriloquy, and bronchophony
- Amphoric breath sounds (low-pitched sound of air moving across a large open cavity)

ETIOLOGY

- The most important factor predisposing to lung abscess is aspiration.
- Following aspiration as a major predisposing factor is periodontal disease.
- Lung abscess is rare in an edentulous person.
- Approximately 90% of lung abscesses are caused by anaerobic microorganisms (*Bacteroides fragilis, Fusobacterium nucleatum*, peptostreptococci, microaerophilic streptococci). Pulmonary actinomycosis will also generate lung abscess.
- In most cases anaerobic infection is mixed with aerobic or facultative anaerobic organisms (*S. aureus, E. coli, K. pneumoniae, P. aeruginosa*).
- Parasitic organisms including *Paragonimus westermani* and *Entamoeba histolytica*.
- Fungi including *Aspergillus, Cryptococcus, Histoplasma, Blastomyces*, and *Coccidioides* spp.
- Immunocompromised hosts may become infected with *Aspergillus*, mycobacteria, *Nocardia, Legionella micdadei*, and *Rhodococcus equi*.

❗ DIAGNOSIS

Lung abscess may be primary or secondary.
- Primary lung abscess refers to infection from normal host organisms within the lung (e.g., aspiration, pneumonia).
- Secondary lung abscess results from other preexisting conditions (e.g., endocarditis, underlying lung cancer, pulmonary emboli).

Lung abscess may be acute or chronic.
- Acute lung abscess is present if symptoms are of less than 4 to 6 wk.
- Chronic lung abscess is present if symptoms last longer than 6 wk.

DIFFERENTIAL DIAGNOSIS

The differential diagnosis is similar to that for cavitary lung lesions:
- Bacterial (anaerobic, aerobic, infected bulla, empyema, actinomycosis, tuberculosis)
- Fungal (histoplasmosis, coccidioidomycosis, blastomycosis, aspergillosis, cryptococcosis)
- Parasitic (amebiasis, echinococcosis)

- Malignancy (primary lung carcinoma, metastatic lung disease, lymphoma, Hodgkin's disease)
- Wegener's granulomatosis, sarcoidosis, endocarditis, and septic pulmonary emboli

WORKUP

- The workup of a patient with lung abscess attempts to elicit a primary or a secondary cause.
- Blood tests are not specific in diagnosing lung abscesses.
- Most diagnoses are made from imaging studies; however, to diagnose a specific cause bacteriologic studies are needed.

LABORATORY TESTS

- CBC with leukocytosis
- Bacteriologic studies
  1. Sputum Gram stain and culture (commonly contaminated by oral flora)
  2. Percutaneous transtracheal aspiration
  3. Percutaneous transthoracic aspiration
  4. Fiberoptic bronchoscopy using bronchial brushings or bronchoalveolar lavage is the most widely used intervention when trying to obtain diagnostic bacteriologic cultures
- Blood cultures on some occasions (<30%) may be positive
- If an empyema is present, obtaining empyema fluid via thoracentesis may isolate the organism

IMAGING STUDIES

- Chest x-ray makes the diagnosis of lung abscess showing the cavitary lesion with an air fluid level.
- Lung abscesses are most commonly found in the posterior segment of the right upper lobe.
- Chest CT scan can localize and size the lesion and assist in differentiating lung abscesses from other pathologic processes (e.g., tumor, empyema, infected bulla, etc.) (Fig. 1-3).

❗ TREATMENT

NONPHARMACOLOGIC THERAPY

- Oxygen therapy
- Postural drainage
- Respiratory therapy maneuvers

ACUTE GENERAL Rx

- Penicillin 1 to 2 million units IV q4h until improvement (e.g., afebrile, decrease in sputum production, etc.) followed by penicillin VK 500 mg PO qid for the next 2 to 3 wk but usually requiring longer 6- to 8-wk courses.
- Metronidazole is given with penicillin at doses of 7.5 mg/kg IV q6h followed by PO 500 mg bid to qid dosing.
- Clindamycin is an alternative choice if concerned about penicillin-resistant organisms. The dose is 600 mg IV q8h until improvement followed by 300 mg to 600 mg PO q6h.

TABLE 1-1	Risk Factors for Aspiration Pneumonia and Lung Abscess
Increased bacterial inoculum	Periodontal disease, gingivitis, tonsillar or dental abscess, drugs that decrease gastric acidity
Impairment of consciousness	Drugs, alcohol, general anesthesia, metabolic encephalopathy, coma, shock, cerebrovascular accident, cardiopulmonary arrest, seizures, surgery, trauma
Impaired cough and gag reflexes	Vocal cord paralysis, intratracheal anesthesia, endotracheal tube, tracheostomy, myopathy, myelopathy, other neurologic disorders
Impairment of esophageal function	Diverticula, achalasia, strictures, disorders of gastrointestinal motility, neoplasm, tracheoesophageal fistula, pseudobulbar palsy
Emesis	Nasogastric tube, gastric dilatation, ileus, intestinal obstruction

From Cohen J, Powderly WG: *Infectious diseases*, ed 2, St Louis, 2004, Mosby.

CHRONIC Rx
- Bronchoscopy to assist with drainage and/or diagnosis is indicated in patients who fail to respond to antibiotics or if there is suspected underlying malignancy.
- Surgery is indicated on rare occasions (<10%) in patients with complications of lung abscess (see "Comments").

DISPOSITION
- More than 95% of patients are cured with the use of antibiotics alone.
- Complications of lung abscesses include:
  1. Empyema
  2. Massive hemoptysis
  3. Pneumothorax
  4. Bronchopleural fistula
- Mortality is low in community-acquired lung abscess (2.5%).
- Hospital-acquired lung abscess carries a high mortality rate (65%).

REFERRAL
If lung abscess is present, consultation with pulmonary and infectious disease specialist is recommended.

PEARLS & CONSIDERATIONS

COMMENTS
- Complications of lung abscesses include:
  1. Empyema
  2. Bronchopleural fistula
  3. Hepatobronchial fistula
  4. Brain abscess
  5. Bronchiectasis
- Refractory cases are usually the result of:
  1. Large cavity size (>6 cm)
  2. Recurrent aspiration
  3. Thick-walled cavities
  4. Underlying lung carcinoma
  5. Empyema formation
- Necrotizing pneumonia is similar to a lung abscess but differs in size (<2 cm in diameter) and number (usually multiple suppurative cavitary lesions).

SUGGESTED READINGS
available at www.expertconsult.com

AUTHORS: **GLENN G. FORT, M.D., M.P.H.,** and **DENNIS J. MIKOLICH, M.D.**

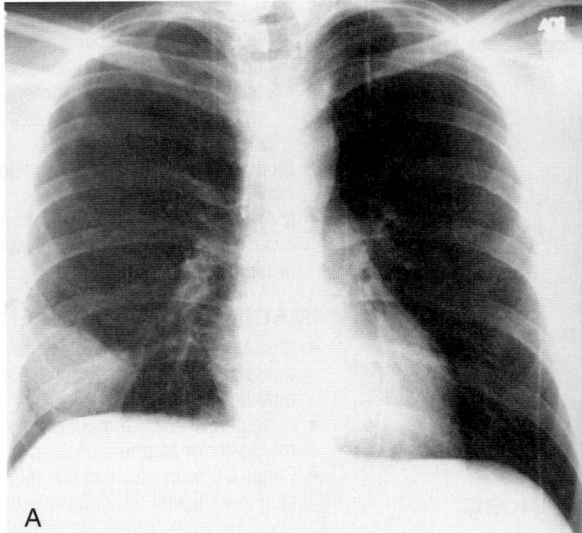
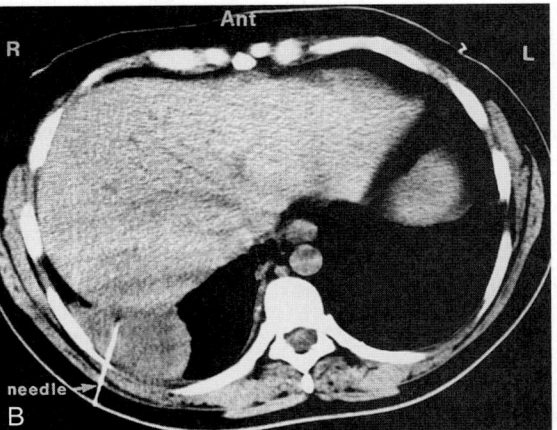

FIGURE 1-3 Lung abscess. On a chest radiograph, a lung abscess may look to be a solid rounded lesion **(A)**, or, if it has a connection with the bronchus, there may be an air fluid level in a thick-walled cavitary lesion. CT scanning **(B)** can be used to localize the lesion and to place a needle for drainage and aspiration of contents for culture. (From Mettler FA [ed]: *Primary care radiology,* Philadelphia, 2000, WB Saunders.)

BASIC INFORMATION

DEFINITION

Pelvic abscess is an acute or chronic infection, most commonly involving the pelvic viscera. Treatment and possible cure require directed therapy that will involve antibiotic therapy and, if medical therapy fails, subsequent surgical therapy. There are four categories based on etiologic factors:

- Ascending infection, spreading from cervix through endometrial cavity to adnexa, forming a tuboovarian complex
- Infection occurring in the puerperium, which spreads to the adnexa from the endometrium or myometrium by a hematogenous or lymphatic route
- Abscess complicating pelvic surgery
- Involvement of the pelvic viscera as a result of spread from contiguous organs, such as appendicitis or diverticulitis

SYNONYMS

Tuboovarian abscess (TOA)
Vaginal cuff abscess

ICD-9CM CODES
614.2 Salpingitis and oophoritis not specified as acute, subacute, or chronic

EPIDEMIOLOGY & DEMOGRAPHICS

INCIDENCE:
- 34% of hospitalized patients with pelvic inflammatory disease
- 1% to 2% of patients undergoing hysterectomy, most with vaginal approach
- Peak incidence third to fourth decade

RISK FACTORS: Same risk factors as for pelvic inflammatory disease, although in 30% to 50% of patients there is no prior history of salpingitis before abscess forms.

PHYSICAL FINDINGS & CLINICAL PRESENTATION

- Abdominal or pelvic pain (90%)
- Fever or chills (50%)
- Abnormal bleeding (21%)
- Vaginal discharge (28%)
- Nausea (26%)
- Up to 60% to 80% present in the absence of fever or leukocytosis; absence of these findings should not rule out diagnosis

ETIOLOGY

- Mixed flora of anaerobes, aerobes, and facultative anaerobes, such as *Escherichia coli*, *Bacteroides fragilis*, *Prevotella* spp., aerobic streptococci, and *Peptococcus* and *Peptostreptococcus* spp.
- *Nesseria gonorrhoeae* and *Chlamydia* are the major etiologic bacteria in cervicitis and salpingitis but are rarely found in abscess cavity cultures.

- In elderly patients consider diverticular disease.

DIAGNOSIS

DIFFERENTIAL DIAGNOSIS

- Pelvic neoplasms, such as ovarian tumors and leiomyomas.
- Inflammatory masses involving adjacent bowel or omentum, such as ruptured appendicitis or diverticulitis.
- Pelvic hematomas, as may occur after cesarean section or hysterectomy.
- Section III describes the diagnostic approach to patients with a pelvic mass; the differential diagnosis of pelvic mass is described in Section II.
- The differential diagnosis of pelvic pain is described in Section II.
- Sonogram or CT scan: commonly used due to associated pain and guarding, resulting in a suboptimal abdominal or pelvic examination.
- Most common cause of preventable death: physician delay in diagnosis.

LABORATORY TESTS

- CBC with differential
- Aerobic as well as anaerobic cultures of cervix, blood, urine, sputum, peritoneal cavity (if entered), and abscess cavity before starting antibiotics
- Pregnancy test in patients of reproductive age

IMAGING STUDIES

- Sonogram: noninvasive, inexpensive study to confirm diagnosis, estimate size of abscess, and monitor response to therapy; sensitivity >90%
- CT scan: used for both diagnosis and therapy (CT-guided drainage)
  1. Useful where sonogram provides insufficient information, as with intraabdominal abscesses
  2. Success rate with CT-guided abscess drainage: unilocular, 90%; multilocular, 40%

TREATMENT

Major concerns:
1. Desire for future fertility
2. Likelihood of rupture of abscess, with resulting peritonitis, septic shock, and morbid sequelae

ACUTE GENERAL Rx

- Clinical quandary is whether patient requires immediate surgery (uncertain diagnosis or suspicion of rupture) or management with IV antibiotics, reserving surgery for those with inadequate clinical response (e.g., 48 to 72 hr of therapy, with persistent fever or leukocytosis, increasing size of mass, or suspicion of rupture)

- Early surgery may be needed in those with large adnexal masses (>8 cm), or in immunocompromised patients
- Antibiotic combinations:
  1. Clindamycin 900 mg IV q8h or metronidazole 500 mg IV q6-8h plus gentamicin either 5 to 7 mg/kg q24h or 1.5 mg/kg q8h
  2. Alternatives: ampicillin sulbactam 3 g IV q6h or cefoxitin 2 g IV q6h or cefotetan 2 g IV q12h plus doxycycline 100 mg IV q12h
- During medical management, high index of suspicion for acute rupture, such as acute worsening of abdominal pain or new-onset tachycardia and hypotension, mandating immediate surgical intervention after patient stabilization
- Surgical options:
  1. Laparoscopy with drainage and irrigation
  2. Transvaginal colpotomy (abscess must be midline, dissect rectovaginal septum, and be adherent to vaginal fornix)
  3. Laparotomy, including total abdominal hysterectomy with bilateral salpingo-oophorectomy or unilateral salpingo-oophorectomy
  4. Evidence of ruptured tuboovarian abscess is a surgical emergency

DISPOSITION

- Of patients treated with medical therapy, response in 75%, with a 50% pregnancy rate. Pregnancy rate decreases with recurrent episodes.
- No response in 30% to 40%; can be treated with either CT-guided drainage or surgical intervention, keeping in mind that unilateral adnexectomy may give equal chance of cure versus hysterectomy, yet preserve reproductive potential.

REFERRAL

If patient has a tuboovarian abscess, refer to gynecologist.

PEARLS & CONSIDERATIONS

COMMENTS

If *Actinomyces* species is isolated from culture, treatment with penicillin is required for an extended period (6 wk to 3 mo).

SUGGESTED READINGS
available at www.expertconsult.com

AUTHORS: **SCOTT J. ZUCCALA, D.O.,** and **RUBEN ALVERO, M.D.**

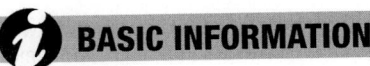

DEFINITION

A perirectal abscess is a localized inflammatory process that can be associated with infections of soft tissue and anal glands based on anatomic location. Perianal and perirectal abscesses may be simple or complex, causing suppuration. Infections in these spaces may be classified as superficial perianal or perirectal with involvement in the following anatomic spaces: ischiorectal, intersphincteric, perianal, and supralevator (Fig. 1-4).

SYNONYMS

Rectal abscess
Perianal abscess
Anorectal abscess

ICD-9CM CODES
566 Perirectal abscess

EPIDEMIOLOGY & DEMOGRAPHICS

INCIDENCE (IN U.S.): Commonly encountered
PREDOMINANT SEX: Male > female
PREDOMINANT AGE: All ages
PEAK INCIDENCE: Not seasonal; common
GENETICS: None known

PHYSICAL FINDINGS & CLINICAL PRESENTATION

- Localized perirectal or anal pain—often worsened with movement or straining
- Perirectal erythema or cellulitis
- Perirectal mass by inspection or palpation

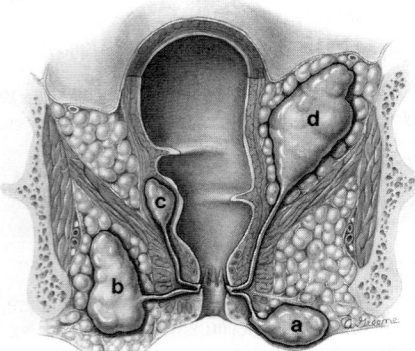

FIGURE 1-4 Common sites of anorectal abscesses: perianal (**a**), ischiorectal (**b**), intersphincteric (**c**), and supralevator (**d**). (From Noble J [ed]: *Textbook of primary care medicine,* ed 2, St Louis, 1996, Mosby.)

- Fever and signs of sepsis with deep abscess
- Urinary retention

ETIOLOGY

- Polymicrobial aerobic and anaerobic bacteria involving one of the anatomic spaces (see "Definition"), often associated with localized trauma
- Microbiology: most bacteria are polymicrobial, mixed enteric and skin flora
- Predominant anaerobic bacteria:
  1. *Bacteroides fragilis*
  2. *Peptostreptococcus* spp.
  3. *Prevotella* spp.
  4. *Porphyromonas* spp.
  5. *Clostridium* spp.
  6. *Fusobacterium* spp.
- Predominant aerobic bacteria:
  1. *Staphylococcus aureus*
  2. *Streptococcus* spp.
  3. *Escherichia coli*
  4. *Enterococcus* spp.

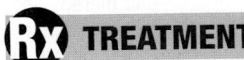

DIAGNOSIS

Many patients will have predisposing underlying conditions including:
- Malignancy or leukemia
- Immune deficiency
- Diabetes mellitus
- Recent surgery
- Steroid therapy

DIFFERENTIAL DIAGNOSIS

- Neutropenic enterocolitis
- Crohn's disease (inflammatory bowel disease)
- Pilonidal disease
- Hidradenitis suppurativa
- Tuberculosis or actinomycosis; Chagas' disease
- Cancerous lesions
- Chronic anal fistula
- Rectovaginal fistula
- Proctitis—often STD-associated, including: syphilis, gonococcal, chlamydia, chancroid, condylomata acuminata
- AIDS-associated: Kaposi's sarcoma, lymphoma, CMV

WORKUP

- Examination of rectal, perirectal/perineal areas
- Rule out necrotic process and crepitance suggesting deep tissue involvement
- Local aerobic and anaerobic culture

- Blood cultures if toxic, febrile, or compromised
- Possible sigmoidoscopy

IMAGING STUDIES

Usually not indicated unless extensive disease abscess but can include CT

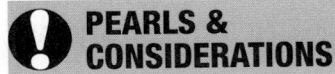

TREATMENT

ACUTE GENERAL Rx

- Incision and drainage of abscess
- Debridement if necrotic tissue
- Rule out need for fistulectomy
- Local wound care—packing
- Sitz baths

Antibiotic treatment: Directed toward coverage for mixed skins and enteric flora

Outpatient—oral:
Amoxicillin/clavulanic acid 875 to 1000 mg bid
Ciprofloxacin 750 mg PO q12h plus metronidazole 500 to 750 mg PO q8h
Clindamycin 150 to 300 mg PO q8h
Inpatient—intravenous:
Ampicillin/sulbactam 1.5 to 3 gm IV q6h
Cefotetan 1 to 2 gm IV q8h
Piperacillin/Tazobactam 3.375 gm IV q6 to 8h
Imipenem 500 to 1000 mg IV q8h

DISPOSITION

Follow-up with a general surgeon or infectious disease physician is often warranted.

REFERRAL

- General surgeon or colorectal surgeon for drainage.
- AIDS specialist may be needed for perirectal complications of HIV infection.
- Gastroenterologist follow-up may be warranted in Crohn's disease with perirectal fistula and other complications.

PEARLS & CONSIDERATIONS

Perirectal abscess may be a presenting manifestation of type 2 diabetes mellitus in older adults. Check the blood sugar in patients to exclude the possibility of unrecognized diabetes mellitus.

SUGGESTED READING
available at www.expertconsult.com

AUTHORS: **GLENN G. FORT, M.D., M.P.H.,** and **DENNIS J. MIKOLICH, M.D.**

BASIC INFORMATION

DEFINITION

Definition from the Federal Child Abuse Prevention and Treatment Act (CAPTA): any recent act or failure to act on the part of a parent or caretaker that results in death, serious physical or emotional harm, sexual abuse or exploitation of a child; or an act or failure to act which presents an imminent risk of serious harm to a child.

- Neglect: failure to provide for the basic needs of a child
  1. Physical neglect: failure to provide necessary food, shelter, and supervision
  2. Medical neglect: failure to provide necessary medical or mental health care
  3. Educational neglect: failure to meet educational needs
  4. Emotional neglect: failure to attend to emotional needs, exposure to domestic violence
- Physical abuse: physical injury inflicted by a parent or caregiver intentionally or in the course of excessive discipline
- Sexual abuse: sexual act inflicted by parent or caretaker; includes exploitation and pornography
- Emotional abuse: pattern of behavior of caretaker toward a child that impairs emotional development. This includes verbal abuse, cruelty, and threats.

SYNONYMS

Child maltreatment syndrome
Physical abuse
Sexual abuse
Battered child syndrome
Shaken baby syndrome
Shaken impact syndrome
Abusive head trauma

ICD-9CM CODES
995.5   Child maltreatment
995.50 Child abuse, unspecified
995.51 Child abuse, emotional or psychological
995.52 Child neglect
995.53 Child abuse, sexual
995.54 Child abuse, physical
995.55 Shaken infant syndrome
995.59 Multiple forms of child abuse

EPIDEMIOLOGY & DEMOGRAPHICS

INCIDENCE (IN U.S.): Any reports of incidence are underestimates because many cases are not recognized or reported. The following data are based on Child Protective Services (CPS) state aggregates. In 2008, roughly 772,000 children were determined to be victims of abuse or neglect.

- Types of abuse by percentage (note the total is greater than 100% since children are often victims of more than one type of abuse).
  1. Neglect: 71.1%
  2. Physical abuse: 16.1%
  3. Sexual abuse: 9.1%
  4. Emotional abuse: 7.3%
  5. Medical neglect: 2.2%
  6. Other: 9% (e.g., abandonment, threats of harm, congenital drug addiction)
- For 2008, an estimated 1740 child deaths were caused by abuse or neglect.
  - Overall annual death rate resulting from abuse or neglect is estimated to be 2.33 deaths/100,000 children.
  - More than 30% of these deaths were due to neglect; 23% were due to physical abuse. Almost 40% were due to multiple forms of maltreatment.
  - 80% of these children were <4 yr of age.
  - Most fatalities were directly caused by one or both parents (71%).
  - Many child abuse fatalities are underreported because of misdiagnosis or variations in state definitions and coding.
- More than 80% of abused children were victimized by one or both of their parents.
- One fifth of adult women report history of molestation or sexual assault as a child or adolescent.

PREDOMINANT SEX:
- There is a slight predominance of girls as victims.
- Infant boys (<1 yr) have the highest death rate: 19.3 per 100,000 boys of the same age versus 17.2 per 100,000 infant girls of the same age.

PREDOMINANT AGE: Youngest children (0 to 3 yr old) have the highest rates of victimization with 33% being younger than the age of 4.

GENETICS: No known genetic factors.

ETIOLOGY

Multiple factors contribute to the incidence. No factor or combination of factors can definitively predict which children will be victimized. Factors contributing to risk of abuse or neglect include the following:
- Parent
  1. Substance abuse
  2. Mental illness
  3. Intellectual impairment
  4. Parental history of being abused as a child
- Child
  1. Low birth weight or prematurity
  2. Chronic physical disability
- Family
  1. Social isolation
  2. Poor parent-child bonding
  3. Stress: unemployment, chronic illness, eviction, arrest, poverty
  4. Domestic violence
- Community/society
  1. Limited transportation
  2. Limited day care
  3. Unsafe neighborhoods
  4. Poverty

DIAGNOSIS

Careful history and physical examination are the most important aspects of the evaluation. Careful documentation of any statements regarding origin of injuries or history of abuse is crucial. Chart and photographic documentation of injuries is also essential. The following are keys to the final diagnosis:

- Patterned bruising (e.g., loop-shaped, square, oval) is indicative of being struck with an object.
- Injury observed is incompatible with the history provided.
- History of injury provided is incompatible with the developmental capabilities of the child.
- Delay in seeking care for a significant injury (e.g., callus formation on a fracture, eschar formation on a burn).
- Bruising is rare in healthy infants and warrants further investigation.
- Multiple significant injuries of different ages.
- Infant with clinically significant head trauma attributed to a trivial cause (e.g., a short fall). Often associated with retinal hemorrhages and skeletal fractures, which are indicative of shaken baby syndrome or abusive head trauma.
- Certain fractures in infants without a history of significant trauma (e.g., motor vehicle accident) are characteristic of abuse: metaphyseal, rib, sternum, scapula, vertebral body.
- Inflicted contact burns are indicated by an impression of the burning object: lighter, iron, cigarette.
- Inflicted immersion burns are indicated by "stocking" burns of the feet or "glove" burns of the hands. Stocking burns are often associated with buttocks/perineal burns from immersion of a minor in a flexed position.
- Most sexual abuse victims will have a normal or nonspecific genital examination. A normal genital examination does not mean the child was not abused. History is the most important part of the diagnosis. Forensic interview by a trained professional is recommended, as is an examination by an experienced health care provider for child and adolescent victims of sexual abuse.
- The identification of a sexually transmitted disease in a prepubertal child who is beyond the neonatal period is suggestive of sexual abuse. Reporting and further careful investigation are warranted. Consult current CDC guidelines and a child sexual abuse expert for further guidance.

DIFFERENTIAL DIAGNOSIS

In all categories, accidental injury is the most common entity to be distinguished from abuse. Accidental injuries are most common over bony prominences: forehead, elbows, knees, shins; soft, fleshy areas are more common for inflicted injury: buttocks, thighs, upper arms.

BRUISING
- Bleeding disorder (idiopathic thrombocytopenic purpura, hemophilia, leukemia, hemorrhagic disease of the newborn, von Willebrand's disease)
- Connective tissue disorder (Ehlers-Danlos syndrome, vasculitis)
- Pigments (Mongolian spots)
- Dermatitis (phytophotodermatitis, nickel allergy)
- Folk treatment (coining, cupping)

BURNS
- Chemical burn
- Impetigo
- Folk treatment (moxibustion)
- Dermatitis (phytophotodermatitis)

INTRACRANIAL HEMORRHAGE
- Bleeding disorder
- Perinatal trauma (should resolve by 4 wk)
- Arteriovenous malformation rupture
- Glutaric aciduria

FRACTURES
- Osteogenesis imperfecta
- Rickets
- Congenital syphilis
- Very low birth weight (osteopenia of prematurity)

SEXUAL ABUSE
- Normal variants
- Lichen sclerosis et atrophicus
- Congenital abnormalities
- Urethral prolapse
- Hemangioma
- Nonsexually acquired infection (group A *Streptococcus, Shigella*)

WORKUP

History and physical examination:
- Careful history from all caretakers and child.
- Scene investigation may be necessary.
- Complete physical examination.
- Sexual abuse: forensic interview and magnified examinations by trained professionals are the standard for evaluation and evidence collection. This is especially important to avoid further psychological or physical trauma to the child.

Laboratory tests for physical abuse:
- Tests performed may vary depending on the severity of abuse and clinical presentation of the child.
- CBC with differential and platelets.
- Prothrombin time, activated partial thromboplastin time.
- Consider closure time (PFA-100), von Willebrand panel.
- Alanine aminotransferase, amylase, urinalysis.

Laboratory tests for sexual abuse:
- If within 72 hr of acute sexual assault/abuse, swabs are obtained for sperm, acid phosphatase, P30, MHS-5 antigen, blood group typing, DNA testing. Also collect samples of foreign hair, blood, saliva, or other tissue if present.
- Per current CDC recommendations, adolescent victims of acute assault should have appropriate specimens collected from sites of penetration or attempted penetration for *Neisseria gonorrheae* and *Chlamydia.* Nucleic acid amplification tests (NAATs) may be used and are preferred. In females, wet mount and culture of vaginal swab for trichomonas should also be done. If there is itching, vaginal discharge or malodor present, wet mount for bacterial vaginosis and candida should also be done. Serum should be obtained for HIV, hepatitis B, and syphilis testing acutely. If

negative, HIV and syphilis testing should be repeated 6, 12, and 24 wk after the assault.
- Child victims (i.e., prepubertal) should have specimens collected if considered high risk for a sexually transmitted infection (STI) per current CDC recommendations. Cervical specimens are not collected and vaginal specimens must be collected with care by an experienced provider to avoid further trauma to the child. Gonorrhea and *Chlamydia* culture is the gold standard for diagnosis and legal purposes. However, many providers now analyze specimens using urine or vaginal NAAT followed by culture confirmation if any positive results are obtained. Any culture testing positive for *N. gonorrheae* should be confirmed by at least two laboratory tests that are based on different principles. Specimens should be collected for gonorrhea and *Chlamydia,* wet mount, and blood for serologic testing (HIV, hepatitis B, syphilis) in the following cases:
  1. Child has a past or current symptom of an STI, such as vaginal discharge, genital ulcer, or vaginal pain
  2. Alleged assailant is known to have an STI or be at high risk for an STI
  3. A sibling or adult in the same household has a known STI
  4. High prevalence of STIs in the community
  5. Evidence of ejaculation or penetration is present on the examination
  6. Child or parent requests testing

IMAGING STUDIES

Physical abuse:
- Radiographic skeletal survey for all children <2 yr; for 2- to 5-yr-olds, done only for severe abuse. Consider repeat skeletal survey in 2 wk if severe physical injury is present.
- Noncontrast head CT scan or MRI for all children <1 yr; for children >1 yr, clinical judgment should be used.
- Head MRI for children with significant abusive head trauma. This is used as an adjunct a few days after initial head CT.
- Abdominal CT scan if indicated by clinical examination or laboratory evaluation.

Rx TREATMENT

ACUTE GENERAL Rx
- Stabilize and treat acute medical injuries.
- Report to Child Protective Services. HIPAA allows reports for suspected child abuse without parental authorization.
- Early report to law enforcement for suspected physical abuse or sexual abuse to allow scene investigation.
- Disposition, once medically stable, is dependent on CPS. The child cannot be returned home if the environment is not safe.
- Physician should remain available to discuss with investigators. This is often critical to determining the outcome of the case and placement of the child.
- Because follow-up of adolescent sexual assault victims can be difficult, many experts

recommend empiric treatment for STIs: gonorrhea, *Chlamydia, Trichomonas,* and bacterial vaginosis. Pregnancy prophylaxis should also be offered. Hepatitis B immunization should be offered if not previously given. HIV prophylaxis is offered in certain situations depending on local epidemiology and type of assault. Consult local infectious disease experts for current recommendations. Repeat examination should be done in 2 wk for all victims of sexual assault, especially if they declined empiric treatment. If empiric treatment was not done, STI testing should be repeated at the 2-week follow-up visit.
- Empiric treatment of child victims of sexual abuse is generally not recommended. This is especially important if NAATs are used for screening for STIs because confirmation is necessary for any positive results. Careful follow-up within 2 wk and treatment based on culture results are indicated. HIV prophylaxis is offered in certain circumstances according to local epidemiology and risk. Consult with a local infectious disease expert for further recommendations.

CHRONIC Rx
- Often depends on CPS and court-ordered interventions
- Treatment of parental mental illness
- Treatment of parental substance abuse, including requirements for random drug testing
- Instruction for parents in behavior management skills, including appropriate limit setting and discipline
- Anger management classes for parents
- Trauma-focused cognitive-behavioral therapy is an evidence-based practice for victims of sexual abuse and exposure to domestic violence; useful to include nonoffending parent/caregiver
- Ongoing individual and family therapy
  - Parent-child interactive therapy is an evidence-based practice that is used with young children with behavioral problems and parent-child relationship problems
  - Child-parent psychotherapy is an evidence-based practice that is for young children (<5 yr) who have experienced a trauma and their caregivers
- May need long-term placement in foster care before it is safe to return home

OUTCOMES
- Victims of chronic abuse and neglect:
  - Have higher rates of mental illness (depression, suicide, posttraumatic stress disorder, eating disorders)
  - Have more cognitive difficulties, often impaired academic performance
  - Are more likely to become aggressive
  - Are more likely to have adverse physical health (cardiovascular disease, cancer, STDs)
- Victims of abusive head trauma:
  - One third die, one third have severe disability, one third appear normal in the short term.

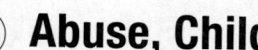
PEARLS & CONSIDERATIONS

PREVENTION

- Home visitation by a specially trained nurse to high-risk families during pregnancy and infancy has shown positive outcomes (Nurse-Family Partnership).
- Anticipatory guidance at health visits to teach normal developmental expectations and appropriate discipline.
- Screening to identify at-risk or abused children.
- Targeted education in the newborn nursery for shaken baby prevention has been shown to be effective.
- Substance abuse prevention and treatment.
- Identification and intervention for domestic violence before children are born.

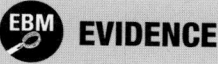 **EVIDENCE**

available at www.expertconsult.com

SUGGESTED READINGS

available at www.expertconsult.com

AUTHOR: **NANCY R. GRAFF, M.D.**

A

Diseases and Disorders

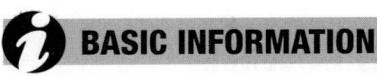

BASIC INFORMATION

DEFINITION

Drug abuse is a recurring pattern of harmful use of a substance despite adverse consequences to work, school, relationships, the legal system, or personal health. This may occur concurrently with or independently from *substance dependence,* in which the impairment or distress is more pervasive and often (though not necessarily) includes physical dependence and withdrawal symptoms (Table 1-2).

SYNONYMS

Substance use disorder
Substance abuse
Addiction

ICD-9CM CODES
Defined by specific substance F10-F19
(DSM-IV code is also defined by specific substance 291-292, 303-305)

EPIDEMIOLOGY & DEMOGRAPHICS

INCIDENCE (IN U.S.): Alcohol or drug dependence: 5% to 10% of population
PREVALENCE (IN U.S.): Approximately 15% of patients in primary care practice have an at-risk pattern of drug and/or alcohol use; lifetime prevalence of any alcohol use disorder: 30%; prescription drug misuse is on the rise with 5% past-year prevalence.
PREDOMINANT SEX: Males > females
PREDOMINANT AGE:
- Problematic use of substances may begin in early life (8 to 10 yr).
- Mean age of onset of problem drinking is approximately 25 yr for men and 30 yr for women.
PEAK INCIDENCE: For most substances: age 15 to 30 yr
DURATION OF CONDITION:
- Men: average >20 yr of heavy drinking
- Women: average 15 yr of heavy drinking
- In general, substance use disorders are chronic and replasing and often progressive

GENETICS: There is evidence of nonspecific genetic factors.

PHYSICAL FINDINGS & CLINICAL PRESENTATION

- Polysubstance use and comorbidity with psychiatric disorders is common.
- History often reveals recurring behavioral problems, such as relationship, work, or legal problems; violence and traumatic injuries; and anxiety, depression, insomnia, and cognitive and memory dysfunction.
- Repeated requests for early refills of controlled substances and obtaining prescriptions from multiple providers should raise concern for prescription drug abuse.
- Physical findings may include injection marks, nasal lesions or recurrent epistaxis, poor dentition, scars or bruises from falls or trauma, and poor nutritional status; signs/symptoms of intoxication or withdrawal are highly suggestive of substance use disorder.

ETIOLOGY

Two models of addiction:
1. Conditioning (reward driven): Substance use is paired with enforcing and triggering stimuli.
2. Homeostatic (self-medicating): Either preexisting abnormalities or drug-induced abnormalities lead to initial or continued use of the drug.

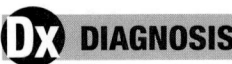 DIAGNOSIS

DIFFERENTIAL DIAGNOSIS

- Psychiatric disorders such as depression, mania, social phobia, or other anxiety disorders may coexist or occur as a consequence of substance abuse.
- Rule out seizure disorder and underlying illness.

WORKUP

- A thorough history is crucial for diagnosis.
- The physician's history-taking style and techniques strongly affect patient's willingness to report use and participate in future treatment activities.
- A structured, nonjudgmental approach is generally preferable:
  1. Ask about alcohol or drug use in the past year.
  2. Use a short screening instrument such as the two-item screen ("In the last year, have you ever consumed alcohol or used drugs more than you meant to? Have you felt you wanted or needed to cut down on your drinking or drug use in the last year?").
  3. Ask about quantity and frequency. For example, the National Institute on Alcohol and Alcoholism declares that problem drinking for men is defined as more than 14 drinks/wk or more than 4 drinks on any one occasion; for women and anyone older than 65 yr, the limits are 7 drinks and no more than 3 on any one occasion.
- Problematic behavior during intoxication or withdrawal is diagnostic.
- Because self-report of substance use and its consequences can be unreliable, obtaining corrobarating information, such as from family members, is often helpful.

LABORATORY TESTS

- Consider toxicology screen or blood alcohol level.
- Elevated mean corpuscular volume and γ-glutamyltransferase are most sensitive indicators of alcohol intake.

IMAGING STUDIES

Not helpful in routine diagnosis and management of substance abuse, but possibly useful in the management of sequelae of substance abuse (e.g., brain imaging to evaluate the alcohol abuse–associated increased risk of subdural hematomas or increased evidence of cerebral atrophy).

TABLE 1-2 Diagnostic Criteria for Dependence and Drug Abuse

Dependence (>3 Needed)	Abuse (>1 for 12 mo)
1. Tolerance	1. Recurrent substance use resulting in failure to fulfill major role obligations at work, school, or home
2. Withdrawal	
3. The substance is often taken in larger amounts over a longer period than intended	2. Recurrent substance use in situations in which it is physically hazardous
	3. Recurrent substance-related legal problems
4. Any unsuccessful effort or a persistent desire to cut down or control substance use	4. Continued substance use despite having persistent or recurrent social or interpersonal problems caused or exacerbated by the effects of the substance
5. A great deal of time is spent in activities necessary to obtain the substance or recover from its effects	5. Never met criteria for dependence
6. Important social, occupational, or recreational activities given up or reduced because of substance use	
7. Continued substance use despite knowledge of having had persistent or recurrent physical or psychological problems that are likely to be caused or exacerbated by the substance	

Rx TREATMENT

NONPHARMACOLOGIC THERAPY

- First assess readiness for change; if precontemplative or contemplative, counsel about risks of use and benefits of abstinence; a motivational interviewing approach has been shown to be effective.
- Nonpharmacologic strategies have the greatest documented efficacy: advice, feedback, goal setting, problem solving, and additional contacts for further assistance.
- Opiate contracts, prohibiting a patient from getting early refills or obtaining opiates from multiple prescribers, should be considered for patients with chronic pain with a medication abuse pattern of medication use.
- Relapse prevention facilitated by avoidance of trigger stimuli or by uncoupling trigger stimuli from substance ingestion.
- Self-help and support groups such as Alcoholics Anonymous, Narcotics Anonymous, and Al-Anon are helpful in achieving and maintaining sobriety.
- Residential or inpatient treatment programs should be a consideration for any individual with contiued or escalating use despite outpatient treatment.

ACUTE GENERAL Rx

- Detoxification is an important first step in substance abuse treatment. Its goals are to facilitate withdrawal and reduce symptoms, initiate abstinence, and refer the patient to ongoing treatment.
- Benzodiazepines, particularly long-acting ones, are safe and effective in acute alcohol withdrawal. One strategy is to give the patient a loading dose of a long-acting benzodiazepine (e.g., 20 mg of diazepam) and then follow the patient clinically. An alternative "symptom-driven" strategy is to follow the patient closely with serial assessments, such as the Clinical Institute Withdrawal Assessment for Alcohol (CIWA) scale, and to dose with 5 to 10 mg of diazepam as needed to treat withdrawal symptoms.
- Beta-blockers and clonidine generally should be avoided in alcohol withdrawal; they may mask markers of the severity of the withdrawal (blood pressure and pulse rate).
- Clonidine alleviates the discomfort of opiate withdrawal. For treatment of opiate withdrawal, prescribe 0.2 mg q8h for 10 to 14 days. Antidiarrheals, ibuprofen, and baclofen

can be used as adjuncts to treat opiate withdrawal symptoms.
- Methadone taper is an effective approach for detoxification in opioid dependence.
- Buprenorphine is a partial μ-opioid receptor agonist that may be used for both detoxification and maintenance in treatment of opioid dependence (see dosing in next section).

CHRONIC Rx

- Naltrexone helps reduce craving for alcohol. Naltrexone 50 mg once daily for 12 wk can be a useful adjunct to substance abuse counseling or rehabilitation programs. Randomized treatment studies are equivocal for long-term outcomes. Naltrexone reduces relapse and the intensity or frequency of any drinking that does occur. It can be hepatotoxic and is contraindicated in opiate users. Intramuscular naltrexone (380 mg monthly) may be considered if adherence is an issue.
- Acamprosate also helps reduce craving for alcohol. Acamprosate 666 mg three times daily may be an effective adjunct to counseling. A recent meta-analysis showed overall benefit with increase in the number of abstinent days.
- Disulfiram (Antabuse) provokes acetaldehyde accumulation after alcohol ingestion, producing a toxic state manifested by nausea, headache, flushing, and respiratory distress. Studies have shown limited efficacy.
- Topiramate may be an alternative treatment for alcoholism. In a recent 14-wk randomized trial topiramate up to 300 mg daily significantly reduced the number of heavy drinking days.
- Methadone maintenance for opiate addiction is effective and involves once-daily dosing of methadone in a controlled setting.
- Buprenorphine as effective as low-dose methadone and may be prescribed by physicians who have completed approved training. For induction, initiate 12 to 24 hr after short-acting opioid use and 24 to 48 hr after long-acting opioid use. Use buprenorphine/naloxone tablets in most patients; buprenorphine only on day 1 for patients with dependence on long-acting opioids. Maximum first-day dosage is 8 to 12 mg of buprenorphine (2 mg buprenorphine q2h for signs of withdrawal). Titrate buprenorphine dose up to 16 mg on day 2 for signs of withdrawal and up to 32 mg daily by end of week 1. Then adjust dosage to minimum needed for maintenance. Naltrexone (oral) may also be

used for maintenance in opioid dependence treatment, though evidence of effectiveness is limited.
- Always combine pharmacotherapy with counseling.
- Treatment of comorbid psychiatric disorders improves outcomes.
- The effect of any intervention wanes after discontinuation of the intervention.

DISPOSITION

- Substance abuse is a chronic relapsing illness, so relapses are best approached as part of the course of the illness, as opposed to as treatment failure.
- The goal of treatment is always abstinence, but success of treatment is measured by return of function, increasing duration between relapses, and prevention of sequelae of use.

REFERRAL

Physicians should refer patients who do not make progress on changing substance use patterns to addiction specialists and/or specialized substance abuse programs. Patients with comorbid psychiatric illness should be referred for mental health care.

! PEARLS & CONSIDERATIONS

- Acute withdrawal from alcohol can become life threatening.
- Withdrawal from opioids can resemble a severe case of the flu.
- A brief intervention (providing information and advising the patient to reduce consumption of alcohol) by the primary care doctor has been demonstrated in randomized trials to reduce drinking in at-risk patients.
- Treatment rates for alcohol use disorders remain low despite available effective treatments.

EBM EVIDENCE

available at www.expertconsult.com

SUGGESTED READINGS

available at www.expertconsult.com

AUTHORS: **OMRI BERGER, M.D.,** and **RADHIKA RAMANAN, M.D., M.P.H.**

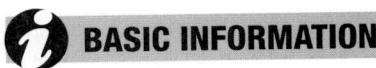

BASIC INFORMATION

DEFINITION

Elder abuse includes abuse commited by someone in a trust relation whether in the community or institutional setting.

- Physical abuse: inflicting physical pain or injury
- Sexual abuse: inflicting nonconsensual sexual activity
- Psychological abuse: inflicting mental anguish, including intimidation, humiliation, or threats
- Financial abuse: improper use of resources, property, or assets without the person's consent
- Neglect: abandonment, failure to fulfill a care-taking obligation, including provision of food, safe shelter, physical health and mental health care, or basic custodial care

SYNONYMS

Battered elder syndrome
Elder mistreatment
Domestic violence in the elderly
Diogenes syndrome

ICD-9CM CODES

995.80 Adult maltreatment, unspecified
995.81 Adult physical abuse
995.82 Adult emotional/psychological abuse
995.83 Adult sexual abuse
995.84 Adult neglect, nutritional
995.85 Other adult abuse and neglect

EPIDEMIOLOGY & DEMOGRAPHICS

INCIDENCE: According to the National Center on Elder Abuse, between 1 and 2 million Americans aged 65 yr and older have been injured, exploited, or mistreated by someone whom they depend on for care.
PEAK INCIDENCE: >75 yr; more recent studies now suggest <75 yr
PREVALENCE:

- 2% to 5% for those older than 65 yr.
- Financial abuse most common form
- 12-month U.S. prevalence rates: emotional abuse 9.0% and 4.6%; physical abuse 0.2% and 1.6%; sexual abuse 0.6%; neglect 0.5%; and financial abuse 3.5% and 5.2%.
- In a study of dementia caregivers in the U.K., one half reported behaving abusively at least some of the time, and one third reported "important" levels of abuse. Verbal abuse was common and physical abuse was rare.
- Elder self-neglect and abuse are associated with increased risk of mortality.
- Adult intimate partner violence perpetrators are significantly more likely to have witnessed intimate partner violence as child than nonperpetrators.

RISK FACTORS (VICTIM):

- Impaired cognition
- Shared living situation
- Social isolation
- Mental or physical dependence
- Female

RISK FACTORS (PERPETRATOR):

- Substance abuse
- Mental illness, particularly depression
- Dependence on the victim
- Being an involuntary caregiver
- History of violence

PHYSICAL FINDINGS & CLINICAL PRESENTATION

- Physical abuse with multiple injuries at various stages with implausible descriptions of their origins.
- Fear, hypervigilance, or withdrawal.
- Evidence of poor nutrition, dehydration, poor hygiene, multiple or neglected pressure ulcers, neglected medical conditions, or evidence of restraint use (bruises around wrists or ankles).
- Toxicologic evidence of unprescribed medications.
- Poor adherence, frequent no-shows, or little contact with health care system.

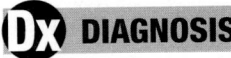

DIAGNOSIS

DIFFERENTIAL DIAGNOSIS

- Advancing dementia
- Depression, substance misuse, or other psychiatric disorder
- Malnutrition from intrinsic causes
- Conscious nonadherence
- Financial hardship
- Falling

WORKUP

1. Ask direct specific questions such as*:
   - "Has anyone close to you called you names or put you down recently?"
   - "Are you afraid of anyone in your life?"
   - "Are you able to use the telephone anytime you want to?"
   - "Has anyone forced you to do things you didn't want to do?"
   - "Has anyone taken things or money that belong to you without your OK?"
   - "Has anyone close to you tried to hurt you or harm you recently?"
2. Interview patient separately from the suspected abuser.
3. Pelvic examination if sexual abuse suspected.
4. Take photographs of physical injuries as legal evidence.

LABORATORY TESTS & IMAGING STUDIES

- Toxicology screens and therapeutic drug monitoring are sometimes helpful.

---

*University of Maine Center on Aging: Elder abuse screening protocol for physicians: lessons learned from the Maine partners for elder protection pilot project, http://www.umaine.edu/mainecenteronaging/documents/elderabusescreeningmanual.pdf)

- Other tests and radiology according to presentation.

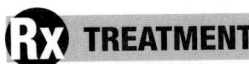

TREATMENT

NONPHARMACOLOGIC THERAPY

- Separate patient and abuser.
- Patient and caregiver may benefit from screening and treatment for substance abuse, mental illness, or cognitive impairment.

ACUTE GENERAL Rx

As indicated for injury or pain relief

DISPOSITION

If the patient's level of disability does not allow independent living, institutionalization may be required. Guidelines vary at the state and county levels regarding guardianship and conservatorship requirements.

REFERRAL

- For outpatients, report to local adult protective services agency. Reporting is mandatory in most states.
- For nursing home patients, report to regional long-term care ombudsman. Reporting is mandatory under federal law.
- In the U.S., the elder care help line is 1-800-677-1116.
- National Center on Elder Abuse: http://www.ncea.aoa.gov.

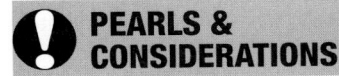

PEARLS & CONSIDERATIONS

COMMENTS

Care should be taken in interacting with the alleged abuser so that access to the victim is not lost.

PREVENTION

- Offer social services (e.g., respite care) for stressed caregivers.
- Make financial arrangements and arrange durable power of attorney for health care and finances while patient is still cognitively intact.

PATIENT & FAMILY EDUCATION

National Center on Elder Abuse: http://www.ncea.aoa.gov
JAMA Patient Page: Hildreth CJ et al: JAMA patient page. Elder abuse, *JAMA* 302(5):588, 2009

SUGGESTED READINGS

available at www.expertconsult.com

AUTHORS: **ROBERT KOHN, M.D.,** and **BREE JOHNSTON, M.D., M.P.H.**

BASIC INFORMATION

DEFINITION

Acetaminophen (APAP) poisoning is a disorder caused by excessive intake of acetaminophen and is manifested by jaundice, nausea, vomiting, and potential death from hepatic necrosis if not treated appropriately.

SYNONYMS

Paracetamol poisoning

ICD-9CM CODES
965.4 Acetaminophen poisoning

EPIDEMIOLOGY & DEMOGRAPHICS

- Acetaminophen is one of the most widely prescribed antipyretics and analgesics in the U.S. Potentially toxic ingestions, both intentional and unintentional, exceed 100,000 cases annually in the U.S.
- APAP toxicity has become the number one cause of acute liver failure in the U.S. (new bullet line)
- Death rate is approximately one in 1000 persons. Nearly 50% of exposures occur in children ≤6 yr.
- Hepatic necrosis is most likely to occur in people who are chronically malnourished, who regularly abuse alcohol, and who are using other potentially hepatotoxic medications.

PHYSICAL FINDINGS & CLINICAL PRESENTATION

- The physical examination may vary depending on the amount of time since ingestion.
- Phase I (0 to 24 hr): Initial symptoms may be mild or absent and may consist of diaphoresis, malaise, nausea, and vomiting.
- Phase II (24 to 72 hr): Right upper quadrant pain, vomiting, somnolence, and increase in transaminases.
- Phase III (72 to 96 hr): Hepatic necrosis with abdominal pain, jaundice, hepatic encephalopathy, coagulopathy, fatality.
- Phase IV (4 days to 3 wk): Complete resolution of symptoms.

ETIOLOGY

- The amount of acetaminophen necessary for hepatic toxicity varies with the patient's body size and hepatic function. It is recommended that APAP intake should not exceed 4 g for adults and 90 mg/kg in children within a 24-hr period.
- Using standardized nomograms calculating the acetaminophen plasma level and the number of hours after ingestion, the clinician can determine potential hepatic toxicity. See the acetaminophen ingestion algorithm in Section III.

DIAGNOSIS

DIFFERENTIAL DIAGNOSIS

- Liver disease from alcohol abuse or hepatitis
- Ingestion of other hepatotoxic substances

WORKUP

Initial workup is aimed at confirming acetaminophen overdose with plasma acetaminophen level and assessment of hepatic damage. A careful history should elicit the time of acetaminophen ingestion, amount, preparation (e.g., extended release) and possibility co-ingestants (see "Laboratory Tests").

LABORATORY TESTS

- Initial laboratory evaluation should include a STAT plasma acetaminophen level with a second level drawn approximately 4 to 6 hr after the initial level. Subsequent levels can be obtained every 2 to 4 hr until the levels stabilize or decline. These levels can be plotted by using the Rumack-Matthew nomogram (see acetaminophen ingestion algorithm [Fig. 3-3] in Section III) to calculate potential hepatic toxicity. The nomogram cannot be used with patients who present >24 h after ingestion, extended release preparations, repeated supratherapeutic ingestions, or when the time of ingestion is unknown.
- Transaminases (AST, ALT), bilirubin level, prothrombin time (INR), blood urea nitrogen, and creatinine should be initially obtained on all patients.
- Serum and urine toxicology screen for other potential toxic substances is also recommended on admission. Screening for infectious hepatitis should also be considered.

TREATMENT

NONPHARMACOLOGIC THERAPY

Consultation with a Poison Control Center is recommended for patients who have ingested a large amount of acetaminophen and/or other toxic substances. A single toxic dose of acetaminophen usually exceeds 7-10 g or 150 mg/kg in the adult.

ACUTE GENERAL Rx

- Hepatotoxicity is defined as any increase in alanine aminotransferase (ALT) or aspartate aminotransferase (AST) >1000 IU/L, and hepatic failure is hepatotoxicity with hepatic encephalopathy. For those who cannot be risk stratified using the nomogram, the American College of Emergency Physicians recommends that N-acetylcysteine be adminis-

tered without delay to those >12 yrs and >8 hr after ingestion at presentation.
- Administer activated charcoal 1g/kg PO if the patient is seen within 1 hr of ingestion or the clinician suspects polydrug ingestion.
- Determine blood levels 4 hr after ingestion; if in the toxic range, start N-acetylcysteine (NAC) either IV (Acetadote) or PO (Mucomyst). Acetylcysteine IV loading dose is 150 mg/kg ×1 diluted in 200 ml D5W over 15 to 60 min. Maintenance dose is 50 mg/kg diluted in 500 ml D5W over 4 hr, followed by 100 mg/kg diluted in 1000 ml D5W over 16 hr. The dose does not require adjustment for renal or hepatic impairment or for dialysis. Total administration time is 21 hours.
- Oral administration is 140 mg/kg PO as a loading dose, followed after 4 hr by 70 mg/kg PO q4h for a total of 17 doses. N-acetylcysteine therapy should be started within 24 hr of acetaminophen overdose. Total administration time is 72 hours.
- Advantages of IV administration include more reliable absorption, fewer doses, and shorter duration of treatment.
- Monitor acetaminophen level; use graph to plot possible hepatic toxicity. Some toxicologists recommend repeating AST/ALT and APAP levels after 12 to 14 hr of IV acetylcysteine infusion and continuing infusion longer than 16 hr if transaminases are elevated or if the serum acetaminophen concentration is measurable.
- Provide adequate IV hydration (e.g., D₅½NS at 150 ml/hr).
- In patients on IV N-acetylcysteine with liver failure, frequent monitoring of vital signs, oxygen saturation by pulse oximetry, AST, and serum creatinine as well as signs of hypoglycemia and infection is essential.
- If acetaminophen level is nontoxic, N-acetylcysteine therapy may be discontinued.

DISPOSITION

Most patients will recover fully without persisting hepatic abnormalities. Hepatic failure is particularly unusual in children <6 yr.

REFERRAL

Psychiatric referral is recommended after intentional ingestions.

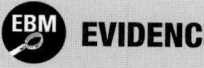

EVIDENCE

available at www.expertconsult.com

SUGGESTED READING

available at www.expertconsult.com

AUTHOR: **TARA M. WAYT, D.O.**

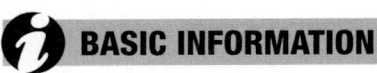

BASIC INFORMATION

DEFINITION

Achalasia is a motility disorder of the esophagus classically characterized by incomplete relaxation of the lower esophageal sphincter (LES) and aperistalsis of esophageal smooth muscle. The result is functional obstruction of the esophagus.

SYNONYMS

Achalasia and cardiospasm
Achalasia (of cardia)
Aperistalsis of esophagus
Megaesophagus
Esophageal achalasia
Esophageal cardiospasm

ICD-9CM CODES
530.0 Achalasia

EPIDEMIOLOGY & DEMOGRAPHICS

- Annual incidence is approximately 0.5 in 100,000 persons.
- Prevalence is <10 per 100,000 persons.
- Although the onset of symptoms may occur at any age, incidence is typically bimodal, 20 to 40 yr, then after 60 yr, with greater incidence in the older group.
- Men and women are affected equally.

PHYSICAL FINDINGS & CLINICAL PRESENTATION

Symptoms:
- Dysphagia with both solids and liquids
- Difficulty belching
- Regurgitation
- Chest pain and/or heartburn
- Globus
- Frequent hiccups
- Vomiting of undigested food
- Symptoms of aspiration such as nocturnal cough; possible dyspnea and pneumonia
Physical findings:
- Focal lung examination abnormalities and wheezing also possible

ETIOLOGY

- Etiology is poorly understood.
- Loss of myenteric nerve fibers in the lower esophageal sphincter and smooth muscle portion of the esophagus. This has been associated with lymphocytic and eosinophilic infiltrates and fibrosis in later stages of disease.
- Loss of intrinsic inhibitory neurons in the myenteric plexus, producing nitric oxide synthase, as well as depletion of networks of interstitial cells of Cajal of the LES, leads to incomplete relaxation.
- This motility disorder may be caused by autoimmune degeneration of the esophageal myenteric plexus because association with the HLA class II antigen DQw1 has been noted. Antimyenteric plexus and other antineural antibodies have also been described.
- Abnormal immune reactions to neurotropic viruses such as varicella zoster, herpes simplex type 1, and measles viruses have been implicated, but the association has not been confirmed.
- Achalasia is also seen in the rare autosomal recessive disorder Allgrove syndrome (achalasia, alacrima, autonomic disturbance, and acetylcholine insensitivity), which has been linked to a gene mutation on chromosome 12q13.

DIAGNOSIS

DIFFERENTIAL DIAGNOSIS

- Primary achalasia:
  - Idiopathic
- Secondary achalasia:
  - Chagas disease
  - Vagal injury or surgery, including fundoplication
- Pseudoachalasia:
  - Esophageal cancer
  - Infiltrating gastric cancer
  - Oat cell and bronchogenic lung cancer
  - Lymphoma
  - Amyloidosis
  - Paraneoplastic syndrome
- Angina
- Bulimia
- Anorexia nervosa
- Gastric bezoar
- Gastritis
- Peptic ulcer disease
- Postvagotomy dysmotility
- Esophageal disease:
  - Gastroesophageal reflux disease
  - Sarcoidosis
  - Amyloidosis
  - Esophageal stricture
  - Esophageal webs and rings
  - Scleroderma
  - Barrett's esophagus
  - Esophagitis
  - Diffuse esophageal spasm

WORKUP

- Physical examination and laboratory analyses to rule out other causes and assess complications
- Imaging studies, manometry, and endoscopy

LABORATORY TESTS

- Assessment of nutritional status
- Complete blood count, ECG, stress test if diagnosis is in doubt
- Serologic assays for trypanosoma cruzi (Chagas disease) in appropriate individuals

IMAGING STUDIES

Barium swallow with fluoroscopy may demonstrate:
- Uncoordinated or absent esophageal contractions
- An acutely tapered contrast column ("bird's beak;" Fig. 1-5)
- Dilation of the distal (smooth muscle portion) esophagus
- Esophageal air fluid level
Manometry is generally required to confirm the diagnosis. In classic achalasia, abnormalities are as follows:
- Low-amplitude disorganized contractions/aperistalsis
- Incomplete or absent LES relaxation after swallow

TABLE 1-3 Esophageal Motor Disorders			
	Achalasia	**Scleroderma**	**Diffuse Esophageal Spasm**
Symptoms	Dysphagia	Gastroesophageal reflux disease	Substernal chest pain (angina-like)
	Regurgitation of nonacidic material	Dysphagia	Dysphagia with pain
Radiographic appearance	Dilated, fluid-filled esophagus	Aperistaltic esophagus	Simultaneous noncoordinated contractions
	Distal *bird-beak* stricture	Free reflux	
		Peptic stricture	
Manometric findings			
Lower esophageal sphincter	High resting pressure	Low resting pressure	Normal pressure
	Incomplete or abnormal relaxation with swallow		
Body	Low-amplitude, simultaneous contractions after swallowing	Low-amplitude peristaltic contractions or no peristalsis	Some peristalsis
			Diffuse and simultaneous nonperistaltic contractions, occasionally high amplitude

- High LES pressure
- A subset of patients with "vigorous achalasia" may have high-amplitude, long-duration, simultaneous esophageal contractions. This term is now felt to be imprecise because of a newer classification of the disease.
- High-resolution manometry, or high-resolution esophageal pressure topography, has recently defined subsets of patients with achalasia who may have different responses to medical or surgical therapies. Unlike classic achalasia (Type I), Type II achalasia shows panesophageal pressurization to greater than 30 mm Hg

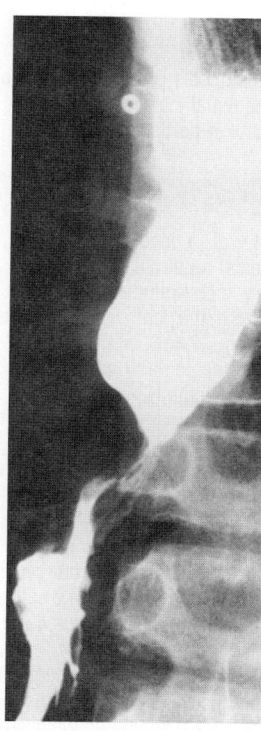

FIGURE 1-5 Classic appearance of achalasia of the esophagus. The dilated esophagus ends in a narrow segment. (From Hoekelman R [ed]: *Primary pediatric care*, ed 3, St Louis, 1997, Mosby.)

on at least two test swallows, and Type III achalasia shows spastic lumen-obliterating contractions of the distal esophagus on at least two test swallows.
- Direct visualization by endoscopy should be performed to exclude other causes of dysphagia, including "functional esophagogastric junction obstruction" and secondary causes of achalasia.

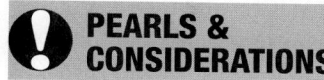 **TREATMENT**

NONPHARMACOLOGIC THERAPY

- The goals of therapy are to decrease LES pressure, relieve symptoms, and prevent progression to a dilated or megaesophagus.
- Pneumatic dilation may benefit 65% to 90% of patients. Esophageal rupture or perforation is a rare complication (2% to 3%) that can be managed conservatively in some stable patients. Multiple sessions may be required.
- Surgical: laparoscopic or, now less commonly, open esophagomyotomy is effective (90%). This approach currently offers the most durable symptom relief. Approximately 35% of patients undergoing surgery will develop reflux disease. As a result, some surgeons will perform a "loose" antireflux repair as part of the surgical procedure. An observational study has suggested that those who have had prior endoscopic treatment before myotomy may not do as well as those who have a primary myotomy.
- Early studies suggest that Type I and Type II patients have better treatment responses to these therapies compared with Type III patients.

GENERAL Rx

- Medications may be useful for short-term symptom relief and in patients with refractory chest pain. They should only be considered in patients unable to receive, or who are scheduled for, more definitive procedures. LES pressure may be lowered by 50% through sublingual use of long-acting nitrates (e.g.,

isosorbide dinitrate 5 to 20 mg) or calcium channel blockers (e.g., nifedipine 10 to 30 mg). Side effects are common and duration of relief tends to be short. Sildenafil was shown to be effective in a few small, short-term studies, but it is generally not recommended.
- Botulinum toxin injection will benefit up to 85% of patients by inhibiting acetylcholine release from cholinergic nerve endings, but up to half of these patients will require repeat injections by 6 months. A few studies have suggested that repeated injections can lead to fibrosis, which may complicate subsequent attempts at surgical therapy.

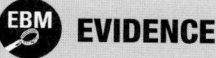 **PEARLS & CONSIDERATIONS**

COMMENTS

- Medication has a limited role in treatment.
- Botulinum toxin is transiently effective in improving symptoms. Pneumatic dilation and surgical myotomy provide more durable long-term responses. Botulinum toxin should be considered primarily in patients too elderly or ill to be considered for these other therapies.
- Surgical myotomy and mechanical dilation are treatments of choice.
- Patients with achalasia may be at long-term risk of squamous cell carcinoma of the esophagus and non–reflux-associated esophagitis. Treated patients may be at long-term risk for reflux esophagitis, Barrett's esophagus, and adenocarcinoma.

EBM EVIDENCE

available at www.expertconsult.com

SUGGESTED READINGS
available at www.expertconsult.com

AUTHOR: **HARLAN G. RICH, M.D.**

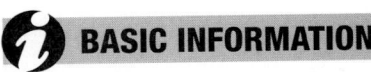

BASIC INFORMATION

DEFINITION

Achilles tendon rupture refers to the loss of continuity of the *tendo Achillis,* usually from attrition.

ICD-9CM CODES
845.09 Achilles tendon rupture

EPIDEMIOLOGY & DEMOGRAPHICS

PREDOMINANT AGE: 30 to 55 yr

PHYSICAL FINDINGS & CLINICAL PRESENTATION

Injury often occurs during an activity that puts great stress on the tendon. Sudden "pop" is often felt followed by weakness and swelling. Sometimes the patient feels like he or she has been shot in the calf.
- Patient walks flat footed and is unable to stand on the ball of the foot.
- Tenderness and hemorrhage are present at the site of injury, and a sulcus is usually palpable but may be obscured by an organizing clot if the examination is delayed.
- Although active plantar flexion is usually lost, some plantar flexion occasionally remains because of the activity of the other posterior compartment muscles.
- Thompson's test is usually positive. Test measures plantar flexion of the foot when the calf is squeezed with the patient kneeling on a chair; normal foot plantar flexes with calf compression, but movement is absent when *tendo Achillis* is ruptured.
- Excessive passive dorsiflexion of the foot is also present on the injured side (Fig. 1-6).

ETIOLOGY

- Relative hypovascularity predisposing to tendon rupture in several tendons (Achilles, biceps, and supraspinatus)
- With advancing age, vascular supply to the tendon further compromised
- Repetitive trauma leading to degeneration of this critical area and weakness
- Rupture of *tendo Achillis* usually 2.5 to 5 cm from the insertion of the tendon into the os calcis
- Most common causative event leading to rupture: sudden dorsiflexion of the plantar flexed foot (landing from a height) or sudden pushing off with the weight on the forefoot
- The tendon may be adversely affected by the use of fluoroquinolone antibiotics

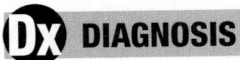

DIAGNOSIS

DIFFERENTIAL DIAGNOSIS

- Incomplete (partial) *tendo Achillis* rupture
- Partial rupture of gastrocnemius muscle, often medial head (previously thought to be "plantaris tendon rupture")

WORKUP

- Clinical diagnosis of complete *tendo Achillis* rupture is usually obvious.
- MRI helpful in partial ruptures.

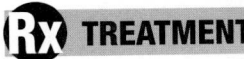

TREATMENT

- Early referral is necessary for open, end-to-end surgical repair.
- If surgery is contraindicated, a short leg cast applied with the foot in equinus may allow healing.
- In cases of neglected rupture, reconstruction is usually indicated.
- Physical therapy is helpful after repair to restore strength and flexibility.
- Bracing is required for partial rupture.

DISPOSITION

- Prognosis for recovery after surgical repair of the acute rupture is good, but recurrence is not uncommon regardless of treatment.
- *Tendo Achillis* must be protected from excessive activity for up to 1 yr.
- Results of reconstruction for neglected cases are worse than with primary repair.
- Return to work with limited weight-bearing is possible in 2 to 4 wk.

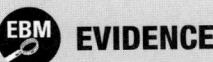

EVIDENCE

available at www.expertconsult.com

SUGGESTED READINGS
available at www.expertconsult.com

AUTHOR: **LONNIE R. MERCIER, M.D.**

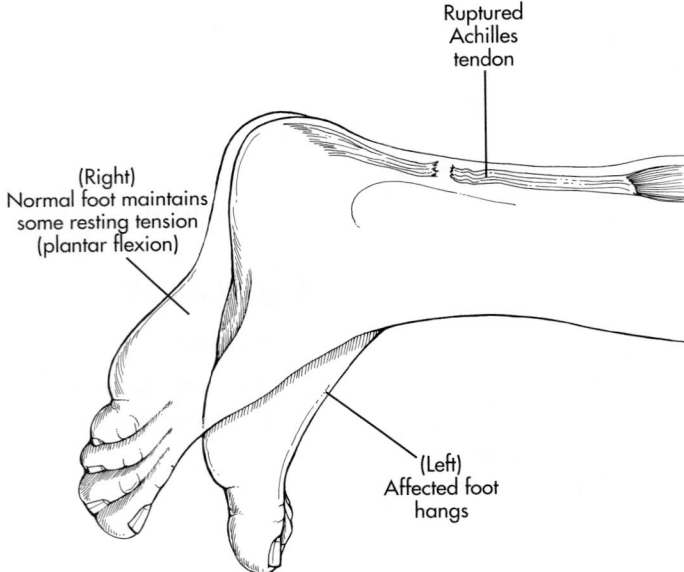

Ruptured Achilles tendon

(Right)
Normal foot maintains some resting tension (plantar flexion)

(Left)
Affected foot hangs

FIGURE 1-6 Observation of Achilles tendon rupture. The patient is asked to lie prone on the examining table with feet hanging off the end. The intact leg retains inherent plantar flexion, whereas on the injured side the foot hangs straight down with gravity. (From Scudieri G [ed]: *Sports medicine: principles of primary care,* St Louis, 1997, Mosby.)

BASIC INFORMATION

DEFINITION

Acne vulgaris is a chronic disorder of the pilosebaceous apparatus caused by abnormal desquamation of follicular epithelium leading to obstruction of the pilosebaceous canal, resulting in inflammation and subsequent formation of papules, pustules, nodules, comedones, and scarring. Acne can be classified by the type of lesion (comedonal, papulopustular, and nodulocystic). The American Academy of Dermatology classification scheme for acne denotes the following three levels:

1. Mild acne: characterized by the presence of comedones (noninflammatory lesions), few papules and pustules (generally <10), but no nodules.
2. Moderate acne: presence of several to many papules and pustules (10 to 40) along with comedones (10 to 40). The presence of >40 papules and pustules along with larger, deeper nodular inflamed lesions (up to five) denotes moderately severe acne (Fig. 1-7).
3. Severe acne: presence of numerous or extensive papules and pustules as well as many nodular lesions.

SYNONYMS

Acne

ICD-9CM CODES
706.1 Acne vulgaris

EPIDEMIOLOGY & DEMOGRAPHICS

- Acne is the most common skin disease in the U.S.
- It is most common in teenagers (highest incidence between ages of 16 and 18 yr).

PHYSICAL FINDINGS & CLINICAL PRESENTATION

- Open comedones (blackheads), closed comedones (whiteheads)
- Greasiness (oily skin)
- Presence of scars from prior acne cysts
- Various stages of development and severity may be present concomitantly
- Common distribution of acne: face, back, and upper chest
- Inflammatory papules, pustules, and ectatic pores

ETIOLOGY

- Overactivity of the sebaceous glands and blockage in the ducts. The obstruction leads to the formation of comedones, which can become inflamed because of overgrowth of *Propionibacterium acnes.*
- Exacerbated by environmental factors (hot, humid, tropical climate), medications (e.g., iodine in cough mixtures, hair greases), industrial exposure to halogenated hydrocarbons.

DIAGNOSIS

DIFFERENTIAL DIAGNOSIS

- Gram-negative folliculitis
- Staphylococcal pyoderma
- Acne rosacea
- Drug eruption
- Sebaceous hyperplasia
- Angiofibromas, basal cell carcinomas, osteoma cutis
- Occupational exposures to oils or grease
- Steroid acne

WORKUP

History and physical examination:
- Inquire about previous treatment
- Careful drug history

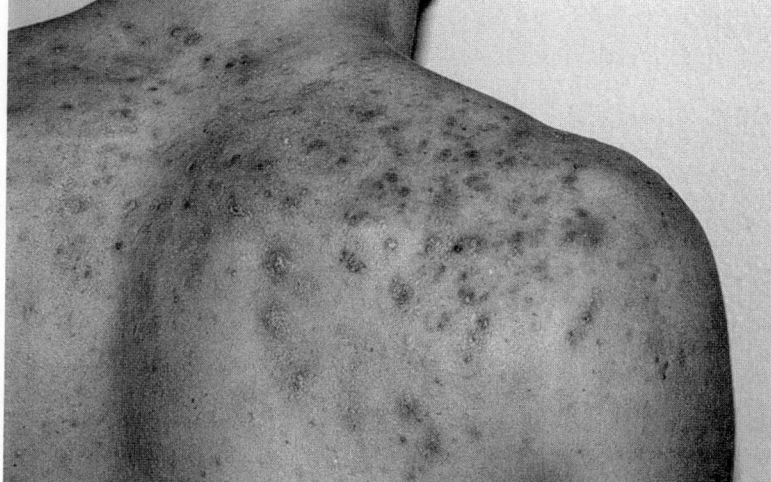

FIGURE 1-7 Acne on back and shoulders. This acne is typically inflammatory and usually needs oral antibiotics or possibly isotretinoin, but the patient may apply topical medication as well. Heat and sweat may aggravate the condition. (From White GM, Cox NH [eds]: *Diseases of the skin*, ed 2, St Louis, 2006, Mosby.)

- Family history, history of cyclic menstrual flares
- History of use of cosmetics and cleansers
- Oral contraceptive use

LABORATORY TESTS

- Laboratory evaluation is generally not helpful.
- Patients who are candidates for therapy with isotretinoin should have baseline liver enzymes, cholesterol, and triglycerides checked because this medication may result in elevation of lipids and liver enzymes.
- A negative serum pregnancy test or two negative urine pregnancy tests should also be obtained in females 1 wk before initiation of isotretinoin; it is also imperative to maintain effective contraception during and 1 mo after therapy with isotretinoin ends because of its teratogenic effects. Pregnancy status should be rechecked at monthly visits.
- If hyperandrogenism is suspected in female patients, levels of dehydroepiandrosterone sulfate, testosterone (total and free), and androstenedione should be measured. For women with regular menstrual cycles, serum androgen measurements generally are not necessary.

TREATMENT

NONPHARMACOLOGIC THERAPY

Blue light (ClearLight therapy system) can be used for treatment of moderate inflammatory acne vulgaris. Light in the violet/blue range can cause bacterial death by a photoreaction in which porphyrins react with oxygen to generate reactive oxygen species, which damage the cell membranes of *P. acnes.* Treatment usually consists of 15-min exposures twice weekly for 4 wk.

ACUTE GENERAL Rx

Treatment generally varies with the type of lesions (comedones, papules, pustules, cystic lesions) and the severity of acne.

- Comedones (noninflammatory acne) can be treated with retinoids or retinoid analogs. Topical retinoids are comedolytic and work by normalizing follicular keratinization. Commonly available agents are Adapalene (Differin, 0.1% gel or cream, applied once or twice daily), tazarotene (Tazorac 0.1% cream or gel applied daily), tretinoin (Retin-A 0.1% cream or 0.025 gel applied once daily), tretinoin microsphere (Retin-A Micro, 0.1% gel, applied at bedtime). Tretinoin is inactivated by ultraviolet light and oxidized by benzoyl peroxide; therefore it should only be applied at night and not used concomitantly with benzoyl peroxide.
- Tretinoin is pregnancy category C and tazarotene is pregnancy category X. Salicylic acid preparations (e.g., Neutrogena 2% wash) have keratolytic and antiinflammatory properties and are also useful in the treatment of comedones. Large, open comedones (blackheads) should be expressed.

- Patients should be reevaluated after 4 to 6 wk. Benzoyl peroxide gel (2.5% or 5%) may be added if the comedones become inflamed or form pustules. The most common adverse effects are dryness, erythema, and peeling. Topical antibiotics (erythromycin, clindamycin lotions or pads) can also be used in patients with significant inflammation. They reduce *P. acnes* in the pilosebaceous follicle and have some antiinflammatory effects. The combination of 5% benzoyl peroxide and 3% erythromycin (Benzamycin) or 1% clindamycin with 5% benzoyl peroxide (BenzaClin) is highly effective in patients who have a mixture of comedonal and inflammatory acne lesions.
- Fixed-dose combinations of clindamycin phosphate 1.2% and tretinoin 0.025% are available (Veltin gel, Ziana) and are more effective than either product used alone; however, they are much more expensive than the individual generic components.
- Pustular acne can be treated with tretinoin and benzoyl peroxide gel applied on alternate evenings; drying agents (sulfacetamide-sulfa lotions [Novacet, Sulfacet]) are also effective when used in combination with benzoyl peroxide; oral antibiotics (doxycycline 100 mg qd or erythromycin 1 g qd given in 2 to 3 divided doses) are effective in patients with moderate to severe pustular acne. Patients not responding well to these antibiotics can be switched to minocycline 50 to 100 mg bid; however, this medication is more expensive.
- Patients with nodular cystic acne can be treated with systemic agents: antibiotics (erythromycin, tetracycline, doxycycline, minocycline), isotretinoin (available on restricted basis), or oral contraceptives. Periodic intralesional triamcinolone (Kenalog) injections by a dermatologist are also effective. The possibility of endocrinopathy should be considered in patients responding poorly to therapy.
- Isotretinoin is indicated for acne resistant to antibiotic therapy and severe acne. It is available only on a restricted basis. Dosage is 0.5 to 1 mg/kg/day in 2 divided doses (maximum of 2 mg/kg/day); duration of therapy is generally 20 wk for a cumulative dose ≥120 mg/kg for severe cystic acne. Before using this medication patients should undergo baseline laboratory evaluation (see "Laboratory Tests"). This drug is absolutely contraindicated during pregnancy because of its teratogenicity. It should be used with caution in patients with history of depression. To prescribe this drug, physicians must be registered members of the manufacturer's System to Manage Accutane-Related Teratogenicity (SMART) program.
- Azelaic acid is a bacteriostatic dicarboxylic acid used to normalize keratinization and reduce inflammation.
- Oral contraceptives reduce androgen levels and therefore sebum production. They represent a useful adjunctive therapy for all types of acne in women and adolescent girls. Commonly used agents are norgestimate/ethinyl estradiol (Ortho Tri-Cyclen) and drosperinone/ethinyl estradiol (Yasmin).

REFERRAL

Referral for intralesional injection and dermabrasion should be considered in patients with severe acne unresponsive to conventional therapy.

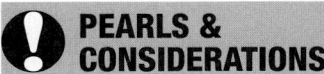 **PEARLS & CONSIDERATIONS**

- Gram-negative folliculitis should be suspected if inflammatory acne worsens after several months of oral antibiotic therapy.
- Acne may worsen during the first 3 to 4 wk of retinoid therapy before improving.

COMMENTS

Indications for systemic therapy of acne are:
- Painful deep papules or nodules
- Extensive lesions
- Active acne with severe scarring or hyperpigmentation
- Patient's morale

Patients should be educated that in most cases acne can be controlled but not cured and that at least 4 to 6 wk of initial therapy should be required before significant improvement is noted.

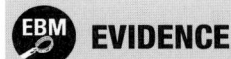 **EVIDENCE**

available at www.expertconsult.com

SUGGESTED READINGS

available at www.expertconsult.com

AUTHOR: **FRED F. FERRI, M.D.**

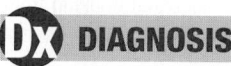

BASIC INFORMATION

DEFINITION

Acoustic neuroma is a benign proliferation of the Schwann cells that cover the vestibular branch of the eighth cranial nerve (CN VIII). Symptoms are commonly a result of compression of the acoustic branch of CN VIII, the facial nerve (CN VII), and the trigeminal nerve (CN V). The glossopharyngeal nerve (CN IX) and vagus nerve (CN X) are less commonly involved. In extreme cases compression of the brain stem may lead to obstruction of cerebrospinal fluid (CSF) outflow and elevated intracranial pressure (ICP).

SYNONYMS

Vestibular schwannoma

ICD-9CM CODES
225.1 Acoustic neuroma

EPIDEMIOLOGY & DEMOGRAPHICS

Annual incidence is approximately one in 100,000 patients per year. There may be a slight female predominance. The tumor most commonly presents in the fifth and sixth decades.

PHYSICAL FINDINGS & CLINICAL PRESENTATION

- Most frequently unilateral hearing loss and/or tinnitus. Also balance problems, vertigo, facial pain (trigeminal neuralgia) and weakness, difficulty swallowing, fullness or pain of the involved ear. Headache may occur.
- With elevated ICP, patients may also have vomiting, fever, and visual changes.
- Hearing loss is the most common presenting complaint and is usually high frequency.

ETIOLOGY

The etiology is incompletely understood, but long-term exposure to acoustic trauma has been implicated. Bilateral acoustic neuromas may be inherited in an autosomal-dominant manner as part of neurofibromatosis type 2. This disease is associated with a defect on chromosome 22q1.

DIAGNOSIS

DIFFERENTIAL DIAGNOSIS

- Benign positional vertigo
- Ménière's disease

- Trigeminal neuralgia
- Cerebellar disease
- Normal-pressure hydrocephalus
- Presbycusis
- Glomus tumors
- Vertebrobasilar insufficiency
- Ototoxicity from medications
- Other tumors:
  - Meningioma, glioma
  - Facial nerve schwannoma
  - Cavernous hemangioma
  - Metastatic tumors

WORKUP

- A detailed neurologic examination with special attention to the cranial nerves is crucial.
- Otoscopic evaluation may help rule out other causes of hearing loss.

LABORATORY TESTS

- Audiometry is useful, often showing asymmetric, sensorineural, high-frequency hearing loss.
- CSF protein may be elevated.

IMAGING STUDIES

- MRI with gadolinium is the preferred test. It can detect tumors as small as 2 mm in diameter.
- CT scan with contrast can detect tumors 1 cm in diameter or larger.
- Treatment decisions should be based on the size of the tumor, rate of growth (older patients tend to have slower growing tumors), degree of neurologic deficit, desire to preserve hearing, life expectancy, age of the patient, and surgical risk. A combination of treatments can also be used.

TREATMENT

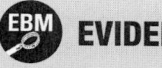

NONPHARMACOLOGIC THERAPY

- Surgery is the definitive treatment. Choice of approach (middle cranial fossa, translabyrinthine, or retromastoid suboccipital) may vary depending on the size of the tumor, amount of residual hearing desired, and degree of surgical risk that can be tolerated. Partial resection is sometimes undertaken to minimize the risk of injury to nearby structures. Intraoperative facial nerve monitoring is recommended.
- Radiation therapy (stereotactic radiotherapy, stereotactic radiosurgery, or proton beam radiotherapy) is useful for tumors <3 cm in

diameter or for those in whom surgery is not an option. Radiotherapy after partial resection has also been used to minimize complications.
- Age alone is not a contraindication to surgery.

ACUTE GENERAL Rx

Not applicable

CHRONIC Rx

Observation with MRI every 6 to 12 mo may be appropriate for frail patients with small tumors, but risk of unrecoverable hearing loss may increase if surgery is delayed.

DISPOSITION

Hearing can be preserved at near-preoperative levels in more than two thirds of patients with small- to medium-sized tumors.

REFERRAL

Prompt referral to an ear-nose-throat specialist or neurosurgeon who is facile with all three surgical approaches is recommended.

PEARLS & CONSIDERATIONS

COMMENTS

- Presents most commonly as unilateral, sensorineural hearing loss.
- Treatment outcomes are generally good, with cure rates approaching 90% at 5 years.
- Of those who are managed with observation only, approximately half have continued enlargement and approximately one fifth eventually have a surgical intervention.

PATIENT/FAMILY EDUCATION

Acoustic Neuroma Association: http://anausa. org.

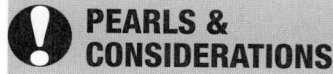

available at www.expertconsult.com

SUGGESTED READINGS
available at www.expertconsult.com

AUTHORS: **SRIVIDYA ANANDAN, M.D.,** and **PAUL A. PIRRAGLIA, M.D., M.P.H.**

BASIC INFORMATION

DEFINITION

Acquired immunodeficiency syndrome (AIDS) is a disorder caused by infection with the human immunodeficiency virus, type 1 (HIV-1), and marked by progressive deterioration of the cellular immune system, leading to secondary infections or malignancies.

SYNONYMS

AIDS

ICD-9CM CODES
042.9 AIDS, unspecified

EPIDEMIOLOGY & DEMOGRAPHICS

INCIDENCE (IN U.S.):
- 27.1 cases/100,000 persons
- Varies widely by location
- 85% of cases in large cities

PREVALENCE (IN U.S.): 62 cases/100,000 persons. 56,000 HIV infections occur each year in the U.S.

PREDOMINANT SEX: 53% of infections occur in men who have sex with men (MSM).

PREDOMINANT AGE: 80% between ages 20 and 40 yr

PEAK INCIDENCE: See "Incidence"

GENETICS:
- Familial disposition: Although there is no proven genetic predisposition, individuals with deletions in the CCR5 gene are immune from infection with macrophage tropic virus (the predominant virus in sexual transmission).
- Congenital infection:
  1. Transmittable from an infected mother to the fetus in utero in as many as 30% of pregnancies.
  2. No specific congenital malformations associated with infection; low birth weight and spontaneous abortion are possible.
- Neonatal infection: transmission possible to the neonate intrapartum or postpartum through breastfeeding.

PHYSICAL FINDINGS & CLINICAL PRESENTATION

- Nonspecific findings: fever, weight loss, anorexia
- Specific syndromes:
  1. Seen in association with opportunistic infection and malignancies, so-called indicator diseases; these include:
     a. Opportunistic infections:
        Disseminated strongyloidiasis
        Disseminated toxoplasmosis, cryptococcosis, histoplasmosis, CMV, herpes simplex, or mycobacterial disease
        Candida esophagitis or bronchopulmonary disease
        Chronic *Cryptosporidia* spp. diarrhea
        Pneumocystis jiroveci pneumonia
        Extensive pulmonary and extrapulmonary tuberculosis
        Recurrent bacterial pneumonia
        Progressive multifocal leukoencephalopathy
     b. AIDS-related neoplasms:
        Kaposi's sarcoma in a person <60 yr of age
        Primary brain lymphoma
        Invasive cervical carcinoma
        High grade B cell non-Hodgkin's lymphoma, Burkitt's lymphoma, undifferentiated non-Hodgkin's lymphoma, or immunoblastic lymphoma
  2. Most common:
     Respiratory infections (*Pneumocystis jiroveci* [formerly known as *Pneumocystis carinii*] pneumonia, TB, bacterial pneumonia, fungal infection)
     CNS infections (toxoplasmosis, cryptococcal meningitis, TB)
     GI (cryptosporidiosis, isosporiasis, cytomegalovirus); Sections II and III describe organisms associated with diarrhea in patients with AIDS
     Eye infections (cytomegalovirus, toxoplasmosis)
     Kaposi's sarcoma (cutaneous or visceral) or lymphoma (nodal or extranodal)
- Possibly asymptomatic
- Diagnosis of AIDS if T-lymphocyte subset analysis demonstrating CD4 cell count <200 or <14% of total lymphocyte in the presence of proven HIV infection even in the absence of other infections
- The various manifestations of HIV infection are described in Section II

ETIOLOGY

- Caused by infection with HIV-1
- Transmitted by heterosexual or male homosexual contact, needle-sharing (during IV drug use), transfusion of contaminated blood or blood products, and from infected mother to fetus or neonate as described previously

DIAGNOSIS

DIFFERENTIAL DIAGNOSIS

- Other wasting illnesses mimicking the non-specific features of AIDS:
  1. TB
  2. Neoplasms
  3. Disseminated fungal infection
  4. Malabsorption syndromes
  5. Depression
- Other disorders associated with dementia or demyelination producing encephalopathy, myelopathy, or neuropathy

WORKUP

Prompt evaluation of respiratory, CNS, and GI complaints

LABORATORY TESTS

- HIV antibody testing
- T-lymphocyte subset analysis: performed to determine the degree of immunodeficiency
- Viral load assay: to plan long-term antiviral therapy consider genotype or phenotype sensitivity testing for patients failing therapy
- CSF examination: for meningitis
- Serologic tests for syphilis, hepatitis B, hepatitis C, and toxoplasmosis
- Genotypic resistance testing: used to assess for primary resistance in naïve patients and secondary resistance in patients failing a regimen
- Eye exam: to evaluate for CMV retinitis in patients with CD4 counts <50 cells/mm^3
- Cryptococcal antigen: part of the evaluation in AIDS patients with CD4 <100 cells/mm^3 who have fever, diffuse pneumonia, or symptoms of meningitis

IMAGING STUDIES

- Cerebral CT for encephalopathy or focal CNS complications (e.g., toxoplasmosis, lymphoma)
- Pulmonary gallium scanning to aid in the diagnosis of *Pneumocystis jiroveci* (*P. carinii*) pneumonia
- Baseline chest x-ray

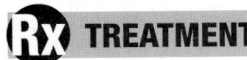

TREATMENT

NONPHARMACOLOGIC THERAPY

- Maintain adequate caloric intake.
- Encourage good oral hygiene, regular dental care.
- Avoid high-risk behaviors that increase the risk of repeated exposure to HIV and other potential pathogens—safer sexual practices, avoid sharing needles, etc.
- Update vaccines—particularly the pneumococcal and hepatitis B vaccine along with annual influenza vaccines.
- Avoid administration of any live attenuated vaccines that may be a risk to these immunocompromised patients.
- When feasible, avoid activities that might increase risk of exposure to opportunistic infections (i.e., cleaning out a cat litter box [toxoplasmosis], getting scratched by a cat [*Bartonella* infections], exposure to pet reptiles [salmonellosis], traveling to developing countries [cryptosporidiosis, tuberculosis], eating undercooked foods and drinking from unsafe water supplies, etc.).

ACUTE GENERAL Rx

Acute management of opportunistic infections and malignancies is reviewed elsewhere in this text under specific AIDS-related disorders.

CHRONIC Rx

For all HIV-infected patients, particularly those meeting the case definition of AIDS:
- Preventive therapy for *Pneumocystis jiroveci* pneumonia and TB (see specific chapters elsewhere in this text). With the advent of modern antiretroviral therapy many patients have experienced substantial restoration of cellular immune function. It has become clear that preventive therapy for *Pneumocystis jiroveci* and *Mycobacterium avium* complex as

well as suppressive therapy for cytomegalo-viral and cryptococcal infection can often be safely withdrawn if the CD4 cell count rises above 200 for at least 6 mo.

- Begin HAART (highly active antiretroviral therapy) when any of the following are present:
  1. Symptomatic HIV infection is associated with any opportunistic infection
  2. CD4 count <200 cells/mm^3
  3. CD4 count <350 cells/mm^3 and before it reaches 200 cells/mm^3, especially if the viral load >30,000 copies/ml
  4. Consider therapy if CD4 count is rapidly decreasing and viral load >100,000 copies/ml
- Antiretroviral therapy employing combinations of nucleoside reverse transcriptase inhibitor (NRTI) agents: zidovudine (AZT), didanosine (DDI), zalcitabine (DDC), lamivudine (3TC), Emtricitabine (FTC), stavudine (D4T), abacavir in addition to protease inhibitors (PI) (saquinavir, indinavir, nelfinavir, agenerase, ritonavir/lopinavir, atazanavir), nonnucleoside reverse transcriptase inhibitors (NNRTI) (nevirapine, delavirdine, efavirenz), or the nucleotide agent tenofovir according to current recommendations based on clinical stage and viral load studies. The protease inhibitor ritonavir should be used, in low dose, in combination with other protease inhibitors to obtain more sustained drug levels. Usual initial dosing regimen consists of two NRTIs and an NNRTI (or a PI). Common regimens include:
  1. Combivir (AZT and 3TC) one tablet by mouth twice a day and efavirenz 600 mg by mouth once daily
  2. Combivir (AZT and 3TC) one tablet by mouth twice a day and ritonavir/lopinavir 3 tablets by mouth twice daily with food
  3. Truvada (tenofovir plus Emtricitabine [FTC]) one tablet once daily and efavirenz 600 mg by mouth once daily

  All these drugs have unique and class-specific side effects and require careful and expert follow-up to achieve optimal antiviral effects, ensure compliance, and maintain efficacy. Antiviral response should be monitored by baseline HIV viral load and CD4 count and repeat measurement at 2 wk and 4 wk into treatment and then periodically (every 3 mo) to ensure viral suppression.
- An approach to evaluating chronic diarrhea in patients with HIV infection, the approach to the acutely ill HIV-infected patient, and the evaluation of respiratory complaints are described in Section III. Approach to a patient with a suspected CNS lesion is also described in Section III.
- Genotypic resistance testing should be strongly considered for any patient failing antiretroviral therapy. Poor adherence to therapy, however, often underlies virologic failure.

DISPOSITION

The outlook for AIDS has changed radically since the advent of HAART therapy from an essentially uniformly fatal disease to a chronic medical illness compatible with long-term survival and remarkably good quality of life. Patients should be aggressively supported in the presence of severe illness as outcomes following ICU admissions remain good. This is accomplished through expert and continuous follow-up, use of highly active antiretroviral drugs, and careful detail to compliance to medications and lifestyle modification.

REFERRAL

All patients with AIDS: to a physician knowledgeable and experienced in the management of the disease and its complications

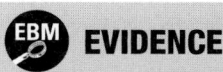 **EVIDENCE**

available at www.expertconsult.com

SUGGESTED READINGS
available at www.expertconsult.com

AUTHORS: **GLENN G. FORT, M.D., M.P.H.,** and **DENNIS J. MIKOLICH, M.D.**

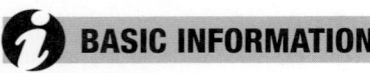

DEFINITION

Acromegaly occurs due to hypersecretion of growth hormone (GH) or increased amounts of insulin-like growth factor I (IGF-I). It is a chronic debilitating disease with an insidious onset.

SYNONYMS

Marie's disease

ICD-9CM CODES
253.0 Acromegaly

EPIDEMIOLOGY & DEMOGRAPHICS

INCIDENCE: Three to four new cases per 1 million persons annually
PREVALENCE: 50 to 60 cases per 1 million persons, with some estimates as high as 90 cases per 1 million persons
PREDOMINANT SEX: No sexual predominance
MEAN AGE AT DIAGNOSIS: Males: 40 yr; females: 45 yr

RISK FACTORS

- Increased mortality rate, primarily from cardiovascular and respiratory causes
- Death in 50% of untreated patients by age 50 yr
- Increased prevalence of colon carcinoma and other malignancies

PHYSICAL FINDINGS & CLINICAL PRESENTATION

- Coarse features resulting from growth of soft tissue
- Coarse, oily skin
- Hands and feet that are spadelike, fleshy, and moist (Fig. 1-8)
- Prognathism, which can give an underbite
- Carpal tunnel syndrome
- Excessive sweating
- Arthralgias and severe osteoarthritis
- History of increased hat, glove, and/or shoe size
- Hypertension
- Skin tags
- Muscle weakness and decreased exercise capacity
- Headache, often severe
- Diabetes mellitus
- Visual field defects

ETIOLOGY

Cause is usually a pituitary adenoma affecting the anterior lobe.

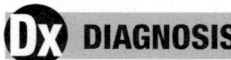

DIFFERENTIAL DIAGNOSIS

Ectopic production of GH-releasing hormone (GHRH) from a carcinoid or other neuroendocrine tumor

WORKUP

1. First screening test: measure serum IGF-I level.
   a. Direct measurement of the GH level is not as useful because it is secreted in a pulsatile fashion and a random level may be falsely normal.
   b. Upper limits of a normal IGF-I level, depending on the assay: >380 ng/ml or 2.5 U/ml.
2. Failure to suppress serum GH to less than 2 ng/ml after 100 g oral glucose is considered conclusive.
   a. Patients may show suppression of GH (paradoxic response).
   b. Patients will not suppress GH to 2 ng/ml or less (typical response in patients with acromegaly).
   c. GHRH level >300 ng/ml is indicative of an ectopic source of GH.

LABORATORY TESTS

- Elevated IGF-I level
- Elevated serum phosphate
- Elevated urine calcium

IMAGING STUDIES

- Imaging studies of choice: MRI of the pituitary and hypothalamus
- CT of the pituitary and hypothalamus sometimes used initially

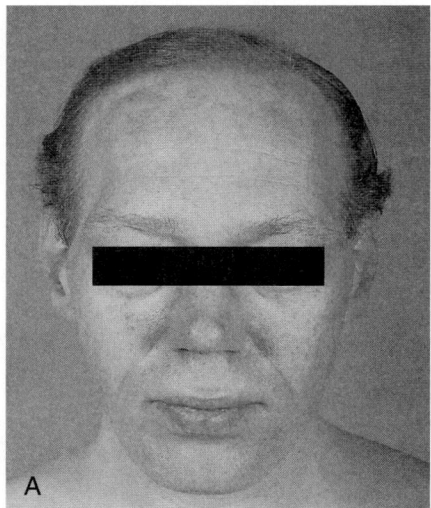
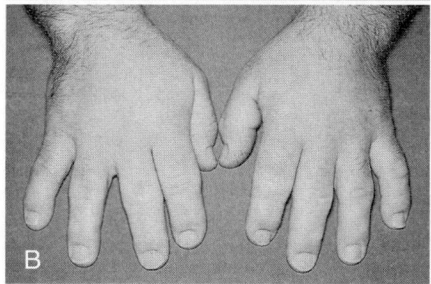

FIGURE 1-8 Typical appearances of acromegaly. A, Face showing enlarged supraorbital ridges, nose, lips, and jaw. **B,** Spade-like hands. (From Souhami RL, Moxham J: *Textbook of medicine,* 4th ed, London, Churchill Livingstone, 2002.)

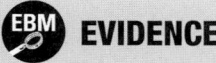

SURGERY

Treatment of choice: transsphenoidal microsurgical adenomectomy

- Surgical failure rate: approximately 13.3% for microadenomas (tumors <10 mm) and 11.1% for macroadenomas (tumors >10 mm confined to the sella)
- Preoperative IGF-I level: indicator of surgical outcome with higher levels associated with surgical failure

RADIOTHERAPY

- Radiotherapy is usually reserved for tumor recurrence or persistence after surgery in patients with resistance to or intolerance of medical treatment
- Major complication: hypopituitarism, which may occur in up to 50% of patients; this complication is more likely in patients who had surgery irradiation

MEDICAL THERAPY

- Indicated when patients have not responded to surgical therapy, when surgery is contraindicated, and in patients waiting for the effects of radiotherapy to begin
- Somastatin receptor ligands: octreotide, lanreotide:
  - Important in the preoperative shrinkage of pituitary tumors and softening of adenomatous tissue.
  - Pegvisomant is a growth hormone receptor antagonist that has shown promising results in the treatment of acromegaly. It is generally used in patients with resistance to or intolerance of somastatin analogues. It should be used in patients who do not have central compressive symptoms and those with resistant diabetes.
  - Dopamine receptor agonists: Bromocriptine, cabergoline: can be used in addition to somastatin receptor ligands.

CHRONIC Rx

Combination of bromocriptine and octreotide may be synergistic, allowing a lower combination dosage than either alone.

DISPOSITION

- Patients receiving radiotherapy need long-term follow-up to monitor the potential development of hypopituitarism.
- Continuation of medical therapy should be based on the normalization of IGF-I levels.

EBM EVIDENCE

available at www.expertconsult.com

SUGGESTED READINGS

available at www.expertconsult.com

AUTHORS: **BETH J. WUTZ, M.D.,** and **RUBEN ALVERO, M.D.**

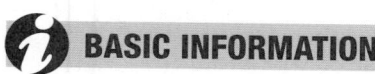

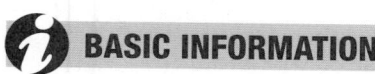 BASIC INFORMATION

DEFINITION

Actinomycosis is an indolent, slowly progressive infection caused by both anaerobic or micro-aerophilic bacteria that normally colonize the mouth, vagina, and colon. Actinomycosis is characterized by the formation of painful abscesses, soft tissue infiltration, and draining sinuses.

SYNONYMS

Actinomyces infection
Lumpy jaw

ICD-9CM CODES
039.9 Actinomycosis

EPIDEMIOLOGY & DEMOGRAPHICS

Geographic distribution:
- Actinomycosis is worldwide in distribution.
- Commonly found as normal flora of the oral cavity (within gingival crevices, tonsillar crypts, periodontal pockets, dental plaques, and carious teeth), pharynx, tracheobronchial tree, gastrointestinal tract, and female urogenital tract.

Incidence and prevalence:
- Incidence 1:300,000.
- Males infected more often than females 3:1.
- Can occur at any age but commonly seen in midlife.
- Incidence has decreased since the 1950s and is attributed to better oral hygiene and antibiotics.

PHYSICAL FINDINGS & CLINICAL PRESENTATION

Actinomycosis can affect any organ. Although not typically considered as opportunistic pathogens, *Actinomyces* species capitalize on tissue injury or mucosal breach to invade adjacent structures in the head and neck regions. As a result, dental infections and oromaxillofacial trauma are common antecedent events. Characteristic manifestations include:
- Cervicofacial disease (most common site):
  1. Occurs in the setting of poor dental hygiene, recent dental surgery, or minor oral trauma
  2. Painful soft tissue swelling commonly seen at the angle of the mandible
  3. Fever, chills, and weight loss
  4. Trismus
  5. Soft tissue facial infection with sinus tract or fistula formation
- Thoracic disease:
  1. Can involve the lungs, pleura, mediastinum, or chest wall.
  2. Presumed secondary to aspiration of *Actinomyces* organisms in patients with poor oral hygiene.
  3. Fever, cough, weight loss, and pleuritic chest pains are common symptoms.
  4. Signs of pneumonia or pleural effusion may be present.
  5. With extension beyond the lungs to mediastinal structures and the chest wall, signs and symptoms of pericarditis, empyema, chest wall sinus drainage, and tracheoesophageal fistula can all occur (Fig. 1-9).

- Abdominal disease:
  1. Occurs most commonly after appendectomy, perforated bowel, diverticulitis, or surgery to the gastrointestinal tract.
  2. Lesions develop most commonly in the ileocecal valve, causing abdominal pain, fever, weight loss, and a palpable mass.
  3. Extension may occur to the liver, causing jaundice and abscess formation.
  4. Sinus tracts to the abdominal wall can occur.
- Pelvic disease:
  1. Commonly occurs by extension from abdominal disease of the ileocecal valve to the right adnexa (80% of cases).
  2. Endometritis.

ETIOLOGY

- Actinomycosis is most commonly caused by *Actinomyces israelii*. Other causes are *A. naeslundii, A. odontolyticus, A. viscosus,* and *A. meyeri.*
- *Actinomyces* are gram-positive, non–spore-forming, filamentous, anaerobic or micro-aerophilic rods.
- Actinomycosis infections are polymicrobial, usually associated with *Streptococcus, Bacteroides, Eikenella corrodens, Enterococcus,* and *Fusobacterium* spp.
- Infects individuals only after entry into disrupted mucosa or tissue injury.

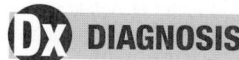 DIAGNOSIS

Isolating the bacteria in the proper clinical setting makes the diagnosis of actinomycosis.

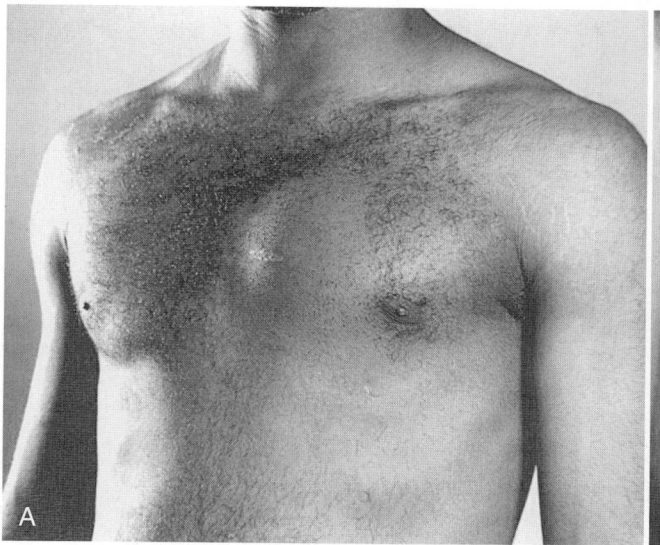
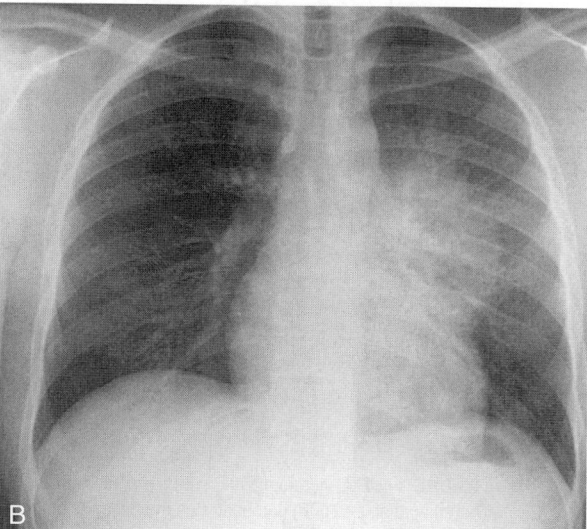

FIGURE 1-9 Thoracic actinomycosis. A, Initial presentation with a bulging mass lesion in the chest wall with a central sinus tract. **B,** The chest radiograph with the associated pulmonary infiltrate. (From Gorbach SL: *Infectious diseases,* ed 2, Philadelphia, 1998, WB Saunders.)

DIFFERENTIAL DIAGNOSIS

- Cervicofacial disease: odontogenic abscesses, brachial cleft cyst
- Pulmonary disease: nocardiosis, botryomycosis, chromomycosis, fungal disease of the lung, tuberculosis
- Intestinal disease: intestinal tuberculosis, ameboma, Crohn's disease, colon cancer
- Pelvic disease: chronic pelvic inflammatory disease, Crohn's disease
- CNS disease: other forms of brain abscess, brain tumors, toxoplasmosis, intracranial hematoma

WORKUP

The workup includes obtaining specimens either by aspirating abscesses, excising sinus tracts, or tissue biopsies. All specimens should be set up to culture anaerobic bacteria and held at least 5 to 7 days.

LABORATORY TESTS

- Isolating "sulfur granules" from tissue specimens or draining sinuses confirms the diagnosis of actinomycosis. *Actinomyces* are noted for forming characteristic sulfur granules in infected tissue but not in vitro. The term *sulfur granule* is a misnomer, reflecting only the yellow color of the granule in pus, because the granules are not composed of any sulfur at all.
  1. Sulfur granules are nests of *Actinomyces* species. Sulfur granules may be macroscopic or microscopic (Fig. 1-10).
  2. Sulfur granules are crushed and stained for identification of *Actinomyces* organisms and may take up to 3 wk to grow in culture media.

IMAGING STUDIES

Imaging studies are useful adjunctive tests in localizing the site and spread of infection.
1. Chest x-ray examination
2. CT scan of the head, chest, abdomen, and pelvic areas is useful

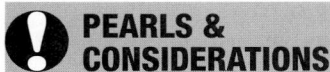 TREATMENT

NONPHARMACOLOGIC THERAPY

- Incision and drainage of abscesses
- Excision of sinus tract

ACUTE GENERAL Rx

- Penicillin 10 to 20 million units per day in 4 divided doses for 4 to 6 wk.
- In penicillin-allergic patients, erythromycin, tetracycline, clindamycin, or cephalosporins (depending on the type of penicillin allergy) are reasonable alternatives.
- Chloramphenicol 50 to 60 mg/kg/day can be used for CNS actinomycosis.

CHRONIC Rx

- Following 4 to 6 wk IV penicillin, oral penicillin V 500 mg PO qid for 6 to 12 mo.
- Treatment of associated microorganisms is not needed.

DISPOSITION

- Clinical actinomycosis, if not treated, spreads to contiguous tissues and structures ignoring tissue planes. Hematogenous spread, although possible, is rare.
- Actinomycosis is very sensitive to antibiotics but requires chronic long-term treatment to prevent relapse.

REFERRAL

If the diagnosis of actinomycosis is suspected, consultation with an infectious disease specialist is suggested. General surgical consultation for excision of sinus tracts and abscess incision and drainage is recommended.

⊘ PEARLS & CONSIDERATIONS

COMMENTS

- There is no person-to-person transmission of *Actinomyces.*
- Isolation of the organism in an asymptomatic individual does not mean the person has actinomycosis. Active symptoms must be present to make the diagnosis.
- Pelvic actinomycosis has been associated with use of an intrauterine device (IUD).
- Actinomycosis can also involve the CNS, causing multiple brain abscesses.

SUGGESTED READINGS

available at www.expertconsult.com

AUTHORS: **GLENN G. FORT, M.D., M.P.H.,** and **DENNIS J. MIKOLICH, M.D.**

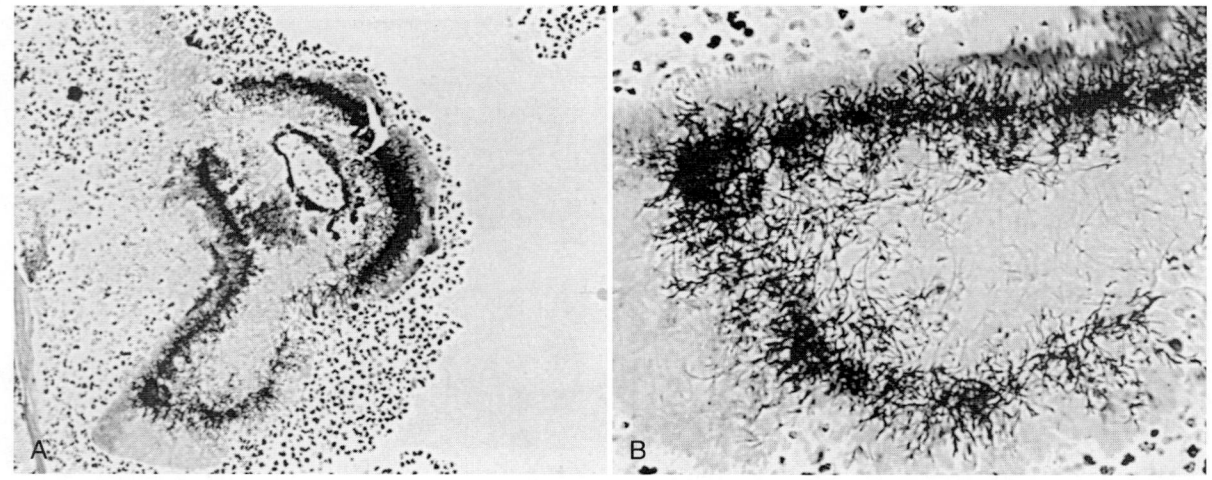

FIGURE 1-10 A, Actinomycotic sulfur granule surrounded by inflammatory cells (Brown-Brenn stain, ×250). **B,** Increased magnification (×1000) demonstrates the delicate, branched filaments of *Actinomyces.* (From Mandell GL [ed]: *Mandell, Douglas, and Bennett's principles and practice of infectious diseases,* ed 6, New York, 2005, Churchill Livingstone.)

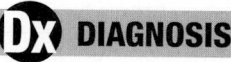

BASIC INFORMATION

DEFINITION

Acute bronchitis is the inflammation of trachea and bronchi.

SYNONYMS

Chest cold

ICD-9CM CODES
466.0 Acute bronchitis

EPIDEMIOLOGY & DEMOGRAPHICS

- Highest incidence in smokers, older adults, and young children and during winter months.
- In the U.S. there are nearly 30 million ambulatory visits annually for cough, leading to more than 12 million diagnoses of "bronchitis."
- Acute lower respiratory tract infection is the most common condition treated in primary care.

PHYSICAL FINDINGS & CLINICAL PRESENTATION

- Cough, usually worse in the morning, often productive; mainly caused by transient bronchial hyperresponsiveness
- Low-grade fever
- Substernal discomfort worsened by coughing
- Postnasal drip, pharyngeal injection
- Rhonchi that may clear after cough, occasional wheezing

ETIOLOGY

- Viral infections are the leading cause of bronchitis (rhinovirus, influenza virus, adenovirus, respiratory syncytial virus)
- Atypical organisms (*Mycoplasma, Chlamydia pneumoniae*)
- Bacterial infections (*Haemophilus influenzae, Moraxella, Streptococcus pneumoniae*)

DIAGNOSIS

DIFFERENTIAL DIAGNOSIS

- Pneumonia
- Asthma
- Sinusitis
- Bronchiolitis
- Aspiration
- Cystic fibrosis
- Pharyngitis
- Cough secondary to medications
- Neoplasm (elderly patients)
- Influenza
- Allergic aspergillosis
- Gastroesophageal reflux disease
- Congestive heart failure (in elderly patients)
- Bronchogenic neoplasm

WORKUP

Seldom necessary (e.g., to rule out pneumonia, neoplasm)

LABORATORY TESTS

Laboratory tests are generally not necessary.

IMAGING STUDIES

Chest x-ray examination is usually reserved for patients with suspected pneumonia, influenza, or underlying chronic obstructive pulmonary disease (COPD) and no improvement with therapy.

TREATMENT

NONPHARMACOLOGIC THERAPY

- Avoidance of tobacco and other pulmonary irritants
- Increased fluid intake
- Use of vaporizer to increase room humidity

ACUTE GENERAL Rx

- Inhaled bronchodilators (e.g., albuterol, metaproterenol) prn for 1 to 2 wk in patients with wheezing or troublesome cough. Inhaled albuterol has been proven effective in reducing the duration of cough in adults with uncomplicated acute bronchitis.
- Cough suppression with dextromethorphan and guaifenesin is commonly recommended; addition of codeine for cough suppression if cough is severe and is significantly interrupting patient's sleep pattern.
- Use of antibiotics (TMP-SMX, amoxicillin, doxycycline, cefuroxime) for acute bronchitis is generally not indicated; should be considered only in patients with concomitant COPD and purulent sputum or in patients unresponsive to prolonged conservative treatment.
- Antibiotics are overused in patients with acute bronchitis (70% to 90% of office visits for acute bronchitis result in treatment with antibiotics); this practice pattern is contributing to increases in resistant organisms.

CHRONIC Rx

Avoidance of tobacco and other pulmonary irritants

DISPOSITION

- Complete recovery within 7 to 10 days in most patients.
- Patients should be informed to expect to have a cough for 10 to 14 days after the visit.

REFERRAL

For pulmonary function testing only in patients with recurrent bronchitis and suspected underlying asthma

PEARLS & CONSIDERATIONS

COMMENTS

- Intervention studies reveal that patient and physician education are effective in reducing the use of antibiotic therapy. No offer or delayed offer of antibiotics for acute uncomplicated lower respiratory tract infection is acceptable, is associated with little difference in symptom resolution, and is likely to reduce antibiotic use and beliefs in the effectiveness of antibiotics.
- It is helpful to refer to acute bronchitis as a "chest cold." Patients should be informed that antibiotics are probably not going to be beneficial and may result in significant side effects.

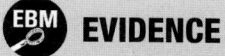 **EVIDENCE**

available at www.expertconsult.com

SUGGESTED READINGS
available at www.expertconsult.com

AUTHOR: **FRED F. FERRI, M.D.**

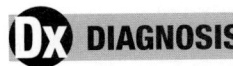

BASIC INFORMATION

DEFINITION

Acute coronary syndrome (ACS) represents a spectrum of clinical disorders that include unstable angina (UA), non–ST-elevation myocardial infarction (NSTEMI), and ST-elevation myocardial infarction (STEMI). While the severity of disease will vary between the three subsets of ACS, they all share a common clinical presentation and pathophysiology. This syndrome is typically caused by atherosclerotic coronary artery disease (CAD). In this spectrum, UA and NSTEMI are represented electrocardiographically by ST-segment depression and T-wave inversion in the appropriate clinical setting (i.e., chest discomfort). NSTEMI would have the addition of positive cardiac biomarkers. STEMI is represented by ST-segment elevation. ACS should be thought of as a continuous spectrum as UA will often progress to a myocardial infarction if left untreated. See Table 1-4.

SYNONYMS

Unstable angina
NSTEMI
STEMI
Acute myocardial infarction

ICD-9CM CODES
410.0 Acute myocardial infarction
411.1 Intermediate coronary syndrome

EPIDEMIOLOGY & DEMOGRAPHICS

INCIDENCE: 1.36 million hospitalizations yearly in the U.S. for ACS; 0.81 million are listed as myocardial infarction, and the remainder are UA. Approximately two thirds of myocardial infarctions are listed as NSTEMI, with the remainder being listed as STEMI. The underling etiology, atherosclerotic CAD, is the number one cause of mortality.
PREDOMINANT SEX AND AGE: In evaluating chest pain, male gender and older age are important clinical factors that can identify ACS as a potential cause. The 2005 overall death rate from cardiovascular disease was 278.9 per 100,000. The rates were 324.7 per 100,000 for white males, 438.4 per 100,000 for black males, 230.4 per 100,000 for white females, and 319.7 per 100,000 for black females.
RISK FACTORS: Hypertension, diabetes mellitus, dyslipidemia, tobacco use, family history of premature CAD (CAD in male first-degree relative <55 yr, female <65 yr). Presence of these risk factors causes damage to the vascular endothelium and progression of atherosclerotic coronary artery plaques.

PHYSICAL FINDINGS & CLINICAL PRESENTATION

- Symptoms often, but not always, include chest discomfort described as a pressure that may radiate to the left arm, neck, jaw, or back. Typical angina is substernal in location, brought on by emotional or physical stress, and relieved with rest and/or nitroglycerin.
- Women and the elderly often have an atypical presentation for ACS.
- Angina is considered unstable if it is new onset (<2 mo), increasing in frequency (crescendo pattern), or occurring at rest (typically lasting >20 min).
- "Anginal equivalents" may include dyspnea, nausea, vomiting, and fatigue.
- ECG for UA and NSTEMI may reveal ST-segment depression and/or T-wave inversion. ECG for definition of STEMI will reveal at least 1 mm ST-segment elevation in two contiguous leads in the appropriate clinical setting.
- Physical exam findings alone are insufficient for the diagnosis of ACS. It is however important to assess the patient's hemodynamic stability and volume status. The patient may be diaphoretic and tachycardic. Signs of heart failure may be present, which include elevated JVP, presence of an S3 gallop, and peripheral edema.

ETIOLOGY

Atherosclerotic CAD is the underlying etiology. The hallmark of ACS is the vulnerable atherosclerotic plaque, which typically has a thin cap and a large lipid core. This vulnerable plaque ultimately ruptures, which leads to platelet activation and aggregation, leading to thrombus formation. STEMI typically results from complete thrombotic occlusion of a coronary artery, whereas UA and NSTEMI often have partial occlusion. Angiographically, it is often the intermediate coronary artery lesions (50% diameter vessel stenosis) that lead to subtotal or total vessel occlusion in two thirds of STEMI cases.

DIAGNOSIS

DIFFERENTIAL DIAGNOSIS

Chest pain mimicking ACS may be the result of various underlying disorders, some of which are also accompanied by ECG changes and/or cardiac biomarker release. Examples include acute pulmonary embolism, acute aortic dissection, pericarditis, myocarditis, costochondritis, pneumonia, tension pneumothorax, perforating, ulcer, or Boerhaave syndrome.

WORKUP

Focused history and physical exam, 12-lead ECG, cardiac biomarkers, and chest radiograph (CXR). Initial biomarkers may not be positive. Often serial biomarkers are drawn every 6 to 8 hr for a total of three sets for the purposes of ruling out MI, or until peak to determine the severity of an established MI. Echocardiogram may reveal new regional wall motion abnormalities.

LABORATORY TESTS

- Cardiac biomarkers, which include creatine kinase (CK), its MB isoenzyme, myoglobin, and troponin I or T will be positive in the setting of NSTEMI or STEMI. See Figure 1-11 for timing of release of each biomarker.
- BNP may also be helpful in patients with heart failure.
- A complete fasting lipid panel should be obtained during the hospital admission.

TABLE 1-4   Acute Coronary Syndromes

	Spectrum of ACS		
	Unstable Angina	**NSTEMI**	**STEMI**
Chest discomfort	+	+	+
Cardiac biomarkers	−	+	+
ECG changes	TWI and/or ST depression	TWI and/or ST depression	ST elevation
Pathophysiology	Partial/transient thrombotic occlusion	Partial/transient thrombotic occlusion	Complete thrombotic occlusion

ACS, Acute coronary syndrome; *ECG*, electrocardiogram; *NSTEMI*, non–ST-segment elevation myocardial infarction; *STEMI*, ST-segment myocardial infarction; *TWI*, T-wave inversion.

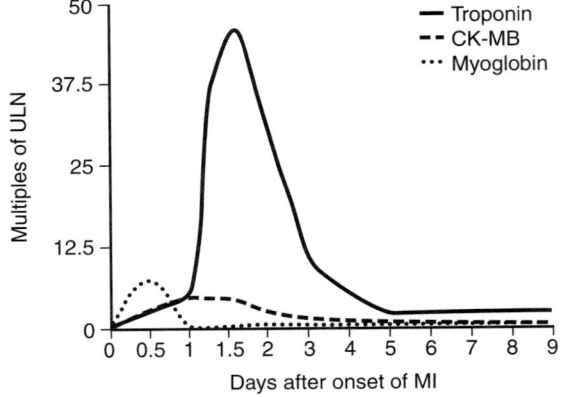

FIGURE 1-11 Timing of release of cardiac biomarkers in ACS. *ULN,* Upper limit of normal; *MI,* myocardial infarction. (Modified from Shapiro BP, Jaffe AS: Cardiac biomarkers. In: Murphy JG, Lloyd MA [eds]: *Mayo Clinic cardiology: concise textbook,* ed 3, Rochester, MN: Mayo Clinic Scientific Press and New York, 2007, Informa Healthcare USA, pp 773-780; and Anderson JL, et al: *J Am Coll Cardiol* 50:e1-e157, 2007, Fig. 5.)

IMAGING STUDIES

- CXR to assist in evaluating for volume status and for other possible causes of chest discomfort.
- In patients where ECG and cardiac biomarkers are nondiagnostic but the suspicion for ACS is high given the history, an echocardiogram may be helpful to assess left ventricular (LV) function and regional wall motion abnormalities.
- Cardiac stress testing (treadmill ECG, imaging stress studies using echocardiography or nuclear modalities) may further help to diagnose and risk stratify these patients.
- Coronary angiogram/cardiac catheterization will reveal coronary artery luminal irregularities/stenotic lesions.

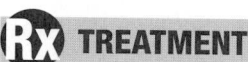 **TREATMENT**

The overall goal for UA and NSTEMI is to relieve myocardial ischemia and to prevent recurrent cardiovascular events. Antithrombotic therapy is needed to reduce thrombus burden, prevent further thrombosis, and improve coronary artery flow. Revascularization is typically needed to prevent further events and improve flow. For STEMI, the goal is immediate reperfusion therapy, whether it is chemical (i.e., thrombolysis) or mechanical (i.e., percutaneous coronary intervention (PCI)). STEMI patients presenting to a hospital with PCI capability should be treated with primary PCI within 90 min of first medical contact (Figs. 1-12 and 1-13).

NONPHARMACOLOGIC THERAPY

- STEMI is a medical emergency and requires immediate reperfusion therapy with the best outcomes being with cardiac catheterization with primary PCI. Guidelines call for a goal door-to-balloon time of ≤90 min.

- Patients with UA or NSTEMI should be risk stratified in conjunction with the Cardiology consult service. Risk scores such as the TIMI and GRACE scores can be used to decide between an early invasive versus an initial conservative management strategy. An early invasive strategy is overall associated with better outcomes and involves cardiac catheterization followed by revascularization with PCI or coronary artery bypass grafting (CABG) within 4 to 24 hr of presentation. An initial conservative strategy involves aggressive medical management and revascularization only if ischemia recurs or is documented on noninvasive testing. This should only be reserved for selected patients with low risk scores (TIMI score 0-2).
- Bed rest and continuous ECG monitoring is recommended for all ACS patients. Supplemental oxygen should be administered to patients with signs of hypoxia or respiratory distress. Finger pulse oximetry should be utilized to assess arterial oxygen saturation.

ACUTE GENERAL Rx

- All patients with ACS should receive full dose aspirin for its antiplatelet effects and medical therapy with the statin class of drugs regardless of LDL level, unless contraindicated.
- Beta-blocker therapy reduces ischemia by decreasing myocardial oxygen demand and should be initiated within 24 hr of onset of ACS unless signs or symptoms of heart failure are present or arrhythmias preclude its use. Oral administration, titrated to a heart rate of 50-60 beats per min, is preferred. Intravenous beta-blockers should not be administered to STEMI patients who have any of the following: (1) signs of heart failure, (2) evidence of a low output state, (3) increased risk for cardiogenic shock, or (4) other rela-

tive contraindications to beta-blockade (PR interval >0.24 sec, 2nd- or 3rd-degree heart block, active asthma, or reactive airway disease).
- Nitroglycerin is a vasodilator that should be administered to relieve chest discomfort in all ACS patients. It can be administered sublingually at first, followed by intravenously if symptoms persist. In the setting of an inferior STEMI, it is wise to rule out a right ventricular (RV) infarct with a right-sided ECG prior to the administration of nitroglycerin. This is because RV infarcts are preload dependent and nitroglycerin decreases preload through venodilation, which leads to hypotension in this setting. This can be corrected with discontinuing nitroglycerin and starting intravenous fluids. Nitroglycerin provides no mortality benefit in ACS patients.
- Calcium channel blockers (nondihydropyridine) may be used in patients with persisting or recurrent symptoms, despite treatment with beta-blockers and nitroglycerin. They work by causing coronary vasodilation and decreasing myocardial oxygen demand. They are useful when beta-blockers are contraindicated or in Prinzmetal variant angina. Calcium channel blockers should not be used in cases of severe LV dysfunction or pulmonary edema.
- Once a diagnosis has been established, morphine is reasonable to relieve chest pain if nitroglycerin is inadequate or contraindicated. Morphine can be used for pain management. Close monitoring of blood pressure and respiratory rate is recommended.
- Patients routinely taking NSAIDs (except for aspirin), both nonselective as well as COX-2 selective agents, prior to STEMI should have those agents discontinued at the time of presentation with STEMI because of the in-

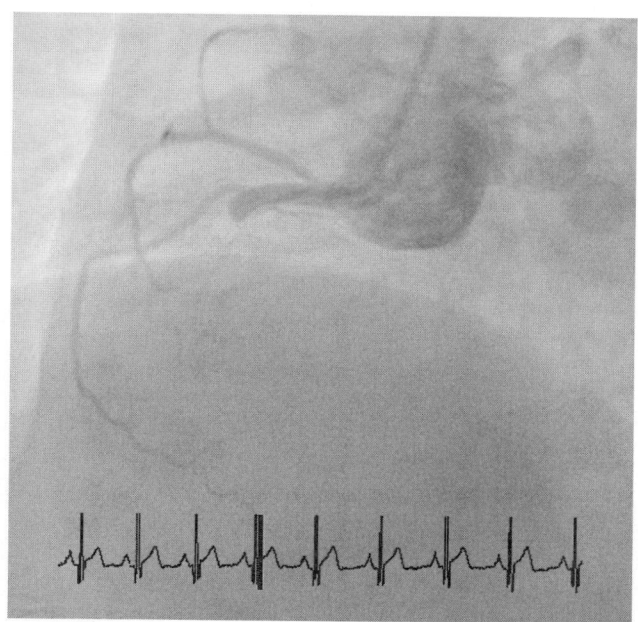

FIGURE 1-12 Right coronary artery totally occluded proximally during STEMI.

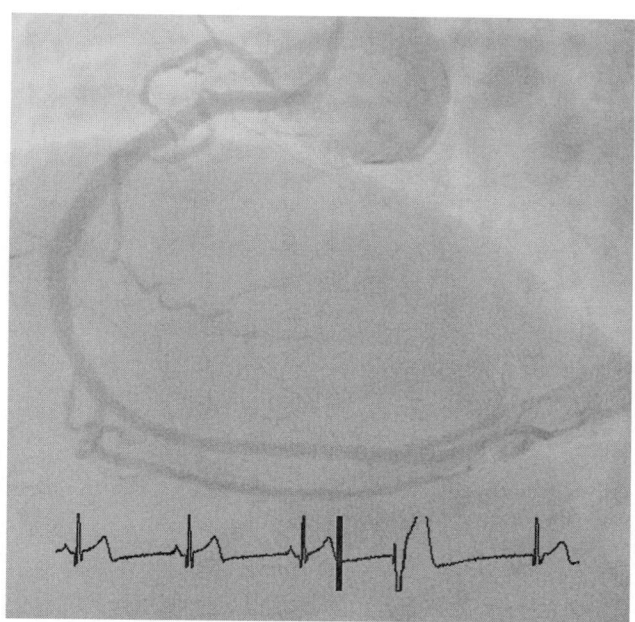

FIGURE 1-13 Right coronary artery after successful percutaneous coronary artery stenting during STEMI.

creased risks of mortality, reinfarction, hypertension, heart failure, and myocardial rupture associated with their use.

- ACE inhibitors may be added and should be used within 24 hr of onset of ACS in all patients with depressed LV function (EF <40%) or pulmonary vascular congestion. Angiotensin receptor blockers (ARB) should be used in patients who are ACE inhibitor intolerant.
- Antithrombotic therapy is critical in treating the underlying pathophysiology of ACS. This consists of administering antiplatelet and anticoagulant agents.
- Antiplatelet agents inhibit platelet activation and aggregation. Aspirin is a cyclooxygenase inhibitor that blocks platelet aggregation and should be administered to all ACS patients without contraindications at an initial dose of 162 mg to 325 mg. Clopidogrel is a thienopyridine agent that inhibits platelet activation and aggregation. It should be administered in all ACS patients, with the timing dependent on the clinical scenario and management strategy. It requires a loading dose of 300 mg to 600 mg followed by 75 mg daily. It should be discontinued at least 5 days prior to CABG. Other antiplatelet agents that can be substituted instead of clopidogrel include prasugrel and ticlopidine. Glycoprotein IIb/IIIa inhibitors (eptifibitide or abciximab) are given intravenously and are effective at blocking the final pathway of platelet aggregation. As a rule, all ACS patients should have two antiplatelet agents on board.
- Anticoagulant agents should be administered to all ACS patients. Options include either unfractionated heparin or low-molecular-weight heparin or direct thrombin inhibitors such as bivalirudin. As with antiplatelet agents, the choice of anticoagulant depends on management strategy and institution pro-

tocols. For STEMI, fondaparinux can be used for anticoagulation. It has been shown to decrease bleeding complications as compared with either unfractionated heparin or low-molecular-weight heparin.

- Some of the disadvantages are that it is difficult to monitor. It has a long half-life (15 hr), and thrombosis on catheters has been noted when using only fondaparinux in the cath lab.

CHRONIC Rx

- Post-ACS medical therapy involves aspirin, statin, beta-blocker, and clopidogrel.
- ACE inhibitors may be added to treat hypertension and should be used in all patients with depressed LV function (EF <40%) or pulmonary vascular congestion. Angiotensin receptor blockers (ARB) should be used in patients who are ACE inhibitor intolerant.
- Eplerenone, an aldosterone receptor blocker, should be considered in post-MI patients with LV EF ≤40% and evidence of congestive heart failure.
- Aggressive risk factor management remains crucial for secondary prevention of future events.

REFERRAL

- All ACS patients should be cared for in conjunction with the Cardiology consult service.
- When appropriate, referral to a Cardiac Surgeon may be necessary for CABG.

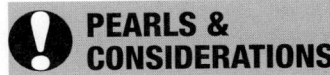

COMMENTS

- ACS is common and a leading cause of mortality in the U.S.

- Its diagnosis hinges on the basics—history and physical, ECG, biomarkers, and CXR.
- Remember the potentially fatal non-ACS causes of chest discomfort, which include acute pulmonary embolism and acute ascending aortic dissection.
- STEMI patients presenting to a hospital with PCI capability should be treated with primary PCI within 90 min of first medical contact.
- STEMI patients presenting to a hospital without PCI capability and who cannot be transferred to a PCI center and undergo PCI within 90 min of first medical contact should be treated with fibrinolytic therapy within 30 min of hospital presentation unless fibrinolytic therapy is contraindicated.

PREVENTION

- Primary prevention of ACS is based on recognizing the major risk factors for CAD and treating them as appropriate.
- Patients with depressed LV function (ejection fraction <35%) at least 40 days after an acute MI benefit from implantation of an implantable cardioverter defibrillator (ICD) for the prevention of sudden cardiac death.

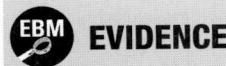 **EVIDENCE**

available at www.expertconsult.com

SUGGESTED READINGS

available at www.expertconsult.com

AUTHORS: **NAUMAN SIDDIQI, M.D.,** and **PRANAV M. PATEL, M.D.**

BASIC INFORMATION

DEFINITION

Acute respiratory distress syndrome (ARDS) is a form of noncardiogenic pulmonary edema that results from acute damage to the alveoli. It is characterized by acute diffuse infiltrative lung lesions with resulting interstitial and alveolar edema, severe hypoxemia, and respiratory failure. The definition of ARDS includes the following three components:

1. A ratio of Pao_2 to Fio_2 ≤200 regardless of the level of positive end expiratory pressure (PEEP)
2. The detection of bilateral pulmonary infiltrates on frontal chest radiograph
3. Absence of congestive heart failure (pulmonary artery wedge pressure [PAWP] ≤18 mm Hg or no clinical evidence of elevated left atrial pressure on the basis of chest radiograph or other clinical data)

The cardinal feature of ARDS, refractory hypoxemia, is caused by formation of protein-rich alveolar edema after damage to the integrity of the lung's alveolar-capillary barrier.

SYNONYMS

ARDS
Adult respiratory distress syndrome

ICD-9CM CODES
518.82 Acute respiratory distress syndrome

EPIDEMIOLOGY & DEMOGRAPHICS

- More than 150,000 ARDS cases per year in the U.S.
- Incidence is 1.5 to 8.3 cases per 100,000 per year.
- Approximately 50% of patients who develop ARDS do so within 24 hours of the inciting event. Mortality rate is 40% to 50%.

PHYSICAL FINDINGS & CLINICAL PRESENTATION

- Signs and symptoms
  1. Dyspnea
  2. Chest discomfort
  3. Cough
  4. Anxiety
- Physical examination
  1. Tachypnea
  2. Tachycardia
  3. Hypertension
  4. Coarse crepitations of both lungs
  5. Fever may be present if infection is the underlying etiology

ETIOLOGY

- Sepsis (>40% of cases)
- Aspiration: near drowning, aspiration of gastric contents (>30% of cases)
- Trauma (>20% of cases)
- Multiple transfusions, blood products
- Drugs (e.g., overdose of morphine, methadone, heroin; reaction to nitrofurantoin)
- Noxious inhalation (e.g., chlorine gas, high O_2 concentration)
- Postresuscitation
- Cardiopulmonary bypass
- Pneumonia
- Burns
- Pancreatitis
- A history of chronic alcohol abuse significantly increases the risk of developing ARDS in critically ill patients

DIAGNOSIS

DIFFERENTIAL DIAGNOSIS

- Cardiogenic pulmonary edema
- Viral pneumonitis
- Lymphangitic carcinomatosis

WORKUP

The search for an underlying cause should focus on treatable causes (e.g., infections such as sepsis or pneumonia)

- Arterial blood gases (ABGs)
- Hemodynamic monitoring
- Bronchoalveolar lavage (selected patients)

LABORATORY TESTS

- ABGs:
  1. Initially: varying degrees of hypoxemia, generally resistant to supplemental oxygen
  2. Respiratory alkalosis, decreased Pco_2
  3. Widened alveolar-arterial gradient
  4. Hypercapnia as the disease progresses
- Bronchoalveolar lavage:
  1. The most prominent finding is an increased number of polymorphonucleocytes.
  2. The presence of eosinophilia has therapeutic implications because these patients respond to corticosteroids.
- Blood and urine cultures

IMAGING STUDIES

Chest radiograph (Fig. 1-14).

- The initial chest radiograph might be normal in the initial hours after the precipitating event.
- Bilateral interstitial infiltrates are usually seen within 24 hr; they often are more prominent in the bases and periphery.
- "White out" of both lung fields can be seen in advanced stages.
- CT scan of chest: diffuse consolidation with air bronchograms, bullae, pleural effusions. Pneumomediastinum and pneumothoraces may also be present.

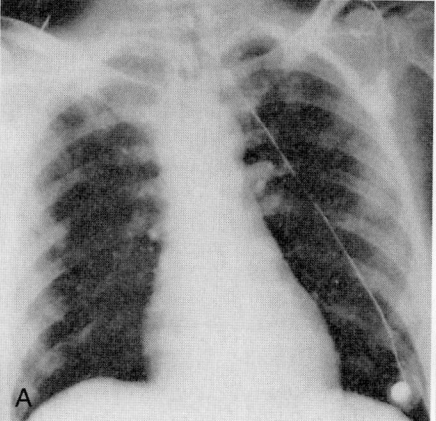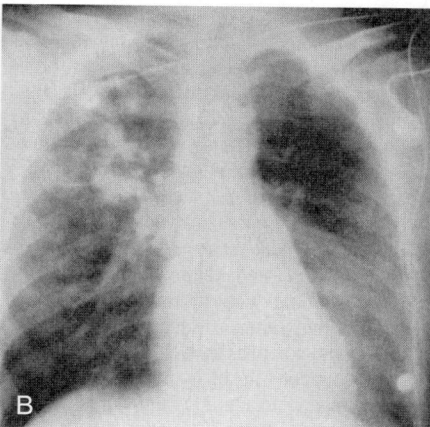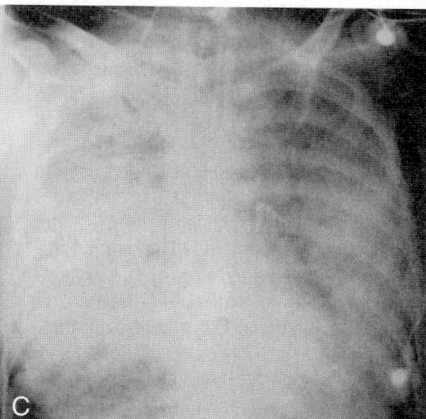

FIGURE 1-14 Acute respiratory distress syndrome. The x-ray of the young man who had sustained severe trauma and blood loss in a road traffic accident; the limbs cover a period of 5 days from a relatively normal x-ray. **A,** To bilateral infiltrates. **B,** To bilateral "white out." **C,** Accompanied by severe hypoxamia. A Swan-Ganz catheter for measurement of pulmonary artery "wedge" pressure (as a reflection of left atrial pressure can be seen in situ on x-ray (**C**). The patient died shortly after the last film. (From Souhami RL, Moxham J: *Textbook of medicine,* ed 4, London, Churchill Livingstone, 2002.)

Rx TREATMENT

NONPHARMACOLOGIC THERAPY

Hemodynamic monitoring:

- Can be used for the initial evaluation of ARDS (in ruling out cardiogenic pulmonary edema) and its subsequent management. Recent studies, however, have shown that clinical management involving the early use of pulmonary artery catheters in patients with ARDS did not significantly affect mortality and morbidity rates.
- Although no dynamic profile is diagnostic of ARDS, the presence of pulmonary edema, a high cardiac output, and a low pulmonary capillary wedge pressure (PCWP) is characteristic of ARDS.
- It is important to remember that partially treated intravascular volume overload and flash pulmonary edema can have the hemodynamic features of ARDS; filling pressures can also be elevated by increased intrathoracic pressures or with fluid administration; cardiac function can be depressed by acidosis, hypoxemia, or other factors associated with sepsis.

Ventilatory support: mechanical ventilation is generally necessary to maintain adequate gas exchange (see Section III). A low tidal volume and low plateau pressure ventilator strategy are recommended to avoid ventilator-induced injury. Assist-control is generally preferred initially with the following ventilator settings:

- FiO_2 1.0 (until a lower value can be used to achieve adequate oxygenation). When possible, minimize oxygen toxicity by maintaining FiO_2 at <60%.
- Tidal volume: Set initial tidal volume at 6 ml/kg of predicted body weight (PBW = 50.0 + 0.91 [height: 152.4 cm] for men, PBW = 45.5 + 0.91 [height: 152.4 cm] for women). The concept of using PBW is based on the fact that lung size depends most strongly on height and sex; PBW normalizes the tidal volume to lung size. Aim to maintain plateau pressure (Pplat) at <30 mm Hg.
- PEEP 5 cm H_2O or greater (to increase lung volume and keep alveoli open). PEEP should be applied in small increments of 3 to 5 cm H_2O (up to a maximum of 15 cm H_2O) to achieve acceptable arterial saturation (>0.9) with nontoxic FiO_2 values (<0.6) and acceptable airway plateau pressures (>30 to 35 cm H_2O). It is important to remember that an increase in PEEP may lower cardiac output and, despite improvement in PaO_2, may actually have a negative effect on tissue oxygenation (the major determinants of tissue oxygenation are hemoglobin, percent saturation, and cardiac output). The optimal level of PEEP remains unestablished. Although higher levels of PEEP may help prevent life-threatening hypioxemia and be associated with lower hospital mortality in patients meeting criteria for ARDS such benefit is unlikely in patients with less severe lung injury and a strategy of treating such patients with high PEEP levels may be harmful.
- Inspiratory flow: 60 L/min.

- Ventilatory rate: high ventilatory rates of 18 to 24 breaths/min are often necessary in patients with ARDS because of their increased physiologic dead space and smaller lung volumes. Patients must be monitored for excessive intrathoracic gas trapping (auto-PEEP or intrinsic PEEP) that can depress cardiac output.
- Sedation: GABA receptor agonists (including propofol and benzodiazepines such as midazolam) have traditionally been the most commonly administered sedative drugs for ICU patients. Recent trials indicate that the alpha-2 agonist dexmedetomidine may have distinct advantages. At comparable sedation levels, dexmedetomidine-treated patients spent less time on ventilator, experienced less delirium, and developed less tachycardia and hypertension. The most notable adverse effect of dexmedetomidine was bradycardia.

ACUTE GENERAL Rx

Identify and treat precipitating conditions:

- Blood and urine cultures and trial of antibiotics in presumed sepsis (routine administration of antibiotics in all cases of ARDS is not recommended).
- Prompt repair of bone fractures in patients with major trauma.
- Bowel rest and crystalloid resuscitation in pancreatitis.
- Fluid management: optimal fluid and hemodynamic management of patients with ARDS is patient specific; in general, administration of crystalloids is recommended if a downward trend in PCWP is associated with diminished cardiac index, resulting in prerenal azotemia, oliguria, and relative tachycardia. On the other hand, if PCWP increases with little or no change in cardiac index, one should begin diuretic therapy and use low-dose dopamine (2 to 4 μg/kg/min) to maintain natriuresis and support adequate renal flow.
- Positioning the patient: changes in position can improve oxygenation by improving the distribution of perfusion to ventilated lung regions; repositioning (lateral decubitus positioning) should be attempted in patients with hypoxemia that is not responsive to other medical interventions. Placing patients with moderate and severe hypoxemia in a prone position may improve their oxygenation but does not provide significant survival benefit
- Corticosteroids: routine use of corticosteroids in ARDS is not recommended; corticosteroids may be beneficial in patients with many eosinophils in the bronchoalveolar lavage fluid. Systemic infections should be ruled out or adequately treated before administration of corticosteroids. Use of methylprednisolone has not been shown to increase the rate of infectious complications but is associated with a higher rate of neuromuscular weakness. In addition, starting methylprednisolone therapy more than 2 wk after the onset of ARDS may increase the risk of death.
- Nutritional support: nutritional support, preferably administered by the enteral route, is necessary to maintain adequate colloid oncotic pressure sand intravascular volume. The inclusion of eicosapentaenoic acid from fish oil may

be beneficial in improving ventilation requirements and length of stay in patients with ARDS.

- Tracheostomy: tracheostomy is warranted in patients requiring >2 wk of mechanical ventilation; discussion regarding tracheostomy should begin with patient (if alert and oriented) and family members/legal guardian after 5 to 7 days of ventilatory support.
- Some form of deep vein thrombosis prophylaxis is indicated in all patients with ARDS.
- Stress ulcer prophylaxis with sucralfate suspension (by nasogastric tube), or IV proton pump inhibitors or H_2 blockers.
- The use of surfactant remains controversial. Patients who receive surfactant have a greater improvement in gas exchange in the initial 24-hour period than patients who receive standard therapy alone; however, the use of exogenous surfactant does not improve survival.

DISPOSITION

- Prognosis for ARDS varies with the underlying cause. Prognosis is worse in patients with chronic liver disease, nonpulmonary organ dysfunction, sepsis, and advanced age.
- Elevated values of dead space fraction ([$PaCO_2$ − $PeCO_2$]/$PaCO_2$; normal is <0.3) is associated with an increased risk of death.
- In ARDS, the percentage of potentially recruitable lung is variable and associated with the response to PEEP.
- Overall mortality rate varies between 32% and 45%. Most deaths are attributable to sepsis or multiorgan dysfunction rather than primary respiratory causes.
- Recent trials have shown that as compared with the current standard of care, a ventilator strategy using esophageal measures to estimate the transpulmonary pressure significantly improves oxygenation and compliance. Further trials will determine if this approach should be widely adapted.
- Preliminary trials involving early administration of a neuromuscular blocking agent (cisatracurium) in patients with severe ARDS have shown improvement in the adjusted 90-day survival and increase in the time off the ventilator without increase in muscle weakness.
- Strategies for treatment of life-threatening refractory hypoxemia (prone positioning, inhaled nitric acid, extracorporeal membrane oxygenation, high-frequency oscillatory ventilation, recruitment maneuvers) may improve oxygenation, but their impact on mortality remains unproven.

REFERRAL

Surgical referral for tracheostomy (see "Acute General Rx").

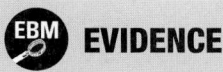 **EVIDENCE**

available at www.expertconsult.com

SUGGESTED READINGS
available at www.expertconsult.com

AUTHOR: **FRED F. FERRI, M.D.**

BASIC INFORMATION

DEFINITION

Addison disease is characterized by inadequate secretion of corticosteroids resulting from partial or complete destruction of the adrenal glands.

SYNONYMS

Primary adrenocortical insufficiency
Adrenal insufficiency

ICD-9CM CODES
255.4 Addison disease

EPIDEMIOLOGY & DEMOGRAPHICS

PREVALENCE: Five cases/100,000 persons
PREDOMINANT SEX: Female/male ratio of 2:1

PHYSICAL FINDINGS & CLINICAL PRESENTATION

- Addison disease may present insidiously with nonspecific symptoms. A high index of suspicion is required for diagnosis. About half of patients may present acutely with adrenal crises
- Hyperpigmentation of skin and mucous membranes is a cardinal sign of Addison disease: more prominent in palmar creases, buccal mucosa, pressure points (elbows, knees, knuckles), perianal mucosa, and around areolas of nipples
- Hypotension, postural dizziness
- Generalized weakness, chronic fatigue, malaise, anorexia
- Amenorrhea and loss of axillary hair in females

ETIOLOGY

- Autoimmune destruction of the adrenal glands (80% of cases)
- Tuberculosis (TB) (15% of cases)
- Carcinomatous destruction of the adrenal glands, lymphoma
- Adrenal hemorrhage (anticoagulants, trauma, coagulopathies, pregnancy, sepsis)
- Adrenal infarction (antiphospholipid syndrome, arteritis, thrombosis)
- AIDS (adrenal insufficiency develops in 30% of patients with AIDS, often cytomegalovirus [CMV] adrenalitis)
- Other: sarcoidosis, amyloidosis, hemochromatosis, Wegener's granulomatosis, postoperative, fungal infections (candidiasis, histoplasmosis)

DIAGNOSIS

DIFFERENTIAL DIAGNOSIS

Sepsis, hypovolemic shock, acute abdomen, apathetic hyperthyroidism in the elderly, myopathies, gastrointestinal malignancy, major depression, anorexia nervosa, hemochromatosis, salt-losing nephritis, chronic infection

WORKUP

- If the clinical picture is highly suggestive of adrenocortical insufficiency, the diagnosis can be made with the rapid adrenocorticotropic hormone (ACTH) test:
  1. Give 250 mcg ACTH (Sinachten, tetracosatrin) by IV push and measure cortisol levels at 0, 30, and 60 min.
  2. An increase in serum cortisol level to peak concentration >500 nmol/L (18 mcg/dl) indicates a normal response. Cortisol level <18 mcg/dl at 30 or 60 min is suggestive of adrenal insufficiency.
  3. Measure plasma ACTH. A high ACTH level confirms primary adrenal insufficiency.
- Critical illness-related corticosteroid insufficiency (e.g., in sepsis) is best established with the 1 mcg ACTH stimulation test in which cortisol levels are measured at baseline and 30 min after administration of ACTH. A level <25 mcg/dl (690 nmol/L) or an increment over baseline of <9 mcg (250 nmol/L) represents an inadequate adrenal response.
- Secondary adrenocortical insufficiency (caused by pituitary dysfunction) can be distinguished from primary adrenal insufficiency by the following:
  1. Normal or low plasma ACTH level after rapid ACTH
  2. Absence of hyperpigmentation
  3. No significant impairment of aldosterone secretion (because aldosterone secretion is under control of the renin-angiotensin system)
  4. Additional evidence of hypopituitarism (e.g., hypogonadism, hypothyroidism)

LABORATORY TESTS

- Hyponatremia, hyperkalemia
- Decreased glucose
- Increased BUN/creatinine ratio (prerenal azotemia)
- Mild normocytic, normochromic anemia, neutropenia, lymphocytosis, eosinophilia (significant dehydration may mask hyponatremia and anemia), hypercalcemia, metabolic acidosis
- A morning cortisol level >500 mmol/L (18 micrograms/dl) generally excludes the diagnosis whereas a level <165 mmol/L (6 micrograms/dl) is suggestive of Addison disease and requires further evaluation (see Workup)
- Useful tests in evaluating the cause of Addison disease are: PPD (rule out TB), adrenal cortex antibodies and 21-hydroxylase antibodies (rule out autoimmune Addison disease), plasma very long chain fatty acids (rule out adrenoleukodystrophy)

IMAGING STUDIES

- Chest radiograph may reveal a small heart.
- Abdominal radiograph: adrenal calcifications may be noted if the adrenocortical insufficiency is secondary to TB or fungal infection.
- Abdominal CT scan: small adrenal glands generally indicate either idiopathic atrophy or longstanding TB, whereas enlarged glands are suggestive of early TB or potentially treatable diseases.

TREATMENT

NONPHARMACOLOGIC THERAPY

- Perform periodic monitoring of serum electrolytes, vital signs, and body weight; liberal sodium intake is suggested.
- Periodic measurement of bone density may be helpful in identifying patients at risk for the development of osteoporosis.
- Patients should carry a MedicAlert bracelet and an emergency pack containing hydrocortisone 100 mg ampule, syringe, and needle.
- Patients and partners should be educated on how to give IM injection in case of vomiting or coma.

ACUTE GENERAL Rx

- Addisonian crisis is an acute complication of adrenal insufficiency characterized by circulatory collapse, dehydration, nausea, vomiting, hypoglycemia, and hyperkalemia.
  1. Draw plasma cortisol level; do not delay therapy while waiting for confirming laboratory results.
  2. Administer hydrocortisone 100 mg IV immediately, followed by 100 to 200 mg of hydrocortisone every 24 hours divided into 3 or 4 doses; if patient shows good clinical response, gradually taper dosage and change to oral maintenance dose (usually prednisone 7.5 mg/day).
  3. Provide adequate volume replacement with D_5NS solution until hypotension, dehydration, and hypoglycemia are completely corrected. Large volumes (2 to 3 L) under continuous cardiac monitoring may be necessary in the first 2 to 3 hr to correct the volume deficit and hypoglycemia and to avoid further hyponatremia.
- Identify and correct any precipitating factor (e.g., sepsis, hemorrhage).

CHRONIC Rx

- Give hydrocortisone 15 to 20 mg PO every morning and 5 to 10 mg in late afternoon or prednisone 5 mg in morning and 2.5 mg hs.
- Give oral fludrocortisone 0.05 mg/day to 0.20 mg/day: this mineralocorticoid is necessary if the patient has primary adrenocortical insufficiency. The dose is adjusted based on the serum sodium level and the presence of postural hypotension or marked ortho-stasis.
- Instruct patients to increase glucocorticoid replacement in times of stress and to receive parenteral glucocorticoids if diarrhea or vomiting occurs. Typical supplementation varies from 25 mg PO qd of hydrocortisone for minor medical and surgical stress to 50 to 100 mg IV hydrocortisone q8h for sepsis-induced hypotension or shock.
- The administration of dehydroepiandrosterone 50 mg PO qd improves well-being and sexuality in women with adrenal insufficiency.

SUGGESTED READINGS
available at www.expertconsult.com

AUTHOR: **FRED F. FERRI, M.D.**

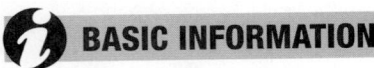

BASIC INFORMATION

DEFINITION

Although defining alcoholism precisely is impossible, among the commonly used screening instruments for this disorder are the CAGE questionnaire, short Michigan Alcoholism Screening Test (SMAST), National Council on Alcoholism criteria, and DSM-IV-R criteria. Moderate drinking has been defined as two standard drinks (e.g., 12 oz of beer) per day and one drink per day for women and persons older than 65 yr. Although not generally included under the alcoholism topic, hazardous or at-risk drinking should also be considered. For men, *at-risk drinking* is defined as more than 14 drinks/wk or more than 4 drinks/occasion. For women, at-risk drinking is defined as approximately half that given for men.

The American Psychiatric Association defines diagnostic criteria for *alcohol withdrawal* as follows:
A. Cessation of (or reduction in) alcohol use that has been heavy and prolonged.
B. Two (or more) of the following, developing within several hours to a few days after criterion A:
    1. Autonomic hyperactivity (e.g., sweating or pulse rate >100 beats/min)
    2. Increased hand tremor
    3. Insomnia
    4. Nausea and vomiting
    5. Transient visual, tactile, or auditory hallucinations or illusions
    6. Psychomotor agitation
    7. Anxiety
    8. Grand mal seizures
C. The symptoms in criterion B cause clinically significant distress or impairment in social, occupational, or other important areas of functioning.

The symptoms are not attributable to a general medical condition and are not better accounted for by another mental disorder.

SYNONYMS

Alcohol abuse
Substance abuse

ICD-9CM CODES
303.9 Alcoholism

EPIDEMIOLOGY & DEMOGRAPHICS

INCIDENCE (IN U.S.):
- The clinical history suggests alcohol problems in 15% to 20% of patients in primary care and hospitalized patients. In the U.S., alcohol abuse generates nearly $185 billion in annual economic costs. An estimated 8 million adults in the U.S. have alcohol dependence.
- 20% achieve abstinence without help; 70% achieve sobriety for 1 yr.

PREVALENCE (IN U.S.): 7% of population ≥18 yr

PREDOMINANT SEX:
- Lifetime risk for males 8% to 10%
- Lifetime risk for females 3% to 5%

PEAK INCIDENCE: 20 to 40 yr. The most common age range for initial treatment of alcohol dependence is 35 to 45 yr. However, the peak period for meeting alcohol dependence criteria is ≥10 years earlier.

GENETICS: More common with a family history of alcoholism and in patients of Irish, Scandinavian, and Native American descent

PHYSICAL FINDINGS & CLINICAL PRESENTATION

- Recurring minor trauma
- Gastrointestinal bleeding from gastritis and/or varices
- Pancreatitis (acute and chronic)
- Liver disease
- Odor of alcohol on breath
- Tremulousness
- Tachycardia
- Peripheral neuropathy
- Recent memory loss

ETIOLOGY

- Social and genetic factors important
- Risk factors:
    1. Broken homes
    2. Unemployment
    3. Divorce
    4. Recurrent depression
    5. Addiction to another substance, including tobacco

DIAGNOSIS

WORKUP

- Several screening tests (CAGE, AUDIT, TWEAK, CRAFFT, SMAST) are available. The four-item CAGE (feeling need to Cut down, Annoyed by criticism, Guilty about drinking, and need for an Eye-opener in the morning) is the most popular screening test in primary care. A positive response should lead to further questioning. The sensitivity of the CAGE ranges from 43% to 94% and its specificity ranges from 70% to 97%. The five-item TWEAK scale (Tolerance, Worry, Eye-openers, Amnesia, [K] cut down) and the T-ACE questionnaire (Tolerance, Annoyance, Cut down, Eye-opener) are designed to screen pregnant women for alcohol misuse. They detect lower levels of alcohol consumption that may pose risks during pregnancy. The CRAFFT questionnaire (riding in Car with someone who was drinking, using alcohol to Relax, using alcohol while Alone, Forgetfulness, criticism from Friends and Family, Trouble) is useful as a screening tool for adolescents. Its sensitivity is 92% and specificity 64% for alcohol abuse. Single-question screening about alcohol consumption in a day ("When was the last time you had more than X drinks in a day?" [where X = 5 for men and 4 for women]) with the threshold set at "in the past 3 months" is 85% sensitive and 70% specific in men and 82% and 70% in women for unhealthy alcohol use.
- Blood studies (see later section).

LABORATORY TESTS

- Lab tests alone do not accurately detect alcohol problems but can help identify medical complications related to alcohol use, such as pancreatitis or cirrhosis.
- Gamma-glutamyltransferase (GGTP), generally elevated
- Liver transaminases (alanine aminotransferase [ALT], aspartate aminotransferase [AST]), often elevated, may be normal or low in advanced liver disease
- Low albumin level, hypophosphatemia, hypomagnesemia from malnutrition
- Complete blood count (CBC) reveals elevated mean corpuscular volume from toxic effect of alcohol on erythrocyte development in nutritional deficiencies
- Stool for occult blood may be positive as a result of gastritis or variceal bleeding

IMAGING STUDIES

Indicated only with a history of trauma. CT or ultrasound of abdomen may reveal fatty liver or cirrhosis in advanced stages.

TREATMENT

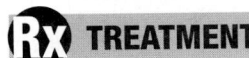

NONPHARMACOLOGIC THERAPY

- Twelve-step facilitation, cognitive behavioral therapy, and motivational enhancement therapy improve the chances of recovery in patients with alcohol abuse and dependence.
- Depression, if present, should be treated at same time alcohol is withdrawn.

ACUTE GENERAL Rx

Alcohol withdrawal syndrome (AWS) occurs when a person stops ingesting alcohol after prolonged consumption. It can result in four possible clinical patterns depending on the severity of the patient's alcohol abuse and the time from the patient's previous alcohol ingestion. Blood ethanol level decreases by ~20 mg/dl/hr (Fig. 1-15) in a normal person. Although discussed separately, these withdrawal states blend together in real life.

1. **Tremulous state** (early alcohol withdrawal, "impending DTs," "shakes," "jitters").
    a. Time interval: usually occurs 6 to 8 hr after the last drink or 12 to 48 hr after reduction of alcohol intake; becomes most pronounced at 24 to 36 hr.
    b. Manifestation: tremors, mild agitation, insomnia, tachycardia; symptoms are relieved by alcohol.
    c. Detoxification can be in the outpatient (ambulatory) or inpatient setting. Candidates for outpatient detoxification should have a reasonable support system (e.g., reliable contact person) who can monitor progress and lack of any significant comorbid conditions (e.g., suicide risk, seizure disorder, coexisting benzodiazepine dependence, prior unsuccessful outpatient detoxification, pregnancy, cirrhosis) or risk factors for severe withdrawal (age >40 yr, drinking >100 g of ethanol daily [e.g., 1 pint of liquor or eight 12-oz cans

of beer, random blood alcohol concentration >200 mg/dl]).
d. Inpatient treatment:
(1) Admit to medical floor (private room); monitor vital signs q4h; institute seizure precautions; maintain adequate sedation.
(2) Administer lorazepam as follows:
(a) Day 1: 2 mg PO q4h while awake and not lethargic.
(b) Day 2: 1 mg PO q4h while awake and not lethargic.
(c) Day 3: 0.5 mg PO q4h while awake and not lethargic.
(d) NOTE: Hold sedation for lethargy or abnormal vital or neurologic signs. The preceding doses are only guidelines; it is best to titrate the dose case by case.
(3) In patients with mild to moderate withdrawal and without history of seizures, individualized benzodiazepine administration (rather than a fixed-dose regimen) results in lower benzodiazepine administration and avoids unnecessary sedation. The Clinical Institute Withdrawal Assessment Scale for Alcohol, Revised (CIWA-Ar) scale can be used to measure the severity of alcohol withdrawal. It consists of 10 items: nausea; tremor; autonomic hyperactivity; anxiety; agitation; tactile, visual, and auditory disturbances; headache; and disorientation. Each item is assigned a score from 0 to 7. For example, in the "agitation" category 0 indicates normal activity, and 7 indicates that the patient constantly thrashes about. For the category of "tremor," 0 indicates that tremor is not present and 7 tremor is severe, even with arms not extended. The maximum total score is 67. Patients with mild AWS symptoms (CIWA-Ar score < 8 to 10 can be monitored on an outpatient basis. Benzodiazepines are recommended in patients with substantial withdrawal symptoms (CIWA-Ar score >12). Patients with

CIWA-Ar score of ≥15 should be admitted to detox unit. In-patient treatment is also recommended for patients with history of withdrawal seizures and for those with suicidal ideation and significant comorbidities.
(4) Beta-adrenergic blockers: beta-blockers are useful for controlling blood pressure and tachyarrhythmias. However, they do not prevent progression to more serious symptoms of withdrawal and, if used, should not be administered alone but in conjunction with benzodiazepines. Beta-blockers should be avoided in patients with contraindications to their use (e.g., bronchospasm, bradycardia, or severe congestive heart failure). Centrally acting alpha-adrenergic agonists such as clonidine ameliorate symptoms in patients with mild to moderate withdrawal but do not reduce delirium or seizures.
(5) Vitamin replacement: thiamine 100 mg IV or IM for at least 5 days plus oral multivitamins. The IV administration of glucose can precipitate Wernicke's encephalopathy in alcoholics with thiamine deficiency; therefore thiamine administration should precede IV dextrose.
(6) Hydration PO or IV (high-caloric solution): if IV, glucose with Na^+, K^+, Mg^{2+}, and phosphate replacement prn.
(7) Laboratory studies.
(a) CBC, platelet count, INR.
(b) Electrolytes, glucose, blood urea nitrogen, creatinine.
(c) GGTP, ALT, AST.
(d) Phosphorus and magnesium.
(e) Serum vitamin B12 and folic acid (if megaloblastic features in blood smear).
(8) Diagnostic imaging: generally not necessary; if subdural hematoma is suspected (evidence of trauma, persistent lethargy), a CT scan should be ordered.

(9) Social rehabilitation: group therapy such as Alcoholics Anonymous; identification and treatment of social and family problems should be initiated during the patient's hospital stay.
2. Alcoholic hallucinosis:
a. Manifestations: hallucinations usually are auditory, but hallucinations occasionally are visual, tactile, or olfactory; usually there is no clouding of sensorium as in delirium (clinical presentation may be mistaken for an acute schizophrenic episode). Disordered perceptions become most pronounced after 24 to 36 hr of abstinence.
b. Treatment: same as for DTs (see "withdrawal seizures").
3. Withdrawal seizures ("rum fits"):
a. Time interval: usually occurs 7 to 30 hr after cessation of drinking, with a peak incidence between 13 and 24 hr.
b. Manifestations: generalized convulsions with loss of consciousness; focal signs are usually absent; consider further investigation with CT scan of head and electroencephalography if clearly indicated (e.g., presence of focal neurologic deficits, prolonged postictal confusion state). In addition, in a febrile patient who is having a seizure or altered mental state, a lumbar puncture is necessary.
c. Treatment:
(1) Diazepam 2.5 mg/min IV until seizure is controlled (check for respiratory depression or hypotension) may be beneficial for prolonged seizure activity; IV lorazepam 1 to 2 mg q2h can be used in place of diazepam. Withdrawal seizures generally are self-limited and treatment is not required; the use of phenytoin or other anticonvulsants for short-term treatment of alcohol withdrawal seizures is not recommended.
(2) Thiamine 100 mg IV, followed by IV dextrose, should also be administered.
(3) Electrolyte imbalances (increased Mg^{2+}, decreased K^+, increased or decreased Na^+, decreased PO_4^{3-}) that may exacerbate seizures should be corrected.
4. DTs:
a. Time interval: variable; usually occurs within 1 wk after reduction or cessation of heavy alcohol intake and persists for 1 to 3 days. Peak incidence is 72 hr and 96 hr after the cessation of alcohol consumption.
b. Manifestations: profound confusion, tremors, vivid visual and tactile hallucinations, autonomic hyperactivity; this is the most serious clinical presentation of alcohol withdrawal (mortality rate is approximately 15% in untreated patients).
c. Treatment
(1) Admission to a detoxification unit where patient can be observed closely.

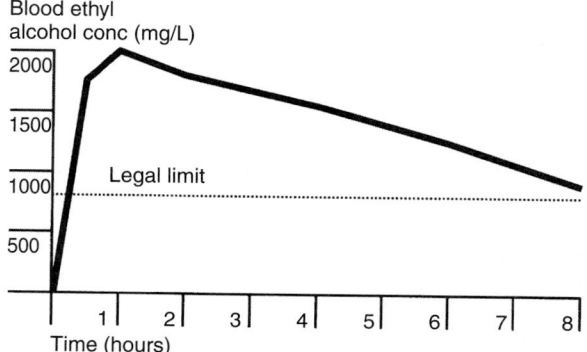

FIGURE 1-15 Blood concentrations after oral administration of ethyl alcohol (2 ml/kg) The concentration declines in a zero-order fashion at an average rate of 190 mg/L each hour. (From Souhami RL, Moxham J: *Textbook of medicine*, ed 4, London, Churchill Livingstone, 2002, Figure 1-12.)

(2) Vital signs q30min (neurologic signs, if necessary).

(3) Use of lateral decubitus or prone position if restraints are necessary

(4) NPO: nasogastric tube for abdominal distention may be necessary but should not be routinely used.

(5) Laboratory studies: same as for early alcohol withdrawal.

(6) Vigorous hydration (4 to 6 L/day): IV with glucose (Na^+, K^+, PO_4^{3-} and Mg^{2+} replacement).

(7) Vitamins: thiamine 100 mg IV qd. The initial dose of thiamine should precede the administration of IV dextrose; multivitamins (may be added to the hydrating solution).

(8) Sedation: control of agitation should be achieved with rapid-acting sedative-hypnotic agents in adequate doses to maintain light somnolence for the duration of delirium.

  (a) Initially: lorazepam 2 to 5 mg IM/IV repeated prn.

  (b) Maintenance (individualized dosage): chlordiazepoxide, 50 to 100 mg PO q4-6h, lorazepam 2 mg PO q4h, or diazepam 5 to 10 mg PO tid; withhold doses or decrease subsequent doses if signs of oversedation are apparent.

  (c) Midazolam is also effective for managing DTs. Its rapid onset (sedation within 2 to 4 min of IV injection) and short duration of action (approximately 30 min) make it an ideal agent for titration in continuous infusion.

(9) Treatment of seizures (as previously described).

(10) Diagnosis and treatment of concomitant medical, surgical, or psychiatric conditions.

CHRONIC Rx

- See "Referral."
- Pharmacotherapies for alcoholism include:
  - ○ Acamprosate is a synthetic compound with a chemical structure similar to the neurotransmitter gamma-aminobutyric acid and the amino acid neuromodulator taurine. Its mechanism of action is not completely understood. It is indicated for the maintenance of abstinence from alcohol in patients with alcohol dependence who are abstinent at treatment initiation. It should be used only as part of a comprehensive psychosocial treatment program. It does not cause a disulfiram-like reaction as a result of ethanol ingestion. Dose is two 333-mg tablets tid. Treatment should be initiated as soon as possible after the period of alcohol withdrawal, when the patient has achieved abstinence, and should be maintained if the patient relapses.
  - ○ The long-acting opiate antagonist naltrexone inhibits the rewarding effects of alcohol. The starting dose is 25 mg/day, increased to 50 mg PO qd after 1 wk. An extended-release, once-monthly injection of naltrexone is also available and can be used along with psychosocial support to maintain alcohol abstinence. In patients with opioid dependence, naltrexone can precipitate acute withdrawal syndrome and should not be used at least 7 days from last opioid use.
  - ○ Disulfiram (Antabuse). Dosage is 500 mg max qd for 1 to 2 wk, then 125 to 500 mg qd. It interferes with the metabolism of alcohol by inhibiting aldehyde dehydrogenase, causing an accumulation of acetaldehyde. It produces unpleasant symptoms (nausea, flushing, elevated blood pressure, headache, weakness) when alcohol is ingested. It is an older drug that is now rarely used.

DISPOSITION

See "Referral."

REFERRAL

- To Alcoholics Anonymous or Adult Children of Alcoholics
- Family members to Al-Anon or Al-A-Teen
- Many cities have Salvation Army Adult Rehabilitation centers; all patients accepted, regardless of ability to pay

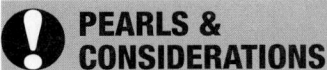

COMMENTS

- Relative indications for inpatient alcohol detoxification are as follows: history of DTs or withdrawal seizures, severe withdrawal symptoms, concomitant psychiatric or medical illness, pregnancy, multiple previous detoxifications, recent high levels of alcohol consumption, and lack of reliable support network.
- Detoxification is not a stand-alone treatment but should serve as a bridge to a formal treatment program for alcohol dependence.
- The cure rate for alcoholism is highly disappointing, regardless of the modality. Only those who want to be helped will be helped. An effective strategy for the primary care physician is a prominently displayed sign in the office that states, "If you think you consume too many alcoholic beverages, please discuss it with me." Those who do open up the discussion can be given the facts in a nonjudgmental way and often can be helped. All too often problem drinkers lie on the questionnaire until they face a life-threatening health issue—and even then denial often reigns supreme.
- In a recent clinical trial, patients receiving medical management with naltrexone (100 mg/day), combined behavioral intervention (CBI), or both fared better on drinking outcomes, whereas acamprosate showed no evidence of efficacy, with or without CBI. No combination produced better efficacy than naltrexone or CBI alone in the presence of medical management.

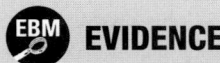 **EVIDENCE**

available at www.expertconsult.com

SUGGESTED READINGS
available at www.expertconsult.com

AUTHOR: **FRED F. FERRI, M.D.**

BASIC INFORMATION

DEFINITION

Alopecia is the term used to describe involuntary hair loss, typically on the scalp or beard, but possibly over the entire body. *Nonscarring alopecia* is hair loss without clinically apparent scarring, inflammation, or skin atrophy. *Scarring alopecia* is characterized by hair loss accompanied by tissue destruction in the form of scarring, inflammation, and/or skin atrophy.

SYNONYMS

Hair loss
Balding

ICD-9CM CODES	
704.0	Alopecia
704.01	Alopecia Areata
704.02	Telogen Effluvium

EPIDEMIOLOGY & DEMOGRAPHICS

INCIDENCE: Depends on etiology, for example:
- Alopecia areata affects 1% of the U.S. population by age 50 yr.
- Androgenetic alopecia affects females << males but affects up to 40% of females by age 60, increasing after menopause.

GENETICS: Depends on etiology, for example:
- Androgenetic alopecia is autosomal dominant ± polygenic and can be inherited from one or both parents
- Certain scarring alopecias are more predominant in people with coarser hair.

ETIOLOGY
NONSCARRING
- Failure of follicle production
- Hair shaft abnormality
- Pattern hair loss, i.e., androgenetic alopecia
- Hair breakage, i.e., trichotillomania, traction alopecia, cosmetic overprocessing
- Problem with cycling (excess shedding), i.e., telogen effluvium, anagen effluvium, loose anagen syndrome, alopecia areata, syphilis

SCARRING
- Infectious: tinea capitis with inflammation (kerion), bacterial folliculitis as in dissecting folliculitis and folliculitis decalvans
- Neoplasm: alopecia mucinosa in cutaneous T cell lymphoma or alopecia neoplastica due to metastatic carcinoma (breast cancer)
- Autoimmune: chronic cutaneous lupus erythematosus
- Congenital

CLINICAL FEATURES

HISTORY: A careful history must be taken and should include time course for hair loss, the pattern of hair loss, any recent change in life situation/stresses, any associated medical conditions, new medications, any family history of hair loss, and other skin/nail symptoms.

PHYSICAL EXAMINATION:
- General: patient's emotional response to hair loss
- Hair/skin:
  - Hair thinning/loss
  - May have fine downy hairs also referred to as vellous hairs
  - Skin may show changes consistent with inflammation, infection, and/or atrophy
  - Women may show virilization
  - Exclamation point hairs can be seen in alopecia areata (Fig. 1-16)
  - Broken hairs of different length may be seen in traumatic alopecia
  - Hairs that crack or crumble with palpation most often signify shaft damage due to overprocessing

DIAGNOSIS

WORKUP

- Hair pull—no shower for 24 hr, scalp with ~60 hairs is gently pulled, <6 hairs pulled is normal and more is suggestive of telogen effluvium, look for telogen bulbs on recovered hairs
- Punch biopsy—send two punches: one for vertical and one for horizontal sectioning for histopathologic analysis preferably by a dermatopathologist

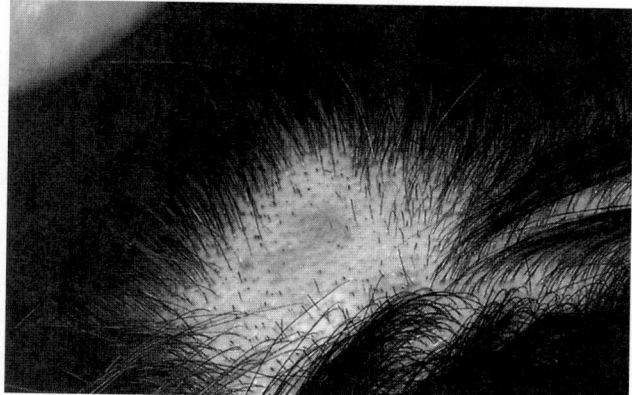

FIGURE 1-16 Alopecia areata. A distinctive feature of alopecia areata is the presence of shortened "exclamation mark" hairs, which taper markedly where they emerge from the scalp. (From Souhami RL, Moxham J: *Textbook of medicine,* ed 4, London, 2002, Churchill Livingstone.)

LABORATORY TESTS

Initiate laboratory studies if not clear based on clinical presentation:
- CBC—rule out Fe deficiency
- Total Fe/ferritin—rule out subclinical Fe deficiency
- TSH—rule out underlying thyroid disease
- ANA—screen for autoimmune disease
- RPR—rule out cutaneous syphilis if history suggestive of increased risk

DIFFERENTIAL DIAGNOSIS
NONSCARRING

- *Telogen effluvium:* This type of alopecia is usually diffuse thinning that follows significant life stress (death of loved one, high fever, severe infection, crash dieting) or change in hormones (postpartum, change in or cessation of oral contraceptives). Patient often presents with a bag of hair that has fallen out. This is caused by a large number of anagen (growing) hairs entering telogen (dying phase) simultaneously. Telogen effluvium is more common in women.
- *Androgenetic alopecia:* Gradual thinning of hair and a trend toward finer hair, which in men has a typical pattern of receding anterior bitemporal hairline resulting in an M-shaped pattern and in women has a typical pattern of thinning along crown with or without frontotemporal thinning. This type of thinning is due to a combination of genetic predisposition and androgenic conversion of hair follicles into vellus-like follicles.
- *Alopecia areata:* Patches of hair loss, typically 2-5 cm in diameter, with normal-appearing skin (including presence of follicular openings) at the base as well as occasional "exclamation point hairs," which are evidence of hair breaking off. Fingernails may show fine pitting. On biopsy, lymphocytes surround the hair bulb "like a swarm of bees," evidence of the autoimmune etiology.
  - AA Universalis (AAU)—generalized loss of body hair
  - AA Totalis (AAT)—complete loss of scalp hair
- *Tinea:* This type of hair loss is evident in round patches, possibly with scarring, erythema and lymphadenopathy. This is the more common type of hair loss in children. Diagnosis can be made by scraping the erythematous edge and placing the scraping with KOH under a microscope to check for hyphae. Woods lamp only fluoresces if tinea is caused by *Microsporum* spp.; however, the more common (in the U.S.) *Trichophyton* spp. does not fluoresce. If a kerion (severe alopecia associated with bogginess) is present. it may cause scarring.
- *Traumatic alopecia:* This type of hair loss is in a pattern consistent with breaking off of hairs due to traction (hair pulling) or chemical agents (hair straightening or permanent). Etiology usually becomes apparent with careful history taking and visualizing the pattern of hair loss.

SCARRING

- *Lichen planus:* The hair loss associated with LP is typically associated with scaling and atrophy of pruritic, painful skin underlying the hair loss. This hair loss is more common in middle aged women. While there are numerous variations in clinical presentation, the general clinical picture is one of a chronic inflammatory condition of the skin, nails, mucous membranes and/or hair. The typical skin lesions are flat topped, violaceous lesions with white lines (Wickham's striae), while the typical oral lesions are milky white.
- *Chronic cutaneous (discoid) lupus erthematosus:* This type of hair loss frequently is evident in well-demarcated, erythematous plaques in chronically sun-exposed areas of skin. Lesions exhibit hypopigmentations or hyperpigmentations, atrophy, erythema, and scaling. It may be present concurrently with SLE or be the first presenting symptom of SLE, but in most cases it is a purely cutaneous condition.
- *Tinea with kerion:* A kerion represents an exuberant delayed type hypersensitivity reaction to the tinea capitis, resulting in one (or many) inflamed boggy plaque(s) on the scalp depending on the severity of the infection.

Rx TREATMENT

- *Telogen effluvium:* Stop insulting stress/medication and in 3-4 mo anagen recurs; hair density should be normalized by 12 mo. Multiple medications have been shown to be an inciting factor and one should consider stopping them (these include but are not limited to enalapril, colchicine, levodopa, metoprolol, propranolol, oral contraceptives, and lithium). Full regrowth is expected in most cases.
- *Androgenetic alopecia:* For men, the most likely first line treatment is oral finesteride (type II 5a-reductase inhibitor) which leads to lower levels of dihydrotestosterone. This leads to hair regrowth in about 6 mo, but with cessation, hair returns to pattern of loss within 12 mo. Topical minoxidil can be useful in partially restoring lost hair in both men and women. In woman with elevated androgens, antiandrogens such as spironolactone, flutamide, and cimetidine may be considered. Other options include surgical intervention with hair transplantation or hair flaps or the use of a hairpiece.
- *Alopecia areata:* Spontaneous remission occurs in patchy AA, but less commonly in AAT or AAU. Glucocorticoids (GCs) are the mainstay of treatment but have little effect on the long-term outcome of hair loss—topical GC for small patches, intralesional injection of high-potency GC, and even systemic steroids can all be temporarily effective but at the cost of glucocorticoid exposure. Induction of allergic contact dermatitis using short contact anthralin therapy or squaric acid sensitization can be effective but tends to have significant local discomfort, limiting its use. Topical photochemotherapy has shown some beneficial outcomes with alopecia areata. Photochemotherapy to the entire body is effective ~30% of the time.
- *Tinea capitis:* To effectively treat tinea capitis, oral antifungal agents must be used. Griseofulvin is considered the drug of choice in the U.S., and the recommended time course is 6 wk to several months. Other oral agents to consider include terbinafine, itraconazole, fluconazole, or ketaconazole. If there is a kerion (area of boggy, purulent inflammation underlying the area of hair loss), the patient is at increased risk for scarring alopecia due to likely bacterial superinfection and a short course of oral steroids and treatment with an oral antibiotic must be considered.
- *Traumatic alopecia:* First priority is stopping inciting activity/agent, which ideally will lead to gradual resolution of hair loss and hair regrowth.
- *Lichen planus:* Associated hair loss is often permanent, however, for symptomatic control of itching and pain; topical or oral glucocorticoids may be considered.
- *Chronic cutaneous discoid erythematosus:* The best prevention is sun protection, with SPF lotion. Treatment options center around the cautious use of topical or intralesional glucocorticoids. Hydroxychloroquinone and retinoids are also used with caution.

REFERRAL

Dermatology

PATIENT/FAMILY EDUCATION

Alopecia areata: www.naaf.org

SUGGESTED READING

available at www.expertconsult.com

AUTHORS: **MARGARET LEKANDER, M.D.,**
AMITY RUBEOR, D.O., and **GLADYS TELANG, M.D.**

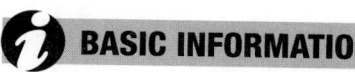

BASIC INFORMATION

DEFINITION

Alpha-1-antitrypsin deficiency is a genetic deficiency of the protease inhibitor alpha-1-antitrypsin that results in a predisposition to pulmonary emphysema and hepatic cirrhosis.

SYNONYMS

AAT

ICD-9CM CODES

277.6 Alpha-1-antitrypsin deficiency

EPIDEMIOLOGY & DEMOGRAPHICS

- Accounts for approximately 2% of chronic obstructive pulmonary disease (COPD) cases in Americans
- Inherited as an autosomal codominant disorder
- Most frequent mutation is in the *SERPINA 1* gene (previously known as *PI* gene)
- Most common alleles are:
  - normal "M" allele (95% frequency in the U.S.)
  - deficient variant "Z" allele (1% to 2%)
  - deficient variant "S" allele (2% to 3%)
- Severe deficiency is most commonly due to homozygotes ZZ
- Risk of COPD is increased with SZ genotype, especially in those who smoke
- Risk of lung disease in heterozygotes (MZ) is uncertain
- One in 10 individuals of European descent carries one of two mutations that may result in partial alpha-1-antitrypsin deficiency

PHYSICAL FINDINGS & CLINICAL PRESENTATION

- Physical findings and clinical presentation are varied and depend on phenotype (see "Etiology")
- Most often affects the lungs but can also involve liver and skin
- Classically associated with early-onset, severe, lower-lobe predominant panacinar emphysema; bronchiectasis may also be seen
- Symptoms are similar to "typical" COPD presentation (dyspnea, cough, sputum production)
- Liver involvement includes neonatal cholestasis, cirrhosis in children and adults, and primary carcinoma of the liver
- Panniculitis is the major dermatologic manifestation

ETIOLOGY

- Degree of alpha-1-antitrypsin deficiency depends on phenotype.
- "MM" represents the normal genotype and is associated with alpha-1-antitrypsin levels in the normal range.
- Mutation most commonly associated with emphysema is Z, with homozygote (ZZ) resulting in approximately 85% deficit in plasma alpha-1-antitrypsin concentrations.
- Development of emphysema is believed to result from an imbalance between the proteolytic enzyme elastase, produced by neutrophils, and alpha-1-antitrypsin, which normally protects lung elastin by inhibiting elastase.
- Deficiency of alpha-1-antitrypsin increases risk of early-onset emphysema, but not all alpha-1-antitrypsin deficient individuals will develop lung disease.
- Smoking increases risk and accelerates onset of COPD.
- Liver disease is caused by pathologic accumulation of alpha-1-antitrypsin in hepatocytes.
- Similar to lung disease, skin involvement is thought to be attributable to unopposed proteolysis in skin.

DIAGNOSIS

DIFFERENTIAL DIAGNOSIS

See "COPD."
See "Cirrhosis."

WORKUP

- Suspicion for alpha-1-antitrypsin deficiency usually results from emphysema developing at an early age and with basilar predominance of disease.
- Suspicion for alpha-1-antitrypsin deficiency resulting in liver disease or skin involvement may arise when other more common etiologies are excluded.

LABORATORY TESTS

- Serum level of alpha-1-antitrypsin can confirm or reject suspicion of deficiency.
- Investigate possibility of abnormal alleles with genotyping.
- Pulmonary function testing is generally consistent with "typical" COPD.

IMAGING STUDIES

- Chest x-ray shows characteristic emphysematous changes at lung bases.
- High-resolution chest CT usually confirms the lower-lobe predominant emphysema and may also show significant bronchiectasis.

TREATMENT

NONPHARMACOLOGIC THERAPY

- Avoidance of smoking is paramount.
- Avoidance of other environmental and occupational exposures that may increase risk of COPD.

ACUTE GENERAL Rx

Acute exacerbations of COPD from alpha-1-antitrypsin deficiency are treated in a similar fashion to "typical" COPD exacerbations.

CHRONIC Rx

- The goal of treatment in alpha-1-antitrypsin deficiency is to increase serum alpha-1-antitrypsin levels above a minimum, "protective" threshold.
- Although several therapeutic options are under investigation, IV administration of pooled human alpha-1-antitrypsin is currently the only approved method to raise serum alpha-1-antitrypsin levels. AAT augmentation therapy has been approved by the FDA for patients with AAT deficiency (defined as a protein level <11 μmol/L) who have COPD. Augmentation therapy is expensive ($60,000 to $150,000/year) and requires lifelong treatment. However, given the cost and a lack of evidence of clinical benefit, a 2010 Cochrane Collaboration review noted that augmentation therapy with alpha-1-antitrypsin cannot be recommended.
- Organ transplantation for patients with end-stage lung or liver disease is also an option.

DISPOSITION

- Prognosis of patients with alpha-1-antitrypsin deficiency will depend on phenotype and level of deficiency.
- Among patients with severe alpha-1-antitrypsin deficiency, the most common underlying causes of death are emphysema (72%) and cirrhosis (10%).

REFERRAL

- Referral to specialists with experience in AAT deficiency is preferred
- Pulmonary and hepatology referrals for advanced lung and liver disease, or if replacement therapy is contemplated (e.g., moderate-severe lung disease)
- Lung and liver transplantation in suitable cases

PEARLS & CONSIDERATIONS

- The liver damage arising from the mutation is not from a deficiency in alpha-1-antitrypsin but from a pathologic accumulation of alpha-1-antitrypsin in hepatocytes.
- Consider alpha-1-antitrypsin deficiency in patients presenting with lower-lobe predominant emphysema; in most smokers without alpha-1-antitrypsin deficiency, emphysema predominates in the upper lobes.
- Alpha-1-antitrypsin deficiency is believed to be under-recognized.
- The American Thoracic Society and the European Respiratory Society recommend testing for AAT deficiency in all patients with COPD, emphysema, or asthma with irreversible obstruction, whereas the Global Initiative for Chronic Obstructive Lung Disease only recommends testing for those with early-onset COPD (age <45 yr) or a strong family history of COPD.

EBM EVIDENCE

available at www.expertconsult.com

SUGGESTED READINGS

available at www.expertconsult.com

AUTHOR: **JOSEPH A. DIAZ, M.D.**

BASIC INFORMATION

DEFINITION

Altitude sickness refers to a spectrum of illnesses related to hypoxemia occurring during rapid ascension to high altitudes. Common acute syndromes occurring at high altitudes include acute mountain sickness (AMS), high-altitude pulmonary edema (HAPE), and high-altitude cerebral edema (HACE).

SYNONYMS

Acute mountain sickness
High-altitude pulmonary edema
High-altitude cerebral edema

ICD-9CM CODES
289 Mountain sickness, acute
993.2 High altitude, effects

EPIDEMIOLOGY & DEMOGRAPHICS

- More than 30 million people are at risk of developing altitude sickness.
- AMS is the most common of the altitude diseases.
  - Approximately 40% to 50% of people ascending to 14,000 ft (4200 m) from lowland living develop AMS.
- HAPE generally arises in people who rapidly ascend to 12,000 to 13,000 ft (3600 to 3900 m); however, it has been reported at altitudes as low as 8000 ft.
- Men are five times more likely to develop HAPE than are women.
- AMS and HACE affect men and women equally.

PHYSICAL FINDINGS & CLINICAL PRESENTATION

AMS
- Occurs within hours to a few days after rapid ascent over 8000 ft (2500 m)
- Headache is the most common symptom
- Dizziness and lightheadedness
- Nausea, vomiting, and loss of appetite
- Fatigue
- Sleep disturbance from an exaggerated hyperventilatory phase of Cheyne-Stokes respiration in response to hypoxemia and alkalosis
- AMS can evolve into HAPE and HACE

HAPE (Fig. 1-17)
- Typically occurs 2 to 4 days after ascent over 8000 ft (2500 m).
- Dyspnea
- Dry cough or cough with frothy rust- or pink-tinged sputum
- Chest tightness
- Tachycardia, tachypnea, rales, cyanosis

HACE
- Usually presents several days after AMS
- Confusion, irritability, drowsiness, stupor, hallucinations
- Headache, nausea, vomiting
- Ataxia, paralysis, and seizures
- Coma and death may develop within hours of the first symptoms

ETIOLOGY

- During ascension to altitudes above sea level, the atmospheric pressure decreases. Although the percentage of oxygen in the air remains the same, the partial pressure of oxygen decreases with increased altitude. This can cause hypoxemia. Figure 1-18 illustrates the effect of altitude on alveolar PaO_2 and oxygen saturation.
- The body responds to low oxygen partial pressures through a process of acclimatization (see "Comments").

DX DIAGNOSIS

Made by clinical presentation and physical findings.

DIFFERENTIAL DIAGNOSIS

- Dehydration
- Carbon monoxide poisoning
- Hypothermia
- Infection
- Substance abuse
- Congestive heart failure
- Pulmonary embolism
- Cerebrovascular accident

WORKUP

Typically the diagnosis is self-evident after history and physical examination. Laboratory tests and imaging studies help monitor cardiopulmonary and central nervous system status in patients admitted to the intensive care unit for pulmonary and/or cerebral edema. In patients with HAPE occurring at lower altitudes (<8000 ft), an evaluation of preexisting pulmonary hypertension or a left-to-right shunt should be considered.

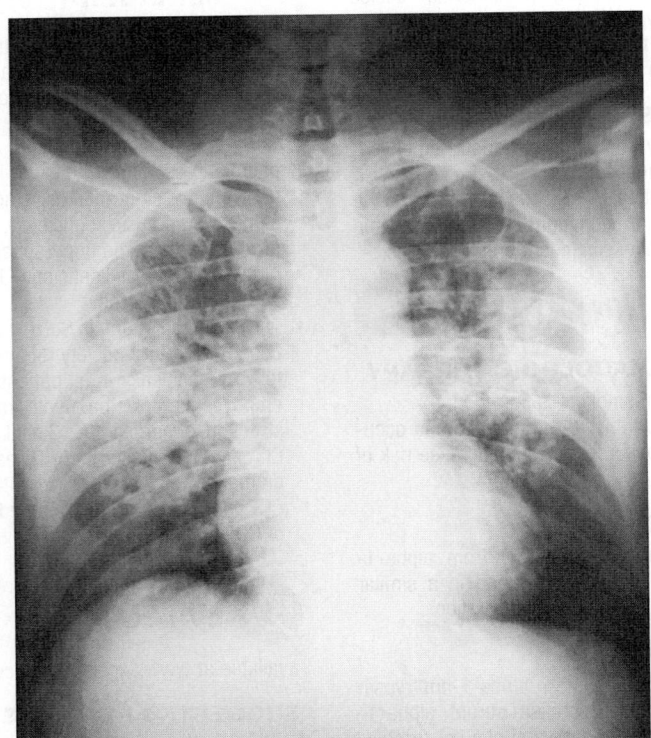

FIGURE 1-17 Chest radiograph showing high-altitude pulmonary edema. (From Strauss RH [ed]: *Sports medicine,* ed 2, Philadelphia, 1991, WB Saunders.)

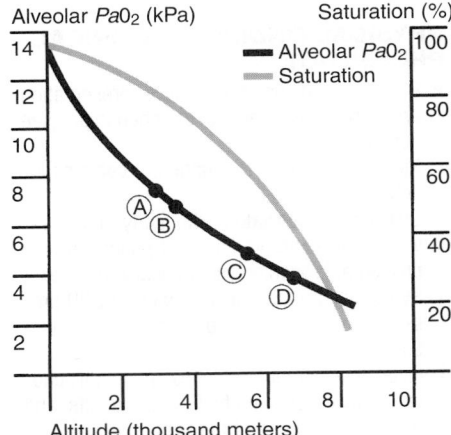

FIGURE 1-18 Effect of altitude on alveolar PaO_2 and oxygen saturation. Because of the steep slope of the oxygen dissociation curve, increasing altitude above 5000 m causes a precipitous fall in saturation. In an unacclimated person, acute change occurs at, **A,** 3000 m (10,000 ft)—slightly impaired memory and judgment, increased heart rate, abdominal cramps and nausea; **B,** 3500 m (12,000 ft)—headache, nausea, diminished visual acuity, and possible pulmonary edema; **C,** 5500 m (18,000 ft)—impaired consciousness after several hours in many people; and **D,** 6750 m (22,000 ft)—loss of consciousness. (From Souhami RL, Moxham J: *Textbook of medicine,* ed 4, London, 2002, Churchill Livingstone.)

LABORATORY TESTS

Not useful

IMAGING STUDIES

- Chest x-ray examination showing Kerley B-lines and patchy edema (see Fig. 1-17)
- CT scan of the head showing diffuse or patchy edema

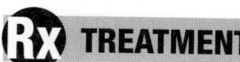 **TREATMENT**

NONPHARMACOLOGIC THERAPY

- Stop the ascent to allow acclimatization or start to descend until symptoms have resolved.
- Oxygen 4 to 6 L/min is used for severe AMS, HAPE, and HACE.
- Portable hyperbaric bags are useful if available at the site.
- Altitude can cause diuresis that may be mediated by enhanced release of atrial natriuretic peptide. When coupled with the increased fluid loss through increased ventilation, there is a higher risk for dehydration, and adequate hydration should be maintained.

ACUTE PHARMACOLOGIC Rx

- Nonsteroidal anti-inflammatory drugs or aspirin is effective in treating headaches in AMS.
- Acetazolamide 125 to 250 mg PO bid has been effective for both prevention and acute therapy in patients with AMS and HAPE.
- Nifedipine 10 mg sublingual followed by long-acting nifedipine 30 mg bid is used for patients with HAPE who cannot descend immediately.
- Dexamethasone 4 mg PO every 6 hr is used in patients with severe AMS, HAPE, or HACE.

CHRONIC Rx

Prevention is the most prudent therapy.
1. Slow, staged ascent to avoid altitude sickness.
2. Start the ascent below 8000 feet.
3. Ascend 1000 feet/day (300 m/day).
4. Spend two nights at the same altitude every 3 days.
5. Sleep at lower heights than the altitude climbed ("climb high, sleep low").

6. Prophylactic therapy with acetazolamide up to 750 mg daily and/or dexamethasone 8 to 16 mg daily decreases the risk of developing AMS (combination may have additive benefit). The drugs should be used until acclimatization occurs.
7. Prophylactic inhalation of a β-adrenergic agonist, salmeterol 125 mcg q12h, or the use of slow-release nifedipine 20 mg bid have both been shown to reduce the risk of HAPE in susceptible individuals.
8. Tadalafil, a long-acting phosphodiesterase inhibitor, has recently been shown to decrease the incidence of HAPE in susceptible individuals.
9. The over-the-counter herbal supplement Ginkgo biloba has gained interest in AMS prophylaxis, primarily because of its low adverse effect profile. However, recent randomized clinical trials have failed to show benefit compared with placebo.

DISPOSITION

- AMS improves over a period of 2 to 3 days.
- HAPE is the most common cause of death among patients with altitude illnesses.
- More than 60% of patients with HAPE will have recurrence of symptoms on subsequent climbs.
- Neurologic deficits may persist for weeks but eventually resolve. If coma occurs, prognosis is poor.

REFERRAL

Cardiology and neurology referrals are made in patients with pulmonary edema and central nervous system findings, respectively.

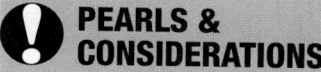 **PEARLS & CONSIDERATIONS**

COMMENTS

- Acclimatization is the process in which an individual who normally resides at low altitude adapts to hypobaric hypoxia to improve tolerance and performance at higher altitude. These mechanisms include:
  1. An increase in respiratory rates and tidal volume. This hyperventilation allows lowering of arterial carbon dioxide to preserve oxygen delivery, even at extreme altitudes.

2. An early increase in heart rate and stroke volume to improve oxygen delivery. After 1 wk, both parameters decrease because of diuresis and lower catecholamine levels.
  3. Pulmonary hypertension develops in response to hypoxemia, resulting in improvement of the ventilation-perfusion mismatch but may be maladaptive and lead to the development of HAPE.
  4. Cerebral vasodilation to increase blood flow to the brain.
  5. Rise in hemoglobin and hematocrit. This is a long-term process that takes up to 1 wk to occur in response to the need for improved oxygen delivery.
- Adaptation to altitude is different from acclimatization and refers to physiologic differences in permanent residents at high altitude (e.g., an increased oxygen diffusion capacity).
- Risk factors for the development of altitude sicknesses are:
  1. Rapid ascent
  2. Previous history of altitude sickness
  3. Strenuous exertion on arrival
  4. Obesity
  5. Male gender
- Physical fitness is not protective against high-altitude illness.
- HAPE is characterized by elevated pulmonary pressures, resulting in protein-rich, hemorrhagic exudates into the lung alveoli.
- Both dexamethasone and tadalafil decrease systolic pulmonary artery pressure and may reduce the incidence of HAPE in adults with a history of HAPE. Dexamethasone prophylaxis may also reduce the incidence of AMS in these adults.
- Descent is mandatory for all persons with high-altitude cerebral or pulmonary edema.

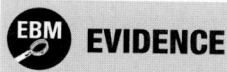 **EVIDENCE**

available at www.expertconsult.com

SUGGESTED READINGS

available at www.expertconsult.com

AUTHORS: **RICHARD REGNANTE, M.D.,** and **PAUL GORDON, M.D.**

Diseases and Disorders

A

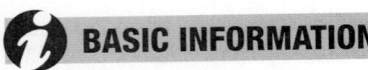

BASIC INFORMATION

DEFINITION

Dementia is a syndrome characterized by progressive loss of previously acquired cognitive skills including memory, language, insight, and judgment. Alzheimer's disease (AD) is believed to account for the majority (50% to 75%) of all cases of dementia.

ICD-9CM CODES
331.0 Alzheimer's disease
290.0 Senile dementia, uncomplicated

EPIDEMIOLOGY & DEMOGRAPHICS

INCIDENCE: Risk doubles every 5 yr after the age of 65; above the age of 85 the incidence is about 8%.
PREVALENCE: Currently an estimated 5.5 million Americans have AD; 7% between the ages of 65 and 74, 53% between 75 and 84, and 40% at 85 years and older.
PREDOMINANT SEX: Female

PHYSICAL FINDINGS & CLINICAL PRESENTATION

- Spouse or other family member, usually not the patient, notes insidious memory impairment.
- Patients have difficulties learning and retaining new information and handling complex tasks (e.g., balancing the checkbook), and have impairments in reasoning, judgment, spatial ability, and orientation (e.g., difficulty driving, getting lost away from home).
- Behavioral changes, such as mood changes and apathy, may accompany memory impairment. In later stages patients may develop agitation and psychosis.
- Atypical presentations include early and severe behavioral changes, focal findings on examination, parkinsonism, hallucinations, falls, or onset of symptoms younger than the age of 65.

DIAGNOSIS

There is no definitive imaging or laboratory test for the diagnosis of AD; rather, diagnosis is dependent on clinical history, a thorough physical and neurologic examination, and use of reliable and valid diagnostic criteria (i.e., DSM-IV or NINDCS-ADRDA) such as the following:

- Loss of memory and one or more additional cognitive abilities (aphasia, apraxia, agnosia, or other disturbance in executive functioning)
- Impairment in social or occupational functioning that represents a decline from a previous level of functioning and results in significant disability
- Deficits that do not occur exclusively during the course of delirium
- Insidious onset and gradual progression of symptoms
- Cognitive loss documented by neuropsychologic tests

- No physical signs, neuroimaging, or laboratory evidence of other diseases that can cause dementia (i.e., metabolic abnormalities, medication or toxin effects, infection, stroke, Parkinson's disease, subdural hematoma, or tumors)

Patients with isolated memory loss who lack functional impairment at home or work do not meet criteria for dementia but may have a mild cognitive impairment (MCI). Identifying patients with MCI is important because patients with MCI may have a slightly higher rate of progression to dementia.

DIFFERENTIAL DIAGNOSIS

- Cancer (brain tumor, meningeal neoplasia)
- Infection (AIDS, neurosyphilis, PML)
- Toxic/metabolic (EtOH, hypothyroidism, B12 deficiency, mercury exposure, drug effects)
- Organ failure (dialysis dementia, Wilson's disease)
- Vascular disorder (multiple strokes, severe small vessel changes, chronic vasculitides, or chronic subdural hematoma)
- Depression (pseudodementia)

WORKUP

HISTORY & GENERAL PHYSICAL EXAMINATION:

- Medication lists should always be reviewed for drugs or home remedies that may cause mental status changes.
- Patients should be screened for depression, because it can sometimes mimic dementia but also often occurs as a coexisting condition and should be treated.
- On examination, look for signs of metabolic disturbance, presence of psychiatric features, or focal neurologic deficits.

MENTAL STATUS TESTING: Brief mental status testing can be done easily and quickly in the office. Most commonly used is the Folstein Mini-Mental State Examination (MMSE). The MMSE is widely available in many reference books and on the Internet. An MMSE score <24 (scores range from 0 to 30, with lower scores reflecting poorer performance) suggests cognitive impairment; however, the MMSE is not sensitive enough to detect mild dementia or dementia in patients with high baseline IQ. Scores may be spuriously low in patients with limited education, poor motor function, African American or Hispanic ethnicity, poor language skills, or impaired vision. The MMSE is perhaps most useful to follow AD patients for long-term outcomes.

Mental status testing should include tests that assess the following cognitive functions:

- Orientation: ask the patient to give the day, date, month, year, and place and to name the current president.
- Attention: ask the patient to recite the months of the year forward and in reverse.
- Verbal recall: ask the patient to remember four items; test for recall after a 1- and 5-min delay.
- Language: ask the patient to write and then read a sentence; have the patient name both common and less common objects.
- Visual-spatial: ask the patient to draw a clock and to set the hands of the clock at 11:10.

Patients with AD typically have trouble with verbal recall, plus visual-spatial or language deficits. Attention is usually preserved until the late stages of AD, so consider alternate diagnoses in patients who perform poorly on tests of attention.

LABORATORY TESTS

- CBC
- Serum electrolytes
- Glucose
- BUN/creatinine
- Liver and thyroid function tests
- Serum vitamin B_{12}
- Syphilis serology (RPR)
- HIV screening as appropriate
- Lumbar puncture if history or signs of cancer, infectious process, or when the clinical presentation is unusual (i.e., rapid progression of symptoms)
- EEG if there is history of seizures, episodic confusion, rapid clinical decline, or suspicion of Creutzfeldt-Jakob disease
- Measurement of apolipoprotein E genotyping, CSF tau and amyloid, and functional imaging including positron emission tomography (PET) or single proton emission computed tomography (SPECT) are not routinely indicated
- Brain biopsy (usually reserved for diagnoses such as prion disease, certain vasculitides)

IMAGING STUDIES

- CT scan or MRI to rule out hydrocephalus and mass lesions, including subdural hematoma
- Florbetapir-PET imaging of the brain correlates with the presence and density of beta-amyloid

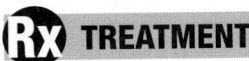 TREATMENT

NONPHARMACOLOGIC THERAPY

- Patient safety, including risks associated with impaired driving, wandering behavior, leaving stoves unattended, and accidents, must be addressed with the patient and family early and appropriate measures implemented.
- Wandering, hoarding or hiding objects, repetitive questioning, withdrawal, and social inappropriateness often respond to behavioral therapies.

ACUTE GENERAL Rx
None

CHRONIC Rx

1. Symptomatic treatment of memory disturbance (Table 1-5):
   a. Cholinesterase inhibitors (ChEls):
      FDA approved for the treatment of mild to moderate AD. Common side effects include nausea, diarrhea, and anorexia and may be bothersome enough to require a slower escalation of dosage or switching to another agent.
   b. NMDA receptor antagonist: memantine (Namenda)
      FDA approved for the treatment of moderate to severe AD. Common side effects include constipation, dizziness,

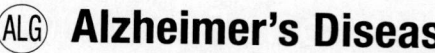

A

or headache. Memantine is contraindicated in patients with renal insufficiency or history of seizures.

2. Symptomatic treatment of neuropsychiatric and behavioral disturbances (Table 1-6): Depression, agitation, delusions, or hallucinations may respond to medications.

DISPOSITION & REFERRAL

- Patients with complex or atypical presentations or challenging management issues should be referred to a neurologist or another specialist with expertise in dementia.
- Family education and support may help reduce need for skilled nursing facility, and reduce caregiver stress, depression, and burnout.

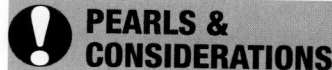

The physician should make a thorough search for the treatable causes of dementia. Current American Academy of Neurology practice parameters recommend:

- Treat cognitive symptoms of AD with ChEIs.
- Treat agitation, psychosis, and depression.
- Encourage caregivers to participate in educational programs and support groups.

COMMENTS

- Ginkgo biloba is marketed widely as effective in delaying cognitive impairment; however, trials have shown that it is not effective in reducing the incidence of Alzheirmer dementia or dementia overall.
- Lower plasma beta-amyloid 42/40 is associated with greater cognitive decline among elderly persons without dementia over 9 yrs, and this association is stronger among those with low measures of cognitive reserve.
- The *APOE* genotype provides information on the risk for AD, but the genotyping of patients raises ethical and emotional concerns. Because the benefits of genetic testing are often modest, and the tests themselves often imprecise in identifying risk, the test is generally discouraged. Recent trials, however, reveal that the disclosure of *APOE* genotyping results to adult children of patients with AD did not result in significant short-term psychological risks. Test-related distress was reduced among those who learned that they were *APOE*4 negative. Persons with high levels of emotional distress before undergoing genetic testing are more likely to have emotional difficulties after disclosure.

For additional information for patients, families, and clinicians, contact the following organizations:

- Alzheimer's Association (www.alz.org; 800-272-3900)
- Alzheimer's Disease Education and Referral Center (http://www.nia.nih.gov/Alzheimers; 800-438-4380)

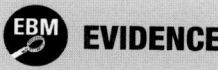

available at www.expertconsult.com

SUGGESTED READINGS
available at www.expertconsult.com

AUTHOR: **TAMARA G. FONG, M.D., PH.D.**

TABLE 1-5 Symptomatic Treatment of Memory Disturbance

	Initial Dose	Target Dose
Donepezil (Aricept)	5 mg qd for 4-6 weeks	10 mg qd
Rivastigmine (Exelon)	1.5 mg bid with food, increase by 1.5 mg bid weekly	3 to 6 mg bid
Galantamine (Reminyl)	4 mg bid with food, increase by 4 mg bid every 4 weeks	8 to 12 mg bid
Memantine (Namenda)	5 mg qd, increase by 5 mg weekly	10 mg bid

TABLE 1-6 Treatment of Behavioral and Neuropsychiatric Symptoms

	Initial Dose	Maximum Dose
Atypical antipsychotics		
Olanzapine (Zyprexa)	2.5 mg qd to bid, may increase by 2.5 mg as needed	7.5 mg bid
Quetiapine (Seroquel)	25 mg bid, may increase by 25 mg every 2 days	250 mg tid
Antidepressants		
Sertraline (Zoloft)	25-50 mg qd, may increase by 25 mg every week	200 mg qd
Citalopram (Celexa)	10 mg qd, may increase after 1 week	20 mg qd

Diseases and Disorders

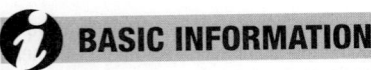

BASIC INFORMATION

DEFINITION

Amaurosis fugax (AF) is a temporary loss of monocular vision caused by transient retinal ischemia.

ICD-9CM CODES
362.34 Amaurosis fugax

EPIDEMIOLOGY & DEMOGRAPHICS

INCIDENCE (IN U.S.): An uncommon but important presentation of carotid artery disease
PEAK INCIDENCE: ≥55 yr

PHYSICAL FINDINGS & CLINICAL PRESENTATION

- Onset is sudden, typically lasting seconds to minutes, and often accompanied by scotomas such as a shade or curtain being pulled over the front of the eye (usually downward).
- Vision loss can be complete or quadrantic.
- Acute stage: cholesterol emboli may be seen in retinal artery (Hollenhorst plaque): carotid bruits or other evidence of generalized atherosclerosis.
- If embolus is cardiac in origin, atrial fibrillation is often present.

ETIOLOGY

- Usually embolic from the internal carotid artery or the heart
- May also be caused by vasculitis, such as giant cell arteritis (GCA), or hyperviscosity syndromes, such as sickle cell disease, that cause ischemia in the vascular territory of the ophthalmic artery

DIAGNOSIS

DIFFERENTIAL DIAGNOSIS

- Retinal migraine: in contrast to amaurosis, the onset of visual loss develops more slowly, usually over 15 to 20 min.
- Transient visual obscurations occur in the setting of papilledema; intermittent rises in intracranial pressure briefly compromise optic disc perfusion and cause transient visual loss lasting 1 to 2 seconds. The episodes may be binocular. If the visual loss persists at the time of evaluation (i.e., vision has not yet recovered), then the differential diagnosis should be broadened to include:
  - Anterior ischemic optic neuropathy: arteritic (classically GCA) or nonarteritic
  - Central retinal vein occlusion

WORKUP

- Workup should focus on embolic sources, but GCA should always be considered.
- Careful examination of retina; embolus may be visible and confirm the diagnosis (Fig. 1-19).
- Auscultation of arteries for carotid bruits.
- Examination of all pulses and for temporal artery tenderness.
- Inquire about symptoms of GCA (scalp tenderness, jaw claudication).
- Examine for signs of hemispheric stroke resulting from intracranial aneurysm (contralateral limb and facial weakness or sensory loss, aphasia, etc.).

LABORATORY TESTS

- Complete blood count with erythrocyte sedimentation rate and C-reactive protein.
- Serum chemistries, including lipid profile.
- ECG and possibly cycling cardiac enzymes.
- Hypercoagulable workup is discretionary based on younger age and history.

IMAGING STUDIES

- Carotid Doppler imaging followed by MR or CT angiography as indicated.
- Transthoracic echocardiography is indicated to screen for embolization in patients with evidence of heart disease and in patients without an evident source for transient neurologic deficit. Transesophageal echocardiography is more sensitive for detecting cardiac sources of embolization (ventricular mural thrombus, atrial appendage, patent foramen ovale, aortic arch).
- Consider MRI of the brain with diffusion-weighted imaging to look for infarcts.

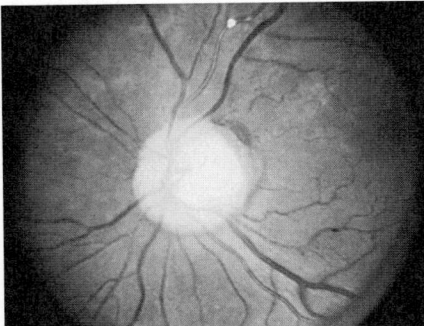

FIGURE 1-19 A cholesterol crystal embolus lodged at an arterial bifurcation. (From Stein JH [ed]: *Internal medicine,* ed 5, St Louis, 1998, Mosby.)

TREATMENT

NONPHARMACOLOGIC THERAPY

- Diet (decrease saturated fatty acids and high-cholesterol foods)
- Exercise
- Cessation of tobacco use

ACUTE GENERAL Rx

- Investigate as an emergency.
- Give aspirin if etiology is presumed embolic.
- If GCA is suspected, start prednisone and refer for temporal artery biopsy within 48 hr (see Giant Cell Arteritis in Section I).

CHRONIC Rx

- Reduce risks by carotid endarterectomy if stenosis >70%. Stenting may be performed in high-risk surgical candidates.
- Control hypertension and manage vascular risk factors.
- Antiplatelet therapy.
- Consider starting an HMG-CoA reductase inhibitor.

DISPOSITION

Among patients with >50% carotid stenosis who do not undergo carotid endarterectomy, those who present with transient monocular blindness have an approximate 10% risk of stroke in 3 yr compared with an approximate 20% risk in patients who present with a hemispheric transient ischemic attack (TIA).

REFERRAL

- Recommend referral to a neurologist for an evaluation and workup.
- If significant carotid stenosis, consider carotid endarterectomy or carotid stenting for the following:
  1. High-grade (≥70%) stenosis
  2. Multiple TIAs despite medical therapy in the setting of high-grade or ulcerative disease

PEARLS & CONSIDERATIONS

- Cholesterol emboli in retinal arteries on funduscopy confirm the diagnosis.
- Recognize that transient visual loss has multiple other causes.

SUGGESTED READING

available at www.expertconsult.com

AUTHOR: **SEAN I. SAVITZ, M.D.**

BASIC INFORMATION

DEFINITION

Amblyopia refers to a decrease in vision in one or both eyes in the presence of an otherwise normal ophthalmologic examination.

SYNONYMS

Deprivation amblyopia
Occlusion amblyopia
Strabismus amblyopia
Refractive amblyopia
Organic or toxic amblyopias
Lazy eye

ICD-9CM CODES
368.00 Amblyopia

EPIDEMIOLOGY & DEMOGRAPHICS

INCIDENCE (IN U.S.): 1% to 4% of the general population
PREVALENCE (IN U.S.): High incidence in premature infants with drug-dependent mothers and in neurologically impaired children
PREDOMINANT SEX: None
PREDOMINANT AGE: Childhood
PEAK INCIDENCE: Childhood

PHYSICAL FINDINGS & CLINICAL PRESENTATION

Decreased vision using best refraction in the presence of normal corneal, lens, retinal, and optic nerve appearance (Fig. 1-20)

ETIOLOGY

- Visual deprivation
- Strabismus
- Occlusion with patching
- Refractive error organic lesions in the nervous system
- Toxins

DIAGNOSIS

DIFFERENTIAL DIAGNOSIS

- Central nervous system (CNS) disease (brainstem)
- Optic nerve disorders
- Corneal or other eye diseases
- Retinal disorders

WORKUP

- Complete eye examination to find cause of amblyopia or deprivation of vision. Referral to an ophthalmologist is recommended for any child with a visual acuity in either eye of ≤20/40 at age 3 to 5 yr or worse at age ≥6 yr or a two-line difference in acuity between eyes.
- Motility evaluation.

LABORATORY TESTS

Usually none

IMAGING STUDIES

Usually not necessary unless central nervous system (CNS) lesion suspected

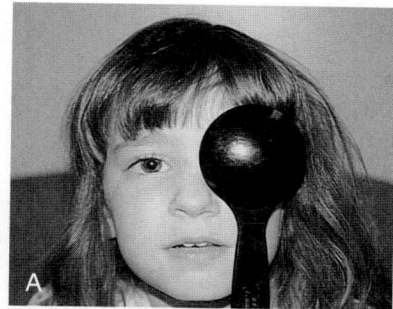
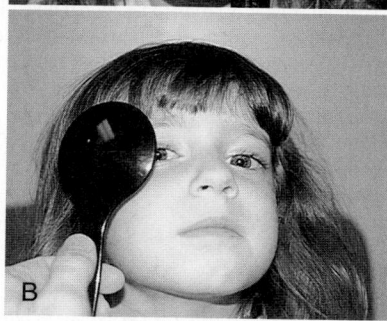

FIGURE 1-20 A, This child happily fixes with her right eye and does not object if the left eye is covered. **B,** When the right eye is covered she moves her head away and tries to remove the cover, demonstrating a fixation preference for the right eye and amblyopia of the left eye. (From Hoekelman R [ed]: *Primary pediatric care,* ed 3, St Louis, 1997, Mosby.)

TREATMENT

NONPHARMACOLOGIC THERAPY

- Glasses or prisms to align eyes with minor deviations and improve vision.
- Patches, mechanical versus atropine: patching and atropine both work. Atropine 1% is used daily for 6 mo; patching is used 6 hr/day for 6 mo. Patching may be more effective; 50% get best vision improvement by 16 wk.
- Removal of the cause of the amblyopia if possible.
- Surgery to align the eyes or remove obstruction to vision.

CHRONIC Rx

- Patching or optics, including prisms and atropine, most effective in 3- to 7-yr-olds only; minimal or no help after 7 yr
- Levodopa/carbidopa has been reported as effective in improving visual acuity in patients with amblyopia younger than 8 yrs; however, it is not known how long the effect lasts or whether it is reversible.

DISPOSITION

Immediate patching, alternating eyes daily

REFERRAL

To ophthalmologist if vision is compromised

PEARLS & CONSIDERATIONS

COMMENTS

- The earlier the referral, the better the outcome.
- The success of therapy is highly dependent on treatment compliance.
- Amblyopia causes unilateral vision loss in 2% to 4% of the population.

EVIDENCE

available at www.expertconsult.com

SUGGESTED READING

available at www.expertconsult.com

AUTHOR: **MELVYN KOBY, M.D.**

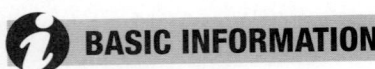

DEFINITION

Amebiasis is an infection caused by the protozoal parasite *Entamoeba histolytica*. Although primarily an infection of the colon, amebiasis may cause extraintestinal disease, particularly liver abscess.

SYNONYMS

Amebic dysentery (when severe intestinal infection)

ICD-9CM CODES
006.9 Amebiasis

EPIDEMIOLOGY & DEMOGRAPHICS

INCIDENCE (IN U.S.): Highest in institutionalized patients, sexually active homosexual men
PREVALENCE (IN U.S.): 4% (80% of infections asymptomatic)
PREDOMINANT SEX:
- Equal sex distribution in general
- Striking male predominance of liver abscess
PREDOMINANT AGE: Second through sixth decades
PEAK INCIDENCE: Peaks at age 2 to 3 yr and >40 yr
GENETICS: Infection more likely to be fulminant in young infants

PHYSICAL FINDINGS & CLINICAL PRESENTATION

- Often nonspecific
- Approximately 20% of cases symptomatic
  1. Diarrhea, which may be bloody
  2. Abdominal and back pain
- Abdominal tenderness in 83% of severe cases
- Fever in 38% of severe cases
- Hepatomegaly, RUQ tenderness, and fever in almost all patients with liver abscess (may be absent in fulminant cases)

ETIOLOGY

- Caused by the protozoal parasite *E. histolytica* (Fig. 1-21)
- Transmission by the fecal-oral route
- Infection usually localized to the large bowel, particularly the cecum where a localized mass lesion (ameboma) may form
- Extraintestinal infection in which the organism invades the bowel mucosa and gains access to the portal circulation

DIAGNOSIS

DIFFERENTIAL DIAGNOSIS

- Severe intestinal infection possibly confused with ulcerative colitis or other infectious enterocolitis syndromes, such as those caused by *Shigella, Salmonella, Campylobacter,* or invasive *Escherichia coli*
- In elderly patients: ischemic bowel possibly producing a similar picture

WORKUP

- Three stool specimens over a period of 7 to 10 days to exclude the diagnosis (sensitivity 50% to 80%)
- Concentration and staining the specimen with Lugol's iodine or methylene blue to increase the diagnostic yield
- Available culture (rarely necessary in routine cases)

LABORATORY TESTS

- Stool examination is generally reliable.
- Mucosal biopsy is occasionally necessary.
- Serum antibody may be detected and is particularly sensitive and specific for extraintestinal infection or severe intestinal disease.
- Aspiration of abscess fluid is used to distinguish amebic from bacterial abscesses.

IMAGING STUDIES

Abdominal imaging studies (sonography or CT scan) to diagnose liver abscess

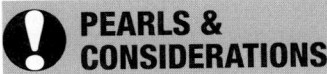

TREATMENT

ACUTE GENERAL Rx

- Metronidazole (750 mg PO tid for 10 days) is used in the treatment of mild to severe intestinal infection and amebic liver abscess; it may be administered intravenously when necessary.
- Follow with iodoquinol (650 mg PO tid for 20 days) to eradicate persistent cysts.

- For asymptomatic patients with amebic cysts on stool examination, use iodoquinol or paromomycin (500 mg PO tid for 7 days).
- Avoid antiperistaltic agents in severe intestinal infections to avoid risk of toxic megacolon.
- Liver abscess is generally responsive to medical management but surgical intervention indicated for extension of liver abscess into pericardium or for toxic megacolon.

DISPOSITION

Host immunity incomplete and reinfection rate high for patients remaining at risk

REFERRAL

- For consultation with infectious diseases specialist for extraintestinal infection or persistent or relapsing intestinal infection
- For surgical consultation:
  1. For toxic megacolon
  2. For impending rupture of or extension of liver abscess into adjacent structures

PEARLS & CONSIDERATIONS

COMMENTS

Infection with other intestinal parasites, particularly *Giardia lamblia,* may coexist with amebiasis.

SUGGESTED READINGS
available at www.expertconsult.com

AUTHORS: **GLENN G. FORT, M.D., M.P.H.,** and **DENNIS J. MIKOLICH, M.D.**

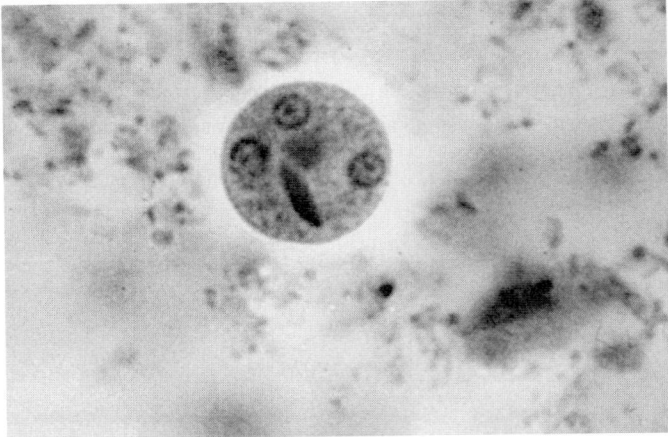

FIGURE 1-21 Mature cyst of *Entamoeba histolytica.* Three of the four nuclei are seen in the plane of focus of this photomicrograph. (From Mandell GL [ed]: *Mandell, Douglas, and Bennett's principles and practice of infectious diseases,* ed 6, New York, 2005, Churchill Livingstone.)

BASIC INFORMATION

DESCRIPTION

Amenorrhea means absence of menstruation. It is classified as either primary or secondary depending on whether the patient has had previous menstrual cycles.

- Primary amenorrhea is defined as the absence of menses by age 16 in the presence of secondary sexual characteristics. However, in the absence of these secondary sexual features by the age of 13 to 14 years, one should begin the workup for primary amenorrhea.
- Secondary amenorrhea is the absence of menses for more than six months in a patient who has had previous normal progesterone withdrawal cycles.

ICD-9CM CODES
626.0 Absence of menstruation

EPIDEMIOLOGY & DEMOGRAPHICS

- Incidence of primary amenorrhea and secondary amenorrhea in the U.S. is <1% and 5% to 7%, respectively.
- It has no racial or ethnic predilection.

ETIOLOGY

- Physiologic amenorrhea
  1. Pregnancy
  2. Lactation
  3. Menopause
- Pathologic amenorrhea
  A. Primary amenorrhea
    1. Hypergonadotropic hypogonadism
       a. Turner syndrome
       b. Pure gonadal dysgenesis
       c. Autoimmune oophoritis
       d. 17, 20-desmolase deficiency or 17-hydroxylase deficiency
       e. Galactosemia
    2. Eugonadism
       a. Müllerian agnesis
       b. Transverse vaginal septum
       c. Imperforate hymen
       d. Androgen insensitivity syndrome (AIS) (1%)
       e. 5-alpha reductase deficiency
       f. PCOS
       g. Adult-onset congenital adrenal hyperplasia (CAH)
       h. Cushing's syndrome
       i. Hypothyroidism
    3. Hypogonadotrophic hypogonadism
       a. Constitutional delay
       b. Hypothalamic disorders
       c. Pituitary diseases
       d. Other CNS diseases
  B. Secondary amenorrhea
    1. Ovarian diseases
       a. PCOS
       b. Iatrogenic (oophorectomy, S/P radiation)
       c. Premature ovarian failure (POF)
       d. Ovarian tumors

    2. Hypothalamic dysfunction
       a. Functional (eating disorders, exercise, stress)
       b. Congenital GNRH deficiency
       c. Infiltrative diseases (sarcoidosis, histiocytosis, lymphoma)
    3. Pituitary diseases
       a. Hyperprolactinemia (drug induced, hypothyroidism, prolactinoma)
       b. Craniopharyngiomas
       c. Empty sella syndrome
       d. Sheehan's syndrome
       e. S/P radiation
       f. Infiltrative diseases
    4. Uterine diseases
       Asherman's syndrome
    5. Others
       Hypothyroidism, Cushing's syndrome, adult-onset congenital adrenal hyperplasia, drug induced (Lupron Depot, Depo-Provera, progesterone IUD, danazol, etc.), chronic illnesses

PHYSICAL FINDINGS & CLINICAL PRESENTATION

- Turner's syndrome
  - Mostly present with primary amenorrhea unless mosaic
  - Short stature
  - Epicanthic folds
  - Low set ears
  - High arched palate
  - Micrognathia
  - Sensorineural hearing loss
  - Otitis media
  - Webbing of the neck
  - Pigmented nevi
  - Square/shield chest
  - Widely spaced nipples
  - Absent breast development
  - Bicuspid aortic valve
  - Coarctation of aorta
  - Cubit valgus
  - Short fourth metacarpal
  - Hyperconvex nails
  - Leg edema
  - Renal abnormalities
  - Autoimmune disorders including thyroiditis
  - Diabetes mellitus
- Pure gonadal dysgenesis
  - Unlike Turner's syndrome has no dysmorphic features
- Müllerian agnesis
  - Sporadic inheritance
  - Primary amenorrhea
  - Normal breast development
  - Normal pubic and axillary hair
  - Normal female external genitalia
  - Absent uterus and upper part of vagina
  - Ovary present
  - Renal and vertebral anomalies
- Vaginal septum and imperforate hymen
  - Primary amenorrhea
  - Progressive cyclic lower abdominal pain
  - Imperforate hymen or vaginal septum on pelvic examination
  - Perirectal fullness from hematocolpos

- Androgen insensitivity syndrome
  - Primary amenorrhea
  - X-linked recessive inheritance
  - Normal breast development
  - Absent pubic and axillary hair
  - Testis may be present in the groin or inguinal canal
  - Uterus and vagina absent
  - No associated renal or vertebral anomalies
- Adult-onset congenital adrenal hyperplasia
  - Commonly seen in Ashkenazi Jewish, Inuit Native American, French Canadian, Mexican population
  - Mimics the presentation of PCOS
  - Features of hyperandrogenism (virilization, hirsutism, acne)
  - Hypertension
- 5-alpha reductase deficiency
  - Primary amenorrhea
  - Undergo striking virilization at puberty
- PCOS
  - Usually present with secondary amenorrhea and oligomenorrhea
  - Features of hyperandrogenism
  - Obesity
  - Infertility
- Cushing's syndrome (rare disorder, prevalence 1/1,000,000)
  - Secondary amenorrhea
  - Features of hyperandrogenism
  - Abnormal fat distribution (buffalo hump, spider legs, significant central obesity)
  - Abdominal striae
  - Easy bruising
  - Hypertension
  - Proximal muscle weakness
- Hypothyroidism
  - Secondary amenorrhea
  - Lethargy
  - Constipation
  - Decreased appetite
  - Weight gain
  - Cold intolerance
  - Hair loss
  - Dry skin
  - Hypotension
  - Bradycardia
- Premature ovarian failure
  - Secondary amenorrhea prior to the age of 40
  - History of oophorectomy or pelvic radiation or chemotherapy
  - Vasomotor symptoms
  - Dry, thin vaginal mucosa without rugosity
- Hyperprolactinemia
  - Usually present with secondary amenorrhea
  - History of use of drugs such as antipsychotics, OC pills, antidepressants, antihypertensives, H_2 blockers, opioids, etc.
  - Pituitary adenomas may be associated with headache, vomiting, vision changes
  - Galactorrhea
- Sheehan's syndrome
  - History of secondary amenorrhea following postpartum hemorrhagia
  - Failure of lactation
  - Other features of hypopituitarism

- Asherman's syndrome
  - History of D&C
  - Secondary amenorrhea
  - Recurrent miscarriage/infertility
- Functional hypothalamic disorders
  - Usually present with secondary amenorrhea
  - History of eating disorders, severe exercise or stress
  - Use of street drugs
- Kallmann's syndrome
  - Usually present with anosmia

Dx DIAGNOSIS

- First step in the workup of amenorrhea is to rule out pregnancy by serum/urine pregnancy test.
- Diagnostic workup depends on history and physical.
- Primary amenorrhea:
  - Pelvic ultrasonography or MRI to detect any anatomic abnormalities of uterus, cervix, ovaries, or vagina. At times examination under anesthesia is needed to assess the pelvic organs.
  - Karyotyping (46,XX in Müllerian agenesis; 46,XY in AIS; 45,XO in Turner's syndrome) is done when uterus is absent or Turner's syndrome is suspected.
  - Serum FSH, TSH/FT4, prolactin, estradiol: FSH>40 mlU/ml along with estradiol <20 pg/ml is indicative of ovarian insufficiency. Prolactin >200 ng/ml is suggestive of prolactinoma.
  - Check serum testosterone (male range in AIS; female range in Müllerian agenesis) when uterus is absent or in presence of features of hyperandrogenism.
  - 17 alpha hydroxyprogesterone level in presence of features of hyperandrogenism to rule out CAH. In addition to low level of 17 alpha hydroxyprogesterone, these patients have elevated level of serum progesterone and deoxycorticosterone, hypernatremia, and hypokalemia.
  - MRI of head in presence of:
    Primary hypogonadotrophic hypogonadism.
    Hyperprolactinemia.
    Visual field defects.
    Headaches.
    Signs of hypothalamic-pituitary dysfunction.
- Secondary amenorrhea:
  - Serum FSH, TSH/FT4, prolactin, estradiol: Low serum FSH with low estradiol indicates secondary (hypogondotrophic) hypogonadism.
    High serum FSH with low estradiol suggests primary (hypergonadotrophic) hypogonadism.
    Progesterone withdrawal bleeding.
    10 mg medroxyprogesterone is given for 10 days.
    Withdrawal bleeding suggests euestrogenic anovulation in presence of normal endorgan (outflow tract) and ovarian function.

- Estrogen-progesterone withdrawal bleeding:
  In the absence of progesterone withdrawal bleeding, the patients are exposed to 25 to 35 days of estrogen (0.625-2.5 mg Premarin daily) followed by 10 days of medroxyprogesterone.
  Withdrawal bleeding indicates hypogonadism.
  Absence of bleeding indicates defects with endorgan (e.g., Asherman's syndrome).
  - Serum LH, testosterone and DHEA-S:
    When features of hyperandrogenism seen these tests are ordered.
    Serum testosterone > 200 ng/ml suggests androgen-producing adrenal or ovarian tumors. This level may be mildly elevated in patients with PCOS.
    DHEA-S >700 mcg/dl suggest adrenal origin over ovarian.
    LH/FSH ratio >2 in patient with PCOS.
  - Pelvic ultrasound when PCOS or ovarian tumor suspected.
  - Abdominal CT when adrenal tumor suspected.
  - MRI of head when indicated.
  - HSG, sonohysterography, or diagnostic hysteroscopy in patients with suspected Asherman's syndrome.
  - Karyotyping is indicated when POF occurs before the age of 30.
  - Other tests which are rarely needed:
    Serum transferrin when hemochromatosis is suspected.
    Serum ACE when sarcoidosis is suspected.

Rx TREATMENT

- The treatment of amenorrhea depends on the etiology, as well as the aims of the patient, such as a desire to treat hirsutism or to become pregnant.
- In the absence of pregnancy, withdrawal bleeding may be induced in the majority of patients with amenorrhea using 5 to 10 mg of medroxyprogesterone for 10 days.
- Estrogen replacement along with calcium and vitamin D should be instituted in essentially every patient with hypogonadism to avoid osteoporosis. Women with a uterus require continuous or intermittent progesterone administration to protect against endometrial hyperplasia or cancer. Frequently, it is easiest to prescribe combination oral contraceptive pills. For most patients, continuation until ~50 years, the usual age of menopause, seems reasonable. Young women in whom secondary sex characteristics have failed to develop fully should be exposed initially to very low dose estrogen (0.3 mg of conjugated equine estrogen) given unopposed daily for 6 mo with incremental dose increases at 6-mo intervals until the required maintenance dose is achieved. Cyclic progesterone therapy, 12 to 14 days per month, should be instituted once vaginal bleeding ensues.
- If possible, patients with anatomic abnormalities will require surgical correction. Cre-

ation of a new vagina for patients with Müllerian agenesis is usually delayed until the woman is emotionally mature and ready to participate in the postoperative care required to maintain vaginal patency. However, if adequate correction is impossible, pregnancy will often require a surrogate to carry a gestation. One should not forget to look for the associated urogenital anomalies in these patients and, when present, treat them appropriately.
- In patients with androgen insensitivity syndrome, the incidence of gonadal malignancy is 22%. However, it rarely occurs before the age of 20. Gonadectomy is performed by laparoscopy following breast development and the attainment of adult stature. In the absence of a uterus these individuals only need estrogen replacement without progesterone.
- Women with adult-onset CAH may be treated with low-dose corticosteroids in addition to sex steroids to partially block ACTH stimulation of adrenal function and thereby decrease overproduction of adrenal androgens.
- Patients with POF will need estrogen and progesterone replacement. If POF cannot be corrected, these patients will require in vitro fertilization using donor oocytes to conceive. These patients have an increased risk of osteoporosis and heart disease. It can also be associated with autoimmune disorders such as hypothyroidism, Addison's disease, and diabetes mellitus. Therefore, fasting blood glucose, TSH, and, if clinically appropriate, morning cortisol should be measured. In the presence of a Y chromosome, removal of gonadal tissue is recommended at the time of diagnosis to avoid gonadal tumors.
- Hypothyroidism should be treated with thyroid replacement.
- Hyperprolactinemia is treated by avoiding the culprit drugs or by giving dopamine agonists, such as bromocriptine or cabergoline. Pituitary adenomas rarely require surgery but may be performed if secondary deficits such as visual changes are observed, when they are resistant to medical therapy, or the lesion is rapidly growing.
- Treatment of hypothalamic amenorrhea depends on the etiology. Patients with eating disorders or who exercise excessively will require behavioral modification and nutritional counseling. Elite athletes may choose not to alter their exercise regimens and will therefore require estrogen treatment and prevention of osteoporosis. When associated with infertility, ovulation induction with clomiphene citrate, exogenous gonadotropins, or pulsatile GNRH therapy should be offered.
- The primary treatment of PCOS is weight loss through diet and exercise. Other treatment options include:
  1. Use of OC pills or cyclic progestational agents to help maintain a normal endometrium.
  2. Insulin-sensitizing agents such as metformin to reduce insulin resistance and improve ovulatory function.

3. Oral contraceptives and/or spironolactone to treat hyperandrogenism.
4. Clomiphene citrate to induce ovulation.
- In patients with Asherman's syndrome, hysteroscopic lysis of intrauterine adhesions is followed by administration of long-term exogenous estrogen to stimulate regrowth of endometrial tissue.
- Geneticist consult is given in patients with hereditary causes of amenorrhea.
- Psychiatrist consult is needed in patients with major depression, anorexia nervosa, bulimia nervosa, or other major psychiatric disorders.

COMPLICATIONS
- Osteoporosis
- Endometrial hyperplasia and uterine cancer
- Infertility

PROGNOSIS
Depends on the primary cause of amenorrhea

PATIENT EDUCATION
- Patients with amenorrhea should be reassured that this is, in and of itself, not a concern.
- All women with an intact endometrium should understand the risks of unopposed estrogen action, whether the estrogen is exogenous such as through hormone therapy, or endogenous such as PCOS.
- Hypoestrogenic women should be counseled about the importance of estrogen replacement to protect against bone loss.
- Potential for future child bearing should be discussed.

SUGGESTED READINGS
available at www.expertconsult.com

AUTHOR: **HEMANT K. SATPATHY, M.D.**

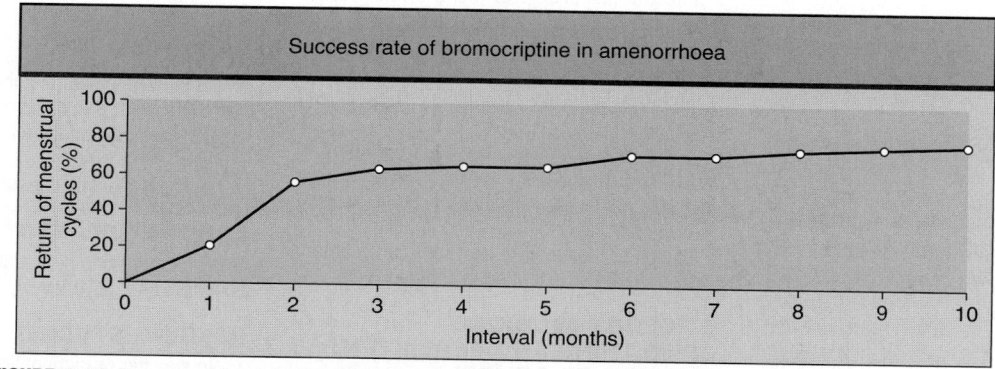

FIGURE 1-22 Success rate of bromocriptine in amenorrhea. If hyperprolactinemia is the cause of amenorrhea, the chances of restoring normal gonadal function with bromocriptine are very good. After 1 month of treatment, one woman in four will return to normal menstrual cycling; within 2 months, this number will increase to six out of 10; and after 10 months, eight out of 10 women will be menstruating normally. Most of the remaining 20% have had pituitary surgery and irradiation therapy and are gonadotropin-deficient. (Besser CM, Thorner MO: *Comprehensive Clinical Endocrinology*, ed 3, 2002, Mosby.)

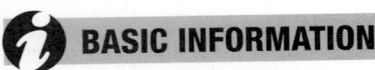

BASIC INFORMATION

The word "amnesia" is derived from the Greek word *amnéstia* meaning "forgetfulness."

DEFINITION

The acquired inability to learn new, or recall previously learned information. The impairment compromises social and occupational functioning. It is caused by an identifiable medical condition or by persisting effects of a substance. Disorder is not caused by delirium or dementia. It may be transient or chronic.

SOME WELL-KNOWN AMNESTIC DISORDERS

Korsakoff syndrome
Transient global amnesia

ICD-9CM CODES
780.9 Amnesia (retrograde); memory disturbance, loss or lack

DSM-IV-TR CODES
294.0 Amnestic disorder due to . . . [indicate the general medical condition]
294.8 Amnestic disorder NOS

EPIDEMIOLOGY & DEMOGRAPHICS

INCIDENCE: Data not available on true incidence or lifetime risk of most amnestic disorders. Transient global amnesia has an incidence in the general population of 23 to 50 per 100,000 population over age 50.
PREDOMINANT AGE: Variable, depending on causative pathology. Transient global amnesia onset usually after age 50 years. Korsakoff syndrome usually presents in patients after the age of 40.
GENETICS: Genetic defect for thiamine metabolism has been described in Korsakoff syndrome.

PHYSICAL FINDINGS & CLINICAL PRESENTATION

HISTORY
- Diagnosis depends on history.
- The inability to learn new or recall previously learned information is the key feature of this disorder.
- The Mini-Mental State Examination is useful. Patients unable to recall events that transpire during the interview but may have a normal digit span and be able to attend to the conversation.
- Neuropsychiatric testing demonstrates specific memory impairments in absence of other cognitive deficits
- Patients are unable to recall events subsequent to the onset of the amnesia.
- Individuals may learn new motor tasks but are unable to recall those learning experiences.
- Amnesia generally is both anterograde and retrograde.
- Commonly, patients are disoriented to time and place. Most lack insight while others may have insight but appear indifferent. Some present with personality change or confabulation.
- Clinico-anatomical correlations of memory disorders are described in Table 1-7.

ETIOLOGY (MEDICAL CONDITIONS AND PERSISTENT EFFECTS OF DRUGS)

The etiology can be either medical or due to the persistent effects of a substance/chemical.
- Traumatic brain injury
- Focal tumors or infarction
- Herpes simplex encephalitis
- Cerebral anoxia
- Korsakoff syndrome (thiamine deficiency)
- Carbon monoxide poisoning
- Transient amnesia may arise from concussion, acute intoxication, anesthesia, medications, seizures, transient global amnesia, and electroconvulsant therapy

- Persistent effects of drugs (note that this must not be because of acute effects of intoxication or withdrawl)

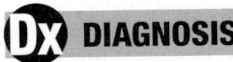

DIAGNOSIS

DIFFERENTIAL DIAGNOSIS

- Dementia
- Delirium
- Major depression
- Minimal cognitive impairment
- Dissociative amnesia
- Memory impairment in substance intoxication or withdrawal
- Malingering
- Factitious disorder

WORKUP

- Complete medical history and mental status testing, with emphasis on identifying underlying medical condition and/or history of drug use
- Neuropsychological testing

LABORATORY TESTS

Tests to determine potential underlying medical condition (e.g., B12 levels, TSH, brain imaging).

IMAGING STUDIES

- No specific or diagnostic features of amnestic disorder are detectable on imaging.
- Brain MRI indicates specific atrophy in diencephalic structures in Korsakoff syndrome and in the hippocampus in hypoxic amnesia.
- Neuroradiological examination with MRI is valuable in the diagnosis of acute Wernicke's encephalopathy.
- Brain MR diffusion-weighted imaging may show hippocampal lesions in transient global amnesia.

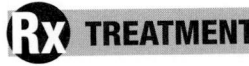

TREATMENT

Treatment is as diverse as the medical conditions causing it!

NONPHARMACOLOGIC THERAPY

- Cognitive rehabilitation to promote recovery from brain injury may be helpful.
- Supervised living to ensure appropriate long-term care.

ACUTE GENERAL Rx

Initial treatment directed to the underlying etiology. Generally, transient global amnesia has full remission of symptoms. Korsakoff, on the other hand, is not usually improved significantly, even after administration of thiamine.

CHRONIC Rx

No known effective treatments to reverse or ameliorate memory deficits.

DISPOSITION

Amnesias may be chronic or transient depending upon etiology.

REFERRAL

Refer for neuropsychological testing.

TABLE 1-7 Clinico-Anatomical Correlations of Memory Disorders

Anatomic Site of Damage	Memory Finding	Other Neurological and Medical Findings
Frontal lobe	Lateralized deficits in working memory—right: spatial defects, left: verbal defects, impaired recall with spared recognition	Personality change Perseveration Chorea, dystonia Bradykinesia, tremor, rigidity
Basal forebrain	Domain-independent declarative memory deficits	
Ventromedial cortex	Frontal lobe-type declarative memory deficits	Upper visual field defects
Hippocampus and parahippocampal cortex	Bilateral lesions yield global amnesia, unilateral lesions show lateralization of deficits—left: verbal deficits; right: spatial deficits	Myoclonus Depressed level of consciousness Cortical blindness Autonomations
Fornix	Global amnesia	
Mammillary bodies	Declarative memory deficits	Confabulation, ataxia, nystagmus, signs of alcohol withdrawal
Dorsal and medial dorsal nucleus thalamus	Declarative memory deficits	Confabulation
Anterior thalamus	Declarative memory deficits	
Lateral temporal cortex	Deficits in autobiographical memory	

From Goetz CG, Pappert EJ: *Textbook of clinical neurology*, Philadelphia, 1999, WB Saunders.

⊘ PEARLS & CONSIDERATIONS

COMMENTS

In Korsakoff syndrome, anterograde amnesia (disturbance in acquisition of new information) is more prominent than retrograde amnesia (problems remembering old information).

PREVENTION

Cases of amnestic disorder due to trauma are usually not preventable. Refraining from abuse of alcohol and other drugs prevents substance induced amnestic disorder, and high-dose thiamine has been shown to prevent Korsakoff syndrome.

PATIENT & FAMILY EDUCATION

Respite care and in-home services for family caregivers

SUGGESTED READINGS

available at www.expertconsult.com

AUTHORS: **MITCHELL D. FELDMAN, M.D., M.PHIL.,** and **WASIM RASHID, M.D.**

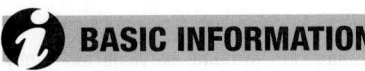

DEFINITION

The term *amyloidosis* refers to a heterogenous group of disorders that are all characterized by the deposition of an amorphous, extracellular fibrillar protein in various organs and tissues of the body. It has the following subtypes:

- Primary amyloidosis (AL)
- Secondary amyloidosis (AA)
- Hereditary amyloidosis
- Localized amyloidosis

ICD-9CM CODES
277.3 Amyloidosis

EPIDEMIOLOGY & DEMOGRAPHICS

INCIDENCE (IN U.S.): Between 1500 and 3500 new cases are diagnosed annually. The most common type is AL.
PREVALENCE: Amyloidosis primarily affects men between the ages of 60 and 70 yr.

PHYSICAL FINDINGS & CLINICAL PRESENTATION

- The most common presenting symptoms of amyloidosis are fatigue, dyspnea, edema, paresthesias, and weight loss. Other findings depend on organ system involvement.
- Signs and symptoms of nephrotic syndrome may be present with renal involvement.
- Fatigue and dyspnea may occur with pulmonary involvement.
- GI involvement is uncommon but presents with diarrhea, nausea, abdominal pain, and macroglossia.
- Patients with cardiac involvement have an infiltrative cardiomyopathy and present with a preserved ejection fraction (EF) and diastolic dysfunction.
- Patients may present with bleeding problems caused by either Factor X deficiency or fragile blood vessels caused by infiltration by amyloid. Bleeding around the eyes (raccoon eyes) is a characteristic finding.
- Involvement of the nervous system presents with peripheral neuropathy, muscle weakness, numbness, syncope, or dizziness. Associated autonomic neuropathy can also cause severe disabling symptoms.

ETIOLOGY

The deposition of an amorphous, extracellular fibrillar protein in various tissues that stains with Congo red is the common underlying mechanism, but there are important differences among various subtypes:

- AL is associated with an underlying clonal plasma cell disorder making an abnormal light chain protein with possible deposition in multiple organ system.
- AA has no underlying plasma cell disorder and is a consequence of longstanding systemic inflammation (e.g., tuberculosis, leprosy, malaria, untreated syphilis).
- Localized amyloidosis results from localized synthesis of fibrillar material with no underlying plasma cell disorder.
- Familial amyloidosis is another subtype, with the most common form resulting from mutation of transthretin gene *(TTR)*.

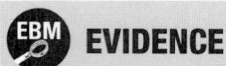 **DIAGNOSIS**

DIFFERENTIAL DIAGNOSIS

Differential diagnosis varies depending on the organ involvement:

- Renal involvement (toxin- or drug-induced necrosis, glomerulonephritis, renal vein thrombosis)
- Interstitial lung disease (sarcoidosis, connective tissue disease, infectious causative factors)
- Restrictive cardiomyopathy (endomyocardial fibrosis, viral myocarditis)
- Carpal tunnel (rheumatoid arthritis, hypothyroidism, overuse)
- Peripheral neuropathy (alcohol abuse, vitamin deficiencies, diabetes mellitus)

WORKUP

Workup consists of performing blood and urine tests to look for abnormal light chain in urine or blood, performing various tests to look for target organ damage, and getting histologic confirmation by doing a fat pad and bone marrow biopsy and then performing Congo red staining on that.

LABORATORY TESTS

- Immunofixation of serum and urine to look for immunoglobulin light chain is a sensitive screening test
- CBC, blood urea nitrogen (BUN)/creatinine, liver function tests, thyroid functions, and urine for albumin
- Histologic confirmation is necessary with a fat pad and bone marrow biopsy with Congo red staining to establish a diagnosis
- If a noninvasive fat pad biopsy does not establish a diagnosis, then a biopsy of the affected organ may be needed

IMAGING STUDIES

- Two-dimensional Doppler echocardiography to study diagnostic filling is useful to evaluate for cardiac involvement.
- Nuclear imaging with technetium-labeled aprotinin may detect cardiac amyloidosis. Serum amyloid P component (SAP) scintigraphy has high sensitivity for the detection of amyloid deposits in liver, spleen, kidneys, adrenal glands, and bones.

TREATMENT

ACUTE GENERAL Rx

- The goal of therapy is to decrease the production of the amyloidogenic light chain with therapy directed at the clonal plasma cells.
- All agents used to treat multiple myeloma are effective against AL including melphalan, prednisone, oral dexamethasone, systemic chemotherapy like cyclophosphamide, doxorubicin (Adriamycin), and more recently immunomodulatory compounds (IMiDs) molecules like thalidomide or lenalidomide, but none has shown to be superior to melphalan and prednisone, which remain the treatment of choice.
- Anti-tumor necrosis factor drugs may be useful to treat kidney amyloid A amyloidosis but may increase the risk and severity of infection.
- In highly selected patients with preserved organ function, autologous bone marrow transplant can have good results.
- Patients who experience development of renal failure can be supported with hemodialysis or renal transplant.
- Liver transplantation has been used successfully in patients with familial amyloidosis.
- Recognition and treatment of the underlying disorder is needed for secondary amyloidosis.

DISPOSITION

Prognosis is determined primarily by the presence or absence of cardiac involvement and the form of amyloidosis:

- In patients with endomyocardial biopsy-documented cardiac amyloidosis, longer-term survival is more strongly associated with NYHA functional class compared with ECG or echocardiography variables.
- In AA, eradication of the predisposing disease slows and can occasionally reverse the progression of amyloid disease. Median survival after diagnosis is 133 mo.
- Patients with familial amyloidotic polyneuropathy generally have a prolonged course lasting 10 to 15 yr.
- Amyloidosis associated with immunocytic processes carries the worst prognosis (life expectancy <1 yr).
- The progression of amyloidosis associated with renal hemodialysis can be improved with newer dialysis membranes that can pass beta 2-microglobulin.
- Median survival in patients with overt CHF is ~6 mo; it is 30 mo without CHF.
- Serum uric acid has a prognostic value in primary systemic amyloidosis. Patients with uric acid levels >8 mg/dl have a median overall survival of 9 mo from diagnosis compared with 20.3 mo for those with lower levels.

EBM **EVIDENCE**

available at www.expertconsult.com

SUGGESTED READINGS
available at www.expertconsult.com

AUTHORS: **BILAL H. NAQVI, M.D.,** and **FRED F. FERRI, M.D.**

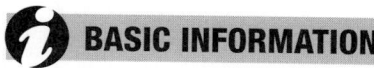 **BASIC INFORMATION**

DEFINITION

Amyotrophic lateral sclerosis (ALS) is a progressive, degenerative neuromuscular condition of undetermined etiology affecting corticospinal tracts and anterior horn cells, resulting in dysfunction of both upper motor neurons (UMN) and lower motor neurons (LMN), respectively.

SYNONYMS

Lou Gehrig's Disease

ICD-9CM CODES
335.20 Amyotrophic lateral sclerosis

EPIDEMIOLOGY & DEMOGRAPHICS

INCIDENCE: 0.5 to 2 cases per 100,000 persons. Onset is usually between the ages of 50 and 70 yr. Male/female ratio is 2:1.
PREVALENCE: Five in 100,000 persons

PHYSICAL FINDINGS & CLINICAL PRESENTATION

- LMN signs (weakness, hypotonia, wasting, fasciculations, hypoflexia or areflexia).
- UMN signs (loss of fine motor dexterity, spasticity, extensor plantar responses, hyperreflexia, clonus).
- Preservation of extraocular movements, sensation, bowel and bladder function.
- Dysarthria, dysphagia, pseudobulbar affect, frontal lobe dysfunction.
- Respiratory insufficiency typically occurs late in the disease.
- ALS comprises approximately 90% of adult-onset motor neuron diseases. Other presentations of motor neuron disease include progressive muscular atrophy, primary lateral sclerosis, progressive bulbar palsy, progressive pseudobulbar palsy, and ALS-parkinsonism-dementia complex.

ETIOLOGY

- 90% to 95% of all cases are sporadic; of the familial cases, 10% to 20% are associated with a genetic defect in the copper-zinc superoxide dismutase enzyme.

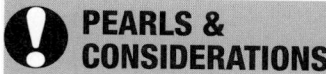 **DIAGNOSIS**

DIFFERENTIAL DIAGNOSIS

- Multifocal motor neuropathy with conduction block
- Cervical spondylotic myelopathy with polyradiculopathy
- Spinal stenosis with compression of lumbosacral nerve roots
- Chronic inflammatory demyelinating polyneuropathy with central nervous system lesions
- Syringomyelia
- Syringobulbia
- Foramen magnum tumor
- Meningeal carcinomatosis
- Spinal muscular atrophy
- Polyglucosan body disease
- Bulbospinal muscular atrophy (Kennedy disease)
- Monomyelic amyotrophy
- ALS-like syndromes have been reported in the setting of lead intoxication, HIV, hyperparathyroidism, hyperthyroidism, lymphoma, and B_{12} deficiency.

WORKUP

- Electromyography and nerve conduction studies (El Escorial criteria)
- Assessment of respiratory function (forced vital capacity [FVC], negative inspiratory force)

LABORATORY TESTS

- Vitamin B_{12}, thyroid function, parathyroid hormone, HIV may be considered.
- Serum protein and immunofixation electrophoresis.
- DNA studies for SMA or bulbospinal atrophy, hexosaminidase levels in pure LMN syndrome.
- 24-hour urine for heavy metals if indicated.

IMAGING STUDIES

- Craniospinal neuroimaging contingent on clinical scenario
- Modified barium swallow to evaluate aspiration risk

TREATMENT

NONPHARMACOLOGIC THERAPY

- Noninvasive positive-pressure ventilation may improve quality of life and may increase tracheostomy-free survival in patients with respiratory difficulty (defined by orthopnea or FVC 50% of predicted).
- Percutaneous endoscopic gastrostomy (PEG) tube placement improves nutritional intake, promotes weight stabilization, and eases medication administration. Some studies suggest PEG placement may prolong life 1 to 4 mo, particularly when placed before FVC falls to ≤50% of predicted value.
- Nutrition, speech therapy, physical and occupational therapy services.
- Suction device for sialorrhea.
- Communication may be eased with computerized assistive devices.

- Early discussion of living will, resuscitation orders, desire for PEG and tracheostomy, potential long-term care options.
- Encourage contact with local support groups.

ACUTE GENERAL Rx

Riluzole (Rilutek), a glutamate antagonist, is the only FDA-approved medication known to extend tracheostomy-free survival in patients with ALS. Dosage is 50 mg q12h, at least 1 hr before or 2 hr after meals. It is shown to prolong survival by 2 to 3 months. Manufacturer recommends checking alanine aminotransferase (ALT) once a month for 3 months initially, followed by once every 3 months until the first year of therapy is completed. ALT should be checked periodically thereafter.

CHRONIC Rx

- Sialorrhea may respond to either glycopyrrolate or amitriptyline (consider either propranolol or metoprolol if secretions are thick). Botulinum toxin may be effective in medically refractory cases.
- Spasticity may be treated pharmacologically with baclofen, tizanidine, clonazepam.
- Pseudobulbar affect may improve with amitriptyline, sertraline (Zoloft), or dextromethorphan/quinine.

DISPOSITION

- Mean duration of symptoms is 3 to 5 yr.
- Approximately 20% of patients survive >5 yr.

REFERRAL

- Referral to a neurologist experienced in neuromuscular disease is recommended to confirm the diagnosis. One prospective, population-based study suggested improved survival in subjects treated in a multidisciplinary clinic.
- Gastrointestinal referral for PEG placement is recommended while FVC remains >50% to minimize morbidity attributable to risks inherent to the procedure.

PEARLS & CONSIDERATIONS

- Patient-physician communication is an integral and essential part in both the initial diagnosis and subsequent treatment of ALS.
- A multidisciplinary approach to supportive care may lead to an improved level of daily functioning and foster an increased sense of independence.

SUGGESTED READINGS
available at www.expertconsult.com

AUTHOR: **TAYLOR HARRISON, M.D.**

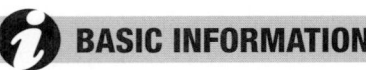

BASIC INFORMATION

DEFINITION

An anaerobic infection is caused by one of a group of bacteria that requires a reduced oxygen tension for growth.

ICD-9CM CODES
See specific condition.

PHYSICAL FINDINGS & CLINICAL PRESENTATION

- May occur at any site, but most are anatomically related to mucosal surfaces
- Should be suspected when there is foul-smelling tissue, soft tissue gas, necrotic tissue, or abscesses
- Head and neck
  1. Odontogenic infections from dental or soft tissue possibly progressing to periapical abscesses, at times extending to bone
  2. Both anaerobic and aerobic pathogens in chronic sinusitis, chronic mastoiditis, peritonsillar abscess, and chronic otitis media
  3. Complications: deep neck space infections, brain abscesses, mediastinitis
- Pleuropulmonary
  1. May involve anaerobes present in the oropharynx
  2. Aspiration more common in persons with altered mental status or seizures
  3. Anaerobic bacteria more likely in those with gingivitis or periodontitis
  4. Manifestations: necrotizing pneumonia, empyema, lung abscess
- Intraabdominal
  1. Disruption of intestinal integrity leading to infection involving anaerobic bacteria
  2. Bacteria from colonic neoplasm, perforated appendicitis, diverticulitis, or bowel surgery, causing bacteremia, peritonitis, at times intraabdominal abscesses
  3. Resulting infections usually mixed, containing both anaerobes and aerobes
- Female genital tract
  1. Anaerobes in bacterial vaginosis, salpingitis, endometritis, pelvic abscesses, septic abortion; infections tend to be mixed
  2. Possible pelvic thrombophlebitis when resolving pelvic infection is accompanied by new or persistent fever
- Other anaerobic infections
  1. Skin and soft tissue infection at any site
  2. More commonly associated infections: synergistic gangrene, bite wound infections, infected decubitus ulcers
  3. Clinical significance of anaerobes in diabetic foot infections unclear
  4. Anaerobic bacteremia uncommon with source usually intraabdominal, followed by female genital tract, pleuropulmonary, and head and neck infections
  5. Osteomyelitis especially when associated with decubitus ulcers or vascular insufficiency
  6. Facial bone osteomyelitis from adjacent infections of the teeth or sinuses

ETIOLOGY

- Most commonly endogenous, arising from bacteria that normally line mucosal surfaces
- Disruption of mucosal barriers resulting from various conditions (trauma, ischemia, surgery, perforation), with infection occurring when organisms gain access to normally sterile sites, causing tissue destruction and abscess formation
- Synergy between different anaerobes or between anaerobes and aerobes important

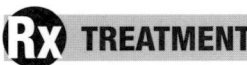

DIAGNOSIS

DIFFERENTIAL DIAGNOSIS

- Primary differential possibility is an aerobic bacterial infection without the presence of anaerobic bacteria.
- Ischemic necrosis without accompanying anaerobic infection (or "dry" gangrene [noninfected necrosis] vs. "wet" gangrene [infected tissue with anaerobic infection]).

WORKUP

- Specimens submitted for anaerobic culture should be processed within 30 min and may take up to 5 to 7 days to grow
- Large volume of material more likely to have significant growth; swabs less efficient for transporting infected material
- Blood cultures—preferably before antibiotic administration

LABORATORY TESTS

- Elevated WBC count, with extremely high WBC counts sometimes seen with pseudomembranous colitis
- Positive stool *C. difficile* toxin A and B assay
- Increased lactate levels in ischemia or perforation
- Possible positive blood or wound cultures, but failure to grow anaerobes in culture may be common, attributed to inadequate culturing techniques or fastidious organisms

IMAGING STUDIES

- Plain film of an affected area to show gas in tissues, free air resulting from a perforated viscus, or an air/fluid level inside an abscess
- Ultrasound, CT scan, or MRI to reveal abscesses or tissue destruction

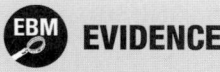

TREATMENT

NONPHARMACOLOGIC THERAPY

- Removal of necrotic tissue
- Drainage of abscesses (accomplished by CT scan–guided percutaneous drainage)

ACUTE GENERAL Rx

Oral antibiotics with anaerobic activity: clindamycin, metronidazole, and chloramphenicol
- Broader spectrum of activity with amoxicillin/clavulanate
- Penicillin VK in odontogenic infections
- Oral metronidazole for *C. difficile*–associated diarrhea, with oral vancomycin used for severe, recurrent, or recalcitrant infections

Parenteral antibiotics for more serious illness
- IV clindamycin, metronidazole, and chloramphenicol
- Cephalosporins (anaerobic or mixed infections): cefoxitin and cefotetan
- Extended-spectrum penicillins (e.g., piperacillin) and combination beta-lactamase plus beta-lactamase inhibitor drugs (e.g., clavulanic acid, sulbactam, tazobactam)
  1. Significant anaerobic activity, plus various degrees of broad-spectrum coverage
  2. Include ampicillin/sulbactam, ticarcillin/clavulanate, and piperacillin/tazobactam
- Imipenem or other carbapenems, such as meropenem or ertapenem, which are broad-spectrum agents with extensive anaerobic activity
- Actinomycosis treated with penicillin for 6 to 12 mo
- SMX/TMP and fluoroquinolones are generally ineffective, but some newer quinolones (e.g., moxifloxacin) have inhibitory activity against anaerobes

DISPOSITION

It is essential that all necrotic debris be removed when treating an anaerobic infection or it will recur; follow-up is critically important to ensure resolution of the process.

REFERRAL

Refer to a surgeon if drainage is required; infectious disease consultation may be useful in complicated patients or if treatment regimen is failing or slow to respond.

EBM EVIDENCE

available at www.expertconsult.com

SUGGESTED READING

available at www.expertconsult.com

AUTHORS: **GLENN G. FORT, M.D., M.P.H.,** and **DENNIS J. MIKOLICH, M.D.**

BASIC INFORMATION

DEFINITION

A fissure is a tear in the epithelial lining of the anal canal (i.e., from the dentate line to the anal verge).

SYNONYMS

Anorectal fissure
Anal ulcer

ICD-9CM CODES

565.0 Anal fissure

EPIDEMIOLOGY & DEMOGRAPHICS

PREDOMINANT SEX: Occurs in men more than women. Women are more likely to have anterior fissure than men (10% vs. 1%, respectively). Common in women before and after childbirth.
PREDOMINANT AGE: Can occur at any age. Most common in young and middle-aged adults. Most common cause of rectal bleeding in infants.

PHYSICAL FINDINGS & CLINICAL PRESENTATION

With separation of the buttocks will see a tear in the posterior midline or, less frequently, in the anterior midline (Fig. 1-23)
- Acute anal fissure:
  1. Sharp burning or tearing pain exacerbated by bowel movements
  2. Bright-red blood on toilet paper, a streak of blood on the stool or in the water

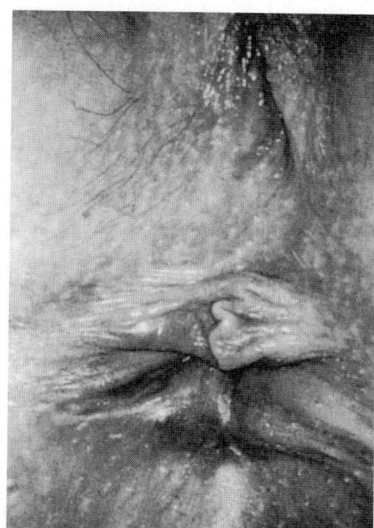

FIGURE 1-23 Lateral anal fissure. (In Seidel HM et al: *Mosby's guide to physical examination,* ed 3, St Louis, 1995, Mosby. Courtesy Gershon Efron, MD, Sinai Hospital of Baltimore.)

- Chronic anal fissure:
  1. Pruritus ani
  2. Pain seldom present
  3. Intermittent bleeding
  4. Sentinel tag at the caudal aspect of the fissure, hypertrophied anal papilla at the proximal end
- Underlying disease possible if the fissure:
  1. Is ectopically located
  2. Extends proximal to the dentate line
  3. Is broad-based or deep
  4. Is especially purulent

ETIOLOGY

- Most initiated after passage of a large, hard stool
- May result from frequent defecation and diarrhea
- Bacterial infections: tuberculosis (TB), syphilis, gonorrhea, chancroid, lymphogranuloma venereum
- Viral infections: herpes simplex virus, cytomegalovirus, human immunodeficiency virus
- Inflammatory bowel disease (IBD): Crohn's disease, ulcerative colitis
- Trauma: surgery (hemorrhoidectomy), foreign bodies, anal intercourse
- Malignancy: carcinoma, lymphoma, Kaposi sarcoma

DIAGNOSIS

DIFFERENTIAL DIAGNOSIS

- Proctalgia fugax
- Thrombosed hemorrhoid

WORKUP

- Digital rectal examination after lubricating the entire anus with anesthetic jelly (i.e., 2% lidocaine) and waiting 5 to 10 min
- Anoscopy
- Proctosigmoidoscopy to exclude inflammatory or neoplastic disease
- Biopsy if doubt exists about the etiology of the condition
- All studies done under adequate anesthesia

IMAGING STUDIES

- Colonoscopy or barium enema if diagnosis of IBD or malignancy is suspected
- Small-bowel series occasionally obtained for similar reasons
- Biopsy to reveal caseating granuloma if TB is suspected
- Wet prep with darkfield examination to demonstrate treponemes if syphilis is suspected

TREATMENT

NONPHARMACOLOGIC THERAPY

- Sitz baths
- High-fiber diet
- Increased oral fluid intake

ACUTE GENERAL Rx

- Bulk-producing agent (e.g., Metamucil) or stool softener
- Local anesthetic jelly (may exacerbate pruritus ani)
- Nitroglycerin ointment
- Suppositories *not* recommended
- Surgery

CHRONIC Rx

- Surgery: lateral internal anal sphincterotomy. It is a more durable treatment for chronic anal fissure compared with topical nitroglycerin therapy and does not compromise long-term fecal continence
- Topical glyceryl trinitrate ointment
- Injection of botulinum toxin (an injection into each side of the internal anal sphincter) is effective in healing chronic anal fissures in more than 90% of patients

DISPOSITION

Outpatient surgery

REFERRAL

- If fissure does not resolve with conservative therapy in 4 to 6 wk
- If patient prefers surgery for acute fissure
- If patient has chronic fissure

PEARLS & CONSIDERATIONS

COMMENTS

HIV-positive patients should be referred to clinicians who are well versed in the myriad infectious and neoplastic conditions that masquerade as anal ulcers in these patients.

EVIDENCE

available at www.expertconsult.com

SUGGESTED READINGS

available at www.expertconsult.com

AUTHORS: **GEORGE T. DANAKAS, M.D.,** and **RUBEN ALVERO, M.D.**

BASIC INFORMATION

DEFINITION

Anaphylaxis is a sudden-onset, life-threatening event characterized by bronchospasm in conjunction with hemodynamic changes. Its clinical presentation may include respiratory, cardiovascular, and cutaneous manifestations.

SYNONYMS

Anaphylactoid reaction is closely related to anaphylaxis. It is caused by release of mast cells and basophil mediators triggered by non–IgE–mediated events.

ICD-9CM CODES	
995.0	Anaphylactic shock
995.60	Anaphylaxis due to food
999.4	Anaphylaxis due to immunization
977.9	Anaphylaxis due to drugs
989.5	Anaphylaxis following stings

EPIDEMIOLOGY & DEMOGRAPHICS

INCIDENCE: From 20,000 to 50,000 persons each year in the U.S. Anaphylaxis rates are 0.0004% for food, 0.7% to 10% for penicillin, 0.22% to 1% for radiocontrast media, and 0.5% to 5% after insect stings. An estimated 1 in every 3000 inpatients in U.S. hospitals develops an anaphylactic reaction. Annual mortality is 500 to 1000 persons per year in the U.S.

PHYSICAL FINDINGS & CLINICAL PRESENTATION

- Urticaria, pruritus, skin flushing, angioedema, weakness, dizziness
- Dyspnea, cough, malaise, difficulty swallowing
- Wheezing, tachycardia, diarrhea
- Hypotension, vascular collapse

ETIOLOGY

Anaphylaxis results from sudden systematic release of histamine, tryptase, and other inflammatory mediators from basophils and mast cells. This causes swelling of the mucus membranes and the urticarial rash on the skin. Virtually any substance may induce anaphylaxis in a given individual.

- Commonly implicated medications are: antibiotics, especially penicillins, insulin, allergen extracts, opiates, vaccines, NSAIDs, contrast media, streptokinase
- Foods and food additives, nuts, egg whites, shellfish, fish, milk, fruits, and berries
- Blood products, plasma, immunoglobulin, cryoprecipitate, whole blood
- Venoms such as snake venom, fire ant venom, bee sting (*Hymenoptera* stings)
- Latex

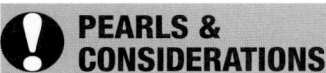 **DIAGNOSIS**

DIFFERENTIAL DIAGNOSIS

- Endocrine disorders (carcinoid, pheochromocytoma)
- Globus hystericus, anxiety disorder
- Systemic mastocytosis
- Pulmonary embolism, serum sickness, vasovagal reactions
- Severe asthma (the key clinical difference is the abrupt onset of symptoms in anaphylaxis without a history of progressive worsening of symptoms)
- Septic shock or other form of shock
- Airway foreign body

WORKUP

Workup is aimed at eliminating other conditions that may mimic anaphylaxis (e.g., vasovagal syncope may be differentiated by the presence of bradycardia as opposed to the tachycardia seen in anaphylaxis; the absence of hypoxemia in arterial blood gas [ABG] analysis may be useful to exclude pulmonary embolism or foreign body aspiration).

LABORATORY TESTS

- Laboratory evaluation is generally not helpful because the diagnosis of anaphylaxis is clinical.
- ABG analysis may be useful to exclude pulmonary embolism, status asthmaticus, and foreign body aspiration.
- Elevated serum and urine histamine levels can be useful for diagnosis of anaphylaxis, but these tests are not commonly available.

IMAGING STUDIES

Generally not helpful.

- Chest radiograph and evaluation for epiglottitis are indicated in patients with acute respiratory compromise.
- ECG should be considered in all patients with sudden loss of consciousness or reports of chest pains or dyspnea and in any elderly patient.

TREATMENT

NONPHARMACOLOGIC THERAPY

- Establish and protect airway. Provide supplemental O_2 if indicated.
- IV access should be rapidly established, and IV fluids (i.e., saline) should be administered. The patient should be placed supine or in Trendelenburg position if hemodynamically unstable.
- Cardiac monitoring is recommended.

ACUTE GENERAL Rx

- Epinephrine should be rapidly administered as an SC or IM injection at a dose of 0.01 ml/kg of aqueous epinephrine 1:1000 (maximum adult dose, 0.3 to 0.5 ml). The dose may be repeated approximately q5 to 10min if there is persistence or recurrence of symptoms. Endotracheal epinephrine should be considered if IV access is not possible during life-threatening reactions.
- Administration of H_1 and H_2 receptor antagonists is also recommended in the initial treatment of anaphylaxis.
  1. Administer diphenhydramine 25 to 50 mg IV or IM.
  2. Cimetidine 300 mg IV over 3 to 5 min, or ranitidine 50 mg IV, should be given initially; subsequent doses of H_1 and H_2 blockers can be given orally q6h for 48 hr.
- Corticosteroids are not useful in the acute episode because of their slow onset of action; however, they should be administered in most cases to prevent prolonged or recurrent anaphylaxis. Commonly used agents are hydrocortisone sodium succinate 250 to 500 mg IV q4 to 6h in adults (4 to 8 mg/kg for children) or methylprednisolone 40 to 250 mg IV in adults (1 to 2 mg/kg in children).
- Aerosolized β-agonists (e.g., albuterol, 2.5 mg, repeat prn 20 min) are useful to control bronchospasm.
- Additional useful agents in specific circumstances: atropine for refractory bradycardia, dopamine for refractory hypotension (despite volume expansion), and glucagon in patients on β-blocking drugs.

PEARLS & CONSIDERATIONS

COMMENTS

- Patient education regarding the nature of the illness and preventive measures is recommended. A documented history of previous anaphylactic episodes or known anaphylaxis triggers is the most reliable method of identifying individuals at risk.
- Prescription for prefilled epinephrine syringe (EpiPen) should be given, and the patient should be instructed on the use of this emergency kit in case of recurrent anaphylactic episodes.
- Patients should also be advised to carry or wear a MedicAlert ID describing substances that have caused anaphylaxis.
- Avoidance of radiologic contrast is also recommended in those who have had a prior reaction.
- Venom immunotherapy immediately after a sting is effective and recommended for up to 5 yr after the anaphylactic incident.

SUGGESTED READING
available at www.expertconsult.com

AUTHOR: **TARA M. WAYT, D.O.**

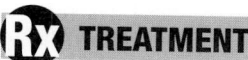

BASIC INFORMATION

DEFINITION

The anemia of chronic disease refers to mild to moderately severe anemias (with hemoglobin [Hb] ranging from 7-12 g/dl), associated with chronic infections and inflammatory disorders, and some malignancies. Anemia of chronic disease may also refer to normal total body iron stores with low circulating iron (<60 mcg/dl).

SYNONYMS

Anemia of inflammation

ICD-9CM CODES
285.21 Anemia in chronic kidney disease
285.22 Anemia in neoplastic disease
285.29 Anemia of other chronic illness
285.3 Antineoplastic chemotherapy induced anemia (effective October 1, 2009)
281.9 Unspecified deficiency anemia

EPIDEMIOLOGY & DEMOGRAPHICS

PREVALENCE: The prevalence rate in the elderly ranges from 8% to 44%, with the greatest prevalence in men 85 yr and older.
- Second-most prevalent anemia after iron deficiency anemia
- Perhaps one third of elderly adults with anemia suffer from anemia of chronic disease, anemia of chronic renal failure, or both
  - 11% of men and 10.2% of women age 65 to 85 yr
  - >20% of adults older than 85 yr

PREDOMINANT SEX AND AGE: Male sex >85 yr of age

RISK FACTORS:
- Chronic inflammatory conditions like autoimmune disorders (e.g., rheumatoid arthritis, systemic lupus erythematosus, vasculitis and sarcoidosis, inflammatory bowel disease [Crohn's disease/ulcerative colitis])
- Neoplasia (both hematologic cancer and solid tumors)
- Renal insufficiency/chronic kidney disease
- Infection (acute/chronic—viral, bacterial, parasitic, and fungal)
- Chronic rejection (graft vs. host disease) after solid-organ transplantation

PHYSICAL FINDINGS & CLINICAL PRESENTATION

Most patients are asymptomatic but may have general findings like skin pallor and conjunctival pallor.

ETIOLOGY

It is caused by several mechanisms (e.g., erythrocyte survival, increased uptake and retention of iron within cells of the reticuloendothelial system, inadequate transfer of iron from the reticuloendothelial system, limited availability of iron from erythroid progenitor cells, iron-restricted erythropoiesis.

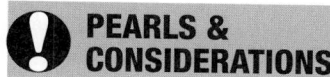

DIAGNOSIS

DIFFERENTIAL DIAGNOSIS

Iron deficiency anemia
Other causes of normocytic anemia
    Red blood cell loss or destruction
        Acute blood loss
        Hypersplenism
        Hemolysis
    Decreased red blood cell production
        Primary causes
            Marrow hypoplasia or aplasia
            Myelopathies
            Myeloproliferative disease
            Pure red blood cell aplasia
        Secondary causes
            Chronic renal failure
            Liver disease
            Endocrine deficiencies states
            Sideroblastic anemia

WORKUP

Detailed history and physical examination

LABORATORY TESTS

CBC, reticulocyte count, reticulocyte index and pheripheral smear, serum iron levels, total iron-binding capacity, percentage saturation, and ferritin and erythropoietin level, and sometimes even bone marrow biopsy. Usual findings are as follows:
- Hb levels (typically): 8 to 9.5 g/dl
- Low reticulocyte count (reflecting ineffective erythropoiesis)
- Low serum iron concentration (also low in iron deficiency anemia)
- Low transferrin saturation (also low in iron deficiency anemia)
- Serum ferritin (marker of iron storage) normal or increased[1]
  - Acute inflammatory states may mimic the hematologic profile of anemia of chronic disease
- Soluble transferrin receptor levels remain within normal limits (decreased in and deficiency anemia)
  - Transferrin receptor assay can distinguish iron deficiency anemia from anemia of chronic disease, even in patients with rheumatologic or other inflammatory disorders; number of transferrin receptors increased in iron deficiency anemia and normal in anemia of chronic disease; enzyme-linked immunosorbent assay (ELISA) testing seems as reliable as bone marrow aspiration
- Erythropoietin level
  - Levels become increased only when Hb <10 g/dl
- Mean corpuscular volume (MCV): 81 to 99 femtoliter (fl)

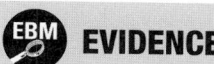

TREATMENT

Treat the underlying disorder/disease.

ACUTE GENERAL Rx

Blood transfusion usually reserved for severe anemia (Hb level <8.0 g/dl) or life-threatening anemia (Hb level <6.5 g/dl), particularly if complicated with ongoing bleeding. Increases survival rates in patients with anemia with myocardial infarction.

CHRONIC Rx

FDA-approved uses of erythropoiesis-stimulating agents epoetin alfa (Epogen, Procrit) and darbepoetin alfa (Aranesp):
- Treatment of anemia with target Hb level ≤12 g/dl in the following patients:
  - Patients with chronic kidney failure
  - Cancer patients receiving chemotherapy
  - Patients with HIV infection who are taking zidovudine

REFERRAL

Hematology and oncology

PEARLS & CONSIDERATIONS

COMMENTS

The anemia of inflammation, which also includes anemia of critical illness, is a condition that presents similarly to anemia of chronic disease but develops within days of the onset of illness. An anemia similar to anemia of inflammation is seen in some elderly patients in the absence of identifiable chronic disease.

PREVENTION

Consider checking Hb levels or CBC in patients with renal failure, cancer, or other chronic disease for screening purposes.

PATIENT/FAMILY EDUCATION

Am Fam Physician 2000 Nov 15;62(10):2264
http://www.mdconsult.com/das/patient/view/0/10041/32120.html/top (English version)
http://www.mdconsult.com/das/patient/view/0/10041/32121.html/top (Spanish version)

EVIDENCE

available at www.expertconsult.com

SUGGESTED READINGS

available at www.expertconsult.com

AUTHOR: **NADIA MUJAHID, M.D.**

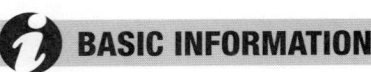

BASIC INFORMATION

DEFINITION
Aplastic anemia is a bone marrow failure syndrome defined by peripheral blood pancytopenia and hypocellular bone marrow.

SYNONYMS
Refractory anemia
Hypoplastic anemia

ICD-9CM CODES
284.9 Aplastic anemia
284.8 Acquired aplastic anemia
284.0 Congenital aplastic anemia

EPIDEMIOLOGY & DEMOGRAPHICS
INCIDENCE: The annual incidence of aplastic anemia is 2 cases per million.
PREDOMINANT SEX AND AGE: The incidence has two peaks, with most patients presenting between age 15 and 25 or after 60 yr.

PHYSICAL FINDINGS & CLINICAL PRESENTATION
- Mucosal bleeding, easy bruising, petechiae or heavy menstrual bleeding is seen secondary to thrombocytopenia.
- Fatigue, lassitude, skin pallor, exertional dyspnea, or palpitations are seen secondary to anemia.
- Infection is an uncommon presentation, but neutropenia may lead to fever and sore throat.
- Various physical manifestations like short stature, skeletal or nail changes may be seen in congenital forms of aplastic anemia.

ETIOLOGY
- In most patients with idiopathic aplastic anemia, bone marrow failure results from immunologically mediated, active destruction of blood-forming cells by lymphocytes.
- Mutations in *TERT,* the gene for the RNA component of telomerase, cause short telomerases in congenital aplastic anemia and in some cases of apparently acquired hematopoietic failure. In patients with severe aplastic anemia receiving immunosuppressive therapy, telomere length is unrelated to response but is associated with risk of relapse, clonal evolution, and overall survival.

- Common etiologic factors in acquired aplastic anemia include:
  - Toxins (e.g., benzene, insecticides)
  - Drugs (e.g., felbamate [Felbatol], cimetidine, NSAIDS, antiepileptics, gold salts, chloramphenicol, sulfonamides, trimethadione, quinacrine, phenylbutazone)
  - Ionizing irradiation
  - Infections (e.g., hepatitis C, HIV, Epstein-Barr virus, parvovirus B_{19})
- Inherited aplastic anemia
  - Fanconi's anemia
  - Reticular dysgenesis
  - Dyskeratosis congenita
  - Nonhematologic syndromes (Down syndrome, etc.)
  - Shwachman-Diamond syndrome
- Pregnancy
- Idiopathic

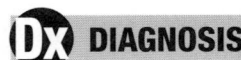

DIAGNOSIS

DIFFERENTIAL DIAGNOSIS
- Bone marrow infiltration from lymphoma, carcinoma, myelofibrosis
- Severe infection
- Hypoplastic myelodysplastic syndrome or hypoplastic acute myeloid leukemia in adults
- Hypersplenism
- Hairy cell leukemia

WORKUP
- Diagnostic workup consists primarily of bone marrow aspiration and biopsy, and laboratory evaluation (CBC and examination of blood film).
- Bone marrow examination generally shows paucity or absence of erythropoietic and myelopoietic precursor cells; patients with pure red cell aplasia demonstrate only absence of red blood cell (RBC) precursors in the marrow.

LABORATORY TESTS
- CBC reveals pancytopenia. Macrocytosis and toxic granulation of neutrophils may also be present. Isolated cytopenias may occur in the early stages.
- Reticulocyte count reveals reticulocytopenia.
- Additional initial laboratory evaluation should include Ham test to exclude paroxysmal nocturnal hemoglobinuria and testing for hepatitis C.

IMAGING STUDIES
MRI with spin-echo sequence is helpful in the study of bone marrow disease, and the high fat content of an aplastic marrow can be easily seen on MRI.

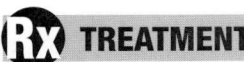

TREATMENT

NONPHARMACOLOGIC THERAPY
Discontinue any offending drugs or agents.

ACUTE GENERAL Rx
- Aggressive treatment of neutropenic fevers with parenteral broad-spectrum antibiotics.
- Administer platelet and RBC transfusions as needed; however, it is important to avoid transfusions in patients who are candidates for bone marrow transplantation.
- A treatment algorithm for aplastic anemia is described in Section III.

CHRONIC Rx
- Allogenic bone marrow transplantation (ABMT) from a human leukocyte antigen (HLA)–matched sibling donor is curative.
- Patients who do not have a matched sibling can be treated with a matched unrelated transplant, but the mortality rate is higher.
- Immunosuppressive therapy with anti-thymocyte globulin (ATG) is an effective alternate treatment for patients who are not candidates for ABMT.
- Other immunosuppressive agents such as cyclosporin, cyclophosphamide, or corticosteroids also have a role in the treatment of aplastic anemia.
- Androgens such as danazol are effective second-line agents.

DISPOSITION
- The most recent update of the European Group for Bone Marrow Translanlation long-term survival rate has been reported to be 80%.
- Graft rejection and graft-versus-host disease are the major complications of ABMT.

REFERRAL
Hematology referral is indicated in all patients with aplastic anemia.

SUGGESTED READINGS
available at www.expertconsult.com

AUTHORS: **BILAL H. NAQVI, M.D.,** and **FRED F. FERRI, M.D.**

BASIC INFORMATION

DEFINITION

Autoimmune hemolytic anemia (AIHA) is anemia secondary to premature destruction of red blood cells (RBCs) caused by the binding of autoantibodies and/or complement to RBCs.

ICD-9CM CODES
283.0 Autoimmune hemolytic anemia

EPIDEMIOLOGY & DEMOGRAPHICS

Predominant sex and age: most common in women <50 yr.

PHYSICAL FINDINGS & CLINICAL PRESENTATION

- Pallor, jaundice.
- Tachycardia with a flow murmur may be present if anemia is pronounced.
- Most common presentation is dyspnea and fatigue.
- Patients with intravascular hemolysis may present with dark urine and back pain.
- The presence of hepatomegaly and/or lymphadenopathy suggests an underlying lymphoproliferative disorder or malignancy; splenomegaly may indicate hypersplenism as a cause of hemolysis.

ETIOLOGY

- Warm antibody mediated: immunoglobulin (Ig) G (often idiopathic or associated with leukemia, lymphoma, thymoma, myeloma, viral infections, and collagen-vascular disease)
- Cold antibody mediated: IgM and complement in majority of cases (often idiopathic; at times associated with infections, lymphoma, or cold agglutinin disease)
- Drug induced: three major mechanisms:
  1. Antibody directed against Rh complex (e.g., methyldopa)
  2. Antibody directed against RBC-drug complex (hapten induced; e.g., penicillin)
  3. Antibody directed against complex formed by drug and plasma proteins; the drug-plasma protein-antibody complex causes destruction of RBCs (innocent bystander; e.g., quinidine)

DIAGNOSIS

DIFFERENTIAL DIAGNOSIS

- Hemolytic anemia caused by membrane defects (paroxysmal nocturnal hemoglobinuria, spur cell anemia, Wilson disease)
- Non–immune mediated (microangiopathic hemolytic anemia, hypersplenism, cardiac valve prosthesis, giant cavernous hemangiomas, march hemoglobinuria, physical agents, infections, heavy metals, certain drugs [nitrofurantoin, sulfonamides])

WORKUP

Evaluation consists primarily of laboratory evaluation to confirm hemolysis and exclude other causes of the anemia. Although most cases of AIHA are idiopathic, potential causes should always be sought. Section III describes an algorithm for evaluation of suspected hemolytic anemia.

LABORATORY TESTS

- Initial laboratory tests: complete blood count (anemia), reticulocyte count (elevated), liver function studies (elevated indirect bilirubin, lactate dehydrogenase), evaluation of peripheral smear, Coombs test (positive direct Coombs test indicates presence of antibodies or complement on the surface of RBCs; positive indirect Coombs test implies presence of anti-RBC antibodies freely circulating in the patient's serum), haptoglobin level (decreased)
- IgG antibody and IgM antibody
- Hepatitis serology, antinuclear antibody
- Urinary tests may reveal hemosiderinuria or hemoglobinuria

IMAGING STUDIES

- Chest radiograph
- CT scan of chest and abdomen to rule out lymphoma should be considered

TREATMENT

NONPHARMACOLOGIC THERAPY

- Discontinuation of any potentially offensive drugs
- Plasmapheresis exchange transfusion for severe life-threatening cases only
- Avoid cold exposure in patients with cold antibody

ACUTE GENERAL Rx

- Prednisone 1 to 2 mg/kg/day in divided doses initially in warm antibody autoimmune hemolytic anemia. Corticosteroids are generally ineffective in cold antibody autoimmune hemolytic anemia.
- Splenectomy in patients responding inadequately to corticosteroids when RBC sequestration studies indicate splenic sequestration.
- Immunosuppressive drugs and/or immunoglobulins only after both corticosteroids and splenectomy (unless surgery is contraindicated) have failed to produce an adequate remission.
- Danazol, typically used in conjunction with corticosteroids (may be useful in warm antibody autoimmune hemolytic anemia).
- Immunosuppressive drugs (azathioprine, cyclophosphamide) may be useful in warm antibody autoimmune hemolytic anemia but are indicated only after both corticosteroids and splenectomy (unless surgery is contraindicated) have failed to produce an adequate remission.

DISPOSITION

Prognosis is generally good unless anemia is associated with underlying disorder with a poor prognosis (e.g., leukemia, myeloma).

REFERRAL

- Hematology referral in all cases of AIHA
- Surgical referral for splenectomy in refractory cases

PEARLS & CONSIDERATIONS

COMMENTS

- The direct Coombs test (also known as the direct antiglobulin test) demonstrates the presence of antibodies or complement on the surface of RBCs and is the hallmark of autoimmune hemolysis.
- Warm AIHA is often associated with autoimmune diseases, whereas cold AIHA often follows viral infections (e.g., mononucleosis) and *Mycoplasma pneumoniae* infections.
- HIV can induce both warm and cold AIHA.

SUGGESTED READINGS
available at www.expertconsult.com

AUTHOR: **FRED F. FERRI, M.D.**

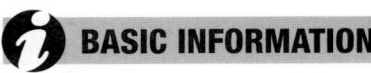
DEFINITION

Iron deficiency anemia is anemia resulting from inadequate iron supplementation or excessive blood loss.

ICD-9CM CODES
280.9 Iron deficiency anemia
648.2 Iron deficiency anemia complicating pregnancy

EPIDEMIOLOGY & DEMOGRAPHICS

- Dietary iron deficiency occurs often in infants as a result of unsupplemented milk diets. It is also commonly seen in women during their reproductive years, as a result of heavy menstrual periods, and during pregnancy (increased demand).
- Iron deficiency is the most common nutritional deficiency worldwide.
- The prevalence of iron deficiency is greatest among toddlers ages 1 to 2 yr (7%) from inadequate intake and female individuals ages 12 to 49 yr (9% to 16%) from menstrual losses.
- The prevalence of iron deficiency is 2% in adult men, 9% to 12% in non-Hispanic white women, and 20% in black and Mexican American women.
- GI cancer is diagnosed in 10% of elderly patients with iron deficiency anemia.

PHYSICAL FINDINGS & CLINICAL PRESENTATION

- Most patients have normal examination results.
- Skin pallor and conjunctival pallor may be present.
- Signs and symptoms specific for iron deficiency are koilonychias, pica, pagophagia, and blue sclera.
- Patients with severe anemia can have palpitations, headache, weakness, dizziness, and easy fatigability.

ETIOLOGY

- Blood loss from GI or menstrual bleeding (genitourinary blood loss less often the cause)
- Dietary iron deficiency (rare in adults)
- Poor iron absorption in patients with gastric or small-bowel surgery
- Repeated phlebotomy
- Increased requirements (e.g., during pregnancy)
- Other: traumatic hemolysis (abnormally functioning cardiac valves), idiopathic pulmonary hemosiderosis (iron sequestration in pulmonary macrophages), paroxysmal nocturnal hemoglobinuria (intravascular hemolysis)
- The most common cause worldwide is hookworm infection

DIAGNOSIS

DIFFERENTIAL DIAGNOSIS
(Table 1-8)
- Anemia of chronic disease
- Sideroblastic anemia
- Thalassemia trait
- Lead poisoning

WORKUP

Diagnostic workup consists primarily of laboratory evaluation. Most patients with iron deficiency anemia are asymptomatic in the early stages. With progressive anemia, the major symptoms are fatigue, dizziness, exertional dyspnea, pagophagia (ice eating), and pica. Patient history may also suggest GI blood loss (melena, hematochezia, hemoptysis).

LABORATORY TESTS

- Laboratory results vary with the stage of deficiency.
- Absent iron marrow stores and decreased serum ferritin are the initial abnormalities.
- Decreased serum iron and increased total iron-binding capacity (TIBC) are the next abnormalities.
- Hypochromic microcytic anemia is present with significant iron deficiency.
- Peripheral smear in patients with iron deficiency generally reveals microcytic hypochromic red blood cells (RBCs) with a wide area of central pallor, anisocytosis, and poikilocytosis when severe.
- Laboratory abnormalities consistent with iron deficiency are low serum ferritin level, increased RBC distribution width with values generally >15, low mean corpuscular volume, low mean corpuscular hemoglobin, increased TIBC, and low serum iron.
- In patients diagnosed with iron deficiency anemia, a GI workup including an upper endoscopy and colonoscopy is necessary to look for source of iron loss.

TREATMENT

The goal of therapy is to supply sufficient iron to correct the low hemoglobin and replenish iron stores.

NONPHARMACOLOGIC THERAPY

Patients should be instructed to consume foods that contain large amounts of iron, such as liver, red meat, and legumes.

ACUTE GENERAL Rx

- Treatment consists of ferrous sulfate 325 mg PO daily for at least 6 mo. Calcium supplements can decrease iron absorption; therefore, these two medications should be staggered.
- Parenteral iron therapy is reserved for patients with poor tolerance, noncompliance with oral preparations, or malabsorption.
- Transfusion of packed RBCs is indicated in patients with severe symptomatic anemia (e.g., angina) or life-threatening anemia.

CHRONIC Rx

Patients should be instructed to continue their iron supplements for at least 6 mo or longer to correct depleted body iron stores.

TABLE 1-8 Differential Diagnosis of Iron Deficiency: Clinical and Laboratory Features

History/Physical Examination	Iron	Total Iron-Binding Capacity	Ferritin	Smear	Red Cell Distribution Width	Marrow Iron
Iron Deficiency						
Bleeding Pica Angular cheilosis Koilonychia Dysphagia	↓	↑	↓	Microcytosis Hypochromia Pencil shapes	↑	Absent
Anemia of Chronic Disease						
Chronic infection or inflammation	↓	↓	↑	RBC normal (1/4 microcytosis)	Normal	↑ (in reticuloendothelial system, not RBC precursors)
Thalassemia Trait						
Family history Splenomegaly (±)	Normal/↑	Normal	↑	Microcytosis Targets Hypochromia	Normal	↑

RBC, Red blood cells.
Carlson KJ et al: *Primary care of women*, ed 2, St Louis, 2002, Mosby.

DISPOSITION

Most patients respond rapidly to iron supplementation with improvement in CBC and general well-being. GI side effects from oral iron therapy are common and may require decreased dosage to once every other day or to change to parenteral iron.

REFERRAL

GI referral for evaluation of GI malignancy is recommended in all patients with iron deficiency and suspected GI blood loss.

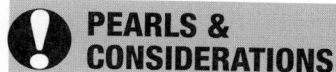

COMMENTS

- Iron deficiency may impair aerobic performance and worsen symptoms in patients with heart failure. Treatment with IV ferric carboxymaltose in patients with chronic heart failure and iron deficiency has been shown to improve symptoms, quality of life, and functional capacity.
- If the diagnosis of iron deficiency anemia is made, locating the suspected site of iron loss is mandatory.

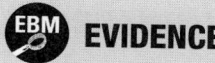

available at www.expertconsult.com

SUGGESTED READINGS

available at www.expertconsult.com

AUTHORS: **BILAL H. NAQVI, M.D.,** and **FRED F. FERRI, M.D.**

A

Diseases and Disorders

I

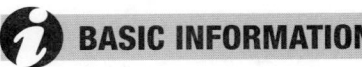

BASIC INFORMATION

DEFINITION

Pernicious anemia (PA) is an autoimmune disease resulting from antibodies against intrinsic factor and gastric parietal cells.

SYNONYMS

Megaloblastic anemia resulting from vitamin B_{12} deficiency

ICD-9CM CODES
281.0 Pernicious anemia

EPIDEMIOLOGY & DEMOGRAPHICS

- Increased incidence in females and older adults (diagnosis is unusual before age 35 yr)
- The overall prevalence of undiagnosed PA after age 60 yr is 1.9%
- Prevalence is highest in women (2.7%), particularly in black women (4.3%)
- Increased incidence of autoimmune disease (e.g., type 1 diabetes mellitus, Graves disease, Addison disease), *Helicobacter pylori* infection

PHYSICAL FINDINGS & CLINICAL PRESENTATION

- Mucosal pallor, glossitis
- Peripheral sensory neuropathy with paresthesias initially and absent reflexes in advanced cases
- Loss of joint position sense, pyramidal or long track signs
- Possible splenomegaly and mild hepatomegaly
- Generalized weakness and delirium/dementia

ETIOLOGY

- Gastric/antiparietal cell antibodies in >70% of patients; antiintrinsic factor antibodies in >50% of patients
- Atrophic gastric mucosa
- Inborn errors of cobalamin-cofactor synthesis are rare. The cobalamin gene *(cblD)* is localized to human chromosome 2q23.2. Mutations in the gene designated MMADHC (methylmalonic aciduria, cblD type, and homocystinuria) are responsible for the cblD defect in vitamin B_{12} metabolism.
- An etiopathophysiologic classification of cobalamin deficiency is described in Section II.

DIAGNOSIS

DIFFERENTIAL DIAGNOSIS

- Nutritional vitamin B_{12} deficiency
- Malabsorption
- Chronic alcoholism (multifactorial)
- Chronic gastritis related to *H. pylori* infection
- Folic acid deficiency
- Myelodysplasia

WORKUP

- The clinical presentation of pernicious anemia varies with the stage. Initially, patients may be asymptomatic. In advanced stages patients may have impaired memory, depression, gait disturbances, paresthesias, and reports of generalized weakness.
- Investigation consists primarily of laboratory evaluation.
- Endoscopy and biopsy for atrophic gastritis may be performed in selected cases.
- Diagnosis is crucial because failure to treat may result in irreversible neurologic deficits.

LABORATORY TESTS

- Complete blood count generally reveals macrocytic anemia and leukopenia with hypersegmented neutrophils.
- Mean corpuscular volume (MCV) is generally significantly elevated in the advanced stages.
- Reticulocyte count is low to normal.
- Falsely low serum cobalamin levels can occur in patients with severe folate deficiency, in patients using high doses of ascorbic acid, and when cobalamin levels are measured after nuclear medicine studies (radioactivity interferes with cobalamin radioimmunoassay measurement).
- Falsely high normal levels in patients with cobalamin deficiency can occur in severe liver disease or chronic granulocytic leukemia.
- The absence of anemia or macrocytosis does not exclude the diagnosis of cobalamin deficiency. Anemia is absent in 20% of patients with cobalamin deficiency, and macrocytosis is absent in >30% of patients at the time of diagnosis. It can be blocked by concurrent iron deficiency or anemia of chronic disease and may be masked by thalassemia trait.
- Schilling test is abnormal in part I; part II corrects to normal after administration of intrinsic factor.
- Laboratory tests used for detecting cobalamin deficiency in patients with normal vitamin B_{12} levels include serum and urinary methylmalonic acid level (elevated), total homocysteine level (elevated), intrinsic factor antibody (positive).
- An increased concentration of plasma methylmalonic acid does not predict clinical manifestations of vitamin B_{12} deficiency and should not be used as the only marker for diagnosis of B_{12} deficiency.
- Additional laboratory abnormalities can include elevated lactate dehydrogenase, direct hyperbilirubinemia, and decreased haptoglobin.

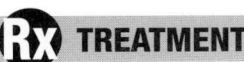

TREATMENT

NONPHARMACOLOGIC THERAPY

Avoid folic acid supplementation without proper vitamin B_{12} supplementation.

ACUTE GENERAL Rx

Traditional therapy of a cobalamin deficiency consists of IM injections of vitamin B_{12} 1000 mcg/wk for the initial 4 to 6 wk followed by 1000 mcg/mo IM indefinitely. When hematologic parameters have returned to normal range, intranasal cyanocobalamin may be used in place of IM cyanocobalamin. The initial dose of intranasal cyanocobalamin (Nascobal) is 1 spray (500 mcg) in one nostril once per week. Cost generally exceeds $120/mo. Monitor response and increase dose if serum B_{12} levels decline. Consider return to intramuscular vitamin B_{12} supplementation if decline persists.

CHRONIC Rx

Parenteral vitamin B_{12} 1000 mcg/mo or intranasal cyanocobalamin 500 mcg/wk (see "Acute General Rx") for the remainder of life

DISPOSITION

Anemia generally resolves with appropriate treatment. Neurologic deficits, if present at diagnosis, may be permanent.

REFERRAL

Gastrointestinal referral for endoscopy on diagnosis of pernicious anemia and surveillance endoscopy every 5 yr to rule out gastric carcinoma

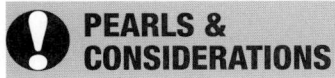

PEARLS & CONSIDERATIONS

COMMENTS

- Patients must understand that therapy is lifelong.
- Self-injection of vitamin B_{12} may be taught in selected patients. Cost of monthly injection is less than $5.
- Oral cobalamin (1000 to 2000 mcg/day) has been reported as also being effective in mild cases of pernicious anemia because approximately 1% of an oral dose is absorbed by passive diffusion, a pathway that does not require intrinsic factor. Cost for 1 mo of therapy is approximately $5.

SUGGESTED READING
available at www.expertconsult.com

AUTHOR: **FRED F. FERRI, M.D.**

BASIC INFORMATION

DEFINITION

Sideroblastic anemia is a heterogenous group of blood disorders whose two distinctive features are ring sideroblasts in the bone marrow (abnormal erythroblasts with excessive iron accumulation in the mitochondria) and impaired heme biosynthesis. They are classified as hereditary, acquired, and reversible.

SYNONYMS

Hereditary sideroblastic anemias
Acquired idiopathic sideroblastic anemia (AISA)
Reversible sideroblastic anemias

ICD-9CM CODES
285.0 Sideroblastic anemia

EPIDEMIOLOGY & DEMOGRAPHICS

- Sex-linked; primarily affects males.
- AISA affects middle-aged and older adults.

PHYSICAL FINDINGS & CLINICAL PRESENTATION

The symptoms for sideroblastic anemia are the same for any anemia and iron overload:
- Fatigue, weakness, palpitations, shortness of breath, headaches, irritability, and chest pain.
- Physical findings may include pallor, tachycardia, hepatosplenomegaly, S3 gallop, jugular vein distension, and rales.

ETIOLOGY

- The hereditary forms can be X-linked, autosomal dominant or autosomal recessive.
- Acquired forms may be associated with chemotherapy or irradiation.
- Refractory anemia with ringed sideroblast develops as a subtype of myelodysplacia.
- Reversible sideroblastic anemia can be caused by alcohol, isoniazid, pyrazinamide, cycloserine, chloramphenicol, or copper deficiency.

DIAGNOSIS

The principle feature is indolent and progressive, mild, lifelong anemia that goes unnoticed. Symptoms of iron overload may lead to discovery of the underlying disorder. The history and clinical findings, together with typical laboratory findings, usually permit accurate diagnosis of each type of sideroblastic anemia. The molecular defects can be identified in several hereditary forms and in some patients with AISA.

DIFFERENTIAL DIAGNOSIS

- Sideroblastic anemia must be differentiated from other causes of microcytic hypochromic anemia: iron deficiency anemia, thalassemia, anemia of chronic disease, and lead poisoning.
- Tissue iron overload from sideroblastic anemia may act similar to hereditary hemochromatosis with liver cirrhosis, diabetes, congestive heart failure, or cardiac arrhythmias.

WORKUP

Laboratory evaluation: complete blood count, iron studies, free erythrocyte protoporphyrin level (FEP); MRI, bone marrow aspiration, and liver biopsy.

LABORATORY TESTS

- Hypochromic microcytic anemia for the hereditary type and normo or macrocytic anemia for AISA.
- High serum iron levels, low transferrin along with increased transferrin saturation and high serum ferritin.
- Peripheral smear: dimorphic large and small cells revealing Pappenheimer bodies or siderocytes when stained for iron.
- Bone marrow shows the classic ringed sideroblasts not seen in normal bone marrow tissue (Fig. 1-24). The ringed sideroblasts represent iron storage in the mitochondria of normoblasts.
- In transfusion-dependent anemias, monitoring of ferritin and transferrin saturation levels is recommended despite minimal transfusion needs to avoid iron overload.
- Features of infective erethropoeisis like increase in bilirubin concentration, decrease in hepatoglobin, increase in LDH, and normal or increase in reticulocyte no is seen.

TREATMENT

Treatment is directed at controlling symptoms of anemia and preventing organ damage from iron overload.

NONPHARMACOLOGIC THERAPY
Avoid alcohol

ACUTE GENERAL Rx

- A trial of pyridoxine (100-200 mg) is indicated for all patients with hereditary sideroblastic anemia.
- 25% to 50% may show full or partial response to pyridoxine.
- Patients who do not respond will need to be treated with blood transfusion.
- Chelation therapy is needed for patients with transfusion-dependant anemia to prevent complications of iron overload.
- Erythropoietin and granulocyte colony-stimulating factor may show some success in treating MDS-associated refractory anemia with ringed sideroblast.
- Secondary sideroblastic anemia caused by medication can be reversed by withdrawing the medication and administering vitamin B_6 (50 to 200 mg/day).

CHRONIC Rx

- Organ dysfunction resulting from iron overload will require periodic phlebotomy to keep serum ferritin level <500 mcg/L.
- Iron chelating therapy for patients with moderately severe anemia in those who require regular red cell transfusion: deferoxamine continuous infusion or the oral agent deferasirox (EXJADE)
- Splenectomy should be avoided at all costs.

DISPOSITION

In patients with anemia alone, life expectancy is normal. In patients dependent on blood transfusions, morbidity from iron overload can be expected. Some patients with acquired sideroblastic anemia develop leukemia. There are two types of AISA:
1. Pure sideroblastic anemia: with dysplasia confined to the erythroid cell lineage; survival similar to age-matched controls; no incidence of leukemic transformation.
2. Refractory anemia with ringed sideroblasts: dysplastic features involving the red cell lineage, granulopoiesis and/or megakaryopoiesis; approximately 5% will develop acute leukemia. Erythropoietin and granulocyte colony-stimulating factor therapy do not change survival.

REFERRAL

- Hematology.
- Families with severe forms of hereditary sideroblastic anemia should receive genetic counseling.

PEARLS & CONSIDERATIONS

- Sideroblastic anemia can be thought of as an iron-loading anemia secondary to defective heme synthesis.
- A predisposition to leukemia evolution has not been observed in patients with hereditary forms.
- Symptoms rather than an absolute hemoglobin level or hematocrit should guide transfusion therapy.

COMMENTS

Vitamin B_6, or pyridoxal phosphate, is a required cofactor in heme synthesis, and drugs such as isoniazid, cycloserine, and pyrazinamide can inhibit its function.

SUGGESTED READINGS
available at www.expertconsult.com

AUTHOR: **BILAL H. NAQVI, M.D.**

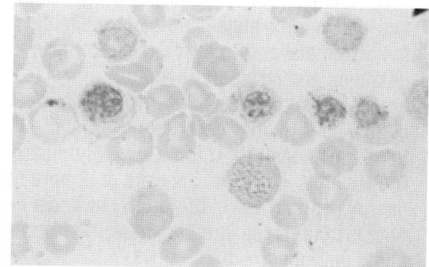

FIGURE 1-24 Prussian blue iron stain of the bone marrow shows ringed sideroblasts. (From Goldman L, Ausiello D [eds]: *Cecil textbook of medicine*, ed 22, Philadelphia, 2004, WB Saunders.)

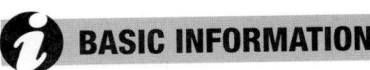

DEFINITION

An abdominal aortic aneurysm (AAA) is a permanent localized dilation of the abdominal aortic artery to at least 1.5 times the diameter measured at the level of the renal arteries; or exceeding the normal diameter of the abdominal aorta by >50%. The normal diameter at the renal arteries is 2.0 cm (range, 1.4 to 3.0 cm), and a diameter >3.0 cm is generally considered aneurysmal.

SYNONYMS

AAA

ICD-9CM CODES
441.4 Aneurysm, abdominal (aorta)
441.3 Ruptured abdominal aortic aneurysm

EPIDEMIOLOGY & DEMOGRAPHICS

- AAA is predominantly a disease of older adults, affecting men more than women (4:1).
- The prevalence rate ranges from 4% to 9% in men >60 yr.
- Clinically important AAAs >4.0 cm are present in 1% of men ages 55 to 64 yr, and the prevalence rate increases by 2% to 4% per decade thereafter.
- Approximately 15,000 deaths/yr in the U.S. are attributed to AAA.
- The peak incidence is among males ~70 yr of age, the prevalence among males over 60 yr totals 2% to 6%. The frequency is much higher in smokers than in nonsmokers (8:1), and the risk decreases slowly after smoking cessation.
- AAA is 4-6 times more common in male siblings of known patients, with a risk of 20% to 30%.
- Rupture of the AAA occurs in 1% to 3% of men aged 65 or more. Rupture is the tenth-leading cause of death in men >55 yr. Mortality from rupture is 70% to 95%.
- Risk factors for AAA are similar to other atherosclerotic cardiovascular diseases, including smoking, hypertension, hyperlipidemia, male sex, peripheral vascular disease, and family history of AAA.

PHYSICAL FINDINGS & CLINICAL PRESENTATION

- Most aneurysms are asymptomatic and incidentally discovered on imaging studies; however, symptomatic aneurysms are at an increased risk for rupture
- Physical examination has a sensitivity of 76% for detecting AAAs >5 cm and only 29% for AAAs 3.0 to 3.9 cm
- Pulsatile epigastric mass that may or may not be tender
- Abdominal pain radiating to the back, flank, and groin
- Abdominal bruits can be present in case of renal or visceral arterial stenosis
- Early satiety, nausea, and vomiting caused by compression of adjacent bowel
- Venous thrombosis from iliocaval venous compression
- Discoloration and pain of the feet from distal embolization of the thrombus within the aneurysm
- Flank and groin pain from ureteral obstruction and hydronephrosis
- Rupture presents as shock, organ hypoperfusion, and abdominal distention
- Rare presentations include hematemesis or melena associated with abdominal and back pain in patients with aortoenteric fistulas
- Aortocaval fistulas may also form and produce loud abdominal bruits

ETIOLOGY

- Atherosclerotic (degenerative or nonspecific)
- Genetic: high familial prevalence rate is notable in male individuals. Unclear as to the nature of the genetic disorder, but may be linked to alpha-1-antitrypsin deficiency or X-linked mutation. Connective tissue disorders, such as Marfan syndrome and Ehlers-Danlos syndrome, have also been strongly associated with AAA. Familial clusters are common, and genetic defects in elastin and collagen degradation by proteases such as plasmin, matrix metalloproteinases, and cathepsin S and K can be seen
- Traumatic injury
- Tobacco use: >90% of people who develop an AAA have smoked at some point in their life
- Cystic medial necrosis (Marfan syndrome)
- Arteritis, inflammatory
- Mycotic, infected (syphilis)

NATURAL HISTORY

- Understanding the natural history of AAA is important in its management. The likelihood that an aneurysm will rupture is largely influenced by aneurysm diameter, rate of expansion, and sex. Other factors associated with increased risk for rupture include continued smoking, uncontrolled hypertension, and increased wall stress.
- AAA tend to develop in the infrarenal aorta. The diameter of the aorta decreases from the root to the distal abdominal aorta. The distal portion also contains less elastin.
- Higher tension in the abdominal aorta (together with histopathologic changes such as accumulation of foam cells, cholesterol crystals and matrix metalloproteinases) renders the abdominal aortic wall more susceptible to dilatation and subsequent rupture.
- The 5-yr rupture rate of asymptomatic AAAs is 25% to 40% for aneurysms >5.0 cm, 1% to 7% for AAAs of 4.0 to 5.0 cm, and nearly 0% for AAAs <4.0 cm. The rate of rupture of aneurysms that were 4.0 to 5.5 cm in diameter is four times greater in women compared with men.
- Mortality rate after rupture is >90% because most patients do not reach the hospital in time for surgical repair. Of those who reach the hospital, the mortality rate is still 50% compared with the 1% to 4% mortality rate for elective repair of a nonruptured AAA.

DIFFERENTIAL DIAGNOSIS

Almost 75% of AAAs are asymptomatic and are discovered on routine examination or serendipitously when ordering studies for other symptoms. Diagnosis of AAA should be considered in the differential of the following conditions:
- Abdominal pain
- Back pain
- Pulsatile abdominal mass

IMAGING STUDIES (Fig. 1-25)

- Plain radiographs may show the outline of an aneurysm in calcified aortas. This is an insensitive test for diagnosing AAA.
- Abdominal ultrasound is nearly 100% accurate in identifying an aneurysm and estimating the size to within 0.3 to 0.4 cm. It is not accurate in estimating the extension to the renal arteries or the iliac arteries.
- CT scan is recommended for preoperative aneurysm imaging and estimates the size of the AAA to within 0.3 mm. There are no false-negative results, and the scan can localize the extent to renal vessels with more precision than ultrasound. CT can also detect the integrity of the wall and exclude rupture.
- Magnetic resonance angiography may also be used and is at least as accurate as CT.
- Angiography gives detailed arterial anatomy, localizing the aneurysm relative to the renal and visceral arteries. This is the definitive preoperative study before surgery.

NONPHARMACOLOGIC THERAPY

- Despite lack of data substantiating reduction in expansion rate through treatment of cardiac risk factors, nonpharmacologic treatment continues to focus on risk factor modification (most importantly smoking cessation, diet, and exercise).
- Serial studies have shown that expansion rates are faster in current smokers than in former smokers.
- Definitive treatment depends on the size of the aneurysm (see "Chronic Rx").

ACUTE GENERAL Rx

- AAA rupture is an emergency.
- Emergent open repair is the traditional method of treatment. However, more centers are increasingly using endovascular repair for patients who fit certain anatomic and physiologic criteria.

CHRONIC Rx

- Blood pressure and fasting lipids should be monitored and controlled as recommended for patients with atherosclerotic disease. Anti-hyperlipidemic agents such as the statin family of drugs should be prescribed unless contraindications are present.
- The most commonly used predictor of rupture is the maximum diameter of the AAA.

A

- Monitoring by ultrasound or CT scan should be performed every 6 to 12 months for AAAs measuring 4.0 to 5.4 cm. In patients with AAAs smaller than 4.0 cm, every 2 to 3 yr is reasonable.
- Beta-blocker therapy may have a role in slowing AAA expansion rates, but conclusive evidence is still lacking.
- Antibiotics such as doxycycline and roxithromycin have potential to limit the growth of AAAs, as shown in small human studies with promising results.
- Surgical repair to eliminate the risk for rupture should be performed for patients with infrarenal or juxtarenal AAA of approximately 5.5 cm. Repair is possibly beneficial for AAAs of 5.0 to 5.4 cm.

- Intervention is not recommended for asymptomatic infrarenal or juxtarenal AAAs <5.0 cm in men or 4.5 cm in women.
- For the high-risk patient, percutaneous, endovascular, stent-anchored grafts placed with the patient under local anesthesia have provided an alternative approach (Fig. 1-26).
- Randomized trials have shown that endovascular repair of AAA is associated with a significantly lower operative mortality than open surgical repair but it has increased rates of graft-related complications, increased rates of reintervention, and is more costly. There are no differences in total mortality or aneurysm-related mortality in the long term between endovascular repair and open surgical repair.

REFERRAL

Vascular surgical referral should be made in asymptomatic patients with AAAs that are approximately 4.0 cm or in rapidly expanding aneurysms of 0.6 to 0.8 cm/yr, especially if symptoms are present.

PEARLS & CONSIDERATIONS

- The U.S. Preventive Services Task Force recommends one-time screening for AAA by ultrasonography in men age 65 to 75 yr who have ever smoked.
- Repairing AAAs smaller than 5.5 cm has not been shown to improve survival.
- Endovascular repair is associated with lower operative mortality than open repair, and similar mid-term and long-term mortality. It has not been shown to improve overall survival in patients unfit for open repair, but is associated with lower aneurysm-related mortality compared with no repair.

COMMENTS

- Most AAAs are infrarenal.
- Surgical risk is increased in patients with coexisting coronary artery disease, pulmonary disease, liver cirrhosis, or chronic renal failure. Evaluation for ischemia and aggressive perioperative hemodynamic monitoring help identify high-risk patients and decrease postoperative complications.
- It is estimated that AAAs <5 cm expand at a rate of 0.4 cm/yr.

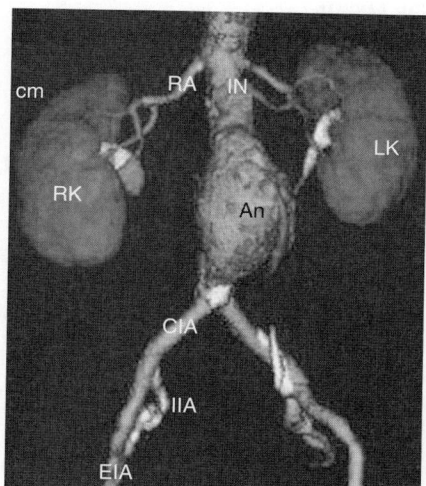

FIGURE 1-25 Three-dimensional CT image illustrates the presence of an infrarenal abdominal aortic aneurysm. *An,* Aneurysm; *CIA,* common iliac artery; *EIA,* external iliac artery; *IIA,* internal iliac artery; *IN,* infrarenal neck; *LK,* left kidney; *RA,* renal artery; *RK,* right kidney. (From Townsend CM et al [eds]: *Sabiston Textbook of Surgery,* ed 17, Philadelphia, 2004, Saunders.)

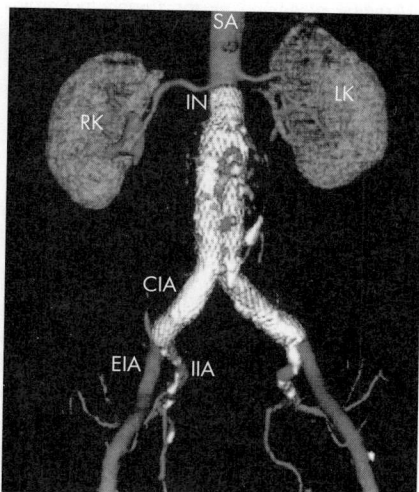

FIGURE 1-26 Endovascular abdominal aortic aneurysm repair involves aneurysm exclusion with an endoluminal aortic stent-graft introduced remotely, usually through the femoral artery. An endovascular graft extends from the infrarenal aorta to both common iliac arteries, preserving the flow to the internal iliac arteries. *CIA,* Common iliac artery; *IIA,* internal iliac artery; *IN,* infrarenal aortic neck; *LK,* left kidney; *RK,* right kidney; *SA,* suprarenal aorta. (From Townsend CM et al [eds]: *Sabiston textbook of surgery,* ed 17, Philadelphia, 2004, Saunders.)

EVIDENCE

available at www.expertconsult.com

SUGGESTED READINGS

available at www.expertconsult.com

AUTHORS: **NAUMAN SIDDIQI, M.D.,** and **PRANAV M. PATEL, M.D.**

Diseases and Disorders

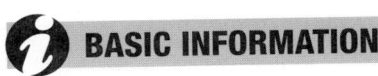

BASIC INFORMATION

DEFINITION

Angina pectoris is a term used to describe a syndrome, typically characterized by chest discomfort, that is caused by myocardial ischemia. This is most commonly related to atheromatous plaque in the coronary arteries; however, myocardial ischemia may occur in the absence of obstructive CAD. Any situation that causes an imbalance in myocardial oxygen supply and demand can cause an angina syndrome. Myocardial ischemia can be asymptomatic (silent ischemia), particularly in diabetics. Angina can be classified as follows:

1. Chronic (stable):
   - Usually follows a precipitating event (e.g., climbing stairs, sexual intercourse, a heavy meal, emotional stress, cold weather).
   - Generally same severity as previous attacks; relieved by rest or by the customary dose of nitroglycerin.
   - Caused by a fixed coronary artery obstruction secondary to atherosclerosis. The presence of one or more obstructions in major coronary arteries is likely; the severity of stenosis is usually >70%.
2. Unstable (rest or crescendo, coronary syndrome):
   - Recent onset
   - Increasing severity, duration, or frequency of chronic angina
   - Occurs at rest or with minimal exertion
3. Prinzmetal's variant:
   - Occurs at rest
   - Manifests electrocardiographically as episodic ST-segment elevations
   - Caused by coronary artery spasms with or without superimposed coronary artery disease (CAD)
   - Patients also more likely to develop ventricular arrhythmias
4. Microvascular angina (syndrome X):
   - Refers to patients with normal coronary angiograms and no coronary spasm but chest pain resembling angina and positive exercise test.
   - Defective endothelium-dependent dilation in the coronary microcirculation contributing to the altered regulation of myocardial perfusion and the ischemic manifestations in these patients.
   - Patients with chest pain and normal or nonobstructive coronary angiograms are predominantly women, and many have a prognosis that is not as benign as commonly thought (2% risk of death or myocardial infarction [MI] at 30 days of follow-up).
5. Other:
   - Angina due to aortic stenosis and idiopathic hypertrophic subaortic stenosis, cocaine-induced coronary vasoconstriction.
6. Refractory angina:
   - Refers to patients who, despite optimal medical therapy, have both angina and objective evidence of ischemia and are not considered candidates for revascularization.
   - Current FDA-approved therapies consist of enhanced external counterpulsation; transcutaneous electrical nerve stimulation; and invasive therapies such as spinal cord stimulation, transmyocardial revascularization, and percutaneous myocardial revascularization. Although some of these therapies may improve symptoms and quality of life, they have not been shown to improve mortality rate.

FUNCTIONAL CLASSIFICATION

It is helpful to grade the severity of stable angina using a grading system and the most commonly adopted is that of the Canadian Cardiovascular Society.

- Grading of angina by the Canadian Cardiovascular Society Classification System:
  - Class I: ordinary physical activity does not cause angina, such as walking, climbing stairs. Angina occurs with strenuous, rapid, or prolonged exertion at work or recreation.
  - Class II: Slight limitation of ordinary activity. Angina occurs on walking or climbing stairs rapidly; walking uphill; walking or stair climbing after meals, in cold, in wind, or under emotional stress; or only during the few hours after awakening. Angina occurs on walking more than two level blocks and climbing more than one flight of ordinary stairs at a normal pace and in normal condition.
  - Class III: Marked limitations of ordinary physical activity. Angina occurs on walking one to two level blocks and climbing one flight of stairs in normal conditions and at a normal pace.
  - Class IV: Inability to carry on any physical activity without discomfort; anginal symptoms may be present at rest.

ICD-9CM CODES

411.1 Angina, stable
413 Angina pectoris
413.1 Prinzmetal's angina
413.9 Angina, unspecified

EPIDEMIOLOGY & DEMOGRAPHICS

- Angina is most common in middle-aged and elderly men.
- Women are usually affected after menopause.
- Prevalence of angina pectoris in people older than 30 yr is >3%.
- Within 12 mo of initial diagnosis, 10% to 20% of patients with diagnosis of stable angina progress to MI or unstable angina.

PHYSICAL FINDINGS & CLINICAL PRESENTATION

- Although there is significant individual variation, most patients report substernal chest pain (pressure, tightness, heaviness, sharp pain, sensation similar to intestinal gas or dysphagia).
- The pain is of short duration (typically <10 min); nonpleuritic; and often accompanied by shortness of breath, nausea, diaphoresis, and numbness or pain in the left arm, jaw, or shoulder. Ischemic pain of more than 30 minutes duration should raise concern for possible myocardial infarction.
- Women are more likely to report atypical chest pain or discomfort compared with men and an atypical presentation does not increase the likelihood of coronary artery disease as it does in men.
- The elderly diabetics may report symptoms other than chest pain, such as dyspnea, fatigue, or diaphoresis.

ETIOLOGY

UNCONTROLLABLE RISK FACTORS FOR ANGINA:
- Advanced age
- Male sex
- Genetic predisposition

MODIFIABLE RISK FACTORS FOR ANGINA:
- Smoking (risk is almost double).
- Hypertension (risk is double if systolic blood pressure is >180 mm Hg).
- Hyperlipidemia.
- Impaired glucose tolerance or diabetes mellitus.
- Obesity (weight >30% over ideal). A higher body mass index during childhood is also associated with an increased risk of coronary heart disease (CHD) in adulthood.
- Hypothyroidism.
- Left ventricular hypertrophy (LVH).
- Sedentary lifestyle.
- Oral contraceptive use.
- Cocaine use (cocaine is used by >5 million Americans regularly and is responsible for >64,000 emergency department [ED] evaluations yearly to rule out myocardial ischemia).
- Metabolic syndrome.
- The development of coronary artery calcium is associated with an increased risk of MI.
- Long-term use of nonsteroidal antiinflammatory drugs is associated with increased cardiovascular risk.
- Exposure to air pollution from traffic (dilute diesel exhaust) promotes myocardial ischemia and is associated with adverse cardiovascular events.
- Low serum folate levels. (Folate is required for conversion of homocysteine to methionine. Hyperhomocysteinemia has a toxic effect on vascular endothelium and interferes with proliferation of arterial wall smooth muscle cells. Folate deficiencies are associated with an increased risk of fatal CHD.)
- Elevated homocysteine levels. Elevated plasma homocysteine level is a strong and independent risk factor for CHD events, especially in patients with type 2 diabetes mellitus. Trials lowering homocysteine levels have, however, been disappointing because lowering therapy with folate did not prevent cardiovascular events among patients with coronary disease.

- Elevated levels of highly sensitive C-reactive protein (hs-CRP, cardio CRP).
- Depression.
- Vasculitis.
- Elevated levels of lipoprotein-associated phospholipase A_2.
- Elevated fibrinogen levels.
- Low level of red blood cell glutathione peroxidase-1 activity.

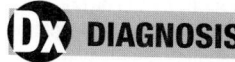 **DIAGNOSIS**

DIFFERENTIAL DIAGNOSIS

Noncardiac pain mimicking angina may be caused by:

- Pulmonary diseases (pulmonary hypertension, pulmonary embolism, pleurisy, pneumothorax, pneumonia)
- Gastrointestinal disorders (peptic ulcer disease, pancreatitis, esophageal spasm or spontaneous esophageal muscle contraction, esophageal reflux, cholecystitis, cholelithiasis)
- Musculoskeletal conditions (costochondritis, chest wall trauma, cervical arthritis with radiculopathy, muscle strain, myositis)
- Acute aortic dissection
- Herpes zoster
- Anxiety disorder

WORKUP

- In patients with chest pain, the probability of CAD should be estimated on the basis of patient age, sex, cardiovascular risk factors, and pain characteristics.
- The most important diagnostic factor is the history. Chest pain or left arm pain or discomfort occurring with exertion and relieved by rest in a patient with cardiovascular risk factors is consistent with a high likelihood of CAD.
- In assessing the likelihood of underlying CAD is it helpful to classify the chest pain as typical angina, atypical angina, and noncardiac chest pain. *Typical angina* will have the following three features: substernal chest discomfort of typical quality and duration, provoked by exertion or emotional stress, and relieved by rest and/or NTG. *Atypical angina* will have two of the above three features and *noncardiac chest pain* will have none of the above features.
- The physical examination is of little diagnostic help and may be completely normal in many patients, although certain findings may be helpful in the assessment of the patient with suspected stable CAD. The presence of hypertension, arcus senilis, xanthelasma, carotid or peripheral bruits, a prominent S4 are all physical signs that could raise concern for the presence of CAD. A murmur of mitral regurgitation may be a marker of an ischemic cardiomyopathy or transient ischemia. A murmur suggestive of hypertrophic cardiomyopathy or aortic stenosis may suggest a cause of angina other than CAD. A normal resting ECG is not unusual in a patient with stable angina pectoris. A normal or nondiag-

nostic ECG during an episode of chest pain also does not exclude the presence of coronary artery disease. 1-6% of patients with acute myocardial infarction will have a nondiagnostic ECG.Patients with intermediate likelihood of CAD and angina should undergo risk stratification through further testing. If the patient is physically capable to perform physical exercise, further testing should be with exercise stress testing because of the important prognostic information obtained from exercise performance and the hemodynamic response. The value of further testing is greatest in patients who have an intermediate risk of CAD, as patients in a low risk or high risk category or more likely to have a false positive or false negative result respectively. An exercise test with electrocardiographic monitoring alone (without imaging) is recommended in patients with intermediate probability of CAD and a normal resting electrocardiogram and the ability to exercise. Stress echocardiography or stress testing with myocardial perfusion imaging may be employed when baseline electrocardiographic abnormalities are present that render the electrocardiographic response to exercise uninterpretable. Stress echocardiography has the advantage of higher specificity and a lower cost. Stress radionuclide perfusion imaging has a higher sensitivity, particularly for single vessel coronary disease, and has a higher technical success rate. When the patient is unable to exercise adequately pharmacologic testing may be used with these imaging modalities (dobutamine, dipyridamole, adenosine).
- A very good predictor of risk for a patient with stable angina is the Duke treadmill score, which incorporates the patient's functional status (METS or time in minutes during the Bruce protocol), ST-segment depression, and an angina index. Patients with favorable Duke scores have a 5-yr survival of >97% and this is independent of other factors such as coronary anatomy and LV function.
- Although invasive, coronary angiography remains the gold standard for the identification of clinically significant CAD. Coronary magnetic resonance angiography can also detect CAD of the proximal and middle segments. This noninvasive approach, where available, can be used to reliably identify (or rule out) left main coronary artery or three-vessel disease.
- Multidetector computed tomography (MDCT) is a newer screening modality for CAD. Its advantages are its speed, safety, and low cost compared with angiography. It has high sensitivity and negative predictive value. Its limitations are as follows: limited to patients with a regular rhythm and slow rates, poor image in morbidly obese patients, inaccurate visualization of the coronary artery within a stent, and decreased diagnostic accuracy in older patients from the prevalence and severity of coronary calcifications with increasing age. Its routine use in clinical practice is not justified. However, it may be useful in

excluding coronary disease in selected patients in whom a false-positive result or inconclusive stress test is suspected.

LABORATORY TESTS

- Initial laboratory tests in patients with chronic stable angina should include hemoglobin, fasting glucose, and fasting lipid panel.
- A resting electrocardiogram should be obtained during pain and when the patient is free of any discomfort. A normal resting electrocardiogram is not unusual in patients with chronic stable angina; in patients who present with chest pain, 1% to 6% that have an acute MI will have a normal or nondiagnostic electrocardiogram.
- Cardio-CRP (hs-CRP): elevation of cardio-CRP is a relatively moderate predictor of CHD, and it adds prognostic information to that conveyed by the Framingham risk score. However, based on current data, it may be premature to adapt widespread assessment of cardio-CRP.
- Measurement of total cholesterol, low-density lipoprotein cholesterol (LDL-C), high-density lipoprotein cholesterol (HDL-C), and fasting serum triglycerides is recommended for cardiovascular screening. NonHDL-C and the ratio of total cholesterol to HDL-C and measurements of apolipoprotein fractions (e.g., apolipoprotein B100, apolipoprotein A1) can also be used to estimate cardiovascular risk.

IMAGING STUDIES

- Echocardiography is indicated in patients with systolic murmur suggestive of aortic stenosis, mitral valve prolapse, or hypertrophic cardiomyopathy. It is also useful in the detection of ischemia-induced regional wall motion abnormalities or mitral regurgitation. Echocardiography combined with treadmill exercise (stress echo) or pharmacologic stress with dobutamine can be used to detect regional wall abnormalities that occur during myocardial ischemia associated with CAD.
- Coronary angiography is performed to define the location and extent of coronary disease; this is indicated in selected patients who are candidates for coronary artery bypass graft (CABG) surgery or angioplasty.
- Noninvasive methods for assessing myocardial viability to predict which patients will have increased left ventricular ejection fraction and improved survival after revascularization include positron-emission tomography, dobutamine echocardiography, multidetector CT, and contrast-enhanced MRI. Cardiac CT is useful for the detection of subclinical CAD in asymptomatic patients with an intermediate Framingham 10-year risk estimate of 10% to 20%. It detects and quantifies coronary calcium and evaluates the lumen and wall of the coronary artery. The calcium score is a strong predictor of incident CHD and provides predictive information beyond that provided by standard risk factors. While coronary artery calcium score (CACS) is a promising tool, CT

cost and radiation exposure are limiting factors to recommending widespread routine use of this marker. Cardiac MRI, in addition to its use for diagnosis of arrhythmogenic right ventricular dysplasia, can also be used to assess myocardial perfusion and viability as well as function. Additional studies are needed to determine the cost effectiveness of these studies in patients with ischemic cardiomyopathy.

Rx TREATMENT

NONPHARMACOLOGIC THERAPY

- Aggressive modification of preventable risk factors (weight reduction in obese patients, regular aerobic exercise program, correction of folate deficiency, low-cholesterol and low-sodium diet, cessation of tobacco use).
- Diets using nonhydrogenated unsaturated fats as the predominant form of dietary fat, whole grains as the main form of carbohydrates, an abundance of fruits and vegetables, and adequate omega-3 fatty acids are optimal for prevention of CHD.
- Correction of possible aggravating factors (e.g., anemia, hypertension, diabetes mellitus, hyperlipidemia, thyrotoxicosis). Blood transfusion in the setting of acute coronary syndromes is associated with higher mortality rates. Use caution regarding the routine use of blood transfusions to maintain arbitrary hematocrit levels in stable patients with ischemic heart disease.

PHARMACOLOGIC THERAPY

The major classes of antiischemic agents are nitrates, beta-adrenergic blockers, calcium channel blockers, aspirin, and heparin; they can be used alone or in combination.

- Nitrates cause venodilation and relaxation of vascular smooth muscle; the decreased venous return from venodilation decreases diastolic ventricular wall tension (preload) and thereby reduces mechanical activity (and myocardial oxygen consumption) during systole. Relaxation of vascular smooth muscle increases coronary blood flow and reduces systemic pressure. Tolerance to nitrates can be minimized by avoiding sustained blood levels with a daily nitrate-free period (e.g., omission of bedtime dose of oral isosorbide dinitrate or 12 hr on/12 hr off transdermal nitroglycerin therapy). Nitrates are relatively contraindicated in patients with hypertrophic obstructive cardiomyopathy, and should also be avoided in patients with severe aortic stenosis. Nitrates should not be used within 24 hr of sildenafil (Viagra) or vardenafil (Levitra) or within 48 hr of tadalafil (Cialis) because of the potential for hypotension.
- Beta-adrenergic blockers achieve their major antianginal effect by decreasing myocardial oxygen consumption by reducing heart rate and systolic blood pressure. Absent contraindications, they should be regarded as initial therapy for stable angina for all patients. Their dose should generally be adjusted to reduce the resting heart rate to 50 to 60 beats/min.
- Calcium channel blockers dilate coronary and systemic arteries, increase coronary blood flow, and decrease myocardial oxygen consumption. They play a major role in preventing and terminating myocardial ischemia induced by coronary artery spasm. They are particularly effective in treating microvascular angina. Short-acting calcium channel blockers should be avoided. Calcium channel blockers should generally also be avoided after complicated MI (congestive heart failure [CHF]) and in patients with CHF secondary to systolic dysfunction (unless necessary to control heart rate).
- Aspirin: use of aspirin reduces cardiovascular mortality and morbidity rates by 20% to 25% among patients with CAD. Initial dose is at least 160 mg/day followed by 81 to 325 mg/day. Aspirin inhibits the enzyme cyclooxygenase and synthesis of thromboxane A_2 and reduces the risk of adverse cardiovascular events by 33% in patients with unstable angina. Patients intolerant to aspirin can be treated with the antiplatelet agent clopidogrel.
- Clopidogrel is a thienopyridine, which acts by irreversibly blocking the P2Y12 adenosine diphosphate receptor on the platelet surface, thereby interrupting platelet activation and aggregation.
- Use of lipid-lowering drugs is recommended in patients with CAD and in patients with hyperlipidemia refractory to diet and exercise. Among patients who have recently had an acute coronary syndrome, an intensive lipid-lowering statin regimen to reduce LDL cholesterol to <70 mg/dl is a reasonable treatment objective. Statins also decrease the level of the inflammatory marker hs-CRP independently of the magnitude of change in lipid parameters.
- ACE inhibition (e.g., ramipril 10 mg/day) has been shown to be effective in reducing cardiovascular death, MI, and stroke in patients who are at risk for or who had vascular disease (without heart failure). Currently evidence for routine use of ACEs in chronic stable angina is insufficient.
- Ranolazine is a newer agent indicated for treatment of chronic angina that is inadequately controlled with other antianginals. It represents a new class of drugs known as *metabolic modulators*. Its exact mechanism of action is unknown. It seems to increase the efficiency of energy production in the heart, maintaining cardiac function. Its antianginal and antiischemic effects do not depend on reductions in heart rate or blood pressure. It is labeled for use in combination with beta-blockers, amlodipine, or nitrates in patients without an adequate antianginal response to those agents. Side effects include prolongation of QT interval.

REFERRAL

Revascularization:
- Revascularization includes either percutaneous coronary intervention (balloon angioplasty and stenting) or CABG.
- CABG surgery is recommended for patients with left main coronary disease, for those with symptomatic three-vessel disease, and for those with LVEF <40% and critical (>70% stenosis) in all three major coronary arteries. Surgical therapy improves prognosis, particularly in diabetic patients with multivessel disease. Compared with percutaneous coronary intervention (PCI), CABG is more effective in relieving angina and leads to fewer repeated revascularizations but has a higher risk for procedural stroke. Survival to 10 years is similar for both procedures.

Angioplasty and coronary stents:
- PCI should be considered for patients with one- or two-vessel disease that does not involve the main left coronary artery and in whom ventricular function is normal or near normal. PCI has an established place in treating angina but is not superior to intensive medical therapy to prevent MI and death in symptomatic or asymptomatic patients. Patients selected for PCI should also be candidates for CABG. The types of lesions best suited for angioplasty are proximal lesions, noncalcified, concentric, and preferably less than 5 mm (should not exceed 10 mm). Approximately 80% of patients show immediate benefit after PCI. The development of coronary stents has increased the number of patients who can be treated in the cardiac laboratory. Cardiac stents are currently used in nearly 95% of all PCI lesions. The rate of restenosis may be reduced by placing a stent electively in primary atheromatous lesions. In patients with symptomatic isolated stenosis of the proximal left anterior descending artery, stenting has advantages over standard coronary angioplasty in that it is associated with both a lower rate of restenosis and a better clinical outcome. The major limitations of stenting are subacute thrombosis, restenosis within the stent, bleeding complications when anticoagulants are used after stenting, and higher cost. The combination of aspirin and clopidogrel is effective in preventing coronary stent thrombosis. Vitamin therapy to lower homocysteine levels has been recommended by some for the prevention of restenosis after coronary angioplasty; however, recent reports indicate that the administration of folate, vitamin B_6, and vitamin B_{12} after coronary stenting may increase the risk of in-stent restenosis and the need for target-vessel revascularization. Regarding the use of various drug-eluting coronary stents, there are no significant differences in clinical outcomes between patients receiving sirolimus- and paclitaxel-eluting stents.

❗ PEARLS & CONSIDERATIONS

COMMENTS

- Although nitrate responsiveness is usually an integral part of a diagnostic strategy for chronic stable chest pain, recent reports question its value and conclude that in a general population admitted for chest pain, relief of pain after nitroglycerin treatment does not predict active CAD and should not be used to guide diagnosis in the acute care setting.
- CABG is associated with higher long-term survival rates and lower rates of repeat revascularization than PCI and stenting; however, patients often prefer stenting because it is less invasive, involves a shorter hospital stay, and has a lower in-hospital mortality rate.
- Section III describes an algorithm for the surgical management of ischemic cardiomyopathy.

EBM EVIDENCE

available at www.expertconsult.com

SUGGESTED READINGS

available at www.expertconsult.com

AUTHORS: **DAVID J. FORTUNATO, M.D., F.A.C.C.,** and **FRED F. FERRI, M.D.**

A

Diseases and Disorders

I

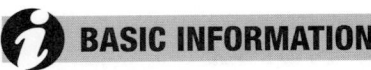

BASIC INFORMATION

DEFINITION

- The mucocutaneous swelling caused by the release of vasoactive mediators is called urticaria and angioedema.
- Urticaria causes edema of the superficial dermis.
- Angioedema involves the deep layers of the dermis and the subcutaneous tissue.

SYNONYMS

Angioneurotic edema
HAE (hereditary angiodema)

ICD-9CM CODES
995.1 Angioedema (allergic)
277.6 Angioedema (hereditary)

EPIDEMIOLOGY & DEMOGRAPHICS

INCIDENCE: 100 to 3000/100,000 persons (for urticaria and angioedema)
LIFETIME PREVALENCE: Approximately 20% of the population experiences urticaria and/or angioedema at some time during life. The prevalence of hereditary angioedema is 1 case per 50,000 persons.
DEMOGRAPHICS:
Race: Slightly more common among African Americans.
Sex: More occurrences in women than men. Angioedema commonly occurs after adolescence in the third decade of life.
Angioedema can occur together with urticaria (40%) or alone (20%); the remaining 40% have urticaria alone.

PHYSICAL FINDINGS & CLINICAL PRESENTATION

- Angioedema may be acute or chronic.
  1. Acute angioedema is defined as symptoms lasting 6 wk.
  2. Chronic angioedema is defined as symptoms lasting >6 wk.
- Urticaria is commonly known as "hives" and is:
  1. Pruritic
  2. Palpable and well demarcated
  3. Erythematous
  4. Millimeters to centimeters in size
  5. Multiple in number
  6. Fades within 12 to 24 hr
  7. Reappears at other sites
- Angioedema is characterized by the following:
  1. Nonpruritic
  2. Burning
  3. Not well demarcated
  4. Involves eyelids (Fig. 1-27), lips, tongue, and extremities
  5. Can involve the upper airway, causing respiratory distress
  6. Can involve the gastrointestinal tract, leading to cyclic abdominal pain, nausea, vomiting, and diarrhea
  7. Resolves slowly

ETIOLOGY

- Angioedema, with or without urticaria, is classified as acquired (allergic or idiopathic) or hereditary.
- Angioedema is primarily caused by mast cell activation and degranulation with release of vasoactive mediators (e.g., histamine, serotonin, bradykinins), resulting in postcapillary venule inflammation, vascular leakage, and edema in the deep layers of the dermis and subcutaneous tissue.
- Pathologically, angioedema has both immunologic- and nonimmunologic-mediated mechanisms.
  1. Immunoglobulin E–mediated angioedema may result from antigen exposure (e.g., foods [milk, eggs, peanuts, shellfish, tomatoes, chocolate, sulfites] or drugs [penicillin, aspirin, nonsteroidal anti-inflammatory drugs, phenytoin, sulfonamides, recombinant tissue plasminogen activator]).
  2. Complement-mediated angioedema involving immune complex mechanisms can also lead to mast cell activation that manifests as serum sickness.
  3. Hereditary angioedema is an autosomal-dominant disease caused by a deficiency of or mutation in C1 esterase inhibitor (C1-INH). C1-INH is a protease inhibitor normally present in high concentrations in the plasma. C1-INH serves many functions, one of which is to inhibit plasma kallikrein, a protease that cleaves kininogen and releases bradykinin. Deficient C1-INH activity results in excess concentration of kininogen and the subsequent release of kinin mediators.
  4. Acquired angioedema is usually associated with other diseases, most commonly B-cell lymphoproliferative disorders, but may also result from the formation of autoantibodies directed against C1 inhibitor protein.
  5. Other causes of angioedema include infection (e.g., herpes simplex, hepatitis B, Coxsackie A and B, Streptococcus, Candida, Ascaris, and Strongyloides), insect bites and stings, stress, physical factors (e.g., cold, exercise, pressure, and vibration), connective tissue diseases (e.g.,

systemic lupus erythematosus, Henoch-Schönlein purpura), and idiopathic causes. Angiotensin-converting enzyme (ACE) inhibitors can increase kinin activity and lead to angioedema.

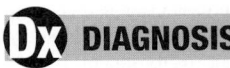

DIAGNOSIS

A detailed history and physical examination usually establish the diagnosis of angioedema. Extensive laboratory testing is of limited value.

DIFFERENTIAL DIAGNOSIS

- Cellulitis
- Arthropod bite
- Hypothyroidism
- Contact dermatitis
- Atopic dermatitis
- Mastocytosis
- Granulomatous cheilitis
- Bullous pemphigoid
- Urticaria pigmentosa
- Anaphylaxis
- Erythema multiforme
- Epiglottitis
- Peritonsillar abscess

WORKUP

- An extensive workup searching for the cause of angioedema is often unrevealing (90%).
- Workup, including diagnostic blood tests and allergy testing, is performed according to results of the history and physical examination.

LABORATORY TESTS

- Complete blood count, erythrocyte sedimentation rate, and urinalysis are sometimes helpful as part of the initial evaluation.
- Stools for ova and parasites.
- Serology testing.
- C4 levels are usually reduced in acquired and hereditary angioedema (occurring without urticaria). If C4 levels are low, C1-INH levels and activity should be obtained. There are isolated reports of hereditary angioedema with normal C4 levels but reduced C1-INH levels.
- Skin and radioallergosorbent testing may be done if food allergies are suspected.

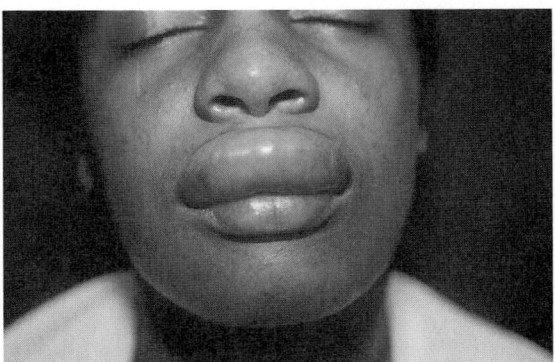

FIGURE 1-27 Angioedema of the upper lip, with severe swelling of deeper tissues. (From Goldstein BG, Goldstein AO: *Practical dermatology,* ed 2, St Louis, 1997, Mosby.)

- Skin biopsy is usually done in patients with chronic angioedema refractory to corticosteroid treatment.

Rx TREATMENT

NONPHARMACOLOGIC THERAPY
- Eliminate the offending agent
- Avoid triggering factors (e.g., cold, stress)
- Cold compresses to affected areas

ACUTE GENERAL Rx
- Acute life-threatening angioedema involving the larynx is treated with:
  1. Epinephrine 0.3 mg in a solution of 1:1000 given SC
  2. Diphenhydramine 25 to 50 mg IV or IM
  3. Cimetidine 300 mg IV or ranitidine 50 mg IV
  4. Methylprednisolone 125 mg IV
- Mainstay therapy in nonhereditary angioedema is H_1 antihistamines
  1. Diphenhydramine 25 to 50 mg q6h
  2. Chlorpheniramine 4 mg q6h
  3. Hydroxyzine 10 to 25 mg q6h
  4. Cetirizine 5 to 10 mg qd
  5. Loratadine 10 mg qd
  6. Fexofenadine 60 mg qd
- H_2 antihistamines can be added to H_1 antihistamines
  1. Ranitidine 150 mg bid
  2. Cimetidine 400 mg bid
  3. Famotidine 20 mg bid
- Tricyclic antidepressants
  1. Doxepin 25 to 50 mg qd
- Corticosteroids are rarely required for symptomatic relief of acute angioedema.

- Antihistamines are probably ineffective in acute hereditary angioedema.
- Purified plasma-derived C1-INH replacement therapy is effective and safe in treating acute attacks of hereditary angioedema caused by C1 inhibitor deficiency. Cost is a limiting factor. Available C1 esterase inhibitors are Cinryze and Berinert
- The recombinant protein kallikrien inhibitor ecallantide is also effective for acute attacks of HFA but also very expensive.

CHRONIC Rx
- Chronic angioedema is treated as described under "Acute General Rx."
- Corticosteroids are used more often in chronic nonhereditary angioedema.
- Prednisone 1 mg/kg/day for 5 days and then tapered over a period of weeks.
- Androgens (danazol, stanozolol, oxandrolone, methyltestosterone) and antifibrinolytic agents are used for the treatment of chronic hereditary angioedema, which does not respond to antihistamines or corticosteroids. C1-INH replacement therapy was approved by the FDA in 2008 . Available agents are Cinryze and Berinert,. Icatibant is a new bradykinin-receptor antagonist in hereditary angioedema currently undergoing trials.

DISPOSITION
- Antihistamines achieve symptomatic relief in more than 80% of patients with nonhereditary acute angioedema.
- In chronic nonhereditary angioedema, corticosteroids are given in addition to antihistamines.

- A small percentage of people will have recurrence of symptoms after steroid treatment.
- Chronic angioedema can last for months and even years.

REFERRAL
Dermatology consultation is recommended in patients with chronic angioedema, hereditary angioedema, and recurring angioedema.

PEARLS & CONSIDERATIONS

ACE inhibitors can cause angioedema up to many months after initiation. There are multiple case reports and case series of angiotensin receptor blocker–induced angioedema, although the risk is substantially less than that of ACE inhibitors.

COMMENTS
- Identifying a cause for angioedema in patients is often difficult and met with frustration.
- Chronic angioedema, unlike acute angioedema, is rarely caused by an allergic reaction.

SUGGESTED READINGS
available at www.expertconsult.com

AUTHOR: **MEL L. ANDERSON, M.D.**

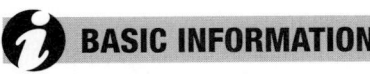

BASIC INFORMATION

DEFINITION

Ankle fractures involve the lateral, medial, or posterior malleolus of the ankle and may occur either alone or in some combination. Associated ligamentous injuries are included.

ICD-9CM CODES
824.8 Ankle fracture (malleolus) (closed)
824.2 Lateral malleolus fracture (fibular)
824.0 Medial malleolus fracture (tibial)

PHYSICAL FINDINGS & CLINICAL PRESENTATION

- Deformity usually depends on extent of displacement
- Pain, tenderness, and hemorrhage at the site of injury
- Gentle palpation of ligamentous structures (especially deltoid ligament) to determine the extent of soft tissue injury
- Evaluation of distal neurovascular status; results recorded

ETIOLOGY

- The ankle depends on its ligamentous and bony support for stability. The joint, or *mortise,* is an inverted U with the dome of the talus fitting into the medial and lateral malleoli. The posterior margin of the tibia is often called the *third* or *posterior malleolus.*
- Most common ankle fractures are the result of eversion or lateral rotation forces on the talus (in contrast with common sprains, which are usually caused by inversion).

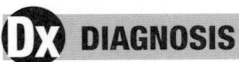

DIAGNOSIS

The diagnosis is usually established on the basis of the nature of the injury, the presence of typical findings of bony tenderness with swelling, and abnormal imaging studies.

DIFFERENTIAL DIAGNOSIS

- Ankle sprain
- Avulsion fracture of hindfoot or metatarsal

IMAGING STUDIES

Standard AP and lateral views accompanied by an AP taken 15° internally rotated. The last view is taken to properly visualize the mortise.

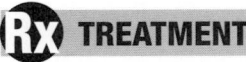

TREATMENT

All fractures: elevation and ice to control swelling for 48 to 72 hr.

ACUTE GENERAL Rx

- Clinical and roentgenographic assessment of the status of the ankle mortise and stability of the injury is mandatory to determine treatment.
- There is potential for displacement if both sides of the joint are significantly injured (e.g., fracture of the lateral malleolus with deltoid ligament injury).
- Deviation of the position of the talus in the mortise could lead to traumatic arthritis.
- If there is no widening of the ankle mortise, many injuries can be safely treated with simple casting without reduction:
  1. Undisplaced or avulsion fractures of either malleolus below the ankle joint line:
     a. Stability of the joint is not compromised and a short leg walking cast or ankle support is sufficient.
     b. Weight bearing is allowed as tolerated.
     c. In 4 to 6 wk, protection may be discontinued.
  2. Isolated undisplaced fractures of the medial, lateral, or posterior malleolus:
     a. Usually stable and require only the application of a short leg walking cast with the ankle in the neutral position or fracture cast boot.
     b. Immobilization should be continued for 8 wk.
     c. Fracture line of lateral malleolus may persist roentgenographically for several months, but immobilization beyond 8 wk is usually unnecessary.
     d. Undisplaced bimalleolar fractures are treated with a long leg cast flexed 30 degrees at the knee to prevent motion and displacement of the fracture fragments. In 4 wk, a short leg walking cast may be applied for an additional 4 wk.
  3. Isolated fractures of the lateral malleolus that are slightly displaced:
     a. May be treated with casting if no medial injury is present.
     b. A below-knee walking cast is applied with ankle in the neutral position; weight bearing is allowed as tolerated.
     c. Six wk of immobilization is sufficient.
     d. If medial tenderness is present, suggesting deltoid ligament rupture, a carefully molded cast may suffice if weight bearing is not allowed and the patient is followed up closely for signs of instability, especially after swelling recedes. If significant widening of the medial ankle mortise (increase in the "medial clear space") develops as a result of lateral displacement of the talus, referral for possible reduction is indicated.
     e. If signs of instability are already present at initial examination (widening of the medial clear space with medial tenderness), referral is indicated.
  4. Undisplaced fracture of the distal fibular epiphysis:
     a. Often diagnosed clinically.
     b. There is tenderness over the epiphyseal plate.
     c. Roentgenographic findings are often negative.
     d. A short leg walking cast or fracture boot is applied for 4 wk.
     e. Growth disturbance is rare.
  5. Isolated posterior malleolar fractures involving less than 25% of the joint surface on the lateral roentgenogram:
     Safely treated by applying a short leg walking cast or fracture brace. (Fractures involving >25% of the weight-bearing surface should be referred because of the potential for instability and subsequent traumatic arthritis.)

CHRONIC Rx

- Early motion is encouraged through a home exercise program.
- Protection from reinjury is appropriate for 4 to 6 wk after cast or brace removal.
- Temporary increase in lower extremity swelling that frequently occurs after short leg cast removal may benefit from the use of support hose.

DISPOSITION

Significant factors involved in the development of traumatic arthritis:
- Amount of joint trauma at the time of injury
- Eventual position of the talus in the mortise

Fracture nonunion is uncommon unless displacement is significant.

REFERRAL

Orthopedic consultation for:
- Unstable ankle joint
- Widened ankle mortise
- Posterior malleolar fracture over 25% of joint with incongruity
- Marked displacement of fracture fragment

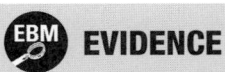

EVIDENCE

available at www.expertconsult.com

SUGGESTED READINGS

available at www.expertconsult.com

AUTHOR: **LONNIE R. MERCIER, M.D.**

BASIC INFORMATION

DEFINITION

An ankle sprain is an injury to the ligamentous support of the ankle. Most (85%) involve the lateral ligament complex (Fig. 1-28). The anterior inferior tibiofibular (AITF) ligament, deltoid ligament, and interosseous membrane may also be injured. Damage to the tibiofibular syndesmosis is sometimes called a *high sprain* because of pain above the ankle.

ICD-9CM CODES
845.00 Sprain, ankle or foot

EPIDEMIOLOGY & DEMOGRAPHICS

PREVALENCE: One case/10,000 people each day
PREDOMINANT SEX: Varies according to age and level of physical activity

PHYSICAL FINDINGS & CLINICAL PRESENTATION

- Often a history of a "pop"
- Variable amounts of tenderness and hemorrhage
- Possible abnormal anterior drawer test (pulling the plantar flexed foot forward to determine if there is any abnormal increase in forward movement of the talus in the ankle mortise) (Fig. 1-29)
- Inversion sprains: tender laterally; syndesmotic injuries: area of tenderness is more anterior and proximal
- Evaluation of motor function (Fig. 1-30)

ETIOLOGY

- Lateral injuries usually result from inversion and plantar flexion injuries.
- Eversion and rotational forces may injure the deltoid or AITF ligament or the interosseous membrane.

Dx DIAGNOSIS

DIFFERENTIAL DIAGNOSIS

- Fracture of the ankle or foot, particularly involving the distal fibular growth plate in the immature patient
- Avulsion fracture of the fifth metatarsal base

WORKUP

- History and clinical examination are usually sufficient to establish the diagnosis.
- Plain radiographs are always needed.

IMAGING STUDIES

Roentgenographic evaluation:
1. Usually normal but always performed
2. Should include the fifth metatarsal base
3. All minor avulsion fractures noted
Varying opinions on the usefulness of arthrograms, tenograms, and stress films

Rx TREATMENT

ACUTE GENERAL Rx

- Ankle sprains are often graded I, II, or III, according to severity, with grade III injury implying complete rupture. The first line of treatment is described by the mnemonic *RICE:*
  - *R*est
  - *I*ce
  - *C*ompression
  - *E*levation
- Varying opinions regarding the initial use of NSAIDs
- In 48 to 72 hr, active range of motion and weight bearing as tolerated
- In 4 to 5 days, exercise against resistance added
- Possible cast immobilization for some patients who require early independent walking; short leg orthoses also available for the same purpose

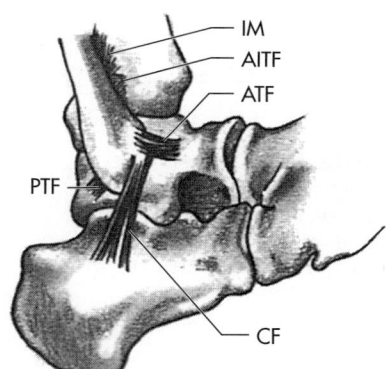

FIGURE 1-28 The lateral ankle ligaments, anterior and posterior talofibular *(ATF, PTF)* and calcaneofibular *(CF)*. Also shown are the anterior inferior tibiofibular ligament *(AITF)* and the beginning of the interosseous membrane *(IM)*. (From Mercier LR [ed]: *Practical orthopaedics,* ed 4, St Louis, 1995, Mosby.)

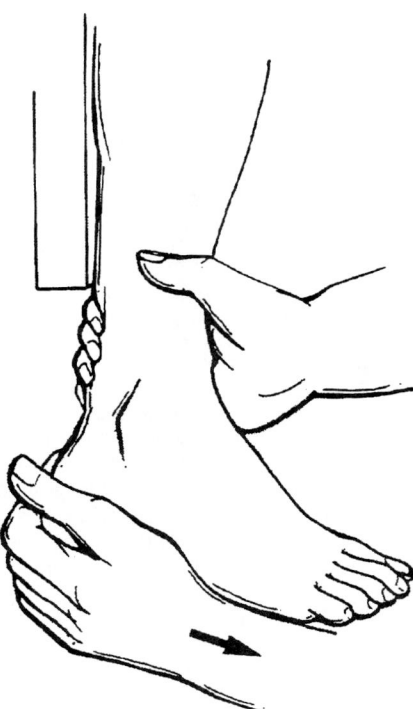

FIGURE 1-29 Anterior drawer test of the ankle (tests the integrity of the anterior talofibular ligament). (From Brinker MR, Miller MD: *Fundamentals of orthopaedics,* Philadelphia, 1999, WB Saunders.)

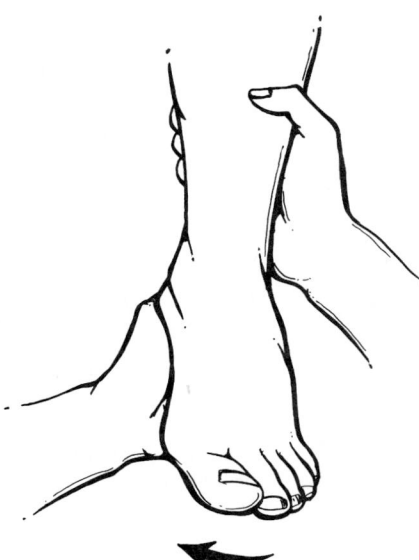

FIGURE 1-30 Talar tilt test (inversion stress) of the ankle (tests the integrity of the anterior talofibular ligament and the calcaneofibular ligament). (From Brinker MR, Miller MD: *Fundamentals of orthopaedics,* Philadelphia, 1999, WB Saunders.)

- Surgery is rarely recommended, even for grade III sprains; reports of equally satisfactory outcomes with nonsurgical treatment

CHRONIC Rx

- Lateral heel and sole wedge to prevent inversion
- Protective taping or bracing during vigorous activities (Fig. 1-31)
- Strengthening exercises

DISPOSITION

- Lateral sprains of any severity may cause lingering symptoms for weeks and months.
  1. Some syndesmotic sprains take even longer to heal.
  2. Heterotopic ossification may even develop in the interosseous membrane, but long-term results do not seem to be affected by such ossification.

- Continuing lateral symptoms may require surgical reconstruction, although late traumatic arthritis or long-term instability is rare regardless of treatment.

REFERRAL

For orthopedic consultation for patients who do not respond to conservative treatment

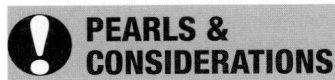

COMMENTS

If healing seems delayed (more than 6 wk), the following conditions should be considered:
1. Talar dome fracture
2. Reflex sympathetic dystrophy
3. Chronic tendinitis

4. Peroneal tendon subluxation
5. Other occult fracture
6. Peroneal weakness (poor rehabilitation)
7. A "high" (syndesmotic) sprain
Repeat plain roentgenograms, bone scan, or MRI may be indicated.

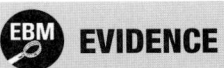

available at www.expertconsult.com

SUGGESTED READINGS
available at www.expertconsult.com

AUTHOR: **LONNIE R. MERCIER, M.D.**

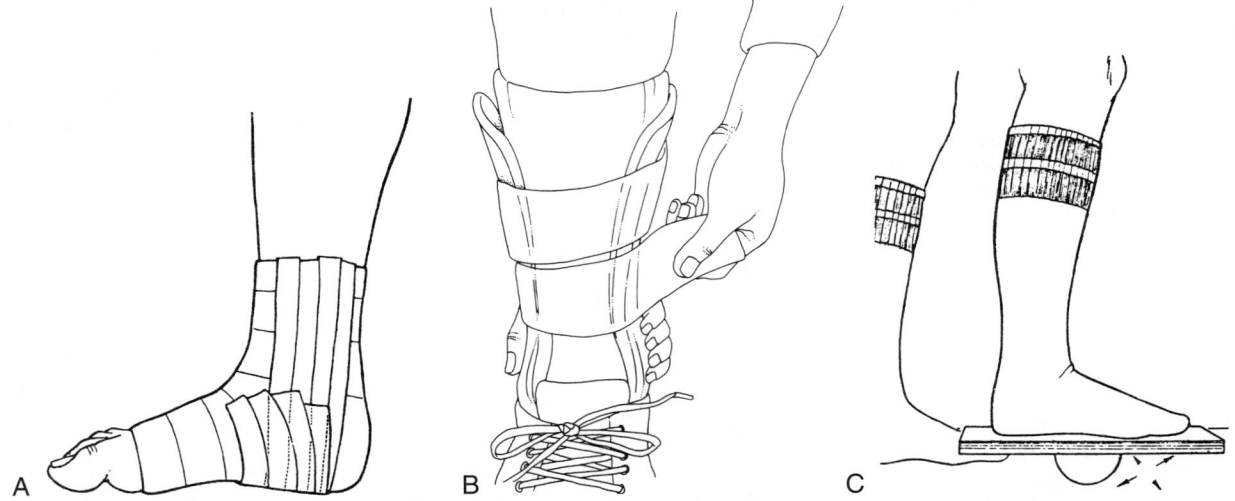

FIGURE 1-31 A, The most effective method of supporting most acute ankle sprains is by using an ACE wrap (BD, Franklin Lakes, NJ) reinforced with 1-inch medial and lateral tape strips. The anterior and posterior aspects of the ankle are left free to allow the patient to flex and extend the ankle. The patient is encouraged to bear weight with crutches. **B,** Diagram of an air splint. Straps are adjusted to heel size, the lower straps are wrapped about the ankle, and the side extensions are centered. The splint is then pressurized and straps adjusted until comfortable support and pressure are attained. **C,** As the ankle pain subsides, about the third to fifth day, balancing exercises can begin to allow the patient to regain ankle proprioception and avoid recurrent instability problems. (From Jardon OM, Mathews MS: Orthopedics. In Rakel RE [ed]: *Textbook of family practice,* ed 5, Philadelphia, 1995, WB Saunders.)

BASIC INFORMATION

DEFINITION

Ankylosing spondylitis is a type of inflammatory arthritis involving the sacroiliac joints and axial skeleton characterized by ankylosis and enthesitis (inflammation at tendon insertions). It is one of a family of overlapping syndromes called seronegative spondyloarthropathies that includes reactive arthritis (Reiter syndrome), psoriatic spondylitis, and enteropathic arthritis.

SYNONYMS

Marie-Strümpell disease

ICD-9CM CODES
720.0 Ankylosing spondylitis

EPIDEMIOLOGY & DEMOGRAPHICS

PREVALENCE: Between 0.1% and 1% of the population
PREDOMINANT AGE AT ONSET: 15 to 35 yr
PREDOMINANT SEX: Male/female ratio 2 to 3:1

PHYSICAL FINDINGS & CLINICAL PRESENTATION

- Prolonged morning back stiffness of insidious onset lasting more than 3 mo
- Bilateral sacroiliac tenderness (sacroiliitis)
- Limited lumbar spine motion (Fig. 1-32)

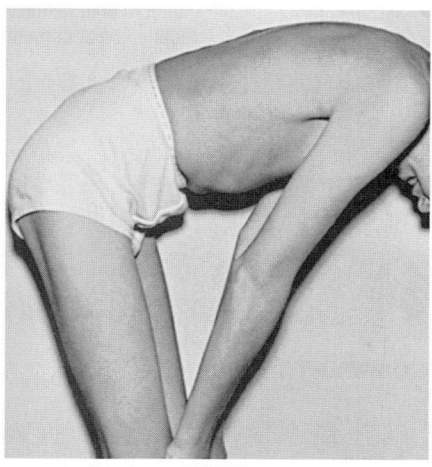

FIGURE 1-32 Loss of lumbodorsal spine mobility in a boy with ankylosing spondylitis. The lower spine remains straight when the patient bends forward. (From Behrman RE: *Nelson textbook of pediatrics,* 17th ed, Philadelphia, 2005, WB Saunders.)

- Tenderness at tendon insertion sites, especially the Achilles tendons and plantar fascia
- Loss of chest expansion reflecting rib cage involvement
- Occasionally, peripheral joint arthritis, usually involving the large joints of the lower extremities
- Extraskeletal manifestations may affect the cardiovascular system (aortic insufficiency), lungs (pulmonary fibrosis), and eye (uveitis)

ETIOLOGY

Genetic factors, particularly *HLA-B27*, play an important role in susceptibility to the spondyloarthropathies. Infectious triggers have been implicated in some cases. Tumor necrosis factor is important in the inflammatory response.

DIAGNOSIS

DIFFERENTIAL DIAGNOSIS

- Diffuse idiopathic skeletal hyperostosis (Forestier disease)
- Noninflammatory back pain (A clinical algorithm for the evaluation of back pain is described in Section III)

LABORATORY TESTS

- Elevated sedimentation rate, C-reactive protein
- Mild hyperchromic anemia
- HLA/B27 antigen is not useful in the evaluation of noninflammatory back pain because it is present in up to 8% to 10% of the normal population.
- Demonstration of inflammatory sacroiliitis by radiography or MRI is essential for diagnosis

IMAGING STUDIES

- Classic features are those of bilateral sacroiliitis on radiographs of the pelvis.
- Vertebral bodies lose anterior concave shape and become square
- With progression, calcification of the annulus fibrosis and paravertebral ligaments develop, giving rise to the so-called bamboo spine.
- MRI may be useful in detecting early inflammatory lesions and is especially helpful when the history is suggestive but radiographs are equivocal.

TREATMENT

NONPHARMACOLOGIC THERAPY

- Exercises primarily to maintain flexibility and aerobic activity are important
- Postural training
  1. Patients must be instructed spinal extension exercises to avoid fusion in a flexed position
  2. Sleeping should be in the supine position on a firm mattress; pillows should not be placed under the head or knees.

CHRONIC Rx

- NSAIDs: indomethacin is often successful in relieving symptoms; newer nonsteroidal agents may be used as well.
- Sulfasalazine may be efficacious in some patients, especially for peripheral arthritis
- Tumor necrosis factor (TNF) antagonists such as etanercept, infliximab and adalimumab have been shown to very effective for relieving symptoms of spinal inflammatory arthritis in numerous controlled studies. Anti-TNF therapy sometimes results in dramatic improvement in symptoms, range of motion of the spine, and in quality of life for these patients.

DISPOSITION

Most patients have a normal life span but many suffer significant disability from loss of spinal mobility

REFERRAL

All patients with seronegative spondyloarthropathy should be referred to a rheumatologist for consideration of anti-TNF therapy

PEARLS & CONSIDERATIONS

A family history of seronegative spondyloarthropathy increases the specificity of testing for *HLA-B27*

EVIDENCE

available at www.expertconsult.com

SUGGESTED READINGS

available at www.expertconsult.com

AUTHOR: **BERNARD ZIMMERMANN, M.D.**

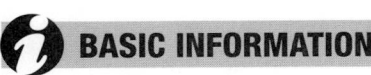

BASIC INFORMATION

DEFINITION

A fistula is an inflammatory tract with a secondary (external) opening in the perianal skin and a primary (internal) opening in the anal canal at the dentate line. It originates in an abscess in the intersphincteric space of the anal canal. Fistulas can be classified as follows:

1. Intersphincteric: fistula track passes within the intersphincteric plane to the perianal skin (most common)
2. Transsphincteric: fistula track passes from the internal opening, through the internal and external sphincter, and into the ischiorectal fossa to the perianal skin (frequent)
3. Suprasphincteric: after passing through the internal sphincter, fistula tract passes above the puborectalis and then tracts downward, lateral to the external sphincter, into the ischiorectal space to the perianal skin (uncommon); if abscess cavity extends cephalad, a supralevator abscess possibly palpable on rectal examination
4. Extrasphincteric: fistula tract passes from the rectum, above the levators, through the levator muscles to the ischiorectal space and perianal skin (rare)

With a horseshoe fistula, the tract passes from one ischiorectal fossa to the other behind the rectum.

SYNONYMS

Fistula-in-ano

ICD-9CM CODES
565.1 Anal fistula

EPIDEMIOLOGY & DEMOGRAPHICS

- Common in all ages
- Occurs equally in men and women
- Associated with constipation
- Pediatric age group: more common in infants; boys more than girls

PHYSICAL FINDINGS & CLINICAL PRESENTATION

- Acute stage: perianal swelling, pain, and fever
- Chronic stage: history of rectal drainage or bleeding; previous abscess with drainage
- Tender external fistulous opening, within 2 to 3 cm of the anal verge, with purulent or serosanguineous drainage on compression; the greater the distance from the anal margin, the greater the probability of a complicated upward extension
- Goodsall's rule:
  1. Location of the internal opening related to the location of the external opening.

2. With external opening anterior to an imaginary line drawn horizontally across the midpoint of the anus: fistulous tract runs radially into the anal canal.
3. With opening posterior to the transanal line: tract is usually curvilinear, entering the anal canal in the posterior midline.
4. Exception to this rule: an external, anterior opening that is >3 cm from the anus. In this case the tract may curve posteriorly and end in the posterior midline.

- If perianal abscess recurs, presence of a fistula is suggested

ETIOLOGY

- Most common: nonspecific cryptoglandular infection (skin or intestinal flora)
- Fistulas more common when intestinal microorganisms are cultured from the anorectal abscess
- Tuberculosis
- Lymphogranuloma venereum
- Actinomycosis
- Inflammatory bowel disease (IBD): Crohn's disease, ulcerative colitis
- Trauma: surgery (episiotomy, prostatectomy), foreign bodies, anal intercourse
- Malignancy: carcinoma, leukemia, lymphoma
- Treatment of malignancy: surgery, radiation

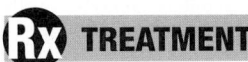 DIAGNOSIS

DIFFERENTIAL DIAGNOSIS

- Hidradenitis suppurativa
- Pilonidal sinus
- Bartholin's gland abscess or sinus
- Infected perianal sebaceous cysts

WORKUP

- Digital rectal examination:
  1. Assess sphincter tone and voluntary squeeze pressure
  2. Determine the presence of an extraluminal mass
  3. Identify an indurated track
  4. Palpate an internal opening or pit
- Gentle probing of external orifice to avoid creating a false tract; 50% do not have clinically detectable opening
- Anoscopy
- Proctosigmoidoscopy to exclude inflammatory or neoplastic disease
- All studies done under adequate anesthesia

LABORATORY TESTS

- Complete blood count
- Rectal biopsy if diagnosis of IBD or malignancy suspected; biopsy of external orifice is useless

IMAGING STUDIES

- Colonoscopy or barium enema if:
  1. Diagnosis of IBD or malignancy is suspected
  2. History of recurrent or multiple fistulas
  3. Patient <25 yr
- Small bowel series: occasionally obtained for reasons similar to above
- Fistulography: unreliable but may be helpful in complicated fistulas

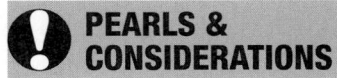 TREATMENT

NONPHARMACOLOGIC THERAPY

Sitz baths

ACUTE GENERAL Rx

- Treatment of choice: surgery
- Broad-spectrum antibiotic given if:
  1. Cellulitis present
  2. Patient is immunocompromised
  3. Valvular heart disease present
  4. Prosthetic devices present
- Stool softener/laxative

CHRONIC Rx

- Surgery
- Surgical goals are as follows:
  1. Cure the fistula
  2. Prevent recurrence
  3. Preserve sphincter function
  4. Minimize healing time
- Methods for the management of anal fistulas: fistulotomy, setons, rectal advancement flaps, colostomy

DISPOSITION

Outpatient surgery

REFERRAL

Refer to a surgeon with expertise in this area

PEARLS & CONSIDERATIONS

COMMENTS

- HIV-positive and diabetic patients with perirectal abscesses/fistulas are true surgical emergencies.
- Risk of septicemia, Fournier's gangrene, and other septic complications make immediate drainage imperative.

SUGGESTED READINGS
available at www.expertconsult.com

AUTHORS: **GEORGE T. DANAKAS, M.D.,** and **RUBEN ALVERO, M.D.**

BASIC INFORMATION

DEFINITION

Anorexia nervosa is a psychiatric disorder characterized by abnormal eating behavior, severe self-induced weight loss, and a specific psychopathology (see "Workup").

ICD-9CM CODES
307.1 Anorexia nervosa

EPIDEMIOLOGY & DEMOGRAPHICS

INCIDENCE/PREVALENCE (IN U.S.):
- Anorexia nervosa occurs in 0.2% to 1.3% of the general population, with an annual incidence of 5 to 10 cases per 100,000 persons.
- Participation in activities that promote thinness (athletics, modeling) is associated with a higher incidence of anorexia nervosa.

PREDOMINANT SEX: Female/male ratio is 9:1. Approximately 0.5% to 1% of women between the ages of 15 and 30 yr have anorexia nervosa.

PREDOMINANT AGE: Adolescence to young adulthood is the predominant age. Mean age of onset is 17 yr. Approximately 0.5% to 1% of college-aged women have anorexia nervosa.

PHYSICAL FINDINGS & CLINICAL PRESENTATION

Primary care physicians must be skilled at recognizing this disorder because patients with mild cases usually present with nonspecific symptoms such as asthenia, cold intolerance, lack of energy, or dizziness. The physical examination may be normal in the early stages or in mild cases. Patients with moderate to severe anorexia have the following physical characteristics:
- Patient is emaciated and bundled in clothing.
- Skin is dry and has excessive growth of lanugo. Skin may also be yellow-tinged from carotenodermia.
- Brittle nails, thinning scalp hair are present.
- Bradycardia, hypotension, hypothermia, and bradypnea are common.
- Female fat distribution pattern is no longer evident.
- Axillary and pubic hair is preserved.
- Peripheral edema may be present.

ETIOLOGY

- Etiology is unknown, but probably multifactorial (sociocultural, psychologic, familial, and genetic factors).
- A history of sexual abuse has been reported in as many as 50% of patients with anorexia nervosa.
- Psychologic factors: anorexics often have an incompletely developed personal identity. They struggle to maintain a sense of control over their environment, they usually have a low self-esteem, and they lack the sense that they are valued and loved for themselves.

DIAGNOSIS

DIFFERENTIAL DIAGNOSIS

- Other eating disorders (see Table 1-9)
- Depression with loss of appetite
- Schizophrenia
- Conversion disorder
- Occult carcinoma, lymphoma
- Endocrine disorders: Addison disease, diabetes mellitus, hypothyroidism or hyperthyroidism, panhypopituitarism
- Gastrointestinal disorders: celiac disease, Crohn disease, intestinal parasitosis
- Infectious disorders: AIDS, tuberculosis
- A clinical algorithm for the evaluation of anorexia is described in Section III

WORKUP

- A diagnosis can be made by using the following DSM-IV diagnostic criteria for anorexia nervosa:
  1. Refusal to maintain body weight (BW) at or above a minimally normal weight for age and height (e.g., weight loss leading to maintenance of BW <85% of that expected or failure to make expected weight gain during a period of growth, leading to BW <85% of that expected)
  2. Intense fear of gaining weight or becoming fat, even though underweight
  3. Disturbance in the way in which BW or shape is experienced, undue influence of BW or shape on self-evaluation, or denial of the seriousness of the current low BW
  4. In postmenarchal females, amenorrhea—that is, the absence of at least three consecutive menstrual cycles (A woman is considered to have amenorrhea if her periods occur only after hormone administration, such as estrogen.)

Specify type:
Restricting type: During the current episode of anorexia nervosa, the person has not regularly engaged in binge eating or purging behavior (i.e., self-induced vomiting or the misuse of laxatives, diuretics, or enemas).

Binge-eating/purging type: During the current episode of anorexia nervosa, the person has regularly engaged in binge eating or purging behavior (i.e., self-induced vomiting or the misuse of laxatives, diuretics, or enemas).

- The SCOFF questionnaire is a screening tool for eating disorders used in England. It consists of the following five questions:
  1. Do you make yourself *s*ick because you feel full?
  2. Have you lost *c*ontrol over how much you eat?
  3. Have you lost more than *o*ne stone (approximately 6 kg) recently?
  4. Do you believe yourself to be *f*at when others say you are thin?
  5. Does *f*ood dominate your life?
- A positive response to two or more questions has a reported sensitivity of 100% for anorexia and bulimia and an overall specificity of 87.5%.
- In college-aged women a positive response to any of the following screening questions also warrants further evaluation:
  1. How many diets have you been on in the past year?
  2. Do you think you should be dieting?
  3. Are you dissatisfied with your body size?
  4. Does your weight affect the way you think about yourself?
- Baseline ECG should be performed on all patients with anorexia nervosa. Routine monitoring of patients with prolonged QT interval is necessary; sudden death in these patients is often caused by ventricular arrhythmias related to QT interval prolongation.
- A dual-energy x-ray absorptiometry (DEXA) scan to screen for osteopenia should be considered after 6 mo of amenorrhea in patients suspected of anorexia nervosa.

LABORATORY TESTS

- In mild cases, laboratory findings may be completely normal.
- Endocrine abnormalities:
  1. Decreased follicle-stimulating hormone, luteinizing hormone, T_4, T_3, estrogens, urinary 17-OH steroids, estrone, and estradiol
  2. Normal free T_4, thyroid-stimulating hormone
  3. Increased cortisol, growth hormone, rT_3, T_3RU
  4. Absence of cyclic surge of luteinizing hormone
- Leukopenia, thrombocytopenia, anemia, reduced erythrocyte sedimentation rate, reduced complement levels, and reduced CD4 and CD8 cells may be present.
- Metabolic alkalosis, hypocalcemia, hypokalemia, hypomagnesemia, hypercholesterolemia, and hypophosphatemia may be present.
- Increased plasma β-carotene levels are useful to distinguish these patients from others on starvation diets.

TABLE 1-9 Diagnostic Features of Eating Disorders

Anorexia nervosa	Body weight willfully maintained below normal level
	Abnormal perception of body morphology
	Intense fear of weight gain
	Amenorrhea
Bulimia nervosa	Large uncontrolled eating binges at least twice weekly
	Inappropriate compensatory behavior (e.g., vomiting, purging)
Binge eating disorder	Large uncontrolled eating binges at least twice weekly
	No regular inappropriate compensatory disorders
	Marked distress about binges

From Besser CM, Thorner MO: *Comprehensive clinical endocrinology*, ed 3, 2002, Mosby.

(Rx) TREATMENT

NONPHARMACOLOGIC THERAPY

- A multidisciplinary approach with psychologic, medical, and nutritional support is necessary.
- A goal weight should be set and the patient should be initially monitored at least once a week in the office setting. The target weight is 100% of ideal BW for teenagers and 90% to 100% for older patients.
- Weight gain should be gradual (1 to 3 lb/wk) to prevent gastric dilation. Begin with 800 to 1200 kcal in frequent small meals (to avoid bloating sensation), then increase calories to 1500 to 3000 depending on height and age.
- Add, as necessary, vitamin and mineral supplements.
- In severe cases, total parenteral nutrition must be used (starting at 800 to 1200 kcal/day).
- Electrolyte levels should be strictly monitored.
- Mealtime should be a time for social interaction, not confrontation.
- Postprandially, sedentary activities are recommended. The patient's access to a bathroom should be monitored to prevent purging.

ACUTE GENERAL Rx

- Criteria to decide on the appropriate initial course of treatment for patients with anorexia nervosa are usually based on the presence of complications, percentage of ideal BW, and severity of body image distortion.
- Outpatient treatment is adequate for most patients.
- Indications for hospitalization are described under "Referral" section.
- Medically stable patients who are within 85% of ideal BW can be followed up by the primary care physician at 3- or 4-wk intervals, which can be lengthened as the patient improves.
- Pharmacologic treatment generally has no role in anorexia nervosa unless major depression or another psychiatric disorder is present. SSRIs can be used to alleviate the depressed mood and moderate obsessive-compulsive behavior in some individuals.

CHRONIC Rx

- Psychotherapy continued for years and focused specifically on self-image, family and peer interactions, and relapse prevention is an integral part of a successful recovery.
- Family therapy is also recommended, especially in younger patients.

DISPOSITION

- The long-term prognosis is generally poor and marked by recurrent exacerbations. The percentage of patients with anorexia nervosa who fully recover is modest. Most patients continue to have a distorted body image, disordered eating habits, and psychic difficulties.
- Most patients with anorexia nervosa will recover menses within 6 mo of reaching 90% of their ideal BW. It is important to note that patients with anorexia nervosa can become pregnant despite amenorrhea.
- Mortality rates vary from 5% to 20% and are six times that of peers without anorexia. Frequent causes of death are electrolyte abnormalities, starvation, or suicide.
- Factors that predict improved outcome in patients with eating disorders include early age at diagnosis, brief interval before initiation of treatment, good parent-child relationships, and having other healthy relationships with friends or therapists.
- A prolonged QT interval is a marker for risk of sudden death.

REFERRAL

Hospitalization should be considered in the following situations:

1. Severe dehydration or electrolyte imbalance
2. ECG abnormalities (prolonged QT interval, arrhythmias)
3. Significant physiologic instability (hypotension, orthostatic changes)
4. Intractable vomiting, purging, or bingeing
5. Suicidal thoughts
6. Weight loss exceeding 30% of ideal BW and unresponsiveness to outpatient treatment
7. Rapidly progressing weight loss (>2 lb in a week)
8. Failure to progress in nutritional rehabilitation in outpatient treatment

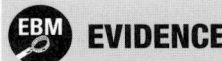 **EVIDENCE**

available at www.expertconsult.com

SUGGESTED READINGS
available at www.expertconsult.com

AUTHOR: **FRED F. FERRI, M.D.**

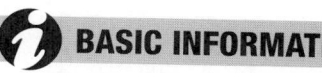

BASIC INFORMATION

DEFINITION

Anoxic brain injury is cerebral ischemic injury due to decreased oxygen or blood flow to the brain typically caused by interruption of cardiac circulation or respiratory failure.

SYNONYMS

Hypoxic-ischemic injury

ICD-9CM CODES
348.1 Anoxic brain damage

EPIDEMIOLOGY & DEMOGRAPHICS

INCIDENCE: 492,000 out-of-hospital cardiac arrests per year in the U.S.; however, reported incidence varies with criteria used for diagnosis.
PREVALENCE: The vegetative state varies from 40 to 168 per 1 million population depending on definition used; recovery is rare after 3 months with life expectancy lasting 2 to 5 years.
RISK FACTORS: For ischemia/hypoxia, include HTN, hyperlipidemia, tobacco use, and physical inactivity.

PHYSICAL FINDINGS & CLINICAL PRESENTATION

- Variable presentation depending on degree of insult
- Minimally conscious state: altered consciousness with normal sleep-wake cycles and intermittent interaction with the environment such as intermittently following simple commands, producing purposeful behavior, and maintaining visual tracking
- Vegetative state: loss of cognitive awareness and ability to interact with environment but maintain normal sleep-wake cycles
- Coma: pathologic loss of awareness and ability to interact with the environment
- Brain death syndrome: irreversible loss of cortical and brainstem function manifesting as loss of awareness, cranial reflexes, and motor response, isoelectric EEG

ETIOLOGY

- Ischemia (decreased cerebral perfusion): myocardial infarction, hemorrhage, shock
- Hypoxia (decreased oxygenation): drowning, strangulation, aspiration, carbon monoxide poisoning

DIAGNOSIS

DIFFERENTIAL DIAGNOSIS

- Potentially reversible forms of stupor and coma: hypoglycemia, hepatic encephalopathy, uremia, thyrotoxicosis, other metabolic disturbances

WORKUP

- Avoid misdiagnosis of reversible causes of coma by repeating clinical and lab tests. Hypothermia, alcohol intoxication, anesthesia, other pharmacologic agents, and other metabolic disturbances may cause stupor but represent reversible causes, which allows potential for recovery.

LABORATORY TEST(S)

Urine drug screen, serum metabolic profile, ammonia, complete blood count, coagulation panel, fingerstick glucose, arterial blood gas, blood alcohol panel, serum neuron specific enolase (if available)

IMAGING STUDIES

- Imaging is usually unrevealing within first 24 hr of an anoxic event.
- CT head without contrast (Figure 1-33): obtain 24 hr after anoxic event to evaluate for stroke, trauma, or hemorrhage
- MRI brain (Figure 1-34): obtain if CT head scan unrevealing
- EEG: to assess for nonconvulsive status epilepticus
- SSEP (somatosensory evoked potentials): obtain 48 hr after anoxic event; poor bilateral cortical response is associated with poor prognosis

TREATMENT

NONPHARMACOLOGIC THERAPY

- Hypothermia: evidence suggests inducing hypothermia 32-34° C for 24 hr reduces metabolic need, which may improve prognosis
- Complications from hypothermia include bradycardia, hemodynamic instability, coagulopathy, infection, hyperglycemia, and hypokalemia; therefore, its use is contraindicated in certain situations.
- Hypothermia is contraindicated in patients with active hemorrhage, hemodynamic instability, sepsis, or trauma.
- Indication for hypothermia: patients who have been resuscitated from a cardiac arrest with VF/VT as the presenting rhythm
- Hyperbaric oxygen in carbon monoxide poisoning

ACUTE GENERAL Rx

- Supportive care to prevent further injury: ABCs, secure airway, and initiate cardiopulmonary resuscitation if indicated
- Control seizures with antiepileptic medications (may need midazolam or propofol drip if severe uncontrolled seizures).
- Treat myoclonus with clonazepam 8-12 mg daily in divided doses.

CHRONIC Rx

- Maintain adequate nutrition and infection precautions, and provide DVT and gastric ulceration prophylaxis.
- Physical, occupational, and speech therapy as indicated per prognosis and patient ability
- May consider withdrawal of treatment per prognosis, family consultation, and respect for autonomy and dignity of the patient

DISPOSITION

Varies per extent of insult from acute rehabilitation to long-term care facility to return to home

REFERRAL

Referral to a neurologist is appropriate for definitive prognostication.

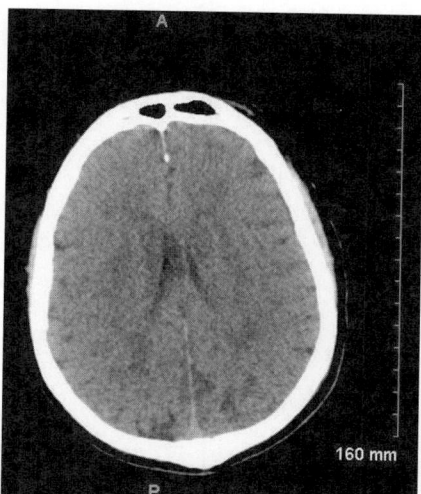

FIGURE 1-33 CT without contrast of a patient 1 day after PEA showing diffuse sulci effacement and loss of gray-white matter differentiation indicating cerebral edema. Diffuse white and gray matter hypodensities are also present. The patient remained comatose and life support was eventually withdrawn.

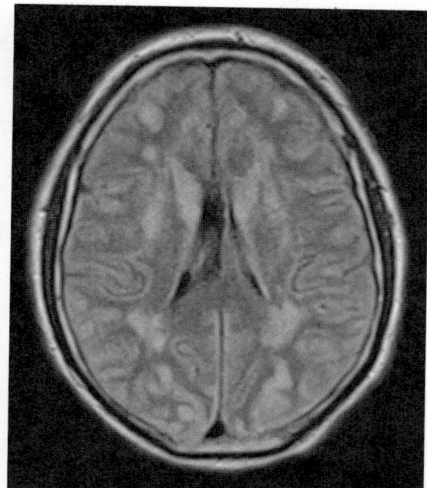

FIGURE 1-34 MRI FLAIR (Fluid attenuated inversion recovery) of a patient 1 day after PEA showing bilateral multiple cortical, subcortical, gray and white hyperintensities. The patient remained comatose and life support was eventually withdrawn.

TABLE 1-10 Predictors of Poor Prognosis

Time from Onset of Anoxic Event	Clinical Exam
Initial exam	Pupils do not react to light (reflex absent)
24 hr	Eye movements are not roving conjugate or orienting and motor response is not better than flexor
72 hr	Motor response is not better than flexor
1 wk	Eye movements are not roving conjugate or orienting, no spontaneous eye opening, no following of commands
2 wk	No normal oculocephalic response, no following of commands, no spontaneous eye opening, and eye opening not improved by at least two grades

Composed from data presented in Levy DE et al: Predicting outcome from hypoxic-ischemic coma, *JAMA* 253(10):1420-1426, 1985.

TABLE 1-11 Predictors of Good Prognosis

Time from Onset of Anoxic Event	Clinical Exam
Initial exam	Pupils react to light (reflex present), motor response flexor or extensor, and eye movements spontaneous roving conjugate or orienting
24 hr	Motor response withdrawal or better, and eye opening improved at least 2 grades
72 hr	Motor response withdrawal or better and normal spontaneous eye movements present
1 wk	Follows commands
2 wk	Normal oculocephalic response

Composed from data presented in Levy DE et al: Predicting outcome from hypoxic-ischemic coma, *JAMA* 253(10):1420-1426, 1985.

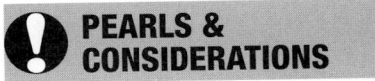

PEARLS & CONSIDERATIONS

COMMENTS
When assessing prognosis, use caution if patient is being treated with anesthetic agents or depressants including anticonvulsants. Refer to Tables 1-10 and 1-11 for indicators of prognosis.

PREVENTION
CPR, risk factor modification, induced hypothermia

PATIENT/FAMILY EDUCATION
Consult with family members regularly and provide accurate assessment of prognosis.

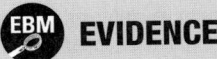 **EVIDENCE**

available at www.expertconsult.com

SUGGESTED READINGS

available at www.expertconsult.com

AUTHOR: **ALEXANDRA BOSKE, M.D.**

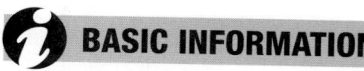

BASIC INFORMATION

DEFINITION

Anthrax is an acute infectious disease caused by the spore-forming bacterium *Bacillus anthracis.*

ICD-9CM CODES
022.0 Cutaneous anthrax
022.1 Inhalation anthrax
022.2 Gastrointestinal anthrax
022.3 Sepsis from anthrax

EPIDEMIOLOGY & DEMOGRAPHICS

- Anthrax most commonly occurs in hoofed animals and can only incidentally infect human beings who come in contact with infected animals or animal products. Between 20,000 and 100,000 cases of cutaneous anthrax occur worldwide annually. In the U.S. the annual incidence was about 130 cases before 2001.
- Until the recent bioterrorism attack in 2001, most cases of anthrax occurred in industrial environments (contaminated raw materials used in manufacturing process) or in agriculture.
- In 2001 there were more than 20 confirmed cases of anthrax resulting from bioterrorism, most of which were associated with handling of contaminated mail. Inhalation anthrax is the most lethal form of anthrax and results from inspiration of 8000 to 50,000 spores of *B. anthracis.* Before 2001 there had not been a case of inhalation anthrax in the U.S. for 20 years.
- Direct person-to-person spread of anthrax is extremely unlikely, if it occurs at all; therefore there is no need to immunize or treat contacts of persons ill with anthrax, such as household contacts, friends, or co-workers, unless they also were exposed to the same source of infection.

PHYSICAL FINDINGS & CLINICAL PRESENTATION

Symptoms of disease vary depending on how the disease was contracted but usually occur within 7 days after exposure. The serious forms of human anthrax are inhalation anthrax, cutaneous anthrax, and gastrointestinal anthrax.

- **Inhalation anthrax** begins with a brief prodrome resembling a viral respiratory illness followed by development of hypoxia and dyspnea, with radiographic evidence of mediastinal widening. Host factors, dose of exposure, and chemoprophylaxis may affect the duration of the incubation period. Initial symptoms include mild fever, muscle aches, and malaise and may progress to respiratory failure and shock; meningitis often develops.
- **Cutaneous anthrax** is characterized by a skin lesion evolving from a papule, through a vesicular stage, to a depressed black eschar. The incubation period ranges from 1 to 12 days. The lesion is usually painless, but patients also may have fever, malaise, headache, and regional lymphadenopathy. The eschar dries and falls off in 1 to 2 wk with little scarring.
- **Gastrointestinal anthrax** is characterized by severe abdominal pain followed by fever and signs of septicemia. Bloody diarrhea and signs of acute abdomen may occur. This form of anthrax usually follows after eating raw or undercooked contaminated meat and can have an incubation period of 1 to 7 days. Gastric ulcers may occur and may be associated with hematemesis. Oropharyngeal and abdominal forms of the disease have been described. Involvement of the pharynx is usually characterized by lesions at the base of the tongue, dysphagia, fever, and regional lymphadenopathy. Lower bowel inflammation typically causes nausea, loss of appetite, and fever followed by abdominal pain, hematemesis, and bloody diarrhea.

ETIOLOGY

The disease is caused by *B. anthracis,* a gram-positive, spore-forming bacillus. It is aerobic, nonmotile, nonhemolytic on sheep's blood agar and grows readily at temperature of 37° C, forming large colonies with irregularly tapered outgrowths (a Medusa's head appearance). In the host it appears as single organisms or chains of two or three bacilli.

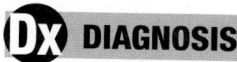

DIAGNOSIS

DIFFERENTIAL DIAGNOSIS

- Inhalation anthrax must be distinguished from influenza-like illness (ILI) and tularemia. Most cases of ILI are associated with nasal congestion and rhinorrhea, which are unusual in inhalation anthrax. Additional distinguishing factors are the usual absence of abnormal chest radiograph in ILI (see below).
- Cutaneous anthrax should be distinguished from staphylococcal disease, ecthyma, ecthyma gangrenosum, plague, brown recluse spider bite, and tularemia.
- The differential diagnosis of gastrointestinal anthrax includes viral gastroenteritis, shigellosis, and yersiniosis.

LABORATORY TESTS

- Presumptive identification is based on Gram stain of material from skin lesion, CSF, or blood showing encapsulated gram-positive bacilli.
- Confirmatory tests are performed at specialized laboratories. Virulent strains grow on nutrient agar in the presence of 5% CO_2. Susceptibility to lysis by gamma phage and DFA staining of cell-wall polysaccharide antigen are also useful confirmatory tests.
- Nasal swab culture to determine inhalation exposure is of limited diagnostic value. A negative result does not exclude the possibility of exposure. It may be used by public health officials to assist in epidemiologic investigations of exposed persons to evaluate the dispersion of spores.
- Serologic testing by enzyme-linked immunosorbent assay (ELISA) can confirm the diagnosis.
- A skin test (Anthracin test) that detects anthrax cell-mediated immunity is also available in specialized laboratories.

IMAGING STUDIES

Chest radiographs usually reveal mediastinal widening. Additional findings include infiltrates and pleural effusion.

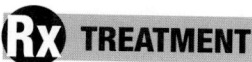

TREATMENT

NONPHARMACOLOGIC Rx

IV hydration and ventilator support may be necessary with inhalation anthrax.

ACUTE GENERAL Rx

- Most naturally occurring *B. anthracis* strains are sensitive to penicillin. The FDA has approved penicillin, doxycycline, and ciprofloxacin for the treatment of inhalational anthrax infection.
- Table 1-12 describes a treatment protocol for inhalation anthrax.
- Initial postexposure prophylaxis therapy in adults is with ciprofloxacin, 500 mg PO bid, or doxycycline 100 mg bid. The total duration of treatment is 60 days.
- A single dose of raxibacumab, a human monoclonal antibody directed against protective antigen, a component of the anthrax toxin, has been reported effective in improving survival in rabbits and monkeys with symptomatic inhalational anthrax.

DISPOSITION

- Case fatality estimates for inhalation anthrax are extremely high (>90%).
- The case fatality rate for cutaneous anthrax is 20% without and <1% with antibiotic treatment.
- The case fatality rate for gastrointestinal anthrax is estimated to be 25% to 60%.

REFERRAL

Consultation with an infectious disease specialist is recommended in all cases of anthrax. Local and state authorities should also be notified of suspected cases of anthrax.

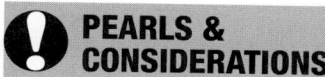

PEARLS & CONSIDERATIONS

COMMENTS

- Postexposure prophylaxis: If the exposure to *B. anthracis* is confirmed and anthrax vaccine is available, 3 doses of the vaccine should be given at 0, 2, and 4 wk, and antibiotics should be continued throughout the 4-wk period. If vaccine is not available, antibiotics should be continued for 60 days.

- Preexposure vaccination is limited to groups at risk for repeated exposures to *B. anthracis* spores, such as bioterrorism level-B laboratories and workers who will be making repeated entries into known *B. anthracis* spore-contaminated areas.
- The U.S. anthrax vaccine is an inactivated cell-free product licensed to be given in a 6-dose series.

SUGGESTED READINGS
available at www.expertconsult.com

AUTHOR: **FRED F. FERRI, M.D.**

TABLE 1-12   Inhalation Anthrax Treatment Protocol[a,b]

Category	Initial Therapy (IV)[c,d]	Duration
Adults	Ciprofloxacin 400 mg q12h[a] **or** Doxycycline 100 mg q12h[f] **and** One or two additional antimicrobials[d]	IV treatment initially.[e] Switch to oral antimicrobial therapy when clinically appropriate: Ciprofloxacin 500 mg PO bid **or** Doxycycline 100 mg PO bid Continue for 60 days (IV and PO combined)[g]
Children	Ciprofloxacin 10-15 mg/kg q12h[h,i] **or** Doxycycline[f,j]: >8 yr and >45 kg: 100 mg q12h >8 yr and ≤45 kg: 2.2 mg/kg q12h ≤8 yr: 2.2 mg/kg q12h **and** One or two additional antimicrobials[d]	IV treatment initially.[e] Switch to oral antimicrobial therapy when clinically appropriate: Ciprofloxacin 10-15 mg/kg PO q12h[i] **or** Doxycycline[j]: >8 yr and >45 kg: 100 mg PO bid >8 yr and ≤45 kg: 2.2 mg/kg PO bid ≤8 yr: 2.2 mg/kg PO bid Continue for 60 days (IV and PO combined)[g]
Pregnant women[k]	Same for nonpregnant adults (the high death rate from the infection outweighs the risk posed by the antimicrobial agent)	IV treatment initially. Switch to oral antimicrobial therapy when clinically appropriate.[b] Oral therapy regimens same for nonpregnant adults.
Immunocompromised persons	Same for nonimmunocompromised persons and children	Same for nonimmunocompromised persons and children

From *MMWR Morb Mortal Wkly Rep* 5:987, 2001.
[a]For gastrointestinal and oropharyngeal anthrax, use regimens recommended for inhalational anthrax.
[b]Ciprofloxacin or doxycycline should be considered an essential part of first-line therapy for inhalational anthrax.
[c]Steroids may be considered as an adjunct therapy for patients with severe edema and for meningitis based on experience with bacterial meningitis of other etiologies.
[d]Other agents with in vitro activity include rifampin, vancomycin, penicillin, ampicillin, chloramphenicol, imipenem, clindamycin, and clarithromycin. Because of concerns of constitutive and inducible beta-lactamases in *Bacillus anthracis,* penicillin and ampicillin should not be used alone. Consultation with an infectious disease specialist is advised.
[e]Initial therapy may be altered based on clinical course of the patient; one or two antimicrobial agents (e.g., ciprofloxacin or doxycycline) may be adequate as the patient improves.
[f]If meningitis is suspected, doxycycline may be less optimal because of poor central nervous system penetration.
[g]Because of the potential persistence of spores after an aerosol exposure, antimicrobial therapy should be continued for 60 days.
[h]If IV ciprofloxacin is not available, oral ciprofloxacin may be acceptable because it is rapidly and well absorbed from the gastrointestinal tract with no substantial loss by first-pass metabolism. Maximum serum concentrations are attained 1 to 2 hr after oral dosing but may not be achieved if vomiting or ileus is present.
[i]In children, ciprofloxacin dosage should not exceed 1 g/day.
[j]The American Academy of Pediatrics recommends treatment of young children with tetracyclines for serious infections (e.g., Rocky Mountain spotted fever).
[k]Although tetracyclines are not recommended during pregnancy, their use may be indicated for life-threatening illness. Adverse effects on developing teeth and bones are dose related; therefore doxycycline might be used for a short time (7 to 14 days) before 6 mo of gestation.

BASIC INFORMATION

DEFINITION

The antiphospholipid antibody syndrome (APS) is characterized by arterial or venous thrombosis and/or pregnancy morbidity *and* the presence of at least one type of antiphospholipid antibody (aPL). aPL are antibodies directed against serum proteins bound to anionic phospholipids. Three types of aPL have been characterized:
- Lupus anticoagulants
- Anticardiolipin antibodies
- Anti-β_2-glycoprotein-1 antibodies
  Primary APS occurs alone and secondary APS is in association with systemic lupus erythematosus (SLE), other rheumatic disorders, or certain infections or medications. APS can affect all organ systems and includes venous and arterial thrombosis, recurrent fetal losses, and thrombocytopenia.

ICD-9CM CODES
795.79 Antiphospholipid antibody syndrome

EPIDEMIOLOGY & DEMOGRAPHICS

PREVALENCE:
- 1% to 5% of healthy individuals have anticardiolipin (ACL) and lupus anticoagulant (LA) antibodies.
- 12% to 30% of patients with SLE have ACL antibodies and 15% to 34% have LA antibodies.

PREDOMINANT AGE: Young to middle-age adults.

RISK FACTORS:
- Underlying SLE and collagen-vascular diseases; other autoimmune disorders including rheumatoid arthritis, Sjögren's syndrome, Behçet's syndrome, and idiopathic thrombocytopenic purpura; AIDS.
- Most individuals are otherwise healthy and have no underlying medical condition.
- Several studies assessing presence of aPL in patients with cardiovascular and cerebrovascular disease have found a higher than expected prevalence of antibody.

GENETICS: Some APS-positive families exist, and human leukocyte antigen (HLA) studies have suggested associations with HLA DR7, DR4, and Dqw7+Drw53.

PHYSICAL FINDINGS & CLINICAL PRESENTATION
- Thrombosis: Patients with APS are at risk for both venous and arterial thromboses. Venous thromboses are more common, occurring as the initial manifestation of APS in ~30% of APS patients. Of all patients with venous thrombosis, 5% to 20% have aPL. The most common site for deep vein thrombosis is the calf, but thromboses may also occur in the renal, hepatic, axillary, subclavian, vena cava, and retinal veins. The most common site of arterial thrombosis is the cerebral vessels, followed by the coronary, renal, mesenteric, and bypass arteries. Recurrent thrombosis is common with APS.

- Common involved organ systems:
  - Central nervous system: stroke, transient ischemic attack, migraine, multiinfarct dementia, epilepsy, movement disorders, transverse myelopathy, depression, and Guillain-Barré syndrome, migraine
  - Pulmonary: pulmonary embolism and infarction, pulmonary hypertension, acute respiratory distress syndrome, intraalveolar pulmonary hemorrhage, a postpartum syndrome characterized by fever, pleuritic chest pain, dyspnea, and patchy infiltrates with pleural effusion on chest radiograph.
  - Cardiology: Libman-Sacks endocarditis, intracardiac thrombosis, coronary artery disease, myocardial infarction.
  - Gastrointestinal: abdominal pain, gastrointestinal bleed secondary to ischemia, splenic or pancreatic infarction, hepatic vein thrombosis, Budd-Chiari syndrome (second most common cause of syndrome).
  - Renal: proteinuria, acute renal failure, hypertension, renal infarct, renal artery or vein thrombosis, postpartum hemolytic-uremic syndrome.
  - Hematology: thrombocytopenia, hemolytic anemia.
  - Endocrine: Addison's disease secondary to adrenal hemorrhage and, less frequently, thrombosis.
  - Cutaneous: livedo reticularis, cutaneous necrosis, skin ulcerations, gangrene of digits.
  - Obstetrics: recurrent spontaneous abortion, premature delivery or fetal growth retardation.
- Catastrophic APS (CAPS) (Table 1-13): rapidly progressive multiorgan thrombotic disease. 1% of APS is CAPS, ~45% of CAPS do not present as APS initially. 50% mortality in CAPS. To make the diagnosis of catastrophic APS, four criteria must be satisfied:
  1. Evidence of involvement of ≥3 organs, systems, and/or tissues
  2. Development of manifestations simultaneously or in ≤1 week
  3. Confirmation by histopathology of small-vessel occlusion in at least one organ or tissue
  4. Laboratory confirmation of the presence of aPL

ETIOLOGY
- aPL react with negatively charged phospholipids.
- Possible mechanisms of thrombosis include effects of aPL on platelet membranes, endothelial cells, and clotting components such as prothrombin, protein C or S.
- Recently shown that prephospholipids are not immunogenic and that a binding protein (β_2-glycoprotein I) may be the key immunogen in the APS.

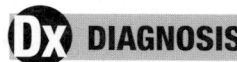 DIAGNOSIS

DIFFERENTIAL DIAGNOSIS

Other hypercoagulable states (inherited or acquired)
- Inherited: ATIII, protein C, S deficiencies, factor V Leiden, prothrombin gene mutation
- Acquired: heparin-induced thrombocytopenia, myeloproliferative syndromes, cancer, hyperviscosity
- Hyperhomocysteinemia
- Nephrotic syndrome

WORKUP

Diagnostic criteria of APS include at least one clinical criterion and at least one laboratory criterion.
- Clinical:
  1. Venous, arterial, or small vessel thrombosis *or*
  2. Morbidity with pregnancy defined as
     - Fetal death at ≥10 wk's gestation *or*
     - ≥1 premature births before 34 wk's gestation secondary to eclampsia, preeclampsia, or severe placental insufficiency *or*
     - ≥3 unexplained consecutive spontaneous abortions at <10 wk's gestation
- Laboratory:
  1. IgG and/or IgM anticardiolipin antibody in medium or high titers *or*
  2. Lupus anticoagulant activity found *or*
  3. Anti-β_2-glycoprotein-1 IgM or IgG antibodies found on ≥2 occasions, at least 12 wk apart

LABORATORY TESTS

Laboratory testing of ACL and LA antibodies indicated in:
- Patient with underlying SLE or collagen-vascular disease with thrombosis

TABLE 1-13 Differential Diagnosis of Catastrophic Antiphospholipid Syndrome

Laboratory Abnormalities	CAPS	TTP	DIC
Microangiopathic hemolytic anemia	−	+	+
Thrombocytopenia	+	+	+
Fibrinogen/FDP	Normal/Normal	Normal/Increased	Decreased/Increased
Anticardiolipin antibody	+	−	−
Lupus anticoagulant	+	−	−

DIC, Diffuse intravascular coagulation; *FDP*, fibrinogen degradation products; *TTP*, thrombotic thrombocytopenia purpura.
(From Hochberg MC et al [eds]: *Rheumatology*, ed 3, St Louis, 2003, Mosby.)

- Patient with recurrent, familial, or juvenile deep vein thrombosis (DVT) or thrombosis in an unusual location (mesenteric or cerebral)
- Possibly in patients with lupus or lupuslike disorders in high-risk situations (e.g., surgery, prolonged immobilization, pregnancy)

Abnormal tests include:

- False-positive test for syphilis (RPR/VDRL)
- Lupus anticoagulant activity, demonstrated by prolongation of activated partial thromboplastin time that does not correct with 1:1 mixing study
- Presence of anticardiolipin antibodies (ELISA for anticardiolipin is most sensitive and specific test [>80%])
- Presence of anti–β_2-glycoprotein I antibody

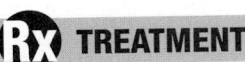

TREATMENT

ACUTE GENERAL Rx

SECONDARY PROPHYLAXIS:

- For positive aPL and venous or arterial thrombosis:
  - Anticoagulation with heparin or low-molecular-weight (LMW) heparin, then lifelong warfarin treatment, INR 2.0 to 3.0
  - Some evidence to support higher INR target or addition of other agents in arterial clots.
- For pregnant women with previously diagnosed APS:
  - Warfarin should be discontinued in early pregnancy secondary to its teratogenic effects.
  - ASA, 81 mg, and unfractionated heparin (UFH) SC or LMW heparin to therapeutic partial thromboplastin time (PTT) or factor Xa levels, respectively.
  - Pregnant patients on LMW heparin should be transitioned to unfractionated heparin prior to delivery as unfractionated heparin is more easily managed in patients who wish to have epidural anesthesia for childbirth due to a shorter half-life and reversibility.

- IVIG, plasmapheresis, hydroxychloroquine, statins, clopidrogel, dipyridamole and rituximab have been used when other treatments have failed.
- For pregnant women with (+) aPL antibodies and a history of <3 spontaneous abortions:
  - ASA 81 mg daily at conception and UFH 5000 to 10,000 IU SC q12h at time of documented viable intrauterine pregnancy (~7 wk's gestation) until 6 wk postpartum.
  - A mid-interval PTT should be checked and should be normal or similar to baseline before therapy.
  - LMW heparin can be used in place of unfractionated heparin and should be titrated to factor Xa levels in the recommended prophylactic range. The combination of ASA 75 mg daily + LMW heparin has been associated with a higher live birth rate when compared to IVIG.
- For pregnant women with (+) aPL antibodies without a history of DVT or pregnancy loss:
  - Consider low-dose UFH or LMW heparin SC, ASA 81 mg, or surveillance.
- For catastrophic APS:
  - Highest survival rate achieved with the combination of anticoagulation, corticosteroids, and IVIG or plasma exchange.
  - Case reports of Rituximab as successful therapy for patients with life-threatening thrombosis refractory to anticoagulation.

CHRONIC Rx

- Anticoagulation with warfarin therapy.
- Immunosuppressive agents such as corticosteroids and cyclophosphamide not effective.
- Limited data suggest that hydroxychloroquine may be effective.

DISPOSITION

- APS patients have a 20% to 70% risk for recurrent thrombosis.

- Initial arterial thrombosis tends to be followed by arterial events, and initial venous thrombosis tends to be followed by venous events.
- Catastrophic APS is associated with a high mortality rate, approaching 50%.
- Incidence of developing catastrophic APS is ~0.8% among APS patients.

REFERRAL

To hematology and/or obstetric medicine when diagnosis is made

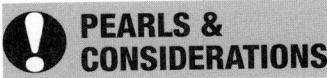

COMMENTS

Cerebral features of SLE may be more related to thrombosis than inflammation and may respond better to anticoagulants than immunosuppression.

PREVENTION

Prophylaxis for asymptomatic patients with (+) aPL without previous thrombosis:

- No routine prophylaxis is recommended.
- Questionable whether ASA 81 mg daily is effective.
- Antithrombotic prophylaxis for major surgery, prolonged immobilization, and pregnancy.
- Avoid oral contraceptive pills in women with (+) aPL.

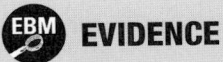 **EVIDENCE**

available at www.expertconsult.com

SUGGESTED READINGS

available at www.expertconsult.com

AUTHORS: **LYNN BOWLBY, M.D.**, and **IRIS TONG, M.D.**

BASIC INFORMATION

DEFINITION

Generalized anxiety disorder (GAD) is most likely to present in combination with other psychiatric and medical conditions. Individuals with GAD commonly present with excessive and disproportionately high levels of anxiety, fear, or worry for most days over at least a 6-mo period. The subjective anxiety must be accompanied by at least three somatic symptoms (e.g., restlessness, irritability, sleep disturbance, muscle tension, difficulty concentrating, or fatigability). GAD cannot be diagnosed if it occurs only in the setting of an active mood disorder, such as depression, or in the setting of an another active anxiety disorder, such as PTSD or panic disorder.

SYNONYMS

Anxiety neurosis (former name for a subset of anxiety disorders)
Chronic anxiety
GAD

ICD-9CM CODE
F41.1

DSM-IV CODE
300.02

EPIDEMIOLOGY & DEMOGRAPHICS

INCIDENCE (IN U.S.): 6% to 9% per year in adult primary care clinics
PEAK INCIDENCE: Chronic condition with onset early in life
PREVALENCE (IN U.S.):
- In general population: prevalence of 5% lifetime
- In primary care setting: 3% (the most common anxiety disorder in this setting)
PREDOMINANT SEX: Women are more frequently affected (2:1 ratio) but may present for treatment less often (3:2 female/male).
PREDOMINANT AGE:
- 30% report onset before age 11
- 50% have onset before age 18
GENETICS: Concordance rates in dizygotic twins and monozygotic twins are not different (0% to 5%)

PHYSICAL FINDINGS & CLINICAL PRESENTATION

- Report of being "anxious" all of their lives.
- Excessive worry, usually regarding family, finances, work, or health.
- Sleep disturbance, particularly early insomnia.
- Muscle tension (typically in the muscles of neck and shoulders) or headache.
- Difficulty concentrating.
- Daytime fatigue.
- GI symptoms compatible with IBS (one third of patients).
- Physical symptoms are the usual reason for seeking medical attention.
- Comorbid psychiatric illness (e.g., dysthymia or major depression) and substance abuse (e.g., alcohol abuse) are frequent.

ETIOLOGY

- Hypotheses include models based on neurotransmitters (catecholamines, indolamines) and developmental psychology.
- Prevalence increased with a family history, increase in stress, history of physical or emotional trauma, and medical illness.

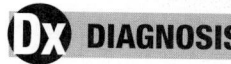 DIAGNOSIS

DIFFERENTIAL DIAGNOSIS

- Wide range of psychiatric and medical conditions:
- Cardiovascular and pulmonary disease, such as cardiac arrhythmias or COPD.
- Hyperthyroidism.
- Substance abuse (e.g., cocaine, amphetamines, and PCP) or withdrawal (e.g., alcohol or benzodiazepines).

WORKUP

- Screening tests may enhance detection. A simple 7-item in-office case finding instrument, the GAD-7, can detect GAD with sensitivity of 89% and specificity of 82%.
- Physical examination: additional laboratory and radiologic workup depend on presenting symptoms.
- Iatrogenic cause should be suspected if anxiety follows recent changes in medication.

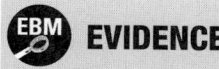 TREATMENT

NONPHARMACOLOGIC THERAPY

- Cognitive-behavioral therapy
- Relaxation training
- Biofeedback
- Psychodynamic psychotherapy

PHARMACOLOGIC THERAPY

- SSRIs/SNRIs
- Azapirones (e.g., buspirone)
- Benzodiazepines (less favored)

ACUTE GENERAL Rx

- Acute treatment is rarely indicated because GAD is a chronic condition.
- If patients are in acute distress, the possibility of another cause, including another anxiety disorder such as panic disorder, should be considered.
- Caution in prescribing benzodiazepines because of the propensity for misuse and dependence. If used, the patient should be educated about the options and the risks.

CHRONIC Rx

- SSRIs and SNRIs (e.g., venlafaxine and duloxetine) are effective typical first-line treatment. Particularly useful if comorbid depression present.
- Buspirone can be effective with minimal potential for tolerance or abuse. May be less effective in patients with previous benzodiazepine exposure and may require a high-dose titration.
- Benzodiazepines can be effective under good supervision; however, tolerance is common, and for this reason they have fallen from a first-line treatment. Benzodiazepines can also create functional impairment.
- Sedating antidepressants may also be useful for initial insomnia secondary to anxious ruminations.

DISPOSITION

- GAD is chronic with periodic exacerbations.
- Treatment is given to reduce level of symptoms. Suicide risk is higher than in the general population.

REFERRAL

- For refractory symptoms.
- For comorbid psychiatric conditions.

EVIDENCE

available at www.expertconsult.com

SUGGESTED READINGS
available at www.expertconsult.com

AUTHORS: **SETH A. BERKOWITZ, M.D.,** and **ILJIE KIM FITZGERALD, M.D., M.S.**

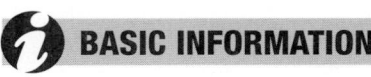

DEFINITION

Aortic dissection is part of a spectrum of aortic pathologies that include intramural hemtoma-sand penetrating atherosclerotic ulcers. Aortic dissection occurs when blood passes through an intimal tear, separating the intima from the medial layers and creating a false lumen. Intramural hematoma (IMH) occurs when the vasa vasorum ruptures within the medial wall. IMH does not involve an intimal tearing unless a dissection develops. One third of IMH will transform into aortic dissection. Penetrating atherosclerotic ulcers destroy the aortic intima and dissect into the aortic media,resulting in the formation of a pseudoaneurysm. Unlike aortic dissection, penetrating ulcers occur on the basis of extensive atherosclerosis in the aortic intima.

SYNONYMS

Dissecting aortic aneurysm

ICD-9CM CODES
441.00 Aortic dissection
444.01 Aortic dissection, thoracic

EPIDEMIOLOGY & DEMOGRAPHICS

PREDOMINANT SEX AND AGE: Males > females (ratio 3:1), ages 60 to 80 yr; mean, 63 yr
INCIDENCE: Approximately 2000 cases per year; thirteenth-leading cause of death in U.S.
RISK FACTORS:
- Hypertension (found in up to 72% of patients with aortic dissection).
- Age
- Atherosclerosis
- Family history of aortic aneurysms/dissection
- History of cardiac surgery, intraaortic catheterization
- Disorders of collagen (Marfan syndrome, Ehlers-Danlos syndrome)

- Vascular inflammation (giant cell arteritis, Takayasu arteritis, rheumatoid arthritis, syphilitic aortitis)
- Aortic coarctation, bicuspid aortic valve
- Turner's syndrome
- Cocaine abuse
- Trauma

CLASSIFICATION

Aortic dissection **is generally** classified according to anatomical location (Fig. 1-35):
- DeBakey: type I ascending and descending aorta, type II ascending aorta, type III descending aorta
- Stanford: type A ascending aorta (proximal), type B descending aorta (distal) (Fig. 1-36)
  Aortic dissection can also be classified by acuity of presentation (acute or chronic), based on the time of onset.

PHYSICAL FINDINGS & CLINICAL PRESENTATION

- Sudden onset of severe sharp, tearing, or ripping chest pain
- Anterior chest pain (ascending dissection)
- Back pain, abdominal pain (descending dissection)
- Syncope, congestive heart failure (CHF), malperfusion may occur
- Most present with severe hypertension, 25% with hypotension (systolic blood pressure <100 mm Hg), which can indicate bleeding, cardiac tamponade, or severe aortic regurgitation
- Pulse and blood pressure differentials (>20 mm Hg between arms) in 9% to 30% of cases, caused by partial compression of subclavian arteries
- Aortic regurgitation in 18% to 50% of cases of proximal dissection, often with diastolic decrescendo murmur

- Myocardial ischemia caused by coronary artery occlusion
- Stroke in 5% to 10% of patients
- Horner syndrome
- Vocal cord paralysis/hoarse voice

ETIOLOGY

Aortic dissection shares a common pathway of cystic medial necorsis with abdominal aortic aneurysm formation. Genetics, in addition to other risk factors listed above, contribute to the development of aortic dissection.

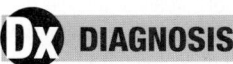
DIAGNOSIS

DIFFERENTIAL DIAGNOSIS

- Known as the great imitator: PE, ACS, aortic stenosis/insufficiency, nondissecting aneurysm, pericarditis, cholecystitis, peptic ulcer disease, pancreatitis, musculoskeletal pain
- Acute MI needs to be ruled out.
- Consider aortic dissection in patients with unexplained stroke, chest pain, syncope, acute onset CHF, abdominal pain, back pain, and malperfusion of extremities or internal organs.

LABORATORY TESTS

- ECG: helpful to rule out MI, although dissection can lead to coronary ischemia
- D-dimer has a 100% negative predictive value but lacks specificity in the setting in acute aortic dissection.
- Three biomarkers with different diagnostic windows, can be used in the diagnosis of aortic dissection.
- Smooth muscle myosin heavy chain protein (released from damaged medial smooth muscle) can be used to detect proximal aortic dissections (91% sensitivity and 93% speci-

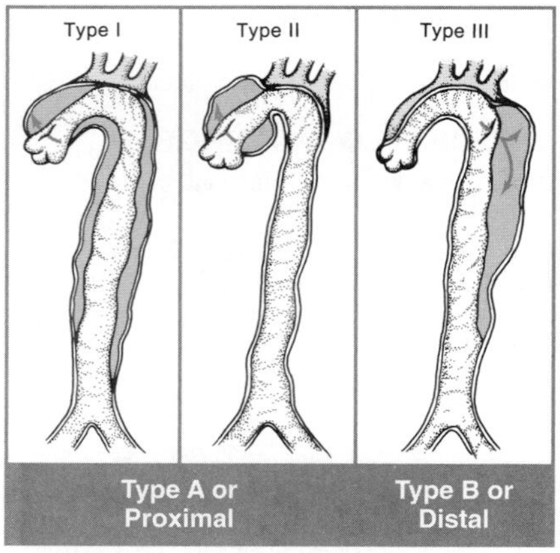

FIGURE 1-35 Classification systems for aortic dissection. (From Isselbacher EM et al: Disease of the aorta. In Braunwald E [ed]: *Heart disease: a textbook of cardiovascular medicine,* ed 5, Philadelphia, 1997, WB Saunders.)

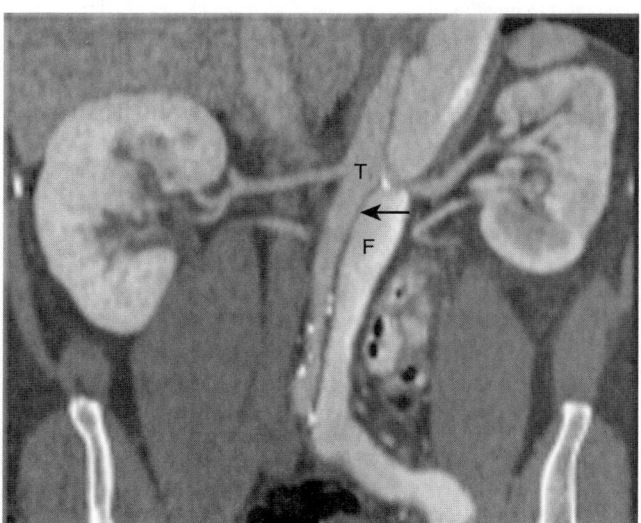

FIGURE 1-36 Computed tomographic angiogram of the aorta shows type B aortic dissection. The intimal flap (*arrow*) separates the two lumen (T) from the false lumen (F) and compromises blood flow to the right kidney, causing renal atrophy and cortical thinning. (Image courtesy of Bart Domatch, M.D., Radiology Department, University of Texas Southwestern Medical Center, Dallas, TX; from Andreoli TE et al: *Andreoli and Carpenter's Cecil essentials of medicine,* ed 8, Philadelphia, 2010, WB Saunders.)

ficity). Myosin heavy chains will peak within 3 hr of dissection and clear within 24 hr of aortic injury.

- CK-BB isoenzyme also peaks within 6 hr of dissection.
- Calponin, a smooth muscle troponin counterpart, increases in aortic dissection with a wider diagnostic window when compared to smooth mucle myosin heavy chain and CK-BB.
- C-reactive protein, fibrinogen, and elastin fragments are under investigation

IMAGING STUDIES

- Chest radiograph may show widened mediastinum (62%) and displacement of aortic intimal calcium.
- Although the diagnostic sensitivity of transthoracic echocardiography is suboptimal, it is useful in assessing potential high risk features or complications, such as pericardial effusion, and making other potential diagnoses. A negative transthoracic echocardiography, however, does not exclude aortic dissection.
- Transesophageal echocardiography (TEE) is study of choice in unstable patients with Type A dissection but is operator dependent.
- MRI has the highest sensitivity and specificity but limited availability; not suitable for unstable patients; contraindicated with pacemakers, metal devices.
- Multidetector CT is considered the gold standard; least operator dependent but involves intravenous contrast.
- TEE, MRI, multidetector CT are imaging modalities of choice. Sensitivities (98% to 100%) and specificities (95% to 98%) nearly equal in skilled hands. Test of choice depends on clinical circumstances and availability.
- With medium or high pretest probability, a second diagnostic test should be done if the first is negative.
- Coronary computed tomographic angiography (CTA) may be an alternative and useful diagnostic study when evaluating for pulmo-

nary embolism, acute coronary syndrome, and aortic dissection.
- Aortography rarely done now.

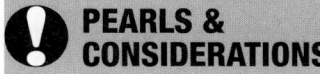 **TREATMENT**

ACUTE GENERAL Rx

- Admit to ICU for monitoring.
- Target SBP 100 to 120 mm Hg or as low as tolerated; heart rate <60 beats/min to reduce aortic wall stress.
- IV beta-blockers are cornerstones of treatment.
- Propanolol 1 mg every 3 to 5 min; metoprolol 5 mg IV every 5 min; or labetalol 20 mg IV, then 20 to 80 mg every 10 min, followed by nitroprusside 0.3 to 10 mg/kg/min.
- Nitroprusside should not be used without beta-blockade because vasodilation can induce reflex sympathetic stimulation and increased aortic sheer stress.
- IV calcium channel blockers with negative inotropy may be used if beta-blockers are contraindicated.
- Pain control, often with morphine.
- Multiple medications may be needed.
- Proximal dissections require emergent surgery to prevent rupture or pericardial effusion.
- Distal dissections are usually treated medically unless distal organ involvement or impending rupture occurs.
- Endovascular repair is feasible for both acute aortic dissection and coronary artery disease. Literature has shown favorable short- and mid-term outcomes. However, long-term outcome data are still under investigation.

CHRONIC Rx

- Chronic aortic dissection (>2 wk) managed with aggressive blood pressure control: target <120/80 mm Hg in most patients.
- Target low-density lipoprotein <70 mg/dl.
- Minimize strenuous physical activity.
- Serial imaging of the aorta, usually with contrast CT.

- Endovascular repair in chronic type B dissection should be considered when the aortic diameter exceeds 5.5-6.0 cm, when there is uncontrolled pain or blood pressure, or when there is rapid growth of the dissecting aneurysm (>1 cm per year).

DISPOSITION

- 85% mortality rate within 2 wk if untreated.
- Proximal dissection is a surgical emergency. Time is critical; mortality rate is 1% to 3% per hour.
- Overall, in-hospital mortality rate is 30% with proximal dissections and 10% with distal dissections.

REFERRAL

For ICU management and surgery

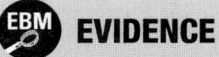 **PEARLS & CONSIDERATIONS**

- Blood pressure control is essential; beta-blocker is first-line medication.
- Proximal dissection is a surgical emergency.
- Cardiac tamponade is not uncommon in patients with acute Type A aortic dissection. Syncope, altered mental status, and a widened mediastinum on chest radiograph on presentation suggest tamponade which warrants urgent operative therapy.
- Surgery for acute Type A aortic dissection in patients ≥70 yr can be performed with acceptable outcomes.

EBM EVIDENCE

available at www.expertconsult.com

SUGGESTED READINGS
available at www.expertconsult.com

AUTHORS: **LYNN BOWLBY, M.D.,** and **ABDULRAHMAN ABDULBAKI, M.D.**

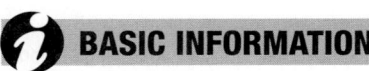

BASIC INFORMATION

DEFINITION
Aortic regurgitation is retrograde blood flow into the left ventricle from the aorta as a result of an incompetent aortic valve.

SYNONYMS
Aortic insufficiency
AI
AR

ICD-9CM CODES
424.1 Aortic valve disorders

EPIDEMIOLOGY & DEMOGRAPHICS
- Prevalence ranges from 4.9% to 10% and increases with age.
- The most common cause of isolated severe aortic regurgitation is aortic root dilation.
- Infectious endocarditis is the most frequent cause of acute aortic regurgitation.

PHYSICAL FINDINGS & CLINICAL PRESENTATION
The clinical presentation varies depending on whether aortic insufficiency is acute or chronic. Chronic aortic insufficiency is well tolerated (except when secondary to infective endocarditis), and the patients remain asymptomatic for years. Common manifestations after significant deterioration of left ventricular function are dyspnea on exertion, syncope, chest pain, and congestive heart failure (CHF). Acute aortic insufficiency manifests primarily with hypotension caused by a sudden fall in cardiac output. A rapid rise in left ventricular diastolic pressure results in a further decrease in coronary blood flow.

Physical findings in chronic aortic insufficiency include the following:
- Widened pulse pressure (markedly increased systolic blood pressure, decreased diastolic blood pressure).
- Bounding pulses, head "bobbing" with each systole (de Musset's sign); "water hammer" or collapsing pulse (Corrigan's pulse) can be palpated at the wrist or on the femoral arteries ("pistol shot" femorals) and is caused by rapid rise and sudden collapse of the arterial pressure during late systole; capillary pulsations (Quincke's pulse) may occur at the base of the nail beds.
- A to-and-fro Duroziez murmur may be heard over femoral arteries with slight compression.
- Popliteal systolic pressure is increased over brachial systolic pressure ≥40 mm Hg (Hill's sign).
- Cardiac auscultation reveals:
  1. Displacement of cardiac impulse downward and to the patient's left
  2. S_3 heard over the apex
  3. Decrescendo, blowing diastolic murmur heard along left sternal border
  4. Low-pitched apical diastolic rumble (Austin-Flint murmur)—the precise etiology of the murmur is uncertain, but it is generally believed to be related to increased velocity of mitral inflow consequent to the aortic regurgitation.
  5. Early systolic ejection sound and systolic ejection murmur.

In patients with acute aortic insufficiency both the wide pulse pressure and the large stroke volume are absent. A short blowing diastolic murmur may be the only finding on physical examination.

ETIOLOGY
- Infective endocarditis
- Rheumatic fibrosis (most common cause in developing countries)
- Trauma with valvular rupture
- Congenital bicuspid aortic valve (most common cause in U.S.)
- Myxomatous degeneration
- Annuloaortic ectasia
- Syphilitic aortitis
- Ankylosing spondylitis
- Systemic lupus erythematosus (SLE)
- Aortic dissection
- Fenfluramine, dexfenfluramine, pergolide, cabergoline
- Takayasu's arteritis, granulomatous arteritis

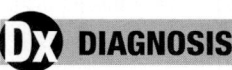

DIAGNOSIS

DIFFERENTIAL DIAGNOSIS
- Patent ductus arteriosus, pulmonary regurgitation, and other valvular abnormalities
- The differential diagnosis of cardiac murmurs is described in Section II

WORKUP
- Echocardiogram, chest radiograph, ECG, and cardiac catheterization (selected patients)
- Medical history and physical examination focused on the following clinical manifestations:
  1. Dyspnea on exertion
  2. Syncope
  3. Chest pain
  4. CHF

IMAGING STUDIES
- Chest radiography:
  1. Left ventricular hypertrophy (chronic aortic regurgitation)
  2. Aortic dilation
  3. Normal cardiac silhouette with pulmonary edema: possible in patients with acute aortic regurgitation
- ECG: left ventricular hypertrophy (LVH).
- Echocardiography is the main imaging modality to diagnose aortic regurgitation and assess left ventricular size and function. Quantification of the severity of regurgitation can be made either qualitatively or quantitatively by effective regurgitant orifice area (severe if >0.30 cm^2) and/or regurgitant volume (severe if >60 ml per beat).
- Cardiac catheterization in selected patients to assess degree of left ventricular dysfunction, to assess the degree of aortic regurgitation when echocardiographic parameters are inclusive, and determine if there is coexistent coronary artery disease.

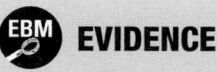

TREATMENT

NONPHARMACOLOGIC THERAPY
- Avoidance of competitive sports and heavy weight lifting if the aortic regurgitation is severe.
- Salt restriction
- In 2007, the AHA guidelines for prevention of infectious endocarditis were revised and routine antibiotic prophylaxis to undergo dental or other invasive procedures is no longer recommended, unless the patient has prior endocarditis.

ACUTE GENERAL Rx
MEDICAL:
- Angiotensin-converting enzyme (ACE) inhibitors, diuretics, and sodium restriction for CHF; nitroprusside in patients with acute aortic regurgitation
- Long-term vasodilator therapy with ACE inhibitors in patients who are not candidates for valve replacement, in asymptomatic patients with severe aortic regurgitation and normal left ventricular function, or asymptomatic patients with severe aortic regurgitation and left ventricular dysfunction.

SURGICAL: Reserved for:
- Symptomatic patients with chronic aortic regurgitation despite optimal medical therapy
- Patients with acute aortic regurgitation (i.e., infective endocarditis) producing left ventricular failure
- Evidence of systolic dysfunction:
  1. Echocardiographic end systolic dimension >55 mm
  2. Echocardiographic end diastolic dimension >75 mm
  3. Left ventricular ejection fraction of 50% or less
- Evidence of heart failure.

EVIDENCE
available at www.expertconsult.com

SUGGESTED READINGS
available at www.expertconsult.com

AUTHORS: **DAVID J. FORTUNATO, M.D., F.A.C.C.,** and **FRED F. FERRI, M.D.**

BASIC INFORMATION

DEFINITION

Aortic stenosis is obstruction to systolic left ventricular outflow across the aortic valve. Symptoms appear when the valve orifice decreases to $<1\ cm^2$ (normal orifice is $3\ cm^2$). The stenosis is considered severe when the orifice is $<0.5\ cm^2/m^2$ or the pressure gradient is ≥ 50 mm Hg.

SYNONYMS

Aortic valvular stenosis
AS

ICD-9CM CODES
424.1 Aortic valvular stenosis

EPIDEMIOLOGY & DEMOGRAPHICS

- Aortic stenosis is the most common valve lesion in adults in Western countries.
- Calcific stenosis (most common cause in patients >60 yr) occurs in 75% of patients.

PHYSICAL FINDINGS & CLINICAL PRESENTATION

- Rough, loud, systolic, diamond-shaped murmur best heard at base of heart and transmitted into neck vessels; often associated with a thrill or ejection click; may also be heard well at the apex.
- Absence or diminished intensity of sound of aortic valve closure (in severe aortic stenosis).
- Late, slow-rising carotid upstroke with decreased amplitude.
- Strong apical pulse.
- Narrowing of pulse pressure in later stages of aortic stenosis.
- Some patients with aortic stenosis experience bleeding into their GI tract or skin. This is caused by an acquired defect in von Willebrand factor. Aortic valve replacement restores normal hemostasis.

ETIOLOGY

- Progressive stenosis of congenital bicuspid valve (found in 1% to 2% of population)
- Idiopathic calcification of the aortic valve
- Congenital (major cause of aortic stenosis in patients <30 yr)
- Rheumatic inflammation of aortic valve is rare as a cause of isolated AS in the U.S.

DIAGNOSIS

DIFFERENTIAL DIAGNOSIS

- Hypertrophic cardiomyopathy
- Mitral regurgitation
- Ventricular septal defect
- Aortic sclerosis. Aortic stenosis is distinguished from aortic sclerosis by the degree of valve impairment. In aortic sclerosis, the valve leaflets are abnormally thickened but obstruction to outflow is minimal.

WORKUP

- Echocardiography.
- Chest radiographs, ECG.
- Laboratory: B-type natriuretic peptide or N-terminal pro-B-type natriuretic peptide

(NT-proBNP) correlates with the mean pressure gradient, aortic valve area, and functional status. It is a useful biochemical marker to evaluate severity of aortic stenosis (AS), monitor disease progression at an early stage, and decide on the optimal time for aortic valve replacement. An increased level of BNP correlates with severity of AS and New York Heart Association functional class.
- Cardiac catheterization in selected patients (see "Imaging Studies")
- Medical history focusing on symptoms and potential complications:
  1. Angina
  2. Syncope (particularly with exertion)
  3. Congestive heart failure (CHF)
  4. GI bleeding: in patients with associated hemorrhagic telangiectasia (AVM)
- Section III describes an algorithm for evaluation of suspected aortic stenosis

IMAGING STUDIES

- Chest x-ray:
  1. Poststenotic dilation of the ascending aorta
  2. Calcification of aortic cusps
  3. Pulmonary congestion (in advanced stages of aortic stenosis)
- ECG:
  1. Left ventricular hypertrophy (found in >80% of patients)
  2. ST-T wave changes
  3. Atrial fibrillation: frequent
- Doppler echocardiography: thickening of the left ventricular wall; if the patient has valvular calcifications, multiple echoes may be seen from within the aortic root and there is poor separation of the aortic cusps during systole. Gradient across the valve can be estimated but is less precise than with cardiac catheterization.
- Cardiac catheterization: indicated in symptomatic patients; it confirms the diagnosis and estimates the severity of the disease by measuring the gradient across the valve, allowing calculation of the valve area. It also detects coexisting coronary artery stenosis that may need bypass at the same time as aortic valve replacement.

TREATMENT

NONPHARMACOLOGIC THERAPY

- Strenuous activity should be avoided
- Sodium restriction if CHF is present

GENERAL Rx
MEDICAL:

- Diuretics and sodium restriction are needed if CHF is present; digoxin is used only to control rate of atrial fibrillation.
- ACE inhibitors are relatively contraindicated.
- Beta-blockers may be useful to control rate of atrial fibrillation. In 2007, the AHA guidelines for prevention of infectious endocarditis were revised and routine antibiotic prophylaxis to undergo dental or other invasive procedures is no longer recommended, unless the patient has prior endocarditis.

SURGICAL:

- Valve replacement is the treatment of choice in symptomatic patients because the 5-yr mortality rate after onset of symptoms is extremely high, even with optimal medical therapy. Valve replacement is indicated if cardiac catheterization establishes a pressure gradient >50 mm Hg and valve area $<1\ cm^2$. Percutaneous approach to implant prosthetic aortic valve has evolved as a viable option for patients with severe symptomatic aortic valve stenosis. Limiting factors are vascular and mechanical complications and operator inexperience
- Percutaneous aortic balloon valvuloplasty serves best as palliative therapy in severely symptomatic patients and as a bridge to surgery in hemodynamically unstable adult patients. It is not an option in patients who are good candidates for surgical valve replacement.
- Percutaneous heart valve replacement (PHVR) is an emerging catheter-based technology that allows for implantation of a prosthetic valve without open heart surgery. Transcatheter aortic-valve implantation (TAVI) has been shown to reduce the death rate in patients with severe aortic stenosis and coexisting conditions who are not candidates for surgical replacement of the aortic valve.

DISPOSITION

- The presence of even mild symptoms is an indicator of poor survival for patients with aortic stenosis. The 5-yr survival rate in adults is 40%.
- The average duration of symptoms before death is angina, 60 mo; syncope, 36 mo; CHF, 24 mo.
- Approximately 75% of patients with symptomatic aortic stenosis will be dead 3 yrs. after onset of symptoms unless the aortic valve is replaced.

REFERRAL

- Surgical referral for valve replacement in symptomatic patients. The risk of aortic valve replacement is greater than any potential benefit for truly asymptomatic patients. There are studies that are examing the presence of moderate or severe valvular calcification, together with a rapid increase in aortic jet velocity and elevated BNP, to identify patients with a very poor prognosis who should be considered for early valve replacement rather than have surgery delayed until symptoms develop.
- Surgical mortality rate for valve replacement is 3% to 5%; however, it varies with patient's age (>8% in patients >75 yr).
- Balloon valvuloplasty is useful in infants and children or poor surgical candidates who do not have calcified valve apparatus; it can be done as an intermediate procedure to stabilize high-risk patients before surgery.

EVIDENCE

available at www.expertconsult.com

SUGGESTED READINGS
available at www.expertconsult.com

AUTHORS: **DAVID J. FORTUNATO, M.D., F.A.C.C.,** and **FRED F. FERRI, M.D.**

BASIC INFORMATION

DEFINITION

Appendicitis is the acute inflammation of the appendix.

ICD-9CM CODES
540.9 Appendicitis
540.0 Appendicitis with generalized peritonitis

EPIDEMIOLOGY & DEMOGRAPHICS

- Appendicitis occurs in 10% of the population, most commonly between the ages of 10 and 30 yr.
- More than 250,000 appendectomies are performed in the U.S. each year.
- It is the most common abdominal surgical emergency.
- Incidence of appendicitis has declined over the past 30 yr.
- Male/female ratio is 3:2 until mid-20s; it equalizes after age 30 yr.

PHYSICAL FINDINGS & CLINICAL PRESENTATION

- In children with abdominal pain, fever is the single most useful sign associated with appendicitis. Vomiting, rectal tenderness, and rebound tenderness along with fever are more indicative of appendicitis in children than in adults.
- Abdominal pain: initially the pain may be epigastric or periumbilical in nearly 50% of patients; it subsequently localizes to the right lower quadrant within 12 to 18 hr. Pain can be found in back or right flank if appendix is retrocecal or in other abdominal locations if there is malrotation of the appendix.
- Pain with right thigh extension *(psoas sign)*, low-grade fever: temperature may be >38° C if there is appendiceal perforation.
- Pain with internal rotation of the flexed right thigh (obturator sign) is present.
- Right lower quadrant (RLQ) pain on palpation of the left lower quadrant (LLQ) *(Rovsing's sign)*: physical examination may reveal right-sided tenderness in patients with pelvic appendix.
- Point of maximum tenderness is in the RLQ *(McBurney's point)*.
- Nausea, vomiting, tachycardia, cutaneous hyperesthesias at the level of T12 can be present.

ETIOLOGY

Obstruction of the appendiceal lumen with subsequent vascular congestion, inflammation, and edema; common causes of obstruction are:
- Fecaliths: 30% to 35% of cases (most common in adults)
- Foreign body: 4% (fruit seeds, pinworms, tapeworms, roundworms, calculi)
- Inflammation: 50% to 60% of cases (submucosal lymphoid hyperplasia [most common etiology in children, teens])
- Neoplasms: 1% (carcinoids, metastatic disease, carcinoma)

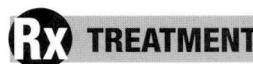 DIAGNOSIS

DIFFERENTIAL DIAGNOSIS

- Intestinal: regional cecal enteritis, incarcerated hernia, cecal diverticulitis, intestinal obstruction, perforated ulcer, perforated cecum, Meckel's diverticulitis
- Reproductive: ectopic pregnancy, ovarian cyst, torsion of ovarian cyst, salpingitis, tuboovarian abscess, mittelschmerz, endometriosis, seminal vesiculitis
- Renal: renal and ureteral calculi, neoplasms, pyelonephritis
- Vascular: leaking aortic aneurysm
- Psoas abscess
- Trauma
- Cholecystitis
- Mesenteric adenitis

WORKUP

Patients with RLQ pain, nausea, vomiting, anorexia, and RLQ rebound tenderness should undergo prompt clinical and laboratory evaluation. Imaging studies are generally not necessary in typical appendicitis and generally reserved for patients with an equivocal likelihood of appendicitis. They are useful when the diagnosis is uncertain. Laparoscopy may be useful as both a diagnostic and a therapeutic modality.

LABORATORY TESTS

- Complete blood count with differential reveals leukocytosis with a left shift in 90% of patients with appendicitis. Total white blood cell (WBC) count is generally lower than 20,000/mm^3. Higher counts may be indicative of perforation. Less than 4% have a normal WBC and differential. A WBC count <10,000/mm^3 decreases the likelihood of appendicitis. Low hemoglobin and hematocrit levels in an older patient should raise suspicion for GI tract carcinoma.
- Microscopic hematuria and pyuria may occur in <20% of patients.

IMAGING STUDIES

- CT of the abdomen/pelvis without contrast has a sensitivity of >90% and an accuracy >94% for acute appendicitis. A distended appendix, periappendiceal inflammation, and a thickened appendiceal wall are indicative of appendicitis.
- Ultrasonography has a sensitivity of 75% to 90% for the diagnosis of acute appendicitis, although it is highly operator dependent and difficult in patients with large body habitus. Ultrasound is useful, especially in pregnancy and in younger women when diagnosis is unclear. Normal ultrasonographic findings should not deter surgery if the history and physical examination are indicative of appendicitis.

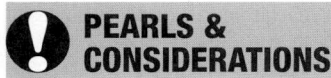 TREATMENT

NONPHARMACOLOGIC THERAPY

- Nothing by mouth
- Do not administer analgesics or antibiotics until the diagnosis is made (may mask signs of peritonitis)

ACUTE GENERAL Rx

- Urgent appendectomy (laparoscopic or open), correction of fluid and electrolyte imbalance with vigorous IV hydration and electrolyte replacement
- IV antibiotic prophylaxis to cover gram-negative bacilli and anaerobes (ampicillin-sulbactam 3 g IV q6h or piperacillin-tazobactam 4.5 g IV q8h in adults)

PEARLS & CONSIDERATIONS

COMMENTS

- Perforation is common (20% in adult patients). Indicators of perforation are pain lasting >24 hr, leukocytosis >20,000/mm^3, temperature >102° F, palpable abdominal mass, and peritoneal findings.
- In general, prognosis is excellent. Mortality rate is <1% in young adults without complications; however, it exceeds 10% in elderly patients with ruptured appendix.
- In approximately 20% of patients who undergo exploratory laparotomy because of suspected appendicitis, the appendix is normal.

SUGGESTED READINGS
available at www.expertconsult.com

AUTHOR: **FRED F. FERRI, M.D.**

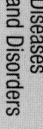

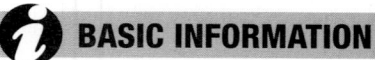

BASIC INFORMATION

DEFINITION

Arrhythmogenic right ventricular dysplasia (ARVD) is a disorder characterized by replacement of the normal myocardium by fibrofatty tissue, RV myocyte loss, and RV wall thinning. It is defined clinically by life-threatening ventricular arrhythmias in otherwise healthy young people.

SYNONYMS

Arrhythmogenic right ventricular cardiomyopathy

ICD-9CM CODES:
427.1 Paroxysmal ventricular tachycardia
425.4 Other primary cardiomyopathies
427.89 Other specified cardiac dysrhythmias

ICD-10 CODES:
I47.2 Paroxysmal ventricular tachycardia
I42.8 Other cardiomyopathies
I49.8 Other specified cardiac arrhythmias

EPIDEMIOLOGY & DEMOGRAPHICS

INCIDENCE: ARVD comprises 2% of sudden cardiac arrest cases.
PREVALENCE: 1:5000 persons
PREDOMINANT SEX AND AGE: Men <35 yr old
RISK FACTORS: Family history of ARVD
GENETICS:
- Autosomal dominant with variable penetrance, and polymorphic phenotypic expression
- Desmosomal dysfunction
- 11 subtypes of ARVD are identified based on the involved genes.

PHYSICAL FINDINGS & CLINICAL PRESENTATION

- Suspect when young males present with syncope, sudden cardiac arrest, ventricular tachycardia, premature ventricular beats originating from the right ventricle, or, less commonly, signs and symptoms of right heart failure.Symptoms vary and range from palpitations, dizziness, and syncope to atypical chest pain, dyspnea, and fatigue.
- Cardiac arrest after physical exertion may be the initial presentation.
- Physical examination will be normal in most patients. Widely split S2 is an important diagnostic clue.

ETIOLOGY

ARVD is characterized by progressive replacement of the right ventricular myocardium with fibrofatty tissue

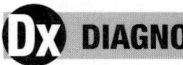

DIAGNOSIS

- Diagnosis is made when two major criteria, one major and two minor, or four minor criteria are met.
- See Table 1-14 for diagnostic criteria.

DIFFERENTIAL DIAGNOSIS

- Cardiomyopathy with involvement of the right ventricle
- Uhl's anomaly: rare anomaly that presents mainly in childhood with signs and symptoms and right heart failure. Uhl's anomaly is characterized by a paper thin right ventricle resulting from death of the myocytes throughout the right ventricle
- Idiopathic RV tachycardia
- Left dominant arrhythmogenic cardiomyopathy

WORKUP

- Resting ECG will have diagnostic findings in 50% to 90% of patients with ARVD. These changes include T-wave inversions in anterior precordial leads V_1-V_6, epsilon waves (Fig. 1-37), and *ventricular tachycardia* (VT) with left bundle branch block pattern.
- Endomyocardial biopsy is the preferred method for diagnosis of ARVD. It has specificity of 92%, but it lacks sensitivity (<20%).
- Electrophysiologic study is important to identify delayed potentials that can lead to tachycardiac events.

TABLE 1-14 Criteria for the Diagnosis of Arrhythmogenic Right Ventricular Dysplasia

Global and/or regional dysfunction and structural alterations

Major
Severe dilatation and reduction of right ventricular ejection fraction with no (or only mild) left ventricular impairment
Localized right ventricular aneurysms
Severe segmental dilatation of the right ventricle

Minor
Mild global right ventricular dilatation and/or ejection fraction with a normal left ventricle
Mild segmental dilatation of the right ventricle
Regional right ventricular hypokinesis

Tissue characterization of the walls

Major
Fibrofatty replacement of myocardium on endomyocardial biopsy

ECG repolarization abnormalities

Minor
Inverted T waves in the right precordial leads (V_2 and V_3) in patients older than 12 yr and in the absence of right bundle branch block

ECG depolarization/conduction abnormalities

Major
Epsilon waves or localized prolongation (greater than 110 ms) of the QRS complex in right precordial leads (V_1 through V_3)

Minor
Late potentials visible on signal-averaged ECG

Arrhythmias

Minor
Sustained or nonsustained left bundle branch block type VT documented on ECG, Holter monitoring, or during exercise stress testing
Frequent ventricular extrasystoles (more than 1000 per 24 hr on Holter monitoring)

Family history

Major
Familial disease confirmed at autopsy or surgery

Minor
Family history of premature sudden death (younger than 35 yr) caused by suspected ARVD/C
Family history (clinical diagnosis based on present criteria)

The diagnosis of ARVD is made if one of the following is met: two major criteria, one major and two minor criteria, or four minor criteria.
ARVD, Arrhythmogenic right ventricular dysplasia; *ARVD/C,* arrhythmogenic right ventricular dysplasia/cardiomyopathy; *ECG,* electrocardiography; *VT,* ventricular tachycardia.
(From *Am Fam Physician* 73[8]:1391-1398, 2006.)

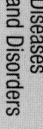

Diseases and Disorders

- Routine immunohistochemical analysis of a conventional endomyocardial-biopsy sample appears to be a highly sensitive and specific diagnostic test for arrhythmogenic right ventricular cardiomyopathy.

IMAGING STUDIES

- MRI is a noninvasive method to detect structural changes and regional dysfunction. Cardiac MRI (CMR) is the most sensitive method

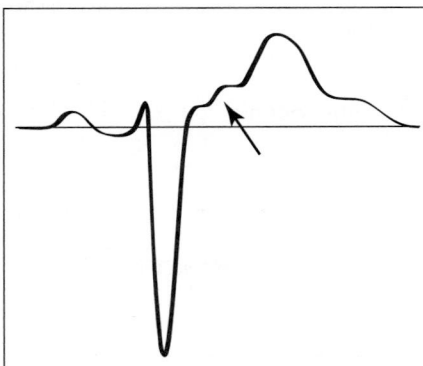

FIGURE 1-37 Epsilon waves are small deflection just beyond the QRS complex. Best visualized in leads V_1-V_3. Any potential in leads V_1-V_3 that exceeds the QRS in leads V6 by more than 25 millisecond should be considered epsilon wave. (From Anderson EL: Arrhythmogenic right ventricular dysplasia, *Am Fam Physician* 73(8):1391-1398, 2006.)

to detect ARVD, but has high false-positive rates.

- Echocardiography will show right ventricular dilatation with regional wall motion abnormalities that varied with the severity of the disease.
- Other imaging modalities used for evaluation of suspected ARVD include signal averaged ECG, Holter monitor, stress test, and radionuclide ventriculography

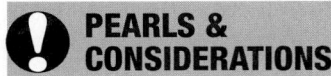

TREATMENT

No definitive therapy is available. Treatment goal is to prevent sudden cardiac death.

NONPHARMACOLOGIC THERAPY

- Avoidance of activity that may trigger tachycardia
- Right ventriculotomy
- Cardiac transplantation

ACUTE GENERAL Rx

Intravenous (IV) amiodarone has been proved to be effective in terminating VT.

CHRONIC Rx

- Antiarrhythmic therapy with sotalol, amiodarone, propafenone, beta-blocker alone or in combination can be used
- Radiofrequency ablation is used in cases of refractory VT, frequent tachycardia after defi-

brillator placement, or localized arrhythmia sites

- Implantable cardioverted defibrillator

REFERRAL

- Early cardiology and electrophysiology referral
- Consider referring for genetic counseling

PEARLS & CONSIDERATIONS

PREVENTION

Test first-degree relatives if there is a positive history of sudden cardiac death or death at an early age.

EDUCATION

Patient handout can be found in *American Family Physician* (American Academy of Family Physicians: Information from your family doctor. Arrhythmogenic right ventricular dysplasia: what you should know. *Am Fam Physician* 73(8):1401, 2006).

SUGGESTED READINGS

available at www.expertconsult.com

AUTHORS: **ABDULRAHMAN ABDULBAKI, M.D.,** and **NADIA MUJAHID, M.D.**

BASIC INFORMATION

DEFINITION

The prototype of granulomatous arthritis is tuberculous arthritis. Atypical mycobacteria, sarcoidosis, and sporotrichosis can cause granulomatous involvement of the synovium, but these entities are much less common.

SYNONYMS

Tuberculous arthritis
Pott's disease

ICD-9CM CODES
711.40 Arthropathy associated with other bacterial disease
730.88 Other infection involving bone

EPIDEMIOLOGY & DEMOGRAPHICS

INCIDENCE (IN U.S.): Unknown
PEAK INCIDENCE: No seasonal predilection
PREVALENCE (IN U.S.): Unknown
PREDOMINANT SEX: Male = female
PREDOMINANT AGE: Rare in childhood

PHYSICAL FINDINGS & CLINICAL PRESENTATION

- Often no constitutional symptoms (fever and weight loss)
- Possibly no clinical or radiographic evidence of pulmonary TB
- Spinal infection most often in the thoracic or upper lumbar area, with back pain as the most common symptom
- Considerable local muscle spasm possible
- Kyphosis and neurologic symptoms resulting from spinal cord compression in advanced disease
- Chronic monoarticular arthritis in the peripheral joints
- Single joint involved in 85% of patients
- Pain, swelling, limitation of motion, and joint stiffness less dramatic than in acute bacterial arthritis; possibly present for months to years
- Seen more often in persons from developing countries, elderly patients, and hemodialysis patients

ETIOLOGY

- Hematogenous spread of organisms from a distant site of infection or by direct spread from bone
- Most commonly affected area: 50% of cases in the spine; next most commonly affected area: large joints (knee and hip)
- Primary infection beginning in the lungs and spreading to the highly vascular synovium

- Tuberculous osteomyelitis commonly involving an adjacent joint
- In peripheral joints, a granulomatous reaction in the synovium causing joint effusion and eventual destruction of underlying bone
- In the spine, infection of the intervertebral disk spreading to adjacent vertebrae
- Osteomyelitis of vertebrae causing collapse, kyphosis, or gibbous deformity, and possibly paraspinal "cold" abscess

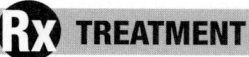 **DIAGNOSIS**

DIFFERENTIAL DIAGNOSIS

- Sarcoidosis
- Fungal arthritis
- Metastatic cancer
- Primary or metastatic synovial tumors

WORKUP

- High index of suspicion needed
- Gold standard: synovial biopsy
- Joint aspiration and culture of the synovial fluid performed while awaiting biopsy
- Positive synovial fluid smear for acid-fast bacilli in 20% of cases; positive culture in 80%
- Elevated synovial fluid protein, low glucose
- Considerable variation in synovial fluid WBC count, but values of 10,000 to 20,000 cells/mm^3 typical; may be predominantly polymorphonuclear leukocytes
- Usually positive tuberculin skin test
- Anergy in elderly patients or in advanced disease
- In spinal infections, percutaneous or open biopsy to obtain accurate C&S data

LABORATORY TESTS

Peripheral WBC count and ESR are elevated but nonspecific.

IMAGING STUDIES

- Plain radiographs of the affected joint
  1. Typically demonstrate bony destruction with little new bone formation
  2. Osteopenia and soft tissue swelling in early infections
  3. Later, erosions at the joint margins
  4. In the spine, disk space narrowing with vertebral collapse (wedging) causing characteristic kyphosis
- CT scan: useful in early diagnosis of infections of the spine and to detect paraspinal abscess
- Technetium and gallium scintigraphic scans: may be positive, but do not permit differentiation from inflammation or osteoarthritis

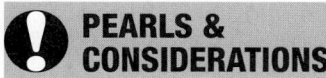 **TREATMENT**

NONPHARMACOLOGIC THERAPY

Encourage range-of-motion exercises of the affected joint to prevent contractures.

ACUTE GENERAL Rx

- Combination chemotherapy
  1. If sensitive TB suspected, give isoniazid 5 mg/kg/day (maximum 300 mg/day) plus rifampin 10 mg/kg/day (maximum 600 mg/day) for at least 6 mo and pyrazinamide 15 to 30 mg/kg/day (maximum 2 g/day) for at least the first 2 mo plus ethambutol 15 to 25 mg/kg/day until sensitivity results are available.
  2. Most patients are treated successfully with chemotherapy alone.
  3. Urgent surgical intervention is necessary if spinal cord compression causes neurologic changes.
- Surgical debridement in cases of extensive bone involvement

CHRONIC Rx

In longstanding extensive disease, arthrodesis of weight-bearing joints

DISPOSITION

Loss of cartilage and destruction of underlying bone if treatment is not initiated promptly

REFERRAL

- To a physician experienced in the management of TB
- For consultation with an infectious diseases specialist if drug resistance is suspected or documented
- For neurosurgical and/or orthopedic consultation if neurologic impairment suspected

! **PEARLS & CONSIDERATIONS**

COMMENTS

As TB has become less prevalent in the U.S. in the last 10 yr, TB arthritis and osteomyelitis have also become less common.

SUGGESTED READINGS
available at www.expertconsult.com

AUTHORS: **GLENN G. FORT, M.D., M.P.H.,** and **DENNIS J. MIKOLICH, M.D.**

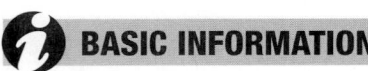

BASIC INFORMATION

DEFINITION

Bacterial arthritis is a highly destructive form of joint disease most often caused by hematogenous spread of organisms from a distant site of infection. Direct penetration of the joint as a result of trauma or surgery and spread from adjacent osteomyelitis may also cause bacterial arthritis. Any joint in the body may be affected.

SYNONYMS

Septic arthritis
Pyogenic arthritis

ICD-9CM CODES
711 Pyogenic arthritis, site unspecified

EPIDEMIOLOGY & DEMOGRAPHICS

INCIDENCE (IN U.S.): Unknown
PEAK INCIDENCE:
- Gonococcal arthritis: young adults
- Other bacterial causes: all ages

PREVALENCE (IN U.S.): Unknown
PREDOMINANT SEX: Gonococcal arthritis in females
PREDOMINANT AGE: Gonococcal arthritis in sexually active adults

PHYSICAL FINDINGS & CLINICAL PRESENTATION

- Hallmark: acute onset of a swollen, painful joint
- Limited range of motion of the joint
- Effusion, with varying degrees of erythema and increased warmth around the joint
- Single joint affected in 80% to 90% of cases of nongonococcal arthritis
- Gonococcal dermatitis-arthritis syndrome
  1. Typical pattern is a migratory polyarthritis or tenosynovitis
  2. Small pustules on the trunk or extremities
- Febrile patient at presentation
- Most commonly affected joints in adult: knee and hip, but any joint may be involved; in children: hip

ETIOLOGY

- Bacteria spread from another locus of infection
  1. Highly vascular synovium is invaded by hematogenously spread bacteria.
  2. WBC enzymes cause necrosis of synovium, cartilage, and bone.
  3. Extensive joint destruction is rapid if infection is not treated with appropriate IV antibiotics and drainage of necrotic material.
- Predisposing factors: rheumatoid arthritis, prosthetic joints, advanced age, immunodeficiency

- The most common nongonococcal organisms are *Staphylococcus aureus,* β-hemolytic streptococci, and gram-negative bacilli
- Staphylococci (*S. aureus* and coagulase-negative staphylococcus species) account for >50% of prosthetic-hip and prosthetic-knee infections. *S. aureus* is very common in patients with rheumatoid arthritis.

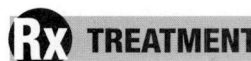

DIAGNOSIS

DIFFERENTIAL DIAGNOSIS

- Gout
- Pseudogout
- Trauma
- Hemarthrosis
- Rheumatic fever
- Adult or juvenile rheumatoid arthritis
- Spondyloarthropathies such as reactive arthritis (Reiter's syndrome)
- Osteomyelitis
- Viral arthritides
- Septic bursitis
- Lyme disease

WORKUP

- Joint aspiration, Gram stain, and culture of the synovial fluid
- Immediate arthrocentesis before other studies are undertaken or antibiotics instituted

LABORATORY TESTS

- Joint fluid analysis
  1. Synovial fluid leukocyte count is usually elevated >50,000 cells/mm^3 with >80% polymorphonuclear cells.
  2. Counts are highly variable, with similar findings in gout, pseudogout, or rheumatoid arthritis.
  3. The differential diagnosis of synovial fluid abnormalities is described in Section III.
  4. A PCR for Lyme disease on synovial fluid is best test to diagnose Lyme arthritis.
- Blood cultures
- Culture of possible extraarticular sources of infection
- Elevated peripheral WBC count and ESR (nonspecific)

IMAGING STUDIES

- X-ray of the affected joint to rule out osteomyelitis
- CT scan for early diagnosis of infections of the spine, hips, and sternoclavicular and sacroiliac joints
- Technetium and gallium scintigraphic scans (positive, but do not permit differentiation of infection from inflammation)
- Indium-labeled WBC scans (less sensitive, but more specific)

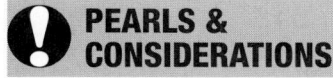

TREATMENT

NONPHARMACOLOGIC THERAPY

- Affected joints aspirated daily to remove necrotic material and to follow serial WBC counts and cultures
- If no resolution with IV antibiotics and closed drainage: open debridement and lavage, particularly in nongonococcal infections
- Prevention of contractures:
  1. After acute stage of inflammation, range-of-motion exercises of the affected joint
  2. Physical therapy helpful

ACUTE GENERAL Rx

- IV antibiotics immediately after joint aspiration and Gram stain of the synovial fluid
- For infections caused by gram-positive cocci: penicillinase-resistant penicillin, such as nafcillin (2 g IV q4h), unless there is clinical suspicion of methicillin-resistant *Staphylococcus aureus,* in which case use vancomycin (1 g IV q12h)
- Infections caused by gram-negative bacilli: treated with a third-generation cephalosporin or an antipseudomonal penicillin plus an aminoglycoside, pending C&S results
- For suspected gonococcal infection, including young adults when the synovial fluid Gram stain is nondiagnostic: ceftriaxone 1 g IV q24h

CHRONIC Rx

See indications for surgical drainage.

DISPOSITION

- With prompt treatment, complete resolution is expected.
- Delay in treatment may result in permanent destruction of cartilage and loss of function of the affected joint.

REFERRAL

To an orthopedist for open drainage if the infected joint fails to improve on appropriate antibiotics and closed aspiration

PEARLS & CONSIDERATIONS

COMMENTS

Any patient with acute monoarticular arthritis should undergo an urgent joint aspiration to rule out septic arthritis, even if there is a history of gout.

SUGGESTED READINGS
available at www.expertconsult.com

AUTHORS: **GLENN G. FORT, M.D., M.P.H.,** and **DENNIS J. MIKOLICH, M.D.**

BASIC INFORMATION

DEFINITION

Psoriatic arthritis is an inflammatory arthropathy occurring in association with skin psoriasis and generally in the absence of rheumatoid factor. It is often included in a class of disorders called the *seronegative spondyloarthropathies*, a family of diseases characterized by inflammation of the spine, peripheral joints and enthesial sites. (sites of insertion of tendon into bone)

ICD-9CM CODES
696.0 Psoriatic arthritis

EPIDEMIOLOGY & DEMOGRAPHICS

PREVALENCE: 0.1% to 0.2% overall, variable estimates of 7% to 30% of patients with psoriasis (psoriasis incidence varies by population but overall estimated prevalence of 1% to 2% of general population)
PREDOMINANT SEX: Equal male:female sex distribution of 1:1
PREDOMINANT AGE: Symptom onset generally age 30 to 55 yr

PHYSICAL FINDINGS & CLINICAL PRESENTATION

- Variably arthritis, dactylitis, spondylitis, and enthesitis occur in the setting of known psoriasis although joint symptoms may predate skin psoriasis in ~15% of patients.
  - Arthritis is inflammatory in nature, commonly characterized by prolonged morning stiffness, joint erythema, warmth, or swelling including joint effusions.
- Distribution of joint involvement follows five classically described patterns (Table 1-15)
- Often more than one classical pattern will occur simultaneously and patterns can evolve over time in an individual patient.
- Dactylitis refers to diffuse swelling of a digit, either finger or toe, which is typically the result of inflammation in both small joints of the digit as well as associated tenosynovitis of digital tendons. Dactylitis is common in psoriatic arthritis and occurs in approximately 30% to 40% of patients during the course of disease.
- Enthesitis commonly occurs at the Achilles tendon insertion into the calcaneous as well as the insertion of the plantar fascia. Findings

on physical exam may include swelling and tenderness.
- Dystrophic changes of the nails (pitting, onycholysis) may occur in association with joint inflammation in involved digits.
- Spondyloarthritis may include sacroiliitis as well as inflammation of the axial spine, but is generally less likely to cause contiguous fusion to the extent seen in ankylosing spondylitis.

ETIOLOGY
Unknown.

DIAGNOSIS

DIFFERENTIAL DIAGNOSIS
- Rheumatoid arthritis
- Erosive osteoarthritis
- Crystal arthritis including gout and pseudogout.
- Other seronegative spondyloarthropathies including reactive arthritis, enteropathic arthritis, and ankylosing spondylitis.
- The differential diagnosis of spondyloarthropathies is described in Section III

WORKUP
- Diagnosis generally made on clinical grounds based on history, exam and radiographic findings given lack of specific lab findings.
- Early diagnosis may be difficult to establish when the arthritis develops before skin lesions appear.

LABORATORY TESTS
- No specific/diagnositic lab tests.
- Acute phase reactants such as ESR and CRP may be elevated although less commonly than in patients with rheumatoid arthritis.

- Anemia of chronic disease may be seen.
- RF, while generally negative, can be present in ~10% of patients.
- *HLA B27* is significantly more common in patients with axial inflammation (note that *HLA B27* positivity is present in up to 8% of general population)
- Arthrocentesis of active joint generally demonstrates inflammatory synovial fluid and absence of crystals.

IMAGING STUDIES
- Radiographic findings of involved joints may include soft tissue swelling, joint space narrowing, subluxation, erosive changes, and new bone formation such as periostitis and fusion.
- Severe digital erosive change with adjacent heterotopic bone formation may give rise to "pencil in cup" deformity seen in arthritis mutilans.
- Findings in patients with spondylitis may include sacroiliitis and development of vertebral syndesmophytes that often bridge adjacent vertebral bodies.
- Musculoskeletal ultrasound may be helpful in the evaluation of an inflamed enthesis or joint.
- MRI may be helpful in the evaluation of sacroiliitis or spinal involvement.

TREATMENT

ACUTE GENERAL Rx
- NSAIDs may be used for mild symptoms or limited involvement.
- Intra-articular corticosteroid injections can be used as adjunctive therapy in involved joints.

TABLE 1-15 The Moll and Wright Classification of Psoriatic Arthritis

Arthritis with distal interphalangeal joint involvement predominant (Fig. 1-38)

Arthritis mutilans

Symmetric polyarthritis—indistinguishable from RA

Asymmetric oliogoarticular arthritis

Predominant spondylitis

From Hochberg M et al: *Rheumatology,* ed 3, St Louis, 2003, Mosby, p. 1242, Table 110.4.

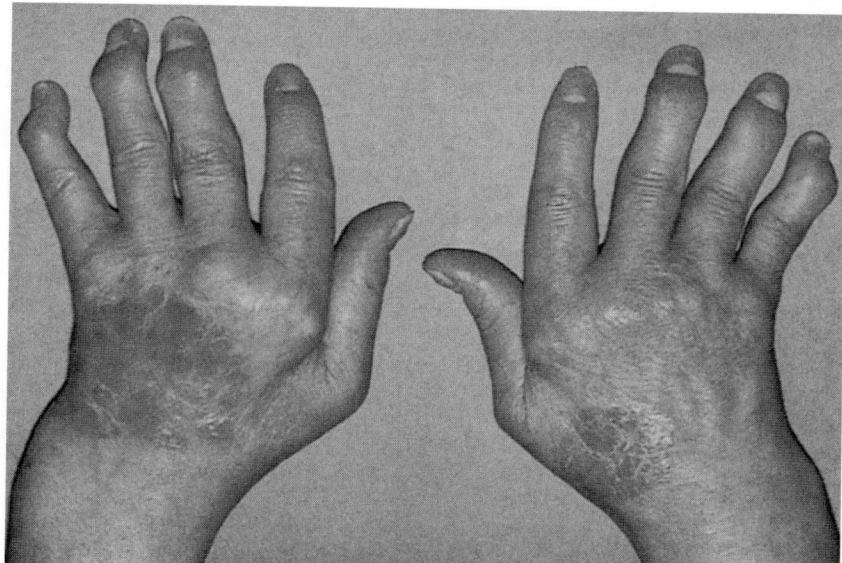

FIGURE 1-38 The hands of a woman with symmetric polyarthritis. Initially, this was indistinguishable from rheumatoid disease, but note the distal interphalangeal joint involvement, which is uncommon in rheumatoid arthritis, as well as the skin psoriasis. (From Klippel J et al [eds]: *Primary care rheumatology,* London, 1999, Mosby.)

CHRONIC Rx

- NSAIDs for mild or limited disease.
- In patients with several sites of active peripheral disease, elevated acute phase reactants, or with evidence of erosive changes on imaging, traditional DMARDs such as methotrexate, sulfasalazine, and leflunamide should be considered early in disease.
- In patients with peripheral arthritis who fail to respond to traditional DMARD therapy, additional therapy with a tumor necrosis factor (TNF) inhibitor should be considered.
- In patients with predominant axial disease not responsive to NSAIDs, anti-TNF therapy should be considered for initial disease modifying therapy.

REFERRAL

Rheumatology for confirmation of diagnosis and management.

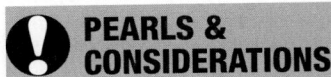

PEARLS & CONSIDERATIONS

- Patients frequently have a positive family history of psoriasis or psoriatic arthritis.
- Severity of skin psoriasis and activity of inflammatory arthritis is frequently discordant.

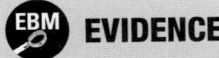 **EVIDENCE**

available at www.expertconsult.com

SUGGESTED READING

available at www.expertconsult.com

AUTHOR: **HARALD A. HALL, M.D.**

BASIC INFORMATION

DEFINITION

Asbestosis is a slowly progressive diffuse interstitial fibrosis resulting from dose-related inhalation exposure to fibers of asbestos.

ICD-9CM CODES
501 Asbestosis

EPIDEMIOLOGY & DEMOGRAPHICS

- Five to 10 new cases per 100,000 persons per year in U.S.
- Prolonged interval (20 to 30 yr) between exposures to inhaled fibers and clinical manifestations of disease
- Most common in workers involved in the primary extraction of asbestos from rock deposits and in those involved in the fabrication and installation of products containing asbestos (e.g., naval shipyards in World War II; installation of floor tiles, ceiling tiles, acoustic ceiling coverings, wall insulation, and pipe coverings in public buildings)

PHYSICAL FINDINGS & CLINICAL PRESENTATION

- Insidious onset of shortness of breath with exertion is usually the first sign of asbestosis.
- Dyspnea becomes more severe as the disease advances; with time, progressively less exertion is tolerated.
- Cough is frequent and usually paroxysmal, dry, and nonproductive.
- Scant mucoid sputum may accompany the cough in the later stages of the disease.
- Fine end-respiratory crackles (rales, crepitations) are heard more predominantly in the lung bases.
- Digital clubbing, edema, jugular venous distention are present.

ETIOLOGY

Inhalation of asbestos fibers

DIAGNOSIS

DIFFERENTIAL DIAGNOSIS

- Silicosis
- Siderosis, other pneumonoconioses
- Lung cancer
- Atelectasis

WORKUP

Documentation of exposure history, diagnostic imaging, pulmonary function testing

LABORATORY TESTS

- Generally not helpful
- Possible mild elevation of erythrocyte sedimentation rate (ESR), positive antinuclear antibody (ANA) and rheumatoid factor (RF) (these tests are nonspecific and do not correlate with disease severity or activity)
- Pulmonary function testing: decreased vital capacity, decreased total lung capacity, decreased carbon monoxide gas transfer
- Arterial blood gases: hypoxemia, hypercarbia in advanced stages

IMAGING STUDIES

Chest radiograph (Fig. 1-39):
- Small, irregular shadows in lower lung zones.
- Thickened pleura, calcified plaques (present under diaphragm and lateral chest wall).
- CT scan of chest confirms diagnosis. Typical findings on high-resolution CT of the chest include increased interstitial markings found mainly at the bases. As the disease progresses, honeycombing is noted.

TREATMENT

NONPHARMACOLOGIC THERAPY

- Smoking cessation, proper nutrition, exercise program to maximize available lung function
- Home oxygen therapy prn
- Removal of patient from further asbestos fiber exposure

GENERAL Rx

- Prompt identification and treatment of respiratory infections

- Supplemental oxygen on a prn basis
- Annual influenza vaccination, pneumococcal vaccination

DISPOSITION

- There is no specific treatment for asbestosis.
- Death is usually from respiratory failure from cor pulmonale.
- Patients with asbestosis have increased risk for mesotheliomas, lung cancer, and tuberculosis. Recent reports indicate that the risk of asbestos-induced lung cancer may be overestimated.
- Survival in patients after development of mesothelioma is 4 to 6 yr.

REFERRAL

To pulmonologist initially

PEARLS & CONSIDERATIONS

COMMENTS

Patient information on asbestosis can be obtained from the American Lung Association, 1740 Broadway, New York, NY 10019.

SUGGESTED READINGS

available at www.expertconsult.com

AUTHOR: **FRED F. FERRI, M.D.**

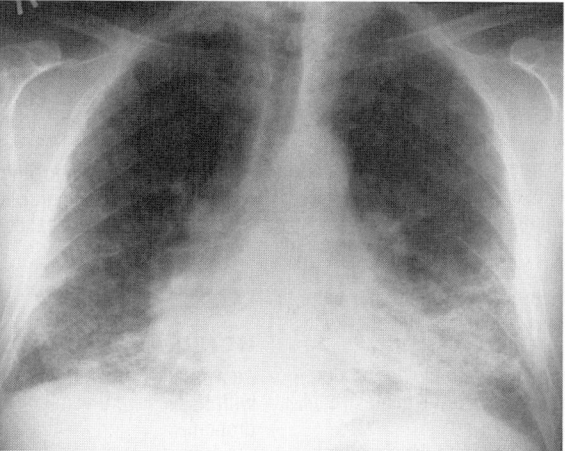

FIGURE 1-39 Asbestosis. Posteroanterior radiograph shows coarse linear opacities at both lung bases obscuring the cardiac borders. (From McLoud TC: *Thoracic radiology: the requisites,* St Louis, 1998, Mosby.)

A

Diseases and Disorders
I

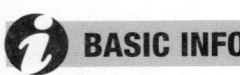

BASIC INFORMATION

DEFINITION

Ascariasis is a parasitic infection caused by the nematode *Ascaris lumbricoides.* The majority of those infected are asymptomatic; however, clinical disease may arise from pulmonary hypersensitivity, intestinal obstruction, and secondary complications.

SYNONYMS

Round worms
Worms

ICD-9CM CODES
127.0 Ascariasis

EPIDEMIOLOGY & DEMOGRAPHICS

INCIDENCE (IN U.S.):
- Unknown
- Three times the infection rates found in blacks as in whites

PEAK INCIDENCE: Unknown

PREVALENCE (IN U.S.): Estimated at 4 million, the majority of which live in the rural southeastern part of the country

PREDOMINANT SEX: Both sexes probably equally affected, with a possible slight female preponderance

PREDOMINANT AGE: Most common in children, with estimated mean age of approximately 5 yr based on surveys in highly endemic areas

NEONATAL INFECTION: Probable transmission, though not specifically studied

PHYSICAL FINDINGS & CLINICAL PRESENTATION

- Occurs approximately 9 to 12 days after ingestion of eggs (corresponding to the larva migration through the lungs)
- Nonproductive cough
- Substernal chest discomfort
- Fever
- In patients with large worm burdens, especially children, intestinal obstruction associated with perforation, volvulus, and intussusception
- Migration of worms into the biliary tree giving clinical appearance of biliary colic and pancreatitis as well as acute appendicitis with movement into that appendage
- Rarely, infection with *A. lumbricoides* producing interstitial nephritis and acute renal failure
- In endemic areas in Asia and Africa, malabsorption of dietary proteins and vitamins as a consequence of chronic worm intestinal carriage

ETIOLOGY

- Transmission is usually hand to mouth, but eggs may be ingested via transported vegetables grown in contaminated soil.
- Eggs are hatched in the small intestine, with larvae penetrating intestinal mucosa and migrating via the circulation to the lungs.
- Larval forms proceed through the alveoli, ascend the bronchial tree, and return to the intestines after swallowing, where they mature into adult worms.
- Estimated time until the female adult worm begins producing eggs is 2 to 3 mo.
- Eggs are passed out of the intestines with feces.
- Within human host, adult worm lifespan is 1 to 2 yr.

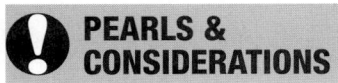

DIAGNOSIS

DIFFERENTIAL DIAGNOSIS

Radiologic manifestations and eosinophilia to be distinguished from drug hypersensitivity and Löffler's syndrome

LABORATORY TESTS

- Examination of the stool for *Ascaris* ova
- Expectoration or fecal passage of adult worm
- Eosinophilia: most prominent early in the infection and subsides as the adult worm infestation established in the intestines
- Anti-ascaris IgG4 blood levels by ELISA is a sensitive and specific marker of infection and may be useful in the evaluation of treatment
- Malondialdehyde levels clearly increase in patients infected with *A. lumbricoides*

IMAGING STUDIES

- Chest x-ray examination to reveal bilateral oval or round infiltrates of varying size (Löffler's syndrome); NOTE: infiltrates are transient and eventually resolve.
- Plain films of the abdomen and contrast studies to reveal worm masses in loops of bowel.
- Ultrasonography and endoscopic retrograde cholangiopancreatography (ERCP) to identify worms in the pancreaticobiliary tract.

TREATMENT

NONPHARMACOLOGIC THERAPY

Aggressive IV hydration, especially in children with fever, severe vomiting, and resultant dehydration

ACUTE GENERAL Rx

- Mebendazole (Vermox)
  1. Drug of choice for intestinal infection with *A. lumbricoides*
  2. 100 mg PO tid given for 3 days or 500 mg as a single dose
- Albendazole, given as a single 400-mg dose PO
- Both mebendazole and albendazole are contraindicated in pregnancy
- Pyrantel pamoate (Antiminth)
  1. Given at a dose of 11 mg/kg PO (maximum dose of 1 g/day)
  2. Considered safe for use in pregnant women
- Piperazine citrate
  1. Recommended in cases of intestinal or biliary obstruction
  2. Administered as a syrup, given via nasogastric tube, a 150 mg/kg loading dose, followed by six doses of 65 mg/kg q12h
  3. Considered safe in pregnancy, but cannot be given concurrently with chlorpromazine
- Complete obstruction should be managed surgically

DISPOSITION

Overall prognosis is good. Patients should be reevaluated in 2 to 3 months. Reinfection is common.

REFERRAL

- To gastroenterologist in cases of visualized pancreaticobiliary tract or appendiceal obstruction
- To surgeon in cases of complete obstruction or suspected secondary complication (e.g., perforation or volvulus)

PEARLS & CONSIDERATIONS

COMMENTS

- Hepatic abscess, containing both viable and dead worms, complicating *Ascaris*-induced biliary duct disease has been documented.
- Given the known transmission of the parasite, routine hand washing and proper disposal of human waste would significantly decrease the prevalence of this disease.

SUGGESTED READINGS

available at www.expertconsult.com

AUTHORS: **GLENN G. FORT, M.D., M.P.H.,** and **DENNIS J. MIKOLICH, M.D.**

BASIC INFORMATION

DEFINITION

Ascites is the accumulation of excess fluid in the peritoneal cavity, most commonly caused by liver cirrhosis.

SYNONYMS

Fluid in peritoneal cavity
Hydroperitoneum
Hydroperitonia
Hydrops abdominis

ICD-9CM CODES
789.5 Ascites
568.82 Peritoneal effusion (chronic)

EPIDEMIOLOGY & DEMOGRAPHICS

Ascites is the most common complication of cirrhosis. Ascites occurs in 50% of individuals with cirrhosis within 10 yr of diagnosis. Cirrhosis is the cause of 75% of cases of ascites. Other causes include malignancy, heart failure, tuberculosis, pancreatitis, nephrotic syndrome, and Budd-Chiari syndrome.

CLINICAL PRESENTATION

- Important information to elicit within history:
  - Viral hepatitis
  - Alcoholism
  - Increasing abdominal girth
  - Increasing lower extremity edema
  - Intravenous drug use
  - Sexual history (i.e., men who have sex with men)
  - History of transfusions
- Important physical exam findings:
  - Bulging flanks
  - Flank dullness to percussion
  - Fluid wave on abdominal exam
  - Lower extremity edema
  - Shifting dullness on abdominal exam
  - Physical signs associated with liver cirrhosis: spider angiomas, jaundice, loss of body hair, Dupuytren's contracture, muscle wasting, bruising, palmar erythema, gynecomastia, testicular atrophy, hemorrhoids, and caput medusae

ETIOLOGY

Pathophysiology of ascites: increased hepatic resistance to portal flow leads to portal hypertension. The splanchnic vessels respond by increased secretion of nitric oxide, causing splanchnic artery vasodilation. Early in the disease increased plasma volume and increased cardiac output compensate for this vasodilation. However, as disease progresses the effective arterial blood volume decreases, causing sodium and fluid retention through activation of the renin-angiotensin system. The change in capillary pressure causes increased permeability and retention of fluid in the abdomen.

DIAGNOSIS

DIFFERENTIAL DIAGNOSIS

- Chronic parenchymal liver disease, leading to portal hypertension
- Peritoneal carcinomatosis
- Congestive heart failure
- Peritoneal tuberculosis
- Nephrotic syndrome
- Pancreatitis

LABORATORY TESTS

- Initial evaluation should always include:
  - Diagnostic paracentesis. Laboratory tests on this fluid should include a CBC with differential, albumin, total protein, culture and Gram stain. Optional tests on paracentesis fluid include amylase, LDH, acid-fast bacilli, and glucose levels.
  - AST, ALT, total and direct bilirubin, albumin, alkaline phosphatase, GGTP
  - CBC, coagulation studies
  - Electrolytes, BUN, creatinine
- A serum to ascites albumin gradient (SAAG) should be calculated in all patients. If the SAAG is greater than 1.1, the cause of ascites can be attributed to portal hypertension. If SAAG is less than 1.1, a non–portal hypertension etiology of ascites must be sought.

IMAGING STUDIES

- Endoscopy of the upper GI tract to evaluate for esophageal varices if ascites is secondary to portal hypertension.
- Abdominal ultrasound is the most sensitive measure for detecting ascitic fluid; a CT or MRI scan is a viable alternative.
- Liver biopsy in selected patients (i.e., those with portal hypertension of uncertain etiology).

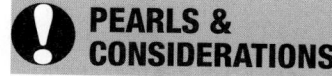

TREATMENT

NONPHARMACOLOGIC THERAPY

- Sodium-restricted diet (less than 2 grams per day).
- Fluid restriction to 1 liter per day in patients with hyponatremia (sodium less than 120 to 130).

ACUTE GENERAL Rx

- Patients with moderate-volume ascites causing only moderate discomfort may be treated on an outpatient basis with the following diuretic regimen: spironolactone 50 to 200 mg qd or amiloride 5 to 10 mg qd. Add furosemide (Lasix) 20 to 40 mg/day in the first several days of treatment, monitoring renal functions carefully for signs of prerenal azo-temia (in patients without edema, goal weight loss is 300 to 500 g/day; in patients with edema it is 800 to 1000 g/day).
- Patients with large-volume ascites causing marked discomfort or decrease in activities of daily living may also be treated as outpatients if there are no complications. There are two options for treatment in these patients: (1) large-volume paracentesis or (2) diuretic therapy until loss of fluid is noted (maximum spironolactone 400 mg qd and furosemide [Lasix] 160 mg qd). No difference in long-term mortality rate was found; however, paracentesis is faster, more effective, and associated with fewer adverse effects.

CHRONIC Rx

5% to 10% of patients with large-volume ascites will be refractory to high-dose diuretic treatment. Treatment strategies include repeated large-volume paracentesis with infusion of albumin every 2 to 4 wk or placement of a transjugular intrahepatic portosystemic shunt (TIPS).

DISPOSITION

Monitor closely for worsening liver function, development of spontaneous bacterial peritonitis (SBP).

REFERRAL

Referral to gastroenterology with ascites

PEARLS & CONSIDERATIONS

COMMENTS

Prevalence of SBP in patients with ascites ranges between 10% and 30%. Presence of at least 250 neutrophils per cubic millimeter of ascitic fluid is diagnostic. Gram negatives such as *E. coli* are the most common isolates. Third-generation cephalosporins are the treatment of choice. By 1 year, 70% of patients have recurrence of SBP and may be prophylaxed with quinolones.

PREVENTION

Prevention of liver cirrhosis through avoidance of long-term use of alcohol, immunization against hepatitis A and B, and treatment of hepatitis C

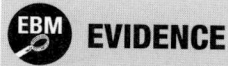

EVIDENCE

available at www.expertconsult.com

SUGGESTED READINGS

available at www.expertconsult.com

AUTHORS: **JOANNE M. SILVIA, M.D.,** and **PAUL F. GEORGE, M.D.**

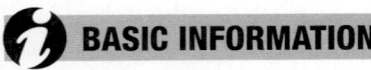

DEFINITION

Aseptic necrosis is cell death in components of bone: hematopoietic fat marrow and mineralized tissue. Osteonecrosis is not a specific disease entity but a final common pathway to several disorders that impair blood supply to the femoral head and other locations.

SYNONYMS

Osteonecrosis
Avascular necrosis

ICD-9CM CODES

733.40 Aseptic necrosis
733.43 Aseptic necrosis of femoral condyle
733.42 Aseptic necrosis of femoral head
733.41 Aseptic necrosis of humeral head
733.44 Aseptic necrosis of talus

EPIDEMIOLOGY & DEMOGRAPHICS

- 15,000 new cases per year in the U.S.
- Associated conditions:
  1. Corticosteroid treatment: 35%
  2. Alcohol abuse: 22%
  3. Idiopathic and other: 43%
- Common sites involved
  1. Femoral head
  2. Femoral condyle
  3. Humeral head
  4. Navicular and lunate wrist bones
  5. Talus

PHYSICAL FINDINGS & CLINICAL PRESENTATION

- May be asymptomatic
- Pain in the involved area exacerbated by movement or weight bearing
- Decreased range of motion as the disease progresses
- Functional limitation

ETIOLOGY

Final common pathway of conditions that lead to impairment of the blood supply to the involved bone.
Stages:
- Stage 0
  - Asymptomatic
  - Normal imaging
  - Histologic findings only (i.e., silent osteonecrosis)
- Stage 1
  - Asymptomatic or symptomatic
  - Normal radiographs and CT scan
  - Abnormal bone scan or MRI
- Stage 2
  - Abnormal radiographs or CT scan, including linear sclerosis, focal bead mineralization, cysts; however, the overall architecture of the involved bone is normal

- Stage 3
  - Early evidence of mechanical bone failure (subchondral fracture), but the overall shape of the bone is still intact
- Stage 4
  - Flattening or collapse of the bone
- Stage 5
  - Joint space narrowing
- Stage 6
  - Extensive joint destruction

DIAGNOSIS

DIFFERENTIAL DIAGNOSIS

- None in late stages
- Early: any condition causing focal musculoskeletal pain, including arthritis, bursitis, tendinitis, myopathy, neoplastic bone and joint diseases, traumatic injuries, pathologic fractures

IMAGING STUDIES (Fig. 1-40)

1. Radiography: insensitive early in the course. The earliest changes include diffuse osteopenia, areas of radiolucency with sclerotic border, and linear sclerosis. Later, a subchondral lucency (crescent sign) indicates subchondral fracture. More advanced cases reveal flattening, collapsed bone, and abnormal bone contour. In late disease, osteoarthritic changes are seen.
2. Bone scan:
   - Early: "cold" area.
   - Later: increased radionuclide uptake as a result of remodeling.
   - Sensitivity in early disease is only 70% and specificity is poor.
3. CT scan: may reveal central necrosis and area of collapse before those are visible on radiographs.
4. MRI: the most sensitive technology to diagnose early aseptic necrosis. The first sign is

a margin of low signal. An inner border of high signal associated with a low-signal line is specific of aseptic necrosis ("double line sign"). Sensitivity is 75% to 100%.

TREATMENT

PREVENTION

- Manage etiologic conditions
- Minimize corticosteroid use

NONPHARMACOLOGIC THERAPY

- Core decompression: effectiveness 35% to 95% in early phases
- Bone grafting
- Osteotomies
- Joint replacement

ACUTE GENERAL Rx

- Decrease weight bearing of affected area.
- Pulsing electromagnetic fields applied externally (still experimental).
- Peripheral vasodilators (e.g., dihydroergotamine) (unproven).

PROGNOSIS

- When diagnosed at an early stage treatment is appropriate in all cases because 85% to 90% can be expected to progress to a more advanced stage.
- Contralateral joint involvement is common (30% to 70%).

SUGGESTED READINGS

available at www.expertconsult.com

AUTHOR: **FRED F. FERRI, M.D.**

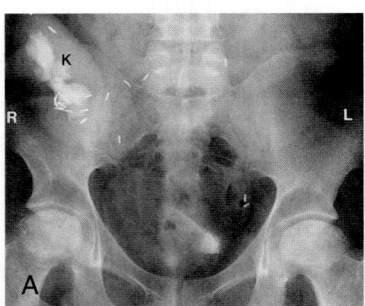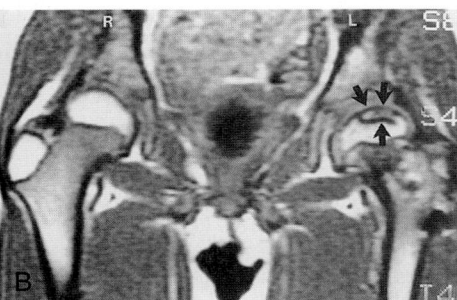

FIGURE 1-40 Aseptic necrosis of the hips. A, Aseptic necrosis can occur from a number of causes, including trauma and steroid use. In this patient, an anteroposterior view of the pelvis shows a transplanted kidney (K) in the right iliac fossa. Use of steroids has caused this patient to have bilateral aseptic necrosis. The femoral heads are somewhat flattened, irregular, and increased in density. **B,** Aseptic necrosis in a different patient is demonstrated on an MRI scan as an area of decreased signal *(arrows)* in the left femoral head. This is the most sensitive method for detection of early aseptic necrosis. (From Mettler FA [ed]: *Primary care radiology,* Philadelphia, 2000, WB Saunders.)

BASIC INFORMATION

DEFINITION

Aspergillosis refers to several forms of a broad range of illnesses caused by infection with *Aspergillus* species.

ICD-9CM CODES
117.3 Aspergillosis
117.3 Aspergillosis with pneumonia
117.3 *Aspergillus* infection (*A. flavus, fumigatus, terreus*)

EPIDEMIOLOGY & DEMOGRAPHICS

INCIDENCE & PREVALENCE:
- *Aspergillus* species are ubiquitous in the environment internationally and occur as a mold found in soil.
- Cause a variety of illness from hypersensitivity pneumonitis to disseminated overwhelming infection in immunosuppressed patients.
- Frequently cultured from hospital wards from unfiltered outside air circulating through open windows as well as water sources.
- Reach the patient by airborne conidia (spores) that are small enough (2.5 to 3 μm) to reach the alveoli on inhalation.
- Can invade the nose, paranasal sinuses, external ear, or traumatized skin.

RISK FACTORS:
- The clinical syndrome depends on the underlying lung architecture, the host's immune response, and the degree of inoculum.
- Incidence of invasive aspergillosis is increasing with advances in the treatment of life-threatening diseases, such as aggressive chemotherapy or bone marrow and organ transplantation. It also can rarely occur in normal hosts, especially associated with influenza A. Liver and lung transplant recipients are at highest risk for pulmonary disease.
- Patients with AIDS and a CD4 count <50 mm³ have an increased susceptibility to invasive aspergillosis.

ETIOLOGY
- *A. fumigatus* is the usual cause.
- *A. flavus* is the second most important species, particularly in invasive disease of immunosuppressed patients and in lesions beginning in the nose and paranasal sinuses. *A. niger* can also cause invasive human infection.

ALLERGIC ASPERGILLOSIS
- Is a hypersensitivity pneumonitis.
- Presents as cough, dyspnea, fever, chills, and malaise typically 4 to 8 hr after exposure.
- Repeated attacks can lead to granulomatous disease and pulmonary fibrosis.

ALLERGIC BRONCHOPULMONARY ASPERGILLOSIS (ABPA):
- Symptoms occur most commonly in atopic individuals during the third and fourth decades of life.
- Hypersensitivity reaction to *Aspergillus* fungal antigens present in the bronchial tree.
- Results from an initial type I (immediate hypersensitivity) and type III reactions (immune complexes).
- Underdiagnosed pulmonary disorder in patients with asthma and cystic fibrosis (reported prevalence in asthmatic patients varies from 6% to 28% and in cystic fibrosis 6% to 25%).

ASPERGILLOMAS ("FUNGUS BALLS"):
- In the absence of invasion or significant immune response, *Aspergillus* can colonize a preexisting cavity, causing pulmonary aspergilloma.
- Forms masses of tangled hyphal elements, fibrin, and mucus.
- Patients typically have a history of chronic lung disease, tuberculosis, sarcoidosis, or emphysema.
- Manifests commonly as hemoptysis.
- Many are asymptomatic.

INVASIVE ASPERGILLOSIS:
- Patients with prolonged and profound granulocytopenia or impaired phagocytic function are predisposed to rapidly progressive *Aspergillus* pneumonia.
- Typically a necrotizing bronchopneumonia, ranging from small areas of infiltrate to intensive bilateral hemorrhagic infarction.
- Most common presentation: unremitting fever and a new pulmonary infiltrate despite broad-spectrum antibiotic therapy in an immunosuppressed patient.
- Dyspnea and nonproductive cough are common; sudden pleuritic pain and tachycardia, sometimes with a pleural rub, may mimic pulmonary embolism; hemoptysis is uncommon.
- Chest radiograph (CXR) may reveal patchy bronchopneumonic, nodular densities, consolidation, or cavitation. High-resolution CT scan is more sensitive and specific than CXR in neutropenic patients.
- Immunocompromised patients: invasive pulmonary *Aspergillus* (IPA) generally is acute and evolves over days to weeks; less commonly, patients with normal or only mild abnormalities of the immune system may develop a more chronic, slowly progressive form of IPA.

EXTRAPULMONARY DISSEMINATION:
- Cerebral infarction from hematogenous dissemination may occur in immunosuppressed individuals.
- Abscess formation from direct extension or invasive disease in the sinuses.
- Esophageal or gastrointestinal ulcerations may occur in the immunosuppressed host.
- Fatal perforation of the viscus or bowel infarction may occur.
- Necrotizing skin ulcers involving the extremities (Fig. 1-41).
- Osteomyelitis.
- Endocarditis in patients who have recently undergone open heart surgery.
- Infection of an implantable cardioverter-defibrillator has been reported.

DIAGNOSIS

DIFFERENTIAL DIAGNOSIS
- Tuberculosis
- Cystic fibrosis
- Carcinoma of the lung
- Eosinophilic pneumonia
- Bronchiectasis
- Sarcoidosis
- Lung abscess

WORKUP
Physical examination and laboratory data

LABORATORY TESTS
ABPA:
- Peripheral blood eosinophilia and an elevated total serum immunoglobulin E (IgE) level.
- Skin test with *Aspergillus* antigenic extract is usually positive but nonspecific.
- *Aspergillus* serum precipitating antibody is present in 70% to 100% of cases.
- Sputum cultures may be positive for *Aspergillus* spp. but are nonspecific.

ASPERGILLOMAS:
- Sputum culture
- Serum precipitating antibody

Invasive aspergillosis: definitive diagnosis requires the demonstration of tissue invasion (i.e.,

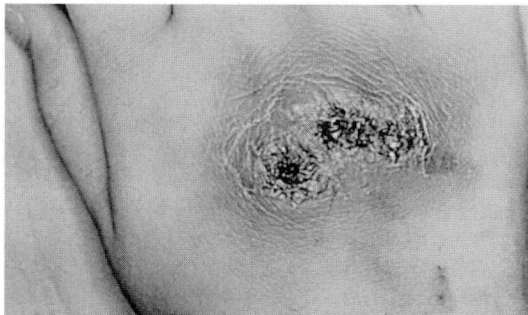

FIGURE 1-41 Cutaneous aspergillosis in a patient with acute leukemia and marked neutropenia. The lesion developed at the site where a steel needle had been left for several days of intravenous infusion. (From Mandell GL [ed]: *Mandell, Douglas, and Bennett's principles and practice of infectious diseases,* ed 6, New York, 2005, Churchill Livingstone.)

septate, acute angle branching hyphae) or a positive culture from the tissue obtained by an invasive procedure such as transbronchial biopsy.

- Sputum and nasal cultures: in high-risk patients a positive culture is strongly suggestive of invasive aspergillosis.
- Serology: the *Platelia Aspergillus* ELISA assay detects a circulating fungal antigen, galactomannan, and is used in some centers in neutropenic patients and for those undergoing stem cell transplantation.
- Blood cultures: usually negative.
- Lung biopsy is necessary for definitive diagnosis.
- Biopsy and culture of extrapulmonary lesions.
- Real-time polymerase chain reaction tests are investigational.

IMAGING STUDIES
ABPA:
- CXRs show a variety of abnormalities, from small, patchy, fleeting infiltrates (commonly in the upper lobes) to lobar consolidation or cavitation.
- A majority of patients eventually develop central bronchiectasis.

ASPERGILLOMAS: CXR or CT scans usually show the characteristic intracavity mass partially surrounded by a crescent of air (Fig. 1-42).

INVASIVE ASPERGILLOSIS: CXR and CT scanning may reveal cavity formation.

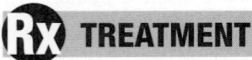 **TREATMENT**

ACUTE GENERAL Rx
ABPA:
- Prednisone (0.5 to 1 mg/kg PO) until the CXR has cleared, followed by alternate-day therapy at 0.5 mg/kg PO (3 to 6 mo).
- If a patient is corticosteroid dependent, prophylaxis for the prevention of *Pneumocystis jiroveci* infection and maintenance of bone mineralization should be considered.

- Bronchodilators and physiotherapy.
- Serial CXR and serum IgE useful in guiding treatment.
- Itraconazole 200 mg PO bid for 4 to 6 mo, then taper over 4 to 6 mo may be considered as a steroid-sparing agent or if steroids are ineffective.

ASPERGILLOMAS:
- Controversial and problematic; the optimal treatment strategy is unknown.
- Up to 10% of aspergillomas may resolve clinically without overt pharmacologic or surgical intervention.
- Observation for asymptomatic patients.
- Surgical resection/arterial embolization for those patients with severe hemoptysis or life-threatening hemorrhage.
- For those patients at risk for marked hemoptysis with inadequate pulmonary reserve, consider itraconazole 200 to 400 mg/day PO.

INVASIVE ASPERGILLOSIS:
- The guidelines of the Infectious Diseases Society of America recommend the use of voriconazole as the primary therapy for invasive aspergillosis. Voriconazole dose is 6 mg/kg IV bid followed by 4 mg/kg IV q12h or 200 mg PO q12h for body weight >40 kg but 100 mg PO q12h for body weight <40 kg.
- Amphotericin B 0.8 to 1.2 mg/kg IV qd to total dose of 2 to 2.5 g; itraconazole 200 to 400 mg/d PO × 1 yr.
- Amphotericin B lipid complex (ABLC) 5 mg/kg IV qd in those intolerant of or refractory to amphotericin B.
- Amphotericin B colloidal dispersion (ABCD) 3 to 6 mg/kg IV qd; stepwise approach in those who have not responded to amphotericin B.
- Liposomal amphotericin B (L-AMB) 3 to 5 mg/kg IV qd; stepwise approach is indicated as empiric therapy for presumed fungal infection in febrile neutropenic patients who are refractory to or intolerant of amphotericin B.

- Itraconazole 200 mg IV bid × 4 doses followed by 200 mg IV qd or 200 mg tid for 4 days, then 200 mg PO bid—first-line therapy if not taking p450 inducers. Levels may be obtained to ensure compliance and adequate absorption. Approved only for salvage therapy in the United States at this time.
- Posaconazole 200 mg PO tid with food or liquid nutritional supplement to enhance absorption is approved in the European Union, but in the United States is approved only for prophylaxis in leukemic neutropenic patients, those with myelodysplasia, or those who have undergone allogeneic hematopoietic stem cell transplantation; ravuconazole is currently under investigation.
- Caspofungin (Candigas) is the first of a new class of antifungals, the echinocandins, approved for the treatment of invasive aspergillosis in patients who do not respond to or are unable to tolerate other antifungal drugs. Starting dose 70 mg IV over 1 hr on day 1, then 50 mg IV qd thereafter (reduce to 35 mg IV qd in cases with moderate hepatic insufficiency). Can switch to oral voriconazole after 2 to 3 wk if the response is favorable. Micafungin 150 mg IV qd is another alternative.
- Because azoles and echinocandins target different cellular sites, combination therapy may have additive activity against *Aspergillus* species. Although still under investigation, some bone marrow transplant units use caspofungin and voriconazole as the preferred initial treatment, especially in patients receiving high-dose corticosteroids.
- Cytokine therapy may offer future treatment options in conjunction with the currently available antifungals.

REFERRAL
To an infectious diseases specialist

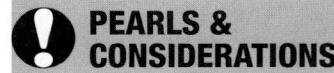 **PEARLS & CONSIDERATIONS**

- Unlike fluconazole, the potential for drug-drug interactions with voriconazole is high.
- Agitation of hospital buildings by renovations or repairs may increase the incidence of *Aspergillus* infections in immunosuppressed individuals.
- Breakthrough zygomycosis infection may occur with voriconazole treatment.
- *A. terreus* is clinically resistant to amphotericin B.

SUGGESTED READINGS
available at www.expertconsult.com

AUTHOR: **SAJEEV HANDA, M.D.**

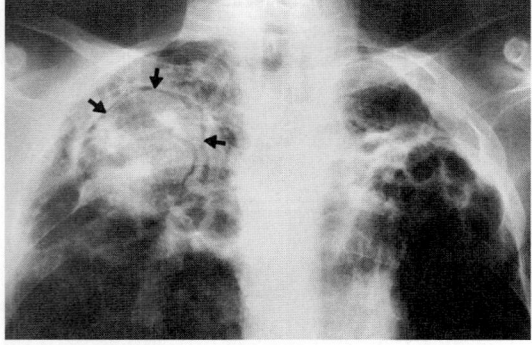

FIGURE 1-42 Fungus ball or mycetoma caused by *Aspergillus*. Coned-down posteroanterior view of the chest of a patient with biapical fibrocavitary tuberculosis accompanied by volume loss. There is a mass in a large right upper-lobe cavity with air dissecting into the cavity producing "air crescents" *(arrows)*. (From McLoud TC: *Thoracic radiology: the requisites,* St Louis, 1998, Mosby.)

BASIC INFORMATION

DEFINITION

The National Asthma Education and Prevention Program (NAEPP) guidelines define asthma as "a chronic inflammatory disease of the airways in which many cells and cellular elements play a role: in particular mast cells, neutrophils, eosinophils, T lymphocytes, macrophages, and epithelial cells. In susceptible individuals, this inflammation causes recurrent episodes of coughing (particularly at night or early in the morning), wheezing, breathlessness, and chest tightness. The episodes are usually associated with widespread but variable airflow obstruction that is reversible either spontaneously or as a result of treatment." *Status asthmaticus* can be defined as a severe continuous bronchospasm.

SYNONYMS

Bronchospasm
Reactive airway disease
Bronchial asthma

ICD-9CM CODES
493.9 Asthma, unspecified
493.1 Intrinsic asthma
493.0 Extrinsic asthma

EPIDEMIOLOGY & DEMOGRAPHICS

- Asthma affects 5% to 12% of the population and accounts for more than 450,000 hospitalizations and nearly 2 million emergency department visits yearly in the U.S.
- It is more common in children (10% of children, 5% of adults).
- 50% to 80% of children with asthma develop symptoms before 5 yr of age.
- Overall asthma mortality rate in the U.S. is 20 per 1 million persons.
- The population of seniors with asthma is increasing rapidly in the U.S. These patients have a high level of morbidity and mortality from their asthma.

PHYSICAL FINDINGS & CLINICAL PRESENTATION

Physical examination varies with the stage and severity of asthma and may reveal only increased inspiratory and expiratory phases of respiration. Physical examination during status asthmaticus may reveal:
- Tachycardia and tachypnea
- Use of accessory respiratory muscles
- Pulsus paradoxus (inspiratory decline in systolic blood pressure >10 mm Hg)
- Wheezing: absence of wheezing (silent chest) or decreased wheezing can indicate worsening obstruction
- Mental status changes: generally secondary to hypoxia and hypercapnia and constitute an indication for urgent intubation
- Paradoxic abdominal and diaphragmatic movement on inspiration (detected by palpation over the upper part of the abdomen in a semirecumbent position): important sign of impending respiratory crisis, indicates diaphragmatic fatigue
- The following abnormalities in vital signs are indicative of severe asthma:
  1. Pulsus paradoxus >18 mm Hg
  2. Respiratory rate >30 breaths/min
  3. Tachycardia with heart rate >120 beats/min

ETIOLOGY

- Symptoms are more commonly due to specific (aeroallergens) or nonspecific (dust, cigarette smoke, fumes, cold air, exercise, etc.) exposures.
- Traditionally, intrinsic asthma was described as occurring in patients who have no history of allergies possibly triggered by upper respiratory infections or psychologic stress and extrinsic asthma (allergic asthma) brought on by exposure to allergens (e.g., dust mites, cat allergen, industrial chemicals).
- Exercise-induced asthma: seen most frequently in adolescents; manifests with bronchospasm after beginning exercise and improves with discontinuation of exercise.
- Drug-induced asthma: often associated with use of NSAIDs, β-blockers, sulfites, and certain foods and beverages.
- There is a strong association of the *ADAM 33* gene with asthma and bronchial hyperresponsiveness.
- Experimental, genetic, and clinical studies support an important role for Th2 immune pathways in the pathogenesis of severe asthma.

DIAGNOSIS

DIFFERENTIAL DIAGNOSIS

- CHF
- COPD
- Pulmonary embolism (in adult and elderly patients)
- Foreign body aspiration (most frequent in younger patients)
- Pneumonia and other upper respiratory infections
- Rhinitis with postnasal drip
- TB
- Hypersensitivity pneumonitis
- Anxiety disorder
- Wegener's granulomatosis
- Diffuse interstitial lung disease

WORKUP

- The clinician should evaluate for environmental causes (e.g., house dust mites, indoor pets) and exposure to other allergens such as tobacco smoke. For symptomatic adults and children aged >5 yr who can perform spirometry, asthma can be diagnosed after a medical history and physical examination documenting an episodic pattern of respiratory symptoms and from spirometry that indicates partially reversible airflow obstruction (>12% increase and 200 ml in forced expiratory volume in 1 sec [FEV_1] after inhaling a short bronchodilator or receiving a short [2 to 3 wk] course of oral corticosteroids). For children aged <5 yr, spirometry is generally not feasible. Young children with asthma symptoms should be treated as having suspected asthma once alternative diagnoses are ruled out.
- The degree of reversibility measured by spirometry correlates with airway obstruction, and patients with a high degree of reversibility have a greater risk of irreversible airflow obstruction in subsequent years.
- Section III describes an algorithm for diagnosing asthma.
- After diagnosis severity of asthma should be classified during the initial assessment before initiating therapy. The following questions from Asthma Control and endorsed by the American Lung Association are important in assessing patients with asthma:
  1. Has your asthma prevented normal activities at home or work?
  2. Have you had shortness of breath in the past 4 wk?
  3. Has your asthma kept you awake at night?
  4. How often have you used your asthma inhaler in the last 4 weeks?
  5. Overall, how have kept your asthma in control in the last 4 weeks?
- Once therapy is initiated, the emphasis for clinical management is changed to the assessment of asthma control. The level of asthma control should be used to guide decisions either to maintain or adjust therapy.
- Schedule visits at 2- to 6-wk intervals for patients who are just starting therapy or who require a step up in therapy to achieve or regain asthma control. Schedule visits at 1- to 6-mo intervals, after asthma control is achieved, to monitor whether asthma control is maintained. The interval will depend on factors such as the duration of asthma control or the level of treatment required. Consider scheduling visits at 3-mo intervals if step-down therapy is anticipated.

LABORATORY TESTS

Laboratory tests are usually not necessary and the results can be normal if obtained during a stable period.
- Arterial blood gases (ABGs) can be used during acute bronchospasm in staging the severity of an asthmatic attack:
  - Mild: decreased Pao_2 and $Paco_2$, increased pH
  - Moderate: decreased Pao_2, normal $Paco_2$, normal pH
  - Severe: marked decreased Pao_2, increased $Paco_2$, and decreased pH
- Complete blood count: leukocytosis with left shift may indicate the existence of bacterial infection.
- Spirometry is recommended at the initial assessment and at least every 1 to 2 yr after treatment is initiated and when the symptoms and peak expiratory flow have stabilized. Spirometry as a monitoring measure

may be performed more frequently, if indicated, based on severity of symptoms and the disease's lack of response to treatment.

- Pulmonary function studies: during acute severe bronchospasm, FEV$_1$ is <1 L and peak expiratory flow rate (PEFR) <80 L/min.

IMAGING STUDIES

- Chest x-ray: usually normal, may show evidence of thoracic hyperinflation (e.g., flattening of the diaphragm, increased volume over the retrosternal air space).
- ECG: tachycardia, nonspecific ST-T wave changes are common during an asthma attack; may also show cor pulmonale, right bundle-branch block, right axial deviation, counterclockwise rotation.

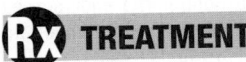 **TREATMENT**

NONPHARMACOLOGIC THERAPY

- Avoidance of triggering factors (e.g., salicylates, sulfites), environmental or occupational triggers
- Encouragement of regular exercise (e.g., swimming)
- Patient education regarding warning signs of an attack and proper use of medications (e.g., correct use of inhalers)

GENERAL Rx

- The 2007 NAEPP guidelines (see Tables 1-16 to 1-24) broadly classify treatment options by age: 0 to 4 yr, 5 to 11 yr, and >12 yr. When asthma symptoms are mild, short-lived, or infrequent, use of short-acting beta-selective adrenergic agonists (SABA) administered by inhalation is the most effective therapy for quick relief of asthmatic symptoms. They are recommended for use only as needed for relief of symptoms or before anticipated exposure to known triggers such as exercise. When symptoms become more frequent or more severe, step-up treatment includes use of an inhaled steroid or leukotriene receptor antagonist (LTRA). If symptoms persist, recommendations include use of long-acting beta-agonist (LABA) or LTRA plus inhaled steroid. If asthma control remains inadequate, additional treatment consists of inhaled steroid plus LABA plus LTM. The addition of omalizumab, an anti-IgE monoclonal antibody, is indicated for the treatment of moderate and severe persistent asthma refractory to other treatment noted earlier. It is administered subcutaneously every 2 or 4 wk. This medicine is expensive ($10,000 to $30,000/yr). Patients should be closely monitored in the first month because omalizumab

can result in allergic reactions (anaphylaxis) in 1 to 2 patients/1000.
Treatment of *status asthmaticus* is as follows:

- Oxygen generally started at 2 to 4 L/min by nasal cannula or Venti-Mask at 40% Fio$_2$; further adjustments are made according to the ABGs.
- Bronchodilators: Initiate treatment with high-dose short-acting beta-2 adrenergic agonist plus ipratropium bromide administered by means of a nebulizer every 20 min. Use of a metered-dose inhaler with valved holding chamber may be acceptable for patients with mild-to-moderate exacerbations.
- Albuterol nebulizer solution (0.63 mg/3 ml, 1.25 mg/3 ml, 2.5 mg/3 ml, or 5.0 mg/ml): 2.5 to 5 mg every 20 min over the first hr, then 2.5-10 mg every 1-4 hr as needed or 10-15 mg/hr continuously. Other useful medications are level-buterol nebulizer solution (0.31 mg/3 ml, 0.63 mg/3 ml, 1.25 mg/3 ml), and ipratropium nebulizer solution (0.25/ml [0.025%]).
- Corticosteroids:
  1. Early administration is advised, particularly in patients using steroids at home.
  2. Patients may be started on systemic corticosteroids: methylprednisolone, prednisone, or prednisolone may be used. Dose range is from 40-80 mg/day in one or two

---

TABLE 1-16 Classifying Asthma Severity and Initiating Treatment in Youths ≥12 Yr and Adults (Assessing severity and initiating treatment for patients who are not currently taking long-term control medications)

Components of Severity		Intermittent	CLASSIFICATION OF ASTHMA SEVERITY (≥12 yr) PERSISTENT Mild	Moderate	Severe
Impairment Normal FEV$_1$/FVC: 8-19 yr 85% 20-39 yr 80% 40-59 yr 75% 60-80 yr 70%	Symptoms	≤2 days/wk	>2 days/wk but not daily	Daily	Throughout the day
	Nighttime awakenings	≤2×/mo	3-4×/mo	>1×/wk but not nightly	Often 7×/wk
	Short-acting beta$_2$-agonist use for symptom control (not prevention of EIB)	≤2 days/wk	>2 days/wk but not daily, and not more than 1× on any day	Daily	Several times per day
	Interference with normal activity	None	Minor limitation	Some limitation	Extremely limited
	Lung function	Normal FEV$_1$ between exacerbations FEV$_1$ >80% predicted FEV$_1$/FVC normal	FEV$_1$ >80% predicted FEV$_1$/FVC normal	FEV$_1$ >60% but <80% predicted FEV$_1$/FVC reduced 5%	FEV$_1$ <60% predicted FEV$_1$/FVC reduced >5%
Risk	Exacerbations requiring oral systemic corticosteroids	0-1 per yr	≥2 per yr ⟶		
		⟵ Consider severity and interval since last exacerbation. Frequency and severity may fluctuate ⟶ over time for patients in any severity category. Relative annual risk of exacerbations may be related to FEV$_1$.			
Recommended Step for Initiating Therapy		Step 1	Step 2	Step 3	Step 4 or 5 and consider short course of oral systemic corticosteroids
		In 2-6 wk, evaluate level of asthma control that is achieved and adjust therapy accordingly.			

The stepwise approach is meant to assist, not replace, the clinical decision-making required to meet individual patient needs.
Level of severity is determined by assessment of both impairment and risk. Assess impairment domain by patient's/caregiver's recall of previous 2-4 wk and spirometry. Assign severity to the most severe category in which any feature occurs.
At present, there are inadequate data to correspond frequencies of exacerbations with different levels of asthma severity. In general, more frequent and intense exacerbations (e.g., requiring urgent, unscheduled care, hospitalization, or ICU admission) indicate greater underlying disease severity. For treatment purposes, patients who had ≥2 exacerbations requiring oral systemic corticosteroids in the past year may be considered the same as patients who have persistent asthma, even in the absence of impairment levels consistent with persistent asthma.
To access the complete *Expert Panel Report 3: Guidelines for the Diagnosis and Management of Asthma*, go to www.nhlbi.nih.gov/guidelines/asthma/asthgdln.pdf.
EIB, Exercise-induced bronchospasm; *FEV$_1$*, forced expiratory volume in 1 second; *FVC*, forced vital capacity; *ICU*, intensive care unit.
From National Asthma Education and Prevention Program: *Expert panel report 3: Guidelines for diagnosis and management of asthma*, National Institutes of Health, National Heart, Lung, and Blood Institute, August 2007, NIH publication 08-4051.

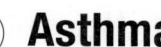

A

divided doses, generally given until peak expiratory flow reaches 70% of predicted value.

3. Generally for corticosteroid courses < 1 week there is no need to taper the dose

- IV hydration: judicious use is necessary to avoid congestive heart failure in elderly patients. Aggressive IV hydration is not recommended
- IV antibiotics are indicated when there is suspicion of bacterial infection (e.g., infiltrate on chest radiograph, fever, or leukocytosis).
- Intubation and mechanical ventilation are indicated when previous measures fail to produce significant improvement.
- Discharge home from the emergency department is appropriate if the FEV$_1$ or PEF after treatment is 70% or greater of the personal best or predicted value and if there is sustained improvement in lung function and symptoms for at least 1 hr.

REFERRAL

Box 1-1 describes indications for referral to an asthma specialist.

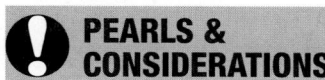

PEARLS & CONSIDERATIONS

COMMENTS

- The differentiation of asthma from COPD can be challenging. A history of atopy and intermittent, reactive symptoms points toward a diagnosis of asthma, whereas smoking and advanced age are more indicative of COPD. Spirometry is useful in distinguishing asthma from COPD.
- In all asthma patients it is important to treat or prevent comorbid conditions (e.g., rhinosinusitis, vocal cord dysfunction, gastroesophageal reflux disease). However, despite the presumed association between asthma and GERD trials of PPIs in patients with poorly controlled asthma did not reveal any beneficial effects.
- Inhaled low-dose corticosteroids are the single most effective therapy for adult patients with asthma who require more than an occasional use of short-acting beta-2 agonists to control their asthma.
- Leukotriene modifiers/receptor agonists represent a reasonable alternative in adults unable or unwilling to use corticosteroids; however, these agents are less effective than monotherapy with inhaled corticosteroids.
- Use of long-acting beta-agonists (LABAs) alone without use of a long-term asthma medication, such as an inhaled corticosteroid, is contraindicated. LABAs should also not be used in patients whose asthma is adequately controlled on low- or medium-dose inhaled corticosteroids. Continued sue of LABAs may cause down-regulation of the

TABLE 1-17 Assessing Asthma Control and Adjusting Therapy in Youths ≥12 Yr and Adults

Components of Control		CLASSIFICATION OF ASTHMA CONTROL (≥12 yr)		
		Well Controlled	Not Well Controlled	Very Poorly Controlled
Impairment	Symptoms	≤2 days/wk	>2 days/wk	Throughout the day
	Nighttime awakenings	≤2×/mo	1-3×/wk	≥4/wk
	Interference with normal activity	None	Some limitation	Extremely limited
	Short-acting beta$_2$-agonist use for symptom control (not prevention of EIB)	≤2 days/wk	>2 days/wk	Several times per day
	FEV$_1$ or peak flow	>80% predicted/personal best	60%-80% predicted/personal best	<60% predicted/personal best
	Validated questionnaires			
	ATAQ	0	1-2	3-4
	ACQ	≤0.75*	≥1.5	N/A
	ACT™	≥20	16-19	≤15
Risk	Exacerbations requiring oral systemic corticosteroids	0-1 per yr	≥2 per yr	
		Consider severity and interval since last exacerbation		
	Progressive loss of lung function	Evaluation requires long-term follow-up care		
	Treatment-related adverse effects	Medication side effects can vary in intensity from none to very troublesome and worrisome. The level of intensity does not correlate to specific levels of control but should be considered in the overall assessment of risk.		
Recommended Action for Treatment		Maintain current step. Regular follow-up every 1-6 mo to maintain control. Consider step down if well controlled for at least 3 mo.	Step up 1 step and Reevaluate in 2-6 wk. For side effects, consider alternative treatment options.	Consider short course of oral systemic corticosteroids. Step up 1-2 steps. Reevaluate in 2 wk. For side effects, consider alternative treatment options.

The stepwise approach is meant to assist, not replace, the clinical decision-making required to meet individual patient needs.

The level of control is based on the most severe impairment or risk category. Assess impairment domain by patient's recall of previous 2-4 wk and by spirometry or peak flow measures. Symptom assessment for longer periods should reflect a global assessment, such as inquiring whether the patient's asthma is better or worse since the last visit.

At present, there are inadequate data to correspond frequencies of exacerbations with different levels of asthma control. In general, more frequent and intense exacerbations (e.g., requiring urgent, unscheduled care, hospitalization, or ICU admission) indicate poorer disease control. For treatment purposes, patients who had ≥2 exacerbations requiring oral systemic corticosteroids in the past year may be considered the same as patients who have not-well-controlled asthma, even in the absence of impairment levels consistent with not-well-controlled asthma.

Validated questionnaires for the impairment domain (the questionnaires do not assess lung function or the risk domain)
 - ATAQ = Asthma Therapy Assessment Questionnaire
 - ACQ = Asthma Control Questionnaire (user package may be obtained at www.qoltech.co.uk or juniper@qoltech.co.uk)
 - ACT = Asthma Control Test™
 - Minimal Important Difference: 1.0 for the ATAQ; 0.5 for the ACQ; not determined for the ACT

Before step up in therapy:
 - Review adherence to medication, inhaler technique, environmental control, and comorbid conditions
 - If an alternative treatment option was used in a step, discontinue and use the preferred treatment for that step

*ACQ values of 0.76-1.4 are indeterminate regarding well-controlled asthma.

EIB, Exercise-induced bronchospasm; *FEV$_1$*, forced expiratory volume in 1 second; *ICU*, intensive care unit.

The Asthma Control Test is a trademark of QualityMetric Incorporated.

From National Asthma Education and Prevention Program: *Expert panel report 3: Guidelines for diagnosis and management of asthma*, National Institutes of Health, National Heart, Lung, and Blood Institute, August 2007, NIH publication 08-4051.

TABLE 1-18 Stepwise Approach for Managing Asthma in Youths ≥12 Yr and Adults

Intermittent Asthma	**Persistent Asthma: Daily Medication** Consult with asthma specialist if step 4 care or higher is required. Consider consultation at step 3.

Step 6
Preferred:
High-dose ICS
+ LABA
+ oral
corticosteroid

AND

Consider
omalizumab
for patients who
have allergies

Step 5
Preferred:
High-dose ICS
+ LABA

AND

Consider
omalizumab
for patients who
have allergies

Step 4
Preferred:
Medium-dose ICS
+ LABA

Alternative:
Medium-dose ICS
+ either LTRA,
theophylline,
or zileuton

Step 3
Preferred:
Low-dose ICS
+ LABA

OR

Medium-dose ICS

Alternative:
Low-dose ICS +
either LTRA,
theophylline,
or zileuton

Step 2
Preferred:
Low-dose ICS

Alternative:
Cromolyn, LTRA,
nedocromil,
or theophylline

Step 1
Preferred:
SABA prn

Step up if needed

(first, check
adherence,
environmental
control, and
comorbid
conditions)

**Assess
control**

Step down
if possible

(and asthma is
well controlled
at least 3 months)

Each step: Patient education, environmental control, and management of comorbidities
Steps 2-4: Consider subcutaneous allergen immunotherapy for patients who have allergic asthma

Quick-Relief Medication for All Patients
• SABA as needed for symptoms. Intensity of treatment depends on severity of symptoms: up to 3 treatments at 20-minute intervals as needed. Short course of oral systemic corticosteroids may be needed.
• Use of SABA >2 days a week for symptom relief (not prevention of EIB) generally indicates inadequate control and the need to step up treatment.

The stepwise approach is meant to assist, not replace, the clinical decision-making required to meet individual patient needs.
If alternative treatment is used and response is inadequate, discontinue it and use the preferred treatment before stepping up.
Zileuton is a less desirable alternative due to limited studies as adjunctive therapy and the need to monitor liver function. Theophylline requires monitoring of serum concentration levels.
In step 6, before oral systemic corticosteroids are introduced, a trial of high-dose ICS + LABA + either LTRA, theophylline, or zileuton may be considered, although this approach has not been studied in clinical trials.
Steps 1, 2, and 3 preferred therapies are based on Evidence A; step 3 alternative therapy is based on Evidence A for LTRA, Evidence B for theophylline, and Evidence D for zileuton. Step 5 preferred therapy is based on Evidence B. Step 6 preferred therapy is based on (EPR-2 1997) and Evidence B for omalizumab.
Immunotherapy for steps 2-4 is based on Evidence B for house-dust mites, animal danders, and pollens; evidence is weak or lacking for molds and cockroaches. Evidence is strongest for immunotherapy with single allergens. The role of allergy in asthma is greater in children than in adults.
Clinicians who administer immunotherapy or omalizumab should be prepared and equipped to identify and treat anaphylaxis that may occur.
This information is directly abstracted from the 2007 NAEPP *Expert Panel Report 3: Guidelines for the Diagnosis and Management of Asthma* and is not intended to promote or endorse any of the listed products.
To access the complete *Expert Panel Report 3: Guidelines for the Diagnosis and Management of Asthma,* go to www.nhlbi.nih.gov/guidelines/asthma/asthgdln.pdf.
ICS, Inhaled corticosteroid; *LABA,* inhaled long-acting beta₂-agonist; *LTRA,* leukotriene receptor antagonist; *SABA,* inhaled short-acting beta₂-agonist.
From National Asthma Education and Prevention Program: *Expert panel report 3: Guidelines for diagnosis and management of asthma,* National Institutes of Health, National Heart, Lung, and Blood Institute, August 2007, NIH publication 08-4051.

BOX 1-1 Possible Indications for Referral to an Asthma Specialist

Severe, acute asthma that has caused loss of consciousness, hypoxia, respiratory failure, convulsions, or near death
Poorly controlled asthma as indicated by admission to a hospital, frequent need for emergency care, need for oral corticosteroids, absence from school or work, disruption of sleep, interference with quality of life
Severe, persistent asthma requiring step 4 care (consider for patients who require step 3 care)
Patient <3 yr who requires step 3 or 4 care (consider for patient <3 yr who requires step 2 care)
Requirement for continuous oral corticosteroids or high-dose inhaled corticosteroids or more than two short courses of oral corticosteroids within 1 yr

Need for additional diagnostic testing such as allergy skin testing, rhinoscopy, provocative challenge, complete pulmonary function testing, bronchoscopy
Consideration for immunotherapy
Need for additional education regarding asthma, complications of asthma and treatment of asthma, problems with adherence to management recommendations, or allergen avoidance
Uncertainty of diagnosis
Complications of asthma, including sinusitis, nasal polyposis, aspergillosis, severe rhinitis, vocal cord dysfunction, gastroesophageal reflux

Modified from National Asthma Education and Prevention Program, National Heart, Lung, and Blood Institute: *Expert Panel Report 2: guidelines for the diagnosis and management of asthma,* Bethesda, MD, 1997, National Institutes of Health, NIH publication No 97-4051.

TABLE 1-19 Classifying Asthma Severity and Initiating Treatment in Children 5-11 Yr (Assessing severity and initiating treatment in children who are not currently taking long-term control medications)

Components of Severity		CLASSIFICATION OF ASTHMA SEVERITY (5-11 yrs of age)			
			PERSISTENT		
		Intermittent	Mild	Moderate	Severe
Impairment	Symptoms	≤2 days/wk	>2 days/wk but not daily	Daily	Throughout the day
	Nighttime awakenings	≤2×/mo	3-4×/mo	>1×/wk but not nightly	Often 7×/wk
	Short-acting beta₂-agonist use for symptom control (not prevention of EIB)	≤2 days/wk	>2 days/wk but not daily	Daily	Several times per day
	Interference with normal activity	None	Minor limitation	Some limitation	Extremely limited
	Lung function	Normal FEV₁ between exacerbations			
		FEV₁ >80% predicted	FEV₁ = >80% predicted	FEV₁ = 60%-80% predicted	FEV₁ <60% predicted
		FEV₁/FVC >85%	FEV₁/FVC >80%	FEV₁/FVC = 75%-80%	FEV₁/FVC <75%
Risk	Exacerbations requiring oral systemic corticosteroids	0-1 per yr	≥2 per yr ──		
		←─── Consider severity and interval since last exacerbation. Frequency and severity may fluctuate over ───→ time for patients in any severity category.			
		Relative annual risk of exacerbations may be related to FEV₁.			
Recommended Step for Initiating Therapy		Step 1	Step 2	Step 3, medium-dose ICS option	Step 3, medium-dose ICS option, or Step 4
				and consider short course of oral systemic corticosteroids	
		In 2-6 wk, evaluate level of asthma control that is achieved and adjust therapy accordingly.			

The stepwise approach is meant to assist, not replace, the clinical decision-making required to meet individual patient needs.

Level of severity is determined by both impairment and risk. Assess impairment domain by patient's/caregiver's recall of previous 2-4 wk and spirometry. Assign severity to the most severe category in which any feature occurs.

At present, there are inadequate data to correspond frequencies of exacerbations with different levels of asthma severity. In general, more frequent and intense exacerbations (e.g., requiring urgent, unscheduled care, hospitalization, or ICU admission) indicate greater underlying disease severity. For treatment purposes, patients who had ≥2 exacerbations requiring oral systemic corticosteroids in the past year may be considered the same as patients who have persistent asthma, even in the absence of impairment levels consistent with persistent asthma.

EIB, Exercise-induced bronchospasm; *FEV₁*, forced expiratory volume in 1 second; *FVC*, forced vital capacity; *ICU*, intensive care unit.

From National Asthma Education and Prevention Program: *Expert panel report 3: Guidelines for diagnosis and management of asthma*, National Institutes of Health, National Heart, Lung, and Blood Institute, August 2007, NIH publication 08-4051.

TABLE 1-20 Assessing Asthma Control and Adjusting Therapy in Children 5-11 Yr

Components of Control		CLASSIFICATION OF ASTHMA CONTROL (5-11 yrs of age)		
		Well Controlled	Not Well Controlled	Very Poorly Controlled
Impairment	Symptoms	≤2 days/wk but not more than once on each day	>2 days/wk or multiple times on ≤2 days/wk	Throughout the day
	Nighttime awakenings	≤1×/mo	≥2×/mo	≥2×/wk
	Interference with normal activity	None	Some limitation	Extremely limited
	Short-acting beta₂-agonist use for symptom control (not prevention of EIB)	≤2 days/wk	>2 days/wk	Several times per day
	Lung function			
	FEV₁ or peak flow	>80% predicted/personal best	60%-80% predicted/personal best	<60% predicted/personal best
	FEV₁/FVC	>80% predicted	75%-80%	<75% predicted
Risk	Exacerbations requiring oral systemic corticosteroids	0-1 per yr	≥2 per yr	
		Consider severity and interval since last exacerbation		
	Reduction in lung growth	Evaluation requires long-term follow-up care		
	Treatment-related adverse effects	Medication side effects can vary in intensity from none to very troublesome and worrisome. The level of intensity does not correlate to specific levels of control but should be considered in the overall assessment of risk.		
Recommended Action for Treatment		Maintain current step. Regular follow-up every 1-6 mo. Consider step down if well controlled for at least 3 mo.	Step up 1 step and Reevaluate in 2-6 wk. For side effects, consider alternative treatment options.	Consider short course of oral systemic corticosteroids. Step up 1-2 steps. Reevaluate in 2 wk. For side effects, consider alternative treatment options.

The stepwise approach is meant to assist, not replace, the clinical decision-making required to meet individual patient needs.

The level of control is based on the most severe impairment or risk category. Assess impairment domain by patient's/caregiver's recall of previous 2-4 wk and by spirometry or peak flow measures. Symptom assessment for longer periods should reflect a global assessment such as inquiring whether the patient's asthma is better or worse since the last visit.

At present, there are inadequate data to correspond frequencies of exacerbations with different levels of asthma control. In general, more frequent and intense exacerbations (e.g., requiring urgent, unscheduled care, hospitalization, or ICU admission) indicate poorer disease control. For treatment purposes, patients who had ≥2 exacerbations requiring oral systemic corticosteroids in the past year may be considered the same as patients who have persistent asthma, even in the absence of impairment levels consistent with persistent asthma.

Before step up in therapy:

- Review adherence to medications, inhaler technique, environmental control, and comorbid conditions.
- If an alternative treatment option was used in a step, discontinue it and use preferred treatment for that step.

EIB, Exercise-induced bronchospasm; *FEV₁*, forced expiratory volume in 1 second; *ICU*, intensive care unit.

From National Asthma Education and Prevention Program: *Expert panel report 3: Guidelines for diagnosis and management of asthma*, National Institutes of Health, National Heart, Lung, and Blood Institute, August 2007, NIH publication 08-4051.

A

Diseases and Disorders

I

TABLE 1-21   Stepwise Approach for Managing Asthma in Children 5-11 Yr

Intermittent Asthma	Persistent Asthma: Daily Medication
	Consult with asthma specialist if step 4 care or higher is required. Consider consultation at step 3.

Step 1
Preferred:
SABA prn

Step 2
Preferred:
Low-dose ICS

Alternative:
Cromolyn, LTRA, nedocromil, or theophylline

Step 3
Preferred:
Low-dose ICS + either LABA, LTRA, or theophylline

OR

Medium-dose ICS

Step 4
Preferred:
Medium-dose ICS + LABA

Alternative:
Medium-dose ICS + either LTRA or theophylline

Step 5
Preferred:
High-dose ICS + LABA

Alternative:
High-dose ICS + either LTRA or theophylline

Step 6
Preferred:
High-dose ICS + LABA + oral corticosteroid

Alternative:
High-dose ICS + either LTRA or theophylline + oral systemic corticosteroid

Step up if needed

(first, check adherence, inhaler technique, environmental control, and comorbid conditions)

Assess control

Step down if possible

(and asthma is well controlled at least 3 months)

Each step: Patient education, environmental control, and management of comorbidities
Steps 2-4: Consider subcutaneous allergen immunotherapy for patients who have allergic asthma

Quick-Relief Medication for All Patients
- SABA as needed for symptoms. Intensity of treatment depends on severity of symptoms: up to 3 treatments at 20-minute intervals as needed. Short course of oral systemic corticosteroids may be needed.
- Caution: Increasing use of SABA or use >2 days a week for symptom relief (not prevention of EIB) generally indicates inadequate control and the need to step up treatment.

The stepwise approach is meant to assist, not replace, the clinical decision-making required to meet individual patient needs.
If alternative treatment is used and response is inadequate, discontinue it and use the preferred treatment before stepping up.
Theophylline is a less desirable alternative due to the need to monitor serum concentration levels.
Step 1 and step 2 medications are based on Evidence A. Step 3 ICS + adjunctive therapy and ICS are based on Evidence B for efficacy of each treatment and extrapolation from comparator trials in older children and adults—comparator trials are not available for this age group; steps 4-6 are based on expert opinion and extrapolation from studies in older children and adults.
Immunotherapy for steps 2-4 is based on Evidence B for house-dust mites, animal danders, and pollens; evidence is weak or lacking for molds and cockroaches. Evidence is strongest for immunotherapy with single allergens. The role of allergy in asthma is greater in children than in adults. Clinicians who administer immunotherapy should be prepared and equipped to identify and treat anaphylaxis that may occur.
This information is directly abstracted from the 2007 NAEPP *Expert Panel Report 3: Guidelines for the Diagnosis and Management of Asthma* and is not intended to promote or endorse any of the listed products.
ICS, Inhaled corticosteroid; *LABA,* inhaled long-acting beta₂-agonist; *LTRA,* leukotriene receptor antagonist; *SABA,* inhaled short-acting beta₂-agonist.
From National Asthma Education and Prevention Program: *Expert panel report 3: Guidelines for diagnosis and management of asthma*, National Institutes of Health, National Heart, Lung, and Blood Institute, August 2007, NIH publication 08-4051.

TABLE 1-22 Classifying Asthma Severity and Initiating Treatment in Children 0-4 Yr
(Assessing severity and initiating treatment in children who are not currently taking long-term control medications)

Components of Severity		Intermittent	CLASSIFICATION OF ASTHMA SEVERITY (0-4 yrs of age) PERSISTENT		
			Mild	Moderate	Severe
Impairment	Symptoms	≤2 days/wk	>2 days/wk but not daily	Daily	Throughout the day
	Nighttime awakenings	0	1-2×/mo	3-4×/mo	>1×/wk
	Short-acting beta₂-agonist use for symptom control (not prevention of EIB)	≤2 days/wk	>2 days/wk but not daily	Daily	Several times per day
	Interference with normal activity	None	Minor limitation	Some limitation	Extremely limited
Risk	Exacerbations requiring oral systemic corticosteroids	0-1 per yr	≥2 exacerbations in 6 mo requiring oral systemic corticosteroids, or ≥4 wheezing episodes/1 yr lasting >1 day AND risk factors for persistent asthma.		
			←——— Consider severity and interval since last exacerbation. ———→ Frequency and severity may fluctuate over time. Exacerbations of any severity may occur in patients in any severity category.		
Recommended Step for Initiating Therapy		Step 1	Step 2	Step 3 and consider short course of oral systemic corticosteroids	
			In 2-6 wk, depending on severity, evaluate level of asthma control that is achieved. If no clear benefit is observed in 4-6 wk, consider adjusting therapy or alternative diagnoses.		

The stepwise approach is meant to assist, not replace, the clinical decision-making required to meet individual patient needs.
Level of severity is determined by assessment of both impairment and risk. Assess impairment domain by patient's/caregiver's recall of previous 2-4 wk. Symptom assessment for longer periods should reflect a global assessment such as inquiring whether the patient's asthma is better or worse since the last visit. Assign severity to the most severe category in which any feature occurs.
At present, there are inadequate data to correspond frequencies of exacerbations with different levels of asthma severity. For treatment purposes, patients who had ≥2 exacerbations requiring oral systemic corticosteroids in the past six months, or ≥4 wheezing episodes in the past year, and who have risk factors for persistent asthma may be considered the same as patients who have persistent asthma, even in the absence of impairment levels consistent with persistent asthma.
To access the complete Expert Panel Report 3: Guidelines for the Diagnosis and Management of Asthma, go to www.nhlbi.nih.gov/guidelines/asthma/asthgdln.pdf.
EIB, Exercise-induced bronchospasm.
From National Asthma Education and Prevention Program: *Expert panel report 3: Guidelines for diagnosis and management of asthma,* National Institutes of Health, National Heart, Lung, and Blood Institute, August 2007, NIH publication 08-4051.

TABLE 1-23 Assessing Asthma Control and Adjusting Therapy in Children 0-4 Yrs of Age

Components of Control		CLASSIFICATION OF ASTHMA CONTROL (0-4 yrs of age) Well Controlled	Not Well Controlled	Very Poorly Controlled
Impairment	Symptoms	≤2 days/wk	>2 days/wk	Throughout the day
	Nighttime awakenings	≤1×/mo	>1×/mo	>1×/wk
	Interference with normal activity	None	Some limitation	Extremely limited
	Short-acting beta₂-agonist use for symptom control (not prevention of EIB)	≤2 days/wk	>2 days/wk	Several times per day
Risk	Exacerbations requiring oral systemic corticosteroids	0-1 per yr	2-3 per yr	>3 per yr
	Treatment-related adverse effects	Medication side effects can vary in intensity from none to very troublesome and worrisome. The level of intensity does not correlate to specific levels of control but should be considered in the overall assessment of risk.		
Recommended Action for Treatment		Maintain current step. Regular follow-up every 1-6 mo. Consider step down if well controlled for at least 3 mo.	Step up 1 step. Reevaluate in 2-6 wk. If no clear benefit in 4-6 wk, consider alternative diagnoses or adjusting therapy. For side effects, consider alternative treatment options.	Consider short course of oral systemic corticosteroids. Step up 1-2 steps. Reevaluate in 2 wk. If no clear benefit in 4-6 wk, consider alternative diagnoses or adjusting therapy. For side effects, consider alternative treatment options.

The stepwise approach is meant to assist, not replace, the clinical decision-making required to meet individual patient needs.
The level of control is based on the most severe impairment or risk category. Assess impairment domain by caregiver's recall of previous 2-4 wk. Symptom assessment for longer periods should reflect a global assessment such as inquiring whether the patient's asthma is better or worse since the last visit.
At present, there are inadequate data to correspond frequencies of exacerbations with different levels of asthma control. In general, more frequent and intense exacerbations (e.g., requiring urgent, unscheduled care, hospitalization, or ICU admission) indicate poorer disease control. For treatment purposes, patients who had ≥2 exacerbations requiring oral systemic corticosteroids in the past year may be considered the same as patients who have not-well-controlled asthma, even in the absence of impairment levels consistent with not-well-controlled asthma.
Before step up in therapy:
– Review adherence to medications, inhaler technique, and environmental control.
– If an alternative treatment option was used in a step, discontinue it and use preferred treatment for that step.
EIB, Exercise-induced bronchospasm; *ICU,* intensive care unit.
From National Asthma Education and Prevention Program: *Expert panel report 3: Guidelines for diagnosis and management of asthma,* National Institutes of Health, National Heart, Lung, and Blood Institute, August 2007, NIH publication 08-4051.

beta-2 receptor with loss of the bronchoprotective effect from from rescue therapy with a short-acting beta-2 agonist.
- Patients who remain symptomatic despite inhaled corticosteroids benefit from the addition of long-acting beta-2 agonists.
- Therapy with with systemic corticosteroids accelerates the resolution of acute asthma and reduces the risk of relapse. There is no evidence that doses >50-100 mg prednisone equivalent are beneficial.
- In patients with allergies and elevated serum immunoglobulin (Ig) E levels, use of anti-IgE therapy is beneficial.

- Bronchial thermoplasty (Alair System) may be used to reduce airway smooth muscle mass and widen the airway in adult patients with severe persistent asthma not well controlled with inhaled corticosteroids and long-acting beta-2 agonists. It requires the insertion of a catheter via bronchoscopy and use of a radiofrequency controller.
- Biological modifiers of the Th2 immune pathways (neutralizing monoclonal antibodies, receptor antagonists, soluble receptors) are potential options for the development of new treatments of severe asthma.

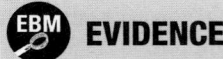

EVIDENCE

available at www.expertconsult.com

SUGGESTED READINGS

available at www.expertconsult.com

AUTHOR: **FRED F. FERRI, M.D.**

TABLE 1-24 Stepwise Approach for Managing Asthma in Children 0-4 Yr

Intermittent Asthma	Persistent Asthma: Daily Medication
	Consult with asthma specialist if step 3 care or higher is required. Consider consultation at step 2.

Step 1
Preferred:
SABA prn

Step 2
Preferred:
Low-dose ICS

Alternative:
Cromolyn or montelukast

Step 3
Preferred:
Medium-dose ICS

Step 4
Preferred:
Medium-dose ICS + either LABA or montelukast

Step 5
Preferred:
High-dose ICS + either LABA or montelukast

Step 6
Preferred:
High-dose ICS + either LABA or montelukast

Oral systemic corticosteroid

Step up if needed
(first, check adherence, inhaler technique, and environmental control)

Assess control

Step down if possible

(and asthma is well controlled at least 3 months)

Patient Education and Environmental Control at Each Step

Quick-Relief Medication for All Patients
- SABA as needed for symptoms. Intensity of treatment depends on severity of symptoms.
- With viral respiratory infection: SABA q 4-6 hours up to 24 hours (longer with physician consult). Consider short course of oral systemic corticosteroids if exacerbation is severe or patient has history of previous severe exacerbations.
- Caution: Frequent use of SABA may indicate the need to step up treatment. See text for recommendations on initiating daily long-term-control therapy.

The stepwise approach is meant to assist, not replace, the clinical decision-making required to meet individual patient needs.
If alternative treatment is used and response is inadequate, discontinue it and use the preferred treatment before stepping up.
If clear benefit is not observed within 4-6 wk and patient/family medication technique and adherence are satisfactory, consider adjusting therapy or alternative diagnosis.
Studies on children 0-4 yr are limited. Step 2 preferred therapy is based on Evidence A. All other recommendations are based on expert opinion and extrapolation from studies in other children.
This information is directly abstracted from the 2007 NAEPP *Expert Panel Report 3: Guidelines for the Diagnosis and Management of Asthma* and is not intended to promote or endorse any of the listed products.
ICS, Inhaled corticosteroid; *LABA*, inhaled long-acting beta₂-agonist; *SABA*, inhaled short-acting beta₂-agonist.
From National Asthma Education and Prevention Program: *Expert panel report 3: Guidelines for diagnosis and management of asthma*, National Institutes of Health, National Heart, Lung, and Blood Institute, August 2007, NIH publication 08-4051.

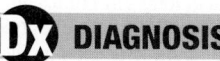

BASIC INFORMATION

DEFINITION

Astrocytoma is a type of neuroepithelial tumor that arises from glial precursor cells (astrocytes, oligodendrocytes, ependymal cells, epithelial cells of the choroids plexus, and others). Astrocytoma arises from astrocytes within the central nervous system (CNS). They are commonly graded by the World Health Organization (WHO) or the Saint Anne–Mayo grading system.

The WHO grades astrocytomas as follows:
- Grade I: pilocytic astrocytoma
- Grade II: low-grade astrocytoma (LGA), fibrillary infiltrating astrocytoma
- Grade III: anaplastic astrocytoma
- Grade IV: glioblastoma multiforme (GBM)
- Grades III and IV are considered high-grade astrocytomas (HGAs) or malignant.

Kernohan system grades astrocytomas based on histologic features: cellularity, mitoses, pleomorphism, vascularity, and necrosis. It has proved to be of prognostic value.
- Grade I: increased cellularity
- Grade II: greater cellularity than grade I plus pleomorphism
- Grade III: greater cellularity and pleomorphism than grade II plus vascular proliferation
- Grade IV: all the above, plus necrosis and pseudopalisading

SYNONYMS

Astroglial neoplasms

ICD-9CM CODES
191.9 Astrocytoma, unspecified site

EPIDEMIOLOGY & DEMOGRAPHICS

- According to SEER registry, the incidence of primary CNS tumor is 2.2 to 8.3/100,000 persons and about 30% of these tumors are astrocytomas.
- Astrocytomas can be found at all ages, with an early peak from birth to 4 yr, followed by a trough between the ages of 15 and 24 yr, and then a steady increase in incidence.
- Male/female ratio is 2:1.
- In adults, glioblastoma is the most common brain tumor.
- In children, astrocytomas are the second most common primary brain tumor and medulloblastoma is the most common.
- LGAs represent approximately 25% of all CNS gliomas in children.
- Peak age of incidence for juvenile pilocytic astrocytomas is 5 to 14 yr.
- Peak age of incidence for glioblastoma is 45 to 70 yr.

GENETICS:

- Alteration of *p53*, a tumor-suppressor gene encoded by the *TP53* gene on chromosome 17, plays a key role in the development of a large number of adult astrocytomas.
- Genetic abnormalities occur in a stepwise manner with accumulation of multiple abnormalities leading to dedifferentiation and transformation into higher grade.
- Abnormalities of the cell cycle regulatory complex that includes p16, cdk6/cyclinD1, cdk4/cyclinD1, and loss of chromosome 9P that targets the CDKN2A locus is thought to play an important role in progression to grade III astrocytoma.
- Transformation to GBM is the result of multiple mitogenic effects, with deregulation of p16-CDK4D1-pRb pathway being an important component. Loss of chromosome 10, which targets the PTEN tumor-suppressor gene, is also a frequent finding.

PHYSICAL FINDINGS & CLINICAL PRESENTATION

The presenting symptoms of astrocytoma depend, in part, on the location of the lesion and its rate of growth. Astrocytomas classically present with any one or more of the following features:
- Headache (less frequent)
- New-onset partial or generalized seizures (>50%)
- Nausea and vomiting
- Focal neurologic deficit (cranial nerve palsy, hemiplegia, ataxia)
- Change in mental status
- Papilledema (rare)

ETIOLOGY

- The specific etiology of astrocytoma is unknown.
- The only proven risk factor for development of astrocytoma has been significant exposure to ionizing radiation.
- Other risk factors, such as increased exposure to certain chemicals (petroleum, solvents, lead, pesticides and herbicides), have been proposed but not proved.

DIAGNOSIS

A provisional diagnosis of astrocytoma is made on clinical grounds and radiographic imaging studies. Tissue pathology is needed to establish the diagnosis and to grade the astrocytoma.

DIFFERENTIAL DIAGNOSIS

The differential diagnosis is vast and includes any cause of headache, seizures, change in mental status, and focal neurologic deficits.

WORKUP

- A CT scan or MRI of the head makes the diagnosis of an intracranial brain tumor. However, tissue is needed to establish a diagnosis of astrocytoma.
- Stereotactic biopsy under CT or MRI guidance has been shown to be a relatively safe and accurate method for diagnosis of LGA.
- In the presence of mass effect, either clinically or radiologically, craniotomy with open biopsy and tumor debulking is more appropriate than stereotactic biopsy to establish a tissue diagnosis.

LABORATORY TESTS

Blood tests are not specific.

IMAGING STUDIES

- MRI (Fig. 1-43) is the diagnostic imaging study of choice. MRI with contrast and magnetic resonance angiography are used to locate the margins of the tumor, distinguish vascular masses from tumors, detect LGAs not seen by CT scan, and provide clear views of the posterior fossa.
- Newer imaging modalities like magnetic resonance spectroscopy, dynamic enhance MRI, diffusion perfusion MRI, and functional MRI may lead to improved tumor delineation and functional mapping, and provide information to facilitate resection.

TREATMENT

ACUTE GENERAL Rx

- Once a clinical diagnosis is made on imaging and there is evidence of edema, patients should be started on dexamethasone 10 mg intravenously (IV) followed by 4 mg IV q6h.

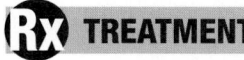

FIGURE 1-43 MR image of a low-grade astrocytoma, demonstrating a hypointense right temporal lesion without contrast enhancement on T1 and hyperintense signal on T2. (From Goetz CG, Pappert EJ: *Textbook of clinical neurology*, Philadelphia, 1999, Saunders.)

- If there is increased intracranial pressure and impending herniation, patient should be started on IV mannitol, and mechanical ventilation with hyperventilation should be considered if there is depressed consciousness.
- Surgery remains the initial treatment of almost all astrocytomas, particularly if the tumor is in an anatomically accessible location. Surgery helps in the following ways:
  1. Establishing a pathologic diagnosis and providing information on grade
  2. Debulking the tumor
  3. Alleviating intracranial pressure
- Grade I astrocytomas are usually circumscribed, and complete resection is possible with a high likelihood of long-term remission.
- In grade II astrocytomas, the extent of surgical resection and amount of postoperative residual disease is an important variable for time to first relapse. Randomized trials have shown that postoperative radiotherapy in grade II astrocytoma increases progression-free survival (PFS), but no increase in median survival occurs.
- In grade III and grade IV astrocytomas, gross total resection is the initial treatment of choice. Patients with no residual enhancing tumor have a longer median survival (17.9 vs 12.9 mo; $P <0.001$) than patients with residual tumor.
- Use of radiation after surgery in HGAs has shown a clear benefit of survival.
- In a randomized trial of patients with GBM, radiation with concurrent temozolomide followed by six cycles of adjuvant temozolomide increases median and overall survival, and this is considered the standard of care for patients with GBM.

CHRONIC Rx

- Attempt at resection again should be considered in all types of astrocytomas on relapse if possible and in grade I astrocytomas can lead to long-term remissions.
- Radiation therapy can be considered in the relapsed setting in grade II astrocytomas if not given in the adjuvant setting. Chemotherapy has been tried but has no proven role in these tumors.
- Chemotherapy in anaplastic astrocytomas that have relapsed after radiation does have a role, and the active agents are nitrosourea-based regimen and temozolomide. Grade III anaplastic astrocytomas that have 1p and 19q deletions are especially sensitive to chemotherapy.
- Chemotherapy is used in patients with GBM on relapse, but efficacy is limited. Temozolomide is the most commonly used agent, but radiologic response is in the 5% to 10% range. Recently, a number of phase II trials have shown the efficacy of the combination of inrinotecan and avastin with response rates in the 30% range and have provided a new option in the treatment of GBMs.
- Patients presenting with seizures should be treated with anticonvulsants.

DISPOSITION

- Approximately 10% to 35% of astrocytomas (usually grade I pilocytic astrocytomas) are amenable to complete surgical excision and cure. WHO grade I astrocytomas usually do not progress to higher grade tumors.
- Grade II astrocytomas have a median survival of 7.7 yr if they are low risk and 3.2 yr if they are high risk.
- Grade III astrocytomas have a 3-yr survival rate of 55%.
- Median survival for patients with GBM is about 1 yr. Median survival of patients with GBM treated with supportive care is approximately 14 wk. This increases to 20 wk with surgical resection alone, 36 wk with surgery plus x-ray therapy, and 40 to 50 wk with the addition of adjuvant chemotherapy.

REFERRAL

A team of specialty consultations is indicated in patients diagnosed with astrocytoma. A neurosurgeon, radiation oncologist, and neurooncologist are all needed to assist in establishing the diagnosis and to provide immediate and follow-up treatment.

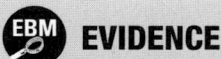 **EVIDENCE**

available at www.expertconsult.com

SUGGESTED READINGS

available at www.expertconsult.com

AUTHOR: **BILAL H. NAQVI, M.D.**

BASIC INFORMATION

DEFINITION

Ataxia telangiectasia (AT) is a rare autosomal recessive disorder of childhood that results from defective DNA repair mechanisms. AT is a multisystemic disease characterized by progressive cerebellar ataxia, choreoathetosis, oculocutaneous telangiectasias (Fig. 1-44), frequent infections, increased sensitivity to ionizing radiation, and predisposition to malignancies.

ICD-9CM CODES
334.8 Ataxia telangiectasia

EPIDEMIOLOGY & DEMOGRAPHICS

INCIDENCE: 1/40,000 live births; it is estimated that 1.4% to 2% of whites in the United States carry one defective AT gene
PEAK INCIDENCE: Childhood
PREDOMINANT SEX: Sexes are equally affected.
GENETICS: Condition is autosomal recessive defective gene, designated ATM (for At Mutated), has been mapped to chromosome 11q22.3. The gene product, which is expressed in all tissues, encodes a large protein that is a member of the phosphatidylinositol-3 kinases and another region similar to DNA repair genes.

PHYSICAL FINDINGS & CLINICAL PRESENTATION

- Children show normal early development until they start to walk, when gait and truncal ataxia become apparent. They soon experience development of polyneuropathy, progressive apraxia of eye movements and slurred speech, choreoathetosis, mild diabetes mellitus, delayed physical and sexual development, and signs of premature aging (graying of the hair).
- Children with AT experience deterioration of motor skills; by the second decade of life, most patients rely on wheelchairs for at least part of the day. Progressive oromotor difficulties also develop over time, placing patients at risk for aspiration.

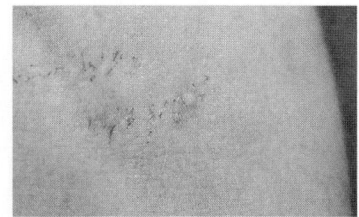
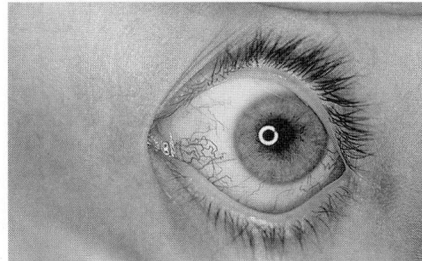

FIGURE 1-44 Ataxia telangiectasia. (From Callen JP [ed]: *Color atlas of dermatology,* ed 2, Philadelphia, 2000, WB Saunders.)

- Telangiectasias, which may be delayed in appearance, occur primarily in the bulbar conjunctivae, over the surface of the ears and cheeks, on exposed parts of the neck, on the bridge of the nose, and in the flexor creases of the forearms.
- Immunodeficiencies occur in 60% to 80% of individuals with AT. Impaired humoral and cellular immunity lead to recurrent sinopulmonary infections in about 70% of children.
- Beyond 10 yr of age, incidence rate is 1% per yr; overall risk rate is 10% to 20%, of which 85% of cases are leukemia and lymphoma. Predisposition to other cancers (such as breast cancer) may also exist, which is thought to be due to the phosphorylation of the tumor-suppressor/breast cancer susceptibility gene *BRCA1* by *ATM*.
- Typically, individuals with AT have normal intelligence. Deterioration of speech is typically noted after the age of 5 to 8 yr. Slow motor and verbal responses may make traditional timed assessments inaccurate.
- Heterozygotes/carriers of the *ATM* gene are thought to have none of the classic manifestations of AT; however, they may have a greater incidence of malignancy at a younger age.

ETIOLOGY

- Cytogenetics show a 7;14 translocation in 5% to 15% of individuals with AT. Cloning and sequencing has identified the *ATM* gene (ataxia telangiectasia, mutated), which is a protein kinase that is missing or defective. This delays accumulation of the tumor-suppressor p53 in response to DNA damage, thereby increasing the risk for cancer. Cells are susceptible to damage by ionizing radiation or chemotherapeutic agents that cause double-stranded DNA breakages.

DIAGNOSIS

DIFFERENTIAL DIAGNOSIS: Early-onset ataxia:
- Friedreich's ataxia
- Abetalipoproteinemia (Bassen-Kornzweig syndrome)
- Acquired vitamin E deficiency
- Early-onset cerebellar ataxia with retained reflexes (EOCA)
- Ataxia-ocular apraxia type 1 (AOA1)
- Ataxia-ocular apraxia type 2 (AOA2)

WORKUP

Diagnosis relies on the constellation of clinical findings, including ataxia and speech changes, as well as family history and neuroimaging studies.

LABORATORY TESTS

- Patients should be evaluated for serum immunoglobulin levels (IgA, IgG, IgE, and IgG subclasses) to evaluate for immunoglobulin deficiency, and α-fetoprotein, which is increased in more than 95% of patients over the age of 8 mo.
- Prenatal testing is available. Fibroblasts can be screened for abnormal sensitivity to ionizing radiation.
- Immunoblotting for ATM protein can be done. This determines whether ATM protein is present in cells; approximately 90% of individuals will have no detectable ATM protein.

IMAGING STUDIES

CT or MRI scans will show cerebellar atrophy but may not be obvious in very young children.

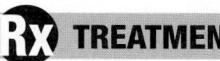
TREATMENT

- There is no proven disease-specific treatment available to delay the progressive ataxia, dysarthria, and oculomotor apraxia. Treatment remains supportive.
- Surveillance for infections and neoplasms is ongoing. Individuals with frequent and severe infections may benefit from intravenous immunoglobulin to supplement immune system.
- The cloning and sequencing of the gene for AT has opened several avenues for intervention, including gene therapy, targeted pharmacologic intervention, and direct protein replacement.

NONPHARMACOLOGIC THERAPY

- Minimize radiation as it may induce further chromosomal damage and lead to neoplasms. Even diagnostic x-rays should be limited because of the theoretical risk that radiation may lead to chromosomal breakages.
- Physical and occupational therapy to maintain flexibility and minimize contractures.

COMPLEMENTARY AND ALTERNATIVE MEDICINE

- Antioxidant treatment with vitamin E is often given empirically, though it has not been formally tested. α-Lipoic acid crosses the blood-brain barrier and may, therefore, have some advantage.

DISPOSITION

- The expected life span has increased considerably; most individuals now live beyond 25 yr of age and some into the fourth and fifth decades of life.

REFERRAL

- Immunology
- Neurology
- Physical and occupational therapy
- Genetic counselor

PEARLS & CONSIDERATIONS

COMMENTS

- Most common cause of hereditary ataxia
- Defect in DNA repair
- Predisposition to frequent infections, malignancies, and sensitivity to ionizing radiation

PATIENT/FAMILY EDUCATION

Ataxia Telangiectasia Children's Project: www.atcp.org
National Ataxia Foundation (NAF): www.ataxia.org

SUGGESTED READINGS
available at www.expertconsult.com

AUTHOR: **NICOLE J. ULLRICH, M.D., PH.D.**

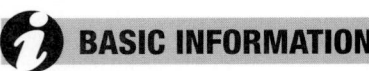

BASIC INFORMATION

DEFINITION

Atelectasis is the collapse of lung volume.

ICD-9CM CODES
518.0 Atelectasis

EPIDEMIOLOGY & DEMOGRAPHICS

- Occurs frequently in patients receiving mechanical ventilation with higher FiO_2
- Dependent regions of the lung are more prone to atelectasis: they are partially compressed, they are not as well ventilated, and there is no spontaneous drainage of secretions with gravity

PHYSICAL FINDINGS & CLINICAL PRESENTATION

- Decreased or absent breath sounds
- Abnormal chest percussion
- Cough, dyspnea, decreased vocal fremitus and vocal resonance
- Diminished chest expansion, tachypnea, tachycardia

ETIOLOGY

- Mechanical ventilation with higher FiO_2
- Chronic bronchitis
- Cystic fibrosis
- Endobronchial neoplasms
- Foreign bodies
- Infections (e.g., TB, histoplasmosis)
- Extrinsic bronchial compression from neoplasms, aneurysms of ascending aorta, enlarged left atrium
- Sarcoidosis
- Silicosis
- Anterior chest wall injury, pneumothorax
- Alveolar injury (e.g., toxic fumes, aspiration of gastric contents)
- Pleural effusion, expanding bullae
- Chest wall deformity (e.g., scoliosis)
- Muscular weaknesses or abnormalities (e.g., neuromuscular disease)
- Mucus plugs from asthma, allergic bronchopulmonary aspergillosis, postoperative state

DIAGNOSIS

DIFFERENTIAL DIAGNOSIS

- Neoplasm
- Pneumonia
- Encapsulated pleural effusion
- Abnormalities of brachiocephalic vein and the left pulmonary ligament

WORKUP

- Chest radiograph (Fig. 1-45)
- CT scan and fiberoptic bronchoscopy (selected patients)

IMAGING STUDIES

- Chest radiograph will confirm diagnosis.
- CT scan is useful in patients with suspected endobronchial neoplasm or extrinsic bronchial compression.
- Fiberoptic bronchoscopy (selected patients) is useful for removal of foreign body or evaluation of endobronchial and peribronchial lesions.

TREATMENT

NONPHARMACOLOGIC THERAPY

- Deep breathing, mobilization of the patient
- Incentive spirometry
- Tracheal suctioning
- Humidification
- Chest physiotherapy with percussion and postural drainage

ACUTE GENERAL Rx

- Positive-pressure breathing (continuous positive airway pressure by face mask, positive end-expiratory pressure for patients on mechanical ventilation)
- Use of mucolytic agents (e.g., acetylcysteine [Mucomyst])
- Recombinant human DNase (dornase alpha) in patients with cystic fibrosis
- Bronchodilator therapy in selected patients

CHRONIC Rx

- Chest physiotherapy
- Humidification of inspired air
- Frequent nasotracheal suctioning

DISPOSITION

Prognosis varies with the underlying etiology

REFERRAL

- Bronchoscopy for removal of foreign body or plugs unresponsive to conservative treatment
- Surgical referral for removal of obstructing neoplasms

PEARLS & CONSIDERATIONS

COMMENTS

Patients should be educated that frequent changes of position are helpful in clearing secretions. Sitting the patient upright in a chair is recommended to increase both volume and vital capacity relative to the supine position.

AUTHOR: **FRED F. FERRI, M.D.**

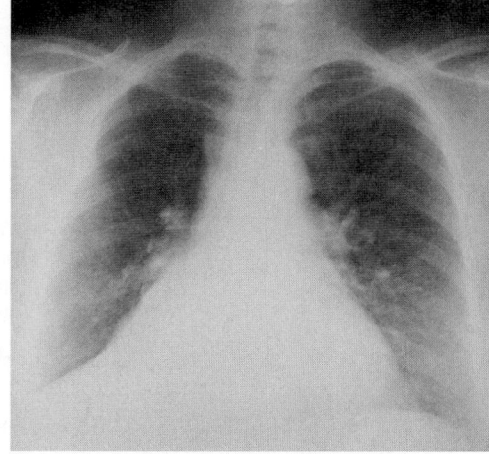

FIGURE 1-45 Right middle and right lower lobe atelectasis that silhouettes the diaphragm and the right heart border. (From Specht N [ed]: *Practical guide to diagnostic imaging,* St Louis, 1998, Mosby.)

A

 BASIC INFORMATION

DEFINITION

Atopic dermatitis is a genetically determined eczematous eruption that is pruritic, symmetric, and associated with personal family history of allergic manifestations (atopy).

SYNONYMS

Eczema
Atopic neurodermatitis
Atopic eczema

ICD-9CM CODES
691.8 Atopic dermatitis

EPIDEMIOLOGY & DEMOGRAPHICS

- Incidence is between 5 and 25 cases/1000 persons.
- Highest incidence is among children (10% to 20%). It accounts for 4% of acute care pediatric visits. It affects 1% to 3% of the adult population.
- Onset of disease before age 5 yr in 85% of patients.
- More than 50% of children with generalized atopic dermatitis develop asthma and allergic rhinitis by age 13 yr.
- Concordance in monozygotic twins is 77%.

PHYSICAL FINDINGS & CLINICAL PRESENTATION

- There are no specific cutaneous signs for atopic dermatitis, and there is a wide spectrum of presentations ranging from minimal flexural eczema to erythroderma.
- The primary lesions are a result of itching caused by severe and chronic pruritus. The repeated scratching modifies the skin surface, producing lichenification, dry and scaly skin, and redness.
- The lesions are typically on the neck, face, upper trunk, and bends of elbows and knees (symmetric on flexural surfaces of extremities).
- There is dryness, thickening of the involved areas, discoloration, blistering, and oozing.
- Papular lesions are frequently found in the antecubital and popliteal fossae.
- In children, red scaling plaques are often confined to the cheeks and the perioral and perinasal areas.
- Inflammation in the flexural areas and lichenified skin is a very common presentation in children.
- Constant scratching may result in areas of hypopigmentation or hyperpigmentation (more common in blacks).
- In adults, redness and scaling in the dorsal aspect of the hands or about the fingers are the most common expression of atopic dermatitis; oozing and crusting may be present.
- Secondary skin infections may be present (*Staphylococcus aureus,* dermatophytosis, herpes simplex).

ETIOLOGY

Unknown; elevated T-lymphocyte activation, defective cell immunity, and B cell IgE overproduction may play a significant role.

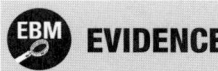 **DIAGNOSIS**

DIFFERENTIAL DIAGNOSIS

- Scabies
- Psoriasis
- Dermatitis herpetiform
- Contact dermatitis
- Photosensitivity
- Seborrheic dermatitis
- Candidiasis
- Lichen simplex chronicus
- Other: Wiskott-Aldrich syndrome, PKU, ichthyosis, HIV dermatitis, nonnummular eczema, histiocytosis X, malignancies (T-cell lymphoma/Mycosis fungoides), Letterer-Siwe disease), graft-versus-host disease, metabolic and nutritional deficiencies (zinc, niacin, pyridoxine deficiencies)

WORKUP

Diagnosis is based on the presence of three of the following major features and three minor features.

MAJOR FEATURES:
- Pruritus
- Personal or family history of atopy: asthma, allergic rhinitis, atopic dermatitis
- Facial and extensor involvement in infants and children
- Flexural lichenification in adults

MINOR FEATURES:
- Elevated IgE
- Eczema-perifollicular accentuation
- Recurrent conjunctivitis
- Ichthyosis
- Nipple dermatitis
- Wool intolerance
- Cutaneous *S. aureus* infections or herpes simplex infections
- Food intolerance
- Hand dermatitis (nonallergic irritant)
- Facial pallor, facial erythema
- Cheilitis
- White dermographism
- Early age of onset (after 2 mo of age)

LABORATORY TESTS

- Lab tests are generally not helpful.
- Elevated IgE levels are found in 80% to 90% of atopic dermatitis.
- Blood eosinophilia correlates with disease severity.

Rx **TREATMENT**

NONPHARMACOLOGIC THERAPY

- Clip nails to decrease abrasion of skin
Avoidance of triggering factors:
- Sudden temperature changes, sweating, low humidity in the winter

- Contact with irritating substance (e.g., wool, cosmetics, some soaps and detergents, tobacco)
- Foods that provoke exacerbations (e.g., eggs, peanuts, fish, soy, wheat, milk)
- Stressful situations
- Allergens and dust
- Excessive hand washing

GENERAL Rx

- Emollients can be used to prevent dryness. Severely affected skin can be optimally hydrated by occlusion in addition to application of emollients.
- Topical corticosteroids (e.g., 1% to 2.5% hydrocortisone) may be helpful and are generally considered first line therapy. Use intermediate-potency steroids (e.g., triamcinolone, fluocinolone) for more severe cases and limit potent corticosteroids (e.g., betamethasone, desoximetasone, clobetasol) to severe cases.
- The topical immunomodulators pimecrolimus and tacrolimus are especially useful for treatment of the face and intertriginous sites, where steroid-induced atrophy may occur. However, due to concerns about carcinogenic potential, the FDA recommends limiting their use for short periods in patients who are intolerant or unresponsive to other treatments. Pimecrolimus cream 1% is applied bid and has antiinflammatory effects secondary to blockage of activated T-cell cytokine production. Tacrolimus ointment (0.03% or 0.1%) applied bid is a macrolide that suppresses humoral and cell-mediated immune responses.
- Oral antihistamines (e.g., hydroxyzine, diphenhydramine) are effective in controlling pruritus and inducing sedation, restful sleep, and prevention of scratching during sleep. Doxepin and other tricyclic antidepressants also have antihistamine effect, induce sleep, and reduce pruritus.
- Oral prednisone, IM triamcinolone, Goeckerman regimen, PUVA are generally reserved for severe cases.
- Methotrexate, cyclosporine azathioprine, and systemic corticosteroids are sometimes tried for recalcitrant disease in adults.

DISPOSITION

- Resolution occurs in approximately 70% of patients by adulthood.
- Most patients have a course characterized by remissions and intermittent flares.

EBM **EVIDENCE**

available at www.expertconsult.com

SUGGESTED READINGS
available at www.expertconsult.com

AUTHOR: **FRED F. FERRI, M.D.**

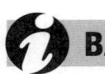 **BASIC INFORMATION**

DEFINITION
Atrial fibrillation (AF) is a supraventricular tachyarrhythmia characterized by uncoordinated atrial activation with resultant deterioration in atrial mechanical function and often times irregular and rapid ventricular conduction The ventricular rate is dependent on the conduction properties of the atrioventricular node, which can be influenced by vagal/sympathetic tone, medications, or disease of the atrioventricular node.

Multiple classification schemes have been used in the past to characterize AF. The current classification scheme (divided into three major types) used by the ACC/AHA guideline committee is as follows:
- **Paroxysmal atrial fibrillation:** 2 or more episodes that terminate spontaneously within 7 days
- **Persistent atrial fibrillation:** lasting > 7 days.
- **Permanent atrial fibrillation:** lasting > 1 yr

SYNONYMS
AF
PAFA-fib
A-fib

ICD-9CM CODES
427.31 Atrial fibrillation

EPIDEMIOLOGY & DEMOGRAPHICS
- The prevalence of AF increases with age, from 0.1% in adults <55 yr old to 9% of those ≥80 yr old.
- The prevalence of AF is increasing and is greater in men than in women.
- AF affects 2.3 million people in the U.S. and is a major cause of stroke (fivefold increased risk).
- Chronic AF develops in 25% of patients 5 yr after paroxysmal AF.
- AF is associated with higher rates of heart failure.

PHYSICAL FINDINGS & CLINICAL PRESENTATION
Clinical presentation is variable:
- Palpitations, dizziness, or lightheadedness
- Fatigue, weakness, or impaired exercise tolerance
- Angina
- Dyspnea
- Some patients are asymptomatic
- Cardiac auscultation revealing irregularly irregular rhythm

ETIOLOGY
- Vascular causes: hypertensive heart disease, increased pulse pressure (calculated as the difference between systolic and diastolic pressure), a reflection of aortic stiffness
- Valvular heart disease
- Pulmonary causes: pulmonary embolism, chronic obstructive pulmonary disease, obstructive sleep apnea, carbon monoxide poisoning
- Structural cardiac disease: pericarditis, myocarditis, cardiomyopathy, congestive heart failure, coronary artery disease, myocardial infarction, congenital heart disease (especially those that lead to atrial enlargement such as atrial septal defect), tachycardia-bradycardia syndrome
- Arrhythmias: atrial tachycardia, Wolff-Parkinson-White syndrome
- Endocrine: thyrotoxicosis, hyperthyroidism or subclinical hyperthyroidism, pheochromocytoma, obesity
- Surgery: both cardiac and noncardiac
- Electrolytes: hypokalemia, hypomagnesemia
- Systemic stress: fever, anemia, hypoxia, sepsis, infections (e.g., pneumonia)
- Medications/toxins: digitalis, adenosine, theophylline, amphetamines, cocaine, antihistamines, alcohol abuse and/or withdrawal, caffeine, steroidal anti-inflammatory drugs (SAIDs), non-steroidal anti-inflammatory drugs (NSAIDs)
- Frequency of vigorous exercise is associated with an increased risk of developing AF in young men and joggers.
- Porphyrias have been associated with autonomic dysfunction and increased risk of AF.

 DIAGNOSIS

DIFFERENTIAL DIAGNOSIS
- Multifocal atrial tachycardia
- Atrial flutter
- Frequent atrial premature beats

WORKUP
New-onset AF: ECG, echocardiogram, Holter monitor (selected patients), and laboratory evaluation

LABORATORY TESTS
- Thyroid-stimulating hormone, free T_4
- Serum electrolytes
- Toxicity screen

IMAGING STUDIES
- ECG (see Fig. 1-46 for atrial flutter and fibrillation)
  - Absence of P waves
  - Fibrillatory or f waves at the isoelectric baseline with varying amplitude, morphology, and intervals
  - Irregular ventricular rate
- Echocardiography to rule out structural heart disease (evaluate ventricular size, thickness, and function, atrial size, and valve function)
- Holter monitor: useful only in selected patients to evaluate paroxysmal AF

TREATMENT

NONPHARMACOLOGIC THERAPY
- Avoidance of alcohol in patients with suspected excessive alcohol use
- Avoidance of caffeine and nicotine
- Treatment of underlying source/cause, if any found
- The Maze surgical procedure, with its recent modifications creating electrical barriers to the macroreentrant circuits that are believed to underlie AF, is being performed with good results in several medical centers (preservation of sinus rhythm in >95% of patients without the use of long-term antiarrhythmic medication). Success rates are higher in paroxysmal than in persistent or permanent atrial fibrillation. It is important to understand that ablation therapy will not eliminate the need to take anticoagulant drugs. Even after ablation, patients with AF face increased risk of thromboembolic events and most electrophysiologists suggest lifelong anticoagulation. Although catheter-based radiofrequency ablation is no longer considered experimental, it is not the first-line treatment for most patients. Clear indications for catheter ablation remain undefined. In general, surgery is reserved for patients with rapid heart rate refractory to pharmacologic therapy or those who cannot tolerate pharmacologic therapy.
- Pulmonary vein ablation for chronic AF: Sinus rhythm can be maintained long term in the majority of patients with chronic AF by circumferential pulmonary vein ablation, independently of the effects of antiarrhythmic drug therapy, cardioversion, or both. The American College of Cardiology/American Heart Association/European Society of Cardiology (ACC/AHA/ESC) guidelines state that catheter ablation is a reasonable alternative to medical therapy to prevent recurrent AF in symptomatic patients in the absence of significant left atrial enlargement (class 2A recommendation).
- Pulmonary vein isolation is being increasingly used to treat AF in patients with heart failure. Trials have shown that pulmonary vein isolation is superior to AV node ablation with biventricular pacing in patients with heart failure who have drug-refractory AF

ACUTE GENERAL Rx
New-onset AF:
- If the patient is hemodynamically unstable (hypotension, congestive heart failure or angina), perform synchronized cardioversion after immediate conscious sedation with a rapid short-acting sedative (e.g., midazolam). The likelihood of cardioversion-related clinical thromboembolism is low in patients with AF lasting <48 hr. Patients with AF lasting >2 days have a 5% to 7% risk for clinical thromboembolism if cardioversion is not preceded by several weeks of warfarin therapy. However, if transesophageal echocardiography reveals no atrial thrombus, cardioversion may be performed safely after anticoagulation has been achieved. Anticoagulant therapy should be continued for at least 1 mo after cardioversion to minimize the incidence of adverse thromboembolic events. It can be stopped after one month as long as AF has not recurred.

- If the patient is hemodynamically stable, a rate-control strategy is typically pursued initially. Treatment options include the following:
  1. Diltiazem 0.25 mg/kg (maximum of 25 mg) given intravenously (IV) over 2 min followed by a second dose of 0.35 mg/kg (maximum of 25 mg) 15 min later if the rate is not slowed to <100 beats/min. May then follow with IV infusion 10 mg/hour (range, 5 to 15 mg/hour) to achieve a resting heart rate of <100 beats/min. Onset of action after IV administration is usually within 3 min, with peak effect most often occurring within 10 min. After the ventricular rate is slowed, the patient can be changed to oral diltiazem 60 to 90 mg q4 to 6h.
  2. Verapamil 2.5 to 5 mg IV initially, then 5 to 10 mg IV 10 min later if the rate is still not slowed to <100 beats/min. After the ventricular rate is slowed, the patient can be changed to oral verapamil 80 to 120 mg q6 to 8h. Main concern is hypotension with this medication.
  3. Esmolol, metoprolol, and atenolol are beta-blockers available in IV preparations that can be used in AF.
  4. Digoxin is not a potent atrioventricular nodal blocking agent, has a potential for toxicity and, therefore, cannot be relied on for acute control of the ventricular response, unless the patient is hypotensive or has a low left ventricular systolic function. When used, give 0.5 mg IV loading dose (slow), then 0.25 mg IV 6 hr later. A third dose may be needed after 6 to 8 hr; daily dose varies from 0.125 to 0.25 mg (decrease dosage in patients with renal insufficiency and elderly patients) depending on the heart rate and signs/symptoms of digoxin toxicity.
- All atrioventricular nodal blocking agents should be avoided in patients with Wolff-Parkinson-White syndrome and AF because they may increase the frequency of atrioventricular conduction through the accessory pathway. Procainamide is the preferred pharmacologic agent in these patients.
- In the acute setting, pharmacologic cardioversion is less commonly used than electrical cardioversion.

CHRONIC Rx

- For patients without symptomatic AF, rate-control strategy with calcium channel blockers, beta-blockers, or digoxin is a reasonable option. Lenient rate control is not inferior to strict rate control for preventing cardiovascular morbidity and mortality in patients with permanent atrial fibrillation. In patients with symptomatic AF or with difficult to control heart rate, attempt should be made to maintain sinus rhythm with antiarrhythmic agents.

Options of antiarrhythmic agents include amiodarone, dofetilide, flecainide, propafenone, procainamide, or sotalol. The decision of which strategy to follow should be best made in consultation with cardiology.
- The decision whether to pursue long-term anticoagulation with warfarin must be made in light of the patient's risk for a cardioembolic event vs. risk for a bleeding event. The CHADS2 scoring system is a well-validated model that estimates the risk for stroke in patients with AF based on clinical risk factors (congestive heart failure, hypertension (HTN), age ≥75 yr, and diabetes, which are 1 point each, or ischemic stroke and transient ischemic attack [TIA], which are 2 points each if present). Patients with a CHADS2 score of 0 are considered low risk, 1 to 2 are considered moderate risk, and ≥3 are considered high risk. The ACC/AHA recommends long-term anticoagulation with warfarin in all patients with a prior TIA or stroke (unless contraindicated) and in patients with more than one risk factor for thromboembolism that is not TIA/stroke.
- Anticoagulation with warfarin is generally not recommended in patients with CHADS2 score of zero. For patients with CHADS2 score of 1 who do not want to undergo anticoagulation, low-dose aspirin is an appropriate alternative in these patients.
- For patients in whom anticoagulation with warfarin is contraindicated, aspirin plus clopidogrel has been shown to be of similar benefit in reducing thromboembolic events as warfarin with a similar bleeding risk.
- Dabigatran (Pradaxa) is an FDA-approved direct thrombin inhibitor indicated to reduce the risk of stroke and systemic embolism in patients with non-valvular atrial fibrillation. Unlike warfarin, it does not reduce periodic lab tests monitoring. Dabigatran can increase the risk of bleeding and can cause significant and sometimes fatal bleeding. In the RE-LY® trial, life-threatening bleeding occurred at an annualized rate of 1.5% and 1.8% for dabigatran 150 mg/day and warfarin, respectively. When converting patients from warfarin to dabigatran, discontinue warfarin and start dabigatran when the INR is below 2.0.

DISPOSITION
Factors associated with maintenance of sinus rhythm after cardioversion include:
- Left atrium diameter <60 mm
- Absence of mitral valve disease
- Short duration of AF

REFERRAL
Refer to a cardiologist those patients in whom antiarrhythmic therapy or catheter-based/surgical intervention is being considered.

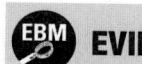 **PEARLS & CONSIDERATIONS**

COMMENTS
The American Academy of Family Physicians and the American College of Physicians provide the following recommendations for the management of newly detected AF:
- Rate control with chronic anticoagulation is the recommended strategy for the majority of asymptomatic patients with chronic AF. Rhythm control has not been shown to be superior to rate control (with chronic anticoagulation) in reducing morbidity and mortality, and may be inferior in some patient subgroups to rate control. Rhythm control is appropriate when based on other special considerations, such as patient symptoms, exercise tolerance, and patient preference.
- Patients with AF should receive chronic anticoagulation with adjusted-dose warfarin, unless they are at low risk for stroke as stated earlier or have specific contraindications to the use of warfarin (thrombocytopenia, recent trauma or surgery, alcoholism).
- For patients with AF, the following drugs are recommended for their demonstrated efficacy in rate control during exercise and while at rest: atenolol, metoprolol, diltiazem, and verapamil (drugs listed alphabetically by class). Digoxin is effective only for rate control at rest and, therefore, should be used only as a second-line agent for rate control in AF.
- For patients who elect to undergo acute cardioversion to achieve sinus rhythm in AF, both direct-current cardioversion and pharmacologic conversion are appropriate options in an otherwise healthy patient.
- Both transesophageal echocardiography with short-term prior anticoagulation followed by early acute cardioversion (in absence of intracardiac thrombus) with postcardioversion anticoagulation vs. delayed cardioversion with preanticoagulation and postanticoagulation are appropriate management strategies for patients who elect to undergo cardioversion.

EBM EVIDENCE
available at www.expertconsult.com

SUGGESTED READINGS
available at www.expertconsult.com

AUTHORS: **JOSHUA R. SILVERSTEIN, M.D., FRED F. FERRI, M.D.,** and **WEN-CHIH WU, M.D.**

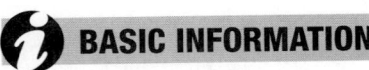

DEFINITION

Atrial flutter is characterized by an atrial macro-reentrant circuit (typically in the right atrium) leading to regular atrial depolarizations, typically at a rate of 250 to 350 beats/min. There is typically 2:1 (or less) conduction through the atrioventricular node resulting in heart rates close to 150 beats/min. The atrial impulses may be conducted at a constant rate through the atrioventricular node resulting in a regular rhythm, or the atrial impulses may be conducted at a variable rate resulting in an irregular rhythm.

ICD-9CM CODES
427.32 Atrial flutter

EPIDEMIOLOGY & DEMOGRAPHICS

- Atrial flutter is the second most common atrial tachyarrhythmia after atrial fibrillation, with an estimated 200,000 new cases annually in the U.S.
- Atrial flutter is common during the first week after open-heart surgery.
- Atrial flutter is more common in men than women.
- Atrial flutter is typically seen in patients with underlying structural heart disease.

PHYSICAL FINDINGS & CLINICAL PRESENTATION

- Palpitations
- Dizziness, lightheadedness, syncope, or near syncope
- Angina
- Congestive heart failure
- Embolic phenomena from intracardiac thrombus

ETIOLOGY

- Rheumatic heart disease
- Congenital heart disease
- Left ventricular dysfunction
- Acute myocardial infarction (rarely)
- Thyrotoxicosis
- Pulmonary embolism
- Mitral valve disease
- Cardiac surgery
- Chronic obstructive pulmonary disease
- Obesity
- Pericarditis
- Atrial flutter can also occur spontaneously or as a result of organization of atrial fibrillation from antiarrhythmic therapy

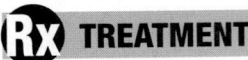

DIFFERENTIAL DIAGNOSIS

- Atrial fibrillation
- Paroxysmal atrial tachycardia

WORKUP

- ECG
- Laboratory evaluation

LABORATORY TESTS

- Thyroid function studies
- Serum electrolytes

IMAGING STUDIES

ECG (Fig. 1-46)
- Absence of P waves
- Regular, "sawtooth," or "F (flutter)" wave pattern in the isoelectric baseline, best seen in leads II, III, and AVF
- There is rarely 1:1 atrioventricular (AV) conduction in atrial flutter (unless preexcitation is present). Rather, AV conduction is usually in a 2:1, 3:1, or 4:1 fashion, with corresponding usual ventricular rates of 150, 100, or 75 beats/min, respectively (assuming an atrial rate of 300 beats/min)
- Echocardiography to evaluate for structural heart disease (ventricular size, thickness, and function, atrial size, and valve function)

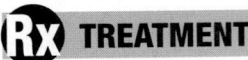

NONPHARMACOLOGIC THERAPY

- Valsalva maneuver or carotid sinus massage usually slows the ventricular rate (increases grade of AV block) and may make flutter waves more evident. Adenosine may be similarly helpful.
- Direct current cardioversion is the treatment of choice for acute management of atrial flutter associated with hemodynamic instability or debilitating symptoms such as angina or congestive heart failure. Electrical cardioversion is typically successful at low energy levels (20 to 25 J). Sedation of a conscious patient is highly recommended before cardioversion is performed. The use of external defibrillators with biphasic waveforms decreases the amount of energy required for cardioversion and improves cardioversion success rate.
- Overdrive pacing in the atrium may also terminate atrial flutter. This method is especially useful in patients who have recently undergone cardiac surgery and still have temporary atrial pacing wires.
- Radiofrequency ablation to interrupt the atrial flutter is highly effective for patients with chronic or recurring atrial flutter and is generally considered first-line therapy in those with recurrent episodes of atrial flutter.

ACUTE GENERAL Rx

- Treatment choices are based on clinical circumstances. If the patient is unstable, proceed directly to electrical cardioversion.
- In the hemodynamically stable patient, proceed with rate control or rhythm control strategy.
- AV blocking agents such as calcium channel blockers, beta-blockers, or digitalis may all be used for rate control. Atrial flutter may spontaneously convert to normal sinus rhythm with this strategy.

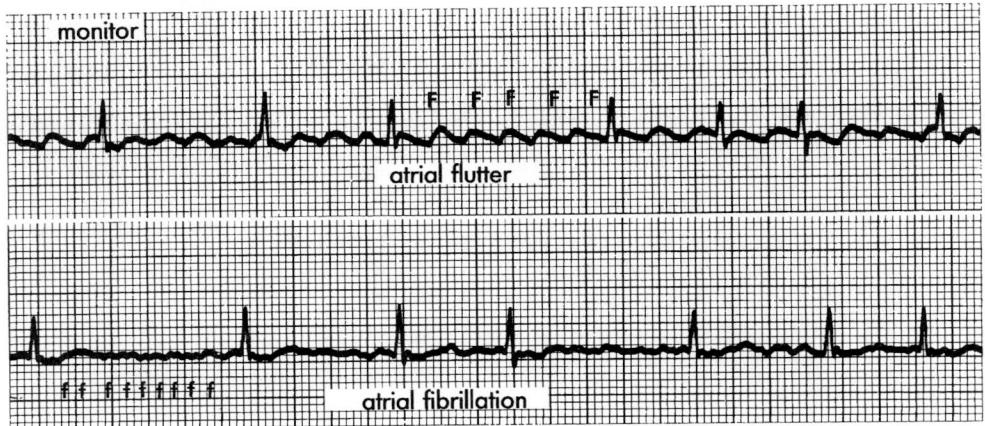

FIGURE 1-46 Atrial flutter and fibrillation. Notice the sawtooth waves with atrial flutter *(F)* and the irregular fibrillatory waves with atrial fibrillation *(f)*. (From Goldberger AL [ed]: *Clinical electrocardiography,* ed 5, St Louis, 1994, Mosby.)

A

- In general, atrial flutter is more difficult to rate control than atrial fibrillation.
- Ibutilide is the first-line medication for chemical cardioversion of atrial flutter in patients with normal systolic function and QT intervals.

CHRONIC Rx

- Fewer data exist to decide on the choice of rate control vs. rhythm control in patients with atrial flutter. There are several options to help maintain sinus rhythm after cardioversion of atrial flutter, such as dofetilide, amiodarone, flecainide, propafenone, or sotalol. The choice of antiarrhythmic therapy is, in part, dictated by the presence or absence of underlying structural heart disease. In patients who have chronic atrial flutter, rate control (to rates as physiologic as possible) can be achieved using AV blocking agents, to prevent occurrence of tachycardia-mediated cardiomyopathy.
- Although data are much less convincing than in atrial fibrillation, current consensus is to treat atrial flutter similar to atrial fibrillation in terms of the risk for thromboembolic events and the need for anticoagulation. In this case, CHADS2 scoring system (see "Atrial Fibrillation") can be used to risk-stratify patients for their need to stay on long-term anticoagulation.

DISPOSITION

More than 85% of patients convert to regular sinus rhythm after cardioversion with as little as 25 to 50 J.

REFERRAL

Refer patients who are considered for rhythm control of atrial flutter to cardiologists, especially patients who are candidates for radiofrequency ablation.

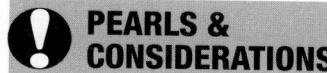

COMMENTS

- Atrial flutter has a stroke risk at least as high as atrial fibrillation and carries a greater risk for subsequent development of atrial fibrillation than in the general population.
- Anticoagulation should be considered for all patients whose CHADS2 score is ≥2.
- Anticoagulation with warfarin is generally not recommended in patients with CHADS2 score of zero. For patients with CHADS2 score of 1 who do not want to undergo anticoagulation, low-dose aspirin is an appropriate alternative in these patients.

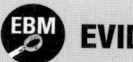 **EVIDENCE**

available at www.expertconsult.com

SUGGESTED READINGS

available at www.expertconsult.com

AUTHORS: **JOSHUA R. SILVERSTEIN, M.D.,
FRED F. FERRI, M.D.,** and **WEN-CHIH WU, M.D.**

Diseases
and Disorders

I

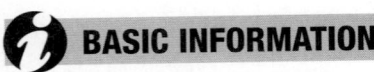 **BASIC INFORMATION**

DEFINITION
Atrial myxoma is a benign neoplasm of mesenchymal origin and is the most common primary tumor of the heart.

SYNONYMS
Cardiac myxoma

ICD-9CM CODES
212.7 Benign neoplasm, heart

EPIDEMIOLOGY & DEMOGRAPHICS
- Primary cardiac tumors are extremely rare, with an autopsy frequency of 0.001% to 0.03%. The most frequent cardiac tumors are metastases, occurring 30 times more frequently than primary tumors.
- Benign atrial myxomas account for 70% of all primary tumors of the heart. The remaining 30% are composed of a variety of benign and malignant tumors.
- 65% of sporadic cases occur in females.
- Average age of incidence of sporadic cases is 30 to 50 yr but can occur at any age.
- Average age of incidence of familial cases is 25 yr.

PHYSICAL FINDINGS & CLINICAL PRESENTATION
Patients with atrial myxomas characteristically present in one of three ways:
1. Atrioventricular valve obstruction (e.g., mitral or tricuspid valve): dyspnea, orthopnea, paroxysmal nocturnal dyspnea, edema, dizziness, syncope, elevated jugular venous pressure, widely split loud S2, secondary pulmonary hypertension, murmurs of regurgitation (holosystolic) or stenosis (rumbles), third heart sound "tumor plop," atrial fibrillation, and sudden death (rarely)
2. Systemic embolization: leading to cerebrovascular accidents, pulmonary embolism, paradoxical embolism
3. Constitutional symptoms: fever, weight loss, arthralgias, Raynaud's phenomenon

ETIOLOGY
- Most cases (90%) of atrial myxomas are sporadic with no known cause
- In the remaining 10% of cases, a familial pattern occurs having an autosomal-dominant transmission, known as the Carney complex or syndrome myxoma (cardiac and noncardiac myxomas, pigmented nevi, endocrine tumors, and schwannomas)

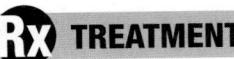 **DIAGNOSIS**

DIFFERENTIAL DIAGNOSIS
- Primary valvular diseases: mitral stenosis, mitral regurgitation, tricuspid stenosis, tricuspid regurgitation
- Pulmonary hypertension
- Endocarditis
- Vasculitis
- Atrial thrombus
- Pulmonary embolism
- Cerebrovascular accidents
- Collagen-vascular disease
- Carcinoid heart disease

WORKUP
A high index of suspicion is needed because the clinical manifestations are nonspecific and similar to many common cardiovascular and pulmonary diseases.

LABORATORY TESTS
Although not very specific, the following laboratory findings may be abnormal in patients with atrial myxomas:
- Complete blood count: anemia, polycythemia, thrombocytopenia may occur
- Erythrocyte sedimentation rate, C-reactive protein, and serum immunoglobulins are commonly elevated
- Electrocardiogram: left or right atrial enlargement, atrial fibrillation, premature ventricular depolarizations, or ventricular tachycardia

IMAGING STUDIES
- Echocardiography: initial test of choice in suspected cases of atrial myxoma
- Chest radiograph: altered cardiac contour and chamber enlargement
- Transesophageal echocardiography: may better define cardiac masses not clearly visualized by transthoracic echocardiography
- CT: often used for diagnosis; defines tumor extension and evaluates adjacent cardiac structures
- MRI: delineates size, shape, and tissue characteristics, helping distinguish thrombus from tumor
- Cardiac catheterization: will show neovascularization in 50% of the cases and may be required to rule out concomitant coronary artery disease in anticipation of surgical excision

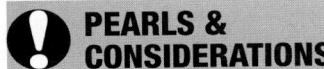 **TREATMENT**

ACUTE GENERAL THERAPY
- Surgical excision is the treatment of choice
- Surgery should be done promptly because systemic embolization and/or sudden death can occur while waiting for the procedure

CHRONIC Rx
Postoperative arrhythmias and conduction abnormalities were present in 26% of patients and can be treated accordingly.

DISPOSITION
- Surgical results have reported a 95% survival rate after a follow-up of 3 yr.
- Careful follow-up is necessary because up to 5% of sporadic cases and 20% of familial cases of atrial myxoma may recur within the first 6 yr after surgery.
- Sudden death in untreated patients may occur in up to 15%, resulting from coronary or systemic embolization or obstruction of the mitral or tricuspid valve.

REFERRAL
- Consultation with a cardiologist is recommended.
- Once the presence of cardiac tumor is confirmed, consultation with a cardiovascular surgeon is needed for prompt surgical excision.

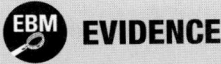 **PEARLS & CONSIDERATIONS**

- Approximately two thirds of patients present with cardiovascular symptoms, specifically dyspnea, often suggestive of valvular obstruction.
- Nearly one third of patients have evidence of systemic embolization.

COMMENTS
Annual echocardiograms should be performed to monitor for recurrence of atrial myxomas after surgical excision.

EBM **EVIDENCE**

available at www.expertconsult.com

SUGGESTED READINGS
available at www.expertconsult.com

AUTHORS: **ROBERTO PACHECO, M.D.,**
FRED F. FERRI, M.D., and **WEN-CHIH WU, M.D.**

BASIC INFORMATION

DEFINITION

Atrial septal defect (ASD) is an abnormal opening in the atrial septum that allows blood flow between the atria. It should be distinguished from patent foramen ovale, which is a persistent patency of the flaplike communication in which the septum primum covering the fossa ovalis overlaps the superior limbic band of the septum secundum. There are several forms (Fig. 1-47):

- Ostium primum: This type of ASD represents a deficiency of the endocardial cushion contribution to the atrial septum. It usually involves the atrioventricular valves.
- Ostium secundum: This is the most common form; it represents a deficiency of the septum primum or a septum secundum, or both. This defect most often occurs in the region of the fossa ovalis.
- Sinus venosus defect: This defect is located at the junction of the right atrium and superior vena cava, and is not a "true ASD" as it does not involve the true atrial septum. In a sinus venusus defect, the wall separating the pulmonary veins and the right atrium is deficient, causing a left-to-right shunt. Most commonly this defect involves the right upper pulmonary vein, which is still connected to the left atrium, but the drainage is anomalous. Less commonly, the right lower pulmonary vein is involved.
- Coronary sinus septal defect (unroofed coronary sinus): This defect results when the wall separating the coronary sinus from the left atrium is deficient, causing a right-to-left shunt. This is not a "true ASD" because it is not a defect in the atrial septum. This defect is often associated with a persistent left superior vena cava.

SYNONYMS

ASD

ICD-9CM CODES
429.71 Atrial septal defect

EPIDEMIOLOGY & DEMOGRAPHICS

- 80% of cases of ASD involve persistence of ostium secundum
- Incidence is greater in female sex
- Accounts for 8% to 10% of congenital heart abnormalities

PHYSICAL FINDINGS & CLINICAL PRESENTATION

- Pansystolic murmur best heard at apex secondary to mitral regurgitation (ostium primum defect)
- Widely split S2
- Visible and palpable pulmonary artery pulsations
- Ejection systolic flow murmur (pulmonary valve flow murmur)
- Diastolic rumble (atrioventricular valve flow murmur)
- Prominent right ventricular (RV) impulse
- Increased jugular venous pressure (with RV failure)
- Cyanosis and clubbing (severe cases)
- Exertional dyspnea
- Patients with small defects: generally asymptomatic

ETIOLOGY

Unknown

DIAGNOSIS

DIFFERENTIAL DIAGNOSIS

- Primary pulmonary hypertension
- Pulmonary stenosis
- Rheumatic heart disease
- Mitral valve prolapse
- Cor pulmonale

WORKUP

- ECG:
  - Ostium primum defect: left axis deviation, incomplete or total right bundle branch block, prolongation of PR interval
  - Sinus venous defect: left axis deviation, abnormal P axis
  - Ostium secundum defect: right axis deviation, incomplete or total right bundle branch block
- Chest x-ray examination
- Echocardiography
- Cardiac catheterization
- Cardiac magnetic resonance imaging (MRI), CT, or both

IMAGING STUDIES

- Chest x-ray examination: cardiomegaly, enlargement of right atrium and right ventricle, increased pulmonary vascularity, small aortic knob

- Echocardiography with saline bubble contrast and Doppler flow studies: may demonstrate the size of the defect, the direction of shunting, presence of anomalous pulmonary return (in sinus venosus ASD), right heart volume overload, and pulmonary artery pressures; transesophageal echocardiography is much more sensitive than transthoracic echocardiography in identifying sinus venous defects and is preferred by some for the initial diagnostic evaluation
- Cardiac catheterization: not usually a diagnostic necessity; is useful unless the coronaries need to be assessed before surgery
- Cardiac MRI and CT: may be useful if echo is not diagnostic; MRI is gold standard for assessing RV size and function, and it can determine whether the right-sided chambers are, in fact, enlarged; it is also good to assess pulmonary venous return; cardiac CT can offer similar information

TREATMENT

NONPHARMACOLOGIC THERAPY

- Symptomatic patients should avoid strenuous activity.
- Patients with small shunts (<10 mm) without pulmonary artery hypertension and normal RV size are generally asymptomatic and require no medical therapy. Routine assessment of these patients includes symptoms, arrhythmias, and embolic events. A repeat echocardiogram should be obtained every 2 to 3 years to assess RV size and function, and pulmonary pressure.

GENERAL Rx

- Children and infants: Closure of ASD before age 10 yr is indicated if pulmonary to systemic flow ratio is >1.5:1.
- Small ASDs with a diameter of <5 mm and no evidence of RV volume overload do not impact the natural history of the individual and thus may not require closure unless associated with paradoxical embolism.
- Closure of an ASD either percutaneously or surgically is indicated for right atrial and RV enlargement with or without symptoms.
- A sinus venosus, coronary sinus, or primum ASD should be repaired surgically rather than by percutaneous closure.
- Surgical closure of secundum ASD is reasonable when concomitant surgical repair/

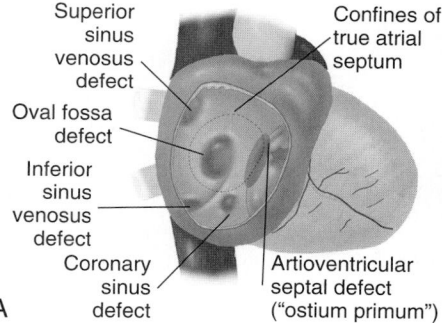

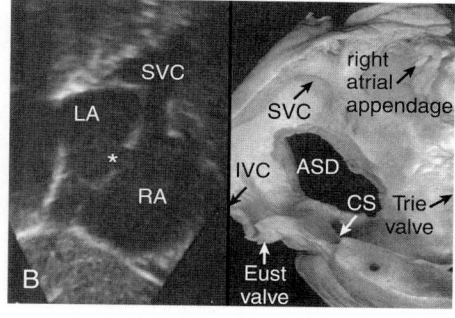

FIGURE 1-47 A, Schematic diagram outlining the different types of interatrial shunting that can be encountered. Note that only the central defect is suitable for device closure. **B,** Subcostal right anterior oblique view of a secundum atrial septal defect (asterisk) that is suitable for device closure. The right panel is a specimen as seen in a similar view, outlining the landmarks of defect. (From Zipes DP et al [eds]: *Braunwauld's heart disease,* ed 7, Philadelphia, 2005, Elsevier.)

A

replacement of a tricuspid valve is considered or when the anatomy of the defect precludes the use of a percutaneous device.

- Closure of an ASD, either percutaneously or surgically, may be considered in the presence of net left-to-right shunting, pulmonary artery pressure less than two-thirds systemic levels, PVR less than two-thirds systemic vascular resistance, or when responsive to either pulmonary vasodilator therapy or test occlusion of the defect (patients should be treated in conjunction with providers who have expertise in the management of pulmonary hypertensive syndromes).
- Concomitant maze procedure may be considered for intermittent or chronic atrial tachyarrhythmias in adults with ASDs.
- Patients with severe irreversible PAH and no evidence of a left-to-right shunt should not undergo ASD closure.
- Closure of an ASD, either percutaneously or surgically, is reasonable in the presence of:
  ○ Paradoxical embolism (Class 2a indication)
  ○ Documented orthodeoxia-platypnea (Class 2a indication)
- Percutaneous catheter device closure is advocated in patients with secundum ASDs (with proper size and location), with ~95% success rate. A combination of low-dose aspirin and clopidogrel is usually prescribed for 3 mo after the procedure to prevent thrombus formation.

DISPOSITION
- Mortality rate is high in patients with significant ostium primum defect if left untreated.
- Patients with small shunts (<10 mm) have a normal life expectancy.
- Basic preoperative assessment for ACHD patients should include systemic arterial oximetry, an ECG, chest radiograph, TTE, and blood tests for full blood count and coagulation screen.
- Intracardiac shunts are considered moderate risk for preoperative evaluation for non-cardiac prcedure. High risk features include severe systolic dysfunction (EF <35%), severe pulmonary hypertension whether primary or secondary, cyanotic heart disease, or severe left side outlet obstruction.
- Annual clinical follow-up is recommended for patients postoperatively if their ASD was repaired as an adult and the following conditions persist or develop: PAH, Atrial arrhythmias, RV or LV dysfunction, Coexisting valvular or other cardiac lesions.
- Preoperative atrial fibrillation is a risk factor for immediate postoperative and long-term atrial fibrillation. Patients with a repaired ASD still have an increased risk for development of atrial fibrillation that directly correlates with the age at which the defect is corrected (later correction = greater risk).
  ○ After closure, anticipated benefits include improved functional status and exercise capacity, improved survival after closure as a child, improved quality of life, prevention of right-heart failure, and prevention of pulmonary arterial hypertension.
  ○ Potential mid- to long-term complications after ASD closure in adulthood include tachyarrhythmias (atrial fibrillation or atrial flutter), bradyarrhythmias (sinus node dysfunction or heart block), stroke (greater risk in older patients), residual ASDs (small usually close spontaneously, large may be because of patch dehiscence), right-heart failure or pulmonary artery hypertension (risk is inversely related to age at time of closure), left atrioventricular valve regurgitation or subaortic stenosis (usually in patients with primum ASDs), device migration/erosion, and pulmonary venous congestion (uncommon).
  ○ Pregnancy is usually well tolerated in women with ASDs. Follow-up is recommended because of small risk for paradoxical embolus, stroke, arrhythmia, and heart failure. If known, ASDs should be closed before pregnancy if indicated. The sole contraindication to pregnancy in women with an ASD is severe pulmonary arterial hypertension.
- In regard to infective endocarditis prophylaxis for dental procedures,
  ○ Prophylaxis is not indicated for ASDs.
  ○ Prophylaxis is indicated for a completely repaired ASD, or any congenital heart disease with prosthetic material during the first 6 mo after the procedure.
  ○ Prophylaxis is indicated for repaired ASDs, or any congenital heart defect with residual defects at the site or adjacent to the site of a prosthetic patch or prosthetic device (both of which inhibit endothelialization).

The estrogen-containing oral contraceptive pill is not recommended in ACHD patients at risk of thromboembolism, such as those with cyanosis related to an intracardiac shunt, atrial fibrillation, severe PAH, or Fontan repair.

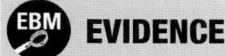 **EVIDENCE**

available at www.expertconsult.com

SUGGESTED READINGS
available at www.expertconsult.com

AUTHORS: **SCOTT COHEN, M.D.,
ABDULRAHMAN ABDULBAKI,
FRED F. FERRI, M.D.,** and **WEN-CHIH WU, M.D.**

BASIC INFORMATION

DEFINITION

Attention deficit/hyperactivity disorder (ADHD) is a chronic disorder of attention and/or hyperactivity-impulsivity. Symptoms must be present before 7 yr of age, last at least 6 mo, and cause functional impairment in multiple settings.

SYNONYMS

Hyperactivity
Hyperkinetic disorder
Attention deficit disorder (ADD)

ICD-9CM CODES
ICD-9: 314.XX
ICD-10: F90.X

EPIDEMIOLOGY & DEMOGRAPHICS

PEAK INCIDENCE: Diagnosis is usually first made in school-aged children (6 to 9 yr).
PREVALENCE: 8% to 10% of school-aged children and 2% to 5% of adults
PREDOMINANT SEX: Among children, male predominance with ratio of 2:1 to 4:1. Among adults, ratio is closer to 1:1 (sex difference may reflect referral bias).
PREDOMINANT AGE: Some symptoms must occur before age 7 yr. Symptoms (especially hyperactivity) tend to diminish with age. Up to 70% continue to meet criteria in adolescence, and an estimated 40% to 65% have some symptoms in adulthood.
GENETICS: Strong polygenetic component. First-degree relatives of ADHD patients have 5 times greater risk of ADHD relative to controls. Studies suggest potential involvement of several genes, including those associated with dopamine metabolism and transmission.
RISK FACTORS: Possible environmental and epidemiologic risk factors include in utero tobacco/drug exposure or hypoxia, low birth weight, prematurity, pregnancy, lead exposure (though most children with elevated lead levels do not develop ADHD), family dysfunction, low socioeconomic status.

PHYSICAL FINDINGS & CLINICAL PRESENTATION

- Three types:
  1. Predominantly inattentive: difficulty organizing, planning, remembering, concentrating, starting/completing tasks; symptoms may not be present during preferred activities.
  2. Predominantly hyperactive-impulsive: edgy/restless, talkative, disruptive/intrusive, disinhibited, impatient.
  3. Combined.
- Usually diagnosed in elementary school when achievement is compromised and behavioral problems are not tolerated. Children with academic underproductivity, problems with peer and family relations, or discipline issues are often referred for evaluation.
- Up to 50% may have associated disorders such as psychiatric diagnoses (oppositional defiant disorder, conduct disorder, depression, anxiety), learning disabilities, or substance abuse.
- In adults, hyperactivity is less common, but restlessness, edginess, and difficulty relaxing are often seen. Disorganization and difficulty completing tasks are other common complaints.

ETIOLOGY

Strongest evidence exists for genetic inheritance. Other theories include abnormal metabolism of brain catecholamines, structural brain abnormalities, and environmental factors (see earlier).

DIAGNOSIS

DIFFERENTIAL DIAGNOSIS

- Medical: visual/hearing impairment, seizure disorder, head injury, sleep disorder, medication interactions, mental retardation, developmental delay, thyroid abnormalities, lead toxicity.
- Psychiatric: depression, bipolar disorder, anxiety, obsessive-compulsive disorder, conduct disorder, posttraumatic stress disorder, and substance abuse.
- Psychosocial: mismatch of learning environment with ability, family dysfunction, abuse/neglect.

WORKUP

- Clinical interview should include assessment of symptoms and impact on work/school and relationships; developmental history; personal and family psychiatric history, including substance abuse; social history, including family dysfunction; medical history.
- Physical examination should be performed to investigate medical causes for symptoms, coexisting conditions, and contraindications to treatment.
- Many patients will not display symptoms during an office visit and may underreport or overreport symptoms. Therefore information from collateral sources (parents, partners, teachers) is crucial to diagnosis.
- Self-rating scales and standardized symptom-specific questionnaires from collateral sources can help diagnose and assess response to treatment.
- Laboratory or imaging studies should be undertaken only if indicated by history or physical examination.
- Ancillary testing (e.g., IQ/achievement testing, language evaluation, and mental health assessment) may be indicated based on clinical findings and may require referral.

TREATMENT

NONPHARMACOLOGIC THERAPY

- The majority of studies comparing the efficacy of pharmacologic vs nonpharmacologic interventions demonstrate the superiority of pharmacologic treatments.
- Studies on combined treatments have not shown significant improvements in core ADHD symptoms when behavioral treatments are added to stimulant medications. However, improvements in related areas of concern such as parent-child relations, aggressiveness, teacher-rated social skills, and reaching achievement have been seen in combined treatment groups.
- Prevailing opinion favors a multimodal approach in which nonpharmacologic therapies can be used to target comorbid conditions or behaviors that have not responded to medication.
- Behavioral therapy alone is often considered when symptoms and impairment are mild, if parents are opposed to or patients cannot tolerate medications, or if there is uncertainty or disagreement about the diagnosis (e.g., between parents and teachers).
- Educational interventions are recommended, particularly in the setting of learning disabilities. Children with ADHD are entitled to reasonable educational accommodations under a 504 Plan or the Individuals with Disabilities Education Act.
- Behavioral interventions (e.g., goal setting and rewards systems) show short-term efficacy and are endorsed by most national organizations (e.g., American Academy of Pediatrics, American Medical Association). Time management and organizational skills appear useful.
- Psychotherapy (cognitive behavioral, group, social skills, and parent training) may be beneficial, particularly with coexisting psychiatric disease.
- Many support and advocacy groups provide education and other resources (e.g., Children and Adolescents with ADHD, National ADD Association, American Academy of Child and Adolescent Psychiatry).

ACUTE GENERAL Rx

- Most studies on treatment of ADHD are performed in children; limited data available on adults.
- Mainstay of treatment is stimulant medications. Second-line therapies include antidepressants and alpha-agonists.
- Stimulants:
  1. Release or block uptake of dopamine and norepinephrine.
  2. Include short- and long-acting methylphenidate, dextroamphetamine, and dextroamphetamine/amphetamine combinations (mixed amphetamine salts). A methylphenidate patch is also available.
  3. All stimulants equally effective; however, not all patients improve with stimulants. Patients who do not respond well to one stimulant may respond to another.
  4. Do not cause euphoria or lead to addiction when taken as directed.
  5. Improve cognition, inattention, impulsiveness/hyperactivity, and driving skills. Limited impact on academic performance, learning, and emotional problems.

6. Side effects are usually mild, reversible, and dose dependent, including anorexia, weight loss, sleep disturbances, increased heart rate and blood pressure, irritability, moodiness, headache, onset or worsening of motor tics, reduction of growth velocity (but not adult height). Do not worsen seizures in patients on adequate anticonvulsant therapy. Rebound of symptoms can occur with withdrawal of medication.

- Atomoxetine (Strattera):
  1. Selective norepinephrine reuptake inhibitor.
  2. Generally felt to be less effective than stimulants, but a useful alternative in patients who have not tolerated or responded to stimulants or in the setting of patient or family substance abuse.
  3. Efficacy and safety of long-term use has not been studied. Reports of behavioral abnormalities and increased suicidality in children and adolescents.
  4. Side effects: gastrointestinal upset, sleep disturbance, decreased appetite, dizziness, sexual side effects in men. Cardiovascular side effects have also been reported.
  5. There have been rare reports of severe liver injury in adults and children.
- Antidepressants (bupropion, imipramine, nortriptyline):
  1. May be useful in patients with coexisting psychiatric disorders.

2. Studies comparing efficacy versus stimulants are inconclusive.
3. Side effects: arrhythmias, anticholinergic effects, lowering of seizure threshold.

- Use of medications, particularly stimulants (which are monitored under the Controlled Substance Act), requires frequent monitoring.
- Stimulants have been associated with cardiovascular events and death. Patients should be carefully evaluated for cardiovascular disease before beginning therapy and be periodically monitored, including blood pressure checks, while they are treated. Routine, pretreatment screening with ECGs is not currently recommended by the American Academy of Pediatrics or the American Academy of Child and Adolescent Psychiatry.
- An extended-release oral formulation of guanfacine hydrochloride (Intuniv), a selective alpha$_{2A}$ adrenergic agonist, has been approved by the FDA for treatment of ADHD in children ages 6 to 17 yrs.

DISPOSITION

- Although symptoms may change over time, for many patients ADHD represents a chronic condition that requires lifelong management.
- Patients are at higher risk for academic underachievement, lower socioeconomic status, work and relationship difficulties, high-risk behavior, and psychiatric comorbidities.

REFERRAL

- Diagnosis complicated by difficult-to-treat comorbid psychiatric conditions, developmental disorders, or mental retardation
- Lack of adequate response to stimulants/atomoxetine

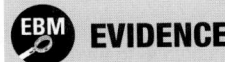

- The World Health Organization's Adult Self-Report Scale (ASRS) v1.1 has good sensitivity and adaptability to the primary care setting.
- Among adults with persistent ADHD symptoms treated with medication, trials have shown that the use of cognitive behavioral therapy compared with relaxation with educational support resulted in improved ADHD symptoms, which were maintained at 12 mos.

EBM **EVIDENCE**

available at www.expertconsult.com

SUGGESTED READINGS

available at www.expertconsult.com

AUTHORS: **EMILY R. KATZ, M.D.,** and **MITCHELL D. FELDMAN, M.D., M.PHIL.**

BASIC INFORMATION

DEFINITION

Autism spectrum disorders (ASD) encompass a spectrum of developmental disorders characterized by marked social impairment. There is usually impairment in several additional domains, including the language and communication. Stereotypic behavior and sensory issues (i.e., hypersensitivity, hyposensitivity) also are prominent. Onset is typically before age 3 yr. and may be diagnosed as early as 15-18 mo of age. In rare cases, a child may be observed to develop normally to 18-24 mo and be diagnosed with autism at 30-36 mo.

SYNONYMS

ASD
Autism
Early infantile autism
Childhood autism
Kanner's autism
Asperger disorder
Pervasive developmental disorder

ICD-9CM CODES
F84.0   Autistic disorder

DSM-IV-TR CODES
299.00 Autistic disorder
299.80 Asperger's disorder
299.80 Pervasive developmental disorder
        NOS

EPIDEMIOLOGY & DEMOGRAPHICS

INCIDENCE (IN U.S.): Autism spectrum disorder afflicts 1% of children in the U.S.
PREVALENCE: 1:166 to 1:250
PREDOMINANT SEX: Male:female ratio of 2.1 to 6.5:1.0
PREDOMINANT AGE: Lifelong
PEAK INCIDENCE: Before age 3 yr
GENETICS:
- Autism is highly heritable with a heritability index of .90.
- De novo mutations account for 10% to 20% of autism spectrum disorder cases. Active research into common biologic mechanisms underlying autism spectrum disorders (including defective synaptic function) has identified chromosomal abnormalities in 6 major genes with as many as 20-30 additional genes in contributory roles, including glutamate-related genes.
- 5% risk rate for siblings of an affected individual, unless fragile X syndrome is determined as the pathway, increasing the risk rate to 50%.
- 70% to 95% concordance for classic autism in monozygotic twins and 5% for dizygotic pairs.

PHYSICAL FINDINGS & CLINICAL PRESENTATION

- Common triad of marked impairment in social interactions, impaired and atypical verbal and nonverbal communication, and repetitive and usual behavior or play
- Marked impairment in the understanding and use of both verbal and nonverbal communication
- Stereotypic behavior or language (i.e., echolalia)
- Perceptual hypersensitivity and avoidance of novel stimuli

ETIOLOGY

- Majority of cases are not associated with a comorbid medical condition.
- Significant increase in comorbid seizure disorder (25%) and developmental delay (75%).
- Autism is sometimes associated with other neurologic conditions (e.g., encephalitis, cytomegalovirus, toxoplasmosis, tuberous sclerosis, phenylketonuria [PKU], fragile X syndrome), suggesting that it also may result from nonspecific neuronal injury.
- Several studies have shown that there is no association between immunizations (specifically MMR vaccine) or thimerosal-containing vaccines and autism.

DIAGNOSIS

DIFFERENTIAL DIAGNOSIS

- Rett's syndrome: occurs in females; follows a brief period of normal development (i.e., 12-15 mo; characterized by severe neurodevelopmental regression including head growth deceleration, loss of purposeful use of hands, hyperventilation (risk of aerophagia), and motor incoordination
- Childhood disintegration disorder: normal development until age 4 yr, followed by marked neurodevelopmental and behavioral regression beginning with loss of bladder and bowel control
- Childhood-onset schizophrenia: follows period of normal development
- Asperger's syndrome: lacks the language and cognitive deficits characteristic of autism
- Isolated symptoms of autism: when occurring in isolation, defined as disorders (i.e., Phelan-Mcdermid syndrome, Aciardi syndrome, selective mutism, expressive language disorder, mixed receptive-expressive language disorder, stereotypic movement disorder, severe-to-profound intellectual disability [aka mental retardation])

WORKUP

- Rule out underlying medical condition Including genetic mental retardation syndromes
- Administer age-appropriate diagnostic instruments based on questionnaires and observation noting scales. Validated autism spectrum disorder–specific screening tools are available for children age ≥18 mo (e.g., Modified Checklist for Autism in Toddlers, Childhood Autism Rating Scale; Autism Diagnostic Observation Scale; Autism Diagnostic Interview-Revised; PDDST-III; Asperger's Syndrome Diagnostic Scale; Gilliam Asperger's Diagnostic Scale) and are being developed for younger children. General developmental screening tools are currently used in children <18 mo.

LABORATORY TESTS

- PKU screen (usually done at birth in the U.S.)
- Lead exposure screening
- Audiology testing for young children with autism spectrum disorders; school-based hearing screening may be sufficient in older children with autism spectrum disorders and without significant language or learning deficits
- Karyotype, microarray analysis, and DNA testing for fragile X syndrome in both boys and girls

IMAGING STUDIES

- EEG to diagnose coexisting seizure disorder if seizure is suspected or if language regression is present (i.e., Landau-Kleffner syndrome)
- Brain MRI if tuberous sclerosis or Aciardi syndrome (colossal agenesis) is suspected

TREATMENT
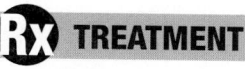

NONPHARMACOLOGIC THERAPY

- Consistent behavioral training program in both the home and school environments
- A number of programs are currently used; many are based on applied behavioral analysis (ABA), others include Pivotal response training (PRT) and Floortime.
- Special educational program focused on language and social and life skills development
- Highly structured home environment
- Education for families and teachers; the Autism Speaks™ website may be helpful in this regard: http://www.autismspeaks.org/about_us.php

ACUTE GENERAL Rx

- Obsessive or ritualistic behaviors: selective serotonin reuptake inhibitors (SSRIs), atypical antipsychotics, valproic acid
- Aggression, irritability, self-injury: atypical antipsychotic agents (e.g., risperidone), α-agonists, anticonvulsant mood stabilizers, SSRIs, beta-blockers
- Hyperactivity, impulsivity, inattention: stimulants, alpha-agonists, atypical antipsychotics
- Anxiety: SSRIs, buspirone, mirtazapine
- Bipolar, mood lability: valproic acid, carbamazepine, lithium
- Depression: SSRIs, mirtazapine

CHRONIC Rx

- Extended use of medications used for acute management of co-morbid psychiatric disorder.
- Pharmacotherapy is palliative, not curative of ASD

DISPOSITION

- Most children will require some degree of assistance as adults.
- With early diagnosis and proper treatment/support, children with Asperger's syndrome may experience fair to very good outcomes despite ongoing symptoms.

- Poorer outcomes include a lack of joint attention by age 4 yr, a lack of functional speech by age 5 yr, intellectual disability, seizures, comorbid medical or psychiatric syndromes, and severe autistic symptoms.
- Better outcomes (associated with early identification and treatment,) cognitive and behavioral capacity for inclusion in regular education settings with typically developing peers.

REFERRAL

Assistance may be needed in diagnosis (child psychiatrist, clinical psychologist, geneticist, pediatric neurologist, developmental pediatrician), management (speech language pathologist, occupational therapist), parental teaching (psychiatric social worker), or intervention with the school system (educational advocate, attorney).

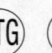 **PEARLS & CONSIDERATIONS**

- There is no scientific evidence of a relation between childhood vaccination and the development of autism.
- The Center for Autism & Developmental Disabilities at Bradley Hospital, an affiliate of the Brown Medical School, is the larget and most comprehensive treatment program in the U.S. for children with ASD and comorbid psychiatric illness (www.bradleyhospital.org).

- University of California Davis M.I.N.D. Institute is devoted to the study of autism (http://www.ucdmc.ucdavis.edu/mindinstitute).

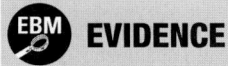 **EVIDENCE**

available at www.expertconsult.com

SUGGESTED READINGS

available at www.expertconsult.com

AUTHORS: **MITCHELL D. FELDMAN, M.D., M.PHIL.,** and **ROWLAND P. BARRETT, PH.D.**

BASIC INFORMATION

DEFINITION

Babesiosis is a tick-transmitted protozoan disease of animals, caused by intraerythrocytic parasites of the genus *Babesia*. Humans are incidentally infected, resulting in a nonspecific febrile illness. The disease can be severe in immunocompromised hosts.

ICD-9CM CODES
088.82 Babesiosis

EPIDEMIOLOGY & DEMOGRAPHICS

INCIDENCE (IN U.S.): Unknown
PREVALENCE (IN U.S.):
- In areas of high endemicity, seropositivity ranging from 9% (Rhode Island) to 21% (Connecticut)
- Highest number of reported cases in New York

PREDOMINANT SEX: Males (most likely through increased exposure to vectors during recreational or occupational activities)
PREDOMINANT AGE: Severity apparently increasing with age >40 yr
PEAK INCIDENCE: Spring and summer months, May through September
GENETICS: None known
CONGENITAL INFECTION: At least one case of probable vertical transmission
NEONATAL INFECTION: At least two cases of perinatal transmission
BLOOD TRANSFUSION: Many instances

PHYSICAL FINDINGS & CLINICAL PRESENTATION

- Incubation period 1 to 4 wk, or 6 to 9 wk in transfusion-associated disease
- Gradual onset of irregular fever, chills, diaphoresis, headache, myalgia, arthralgia, fatigue, and dark urine
- On physical examination: petechiae, frank or mild hepatosplenomegaly, and jaundice
- Infection with *B. divergens* (Europe) producing a more severe illness with a rapid onset of symptoms and increasing parasitemia progressing to massive intravascular hemolysis and renal failure

ETIOLOGY

- Vector: Deer tick, *Ixodes scapularis* (also known as *I. dammini*)
  1. Feeds on rodents during the spring and summer while in its larval and nymphal stages and on deer as an adult
  2. Requires a blood meal to mature to each stage, hence human infection
  3. During the warmer months in endemic areas, humans are readily infected while engaging in outdoor activities
- *B. microti* and *B. divergens* account for most human infections.
- In the U.S., cases caused by *B. microti* are acquired on offshore islands of the northeastern coast, including Nantucket Island, Cape

Cod, and Martha's Vineyard in Massachusetts; Block Island in Rhode Island; and Long Island, Fire Island, and Shelter Island in New York; as well as the nearby mainland including Connecticut and New Jersey.
- Sporadic cases reported from California, Georgia, Maryland, Minnesota, Virginia, Wisconsin, and most recently the WA-1 strain from Washington State and the MO-1 strain from Missouri.
- *B. divergens* is implicated in human disease in Europe, where the disease remains rare and predominantly associated with asplenia.
- Majority of cases are asymptomatic.
- May be transmissible by transfusion, through platelets and erythrocytes.
- Mixed infections (*B. microti* and *Borrelia burgdorferi*, the causative agent of Lyme disease) are estimated to occur in 10% (Rhode Island and Connecticut) to 60% (New York) of cases.

DIAGNOSIS

DIFFERENTIAL DIAGNOSIS

- Amebiasis
- Ehrlichiosis
- Hepatic abscess
- Leptospirosis
- Malaria
- Salmonellosis, including typhoid fever
- Acute viral hepatitis
- Hemorrhagic fevers

WORKUP

Should be suspected in any febrile patient living or traveling in an endemic area, irrespective of exposure history to ticks or tick bites, especially if asplenic

LABORATORY TESTS

- CBC to reveal mild to moderate pancytopenia
- Abnormally elevated serum chemistries, including creatinine, liver function profile, lactate dehydrogenase, and indirect and total bilirubin levels; hepatoglobin is low.
- Urinalysis to reveal proteinuria and hemoglobinuria
- Examination of Giemsa- or Wright-stained thin blood films for intraerythrocytic parasites
  1. In its classic, though infrequently seen, form a "tetrad" or "Maltese Cross" composed of four daughter cells attached by cytoplasmic strands is observed (Fig. 1-48).
  2. More commonly, smaller forms composed of a single chromatin dot are eccentrically located within bluish cytoplasm.
  3. Parasitized erythrocytes may be multiply infected but not enlarged.
- Babesial DNA by polymerase chain reaction (PCR) has comparable sensitivity and specificity to microscopic analysis of thin blood smears.
- Diagnosis achieved serologically by indirect immunofluorescence assay (IFA) is specific for *B. microti*.
  1. Assay is hampered by the inability to distinguish between exposed patients and those who are actively infected.
  2. Titer of ≥1:64 is indicative of seropositivity, whereas one ≥1:256 is considered diagnostic of acute infection.
  3. Immunoglobulin M indirect immunofluorescent-antibody test may be highly sensitive and specific for diagnosis.

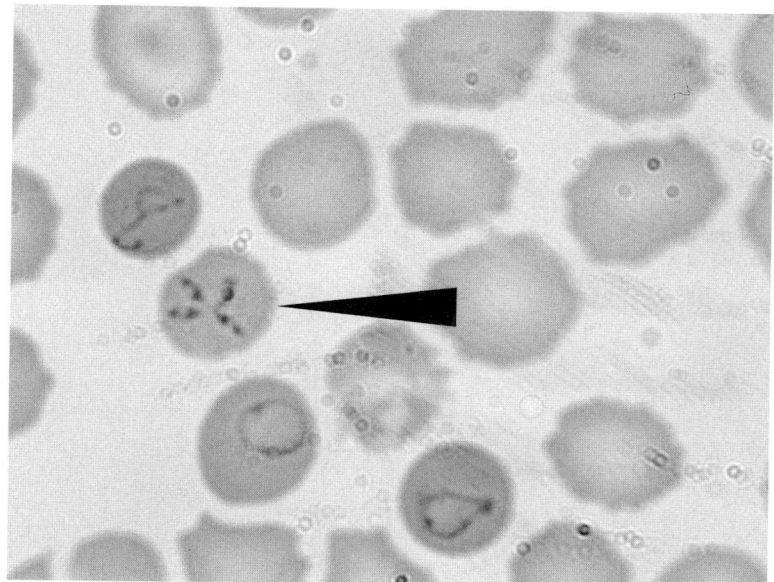

FIGURE 1-48 *Babesia* **spp.** Single and multiple intraerythrocytic parasites can be seen. The *arrow* marks a typical Maltese cross. (From Cohen J, Powderly WG: *Infectious diseases*, ed 2, St Louis, 2004, Mosby.)

TREATMENT

NONPHARMACOLOGIC THERAPY
Supportive care with adequate hydration

ACUTE GENERAL Rx
- In patients with intact spleens: predominantly asymptomatic or if symptomatic, generally self-limited
- Therapy reserved for the severely ill patient, especially if asplenic, elderly, or immunosuppressed
- Combination of quinine sulfate 650 mg PO tid plus clindamycin 600 mg PO tid (600 mg parenterally qid) taken for 7 to 10 days: effective but may not eliminate parasites
- Combination of atovaquone 750 mg q12h and azithromycin 500 mg on day 1 and 250 mg per day thereafter for 7 days appears to be as effective as a regimen of clindamycin and quinine with fewer adverse reactions
- Severely ill patients are hospitalized and treated with clindamycin and quinine
- Exchange transfusions in addition to antimicrobial therapy: successful treatment for severe infections in asplenic patients associated with high levels of *B. microti* or *B. divergens* parasitemia
- Relapsed and immunocompromised patients may require a longer duration of therapy

DISPOSITION
Prognosis is usually good and fatal outcomes are rare.

REFERRAL
- For prompt consultation with an infectious disease specialist if the diagnosis is acutely suspected, especially in the asplenic, elderly, or immunocompromised patient
- For hospitalization for the severely ill patient who may require exchange transfusions in addition to antibiotic therapy

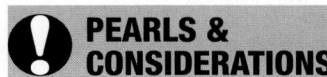 PEARLS & CONSIDERATIONS

COMMENTS
- Prevention of babesiosis in asplenic or immunocompromised hosts is best achieved by avoidance of areas where the vector is endemic, especially May through September.
- If residence or travel in endemic areas is unavoidable, advise patients to perform daily cutaneous self-examination, wear light-colored clothing (to facilitate removal of ticks), tuck pants into socks, and apply tick repellent (diethyltoluamide and dimethylphthalate) to skin or clothing.
- Advise a daily inspection for ticks in family pets (e.g., cats and dogs).
- Infection with *B. divergens,* especially in the asplenic patient, is often fatal.
- Concurrent babesiosis and Lyme disease has been documented—check for combined infection in severely ill patients.
- Clindamycin and quinine has been successfully used to treat babesiosis during the third trimester of pregnancy without incurring apparent adverse effect on the fetus.

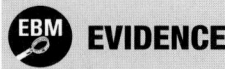 EVIDENCE
available at www.expertconsult.com

SUGGESTED READINGS
available at www.expertconsult.com

AUTHOR: **PATRICIA CRISTOFARO, M.D.**

BASIC INFORMATION

DEFINITION

Baker's cyst is a fluid-filled popliteal bursa located along the medial border of the popliteal fossa.

SYNONYMS

Popliteal cyst

ICD-9CM CODES
727.51 Baker's cyst (knee)

EPIDEMIOLOGY & DEMOGRAPHICS

- Occurs at all ages.
- Incidence is unknown.
- Between 2% and 6% of all patients believed to have clinical deep venous thrombosis (DVT) have symptomatic Baker's cysts.
- Approximately 5% of MRIs of the knees reveal popliteal cysts.

PHYSICAL FINDINGS & CLINICAL PRESENTATION

- Pain in the popliteal space
- Knee swelling
- Leg edema
- Prominence of the popliteal fossa
- Decreased range of motion of the knee
- Locking of the knee
- Foucher's sign: The cyst becomes hard with knee extension and soft with knee flexion.
- Neuropathic lancinating pains radiating from the knee down the back of the leg
- Presence of associated DVT

ETIOLOGY

- Believed to represent fluid distention of the bursal sac separating the semimembranous tendon from the medial head of the gastrocnemius.
- May represent a true cyst but more often results from the posterior herniation of a tense knee effusion. Thus a Baker's cyst usually denotes increased intraarticular pressure from underlying joint disease.
- In children, Baker's cysts are believed to result from trauma and irritation of the knee.
- In adults, Baker's cysts are usually associated with pathologic changes of the knee joint, such as the following:
  ○ Rheumatoid arthritis (RA)
  ○ Osteoarthritis of the knee
  ○ Meniscal tears
  ○ Patellofemoral chondromalacia
  ○ Fracture
  ○ Gout
  ○ Pseudogout
  ○ Infection (tuberculosis)

DIAGNOSIS

Baker's cyst frequently mimics DVT and is sometimes referred to as *pseudothrombophlebitis syndrome.*

DIFFERENTIAL DIAGNOSIS

- DVT
- Popliteal aneurysm
- Abscess
- Tumor
- Lymphadenopathy
- Varicosity
- Ganglion

WORKUP

Anyone suspected of having a popliteal cyst should undergo imaging studies to exclude other causes.

LABORATORY TESTS

Blood tests are not specific in the diagnosis of Baker's cysts.

IMAGING STUDIES

- Plain radiographs (AP and lateral views) may show calcification in a solid tumor or in the posterior meniscal area.
- Ultrasound is safe, portable, cost effective, and excludes other clinically important causes of popliteal fossa pathology, including DVT.
- MRI of the knee identifies coexisting joint pathology (e.g., osteoarthritis, torn meniscus).

TREATMENT

NONPHARMACOLOGIC THERAPY

- Rest
- Strenuous activity avoidance
- Knee immobilization necessary in some cases

ACUTE GENERAL Rx

- Nonsteroidal antiinflammatory drugs, ibuprofen 400 to 800 mg PO tid or naproxen 250 to 500 mg PO bid, can be used to treat Baker's cyst caused by RA, gout, and pseudogout.
- Intraarticular injection or injection of the cyst with corticosteroids, triamcinolone acetonide 40 mg, is sometimes tried.

CHRONIC Rx

- The majority of Baker's cysts are successfully treated conservatively.

- Surgical procedures addressing the underlying cause include:
  1. Arthroscopic surgery to remove loose cartilaginous fragment
  2. Partial or total meniscectomy
  3. Open excision of the cyst (Fig. 1-49)

DISPOSITION

- Baker's cyst may spontaneously resolve without treatment.
- Complications of Baker's cysts include:
  1. Rupture
  2. DVT
  3. Nerve impingement

REFERRAL

Rheumatology or orthopedics if surgery is contemplated

PEARLS & CONSIDERATIONS

- Popliteal cysts were first described in 1840 by Adams, but it is Baker's writing about disease of the knee joint in 1877 that gave rise to the eponym Baker's cyst.
- A Baker's cyst may serve as a protective mechanism for the knee. Intrinsic intraarticular disorders cause joint effusion. The knee effusion is displaced into the Baker's cyst, thus reducing potentially destructive pressure in the joint space.

COMMENTS

Baker's cyst and DVT can coexist. It is imperative to exclude the diagnosis of DVT before discharging the patient.

SUGGESTED READINGS
available at www.expertconsult.com

AUTHORS: **RICHARD REGNANTE, M.D.,** and **IMMAD SADIQ, M.D.**

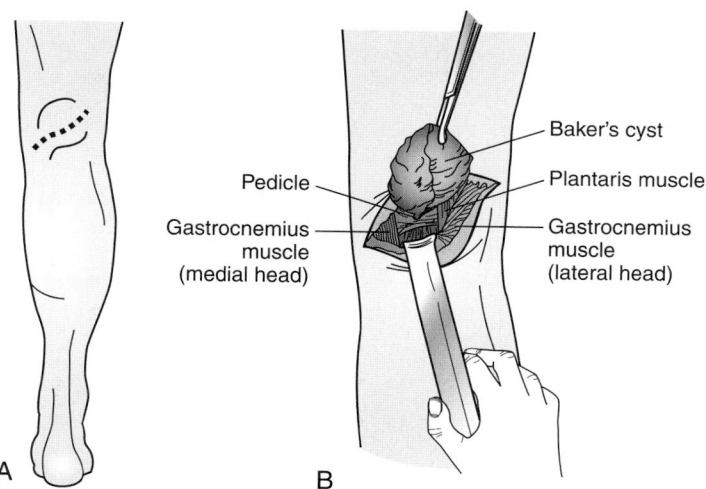

FIGURE 1-49 Removal of midline Baker's cyst. A, Skin incision. B, After being exposed, pedicle is clamped, ligated, divided, and inverted. (Redrawn and modified from Meyerding HW, Van Demark GE: Posterior hernia of the knee, *JAMA* 122:858, 1943.)

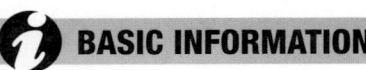

BASIC INFORMATION

DEFINITION
Balanitis is an inflammation of the superficial tissues of the penile head.

ICD-9CM CODES
112.2 Balanitis

EPIDEMIOLOGY & DEMOGRAPHICS
INCIDENCE (IN U.S.): Unknown
PREVALENCE (IN U.S.): Unknown
PREDOMINANT SEX: Exclusive to males
PEAK INCIDENCE: All ages, especially in sexually active men

PHYSICAL FINDINGS & CLINICAL PRESENTATION
- Itching and tenderness
- Pain, dysuria, and local edema
- Rarely, ulceration and lymph node enlargement
- Severe ulcerations leading to superimposed bacterial infections
- Inability to void: unusual, but a more distressing and serious complication

ETIOLOGY
- Poor hygiene, causing erosion of tissue with erythema and promoting growth of *Candida albicans*
- Sexual contact, urinary catheters, and trauma
- Allergic reactions to condoms or medications

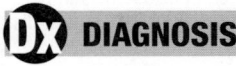 DIAGNOSIS

DIFFERENTIAL DIAGNOSIS
- Leukoplakia
- Reiter's syndrome
- Lichen planus
- Balanitis xerotica obliterans
- Psoriasis
- Carcinoma of the penis
- Erythroplasia of Queyrat
- Nodular scabies

WORKUP
- Sexually active males: assessment for evidence of other sexually transmitted diseases
- Biopsy if lesions do not heal

LABORATORY TESTS
- VDRL
- Serum glucose
- Wet mount
- KOH prep
- Microbial culture

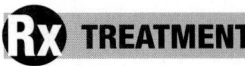 TREATMENT

NONPHARMACOLOGIC THERAPY
- Maintenance of meticulous hygiene
- Retraction and bathing of prepuce several times a day
- Warm sitz baths to ease edema and erythema
- Consideration of circumcision, especially when symptoms are severe or recurrent
- With Foley catheters, strict catheter care strongly advised

ACUTE GENERAL Rx
- Fluconazole 150 mg PO × 1 or itraconazole 200 mg PO bid × 1 day
- Clotrimazole 1% cream applied topically twice daily to affected areas
- Bacitracin or Neosporin ointment applied topically 4 times daily
- With more severe bacterial superinfection: cephalexin 500 mg PO qid
- Topical corticosteroids added 4 times daily if dermatitis severe
- Patients with suspected urinary tract infections: trimethoprim-sulfa DS twice daily or ciprofloxacin 500 mg PO bid after obtaining appropriate cultures

DISPOSITION
Balanitis is often self-limited and usually responds to conservative therapy; if it does not improve, consider circinate balanitis (Reiter's syndrome), nodular scabies, and primary skin lesions including skin carcinoma.

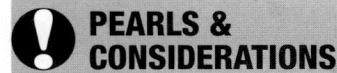 PEARLS & CONSIDERATIONS

Don't forget about nodular scabies involving the prepubic area—examine the region carefully for burrows and tracks of *Sarcoptes scabiei*.

REFERRAL
- For surgical evaluation for circumcision if symptoms are recurrent, especially if phimosis or meatitis occurs (NOTE: Severe phimosis with an inability to void may require prompt slit drainage.)
- For biopsy to rule out other diagnosis such as premalignant or malignant lesions if lesions are not healing

SUGGESTED READINGS
available at www.expertconsult.com

AUTHORS: **GLENN G. FORT, M.D., M.P.H.,** and **DENNIS J. MIKOLICH, M.D.**

BASIC INFORMATION

DEFINITION

Barrett's esophagus occurs when the squamocolumnar junction is displaced proximal to the gastroesophageal junction, and the squamous lining of the lower esophagus is replaced by metaplastic columnar epithelium, which predisposes to the development of cancer. Intestinalized epithelium is no longer considered essential for the diagnosis. The condition is associated with an increased risk (~0.5%/yr) for development of adenocarcinoma of the esophagus.

SYNONYMS

Esophagus, Barrett's
Esophagus, columnar-lined
Ulcer, Barrett's

ICD-9CM CODES
530.85 Barrett's esophagus

EPIDEMIOLOGY & DEMOGRAPHICS

- Male:female ratio of 4:1
- Mean age of onset is 40 yr, with a mean age range of diagnosis of 55 to 60 yr
- Occurs more frequently in white and Hispanic individuals than in African American individuals, with a ratio of 10 to 20:1
- Mean prevalence of 5% to 15% in patients undergoing endoscopy (EGD) for symptoms of gastroesophageal reflux disease (GERD)
- Obesity may be an independent risk factor
- Prevalence rate in asymptomatic cohorts ranges from 5% to 25%

CLINICAL PRESENTATION

SYMPTOMS:
- Chronic heartburn
- Dysphagia with solid food
- May be an incidental finding on EGD in patients without reflux symptoms
- Less frequent: chest pain, hematemesis, melena
- Patients may be asymptomatic

PHYSICAL FINDINGS:
- Nonspecific; can be completely normal
- Epigastric tenderness on palpation

ETIOLOGY

- Metaplasia is thought to result from reepithelialization of esophageal tissue injured as a result of chronic GERD.
- Patients with Barrett's esophagus tend to have more severe esophageal motility disturbances (decreased lower esophageal sphincter pressure, ineffective peristalsis) and greater esophageal acid exposure on 24-hour pH monitoring.
- Intraesophageal bile reflux may also play a role in the pathogenesis.
- Familial clustering of GERD and Barrett's esophagus suggests a genetic predisposition, but no gene has yet been identified. Early data suggest that patients who develop Barrett's are genetically predisposed to a severe inflammatory response to GERD.

- Progression from metaplasia to carcinoma is associated with changes in gene structure and expression, including the Caudal-related homeobox family of transcription factors (CDX1 and CDX2), and the tumor suppressors p16 (CDKN2A) and TP53.

DIAGNOSIS

DIFFERENTIAL DIAGNOSIS

- GERD, uncomplicated
- Erosive esophagitis
- Gastritis
- Peptic ulcer disease
- Angina
- Malignancy
- Stricture or Schatzki's ring

WORKUP

- EGD with biopsy is necessary for diagnosis.
- Wireless esophageal capsule endoscopy may detect Barrett's, but with a lower sensitivity and specificity than EGD.

- Imaging studies are nonspecific and insensitive for the diagnosis.
- Diagnosis requires the presence of metaplastic columnar epithelium proximal to the gastroesophageal junction (Fig. 1-50). Longer segment Barrett's esophagus is more readily diagnosed.
- Intestinal metaplasia of the gastric cardia is not Barrett's esophagus and does not have the same risk for malignancy.
- The Practice Parameters Committee of the American College of Gastroenterology (ACG) has suggested that the highest yield for Barrett's esophagus screening is in older (age >50 yr) white men with longstanding heartburn. General population screening is not currently recommended. The benefit of screening in high-risk populations is not established. Although screening has become standard of practice in some communities, the effectiveness of screening using current techniques is controversial because it may not improve mortality rates from adenocarcinoma or be cost-effective.

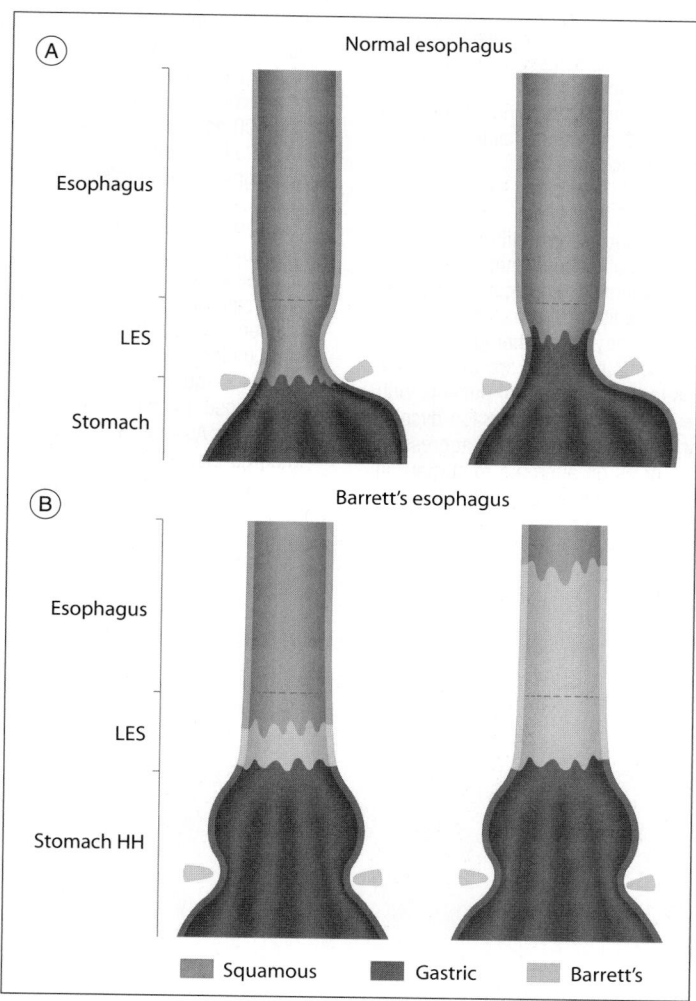

FIGURE 1-50 Anatomic landmarks of the normal LES region **(A)** and of Barrett's esophagus **(B).** Note that gastric mucosa is very common and normal in the LES region and that in Barrett's esophagus, the squamocolumnar junction is not only proximally displaced within the tubular esophagus, but that the intervening mucosa is composed of intestinalized Barrett's metaplastic epithelium, noted in red (HH, hiatal hernia) (From Silverburg SG: *Principles of practice of surgical pathology and cytopathology,* ed 4, New York, 2006.)

- Screening for *Helicobacter pylori* infection in patients with GERD and Barrett's esophagus is not recommended.

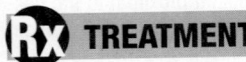 **TREATMENT**

Goal is to control GERD symptoms and maintain healed mucosa.

NONPHARMACOLOGIC THERAPY

Lifestyle modifications; elevating head of bed; avoiding chocolate, tobacco, caffeine, mints, and certain drugs (see "Gastroesophageal Reflux Disease")

ACUTE GENERAL Rx

- Proton pump inhibitors are the most effective treatment for GERD. Chronic acid suppression is often necessary to control symptoms and promote healing.
- Adequate control of GERD symptoms in patients with Barrett's esophagus may not completely control intraesophageal acid exposure. Some studies suggest that normalization of intraesophageal acid exposure may either lead to regression of Barrett's esophagus or reduce the risk for dysplasia, although overall, the data are inconsistent.
- If patient is asymptomatic and incidentally found to have Barrett's esophagus, medication use may be considered.

CHRONIC Rx

- When GERD is controlled by either medical or surgical therapy, ablation of metaplastic epithelium usually leads to replacement by normal squamous epithelium. Thermal ablation techniques, photodynamic therapy, and endoscopic mucosal resection are all possible approaches to the treatment of patients with Barrett's esophagus and high-grade dysplasia, either in conjunction with aggressive surveillance or as an alternate to surgery in poor operative candidates. Radiofrequency ablation and cryotherapy are newer techniques currently being evaluated for the complete eradication of both dysplasia and intestinal metaplasia and reduced risk for disease progression.. All these options run the risk for residual or buried metaplasia. Because only a minority of patients with Barrett's esophagus progress to high-grade dysplasia or carcinoma, these techniques cannot be currently recommended in patients with Barrett's esophagus without dysplasia. Additional studies will need to show that radiofrequency ablation and cryotherapy reduce or eliminate the need for surveillance endoscopy and/or the risk for cancer, and that they are cost-effective in the long term.
- Antireflux surgery may be considered for management of GERD and associated sequelae. Patients should still have endoscopic surveillance of their esophagus. Surgical resection is offered for multifocal high-grade dysplasia or carcinoma.

DISPOSITION

- Overall, increased risk for adenocarcinoma of the esophagus in patients with Barrett's esophagus may be as high as 100 times that of the general population.
- Corresponds to 500 cancers per yr per 100,000 persons with Barrett's esophagus.
- The lifetime cancer risk for patients with nondysplastic Barrett's esophagus is ~5% to 8%.
- Frequency of monitoring is controversial; no studies have proved that surveillance increases life expectancy.
- American College of Gastroenterology recommends that patients with Barrett's esophagus undergo surveillance EGD and systematic four-quadrant biopsy at intervals determined by the presence and grade of dysplasia. All mucosal abnormalities should undergo biopsy. Patients who have had two consecutive EGDs showing no dysplasia should have follow-up every 3 yr. Patients with low-grade dysplasia should have extensive mucosal sampling within 6 mo and follow-up every year. Patients with high-grade dysplasia should have expert confirmation and extensive mucosal sampling. High-grade dysplasia with visible mucosal irregularities should be removed by endoscopic mucosal resection. Consider intensive surveillance every 3 mo for patients with focal high-grade dysplasia. Patients with multifocal high-grade dysplasia or carcinoma should be considered for resection or ablation if not an operative candidate.
- Patients should be treated aggressively for GERD before surveillance.

REFERRAL

- Consider EGD with biopsy in patients (particularly white men >50 yr old) with chronic GERD who have not had previous EGD.
- Refer patients with GERD for evaluation if "red flag" symptoms are present (dysphagia, odynophagia, weight loss, vomiting, early satiety, GI bleeding, iron deficiency).
- Refer for surveillance those with biopsy-proven Barrett's esophagus.
- For those with high-grade dysplasia, refer for intensive surveillance or esophageal resection; ablative therapy may be considered as part of a research protocol or if patient is not an operative candidate.

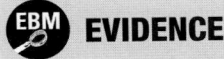 **EVIDENCE**

available at www.expertconsult.com

SUGGESTED READINGS
available at www.expertconsult.com

AUTHOR: **HARLAN G. RICH, M.D.**

BASIC INFORMATION

DEFINITION

Bartter's syndrome is a group of renal tubular disorders characterized by metabolic alkalosis, hypokalemia, hyperplasia of the juxtaglomerular apparatus, hyperreninemic hyperaldosteronism, and hypercalciuria.

SYNONYMS

Hypokalemic alkalosis with hypercalciuria

ICD-9CM CODES
255.13 Bartter's Syndrome

EPIDEMIOLOGY & DEMOGRAPHICS

Classic Bartter's syndrome can present with symptoms at 2 yr of age or younger. Neonatal Bartter's syndrome can be diagnosed at birth or even prenatally. The true incidence in the U.S. is not known. Incidence is similar in males and in females.

CLINICAL PRESENTATION

- Neonatal Bartter's syndrome involves maternal polyhydramnios, frequent preterm delivery, fetal polyuria, and FTT.
- Classic Bartter's syndrome may include a history of maternal polyhydramnios and premature delivery. The following features are characteristic:
  - Polyuria
  - Polydipsia
  - Hypokalemia
  - Metabolic alkalosis
  - Hypercalciuria
  - Plasma magnesium is normal or mildly reduced.
  - Patients are normotensive or have low blood pressure.
  - Patients do not have edema.

- Growth retardation remains a major complication in children with primary tubular disorders, despite treatment.

ETIOLOGY

- Disorder of chloride reabsorption in the thick ascending loop of Henle.
- The multiple and complex functions of the renal tubule in regulating water, electrolyte, and mineral homeostasis make it prone to numerous genetic abnormalities resulting in malfunction. Bartter's syndrome is caused by different genetic mutations that manifest in a similar phenotype (Table 1-25).

DIAGNOSIS

DIFFERENTIAL DIAGNOSIS

- Diuretic abuse
- Surreptitious vomiting
- Gitelman's syndrome
- Autosomal dominant hypocalcemia
- Hyperprostaglandin E syndrome

WORKUP

- Classic Bartter's syndrome is usually a diagnosis of exclusion.
- Vomiting associated with a low urine chloride and scarring of the dorsum of the hand and dental erosions suggests bulimia nervosa.
- Diuretic abuse can only be excluded by a urinary assay for diuretics.

LABORATORY TESTS

- Serum sodium, potassium, chloride, bicarbonate, calcium, magnesium, phosphorus.
- Urine calcium, chloride, assay for diuretics as above.
- Serum pH can be confirmed by performing ABG.
- Genetic diagnosis is possible, but not widely available

IMAGING STUDIES

- Renal ultrasonography may show nephrocalcinosis, hydronephrosis, and hydroureter in neonatal Bartter's syndrome.
- Classic signs of hypokalemia may be present on ECG.

TREATMENT

ACUTE GENERAL Rx

Neonatal Bartter's syndrome requires correction of electrolyte imbalance and volume depletion.

CHRONIC Rx

- Patients are generally treated with oral potassium and magnesium supplementation. though achievement of normal serum potassium and magnesium levels is often difficult.
- Nonsteroidal anti-inflammatory drugs (NSAIDs) combined with potassium-sparing diuretics such as spironolactone/amiloride have been used effectively in the treatment of Bartter's. ACE inhibitors have also been used.

REFERRAL

Consultation with nephrology facilitates diagnosis and management of this condition.

PEARLS & CONSIDERATIONS

COMMENTS

- Just as Bartter's looks like loop diuretic use from the point of view of laboratory testing, Gitelman's syndrome appears identical to thiazide use.
- High urine calcium is the best way to distinguish Bartter's from Gitelman's syndrome.
- Serum magnesium differences have been described but are likely to be low in both syndromes and are probably not useful in distinguishing these syndromes.

PATIENT/FAMILY EDUCATION

- Foods with high potassium content should be emphasized in dietary education.
- Patients with Bartter's syndrome are more vulnerable to volume depletion due to potassium derangement during exercise and exposure.
- Genetic counseling may be indicated.

SUGGESTED READINGS
available at www.expertconsult.com

AUTHOR: **JONATHAN BURNS, M.A., M.D.**

TABLE 1-25 Various Bartter Syndromes

	Type 1	Type 2	Type 3	Type 4	Type 5
Gene name	SLC12A1	KCNJ1	CLCNKB	BSND	CASR
Protein name	NKCC2	ROMK	CLCNKB	Barttin	CaR
Major symptoms	Polyuria, hypocalcemia	As for type 1	Variable	As for type 1	—
Seizures	Dehydration	—	Mild to severe	+ Deafness	—
Urine Ca^{2+}	↑	↑	↑	↑	↑
Urine Mg^{2+}	↓	↓	↓	↓	↓
Nephrocalcinosis	+++	+++	±	—	+++

Ca^{2+}, Calcium; Mg^{2+}, magnesium.
From Andreoli TE et al: *Andreoli and Carpenter's Cecil essentials of medicine*, ed 8, Philadelphia, 2010, Saunders.

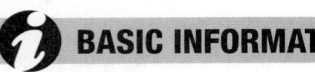

BASIC INFORMATION

DEFINITION

Basal cell carcinoma (BCC) is a malignant tumor of the skin arising from basal cells of the lower epidermis and adnexal structures. It may be classified as one of six types: nodular, superficial, pigmented, cystic, sclerosing or morpheaform, and nevoid. The most common type is nodular (21%); the least common is morpheaform (1%). A mixed pattern is present in approximately 40% of cases. BCC advances by direct expansion and destroys normal tissue.

SYNONYMS

BCC

ICD-9CM CODES
179.9 Basal cell carcinoma, site unspecified
173.3 Basal cell carcinoma, face
173.4 Basal cell carcinoma, neck, scalp
173.5 Basal cell carcinoma, trunk
173.6 Basal cell carcinoma of the limb
173.7 Basal cell carcinoma, lower limb

EPIDEMIOLOGY & DEMOGRAPHICS

- Most common cutaneous neoplasm
- 85% of cases appear on the head and neck region
- Most common site: nose (30%)
- Increased incidence with age >40 yr
- Increased incidence in men

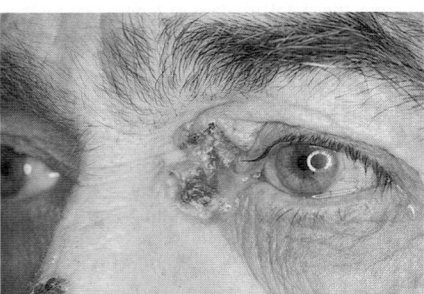

FIGURE 1-51 Basal cell carcinoma. Note rolled translucent border and central ulceration in typical facial location. (From Noble J et al: *Textbook of primary care medicine,* ed 3, St Louis, 2001, Mosby.)

- Risk factors: fair skin, increased sun exposure, use of tanning salons with ultraviolet A or B radiation, history of irradiation (e.g., Hodgkin's disease), personal or family history of skin cancer, impaired immune system

PHYSICAL FINDINGS & CLINICAL PRESENTATION

Variable with the histologic type:
- Nodular: dome-shaped, painless lesion that may become multilobular and frequently ulcerates (rodent ulcer); prominent telangiectatic vessels are noted on the surface. Border is translucent, elevated, pearly white (Fig. 1-51). Some nodular BCCs may contain pigmentation, giving an appearance similar to a melanoma.
- Superficial: circumscribed, scaling, black appearance with a thin, raised, pearly-white border; a crust and erosions may be present. Occurs most frequently on the trunk and extremities.
- Morpheaform: flat or slightly raised yellowish or white appearance (similar to localized scleroderma); appearance similar to scars; surface has a waxy consistency.

DIAGNOSIS

DIFFERENTIAL DIAGNOSIS

- Keratoacanthoma
- Melanoma (pigmented BCC)
- Xeroderma pigmentosa
- Basal cell nevus syndrome
- Molluscum contagiosum
- Sebaceous hyperplasia
- Psoriasis

WORKUP

Biopsy to confirm diagnosis

TREATMENT

Variable with tumor size, location, and cell type:
- Excision surgery: preferred method for large tumors with well-defined borders on the legs, cheeks, forehead, and trunk.
- Mohs' micrographic surgery: preferred for lesions in high-risk areas (e.g., nose, eyelid), very large primary tumors, recurrent BCCs,

and tumors with poorly defined clinical margins.
- Electrodesiccation and curettage: useful for small (<6 mm) nodular BCCs.
- Cryosurgery with liquid nitrogen: useful in BCCs of the superficial and nodular types with clearly definable margins; no clear advantages over the other forms of therapy; generally reserved for uncomplicated tumors.
- Radiation therapy: generally used for BCCs in areas requiring preservation of normal surrounding tissues for cosmetic reasons (e.g., around lips); also useful in patients who cannot tolerate surgical procedures or for large lesions and surgical failures.
- Imiquimod 5% cream can be used for treatment of small, superficial BCCs of the trunk and extremities. Efficacy rate is approximately 80%. Its main advantage is lack of scarring, which must be weighed against higher cure rates with surgical intervention.
- GDC-0449, an orally active small molecule that targets the hedgehog pathway, appears to have antitumor activity in locally advanced or metastatic basal-cell carcinoma.

DISPOSITION

- More than 90% of patients are cured; however, periodic evaluation for at least 5 yr is necessary because of increased risk of recurrence of another BCC (>40% risk within 5 yr of treatment).
- A lesion is considered low risk if it is <1.5 cm in diameter, is nodular or cystic, is not in a difficult-to-treat area (H zone of face), and has not been previously treated.
- Nodular and superficial BCCs are the least aggressive.
- Morpheaform lesions have the highest incidence of positive tumor margins (>30%) and the greatest recurrence rate.

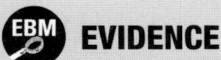

EVIDENCE

available at www.expertconsult.com

SUGGESTED READING

available at www.expertconsult.com

AUTHOR: **FRED F. FERRI, M.D.**

BASIC INFORMATION

DEFINITION

A bedbug's bite is a wound caused by the penetration of the bedbug mouthpiece into the skin as the insect feeds on blood from vessels or extravasated blood from the damaged surrounding tissue. The saliva of the bedbug contains pharmacologically active substances responsible for a spectrum of undesirable skin reactions depending on the individual.

SYNONYMS

Insect bite
Bedbug *Cimex lectularius* bite

ICD-9CM CODES

919.4 Insect bite w/o infection (may also code based on bite location)

EPIDEMIOLOGY & DEMOGRAPHICS

- Traditionally, bedbugs were considered more common in poorer areas, but they are now increasingly found in areas of frequent travel.
- Bedbug infestations may spread among multifamily and institutional facilities with shared walls and are consequently difficult to eradicate.
- Reports of bedbug infestations have increased dramatically in the U.S., as well as worldwide, likely because of the decreased use of pesticides and increased international travel.
- Bedbugs are attracted to carbon dioxide gas and warm bodies.
- Bedbugs do not have a preference for specific age groups, ethnicity, or sex.
- Studies have shown increased sensitivity of cutaneous reaction in previous bite victims.

PHYSICAL FINDINGS AND CLINICAL PRESENTATION

- Firm, purpuric or erythematous macules, urticaria, or bullae may be present. Bites are often inflammatory and pruritic, although bedbug-naive individuals may be asymptomatic to their first bites.
- Bite may have a central hemorrhagic punctum.
- Victim may observe a linear series of three bites ("breakfast, lunch, and dinner").
- As bedbug bites usually do not penetrate clothing, bite distribution is generally on areas of exposed skin. Otherwise, there is no preferential distribution.

ETIOLOGY

- The *Cimex lectularius* species, also known as the common bedbug, feeds on mammals and birds. *Cimex hemipterus* is a tropical species that bites mostly humans, and hybrid species of the two insects exist. Both generally feed nocturnally on the blood of sleeping humans. The adult bedbug is wingless and about 5 to 7 mm in length. It has a modified mouthpart for piercing and sucking that usually leaves a bite mark of papular urticarial presentation to exposed areas of skin. Bedbugs have weak appendages for latching on to their hosts and are not usually transported from person to person.
- The saliva of the bedbug contains nitrophorin that enables vasodilation, an anticoagulant that interferes with production of coagulation Factor Xa, a salivary apyrase that inhibits platelet aggregation, and an anesthetic. Consequently, the host often does not feel the bite until the effects have worn off.

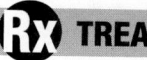 DIAGNOSIS

DIFFERENTIAL DIAGNOSIS

Scabies, flea and mite bites, vesicular disorders, delusional parasitosis, dermatitis herpetiformis, pemphigus herpetiformis, ecthyma, drug eruptions

WORKUP

- Workup begins with history and physical for clinical symptoms and environmental findings.
- Victims should carefully scrutinize the bedroom for signs of bedbug infestation. One may encounter fecal smears or flecks of blood on bed linens, inside furniture cracks and crevices, and behind peeling wallpaper. Bedbugs may travel as far as 20 feet for a meal. Densely infested rooms may also have a distinctive, pungent, soda syrup–like odor.

LABORATORY TESTS

- No specific tests recommended except for identification of the insect.
- The histology of bedbug bites is similar to other insect bites. Perivascular infiltrate of lymphocytes, histiocytes, eosinophils, and mast cells are seen within the upper dermis. One may also observe collagen bundles with interstitial eosinophils, dermal edema, and extravasated erythrocytes.

IMAGING STUDIES

None

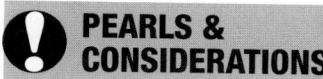 TREATMENT

- Treatment of bites is often not necessary. Bites may self-resolve within a week for milder cases and a few weeks for more severe cases.
- Topical glucocorticoids or systemic antihistamines are appropriate in patients with severe pruritus from the bedbug bite.
  - triamcinolone cream 0.1%, apply thin film to affected areas bid
  - chlorpheniramine 4 mg PO hs (adults), 2 mg PO hs (children)
- Insecticides may be effective in eradicating the bedbug, but growing resistance has been seen and multi-insecticide therapy is recommended.
  - Use permethrin spray for clothing and bedsheets or bednets
  - Diethyltoluamide (DEET): Be wary of toxic levels in children when used at high concentrations.
  - Deltamethrin and chlorfenapyr are two common insecticides used.
  - Please consult a pest control professional for safe eradication.

NONPHARMACOLOGIC THERAPY

Vacuuming is effective in removing bedbugs but does not remove the eggs. Wash bedsheets and clothing in hot water with detergent with at least 20 minutes in a dryer. Bedbugs have a high thermal death point of 45° C and also may survive at temperatures as low as 7° C. Coating bedposts with antifriction or adhesive substances such as petrolatum or duct tape may hinder bedbugs from gaining access to the bed.

ACUTE GENERAL Rx

Immunologic response is dependent on immunocompetence and individual sensitivity to the salivary components of the bedbug bite. Often, patients with papular urticaria have IgG antibodies to specific bedbug proteins. IgE antibodies may also mediate bullae formation. Anaphylaxis and death from bites is rare but documented in literature.

DISPOSITION

Patient may resume normal activity and lifestyle. Travelers should inspect their clothing and suitcases before returning home.

BEDBUGS AS POTENTIAL VECTORS

The bedbug has been studied extensively as a potential vector for human pathogens such as HIV and viral hepatitis, as well as many other diseases. To date, there is no evidence of transmission from an infected bedbug to a human.

PEARLS & CONSIDERATIONS

COMMENTS

- Bedbugs are an increasing source of anguish and frustration for humans, and clinicians should evaluate for signs of stress and depression.
- A combination of chemical and physical intervention is often necessary for complete eradication. All hiding areas must be carefully inspected and cleaned. Treatment may include pesticides plus laundering, heat, freezing, and vacuuming.

SUGGESTED READINGS

available at www.expertconsult.com

AUTHOR: **STEPHANIE W. CHOW, M.D.**

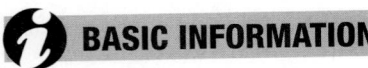

BASIC INFORMATION

DEFINITION

Behçet's disease is a chronic, relapsing, inflammatory disorder characterized by the presence of recurrent oral aphthous ulcers, genital ulcers, uveitis, and skin lesions (Figs. 1-52 and 1-53).

SYNONYMS

Behçet's syndrome

ICD-9CM CODES
136.1 Behçet's syndrome

EPIDEMIOLOGY & DEMOGRAPHICS

PREVALENCE:
- Behçet's disease is observed in two different geographic locations.
  1. One region consists of Eastern Asia, Turkey, and the Mediterranean basin.
     - Prevalence ranges from 13 to 17 cases per 100,000 persons.
     - Turkey has the highest prevalence at up to 300 cases per 100,000 persons.
  2. The second region consists of North America and Northern Europe.
     - Prevalence ranges from 0.5 to 17 cases per 100,000 persons. Germany has the greatest prevalence.
     - Prevalence of Behçet's disease in the U.S. is 6.6 cases per 100,000 persons.
- In these regions, the prevalence of HLA-B51 is greater in patients with Behçet's disease.

PREDOMINANT SEX: Equal sex distribution

GENETICS: No clear pattern of inheritance can be determined. Familial disease was noted in 15% of affected children.

PHYSICAL FINDINGS & CLINICAL PRESENTATION

- Behçet's disease typically affects individuals in the third to fourth decade of life and primarily presents with painful aphthous oral ulcers. The ulcers occur in crops measuring 2 to 12 mm and are found on the mucous membrane of the cheek, gingiva, tongue, pharynx, and soft palate.
- Genital and perianal ulcers are similar to the oral ulcers. They may result in scarring.
- Decreased vision secondary to uveitis, keratitis, and retinal artery occlusion with ischemia may be followed by neovascularization, vitreous hemorrhage and contraction, glaucoma, and retinal detachment. Younger male individuals are at greater risk for ocular involvement.
- Skin findings (41% to 97%) include nodular lesions, which are histologically divided to erythema nodosum-like lesions, pseudofolliculitis, papulopustular lesions, acneform nodules, or pyoderma gangrenosum-like lesions (cutaneous aphthosis).
- Intermittent, symmetric oligoarthritis (40% to 70%) is the most common; ankylosing spondylitis or arthralgias may occur.
- Central nervous system (CNS; 30% in U.S. and 5% in Turkey) meningeal findings including headache, fever, and stiff neck can occur. Cerebellar ataxia, pseudobulbar palsy, and dementia occur with involvement of the brainstem.
- Vascular involvement (25% to 30%), arterial and venous, of all sizes may cause systemic arterial vasculitis (aneurysms and occlusions), pulmonary artery vasculitis, venous occlusions (including superficial, deep, cerebral, portal, and mesenterial veins), pulmonary embolus, right ventricle thrombosis, and Budd-Chiari syndrome.
- GI involvement is more common in Japanese individuals; ulcerative lesions primarily involve distal ileum and cecum, but any region can be affected. GI lesions tend to perforate or bleed and may recur after surgery.

ETIOLOGY

The etiology of Behçet's disease is unknown. An immune-related vasculitis, a perivascular inflammation, or both are thought to lead to many of the manifestations of Behçet's disease. Multiple triggers for this process have been investigated, including herpes simplex virus infection, streptococcal antigen, and others.

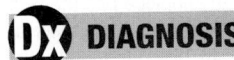

DIAGNOSIS

According to the International Study Group for Behçet's disease, the diagnosis of Behçet's disease is established when oral ulcerations recur at least three times in one 12-mo period plus at least two of the following conditions in the absence of other systemic diseases:
- Recurrent genital ulceration
- Eye lesions
- Skin lesions
- Positive pathergy test (erythematous papules or pustules [>2 mm in diameter] at sterile needle injection sites after 24 to 48 hours)

DIFFERENTIAL DIAGNOSIS

- Inflammatory bowel disease (ulcerative colitis and Crohn's disease)
- Sprue disease
- Herpes simplex infection
- Benign aphthous stomatitis
- Cyclic neutropenia
- Acquired immune deficiency syndrome (AIDS)
- Systemic lupus erythematosus
- Reiter's syndrome
- Ankylosing spondylitis
- Hypereosinophilic syndrome
- Sweet's syndrome
- Lichen planus
- Pemphigoid

WORKUP

The diagnosis of Behçet's disease is a clinical diagnosis. Laboratory tests and x-ray imaging may be helpful in working up the complications of Behçet's disease or excluding other diseases in the differential.

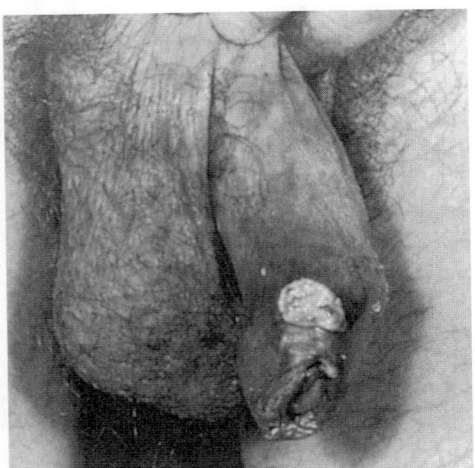

FIGURE 1-52 Behçet's syndrome. Painful preputial ulcer in a male patient with superficial thrombophlebitis, oral ulcers, and bowel vasculitis. (From Canoso J: *Rheumatology in primary care,* Philadelphia, 1997, WB Saunders.)

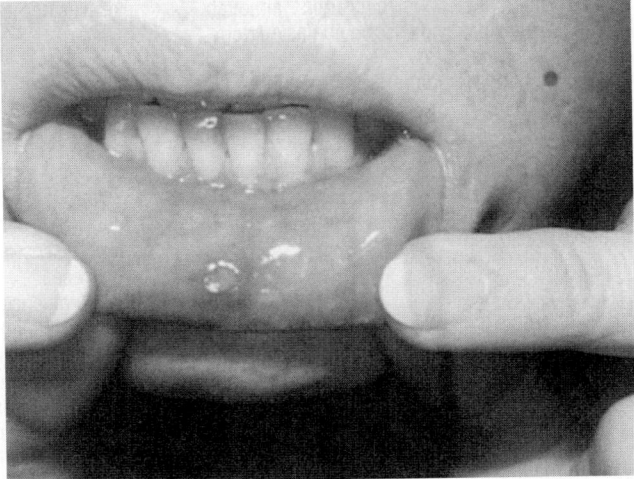

FIGURE 1-53 Behçet's syndrome. Painful aphthous inner lower lip ulcer in a 30-yr-old Chinese woman with relapsing oral and genital ulcers and uveitis. She responded well to low-dose prednisone plus colchicine. (From Canoso J: *Rheumatology in primary care,* Philadelphia, 1997, WB Saunders.)

LABORATORY TESTS

No diagnostic laboratory tests for Behçet's disease exist. The measurements of T cell proliferative response to heat shock protein (HSP) and impaired fibrinolytic activity have been proposed for the diagnosis of Behçet's disease, but the value of testing has not been confirmed.

IMAGING STUDIES

CT scan, MRI, and angiography are useful for detecting CNS and vascular lesions.

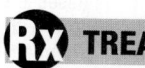 **TREATMENT**

Treatment is directed at the patient's clinical presentation and complications (e.g., mucocutaneous lesions, ocular lesions, arthritis, GI, CNS, or vascular lesions).

NONPHARMACOLOGIC THERAPY

Supportive care and rest during flares, and moderate exercises such as swimming or walking when symptoms improve or disappear

ACUTE GENERAL Rx

- Oral and genital ulcers:
  1. Topical and intralesional corticosteroids (e.g., triamcinolone acetonide ointment applied tid)
  2. Tetracycline tablets 250 mg dissolved in 5 cc water and applied to the ulcer for 2 to 3 min
  3. Colchicine 0.5 to 1.5 mg/day PO
  4. Thalidomide 100 to 300 mg PO daily
  5. Dapsone 100 mg PO daily
  6. Pentoxifylline 300 mg/day PO
  7. Azathioprine 1 to 2.5 mg/kg/day PO
  8. Methotrexate 7.5 to 25 mg/wk PO or intravenously

  9. Interferon alfa-2a and interferon alfa-2b (generally given 3 to 19 million units three times weekly)
- Ocular lesions:
  1. Anterior uveitis is treated by an ophthalmologist with topical corticosteroids (e.g., betamethasone drops 1 to 2 drops tid); topical injection with dexamethasone 1 to 1.5 mg has also been tried
  2. Infliximab 5 mg/kg single dose
  3. Cyclosporine A (5 mg/kg/day) with or without prednisone or azathioprine 1 to 2.5 mg/kg/day PO
- CNS disease:
  1. Chlorambucil 0.1 mg/kg/day is used in the treatment of posterior uveitis, retinal vasculitis, or CNS disease; patients not responding to chlorambucil can be tried on cyclosporine 5 to 7 mg/kg/day.
  2. In CNS vasculitis, cyclophosphamide 2 to 3 mg/kg/day is used. Prednisone can be used as an alternative.
- Arthritis:
  1. NSAIDs (e.g., ibuprofen 400 to 800 mg tid PO or indomethacin 50 to 75 mg/day PO)
  2. Sulfasalazine 1 to 3 g/day PO is an alternative treatment
- GI lesions:
  1. Sulfasalazine 1 to 3 g/day PO
  2. Prednisone 40 to 60 mg/day PO
- Vascular lesions:
  1. Prednisone 40 to 60 mg/day PO
  2. Cytotoxic agents as mentioned previously
  3. Heparin 5000 to 20,000 U/day followed by oral warfarin

CHRONIC Rx

- Chronic therapy is usually continued for approximately 1 yr after remission.

- Surgery may be indicated in patients with complications of bowel perforation, vascular occlusive disease, and aneurysm formation.

DISPOSITION

- The aphthous oral ulcers last 1 to 2 wk, recurring more frequently than genital ulcers.
- 25% of Japanese patients with ocular lesions become blind.
- The disease course is unpredictable.
- The morbidity of Behçet's disease comes primarily from ocular and cutaneous involvement; however, mortality relates primarily to large-size vessel involvement and CNS diseases.

REFERRAL

If the diagnosis of Behçet's disease is suspected, a referral to dermatology, rheumatology, and ophthalmology is indicated because the disease is so rare.

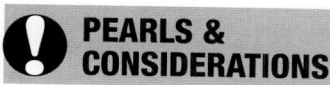 **PEARLS & CONSIDERATIONS**

COMMENTS

- The pathergy test refers to the formation of an erythematous papule or pustule of ≥2 mm after oblique insertion of a sterile 20- or 25-gauge needle into the skin after 24 to 48 hours.
- Because of the rarity of this disease, data from controlled, prospective, randomized clinical trials are lacking.

SUGGESTED READINGS
available at www.expertconsult.com

AUTHOR: **MONZR M. AL MALKI, M.D.**

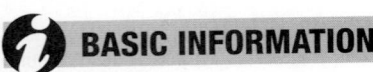

BASIC INFORMATION

DEFINITION

Acute peripheral facial (seventh) nerve palsy

SYNONYMS

Idiopathic facial paralysis

ICD-9CM CODES
351.0

EPIDEMIOLOGY & DEMOGRAPHICS

INCIDENCE: 20-30 cases per 100,000
PEAK INCIDENCE: People >70 yr and pregnant females, especially during the third trimester and/or 1 wk postpartum
PREDOMINANT SEX AND AGE: Sexes are equally affected. Median age is 40 yr.
RISK FACTORS: Diabetes, older age, pregnancy.

PHYSICAL FINDINGS & CLINICAL PRESENTATION

- Dependent on location of facial nerve injury. Onset is usually acute to subacute over hours of unilateral facial paralysis with maximal weakness at 3 wk. One third of patients demonstrated incomplete paralysis, whereas the remaining two thirds had complete paralysis. Recovery is present within the first 6 mo.
- Based on the following criteria: Diffuse facial nerve involvement depicted by paralysis of the facial muscles, along with variable involvement of taste over the anterior two thirds of the tongue or altered secretion of the lacrimal and salivary glands.
  - The degree of involvement is dependent on proximity of facial nerve involvement and involvement of associated branches.

ETIOLOGY

Most cases of Bell's palsy are thought to be secondary to a viral inflammatory/immune mechanism of injury. Herpes simplex virus is thought to be the most common viral pathogen, followed by herpes zoster. Other infectious causes include EBV, CMV, adenovirus, rubella, and mumps.

DIAGNOSIS

DIFFERENTIAL DIAGNOSIS

- Lyme disease: Facial nerve palsy is the most common cranial neuropathy associated with Lyme meningitis. May be unilateral or bilateral.
- HIV
- Ramsay-Hunt syndrome: Facial nerve paralysis associated with ipsilateral zoster oticus
- Parotid gland tumors
- Trauma/temporal bone fracture
- Meningeal processes
  - Infectious: Lyme (mentioned earlier), HIV, syphilis, leprosy, tuberculosis

- Inflammatory: sarcoid, Sjögren, Guillain-Barré syndrome
  - Carcinomatous: breast, lung, lymphoma
- Congenital: Mobius syndrome
- Melkerson-Rosenthall syndrome:
- Brainstem stroke: Affecting the nucleus or fascicle of the seventh nerve

WORKUP

Typically not indicated for most cases because it is a clinical diagnosis based on historical and examination details. May be necessary in those patients with complete injury or lack of any recovery or in whom the diagnosis of Bell's palsy is uncertain.

LABORATORY TESTS

Not typically recommended. However, if the diagnosis of Bell's palsy versus facial nerve paralysis from secondary causes is in question (especially if the facial paralysis is bilateral), the following are reasonable:
- Lyme antibody followed by Western blot for positive cases
- ACE level
- Glycosylated hemoglobin
- HIV
- VDRL
- ESR

ELECTRODIAGNOSTIC TESTING

May be performed 2 wk after onset to assess prognosis. Facial motor response remains normal for the first 3 days following injury and then rapidly decreases depending on severity of lesion. Facial motor study may be performed at 10 days and compared to contralateral side. A motor response that is 10% the amplitude of the unaffected side has been defined as a critical value in one study in which recovery was poor when associated with 90% degeneration. EMG can be used to visualize any motor units in the affected muscles that would assess the integrity of the facial nerve.

IMAGING STUDIES

Not usually indicated.
- Brain MRI in certain cases where the temporalis branch is spared of the facial nerve resulting in the patient able to wrinkle the forehead
- Brain MRI with gadolium: Indicated when other cranial nerve palsies are present or in whom a meningeal process is suspected
- CT temporal bone: Trauma cases or indicated in those cases where the facial paralysis is complete and the surgeon is considering decompression.

TREATMENT

NONPHARMACOLOGIC THERAPY

- Reassurance that most patients have a full recovery and that the patient did not sustain a stroke.

- Eye patch: To prevent corneal drying/abrasion and subsequent ulceration.
  - Lacrilube to eye at night and artificial tears during the day.

ACUTE GENERAL Rx

- Typically consists of steroids (based on early findings of inflammation and swelling during decompression studies) and antiviral therapy (predicated on findings of herpes simplex virus in the endoneurial fluid)
- Two high-quality randomized trials assessed efficacy of early (<72 hr) treatment with glucocorticoids alone, antiviral treatment alone, and combination therapy of Bell's palsy. Glucocorticoid treatment alone was effective, while antiviral therapy showed no benefit when given either alone or with concomitant glucocorticoid therapy.
  - Largest study compared prednisolone (60 mg daily) versus valacyclovir (1000 mg 3 times daily × 7 days) versus combination therapy versus placebo with 72 hr of presentation.
  - At 1-year follow-up, time to recovery was shorter in prednisolone-treated group, while valacyclovir therapy efficacy did not differ from placebo. No added benefit was seen with combination therapy.
- Treatment guidelines, in lieu of above, recommend prednisone 60 to 80 mg/day for 1 wk.
  - Some authors still recommend treatment with valacyclovir (1000 mg 3 times daily for 1 wk) despite lack of clinical evidence.
- Surgical decompression: Not currently recommended.
  - AAN Practice Parameter (2001) concluded there was insufficient evidence to make any recommendation regarding surgical decompression for Bell's palsy.

CHRONIC Rx

Botulinum toxin may be used in cases of hemifacial spasm.

DISPOSITION

- 71% of patients had complete recovery.
- 85% show recovery at 3 wk.
- 13% had slight sequelae.
- 16% had residual weakness, synkinesis, or contracture.
- Prognosis is favorable if recovery is seen within the first 3 wk.
- Recurrence rate is 7%. Average time to recurrence was 10 yr.

REFERRAL

- Neurologist if clinical diagnosis is in question
- Ophthalmologist if concern for corneal abrasion or ulceration

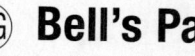

PEARLS & CONSIDERATIONS

COMMENTS

- Assess wrinkling of forehead (Fig. 1-54). If present on affected side, need to ensure that the facial weakness is not central.
- Assess for other cranial nerve deficits or long-tract signs because brainstem fascicular lesions of the seventh nerve can show peripheral facial pattern of weakness.

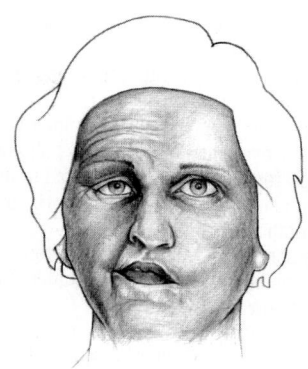

FIGURE 1-54 The patient with Bell's palsy (facial nerve palsy) will demonstrate an unwrinkled forehead, widely opened eyes (with weakness of eyelid color), flattening of the nasolabial fold, and a droop of the corner of the mouth. (From Remmel KS et al: *Handbook of symptom-oriented neurology,* ed 3, St Louis, 2002, Mosby.)

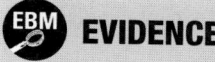 **EVIDENCE**

available at www.expertconsult.com

SUGGESTED READING

available at www.expertconsult.com

AUTHOR: **JOHN SLADKY, M.D.**

B

Diseases and Disorders

I

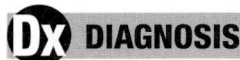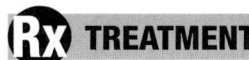

BASIC INFORMATION

DEFINITION

This is a common cause of anterior shoulder pain characterized by an inflammatory process that involves the long head of the biceps tendon as well as its sheath within the bicipital groove. The tendon involvement can be intra-articular from its attachment to the superior glenoid labrum as it runs across the glenohumeral joint and extra-articular as it runs in the bicipital or intertubercular groove (Fig. 1-55).

SYNONYMS

Bicipital tendonitis
Bicipital tenosynovitis
Biceps tendinosis

ICD-9-CM CODES

726.12 Bicipital tenosynovitis

EPIDEMIOLOGY & DEMOGRAPHICS

INCIDENCE: 41% of complete rotator cuff tears have concomitant biceps tendonitis
PREVALENCE: Common but prevalence uncertain
PREDOMINANT AGE: 18 to 35 yr old
RISK FACTORS: Athletes involved in throwing sports, swimming, contact sports, weight lifting, gymnastics, martial arts, repetitive overhead movements among carpenters, electricians, mechanical wheelchair users

PHYSICAL FINDINGS & CLINICAL PRESENTATION

- Pain referred to the anterior shoulder
- Pain that worsens at night
- A history of trauma may or may not be present
- Pain on lifting, pulling, and repetitive overhead reaching
- Most common physical exam finding is tenderness over bicipital groove by palpating the biceps tendon 3 to 6 cm below the anterior acromion and felt most easily in 10° of internal rotation
- Yergason's test—pain on biceps tendon area on resisted supination of pronated forearm with elbow at 90 degrees
- Speed's test—pain on the biceps tendon area on resisted forward flexion of the shoulder with elbows and arms fully supinated and extended

ETIOLOGY

- Primary—of unknown cause and the inflammation is specific to the intertubercular groove without any associated shoulder pathology
- Secondary—associated with other pathologic conditions such as rotator cuff disease, impingement syndrome, SLAP (Superior Labrum from Anterior to Posterior) injuries, presence of spurs or any systemic inflammatory disease involving the shoulders

DIAGNOSIS

DIFFERENTIAL DIAGNOSIS

- Impingement syndrome
- Rotator cuff tendonitis
- Subacromial bursitis
- Rotator cuff tears
- SLAP injuries
- Adhesive capsulitis
- Acromioclavicular joint arthritis
- Glenohumeral joint arthritis
- Cervical radiculopathy
- Coracoid impingement
- Brachial plexus neuritis

WORKUP

May proceed to imaging modalities

IMAGING STUDIES

- X-ray plain films are usually normal in primary tendinopathy; special views of the bicipital groove may demonstrate presence of spurs
- Musculoskeletal ultrasound evaluates dynamic movements of the biceps tendon; it is 49% sensitive but 91% to 97% specific; use in both diagnosis and treatment
- CT/MRI Arthrography are early techniques used to reliably identify shoulder pathology
- MRI is a non-invasive way of getting detailed images of the biceps tendon and other shoulder structures such as the superior labrum and rotator cuff structures and identify pathologies that may or may not coexist
- Arthroscopy is the gold standard technique for diagnosis and treatment.

TREATMENT

It is often necessary to establish whether the tendonitis is primary or secondary to address certain aspects of the treatment. Initial conservative treatment is usually very successful.

NONPHARMACOLOGIC THERAPY

Ice, rest from overhead physical activities, physical therapy after acute phase

ACUTE GENERAL Rx

Nonsteroidal anti-inflammatory drugs (NSAIDs) are good adjuncts to treatment that expedites the recovery process by decreasing edema, inflammation, and pain.

CHRONIC Rx

- If with persistent pain or severe night symptoms that fail to resolve after 6 to 8 wk of conservative treatment, corticosteroid injections may be considered
- Injection into the tendon sheath, with care not to inject into the biceps tendon, may have good to excellent results; best done under ultrasound guidance
- Subacromial steroid injections can address tendonitis secondary to impingement
- Glenohumeral joint injection delivers the steroids directly to the intra-articular portion of the biceps that is often irritated
- Gradual biceps and rotator cuff strengthening with physical therapy if symptoms have decreased
- Low-power laser therapy has reported beneficial effects but disputes exist

DISPOSITION

- Usually self-limited with conservative measures

FIGURE 1-55 Anatomic location of the long head of the biceps tendon with surrounding structures of the shoulder. (Illustration printed in Roberts et al: *Clinical procedures in emergency medicine*, ed 5, 2009, Saunders.)

Site of inflammation
Bursa
Greater tuberosity of the humerus
Biceps tendon
Bicipital groove
Biceps
Lesser tuberosity of the humerus
Scapula

- If pain persists after 3 mo, referral to orthopedic surgery
- Surgical options are tendon debridement, release of constricted synovial sheath, tenodesis, or tenotomy.
- Tenodesis is done by moving the attachment to relieve pressure of the irritated tendon; results to better strength and cosmesis but requires longer rehab; consider for younger active patients
- Tenotomy consists of cutting the long head of the biceps tendon prior to its intra-articular superior labral insertion; technically simple procedure with short rehabilitation but deformity, weakness and cramping may occur; consider for older patients
- Can progress to tendon rupture resulting to a "Popeye deformity" (Fig. 1-56)

REFERRAL

- Refer to physical therapy early in the phase of conservative treatment
- Refer to orthopedics if symptoms persist beyond 3 to 4 mo

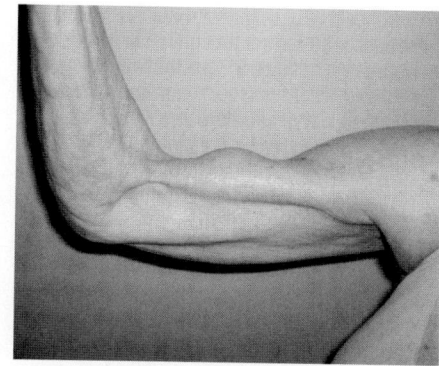

FIGURE 1-56 Popeye deformity after a biceps tendon rupture. (Illustration borrowed from Fernandez et al FIGURE 4, PAGE 7. Seminarios de la Fundación Española de Reumatologia Maniobras exploratorias del hombro doloros martes, 13 jul 2010, Elsevier.)

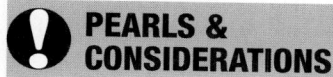

❗ PEARLS & CONSIDERATIONS

COMMENTS

A complete rotator cuff tear almost always involves the biceps tendon as its intra-articular portion gets exposed to the overlying acromion, which causes further impingement and pain.

PREVENTION

After corticosteroid injection, patient should not return immediately to vigorous physical activities that could potentially progress into a biceps tendon complete tear.

SUGGESTED READINGS

available at www.expertconsult.com

AUTHOR: **CRISOSTOMO R. BALIOG, JR., M.D.**

B

Diseases and Disorders

I

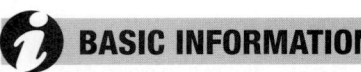

BASIC INFORMATION

DEFINITION

Bipolar disorder is an episodic, recurrent, and frequently progressive condition in which the afflicted individual experiences at least one episode of mania, characterized by at least 1 wk of continuous symptoms of elevated, expansive, or irritable mood, in association with three or four of the following symptoms:
- Decreased need for sleep
- Grandiosity
- Pressured speech
- Subjective or objective flight of ideas
- Distractibility
- Increased level of goal-directed activity
- Problematic behavior

Most individuals with bipolar disorder also experience one or more episodes of major depression over their lifetimes or have symptoms of a depressive episode commingled with those of mania (mixed episode).

SYNONYMS

Manic-depression
Cycloid psychosis

ICD-9CM CODES
296.4-6 Circular manic, circular depressed, circular type mixed

EPIDEMIOLOGY & DEMOGRAPHICS

INCIDENCE: 0.016% to 0.021%
PREVALENCE (IN U.S.): 0.4% to 1.6%; bipolar spectrum disorders: 2.8% to 6.5%
PREDOMINANT SEX: Equal distribution among male and female
PREDOMINANT AGE: Lifelong condition with age of onset 14 to 30 yr
PEAK INCIDENCE: Onset in 20s
GENETICS:
- Concordance rates for monozygotic twins: 0.7 to 0.8; for dizygotic twins: 0.2
- Risk of affective disorder in offspring with one affected parent with bipolar disorder: 27% to 29%; with two affected parents: 50% to 74%
- Heritability estimate of 0.85
- No specific causal mutations have been identified. Genome-wide association analyses have suggested a role for *ANK3, CACNA1C.* and a gene at 3p21.1 and implicated ion channelopathies in pathogenesis of bipolar disorder.

PHYSICAL FINDINGS & CLINICAL PRESENTATION

- Mania associated with:
  - Psychomotor activation that is usually goal directed but not necessarily productive
  - Increase in goal-directed activity and excessive involvement in activities leading to unexpected adverse outcomes
  - Elevated, euphoric, and frequently labile mood
  - Decreased need for sleep
  - Flight of ideas with rapid, loud, pressured speech

- Psychosis may occur, with delusions, hallucinations, and formal thought disorder
- Depressive episodes resembling major depressive disorder (see "Depression, Major"); however, atypical features (hypersomnia, weight gain) may be present
- Mixed states, characterized by activation, irritability, and dysphoria, also possible

KEY DIAGNOSTIC CRITERIA DISTINGUISHING BIPOLAR I DISORDER FROM BIPOLAR II DISORDER*:

Manic episode (Bipolar I Disorder)
- Distinct period during which there is an abnormally and persistently elevated, expansive, or irritable mood lasting at least 1 wk (or less if hospitalization is required)
- Must be accompanied by at least three of the following symptoms (four if mood is only irritable): inflated self-esteem or grandiosity, decreased need for sleep, pressured speech, racing thoughts, distractibility, increased involvement in goal-directed activity or psychomotor agitation, excessive involvement in pleasurable activities with a high potential for painful consequences
- Symptoms do not meet criteria for a mixed episode
- Disturbance must be sufficiently severe to cause marked impairment in social or occupational functioning or to require hospitalization, or it is characterized by the presence of psychotic features
- Symptoms not due to direct physiological effect of medication, general medication condition, or substance abuse

Hypomanic episode (Bipolar II Disorder)
- Distinct period during which there is an abnormally and persistently elevated, expansive, or irritable mood lasting at least 4 days
- Must be accompanied by at least three of the following symptoms (four if mood is only irritable): inflated self-esteem or grandiosity, decreased need for sleep, pressured speech, racing thoughts, distractibility, increased involvement in goal-directed activity or psychomotor agitation, excessive involvement in pleasurable activities with a high potential for painful consequences
- Hypomanic episodes must be clearly different from the person's usual nondepressed mood, and there must be a clear change in functioning that is not characteristic of the person's usual functioning
- Changes in mood and functioning must be observable by others. In contrast to a manic episode, a hypomanic episode is not severe enough to cause marked impairment in social or occupational functioning or to require hospitalization, and there are no psychotic features
- Symptoms not due to direct physiological effect of medication, general medication condition, or substance abuse

---

*Criteria are from the American Psychiatric Association, *Diagnostic and statistic manual of mental disorders,* 4th ed. rev.: *DSM-IV-R,* Washington, DC: 2000, American Psychiatric Association.

ETIOLOGY

Hypotheses:
1. Abnormalities of receptor and membrane function
2. Alteration of cAMP, MAP kinase, protein kinase C, arachidonic acid cascade, and glycogen synthase kinase-3 signal transduction pathways
3. Alteration in cell survival pathways

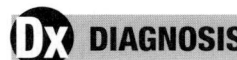

DIAGNOSIS

DIFFERENTIAL DIAGNOSIS

- Secondary manias caused by medical disorders (e.g., hyperthyroidism, AIDS, stroke, Cushing syndrome).
- First onset of mania after age 50 yr suggestive of secondary mania.
- Less severe, and possibly distinct, conditions of bipolar type II and cyclothymia
- Comorbid substance abuse or dependency may confound diagnosis and treatment.
- Presentation can be confused with schizophrenia or paranoid psychosis.

WORKUP

- History
- Physical examination
- Mental status examination
- Mood Disorder Questionnaire (MDQ)

LABORATORY TESTS

Because of high rate of secondary manias, initial evaluation to confirm health of all major organ systems (routine chemistries, complete blood count, urinalysis, sedimentation rate)

IMAGING STUDIES

- Consider brain imaging if late onset or if neurologic examination is abnormal.
- Neuroimaging may show evidence of ventricular enlargement or increased white matter hyperintensities; changes in amygdala, frontal cortex, and striatal volume also reported.

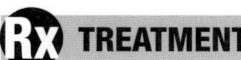

TREATMENT

NONPHARMACOLOGIC THERAPY

- Cognitive-behavioral and family-focused psychoeducational psychotherapy to help patients cope with consequences of the disease, improve adherence with medications, and identify possible environmental triggers
- Bright light therapy in the northern latitudes in individuals exhibiting a seasonal pattern of winter depression
- Lifestyle "regularization"

ACUTE GENERAL Rx

- First-line agents for acute mania: lithium 1500 to 1800 mg/day (0.8 to 1.2 mEq/L), valproate 1000 to 1500 mg/day (50 to 125 ng/ml), carbamazepine 600 to 800 mg/day (4 to 12 micrograms/ml), oxcarbazepine 900 to 2400 mg/day, olanzapine 10 to 20 mg/day, risperidone 2 to 4 mg/day, quetiapine 350 to

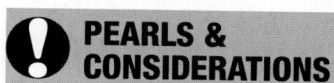 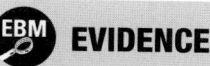

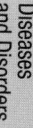

800 mg/day, ziprasidone 80 to 120 mg/day, or aripiprazole 10 to 30 mg/day.
- Useful adjuncts to acute treatment: benzodiazepines: lorazepam 1 to 2 mg q4h, clonazepam 1 to 2 mg q4h.
- Traditional antidepressants can induce manic episodes and exacerbate mania in mixed episodes.
- Lamotrigine can have acute antidepressant benefit, but appears more effective in prophylaxis of future episodes.

CHRONIC Rx

- Goal of long-term treatment: prevention of relapse or episode recurrence
- Best agents for prophylaxis of mania: lithium, valproate, and olanzapine (carbamazepine/oxcarbazepine possibly beneficial)
- Best agents for prophylaxis of depression: lamotrigine and lithium
- Role of atypical antipsychotics in maintenance unclear
- Long-term use of antidepressants: frequently destabilizes patient and leads to more frequent relapses

DISPOSITION

- Course is variable.
- More than 90% of patients having a single manic episode are likely to experience others.
- Uncontrolled manic or depressive episodes can lead to additional episodes.
- Lithium shown to specifically decrease suicidal risk.
- Psychosocioeconomic consequences of both mania and depression can be severe and disabling.

REFERRAL

- If use of antidepressant contemplated
- If patient is severely manic, rapid cycling, or suicidal or is in a bipolar, mixed episode

PEARLS & CONSIDERATIONS

COMMENTS

- All patients presenting with depression should be asked about past personal and family history of mania and hypomania; 70% of bipolar patients have previously been misdiagnosed.

- Prompt recognition of the earliest signs of mania in a given individual (e.g., decreased need for sleep, increased rate of speech) allows earlier intervention and a better likelihood of preventing a full episode.
- Bipolar disorder in children frequently manifests as behavioral disinhibition, but current consensus indicates that the condition is overdiagnosed in this age group.
- Patients treated with atypical antipsychotic agents should be carefully monitored for development of metabolic syndrome.

PATIENT/FAMILY EDUCATION

Information available at www.NMHA.org/ and www.dbsalliance.org/.

EVIDENCE

available at www.expertconsult.com

SUGGESTED READINGS

available at www.expertconsult.com

AUTHOR: **VICTOR I. REUS, M.D.**

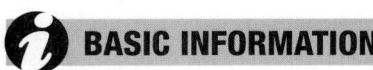

BASIC INFORMATION

DEFINITION

A bite wound can be animal or human, accidental or intentional.

ICD-9CM CODES
879.8 Bite wound, unspecified site

EPIDEMIOLOGY & DEMOGRAPHICS

- Bite wounds account for 1% of emergency department visits.
- More than 1 million bites occur in human beings annually in the U.S.
- Dog bites account for 85% to 90% of all bites and result in 10 to 20 fatalities yearly in the U.S.; cat bites account for 10% to 20%. The animal typically is owned by the victim.
- Infection rates are highest for cat bites (30% to 50%), followed by human bites (15% to 30%) and dog bites (5%).
- The extremities are involved in 75% of bites.

PHYSICAL FINDINGS & CLINICAL PRESENTATION

- The appearance of the bite wound is variable (e.g., puncture wound, tear, avulsion).
- Cellulitis, lymphangitis, and focal adenopathy may be present in infected bite wounds.
- Patient may have fever and chills.

ETIOLOGY

- Increased risk of infection: human and cat bites, closed-fist injuries, wounds involving joints, puncture wounds, face and lip bites, bites with skull penetration, bites in immunocompromised hosts
- Most frequent infecting organisms:
  1. *Pasteurella* spp.: responsible for majority of infections within 24 hr of dog *(P. canis)* and cat *(P. multocida, P. septica)* bites
  2. *Capnocytophaga canimorsus* (formerly DF-2 bacillus): a gram-negative organism responsible for late infection, usually after dog bites
  3. Gram-negative organisms *(Pseudomonas, Haemophilus)*: often found in human bites
  4. *Streptococcus* spp., *Staphylococcus aureus*
  5. *Eikenella corrodens* in human bites

DIAGNOSIS

DIFFERENTIAL DIAGNOSIS

- Bite from a rabid animal (often the attack is unprovoked)
- Factitious injury

WORKUP

- Determination of the time elapsed since the patient was bitten, status of rabies immunization of the animal, and underlying medical conditions that might predispose the patient to infection (e.g., DM, immunodeficiency)
- Documentation of bite site, notification of appropriate authorities (e.g., police department, animal officer)

LABORATORY TESTS

- Generally not necessary
- Hct if there has been significant blood loss
- Wound cultures (aerobic and anaerobic) if there is evidence of sepsis or victim is immunocompromised; cultures should be obtained before irrigation of the wound but after superficial cleaning

IMAGING STUDIES

Radiographs are indicated when bony penetration is suspected or if there is suspicion of fracture or significant trauma; they are also useful for detecting foreign bodies (when suspected).

TREATMENT

NONPHARMACOLOGIC THERAPY

- Local care with debridement, vigorous cleansing, and saline irrigation of the wound; debridement of devitalized tissue
- High-pressure irrigation to clean bite wound and ensure removal of contaminants (e.g., use saline solution with a 30- to 35-ml syringe equipped with a 20-gauge needle or catheter with tip of syringe placed 2 to 3 cm above the wound)
- Avoid blunt probing of wounds (increased risk of infection)
- If the animal is suspected to be rabid: infiltrate wound edges with 1% procaine hydrochloride, swab wound surface vigorously with cotton swabs and 1% Benz alcuronium solution or other soap, and rinse wound with normal saline

ACUTE GENERAL Rx

- Avoid suturing of hand wounds and any wounds that appear infected
- Puncture wounds should be left open
- Give antirabies therapy and tetanus immune globulin (250 to 500 units IM in limb contralateral to toxoid) and toxoid (adult or child older than 5 yr: 0.5 ml DT given IM, child <5 yr 0.5 ml DPT IM) as needed

- Use empiric antibiotic therapy in high-risk wounds (e.g., cat bite, hand bites, face bites, genital area bites, bites with joint or bone penetration, human bites, immunocompromised host): amoxicillin-clavulanate 875 to 1000 mg bid for 7 days or cefuroxime 500 mg bid for 7 days
- In hospitalized patients, IV antibiotics of choice are cefoxitin 1 to 2 g q6h, ampicillin-sulbactam 1.5 to 3 g q6h, ticarcillin-clavulanate 3 g q6h, or ceftriaxone 1 to 2 g q24h
- Penicillin allergy: animal bite (doxycycline or moxifloxacin or trimethoprim/sulfamethoxazole with either clindamycin or metronidazole); human bite (moxifloxacin plus clindamycin trimethoprim/sulfamethoxazole plus metronidazole)
- Prophylactic therapy for persons bitten by others with HIV and hepatitis B (see Section V)

DISPOSITION

- Prognosis is favorable with proper treatment.
- Important prognostic factors are type and depth of wound, which compartments are entered, and pathogenicity of inoculated bacteria.
- Punctures that are difficult to irrigate adequately, carnivore bites over vital structures (arteries, nerves, joints), and tissue crushing that cannot be debrided have a worse prognosis.
- In general, human bites have a higher complication and infection rate than do animal bites.
- Nearly 50% of the anaerobic gram-negative bacilli isolated from human bite wounds may be penicillin resistant and beta-lactamase positive.

REFERRAL

- Hospitalization and IV antibiotic therapy for infected human bites; bites with injury to joints, nerves, or tendons; or any animal bites unresponsive to oral therapy.
- Human bites with tendon involvement should go to operating room for washout.
- In the outpatient setting, bite wounds should be reevaluated within 48 hr to assess for signs of infection.

SUGGESTED READING
available at www.expertconsult.com

AUTHOR: **FRED F. FERRI, M.D.**

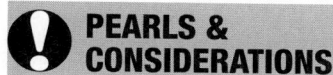

BASIC INFORMATION

DEFINITION

There are two major classes of arthropods: insects and arachnida. This chapter focuses on the class arachnida. Arachnid bites consist of bites caused by:
- Spiders
- Scorpions
- Ticks

ICD-9CM CODES

E905.1 Venomous spiders (black widow spider, brown spider, tarantula)
E905.2 Scorpion
989.5 Bites of venomous snakes, lizards, and spiders; tick paralysis
E906.4 Bite of nonvenomous arthropod; insect bite NOS

EPIDEMIOLOGY & DEMOGRAPHICS

- Spiders—ubiquitous; only three types potentially significantly harmful:
  1. Sydney funnel web spider—Australia
  2. Black widow—worldwide (excluding Alaska)
  3. Brown recluse—most common (South Central U.S.)
- Scorpions—various warm climates: Africa, Central South America, Middle East, India; Texas, New Mexico, California, and Nevada in the U.S.
- Ticks—woodlands

PHYSICAL FINDINGS & CLINICAL PRESENTATION

Spiders:
- Sydney funnel web—natracotoxin toxin
  1. Piloerection, muscle spasms leading to tachycardia, hypertension, increased intracranial pressure, coma
- Black widow—females toxic
  1. Initial reaction: local swelling, redness (two fang marks) leading to local piloerection, edema, urticaria, diaphoresis, lymphangitis
  2. Pain in limb leading to rest of body (chest pain, abdominal pain), compartment syndrome
- Brown recluse
  1. Minor sting or burn.
  2. Wound may become pruritic and red with a blanched center with vesicle. Can necrose, especially in fatty areas. Leaves eschar, which sloughs and leaves ulcer; can take months to heal.
  3. Systemic symptoms: headache, fever, chills, gastrointestinal upset, hemolysis, renal tubular necrosis, disseminated intravascular coagulation possible.

Scorpions:
- Sting leading to sympathetic and parasympathetic stimulation: hypertension, bradycardia, vasoconstriction, pulmonary edema, reduced coronary blood flow, priapism, inhibition of insulin
  - Also possible: tachycardia, arrhythmia, vasodilation, bronchial relaxation, excessive salivation, vomiting, sweating, bronchoconstriction, pancreatitis.
  - Clinically significant scorpion envenomation by Centruroides sculpturatus produces a severe neuromotor syndrome and respiratory insufficiency that often requires ICU admission.

Ticks: U.S., Europe, Asia
- Very small (<1 mm). Must be attached >36 hr to transmit disease.
- Lyme disease—most common
  1. Early: erythema migrans in 60% to 80% of cases
  2. 7 to 10 days: mild to moderate constitutional symptoms—disseminated—secondary skin lesions, fever, adenopathy, constitutional symptoms, facial palsy, peripheral neuropathy, lymphocytic meningitis, meningoencephalitis, cardiac manifestations (heart block)
  3. Late: chronic arthritis, dermatitis, neuropathy, keratitis
- Babesiosis (see "Babesiosis")
- Ehrlichiosis/Anaplasmosis (see "Babesiosis" and "Lyme Disease")

DIAGNOSIS

DIFFERENTIAL DIAGNOSIS

- Cellulitis
- Urticaria

Other tick-borne illnesses:
- Babesiosis
- Tick-borne relapsing fever
- Tularemia
- Rocky Mountain spotted fever
- Ehrlichiosis/anaplasmosis
- Colorado tick fever
- Tick paralysis
- Community-acquired cutaneous methicillin-resistant Staphylococcus aureus

WORKUP

Physical examination: thorough skin examination may reveal fang marks, attached ticks, black eschar.

TREATMENT

ACUTE GENERAL Rx

Spiders:
- Sydney funnel web
  1. Pressure, immediate immobilization, supportive care, antivenin.
- Black widow
  1. Treatment based on severity of symptoms; bite is rarely fatal.
  2. All should receive oxygen, IV, cardiac monitor, tetanus prophylaxis.
  3. Symptomatic/supportive therapy.
  4. 10% calcium gluconate for muscle cramps (controversial).
  5. Antivenin only for more severe reactions; it carries a risk of anaphylaxis.
     - Dose: one vial in 100 ml 0.9% saline over 20 to 30 min.
     - Skin test before use.
     - Give antihistamines with use.
- Brown recluse
  1. Pain management, tetanus, supportive treatment.
  2. No consensus regarding best treatment; some evidence for hyperbaric oxygen.

Scorpions:
- Fluids, supportive care, species-specific antivenin (equine based, risk of serum sickness) is controversial.
- IV administration of scorpion-specific F(ab')2 antivenom has been reported effective in resolving the clinical syndrome within 4 hours and reducing the need for concomitant sedation with midazolam and reducing the levels of circulating unbound venom.

Ticks:
- Prophylactic: tick >36 hr: single dose of doxycycline 200 mg
- Early localized disease
  1. Treatment of choice in children: amoxicillin for 14 days.
  2. Doxycycline preferred in patients with possible concurrent ehrlichiosis.
  3. Early disseminated: treatment depends on manifestation.
  4. Late disease: may require longer term or IV therapy; controversial for neurologic disease (see "Lyme disease").

DISPOSITION

- For patients with systemic reactions, send home with emergency epinephrine kit.
- If severe or anaphylactic reaction, admit and observe for 48 hr for cardiac, renal, or neurologic problems.

REFERRAL

For patients with systemic reactions, refer to allergist for immunotherapy; 95% to 98% effective in preventing anaphylaxis.

PEARLS & CONSIDERATIONS

Identification of spider should not be based on patient history (many lookalikes); spider should be brought to medical facility to be identified. Bedbugs becoming more prevalent, repeated exposure increases severity of reaction.

SUGGESTED READINGS

available at www.expertconsult.com

AUTHOR: **GAIL M. O'BRIEN, M.D.**

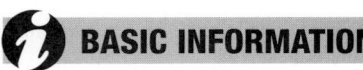

BASIC INFORMATION

DEFINITION

Most stinging insects belong to the Hymenoptera order and include yellow jackets (most common cause of reactions), hornets, bumblebees, sweat bees, wasps, harvester ants, fire ants, and the Africanized honey bee ("killer bee"). Brown recluse spiders, although not insects, are another common cause of bites (see "Bites and Stings, Arachnids"). The usual effect of a sting is intense local pain, some immediate erythema, and often a small area of edema from the injecting venom. Allergic reactions can be either local or generalized, leading to anaphylactic shock. The majority of reactions occur within the first 6 hr after the sting or bite, but a delayed presentation may occur up to 24 hr.

SYNONYMS Venom allergy

ICD-9CM CODES
989.5 Stings (bees, wasps)
989.5 Bites (fire ant, brown recluse spider)

EPIDEMIOLOGY & DEMOGRAPHICS

PREVALENCE (OF BEE STINGS AND INSECT BITES):
- Unknown.
- From 0.5% to 3.3% of the population is allergic to the venom of one or more stinging insects.
- Most anaphylactic reactions occur during summer months in those most likely to be exposed, including children, males, outdoor workers.
- Approximately half of fatal reactions occur without prior allergic response.
- Bites by fire ants and brown recluse spiders are less likely to cause systemic disease.

INCIDENCE (IN U.S.): Forty to 100 people die each year from insect sting anaphylaxis; anaphylaxis occurs more often within 10 to 30 min of a sting. Delayed reactions are rare, occurring only in <0.3% of stings.

PHYSICAL FINDINGS & CLINICAL PRESENTATION

Stings:
- Cutaneous: the skin is the most common site of an allergic reaction. Manifestations include flushing, urticaria, pruritus, and angioedema.
- Respiratory: hoarseness, difficulty speaking, choking, throat tightness or tingling may progress to stridor, laryngeal edema, laryngospasm, and bronchoconstriction. This is the leading cause of anaphylactic death.
- Cardiovascular: tachycardia, hypotension, and arrhythmia can progress to profound hypovolemic shock. Myocardial infarction is rare. Cardiac manifestations are the second leading cause of death from anaphylaxis.
- Other symptoms: abdominal pain, nausea, vomiting, and diarrhea.

Fire ant bites:
- Initial wheal and flare response.
- Subsequent development of circularly arrayed blisters within 24 hr.
- Blisters may develop appearance of pustules, but they are not infected.

ETIOLOGY

Stings:
- Most systemic reactions to insect stings are classic immunoglobin E (IgE)–mediated reactions.
- Reactions occur in previously sensitized patients who have produced high titers of IgE antibody to insect venom antigens.
- Sensitization to wasp venom requires only a few stings and can occur after a single sting.
- Sensitization to bee venom occurs mainly in people who have been stung frequently by bees.

Bites:
- Fire ant venom contains proteins toxic to the skin.

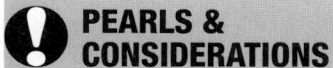

DIAGNOSIS

DIFFERENTIAL DIAGNOSIS

- Stings: cellulitis, bites
- Bites: stings, cellulitis

WORKUP

History is essential for accurate diagnosis including timing of sting or bite and type of insect (bee, wasp, spider, or ant) if known.

LABORATORY TESTS

- Skin test: either skin prick test or intradermal method with fire ant or hymenoptera venom.
- Venom skin tests and occasionally radioallergosorbent tests (RAST) to provide additional information.

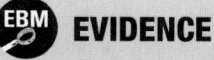

TREATMENT

ACUTE GENERAL Rx

Sting:
- Removal of the stinger most easily performed with a flat tool such as a credit card, followed by cleansing and application of ice.
- Treatment with oral antihistamines and nonsteroidal antiinflammatory medications for limited reactions. Topical corticosteroids may provide some relief of inflammation.
- Patients with previous reactions or multiple stings to the mouth or neck should be evaluated in an emergency department.
- Larger swellings may benefit from oral steroids.
- Generalized reactions should be treated with epinephrine. Antihistamines, oxygen, IV corticosteroids, beta-agonists, pressors, and IV fluids may also be beneficial for anaphylaxis.

Bite:
- Supportive care
- Application of ice
- Surveillance for secondary infection

DISPOSITION

Sting:
- Prognosis for a limited reaction is excellent.
- Subsequent anaphylaxis may occur in 35% to 65% of patients stung again.
- There is no evidence that the next sting will necessarily cause a more severe reaction. The reasons for the variable outcome include patient's age, comorbidities, time elapsed since prior exposure, dose of venom injected, and site of sting.
- Patients with a history of sting allergies should carry syringes preloaded with epinephrine (EpiPen) and oral antihistamines to take if they are stung again.
- Patients should seek additional medical care after using an autoinjector.
- Patients at risk should wear shoes and socks outdoors, remove nests near homes, keep food containers closed, and avoid wearing perfume or flowered print clothing.

Bite:
- Prognosis for fire ant bite is excellent.
- Large lesions from brown recluse spider bites may take months to heal.

REFERRAL

- Consider a referral to an allergist for venom immunotherapy (VIT).
- Risk of subsequent anaphylaxis with immunotherapy falls to <3%.
- VIT for 3 to 5 yr induces long-term protection in most patients.

PEARLS & CONSIDERATIONS

Hypersensitivity to stings is common. Reactions range from local nonallergic reaction to venom to life-threatening anaphylaxis. Venom-specific immunotherapy is highly effective in decreasing subsequent anaphylaxis. Although venom immunotherapy is currently indicated only for systemic reactions, investigation is underway to assess efficacy for prevention of large local reactions, which can result in significant morbidity.

EVIDENCE

available at www.expertconsult.com

SUGGESTED READINGS
available at www.expertconsult.com

AUTHOR: **JENNIFER JEREMIAH, M.D.**

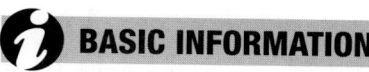

BASIC INFORMATION

DEFINITION

Injury resulting from snake biting a human.

ICD-9CM CODES
989.5 Venomous poisoning

EPIDEMIOLOGY & DEMOGRAPHICS

- 45,000 snakebites occur annually in the U.S. Of the 4000-6000 caused by poisonous snakes, approximately 5 to 12 result in fatality (i.e., <1% to 2%). Children, the elderly, and those in whom treatment has been delayed are at highest risk.
- In the U.S., at least one species of poisonous snake has been identified in every state except Alaska, Hawaii, and Maine (Fig. 1-57). The majority of venomous snakes are members of the family Crotalidae, which includes rattlesnakes, copperheads, and cottonmouths. The Elapidae family, which includes the coral snake, accounts for the remainder. Coral snakes account for less than 1% of venomous snakebites in the US.

PHYSICAL FINDINGS & CLINICAL PRESENTATION

In addition to local tissue injury, envenomation may affect the renal, neurologic, gastrointestinal, vascular, and coagulation systems. Symptoms vary widely depending on type of envenomation. Species-specific signs and symptoms follow.

CROTALIDAE (PIT VIPERS): Signs and symptoms:
- Fang punctures (see "Diagnosis")
- Pain within 5 min
- Edema within 30 min
- Erythema of site and adjacent tissues/serous or hemorrhagic bullae, ecchymosis and/or lymphangitis over the ensuing hours

If no edema or erythema is manifested within 8 hr after a confirmed Crotalid snakebite, it is safe to assume envenomation did not occur. (Roughly 25% of cases do not involve envenomation.) In general, rattlesnake bites are more severe than those of the other snakes in the Crotalid family.

Systemic manifestations may include:
- Mild to moderate manifestations: nausea/vomiting, perioral paresthesias, metallic taste, tingling of fingers or toes (especially with rattlesnake bites), and/or fasciculations (local or generalized).
- Severe manifestations: hypotension (due to increased vascular permeability), mental status change, respiratory distress, tachycardia, acute renal failure, rhabdomyolysis, and coagulopathies including intravascular hemolysis and disseminated intravascular coagulation.

ELAPIDAE (CORAL SNAKES): Signs and symptoms:
- Local symptoms are far less pronounced (little or no pain/swelling immediately after the bite).
- Systemic symptoms predominate, but onset may be delayed for up to 12 hr. Examples include:
  - Cranial nerve palsies featuring ptosis, dysphagia, or dysarthria
  - Tremors
  - Intense salivation
  - Loss of DTRs and respiratory depression (late manifestations)

ETIOLOGY

- The majority of victims are young men who purposefully attempt to handle or harm a snake that formerly had no intention of biting them.
- Victims are frequently intoxicated at the time of the bite.

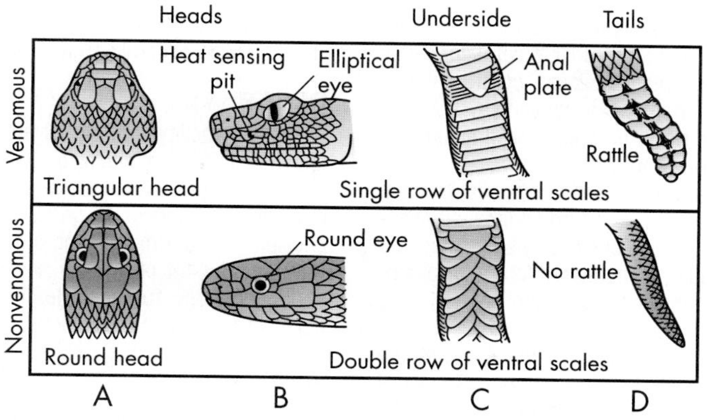

DIAGNOSIS

DIFFERENTIAL DIAGNOSIS

- Harmless snakebite
- Scorpion bite
- Insect bite
- Cellulitis
- Laceration or puncture wound
- Necrotizing fasciitis

NOTE: Harmless snakebites are usually characterized by 4 rows of small scratches (teeth in upper jaw) separated from two rows of scratches (teeth in lower jaw). This is in distinction to venomous snakebites, which should have paired puncture wounds produced by the snake's fangs, whether other teeth marks are noted.

WORKUP

An estimated 25% of venomous snakebites do not result in envenomation, but all cases of suspected envenomation should be observed 8 hr or longer:
- Determine the severity of envenomation using clinical and laboratory evaluation.
- A nonstandardized classification system for grading envenomations was developed by Russell in 1964:
  - Minimal: confined to the site of the bite, no significant systemic symptoms or signs, no laboratory abnormalities
  - Moderate: manifestations extend beyond the site of the bite, but no life-threatening systemic symptoms
  - Severe: extensive limb involvement, severe systemic symptoms and signs, or significant laboratory abnormalities (including abnormal coagulation studies)

Determination of severity is based on the most severe symptom, sign, or laboratory result. Continual reassessment is indicated throughout the observation period because grading may change.

LABORATORY TESTS

- For all suspected envenomations, obtain CBC (with peripheral smear and platelet count), DIC screen (PT/INR, PTT, fibrinogen, fibrin degradation products, D-dimer), ECG, serum electrolytes, BUN, Cr, and urinalysis.
- For more severe bites, consider LFTs, sedimentation rate, creatine kinase (rule out rhabdomyolysis), ABG, and type and crossmatch.
- Other: consider CXR in cases with severe envenomation or in patients >40 yr with underlying cardiopulmonary disease; x-ray of bite site for retained fangs (poor sensitivity); head CT if concern is raised for intracranial hemorrhage.

TREATMENT

ACUTE GENERAL Rx

IN THE FIELD: For a suspected snakebite:
- Transport immediately to nearest medical facility. No treatments in the field should delay travel to the nearest facility where an antivenom can be given if necessary.
- Immobilize affected part below level of the heart.
- Remove any constricting items. Local pressure has been advocated for elapid bites, particularly in Australia, as a means of delaying absorption of neurotoxins. However, crotalid bites are far more common in the U.S., and these frequently have tissue-necrosing venom, which will yield more damage with

---

Heads / Underside / Tails

Venomous

Heat sensing pit — Elliptical eye — Anal plate — Rattle

Triangular head — Single row of ventral scales

Nonvenomous

Round eye — Round head — Double row of ventral scales — No rattle

A   B   C   D

FIGURE 1-57 Comparison of pit vipers and nonvenomous snakes. Rattle in **D** (*top* panel) applies to rattlesnakes only. (**A** to **D**, From Sullivan JB et al: North American venomous reptile bites. In Auerbach PS [ed]: *Wilderness medicine: management of wilderness and environmental emergencies,* ed 3, p. 684, St Louis, 1995, Mosby.)

local pressure. Thus, as with incision and suction techniques, use by those without specialized training in snakebite management is discouraged.

- Do not apply ice; keep victim warm.
- Avoid alcohol, stimulants (caffeine), or agents that can suppress mental status.

IN THE HOSPITAL:

- Record vital signs: BP, HR, T, RR, and O_2 sat
- Establish intravenous access.
- Obtain time of bite and description of snake if possible.
- Obtain and initiate reconstitution of appropriate antivenom. (Antivenoms are typically supplied in powder form and must be reconstituted before administration. If using older antivenoms, this process can take up to 1 hr, so it is recommended that it be initiated as soon as the patient arrives in the ED).
  - Inspect site of bite for fang marks, local symptoms.
  - Delineate margins of erythema/edema with a marker.
  - Measure circumference of bitten part at 2 or more proximal sites and compare with unaffected limb; repeat every 15 to 20 min; assess for extension of erythema/edema.
  - Neurologic examination.
  - Gauge the severity of the bite and decide whether administration of antivenom is necessary.
  - Obtain past medical history; ask about allergies to horse serum in those previously treated for snake bite.
  - For minimal envenomation without progressive manifestations:
    1. Clean and immobilize affected part.
    2. Immunize against tetanus.
    3. Observe patient for at least 8 hr. If, at the end of this interval, local and systemic sequelae are absent and lab values remain normal, the likelihood of significant envenomation is low, and the patient can be discharged from the acute setting.
- Patients who have progressive symptoms (local or systemic) or moderate to severe envenomation should be considered for antivenom. The high incidence of allergic reactions using horse serum antivenoms was sited in the past arguing against its use in less severe cases but newer antivenoms derived from sheep serum are less allergenic and may be suitable even for mild envenomations.
- Contact Poison Control: 1-800-222-1222

Once the decision is made to use antivenom:

- Prepare epinephrine 0.5 to 1.0 mg (0.5-1 ml of a 1:1000 solution) to be administered subcutaneously (SQ) in case of a hypersensitivity reaction to the antivenom. Some studies advocate the use of empiric prophylactic SQ epinephrine, but further study is needed. Empiric prophylactic antihistamines have not been shown to prevent reactions.

ANTIVENOM TREATMENT OF CROTALID (RATTLESNAKE, PIT VIPER, COPPERHEAD, COTTONMOUTH) ENVENOMATIONS

- Most centers now have sheep immunoglobulin-based antivenom (Crofab) for crotalid bites. Sheep-based antivenoms are very safe, but repeat administration may be necessary owing to a short half-life.
  - An initial IV loading dose of 4-6 vials (depending on the size and age of the patient and the severity of the bite) is infused over 60 min. The infusion should be given very slowly for the first 10 min to watch for allergic reaction.
  - If the patient has not responded after 1 hr, a repeat dose of 4-6 vials is indicated.
- Because of the short half-life of sheep-based antivenom, relapse may occur in up to two thirds of patients after an initial response. Consequently, it is recommended that three maintenance doses—each consisting of 2 vials—be given at 6, 12, and 18 hr following the patient's initial response to the loading dose.
- The manufacturer of Crofab maintains a 24/7 hotline: 877-377-3784
- Antivenin Crotalidae Polyvalent horse serum is no longer produced but may still be available at some pharmacies. It should be given as follows:
  - Mild symptoms: 5 vials
  - Moderate symptoms: 10 vials
  - Severe symptoms: 15 vials
  - Shock: 20 vials

ANTIVENOM TREATMENT OF ELAPIDAE (CORAL SNAKE) ENVENOMATIONS

- Production of horse serum–based coral snake antivenom was discontinued in 2006 (horse serum–based antivenoms are being phased out due to much higher risk of hypersensitivity). All stock is expired as of October 31, 2008, except for lot 4030026, which received a 2-yr extension until October 31, 2010. After that date, one option will be to seek compassionate release of expired stock in conjunction with your local Poison Control Center. Prior experience suggests that translucent samples are more likely to have retained potency than cloudy samples. A potent, safe, sheep-based antivenom for elapid bites exists and is being used internationally but is not yet approved in the U.S. Another option is to contact a zoo that cares for exotic snakes and obtain Mexican coral snake or Australian Tiger snake antivenom, although efficacy for North American coral snake envenomation is unproved.
- For confirmed coral snake bites, antivenom should be administered immediately if available. If coral snake bite is only suspected, the patient should be monitored for 12 hr for evidence of envenomation, and treated if it occurs.
- If there are no systemic symptoms at the time of administration, start with 3 vials. If symptoms evolve, repeat with 5 vials.

- If systemic symptoms are already present, an initial dose of 6-10 vials is recommended.

TREATMENT OF NONNATIVE (EXOTIC) SNAKE BITES

- For bites by exotic or nonnative snakes, contact a poison control center or your local zoo. (Zoos with exotic snakes are required to maintain a supply of snake-specific antivenom on their premises.)

Other considerations:

- Initial dose of antivenom should be repeated until progression of symptoms has abated, but observation of bitten part should be continued for another 48 hr.
- Dosage of antivenom is based on typical envenomation rather than age or weight, so dose is the same for children and adults.
- Pregnancy is not a contraindication to antivenom. The rate of miscarriage is significantly lower in pregnant patients treated with antivenom.
- Immunize against tetanus if no booster within past 5 yr; if never immunized, give immunoglobulin as well as toxoid.
- Manage pain as needed (acetaminophen, codeine, morphine).
- Avoid sedation in Mojave rattlesnake, Eastern diamondback rattlesnake, and coral snake bites as all can have more systemic than local effects.
- Antibiotics reserved for moderate to severe contamination or definite infection; broad-spectrum coverage to include gram negatives preferred (i.e., amp-sulbactam or quinolone derivatives).
- Antivenom is most effective when given within 4 hr of the bite and least effective if delayed beyond 12 hr. Systemic symptoms (coagulopathy, CNS effects, etc.) respond better to treatment than do local symptoms (erythema/edema, bullae, etc.).
- Although local wound effects can be severe, wound management should not take precedence over antivenom administration. Some studies suggest that even in the case of compartment syndrome, antivenom may be more effective than fasciotomy, although both may be necessary.

DISPOSITION

Prognosis is good with prompt evaluation and treatment. All patients who receive antivenom should be monitored in an ICU setting.

REFERRAL

To medical facility with ICU for administration of antivenom. The approach to snakebites should be multidisciplinary and may include surgery for management of wounds, orthopedic surgery for possible compartment syndrome, hematology for management of anemia and coagulopathy, and nephrology for possible renal failure. All cases of snake bites should also be reported to Poison Control and the local health department as data are limited.

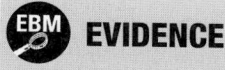

PEARLS & CONSIDERATIONS

COMPLICATIONS

- Allergic reactions were very frequent with horse serum antivenoms, up to 20% anaphylaxis and the majority of patients suffering some degree of serum sickness.
- Anaphylaxis occurs within 30 minutes and should be treated by immediately stopping the infusion to manage the symptoms of anaphylaxis, including epinephrine, SQ or IM initially and IV if needed, diphenhydramine IV and hydrocortisone IV. If the anaphylactic symptoms can be managed and the envenomation is severe, the infusion can then be resumed.
- The most frequent complication of treated envenomations is serum sickness; occurs 7 to 14 days after antivenom administration and is characterized by fever, rash, arthralgias, and lymphadenopathy. It can be treated with PO prednisone 60 mg/day, tapered over 7 to 10 days.
- Injuries also result from:
  - Tourniquet placement, which should be avoided
  - Ice application (cryotherapy), which can worsen tissue damage
- National Poison Control hotline: 800-222-1222

B

EBM EVIDENCE

available at www.expertconsult.com

SUGGESTED READINGS

available at www.expertconsult.com

AUTHOR: **LAURA H. McPEAKE, M.D.**

Diseases and Disorders

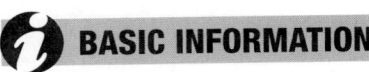

BASIC INFORMATION

DEFINITION

Bladder cancer is a heterogeneous spectrum of neoplasms ranging from non–life-threatening, low-grade, superficial papillary lesions to high-grade invasive tumors, which often have metastasized at the time of presentation. It is a field change disease in which the entire urothelium from the renal pelvis to the urethra may be susceptible to malignant transformation. The three types of bladder cancer are transitional cell carcinoma (TCCa), squamous cell carcinoma, and adenocarcinoma.

ICD-9CM CODES	
Primary:	188.9
Secondary:	198.1
CIS:	233.7
Benign:	223.3
Uncertain behavior:	236.7
Unspecified:	239.4

EPIDEMIOLOGY & DEMOGRAPHICS

Each year approximately 54,000 new cases are diagnosed and more than 12,000 deaths are attributed to bladder cancer. Overall, bladder cancer is the sixth most prevalent malignancy in the U.S.

Until 1990, the incidence of bladder cancer in the U.S. was rising. Since 1990, the incidence of bladder cancer is decreasing at a rate of 0.8% per year (1.2% among men and 0.4% among women).

PREDOMINANT SEX: In males, it is the fourth most common cancer, accounting for 10% of all cancers. In females, it is the eighth most common cancer, accounting for 4% of all cancers.

RISK: The lifetime risk of developing bladder cancer is 2.8% in white males, 0.9% in black males, 1% in white females, and 0.6% in black females.

Smoking:

- Users of "black" tobacco in place of "blond" tobacco have a twofold to threefold increase in developing bladder cancer.
- Smoking risk is based on consumption:
  - A twofold to threefold increase for subjects smoking at least 10 cigarettes per day
  - The risk increases again when the daily consumption rises above 40 to 60 cigarettes per day
- Smokers of low-tar and nicotine cigarettes have a lower risk when compared with higher tar and nicotine cigarettes.
- Those who smoke unfiltered cigarettes have a 50% increased risk of bladder cancer compared with those who smoke filtered cigarettes.
- Pipe smokers have a lower risk of bladder cancer compared with cigarette smokers.
- Cigars, snuff, and chewing tobacco, although implicated in nonurologic cancers, are not believed to influence bladder cancer risk.

Diet:

- Diets rich in beef, pork, and animal fat increase risk of bladder cancer.

- There is no indication that consumption of non-beer alcoholic drinks contributes to bladder cancer development.
- Beer consumption has been linked to bladder cancer development as a result of the presence of nitrosamines in the beer. Nitrosamines have also been implicated in the development of rectal cancer.
- Drinking coffee is not believed to contribute to bladder cancer risk. There is additional evidence that coffee consumption is protective for colorectal cancers, possibly by diminishing fecal transit time.

PEAK INCIDENCE: Incidence increases with age: higher after age 60 yr, uncommon younger than 40 yr.

GENETICS: It is thought to be multifactorial in etiology, involving both genetic and environmental interactions. Overall, approximately 20% to 25% of the male population in the U.S. with bladder cancer is estimated to have the disease as a result of occupational exposure.

DISTRIBUTION: In North America, transitional cell carcinomas comprise 93%, squamous cell carcinomas comprise 6%, and adenocarcinomas account for 1% of bladder cancers.

PATHOGENESIS: Two pathways exist for bladder cancer (TCCa):

1. Papillary superficial disease occasionally leading to invasive cancer (75%)
2. Carcinoma-in-situ (CIS) and solid invasive cancer with high risk of disease progression (25%)

Two distinct forms of "superficial cancer" exist:

1. T_a: Papillary low-grade tumor with a high rate of recurrence; disease progression occurs in 5%.
2. T_1: Higher grade papillary tumor that infiltrates the lamina propria; often associated with flat CIS that may involve the urothelium diffusely. Disease progression occurs in 30% to 50%.

Subdivided into:

- T_{1a}: Penetration of tumor up to the muscularis mucosa; disease progression in 5.3%
- T_{1b}: Penetration of tumor through the muscularis mucosa; disease progression 53%

Flat CIS:

- Entirely different and separate pathway of cancer development whose mechanism is manifested by dysplasia, which leads to the occurrence of poorly differentiated malignant cells that replace or undermine the normal urothelium and extend along the plane of the bladder wall. It penetrates the basement membrane and lamina propria in 20% to 30% of cases and is associated with the development of solid tumor growth. A defect in chromosome 17p53 occurs in 50% of the cases.

At presentation, 72% of cancers are localized to the bladder, 20% of the cancers extend to the regional lymph nodes, and 3% present with distant metastases. Eighty percent of superficial TCCa recur, with up to 30% progressing to a higher stage or grade. Younger patients most commonly develop low-grade papillary noninvasive TCCa and are less likely to have recurrences when compared with older patients with

similar lesions. Involvement of the upper tracts with tumor occurs in 25% to 50% of the cases.

STAGING (BASED ON THE TNM SYSTEM):

T_0	No tumor in specimen
T_{is}	CIS
T_a	Papillary TCCa noninvasive
T_1	Papillary TCCa into lamina propria
T_2	TCCa invasive of superficial muscle
T_{3a}	Invasive of deep muscle
T_{3b}	Invasive of perivesical fat
T_{4a}	Invasive of adjacent pelvic organ
T_{4b}	Invasive of pelvic wall with fixation

Invasive of nodal status:

N_0	No nodal involvement
N_{1-3}	Pelvic nodes
N_4	Nodes above bifurcation
N_x	Unknown

Invasive of metastatic status:

M_0	No distant metastases
M_1	Distant metastases
M_x	Unknown

MOLECULAR EPIDEMIOLOGY: TCCa is usually a field change disease with tumors arising at different times and sites in the urothelium, suggesting a polyclonal etiology of bladder cancer. Bladder cancers have been associated with abnormalities on chromosomes 1, 4, 11, 5, 7, 3, 9, 21, 18, 13, 8; with alterations in suppressor genes *P53*, retinoblastoma gene, and *P16*; and with alterations on oncogenes H-ras and epidermal growth factor receptor.

PHYSICAL FINDINGS & CLINICAL PRESENTATION

- Gross, painless hematuria
- Microhematuria
- Frequency, urgency, occasional dysuria

With locally invasive to distant metastatic disease, the presentation can include:

- Abdominal pain
- Flank pain
- Lymphedema
- Renal failure
- Anorexia
- Bone pain

ETIOLOGY

Bladder cancer is a potentially preventable disease associated with specific etiologic factors:

- Cigarette smoking is associated with 25% to 65% of cases. The risk of developing a TCCa is two to four times higher in smokers than in nonsmokers, and that risk persists for many years, being equal to nonsmokers only after 12 to 15 yr of smoking abstinence. Smoking tobacco is associated with tumors that are characterized by higher histologic grade, increased tumor stage, increase in the numbers of tumor present, and increased tumor size.
- Occupational exposures: dye workers, textile workers, tire and rubber workers, petroleum workers.
- Chemical exposure: O-toluidine, 2-naphthylamine, benzidine, 4-amino-biphenyl, and nitrosamines.
- Exposure to herpes papilloma virus type 16.

Squamous carcinomas are associated with:

- Schistosomiasis
- Urinary calculi

B

I

- Indwelling catheters
- Bladder diverticula

Miscellaneous causes:
- Phenacetin abuse
- Cyclophosphamide
- Pelvic irradiation
- Tuberculosis

Adenocarcinomas are associated with:
- Exstrophy
- Endometriosis
- Neurogenic bladder
- Urachal abnormalities
- As a secondary site for distant metastases from other organs (e.g., colon cancer)

Dx DIAGNOSIS

- History and physical examination.
- Urinalysis.
- Cystoscopy with bladder barbotage and biopsy. Fluorescence cystoscopy offers improvement in the detection of flat neoplastic lesions such as carcinoma in situ.
- Transurethral resection of bladder tumor(s).
- There is insufficient evidence to determine whether a decrease in mortality rate from bladder cancer occurs with hematuria testing, urinary cytology, or a variety of other tests on exfoliated urinary cells or other substances.
- In addition to urinary cytology and bladder barbotage, BTA, NMP22, and fibrin degradation products have been approved by the FDA as bladder cancer tumor markers. No marker has general, widespread acceptance because the results are affected by the presence of stents, recent urologic manipulation, stones, infection, bowel interposition, and prostatitis, creating false-positive results.

DIFFERENTIAL DIAGNOSIS

- Urinary tract infection
- Frequency-urgency syndrome
- Interstitial cystitis
- Stone disease
- Endometriosis
- Neurogenic bladder

LABORATORY TESTS

- Urine cytology.
- Urine telomerase: telomerase activity in voided urine or bladder washings determined by the telomeric repeat amplification protocol (TRAP) assay. This test has been reported to accurately detect the presence of bladder tumors in men. It represents a potentially useful noninvasive diagnostic innovation for bladder cancer detection in high-risk groups such as habitual smokers or in symptomatic patients.

RADIOLOGIC TESTS

- IVP, renal ultrasound, retrograde pyelography, CT scan, and MRI.
- One or a combination of studies can be used. In the absence of skeletal symptoms, bone scan is not recommended.

Rx TREATMENT

NONPHARMACOLOGIC THERAPY

- Initially, transurethral resection of bladder tumor (TURBT) (Fig. 1-58)
- Loop biopsy of the prostatic urethra if high-grade TCCa is suspected
- If superficial disease, follow-up protocol with repeat TURBT and/or the use of intravesical agents is recommended
- For advanced bladder cancer, radical cystectomy with urethrectomy (unless orthotopic diversion is planned) and either ileal loop conduit or orthotopic diversion

BLADDER PRESERVATION APPROACHES: After cystectomy for muscle invasive disease, 50% or more of the patients will develop metastases. Most patients develop metastases at distant sites, a third relapse locally. Bladder preservation management is offered in individuals who refuse surgery or who might not be suitable radical cystectomy patients. Bladder-sparing protocols include extensive TURBT or partial cystectomy with external-beam or interstitial radiotherapy and systemic chemotherapy. Radiotherapy as a single treatment modality is not

effective. The best predictor of successful bladder preservation is a complete response after the combination of initial TURBT and two cycles of CMV (cisplatin, methotrexate, vinblastine) chemotherapy used with stages T$_2$ to T$_{3a}$.

INDICATIONS FOR PARTIAL CYSTECTOMY:
- Tumor within a bladder diverticulum
- Solitary, primary, and muscle-invasive or high-grade lesion of a region of the bladder that allows complete excision with adequate surgical margins
- Inability to adequately resect tumor by TURBT alone because of size or location
- Tumor overlying a ureteral orifice requiring ureteral reimplantation
- Biopsy of a radiation-induced ulceration
- Palliation of severe local symptoms
- Patient refusal of urinary diversion
- Poor-risk patient who is not a diversion candidate

CONTRAINDICATIONS:
- Multiple tumors
- CIS
- Cellular atypia on biopsy
- Prostatic invasion
- Invasion of the trigone
- Inability to achieve adequate surgical margins
- Prior radiotherapy
- Inability to maintain adequate bladder volume after resection
- Evidence of extravesical tumor extension
- Poor surgical risk

ACUTE GENERAL Rx
INDICATIONS FOR INTRAVESICAL CHEMOTHERAPY:
- High-grade tumor
- Tumor size >5 cm
- Tumor multiplicity
- Presence of CIS
- Positive urinary cytologic findings after a resection
- Incomplete tumor resection

Intravesical agents: thiotepa, Adriamycin, mitomycin C, AD-32, BCG, interferon, bropirimine, Epodyl, interleukin-2, and keyhole-limpet hemocyanin. Photodynamic therapy with hematoporphyrin derivatives has also been used.

INDICATIONS FOR CYSTECTOMY:
- Large tumors not amenable to complete TURBT
- High-grade tumor
- Multiple tumors with frequent recurrences
- Diffuse CIS not responsive to intravesical chemotherapy
- Prostatic urethra involvement
- Irritative bladder symptoms with upper tract deterioration
- Muscle-invasive disease
- Disease outside the bladder

SYSTEMIC CHEMOTHERAPY: Used as neoadjuvant and adjuvant therapy for systemic disease. The most effective agents are cisplatin, methotrexate, vinblastine, Adriamycin (MVAC). Other agents include mitoxantrone, vincristine, etoposide (VP16), 5-fluorouracil, ifosfamide, Taxol, gemcitabine, Piritrexim, and gallium nitrate.

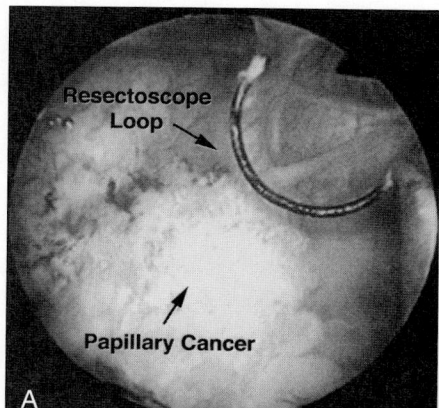

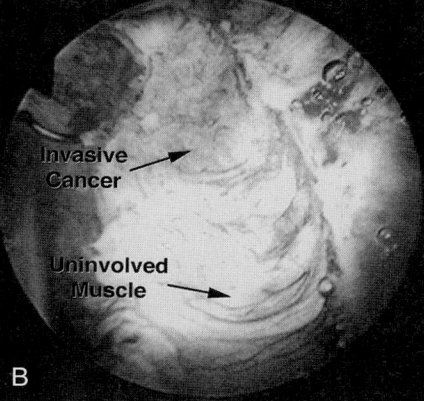

FIGURE 1-58 A, Papillary bladder cancer in right lower aspect of photo with resection loop poised to begin transurethral resection. **B,** Demonstration of grossly uninvolved muscularis propia (*bottom*) and cancer grossly invading the bladder wall (*top*). (From Abeloff MD: *Clinical oncology*, ed 3, Philadelphia, 2004, Elsevier.)

Chemotherapy in combination can provide palliation and modest survival benefit.

RADIOTHERAPY: Conflicting reports suggest that superficial bladder cancer is more sensitive to radiotherapy. Squamous changes within the tumor and secretion of human chorionic gonadotropin by the lesion are associated with poor response to radiotherapy. Only 20% to 30% of patients with invasive bladder cancer can be cured by external-beam radiation therapy alone. It is used in combination with surgery or with systemic agents to treat bladder cancer primarily in patients who are not surgical candidates or who refuse surgery.

CHRONIC Rx

FOLLOW-UP RECOMMENDATIONS FOR SUPERFICIAL BLADDER CANCER:

- Cystoscopy, bladder barbotage, and bimanual examination every 3 mo for 2 yr, then every 6 mo for 2 yr, and annually thereafter.
- Upper tract studies are based on the risk of upper tract tumor development, generally every 2 to 5 yr.

FOLLOW-UP RECOMMENDATIONS FOR ADVANCED DISEASE:

Bladder preservation:

- Cystoscopy, barbotage, bimanual examination, biopsy (when indicated), every 3 mo for 2 yr, then every 6 mo for 2 yr, yearly thereafter
- CT scan of abdomen and pelvis every 6 mo for 2 yr in addition to chest x-ray examination, liver function testing, and serum creatinine

Cystectomy with ileal loop/orthotopic bladder:

- Neobladder endoscopy and IVP yearly
- CT scan of abdomen and pelvis every 6 mo for 2 yr in addition to chest x-ray examination, liver function tests, and serum creatinine
- Loopogram every 6 mo for 2 yr, then annually

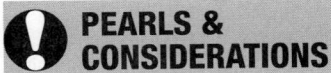

PEARLS & CONSIDERATIONS

COMMENTS

- The most useful prognostic parameters for bladder tumor recurrence and subsequent cancer progression are tumor grade, depth of tumor penetration, multifocal tumors, frequency of recurrence, tumor size, CIS, lymphatic invasion, papillary or solid tumor configuration.
- Box 1-2 describes the American Urological Association Guideline Recommendations for bladder cancer.

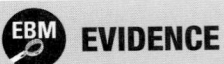 **EVIDENCE**

available at www.expertconsult.com

SUGGESTED READINGS

available at www.expertconsult.com

AUTHORS: **PHILIP J. ALIOTTA, M.D., M.S.H.A.,** and **RUBEN ALVERO, M.D.**

BOX 1-2 American Urological Association Guideline Recommendations

For all index patients:
- Standard: Physicians should discuss with the patient the treatment options and the benefits and harms, including side effects, of intravesical treatment.

For a patient who presents with an abnormal growth on the urothelium but who has not yet been diagnosed with bladder cancer:
- Standard: If the patient does not have an established histologic diagnosis, a biopsy should be obtained for pathologic analysis.
- Standard: Under most circumstances, complete eradication of all visible tumors should be performed.
- Standard: If bladder cancer is confirmed, periodic surveillance cystoscopy should be performed.
- Option: An initial single dose of intravesical chemotherapy may be administered immediately postoperatively.

For a patient with small volume, low-grade Ta bladder cancer:
- Recommendation: An initial single dose of intravesical chemotherapy may be administered immediately postoperatively.

For a patient with multifocal and/or large volume, histologically confirmed, low-grade Ta or a patient with recurrent low-grade Ta bladder cancer:
- Recommendation: An induction course of intravesical therapy with bacillus Calmette-Guérin or mitomycin C is recommended for the treatment of these patients with the goal of preventing or delaying recurrence.
- Option: Maintenance bacillus Calmette-Guérin or mitomycin C may be considered.

For a patient with initial histologically confirmed high-grade Ta, T1, and/or carcinoma in situ bladder cancer:
- Standard: For patients with lamina propria invasion (T1) but without muscularis propria in the specimen, repeat resection should be performed prior to additional intravesical therapy.
- Recommendation: An induction course of bacillus Calmette-Guérin followed by maintenance therapy is recommended for treatment of these patients.
- Option: Cystectomy should be considered for initial therapy in select patients.

For a patient with high-grade Ta, T1, and/or carcinoma in situ bladder cancer that has recurred after prior intravesical therapy:
- Standard: For patients with lamina propria invasion (T1) but without muscularis propria in the specimen, repeat resection should be performed prior to additional intravesical therapy.
- Recommendation: Cystectomy should be considered as a therapeutic alternative for these patients.
- Option: Further intravesical therapy may be considered for these patients.

From the American Urological Association, Guideline Division, http://www.auanet.org.

BASIC INFORMATION

DEFINITION

Blastomycosis is a systemic pyogranulomatous disease caused by a dimorphic fungus, *Blastomyces dermatitidis*.

ICD-9CM CODES
116.0 Blastomycosis

EPIDEMIOLOGY & DEMOGRAPHICS

INCIDENCE & PREVALENCE:
- Most patients reside in the southeastern and south central states, especially those bordering the Mississippi and Ohio River valleys, the Midwestern states, and Canadian provinces bordering the Great Lakes.
- Rare cases reported outside the U.S.

RISK FACTORS:
- Widely disseminated disease is most common in immunocompromised hosts, especially those with acquired immunodeficiency syndrome (AIDS).
- Initial infections result from inhalation of conidia into the lungs, although primary cutaneous blastomycosis has been reported after dog bites.

PHYSICAL FINDINGS & CLINICAL PRESENTATION

- Acute infection: <50% symptomatic, median incubation 30 to 45 days. Symptoms are nonspecific: mimic influenza or bacterial infection with abrupt onset of myalgias, arthralgias, chills and fever; transient pleuritic pain, cough that is initially nonproductive. Resolution within 4 wk is usual.
- Chronic or recurrent infection: indolent, progressive; includes pulmonary or extrapulmonary disease.

PULMONARY MANIFESTATIONS: Symptoms and signs of chronic pneumonia: productive cough, hemoptysis, pleuritic chest pain, weight loss, low-grade pyrexia

EXTRAPULMONARY MANIFESTATIONS:
1. Cutaneous: most common; may occur with or without pulmonary disease. Two different lesions:
   - *Verrucous:* beginning as a small papulopustular lesion on exposed body areas that may develop into an eschar with peripheral microabscesses (Fig. 1-59)
   - *Ulcerative:* Subcutaneous nodules (cold abscesses) and rarely cutaneous inoculation blastomycosis may occur
2. Bone and joint: 10% to 50% have osteolytic lesions; affects long bones, vertebrae, and ribs; lesions may present with contiguous soft tissue abscess or draining sinus that spreads to a joint, resulting in pyarthrosis
3. Genitourinary: 10% to 30%; prostatic involvement is most common and may present as obstruction; epididymis and testes may also be affected
4. Central nervous system: 5% normal host; 40% AIDS patients; meningitis and abscess formation

ETIOLOGY

Blastomyces dermatitidis exists in warm, moist soil that is rich in organic material. When these microfoci are disturbed, the aerosolized spores or conidia are inhaled into the lungs. Disease at other sites is a result of dissemination from the initial pulmonary infection; the latter may be acute or chronic.

DIAGNOSIS

DIFFERENTIAL DIAGNOSIS

PULMONARY INFECTION:
- Tuberculosis
- Bronchogenic carcinoma
- Histoplasmosis
- Bacterial pneumonia

CUTANEOUS INFECTION:
- Bromoderma
- Pyoderma gangrenosum
- *Mycobacterium marinum* infection
- Squamous cell carcinoma
- Giant keratoacanthoma

WORKUP

- Physical examination and laboratory data
- Definitive diagnosis established by culture

LABORATORY TESTS

- Presumptive diagnosis can be made by visualizing the distinctive yeast forms in clinical specimens
- Culture: on Sabouraud medium or more enriched media
  1. Aspirated material from abscesses
  2. Skin scrapings
  3. Prostatic secretions (urine culture with prostatic massage)
- Direct examination of specimens
  1. Wet preparation with 10% KOH (Fig. 1-60)
  2. Histopathology: typically demonstrates pyogranulomas; yeast identification requires special stains
- A commercial test for *Blastomyces* antigen in specimens of urine, blood, and other fluids is available

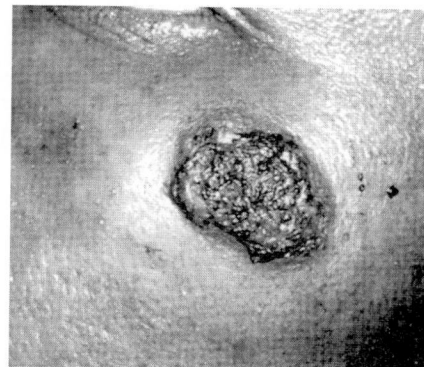

FIGURE 1-59 The typical verrucous skin lesion of blastomycosis on the cheek. Note the circumscribed edges. (From Mandell GL, Bennett JE, Dolin R: *Principles and practice of infectious diseases,* ed 6, Philadelphia, 2005, Elsevier.)

- Serologic tests: a negative test cannot exclude blastomycosis, and a positive titer should not be an indication to start treatment

IMAGING STUDIES

In chronic disease, chest radiographic findings are nonspecific, but lobar or segmental alveolar infiltrates, especially of the upper lobes, are most common and may progress to cavitation.

TREATMENT

ACUTE BLASTOMYCOSIS GENERAL Rx

- Treatment remains controversial for acute pulmonary blastomycosis.
- Because the acute form may be benign and self-limited, patients may be closely observed.
- Some patients progress to chronic infection with significant morbidity and therefore may require treatment.
- Patients who are immunocompromised or who have extrapulmonary disease or progressive pulmonary disease should be treated.

PULMONARY BLASTOMYCOSIS

- Amphotericin B (AmB) lipid formulation 3 to 5 mg/kg/day or AmB deoxycholate at 0.7 to 1 mg/kg/day for 1 to 2 wk or until improvement is noted, followed by oral itraconazole 200 mg PO tid for 3 days and then 200 mg PO bid for a total of 6 to 12 mo.
- Itraconazole 200 mg PO tid for 3 days and then once or bid for 6 to 12 mo for mild to moderate diseases.
- Fluconazole 400 to 800 mg PO once a day for those intolerant to itraconazole.

DISSEMINATED EXTRAPULMONARY BLASTOMYCOSIS

- Lipid formulation AmB 3 to 5 mg/kg/day or AmB dexoycholate 0.7 to 1 mg/kg/day for 1 to 2 wk or until improvement is noted followed by oral itraconazole 200 mg PO tid for 3 days and then 200 mg PO bid for a total of at least 12 mo for moderately severe to severe disease

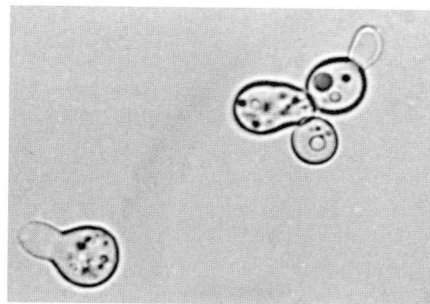

FIGURE 1-60 Yeast cells of *Blastomyces dermatitidis* in wet smear (×1000). (From Mandell GL, Bennett JE, Dolin R: *Principles and practice of infectious diseases,* ed 6, Philadelphia, 2005, Elsevier.)

- Itraconazole 200 mg PO tid for 3 days and then once or bid for 6 to 12 mo for mild to moderate diseases

CENTRAL NERVOUS SYSTEM BLASTOMYCOSIS

AmB lipid formulation at a dosage of 5 mg/kg/day over 4 to 6 wk followed by either fluconazole 800 mg/day or itraconazole 200 mg PO two to three times per day or voriconazole 200 to 400 mg PO twice a day for at least 12 mo and until resolution of CSF abnormalities.

BLASTOMYCOSIS IN IMMUNOSUPPRESSED INDIVIDUALS

- AmB as a lipid formulation 3 to 5 mg/kg/day or AmB deoxycholate 0.7 to 1 mg/kg/day for 1 to 2 wk or until improvement is noted followed by itraconazole 200 mg PO tid for 3 days and then bid as step-down therapy for at least 12 mo. Lifelong suppressive therapy with oral itraconazole 200 mg/day may be required.
- Serum itraconazole levels should be determined in all patients after they have received treatment with this agent for 2 wk.
- Surgery may be indicated for drainage of large abscesses.

DISPOSITION

- Before antifungal therapy, the disease had a progressive course with eventual extrapulmonary disease and a mortality rate >60%.
- Relapse rate for patients treated with AmB is 5%; relapse is more common in AIDS patients.

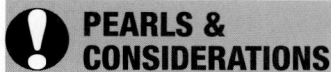

PEARLS & CONSIDERATIONS

- *Blastomyces dermatitidis* may mimic other diseases.
- Colonization does not occur as with *Candida* and *Aspergillus* species.

SUGGESTED READINGS
available at www.expertconsult.com

AUTHOR: **SAJEEV HANDA, M.D.**

BASIC INFORMATION

DEFINITION

Blepharitis is an acute or, most often, chronic inflammation of the eyelid margins that is often refractory to treatment.

SYNONYMS

Eye lid infection or inflammation
Eczema of the eye lids
Dermatoblepharitis
Angular blepharitis

ICD-9CM CODES
373.0 Blepharitis

EPIDEMIOLOGY & DEMOGRAPHICS

- Common in children, particularly those with atopic dermatitis and eczema
- Adults with seborrhea involving the eyelids

PHYSICAL FINDINGS & CLINICAL PRESENTATION

- Chronically infected lids are usually diffusely erythematous, with collarettes (fibrin exudate) at the base of the lashes (Fig. 1-61).

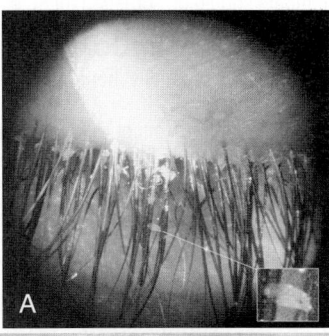
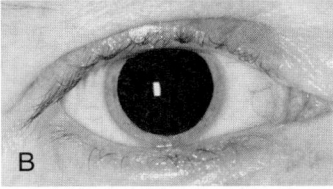

FIGURE 1-61 A, Seborrheic blepharitis. The typical scales (scurf) are translucent and easily removed. **B,** Staphylococcal blepharitis showing the typical lid margin erythema and discharge. (From Palay D [ed]: *Ophthalmology for the primary care physician,* St Louis, 1997, Mosby.)

- Lid margins thicken over time, with associated loss of eyelashes (madarosis), misdirected growth of lashes (trichiasis), and overflow or inspissation of the meibomian glands.
- Associated conjunctivitis with erythema, edema but no discharge.
- Chalazia may develop.
- Superficial punctate erosions of the inferior corneal epithelium are common.
- More severe findings, such as corneal pannus, ulcerative keratitis, or lid ectropion, are less common.

ETIOLOGY

Multiple: bacterial and nonbacterial causes
- Staphylococcal infection most common but streptococcal, Moraxella, and other bacterial infections; viral infections (e.g., herpes simplex, herpes zoster, *Molluscum contagiosum*); and a number of ecoparasites, including pediculosis, may cause blepharitis
- Seborrheic dermatitis
- Rosacea
- Dry eye (keratoconjunctivitis sicca): decrease in tear volume
- Meibomian gland dysfunction
- Two categories of blepharitis:
  1. Anterior blepharitis, most often associated with staphylococcal infection or seborrheic dermatitis
  2. Posterior blepharitis, associated with meibomian gland dysfunction

NOTE: Blepharitis patients have normal skin microflora in greater amounts (mostly *S. epidermidis* and *P. acnes*). (*S. aureus* and *S. epidermidis* can be cultured in 10% to 35% and 90% to 95% of healthy persons, respectively.)

DIAGNOSIS

DIFFERENTIAL DIAGNOSIS

- Keratoconjunctivitis sicca
- Eyelid malignancies
- Herpes simplex blepharitis
- Molluscum contagiosum
- Phthiriasis palpebrarum
- Phthirus pubis (pubic lice)
- Demodex folliculorum (transparent mites)
- Allergic blepharitis

WORKUP

Scrapings of the eyelids to show polymorphonuclear leukocytes and gram-positive cocci

LABORATORY TESTS

Eyelid cultures and antibiotic sensitivity testing (usually not done unless patient fails to respond to initial treatment regimen)

TREATMENT

B

NONPHARMACOLOGIC THERAPY

- Alkaline soaps may be beneficial; alcohol and some detergents remove surface lipids and microflora.
- Hot compresses applied to closed lids for 5 to 10 min: heat loosens debris from lid margins and increases meibomian gland fluidity.
- Firm massage of the lid margins to enhance the flow of secretions from glands, followed by cleansing of the lids with cotton-tipped applicators dipped in a 50:50 mixture of baby shampoo and water.
- Lashes and lid margins scrubbed vigorously while the eyelids are closed, followed by thorough rinsing.
- Following local massage and cleansing, the mainstay of treatment is application of topical antibiotic ointment to the eyelid margins.
  1. Most effective topical antibiotics include bacitracin, erythromycin, aminoglycoside and fluoroquinolone ophthalmic ointments.
  2. Ointment is applied 1 to 4 times daily, depending on the severity, for 1 to 2 wk, followed by once daily, at bedtime, for another 4 to 8 wk until all signs of inflammation have disappeared.

For patients with rosacea:
1. Tetracycline 250 mg orally 4 times daily or doxycycline 100 mg orally bid along with local treatment for several months

Recalcitrant cases with antibiotic resistance:
1. Vancomycin eye drops 1%
2. Ciprofloxacin or ofloxacin eyedrops

CHRONIC Rx

By definition, this is a chronic condition for which there is frequently no cure.

Some newer agents being evaluated are antioxidant flavonoid-type compounds (resveratrol, silymarin); azelaic acid and glycolic acid (antikeratinizing effects); and adapalene gel (anti-inflammatory properties and an antiproliferative effect on keratinocytes).

DISPOSITION

This condition may be refractory to treatment.

REFERRAL

To an ophthalmologist if patient fails to respond to local therapy.

SUGGESTED READINGS
available at www.expertconsult.com

AUTHORS: **GLENN G. FORT, M.D., M.P.H.,** and **DENNIS J. MIKOLICH, M.D.**

Diseases and Disorders

I

BASIC INFORMATION

DEFINITION

Body dysmorphic disorder (BDD) is a somatoform disorder characterized by preoccupation with a slight or imagined defect in physical appearance that causes clinically significant distress or impairment in social, occupational, or other important areas of functioning. The appearance preoccupations are not restricted to concerns with body fat or weight in an individual with an eating disorder.

SYNONYMS

Dysmorphophobia

ICD-9CM CODES
300.7

DSM-IV CODES
300.7

EPIDEMIOLOGY & DEMOGRAPHICS

- Affects 1% to 2.4% of the general population
- Prevalence among cosmetic surgery patients (in most studies) is 7% to 15%.
- Prevalence among dermatology patients is 9% to 12%.
- Onset most commonly in adolescence
- Slightly higher prevalence among females

PHYSICAL FINDINGS & CLINICAL PRESENTATION

- Excessive preoccupation (obsession) with a perceived defect(s) in appearance that is not observable or appears slight to others. Any part of the body may be a focus of concern, although skin, hair, and nose concerns are most common. Most patients are preoccupied with multiple body areas.
- The patient usually appears physically normal; if a defect is present, it is slight, and the patient's reaction to it is.
- Most patients have poor insight or are delusional regarding the defects.
- Nearly all patients engage in repetitive behaviors such as frequent mirror checking, excessive grooming, camouflaging, skin picking, reassurance seeking, and repeatedly measuring or feeling the perceived defect.
- Nearly all experience impairment in psychosocial functioning and quality of life.
- Suicidal ideation, suicide attempts, and completed suicide appear common.

- Commonly co-occurring mental disorders are major depressive disorder, substance use disorders, social phobia, obsessive-compulsive disorder (OCD), and personality disorder.

ETIOLOGY

Likely multifactorial, with both genetic and environmental risk factors (e.g., teasing). Neuropsychological and fMRI studies indicate abnormalities in visual processing consisting of excessive focus on details rather than larger configural elements of visual stimuli.

DIAGNOSIS

Psychiatric interview
- Ask:
  1. Are you very worried about your appearance in any way? *OR:* Are you unhappy with how you look?
  2. Does this concern with your appearance preoccupy you?
  3. How much distress does this concern cause you?
  4. What effect does this concern have on your life?

DIFFERENTIAL DIAGNOSIS

- Often undiagnosed because of patient's reluctance to divulge symptoms due to shame and fear of being misunderstood (e.g., considered vain).
- OCD.
- Eating disorder
- Social phobia.
- Hypochondriasis.

WORKUP

Clinical evaluation focused on BDD symptoms and associated impairment in functioning.

TREATMENT

NONPHARMACOLOGIC THERAPY

- CBT, with a focus on cognitive restructuring, exposure and response prevention.
- Do not try to talk patients out of their concern; it is ineffective.
- Avoid cosmetic procedures.

ACUTE GENERAL Rx

Precautions/hospitalization if actively suicidal

CHRONIC Rx

- SSRIs are medication of choice; relatively high doses often needed.
- Other agents (e.g., neuroleptics, tricyclic antidepressants other than clomipramine) do not appear as beneficial.
- CBT recommended with or without SSRI.
- Support groups if available.

DISPOSITION

- Untreated BDD tends to be chronic and can lead to social isolation, school dropout, major depression, unnecessary surgery, and even suicide.
- With correct diagnosis and treatment, a majority improve.

REFERRAL

Refer for psychiatric evaluation and treatment if diagnosis is suspected.

PEARLS & CONSIDERATIONS

- In clinical settings, more than 60% have co-occurring major depressive disorder.
- Reassurance is rarely helpful.
- Patients often have an unrealistic expectation of improvement with plastic surgery, dermatologic treatment. and other cosmetic procedures.
- All patients should be screened for suicidality.

PATIENT/FAMILY EDUCATION

- Family members usually benefit from psychoeducation.
- Family support and encouragement of appropriate treatment is important.
- Phillips KA: *Understanding Body Dysmorphic Disorder: An Essential Guide.* Oxford University Press, 2009
- http://www.BDDProgram.com (http://www.rhodeislandhospital.org/RIH/Services/MentalHealth/Bodylmage/default.htm)
- Body Dysmorphic Disorder Central: http://www.BDDCentral.com

SUGGESTED READINGS
available at www.expertconsult.com

AUTHOR: **KATHARINE A. PHILLIPS, M.D.**

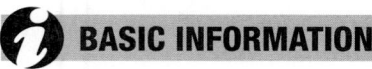

BASIC INFORMATION

DEFINITION

Primary malignant bone tumors are invasive and anaplastic and have the ability to metastasize. Most arise from the marrow (myeloma), but tumors may develop from bone, cartilage, fat, and fibrous tissues. Leukemia and lymphoma are excluded from this discussion.

FIBROSARCOMA AND LIPOSARCOMA: Extremely rare. They are similar to tumors arising in soft tissue.

OSTEOSARCOMA: A rare primary malignant tumor of bone characterized by malignant tumor cells that produce osteoid or bone. Several variants have been described: parosteal sarcoma, periosteal sarcoma, multicentric, and telangiectatic forms.

CHONDROSARCOMA: A malignant cartilage tumor that may develop primarily or secondarily from transformation of a benign osteocartilaginous exostosis or enchondroma.

EWING'S SARCOMA: A malignant tumor of unknown histogenesis.

MULTIPLE MYELOMA: A neoplastic proliferation of plasma cells.

SYNONYMS

Multiple myeloma:
1. Plasma cell myeloma
2. Plasmacytoma

ICD-9CM CODES	
203.0	Multiple myeloma
170.9	Neoplasm, bone (periosteum), primary malignant
M9180/3	Osteosarcoma
N9220/3	Chondrosarcoma
M9260/3	Ewing's sarcoma

EPIDEMIOLOGY & DEMOGRAPHICS

MULTIPLE MYELOMA:
- The most common tumor in bone
- Age at onset: usually >40 yr
- Male/female ratio of 2:1

OSTEOGENIC SARCOMA:
- Average age at onset: 10 to 20 yr
- Males afflicted more often than females
- Parosteal sarcoma in older patients

CHONDROSARCOMA:
- Age at onset: 40 to 60 yr
- Male/female ratio of 2:1

EWING'S SARCOMA: Age at onset: 10 to 15 yr

PHYSICAL FINDINGS & CLINICAL PRESENTATION

MULTIPLE MYELOMA:
- May present as a systemic process or, less commonly, as a "solitary" lesion

- Early manifestations: anorexia, weight loss, and bone pain; majority of cases present initially with back pain that often leads to the detection of a destructive skeletal lesion
- Other organ systems eventually become involved, resulting in more bone pain, anemia, renal insufficiency, and/or bacterial infections, usually as a result of the dysproteinemia typical of this disorder
- Possible secondary amyloidosis, leading to cardiac failure or nephrotic syndrome

OSTEOSARCOMA:
- Most originating in the metaphysis
- 50% to 60% around the knee
- Possible pain and swelling, but otherwise healthy patient
- Osteosarcoma in conjunction with Paget's disease, manifested primarily as a sudden increase in bone pain

CHONDROSARCOMA:
- Tumor most commonly involving the pelvis, upper femur, and shoulder girdle
- Painful swelling

EWING'S SARCOMA:
- Painful soft tissue mass often present
- Possibly increased local heat
- Midshaft of a long bone usually affected (in contrast to other tumors)
- Weight loss, fever, and lethargy

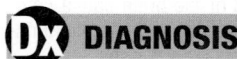

DIAGNOSIS

DIFFERENTIAL DIAGNOSIS
- Osteomyelitis
- Metastatic bone disease

LABORATORY TESTS
- Slightly elevated alkaline phosphatase in osteosarcoma
- In Ewing's sarcoma: reflective of systemic reaction; include anemia, an increase in white blood cell count, and an elevated sedimentation rate
- In multiple myeloma:
  1. Bence Jones protein in the urine
  2. Anemia and elevated sedimentation rate
  3. Characteristic dysproteinemia on serum protein electrophoresis
  4. Diagnostic feature: peak in the electrophoretic pattern suggestive of a monoclonal gammopathy
  5. Rouleaux formation in the peripheral blood smear
  6. Often presence of hypercalcemia, but alkaline phosphatase levels usually normal

IMAGING STUDIES
- Classic osteogenic sarcoma penetrates the cortex early in many cases.
  1. A blastic (dense), lytic (lucent), or mixed response may be seen in the affected bone.
  2. An aggressive perpendicular sunburst pattern may be present as a result of periosteal reaction, and peripheral Codman's triangles are often noted.
  3. Margins of the tumor are poorly defined.
- Speckled calcifications in a destructive radiolucent lesion are usually suggestive of chondrosarcoma.
- Ewing's sarcoma is characterized radiographically by mottled, irregular destructive changes with periosteal new bone formation. The latter may be multilayered, producing the typical "onion skin" appearance.
- Typical roentgenographic finding in multiple myeloma is the "punched out" lesion with sharply demarcated edges.
  1. Multiple lesions are usual.
  2. Diffuse osteoporosis may be the only finding in many cases.
  3. Pathologic fractures are common.

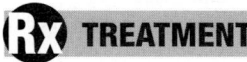

TREATMENT

The evaluation and treatment of malignant bone tumors are complicated. Diagnostic studies and treatment should be supervised by an orthopedic cancer specialist and oncologist.

DISPOSITION
- In the past 20 yr, dramatic improvements have been made in the treatment protocols for osteosarcoma with the use of adjuvant multidrug regimens and limb-sparing surgery.
- Prognosis of multiple myeloma remains poor despite new therapies.
- Prognosis for Ewing's sarcoma has improved with a combination of chemotherapy, local resection, and radiation therapy.
- Chondrosarcomas are not sensitive to chemotherapy or radiation, and prognosis depends on the grade of the tumor and the ability to obtain an adequate resection.

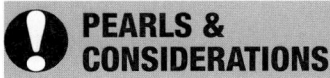

PEARLS & CONSIDERATIONS

Early diagnosis is important because most tumors have not metastasized at the time of initial presentation.

SUGGESTED READINGS
available at www.expertconsult.com

AUTHOR: **LONNIE R. MERCIER, M.D.**

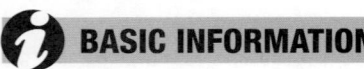

BASIC INFORMATION

DEFINITION

Borderline personality disorder (BPD) is characterized by a pervasive pattern of instability in interpersonal relationships, self-image, affect regulation, and impulse control that causes significant subjective distress or impairment of functioning. The individual must meet five or more of the following criteria:

1. Frantic efforts to avoid real or imagined abandonment
2. Unstable and intense personal relationships characterized by alternating between extremes of idealization and devaluation
3. Identity disturbance characterized by an unstable self-image
4. Impulsivity in at least two areas that are potentially self-damaging (e.g., overspending, sex, substance abuse, binge eating, reckless driving)
5. Recurrent suicidal behavior, gestures, threats, or self-mutilating behavior
6. Affective instability due to a marked reactivity of mood
7. Chronic feelings of emptiness
8. Inappropriate, intense anger or difficulty controlling anger
9. Transient, stress-related paranoid ideation or severe dissociative symptoms

ICD-9CM CODES
301.83 Borderline personality

EPIDEMIOLOGY & DEMOGRAPHICS

PREVALENCE: Affects approximately 1% to 2% of the general population and up to 10% of psychiatric outpatients
PREDOMINANT SEX: Female (3:1)
PREDOMINANT AGE: 20s
GENETICS: BPD is five times as likely if disorder is present in a first-degree relative. Increased prevalence of mood disorders and substance abuse disorders also found in first-degree relatives.
RISK FACTORS: Association with childhood physical, sexual, or emotional abuse and/or neglect

PHYSICAL FINDINGS & CLINICAL PRESENTATION

- No specific associated physical findings.
- Mental status examination may reveal affective lability.
- Clinical presentation may reveal the following:
  - A pervasive sense of loneliness and emptiness.
  - Underlying negative affect with dysphoria.
  - High frequency of multiple psychiatric disorders, especially posttraumatic stress disorder (PTSD), mood disorders, and substance use disorders. Intense emotions with difficulty returning to emotional baseline.
  - All-or-nothing, either/or cognitive style that is represented by a phenomenon known as "splitting," in which patient sees situations or people as all good or all bad.
  - Difficulty in maintaining commitment to long-term goals; history of numerous stormy relationships and multiple jobs.
  - Reacts with rage, panic, despair to actual or perceived abandonment; may present with suicidality or self-mutilating behavior in response to recent stressor.
  - Attempts to block the experience of pain, which may induce feelings of derealization, depersonalization, changes in consciousness, and/or brief psychotic reactions with delusions and hallucinations.
  - Substance use, gambling, overspending, eating binges, and/or self-mutilation as a way to escape intensely painful affect.
- Some patients may display psychotic symptoms.

ETIOLOGY

- Interaction of psychosocial adversity plus genetic factors
- Hypotheses:
  1. Genetic: increased risk if first-degree relative with BPD.
  2. Biologic: abnormalities in limbic system and other areas of the brain cause emotional dysregulation. Serotonergic functioning appears to be disturbed.
  3. Environmental: history of childhood abuse or neglect.

DIAGNOSIS

DIFFERENTIAL DIAGNOSIS

- Histrionic and narcissistic personality disorders share some common features.
- Dysthymia and other depressive disorders: requires a stability of affective symptoms not seen in BPD.
- Bipolar disorder: mood changes in BPD often triggered by stressors and less sustained than in bipolar disorder. Many patients with BPD are incorrectly diagnosed with bipolar disorder.
- Substance abuse or dependence: often induces impulsive, emotionally labile behavior.
- Posttraumatic stress disorder (PTSD): individuals with BPD often have history of trauma but do not avoid the feared stimulus or reexperience the trauma, as with PTSD.
- Mild cases of schizophrenia may superficially resemble BPD.

WORKUP

- History (helpful to gather collateral information from family and friends)
- Physical examination
- Mental status examination

LABORATORY TESTS

- Toxicology screen; substance use is common and can mimic features of personality disorders.
- Screen for HIV and other sexually transmitted illnesses.

IMAGING STUDIES

Structural and functional MRI demonstrate amygdala hyperactivity and reduced hippocampus volume. PET scans reveal reduced metabolism in prefrontal cortex. Recent PET research reveals dysregulation of endogenous opioid function. Imaging is not recommended as part of routine evaluation.

TREATMENT

NONPHARMACOLOGIC THERAPY

Dialectical behavior therapy (DBT) and mentalization-based therapy, variations of cognitive behavior therapy (CBT), and transference-focused psychotherapy, a type of psychodynamic therapy, have the most empirical support from randomized trials. The goal of DBT is to help patients control impulses and angry outbursts and to develop social skills. The emphasis of mentalization treatment is to teach patients to stand outside of their feelings and observe emotions in oneself and others. The focus of transference-focused psychotherapy is on examining the affect-laden themes that emerge in the relationship between patient and therapist.

ACUTE GENERAL Rx

Low-dose antipsychotics to control impulsivity, brief psychotic episodes.

CHRONIC Rx

- Medications have low-to-moderate effectiveness and are most effective in improving symptoms of impulsivity, mood instability, and self-destructive behavior. Effectiveness only studied for the first 3 mo of treatment.
- SSRIs if concurrent mood disorder. Higher doses may be required than for major depression.
- Low-dose antipsychotics.
- Mood stabilizers (lithium, valproate, carbamazepine, topiramate).
- In preliminary studies, omega-3 fatty acids improve irritability.

DISPOSITION

- Course is variable. The most unstable period is typically in early adulthood; the majority achieve greater stability in social/occupational functioning later in life but often continue with difficulty maintaining intimate relationships.
- No evidence of progression to schizophrenia, but there is a high incidence of concurrent major depression and other Axis I disorders.

REFERRAL

- Referral to mental health specialist:
  - For diagnosis and management.
  - Use of pharmacotherapy
  - Patient is severely impaired or suicidal

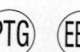
B

PEARLS & CONSIDERATIONS

COMMENTS

- Consider frequent, brief, scheduled visits for needy, demanding, or somaticizing patients with BPD.
- Validate the patient's feelings while stating the expectation of behavior control.
- Be matter-of-fact; avoid expressing extreme emotions.
- Be alert to the risk of suicide and assess suicide risk often.
- Convey a demeanor of competence but openly acknowledge minor errors.
- Have a low threshold for seeking psychiatric consultation.

PREVENTION

- There are no known ways to prevent BPD (or other personality disorders).
- Suicidality should be actively and consistently monitored.
- Benzodiazepines, narcotic analgesics, and other drugs with potential for dependency should be used rarely and with great caution, due to impaired impulse control and risk of addictive behavior.
- Patients should be asked frequently and in detail about parenting practices. Low frustration tolerance, externalization of blame for psychological distress, and impaired impulse control put children at risk for neglect or abuse.

PATIENT & FAMILY EDUCATION

National Alliance for the Mentally Ill (NAMI; http://www.nami.org) provides patient information, online chat groups, and information on support groups throughout the U.S. for people with BPD and their families.

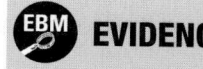 **EVIDENCE**

available at www.expertconsult.com

SUGGESTED READINGS

available at www.expertconsult.com

AUTHORS: **MITCHELL D. FELDMAN, M.D., M.PHIL.,** and **MARK ZIMMERMAN, M.D.**

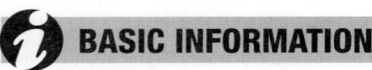

BASIC INFORMATION

DEFINITION

Botulism is an illness caused by a neurotoxin produced by *Clostridium botulinum.* Three types of disease can occur: foodborne botulism, wound botulism, and infant intestinal botulism. Recent concern has increased about a possible fourth type of disease: inhalational botulism, which does not occur naturally, but may occur as a result of bioterrorism.

SYNONYMS

Clostridium botulinum food poisoning
Botulinum toxin food poisoning
Wound botulism
Infantile botulism

ICD-9CM CODES
005.1 Botulism

EPIDEMIOLOGY & DEMOGRAPHICS

INCIDENCE (IN U.S.): Approximately 24 cases/yr of foodborne illness, 3 cases/yr of wound botulism, and 71 cases/yr of infant botulism

PHYSICAL FINDINGS & CLINICAL PRESENTATION

- Symptoms usually begin 12 to 36 hr following ingestion.
- Severity of illness is related to the quantity of toxin ingested.
- Significant findings:
  1. Cranial nerve palsies, with ocular and bulbar manifestations being most frequent (diplopia, ophthalmoplegia, ptosis, dysphagia, dysarthria, fixed and dilated pupils, and dry mouth)
  2. Usually bilateral nerve involvement that may progress to a descending flaccid paralysis
  3. Typically, absence of sensory findings; sensorium intact
  4. GI symptoms (nausea, vomiting, diarrhea, or cramps)
  5. Usually no fever
- Wound botulism
  1. Occurs mostly in injecting drug users (subcutaneous heroin injection—"skin popping") or with traumatic injury.
  2. Presentation is similar to that of foodborne disease, except for a longer incubation period and the absence of GI symptoms.
  3. Wound infection is not always apparent, but injection sites frequently reveal cellulitis, draining pus, or abscess formation.

ETIOLOGY

- Cause is one of several types of neurotoxins (usually A, B, or E) produced by *C. botulinum,*

an anaerobic, gram-positive bacillus. Spore production guarantees survival of the organism in extreme conditions. Botulinum toxin is the most powerful neurotoxin known.
- Disease results from absorption of toxin into the circulation from a mucosal surface or wound. Botulinum toxin does not penetrate intact skin.
- In foodborne variety, disease is caused by ingestion of preformed toxin. Although rapidly inactivated by heat, the toxin can survive the proteolytic environment of the stomach.
- In wound botulism, toxin is elaborated by organisms that contaminate a wound. Most cases reported are from California.
- In infant botulism, toxin is produced by organisms in the GI tract.
- Inhalational botulism has been demonstrated experimentally in primates. This manufactured form results from aerosolized toxin and has been attempted by bioterrorists.

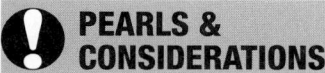

DIAGNOSIS

DIFFERENTIAL DIAGNOSIS

- Myasthenia gravis
- Guillain-Barré syndrome
- Tick paralysis
- CVA

WORKUP

- Search made for toxin and the organism (see "Laboratory Tests")
- Electrophysiologic studies (e.g., EMG) may aid in the diagnosis

LABORATORY TESTS

- Samples of food and stool are cultured for the organism.
- Food, serum, and stool are sent for toxin assay.

TREATMENT

NONPHARMACOLOGIC THERAPY

- Supportive care with intubation if respiratory failure occurs
- Debridement of the wound in wound botulism

ACUTE GENERAL Rx

- Give trivalent equine serum botulinum antitoxin as early as possible. Once a clinical diagnosis is made, antitoxin should be administered before laboratory confirmation.
  1. Give one vial by IM injection and one vial IV.
  2. The antitoxin is available from the Centers for Disease Control and Prevention [(404) 639-2206 or (404) 639-2888]; it is derived from horse serum, so there is a

significant incidence of serum sickness. A human-derived antitoxin immunoglobin is now available for infants less than 1 yr of age (BIG-IV).
  3. Skin testing (conjunctival instillation and observation for 15 min), and possible desensitization, is recommended before treatment.
- Give wound botulism patients penicillin 2 million U IV q4h.
- Babies with infantile intestinal botulism may benefit from a cathartic to mechanically clear the number of *C. botulinum* vegetative forms and spores residing in the gastrointestinal tract.

CHRONIC Rx

- Supportive
- Rehabilitation/physical therapy

DISPOSITION

- Highest mortality in the first case in an outbreak, with subsequent cases receiving rapid treatment
- Complete recovery for most individuals (this may take several weeks in severely affected individuals)

REFERRAL

Immediate for all cases to an ER and an infectious disease consultant

PEARLS & CONSIDERATIONS

COMMENTS

- Routine cooking inactivates the toxin, but spores are resistant to environmental factors. At room temperature, spores can germinate and produce toxin.
- Most outbreaks are associated with home-canned foods, especially vegetables.
- Patients must be closely monitored for progression to respiratory paralysis.
- There is increasing concern over the potential use of botulinum toxin as a biologic weapon, either by the enteric route or by aerosolization.
- Notify public health authorities immediately to alert other health care services of possible additional cases and to initiate investigation into cause and scope of outbreak.
- Recent botulism food recalls have involved canned chili, cut green beans, and olives.

SUGGESTED READINGS
available at www.expertconsult.com

AUTHORS: **GLENN G. FORT, M.D., M.P.H.,** and **DENNIS J. MIKOLICH, M.D.**

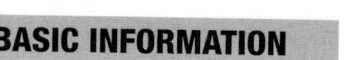

BASIC INFORMATION

DEFINITION

Brain metastases spread to the brain from cancer originating in other organs. Brain metastases are the most common intracranial tumors in adults and account for more than one half of brain tumors.

SYNONYMS

ICD-9CM CODES
198 Secondary neoplasm of other specified sites

EPIDEMIOLOGY & DEMOGRAPHICS

INCIDENCE: In the United States, an estimated 98,000 to 170,000 new cases occur each year, which represents 24% to 45% of all cancer patients. The prevalence is thought to be 120,000 to 140,000/yr. Incidence is significantly higher in autopsy series, where 20% of patients with systemic disease have brain metastases.
PREDOMINANT SEX AND AGE: In patients with systemic malignancies, brain metastases occur in 10% to 30% of adults and 6% to 10% of children. About 60% of patients ages 50 to 70. Gender does not affect the incidence of brain metastases.
RISK FACTORS: In adults, the most common primary tumors accounting for brain metastases are carcinomas, including lung, breast, kidney, and colorectal cancers, and melanoma. In children, the most common are sarcomas, neuroblastoma, and germ cell tumors. Incidence is increasing, which is thought to be related to advances in systemic treatment efficacy.

PHYSICAL FINDINGS & CLINICAL PRESENTATION

- Brain metastases are highly variable and should be suspected in any cancer patient who develops acute neurologic signs or symptoms. Neurologic symptoms, however, are common in patients with systemic cancer; in an analysis of more than 800 patients with neurologic symptoms, brain metastases were found in only 16%.
- Most frequent symptoms:
  - Headache occurs in 40% to 50% of patients with brain metastases. Frequency is higher with metastases located in the posterior fossa, which may result in obstructive hydrocephalus. Associated nausea, vomiting, focal neurologic signs, and worsening with position are suggestive of a possible intracranial lesion as the headache etiology.
  - Focal neurologic signs/symptoms are the presenting symptom in 20% to 40% of patients. Hemiparesis is the most frequent complaint.
  - Cognitive dysfunction, including memory problems and/or mood/personality changes, is the presenting problem in 30% to 45% of patients.
  - The frequency of seizures in patients with metastatic brain tumor is 30% to 40%.
  - Acute stroke secondary to hemorrhage into a metastasis, hypercoagulability, or local vascular invasion accounts for 5% to 10% of patients.

ETIOLOGY

The most common mechanism of metastasis to the brain is by hematogenous spread. (Patchell). To successfully metastasize, tumor cells have to gain access to the circulation, pass through the local microvasculature, extravasate into the organ parenchyma, and reestablish themselves at the secondary site. The most common location is at the junction of the gray and white matter; blood vessels decrease in diameter in these regions, which is thought to act like a trap for clumps of tumor cells. Different tumor types have a predilection for metastasis in different regions of the brain. For example, metastases of small cell lung carcinoma are equally distributed in all regions, whereas pelvic (prostate and uterine) and gastrointestinal tumors more commonly metastasize to the posterior fossa.

DIAGNOSIS

DIFFERENTIAL DIAGNOSIS

- Primary brain tumor
- Infection: abscess/fungal disease
- Progressive multifocal leukoencephalopathy
- Demyelinating disease: multiple sclerosis, postinfectious encephalomyelitis
- Cerebral infarction/bleeding
- Effects of treatment, such as radiation necrosis

LABORATORY TESTS

- Routine laboratory studies are not typically helpful.
- Lumbar puncture is generally contraindicated due to increased intracranial pressure.
- Brain biopsy is necessary in some cases for a definitive diagnosis, particularly in the case of unknown primary tumor.

IMAGING STUDIES

- MRI with and without contrast is the imaging study of choice. MRI is superior to CT scanning to evaluate the meninges, subarachnoid space, and posterior fossa, and for defining relation to major intracranial vessels. MRI also helps to differentiate from other lesions. Important features on MRI that suggest brain metastases include: presence of multiple lesions, localization at the junction of the gray and white matter, circumscribed margins, large amounts of vasogenic edema.
- MRI spectroscopy and PET are useful to delineate tumor from non-tumor or from radiation necrosis.
- Newer experimental imaging studies, such as receptor-targeted and ligand-based molecular imaging, are on the horizon.

- Patients without a known primary tumor. In about 80% of patients, brain metastases develop after the diagnosis of systemic cancer. In the remaining patients, brain metastases are diagnosed synchronously (at the same time as) or before the primary tumor is found. In patients without a known primary tumor, the lung should be the primary focus of evaluation. Other frequent sites include melanoma, colon cancer, and breast cancer. PET scan may be useful in these patients to help identify the primary tumor or to identify other sites of metastatic disease—these latter sites might also be more amenable to biopsy.

TREATMENT

- The manamagent of patients with brain metastases is strongly influenced by the overall prognosis and may include treatments targeted at the metastases, management and prevention of complications (seizures, edema), and treatment of systemic malignancy, where appropriate.
- In patients considered to have a favorable prognosis, treatment focuses on eradication or control of the brain metastases. Approaches include surgical resection and radiation therapy.
- In patients with poor prognosis, treatment focuses on symptom control.

ACUTE GENERAL Rx

- Steroids are used to reduce peritumoral edema and increased intracranial pressure.
- The type of seizure guides treatment. Prophylactic treatment for seizure is not necessary in patients with no prior history of seizure.
- Anticoagulants are sometimes used to prevent venous thromboembolic disease.

CHRONIC Rx

- Radiation therapy has become the mainstay of treatment for brain metastases, including whole brain radiation therapy and stereotactic radiosurgery (SRS).
- For highly chemosensitive tumors, chemotherapy has been integrated into the primary management of patients with disseminated disease.
- For other tumors (e.g., small cell and non-small cell lung cancers, breast cancer, melanoma) systemic chemotherapy or molecularly targeted agents may be of palliative value when surgery, whole brain radiation therapy, and SRS have failed or are inappropriate. In most cases, two to three agents in combination and in conjunction with whole brain radiation therapy is used.

DISPOSITION

- The median survival of patients who receive supportive care and are treated with corticosteroids only is approximately 1 to 2 mo.
- Key prognostic factors are performance status, extent of systemic disease, and age.

Most favorable outcome is found in patients with Karnofsky performance score >70, age younger than 70 yr, no systemic disease or local control of primary tumor without extra-cranial metastases, and female gender. In this group, median survival is estimated at 7.1 mo.

REFERRAL

Treatment involves a multispecialty team. Consultations from oncology, neurosurgery, neurology, radiation oncology, psychiatry, and physical therapy are all warranted.

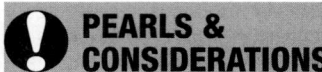

COMMENTS

Brain metastases are the most common intracranial tumors in adults, accounting for more than half. Lung cancer, melanoma, renal cell carcinoma, and breast cancer are the most common primary brain tumors that metastasize to the brain. MRI is the most reliable imaging modality. Patient treatment depends upon the overall prognosis.

PATIENT/FAMILY EDUCATION

American Brain Tumor Association (http://www.abta.org)
National Brain Tumor Society (http://www.braintumor.org)

SUGGESTED READINGS

available at www.expertconsult.com

AUTHOR: **NICOLE J. ULLRICH, M.D., PH.D.**

BASIC INFORMATION

DEFINITION

Brain neoplasms are a diverse group of primary (nonmetastatic) tumors arising from one of many different cell types within the central nervous system (CNS). Specific tumors subtypes and prognosis depend on the tumor cell of origin and pattern of growth.

SYNONYMS

Low-grade glioma
Glioneuronal tumor
Meningioma
Primary brain tumor

ICD-9CM CODES
225.0 Brain neoplasm (benign)
239.2 Brain neoplasm (unspecified)

EPIDEMIOLOGY & DEMOGRAPHICS

INCIDENCE: Approximately 18.2 cases/100,000 persons per yr for all primary brain tumors (Table 1-26). Incidence of primary nonmalignant tumors ranged from 6.3 to 16.68 cases/100,000 persons per yr from 2004 to 2005. Primary brain neoplasms account for ~2% of all cancers, with a disproportionate share of cancer morbidity and mortality. It is the most common cause of cancer death in children up to 15 yr.
PEAK INCIDENCE: Depends on histology, though highest peak at ~age 50 yr
PREDOMINANT SEX AND AGE: Slight male preponderance (8.0 vs. 5.5/100,000 person/yr)
GENETICS: Most primary CNS neoplasms are sporadic; 5% is associated with hereditary syndromes that predispose to neoplasia. The most common of these include:
- Li-Fraumeni syndrome: *p53* mutation on chromosome 17q13, gliomas
- Von Hippel-Lindau: VHL, chromosome 3p25, hemangioblastoma
- Tuberous sclerosis: TSC1/TSC2 (chromosome 9q34/16p13), subependymal giant cell astrocytoma
- Neurofibromatosis type 1: NF1, chromosome 17q11, neurofibroma, optic nerve glioma, low-grade glioma
- Neurofibromatosis type 2: NF2, chromosome 22q12, schwannoma, meningioma, ependymoma
- Retinoblastoma: pRB, chromosome 13q, retinoblastoma
- Gorlin's syndrome: chromosome 9q31, desmoplastic medulloblastoma

RISK FACTORS: Exposure to ionizing radiation has been implicated in meningiomas, gliomas, and nerve sheath tumors. No convincing evidence has shown a link with trauma, occupation, diet, or electromagnetic fields.

PHYSICAL FINDINGS & CLINICAL PRESENTATION

- In general, the location, size, and rate of growth will determine the symptoms and signs of a brain tumor.
- Headache is common and is the worst symptom in nearly half of all patients. Symptoms of intracranial pressure may also be present, including nausea and vomiting. Headache may be localizing. Papilledema is suggestive of obstructive hydrocephalus.
- Seizures occur in 33% of patients and are among the most common symptoms, particularly with brain metastases and low-grade gliomas. The type of seizure and clinical presentation depends on location. Seizures are more common in low-grade compared with high-grade gliomas. It is thought that patients with seizures typically have smaller tumors at time of diagnosis compared with those with other symptoms, because the onset of seizures prompts an imaging study, leading to an earlier diagnosis.
- Focal neurologic signs and symptoms, including muscle weakness, sensory changes, or visual disturbances are also quite frequent. In addition, cognitive dysfunction, accompanied by changes in memory or personality change, may be recounted, often in retrospect.

ETIOLOGY

Most cases are idiopathic, though specific chromosomal abnormalities have been implicated in some tumor types.

DIAGNOSIS

- Most common tumors in children: low-grade astrocytoma, medulloblastoma, ependymoma
- Most common adult tumors: glioblastoma multiforme, anaplastic astrocytoma, meningioma

LABORATORY

- Ultimately, only histologic examination can provide the exact diagnosis. Information may also be gleaned from additional features such as proliferative index, immunohistochemical stains, and electron microscopy.
- The current classification schema for gliomas is based on pathologic and microscopic criteria.
- Genetic analysis of tumors is rapidly becoming important for genetic classification, stratification of treatments, and predicting outcome. Different subtypes of gliomas have distinct gene-expression profiles, which can be distinguished from one another and from normal tissue; these differences typically involve pathways of cell proliferation, energy metabolism, and signal transduction. In adults, global expression profiling identified differences in 360 genes between low-grade and high-grade tumors.

DIFFERENTIAL DIAGNOSIS

- Stroke/cerebral hemorrhage
- Abscess/parasitic cyst
- Demyelinating disease: multiple sclerosis, postinfectious encephalomyelitis
- Metastatic tumors
- Primary CNS lymphoma

WORKUP

- Neuroimaging studies and pathologic sampling are the most important diagnostic modalities in evaluation of brain tumors and may be critical for preoperative planning.

IMAGING STUDIES

- MRI with gadolinium enhancement is highly sensitive, though CT scanning is useful if calcification or hemorrhage suspected. MRI permits visualization of the tumor, as well as the relation to the surrounding tissue. Enhancing tumor can be distinguished from surrounding edema. Low-grade tumors often present as an infiltrating lesion without mass effect. MRI is superior to CT scanning to evaluate the meninges, subarachnoid space,

TABLE 1-26 Frequency of Primary CNS Tumors

CHILDREN (0-14 YEARS)		ADULTS (≥15 YEARS)	
Type	Percentage	Type	Percentage
Glioblastoma	20	Glioblastoma	50
Astrocytoma	21	Astrocytoma	10
Ependymoma	7	Ependymoma	2
Oligodendroglioma	1	Oligodendroglioma	3
Medulloblastoma	24	Medulloblastoma	2
Neuroblastoma	3	Neurilemmoma	2
Neurilemmoma	1	Pituitary adenoma	4
Craniopharyngioma	5	Craniopharyngioma	1
Meningioma	5	Meningioma	17
Teratoma	2	Pinealoma	1
Pinealoma	2	Hemangioma	2
Hemangioma	3	Sarcoma	1
Sarcoma	1		
Others	5	Others	5
Total	100	Total	100

From Goetz CG, Pappert EJ: *Textbook of clinical neurology*, Philadelphia, 1999, Saunders.

and posterior fossa, and for defining relation to major intracranial vessels.

- Magnetic resonance spectroscopy is increasingly being used as a diagnostic tool to define metabolic composition of an area of interest and may be useful to contrast areas of tumor progression from radiation necrosis. N-acetylaspartate is often decreased in brain tumors, whereas choline, a component of cell membranes, is increased because of high cellular turnover.
- PET scan is helpful to distinguish neoplastic lesions (with high rate of metabolism) from other lesions such as demyelination or radiation necrosis (with a much lower metabolic rate). Such lesions take up greater amounts of glucose than surrounding tissues or tumors with slower metabolic rates. May be useful to help map functional areas of the brain before surgery or radiation.
- Functional MRI is now used as an adjunct in perioperative planning for patients whose lesion is in vital regions, such as those responsible for speech, language, and motor control.

Rx TREATMENT

NONPHARMACOLOGIC THERAPY

- Maximal surgical removal or debulking is the initial treatment of choice and provides tissue for diagnosis and molecular characterization. Maximal safe resection is often favored with a trend toward improved survival with this approach.
- Biopsy alone is performed if the tumor is located in eloquent regions of brain or is inaccessible; this is essential for histopathologic diagnosis. Biopsy can be performed under CT or MRI guidance using stereotactic localization.
- If the tumor is benign (e.g., meningioma, acoustic neuroma), often no further therapy is required.

ACUTE GENERAL Rx

Antiseizure medications have been used perioperatively and to control seizures resulting from focal lesions. Prophylactic use of anticonvulsants is not typically recommended without clear history of seizures.

CHRONIC Rx

- Chemotherapy (combination or single agent) may be used before, during, or after surgery and radiation therapy. (In children, chemotherapy is often used to delay radiation therapy.) Radiosensitizers may help increase the therapeutic effect of radiation therapy.
- Radiation is useful for certain types of tumors and is often used if there is residual tumor after surgery; conventional radiation uses external beams over a period of weeks, whereas stereotactic radiosurgery delivers a single, high dose of radiation to a well-defined area (usually <1 cm). Long-term effects of radiation therapy include radiation necrosis (particularly of white matter), blood vessel hyalinization, and secondary tumors (usually meningiomas, sarcomas, and malignant astrocytomas).
- Experimental therapies are continually in development and are typically based on molecular characterization of tumors and small molecule blockers of signal transduction cascades. Some of these therapies involve antisense molecules, biologic agents, immunotherapies, or angiogenesis inhibitors. Intratumoral drug infusions and convection-enhanced delivery of novel agents are currently under study.

DISPOSITION

- Tumor histology/histologic diagnosis (World Health Organization [WHO] grading system), including number of mitoses, capillary endothelial proliferation, and necrosis (*Note:* There can be a high degree of morbidity based on tumor location, even with more benign histology.)

- In general, younger age, high performance status, and lower pathologic grade have more favorable prognosis. For all histologic subtypes of brain tumors, pediatric and young adult patients have a better survival rate.

REFERRAL

- All cases warrant evaluation by an oncologist and neurosurgeon.
- Patients should be evaluated for physical and occupational therapy.
- Children should undergo neuropsychologic evaluations and screening for learning disabilities.

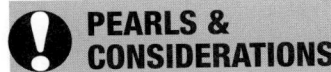

PEARLS & CONSIDERATIONS

COMMENTS

In general, younger age, high performance status, and lower pathologic grade have more favorable prognosis. For all histologic subtypes of brain tumors, pediatric and young adult patients have a better survival.

PATIENT/FAMILY EDUCATION

American Brain Tumor Association
National Brain Tumor Society (http://www.braintumor.org)

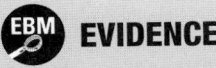

available at www.expertconsult.com

SUGGESTED READINGS
available at www.expertconsult.com

AUTHOR: **NICOLE J. ULLRICH, M.D., PH.D.**

BASIC INFORMATION

DEFINITION

Brain neoplasms are a diverse group of primary (nonmetastatic) tumors arising from one of the many different cell types within the central nervous system. Malignant brain tumors are defined by histopathologic features and a rapidly progressive pattern of growth. Glioblastoma is the most common primary brain tumor in adults, accounting for 50% to 60% of primary brain tumors.

SYNONYMS

Glioblastoma
GBM

ICD-9CM CODES
191.9

EPIDEMIOLOGY & DEMOGRAPHICS

INCIDENCE: Annual incidence rate of glioblastoma is approximately 2 to 3 cases/100,000 persons. High-grade/malignant astrocytomas are slightly more common in whites than in blacks, Latinos, and Asians.
PREDOMINANT SEX AND AGE: Glioblastoma is slightly more common in men than women with a male:female ratio of 3:2. Peak incidence is between 45 and 70 yr. Approximately 10% of glioblastomas occur in children.
PEAK INCIDENCE: High-grade gliomas, such as anaplastic astrocytoma and glioblastoma, tend to originate in the fourth to fifth decade of life and beyond.
RISK FACTORS: Prior radiation may increase risk for primary brain tumor.
GENETICS: Malignant progression is associated with inactivation of *PTEN* tumor-suppressor gene and amplification of epidermal growth factor receptor (*EGFR*) gene.

PHYSICAL FINDINGS & CLINICAL PRESENTATION

- In general, the location, size, and rate of growth will determine the symptoms and signs. Clinical history of patients with glioblastoma is typically brief, <3 mo in the majority of patients with primary glioblastoma.
- Most frequent symptoms include:
  - Headache occurs in the majority of cases. The headache can be localizing or may result from increased intracranial pressure.
  - Seizures occur in 30% to 60% depending on tumor location and grade.
  - Symptoms and signs of hydrocephalus and raised intracranial pressure (headache, vomiting, clouding of consciousness, papilledema).
  - Other symptoms seen in 20% or more of patients include memory loss, focal motor weakness, visual changes, language deficits, and cognitive disturbances or memory changes.

ETIOLOGY

- Glioblastomas are classified as primary or secondary. Primary glioblastoma constitutes the majority of cases (60%) in adults older than 50 yr and are considered de novo tumors. Secondary glioblastoma typically involves malignant progression from a lower grade (grade II or III) glioma. Overexpression of *EGFR* gene occurs in 40% to 50% of primary glioblastoma cases. Loss of heterozygosity on chromosome 10q occurs in 60% to 90% of both primary and secondary glioblastoma cases and is associated with poor prognosis. The pathway involving mutations of the tumor-suppressor gene *p53* is typically associated with secondary glioblastoma. Other genetic mutations have also been recognized as potential contributors in the pathogenesis of glioblastoma, including *PTEN* and *MDM2*.

DIAGNOSIS

DIFFERENTIAL DIAGNOSIS

- Stroke
- Arteriovenous malformations
- Abscess/parasitic cyst (neurocysticercosis)
- Demyelinating disease: multiple sclerosis, postinfectious encephalomyelitis
- Metastatic tumors
- Primary central nervous system lymphoma

LABORATORY TESTS

- Routine laboratory studies are not typically helpful.
- Lumbar puncture is generally contraindicated; cerebrospinal fluid studies do not add much specific additional information for the diagnosis for glioblastoma.
- Ultimately, only a histologic examination can provide the exact diagnosis. Information may also be gleaned from additional features such as proliferative index, immunohistochemical stains, and electron microscopy, as well as molecular markers.

IMAGING STUDIES (Fig. 1-62)

- MRI with and without contrast is the imaging study of choice, though CT scanning is useful if calcification or hemorrhage is suspected. MRI permits visualization of the tumor, as well as the relation to the surrounding tissue. Enhancing tumor can be distinguished from surrounding edema. MRI is superior to CT scanning to evaluate the meninges, subarachnoid space, and posterior fossa, and for defining relation to major intracranial vessels.
- Magnetic resonance spectroscopy (MRS) is increasingly being used as a diagnostic tool to define metabolic composition of an area of interest and may be useful to contrast areas of tumor progression from radiation necrosis. N-acetylaspartate, a marker of neurons, is often decreased in brain tumors, whereas choline, a component of cell membranes, is increased because of high cellular turnover.
- PET scan is helpful to distinguish neoplastic lesions (with high rate of metabolism) from other lesions such as demyelination or radiation necrosis (with a much lower metabolic rate). Such lesions take up greater amounts of glucose than surrounding tissues or tumors with slower metabolic rates. May also aid in preoperative planning to increase diagnostic yield and to help map functional areas of the brain before surgery.
- Functional MRI is now used as an adjunct to in perioperative planning for patients whose lesion is in vital regions, such as those responsible for speech, language, and motor control.

TREATMENT

- Current standard-of-care therapies include surgery, radiation, and palliative chemotherapy, which have significant adverse effects and limited efficacy. Median time to recurrence after standard therapy is 6.9 mo.

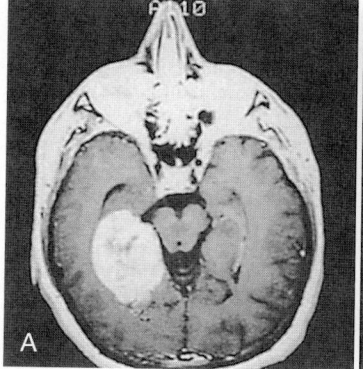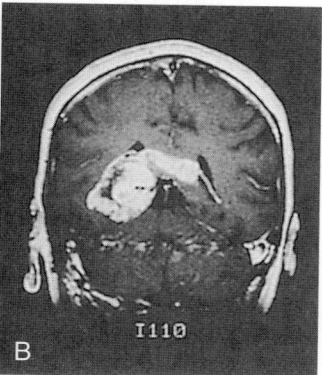

FIGURE 1-62 Glioblastoma multiforme. Axial (**A**) and coronal (**B**) postcontrast enhanced T1-weighted image showing a large homogenously contrast-enhancing mass in the right medial temporal lobe with extension across the midline. (From Specht N [ed]: *Practical guide to diagnostic imaging,* St Louis, 1998, Mosby.)

NONPHARMACOLOGIC THERAPY
- Maximal surgical removal or debulking is the initial treatment of choice.
- Biopsy alone is performed if the tumor is located in eloquent regions of brain or is inaccessible; this is essential for histopathologic diagnosis. Biopsy can be performed under CT or MRI guidance using stereotactic localization.

ACUTE GENERAL Rx
- Steroids are used to reduce edema and may also be used perioperatively or during radiation therapy.
- Antiseizure medications have been used perioperatively and to control seizures resulting from focal lesions. Prophylactic use of anticonvulsants is not typically recommended without clear history of seizures.

CHRONIC Rx
- Even patients with a gross total resection of tumor have a high recurrence rate. Radiation therapy improves local control and overall survival after surgery.
- Chemotherapy (combination or single agent) may be used before, during, or after surgery and radiation therapy. (In children, chemotherapy is often used to delay radiation therapy.) Radiosensitizers may help increase the therapeutic effect of radiation therapy.
- Experimental therapies are continually in development and are typically based on molecular characterization of tumors and small molecule blockers of signal transduction cascades. Some of these therapies involve antisense molecules, biologic agents, immunotherapies, or angiogenesis inhibitors. Intratumoral drug infusions and convection-enhanced delivery of novel agents are currently under study.

DISPOSITION
- The most important prognostic factors are extent of resection, patient age, tumor grade/histology, and performance status. In general, younger age, high performance status, and lower pathologic grade have more favorable prognosis. For all histologic subtypes of brain tumors, pediatric and young adult patients have a better survival.
- Terminal events typically result from increased intracranial pressure.

REFERRAL
Treatment involves a multispecialty team. Consultations from oncology, neurosurgery, neurology, radiation oncology, psychiatry, and physical therapy are all warranted.

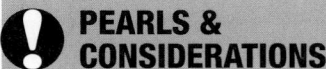 **PEARLS & CONSIDERATIONS**

COMMENTS
Glioblastoma distinguished pathologically by the presence of vascular proliferation and necrosis. The most important prognostic factors are age, tumor grade, and performance status. The extent of surgical resection also appears to impat prognosis.

PATIENT/FAMILY EDUCATION
American Brain Tumor Association
National Brain Tumor Society (http://www.braintumor.org)

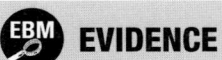 **EVIDENCE**
available at www.expertconsult.com

SUGGESTED READINGS
available at www.expertconsult.com

AUTHOR: **NICOLE J. ULLRICH, M.D., PH.D.**

ℹ️ BASIC INFORMATION

DEFINITION

The term *breast cancer* refers to invasive carcinoma of the breast, whether ductal or lobular.

SYNONYMS

Carcinoma of the breast

ICD-9CM CODES
174.9 Malignant neoplasm female breast

EPIDEMIOLOGY & DEMOGRAPHICS

- Nearly exclusively the disease of women, with only 1% of breast cancers in males
- Steady increase in its incidence in the U.S., with 205,000 new patients annually
- Annual mortality of 40,000
- Risk steadily increases with age
- Genetically defined group of women with *BRCA-1* or *BRCA-2* genes identified to carry lifetime risk as high as 85%

PHYSICAL FINDINGS & CLINICAL PRESENTATION

- Increasing number of small breast cancers found by mammograms
- Patients usually completely free of physical findings
- Palpable tumors possibly as small as 1 cm or even smaller
- Size of the mass and its location measured and documented
- Skin and/or nipple retraction and skin edema, erythema, ulcer, satellite nodule
- Nodal enlargement in axilla and supraclavicular areas
- Advanced disease: clinical signs of pleural effusion and/or hepatomegaly
- Rare instances: clear, serous, or bloody discharge only symptom
- Nipple evaluation (see "Paget's Disease of the Breast")

ETIOLOGY

- Precise mechanism of carcinogenesis not understood
- Possibly interaction of ovarian estrogen, non-ovarian estrogen, estrogens of exogenous origin with breast tissue of varied carcinogenic susceptibility to develop cancer
- Other known or suspected variables: childbearing, breastfeeding practice, diet, physical activities, body mass, alcohol intake
- Have identified families with known high risk
- Women with *BRCA-1* and *BRCA-2* genes associated with high risk

𝐃𝐱 DIAGNOSIS

DIFFERENTIAL DIAGNOSIS

The following nonmalignant breast lesions can simulate breast cancer on both physical and mammogram examinations:
- Fibrocystic changes
- Fibroadenoma
- Hamartoma

WORKUP

- Physical examination:
  1. Mass detected by patient or medical professional: workup required
  2. Negative mammogram: breast cancer not ruled out
  3. Sonogram: to demonstrate mass to be cyst, usually eliminating need for further workup
  4. Screening with both MRI and mammography might rule out cancerous lesions better than mammography alone in women who are known or likely to have an inherited predisposition to breast cancer
- To establish diagnosis:
  1. Positive aspiration cytology on a clinically and mammographically malignant mass—highly accurate but still requires open biopsy confirmation
  2. Stereotactic core needle biopsy diagnosis: Stereotactic- and ultrasonography-guided core-needle biopsy procedures seem to be almost as accurate as open surgical biopsy with lower complication rates. They are reliable with invasive carcinoma identified, but negative or equivocal results require careful evaluation
  3. Atypical hyperplasia or in situ carcinoma found by core needle biopsy: open surgical biopsy confirmation still required
  4. Excisional or incisional biopsy: establishes diagnosis

  NOTE: Do not rely on negative mammogram or negative aspiration cytology findings to exclude malignancy. Make appropriate referral. Obtain imaging studies such as bone scan, chest x-ray examination, CT scan of abdomen, or CT scan of liver.
- Breast radiologic evaluation and an algorithm for breast cancer screening and evaluation are described in Section III. The differential diagnosis of breast lumps is described in Section II.

IMAGING STUDIES

Mammograms (Fig. 1-63): 30% to 50% of breast cancers detected by screening mammograms only as a spiculated mass, a mass with or without microcalcifications, or a cluster of microcalcifications. MRI is an excellent modality that is particularly useful in patients with breast implants and when there is a strong family history of breast cancer.

℞ TREATMENT

NONPHARMACOLOGIC THERAPY

- Early breast cancer: primarily surgical or surgical and radiotherapeutic
- Choice in 60% to 70% of women between modified mastectomy and breast-conserving treatment, which consists of lumpectomy, axillary staging with sentinel node biopsy or axillary dissection, and breast irradiation
- Recent trials reveal that among patients with limited sentinel lymph nodes (SNL), metastatic breast cancer treated with breast conservation and systematic therapy, the use of sentinel lymph node dissection (SNLD) alone compared with axillary lymph node dissection (ALND) did not result in inferior survival

ACUTE GENERAL Rx

- May require adjuvant chemotherapy or endocrine therapy. Standard chemotherapy consists of either cyclophosphamide, methotrexate, and fluorouracil or cyclophosphamide plus doxorubicin. Endocrine therapy is recommended after chemotherapy in patients with hormone-receptor positive tumors.

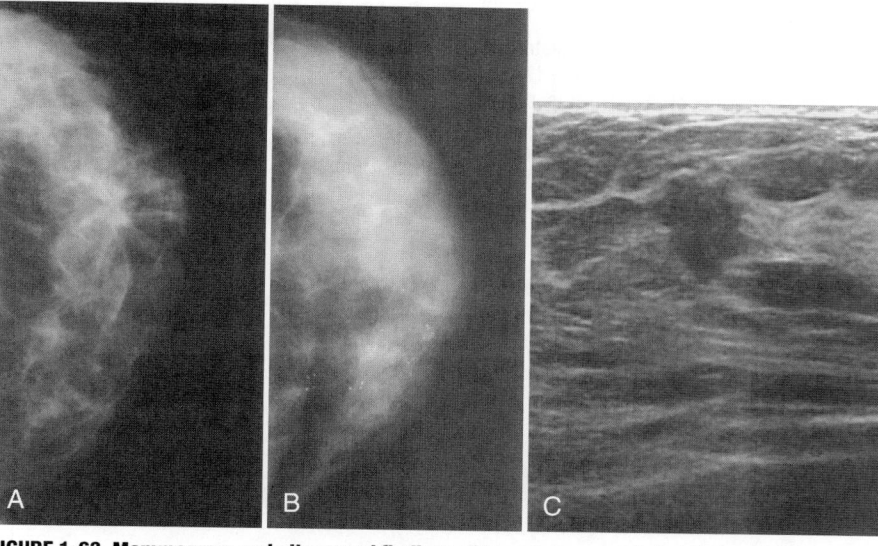

FIGURE 1-63 Mammogram and ultrasound findings of breast disease. A, A stellate mass in the breast. The combination of a density with spiculated borders and distortion of surrounding breast architecture suggests a malignancy. **B,** Clustered microcalcification. Fine, plemorphic, and linear calcifications that cluster together suggest the diagnosis of ductal carcinoma in situ (DCIS). **C,** An ultrasound image of breast cancer. The mass is solid, containing internal echoes, and displaying an irregular border. Most maligant lesions are taller than they are wide. (From Townsend CM et al [eds]: *Sabiston textbook of surgery,* ed 17, Philadelphia, 2004, Saunders.)

- Weekly paclitaxel after standard adjuvant chemotherapy with doxorubicin and cyclophosphamide improves disease-free and overall survival in women with breast cancer. However, patients with *HER2*-negative, estrogen-receptor–positive, node-positive breast cancer may gain little benefit from administration of paclitaxel after adjuvant chemotherapy with doxorubicin plus cyclophosphamide.
- Initial therapy of metastatic breast cancer with paclitaxel plus bevacizumab prolongs progression-free survival, but not overall survival. The FDA has recommended removal of the indication for use of bevacizumab in breast cancer patients.
- Evaluation and treatment by medical oncologist.

CHRONIC Rx

Follow-up required after proper treatment of primary breast cancer includes:
- Periodic clinical evaluations as delineated by medical oncologist or surgeon
- Annual mammograms
- Other tests as indicated
- Patient instruction in monthly breast self-examination technique

DISPOSITION

- Prognosis after curative therapy: depends on size of tumor, extent of nodal metastasis, and pathologic grade of tumor
  1. Patient with 1-cm tumor with no axillary node metastasis: 10-yr disease-free survival rate of 90%
  2. Patient with 3-cm tumor with metastasis in four nodes: 10-yr disease-free survival rate of 15% if no systemic adjuvant therapy given
  3. Outlook for most patients is between these extremes
- Systemic adjuvant therapy: improves prognosis significantly
- Isolated tumor cells or micrometastases in regional lymph nodes is associated with a reduced 5-yr rate of disease-free survival among women with favorable early-stage breast cancer who do not receive adjuvant therapy. Survival is improved in patients with isolated tumor cells or micrometastases who received adjuvant therapy.
- Retrospective analyses suggest that occult lymph-node metastases are an important

prognostic factor for disease recurrence of survival among patients with breast cancer; however, recent trials indicate that the magnitude of the difference in outcome at 5 yrs is small (1.2 percentage points). These data do not favor a clinical benefit of additional evaluation (including immunohistochemical analysis) of initially negative sentinel nodes in patients with breast cancer.
- The addition of zoledronic acid to adjuvant endocrine therapy improves disease-free survival in premenopausal patients with estrogen-responsive early breast cancer.

REFERRAL

Referral is necessary as soon as breast cancer is suspected.

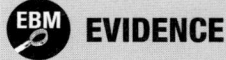 **PEARLS & CONSIDERATIONS**

Breast cancer in pregnancy and lactation:
1. Frequency in women 40 yr or younger reported to be 15%
2. May carry worse prognosis because disease discovery delayed by engorged and nodular breast changes and/or because disease progression more rapid in pregnancy
3. Survival rates similar to those for nonpregnant early-stage breast cancer patients in same age group
4. Mass usually found by patient or obstetrician
5. Expedient workup recommended, including mammography and sonography
6. Diagnosis to be made without delay
7. Choice of mastectomy or lumpectomy with axillary dissection for treatment
8. Adjuvant chemotherapy delayed until third trimester or after delivery
9. Irradiation to breast after lumpectomy delayed until after delivery

Ductal carcinoma in situ (DCIS, intraductal carcinoma):
1. Discovered by mammogram as cluster of microcalcifications and/or density
2. Presents less often as a palpable mass or nipple discharge
3. Before mammogram screening, DCIS accounted for 1% of all breast cancers
4. Now 15% to 20% or even higher proportion have DCIS

5. Formerly treated with mastectomy, now lumpectomy
6. Cure rates 98% to 99%
7. No axillary dissection required
8. With radiation, breast recurrences reduced
9. Mastectomy possibly required with extensive and/or high-grade DCIS
10. Systemic adjuvant treatment is not indicated

Inflammatory carcinoma:
1. Rare but rapidly progressive and often lethal form of breast cancer
2. Presents as erythematous and edematous breast resembling mastitis
3. Biopsy required, including skin
4. Treatment with combination chemotherapy followed by surgery and radiation therapy
5. Prognosis once dismal, now 5-yr disease-free survival in 50% of patients

COMMENTS

- The U.S. Preventive Services Task Force (USPSTF) now recommends against automatic "routine" screening of younger women (age range 40 to 49). The task force recommends biennal screening mammography for all middle-aged women (age range 50 to 74). It also states that current evidence is insufficient to assess the benefits and harms of screening mammography in older women (aged 75 and older). The task force also discourages women from performing breast self-examination. Several other U.S. organizations however still recommend annual screening beginning at age 40. This creates anxiety and confusion in the general public. Physicians and patients should follow the guideline that is most reflective of their preferences and misconceptions.
- Breast radiologic evaluation, evaluation of nipple discharge, and evaluation of palpable mass are described in Section III.

EBM EVIDENCE

available at www.expertconsult.com

SUGGESTED READINGS

available at www.expertconsult.com

AUTHORS: **TAKUMA NEMOTO, M.D.,** and **RUBEN ALVERO, M.D.**

BASIC INFORMATION

DEFINITION

Breech presentation occurs when the fetal longitudinal axis is such that the cephalic pole occupies the uterine fundus (Fig. 1-64). Three types exist, with respective percentages at term: frank (48% to 73%, flexed hips, extended knees), complete (4.6% to 11.5%, flexed hips and knees), and footling (12% to 38%, hips extended).

ICD-9CM CODES
652.2 Breech presentation without mention of version

EPIDEMIOLOGY & DEMOGRAPHICS

INCIDENCE: Gestational age dependent: 3% to 4% overall, 14% at 29 to 32 wk, 33% at 21 to 24 wk

PERINATAL MORTALITY: 9% to 25%, or three to five times increase over vertex presentation at term. When corrected for the associated increase in congenital anomalies and complications of prematurity, the morbidity and mortality rates approach those of the vertex presentation at term regardless of route of delivery.

PHYSICAL FINDINGS & CLINICAL PRESENTATION

- Lack of presenting part on vaginal examination
- Fetal heart tones heard above the umbilicus
- Leopold maneuvers revealing mobile fetal part in the uterine fundus

ETIOLOGY

- Abnormal placentation (fundal), uterine anomalies (fibroids, septa), pelvic or adnexal masses, alterations in fetal muscular tone, or fetal malformations
- Associated conditions: trisomy 13, 18, 21; Potter syndrome; myotonic dystrophy; prematurity

DIAGNOSIS

DIFFERENTIAL DIAGNOSIS

Vertex, oblique, or transverse lie

WORKUP

- Determine reason for breech presentation, history of uterine anomalies, gestational age, or associated fetal congenital anomalies
- Assess fetal status by continuous fetal heart rate monitoring or ultrasound
- Assess pelvis to determine feasibility of vaginal delivery
- Assess risk for safety of vaginal versus abdominal delivery

IMAGING STUDIES

Ultrasound to evaluate for:
- Fetal anomalies, such as hydrocephalus
- Placental location
- Position of fetal head relative to spine (check for hyperextension)
- Estimated fetal weight (2500 to 3800 g)
- Type of breech (frank, complete, footling)

TREATMENT

ACUTE GENERAL Rx

- Vaginal delivery in selected patients (see "Comments" section): allow maternal expulsive forces to deliver fetus until scapula visible (avoiding traction); with flexion and/or Piper forceps, deliver fetal head
- Perform cesarean section (see "Comments")
- External cephalic version: success 60% to 75% after 37 wk, contraindicated with placental abruption, low-lying placenta, maternal hypertension, previous uterine incision, multiple gestation, nonreassuring fetal status
- Adequate pelvic/cervical relaxation essential for vaginal breech (i.e., need anesthesia in-room during birth [delivery] with uterine relaxants on hand [nitroglycerin, terbutaline])

COMPLICATIONS

- Head entrapment: leading cause of death (with the exception of anomalous fetuses), 88 cases per 1000 deliveries; avoid by maintaining flexion of fetal head, use of Piper forceps or Dührssen's incisions. Avoid hyperextension of head during delivery.
- Cord prolapse: usually occurs late in the course of labor. Incidence depends on type of breech: frank (0.5%), complete (4% to 5%), footling (10%).
- Nuchal arm: arm extended above fetal head, occurs when there is undue traction before delivery of fetal scapulas. Treatment depends on bringing trapped arm across infant's face.

DISPOSITION

If confounding variables are corrected for, such as prematurity and associated congenital anomalies (6.3% of breeches vs. 2.4% in general population), route of delivery plays a less important role in fetal outcome than previously believed.

REFERRAL

An obstetrician trained in delivery of the vaginal breech is a prerequisite for attempting vaginal route, although it must be explained to the patient that with cesarean section certain risks (such as hyperextension of the fetal head with resultant spinal cord injury) may be minimized but not eliminated.

PEARLS & CONSIDERATIONS

COMMENTS

In general, for breech presentation, mortality rate is increased 13-fold and morbidity sevenfold. The main reasons are an increase in congenital anomalies, perinatal hypoxia, birth injury, and prematurity.

There is no contraindication to induction of labor in the breech presentation, and labor is not prohibited in a primigravida.

CRITERIA FOR TRIAL OF LABOR:
- Estimated fetal weight 2000 to 3800 g
- Frank breech
- Adequate pelvis
- Flexed fetal head
- Continuous fetal monitoring
- Normal progress of labor
- Bedside availability of anesthesia and capability for immediate cesarean section
- Informed consent
- Obstetrician trained in vaginal breech delivery

CRITERIA FOR CESAREAN SECTION:
- Estimated fetal weight <1500 g or >4000 g
- Footling presentation (20% risk of cord prolapse, usually late in course of labor)
- Inadequate pelvis
- Hyperextended fetal head (21% risk of spinal cord injury)
- Nonreassuring fetal status
- Abnormal progress of labor
- Lack of trained obstetrician

AUTHORS: **SCOTT J. ZUCCALA, D.O.,** and **RUBEN ALVERO, M.D.**

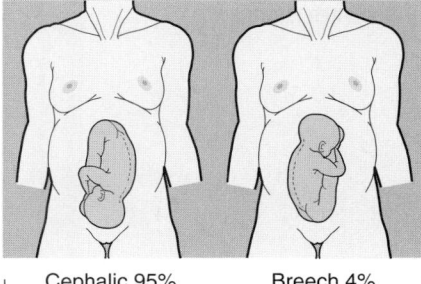

Cephalic 95%	Breech 4%

Longitudinal lie 99%

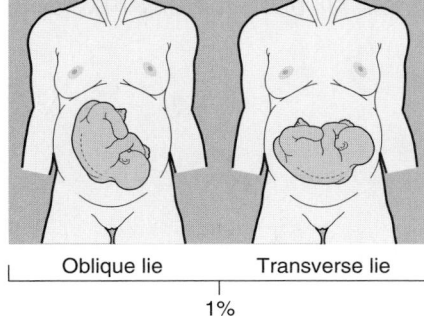

Oblique lie	Transverse lie

1%

FIGURE 1-64 Fetal lie at term. (Drife J, Magowan B: *Clinical obstetrics and gynecology,* Philadelphia, 2004, Saunders.)

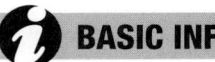

DEFINITION

Bronchiectasis is the abnormal dilation and destruction of bronchial walls, which may be congenital or acquired.

ICD-9CM CODES
494.0 Bronchiectasis

EPIDEMIOLOGY & DEMOGRAPHICS

- Cystic fibrosis is responsible for nearly 50% of all cases of bronchiectasis.
- Acquired primary bronchiectasis is uncommon because of rapid diagnosis of pulmonary infections and frequent use of antibiotics.
- Effective childhood immunizations have led to a significant decrease in the incidence of bronchiectasis resulting from pertussis.

PHYSICAL FINDINGS & CLINICAL PRESENTATION

- Moist crackles at lung bases
- Cough with expectoration of large amount of purulent sputum
- Fever, night sweats, generalized malaise, weight loss
- Hemoptysis
- Halitosis, skin pallor
- Clubbing (infrequent)

ETIOLOGY

- Cystic fibrosis
- Lung infections (pneumonia, lung abscess, TB, fungal infections, viral infections)
- Abnormal host defense (panhypogammaglobulinemia, Kartagener's syndrome, AIDS, chemotherapy)
- Localized airway obstruction (congenital structural defects, foreign bodies, neoplasms)
- Inflammation (inflammatory pneumonitis, granulomatous lung disease, allergic aspergillosis)

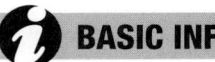 **DIAGNOSIS**

DIFFERENTIAL DIAGNOSIS

- TB
- Asthma
- Chronic bronchitis or chronic sinusitis
- Interstitial fibrosis
- Chronic lung abscess
- Foreign body aspiration
- Cystic fibrosis
- Lung carcinoma

LABORATORY TESTS

- Sputum for Gram stain, culture and sensitivity, and acid-fast bacteria
- Complete blood count with differential (leukocytosis with left shift, anemia)
- Serum protein electrophoresis to evaluate for hypogammaglobulinemia
- Antibody test for aspergillosis
- Sweat test in patients with suspected cystic fibrosis

IMAGING STUDIES

- Chest radiograph: hyperinflation, crowded lung markings, small cystic spaces at the base of the lungs (Fig. 1-65).
- High-resolution CT scan of the chest has become the best tool to detect cystic lesions and exclude underlying obstruction from neoplasm. The CT study should be a noncontrast study with the use of 1- to 1.5-mm window every 1 cm with acquisition time of 1 sec. Typical findings on CT include dilation of airway lumen, lack of tapering of an airway toward periphery, ballooned cysts at the end of bronchus, and varicose constrictions along airways.
- Bronchoscopy may be helpful to evaluate hemoptysis, rule out obstructive lesions, and remove mucus plugs.

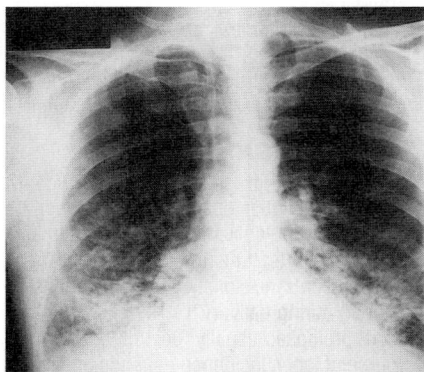

FIGURE 1-65 Extensive bilateral basal bronchiectasis. (Souhami RL, Moxham J: *Textbook of medicine*, ed 4, London, 2002, Churchill Livingstone.)

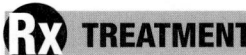

NONPHARMACOLOGIC THERAPY

- Postural drainage (reclining prone on a bed with the head down on the side) and chest percussion with use of inflatable vests or mechanical vibrators applied to the chest may enhance removal of respiratory secretions.
- Adequate hydration.
- Supplemental oxygen for hypoxemia.

ACUTE GENERAL Rx

- Antibiotic therapy is based on the results of sputum, Gram stain, and culture and sensitivity; in patients with inadequate or inconclusive results, empiric therapy with amoxicillin/clavulanate 500 mg to 875 mg q12h, TMP-SMX q12h, doxycycline 100 mg bid, or cefuroxime 250 mg bid for 10 to 14 days is recommended.
- Bronchodilators are useful in patients with demonstrable airflow obstruction.

CHRONIC Rx

- Avoidance of tobacco
- Maintenance of proper nutrition and hydration
- Prompt identification and treatment of infections
- Pneumococcal vaccination and annual influenza vaccination

DISPOSITION

Prognosis is variable with severity of the disease and underlying etiology of bronchiectasis.

REFERRAL

Surgical referral for partial lung resection in patients with localized severe disease unresponsive to medical therapy or in patients with massive hemoptysis

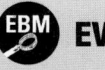 **EVIDENCE**

available at www.expertconsult.com

SUGGESTED READING
available at www.expertconsult.com

AUTHOR: **FRED F. FERRI, M.D.**

BASIC INFORMATION

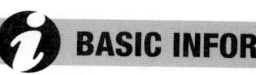

DEFINITION

Brucellosis is a zoonotic infection caused by one of four species of *Brucella*. It commonly presents as a nondescript febrile illness.

SYNONYMS

Malta fever, undulant fever
Bang's disease

ICD-9CM CODES
023.9 Brucellosis

EPIDEMIOLOGY & DEMOGRAPHICS

INCIDENCE (IN U.S.): About 100 cases/yr (may be underreported)
PREDOMINANT SEX: Male
PREDOMINANT AGE: Adult
CONGENITAL INFECTION: Recent evidence suggests a high rate of spontaneous abortions in untreated pregnant women during the first and second trimesters.
NEONATAL INFECTION: Can occur if mother is infected during pregnancy.

PHYSICAL FINDINGS & CLINICAL PRESENTATION

- Incubation period is 1 wk to 3 mo.
- Patients may be asymptomatic or have non-specific symptoms such as fever, sweats, malaise, weight loss, depression, arthralgia, and arthritis.
- Fever is the most common finding.
- Hepatomegaly, splenomegaly, or lymphadenopathy is possible.
- Localized disease includes endocarditis, meningitis, spondylitis, sacroiliitis, and osteomyelitis (especially vertebral).

Chronic hepatosplenic suppurative brucellosis (CHSB) presents with hepatic or splenic abscesses. This form is thought to be a reactivation and can occur years after the acute infection.

ETIOLOGY

- Caused by infection with *Brucella* species:
  1. Most commonly *B. melitensis,* but also *suis, abortus,* or *canis*
  2. A small, gram-negative coccobacillus

- Acquired through ingestion of organisms (unpasteurized goat or cow's milk), breaks in the skin, or by inhalation.
- Most cases occur after exposure to animals (sheep, goats, swine, cattle, or dogs), or animal products (i.e., milk, hides, tissue).
- Most cases (in U.S.) occur in men with occupational exposure to animals (farmers, ranchers, laboratory workers, veterinarians, abattoir workers).
- Laboratory workers, especially those in microbiology, are also at increased risk. Guidelines for postexposure prophylaxis are available from *MMWR Surveill Summ* 57:39, 2009.

DIAGNOSIS

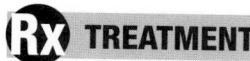

DIFFERENTIAL DIAGNOSIS

Many febrile conditions without localizing manifestations (i.e., TB, endocarditis, typhoid fever, malaria, autoimmune diseases)

WORKUP

- Cultures of blood, bone marrow, or other tissue (lymph node, liver) should be sent and held for 4 wk, because *Brucella* spp. grow slowly in vitro.
- Granulomas on biopsy are suggestive of diagnosis.

LABORATORY TESTS

- WBC count: normal or low
- Serology:
  1. Serum agglutination test (SAT) to detect antibodies to *B. abortus, melitensis,* and *suis.* Positive tests warrant confirmatory testing with specific Brucella agglutination tests.
  2. Specific antibody test to identify antibodies to *B. canis.*
  3. False-negative SAT possibly resulting from a prozone effect.
  4. PCR (polymerase chain reaction) for *Brucella* spp. specific 16S rRNA or DNA sequences are increasingly used for the diagnosis of brucellosis from blood, tissue samples, and bone marrow.

IMAGING STUDIES

- Radiographs to show splenic or hepatic calcifications in chronic disease
- Bone scan, MRI, and radiographs of the spine to suggest osteomyelitis
- Ultrasound or CT scan of the abdomen to show an enlarged liver or spleen
- Echocardiogram to reveal vegetations in endocarditis

TREATMENT

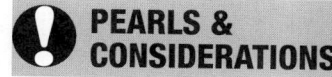

NONPHARMACOLOGIC THERAPY

- Drainage of abscesses
- Valve replacement for endocarditis

ACUTE GENERAL Rx

Combination antibiotics required:
Major options:
- Doxycycline 100 mg PO bid for 6 wk plus streptomycin 1 g IM qd for the first 14-21 days.
Alternative therapies:
- Doxycycline 100 mg PO bid plus rifampin 600 to 900 mg PO qd for 6 wk.
- Sulfamethoxazole 800 mg/trimethoprim 160 mg one DS tablet PO qid, ciprofloxacin 500 mg bid for 6 wk along with doxycycline or rifampin as an alternative regimen.
- Courses <6 wk are associated with higher relapse rates; longer courses are recommended for complicated disease (e.g., osteomyelitis, endocarditis, and neurobrucellosis).

DISPOSITION

- Relapse is possible weeks to months after the completion of therapy.
- Reactivation with CHSB has been reported up to 35 yr after initial illness.

REFERRAL

For all cases to an infectious disease specialist

PEARLS & CONSIDERATIONS

COMMENTS

- Alert the microbiology laboratory to the possibility of *Brucella* spp. (prolonged incubation needed and biohazard for laboratory personnel).
- Do not use doxycycline in children or pregnant women.
- Avoid aminoglycosides in pregnant women.
- Fluoroquinolones have good in vitro activity against *Brucella* spp. and are under study as components of complex regimens. Monotherapy is not effective.

EVIDENCE

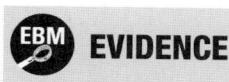

available at www.expertconsult.com

SUGGESTED READINGS

available at www.expertconsult.com

AUTHOR: **PATRICIA CRISTOFARO, M.D.**

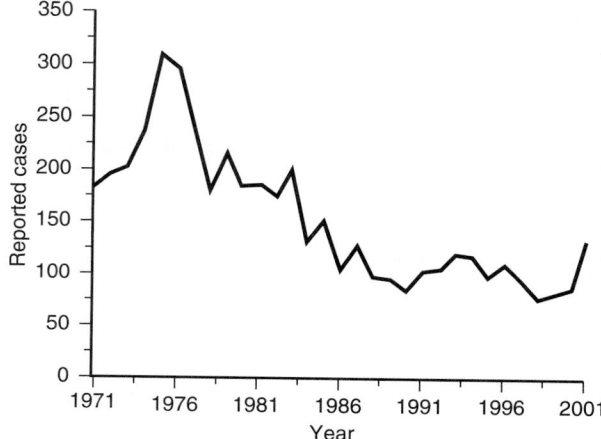

FIGURE 1-66 Cases of human brucellosis reported annually (1971–2001) to the Centers of Disease Control and Prevention. After peaking at more than 300 cases in 1975, the number of brucellosis cases has declined and, for the past 10 years, has remained relatively stable at approximately 100 cases per year. (From Centers for Disease Control and Prevention. Summary of notifiable diseases, United States, 2001. *MMWR Morb Mortal Wkly Rep* 50:53, 2001.) (Mandell GL, Bennett JE, Dolin R: *Principles and Practice of Infectious Diseases,* ed 6, Philadelphia, 2005, Elsevier.)

BASIC INFORMATION

DEFINITION

Genetic disease characterized by a specific electrocardiogram (ECG) pattern and increased risk of sudden cardiac death (SCD) in individuals with structurally normal hearts.

ICD-9-CM CODES
746.89 Other specified congenital anomalies of heart

EPIDEMIOLOGY & DEMOGRAPHICS

INCIDENCE: 5:100,000 people. Thought to be accountable for ~20% of sudden deaths in patients with structurally normal hearts.
PREVALENCE: Up to 0.4% (US)
PREDOMINANT SEX AND AGE: Males (4:1), ages 18 to 65 typically (although can manifest in children)
GENETICS: Autosomal dominant with variable expression. *SCN5A* mutation (15-20%) (alpha subunit of cardiac sodium channel gene). Other mutations have been identified. Only ~35% of cases of Brugada have been linked to an actual gene mutation.
RISK FACTORS: First degree relatives with the disease

PHYSICAL FINDINGS & CLINICAL PRESENTATION

- Physical exam is usually benign
- Classic ECG finding is right bundle branch block (RBBB) pattern with persistent ST elevation of cove-like morphology and T-wave inversion in the anterior leads (V_1-V_3)
- Often an incidental finding diagnosed from a typical ECG pattern
- Palpitations
- Syncope from ventricular tachycardia (VT)
- Sudden cardiac arrest (SCA) from ventricular fibrillation (VF) that was successfully resuscitated
- SCD may be the initial presentation in up to one third of patients.
- There are three types of ECG pattern. Type 1 is the most common and characteristic (Fig. 1-67).
- ECG pattern can be transient and may be provoked (sodium channel blockers, vagal maneuvers, increased alpha-adrenergic tone, beta-blockers, tricyclic or tetracyclic antidepressants, fever, hypokalemia, hyperkalemia, hypercalcemia, and alcohol and cocaine toxicity)

ETIOLOGY

Genetic abnormality(ies) leading to dysfunction of ion channels in myocardium (most commonly sodium channels), which can result in fatal ventricular arrhythmias

DIAGNOSIS

Consensus report from the Study Group on the Molecular Basis of Arrhythmias of the European Society of Cardiology (2002).
- Presence of Type I ECG in ≥2 leads in right precordium (V_1-V_3) and at least one of the following:
  - Documented ventricular fibrillation
  - Self-terminating polymorphic VT
  - Family history of SCD at <45 yr
  - Type 1 ST-segment elevation (Fig. 1-67) in family members
  - Electrophysiologic inducibility of VT
  - Unexplained syncope suggestive of a tachyarrhythmia
  - Nocturnal agonal respiration
- Presence of Type II or III ECG (Fig. 1-67) that converts into Type I ECG following sodium channel blocker challenge AND one of the features previously described.

DIFFERENTIAL DIAGNOSIS

- Long QT syndrome
- Sudden unexpected noctural death syndrome (SUNDS)
- Commotio cordis (disruption of heart rhythm as a result of trauma to the precordium)
- Preexcitation syndrome

WORKUP

- Cardiology consult is strongly recommended if Brugada syndrome is suspected.
- Detailed history with emphasis for history of syncope, cardiac arrest, SCD in family
- 2D echocardiogram
- Electrophysiological study may be indicated.
- First degree relatives should obtain ECG and evaluated for symptoms.

LABORATORY TESTS

None required. Currently, the presence of *SCN5A* mutation is not considered a diagnostic criterion.

IMAGING STUDIES

2D echocardiogram

TREATMENT

There is no definitive treatment for this condition. However, there is some evidence that quinidine may reduce event rates.

NONPHARMACOLOGIC THERAPY

Implantable cardioverter-defibrillator (ICD) can prevent SCD in patients with Brugada syndrome. However, selecting which patients should receive an ICD is challenging.

ACUTE GENERAL Rx

Stabilization of ventricular arrhythmia if present; otherwise, none.

DISPOSITION

If patient has had recent high-risk symptoms (syncope, SCA/SCD), they should be admitted for an inpatient evaluation. If no recent high-risk symptoms, then an outpatient referral to cardiology is reasonable.

REFERRAL

Consultation with cardiology is strongly recommended if Brugada syndrome is suspected.

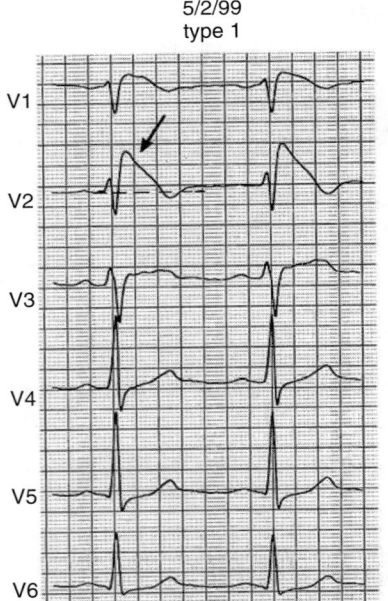
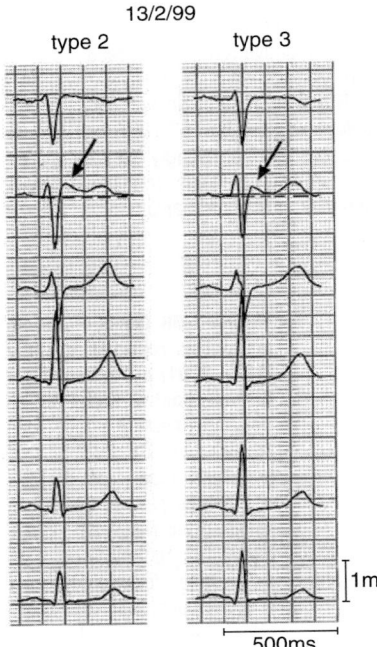

FIGURE 1-67 ECG changes in Brugada syndrome. ST elevation occurs in the anterior precordial leads, leads V_1 and V_2. Type 1 (coved) ECGs with 1 mV of ST elevation have the most prognostic significance. (From Wilde AA, Strickberger SA et al: *J Am Coll Cardiol* 47:473-484, 2006, Fig. 3.)

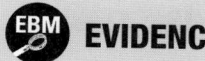
ⓘ PEARLS & CONSIDERATIONS

COMMENTS

- The classic ecg changes in Brugada syndrome can be transient and are often provokable.
- Up to one third of patients with Brugada syndrome initially present with SCD/SCA.
- Only ~35% of cases of Brugada Syndrome have an identified genetic abnormality.

PREVENTION

Identification of patients with Brugada syndrome and appropriate screening of family members is paramount to the prevention of SCD.

PATIENT/FAMILY EDUCATION

Immediate family members should be notified and be screened for Brugada syndrome.

EBM EVIDENCE

available at www.expertconsult.com

SUGGESTED READINGS

available at www.expertconsult.com

AUTHORS: **PHILIP LEE, M.D.**, and **WEN-CHIH WU, M.D.**

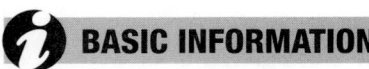

DEFINITION

Forcible clenching or grinding of the teeth during sleep or wakefulness, often leading to damage of the teeth.

ICD-9CM CODES
306.8 Bruxism

EPIDEMIOLOGY & DEMOGRAPHICS

- Occurs in 15% of children and 75% of adults
- Familial cases have occasionally been described.
- Bruxism often presents between age 10 and 20 yr but may persist throughout life.
- Nocturnal bruxism is noted most often during stages I and II NREM sleep and REM sleep.

PHYSICAL FINDINGS & CLINICAL PRESENTATION

Complaints of grinding of teeth from a sleep partner or members of the family are common. In many cases the masticatory system will adapt to the phenomenon, but in severe cases nearly every part of the masticatory system may be damaged. Excessive wearing of dentition is the most common physical finding. Tender or hypoatrophied masticatory muscles may also be observed.

ETIOLOGY

- Cause is controversial.
- Possible causes include occlusal discrepancies, anatomy of the bony structures of the orofacial region, part of the sleep arousal response, disturbances of the central dopaminergic system, smoking, alcohol, drugs, stress, and personality.

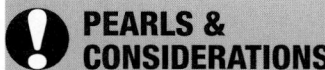 **DIAGNOSIS**

DIFFERENTIAL DIAGNOSIS

- Dental compression syndrome
- Temporomandibular joint disorders
- Chronic orofacial pain disorders
- Oral motor disorders
- Malocclusion

WORKUP

- History should have an emphasis on sleep habits, including excessive snoring, pain in the temporal mandibular region, interview with close family members, health habits, personality quirks.
- Physical examination of the teeth and masticatory muscles is mandatory.
- Sleep studies in selected cases may be helpful.

LABORATORY TESTS

None indicated unless a systemic disease is suspected (e.g., infection, autoimmune disorder)

IMAGING STUDIES

X-ray studies of teeth and temporomandibular joints

TREATMENT

NONPHARMACOLOGIC THERAPY

Biofeedback, psychological counseling, and elimination of harmful health habits have been used with limited success.

GENERAL Rx

- Oral splints (Fig. 1-68); nightguard to protect teeth may be useful
- Correction of malocclusion

- Pain management (e.g., gabapentin, ibuprofen)
- Medication to relieve anxiety and improve sleep (e.g., benzodiazepine or trazodone at bedtime)
- Local injections of botulinum toxin into masseter muscles to prevent dental and temporomandibular joint complications

DISPOSITION

Referral to dentist mandatory if damage to teeth evident

PEARLS & CONSIDERATIONS

- Like any poorly understood disease, treatment is often unsatisfactory and subject to quackery.
- Both diurnal and nocturnal bruxism may be associated with various movement and degenerative disorders (e.g., Huntington disease, oromandibular dystonia) and are quite common in children with cerebral palsy and mental retardation.

SUGGESTED READINGS

available at www.expertconsult.com

AUTHOR: **FRED F. FERRI, M.D.**

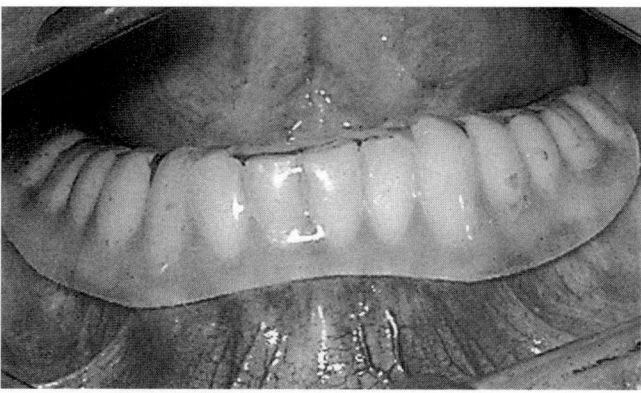

FIGURE 1-68 Occlusal splint. (From Hochberg MC et al [eds]: *Rheumatology,* ed 3, St Louis, 2003, Mosby.)

ℹ️ BASIC INFORMATION

DEFINITION

Budd-Chiari syndrome (BCS) is a rare disease defined by the obstruction of hepatic venous outflow anywhere from the small hepatic veins to the junction of the inferior vena cava (IVC) and the right atrium. Primary BCS is defined by endoluminal obstruction as seen in thromboses or webs. Secondary BCS occurs when the obstruction is caused by compression or invasion by a lesion originating outside the veins (tumor, abscess, cyst, etc.). It can also be a postoperative complication of orthotopic liver transplantation.

SYNONYMS

Hepatic vein thrombosis
Obliterative endophlebitis of the hepatic veins
IVC thrombosis (obliterative hepatocavopathy)

ICD-9CM CODES
453.0 Budd-Chiari syndrome

EPIDEMIOLOGY & DEMOGRAPHICS

INCIDENCE: 1/2.5 million persons per yr
PREDOMINANT SEX: In Western countries, women are more commonly affected
PREDOMINANT AGE: Presentation is usually in the third and fourth decades of life.

PHYSICAL FINDINGS & CLINICAL PRESENTATION

Clinical presentation and characteristics vary with geography. In Africa and South Asia, intravascular webs are more often associated with IVC thrombosis with a stronger association with subsequent hepatocellular carcinoma. In the U.S., BCS is more commonly associated with primary myeloproliferative disorders and underlying hypercoagulable states. Underlying factors that contribute to BCS can be identified in ~85% of cases, and multiple causative factors are identified in 50% of cases.

- Need two of three hepatic veins to be compromised to see clinical manifestations.
- Variable according to the degree, location, acuity of obstruction, and presence of collateral circulation:
  - Fulminant/acute (20%): severe right upper quadrant abdominal pain, fever, nausea, vomiting, jaundice, hepatomegaly, ascites, marked elevation in serum aminotransferases, elevation of alkaline phosphatase to 300 to 400 IU/L, decrease in coagulation factors, and encephalopathy within 8 wk of onset of jaundice; early recognition and treatment are essential for survival
  - Subacute/chronic (60%): vague abdominal discomfort, gradual progression to caudate lobe hypertrophy with atrophy of the rest of the liver, portal hypertension with or without cirrhosis and its sequelae, ascites, lower extremity edema, esophageal varices, splenomegaly, coagulopathy, hepatorenal syndrome in up to half of patients, hepatopulmonary syndrome in up to 28% of patients, and rarely, encephalopathy

  - Asymptomatic (5% to 20%): usually discovered incidentally by abnormal liver function tests

ETIOLOGY

- Primary myeloproliferative diseases: 20% to 53%
  - Polycythemia vera, responsible for 10% to 40% of cases
  - Essential thrombocythemia and idiopathic myelofibrosis are less common causes
  - *JAK2* mutations associated with many myeloproliferative disorders are now being implicated in cases of idiopathic BCS
- Hypercoagulable states (inherited and acquired): often coexist with other causes, 30% to 65%
  - Factor V Leiden (25%)
  - Factor II gene mutation (5%)
  - Anticardiolipin antibodies (25%)
  - Hyperhomocysteinemia (22%)
  - Paroxysmal nocturnal hemoglobinuria (19%)
- Protein C deficiency, protein S deficiency, and antithrombin III deficiency are difficult to interpret because of acute thrombus and liver disease; need familial studies to prove
- Heterozygosity for G20210A prothrombin gene mutation or methylene-tetrahydrofolate reductase (MTHFR) mutation may be seen in BCS
- Pregnancy and oral contraceptive pills
- Rare but reported: sickle cell anemia, infections with liver abscess, hydatid cyst (echinococcosis), schistosomiasis, malignancies, sarcoidosis, Behçet's disease (<5%), IVC membrane/congenital web, abdominal trauma, ulcerative colitis, celiac disease, idiopathic (10% to 20%)

🩺 DIAGNOSIS

DIFFERENTIAL DIAGNOSIS

- Hepatitis from ischemia, viral infection, toxin, alcohol
- Cholecystitis
- Hepatic venoocclusive disease (sinusoidal obstruction syndrome)
- Congestive hepatopathy, also known as *cardiac cirrhosis,* from tricuspid regurgitation, right atrial myxoma, constrictive pericarditis
- Cirrhosis from any etiology

LABORATORY TESTS

- Assessment of liver injury and function: serum aminotransferases, alkaline phosphatase, prothrombin time (PT), albumin, bilirubin
- Exclusion of another form of liver disease: viral hepatitis panel, autoantibodies (antinuclear antibody, anti–smooth muscle antibody, anti-mitochondrial antibody), serum iron, transferrin saturation, ferritin, ceruloplasmin, and α-1 antitrypsin
- Ascites protein content >3.0 g/dl and serum ascites albumin gradient ≥1.1 g/dl are suggestive of ascites from BCS, cardiac or pericardial disease

- Evaluation for underlying myeloproliferative disorder and hypercoagulable state: CBC, bone marrow biopsy, tests for hypercoagulable states (Factor V Leiden, prothrombin gene G20210A mutation, protein C, protein S, and antithrombin deficiencies, antiphospholipid antibodies, hyperhomocystinemia, paroxysmal nocturnal hemoglobinuria, and MTHFR C677T mutation); protein C, protein S, and antithrombin deficiencies may be difficult to interpret in the setting of liver dysfunction, but levels <20% of normal are suggestive of a true deficiency; thrombophilia screening for the JAK2 V617F mutation may be useful

IMAGING STUDIES

- Diagnosis of BCS is made by radiographic imaging.
- Ultrasound and color and pulsed Doppler are the first-line tests. Diagnostic sensitivity and specificity are 85% to 90%. Findings include large hepatic vein with an absent flow signal, or with reversed or turbulent flow; large intrahepatic collateral vessels; enlarged, stenotic, or tortuous hepatic veins; and caudate lobe hypertrophy.
- MRI with gadolinium contrast—better than contrast-enhanced CT (Fig. 1-69), with a sensitivity and specificity of approximately 90%—is the second-line test. Findings include obstructed hepatic veins or IVC, large, intrahepatic, or subcapsular collaterals, and caudate lobe hypertrophy. Three-dimensional contrast-enhanced magnetic resonance angiography rivals hepatic venography in sensitivity.
- CT image reconstruction of vasculature is becoming available.
- Venography: This is not essential for diagnosis, but when done with measurement of pressure gradients is mainly indicated to predict success of percutaneous or surgical shunt intervention. Confirms the pathognomonic web pattern caused by collateral venous flow.
- Liver biopsy: This is not necessary to diagnose BCS but may be helpful in patients with cirrhosis in whom the diagnosis remains un-

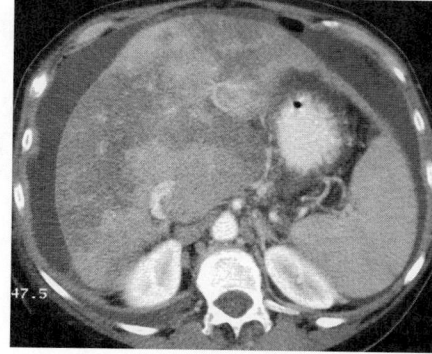

FIGURE 1-69 CT scan of Budd-Chiari syndrome.
The appearances are not immediately diagnostic for the nonexpert, and infiltrative disease is sometimes suspected. (From Forbes A et al [eds]: *Atlas of clinical gastroenterology,* ed 3, 2005, Mosby.)

certain and critical for differentiating from hepatic venoocclusive disease. Findings include hepatic congestion, hepatocyte necrosis and fibrosis in centrilobular areas, and compensatory nodular regenerative hyperplasia with progression to fibrosis and cirrhosis. In advanced BCS, may also see infarction caused by concomitant thrombosis of the intrahepatic, extrahepatic, and portal veins.

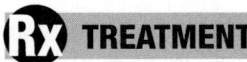

NONPHARMACOLOGIC THERAPY

- Goal of therapy is decompression of hepatic congestion.
- In general, therapeutic procedures should be introduced by order of increasing invasiveness based on response/failure to therapy rather than disease severity.
- Hypercoagulable states should be investigated in all patients.

ACUTE GENERAL Rx

- Anticoagulation, first with low-molecular-weight heparin (LMWH), followed by warfarin, even in the absence of an underlying hypercoagulable disorder
- In situ thrombolysis: can be successful when performed in recently thrombosed veins, and high blood flow can be restored by angioplasty or stenting
- Balloon angioplasty: complicated by 50% restenosis rate
- Stenting: may improve long-term patency rates to 90%, but if placed above the intrahepatic IVC, may complicate future liver transplantation
- Transjugular intrahepatic portosystemic shunt (TIPS) has been increasingly used in recent years; usually performed in patients with no improvement on anticoagulation therapy; TIPS has replaced surgical shunting as the most common invasive therapeutic procedure
- Surgical portal systemic shunts: feasibility depends on technical factors, as well as on locating a center with well-trained surgeons

- Liver transplant may be indicated in patients with fulminant hepatic failure and in patients who fail to respond to TIPS
- Supportive measures

CHRONIC Rx

- Lifelong anticoagulation: Warfarin therapy with a target international normalized ratio of (INR) 2 to 3 lessens, but does not completely prevent, recurrence.
- In patients with an underlying myeloproliferative disorder, treatment with hydroxyurea and aspirin, or anagrelide, may be given instead of traditional anticoagulation.
- Treat liver dysfunction and complications related to portal hypertension, such as ascites.
- Invasive interventions should be reserved for symptomatic patients who do not improve with medical therapy.
- Manage shunt thrombosis, which is a common complication.
- Liver transplantation is another treatment option.
- Monitor for development of hepatocellular carcinoma and transformation of myeloproliferative disease in patients with longstanding, well-controlled BCS.

DISPOSITION

Prognosis is variable and depends on multiple factors, including time to recognition and treatment, etiology, acuity, the type of intervention, and the condition of the patient at the time of treatment. Overall mortality rates are decreasing with the use of anticoagulation and early diagnosis of asymptomatic cases. Survival rates have been reported as 77%, 65%, and 57% at 1, 5, and 10 yr from diagnosis. A prognostic index called the *Rotterdam BCS Index* has been described: $1.27 \times$ Encephalopathy $+ 1.04 \times$ Ascites $+ 0.72 \times$ PT $+ 0.004 \times$ Bilirubin. Encephalopathy and ascites are scored as 1 for present or 0 as absent, and PT is scored as greater (1) or less than (0) an INR of 2.3. An in-

dex of <1.1 correlates to low risk (5-yr survival rate, 89%), 1.1 to 1.5 with intermediate risk (5-yr survival rate, 74%), and >1.5 with high risk (5-yr survival rate, 42%).

REFERRAL

Fulminant presentations should immediately be referred to a center capable of liver transplantation. All cases benefit from referral to a hepatologist, a hematologist, an interventional radiologist, and a surgeon specializing in hepatobiliary disease.

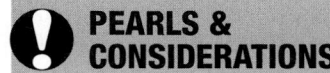

COMMENTS

- Look for one or more underlying causes, especially hypercoagulable or hematologic disorders.
- Myeloproliferative disorders are most common.
- Diagnosis relies on imaging, beginning with Doppler ultrasound.
- Treatment with anticoagulation comes first, followed by invasive interventions as needed.
- Referral for liver transplantation may be necessary.
- Prognosis depends on presence of ascites, encephalopathy, PT, and serum bilirubin levels.

PREVENTION

In the setting of known risk factors, such as a hypercoagulable state or myeloproliferative disorder, any additional risks, such as smoking or oral contraceptive therapy, should be avoided.

SUGGESTED READINGS
available at www.expertconsult.com

AUTHOR: **KITTICHAI PROMRAT, M.D.**

BASIC INFORMATION

DEFINITION

Bulimia nervosa is a prolonged illness characterized by a specific psychopathology.

ICD-9CM CODES
783.6 Bulimia

EPIDEMIOLOGY & DEMOGRAPHICS

INCIDENCE/PREVALENCE: Affects 1% to 3% of female adolescents and young adults
PREDOMINANT SEX: Female/male ratio of 10:1
PREDOMINANT AGE: Adolescence to young adulthood; mean age of onset: 17 yr

PHYSICAL FINDINGS & CLINICAL PRESENTATION

- Parotid and salivary gland swelling
- Scars on the back of the hand and knuckles (Russell sign) from rubbing against the upper incisors when inducing vomiting
- Eroded enamel, particularly on the lingual surface of the upper teeth; pyorrhea and other gum disorders possible
- Petechial hemorrhages of the cornea, soft palate, or face possibly noted after vomiting
- Loss of gag reflex, well-developed abdominal musculature
- Often no emaciation; normal physical examination possible

ETIOLOGY

- Etiology is unknown but likely multifactorial (sociocultural, psychologic, familial factors).
- Bulimia is much more common in Western societies, where there is a strong cultural pressure to be slender.
- According to the American Psychiatric Association, patients with eating disorders display a broad range of symptoms that occur along a continuum between those of anorexia nervosa and bulimia.

DIAGNOSIS

DIFFERENTIAL DIAGNOSIS

- Schizophrenia
- Gastrointestinal disorders
- Neurologic disorders (seizures, Kleine-Levin syndrome, Klüver-Bucy syndrome)
- Brain neoplasms
- Psychogenic vomiting

WORKUP

- The following questions are useful to screen patients for bulimia:
  1. "Are you satisfied with your eating habits?"
  2. "Do you ever eat in secret?"
- Answering "no" to the first question and/or "yes" to the second question has 100% sensitivity and 90% specificity for bulimia. The SCOFF questionnaire can also be used as a screening tool for eating disorders (see Anorexia Nervosa).
- A diagnosis can be made using the following DSM-IV diagnostic criteria for bulimia nervosa:
  1. Recurrent episodes of binge eating (rapid consumption of a large amount of food in a discrete period)
  2. A feeling of lack of control over eating behavior during the eating binges
  3. Self-induced vomiting, use of laxatives or diuretics, strict dieting or fasting, or rigorous exercise to prevent weight gain
  4. A minimum of two binge-eating episodes a week for at least 3 mo
  5. Persistent overconcern with body shape and weight

LABORATORY TESTS

- Electrolyte abnormalities from vomiting (hypokalemia and metabolic alkalosis) or diarrhea from laxative abuse (hypokalemia and hyperchloremic metabolic acidosis)
- Hyponatremia, hypocalcemia, hypomagnesemia (caused by laxative abuse)
- Elevated cortisol, decreased luteinizing hormone, decreased follicle-stimulating hormone

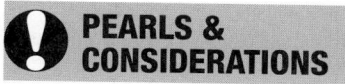

TREATMENT

NONPHARMACOLOGIC THERAPY

- Cognitive behavioral therapy, particularly interpersonal therapy to control abnormal behaviors
- Use of food diaries, nutritional counseling, and planning meals at least 1 day in advance are useful measures to counter abnormal eating behaviors
- Correction of electrolyte abnormalities

ACUTE GENERAL Rx

- Selective serotonin reuptake inhibitors are generally considered to be the safest medication option in these patients. They are useful in severely depressed patients and in those who do not benefit from cognitive behavioral therapy.

- Prompt recognition and treatment of complications:
  1. Ipecac cardiotoxicity from laxative abuse
  2. Electrolyte abnormalities (see "Laboratory Tests")
  3. Esophagitis and Mallory-Weiss tears; esophageal rupture from repeated vomiting
  4. Aspiration pneumonia and pneumomediastinum
  5. Menstrual irregularities (including amenorrhea)
  6. Gastrointestinal abnormalities: acute gastric dilatation, pancreatitis, abdominal pain, constipation

CHRONIC Rx

- Psychotherapy continued for years and focused specifically on self-image and family and peer interactions is an integral part of successful recovery.
- Family therapy is also recommended, especially in younger patients.

DISPOSITION

Course is variable and marked by frequent recurrence of exacerbations.

REFERRAL

- In addition to the primary care physician, the multidisciplinary team should include a dietician, a psychiatrist, and a family therapist.
- Hospitalization should be considered for patients with severe electrolyte abnormalities or those with suicidal thoughts.

PEARLS & CONSIDERATIONS

COMMENTS

- Bulimia has a close association with depression, bipolar disorder, obsessive-compulsive disorder, alcoholism, and substance abuse.
- Bulimia should be considered in all patients (especially adolescents) with unexplained hypokalemia and metabolic alkalosis.

EVIDENCE

available at www.expertconsult.com

SUGGESTED READINGS
available at www.expertconsult.com

AUTHOR: **FRED F. FERRI, M.D.**

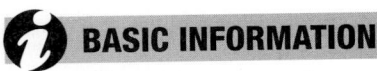

DEFINITION

Bullous pemphigoid is an autoimmune, subepidermal blistering disease commonly seen in the elderly. A related entity is cicatricial pemphigoid, which predominantly affects the mucous membranes.

SYNONYMS

Pemphigoid

ICD-9CM CODES
694.5 Pemphigoid

EPIDEMIOLOGY & DEMOGRAPHICS

- Occurs most commonly in people older than 60 yr, with peak incidence in those aged ≥80 yr
- Incidence is approximately 10 cases per 1 million persons
- No gender or racial predilection
- Most common of the autoimmune bullous dermatoses

PHYSICAL FINDINGS & CLINICAL PRESENTATION

HISTORY:
- Skin lesions typically start as eczematous or urticarial plaques on the extremities and are often very pruritic
- Taut blisters can form within 1 wk to several months

PHYSICAL FINDINGS:
- Anatomic distribution
  1. Flexor surfaces of the arms and legs, groin, axilla, chest, and abdomen; generally spares the head and neck
  2. Rare involvement of mucous membranes
- Lesion configuration
  1. May be localized to the extremities or generalized
  2. Lesions irregularly grouped but may sometimes be serpiginous (Fig. 1-70)
- Lesion morphology
  1. Taut blisters (bullae) measuring 5 mm to 2 cm in diameter filled with clear or bloody fluid on either normal or erythematous skin are characteristic
  2. Heal without scarring but may leave postinflammatory hyperpigmentation

ETIOLOGY

- Autoimmune disease with immunoglobulin (Ig) G and/or C3 complement targeting hemidesmosomal antigens located in the epidermal basement membrane zone
- Drug-induced pemphigoid, although rare, can occur in patients taking penicillamine, furosemide, captopril, penicillin, or sulfasalazine

 DIAGNOSIS

Skin biopsy aids in the diagnosis, and specimens should be sent for routine histochemical staining and direct immunofluorescence.

DIFFERENTIAL DIAGNOSIS

- Cicatricial pemphigoid
- Epidermolysis bullosa acquisita
- Pemphigus
- Linear IgA disease

LABORATORY TESTS

- Histology of lesional skin shows a subepidermal blister with a superficial inflammatory infiltrate, often with numerous eosinophils
- Indirect immunofluorescence detects anti–basement membrane antibodies in 70% of patients with bullous pemphigoid.
- Direct immunofluorescence of perilesional skin shows C3 and IgG linearly arranged along the epidermal basement membrane.
- Approximately half of patients will have a peripheral blood eosinophilia.

TREATMENT

Bullous pemphigoid may be a self-limited disease, but its course may last from months to years. Treatment is based on the degree of disease involvement and the rate of disease progression.

NONPHARMACOLOGIC THERAPY

- Mild soaps with emollients to wet skin after bathing
- Topical antipruritic creams

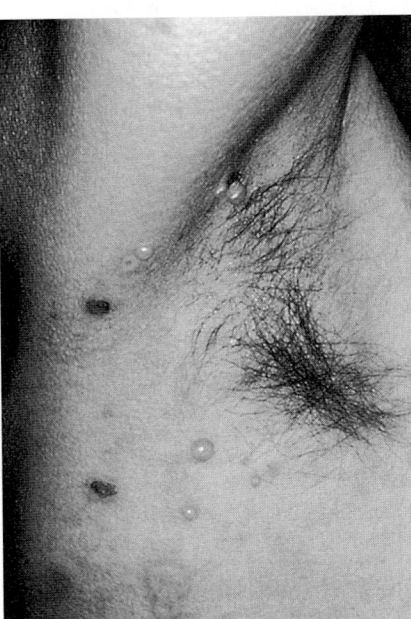

FIGURE 1-70 Bullous pemphigoid. Note intact bullae with erosions in a flexural distribution. (From Goldstein BG, Goldstein AO: *Practical dermatology*, ed 2, St Louis, 1997, Mosby.)

ACUTE GENERAL Rx

Localized disease:
- Potent topical steroids (e.g., clobetasol) until blistering ceases with gradual tapering over several weeks
- Oral antihistamines to control pruritus

Generalized disease:
- Mainstay of therapy is prednisone, usually beginning with a minimal dose of 1 mg/kg/day
- Steroid-sparing agents, such as azathioprine or mycophenolate mofetil, may be started with prednisone or shortly after prednisone therapy is initiated and may be continued once prednisone is discontinued
- Tetracyclines
- Low-dose methotrexate has recently been suggested to be an optimal therapy in the elderly
- Rituximab, a monoclonal antibody to CD20, has been used for treatment-refractory bullous pemphigoid

CHRONIC Rx

- Prednisone combined with steroid-sparing agents with the goal of limiting oral corticosteroid intake
- Other immunosuppressive agents, such as cyclophosphamide or cyclosporine, are occasionally used

DISPOSITION

Mortality rates are estimated at between 10% and 40% after 1 yr. Patients with widespread disease requiring immunosuppressive therapy and with other comorbidities are at highest risk for complications from the disease Approximately 50% of treated patients experience remission within 2 to 6 yr.

REFERRAL

Dermatology

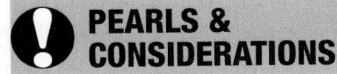 PEARLS & CONSIDERATIONS

COMMENTS

- Bullous pemphigoid is mainly a disease of elderly persons and should be suspected in older persons with chronic pruritic eruptions and in those patients who have new-onset taut vesicles and bullae
- Not believed to represent a paraneoplastic process.

SUGGESTED READINGS
available at www.expertconsult.com

AUTHORS: **JESSICA RISSER, M.D., M.P.H.,** and **KACHIU LEE, B.A.**

ℹ BASIC INFORMATION

DEFINITION

Burning mouth syndrome (BMS) is characterized by burning pain in the tongue or oral mucous membranes, usually occurring without any identifiable precipitating factor. Affected patients may also complain about bitter or metallic taste, dry mouth, and alterations in taste.

SYNONYMS

Scalded mouth syndrome
Glossodynia
Glossopyrosis

ICD-9CM CODES
529.6 Glossodynia

EPIDEMIOLOGY & DEMOGRAPHICS

- Most prevalent in postmenopausal women; reported in 10% to 40% of women presenting for treatment of menopausal symptoms.
- Exact figures are difficult to ascertain, but likely <1% of the general population.
- Typically occurs in middle-aged or older adults.

PHYSICAL FINDINGS & CLINICAL PRESENTATION

- For the majority of patients, the onset of pain is spontaneous without an identifiable precipitating factor.
- One third of patients relate the time of onset to a dental procedure, recent illness, or medication.
- Often persists for many years.
- The burning sensation often occurs in more than one oral site, most frequently in the anterior two thirds of the tongue, the anterior hard palate, and the lower lip mucosa.
- Pain is often absent at night but will increase in severity progressively throughout the day.
- Associated with sleep disturbances as well as difficulty falling asleep.
- Also associated with mood changes such as irritability, anxiety, and depression.
- Up to two thirds of patients report a spontaneous partial recovery within 6 to 7 years from onset with the pain changing from constant to intermittent.

ETIOLOGY

Because of its complex clinical picture, many different hypotheses have been suggested for its etiology. Possible causes include:

- Psychologic dysfunction: many patients concomitantly have personality or mood changes,

report more adverse life events, somatization, anxiety, and depression.
- Chronic pain conditions, such as headaches.
- Local irritants such as smoking.
- Dry mouth: however, most salivary flow rate studies in affected patients have not shown a decrease in unstimulated or stimulated salivary flow.
- Oral candidal infections.
- Medications: e.g., angiotensin-converting enzyme (ACE) inhibitors.
- Nerve damage.
- Nutritional deficiencies: iron, zinc, folate, and vitamin B.

There may be an association between supertasters (those with enhanced ability to taste) and those with BMS due to their increased density of taste buds that are surrounded by bundles of trigeminal nerve neurons.

Dx DIAGNOSIS

DIFFERENTIAL DIAGNOSIS

- Mucosal disease such as lichen planus or candidiasis
- Nutritional deficiency in zinc, iron, folate, or vitamins B1, B2, B6, B9, B12
- Dry mouth from Sjögren's syndrome or after chemo/radiation therapy
- Cranial nerve injury
- Medication effect

WORKUP

- Clinical history is the most important in diagnosing BMS.
- Very important to rule out other pathologic conditions first.

LABORATORY TESTS

There is no test for BMS, but consider testing for vitamin B or zinc deficiency.

Rx TREATMENT

NONPHARMACOLOGIC THERAPY

Formal psychotherapy and cognitive behavior therapy have been helpful for some patients.

Capsaicin (hot pepper powder) can be used as a topical desensitizing agent.

- Rinse mouth with 1 tsp of a 1:2 solution of hot pepper and water; increase strength of

capsaicin as tolerated to a maximum 1:1 dilution.

ACUTE GENERAL Rx

There is no known cure for BMS so many different treatment methods may have to be tried before finding one or a combination that is helpful to the patient.

Treatment options include:
- Low-dose benzodiazepines:
  - Clonazepam (Klonopin) 0.25 to 2 mg/day; start with 0.25 mg qhs and increase dose q 4 to 7 days until oral burning is relieved or side effects
  - Chlordiazepoxide (Librium) 10 to 30 mg/day; start with 5 mg qhs and increase dose q 4 to 7 days until oral burning is relieved or side effects
- Low-dose tricyclic antidepressants:
  - Amitriptyline or nortriptyline 10 to 150 mg/day; start with 10 mg qhs and increase dose by 10 mg q 4 to 7 days.
- Low-dose gabapentin (Neurontin) 300 to 1600 mg/day; start with 100 mg qhs and increase dose by 100 mg q 4 to 7 days (take in divided doses).

COMPLEMENTARY AND ALTERNATIVE MEDICINE

- Antioxidant alpha lipoic acid
- Relaxation programs, massage, or acupuncture

REFERRAL

To a subspecialist in this area, such as a dentist or ENT, if initial therapy fails to resolve symptoms.

❗ PEARLS & CONSIDERATIONS

COMMENTS

Burning mouth syndrome is a rare but possibly debilitating disease. Other diseases should be ruled out.

SUGGESTED READINGS
available at www.expertconsult.com

AUTHOR: **MADHAVI SHAH, M.D.**

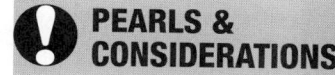

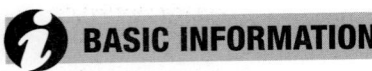

BASIC INFORMATION

DEFINITION
Burn injuries include thermal injuries (flames, scalds, cigarettes), as well as chemical, electrical, and radiation burns.

SYNONYMS
Thermal injury

ICD-9CM CODES
942-949 (by region, % burn)

EPIDEMIOLOGY & DEMOGRAPHICS
PREVALENCE (IN U.S.): Burn injuries account for approximately 500,000 emergency department visits, 40,000 hospitalizations, and 4000 deaths annually.
PREDOMINANT SEX: Occur in males more often than females

PHYSICAL FINDINGS & CLINICAL PRESENTATION
- Burns are defined by surface area and depth of skin involved.
- First-degree burns (superficial) involve the epidermis only and appear painful and red.
- Second-degree burns involve the dermis and appear blistered, moist, and red with two-point discrimination intact (superficial partial-thickness) or red and blanched white with only sensation of pressure intact (deep partial thickness).
- Third-degree burns (full-thickness) extend through the dermis with associated destruction of hair follicles and sweat glands. The skin is charred, pale, painless, and leathery. These burns are caused by flames, immersion scalds, and chemical and high-voltage injuries.

DIAGNOSIS

CLASSIFICATION
Burns are classified by extent of the burn or total burn surface area (TBSA). The TBSA is best classified by using age-specific burn charts and the "rules of nines" (Fig. 1-71).
Major burns: Partial-thickness burns ≥25% TBSA (or 20% if younger than 10 yr or older than 50 yr); full-thickness burns ≥10% TBSA; burns crossing major joints or involving the hands, face, feet, or perineum; electrical or chemical burns; those complicated by inhalation injury or involving high-risk patients (extremes of age/comorbid diseases)
Moderate burns: Partial-thickness burns ≥15% to 25% TBSA (or 10% in children and adults); full-thickness burns ≥2% to 10% TBSA and not involving the specific conditions of major burns
Minor burns: Partial-thickness burns <15% TBSA or full-thickness burns <2% TBSA

LABORATORY STUDIES
- CBC, electrolytes, BUN, creatinine, and glucose
- Serial ABG and carboxyhemoglobin if smoke inhalation suspected
- Urinalysis, urine myoglobin, and CPK levels if concern for rhabdomyolysis

IMAGING STUDIES
Chest radiograph and bronchoscopy if smoke inhalation suspected

TREATMENT

ACUTE GENERAL Rx
- Establish airway: inspect for inhalation injury and intubate for suspected airway edema (often seen 12 to 24 hr later); supplemental O2
- Remove jewelry and clothing and place one or two large-bore peripheral IVs (if TBSA >20%)
- The primary goal for severely burned patients' resuscitation is prevention of ischemia by maintaining organ perfusion and restoring the deficit of sodium lost from the extracellular space. The hypertonic lactate saline (HLS) solutions with mild concentration of sodium have been used in some burn centers to maintain plasma volume without using larger fluid volumes. Fluid resuscitation with Ringer's lactate at 2 to 4 ml/kg per %TBSA per 24 hr with half the calculated fluid given in the first 8 hr is an effective modality in severe burns.
- Foley catheter and NG tube (20% of patients develop an ileus)
- Tetanus update
- Treat pain and anxiety
- Stress ulcer prophylaxis in high-risk patients
- Address adequate nutritional support
- ECG monitoring for high-voltage burns given increased risk for arrhythmias

- Routine systemic prophylactic antibiotic treatment is not recommended for the prevention of burn wound infections; however, burn victims should be considered immunosuppressed. Of note, early use of topical antibiotics such as silver sulfadiazine has been associated with decreased incidence of burn infections.

BURN WOUND Rx
First-degree burns (e.g., sunburns):
- Can be treated with cool compresses, antihistamines, emollients, and, at times, a rapidly tapering dose of steroids.

Second-degree and third-degree burns:
- Wash burned skin with cool tap water or saline (15° to 25° C; immerse approximately 30 min if able) and cleanse with mild soap. Ice or ice water may increase tissue injury and should not be used.
- Sharp debridement of ruptured blisters (except palms and soles). Leave unruptured blisters intact.
- Several approaches to burn dressings after cleansing and debriding:
  1. Apply thin layer of antibiotic ointment (silver sulfadiazine can be used unless sulfa allergy or facial burn) and cover with a nonadherent dressing (e.g., Telfa or petroleum-soaked gauze) followed by a sterile gauze wrap. Wash wound and change dressing when dressing soaked.
  2. Apply saline-soaked gauze (Xeroform, Owen's), cover with 4 × 4 dressing and a bulky absorbent dressing such as Kerlex. Reevaluate in 5 to 7 days.
  3. Apply occlusive dressing (DuoDerm, Tega-sorb), remove in 7 to 10 days.
- Specialized care, such as excision and autografting, is required for some deep second-degree and most third-degree burns.

DISPOSITION
- Respiratory injury, sepsis, and multiorgan failure may complicate severe burns.
- Scarring can be expected in many second-degree and all third-degree burns.

REFERRAL
Major and some moderate burns require referral to specialized burn centers for surgical debridement, grafting evaluation, and rehabilitation.

PEARLS & CONSIDERATIONS

COMMENTS
Burn victims must be reassessed frequently because the patient's condition can change significantly in the first 24 to 72 hr.

EVIDENCE
available at www.expertconsult.com

SUGGESTED READINGS
available at www.expertconsult.com

AUTHORS: **SRIVIDYA ANANDAN, M.D.,** and **MICHELLE STOZEK ANVAR, M.D.**

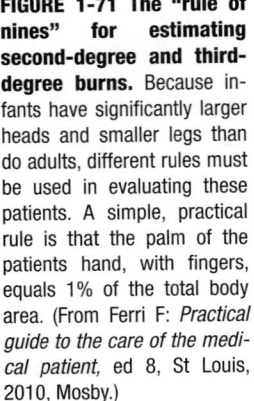
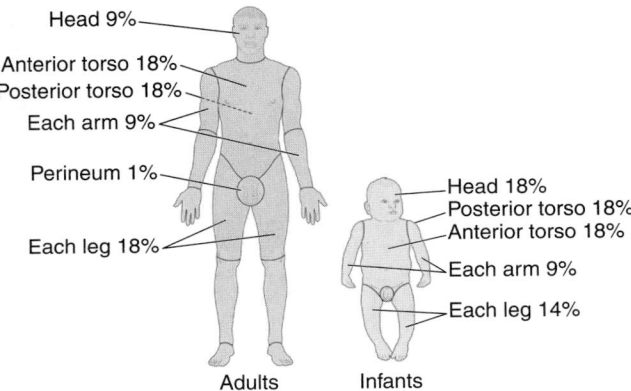

FIGURE 1-71 The "rule of nines" for estimating second-degree and third-degree burns. Because infants have significantly larger heads and smaller legs than do adults, different rules must be used in evaluating these patients. A simple, practical rule is that the palm of the patients hand, with fingers, equals 1% of the total body area. (From Ferri F: *Practical guide to the care of the medical patient,* ed 8, St Louis, 2010, Mosby.)

Head 9%
Anterior torso 18%
Posterior torso 18%
Each arm 9%
Perineum 1%
Each leg 18%

Head 18%
Posterior torso 18%
Anterior torso 18%
Each arm 9%
Each leg 14%

Adults   Infants

BASIC INFORMATION

DEFINITION

Bursitis is an inflammation of a bursa and is usually aseptic. A *bursa* is a closed sac lined with a synovial-like membrane that sometimes contains fluid that is found or that develops in an area subject to pressure or friction.

SYNONYMS

Housemaid's knee (prepatellar bursitis)
Weaver's bottom (ischial gluteal bursitis)
Baker's cyst (gastrocnemius-semimembranosus bursa)

ICD-9CM CODES
726.19 Subacromial bursitis
726.33 Olecranon bursitis
726.5 Ischiogluteal bursitis (hip)
726.5 Iliopsoas bursitis (hip)
726.61 Anserine bursitis
726.5 Trochanteric bursitis
726.65 Prepatellar bursitis
727.51 Baker's cyst
726.79 Retrocalcaneal bursitis

PHYSICAL FINDINGS & CLINICAL PRESENTATION

- Swelling, especially if bursa is superficial (olecranon, prepatellar)
- Local tenderness with pain on pressure against bursa
- Pain with joint movement
- Referred pain
- Palpable occasional fibrocartilaginous bodies (most common in olecranon and prepatellar bursae)

ETIOLOGY

- Acute trauma
- Repetitive trauma
- Sepsis
- Crystalline deposit disease
- Rheumatoid arthritis

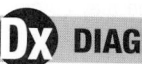

DIAGNOSIS

DIFFERENTIAL DIAGNOSIS

- Degenerative joint disease
- Tendinitis (sometimes occurs in conjunction with bursitis)
- Cellulitis (if bursitis is septic)
- Infectious arthritis

WORKUP

Aspiration with Gram stain and C&S if infection suspected

IMAGING STUDIES

- Plain radiography to rule out other potential or coexisting bone or joint problems (Fig. 1-72)
- MRI

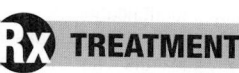

TREATMENT

NONPHARMACOLOGIC THERAPY

- If chronic, elimination of cause of pressure or irritation
- Use of relief pads, avoidance of direct pressure
- Rest
- Elevation
- Ice for acute trauma

ACUTE GENERAL Rx

- Septic:
  1. Appropriate antibiotic coverage and drainage
  2. Aspiration of purulent fluid with a large-bore needle (if there is no rapid clinical response, incision and drainage are indicated)
- Nonseptic:
  1. Aspiration of blood from acute trauma
  2. Application of compression dressing

CHRONIC Rx

- Aspiration if excessive fluid volume present, followed by application of compression dressing to prevent fluid reaccumulation (repeat aspiration may be required)
- Steroid injection into bursa (1 ml of triamcinolone, 40 mg, mixed with 1 to 3 ml of Xylocaine depending on size of bursa)
- NSAIDs

DISPOSITION

- Many bursal sacs "dry up" eventually.
- Nonsurgical treatment is effective in most cases.

REFERRAL

For orthopedic consultation to assist in treatment of sepsis or for excision of chronic enlarged bursa when indicated

PEARLS & CONSIDERATIONS

COMMENTS

- Injection of trochanteric bursa may require spinal needle in a large patient.
- Sterile bursae should not be incised and drained because a chronic draining sinus tract may develop.
- Involvement of the iliopsoas bursa may cause groin pain, although the diagnosis is difficult to make because of the inaccessibility of the area to direct examination. (This also makes steroid injection impossible even if the diagnosis could be established.)

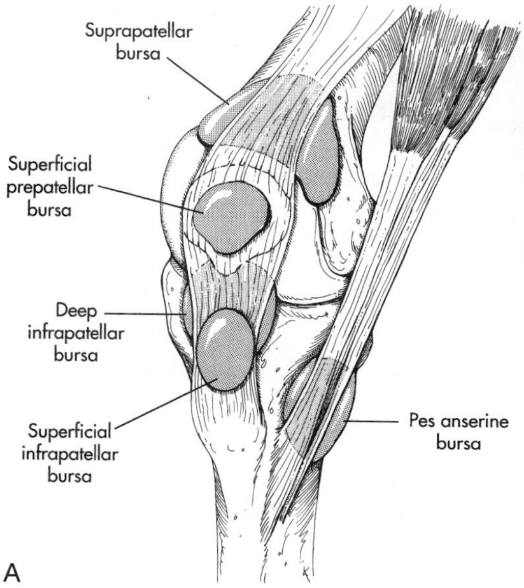

SUGGESTED READINGS
available at www.expertconsult.com

AUTHOR: **LONNIE R. MERCIER, M.D.**

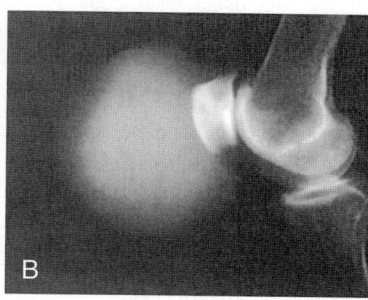
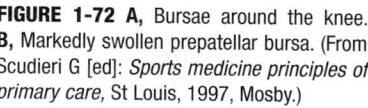
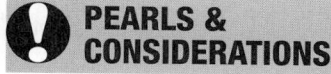

Suprapatellar bursa

Superficial prepatellar bursa

Deep infrapatellar bursa

Superficial infrapatellar bursa

Pes anserine bursa

A

FIGURE 1-72 A, Bursae around the knee. **B,** Markedly swollen prepatellar bursa. (From Scudieri G [ed]: *Sports medicine principles of primary care,* St Louis, 1997, Mosby.)

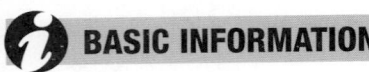

BASIC INFORMATION

DEFINITION

Candidiasis is an inflammatory process involving the vulva or the vagina caused by superficial invasion of epithelial cells by *Candida* species.

SYNONYMS

Moniliasis
Thrush

ICD-9CM CODES	
112.1	Moniliasis
112.0	Thrush
112	Candidosis

EPIDEMIOLOGY & DEMOGRAPHICS

- This is the second most common form of vaginitis in the U.S.; 75% of women will have at least one episode of vulvovaginal candidiasis (VVC) during their childbearing years and approximately 45% will have a second attack. A small subpopulation of <5% of adult women has recurrent, often intractable episodes. *Candida* may be isolated in up to 20% of asymptomatic women of childbearing age.
- Factors that predispose to development of symptomatic VVC include pregnancy, antibiotic use, and diabetes. Antibiotic use disturbs normal vaginal flora and allows overgrowth of fungi; pregnancy and diabetes are associated with decrease in cell-mediated immunity.
- Factors associated with increased rates of asymptomatic vaginal colonization: pregnancy, high-estrogen oral contraceptives, uncontrolled diabetes mellitus, treatment at sexually transmitted disease clinics.

UNCOMPLICATED VVC

- Infrequent VVC
- Mild-to-moderate vaginitis and candida
- Likely to be *C. albicans*
- Nonimmunocompromised women

COMPLICATED VVC

- Recurrent VVC
- Severe VVC
- Non-*albicans* candidiasis
- Women with uncontrolled diabetes, immunosuppression, or pregnancy

PHYSICAL FINDINGS & CLINICAL PRESENTATION

Symptoms of VVC consist of:
- Vulvar pruritus with vaginal discharge that typically resembles cottage cheese.
- Erythema and edema of labia and vulvar skin; possible discrete papular peripheral lesions (satellite lesions).
- Vagina may be erythematous with an adherent, whitish discharge.
- Cervix may appear normal.

- Symptoms characteristically exacerbated in the week preceding menses with some relief after onset of menstrual flow.

ETIOLOGY

- *Candida* are dimorphic fungi (spores and mycelial forms).
- *C. albicans* is responsible for 85% to 90% of vaginal yeast infections.
- *C. glabrata*, *C. tropicalis* (non-*albicans* species) also cause vaginitis and may be more resistant to conventional therapy.

DIAGNOSIS

DIFFERENTIAL DIAGNOSIS

- Bacterial vaginosis
- Trichomoniasis

WORKUP

- Usually normal vaginal pH (<4.5).
- Budding yeast forms or mycelia will appear in as many as 80% of cases. Saline wet prep of vaginal secretions usually is normal; may be increased in inflammatory cells in severe cases.
- Whiff test negative (KOH).
- 10% KCl useful and more sensitive than wet mount for microscopic identification.
- Can make a presumptive diagnosis based on symptomatology in the absence of microscopy-proven fungal elements if the pH and wet prep are normal. Fungal culture is recommended to confirm diagnosis.
- In chronic/recurrent VVC, burning replaces itching as prominent symptom. Confirm diagnosis with direct microscopy and culture. Many may actually have chronic or atrophic dermatitis. Test for HIV.

LABORATORY TESTS

If sending cultures, send on Nickerson's media or semiquantitative Slide-Stix cultures. There is no reliable serologic technique for diagnosis.

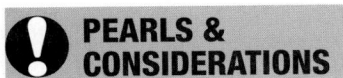 TREATMENT

ACUTE GENERAL Rx (UNCOMPLICATED VVC)

ORAL FLUCONAZOLE:
- 150-mg single PO dose

TOPICAL BUTOCONAZOLE:
- 2% vaginal cream 5 g intravaginally for 3 days
- Butoconazole (sustained release) 5 g intravaginally for 1 dose

TOPICAL CLOTRIMAZOLE
- 1% cream 5 g intravaginally for 7 to 14 days
- 100-mg vaginal tablet for 7 days
- 100-mg vaginal tablets, 2 tablets for 3 days
- 500-mg vaginal tablet, single dose

TOPICAL MICONAZOLE:
- 2% cream 5 g intravaginally for 7 days
- 200-mg vaginal suppository for 3 days
- 100-mg vaginal suppository for 7 days

TOPICAL TIOCONAZOLE:
- 6.5% ointment 5 g intravaginally, single dose

TOPICAL TERCONAZOLE:
- 0.4% cream 5 g intravaginally for 7 days
- 0.8% cream 5 g intravaginally for 3 days
- 80-mg suppository for 3 days

(COMPLICATED VVC)
- 150 mg fluconazole orally, repeat in 3 days
- Recurrent VVC: 7 to 14 days of topical therapy
- Maintenance regimen:
  1. Clotrimazole: 500-mg vaginal suppositories once weekly
  2. Ketoconazole: 100 mg qd
  3. Fluconazole: 100 to 150 mg orally once weekly
  4. Itraconazole 400 mg/mo or 100 mg/day
  5. Continue one of the above regimens for 6 mo

(COMPROMISED HOST)
- Treat with traditional antimycotics for at least 7 to 14 days
- Pregnancy: topical azoles recommended for 7 days
- Women with HIV: fluconazole 200 mg/wk
- Not usually a sexually transmitted disease

CHRONIC Rx

Ketoconazole 400 mg PO qd or fluconazole 200 mg PO qd until symptoms resolve. Then maintenance on prophylactic doses of these agents for 6 mo (ketoconazole 100 mg/day, fluconazole 150 mg/wk).

DISPOSITION

If chronic or recurrent, consider screening for diabetes, HIV, or other immune deficiencies.

PEARLS & CONSIDERATIONS

COMMENTS

- Azoles are more effective than nystatin. Symptoms usually take 2 to 3 days to resolve. Adjunctive treatment with weak topical steroid such as 1% hydrocortisone cream may help with relief of symptoms.
- Creams and suppositories are oil based and may weaken latex condoms and diaphragms.
- Invasive candidosis is discussed in the EBM section.

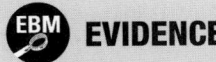 EVIDENCE

available at www.expertconsult.com

SUGGESTED READINGS
available at www.expertconsult.com

AUTHORS: **MARIA A. CORIGLIANO, M.D.,** and **RUBEN ALVERO, M.D.**

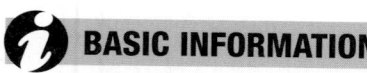

BASIC INFORMATION

DEFINITION

Carbon monoxide (CO) is a colorless, odorless, tasteless, nonirritating gas. When inhaled it produces toxicity by causing cellular hypoxia and damage.

ICD-9CM CODES
986 Carbon monoxide poisoning

EPIDEMIOLOGY & DEMOGRAPHICS

- A leading cause of accidental and intentional poisoning in the U.S.
- CO poisoning is seen more frequently during the fall and winter months in cold climates. Frequently seen after storm-related power outages, mostly due to the use of portable gasoline-powered electrical generators.
- In adults, 20% of CO poisonings occur in occupational settings.

PHYSICAL FINDINGS & CLINICAL PRESENTATION

- Depends on the severity and duration of exposure. The brain and heart are most sensitive to CO poisoning.
- Presentation is often nonspecific and may be mistaken for a flulike illness.
- Mild to moderate poisoning may present with headache, malaise, dizziness, nausea, dyspnea, difficulty concentrating, confusion, and blurred vision. Patients may have tachypnea and tachycardia.
- Severe poisoning may present with hypotension, arrhythmias, myocardial ischemia, pulmonary edema, lethargy, ataxia, loss of consciousness, seizure, coma, or rarely, cherry-red skin.
- Severity of poisoning does not correlate with carboxyhemoglobin (COHgb) levels.
- Delayed neurologic sequelae may develop days to weeks after apparent recovery from acute poisoning. Patients may present with neurologic or psychiatric symptoms (cognitive deficits, memory loss, personality

changes, movement disorders, Parkinson's, psychosis, neurologic deficits).

ETIOLOGY

- CO results from the incomplete combustion of carbon-containing compounds. CO poisoning occurs from inhaling smoke from fires, motor vehicle exhaust, or the burning of fuel (oil, wood, coal, natural gas) in poorly functioning or improperly ventilated devices (heating systems, stoves/grills, portable generators, etc.). Methylene chloride (paint stripper) fumes are converted to CO by the liver.
- CO toxicity results from tissue hypoxia and direct CO-mediated damage at the cellular level. This may explain why COHgb levels alone are not predictive of clinical toxicity. The mechanisms of CO toxicity are not completely understood.
- CO impairs oxygen delivery. CO binds hemoglobin with an affinity 250 times greater than oxygen, displacing oxygen from hemoglobin and decreasing the oxygen-carrying capacity of blood. By binding to hemoglobin, CO changes the structure of the hemoglobin molecule and decreases oxygen release to tissue.
- CO also interferes with peripheral oxygen utilization. It binds to other heme-containing proteins including cytochromes and myoglobin. Cellular respiration is depressed by inhibition of the mitochondrial cytochrome oxidase system. By binding to myoglobin, CO decreases its ability to use and store oxygen.
- Neurologic toxicity is not explained by hypoxia alone and is related to the complex intracellular actions of CO. CO precipitates an inflammatory cascade that results in oxidative damage and brain lipid peroxidation.

DIAGNOSIS

DIFFERENTIAL DIAGNOSIS

- Viral syndromes
- Cyanide, hydrogen sulfide
- Methemoglobinemia
- Amphetamines and derivatives
- Cocaine, phencyclidine (PCP)

- Cyclic antidepressants
- Phenothiazines
- Theophylline

WORKUP

History (duration and source of CO exposure, loss of consciousness), physical examination (detailed neurologic examination), laboratory and imaging tests

LABORATORY TESTS

- COHgb level (measured by co-oximetry of blood gas sample): COHgb level >3% in nonsmokers confirms exposure. Heavy smokers may have baseline levels of up to 10%. Levels may be low if the patient has already received supplemental oxygen or if delay occurs between exposure and testing.
- Direct measurement of arterial oxyhemoglobin (by co-oximetry): Pulse oximetry and arterial blood gas (ABG) may be falsely normal because neither measures oxygen saturation of hemoglobin directly. Pulse oximetry is inaccurate because of the similar absorption characteristics of oxyhemoglobin and COHgb. An ABG is inaccurate because it measures oxygen dissolved in plasma (which is not affected by CO) and then calculates oxygen saturation of hemoglobin.
- Electrolytes, glucose, BUN, creatinine, cardiac biomarkers, ABG (lactic acidosis and rhabdomyolysis may develop), CBC (polycythemia from hypoxia in chronic CO poisoning).
- ECG (ischemia, arrhythmia).
- Pregnancy test (fetus at high risk).
- Consider toxicology screen.

IMAGING STUDIES

- Chest radiograph (noncardiogenic edema)
- CT, MRI if neurologic abnormalities are present

TREATMENT

ACUTE GENERAL Rx

- Remove from site of CO exposure.
- Ensure adequate airway.
- Continuous ECG monitor.
- Fetal monitoring if pregnant.
- 100% oxygen by nonrebreather mask or endotracheal tube (decreases half-life of COHgb from 4 to 6 hr to 60 to 90 min) until COHgb level is <10% and patient is asymptomatic. Fig. 1-73 illustrates the effects of oxygen on the dissociation of CO from carboxyhemoglobin.
- Hyperbaric oxygen (2.5 to 3 atm).
  - Decreases half-life of COHgb to 20 to 30 min; increases amount of oxygen dissolved in plasma. It also reduces CO binding to other heme-containing proteins.
  - Questionable beneficial effect over normobaric oxygen
  - May reduce incidence of neurologic sequelae of CO poisoning
  - Consider for individuals with:
    1. Severe intoxication (COHgb >25%, history of loss of consciousness, neu-

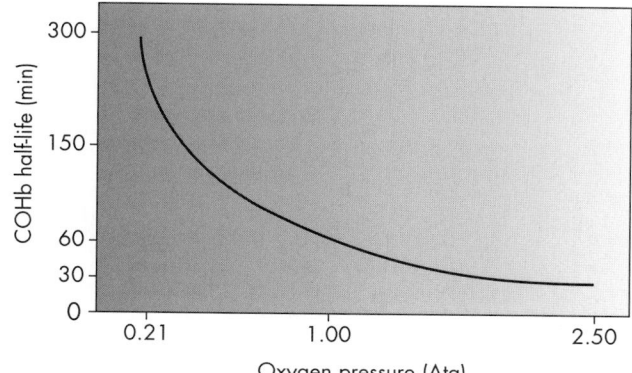

FIGURE 1-73 The effects of oxygen on the dissocation of CO from carboxyhemoglobin (COHb). Oxygen breathing at 1.0 atm decreases the half-life of COHb to 60 min from approximately 300 min, allowing most of the COHb to be removed from the body within 90 min. (From Auerbach P: *Wilderness medicine*, ed 4, St Louis, 2001, Mosby.)

rologic symptoms or signs, cardiovascular compromise, severe metabolic acidosis)

2. Pregnant women with COHgb >20% or signs of fetal distress. CO elimination is slower in fetus than mother, fetal Hgb has greater affinity for CO than adult Hgb

  ○ Should be instituted quickly if deemed necessary

- Consider concomitant poisoning with other toxic/irritant gases that may be present in smoke (e.g., cyanide) or thermal injury to airway. Toxic effects of CO and cyanide are synergistic.
- Identify source of exposure and determine if poisoning was accidental.

DISPOSITION

- Patients with mild accidental poisoning can be treated in an ambulatory setting. Those with moderate/severe poisoning or coexisting illness require hospitalization.

- Survivors of severe poisoning are at 14% to 40% risk for neurologic sequelae.
  ○ Deficits are usually apparent within 3 wk of poisoning but may present months later.
  ○ Risk of developing sequelae is greater if patient lost consciousness during acute poisoning and with older age.
  ○ Brain MRI may reveal changes; damage is seen most often in the globus pallidus and deep white matter
  ○ Recovery may occur over months to years.
- CO-mediated cardiac damage is associated with increased long-term mortality rate.
- High risk of fetal demise.

REFERRAL

- U.S. Poison Control Network: 1-800-222-1222
- Hyperbaric unit; facilities are listed on the Undersea & Hyperbaric Medical Society website (www.uhms.org)
- Psychiatric evaluation if intentional poisoning

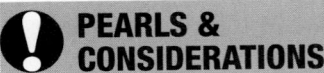

- Severity of poisoning and prognosis do not correlate with COHgb levels.
- Neuropsychometric testing is an objective measure of cognitive function but is not universally used.
- Contact local Fire Department to assess environment and identify source of CO.

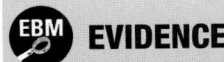 **EVIDENCE**

available at www.expertconsult.com

SUGGESTED READINGS
available at www.expertconsult.com

AUTHOR: **SUDEEP KAUR AULAKH, M.D.**

ⓘ BASIC INFORMATION

DEFINITION

Carcinoid syndrome is a symptom complex characterized by paroxysmal vasomotor disturbances, diarrhea, and bronchospasm. It is caused by the action of amines and peptides (serotonin, bradykinin, histamine) produced by tumors arising from neuroendocrine cells.

SYNONYMS

Flush syndrome
Argentaffinoma syndrome

ICD-9CM CODES
259.2 Carcinoid syndrome

EPIDEMIOLOGY & DEMOGRAPHICS
INCIDENCE:
- Carcinoid tumors are found incidentally in 0.5% to 0.75% of autopsies.
- Carcinoid tumors are principally found in the following organs: appendix (40%); small bowel (20%; 15% in the ileum); rectum (15%); bronchi (12%); esophagus, stomach, and colon (10%); and ovary, biliary tract, and pancreas (3%).
- The incidence of carcinoids is 2.47 to 4.48/100,000, depending on race and sex, and is highest in black men. The overall incidence has increased over the last 30 years due in part to improved diagnostic modalities.

PHYSICAL FINDINGS & CLINICAL PRESENTATION

- Cutaneous flushing (75% to 90%)
  1. The patient usually has red-purple flushes starting in the face, then spreading to the neck and upper trunk.
  2. The flushing episodes last from a few minutes to hours (longer lasting flushes may be associated with bronchial carcinoids).
  3. Flushing may be triggered by emotion, alcohol, or foods or may occur spontaneously.
  4. Dizziness, tachycardia, and hypotension may be associated with the cutaneous flushing.
- Diarrhea (>70%): often associated with abdominal bloating and audible peristaltic rushes
- Intermittent bronchospasm (25%): characterized by severe dyspnea and wheezing
- Facial telangiectasia
- Tricuspid insufficiency, pulmonic stenosis from carcinoid heart lesions

ETIOLOGY

- Carcinoid syndrome is caused by neoplasms originating from neuroendocrine cells.
- Carcinoid tumors do not usually produce the syndrome unless liver metastases are present or the primary tumor does not involve the gastrointestinal tract.

Ⓓ DIAGNOSIS

DIFFERENTIAL DIAGNOSIS

- Flushing: Carcinoid syndrome must be distinguished from idiopathic flushing (IF); patients with IF more often are female, are younger, and have a longer duration of symptoms; palpitations, syncope, and hypotension occur primarily in patients with IF. Additional causes of flushing that need to be ruled out are menopause, medications (niacin, nitrates), alcohol, renal cell carcinoma, medullary cancer of thyroid, VIPoma, mastocytosis, and chronic use of food additives (nitrites, sulfites)
- Diarrhea: IBD, IBS, laxative abuse, infectious colitis
- Bronchospasm: Asthma, foreign body, GERD, lung neoplasm

LABORATORY TESTS

- The biochemical marker for carcinoid syndrome is increased 24-hr urinary 5-hydroxyindoleacetic acid, a metabolite of serotonin (5-hydroxytryptamine).
- False elevations can be seen with ingestion of certain foods (bananas, pineapples, eggplant, avocados, walnuts) and certain medications (acetaminophen, caffeine, guaifenesin, reserpine); therefore patients should be on a restricted diet and avoid these medications when the test is ordered.
- Falsely low results can occur with use of alcohol, aspirin, MAO inhibitors, and St. John's wort.
- Liver function studies are an unreliable indicator of liver involvement.

IMAGING STUDIES

- Chest x-ray is useful to detect bronchial carcinoids.
- CT scan of abdomen or a liver and spleen radionuclide scan is useful to detect liver metastases (palpable in >50% of cases).
- Iodine-123–labeled somatostatin can detect carcinoid endocrine tumors with somatostatin receptors.
- Scanning with radiolabeled octreotide can visualize previously undetected or metastatic lesions.

Ⓡ TREATMENT

NONPHARMACOLOGIC THERAPY

Avoidance of ethanol ingestion (may precipitate flushing)

GENERAL Rx

- Surgical resection of the tumor can be curative if the tumor is localized or palliative and results in prolonged asymptomatic periods if metastases are present. Surgical manipulation of the tumor can, however, cause severe vasomotor abnormalities and bronchospasm (carcinoid crisis).
- Percutaneous embolization and ligation of the hepatic artery can decrease the bulk of the tumor in the liver and provide palliative treatment of tumors with hepatic metastases.
- Cytotoxic chemotherapy: combination chemotherapy with 5-fluorouracil and streptozocin can be used in patients with unresectable or recurrent carcinoid tumors; however, it has only limited success.
- Control of clinical manifestations:
  1. Somatostatin analogues (octreotide and lancreotide) are effective for both flushing and diarrhea in most patients. Interferon alfa may be useful as an additive therapy for persistent symptoms despite use of somatostatin analogues; however, data remains inconclusive.
  2. Flushing may be controlled by the combination of H_1- and H_2-receptor antagonists (e.g., diphenhydramine 25 to 50 mg PO q6h and ranitidine 150 mg bid).
  3. Diarrhea may respond to diphenoxylate with atropine (Lomotil).
  4. Bronchospasm can be treated with aminophylline and/or albuterol.
- Nutritional support: supplemental niacin therapy may be useful to prevent pellagra because the tumor uses dietary tryptophan for serotonin synthesis, resulting in a nutritional deficiency in some patients.
- Interferon alfa may be useful as an additive to control symptoms unresponsive to somatostatin analogues.
- Echocardiography and monitoring for right-sided congestive heart failure are recommended for patients with unresectable disease because endocardial fibrosis, involving predominantly the endocardium, chordae, and valves of the right side of the heart, can occur.

DISPOSITION

Carcinoids of the appendix and rectum have a low malignancy potential and rarely produce the clinical syndrome; metastases are also uncommon if the size of the primary lesion is <2 cm in diameter.

Ⓔ EVIDENCE

available at www.expertconsult.com

AUTHOR: **FRED F. FERRI, M.D.**

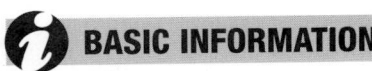

BASIC INFORMATION

DEFINITION

Cardiac tamponade is a life-threatening condition where an accumulation of fluid within the pericardial sac impairs filling of the ventricles during diastole and causes a decline in cardiac output.

ICD-9CM CODES
423.9 Unspecified diseases of the pericardium

PHYSICAL FINDINGS & CLINICAL PRESENTATION

- Chest pain
- Tachypnea/dyspnea
- Beck's triad
  1. Absolute or relative hypotension
  2. Elevated jugular venous pressure (with prominent *x* descent and blunted *y* descent)
  3. Muffled heart sounds
- Tachycardia (except in uremia or hypothyroid patients)
- Pulsus paradoxus (decrease in systolic arterial pressure of 10 mm Hg or more during normal inspiration while in normal sinus rhythm)
- Pericardial friction rub may be present
- Reduced or absent apical cardiac impulse

ETIOLOGY

Acute (rapidly accumulating pericardial effusion leading to cardiac tamponade): does not need a large amount of effusion to cause tamponade
- Penetrating trauma
- Aortic dissection
- Post-infarction myocardial rupture and/or hemorrhagic pericarditis
- Iatrogenic (central line and pacemaker insertions, post–coronary bypass surgery or post–percutaneous coronary intervention)
Subacute or chronic (effusion is usually large):
- Malignancy (e.g., lung, breast, lymphoma)
- Viral pericarditis (e.g., Coxsackie, human immunodeficiency virus)
- Bacterial, fungal, or tuberculous pericarditis
- Uremia
- Hypothyroidism/myxedema (rare)
- Collagen vascular disease (e.g., lupus, rheumatoid arthritis, scleroderma)
- Radiation
- Idiopathic

DIAGNOSIS

Cardiac tamponade is a clinical diagnosis made at the bedside from history and physical examination. The echocardiogram will help confirm or reject the clinical diagnosis. Tamponade can be confirmed invasively by the measurement of elevated intrapericardial pressures with an intrapericardial catheter and right-sided heart catheterization. Typical findings are diastolic equalization of pressures, usually ranging from 15 to 30 mm Hg (diastolic pulmonary artery pressure = right ventricular diastolic pressure = right atrial pressure = intrapericardial pressure) and lowering of the intrapericardial pressure with fluid drainage. Thereafter, the underlying etiology must be determined with specific laboratory work (see "Laboratory Tests" below).

DIFFERENTIAL DIAGNOSIS

Other conditions that can also lead to elevated jugular venous pressure, decreased systemic pressure, and pulsus paradoxus include:
- Chronic obstructive pulmonary disease
- Constrictive pericarditis
- Restrictive cardiomyopathy
- Right ventricular infarction
- Pulmonary embolism
- Chronic biventricular heart failure

LABORATORY TESTS

- Electrolytes, blood urea nitrogen, creatinine, erythrocyte sedimentation rate, thyroid function tests, antinuclear antibody, rheumatoid factor, PPD, blood cultures, viral titers, and pericardial fluid analysis and cultures
- Possible 12-lead ECG findings:
  - Sinus tachycardia
  - PR depression and/or diffuse ST elevations if acute pericarditis is present
  - Electrical alternans
  - Low voltage if massive effusion is present

IMAGING STUDIES

- Chest radiograph (enlarged cardiac silhouette with clear lung fields)
- Chest CT (may overestimate size of the effusion)
- Echocardiogram (pericardial effusion, diastolic collapse of the right atrium and/or the right ventricle, mitral and tricuspid valve inflow variation with respiration, and a plethoric inferior vena cava)

TREATMENT

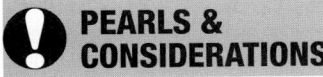

NONPHARMACOLOGIC THERAPY

- Cardiac tamponade should be treated emergently.
- Avoid drugs that reduce preload (e.g., nitrates, diuretics).
- Large pericardial effusions without hemodynamic compromise (tamponade) can be managed conservatively with careful monitoring, treatment of the underlying cause, and frequent serial surveillance echocardiography.

ACUTE GENERAL Rx

- Aggressive intravascular volume expansion (saline or blood)
- Emergency pericardial fluid removal by pericardiocentesis or surgical pericardiotomy by way of the subxiphoid pericardial window
- Pericardiocentesis should be performed under fluoroscopic or echocardiographic guidance when available
- Inotropic or vasopressor support if above measures cannot be performed immediately

CHRONIC Rx

- Depends on etiology.
- Pericardiocentesis with draining catheter: the catheter can be left inside the pericardium to allow continued drainage for 24 to 4 hr. If residual fluid still persists with hemodynamic compromise, surgical drainage should be sought. In the absence of hemodynamic compromise or significant residual fluid, discontinuation of the draining catheter can be done with periodic postprocedure echocardiographic monitoring of reaccumulation (e.g., 24 hr, 7 days, 30 days, 3 mo, 6 mo, 12 mo) depending on the etiology and rate of reaccumulation.
- Other surgical drainage procedures include:
  1. Subxiphoid pericardiotomy drainage
  2. Limited pericardiectomy draining the pericardial fluid into the left hemithorax
  3. Complete pericardiectomy, especially in patients with effusive-constrictive pericarditis or bacterial pericarditis (see "Pearls & Considerations" below).

DISPOSITION

The prognosis of cardiac tamponade depends on the underlying cause.

REFERRAL

- Emergent cardiology consultation should be made if cardiac tamponade is suspected.
- Cardiothoracic surgery consultation should also be considered if surgical pericardial drainage is indicated.

PEARLS & CONSIDERATIONS

- Cardiac tamponade should always be considered during pulseless electrical activity arrest and may require emergent pericardiocentesis.
- Evaluation for pulsus paradoxus should always be performed during normal respiration because deep inspiration may render a false positive finding.
- Strong consideration should be given to performing early pericardiocentesis in patients who have pericardial effusion associated with bacterial pneumonia or empyema because the incidence of bacterial pericarditis is especially high in this clinical situation and the subsequent development of cardiac tamponade and severe chronic constrictive pericarditis occurs frequently.

COMMENTS

As little as 100 ml of fluid can lead to acute cardiac tamponade, whereas with gradual accumulation, the pericardial sac can hold up to 5 L of fluid before tamponade occurs.

EVIDENCE

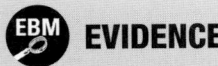

available at www.expertconsult.com

SUGGESTED READINGS
available at www.expertconsult.com

AUTHORS: **SCOTT COHEN, M.D., GAURAV CHOUDHARY, M.D.,** and **ROBERTO PACHECO, M.D.**

BASIC INFORMATION

DEFINITION

Dilated cardiomyopathy describes a group of diseases involving the myocardium and characterized by myocardial dysfunction that is not primarily the result of hypertension, coronary atherosclerosis, valvular dysfunction, or congenital or other structural heart disease. As a result, the heart is enlarged and the ventricles are dilated with impaired systolic function.

SYNONYMS

Congestive cardiomyopathy

ICD-9CM CODES
425.4 Other primary cardiomyopathies

EPIDEMIOLOGY & DEMOGRAPHICS

- The prevalence rate of dilated cardiomyopathy in the general adult population is approximately 1%.
- Incidence increases with age and approaches 10% at age 80 yr.
- It is the most common cardiomyopathy in the young accounting for 25% of cases.

PHYSICAL FINDINGS & CLINICAL PRESENTATION

Classical symptoms of heart failure may be absent. When present, findings are indistinguishable from other heart failure syndromes, including:
- Increased jugular venous pressure
- Narrow pulse pressure
- Pulmonary rales, hepatomegaly, peripheral edema
- S3, S4
- Mitral regurgitation, tricuspid regurgitation (less common)

ETIOLOGY

In approximate order of occurrence:
- Idiopathic (often a viral infection that cannot be confirmed)
- Infections (viral [Coxsackie B, adenovirus, parvovirus, HIV], rickettsial, mycobacterial, toxoplasmosis, trichinosis, Chagas' disease)
- Alcoholism (15% to 40% of all cases in Western countries)

- Uncontrolled tachyarrhythmia ("tachycardia-mediated")
- Peripartum (greatest risk from last trimester of pregnancy to 6 mo postpartum)Chemotherapeutic (anthracycline, doxorubicin, danorubicin) or pharmacologic agents (antiretrovirals, phenotiazines)
- Substance abuse (cocaine, heroin, organic solvents "glue-sniffer's heart")
- Postmyocarditis
- Toxins (cobalt, lead, phosphorus, carbon monoxide, mercury)
- Collagen-vascular disease (systemic lupus, rheumatoid arthritis, polyarteritis, dermatomyositis, sarcoidosis)
- Heredofamilial neuromuscular disease (e.g., muscular dystrophy)
- Excess hormones (acromegaly, osteogenesis imperfecta, myxedema, thyrotoxicosis, diabetes)
- Hematologic (e.g., sickle cell anemia, hemochromatosis)

DIAGNOSIS

Dilated cardiomyopathy is a diagnosis of exclusion, made after ruling out other potential causes of myocardial dysfunction.

DIFFERENTIAL DIAGNOSIS

- Coronary atherosclerosis, that is, left ventricular dysfunction secondary to ischemia and/or myocardial infarction
- Valvular dysfunction (especially aortic and mitral regurgitation)
- Other cardiomyopathies (restrictive, hypertrophic)
- Pulmonary disease (embolism, obstructive, restrictive)
- Pericardial abnormalities (constrictive pericarditis, tamponade)
- Anemia
- Hypothyroidism/myxedema

WORKUP

- Chest x-ray examination, ECG, echocardiogram; myocardial biopsy is not routinely recommended, unless acute myocarditis requiring immunosuppressive therapy is considered (e.g., giant cell myocarditis)

- Medical history with emphasis on the following symptoms:
  - Dyspnea on exertion, orthopnea, paroxysmal nocturnal dyspnea.
  - Palpitations.
  - Systemic and pulmonary embolism.
- Persistently increased cardiac troponin T levels are a marker of poor outcome in cardiomyopathy patients

IMAGING STUDIES

Chest x-ray:
- Cardiac silhouette enlargement (sometimes massive)
- Interstitial pulmonary edema (Kerley B lines, cephalization of vasculature), pleural effusion (may appear as unilateral, most often on the right side)

ECG:
- Left ventricular (LV) hypertrophy with ST-T wave changes
- Right or left bundle branch block
- Arrhythmias (atrial fibrillation, premature ventricular or atrial contractions, ventricular tachycardia)

Echocardiogram:
- Low ejection fraction with global hypokinesis
- Four-chamber enlargement (LV enlargement usually predominates)
- Mitral or tricuspid regurgitation (due to incomplete leaflet closure caused by ventricular dilatation)

TREATMENT

NONPHARMACOLOGIC THERAPY

- Treatment of underlying disease (systemic lupus, alcoholism)
- Dietary sodium restriction (<2 g/day).
- Exercise training has been shown to be associated with reduced risk for hospitalization and death in patients with history of heart failure in limited trials; enrollment in a formal cardiac rehabilitation program may be beneficial in improving patient's functional status

ACUTE GENERAL Rx

- Diuretics are indicated for all patients with current symptoms or history of heart failure and reduced left ventricular ejection fraction (LVEF) with evidence of volume overload (peripheral edema, orthopnea, paroxysmal nocturnal dyspnea).
- ACE inhibitors (and angiotensin receptor blockers) have been shown to have favorable effects on ventricular remodeling in patients with cardiomyopathy and a demonstrable mortality benefit in these patients. Therefore they are recommended in all patients with reduced LV systolic function, regardless of symptoms, unless specific contraindications exist.
- Beta-blockers (in particular, carvedilol, long-acting metoprolol, and bisoprolol) work by inhibiting the adverse effects of the sympathetic nervous system in patients with ventricular systolic dysfunction, and have likewise shown a mortality benefit in patients with LV systolic

TABLE 1-27 Factors Associated with an Adverse Outcome in Dilated Cardiomyopathy

Clinical	Noninvasive	Invasive
NYHA Class III/IV	Low LV ejection fraction	High LV filling pressures
Increasing age	Marked LV dilation	
Low-exercise peak oxygen consumption	Low LV mass	
Marked intraventricular conduction delay	≥Moderate mitral regurgitation	
Complex ventricular arrhythmias	Abnormal diastolic function	
Abnormal signal-averaged ECG	Abnormal contractile reserve	
Evidence of excessive sympathetic stimulation	Right ventricular dilation or dysfunction	
Protodiastolic gallop (S3)		

ECG, Electrocardiogram; *LV*, left ventricular; *NYHA*, New York Heart Association.
From Zipes DP et al [eds]: *Braunwauld's heart disease*, ed 7, Philadelphia, 2005, Elsevier.

dysfunction; they should be used unless specifically contraindicated.

- Additional medical therapies (aldosterone antagonists, hydralazine/nitrates, digitalis) can be considered in certain patient subpopulations with persistent symptoms on otherwise optimal medical management.
- Patients with associated coronary atherosclerosis (angina, ECG changes, reversible defects on myocardial perfusion imaging) may benefit from percutaneous or surgical revascularization.

DISPOSITION

- Annual mortality rate is 20% in patients with moderate heart failure, and it exceeds 50% in patients with severe heart failure. Once symptomatic, hospitalizations are frequent and readmission rates are high (>50% at 3 mo). A multispecialty treatment approach (e.g., primary care, cardiology, nutrition, cardiac rehabilitation) is recommended.
- Factors associated with an adverse outcome in dilated cardiomyopathy are described in Table 1-27.

REFERRAL

- Patients with dilated cardiomyopathy are at increased risk for ventricular arrhythmias and sudden cardiac death. Implantation of a cardiac defibrillator for primary prevention of sudden cardiac death can be considered for patients with LVEF < 35% on optimal medical therapy regardless of symptom status.
- Patients with LVEF < 35%, bundle branch block on ECG (QRS ≥ 0.12 sec), and persistent heart failure symptoms may benefit from cardiac resynchronization therapy via a biventricular pacemaker.
- Consider heart transplantation for relatively young patients (there is no precise age threshold) free of other significant comorbid conditions who are unresponsive to medical therapy. Dilated cardiomyopathy is the reason for 45% of all heart transplantations in the U.S.

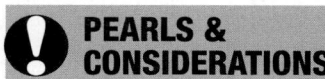

COMMENTS

- Patients should be encouraged to restrict or eliminate alcohol and reduce sodium intake (<2 g daily).

- Patients may benefit from daily weight checks as a means of early detection of volume overload and decompensated heart failure.
- Vulnerability to cardiomyopathy among chronic alcohol abusers is partially genetic and related to the presence of the ACE DD genotype.
- Idiopathic dilated cardiomyopathy is often familial, and apparently healthy relatives may have latent, early, or undiagnosed disease. Echocardiographic evaluation of family members is recommended.

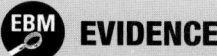

EVIDENCE

available at www.expertconsult.com

SUGGESTED READINGS

available at www.expertconsult.com

AUTHORS: **GABRIEL A. DELGADO, M.D.,**
FRED F. FERRI, M.D., and
DAVID J. FORTUNATO, M.D., F.A.C.C.

BASIC INFORMATION

DEFINITION

Cardiomyopathy describes a group of diseases that involve the myocardium and are characterized by myocardial dysfunction that is not primarily the result of hypertension, coronary atherosclerosis, valvular dysfunction, congenital, or other structural heart disease. Hypertropic cardiomyopathy (HCM) is a primary myocardial disorder characterized by disorganized myocyte architecture and severe thickening (hypertrophy) of the left ventricular wall out of proportion to the resistance to ventricular contraction (afterload). The interventricular septum is the most common site of enlargement, though hypertrophy may involve other focal regions or may be concentric. HCM may result in hemodynamically significant obstruction within the left ventricular outflow tract (LVOT) and/or impairment of the diastolic function of the left ventricle.

SYNONYMS

HCM
Hypertrophic cardiomyopathy
Idiopathic hypertrophic subaortic stenosis (IHSS)
Hypertrophic obstructive cardiomyopathy (HOCM)
Asymmetric septal hypertrophy (ASH)

ICD-9CM CODES
425.4	Cardiomyopathy, hypertrophic nonobstructive
425.1	Cardiomyopathy, hypertrophic obstructive
746.84	Cardiomyopathy, hypertrophic congenital

EPIDEMIOLOGY & DEMOGRAPHICS

- The most common form of the disease is familial (60% to 70% of cases) and it follows an autosomal dominant inheritance pattern with variable expression.
- Spontaneous mutations can also occur, accounting for approximately 20% of cases. It is otherwise indistinguishable from the familial form.
- A variant form seen in the elderly (5% to 10% of cases) has a better prognosis and it is not typically associated with sudden cardiac death.
- The familial form is usually diagnosed in young patients. It is mapped to chromosome 14q and is caused by a missense mutation in multiple genes (>200 identified) causing a single amino acid substitution in one of the contractile proteins of the cardiac sarcomere.
- Prevalence in the general population is 1 in 500 (one of the most common genetically transmitted cardiovascular diseases).
- In Japan 25% of cases are due to a variant (Yamaguchi's apical HCM), in which only the apex is affected, and there is no LVOT obstruction. It is rare outside of Japan (1% to 2%).
- It is the most common cause of sudden cardiac death in young athletes.

PHYSICAL FINDINGS & CLINICAL PRESENTATION

HCM may be suspected on the basis of abnormalities found on physical examination. Classic findings include:

- Harsh, systolic, crescendo–decrescendo murmur at the left sternal border or apex. The murmur increases with maneuvers that decrease venous return or LV size (Valsalva, standing), and decreases with those that increase venous return or afterload (squatting, hand grip, post-Valsalva release).
- Paradoxic splitting of S2 (if left ventricular obstruction is present).
- S4 may be present.
- Double or triple LV apical impulse ("triple ripple": atrial contraction, early rapid ejection, and late slow ejection).
- Pulsus bisferens (double pulsation on palpation of the carotid pulse).

Increased obstruction can occur with:
- Drugs: digitalis, β-adrenergic stimulators (isoproterenol, dopamine, epinephrine), nitroglycerin, vasodilators, diuretics, alcohol
- Hypovolemia
- Tachycardia
- Valsalva maneuver
- Standing position

Decreased obstruction is seen with:
- Drugs: β-adrenergic blockers, calcium channel blockers, disopyramide, α-adrenergic stimulators
- Volume expansion
- Bradycardia
- Hand-grip exercise
- Squatting position
- Release phase of the Valsalva maneuver

Clinical manifestations are as follows:
- Dyspnea
- Syncope (usually seen with exercise)
- Angina
- Palpitations

ETIOLOGY

- Genetic: Autosomal dominant trait with variable penetrance caused by mutations in multiple genes encoding proteins of the cardiac sarcomere. To date, >200 mutations have been identified.
- Sporadic occurrence.

DIAGNOSIS

DIFFERENTIAL DIAGNOSIS

- Hypertensive heart disease
- Valvular disease, especially aortic stenosis
- Cardiac amyloidosis
- Fabry disease
- Athlete's heart

WORKUP

- ECG is abnormal in 90% to 95% of patients, although there are no pathognomonic findings. Typical findings include:
  - LV hypertrophy (abnormally tall R waves in the precordial leads)
  - Abnormal Q waves in lateral and inferior leads
  - T wave inversions (associated with the apical hypertrophy predominant variant)
- Echocardiography is usually diagnostic as the majority of patients have significant LV hypertrophy. (See "Imaging Studies" for details.)
- 24-hour Holter monitor to screen for potentially lethal ventricular arrhythmias (principal cause of syncope or sudden death in obstructive cardiomyopathy) should be performed at diagnosis and annually afterward as part of routine follow-up regardless of symptoms.
- In the absence of significant LVOT obstruction, exercise testing is indicated at diagnosis and annually afterward to evaluate for symptoms and response to exercise. A drop in systolic blood pressure with exercise is a marker of poor prognosis and it is one of the indicators for referral for myotomy/myomectomy.
- Screening for sarcomere protein gene mutations in family members of patients with HCM can identify a broad subgroup of patients with increased propensity toward long-term impairment of left ventricular function and adverse outcome, irrespective of the myofilament (thick, intermediate, or thin) involved.

IMAGING STUDIES

- Chest x-ray may be normal or show cardiomegaly.
- Two-dimensional echocardiography is used to establish the diagnosis and assess the severity of obstruction when present. Most patients (up to 95%) will have asymmetric (ratio of septum thickness to left ventricular wall thickness >1.31) LV wall hypertrophy of >15 mm. Symmetric LV hypertrophy is less common. The septum is most often affected, followed by the left ventricular mid-cavity and apex. In addition, 25% to 30% of patients will manifest systolic anterior motion of the anterior leaflet of the mitral valve, causing obstruction of the LVOT. Two-dimensional strain imaging echocardiography is useful for differentiation of hypertrophic cardiomyopathy and cardiac amyloidosis from other causes of ventricular wall thickening. This technique, however, is not widely available.
- Cardiac MRI may be of diagnostic value when echocardiographic studies are technically inadequate. MRI is also useful in identifying unusual segmental hypertrophy undetectable by standard echocardiography.

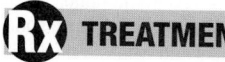 TREATMENT

NONPHARMACOLOGIC THERAPY

- Avoid volume depletion: HCM patients experience decrease in stroke volume and consequent increase in left ventricular outflow gradient on exercise. This may lead to hypotension, dizziness, and syncope.
- Exercise restriction: the risk of sudden cardiac death is increased by exercise in HCM patients. Participation in competitive sports and intense physical activity should be avoided.

- Advise avoidance of alcohol: alcohol use (even in small amounts) may result in increased obstruction of the left ventricular outflow tract.

GENERAL Rx

- Therapy for HCM is directed at blocking the effect of catecholamines that can exacerbate the dynamic left ventricular outflow tract obstruction and avoiding vasodilator or diuretic agents that can also worsen the obstruction.
- Beta-blockers: The beneficial effects of beta-blockers on symptoms (principally dyspnea and chest pain) and exercise tolerance appear to be largely a result of a decrease in the heart rate with consequent prolongation of diastole and increased passive ventricular filling. By reducing the inotropic response, beta-blockers may also reduce myocardial oxygen demand and decrease the outflow gradient during exercise, when sympathetic tone is increased.
- The nondihydropiridine calcium channel blockers (verapamil, diltiazem) can also decrease left ventricular outflow obstruction through a mechanism similar to beta-blockers. However, they are mainly second-line agents used in patients who cannot tolerate beta-blockers. They should be used with caution in patients with symptomatic obstruction. Administration in the hospital setting is recommended in these patients.
- Disopyramide is an antiarrhythmic that is also a negative inotrope, resulting in further decrease in outflow gradient. It is sometimes used in combination with beta-blockers.
- Prophylactic antibiotics before dental, GI, and genitourinary procedures are no longer recommended according to the 2007 American Heart Association (AHA) guidelines.
- Avoid use of digitalis, diuretics, nitrates, and vasodilators.
- Dual-chamber pacing has been recommended for hemodynamic and symptomatic benefit in patients with drug-resistant hypertrophic obstructive cardiomyopathy; however, it has not been shown to result in significant improvement in objective measures of exercise capacity.
- Implantable cardiac defibrillators (ICDs) are a safe and effective therapy in HCM patients prone to ventricular arrhythmias. In their practice guidelines, the major cardiology societies (AHA/ACC/HRS) give a strong recommendation (Class I) for ICD implantation in all patients with HCM who have had an episode of sustained ventricular tachycardia or fibrillation. In addition, they endorse the prophylactic placement of an ICD (Class IIa recommendation) for patients with one or more of the major risk factors for sudden cardiac death (outlined in "Disposition").

DISPOSITION

HCM is not a static disease. Some adults may experience subtle regression in wall thickness, whereas others (~5% to 10%) paradoxically evolve into an end-stage cardiomyopathy resembling dilated cardiomyopathy, characterized by cavity enlargement, left ventricular wall thinning, and systolic dysfunction. Patients with HCM are at increased risk for sudden death, especially if onset of symptoms began during childhood. Severe left ventricular outflow obstruction at rest is also a strong, independent predictor of severe symptoms of heart failure and death. Adult patients can be considered low risk if they have no symptoms or mild symptoms, and also if they have none of the following:

- A family history of premature death caused by HCM
- Nonsustained ventricular tachycardia during Holter monitoring
- A marked outflow tract gradient (≥50 mm Hg)
- Substantial hypertrophy (>20 mm)
- Marked left atrial enlargement
- Abnormal blood pressure response during exercise

REFERRAL

- Surgical treatment (myotomy-myectomy involving resection of the basal septum) is reserved for patients who have both a large outflow gradient (≥50 mm Hg) and severe symptoms of heart failure unresponsive to medical therapy. The risk for sudden death from arrhythmias is not altered by surgery. When this operation is performed by experienced surgeons in tertiary referral centers, the operative mortality rate is <2%, and many patients are able to achieve near-normal exercise capacity after surgery.
- Nonsurgical reduction of the interventricular septum can be done in patients with HCM refractory to pharmacologic treatment who are not candidates for myomectomy due to high surgical risk. This technique involves the injection of ethanol in a septal perforator branch of the left anterior descending coronary artery, producing a controlled myocardial infarction of the interventricular septum, and thereby reducing septal mass and consequently the left ventricular outflow tract gradient. This method may lead to improvement in both subjective and objective measures of exercise capacity, but results are not as effective as surgery and are associated with a high incidence of heart block, requiring permanent pacing in approximately one fourth of patients and/or recurrence of obstruction and symptoms.

PEARLS & CONSIDERATIONS

COMMENTS

- Screening of first-degree relatives with two-dimensional echocardiography and ECG is indicated, particularly if adverse HCM-related events have occurred in the family. Annual screening is recommended for all first-degree family members from age 12 to 18 yr. Afterward, periodic screening of first-degree adult family members at 5-yr intervals is recommended because hypertrophy may not be detected until the sixth decade of life. It is advisable to have a trained clinical genetic counselor see the patient and obtain consent before genetic testing.
- Future screening techniques may involve identification of mutations in the gene encoding the sarcomeric proteins. The most common sarcomeric subtype is MYBPC3-HCM, affecting one in five patients. Clinical predictors of positive genotype, such as the presence of ventricular arrhythmias, age at diagnosis, degree of left ventricular wall hypertrophy, and family history of HCM, may aid in patient selection for genetic testing and increase the yield of cardiac sarcomere gene screening. However, given the genetic polymorphism of HCM, genetic testing is still limited by its variable sensitivity and specificity, limited availability, and high cost. Its role in routine practice is still unclear.
- The mortality rate in HCM is approximately 1% to 2%.
- It is important to remember that HCM is predominantly a nonobstructive disease (75% of patients do not have a sizable resting outflow tract gradient) and that lethal ventricular arrhythmias can occur in the absence of obstruction or symptoms.
- Myocardial fibrosis is a hallmark of hypertrophic cardiomyopathy. Biomarkers of collagen metabolism such as serum C-terminal propeptide of type I procollagen (PICP) are significantly higher in mutation carriers without left ventricular hypertrophy and in subjects with overt hypertrophic cardiomyopathy than in controls indicating that a probiotic state precedes the development of hypertrophy of fibrosis identifiable with cardiac MRI.

EVIDENCE

available at www.expertconsult.com

SUGGESTED READINGS

available at www.expertconsult.com

AUTHORS: **GABRIEL A. DELGADO, M.D.,**
FRED F. FERRI, M.D., and
DAVID J. FORTUNATO, M.D., F.A.C.C.

BASIC INFORMATION

DEFINITION

Cardiomyopathy, in general, describes a group of diseases involving the myocardium and characterized by myocardial dysfunction that is not primarily the result of hypertension, coronary atherosclerosis, valvular dysfunction, congenital, or other structural heart disease. Restrictive cardiomyopathy is characterized by decreased ventricular compliance, with impaired ventricular filling (of either or both ventricles) and generally normal systolic function.

ICD-9CM CODES
425.4 Other primary cardiomyopathies

EPIDEMIOLOGY & DEMOGRAPHICS

- Relatively uncommon cardiomyopathy, accounting for 5% of all primary myocardial diseases
- Most frequently caused by amyloidosis (Fig. 1-74), myocardial fibrosis (following open heart surgery, transplantation or radiation).
- Patients classified as having "idiopathic" restrictive cardiomyopathy may have mutations in the gene for cardiac troponin I, and restrictive cardiomyopathy may represent an overlap with hypertrophic cardiomyopathy in many familial cases.

PHYSICAL FINDINGS & CLINICAL PRESENTATION

Restrictive cardiomyopathy presents with symptoms of progressive left-sided and right-sided heart failure:
- Fatigue, weakness (caused by low output as patients are unable to augment cardiac output by increasing heart rate without compromising ventricular filling).

- Progressively worsening exercise intolerance and dyspnea.
- Anginal chest pain can be seen (particularly in patients with amyloidosis) from myocardial compression of small coronaries.
- Palpitations (atrial fibrillation is common), dizziness or syncope (from heart block).
- Edema, ascites, hepatomegaly, distended neck veins.
- Kussmaul's sign may be present (rise, or failure to fall, of the jugular venous on inspiration).
- On auscultation: murmurs of mitral or tricuspid regurgitation may be heard; an S3 may be present but an S4 almost never is (likely due to infiltration of the atria).
- Apical impulse may be palpable (can help distinguish it from constrictive pericarditis).

ETIOLOGY

Disease may be classified according to pathophysiologic processes:
Infiltrative:
- ○ Amyloidosis (most common overall)
- ○ Sarcoidosis (usually results in a dilated cardiomyopathy with regional wall motion abnormalities)
Noninfiltrative:
- ○ Idiopathic (familial subtypes may have genetic overlap with hypertrophic cardiomyopathy)
- ○ Scleroderma
- ○ Diabetic cardiomyopathy
- ○ Pseudoxanthoma elasticum
Storage diseases:
- ○ Hemochromatosis (unusual as it is commonly associated with a dilated cardiomyopathy)
- ○ Glycogen or other storage diseases (Gaucher, Hurler, Fabry—all rare)

Endomyocardial:
- ○ Endomyocardial fibrosis
- ○ Hypereosinophilic syndrome (Loeffler's)
- ○ Carcinoid heart disease
- ○ Radiation
- ○ Metastatic cancers
- ○ Drug related (anthracyclines, serotonin, ergotamine, busulfan, methylsergide)

DIAGNOSIS

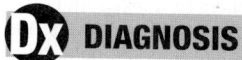

DIFFERENTIAL DIAGNOSIS

- Constrictive pericarditis (see Table 1-28)
- Valvular dysfunction (especially aortic stenosis)
- Hypertrophic cardiomyopathy
- Hypertension
- Coronary atherosclerosis
- Chronic lung disease

WORKUP

- Blood count (to identify eosinophilia), chest x-ray examination, ECG, echocardiogram.
- Cardiac catheterization, magnetic resonance imaging, and computed tomography (selected cases)
- Aspiration biopsy of subcutaneous fat to detect amyloidosis.
- Brain natriuretic peptide (BNP) serum levels: there is data suggesting that BNP levels are markedly elevated in restrictive cardiomyopathy but near normal in patients with constrictive pericarditis, despite nearly identical clinical and hemodynamic features.

IMAGING STUDIES

- Chest x-ray:
  - ○ Ranges from normal cardiomediastinal silhouette to moderate cardiomegaly (primarily because of biatrial enlargement).
  - ○ Evidence of heart failure may be present.
  - ○ Presence of pericardial calcification favors alternate diagnosis of constrictive pericarditis.
- ECG:
  - ○ Nonspecific ST-T wave abnormalities are the most common finding. Voltage may be low in infiltrative etiologies such as amyloidosis.
  - ○ Frequent atrial and ventricular ectopy are often present. Atrial fibrillation may be present.
  - ○ High-degree atrioventricular block, intraventricular conduction delay may be seen in advanced cases.
- Echocardiogram:
  - ○ Biatrial enlargement almost always present.
  - ○ Wall thickness depends on etiology, often normal but may be thickened in infiltrative disease such as amyloidosis.
  - ○ Ventricular chamber sizes and systolic function are often normal or reduced.
  - ○ Echo Doppler shows evidence of diastolic dysfunction.
- Cardiac catheterization:
  - ○ Characteristic hemodynamic finding is a dip and plateau, or square-root sign in the left ventricular tracing, where deep and

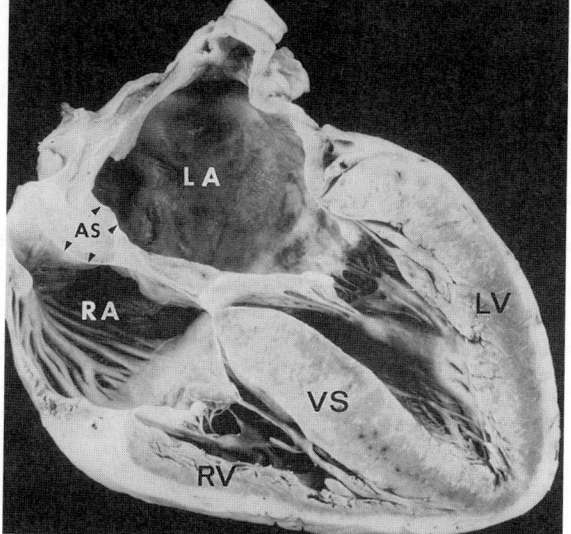

FIGURE 1-74 Necropsy specimen of an amyloid heart demonstrating the thickened ventricular septum *(VS)*, atrial septum *(AS)*, and free wall of the left ventricle *(LV)* and right ventricle *(RV)*, and the dilated left atrium *(LA)*. *RA,* Right atrium. (Courtesy Dr. William Edwards, Mayo Clinic, Rochester, MN. From Goldman L, Ausiello D [eds]: *Cecil textbook of medicine,* ed 22, Philadelphia, 2004, WB Saunders.)

rapid decline in ventricular pressure at the onset of diastole is immediately followed by rapid rise and plateau in early diastolic phase. To distinguish restrictive cardiomyopathy from constrictive pericarditis:

Constrictive pericarditis: Usually involves both ventricles and leads to equalization of diastolic pressures between all four cardiac chambers to within 5 mm Hg.

Restrictive cardiomyopathy: Impairs the left ventricle more than the right, often with left-sided end-diastolic pressures of 5 mm Hg greater than the right. The presence of increased pulmonary arterial systolic pressures is also suggestive of restrictive disease.

- Cardiac computed tomographic scan may be helpful to identify a thickened and calcified pericardium, consistent with constrictive pericarditis.
- Magnetic resonance imaging may also be useful to distinguish restrictive cardiomyopathy from constrictive pericarditis (thickness of the pericardium less than 5 mm in the latter).

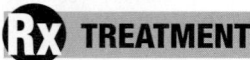 **TREATMENT**

NONPHARMACOLOGIC THERAPY

Congestive symptoms may respond to dietary sodium restriction (<2 g/day).

ACUTE GENERAL Rx

Treatment of volume overload and heart failure symptoms with diuretic therapy.

CHRONIC Rx

- Treatment involves management of the underlying disease if it exists (hemochromatosis may respond to repeated phlebotomy to decrease iron deposition in the heart, sarcoidosis may respond to corticosteroid therapy, and eosinophilic cardiomyopathy may respond to corticosteroid and cytotoxic drugs). There is no effective therapy for other causes of restrictive cardiomyopathy.
- Overall, the goal of treatment is to reduce symptoms by decreasing filling pressures while preserving cardiac output. Since there is currently no drug available to specifically act on myocardial relaxation, therapy centers on low-dose diuretics to lower the preload.
- Beta-blockers or calcium channel blockers have not been demonstrated to improve symptoms or alter the course of disease.
- ACE inhibitors (or angiotensin receptor blockers [ARBs]) should be avoided in patients with amyloidosis as they are poorly tolerated. Even small doses can trigger profound hypotension (probably due to associated autonomic neuropathy).
- Atrial fibrillation is common and patients with it or with a history of embolization should be anticoagulated. Tachycardia (of any cause) is poorly tolerated and a common cause of de-

compensation. Rate control is of paramount importance. Cardioversion in case of rapid atrial fibrillation should be considered. Of note, digoxin should be used with caution as it is potentially arrhythmogenic (particularly in patients with amyloidosis).
- Fibrosis of the cardiac conduction system may result in complete heart block presenting as dizziness or syncope (especially in amyloidosis) and pacemaker implantation may be required.
- The course of restrictive cardiomyopathy is variable and depends on the underlying etiology. Death usually results from heart failure or arrhythmias, and interventions aimed at addressing these are recommended.

DISPOSITION

Prognosis varies with the etiology of the cardiomyopathy but is poor overall as disease is rarely detected before advanced stages.

REFERRAL

Cardiac transplantation can be considered in patients with refractory symptoms and idiopathic or familial restrictive cardiomyopathies.

SUGGESTED READINGS

available at www.expertconsult.com

AUTHORS: **GABRIEL A. DELGADO, M.D., FRED F. FERRI, M.D.,** and **DAVID J. FORTUNATO, M.D., F.A.C.C.**

TABLE 1-28 Differentiation between Restrictive Cardiomyopathy and Constrictive Pericarditis

Type of Evaluation	Restrictive Cardiomyopathy	Constrictive Pericarditis
Physical examination	Kussmaul sign present Apical impulse may be prominent Regurgitant murmurs are common	Kussmaul sign may be present Apical impulse usually not palpable Pericardial knock may be present
Electrocardiography	Low QRS voltage (especially in amyloidosis) Pseudoinfarction pattern Bundle branch blocks AV conduction disturbances Atrial fibrillation	Low QRS voltage Repolarization abnormalities
Chest radiography		Calcification of the pericardium may be present
Echocardiography	Marked enlargement of the atria Increased wall thickness (especially in amyloidosis)	Atria usually of normal size Normal wall thickness Pericardial thickening may be seen
Doppler echocardiography	Restrictive mitral inflow (dominant E wave with short deceleration time) No significant variation of transvalvular velocities with respiration (<10%) Reversal of forward flow in hepatic veins during inspiration	Restrictive mitral inflow (dominant E wave with short deceleration time) Increased velocity of RV filling and decreased velocity of LV filling with inspiration; opposite with expiration; variation in velocity exceeds 15% Reversal of forward flow in hepatic veins during expiration
Cardiac catheterization	Prominent atrial x and y descents (w sign) Dip-and-plateau appearance of ventricular diastolic pressure Diastolic pressures increased but not equalized (LV diastolic pressure higher than RV diastolic pressure)	Prominent atrial x and y descents (w sign) Dip-and-plateau appearance of ventricular diastolic pressure Increase and equalization of diastolic pressures Discordance of RV and LV peak systolic pressures (with inspiration, RV systolic pressure increases and LV systolic pressure decreases)
Endomyocardial biopsy	May reveal specific cause of restrictive cardiomyopathy	No specific findings on endomyocardial biopsy Pericardial biopsy may reveal abnormality
Computed tomography, magnetic resonance imaging		Pericardial thickening

AV, Atrioventricular; *LV,* left ventricular; *RV,* right ventricular.
Andreoli TE et al [eds]: *Andreoli and Carpenter's Cecil essentials of medicine,* ed 8, Philadelphia, 2010, Elsevier Saunders.

BASIC INFORMATION

DEFINITION

Syndrome characterized by transient systolic dysfunction and ballooning of the apical and/or mid segments of the left ventricle that mimics myocardial infarction (MI) but in the absence of obstructive (≤70% for the three epicardial coronary vessels or ≤50% for left main) coronary artery disease that can explain the wall motion abnormality. Typically, but not always, it is preceded by severe illness or intense stress.

SYNONYMS

Takotsubo cardiomyopathy
Apical ballooning syndrome
Broken heart syndrome

ICD-9CM CODES
429.83

EPIDEMIOLOGY & DEMOGRAPHICS

INCIDENCE: Uncertain, although increasingly reported
PREVALENCE: Small studies suggest a prevalence of 1.2% to 2.2% of all patients presenting with suspected acute coronary syndrome (ACS)
PREDOMINANT SEX AND AGE: Most common in women aged 60 to 76 yr
RISK FACTORS: Frequently, but not always, triggered by severe medical illness or intense emotional or physical stress (death of loved ones, domestic abuse, heated arguments, financial hardships, etc.)

PHYSICAL FINDINGS & CLINICAL PRESENTATION

Similar to acute MI (chest pain, electrocardiographic changes, shock, elevated cardiac biomarkers).

ETIOLOGY

Not well understood. Hypotheses include excessive catecholamine release, coronary artery spasm, and/or microvascular disease. Unknown why women are more commonly affected or why the apex and/or mid cavity are affected.

DIAGNOSIS

Mayo Clinic proposed criteria (2008): All 4 criteria required to make diagnosis.

- Transient hypokinesis, akinesis or dyskinesis of the left ventricular mid segments with or without apical involvement (Fig. 1-75). The regional wall motion abnormalities typically extend beyond a single epicardial coronary distribution. A stressful trigger is often, but not always present.
- Absence of obstructive coronary disease or angiographic evidence of acute plaque rupture.
- New electrocardiographic abnormalities (either ST-segment elevation and/or T-wave inversion) or modest elevation in cardiac troponin.
- Absence of pheochromocytoma or myocarditis.

DIFFERENTIAL DIAGNOSIS

- Acute MI
- Cardiac syndrome X
- Prinzmetal's angina
- Myocarditis
- Cocaine abuse

WORK-UP

- Should be suspected in postmenopausal women who present with suspected ACS after intense stress.
- Cardiology consult should be immediately obtained
- Significant CAD should be ruled out as an etiology of the cardiomyoapthy, usually by coronary catheterization.

LABORATORY TESTS

Cardiac biomarkers are often elevated, but typically less than MI

IMAGING STUDIES

Typically diagnosed in the catheterization lab during left ventriculography, although echocardiography can also show the characteristic apical ballooning.

TREATMENT

There are no randomized data, but treatment includes treatment for systolic dysfunction (beta blockers, ACE inhibitors, diuretics). Patients who are in shock should get urgent echocardiography to determine if left ventricular outflow tract (LVOT) obstruction is present.

NONPHARMACOLOGIC THERAPY

Patients in shock without significant LVOT obstruction may benefit from an intra-aortic balloon pump (IABP).

ACUTE GENERAL Rx

- Patients who are hemodynamically stable should be started on a beta-blocker, ACE inhibitor, and diuretic if needed.
- Patients who are in shock and have significant LVOT obstruction may benefit from cautious fluid resuscitation (if no significant pulmonary congestion), beta-blockers (can lessen obstruction). The use of IABP in this case is controversial due to the potential worsening of LVOT obstruction.
- If patients are in shock and there is no significant LVOT obstruction, inotropic support may be helpful.

CHRONIC Rx

Continued medical therapy for systolic dysfunction and repeat echocardiography (in 4 to 6 wk) to ensure normalization of systolic function (most patients normalize by this time). Duration of medical therapy is debatable.

DISPOSITION

Typically a diagnosis of exclusion.

REFERRAL

Should be followed by a cardiologist.

PEARLS & CONSIDERATIONS

COMMENTS

The term *takotsubo* is the Japanese name for an octopus trap (*tako-tsubo*), which has a similar shape of the LV in systole during a left ventriculogram (Fig. 1-75).

PREVENTION

Minimizing stress may reduce incidence but no data to support this.

EVIDENCE

available at www.expertconsult.com

SUGGESTED READINGS

available at www.expertconsult.com

AUTHORS: **PHILIP LEE, M.D.,** and **WEN-CHIH WU, M.D.**

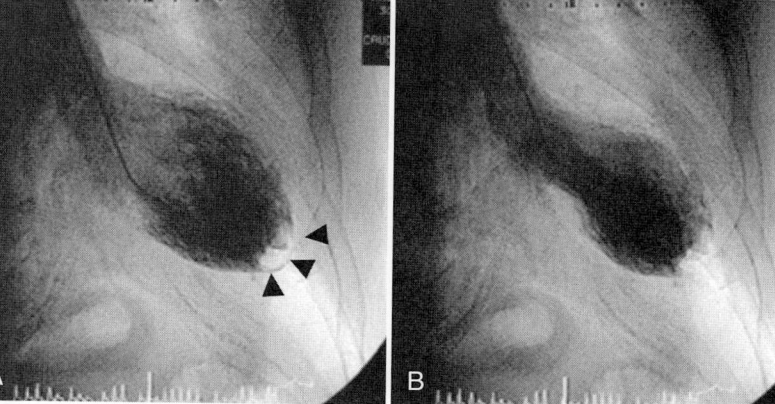

FIGURE 1-75 Left ventriculogram showing apical ballooning characteristic of stress-induced cardiomyopathy. (From Mitsuma W et al: *JACC* 51(1):cover, 2008.)

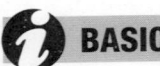

BASIC INFORMATION

DEFINITION

Light-headedness, dizziness, presyncope, or syncope in a patient with carotid sinus hypersensitivity is defined as carotid sinus syndrome (CSS). Carotid sinus hypersensitivity is the exaggerated response to carotid stimulation resulting in bradycardia, hypotension, or both. CSS is often considered a variant of neurocardiogenic syncope.

SYNONYMS

Carotid sinus syncope
CSS
Carotid sinus hypersensitivity

ICD-9CM CODES
337.0 Idiopathic peripheral autonomic neuropathy
780.2 Syncope or collapse

EPIDEMIOLOGY & DEMOGRAPHICS

- Carotid sinus hypersensitivity accounts for 10% to 20% of presyncopal and syncopal episodes.
- Carotid sinus hypersensitivity is frequently associated with atherosclerosis and diabetes mellitus.
- Incidence increases with age, with an average age of onset at 61 to 74 yr.
- Men are affected more often than women (2:1).
- Carotid sinus syndrome is rarely found in patients younger than 50 yr.

PHYSICAL FINDINGS & CLINICAL PRESENTATION

- Usually associated with sudden neck movements or tight-fitting collars
- Usually associated with prodrome of nausea, warmth, pallor, or diaphoresis
- Light-headedness or presyncopal symptoms
- Syncope

Properly performed carotid sinus massage (CSM) at the bedside is diagnostic. This maneuver can elicit three types of responses in patients with carotid sinus hypersensitivity (see "Diagnosis").

1. CSM should be performed with the patient in the supine and upright position while monitoring the patient's blood pressure by cuff and heart rate by ECG.
2. CSM should be performed on only one carotid artery at a time.
3. Vigorous circular pressure is applied over one carotid artery at the level of the cricoid cartilage for approximately 5 to 10 sec and repeated on the opposite side if no effect is produced.
4. Contraindications to CSM include the presence of carotid artery bruits, documented carotid artery stenosis >70%, history of stroke or transient ischemic attack <3 mo, history of myocardial infarction <6 mo, history of serious ventricular arrhythmia, or prior carotid endarterectomy.
5. Complications of transient visual disturbance or transient paresis occur in <1% of patients.

ETIOLOGY

- Idiopathic
- Head and neck tumors (e.g., thyroid)
- Significant lymphadenopathy
- Carotid body tumors
- Prior neck surgery

DIAGNOSIS

- The diagnosis of CSS is made when carotid sinus hypersensitivity is demonstrated by CSM and no other cause of syncope is identified.
- CSM can elicit three types of responses diagnostic of carotid sinus hypersensitivity:
  1. Cardioinhibitory type: CSM producing (1) asystole for at least 3 sec in the absence of symptoms or (2) reproduction of symptoms occurring with a decline in heart rate of 30% to 40% or asystole of up to 2 sec in duration. Symptoms should not recur when CSM is repeated after atropine infusion.
  2. Vasodepressor type: CSM producing (1) a decrease in systolic blood pressure of 50 mm Hg in the absence of symptoms or 30 mm Hg in the presence of neurologic symptoms; (2) no evidence of asystole; or (3) neurologic symptoms that persist after infusion of atropine.
  3. Mixed type: CSM producing both types of responses.

DIFFERENTIAL DIAGNOSIS

All causes of syncope

WORKUP

- CSS is a diagnosis of exclusion.
- Exclude other causes of syncope or presyncope: detailed history, physical examination including orthostatic vital signs, ECG. Other tests should be considered depending on the clinical setting.

TREATMENT

NONPHARMACOLOGIC THERAPY

Avoid applying neck pressure from tight collars, shaving, or rapid head turning.

ACUTE GENERAL Rx

Treatment will vary according to the type of carotid hypersensitivity response and symptoms present (see "Chronic Rx").

CHRONIC Rx

Therapy is divided into three classes: medical, surgical (carotid denervation), and cardiac pacing. Surgical therapy has been largely abandoned except in cases of compressing tumors or masses responsible for CSS.

For infrequent and mildly symptomatic carotid sinus hypersensitivity of either the cardioinhibitory or vasodepressor type, treatment is generally not necessary.

For symptomatic patients with a cardioinhibitory response to CSM:
- A dual-chamber permanent pacemaker is a class I indication.

For symptomatic patients with a vasodepressor response to CSM:
- Sympathomimetics: midorine 2.5 to 10 mg tid
- Serotonin-specific reuptake inhibitors
- Fludrocortisone
- Elastic knee-high or thigh-high stockings
- Carotid sinus denervation

For symptomatic patients with CSS with a mixed response to CSM:
- Combination of dual-chamber permanent pacemaker and agents used to treat vasodepressor response

DISPOSITION

- Up to 50% of the patients have recurrent symptoms.
- No increased mortality rate in patients with idiopathic CSS compared with the general population.

REFERRAL

Cardiology referral is indicated if cardiac testing, such as tilt-table test, or pacemaker placement is being considered.

Neurology referral is indicated if neurologic causes of syncope are suggested by history or physical examination findings.

PEARLS & CONSIDERATIONS

CSS accounts for syncope in 6% to 14% of patients.

The most common type of CSS is cardioinhibitory, followed by mixed and vasodepressor responses.

COMMENTS

Prognosis depends on the underlying cause.

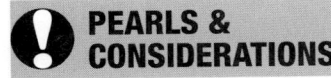

SUGGESTED READINGS
available at www.expertconsult.com

AUTHORS: **SCOTT BRANCATO, M.D.,**
WEN-CHIH WU, M.D., and
ALEXANDER G. TRUESDELL, M.D.

BASIC INFORMATION

DEFINITION

Carotid stenosis is narrowing of the arterial lumen within the carotid artery that is typically a result of atherosclerosis.

SYNONYMS

Atherosclerotic disease of the carotid artery

ICD-9CM CODES
433.1 Carotid stenosis

EPIDEMIOLOGY & DEMOGRAPHICS

INCIDENCE: 2.2 to 8/1000 persons per yr
PREVALENCE: 1.1 to 77/100,000 persons; it is estimated that 5/1000 persons aged 50 to 60 yr and 100/1000 persons >80 yr have carotid stenosis >50%. (*Note:* The incidence of carotid stenosis is unknown as screening is not routine. However, the incidence of transient ischemic attack [TIA], a common presenting symptom of carotid stenosis, is well known.)
PREDOMINANT SEX AND AGE: Male:female ratio of 2:1; more common in whites than African Americans and Asians
PEAK INCIDENCE: Peak incidence is between 50 and 60 yr of age.
GENETICS: Multifactorial; twin studies (monozygous vs. dizygous) suggest a familial influence
RISK FACTORS: Hypertension, dyslipidemia, diabetes mellitus, and smoking are the four major risk factors.

PHYSICAL FINDINGS & CLINICAL PRESENTATION

Patients with carotid stenosis are often asymptomatic, but many have presence of a carotid bruit or TIA.

- Carotid bruit: In general, the presence of a carotid bruit is a better indicator of generalized atherosclerosis and as such, is a better predictor of ischemic heart disease than future stroke.
- TIA: Carotid stenosis is classically heralded by ipsilateral transient monocular blindness (Amaurosis fugax), contralateral numbness or weakness, contralateral homonymous hemianopsia, aphasia, or *syncope (if bilateral disease is present)*.

ETIOLOGY

- Atherosclerosis (most common by far)
- Aneurysm
- Arteritis
- Carotid dissection
- Fibromuscular dysplasia
- Postradiation necrosis
- Vasospasm

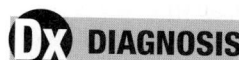

DIAGNOSIS

DIFFERENTIAL DIAGNOSIS

Aneurysm, arteritis, and carotid dissection

WORKUP

Systematic history, examination, and diagnostic studies to assess for carotid stenosis and other risk factors of TIA

LABORATORY TESTS

CBC, basic metabolic panel, fasting lipid profile, prothrombin time/international normalized ratio, activated partial thromboplastin time, C-reactive protein

IMAGING STUDIES

- Four imaging modalities exist for the evaluation of carotid stenosis (see Table 1-29).
- General guidelines state that patients who have neurologic sequelae suggestive of carotid stenosis should be screened via carotid duplex. If carotid stenosis is suspected on carotid duplex, but inconclusive, magnetic resonance angiography, computed tomography angiography, or angiography should be obtained to confirm the degree of stenosis (Fig. 1-76).

TREATMENT

NONPHARMACOLOGIC THERAPY

Carotid endarterectomy (CEA) and carotid angioplasty and stenting (CAS) are available.
CEA—several studies have proved the efficacy of this procedure. The selection of surgical candidates should be guided primarily by the presence or absence of symptoms and the degree of stenosis.
Asymptomatic patients: Four major trials have investigated the benefit of CEA in an asymptomatic patient with carotid stenosis: Carotid Artery Surgery Asymptomatic Narrowing Operation vs Aspirin (CASANOVA), Veterans Affairs Cooperative Study Group, Asymptomatic Carotid Atherosclerosis Study (ACAS), and Asymptomatic Carotid Surgery Trial (ACST). In addition, a meta-analysis was subsequently performed.
Pearls:
  Most studies have shown that a benefit from CEA in asymptomatic patients is not seen until 2 yr after surgery.
  CEA should be considered in asymptomatic patients only if the perioperative risk for stroke and death at the given surgical institution is less than 3%.
  The studies failed to show a benefit in the presence of contralateral carotid occlusion.
Recommendations for asymptomatic patients with carotid stenosis:
  CEA should be considered in patients between the ages of 40 and 75 yr with asymptomatic 60% to 99% stenosis if their life expectancy is greater than 5 yr and the perioperative stroke and mortality rates are <3%.

TABLE 1-29 Imaging Modalities for Carotid Stenosis

Imaging Modality	Benefit	Drawback
Cerebral angiography	• Gold standard • Assesses plaque morphology • Assesses presence of collaterals	• Invasive • High cost • 4% incidence rate of complications • 1% incidence rate of serious complications or death
Carotid duplex	• Sensitive in detecting high-grade stenosis (>70%) • Less invasive • Lower cost	• Can be limited by body habitus • Technician dependent • Overestimates degree of stenosis
Magnetic resonance angiography (MRA)	• Sensitive in detecting high-grade stenosis (>70%) • Less operator dependent	• Overestimates degree of stenosis • Cannot be performed in patients who are critically ill, unable to tolerate supine positioning, have pacemaker or other ferromagnetic hardware, or are claustrophobic* • Expensive • Takes much longer to obtain compared with other modalities
Computed tomography angiography (CTA)	• Sensitive for high-grade stenosis	• Contraindicated in patients with serum creatinine concentration >1.5 mg/dl

*One study revealed that ~17% of patients are unable to tolerate MRA secondary to claustrophobia or are unable to lie still for procedure.

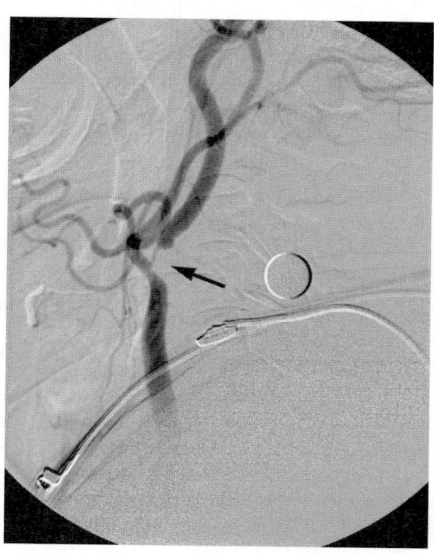

FIGURE 1-76 Conventional angiography demonstrating severe stenosis of the internal carotid artery at the bifurcation.

All patients undergoing CEA should be started on aspirin (ASA; 81 or 325 mg daily) before surgery and should be continued indefinitely. Although variations exist among surgeons, aspirin is typically continued during the perioperative period.

Symptomatic patients: Two major trials (North American Symptomatic Carotid Endarterectomy Trial [NASCET] and European Carotid Surgery Trial [ECST]) and subsequent pooled analysis have shown the benefit of CEA in patients with symptomatic carotid stenosis.

Pearls:

There is improved outcome in patients with mild stroke or TIA if surgical treatment is within 2 wk of the symptomatic event.

Men seem to benefit more when compared with women.

CEA does not appear to be beneficial in women with 50% to 69% stenosis.

Despite increased perioperative risk, patients with contralateral carotid occlusion who undergo CEA have benefit in terms of stroke and death rate when compared with patients undergoing medical management alone.

Recommendations:

CEA is recommended for recently symptomatic patients with 70% to 99% stenosis if their life expectancy is >5 yr and perioperative risk for mortality is <6%. Number needed to treat (NNT) at 5 yr = 6.3.

CEA is beneficial for recently symptomatic men with 50% to 69% stenosis if their life expectancy is >5 yr and perioperative risk of mortality is <6%. NNT at 5 yr = 22.

Medical management is recommended for patients with stenosis <50%.

ASA (81 or 325 mg daily) should be initiated before CEA and continued after surgery.

CAS (stenting) is a less invasive alternative to CEA. Four major studies have compared stenting and CEA (Stent-Protected Angioplasty vs. Carotid Endarterectomy [SPACE], endarterectomy vs. stenting in patients with symptomatic severe carotid stenosis [EVA-3S], Stenting and Angioplasty with Protection in Patients at High Risk for Endarterectomy [SAPPHIRE]), and Carotid Revascularization Endarterectomy Versus Stenting [CREST].

Recommendations:

CAS may be considered for symptomatic patients with >70% carotid stenosis who have either difficult surgical access or medical risk that increases the risk of surgery (those with severe cardiac or pulmonary disease, contralateral carotid occlusion, prior neck surgery, prior neck irradiation, contralateral laryngeal nerve palsy, recurrent stenosis after prior CEA, age >0 yr).

CAS should be considered only if operators have periprocedural morbidity and mortality rates between 4% and 6%.

ASA should be given before procedure and indefinitely after procedure.

Clopidogrel should be given for 6 mo to 2 yr after stent placement or continued indefinitely depending on individual circumstances.

Risk for CAS:

Minor or major stroke related to hyperperfusion syndrome, periprocedural bradycardia, hypotension, and restenosis. Hyperfusion syndrome 1.1% Restenosis: 0.5% to 2%

Stenting vs. Endarterectomy for Treatment of Carotid Artery Stenosis

The large CREST study, published in 2010, demonstrated no difference in primary outcomes (stroke, myocardial infarction or death in the periprocedural period or ipsilateral stroke within four years following randomization).

Individual results, however, may depend on factors such as the surgeon's experience and skill, and age of the patient with older patients (>70 yr) possibly doing better with CEA.

ACUTE GENERAL Rx

General medical therapy should be aimed at risk factor reduction. As stated earlier, the major risk factors for carotid stenosis are hypertension (HTN), diabetes mellitus (DM), dyslipidemia (HL), and smoking.

Antiplatelet therapy:

Three antiplatelet options are available for patients with carotid stenosis: ASA, ASA plus dipyridamole, and clopidogrel.

DISPOSITION

Disposition and prognosis depend on several variables (Table 1-30): the degree of stenosis, the presence of symptoms, medication compliance, and the type of intervention (if any).

REFERRAL

Patients with carotid stenosis should be referred to a neurologist with vascular neurology experience.

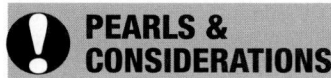

PEARLS & CONSIDERATIONS

There are ongoing studies concerning the best treatment of patients with carotid artery stenosis. Based on the results of these studies, guidelines may change rapidly.

SPECIAL CONSIDERATION

Some studies have shown that in patients with bilateral hemodynamically significant stenosis (>70%), reduction of blood pressure resulted in worse outcome in terms of stroke. These patients would likely be candidates for CEA.

Carotid artery occlusion (100% blockage), for which there is no routine treatment, is being reexamined in the national Carotid Occlusion Surgery Study (http://www.cosstrial.org). Consider referring symptomatic carotid occlusion patients for consideration of this study.

PREVENTION

Prevention of carotid stenosis should be guided at pursuing a healthy lifestyle and management of risk factors for development of atherosclerosis.

PATIENT/FAMILY EDUCATION

Patients should be counseled on pursuing a healthy lifestyle to include exercise and smoking cessation. In addition, patients should take an active role in controlling blood pressure and blood glucose. Further educational materials can be found online at: http://www.strokecenter.org/education.

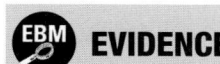 **EVIDENCE**

available at www.expertconsult.com

SUGGESTED READINGS

available at www.expertconsult.com

AUTHOR: **JOSEPH R. OWENS, M.D.**

TABLE 1-30 Carotid Stenosis Management			
Degree of Carotid Stenosis	**<50%**	**50%-69%**	**70%-99%**
Asymptomatic	• Medical management	• Men: CEA if stenosis >60% and age <75 yr; otherwise, medical management • Women: medical management	• Men <75 yr: CEA • Women: medical management
Symptomatic	• Medical Management	• Men: CEA • Women: medical management	• Men: CEA • Women: CEA

CEA, Carotid endarterectomy.

BASIC INFORMATION

DEFINITION

Carpal tunnel syndrome is a compressive neuropathy of the median nerve as it passes under the transverse carpal ligament at the wrist (Fig. 1-77). It is the most common entrapment neuropathy.

ICD-9CM CODES
354.0 Carpal tunnel syndrome

EPIDEMIOLOGY & DEMOGRAPHICS

PREVALENT AGE: 30 to 60 yr (bilateral up to 65%)

PREVALENT SEX: Females are affected two to five times as often as males.

PHYSICAL FINDINGS & CLINICAL PRESENTATION

- Pain, paresthesia in first through lateral fourth fingers, worse at night
- Tinel's sign at wrist: tapping lightly over the median nerve on the volar surface of the wrist produces a tingling sensation radiating from the wrist to the hand
- Phalen's sign: reproduction of symptoms after 1 min of gentle, unforced wrist flexion
- Carpal compression test: direct pressure over the patient's carpal tunnel for 30 sec elicits symptoms
- Hand elevation test: raising hands above head for 1 min reproduces symptoms

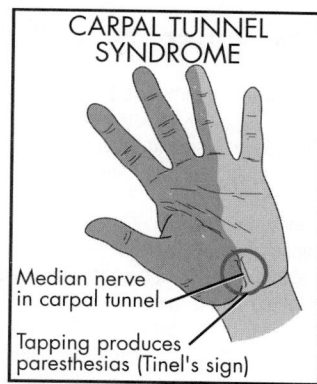

FIGURE 1-77 Distribution of pain and/or paresthesias *(dark-shaded area)* when the median nerve is compressed by swelling in the wrist (carpal tunnel). (From Arnett FC: Rheumatoid arthritis. In Andreoli TE [ed]: *Cecil essentials of medicine,* ed 6, Philadelphia, 2005, WB Saunders.)

- Thenar atrophy in longstanding cases with weakness of thumb abduction and opposition

ETIOLOGY

- Idiopathic in most cases
  - Increased intracarpal tunnel pressure
  - Ischemia, friction, or angulation of median nerve
- Space-occupying lesions in carpal tunnel (tenosynovitis, ganglia, aberrant muscles)
- Can be associated with diabetes, hypothyroidism, pregnancy, connective tissue diseases, acromegaly, amyloidosis
- Repetitive strain or job-related mechanical overuse may be a risk factor
- Crystal-induced rheumatic disorders

DIAGNOSIS

DIFFERENTIAL DIAGNOSIS

- Cervical radiculopathy
- Chronic tendinitis
- Other arthritides
- Reflex sympathetic dystrophy
- Brachial plexopathy
- Polyneuropathy
- Other entrapment neuropathies
- Traumatic wrist injuries

IMAGING STUDIES

Carpal tunnel syndrome is a clinical diagnosis but imaging may assist workup in uncertain situations. High-resolution ultrasound has been found to be very effective in supporting the diagnosis. Roentgenograms or MRI may be helpful in ruling out other conditions.

ELECTRODIAGNOSTIC STUDIES

Nerve conduction velocity tests demonstrate impaired sensory conduction across the carpal tunnel. Electromyography may show active denervation muscle potentials.

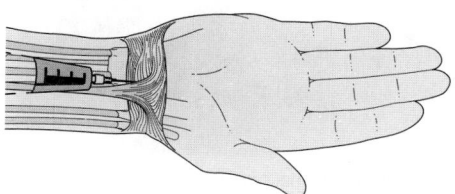

FIGURE 1-78 Injection of the carpal tunnel. (From Hochberg MC et al [eds]: *Rheumatology,* ed 3, St Louis, 2003, Mosby.)

TREATMENT

ACUTE GENERAL Rx

- Activity modification
- Nocturnal wrist splint
- No evidence for effectiveness of NSAIDs
- Corticosteroid injection of carpal canal on ulnar side of palmaris longus tendon proximal to wrist crease (Fig. 1-78)
- Low-dose oral corticosteroids
- Short-term benefit from ultrasound therapy
- Ergonomic keyboards (vs. standard keyboards)

DISPOSITION

Clinical course may have remissions and exacerbations. Some may progress from intermittent to persistent sensory complaints, then later to develop motor symptoms. In pregnancy, symptoms usually resolve spontaneously weeks after delivery.

REFERRAL

Surgical referral needed if conservative treatment fails. It is usually reserved for severe symptoms or presence of weakness/thenar atrophy. Surgery (sectioning of transverse carpal ligament) to release pressure on the median nerve is done by open or endoscopic approach, with good long-term results.

PEARLS & CONSIDERATIONS

- Carpal tunnel syndrome sensory changes spare the thenar eminence. This distinctive pattern occurs because the palmar sensory cutaneous branch of the median nerve arises proximal to the wrist, passing over, rather than through the tunnel.
- Role of repetitive hand or wrist use and workplace factors in the development of carpal tunnel syndrome remains controversial.

EVIDENCE

available at www.expertconsult.com

SUGGESTED READINGS

available at www.expertconsult.com

AUTHOR: **CANDICE YUVIENCO, M.D.**

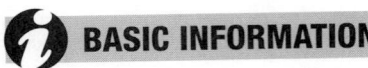

BASIC INFORMATION

DEFINITION

Cataracts are the clouding and opacification of the normally clear crystalline lens of the eye. The opacity may occur in the cortex, the nucleus of the lens, or the posterior subcapsular region, but it is usually in a combination of areas.

SYNONYMS

Congenital cataracts (e.g., from rubella)
Metabolic cataracts (e.g., caused by diabetes)
Collagen-vascular disease cataracts (caused by lupus)
Hereditary cataracts
Age-related senile cataracts
Traumatic cataracts
Toxic or drug-induced cataracts (e.g., caused by steroids)
Lenticular opacities

ICD-9CM CODES
366 Cataract

EPIDEMIOLOGY & DEMOGRAPHICS

INCIDENCE (IN U.S.): Most common cause of treatable blindness; cataract removal is the most frequent surgical procedure in patients >65 yr (1.3 million operations per year, with an annual cost of approximately $3 billion). By year 2020 more than 30 million Americans will have cataracts. Of Americans >40 yr, 20.5 million (17.2%) have cataracts. Of these, 5% have had surgery.
PEAK INCIDENCE:
- In early life: congenital and hereditary causes predominant; consider drug related and trauma
- In older age group: senile cataracts (after 40 yr)

PREDOMINANT AGE: Elderly; some stage of cataract development is present in >50% of persons 65 to 74 yr and in 65% of those >75 yr. Lens clouding begins at 39 to 40 yr and then usually progresses either slowly or rapidly depending on individual and health.
GENETICS: Hereditary with syndromes such as galactosemia, homocystinuria, diabetes

PHYSICAL FINDINGS & CLINICAL PRESENTATION

Cloudiness and opacification of the crystalline lens of the eye (Fig. 1-79)

ETIOLOGY
- Heredity
- Trauma
- Toxins
- Age related
- Drug related (e.g., statins)
- Congenital
- Inflammatory
- Diabetes
- Collagen vascular disease

DIAGNOSIS

DIFFERENTIAL DIAGNOSIS
- Corneal lesions
- Retinal lesions, detached retina, tumors
- Vitreous disease, chronic inflammation

WORKUP
- Complete eye examination, including slit lamp examination, funduscopic examination, and brightness acuity testing
- Complete physical examination for other underlying causes

LABORATORY TESTS
- Rarely, urinary amino acid screening and central nervous system imaging studies with congenital cataracts
- Fasting glucose in young adults with cataracts
- Diabetes, collagen vascular disease, other metabolic diseases in younger patients
- Genetic and hereditary evaluation

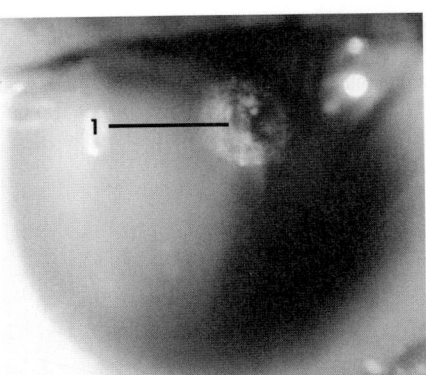

FIGURE 1-79 The central location of a posterior subcapsular cataract *(1)*. (From Palay D [ed]: *Ophthalmology for the primary care physician,* St Louis, 1997, Mosby.)

TREATMENT

There is no evidence that antioxidants or drugs will slow or treat cataracts.

NONPHARMACOLOGIC THERAPY
- Wait until vision is compromised before doing surgery.
- Surgery is indicated when corrected visual acuity in the affected eye is >20/30 in the absence of other ocular disease; however, surgery may be justified when visual acuity is better in specific situations (especially disabling glare, monocular diplopia). Surgery indicated when vision in one eye is greatly different from the other and affects the patient's life.

ACUTE GENERAL Rx

None necessary except when acute glaucoma or inflammation occurs

CHRONIC Rx
- Change glasses as cataracts develop.
- Myopia is common, and glasses can be adjusted until surgery is contemplated.

DISPOSITION

Refer if sight is compromised or the eye is red or inflamed.

REFERRAL

Refer to ophthalmologist for evaluation for extraction when vision is compromised (see "Nonpharmacologic Therapy").

PEARLS & CONSIDERATIONS

- Patients want to know five things about cataracts:
  1. Chance for vision improvement
  2. When vision will improve
  3. Risk from surgery
  4. Effect of surgery
  5. Types of complications
- Men planning cataract surgery should, if possible, avoid use of alpha blockers until after surgery has been completed. The risk of intraoperative floppy iris syndrome is substantial among men taking tamsulosin, ranging from about 43% to 90%.

EVIDENCE

available at www.expertconsult.com

SUGGESTED READINGS
available at www.expertconsult.com

AUTHOR: **MELVYN KOBY, M.D.**

BASIC INFORMATION

DEFINITION

Cat-scratch disease (CSD) is a syndrome consisting of gradually enlarging regional lymphadenopathy occurring after contact with a feline. Atypical presentations are characterized by a variety of neurologic manifestations as well as granulomatous involvement of the eye, liver, spleen, and bone. The disease is usually self-limiting, and recovery is complete; however, patients with atypical presentations, especially if immunocompromised, may suffer significant morbidity and mortality.

SYNONYMS

Cat-scratch fever
Benign inoculation lymphoreticulosis
Nonbacterial regional lymphadenitis

ICD-9CM CODES
078.3 Cat-scratch disease

EPIDEMIOLOGY & DEMOGRAPHICS

PREVALENCE: Unknown
INCIDENCE (IN U.S.):
- Unknown
- Majority of reported cases in children
PEAK INCIDENCE: August through January
GENETICS: Unknown

PHYSICAL FINDINGS & CLINICAL PRESENTATION

- Classic, most common finding: regional lymphadenopathy occurring within 2 wk of a scratch or contact with felines; usually a new kitten in the household
- Tender, swollen lymph nodes most commonly found in the head and neck, followed by the axilla and the epitrochlear, inguinal, and femoral areas
- Erythematous overlying skin, showing signs of suppuration from involved lymph nodes
- On careful examination; evidence of cutaneous inoculation in the form of a nonpruritic, slightly tender pustule or papule
- Fever in most patients
- Malaise and headache in fewer than a third of patients
- Atypical presentations in fewer than 15% of cases
  1. Usually in association with lymphadenopathy and a low-grade or frank fever ($>101°$ F, $>38.3°$ C)
  2. Include granulomatous involvement of the conjunctiva (Parinaud's oculoglandular syndrome) and focal masses in the liver, spleen, and mesenteric nodes
- CNS involvement: neuroretinitis, encephalopathy, encephalitis, transverse myelitis, seizure activity, and coma
- Osteomyelitis in adults and children

ETIOLOGY

- Major cause: *Bartonella henselae*, possibly *Afipia felis* and *B. clarrigeiae*

- Mode of transmission: predominantly by direct inoculation through the scratch, bite, or lick of a cat, especially a kitten
- Limited evidence in support of an arthropod (flea) as an alternative vector of infection arising from bacteremic felines
- Rarely, associated with dogs, monkeys, and inanimate objects with which a feline has been in recent contact
- Approximately 2 wk after introduction of the bacteria into the host, regional lymphatic tissues displaying granulomatous infiltration associated with gradual hypertrophy
- Possible dissemination to distant sites (e.g., liver, spleen, and bone), usually characterized by focal masses or discrete parenchymal lesions

DIAGNOSIS

DIFFERENTIAL DIAGNOSIS

Granulomas of this syndrome must be differentiated from those associated with:
- Tularemia
- Tuberculosis or other myobacterial infections
- Brucellosis
- Sarcoidosis
- Sporotrichosis or other fungal diseases
- Toxoplasmosis
- Lymphogranuloma venereum
- Benign and malignant tumors such as lymphoma

WORKUP

Diagnosis should be considered in patients who present with a predominant complaint of gradually enlarging regional (focal) lymphadenopathy, often with fever and a recent history of having contact with a cat. A primary ulcer at the site of the cat scratch may or may not be present at the time lymphadenopathy becomes manifest.

LABORATORY TESTS

- CSD skin test is no longer used for clinical purposes.
- Biopsied lymph node histology consistent with CSD.
- Enhanced culture techniques and serologies augment establishment of the diagnosis. An IFA *Bartonella* serology is commercially available. A PCR is used in research settings.
- Histopathologically, Warthin-Starry silver stain has been used to identify the bacillus.
- Routine laboratory findings:
  1. Mild leukocytosis or leukopenia
  2. Infrequent eosinophilia
  3. Elevated ESR or CRP
- Abnormalities of bilirubin excretion and elevated hepatic transaminases are usually secondary to hepatic obstruction by granuloma, mass, or lymph node.
- In patients with neurologic manifestations, lumbar puncture usually reveals normal CSF, although there may be a mild pleocytosis and modest elevation in protein.

TREATMENT

NONPHARMACOLOGIC THERAPY

- Warm compresses to the affected nodes
- In cases of encephalitis or coma: supportive care

ACUTE GENERAL Rx

- There is no consensus over therapy, especially as the disease is self-limited in a majority of cases.
- It would be prudent to treat severely ill patients, especially if immunocompromised, with antibiotic therapy, because these patients tend to suffer dissemination of infection and increased morbidity.
- *Bartonella* is usually sensitive to a 5-day course of azithromycin, or alternatively aminoglycosides, tetracycline, and the quinolones can be used.
- When the isolate is proven by culture, the patient should receive antibiotic therapy as directed by the obtained susceptibilities.
- Antipyretics and NSAIDs may also be used.

DISPOSITION

Overall prognosis is good.

REFERRAL

- To an appropriate subspecialist to evaluate specific lesions
- For diagnostic aspiration or excision in presence of regional lymphadenopathy, bone lesions, and mesenteric lymph nodes and organs
- To ophthalmologist for ocular granulomas
  1. Usually diagnosed clinically
  2. Rarely require excision

PEARLS & CONSIDERATIONS

COMMENTS

- A presentation of this syndrome, especially in patients with HIV infection or impaired cellular immunity, may be fever of unknown origin.
- Hepatic and splenic granulomas, coronary valve infections may offer few physical clues to diagnosis, emphasizing the need for a complete history.
- CSD should be considered in the differential diagnosis of school-aged children presenting with status epilepticus.
- Chronically immunocompromised patients considering the acquisition of a young feline should be made aware of the possible risk of infection.
- No signs of illness may be apparent in bacteremic kittens.

SUGGESTED READINGS

available at www.expertconsult.com

AUTHORS: **GLENN G. FORT, M.D., M.P.H.,** and **DENNIS J. MIKOLICH, M.D.**

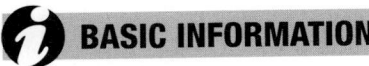

BASIC INFORMATION

DEFINITION

Cavernous sinus thrombosis (CST) is a late complication of facial or paranasal sinus infection, resulting in thrombosis of the cavernous sinus and inflammation of its surrounding anatomic structures, including cranial nerves III, IV, V (ophthalmic and maxillary branch), and VI, and the internal carotid artery.

SYNONYMS

Intracranial venous sinus thrombosis or thrombophlebitis

ICD-9CM CODES
325 Phlebitis and thrombophlebitis of intracranial venous sinuses

EPIDEMIOLOGY & DEMOGRAPHICS

- Cavernous sinus thrombosis is rare in the postantibiotic era.
- Before antibiotics the mortality rate was 80% to 100%.
- With antibiotics and early diagnosis, mortality rates have fallen to ~20%.
- Reported morbidity rates have also declined from between 50% and 70% to only 22% with advances in imaging modalities and aggressive medical care.

PHYSICAL FINDINGS & CLINICAL PRESENTATION

- Can be either an acute and fulminant disease or an indolent and subacute presentation.
- Headache, though not specific, is the most common presenting symptom and may precede fever and periorbital edema by several days. Elderly patients, however, may only demonstrate alteration in mental status without antecedent headache. A classic presentation is abrupt onset of unilateral periorbital edema progressing to bilateral eye involvement, headache, photophobia, and proptosis. These signs and symptoms are related to the anatomic structures affected within the cavernous sinus, notably cranial nerves III to VI, as well as impaired venous drainage from the orbit and the eye.

Other common signs and symptoms include:
- Ptosis
- Chemosis
- Cranial nerve palsies (III, IV, V, VI)
  1. Sixth nerve palsy is the most common (abducens nerve is located medially in the cavernous sinus and is surrounded by blood, making it more susceptible to inflammatory changes).
  2. Hypoesthesia or hyperesthesia of the ophthalmic and maxillary branch of the fifth nerve is common. Periorbital sensory loss and impaired corneal reflex may be noted.
- Papilledema, retinal hemorrhages, and decreased visual acuity to blindness may occur from venous congestion within the retina.

- Pupil may be dilated and sluggishly reactive.
- Fever, tachycardia, and sepsis may be present.
- Headache with nuchal rigidity and changes in mental status may occur.
- Infection can spread to the contralateral cavernous sinus through the intercavernous sinuses within 24 to 48 hr of initial presentation.

ETIOLOGY

- CST most commonly results from contiguous spread of an infection from the sinuses (sphenoid, ethmoid, or frontal) or the medial third of the face (areas around the eyes and nose that drain to the ophthalmic vein). Nasal furuncles are the most common facial infection to produce this complication. Less-common primary sites of infection include dental abscess, tonsils, soft palate, middle ear, or orbit (orbital cellulitis).
- CST also can result from hematogenous spread of infection to the cavernous sinus by the superior and inferior ophthalmic veins or through the lateral and sigmoid sinuses. It can spread in a retrograde direction depending on the pressure gradients, because the dural sinuses are valveless.
- *Staphylococcus aureus* is the most common infectious microbe, found in 60% to 70% of the cases.
- *Streptococcus* is the second leading cause.
- Gram-negative rods and anaerobes may also lead to cavernous sinus thrombosis.
- Rarely, *Aspergillus fumigatus* and mucormycosis cause CST.

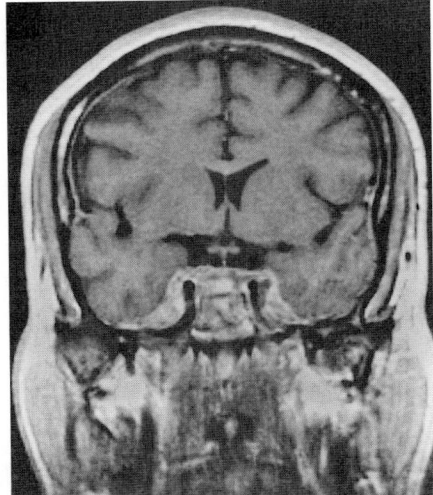

FIGURE 1-80 Contrast-enhanced MRI scan of the head in the sagittal projection of a 29-year-old man with sinus congestion and headache. There is non-uniform signal intensity of the cavernous venous sinuses, indicating cavernous sinus thrombosis. The sphenoid, ethmoidal, and maxillary paranasal sinuses also demonstrated abnormal signal intensity. (Cohen J, Powderly WG: *Infectious diseases,* ed 2, St Louis, 2004, Mosby.)

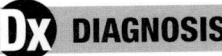 **DIAGNOSIS**

- The diagnosis of CST is made by clinical suspicion and confirmed by appropriate imaging studies.
- Proptosis, ptosis, chemosis, and cranial nerve palsy beginning in one eye and progressing to the other eye establish the diagnosis.

DIFFERENTIAL DIAGNOSIS

- Orbital or periorbital cellulitis
- Internal carotid artery aneurysm or fistula
- Cerebrovascular disease
- Migraine headache
- Allergic blepharitis
- Thyroid ophthalmopathy
- Orbital neoplasm
- Meningitis
- Epidural and subdural infections
- Epidural and subdural hematoma
- Subarachnoid hemorrhage
- Acute angle-closure glaucoma
- Trauma

WORKUP

CST is a clinical diagnosis, with laboratory tests and imaging studies confirming the clinical impression.

LABORATORY TESTS

- Complete blood count, erythrocyte sedimentation rate, blood cultures, and sinus cultures help establish and identify an infectious primary source.
- Lumbar puncture (LP) helps to distinguish CST from more localized processes (e.g., sinusitis, orbital cellulites). LP reveals inflammatory cells in 75% of cases. In half of these cases, the cerebrospinal fluid profile is typical for a parameningeal focus (high white blood cells with polymorphonuclear and/or mononuclear cells, normal glucose, normal protein, culture negative), and in one third may be similar to that of a bacterial meningitis.

IMAGING STUDIES

- Contrast-enhanced CT or MRI venography can show evidence of CST.
- Noncontrast CT scan of the head and orbits may demonstrate increased density in the region of the cavernous sinus but has relatively low sensitivity. Contrast-enhanced CT scan may reveal underlying sinusitis, thickening of the superior ophthalmic vein, and irregular filling defects within the cavernous sinus; however, findings may be normal early in the disease course.
- MRI with gadolinium (Fig. 1-80), including magnetic resonance angiography, is more sensitive than CT scan and is the imaging study of choice to diagnose CST. Findings may include deformity of the internal carotid artery within the cavernous sinus and an obvious signal hyperintensity within thrombosed vascular sinuses on all pulse sequences.
- Cerebral angiography can be performed, but it is invasive and not very sensitive.

- Orbital venography is difficult to perform, but it is excellent in diagnosing occlusion of the cavernous sinus.

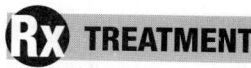 **TREATMENT**

NONPHARMACOLOGIC THERAPY

Recognizing the primary source of infection (i.e., facial cellulitis, middle ear, and sinus infections) and treating the primary source expeditiously is the best way to prevent CST.

ACUTE GENERAL Rx

- Appropriate therapy should take into account the primary source of infection as well as possible associated complications such as brain abscess, meningitis, or subdural empyema.
- Broad-spectrum intravenous antibiotics are used as empiric therapy until a definite pathogen is found. Treatment should include a penicillinase-resistant penicillin at maximum dose plus a third- or fourth-generation cephalosporin:
  1. Nafcillin (or oxacillin) 2 g IV q4h plus either ceftriaxone (2 g q12h) or cefepime (2 g q8 to 12h).
  2. Metronidazole 500 mg IV q6h should be added if anaerobic bacterial infection is suspected (dental or sinus infection).
- Vancomycin (1 g q12h with normal renal function) may be substituted for nafcillin if significant concern exists regarding infection by methicillin-resistant *Staphylococcus aureus* or resistant *Streptococcus pneumoniae*.
- Anticoagulation with heparin is controversial. Cerebral infarction or intracranial hemorrhage should first be ruled out by noncontrast CT scan before initiating heparin therapy. Early heparinization has been suggested in patients with unilateral cavernous sinus thrombosis to prevent clot propagation. Coumadin therapy should be avoided in the acute phase of the illness but should ultimately be instituted to achieve an INR of 2 to 3 and continued until the infection, symptoms, and signs of CST have resolved or significantly improved. A nonrandomized prospective cohort study found treatment with low-molecular weight heparin led to more functional independence at 6 mo without significant differences in complete recovery and mortality compared to unfractionated heparin.
- Steroid therapy is also controversial but may prove helpful in reducing cranial nerve dysfunction or when progression to pituitary insufficiency occurs. Corticosteroids should only be instituted after appropriate antibiotic coverage. Dexamethasone 10 mg q6h is the treatment of choice.
- Emergent surgical drainage with sphenoidotomy is indicated if the primary site of infection is believed to be the sphenoid sinus.

CHRONIC Rx

- Patients with CST are usually treated with prolonged courses (3 to 4 wk) of IV antibiotics. If there is evidence of complications such as intracranial suppuration, 6 to 8 wk of total therapy may be warranted.
- All patients should be monitored for signs of complicated infection, continued sepsis, or septic emboli while antibiotic therapy is being administered.

DISPOSITION

- CST can be a life-threatening, rapidly progressive infectious disease with high morbidity and mortality rates (30%) despite antibiotic use. Morbidity and mortality rates are increased in cases of sphenoid sinus infection.
- Complications of untreated CST include extension of thrombus to other dural sinuses, carotid thrombosis with concomitant strokes, subdural empyema, brain abscess, or meningitis. Septic embolization may also occur to the lungs, resulting in acute respiratory distress syndrome, pulmonary abscess, empyema, and pneumothorax.
- Thirty percent of treated patients develop long-term sequelae, including cranial nerve palsies, blindness, pituitary insufficiency, and hemiparesis.

REFERRAL

If CST is suspected, it should be considered a medical emergency. Depending on the primary site of infection, appropriate consultation should be made (i.e., ear-nose-throat, ophthalmology, and infectious disease).

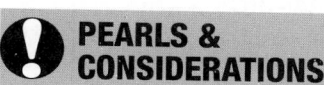 **PEARLS & CONSIDERATIONS**

COMMENTS

Realizing the cavernous sinus lies just above and lateral to the sphenoid sinus and drains the middle portion of the face by the superior and inferior ophthalmic veins and knowing that cranial nerves III, IV, V, and VI pass alongside or through the cavernous sinus make the clinical findings and diagnosis easier to understand.

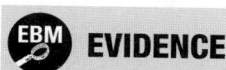 **EVIDENCE**

available at www.expertconsult.com

SUGGESTED READINGS

available at www.expertconsult.com

AUTHORS: **MARK F. BRADY, M.D., M.P.H.,** and **WEN Y. WU-CHEN, M.D.**

C

Diseases and Disorders

I

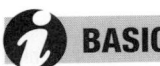

BASIC INFORMATION

DEFINITION

Celiac disease is a chronic autoimmune disease characterized by malabsorption and diarrhea precipitated by ingestion of food products containing gluten.

SYNONYMS

Gluten-sensitive enteropathy
Celiac sprue
Nontropical sprue

ICD-9CM CODES
579.0 Celiac disease

EPIDEMIOLOGY & DEMOGRAPHICS

- The prevalence of celiac disease is 1% in the general population in North America and Western Europe and 5% in high-risk groups such as first-degree relatives of persons with the disease.
- Incidence is highest during infancy and the first 36 mo of life (after introduction of foods containing gluten), in the third decade (frequently associated with pregnancy and severe anemia during pregnancy), and in the seventh decade.
- There is a slight female predominance.

PHYSICAL FINDINGS & CLINICAL PRESENTATION

- Physical examination may be entirely within normal limits.
- Weight loss, dyspepsia, short stature, and failure to thrive may be noted in children and infants.
- Weight loss, fatigue, and diarrhea are common in adults.
- Abdominal pain, nausea, and vomiting are unusual.
- Pallor as a result of iron-deficiency anemia is common.
- Atypical forms of the disease are being increasingly recognized and include osteoporosis, short stature, anemia, infertility, and neurologic problems. Manifestations of calcium deficiency, such as tetany and seizures, are rare and can be exacerbated by coexistent magnesium deficiency.
- Angular cheilitis, aphthous ulcers, atopic dermatitis, and dermatitis herpetiformis are frequently associated with celiac disease.

ETIOLOGY

- Celiac sprue is considered an autoimmune-type disease, with tissue transglutaminase (tTG) suggested as a major autoantigen. It results from an inappropriate T-cell–mediated immune response against ingested gluten in genetically predisposed individuals who carry either *HLA-DQ2* or *HLA-DQ8* genes. There is sensitivity to gliadin, a protein fraction of gluten found in wheat, rye, and barley. In patients with celiac disease, immune responses to gliadin fractions promote an inflammatory reaction, mainly in the upper small intestine, manifested by infiltration of the lamina propria and the epithelium with chronic inflammatory cells and villous atrophy.

- Timing of introduction of gluten into the infant diet is associated with the appearance of celiac disease in children at risk. Children initially exposed to gluten in the first 3 mo of life have a fivefold increased risk.

DIAGNOSIS

Diagnostic criteria for celiac disease require at least four out of five or three out of four if the HLA genotype is not performed:
1. Typical symptoms of celiac disease
2. Positivity of serum celiac disease Ig A class autoantibodies at high titer
3. *HLA-DQ2* or *HLA-DQ8* genotypes
4. Celiac enteropathy at the small intestinal biopsy
5. Response to gluten-free diet

DIFFERENTIAL DIAGNOSIS

- Inflammatory bowel disease
- Laxative abuse
- Intestinal parasitic infestations
- Other: irritable bowel syndrome, tropical sprue, chronic pancreatitis, Zollinger-Ellison syndrome, cystic fibrosis (children), lymphoma, eosinophilic gastroenteritis, short bowel syndrome, Whipple's disease

LABORATORY TESTS

- Iron-deficiency anemia (microcytic anemia, low ferritin level).
- Folic acid deficiency.
- Vitamin B12 deficiency, hypomagnesemia, hypocalcemia.
- IgA tTG antibody by enzyme-linked immunosorbent assay (tissue transglutaminase [tTG] test) is the best screening serologic test for celiac sprue. IgA antiendomysial antibodies (EMA) test is also a good screening test for celiac disease, except in the case of patients with IgA deficiency.
- Biopsy of the small bowel, considered the gold standard, has been questioned as a reliable and conclusive test in all cases. It may be reasonable in children with significant elevations of tTG levels (>100 U) to first try a gluten-free diet and consider biopsy in those who do not improve with diet.
- The HLA-DQ2 allele is identified in >90% of patients with celiac disease, and HLA-*DQ8* is identified in most of the remaining patients. These genes occur in only 30% to 40% of the general population. Their greatest diagnostic value is in their negative predictive value, making them useful when negative in ruling out the disease.

IMAGING STUDIES

Capsule endoscopy can be used to evaluate mucosa of the small intestine, especially if future innovations will allow mucosal biopsy.

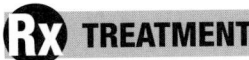

TREATMENT

NONPHARMACOLOGIC THERAPY

Patients should be instructed on a gluten-free diet (avoidance of wheat, rye, and barley). Safe grains (gluten-free) include rice, corn, oats, buckwheat, millet, amaranth, quinoa, sorghum, and teff (an Ethiopian cereal grain).

GENERAL Rx

- Correct nutritional deficiencies with iron, folic acid, calcium, and vitamin B12 as needed.
- Prednisone 20 to 60 mg qd gradually tapered is useful in refractory cases.
- Lifelong gluten-free diet is necessary.

DISPOSITION

- Prognosis is good with adherence to a gluten-free diet. Rapid improvement is usually seen within a few days of treatment.
- Serial antigliadin or antiendomysial antibody tests can be used to monitor the patient's adherence to a gluten-free diet.
- Repeat small-bowel biopsy after treatment generally reveals significant improvement. It is also useful to evaluate for increased risk of small-bowel T-cell lymphoma in these patients, especially untreated patients.

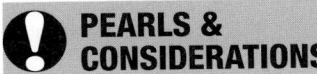

PEARLS & CONSIDERATIONS

COMMENTS

- Some experts recommend a repeat biopsy only in selected patients who have an unsatisfactory response to a strict gluten-free diet.
- Celiac disease should be considered in patients with unexplained metabolic bone disease, osteoporosis, or hypocalcemia, because gastrointestinal symptoms absent or mild. Clinicians should also consider testing children and young adults for celiac disease if unexplained weight loss, abdominal pain or distention, or chronic diarrhea present.
- The prevalence of celiac disease in patients with dyspepsia is twice that of the general population. Screening for celiac disease should be considered in all patients with persistent dyspepsia.
- Patients with celiac disease have an overall risk of cancer that is almost twice that of the general population. The risk of adenocarcinoma of the small intestine is increased manifold compared with the risk in the general population. Celiac disease is also associated with an increased risk for non-Hodgkin's lymphoma, especially of T-cell type and primarily localized in the gut. Lymphoma is 4 to 40 times more common, and death from lymphoma is 11 to 70 times more common in patients with celiac disease.
- In adult patients presenting with abdominal pains, IgA antitissue transglutaminase antibodies and IgA antendomysial antibodies have a high sensitivity and specificity for diagnosing celiac disease.

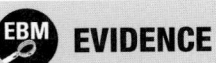 **EVIDENCE**

available at www.expertconsult.com

SUGGESTED READINGS
available at www.expertconsult.com

AUTHOR: **FRED F. FERRI, M.D.**

BASIC INFORMATION

DEFINITION

Cellulitis is a superficial inflammatory condition of the skin and underlying tissues characterized by erythema, warmth, and tenderness of the involved area.

SYNONYMS

Erysipelas (cellulitis generally caused by group A β-hemolytic streptococci)

ICD-9CM CODES
682.9 Cellulitis

EPIDEMIOLOGY & DEMOGRAPHICS

- Occurs most frequently in diabetics, immunocompromised hosts, and patients with venous and lymphatic compromise.
- Frequently found near skin breaks (trauma, surgical wounds [surgical site infections develop in 2% to 5% of all surgical procedures], ulcerations, tinea infections). Edema, animal or human bites, subadjacent osteomyelitis, and bacteremia are potential sources of cellulitis.

PHYSICAL FINDINGS & CLINICAL PRESENTATION

Variable with the causative organism:
- Erysipelas: superficial-spreading, warm, erythematous lesion distinguished by its indurated and elevated margin; lymphatic involvement and vesicle formation are common.
- Staphylococcal cellulitis: area involved is erythematous, hot, and swollen; differentiated from erysipelas by nonelevated, poorly demarcated margin; local tenderness and regional adenopathy are common; up to 85% of cases occur on the legs and feet.
- *Haemophilus influenzae* cellulitis: area involved is a blue-red/purple-red color; occurs mainly in children; generally involves the face in children and the neck or upper chest in adults.
- *Vibrio vulnificus:* larger hemorrhagic bullae, cellulitis, lymphadenitis, myositis; often found in critically ill patients in septic shock.

ETIOLOGY

- Group A β-hemolytic streptococci (may follow a streptococcal infection of the upper respiratory tract). β-hemolytic streptococci are implicated in most cases of nontraumatic cellulitis.
- Staphylococcal cellulitis: Diabetics, athletes, men who have sex with men, people living in public housing, and incarcerated men are at greater risk for methicillin-resistant *S. aureus* (MRSA) infection. A community-acquired MRSA strain, USA 300, is replacing nosocomial strains of MRSA in hospitals.
- IV drug use: MRSA, *P. aeruginosa.*
- *V. vulnificus:* higher incidence in patients with liver disease (75%) and in immunocompromised hosts (corticosteroid use, diabetes mellitus, leukemia, renal failure). *V. vulnificus* infection is the leading cause of death related to seafood consumption in the United States.
- *Erysipelothrix rhusiopathiae:* common in people handling poultry, fish, or meat.
- *Aeromonas hydrophila:* generally occurs in contaminated open wounds in fresh water.
- Fungi *(Cryptococcus neoformans):* may be present in immunocompromised granulopenic patients.
- Gram-negative rods *(Serratia, Enterobacter, Proteus, Pseudomonas):* may be present in immunocompromised or granulopenic patients.
- Hot tub exposure: *P. aeruginosa;* fish tank exposure: *Mycobacterium marinum.*
- Bites: Human *(eikenella corrodens),* dog *(P. multicida, C. canimorsus),* cat *(P. multicida),* rat *(Streptobacillus moniliformis).*

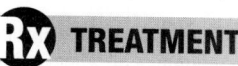 **DIAGNOSIS**

DIFFERENTIAL DIAGNOSIS

- Necrotizing fasciitis (reddish-purple discoloration of skin, rapid increase in size, woody induration and pale appearance rather then erythema, violaceous bullae, pain out of proportion to appearance, sepsis)
- Deep vein thrombosis
- Peripheral vascular insufficiency
- Paget disease of the breast
- Thrombophlebitis
- Acute gout
- Psoriasis
- Candida intertrigo
- Pseudogout
- Osteomyelitis
- Insect bite
- Fixed drug eruption
- Lymphedema
- Contact dermatitis
- Olecranon bursa infection
- Herpetic whitlow, early herpes zoster (before blisters)
- Erythema migrans (Lyme disease)
- Rare: *Vaccinia* vaccination, Kawasaki disease, pyoderma gangrenosum, Sweet syndrome, carcinoma erysipeloides, anaerobic myonecrosis, erythromelalgia, eosinophilic cellulitis (Well's syndrome), familial Mediterranean fever

LABORATORY TESTS

- Gram stain and culture (aerobic and anaerobic):
  1. Aspirated material from:
     a. Advancing edge of cellulitis
     b. Any vesicles
  2. Swab of any drainage material
  3. Punch biopsy (in selected patients)
- Blood cultures in hospitalized patients, in patients who have cellulitis superimposed on lymphedema, in patients with buccal or periorbital cellulitis, and in patients suspected of having a salt-water or fresh-water source of infection. Bacteremia is uncommon in cellulitis (positive blood cultures in only 4% of patients).
- Anti-streptolysin O (ASLO) titer (in suspected streptococcal disease)

Despite the previous measures, the cause of cellulitis remains unidentified in most patients. Patients with recurrent lower-extremity cellulites should be inspected for tinea pedis. If found it should be treated.

IMAGING STUDIES

CT or MRI in patients with suspected necrotizing fasciitis (deep-seated infection of the subcutaneous tissue that results in the progressive destruction of fascia and fat).

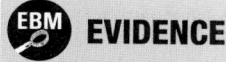 **TREATMENT**

NONPHARMACOLOGIC THERAPY

Immobilization and elevation of the involved limb. Cool sterile saline dressings to remove purulence from any open lesion. Support stockings in patients with peripheral edema.

ACUTE GENERAL Rx

Erysipelas:
- PO: dicloxacillin 500 mg PO q6h
- IV: cefazolin 1 g q6 to 8h or nafcillin 1.0 or 1.5 g IV q4 to 6h

NOTE: Use erythromycin, clindamycin, or vancomycin in patients allergic to penicillin.
Staphylococcal cellulitis:
- PO: dicloxacillin 250 to 500 mg qid
- IV: nafcillin 1 to 2 g q4 to 6h
- Cephalosporins (cephalothin, cephalexin, cephradine) also provide adequate antistaphylococcal coverage, except for MRSA.
- Trimethoprim-sulfamethoxazole (Bactrim DS 1 PO bid) may be appropriate in mild MRSA infections. Use vancomycin 1.0 to 2.0 g IV qd or linezolid 0.6 g IV q12h in patients allergic to penicillin or cephalosporins and in patients with moderate/severe MRSA. Daptomycin (Cubicin), a cyclic lipopeptide, can be used as an alternative to vancomycin for complicated skin and skin structure infections. Usual dose is 4 mg/kg IV given over 30 min every 24 hr. Telavancin is a new glycopeptide derivative of vancomycin effective for gram-positive skin and skin structure infections, including those caused by MRSA. Ceftaroline fosamil (Teflaro) is a new IV cephalosporin also effective against MRSA.

H. influenzae cellulitis:
- PO: cefixime or cefuroxime
- IV: cefuroxime or ceftriaxone

Vibrio vulnificus:
- Doxycycline 100 mg IV bid plus ceftazidime 2 g IV q8h or IV ciprofloxacin 400 mg bid. Mild cases can be treated with oral antibiotics (doxycycline 100 mg bid plus ciprofloxacin 750 mg bid).
- IV support and admission into intensive care unit (mortality rate >50% in septic shock).

E. rhusiopathiae:
- Penicillin

A. hydrophila:
- Aminoglycosides
- Chloramphenicol
- Complicated skin and skin structure infections in hospitalized patients can be treated with daptomycin (Cubicin) 4 mg/kg IV q24h

EBM **EVIDENCE**

available at www.expertconsult.com

SUGGESTED READINGS

available at www.expertconsult.com

AUTHOR: **FRED F. FERRI, M.D.**

C

Diseases and Disorders

I

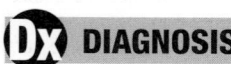
BASIC INFORMATION

DEFINITION
Cerebral palsy (CP) is a group of disorders of the central nervous system characterized by aberrant control of movement or posture, present since early in life and not the result of a progressive or degenerative disease.

SYNONYMS
Little's disease
Congenital static encephalopathy
Congenital spastic paralysis
CP

ICD-9CM CODES
343 Infantile cerebral palsy

EPIDEMIOLOGY & DEMOGRAPHICS
INCIDENCE (IN U.S.): 2 to 2.5 persons per 1000 live births
PREDOMINANT SEX: Males and females affected equally
PREDOMINANT AGE: Diagnosis typically made at 3 to 5 yr

PHYSICAL FINDINGS & CLINICAL PRESENTATION
- Monoplegia, diplegia, quadriplegia, hemiplegia
- Often hypotonic in newborn period, followed by development of hypertonia
- Spasticity
- Athetosis
- Delay in motor milestones
- Hyperreflexia
- Seizures
- Mental retardation

ETIOLOGY
Multifactorial, including low birth weight, congenital malformation, asphyxia, multiple gestation, intrauterine exposure to infection, neonatal stroke, hyperbilirubinemia and maternal thyroid malfunction

DIAGNOSIS

A motor deficit is always present. The usual presenting complaint is that child is not reaching motor milestones at the appropriate age.

Medical history establishes that the child is not losing function. This history, combined with a neurologic examination establishing that motor deficit is due to a cerebral abnormality, establishes the diagnosis of CP. Serial examinations may be necessary if the history is unreliable.

DIFFERENTIAL DIAGNOSIS
Other causes of neonatal hypotonia include muscular dystrophies, spinal muscular atrophy, Down syndrome, and spinal cord injuries.

WORKUP
- Laboratory tests are not necessary to establish the diagnosis.
- Workup is helpful for assessment of recurrence risk, implementation of prevention programs, and medicolegal purposes.

LABORATORY TESTS
- Metabolic and genetic testing should be considered if on follow-up the child has (1) evidence of deterioration or episodes of metabolic decompensation, (2) no etiology determined by neuroimaging, (3) family history of childhood neurologic disorder associated with CP, or (4) developmental malformation on neuroimaging.
- If previous stroke seen on neuroimaging, consider evaluation for coagulopathy.
- An EEG should be obtained when a child with CP has a history suggestive of seizures.
- Children with CP should be screened for ophthalmologic and hearing impairments, as well as speech and language disorders. Nutrition, growth, and swallowing function should be monitored.

IMAGING STUDIES
- Neuroimaging is recommended if the etiology has not been established previously, for example by perinatal imaging.
- MRI, when available, is preferred to CT scanning because of higher yield in suggesting an etiology and timing of the insult leading to CP.

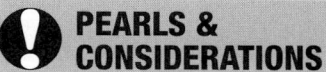
TREATMENT

NONPHARMACOLOGIC THERAPY
- Physical therapy, occupational therapy, and speech therapy.
- Orthotics and casting are used to increase musculotendinous length.

ACUTE GENERAL Rx
If present, treatment of seizures

CHRONIC Rx
- Treatment of seizures, as directed by seizure type.
- Medical treatment of spasticity includes baclofen (oral and intrathecal), as well as botulinum toxin A.
- Surgical treatments of spasticity include dorsal rhizotomy, tendon lengthening, and osteotomy.

DISPOSITION
Most children with cerebral palsy live at home. Those children with severely impaired mobility or other disabilities often live in chronic-care nursing facilities.

REFERRAL
If the child has difficulty with spasticity, physical medicine and rehabilitation referrals are especially helpful.

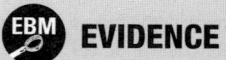
PEARLS & CONSIDERATIONS

- In full-term infants, there is usually no history of traumatic delivery.
- Compared with delivery at 40 wks' gestation, delivery at 37 or 38 wks or at 42 wks or later was associated with an increased risk of CP.
- There is strong data for the utilization of magnesium sulfate to lower the risk of cerebral palsy among the survivors of early preterm birth. In the U.S., the use of magnesium sulfate for fetal neuroprotection has the potential to prevent 1000 cases of handicapping cerebral palsy annually.

EVIDENCE
available at www.expertconsult.com

SUGGESTED READINGS
available at www.expertconsult.com

AUTHOR: **MAITREYI MAZUMDAR, M.D., M.P.H., M.SC.**

BASIC INFORMATION

DEFINITION

Cerebral vasculitis refers to a group of heterogenous disorders characterized by pathologic inflammation and leukocytoclastic changes in the blood vessel walls.

SYNONYMS

Central nervous system angiitis/cerebral arteritis

EPIDEMIOLOGY & DEMOGRAPHICS

INCIDENCE: Average annual incidence rate is 2.4 cases per 1,000,000 person-yr.
PEAK INCIDENCE: Fourth decade of life
PREDOMINANT SEX: Males are affected twice as often as females.
PREDOMINANT AGE: Usual age of presentation is in the third and fourth decades of life, but can present in age ranging from 17 to 70 yr.
GENETICS: Multifactorial
RISK FACTORS: Infections, connective tissue disorders, systemic vasculitis, and substance abuse are the prominent risk factors for secondary cerebral vasculitis.
CLASSIFICATION:
- Primary cerebral vasculitis/primary angiitis of the central nervous system (CNS): Is due to primary involvement of the blood vessels in brain or spinal cord. It does not involve blood vessels or organs beyond the CNS.
- Secondary CNS vasculitis (Table 1-31): Is secondary involvement of the brain or spinal cord blood vessels by a systemic disorder such as systemic vasculitis, connective tissue disorders, infections, malignancy, or substance abuse.

PHYSICAL FINDINGS & CLINICAL PRESENTATION

- The range of manifestations of cerebral vasculitis is diverse. It can present with nonspecific symptoms like weight loss, lethargy, vomiting, headache, and confusion in the early course of the disease. As the disease progresses, multifocal neurologic deficits appear in 80% of the patients.
- Clinical presentations of primary vasculitis can mimic atypical multiple sclerosis, predominantly relapsing and remitting course. Stroke can occur in 40% of the patients; transient ischemic attacks have been reported in 30% to 50% of patients. Aphasia and visual field deficits are commonly seen as well. Seizures have been reported in 25% of the patients. Other common presentations include intracerebral hemorrhage (11%) and intracranial space-occupying lesions (15%).
- Most of the cases of secondary vasculitis present with stroke-like symptoms. Sjögren's syndrome and Behçet's disease can present with variety of symptoms including multiple sclerosis–like presentation, seizures, movement disorders, encephalopathy, dementia, and aseptic meningitis.

ETIOLOGY

The exact etiology of primary cerebral vasculitis is unknown. It has been associated with various infectious agents such as herpes zoster, mycoplasma, HIV, and unknown viruses. Amyloid angiopathy has been described with primary cerebral vasculitis.

DIAGNOSIS

DIFFERENTIAL DIAGNOSIS

- Reversible cerebral vasoconstriction syndromes
- Intracranial vessels atherosclerosis
- Cerebral emboli
- Intravascular lymphoma
- Sarcoidosis

TABLE 1-31 Common Causes of Secondary Cerebral Vasculitis and Associated Features

Giant cell arteritis/Takayasu's arteritis	"Pulseless disease," fever, weight loss, syncope, visual field defects
Polyarteritis nodosa	Fever, weight loss, arthralgia, renal failure, myocardial infarction
Churg-Strauss syndrome	Asthma-like features followed by multiple-organ system involvement including GI, skin, kidneys, CNS, heart
Wegener's granulomatosis	Rhinitis, epistaxis, hemoptysis, hematuria, chronic renal failure
Behçet's disease	Oral ulcers, genital ulcers, skin lesions, uveitis, iritis
Systemic lupus erythematosus	Malar rash, oral ulcers, photosensitivity, arthralgia, renal failure, anemia, ANA positive
Rheumatoid arthritis	Arthritis involving hand joints, radiological evidence of joint erosion, rheumatoid factor positive
Sjögren's syndrome	Dry mouth, dry eyes, involvement of lung, liver, pancreas, joints
Lymphoma	Fever, weight loss, night sweats, lymph node enlargement, hepatosplenomegaly

- Cerebral autosomal dominant arteriopathy with subcortical infarcts and leukoencephalopathy (CADASIL)

WORKUP

Brain biopsy (nondominant temporal lobe tip along with overlying leptomeninges) is the gold standard for the diagnosis of cerebral vasculitis. Cerebral angiography also supports the diagnosis of CNS vasculitis but has low sensitivity and specificity (Fig. 1-81).

LABORATORY TESTS

Cerebrospinal fluid analysis should be part of the workup for diagnosis of cerebral vasculitis (common findings include increased opening pressure, raised proteins, lymphocytic pleocytosis, negative cultures).

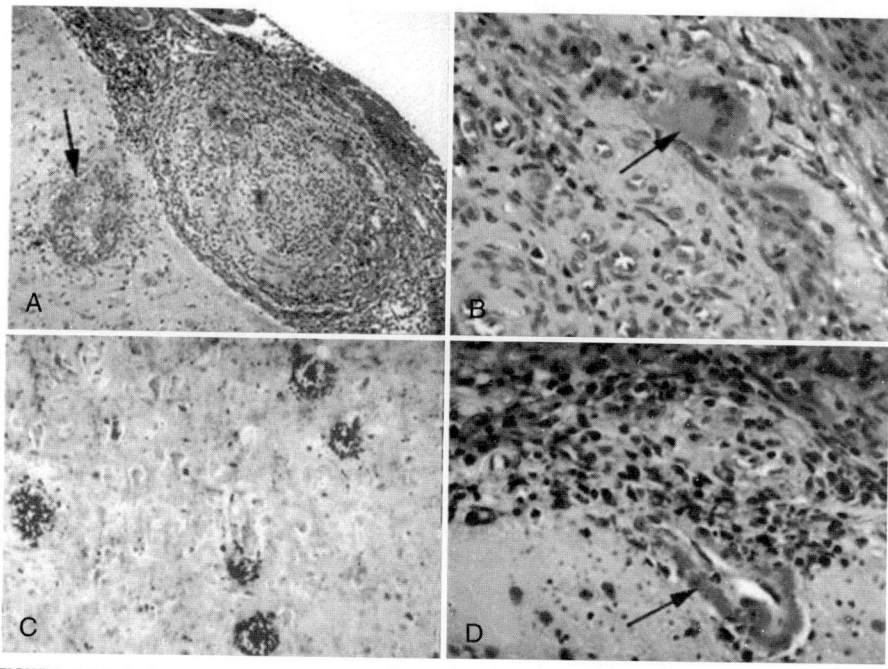

FIGURE 1-81 A, Low-power hematoxylin and eosin stain ($10\times$) demonstrates diffuse inflammation in the leptomeninges with infiltration of lymphocytes, eosinophils, and macrophages with destruction of the vessel wall. **B,** A multinucleated giant cell *(arrow)*. **C,** Multiple neuritic plaques are seen on this silver stain. **D,** Congo red stain demonstrating the presence of amyloid within a vessel wall *(arrow)*. (From Jacobs DA et al: Primary central nervous system angiitis, amyloid angiopathy and Alzheimer's pathology presenting with Balint's syndrome, *Surv Ophthalmol* 49(4):454-459, 2004, Elsevier Inc.)

Basic laboratory testing should include CBC with differential, blood urea nitrogen and serum creatinine, hepatic functions and enzymes, erythrocyte sedimentation rate, C-reactive protein, and urine analysis.

Specific tests for systemic causes include ANA, rheumatoid factor, anti–double-stranded DNA, anti SS-A, anti SS-B, anti–neutrophil cytoplasmic antibody (ANCA), complement 3 and 4, cryoglobulins, serum immunoglobulins, HIV testing, and blood cultures.

IMAGING STUDIES

Magnetic resonance imaging (MRI) is the neuroimaging of choice. Abnormal findings are seen in 90% to 100% of the patients. Cerebral cortex, deep white and gray matter changes are commonly reported (Fig. 1-82).

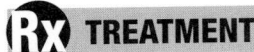

No prospective studies suggesting specific guidelines for treatment of cerebral vasculitis are available. Most of the treatment is similar to the therapies used for other systemic vasculitis.

NONPHARMACOLOGIC THERAPY

Patients with permanent deficits are provided with physical and occupational therapy.

ACUTE GENERAL Rx

If cerebral vasculitis is suspected, after ruling out infections, empiric therapy with glucocorticoids is started while the workup is completed. Intravenous pulse glucocorticoid, methylprednisolone 1 g daily is given for 3 days, if patient has immediate life-threatening condition; otherwise, oral prednisone is started at 1 mg/kg/day.

CHRONIC Rx

Oral prednisone is continued at high dose (1 mg/kg/day) for 4 to 6 wk and then tapered over 12 mo. As a part of remission induction strategy, cyclophosphamide is given orally daily for 3 to 6 mo, then switched to milder and relatively safer immunosuppressants like azathioprine, methotrexate, or mycophenolate for 2 to 3 yr.

DISPOSITION

Course and prognosis of the disease is variable. It depends on the extent of neurologic involvement, severity of deficits, and response to treatment. Neurologic deficits may resolve acutely, slowly, or not at all. Some patients have symptomatic improvement with resolution of headache or altered mental status. Some have improvement in laboratory values, and others have improved MRI scans.

REFERRAL

Refer to neurology if diagnosis is uncertain or patients have neurologic deficits of uncertain etiology, at younger age, or with headaches not responding to medical therapy.

Refer to neurosurgery for brain biopsy.

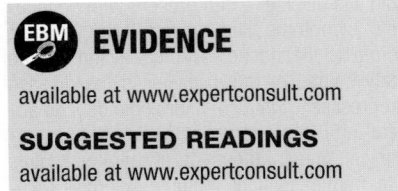

COMMENTS

Cerebral vasculitis is a rare disorder that is difficult to identify because of variable presentation. Early recognition of the clinical symptoms and signs is important to prevent long-term morbidity and mortality. Response to the treatment should be assessed periodically by repeated evaluation of the clinical symptoms, examination, and neuroimaging.

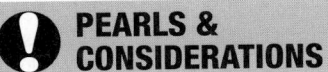

available at www.expertconsult.com

SUGGESTED READINGS
available at www.expertconsult.com

AUTHOR: **FARIHA ZAHEER, M.D.**

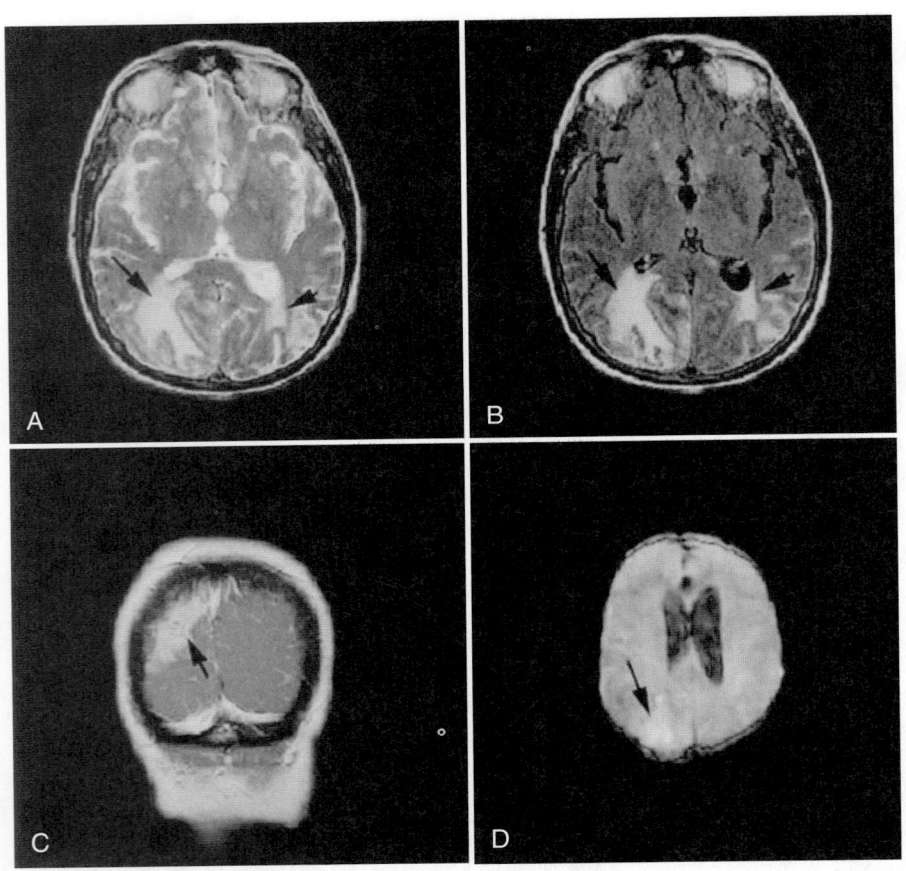

FIGURE 1-82 A, Axial T2-weighted image shows abnormal signal in bilateral parietooccipital lobes, greater on the right than left *(arrows).* **B,** Axial fluid attenuated inversion recovery image further delineating the extent of bilateral parietooccipital lesions *(arrow).* **C,** Coronal T1-gadolinium study demonstrating nodular leptomeningeal enhancement in the lesion *(arrow).* **D,** Diffusion-weighted magnetic resonance imaging shows bright signal in the right parietooccipital region, suggesting ischemic changes *(arrow).* (From Jacobs DA et al: primary central nervous system angiitis, amyloid angiopathy and Alzheimer's pathology presenting with Balint's syndrome, *Surv Ophthalmol* 49(4):454-459, 2004, Elsevier Inc.)

BASIC INFORMATION

DEFINITION

Cervical cancer is penetration of the basement membrane and infiltration of the stroma of the uterine cervix by malignant cells.

ICD-9CM CODES
180 Malignant neoplasm of cervix uteri

EPIDEMIOLOGY & DEMOGRAPHICS

INCIDENCE: There are approximately 15,000 new cases annually, with 4000 to 5000 associated deaths. The U.S. has an age-adjusted mortality rate of 2.6 per 100,000 persons for cervical cancer.
PREDOMINANCE: Higher incidence rates occur in developing countries. Among the U.S. population, Hispanics have a higher incidence than African Americans, who likewise have a higher incidence than whites.
RISK FACTORS: Smoking, early age at first intercourse, multiple sexual partners, immunocompromised state, nonbarrier methods of birth control, infection with high-risk human papillomavirus (HPV; types 16 and 18), and multiparity.

PHYSICAL FINDINGS & CLINICAL PRESENTATION

- Unusual vaginal bleeding, particularly postcoital
- Vaginal discharge and/or odor
- Advanced cases may present with lower extremity edema or renal failure
- In early stages there may be little or no obvious cervical lesion; more advanced cases may present with large, bulky, friable lesions encompassing the majority of the vagina

ETIOLOGY

- Dysplastic cells progress to invasive carcinoma.
- Believed to be linked to the presence of HPV 16, 18, 45, and 56 by interaction of E6 oncoprotein on p53 gene product.
- There may be an association with past infection with *Chlamydia trachomatis*.

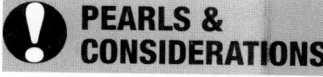 **DIAGNOSIS**

DIFFERENTIAL DIAGNOSIS

- Cervical polyp or prolapsed uterine fibroid
- Preinvasive cervical lesions
- Neoplasia metastatic from a separate primary neoplasia

WORKUP

- Thorough history and physical examination.
- Pelvic examination with careful rectovaginal examination.
- Compared with Pap testing, HPV testing has a greater sensitivity for the detection of cervical intraepithelial neoplasia. The addition of an HPV test to the Pap test to screen women in their mid-30s for cervical cancer reduces the incidence of grade 2 or 3 cervical intraepithelial neoplasia or cancer detected by subsequent screening examinations.
- Colposcopy with directed biopsy and endocervical curettage.
- FIGO staging of cervical cancer is described in Table 1-32.

LABORATORY TESTS

- Complete blood count, chemistry profile
- Squamous cell carcinoma antigen in research setting
- Carcinoembryonic antigen

IMAGING STUDIES

- Chest x-ray
- Depending on stage, may need cystoscopy, sigmoidoscopy or barium enema, CT scan or MRI, lymphangiography
- Intravenous pyelogram

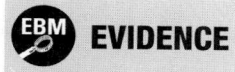 **TREATMENT**

NONPHARMACOLOGIC THERAPY

- FIGO stage IA: cone biopsy or simple hysterectomy
- FIGO stage IB or IIA: type III radical hysterectomy and pelvic lymphadenectomy or pelvic radiation therapy

- Advanced or bulky disease: multimodality therapy (radiation, chemotherapy, and/or surgery); platinum use before radiation therapy

ACUTE GENERAL Rx

In advanced cases cervical cancer may present with massive and acute vaginal bleeding requiring volume and blood replacement, vaginal packing or other hemostatic modalities, and/or high-dose local radiotherapy.

CHRONIC Rx

- Physical examination with Pap smear every 3 mo for 2 yr, every 6 mo during the third to fifth year, and annually thereafter
- Chest x-ray examination annually

DISPOSITION

Five-year survival varies by stage:
- Stage I: 60% to 90%
- Stage II: 40% to 80%
- Stage III: <60%
- Stage IV: <15%
  Early detection by Pap smear is imperative to long-term improvements in survival.

REFERRAL

Gynecologic oncologist for all invasive disease

PEARLS & CONSIDERATIONS

Gardasil is a vaccine indicated in girls and women aged 9 to 26 yr for the prevention of cervical cancer caused by HPV types 6, 11, 16, and 18. In October 2009, the Food and Drug Administration approved the use of Gardasil for boys and men aged 9 to 26 yr as well.

EBM EVIDENCE

available at www.expertconsult.com

SUGGESTED READINGS

available at www.expertconsult.com

AUTHORS: **GIL M. FARKASH, M.D.,** and **RUBEN ALVERO, M.D.**

TABLE 1-32 FIGO Staging of Cervical Cancer

Stage	Invasion	Prognosis 5-yr Survival	Treatment
1$_{A1}$	Depth of invasion up to 3 mm and width up to 7 mm (includes early stromal invasion of up to 1 mm)	84-90% if tumor < 3 cm; 85% will have negative pelvic nodes and 95% of these patients will be 'cured'	Local excision; if margins of a cone clear (i.e., no residual tumor or CIN) then conization is adequate, with no need for pelvic lymphadenectomy
1$_{A2}$	Depth of invasion between 3 and 5 mm (i.e., 3.1-5 mm) and width up to 7mm		Simple hysterectomy and pelvic lymphadenectomy
1$_{B1}$	Tumor confined to cervix and diameter less than 4 cm	66% if tumor > 3 cm	Radical hysterectomy or radiotherapy
1$_{B2}$	Tumor confined to cervix and diameter more than 4 cm		Radical hysterectomy or radiotherapy
II$_A$	Upper 1/3 vagina	62%	Radical hysterectomy or radiotherapy
II$_B$	Upper 2/3 of vagina plus parametrial disease		Radiotherapy ± chemotherapy
III$_A$	Lower 1/3 vagina	40%	Radiotherapy ± chemotherapy
III$_B$	Pelvic sidewall and/or hydronephrosis		Radiotherapy ± chemotherapy
IV$_A$	Bladder, rectum	15%	Radiotherapy ± chemotherapy
IV$_B$	Beyond pelvis		Radiotherapy ± chemotherapy

From Drife J, Magowan B: *Clinical obstetrics and gynecology*, Philadelphia, 2004, Saunders.

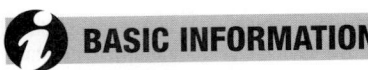

DEFINITION

Cervical disk syndromes refer to diseases of the cervical spine resulting from disk disorder, either herniation or degenerative change (spondylosis). When posterior osteophytes compress the anterior spinal cord, lower extremity symptoms may result, a condition called *cervical spondylotic myelopathy*.

ICD-9CM CODES

722.4 Degenerative intervertebral cervical disk
722.71 Degenerative cervical disk with myelopathy

EPIDEMIOLOGY & DEMOGRAPHICS

PREVALENCE: 10% of general adult population (symptoms in 50% of population at some time in their life)
PREDOMINANT SEX: Males and females affected equally
PREDOMINANT AGE: 30 to 60 yr

PHYSICAL FINDINGS & CLINICAL PRESENTATION

- Neck pain, radicular symptoms, or myelopathy, either alone or in combination
- Limited neck movement
- Pain with neck motion, especially extension
- Referred unilateral interscapular pain, resulting in a local trigger point
- Radicular arm pain (usually unilateral), numbness, and tingling possible, most commonly involving the C6 (C5-C6 disk) or C7 (C6-C7 disk) nerve root
- Weakness and reflex changes (C6, biceps; C7, triceps)
- Myelopathy, possibly resulting in gait disturbance, weakness, and even spasticity
- Sensory examination usually not helpful

ETIOLOGY

Unknown

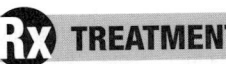

DIFFERENTIAL DIAGNOSIS

- Rotator cuff tendinitis
- Carpal tunnel syndrome
- Thoracic outlet syndrome
- Brachial neuritis

A differential diagnosis for evaluation of neck pain is described in Section II.

WORKUP

In most cases, the diagnosis can be established on a clinical basis alone.

Cervical Disk Syndrome in Section III describes an algorithm for a workup of suspected cases.

IMAGING STUDIES

- Plain roentgenograms within the first few weeks
  1. Usually normal in soft disk herniation
  2. With chronic degenerative disk disease, usually loss of height of the disk space, anterior and posterior osteophyte formation, and encroachment on the intervertebral foramen by osteophytes
- Myelography, CT scanning, and MRI indicated in patients whose symptoms do not resolve or when other spinal pathology suspected
- Electrodiagnostic studies to confirm the diagnosis or rule out peripheral nerve disorders

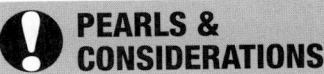

NONPHARMACOLOGIC THERAPY

- Rest and cervical collar if needed
- Local modalities such as heat
- Physical therapy (Fig. 1-83)
- Avoid extreme range-of-motion exercises in degenerative disk disease

ACUTE GENERAL Rx

- Nonsteroidal anti-inflammatory drugs
- "Muscle relaxants" for their sedative effect
- Analgesics as needed
- Epidural steroid injection for radicular pain

DISPOSITION

- Usually improves with time
- Surgical intervention in <5%

REFERRAL

Orthopedic or neurosurgical consultation for intractable pain or neurologic deficit

PEARLS & CONSIDERATIONS

Myelopathy from cervical spondylosis is the most common cause of acquired spastic paralysis in the adult and is usually progressive. Whether to intervene surgically is a complicated decision in these patients.

COMMENTS

- Pain relief with physical therapy seems anecdotal and short lived; any overall improvement usually parallels what would have probably occurred naturally.
- Sometimes carpal tunnel syndrome and cervical radiculopathy occur together; this is called *double-crush syndrome* and results from nerve compression at two separate levels. Proximal compression may decrease the ability of the nerve to tolerate a second, more distal compression.
- Surgical intervention is indicated primarily for relief of radicular pain caused by nerve root compression or for the treatment of myelopathy; it is generally not helpful when the chief complaint is neck pain alone.
- In many cases of cervical spondylosis with myelopathy, the lower extremity symptoms are much more disabling than the neck symptoms, a situation that can cause some difficulty in determining their etiology.

SUGGESTED READINGS

available at www.expertconsult.com

AUTHOR: **LONNIE R. MERCIER, M.D.**

FIGURE 1-83 Isometric neck exercises. A, The hand is placed against the side of the head slightly above the ear, and pressure is gradually increased while resisting with the neck muscles and keeping the head in the same position. The position is held 5 sec, relaxed, and repeated five times. **B,** The exercise is performed on the other side and then from the back and front **(C).** The exercise should be performed three to four times daily. (From Mercier LR [ed]: *Practical orthopedics,* ed 4, St Louis, 1995, Mosby.)

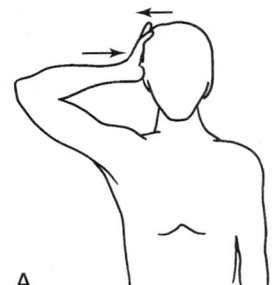
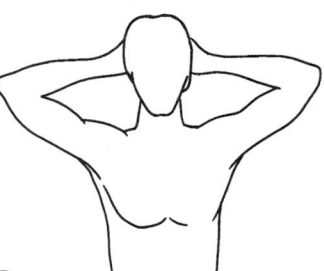
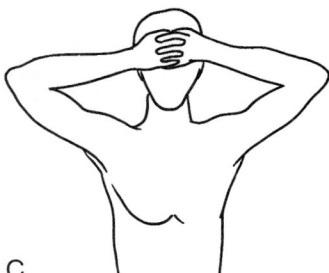

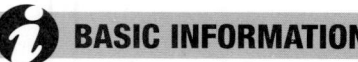 **BASIC INFORMATION**

DEFINITION

Cervical dysplasia refers to atypical development of immature squamous epithelium that does not penetrate the basement epithelial membrane. Characteristics include increased cellularity, nuclear abnormalities, and increased nuclear:cytoplasm ratio. A progressive polarized loss of squamous differentiation exists beginning adjacent to the basement membrane and progressing to the most advanced stage (severe dysplasia), which encompasses the complete squamous epithelial layer thickness. The revised 2001 Bethesda System terminology was used in a National Institutes of Health consensus conference, sponsored by the American Society for Colposcopy and Cervical Pathology (ASCCP) and its partner professional organizations in 2006. The conference updated therapeutic options for women based on studies such as the **A**SC-US (atypical squamous cells of undetermined significance)/**L**SIL (low-grade squamous intraepithelial lesions) **T**riage **S**tudy (ALTS) that appeared after revision of the Bethesda classification.v

BETHESDA 2001 UPDATED CLASSIFICATION:

The Bethesda 2001 System was the result of a year-long iterative process held to update the original 1991 system and to broaden participation in the consensus process, clarify reporting of abnormalities and incorporating data that had been collected since the initial system was created.

The reporting system includes the following areas:

Specimen adequacy: The system defines the specimen as either satisfactory for evaluation or unsatisfactory and then specifies the reason for inadequacy if necessary.

General categorization (optional): This serves to triage the specimen into normal finding (negative for intraepithelial lesion or malignancy) or identifies it as an "epithelial abnormality." The descriptions are meant to be mutually exclusive.

Interpretation/result: Makes a distinction between "interpretation" and "diagnosis" of the specimen so that the interpretation may be incorporated into the overall clinical context for the particular patient being evaluated.

Negative for intraepithelial lesion or malignancy: In this screening test, no intraepithelial lesion or malignancy is identified. Non-neoplastic findings such as organisms or reactive cellular findings may be specified but are still considered to be a negative result.

Epithelial cell abnormalities:
Squamous cell:
Atypical squamous cell (ASC) of undetermined significance (ASC-US) emphasizing the unusual but still possible association with underlying cervical intraepithelial neoplasia (CIN) II/III and extremely rare possibility of squamous cell carcinoma
ASC cannot exclude high-grade squamous intraepithelial lesion (HSIL)

(ASC-H), suggesting a risk for CIN II/III that is intermediate between ASC-US and HSIL
Low-grade squamous intraepithelial lesion (LSIL) suggests a transient viral infection with a greater likelihood for regression, more likely to encompass human papillomavirus (HPV) infection and CIN I histologically
HSIL suggestive of a more persistent viral infection and with a greater risk for progressive disease, more likely to encompass CIN II/III and carcinoma in situ (CIS) histologically
Squamous cell carcinoma
Glandular cell
Atypical glandular cells (should specify endocervical, endometrial, or not otherwise specified)
Atypical glandular cell, favor neoplasia (should specify endocervical or not otherwise specified)
Endocervical adenocarcinoma in situ (AIS)
Adenocarcinoma
Other: Endometrial cells in a woman ≥40 yr of age. Because menopausal status is sometimes uncertain, age was chosen to discriminate women who might, with the findings of endometrial cells on cytology, warrant further evaluation with endometrial sampling

KEY POINTS:

1. The cytologic distinction of low grade (LSIL) and high grade (HSIL) do not necessarily equate to the histologic classifications CIN I and CIN II/III.
2. The 2006 conference notes that one cytologic abnormality can have different histologic risk in different women and highlights "special populations" such as adolescent and young women, and those women who are pregnant. In young women, spontaneous HPV clearance rates are exceptionally high; therefore, it is worthwhile to defer aggressive evaluative and therapeutic steps to assess whether spontaneous remission has taken place. In pregnant women, colposcopy may be deferred if the patient is at low risk for invasive cancer, and therapy should take place only if there is a strong suspicion for carcinoma.
3. DNA testing for high-risk HPV types is incorporated into the evaluation and treatment algorithms for women with cytologic cervical abnormalities.

Histologically, a two-tiered system is developed in this guideline that distinguishes between the lower risk CIN I and higher risk CIN II/III diagnoses.

ICD-9CM CODES
622.1 Dysplasia of cervix (uteri)

EPIDEMIOLOGY & DEMOGRAPHICS

PREDOMINANT AGE:

• Dysplasia: peak age, 26 yr (3600 cases/ 100,000 persons)

• CIS: peak age, 32 yr (1100 cases/100,000 persons)
• Invasive cancer: peak age >60 yr (800 cases/100,000 persons)

PEAK INCIDENCE:

• Age 35 yr
• Abnormal Pap smear rate revealing dysplasia approximates 2% to 5% depending on population risk factors and false-negative rate variance
• False-negative rate approaching 40%
• Average age-adjusted incidence of severe dysplasia is 35 cases/100,000 persons

PHYSICAL FINDINGS & CLINICAL PRESENTATION

• Cervical lesions associated with dysplasia often are not visible to the naked eye; therefore, physical findings are best viewed by colposcopy of a 3% acetic acid–prepared cervix.
• Patients evaluated by colposcopy are identified by abnormal cervical cytology screening from Pap smear screening.
• Colposcopic findings:
  1. Leukoplakia (white lesion seen by the unaided eye that may represent condyloma, dysplasia, or cancer)
  2. Acetowhite epithelium with or without associated punctation, mosaicism, abnormal vessels
  3. Abnormal transformation zone (abnormal iodine uptake, "cuffed" gland openings)

ETIOLOGY

• Strongly associated and initiated by oncogenic HPV infection (high-risk HPV types are 16, 18, 31, 33, 35, 45, 51, 52, 56, and 58; low-risk HPV types are 6, 11, 42, 43, and 44)
• Risk factors:
  ○ Any heterosexual coitus
  ○ Coitus during puberty (transformation-zone metaplasia peak)
  ○ Diethyl stilbestrol exposure
  ○ Multiple sexual partners
  ○ Lack of prior Pap smear screening
  ○ History of STD
  ○ Other genital tract neoplasia
  ○ HIV
  ○ Tuberculosis
  ○ Substance abuse
  ○ "High-risk" male partner (HPV)
  ○ Low socioeconomic status
  ○ Early first pregnancy
  ○ Tobacco use
  ○ HPV

Dx **DIAGNOSIS**

DIFFERENTIAL DIAGNOSIS

• Metaplasia
• Hyperkeratosis
• Condyloma
• Microinvasive carcinoma
• Glandular epithelial abnormalities
• AIS
• Vulvar intraepithelial neoplasm

- Vaginal intraepithelial neoplasm
- Metastatic tumor involvement of the cervix

WORKUP

- Periodic history and physical examination (including cytologic screening) depending on age, risk factors, and history of preinvasive cervical lesions
- Consider screening for sexually transmitted disease (gonorrhea, chlamydia, herpes, HIV, HPV)
- Abnormal cytology (HSIL/LSIL, initial ASC/ASC-US/ASC-H in high-risk patients, recurrent in low-risk/postmenopausal patients) and grossly evident suspicious lesions; refer for colposcopy and possible directed biopsy/endocervical curettage (ECC) (examination should include cervix, vagina, vulva, and anus)
- For glandular cell abnormalities (AGCs): refer for colposcopy and possible directed biopsy/ECC, and consider endometrial sampling
- In pregnancy: abnormal cytology followed by colposcopy in the first trimester and at 28 to 32 wk; only high-grade lesions suspect for cancer biopsied; ECC contraindicated

LABORATORY TESTS

- Gonorrhea, Chlamydia to rule out STD
- Pap cytology screening (requires appropriate sampling, preparation, cytologist interpretation, and reporting)
- Colposcopy and directed biopsy, ECC for indications (see "Workup")
- HPV DNA typing if identified abnormal cytology
- As compared with Pap testing, HPV testing has greater sensitivity for the detection of intraepithelial neoplasia

IMAGING STUDIES

- Cervicography
- Computer-enhanced Pap cytology screening (e.g., PAPNET)

MANAGEMENT

Refer to the literature for a more comprehensive approach. The following treatment paradigms give a general outline for care. Where identified below, HPV status refers to oncogenic types (e.g., 16, 18, 31, 33, 35, 45, 51, 52, 56, 58)

- ASC-US: Patients with ASC-US who are HPV negative can repeat cytologic screen in 12 mo. Women who have oncogenic HPV type should have colposcopy performed. Adolescent women should not have HPV testing performed and can be followed with cytologic screen, with colposcopy performed if ASC-US persists after 24 mo or if HSIL is found. Pregnant women can be followed as with nonpregnant women; but if colposcopy is recommended, it can be deferred until at least 6 wk after delivery. Pregnant women should not have endocervical curettage performed.
- ASC-H: Patients with ASC-H should have a colposcopic evaluation.
- LSIL: Colposcopy with endocervical biopsy is recommended for women with LSIL. Adolescent women with LSIL may be followed with

cytology at 12 and 24 mo, and referred for colposcopy if they retain a finding of ASC-US or greater. Postmenopausal women may have DNA testing and be referred for colposcopy if this test is positive for oncogenic HPV type. Pregnant women should have colposcopy, but this procedure may be deferred until the patient is postpartum, particularly if there is no other clinical suspicion for higher grade lesions.

- HSIL: Either colposcopy with endocervical curettage or immediate loop electrosurgical excision procedures (LEEPs) are acceptable with HSIL. If CIN II/III is not found by either method, the patient may followed colposcopically or a LEEP performed if only colposcopy was initially used. If CIN II/III is identified by adequate colposcopy, a LEEP or ablation may be performed. Adolescent girls in whom CIN II/III is not identified may be observed by colposcopy and cytology at 6-mo intervals up to 24 mo. If CIN II/III persists for 24 mo, then the adolescent girl may be treated by excisional or ablative therapy. Pregnant women should have colposcopy and biopsies performed where CIN II/III or cancer is suspected. Colposcopy should be performed 6 wk or later after delivery when CIN II/III is not found antepartum.
- AGC/AIS: Colposcopy with endocervical biopsy should be performed in these women. In women older than 35 and in women with high risk for endometrial hyperplasia or carcinoma (oligo-ovulation, unscheduled bleeding), an endometrial biopsy should also be performed. Pregnant women should also be colposcoped, but endocervical and endometrial curettings should not be performed during the gestation.

DISPOSITION

- Because of the large number of women in high-risk groups, the prevalence of HPV, and the high false-negative Pap smear rate, routine Pap smear screening should be strongly encouraged for all women, especially those with a history of cervical dysplasia. The addition of an HPV test to the Pap test reduces the incidence of CIN II or III, or cancer detected by subsequent screening.
- Success rates for treatment approach 80% to 90%.
- Detection of persistence of recurrence requires careful follow-up.
- Cervical treatment possibly results in infertility (cervical stenosis or incompetence), which requires careful consideration and discretion for use of LEEP and cone biopsy.
- Appropriate counseling and informed consent are needed when considering any form of management of cervical dysplasia.

REFERRAL

- Patients with abnormal Pap cytology should not be monitored by repeat Pap smear screening.
- Patients with identified abnormal cytology should be evaluated by a skilled colposcopist (defined as documented didactic and precep-

torship training, including 50 cases of identified pathology, ongoing colposcopy activity with a minimum of 2 cases/wk, quality-assurance log, and periodic continuing medical education).

- If treatment is required, patient should be referred to a gynecologist or gynecologic oncologist skilled in the diagnosis and treatment of preinvasive cervical disease.

⚠ PEARLS & CONSIDERATIONS

COMMENTS

- Testing for human papillomavirus by Hybrid capture 2 DNA test will identify 91% of the small proportion of women with post-treatment residual or recurrent disease, but 30% of all women who are tested will test positive and need colposcopy.
- Gardasil is a vaccine indicated in girls and women aged 9 to 26 yr for the prevention of CIN caused by HPV types 6, 11, 16, and 18.
- ACOG cervical cytology screening recommendations are as follows:
  1. Cervical cancer screening should begin at age 21 regardless of age at onset of sexual activity
  2. Cervical cytology screening from age 21 to 29 is recommended every 2 years but should be more frequent in women who are HIV-positive, are immunosuppressed, were exposed in utero to diethylstilbestrol, or have been treated for intraepithelial neoplasia (CIN) 2,3 or cervical cancer.
  3. Women age 30 or over who have 3 consecutive negative screens and who do not fit the above criteriafor more frequent screening may be tested every 3 years. Co-testing with cervical cytology and high-risk HPV typing is also appropriate; if both tests are negative, re-screening in 3 years is warranted
  4. Cervical cancer screening is unnecessary in women who have undergone hysterectomies for benign disease and who have no histories of CIN
  5. Discontinuation of screening after age 65 or 70 is reasonable in women with 3 or more negative consecutive tests and no cervical abnormalities during the previous decade.
  6. Women with histories of CIN 2, 3, or cancer should undergo annual screening for 20 years after treatment
  7. HPV vaccination does not change these recommendations

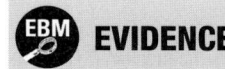 **EVIDENCE**

available at www.expertconsult.com

SUGGESTED READINGS

available at www.expertconsult.com

AUTHORS: **DENNIS M. WEPPNER, M.D.,** and **RUBEN ALVERO, M.D.**

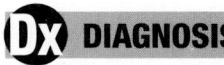

BASIC INFORMATION

DEFINITION

A cervical polyp is a growth protruding from the cervix or endocervical canal. Polyps that arise from the endocervical canal are called *endocervical polyps*. If they arise from the ectocervix, they are called *cervical polyps*.

ICD-9CM CODES
622.7 Mucous polyp of cervix

EPIDEMIOLOGY & DEMOGRAPHICS

Cervical polyps are found in approximately 4% of all gynecologic patients. They most commonly present in perimenopausal and multigravida women between the ages of 30 and 50 yr. Endocervical polyps are more common than cervical polyps and are almost always benign (Fig. 1-84). Malignant degeneration is extremely rare.

PHYSICAL FINDINGS & CLINICAL PRESENTATION

Polyps may be single or multiple and vary in size from being extremely small (a few mm) to large (4 cm). They are soft, smooth, and reddish-purple to cherry-red in color. They bleed easily when touched. Very large polyps can cause some cervical dilation. There may be vaginal discharge associated with cervical polyps if the polyp has become infected.

ETIOLOGY
- Most unknown
- Inflammatory
- Traumatic
- Pregnancy

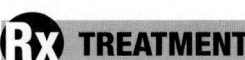

DIAGNOSIS

DIFFERENTIAL DIAGNOSIS
- Endometrial polyp
- Prolapsed myoma
- Retained products of conception
- Squamous papilloma
- Sarcoma
- Cervical malignancy

WORKUP

Polyps are most commonly asymptomatic and are usually found at the time of annual gynecologic pelvic examination. Polyps are also found in women who present for evaluation of intermenstrual or postcoital bleeding and for profuse vaginal discharge. Polyps are generally painless. Unless a patient has a bleeding abnormality that necessitates evaluation by a physician, polyps would go undiagnosed until the next Pap smear was obtained.

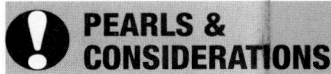

TREATMENT

NONPHARMACOLOGIC THERAPY

Simple surgical excision can be done in the office. The physician should be prepared for bleeding, which can easily be controlled with silver nitrate or Monsel's solution. Most commonly a polyp is excised by grasping it at the stalk with a sponge forceps or similar device and twisting it off. Polyps can also be excised by electrocautery or, in the case of very large polyps, in an outpatient surgical suite. Sexual intercourse and tampon use are to be avoided until the patient's follow-up visit. Douching is not to be performed.

ACUTE GENERAL Rx

Generally no medication is needed.

CHRONIC Rx

Patient is followed up in 2 wk for recheck of the surgical excision site unless there is active bleeding, in which case she would be seen immediately. The cervix should be checked at the patient's routine gynecologic visits.

DISPOSITION

Because these are almost always benign, no further treatment is usually needed. Annual gynecologic examinations should be performed to check for any regrowths.

REFERRAL

To a gynecologist for removal of polyps

PEARLS & CONSIDERATIONS

COMMENTS

A Pap smear should be obtained before removing the polyp. If an abnormal Pap smear is obtained, it is highly probable that the cause will be the polyp. If a colposcopic evaluation is needed, this should also be performed. During pregnancy the cervix is highly vascularized. If the polyps are stable and benign appearing, they should be observed during the pregnancy and removed only if they cause bleeding.

SUGGESTED READINGS
available at www.expertconsult.com

AUTHORS: **GEORGE T. DANAKAS, M.D.,** and **RUBEN ALVERO, M.D.**

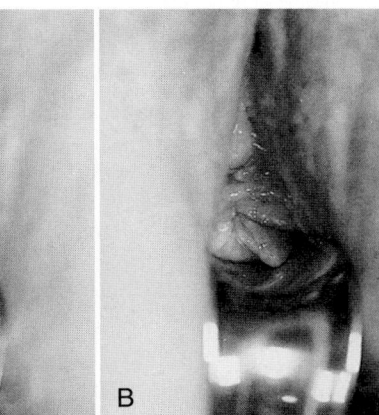

FIGURE 1-84 A, Fibroid polyp protruding through the external cervical os. **B,** Small endocervical polyp. (From Symonds EM, Macpherson MBA: *Color atlas of obstetrics and gynecology,* St Louis, 1994, Mosby.)

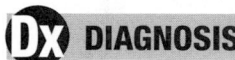 BASIC INFORMATION

DEFINITION

Cervicitis is an infection of the cervix. It may result from direct infection of the cervix, or it may be secondary to uterine or vaginal infection.

SYNONYMS

Endocervicitis
Ectocervicitis
Mucopurulent cervicitis

ICD-9CM CODES	
616.0	Cervicitis
098.15	Acute gonococcal cervicitis
079.8	Chlamydia infection

EPIDEMIOLOGY & DEMOGRAPHICS

Cervicitis accounts for 20% to 25% of patients with abnormal vaginal discharge. It is most common in adolescents, but it can be found in any sexually active woman. Practicing unsafe sex with multiple partners increases the risk of developing cervicitis as well as other sexually transmitted diseases.

PHYSICAL FINDINGS & CLINICAL PRESENTATION

Cervicitis is usually asymptomatic or associated with mild symptoms. Copious purulent or mucopurulent vaginal discharge (Fig. 1-85), pelvic pain, and dyspareunia may be present if cervicitis is severe. The cervix can be erythematous and tender on palpation during bimanual examination. The cervix may also bleed easily when obtaining cultures or a Pap smear. Patients may have postcoital bleeding.

ETIOLOGY

- *Chlamydia trachomatis*
- Trichomonas
- *Neisseria gonorrhoeae*
- Herpes simplex
- *Trichomonas vaginalis*
- Human papillomavirus

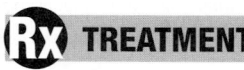 DIAGNOSIS

DIFFERENTIAL DIAGNOSIS

- Carcinoma of the cervix
- Cervical erosion
- Cervical metaplasia

WORKUP

The patient usually presents with a vaginal discharge or history of postcoital bleeding. Otherwise the patient is asymptomatic and diagnosed during routine examination. On examination there is gross visualization of yellow, mucopurulent material on the cotton swab.

LABORATORY TESTS

A finding of leukorrhea (>10 WBC per high-power field on microscopic examination of vaginal fluid) has been associated with chlamydial and gonococcal infection of the cervix. Positive Gram stain is found. Nucleic acid amplification tests (NAAT) should be used for diagnosing *C. trachomitis* and *N. gonorrhoeae* in women with cervicitis; this testing can be performed in either vaginal, cervical, or uterine samples. Use a wet mount to look for trichomonads, but because the sensitivity of microscopy to detect *T. vaginalis* is relatively low (~50%), symptomatic women with cervicitis and negative microscopy for trichomonads should re-ceive further testing with culture. Obtain a Pap smear. HIV testing is recommended in all patients with supposed cervicitis. Although HSV-2 infection has been associated with cervicitis, the utility of specific testing (i.e., culture or serologic testing) for HSV-2 in this setting is unknown.

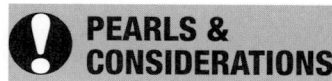 TREATMENT

NONPHARMACOLOGIC THERAPY

- Cervicitis is treated in an outpatient setting. Safe sex should be practiced with the use of condoms.
- Partners should be treated in all cases of infection proven by culture.

ACUTE GENERAL Rx

Because *Chlamydia* and *N. gonorrhoeae* cause >50% of cases of infectious cervicitis, if it is suspected treat without waiting for test results. Administer ceftriaxone 125-mg IM single dose followed by azithromycin 1-g single dose or doxycycline 100 mg PO bid for 7 days. If the patient is pregnant, treat with azithromycin 1-g single dose instead of using doxycycline, which is contraindicated in pregnant or nursing mothers. If *Trichomonas* is the etiologic agent, treat with metronidazole 2-g single dose. For herpes, treat with acyclovir 200 mg PO five times daily for 7 days.

DISPOSITION

Cervicitis responds well to antibiotics. Possible complications to watch for are a subsequent pelvic inflammatory disease (PID) and infertility (found in 5% to 10% of patients). Repeat cultures should be performed after treatment. Sexual relations can be resumed after negative cultures.

REFERRAL

If subsequent PID develops, consider hospital admission for IV antibiotics.

⊘ PEARLS & CONSIDERATIONS

COMMENTS

Management of sex partners of women tested for cervicitis should be appropriate for the identified or suspected STD.

SUGGESTED READINGS

available at www.expertconsult.com

AUTHORS: **GEORGE T. DANAKAS, M.D.,** and **RUBEN ALVERO, M.D.**

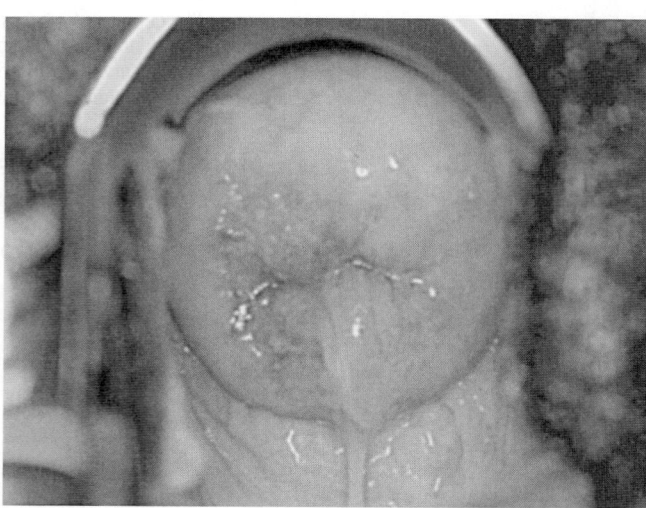

FIGURE 1-85 Colposcopy of a woman with mucopurulent cervicitis and purulent discharge from endocervical os. (Courtesy Dr. David Soper, Richmond, VA. From Mandell GL [ed]: *Mandell, Douglas, and Bennett's principles and practice of infectious diseases,* ed 6, New York, 2005, Churchill Livingstone.)

BASIC INFORMATION

DEFINITION

Chagas' disease is an infection caused by the protozoan parasite *Trypanosoma cruzi*. This is a vector-borne disease transmitted by reduviid bugs from multiple wild and domesticated animal reservoirs. The disease is characterized by an acute nonspecific febrile illness that may be followed, after a variable latency period, by chronic cardiac, GI, and neurologic sequelae.

SYNONYMS

American trypanosomiasis

ICD-9CM CODES
086.2 Chagas' disease

EPIDEMIOLOGY & DEMOGRAPHICS

INCIDENCE (IN U.S.):
- Five cases of autochthonous transmission in California and Texas
- In the last 2 decades, six cases of laboratory-acquired infection, three cases of transfusion-associated transmission, and nine cases of imported disease reported to the Centers for Disease Control and Prevention (none of the imported cases involving returning tourists)
- Infection has been transmitted by organ transplantation

PREVALENCE (IN U.S.): Based on regional seroprevalence studies in Hispanic blood donors, it is estimated that between 50,000 and 100,000 persons infected with *T. cruzi* are currently residing in the U.S.

PREDOMINANT SEX: Male = female
PREDOMINANT AGE:
- In highly endemic areas, mean age of acute infection: approximately 4 yr
- Variable age distribution for both types of chronic disease, depending on geography
- Mean age of onset: usually between 35 and 45 yr

PEAK INCIDENCE: Unknown
GENETICS:
Congenital infection: Congenital transmission has been documented with attendant high fetal mortality and morbidity in surviving infants.
Neonatal infection: In rural areas, within substandard housing, transmission is likely to occur.

PHYSICAL FINDINGS & CLINICAL PRESENTATION

- Inflammatory lesion that develops about 1 wk after contamination of a break in the skin with infected insect feces (chagoma)
  1. Area of induration and erythema
  2. Usually accompanied by local lymphadenopathy
- Presence of Romaña's sign, which consists of unilateral painless palpebral and periocular edema, when conjunctiva is portal of entry
- Constitutional symptoms of fever, fatigue, and anorexia, along with edema of the face and lower extremities, generalized lymphadenopathy, and mild hepatosplenomegaly after the appearance of local signs of disease
- Myocarditis in a small portion of patients, sometimes with resultant CHF
- Uncommonly, CNS disease, such as meningoencephalitis, which carries a poor prognosis
- Symptoms and signs of disease persisting for weeks to months, followed by spontaneous resolution of the acute illness; patient then in the indeterminate phase of the disease (asymptomatic with attendant subpatent parasitemia and reactive antibodies to *T. cruzi* antigens)
- Chronic disease may become manifest years to decades after the initial infection:
  1. Most common organ involved: heart, followed by GI tract, and to a much lesser extent the CNS
     a. Cardiac involvement takes the form of arrhythmias or cardiomyopathy, but rarely both.
     b. Cardiomyopathy is bilateral but predominantly affects the right ventricle and is often accompanied by apical aneurysms and mural thrombi.
     c. Arrhythmias are a consequence of involvement of the bundle of His and have been implicated as the leading cause of sudden death in adults in highly endemic areas.
     d. Right-sided heart failure, thromboembolization, and rhythm disturbances associated with symptoms of dizziness and syncope are characteristic.
  2. Patients with megaesophagus: dysphagia, odynophagia, chronic cough, and regurgitation, frequently resulting in aspiration pneumonitis
  3. Megacolon: abdominal pain and chronic constipation, which, when severe, may lead to obstruction and perforation
  4. CNS symptoms: most often secondary to embolization from the heart or varying degrees of peripheral neuropathy

ETIOLOGY

- *T. cruzi*
  1. Found only in the Americas, ranging from the southern U.S. to southern Argentina
  2. Transmitted to humans by various species of bloodsucking reduviid ("kissing") insects, primarily those of the genera *Triatoma, Panstrongylus,* and *Rhodnius*
  3. Usually found in burrows and trees where infected insects transmit the parasite to natural reservoirs (e.g., opossums and armadillos)
  4. Intrusion into enzootic areas for farmland, allowing insects to take up residence in rural dwellings, thus including humans and domestic animals in the cycle of transmission
  5. Initial infection of insects by ingesting blood from animals or humans that have circulating flagellated trypanosomes (trypomastigotes)
  6. Multiplication in the insect midgut as epimastigotes, then differentiation into metacyclic trypomastigotes discharged with the feces during subsequent blood meals (Fig. 1-87)
  7. Transmission to the second mammalian host through contamination of mucous membranes, conjunctivae, or wounds with insect feces containing infected forms
- In the vertebrate host
  1. Movement of parasites into various cell types, intracellular transformation into amastigotes, and thereafter differentiation into trypomastigotes
  2. Following rupture of the cell membrane, parasitic invasion of local tissues or hematogenous spread to distant sites, maintaining a parasitemia infective for vectors
- In addition to insect vectors, *T. cruzi* is transmitted through blood transfusions, transplacentally, and, occasionally, secondary to laboratory accidents or ingestion

DIAGNOSIS

DIFFERENTIAL DIAGNOSIS

Acute disease
- Early African trypanosomiasis
- New World cutaneous and mucocutaneous leishmaniasis

Chronic disease
- Idiopathic cardiomyopathy
- Idiopathic achalasia
- Congenital or acquired megacolon

WORKUP

Principal considerations in diagnosis:
- A history of residence where transmission is known to occur
- Recent receipt of a blood product while in an endemic area
- Occupational exposure in a laboratory

LABORATORY TESTS

For acute diagnosis:
- Demonstration of *T. cruzi* in wet preparations of blood (Fig. 1-86), buffy coat, or Giemsa-stained smears

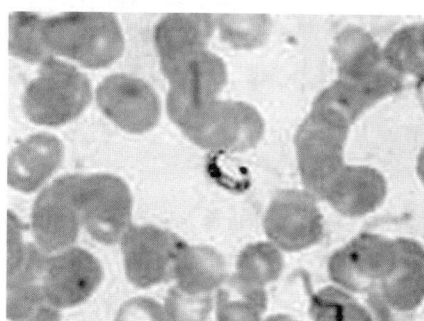

FIGURE 1-86 *T. cruzi* in human blood film. The causative agent occurs in blood films characteristically as short C-shaped or S-shaped trypomastigotes with a prominent kinetoplast. It is otherwise monomorphic *(Giemsa × 950).* (From Hoffmann R et al: *Hematology: basic principles and practice,* ed 5, Philadelphia, 2009, Churchill Livingstone.)

- Xenodiagnosis, a technique involving laboratory-reared insect vectors fed on subjects with suspected infection thereafter examined for parasites, and culture of body fluids in liquid media to establish diagnosis
  1. Hampered by the length of time required for completion
  2. Of limited use in clinical decision making with regard to drug therapy
  3. Although xenodiagnosis and broth culture are considered to be more sensitive than microscopic examination of body fluids, sensitivities may not exceed 50%
- Recent advances in serologic testing include immunoblot assay, in situ indirect fluorescent antibody, PCR-based techniques, and an immunochromatographic assay (Chagas Stat Pak)

For chronic *T. cruzi* infection:

- Traditional serologic tests including: complement fixation (CF), indirect immunofluorescence (IIF), indirect hemagglutination, and enzyme-linked immunosorbent assay (ELISA)
- Serologic tests have variable sensitivity and specificity and frequent false-positive results
- Saliva ELISA may be useful as a screening diagnostic test in epidemiologic studies of chronic trypanosomiasis infection in endemic areas

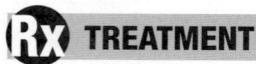 **TREATMENT**

NONPHARMACOLOGIC THERAPY

- Chronic chagasic heart disease: mainly supportive

- Megaesophagus: symptoms usually amenable to dietary measures or pneumonic dilation of the esophagogastric junction
- Chagasic megacolon: in its early stages responsive to a high-fiber diet, laxatives, and enemas

ACUTE GENERAL Rx

It is now recommended that all patients, acute, indeterminant, and chronic be treated with antiparasitic therapy.

A single course of each of the medications below is thought to offer an approximately 50% cure rate.

Nifurtimox (Lampit, Bayer 2502):

- Only drug available in the U.S. for the treatment of acute, congenital, or laboratory-acquired infection
- Recommended oral dosage for adults: 8 to 10 mg/kg/day given in 3 to 4 divided daily doses and continued for 90 to 120 days
- Parasitologic cure in approximately 50% of those treated; should be begun as early as possible

Benznidazole, a nitroimidazole derivative:

- Has demonstrated similar efficacy as nifurtimox in limited trials
- Recommended oral dosage: 5 to 7 mg/kg/day for 30 to 90 days

CHRONIC Rx

- In patients with indeterminate phase or chronic disease: Some evidence of benefit in a recent uncontrolled trial with benznidazole in patients with chagasic cardiomyopathy

- In patients exhibiting bradyarrhythmias: pacemakers
- In individuals with congestive heart failure:
  1. Treat with standard modalities for dilated, right-sided, cardiomyopathic disease.
  2. Cardiac transplant is an option for end-stage cardiomyopathy; moreover, reactivation rate found to be low and amenable to therapy without subsequent infection of the allograft.
  3. Myotomy or esophageal resection is reserved for patients with advanced disease.
- In advanced chagasic megacolon associated with chronic fecal impaction, perforation, or, less commonly, volvulus: surgical resection

DISPOSITION

Based on few prospective studies, most patients infected with *T. cruzi* will not develop symptomatic Chagas' disease.

REFERRAL

- For consultation with an infectious disease specialist or communication with the Centers for Disease Control and Prevention when the disease is acutely suspected
- To a cardiologist for pacemaker implantation for patients with bradyarrhythmias
- To a surgeon for symptomatic disease with chagasic megaesophagus or megacolon

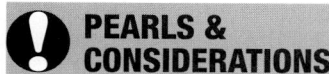 **PEARLS & CONSIDERATIONS**

COMMENTS

- In recipients of solid organ or bone marrow transplants, patients with AIDS, or those receiving chemotherapy, there may be reactivation of indeterminate phase disease.
- Mortality predictors associated with chagasic cardiomyopathy include CHF, QT-interval dispersion, left ventricular (LV) end-systolic dimension, the presence of pathological Q waves, frequent PVCs, and isolated LAFB on ECG.
- Chagasic esophageal disease has an increased incidence of esophageal malignancy.
- The use of pyrethroid-impregnated curtains may represent an option for the reduction or elimination of Chagas' disease transmission in certain endemic areas.

SUGGESTED READINGS
available at www.expertconsult.com

AUTHOR: **PATRICIA CRISTOFARO, M.D.**

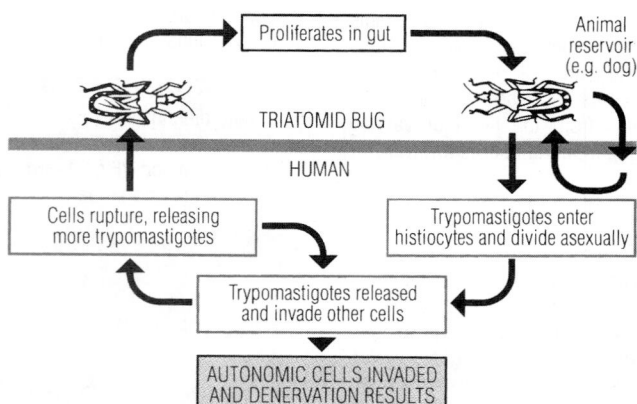

FIGURE 1-87 Lifecycle of *Trypanosoma cruzi*. (From Souhami RL, Mozham J: *Textbook of medicine*, ed 4, London, 2002, Churchill Livingstone.)

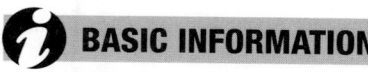

BASIC INFORMATION

DEFINITION

Chancroid is a sexually transmitted disease characterized by painful genital ulceration and inflammatory inguinal adenopathy.

SYNONYMS

Soft chancre
Ulcus molle

ICD-9CM CODES
099.0 Chancroid

EPIDEMIOLOGY & DEMOGRAPHICS

- Exact incidence is unknown. The prevalence of chancroid has declined in the United States. When infection occurs, it is usually associated with sporadic outbreaks.
- Occurs more frequently in men (male/female ratio of 5:1 to 10:1).
- Clinical infection is rare in women.
- There is a higher incidence in uncircumcised men and in tropical and subtropical regions.
- Incubation period is 4 to 7 days but may take up to 3 wk.
- High incidence of HIV infection associated with chancroid.

PHYSICAL FINDINGS & CLINICAL PRESENTATION

- One to three extremely painful ulcers (Fig. 1-88) accompanied by tender inguinal lymphadenopathy (especially if fluctuant). The chancre is typically soft in comparison with the hard, painless chancre of syphilis

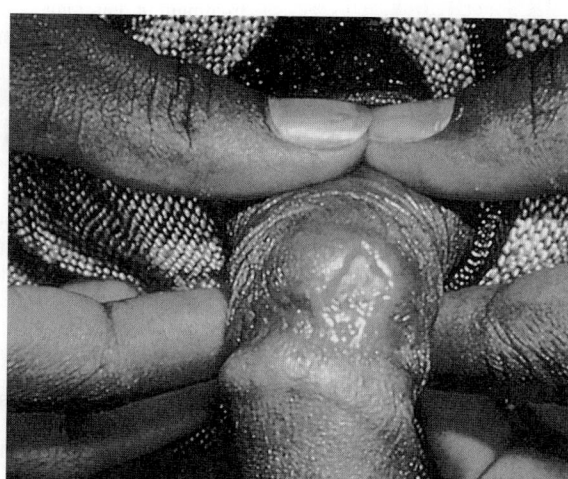

FIGURE 1-88 Chancroid. Note shaggy, ragged-edged ulcer with edema and exudative base. (Courtesy Beverly Sanders. From Goldstein B [ed]: *Practical dermatology,* ed 2, St Louis, 1997, Mosby.)

- May present with inguinal bubo and several ulcers
- In women: initial lesion in the fourchette, labia minora, urethra, cervix, or anus; inflammatory pustule or papule that ruptures, leaving a shallow, nonindurated ulceration, usually 1- to 2-cm diameter with ragged, undermined edges
- Unilateral lymphadenopathy develops 1 wk later in 50% of patients

ETIOLOGY

Haemophilus ducreyi, a bacillus

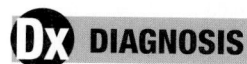

DIAGNOSIS

DIFFERENTIAL DIAGNOSIS

- Other genitoulcerative diseases such as syphilis, herpes, lymphogranuloma venereum (LGV), granuloma inguinale.
- A clinical algorithm for the initial management of genital ulcer disease is described in Section III.

WORKUP

Diagnosis based on history and physical examination is often inadequate. Must rule out syphilis in women because of the consequences of inappropriate therapy in pregnant women. Base initial diagnosis and treatment recommendations on clinical impression of appearance of ulcer and most likely diagnosis for population. Definitive diagnosis is made by isolation of organism from ulcers by culture or Gram stain. Special culture media for *H. ducreyi*; is not widely available commercially and even when these media are used, sensitivity is <80%.

LABORATORY TESTS

Darkfield microscopy, RPR, HSV cultures, *H. ducreyi* culture, HIV testing recommended

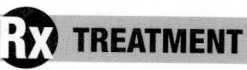

TREATMENT

NONPHARMACOLOGIC THERAPY

Fluctuant nodes should be aspirated through healthy adjacent skin to prevent formation of draining sinus. Incision and drainage not recommended because it delays healing. Use warm compresses to remove necrotic material.

ACUTE GENERAL Rx

- Azithromycin 1 g PO (single dose) *or*
- Ceftriaxone 250 mg IM (single dose) *or*
- Ciprofloxacin 500 mg PO bid for 3 days *or*
- Erythromycin 500 mg PO qid for 7 days

NOTE: Ciprofloxacin is contraindicated in patients who are pregnant, lactating, or <18 yr.

- HIV-infected patients may need more prolonged therapy

DISPOSITION

- All sexual partners should be treated with a 10-day course of one of the regimens (see "Acute General Rx").
- Patients should be reexamined 3 to 7 days after initiation of therapy. Ulcers should improve symptomatically within 3 days and objectively within 7 days after initiation of successful therapy.

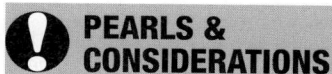

PEARLS & CONSIDERATIONS

COMMENTS

- In the U.S. herpes simplex-1 and syphilis are the most common causes of genital ulcers, followed by chancroid, LGV, and granuloma inguinale.
- The combination of a painful genital ulcer and tender suppurative inguinal adenopathy suggests the diagnosis of chancroid.

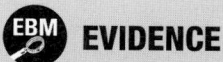

EVIDENCE

available at www.expertconsult.com

SUGGESTED READINGS
available at www.expertconsult.com

AUTHORS: **MARIA A. CORIGLIANO, M.D.,** and **RUBEN ALVERO, M.D.**

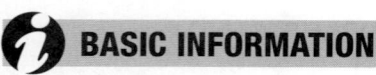

BASIC INFORMATION

DEFINITION

Charcot-Marie-Tooth disease (CMT) is a heterogeneous group of noninflammatory inherited peripheral neuropathies characterized by chronic motor and sensory polyneuropathy. It is the most common inherited disorder of the peripheral nervous system (see also "Neuropathy, Hereditary").

SYNONYMS

Peroneal muscular atrophy
Hereditary motor and sensory neuropathy (HMSN)

ICD-9CM CODES
356.1 Charcot-Marie-Tooth disease, paralysis, or syndrome

EPIDEMIOLOGY & DEMOGRAPHICS

PREVALENCE: 1:3,300
PREDOMINANT AGE: Onset usually 10 to 20 yr, and infants may be symptomatic.
GENETICS: Transmission may be autosomal dominant, autosomal recessive, or X-linked, with some sporadic cases reported. At least 43 CMT genes are known. Duplication of *peripheral myelin protein 22* (PMP22) is the most common cause of CMT.

PHYSICAL FINDINGS & CLINICAL PRESENTATION

- Wide variation in clinical presentation, but affected individuals in a family tend to have similar symptoms
- Symmetric, slowly progressive distal motor neuropathy resulting in weakness and atrophy in legs, often progresses to involve hands
- High-arched feet (pes cavus) and hammer toes
- Atrophy of the lower legs producing a stork-like appearance (muscle wasting does not involve the upper legs) (Fig. 1-89)
- Nerve enlargement
- Mild to moderate distal sensory loss; uncommonly can have painful paresthesias
- Decreased proprioception and weakness of ankle dorsiflexors often interfere with balance and gait (steppage gait)
- Depressed or absent deep tendon reflexes in many cases
- Hearing loss and hip dysplasia are under-recognized manifestations
- Ambulation usually maintained throughout life

ETIOLOGY

Genetic abnormalities cause defects in either peripheral nerve myelination, or result in axonal degeneration.

DIAGNOSIS

DIFFERENTIAL DIAGNOSIS

- Other inherited neuropathies
- Acquired peripheral neuropathies such as toxic, metabolic, infectious, endocrine, inflammatory, immune-mediated, and nutritional polyneuropathies

WORKUP

- Clinical diagnosis is based on family history, characteristic presentation, and findings on physical and detailed neurologic examination.

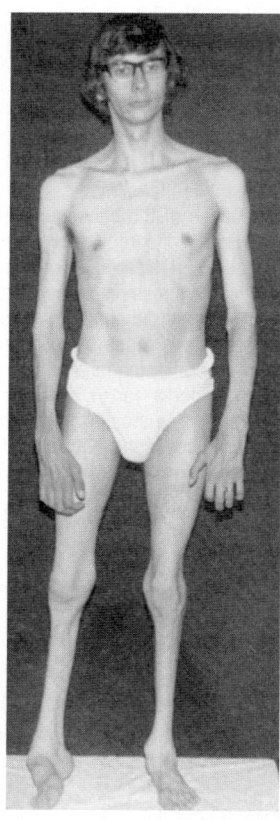

FIGURE 1-89 Patient with Charcot-Marie-Tooth disease showing marked wasting of calf muscles and intrinsic foot muscles. (From Dubowitz V: *Muscle disorders in childhood,* London, 1995, WB Saunders. In Goetz CG: *Textbook of clinical neurology,* Philadelphia, 1999, WB Saunders.)

- Electrophysiologic studies are often diagnostic, and may help define various subtypes of CMT along with clinical and genetic findings.
- Occasionally sural nerve biopsy is helpful in establishing diagnosis.

TREATMENT

ACUTE GENERAL Rx

- Symptomatic and supportive, managed by multidisciplinary team including physical and occupational therapy.
- Special shoes with good ankle support, ankle/foot orthoses (AFO).
- Some require crutches/cane for gait stability; <5% need wheelchair.
- Daily heel cord stretching exercises and hand grip exercises.
- Musculoskeletal pain may respond to acetaminophen or NSAIDs; neuropathic pain may respond to tricyclic antidepressants or drugs such as carbamazepine or gabapentin.

CHRONIC Rx

Occasionally, orthopedic surgery is required to correct severe pes cavus deformity or hip dysplasia. Avoiding obesity is essential as it makes walking difficult; avoiding potentially toxic medications is also important, particularly Vinca alkaloids.

DISPOSITION

- Disability is usually compatible with a long life.
- 10% to 20% of patients are asymptomatic.

REFERRAL

- Orthopedic consultation for bracing and treatment of deformity
- Genetic counseling and family planning

PEARLS & CONSIDERATIONS

COMMENTS

Patient information on Charcot-Marie-Tooth disease is available from the Muscular Dystrophy Association, 3300 East Sunrise Drive, Tucson, AZ 85718; phone (520) 529-2000.

SUGGESTED READINGS

available at www.expertconsult.com

AUTHOR: **CANDICE YUVIENCO, M.D.**

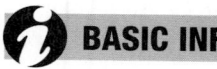

DEFINITION

Charcot's joint is a chronic, often devastating, progressive joint degeneration seen most commonly in peripheral weight-bearing joints and vertebrae, which develops as a result of the loss of normal sensory innervation of the joint. It was described by Charcot as a result of tabes dorsalis.

SYNONYMS

Neuropathic arthropathy

ICD-9CM CODES
094.0 Charcot's arthropathy

EPIDEMIOLOGY & DEMOGRAPHICS

PREVALENCE:
- One case per 750 patients with diabetes mellitus; five cases per 100 of those with peripheral neuropathy (foot is most commonly involved)
- 20% to 40% of patients with syringomyelia (shoulder, elbow, and wrist are most commonly involved).
- 5% to 10% of patients with tabes dorsalis; usually >60 yr (spine, hip, knee, and ankle are most commonly involved).
- Average age of onset is 50 to 60 yr.
- No definite sex predilection.

PHYSICAL FINDINGS & CLINICAL PRESENTATION

Neuropathic joint disease is relatively painless, often despite considerable destruction. The tarsometatarsal and tarsal joints of the foot and ankle are most commonly involved.
- Initial presentation is with a diffusely warm, swollen, and occasionally erythematous joint.
- Possible progression of joint instability; palpable osseous debris; crepitus common.
- Frank dislocation leading to bony deformity often found, especially in more superficial joints.

ETIOLOGY

Predisposing factors in the Charcot process include peripheral sensorimotor neuropathy, autonomic neuropathy, intact peripheral circulation and trauma, which is usually subtle or even unnoticed.

The most widely accepted theory is the "neurotraumatic" theory:
- Impairment and loss of joint sensitivity decrease the protective mechanism around the joint.
- Rapid destruction occurs when fracture dislocation and bone fragmentation and resorption lead to joint disorganization.
- Chronic inflammation and repetitive effusions develop, eventually contributing to joint instability and incongruity.

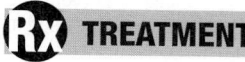

DIFFERENTIAL DIAGNOSIS
- Osteomyelitis
- Cellulitis
- Abscess
- Infectious arthritis
- Osteoarthritis
- Rheumatoid and other inflammatory arthritides (particularly gout)

WORKUP

Diagnosis is challenging, particularly in early stages, and requires a high index of suspicion.
- An underlying neurologic disorder must always be present.
- Diabetes mellitus with peripheral neuropathy is the most common cause (Fig. 1-90).
- Syringomyelia, tabes dorsalis, Charcot-Marie-Tooth disease, congenital indifference to pain, alcoholism, poliomyelitis, syphilis, leprosy, familial amyloid neuropathy, spinal or peripheral nerve surgery, trauma, and spinal dysraphism can all lead to the disorder.

LABORATORY TESTS

In questionable cases, aspiration, sometimes including biopsy, to rule out sepsis

IMAGING STUDIES

Plain roentgenography:
- Sufficient to establish diagnosis in most cases, especially if etiology is known.
- Findings: variable degrees of destruction and dislocation.

- In cases of x-ray evidence of bone destruction and an open wound, osteomyelitis is ruled out with either a leukocyte-labeled bone scan or MRI.

TREATMENT

The mainstay of therapy is early offloading, protection, and stabilization.

ACUTE GENERAL Rx
- Protection of effusions, sprains, and fractures until all hyperemic response has resolved
- Total contact casts, braces, special shoes with molded inserts, and elevation of the extremity
- Patient education with avoidance of weight bearing when lower extremity joints are involved
- Pharmacologic: bisphosphonates (Pamidronate studied) shown to reduce disease activity and bone turnover markers
- Surgery: only limited value

DISPOSITION

Once the full-blown neuropathic joint has developed, treatment is difficult. Deformity and joint instability cause major morbidity and often lead to infection, ulceration, and eventual amputation.

SUGGESTED READINGS
available at www.expertconsult.com

AUTHOR: **LONNIE R. MERCIER, M.D.**

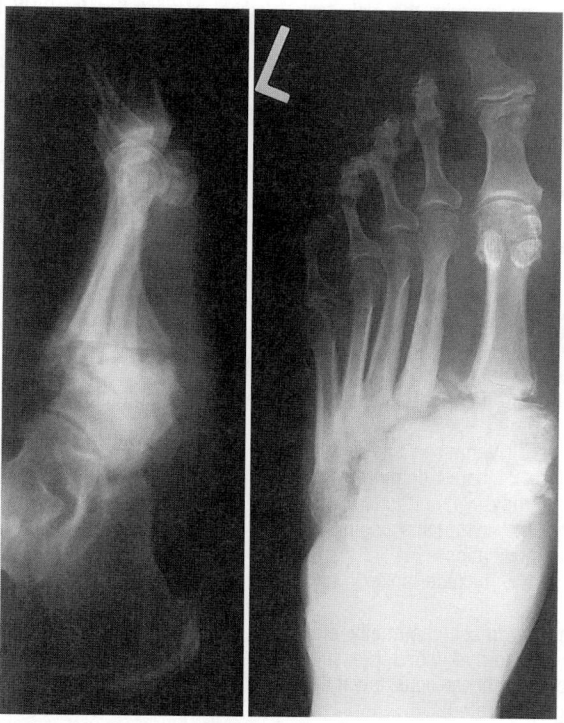

FIGURE 1-90 Diabetes mellitus and neuropathic arthritis. Note lateral displacement of metatarsals *(left)* and fragmentation and osseous debris *(right)*. (From Goldman L, Ausiello D [eds]: *Cecil textbook of medicine,* ed 22, Philadelphia, 2004, WB Saunders.)

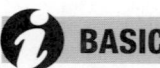

BASIC INFORMATION

DEFINITION

Chemotherapy-induced nausea and vomiting (CINV) refers to adverse effects of drugs used to treat cancer. There are three recognized subtypes: acute-phase CINV, where nausea and vomiting begin minutes to hours after administration of the drug(s); delayed-phase CINV, where symptoms can begin or return 24 hours or more after taking the medication(s); and anticipatory CINV, where nausea and vomiting begin before receiving treatment.

SYNONYMS

Drug-induced nausea and vomiting
Chemotherapy-induced emesis

ICD-9CM CODES
787.01 Nausea with vomiting
787.02 Nausea alone
787.03 Vomiting alone
E933.1 Adverse effect of antineoplastic and immunosuppressive drugs
V58.11-V58.12 Encounter for antineoplastic chemotherapy and immunotherapy

EPIDEMIOLOGY & DEMOGRAPHICS

- The patient's risk for development of nausea and vomiting is most strongly dependent on the drugs used.
- With certain medications, nausea and vomiting will occur in almost 100% of patients. With other drugs, the risk for symptoms can be as low as 10%.
- Symptoms may be dose dependent (the higher the dose, the greater the risk for symptoms).
- CINV is more likely to affect female and younger patients.
- Those patients expecting CINV from medications are more likely to have it (anticipatory emesis).
- Those patients with a history of alcohol consumption are at lower risk.
- Patients with a history of motion sickness are at greater risk.

PHYSICAL FINDINGS & CLINICAL PRESENTATION

- For acute-phase CINV, nausea and vomiting start within minutes to hours after receiving chemotherapy.
- For delayed-phase CINV, nausea and vomiting begin or return 24 hours or more after receiving chemotherapy.
- With anticipatory CINV, symptoms begin before receiving the medication.
- Other symptoms may include anxiety and lightheadedness.
- Physical findings are most commonly elevated pulse and abnormal blood pressure (high if the person is highly anxious, low if the patient is getting dehydrated).

- Symptoms such as diarrhea, fever, headache, and abdominal pain may suggest an etiology of symptoms other than chemotherapy; physical examination findings such as increased blood pressure, abdominal tenderness, or focal neurologic deficits may suggest symptoms caused by cancer progression or other acute illness such as infection.

ETIOLOGY

CINV is probably the result of chemotherapy drugs acting in two places: in the gastrointestinal tract directly and in the vomiting center of the brain. In both areas, nausea and vomiting are mediated by the actions of certain neurotransmitters, with serotonin, dopamine, and neurokinin being the most important.

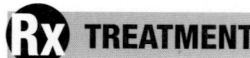

DIAGNOSIS

DIFFERENTIAL DIAGNOSIS

- The two main considerations are progression of cancer and infection
- Intestinal/gastric: obstruction or partial obstruction of the digestive tract from tumor
- Neurologic: metastases to the brain causing vomiting; infiltration of nerves affecting the digestive tract
- Infectious: acute bacterial, viral, or parasitic infectious of the digestive tract causing symptoms (usually diarrhea will be present)
- Renal: dehydration leading to kidney failure, causing a worsening of nausea and vomiting

WORKUP

No workup is indicated if patient's symptoms and timeframe of nausea and vomiting fit the usual presentation for CINV. If other symptoms or unexpected physical examination findings are present, then other causes need to be ruled out. A combination of blood work and imaging may be helpful.

LABORATORY TESTS

- If the onset of symptoms is not typical for CINV, then blood tests such as a CBC, liver tests, and kidney tests may be indicated.
- Stool studies looking for infections from bacteria or parasites may be ordered if diarrhea is also present.

IMAGING STUDIES

- Abdominal radiographs may be ordered to look for obstruction of the digestive tract but will not give any information about tumor progression.
- Abdominal CT scan will give more detailed information about cancer in the proximity of the digestive tract and whether obstruction of the digestive tract is present.
- Brain CT scan or magnetic resonance imaging (MRI) will give information about possible metastases to the brain.

TREATMENT

- Treatment depends on the likelihood of a given drug or drug regimen to cause CINV and is preventative in nature.
- For those medications with a high probability of causing CINV, a combination of antinausea medications has proved to be highly effective.
- Which combination of drugs is used and for how many days is dependent on the chemotherapy regimen used.
- The most common combination includes a serotonin-receptor antagonist (ondansetron, granisetron, dolasetron, tropisetron, or palonosetron), a corticosteroid (methylprednisolone or dexamethason), and a neurokinin-1 receptor antagonist (aprepitant).
- Many other drugs are available, such as prochlorperazine, metochlopramide, haloperidol, and marinol, but most are less effective and have greater potential for adverse effects.
- Benzodiazepines (usually lorazepam) may help in patients with high anxiety levels leading to anticipatory CINV.
- Patients with uncontrolled symptoms may require hospitalization for supportive care including intravenous fluids.

NONPHARMACOLOGIC THERAPY

For those patients with a significant anxiety component to their CINV, behavior therapy may help.

DISPOSITION

Although CINV is one of the most feared complications of cancer therapy, its treatment has been revolutionized in the last 20 years, with most patients achieving adequate symptom control.

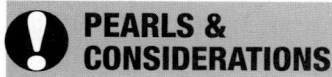

PEARLS & CONSIDERATIONS

COMMENTS

- Aggressive attempts to control the acute phase of CINV are the key to symptom control. Prevention of the acute phase has led to much greater control of the delayed phase, which, in turn, has greatly decreased the incidence of anticipatory CINV.
- Prevention of symptoms is much easier to achieve than controlling/treating symptoms once they have begun.

SUGGESTED READINGS
available at www.expertconsult.com

AUTHOR: **CHARLES WOLFF, M.D.**

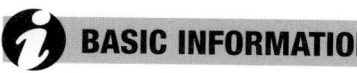

BASIC INFORMATION

DEFINITION

Genital infection with *Chlamydia trachomatis* may result in urethritis, epididymitis, cervicitis, and acute salpingitis, but often it is asymptomatic in women (see "Pelvic Inflammatory Disease"). In men, urethritis, mucopurulent discharge, dysuria, and urethral pruritus are noted.

ICD-9CM CODES
597.80 Urethritis
604.0   Epididymitis
616.0   Cervicitis
381.51 Acute salpingitis

EPIDEMIOLOGY & DEMOGRAPHICS

- *Chlamydia trachomatis* is the most common sexually transmitted disease in the U.S. More than 4 million infections occur annually, although the exact number is unknown because reporting is not required in all states. Occurrence is common worldwide and has been increasing steadily over the last 2 decades in the U.S., Canada, Australia, and Europe.
- Most women with endocervical or urethral infections are asymptomatic.
- Up to 45% of cases of gonococcal infection may have concomitant chlamydial infection.
- Infertility or ectopic pregnancy can result as a complication from symptomatic or asymptomatic chronic infections of the endometrium and fallopian tubes.
- Conjunctival and pneumonic infection of the newborn may result from infection in pregnancy.
- In men 15% to 55% of cases are caused by *C. trachomatis*. Complications of nongonococcal urethritis in men infected with *C. trachomatis* include epididymitis and Reiter's syndrome.

PHYSICAL FINDINGS & CLINICAL PRESENTATION

Clinical manifestations may be similar to those of gonorrhea: mucopurulent endocervical discharge, with edema, erythema, and easily induced endocervical bleeding caused by inflammation of endocervical columnar epithelium. Less-frequent manifestations may include bartholinitis, urethral syndrome with dysuria and pyuria, and perihepatitis (Fitz-Hugh–Curtis syndrome).

ETIOLOGY
- *Chlamydia trachomatis,* serotypes D through K
- Obligate, intracellular bacteria

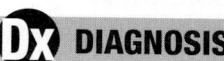

DIAGNOSIS

DIFFERENTIAL DIAGNOSIS

Gonorrhea, nongonococcal urethritis (nonchlamydial etiologies)

WORKUP

Diagnosis based on laboratory demonstration of evidence of infection in intraurethral or endocervical swab by various tests. The intracellular organism is less readily recovered from the discharge.

LABORATORY TESTS

- Cell culture is the reference method for diagnosis (single culture sensitivity 80% to 90%), but it is labor intensive and takes 48 to 96 hr; it is not suited for large screening programs.
- Nonculture methods:
  - Direct fluorescent antibody tests
  - Enzyme immunoassay
  - DNA probes
  - Polymerase chain reaction (PCR)
- With the exception of PCR, the other tests are probably less specific than cell culture and may yield false-positive results.
- Because this is an intracellular organism, purulent discharge is not an appropriate specimen. An adequate sample of infected cells must be obtained.
- Ten white blood cells per high-power field.

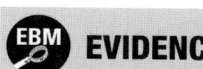

TREATMENT

ACUTE GENERAL Rx

Nongonococcal urethritis, urethritis, cervicitis, conjunctivitis (except for lymphogranuloma venereum):
- Azithromycin 1 g PO × 1 *or*
- Doxycycline 100 mg PO bid for 7 days
- Alternatives
  1. Erythromycin base 500 mg PO qid for 7 days *or*
  2. Erythromycin ethylsuccinate 800 mg PO qid for 7 days *or*
  3. Ofloxacin 300 mg PO bid for 7 days
  4. Levofloxacin 500 mg PO qd for 7 days
Infection in pregnancy:
- Erythromycin base 500 mg PO qid for 7 days *or*
- Amoxicillin 500 mg PO tid for 7 days
Alternatives:
  1. Erythromycin base 250 mg PO qid for 7 days *or*
  2. Erythromycin ethylsuccinate 800 mg PO qid for 7 days *or*
  3. Erythromycin ethylsuccinate 400 mg PO qid for 14 days *or*
  4. Azithromycin 1 g PO (single dose)
NOTE: Doxycycline and ofloxacin are contraindicated in pregnancy. Safety and efficacy of azithromycin are not established in pregnancy and lactation, although preliminary data indicate that it may be safe and effective. Erythromycin estolate is contraindicated in pregnancy because of drug-related hepatotoxicity.
FOLLOW-UP: Reculture after therapy completion and refer partners for evaluation and treatment.
RECURRENT AND PERSISTENT URETHRITIS: Retreat noncompliant patients with the above regimens. If patient was initially compliant, recommended regimens: metronidazole 2 g PO in single dose plus erythromycin base 500 mg PO qid for 7 days or erythromycin ethylsuccinate 800 mg PO qid for 7 days.

CLINICAL PEARL

When treating *Chlamydia,* it is best to assume concomitant gonorrhea because co-infection is common. Combination of cetriaxone 125 mg IM single dose plus azithromycin 1 g PO single dose will treat both.

REFFERAL

Refer to infectious disease specialist if persistent infection or gynecologist if salpingitis is suspected.

EBM EVIDENCE

available at www.expertconsult.com

SUGGESTED READINGS
available at www.expertconsult.com

AUTHORS: **MARIA A. CORIGLIANO, M.D.,** and **RUBEN ALVERO, M.D.**

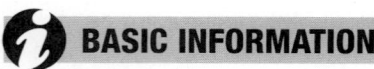

BASIC INFORMATION

DEFINITION

Cholangitis refers to an inflammation and/or infection of the hepatic and common bile ducts associated with obstruction of the common bile duct.

SYNONYMS

Biliary sepsis
Ascending cholangitis
Suppurative cholangitis

ICD-9CM CODES
576.1 Cholangitis

EPIDEMIOLOGY & DEMOGRAPHICS

INCIDENCE (IN U.S.): Complicates approximately 1% of cases of cholelithiasis
PEAK INCIDENCE: Seventh decade
PREVALENCE (IN U.S.): 2 cases/1000 hospital admissions
PREDOMINANT SEX:
- Females, for cholangitis secondary to gallstones
- Males, for cholangitis secondary to malignant obstruction and HIV infection

PREDOMINANT AGE: Seventh decade and older; unusual <50 yr of age

PHYSICAL FINDINGS & CLINICAL PRESENTATION

- Usually acute onset of fever, abdominal pain (RUQ), and jaundice (Charcot's triad)
- All signs and symptoms in only 50% to 85% of patients
- Often, dark coloration of the urine resulting from bilirubinuria
- Complications:
  1. Bacteremia (50%) and septic shock
  2. Hepatic abscess and pancreatitis

ETIOLOGY

Obstruction of the common bile duct causing rapid proliferation of bacteria in the biliary tree
- Most common cause of common bile duct obstruction: stones, usually migrated from the gallbladder
- Other causes: prior biliary tract surgery with secondary stenosis, tumor (usually arising from the pancreas or biliary tree), and parasitic infections from *Ascaris lumbricoides* or *Fasciola hepatica*
- Iatrogenic after contamination of an obstructed biliary tree by endoscopic retrograde cholangiopancreatoscopy (ERCP) or percutaneous transhepatic cholangiography (PTC)
- Primary sclerosing cholangitis (PSC)
- HIV-associated sclerosing cholangitis: associated with infection by CMV, *Cryptospo-*

ridium, Microsporidia, and *Mycobacterium avium* complex

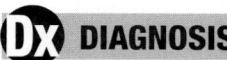

DIAGNOSIS

DIFFERENTIAL DIAGNOSIS

- Biliary colic
- Acute cholecystitis
- Liver abscess
- Peptic ulcer disease (PUD)
- Pancreatitis
- Intestinal obstruction
- Right kidney stone
- Hepatitis
- Pyelonephritis

WORKUP

- Blood cultures
- CBC
- Liver function tests

LABORATORY TESTS

- Usually, elevated WBC count with a predominance of polymorphonuclear forms
- Elevated alkaline phosphatase and bilirubin in chronic obstruction
- Elevated transaminases in acute obstruction
- Positive blood cultures in 50% of cases, typically with enteric gram-negative aerobes (e.g., *E. coli, Klebsiella pneumoniae*), enterococci, or anaerobes

IMAGING STUDIES

- Ultrasound:
  1. Allows visualization of the gallbladder and bile ducts to differentiate extrahepatic obstruction from intrahepatic cholestasis
  2. Insensitive but specific for visualization of common duct stones
- CT scan:
  1. Less accurate for gallstones
  2. More sensitive than ultrasound for visualization of the distal part of the common bile duct
  3. Also allows better definition of neoplasm
- ERCP:
  1. Confirms obstruction and its level
  2. Allows collection of specimens for culture and cytology
  3. Indicated for diagnosis if ultrasound and CT scan are inconclusive
  4. May be indicated in therapy (see "Treatment")

TREATMENT

NONPHARMACOLOGIC THERAPY

Biliary decompression
- May be urgent in severely ill patients or those unresponsive to medical therapy within 12 to 24 hr

- May also be performed semielectively in patients who respond
- Options:
  1. ERCP with or without sphincterotomy or placement of a draining stent
  2. Percutaneous transhepatic biliary drainage for the acutely ill patient who is a poor surgical candidate
  3. Surgical exploration of the common bile duct

ACUTE GENERAL Rx

- Nothing by mouth
- Intravenous hydration
- Broad-spectrum antibiotics directed at gram-negative enteric organisms, anaerobes, and enterococcus such as ampicillin/sulbactam or piperacillin/tazobactam; if infection is nosocomial, post-ERCP, or the patient is in shock, broaden antibiotic coverage.

CHRONIC Rx

Repeated decompression may be necessary, particularly when obstruction is related to neoplasm.

DISPOSITION

Excellent prognosis if obstruction is amenable to definitive surgical therapy; otherwise relapses are common.

REFERRAL

- To biliary endoscopist if obstruction is from stones or a stent needs to be placed
- To interventional radiologist if external drainage is necessary
- To a general surgeon in all other cases
- To an infectious disease specialist if blood cultures are positive or the patient is in shock or otherwise severely ill

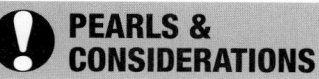

PEARLS & CONSIDERATIONS

- Cholangitis is a life-threatening form of intra-abdominal sepsis, though it may appear to be rather innocuous at its onset.
- Antibiotics alone will not resolve cholangitis in the presence of biliary obstruction because high intrabiliary pressures prevent antibiotic delivery. Decompression and drainage of the biliary tract to alleviate the obstruction with antimicrobial therapy is the therapy of choice.

SUGGESTED READINGS
available at www.expertconsult.com

AUTHORS: **GLENN G. FORT, M.D., M.P.H.,** and **DENNIS J. MIKOLICH, M.D.**

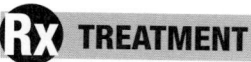 **BASIC INFORMATION**

DEFINITION

Cholecystitis is acute or chronic inflammation of the gallbladder generally caused by gallstones (>95% of cases).

SYNONYMS

Gallbladder attack

ICD-9CM CODES
575.0 Acute cholecystitis
574.0 Calculus of the gallbladder with acute cholecystitis
575.1 Cholecystitis without mention of calculus

EPIDEMIOLOGY & DEMOGRAPHICS

- Acute cholecystitis occurs most commonly in women during the fifth and sixth decades. Approximately 120,000 cholecystectomies are performed for acute cholecystitis annually in the U.S.
- The incidence of gallstones is 0.6% in the general population and much higher in certain ethnic groups (>75% of Native Americans by age 60 yr). Most patients with gallstones are asymptomatic. Of such patients, biliary colic develops in 1% to 4% annually.

PHYSICAL FINDINGS & CLINICAL PRESENTATION

- Pain and tenderness in the right hypochondrium or epigastrium; pain possibly radiating to the infrascapular region
- Palpation of the right upper quadrant (RUQ) eliciting marked tenderness and stoppage of inspired breath (Murphy's sign)
- Guarding
- Fever (33%)
- Jaundice (25% to 50% of patients)
- Palpable gallbladder (20% of cases)
- Nausea and vomiting (>70% of patients)
- Fever and chills (>25% of patients)
- Medical history often revealing ingestion of large, fatty meals before onset of pain in the epigastrium and RUQ

ETIOLOGY

- Gallstones (>95% of cases)
- Ischemic damage to the gallbladder, critically ill patient (acalculous cholecystitis)
- Infectious agents, especially in patients with AIDS (cytomegalovirus, *Cryptosporidium*)
- Strictures of the bile duct
- Neoplasms, primary or metastatic
- Risk factors for cholelithiasis include age, obesity, female sex, rapid weight loss, ethnicity/race (Native American), use of contraceptives, pregnancy, diabetes mellitus, hemolysis, total parenteral nutrition, biliary parasites

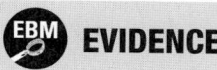 **DIAGNOSIS**

DIFFERENTIAL DIAGNOSIS

- Hepatic: hepatitis, abscess, hepatic congestion, neoplasm, trauma

- Biliary: neoplasm, stricture, sphincter of Oddi dysfunction
- Gastric: pelvic ulcer disease, neoplasm, alcoholic gastritis, hiatal hernia, non-ulcer dyspepsia
- Pancreatic: pancreatitis, neoplasm, stone in the pancreatic duct or ampulla
- Renal: calculi, infection, inflammation, neoplasm, ruptured kidney
- Pulmonary: pneumonia, pulmonary infarction, right-sided pleurisy
- Intestinal: retrocecal appendicitis, intestinal obstruction, high fecal impaction, irritable bowel syndrome (IBS), inflammatory bowel disease (IBD)
- Cardiac: myocardial ischemia (particularly involving the inferior wall), pericarditis
- Cutaneous: herpes zoster
- Trauma
- Fitz-Hugh-Curtis syndrome (perihepatitis), ruptured ectopic pregnancy
- Subphrenic abscess
- Dissecting aneurysm
- Nerve root irritation caused by osteoarthritis of the spine

WORKUP

Workup consists of detailed history and physical examination coupled with laboratory evaluation and imaging studies. No single clinical finding or laboratory test is sufficient to establish or exclude cholecystitis without further testing.

LABORATORY TESTS

- Leukocytosis (12,000 to 20,000) is present in >70% of patients.
- Elevated alkaline phosphatase, ALT, AST, bilirubin; bilirubin elevation >4 mg/dl is unusual and suggests presence of choledocholithiasis.
- Elevated amylase may be present (consider pancreatitis if serum amylase elevation exceeds 500 U).

IMAGING STUDIES

- Ultrasound of the gallbladder is the preferred initial test; it will demonstrate the presence of stones and also dilated gallbladder with thickened wall and surrounding edema in patients with acute cholecystitis.
- Nuclear imaging (HIDA scan) is useful for diagnosis of cholecystitis when sonogram is inconclusive: sensitivity and specificity exceed 90% for acute cholecystis. This test is only reliable when bilirubin is <5 mg/dl. A positive test result (absence of gallbladder filling within 60 min after the administration of tracer) will demonstrate obstruction of the cystic or common hepatic duct; the test will not demonstrate the presence of stones.
- CT scan of abdomen is useful in cases of suspected abscess, neoplasm, or pancreatitis.
- Plain radiograph of the abdomen generally is not useful because <25% of stones are radiopaque.

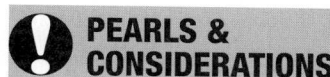 **TREATMENT**

NONPHARMACOLOGIC THERAPY

Provide IV hydration; withhold oral feedings.

ACUTE GENERAL Rx

- Laparoscopic cholecystectomy is considered the treatment of choice for most patients. The rate of conversion to open cholecystectomy is higher when laparoscopic cholecystectomy is performed for acute cholecystitis rather than for uncomplicated cholelithiasis; conservative management with IV fluids and antibiotics (ampicillin-sulbactam [Unasyn] 3 g IV q6h or piperacillin-tazobactam [Zosyn] 4.5 g IV q8h) may be justified in some high-risk patients to convert an emergency procedure into an elective one with a lower mortality rate.
- Endoscopic retrograde cholangiopancreatoscopy with sphincterectomy and stone extraction can be performed in conjunction with laparoscopic cholecystectomy for patients with choledochal lithiasis; approximately 7% to 15% of patients with cholelithiasis also have stones in the common bile duct.

DISPOSITION

- Prognosis is good; elective laparoscopic cholecystectomy can be performed as outpatient procedure.
- Hospital stay (when necessary) varies from overnight with laparoscopic cholecystectomy to 4 to 7 days with open cholecystectomy.
- Complication rate is approximately 1% (hemorrhage and bile leak) for laparoscopic cholecystectomy and <0.5% (infection) with open cholecystectomy.

REFERRAL

Surgical referral in all patients with acute cholecystitis

PEARLS & CONSIDERATIONS

COMMENTS

- Patients should be instructed that stones may recur in bile ducts.
- Gallbladder aspiration, in which all fluid visualized by ultrasound is aspirated, represents a nonsurgical treatment when patients who are at high operative risk develop acute cholecystitis. Salvage cholecystectomy is reserved for nonresponders.

EBM EVIDENCE

available at www.expertconsult.com

SUGGESTED READING

available at www.expertconsult.com

AUTHOR: **FRED F. FERRI, M.D.**

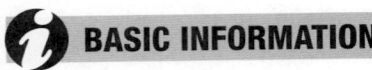

BASIC INFORMATION

DEFINITION

Cholelithiasis is the presence of stones in the gallbladder.

SYNONYMS

Gallstones

ICD-9CM CODES
574.2 Calculus of the gallbladder without mention of cholecystitis
574.0 Calculus of the gallbladder with acute cholecystitis

EPIDEMIOLOGY & DEMOGRAPHICS

- Gallstone disease can be found in 12% of the U.S. population. Of these, 2% to 3% (500,000 to 600,000) are treated with cholecystectomies each year.
- Annual medical expenditures for gallbladder surgeries in the U.S. exceed $5 billion.
- Incidence of gallbladder disease increases with age. Highest incidence is in the fifth and sixth decades. Predisposing factors for gallstones are female sex, pregnancy, age >40 yr, family history of gallstones, obesity, ileal disease, oral contraceptives, diabetes mellitus, rapid weight loss, estrogen replacement therapy.
- Patients with gallstones have a 20% chance of developing biliary colic or its complications at the end of a 20-yr period.

PHYSICAL FINDINGS & CLINICAL PRESENTATION

- Physical examination is entirely normal unless patient is having biliary colic; 80% of gallstones are asymptomatic.
- Typical symptoms of obstruction of the cystic duct include intermittent, severe, cramping pain affecting the right upper quadrant.
- Pain occurs mostly at night and may radiate to the back or right shoulder. It can last from a few minutes to several hours.

ETIOLOGY

- 75% of gallstones contain cholesterol and are usually associated with obesity, female sex, and diabetes mellitus; mixed stones are most common (80%); pure cholesterol stones account for only 10% of stones.
- 25% of gallstones are pigment stones (bilirubin, calcium, and variable organic material) associated with hemolysis and cirrhosis. These tend to be black-pigmented stones that are refractory to medical therapy.
- 50% of mixed-type stones are radiopaque.

DIAGNOSIS

DIFFERENTIAL DIAGNOSIS

- Pelvic ulcer disease
- Gastroesophageal reflux disease
- Irritable bowel disease
- Pancreatitis
- Neoplasms
- Nonnuclear dyspepsia
- Inferior wall myocardial infarction
- Hepatic abscess

LABORATORY TESTS

Generally normal unless patient has biliary obstruction (elevated alkaline phosphatase, bilirubin).

IMAGING STUDIES

- Ultrasound of the gallbladder will detect small stones and biliary sludge (sensitivity, 95%; specificity, 90%); the presence of dilated gallbladder with thickened wall is suggestive of acute cholecystitis.
- Nuclear imaging (HIDA scan) can confirm acute cholecystitis (>90% accuracy) if gallbladder does not visualize within 4 hr of injection and the radioisotope is excreted in the common bile duct.
- Common bile duct stones can be detected noninvasively by magnetic resonance cholangiopancreatography or invasively by endoscopic retrograde cholangiopancreatography (ERCP) and intraoperative cholangiography.

TREATMENT

NONPHARMACOLOGIC THERAPY

Lifestyle changes (avoidance of diets high in polyunsaturated fats, weight loss in obese patients; however, avoid rapid weight loss)

ACUTE GENERAL Rx

- The management of gallstones is affected by the clinical presentation.
- Asymptomatic patients do not require therapeutic intervention.
- Surgical intervention is generally the ideal approach for symptomatic patients. Laparoscopic cholecystectomy is generally preferred over open cholecystectomy because of the shorter recovery period and lower mortality rate. Between 5% and 26% of patients undergoing elective laparoscopic cholecystectomy will require conversion to an open procedure. Most common reason is the inability to clearly identify the biliary anatomy.
- Laparoscopic cholecystectomy after endoscopic sphincterectomy is recommended for patients with common bile duct stones and residual gallbladder stones. Where possible, single-stage laparoscopic treatments with removal of duct stones and cholecystectomy during the same procedure are preferable.
- Patients who are not appropriate candidates for surgery because of coexisting illness or patients who refuse surgery can be treated with oral bile salts: ursodiol (Actigall) 8 to 10 mg/kg/day in two to three divided doses for 16 to 20 mo, or chenodiol (Chenix) 250 mg bid initially, increasing gradually to a dose of 60 mg/kg/day. Candidates for oral bile salts are patients with cholesterol stones (radiolucent, noncalcified stones), with a diameter of ≤15 mm and having three or fewer stones. Candidates for medical therapy must have a functioning gallbladder and must have absence of calcifications on CT scans.
- Direct solvent dissolution with methyl *tert*-butyl ether (MTBE) is rarely used. Administration of the solvent is either through percutaneous transhepatic placement of a catheter into the gallbladder or endoscopic retrograde catheter placement with subsequent continuous infusion and aspiration of the solvent either manually or by automatic pump system.
- Extracorporeal shock wave lithotripsy (ESWL) is another form of medical therapy. It can be used in patients with stone diameter of ≤3 cm and having three or fewer stones.

DISPOSITION

- Recurrence rate after bile acid treatment is approximately 50% in 5 yr. Periodic ultrasound is necessary to assess the effectiveness of treatment.
- Gallstones recur after dissolution therapy with MTBE in >40% of patients within 5 yr.
- After ESWL, stones recur in approximately 20% of patients after 4 yr.
- Patients with at least one gallstone <5 mm in diameter have a greater than fourfold increased risk of presenting with acute biliary pancreatitis. A policy of watchful waiting in such cases is generally unwarranted.
- A potential serious complication of gallstones is acute cholangitis. ERCP and endoscopic sphincterectomy followed by interval laparoscopic cholecystectomy are effective in acute cholangitis.

SUGGESTED READINGS
available at www.expertconsult.com

AUTHOR: FRED F. FERRI, M.D.

BASIC INFORMATION

DEFINITION

Cholera is an acute diarrheal illness caused by *Vibrio cholerae.*

ICD-9CM CODES
001.0 Cholera

EPIDEMIOLOGY & DEMOGRAPHICS

INCIDENCE (IN U.S.): Previously, approximately 50 cases per yr, mostly in travelers returning from endemic areas. From 1995 to 2003, 68 cases reported, 44 (65%) of which were acquired outside the U.S. 9% were acquired from seafood from the Gulf Coast waters.

PEAK INCIDENCE:
- None in the U.S.
- Summer and fall in endemic areas

PREDOMINANT SEX: None

PREDOMINANT AGE: In nonendemic areas, attack rates are equal in all age groups. In epidemic areas, children over the age of 2 yr are most commonly infected. Neonatal infection: illness is uncommon before the age of 2 yr, likely because of passive immunity.

PHYSICAL FINDINGS & CLINICAL PRESENTATION

Infection may result in asymptomatic illness or a mild diarrhea. The classic illness is described as the abrupt onset of voluminous watery diarrhea, which may lead to severe dehydration, acidosis, shock, and death. Vomiting may occur early in the illness, but fever and abdominal pain are usually absent. The typical "rice water" stools are pale with flecks of mucus and contain no blood. Muscle cramps may be prominent and are the result of loss of fluid and electrolytes. Untreated illness results in hypovolemic shock, and death may occur in hours to days. With adequate fluid and electrolyte repletion, cholera is a self-limited illness that resolves in a few days. The use of antimicrobials can shorten the course of illness.

ETIOLOGY

The organism responsible for this illness is one of several strains of *V. cholerae.* Most infections result from the 01 serotype, the El Tor biotype. In the U.S., one outbreak occurred from the ingestion of illegally imported crab, and sporadic infection has been associated with the consumption of contaminated shellfish in Gulf Coast states. Most cases are seen in returning travelers. Transmission during epidemics is the result of the ingestion of contaminated water and, in some instances, contaminated food.

DIAGNOSIS

DIFFERENTIAL DIAGNOSIS

- Mild illness may mimic gastroenteritis resulting from a variety of etiologies.
- Sudden, voluminous diarrhea causing marked dehydration is uncommon in other illnesses.

WORKUP

Stool should be sent for culture and microscopy. Treatment should not be delayed while awaiting culture results.

LABORATORY TESTS

- WBC may be elevated, and hemoglobin may be increased as a result of hemoconcentration.
- Elevated BUN and creatinine suggests prerenal azotemia. Hypoglycemia may occur. Stool cultures on appropriate media may grow the organism. Wet mount of stool under dark field or phase contrast microscopy shows organisms with characteristic darting motility.

TREATMENT

NONPHARMACOLOGIC THERAPY

The mainstay of therapy is adequate fluid and electrolyte replacement (see Table 1-33). This can usually be achieved using oral rehydration solutions containing salts and glucose. Some patients may require intravenous fluid and electrolyte replacement.

ACUTE GENERAL Rx

- Antimicrobial therapy can decrease shedding of fluid and organisms and can shorten the course of illness:
  1. Doxycycline 100 mg PO bid for 5 days *or*
  2. Ciprofloxacin 1 g as a single dose *or*
  3. Azithromycin two 500-mg tablets PO as a single dose
- Resistance to SMX-TMP is increasing in travel-associated infections and is no longer recommended.
- Zinc supplementation may be helpful in children.

CHRONIC Rx

It is likely that asymptomatic chronic carriers exist; however, because they are difficult to identify, and their role in transmission of disease appears to be rather limited, there is no recommendation for treatment of these individuals.

DISPOSITION

The mortality of adequately hydrated patients is less than 1%.

REFERRAL

If more than mild illness occurs

REPORTING

In the U.S., all cases of cholera must be reported to the local and state health departments. Bacterial isolates must be sent to the state health department and the CDC.

PEARLS & CONSIDERATIONS

COMMENTS

- There is currently no indication for vaccination of travelers to endemic areas. The risk of infection is small, protection from available vaccines is limited, and side effects are prominent and frequent.
- Doxycycline should not be used to treat children or pregnant women.
- A recent study indicates a single dose treatment strategy with azithromycin is significantly better than ciprofloxacin for the management of cholera.

EVIDENCE

available at www.expertconsult.com

SUGGESTED READINGS

available at www.expertconsult.com

AUTHORS: **PATRICIA CRISTOFARO, M.D.,** **GLENN G. FORT, M.D., M.P.H.,** and **DENNIS J. MIKOLICH, M.D.**

TABLE 1-33 Electrolyte Concentration of Cholera Stools and Common Solutions Used for Treatment

	ELECTROLYTE AND GLUCOSE CONCENTRATION (mmol/L)				
	Na⁺	Cl⁻	K⁺	HCO₃⁻	Glucose
Cholera stool					
Adults	130	100	20	44	
Children	100	90	33	30	
Intravenous solutions					
Ringer's lactate	130	109	4	28*	0
Dhaka	133	98	13	48	0
Normal saline	154	154	0	0	0
Peru polyelectrolyte	90	80	20	30	111
WHO ORS	90	80	20	30†	111

*Ringer's lactate does not contain HCO_3^-; it has lactate instead.
†Bicarbonate is replaced by trisodium citrate, which persists longer than bicarbonate in sachets.
WHO ORS, World Health Organization oral rehydration solution.
From Mandell GL et al: *Principles and practice of infectious diseases,* ed 6, Philadelphia, 2005, Elsevier.

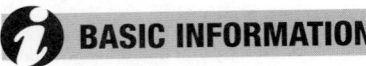

BASIC INFORMATION

DEFINITION

Chronic fatigue syndrome (CFS) is characterized by four or more of the following symptoms, present concurrently for at least 6 mo:
- Impaired memory or concentration
- Sore throat
- Tender cervical or axillary lymph nodes
- Muscle pain
- Multijoint pain
- New headaches
- Unrefreshing sleep
- Postexertion malaise

SYNONYMS

Yuppie flu
CFS
Chronic Epstein-Barr syndrome

ICD-9CM CODES
780.7 Chronic fatigue syndrome
300.8 Neurasthenia

EPIDEMIOLOGY & DEMOGRAPHICS

PREVALENCE IN U.S.: 10 to 300 cases per 100,000 persons
PREDOMINANT AGE: Young adulthood and middle age
PREDOMINANT SEX: Females affected more often than males

PHYSICAL FINDINGS & CLINICAL PRESENTATION
- There are no physical findings specific for CFS.
- The physical examination may be useful to identify fibromyalgia and other rheumatologic conditions that may coexist with CFS.

ETIOLOGY
- The etiology of CFS is unknown.
- Many experts suspect that a viral illness may trigger certain immune responses that lead to the various symptoms. Most patients often report the onset of their symptoms with a flulike illness.

DIAGNOSIS

DIFFERENTIAL DIAGNOSIS
- Psychosocial depression, dysthymia, anxiety-related disorders, and other psychiatric diseases

- Infectious diseases (subacute bacterial endocarditis, Lyme disease, fungal diseases, mononucleosis, HIV, chronic hepatitis B or C, TB, chronic parasitic infections)
- Autoimmune diseases: SLE, myasthenia gravis, multiple sclerosis, thyroiditis, RA
- Endocrine abnormalities: hypothyroidism, hypopituitarism, adrenal insufficiency, Cushing's syndrome, diabetes mellitus, hyperparathyroidism, pregnancy, reactive hypoglycemia
- Occult malignant disease
- Substance abuse
- Systemic disorders: chronic renal failure, chronic obstructive pulmonary disease, cardiovascular disease, anemia, electrolyte abnormalities, liver disease
- Other: inadequate rest, sleep apnea, narcolepsy, fibromyalgia, sarcoidosis, medications, toxic agent exposure, Wegener's granulomatosis

LABORATORY TESTS
- No specific laboratory tests exist for diagnosing CFS. Initial laboratory tests are useful to exclude other conditions that may mimic or may be associated with CFS.
  1. Screening laboratory tests: CBC, ESR, ALT, total protein, albumin, globulin, alkaline phosphatase, calcium, phosphorus, glucose, BUN, creatinine, electrolytes, TSH, and urinalysis are useful.
  2. Serologic tests for Epstein-Barr virus, *Candida albicans,* human herpesvirus 6, and other studies for immune cellular abnormalities are not useful; these tests are expensive and generally not recommended.
- Other tests may be indicated depending on the history and physical examination (e.g., ANA, RF in patients presenting with joint complaints or abnormalities on physical examination, Lyme titer in areas where Lyme disease is endemic).

IMAGING STUDIES

Generally not recommended unless history and physical examination indicate specific abnormalities (e.g., chest radiography in any patient suspected of TB or sarcoidosis)

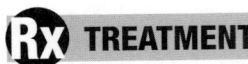 TREATMENT

NONPHARMACOLOGIC THERAPY
- Patients should be reassured that the illness is not fatal and that most patients improve over time.
- An initially supervised exercise program to preserve and increase strength is beneficial for most patients and can improve symptoms.

GENERAL Rx

Therapy is generally palliative. The following medications may be helpful; however, evidence is conflicting:
- Antidepressants: The choice of antidepressant varies with the desired side effects. Patients with difficulty sleeping or fibromyalgia-like symptoms may benefit from low-dose tricyclics (doxepin 10 mg hs or amitriptyline 25 mg qhs). When sedation is not desirable, low-dose SSRIs (paroxetine 20 mg qd) often help alleviate fatigue and associated symptoms.
- NSAIDs can be used to relieve muscle and joint pain and headaches.

"Alternative" medications (herbs, multivitamins, nutritional supplements) are very popular with many CFS patients but are generally not very helpful.

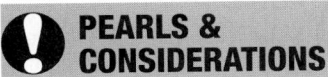

PEARLS & CONSIDERATIONS

COMMENTS
- In CFS the symptoms are serious enough to reduce daily activities by >50% in the absence of any other medically identifiable disorders.
- Moderate to complete recovery at 1 yr occurs in 22% to 60% of patients with CFS.

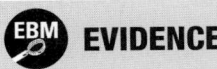 EVIDENCE

available at www.expertconsult.com

SUGGESTED READING
available at www.expertconsult.com

AUTHOR: **FRED F. FERRI, M.D.**

C

BASIC INFORMATION

DEFINITION

Symmetric proximal and distal weakness with associated sensory loss along with reduced or absent reflexes for >2 mo

SYNONYMS

Chronic inflammatory demyelinating polyneuropathy

Chronic inflammatory demyelinating polyradiculoneuropathy

ICD-9CM CODES
357.81 Chronic inflammatory demyelinating polyneuritis

EPIDEMIOLOGY & DEMOGRAPHICS

PREVALENCE: 0.5/100,000 children; 1 to 2/100,000 adults

PREDOMINANT SEX AND AGE: Slightly higher in males

RISK FACTORS: Association with certain systemic medical conditions (see under differential diagnosis below), but association is unclear

PHYSICAL FINDINGS & CLINICAL PRESENTATION

Characterized by occurrence of symmetrical weakness in both proximal and distal muscles that progressively increases over 2 mo. It is associated with impaired sensation, postural instability, reduced or absent deep-tendon reflexes, and variable craniofacial-bulbar involvement.

ETIOLOGY

Immune-mediated disorder emerging from interplay of both cell-mediated and humoral immune responses directed against incompletely characterized peripheral nerve antigens. May also be associated with various concurrent illnesses (Table 1-34), although the pathogenetic significance is unclear.

DIAGNOSIS

There is no universal consensus regarding diagnostic criteria for CIDP. The three most widely used are the American Academy of Neurology (AAN), Saperstein, and Inflammatory Neuropathy Cause and Treatment (INCAT) criteria.

- The AAN and INCAT criteria are the least stringent regarding clinical criteria and require motor and sensory function in one limb, whereas the Saperstein criteria are more stringent requiring both symmetrical proximal and distal weakness.
  - Therefore, a patient with DADS (distal acquired demyelinating symmetric neuropathy) could fulfill AAN and INCAT criteria for CIDP.
- All require cerebral spinal fluid analysis to assess for albuminocytologic dissociation.
- Nerve conduction study (NCS): All require some features of demyelination including prolonged distal latencies and F-waves, slowed velocities, and at least one nerve demonstrating partial conduction block (feature of acquired demyelination).
- INCAT criteria do not require a nerve biopsy.
- See Table 1-34 for complete review of differences.

DIFFERENTIAL DIAGNOSIS

- Other demyelinating neuropathies such as:
  - Distal acquired demyelinating symmetric neuropathy (DADS)
  - Multifocal motor neuropathy (MMN)
  - Multifocal acquired demyelinating sensory and motor neuropathy (MADSAM; Lewis-Sumner syndrome)
- Inherited neuropathies: family history, genetic testing and lack of acquired demyelinating features on NCS will help differentiate it from CIDP

- Metabolic neuropathies: diabetes, uremia
- Paraneoplastic neuropathy: associated with lymphoma or carcinoma
- Neuropathy associated with monoclonal gammopathy: associated with osteosclerotic myeloma, MGUS and Waldenstrom's macroglobulinemia.
- Neuropathy associated with infectious diseases: HIV and leprosy
- Neuropathy associated with systemic inflammatory or immune-mediated diseases:
  - Sarcoidosis
  - Amyloidosis
  - Vasculitis: PAN, Behcet's, Sjögren's, cryoglobulinemia, lupus, Castleman's disease, Wegener's, Churg-Strauss
- Toxic neuropathies: ETOH, acrylamide, drugs (platinum-based agents, amiodarone, tacrolimus, perhexilene)

WORKUP

Nerve conduction studies and EMG to assess for demyelinating polyneuropathy with features of acquired demyelination (temporal dispersion and conduction block (Fig. 1-91)

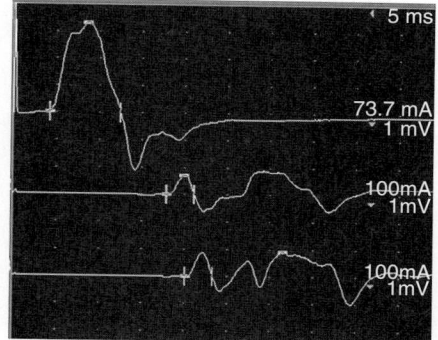

FIGURE 1-91 Conduction block.

TABLE 1-34 Diagnostic Criteria

Feature	AAN (American Academy of Neurology) Criteria	Saperstein Criteria	INCAT (Inflammatory Neuropathy Cause and Treatment) Criteria
Clinical involvement	Motor dysfunction, sensory dysfunction of >1 limb or both	Major: Symmetric proximal and distal weakness; minor: exclusively symmetrical distal weakness or sensory loss	Progressive or relapsing motor and sensory dysfunction of >1 limb
Time course	≥2 mo	≥2 mo	≥2 mo
Reflexes	Reduced or absent	Reduced or absent	Reduced or absent
Electrodiagnostics	Any 3 of the following 4 criteria: partial conduction block (CB) of ≥1 motor nerve, reduced velocity of ≥2 motor nerve, prolonged distal latency of ≥2 motor nerves, or prolonged F-waves of ≥2 motor nerves	2 of the 4 AAN electrodiagnostic criteria	Partial conduction block of ≥2 motor nerves and abnormal conduction velocity or distal Latency or F-wave latency in 1 other nerve; or, in the absence of partial conduction block, abnormal conduction velocity, distal latency, or F-wave latency in 3 motor nerves; or electrodiagnostic abnormalities indicating demyelination in 2 nerves and histologic evidence of demyelination
CSF analysis	WBC count <10, negative CSF VDRL, and elevated protein (supportive)	Protein >45, WBC <10 (supportive)	CSF recommended but not mandatory
Biopsy findings	Evidence of demyelination and remyelination	Predominant features of demyelination; inflammation (not required)	Not mandatory (except in cases with electrodiagnostic abnormalities in only 2 motor nerves)

LABORATORY TESTS

- CSF analysis to assess for albumin-cytologic dissociation (i.e., elevated protein with normal cell count), along with appropriate laboratory studies to exclude associated conditions.
- Nerve biopsy specimens (rarely done now) also reveal signs of demyelination with variable degrees of inflammation and secondary axonal loss.

IMAGING STUDIES

MRI with/without gadolinium may show enlargement and enhancement of the proximal nerve root segments, respectively (Figs. 1-92 and 1-93)

TREATMENT

Therapies are directed at blocking the underlying immune processes to arrest demyelination and inflammation and to prevent secondary axonal degeneration. The most widely used forms of immunomodulatory therapy are IV immunoglobulin (IVIg), plasmapheresis/plasma exchange (PE), and corticosteroids. There is no difference in efficacy between these three modalities of treatment. Azathioprine, myocophenylate mofetil, cyclophosphamide, Rituximab, and cyclosporine may be used as secondary agents.

NONPHARMACOLOGIC THERAPY

Orthotics/braces for significant distal weakness

ACUTE GENERAL Rx

IVIg 2 g/kg divided over 2 to 5 days; plasmapheresis (5 to 6 exchanges)

CHRONIC Rx

- Oral prednisone (1 mg/kg daily starting dose). Typically changed to every other day after 1 mo or when strength plateaus. Reduce by 10 mg every month until 20 mg every other day. Then reduce by 5 mg/mo. Get tuberculin skin test prior to administration. Treat with calcium and vitamin D; low-sodium/high-protein diet, routine ophthalmologic evaluation for cataract and glaucoma screening, and surveillance for diabetes and GERD symptoms/signs.
- IVIg: 0.4 to 1 g/kg administered monthly. Check baseline IgA level. Check renal function panel and survey for hypercoagulable states and development of headache.
- Mycophenylate mofetil: Start 500 mg bid and increase in 2 to 4 wk to 1 g bid (check CBC, LFTs, and CBC monthly for first 3 mo, then every 3 mo thereafter). May cause GI upset.
- Imuran: Start 25 to 50 mg bid and increase in 4 wk to 100 mg bid (check baseline LFTs and CBC for first 3 mo, then every 3 mo thereafter). Watch for idiosyncratic reaction of fever, GI upset. If occurs, cannot re-challenge patient.

DISPOSITION

- In one series, 90% of patients with CIDP improved. However, relapse rate was approximately 50%. In Mayo Clinic series, 64% of the patients were either improved or in remission and able to work. 8% were ambulatory but unable to work, 11% were bedridden or wheelchair bound, and 11% died from the disease.
- Patients with CIDP associated with IgM monoclonal gammopathy often respond poorly to treatment.
- Younger age, female gender, and relapsing-remitting course may portend a more favorable prognosis.

REFERRAL

- Neurologist, physical therapy/occupational therapy, orthotics

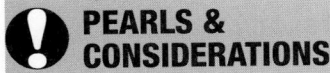 PEARLS & CONSIDERATIONS

- Patients are compliant with Imuran treatment if MCV > 100.
- Always place PPD prior to initiation of steroid treatment.
- Consider Bactrim 3 times weekly in patients concomitant with steroids and other immunosuppressant agent for *Pneumocystis* pneumonia prophylaxis (especially in patients with coexisting lung disease).
- NCS: Look for acquired features of demyelination
  - Conduction block
  - Temporal dispersion
- CSF: Albuminocytological dissociation; high CSF protein with normal cell count.

PATIENT/FAMILY EDUCATION

CIDP is a chronic illness usually characterized by a relapsing-remitting course that typically responds well to treatment. Early referral to a neurologist is important, and education on steroid side effects and mitigating factors is paramount.

EVIDENCE

available at www.expertconsult.com

SUGGESTED READINGS

available at www.expertconsult.com

AUTHOR: **JOHN SLADKY, M.D.**

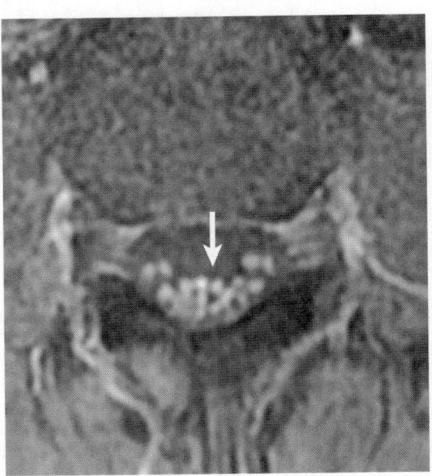

FIGURE 1-92 Contrast-enhanced MRI shows enhancement of nerve roots.

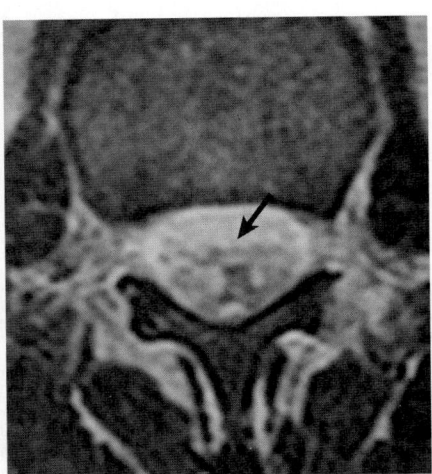

FIGURE 1-93 T2-weighted axial MRI shows enlarged nerve roots.

BASIC INFORMATION

DEFINITION

- Chronic obstructive pulmonary disease (COPD) is an inflammatory respiratory disease caused by exposure to tobacco smoke. It is characterized by the presence of airflow limitation that is not fully reversible. The pathophysiology of COPD is related to chronic airway irritation, mucus production, and pulmonary scarring. Traditionally, COPD was described as encompassing *emphysema,* characterized by loss of lung elasticity and destruction of lung parenchyma with enlargement of air spaces, and *chronic bronchitis,* characterized by obstruction of small airways and productive cough >3 mo for more than 2 successive yr. These terms are no longer included in the formal definition of COPD, although they are still used clinically.
- Patients with COPD have also been classically subdivided in two major groups based on their appearance:
  1. *Blue bloaters* are patients with chronic bronchitis; the name is derived from the bluish tinge of the skin (as a result of chronic hypoxemia and hypercapnia) and from the frequent presence of peripheral edema (from cor pulmonale); chronic cough with production of large amounts of sputum is characteristic.
  2. *Pink puffers* are patients with emphysema; they have a cachectic appearance but pink skin color (adequate oxygen saturation); shortness of breath is manifested by pursed-lip breathing and use of accessory muscles of respiration.

SYNONYMS

COPD
Emphysema
Chronic bronchitis

ICD-9CM CODES
496   COPD
492.8 Emphysema

EPIDEMIOLOGY & DEMOGRAPHICS

- COPD affects 16 million Americans and is responsible for >80,000 deaths annually.
- COPD is the fourth leading cause of death in the U.S. and is expected to become the third leading cause of death by 2020.
- Highest incidence is in males >40 yr.
- 16 million office visits, 500,000 hospitalizations, 120,000 deaths annually, and >$18 billion in direct health care costs annually can be attributed to COPD.

PHYSICAL FINDINGS & CLINICAL PRESENTATION

- Cyanosis, chronic cough (usually productive but may be intermittent and may be unproductive), tachypnea, tachycardia.
- Dyspnea (persistent, progressive), pursed-lip breathing with use of accessory muscles for respiration, decreased breath sounds, wheezing.
- Chronic sputum production.
- Chest wall abnormalities (hyperinflation, "barrel chest," protruding abdomen).
- Flattening of diaphragm.
- Acute exacerbation of COPD is mainly a clinical diagnosis and generally manifests with worsening dyspnea, increase in sputum purulence, and increase in sputum volume.

ETIOLOGY

- Tobacco exposure
- Occupational exposure to pulmonary toxins (e.g., dust, noxious gases, vapors, fumes, cadmium, coal, silica). The industries with the highest exposure risk are plastics, leather, rubber, and textiles.
- Atmospheric pollution.
- Alpha-1-antitrypsin deficiency (rare; <1% of COPD patients).

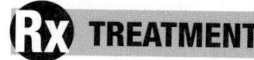

DIAGNOSIS

DIFFERENTIAL DIAGNOSIS

- Congestive heart failure
- Asthma
- Tuberculosis, other respiratory infections
- Bronchiectasis
- Cystic fibrosis
- Neoplasm
- Pulmonary embolism
- Obliterative bronchiolitis
- Diffuse panbronchiolitis
- Sleep apnea, obstructive
- Hypothyroidism <50% predicted

WORKUP

Chest x-ray (seldom diagnostic but useful to exclude alternative diagnosis [CHF, TB]), pulmonary function testing (spirometry), oxygen saturation, blood gases (in selected patients with $FEV_1 < 50\%$ predicted or with acute exacerbation). Alpha-1-antitrypsin deficiency screening may be useful in Caucasians.

LABORATORY TESTS

- CBC: may reveal leukocytosis with left shift during acute exacerbation.
- Sputum may be purulent with bacterial respiratory tract infections. Sputum staining and cultures are usually reserved for cases refractory to antibiotic therapy.
- Arterial blood gases: normocapnia, mild to moderate hypoxemia may be present.
- Spirometry pulmonary function testing (PFT) with measurement of forced vital capacity (FVC) and forced expiratory volume in 1 s (FEV_1). Spirometry reveals that the primary physiologic abnormality in COPD is an accelerated decline in FEV_1 from the normal rate in adults >30 yr of approximately 30 ml/yr to nearly 60 ml/yr. PFT results in COPD reveal abnormal diffusing capacity, increased total lung capacity and/or residual volume, and fixed reduction in FEV_1 in patients with emphysema; normal diffusing capacity and reduced FEV_1 are found in patients with chronic bronchitis. PFTs can be used to estimate disease severity in COPD as follows (where FEV is forced vital capacity):
  - Mild COPD: $FEV_1/FVC < 0.70$; $FEV_1 \geq 80\%$ of predicted
  - Moderate COPD: $FEV_1/FVC < 0.70$; FEV_1 50% to 79% of predicted
  - Severe COPD: $FEV_1/FVC < 0.70$; FEV_1 30% to 49% of predicted
  - Very severe COPD $FEV_1/FVC < 0.70$; $FEV_1 < 30\%$ of predicted or < 50% of predicted with chronic respiratory failure ($SaO_2 < 88\%$)
- Patients with COPD can generally be distinguished from asthmatics by their incomplete response to albuterol (change in FEV_1 <200 ml and 12%) and absence of an abnormal bronchoconstrictor response to methacholine or other stimuli. However, nearly 40% of patients with COPD respond to bronchodilators.

IMAGING STUDIES

Chest x-ray:
- Hyperinflation with flattened diaphragm, tenting of the diaphragm at the rib, and increased retrosternal chest space (Fig. 1-94)
- Decreased vascular markings and bullae in patients with emphysema
- Thickened bronchial markings and enlarged right side of the heart in patients with chronic bronchitis

TREATMENT

NONPHARMACOLOGIC THERAPY

- Weight loss in obese patients.
- Avoidance of tobacco and elimination of air pollutants.

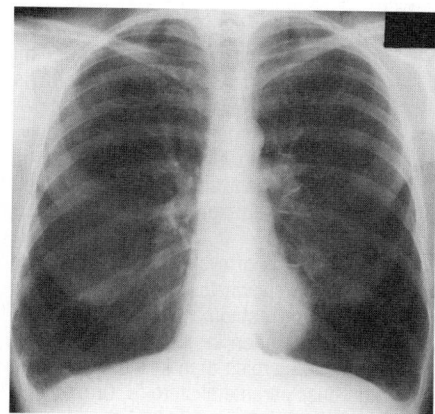

FIGURE 1-94 Severe diffuse emphysema. The posteroanterior chest radiograph shows the right hemidiaphragm to be flattened and located below the anterior aspect of the eighth rib. Left lung parenchyma is seen between the heart and the left hemidiaphragm. Arterial depletion is present in the lung bases. (From Grainger RG et al [eds]: *Grainger & Allison's diagnostic radiology,* ed 4, Philadelphia, 2001, Churchill Livingstone.)

- Supplemental oxygen, usually through a face mask, to ensure oxygen saturation >90% as measured by pulse oximetry.
- Pulmonary clearing: careful nasotracheal suction is indicated only in patients with excessive secretions and an inability to expectorate. Mechanical percussion of the chest as applied by a physical or respiratory therapist is ineffective with acute exacerbations of COPD.
- Pulmonary rehabilitation should be considered in COPD patients who remain symptomatic despite optimal medical management. Medicare will cover up to 36 sessions of pulmonary rehabilitation in COPD patients.

GENERAL Rx

- Pharmacologic treatment should be administered in a stepwise approach according to the severity of disease and patient's tolerance for specific drugs.
  - Bronchodilators improve symptoms, quality of life, and exercise tolerance, and decrease incidence of exacerbations.
  - Short-acting beta-2 agonists (e.g., albuterol metered-dose inhaler 1 to 2 puffs q4 to 6h prn) or short-acting anticholinergic agents (e.g., ipratropium inhaler 2 puffs qid) are acceptable in patients with mild, variable symptoms. Anticholinergics are also effective and are available in combination with albuterol (Combivent). Long-acting inhaled agents are preferred in patients with mild to moderate or continuous symptoms. Tiotropium (Spiriva handihaler) is an excellent long-acting bronchodilator. It is very effective for long-term, once-a-day use.
  - Addition of inhaled steroids (fluticasone, budesonide, triamcinolone) is used to reduce exacerbations in patients with moderate to severe COPD.
- Acute exacerbation of COPD can be treated with:
  - Aerosolized beta-2 agonists (e.g., metaproterenol nebulizer solution 5% 0.3 ml or albuterol nebulized 5% solution 2.5 to 5 mg).
  - Anticholinergic agents, which have equivalent efficacy to inhaled beta-adrenergic agonists. Inhalant solution of ipratropium bromide 0.5 mg can be administered every 4 to 8 hr.
  - Short courses of systemic corticosteroids have been shown to improve spirometric and clinical outcomes. Treatment failure occurs less often in patients who receive low-dose steroids than in those receiving high-dose parenteral steroids. Oral prednisone 40 mg/day for 10 to 14 days is generally effective. Courses of treatment that are extended for >14 days confer no added benefit and increase the risk of adverse events.
  - Use of noninvasive positive pressure ventilation (NIPPV) decreases the risk of endotracheal intubation and decreases intensive care unit admission rates. Contraindications

to its use are uncooperative patient, decreased level of consciousness, hemodynamic instability, inadequate mask fit, and severe respiratory acidosis. Increased airway pressure can be delivered by using inspiratory positive airway pressure, continuous positive airway pressure, or bilevel positive airway pressure, which combines the other modalities. When using NIPPV, the nasal mask is usually tolerated the best; however, patients must be instructed to keep their mouths closed while breathing with the nasal apparatus. Oxygen can be delivered at 10 to 15 L/min and started in spontaneous ventilation mode with an initial expiratory positive airway pressure setting of 3 to 5 cm H_2O and an inspiratory positive airway pressure setting of up to 10 cm H_2O. Adjustments in these settings should be made in 2-cm H_2O increments. It is important to monitor patients with frequent vital signs measurements, arterial blood gases, or pulse oximetry. Intubation and mechanical ventilation may be necessary if previous measures fail to provide improvement.
  - The role of inhaled corticosteroids (ICS) in COPD is controversial. Although some trials have demonstrated mild improvement in patients' symptoms and decreased frequency of exacerbations, most pulmonologists believe that these drugs are ineffective in most patients with COPD but should be considered for patients with moderate to severe airflow limitation who have persistent symptoms despite optimal bronchodilator therapy. ICS therapy does not affect 1-yr all-cause mortality among patients with COPD and is associated with a higher risk of pneumonia.
  - IV aminophylline administration is controversial and generally not recommended. When used, serum levels should be closely monitored (keep level 8 to 12 mcg/ml) to minimize risks of tachyarrhythmias.
- Approximately 50% of COPD exacerbations are caused by bacterial infection. Antibiotics are indicated in suspected respiratory infection (e.g., increased purulence and volume of phlegm).
  - *Haemophilus influenzae* and *Streptococcus pneumoniae* are frequent causes of acute bronchitis.
  - Oral antibiotics of choice are azithromycin, levofloxacin, amoxicillin-clavulanate, trimethoprim-sulfamethoxazole, doxycycline, and cefuroxime.
  - The use of antibiotics is beneficial in exacerbations of COPD presenting with increased dyspnea and sputum purulence (especially if the patient is febrile).
- Guaifenesin may improve cough symptoms and mucus clearance; however, mucolytic medications are generally ineffective. Their benefits may be greatest in patients with more advanced disease.
- Lung volume reduction surgery has been proposed as a palliative treatment for severe

emphysema. Overall it increases the chance of improved exercise capacity but does not confer a survival advantage over medical therapy. It is most beneficial in patients with both predominantly upper-lobe emphysema and low baseline exercise capacity.
- In patients with end-stage emphysema who have an FEV1 <25% of predicted normal value after administration of bronchodilator and additional complications such as severe hypoxemia, hypercapnia and pulmonary hypertension single-lung transplantation should be considered a surgical option.
- Trials involving endobronchial valves that allow air to escape from a pulmonary lobe but not to enter it have been done to improve lung function by reducing lobar volume in patients with advanced heterogeneous emphysema. Results have shown modest improvements in lung function, symptoms, and exercise tolerance, but more frequent exacerbations of COPD. Other complications included pneumonia and hemoptysis postimplantation.

DISPOSITION

- After the initial episode of respiratory failure, 5-yr survival is approximately 25%.
- Development of cor pulmonale or hypercapnia and persistent tachycardia are poor prognostic indicators.

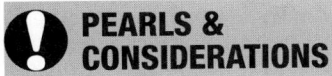

PEARLS & CONSIDERATIONS

COMMENTS

- All patients with COPD should receive pneumococcal vaccine and yearly influenza vaccine.
- Early antibiotic administration is associated with improved outcomes among patients hospitalized for acute exacerbations of COPD regardless of the risk of treatment failure.
- In assessing the severity of COPD, the FEV_1 is limited by the fact that it does not take into account the systemic manifestations of COPD. The BODE index (*b*ody mass index, degree of *o*bstruction, *d*yspnea, and *e*xercise capacity) has been proposed as a multidimensional scale to better assess the morbidity and mortality associated with COPD. It is better than the FEV_1 at predicting the risk of death from any cause and from respiratory causes among patients with COPD.

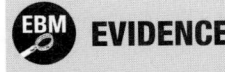

EVIDENCE

available at www.expertconsult.com

SUGGESTED READINGS

available at www.expertconsult.com

AUTHOR: **FRED F. FERRI, M.D.**

BASIC INFORMATION

DEFINITION

Chronic pain is pain that persists for longer than the expected time frame or that is associated with progressive, nonmalignant disease. Pain is an unpleasant sensory and emotional experience associated with actual or potential tissue damage or described in terms of such damage. The perception of pain is influenced by physiologic, psychological, and social factors.

SYNONYMS

Nonmalignant chronic pain

ICD-9CM CODES	
338.29	Chronic Pain
338.4	Chronic Pain Syndrome
780.96	Generalized Pain
304.7x/304.8x	Opioid Dependence

EPIDEMIOLOGY & DEMOGRAPHICS

Estimates of the prevalence of chronic pain in the United States vary widely. Data from one national survey (1999–2002 National Health and Nutrition Examination Survey [NHANES]) reported a prevalence of chronic regional and widespread pain of 11% and 3.6%, respectively, while the National Center for Health Statistics estimates that 32.8% of the U.S. population suffers from some form of chronic pain. Chronic pain is the third leading cause of physical impairment in the U.S., and related costs are estimated to be tens of billions annually. Patients with chronic pain may also experience changes in mood, depression, sleep disturbances, and fatigue, and decreased overall physical functioning.

CLINICAL PRESENTATION

- History: Comprehensive patient assessment, including history of present illness (cause of pain, location timing, characteristics, exacerbating/relieving factors, triggers, past therapies (pharmacologic and nonpharmacologic and outcomes of these therapies), medical history, family and social history, psychiatric history, substance use history, allergies, and current medications, should be performed on initial evaluation.
- Pain assessment should be performed at each visit; includes pain intensity (1 to 10), response to medication, attributes of pain, and assessment of function (cognitive, emotional, employment, sleep, mobility, and self-care). Standardized templates for both initial and follow-up pain assessment have been developed by various organizations. The website Pain Treatment Topics contains many of these assessment tools (http://pain-topics.org/clinical_concepts/assess.php).
- Physical examination: Directed at systems affected by pain and neurologic examination.

ETIOLOGY

Chronic pain can generally be categorized as originating from one of five etiologies: musculo-skeletal, neuropathic, inflammatory, mechanical, or mixed. Chronic pain may include such diagnoses as headache, low back pain, previous trauma, arthritis, neurogenic (e.g., trigeminal neuralgia), psychogenic (related to depression or anxiety), fibromyalgia, reflex sympathetic dystrophy, myofascial pain syndrome, phantom limb pain, idiopathic, or unknown.

DIAGNOSIS

DIFFERENTIAL DIAGNOSIS

- Based on proposed etiology.
- Depression and anxiety disorders can be both a cause and a result of chronic pain, so temporal association of these disorders is important.

WORKUP

- Laboratory testing, imaging studies, and/or electromyographic studies should be used when etiology of chronic pain is unknown or unclear, when comorbidities are suspected, and as the history and physical examination direct.
- Consider use of random urine drug screens or other tests to screen for presence of illegal drugs, unreported prescribed medications, or alcohol use.

TREATMENT

- Studies increasingly support the application of a multidisciplinary approach that ad-dresses the multiple facets of pain (e.g., physical, psychologic, social aspects).
- Therapeutic goal is the reduction of pain (elimination of chronic pain is generally unlikely and providers need to discuss these limitations with patients at outset).

NONPHARMACOLOGIC THERAPY

- Exercise
- Modalities: heat therapy, cold therapy, transcutaneous electrical nerve stimulation (TENS) units, cognitive behavioral therapy, psychological counseling, and physical therapy
- Electrostimulation therapy: TENS units
- Behavioral therapies: cognitive behavioral therapy, hypnosis, biofeedback, relaxation therapy
- Music therapy (in conjunction with other types of therapy)
- Surgery

ACUTE GENERAL Rx

- Short-acting anti-inflammatory and analgesic medications (e.g., acetaminophen/NSAIDs/opioids)
- Trigger point or joint injections (immediate anesthetic plus long-acting corticosteroids)
- Epidural steroid injections
- Nerve blocks

CHRONIC Rx

- Pain management with long-acting pharmacologic agents is considered a key aspect of therapy but is often underused. Fig. 1-95 illustrates a strategy for pharmacologic man-

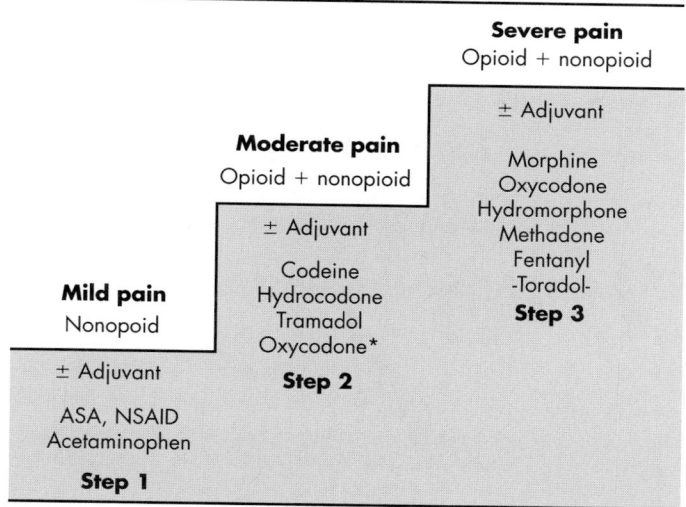

WHO ANALGESIC LADDER

Severe pain
Opioid + nonopioid

± Adjuvant

Morphine
Oxycodone
Hydromorphone
Methadone
Fentanyl
-Toradol-

Step 3

Moderate pain
Opioid + nonopioid

± Adjuvant

Codeine
Hydrocodone
Tramadol
Oxycodone*

Step 2

Mild pain
Nonopoid

± Adjuvant

ASA, NSAID
Acetaminophen

Step 1

• Advance up the ladder if pain persists

FIGURE 1-95 Strategy for pharmacologic management of pain using the World Health Organization (WHO) analgesic ladder. Multiagent therapy is usually required for optimal pain management. Patients with mild pain should be started on a nonopioid analgesic, and those with moderate pain on a step 2 opioid. Many patients can benefit from the addition of a nonopioid to the opioid (e.g., for bone pain) or an adjuvant agent to the opioid (e.g., for neuropathic pain). If this combination does not produce adequate relief or the patient has severe pain, step 3 opioids should be started initially. Toradol (Ketorolac) is a nonsteroidal anti-inflammatory drug (NSAID) with the pain-relieving potency of a step 3 opioid. Many patients can benefit from the addition of nonopioid analgesics or adjuvants, if indicated. *ASA*, Aspirin. (From Hoffman R et al: *Hematology, basic principles and practice*, ed 5, Philadelphia, 2009, Churchill Livingstone.)

agement of pain using the World Health Organization (WHO) analgesic ladder.

- Long-acting NSAIDs.
- Sustained-release opioids (used for moderate to severe pain that has failed other therapeutic interventions) oxycodone, morphine SR, methadone (use with caution), or Duragesic patch; short-acting opioids can be used in conjunction with these agents for management of breakthrough pain. Conversion to a long-acting opioid should be based on an equianalgesic conversion (http://www.acpinternist.org/archives/2008/01/extra/pain_charts.pdf).
- Antidepressants (tricyclic and selective serotonin reuptake inhibitor).
- Anticonvulsant medications particularly helpful for neuropathic conditions (e.g., carbamazepine, valproic acid, gabapentin, pregabalin).
- Implantable methods epidural and intrathecal drug delivery systems, dorsal column stimulators.

COMPLEMENTARY & ALTERNATIVE MEDICINE

Acupuncture and massage (evidence based for some indications). Acupuncture is most likely to benefit patients with low back pain, neck pain, chronic idiopathic or tension headache, migraine, and knee osteoarthritis.

REFERRAL

- Pain medicine specialist or multidisciplinary pain clinic: useful when primary therapies fail, in patients with complex pain conditions, or for invasive therapies

- Consider referral to an addiction specialist if patient has a history of substance abuse or addiction
- Psychiatry/psychologic services for counseling, if needed

PEARLS & CONSIDERATIONS

- Patient consent should be obtained in the form of a written treatment agreement before initiating treatment. This agreement should outline the goals of therapy, use of a single provider or treatment team and a single pharmacy, limitations on dose and number of prescribed medications, prohibition on use with alcohol or sedating medications, keeping medication safe and secure, prohibition on selling or sharing medication, limitations on refills, compliance with all components of the treatment plan, the role of drug screening, and consequences of nonadherence.
- Follow-up assessment should occur every 1 to 6 mo and include a complete pain assessment (see earlier), review of the type of long-acting analgesic used and dosage, use of breakthrough analgesics, side effects and their management, use of nonpharmacologic therapies, and adjunct medication use.

COMMENTS

- Medication dependence and addiction should not be confused. Most patients receiving

chronic opioid therapy can become dependent on these medications for pain relief but opioid addiction does not occur. Patients exhibiting signs of addiction often will seek escalating doses of medication, request refills of prescriptions earlier than planned, and engage in drug-seeking activities (e.g., emergency department visits between prescriptions, seeking multiple prescriptions).

- Side effects need not preclude use of opioid medications and should be anticipated. Antiemetics can aid in controlling nausea. Constipation can be managed with stool softeners and laxatives.

PATIENT/FAMILY EDUCATION

National Pain Foundation
(http://www.painconnection.org)
American Pain Foundation
(http://www.painfoundation.org)
National Institutes of Health
(http://www.nih.gov)

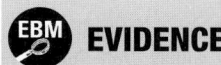

EVIDENCE

available at www.expertconsult.com

SUGGESTED READINGS

available at www.expertconsult.com

AUTHOR: **ANNGENE A. GIUSTOZZI, M.D., M.P.H., F.A.A.F.P.**

BASIC INFORMATION

DEFINITION

Churg-Strauss syndrome (CSS) refers to a systemic granulomatous vasculitis accompanied by severe asthma (core clinical feature) and hypereosinophilia (HES).

SYNONYMS

Allergic angiitis
Allergic granulomatosis

ICD-9CM CODES
446.4 Angiitis, allergic granulomatous

EPIDEMIOLOGY & DEMOGRAPHICS

- Overall incidence of 2.4 cases per 1 million persons in the U.S. Among asthma patients, the annual incidence of CSS is estimated to average 34.6 per 1 million patients.
- Usually occurs at a mean age of 50 yr but may present as young as 4 yr or in the elderly
- Slight male/female predominance (1.3:1).
- With treatment, 1-year survival is approximately 90% and 5-year survival is 62%.

PHYSICAL FINDINGS & CLINICAL PRESENTATION

The clinical picture of CSS typically consists of three partially overlapping phases, which may or may not be sequential:
1. Prodromal phase:
   - Severe adult-onset asthma, with or without allergic rhinitis, sinusitis, headache, cough, and wheezing
   - Precedes development of systemic vasculitis by several years
2. Eosinophilic/tissue infiltration phase:
   - Peripheral eosinophilia and eosinophilic infiltration of the lungs, myocardium, and gastrointestinal (GI) tract, with or without granulomas
   - Signs and symptoms of cough, fever, anorexia, weight loss, sweats, malaise, nausea, vomiting, abdominal pain, and diarrhea
3. Systemic vasculitic phase:
   - Development of necrotizing vasculitis that is clinically apparent primarily in peripheral nerves, skin, and kidneys
   - Any organ can be affected, with skin involvement present in 50% to 67% of patients

Skin involvement is divided into three categories:
1. Erythematous maculopapules (can resemble erythema multiforme)
2. Hemorrhagic lesions (associated with wheals)
3. Cutaneous and subcutaneous nodules

ETIOLOGY

- Etiology unknown, but believed to be an autoimmune-mediated process
- Triggering factors implicated in CSS include inhaled allergens, vaccinations, infections, and drugs such as macrolides (see "Comments").

DIAGNOSIS

- Clinical findings and biopsy showing eosinophilic vasculitis
- The American College of Rheumatology (ACR) has established the criteria for CSS diagnosis in patients without vasculitis:
  - Asthma
  - Eosinophilia >10% of white blood cell count
  - Mononeuropathy or polyneuropathy
  - Migratory pulmonary infiltrates
  - Paranasal sinus abnormalities
  - Extravascular eosinophils on biopsy

The presence of any four or more of the six criteria yields a sensitivity of 85% and a specificity of 99.7%. For patients with vasculitis, the presence of asthma and eosinophilia was 90% sensitive and 99% specific for CSS.

DIFFERENTIAL DIAGNOSIS

- Polyarteritis nodosa (PAN)
- Wegener's granulomatosis (WG)
- Goodpasture syndrome
- Loeffler syndrome
- Hypereosinophilia syndrome
- Rheumatoid arthritis
- Leukocytoclastic vasculitis

Although similar and at times grouped with patients with PAN or WG, CSS differs in that:
- CSS vasculitis involves small-sized arteries, veins, and venules
- CSS, unlike PAN, predominantly involves the lung. Other organs affected include heart, GI system, central nervous system, kidney, and skin
- Kidney involvement is much less common in CSS than in WG. Pulmonary lesions in WG usually involve the upper respiratory tract rather than the peripheral lung parenchyma in CSS
- CSS shows necrotizing vasculitis along with eosinophilic granulomas

LABORATORY TESTS

- Complete blood count with differential: eosinophilia >10% is an American College of Rheumatology (ACR) diagnostic criterion
- Blood urea nitrogen and creatinine may be mildly elevated, suggesting renal involvement
- Urinalysis may show mild hematuria and proteinuria.
- 24-hour urine for protein; greater than 1 g/day is a poor prognostic factor
- Perinuclear antineutrophilic cytoplasmic antibody (ANCA) is found in 13% to 70% of patients. Negative ANCA does not rule out CSS
- Stools may be positive for occult blood (enteric involvement during eosinophilic phase)
- Elevation of aspartate aminotransferase, alanine aminotransferase, and creatine phosphokinase may indicate liver or muscle (skeletal or cardiac) involvement
- Rheumatoid factor and antinuclear antibody may be positive. Erythrocyte sedimentation rate is usually elevated
- Biopsy helps confirm the diagnosis. Surgical lung biopsy is the gold standard. Transbronchial biopsy is rarely helpful. Necrotizing vasculitis and extravascular necrotizing granulomas, usually with eosinophilic infiltrates, are suggestive of CSS. The presence of eosinophils in extravascular tissues is most specific for CSS

IMAGING STUDIES

- Chest radiograph is abnormal in eosinophilic and vasculitic phases: asymmetrical bilateral patchy migratory infiltrates, interstitial lung disease, or nodular infiltrates (Fig. 1-96). Small pleural effusions are found in 29% of cases
- Lung lesions in CSS are noncavitating, as opposed to those in WG
- Paranasal sinus films may reveal sinus opacification, which is an ACR diagnostic criterion
- Angiography is sometimes done in patients with mesenteric ischemia or renal involvement

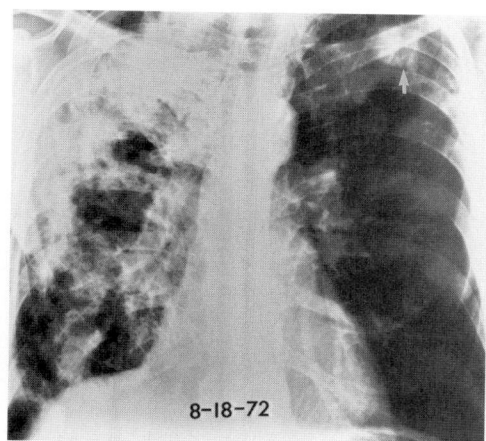

FIGURE 1-96 Allergic angiitis and granulomatosis. Posteroanterior chest radiograph demonstrates peripheral air space consolidation in the right lung and a nodule *(arrow)* in the left upper lobe in this asthmatic patient. (From McLoud TC [ed]: *Thoracic radiology: the requisites,* St Louis, 1998, Mosby.)

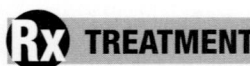 **TREATMENT**

NONPHARMACOLOGIC THERAPY

Oxygen therapy in severe asthmatic exacerbations

PHARMACOLOGIC THERAPY

The following five factors suggest poor prognosis (five-factor score) and determine the aggressiveness of the immune suppressive therapy:
1. Proteinuria >1 g/day
2. Creatinine >1.58 mg/dl
3. Cardiomyopathy
4. GI tract involvement
5. Central nervous system involvement

ACUTE GENERAL Rx

- Corticosteroids are the treatment of choice if no poor prognostic factors are present. Prednisone 1 mg/kg/day is the starting dose and is continued for 6 to 12 wk and then tapered to 10 mg/day at 1 yr as clinical disease resolves. Response to steroids may be dramatic. Patients with extensive disease may require IV corticosteroids.
- A drop in the patient's eosinophil count and the erythrocyte sedimentation rate indicates a response to treatment. ANCA does not reliably correspond with disease activity.

CHRONIC Rx

- In patients with one or more poor prognostic factors, immunosuppressant agents (cyclophosphamide 1 to 2 mg/kg/day) are used with corticosteroids as first-line therapy. Limit duration of cyclophosphamide to a maximum of 6 mo.
- In patients who do not respond to corticosteroid treatment or in CSS relapse, cyclophosphamide therapy is indicated as a second-line therapy.
- Azathioprine (2 mg/kg/day) or high-dose intravenous immunoglobulin has shown benefit in patients with severe disease and in patients unresponsive to corticosteroids.

- Corticosteroids, in combination with interferon-alpha, have also been used in refractory cases but may be difficult to tolerate.
- Patients with persistent symptoms of asthma will require long-term corticosteroids even if vasculitis is no longer present.
- Maintenance therapy using methotrexate (15 to 25 mg/wk) or azathioprine (2 mg/kg/day) is an alternative to cyclophosphamide.

DISPOSITION

- Clinical remission is obtained in more than 90% of patients after treatment. Relapse is common on cessation of therapy (approximately 26%).
- 5-yr survival rate with treatment is between 60% and 90% and decreases to 50% at 7 yr. Asthma generally remains persistent, and ischemic damage to peripheral nerves can be permanent.
- The 5-yr survival rate of untreated CSS is 25%.
- Death usually occurs from progressive refractory vasculitis, myocardial involvement (approximately 50% of deaths), or severe GI involvement (mesenteric ischemia, pancreatitis).

REFERRAL

- A pulmonary referral for diagnosis and management is appropriate.
- Patients should be followed up closely by rheumatology. Patients usually need long-term immunosuppressive medications.

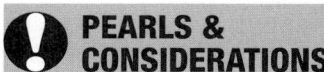 **PEARLS & CONSIDERATIONS**

COMMENTS

- CSS is a rare disease that is less common than other ANCA-associated vasculitides
- CSS is distinguished from other vasculitides by the nearly universal presence of adult-onset asthma that typically precedes all other symptoms. Family history is often negative for allergies or asthma
- Up to 77% of patients in the prodromal phase of CSS require oral steroids for asthma control
- Patients often have constitutional symptoms of weight loss, fever, and malaise before specific organ involvement is clinically evident
- Peripheral nerve involvement from vasculitis of the vasa vasorum commonly manifests as mononeuritis multiplex. Patients may present with sudden foot or wrist drop, along with sensory deficits in the distribution of one or more distal nerves
- Most patients with GI involvement are symptomatic. Gastroenteritis, acute abdomen, cholecystitis, hemorrhage, bowel perforation, and mesenteric ischemia have all been reported in patients with CSS
- Most patients with CSS respond to corticosteroid treatment and do not require cytotoxic therapy
- Symptoms of CSS typically appear as oral corticosteroids are being decreased or discontinued for the treatment of asthma and not triggered by leukotriene receptor-1 antagonists, as previously reported
- Compared to WG, patients more often present with history of atopy, asthma, or allergic rhinitis. When present, eosinophilia in CSS is often >1000 eosinophils/mm^3 compared with WG, where eosinophilia is much milder (<500 eosinophils/mm^3)
- The heart is involved in up to 60% of patients with CSS and represents a major cause of mortality

SUGGESTED READINGS
available at www.expertconsult.com

AUTHORS: **KACHIU LEE, B.A.,** and **JESSICA RISSER, M.D., M.P.H.**

BASIC INFORMATION

DEFINITION

Cirrhosis is defined histologically as the presence of fibrosis and regenerative nodules in the liver. It can be classified as micronodular, macronodular, or mixed; however, each form may be seen in the same patient at different stages of the disease. Cirrhosis manifests clinically with portal hypertension, hepatic encephalopathy, and variceal bleeding.

ICD-9CM CODES
571.5 Cirrhosis of the liver
571.2 Cirrhosis of the liver secondary to alcohol

EPIDEMIOLOGY & DEMOGRAPHICS

- Cirrhosis is the eleventh leading cause of death in the U.S. (9 per 100,000 persons annually).
- Alcohol abuse and viral hepatitis are the major causes of cirrhosis in the U.S.

PHYSICAL FINDINGS & CLINICAL PRESENTATION

SKIN: Jaundice, palmar erythema (alcohol abuse), spider angiomata, ecchymosis (thrombocytopenia or coagulation factor deficiency), dilated superficial periumbilical vein (caput medusae), increased pigmentation (hemochromatosis), xanthomas (primary biliary cirrhosis), and needle tracks (viral hepatitis). Cutaneous lesions often accompany cirrhosis and can be found in >40% of people with chronic alcoholism.
EYES: Kayser-Fleischer rings (corneal copper deposition seen in Wilson's disease; best diagnosed with slit lamp examination), scleral icterus
BREATH: Fetor hepaticus (musty odor of breath and urine found in cirrhosis with hepatic failure)
CHEST: Possible gynecomastia in men
ABDOMEN: Tender hepatomegaly (congestive hepatomegaly), small, nodular liver (cirrhosis), palpable, nontender gallbladder (neoplastic extrahepatic biliary obstruction), palpable spleen (portal hypertension), venous hum auscultated over periumbilical veins (portal hypertension), ascites (portal hypertension, hypoalbuminemia)
RECTAL EXAMINATION: Hemorrhoids (portal hypertension), guaiac-positive stools (alcoholic gastritis, bleeding esophageal varices, peptic ulcer disease, bleeding hemorrhoids)
GENITALIA: Testicular atrophy in males (chronic liver disease, hemochromatosis)
EXTREMITIES: Pedal edema (hypoalbuminemia, failure of right side of the heart), arthropathy (hemochromatosis)
NEUROLOGIC: Flapping tremor, asterixis (hepatic encephalopathy), choreoathetosis, dysarthria (Wilson's disease)

ETIOLOGY

- Alcohol abuse
- Secondary biliary cirrhosis, obstruction of the common bile duct (stone, stricture, pancreatitis, neoplasm, sclerosing cholangitis)
- Drugs (e.g., acetaminophen, isoniazid, methotrexate, methyldopa)
- Hepatic congestion (e.g., CHF, constrictive pericarditis, tricuspid insufficiency, thrombosis of the hepatic vein, obstruction of the vena cava)
- Primary biliary cirrhosis
- Hemochromatosis
- Chronic hepatitis B or C
- Wilson's disease
- Alpha-1-antitrypsin deficiency
- Infiltrative diseases (amyloidosis, glycogen storage diseases, hemochromatosis)
- Nutritional: jejunoileal bypass
- Others: parasitic infections (schistosomiasis), idiopathic portal hypertension, congenital hepatic fibrosis, systemic mastocytosis, autoimmune hepatitis, hepatic steatosis, inflammatory bowel disease (IBD)

DIAGNOSIS

WORKUP

In addition to an assessment of liver function, the evaluation of patients with cirrhosis should also include an assessment of renal and circulatory function. Diagnostic workup is aimed primarily at identifying the most likely cause of cirrhosis. The history is extremely important:
- Alcohol abuse: alcoholic liver disease
- History of hepatitis B (chronic active hepatitis, primary hepatic neoplasm, or hepatitis C)
- History of IBD (primary sclerosing cholangitis)
- History of pruritus, hyperlipoproteinemia, and xanthomas in a middle-aged or elderly woman (primary biliary cirrhosis)
- Impotence, diabetes mellitus, hyperpigmentation, arthritis (hemochromatosis)
- Neurologic disturbances (Wilson's disease, hepatolenticular degeneration)
- Family history of "liver disease" (hemochromatosis [positive family history in 25% of patients], alpha-1-antitrypsin deficiency)
- History of recurrent episodes of right upper quadrant pain (biliary tract disease)
- History of blood transfusions, IV drug abuse (hepatitis C)
- History of hepatotoxic drug exposure
- Coexistence of other diseases with immune or autoimmune features (immune thrombocytopenic purpura, myasthenia gravis, thyroiditis, autoimmune hepatitis)

LABORATORY TESTS

- Decreased hemoglobin and hematocrit, elevated mean corpuscular volume, increased blood urea nitrogen (BUN) and creatinine (the BUN may also be "normal" or low if the patient has severely diminished liver function), decreased sodium (dilutional hyponatremia), and decreased potassium (as a result of secondary aldosteronism or urinary losses). Evaluation of renal function should also include measurement of urinary sodium and urinary protein from 24-hr urine collection.
- Decreased glucose in a patient with liver disease, indicating severe liver damage.
- Other laboratory abnormalities:
  - Alcoholic hepatitis and cirrhosis: possible mild elevation of alanine aminotransferase (ALT) and aspartate aminotransferase (AST), usually <500 IU; AST > ALT (ratio > 2:3).
  - Extrahepatic obstruction: possible moderate elevations of ALT and AST to levels <500 IU.
  - Viral, toxic, or ischemic hepatitis: extreme elevations (>500 IU) of ALT and AST.
  - Transaminases may be normal despite significant liver disease in patients with jejunoileal bypass operations or hemochromatosis or after methotrexate administration.
  - Alkaline phosphatase elevation can occur with extrahepatic obstruction, primary biliary cirrhosis, and primary sclerosing cholangitis.
  - Serum lactate dehydrogenase is significantly elevated in metastatic disease of the liver; lesser elevations are seen with hepatitis, cirrhosis, extrahepatic obstruction, and congestive hepatomegaly.
  - Serum gamma-glutamyl transpeptidase is elevated in alcoholic liver disease and may also be elevated with cholestatic disease (primary biliary cirrhosis, primary sclerosing cholangitis).
  - Serum bilirubin may be elevated; urinary bilirubin can be present in hepatitis, hepatocellular jaundice, and biliary obstruction.
  - Serum albumin: significant liver disease results in hypoalbuminemia.
  - Prothrombin time/INR: elevation in patients with liver disease indicates severe liver damage and poor prognosis.
  - Presence of hepatitis B surface antigen implies acute or chronic hepatitis B.
  - Presence of antimitochondrial antibody suggests primary biliary cirrhosis, chronic hepatitis.
  - Elevated serum copper, decreased serum ceruloplasmin, and elevated 24-hr urine may be diagnostic of Wilson's disease.
  - Protein immunoelectrophoresis may reveal decreased α-1 globulins (alpha-1-antitrypsin deficiency), increased IgA (alcoholic cirrhosis), increased IgM (primary biliary cirrhosis), increased IgG (chronic hepatitis, cryptogenic cirrhosis).
  - An elevated serum ferritin and increased transferrin saturation are suggestive of hemochromatosis.
  - An elevated blood ammonia suggests hepatocellular dysfunction; serial values, however, are generally not useful in monitoring patients with hepatic encephalopathy because there is poor correlation between blood ammonia level and degree of hepatic encephalopathy.
  - Serum cholesterol is elevated in cholestatic disorders.
  - Antinuclear antibodies (ANA) may be found in autoimmune hepatitis.

- Alpha fetoprotein: levels >1000 pg/ml are highly suggestive of primary liver cell carcinoma.
- Hepatitis C viral testing identifies patients with chronic hepatitis C infection.
- Elevated level of serum globulin (especially gamma-globulins) and positive ANA test may occur with autoimmune hepatitis.

IMAGING STUDIES

- Ultrasonography is the procedure of choice for detecting gallstones and dilation of common bile ducts.
- CT scan is useful for detecting mass lesions in liver and pancreas, assessing hepatic fat content, identifying idiopathic hemochromatosis, diagnosing Budd-Chiari syndrome early, assessing dilation of intrahepatic bile ducts, and detecting varices and splenomegaly.
- MRI can be used to identify hemangiomas.
- Technetium-99m sulfur colloid scanning is rarely used but can be useful for diagnosing cirrhosis (there is a shift of colloid uptake to the spleen and bone marrow), identifying hepatic adenomas (cold defect is noted), and diagnosing Budd-Chiari syndrome (there is increased uptake by the caudate lobe).
- Endoscopic retrograde cholangiopancreatography can be used for diagnosing periampullary carcinoma and common duct stones; it is also useful in diagnosing primary sclerosing cholangitis.
- Percutaneous transhepatic cholangiography is useful when evaluating patients with cholestatic jaundice and dilated intrahepatic ducts by ultrasonography; presence of intrahepatic strictures and focal dilation is suggestive of primary sclerosing cholangitis.
- Percutaneous liver biopsy is useful in evaluating hepatic filling defects; diagnosing hepatocellular disease or hepatomegaly; evaluating persistently abnormal liver function tests; and diagnosing hemachromatosis, primary biliary cirrhosis, Wilson's disease, glycogen storage diseases, chronic hepatitis, autoimmune hepatitis, infiltrative diseases, alcoholic liver disease, drug-induced liver disease, and primary or secondary carcinoma.

 TREATMENT

NONPHARMACOLOGIC THERAPY

- Avoid any hepatotoxins (e.g., ethanol, acetaminophen), improve nutritional status
- Transjugular intrahepatic porto-systemic shunt (TIPS) in patients with recurrent variceal hemorrhage despite optical medical therapy. Early use of TIPS is associated with significant reductions in treatment failure and in mortality in patients with cirrhosis who are hospitalized for acute variceal bleeding and are at high risk for treatment failure.

GENERAL Rx

- Beta-blockers with or without nitrates in patients with cirrhosis and variceal hemorrhage.
- Pruritus due to liver disease may be treated with cholestyramine 4 g/day initially. Dose can be increased to 24 g/day as needed
- Remove excess body iron with phlebotomy and deferoxamine in patients with hemochromatosis.
- Remove copper deposits with d-penicillamine in patients with Wilson's disease.
- Long-term ursodiol therapy will slow the progression of primary biliary cirrhosis. It is, however, ineffective in primary sclerosing cholangitis.
- Glucocorticoids (prednisone 20 to 30 mg/day initially or combination therapy or prednisone and azathioprine) is useful in autoimmune hepatitis.
- Liver transplantation may be indicated in otherwise healthy patients (age <65 yr) with sclerosing cholangitis, chronic hepatitis cirrhosis, or primary biliary cirrhosis with prognostic information suggesting <20% chance of survival without transplantation. Contraindications to liver transplantation are AIDS, most metastatic malignancies, active substance abuse, uncontrolled sepsis, and uncontrolled cardiac or pulmonary disease.
- Treatment of complications of portal hypertension (ascites, esophagogastric varices, hepatic encephalopathy, and hepatorenal syndrome).

DISPOSITION

- Prognosis varies with the etiology of the patient's cirrhosis and whether there is ongoing hepatic injury. Regression of cirrhosis has been demonstrated after antiviral therapy in some patients with chronic hepatitis C. Regression is associated with decreased disease-related morbidity and improved survival. Mortality rate exceeds 0% in patients with hepatorenal syndrome.
- If advanced cirrhosis is present and transplantation is not feasible, survival is 1 to 2 yr.

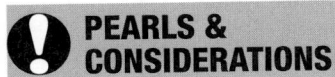 **PEARLS & CONSIDERATIONS**

COMMENTS

- Thrombocytopenia and advanced Child-Pugh cases (see Table 1-35) are associated with the presence of varices. These factors are useful to identify cirrhotic patients who benefit most from referral for endoscopic screening for varices.
- A combination of endoscopic and drug therapy reduces overall and variceal rebleeding in cirrhosis more than either therapy alone.

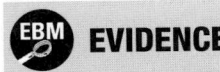 **EVIDENCE**

available at www.expertconsult.com

SUGGESTED READINGS

available at www.expertconsult.com

AUTHOR: **FRED F. FERRI, M.D.**

TABLE 1-35 Child Pugh Staging Criteria

	CHILD PUGH SCORE		
Criteria	**1 point**	**2 points**	**3 points**
Total serum bilirubin (mg/dl)	<2	2-3	>3
Serum albumin (g/dl)	>3.5	2.8-3.5	<2.8
INR	<1.70	1.71-2.20	>2.20
Ascites	No ascites	Ascites controlled	Ascites not controlled
Encephalopathy	No encephalopathy	Encephalopathy controlled	Encephalopathy not controlled

INTERPRETATION OF CHILD PUGH SCORES			
	Points	**Life expectancy**	**Perioperative mortality**
Child Class A	5-6	15-20 yr	10%
Child Class B	7-9	Candidate for liver transplant	30%
Child Class C	10-15	1-3 yr	82%

BASIC INFORMATION

DEFINITION

Primary biliary cirrhosis (PBC) is a chronic, variably progressive cholestatic liver disease most often affecting women and characterized by destruction of the small intrahepatic bile ducts leading to portal inflammation, fibrosis, cirrhosis, and ultimately, liver failure.

SYNONYMS

Biliary cirrhosis
Nonsuppurative destructive cholangitis
Autoimmune cholangiopathy

ICD-9CM CODES
571.6 Biliary cirrhosis
698 Pruritus
780.7 Malaise and Fatigue

EPIDEMIOLOGY & DEMOGRAPHICS

INCIDENCE:
- PBC affects all races and accounts for 0.6% to 2% of deaths from cirrhosis worldwide.
- Annual incidence rates range from 0.7 to 49 cases per million.

PREVALENCE: Prevalence is greatest in the U.K., Scandinavia, Canada, and the U.S., and varies tremendously by geographic areas, ranging from 6.7 to 402 cases per million.

PREDOMINANT SEX: Female to male ratio of up to 10:1.

PREDOMINANT AGE: Onset typically occurs between the ages of 30 and 65 yr, and it is uncommon before age 25 yr.

GENETICS:
- Although there are no clearly identified genetic factors associated with PBC, there is a clear familial occurrence. Prevalence among first-degree relatives is 5% to 6%, and 1% to 6% of all patients have at least one affected family member. The concordance rate among monozygotic twins is 63%.
- Up to 84% of patients with PBC have at least one other autoimmune disorder, such as thyroiditis, Sjögren's syndrome, rheumatoid arthritis, Raynaud's phenomenon, or scleroderma. A variant form of PBC exists as an overlap syndrome with autoimmune hepatitis (AIH).

ETIOLOGY

- Although the cause of PBC remains unknown, it is believed to be attributable to an environmental insult that modifies mitochondrial proteins triggering persistent T lymphocyte–mediated attack on intralobular bile duct epithelial cells in genetically susceptible individuals.
- PBC is associated with the DRB1*08 family of alleles, but there is a great deal of variation among ethnicities.
- Possible environmental triggers include cigarette smoking, urinary tract infections, reproductive hormone replacement, nail polish, and toxic waste sites, as well as xenobiotics in animal models of PBC.

- Recent studies have identified a peptide, an enzyme complex subunit (PDC-E2) in the mitochondrial membrane, as a major autoantigen in the early pathogenesis of PBC. Patients with PBC have a tenfold increased concentration of cytotoxic CD8$^+$ lymphocytes recognizing this peptide in their livers compared with their blood, and anti–mitochondria antibodies (AMA), especially the PDC-E2 subunit, are the serologic hallmark of this disease. In addition, bile duct epithelial cells handle PDC-E2 in a unique way that exposes them to immune-mediated attack by PDC-E2–oriented cytotoxic T cells. Future therapies may be specific immunomodulation directed at these peptides.
- In addition to the T lymphocyte–mediated direct destruction of small bile ducts, secondary damage to hepatocytes results from the accumulation of noxious substances such as bile acids.

PHYSICAL FINDINGS & CLINICAL PRESENTATION

Clinical stages:
- Asymptomatic
- Symptomatic
- Cirrhotic
- Hepatic failure

Symptoms:
- 50% to 60% of patients may be asymptomatic; 40% to 100% of these patients will develop symptoms, and nearly 25% of symptomatic patients at diagnosis will progress to liver failure within 10 yr without treatment.
- Fatigue (78% of patients) and pruritus (20% to 70% of patients) are the usual presenting symptoms.
- Pruritus is worse at night, under constricting, coarse garments; in association with dry skin; and in hot, humid weather. The cause is unknown; it is no longer believed to be a result of the retention of bile acids in skin. Pruritus may first occur during pregnancy but is distinguished from pruritus of pregnancy because it persists into the postpartum period and beyond.
- Other common symptoms include hepatomegaly, jaundice, unexplained right upper quadrant pain (10%), splenomegaly, manifestations of portal hypertension, sicca symptoms, and scleroderma-like lesions.
- Musculoskeletal complaints caused by inflammatory arthropathy in 40% to 70% of patients: 5% to 10% experience development of chronic rheumatoid arthritis and 10% experience development of "arthritis of PBC."
- Steatorrhea may be seen in advanced disease.

Physical:
- Variable: Results depend on stage of disease at time of presentation; patients at the early stage may be completely unaffected.
- Excoriations may be present.
- Hepatomegaly (70%) and splenomegaly (initially 35%) may be present in more advanced disease.

- Xanthomas and jaundice appear in advanced disease. Kayser-Fleischer rings are rare and result from copper retention.
- Late physical findings mirror those of cirrhosis: spider nevi, temporal and proximal limb wasting, ascites, and edema.

DIAGNOSIS

The diagnosis of PBC can be established when two of the following three criteria are met.
- Positive serum AMA, titer >1:40
- Biochemical evidence of cholestasis (mainly alkaline phosphatase elevation)
- Characteristic liver histology: nonsuppurative destructive cholangitis and destruction of interlobular bile ducts

DIFFERENTIAL DIAGNOSIS

- Drug-induced cholestasis
- PBC-AIH overlap syndrome: reported in almost 10% of adults with AIH or PBC; transition from stable PBC to AIH and vice versa also seen
- Other etiologies of chronic liver disease and cirrhosis, such as alcoholic cirrhosis, chronic viral hepatitis, primary sclerosing cholangitis, AIH, sarcoidosis, chemical/toxin-induced cirrhosis, other hereditary or familial disorders (e.g., cystic fibrosis, α-1-antitrypsin deficiency)
- Biliary obstruction

WORKUP

History, physical examination, laboratory evaluation, liver biopsy

LABORATORY TESTS

- AMAs found in 95% of patients with PBC and are 98% specific.
- Antinuclear antibodies (ANAs) and anti–smooth muscle antibody (AMA) found in approximately 50% of patients. In approximately 5% of patients, AMAs are absent or present only in low titer (AMA-negative PBC). Nearly all of these patients have ANA or anti–smooth muscle antibodies, or both.
- Cholestatic pattern of liver biochemical markers, that is, markedly increased alkaline phosphatase (of hepatic origin).
- γ-Glutamyl transpeptidase is increased.
- Serum IgM levels are increased (lower in AMA-negative PBC).
- Bilirubin level is normal early; increases with disease progression (direct and indirect) in 60% of patients. Increased serum bilirubin level is a poor prognostic sign.
- Aminotransferase level may be normal and, if increased, is rarely more than five times the upper limit of normal.
- Markedly increased serum lipids in more than 50% of patients. Total cholesterol may exceed 1000 mg/dl. No increased risk for death from atherosclerosis seen, possibly because of high levels of LP-X, an antiatherogenic low-density lipoprotein particle, very-high-density lipoprotein levels, and low serum levels of lipoprotein(a).

- Percutaneous liver biopsy confirms or rules out the diagnosis, allows staging, but is not essential to initiate medical therapy in patients with typical liver chemistry and positive AMA test.
- Histology is not uniform, so histologic stage is based on the most advanced lesion present.
  - Stage I: Lymphocytic infiltration of the epithelial cells of the small bile ducts with granuloma-like lesions, limited to portal triads
  - Stage II: Extension of inflammatory cells to periportal parenchyma, invasion by foamy macrophages, and development of biliary piecemeal necrosis
  - Stage III: Fibrous septa link portal triads
  - Stage IV: Frank cirrhosis; hyaline deposits and accumulation of stainable copper are also seen

IMAGING STUDIES

If history, physical examination, blood tests, and liver biopsy are all consistent with PBC, neither imaging nor cholangiography is necessary.

PROGNOSIS

- Median survival was 10 yr but may be getting longer with earlier diagnosis and initiation of treatment.
- Mean time of progression from stage I or II disease to cirrhosis with no medical treatment is 4 to 6 yr.
- Neither presence nor titer of antimitochondrial antibodies predicts survival, disease progression, or response to therapy.
- Prognostic laboratory measures: Serum bilirubin is most important.
- Response to ursodiol therapy can be prognostic: Patients with a decrease in alkaline phosphatase level of at least 40% or to the reference range after 1 yr of treatment with ursodeoxycholic acid (UDCA) may have a prognosis similar to an age-matched healthy population. Similarly, the Mayo Risk score, a predictor of short-term survival probability (http://www.mayoclinic.org/gi-rst/mayo-model1.html), can also reliably predict life expectancy when calculated after 6 mo of ursodiol therapy.
- Poorer prognosis exists with jaundice, advanced histologic stage, advanced age, edema, coagulopathy, and ascites.

Rx TREATMENT

- Treatment is according to the clinical stage of the disease.
- Asymptomatic stage: Follow bilirubin every 3 mo. Once liver function test results become abnormal, begin UDCA at 13 to 15 mg/kg/day in a twice-daily divided dose regardless of histologic stage. Side effects may include weight gain of approximately 5 lbs during the first 1 to 2 yr and, less commonly, thinning of hair and loose stools. Watch for interactions with cholestyramine and other bile-acid sequestrants, as well as antacids, which may interfere with UDCA absorption. Efficacy is best if started during stage I or II disease but should be started at any stage of disease. Lifelong therapy is currently recommended, but benefits are still observed if therapy is interrupted and restarted.
- Treatment also includes treatment of associated conditions such as pruritus, osteoporosis, increased low-density lipoprotein level, and any eventual complications of cirrhosis.
- 20% of patients will not respond to medical therapy and will proceed to liver transplantation, which is the only definitive treatment for this disease.

ACUTE GENERAL Rx

- Symptomatic stage: Goals of treatment are resolution of pruritus, decrease of alkaline phosphatase levels, and delay of progression to liver failure.
- Ursodiol can significantly improve bilirubin and alkaline phosphatase levels, prolong survival without liver transplantation, and delay progression of liver fibrosis and development of portal hypertension.
- The addition of colchicine (0.6 mg bid) or methotrexate (15 mg/wk) has not been found to be of benefit in controlled trials.
- Prednisone, azathioprine, penicillamine, and cyclosporine are no longer used because of limited efficacy and significant toxicity.
- For the pruritus of PBC, cholestyramine resin (4 g/dose; maximum, 16 g/day) reduces pruritus in most patients but must be given at least 2 to 4 hr apart from ursodiol to avoid reducing the efficacy of that drug. Antihistamines at bedtime help nighttime symptoms. Rifampin (150 to 300 mg bid) or oral opiate antagonists such as naltrexone (50 mg daily) can be used for pruritus refractory to bile acid sequestrants. Intractable pruritus can be an indication for liver transplantation.

CHRONIC Rx

- Management of Sicca syndrome: Artificial tears can be used initially for dry eyes. Saliva substitutes can be used for xerostomia and dysphagia; pilocarpine or cevimeline for refractory cases. Moisturizers can be given for vaginal dryness.
- Treatment for osteopenia/osteoporosis: Patients with PBC should be provided 1000 to 1500 mg calcium and 1000 IU of vitamin D daily in the diet and as supplements if needed. Alendronate (70 mg weekly) should be considered if patients are osteopenic in the absence of acid reflux or known varices.
- Hyperlipidemia is common in patients with cholestatic liver disease. Statins are safe in patients who may need treatment even if liver chemistry is abnormal.
- Vitamin A, K, and E deficiencies can be clinically important in advanced cases and respond to oral replacement.
- Upper endoscopy to assess for varices should be done every 2 to 3 yr in patients with cirrhosis or Mayo risk score >4.1. Nonselective beta-blockers or endoscopic banding can be considered for prevention of variceal hemorrhage.
- Regular screening for hepatocellular carcinoma with ultrasound and α-fetoprotein every 6 to 12 mo is recommended for patients with cirrhosis.
- Liver transplantation is the only effective treatment for patients with liver failure. Indications for transplantation include hepatic decompensation (ascites, encephalopathy, jaundice), hepatocellular carcinoma fulfilling Milan criteria (see "Hepatocellular Carcinoma"), and intractable pruritus.
- The outcome of liver transplantation for patients with PBC is more favorable than that of nearly all other liver disease categories. The survival rates are 85% to 90% and 80% to 85% at 1 and 5 yr, respectively. Although recurrent disease may develop in 20% to 25% of patients after liver transplantation over 10 yr, patient and graft survival is usually not affected.

DISPOSITION

Definitive treatment requires liver transplantation; survival is 7 to 16 yr depending on symptoms at time of diagnosis.

REFERRAL

Gastroenterology and/or hepatology for treatment, evaluation for liver transplantation, and management of portal hypertension

ⓘ PEARLS & CONSIDERATIONS

- Anti–mitochondrial antibody (AMA) is the serologic hallmark of PBC.
- The prototypical patient with PBC is a middle-aged, white woman reporting fatigue and pruritus.
- Ursodiol should be started as soon as liver biochemical markers begin to increase and is most effective when started early in the course of the disease.
- Associated illnesses must be detected and treated.
- Liver transplantation is the only effective treatment for PBC with end-stage liver failure.

SUGGESTED READINGS
available at www.expertconsult.com

AUTHOR: **KITTICHAI PROMRAT, M.D.**

BASIC INFORMATION

DEFINITION

Claudication refers to reproducible discomfort of muscles brought on by exertion and relieved with rest. It is caused by poor circulation of the blood to the affected muscle groups usually from arterial atherosclerotic stenosis to the affected area. This intermittent vascular claudication is most common in the calves and lower extremities but it can also affect the upper extremities.

SYNONYMS

Intermittent claudication

ICD-9CM CODES
443.9   Peripheral vascular disease, unspecified
440.21 Intermittent claudication due to atherosclerosis

EPIDEMIOLOGY & DEMOGRAPHICS

- The prevalence is 2% to 4% in the general population, increasing with age particularly after age 40 yr.
- The risk factors associated with development of intermittent claudication are similar to coronary artery disease. Increasing age, cigarette smoking, and diabetes mellitus are the strongest risk factors, followed by hypertension and dyslipidemia. Nontraditional risk factors include race/ethnicity, with African American patients being at higher risk. In addition, chronic renal disease, metabolic syndrome, and patients with elevated levels of C-reactive protein, lipoprotein(a), and homocysteine should also be considered.
- There is a strong association among peripheral artery disease (PAD), carotid artery stenosis, and cardiovascular disease.
- In 2005, the American College of Cardiology/American Heart Association (ACC/AHA) guidelines suggested the following distribution of clinical presentation of PAD in patients >50 yr of age:
  ○ Asymptomatic: 20% to 50%
  ○ Atypical leg pain: 40% to 50%
  ○ Classic claudication: 10% to 35%
  ○ Critical limb ischemia: 1% to 2%

PHYSICAL FINDINGS & CLINICAL PRESENTATION

- The severity of claudication symptoms varies with severity of stenoses, collateral blood supply, and exertional demand.
- Classic symptoms include calf pain brought on by exertion, causing patient to stop exertion and pain resolves within 10 min of rest. Claudication can present in buttock and hip, thigh, calf, or foot, with one or more of the following findings:
  ○ Diminished or absent pedal pulses, with cool skin temperature
  ○ Bruit over the distal aorta, iliac, or femoral arteries
  ○ Pallor of the distal extremities on elevation
  ○ Rubor with prolonged capillary refill on dependency
  ○ Trophic changes, including hair/nail loss and muscle atrophy
  ○ Nonhealing ulcers, necrotic tissue, and gangrene
  ○ Weakness, numbness, or heaviness in the lower extremities
- Location of pain usually corresponds to analogous anatomy:
  ○ Buttock and hip: aortoiliac disease
  ○ Thigh: aortoiliac or common femoral artery
  ○ Upper two thirds of calf: superficial femoral artery
  ○ Lower one third of calf: popliteal artery
  ○ Foot: tibial or peroneal artery

ETIOLOGY

The primary cause of claudication is peripheral atherosclerosis, resulting in inability to supply enough blood to meet the metabolic demand of limb muscles.

DIAGNOSIS

DIFFERENTIAL DIAGNOSIS

- Spinal stenosis (neurogenic or pseudoclaudication)
- Musculoskeletal disorders: arthritis or myositis
- Degenerative osteoarthritic joint disease, predominantly of the lumbar spine and hips
- Compartment or popliteal artery entrapment syndrome
- Peripheral neuropathy
- Atheromatous embolization and deep venous thrombosis
- Vasculitis: thromboangiitis obliterans, takayasu, or giant cell arteritis

WORKUP

History and physical findings suggest the diagnosis of claudication. Noninvasive studies help confirm the diagnosis.
- Measurement of resting ankle–brachial index (ABI): the ratio of highest ankle systolic pressure to brachial systolic pressure. A normal ABI is 0.90 to 1.40. A low ABI has been shown to be an independent predictor of mortality.
- The severity of PAD is based on the ABI at rest and during treadmill exercise (1 to 2 mi/hr, 5 min, or symptom limited). ABI does not define the level of obstructive disease, it only correlates with the severity of perfusion. It is classified as follows:
  ○ Mild: ABI at rest 0.71 to 0.0 or ABI during exercise 0.50 to 0.0
  ○ Moderate: ABI at rest 0.41 to 0.70 or ABI during exercise 0.20 to 0.50
  ○ Severe: ABI at rest <0.40 or ABI during exercise <0.20
- Segmental systolic pressures are measured from thigh, calf, ankle, metatarsal, and toes. Normally, there should not be >20 mm Hg difference in pressures between adjacent segments. If the gradient is >20 mm Hg, significant narrowing is suspected in the intervening segment.
- Both ABI and segmental pressures can be taken before and after exercise for objective characterization of severity of claudication symptoms.
- ABI >1.3 may represent significant PAD. In such cases, measuring a toe–brachial index can increase the sensitivity of testing, as highly calcified arteries are not compressible and may have a normal or increased ABI. A toe–brachial index <0.7 is considered abnormal.

IMAGING STUDIES

- Duplex ultrasound can be used to assess occlusion location, length, and patency of the distal arterial system or prior vein grafts. Ultrasound is a great noninvasive modality for routine monitoring after revascularization.
- Magnetic resonance angiography (MRA) and spiral CT angiography are effective modalities for imaging of the aorta and peripheral lower extremity arteries above the knee. MRA has almost replaced catheter-based angiography, with 90% sensitivity and 97% specificity in identification of hemodynamically significant stenoses in the lower extremities.
- Angiography (Fig. 1-97) remains the gold standard for diagnosing peripheral arterial occlusion, especially below the knee, and before revascularization.

TREATMENT

NONPHARMACOLOGIC THERAPY

- Smoking cessation is vital.
- Aggressive risk factor modification for hypertension, dyslipidemia and diabetes mellitus, including diet and weight loss counseling.
- Walking 30 to 60 min/day, at least 3 times per week at approximately 2 mi/hr to near-maximal pain for 6 mo is recommended.
- New prospective data point to intermittent pneumatic compression as a promising adjunctive therapy.

ACUTE GENERAL Rx

Revascularization by endovascular or surgical approach is usually reserved for patients with symptoms refractory to medical therapy or impending ischemic limb loss.

CHRONIC Rx

- Aspirin 75 to 325 mg daily; thienopyridines (clopidogrel and ticlodipine) can be considered as alternatives, especially for those intolerant of aspirin. There is no current data to support combination treatment (CHARISMA trial) or treatment with newer agents such as Prasugrel.
- Cilostazol 100 mg bid may be used in conjunction with aspirin or clopidogrel. It has been shown to increase walking distance by 50% to 67% in symptomatic patients.
- Individuals with intermittent claudication who are offered the option of endovascular or surgical therapies should:
  ○ Be provided information regarding supervised claudication exercise therapy and pharmacotherapy

○ Receive comprehensive risk factor modification and antiplatelet therapy
○ Have a significant disability, either being unable to perform normal work or having serious impairment of other activities important to the patient
○ Have lower extremity PAD lesion anatomy such that the revascularization procedure would have low risk and a high probability of initial and long-term success
- Revascularization is indicated in patients with refractory rest pain or claudication that limits their lifestyle, results in non-healing ulcers or gangrene, and in a select group of patients with functional disability. Common procedures include:
○ Aorto-iliofemoral reconstruction or bypass or infrainguinal bypass (e.g., femoropopliteal, femorotibial)
○ Angioplasty, often with stenting, is used primarily on short, discrete stenotic lesions in the iliac or femoropopliteal arteries

COMPLEMENTARY & ALTERNATIVE MEDICINE

- A meta-analysis found that over 12 to 24 wk, Ginkgo biloba increased pain-free walking distance by 34 m compared with placebo, although the benefit is not well established according to ACC/AHA guidelines.
- Naftidrofuryl, a serotonin receptor inhibitor, available in Europe, has shown some efficacy in improving claudication symptoms.
- Estrogen replacement therapy, propionyl-L-carnitine, L-arginine, oral vasodilators, prostaglandins, and chelation therapy are ineffective in the treatment of intermittent claudication.

DISPOSITION

- Intermittent claudication progressing to an ischemic leg or limb loss is unusual, especially if maintaining conservative treatments of risk factor modification, exercise, and smoking cessation.
- The 5-yr risk for development of ischemic ulceration in patients treated for diabetes and with ABI <0.5 was 30% compared with only 5% in patients with neither characteristic.

REFERRAL

Consultation with physicians specializing in vascular medicine is recommended in the patient with threatened limb loss, rest pain, nonhealing ulcers, functional disability from pain, and gangrene.

PEARLS & CONSIDERATIONS

- Approximately 70% of patients with peripheral vascular disease will have concomitant coronary artery disease.
- Beta-blockers may worsen claudication symptoms in some patients, although their underuse is associated with excess cardiovascular death. Patients with intermittent claudication are less likely to receive beta-blocker therapy after an initial myocardial infarction. Those who did not receive this treatment have at least a significant threefold higher mortality.
- Patients with peripheral vascular disease may benefit from secondary cardiovascular prevention with clopidogrel versus aspirin more so than other high-risk patients (CAPRIE trial).

COMMENTS

- Claudication is a marker for generalized atherosclerosis. This group of patients has a greater risk for death from cardiovascular events than from limb loss. Patients with claudication experience diminished overall quality of life similar to patients with diagnosed coronary or cerebrovascular disease.
- The ABI is more closely associated with leg function in persons with peripheral arterial disease than is intermittent claudication or other leg symptoms.

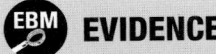 **EVIDENCE**

available at www.expertconsult.com

SUGGESTED READINGS
available at www.expertconsult.com

AUTHORS: **AMANDA M. DONOHUE, D.O.,** and **PRANAV M. PATEL, M.D.**

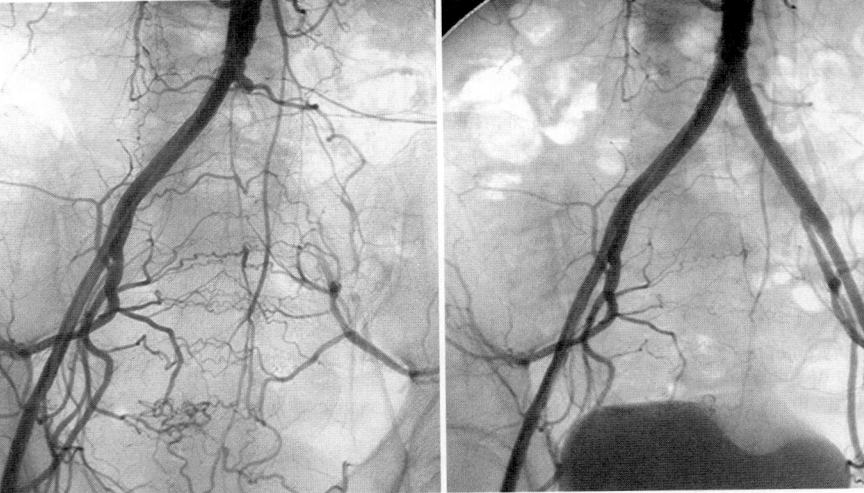

FIGURE 1-97 Angiogram of the distal abdominal aorta and iliac arteries demonstrates an occluded left common iliac artery with extensive collateral circulation from contralateral internal iliac artery *(left panel),* which resolved after successful stent implantation *(right panel).* (Images courtesy of Bart Domatch, MD, Radiology Department, University of Texas Southwestern Medical Center, Dallas, Texas. From Andreoli TE et al: *Andreoli and Carpenter's Cecil essentials of medicine,* ed 8, Philadelphia, 2010, Elsevier/Saunders.)

BASIC INFORMATION

DEFINITION

Clostridium difficile infection (CDI) is the occurrence of diarrhea and bowel inflammation associated with antibiotic use. CDI can manifest clinically in several forms ranging from fulminant diarrhea and leukocytosis associated with pseudomembranous colitis, mild to severe acute diarrhea, short-term colonization seen typically in health care facilities, and recurrent CDI with 60 days after initial treatment occurring in 20% to 30% of cases.

SYNONYMS

Antibiotic-induced colitis
Pseudomembranous colitis
CDI

ICD-9CM CODES
008.45 *Clostridium difficile*, pseudomembranous colitis

EPIDEMIOLOGY & DEMOGRAPHICS

- Cephalosporins are the most frequent offending agent in pseudomembranous colitis because of their high rates of use.
- The antibiotic with the highest incidence is clindamycin (10% incidence of pseudomembranous colitis with its use).
- Since 1996, the incidence of clostridium difficile infection has more than doubled. *Clostridium difficile* is responsible for approximately 3 million cases of diarrhea and colitis in the U.S. every year.

PHYSICAL FINDINGS & CLINICAL PRESENTATION

- Abdominal tenderness (generalized or lower abdominal)
- Fever
- In patients with prolonged diarrhea, poor skin turgor, dry mucous membranes, and other signs of dehydration may be present

ETIOLOGY

Risk factors for *C. difficile* (the major identifiable agent of antibiotic-induced diarrhea and colitis):

- Administration of antibiotics: can occur with any antibiotic, but occurs most frequently with clindamycin, ampicillin, cephalosporins, and fluoroquinolone
- Prolonged hospitalization
- Advanced age
- Abdominal surgery
- Underlying disease (malignancy, renal failure, debilitated status)
- Hospitalized, tube-fed patients are at risk for *C. difficile*–associated diarrhea. Clinicians should consider testing for *C. difficile* in tube-fed patients with diarrhea unrelated to the feeding solution.
- PPI and H_2 blocker therapy increases risk of CDI and recurrent CDI

DIAGNOSIS

The clinical signs of pseudomembranous colitis generally include diarrhea, fever, and abdominal cramps after use of antibiotics.

DIFFERENTIAL DIAGNOSIS

- Gastrointestinal bacterial infections (e.g., *Salmonella, Shigella, Campylobacter, Yersinia*)
- Enteric parasites (e.g., *Cryptosporidium, Entamoeba histolytica*)
- Inflammatory bowel disease
- Celiac sprue
- Irritable bowel syndrome
- Ischemic colitis
- Antibiotic intolerance

WORKUP

- All patients with diarrhea accompanied by current or recent antibiotic use should be tested for *C. difficile* (see below).
- Sigmoidoscopy (without cleansing enema) may be necessary when the clinical and laboratory diagnosis is inconclusive and the diarrhea persists.
- In antibiotic-induced pseudomembranous colitis, the sigmoidoscopy often reveals raised white-yellow exudative plaques adherent to the colonic mucosa (Fig. 1-98).

LABORATORY TESTS

- *C. difficile* toxin can be detected by cytotoxin tissue-culture assay (cytotoxin assay, gold standard for identifying *C. difficile* toxin in stool specimen). This test is difficult to perform and results are not available for 24 to 48 hr. A more useful test is the enzyme-linked immunosorbent assay for *C. difficile* toxins A and B. The latter is used most widely in the clinical setting. It has a sensitivity of 85% and a specificity of 100%.
- Fecal leukocytes (assessed by microscopy or lactoferrin assay) are generally present in stool samples.
- Complete blood count usually reveals leukocytosis. A sudden increase in white blood cells to >30,000/mm^3 may be indicative of fulminant colitis.

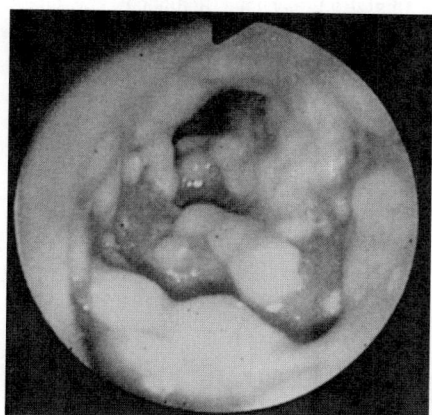

FIGURE 1-98 Pseudomembranous plaques seen with colonoscopy in a patient with *Clostridium difficile*–associated pseudomembranous colitis. (From Gorbach SL: *Infectious diseases*, ed 2, Philadelphia, 1998, WB Saunders.)

IMAGING STUDIES

Abdominal film (flat plate and upright) is useful in patients with abdominal pain or evidence of obstruction on physical examination.

TREATMENT

NONPHARMACOLOGIC THERAPY

- Discontinue offending antibiotic
- Fluid hydration and correction of electrolyte abnormalities
- Probiotics to restore natural defense mechanisms may be useful as adjuvant therapy; however, evidence is limited

ACUTE GENERAL Rx

- Metronidazole 500 mg PO qid for 10 to 14 days.
- Vancomycin 125 mg PO qid for 10 to 14 days in cases resistant to metronidazole. However, vancomycin may be considered as first-line therapy in hospitalized patients who are seriously ill.
- Cholestyramine 4 g PO qid for 10 days in addition to metronidazole to control severe diarrhea (avoid use with vancomycin).
- When parenteral therapy is necessary (e.g., patient with paralytic ileus), IV metronidazole 500 mg qid can be used. It can also be supplemented with vancomycin 500 mg by nasogastric tube with intermittent clamping or retention enema.
- IV tigecycline (a broad-spectrum antibiotic used for skin or soft-tissue infection) can be used as adjunctive or alternative therapy for severe refractory *C. difficile* toxin infection.
- The addition of monoclonal antibodies against *C. difficile* toxins to antibiotic agents has been shown to reduce the recurrence of *C. difficile* infection.
- Recent trials with fidaxomicin, a newer antibiotic, have shown non-inferiority to vancomycin and a lower rate of CDI recurrence.

CHRONIC Rx

Judicious future use of antibiotics to prevent recurrences (e.g., avoid prolonged antibiotic therapy)

DISPOSITION

- Most patients recover completely with appropriate therapy. Fever resolves within 48 hr and diarrhea within 4 to 5 days. Overall mortality rate is 1% to 2.5% but exceeds 10% in untreated patients.
- Hospital-acquired CDI is independently associated with an increased risk of in-hospital death.

SUGGESTED READINGS
available at www.expertconsult.com

AUTHOR: **FRED F. FERRI, M.D.**

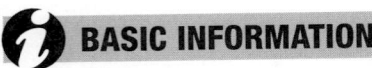

BASIC INFORMATION

DEFINITION

Cocaine is an alkaloid derived from the coca plant *Erythroxylum coca,* native to South America, which contains approximately 0.5% to 1% cocaine. The drug produces physiologic and behavioral effects when administered orally, intranasally, intravenously, or by inhalation after smoking. Cocaine has potent pharmacologic effects on dopamine, norepinephrine, and serotonin neurons in the central nervous system (CNS) involving alteration and blockade of cellular membrane transport and prevention of reuptake. Cocaine's second action involves the blockage of voltage-gated sodium ion membrane channels, which is responsible for its anesthetic effect. The mechanisms by which cocaine may induce myocardial ischemia or infarction are described in Fig. 1-99.

SYNONYMS

Cocaine hydrochloride: topical solution (FDA approved as a topical anesthetic)

Freebase: aqueous solution of cocaine hydrochloride converted to a more volatile base state by the addition of alkali, thereby extracting the cocaine base in a residue or precipitate

Crack: potent, purified smokable form; produces effects similar to those of intravenous administration

Street names include Bernice, Bernies, C, Cadillac or Champagne of drugs, Carrie, Cecil, Charlie, Coke, Dust, Dynamite, Flake, Gin, Girl, Gold dust, Green gold, Jet, Powder, Star dust, Paradise, Pimp's drug, Snowflake, Stardust, White girl

Liquid lady = alcohol + cocaine

Speedball = heroin + cocaine

Street measures: hit (2 to 200 mg), snort, line, dose, spoon (approximately 1 g)

ICD-9CM CODES
304.2 Cocainism

EPIDEMIOLOGY & DEMOGRAPHICS

- The 1993 National Household Survey on Drug Abuse estimated that 4.5 million Americans used cocaine in 1992, with 1.3 million reporting use at least monthly. By 1998 this had not significantly changed.
- Between 1993 and 1994, intravenous cocaine and heroin abusers accounted for a major new group of persons with HIV in several metropolitan areas.
- In 1999 an estimated 25 million Americans admitted that they used cocaine at least once—3.7 million the previous year and 1.5 million currently. It is the most frequent cause of drug-related death reported by medical examiners and is increasing more sharply in women than in men.
- The 2006 National Survey on Drug Use and Health indicates that there were 2.4 million users aged ≥12 yr, which was the same in 2005 but greater than in 2002, when there were an estimated 2 million.
- The 2007 National Survey on Drug Use and Health indicates that there were 2.1 million users aged 12 yr or older.

PHYSICAL FINDINGS & CLINICAL PRESENTATION

PHASE I:
- CNS: euphoria, agitation, headache, vertigo, twitching, bruxism, unintentional tremor
- Nausea, vomiting, fever, hypertension, tachycardia

PHASE II:
- CNS: lethargy, hyperreactive deep tendon reflexes, seizures (status epilepticus)
- Sympathetic overdrive: tachycardia, hypertension, hyperthermia
- Incontinence

PHASE III:
- CNS: flaccid paralysis, coma, fixed dilated pupils, loss of reflexes
- Pulmonary edema
- Cardiopulmonary arrest

Psychologic dependence manifests with habituation, paranoia, and hallucinations (cocaine "bugs"):

CNS: Cerebral ischemia and infarction, cerebral arterial spasm, cerebral vasculitis, cerebral vascular thrombosis, subarachnoid hemorrhage, intraparenchymal hemorrhage, seizures, cerebral atrophy, movement disorders

Cardiac: Acute myocardial ischemia and infarction, arrhythmias and sudden death, dilated cardiomyopathy and myocarditis, infective endocarditis, aortic rupture

Pulmonary: Inhalation injuries (secondary to smoking crack cocaine): cartilage and nasal septal perforation, oropharyngeal ulcers; immunologically mediated diseases: hypersensitivity pneumonitis, bronchiolitis obliterans; pulmonary vascular lesions and hemorrhage, pulmonary infarction, pulmonary edema secondary to left ventricular failure, pneumomediastinum, and pneumothorax

Gastrointestinal: Gastroduodenal ulceration and perforation; intestinal infarction or perforation, colitis

Renal: Acute renal failure secondary to rhabdomyolysis and myoglobinuria; renal infarction; focal segmental glomerulosclerosis

Obstetric: Placental abruption, low infant weight, prematurity, microcephaly

Psychiatric: Anxiety, depression, paranoia, delirium, psychosis, suicide

ETIOLOGY

Cocaine may be absorbed through different routes with varying degrees of speed:
- Nasal insufflation/snorting: 2.5 min
- Smoking: <30 sec
- Oral: 2 to 5 min
- Mucosal: <20 min
- Intravenous injection: <30 sec

DIAGNOSIS

DIFFERENTIAL DIAGNOSIS

- Methamphetamine ("speed") abuse
- Methylenedioxyamphetamine ("ecstasy") abuse
- Cathione ("khat") abuse
- Lysergic acid diethylamide (LSD) abuse

WORKUP

Physical examination and laboratory evaluation

LABORATORY TESTS

- Toxicology screen (urine): cocaine is metabolized within 2 hr by the liver to major metabolites, benzoylecgonine and ecgonine methyl ester, which are excreted in the urine. Metabolites can be identified in urine within 5 min of IV use and up to 48 hr after oral ingestion.
- Blood: CBC, electrolytes, glucose, BUN, creatinine, calcium.
- Arterial blood gas analysis.
- ECG.
- Serum creatinine kinase and troponin concentration.

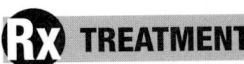

TREATMENT

There is no specific antidote and, at present, no drug therapy is uniquely effective in treating cocaine abuse and dependence. In addition, adulterants, contaminants, and other drugs may be admixed with street cocaine. Amantadine may provide effective treatment for cocaine-dependent patients with severe cocaine withdrawal symptoms, as well as the other dopamine agonist bromocriptine (1.5 mg PO tid), which may alleviate some of the symptoms of craving associated with acute cocaine withdrawal.

ACUTE GENERAL Rx

Acute cocaine toxicity requires following advanced poisoning treatment and life support. A suspected "body packer" should have an abdominal radiograph to detect the continued presence of cocaine-containing condoms in the intestinal tract. If present, gentle catharsis with charcoal and mineral oil should be performed with ICU admission and monitoring.

SPECIFIC TREATMENT

INHALATION: Wash nasal passages

AGITATION:
- Check STAT glucose
- Diazepam 15 to 20 mg PO or 2 to 10 mg IM or IV for severe agitation

HYPERTHERMIA:
- Check rectal temperature, creatine kinase, electrolytes
- Monitor with continuous rectal probe; bring temperature down to 101° F within 30 to 45 min

RHABDOMYOLYSIS:
- Vigorous hydration with urine output at least 2 ml/kg
- Mannitol or bicarbonate for rhabdomyolysis resistant to hydration

SEIZURE MANAGEMENT (STATUS EPILEPTICUS):
- Diazepam 5 to 10 mg IV over 2 to 3 min; may be repeated every 10 to 15 min.
- Lorazepam 2 to 3 mg IV over 2 to 3 min; may be repeated.
- Phenytoin loading dose 15 to 18 mg/kg IV at a rate not to exceed 25 to 50 mg/min under cardiac monitoring.

Diseases
and Disorders

I

- Phenobarbital loading dose 10 to 15 mg/kg IV at a rate of 25 mg/min; an additional 5 mg/kg may be given in 30 to 45 min if seizures are not controlled.
- For refractory seizures, consider:
  1. Pancuronium 0.1 mg/kg IV
  2. Halothane general anesthesia
  3. Both require EEG monitoring to determine brain seizure activity.

HYPERTENSION: Cocaine-induced hypertension usually responds to benzodiazepines. If this fails:
- Consider arterial line for continuous blood pressure monitoring
- Avoid the use of calcium channel blockers because they may potentiate the incidence of seizures and death, especially in body packers.
- The use of beta-blockers may exacerbate cocaine-induced vasoconstriction.

- Phentolamine (unopposed adrenergic effects) or nitroglycerin may be required.
- If diastolic pressure >120 mm Hg: hydralazine hydrochloride 25 mg IM or IV; may repeat q1h.
- If hypertension is uncontrolled or hypertensive encephalopathy is present: sodium nitroprusside initially at 0.5 µg/kg/min not to exceed 10 µg/kg/min.

CHEST PAIN:
- Chest radiograph, ECG, cardiac enzymes.
- Benzodiazepines for agitation.
- Acetylsalicylic acid and nitroglycerin for ischemic pain. (Aspirin is contraindicated if dissection is suspected.)
- Percutaneous transluminal coronary angioplasty possibly better than thrombolysis for cocaine-associated myocardial infarction.

- The use of beta-adrenergic blockers remains controversial because of the unopposed alpha-adrenergic effects of cocaine.
- If beta-blockers are to be used, this should be preceded by administration of phentolamine to prevent unopposed alpha adrenergic stimulation.

VENTRICULAR ARRHYTHMIAS:
- Antiarrhythmic agents should be used with caution during the early period after cocaine exposure as a result of their proarrhythmic and proconvulsant effects.
- Propranolol 1 mg/min IV for up to 6 mg.
- Lidocaine 1.5 mg/kg IV bolus followed by IV infusion (controversial: may be proarrhythmic and proconvulsant).
- Termination of ventricular arrhythmias may be resistant to lidocaine and even cardioversion.
- $NaHCO_3^-$ is under investigation in cocaine-mediated conduction abnormalities and rhythm disturbances.

DISPOSITION

Although many patients who use cocaine may not require treatment because of the short half-life of the drug, others may require specific treatment for possible cocaine-related complications.

REFERRAL

Consider psychotherapy or behavioral therapy once stable.

PEARLS & CONSIDERATIONS

- Cocaine-induced vasoconstriction may be exacerbated by the use of selective and nonselective beta-adrenergic blocking agents.
- The use of lidocaine in treating ventricular arrhythmias may precipitate seizures and further arrhythmias.

SUGGESTED READINGS
available at www.expertconsult.com

AUTHOR: **SAJEEV HANDA, M.D.**

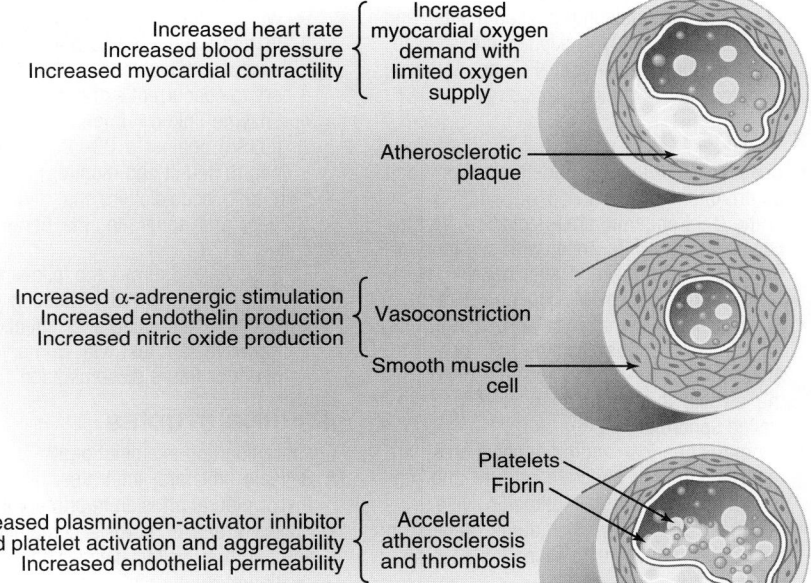

Increased heart rate
Increased blood pressure
Increased myocardial contractility
} Increased myocardial oxygen demand with limited oxygen supply

Atherosclerotic plaque

Increased α-adrenergic stimulation
Increased endothelin production
Increased nitric oxide production
} Vasoconstriction

Smooth muscle cell

Platelets
Fibrin

Increased plasminogen-activator inhibitor
Increased platelet activation and aggregability
Increased endothelial permeability
} Accelerated atherosclerosis and thrombosis

Atherosclerotic plaque

FIGURE 1-99 The mechanisms by which cocaine may induce myocardial ischemia or infarction. Cocaine may cause increase in the determinants of myocardial oxygen demand when oxygen supply is limited (top), when intense vasoconstriction of the coronary arteries occurs (middle), or when accelerated atherosclerosis and thrombosis are present (bottom). (Andreoli TE, Benjamin IJ, Griggs RC, Wings EJ: *Andreoli and Carpenter's Cecil essentials of medicine,* 8th ed, Philadelphia, Saunders, 2010.)

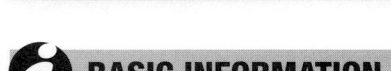
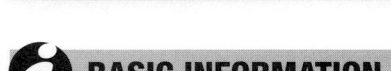

BASIC INFORMATION

DEFINITION

Coccidioidomycosis is an infectious disease caused by the fungus *Coccidioides immitis.* It is usually asymptomatic and characterized by a primary pulmonary focus with infrequent progression to chronic pulmonary disease and dissemination to other organs.

SYNONYMS

San Joaquin Valley fever

ICD-9CM CODES
114.0 Coccidioides pneumonia
114.1 Cutaneous or extrapulmonary (primary) coccidioidomycosis
114.3 Disseminated or prostate coccidioidomycosis
114.5 Pulmonary coccidioidomycosis
114.2 Coccidioidal meningitis
114.4 Chronic coccidioidomycosis

EPIDEMIOLOGY & DEMOGRAPHICS

INCIDENCE (IN U.S.): Estimated annual infection rate 100,000 persons, predominantly in southwest U.S.
PEAK INCIDENCE: Unknown
PREVALENCE: Unknown
PREDOMINANT SEX: Males, between the ages of 25 and 55 yr
Clinical disease more severe in older children and adults

PHYSICAL FINDINGS & CLINICAL PRESENTATION

- The clinical manifestations vary widely according to the host, the severity of the illness, and location of dissemination.
- Asymptomatic infections or illness consistent with a nonspecific upper respiratory tract infection in at least 60%.
- Symptoms of primary infection—cough, malaise, fever, chills, night sweats, anorexia, weakness, and arthralgias (desert rheumatism)—in remaining 40% within 3 wk of exposure.
- Erythema nodosum and erythema multiforme more common in women.
- Scattered rales and dullness on percussion.
- Spontaneous improvement within 2 wk of illness, with complete recovery usual.
- Pulmonary nodules and cavities in <10% of those patients with primary infection; half of these patients asymptomatic.
- In a small portion of these patients: a progressive pneumonitis, often with a fatal outcome.
- Immunocompromised or diabetic patients may progress to chronic pulmonary disease.
- Over many years, granulomas rupture, leading to new cavity formation and continued fibrosis, often accompanied by hemoptysis.
- Disseminated or extrapulmonary disease in approximately 0.5% of acutely infected patients.
  1. Early signs of probable dissemination: fever, malaise, hilar adenopathy, and ele-

vated ESR persisting in the setting of primary infection.
  2. Most organs are susceptible to dissemination, with heart and GI tract generally spared.
- Musculoskeletal involvement: bone lesions often unifocal, ribs, long bones, and vertebral lesions are common.
  1. Joint lesions predominantly unifocal, most commonly involving the ankle and knee, and often accompanying adjacent sites of osteomyelitis.
- Meningeal involvement: headache, fever, weakness, confusion, lethargy, cranial nerve defects, seizures; meningeal signs often minimal or absent.
- Cutaneous involvement: variable lesions—pustules, papules, plaques, nodules, ulcers, abscesses, or verrucous proliferative lesions.
  1. Dissemination and fatal outcomes most common in men, pregnant women, neonates, immunocompromised hosts, and individuals of dark-skinned races, especially those of African, Filipino, Mexican, and Native American ancestry.

ETIOLOGY

- *Coccidioides immitis* is endemic to North and South America.
- In the U.S., endemic areas coincide with the Lower Sonoran Life Zone, with semiarid climate, sparse flora, and alkaline soil in Arizona, California, New Mexico, and Texas.
- Fungus exists in the mycelial phase in soil, having barrel-shaped hyphae (arthroconidia). Arthrospores are aerosolized and deposit in the alveoli, then fungus converts to thick-walled spherule.
- Internal spherical spores (endospores) are released through spherule rupture and mature into new spherules (parasitic cycle).
- Fungus incites a granulomatous reaction in host tissue, usually with caseation necrosis.

DIAGNOSIS

DIFFERENTIAL DIAGNOSIS

- Acute pulmonary coccidioidomycoses:
  1. Community-acquired pneumonias caused by *Mycoplasma* and *Chlamydia*
  2. Granulomatous diseases, such as *Mycobacterium tuberculosis* and sarcoidosis
  3. Other fungal diseases, such as *Blastomyces dermatitidis* and *Histoplasma capsulatum*
- Coccidioidomas: true neoplasms

WORKUP

Suspected in patients with a history of residence or travel in an endemic area, especially during periods favorable to spore dispersion (e.g., dust storms and drought followed by heavy rains)

LABORATORY TESTS

- CBC to reveal eosinophilia, especially with erythema nodosum
- Routine chemistries: usually normal but may reveal hyponatremia

- Elevated serum levels of IgE; associated with progressive disease
- CSF cell counts and chemistry: pleocytosis with mononuclear cell predominance associated with hypoglycorrhachia and elevated protein level
- Definitive diagnosis based on demonstration of the organism by culture from body fluids or tissues
  1. Greatest yield with pus, sputum, synovial fluid, and soft tissue aspirations, varying with the degree of dissemination
  2. Possible positive cultures of blood, gastric aspirate, pleural effusion, peritoneal fluid, and CSF, but less frequently obtained
- Serologic evaluations
  1. Latex agglutination and complement fixation
  2. Elevated serum complement-fixing antibody (CFA) titers ≥1:32 strongly correlated with disseminated disease, except with meningitis where lower titers seen
  3. In meningeal disease: CFA detected in CSF except with high serum CFA titers secondary to concurrent extraneural disease
  4. Enzyme-linked immunosorbent assay (ELISA) against a 33-kDa spherule antigen to detect and monitor CNS disease
- Skin test: coccidioidin, the mycelial phase antigen, and spherulin, the parasitic phase antigen
  1. Positive (>5 mm) 1 mo following onset of symptomatic primary infection
  2. Useful in assessing prior infection
  3. Negative skin test with primary infection: latent or future dissemination

IMAGING STUDIES

Chest radiograph examination:
- Reveals unilateral infiltrates, hilar adenopathy, or pleural effusion in primary infection
- Shows areas of fibrosis containing usually solitary, thin-walled cavities that persist as residua of primary infection
- Possible coccidioidoma, a coinlike lesion representing a healed area of previous pneumonitis

TREATMENT

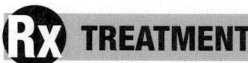

NONPHARMACOLOGIC THERAPY

- Supportive care in mild symptomatic disease
- In patients with extrapulmonary manifestations involving draining skin, joint, and soft tissue infection: local wound care to avoid possible bacterial superinfection

ACUTE GENERAL Rx

- In general, drug therapy is not required for patients with asymptomatic pulmonary disease and most patients with mild symptomatic primary infection.
- Chemotherapy is indicated under the following circumstances:
  1. Severe symptomatic primary infection
  2. High serum CFA titers
  3. Persistent symptoms >6 wk
  4. Prostration

C

Diseases and Disorders

5. Progressive pulmonary involvement
6. Pregnancy
7. Infancy
8. Debilitation
9. Concurrent illness (e.g., diabetes, asthma, COPD, malignancy)
10. Acquired or induced immunosuppression
11. Racial group with known predisposition for disseminated disease

- Fluconazole
  1. Most commonly, oral therapy with 400 mg/day up to 1.2 g/day appears to be the drug of choice for meningeal and deep-seated mycotic infections.
  2. In patients with AIDS, fluconazole may be considered the drug of choice for initial and maintenance therapy.
  3. All patients with coccidioidal meningitis should continue azole therapy indefinitely.
- Itraconazole
  1. 400 to 600 mg/day achieves 90% response rate in bone, joint, soft tissue, lymphatic, and genitourinary infections.
  2. Itraconazole may be more efficacious than fluconazole in the treatment of skeletal (bone) infections.
- Posaconazole is a new triazole that has recently been approved for use for systemic mycoses such as coccidioidomycosis; its relative efficacy compared to other agents will need additional clinical study.
- For pulmonary infections, treatment with either fluconazole or itraconazole, given for 6 to 12 wk, appears to be equal in efficacy.
- Amphotericin B is the classic therapy for disseminated extraneural disease, dose 0.6 to 1 mg/kg/day, qd for the first week then 0.8 mg/kg every other day, for a total dose of 1 to 2.5 g or until clinical and serologic remission is accomplished.
  1. Local instillation into body cavities such as sinuses, fistulae, and abscesses has been adjunct to therapy.
  2. Liposomal amphotericin B is probably equally effective.
  3. Duration of therapy for extraneural disease is undefined but probably about 1 yr.

- With meningeal disease: fluconazole 400 to 1000 mg PO q24h indefinitely
  1. Intrathecal amphotericin B is the alternate treatment modality, given alone or preceding the use of oral agents.
  2. Begin in doses of 0.01 to 0.025 mg/day, gradually increasing the dose as tolerated, to 0.5 mg/day with the patient in Trendelenburg's position.
  3. If given via Ommaya reservoir, as in ventriculitis, dose may be increased to 1.5 mg/day if tolerated.
  4. Concomitant parenteral therapy with amphotericin B is used for simultaneous extraneural disease as standard doses and with purely meningeal disease in smaller doses, although not strictly indicated.
  5. Intrathecal therapy is usually given three times a week for at least 3 mo, then discontinued or gradually tapered until once every 6 wk through 1 yr of therapy.
  6. Patients need routine monitoring of CSF, CFA, cell count, and chemistries for at least 2 yr following cessation of therapy.
- For osteomyelitis, soft tissue closed-space infections, and pulmonary fibrocavitary disease: surgical debridement, drainage, or resection, respectively, in addition to oral azole therapy or parenteral administration of amphotericin B.

CHRONIC Rx

For chronically immunocompromised patients, lifelong therapy with oral azoles or amphotericin B

DISPOSITION

- Prognosis for primary symptomatic infection is good.
- Immunocompromised patients are most likely to have disseminated disease and higher morbidity and mortality.

REFERRAL

- To surgeon for the evaluation of chronic hemoptysis, enlarging cavitary lesions despite chemotherapy and intrapleural rupture, os-

teomyelitis, and other synovial or soft tissue closed space infections
- For neurosurgical consultation in patients with meningeal disease to establish the delivery route of intrathecal drug therapy

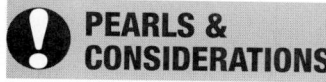 **PEARLS & CONSIDERATIONS**

COMMENTS

- Although coccidioidomycosis is a great imitator, a diagnosis will become apparent if a high degree of suspicion is maintained and appropriate testing (serologic testing, cultures, and histology) is performed.
- Infected body fluids contained within a closed moist environment (e.g., sputum in a specimen cup) provide the opportunity for the fungus to revert to its hyphal form whereby spores may be made airborne on opening of the container. This is a biohazard for laboratory personnel. Purulent drainage into a cast, allowing conversion of fungus to the saprophytic phase, has been responsible for acute disease when the cast was opened and the spores were unintentionally made airborne.
- Patients with a remote history of exposure, especially if immunosuppressed by medication or disease, may reactivate primary disease and suffer rapid dissemination.
- Although cardiac disease is rare, constrictive pericarditis in the setting of disseminated coccidioidomycosis has been documented and is potentially fatal.
- Organ transplant recipients may develop disease if the transplant donor has unrecognized active coccidioidomycosis at the time of death.

SUGGESTED READINGS
available at www.expertconsult.com

AUTHORS: **GLENN G. FORT, M.D., M.P.H.,** and **DENNIS J. MIKOLICH, M.D.**

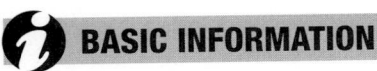

BASIC INFORMATION

DEFINITION
Acute, self-limited febrile illness caused by infection with a Coltivirus.

ICD-9CM CODES
066.1 Colorado tick fever

EPIDEMIOLOGY & DEMOGRAPHICS
- Incidence: approximately 330 cases reported per year in the U.S.
- Demographics: children and adults of both genders.
- Geography: Rocky Mountains at elevations of 4000 to 10,000 feet. Sporadic cases have been reported from areas of California outside the range of *Dermacentor andersoni*.
- Colorado has the highest incidence (Fig. 1-100).

PHYSICAL FINDINGS & CLINICAL PRESENTATION
- Incubation: 3 to 4 days is usual but can be up to 14 days
- First symptoms: fever, chills, severe headache, severe myalgias, and hyperesthetic skin
- Initial signs and symptoms:
  1. Tick bite
  2. Fever and chills
  3. Headache
  4. Myalgias
  5. Weakness
  6. Prostration and indifference
  7. Injected conjunctivae
  8. Erythematous pharyngitis
  9. Lymphadenopathy
  10. Maculopapular or petechial rash

These first symptoms last for 1 wk or less but 50% of patients have a febrile relapse 2 to 3 days after an initial remission. Weakness and fatigue may persist for several months after the acute phase(s). This chronic phase is more likely in older patients.

In children, 5% to 10% of cases are complicated by aseptic meningitis. In adults, rare complications include pneumonia, hepatitis, myocarditis, and epididymo-orchitis. Vertically transmitted fetal infection is possible.

ETIOLOGY
- Infectious agent: Coltiviruses; 7 species, including three in the U.S.
- Vector: wood tick, *D. andersoni*.
- Pathogenesis: human transmission occurs by tick bite. Tick season spans from March to September. The virus infects marrow erythrocytic precursors, explaining the protracted disease course because viremia lasts for the lifespan of the infected red blood cell.

DIAGNOSIS

DIFFERENTIAL DIAGNOSIS
- Rocky Mountain spotted fever
- Influenza
- Leptospirosis

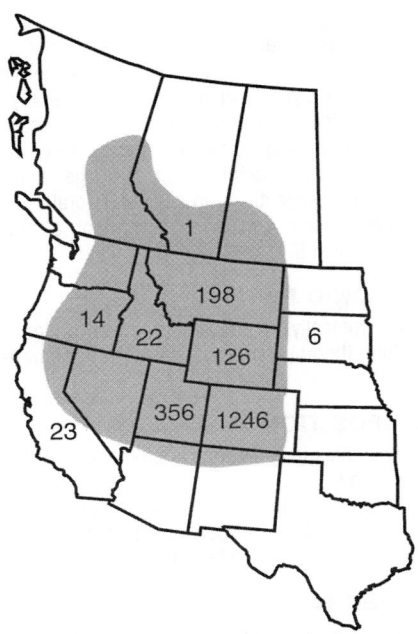
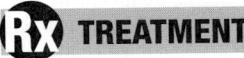

FIGURE 1-100 Geographic distribution of *Dermacentor andersoni* (wood ticks) and reported cases of Colorado tick fever, 1990-1996, United States and Canada. (From Mandell GL: *Mandell, Douglas, and Bennett's principles and practice of infectious diseases*, ed 6, New York, 2005, Churchill Livingstone.)

- Infectious mononucleosis
- CMV infection
- Pneumonia
- Hepatitis
- Meningitis
- Endocarditis
- Scarlet fever
- Measles
- Rubella
- Typhus
- Lyme disease
- Immune thrombocytopenic purpura (ITP)
- Thrombotic thrombocytopenic purpura (TTP)
- Kawasaki disease
- Toxic shock syndrome
- Vasculitis

WORKUP
Consider Colorado tick fever in the presence of the above symptoms associated with travel to an endemic area coupled with a history of tick exposure.

LABORATORY TESTS
- Complete blood count
  1. Leukopenia
  2. Atypical lymphocytes
  3. Moderate thrombocytopenia
- Virus identification in red blood cells by indirect immunofluorescence
- Serology with enzyme-linked immunosorbent assay, neutralization, or complement fixation

TREATMENT
- No specific therapy, although Coltiviruses are sensitive to ribavirin
- Bedrest, fluids, acetaminophen
- Avoid aspirin because of thrombocytopenia
- Prevention: tick avoidance measures

SUGGESTED READINGS
available at www.expertconsult.com

AUTHOR: **FRED F. FERRI, M.D.**

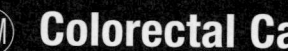

BASIC INFORMATION

DEFINITION

Colorectal cancer (CRC) is a neoplasm arising from the luminal surface of the large bowel; locations include descending colon (40% to 42%), rectosigmoid and rectum (30% to 33%), cecum and ascending colon (25% to 30%), and transverse colon (10% to 13%).

ICD-9CM CODES
154.0 Colorectal cancer

EPIDEMIOLOGY & DEMOGRAPHICS

- CRC is the second leading cause of cancer deaths in the U.S. (>160,000 new cases and >55,000 deaths/yr).
- Peak incidence is in the seventh decade of life. The lifetime risk for development of CRC is 1 in 17, with 90% of cases occurring after age 50 yr.
- 50% of rectal cancers are within reach of the examiner's finger, and 50% of colon cancers are within reach of the flexible sigmoidoscope.
- CRC accounts for 14% of all cases of cancer (excluding skin malignancies) and 14% of all yearly cancer deaths.
- Risk factors:
  - Hereditary polyposis syndromes
    Familial polyposis (high risk)
    Gardner's syndrome (high risk)
    Turcot's syndrome (high risk)
    Peutz-Jeghers syndrome (low to moderate risk)
  - Inflammatory bowel disease (IBD), both ulcerative colitis and Crohn's disease
  - Family history of "cancer family syndrome"
  - Heredofamilial breast cancer and colon carcinoma
  - History of previous colorectal carcinoma
  - Women undergoing irradiation for gynecologic cancer
  - First-degree relatives with colorectal carcinoma
  - Age >40 yr
  - Possible dietary factors (diet high in fat or meat, beer drinking, reduced vegetable consumption); prolonged high consumption of red and processed meat may increase the risk for cancer of the large intestine
  - Hereditary nonpolyposis colon cancer (HNPCC): autosomal dominant disorder characterized by early age of onset (mean age, 44 yr) and right-sided or proximal colon cancers, synchronous and metachronous colon cancers, mucinous and poorly differentiated colon cancers; accounts for 1% to 5% of all cases of CRC
  - Previous endometrial or ovarian cancer, particularly when diagnosed at an early age

PHYSICAL FINDINGS & CLINICAL PRESENTATION

- Physical examination may be completely unremarkable.
- Digital rectal examination can detect approximately 50% of rectal cancers.
- Palpable abdominal masses may indicate metastasis or complications of colorectal carcinoma (abscess, intussusception, volvulus).
- Abdominal distention and tenderness are suggestive of colonic obstruction.
- Hepatomegaly may be indicative of hepatic metastasis.

ETIOLOGY

CRC can arise through two mutational pathways: microsatellite instability or chromosomal instability. Germline genetic mutations are the basis of inherited colon cancer syndromes; an accumulation of somatic mutations in a cell is the basis of sporadic colon cancer.

DIAGNOSIS

DIFFERENTIAL DIAGNOSIS

- Diverticular disease
- Strictures
- IBD
- Infectious or inflammatory lesions
- Adhesions
- Arteriovenous malformations
- Metastatic carcinoma (prostate, sarcoma)
- Extrinsic masses (cysts, abscesses)

WORKUP

The clinical presentation of colorectal malignancies is initially vague and nonspecific (weight loss, anorexia, malaise). It is useful to divide colon cancer symptoms into those usually associated with the right side of the colon and those commonly associated with the left side of the colon because the clinical presentation varies with the location of the carcinoma.

- Right side of colon:
  - Anemia (iron deficiency from chronic blood loss).
  - Dull, vague, and uncharacteristic abdominal pain may be present, or patient may be completely asymptomatic.
  - Rectal bleeding is often missed because blood is mixed with feces.
  - Obstruction and constipation are unusual because of large lumen and more liquid stools.
- Left side of colon:
  - Change in bowel habits (constipation, diarrhea, tenesmus, pencil-thin stools).
  - Rectal bleeding (bright red blood coating the surface of the stool).
  - Intestinal obstruction is frequent because of small lumen.

Early diagnosis of patients with surgically curable disease (Dukes A/B) is necessary because survival time is directly related to the stage of the carcinoma at the time of diagnosis. Appropriate screening recommendations are discussed in Section V.

CLASSIFICATION AND STAGING

Dukes and UICC classification for CRC:
A. Confined to the mucosa-submucosa (stage I)
B. Invasion of muscularis propria (stage II)
C. Local node involvement (stage III)
D. Distant metastasis (stage IV)

TNM Classification:

Stage	TNM classification
I	T1-2, N0, M0
IIA	T3, N0, M0
IIB	T4, N0, M0
IIIA	T1-2, N1, M0
IIIB	T3-4, N1, M0
IIIC	T(any), N2, M0
IV	T(any), N(any), M1

LABORATORY TESTS

- Positive fecal occult blood test (FOBT): Many primary care physicians use single digital FOBT as their primary screening test for CRC. Single FOBT has low specificity for detecting human hemoglobin, is a poor screening method for CRC (sensitivity, 4.9%), and is inappropriate as the only test because negative results do not decrease the odds of advanced neoplasia. The American College of Gastroenterology recommends fecal immunochemical test as a replacement for guaiac-based FOBT for CRC detection. Annual Hemoccult SENSA and fecal DNA testing every 3 yr are alternative cancer detection tests.
- Microcytic anemia on CBC may be indicative of chronic blood loss.
- Increased plasma carcinoembryonic antigen (CEA) level: CEA should not be used as a screening test for CRC because it can be increased in patients with many other conditions (smoking, IBD, alcoholic liver disease). A normal CEA result does not exclude the diagnosis of CRC.
- Liver function tests should be ordered.

IMAGING STUDIES

- Colonoscopy with biopsy (primary assessment tool): The American College of Physicians recommends that patients should be offered a colonoscopy beginning at age 50 yr and repeated every 10 yr in average-risk patients. Screening is recommended in African Americans beginning at 45 yr of age. Persons with only one first-degree relative with CRC or advanced adenomas diagnosed at 60 yr or older may be screened as at average risk. A family history of small tubular adenomas in first-degree relatives is not considered to increase the risk for CRC. The U.S. Preventive Services Task Force guidelines state that screening should not be routinely recommended in persons older than 75 yr, and it should be not recommended at all in persons older than 85 yr. If persons between the ages of 75 and 85 yr have never undergone screening, the decision about screening should be individualized according to health status. Table 1-36 describes colorectal cancer screening and surveillance recommendations.

- Computed tomography colonoscopy (CTC) virtual colonoscopy (VC) uses helical (spiral) CT scanning to generate a two- or three-dimensional virtual colorectal image. CTC does not require sedation; but, like optical colonoscopy, it requires some bowel preparation (either bowel cathartics or ingestion of iodinated contrast medium with meals during the 48 hr before CT) and air insufflation. It also involves substantial exposure to radiation. In addition, patients with lesions detected by VC will require traditional colonoscopy. Compared with colonoscopy, CTC sensitivity for detection of polyps >10 mm ranges from 70% to 96%, and specificity ranges from 72% to 96%. CTC has replaced double-contrast barium enema as the radiographic screening alternative when patients decline colonoscopy.
- Capsule endoscopy allows visualization of the colonic mucosa but is not recommended as a screening procedure because its sensitivity for detecting colonic lesions is low compared with colonoscopy.
- CT scanning of the abdomen, pelvis, and chest assists in preoperative staging.
- PET scanning can display functional information and is accurate in the detection of CRC and its distant metastases. Combined PET/CT scanners are increasingly more available, and are useful to detect and characterize malignant lesions. Colonography composed of a combined modality of PET and CT is a newer diagnostic modality that can provide whole-body tumor staging in a single session.

Rx TREATMENT

GENERAL Rx

- Surgical resection: 70% of CRCs are resectable for cure at presentation; 45% of patients are cured by primary resection. Stage I and II tumors are curable by surgical resection, and up to 73% of cases of stage III can be cured by surgery combined with adjuvant chemotherapy.
- The backbone of chemotherapy treatment of CRC is fluorouracil (FU). Leucovorin (folinic acid) enhances the effect of FU and is given concomitantly. Adjuvant chemotherapy with combination of 5-FU and levamisole substantially increases cure rates for patients with stage III colon cancer and should be considered standard treatment for all such patients and selected patients with high-risk stage II colon cancer (adherence of tumor to an adjacent organ, bowel perforation, or obstruction).
- Radiation therapy is a useful adjunct to FU and leucovorin therapy for stage II or III rectal cancers.
- When given as adjuvant therapy after a complete resection in stage III disease, FU increases overall 5-yr survival rate from 51% to 64%. The use of adjuvant FU in stage II disease (no involvement of regional nodes) is controversial because 5-yr overall survival is 80% for treated or untreated patients, and the addition of FU only increases the probability of a 5-yr disease-free interval from 72% to 76%. For patients with standard-risk stage III tumors (e.g., involvement of one to three

regional lymph nodes), both FU alone and FU with oxaliplatin (Eloxatin, an inhibitor of DNA synthesis) are reasonable choices. In general, reversible peripheral neuropathy is the main side effect of FU plus oxaliplatin. The oral fluoropyrimidine capecitabine (Xeloda) is a prodrug that undergoes enzymatic conversion to FU. It is an effective alternative to IV FU as adjuvant treatment for stage III colon cancer because it has a lower incidence of mouth sores and bone marrow suppression. It does, however, have an increased incidence of palmar-plantar erythrodysesthesia (hand-foot syndrome).
- Irinotecan (Camptosar), a potent inhibitor of topoisomerase I, a nuclear enzyme involved in the unwinding of DNA during replication, can be used to treat metastatic CRC refractory to other drugs, including 5-FU; it may offer a few months of palliation but is expensive and is associated with significant toxicity.
- Oxaliplatin (Eloxatin), a third-generation platinum derivative, can be used in combination with FU and leucovorin (FL) for patients with metastatic CRC whose disease has recurred or progressed despite treatment with FL plus irinotecan. FL plus oxaliplatin should be considered for high-risk patients with stage III cancers (e.g., more than three involved regional nodes [N2] or tumor invasion beyond the serosa [T4 lesion]).
- Laboratory studies have identified molecular sites in tumor tissue that may serve as specific targets for treatment by using epidermal growth factor receptor (EGFR) antagonists and angiogenesis inhibitors. The monoclonal antibodies cetuximab (Erbitux), panitumumab (Vectibix), and bevacizumab (Avastatin) have been approved by the FDA for advanced CRC. Bevacizumab is an angiogenesis inhibitor that binds and inhibits the activity of human vascular endothelial growth factor. Cetuximab and panitumumab are EGFR blockers that inhibit the growth and survival of tumor cells that overexpress EGFR. Cetuximab has synergism with irinotecan, and its addition to irinotecan in patients with advanced disease resistant to irinotecan increases the response rate from 10% when cetuximab is used alone to 22% with combination of cetuximab and irinotecan. The addition of bevacizumab to FL in patients with advanced CRC has been reported to increase the response rate from 17% to 40%. Severe dermatologic toxicity can occur with both cetuximab and panitumumab.
- The liver is generally the initial and most common site of CRC metastases. Resection of metastases limited to the liver is curative in more than 30% of selected patients. In patients who undergo resection of liver metastases, postoperative treatment with a combination of hepatic arterial infusion of floxuridine and IV FU improves the outcome at 2 yr. Trials comparing hepatic resection (HR) and radiofrequency ablation (RFA) in the treatment of solitary colorectal liver metastases reveal that HR has better outcome; however, in tumors <3 cm, RFA can be recom-

TABLE 1-36 Colorectal Cancer (CRC) Screening and Surveillance Recommendations

Indication	Recommendations

Average risk	Beginning at age 50 yr:
	  Colonoscopy every 10 yr
	  Computed tomographic colonography every 5 yr
	  Flexible sigmoidoscopy every 5 yr
	  Double-contrast barium enema every 5 yr
	  (Stool blood testing annually or stool DNA testing acceptable but not preferred)

One or two first-degree relatives with CRC at any age or adenoma at age < 60 yr	Colonoscopy every 5 yr beginning at age 40 yr, or 10 yr younger than earliest diagnosis, whichever comes first
Hereditary nonpolyposis colorectal cancer	Genetic counseling and screening† Colonoscopy every 1 to 2 years beginning at age 25 yr and then yearly after age 40 yr‡
Familial adenomatous polyposis and variants	Genetic counseling and testing† Flexible sigmoidoscopy yearly beginning at puberty‡
Personal history of CRC	Colonoscopy within 1 yr of curative resection; repeat at 3 yr and then every 5 yr if normal
Personal history of colorectal adenoma	Colonoscopy every 3 to 5 yr after removal of all index polyps
Inflammatory bowel disease	Colonoscopy every 1 to 2 yr beginning after 8 yr of pancolitis or after 15 yr if only left-sided disease

*Recommendations proposed by the American Cancer Society and U.S. Multi-Society Task Force on Colorectal Cancer; recommendations for average-risk patients also endorsed by the American College of Radiology.
†Whenever possible, affected relatives should be tested first because of potential false-negative results.
‡Screening recommendation for individuals with positive or indeterminate tests as well as for those who refuse genetic testing.
From Andreoli TE et al: *Andreoli and Carpenter's Cecil essentials of medicine*, ed 8, Philadelphia, 2010, Elsevier/Saunders.

mended in patients who are not surgical candidates due to comorbidities or when the liver met is poorly localized anatomically.

CHRONIC Rx

Follow-up is indicated with:
- Physician visits with a focus on the clinical and disease-related history, directed physical examination guided by this history, coordination of follow-up, and counseling every 3 to 6 mo for the first 3 yr, then decreased frequency thereafter for 2 yr
- Colonoscopy yearly for the initial 2 yr, then every 3 yr
- Baseline CEA level should be obtained; if elevated, it can be used after surgery as a measure of completeness of tumor resection or to monitor tumor recurrence. If used to monitor tumor recurrence, CEA should be obtained every 3 to 6 mo for up to 5 yr. The role of CEA for monitoring patients with resected colon cancer has been questioned because of the small number of cures attributed to CEA monitoring despite the substantial cost in dollars and physical and emotional stress associated with monitoring.

DISPOSITION

The 5-yr survival rate varies with the stage of the carcinoma:
- Dukes:
  - Dukes A 5-yr survival rate >80%
  - Dukes B 5-yr survival rate 60%
  - Dukes C 5-yr survival rate 20%
  - Dukes D 5-yr survival rate 3%
- TNM classification:

Stage	TNM Classification	5-yr Survival Rate
I	T1-2, N0, M0	>90%
IIA	T3, N0, M0	60-85%
IIB	T4, N0, M0	60-85%
IIIA	T1-2, N1, M0	25-65%
IIIB	T3-4, N1, M0	25-65%
IIIC	T(any), N2, M0	25-65%
IV	T(any), N(any), M1	5-7%

- Overall 5-yr disease-free survival rate has increased from 50% to 63% during the past two decades.
- High-frequency microsatellite instability in CRC is independently predictive of a relatively favorable outcome and reduces the likelihood of metastases.

- In patients with Dukes C (stage III) CRC, there is improved 5-yr survival among women treated with adjuvant chemotherapy (53% with chemotherapy vs. 33% without) and among patients with right-sided tumors treated with adjuvant chemotherapy.
- Retention of 19q alleles in microsatellite-stable cancers and mutation of the gene for the type I receptor for tumor growth factor B1 in cancers with high levels of microsatellite instability point to a favorable outcome after adjuvant chemotherapy with FU-based regimens for stage II colon cancer.
- Expression patterns of microRNA are systemically altered in colon adenocarcinomas. High miR-21 expression is associated with poor survival and poor therapeutic outcome.
- Guanylyl cyclase 2 C (GUCY2C) has been identified as a marker expressed by colorectal tumors that could reveal occult metastases in lymph nodes. Expression of GUCY2C in histologically negative lymph nodes appears to be independently associated with time to recurrence and disease-free survival in patients with lymph nodes free of tumor cells by histopathology (pNO) in CRC.
- Regular aspirin use after the diagnosis of CRC has been reported to be associated with lower risk for CRC-specific and overall mortality, especially among individuals with tumors that overexpress cyclooxygenase-2.

REFERRAL

- Surgical referral for resection
- Oncology referral for adjuvant chemotherapy in selected patients
- Radiation oncology referral for patients with stage II or III rectal cancers

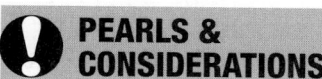

PEARLS & CONSIDERATIONS

COMMENTS

- Metastases of tumor cells to regional lymph nodes is the single most important prognostic factor in patients with colon cancer.
- Decreased fat intake to 30% of total energy intake, increased fiber, and fruit and vegetable consumption may reduce CRC risk. Recent literature reports, however, do not support a protective effect from dietary fiber against CRC in women.

- Chemoprophylaxis with aspirin (81 mg/day) reduces the incidence of colorectal adenomas in persons at risk.
- Statins inhibit the growth of colon cancer lines. Use of statins is associated with a 47% relative reduction in the risk for CRC. Additional trials are necessary to investigate the overall benefits of statins in preventing CRC.
- The National Cancer Institute has published consensus guidelines for universal screening for HNPCC in patients with newly diagnosed CRC. Tumors in mutation carriers of HNPCC typically exhibit microsatellite instability, a characteristic phenotype caused by expansion or contraction of short nucleotide repeat sequences. These guidelines (Bethesda Guidelines) are useful for selective patients for microsatellite instability testing. Screening patients with newly diagnosed CRC for HNPCC is cost effective, especially if the benefits to their immediate relatives are considered.
- Expression of guanylyl cyclase C mRNA in lymph nodes is associated with recurrence of CRC in patients with stage II disease. Analysis of guanylyl cyclase mRNA expression by reverse transcription polymerase chain reaction may be useful for CRC staging.
- The use of either annual or biennial FOBT significantly reduces the incidence of CRC.
- The detection of mutations in the *APC* gene from stool samples is a promising new modality for early detection of colorectal neoplasms.
- KRAS mutations are consistently associated with reduced overall and progression-free survival and increased treatment failure. Rates among patients with advanced colorectal cancer treated with anti-EGFR antibodies.

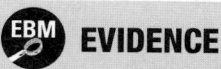

(EBM) EVIDENCE

available at www.expertconsult.com

SUGGESTED READINGS

available at www.expertconsult.com

AUTHOR: **FRED F. FERRI, M.D.**

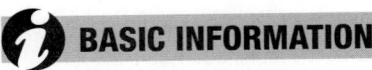

DEFINITION

Complex regional pain syndrome (CRPS) type 1 or reflex sympathetic dystrophy (RSD) is a pain disorder characterized by constant and intense limb pain associated with vasomotor and sudomotor abnormalities that occurs without a definable nerve lesion. RSD or CRPS type 1 should be distinguished from CRPS type 2, which refers to pain disorders in which a definable nerve lesion exists.

SYNONYMS

CRPS type 1
Reflex sympathetic dystrophy
Causalgia (or CRPS type 2)
Shoulder-hand syndrome
Sudeck's atrophy
Posttraumatic pain syndrome
RSD

ICD-9CM CODES

337.20 Dystrophy sympathetic (posttraumatic) (reflex)

EPIDEMIOLOGY & DEMOGRAPHICS

- First described by Mitchell et al during the American Civil War.
- The incidence and prevalence are not known.
- Usually initiated by trauma, mostly after orthopedic procedures, especially those on the extremities.
- Can occur in adults or children.
- Often associated with psychiatric and emotional lability, anxiety, and depression.

PHYSICAL FINDINGS & CLINICAL PRESENTATION

RSD is divided into three stages:
- Acute stage (occurring within hours to days after the injury)
  1. Burning or aching pain occurring over the injured extremity
  2. Hyperalgesia (exquisitely sensitive to touch)
  3. Edema
  4. Dysthermia
  5. Increased hair and nail growth
- Dystrophic stage (3 to 6 mo after the injury)
  1. Burning pain radiating both distally and proximally from the site of injury
  2. Brawny edema
  3. Hyperhidrosis
  4. Hypothermia and cyanosis
  5. Muscle tremors and spasms
  6. Increased muscle tone and reflexes
- Atrophic stage (6 mo after injury)
  1. Spread of pain proximally
  2. Cold, pale cyanotic skin
  3. Trophic skin changes with subcutaneous atrophy
  4. Fixed joints
  5. Contractures

ETIOLOGY

- The cause is unknown. It is thought to represent dysfunction of the sympathetic nervous system.
- Any injury can precipitate RSD, including:
  1. Crush blunt trauma, burns, frostbite
  2. Surgery
  3. Parkinson's disease
  4. Cerebrovascular accident
  5. Myocardial infarction
  6. Osteoarthritis, cervical and lumbar disk disease
  7. Carpal tunnel and tarsal tunnel syndrome
  8. Diabetes
  9. Hyperthyroidism
  10. Isoniazid therapy

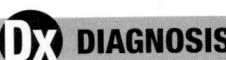 **DIAGNOSIS**

The diagnosis is primarily clinical, based on the patient's history and physical presentation.

DIFFERENTIAL DIAGNOSIS

The differential diagnosis includes all the causes mentioned under "Etiology."

WORKUP

- No workup is needed because there are no specific diagnostic tests establishing the diagnosis.
- Electrophysiologic testing is useful to identify patients with type 2 CRPS.
- Long-term skin temperature measurements can be used as a diagnostic test.

LABORATORY TESTS

Blood tests are not specific.

IMAGING STUDIES

- No imaging studies are diagnostic. Three-phase bone imaging may be helpful.
- Autonomic testing, although not commonly done, has been proposed.
  1. Measuring resting sweat output
  2. Measuring resting skin temperature
  3. Quantitative sudomotor axon reflex test
- Radiograph studies of the affected limb may show osteoporosis from disuse.

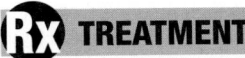 **TREATMENT**

Treatment is aimed at relieving the pain and improving disuse atrophy with physical therapy.

NONPHARMACOLOGIC THERAPY

- Physical therapy
- Transcutaneous nerve stimulation

ACUTE GENERAL Rx

- The following has been tried for neuropathic pain relief:
  1. Amitriptyline 10 mg to 150 mg qid
  2. Phenytoin 300 mg qid
  3. Carbamazepine 100 mg bid

  4. Calcium channel blockers, nifedipine extended release 30 to 60 mg qid
  5. Prednisone 60 to 80 mg qid for 2 wk and then tapered over 1 to 2 wk to a maintenance dose of 5 mg qid for 2 to 3 mo
  6. Vitamin C 500 mg daily for 50 days after wrist fracture can decrease the occurrence of CRPS
  7. Gabapentin 300 mg daily up to 3 times a day
- Regional nerve block that provides a perioperative sympathectomy may be advantageous for patients with a history of CRPS who require orthopedic surgery.
- Because CRPS type 2 is the result of a definable nerve lesion, using a surgical technique that minimizes the risk of nerve damage is important.

CHRONIC Rx

- Stellate ganglion and lumbar sympathetic blocks can be tried.
- Intravenous alpha-adrenergic blockade with phentolamine may predict response to subsequent sympatholytic treatment.
- Surgical sympathectomy.
- Surgical correction can be performed for severe foot and ankle contracture.
- Recent trials have shown that intravenous immunoglobulin (IVIG 0.5 g/mg) can reduce pain in refractory complex regional pain syndrome.

DISPOSITION

Spontaneous remission can occur after several weeks to months.

REFERRAL

RSD is a very difficult diagnosis to make and referral to either rheumatology, neurology, orthopedic, or psychiatry specialists is recommended.

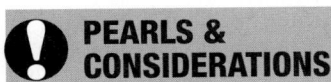 **PEARLS & CONSIDERATIONS**

COMMENTS

- RSD is a common clinical entity without clear definition, pathophysiologic features, or treatment.
- Pain is the most disabling symptom for most patients and is usually out of proportion to the extent of the injury.

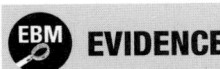 **EVIDENCE**

available at www.expertconsult.com

SUGGESTED READINGS
available at www.expertconsult.com

AUTHOR: **JORGE A. VILLAFUERTE, M.D.**

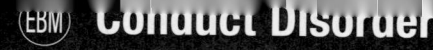
C

 BASIC INFORMATION

DEFINITION

Conduct disorder (CD) is defined by a combination of antisocial acts. It is classified under the DSM-IV-R category of illnesses labeled as "disorders usually first diagnosed in infancy, childhood or adolescence," and it is a "disruptive behavior disorder." The essential feature is a repetitive and persistent pattern of behavior in which either the basic rights of others are violated and/or major age-appropriate societal rules are violated. The DSM-IV-R lists 15 possible behavioral manifestations of CD, grouped into four categories: aggression to people and animals, destruction of property, deceitfulness or theft, and serious violations of rules. Three of the 15 behaviors are required to have occurred in the last 12 months and one behavior must have occurred in the last 6 mo. Specifiers describe the age of onset and the severity of the disorder. CD represents a heterogeneous group with respect to presentation, etiology, severity, and course.

ICD-10-CM CODES
F90, F91, F92/312

EPIDEMIOLOGY & DEMOGRAPHICS

INCIDENCE: 1% (12-mo span, National Comorbidity Survey-Replication [NCS-R])
PREVALENCE: Approximately 1% to 16%; NCS-R: 9%. Disruptive behavior disorders are considered the most common reason for referral of children to mental health providers. There is wide variation in documented prevalence rates when subgroups are considered (i.e., gender, age, neighborhood, acts of physical aggression, acts of rule breaking). Subtypes characterized by rule violations, deceit, and theft are more prevalent than subtypes characterized by aggression.
PREDOMINANT SEX: More common in males (4:1 preadolescence and 2:1 postadolescence). It is unclear if CD females are underrepresented, as diagnostic criteria were validated on male samples. Nonconfrontational aggression and promiscuity are examples of possible gender-specific criteria that, at this time, have unknown predictive validity.
PREDOMINANT AGE: Most common onset in early adolescence. Median age of onset is 11 yr.
GENETICS: Meta-analyses of twin and adoption studies report a heritability estimate of approximately 50%.
RISK FACTORS: Factors associated with illness onset include parental criminality, hostile parenting, perinatal complications, low IQ, impulsivity, and overcrowded neighborhoods. Factors associated with poor prognosis include early onset, more severe behaviors, attention deficit hyperactivity disorder (ADHD), and substance abuse.

PHYSICAL FINDINGS & CLINICAL PRESENTATION

- Severity often increases with age (i.e., lying and truancy to sexual assault and robbery).
- Aggressive youth are more likely to interpret as negative or hostile the intent of neutral others and are more likely to believe that conflict can be adequately resolved via aggression.
- Poor frustration tolerance, irritability, temper outbursts, and recklessness are often associated with CD.

ETIOLOGY

- Estimated population variance in antisocial behavior accounted for by:
  - Genes: 50%
  - Environmental factors shared among family members: 20%
  - Environmental factors unshared among family members: 20% to 30%

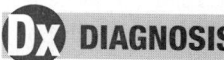 **DIAGNOSIS**

DIFFERENTIAL DIAGNOSIS

- DSM-IV-R: Oppositional defiant disorder, mood disorder, adjustment disorder, ADHD, antisocial personality disorder (for those over age 18), mental retardation, post traumatic stress disorder and/or V code: child or adolescent antisocial behavior
- ICD 10 ("Mixed Disturbances"): depressive conduct disorder and hyperkinetic conduct disorder
- Adaptive behavior or subcultural delinquency
- Rule out medical etiologies based on review of presenting symptoms (i.e., steroid intoxication, endocrine abnormality)

WORKUP

- Diagnostic criteria are based on observable objective behaviors. Youth may minimize antisocial acts; therefore, collateral data resources are essential.
- Evaluate for common potentially treatable comorbidities such as substance abuse, ADHD, and cognitive impairments, including learning disorders.

LABORATORY TESTS

- Consider urine toxicology for possible substance use comorbidity.
- Slow resting heart rate is the most replicated of all biologic markers for conduct problems. However, there is no established clinical cutoff for "slow" heart rate.

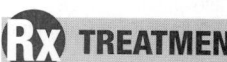 **TREATMENT**

Treatment that is multitarget and multimodal is often indicated. Treatment is most ideally initiated when the breadth of the individual's needs (comorbidity, psychosocial impairments, high-risk behaviors) are considered with respect to the community's treatment resources.

NONPHARMACOLOGIC THERAPY

- Parent management training
- Problem solving skills training: social skills, conflict resolution, anger management, impulse control, vocational
- Functional family therapy
- Multisystemic therapy
- Other: cognitive behavioral therapy for comorbidity

PHARMACOLOGIC THERAPY

Treat the presumed underlying etiology of the most functionally impairing behavior.

DISPOSITION

- Approximately half of those with early onset of CD persist with antisocial behaviors into adulthood. There is no reliable way to predict which 50% will persist.
- Approximately half of those with early onset of CD do not develop antisocial personality disorder in adulthood. This subgroup appears to become depressed, anxious, and socially isolated adults.
- Approximately 85% of those with adolescent onset of CD do not demonstrate lifetime persistent violence, convictions, and incarcerations. However, adult prognosis may often include substance abuse and crimes that go largely undetected.

REFERRAL

Due to the high rate of comorbidities and pervasive psychosocial impairment, a high level of broad treatment services is often necessary. Treatment most often requires referral into the mental health community.

 **PEARLS & CONSIDERATIONS**

COMMENTS

- DSM-V is due to be published in 2012.
  - Consideration is being given to adding a new subtype to conduct disorder: high versus low callous unemotional traits. Those with CD who have callous unemotional traits are suggested to have a stronger genetic risk and more severe aggression, and may be less responsive to typical parental socialization practices as a result of their insensitivity to punishment and insensitivity to distress cues from others.
  - Consideration is also being given to the introduction of a separate mood disorder with disruptive behavioral manifestations. The nomenclature that is proposed is "behavioral dysregulation disorder with dysphoria."
- Expect 30% treatment noncompliance rate.
- Clinical pitfall: overdiagnosis and undertreatment.
- Due to the high rate of comorbidity of substance abuse and depression, educate youth who are treated with SSRIs regarding serotonin syndrome and other commonly abused serotonergic substances such as ecstacy, dextromethorphan, cocaine, and stimulants.

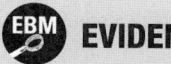 **EVIDENCE**

available at www.expertconsult.com

SUGGESTED READINGS
available at www.expertconsult.com

AUTHOR: **SARAH L. XAVIER, D.O.**

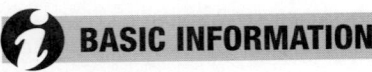

BASIC INFORMATION

DEFINITION

Condyloma acuminatum is a sexually transmitted viral disease of the vulva, vagina, and cervix caused by the human papillomavirus (HPV). 90% of genital warts are caused by HPV 6 or 11.

SYNONYMS

Genital warts
Venereal warts
Anogenital warts

ICD-9CM CODES

078.11 Condyloma acuminatum

EPIDEMIOLOGY & DEMOGRAPHICS

- Seen mostly in young adults, with a mean age of onset of 16 to 25 yr
- A sexually transmitted disease spread by skin-to-skin contact
- Highly contagious, with 25% to 65% of sexual partners developing it
- Virus shed from both macroscopic and microscopic lesions
- Average incubation time is 2 mo (range, 1 to 8 mo)
- Predisposing conditions: diabetes, pregnancy, local trauma, and immunosuppression (e.g., transplant recipients, those with HIV infection)

PHYSICAL FINDINGS & CLINICAL PRESENTATION

- Usually found in genital area but can be present elsewhere
- Lesions usually in similar positions on both sides of perineum
- Initial lesions pedunculated, soft papules about 2 to 3 mm in diameter, 10 to 20 mm long; may occur as single papule or in clusters
- Size of lesions varies from pinhead to large cauliflower-like masses
- Usually asymptomatic, but if infected can cause pain, odor, or bleeding
- Vulvar condyloma more common than vaginal and cervical
- Four morphologic types: condylomatous, keratotic, papular, and flat warts
- Intra-anal warts are observed predominantly in persons who have had receptive anal intercourse.

ETIOLOGY

- HPV DNA types 6 and 11 usually found in exophytic warts and have no malignant potential
- HPV types 16 and 18 usually found in flat warts and are associated with increased risk of malignancy

- Recurrence associated with persisting viral infection of adjacent normal skin in 25% to 50% of cases

DIAGNOSIS

DIFFERENTIAL DIAGNOSIS

- Abnormal anatomic variants or skin tags around labia minora and introitus
- Dysplastic warts

WORKUP

- Colposcopic examination of lower genital tract from cervix to perianal skin with 3% to 5% acetic acid
- Biopsy of vulvar lesions that lack the classic appearance of warts and that become ulcerated or do not respond to treatment
- Biopsy of flat, white, or ulcerated cervical lesions

LABORATORY TESTS

- Pap smear
- Cervical cultures for *Neisseria gonorrhoeae* and *Chlamydia*
- Serologic test for syphilis
- HIV testing offered
- Wet mount for trichomoniasis, *Candida albicans,* and *Gardnerella vaginalis*
- Testing for diabetes (blood glucose)

TREATMENT

NONPHARMACOLOGIC THERAPY

- Keep genital area dry and clean.
- If present, keep diabetes well controlled.
- Advise use of condoms to prevent spread of infection to sexual partner.

ACUTE GENERAL Rx

Factors that influence selection of treatment include wart size, wart number, anatomic site of wart, wart morphology, patient preference, cost of treatment, convenience, adverse effects, and provider experience.
Keratolytic agents:
- Podophyllin (Podofilox 0.5% solution or gel)
  - Acts by poisoning mitotic spindle and causing intense vasospasm
  - Applied directly to lesion weekly and washed off in 6 hr
  - Used in minimal vulvar or anal disease
  - Applied cautiously to nonkeratinized epithelial surfaces
  - Contraindicated in pregnancy
  - Discontinued if lesions do not disappear in 6 wk; switch to other treatment
- Sinecatechin 15% ointment
  - Applied tid (0.5 cm strand of ointment to each wart)
  - Should not be continued longer than 16 wk

- Trichloroacetic acid (30% to 80% solution)
  - Acts by precipitation of surface proteins
  - Applied twice monthly to lesion
  - Indicated for vulvar, anal, and vaginal lesions; can be used for cervical lesions
  - Less painful and irritating to normal tissue than podophyllin
- Fluorouracil
  - Causes necrosis and sloughing of growing tissue
  - Can be used intravaginally or for vulvar, anal, or urethral lesions
  - Better tolerated; 3 g (two thirds of vaginal applicator) applied weekly for 12 wk
  - Possible vaginal ulceration and erythema
  - Patient's vagina examined after four to six applications
  - 80% cure rate
Physical agents:
- Cryotherapy with liquid nitrogen or cryoprobe
  - Can be used weekly for 3 to 6 wk
  - 62% to 79% success rate
  - Not suitable for large warts
- Laser therapy
  - Done by physician with necessary expertise and equipment
  - Painful; requires anesthesia
- Electrocautery or excision
  - For recurrent, very large lesions
  - Local anesthesia needed
Immunotherapy:
- Interferon
  - Injected intralesionally at a dose of 3 million U/m^2 three times weekly for 8 wk
  - Side effects: fever, chills, malaise, headache
- Imiquimod 5% cream at hs, 3× wk up to 16 wk increases wart clearance after 3 mo
- Interferon, topical: increases wart clearance at 4 wk

DISPOSITION

- Follow-up exam every 6 to 12 mo, as needed.
- Correct and consistent male condom use might lower the chances of giving or getting genital HPV, but such use is not fully protective because HPV can infect areas that are not covered by a condom.

EBM EVIDENCE

available at www.expertconsult.com

SUGGESTED READING

available at www.expertconsult.com

AUTHORS: **GEORGE T. DANAKAS, M.D.,** and **RUBEN ALVERO, M.D.**

BASIC INFORMATION

DEFINITION

Congenital adrenal hyperplasia (CAH) is a spectrum of disorders resulting from a deficiency or complete lack of one of the enzymes in the cortisol synthesis pathway. These autosomal-recessive genetic disorders are usually characterized by cortisol deficiency and virilization, with or without salt wasting.

SYNONYMS

21-hydroxylase deficiency (equivalent to CYP21A2 deficiency)
11β-hydroxylase deficiency
3β-hydroxysteroid dehydrogenase deficiency
17-hydroxylase deficiency
Lipoid adrenal hyperplasia
Adrenal virilism
Adrenogenital syndrome
Virilizing adrenal hyperplasia

ICD-9CM CODES
255.2 Adrenogenital disorders; hyperplasia, congenital adrenal

EPIDEMIOLOGY & DEMOGRAPHICS

- About 95% of cases of CAH are caused by 21-hydroxylase deficiency, of which two thirds are the salt-wasting form.
- Autosomal recessive inheritance.
- The "classic" form presents in childhood, nonclassic is mild or late onset.
- Incidence is estimated at about 1 in 16,000 live births in North America (Hispanic > American Indian > white > black > Asian).
- Most common cause of ambiguous genitalia in 46X,X females.

CLINICAL PRESENTATION

"Classic" salt-wasting form (impaired cortisol and aldosterone synthesis):
- Adrenal crisis in first weeks of life with vomiting, poor weight gain, lethargy, dehydration, hyponatremia, hyperkalemia, and elevated plasma renin.
- Females are born with ambiguous genitalia that often leads to diagnosis before adrenal crisis occurs.
- Males may have greater penile size and smaller testes than expected during childhood. Males may also develop adrenal rests, or ectopic islands of adrenal cortical tissue in the testes, in childhood and may experience infertility as adults.
- If patients survive infancy, their overall life expectancy is not compromised.
- Both males and females may exhibit rapid growth in childhood (due to early epiphyseal closure, which then results in short stature in adulthood).
- Precocious puberty is common in both males and females.

"Classic" non-salt-wasting or simple virilizing form (impaired cortisol synthesis only):
- Females present with ambiguous genitalia at birth.
- The normal appearance of male genitalia in the simple virilizing form makes this a difficult diagnosis in male infants.
- Characterized by precocious puberty, short stature, and testicular adrenal rests, as in the salt-wasting form.

"Nonclassic" or mild, late-onset form (varying degrees of androgen excess):
- Usually presents in adolescence or adulthood and is not detected on newborn screening.
- Often asymptomatic but can be associated with mild virilization.

- PCOS-like symptoms occur in women (hirsutism, oligomenorrhea, acne, infertility, insulin resistance, abnormal menses).
- Associated with infertility in males.

ETIOLOGY

In 21-hydroxylase deficiency, the pathways for aldosterone production (from the conversion of progesterone to deoxycorticosterone) and cortisol production (from the conversion of 17-hydroxyprogesterone to 11-deoxycortisol) by the cP450 enzyme 21-hydroxylase are interrupted. The production of ACTH is thus stimulated by a negative feedback mechanism, leading to adrenal hyperplasia and mineralocorticoid deficiency as the intermediaries in aldosterone and cortisol synthesis are shunted to the androgen biosynthesis pathway (Fig. 1-101, A and B). A recombination event between the active CYP21A2 gene on chromosome 6p21.3 and the CYP21A1 pseudogene is thought to create the deficient 21-hydroxy-lase enzyme.

DIAGNOSIS

DIFFERENTIAL DIAGNOSIS

- Precocious puberty
- Polycystic ovarian syndrome (PCOS)
- Androgen resistance syndromes
- Pseudohermaphroditism
- Mixed gonadal dysgenesis
- Testicular carcinoma
- Leydig cell tumors
- Adrenocortical carcinoma
- Addison's disease
- Pituitary adenoma

LABORATORY TESTS

- Prenatal: chorionic villus sampling for genetic testing or measurement of 17-hydroxyprogesterone

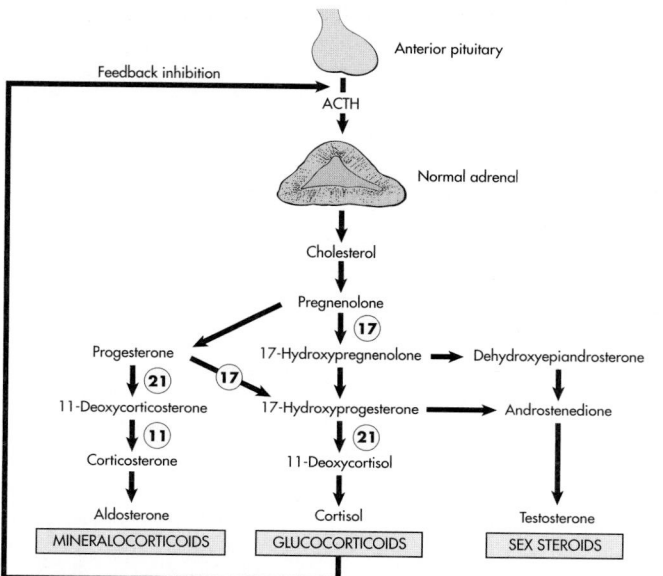
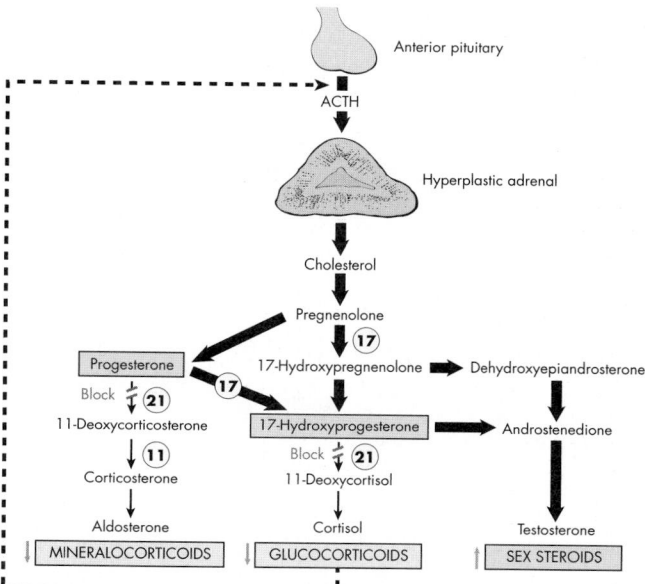

FIGURE 1-101 A, Normal adrenal steroidogenesis. **B,** Consequences of C-21 hydroxylase deficiency. (From Cotran R et al [eds]: *Robbins pathologic basis of disease,* ed 6, Philadelphia, 1999, WB Saunders, p 1158.)

- Neonates, children, and adults: dehydroepi-androsterone sulfate (DHEA-S, DS) and androstenedione will be increased. Elevated 17-hydroxyprogesterone levels >242 ng/dl confirms classic 21-hydroxylase deficiency (higher cutoffs needed for preterm infants). ACTH stimulation test may be required to confirm nonclassic CAH. Also consider obtaining adrenal androgen profile, electrolytes, BUN, Cr, plasma renin activity, and 21-hydroxylase genotyping. Cortisol levels are too variable to be of use.
- Many states include 17-hydroxyprogesterone levels in newborn screen.

IMAGING STUDIES

- Abdominal ultrasound to evaluate adrenal glands can accelerate diagnosis.
- Ultrasound to identify a uterus in cases of ambiguous genitalia.
- Ultrasound is preferred to rule out testicular adrenal rest tumors (found in classic and nonclassic forms) and should be done beginning in adolescence.

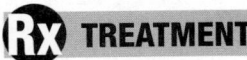

NONPHARMACOLOGIC THERAPY

- Surgical correction of ambiguous genitalia is recommended by 6 months.
- Monitoring: serum 17-hydroxyprogesterone and androstenedione, renin, electrolytes, blood pressure, bone age and density, Tanner staging, growth velocity, weight.
- Bilateral laparoscopic adrenalectomy with lifelong glucocorticoid and mineralocorticoid replacement (controversial).

- Gene therapy (hypothetical).
- Psychological counseling.

CHRONIC Rx

- Glucocorticoids to partially suppress adrenal androgen secretion. During periods of physiologic stress may need to be doubled or tripled.
  - Children: hydrocortisone 15 to 20 mg/m²/day in 3 divided doses (minimizes the risk of iatrogenic short stature found in other corticosteroids with longer half-lives).
  - Adolescents/adults: dexamethasone 0.25 to 0.75 mg PO QHS (also use to treat adrenal rests) or prednisone 5 to 7.5 mg/day in 2 divided doses.
- Mineralocorticoids to normalize electrolytes and plasma renin activity.
  - Infants up to 6 months: fludrocortisone 0.1 to 0.3 mg daily in 2 divided doses but occasionally up to 0.4 mg daily. Often require 1 to 3 g sodium chloride supplementation.
  - Children: fludrocortisone: 0.05 to 0.1 mg daily.
  - Adolescents/adults: fludrocortisone 0.1 to 0.2 mg daily (may decrease glucocorticoid requirement).
- Treatment of simple virilizing form: similar to salt-wasting form but mineralocorticoid replacement is unnecessary.
- Treatment of nonclassic form:
  - In adolescent and adult women: oral contraceptives, glucocorticoids, and/or antiandrogens.
  - In children and adult males, usually no treatment is necessary.

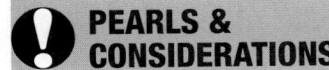

COMMENTS

- Consider the diagnosis of classic salt-wasting CAH in infants with failure to thrive.
- There is believed to be an increased prevalence of CAH in patients diagnosed with adrenal "incidentalomas"—adrenal gland lesions detected unexpectedly on imaging, usually by MRI or CT scanning.
- Cushing's syndrome may result from over-treatment of CAH with glucocorticoids.
- Treatment of CAH in pregnancy with dexamethasone will confound newborn screening for 17-hydroxyprogesterone such that these infants should be screened 1 to 2 wk postpartum.
- Patients with CAH may suffer from gender identity disorders and sexual dysfunction.

PREVENTION

- Prenatal: Early CVS sampling. Use of dexamethasone 20 to 25 μg/kg daily beginning at 5- to 8-wk gestation for female fetuses only is controversial because long-term studies are unavailable.
- Neonatal screening.
- Genetic counseling.

SUGGESTED READINGS

available at www.expertconsult.com

AUTHOR: **ELIZABETH BROWN, M.D.**

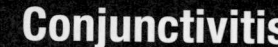
C

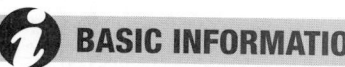 **BASIC INFORMATION**

DEFINITION

The term *conjunctivitis* refers to an inflammation of the conjunctiva resulting from a variety of causes, including allergies and bacterial, viral, and chlamydial infections.

SYNONYMS

"Red eye"
Pink eye
Acute conjunctivitis
Subacute conjunctivitis
Chronic conjunctivitis
Purulent conjunctivitis
Pseudomembranous conjunctivitis
Papillary conjunctivitis
Follicular conjunctivitis
Newborn conjunctivitis

ICD-9CM CODES
372.30 Conjunctivitis, unspecified

EPIDEMIOLOGY & DEMOGRAPHICS

INCIDENCE (IN U.S.): 1.6% to 12% in *newborns*
PREVALENCE (IN U.S.):
- Allergic conjunctivitis, the most common form of ocular allergy, is usually associated with allergic rhinitis and may be seasonal or perennial.
- Bacterial or viral conjunctivitis is often seasonal and can be extremely contagious.

PREDOMINANT AGE: Occurs at *any* age. Most cases in adults are due to viral infection. Children are more prone to develop bacterial conjunctivitis than viral forms.
PEAK INCIDENCE: More common in the fall, when *viral* infections and pollens increase

PHYSICAL FINDINGS & CLINICAL PRESENTATION

- Infection and chemosis of conjunctivae with discharge (Fig. 1-102). Gluing of the eyelids and no itching is more indicative of a bacterial cause.
- Cornea is clear or can be involved.
- Vision is often normal but can be blurred.

ETIOLOGY

- Bacterial: *Haemophilus influenzae, Streptococcus pneumoniae,* and *Moraxella catarrhalis* in children; *Staphylococcus* species in

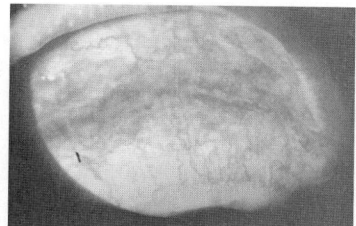

FIGURE 1-102 Conjunctival infection from viral conjunctivitis. (From Marx JA [ed]: *Rosen's emergency medicine,* ed 5, St Louis, 2002, Mosby.)

adults. Gram-negative infections are more common in contact lens wearers. Gonococcal ophthalmia neonatorum is caused by *Neisseria gonorrhoeae* acquired by exposure of the neonatal conjunctivae to infected cervicovaginal secretions during delivery.
- Viral.
- Chlamydial.
- Allergic.
- Traumatic.

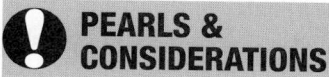 **DIAGNOSIS**

DIFFERENTIAL DIAGNOSIS

- Acute glaucoma
- Corneal lesions
- Acute iritis
- Episcleritis
- Scleritis
- Uveitis
- Canalicular obstruction

WORKUP

- History and physical examination
- Reports of itching, pain, and visual changes

LABORATORY TESTS

Cultures are useful if not *successfully* treated with antibiotics; initial culture is usually not necessary.

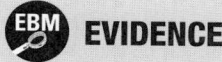 **TREATMENT**

NONPHARMACOLOGIC THERAPY

- Warm compresses if infective conjunctivitis.
- Cold compresses if irritative or allergic conjunctivitis.
- Contact lenses should be taken out until an infection is completely resolved. Nondisposable lenses should be cleaned thoroughly as recommended by the manufacturer, and a new lens case should be used. Disposable contact lenses should be thrown away.

ACUTE GENERAL Rx

- Antibiotic drops (e.g., levofloxacin, ofloxin, ciprofloxacin, tobramycin, gentamicin ophthalmic solution, 1 or 2 drops q2 to 4h) are indicated for suspected bacterial conjunctivitis.
- Caution: be careful with ophthalmic corticosteroid treatment and avoid unless sure of diagnosis; corticosteroids can exacerbate infections and have been associated with increased intraocular pressure and cataract formation.
- An oral antihistamine (cetirizine, loratadine, desloratadine, or fexofenadine) is effective in relieving itching.
- Mast cell stabilizers (e.g., cromolyn [4%, 1 to 2 drops q4 to 6h], lodoxamide [0.1%, 1 to 2 drops qid]) are effective for allergic conjunctivitis. Others include Elestat, Optivar, and Patanol.
- Bepotastine 1.5% ophthalmic solution is an H1-antihistamine effective for topical treatment of itching associated with allergic con-

junctivitis. The topical NSAID ketorolac (0.5%, 1 drop qd) is also useful in allergic conjunctivitis.
- Antihistamine/decongestant combinations such as pheniramine/naphazoline (Visine A), available over the counter, are more effective than either agent alone but have a short duration and can result in rebound vasodilatation with prolonged use. Others include Naphcon-A, Albacon-A, and Opcon-A.

CHRONIC Rx

- Depends on cause.
- If allergic, nonsteroidals such as Voltaren, Acular, and Xibrom ophthalmic solution; mast cell stabilizers such as Elestat, Alocril, Patanol, and Zaditor are useful for improving ocular itching in patients with allergic conjunctivitis.
- If an infection, use antibiotic drops (see "Acute General Rx").
- Dry eyes need artificial tears (Restasis) or lacrimal duct plugs when indicated.

DISPOSITION

Follow carefully for the first 2 wk to ensure secondary complications do not occur. Otitis media can develop in 25% of children with *Hemophilus influenzae* conjunctivitis. Bacterial keratitis occurs in 30/1000 contact lens wearers.

REFERRAL

To ophthalmologist if symptoms are refractory to initial treatment. Indications for urgent referral are severe eye pain or headache, photophobia, decreased vision, and contact lens use.

PEARLS & CONSIDERATIONS

COMMENTS

- Red eyes are not simply conjunctivitis when the patient has significant pain or loss of sight. However, it is usually safe to treat pain-free eyes and the normal seeing red eye with lid hygiene and topical treatment.
- Use caution with patients wearing soft contact lenses, infants, and the elderly.
- Do not use steroids indiscriminately; use only when the diagnosis is certain.
- Bacterial conjunctivitis is generally self-limiting. Over 60% of persons will improve with placebo within 2 to 5 days.

EBM EVIDENCE

available at www.expertconsult.com

AUTHOR: **MELVYN KOBY, M.D.**

Diseases and Disorders

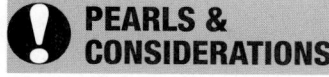

BASIC INFORMATION

DEFINITION

Contact dermatitis is an acute or chronic skin inflammation, usually eczematous dermatitis resulting from exposure to substances in the environment. It can be subdivided into "irritant" contact dermatitis (nonimmunologic physical and chemical alteration of the epidermis) and "allergic" contact dermatitis (delayed hypersensitivity reaction).

SYNONYMS

Irritant contact dermatitis
Allergic contact dermatitis

ICD-9CM CODES

692 Contact dermatitis and other eczema

EPIDEMIOLOGY & DEMOGRAPHICS

- 20% of all cases of dermatitis in children are caused by allergic contact dermatitis.
- Rhus dermatitis (poison ivy, poison oak, and poison sumac) is responsible for most cases of contact dermatitis.
- Frequent causes of irritant contact dermatitis are soaps, detergents, and organic solvents.
- Chemical irritants (e.g., cutting fluids used in machining, solvents) account for most cases of irritant contact dermatitis. Occupational skin diseases are second only to traumatic injuries as the most common types of occupational disease.

PHYSICAL FINDINGS & CLINICAL PRESENTATION

Clinical presentation varies with the responsible agent and affected area of skin.

IRRITANT CONTACT DERMATITIS:
- Mild exposure may result in dryness, erythema, and fissuring of the affected area (e.g., hand involvement in irritant dermatitis caused by exposure to soap, genital area involvement in irritant dermatitis caused by prolonged exposure to wet diapers).
- Eczematous inflammation may result from chronic exposure.

ALLERGIC CONTACT DERMATITIS:
- Poison ivy dermatitis can present with vesicles and blisters; linear lesions (as a result of dragging of the resins over the surface of the skin by scratching) are a classic presentation.
- The pattern of lesions is asymmetric; itching, burning, and stinging may be present.
- The involved areas are erythematous, warm to touch, swollen, and may be confused with cellulitis.

ETIOLOGY

- Irritant contact dermatitis: cement (construction workers), rubber, ragweed, malathion (farmers), orange and lemon peels (chefs, bartenders), hair tints, shampoos (beauticians), rubber gloves (medical, surgical personnel)
- Allergic contact dermatitis: poison ivy, poison oak, poison sumac, rubber (shoe dermatitis), nickel (jewelry), balsam of Peru (hand and face dermatitis), neomycin, formaldehyde (cosmetics)

DIAGNOSIS

DIFFERENTIAL DIAGNOSIS

- Impetigo
- Lichen simplex chronicus
- Atopic dermatitis
- Nummular eczema, dyshidrotic eczema
- Seborrheic dermatitis
- Inverse psoriasis, palmoplantar psoriasis
- Scabies
- Tinea pedis

WORKUP

- Medical history: gradual onset versus rapid onset, number of exposures, clinical presentation, occupational history.
- Physical examination: contact dermatitis in the neck may be caused by necklaces, perfumes, after-shave lotion. Involvement of the axillae is often secondary to deodorants, clothing. Face involvement can occur with cosmetics, airborne allergens, aftershave lotion.

LABORATORY TESTS

- Patch testing has a sensitivity and specificity of 70% to 80%. It is useful to confirm the diagnosis of contact dermatitis; it is indicated only when inflammation persists despite appropriate topical therapy and avoidance of suspected causative agent; patch testing should not be used for irritant contact dermatitis because this is a nonimmunologic-mediated inflammatory reaction.
- Dermoscopy and microscopy when suspecting scabies and mites.
- A potassium hydroxide (KOH) preparation may be useful if suspecting tinea or *Candida* infection.

TREATMENT

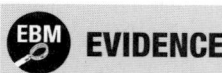

NONPHARMACOLOGIC THERAPY

Avoidance of suspected allergens

ACUTE GENERAL Rx

- Removal of the irritant substance by washing the skin with plain water or mild soap within 15 min of exposure is helpful in patients with poison ivy, poison oak, or poison sumac dermatitis.
- Cold or cool water compresses for 20 to 30 min 5 to 6 times a day for the initial 72 hr are effective during the acute blistering stage.
- Topical steroids (clobetasol 0.05%, triamcinolone 0.1%) are effective for acute localized allergic contact dermatitis lesions. Lower potency topical steroids are preferred on face, anogenital regions and flexural surfaces to minimize risk of skin atrophy. Oral corticosteroids (e.g., prednisone 20 mg bid for 6 to 10 days) are generally reserved for severe, widespread dermatitis.
- IM steroids (e.g., Kenalog) are used for severe reactions and in patients requiring oral corticosteroids but unable to tolerate PO.
- Oral antihistamines (e.g., hydroxyzine 25 mg q6h) will control pruritus, especially at night; calamine lotion is also useful for pruritus; however, it can lead to excessive drying.
- Colloidal oatmeal (Aveeno) baths can also provide symptomatic relief.
- Patients with mild to moderate erythema may respond to topical steroid gels or creams.
- Patients with shoe allergy should change their socks at least once a day; use of aluminum chloride hexahydrate in a 20% solution (Drysol) qhs will also help control perspiration.
- Use hypoallergenic surgical gloves in patients with rubber and surgical glove allergy.

DISPOSITION

Allergic contact dermatitis generally resolves within 2 to 4 wk if reexposure to allergen is prevented.

REFERRAL

For patch testing in selected patients, see "Laboratory Tests."

PEARLS & CONSIDERATIONS

COMMENTS

Commercially available corticosteroid dose packs should be avoided, because they generally provide an inadequate amount of medication.

EVIDENCE

available at www.expertconsult.com

SUGGESTED READING

available at www.expertconsult.com

AUTHOR: FRED F. FERRI, M.D.

BASIC INFORMATION

DEFINITION

Contraception refers to the various modalities that a sexually active couple use to prevent pregnancy. These options can be either medical or nonmedical and used by men or women or both. The options are as follows:

- No contraception: failure rate 5% both typical use and perfect use
- Abstinence
  - 12.4% of unmarried men
  - 13.2% of unmarried women
  - More frequently practiced before age 17 yr
  - No intercourse experienced by 13% of women ages 30 to 34 yr
  - Failure rate 0%
- Withdrawal
  - Used in only 2% of sexually active women
  - Failure rate with perfect use, 4%; with typical use, 19%
- Rhythm method (natural family planning)
  - Failure rate with perfect use, 1% to 9%; with typical use, 20%
  - Symptothermal type: mucus method and ovulation pain combined with basal body temperature
  - Ovulation (Billings' method): takes into account mucus quality
  - Basal body temperature method: uses biphasic temperature chart
  - Lactation amenorrhea method: effective in fully breastfeeding women, especially 70 to 100 days after delivery; depends on number of feedings per day
- Barriers
  - Diaphragm and cervical cap: failure rate 5% to 9% in nulliparous women, 20% in multiparous women
  - Female condom: failure rate with perfect use, 5.1%; with typical use, 12.4%; FDA labeling states 25% failure rate
  - Male condom: failure rate with perfect use, 3%; with typical use, 12%
  - Spermicides (aerosols, foam, jellies, creams, tabs): failure rate with perfect use, 3%; with typical use, 21%
- Oral contraceptives
  - Failure rate with perfect use, <1%; with typical use, 3%
  - Come in combinations of estrogen/progestin or as progestin only
- Hormonal implants and injectables
  - Implanon (etonogestrel) implant 2-yr cumulative pregnancy rate 0.05%
  - Depo-Provera: failure rate 0.3% in first year of use
  - Lunelle failure rate 0.2% in first year
  - Nestorone-releasing single implant: not yet available
  - Jadelle implant: Succesor to the Norplant implant, which has been discontinued in the U.S. The Jadelle implant is not available in the U.S.
- Mini pill (progesterone only pill)
  - Failure rate with typical use, 1.1% to 13.2%

- With perfect use, 5 pregnancies per 1000 women
- Emergency postcoital contraception
  - Decreases pregnancy rate by 75% with women treated immediately postcoitally
  - Involves dedicated hormonal (Plan B, which contains levonorgestrel) use or intrauterine device (IUD) insertion
- IUD (available over the counter in some states)
  - Progestasert: failure rate with perfect use, 2%; with typical use, 3%
  - Copper T (30-A): failure rate with perfect use, 0.8%; with typical use, 3%
  - Levonorgestrel Intrauterine System (Mirena)
    - 1-yr failure rate, 1%
    - 5-yr cumulative failure rate, 0.71 per 100 women
- Female sterilization (tubal ligation): failure rate with perfect use, 0.2%; with typical use, 3%
- Male sterilization (vasectomy): failure rate of 0.1% in first year
- Vaginal ring (Nuva ring): failure rate pearl index 0.77
- Contraceptive patch (Ortho Evra): failure rate 0.4% to 0.7%

SYNONYMS

Birth control
Family planning

ICD-9CM CODES

V25.01	Oral contraceptives
V25.02	Other contraceptive measures
V25.09	Family planning
V25.1	IUD
V25.2	Sterilization

DIAGNOSIS

WORKUP

- Thorough medical history
- Thorough surgical history
- Obstetric history (fertility desired?)
- Gynecologic history, including:
  - History of previous sexually transmitted diseases
  - Number of partners
  - Previous difficulties with contraception
  - Frequency of intercourse
- Family history

LABORATORY TESTS

- Pap smear
- Cultures, aerobic and *Chlamydia*
- Pregnancy test if suspected pregnancy
- Lipid profile if family history of premature vascular event

TREATMENT

NONPHARMACOLOGIC THERAPY

- Male condoms
  - 95% latex (rubber), 5% skin or natural membrane

- Proper use: place on an erect penis and leave ½-inch empty space at the tip of the condom; use with non–oil-based lubricants
  - Effectiveness increased when used with spermicides
- Female condoms
  - Composed of polyurethane, with one end open and one end closed
  - Proper use: place closed end over cervix, open end hanging out of vagina to cover penis and scrotum
  - Highly effective against HIV
- Spermicides
  - Types: nonoxynol, octoxynol
  - Forms: jellies, creams, foams, suppositories, tablets, soluble films
  - Proper use: put in immediately before intercourse; may be used with other barrier methods
- Diaphragm and cervical cap
  - Must be fitted by practitioner, used with contraceptive gels, and refitted with weight gain or loss
  - Diaphragm sizes: 50 to 5 mm; cervical cap sizes 22, 25, 2, and 31 mm
  - Proper use of diaphragm: put in immediately before intercourse and keep in for 6 hr after intercourse; must not remain in the vagina for longer than 24 hr
  - Proper use of cervical cap: fit over the cervix exactly; must not remain in place for longer than 48 hr
- Lactation amenorrhea method
  - Depends on number of feedings per day; effective as birth control for 6 mo if 15 or more feedings, lasting 10 min each, are accomplished daily
  - Not a common practice in the U.S.
- Withdrawal
  - Withdrawal of the penis from the vagina before ejaculation
  - Depends on self-control
- Rhythm method
  - Depends on awareness of physiology of male and female reproductive tracts
  - Sperm viable in vagina for 2 to 7 days
  - Ovum life span 24 hr
- Sterilization
  - Male:
    - Vasectomy to interrupt vas deferens and block passage of sperm to seminal ejaculate
    - Scalpel and nonscalpel techniques available
    - More easily performed procedure than female sterilization and does not require general anesthesia
  - Female:
    - Leading method of birth control in U.S. in women older than 30 yr
    - Interrupts fallopian tubes, blocking passage of ovum proximally and sperm distally through tube
    - Several types; modified Pomeroy done during cesarean section or laparoscopic done in nonpregnant females most common

- Essure-tubal occlusion through hysteroscopic placement of micro-inserts into the fallopian tubes.

ACUTE GENERAL Rx

- Combination oral contraceptives
  - Taken daily for 21 days, pill-free interval of 7 days
  - Less than 50 mcg ethynyl estradiol in most common combination oral contraceptives; progestins most commonly used in combination pills are norethindrone, levonorgestrel, norgestrel, norethindrone acetate, ethynodiol diacetate, norgestimate, or desogestrel; triphasic combination oral contraceptives (give varying doses of progestin and estrogens throughout cycle); monophasic oral contraceptives: offer same dose of progestin and estrogen throughout cycle, taken daily at same time; estrophasic pill (constant progesterone with variation of estrogen throughout the cycle)
  - If pill taken with antibiotics, efficacy affected by inadequate gastrointestinal absorption in most cases; only rifampin truly reduces pill's effectiveness
  - Increased body weight decreases effectiveness
- Mini pill
  - Progestin only; taken without a break
  - Causes much irregular bleeding because of the lack of estrogen effect on the lining of the uterus
- Hormonal implants and injectables
  - Implanon
    - Single etonorgestrel secreting device that is inserted underneath the skin
    - Among the most effective contraceptive available
    - Approved by FDA in 2006 and effective over three-yr period
  - Depo-Provera
    - Medroxyprogesterone acetate given every 3 mo in IM injection form
    - Major side effect: irregular bleeding
    - Fertility return possibly delayed up to 1 mo after discontinuation
  - Lunelle: monthly injectable administered intramuscularly. Contains 0.5 ml aqueous, 5 mg estradiol cypionate and 25 mg medroxyprogesterone acetate

- Postcoital contraception
  - Done on emergency basis, usually as a result of noncompliance with birth control or failure of birth control (e.g., condom breakage) at the time of ovulation
  - Methods:
    - Hormonal methods
      - Levonorgestrel is available either as two 0.75 mg tablets taken 12 hr apart (next choice) or as a 1.5 mg tablet taken once (Plan B, one step). It is indicated for emergency contraception to be used within 72 hr after unexpected intercourse. It can be obtained OTC by women ≥17 yr of age and by prescription by younger patients
      - Ulipristal (ELLA) is a progesterone-receptor agonist/antagonist available by prescription only. It is a 30-mg, single-dose tablet and can be taken up to 5 days after unexpected intercourse
    - Copper IUD insertion within 5 days of coitus
- IUD
  - Device inserted into uterus to prevent sperm and ovum from uniting in fallopian tube
  - Types available in the U.S.:
    - Progestasert a T-shaped device that is an ethylene vinyl acetate copolymer T; vertical stem contains 38 mg progesterone and must be changed yearly
    - ParaGard (Copper T/30-A): a polyethylene T wrapped with a fine copper wire effective for 10 yr
    - Mirena Levonorgestrel Intrauterine System (LNGIUS): a T-shaped system with a chamber that contains levonorgestrel. Releases 20 mcg/day; is effective for 5 yr
- Vaginal ring (NuvaRing)
  - Provides daily dose of 120 mcg of etonogestrel and 15 mcg ethinyl estradiol
  - Stays in vagina 3 wk and is removed the fourth for a contraceptive free interval analogous to the placebo pills in oral contraceptive pills
  - Increased body weight decreases effectiveness

- Contraceptive patch (Evra)
  - Provides low daily dose of steroids
  - Releases a progestin and estrogen (ethinyl estradiol)
  - Patch size 20 cm^2
  - Each patch contains 6 mg norelgestromin and delivers an estimated continuous systemic dose of 150 mcg norelgestromin and 20 mcg of ethinyl estradiol; common dose 250 mcg/day progestin and 25 mcg/day estrogen
  - Worn 3 out of 4 wk
  - Increased body weight decreases effectiveness

CHRONIC Rx

- With all the previously mentioned types of birth control, patient is followed up at least yearly, or as necessary, if problems arise.
- Full history, physical examination, and Pap smear, including cultures when needed, are performed yearly.
- Patients with medical problems are followed up approximately every 6 mo when taking hormonal therapy.

DISPOSITION

- Follow yearly or more frequently according to patient's side effects.
- Tailor birth control to patient according to different needs or side effects present at different times in life. Effective counseling also requires an understanding of a woman's preference and medical risks, benefits, side effects, and contraindications of each contraceptive method.

REFERRAL

With hormonal contraception, if neurologic or cardiac symptoms arise, stop method immediately, evaluate, and refer to internist when appropriate.

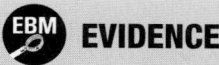 **EVIDENCE**

available at www.expertconsult.com

SUGGESTED READING

available at www.expertconsult.com

AUTHORS: **MARIA A. CORIGLIANO, M.D.,** and **RUBEN ALVERO, M.D.**

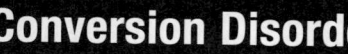

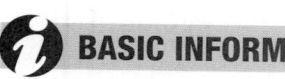 **BASIC INFORMATION**

DEFINITION

Conversion disorder is a diagnosis of exclusion that presents with one or more symptoms that affects voluntary motor or sensory function. The symptoms are not due to a neurologic or other general medical condition, or to the effects of a substance, or a culturally sanctioned behavior or experience. Conversion disorder is usually characterized by a single symptom that is sporadic, such as paralysis, blindness, numbness, or the inability to speak, and is presumed to be preceded by a psychological conflict or stressor that may or may not be remembered and may have happened recently or in the distant past. The conversion symptom is presumed to express and manage the psychological distress, or "convert" the distress into a physical symptom. There is no well validated neurobiological model for conversion disorder, but advances in neuroscience and neuroimaging may reveal new etiologies in the future. The symptom or deficit is not intentionally produced, distinguishing conversion disorder from factitious disorder or malingering.

SYNONYMS

Dissociative conversion
Hysterical conversion
Hysteria
Medically unexplained symptom
Psychogenic, nonorganic, or functional symptoms

ICD-10
Dissociative (Conversion) Disorders

EPIDEMIOLOGY & DEMOGRAPHICS

- Incidence estimated at 5 to 10/100,000 in general population, 20 to 100/100,000 in hospital inpatients
- All ages, including early childhood
- Affects women more than men (ratios range from 2:1 to 5:1)
- Highest in rural areas, among undereducated, and in lower socioeconomic classes
- Associated with axis I (depression more than anxiety) and axis II disorders (most commonly histrionic, passive dependent, and passive aggressive)

PHYSICAL FINDINGS & CLINICAL PRESENTATION

- Presents with a motor symptom (e.g., paralysis, aphonia, difficulty swallowing), a sensory symptom (loss of sensation, double vision, blindness, deafness), a psychogenic seizure, or "mixed" (symptoms from more than one category).
- Symptoms tend to occur in isolation (compared with multisystem involvement in somatization disorder).
- The symptoms or signs persist whether the patient is observed or unobserved, though are typically worse when the patient is attentive to them.
- May last from hours to years and tends to be sporadic.

- May occur in the context of documented medical illness (e.g., a patient with epileptic seizure may also have psychogenic seizure).
- May have comorbid axis I or axis II disorders, commonly depression, panic attacks, generalized anxiety, and PTSD.

ETIOLOGY

- Complex interplay of neurologic and psychologic factors is not well-understood.
- Presumed to be preceded by psychological conflict or stressor that is completely or partially unconscious.
- Functional brain imaging studies suggest alterations in processing of sensory and motor signals.

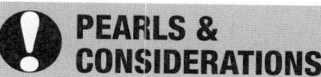 **DIAGNOSIS**

DIFFERENTIAL DIAGNOSIS

Broad differential diagnosis depending on presenting signs and symptoms, including multiple sclerosis, CNS neoplasm, myasthenia gravis, Guillain-Barré syndrome, amyotrophic lateral sclerosis, Parkinson's disease, seizure disorder, systemic lupus erythematosus, spinal cord compression, intracerebral infarct, drug-induced dystonia, and HIV.

WORKUP

Thorough history and physical examination, including careful neurologic examination

LABORATORY TESTS

- No gold standard diagnostic tests exist; no single finding is pathognomonic.
- Laboratory tests or procedures may be needed to rule out other etiologies (e.g., EEG for seizures, EMG for lower motor neuron paralysis, optokinetic drum test in blindness).

IMAGING STUDIES

As indicated by presenting signs and symptoms

Rx **TREATMENT**

NONPHARMACOLOGIC THERAPY

- No good evidence exists demonstrating the efficacy of any treatment.
- Cognitive behavioral therapy is often the treatment of choice, although evidence is mixed.
- A long tradition of psychodynamic therapy exists but has not been validated by controlled trials.
- Treatment success has been associated with a caring, long-term relationship between patient and physician and a safe, nonconfrontational approach, with the exception of psychogenic seizure for which empathic confrontation and acceptance of disease is advocated as a foundation of treatment.
- Physical and occupational therapy can help "retrain" the patient in normal behaviors and is important for maintaining strength and function in extended cases of paralysis.
- Studies have shown no additional benefit to hypnosis, although case records describe treatment with hypnosis.

ACUTE GENERAL Rx

- Antidepressants may be helpful for underlying mood or anxiety disorders.
- Longstanding symptoms may require inpatient treatment.

CHRONIC Rx

See "Nonpharmacologic Therapy" and "Acute General Rx."

DISPOSITION

Long-term follow-up essential for recurrent conversion symptoms and underlying mood disorders.

REFERRAL

To rule out other psychiatric disorders and for psychotherapy.

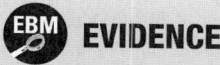 **PEARLS & CONSIDERATIONS**

COMMENTS

- Three modifications have been proposed for the diagnostic criteria DSM-5: the removal of the requirement that the clinician establish that 1) the patient is not feigning or 2) that there is an associated psychological stressor, as both of these can be difficult and sometimes impossible to demonstrate; 3) the importance of positive neurological evidence, such as the absence of seizure activity on EEG or Hoovers sign for motor weakness.
- Good prognostic factors: sudden onset, presence of psychological stressors at onset, short duration between diagnosis and treatment, high level of intelligence, absence of other psychiatric or medical disorders.
- Poor prognostic factors: severe disability, long duration of symptoms, age >40 yr at onset, and convulsions or paralysis as presenting symptoms.
- Differentiation between conversion, somatization, dissociative, factitious, and malingering disorders, as well as organic versus functional etiologies, may be challenging.
- Studies show an association between sexual trauma and conversion symptoms, although evidence does not support causality because of confounding and methodological factors.
- Although not well demonstrated, some argue that conversion and somatized symptoms are more prevalent in cultures without an articulated concept of affective disorder or in which mental illness is highly stigmatized.

EBM **EVIDENCE**

available at www.expertconsult.com

SUGGESTED READINGS
available at www.expertconsult.com

AUTHOR: **KAILA COMPTON, M.D., PH.D.**

C

Diseases and Disorders

I

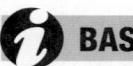

DEFINITION

Cor pulmonale is an alteration in the structure and function of the right ventricle from pulmonary hypertension caused by diseases of the lungs or pulmonary vasculature. It is a state of cardiopulmonary dysfunction that may result from multiple etiologies rather than a specific disease state. Right-sided heart failure resulting from primary disease of the left heart and congenital heart disease are not considered in this disorder.

SYNONYMS

Acute cor pulmonale
Chronic cor pulmonale

ICD-9CM CODES
415.0 Cor pulmonale, acute
416.9 Cor pulmonale, chronic

ETIOLOGY

Most conditions that cause cor pulmonale are chronic. Acute cor pulmonale is often life threatening but transient. For example, acute pulmonary embolus may present with acute cor pulmonale, cardiogenic shock, or death, but if the patient survives the initial event, then the right ventricle often recovers and cor pulmonale is no longer existent after several weeks.

Mechanisms leading to pulmonary hypertension and predisposing to the development of cor pulmonale include:
- Pulmonary vasoconstriction resulting from any condition causing alveolar hypoxia and/or acidosis
- Anatomic reduction of the pulmonary vascular bed (e.g., emphysema, interstitial lung disease, pulmonary emboli)
- Increased blood viscosity (e.g., polycythemia vera, Waldenström's macroglobulinemia)

PHYSICAL FINDINGS & CLINICAL PRESENTATION

No symptoms are specific for cor pulmonale. Typically, the symptoms depend on the underlying disease process. The symptoms are most often a result of right ventricular failure:
- Dyspnea, fatigue, chest pain, or syncope with exertion (from pulmonary hypertension)
- Right upper quadrant abdominal pain and anorexia (from passive hepatic congestion)
- Hoarseness (caused by compression of the left recurrent laryngeal nerve by dilation of the main pulmonary artery; known as *Ortner's syndrome*)
- Signs of right ventricular failure: jugular venous distention, peripheral edema, hepatic congestion, ascites, and a right ventricular third heart sound
- Signs of associated tricuspid regurgitation: holosystolic murmur heard best along the left parasternal border (augments during inspiration), prominent V-wave on jugular venous pulse, and pulsatile hepatomegaly (in severe tricuspid regurgitation)

- Pulmonary hypertension will increase the intensity of the pulmonic component of S2, which may be narrowly split
- Rarely, cough and hemoptysis

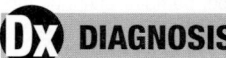

WORKUP

Search for an underlying pulmonary process resulting in pulmonary hypertension:
- Left ventricular dysfunction should be excluded in initial assessment.
- 80% to 90% of cor pulmonale cases are attributable to chronic obstructive pulmonary disease (COPD).
- Consideration of alveolar hypoventilation, chronic thromboembolic disease, and neuromuscular disease should be given in the absence of parenchymal lung disease.

LABORATORY TESTS
- Complete blood count may show erythrocytosis from chronic hypoxia.
- Arterial blood gas levels confirm hypoxemia and acidosis or hypercapnia.
- Pulmonary function tests.

IMAGING STUDIES
- Chest radiograph may show underlying pulmonary disease and evidence of pulmonary hypertension (e.g., enlargement of the pulmonary arteries or right atrium and right ventricular dilation) (Fig. 1-103).
- ECG may reveal right ventricular hypertrophy, right atrial enlargement (P-pulmonale), right-axis deviation, or incomplete/complete right bundle branch block.

- Echocardiogram to detect right ventricular enlargement and/or hypertrophy and estimate pulmonary artery pressure.
- Radionuclide ventriculography to measure right ventricular ejection fraction, which may be reduced.
- Cardiac MRI can accurately measure right ventricular dimensions and function.
- Right-sided heart catheterization measures pulmonary artery pressures and pulmonary vascular resistance. It can also determine response to oxygen or vasodilators.
- Chest CT can assess for pulmonary parenchymal disease and embolus in the pulmonary vasculature.

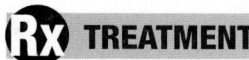

The treatment of cor pulmonale is directed toward the underlying etiology while also reversing hypoxemia, improving right ventricular contractility, decreasing pulmonary artery vascular resistance, and improving pulmonary hypertension

NONPHARMACOLOGIC THERAPY
- Continuous positive airway pressure is used in patients with obstructive sleep apnea.
- Phlebotomy is reserved as adjunctive therapy in patients with polycythemia (hematocrit >55%) who have acute decompensation of cor pulmonale or remain polycythemic despite long-term oxygen therapy. Phlebotomy has been shown to decrease mean pulmonary artery pressure and pulmonary vascular resistance.

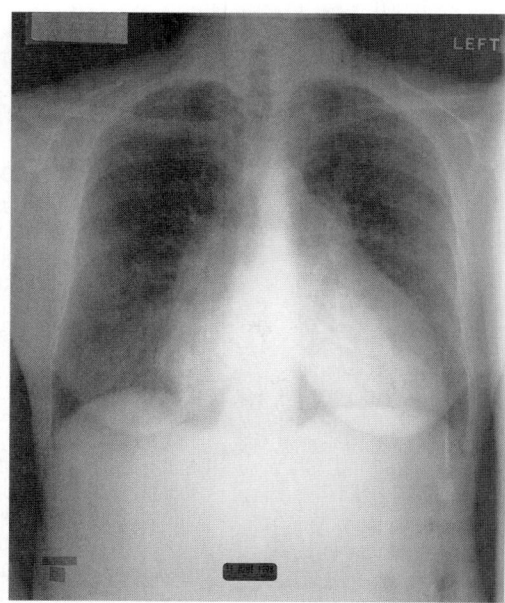

FIGURE 1-103 Chest radiography in a patient with severe intrinsic pulmonary vascular disease demonstrating enlargement of the main pulmonary artery, right ventricle, and right atrium. (From Crawford MH et al [eds]: *Cardiology,* ed 2, St Louis, 2004, Mosby.)

ﬁ .

ACUTE GENERAL Rx

- Pulmonary embolism is the most common cause of acute cor pulmonale (see "Pulmonary Embolism"). The treatment is anticoagulation, hemodynamic support, and consideration of thrombolytics.
- In patients with preexisting cor pulmonale, acute pulmonary illnesses or hypoxia can increase pulmonary hypertension and worsen right ventricular function. The underlying exacerbating conditions should be treated.

CHRONIC Rx

- Long-term oxygen supplementation improves survival in hypoxemic patients with COPD.
- Right ventricular volume overload should be treated with diuretics (e.g., furosemide). However, excessive diuresis can reduce right ventricular filling and decrease cardiac output.
- Theophylline and sympathomimetic amines may improve diaphragmatic excursion, myocardial contraction, and pulmonary artery vasodilation.

- The long-term use of nonselective vasodilators including nitrates, calcium channel blockers, and angiotensin-converting enzyme inhibitors has not resulted in significant survival improvement. This is probably because of a lack of vasoreactivity in patients with COPD as well as the risk of worsening of ventilation/perfusion mismatch and systemic vasodilation. Vasodilators to combat pulmonary hypertension should not be administered empirically in the absence of a right-sided heart catheterization.

DISPOSITION

The level of pulmonary artery pressure in COPD patients with cor pulmonale is a good indicator of prognosis. Right ventricular function may provide additional information.

REFERRAL

Patients with pulmonary disease who have progressed to cor pulmonale should be followed up by a pulmonologist.

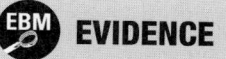 **PEARLS & CONSIDERATIONS**

- There is no differential diagnosis, but rather an evaluation of the patient to identify the underlying cause.
- Prognosis and treatment are related to the underlying cause, whereas the presence of cor pulmonale is merely a marker of the underlying disease severity.

COMMENTS

There is increasing interest in selective pulmonary vasodilators to improve right ventricular heart function in patients with cor pulmonale.

EBM EVIDENCE

available at www.expertconsult.com

SUGGESTED READINGS

available at www.expertconsult.com

AUTHORS: **DOUGLAS W. MARTIN, M.D.,** and **GAURAV CHOUDHARY, M.D.**

C

Diseases and Disorders

I

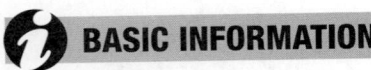
BASIC INFORMATION

DEFINITION
A corneal abrasion is a loss of surface epithelial tissue of the cornea caused by trauma.

SYNONYMS
Corneal erosion
Corneal contusion

ICD-9CM CODES
918.1 Corneal abrasion

EPIDEMIOLOGY & DEMOGRAPHICS
INCIDENCE (IN U.S.): A universal problem
PEAK INCIDENCE: Childhood through active adulthood and older and debilitated patients
PREDOMINANT AGE: Any age

PHYSICAL FINDINGS & CLINICAL PRESENTATION
- Haziness of the cornea
- Disruption of the corneal surface (Fig. 1-104)
- Redness and infection of the conjunctiva
- Pain
- Light sensitivity
- Tearing
- Gritty feeling
- Pain on opening or closing eyes
- Sensation of a foreign body

ETIOLOGY
- Trauma (direct mechanical event)
- Foreign body
- Contact lenses
- Unknown

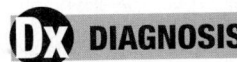
DIAGNOSIS

DIFFERENTIAL DIAGNOSIS
- Acute-angle glaucoma
- Herpes ulcers and other corneal ulcers
- Foreign body in the cornea (be certain it is not a keratitis)

WORKUP
- Fluorescein staining, slit lamp evaluation
- Assessment of visual acuity
- Intraocular pressure
- Rule out corneal laceration
- Rule out other eye pathology

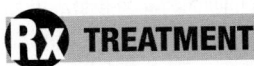
TREATMENT

NONPHARMACOLOGIC THERAPY
- Patching is controversial (see below).
- Bandage.
- Contact lenses.
- Warm compresses.
- Pressure dressing is controversial. Although eye patching traditionally has been recommended in the treatment of corneal abrasions, several studies show that patching does not help and may hinder healing.
- Removal of any foreign particles if present.

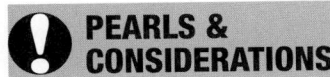
ACUTE GENERAL Rx
- Topical antibiotics such as 10% sulfacetamide or ofloxacin 0.3% solution 2 drops qid.
- Pressure patching of eye with eyelid closed is no longer recommended because it can result in decreased oxygen delivery, increased moisture, and a higher chance of infection.
- Cycloplegics such as 5% homatropine are often prescribed to relieve ciliary muscle spasm; however, their benefit has been questioned and they are no longer routinely recommended.
- Topical nonsteroidal anti-inflammatory drugs (e.g., diclofenac 0.1% or ketorolac 0.5%) 1 drop qid.
- Topical antibiotics to prevent secondary infection.

DISPOSITION
Follow-up in 24 hr and then every 3 days until abrasion has cleared and vision has returned to normal

REFERRAL
To ophthalmologist if patient has no relief within 24 hr or for patients with deep eye injuries, foreign bodies that cannot be removed, or suspected recurrent corneal erosion.

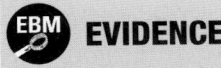
PEARLS & CONSIDERATIONS

COMMENTS
- Never give the patient topical anesthetic to use at home because these can cause decomposition of the cornea and permanent damage.
- Most corneal abrasions heal in 24 to 48 hr and rarely progress to corneal erosion or infection.

EVIDENCE
available at www.expertconsult.com

SUGGESTED READING
available at www.expertconsult.com

AUTHOR: **MELVYN KOBY, M.D.**

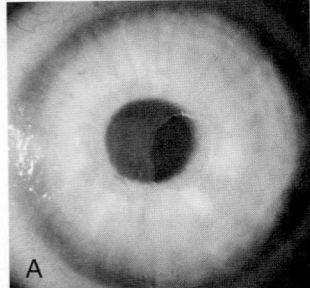
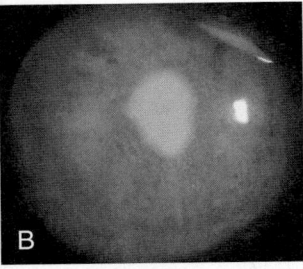

FIGURE 1-104 Corneal epithelial abrasion. A, Epithelial defect without fluorescein highlighting the defect. An irregularity in the otherwise smooth corneal surface is the key to identifying the defect if no fluorescein is available. **B,** Classic fluorescein staining of an epithelial defect. (From Palay D [ed]: *Ophthalmology for the primary care physician,* St Louis, 1997, Mosby.)

BASIC INFORMATION

DEFINITION

Corneal ulceration refers to the disruption of the corneal surface and/or deeper layers caused by trauma, contact lenses infection, degeneration, or other means.

SYNONYMS

Infectious keratitis with ulceration
Bacterial keratitis with ulceration
Viral keratitis with ulceration
Fungal keratitis with ulceration

ICD-9CM CODES

370.0 Corneal ulcer NOS

EPIDEMIOLOGY & DEMOGRAPHICS

INCIDENCE (IN U.S.): Four to six cases per month seen by an average general ophthalmologist
PREVALENCE (IN U.S.): Common
PREDOMINANT SEX: Either
PREDOMINANT AGE: All ages

PHYSICAL FINDINGS & CLINICAL PRESENTATION

- Localized, well-demarcated, infiltrative lesion with corresponding focal ulcer (Fig. 1-105) or oval, yellow-white stromal suppuration with thick mucopurulent exudate and edema. Usually red, angry-looking eye with infiltration in surrounding area of cornea.
- Eye possibly painful, with conjunctival edema and infection.
- Sterile neurotrophic ulcers with tissue breakdown and no pain.

ETIOLOGY

- Complication of contact lens wear, trauma, or diseases such as herpes simplex keratitis or keratoconjunctivitis sicca. Often associated with collagen vascular disease and severe exophthalmus and thyroid disease.
- Viral causes often contagious.

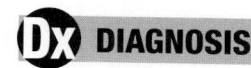 **DIAGNOSIS**

DIFFERENTIAL DIAGNOSIS

- *Pseudomonas* and pneumococcus and other bacterial infection—virulent
- *Moraxella, Staphylococcus, α-Streptococcus* infection—less virulent
- Herpes simplex infection or disease caused by other viruses
- Contact lens ulcers differ

WORKUP

- Fluorescein staining, slit lamp
- Appearance often typical

- Differentiate carefully with contact lens wearers
- Note previous eye surgery or laser vision correction

LABORATORY TESTS

Microscopic examination and culture of scrapings

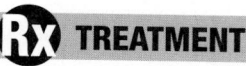 **TREATMENT**

NONPHARMACOLOGIC THERAPY

- Warm compresses
- Bandage contact lenses
- Patching
- Stop contact lens wearing
- Remove eyelid crusting

ACUTE GENERAL Rx

- An ophthalmic emergency
- Intense antibiotic and antiviral therapy
- Nonsteroidal antiinflammatory drugs
- Viroptic/Zymar
- Bacterial infection: subconjunctival cefazolin or gentamicin (topical Zymar, Vigomax, etc.)
- Fungal infection: hospitalization and topical application of antifungal agents
- Herpes: Viroptic and oral therapy

DISPOSITION

Ideally treated by an ophthalmologist if the patient does not rapidly respond to antibiotics (within 24 hr)

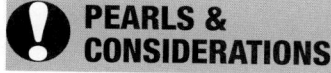 **PEARLS & CONSIDERATIONS**

- Always stop contact lens wearing.
- Always refer ulcers to ophthalmologist.
- Never treat with topical anesthetics or steroids.

COMMENTS

Do not use topical steroids because herpes, fungal, or other ulcers may be aggravated, leading to perforation of the cornea. Antibiotics may delay response and result in overgrowth of nonbacterial (fungal and amoebic) pathogens.

SUGGESTED READINGS

available at www.expertconsult.com

AUTHOR: **MELVYN KOBY, M.D.**

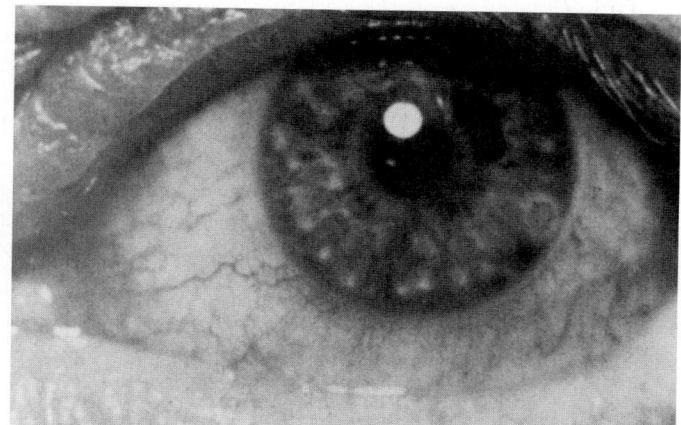

FIGURE 1-105 Peripherally located corneal ulcer. (From Marx JA [ed]: *Rosen's emergency medicine,* ed 5, St Louis, 2002, Mosby.)

BASIC INFORMATION

DEFINITION

Clinical condition characterized by pain and tenderness at costochondral or chondrosternal joints of the anterior chest wall.

SYNONYMS

Anterior chest wall syndrome
Chest wall pain syndrome
Costosternal syndrome
Parasternal chondrodynia

ICD-9CM CODES
733.6 Costochondritis

EPIDEMIOLOGY & DEMOGRAPHICS

PREVALENCE: Fairly common, comprises approximately 28% of undifferentiated noncardiac chest pain patients.
PREDOMINANT SEX: Women > men
PREDOMINANT AGE: >40 yr

PHYSICAL FINDINGS & CLINICAL PRESENTATION

SYMPTOMS:
- Anterior chest wall pain, usually acute, pleuritic, positional, and aggravated by coughing, sneezing, inspiration, or any chest-wall movement.
- In children, especially teenagers, may present as sudden episode of sharp chest pain, with feeling that they cannot take deep breath, but actually improves with deep breathing.
- May radiate to arms and shoulders.

SIGNS:
- Reproducible pain/tenderness of costochondral (second through fifth) or costosternal junction without localized swelling.
- Pain on crossed-chest adduction of arm and backward extension of arm from 90 degrees of abduction signifies pain of musculoskeletal origin.

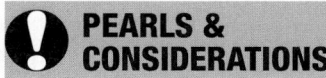 **DIAGNOSIS**

DIFFERENTIAL DIAGNOSIS

- Cardiac pain: primary concern; ischemic chest pain, acute pericarditis, aortic dissection
- Gastrointestinal: gastroesophogeal reflux disease
- Pulmonary embolism, pneumonia, pneumothorax
- Musculoskeletal (Table 1-37): Tietze's syndrome, cervical or thoracic spine disease, fibromyalgia, arthritis
- Involvement of ribs by trauma, infections (*Candida albicans*) or neoplasms (breast cancer, prostate cancer, sarcoma, plasma cell cytoma)
- Psychiatric: panic attack

WORKUP

- A diagnosis of exclusion for chest pain after ruling out more serious conditions. Key to diagnosis are history and physical exam.
- Absence of laboratory or radiographic abnormalities.

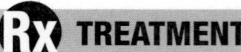 **TREATMENT**

ACUTE GENERAL Rx

- Often self-limiting, so reassurance is important.
- Symptomatic treatment includes local application of heat, minimize activities that aggravate symptoms, stretching exercises for chest-wall muscles, and nonsteroidal antiinflammatory drugs or acetaminophen.
- Refractory cases can be treated with local injections of combined lidocaine/corticosteroid (may be a useful diagnostic and therapeutic tool).
- Recurrent costochondritis may respond to sulfasalazine.

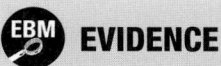 **PEARLS & CONSIDERATIONS**

Presence of costochondritis in a patient with chest pain does not exclude more serious problems including cardiac pain.

EBM **EVIDENCE**

available at www.expertconsult.com

SUGGESTED READINGS
available at www.expertconsult.com

AUTHOR: **ASHA SHRESTHA, M.D.**

TABLE 1-37 Musculoskeletal Chest Pain

Disorder	Clinical Features	Comments
Tietze's syndrome	Painful swelling of usually second or third costal cartilage (usually left).	Less common than costochondritis; usually before 40 years, equal male and female involvement.
Costochondritis	Pain and tenderness but no swelling. Costochondral junctions of ribs 2 to 5. Increased pain with cough and sneeze.	Sometimes associated with headache and hyperventilation.
Seronegative spondyloarthropathy (ankylosing spondylitis)	Sternoclavicular or manubriosternal joint. Worse in morning. Relieved by activity. May be associated with swelling.	Local chest findings usually associated with other symptoms of ankylosing spondylitis such as sacroiliitis. May need HLA-B27 antigen testing.
Cervical, thoracic disc disease	Referred regional pain from affected area. No local swelling. Often aggravated by spine motion and may be accompanied by radicular pain into arm if cervical or along intercostal nerve if thoracic. Symptoms reproduced by Spurling's maneuver (steady pressure to head causing increased axial loading on the nerve root).	May mimic chest disease if spinal complaints are minimal and referred or radicular symptoms predominate.
Fibromyalgia	Widespread pain with other sites involved. Symptoms often change in location. Local tender points but no swelling or objective findings.	Female/male ratio of 9:1. Prevalent age 30-50 yr.
Osteoarthritis, sternoclavicular or manubriosternal joint	Dull, aching local pain with tenderness. Occasional bony joint enlargement with soft tissue swelling.	Crepitus may rarely be present.

BASIC INFORMATION

DEFINITION

Craniopharyngiomas are tumors arising from squamous cell remnants of Rathke's pouch, located in the infundibulum or upper anterior hypophysis.

SYNONYMS

Subset of nonadenomatous pituitary tumors

ICD-9CM CODES

237.0 Craniopharyngioma

EPIDEMIOLOGY & DEMOGRAPHICS

PEAK INCIDENCE: Occurs at all ages; peak during the first 2 decades of life, with a second small peak occurring in the sixth decade.

PREDOMINANT SEX:

- Both sexes are usually equally affected.
- Craniopharyngiomas are the most common nonglial tumors in children and account for 3% to 5% of all pediatric brain tumors.

PHYSICAL FINDINGS & CLINICAL PRESENTATION

- The typical onset is insidious and a 1- to 2-year history of slowly progressive symptoms is common.
- Presenting symptoms are usually related to the effects of a sella turcica mass. Approximately 75% of patients report headache and have visual disturbances.
- The usual visual defect is bitemporal hemianopsia. Optic nerve involvement with decreased visual acuity and scotomas and homonymous hemianopsia from optic tract involvement may also occur.
- Other symptoms include mental changes, nausea, vomiting, somnolence, or symptoms of pituitary failure. In adults, sexual dysfunction is the most common endocrine complaint, with impotence in men and primary or secondary amenorrhea in women. Diabetes insipidus is found in 25% of cases. In children, craniopharyngiomas may present with dwarfism.
- More than 70% of children at the time of diagnosis present with growth hormone deficiency, obstructive hydrocephalus, short-term memory deficits, and psychomotor slowing.

ETIOLOGY

Craniopharyngiomas are believed to arise from nests of squamous epithelial cells that are commonly found in the suprasellar area surrounding the pars tuberalis of the adult pituitary.

DIAGNOSIS

DIFFERENTIAL DIAGNOSIS

- Pituitary adenoma
- Empty sella syndrome
- Pituitary failure of any cause
- Primary brain tumors (e.g., meningiomas, astrocytomas)
- Metastatic brain tumors
- Other brain tumors
- Cerebral aneurysm

LABORATORY TESTS

- Hypothyroidism (low FT_4, FT_3 with high thyroid-stimulating hormone).
- Hypercortisolism (low cortisol) with low adrenocorticotropic hormone.
- Low sex hormones (testosterone, estriol) with low follicle-stimulating hormone and luteinizing hormone.
- Diabetes insipidus (hypernatremia, low urine osmolarity, high plasma osmolarity).
- Prolactin may be normal or slightly elevated.
- Pituitary stimulation tests may be required in some cases.

IMAGING STUDIES

- Visual field testing for bitemporal hemianopsia.
- Skull film.
  - Enlarged or eroded sella turcica (50%)
  - Suprasellar calcification (50%)
- MRI (Fig. 1-106) or head CT. MRI features include a multicystic and solid enhancing suprasellar mass. Hydrocephalus may also be present if the mass is large. CT usually reveals intratumoral calcifications.

TREATMENT

GENERAL Rx

- Surgical resection (curative or palliative).
  - Transsphenoidal surgery for small intrasellar tumors
  - Subfrontal craniotomy for most patients

- Postoperative radiation.
- Intralesional ^{32}P irradiation or bleomycin for unresectable tumors. Long-term complications of radiation include secondary malignancies, optic neuropathy, and vascular injury.

PROGNOSIS

- Operative mortality rate: 3% to 16% (higher with large tumors).
- Postoperative recurrence rate: 30% of cases after total resection and 57% of cases after subtotal resection.
- 5-yr and 10-yr survival: 88% and 76%, respectively, with surgery and radiation.
- The most important factors that correlate with prognosis are the extent of resection and postoperative radiation.

AUTHOR: **FRED F. FERRI, M.D.**

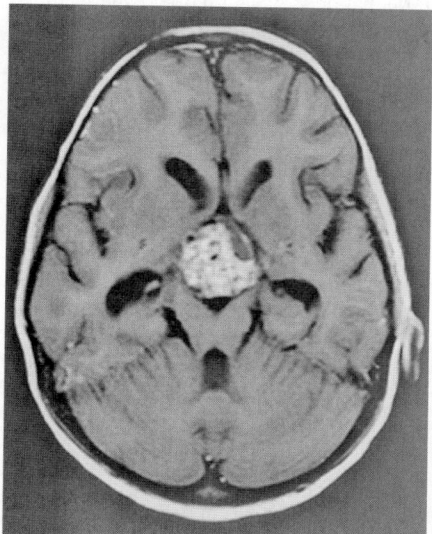

FIGURE 1-106 MRI scan of a craniopharyngioma, demonstrating a cystic contrast-enhancing mass in the suprasellar area extending upward and compressing the hypothalamus. (From Goetz CG: *Textbook of clinical neurology*, Philadelphia, 1999, WB Saunders.)

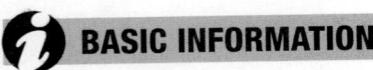 **BASIC INFORMATION**

DEFINITION
Creutzfeldt-Jakob disease (CJD) is a progressive, fatal, dementing illness caused by an infectious protein agent known as a *prion.*

SYNONYMS
Transmissible spongiform encephalopathy
Mad cow disease
Prion disease

ICD-9CM CODES
046.1 Creutzfeldt-Jakob disease

EPIDEMIOLOGY & DEMOGRAPHICS
- Incidence of one per 1 million population per year
- Peak age 60 yr (range, 16 to 82 yr)
- 5% to 10% familial, remaining cases are sporadic; iatrogenic cases (corneal transplants, dura mater allograft, human pituitary extract) are very rare
- Normal prion protein (PRNP) gene found on human chromosome 20
- Methionine and valine distribution on codon 129 of the PRNP determines the six clinical phenotypes of CJD

PHYSICAL FINDINGS & CLINICAL PRESENTATION
- All patients present with cognitive deficits (dementing illness—memory loss, behavioral abnormalities, higher cortical function impairment).
- More than 80% will have myoclonus.
- Pyramidal tract signs (weakness), cerebellar signs (clumsiness), and extrapyramidal signs (parkinsonian features) are seen in more than 50% of the cases.
- Less common features include cortical visual abnormalities, abnormal eye movements, vestibular dysfunction, sensory disturbances, autonomic dysfunction, lower motor neuron signs, and seizures.

ETIOLOGY
Small proteinaceous infectious particle (prion). Noninfectious prion protein (PrP) is a cellular protein found on the surfaces of neurons. Normal function is not known. Protein is converted to protease-resistant and infectious agent by infectious prion protein.

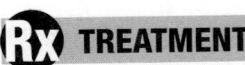 **DIAGNOSIS**

- Definite CJD: Neuropathologically confirmed spongiform encephalopathy in a case of progressive dementia.
- Probable CJD: History of rapidly progressive dementia (<2 yr) with typical EEG and with at least two of the following clinical features: myoclonus, visual or cerebellar dysfunction, pyramidal or extrapyramidal features, akinetic mutism.
- Possible CJD: Same as probable CJD without EEG findings.

DIFFERENTIAL DIAGNOSIS
- Other dementias (Alz, FTD, DLBD, vascular)
- Infectious (viral, HIV, fungal, TB)
- Inflammatory/Autoimmune (CNS vasculitis, Hashimoto's encephalopathy)
- Metabolic (vitamin deficiency, endocrine)
- Cancers (CNS lymphoma, gliomatosis cerebri, paraneoplastic)
A clinical algorithm for the evaluation of dementia is described in Section III, "Dementia."

WORKUP
- Evaluate for treatable causes of dementia (see "Alzheimer's Disease").
- Brain biopsy can be diagnostic, but it is usually not performed because there is no treatment or cure.

LABORATORY TESTS
- Presence of periodic sharp wave complexes on EEG in cases of rapidly progressive dementia has a sensitivity of 67% and a specificity of 86%.
- In cases of probable or possible CJD, presence of the 14,3,3 protein in CSF has a 95% positive predictive value with its absence having a 92% negative predictive value.

IMAGING STUDIES
MRI scan can show areas of restricted diffusion in the basal ganglia and cerebral cortex. MRI diffusion-weighted imaging has a sensitivity of 92.3% and a specificity of 93.8% only in cases of rapidly progressive dementia.

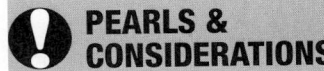 **TREATMENT**

NONPHARMACOLOGIC THERAPY
Full-time caregiver and/or nursing home. Social work can be helpful with end-of-life discussions, family counseling, and optimizing appropriate home services.

ACUTE GENERAL Rx
No known therapy

CHRONIC Rx
No known therapy

DISPOSITION
The disease is fatal. Mean duration of illness is 8 mo (range, 1 to 130 mo). One in 7 survives to 1 yr, and 1 in 30 survives to 2 yr. Better survival found in younger age at onset of disease and female gender.

REFERRAL
- Neurology for evaluation of any rapidly progressive dementia
- Social work

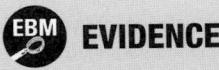 **PEARLS & CONSIDERATIONS**

COMMENTS
- Related diseases in human beings: kuru, fatal familial insomnia, Gerstmann-Sträussler-Scheinker syndrome, new-variant Creutzfeldt-Jakob disease.
- Related diseases in animals: scrapie, bovine spongiform encephalopathy (mad cow disease).

EBM EVIDENCE

available at www.expertconsult.com

SUGGESTED READINGS
available at www.expertconsult.com

AUTHOR: **CHUN LIM, M.D., PH.D.**

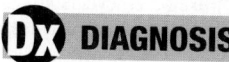 BASIC INFORMATION

DEFINITION

Crohn's disease is an inflammatory disease of the bowel of unknown etiology, most commonly involving the terminal ileum and manifesting primarily with diarrhea, abdominal pain, fatigue, and weight loss.

SYNONYMS

Regional enteritis
Inflammatory bowel disease (IBD)

ICD-9CM CODES
555.9 Crohn's disease, unspecified site
555.0 Crohn's disease, small intestine
555.1 Crohn's disease involving large intestine

EPIDEMIOLOGY & DEMOGRAPHICS
PREVALENCE:
- One case per 1000 persons; most common in whites and Jews
- Crohn's disease affects approximately 380,000 to 480,000 persons in the U.S.
- Incidence: bimodal with a peak in the third decade of life and another in the fifth decade

PHYSICAL FINDINGS & CLINICAL PRESENTATION
- Abdominal tenderness, mass, or distention
- Chronic or nocturnal diarrhea
- Weight loss, fever, night sweats
- Hyperactive bowel sounds in patients with partial obstruction, bloody diarrhea
- Delayed growth and failure of normal development in children
- Perianal and rectal abscesses, mouth ulcers, and atrophic glossitis
- Extraintestinal manifestations: joint swelling and tenderness, hepatosplenomegaly, erythema nodosum, clubbing, tenderness to palpation of the sacroiliac joints

- Symptoms may be intermittent with varying periods of remission

ETIOLOGY

Unknown. Pathophysiologically, Crohn's disease involves an immune system dysfunction.

DX DIAGNOSIS

DIFFERENTIAL DIAGNOSIS
- Ulcerative colitis (see Table 1-38)
- Infectious diseases (tuberculosis, *Yersinia, Salmonella, Shigella, Campylobacter*)
- Parasitic infections (amebic infection)
- Pseudomembranous colitis
- Ischemic colitis in elderly patients
- Lymphoma
- Colon carcinoma
- Diverticulitis
- Radiation enteritis
- Collagenous colitis
- Fungal infections *(Histoplasma, Actinomyces)*
- Gay bowel syndrome (in homosexual patient)
- Carcinoid tumors
- Celiac sprue
- Mesenteric adenitis

LABORATORY TESTS
- Decreased hemoglobin and hematocrit from chronic blood loss, effect of inflammation on bone marrow, and malabsorption of vitamin B12
- Hypokalemia, hypomagnesemia, hypocalcemia, and low albumin in patients with chronic diarrhea
- Vitamin B12 and folate deficiency
- Elevated erythrocyte sedimentation rate
- Positive antisaccharomyces cerevisiae antibodies (ASCA)
- Elevated INR (due to vitamin K malabsorption)
- Fecal calprotectin has been reported as useful in screening of patients with suspected IBD. Based on a pretest probability of 32% in adults, an abnormal calprotectin test results

increases the posttest probability to 91%, and a normal result reduces the probability of IBD to 3%. False elevations may occur with other gastrointestinal diseases such as bacterial, viral, and protozoal causes of infective diarrhea

ENDOSCOPIC EVALUATION

Endoscopic features of Crohn's disease include asymmetric and discontinued disease, deep longitudinal fissures, cobblestone appearance, and presence of strictures. Crypt distortion and inflammation are also present. Granulomas may be present.

IMAGING STUDIES
- Barium imaging studies are essentially outdated examinations. When performed, they reveal deep ulcerations (often longitudinal and transverse) and segmental lesions (skip lesions, strictures, fistulas, cobblestone appearance of mucosa caused by submucosal inflammation); "thumbprinting" is common, and "string sign" in terminal ileum may be noted. Although the diagnosis may be suggested by radiographic studies, it should be confirmed by endoscopy and biopsy when possible.
- CT of abdomen is helpful in identifying abscesses and other complications.
- Magnetic resonance enterography (MRe) is superior to other imaging modalities in its ability to distinguish active from chronic fibrotic disease. It is, however, more expensive.
- In 5% to 10% of patients with IBD, a clear distinction between ulcerative colitis and Crohn's disease cannot be made. In general, Crohn's disease can be distinguished from ulcerative colitis by the presence of transmural involvement and the frequent presence of noncaseating granulomas and lymphoid aggregates on biopsy.

RX TREATMENT

The medical management of Crohn's disease is based on disease activity. According to Hanauer and Sanborn, disease activity can be defined as follows:
- Mild to moderate disease: The patient is ambulatory and able to take oral alimentation. There is no dehydration, high fever, abdominal tenderness, painful mass, obstruction, or weight loss of >10%.
- Moderate to severe disease: Either the patient has not responded to treatment for mild to moderate disease or has more pronounced symptoms, including fever, significant weight loss, abdominal pain or tenderness, intermittent nausea and vomiting, or significant anemia.
- Severe fulminant disease: Either the patient has persistent symptoms despite outpatient steroid therapy or has high fever, persistent vomiting, evidence of intestinal obstruction, rebound tenderness, cachexia, or evidence of an abscess.
- Remission: The patient is asymptomatic or without inflammatory sequelae, including pa-

TABLE 1-38 Differentiating Features

	Ulcerative Colitis	Crohn Disease
Site of involvement	Only involves colon Rectum almost always involved	Any area of the gastrointestinal tract Rectum usually spared
Pattern of involvement	Continuous	Skip lesions
Diarrhea	Bloody	Usually nonbloody
Severe abdominal pain	Rare	Frequent
Perianal disease	No	In 30% of patients
Fistula	No	Yes
Endoscopic findings	Erythematous and friable Superficial ulceration	Aphthoid and deep ulcers Cobblestoning
Radiologic findings	Tubular appearance resulting from loss of haustral folds	String sign of terminal ileum RLQ mass, fistulas, abscesses
Histologic features	Mucosa only Crypt abscesses	Transmural Crypt abscesses, granulomas (about 30%)
Smoking	Protective	Worsens course
Serology	p-ANCA more common	ASCA more common

ASCA, Anti–*Saccharomyces cerevisiae* antibodies; p-ANCA, perinuclear antineutrophil cytoplasmic antibody; RLQ, right lower quadrant.
Andreoli TE et al: *Andreoli and Carpenter's Cecil essentials of medicine*, ed 8, Philadelphia, 2010, Saunders.

tients responding to acute medical intervention.

NONPHARMACOLOGIC THERAPY

- Nutritional supplementation is needed in patients with advanced disease. Total parenteral nutrition may be necessary in selected patients.
- Low-residue diet is necessary when obstructive symptoms are present.
- If diarrhea is prominent, increased dietary fiber and decreased fat in the diet are sometimes helpful.
- Psychotherapy is useful for situational adjustment crises. A trusting and mutually understanding relationship and referral to self-help groups are very important because of the chronicity of the disease and the relatively young age of the patients.
- Avoid oral feedings during acute exacerbation to decrease colonic activity: a low-roughage diet may be helpful in early relapse.

ACUTE GENERAL Rx

- Traditionally, sulfasalazine, 500 mg PO qid initially, increased qd or qod by 1 g until therapeutic dosages of 4 to 6 g/day are achieved, has been used. Individuals with sulfa allergies should avoid sulfasalazine. Folate supplementation is recommended because sulfasalazine inhibits folate absorption. Oral salicylates, such as mesalamine (Asacol, Rowasa), are as effective as sulfasalazine and better tolerated and have become preferred agents despite their higher cost.
- Corticosteroids have been the mainstay for treating moderate to severe active Crohn's disease. Prednisone 40 to 60 mg/day is useful for acute exacerbation. Steroids are usually tapered over approximately 2 to 3 mo. Some patients require a low dose for a prolonged period of maintenance.
- Steroid analogues are locally active corticosteroids that target specific areas of inflammation in the gastrointestinal tract. Budesonide is available as a controlled-release formulation and is approved for mild to moderate active Crohn's disease involving the ileum and/or ascending colon. The adult dose is 9 mg qd for a maximum of 8 wk.
- Immunosuppressants such as azathioprine 150 mg/day, methotrexate, or cyclosporine can be used for severe, progressive disease. In patients with Crohn's disease who enter remission after treatment with methotrexate, a low dose of methotrexate maintains remission.
- Metronidazole 500 mg qid may be useful for colonic fistulas and treatment of mild to moderate active Crohn's disease. Ciprofloxacin 1 g qd has also been found to be effective in decreasing disease activity.
- TNF inhibitors: Infliximab, a chimeric monoclonal antibody targeting tumor necrosis factor-α, is effective in the treatment of enterocutaneous fistulas. This medication can induce clinical improvement in 80% of patients with Crohn's disease refractory to other agents. It can be used in combination with other medications such as azathioprine in patients with severe Crohn's disease. A PPD test should be done before using this medication. Adalimumab and certolizumab are other TNF inhibitors also effective in inducing remissions and may be useful in adult patients with Crohn's disease who cannot tolerate infliximab or have symptoms despite receiving infliximab therapy.
- Natalizumab, a selective adhesion-molecule inhibitor, has been reported to be effective in increasing the rate of remission and response in patients with active Crohn's disease. Recent trials with pegylated antibody fragments in patients with moderate to severe Crohn's disease involving certolizumab pegol revealed a modest improvement in response rates but no significant improvement in remission rates.
- Hydrocortisone enema bid or tid is useful for proctitis.

- Most patients who have anemia associated with Crohn's disease respond to iron supplementation. Erythropoietin is useful in patients with anemia refractory to treatment with iron and vitamins.

CHRONIC Rx

- Monitor disease activity with symptom review and laboratory evaluation (complete blood count and sedimentation rate)
- Liver tests and vitamin B_{12} levels monitored on a yearly basis

DISPOSITION

One tenth of patients have prolonged remission, three quarters have a chronic intermittent disease course, and one eighth have an unremitting course.

REFERRAL

- Surgical referral is needed for complications such as abscess formation, obstruction, fistulas, toxic megacolon, refractory disease, or severe hemorrhage. A conservative surgical approach is necessary because surgery is not curative. Multiple surgeries may also result in short bowel syndrome.

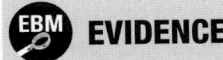

EVIDENCE

available at www.expertconsult.com

SUGGESTED READINGS
available at www.expertconsult.com

AUTHOR: **FRED F. FERRI, M.D.**

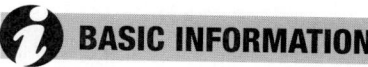

BASIC INFORMATION

DEFINITION

Cryoglobulins are serum immunoglobulins that precipitate when cooled and redissolve when heated. Cryoglobulinemia is a clinical syndrome that results from systemic inflammation caused by cryoglobulin-containing immune complexes. Mixed cryoglobulinemia is a vasculitis of small and medium-sized arteries and veins due to the deposition of complexes of antigen, cryoglobulin, and complement in the vessel walls.

SYNONYMS

Cryoglobulinemic vasculitis
Cryoproteinemia
Mixed cryoglobulinemia
Essential cryoglobulinemia

ICD-9CM CODES
273.2 Cryoglobulinemia, cryoglobulinemic vasculitis (CV), mixed cryoglobulinemia (MC)

EPIDEMIOLOGY & DEMOGRAPHICS

PREVALENCE:
- Prevalence of mixed cryoglobulinemia is approximately 1:100,000
- More than 50% of patients with HCV are found to have mixed cryoglobulinemia
- Three types: I (monoclonal), II (IgM monoclonal and IgG polyclonal), and III (polyclonal)

PREDOMINANT SEX AND AGE: Female:male ratio of 3:1
PREDOMINANT AGE: Mean age reported is 42 to 52 yr
RISK FACTORS: Hepatitis C virus (HCV) infection, connective tissue disorders, lymphoproliferative disorders

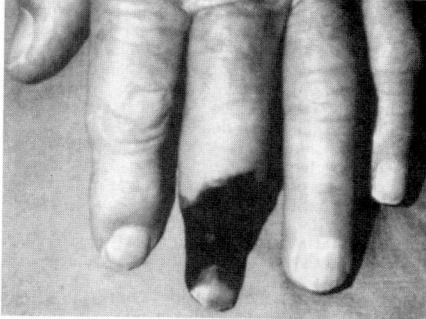

FIGURE 1-107 Cryoglobulinemia. (From Hoffman R et al: *Hematology, basic principles and practice*, ed 5, New York, 2009, Churchill Livingstone, 2009.)

PHYSICAL FINDINGS & CLINICAL PRESENTATION

- Meltzer triad of purpura, arthralgias/myalgia, and weakness
- Other symptoms include dyspnea, cough, numbness, abdominal pain, acrocyanosis
- Hypertension, hepatosplenomegaly, Raynaud's phenomenon, and in severe cases, distal necrosis and ulcerations of lower limbs (Fig. 1-107)

ETIOLOGY

- Intravascular deposition of cryoglobulins leads to ischemic insults in territory supplied by vasa nervorum
- Necrotizing vasculitis caused by cryoglobulin precipitation
- Infections: HCV, mycosis fungoides, HBV, Epstein-Barr virus, cytomegalovirus, *Treponema pallidum, Mycobacterium leprae,* and in post-streptococcal glomerulonephritis
- Lymphoproliferative disorders: chronic lymphocytic leukemia, Waldenström's macroglobulinemia, multiple myeloma
- Connective tissue disorders: rheumatoid arthritis, systemic lupus erythematosus (SLE), scleroderma, Sjögren's syndrome, vasculitis
- Renal diseases including proliferative glomerulonephritis

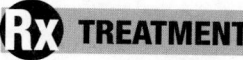 DIAGNOSIS

DIFFERENTIAL DIAGNOSIS

Antiphospholipid syndrome, SLE, lupus, Churg-Strauss syndrome, cirrhosis, glomerulonephritis, Goodpasture syndrome, hemolytic uremic syndrome, hepatitis, lymphoma, sarcoidosis, Waldenström's hypergammaglobulinemia

WORKUP

History and physical examination; laboratory tests; imaging tests depending on patients' presentations

LABORATORY TESTS

- Serum cryoglobulins, rheumatoid factor, serum complement, hepatitis C titers, urinalysis, CBC, ALT, AST, BUN, Creat
- Electromyogram/nerve conduction studies may demonstrate axonal changes and distal muscle denervation
- Sural nerve and skin biopsy

IMAGING STUDIES

Chest x-ray for pulmonary involvement, CT to study for malignancy, and angiography for vasculitis

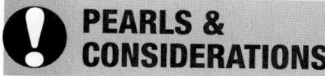 TREATMENT

- Immunosuppressive therapies such as corticosteroids are the mainstay treatment for mixed cryoglobulinemia.

- In patients with HCV, IFN-α can be added. The treatment of HCV-related mixed cryoglobulinemia is difficult due to the multifactorial origin and polymorphism of the syndrome. Therapy is aimed at eradicating the HCV infection, suppressing B-cell clonal expansion and cryoglobulin production and ameliorating symptoms
- Combination of pegylated IFN-α with ribavirin results in 77% remission.
- Variable success rate with plasma exchange, intravenous immunoglobulin, and anti-CD20 (rituximab) treatments

NONPHARMACOLOGIC THERAPY

Avoidance of cold exposure

ACUTE GENERAL Rx

NSAIDS in those with general fatigue and arthralgia; see "Treatment" for further management

DISPOSITION

Overall prognosis is worse with concomitant renal disease. Mean survival rate is ~50% at 10 yr.

REFERRAL

Nephrologist if there is renal involvement, hematologist in those with lymphoproliferative disorders, gastroenterologist/hepatologist in hepatitis, rheumatologist in connective tissue disease cases, and consider clinical immunologist in severe cases.

PEARLS & CONSIDERATIONS

COMMENTS

Always look for underlying causes for cryoglobulinemia.

PREVENTION

Avoidance of cold exposure, avoidance of late complications

PATIENT/FAMILY EDUCATION

Inform patients about early signs/symptoms of cryoglobulinemia so that treatments can be rendered before the development of complications.

SUGGESTED READINGS
available at www.expertconsult.com

AUTHOR: **QUANG P. LE, M.D., M.P.H.**

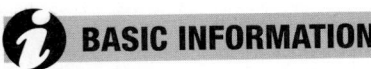

BASIC INFORMATION

DEFINITION

Cryptococcosis is an infection caused by the fungal organism *Cryptococcus neoformans*.

SYNONYMS

C. neoformans var. *neoformans* infection
C. neoformans var. *gatti* infection
C. neoformans var. *grubii* infection

ICD-9CM CODES
117.5 Cryptococcosis

EPIDEMIOLOGY & DEMOGRAPHICS

INCIDENCE (IN U.S.)
- 1 to 2 cases/1 million (non–HIV-infected) persons annually
- 6% to 7% in HIV-infected persons

PEAK INCIDENCE: 20 to 40 yr (parallel to AIDS epidemic)

PREDOMINANT SEX: Equal sex distribution when corrected for HIV status

PREDOMINANT AGE: Less than 2 yr of age; 20 to 40 yr of age

NEONATAL INFECTION: Very uncommon

PHYSICAL FINDINGS & CLINICAL PRESENTATION

- More than 90% present with meningitis; almost all have fever and headache.
- Meningismus, photophobia, mental status changes are seen in approximately 25%.
- Increased intracranial pressure.
- Most common infections outside the CNS:
  1. In the lungs (fever, cough, dyspnea)
  2. In the skin (cellulitis, papular eruption)
  3. In the lymph nodes (lymphadenitis)
  4. Potential involvement of virtually any organ

ETIOLOGY

- Caused by the fungal organism *C. neoformans*

There are 3 varieties of *Cryptococcus spp.* and 4 capsular serotypes: Serotype A is *Cryptococcus neoformans* var. *grubii* and Serotype D is known as *Cryptococcus neoformans* var. *neoformans*. Both cause disease primarily in immunocompromised patients. Serotype B and C are known as *C. neoformans* var. *gatti*. This organism causes disease primarily in normal hosts.

- Infection originates by inhalation into the respiratory tract followed by dissemination to the CNS in most cases, usually without recognizable lung involvement
- Almost always in the setting of AIDS or other disorders of cellular immune function
- Neutropenia alone poses a much lower risk of significant cryptococcal infection

DIAGNOSIS

DIFFERENTIAL DIAGNOSIS

- Subacute meningitis (caused by *Listeria monocytogenes, Mycobacterium tuberculosis, Histoplasma capsulatum,* viruses)

- Intracranial mass lesion (neoplasms, toxoplasmosis, TB)
- Pulmonary involvement confused with *Pneumocystis jiroveci* pneumonia when diffuse or confused with TB or bac-terial pneumonia when focal or involving the pleura
- Skin lesions confused with bacterial cellulitis or molluscum contagiosum

WORKUP

- Lumbar puncture to exclude cryptococcal meningitis.
- CT scan of the head when focal lesion or increased intracranial pressure is suspected.
- Biopsy of enlarged lymph nodes and skin lesions if feasible.

LABORATORY TESTS

- Culture and India ink stain (60% to 80% sensitive in culture-proven cases [Fig. 1-108]) examination of the CSF in all cases when CNS involvement is suspected
- Blood and serum cryptococcal antigen assay (>90% sensitivity and specificity)
- Culture and histologic examination of biopsy material

IMAGING STUDIES

- CT scan or MRI of the head if focal neurologic involvement is suspected
- Chest x-ray examination to exclude pulmonary involvement

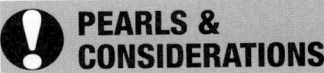

TREATMENT

ACUTE GENERAL Rx

- Therapy for CNS disease is initiated with IV Amphotericin B (0.7 to 1 mg/kg/day) with flucytosine, 100 mg/kg/day (assuming normal renal function), for 2 weeks.
- After stabilization, fluconazole (400 to 800 mg qd PO) for a minimum of 10 wk.
- Alternative: IV fluconazole for initial therapy in patients unable to tolerate amphotericin B.

- If symptomatic increased intracranial pressure, consider therapeutic lumbar taps or intraventricular shunt.

CHRONIC Rx

- Fluconazole (200 to 400 mg PO qd) is highly effective in preventing a relapse in HIV-infected patients; development of resistance may occur. Itraconazole is an alternative agent.
- Immune reconstitution syndrome following the institution of HARRT can cause transient worsening of meningitis and necessitate the use of a short course of corticosteroids.

DISPOSITION

Without maintenance therapy, relapse rate is >50% among AIDS patients.

REFERRAL

- For consultation with infectious diseases specialist in all cases
- For neurologic consultation if level of consciousness is depressed or focal lesion is present

PEARLS & CONSIDERATIONS

Cryptococcal meningitis can be remarkably insidious in nonimmunocompromised patients.

COMMENTS

Cryptococcosis is considered an AIDS-defining infection; thus all patients should be HIV tested.

SUGGESTED READINGS
available at www.expertconsult.com

AUTHORS: **GLENN G. FORT, M.D., M.P.H.,** and **DENNIS J. MIKOLICH, M.D.**

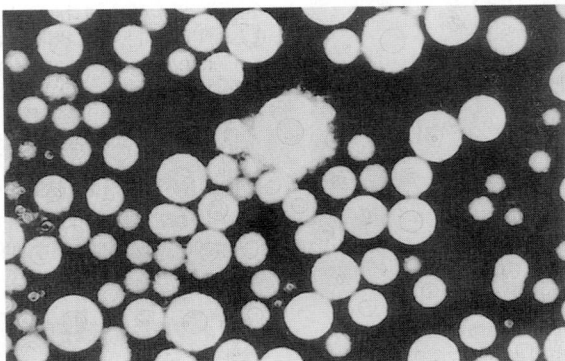

FIGURE 1-108 India ink preparation of cerebrospinal fluid revealing encapsulated cryptococci. Note the large capsules surrounding the smaller organisms. (From Andreoli TE [ed]: *Cecil essentials of medicine,* ed 4, Philadelphia, 1997, WB Saunders.)

BASIC INFORMATION

DEFINITION

Cryptorchidism is the incomplete or improper descent of the testis (testes) into the scrotum during fetal development. Testes that can be manually manipulated into the scrotum and which remain there without traction until cremasteric reflexes are induced are called *retractile*. Testes previously located but no longer palpable in the scrotum are called *ascended testes*.

SYNONYMS

Undescended testis

ICD-9CM CODES
752.51 Cryptorchidism

EPIDEMIOLOGY & DEMOGRAPHICS

- Cryptorchidism is the most common genitourinary disorder of male children.
- Occurs in approximately 30% of premature and 5% of term male infants. In 10%, it can be bilateral.
- Within the first year of life, most cryptorchid testes descend into the scrotum so that incidence becomes approximately 1% in boys.
- Increased rates with premature birth, low birth weight, twins, and family history of cryptorchidism.
- Associated with Kallman's and Prader-Willi syndromes, pituitary hypoplasia, testicular feminization, prune belly syndrome, cystic fibrosis, myelomeningocele, and Reifenstein syndrome.
- With retractile testes there is up to a 32% risk of subsequent ascent leading to an undescended testis.

CLINICAL PRESENTATION

- Typically asymptomatic and is noted incidentally on screening examination. Undescended testes are at risk for testicular torsion and inguinal hernia.
- The testis may be nonpalpable or palpable in a location along the path of normal descent (Fig. 1-109) or less commonly ectopic and located in the perineum, femoral canal, superficial inguinal pouch, suprapubic area, or contralateral hemiscrotum.
- In 80% the undescended testis is palpable in the inguinal canal.
- Associated with infertility and a sevenfold increased risk of testicular cancer. Risk of infertility is the greatest for a child with bilateral intraabdominal testes and longer duration of cryptorchidism.

ETIOLOGY

Normal testicular descent is a complex interplay among mechanical (gubernaculums, vas deferens and testicular vessel length, cremasteric muscles, and abdominal pressure), hormonal (gonadotropin, testosterone, dihydrotestosterone, and mullerian inhibiting substance), and neural (ilioinguinal and genitofemoral nerves) factors.

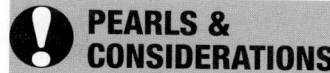 DIAGNOSIS

DIFFERENTIAL DIAGNOSIS

- Retractile testis
- Ascended testis
- Atrophic testis
- Vanished testis

WORKUP

- Physical examination:
  - When done in a warm room with warm hands, can identify presence, absence, and location of palpable testes.
  - Should be done with the patient in the supine, sitting, and standing positions with adequate cremasteric relaxation to differentiate true cryptorchidism from retractile testes.
  - Often associated with an indirect inguinal hernia as the tunica vaginalis fails to close above the testis.
  - An enlarged contralateral testis in the presence of a nonpalpable undescended testis is suggestive of but not definitive for testicular atrophy/absence.
- Hormonal challenge:
  - Human chorionic gonadotropin (hCG) will confirm the presence of functioning testicular tissue and is useful in the setting of bilateral nonpalpable undescended testes.
  - If the follicular stimulating hormone level is three times normal and there is no increase in testosterone in response to hCG, functional testes are absent.

IMAGING

- Ultrasound: sensitivity of 76%, specificity of 100%, accuracy of 84%.
- MRI: sensitivity of 86% and specificity of 79%. CT results are inconsistent.

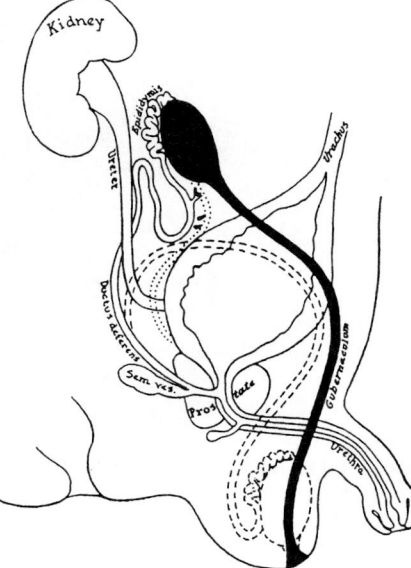

FIGURE 1-109 The path of testicular descent. (Reproduced with permission from Sarnat HB, Sarnat MS: Disorders of muscle in the newborn. In Moss AJ, Stern L [eds]: *Pediatrics update,* ed 4, New York, 1983, Elsevier-North Holland.)

TREATMENT

- Repeat examination at 3 mo of age because many testes will descend spontaneously. Spontaneous descent is rare after 3 mo of age.
- Treatment can be hormonal, surgical, or both.
- Treatment recommended as early as 6 mo and should be completed before 2 yr because histologic changes have been identified as early as age 1.5 yr.
- Earlier orchidopexy may improve testicular function and decrease the risk of testicular cancer. Orchidopexy allows testicular self-examination and detection of testicular cancer should it occur.

HORMONAL Rx

- Results of hCG are variable for undescended testes but good for retractile testes.
- The International Health Foundation recommends biweekly injections of 250 IU hCG for infants, 500 IU for children up to 6 yr, and 100 IU for children 6 yr and older, for a total of 5 wk. Therapy may induce precocious puberty.
- Administration of gonadotropin-releasing hormone before orchiopexy may improve fertility in adulthood.

SURGICAL Rx

- For the palpable undescended testis, orchiopexy, the surgical placement of an undescended testis into the scrotum, is the standard approach, performed between 6 mos and 1 yr of age in a healthy child.
- In the setting of a nonpalpable undescended testis, laparoscopy is recommended to identify the presence or absence of a testis and the location of the testis if present and to determine the length of the testicular vessels.
- A two-stage approach is recommended for an intraabdominal testis with short vessels. The testicular vessels are clipped laparoscopically in the first stage, and the testis is brought into the scrotum in the second stage.

DISPOSITION

- Earlier orchidopexy may decrease the risk of malignancy and infertility.
- Lifelong testicular examinations after puberty.

REFERRAL

Early referral to a pediatric urologist

⊘ PEARLS & CONSIDERATIONS

Regular testicular examinations should be performed in infants and children, particularly those with retractile testes, because ascent of scrotal testis can occur.

SUGGESTED READINGS
available at www.expertconsult.com

AUTHORS: **PAMELA ELLSWORTH, M.D.,** and **IRIS TONG, M.D.**

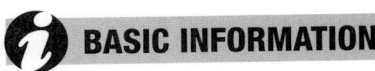

BASIC INFORMATION

DEFINITION

The intracellular protozoan parasite *Cryptosporidium parvum* is associated with gastrointestinal disease and diarrhea, especially in AIDS patients or immunocompromised hosts. It is also associated with sporadic infections and waterborne outbreaks in immunocompetent hosts.

Other species, including *C. hominus, C. felis, C. muris,* and *C. meleagridis,* are now described to be pathogens as well.

SYNONYMS

Cryptosporidiosis

ICD-9CM CODES

007.4 Cryptosporidia infection

EPIDEMIOLOGY & DEMOGRAPHICS

INCIDENCE (IN U.S.):
- Approximately 2% in industrial countries, 5% to 10% in third world countries
- 10% to 20% of HIV patients in U.S. may excrete cyst

PREVALENCE: Worldwide, especially third world countries; associated with poor hygiene as a waterborne pathogen

PREDOMINANT SEX: Male = female

TRANSMISSION:
- Person to person (daycare, family members)
- Animal to person (pets, farm animals)
- Environmental (water-associated outbreaks, including travel associated with swimming in or drinking contaminated water)
- May be significant pathogen causing diarrhea in AIDS

PHYSICAL FINDINGS & CLINICAL PRESENTATION

- Usually limited to gastrointestinal tract
- Diarrhea, severe abdominal pain (2 to 28 days)
- Impaired digestion, dehydration
- Fever, malaise, fatigue, nausea, vomiting
- Pneumonia if aspirated

ETIOLOGY

Cryptosporidium hominis, C. parvum, C. felis, C. muris, C. meleagridis

DX DIAGNOSIS

Clinical presentation of acute gastrointestinal illness, especially associated with HIV or with travel and waterborne outbreaks.

DIFFERENTIAL DIAGNOSIS

- *Campylobacter*
- *Clostridium difficile*
- *Entamoeba histolytica*
- *Giardia lamblia*
- *Salmonella*
- *Shigella*
- Microsporidia
- Cytomegalovirus
- *Mycobacterium avium*

Disease may cause cholecystitis, reactive arthritis, hepatitis, pancreatitis, pneumonia in immunocompromised or HIV-infected patients.

WORKUP

- Stool evaluation looking for characteristic oocyst by modified acid-fast stain (Fig. 1-110).
- Direct immunofluorescence using monoclonal antibodies is the gold standard for stool exams.

Rx TREATMENT

- May be self-limited in normal host—often requiring hydration. Antidiarrhea agents Pepto-Bismol, Kaopectate, or loperamide may give symptomatic relief.
- Pharmacologic treatment with antibiotics has been largely unsatisfactory in AIDS patients. Oocyst excretion reduction has been shown with nitazoxanide 500 mg PO bid for 3 days. If treatment fails, consider a trial of paromomycin, metronidazole, or Bactrim.
- Nitazoxanide elixir has been approved for the treatment of cryptosporidiosis in children ages 1 to 11 yr.
- Biliary cryptosporidiosis can be treated with antiretroviral therapy in the HIV setting.

DISPOSITION

- A self-limited disease in immunocompetent patients with complete recovery over 2 to 3 weeks.

- Chronic arthralgia, headache, malaise, and weakness may persist after cryptosporidial infection even in immunologically normal people.
- If severe and prolonged (>30 days), testing for HIV and other immunocompromised states is appropriate along with a referral to an infectious disease specialist or gastroenterologist.

REFERRAL

- To an infectious disease specialist if symptoms persist and if HIV infection is found
- To a gastroenterologist if chronic malabsorption, or biliary or pancreatic complications occur

PEARLS & CONSIDERATIONS

- Chronic cryptosporidiosis (>30 days of diarrhea from *Cryptosporidium* spp. infection) in a patient with HIV is an AIDS-qualifying opportunistic infection.
- *Cryptosporidium hominis* has a limited host range (humans), whereas *Cryptosporidium parvum* has a wide host range including humans, horses, cattle, other domesticated animals, and wild animals—both species present a similar illness in humans.

SUGGESTED READINGS

available at www.expertconsult.com

AUTHORS: **GLENN G. FORT, M.D., M.P.H.,** and **DENNIS J. MIKOLICH, M.D.**

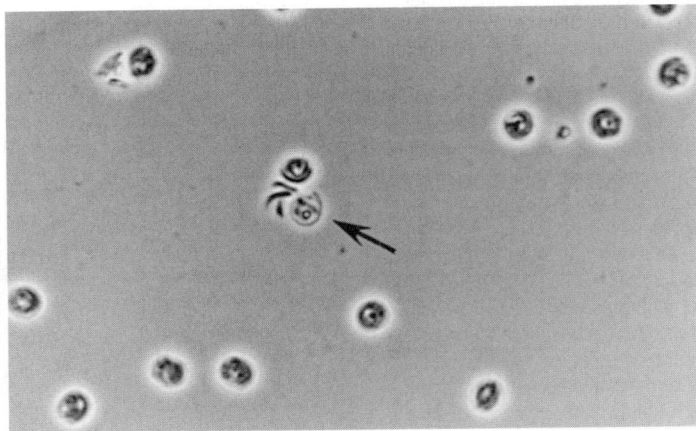

FIGURE 1-110 Human stool-derived *Cryptosporidium* oocysts. Excysting oocyst *(arrow)* is releasing three of its four sporozoites. (Phase-control microscopy ×630.) (From Gorbach SL: *Infectious diseases,* ed 2, Philadelphia, 1998, WB Saunders.)

BASIC INFORMATION

DEFINITION

This is a compression neuropathy of the ulnar nerve as it traverses the cubital tunnel at the elbow. It is the second most common entrapment neuropathy of the upper extremity.

ICD-9CM CODES
354.2 Cubital tunnel syndrome

EPIDEMIOLOGY & DEMOGRAPHICS

Males and females equally affected

PHYSICAL FINDINGS & CLINICAL PRESENTATION

- Paresthesias, numbness along distribution of ulnar nerve (little finger and one half of ring finger); pain is less common
- Positive Tinel's sign at elbow over the ulnar groove—highest negative predictive value
- Positive elbow flexion test (flexion of elbow with wrist extended for 30 sec may reproduce symptoms)
- Pressure provocation test (direct pressure over cubital tunnel for 60 sec elicits symptoms)
- "Scratch collapse" test—positive if temporary loss of external rotation resistance after examiner scratches over the compressed ulnar nerve; due to allodynia
- Signs of old trauma or elbow instability (valgus stress)
- Ulnar nerve may be subluxable over medial epicondyle with elbow motion
- Weakness/atrophy of intrinsic musculature of hand in longstanding cases (Fig. 1-111)
- Intrinsic minus or claw hand, aka Duchenne's sign; due to paralysis of lumbricals and interossei (clawing usually limited to ring and small fingers)
- Masse's sign—hand appears flattened due to hypothenar muscle paralysis
- Wartenberg's sign—due to weakness of adduction of small finger
- Froment's sign—compensation for diminished thumb pinch strength

ETIOLOGY

- Previous trauma, fractures
- Chronic pressure over ulnar groove from occupational stress, unusual elbow positioning
- Cubitus valgus deformity
- Subluxation of ulnar nerve
- Repeated stretching during throwing motion
- Elbow synovitis, osteophytes
- Local muscular hypertrophy
- Increased cubital tunnel pressure, particularly in elbow flexion
- Symptoms develop due to local nerve ischemia

DIAGNOSIS

DIFFERENTIAL DIAGNOSIS

- Tardy ulnar palsy
- Medial epicondylitis
- Other peripheral neuropathies
- Carpal tunnel syndrome
- Cervical radiculopathy
- Ulnar nerve compression at wrist (Guyon's canal)

WORKUP

Diagnosis can usually be established clinically.

IMAGING STUDIES

- Routine roentgenograms may be helpful in ruling out other conditions.
- Electrodiagnostic studies: nerve conduction tests and electromyography are useful to confirm the clinical diagnosis and can help localize site of compression.
- High-resolution ultrasound may be a valuable adjunct to diagnosis, as studies show enlargement of ulnar nerve in patients with cubital tunnel syndrome.

TREATMENT

ACUTE GENERAL Rx

- Activity modification, avoiding prolonged/repetitive flexion
- Elbow pads to relieve pressure, splints limiting flexion
- Physical therapy

DISPOSITION

- There is tendency towards spontaneous recovery with mild/moderate or intermittent symptoms if provocative causes are avoided.
- If muscle atrophy has developed, recovery of strength may be incomplete despite treatment.

REFERRAL

Surgical referral needed in cases of failed medical management. Patients with constant symptoms or muscle atrophy usually require surgical treatment.

PEARLS & CONSIDERATIONS

Patients with cubital tunnel syndrome are 4 times more likely to present with atrophy than those with carpal tunnel syndrome. Surgical decompression has been shown to be successful and may be adequate in most cases. More recently, endoscopic decompression techniques have been described. Ulnar nerve transposition and medial epicondylectomy are other surgical options.

SUGGESTED READINGS
available at www.expertconsult.com

AUTHOR: **CANDICE YUVIENCO, M.D.**

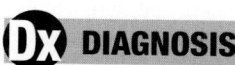

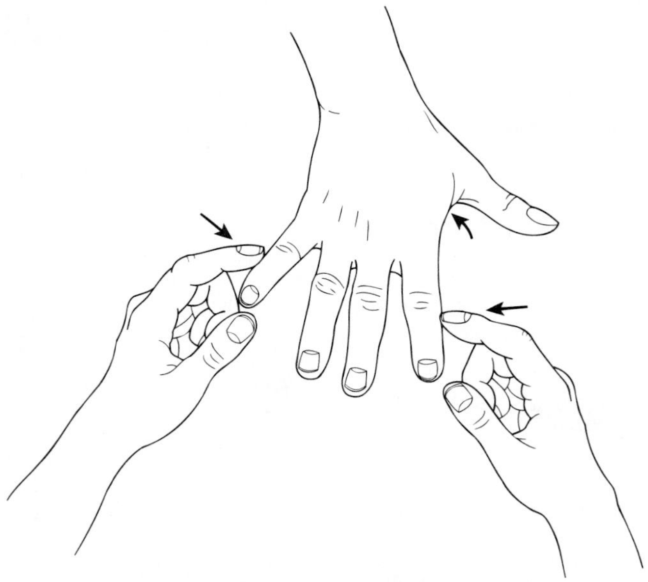

FIGURE 1-111 Testing for intrinsic (ulnar) motor weakness (fanning the fingers against resistance). Always look for atrophy of the first dorsal interosseus *(curved arrow)* when ulnar nerve lesions are suspected. (From Mercier LR: *Practical orthopedics*, ed 5, St Louis, 2000, Mosby.)

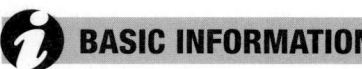 **BASIC INFORMATION**

DEFINITION

- Cushing's syndrome is the occurrence of clinical abnormalities associated with glucocorticoid excess as a result of exaggerated adrenal cortisol production or long-term glucocorticoid therapy.
- Cushing's disease is Cushing's syndrome caused by pituitary adrenocorticotropic hormone (ACTH) excess.

ICD-9CM CODES
255.0 Cushing's disease or syndrome

PHYSICAL FINDINGS & CLINICAL PRESENTATION

- Hypertension
- Central obesity with rounding of the facies (moon facies); thin extremities
- Hirsutism, menstrual irregularities, hypogonadism
- Skin fragility, ecchymoses, red-purple abdominal striae, acne, poor wound healing, hair loss, facial plethora, hyperpigmentation (with ACTH excess)
- Psychosis, emotional lability, paranoia
- Muscle wasting with proximal myopathy

NOTE: The previous characteristics are not commonly present in Cushing's syndrome caused by ectopic ACTH production. Many of these tumors secrete a biologically inactive ACTH that does not activate adrenal steroid synthesis. These patients may have only weight loss and weakness.

ETIOLOGY

- Iatrogenic from long-term glucocorticoid therapy (common)
- Pituitary ACTH excess (Cushing's disease; 60%)
- Adrenal neoplasms (30%)
- Ectopic ACTH production (neoplasms of lung, pancreas, kidney, thyroid, thymus; 10%)

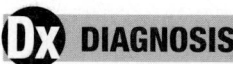 **DIAGNOSIS**

DIFFERENTIAL DIAGNOSIS

- Alcoholic pseudo-Cushing's syndrome (endogenous cortisol overproduction)
- Obesity associated with diabetes mellitus
- Adrenogenital syndrome

WORKUP

- In patients with a clinical diagnosis of Cushing's syndrome the initial screening test is the overnight dexamethasone suppression test:
  1. Dexamethasone 1 mg PO given at 11 PM
  2. Plasma cortisol level measured 9 hr later (8 AM)
  3. Plasma cortisol level <5 mcg/100 ml excludes Cushing's syndrome

- Serial measurements (two or three consecutive measurements) of 24-hr urinary free cortisol and creatinine (to ensure adequacy of collection) are undertaken if overnight dexamethasone test is suggestive of Cushing's syndrome. Persistent elevated cortisol excretion (>300 mcg/24 hr) indicates Cushing's syndrome.
- The low-dose (2 mg) dexamethasone suppression test is useful to exclude pseudo-Cushing's syndrome if the previous results are equivocal. Corticotropic-releasing hormone (CRH) stimulation after low-dose dexamethasone administration (dexamethasone-CRH test) is also used to distinguish patients with suspected Cushing's syndrome from those who have mildly elevated urinary free cortisol level and equivocal findings.
- The high-dose (8 mg) dexamethasone test and measurement of ACTH by radioimmunoassay are useful to determine the etiology of Cushing's syndrome.
  1. ACTH undetectable or decreased and lack of suppression indicate adrenal cause of Cushing's syndrome.
  2. ACTH normal or increased and lack of suppression indicate ectopic ACTH production.
  3. ACTH normal or increased and partial suppression suggest pituitary excess (Cushing's disease).

Bilateral inferior petrosal sinus sampling (BIPSS) can be used to distinguish pituitary Cushing's disease from the ectopic ACTH syndrome.

LABORATORY TESTS

- Hypokalemia, hypochloremia, metabolic alkalosis, hyperglycemia, hypercholesterolemia
- Increased 24-hr urinary free cortisol (>100 mcg/24 hr)

IMAGING STUDIES

- CT scan or MRI of adrenal glands in suspected adrenal Cushing's syndrome
- MRI of pituitary gland with gadolinium is the preferred procedure for localizing a pituitary edema in suspected pituitary Cushing's syndrome
- Additional imaging studies to localize neoplasms of the lung, pancreas, kidney, thyroid, or thymus in patients with ectopic ACTH production

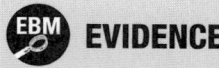 **TREATMENT**

GENERAL Rx

The treatment of Cushing's syndrome varies with its cause:
- Pituitary adenoma: transsphenoidal microadenomectomy is the therapy of choice in adults. Pituitary irradiation is reserved for pa-

tients not cured by transsphenoidal surgery. In children, pituitary irradiation may be considered as initial therapy because 85% of children are cured by radiation. Stereotactic radiotherapy (photon knife or gamma knife) is effective and exposes the surrounding neuronal tissues to less irradiation than conventional radiotherapy. Total bilateral adrenalectomy is reserved for patients not cured by transsphenoidal surgery or pituitary irradiation.
- Adrenal neoplasm:
  1. Surgical resection of the affected adrenal
  2. Glucocorticoid replacement for approximately 9 to 12 mo after the surgery to allow time for the contralateral adrenal gland to recover from its prolonged suppression
- Bilateral micronodular or macronodular adrenal hyperplasia: bilateral total adrenalectomy
- Ectopic ACTH:
  1. Surgical resection of the ACTH-secreting neoplasm
  2. Control of cortisol excess with metyrapone, aminoglutethimide, mifepristone, or ketoconazole
  3. Control of the mineralocorticoid effects of cortisol and 11-deoxycorticosteroid with spironolactone
  4. Bilateral adrenalectomy: a rational approach to patients with indolent, unresectable tumors

DISPOSITION

Prognosis is favorable in patients with surgically amenable disease.

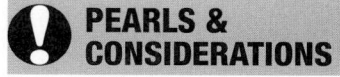 **PEARLS & CONSIDERATIONS**

COMMENTS

- A single midnight serum cortisol level (normal diurnal variation leads to a nadir around midnight) >7.5 mcg/dl has been reported as 96% sensitive and 100% specific for the diagnosis of Cushing's syndrome.
- Screening for multiple endocrine neoplasia type I should be considered in patients with Cushing's disease.

EBM **EVIDENCE**

available at www.expertconsult.com

SUGGESTED READING
available at www.expertconsult.com

AUTHOR: **FRED F. FERRI, M.D.**

BASIC INFORMATION

DESCRIPTION

Cutaneous larva migrans (CLM) is a syndrome defined clinically and parasitologically by subcutaneous larval migration of nematodes. Creeping eruption is the cardinal manifestation. It includes neither diseases in which creeping eruption is due to non-larval forms of parasites nor diseases without creeping eruptions from subcutaneous migration of larval parasites. As animal hookworms are the most common cause, some people use the term "hookworm-related cutaneous larva migrans" (HrCLM) instead. Table 1-39 describes other clinical syndromes associated with unusual helminth infections in humans.

SYNONYMS

Creeping eruption
Plumber's itch
Creeping verminous dermatitis
Sand worm eruption
Duck hunter's itch

ICD-9CM CODES
126.9

EPIDEMIOLOGY & DEMOGRAPHICS

- Commonly seen in tropical and subtropical countries. In U.S. it is most prevalent in southeastern states. Florida tops among these states.
- More often seen in children than adults.
- Has no racial or sexual predilection.
- Peak incidence is seen during rainy season.
- Second to pinworm among helminth infection in developed countries.
- Most common tropically acquired dermatosis.
- Most common imported ectoparasites in travelers returning to U.S. after holiday.

RISK FACTORS

Hobbies and occupations that involve contact with warm, moist, sandy soil
- Tropical/subtropical climate travels
- Barefoot beach goers/sunbathers
- Children playing in sandboxes
- Carpenter, electrician, plumber, farmer, gardener, pest exterminator

ETIOLOGY

- Animal hookworms
- *Ancylostoma Braziliense* (commonest cause)
- *Ancylostoma caninum*
- *Uncinaria stenocephala*
- *Bunostomum phlebotomum*
- *Pelodera strongyloides*
- *Gnathostoma* species
- *Strongyloides stercoralis*
- *Spirurina* species

PATHOGENESIS

The infection is usually acquired via skin contact with the soil or sand contaminated with feces of infected dogs or cats. The filariform larva is the infective form. It penetrates the skin and migrates within the epidermis by releasing protease and hyaluronidase. The inflammatory reaction along the cutaneous tract of their migration results in creeping eruptions. The larvae are believed to lack the collagenase enzymes required to penetrate the basement membrane to invade the dermis. In contrast to cats or dogs, humans are incidental host. Thus the larvae are unable to complete their natural cycles in humans. The larvae die without treatment and are resorbed within weeks to months of invasion. This explains why CLM is a self-limiting disease and rarely has systemic features.

CLINICAL FEATURES

- Often associated with a history of sunbathing, walking barefoot on a beach, or similar activity in a tropical location.
- Incubation period is around 1 to 6 days.
- Intense pruritus at the site of invasion within hours of invasion.
- Many patients report a stinging sensation, which they may misinterpret as a puncture or insect bite.
- Erythematous papules develop at the larval penetration site. Feet, buttocks, and thighs are most commonly affected anatomical locations.
- The most frequent and cardinal finding of HrCLM is *creeping dermatitis* (Fig. 1-112), which takes few days to develop. It is defined as an erythematous, slightly elevated, linear, or serpiginous track that is 3 mm in width and may be up to 15 to 20 cm in length. The mean number of lesions per person varies from 1 to 3. The creeping track associated with the larva migration may extend a few millimeters to few centimeters daily. These eruptions last 2 to 8 wk without treatment.
- Edema and vesicobullous lesions along the course of the larva.
- Rare presentation is hookworm folliculitis. It is characterized by numerous (20-100) follicular, erythematous, and pruritic papules and pustules, located mainly in the buttocks. Generally numerous short tracks are seen arising from these follicular lesions.
- In case of rare pulmonary involvement, dry cough and wheezing develop a week after the dermal invasion.

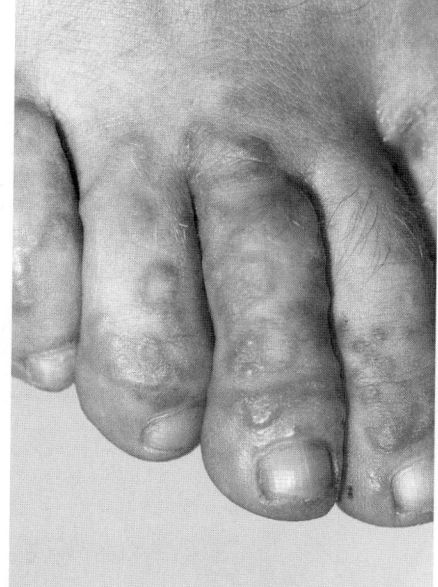

FIGURE 1-112 Cutaneous larva migrans ("creeping eruption") due to invasion of infective larvae of the dog hookworm *Ancylostoma caninum.* This condition may be mistaken for infestation with the larvae of ectoparasitic arthopods. The lesions respond rapidly to treatment with Albendazole or Ivermectin. Peters W, Pasvol G: *Tropical medicine and parasitology,* 5th ed, London: Mosby-Wolfe, 2002. (Cohen J, Powderly WG: *Infectious diseases,* ed 2, St Louis, 2004, Mosby.)

TABLE 1-39 Clinical Syndromes Associated with Unusual Helminth Infections in Humans

Clinical Syndrome	Parasite	Usual Host
Visceral larva migrans	Toxocara canis	Canines
	Toxocara cati	Felines
	Baylisascaris procyonis	Raccoons
Eosinophilic gastroenteritis	*Anisakis* spp.	Sea mammals
	Phocanema spp.	Sea mammals
	Ancylostoma caninum	Canines
Cutaneous larva migrans	Ancylostoma braziliense	Canines, felines
	Ancylostoma caninum	Canines, felines
	Uncinaria stenocephala	Canines, felines
Eosinophilic meningitis	Angiostrongylus cantonensis	Rats
	Gnathostoma spinigerum	Felines, other mammals
Pulmonary or cutaneous nodules	*Dirofilaria* spp.	Canines, other mammals
Abdominal angiostrongyliasis	Angiostrongylus costaricensis	Cotton rats
Capillariasis	Capillaria philippinensis	Birds
Diarrhea	Nanophyetus salmincola	Mammals, birds
Swimmer's itch	*Trichobilharzia* spp.	Birds

DX DIAGNOSIS

Diagnosis is made on clinical grounds and history of potential exposure. Clinical characteristics of the creeping trails (length, width, speed of migration, location, duration) help differentiate HrCLM from other causes of creeping dermatitis.

- Blood tests are not necessary for diagnosis. Theoretically, blood test could detect eosinophilia and elevated IgE level.
- Biopsy specimens usually show an eosinophilic inflammatory infiltrate, but not the migratory parasite. For this reason, biopsy is not indicated to establish the diagnosis. Nonetheless, in case of hookworm folliculitis, skin biopsy specimens may reveal nematode larvae in the follicular canal.
- Stool studies and serology are not helpful.
- Radiograph of chest is indicated when migratory pulmonary infiltrates are suspected.
- A new technology, optical coherence tomography, has been found to identify the larva in the epidermis, allowing direct removal.

DIFFERENTIAL DIAGNOSIS

- Superficial thrombophlebitis
- Mondor's disease
- Lichen striatus
- Phytophotodermatitis
- Herpes zoster
- Migratory myiasis
- Scabies
- Loiasis
- Dracunculiasis
- Cercarial dermatitis
- Onchocerciasis
- Dirofilariasis
- Contact dermatitis
- Creeping hair
- Jelly fish stings
- Fascioliasis
- Bacterial folliculitis
- Tenia pedis/corporis
- Impetigo
- Erytherma chronicum migrans of Lyme disease
- Ground itch
- Toxocariasis

RX TREATMENT

- Oral Albendazole and Ivermectin are the first line of drugs.
- Oral administration is preferred in presence of extensive lesions or when topical application fails.
- Topical application should cover the tracks and area covering up to 2 cm from the leading edge.
- Albendazole should be given (400 mg orally per day for 3 to 5 days).
- At times, when oral drugs are contraindicated, topical 10% albendazole creams are applied twice a day for a period of 10 days.
- Ivermectin should be given (200 mcg/kg given as a single dose).
- Thiabendazole should be given (25 to 50 mg/kg divided into twice-daily doses for 2 days).
- Because of its higher side effect profile when given orally, it is more often applied topically (10% to 15% cream or aqueous suspension of 500 mg/5 ml) four times a day for 5 to 10 days.
- Mebendazole should be given (100 mg orally twice for 3 days).
- Cryotherapy with liquid nitrogen is obsolete. It is ineffective as the larva is usually located 1 to 2 cm beyond the visible end of the trail, and the larva is capable of withstanding temperature as low as −21° C for more than 5 minutes. Moreover, this procedure is painful and can lead to chronic ulcerations.
- Specific antihelminthic therapy for pulmonary involvement is generally not required since the illness is usually mild and self-limiting.
- In the case of hookworm folliculitis, treatment is more difficult than traditional form and necessitates repeated courses of oral antihelmintic agents.
- Antihistamines and topical steroids relieve intense pruritus.
- Antibiotics are indicated for bacterial superinfection.
- Generally there should be no attempt to extract the worm.

COMPLICATIONS

- Secondary bacterial infection
- Erythema multiform
- Migratory eosinophilic pneumonitis (Loeffler syndrome)
- Eosinophilic enteritis

PROGNOSIS

Self-limiting benign disease. Even without treatment most cases resolve within 4 to 8 weeks.

PREVENTION

- Prohibit pets such as dogs and cats walking on the beaches in tropical areas.
- Avoid allowing pets in the sandbox.
- Deworm household pets.
- Clean up pet droppings.
- Protective foot wear while walking on the beach.
- Avoiding tropical beaches frequented by dogs and cats.
- When lying on tropical beaches potentially frequented by dogs and cats, areas of sand washed by the tide are preferable to dry sand, and mattresses are preferable to towels.
- Towels and clothes should not touch the ground when hung up for drying.

SUGGESTED READINGS
available at www.expertconsult.com

AUTHOR: **HEMANT K. SATPATHY, M.D.**

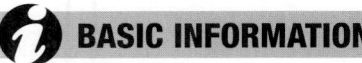 BASIC INFORMATION

DEFINITION

Cystic fibrosis (CF) is an autosomal recessive disorder characterized by dysfunction of exocrine glands.

ICD-9CM CODES
277.0 Cystic fibrosis

EPIDEMIOLOGY & DEMOGRAPHICS

- CF is the most common fatal hereditary disorder of whites in the U.S. (one case per 2500 whites) and second most common life-shortening childhood-onset inherited disorder in the U.S., behind sickle cell disease.
- Median age at diagnosis is 5.3 mo. Median survival is 30 yr.
- Carrier screening is associated with a decrease in incidence of CF.

PHYSICAL FINDINGS & CLINICAL PRESENTATION

- Failure to thrive in children
- Increased anterior/posterior chest diameter
- Basilar crackles and hyperresonance to percussion
- Digital clubbing
- Chronic cough
- Abdominal distention
- Greasy, smelly feces

ETIOLOGY

Chromosome 7 gene mutation (*CFTR* gene) resulting in abnormalities in chloride transport and water flux across the surface of epithelial cells; the abnormal secretions cause obstruction of glands and ducts in various organs and subsequent damage to exocrine tissue (recurrent pneumonia, atelectasis, bronchiectasis, diabetes mellitus, biliary cirrhosis, cholelithiasis, intestinal obstruction, increased risk of gastrointestinal malignancies).

DIAGNOSIS

DIFFERENTIAL DIAGNOSIS

- Immunodeficiency states
- Celiac disease
- Asthma
- Recurrent pneumonia

WORKUP

A diagnosis of CF requires a positive quantitative pilocarpine iontophoresis test with one or more phenotypic features consistent with CF (e.g., chronic suppurative obstructive lung disease, pancreatic insufficiency) or documented CF in a sibling or first cousin.

LABORATORY TESTS

- Pilocarpine iontophoresis (sweat test): diagnostic of CF in children if sweat chloride is >60 mmol/L (>80 mmol/L in adults) on two separate tests on consecutive days. Repeat testing may be necessary because not all infants have sufficient quantities of sweat for reliable testing.
- DNA testing may be useful for confirming the diagnosis and providing genetic information for family members.
- Sputum culture and sensitivity and Gram stain (frequent bacterial infections with *Staphylococcus aureus, Pseudomonas aeruginosa* [most common virulent respiratory pathogen], *Haemophilus influenzae*).
- Low albumin level, increased 72-hr fecal fat excretion.
- Pulse oximetry or arterial blood gases: hypoxemia.
- Pulmonary function studies: decreased total lung capacity, forced vital capacity, pulmonary diffusing capacity.

IMAGING STUDIES

- Chest radiograph: may reveal focal atelectasis, peribronchial cuffing, bronchiectasis, increased interstitial markings, hyperinflation
- High-resolution chest CT scan: bronchial wall thickening, cystic lesions, ring shadows (bronchiectasis)

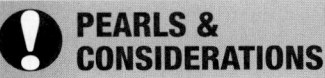 TREATMENT

NONPHARMACOLOGIC THERAPY

- Postural drainage and chest percussion
- Encouragement of regular exercise and proper nutrition
- Psychosocial evaluation and counseling of patient and family members

ACUTE GENERAL Rx

- Antibiotic therapy based on results of Gram stain and culture and sensitivity of sputum (PO quinolones for *Pseudomonas,* cephalosporins for *S. aureus,* IV aminoglycosides plus ceftazidime for life-threatening *Pseudomonas* infections). Inhaled antibiotics (aztreonam or tobramycin) can also be used and can achieve high airway concentration with lower systemic side effects. Macrolides are also active against *Pseudomonas aeruginosa.* A recent study using azithromycin maintenance in children with CF for 6 mo found less use of additional antibiotics and improvement in some aspects of pulmonary function. Additional studies may be necessary to determine if azithromycin should be used as a primary therapy or rescue treatment.
- Bronchodilators for patients with airflow obstruction.
- Long-term pancreatic enzyme replacement.
- Alternate-day prednisone (2 mg/kg) possibly beneficial in children with CF (decreased hospitalization rate, improved pulmonary function); routine use of corticosteroids not recommended in adults; among children with CF who have received alternate-day treatment with prednisone, boys, but not girls, have persistent growth impairment after treatment is discontinued.
- Proper nutrition and vitamin supplementation.
- Recombinant human deoxyribonuclease (DNase [Dornase alpha]) 2.5 mg qd or bid given by aerosol for patients with viscid sputum. It is useful to improve mucociliary clearance by liquefying difficult-to-clear pulmonary secretions. It is, however, very expensive (annual cost to the pharmacist is >$10,000); most beneficial in patients with forced vital capacity values >40% of predicted. Its cost can be decreased by using alternate-day rhDNase therapy.
- Intermittent administration of inhaled tobramycin has been reported beneficial in CF.
- Treatment of impaired glucose tolerance and diabetes mellitus.

CHRONIC Rx

Pneumococcal and influenza vaccination

DISPOSITION

- More than 50% of children with CF live beyond age 20 yr.
- Lung transplantation is the only definitive treatment; 3-yr survival after transplantation exceeds 50%.
- Obstructive azoospermia is present in >98% of postpubertal males.
- The SERPINA Z allele is a risk factor for liver disease in CF. Patients that carry the Z allele are at a greater risk of developing severe liver disease with portal hypertension.

REFERRAL

- For lung transplantation in selected patients. Indications for lung transplantation are FEV$_1$ <30% of predicted, rapidly progressive respiratory deterioration, increasing number of hospital admissions, massive hemoptysis, recurrent pneumothorax, arterial partial pressure of oxygen <55 mm Hg, arterial partial pressure of carbon dioxide >50 mm Hg, multiresistant organisms, wasting. Young female patients should be referred earlier because of overall poor prognosis.
- For screening of family members with DNA analysis.

PEARLS & CONSIDERATIONS

COMMENTS

- Clinicians should think of CF in any patient with bronchiectasis plus any of the following: male infertility, recurrent idiopathic pancreatitis, recurrent nasal polyposis.
- Genetic testing for CF should be offered to adults with a positive family history of CF, to couples currently planning a pregnancy, and to couples seeking prenatal care.
- Inhalation of hypertonic saline (5 ml of 7% sodium chloride qid) has been reported to produce a sustained acceleration of mucus clearance and improved lung function.
- The prevalence of MRSA in the respiratory tract of individuals with CF has increased dramatically over the past decade and is associated with worse survival.

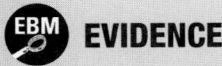 EVIDENCE

available at www.expertconsult.com

SUGGESTED READINGS

available at www.expertconsult.com

AUTHOR: FRED F. FERRI, M.D.

BASIC INFORMATION

DEFINITION

Cysticercosis is an infection caused by the tissue deposition of larval forms of the pork tapeworm *Taenia solium*. *T. solium* cysts, or cysticerci, may accumulate in any human tissue, including the eyes, spinal cord, skin, muscle, heart, and brain.

Central nervous system (CNS) involvement is common and is known as neurocysticercosis. Humans acquire cysticercosis by fecal-oral transmission of *T. solium* eggs from human tapeworm carriers, by ingesting tapeworm eggs or cysts in contaminated food or water. Undercooked pork is the most commonly identified food source. The eggs hatch in the gastrointestinal tract, and the larvae migrate hematogenously to tissues where they encyst, forming cysticerci.

SYNONYMS

Cysticerciasis
Taeniasis
Pork tapeworm

ICD-9CM CODES
123.1 Cysticercosis

EPIDEMIOLOGY & DEMOGRAPHICS

- *T. solium* infection is worldwide in distribution. Tapeworm infection and cysticercosis are endemic in rural, developing countries where pigs are raised as a food source.
- Serologic studies from endemic areas of Latin America have demonstrated seroprevalences of 4% to 24%.
- Neurocysticercosis is the most common cause of acquired epilepsy worldwide and has become an important parasitic disease in the U.S., especially in states with large immigrant populations from countries where the disease is endemic.

PHYSICAL FINDINGS & CLINICAL PRESENTATION

- After ingestion of *T. solium* eggs or cysts, human beings may remain asymptomatic for years.
- The symptoms vary and depend on the location of cysticerci. Cysticerci in muscles and skin may form "cold" nodules, which are usually asymptomatic but may calcify.
- Neurocysticercosis, or the presence of cysts within the brain parenchyma, is usually asymptomatic. Symptoms stem from inflammation associated with the degeneration of cysts.
- Seizures are the most common manifestation of neurocysticercosis, occurring in 70% to 90% of symptomatic cases. Headache is also common.
- Inflammation around degenerating cysts may result in focal encephalitis, vasculitis, chronic meningitis, and cranial nerve palsies.
- In 10% to 20% of cases of neurocysticercosis, cysts lodge within the ventricular system

and result in obstructive hydrocephalus, causing acute intracranial hypertension. This syndrome is related to the location of the parasites in the cerebral ventricles or basal cisterns, blocking the circulation of cerebrospinal fluid, and is caused by the presence of the parasite itself, ependymal inflammation, and/or fibrosis. Death may occur from progressive hydrocephalus, cerebral edema, or intractable seizures.
- Ocular cysticercosis occurs in <5% of infections and is generally asymptomatic. Inflammation in response to degenerating cysticerci may result in chorioretinitis, vasculitis, or retinal detachment, threatening vision.

ETIOLOGY

- *T. solium* has a complex two-host life cycle.
- Human beings are the only definitive host and harbor the adult worm in the intestine (taeniasis). However, both human beings and pigs can serve as intermediate hosts and harbor the larvae or cysticerci (Fig. 1-113).

DIAGNOSIS

DIFFERENTIAL DIAGNOSIS

- Idiopathic epilepsy
- Migraine
- CNS vasculitis
- Primary neoplasia of CNS
- Chronic CNS infections, including toxoplasmosis, coccidioidomycosis, tuberculosis, and cryptococcosis
- Brain abscess
- CNS sarcoidosis, systemic lupus erythematosus (SLE)

WORKUP

Comprehensive clinical history: obtain information on area and sanitary conditions of residence, previous travel, and dietary habits, most importantly consumption of undercooked pork.

LABORATORY TESTS

- Definitive diagnosis is based on the histopathologic demonstration of cysticerci in the tissue involved.
- Peripheral eosinophilia is usually absent.
- Stool examination for ova and proglottids of *T. solium* is insensitive and not specific for the diagnosis of cysticercosis.
- Cerebrospinal fluid (CSF) examination may demonstrate pleocytosis, with lymphocytic or eosinophilic predominance, low glucose, and elevated protein with neurocysticercosis. However, CSF is normal in most cases.
- Serologic testing is supportive of a suspected diagnosis of cysticercosis. An enzyme-linked immunoelectrotransfer blot (EITB) assay is the test of choice for detecting anticysticercal antibodies. This assay uses purified glycoprotein antigens and has higher sensitivity (83% to 100%) and specificity (93% to 98%) than other enzyme-linked antibody (e.g., ELISA) tests. However, the diagnostic performance of the EITB can vary in different patient populations depending on the activity of the cysts

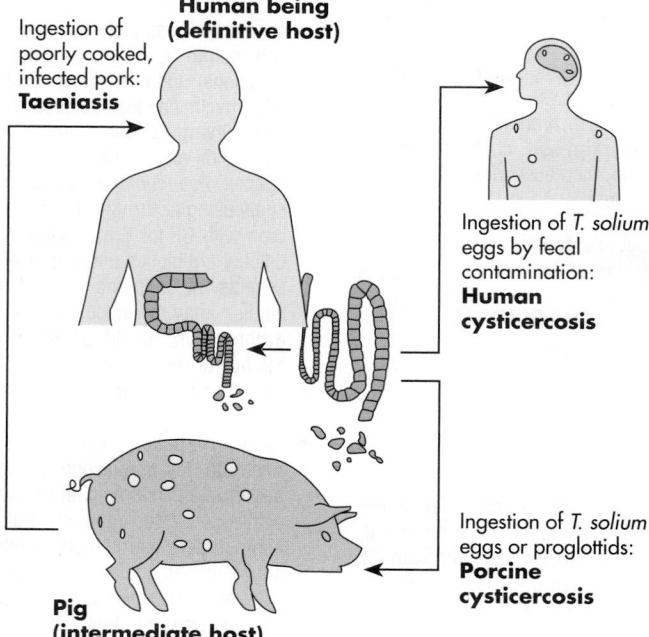

FIGURE 1-113 Cysticercosis is most commonly acquired by ingesting undercooked pork infected with *Taenia solium* cysticerci. Adult worms develop in the small intestine, forming proglottids that produce many fertilized eggs. Eggs and proglottids are intermittently shed in the stools of the persons infected with an adult tapeworm, where they can be ingested by pigs (the intermediate host) or transmitted by fecal-oral contamination to other human beings. In the small intestine of the host, the eggs hatch and release larvae that travel through the bloodstream to various organs, where they develop into fluid-filled cystic larvae within months. Skeletal muscle, subcutaneous tissue, the eyes, and the central nervous system are most commonly invaded.

and number of lesions. Single calcified lesions are more likely to be associated with a false-negative assay result. Antibodies detected by EITB can persist for years after successful therapy limiting the usefulness of this assay in following patients after treatment. EITB can be run on CSF, although its sensitivity is limited.

- Antigen detection tests are also being developed. The antigen-detecting ELISA performs better for CSF samples than for serum samples, but for both specimen types it is less sensitive than the EITB assay. The antigen-detecting ELISA seems to correlate better with viable and nonviable cysts. Furthermore, high antigen levels suggest the presence of subarachnoid neurocysticercosis. This method may be particularly useful in monitoring patients following therapy. Parasite antigen levels usually fall by 3 mo of treatment.
- More recently, amplification of *T. solium* DNA, with the method of polymerase chain reaction, has been achieved (sensitivity 96.7%).

IMAGING STUDIES

- Plain radiographs of the extremities may reveal calcified cysts in patients with soft tissue or muscle involvement.
- For diagnosis of neurocysticercosis, CT and MRI are most commonly used.
- Brain CT has a sensitivity and specificity of 95% and can identify living cysticerci, which appear as hypodense lesions, as well as degenerating cysts, which appear as isodense or hyperdense lesions with surrounding ring of edema. CT is the best method for detecting calcification associated with prior infection, which suggests inactivity.
- Brain MRI is the most accurate technique to assess the extent of infection, location, and evolutionary stage of the parasites. MRI provides detailed images of living and degenerating cysts, perilesional edema, as well as small cysts or those located in the ventricles, brainstem, and cerebellum.

Rx TREATMENT

ACUTE GENERAL Rx

Asymptomatic cysticercosis:
- There is no evidence that administering antiparasitic therapy is beneficial.

Symptomatic cysticercosis:
- Patients with active lesions, with evidence of surrounding edema and/or inflammation, generally warrant treatment with antiparasitics, corticosteroids, and anticonvulsants.
  - Anticonvulsant therapy:
    Patients who have seizures or are considered at risk for recurrent seizures based on imaging should be treated with anticonvulsants.
  - Antiparasitic therapy:
    Pharmacologic therapy is indicated in the treatment of symptomatic patients with multiple viable brain parenchymal cysticerci. However, despite treatment, only 30% to 50% of lesions resolve within 6 mo.
    Calcified cysticerci are inactive and do not warrant antiparasitic treatment.
    Antiparasitic therapy is often unnecessary in patients with single cysts, which are usually self-limited and resolve within 6 mo.
  - Cysticidal therapy:
    Antiparasitic therapy hastens the disappearance of cysts and should initially be given in conjunction with corticosteroids to control the inflammation associated with dying organisms.
    Patients with viable parenchymal or subarachnoid cysts should be treated with albendazole 15 mg/kg/day for 8 days or praziquantel 50 mg/kg/day for 15 days. Antiparasitics should be used cautiously in patients with massive cysticercal infection of the brain parenchyma (≥50 cysts) or cysticercal encephalitis. These patients should be managed initially with corticosteroids, and perhaps mannitol, to control intracranial hypertension. Once the inflammation and the edema have resolved by MRI, antiparasitics can be administered.
    Praziquantel may cause drug interactions with other agents metabolized by the cytochrome p450 systems, including phenytoin and phenobarbital. Furthermore, praziquantel serum levels are decreased by concomitant use of corticosteroids.
    Albendazole has no significant drug interactions with anticonvulsants.
  - Surgical therapy:
    Surgery may be indicated in patients with obstructive hydrocephalus or giant cysts with associated intracranial hypertension.
    Surgical interventions may include craniotomy, with cyst extraction, stereotactic cyst aspiration, and/or ventriculoperitoneal shunt placement to control hydrocephalus.
    Extraparenchymal cysticercosis, including ocular, subarachnoid, and intraventricular disease, carries a poor prognosis and requires a more aggressive approach. When feasible, complete surgical excision of lesions remains the definitive therapy.

CHRONIC Rx

- A recently published study suggests that prolonged antiparasitic therapy does not improve outcomes in patients with neurocysticercosis and seizures. Antiparasitic therapy, in fact, delayed calcification of lesions. Antiepileptic medications may need to be continued indefinitely.
- Rare patients with neurocysticercosis develop chronic or recurrent perilesional inflammation, requiring long-term, high-dose steroid therapy. Methotrexate has been reported to be of use as a steroid-sparing agent in this setting.

DISPOSITION

- In seizure-free, stable neurocysticercosis, outpatient management is appropriate.
- Patients with seizures should be restricted from driving.

REFERRAL

- Infectious diseases consultation
- Neurology consultation in patients with seizures
- Neurosurgical consultation if extraparenchymal neurocysticercosis or obstructive hydrocephalus is present

PREVENTION

- Eradication of taeniasis/cysticercosis is possible with implementation of meat inspection, improvement of pig husbandry, and improvement of socioeconomic conditions in endemic areas.
- A porcine vaccine against *T. solium* has been developed and successfully implemented in Peru, Mexico, and Australia.
- There is currently no human vaccine to prevent tapeworm infection or cysticercosis.

PATIENT & FAMILY EDUCATION

- Pork should be inspected for the presence of cysticerci, which are visible in raw meat.
- Pork must be well cooked.
- Proper disposal of human excreta and handwashing are of utmost importance to break the transmission cycle in households.

SUGGESTED READINGS
available at www.expertconsult.com

AUTHORS: **ELENI PATROZOU, M.D.,** and **STACI A. FISCHER, M.D.**

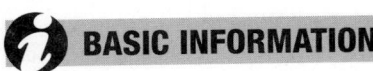

DEFINITION

Infection with cytomegalovirus (CMV), a herpes virus, is common in the general population, with multiple mechanisms for transmission, often during childhood and adolescence. CMV is associated with pregnancy and can be a congenital disease. CMV is also associated with immunocompromised states and may be life threatening.

SYNONYMS

CMV
Heterophil-negative mononucleosis
Cytomegalic inclusion disease virus

ICD-9CM CODES
078.5 CMV infection
771.1 Congenital or perinatal CMV infection
V01.7 Exposure to CMV

EPIDEMIOLOGY & DEMOGRAPHICS

- Seroprevalence is widespread: 40% to 100% antibody positivity in adults.
- Increased infection develops perinatally, in day care exposure, and then during reproductive age, related to sexual activity.

ROUTES OF TRANSMISSION

- Blood transfusions
- Sexually (STDs) via uterus, cervix, and semen
- Perinatally via breast milk
- Transplant of organs—bone marrow, kidneys, liver, heart, or lung

PHYSICAL FINDINGS & CLINICAL PRESENTATION

CHILDREN: Congenital—25% of infected children with symptoms if congenital:
- Petechial rash
- Jaundice and/or hepatosplenomegaly
- Lethargy
- Respiratory distress
- CNS involvement, seizures
Postnatal acquisition:
- CMV mononucleosis
- Pharyngitis, croup, bronchitis, pneumonia
HEALTHY ADULTS:
Common
- May be asymptomatic
- CMV mononucleosis similar to EBV mononucleosis
- Fever—lasting 9 to 30 days—mean of 19 days
Less common
- Exudative pharyngitis
- Lymphadenopathy, hepatitis, splenomegaly
- Interstitial pneumonia (rare)
- Nonspecific rash
- Thrombocytopenia/hemolytic anemia

Rare
- Guillain-Barré syndrome
- Meningoencephalitis
- Myocarditis

IMMUNOSUPPRESSED PATIENTS:
- Febrile mononucleosis
- GI ulcerations, hepatitis, pneumonitis, retinitis, encephalopathy, meningoencephalopathy
- HIV associated—dementia, demyelination, retinitis, acalculous cholecystitis, adrenalitis, diarrhea, enterocolitis, esophagitis
- Diabetes associated with pancreatitis
- Adrenalitis associated with HIV

ETIOLOGY

Cytomegalovirus infection can remain latent, reactive with immunosuppression.

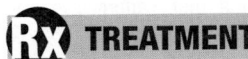
DIAGNOSIS

DIFFERENTIAL DIAGNOSIS

Congenital:
- Acute viral, bacterial, parasitic infections including other congenitally transmitted agents (toxoplasmosis, rubella, syphilis, pertussis, croup, bronchitis)
Acquired:
- EBV mononucleosis
- Viral hepatitis—A, B, C
- Cryptosporidiosis
- Toxoplasmosis
- *Mycobacterium avium* infections
- Human herpesvirus 6
- Acute HIV infection

WORKUP
- Laboratory confirmation combined with clinical findings often with leukopenia, thrombocytopenia, lymphocytosis
- Demonstration of virus in tissue or serologic testing including CMV IgM antibodies, rising titers of complement fixation (CF), and indirect fluorescent antibody (IFA) or anticomplement IFA
- Funduscopic—necrotic patches with white granular component of retina
- Cultures—(viral) human fibroblast from urine, cervical swab, tissue buffy coat
- Biopsy—"owl's eye" inclusion bodies on tissue sample

IMAGING STUDIES
- Chest radiograph—if pneumonitis suspected, consider bronchoscopy
- Endoscopy—if GI involvement
- CT scan/MRI—if CNS involvement

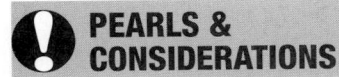
TREATMENT

NONPHARMACOLOGIC THERAPY
- Strict hand washing and standard precautions limit CMV transmission in health care facilities

- Highly active antiretroviral therapy (HAART) in patients with CD4 count <50/mm³ for the goal of CD4 >100/ mm³ for a 3- to 6-mo period

ACUTE GENERAL Rx

For compromised hosts with CMV retinitis or pneumonitis:
- Ganciclovir 5 mg/kg bid IV × 21 days, then 5 mg/kg/day IV, or 1 g PO tid or ocular implant
- Foscarnet 60 mg/kg tid × 3 wk, then 90 mg/kg/day
- Cidofovir 5 mg/kg IV, repeat 1 wk later, then q2 wk IV
- Fomivirsen-salvage therapy for CMV retinitis 300 μg injected into vitreous

DISPOSITION
- CMV infection in patients who are immunocompromised (especially those with AIDS, bone marrow and solid organ transplant recipients, and disorders of cell-mediated immune function) will need expert, long-term follow-up by an infectious disease specialist or immunologist familiar with the care of such patients.
- CMV mononucleosis, hepatitis, pharyngitis, etc. in immunologically normal hosts are usually self-limiting infections requiring no special follow-up plans.

REFERRAL
- To an ophthalmologist if CMV retinitis is present
- To an infectious disease specialist or AIDS specialist for patients who are HIV-positive with CMV disease
- To a cellular immunologist or transplant specialist in the case of CMV infection in a transplant recipient
- To a pediatric infectious disease specialist for congenital CMV infection

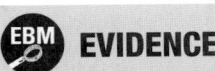
PEARLS & CONSIDERATIONS

CMV is ubiquitous in the environment and is asymptomatically shed by latently infected persons with CMV infection, making it difficult to protect patients who are immunocompromised from acquiring this infection.

EBM EVIDENCE

available at www.expertconsult.com

SUGGESTED READINGS
available at www.expertconsult.com

AUTHORS: **GLENN G. FORT, M.D., M.P.H.,** and **DENNIS J. MIKOLICH, M.D.**

BASIC INFORMATION

DEFINITION
Decubitus ulcers (pressure ulcers) are any damage to the skin and the underlying tissue or both that results from pressure, friction, or shearing forces that usually occur over bony prominences.

SYNONYMS
Pressure ulcers
Pressure sores
Bedsores
Decubiti

ICD-10 CODES
L89 Decubitus ulcers

EPIDEMIOLOGY & DEMOGRAPHICS
- Present in 5% to 10% of patients in all health care settings: hospitals, nursing homes, and home confined.
- Associated with significant morbidity and mortality. One-year mortality rate approaches 40%.
- Pain occurs in two thirds of patients with stage II or greater pressure ulcers.
- Complicated by cellulitis, osteomyelitis, abscesses, and sepsis.

CLINICAL PRESENTATION
A new pressure ulcer staging system was developed in 2007, adding the last two stages.
Stage I: Nonblanchable erythema of intact skin or boggy, mushy feeling of skin
Stage II: Partial-thickness skin loss involving the epidermis, dermis, or both
Stage III: Full-thickness skin loss involving damage or necrosis of subcutaneous tissue that may extend down to, but not through, underlying fascia or muscle
Stage IV: Full-thickness skin loss with extensive destruction and tissue damage to muscle, bone, or supporting structures (e.g., tendons, joint capsule) (Fig. 1-114)
Deep tissue injury: Purple or maroon skin overlying an area of dead tissue (muscle or fat), which usually develops into a stage III or IV.
Unstageable: Ulcer base is covered by slough and eschar and cannot be staged.

ETIOLOGY
Decubitus ulcers are caused by constant, unrelieved pressure in tissues where circulation is diminished, leading to necrosis of the tissues. Shearing and friction forces can also contribute or cause damage to the tissues, leading to an ulcer. Risk factors include malnutrition, bowel or bladder incontinence, and dry or damaged skin.

DIAGNOSIS

DIFFERENTIAL DIAGNOSIS
- Venous stasis ulcers
- Arterial ulcers
- Diabetic ulcers
- Skin cancer
- Cellulitis
- Kennedy ulcers (rapidly progressing ulcers that occur at the end of life)

WORKUP
Describe ulcer, including the stage, location, and size. For stages III and IV, describe the wound bed (epithelialization, granulation tissue, necrotic tissue, eschar); presence of any exudates, including type and amount; depth and wound edges (undermining, sinus tracts, tunneling, or fistulas); any signs of infection (purulent drainage, odor, surrounding cellulitis); and pain. In addition, pressure ulcer risk factors and causes should be reassessed.

LABORATORY TESTS
- Directed at identifying cause of risk factors or any complications arising from the pressure ulcer (e.g., abscess or osteomyelitis).
- Cultures of wound bed are often not helpful and should not be routinely performed.
- Low prealbumin levels may reveal malnutrition.
- Complete blood count if infection is suspected.

IMAGING STUDIES
- Ultrasound not proven to be effective.
- MRI or bone scans may help identify osteomyelitis when clinically suspected.

TREATMENT

PREVENTION
- Identify high-risk patients by using standardized risk assessment scales such as the Braden scale.
- Routine skin inspection and good skin care for high-risk patients.
- Minimize prolonged skin exposure to moisture, urine, or stool.
- Treat dry, cracking skin.
- Use repositioning and pressure-reducing devices (e.g., foam mattresses, low–air loss beds, pillows, or foam wedges when in bed or in a chair).
  - Patient repositioning
    Although there is clinical consensus that repositioning is critical, three randomized controlled trials (RCTs) found no evidence that regular manual repositioning prevented pressure ulcers.
  - Bed surface
    Air-fluidized beds
    a. Two RCTs found that use of air-fluidized beds contributed to the healing of a greater number of ulcers after 15 days compared with standard care.
    b. Systematic review revealed no differences in rate of pressure ulcer healing with use of either alternating-pressure mattresses or low–air loss beds compared with standard care.
    Pressure-relieving overlays
    a. One RCT demonstrated that viscoelastic pad on the operating table significantly reduced incidence of postoperative pressure ulcers compared with a standard operating table.
    b. One RCT found that sheepskin overlays plus standard care compared with standard care alone significantly reduced incidence of pressure sores in elderly patients recuperating from hip fracture.
    Foam alternatives
    a. Four RCTs revealed that foam alternatives versus standard hospital mattresses reduced the incidence of pressure ulcer development in elderly patients in orthopedic hospital wards.
    b. Forty-one RCTs demonstrated that patients lying on standard hospital mattresses are more likely to develop pressure ulcers than those patients lying on higher specification foam mattresses.
- Use adequate support surfaces while in bed or in a chair to prevent "bottoming out" (defined as less than 1 inch between patient and

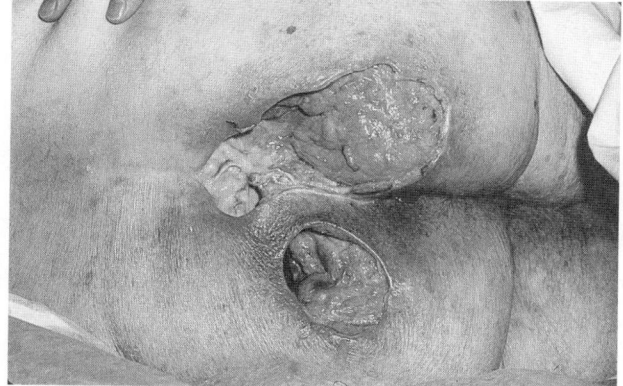

FIGURE 1-114 Natural debridement of pressure injury at 2 wk. (From Tallis R, Fillit H: *Brockelhurst's textbook of geriatric medicine and gerontology*, ed 6, London, 2003, Churchill Livingstone.)

support surface; measured by putting hand under support surface and feeling thickness to patient).
- Recent systematic review of pressure ulcer prevention strategies showed poor methodology in most studies. Use of support surfaces, repositioning, optimized nutrition, and sacral skin moisturizing were most appropriate.

NONPHARMACOLOGIC THERAPY
- Should be cleaned at each dressing change; necrotic tissue should be debrided quickly because it delays wound healing (except for heel ulcers).
- Wound irrigation should not exceed 15 psi and is best done with an 18-gauge angiocatheter.
- No single dressing or product is superior; should be used to keep ulcer bed moist and protect it from urine/stool. Silver dressings (which are felt to be antimicrobial), topical phenytoin, and growth factors should be limited to difficult to heal wounds, chronic ulcers, and extensive burns given their extra cost and limited scientific validation.
- Avoid agents that are cytotoxic to epithelial cells (e.g., iodine, iodophor, sodium hypochlorite, hydrogen peroxide, acetic acid, alcohol).
- Reduce pressure by using foam mattress, dynamic support surface (e.g., low–air loss bed), and frequent repositioning (e.g., q2h).
- Hyperbaric oxygen, ultrasound, ultraviolet, electromagnetic therapy, and low-energy radiation either are ineffective or have not been extensively evaluated for efficacy.
- Negative pressure devices (Vac devices) may help in wounds that have significant drainage. It also may improve healing by promoting angiogenesis, improving tissue perfusion, and decreasing bacterial count. Calcium alginate and foam dressings may also be beneficial for such wounds.
- Correct poor nutrition.
- Minimize urinary and/or fecal contamination.
- Use a standardized assessment tool (e.g., PUSH tool) to monitor wound healing on weekly basis.
- No RCTs have compared debridement versus no debridement in the treatment of pressure ulcers.

- Thirty-two RCTs have compared different debridement agents, but there is insufficient evidence to promote the use of one particular agent.
- One RCT demonstrated ulcers treated with collagenase healed significantly more quickly than those treated with hydrocolloid.
- A meta-analysis and one RCT found significant benefit in rates of healing with use of hydrocolloid dressings versus traditional saline gauze dressings but not over other forms such as hydrogels, foam dressings, or collogenase.
- No benefit was found with honey, nutritional and vitamin supplements, artificial nutrition, or ultrasound therapy.

ACUTE GENERAL Rx
- Pain medications may be necessary because 50% of decubitus ulcers are painful.
- Growth factors appear promising but are second-line treatments if traditional approaches are ineffective.

CHRONIC Rx
- Continue vigilance with pressure reduction because decubitus ulcers can recur with minimal trauma.
- Consider radiological evaluation for infected ulcer bed, occult osteomyelitis, or abscess.

COMPLEMENTARY & ALTERNATIVE MEDICINE
Vitamin C, zinc, and multivitamin supplements may be of benefit to optimize nutrition.

DISPOSITION
- When systematic risk assessments are done and preventive measures are followed, most pressure ulcers can be prevented. Most ulcers heal when appropriate management strategies are followed.
- Stage IV ulcers in high-risk patients (e.g., paraplegics) can take months or years to heal.

REFERRAL
- Physical and occupational therapists to improve bed and chair mobility.

- Wounds with necrotic tissue need referral to persons trained in sharp debridement.
- To plastic surgeons for operative repair for large stage III or IV ulcers that do not respond to optimal care.
- To a specialty wound center for nonhealing ulcers.

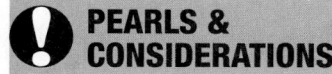

COMMENTS
- Up to 10% of older persons will have a pressure ulcer.
- Because 70% of decubitus ulcers occur in older persons, the approach should be similar to other multifactorial geriatric syndromes with a multidisciplinary team approach. Identify and reduce all modifiable risk factors for pressure ulcers.
- Treat the pain associated with pressure ulcers.
- Proper skin care, use of support surfaces, mobilization, and attention to nutrition are key for prevention and treatment.
- Clinical studies have not revealed if any one dressing product is superior.
- Nonhealing ulcers require assessment for debridement, infection, abscess, and/or referral to a wound center.

PATIENT & FAMILY EDUCATION
- Educate patient and family members on the risk factors for pressure ulcers.
- Encourage mobility and adequate nutritional intake and avoid bed rest.

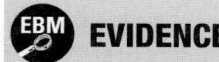

available at www.expertconsult.com

SUGGESTED READINGS
available at www.expertconsult.com

AUTHOR: **LYNN MCNICOLL, M.D., F.R.C.P.C.**

BASIC INFORMATION

DEFINITION
Deep vein thrombosis (DVT) is the development of thrombi in the deep veins of the extremities or pelvis.

SYNONYMS
DVT
Venous thromboembolism (VTE) (VTE includes DVT and pulmonary embolism [PE])
Deep venous thrombosis

ICD-9CM CODES
451.1   Thrombosis of deep vessels of lower extremities
451.83 Thrombosis of deep veins of upper extremities
541.9   Deep vein thrombosis of unspecified site

EPIDEMIOLOGY & DEMOGRAPHICS
- Annual incidence in urban population is 1.6 cases/1000 persons.
- The risk of recurrent thromboembolism is higher among men than women.

PHYSICAL FINDINGS & CLINICAL PRESENTATION
- Pain and swelling of the affected extremity
- In lower extremity DVT: leg pain on dorsiflexion of the foot (Homans' sign)
- Physical examination may be unremarkable in early DVT

ETIOLOGY
The etiology is often multifactorial (prolonged stasis, coagulation abnormalities, vessel wall trauma). The following are risk factors for DVT:
- Prolonged immobilization (≥3 days)
- Postoperative state
- Trauma to pelvis and lower extremities for lower extremity DVT; central line placement for upper extremity DVT
- Birth control pills, high-dose estrogen therapy; conjugated equine estrogen but not esterified estrogen is associated with increased risk of DVT; estrogen plus progestin is associated with doubling the risk of venous thrombosis. The use of bevacizumab is also significantly associated with an increased risk of developing DVT in cancer patients receiving this drug
- Visceral cancer (lung, pancreas, alimentary tract, genitourinary tract)
- Age >60 yr
- History of thromboembolic disease
- Hematologic disorders (e.g., factor V Leiden mutation [FVL], antithrombin III deficiency, protein C deficiency, protein S deficiency, heparin cofactor II deficiency, sticky platelet syndrome, G20210A prothrombin mutation, lupus anticoagulant, dysfibrinogenemias, anticardiolipin antibody, hyperhomocystinemia, concurrent homocystinuria, high levels of factors VIII, XI, and single nucleotide polymorphisms [SNPs] such as CYP4V2)

- Pregnancy and early puerperium
- Obesity (BMI >30)
- Congestive heart failure
- Surgery, fracture, or injury involving lower leg or pelvis
- Plaster cast immobilization
- Surgery requiring >30 min of anesthesia
- Gynecologic surgery (particularly gynecologic cancer surgery)
- Recent travel (within 2 wk, lasting ≥2 hr). Every 2 hr spent traveling increases VTE risk by 18%
- Smoking and abdominal obesity
- Central venous catheter or pacemaker insertion
- Superficial vein thrombosis (10% risk of DVT within 3 mo), varicose veins
- Collagen vascular disease
- Nephrotic syndrome
- Myeloproliferative disorders
- Long-term exposure to particulate air pollution is also associated with altered coagulation function and DVT risk

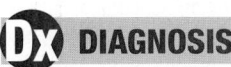 **DIAGNOSIS**

DIFFERENTIAL DIAGNOSIS
- Postphlebitic syndrome
- Superficial thrombophlebitis
- Ruptured Baker's cyst
- Cellulitis, lymphangitis, Achilles tendinitis
- Hematoma
- Muscle or soft tissue injury, stress fracture
- Varicose veins, lymphedema
- Arterial insufficiency
- Abscess
- Claudication
- Venous stasis

WORKUP
- The clinical diagnosis of DVT is inaccurate. Pain, tenderness, swelling, or color changes are not specific for DVT.
- Clinical prediction rules can be used to establish pretest probability of DVT. The Wells prediction rules for DVT and for pulmonary embolism are described in Box 1-3. These rules perform better in younger patients without a history of DVT and in those without comorbidities. In younger patients without associated comorbidities and a low pretest probability using Wells criteria and a negative high-sensitivity D-dimer test, the diagnosis of DVT can be reasonably excluded.
- Compression ultrasonography (CUS) is preferred as the initial study to diagnose DVT in patients with intermediate to high pretest probability. An initial negative test limited to the proximal leg should be repeated after 5 days (if the clinical suspicion of DVT persists) to exclude DVT that is propagating proximally from the calf. Comprehensive ultrasonography (whole-leg CUS) is a more extensive test that examines the deep veins from the inguinal ligament to the level of the malleolus. Recent literature reports indicate that it may be safe to withhold anticoagulation after negative results on comprehensive duplex ultrasonography in nonpregnant patients with a suspected first episode of symptomatic DVT of the leg.

LABORATORY TESTS
- Laboratory tests are not specific for DVT. Baseline prothrombin time (INR), partial thromboplastin time, and platelet count should be obtained on all patients before starting anticoagulation.
- Use of D-dimer assay by ELISA is useful in the management of suspected DVT. The combination of a normal D-dimer study on presentation together with a normal compression venous ultrasound is useful to exclude DVT and generally eliminate the need to do repeat ultrasound at 5 to 7 days. Recent trials indicate that DVT can be ruled out in patients who are clinically unlikely to have DVT and who have a negative D-dimer test. Compressive ultrasonography can be safely omitted in such patients. An algorithm for the diagnosis of deep vein thrombosis is described in Section III.

BOX 1-3 Wells Prediction Rule for Diagnosing Deep Venous Thrombosis: Clinical Evaluation Table for Predicting Pretest Probability of Deep Venous Thrombosis*

Clinical Characteristic	Score
Active cancer (treatment ongoing, within previous 6 mo, or palliative)	1
Paralysis, paresis, or recent plaster immobilization of the lower extremities	1
Recently bedridden >3 days or major surgery within 12 wk requiring general or regional anesthesia	1
Localized tenderness along the distribution of the deep venous system	1
Entire leg swollen	1
Calf swelling 3 cm larger than asymptomatic side (measured 10 cm below tibial tuberosity)	1
Pitting edema confined to the symptomatic leg	1
Collateral superficial veins (nonvaricose)	1
Alternative diagnosis at least as likely as deep venous thrombosis	−2

*Clinical probability: low, ≤0; intermediate, 1-2; high, ≥3. In patients with symptoms in both legs, the more symptomatic leg is used.
    Reprinted from Wells PS et al: Value assessment of pretest probability of deep-vein thrombosis in clinical management, *Lancet* 351:1795-1798, 1997. With permission from Elsevier.

- Laboratory evaluation of young patients with DVT, patients with recurrent thrombosis without obvious causes, and those with a family history of thrombosis should include protein S, protein C, fibrinogen, antithrombin III level, lupus anticoagulant, anticardiolipin antibodies, factor V Leiden, factor VIII, factor IX, and plasma homocysteine levels.

IMAGING STUDIES

Compression ultrasonography (CUS) is generally preferred as the initial study because it is noninvasive and can be repeated serially (useful to monitor suspected acute DVT); it offers good sensitivity for detecting proximal vein thrombosis (in the popliteal or femoral vein). Its disadvantages are poor visualization of deep iliac and pelvic veins and poor sensitivity in isolated or nonocclusive calf vein thrombi. Whole-leg compression ultrasound can generally exclude proximal and distal DVT in a single evaluation. Withholding anticoagulation following a single negative whole-leg CUS is associated with a relatively low risk of venous thromboembolism (3.5 % of inpatients will develop DVT) during a 3-mo follow-up.

Contrast venography is the gold standard for evaluation of DVT of the lower extremity. It is, however, invasive and painful. Additional disadvantages are the increased risk of phlebitis, new thrombosis, renal failure, and hypersensitivity reaction to contrast media; it also gives poor visualization of the deep femoral vein in the thigh and the internal iliac vein and its tributaries.

Magnetic resonance direct thrombus imaging (MRDTI) is an accurate noninvasive test for diagnosis of DVT. It is particularly useful in suspected DVT patients with leg casts, which prevent CVS. Current limitations are its cost and lack of widespread availability.

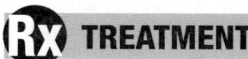 **TREATMENT**

NONPHARMACOLOGIC THERAPY

- Gradual resumption of normal activity. Immobility promotes stasis and propagation of DVT. Patients should get up and walk as tolerated. The theoretical risk that ambulation may dislodge thrombi in the legs, precipitating PE, is unfounded.
- Patient education on anticoagulant therapy and associated risks.

ACUTE GENERAL Rx

- Low-molecular-weight heparin (LMWH) for 4 to 7 days followed by warfarin therapy. Recommended dose of enoxaparin is 1 mg/kg q12h SC and continued for a minimum of 5 days and until a therapeutic INR (2 to 3) has been achieved with warfarin. Once-daily fondaparinux, a synthetic analog of heparin, is also as effective and safe as twice-daily enoxaparin in the initial treatment of patients with symptomatic DVT. Warfarin therapy should be initiated when appropriate (usually within 72 hr of initiation of heparin). A 5-mg loading dose of warfarin is recommended in inpatients because it produces less excess

anticoagulation than does a 10-mg dose; the smaller dose also avoids the development of a potential hypercoagulable state caused by precipitous decreases in levels of protein C during the first 36 hr of warfarin therapy. In the outpatient setting, a warfarin nomogram using 10-mg loading doses may be more effective in reaching a therapeutic INR. Long-term LMWH may be preferable to warfarin in patients with cancer or those whose INR is difficult to control. Dabigatran is a direct oral thrombin inhibitor recently FDA approved. It is as effective as warfarin but does not require laboratory monitoring.
- Outpatient treatment of DVT is appropriate for patients without prior DVT, thrombophilic conditions, or substantial comorbidity, but not for those who are pregnant or likely not to adhere to therapy.
- Exclusions from outpatient treatment of DVT include patients with potential high complication risk (e.g., hemoglobin <7, platelet count <75,000, guaiac-positive stool, recent cerebrovascular accident or noncutaneous surgery, noncompliance).
- Compression stockings are effective in reducing the incidence of postthrombotic syndrome and should be used starting within 1 mo of proximal DVT and for at least 1 yr after diagnosis.
- Insertion of an inferior vena cava filter to prevent pulmonary embolism is recommended in patients with contraindications to anticoagulation.
- Thrombolytic therapy (streptokinase) can be used in rare cases (unless contraindicated) in patients with extensive iliofemoral venous thrombosis and a low risk of bleeding. There are concerns about hemorrhagic complications related to the large doses of thrombolytics required in systemic thrombolysis for DVT (2% to 10% risk of major hemorrhagic complications).
- Other treatment modalities for DVT include surgical tthombectomy and Catheter directed thrombolysis (CDT). Thromboreduction by surgical thrombectomy is effective but invasive and expensive. CDT is also invasive, carries a bleeding risk and will require ICU admission.

CHRONIC Rx

- Conventional-intensity warfarin therapy is more effective than low-intensity warfarin therapy for the long-term prevention of recurrent DVT. The low-intensity warfarin regimen does not reduce the risk of clinically important bleeding.
- The optimal duration of anticoagulant therapy varies with the cause of DVT and the patient's risk factors. The risk of recurrence is low if VTE is provoked by surgery, intermediate if provoked by a nonsurgical risk factor, and high if unprovoked. These risks should determine whether patients with VTE should undergo short-term vs. indefinite treatment.
- Therapy for 3 to 6 mo is generally satisfactory in patients with reversible risk factors (low-risk group). A high D-dimer level mea-

sured after 3 mo of anticoagulation in patients with unprovoked DVT should favor a longer duration of therapy.
- Anticoagulation for at least 6 mo is recommended for patients with idiopathic venous thrombosis or medical risk factors for DVT (intermediate-risk group).
- Indefinite anticoagulation is necessary in patients with DVT associated with active cancer; long-term anticoagulation is also indicated in patients with inherited thrombophilia (e.g., deficiency of protein C or S antibody), antiphospholipid antibody, and those with recurrent episodes of idiopathic DVT (high-risk group).
- Measurement of D-dimer after withdrawal of oral anticoagulation may be useful to estimate the risk of recurrence. In patients with a first unprovoked DVT, positive D-dimer test results after cessation of anticoagulation predict recurrence, regardless of test timing or pt's age. Patients with a first spontaneous DVT and a D-dimer level <250 mg/ml after withdrawal of oral anticoagulation have a low risk of DVT recurrence. Recent trials show that in patients who have completed at least 3 mo of anticoagulation for a first episode of unprovoked DVT and after approximately 2 yr of follow-up, a negative D-dimer result was associated with a 3.5% annual risk of recurrent disease, whereas a positive D-dimer result was associated with an 8.9% annual risk for recurrence.
- The presence of residual thrombosis on ultrasonography when warfarin therapy is discontinued is also associated with an increased risk for subsequent recurrent DVT; a recent trial showed that tailoring the duration of anticoagulation on the basis of the persistence of residual thrombi on ultrasonography may reduce the rate of recurrent DVT. Additional trials are needed before this approach can be adapted for all patients.

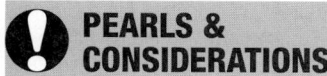 **PEARLS & CONSIDERATIONS**

COMMENTS

- When using heparin, there is a risk of heparin-induced thrombocytopenia (HIT) (with unfractionated more so than with LMWH). Platelet count should be obtained initially and repeated every 3 days while on heparin.
- Prophylaxis of DVT is recommended in all patients at risk (e.g., low-molecular-weight heparin [enoxaparin 30 mg SC bid] after major trauma, post surgery of hip and knee; enoxaparin 40 mg SC qd post–abdominal surgery in patients with moderate to high DVT risk; gradient elastic stockings alone or in combination with intermittent pneumatic compression [IPC] boots following neurosurgery). Graduated compression stockings (GCSs) are effective for preventing air-travel-related DVT and in reducing the risk of DVT in patients hospitalized for conditions other than stroke. The type of GCSs is also important because proximal DVT occurs more often in patients with stroke who

wear below-knee stockings than in those who wear high-length stockings.

- Fondaparinux, a synthetic analog of heparin, can also be used for prevention of DVT after hip fracture surgery, hip replacement, or knee replacement. Initial dose is 2.5 mg SC given 6 to 8 hr postoperatively and continued daily. Its bleeding risk is similar to enoxaparin; however, it is more effective in preventing DVT. Desirudin is an injectable direct thrombin available for prevention of VTG after selective hip arthroplasty. Unlike unfractionated heparin and LMWH, desirudin does not cause HIT.
- The risk of recurrent venous thromboembolism in heterozygous carriers of factor V Leiden and a first spontaneous venous thromboembolism is similar to that of noncarriers of factor V Leiden; therefore, heterozygous patients should receive secondary thromboprophylaxis for a similar length of time as patients without factor V Leiden.
- Approximately 20% to 50% of patients with DVT develop *postthrombotic syndrome* characterized by leg edema, pain, venous ectasia, skin induration, and ulceration. Patients with extensive DVT and those with more severe postthrombotic manifestations 1 month after DVT have poorer long-term outcomes.
- Exercise following DVT is reasonable because it improves flexibility of the affected leg and does not increase symptoms in patients with postthrombotic syndrome.
- Previously undiagnosed cancer is frequent in patients with newly diagnosed DVT. A cancer screening strategy should be considered in all patients with unprovoked venous thromboembolism.
- Vitamin K (1 mg PO or 2 mg IV) can be used to reverse elevated INR (3 to 6) when elective or urgent procedures are needed.

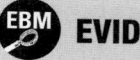

EVIDENCE
available at www.expertconsult.com

SUGGESTED READINGS
available at www.expertconsult.com

AUTHOR: **FRED F. FERRI, M.D.**

D

Diseases
and Disorders

I

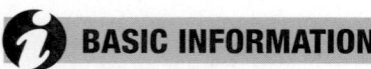

BASIC INFORMATION

DEFINITION

The key to delirium is that it has an acute/subacute onset. The American Psychiatric Association's *Diagnostic and Statistical Manual*, 4th edition (DSM-IV) defines delirium as:

- Disturbance of consciousness (i.e., reduced clarity of awareness about the environment) with reduced ability to focus, sustain, or shift attention.
- A change in cognition (e.g., memory deficit, disorientation, language disturbance) or development of a perceptual disturbance that is not better accounted for by a preexisting, established, or evolving dementia.
- The disturbance develops over a short period of time (usually hours to days) and tends to fluctuate during the course of a day.
- Evidence from the history, physical examination, or laboratory findings indicates that the disturbance is caused by direct physiologic consequences of a general medical condition.

SYNONYMS

Acute confusional state
Acute brain syndrome
Toxic or metabolic encephalopathy

ICD-9CM CODES
780.09 Delirium

EPIDEMIOLOGY & DEMOGRAPHICS

Approximately 10% to 30% of hospitalized patients experience delirium during the course of their treatment, *but* the rates can be even higher, especially in intensive care units where it can affect up to 60% to 80%. Risk factors include extremes of age, severe pain, illicit substance use, surgery, dementia, and kidney or liver failure.

PHYSICAL FINDINGS & CLINICAL PRESENTATION

- Pay particular attention to reversible causes for delirium.
- Start with a careful history, especially including the time course of the symptoms. Symptoms may differ both among and within one patient. Thus history from various caregivers may conflict because delirium implies a mental status that is frequently in flux. Symptoms may include poor attention, sleepiness, agitation, or psychosis. Take notice of new medications, recent surgeries or illnesses, and treatments.
- Next perform a physical examination focusing on signs of infection, dehydration, or chronic disease that may be exacerbated. Vital signs are key. Be sure to include the Mini-Mental Status Exam. There are several other bedside delirium instruments available (confusion assessment method [CAM], delirium rating scale revised [DRS-12-98], clinical assessment of confusion [CAC]). The choice of instrument may be dictated by the disci-

pline of the examiner and the time available; however, the best evidence supports the use of the CAM. It takes 5 min to administer and assesses the presence, severity, and fluctuation of the following delirium features: acute onset, inattention, disorganized thinking, altered level of consciousness, disorientation, memory impairment, perceptual disturbances, psychomotor agitation or retardation, and altered sleep-wake cycle.

ETIOLOGY

Can be multifactorial; often *falls* into one of the following categories:

- Drugs: psychiatric and neurologic, narcotics, anticholinergics, beta-blockers, steroids, nonsteroidal anti-inflammatory drugs, digoxin, cimetidine
- Infection or inflammation: any, including abdominal processes
- Metabolic: kidney or liver failure, thyroid, adrenal or glucose dysregulation, anemia, vitamin deficiency
- Stress: surgery, sleep problems, pain, fever, hypoxia, anesthesia, environmental changes, fecal or urinary retention
- FEN: dysregulation of calcium, magnesium, potassium, or sodium; dehydration; volume overload; altered pH

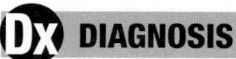 **DIAGNOSIS**

DIFFERENTIAL DIAGNOSIS

- Psychosis
- Dementia
- Depression or mania

LABORATORY TESTS

- Complete blood count, blood urea nitrogen, creatinine, and electrolytes
- Toxicology screen, liver function tests, ammonia
- Thyroid function tests, vitamin B_{12}, and folate levels
- Rapid plasma reagin for syphilis, blood, urine, and spinal culture
- Arterial blood gas measurement

IMAGING STUDIES

- Consider head CT (to look for bleed, trauma, tumor, atrophy, dementia, stroke)
- Chest radiograph (to look for tumor, infection)

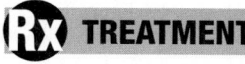 **TREATMENT**

NONPHARMACOLOGIC THERAPY

- The most important consideration is to keep the patient safe by using a variety of methods, including frequent reorientation.
- A quiet, restful, simplified environment with cues to time and location such as clock or calendar are helpful, as well as consistent staff providing both personal and medical care.
- Physical restraints if necessary to ensure safety.

ACUTE GENERAL Rx

- Reverse any treatable cause.
- Haloperidol can be used to control agitation, with doses ranging from 0.25 to 2 mg IM/IV twice daily, repeating the dose every 20 to 30 min until patient has calmed and using lower doses for the elderly.
- Risperidone 0.5 mg twice daily can also be used with a slow increase to desired dose.

CHRONIC Rx

Delirium is not a chronic *condition;* if assessing a more long-term mental status change, consider other diagnoses.

DISPOSITION

Requires frequent *monitoring*, often necessitating hospital level of care to ensure safety and assess etiology.

REFERRAL

Consider neurologic or *psychiatric* consultation if not improved in several days or in complicated cases.

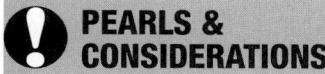 **PEARLS & CONSIDERATIONS**

COMMENTS

Although benzodiazepines are frequently used in hospitalized patients for sedation and are the mainstay of *therapy* for alcohol withdrawal, they must be used with caution in the elderly because they can have a paradoxic effect on agitation.

PREVENTION

- Avoid polypharmacy as much as possible.
- Optimize chronic medical conditions.
- Provide frequent reorientation and a soothing environment for high-risk patients (e.g., lights on during the day, off at night; open curtains during the day so patient can see the weather).
- In patients over 70 without dementia, regular exercise has been associated with lower risk for developing delirium.

PATIENT & FAMILY EDUCATION

Inform about the above *preventative* techniques, especially polypharmacy risks.

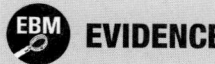 **EVIDENCE**

available at www.expertconsult.com

SUGGESTED READINGS
available at www.expertconsult.com

AUTHOR: **CRISTINA ANTONIO PACHECO, M.D.**

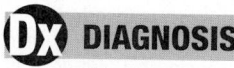

BASIC INFORMATION

DEFINITION

Delirium tremens is overactivity of the central nervous system after cessation of alcohol intake. The time interval is variable; it usually occurs within 1 wk after reduction or cessation of heavy alcohol intake and persists for 1 to 3 days.

SYNONYMS

Alcohol withdrawal syndrome
DTs
Alcoholic delirium

ICD-9CM CODES
291.00 Alcohol withdrawal delirium

EPIDEMIOLOGY & DEMOGRAPHICS

INCIDENCE (IN U.S.): Up to 500,000 cases annually
PEAK INCIDENCE: 30 yr and older
PREDOMINANT SEX: Male
PEAK AGE: Teenage years and older
GENETICS: More common with patients who have relatives who are alcoholics

PHYSICAL FINDINGS & CLINICAL PRESENTATION

- Initially: anxiety, insomnia, tremulousness
- Early: tachycardia, sweating, anorexia, agitation, headache, gastrointestinal distress
- Late: seizures, visual hallucinations, delirium

ETIOLOGY

Alcoholism

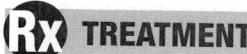

DIAGNOSIS

DIFFERENTIAL DIAGNOSIS

- Coexisting illness
- Trauma
- Drug use

WORKUP

- Frequent rating of symptoms (hallucinations, tremor, sweating, agitation, orientation).
- The Clinical Institute Withdrawal Assessment-Alcohol (CIWA-A) scale can be used to mea-

sure the severity of alcohol withdrawal. It consists of the 10 following items:
1. Nausea
2. Tremor
3. Autonomic hyperactivity
4. Anxiety
5. Agitation
6. Tactile disturbances
7. Visual disturbances
8. Auditory disturbances
9. Headache
10. Disorientation
The maximum score is 67.

LABORATORY TESTS

- Electrolytes (including magnesium, phosphate)
- Close monitoring of glucose levels
- Drug screen (blood and urine)

IMAGING STUDIES

CT scan of head if there is a history of head trauma.

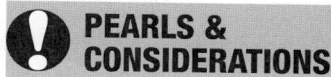

TREATMENT

NONPHARMACOLOGIC THERAPY

Refer to drug rehabilitation program after patient recovers.

ACUTE GENERAL Rx

- Admission to a detoxification unit where patient can be observed closely.
- Vital signs q30min initially (neurologic signs, if necessary).
- Use of lateral decubitus or prone position if restraints are necessary.
- Nothing by mouth: nasogastric tube for abdominal distention may be necessary but should not be routinely used.
- Vigorous hydration (4 to 6 L/day): IV with glucose (Na^+, K^+, PO_4^{-3}, and Mg^{2+} replacement). Use with caution in patients with CHF.
- Vitamins: thiamine 100 mg IV qd. The initial dose of thiamine should precede the administration of IV dextrose; multivitamins (may be added to the hydrating solution).
- Sedation:
  - Initially: lorazepam 2 to 5 mg IM/IV repeated prn
  - Maintenance (individualized dosage): chlordiazepoxide, 50 to 100 mg PO

q4 to 6h, lorazepam 2 mg PO q4h, or diazepam 5 to 10 mg PO tid; withhold doses or decrease subsequent doses if signs of oversedation are apparent.
  - Midazolam is also effective for managing DTs. Its rapid onset (sedation within 2 to 4 min of IV injection) and short duration of action (approximately 30 min) make it an ideal agent for titration in continuous infusion.
- Treatment of seizures: diazepam 2.5 mg/min IV until seizure is controlled (check for respiratory depression or hypotension) may be beneficial for prolonged seizure activity; IV lorazepam 1 to 2 mg q2h can be used in place of diazepam. In general, withdrawal seizures are self-limited and treatment is not required; the use of phenytoin or other anticonvulsants for short-term treatment of alcohol withdrawal seizures is not recommended.
- Diagnosis and treatment of concomitant medical, surgical, or psychiatric conditions.

CHRONIC Rx

Alcoholics Anonymous has the best record in breaking addiction, but the results are still disappointing.

DISPOSITION

Refer to drug rehabilitation program.

REFERRAL

If cardiac arrhythmias are prominent or respiratory distress develops

PEARLS & CONSIDERATIONS

COMMENTS

This is a potentially lethal disease if not carefully treated. Mortality rate is 15% in untreated patients.

SUGGESTED READING
available at www.expertconsult.com

AUTHOR: **FRED F. FERRI, M.D.**

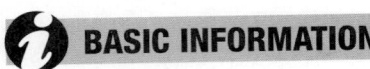

BASIC INFORMATION

DEFINITION

A neurodegenerative disease characterized by dementia preceding mild parkinsonism by 1 yr with other core features including fluctuations in attention and alertness and recurrent visual hallucinations. It characteristically responds to cholinesterase inhibitors, is relative unresponsive to L-dopa, and is very sensitive to neuroleptics.

SYNONYMS

Lewy body dementia
Diffuse Lewy body disease
Lewy body type senile dementia
Cortical Lewy body disease

ICD-9CM CODES
Lewy bodies
331.82 [294.11] with behavioral disturbance
331.82 [294.10] without behavioral
disturbance

EPIDEMIOLOGY & DEMOGRAPHICS

INCIDENCE: Accounts for 10% to 22% of all dementias.
PEAK INCIDENCE: Affects individuals in their sixth decade or older.
PREVALENCE: Estimated 0.7% of individuals older than age 65.
PREDOMINANT SEX AND AGE:
- Sex: Male predominance
- Mean age of onset: 75 yr. On average, 10 yr greater for dementia with Lewy bodies (DLB) than Parkinson's disease (PD).

GENETICS:
- Most cases are sporadic with a discordant among monozygotic twins, which suggests that environment or other epigenetics play a major role in the incidence of DLB.
- Triplication of alpha-synuclein gene (SNCA) was reported in two families with autosomal-dominant inheritance, but a duplication of the same gene was associated in motor PD.

RISK FACTORS:
- Male sex
- Advanced age

PHYSICAL FINDINGS & CLINICAL PRESENTATION

- Importance of recognizing DLB relates to its pharmacologic management, including responsiveness to cholinesterase inhibitors, sensitivity to side effects of neuroleptics, and relative unresponsiveness to L-dopa.
- Insidious onset of dementia with core features of fluctuations in cognition, recurrent visual hallucinations, and extrapyramidal motor symptoms, along with other features either suggestive or supportive of the clinical diagnosis. Refer to Revised Criteria for the Clinical Diagnosis of Dementia with Lewy bodies (McKeith I et al, Neurology 2005).
- Detailed neuropsychological assessment demonstrates a characteristic profile of impairments in visuoperceptual, attentional, and executive functions, which reflects a combination of cortical and subcortical damage.

ETIOLOGY

- SNCA is a protein normally found at the synapse with a role in vesicle production. In its insoluble form, SNCA aggregates into Lewy bodies found at the cortical and subcortical levels.
- Lewy bodies are round, eosinophilic, intracytoplasmic inclusions in the nuclei of neurons.
- Cortical Lewy bodies are found in deep cortical layers of the anterior frontal and temporal lobes, the cingulate gyrus, and insula.
- Just like PD, Lewy bodies also aggregate in the following structures: substantia nigra, locus coeruleus, raphe nuclei, nucleus basalis of Meynert, and brain stem nuclei.

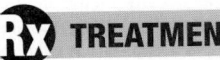

DIAGNOSIS

DIFFERENTIAL DIAGNOSIS

- Similar to Parkinson's disease with dementia, including fluctuation in neuropsychological function, neuropsychiatric features, and extrapyramidal motor features
- Diagnosis of DLB when dementia occurs before or concurrently with extrapyramidal features—arbitrarily set as the "1-yr rule" vs. Parkinson's disease with dementia, which occurs after 1 yr
- Dementia: AD, vascular dementia
- Parkinsonian features: progressive supranuclear palsy, multisystem atrophy, corticobasal degeneration
- Rapidly progressive form: Creutzfeldt-Jakob disease. Lack of cerebellar signs may help distinguish DLB from classic CJD (but not variant form of CJD)
- Psychiatric features: late-onset psychosis or depression with psychotic features
- Hallucinations with fluctuations in consciousness: temporal lobe epilepsy

WORKUP

- Lumbar puncture to rule out underlying chronic infections. Protein 14-3-3 may be present in both DLB and CJD.
- EEG to rule out potential TLE. However, either DLB or TLE may show nonspecific slowing or periodic complexes.

LABORATORY TESTS

- Rule out other potential reversible causes for dementia including:
  - Hormonal dysregulation: thyroid stimulating hormone, free thyroxine
  - Vitamin deficiency: thiamine, cyanocobalamin, folate
  - Vascular risk factors: lipid profile, A1C, homocysteine, syphilis or ApoE genotype

IMAGING STUDIES

- MRI typically shows a relative preservation of the hippocampi and medial temporal lobe volumes (as found in AD) but generalized atrophy and white matter changes.
- Functional imaging including single photon emission computed tomography (SPECT) demonstrates hypoperfusion of the occipital region.

TREATMENT

Patient and caregiver education on benefits, side effects, and limitations of treatment is very important. Based on the preference of the patient and caregiver, a fine balance between psychosis and Parkinsonism features confounds the treatment choices.

NONPHARMACOLOGIC THERAPY

- Social interaction and environmental novelty may improve cognitive dysfunction and psychiatric features often exacerbated by low levels of arousal and attention.
- Physical therapy and mobility aids.

ACUTE GENERAL Rx

Neuroleptic for disabling, persistent psychotic features despite initiation of a cholinesterase inhibitor. A very low dose of an atypical antipsychotic (quetiapine 12.5 mg daily) may be started after patient/caregiver education regarding the sensitivity to neuroleptics.

CHRONIC Rx

- Cholinesterase inhibitors for cognitive and behavioral symptoms. Rivastigmine (6 to 12 mg per day orally or 9.5 mg per day by transdermal patch) showed in RCT a significant reduction in anxiety, delusions, and hallucinations and significantly improved performance on neuropsychological testing.
- Antiparkinson medications for disabling Parkinsonian features. L-dopa is reported to be more effective with fewer side effects than dopamine agonists. Begin at a low dose of L-dopa (25/100 mg tid), and slowly titrate over several weeks as tolerated and according to response.
- Selective-serotonin reuptake inhibitors are commonly used for depression.
- If REM sleep disorder remains disabling (or patient has not responded to an atypical antipsychotic initiated for psychosis), a trial of a low dose clonazepam (0.25 to 0.5 mg) or melatonin (3 mg) at bedtime remains an option.
- Orthostatic hypotension may be aided by nonpharmacologic therapy, such as supportive stockings, or pharmacologically by midodrine and/or fludrocortisone.
- Memantine demonstrated an improvement in clinical global measure and remains well-tolerated but may worsen hallucinations or delusions.
- Avoid anticholinergics (including tricyclic antidepressants) and benzodiazepines.

DISPOSITION

- Survival resembles the progression of AD, but a minority of cases may have a rapid disease course.

- Progression in cognitive decline, similar to AD, by an approximate 10% per year on cognitive testing.

REFERRAL

DLB requires a multidisciplinary approach including the general practitioner, neurologist, neuropsychologist, and/or neuropsychiatrist.

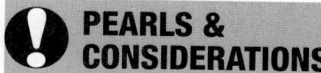

PEARLS & CONSIDERATIONS

COMMENTS

- Typically, the clinical presentation helps differentiate DLB from AD. AD presents with early signs of anterograde episodic memory loss without the benefit of recognition on neuropsychological testing due to cortical atrophy at the medial temporal lobe region.
- Vascular dementia may also present with evidence of frontal-subcortical features but typically without the core features listed in the criteria above.
- Bed partners may report of individuals with DLB "acting out their dreams," sometimes violently, leading to sleeping in separate beds. A history of REM sleep behavior may precede the diagnosis by many years.

PATIENT/FAMILY EDUCATION

- Visual hallucinations (VH) typically consist of innocuous, well-formed, detailed images of animate figures. Unless VH lead to a potential threat to self or others, avoid antipsychotics due to the sensitivity of neuroleptics. Family/friends are often more alarmed by the VH than the patient with DLB.
- Apathy is a common clinical feature of DLB and mimic changes in mood, including depression, or excessive daytime somnolence. These features are often noticed by family/friends.

SUGGESTED READINGS

available at www.expertconsult.com

AUTHORS: **D. BRANDON BURTIS, D.O.,** and **GLEN FINNEY, M.D.**

D

Diseases and Disorders

I

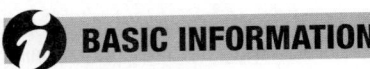

BASIC INFORMATION

DEFINITION

Dengue fever (DF) is an infectious disease endemic in most tropical and subtropical countries (Fig. 1-115). It may be the most widespread arboviral illness worldwide. The causative agent is the dengue virus, a single positive-stranded RNA virus of the Flaviviridae family, which has four distinct but closely related serotypes (DEN-1, DEN-2, DEN-3, DEN-4). Dengue virus is transmitted by the *Aedes* mosquito, principally *Aedes aegypti*.

SYNONYMS

Classic dengue fever
Dengue hemorrhagic fever
Dengue shock syndrome

ICD-9CM CODES
061   Dengue
065.4 Mosquito-borne hemorrhagic fever

EPIDEMIOLOGY & DEMOGRAPHICS

INCIDENCE: Attack rates during epidemics range from 1 to 10/1000.
PEAK INCIDENCE: In hyperendemic countries, rates among children are as high as 22 to 292 per 1000 per yr.
PREVALENCE: Worldwide, more than 50 million cases of dengue infection are diagnosed yearly. DF is confirmed in up to 8% of febrile travelers returning from the tropics.
PREDOMINANT AGE: All ages are susceptible.
RISK FACTORS: Travel to endemic regions. A few locally acquired U.S. cases have been documented in Texas since 1980, in Hawaii during 2001 to 2002, and more recently in Key West, Florida, during 2009 to 2010. The majority of indigenous cases presented as uncomplicated fever and a minor percentage developed dengue hemorrhage fever (DHF) or dengue shock syndrome (DSS).

ETIOLOGY

After bite by infected mosquito, the virus replicates in regional lymph nodes, then spreads by blood and the lymphatic system to other tissues. Incubation period is typically 4 to 7 days (range, 3 to 14 days). Most important risk factors for development of severe disease (DHF/DSS) are age, viral genotype, genetic background of the host, and prior infection. Majority of DHF/DSS cases occur during secondary heterologous (different from first exposure) infection, in which T memory cells from the primary infection are preferentially expanded because of a lower threshold of activation compared with naïve T cells of higher affinity to the current serotype. This results in suboptimal clearance of the virus and quicker, more robust cytokine production leading to changes in vascular permeability and plasma leakage. Severe disease during primary infection is most commonly seen in infants in whom dengue virus-specific antibodies transferred transplacentally from their dengue virus-immune mothers facilitate viral entry into cells through an antibody-dependent enhancement mechanism, increasing viral load and inducing immune activation.

PHYSICAL FINDINGS & CLINICAL PRESENTATION

Clinical presentation ranges from asymptomatic infection to shock syndrome and vary according to age of patient and previous infection with dengue virus.

Symptomatic DF infection can be classified into three categories:
1. Undifferentiated fever
2. Classic DF: characterized by acute febrile illness accompanied by symptoms such as headache, retroorbital pain, fatigue, mild respiratory and gastrointestinal symptoms, and myalgias/arthralgias ("break bone fever"); DF usually follows an incubation period of 3 to 14 days and fever typically lasts 5 to 7 days; physical findings may include a maculopapular rash, lymphadenopathy, pharyngeal erythema, and injected conjunctivae; some patients may experience development of hemorrhagic manifestations with petechiae, purpura, and rarely, epistaxis, gum bleeding, and gastrointestinal bleeding; during pregnancy, DF has been associated with increased risk for premature labor and birth, uterine hemorrhage, intrautero death, neonatal death, and maternofetal transmission
3. DHF/DSS: occurs in less than 3% of infected individuals; early course is similar to presentation of classic dengue, but 4 to 7 days after onset of illness, plasma leakage with hemorrhagic manifestations develops; plasma leakage may result in hypoproteinemia, peripheral edema, ascites, and pleural and cardiac effusions, and is suggested by a hematocrit increase of 20% during course of illness; thrombocytopenia is also a hallmark, with resultant clinical manifestations such as petechiae, echymosis, mucosal hemorrhage, and GI bleeding; may progress to DSS with circulatory collapse, manifested by rapid/weak pulse, profound hypotension, and pulse pressure of <20 mm Hg; warning signs for DHF/DSS include abdominal pain, persistent vomiting, abrupt defervescence, change in mental status, and respiratory distress.

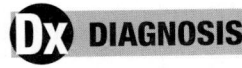

DIAGNOSIS

DIFFERENTIAL DIAGNOSIS

- Influenza
- Measles
- Rubella
- Epstein-Barr virus
- West Nile virus
- HIV conversion
- Malaria
- Typhoid
- Leptospirosis
- Chikungunya
- Rickettsial diseases
- Early severe acute respiratory syndrome
- Other viral hemorrhagic fevers

DHF is defined by the following World Health Organization (WHO) criteria:
1. Fever lasting 2 to 7 days
2. Hemorrhagic tendency (spontaneous bleeding or positive tourniquet test)
3. Thrombocytopenia
4. Evidence of plasma leakage

WORKUP

- Suspicion for DF based on travel, exposure history, and clinical presentation
- Tourniquet test can be performed to look for hemorrhagic manifestations; inflate blood pressure cuff midway between systolic and diastolic blood pressure for 5 min; the test result is positive when more than 20 petechial hemorrhages per square inch are counted on the forearm

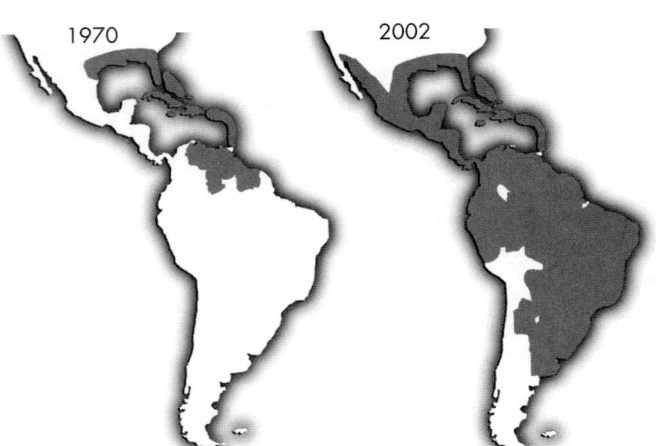

FIGURE 1-115 Distribution of *Aedes aegypti* in the Americas in 1970 (at the end of the mosquito eradication program) and in 2002. (Source: CDC and PAHO; from Mandell GL et al: *Principles and practice of infectious diseases,* ed 6, Philadelphia, 2005, Elsevier.)

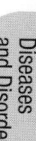

LABORATORY TESTS

- CBC, liver function tests, chemistries
- Additional laboratory tests based on differential diagnoses (e.g., malaria smears, monospot/Epstein-Barr virus titers, HIV testing)
- With compatible exposure history and symptom profile, positive anti–dengue IgM suggests recent infection, whereas positive anti–dengue IgG may indicate past infection
- Confirm diagnosis with a fourfold increase of IgG and IgM between acute (<6 days after illness onset) and convalescence titers; IgM capture enzyme-linked immunosorbent assay (ELISA) commonly used, but test is negative early in the course of disease
- Identification of DENV from serum by reverse transcriptase polymerase chain reaction

IMAGING STUDIES

As dictated by clinical course

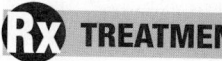

TREATMENT

No specific pharmacologic treatment for dengue.

NONPHARMACOLOGIC THERAPY

- Treatment is based on supportive measures.
- Mortality rate from DHS/DSS is improved by early and correct fluid replacement.

ACUTE GENERAL Rx

- Monitor platelet count and hematocrit at least daily.
- Patients with platelet counts <100,000 have increased risk for DHF and should be monitored as inpatients.

- Hematocrit increase of 20% suggests substantial plasma loss for which patients should be admitted for intensive care and intravenous fluid replacement.
- Fever should be managed with acetaminophen; aspirin and NSAIDs should be avoided because of their anticoagulant properties.

DISPOSITION

- Classic dengue is usually self-limiting and rarely fatal.
- Of an estimated 500,000 cases of DHF/DSS admitted early, the mortality rate is approximately 2.5%.
- Mortality rate for DHF/DSS is as high as 20% without proper treatment but decreases to <1% with prompt recognition and appropriate treatment.

REFERRAL

- Infectious disease consultation for suspicion of DF
- Referral/transfer to center experienced with DHF/DSS if available

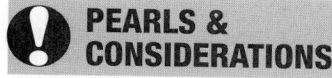

PEARLS & CONSIDERATIONS

COMMENTS

- Health care providers should consider dengue infection in any traveler returning from endemic areas who presents with fever.
- Given the incubation period, dengue infection can be ruled out if onset of symptoms begins 2 wk after individual leaves endemic area.

- Asymptomatic dengue infections are common; however, immunity that results from primary infection increases the risk for DHF/DSS during subsequent infections.
- Serologic testing is complicated by cross-reactions with over flaviviruses (including vaccines for yellow fever and Japanese encephalitis).
- Contact the Dengue Branch at the Centers for Disease Control and Prevention for additional information and testing (http://www.cdc.gov/ncidod/dvbid/misc/db.htm).

PREVENTION

- There is no vaccine for dengue.
- For travelers, the most effective preventive measure is avoidance of mosquito bites by using protective clothing and insect repellents containing DEET.
- *Aedes* mosquitoes primarily bite during the day and typically live in urban areas.

SUGGESTED READINGS

available at www.expertconsult.com

AUTHORS: **VALERIA FABRE, M.D.**, **CLAUDIA RODRIGUEZ CABRERA, M.D.**, and **JOSEPH DIAZ, M.D.**

Diseases and Disorders

D

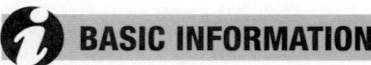

BASIC INFORMATION

DEFINITION

Dependent personality disorder (DPD) is characterized by a pervasive and excessive need to be taken care of that leads to submissive and clinging behavior and fears of separation. DPD begins by early adulthood and causes significant distress or impairment in multiple domains of functioning. Individuals must meet five or more of the following criteria:

1. Difficulty making routine decisions without an excessive amount of advice and reassurance from others.
2. Need others to assume responsibility for most major areas of their life.
3. Difficulty expressing disagreement with others because of fear of loss of support or approval.
4. Difficulty initiating or completing projects on own because of a lack of self-confidence in abilities rather than lack of motivation or energy.
5. Excessive attempts to obtain nurturance and support from others.
6. Feel uncomfortable or helpless when alone because of exaggerated fears of being unable to care for self.
7. Urgently seek another relationship when a close relationship ends.
8. Unrealistically preoccupied with being left to take care of self.

SYNONYMS

None

ICD-9CM CODES
301.6

EPIDEMIOLOGY & DEMOGRAPHICS

PREVALENCE: 0.5% in general population. Dependent traits, as opposed to the disorder itself, are among the most frequently reported in outpatient mental health clinics.
PREDOMINANT SEX: Female (2:1) in clinical settings.

CLINICAL PRESENTATION

- Early onset and chronic course. Impairment is frequently mild.
- On interview, will defer excessively to partner or parent.
- Indecision in routine decisions.
- Depend on a parent or spouse to decide where they should live, work, and recreate and who they should befriend.
- Need for others to function for them goes beyond age-appropriate and situation-appropriate requests for assistance.
- Will agree with objectionable opinions, submit to unreasonable requests, and not express appropriate anger or disappointment

for fear of alienating the person without whom they believe they cannot function.
- Convinced that they are not capable of independent function and present themselves as inept.
- Often do not develop independent living skills, perpetuating their dependency.
- Social relations tend to be limited to those few people on whom the person depends.

ETIOLOGY

Chronic physical illness or separation anxiety disorder may predispose for DPD.

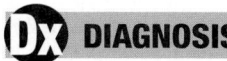

DIAGNOSIS

DIFFERENTIAL DIAGNOSIS

- Dependency and personality changes arising as a consequence of an Axis I disorder.
- Dependency arising as a consequence of a general medical condition.
- Most common comorbid Axis I conditions are major depressive and other mood disorders, anxiety disorders, including social phobia, and adjustment disorder.
- Most common comorbid personality disorders are histrionic, avoidant, and borderline. Each of these disorders is characterized by dependent features. DPD is distinguished by its predominantly submissive, reactive, and clinging behavior.

WORKUP

- History: collateral information is essential to establishing the presence of longstanding interpersonal pattern in multiple domains of the patient's life.
- Physical examination.
- Mental status examination.

LABORATORY TESTS

Tests necessary to rule out medical causes of personality changes

IMAGING STUDIES

Tests necessary to rule out medical causes of personality changes

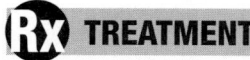

TREATMENT

NONPHARMACOLOGIC THERAPY

- Cognitive-behavioral and psychodynamic psychotherapy to diminish and better contain anxiety and to help patients develop sense of self as competent and requisite assertiveness skills
- Psychodynamic psychotherapy to help develop improved self-concept and interpersonal functioning

ACUTE GENERAL Rx

Benzodiazepines to control highly anxious states

CHRONIC Rx

Selective serotonin reuptake inhibitors (SSRIs) and selective serotonin-norepinephrine reuptake inhibitors (SNRIs) for comorbid depression, social phobia, other anxiety disorders, and agoraphobia

DISPOSITION

- Chronic course; severity is variable
- Impairments often mild
- At increased risk for major depression, social phobia, and other anxiety disorders, including panic and agoraphobia

REFERRAL

- If pharmacotherapy or psychotherapy is contemplated
- If patient's functioning is impaired

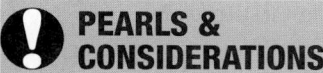

PEARLS & CONSIDERATIONS

COMMENTS

- DPD patients fear illness will lead to abandonment by others.
- This fear of simultaneous helplessness and abandonment intensifies neediness and may lead to dramatic demands for urgent medical attention.
- When physicians do not respond as wanted, angry outbursts may ensue.
- Medical care can also become a means by which dependency needs are met. As a result, some of these patients may unconsciously or consciously prolong their illness for primary gain.
- Physicians often react to the extreme neediness with avoidance or overengagement, leading to burnout.
- Management guidelines:
  1. Overall strategy is to provide reassurance and allay fear of abandonment.
  2. Specific strategies include scheduling frequent visits, noncontingent care (i.e., scheduling visits regardless of whether ill or not).
  3. Establish firm and realistic limits to availability as early as possible in treatment.
  4. Enlist other members of health care team for support.
  5. Encourage patient to develop additional "outside" support systems.

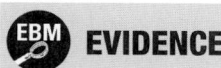

EVIDENCE

available at www.expertconsult.com

SUGGESTED READINGS
available at www.expertconsult.com

AUTHOR: **JOHN Q. YOUNG, M.D., M.P.P.**

BASIC INFORMATION

DEFINITION

Major depression is an episodic, frequently recurring syndrome. The diagnosis requires that five of nine criteria be present for 2 wk. One of these nine criteria must be either a persistent depressed mood or pervasive anhedonia (loss of interest or pleasure in all, or almost all, usual interests or activities). Other symptoms include sleep disturbance (insomnia or hypersomnia), appetite loss/gain or weight loss/gain, fatigue, psychomotor retardation or agitation, difficulty concentrating or indecisiveness, feelings of guilt or worthlessness, and recurrent thoughts of death or suicidal ideation.

SYNONYMS

Unipolar affective disorder
Melancholia
Manic-depressive illness, depressed type
Depressive episode

ICD-9CM CODES
296.2
296.3
311

EPIDEMIOLOGY & DEMOGRAPHICS

LIFETIME RISK (IN U.S.): 10% of men, 20% of women
PREVALENCE (IN U.S.): Point prevalence in a community sample is 3% of men, 4.5% to 9.3% of women, and 1% of children. Prevalence of 20% to 40% in patients with comorbid medical conditions.
PREDOMINANT SEX: Female/male ratio 2:1
PREDOMINANT AGE: 25 to 44 yr; 5% of adolescents
PEAK INCIDENCE: 30 to 40 yr; 13% of postpartum women
GENETICS:
- Clear evidence of familial predominance
- Prevalence is 2 to 3 times greater among first-degree relatives.
- Concordance among monozygotic twins approximately 50%
- No established pattern of inheritance

PHYSICAL FINDINGS & CLINICAL PRESENTATION

- Clinical evaluation facilitated by organizing the major symptoms into four hallmarks: (1) depressed mood, (2) anhedonia, (3) physical symptoms (sleep disturbance, appetite problem, fatigue, psychomotor changes), and (4) psychologic symptoms (difficulty concentrating or indecisiveness, guilt or worthlessness, and suicidal ideation).
- A stressful life event, typically a serious loss, may trigger a depressive episode; however, the presence or absence of identifiable precipitants is irrelevant to the diagnosis.
- Patients often present with somatic complaints such as pain, fatigue, insomnia, dizziness, headache, or gastrointestinal problems.

- May be associated with mood-congruent delusional thinking (paranoid and melancholic themes).
- May be associated with active or passive suicidal ideation.
- Serious misconduct may appear in adolescents.
- May be misdiagnosed in elderly patients, with signs and symptoms attributed to normal aging.

ETIOLOGY

- A heterogeneous group of disorders probably arising from a various etiologies.
- Genetic and family experiences both contribute.
- Significant psychosocial stressors, especially loss, often trigger depression.
- Numerous biologic correlates have been identified, including endocrine and central nervous system factors, though none is considered causative or diagnostic.

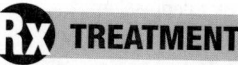 **DIAGNOSIS**

DIFFERENTIAL DIAGNOSIS

- Anxiety disorders, somatoform disorders, obsessive-compulsive disorder, substance abuse, and personality disorders often present with depressive symptoms.
- Important to determine if a depressive episode is part of major depression or part of bipolar disorder.
- Approximately 10% to 15% of depression caused by general medical illnesses, such as Alzheimer's disease, Parkinson's disease, stroke, end-stage renal failure, cardiac disease, HIV infection, and cancer.
- Some medical conditions present as depression (e.g., hypothyroidism, hyperthyroidism or neurosyphilis).
- Premenstrual dysphoric disorder.
- In elderly, depression often coexists with dementia.

WORKUP

- Careful medical history is required
- Physical examination reveals no specific diagnostic signs of depression
- Mental status examination
- Self-report scales can assist in screening.

LABORATORY TESTS

- No laboratory studies are diagnostic.
- The following can assist in ruling out other confounding issues:
  1. Routine blood chemistry evaluation
  2. CBC with differential
  3. Thyroid function studies
  4. Vitamin B_{12} levels

IMAGING STUDIES

With unusual presentations (e.g., associated with new-onset severe headache, focal neurologic signs, a cognitive or sensory disturbance), the following may be performed:

- EEG (diffuse slowing indicates metabolic encephalopathy)
- Anatomic brain imaging (CT scan or MRI)

TREATMENT

NONPHARMACOLOGIC THERAPY

- Good evidence that cognitive-behavioral therapy is as effective as antidepressant medication in achieving significant reduction or remission.
- Problem solving and interpersonal psychotherapies have efficacy rates of 50% to 60%.
- By 12 wk, psychotherapy and medication approaches are equally effective.
- Patients with severe symptoms should generally not be treated by psychotherapy alone.
- Combined psychotherapy and medication more effective than either treatment alone.

ACUTE GENERAL Rx

- Concurrent medical or psychiatric illnesses, history of prior response, cost, and side effects should be considered when selecting initial treatment.
- Antidepressants are effective in approximately 60% to 70% of cases.
- Selective serotonin reuptake inhibitors (SSRIs) generally are first-line.
- According to the STAR-D trial, approximately 30% achieve remission with the first prescribed medication after 3 months of treatment. Another 25% to 30% respond to treatment, but do not achieve remission. Treatment-refractory patients should be switched to another SSRI or to another class of medication, offered adjunctive medication such as bupropion, or referred for evidence-based counseling. Approximately 25% more patients will achieve remission with this secondary intervention.
- Therapy should be continued for 4 to 9 mo after the full remission of symptoms.
- Electroconvulsive therapy is the most effective means available for the treatment of severe, refractory depression.
- Antipsychotic medication should be added for psychotic depression.

CHRONIC Rx

Long-term treatment, in some cases, lifelong recommended for multiple depressive episodes, a severe episode or significant suicidality, or a strong family history of severe depression or bipolar disorder.

DISPOSITION

- Major depression is often a relapsing and remitting illness.
- Physical symptoms predict a favorable response to biologic intervention.
- Additional episodes experienced by >50% after one episode.
- Without treatment, episodes last an average of 6 to 12 mo; risk of recurrence higher without treatment.

REFERRAL

- If treatment refractory
- If patient suicidal or psychotic
- For suspected bipolar depression

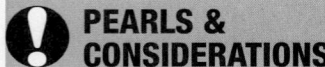

COMMENTS

- All threats of suicide should be taken very seriously. Clinicians can use the mnemonic SAL: Is the method specific? Is it available? Is it lethal?

- Rule out bipolar affective disorder before initiating antidepressant medication.
- Many patients and families reluctant to acknowledge depression because of stigma.
- A two-question screener is as effective as longer instruments. A positive answer to either question warrants a full assessment.
  1. Over the past 2 weeks, have you ever felt down, depressed, or hopeless?
  2. Over the past 2 weeks, have you felt little interest or pleasure in doing things?
- Depression screening programs without treatment programs are unlikely to improve depression outcomes.

- Strict monitoring of patients who initiate antidepressant therapy is necessary both for safety and to ensure optimal treatment.

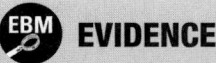

available at www.expertconsult.com

SUGGESTED READINGS
available at www.expertconsult.com

AUTHORS: **MITCHELL D. FELDMAN, M.D., M.PHIL.,** and **MARK ZIMMERMAN, M.D.**

BASIC INFORMATION

DEFINITION

De Quervain's tenosynovitis refers to an inflammatory process of the first dorsal retinacular compartment containing the tendons of the abductor pollicis longus (APL) and extensor pollicis brevis (EPB).

SYNONYMS

Stenosing tenosynovitis of the radial styloid process
Stenosing tenovaginitis of the first dorsal compartment
De Quervain's disease
De Quervain's tendonitis
De Quervain's stenosinig tenosynovitis

ICD-9CM CODES
727.04 Tenosynovitis radial styloid

EPIDEMIOLOGY & DEMOGRAPHICS

- More common in women than in men (10:1)
- Usually occurs between the ages of 30 and 50
- Associated with rheumatoid arthritis
- Seen more frequently in certain occupations involving repetitive wrist motion (e.g., clerical, assembly, and manual labor)

PHYSICAL FINDINGS & CLINICAL PRESENTATION

- Pain over the styloid process of the radius with grasping and isometric thumb abduction
- Swelling compared to the contralateral side
- Tenderness in the anatomic snuffbox
- Positive Finkelstein's test (Fig. 1-116)
- Crepitance

ETIOLOGY

- The cause is usually repetitive use or overuse of the hands (e.g., typing, writing, nailing, new mothers who hold or pick up their babies with poor form, etc.).
- Acute trauma can also cause tenosynovitis of the radial styloid.

DIAGNOSIS

- The diagnosis of de Quervain's tenosynovitis is based on the clinical triad of:
  1. Tenderness over the radial styloid
  2. Swelling over the first dorsal retinacular compartment
  3. Positive Finkelstein's test (see Fig. 1-116)
- Consideration can be given to injecting 1.5 ml of 1% Xylocaine into the tenosynovial sac, and if all three physical signs resolve, the diagnosis is confirmed, allowing for differentiation from carpometacarpal osteoarthritis.

DIFFERENTIAL DIAGNOSIS

- Carpal tunnel syndrome
- Arthritis (e.g., degenerative osteoarthritis or rheumatoid arthritis)
- Gout
- Infiltrative tenosynovitis
- Radiculopathy
- Compression neuropathy (e.g., superficial branch of the radial nerve "bracelet syndrome")
- Infection (e.g., tuberculosis, bacterial)

LABORATORY TESTS

- Erythrocyte sedimentation rate (ESR) is usually normal in patients with de Quervain's tenosynovitis
- Arthrocentesis can be used to rule out gout (crystals) and infection (gram stain and culture of aspirate)

IMAGING STUDIES

- Radiograph studies of the hand if fracture is suspected

TREATMENT

NONPHARMACOLOGIC THERAPY

- Rest
- Splinting (thumb spica)
- Icing
- Physiotherapy

ACUTE GENERAL Rx

- Corticosteroid injection using 20 to 40 mg triamcinolone acetonide and 1% Xylocaine is effective in relieving pain.
- Nonsteroidal anti-inflammatory drugs (NSAIDs) ibuprofen 800 mg tid or naproxen 500 mg bid.

CHRONIC Rx

Surgical release is generally reserved for patients not responding to NSAIDs and corticosteroid injection therapy.

DISPOSITION

- Approximately 90% of patients have relief of symptoms with either single or multiple steroid injections.
- Surgical control of symptoms achieved in 90% of referred cases.
- Complications of surgery include:
  1. Radial nerve damage
  2. Paresthesia (~10%)
  3. Neuroma

REFERRAL

Rheumatologist or orthopedist

PEARLS & CONSIDERATIONS

- Steroid injection is generally recommended after failure of conservative treatment for 2 to 6 wks.
- Pain relief is usually noted within 48 hr with patient becoming asymptomatic by the first or second week after corticosteroid injection.
- If there is no improvement by 6 wk post second corticosteroid injection, referral to an orthopedic hand surgeon is recommended.
- Avoid repetitive activities.

SUGGESTED READINGS

available at www.expertconsult.com

AUTHOR: **MARK F. BRADY, M.D., M.P.H., M.M.S.**

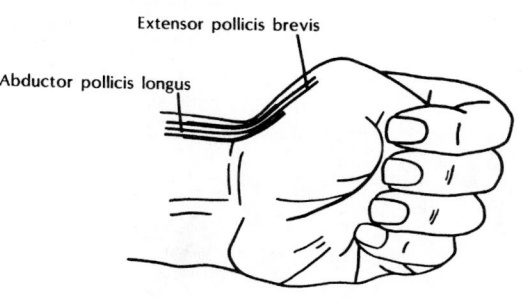
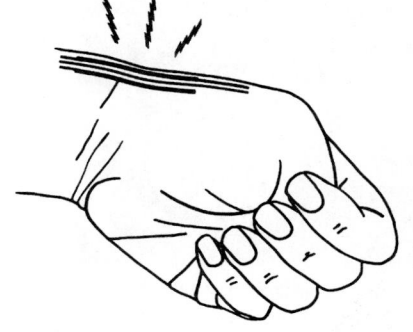

Extensor pollicis brevis

Abductor pollicis longus

FIGURE 1-116 Finkelstein's test is positive in de Quervain's stenosing synovitis. Ulnar flexion of the wrist produces pain over the dorsal compartment containing the extensor pollicis brevis and abductor pollicis longus. (From Noble J [ed]: *Textbook of primary care medicine,* ed 2, St Louis, 1996, Mosby.)

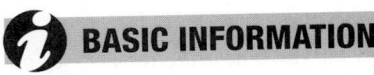

DEFINITION

Dermatitis herpetiformis (DH) is a rare, chronic skin disorder characterized by an intensely burning, pruritic, vesicular rash. It is strongly associated with gluten-sensitive enteropathy. Most, if not all, patients with DH will have gastrointestinal symptoms, whereas approximately 25% of patients with celiac sprue will have DH.

SYNONYMS

None

ICD-9CM CODES
694.0 Dermatitis herpetiformis

EPIDEMIOLOGY & DEMOGRAPHICS

PREVALENCE (IN U.S.): 11.2 cases per 100,000 persons; prevalence for celiac disease is one in 133 adults
PREDOMINANT SEX: Slight male predominance
PREDOMINANT AGE: Third to fifth decades
PREDOMINANT RACE: Rarely seen in blacks/African Americans or Asians
GENETICS: A specific HLA type, DQ2, is present in 90% of patients with celiac disease with or without DH. DQ8 is present in the remaining 10%. DQ2 is present in 16% to 18% of the normal population. Eleven percent of patients with DH have a first-degree relative with either DH or celiac disease.

PHYSICAL FINDINGS & CLINICAL PRESENTATION

- Pruritic, burning vesicles initially, frequently grouped (hence the name "herpetiform") (Fig. 1-117)
- Symmetrically distributed on extensor surfaces: elbows, knees, scalp, nuchal area, shoulder, and buttocks; rarely found in mouth
- May evolve in time to intensely burning urticarial papules, vesicles, and rarely bullae
- Celiac-type enamel defects to permanent teeth found in 53% of patients

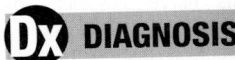

DIAGNOSIS

Diagnosis is confirmed histologically by the demonstration of granular deposition of immunoglobulin (Ig) A at the dermal-epidermal junction, which is specific to the diagnosis of DH.

DIFFERENTIAL DIAGNOSIS

- Linear IgA bullous dermatosis (not associated with gluten-sensitive enteropathy)
- Herpes simplex infection
- Herpes zoster infection
- Bullous erythema multiforme
- Bullous pemphigoid

WORKUP

History of chronic diarrhea and pruritic, vesicular rash highly suggestive of diagnosis

LABORATORY TESTS

- Skin biopsy for immunofluorescence studies. Diagnosis is confirmed by granular IgA deposits at the dermal-epidermal junction. More than 90% will have granular or fibrillar IgA deposits in the dermal papillae. Multiple specimens may be needed to obtain positive findings because of the focal nature of deposits. Biopsies are taken from adjacent normal skin because the diagnostic IgA deposits are usually destroyed by the blistering process.
- Circulating antibody levels
  1. IgA antiendomysial antibody is found:
     a. In 70% of patients with rash and who are not on gluten-free diet and
     b. In 100% of patients with rash and grade 3 to 4 flattening of intestinal mucosa or with untreated celiac disease. Levels decrease to 0% when gluten is avoided for 3 mo.
  2. IgA antigliadin antibodies: found in 66% of patients with DH; also present in patients with pemphigus and pemphigoid
  3. IgA reticulin antibody: found in 36% of patients with DH
  4. IgA antitissue transglutaminase: elevated levels in 75% patients with DH and in 90% to 100% of patients with celiac disease
  5. IgA antiepidermal transglutaminase: elevated in adult patients with DH or celiac disease but may be more specific for DH

TREATMENT

- Spontaneous remission of DH in patients on a normal diet has been described in 10% to 15% of cases.
- Adherence to a gluten-free diet has been associated with sustained remission of DH.
- Patients may be given a trial of pharmacologic therapy if they are extremely uncomfortable. Symptoms are often dramatically relieved within hours or days of initiation of medical therapy.

NONPHARMACOLOGIC THERAPY

- Gluten-free diet: for at least 6 mo, which will allow most patients to begin to decrease or discontinue sulfone therapy (see "Acute General Rx" below). The diet usually needs to be followed for 2 yr before medications can be discontinued. Although intestinal villous architecture improves, symptoms and lesions recur in 1 to 3 wk if a normal diet is resumed. Most patients need to follow the diet indefinitely. Gluten is found in grains, such as wheat, barley, rye, and oats, but not rice or corn.
- A recent small study demonstrated that a gluten-free diet alone was comparable to a gluten-free diet plus dapsone in the treatment of DH.
- Elemental diet: other dietary factors may also be important in DH. Antigens stimulate the production of antibodies, leading to the formation of immune complexes. Most antigens that elicit a humoral immune response are proteins. Thus a diet without full proteins, an elemental diet, is not likely to contain major antigens. A diet of amino acids, fat, and carbohydrates can produce a rapid benefit and allow a decrease in the dosage of dapsone within 2 wk.

ACUTE GENERAL Rx

- Dapsone:
  - Initial dose of 50 mg PO bid. Itching and burning are controlled in 12 to 48 hr and new lesions stop appearing.
  - Adjust dose to the lowest level that provides adequate relief, which can range from 25 to 400 mg/day.
  - Peripheral motor neuropathy, such as paresthesias and weakness of the distal upper and lower extremities and footdrop, can

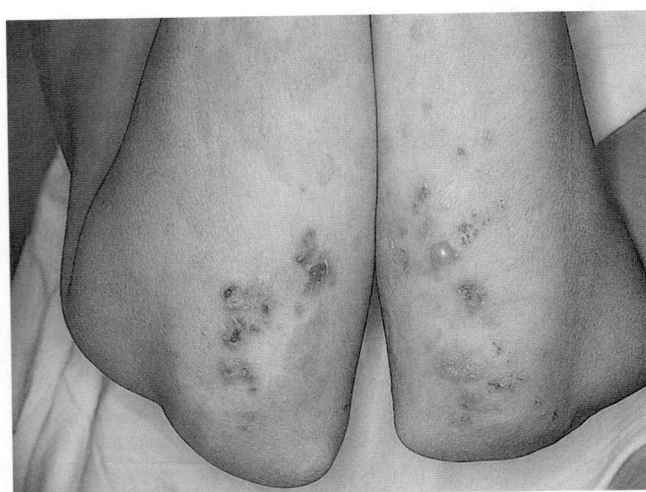

FIGURE 1-117 Dermatitis herpetiformis is an immunologically mediated blistering disease. There is a strong association of dermatitis herpetiformis with HLA-B8, DR3. Gluten-sensitive enteropathy is a common associated finding. The lesions are grouped (herpetiform) and extremely pruritic. (From Callen JP [ed]: *Color atlas of dermatology,* ed 2, Philadelphia, 2000, WB Saunders.)

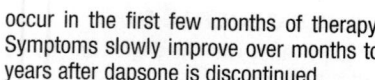
occur in the first few months of therapy. Symptoms slowly improve over months to years after dapsone is discontinued.

- Hemolysis, anemia, and methemoglobinemia occur to some degree in all patients receiving dapsone therapy. Vitamin E 800 IU daily may be helpful in preventing methemoglobinemia. Patients at risk for G6PD deficiency should have levels drawn before initiation because dapsone may cause severe hemolytic anemia in these patients.
- Probenecid blocks the renal excretion of dapsone, and rifampin increases the rate of its clearance.

- Sulfapyridine:
  - Initial dosage 500 to 1500 mg/day.
  - Sulfapyridine is associated with agranulocytosis and aplastic anemia. It also may cause severe hemolysis in patients with G6PD deficiency.
- Sulfasalazine:
  - 500 to 1000 mg bid.
  - Sulfasalazine is metabolized to sulfapyridine and has been demonstrated to be effective in patients who are unable to tolerate dapsone in case reports.
- Tetracycline:
  - Successful treatment has been reported with tetracycline 500 mg PO qd to tid and minocycline 100 mg PO bid. Cessation resulted in a flare of the rash.

- Nicotinamide:
  - Successful treatment has been reported with nicotinamide 500 mg PO bid to tid. Cessation resulted in a flare of the rash.
- Topical steroids: may help but can cause skin irritation and atrophy with prolonged use.
- Nonsteroidal anti-inflammatory drugs and iodide can worsen skin inflammation.

CHRONIC Rx

Gluten-free diet

DISPOSITION

- DH is considered to represent an intolerance to gluten, which requires lifelong avoidance of gluten.
- Some patients may be able to reintroduce gluten into their diet without experiencing a recurrence of DH.
  - A study of 38 patients demonstrated that seven (18%) could resume a normal diet without relapse of cutaneous or gastrointestinal symptoms.
  - Patients who did not relapse after resumption of a normal diet were all diagnosed in childhood, had poor adherence to a gluten-free diet, and were more likely to have been treated with dapsone.
- There is an increased incidence of other autoimmune disorders, including thyroid disease, type 1 diabetes mellitus, systemic lupus erythematosus, vitiligo, and Sjögren's syndrome in patients with DH.
- Small bowel lymphoma and nonintestinal lymphoma have been reported in patients with DH and celiac disease. Patients adhering strictly to a gluten-free diet can reduce their risk of gut-related lymphomas within 5 yr to that of the baseline population.

REFERRAL

To dermatologist for skin biopsy and to nutritionist to educate patients about gluten-free diet

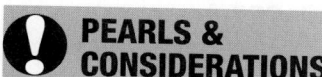 **PEARLS & CONSIDERATIONS**

- Treatment with a gluten-free diet alone was found comparable to dapsone plus a gluten-free diet in a recent small study.
- Maintaining a gluten-free diet has been demonstrated to have a protective effect against the development of lymphoma in patients with celiac disease.

SUGGESTED READINGS

available at www.expertconsult.com

AUTHOR: **IRIS TONG, M.D.**

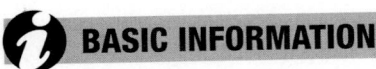

BASIC INFORMATION

DEFINITION

Diabetes insipidus is a polyuric disorder resulting from insufficient production of antidiuretic hormone (ADH) (pituitary [neurogenic] diabetes insipidus) or unresponsiveness of the renal tubules to ADH (nephrogenic diabetes insipidus).

ICD-9CM CODES
253.5 Diabetes insipidus

EPIDEMIOLOGY & DEMOGRAPHICS

GENETICS:
- Nephrogenic diabetes insipidus can be inherited as a sex-linked recessive trait.
- There is also a rare autosomal-dominant form of neurogenic diabetes insipidus.

PHYSICAL FINDINGS & CLINICAL PRESENTATION

- Polyuria: urinary volumes ranging from 2.5 to 6 L/day
- Polydipsia (predilection for cold or iced drinks)
- Neurologic manifestations (seizures, headaches, visual field defects)
- Evidence of volume contractions

NOTE: The physical findings and clinical manifestations are generally not evident until vasopressin secretory capacity is reduced to <20% of normal.

ETIOLOGY

Neurogenic diabetes insipidus:
- Idiopathic
- Neoplasms of brain or pituitary fossa (craniopharyngiomas, metastatic neoplasms from breast or lung)
- Posttherapeutic neurosurgical procedures (e.g., hypophysectomy)
- Head trauma (e.g., basal skull fracture)
- Granulomatous disorders (sarcoidosis or tuberculosis)
- Histiocytosis (Hand-Schüller-Christian disease, eosinophilic granuloma)
- Familial (autosomal dominant)
- Other: interventricular hemorrhage, aneurysms, meningitis, postencephalitis, multiple sclerosis

Nephrogenic diabetes insipidus:
- Drugs: lithium, amphotericin B, demeclocycline, methoxyflurane anesthesia
- Familial: X-linked
- Metabolic: hypercalcemia or hypokalemia
- Other: sarcoidosis, amyloidosis, pyelonephritis, polycystic disease, sickle cell disease, postobstructive, low-protein diets (protein malnourishment)

DIAGNOSIS

DIFFERENTIAL DIAGNOSIS

- Diabetes mellitus, nephropathies
- Primary polydipsia, medications (e.g., chlorpromazine)
- Osmotic diuresis (glucose, mannitol, anticholinergics)
- Psychogenic polydipsia, electrolyte disturbances

WORKUP

- The diagnostic workup is aimed at showing that polyuria is caused by the inability to concentrate urine and determining whether the problem is the result of decreased ADH or insensitivity to ADH. This is done with the water deprivation test:
  - After baseline measurement of weight, ADH, plasma sodium, and urine and plasma osmolarity, the patient is deprived of fluids under strict medical supervision.
  - Frequent (q2h) monitoring of plasma and urine osmolarity follows.
  - The test is generally terminated when plasma osmolarity is >295 mOsm/kg or the patient loses ≥3.5% of initial body weight.
  - Diabetes insipidus is confirmed if the plasma osmolarity is >295 mOsm/kg and the urine osmolarity is <500 mOsm/kg.
  - To distinguish nephrogenic from neurogenic diabetes insipidus, the patient is given 5 U of vasopressin (ADH) and the change in urine osmolarity is measured. A significant increase (>50%) in urine osmolarity after administration of ADH is indicative of neurogenic diabetes insipidus.
- A diagnostic algorithm for diabetes insipidus is described in Section III.

LABORATORY TESTS

- Decreased urinary specific gravity (≤1.005)
- Decreased urinary osmolarity (usually <200 mOsm/kg) even in the presence of high serum osmolality
- Hypernatremia, increased plasma osmolarity, hypercalcemia, hypokalemia

IMAGING STUDIES

MRI of the brain if neurogenic diabetes insipidus is confirmed

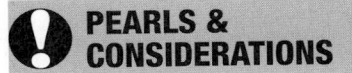

NONPHARMACOLOGIC THERAPY

- Patient education regarding control of fluid balance and prevention of dehydration with adequate fluid intake
- Daily weight

ACUTE GENERAL Rx

Therapy varies with the degree and type of diabetes insipidus.
- Neurogenic diabetes insipidus:
  - Desmopressin acetate (DDAVP) 10 to 40 mcg qd intranasally in one to three divided doses or in tablet form 0.1 or 0.2 mg. Usual oral dose is 0.1 to 1.2 mg/day in two to three divided doses. Desmopressin is also available in injectable form given as 2 to 4 mcg/day SC or IV in two divided doses.
  - Vasopressin tannate in oil: 2.5 to 5 U IM q24 to 72h; useful for long-term management because of its long half-life.
  - In mild cases of neurogenic diabetes insipidus, polyuria may be controlled with HCTZ 50 mg qd (decreases urine volume by increasing proximal tubular reabsorption of glomerular infiltrate).
- Nephrogenic diabetes insipidus:
  - Removal of the underlying cause. However, prolonged lithium therapy can lead to irreversible nephrogenic diabetes insipidus even after lithium therapy is withdrawn.
  - Adequate hydration.
  - Low-sodium diet and chlorothiazide to induce mild sodium depletion. Indomethacin may also be useful to reduce urine volume.

CHRONIC Rx

Patients should be aware of the danger of dehydration and the need for liberal water intake.

REFERRAL

Endocrinology consultation for diagnostic testing

PEARLS & CONSIDERATIONS

COMMENTS

- Patients should be instructed to wear a medical identification tag or bracelet identifying their medical illness.
- In central diabetes insipidus, the use of DDAVP has become the standard of care. Extensive clinical experience has shown it to be both safe and effective in the treatment of this disorder.
- The treatment of nephrogenic diabetes insipidus is more complicated than the central form, and opinion varies among experts in the field. Consultation with a specialist is always recommended in this setting.

SUGGESTED READING
available at www.expertconsult.com

AUTHOR: **FRED F. FERRI, M.D.**

ⓘ BASIC INFORMATION

DEFINITION

- Diabetes mellitus (DM) refers to a syndrome of hyperglycemia resulting from many different causes (see "Etiology"). It can be classified into type 1 and type 2 DM. Because "insulin-dependent" and "non–insulin-dependent" refer to stage at diagnosis, when a person with type 2 diabetes needs insulin, he or she remains labeled as type 2 and is not reclassified to type 1. Table 1-40 provides a general comparison of the two types of DM.
- The American Diabetes Association (ADA) defines DM as follows:
  - A fasting plasma glucose (FPG) $\geq$126 mg/dl, which should be confirmed with testing on a different day; fasting is defined as no caloric intake for at least 8h. The ADA also defines a value <100 mg/dl on fasting blood sugar as the upper limit of normal for glucose; a fasting glucose level between 100 and 126 mg/dl is classified as "impaired fasting glucose" (IFG).
  - Symptoms of hyperglycemia and a casual (random) plasma glucose $\geq$200 mg/dl, random plasma glucose is defined as any time of the day without regard to time since last meal; classic symptoms of hyperglycemia include polyuria, polydipsia, and unexplained weight loss
  - An oral glucose tolerance test (OGTT) $\geq$200 mg/dl in the 2-hour sample; OGTT using glucose load containing the equivalent of 75 g (100 g for pregnant women) anhydrous glucose dissolved in water; furthermore, when results of the OGTT are between 140 and 199 mg/dl, the patient is classified as "impaired glucose tolerance" (IGT)
  - A 2010 update to the ADA Guidelines for Standards of Medical Care in Diabetes included a hemoglobin A$_{1c}$ value $\geq$6.5% within the diagnostic criteria for diabetes mellitus.

SYNONYMS

IDDM (insulin-dependent diabetes mellitus)
NIDDM (non–insulin-dependent diabetes mellitus)
Type 1 diabetes mellitus (insulin-dependent diabetes mellitus)
Type 2 diabetes mellitus (non–insulin-dependent diabetes mellitus)

ICD-9CM CODES

250.0 Diabetes mellitus (NIDDM)
250.1 Insulin-dependent diabetes mellitus without complication (IDDM)

EPIDEMIOLOGY & DEMOGRAPHICS

- DM affects 9% to 10% of the U.S. population. Prevalence rates vary considerably by race/ethnicity.
- Incidence rate increases with age, with 2% in persons age 20 to 44 yr to 18% in persons 65 to 74 yr. Type 2 DM is often present at least 4 to 7 yr before diagnosis.
- Diabetes accounts for 8% of all legal blindness in the United States and is the leading cause of end-stage renal disease (ESRD).
- Patients with diabetes are twice as likely as nondiabetic patients to experience development of cardiovascular disease.

PHYSICAL FINDINGS & CLINICAL PRESENTATION

1. Physical examination varies with the presence of complications and may be normal in early stages
2. Diabetic retinopathy:
   a. Nonproliferative (background diabetic retinopathy):
      (1) Initially: microaneurysms, capillary dilation, waxy or hard exudates, dot and flame hemorrhages, atrioventricular shunts
      (2) Advanced stage: microinfarcts with cotton wool exudates, macular edema
   b. Proliferative retinopathy: characterized by formation of new vessels, vitreal hemorrhages, fibrous scarring, and retinal detachment
3. Cataracts and glaucoma occur with increased frequency in patients with diabetes
4. Peripheral neuropathy: patients often report paresthesias of extremities (feet more than hands); the symptoms are symmetric, bilateral, and associated with intense burning pain (particularly during the night)
   a. Mononeuropathies involving cranial nerves III, IV, and VI, intercostal nerves, and femoral nerves are also common.
   b. Physical examination may reveal:
      (1) Decreased pinprick sensation, sensation to light touch, and pain sensation
      (2) Decreased vibration sense
      (3) Loss of proprioception (leading to ataxia)
      (4) Motor disturbances (decreased deep tendon reflexes [DTRs], weakness and atrophy of interossei muscles); when the hands are affected, the patient has trouble picking up small objects, dressing, and turning pages in a book
      (5) Diplopia, abnormalities of visual fields
5. Autonomic neuropathy:
   a. GI disturbances: esophageal motility abnormalities, gastroparesis, diarrhea (usually nocturnal)

TABLE 1-40   General Comparison of the Two Most Common Types of Diabetes Mellitus

	Type 1	Type 2
Previous terminology	Insulin-dependent diabetes mellitus (IDDM), type I, juvenile-onset diabetes	Non–insulin-dependent diabetes mellitus, type II, adult-onset diabetes
Age of onset	Usually <30 yr, particularly childhood and adolescence, but any age	Usually >40 yr, but any age
Genetic predisposition	Moderate; environmental factors required for expression; 35%-50% concordance in monozygotic twins; several candidate genes proposed	Strong; 60%-90% concordance in monozygotic twins; many candidate genes proposed; some genes identified in maturity-onset diabetes of the young
Human leukocyte antigen associations	Linkage to DQA and DQB, influenced by DRB (3 and 4) (DR2 protective)	None known
Other associations	Autoimmune; Graves' disease, Hashimoto's thyroiditis, vitiligo, Addison's disease, pernicious anemia	Heterogenous group, ongoing subclassification based on identification of specific pathogenic processes and genetic defects
Precipitating and risk factors	Largely unknown; microbial, chemical, dietary, other	Age, obesity (central), sedentary lifestyle, previous gestational diabetes
Findings at diagnosis	85%-90% of patients have one and usually more autoantibodies to ICA512/IA-2/IA-2β, GAD$_{65}$, insulin (IAA)	Possibly complications (microvascular and macrovascular) caused by significant preceding asymptomatic period
Endogenous insulin levels	Low or absent	Usually present (relative deficiency), early hyperinsulinemia
Insulin resistance	Only with hyperglycemia	Mostly present
Prolonged fast	Hyperglycemia, ketoacidosis	Euglycemia
Stress, withdrawal of insulin	Ketoacidosis	Nonketotic hyperglycemia, occasionally ketoacidosis

GAD, Glutamic acid decarboxylase; *IA-2/IA-2β*, tyrosine phosphatases; *IAA*, insulin autoantibodies; *ICA*, islet cell antibody; *ICA512*, islet cell autoantigen 512 (fragment of IA-2).
From Andreoli TE (ed): *Cecil essentials of medicine*, ed 6, Philadelphia, 2005, WB Saunders.

b. Genitourinary (GU) disturbances: neurogenic bladder (hesitancy, weak stream, and dribbling), impotence
c. Orthostatic hypotension: postural syncope, dizziness, light-headedness
6. Nephropathy: pedal edema, pallor, weakness, uremic appearance
7. Foot ulcers: occur in 15% of individuals with diabetes (annual incidence rate, 2%) and are the leading causes of hospitalization; they are usually secondary to peripheral vascular insufficiency, repeated trauma (unrecognized because of sensory loss), and superimposed infections; if a diabetic foot ulcer has been present for weeks and foot pulses are palpable, neuropathy should be considered a major cause; neuropathy can be detected with a simple examination of the lower extremities using a 10-g monofilament to test sensation; prevention of foot ulcers in individual with diabetes includes strict glucose control, patient education, prescription footwear, intensive podiatric care, and evaluation for surgical interventions
8. Neuropathic arthropathy (Charcot's joints): bone or joint deformities from repeated trauma (secondary to peripheral neuropathy; Fig. 1-118)
9. Necrobiosis lipoidica diabeticorum: plaquelike reddened areas with a central area that fades to white-yellow found on the anterior surfaces of the legs (Fig. 1-119); in these areas, the skin becomes very thin and can ulcerate readily

ETIOLOGY
IDIOPATHIC DIABETES:
Type 1 DM: results from beta-cell destruction, usually leading to absolute insulin deficiency
- Hereditary factors:
  1. Islet cell antibodies (found in 90% of patients within the first yr of diagnosis)
  2. Higher incidence of human leukocyte antigen (HLA) types DR3, DR4
  3. 50% concordance rate in identical twins

- Environmental factors: viral infection (possibly Coxsackie virus, mumps virus)
Type 2 DM: results from a progressive insulin secretory defect on the background of insulin resistance
- Hereditary factors: 90% concordance rate in identical twins
- Environmental factor: obesity, sedentary lifestyle, high carbohydrate content in food

DIABETES SECONDARY TO OTHER FACTORS:
- Hormonal excess: Cushing's syndrome, acromegaly, glucagonoma, pheochromocytoma
- Drugs: glucocorticoids, diuretics, oral contraceptives
- Insulin receptor unavailability (with or without circulating antibodies)
- Pancreatic disease: pancreatitis, pancreatectomy, hemochromatosis
- Genetic syndromes: hyperlipidemias, myotonic dystrophy, lipoatrophy
- Gestational diabetes (GDM) (diabetes diagnosed during pregnancy that is not clearly overt diabetes)

Dx DIAGNOSIS

DIFFERENTIAL DIAGNOSIS
- Diabetes insipidus
- Stress hyperglycemia
- Diabetes secondary to hormonal excess, drugs, pancreatic disease

LABORATORY TESTS
- Diagnosis is made on the basis of the following tests:
  1. Fasting glucose ≥126 mg/dl (ADA criterion), should be confirmed by repeated testing on a different day
  2. Non-FPG ≥200 mg/dl and symptoms of DM
  3. OGTT (75-g glucose load for nonpregnant individuals)
  4. Glycosylated hemoglobin (HbA$_{1c}$) ≥6.5% (International Expert Committee [IEC], 2009 recommendation, adopted into 2010 ADA Standard of Care Guidelines)

A$_{1c}$ test should be performed at least two times/yr in diabetic patients who have stable glycemic control and quarterly in patients whose therapy has changed or who are not meeting glycemic goals
5. Testing for prediabetes and diabetes in asymptomatic patients:
   ○ Should be considered in adults of any age who are overweight or obese (body mass index [BMI] >25 kg/m^2) and who have one or more additional risk factors for diabetes. In those who are without these risk factors, testing should begin at age 45 yr.
   ○ If normal, repeat testing should be carried out at least at 3-yr intervals.
6. Detection and diagnosis of gestational diabetes mellitus (GDM)
   ○ Screen for GDM using risk factor analysis and, if appropriate, use of an OGTT
   ○ Women with GDM should be screened for diabetes 6 to 12 wk postpartum and should be followed with subsequent screening for the development of diabetes or prediabetes at least every 3 yr
- Screening for diabetic nephropathy by measurement of microalbuminuria is recommended in all patients with diabetes. It can be accomplished by any of the following three methods:
  1. Measurement of the albumin:creatinine ratio in random spot urine collection. This is the easiest method to administer in the office setting.
  2. Measurement of a 24-hour urine collection for albumin, creatinine clearance.
  3. Timed (4 hours or overnight) urine collection.
- The diagnosis of microalbuminuria (30 to 299 mg/24 hours) should be based on 2 to 3 elevated levels within a 3- to 6-mo period because there is a marked variability in day-to-day albumin excretion and possible transient elevations in urine albumin from short-term hyperglycemia, exercise, severe hypertension, and other illnesses such as

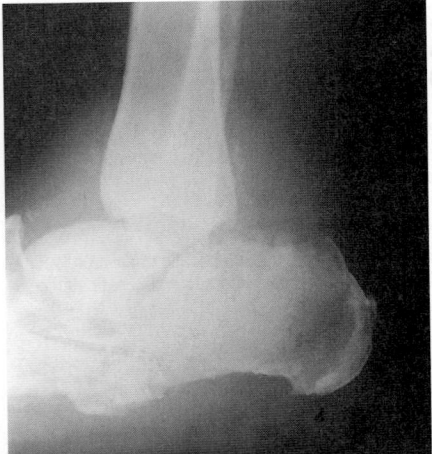

FIGURE 1-118 Diabetic neuropathy of the hindfoot. Destruction of the joint with collapse and fragmentation. (From Hochberg MC et al [eds]: *Rheumatology*, ed 3, St Louis, 2003, Mosby.)

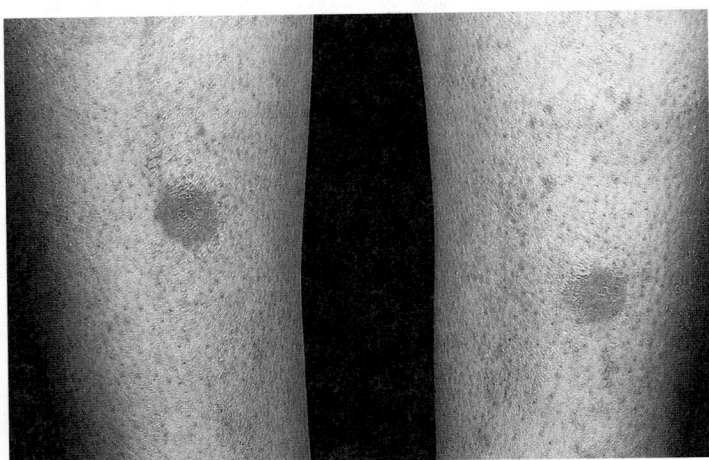

FIGURE 1-119 Necrobiosis lipoidica: symmetrical early lesions with erythema. (Courtesy of the Institute of Dermatology; from McKee PH, Calonje E, Granter SR [eds]: *Pathology of the skin with clinical correlations,* ed 3, St Louis, 2005, Mosby.)

sepsis and congestive heart failure. Patients with overt nephropathy do not need screening for microalbuminuria because the level of protein in the urine is high enough to be detected on routine urinalysis. The albumin to creatinine ratio (ACR) is independently associated with mortality at all levels of estimated glomerular filtration rate (eGFR) in older adults with diabetes and may be particularly helpful for risk stratification.

- A fasting serum lipid panel, serum creatinine, and electrolytes should be obtained yearly on all adult patients with diabetes.
- Self-monitoring of blood glucose (SMBG) is crucial for assessing the effectiveness of the management plan. The frequency and timing of SMBG varies with the needs and goals of each patient. In most patients with type 1 DM and pregnant women taking insulin, SMBG is recommended at least 3 times/day. In patients with type 2 DM not on insulin, recommendations are unclear for SMBG, but testing once or twice/day is acceptable in most patients.
- Screening for thyroid dysfunction (TSH level), Vitamin B_{12} deficiency, and celiac disease should be considered in type 1 diabetes due to the increased frequency of other autoimmune diseases in these individuals.

Rx TREATMENT

ADA and European Association for the Study of Diabetes recommends: "Intervention at the time of diagnosis with metformin in combination with life style changes (diet and exercise) and continuing timely augmentation of therapy with additional agents (including early initiation of insulin therapy) as a means of achieving and maintaining recommended levels of glycemic control of HbA1C <7%." Trials have shown that intensive glucose control reduces the risk for some cardiovascular disease outcomes (such as nonfatal MI) but did not reduce the risk of cardiovascular death or all-cause mortality and increased risk of severe hypoglycemia. It is important to remember that tight glycemic control may burden patients with complex treatment programs, hypoglycemia, weight gain, and costs. Clinicians should individualize HbA1C targets so that they are reasonable and reflect patients' personal and clinical contexts and their informed values and preferences.

NONPHARMACOLOGIC THERAPY

1. Diet
   a. Calories
      (1) The patient with diabetes can be started on 15 calories/lb of ideal body weight; this number can be increased to 20 calories/lb for an active person and 25 calories/lb if the patient does heavy physical labor.
      (2) The calories should be distributed as 45% to 65% carbohydrates, <30% fat, with saturated fat limited to <7% of total calories, and 10% to 30% protein. Daily cholesterol intake should not exceed 300 mg.
      (3) The emphasis should be on complex carbohydrates rather than simple and refined starches, and on polyunsaturated instead of saturated fats in a ratio of 2:1.
   b. Seven food groups
      (1) The exchange diet of the ADA includes bread or starches, meat or proteins, vegetables, fruits, fats, milk, and free foods (e.g., black tea, sugar-free gelatin).
      (2) The name of each exchange is meant to be all-inclusive (e.g., cereal, muffins, spaghetti, potatoes, rice are in the bread group; meats, fish, eggs, cheese, peanut butter are in the protein group).
      (3) The glycemic index compares the increase in blood sugar after the ingestion of simple sugars and complex carbohydrates with the increase that occurs after the absorption of glucose; equal amounts of starches do not give the same increase in plasma glucose (pasta equal in calories to a baked potato causes less of an increase than the potato); thus, it is helpful to know the glycemic index of a particular food product.
      (4) Fiber: Insoluble fiber (bran, celery) and soluble globular fiber (pectin in fruit) delay glucose absorption and attenuate the postprandial serum glucose peak; they also appear to reduce the increased triglyceride level often present in patients with uncontrolled diabetes. A diet high in fiber should be emphasized (20 to 35 g/day of soluble and insoluble fiber).
   c. Other principles
      (1) Modest sodium restriction to 2400 to 3000 mg/day. If hypertension is present, restrict to <2400 mg/day; if nephropathy and hypertension are present, restrict to <2000 mg/day.
      (2) Moderation of alcohol intake recommended (≤2 drinks/day in men, ≤1 drink/day in women).
      (3) Non-nutritive artificial sweeteners are acceptable in moderate amounts.
2. Exercise: increases the cellular glucose uptake by increasing the number of cell receptors. The following points must be considered:
   a. Exercise program must be individualized and built up slowly. Consider beginning with 15 min of low-impact aerobic exercise 3 times per wk and increasing the frequency and duration to 30 to 45 min of moderate aerobic activity (50% to 70% of maximum age predicted heart rate) to 3 to 5 days/wk.
      In the absence of contraindications, resistance training three times per wk should be encouraged.
   b. Insulin is more rapidly absorbed when injected into a limb that is then exercised, and this can result in hypoglycemia.
   c. Vigorous exercise should be avoided in the presence of ketosis in individuals taking insulin and/or insulin secretagogues. Physical activity can result in hypoglycemia if medication dose or carbohydrate consumption is not modified. Ingestion of additional carbohydrates is recommended if pre-exercise glucose levels are <100 mg/dl.
3. Weight loss: to ideal body weight if the patient is overweight
4. Screening for nephropathy, neuropathy, and retinopathy: annual serum creatinine and urine albumin excretion; initial comprehensive eye examination and at least annually thereafter
5. Diabetes self-management education: could also address psychosocial issues
6. Self-monitoring of blood glucose should occur three to four times per day for patients using multiple insulin injections or on insulin pump therapy
7. Perform A1C at least two times a year in patients who are meeting treatment goals and who have stable glycemic control
   ○ A1C quarterly in patients whose therapy has changed or who are not meeting glycemic goals
   ○ The A1c goal for nonpregnant adults in general is <7%

GENERAL Rx

- When the previous measures fail to normalize the serum glucose, oral hypoglycemic agents should be added to the regimen in type 2 DM. Table 1-41 describes commonly used oral hypoglycemic agents.
- The primary mechanism of metformin is to decrease hepatic glucose output. Because metformin does not produce hypoglycemia when used as a monotherapy, it is preferred for most patients. It is contraindicated in patients with severe renal insufficiency with an estimated glomerular filtrate rate <30 ml/min or in patients with significant liver disease.
- Sulfonylureas work best when given before meals because they increase the postprandial output of insulin from the pancreas. All sulfonylureas are contraindicated in patients who are allergic to sulfa.
- Sitagliptin inhibits the enzyme DPP-4, responsible for inactivation and degradation of glucagon-like peptide-1 (GLP-1) and glucose-dependent insulinotropic polypeptide (GIP), which potentiate insulin synthesis, and release and decrease glucagon production.
- Pioglitazone and rosiglitazone increase insulin sensitivity and are useful in addition to other agents in patients with type 2 diabetes, whose hyperglycemia is inadequately controlled. Serum transaminase levels should be obtained before starting therapy and monitored periodically. Glitazones, in general, may increase the risk for heart failure. Rosiglitazone has recently come under increased scrutiny by the FDA after multiple meta-analyses showed an increased incidence of MI associated with the medicine.

TABLE 1-41 Non-Insulin Antidiabetic Agents

	Sulfonylureas	Biguanides	α-Glucosidase Inhibitors	Thiazolidine-diones	Meglitinides	Dipeptidyl Peptidase-4 Inhibitors	Incretin Mimetics	Amylin Analogue
Generic name	Glimepiride, glyburide, glipizide,	Metformin	Acarbose, miglitol	Pioglitazone	Repaglinide, nateglinide	Sitagliptin, saxagliptin	Exenatide	Pramlintide
Mode of action	↑↑ Pancreatic insulin secretion chronically	↓↓HGP; ↓ peripheral IR; ↓ intestinal glucose absorption	Delays PP digestion of carbohydrates and absorption of glucose	↓↓ Peripheral IR; ↑↑ glucose disposal; ↓ HGP	↑↑ Pancreatic insulin secretion acutely	Potentiate insulin synthesis and release	Mimics incretin action by increasing glucose dependent insulin secretion	Amylinomimetic agent; modulates gastric emptying, prevents postprandial glucagon secretion, and promotes satiety
Preferred patient type	Type 2 DM	Overweight, IR, fasting hyperglycemia, dyslipidemia	PP hyperglycemia	Overweight, IR, dyslipidemia, renal dysfunction	PP hyperglycemia	Type 2 DM	DM type 2 as monotherapy or adjunct, overweight	As an adjunct type 1 and type 2 DM

Therapeutic Effects

	Sulfonylureas	Biguanides	α-Glucosidase Inhibitors	Thiazolidine-diones	Meglitinides	Dipeptidyl Peptidase-4 Inhibitors	Incretin Mimetics	Amylin Analogue
↓ HBA$_{1c}$* (%) decrease	1-2	1-2	0.5-1	0.8-1	1-2	0.5	24 wks of monotherapy with 5 mcg reduces HbA1c by 0.7% and 10 mcg reduces by 0.9%	With the start of pramlintide, reduce preprandial, rapid acting or short acting insulin dosages by 50%
↓ FPG* (mg/dl) decrease	50-70	50-80	15-30	25-50	40-80			
↓ PPG* (mg/dl) decrease	~90	80	40-50	—	30			
Insulin levels	↑	—	—	—	↑			
Weight	↑	—/↓	—	—/↑	↑		↓	↓
Lipids	—	↓ LDL ↓↓ TG	—	↑ Large "fluffy" LDL ↓↓ TG ↑ HDL	—			
Side effects	Hypoglycemia	Diarrhea, lactic acidosis	Abdominal pain, flatulence, diarrhea	Heart failure; edema	Hypoglycemia (low-risk)		Hypoglycemia, nausea, vomiting, diarrhea, headache, pancreatitis	Severe hypoglycemia, abdominal pains, loss of appetite, nausea, vomiting, headache, cough
Dose(s)/day	1-2	1-3	1-3	1-2	+−2		Initial: 5 mcg SUBQ twice a day; maintenance: 10 mcg SUBQ twice a day after one month of start of therapy	Type 1 initial: 15 mcg SUBQ prior to major meals; maintenance: titrate 15-mcg increments to 30-60 mcg; type 2 initial 60 mcg SUBQ immediately prior to major meals; maintenance, 120 mcg SUBQ as tolerated
Maximum daily dose	Glimepiride 8 mg, glyburide 20 mg, glipizide 40 mg	2550 mg	150 mg (<60-kg bw), 300 mg (>60-kg bw or above)	45 mg for pioglitazone	16 mg (repaglinide), 360 mg (nateglinide)	Sitagliptin 100 mg; saxagliptin 5 mg	10 mcg SUBQ twice a day	Type 1: 60 mcg as tolerated; type 2: 120 mcg as tolerated
Renal impairment	Glipizide preferred—no adjustment needed	Can be used in creatinine clearance > 30 ml/min	Can be used when serum creatinine < 2 mg/dl	No dose adjustment needed	Repaglinide: CrCl 20-40 ml/min start lower at 0.5 mg, avoid if CrCl < 20 ml/min; Nateglinide: no adjustment needed	50% of the dose when CrCl < 50 ml/min	No dose adjustment needed	No dose adjustment needed when CrCl > 20 ml/min, not studied < 20 ml/min
Optimal administration time	~30 min premeal	After meal	With first bite of meal	With meal (breakfast)	Preferably <15 (0-30 min) pre-meals (omit if no meal)		Within 30-60 min period before meals twice a day	Immediately prior to major meals
Main site of metabolism/ excretion	Hepatic/renal, fecal	Not metabolized/ renal	Only 2% absorbed/fecal	Hepatic/fecal	Hepatic/fecal		Renal	Renal

*Values combined from numerous studies; values are also dose dependent.

↑, Increased; ↓, decreased; —, unchanged; *bw*, body weight; *FPG*, fasting plasma glucose; *HDL*, high-density lipoprotein; *HGP*, hepatic glucose production; *IR*, insulin resistance; *LDL*, low-density lipoprotein; *PP*, postprandial; *PPG*, postprandial plasma glucose; *TG*, triglyceride.

Modified from Andreoli TE (ed): *Cecil essentials of medicine*, ed 6, Philadelphia, 2005, WB Saunders.

- Acarbose and miglitol work by competitively inhibiting pancreatic amylase and small intestinal glucosidases, which delay gastrointestinal absorption of carbohydrates, thereby reducing alimentary hyperglycemia. The major side effects are flatulence, diarrhea, and abdominal cramps.
- Exenatide, a synthetic peptide that stimulates release of insulin from pancreatic beta cells, can be used as adjunctive therapy for patients with type 2 DM. It is an incretin mimetic. Incretins are endogenous proteins that modulate the glycemic response. Exenatide is not indicated in type 1 DM and is contraindicated in patients with severe renal impairment. Starting dose is 5 μg subcutaneously (SC) bid before morning and evening meals.
- Pramlintide, a synthetic analog of human amylin (a hormone synthesized by pancreatic beta cells and cosecreted with insulin in response to food intake) can be used as an adjunctive treatment for patients with type 1 or type 2 DM who inject insulin at mealtime. In type 1 DM, initial dose is 15 μg SC before major meals. In type 2 DM, initial dose is 60 μg before major meals. Nausea is its major side effect.
- Combination therapy of various hypoglycemic agents is commonly used when monotherapy results in inadequate glycemic control.
- Insulin is indicated for the treatment of all type 1 DM and type 2 DM patients whose condition cannot be adequately controlled with diet and oral agents. Recommended therapy for type 1 DM consists of use of multiple dose insulin injections (three to four injections per day of basal and prandial insu-

lin), matching of prandial insulin to carbohydrate intake, premeal blood glucose, and anticipated activity; and in many patients use of insulin analogs (especially if hypoglycemia is a problem). Table 1-42 describes commonly used types of insulin. The risks of insulin therapy include weight gain, hypoglycemia, and in rare cases, allergic or cutaneous reactions. Replacement insulin therapy should mimic normal release patterns. Approximately 50% to 60% of daily insulin can be given as a long-acting insulin (NPH, ultralente, glargine, detemir) injected once or twice daily, the remaining 40% to 50% can be short-acting or rapid-acting to cover mealtime carbohydrates and correct increased current glucose levels. Among long-acting insulins, once-daily bedtime insulin glargine is as effective as once- or twice-daily NPH but has a lower risk for nocturnal hypoglycemia and less weight gain. Insulin detemir is a long-acting insulin analog approved as basal therapy for treatment of DM. It is indicated for use in adults and children in combination with short-acting insulin for type 1 diabetes and oral agents or short-acting insulin for adults with type 2 DM. Unlike NPH insulin, its use has not been associated with weight gain. Short-acting insulins include insulin aspart and insulin lispro, which are more effective in lowering postprandial glucose levels than regular insulin.
- Continuous subcutaneous insulin infusion (CSII, or insulin pump) provides better glycemic control than does conventional therapy and comparable with or slightly better control than multiple daily injections. It should be

considered for diabetes presenting in childhood or adolescence and during pregnancy.
- The Diabetes Control and Complications Trial (DCCT) showed that intensive treatment for glucose control decreases the development and progression of complications of type 1 DM. In this trial, the risks for retinopathy, nephropathy, and neuropathy were decreased by 70%, 54%, and 64%, respectively.
- Low-dose aspirin (ASA; 81 mg/day) to decrease the risk for cerebrovascular disease is beneficial for patients with diabetes older than 50 yr with other risk factors (hypertension, dyslipidemia, smoking, obesity). Low-dose aspirin therapy is reasonable in adults with diabetes and no history of vascular disease, whose 10-yr risk of CHD events is >10%, and who are not at increased risk of bleeding. Aspirin is not indicated for diabetic men younger than 50 and women younger than 60 with no other risk factors (10-yr cardiovascular disease risk <5%).
- Measure fasting lipid profile at least annually in adults with low-risk lipid values (low-density lipoprotein [LDL] cholesterol <100 mg/dl, high-density lipoprotein [HDL] cholesterol >50 mg/dl, and triglycerides <150 mg/dl). All patients with diabetes older than 40 yr with one or more additional risk factors for cardiovascular disease should be on statin therapy together with lifestyle modification regardless of baseline lipid levels. The primary goal is an LDL cholesterol level <100 mg/dl without overt coronary artery disease (CAD), and in patients with overt CAD, a goal of <70 mg/dl is an option. In patients for whom target goals cannot be easily reached on maximal tolerated therapy, an alternative therapeutic goal should be the reduction in LDL of ~30% to 40% from baseline.
- Becaplermin is a recombinant human platelet-derived growth factor useful for diabetic foot ulcers. It is applied as a topical gel to promote wound healing by enhancing the formation of granulation tissue in stage III and IV diabetic peripheral ulcers of the lower extremities.
- Aggressive antihypertensive therapy is recommended to keep systolic blood pressure (BP) <130 and diastolic BP <80 mm Hg. Use of angiotensin-converting enzyme (ACE) inhibitors or angiotensin receptor blockers (ARBs) to decrease albuminuria and for prevention of progression of kidney disease should be considered regardless of presence of hypertension kidney function and serum potassium levels should be closely monitored.
- Bariatric surgery should be considered in adults with BMI >35 kg/m² and type 2 diabetes, especially if the diabetes is difficult to control with lifestyle and pharmacologic therapy.
- Treat hypoglycemia in a conscious person with glucose tab or gel 15 to 20 g, and intramuscular injection of glucagon if unconscious. Patient and family members should be instructed on the administration of glucagon for individuals at significant risk for severe hypoglycemia.

TABLE 1-42 Types of Insulin

Preparation	Brand	Onset (hr)*	Peak (hr)	Duration (hr)†	Route
Insulin Aspart	NovoLog‡	<0.25	1-3	3-5	SC, IV, CSII
Insulin Aspart Protamine/ Insulin Aspart	NovoLog Mix 70/30‡	<0.25	1-4	24	SC
Insulin Detemir	Levemir§	1	None	24	SC
Insulin Glargine	Lantus‡	1.1	None	≥24	SC
Insulin Glulisine	Apidra‡	≤0.25	1	2-4	SC, IV
Insulin Lispro	Humalog‡	<0.25	1	3.5-4.5	SC
Insulin Lispro Protamine/ Insulin Lispro	Humalog Mix 75/25‡	≤0.25	0.5-1.5	24	SC
	Humalog Mix 50/50‡	≤0.25	1	16	SC
Insulin Injection Regular (R)	Humulin R¶	0.5	2-4	6-8	SC, IM, IV
	Novolin N§	0.5	2.5-5	8	SC, IM, IV
Insulin Isophane Suspension (NPH)/Regular Insulin (R)	Humulin 70/30¶	0.5	2-12	24	SC
	Humulin 50/50¶	0.5	3-5	24	SC
	Novolin 70/30§	0.5	2-12	24	SC
Insulin Isophane Suspension (NPH)	Humulin N¶	1-2	6-12	18-24	SC
	Novolin N§	1.5	4-12	24	SC

*Onset for injectable formulations is always for the subcutaneous (SC) route. All times are approximate.
†Maximum effect occurs between these times; actual effect may last longer.
‡Recombinant human insulin analogue (using *E. coli*).
§Recombinant (using *S. cerevisiae*).
Injectable insulins listed are available in a concentration of 100 U/ml; Humulin R, in a concentration of 500 U/ml for SC injection. SC injection only, is available by prescription from Lilly for insulin-resistant patients who are hospitalized or in need of medical supervision.
¶Recombinant (using *E. coli*).
CSII, Continuous subcutaneous infusion; *IM*, intramuscularly; *IV*, intravenously.

DISPOSITION

- Diabetic retinopathy occurs in ~15% of patients with diabetes after 15 yr of diagnosis and increases 1%/yr after diagnosis. Retinal laser photocoagulation and vitrectomy are effective treatment modalities. Prevention is best accomplished by strict glucose and BP control. Early blockade of the renin-angiotensin system has been shown to slow progression of retinopathy in patients with type 1 diabetes.
- The frequency of neuropathy in patients with type 2 diabetes approaches 70% to 80%. It can be subdivided in sensorimotor neuropathy (distal symmetric polyneuropathy, focal neuropathy [diabetic mononeuropathy, mononeuropathy multiplex], diabetic amyotrophy) and autonomic neuropathy (vasomotor neuropathy, GI autonomic neuropathy [gastric atony, diabetic diarrhea or constipation, fecal incontinence], genitourinary autonomic neuropathy [bladder dysfunction, sexual dysfunction], hypoglycemic unawareness, sudomotor neuropathy). Duloxetine, a selective serotonin and norepinephrine reuptake inhibitor, is effective and FDA approved for relief of diabetic peripheral neuropathy. Pregabalin and gabapentin (900 to 3600 mg/day) are also effective for the symptomatic treatment of peripheral neuropathic pain. Topical capsaicin, 5% lidocaine transdermal patches, amitriptyline, and carbamazepine are also modestly effective.
- Diabetic gastroparesis is most often seen in patients who have had diabetes for at least 10 yr and typically have retinopathy, neuropathy, and nephropathy. Major manifestations are postprandial fullness, nausea, vomiting, and bloating. Pharmacologic therapy involves prokinetic agents (metoclopramide). Endoscopic injection of botulinum toxin into the pylorus and gastric electrical stimulation (using f electrodes placed laparoscopically in the muscle wall of the stomach antrum and connected to a neurostimulator) represent newer approaches to nonpharmacologic therapy.
- Nephropathy: The first sign of renal involvement in patients with DM is most often microalbuminuria, which is classified as incipient nephropathy. Without specific intervention, 50% of patients with diabetes with type 1 DM with overt diabetic nephropathy (urine protein ≥300 mg/24 hr) progress to ESRD within

10 yr of onset. More than 75% of type 1 DM and 20% of type 2 DM cases progress t o ESRD over a 20-yr period.
- Infections are generally more common in patients with diabetes because of multiple factors, such as impaired leukocyte function, decreased tissue perfusion secondary to vascular disease, repeated trauma because of loss of sensation, and urinary retention secondary to neuropathy.
- Diabetic ketoacidosis and hyperosmolar nonketotic state are described in detail in Section I.
- Prevention/delay of type 2 diabetes: Patients with IGT or IFG should achieve weight loss of 5% to 10% of body weight and increase physical activity to at least 150 min/wk of moderate activity such as walking.

REFERRAL

- Patients with diabetes should be advised to have annual ophthalmologic examinations. In type 1 DM, ophthalmologic visits should begin within 3 to 5 yr of diagnosis, whereas type 2 DM patients should be seen from disease onset.
- Podiatric care can significantly reduce the rate of foot infections and amputations in patients with DM. Noninfected neuropathic foot ulcers require debridement and reduction of pressure.
- Nephrology consultation in all cases of proteinuria, hyperkalemia, uncontrolled BP, and when GFR has decreased to <30 ml/min/1.73 m^2.

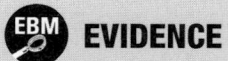

PEARLS & CONSIDERATIONS

COMMENTS

- Because normalization of serum glucose level is the ultimate goal, every patient should measure his or her blood glucose unless contraindicated by senility or blindness.
- For blood glucose monitoring, glucose oxidase strips are used in conjunction with a meter to give a digital reading. The testing can be done once a day, but the time should be varied each day so that over time the serum glucose level before meals and at bedtime can be assessed frequently without pricking the patient's fingers four times daily.

- Underinsured children and those with psychiatric illness are at greater risk for acute complications in type 1 DM and require frequent monitoring and aggressive risk management with diet, exercise, and periodic laboratory evaluation.
- Vascular endothelial growth factor and erythropoietin have been identified as factors involved in angiogenesis in proliferative diabetic retinopathy.
- Significant sustained weight loss using bariatric surgery has been reported as effective in achieving remission of type 2 diabetes in morbidly obese patients. Bariatric surgery may be considered for adults with BMI >35 μg/m^2 and type 2 DM, especially if diabetes or associated comorbidities are difficult to control with lifestyle and pharmacologic therapy.
- Cigarette smoking predicts incident type 2 diabetes. For a smoker at risk for diabetes, smoking cessation should be coupled with strategies for diabetes prevention and early detection.
- Compared with a low-fat diet, a low-carbohydrate, Mediterranean-style diet leads to more favorable changes in glycemic control and coronary risk factors and delayed the need for antihyperglycemic drug therapy in overweight patients with newly diagnosed type 2 diabetes.
- Individuals with impaired fasting glucose (IFG) and/or impaired glucose tolerance (IGT) have a relatively high risk for future development of diabetes and are referred as having "prediabetes." These individuals should not be viewed as having clinical entities in their own right but as having risk factors for diabetes. The same applies to individuals with HBA_{1C} ranging from 5.7% to 6.4%.

EBM EVIDENCE

available at www.expertconsult.com

SUGGESTED READINGS
available at www.expertconsult.com

AUTHORS: **ANTHONY GEMIGNANI, M.D.,**
FRED F. FERRI, M.D., and **WEN-CHIH WU, M.D.**

BASIC INFORMATION

DEFINITION

Diabetic ketoacidosis (DKA) is a life-threatening complication of diabetes mellitus resulting from severe insulin deficiency or insulin resistance with relative insulin deficiency and manifested clinically by severe dehydration and alterations in sensorium.

SYNONYMS

DKA

ICD-9CM CODES
250.1 Diabetic ketoacidosis

EPIDEMIOLOGY & DEMOGRAPHICS

INCIDENCE/PREVALENCE: 6 episodes per 10,000 individuals with diabetes; it accounts for 8% to 29% of all hospital admissions of patients with diabetes
PREDOMINANT AGE: 1 to 25 yr

PHYSICAL FINDINGS & CLINICAL PRESENTATION

- Evidence of dehydration (tachycardia, hypotension, dry mucous membranes, sunken eyeballs, poor skin turgor)
- Altered mental status
- Tachypnea with air hunger (Kussmaul's respiration)
- Fruity breath odor (caused by acetone)
- Lipemia retinalis in some patients
- Possible evidence of precipitating factors (infected wound, pneumonia)
- Abdominal tenderness in some patients

ETIOLOGY

- Metabolic decompensation in individuals with diabetes is frequently precipitated by an infectious process (up to 40%).
- Poor compliance with insulin therapy and severe medical illness (for example, pancreatitis, cardiovascular events) are other common causes.
- Cocaine abuse has been reported as a risk factor for DKA in adult and teenage patients, particularly in patients with multiple admissions.
- Lack of education of primary caregiver (mother, sibling), as well as deficiencies in proper monitoring of blood glucose, correct administration of insulin, supervision of insulin pump maintenance, and monitoring of diabetic caloric restraints are causes of recurrent episodes of DKA.

DIAGNOSIS

DIFFERENTIAL DIAGNOSIS

- Hyperosmolar nonketotic state
- Alcoholic ketoacidosis
- Uremic acidosis
- Metabolic acidosis caused by methyl alcohol or ethylene glycol
- Salicylate poisoning

WORKUP

- Laboratory evaluation (see "Laboratory Tests") to confirm diagnosis and evaluate precipitating factors
- ECG to evaluate electrolyte abnormalities and rule out myocardial ischemia or infarction as a contributing factor

LABORATORY TESTS

- Glucose level demonstrates severe hyperglycemia (serum glucose generally >250 mg/dl)
- Arterial blood gases demonstrate acidosis: arterial pH usually <7.30 with P_{CO_2} <40 mm Hg
- Serum ketonemia (β-hydroxybutyrate > 300 μmol/L), ketonuria, and glycosuria
- Serum electrolytes:
  1. Serum bicarbonate is usually <15 mEq/L.
  2. Serum potassium (K^+) may be low, normal, or high. There is always significant total body potassium depletion regardless of the initial potassium level.
  3. Serum sodium is usually decreased as a result of hyperglycemia, dehydration, and lipemia. Assume 1.6-mEq/L decrease in extracellular sodium for each 100-mg/dl increase in glucose concentration. Initially, a modest degree of hypernatremia is advantageous to help prevent the fast fall of effective plasma osmolality when glycemia is under control.
  4. Calculate the anion gap (AG):

     $$AG = Na^+ - (Cl^- + HCO^-_3)$$

     In DKA, the anion gap is increased (generally >10) because of high levels of ketones; hyperchloremic metabolic acidosis may be present in unusual circumstances when both the glomerular filtration rate and the plasma volume are well maintained.

     Mixed metabolic disturbances demonstrating anion gap metabolic acidosis overlapping with metabolic alkalosis may be present; this is common in patients with DKA with persistent vomiting.
- CBC with differential, urinalysis, and urine and blood cultures to rule out infectious precipitating factor
- Serum calcium, magnesium, and phosphorus; the plasma phosphate and magnesium levels may be significantly depressed and should be rechecked within 24 hours because they may decrease further with correction of DKA
- Blood urea nitrogen and creatinine generally reveal significant dehydration
- Amylase and liver enzymes should be checked in patients with abdominal pain

IMAGING STUDIES

Chest radiographs are helpful to rule out infectious process. The initial chest film may be negative if the patient has significant dehydration. Repeat chest x-ray after 24 hours if pulmonary infection is strongly suspected.

TREATMENT

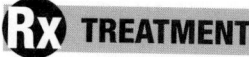

NONPHARMACOLOGIC THERAPY

- Monitor mental status, vital signs, and urine output hourly until improved, then monitor q2 to 4h.
- Monitor electrolytes, renal function, and glucose level (see "Acute General Rx").

ACUTE GENERAL Rx

Fluid replacement (usual deficit is 6 to 8 L):
1. Do not delay fluid replacement until laboratory results have been received. Fluid deficits are typically 100 ml/kg of body weight. The normalization of hypotension is imperative within the initial hour of presentation while avoiding the use of hypotonic fluids. The total fluid administered should not exceed 4 L/m²/24 hours for fear of causing cerebral edema (CE). One rule of thumb is to deliver fluids (deficit and maintenance) over a period of 48 hours if serum osmolality is >360 mOsm/L.
2. The initial fluid replacement should be with 0.9% normal saline (NS) until blood pressure and organ perfusion are restored. In patients with severe hypernatremia (serum sodium >160 mEq/L), 0.45% saline infusion can be used. Careful monitoring for fluid overload is necessary in elderly patients and those with a history of congestive heart failure.
3. The rate of fluid replacement varies with the age of the patient and the presence of significant cardiac or renal disease.
   - The usual rate of infusion is 500 ml to 1 L over the first hour and 300 to 500 ml/hour for the next 12 hours.
   - Continue the infusion at a rate of 200 to 300 ml/hour, using 0.45% NS until the serum glucose level is <300 mg/dl, then change the hydrating solution to D_5W to prevent hypoglycemia, replenish free water, and introduce additional glucose substrate (necessary to suppress lipolysis and ketogenesis).

Insulin administration:
1. The patient should be given an initial loading IV bolus of 0.15 to 0.2 U/kg regular insulin followed by a constant infusion at a rate of 0.1 U/kg/hour (e.g., 25 U of regular insulin in 250 ml of 0.9% saline solution at 70 ml/hour equals 7 U/hour for a 70-kg patient). Insulin replacement should generally not be started until serum potassium is >3.3 mEq/L to prevent life-threatening hypokalemia.
2. Monitor serum glucose hourly for the first 2 hours, then monitor q2 to 4h.
3. The goal is to decrease serum glucose level by 80 mg/dl/hour (after an initial decline because of rehydration); if the serum glucose level is not decreasing at the expected rate, double the rate of insulin infusion.
4. When the serum glucose level approaches 250 mg/dl, decrease the rate of insulin infusion to 2 to 3 U/hour and continue this rate until the patient has received adequate fluid replacement, HCO^-_3 is close to normal, and

ketones have cleared. After target glucose levels are achieved, it usually takes 5 to 7 hours for ketosis to clear. In young children and adolescents who have high growth rate, they have greater levels of human growth hormones so that there is a prolonged time lag for plasma glucose to reach to above levels. Patients with fever or infections and higher metabolic requirements need 15% to 20% more insulin than the usual starting dose.

5. Approximately 30 to 60 min before stopping the IV insulin infusion, administer an SC dose of regular insulin (dose varies with the patient's demonstrated insulin sensitivity); this SC dose of regular insulin is necessary because of the extremely short life of the insulin in the IV infusion.

6. When the patient is able to eat, long-acting insulin such as NPH insulin is given in the morning and/or at bedtime, and shorter-acting insulin such as aspart insulin is administered before each meal by using a sliding scale. In individuals with newly diagnosed diabetes, the total daily dose to maintain metabolic control ranges from 0.5 to 0.8 U/kg/day.

Electrolyte replacement:
- Potassium replacement: the average total potassium loss in DKA is 300 to 500 mEq.
- K^+ can be supplemented as chloride- and phosphate-containing solutions.
  1. The rate of replacement varies with the patient's serum potassium level, degree of acidosis (decreased pH, increased potassium level), and renal function (potassium replacement should be used with caution in patients with renal failure).
  2. As a rule of thumb, potassium replacement may be started when there is no ECG evidence of hyperkalemia (tall, narrow, or tent-shaped T waves; decreased or absent P waves; short QT intervals; widening of QRS complex).
  3. In patients with normal renal function, potassium replacement can be started by adding 20 to 40 mEq KCl/L of IV hydrating solution if serum potassium is 4 to 5 mEq/L, and more if serum potassium level is lower than 4 mEq/L. In patients with severe hypokalemia (potassium <3.3 mEq/L), give 40 mEq/hour potassium until potassium is >3.3 mEq/L.
  4. Monitor serum potassium level hourly for the first 2 hours, then monitor q2 to 4h.
- Phosphate replacement: If the serum PO_4 is <1.5 mEq/L, give 2.5 mg/kg IV over 6 hours

of elemental phosphate. Routine replacement of phosphate (in the absence of laboratory evidence of significant hypophosphatemia) is not indicated. Rapid IV phosphate administration can cause hypocalcemia.
- Magnesium replacement: Replacement is indicated only in the presence of significant hypomagnesemia or refractory hypokalemia.

Bicarbonate therapy:
- Routine use of bicarbonate in DKA is contraindicated because it can worsen hypokalemia and intracellular acidosis, and cause CE. Bicarbonate therapy should be considered only if the arterial pH is <6.9 and HCO^-_3 is <5.
- In these patients, 44 to 88 mEq sodium bicarbonate can be added to 1 L of 0.45% NS q2-4h until pH increases to >7.
- Use of bicarbonate therapy is particularly dangerous in the pediatric population. Children with DKA who have a low $Paco_2$ and high serum urea nitrogen concentration at presentation and who are treated with bicarbonate are at increased risk for CE. Bicarbonate therapy in children with DKA should be limited to those with severe circulatory failure and a high risk for cardiac decompensation resulting from profound acidosis.

PREVENTION

- Provide information/education for teachers, parents, school staff, and caregivers on how to recognize children with undiagnosed diabetes.
- Review sick day management; increase home blood glucose monitoring, education on how to measure urinary or fingerstick ketones, compliance with insulin; and maintain adequate hydration and nutrition.

DISPOSITION

- Average mortality rate in DKA is 5% to 10%.
- In children <10 yr, DKA causes 70% of diabetes-related deaths.
- Cerebral edema (CE) occurs in 1% of episodes of DKA in children and is associated with a mortality rate of 40% to 90%.

REFERRAL

Patients with DKA should be admitted to the intensive care unit. Alert patients who are able to take fluids orally and have mild DKA occasionally can be treated under observation and sent home. The American Diabetes Association admission guidelines are a plasma glucose level >250 mg/dl, with arterial pH <7.30, a serum bicarbonate level <15 mEq/L, and a moderate or greater level of ketones in the serum or urine.

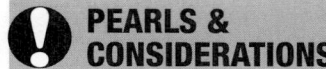

COMMENTS

- Although DKA occurs more commonly in type 1 diabetes mellitus, a significant proportion (>20%) occurs in patients with type 2 diabetes.
- 30% to 40% of DKA admissions involve patients with newly diagnosed diabetes.
- Potential complications of DKA therapy include hypoglycemia, CE, cardiac arrhythmias, shock, myocardial infarction, and acute pancreatitis.
- Risk factors for CE include age <5 yr, high initial BUN reflecting severe prolonged state of dehydration, hyperventilation to a $Paco_2$ of <22 mm Hg, and presenting arterial pH of <7.00. It presents 4 to 8 hours after start of rehydration therapy. Presentation may be abrupt with sudden severe headache, vomiting, sudden hypertension, and obtunded sensorium. First management response to CE is to elevate head of the patient to 30-degree angle, followed by IV mannitol and intubation and hyperventilation, finally cutting back of the maintenance fluid to 75% of the amount required.
- Underinsured children and those with psychiatric illness are at greater risk for DKA.
- Subcutaneous administration of rapid-acting insulin analogues may be reasonable alternatives to IV regular insulin infusion for treating uncomplicated DKA.
- DKA can occur with blood glucose <350 mg/dl in the setting of poor oral intake or pregnancy.
- Ketones can be positive in starvation or with heavy alcohol intake; DKA can coexist with other causes of metabolic acidosis such as lactic acidosis.
- Euglycemic DKA is reported to occur in 1% to 17% of cases; normal or minimally elevated blood sugar levels seen in starvation, especially if insulin is continued or in the presence of severe hepatic disease.
- Use of low-level IV unfractionated herapin has been reported as effective in reducing severe elevations of plasma triglycerides in DKA.

SUGGESTED READINGS
available at www.expertconsult.com

AUTHORS: **ANTHONY GEMIGNANI, M.D.,** **FRED F. FERRI, M.D.,** and **WEN-CHIH WU, M.D.**

BASIC INFORMATION

DEFINITION

Diabetic polyneuropathy is a term used to encompass the various forms of peripheral nerve dysfunction that occur in the setting of diabetes. The most common form of diabetic polyneuropathy is distal symmetric polyneuropathy (DSPN), which is a length-dependent process typically characterized by numbness, tingling, and occasionally, pain that begins in the feet and slowly progresses more proximally. Besides DSPN, in which distal sensory nerves are predominantly involved, diabetes is also associated with autonomic neuropathies, as well as focal or multifocal neuropathies that can lead to proximal and asymmetric presentations.

SYNONYMS

Chronic distal symmetric polyneuropathy
Diabetic peripheral neuropathy

ICD-9CM CODES
250.6 Diabetes with neurological
       manifestations
357.2 Polyneuropathy in diabetes

EPIDEMIOLOGY & DEMOGRAPHICS

PREVALENCE: The true prevalence of diabetic polyneuropathy in its varying forms is unknown, but it is the most common cause of peripheral neuropathy in developed countries. As many as 66% of individuals with diabetes may have some form of neuropathy.

RISK FACTORS: Patients with poor glycemic control and patients with diabetic nephropathy or retinopathy are at increased risk.

PHYSICAL FINDINGS & CLINICAL PRESENTATION

Distal symmetric polyneuropathy (DSPN):
- Patients most commonly experience numbness and tingling, but may also experience feelings of tightness or a sensation of heat or cold.
- Pain is not uncommon, is often worst at night, and can be burning, aching, shooting, or lancinating in nature.
- These symptoms begin in the feet and may slowly ascend over months to years. Symptoms in the hands do not generally occur until symptoms in the lower extremities have reached the level of the knees. In more severe cases, the symptoms can spread to the trunk and head.
- Neurological examination reveals early loss of small-fiber modalities resulting in decreased pinprick and temperature sensation with later involvement of large-fiber modalities leading to a reduction in vibratory and proprioceptive sensation. Ankle reflexes are usually reduced or absent, and more proximal reflexes may also become involved as the neuropathy progresses. Strength is usually normal, but there can be some motor involvement leading to mild weakness and

atrophy which is usually limited to intrinsic foot muscles and ankle dorsiflexors.

OTHER DIABETIC NEUROPATHIES
Autonomic neuropathy:
- Some form of autonomic dysfunction may be present in up to half of diabetic individuals and usually occurs along with a DSPN.
- Symptoms are usually mild and may include difficulty adjusting to changes in light or dryness of the eyes or mouth.
- Gastrointestinal symptoms are common and can include early satiety, bloating, vomiting, constipation, or diarrhea.
- Cardiovascular complications include cardiac arrhythmias and postural hypotension.
- Patients may also have symptoms related to dysfunction of the genitourinary (erectile dysfunction and incontinence) or thermoregulatory (excessive or reduced sweating, intolerance of cold or heat) systems.

Regional diabetic polyneuropathy:
- In contrast to DSPN, the regional diabetic polyneuropathies tend to be subacute in onset, predominantly proximal, and asymmetric or unilateral.
- These usually occur in individuals who also have a DSPN
- The most common presentation is the diabetic lumbosacral radiculoplexus neuropathy, which is also known as diabetic amyotrophy or Bruns-Garland syndrome. Patients usually report acute or subacute onset of severe pain involving the lower back, hip, and thigh. Weakness and atrophy of the affected leg progresses over the course of days to weeks, often predominantly in the anterior thigh. There may also be numbness, tingling, and significant weight loss. Although the initial onset is typically unilateral, asymmetric involvement of the other leg commonly occurs within weeks or months. Progression of weakness usually plateaus within several months, followed by some degree of gradual improvement that can take 2 to 3 yr. The degree of improvement is variable, and many individuals have significant, chronic pain, weakness, or sensory loss.
- Less commonly, involvement of several thoracic nerve roots may cause a thoracoabdominal neuropathy, resulting in pain and numbness in the chest, back, or abdomen. The symptoms are usually in a dermatomal distribution but may mimic more common causes of pain in these areas. There may also be associated weakness of the abdominal muscles.
- The cervical roots and brachial plexus are not usually involved.

Focal diabetic neuropathy:
- These also tend to occur in patients who also have DSPN.
- Diabetic patients are at increased risk for common limb mononeuropathies, particularly median neuropathy at the wrist and ulnar neuropathy at the elbow, but other nerves (femoral, sciatic, or peroneal) may be involved as well.

- A diabetic cranial mononeuropathy usually presents acutely and unilaterally, with or without pain. The examination findings should be limited to dysfunction of a single cranial nerve, usually cranial nerve III, VI, VII, or, less frequently, IV. There is typically significant improvement or complete resolution within several months.

ETIOLOGY

The etiology is unknown but most likely involves a complex interaction of metabolic derangements and microvascular insults that occur in the setting of diabetes.

DIAGNOSIS

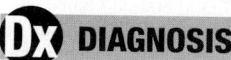

DIFFERENTIAL DIAGNOSIS

Although diabetes is the leading cause of peripheral neuropathy in developed countries, there are many other causes.

WORKUP

- A thorough history and neurologic examination are essential to confirm features consistent with a diabetic polyneuropathy and exclude other features that would suggest alternative diagnoses.
- For some patients, neuropathy may be the presenting feature of previously undiagnosed diabetes.
- Electrodiagnostic evaluation to include nerve conduction studies and electromyography can be helpful in confirming the presence, extent, and severity of a neuropathy.
- Patients with DSPN typically have a reduction of amplitudes and slowing of conduction velocities involving sensory and possibly motor nerves in a length-dependent and symmetric fashion.
- Electromyographic examination of distal muscles may reveal fibrillation potentials, positive sharp waves, and large motor unit action potentials, suggestive of denervation and reinnervation.
- Skin biopsy and nerve biopsy are not necessary in the vast majority of cases.

LABORATORY TESTS

- Fasting blood sugar, hemoglobin A1c, and oral glucose tolerance test should all be considered in patients with peripheral neuropathy without a known history of diabetes.
- A focused laboratory evaluation for other common or potentially treatable causes of neuropathy is also indicated: complete blood cell count, complete metabolic panel to include electrolytes and liver function tests, erythrocyte sedimentation rate, vitamin B_{12} and folate levels, thyroid function tests, serum protein electrophoresis and immunofixation electrophoresis.
- Additional laboratory tests can be considered based on history or exam findings that may suggest other underlying diagnoses: antinuclear antibodies, extractable nuclear antigens, and rheumatoid factor.

IMAGING STUDIES

Imaging is not necessary unless there is concern for an alternate or coexisting process based on the history and examination.

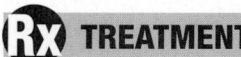 TREATMENT

CHRONIC Rx

- The primary treatment for diabetic polyneuropathy is effective glycemic control as this may improve or at least slow progression of the neuropathy.
- Another aspect of treatment is the symptomatic management of pain and paresthesias
  - Topical agents: Lidocaine 5% patch can be applied to painful areas for 12 hours a day.
  - Anticonvulsants: gabapentin (100 to 1200 mg tid) and pregabalin (50 to 100 mg tid)
  - Antidepressants: amitriptyline (10 to 100 mg qhs), nortriptyline (25 to 150 mg qhs), and duloxetine (60 to 120 mg daily)
  - Tramadol (50 mg qid as needed) can be a useful adjunctive analgesic

DISPOSITION

The distal sensory loss of diabetic polyneuropathy places patients at increased risk of trauma to the extremities with the potential for ulceration and infection which could ultimately necessitate amputation.

REFERRAL

- A neurologist can assist in the diagnosis and management of diabetic polyneuropathy.
- Patients with diabetic polyneuropathy should also be evaluated at least annually by a podiatrist and ophthalmologist

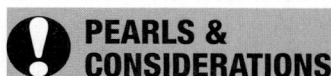 PEARLS & CONSIDERATIONS

COMMENTS

- For many patients, a DSPN or other form of diabetic neuropathy may be the initial presentation of previously undiagnosed diabetes.

- In addition to regular visits with podiatry, patients with diabetic polyneuropathy should be educated on aggressive foot hygiene and the importance of examining their own feet

PATIENT/FAMILY EDUCATION

Website: http://www.mayoclinic.com/health/diabetic-neuropathy/DS01045

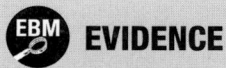 EVIDENCE

available at www.expertconsult.com

SUGGESTED READINGS
available at www.expertconsult.com

AUTHOR: **JEFFREY C. MCCLEAN II, M.D.**

BASIC INFORMATION

DEFINITION

Digoxin, a cardiac glycoside, is used for the treatment of symptomatic heart failure and ventricular rate control in atrial fibrillation.

Chronic digoxin therapy or acute overdose can cause toxicity. Toxicity can occur even when serum levels are within the therapeutic range.

SYNONYMS

Digitalis overdose
Cardiac glycoside toxicity

ICD-9CM CODES
972.1 Digitalis overdose

PHARMACOKINETICS

Steady-state levels (not peak levels) correlate with toxicity; digoxin reaches steady state 6 to 8 hr after ingestion.
BIOAVAILABILITY: Approximately 80%
VOLUME OF DISTRIBUTION: 5 to 7 L/kg, highly tissue bound
HALF-LIFE: 36 hr
EXCRETION: Predominantly renal
THERAPEUTIC LEVEL: 0.5 to 2 ng/ml (0.5 to 0.8 ng/ml suggested in heart failure); check level one week after starting therapy or changing dose. Sample should be drawn at least 6 to 8 hr after last dose.

EPIDEMIOLOGY & DEMOGRAPHICS

- Digoxin toxicity occurs in up to 5% of individuals on therapy.
- Factors that potentiate toxicity (may increase level or modify cardiac sensitivity): advanced age, female gender, renal insufficiency, cardiac or pulmonary disease, drugs that affect elimination (ACE inhibitors, amiodarone, clarithromycin, cyclosporine, diltiazem, erythromycin, itraconazole, NSAIDs, rifampin, spironolactone, SSRIs, tetracyclines, quinidine,

verapamil, and herbal supplements), co-ingestion of cardiotoxic drugs (beta-blockers, calcium channel blockers, tricyclic antidepressants), hypokalemia, hypomagnesemia, hypercalcemia, hypernatremia, acid-base disturbance, hypoxia, hypothyroidism, and volume depletion.

PHYSICAL FINDINGS & CLINICAL PRESENTATION

Cardiac, gastrointestinal, and central nervous systems are affected. Fatigue, malaise, and weakness are common symptoms.
CARDIAC: The most common and often first finding is an increase in premature ventricular complexes. Can present with almost any dysrhythmia or conduction block.
GASTROINTESTINAL: Anorexia, nausea, vomiting, diarrhea, abdominal pain
CENTRAL NERVOUS SYSTEM:
- Headache, dizziness, visual disturbance (flashing lights, halos, blurred vision, change in color perception, decreased visual acuity), confusion, hallucinations, delirium, syncope
- Hyperkalemia often seen in acute poisoning; hypokalemia more common in chronic toxicity

ETIOLOGY

Digoxin reversibly inhibits the function of sodium-potassium adenosine triphosphatase, increasing extracellular K^+ and intracellular Na^+. This reduces the activity of the Na-Ca exchanger, leading to intracellular accumulation of calcium. This results in increased myocardial contractility and cardiac output, the positive inotropic effect associated with digoxin therapy. Cardiac glycosides also decrease the heart rate (effect on SA node) and slow conduction throughout the AV node by increasing parasympathetic tone. Sympathetic activity is decreased at therapeutic levels but increased in toxicity. Enhanced automaticity of cardiac tissue and depressed conduction lead to the extrasystoles and arrhythmias seen in toxicity.

DIAGNOSIS

DIFFERENTIAL DIAGNOSIS

Medications:
- Beta-blockers
- Calcium channel blockers
- Clonidine
- Cyclic antidepressants
- Encainide and flecainide
- Procainamide
- Propoxyphene
- Quinidine
Plants producing digitalis-like glycosides:
- Foxglove
- Oleander
- Lily of the valley
Cardiac conduction abnormalities:
- Sick sinus syndrome
- AV node dysfunction
Electrolyte abnormalities:
- Hyperkalemia

WORKUP

- History: medication changes, herbal supplements, deliberate overdose
- Physical examination

LABORATORY TESTS

- Stat digoxin level (in acute ingestion high levels may not be toxic, as tissue redistribution will occur)
- Electrolytes, BUN, creatinine, magnesium, calcium
- ECG (Figs. 1-120 and 1-121)
- Almost any dysrhythmia can occur, but simultaneous increased automaticity of cardiac tissue and conduction delay in the AV node should raise suspicion. Findings suggestive of toxicity include the following:
  - Frequent premature ventricular complexes, bigeminy
  - Bradydysrhythmias
  - AV block (Mobitz type 1)
  - Atrial tachycardia with AV block

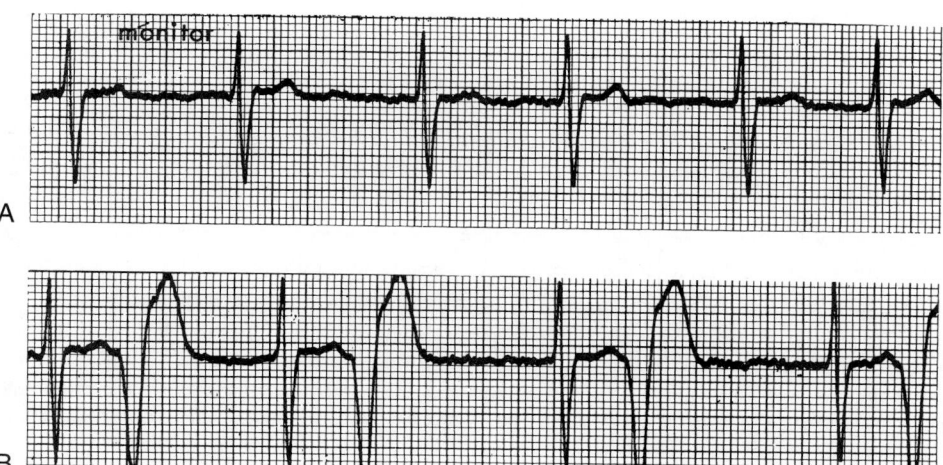

FIGURE 1-120 Ventricular bigeminy caused by digoxin toxicity. Ventricular ectopy is one of the most common signs of digoxin toxicity. The underlying rhythm in **A** is atrial fibrillation. In **B** each normal QRS is followed by a ventricular premature beat. (Reprinted from Goldberger AL [ed]: *Clinical electrocardiography*, ed 5, St Louis, 1994, Mosby.)

- ○ Junctional tachycardia
- ○ Venticular arrhythmias: Bidirectional ventricular tachycardia, ventricular tachycardia, ventricular fibrillation

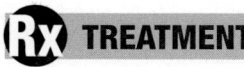

NONPHARMACOLOGIC THERAPY

- Ensure adequate airway
- Cardiac monitor

ACUTE GENERAL Rx

DECREASE TOXICITY:

- Acute poisoning: single dose of activated charcoal if within 2 hr of ingestion.
- Treat hyperkalemia: use caution as this reflects potassium redistribution and not an increase in total body load. As digoxin toxicity is corrected, potassium moves back into the cell and hypokalemia can develop.
- Treat hypokalemia and hypomagnesemia; both potentiate toxicity.
- Digoxin-specific Fab fragments (Digibind or DigiFab):
  1. Specific antibodies that bind to digoxin and to a lesser extent other cardiac glycosides
  2. Initial response usually seen in 30 min, and complete reversal usually occurs within 4 hr
  3. Indications: hyperkalemia ($\geq$5 mEq/L), hemodynamic instability, severe arrhythmias, massive overdose (acute ingestion of $\geq$10 mg digoxin or steady-state serum digoxin level $\geq$6 ng/ml), coingestion of cardiotoxic drugs or plants containing cardiac glycosides
  4. Dosing: 1 vial of Fab fragments binds 0.5 mg of digoxin. Round up when calculating number of vials to administer
     a. Acute ingestion: number of vials = (ingested digoxin [mg] × 0.8)/0.5
     b. Chronic ingestion: number of vials = (serum digoxin level [ng/ml] × weight [kg]/100

  c. If neither the amount ingested nor serum level is known, treat empirically:
     (i) Acute intoxication: 10 vials and repeat if needed
     (ii) Chronic toxicity: 6 vials
     NOTE: Underdosing of Fab fragments may result in rebound toxicity as free digoxin is released from tissue stores.
  5. After use of Fab fragments, the free digoxin level decreases, but the measured digoxin level may increase because most assays measure free and bound digoxin levels. Serum levels are unreliable for days.
  6. Renal elimination: half-life of inactive complex is 15 to 20 hr. In renal failure, consider plasma exchange or plasmapheresis to remove Fab-digoxin complex; theoretically, complexes may dissociate before excretion and toxicity may reoccur.
  7. Class C for pregnancy.
  8. Adverse effects of treatment:
     a. May undo desirable action of digoxin and exacerbate heart failure or increase ventricular response in previously controlled atrial fibrillation.
     b. Hypokalemia: monitor potassium level hourly for several hours.
     c. Allergic reactions (<1%): Skin testing appropriate for high-risk individuals (history of sheep protein allergy or prior use).
- Hemodialysis and hemoperfusion: not useful because of extensive tissue binding and large volume of distribution.

COMPLICATIONS:

Hyperkalemia:
- Sodium bicarbonate
- Glucose and insulin
- Sodium polystyrene sulfonate (Kayexalate)
- Do not use calcium because it may worsen ventricular arrhythmias

Bradycardia and heart block:
- Atropine
- Cardiac pacing: use with caution, may precipitate life-threatening ventricular arrhythmias

Supraventricular and ventricular tachycardia:
- Lidocaine or phenytoin: decrease ventricular automaticity without slowing AV node conduction
- Avoid quinidine, bretylium, procainamide, and verapamil; may increase ventricular arrhythmias/AV node block
- Elective electrocardioversion is relatively contraindicated because it may precipitate ventricular fibrillation

DISPOSITION

- Good with prompt treatment
- Chronic poisoning is associated with higher mortality rate than acute poisoning

REFERRAL

U.S. Poison Control network: 800-222-1222

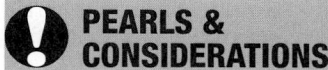

- High index of suspicion is necessary; the signs and symptoms of toxicity often are similar to those of the underlying disease.
- To minimize toxicity, digoxin levels should be checked if the patient's condition changes (e.g., weight loss, worsening renal function) or an interacting drug is started or stopped.
- Hyperkalemia in acute toxicity is suggestive of significant poisoning (reflects the amount of poisoning of Na^+-K^+ ATPase) and is associated with increased mortality rate.
- Falsely elevated digoxin levels may be seen in pregnant women, renal failure, hepatobiliary disease, and CHF due to the presence of an endogenous digoxin-like substance.
- Severe toxicity from ingestion of nondigoxin cardiac glycosides (plants, etc.) may present with low digoxin levels because of low cross-reactivity between these substances and the digoxin assay.

SUGGESTED READINGS

available at www.expertconsult.com

AUTHOR: **SUDEEP KAUR AULAKH, M.D.**

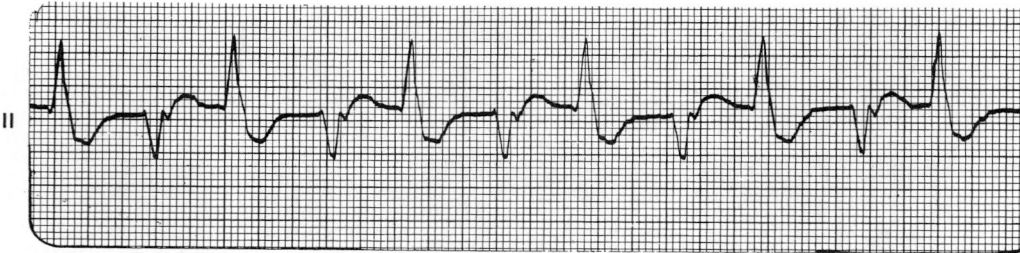

FIGURE 1-121 This digoxin-toxic arrhythmia is a special type of ventricular tachycardia (bidirectional tachycardia) with QRS complexes that alternate in direction from beat to beat. No P waves are present. (Reprinted from Goldberger AL [ed]: *Clinical electrocardiography,* ed 5, St Louis, 1994, Mosby.)

BASIC INFORMATION

DEFINITION

Diphtheria is an infection of the mucous membranes or skin caused by *Corynebacterium diphtheriae*.

SYNONYMS

Pharyngeal diphtheria
Wound diphtheria
Diphtheric cardiomyopathy
Diphtheric polyneuropathy

ICD-9CM CODES
032.9 Diphtheria

EPIDEMIOLOGY & DEMOGRAPHICS

INCIDENCE (IN U.S.): Since 2000 only 5 cases in the U.S. due to widespread vaccination
PREDOMINANT AGE: Adult years (in the U.S.)

PHYSICAL FINDINGS & CLINICAL PRESENTATION

RESPIRATORY DIPHTHERIA:
- Commonly presenting as pharyngitis, but any part of the respiratory tract may be involved, including the nasopharynx, larynx, trachea, or bronchi
- Areas of gray or white exudate coalescing to form a "pseudomembrane" that bleeds when removed
- Possible fever and dysphagia
- Complications: respiratory tract obstruction and pneumonia
- Systemic effects of the toxin: myocarditis and polyneuritis (frequently involving a bulbar distribution), less often nephritis
- Occurs mostly in nonimmune individuals; usually milder and less likely to be complicated in those adequately immunized

CUTANEOUS DIPHTHERIA:
- Usually complicates existing skin lesion (i.e., impetigo or scabies)
- Resembles the underlying condition or presents as a nonhealing ulcer with a grayish membrane

ETIOLOGY

- Caused by *C. diphtheriae,* an aerobic, gram-positive rod
- Transmitted by close contact through droplets of nasopharyngeal secretions
- Symptomatic disease of the respiratory system caused by toxin-producing strains (tox$^+$)
- Systemic effects of toxin: ranging from nausea and vomiting to polyneuropathy, nephritis, myocarditis, and vascular collapse
- Presence of strains not producing toxin (tox$^+$) in the respiratory tract of asymptomatic carriers and in skin lesions of cutaneous diphtheria

DIAGNOSIS

DIFFERENTIAL DIAGNOSIS

- Streptococcal pharyngitis
- Viral pharyngitis
- Mononucleosis

WORKUP

- Presence of a pseudomembrane in the oropharynx suggestive of diagnosis (not always present)
- Gram stains of secretions to show club-shaped organisms, which appear as "Chinese letters"
- Nasolaryngoscopy to identify lesions in the nares, nasopharynx, larynx, or tracheobronchial tree

LABORATORY TESTS

- Cultures of mucosal lesions or of nasal discharge
  1. Positive culture for *C. diphtheriae* confirms the diagnosis.
  2. Laboratory is notified of the suspected diagnosis so that appropriate culture medium (Tinsdale agar) is used.
- Testing of all isolated organisms for toxin production

IMAGING STUDIES

Chest radiograph examination to rule out pneumonia

TREATMENT

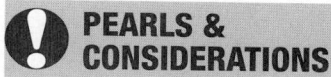

NONPHARMACOLOGIC THERAPY

- Intubation or tracheostomy if signs of respiratory distress occur
- Nasogastric or parenteral nutrition in those with bulbar signs
- ICU monitoring for patients with signs of systemic toxicity
- Cardiac pacing in patients with heart block
- Respiratory isolation

ACUTE GENERAL Rx

- Administration of diphtheria antitoxin once a clinical diagnosis is made
- If tests for hypersensitivity to horse serum are negative: 20,000 to 40,000 units for pharyngeal/laryngeal disease present less than 48 hr, 40,000 to 60,000 units for nasopharyngeal disease, and 80,000 to 120,000 units for greater than 3 days of illness or diffuse neck swelling ("bull-neck") (available via the CDC)
- IV infusion of antitoxin over 60 min
- Serum sickness in 10% of treated individuals; those with hypersensitivity to horse serum should be desensitized before administration of antitoxin
- Antibiotics to eradicate the organism in carriers or patients

- For respiratory diphtheria:
  1. Erythromycin 500 mg qid PO or IV (clarithromycin and azithromycin are acceptable alternatives) or IV penicillin G 25,000 to 50,000 units/kg to a maximum of 1.2 million units bid for 14 days. The course may be completed orally when able.
  2. Carriers or patients with cutaneous disease: erythromycin 500 mg PO qid or IM penicillin.
  3. Patients should be given diphtheria toxoid vaccine during convalescence as disease does not interfere with immunity.

CHRONIC Rx

Antibiotics to limit toxin production and eradicate carrier state, thereby preventing transmission

DISPOSITION

Complete recovery with adequate supportive measures and antitoxin

REFERRAL

- Hospitalization and referral to an infectious disease specialist for all suspected patients
- To an otolaryngologist for evaluation in cases of respiratory diphtheria
- All cases reported to the public health authorities

PEARLS & CONSIDERATIONS

COMMENTS

- Most cases are imported by travelers in epidemic areas, so recent epidemics in Eastern Europe are a cause for concern. A widespread epidemic of diphtheria began in 1990 in the former Soviet Union.
- Vaccination with diphtheria toxoid (attenuated toxin) is safe and effective in the form of DPT or Td; Td boosters should be given to adults every 10 yr. A new formulation of Tdap vaccine with reduced amounts of diphtheria toxoid and acellular pertussis antigens is available; it is well tolerated in clinical trials and provides excellent protection in adolescents and adults.
- According to serologic studies, 20% to 60% of U.S. adults >20 yr of age are susceptible to diphtheria.

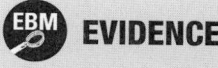 **EVIDENCE**

available at www.expertconsult.com

SUGGESTED READINGS
available at www.expertconsult.com

AUTHOR: **PATRICIA CRISTOFARO, M.D.**

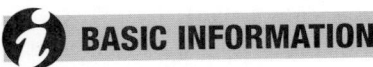

BASIC INFORMATION

DEFINITION

Discoid lupus erythematosus (DLE) refers to a chronic inflammatory autoimmune skin disorder that can lead to significant disfiguration and scarring. It can be associated with systemic lupus erythematosus (SLE).

SYNONYMS

Chronic cutaneous lupus erythematosus (CLE)

ICD-9CM CODES
695.4 Lupus erythematosus erythematodes (discoid) erythematosus (discoid), not disseminated

EPIDEMIOLOGY & DEMOGRAPHICS

- Slightly more common in African Americans than in Asians or whites
- Cutaneous lupus erythematosus is two to three times more likely in women than in men

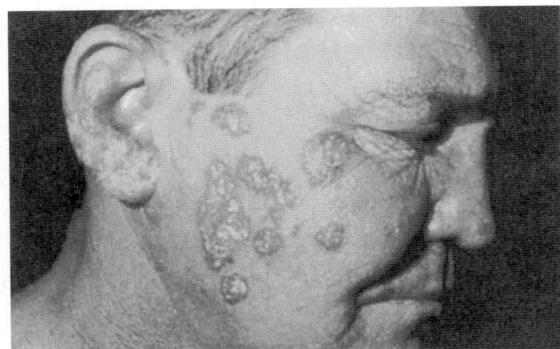

FIGURE 1-122 Scaling plaques with thick scales on the ear and face of a patient with discoid lupus. (Courtesy Department of Dermatology, University of North Carolina at Chapel Hill. From Goldstein BG, Goldstein AO [eds]: *Practical dermatology,* ed 2, St Louis, 1977, Mosby.)

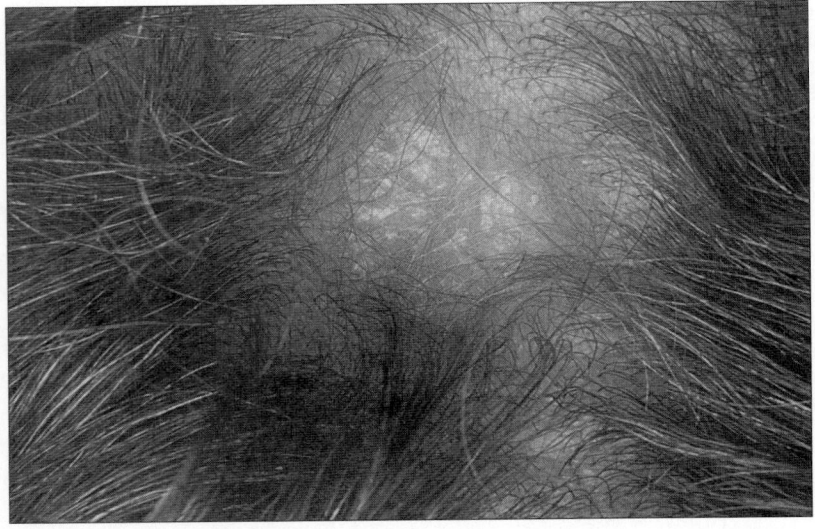

FIGURE 1-123 Discoid lupus erythematosus. There is considerable scaling and conspicuous background erythema. (Courtesy of the Institute of Dermatology, London, UK. From Granter SR [ed]: *Pathology of the skin with clinical correlations,* St Louis, Mosby.)

- Approximately 5% to 10% of patients presenting with DLE will develop SLE; those with widespread, numerous lesions are more likely to progress

PHYSICAL FINDINGS & CLINICAL PRESENTATION

General:
- Early lesions: single or multiple erythematous or violaceous, discrete papules or plaques with scale, often extending into dilated hair follicles (Figs. 1-122 and 1-123)
- Older lesions: peripheral hyperpigmentation with scarring, central depigmentation, and telangiectasia

Anatomic distribution:
- Commonly involves the scalp, face, ears, and extensor surface of the arms
- Mucosal and nail involvement is also possible

Lesion configuration:
- Irregularly grouped, confluent and disfiguring plaques

Lesion morphology:
- Plaque lesions with scale
- Follicular plugging

- Atrophy
- Irreversible, scarring alopecia (34%)
- May be associated with other clinical findings of SLE (e.g., oral ulcers, arthritis, pleuritis, pericarditis)

ETIOLOGY

Unknown, but thought to be an autoimmune-mediated disorder

DX DIAGNOSIS

Clinical findings and skin biopsy are used to establish the diagnosis of DLE

DIFFERENTIAL DIAGNOSIS

Psoriasis, lichen planus or lichen planopilaris, dermatophyte infections, photosensitivity eruption, sarcoidosis, subacute CLE, rosacea, dermatomyositis, cutaneous T-cell lymphoma

LABORATORY TESTS

- Complete blood count is usually normal in isolated DLE, but a small percentage of patients may show low-grade anemia
- Blood urea nitrogen and creatinine are normal in isolated DLE
- Erythrocyte sedimentation rate is elevated in active disease
- Urinalysis may show proteinuria
- Antinuclear antibody positive in 30% to 40% of patients with isolated DLE
- Anti-Ro (SS-A) autoantibodies are present in 1% to 3% of patients
- dsDNA antibodies are uncommon
- Complement levels may be low in rare instances
- Histology of skin reveals hyperkeratosis with follicular plugging, a thickened basement membrane, and a perivascular, interstitial, and appendageal lymphocytic infiltrate

RX TREATMENT

NONPHARMACOLOGIC THERAPY

Avoid sun exposure by using protective clothing and a broad-spectrum sunscreen of SPF >30

ACUTE GENERAL Rx

1. Topical steroids: intermediate- to high-potency steroids are needed; use caution when applying to the face
2. Intralesional steroids: triamcinolone acetonide 2.5 to 5.0 mg/ml with 1% Xylocaine
3. Topical calcineurin inhibitors: pimecrolimus 1% cream and tacrolimus 0.1% ointment
4. Hydroxychloroquine sulfate 400 mg PO qd
5. Avoid use of systemic glucocorticoids in patients with isolated DLE because of risks of side effects

CHRONIC Rx

1. Chloroquine 250 to 500 mg PO qd
2. Auranofin 6 mg/day PO qd or divided bid; after 3 mo, may increase to 9 mg/day divided tid
3. Thalidomide 100 to 300 mg PO before sleep, with water, and >1 hr after meals for refractory CLE

4. Azathioprine 1 mg/kg/day PO for 6 to 8 wk, increase by 5 mg/kg q4 wk until response is seen or dose reaches 2.5 mg/kg/day
5. Dapsone: 100 mg/day

DISPOSITION

If untreated, DLE can lead to significant and permanent atrophy and scarring of the skin.

REFERRAL

Dermatology, rheumatology

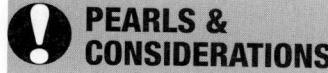 **PEARLS & CONSIDERATIONS**

- Cutaneous lesions account for four of the 11 criteria in the diagnosis of SLE (e.g., malar rash, discoid rash, photosensitivity, and oral ulcers).
- Rarely, patients with DLE may develop non-melanoma skin cancer in areas of disease.

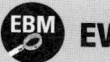 **EVIDENCE**

available at www.expertconsult.com

SUGGESTED READINGS

available at www.expertconsult.com

AUTHORS: **KACHIU LEE, B.A.,** and **JESSICA RISSER, M.D., M.P.H.**

D

Diseases and Disorders

I

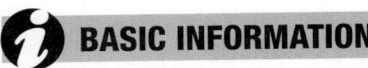

BASIC INFORMATION

DEFINITION

Disseminated intravascular coagulation (DIC) is an acquired thromboembolic disorder characterized by generalized activation of the clotting mechanism, which results in the intravascular formation of fibrin and ultimately thrombotic occlusion of small and midsize vessels.

SYNONYMS

Consumptive coagulopathy
DIC
Defibrination syndrome

ICD-9CM CODES
286.6 Disseminated intravascular coagulation

EPIDEMIOLOGY & DEMOGRAPHICS

More than 50% of cases are associated with gram-negative sepsis or other septicemic infections.

PHYSICAL FINDINGS & CLINICAL PRESENTATION

- Wound site bleeding, epistaxis, gingival bleeding, hemorrhagic bullae
- Petechiae, ecchymosis, purpura
- Dyspnea, localized rales, delirium
- Oliguria, anuria, gastrointestinal bleeding, metrorrhagia

ETIOLOGY

- Infections (e.g., gram-negative sepsis, Rocky Mountain spotted fever, malaria, viral or fungal infection)
- Obstetric complications (e.g., dead fetus, amniotic fluid embolism, toxemia, abruptio placentae, septic abortion, eclampsia, placenta previa, uterine atony)
- Tissue trauma (e.g., burns, hypothermia rewarming)
- Neoplasms (e.g., adenocarcinomas [gastrointestinal, prostate, lung, breast], acute promyelocytic leukemia)
- Quinine, cocaine-induced rhabdomyolysis
- Liver failure
- Acute pancreatitis
- Transfusion reactions
- Respiratory distress syndrome
- Toxins (snake bites, amphetamine overdose)
- Other: systemic lupus erythematosus (SLE), vasculitis, aneurysms, polyarteritis, cavernous hemangiomas

DIAGNOSIS

DIFFERENTIAL DIAGNOSIS

- Hepatic necrosis: normal or elevated Factor VIII concentrations

- Vitamin K deficiency: normal platelet count
- Hemolytic uremic syndrome
- Thrombotic thrombocytopenic purpura
- Renal failure, SLE, sickle cell crisis, dysfibrinogenemias
- HELLP syndrome (*h*emolysis, *e*levated *l*iver function tests, and *l*ow *p*latelets)
- Section III describes an algorithm for the differential diagnosis of deep vein thrombosis

WORKUP

Diagnostic workup includes laboratory screening to confirm the diagnosis and exclude conditions noted in the differential diagnosis. Workup is also aimed at distinguishing DIC progression (acute vs. chronic), chief manifestations (thrombotic or hemorrhagic), and extent (localized or systemic).

LABORATORY TESTS

- Peripheral blood smear generally shows red blood cell fragments (schistocytes) and low platelet count.
- Coagulation factors are consumed at a rate in excess of the capacity of the liver to synthesize them, and platelets are consumed in excess of the capacity of the bone marrow megakaryocytes to release them. Diagnostic characteristics of DIC are decreased fibrinogen level; thrombocytopenia; and increased prothrombin time (PT), partial thromboplastin time (PTT), TT, fibrin split products, and D-dimer.
- Coagulopathy secondary to DIC must be differentiated from that secondary to liver disease or vitamin K deficiency.
  1. Vitamin K deficiency manifests with prolonged PT and normal PTT, TT, platelet, and fibrinogen level; PTT may be elevated in severe cases.
  2. Patients with liver disease have abnormal PT and PTT; TT and fibrinogen are usually normal unless severe disease is present; platelets are usually normal unless splenomegaly is present.
  3. Factors V and VIII are low in DIC, but they are normal in liver disease with coagulopathy.

IMAGING STUDIES

Imaging studies are generally not useful. Chest radiographs may be helpful to exclude infectious processes in patients with pulmonary symptoms such as dyspnea, cough, or hemoptysis.

TREATMENT

NONPHARMACOLOGIC THERAPY

No specific precautions regarding activity level are necessary unless thrombocytopenia is severe.

ACUTE GENERAL Rx

- Correct and eliminate underlying cause (e.g., antimicrobial therapy for infection, removal of necrotic bowel, evacuation of uterus in obstetric emergencies).
- Give replacement therapy with fresh frozen plasma (FFP) and platelets in patients with significant hemorrhage:
  1. FFP 10 to 15 ml/kg can be given with a goal of normalizing International Normalized Ratio.
  2. Platelet transfusions are given when platelet count is <10,000 (or higher if major bleeding is present).
  3. Cryoprecipitate 1 U/5 kg is reserved for hypofibrinogen states.
  4. Antithrombin III treatment may be considered as a supportive therapeutic option in patients with severe DIC. Its modest results and substantial cost are limiting factors.
- Heparin therapy at a dose lower than that used in venous thrombosis (300 to 500 U/hr) may be useful in selected cases to increase neutralization of thrombin (e.g., DIC associated with acute promyelocytic leukemia, purpura fulminans, acral ischemia).

CHRONIC Rx

Follow-up management includes coagulation screening to assess factor replacement therapy. Laboratory abnormalities generally correct with treatment of the underlying disorder. Long-term laboratory monitoring is not required.

DISPOSITION

Mortality rate in severe DIC exceeds 75%. Death generally results from progression of the underlying disease and complications such as acute renal failure, intracerebral hematoma, shock, or cardiac tamponade.

REFERRAL

Hematology consultation is recommended in all cases of DIC.

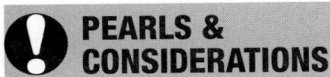

PEARLS & CONSIDERATIONS

COMMENTS

The treatment of chronic DIC is controversial. Low-dose SC heparin and/or combination antiplatelet agents such as aspirin and dipyridamole may be useful.

AUTHOR: **FRED F. FERRI, M.D.**

BASIC INFORMATION

DEFINITION

- Colonic diverticula are herniations of mucosa and submucosa through the muscularis. They are generally found along the colon's mesenteric border at the site where the vasa recta penetrates the muscle wall (anatomic weak point).
- *Diverticulosis* is the asymptomatic presence of multiple colonic diverticula.
- *Diverticulitis* is an inflammatory process or localized perforation of diverticulum.

ICD-9CM CODES
562.10 Diverticulosis of colon
562.11 Diverticulitis of colon

EPIDEMIOLOGY & DEMOGRAPHICS

- Incidence of diverticulosis in the general population is 35% to 50%.
- Diverticulosis is more common in Western countries, affecting >30% of people >40 yr and >50% of people >70 yr.

PHYSICAL FINDINGS & CLINICAL PRESENTATION

- Physical examination in patients with diverticulosis is generally normal.
- Painful diverticular disease can present with LLQ pain, often relieved by defecation; location of pain may be anywhere in the lower abdomen because of the redundancy of the sigmoid colon.
- Diverticulitis can cause muscle spasm, guarding, and rebound tenderness predominantly affecting the LLQ.

ETIOLOGY

Diverticular disease is believed to be secondary to low intake of dietary fiber.

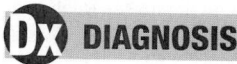

DIAGNOSIS

DIFFERENTIAL DIAGNOSIS

- Irritable bowel syndrome
- IBD
- Carcinoma of colon
- Endometriosis
- Ischemic colitis
- Infections (pseudomembranous colitis, appendicitis, pyelonephritis, PID)
- Lactose intolerance

LABORATORY TESTS

- WBC count in diverticulitis reveals leukocytosis with left shift.
- Microcytic anemia can be present in patients with chronic bleeding from diverticular disease. MCV may be elevated in acute bleeding secondary to reticulocytosis.

PROCEDURES: Colonoscopy should be avoided during acute diverticulitis due to the risk of perforation. It can generally be performed after 6 wk to rule out the presence of cancer and IBD.

IMAGING STUDIES

- A CT scan of the abdomen is recommended as the initial radiologic examination to diagnose acute diverticulitis; It has a sensitivity of 93% to 97% and a specificity approaching 100%. Typical findings are thickening of the bowel wall, fistulas, or abscess formation. CT may also reveal other disease processes (e.g., appendicitis, tubo-ovarian abscess, Crohn's disease) accounting for lower abdominal pain
- Evaluation of suspected diverticular bleeding:
  1. Arteriography if the bleeding is faster than 1 ml/min (advantage: the possible infusion of vasopressin directly into the arteries supplying the bleeding, as well as selective arterial embolization; disadvantages: its cost and invasive nature).
  2. Technetium-99m sulfa colloid
  3. Technetium-99m labeled RBC (can detect bleeding rates as low as 0.12 to 5 ml/min)

TREATMENT

NONPHARMACOLOGIC THERAPY

- Increase in dietary fiber intake and regular exercise to improve bowel function
- NPO and IV hydration in severe diverticulitis; NG suction if ileus or small bowel obstruction is present

ACUTE GENERAL Rx
TREATMENT OF DIVERTICULITIS:

- Mild case: broad-spectrum PO antibiotics (e.g., Ciprofloxacin 500 mg bid to cover aerobic component of colonic flora and metronidazole 500 mg q6h for anaerobes) and liquid diet for 7 to 10 days
- Severe case: NPO and aggressive IV antibiotic therapy
  a. Ampicillin-sulbactam 3 g IV q6h *or*
  b. Piperacillin-tazobactam 4.5 g IV q8h *or*
  c. Ciprofloxacin 400 mg IV q12h plus metronidazole 500 mg IV q6h *or*
  d. Cefoxitin 2 g IV q8h plus metronidazole 500 mg IV q6h
- Life-threatening case: Imipenem 500 mg IV q6h *or* meropenem 1 g IV q8h
- Surgical treatment consisting of resection of involved areas and reanastomosis (if feasible); otherwise a diverting colostomy with reanastomosis performed when infection has been controlled; surgery should be considered in patients with:
  1. Repeated episodes of diverticulitis (two or more)
  2. Poor response to appropriate medical therapy (failure of conservative management)
  3. Abscess or fistula formation
  4. Obstruction
  5. Peritonitis
  6. Immunocompromised patients, first episode in young patient (<40 yr old)
  7. Inability to exclude carcinoma (10% to 20% of patients diagnosed with diverticulosis on clinical grounds are subsequently found to have carcinoma of the colon)

DIVERTICULAR HEMORRHAGE:
1. Bleeding is painless and stops spontaneously in the majority of patients (60%); it is usually caused by erosion of a blood vessel by a fecalith present within the diverticular sac.
2. Medical therapy consists of blood replacement and correction of volume and any clotting abnormalities.
3. Colonoscopic treatment with epinephrine injections, bipolar coagulation, or both may prevent recurrent bleeding and decrease the need for surgery.
4. Surgical resection is necessary if bleeding does not stop spontaneously after administration of 4 to 5 U of PRBCs or recurs with severity within a few days; if attempts at localization are unsuccessful, total abdominal colectomy with ileoproctostomy may be indicated (high incidence of rebleeding if segmental resection is performed without adequate localization).

CHRONIC Rx

Asymptomatic patients with diverticulosis can be treated with a high-fiber diet or fiber supplements.

DISPOSITION

- Most patients with diverticulitis respond well to antibiotic management and bowel rest. Up to 30% of patients with diverticulitis will eventually require surgical management.
- Diverticular bleeding can recur in 15% to 20% of patients within 5 yr.

REFERRAL

GI referral for colonoscopy. Surgical referral when considering resection.

SUGGESTED READING
available at www.expertconsult.com

AUTHOR: **FRED F. FERRI, M.D.**

D

Diseases
and Disorders

I

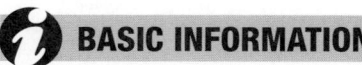

DEFINITION

Down syndrome is a disorder characterized by mental retardation and multiple organ defects that is caused by a chromosomal abnormality (trisomy 21).

SYNONYMS

Trisomy 21

ICD-9CM CODES
758.0 Down Syndrome

EPIDEMIOLOGY & DEMOGRAPHICS

INCIDENCE (IN U.S.): 1 in 800 births
PEAK INCIDENCE: Newborn
PREVALENCE (IN U.S.): 300,000 persons
PREDOMINANT SEX: Male:female ratio of 1.3:1.0
PREDOMINANT AGE: Newborn to early adulthood
GENETICS: Nondisjunction causing trisomy 21

PHYSICAL FINDINGS & CLINICAL PRESENTATION

(Fig. 1-124)
- Microcephaly
- Flattening of occiput and face

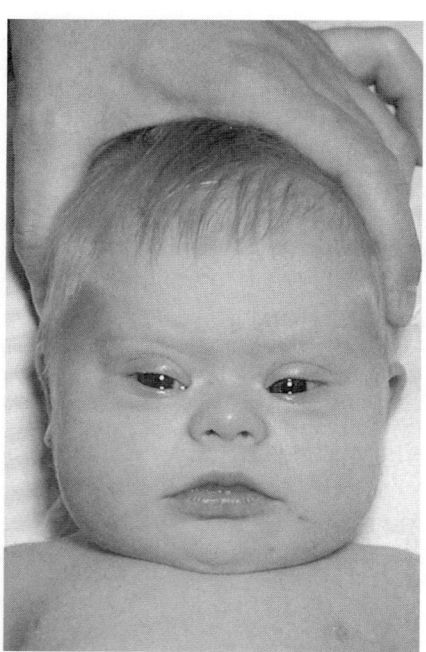

FIGURE 1-124 Down syndrome. Note depressed nasal bridge, epicanthal folds, mongoloid slant of eyes, low-set ears, and large tongue. (From Zitelli BJ, Davis HW: *Atlas of pediatric physical diagnosis*, ed 3, St Louis, 1997, Mosby.)

- Upward slant to eyes with epicanthal folds
- Brushfield spots in iris
- Broad, stocky neck
- Small feet, hands, digits
- Single palmar crease
- Hypotonia
- Short stature
- Associated with congenital heart disease, malformations of the GI tract, cataracts, hypothyroidism, hip dysplasia, obstructive sleep apnea, and myeloproliferative disorders
- About half of children with Down syndrome are born with congenital heart disease, with the most common lesions being atrial septal defect and ventricular septal defect
- Persistent primary congenital hypothyroidism is found in 1 in 141 newborns with Down syndrome, as compared with 1 in 4000 in the general population
- Ophthalmologic disorders increase in frequency with age; >80% of children aged 5 to 12 yr have disorders that need monitoring or intervention, such as refractive errors, strabismus, or cataracts
- Renal and urinary tract abnormalities

ETIOLOGY

Nondisjunction of chromosome 21

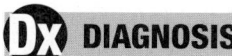
DIAGNOSIS

- Prenatal cytogenic diagnosis by amniocentesis or chorionic villus sampling
- Combined use of serum screening and fetal ultrasound testing for thickened nuchal fold has 85% detection rate with 5% false-positive results
- Postnatal chromosomal karyotype

DIFFERENTIAL DIAGNOSIS

- Congenital hypothyroidism
- Other chromosomal abnormalities

WORKUP

Postnatal chromosomal karyotype

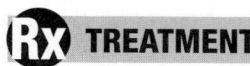
TREATMENT

- Thyroid screen at birth, at age 6 mo, and yearly thereafter
- Echocardiogram in all newborns and cardiac assessment of adolescents for development of mitral valve prolapse
- Treatment consists of vigilant monitoring for comorbid states, such as obesity, hypothyroidism, leukemia, hearing loss, and valvular heart disease
- Prevention of obesity with low-calorie, high-fiber diet
- Auditory brain stem responses in all newborns and aggressive testing for hearing loss in children with chronic otitis media

- Ophthalmologic assessment by age 6 mo for congenital cataracts and annual examinations for monitoring of refractive errors and strabismus
- Regular dental care
- Pelvic examination of women who are sexually active or who have menstrual problems
- Dermatologic issues such as folliculitis can become problematic in adolescents, and require topical antibiotics and careful attention to hygiene

DISPOSITION

Most children with Down syndrome live at home. As these individuals reach adulthood, those with higher functioning sometimes live in supervised settings away from their families.

REFERRAL

Down syndrome clinics use a preventive checklist to anticipate many clinical challenges.

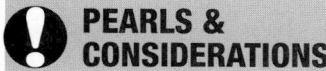
PEARLS & CONSIDERATIONS

COMMENTS

- Screening for atlantoaxial subluxation is controversial.
- Most patients experience neuropathologic changes typical of Alzheimer's disease. Presenting symptoms include seizures, focal neurologic signs, and apathy. If Alzheimer's disease is suspected, screen for treatable diseases such as depression or hypothyroidism.
- This syndrome accounts for approximately one third of moderate-to-severe cases of mental retardation.
- Individuals with Down syndrome have a wide range of function, but all will have decrease in intelligence quotient (IQ) in first decade of life.
- Deficiency of language production relative to other areas of development often causes substantial impairment.
- Individuals with Down syndrome have more behavioral and psychiatric problems than other children, but fewer than other individuals with mental retardation.
- Though increased maternal age is a risk factor, most children with Down syndrome are born to women younger than 35 yr.

SUGGESTED READINGS
available at www.expertconsult.com

AUTHOR: **MAITREYI MAZUMDAR, M.D., M.P.H.**

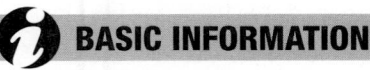

BASIC INFORMATION

DEFINITION

Dumping syndrome refers to a constellation of postprandial symptoms resulting from rapid delivery of hypertonic stomach contents into the small bowel that is most often caused by gastric surgery, such as procedures for peptic ulcer disease and gastric bypass.

SYNONYMS

Postgastrectomy syndrome
Rapid gastric emptying

ICD-9CM CODES

564.2 Postgastric surgery syndromes

EPIDEMIOLOGY & DEMOGRAPHICS

Incidence is 10% of all patients having gastric surgery.
- Vagotomy and pyloroplasty (8.5% to 20%)
- Vagotomy and antrectomy (4% to 27%)
- Subtotal gastrectomy (10% to 40%)
- Parietal cell vagotomy (3% to 5%)
- Gastric bypass surgeries (up to 50%)
- Males and females are affected equally

PHYSICAL FINDINGS & CLINICAL PRESENTATION

1. Early dumping syndrome: symptoms start within 1 hr after eating food:
   - No symptoms in fasting state
   - Nausea, vomiting, and belching
   - Epigastric fullness, cramping, and diarrhea
   - Dizziness, flushing, diaphoresis, and syncope
   - Palpitations and tachycardia
2. Late dumping syndrome: symptoms occurring 1 to 3 hr after eating:
   - Diaphoresis
   - Irritability
   - Difficulty in concentration
   - Tremulousness

ETIOLOGY

Dumping syndrome occurs almost exclusively in patients who have had gastric surgery.
- Systemic symptoms in early dumping syndrome are thought to be partially due to hypovolemia caused by rapid shifts of fluid from the intravascular space into the lumen of the bowel.
- Increase in vasoactive substances related to rapid gastric emptying is thought to play a role in dumping syndrome.
- Late dumping symptoms are thought to be due to reactive hypoglycemia.

DIAGNOSIS

A detailed clinical history and evidence of prior gastric surgery are necessary for the diagnosis.

DIFFERENTIAL DIAGNOSIS

- Pancreatic insufficiency
- Inflammatory bowel disease
- Afferent loop syndromes
- Bile acid reflux after surgery
- Bowel obstruction
- Gastroenteric fistula

WORKUP

Diagnosis is typically made on clinical grounds. In certain clinical settings, where patients exhibit symptoms with no prior history of gastric surgery, oral glucose challenge and imaging studies may be pursued and aid in establishing the diagnosis.

LABORATORY TESTS

Oral glucose challenge test:
- After overnight fasting, oral intake of 50 g of glucose is followed by serial measurements of heart rate, serum glucose, and hydrogen breath test every 15 to 30 min for 3 to 6 hrs. A 30 min hematocrit can also be taken.
- An increase in the heart rate >12 beats/min and a rise in hydrogen breath excretion have a sensitivity of 94% and specificity >92%. An increase of >3% in the 30 min hematocrit is also suggestive of a positive test. A nadir blood glucose <3.3 mmol/L (<59 mg/dl) was present in 75% of late dumpers.

IMAGING STUDIES

- Upper GI series properly defines anatomy.
- Scintigraphic imaging documents rapid gastric emptying and may be useful in patients with dumping syndrome and no prior history of gastric surgery.

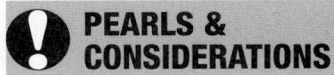

TREATMENT

NONPHARMACOLOGIC THERAPY

- Diet modification
  1. Divide caloric intake over six small meals
  2. Limit fluid intake with meals (try to avoid fluids 30 min before meals and following meals)
  3. Decrease carbohydrate intake and avoid simple sugars
  4. Increase/supplement dietary fibers
  5. Avoid milk/milk products

ACUTE GENERAL Rx

- Acarbose 50 mg PO daily can be tried if dietary modification does not help.
- Octreotide 25 to 50 µg SC 30 min before meals is effective in relieving symptoms of dumping syndrome.
- Pectin and Guar have been used to increase viscosity of intraluminal contents and relieve symptoms from rapid emptying and absorption.

CHRONIC Rx

- Surgery is considered in patients with severe symptoms refractory to the above mentioned dietary and acute general treatment.
- Surgical procedures include: reconstruction of the pylorus, converting Billroth II to a Billroth I anastomosis, and a Roux-en-Y reconstruction.
- In severe cases, can consider depot long acting release octreotide, given as 10 mg intramuscularly every 4 wks for symptom relief.

DISPOSITION

- Dumping syndrome improves with time. Approximately 1% to 2% of patients will continue to have significant symptoms several months after surgery.
- Dietary modification effectively treats the majority of patients.

REFERRAL

- A gastrointestinal specialist consult is recommended in patients suspected of having dumping syndrome.
- If medical management is unsuccessful, a general surgical consultation is warranted.

PEARLS & CONSIDERATIONS

COMMENTS

- The majority of patients usually manifest with early dumping symptoms or combination of early and late symptoms. Few have late dumping symptoms alone.
- Octreotide has an inhibitory effect on the release of insulin and other vasoactive substances released by the gut. It also works by decreasing gastric emptying.

SUGGESTED READINGS

available at www.expertconsult.com

AUTHOR: **MARK F. BRADY, M.D., M.P.H., M.M.S.**

D

Diseases and Disorders

I

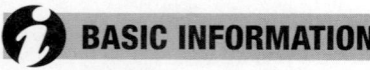

DEFINITION

Dupuytren's contracture is a disease of the palmar fascia characterized by nodular fibroblastic proliferation that often results in progressive contractures of the fascia and flexion deformity of the fingers.

ICD-9CM CODES
728.6 Dupuytren's contracture

EPIDEMIOLOGY & DEMOGRAPHICS

PREVALENCE: Varies depending on nationality
PREVALENT SEX: Male/female ratio of 10:1
PREVALENT AGE: 40 to 60 yr

PHYSICAL FINDINGS & CLINICAL PRESENTATION

- Usually asymptomatic
- Most common complaints: deformity and interference with the use of the hand by the flexed, contracted fingers (Fig. 1-125)
- Process usually begins on the ulnar side of the hand, often starting at the ring finger
- Isolated, painless nodules that eventually harden and mature into a longitudinal cord that extends into the finger
- Lesion often begins in the distal palmar crease
- Overlying skin adherent to the fascia
- Later stages: fibrous cord begins to contract and pull the finger into flexion
- Possible involvement of other fingers, particularly small finger

ETIOLOGY

Unknown. Pathologically, the contracture consists of proliferating vascular tissue that later develops into mature collagen.

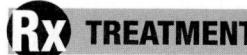 **DIAGNOSIS**

DIFFERENTIAL DIAGNOSIS

- Soft tissue tumor
- Tendon cyst

WORKUP

The typical case is easily diagnosed clinically. Plain radiographs may be useful to rule out bony abnormalities.

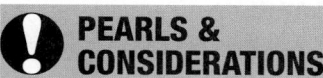 **TREATMENT**

NONPHARMACOLOGIC THERAPY

- Stretching exercises
- Local heat

- Surgical referral is indicated when metacarpophalangeal joint contracture occurs at any degree.
- Surgery is usually performed when the metacarpophalangeal joint contracture exceeds 40 degrees or when the proximal interphalangeal joint contracture exceeds 20 degrees.
- Percutaneous needle aponeurotomy performed in the office represents an alternative to surgery.

DISPOSITION

Rate of development is variable.

REFERRAL

- If joint contracture begins to develop
- For excision of rare nodule that is painful (at any stage)

PEARLS & CONSIDERATIONS

COMMENTS

- Dupuytren's contracture develops earlier and more often in certain families.
- The disorder is more common in Scandinavians; some Northern Europeans have a 25% prevalence after age 60 yr.
- Approximately 5% of patients develop a similar condition elsewhere, such as Peyronie's disease or Ledderhose disease (involvement of the plantar fascia).
- Soft tissue "pads" in the knuckles may also be present.
- Individuals with these additional findings are considered to have Dupuytren's diathesis, and their disease is generally more severe and recurrent.

SUGGESTED READINGS
available at www.expertconsult.com

AUTHOR: **LONNIE R. MERCIER, M.D.**

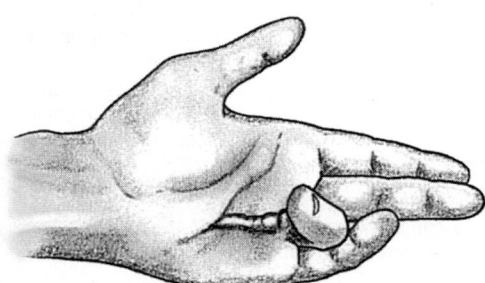

FIGURE 1-125 Dupuytren's contracture. A flexion deformity of the finger is present, with nodular thickening of the fascia to the ring finger.

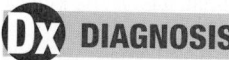

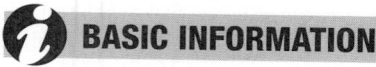

DEFINITION

Dysfunctional uterine bleeding (DUB) describes abnormal uterine bleeding in the absence of disease in the pelvis, pregnancy, or medical illness. Parameters of normal menstrual function are described in Box 1-4. Specific types of abnormal bleeding include the following:

- Hypermenorrhea: excessive bleeding amount during normal duration of regular menstrual cycles
- Hypomenorrhea: decreased bleeding amount in regular menstrual cycles
- Menorrhagia: regular normal intervals, excessive flow and duration
- Metrorrhagia: irregular intervals, excessive flow and duration
- Menometrorrhagia: irregular or excessive bleeding during menstruation and between periods
- Oligomenorrhea: intervals >35 days
- Polymenorrhea: intervals <21 days

SYNONYMS

DUB

ICD-9CM CODES
626	Disorders of menstruation and other abnormal bleeding from female genital tract
626.2	Hypermenorrhea
626.1	Hypomenorrhea
626.2	Menorrhagia
626.6	Metrorrhagia
626.2	Menometrorrhagia
626.1	Oligomenorrhea
626.2	Polymenorrhea

EPIDEMIOLOGY & DEMOGRAPHICS

- Most cases of DUB occur in postmenarchal and perimenopausal age groups.
- During reproductive age, <20% of abnormal bleeding results from anovulatory DUB.

PHYSICAL FINDINGS & CLINICAL PRESENTATION

- A clinical diagnosis of exclusion
- Thorough physical and pelvic examination to exclude the other causes of abnormal bleeding
  1. Includes thyroid, breast, liver, presence or absence of ecchymotic lesions
  2. Patient possibly obese and hirsute (polycystic ovarian disease)
  3. No evidence of any vulvar, vaginal, cervical lesions, uterine (fibroid) or ovarian tumor, urethral caruncle, urethral diverticula, hemorrhoids, anal fissure, colorectal lesions
  4. Bimanual pelvic examination: normal-sized or slightly enlarged uterus

ETIOLOGY

- 90% is caused by anovulation.
- 10% is ovulatory in origin; can be caused by dysfunction of corpus luteum or midcycle bleeding.

- Section II describes the various causes of abnormal uterine bleeding.

DIAGNOSIS

DIFFERENTIAL DIAGNOSIS

- Pregnancy-related cause
- Anatomic uterine causes:
  1. Leiomyomas
  2. Adenomyosis
  3. Polyps
  4. Endometrial hyperplasia
  5. Cancer
  6. Sexually transmitted diseases
  7. Intrauterine contraceptive devices
- Anatomic nonuterine causes:
  1. Cervical neoplasia, cervicitis
  2. Vaginal neoplasia, adhesions, trauma, foreign body, atrophic vaginitis, infections, condyloma
  3. Vulvar trauma, infections, neoplasia, condyloma, dystrophy, varices
  4. Urinary tract: urethral caruncle, diverticulum, hematuria
  5. Gastrointestinal tract: hemorrhoids, anal fissure, colorectal lesions
- Systemic diseases:
  1. Exogenous hormone intake
  2. Coagulopathies: von Willebrand's disease, thrombocytopenia, hepatic failure
  3. Endocrinopathies: thyroid disorder, hypothyroidism and hyperthyroidism, diabetes mellitus
  4. Renal diseases
- Section II describes a differential diagnosis of vaginal bleeding abnormalities.

WORKUP

- A detailed history and thorough physical examination, including a pelvic examination to exclude causes mentioned above.
- Clinical algorithms for the evaluation of vaginal bleeding are described in Section III, "Bleeding, Vaginal."

LABORATORY TESTS

- Complete blood count with platelets; possible iron-deficiency anemia or thrombocytopenia
- Prothrombin; partial thromboplastin and bleeding time if coagulopathy is suspected
- Serum human chorionic gonadotropin
- Chemistry profile, including liver function tests
- Thyroid profile
- Stool testing for occult blood
- Urinalysis for hematuria
- Pap smear

BOX 1-4 Parameters of Normal Menstrual Function

Cycle interval (days)	21-35
Duration of flow (days)	2-8
Blood loss/cycle (ml)	30-80

Carlson KJ, Eisenstat SA, Frigoletto FD, Schiff I: *Primary care of women*, ed 2, St Louis, Mosby, 2002.

- Cultures for gonorrhea and *Chlamydia*
- Serum gonadotropins and prolactin
- Serum androgens
- Endometrial biopsy in women >35 yr or earlier if longstanding history of anovulatory bleeding
- Hysterogram and hysteroscopy

IMAGING STUDIES

- Pelvic ultrasound, including measurement of endometrial thickness
- Fluid contrast ultrasound (also called saline sonogram, sonohysterogram, hydrosonogram, and various other names)

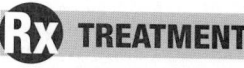

NONPHARMACOLOGIC THERAPY

Increase iron intake in the form of pills and in a diet rich in iron.

ACUTE GENERAL Rx

- Progestational agents (see Box 1-5)
  1. Progesterone in oil, 100 to 200 mg
  2. Medroxyprogesterone acetate, 20 to 40 mg qd for 15 days
  3. Megestrol acetate, 40 to 120 mg daily in divided doses for 15 days
  4. Oral contraceptives: any oral contraceptive pill, 1 tablet qid for 5 to 7 days, followed by 1 tablet low-dose estrogen qd for 21 days; causes withdrawal bleeding; should then be on cyclical Provera or continue on oral contraceptives
- Estrogens
  1. Conjugated estrogen (Premarin) 25 mg IV q4h until bleeding is under control (in cases of severe or life-threatening bleeding); maximum three doses
  2. For prolonged bleeding that is not life threatening: Premarin 1.25 mg (Estrace 2 mg) q4h for 24 hr, followed by Provera to bring on withdrawal bleeding; then sequential regimen of estrogen and progestin (Premarin 1.25 mg qd for 24 days, Provera 10 mg for last 10 days) or oral contraceptives
- Surgical treatment
  1. Dilation and curettage (D&C) and hysteroscopy
  2. Endometrial ablation
  3. Hysterectomy

BOX 1-5 Equivalent Daily Doses of Oral Progestins for the Treatment of Dysfunctional Uterine Bleeding

Medroxyprogesterone acetate (Provera, Cycrin)	10 mg
Micronized progesterone (Prometrium)	400 mg
Norgestrel (Ovrette)	150 µg
Norethindrone acetate (Micronor, Nor-QD)	0.7-1.0 mg

Carlson KJ, Eisenstat SA, Frigoletto FD, Schiff I: *Primary care of women*, ed 2, St Louis, Mosby, 2002.

CHRONIC Rx

- Progestational agents
  - Medroxyprogesterone acetate 10 mg qd for 12 days, then cyclically to induce monthly withdrawal bleeding
  - Norethindrone 2.5 to 10 mg qd for 12 days
  - Depo-Provera 150 mg IM and then 150 mg every 3 mo
  - Oral contraceptives, 1 tablet qd
  - Levonorgestrel-releasing intrauterine device (Mirena)
- Clomiphene citrate: patients with anovulatory bleeding who want to become pregnant

- Others
  - Antiprostaglandins
  - Danazol (rarely used due to side-effect profile)
  - Gonadotropin-releasing hormone analogs (GNRH)
  - Human menopausal gonadotropin (HMG) (desire pregnancy)
  - Tranexamic acid (Lysteda) is an antifibrinolytic agent recently FDA approved for cyclic heavy menstrual bleeding. Dosage in normal renal function is 3900 mg daily (650-mg tablets, 2 tablets tid) for up to 5 days during menses

- Surgical treatment
  1. D&C and hysteroscopy
  2. Endometrial ablation
  3. Hysterectomy

DISPOSITION

Cyclical treatment on birth control pills or Provera for several cycles, then discontinue pill and watch patient for onset of regular menses

REFERRAL

To gynecologist in case of failure of treatment

TABLE 1-43 Management of Dysfunctional Uterine Bleeding

Bleeding Pattern	Cause	Treatment
Ovulatory DUB		
Heavy menstrual bleeding	Imbalance in endometrial prostacyclins and prostaglandins	Nonsteroidal anti-inflammatory drugs Combination oral contraceptive pill Progestin intrauterine device Endometrial ablation
Midcycle spotting	Periovulatory estrogen decline	None
Delayed menses	Persistent corpus luteum	None (rule out pregnancy)
Anovulatory DUB		
Irregular menses	Unopposed estrogen stimulation of endometrium	Combination oral contraceptive pill Cyclic progestins Endometrial ablation
Postmenopausal bleeding	Endometrial atrophy	Hormone replacement therapy Endometrial ablation

DUB, Dysfunctional uterine bleeding.
Carlson KJ, Eisenstat SA, Frigoletto FD, Schiff I: *Primary care of women,* ed 2, St Louis, Mosby, 2002.

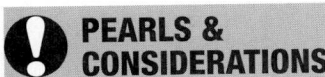

PEARLS & CONSIDERATIONS

COMMENTS

- Table 1-43 describes management options for dysfunctional uterine bleeding.
- Patient education material may be obtained from the American College of Obstetricians and Gynecologists, 409 12th Street SW, Washington, DC 20024-2188; phone 202-638-5577.

EVIDENCE

available at www.expertconsult.com

SUGGESTED READING

available at www.expertconsult.com

AUTHORS: **MANDEEP K. BRAR, M.D.,** and **RUBEN ALVERO, M.D.**

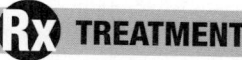

D

I

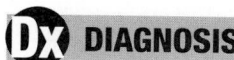 **BASIC INFORMATION**

DEFINITION

Dysmenorrhea is pain with menstruation, usually cramping and usually centered in the lower abdomen. It is defined as *primary dysmenorrhea* when there is no associated organic pathology and *secondary dysmenorrhea* when there is demonstrable organic pathology.

SYNONYMS

Menstrual cramps
Painful periods

ICD-9CM CODES
625.3 Dysmenorrhea

EPIDEMIOLOGY & DEMOGRAPHICS

Approximately 50% of menstruating women are affected by dysmenorrhea, with approximately 10% of them having severe dysmenorrhea with incapacitation for 1 to 3 days/mo. Dysmenorrhea is most common in the age group from 20 to 24 yr, and primary dysmenorrhea usually appears within 6 to 12 mo after menarche.

PHYSICAL FINDINGS & CLINICAL PRESENTATION

- Sharp, crampy, midline, lower abdominal pain without a lower quadrant or adnexal component but possible radiation to the lower back and upper thighs
- Unremarkable pelvic examination in nonmenstruating patient
- Accompanying symptoms: nausea, vomiting, headaches, anxiety, fatigue, diarrhea, fainting, and abdominal bloating
- Cramps usually lasting <24 hr and seldom lasting >2 to 3 days
- Secondary dysmenorrhea: dyspareunia is a common complaint, and bimanual pelvic-abdominal examination may demonstrate uterine or adnexal tenderness, fixed uterine retroflexion, uterosacral nodularity, a pelvic mass, or an enlarged, irregular uterus

ETIOLOGY

Prostaglandin $F_2\alpha$ is the agent responsible for dysmenorrhea. It stimulates uterine contractions and cervical stenosis (narrowing) and increases vasopressin release. Behavior and psychological factors have also been implicated in the etiology of primary dysmenorrhea. Primary

dysmenorrhea only occurs in ovulatory cycles. Secondary dysmenorrhea is usually caused by endometriosis, adenomyosis, leiomyomas and, less commonly, chronic salpingitis, intrauterine device (IUD) use, or congenital or acquired outflow tract obstruction, including cervical stenosis.

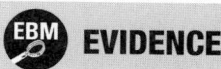 **DIAGNOSIS**

DIFFERENTIAL DIAGNOSIS

- Adenomyosis
- Adhesions
- Allen-Masters syndrome
- Cervical structures or stenosis
- Congenital malformation of müllerian system
- Ectopic pregnancy
- Endometriosis, endometritis
- Imperforate hymen
- IUD use
- Leiomyomas
- Ovarian cysts
- Pelvic congestion syndrome, pelvic inflammatory disease
- Polyps
- Transverse vaginal septum

WORKUP

- Primary dysmenorrhea: characteristic history, physical examination normal with the absence of an identifiable cause of pelvic pain
- Secondary dysmenorrhea: history of onset generally >2 yr after menarche; physical examination may reveal uterine irregularity, cul-de-sac tenderness, or nodularity or pelvic masses

LABORATORY TESTS

- No specific tests diagnostic for dysmenorrhea
- Elevated white blood cell count in the presence of infection
- Human chorionic gonadotropin to rule out ectopic pregnancy

IMAGING STUDIES

- Ultrasound scan of the pelvis to evaluate the presence of leiomyomas, ovarian cysts, or ectopic pregnancy
- Hysterosalpingogram or saline ultrasonography to assess the uterine cavity to rule out endometrial polyps or submucosal or intraluminal leiomyomas

Rx TREATMENT

NONPHARMACOLOGIC THERAPY

- Applying heat to the lower abdomen with hot compresses, heating pads, or hot water bottles seems to offer some relief.
- Other reassurance that this is a treatable condition.

ACUTE GENERAL Rx

- Nonsteroidal anti-inflammatory drugs such as ibuprofen 400 to 600 mg q4 to 6h or naproxen sodium 550 mg q12h, mefenamic acid 500 mg initial dose followed by 250 mg q6h prn, aspirin 650 mg q4 to 6h, or oral contraceptives
- Nifedipine 30 mg qd in difficult cases of dysmenorrhea
- Magnesium supplements have been found likely to be beneficial
- Thiamine supplements may reduce pain
- Secondary dysmenorrhea: treatment directed to the specific underlying condition; surgery may be indicated if pathology is found on physical examination or by imaging

CHRONIC Rx

Acupuncture and transcutaneous electrical nerve stimulation may be tried. In cases in which medical therapy has not worked, laparoscopy or other surgical treatments should be considered depending on the secondary cause of the dysmenorrhea.

DISPOSITION

The majority of patients are satisfactorily treated with good outcomes. Possible chronic complications with primary dysmenorrhea that has not been adequately treated can lead to anxiety and depression. With certain causes of secondary dysmenorrhea, infertility can become a problem.

REFERRAL

If a secondary cause of dysmenorrhea is revealed, refer to the appropriate specialist for further medical or surgical treatment (e.g., gynecologist, pain management center).

EBM EVIDENCE

available at www.expertconsult.com

AUTHORS: **GEORGE T. DANAKAS, M.D.,** and **RUBEN ALVERO, M.D.**

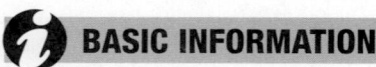

DEFINITION

Persistent and/or recurrent pain associated with sexual intercourse

SYNONYMS

Painful intercourse

ICD-9CM CODES

625.0   Pain associated with female genital organs
302.76   Sexual deviations and disorders with functional dyspareunia, psychogenic dyspareunia

EPIDEMIOLOGY & DEMOGRAPHICS

PREVALENCE: 7% to 60% depending on definition
PREDOMINANT SEX: Female
AT-RISK POPULATION: No consistent findings regarding:
- Age
- Parity
- Educational status
- Race
- Income
- Marital status

RISK FACTORS: Lower:
- Frequency of intercourse
- Levels of desire and arousal
- Orgasmic response
- Physical and emotional satisfaction
- General happiness

HISTORICAL FACTORS:
- Pain parameters
  1. Character
  2. Location (Introital, middle, deep)
  3. Onset
  4. Duration
  5. Timing
  6. Chronicity
  7. Cyclicity
  8. Recurrence
- Gynecologic history
  1. History of STD
  2. History of HSV or HPV
  3. Other sexual dysfunctions
  4. Prior abdominal or gynecologic surgery
  5. Prior pelvic or abdominal radiation
  6. History of endometriosis, fibroids
  7. History of genital or uterine prolapse
  8. History of gynecologic infection
  9. History of pelvic pain
  10. History of menopausal symptoms
  11. Sexual misinformation
- OB history
  1. Lacerations
  2. Episiotomy
- General medical causes
  1. History of chronic diseases
  2. GI or GU symptoms
  3. Medications
  4. History of psychological disorders
  5. History of dermatologic condition
  6. Religious beliefs
  7. Generalized anxiety

PHYSICAL FINDINGS & CLINICAL PRESENTATION

- Primary versus secondary dyspareunia
  1. Latter with history of pain-free coitus
- Visual inspection
  1. Discoloration
  2. Ulcerations
  3. Discharge
  4. Prolapse
  5. Dysplastic changes
  6. Infestations
- Physical examination
  1. Sensitivity to light touch
  2. Tenderness to palpation
  3. Genital prolapse
     a. Uterus
     b. Bladder
     c. Cervix
     d. Vagina
     e. Adnexa
     f. Rectum
     g. Bowel
  4. Ridges, septum
  5. Levator muscle tone
  6. Evidence of previous surgery
  7. Vaginal length, depth, caliber constrictions

ETIOLOGY

- Pathology or alteration or reduction of genital-associated tissue
- Psychosocial factors
- Marital or relationship discord
- History of sexual abuse

Dx DIAGNOSIS

DIFFERENTIAL DIAGNOSIS

- Congenital deformities (septa/agenesis)
- Imperforate hymen
- Menopausal changes
- Atrophic tissue
- Impaired lubrication
- Psychogenic
- Vaginismus
- Inadequate foreplay
- Endometriosis
- Levator ani myalgia
- Chronic pelvic pain
- Previous surgery (posterior colporrhaphy, perineorrhaphy)
  1. Alteration in vaginal length, depth, caliber
  2. Adhesions
- Infectious
  1. Human papillomavirus
  2. Herpes simplex virus
  3. Candidiasis
  4. Tinea cruris
  5. Acute or chronic salpingitis or endometritis
- Pelvic carcinoma
- Previous radiation
- Adnexal attachment or tubal prolapse
- Pelvic tumor
- Uterine prolapse, malposition, enlargement, or retroversion
- Genital prolapse

- Cystocele, rectocele, enterocele
- Urethral or bladder pathology
- Pelvic congestion
- Vulvar vestibulitis
- Postcoital cystitis
- Broad ligament pathology
- Neuroma at the site of previous episiotomy
- Previous sexual abuse
- Vulvodynia
- Contact or allergic dermatitis
- Vitamin A, B, or C deficiency
- Equestrian dyspareunia
- Interstitial cystitis
- Pudendal neuralgia
- Myofascial pain syndrome
- Rectal pathology
- Structural abnormalities or alterations
  1. Muscle
  2. Bone
  3. Ligament

WORKUP

- History and physical examination are key
- If needed:
  1. Colposcopy
  2. Cystoscopy
  3. Consider laparoscopy for unexplained deep dyspareunia

LABORATORY TESTS

- Erythrocyte sedimentation rate
- White blood cell count
- Wet mount
- Cultures
  1. Cervical
     a. Gonorrhea
     b. *Chlamydia*
  2. Vaginal
  3. Lesions
  4. Urine
- Vulva, vaginal, or cervical biopsy
- Pap smear
- Herpes simplex virus antibodies
- Gonadotropin levels

IMAGING STUDIES

Pelvic or abdominal ultrasonography. Transvaginal ultrasonography provides for greater resolution of uterus and ovaries due to proximity to pelvic organs.

Rx TREATMENT

NONPHARMACOLOGIC THERAPY

- Patient education
- Discontinue exacerbating activity and irritants
- Lubrication with coitus
- Coital position changes: female superior position
- Warm or cool soaks
- Reassurance to patient of nonmalignant condition
- Psychosocial interventions
  1. Systemic desensitization techniques
  2. Behavior modification
- Vaginal dilators

- Vaginal muscle exercises and relaxation techniques
- Excision of pathologic tissue
- Surgical correction of altered, reduced, or deformed tissues

ACUTE GENERAL Rx

- Topical lidocaine
- Corticosteroids
- Antiinfective agents
- Trigger point injections
- Massage
- Acupuncture
- Transcutaneous electrical nerve stimulation
- Stress reduction techniques
- Safe sexual practices
- Hormonal replacement therapy
- Antiviral agents
- Intralesional interferon
- Mild analgesics
- Antidepressants

CHRONIC Rx

All the previous plus:
- Set supportive visits as needed
- Oral contraceptives
- Regular sexual activity
- Balanced diet

- Vitamin supplementation
- Proper hygiene

DISPOSITION

Most patients will have a reduction and/or resolution of their symptoms by using the appropriate therapeutic approaches.

REFERRAL

As with other chronic pain conditions, a multidisciplinary approach using the expertise of psychologists, dermatologists, gynecologic surgeons, infectious disease specialists, or urologists is helpful.

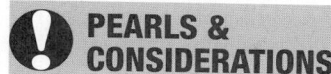

PEARLS & CONSIDERATIONS

- Dyspareunia is a symptom complex resulting from a multitude of etiologies, some of which act simultaneously.
- Uncovering the etiology of dyspareunia is predominantly based on a comprehensive history and physical examination.
- The differential diagnoses can be sorted into superficial, intermediate, and deep dyspareunia categories.

- As with the physical evaluation of any painful condition, attempt—by precise touching (moistened cotton swab), palpation, or applied pressure—to reproduce the patient's chief complaint.
- Performing a one-finger pelvic examination without concurrent abdominal palpation allows a more precise assessment of the source of genital pain.
- Individualize therapy.
- Initiate and maintain an honest diagnosis and compassionate demeanor with the patient and her partner.
- Be open minded, approachable, nonjudgmental, and diligent in your search for a solution to help these often silently suffering patients.

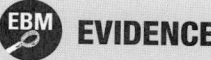

EVIDENCE

available at www.expertconsult.com

SUGGESTED READINGS

available at www.expertconsult.com

AUTHORS: **DAVID I. KURSS, M.D.,** and **RUBEN ALVERO, M.D.**

Diseases and Disorders

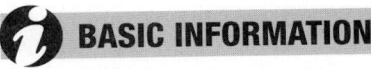 **BASIC INFORMATION**

DEFINITION

Nonulcerative dyspepsia is a term used to describe signs and symptoms of persistent or recurrent dyspepsia centered in the upper abdomen that have no obvious cause or evidence of organic disease

SYNONYMS

Functional dyspepsia
Idiopathic dyspepsia

ICD-9CM CODES
536.8 Nonulcerative dyspepsia

EPIDEMIOLOGY & DEMOGRAPHICS

- Annual prevalence of dyspepsia approximately 25% of population.
- Dyspepsia, GERD, PUD account for 2% to 5% of all primary care visits.

PHYSICAL FINDINGS & CLINICAL PRESENTATION

An international committee of clinical investigators, sponsored by the American Gastroenterological Association (AGA), developed the Rome III criteria in 2006 to define Functional Dyspepsia (nonulcerative dyspepsia) for both research purposes and clinical practice:

Diagnostic criteria* must include:
One or more of the following:
    a. Bothersome postprandial fullness
    b. Early satiation
    c. Epigastric pain
    d. Epigastric burning
AND
No evidence of structural disease (including at upper endoscopy) that is likely to explain the symptoms

ETIOLOGY

The etiology and pathophysiology are still unclear but research is focused on the following factors:
- Abnormalities of gastric motor function—especially in delayed gastric emptying, antral hypomotility, the relationship between low fasting gastric volumes and faster gastric emptying, and lower gastric compliance
- Visceral hypersensitivity
- *Helicobacter pylori* infection
- Psychosocial factors—associated with anxiety and depression

RISK FACTORS

Risk factors include excessive amounts of caffeine, alcohol, or smoking or taking steroids, NSAIDs, or certain other medications, and living in a high *H. pylori* prevalence area.

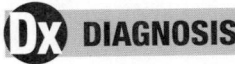 **DIAGNOSIS**

DIFFERENTIAL DIAGNOSIS

Made from the exclusion of other causes of dyspepsia

Other possible etiologies for dyspepsia:
- Peptic ulcer disease
- Gastroesophageal reflux
- Gastric/esophageal/all abdominal cancers
- Biliary tract disease
- Gastroparesis
- Pancreatitis
- Medications (i.e., NSAIDs, erythromycin, steroids)
- Infiltrative diseases of the stomach (i.e., Crohn's or sarcoidosis)
- Metabolic disturbances (i.e., hypercalcemia or hyperkalemia)
- Ischemic bowel disease
- Systemic disorders (i.e., diabetes, thyroid disorders, or connective tissue diseases)

WORKUP

The American Gastroenterological Association and the Maastricht III European consensus reports have similar recommendations.
- The pattern of symptoms overlaps considerably for all types of dyspepsia; therefore, the history and physical should focus on finding specific symptoms that help exclude other causes of dyspepsia.
- The AGA guidelines recommend that patients 55 yr of age or younger without alarm features should receive *H. pylori* testing and treatment, followed by acid suppression if symptoms remain. The European Guidelines also recommend an *H. pylori* test-and-treat approach for all adults in high prevalence areas. In areas with low *H. pylori* prevalence, either a test-and-treat or an acid-suppression strategy may be appropriate.

ENDOSCOPY:

- AGA Guidelines recommend endoscopy for patients older than 55 yr and for younger patients with alarm features (e. g., weight loss, progressive dysphagia, recurrent vomiting, evidence of gastrointestinal bleeding, or family history of cancer) presenting with new-onset dyspepsia. Biopsy specimens should be obtained during endoscopy for *H. pylori* and eradication therapy offered to those who are infected since this may reduce the risk of subsequent peptic ulcer disease and gastric malignancy
- It should be noted that the value of alarm features in younger patients is controversial and endoscopy may add little in younger patients who continue to have symptoms.

LABORATORY TESTS

H. pylori testing, especially in high prevalence areas. Laboratory methods include serology, stool antigen, or urea breath test.
Other lab testing as appropriate.

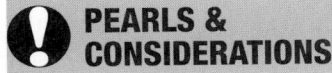 **TREATMENT**

NONPHARMACOLOGIC THERAPY

Controversial and often disappointing. Goal should be to help patients reduce risk or exacerbating factors, accept, diminish, and cope with symptoms rather than seek to totally eliminate them.

ACUTE GENERAL Rx

PHARMACOLOGIC THERAPY: Treatment may depend on the predominant symptoms. Possible approaches, based on predominant symptoms, may include the following:

Predominant Symptom	Possible Etiology	Medication Recommended
Nausea	Motility dysfunction	Prokinetic agent
Bloating	Motility dysfunction	Simethicone and/or prokinetic agent
Pain	Mucosal disease or *H. pylori* infection	Antibiotic trial
Somatic complaints	Psychosocial	Psychotropic medication trial

Medication Categories
- Antacids (i.e., aluminum hydroxide, calcium carbonate)
- Gas-reducing agents, such as those containing simethicone
- H2-receptor antagonists (i.e., cimetidine)
- Proton pump inhibitors (PPIs) (i.e., omeprazole)
- Prokinetic agents (i.e., metoclopramide)
- Antidepressants (i.e., selective serotonin receptor inhibitors)
- *H. pylori* therapy/antibiotic therapy (e.g., clarithromycin + amoxicillin and/or metronidazole + PPI)

CHRONIC RX

Controversy currently exists around the long-term use of PPIs.

COMPLEMENTARY AND ALTERNATIVE THERAPIES

Peppermint and caraway oil may be helpful.

REFERRAL

- Referral to gastroenterology if patient with alarming symptoms (such as GI bleeding, dysphagia, odynophagia, unexplained anemia, change in appetite, and weight loss) or when endoscopy is indicated—although controversy exists about the work-up of younger patients.
- Referral to cardiology if cardiac etiology suspected.

! PEARLS & CONSIDERATIONS

PREVENTION

Avoid excessive amounts of caffeine, alcohol, smoking, or long-term use of steroids and NSAIDs.

PATIENT AND FAMILY EDUCATION

http://www.mayoclinic.com/health/stomach-pain/DS00524

SUGGESTED READINGS
available at www.expertconsult.com

AUTHORS: **JEFFREY BORKAN, M.D., PH.D.,** and **HANNAH VU, D.O.**

---

*Criteria need to be fulfilled for the last months with symptom onset at least 6 mo prior to diagnosis.

(i) BASIC INFORMATION

DEFINITION

The term "dysphagia" is derived from the Greek words dys (with difficulty) and phagia (to eat). It is characterized by abnormal transfer of food from mouth to the stomach, which may involve the oral, pharyngeal, or esophageal stages of swallowing.

ICD-9CM CODES
782.2 Dysphagia

EPIDEMIOLOGY & DEMOGRAPHICS

- This is seen in 10% of individuals above the age of 50 yr. Its prevalence increases with advancing age.
- Nearly 12% of hospitalized patients have symptoms of dysphagia.
- Up to 30% to 60% of nursing home patients have some form of dysphagia.
- Special populations, including patients with head injury, stroke, or Parkinson's disease, have 30% to 50% prevalence of oropharyngeal dysphagia.

ETIOLOGY

- Oropharyngeal
  1. Neuromuscular causes
     - Stroke
     - Parkinson's disease
     - Multiple sclerosis
     - Myasthenia gravis
     - Amyotrophic lateral sclerosis
     - CNS tumors
     - Muscular dystrophy
     - Thyroid dysfunction
     - Polymyositis and dermatomyositis
     - Sarcoidosis
     - Cerebral palsy
     - Head trauma
     - Metabolic encephalopathy
     - Dementia
     - Bell's palsy
  2. Structural causes
     - Oropharyngeal tumors
     - Zenker's diverticulum
     - Infection of pharynx or neck (mucositis from candida, herpes, and CMV)
     - Thyromegaly
     - Prior surgery or radiotherapy
     - Osteophytes and other spinal disorders
     - Proximal esophageal webs
     - Congenital anomalies (e.g., cleft palate)
     - Poor dentition
- Esophageal
  1. Neuromuscular disorders
     - Achalasia
     - Diffuse esophageal spasm
     - Nutcracker esophagus
     - Hypertensive lower esophageal sphincter
     - Ineffective esophageal motility
     - Scleroderma
     - Reflex-associated dysmotility

  2. Structural disorder
     - Peptic stricture
     - Esophageal rings and webs
     - Diverticuli
     - Carcinoma and benign tumors
     - Foreign bodies
     - Vascular compression
     - Mediastinal masses
     - Spinal osteophytes
     - Mucosal injury (from pills, infection, GERD, etc.)

PATHOGENESIS

The inability to swallow is caused either by a problem in strength or coordination of the muscles required to move material from the mouth to stomach or by a fixed obstruction somewhere between the mouth and the stomach.

CLINICAL FEATURES

Oropharyngeal dysphagia
- Problem arises within 2 seconds of initiating the voluntary phase of swallowing.
- Typical symptoms include drooling, spillage of food, postnasal regurgitation, difficulty in initiation of swallowing, sialorrhea, sensation of food stuck in the neck, coughing or choking during swallowing, the need to swallow repeatedly to clear food or fluid from the pharynx, dysphonia, nasal speech, hoarseness of voice, and dysarthria.
- A thorough physical examination including that of the nervous system, oral cavity, and the head/neck is very important in patients with oropharyngeal dysphagia.

Esophageal dysphagia
- Problem usually arises several seconds after swallowing.
- Patients often complain of food being stuck in lower substernal area.
- Dysphagia to solids suggests mechanical obstruction.
- Neuromuscular causes result in dysphagia to both solids and liquids. Particularly, patients with achalasia tend to drink a lot of fluids while eating or apply maneuvers such as straightening the back, raising their arms over their heads, or standing to increase intraesophageal pressure to facilitate the emptying of food into the stomach.
- Oftentimes, ingestion of very cold or very hot foods precipitate the dysphagia associated with neuromuscular disorder.
- Delayed regurgitation of food, heartburn, and chest pain are usually present.
- Weight loss is usually associated with malignancy or achalasia.
- Symptoms are intermittent in patients with esophageal dysphagia from benign causes of structural obstruction or diffuse esophageal spasm. However, it is progressive in patients with peptic stricture, esophageal carcinoma, scleroderma, and achalasia.
- In patients with structural obstruction, when the luminal diameter is more than 18 to 20 mm, they are rarely symptomatic, whereas those with a diameter of less than 13 mm are nearly always symptomatic.

- These patients with esophageal dysphagia usually do not have any characteristic physical findings.

(Dx) DIAGNOSIS

Laboratory evaluation
- CBC
- Thyroid studies
- Nutritional assessment by checking serum protein and albumin levels
- Other studies based on specific clinical conditions

Special studies
- Oropharyngeal dysphagia
  1. Videofluoroscopy is the first test often ordered in evaluation of patients with oropharyngeal dysphagia
  2. Double contrast modified barium swallow study
  3. Fiberoptic flexible nasopharyngeal laryngoscopy is mandatory in all cases when a structural lesion, particularly malignancy, is suspected.
  4. Pharyngeal and upper esophageal manometry (Fig. 1-126) are occasionally of value to predict which patients will have a favorable outcome from cricopharyngeal myotomy or dilatation.
  5. Radiography of head and neck when indicated
- Esophageal dysphagia
  1. Barium esophagography should precede upper endoscopies to identify patients at risk from potential perforation with an endoscopy and to help plan fluoroscopically guided dilatation. It is often the first step in evaluating patients with dysphagia, especially if an obstructive lesion is suspected.
  2. EGD
  3. Esophageal manometry is indicated if no abnormality is identified by barium study or EGD.
  4. Esophageal pH monitoring in patients with suspected reflux disease
  5. Endoscopic ultrasonography
  6. Radiograph, CT, and MRI of chest

DIFFERENTIAL DIAGNOSIS

- Globus pharyngeus
- Odynophagia
- Phagophobia
- GERD

(Rx) TREATMENT

- Treatment should be approached with the help of specialists of multiple disciplines (ENT, head and neck surgeon, radiologist, speech pathologist, physical therapist, dietitian, gastroenterologist, physical medicine and rehabilitation specialist, dentist, neurologist, etc.).
- Goal of therapy is airway protection and maintenance of nutrition.
- Alteration of food consistency, volume, and delivery rate plays a major role.

- The goal of direct therapy is to change swallowing physiology with medical treatment of primary disease, maxillofacial prosthesis, and cricopharyngeal myotomy
- Indirect therapies include exercise programs for tongue coordination and chewing under the guidance of a speech therapist.
- Maintenance of oral feeding often requires compensatory techniques such as chin-tuck position, rotation of head to the affected side, tilting of head to the strong side, and lying on one's back or on one's side during swallowing.
- Some of the voluntary maneuvers applied include supraglottic swallow, effortful swallow, Mendelson maneuver, Shaker exercise, and the Heimlich maneuver.
- Placement of nasogastric tube, jejunostomy tube, or percutaneous endoscopic gastrotomy (PEG) tube is considered for enteral feeding when other measures fail and the patient remains at significant risk for aspiration or nutrition becomes compromised.
- Treatment of associated GERD should not be forgotten.
- Surgery for chronic aspiration may involve tracheostomy, medialization, laryngeal suspension, laryngeal closure, and/or laryngotracheal separation-diversion.
- Other measures include esophageal dilatation, removal of foreign body, esophageal resection, chemotherapy, radiotherapy, endoscopic ablation of tumor, phodynamic therapy, esophageal prosthesis/stents, diverticulectomy, intrasphincteric injection of botulinum toxin, surgical myotomy, and others. Smooth muscle relaxants such as nitrates and calcium channel blockers have been used to effectively treat patients with diffuse esophageal spasm and nutcracker esophagus.
- Several scales have been suggested to determine patients' functional outcome. One of them is the "Swallowing Rating Scale."

COMPLICATIONS

- Dehydration
- Malnutrition
- Aspiration pneumonia
- Airway obstruction
- Death resulting from pulmonary complications

PROGNOSIS

- Depends on the etiology.
- Nursing home patients with oropharyngeal dysphagia and a history of aspiration have an approximately 45% mortality rate over one year.
- All patients, especially the elderly, should take their medications with a full glass of water while in upright position well before bedtime.
- Dysphagia should be considered an alarm symptom, indicating the need for immediate evaluation.

PATIENT EDUCATION

Elderly patients with dysphagia should not attribute their symptoms to aging.

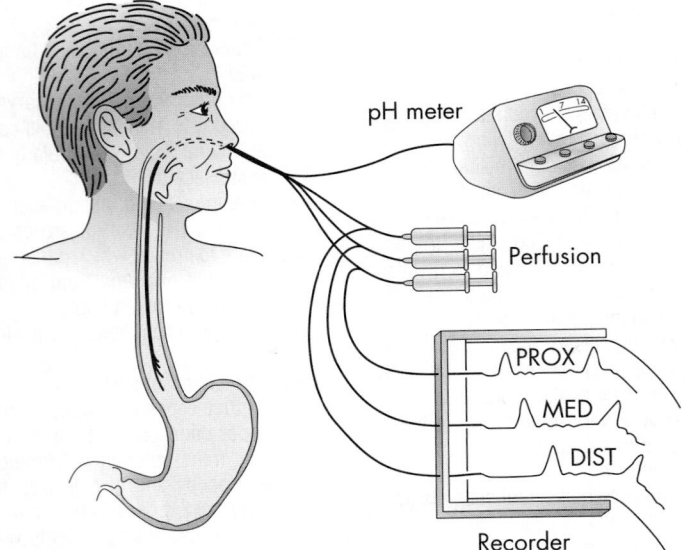

FIGURE 1-126 Combined manometric-pH recording system used in the evaluation of esophageal function. The triple-lumen perfused recording catheter measures intraluminal pressures from three levels in the esophagus. Measurements are made in terms of centimeters from the nostrils to the proximal opening of the recording catheter (PROX). The medial catheter (ED) records pressures 5 cm distal to the proximal opening and the distal catheter (DIST) 5 cm below this. The intraesophageal pH electrode is used to document gastroesophageal reflux. (From Townsend CM et al: *Sabiston textbook of surgery,* ed 17, Philadelphia, 2004, Saunders.).

SUGGESTED READINGS
available at www.expertconsult.com

AUTHOR: **HEMANT K. SATPATHY, M.D.**

BASIC INFORMATION

DEFINITION

Dystonia refers to a group of disorders characterized by involuntary muscle contractions (sustained or spasmodic) that lead to abnormal body movements or postures. Dystonia can be generalized or focal, of early (<20 yr) or late onset, and primary or secondary.

SYNONYMS

Blepharospasm
Oromandibular (orofacial) dystonia
Spasmodic (limb or axial) dystonia
Torticollis
Writer's cramp

ICD-10 CODES
G24   Dystonia
G24.1 Idiopathic familial dystonia
G24.0 Drug induced dystonia
G24.3 Spasmodic torticollis

EPIDEMIOLOGY & DEMOGRAPHICS

PREVALENCE: Estimated at one in 3000 persons.
PREDOMINANT SEX: Cervical dystonia has a 3:2 female preponderance.
PREDOMINANT AGE:
- Onset of focal cervical dystonia is usually in the fifth decade.
- Hereditary forms may have an onset in childhood or adulthood and tend to be more severe.

GENETICS: Autosomal-dominant, autosomal-recessive, and X-linked forms of dystonia have been identified. Ashkenazi Jews are particularly susceptible to primary early-onset dystonia.

CLINICAL PRESENTATION

Focal dystonias produce abnormal sustained muscle contractions in a single region of the body:
- Neck (torticollis): most commonly affected site with a tendency for the head to turn to one side
- Eyelids (blepharospasm): involuntary closure of the eyelids
- Mouth (oromandibular dystonia): involuntary contraction of muscles of the mouth, tongue, or face
- Hand (writer's cramp) (Fig. 1-127)

Generalized dystonia affects multiple areas of the body and can lead to marked joint deformities.

ETIOLOGY

- Exact pathophysiology of primary dystonia is unknown but believed to involve abnormalities of basal ganglia. Specifically, reduced and abnormal patterns of neuronal activity in the basal ganglia result in disinhibition of the motor thalamus and cortex, leading to abnormal movement.
- Fifteen hereditary forms have been described, including the severe progressive form, dystonia musculorum deformans.
- Secondary dystonia results from central nervous system (CNS) disease of the basal ganglia (stroke, demyelination, hypoxia, trauma), Huntington's disease, Wilson's disease, Parkinson syndromes, and lysosomal storage diseases.
- Acute dystonia can occur with drugs that block dopamine receptors, such as phenothiazines or butyrophenones.
- Tardive dyskinesia can result from long-term treatment with antiemetics (e.g., phenothiazines), antipsychotics (e.g., haloperidol), levodopa, anticonvulsants, or ergots.

DIAGNOSIS

DIFFERENTIAL DIAGNOSIS
- Parkinson's disease
- Progressive supranuclear palsy
- Wilson's disease
- Huntington's disease
- Drug effects

WORKUP

History (family history, birth history, trauma, medication use), physical examination

LABORATORY TESTS
- Usually not helpful for diagnosis
- Serum ceruloplasmin if Wilson's disease is suspected

IMAGING STUDIES
- Primary dystonias are generally not associated with structural CNS abnormalities. CT scan or MRI of brain if a CNS lesion is suspected as a cause of secondary dystonia.
- Electrophysiologic testing can provide diagnostic support for the diagnosis.

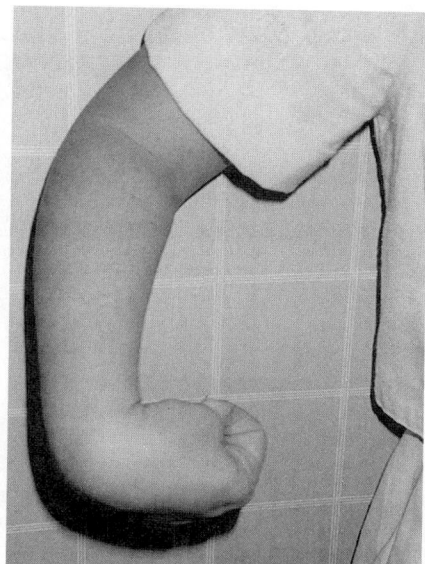

FIGURE 1-127 Focal dystonia of the distal right arm. (From Goldman L, Ausiello D [eds]: *Cecil textbook of medicine,* ed 22, Philadelphia, 2004, WB Saunders.)

TREATMENT

NONPHARMACOLOGIC THERAPY
- Heat, massage, physical therapy to relieve pain
- Splints to prevent contractures

ACUTE GENERAL Rx

For acute dystonic reactions to phenothiazines/butyrophenones, use diphenhydramine 50 mg IV or benztropine 2 mg IV.

CHRONIC Rx
- Pharmacologic treatment is often ineffective.
- Slowly withdraw offending agents.
- Diazepam, baclofen, or carbamazepine may be helpful.
- Intrathecal baclofen is most useful for spastic or truncal dystonia.
- Trihexyphenidyl or benztropine may be helpful in up to 50% of tardive dystonias.
- For generalized dystonia, a trial of carbidopa/levodopa may be beneficial.
- Injections of botulinum toxin into the affected muscles is the standard treatment for focal dystonias. Both type A and type B toxins produced by *Clostridium* botulinum block cholinergic transmission at the neuromuscular junction by inhibiting release of acetylcholine.
- Surgical procedures, including denervation, myectomy, rhizotomy, thalamotomy (pallidotomy), or functional stereotactic surgery may be helpful for severe, refractory cases.
- Deep brain stimulation is becoming more promising, especially for refractory primary generalized dystonias.

DISPOSITION

Spontaneous remission of focal cervical dystonia can occur, but dystonia is generally progressive and pharmacologic therapy is often ineffective.

REFERRAL

Neurology and/or neurosurgery for severe or refractory cases.
Physical therapy for maintaining flexibility.

PEARLS & CONSIDERATIONS

COMMENTS
- Avoid triggers/exacerbating factors.
- Early physical therapy and splinting to prevent contractures.
- Consider botulism injections or deep brain stimulation surgery for severe or refractory dystonia.
- Botulism injections remain the treatment of choice for focal dystonias.

SUGGESTED READINGS
available at www.expertconsult.com

AUTHOR: **LYNN MCNICOLL, M.D., F.R.C.P.C.**

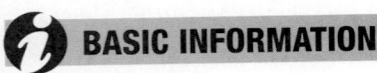

BASIC INFORMATION

DEFINITION

Echinococcosis is a chronic infection caused by the larval stage of several animal cestodes (tapeworms) of the genus *Echinococcus*.

SYNONYMS

Hydatid disease

ICD-9CM CODES
122.9 *Echinococcus* infection

EPIDEMIOLOGY & DEMOGRAPHICS

INCIDENCE (IN U.S.): Seen primarily in immigrants.
PEAK INCIDENCE: Presumed to be acquired in childhood or early adulthood in most cases.
PREVALENCE (IN U.S.): See Incidence
PREDOMINANT SEX: Male = female
PREDOMINANT AGE: 0 to 50 yr of age

PHYSICAL FINDINGS & CLINICAL PRESENTATION

- Signs of an enlarging mass lesion in a visceral site such as the liver, lungs, kidneys, bone, or CNS
- Occasional cyst rupture causing allergic manifestations such as urticaria, angioedema, or anaphylaxis that bring the patient to medical attention
- Incidental discovery of cysts by abdominal or thoracic imaging studies performed for other reasons

ETIOLOGY

- Four species of *Echinococcus*: *E. granulosus*, *E. multilocularis*, *E. oligarthrus,* and *E. vogeli.*
  1. *E. granulosus* is the cause of cystic hydatid disease.
  2. *E. multilocularis* and *E. vogeli* are the causes of alveolar and polycystic disease.
- The disease is transmitted to humans by infected canines (domestic or wild dogs, wolves, foxes) and seen most commonly in livestock-producing areas of the Middle East, Africa, Australia, New Zealand, Europe, and the Americas, including the southwestern U.S.
- Eggs are present in the feces of infected canines; human infection occurs by ingestion of viable eggs in contaminated food.
- It is common in many areas of the world, especially the Middle East.

DIAGNOSIS

DIFFERENTIAL DIAGNOSIS

- Cystic neoplasms
- Abscess (amebic or bacterial)
- Congenital polycystic disease

WORKUP

- Antibody assay
- Imaging study (CT scan, ultrasonography)
- Histologic examination of cyst or contents obtained by aspiration or resection (if possible) to confirm diagnosis

LABORATORY TESTS

Antibody assays (ELISA, Latex agglutination, and Western blot): >90% sensitive and specific for liver cysts, but less accurate for cysts in other sites. A PCR assay is now available for problematic cases.

IMAGING STUDIES

Ultrasonography and/or CT scan:
- Both are extremely sensitive for the detection of cysts, especially in the liver (Fig. 1-128).
- Both lack specificity and are inadequate to establish the diagnosis of echinococcosis with certainty.

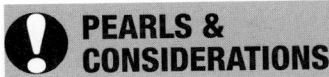

TREATMENT

NONPHARMACOLOGIC THERAPY

- Treatment of choice for echinococcal cysts is surgical resection, when feasible.
- If resection is not feasible, perform percutaneous drainage with instillation of 95% ethanol to prevent dissemination of viable larvae.
- Surgical therapy is followed by medical therapy with albendazole (see "Acute General Rx").

ACUTE GENERAL Rx

For echinococcosis confined to the liver:
- Albendazole (400 mg bid for 28 days followed by 14 days of rest for at least three cycles)
- Mebendazole (50 to 70 mg/kg qd) if albendazole not available

CHRONIC Rx

See "Acute General Rx."

DISPOSITION

- Long-term follow-up is necessary following surgical or medical therapy because of the high incidence of late relapse.
- Antibody assays and imaging studies are repeated every 6 to 12 mo for several years following successful surgical or medical therapy.

REFERRAL

All patients for evaluation for possible surgical resection of cysts

PEARLS & CONSIDERATIONS

COMMENTS

Cyst resection, if indicated, should be performed by surgeons experienced with this procedure.

SUGGESTED READINGS

available at www.expertconsult.com

AUTHORS: **GLENN G. FORT, M.D., M.P.H.,** and **DENNIS J. MIKOLICH, M.D.**

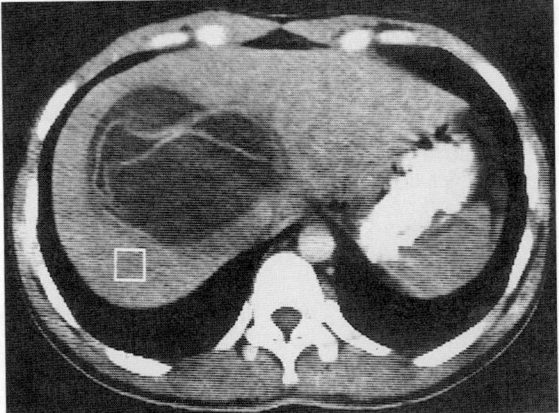

FIGURE 1-128 Computed tomographic scan of an echinococcal cyst in a 25-year-old man, demonstrating the complex structure of the wall and the interior. (From Goldman L, Ausiello D [eds]: *Cecil textbook of medicine,* ed 22, Philadelphia, 2004, WB Saunders.)

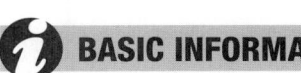

BASIC INFORMATION

DEFINITION
Eclampsia is the occurrence of seizures or coma in a woman with preeclampsia, occurring at >20 wk of gestation or <48 hr postpartum. Atypical eclampsia occurs at <20 wk of gestation or as much as 14 days postpartum.

SYNONYMS
Toxemia
Seizures of pregnancy

ICD-9CM CODES
642.6 Eclampsia

EPIDEMIOLOGY & DEMOGRAPHICS
INCIDENCE: One case per 150 to 3000 pregnancies; 2% to 4% of those with preeclampsia
GENETICS: Increased incidence with a first-degree relative (sister or mother) having had eclampsia
RISK FACTORS: Multifetal gestation (3.6% in twin gestation), molar pregnancy, nonimmune hydrops fetalis, uncontrolled hypertension, preexisting hypertension, renal disease

PHYSICAL FINDINGS & CLINICAL PRESENTATION
- Seizure begins as facial twitching, then spreads to generalized clonicotonic state, with cessation of respiration followed by a postictal period of amnesia, agitation, and confusion.
- 40% have severe hypertension, 40% have mild to moderate hypertension, and 20% are normotensive.
- Generalized edema with rapid weight gain (>2 lb/wk) may be one of the earliest signs of eclampsia.
- Persistent occipital headache and hyperreflexia with clonus occur in 80% of patients with eclampsia; epigastric pain occurs in 20% of these patients.

ETIOLOGY
- Exact etiology unknown.
- Common pathway relates to abnormalities in autoregulation of cerebral blood flow. This may involve transient vasospasm, ischemia, cerebral hemorrhage, and edema occurring by a mechanism involving hypertensive encephalopathy, decreased colloid osmotic pressure, and prostaglandin imbalance.

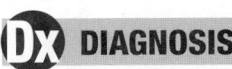

DIAGNOSIS

DIFFERENTIAL DIAGNOSIS
- Preexisting seizure disorder
- Metabolic abnormalities (hypoglycemia, hyponatremia, hypocalcemia)
- Substance abuse
- Head trauma, infection (meningitis, encephalitis)
- Intracerebral bleeding or thrombosis
- Amniotic fluid embolism
- Space-occupying brain lesions or neoplasms
- Pseudoseizure

WORKUP
- Rule out other causes of seizures during pregnancy.
- Atypical presentations such as prolonged postictal state; status epilepticus; gestational age <20 wk or >48 hr postpartum; or signs of meningitis, substance abuse, or severe uncontrolled hypertension should prompt a search for other seizure etiologies.

LABORATORY TESTS
- Proteinuria: severe (49%), mild to moderate (29%), absent (22%)
- HCT: elevated as a result of hemoconcentration
- Platelet count: decreased; LFTs elevated in HELLP syndrome (hemolysis, elevated liver enzymes, and low platelet count)
- BUN and creatinine: elevated with renal involvement
- Serum electrolytes, glucose, calcium, toxicology profile: rule out other causes of seizures
- Hyperuricemia: >6.9 mg/dl found in 70% of eclamptics
- ABG: maternal acidemia and hypoxia

IMAGING STUDIES
- CT scan or MRI indicated in atypical presentation, suspected intracerebral bleeding, or focal neurologic deficit.
- There are abnormal findings, including cerebral edema, hemorrhage, and infarction, in 50% of patients.

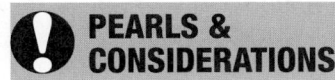

TREATMENT

NONPHARMACOLOGIC THERAPY
- Airway protection (risk of aspiration)
- Supportive care during acute event

ACUTE GENERAL Rx
- Maintain airway, adequate oxygenation, and IV access.
- Fetal resuscitation, involving maternal oxygenation, left lateral positioning, and continuous fetal heart rate monitoring, is needed.
- Magnesium sulfate is the drug of choice. Give magnesium sulfate 6 g IV load over 20 min, then 3 g/hr maintenance, for recurrent seizure prophylaxis. If repeated convulsions, may give an additional 2 g IV over 3 to 5 min. Approximately 10% to 15% of patients will have a second seizure after initial loading dose. Check magnesium level 1 hr after loading dose, then q6h (therapeutic range 4 to 6 mg/dl). Antidote for toxicity is calcium gluconate 10 ml of 10% solution. Phenytoin has been used as an alternative in patients in whom magnesium sulfate is contraindicated (renal insufficiency, heart block, myasthenia gravis, hypoparathyroidism).
- Give sodium amobarbital 250 mg IV over 3 min for persistent seizures.
- Treat blood pressure if >160 mm Hg/110 mm Hg with labetalol 20- to 40-mg IV bolus, hydralazine 10 mg IV, or nifedipine 10 to 20 mg sublingual q20min.
- Evaluate patient for delivery.

CHRONIC Rx
- The first priority is stabilization of the mother in terms of adequate oxygenation, hemodynamics, and laboratory abnormalities, such as associated coagulopathies.
- Cervical status and gestational age should be assessed. If unfavorable cervix and <30 wk of gestation, consider C-section; otherwise consider induction.
- Controlled epidural is the anesthesia of choice for labor or C-section.
- Avoid general anesthesia in uncontrolled hypertension to minimize risk of catastrophic cerebral events.

DISPOSITION
The maternal mortality rate for eclampsia averages 5% to 6%. Morbidity rate is 25%, including placental abruption (10%), maternal apnea with fetal asphyxia, aspiration pneumonia, pulmonary edema (4%), renal failure, cardiopulmonary arrest, and coma.

REFERRAL
Because of the potential for serious permanent maternal and fetal sequelae, all cases should be managed by a team approach of obstetrician, neonatologist, and intensivist.

PEARLS & CONSIDERATIONS

COMMENTS
- Eclampsia antepartum, 50%; intrapartum, 20%; and postpartum, 30%.
- Postseizure there is an associated period of fetal bradycardia from 1 to 9 min; if there is evidence of fetal compromise beyond that time, consider alternative etiologies such as placental abruption (23% incidence).

SUGGESTED READINGS
available at www.expertconsult.com

AUTHORS: **SCOTT J. ZUCCALA, D.O.,** and **RUBEN ALVERO, M.D.**

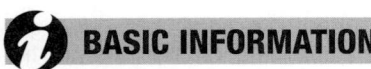

BASIC INFORMATION

DEFINITION

An ectopic pregnancy (EP) occurs when a fertilized ovum implants outside the endometrial lining of the uterus.

SYNONYMS

Abdominal pregnancy (1% to 2%)
Cervical pregnancy (0.5%)
Interstitial pregnancy (2% to 3%)
Ovarian pregnancy (1%)
Tubal pregnancy (97%)

ICD-9CM CODES
633 Ectopic pregnancy

EPIDEMIOLOGY & DEMOGRAPHICS

- 1% to 2% of pregnancies
- 13% of maternal deaths

PREVALENCE (IN U.S.): Increasing number of EPs; 17,800 reported cases in 1970 and 108,000 reported cases in 1992.

RISK FACTORS: Previous salpingitis, previous EP, previous tubal ligation, previous tuboplasty, intrauterine device use, progestin-only pill, assisted reproductive techniques

PHYSICAL FINDINGS & CLINICAL PRESENTATION

- Abdominal tenderness: 95%
- Adnexal tenderness: 87% to 99%
- Peritoneal signs: 71% to 76%
- Adnexal mass: 33% to 53%
- Enlarged uterus: 6% to 30%
- Shock: 2% to 17%
- Amenorrhea or abnormal vaginal bleeding: 75%
- Shoulder pain: 10%
- Tissue passage: 6% to 7%

ETIOLOGY

- Anatomic obstruction to zygote passage
- Abnormalities in tubal motility
- Transperitoneal migration of the zygote

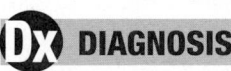

DIAGNOSIS

DIFFERENTIAL DIAGNOSIS

- Corpus luteum cyst
- Rupture or torsion of ovarian cyst
- Threatened or incomplete abortion
- Pelvic inflammatory disease
- Appendicitis
- Gastroenteritis
- Dysfunctional uterine bleeding
- Degenerating uterine fibroids
- Endometriosis

WORKUP

1. The classic presentation of EP includes the triad of abnormal vaginal bleeding, pelvic pain, and an adnexal mass. Consider in all women with abdominopelvic pain and a positive pregnancy test
2. Transvaginal ultrasound
3. Quantitative serum human chorionic gonadotropin level
4. Laparoscopy in equivocal situations and possibly for treatment

LABORATORY TESTS

- Quantitative human chorionic gonadotropin (QhCG): if normal intrauterine pregnancy (IUP), 85% have doubling time of 2 days. If abnormal gestation, will show <66% increase of QhCG within 2 days. However, 13% of ectopic pregnancies have a normal doubling time (see Section III, "Ectopic Pregnancy").
- Progesterone: decreased production in EP; <5 ng/ml strongly predictive of abnormal pregnancy. If >25 ng/ml, strongly predictive of normal IUP.
- Dropping hematocrit associated with tubal rupture, resolving ectopic pregnancy, or abnormal intrauterine pregnancy.
- Leukocytosis.

IMAGING STUDIES

- Ultrasound (Fig. 1-129): presence of an IUP makes EP extremely unlikely. However, if the patient used assisted reproductive technologies, a heterotopic pregnancy (a pregnancy in the uterus as well as in the fallopian tube) is much more likely to occur. A repeat ultrasonographic examination 2 to 7 days after presentation may identify the location of a pregnancy that was not identified on initial ultrasonographic examination.
- If QhCG >6000 mIU/ml, should see IUP on abdominal scan; QhCG >1500 mIU/ml for transvaginal scan. Since transvaginal ultrasonography is overwhelmingly the preferred modality for imaging, the latter value is clearly the discriminatory threshold that is used in diagnosis.
- Findings on ultrasound in EP include:
  1. Empty uterus
  2. Adnexal mass
  3. Cul-de-sac fluid
  4. Fetal sac in tube
  5. Fetal cardiac activity in adnexa

TREATMENT

NONPHARMACOLOGIC THERAPY

Surgery can be performed by laparoscopy if patient is stable or, rarely, by laparotomy if pa-

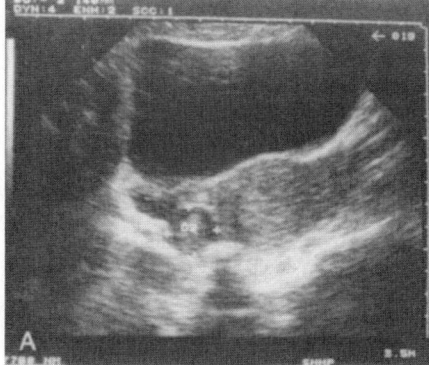

FIGURE 1-129 Ultrasound scan showing ectopic pregnancy. This transabdominal scan shows empty uterus with a complex mass in the right adnexa. The mass measures 21 × 22 mm. (From Greer IA et al: *Mosby's color atlas and test of obstetrics and gynecology*, London, 2001, Harcourt.)

tient is very unstable. Salpingiosis is the direct injection of chemotherapy into the EP by laparoscopy, transvaginal ultrasound, or hysteroscopy.

- Conservative surgery, salpingostomy or segmental resection, depends on tubal location and size of EP.
- Salpingectomy should be considered in the following circumstances:
  1. Ruptured tube
  2. Future fertility not desired
  3. Recurrent EP in the same tube
  4. Uncontrolled hemorrhage

ACUTE GENERAL Rx

- If the patient is stable and compliant, consider medical management with methotrexate. Patient should not have contraindications to methotrexate such as hepatic or renal disease, thrombocytopenia, leukopenia, or significant anemia. There should be no evidence of hemoperitoneum on transvaginal ultrasound. EP should be <3.5 cm mass with QhCG <6,000 to 15,000 mIU/ml, but these are relative contraindications. Presence of cardiac activity in the fetus is also a relative contraindication to methotrexate.
- Most common regimen is methotrexate 50 mg/m^2 of body surface area. May require second dose or surgical intervention if QhCG increases or plateaus (<15% drop) when comparing values from the fourth through seventh day after treatment. Absolute contraindications to methotrexate include breast feeding, preexisting blood dyscrasias, known sensitivity to methotrexate, active pulmonary disease, chronic liver disease, alcoholism, laboratory evidence of immunodeficiency, renal disease, and peptic ulcer disease.

CHRONIC Rx

Persistent EP results from residual trophoblastic tissue or secondary implantation after conservative surgery. There is a 5% incidence of persistent EP with conservative treatment.

DISPOSITION

If diagnosed and treated early (before rupture), prognosis is excellent for good recovery. Monitor QhCG weekly until negative. Use reliable contraception until hCG is negative. With subsequent pregnancies, follow QhCG and perform early ultrasound to confirm IUP. There is a 12% recurrence rate for EP.

REFERRAL

Should obtain gynecologic consultation if EP is suspected.

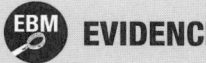 **EVIDENCE**

available at www.expertconsult.com

SUGGESTED READINGS
available at www.expertconsult.com

AUTHORS: **GEORGE T. DANAKAS, M.D.,** and **RUBEN ALVERO, M.D.**

BASIC INFORMATION

DEFINITION

Ehlers-Danlos syndrome (EDS) refers to a group of inherited, clinically variable, and genetically heterogeneous connective tissue disorders. EDS is characterized by skin hyperextensibility, skin fragility, joint laxity, and joint hyperextensibility.

ICD-9CM CODES
756.83 Ehlers-Danlos syndrome

EPIDEMIOLOGY & DEMOGRAPHICS

- The prevalence of EDS is estimated to be approximately one in 5000 births, although it is somewhat higher in African Americans.
- There are six distinct forms of EDS according to the revised classification system established at the Villefranche Consensus Conference, 1997 (see "Physical Findings & Clinical Presentation").
- Classic and hypermobility EDS are most prevalent. Classic EDS accounts for approximately 80% of reported cases.
- Vascular EDS is the most dangerous because it is associated with spontaneous rupture of medium and large arteries and hollow organs, especially the large intestine and uterus; occurs in 4% of patients with EDS. Vascular events typically occur between the third and fifth decade.
- In most cases, transmission is autosomal dominant except for some unclassified forms of EDS (previously known as type V and type IX, which are x-linked; type X is autosomal recessive). The current classification proposes six subtypes based on clinical, biochemical, and molecular characteristics. However, examples of unclassified variants and "overlap phenotypes" are becoming more common.

PHYSICAL FINDINGS & CLINICAL PRESENTATION

- Classic (previously types I and II): patients have moderate-to-severe skin hyperelasticity (easy scarring and bruising ("cigarette-paper scars"); smooth, velvety skin and subcutaneous spheroids (small, firm, cystlike nodules) along shins or forearms, hyperextensibility ("Gorlin's sign": ability to touch tip of tongue to nose [see Fig. 1-130]), and joint hypermobility and dislocation; patients have complications such as hernias, pelvic organ prolapsed, premature arthritis, and cervical insufficiency
- Hypermobility (type III): most frequent form, causing recurrent joint dislocations, often leaving a patient unable to walk; chronic limb/joint pain is a prominent feature; skin involvement is less prominent
- Vascular (type IV): cardinal features include distinctive facial features (pinched nose, thin lips, tight skins hollow cheeks, lobeless ears), acrogeria, thin, translucent skin, excessive bruising, and most importantly, rupture of vessels and viscera including arterial, intestinal, and uterine walls; spontaneous rupture of organs occurs in the sigmoid colon, spleen,

liver, and uterus; facial features are often not prominent in children, and vascular EDS is usually not diagnosed until adulthood
- Kyphoscoliotic (type VI): rare; characterized by marked muscular hypotonia, osteopenia, joint hypermobility, progressive scoliosis, ocular fragility and possible globe rupture, mitral valve prolapse, and aortic dilation
- Arthrochalasia (types VIIA and VIIB): prominent joint hypermobility with subluxations, congenital hip dislocation, skin hyperextensibility, and tissue fragility
- Dermatosparaxis (type VIIC): severe skin fragility with decreased elasticity, bruising, hernias
- Unclassified types: type V—X-linked recessive, similar to classic EDS with skin fragility but less joint hypermobility and bruising; type IX—classic characteristics; type VIII—classic characteristics and severe periodontal disease; type X—mild classic characteristics, mitral valve prolapse; type XI—joint instability

ETIOLOGY

- Defects of collagen in extracellular matrices of multiple tissues (skin, tendons, blood vessels, and viscera) underlie all forms of EDS.
- Classic EDS is associated with defects in type V collagen, corresponding to mutations of COL5A genes.
- Vascular EDS involves a deficiency in type III collagen, and several studies suggest that mutations of gene COL3A1 lead to this deficiency.
- Arthrochalasia EDS results from a defect in type I collagen, caused by mutations in the COL1A1 and COL1A2 genes.

DIAGNOSIS

Diagnosis is based solely on clinical criteria. It is important to identify patients with vascular EDS

because of the grave consequences of the disease.
- Clinical criteria for vascular EDS: two of four major diagnostic criteria establish the diagnosis; $\geq$1 minor criterion supports but is not sufficient to establish the diagnosis.
- Major criteria:
  1. Easy bruising
  2. Arterial, intestinal, or uterine fragility
  3. Thin, translucent skin
  4. Characteristic facial features (thin, delicate, and pinched nose, hollow cheeks, prominent staring eyes): occur in <30% of patients with vascular EDS
- Minor criteria:
  ○ Small joint hypermobility
  ○ Skin hyperextensibility
  ○ Spontaneous pneumothorax/hemothorax
  ○ Tendon or muscle rupture
  ○ Early-onset varicose veins
  ○ Carotid-cavernous fistula
  ○ Talipes equinovarus (clubfoot)

DIFFERENTIAL DIAGNOSIS

- Marfan's syndrome
- Osteogenesis imperfecta
- Autosomal dominant cutis laxa
- Familial joint hypermobility

WORKUP

Diagnosis is based solely on clinical criteria.

LABORATORY TESTS

- Biochemical and gene testing for known molecular defects recommended to confirm the diagnosis in vascular EDS.
- Plain radiographs may reveal calcified nodules along the shin or forearms corresponding to the subcutaneous spheroids.
- Echocardiogram can identify mitral valve prolapse and aortic dilation.

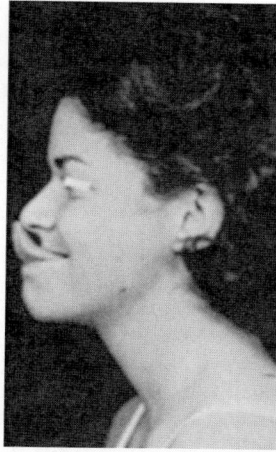
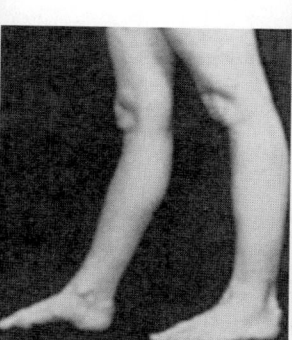
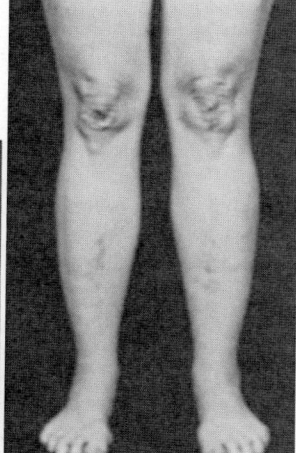

FIGURE 1-130 Ehlers-Danlos syndrome (EDS 1). Tissue elasticity, joint hypermobility, and tissue fragility are demonstrated by the patient's ability to extend her tongue to the tip of her nose (Gorlin's sign), by hyperextensibility at the knee (genu recurvatum), and by characteristic "cigarette paper" or papyracious scars of the knee and tibial skin. (Courtesy of V. McKusick, J. D. From Harris ED, Budd RC, Genovese MC, Firestein GS, Sargent JS, Sledge CB, Ruddy S: *Kelley's textbook of rheumatology,* ed 7, 2005, Saunders.)

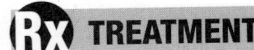 **TREATMENT**

- All patients should receive genetic counseling about the mode of inheritance of their EDS.
- Management of most skin and joint problems should be conservative and preventive. Joint hypermobility and pain in EDS usually does not require surgical intervention. Physical therapy to strengthen muscles is helpful. Surgical repair and tightening of joint ligaments can be performed, but ligaments frequently will not hold sutures. Surgical intervention should be considered on an individual basis.
- For patients with vascular EDS:
  - Special surgical care is required because of increased tissue friability.
  - Patients should be advised to avoid contact sports.
  - Elevated blood pressure should be aggressively treated with beta-blockers, given the risk of arterial dissection.

DISPOSITION

Prognosis varies according to type of EDS. For vascular EDS:

- 25% will have a complication by age 25 yr; >80% will have a complication by age 40 yr.
- Most vascular complications consist of arterial dissections.
- Vascular events typically occur between the third and fifth decade.
- Median age of survival is 48 years. Most deaths are related to arterial rupture.

REFERRAL

Referral to dermatology for skin biopsy to confirm diagnosis of vascular EDS and to cardiology, orthopedic surgery, general surgery, and physical therapy as needed.

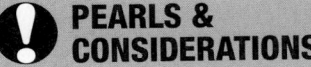 **PEARLS & CONSIDERATIONS**

- Women with vascular EDS should be counseled about the risk of uterine, intestinal, and arterial rupture.
  - Pregnancy is associated with up to a 25% mortality rate; however, successful childbirth is possible.
  - There is a 50% chance that the child will be affected.
- Family members of patients with EDS should be recommended for evaluation for EDS and genetic testing/counseling.

SUGGESTED READINGS
available at www.expertconsult.com

AUTHORS: **AHMAD ISMAIL** and **IRIS TONG, M.D.**

ℹ BASIC INFORMATION

DEFINITION

The clinically significant disorders of ejaculation are failure of emission, retrograde ejaculation, premature ejaculation, hematospermia, and anorgasmia (including delayed orgasm). Failure of emission occurs when semen is not propulsed into the urethra during orgasm, resulting in a dry ejaculate. Retrograde ejaculation is a backward flow of semen into the bladder. Premature ejaculation exists when there is an inability to delay ejaculation such that ejaculation occurs sooner than desired, either before or shortly after penetration, causing distress to either one or both partners. Hematospermia is the appearance of blood in the ejaculate. Anorgasmia is the inability to achieve orgasm, while delayed orgasm is the inability to achieve orgasm in a timely manner.

SYNONYMS

Ejaculatory dysfunction
Retarded ejaculation
Early or rapid ejaculation
Inhibited ejaculation
Anejaculation

ICD-9CM CODES
608.87 Ejaculation, retrograde
608.82 Hematospermia
306.59 Ejaculation, psychogenic
302.75 Ejaculation, premature
302.74 Orgasm inhibited male
(psychosexual)

EPIDEMIOLOGY & DEMOGRAPHICS

Premature ejaculation is the most prevalent male sexual complaint, affecting 20% to 30% of men. Retarded or delayed ejaculation is the least common, least studied, and least understood of the male sexual dysfunctions. Men with ejaculatory dysfunction of any type usually indicate higher levels of relationship stress, sexual dissatisfaction, anxiety about sexual performance, and general health issues, as compared to sexually functional men.

CLINICAL PRESENTATION

- Failure of emission: No ejaculate is expelled either antegrade or retrograde during orgasm. Physical findings may be normal or may reveal nervous system dysfunction (e.g., spinal cord injury); may present with infertility.
- Retrograde ejaculation: Little or no ejaculate is expelled at orgasm. Patients may report cloudy postcoital urine. Physical examination is usually normal; may present with infertility.
- Premature ejaculation: Ejaculation occurs sooner than desired, either before or shortly after penetration. Physical examination is normal. Sexual and psychologic history may be revealing. Patients often incorrectly report erectile dysfunction because they lose the erection after orgasm.
- Hematospermia: bloody ejaculate, may be (but is usually not) associated with pain. Physical findings usually normal; not associated with malignancy.

- Anorgasmia: patient is not able to achieve orgasm despite appropriate stimulation, whereas with delayed orgasm, the patient requires excessive time and/or stimulation to achieve orgasm.

ETIOLOGY

- Retrograde ejaculation may be caused by anatomic abnormalities of the bladder neck, or nerve injury affecting the bladder neck sphincter.
- Either retrograde ejaculation or failure of emission may result from functional abnormalities. These include spinal cord injury, diabetes mellitus, retroperitoneal surgery, transurethral prostate surgery, urethral strictures, alpha-blocker therapy, antipsychotics, multiple sclerosis, peripheral neuropathies, or other neurologic abnormalities.
- The exact etiology of premature ejaculation is unknown, but there is evidence for psychological and biologic contributions.
- Hematospermia may be idiopathic or secondary to infection or inflammation of the genitourinary tract.
- Anorgasmia or delayed orgasm may be caused by medications, particularly serotonin re-uptake inhibitors. Patients with spinal cord injuries may be unable to achieve orgasm. Additional causes include psychogenic factors and dysfunctional sexual techniques.

ⒹⓍ DIAGNOSIS

DIFFERENTIAL DIAGNOSIS

- Erectile dysfunction
- Low seminal fluid volume attributable to hypogonadism or ejaculatory duct obstruction

LABORATORY TESTS

- In the case of a dry or low-volume ejaculate, post-ejaculate urine should be evaluated for spermatozoa to differentiate failure of emission from retrograde ejaculation.
- A urine analysis in the setting of hematospermia can help rule out hematuria. The presence of hematuria requires a hematuria evaluation.
- A fasting blood glucose may be considered if diabetes is suspected as a cause of lack of emission or retrograde ejaculation.

IMAGING STUDIES

Transrectal ultrasound can rule out ejaculatory duct obstruction or absence of the seminal vesicles, if these diagnoses are suspected as a cause of low-volume ejaculate.

℞ TREATMENT

NONPHARMACOLOGIC THERAPY

- Retrograde ejaculation and failure of emission do not require treatment unless fertility is desired.
- Retrograde ejaculation may rarely be converted to antegrade ejaculation if intercourse occurs when the bladder is full. Viable sperm can be recovered from the post-ejaculate

urine and used for intrauterine insemination or in vitro fertilization.
- Premature ejaculation can improve with sex therapy (e.g., 'coronal squeeze' or 'start-and-stop' technique) and effective partner communication. These approaches may be more effective when combined with pharmacologic therapy.
- Although alarming to the patient, idiopathic hematospermia may be followed expectantly.
- Anorgasmia or delayed orgasm caused by serotonin reuptake inhibitors usually improves with withdrawal of the medication or change to another medication. Sexual therapy and counseling can improve anorgasmia or delayed orgasm caused by dysfunctional sexual techniques or psychological issues. Vibratory or electrical stimulation of emission is helpful in selected cases.

ACUTE GENERAL Rx

- Retrograde ejaculation: it is crucial to distinguish between anatomic and functional causes because pharmacologic treatment is only likely to be effective in patients who do not have an anatomic disturbance of the bladder neck. Sympathomimetic medications (phenylpropanolamine, ephedrine, pseudoephedrine) and imipramine may be useful in converting retrograde ejaculation to antegrade ejaculation.
- Failure of emission: may be converted to retrograde ejaculation by oral sympathomimetic therapy.
- Premature ejaculation: selective serotonin reuptake inhibitors (SSRIs) (sertraline, fluoxetine) and clomipramine have shown success in delaying premature ejaculation when taken daily. Recent research has focused on dapoxetine, a short-acting SSRI, which has shown promise as an "on-demand" treatment for premature ejaculation. Topical anesthetics such as lidocaine cream have also been used with limited success.

SURGICAL THERAPY

There is currently no role for surgery for ejaculatory disorders.

DISPOSITION

Prognosis varies with etiology. Ejaculatory dysfunction attributable to sexual techniques or psychological issues can improve with therapy and counseling. Pharmacologic treatment may be helpful in certain cases of premature ejaculation.

REFERRAL

All fertility issues and suspected anatomic problems should be referred to a Urologist. Professional psychotherapy and sex therapy should be considered for some patients. Endocrine input should be considered for patients with diabetes.

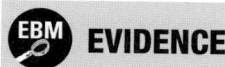 EVIDENCE

available at www.expertconsult.com

SUGGESTED READINGS

available at www.expertconsult.com

AUTHORS: **AKANKSHA MEHTA, M.D.,**
and **MARK SIGMAN, M.D.**

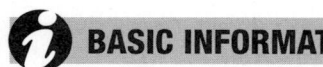

BASIC INFORMATION

DEFINITION

Premature ejaculation is a persistent or recurrent problem in which a male experiences orgasm or ejaculation in the early phases of sexual contact and before he and his partner wish it. Other definitions have emphasized elapsed time after intromission (with durations of 30 sec to several min), number of thrusts, or rate of partner satisfaction. However, no absolute measure is applicable to the diverse numbers of men with this problem.

SYNONYMS

Rapid ejaculation
Early ejaculation
Inadequate ejaculatory control

ICD-9CM CODES
F52.4 Premature ejaculation
(DSM-IV Code 302.75)

EPIDEMIOLOGY & DEMOGRAPHICS

PEAK INCIDENCE: Adolescence and young adulthood
PREVALENCE (IN U.S.):
- 7% to 40% of adult men, most with no underlying physical condition
- Often present more or less since start of sexual life
- Most prevalent sexual disorder in men; more common than low libido and erectile dysfunction

PREDOMINANT AGE: None defined
GENETICS: No identifiable genetic factors

PHYSICAL FINDINGS & CLINICAL PRESENTATION

- Complaint of ejaculation before, upon, or shortly after penetration
- Frequently associated with anxiety related to either sexual activity or more generalized anxiety disorder
- Premature ejaculation caused by a medical condition frequently associated with low desire and/or erectile insufficiency

ETIOLOGY

- Increasingly believed to be a neurobiologic phenomenon particularly related to serotonergic pathway
- Different theoretical frameworks emphasize anxiety related to performance or personal interactions, behavioral concepts of learned expectations related to early experience, or heightened penile sensitivity
- Organic factors are contributory in some individuals (e.g., abdominal or pelvic trauma or surgery, neuropathies, or urologic pathology such as prostatic urethritis)
- Biologic causes include penile hypersensitivity, hyperexcitable ejaculatory reflex, increased sexual arousability, possible endocrinopathy, a genetic predisposition, and central 5-hydroxytryptamine receptor dysfunction

DIAGNOSIS

DIFFERENTIAL DIAGNOSIS

- In young adolescents, premature ejaculation may be normally experienced as a consequence of heightened excitation.
- Distinguish comorbid erectile dysfunction, which may influence management.

WORKUP

- History with a specific emphasis on sexual activities and beliefs
- Factors to be assessed include patient's subjective evaluation, degree of sexual satisfaction, sense of control, and personal or interpersonal distress related to ejaculation
- Collateral information from sexual partner when possible
- Additional history regarding surgery, trauma, and neurologic symptoms
- History of prescribed and recreational drugs (e.g., antidepressants, alcohol, opiates)

LABORATORY TESTS

Urinalysis and urine culture after prostatic massage to rule out prostatic infection

IMAGING STUDIES

None routinely indicated

TREATMENT

NONPHARMACOLOGIC THERAPY

- Behavioral and psychotherapeutic interventions: strongly guided by a specific theoretical framework; inadequate data to suggest the superiority of any particular approach.
- Use of condoms may reduce penile sensitivity, prolonging erection.
- Use of Masters and Johnson's "pause-squeeze" technique (in which 4 sec of moderate pressure is applied to the frenulum to reduce ejaculatory urge) or "stop-start" technique may be helpful for some patients.

ACUTE GENERAL Rx

- Topical anesthetic, such as lidocaine-prilocaine cream and topical eutectic mixture for PE (TEMPE) aerosol spray, increases ejaculatory latency if applied <20 min before intercourse.
- Daily selective serotonin reuptake inhibitors (SSRIs), such as paroxetine (most potent) or sertraline, delay ejaculation. May take several weeks for response to occur. If one SSRI does not work, may try a different SSRI. Clomipramine (tricyclic antidepressant) has also been found to delay orgasm in men. Discontinuation of daily SSRIs often leads to recurrence of premature ejaculation.
- Sildenafil or vardenafil may be useful in delaying ejaculation, especially in premature ejaculation accompanied by erectile dysfunction.

DISPOSITION

There is gradual improvement with age, but it is frequently a chronic, lifelong problem with few spontaneous remissions.

REFERRAL

Behavioral sex therapy or psychotherapy may be helpful; if recurrent prostate infection, referral to urology is indicated.

PEARLS & CONSIDERATIONS

Various psychological risk factors are cited for premature ejaculation, including lack of sexual experience, infrequent sexual intercourse, fear, anxiety, social phobia, relationship problems, and a lack of sexual education.

Treatment should emphasize partner communication, behavioral technique, and topical anesthetics/condoms as first line treatment. If these treatments are ineffective and PE is causing significant distress, consider SSRIs and PDE5 inhibitors.

EVIDENCE

available at www.expertconsult.com

SUGGESTED READINGS
available at www.expertconsult.com

AUTHOR: **NICOLE APPELLE, M.D, M.P.H.**

BASIC INFORMATION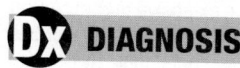

DEFINITION

Injuries or wounds that occur as a result of contact with an electrical current.

ICD-9CM CODES
994.8 Electrical shock, nonfatal

EPIDEMIOLOGY & DEMOGRAPHICS

- Causes approximately 1000 deaths annually, with two thirds occurring in persons between ages 15 and 40 yr.
- Most electrical injuries in children occur at home (e.g., oral burns from electrical appliances).
- Most electrical injuries in adults are occupationally related. It ranks fifth as a cause of occupational death.
- Accounts for 4% to 6.5% of all admissions to burn units.
- Lightning strikes kill on average 100 people annually.
  - Eight of every 10 lightning strike victims are male; 75% of lightning deaths in the U.S. occur in the South and Midwest.
  - 25% of lightning deaths are work related.
- Electronic weapons (stun gun and Taser) are capable of causing fatal cardiac arrhythmias.

PHYSICAL FINDINGS & CLINICAL PRESENTATION

- Cognitive changes: depending on the extent of injury, the patient may be unconscious, seizing, or confused and unable to present a history
- Extensive skin burns (>10% of the body surface)
  1. Located over the entry and exit sites (Fig. 1-131)
  2. Most common entry sites are the hands and skull
  3. Most common exit sites are the heels

4. "Kissing burns" over the flexor creases
5. Oral burns are common in children; bleeding from the labial artery may present 7 to 10 days after the injury
- Asystole or ventricular fibrillation may be the initial cardiac rhythm
- Bone fractures and periosteal burns
- Compartment syndrome from severe muscle tissue damage
- Headaches, memory disturbances
- Weakness and paresthesias
- Otologic injury, conductive hearing loss from tympanic membrane rupture or ossicular disruption
- Rhabdomyolysis and myoglobin-induced acute tubular necrosis
- Vascular injury from coagulation of small vessels or compartment syndrome

ETIOLOGY

- Electricity causes tissue injury by converting electrical energy into heat or by blunt trauma from being thrown from the electrical source or from continuous muscle contraction (tetany).
- The effects of electricity are determined by seven factors: type of current, amount of current, pathway of current, duration, area of contact, resistance of the body, and voltage.
- Tissue damage is greater with higher voltage and longer duration of contact.
- Direct current (DC) contact causes a single muscle contraction, throwing the patient away from the source. Alternating current (AC) contact precipitates a tetanic contraction, not allowing the patient to withdraw from the source and prolonging the duration of contact. AC contact is more ominous than DC contact.
- Electrical injuries are arbitrarily divided into high-voltage (>1000 volts) and low-voltage (<1000 volts) burns. Low-voltage burns involve almost exclusively either the hands or oral cavity. High-voltage injuries have a wide variety of systemic manifestations.

- The entry and exit path of the electrical current determines which tissues are affected.

DIAGNOSIS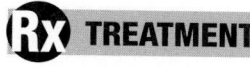

WORKUP

Physical examination may not reveal the extent of damage that has occurred. Detailed testing to determine the extent of internal organ damage is indicated. In lightning injuries, male victims may have scrotal (on the undersurface of the scrotum) and penile burns, which may often be overlooked. Hemorrhage behind the eardrum with or without perforation is not uncommon. An otoscopic examination is indicated in all lightning strike victims.

LABORATORY TESTS

- Complete blood count
- Blood chemistry profile including electrolytes
- Blood urea nitrogen and creatinine
- Arterial blood gas analysis
- Myoglobin
- Creatinine kinase with isoenzyme fractionation
- Urinalysis, including screening for myoglobinuria
- Liver function tests
- Type and cross-match
- ECG

IMAGING STUDIES

- Radiographs: any suspicious area for bone fractures
- CT scan of the head and cervical spine in patients with suspected head injury, coma, or neurologic deficit

TREATMENT

NONPHARMACOLOGIC THERAPY

- At the scene: ensure the electrical power source of injury is turned off before approaching patients.
- Basic and advanced cardiac life support with cervical spine precautions. Prolonged cardiopulmonary resuscitation should be undertaken regardless of the initial cardiac rhythm.
- Cardiac monitoring.
- Oxygen.
- Tetanus prophylaxis.

ACUTE GENERAL Rx

- IV fluids to maintain urine output of 50 to 100 ml/hr (IV hydration should be reassessed with central nervous system expert in patients at risk of developing cerebral edema).
- Alkalinization of the urine (sodium bicarbonate 50 mEq in 1 L of normal saline) in patients with or at risk of myoglobinuria.
- Furosemide 20 to 40 mg PO or IV and/or mannitol 12.5 g/kg/hr may be used to force diuresis.
- Seizures are treated in the standard fashion.
- Treat burns with sulfadiazine silver dressings.

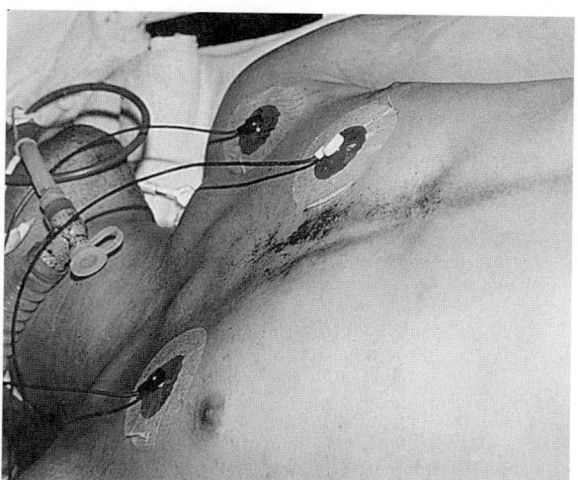

FIGURE 1-131 Linear burns from lightning injury. (From Auerbach P: *Wilderness medicine,* ed 4, St Louis, 2001, Mosby.)

CHRONIC Rx

- Hospitalization is indicated in patients with high-voltage injuries, extensive burns, central nervous system symptoms, myonecrosis (creatine kinase level more than twice normal, high serum myoglobin levels, or myoglobinuria), new cardiac arrhythmia or ECG changes, or any internal organ damage.
- Ophthalmology consultation at the follow-up to screen for cataract formation (occurs within 1 to 24 mo of a high-voltage electrical injury in 5% to 20% of patients).

DISPOSITION

- Patients with severe burns should be transferred to the regional burn center.
- Complications of electrical injuries include:
  1. Infection
  2. Renal failure from rhabdomyolysis
  3. Seizure disorder
  4. Fasciotomies
  5. Amputation
- Delayed neurologic damage may present as ascending paralysis, amyotrophic lateral sclerosis, or transverse myelitis weeks to years after the injury.
- Vascular damage may also present in a delayed fashion.

REFERRAL

- Referrals to general surgery, burn surgery, trauma surgery, orthopedic surgery, and/or critical care specialists as appropriate in any patient that meets hospitalization criteria. Ophthalmology and ear-nose-throat specialist referral may be indicated.
- Plastic surgery is recommended in children with oral burns.

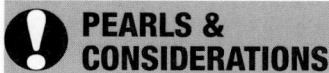

PEARLS & CONSIDERATIONS

COMMENTS

- The size of external skin burns can often underestimate the degree of internal injury.
- Lightning Strike and Electric Shock Survivors International is a support group that serves people from around the world who have sustained an electric injury (http://www.lightning-strike.org).
- Home safety education provided one to one in a clinical setting or at home, especially with the provision of safety equipment, is effective in increasing the range of safety practices.

SUGGESTED READINGS

available at www.expertconsult.com

AUTHORS: **ROBERT M. KIRCHNER, M.D.,** and **PAUL GORDON, M.D.**

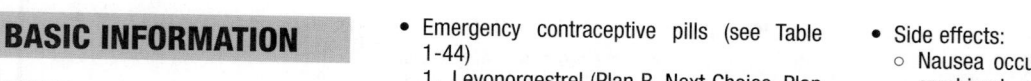

BASIC INFORMATION

DEFINITION

Emergency contraception (EC) can prevent pregnancy soon after unprotected intercourse, sexual assault, or failure or improper use of a birth control method. EC reduces the risk of pregnancy when used up to 120 hr (5 days) after unprotected sex but is more effective if used earlier.

MECHANISM: Current evidence indicates that the primary mechanism of levonorgestrel EC is inhibition or delay of ovulation. Emergency insertion of the copper IUD may prevent fertilization or implantation.

EFFECTIVENESS: Levonorgestrel prevents an estimated 89% of unexpected pregnancies after unprotected intercourse, combined hormonal EC prevents 74%, and the copper IUD prevents 99%.

SYNONYMS

Morning-after pill, postcoital contraception

ICD-9CM CODES
V25.03 Emergency contraceptive counseling and treatment
V25.09 Family planning

EPIDEMIOLOGY & DEMOGRAPHICS

Approximately 49% of all pregnancies and more than 82% of teen pregnancies in the U.S. are unintended. An estimated 1.7 million unintended pregnancies could be prevented annually if emergency contraception use were widespread.

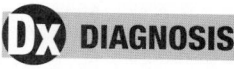 DIAGNOSIS

LABORATORY TESTS

- If there is doubt about whether a patient is already pregnant from intercourse that occurred more than 1 wk previously, a pregnancy test may be helpful. However, there is no need for a pregnancy test before administering EC pills. Delays in administration of the medication will reduce its efficacy. The medications in EC pills will not harm an established pregnancy.
- A pregnancy test should be done before insertion of a copper IUD.

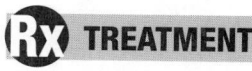 TREATMENT

ACUTE GENERAL Rx

- Administer EC as soon as possible after unprotected intercourse. EC reduces the risk of pregnancy when used up to 120 hr (5 days) after unprotected intercourse but is more effective if used earlier. NOTE: Package inserts for levonorgestrel EC recommend use within 72 hr, but research supports some efficacy up to 120 hr.

- Emergency contraceptive pills (see Table 1-44)
  1. Levonorgestrel (Plan B, Next Choice, Plan B One-Step)
     - Total dose 1.5 mg levonorgestrel
     - A single dose is equally effective and causes no more side effects than two divided doses.
  2. Ulipristal acetate (ella)
     - Available by prescription only
     - Single dose 30 mg ulipristal acetate, a progesterone-receptor modulator
     - FDA-approved for use up to 5 days after unprotected intercourse
     - Appears to be more effective than levonorgestrel for emergency contraception
  3. Combined oral contraceptive pills:
     - Two doses, 12 hr apart, of 100 to 120 mcg ethinyl estradiol and 0.5 to 0.6 mg levonorgestrel (or 1.0 to 1.2 mg norgestrel) per dose.
     - See Table 1-44 for dosing.

- Side effects:
  - Nausea occurs in 50% of women taking combined estrogen-progestin EC pills, vomiting in 20%. Levonorgestrel and ulipristal are associated with much lower incidence of side effects. Side effects resolve within 1 to 2 days. Antinausea medication such as meclizine 25 mg orally is recommended 1 hr before taking combined EC pills.
- Contraindications:
  - Few contraindications to EC exist other than hypersensitivity to the product. EC pills will not affect an established pregnancy.
  - There are no other evidence-based medical contraindications to the use of EC pills. The benefits of EC in preventing pregnancy generally outweigh the theoretical risks for women with contraindications to long-term use of combined hormonal contraception, such as thromboembolic disease, smoking after age 35, heart disease, or liver disease. Levornorgestrel or ulipris-

TABLE 1-44 Emergency Contraceptive Pills Available in the United States

Emergency Contraception Pills

Brand	Dose	Dose
Next Choice[1]	2 pills	1.5 mg levonorgestrel
Plan B[1]	2 pills	1.5 mg levonorgestrel
Plan B One-Step	1 pill	1.5 mg levonorgestrel
Ella	1 pill	30 mg ulipristal acetate

Combined Oral Contraceptive Pills for Emergency Contraception[2]

Brand	First Dose	Second Dose (12 hours later)	Ethinyl Estradiol per Dose (mcg)	Levonorgestrel per Dose (mg)
Aviane	5 orange pills	5 orange pills	100	0.50
Cryselle	4 white pills	4 white pills	120	0.60
Enpresse	4 orange pills	4 orange pills	120	0.50
Jolessa	4 pink pills	4 pink pills	120	0.60
Lessina	5 pink pills	5 pink pills	100	0.50
Levora	4 white pills	4 white pills	120	0.60
Lo/Ovral	4 white pills	4 white pills	120	0.60
LoSeasonique	5 orange pills	5 orange pills	100	0.50
Low-Ogestrel	4 white pills	4 white pills	120	0.60
Lutera	5 white pills	5 white pills	100	0.50
Lybrel	6 yellow pills	6 yellow pills	120	0.54
Nordette	4 light-orange pills	4 light-orange pills	120	0.60
Ogestrel	2 white pills	2 white pills	100	0.50
Portia	4 pink pills	4 pink pills	120	0.60
Quasense	4 white pills	4 white pills	120	0.60
Seasonale	4 pink pills	4 pink pills	120	0.60
Seasonique	4 light-blue-green pills	4 light-blue-green pills	120	0.60
Sronyx	5 white pills	5 white pills	100	0.50
Trivora	4 pink pills	4 pink pills	120	0.50

[1]Package instructions for Plan B and Next Choice recommend 1 pill per dose, 12 hours apart, but research shows similar efficacy and side effects with taking both pills at the same time.
[2]For combined oral contraceptive pills as EC, take two doses, 12 hours apart. The FDA has declared these products safe for use as EC.

tal EC may be preferable to estrogen-containing EC for women with any of these conditions or who are breastfeeding. EC is not indicated for breastfeeding women <6 weeks postpartum as ovulation is extremely unlikely.

- Copper IUD for emergency contraception
  - Emergency insertion of the copper IUD is the most effective option for EC and can be used up to 5 days after unprotected intercourse. This option may be preferable for women who desire effective long-term contraception and have no contraindications to IUD insertion. A pregnancy test should be done before IUD insertion.

CHRONIC Rx

Because EC pills are less effective than other forms of contraception, they are not recommended as an ongoing method of contraception. The copper IUD is highly effective for emergency contraception and can be kept in place to prevent pregnancy for 10 yr.

DISPOSITION

After using EC, for most women menses will occur within 3 days of the expected onset date. If a woman's next expected menses are delayed by more than 1 wk, a pregnancy test should be done.

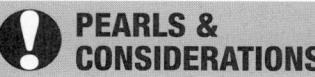

PEARLS & CONSIDERATIONS

COMMENTS

- EC reduces the risk of pregnancy up to 120 hr (5 days) after unprotected intercourse.
- A pregnancy test is not necessary before administering EC pills because the medicines in EC will not harm an existing pregnancy.
- Advanced prescription of EC pills at routine visits may increase timely use of EC and does not decrease the use of more reliable means of contraception.

- Men and women ≥17 can purchase EC pills (Plan B, Next Choice, Plan B One-Step) without a prescription.

PREVENTION

- Patients should begin an effective method of birth control immediately after using EC. Hormonal contraceptives can be started the day after EC is administered. A backup method should be used for 7 days.
- Emergency contraception should be offered to all women after sexual assault.

PATIENT & FAMILY EDUCATION

- Emergency contraception website: http://www.not-2-late.com

SUGGESTED READINGS

available at www.expertconsult.com

AUTHORS: **MELISSA NOTHNAGLE, M.D., M.SC.,** and **JENNIFER BUCKLEY, M.D.**

BASIC INFORMATION

DEFINITION

An accumulation of pus in the pleural space, most often caused by bacterial infection.

SYNONYMS

Infected pleuritis
Infected pleural effusion
Purulent pleural effusion

ICD-9CM CODES

510.9 Empyema Lung

EPIDEMIOLOGY & DEMOGRAPHICS

- Empyema most commonly a complication of bacterial pneumonia, especially in association with pneumococcal or anaerobic infection
- Occur as a complication of thoracic surgery
- Penetrating chest trauma
- Bronchopleural fistulae resulting from malignancy or lung biopsy

PHYSICAL FINDINGS & CLINICAL PRESENTATION

- May be abrupt or chronic and insidious depending on the etiologic agent and host factors.

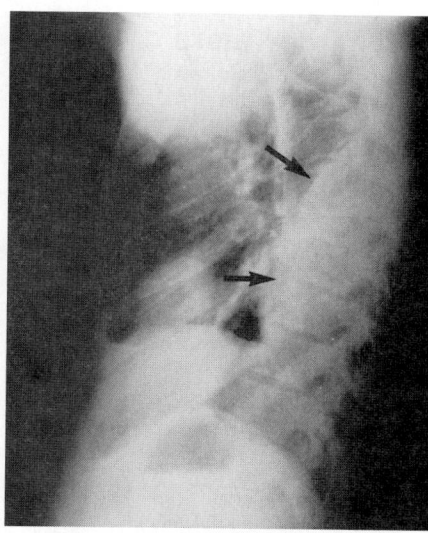

FIGURE 1-132 Empyema. On the lateral chest x-ray, the configuration of the posterior loculated pleural fluid is typical of empyema. The left hemidiaphragm is well seen, with the gastric bubble beneath it. The posterior curve of the right hemidiaphragm is obscured by the empyema. (Souhami RL, Moxham J: *Textbook of medicine*, ed 4, London, 2002, Churchill Livingstone.)

- Typically presents as progressive pleuritic chest pain, persistent fever, and other sustained signs and symptoms of infection.
- In anaerobic empyema, particularly that caused by the actinomycetes, the clinical picture is dominated by systemic symptoms and signs: weight loss, malaise, and low grade fever.
- A slowly enlarging chest wall mass.
- As a complication of thoracic trauma or surgery, empyema typically results from contamination of blood within the pleural space several days following the event.
- The physical findings of empyema are those of pleural effusion. Decreased breath sounds and dullness to percussion over the involved part of the thorax is typical. Systemic signs include fever, tachycardia, leukocytosis, and warmth and erythema over the involved area.

ETIOLOGY

Infection of the lung parenchyma spreading to pleural space caused by
- *Streptococcus pneumoniae*
- *Haemophilus influenzae*
- *Staphylococcus aureus*
- *Legionella* species
- *Mycobacterium tuberculosis*
- *Actinomyces* spp.
- A variety of oral anaerobic bacteria have been cultured in 36% to 37% of empyemas

DIAGNOSIS

DIFFERENTIAL DIAGNOSIS

- Uninfected parapneumonic effusion
- Congestive heart failure
- Malignancy involving the pleura
- Tuberculous pleurisy
- Collagen vascular disease (particularly rheumatoid lung and systemic lupus erythematosus)

LABORATORY TESTS

- Complete blood count; arterial blood gas.
- Blood cultures.
- Pleural fluid analysis in empyema has the characteristics of an exudate with a ratio of pleural fluid to serum protein >0.5 or pleural fluid to serum LDH >0.6. Characteristically, empyema fluid is grossly purulent with visible organisms on Gram stain with glucose <50 mg/dl and pH <7. These findings justify immediate drainage by chest tube or surgery because of the high risk of loculation and progressive systemic infection.

IMAGING STUDIES

- Chest roentgenogram (see Fig. 1-132)
- Lateral decubitus view to establish the presence of free fluid in the pleural space
- Computed tomography to establish the presence of fluid loculation, underlying mass lesions, and other intrathoracic pathology

TREATMENT

NONPHARMACOLOGIC THERAPY

Prompt drainage by thoracostomy (chest tube) or open thoracotomy

ACUTE GENERAL Rx

- Maintenance of drainage until infection controlled.
- Antibiotics directed at suspected or proven bacterial or fungal pathogens.
- Thoracoscopy or instillation of thrombolytic agents (streptokinase or urokinase) may be considered in refractory, loculated empyema.

CHRONIC Rx

- If thorough drainage cannot be accomplished, open thoracotomy with pleural decortication may be required.
- Lung function should be monitored following completion of therapy.

DISPOSITION

Hospitalization with supplemental oxygen with ventilatory support if necessary

REFERRAL

Consultation by infectious diseases, pulmonary, or thoracic surgery specialists as needed.

PEARLS & CONSIDERATIONS

COMMENTS

- Empyema caused by actinomycetes may present with erosion through the chest wall and formation of a fistulous tract.
- Nosocomial infection caused by relatively resistant bacterial or fungal pathogens may result in empyema in patients with indwelling thoracostomy tubes.

SUGGESTED READINGS

available at www.expertconsult.com

AUTHORS: **GLENN G. FORT, M.D., M.P.H.,** and **DENNIS J. MIKOLICH, M.D.**

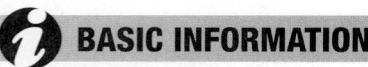

DEFINITION

Acute viral encephalitis is an acute febrile syndrome with evidence of meningeal involvement and of derangement of the function of the cerebrum, cerebellum, or brain stem.

SYNONYMS

Arboviral encephalitis
Brain stem encephalitis
Acute necrotizing encephalitis
Rasmussen encephalitis
Encephalitis lethargica

ICD-9CM CODES
049.9 Viral encephalitis, NOS

EPIDEMIOLOGY & DEMOGRAPHICS

INCIDENCE (IN U.S.): About 20,000 cases/yr are reported to the CDC.
PEAK INCIDENCE: Any age
PREVALENCE (IN U.S.): Unknown
PREDOMINANT SEX: Male = female
PREDOMINANT AGE: Any age
GENETICS: No specific genetic or congenital predisposition

ETIOLOGY

- Can be caused by a host of viruses, with herpes simplex the most common virus identified.
- Arboviruses transmitted by mosquitoes include Eastern equine encephalitis, Western equine encephalitis, St. Louis encephalitis, Venezuelan equine encephalitis, California virus encephalitis, Japanese B encephalitis, Murray Valley and West Nile encephalitis. Tick-borne diseases include Russian spring-summer encephalitis, Powassan encephalitis, and other lesser known agents.
- Also implicated: rabies-causing agents, CMV, Epstein-Barr, varicella-zoster, echo virus, mumps, adenovirus, coxsackie, rubeola, and herpes viruses.
- Meningoencephalitis: acute retroviral infection
- In the U.S., the most commonly identified etiologies are herpes simplex virus, West Nile virus, and the enteroviruses.

PHYSICAL FINDINGS & CLINICAL PRESENTATION

- Initially, fever and evidence of meningeal irritation
- Headache and stiff neck
- Later, development of signs of cortical dysfunction: lethargy, coma, stupor, weakness, seizures, facial weakness, as well as brainstem findings
- Cerebellar findings: ataxia, nystagmus, hypotonia, myoclonus, cranial nerve palsies, and abnormal tendon reflexes
- Patients with rabies: hydrophobia, anxiety, facial numbness, psychosis, coma, or dysarthria
- Rarely, movement disorders, such as chorea, hemiballismus, or dystonia
- Recall of a prodromal viral-like illness (this finding is not at all uniform)

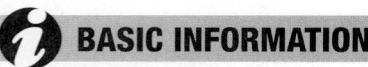

DIFFERENTIAL DIAGNOSIS

- Bacterial infections: brain abscess, toxic encephalopathies, TB
- Protozoal infections
- Behçet's disease
- Lupus encephalitis
- Sjögren's syndrome
- Multiple sclerosis
- Syphilis
- Cryptococcus
- Toxoplasmosis
- Brucellosis
- Leukemic or lymphomatous meningitis
- Other metastatic tumors
- Lyme disease
- Cat-scratch disease
- Vogt-Koyanagi-Harada syndrome
- Mollaret's meningitis

WORKUP

- Lumbar puncture to reveal pleocytosis, usually lymphocytic, although neutrophils may be seen early on
- Usually, elevated CSF protein
- Normal or low CSF glucose
- In herpes simplex encephalitis: RBCs and xanthochromia
- EEG changes showing periodic high-voltage sharp waves in the temporal regions and slow wave complexes suggestive of herpes encephalitis (Fig. 1-133)

- CT scan and MRI to reveal edema and hemorrhage in the frontal and temporal lobes
- Temporal lobe involvement suggests herpes simplex encephalitis
- Basal ganglia and thalami are areas involved as generally seen in Eastern equine encephalitis
- With West Nile infection, MRI changes have shown changes in basal ganglia, thalami, mesial temporal structures, brain stem, and cerebellum
- Arboviral infections suspected during outbreaks in specific areas
- Rising titers of neutralizing antibodies from the acute to the convalescent stage demonstrated but often not helpful in the acutely ill patient
- Polymerase chain reaction that amplifies DNA from the CSF for herpes simplex encephalitis
- Rarely, brain biopsy to assist in the diagnosis; viral culture of cerebral tissue obtained if biopsy done
- Classic herpetic skin lesions suggestive of herpes encephalitis
- In diagnosing arboviral encephalitis:
  1. Presence of antiviral IgM within the first few days of symptomatic disease; detected and quantified by ELISA
  2. Unusual to recover an arbovirus from the blood or CSF

LABORATORY TESTS

- Aside from the lumbar puncture, most other laboratory studies are nonspecific.
- Skin lesions and urine may be cultured for herpes simplex and CMV.

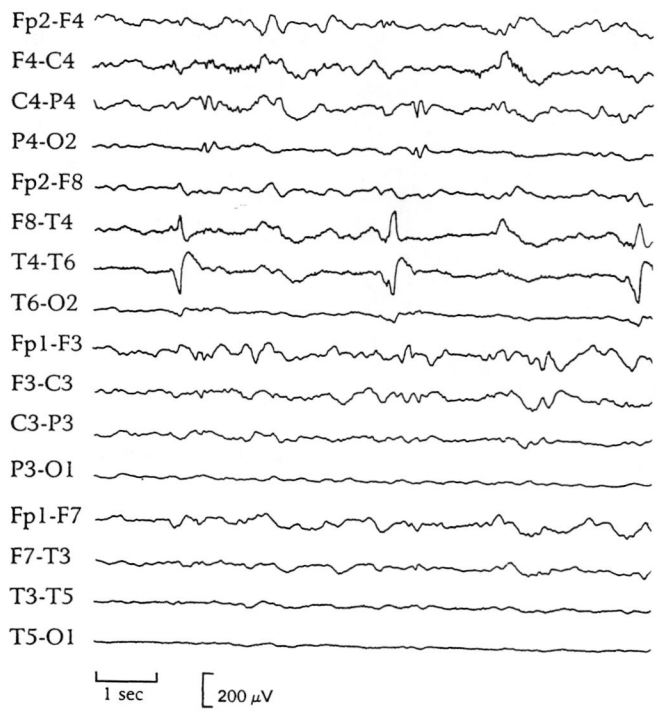

FIGURE 1-133 Repetitive complexes occurring in the right temporal region of a child with herpes simplex encephalitis. (From Goetz CG, Pappert EJ: *Textbook of clinical neurology*, Philadelphia, 1999, Saunders.)

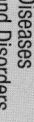

Rx TREATMENT

ACUTE GENERAL Rx

- Supportive care, frequent evaluation, and neurologic examination
- Ventilatory assistance for patients who are moribund or at risk for aspiration
- Avoidance of infusion of hypotonic fluids to minimize the risk of hyponatremia
- For patients who develop seizures: anticonvulsant therapy and follow-up in a critical care setting
- For comatose patients:
  1. Aggressive care to avoid decubitus ulcers, contractures, and DVT
  2. Close attention to weights, input/output, and serum electrolytes
- Acyclovir 30 mg/kg/day IV total dose divided in q8 hour intervals for 14 days for herpes simplex encephalitis
- Short courses of corticosteroids to control brain edema and prevent herniation
- In patients with suspected rabies:
  1. Human rabies immune globulin (HRIG) should be given at a dose of 20 U/kg.
  2. Active immunization may be stimulated by recently developed rabies vaccine, which is grown on a human diploid cell line (HDCV) and has reduced the number of doses needed to five.
  3. If suspect animal is a dog or cat and can be found, observe closely for 10 days to detect rabid behavior; any significant illness in the animal should promptly initiate humane sacrifice of the animal with the brain submitted to local or state health departments for pathology and immunologic testing for rabies. Any wild animal suspected of rabies should be humanely sacrificed, if possible, and submitted for rabies testing immediately.
  4. If signs are seen, animal should be euthanized and its brain examined for signs of rabies.
- No specific pharmacologic therapy for most other viral pathogens

CHRONIC Rx

Some patients may develop permanent neurologic sequelae; these patients will benefit from intensive rehabilitation programs, including physical, occupational, and speech therapy.

DISPOSITION

- Patients with suspected encephalitis of any cause should generally be admitted for initial diagnostic workup and specific treatment (if available).
- Long-term management of patients with significant neurologic sequelae from encephalitis (e.g., memory defects, depression, difficulty with organization of thoughts, movement disorders) may benefit from rehabilitation services, home care, or nursing home placement.

REFERRAL

- To a neurologist for initial workup and management
- To an infectious disease specialist for diagnostic and therapeutic plan
- To a rehabilitation service for long-term evaluation and convalescent services

⚠ PEARLS & CONSIDERATIONS

- West Nile virus encephalitis occurs primarily in elderly patients >65 years of age.
- Rabies may occur months after contact with the rabid animal, and the exposure (especially bat rabies) may have been seemingly insignificant and even inapparent.
- Experimental therapies are worthy of consideration for some forms of viral encephalitis (e.g., immune plasma, ribavirin, interferons), and expert consultation should be obtained early on for possible treatment interventions with promising experimental therapies.

SUGGESTED READINGS
available at www.expertconsult.com

AUTHORS: **GLENN G. FORT, M.D., M.P.H.,** and **DENNIS J. MIKOLICH, M.D.**

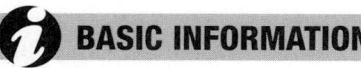

BASIC INFORMATION

DEFINITION

Encephalopathy is a clinical syndrome of global cognitive impairment characterized by impaired arousal, inattention, and disorientation.

SYNONYMS

Delirium, acute confusional state

ICD-9CM CODES	
348.3	Encephalopathy, NOS
348.30	Encephalopathy, unspecified
348.31	Encephalopathy, metabolic
348.39	Encephalopathy, other
349.82	Encephalopathy, toxic

EPIDEMIOLOGY & DEMOGRAPHICS

POINT PREVALENCE: 1.1% of adults in the general population >55 yr, 10% to 40% of hospitalized elderly, and 60% of nursing home patients >75 yr; 100,000 to 200,000 cases annually with anoxic encephalopathy
RISK FACTORS: Age, cancer, AIDS, terminal illness, bone marrow transplant, surgery

PHYSICAL FINDINGS & CLINICAL PRESENTATION

- The essential feature of encephalopathy is the patient's inability to maintain a coherent stream of thought or action.
- The history may often suggest a waxing and waning of the level of arousal and general cognitive ability.
- Because toxins and metabolic disturbances are common causes of encephalopathy, the history should focus on exposure to toxins (especially medications) and symptoms suggesting a concurrent illness such as a urinary tract infection or pneumonia.
- Common to all encephalopathies is a fluctuating level of arousal, poor attention, and disorientation.
- Some patients may appear agitated and others lethargic.
- Delusions (fixed false beliefs) and hallucinations are common.
- Asterixis (negative myoclonus) is extremely common.
- Other physical findings may vary depending on the underlying cause of encephalopathy, such as fever, ascites, jaundice, or tachycardia.

ETIOLOGY

- The final common pathway of all causes of encephalopathy is widespread cortical and subcortical neuronal dysfunction. The causes may be structural or functional.
- Many conditions are reversible and carry a good prognosis if treated in a timely manner.
- Organ failure (e.g., hepatic encephalopathy, hypoxia, hypercapnia, uremia).
- Infection: systemic (e.g., urinary tract, pneumonia) or involving the central nervous system (e.g., meningitis, encephalitis).
- Toxin ingestion or withdrawal (e.g., alcohol, medications, recreational drugs).

- Metabolic disturbances: hyperosmolar states, hypernatremia, hyponatremia, hyperglycemia, hypoglycemia, hypercalcemia, hypophosphatemia, acidosis, alkalosis, inborn errors of metabolism.
- Endocrinopathy: hyperthyroidism, hypothyroidism, Cushing's syndrome, adrenal insufficiency, pituitary failure.
- Neoplasm: tumors of the central nervous system, primary or metastatic. Also effect of distant tumors (e.g., paraneoplastic limbic encephalitis).
- Nutritional deficiency, mostly in alcoholics and chronically ill patients, such as vitamin B_1 deficiency (Wernicke's encephalopathy).
- Seizures: postictal state, nonconvulsive status epilepticus, complex partial seizures, absence seizures.
- Trauma: concussion, contusion, subdural hematoma, epidural hematoma, diffuse axonal injury.
- Vascular: both ischemic and hemorrhagic strokes, vasculitis, venous thrombosis.
- Postanoxic encephalopathy.
- Other: hypertensive encephalopathy, postoperative status, sleep deprivation.

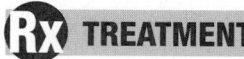

DIAGNOSIS

DIFFERENTIAL DIAGNOSIS

- Dementia: distinguished from encephalopathy by a history of slowly progressive cognitive decline over time (fluctuating cognitive function is rare except in diffuse Lewy body disease).
- Hypersomnia.
- Aphasia: distinguished from encephalopathy by virtue of it representing a specific disorder of language rather than a global disturbance of cognitive function.
- Depression.
- Psychosis: some overlap with encephalopathy because delusions and hallucinations may be common to both.
- Mania.
- Vegetative state from cerebral injury; these patients appear awake (eyes are open) but there is no content to their consciousness.
- Akinetic mutism: these patients do not talk and do not move; there is little fluctuation in their state and there is no asterixis.
- Locked-in syndrome: may be distinguished from encephalopathy by the presence of fixed neurologic deficits (e.g., paralysis of all four limbs).

WORKUP

- Electroencephalography is helpful to confirm the presence of encephalopathy (diffuse slowing) and also to exclude nonconvulsive seizures.
- Chest radiograph to rule out pneumonia.

LABORATORY TESTS

- General chemistry: electrolytes, glucose, creatinine, ammonia, blood urea nitrogen, transaminases, amylase, lipase
- Arterial blood gases
- Complete blood count

- Drug screen and alcohol level (must order ethylene glycol separately if suspected)
- Lumbar puncture if meningitis, encephalitis, or subarachnoid hemorrhage with negative imaging is suspected
- HIV testing
- Endocrine testing: cortisol level, thyroid function test
- Urinalysis and microscopy

IMAGING STUDIES

- CT to rule out bleeding, hydrocephalus, tumors
- MRI with diffusion-weighted images for suspected encephalitis, tumors, and acute strokes
- Magnetic resonance angiography/venography for strokes, arterial dissection, venous thrombosis
- Conventional angiography for central nervous system (CNS) vasculitis and aneurysms

TREATMENT

NONPHARMACOLOGIC THERAPY

The best approach is to treat the underlying toxic or metabolic disturbance. The encephalopathy itself is a symptom of these underlying problems. In general, it is best to avoid treating the symptom of encephalopathy with antipsychotics or sedatives.

GENERAL Rx

- Glucose if hypoglycemia
- Antibiotics in cases of infections (choice of an agent with good CNS penetration in cases of primary CNS infections)
- Insulin in hyperglycemic conditions (e.g., diabetic ketoacidosis, hyperosmolar nonketosis, and sepsis)
- The main approach to hepatic encephalopathy is the use of nonabsorbed disaccharides or antibiotics (alone or in combination) to reduce colony counts of ammonia-producing gut flora and to decrease the systemic absorption of ammonia from the intestinal lumen. Lactulose has been used for decades. Rifaximin is a newer agent. It is a minimally absorbed antibiotic useful in both acute hepatic encephalopathy and to maintain remission from recurrent hepatic encephalopathy in patients with chronic liver disease
- Thiamine (vitamin B_1) and folate replacement when deficiency is suspected
- Anticonvulsants if seizures likely
- Librium or diazepam for delirium tremens (alcohol withdrawal)
- Ensure hemodynamic stability (blood pressure and heart rate)

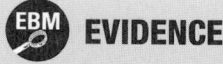 **EVIDENCE**

available at www.expertconsult.com

SUGGESTED READINGS
available at www.expertconsult.com

AUTHOR: **ACHRAF A. MAKKI, M.D., M.SC.**

BASIC INFORMATION

DEFINITION/DIAGNOSTIC CRITERIA (*DSM-IV*, 1994)

Encopresis is the voluntary or involuntary passage of stool in inappropriate places, in children over the developmental age of 4 yr. Occurs at least once per month for at least 3 mo and is not due to the effects of a substance (e.g., laxative) or a general medical condition, *except constipation.*

SYNONYMS

Stool incontinence; soiling

ICD-9CM CODES
787.6 Incontinence of feces
307.7 Encopresis

DSM-IV CODES
787.6 Encopresis With Constipation and Overflow Incontinence
307.7 Encopresis Without Constipation and Overflow Incontinence

EPIDEMIOLOGY & DEMOGRAPHICS

PEAK INCIDENCE: Preschool age (though also occurs during school age and adolescence)
PREVALANCE (IN U.S.): 1.5% to 7.5% of children 4 to 12 yr old
PREDOMINANT SEX: More often in males (estimates range from 1.9:1 to 9:1)

PHYSICAL FINDINGS & CLINICAL PRESENTATION

- Most children are toilet-trained for stool by age 4. Traditionally, in primary encopresis, fecal continence is never fully established; in secondary encopresis, soiling is preceded by a period of fecal continence. However, definitions of "primary" vs. "secondary" do not reliably correlate with etiology or outcome.
- Constipation and withholding of stool are significant factors in 80% to 90% of cases ("retentive encopresis"). In 10% to 20%, constipation is not a factor ("nonretentive" encopresis).
- When constipation is longstanding, soft or liquid stool may flow around the retained feces, resulting in overflow incontinence. This may occur several times per day and mistakenly be interpreted as diarrhea.
- Children may report a lack of awareness of stool passage when longstanding constipation/impaction has resulted in loss of rectal tone and sensation. Furthermore, some children habituate to the odor.

ETIOLOGY

- Approximately 96% of children have bowel movements between three times daily to once every other day. When bowel movements are less frequent, stool becomes drier and harder and much more uncomfortable or painful to pass. Children may avoid the discomfort or pain by avoiding elimination, re-

sulting in worsening constipation and overflow incontinence.
- Constipation may begin gradually as a result of a decrease in elimination frequency, or more acutely after an illness or changes in diet.
- Toilet training practices that increase anxiety may also play a role in stool retention, the development of constipation, and eventual encopresis.

DIAGNOSIS

DIFFERENTIAL DIAGNOSIS

- Hirschsprung's disease
- Endocrine disease (hypothyroidism)
- Cerebral palsy
- Myelomeningocele
- Pseudoobstruction
- Anorectal lesions (rectal stenosis)
- Malformations
- Trauma
- Rectal prolapse
- Celiac disease
- Hypothyroidism
- Medications

WORKUP

- History: frequency of elimination, character of the stool, associated pain, and presence of enuresis (with which it is frequently associated).
- Evaluate for other developmental or psychiatric problems.
- Physical examination: pay particular attention to the abdomen, anus, rectum, and neurologic examination.

LABORATORY TESTS

- Consider thyroid function tests, celiac screening tests, electrolytes, calcium, urinalysis, and urine culture.
- If concerned about the possibility of Hirschprung's disease, obtain rectal biopsy.

IMAGING STUDIES

- Abdominal imaging to determine extent of obstruction or megacolon
- Anorectal manometric studies or barium enema can support suspicion of Hirschsprung's disease

TREATMENT

ACUTE GENERAL Rx

- Disimpaction is anecessary first step, by oral or rectal route (or combination).
- For oral disimpaction, polyethylene glycol or high doses of mineral oil are effective (avoid use of mineral oil in patients at risk for aspiration).
- Adding stimulant laxatives such as senna or bisacodyl can sometimes make oral disimpaction more effective.
- For rectal disimpaction, phosphate soda, saline, or mineral oil enemas are effective.

- When medical workup determines that constipation is not present ("nonretentive encopresis"), consider implementing toilet-training routines or referral to behavioral health provider.

CHRONIC Rx

- Prevent recurrence of constipation with oral stool softeners (e.g., polyethylene glycol, sorbital, or lactulose) or stool libricants (mineral oil).
- In immediate postdisimpaction period (1 mo after acute treatment), stimulant laxatives may be needed because bowel tone remains low; taper use as quickly as possible to avoid dependence.
- Family documentation of stool passage, including location and amount, on a chart or calendar helps inform medication changes and best times for toilet sitting.
- Praise and other small incentives for positive toileting routines and taking medication can help to maintain good bowel habits. Balanced diet and increased fiber intake/supplementation may also help.
- Formal behavioral treatment (education, treatment, adherence and exercises to improve anal sphincter control) increases treatment success. Biofeedback to improve sphincter function is advocated by some, with 1-yr results comparable to behavioral treatment.

DISPOSITION

Encopresis may be self-limited or relatively brief in duration; may require prolonged maintenance therapy. Relapses are common.

REFERRAL

Behavioral family therapy should be considered for patients who do not respond to medical treatment within a few months or who have significant contiubuting psychiatric or family factors.

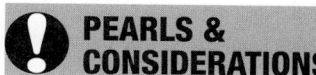

PEARLS & CONSIDERATIONS

- It is crucial to educate parents and children about constipation and encopresis and to defuse negative interactions.
- Emphasize that this can require prolonged maintenance therapy and that relapses are common.

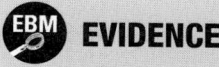

EVIDENCE

available at www.expertconsult.com

SUGGESTED READINGS

available at www.expertconsult.com

AUTHORS: **JACK H. NASSAU, PH.D.,**
WENDY A. PLANTE, PH.D., and
VINCENT A. MUKKADA, M.D.

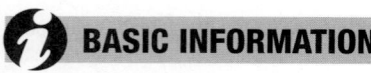
DEFINITION

Infective endocarditis is an infection of the endocardial surface of the heart or mural endocardium.

ACUTE ENDOCARDITIS: Usually caused by *Staphylococcus aureus, Streptococcus pyogenes, Streptococcus pneumoniae,* and *Neisseria* organisms; classic clinical presentation of high fever, positive blood cultures, vascular and immunologic phenomenon

SUBACUTE ENDOCARDITIS: Usually caused by viridans streptococci in the presence of valvular pathology; less toxic, often indolent presentation with lower fevers, night sweats, fatigue

ENDOCARDITIS IN INJECTION DRUG USERS: Often involving *S. aureus* or *Pseudomonas aeruginosa* with variation that may be geographically influenced; tricuspid (Fig. 1-134) or multiple valvular involvement; high mortality rate of 50% to 60%

PROSTHETIC VALVE ENDOCARDITIS (EARLY): Usually caused by *S. aureus* (leading cause of PVE) within 2 mo of valve replacement; other organisms include *S. epidermis,* gram-negative bacilli, diphtheroids, *Candida* organisms

PROSTHETIC VALVE ENDOCARDITIS (LATE): Typically develops >60 days after valvular replacement; involved organisms similar to early prosthetic valve endocarditis, including viridans streptococci, enterococci, and group D streptococci

NOSOCOMIAL ENDOCARDITIS: Secondary to intravenous catheters, TPN lines, pacemakers; coagulase-negative staphylococci, *S. aureus,* and streptococci most common

Non-HACEK gram-negative bacillus endocarditis is not primarily a disease of injection drug users. More than half of all cases are associated with health care contact

SYNONYMS

Bacterial endocarditis
Subacute bacterial endocarditis (SBE)
Endocarditis

ICD-9CM CODES
421.0 Infective endocarditis
996.61 Prosthetic valve endocarditis

EPIDEMIOLOGY & DEMOGRAPHICS

INCIDENCE (IN U.S.): 1.7 to 3.8 cases/100,000 persons/yr
PEAK INCIDENCE: Females: often <35 yr old; males: 45 to 65 yr old
NOSOCOMIAL ENDOCARDITIS: 14% to 28% of cases
PREVALENCE (IN U.S.): 0.3 to 3 cases/1000 hospital admissions
PREDOMINANT SEX: Male > female
PREDOMINANT AGE: 45 to 65 yr

PHYSICAL FINDINGS & CLINICAL PRESENTATION

- Clinical manifestations of infective endocarditis are described in Table 1-45.
- Fever may be variable in presentation; may be high, hectic, or absent.
- Fever, chills, fatigue, and rigors occur in 25% to 80% of patients.
- Heart murmur may be absent in right-sided endocarditis.
- Embolic phenomenon with peripheral manifestations is found in 50% of patients.
- Skin manifestations include petechiae, Osler nodes, splinter hemorrhages, Janeway lesions.
- Splenomegaly is more common with subacute course.

ETIOLOGY

Streptococcal and staphylococcal infections are the most common causes of infective endocarditis. Variation in incidence may occur that is influenced by the patient's risk for developing infection.

ACUTE ENDOCARDITIS:
- *S. aureus*
- *S. pneumoniae*
- Streptococcal species and groups A through G
- *Haemophilus influenzae*

SUBACUTE ENDOCARDITIS:
- Viridans streptococci (alpha-hemolytic)
- *S. bovis*
- Enterococci
- *S. aureus*

ENDOCARDITIS IN INJECTION DRUG USERS:
- *S. aureus*
- *P. aeruginosa*
- *Candida* spp.
- Enterococci

PROSTHETIC VALVE ENDOCARDITIS (EARLY):
- *S. epidermidis*
- *S. aureus*
- Gram-negative bacilli
- Group D streptococci

PROSTHETIC VALVE ENDOCARDITIS (LATE):
- *S. epidermidis*
- Viridans streptococci
- *S. aureus*
- Enterococci and group D streptococci

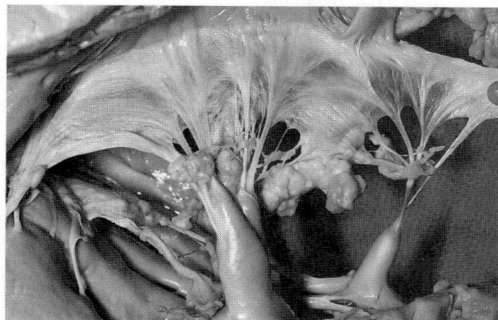

FIGURE 1-134 Tricuspid valve endocarditis. There are large vegetations on the leaflets and the chordae tendineae. (From Crawford MH et al [eds]: *Cardiology,* ed 2, St Louis, 2004, Mosby.)

TABLE 1-45 Clinical Manifestations of Infective Endocarditis Myalgia/Arthralgia

Symptoms	Patients Affected (%)	Signs	Patients (%)
Fever	80	Fever	90
Chills	40	Heart murmur	85
Weakness	40	Changing murmur	5-10
Dyspnea	40	New murmur	3-5
Sweats	25	Embolic phenomenon	>50
Anorexia	25	Skin manifestations	18-50
Weight loss	25	Osler nodes	10-23
Malaise	25	Splinter hemorrhages	15
Cough	25	Petechiae	20-40
Skin lesions	20	Janeway lesion	<10
Stroke	20	Splenomegaly	20-57
Nausea/vomiting	20	Septic complications (e.g., pneumonia, meningitis)	20
Headache	20	Mycotic aneurysms	20
Myalgia/arthralgia	15	Clubbing	12-52
Edema	15	Retinal lesion	2-10
Chest pain	15	Signs of renal failure	10-25
Abdominal pain and delirium/coma	15		
Delirium/coma	10-15		
Hemoptysis	10		
Back pain	10		

From Mandell GL et al: *Principles and practice of infectious diseases,* ed 6, Philadelphia, Elsevier, 2005.

NOSOCOMIAL ENDOCARDITIS:
- Coagulase-negative staphylococci
- *S. aureus*
- Streptococci: viridans, group B, enterococcus

HACEK ORGANISMS:
- Fastidious gram-negative bacilli
- *Haemophilus parainfluenzae*
- *Haemophilus aphrophilus*
- *Actinobacillus actinomycetemcomitans*
- *Cardiobacterium hominis*
- *Eikenella corrodens*
- *Kingella kingae*

RISK FACTORS
- Poor dental hygiene
- Long-term hemodialysis
- Diabetes mellitus
- HIV infection
- Mitral valve prolapse

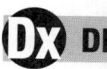 **DIAGNOSIS**

DIFFERENTIAL DIAGNOSIS
- Brain abscess
- FUO
- Pericarditis
- Meningitis
- Rheumatic fever
- Osteomyelitis
- Salmonella
- TB
- Bacteremia
- Pericarditis
- Glomerulonephritis

WORKUP
Physical examination to evaluate for the previous physical findings followed by laboratory testing (see "Laboratory Tests")

LABORATORY TESTS
- Blood cultures: three sets in first 24 hr
- More culturing if patient has received prior antibiotic
- CBC (anemia possibly present, subacute)
- WBC (leukocytosis is higher in acute endocarditis)
- ESR and C-reactive protein (elevated)
- Positive rheumatoid factor (subacute endocarditis)
- False-positive VDRL
- Proteinuria, hematuria, RBC casts

- Electrocardiogram: look for cardiac conduction abnormalities, injury pattern, or evidence of pericarditis—any such new findings are suggestive of myocardial abscess

IMAGING STUDIES
- Echocardiogram: two-dimensional
- Transesophageal echocardiography (TEE): more sensitive in detecting vegetations if two dimensional is negative, especially helpful with prosthetic valves or in detecting perivalvular disease

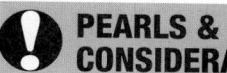 **TREATMENT**

Initial IV antibiotic therapy (before culture results) is aimed at the most likely organism:
- In patients with prosthetic valves or patients with native valves who are allergic to penicillin: vancomycin (1 g IV every 12 hr for 4 wk) plus rifampin 600 mg PO daily and gentamicin (1 mg/kg IV every 8 hr for 2 wk)—assuming normal renal function in adult patients.
- In IV drug users: nafcillin or oxacillin (2 g IV every 4 hr) plus gentamicin (1 mg/kg every 8 hr for 3 to 5 days until blood cultures are negative); if MRSA, vancomycin (1 g IV every 12 hr for 4 wk) plus gentamicin (1 mg/kg every 8 hr for 3 to 5 days until blood cultures are negative).
- In native valve endocarditis with a penicillin-susceptible streptococcal isolate: combination of penicillin (18 to 24 million units/day IV for 4 wk) and gentamicin (1 mg/kg every 8 hr for 2 wk) assuming normal renal function. Extend the gentamicin therapy for 4 wk if a relatively penicillin-resistant strain of streptococcus is isolated (penicillin MIC >0.5 microgram/ml); a penicillinase-resistant penicillin (oxacillin or nafcillin—2 g IV every 4 hr for 4 to 6 wk plus gentamicin 1 mg/kg IV every 8 hr for 3 to 5 days) can be used if acute bacterial endocarditis is present or if *S. aureus* is suspected as one of the possible causative organisms; for HACEK organisms, treat with third-generation cephalosporin (ceftriaxone—2 g IV every 24 hr for 4 to 6 wk).
- Ceftriaxone: 2 g IV every 24 hr and an aminoglycoside (e.g., gentamicin 1 mg/kg IV every 8 hr for 2 wk) effective for *Streptococcus viridans* endocarditis.

- Daptomycin (6 mg/kg/day for 4 to 6 wk) has recently been approved for use in *S. aureus* bacteremia and right-sided endocarditis; may prove useful in MRSA infections.
Antibiotic therapy after identification of the organism should be guided by susceptibility testing—preferably by formal testing by MIC (minimum inhibitory testing).

DISPOSITION
- The patient may need outpatient IV antibiotic therapy, and arrangements need to be made to ensure safe vascular access and continuity of care with outpatient IV therapy team.
- Long-term follow-up is essential after therapy has ended; relapse of endocarditis may occur.
- Prophylaxis with antibiotics will be needed before dental procedures as a previous episode of endocarditis increases the risk of recurrent endocarditis associated with transient bacteremia from dental procedures.

REFERRAL
- To an infectious disease specialist for an optimal antibiotic regimen
- To a cardiologist or a cardiac surgeon if evidence of heart failure, refractory infection, myocardial abscess, valve disruption, or major embolic events occur
- To a dentist or oral surgeon if dental work needs to be conducted with appropriate use of prophylactic antibiotics to prevent recurrent endocarditis

⚠ PEARLS & CONSIDERATIONS

COMMENTS
For endocarditis prophylaxis refer to Section V.

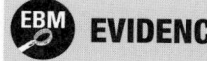 **EVIDENCE**

available at www.expertconsult.com

SUGGESTED READINGS
available at www.expertconsult.com

AUTHORS: **GLENN G. FORT, M.D., M.P.H.,** and **DENNIS J. MIKOLICH, M.D.**

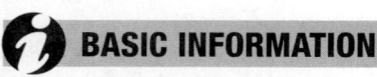

BASIC INFORMATION

DEFINITION

Endometrial cancer (EC) is a malignant transformation of endometrial stroma and/or glands typified by irregular nuclear membranes, nuclear atypia, mitotic activity, loss of glandular pattern, and irregular cell size. The two main histologic subcategories of EC, endometrioid and nonendometrioid EC, show unique molecular aberrations and differing clinical behaviors.

SYNONYMS

Uterine cancer (some forms)
EC

ICD-9CM CODES
182 Malignant neoplasm of body of uterus

EPIDEMIOLOGY & DEMOGRAPHICS

INCIDENCE: 21.2 cases per 100,000 persons; approximately 30,000 new cases annually. It is the most common gynecologic malignancy in the U.S.

PREDOMINANCE: Median age at onset: 60 yr; only 5% occur in women <40 yr

RISK FACTORS: Obesity, diabetes, nulliparity, early menarche and late menopause, unopposed estrogen therapy, tamoxifen use, endometrial atypical hyperplasia

PHYSICAL FINDINGS & CLINICAL PRESENTATION

- Abnormal uterine bleeding or postmenopausal bleeding in 90%
- Pyometra or hematometra
- Abnormal Pap smear

ETIOLOGY

Endogenous or exogenous chronic unopposed estrogen stimulation of the endometrium

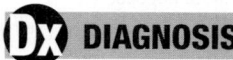

DIAGNOSIS

DIFFERENTIAL DIAGNOSIS

- Atypical hyperplasia
- Other genital tract malignancy
- Polyps
- Atrophic vaginitis
- Granuloma cell tumor
- Fibroid uterus

WORKUP

- Complete history and physical examination
- Endometrial biopsy or dilation and curettage
- Assessment of operative risk
- Staging (Table 1-46)

LABORATORY TESTS

- Complete blood count
- Chemistry profile including liver function tests
- Consider CA-125 level

IMAGING STUDIES

- Chest x-ray examination
- CT scan, and/or pelvic ultrasound
- Endovaginal ultrasound in postmenopausal women with vaginal bleeding

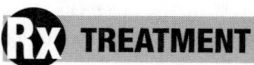

TREATMENT

NONPHARMACOLOGIC THERAPY

- Surgery is the mainstay of treatment, with or without radiation, depending on tumor stage

and grade. Laparoscopic surgery for early-stage endometrial cancer is as safe and effective as laparatomy.
- Surgery generally consists of pelvic washings, total abdominal hysterectomy and bilateral salpingo-oophorectomy, omental biopsy, and selective pelvic and periaortic lymphadenectomy, depending on stage and grade.
- Brachytherapy and/or teletherapy are added in an advanced stage.
- Chemotherapy (cisplatin, Adriamycin) or tamoxifen may also be used.
- Hormonal therapy is an option for some young women with EC who wish to preserve fertility.

ACUTE GENERAL Rx

- A thorough workup should be completed before any therapy for endometrial cancer.
- Surgery is the treatment of choice.

CHRONIC Rx

- Physical and pelvic examination every 3 mo for 2 yr, then every 6 mo for 2 yr, annually thereafter
- Yearly Pap smear
- Hormone replacement (combination) a consideration in low-risk patients (stage I or early stage II)

DISPOSITION

The majority of cases present early, and the 5-yr survival is generally good:

Stage I	75%-100%
Stage II	65%
Stage III	40%
Stage IV	10%

Some histologic types (clear cell, serous papillary) have worse survival rates.

REFERRAL

Refer to a gynecologic oncologist.

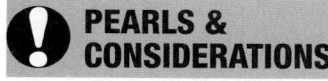

PEARLS & CONSIDERATIONS

COMMENTS

- Estrogen replacement therapy after surgery for endometrial cancer remains controversial. Recent data suggest that it does not increase endometrial cancer recurrence rates.
- Obesity and sedentary lifestyle put endometrial cancer survivors at increased risk for health problems. Even moderate activity is associated with better physical functioning in endometrial cancer survivors

SUGGESTED READINGS
available at www.expertconsult.com

AUTHORS: **GIL M. FARKASH, M.D.,** and **RUBEN ALVERO, M.D.**

TABLE 1-46 FIGO Staging of Endometrical Carcinoma

Stage	Definition	Stage at Presentation	Pelvic Nodes	5-year Survival
I$_A$	Tumor limited to the endometrium			
I$_B$	Growth that has invaded <50% of myometrial thickness	73%	<20%	85%
I$_C$	Growth that has invaded >50% of myometrial thickness			
II$_A$	Endocervical glandular involvement only	11%	20%	65%
II$_B$	Cervical stroma involved			
III$_A$	Invades sero-serosal surface of uterus, ± adnexa, ± positive washings			
III$_B$	Vaginal metastases	13%	35%	40%
III$_C$	Metastases to pelvic or para-aortic nodes			
IV$_A$	Tumor invasion of bladder and/or bowel			
IV$_B$	Distant metastases including intra-abdominal and/or inguinal lymph nodes	3%	50%	10%

Histopathology: degree of differentiation

Uterine adenocarcinoma should be grouped according to the degree of differentiation as follows:

- G1 — 5% or less of a solid growth pattern
- G2 — 6%-50% of a solid growth pattern
- G3 — More than 50% of a solid growth pattern

From Drife J, Magowan B: *Clinical obstetrics and gynecology*, Philadelphia, 2004, Saunders.

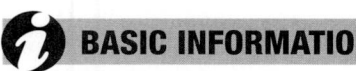

BASIC INFORMATION

DEFINITION

Endometriosis is defined as the presence of functioning endometrial glands and stroma outside the uterine cavity (Fig. 1-135).

ICD-9CM CODES
617.9 Endometriosis

EPIDEMIOLOGY & DEMOGRAPHICS

PREVALENCE:
- In asymptomatic women: 2% to 22%
- Women with dysmenorrhea: 40% to 60%
- Subfertile women: 20% to 30%
- Incidence peaks at approximately 40 yr

MOST COMMON AGE AT DIAGNOSIS: 25 to 29 yr

GENETICS:
- Multifactorial inheritance pattern
- 6.9% occurrence rate in first-degree female relatives

PHYSICAL FINDINGS & CLINICAL PRESENTATION

- Classic triad is dysmenorrhea, dyspareunia, and infertility.
- Presence of pelvic pain not correlated with the total area of endometriosis, type of lesion, or volume of disease, but is correlated with the depth of infiltration.
- Other symptoms include abnormal bleeding (premenstrual spotting, menorrhagia), cyclic abdominal pain, intermittent constipation/diarrhea, dyschezia, dysuria, hematuria, and urinary frequency.
- Rare manifestations: catamenial hemothorax, bloody pleural effusion, massive ascites occurring during menses.
- Most severe discomfort is associated with lesions >1 cm in depth.
- Bimanual examination may reveal tender uterosacral ligaments, cul-de-sac nodularity, induration of the rectovaginal septum, fixed retroversion of the uterus, adnexal mass, and generalized or localized tenderness.

ETIOLOGY

- Reflux and direct implantation theory: retrograde menstruation with implantation of viable endometrial cells to surrounding pelvic structures
- Coelomic metaplasia theory: transformation of multipotential cells of the coelomic epithelium into endometrium-like cells
- Vascular dissemination theory: transport of endometrial cells to distant sites by the uterine vascular and lymphatic systems
- Autoimmune disease theory: disorder of immune surveillance allows growth of endometrial implants

DIAGNOSIS

DIFFERENTIAL DIAGNOSIS

- Ectopic pregnancy
- Acute appendicitis
- Chronic appendicitis
- Pelvic inflammatory disease (PID)
- Pelvic adhesions
- Hemorrhagic cyst
- Hernia
- Psychologic disorder
- Irritable bowel syndrome
- Uterine leiomyomata
- Adenomyosis
- Nerve entrapment syndrome
- Scoliosis
- Muscular/skeletal strain
- Interstitial cystitis

WORKUP

- Thorough history and physical examination, including inquiry about physical and emotional abuse. Defining diagnosis of endometriosis can be made only by histology of lesions that have been removed surgically
- Colonoscopy if rectal bleeding present
- Laparoscopy for definitive diagnosis
- Revised American Fertility Society (renamed American Society for Reproductive Medicine) scale to classify endometriosis (since 1985):
  Stage I   Minimal
  Stage II Mild
  Stage III Moderate
  Stage IV Severe

LABORATORY TESTS

Cancer antigen 125 (CA125):
- Also elevated in ovarian epithelial neoplasm, myomas, adenomyosis, acute PID, ovarian cysts, pancreatitis, chronic liver disease, menstruation, and pregnancy
- CA125 value >35 U/ml: positive predictive value of 0.58 and a negative predictive value of 0.96 for the presence of endometriosis

IMAGING STUDIES

- Ultrasound: for evaluating adnexal mass; ultrasound characteristics may suggest endometriomas versus other benign or malignant ovarian conditions but persistent solid or cystic-solid ovarian masses require definitive tissue diagnosis with laparoscopy.
- MRI:
  1. Highly accurate in detecting endometriomas
  2. Limited sensitivity in detecting diffuse pelvic endometriosis

TREATMENT

NONPHARMACOLOGIC THERAPY

Expectant management (observation for 5 to 12 mo) for stage I or stage II endometriosis-associated infertility. Evaluation should take place if the couple meet the diagnostic criteria for infertility.

ACUTE GENERAL Rx

Nonsteroidal anti-inflammatory drugs for symptomatic relief of dysmenorrhea

CHRONIC Rx

PHARMACOLOGIC MANAGEMENT:
Estrogen-progesterone:
- State of "pseudopregnancy" created by continuous use of combination oral contraceptives for 6 to 12 mo
- Breakthrough bleeding treated by administering conjugated estrogens 1.25 mg/day for 2 wk

Progestins:
- Medroxyprogesterone acetate 10 to 30 mg PO qd and occasionally up to 100 mg PO qd
- Alternatively, 100 mg IM q2wk for four doses, followed by 200 mg IM monthly for 4 mo
- Breakthrough bleeding treated with ethinyl estradiol (20 mcg/day) or conjugated estrogens (1.25 mg/day) for 1 to 2 wk

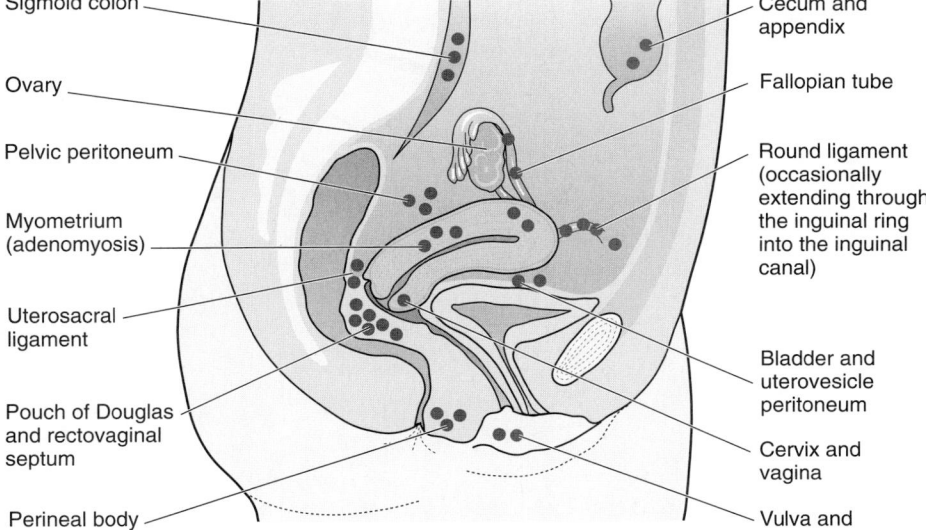

FIGURE 1-135 Common sites for endometriotic deposits in the pelvis. (From Drife J, Magowan B: *Clinical obstetrics and gynecology,* Philadelphia, 2004, Saunders.)

Sigmoid colon
Ovary
Pelvic peritoneum
Myometrium (adenomyosis)
Uterosacral ligament
Pouch of Douglas and rectovaginal septum
Perineal body

Cecum and appendix
Fallopian tube
Round ligament (occasionally extending through the inguinal ring into the inguinal canal)
Bladder and uterovesicle peritoneum
Cervix and vagina
Vulva and Bartholin's gland

E

Diseases and Disorders

- Comparison with danazol: progestins cost less, have a more tolerable side-effect profile, and have comparable efficacy with regard to pain relief and so are often the first-line drug

Gonadotropin-releasing hormone (GnRH) agonists:

- Use usually limited to 6 mo due to hypoestrogenic effects such as osteopenia or osteoporosis
- Leuprolide acetate depot 3.75 mg IM monthly or 11.25 mg IM q3mo or nafarelin 200 mcg nasal puffs bid or goserelin 3.6 mg SC monthly
- As effective as danazol for relief of pelvic pain
- Add-back therapy for protection against vasomotor symptoms and bone loss: norethindrone acetate 5 mg PO qd alone or in combination with conjugated estrogen 0.625 mg PO qd
- Add-back therapy allows gonadotropin-releasing hormone (GnRH) agonist use to be extended to 1 yr based on limited studies available

Alternative therapies for inhibition of estrogen action currently under investigation are:

- Aromatase inhibitors: anastrozole, letrozole
- SERM: raloxifene
- Agents enhancing cell-mediated immunity are cytokines (interleukin-12 and interferon-α2b)
- Immunomodulators (loxoribine, levamisole)
- Anti-inflammatory: pentoxifylline

SURGICAL MANAGEMENT:

Conservative:

- Directed at enhancing fertility or treating pain unresponsive to first-line medical treatment
- Usually accomplished through laparoscopy
- Removal or destruction of endometriotic implants by excision, electrocautery, or laser

- Cystectomy for endometrioma
- Laparoscopic uterosacral nerve ablation for midline pain such as dysmenorrhea or dyspareunia (evidence does not support its use)
- Unless pregnancy is desired, patient is usually started on GnRH agonist therapy immediately after surgery
- For those desiring pregnancy, surgery alone results in significant increase in fertility

Definitive:

- Directed at relieving endometriosis-associated pain
- Total abdominal hysterectomy with bilateral salpingo-oophorectomy and complete excision or ablation of endometriosis
- Thorough abdominal exploration to ensure removal of all disease
- Must be prepared to manage possible gastrointestinal and urinary tract endometriosis
- 90% effective in pain relief; patient must be counseled that pain relief is not guaranteed
- Estrogen replacement therapy (ERT) to be considered in all women undergoing definitive surgical management; after ERT, recurrence rate is 0% to 5% in women with endometriosis confined to the pelvis but 18% in women with bowel involvement

MANAGEMENT OF ENDOMETRIOSIS-ASSOCIATED INFERTILITY:

Conservative surgery:

- Yields significantly increased pregnancy rate than does expectant management, in part because of correction of mechanical factors such as adhesions

Assisted reproductive technologies:

- Can be used to circumvent unknown mechanism of endometriosis-associated infertility
- Superovulation with clomiphene citrate or human menopausal gonadotropins; clomiphene citrate results in threefold pregnancy rate over either danazol or expectant management
- Further improvement with intrauterine insemination combined with superovulation
- In vitro fertilization if above procedures are unsuccessful

DISPOSITION

Tends to recur unless definitive surgery is performed and should be considered a chronic condition

REFERRAL

To a reproductive endocrinologist for advanced surgical management or infertility management

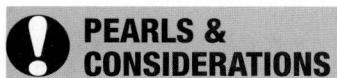

PEARLS & CONSIDERATIONS

COMMENTS

Patient information can be obtained through the following organizations: Endometriosis Association, 8585 North 76th Place, Milwaukee, WI 53223, 414-355-2200 or 800-992-ENDO; Women's Reproductive Health Network, P.O. Box 30167, Portland, OR 97230-9067 or 503-667-7757.

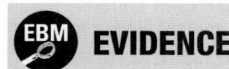

EVIDENCE

available at www.expertconsult.com

SUGGESTED READINGS

available at www.expertconsult.com

AUTHORS: **WAN J. KIM, M.D.,** and **RUBEN ALVERO, M.D.**

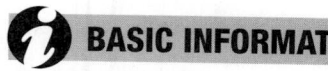

BASIC INFORMATION

DEFINITION

Endometritis is defined as a uterine infection after delivery or abortion.

SYNONYMS

Endomyometritis
Metritis

ICD-9CM CODES

615.9 Endometritis

EPIDEMIOLOGY & DEMOGRAPHICS

- Overall rate of postpartum infection: estimated between 1% and 8%
- Most common genital tract infection after delivery
- Usually presents early in postpartum period; more commonly seen after cesarean section than vaginal delivery; also seen with an incomplete abortion (spontaneous abortion, legal abortion, or illegal abortion)
- More common in preterm deliveries
- Possible after any uterine manipulation in the presence of undiagnosed cervicitis or vaginitis

PHYSICAL FINDINGS & CLINICAL PRESENTATION

- Postpartum oral temperature >37.8° C
- Localized uterine tenderness, purulent or foul lochia; physical examination revealing uterine or parametrial tenderness
- Nonspecific signs and symptoms such as malaise, abdominal pain, chills, and tachycardia

ETIOLOGY

Endometritis is usually associated with multiple organisms: group A or B streptococci, *Staphylococcus aureus* and *Bacteroides* species, *Neisseria gonorrhoeae*, *Chlamydia trachomatis*, enterococci, *Gardnerella vaginalis*, *E. coli*, and *Mycoplasma*.

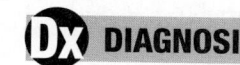

DIAGNOSIS

DIFFERENTIAL DIAGNOSIS

Causes of postoperative or postprocedural infections

WORKUP

Diagnosis based on symptoms of fever, malaise, abdominal pain, uterine tenderness, and purulent, foul vaginal discharge

LABORATORY TESTS

Complete blood count, blood cultures, and uterine culture

IMAGING STUDIES

Ultrasound may be useful if retained products are considered a possible source of infection.

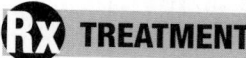

TREATMENT

ACUTE GENERAL Rx

- In treating endometritis after a vaginal delivery, ampicillin 2 g IV q6h plus gentamicin loading dose IV or IM (2 mg/kg of body weight) followed by a maintenance dose (1.5 mg/kg of body weight) q8h are used.
- Regimen should be continued for at least 48 hr after substantial clinical improvement. If response is not adequate, check cultures and treat with appropriate antibiotics (Table 1-47).
- Endometritis after cesarean section should be treated with ampicillin 2 g IV q6h plus gentamicin loading dose IV or IM (2 mg/kg of body weight) followed by a maintenance dose (1.5 mg/kg of body weight) q8h and clindamycin 900 mg IV q8h. If *Chlamydia* is one of the etiologic agents, add doxycycline 100 mg PO bid for completion of a 14-day course of therapy (if breastfeeding, use erythromycin).

CHRONIC Rx

Watch for recurrent infection.

DISPOSITION

With appropriate antibiotic therapy, 95% to 98% cure rate

REFERRAL

For patients who do not respond within 48 to 72 hr of appropriate antibiotic therapy, obtain an infectious disease consult or gynecologic consultation.

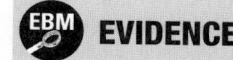

EVIDENCE

available at www.expertconsult.com

AUTHORS: **GEORGE T. DANAKAS, M.D.**, and **RUBEN ALVERO, M.D.**

TABLE 1-47 Identified Causes of Poor Response to Antibiotic Therapy in Patients with Endometritis

Cause	Approximate Prevalence (%)
Infected mass, including abscess, hematoma, septic pelvic thrombophlebitis, pelvic cellulitis, retained placenta	40-50
Resistant organisms, commonly enterococci, in a patient receiving clindamycin-aminoglycoside or a cephalosporin	20
Additional cause, including catheter phlebitis, inadequate dose of antibiotics	10
No cause evident but response to empirical change in antibiotic therapy	20-30

From Gorbach SL: *Infectious diseases*, ed 2, Philadelphia, 1998, WB Saunders.

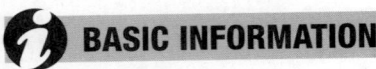

BASIC INFORMATION

DEFINITION

Enuresis refers to the voiding of urine into clothes or in bed that is usually involuntary in individuals who are expected to be continent (>5 yr of age). The diagnosis is made if voiding occurs at least twice a week for 3 mos. Primary enuresis refers to enuresis without a period of continence, whereas secondary enuresis occurs after a period of normal bladder control.

SYNONYMS

Urinary incontinence
Bed-wetting

ICD-9CM CODES
788.36 Nocturnal Enuresis
DMS-IV Code 307.6 Enuresis Primary/
Secondary of
Nonorganic Origin

EPIDEMIOLOGY & DEMOGRAPHICS

PEAK INCIDENCE: Ages 5 to 10 yr
PREVALENCE (IN U.S.):
- Age 5 yr: 7% of males and 3% of females
- Age 10 yr: 3% of males and 2% of females
- Age 18 yr: 1% of males
PREDOMINANT SEX: Twice as many males as females at all ages
PREDOMINANT AGE: By definition, enuresis does not begin before age 5 yr, at which time the prevalence is highest, and decreases steadily thereafter at a rate of approximately 12% to 15% per year.
GENETICS:
- Approximately 75% of children with enuresis have a first-degree relative with enuresis.
- Almost twice as common in monozygotic than dizygotic twins.

PHYSICAL FINDINGS & CLINICAL PRESENTATION

Three enuresis subtypes are defined:
- Nocturnal only: occurs in each sleep stage in proportion to the time spent in the particular stage. May occur during transition from deep sleep to REM.
- Diurnal only: more frequent in girls and rarely after age 9 yr; voiding occurs in early afternoon on school days.
- Combined nocturnal and diurnal; often called complex or complicated enuresis.

ETIOLOGY

- Enuresis often correlates with other maturational delays, particularly language, motor skills, and social development.
- May be related to toilet training issues, stress (secondary enuresis), inability to concentrate urine, altered smooth muscle physiology, or dysfunction of the arousal system.
- Diurnal enuresis associated with a higher rate of urinary tract infections.

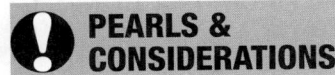

DIAGNOSIS

DIFFERENTIAL DIAGNOSIS

- May be associated with encopresis and sleep disorders such as sleep terrors; much less likely to be a primary psychological disorder.
- Organic causes of enuresis include diabetes mellitus, diabetes insipidus, bladder outlet obstruction, small bladder capacity, detrusor instability, urethral valves, meatal stenosis, cerebral palsy, spina bifida, pelvic mass, impacted stool, sedating medications, nocturnal seizures.

WORKUP

- History and physical examination to rule out anatomic abnormalities. Fluid intake and voiding diaries may be useful.
- Children frequently experience shame, so gentleness and care must be exercised when questioning or examining the child.
- Observation of voiding stream is useful.

LABORATORY TESTS

- Urinalysis with specific gravity and urine culture if white cells or nitrites on analysis.
- Serum studies to rule out diabetes, electrolyte abnormalities, or renal dysfunction.

IMAGING STUDIES

- In complicated cases, sleep studies may be useful.
- If an anatomic abnormality suspected, renal ultrasound or intravenous pyelogram is possibly indicated; MRI of the spine if evidence of abnormalities of lower spine or perineum is found on examination.

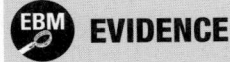

TREATMENT

NONPHARMACOLOGIC THERAPY

Behavioral treatment:
- Alarm and pad technique: up to 80% cure rate, although 30% relapse.
- Scheduled voiding to reduce the frequency of enuretic episodes.
- Star charts to reward child for dry nights.
- Punishment for enuresis is not effective.

ACUTE GENERAL Rx

- Desmopressin (DDAVP) administered intranasally or orally at bedtime significantly reduces the incidence of bedwetting.
- Tricyclic antidepressants (imipramine): efficacy supported by randomized control trials. Use with care in children.
- Serotonin reuptake inhibitors: lack of adequate trials is notable.
- Indomethacin suppositories may reduce normal prostaglandin inhibitory effects on antidiuretic hormone.

DISPOSITION

- After age 5 yr, the rate of spontaneous remissions is approximately 12% to 15% per year.
- The disorder usually resolves by adolescence. However, effective treatment spares considerable misery.
- Fewer than 1% will have enuresis as adults.

REFERRAL

If coexisting, a psychiatric condition complicates the course of treatment.

PEARLS & CONSIDERATIONS

Illness, hospitalization, and family stressors may precipitate recurrent enuresis after a period of dryness.

PATIENT & FAMILY EDUCATION

Bedwetting: Jasper to the Rescue! video available from Disney Educational Productions (http://dep.disney.go.com/educational/index)

EBM EVIDENCE

available at www.expertconsult.com

SUGGESTED READINGS
available at www.expertconsult.com

AUTHORS: **GREGORY K. FRITZ, M.D.,** and **MITCHELL D. FELDMAN, M.D., M.PHIL.**

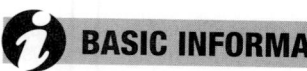

DEFINITION

Eosinophilic fasciitis (EF) is a rare inflammatory disease of the skin and subcutaneous tissue that is initially characterized by pain, edema, and eosinophilia in peripheral blood. This condition starts with symmetrical erythema, edema, and induration of an extremity or trunk and later may progress to sclerosis of the dermis and subcutaneous fascia leading to contractures.

SYNONYMS

Shulman's syndrome
Diffuse fasciitis with eosinophilia

ICD-9CM CODES
728.89 Eosinophilic fasciitis

EPIDEMIOLOGY & DEMOGRAPHICS

- Males and females are affected equally.
- Most common in the fourth and fifth decades.

CLINICAL PRESENTATION

- Initial presentation consists of acute erythema, swelling, and induration of the skin that is accompanied by eosinophilia.
  - Extremities usually symmetrically involved.
  - Upper more commonly affected than lower extremities.
  - Face, fingers, and toes are spared.
  - Sunken veins may be seen when the extremity is elevated (Fig. 1-136). The groove sign marks the borders of different muscle groups.
  - Skin may appear deeply rippled (peau d'orange).
- Arthritis was found in 40% of cases in one series.
- Cranial and peripheral neuropathy (mononeuritis multiplex) may occur.
- Myalgia and weakness are common.

- Hematologic abnormalities are present in 10% of cases, including aplastic anemia, amegakaryocytic thrombocytopenia, myeloproliferative disorders, and hematologic malignancies.
- The presence of Raynaud's phenomenon and visceral involvement is more suggestive of systemic sclerosis or other scleroderma-like disorders than EF.
- Spontaneous resolution or improvement has been reported after 2 to 5 yr.

ETIOLOGY

The etiology is unknown. Most cases are considered idiopathic. Vigorous exercise, initiation of hemodialysis, and infection with *Borrelia burgdorferi* have been suggested as possible causes of EF.

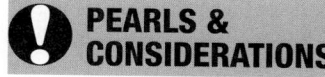

DIFFERENTIAL DIAGNOSIS

- Systemic or localized sclerosis
- Systemic or localized scleroderma
- Scleroderma-like disorders
- Chemical-induced sclerosis
- Generalized lichen sclerosus et atrophicus
- Eosinophilia-myalgia syndrome
- Porphyria cutanea tarda
- Chronic Lyme borreliosis

WORKUP

- Physical examination to confirm characteristic distribution.
- Skin biopsy that penetrates to muscle is optimal for diagnosis:
  - Epidermis is usually normal.
  - Dermis may demonstrate mild inflammation with lymphocytes, histiocytes, plasma cells, and eosinophils with some fibrosis.
  - Moderate inflammation of subcutaneous tissue and sclerosis of fat septa.
  - Muscle demonstrates perivascular mixed inflammatory cell infiltrate.

LABORATORY TESTS

- Peripheral eosinophilia in up to 70% during the acute phase of the disease
- Elevated erythrocyte sedimentation rate (29%)
- Hypergammaglobulinemia (35%)
- Creatine kinase is usually normal even in patients with myalgia
- Occasional thrombocytopenia, anemia
- Serum antinuclear antibodies are negative

IMAGING STUDIES

- MRI may be useful in assessing patients with suspected EF
- Increased T2 signal in the subcutaneous and deep fascia with enhancement of these structures on T1 images after gadolinium administration

Rx TREATMENT

ACUTE GENERAL Rx

- Although no controlled trials exist, corticosteroids (prednisone 1 mg/kg/day) are effective in most patients, but the duration and extent of symptom reduction are variable.
- Hydroxychloroquine is an alternative that may be as effective as steroids.
- In resistant cases, ultraviolet A photochemotherapy, cyclosporine, antithymocyte globulin, methotrexate, D-penicillamine, intravenous immune globulin, and sulfasalazine have been successfully used.

CHRONIC Rx

Surgery is sometimes required to reduce contractures and maintain function.

DISPOSITION

- Prognosis is generally good with frequent spontaneous regression and response to steroids.
- Contractures are common.
- 10% may develop blood dyscrasias.

REFERRAL

To dermatology for biopsy to make definitive diagnosis. Functional impairment requires surgical evaluation.

PEARLS & CONSIDERATIONS

COMMENTS

- EF is a rare inflammatory disorder of unknown etiology with symmetric painful edema and induration of the arms and legs with peripheral eosinophilia.
- Rapid onset, progression, and good response to systemic corticosteroids are characteristic of the disease.
- Prognosis is usually good.

SUGGESTED READINGS

available at www.expertconsult.com

AUTHOR: ETSUKO AOKI, M.D., PH.D.

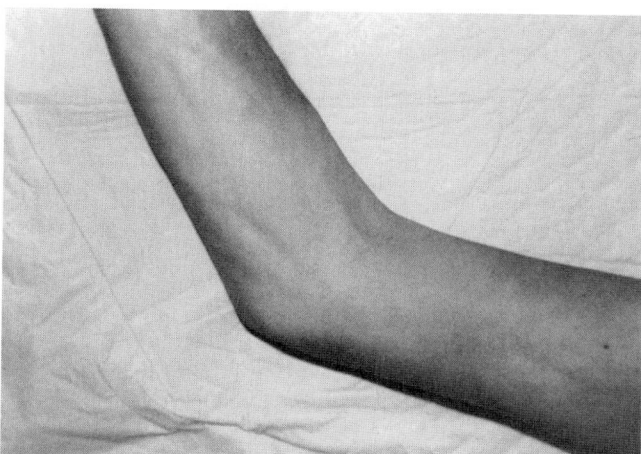

FIGURE 1-136 Eosinophilic fasciitis. This 29-year-old butcher had to stop working because of a generalized painful induration of his skin. Fingers were spared. As he raised his forearms, the collapsed veins appeared as grooves (the "groove sign"), which is pathognomonic of eosinophilic fasciitis. His condition subsided 4 years later, leaving joint contractures. (Reprinted from Canoso J: *Rheumatology in primary care*, Philadelphia, 1997, WB Saunders.)

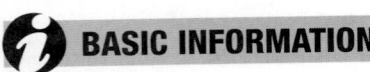

BASIC INFORMATION

DEFINITION

Eosinophilic pneumonias (EPs) are a group of disorders characterized by pulmonary infiltrates, pulmonary parenchymal eosinophilia, and possibly peripheral blood eosinophilia. They manifest by different radiologic and clinical syndromes.

SYNONYMS

Simple pulmonary eosinophilia
Chronic eosinophilic pneumonia
Acute eosinophilic pneumonia
Churg-Strauss syndrome
Idiopathic hypereosinophilic syndrome
Allergic bronchopulmonary aspergillosis
Parasite-induced, fungal-induced, and drug-induced pulmonary eosinophilia

ICD-9CM CODES
518.3 Eosinophilic pneumonia

EPIDEMIOLOGY & DEMOGRAPHICS

Vary depending on the specific cause

PHYSICAL FINDINGS & CLINICAL PRESENTATION

- Fever, cough, and shortness of breath
- Vary depending on the specific cause

ETIOLOGY

SIMPLE PULMONARY EOSINOPHILIA (LÖFFLER'S SYNDROME):

- Transient pulmonary infiltrates
- Symptoms range from asymptomatic to dyspnea and dry cough
- Usually idiopathic
- May be secondary to parasitic infection or drugs (nitrofurantoin, penicillin)
- Remove the offending agent
- If idiopathic and severe symptoms, then give glucocorticoid therapy

IDIOPATHIC ACUTE EP:

- Absence of infection or other cause
- Acute onset of fever, cough, dyspnea (<1 mo); often presents with acute respiratory failure, requiring intensive care
- Erythrocyte sedimentation rate (ESR), C-reactive protein (CRP), and IgE may be elevated but nonspecific
- Bilateral diffuse infiltrates on chest radiograph
- High-resolution CT scan of the chest may demonstrate patchy ground glass with reticular infiltrates; small pleural effusions present in two thirds of cases
- Pleural fluid analysis reveals elevated pH and high eosinophil count
- Hypoxemia (PaO$_2$ <60)
- Lung eosinophilia >25% on bronchoalveolar lavage (BAL)
- Pulmonary function test can demonstrate restrictive dysfunction with reduction in diffusion capacity
- Associations: recent onset of tobacco smoking, World Trade Center dust, Scotchguard

inhalation, tear gas, gasoline, indoor renovation work, multiple medications, firework smoke, cocaine
- Steroids lead to rapid improvement, though there is no consensus about ideal dosing strategy

IDIOPATHIC CHRONIC EP:

- Absence of infection or other cause
- Presentation over weeks to months
- Productive cough, dyspnea, malaise, weight loss, night sweats, and fever (with or without hemoptysis/chest pain)
- Progressive pulmonary infiltrates
- "Photographic negative" pulmonary edema (peripheral alveolar infiltrates) is pathognomonic but only present in 25% of cases; high-resolution CT of the chest may reveal atelectasis, pleural effusions, lymphadenopathy, and septal line thickening
- Blood eosinophilia not always present
- ESR, CRP, platelets, and IgE may be elevated but are nonspecific
- Diagnose by BAL (up to 90% of cases will have 60% eosinophils) or lung biopsy
- Spontaneous remission in 10% of cases
- Treatment with glucocorticoids is rapidly effective
- Relapses are common when glucocorticoids tapered
- Prevalence of patients with asthma

ALLERGIC BRONCHOPULMONARY ASPERGILLOSIS (ABPA):

- Hypersensitivity reaction to *Aspergillus fumigatus*
- Occurs most often in patients with asthma and atopy (up to 13% of the asthma population)
- Fever, flulike symptoms, myalgias, lassitude, persistent cough and wheezing, hemoptysis, and/or expectoration of brown-black mucous plugs
- A patient with chronic asthma with a component of bronchiectasis and pulmonary infiltrates should be evaluated carefully for ABPA
- Chest radiograph: infiltrates (sometimes migratory) and atelectasis, reflecting endobronchial mucous inspissation ("finger in glove")
- Blood and sputum eosinophilia
- Diagnosis by
  1. *Aspergillus* isolation from multiple sputum samples
  2. Positive skin test to *Aspergillus* (Fig. 1-137)
  3. Elevated serum IgE
  4. *Aspergillus*-specific IgE and IgG
  5. Serum eosinophilia >1000 cells/μl

The disease has been characterized by a staging system:
Patients do not necessarily proceed from one stage to another.

Stage I	Acute phase
Stage II	Remission
Stage III	Exacerbation
Stage IV	Glucocorticoid-dependent ABPA
Stage V	End-stage (fibrotic) ABPA

- Treatment: systemic corticosteroids are the mainstay of treatment. Antifungals may provide additional benefit in modulating airway fungal burden and are recommended for use in patients with relapse or glucocorticoid-dependent disease
- Development of bronchiectasis portends a worse prognosis
- Response to therapy and activity of disease may be monitored by measuring IgE levels,

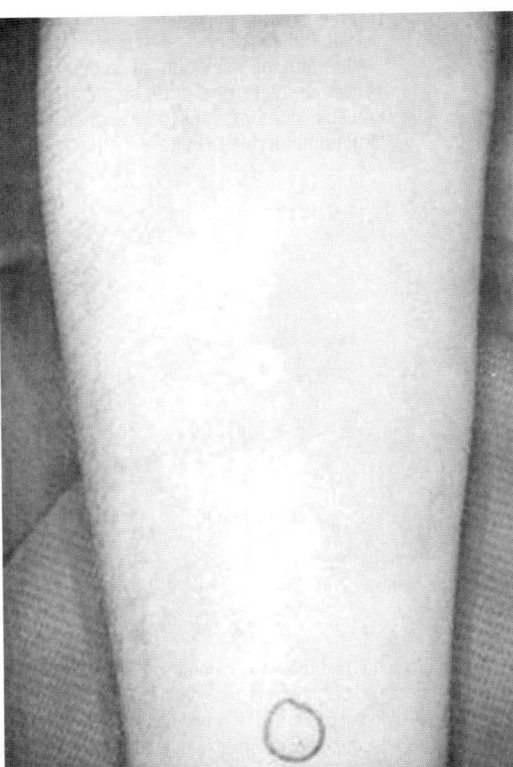

FIGURE 1-137 A positive prick test with *Aspergillus fumigatus* in a patient with allergic bronchopulmonary aspergillosis. The wheal and erythema reaction at 15 min after performing the skin test. (From Fireman P: *Atlas of allergies and immunology*, ed 3, St Louis, 2006, Mosby.

which will decrease by 35% to 50% when a patient is in remission

TROPICAL PULMONARY EOSINOPHILIA:

- Onset of asthma, fever, paroxysmal cough and bronchospasm, marked blood eosinophilia
- Basilar reticulonodular and alveolar infiltrates
- High serum IgE levels
- Presumed etiology: filariasis

PULMONARY VASCULITIS (ALLERGIC GRANULOMATOSIS AND ANGIITIS OR CHURG-STRAUSS SYNDROME):

- Vasculitis and necrotizing granulomatous inflammation that involves many organ systems in the setting of asthma
- Blood eosinophilia and elevated IgE
- Antineutrophilic cytoplasmic antibody may be positive in up to two thirds of patients; antinuclear antibody, rheumatoid factor, and ESR also may be elevated
- Common symptoms include cough, dyspnea, sinusitis, allergic rhinitis; other symptoms depend on other organs involved
- Pulmonary function test may reveal obstructive dysfunction
- Organ and systems involved include lungs, heart (including refractory coronary vasospasm), skin, gastrointestinal, renal, neurologic

HYPEREOSINOPHILIC SYNDROME:

- A disease of persistently elevated eosinophils (>6 mo) with no known cause
- Cardiac problems are the prominent clinical feature with mural thrombi and endocardial/myocardial fibrosis
- Hepatosplenomegaly is common
- Fever, cough, weight loss, wheezing
- Diagnosis of exclusion
- Check echocardiogram
- Treat with steroids if symptoms or cardiac abnormalities

DRUG- OR TOXIN-INDUCED EP:

- Can have several different clinical presentations, including simple pulmonary eosinophilia, chronic, or acute
- Symptoms resolve when offending drug is removed

- Common drug/toxin causes: antibiotics, NSAIDs, amiodarone, bleomycin, captopril, gold salts, iodine, methotrexate, smoke, illicit drugs, radiation exposure
- BAL to exclude infection or other lung disease
- Laboratory evaluation rarely diagnostic

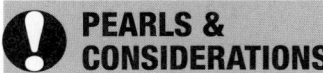

DIAGNOSIS

- Diagnosis varies depending on specific cause of pneumonia
- Usually involves chest radiograph, CT, peripheral eosinophil count, BAL, and possibly lung biopsy

DIFFERENTIAL DIAGNOSIS

- Tuberculosis
- Brucellosis
- Fungal diseases
- Parasitic infection (ascaris, strongyloides)
- Idiopathic pulmonary fibrosis
- Bronchiolitis obliterans and organizing pneumonia
- Radiation pneumonitis
- Bronchogenic carcinoma
- Hodgkin's disease
- Immunoblastic lymphadenopathy
- Rheumatoid lung disease
- Sarcoidosis

WORKUP

Physical examination, laboratory tests, imaging, bronchoscopy

LABORATORY TESTS

- WBC counts are often normal
- Often blood eosinophilia
- Elevated eosinophil count on BAL

IMAGING STUDIES

Chest radiograph may show a variety of infiltrates depending on the cause of EP. CT demonstrates a more characteristic pattern and distribution of parenchymal opacities than chest radiograph.

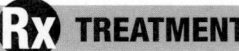

TREATMENT

- Varies depending on the cause.
- Remove offending agent or treat with appropriate antibiotic.
- Steroids may be helpful in many cases; doses and length of treatment depend on etiology of symptoms and response to treatment.
- Supportive respiratory care.

DISPOSITION

Prognosis is good if offending agent can be removed or an infectious etiology treated. Glucocorticoids have a good effect, but relapse often recurs with tapering in chronic idiopathic cases.

REFERRAL

To pulmonologist if a BAL is needed to establish the diagnosis

PEARLS & CONSIDERATIONS

- History (including travel) and physical examination are most important. Temporal association of eosinophilia and pulmonary abnormalities is an important diagnostic clue.
- Coccidioidomycosis and *Aspergillus* can present as eosinophilic lung disease and are important to recognize because steroid therapy can produce progressive infection.
- *Aspergillus* from respiratory specimens does not always indicate true infection and may be colonization.
- Blood eosinophilia $>1 \times 10^9$ eosinophils/L or BAL >25% is helpful in narrowing diagnosis.
- Integrating the clinical, radiologic, and pathologic findings facilitates the initial and differential diagnoses of various eosinophilic lung diseases.

SUGGESTED READINGS
available at www.expertconsult.com

AUTHORS: **CAROLYN J. O'CONNOR, M.D.,** and **KRISTINA KRAMER, M.D.**

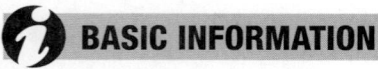

BASIC INFORMATION

DEFINITION

Epicondylitis is inflammation (tendinosis) of the musculotendinous origin of the common extensors at the lateral elbow or the flexor pronator group at the medial elbow.

SYNONYMS

Tennis elbow (lateral epicondylitis)
Golfer's elbow (medial epicondylitis)

ICD-9CM CODES	
726.31	Medial epicondylitis
726.32	Lateral epicondylitis
723.4	Radial nerve neuralgia

EPIDEMIOLOGY & DEMOGRAPHICS

PREVALENCE:
- 10% to 15% of regular (2 hr/wk) tennis players
- Lateral side is involved five times more often than the medial

PREVALENT AGE AND SEX: Affects men and women equally and is more common in persons 40 yr and older

PHYSICAL FINDINGS & CLINICAL PRESENTATION

- Local tenderness over affected epicondyle
- Reproduction of pain by resistance against wrist extension (lateral) (Fig. 1-138) or flexion (medial)

ETIOLOGY

- Unknown
- Overuse probably causing minor tendinous tears, resulting in inflammation
- Posterior interosseous nerve syndrome: compression of this nerve has occasionally been cited as a possible etiology, especially in cases that have not responded to traditional medical and surgical treatment. In this disorder the site of tenderness is 2 to 3 cm distal to the epicondyle.

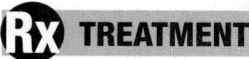

DIAGNOSIS

DIFFERENTIAL DIAGNOSIS

- Cervical radiculopathy
- Intraarticular elbow pathology (osteoarthritis, osteochondritis dissecans, loose body)
- Radial nerve compression
- Ulnar neuropathy
- Medial collateral ligament instability

IMAGING STUDIES

Traction spur or minor soft tissue calcification may be present on plain radiography. Other studies are not usually needed.

TREATMENT

- Rest, restricted activities
- Ice after exercise
- Stretching exercise program
- Nonsteroidal anti-inflammatory drugs (NSAIDs)
- Local steroid/lidocaine injection (Table 1-48; Fig. 1-139)
- Counterforce brace

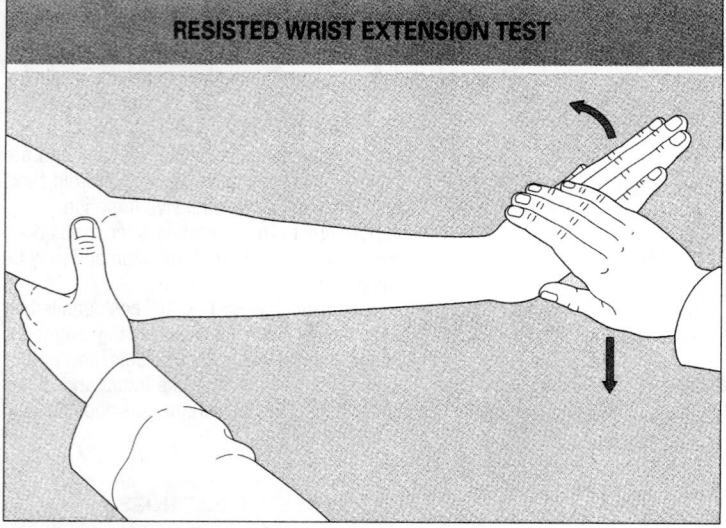

FIGURE 1-138 Resisted wrist extension to test for lateral epicondylitis. The examiner asks the patient to try to extend the wrist but prevents movement by fixing the wrist; this puts tension on the lateral epicondyle without moving the elbow and reproduces the pain of lateral epicondylitis. (From Klippel J et al [eds]: *Primary care rheumatology,* London, 1999, Mosby.)

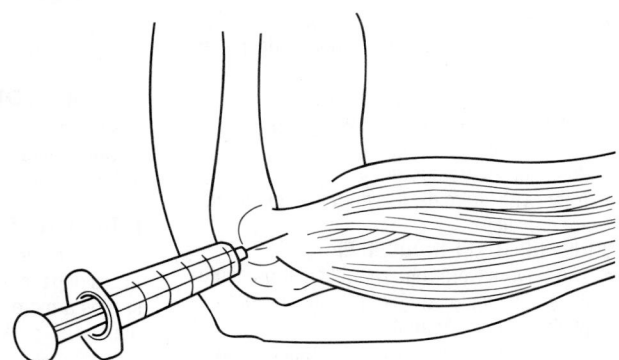

FIGURE 1-139 Soft-tissue injection for lateral epicondylitis. The patient is supine and the elbow is flexed 90 degrees. A 25-gauge needle is used to inject the tender spot, which is usually approximately 1 cm distal to the bony epicondyle. (From Mercier L: *Practical orthopedics,* ed 6, St Louis, 2005, Mosby.)

TABLE 1-48 Guidelines for Common Steroid Injections

Site	Diagnosis	Needle Size (Gauge, Inches)	Anesthetic Volume (ml)
Subacromial bursa	Rotator cuff tendinitis	22, 1½	4-5
Bicipital groove	Biceps tendinitis	22, 1½	2-3
A-C joint	Arthritis	25, 1½	1-2
Lateral medial epicondyle	Epicondylitis	25, ⅝	1.5
First extensor sheath	De Quervain's disease	25, ⅝	1.5
Trochanteric bursa	Tendinitis	22, spinal	4-5
Knee joint	Arthritis	22, 1½	5-10
Knee, soft tissue	Tendinitis	25, 1½	3-4
Plantar fascia	Fasciitis	25, 1½	1.0
Toe metatarsophalangeal	Arthritis	25, ⅝	1.5

From Mercier LR: *Practical orthopedics,* ed 5, St Louis, 2000, Mosby.

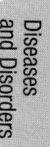

- Proper technique in sports activities
- Intermittent immobilization
- Patients with refractory symptoms may benefit from surgical intervention

DISPOSITION

Disorder is self-limited in most cases. Resolution of symptoms may take months to years.

REFERRAL

- If symptoms do not respond to medical management
- For surgical consideration

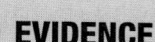 **PEARLS & CONSIDERATIONS**

Concepts are changing regarding the underlying pathology of epicondylitis and similar musculoskeletal conditions, which were always thought to be inflammatory in nature. Many are now considered more degenerative, as evidenced by tissue specimens that lack the cellular changes expected with inflammation.

EVIDENCE

available at www.expertconsult.com

SUGGESTED READINGS

available at www.expertconsult.com

AUTHOR: **LONNIE R. MERCIER, M.D.**

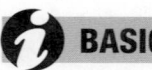

BASIC INFORMATION

DEFINITION

- Epididymitis is an inflammatory reaction of the epididymis caused by either an infectious agent or local trauma. In most cases of acute epididymitis, the testis is also involved in the process, a condition referred to as epididymo-orchitis.
- Epididymitis is considered chronic if lasting ≥6 wk. Chronic epididymitis has been subcategorized into inflammatory chronic epididymitis, obstructive chronic epididymitis, and chronic epididymalgia.

SYNONYMS

Nonspecific bacterial epididymitis
Sexually transmitted epididymitis

ICD-9CM CODES
604.90 Nonvenereal epididymitis
098.0   Gonococcal epididymitis

EPIDEMIOLOGY & DEMOGRAPHICS

INCIDENCE (IN U.S.): Cause of >600,000 visits to physicians per year
PEAK INCIDENCE: Sexually active years
PREDOMINANT SEX: Exclusive to males
PREDOMINANT AGE: All ages affected but usually in sexually active men or older males
CONGENITAL: Congenital urologic structural disorders possibly predisposing to infections

PHYSICAL FINDINGS & CLINICAL PRESENTATION

- Tender swelling of the scrotum with erythema, usually unilateral testicular pain and tenderness
- Dysuria and/or urethral discharge
- Fever and signs of systemic illness (less common)
- Pain and redness on scrotal examination
- Hydrocele or even epididymoorchitis, especially late
- Chronic draining scrotal sinuses with a "beadlike" enlargement of the vas deferens in tuberculous disease

ETIOLOGY

- In young, sexually active men, the most common infectious agents isolated are *N. gonorrhoeae* and *Chlamydia trachomatis.*
- In men >35 yr or with underlying urologic disease:
  1. Gram-negative aerobic rods are predominant.
  2. Similar organisms are found in men following invasive urologic procedures.
  3. Gram-positive cocci are rarely seen in these groups.
  4. Mycobacteria are also a cause of epididymitis.
- Young, prepubertal boys may present with epididymitis caused by coliform bacteria; almost always a complication of underlying urologic disease such as reflux.

- In AIDS patients, CMV and *Salmonella* epididymitis have been described. CMV may have a negative urine culture. Toxoplasmosis should also be considered as a cause of epididymitis in AIDS patients.
- Chronic infectious epididymitis is mostly frequently seen in conditions associated with granulomatous reaction; mycobacterium tuberculosis is the most common granulomatous disease affecting the epididymus.

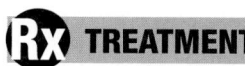

DIAGNOSIS

DIFFERENTIAL DIAGNOSIS

- Orchitis
- Testicular torsion, trauma, or tumor
- Epididymal cyst
- Hydrocele
- Varicocele
- Spermatocele
- Testicular torsion should be considered in all cases.

WORKUP

- Consideration of a full assessment of the urologic tract in patients with bacterial infection, especially if recurrent
- Imaging with sonogram or IVP (possibly procedures of choice)
- If discharge is present: cultures and Gram stain smear of urethral exudate. Gram stain will demonstrate ≥5 WBC per oil immersion field.
- In sexually active men: gonococcal cultures of the throat and rectum possibly of value
- If testicular torsion a consideration: radionuclear imaging
- Examination of first void uncentrifuged urine for leukocytes if the urethral Gram stain is negative. Positive leukocyte esterase test on first-void urine or microscopic examination of first-void urine sediment will demonstrate ≥10 WBC per high power field. A culture and Gram-stained smear of this urine specimen should be obtained along with nucleic acid amplifications studies (ligase chain reaction [LCR]) from urine samples for gonorrhea and *Chlamydia* spp.

LABORATORY TESTS

- Urinalysis and urine culture if dysuria is present or if urinary tract infection is suspected
- VDRL in sexually active men
- PPD placed and chest x-ray viewed if TB suspected
- Rarely, biopsy to assure the diagnosis of tuberculous epididymitis
- HIV testing and counseling

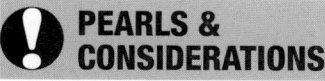

TREATMENT

ACUTE GENERAL Rx

- Ice packs and scrotal elevation for relief of pain
- Analgesia with acetaminophen with or without codeine or NSAIDs

- Antibiotics to cover suspected pathogens. Empiric therapy is indicated before laboratory test results are available
- Recommended regimens are ceftriaxone 250 mg IM in a single dose plus doxycycline 100 mg bid for 10 days. For acute epididymitis most likely caused by enteric organisms, treatment options are levofloxacin 500 mg qd × 10 days or ofloxacin 300 mg bid × 10 days
- Best treatment for older men with gram-negative bacteriuria: ofloxacin 300 mg PO bid for 10 days or levofloxacin 500 mg PO qd for 10 days
- *Pseudomonas* covered by ciprofloxacin PO or IV or cefepime (2 g IV q12h)
- Gentamicin in toxic-appearing patients (1 mg/kg IV q8h following a loading dose of 2 mg/kg): doses must be adjusted for renal function and these agents may be more toxic
- Vancomycin (1 g IV q12h) to cover suspected gram-positive infections
- Surgical aspiration of local abscesses or even open surgical drainage
- Diabetics: especially prone to develop more extensive scrotal infections, including Fournier's gangrene
- Reinforcement of compliance with antibiotics to avoid partial treatment

CHRONIC Rx

- Repair of underlying structural defects is considered especially if infections are severe or recur.
- Surgical repair of reflux in young boys should be undertaken promptly and at a young age when possible.
- Sex partners of patient should be referred for evaluation and treatment.

DISPOSITION

Usually self-limited (≤6 wk duration in most cases)

REFERRAL

- If abscess or chronic structural problems suspected
- If other diagnosis, such as testicular torsion, strongly considered

PEARLS & CONSIDERATIONS

- Recurrent epididymitis in sexually active men is usually related to failure to simultaneously treat sexual partners for STDs.
- Recurrent epididymitis in non-sexually active men is generally related to structural-anatomic defects in the genitourinary system or relapsing disease from inadequate initial treatment or antimicrobial resistance.
- Tuberculous epididymitis fails to respond to seemingly adequate antimicrobial therapy even without characteristic radiographic changes on chest films.

SUGGESTED READINGS
available at www.expertconsult.com

AUTHORS: **GLENN G. FORT, M.D., M.P.H.,** and **DENNIS J. MIKOLICH, M.D.**

BASIC INFORMATION

DEFINITION

Bleeding in the potential space surrounding the brain, between the dura mater and the inner surface of the skull

SYNONYMS

Extradural hematoma/hemorrhage

ICD-9CM CODES

432.0 Nontraumatic extradural hemorrhage
852.5 Extradural hemorrhage following injury without intracranial wound
852.5 Extradural hemorrhage following injury with open intracranial wound

EPIDEMIOLOGY & DEMOGRAPHICS

INCIDENCE: Exact incidence is unknown, however, it is found in 1% to 4% of traumatic head injury cases and 5% to 15% of autopsy series
PREDOMINANT SEX AND AGE: Male > female
PEAK INCIDENCE: Peak incidence among adolescents and young adults
GENETICS: There is a role for genetics in spontaneous (nontraumatic) epidural hematoma caused by coagulopathies and vascular malformations.
RISK FACTORS: Head trauma associated with skull fracture

PHYSICAL FINDINGS & CLINICAL PRESENTATION

- History of head trauma is present.
- Transient loss of consciousness, followed by a "lucid interval" in 47% of cases, where the patient is free of any neurologic signs or symptoms. This is followed by clinical deterioration.

- Signs and symptoms vary depending on severity.
- Symptoms: headache, vomiting, drowsiness, confusion, aphasia, seizures, paralysis, and even coma are found.
- Signs: external signs of skull fracture—lacerations, ecchymoses, cerebrospinal fluid (CSF) rhinorrhea or otorrhea are observed.
- Altered mental status, nuchal rigidity, photophobia, focal neurologic deficit—paralysis of one limb, unequal pupils, decerebrate posture, coma—are seen.

ETIOLOGY

- Traumatic: commonly caused by arterial injury (the middle meningeal artery) but may also be injury of the anterior meningeal artery, a dural arteriovenous (AV) fistula at the vertex, or from venous bleeding
- Nontraumatic: caused by an infection/eroding abscess, coagulopathy, hemorrhagic tumors, vascular malformations, postsurgical procedures, and in special populations (e.g., pregnant women, patients receiving hemodialysis)

DIAGNOSIS

DIFFERENTIAL DIAGNOSIS

In the setting of head trauma: subdural hematoma, subarachnoid hemorrhage, cerebral contusion, brain laceration, diffuse brain swelling

WORKUP

- Imaging is the mainstay of diagnosis.
- Head CT is the test most commonly used due to its simplicity, widespread use and availability. Typical appearance is a "lens shaped," or "lentiform" hyperdensity (Fig. 1-140).
- NOTE: Head CT is not conclusive in 8% of cases due to severe anemia, early scanning, and severe hypotension.

- Brain MRI: more sensitive. Indicated in situations in which there is a strong clinical suspicion but no evidence of epidural hematoma on head CT (Fig. 1-141). Preferred in spinal as opposed to intracranial pathology due to higher resolution.
- Angiography: rarely necessary but may be used to evaluate an underlying vascular lesion.
- Note: lumber puncture (LP) is contraindicated in epidural hematoma due to risk of brain stem herniation.

LABORATORY TESTS

- Laboratory tests are helpful as adjunct to diagnosis but are not the mainstay of diagnosis or treatment.
- CBC may be helpful to evaluate for anemia.
- Other tests: renal functions, electrolytes, liver functions may be helpful depending on the case scenario.

TREATMENT

Acute symptomatic epidural hematoma is a neurologic emergency that requires surgical treatment to prevent permanent brain injury.

NONPHARMACOLOGIC THERAPY

- Burr hole evacuation: this involves drilling a hole in the skull to evacuate the hematoma. It is a lifesaving procedure that is indicated if surgical expertise is limited.
- Craniotomy and hematoma evacuation is the mainstay of treatment. When indicated, identification and ligation of the bleeding vessel.

ACUTE GENERAL Rx

- ABCD: Airway, breathing (may need intubation), circulation, and assess for disability.
- Medical resuscitation maneuvers: head elevation, hyperventilation, monitoring of vital signs and avoidance of hypotension and hyperthermia, sedation if necessary.
- Medications: osmotic diuresis with IV mannitol, antiepileptics may be used to treat or, in some situations, prevent seizures.
- Note: glucocorticoid therapy is *not* indicated following head injury and may be related to increased mortality.
- Evaluation for surgery: nonoperative treatment is only indicated if the patient has no symptoms, no focal neurologic deficit, no coma (Glasgow coma score >8), and epidural hematoma volume is less than 30 ml by CT scan, with clot thickness <15 mm and midline shift of less than 5 mm.
- Nonoperative treatment involves close monitoring, hourly neurologic checks, and serial head CT scans.

CHRONIC Rx

- There is a risk of permanent brain damage whether the disorder is treated or not. Most recovery occurs in the first 6 months with some improvement over 2 years.
- Children recover more quickly.
- Patients should be educated on rehabilitative exercises and to alert medical professionals in the event of new neurologic symptoms.

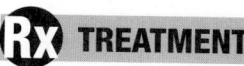

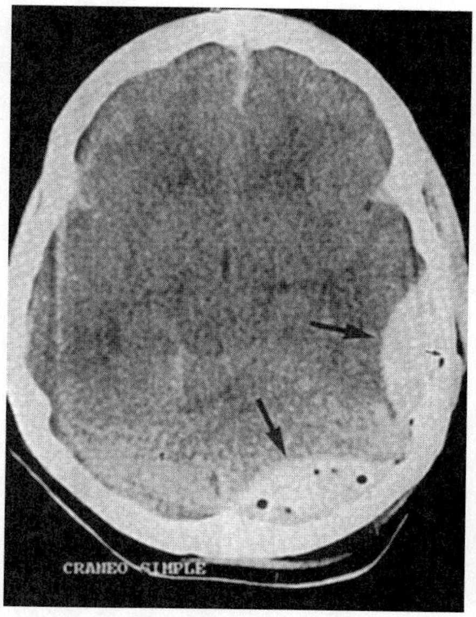

FIGURE 1-140 Head CT showing two epidural hematomas in 23-year-old involved in a motor vehicle accident. Note air bubbles that are a result of linear fracture in the left temporal bone (short arrow).

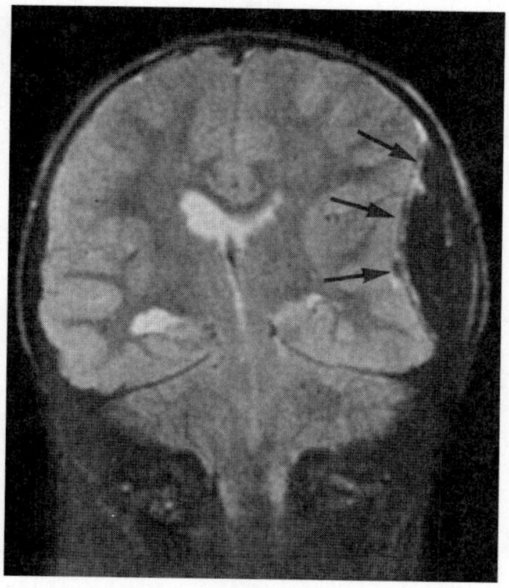

FIGURE 1-141 Epidural hematoma on MRI. Coronal T2-weighted images show hypointense biconvex extraaxial collection in the left temporal region.

- Support and encouragement to patient and family should always be provided.

REFERRAL

Clinical nurse practitioners, pastoral care staff, and social workers to help patients and families are also appropriate.

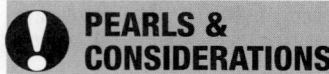

PEARLS & CONSIDERATIONS

- Acute symptomatic epidural hematoma is a neurologic emergency.

- Epidural hematoma should be suspected in any patient with a history of blow to the head leading to a period of loss of consciousness.
- Initial resuscitation is extremely important, but surgery is the mainstay of treatment for acute symptomatic epidural hematoma.

PREVENTION

Should be directed toward preventing head trauma: use of appropriate safety equipment (e.g., helmets, hard hats, safe driving, avoiding to dive into unknown depths)

PATIENT/FAMILY EDUCATION

Online head injury support groups are helpful: www.headinjury.com/linktbisup.htm, www.headinjury.com/, www.dailystrength.org/c/Brain-Injury/support-group.

SUGGESTED READINGS

available at www.expertconsult.com

AUTHOR: **HODA ELTOMI, M.D.**

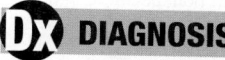

BASIC INFORMATION

DEFINITION

Epiglottitis is a rapidly progressive cellulitis of the epiglottis and adjacent soft tissue structures with the potential to cause abrupt airway obstruction.

SYNONYMS

Supraglottitis
Cherry-red epiglottitis

ICD-9CM CODES
464.30 Epiglottitis

EPIDEMIOLOGY

INCIDENCE (IN U.S.): Highest in young children, 2 to 4 yr
INCIDENCE (IN U.S.): Unknown
PEAK INCIDENCE: Peaks in young boys ages 2 to 4 yr, but it is reported in adults as well
PREDOMINANT SEX: Males

PHYSICAL FINDINGS & CLINICAL PRESENTATION

- Irritability, fever, dysphonia, and dysphagia
- Respiratory distress, with child tending to lean up and forward
- Often, drooling or oral secretions
- Often, presence of tachycardia and tachypnea
- On visualization, edematous and cherry-red epiglottis
- Often, no classic barking cough as seen in croup
- Possibly fulminant course (especially in children), leading to complete airway obstruction

ETIOLOGY

- In children, *Haemophilus influenzae* type b is usual.

- In adults, *H. influenzae* can be isolated from blood and/or epiglottis (about 26% of cases).
- Pneumococci, streptococci, and staphylococci are also implicated.
- Role of viruses in epiglottitis unclear.

DIAGNOSIS

DIFFERENTIAL DIAGNOSIS

- Croup
- Angioedema
- Retropharyngeal or peritonsillar abscess
- Diphtheria
- Foreign body aspiration
- Lingual tonsillitis

WORKUP

- Cultures of blood and urine
- Lateral neck radiograph to show an enlarged epiglottis, ballooning of the hypopharynx, and normal subglottic structures (Fig. 1-142)
  1. Radiographs are of only moderate sensitivity and specificity and take time to perform.
  2. Visualization of the epiglottitis may be safer in adults than in children.
- Cultures of the epiglottitis

LABORATORY TESTS

- CBC: may reveal a leukocytosis with a shift to the left
- Chest radiograph examination: may reveal evidence of pneumonia in close to 25% of cases
- Cultures of blood, urine, and the epiglottis, as noted previously

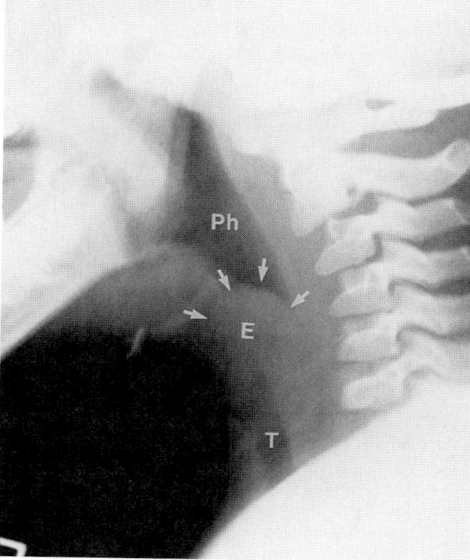

FIGURE 1-142 Epiglottitis. A lateral soft tissue view of the neck shows a ballooned pharynx *(Ph)* with swollen epiglottis *(E)* in the shape of a large thumbprint *(arrows)*. *T*, Trachea. (From Mettler FA [ed]: *Primary care radiology,* Philadelphia, 2000, WB Saunders.)

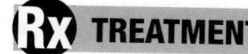

TREATMENT

ACUTE GENERAL Rx

- Maintenance of adequate airway is critical.
- Early placement of an endotracheal or nasotracheal tube in a child is advised.
- Closely follow the adult patient, if no signs of airway obstruction, and defer intubation.
- In children, visualization and intubation are best done in the most controlled environment.
- *H. influenzae* in children is much less common in large part due to the HIB vaccine.
- Use antibiotics such as ceftriaxone (80 to 100 mg/kg/day in two divided doses), cefotaxime (50 to 180 mg/kg/day in four divided doses), or ampicillin (200 mg/kg/day in four divided doses) with chloramphenicol (75 to 100 mg/kg/day in four divided doses).
- If possible, obtain cultures before initiating antibiotics.
- Treat adult patients with similar antibiotic regimens.
- If there is an unvaccinated child at home (or in a day care center) who is >4 yr and living with an index case, give close family contacts of the patient (including adults) rifampin 20 mg/kg/day for 4 days (up to 600 mg/day) for prophylaxis.
- Role of epinephrine or corticosteroids in the management of epiglottitis is not firmly established.

DISPOSITION

Invasive *Haemophilus influenzae* infections and epiglottitis are reportable illnesses; this may be particularly important in recognizing an outbreak in a day care center with unvaccinated children.

REFERRAL

- Close cooperation between the pediatrician or internist, anesthesiologist, and otorhinolaryngologist, especially when epiglottis is visualized and when the patient requires endotracheal intubation
- Best managed in a critical care setting or ICU

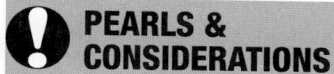

PEARLS & CONSIDERATIONS

The incidence of epiglottitis has diminished markedly since the introduction of the conjugate vaccine against *H. influenzae* serotype B into routine childhood immunization.

SUGGESTED READINGS
available at www.expertconsult.com

AUTHORS: **GLENN G. FORT, M.D., M.P.H.,** and **DENNIS J. MIKOLICH, M.D.**

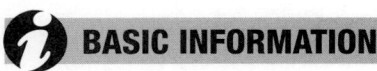

BASIC INFORMATION

DEFINITION

Episcleritis is an inflammation of the episclera, the thin layer of vascular elastic tissue between the sclera and conjunctiva.

ICD-9CM CODES
379.0 Scleritis and episcleritis

EPIDEMIOLOGY & DEMOGRAPHICS

INCIDENCE (IN U.S.): Relatively rare in an ophthalmologic practice
PEAK INCIDENCE: Most common in middle and old age
PREDOMINANT SEX: None
PREDOMINANT AGE: 43 yr

PHYSICAL FINDINGS & CLINIAL PRESENTATION

- Red, vascular injection of conjunctiva with engorged and enlarged blood vessels beneath the conjunctions (Fig. 1-143)
- Pain in area of inflammation that is usually localized

ETIOLOGY

Associated with collagen-vascular diseases, vasculitis, trauma; often nonspecific

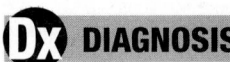

DIAGNOSIS

DIFFERENTIAL DIAGNOSIS

- Acute glaucoma
- Conjunctivitis
- Scleritis
- Subconjunctival hemorrhage
- Congenital or lymphoid masses
- The differential diagnosis of "red eye" is described in Section II

WORKUP

Eye examination, general check-up for collagen-vascular disease or other autoimmune diseases

LABORATORY TESTS

Studies for collagen-vascular disease (e.g., ANA, ESR, RF)

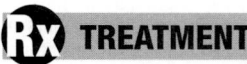

TREATMENT

NONPHARMACOLOGIC THERAPY

Warm compresses

ACUTE GENERAL Rx

- Topical steroids, 1% prednisolone if no glaucoma; nonsteroidals if there is a tendency for glaucoma
- Nonsteroidal anti-inflammatory drugs (NSAIDs): treat underlying systemic disease

CHRONIC Rx

NSAIDs such as Voltaren or Acular qd

DISPOSITION

Close follow-up needed

REFERRAL

To ophthalmologist if patient unresponsive to treatment after a few days

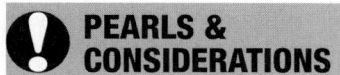

PEARLS & CONSIDERATIONS

COMMENTS

- Often associated with collagen-vascular disease
- Usually related to systemic disease

SUGGESTED READINGS
available at www.expertconsult.com

AUTHOR: **MELVYN KOBY, M.D.**

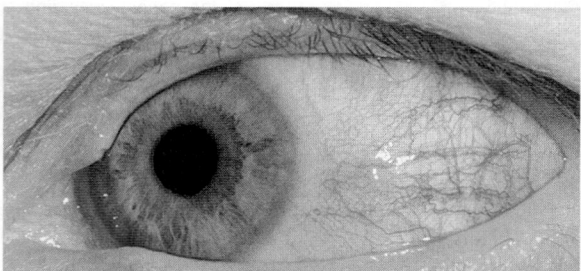

FIGURE 1-143 Nodular episcleritis in a patient with gout. (From Palay D [ed]: *Ophthalmology for the primary care physician,* St Louis, 1997, Mosby.)

Epistaxis

BASIC INFORMATION

DEFINITION

Epistaxis is defined as bleeding from the nose or nasal hemorrhage and is classified as either anterior or posterior.

SYNONYMS

Nosebleed

ICD-9CM CODES
784.7 Epistaxis

EPIDEMIOLOGY & DEMOGRAPHICS

- Epistaxis accounts for one of every 200 emergency department visits in the U.S. annually.
- It increases in frequency after age 20 yr and reaches the highest levels among the elderly population.
- More than 80% of cases of epistaxis are anterior in origin (Little's area) and occur from Kiesselbach's plexus (Fig. 1-144).
- Only 5% of patients with epistaxis have posterior bleeds.

PHYSICAL FINDINGS & CLINICAL PRESENTATION

- Nosebleed
- Hypotension and hemodynamic instability with acute, severe epistaxis

ETIOLOGY

- Approximately 90% of epistaxis events are idiopathic.
- Common identifiable causes are:
  1. Cold, dry environment
  2. Trauma (nose picking, accidents, and physical altercations)
  3. Structural deformities (septal deviations or spurs, chronic perforations)
  4. Inflammatory (rhinosinusitis, nasal polyposis)
  5. Allergies
  6. Foreign bodies in the nasal cavity
  7. Tumors (juvenile angiofibroma)
  8. Irritants
  9. Hypertension
  10. Coagulopathy (hemophilia, von Willebrand's disease, thrombocytopenia)
  11. Osler-Weber-Rendu disease
  12. Renal failure
  13. Drugs: aspirin, nonsteroidal antiinflammatory drugs, warfarin, alcohol, sildenafil, and tadalafil
  14. Blood vessel disorders (connective tissue disease, hereditary hemorrhagic telangiectasia)
  15. Pseudoaneurysm and aneurysm of the internal carotid artery might present as epistaxis

DIAGNOSIS

A good attempt should be made to directly visualize the source of bleeding to confirm the diagnosis and determine the best treatment.

DIFFERENTIAL DIAGNOSIS

Pseudoepistaxis must be ruled out. Common extranasal sites of bleeding that can simulate epistaxis include:
1. Pulmonary hemoptysis
2. Bleeding esophageal varices
3. Tumor bleeding from the pharynx, larynx, or trachea

WORKUP

The workup should include laboratory blood testing to exclude obvious causes. Type and cross in anticipation of transfusion if the bleeding is severe.

LABORATORY TESTS

- Hemoglobin and hematocrit
- Platelet count
- Blood urea nitrogen and creatinine
- Coagulation studies (prothrombin time and partial thromboplastin time)
- Type and crossmatching of blood products

IMAGING STUDIES

Radiographic studies are usually not helpful.

TREATMENT

NONPHARMACOLOGIC THERAPY

- Digital compression or pinching of the lower soft cartilaginous part of the nose for 10 min is the method of choice.
- Use cotton or tissue plug.
- The patient should be sitting and leaning forward, breathing through the mouth, allowing blood to flow out of the nostrils as opposed to bending backward, which would allow the blood to flow down the throat.
- Application of cold compresses to the bridge of the nose to cause a vasoconstrictive effect; the patient may also suck on ice to achieve this effect.

ACUTE GENERAL Rx

Anterior epistaxis:
- Local vasoconstriction is performed by moistening a cotton pledget with either:
  1. 4% lidocaine with 1:1000 epinephrine
  2. 4% lidocaine with 1% phenylephrine (Neo-Synephrine)
  3. 4% lidocaine with 0.05% oxymetazoline (Afrin)
  4. 4% cocaine or cocaine 25% in paraffin base ointment and inserting the pledget into the nasal cavity with bayonet forceps.
- Cauterization with silver nitrate or trichloroacetic acid is performed once hemostasis is achieved.
- Anterior nasal packing is needed when local measures are unsuccessful. Nasal packing is performed under local anesthesia and is done by inserting Vaseline gauze strips in layers from the floor of the nasal cavity to the front entrance of the nasal orifice. Enough pressure is placed to tamponade the epistaxis (Fig. 1-145).
- Other commercially available nasal packing uses sponge packs that expand when exposed to blood or moisture and can be used for anterior epistaxis.

Posterior epistaxis:
- Posterior nasal packing
  1. Commercially available nasal sponge packing can be applied
  2. Rolled gauze technique
- Foley catheter balloon insertion into the nasopharynx can be tried in patients with posterior epistaxis (for the proper technique, see reference)

Newer agents in the treatment of epistaxis:
- Quick clot hemostatic agent, available OTC. When it comes in contact with blood in and around a wound, it absorbs the smaller water molecules from the blood to promote rapid clotting

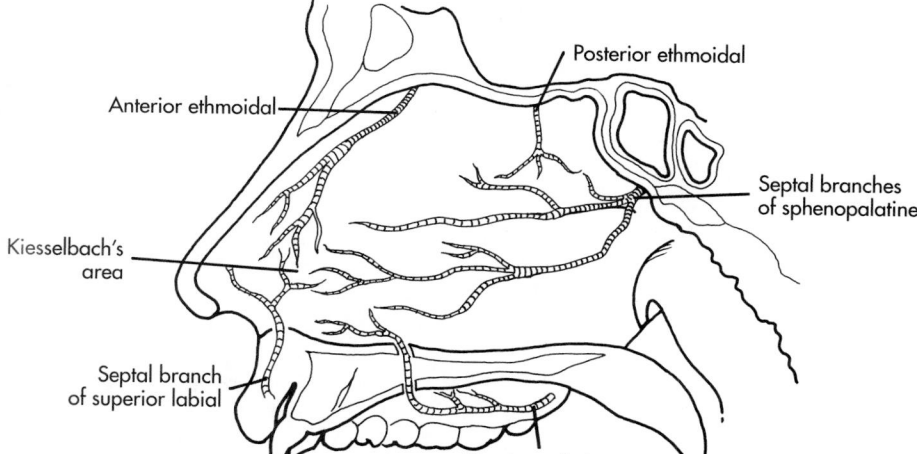

FIGURE 1-144 Kiesselbach's plexus on the anterior septum derives blood supply from the superior labial, descending palatine, and sphenopalatine arteries. (From Noble J: *Primary care medicine,* ed 3, St Louis, 2001, Mosby.)

Labels on figure: Posterior ethmoidal; Anterior ethmoidal; Septal branches of sphenopalatine; Kiesselbach's area; Septal branch of superior labial; Greater palatine

- Floseal hemostatic matrix, a combination of human thrombin, gelatin matrix, and calcium chloride, which are mixed together and placed at bleeding site
- Recombinant Factor VIIa, generally reserved for uncontrolled epistaxis

CHRONIC Rx

- If acute treatment fails to stop the bleeding or the site of bleeding cannot be located, electrocautery or endoscopic cauterization can be used.
- Electrocautery is performed after suitable anesthesia, such as application of a topical anesthetic followed by local anesthetic injection. Only one side of the nasal septum should be cauterized at a time because perforation can result from bilateral cauterization.
- Arterial ligation or embolization has been used in refractory posterior epistaxis.

- For cases involving irritated or inflamed mucosa, a conservative regimen of triamcinolone 0.025%, Nemdyn, Nasalate, or equivalent cream should be applied once a week, combined with nightly application of a small quantity of petroleum jelly to the septum before bedtime.

DISPOSITION

- Most cases of anterior epistaxis from Kiesselbach's plexus can be stopped by nasal compression and local vasoconstriction or cauterization.
- Nasal packing with gauze or sponge can control 90% of anterior epistaxis.
- Anterior and posterior packs are removed in 2 to 3 days. Hospital admission should be considered in patients who cannot be expected to return for prompt follow-up because prolonged packing increases the risk

of pressure necrosis, toxic shock syndrome, sinus infections, and other complications.
- Although rare, epistaxis can lead to death by aspiration of blood, hemodynamic compromise from rapid excessive blood loss, or toxic shock syndrome.

REFERRAL

- If epistaxis cannot be controlled, an ear-nose-throat (ENT) specialist should be called for assistance.
- ENT specialist should be consulted in any patient with posterior epistaxis requiring posterior packing.

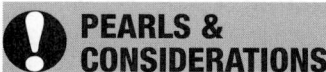

COMMENTS

- Silver nitrate cauterization, if done on both sides of the nasal septum, can lead to septal perforation and should be discouraged.
- If anterior nasal packing is done, broad-spectrum antibiotics (e.g., amoxicillin-clavulanate 250 mg PO tid or trimethoprim-sulfamethoxazole 1 tablet PO bid) are used until the anterior packs are removed. Although it is customary to place patients on antibiotics to prevent sinusitis from obstruction, there is no proof that this is effective.
- Complications of nasal packing include:
  1. Aspiration
  2. Dislodged packing
  3. Infection
  4. Nasal trauma

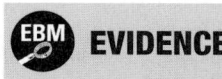

available at www.expertconsult.com

SUGGESTED READINGS

available at www.expertconsult.com

AUTHOR: **TANYA ALI, M.D.**

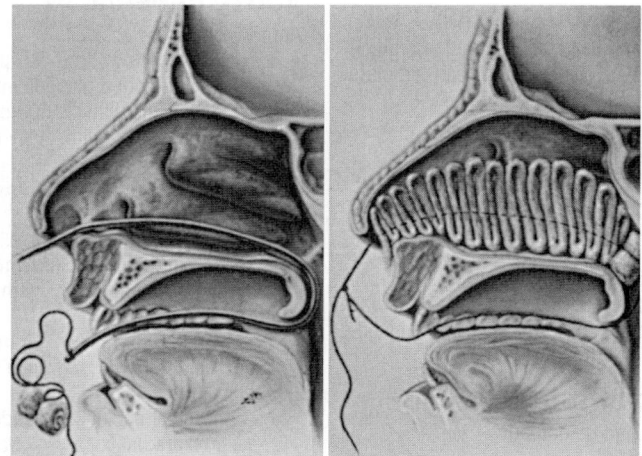

FIGURE 1-145 Packing of the nose for epistaxis with a postnasal pack and an anterior nose pack. (From Boies LR et al: *Fundamentals of otolaryngology: a textbook of ear, nose, and throat diseases,* ed 4, Philadelphia, 1964, WB Saunders.)

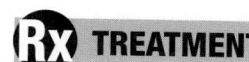

BASIC INFORMATION

DEFINITION

Epstein-Barr virus infection refers to a disease caused by Epstein-Barr virus (EBV), a human herpesvirus.

SYNONYMS

Infectious mononucleosis (IM)
Kissing disease

ICD-9CM CODES
075 Mononucleosis

EPIDEMIOLOGY & DEMOGRAPHICS

INCIDENCE (IN U.S.): 5 cases/100,000 persons per yr of IM
PREDOMINANT SEX: Neither, although peak incidence occurs about 2 yr earlier in women
PREDOMINANT AGE:
- Clinical evidence of IM: occurs most commonly at ages 15 to 24 yr
- EBV infection: occurs earlier in life in lower socioeconomic groups

PHYSICAL FINDINGS & CLINICAL PRESENTATION

- Most EBV infections either are asymptomatic or cause a nonspecific viral illness.
- Incubation period is 1 to 2 mo, possibly followed by a prodrome of anorexia, low-grade fever, malaise, headache, and chills; after several days, clinical triad of pharyngitis, moderate to high fever, and adenopathy may appear, accompanied by fatigue and malaise.
- Pharyngitis is usually the most severe symptom; white or necrotic appearance exudates are common.
- Symmetrical lymphadenopathy is most prominent in the posterior more than anterior cervical region but may be diffuse.
- Splenomegaly (50% of cases) is possible, most commonly during the second week of illness.
- Maculopapular or morbilliform rash is uncommon but will occur in patients who receive ampicillin. Patients may have palatal petechiae, periorbital, or palpebral edema. Mucocutaneous oral hairy leukoplakia (OHL), which is associated with intense EBV replication and the action of EBV-encoded proteins such as latent membrane protein-1, may occur.
- Possible IM presentation: fever and adenopathy without pharyngitis.
- Nausea, vomiting, and anorexia are frequent in patients with IM, probably reflecting mild hepatitis encountered in 90% of infected individuals.
- Although complications such as spleen rupture, airway obstruction, and malignancy may be severe and fatal, they are uncommon and tend to resolve completely.
- Hematologic involvement includes hemolytic or aplastic anemia, thrombocytopenia, thrombotic thrombocytopenic purpura/hemolytic-uremic syndrome, and disseminated intravascular coagulation (DIC). Pneumonia, myocarditis, pancreatitis, mesenteric adenitis, myositis, and glomerulonephritis may occur as well. Nervous system involvement includes Guillain-Barré syndrome, facial nerve palsy, meningoencephalitis, aseptic meningitis, transfer myelitis, peripheral neuritis and optic neuritis.

- IM is usually a self-limited illness. Acute symptoms resolve in 1 to 2 wk, but symptoms of malaise and fatigue often persist for months.
- EBV is related to lymphoproliferative syndromes in transplant recipients and in AIDS patients.
- Increasing evidence showing an association between EBV infection and African Burkitt's, B-cell, T-cell lymphoma, and nasopharyngeal carcinoma.

ETIOLOGY

- EBV is a ubiquitous virus.
- Infection during childhood is much less likely to cause significant illness.
- Frequency of IM in late adolescence is attributed to the onset of social contact between the sexes.
- Close personal contact is usually necessary for transmission, although EBV is occasionally transmitted by blood transfusion; transfer via saliva while kissing may be responsible for many cases.

DIAGNOSIS

DIFFERENTIAL DIAGNOSIS

- Heterophile-negative IM caused by cytomegalovirus (CMV)
- Although clinical presentation similar, CMV more frequently follows transfusion
- Bacterial and viral causes of pharyngitis
- Toxoplasmosis
- Acute retroviral syndrome of HIV
- Lymphoma
- Lyme disease

WORKUP

Heterophile antibody and CBC with blood smear

LABORATORY TESTS

- Increased WBC common, with a relative lymphocytosis of more than 50% and neutropenia are identified.
- Hallmark of IM: atypical lymphocytes of more than 10% (not pathognomonic) are found.
- Mild thrombocytopenia is present.
- Falling hematocrit signals the possibility of splenic rupture or immune hemolytic anemia.
- Elevated hepatocellular enzymes and cryoglobulins are found in most cases.
- Heterophile antibody:
  - As measured by the monospot test, may be positive at presentation or may appear later in the course of illness.
  - Negative test is repeated in 1 wk if clinical suspicion is high.
  - A positive test has been reported with primary HIV infection.
- Viral capsid antigen (VCA) IgG and IgM are rarely used for diagnosis, but better value in children because heterophile antibody is negative in most of children younger than 8 years.
- PCR DNA for CMV is the test of choice in transplant recipients who develop lymphoproliferative syndromes.

IMAGING STUDIES

Chest radiograph examination:
- May rarely show infiltrates
- Possible elevated left hemidiaphragm with splenic rupture

TREATMENT

NONPHARMACOLOGIC THERAPY

- Supportive including rest
- Splenectomy if rupture occurs
- Transfusions for severe anemia or thrombocytopenia

ACUTE GENERAL Rx

- Pharmacologic therapy is not indicated in uncomplicated illness.
- Avoid aspirin due to the risk of Reye's syndrome.
- Avoid ampicillin and amoxicillin as their use can frequently precipitate a nonallergic rash.
- Use of steroids is suggested in patients who have severe thrombocytopenia, hemolytic anemia, impending airway obstruction resulting from enlarged tonsils, or fulminant liver failure. Prednisone 60 to 80 mg PO qd for 3 days, then tapered over 1 to 2 wk.
- Although it may reduce initial viral shedding, there is little evidence to support the use of antiviral agents such as acyclovir in the management of IM.

CHRONIC Rx

An extremely rare, chronic form of IM with persistent fevers and fatigue has been described and should be differentiated from chronic fatigue syndrome, which is not related to EBV.

DISPOSITION

Eventual resolution of all symptoms

REFERRAL

If more than mild illness

PEARLS & CONSIDERATIONS

COMMENTS

Avoidance of contact sports during the first month of illness because splenic rupture can occur even in the absence of clinically detectable splenomegaly.

SUGGESTED READINGS

available at www.expertconsult.com

AUTHOR: **MONZR M. AL MALKI, M.D.**

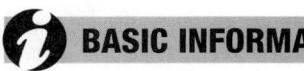

DEFINITION

Erectile dysfunction (ED) is the persistent inability to achieve or sustain a penile erection of adequate rigidity to make intercourse possible or satisfactory.

SYNONYMS

ED
Impotence
Male erectile disorder
Sexual dysfunction (a nonspecific term)

ICD-9CM CODES
F52.2 Male erectile disorder (DSM-IV Code: 302.72 Male erectile disorder)

EPIDEMIOLOGY & DEMOGRAPHICS

PREVALENCE (IN U.S.):
- Increases with age and presence of vascular comorbidities.
- Approximately 7% in the 20s, 18% in the 50s, 25% in the 60s, 80% in the 80s.

PREDOMINANT SEX: By definition, only in males
PREDOMINANT AGE: Increases with age
RISK FACTORS: Coronary artery disease, peripheral vascular disease, hypertension, diabetes mellitus, hypercholesterolemia, numerous medications, alcohol, smoking or drug abuse

PHYSICAL FINDINGS & CLINICAL PRESENTATION

- Psychogenic impotence: inability to obtain erection, inability to obtain or maintain an adequate erection, or the loss of erection before completion of sexual intercourse; nocturnal penile tumescence usually normal
- Organic impotence: inability to obtain an erection or inability to obtain an adequate erection; nocturnal penile tumescence usually abnormal

ETIOLOGY

- Most cases are caused by organic problems related to neurologic, hormonal, or vascular abnormalities or prescription or recreational drugs.
- Psychogenic erectile dysfunction results from mental stress, depression, widower syndrome, and performance anxiety. Characterized objectively by nocturnal and morning erections and otherwise negative test results.
- Vascular disease: History of hypertension (HTN), peripheral vascular disease, ischemic heart disease, diabetes, smoking. In approximately 40% of men >50 yr, the primary cause of ED is related to atherosclerotic disease, diabetes mellitus (DM), neuropathy, or vascular disease.
- Medication side effects: Antihypertensives such as thiazides and clonidine (consider change to ACE inhibitors and calcium channel blockers with lower reported incidence of ED); antiandrogens such as spironolactone, finasteride, ketoconazole; cimetidine; antide-

pressants such as selective serotonin reuptake inhibitors [SSRIs]; and antipsychotics.
- Alcohol and nicotine use.
- Recreational drugs, including cocaine, heroin, amphetamines, and marijuana. These may increase libido but impair performance.
- Hormonal dysfunction such as testosterone deficiency (decreases libido and erection), hypothyroidism or hyperthyroidism, hyperprolactinemia, and adrenal insufficiency.
- Neurogenic causes including spinal cord lesions, cortical lesions, and peripheral neuropathies.
- Pelvic surgeries such as radical prostatectomy or cystectomy.

DIAGNOSIS

DIFFERENTIAL DIAGNOSIS

- A useful tool to diagnose/evaluate ED severity is the Sexual Health Inventory for Men.
- Psychogenic dysfunction distinguished from organic.
- Determine etiology of organic dysfunction.
- ED possible in the setting of another psychiatric condition (e.g., depression or obsessive-compulsive disorder).

WORKUP

- Clinical history should include time course (abrupt onset may correlate with reversible cause such as medication, psychosocial stress, psychiatric complaint), cause (psychogenic vs. organic), and change in libido.
- Report of spontaneous nocturnal or morning erections indicate intact neurologic reflexes and penile blood flow.
- Decreased libido may indicate endocrinologic or psychogenic cause.
- Medical and social history (including partner report) should address cardiac disease symptoms and risk factors (HTN, DM, hyperlipidemia, smoking, and substance abuse), pelvic surgery, medications, and mental health.
- Physical examination to check blood pressure, femoral and peripheral pulses, femoral bruits; gynecomastia; neuronal damage (genital sensation, cremasteric reflex); direct penile damage (e.g., plaque formation such as Peyronie's disease); prostate examination; or testicular atrophy and other secondary sexual characteristics.

LABORATORY TESTS

Screen with fasting glucose. Consider lipid panel, thyroid-stimulating hormone, morning serum testosterone. If decreased testosterone, check prolactin, follicle-stimulating hormone, and luteinizing hormone.

IMAGING STUDIES

Imaging studies are rarely performed except in situations of pelvic trauma or surgery.

OTHER STUDIES

- Nocturnal penile tumescence testing very specific for distinguishing psychogenic versus organic causes.

- Neurogenic etiologies examined by the cremasteric reflex (inner-thigh touch elicits scrotal contraction), the bulbocavernosus reflex, or the pudendal-evoked response.
- Intracorporeal injection of prostaglandin E_1 to distinguish vascular and nonvascular etiologies (erection is achieved in patients with normal vascular systems). If no erection with direct injection of vasoactive substance, consider duplex ultrasound of penile vasculature.

TREATMENT

NONPHARMACOLOGIC THERAPY

- Various psychotherapeutic approaches: cognitive-behavioral therapy preferred; success rates decrease with advancing age and duration of symptoms.
- Psychosexual therapy (sex therapy and couples therapy) is first line for psychogenic ED and for adjunctive therapy in ED from any cause. Therapy is used to address contributing social issues.
- Mechanical vacuum devices (function by drawing blood into corpus cavernosum) are 70% to 90% effective but are difficult to use.
- Incorporate vascular risk factor reduction including counsel on diet, exercise, smoking cessation, ETOH intake and screening/treatment for HTN, insulin resistance, and hypercholesterolemia as appropriate.

ACUTE GENERAL Rx

- First-line treatment: In setting of sexual stimulation, three selective phosphodiesterase type 5 (PDE5) inhibitors prolong nitric oxide–induced vasodilation by increase of intracavernosal cyclic guanosine monophosphate levels. All three PDE5 inhibitors have similar efficacy and tolerability, but tadalafil has a longer duration of action and is less affected by high-fat meals and alcohol. Counsel men on sildenafil or vardenafil to limit high-fat meals and excessive alcohol, as they may impede effectiveness. Sildenafil (Viagra) and vardenafil (Levitra) can be taken 30 to 60 min before sexual activity, and both are effective for about 4 hr. Tadalafil (Cialis) can be taken several hours before sexual activity (although 50% respond within 30 min) and lasts up to 36 hr.
- With PDE5 inhibitors, avoid concomitant use of nitrates (absolute contraindication), drugs that inhibit or induce cytochrome P450 CYP3A4, and drugs that prolong the QT interval. Caution in men on stable alpha adrenergic blocker therapy (commonly used for benign prostatic hypertrophy) because of concern for hypotension; start the lowest dose of PDE5 inhibitor. Caution in men who have had myocardial infarction in the past 6 mo, resting hypotension or uncontrolled hypertension, unstable angina, positive exercise stress test or poor exercise tolerance. Counsel on side effects of headache, flushing, dyspepsia, nasal congestion, changes in color perception, and priapism (rare). Nonarteritic anterior ischemic optic neuropathy is

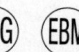

also a rare association with sildenafil and tadalafil. Consider counseling on safe sexual practices when prescribing PDE5 inhibitors.
- Second-line treatment if PDE5 inhibitors fail: intraurethral alprostadil (prostaglandin E_1 [medicated urethral suppository]) applied into meatus of penis before intercourse; or intracavernosal injections of vasodilators (e.g., papaverine or prostaglandin E_1 pellet). Consider combining intraurethral alprostadil with sildenafil.
- Second-line treatment alternative: vacuum constriction pump; has variable satisfaction rate.

CHRONIC Rx

- Psychosexual therapy is helpful as an adjunctive treatment in all cases. Sexual therapists can also re-motivate patients in whom PDE5 inhibitors initially failed.
- Psychogenic impotence: PDE5 inhibitors are effective in patients with depression because tissues, nerves, hormones, and vasculature are normal. Full psychologic evaluation is recommended before starting treatment.
- For men not responding to other approaches: penile prosthesis.
- Testosterone therapy in men with low testosterone (i.e., hypogonadal); must rule out prostate cancer before use.

DISPOSITION

- When ED has an organic cause it does not remit unless the cause is corrected; therefore it is usually a chronic condition.
- Psychogenic-acquired ED will remit spontaneously in 15% to 30% of cases.
- Lifelong ED is usually a chronic and unremitting condition.
- Situational ED may remit with changes in social environment but usually recurs.

REFERRAL

- If psychotherapy, sex therapy, or invasive organic treatment required
- To urology if PDE5 inhibitors fail

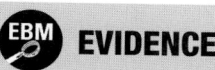 **PEARLS & CONSIDERATIONS**

- Commonly evaluated and treated by primary care physician; refer to urologist if oral therapy fails or surgery is required.
- PDE5 inhibitors are treatment of choice for most causes of ED. Main contraindications are nitrate use and decompensated cardiac disease. Caution in patients on alpha adrenergic blockers and with blood pressures at extreme ends (significant hypotension or hypertension).
- For optimal response, patients should be appropriately informed of proper use, precautions, and adverse effects of PDE5 inhibitors. Try six to eight times at optimal doses before declaring PDE5 inhibitors a failure. Consider switching among the three PDE5 inhibitors if one fails.
- Men with ED are at increased risk of coronary, cerebrovascular, and peripheral vascular diseases. Screening for cardiovascular risk factors should be considered in these patients because symptoms of ED present on average 3 yr prior to symptoms of CAD.

EBM EVIDENCE

available at www.expertconsult.com

SUGGESTED READINGS
available at www.expertconsult.com

AUTHORS: **CINDY LAI, M.D.,** and **NICOLE APPELLE, M.D.**

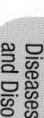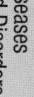
Diseases and Disorders

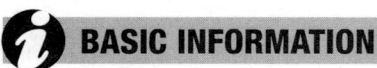

DEFINITION

Erysipelas is a type of cellulitis caused by infection of the superficial layers of the skin and cutaneous lymphatics. Erysipelas is characterized by redness, induration, and a sharply demarcated, raised border.

SYNONYMS

St. Anthony's fire

ICD-9CM CODES
035 Erysipelas

EPIDEMIOLOGY & DEMOGRAPHICS

PREDOMINANT AGE: Occurs most often in the young or old
RISK FACTORS: Patients with impaired lymphatic or venous drainage (mastectomy, saphenous vein harvesting) and immunocompromised patients. Athlete's foot is a common portal of entry.
RECURRENCE RATE: Relatively common

PHYSICAL FINDINGS & CLINICAL PRESENTATION

- Distinctive red, warm, tender skin lesion with induration and a sharply defined, advancing, raised border (Fig. 1-146).
- Most common sites are lower extremities and face.
- Systemic signs of infection (fever) are often present.
- Vesicles or bullae may develop.
- After several days lesions may appear ecchymotic.
- After 7 to 10 days desquamation of affected area may occur.

ETIOLOGY

- Usually group A β-hemolytic streptococci
- Less often group B, C, or G streptococci
- Rarely *Staphylococcus aureus*

COMPLICATIONS

- Abscess
- Necrotizing fasciitis
- Thrombophlebitis
- Gangrene
- Metastatic infection

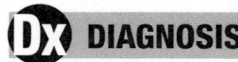 **DIAGNOSIS**

DIFFERENTIAL DIAGNOSIS

- Other types of cellulitis
- Necrotizing fasciitis
- Deep vein thrombosis
- Contact dermatitis
- Erythema migrans (Lyme's disease)
- Insect bite
- Herpes zoster
- Erysipeloid
- Acute gout
- Pseudogout

WORKUP

History, physical examination, and laboratory evaluation

LABORATORY TESTS

Diagnosis is usually made by characteristic clinical setting and appearance.

- Complete blood count and white blood cell count often elevated
- Blood cultures positive in 5% of patients
- Gram stain and culture of any drainage from skin lesions
- Culture of aspirated fluid from leading edge of skin lesion has low yield

IMAGING STUDIES

- Duplex ultrasound for patients suspected of having deep vein thrombosis
- CT scan or MRI for patients with suspected necrotizing fasciitis

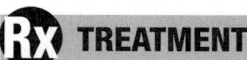 **TREATMENT**

NONPHARMACOLOGIC THERAPY

- Elevation of the affected limb
- Warm compresses

ACUTE GENERAL Rx

Typical erysipelas of extremity in nondiabetic patient:
- PO: penicillin V 250 mg to 500 mg qid
- IV: penicillin G (aqueous) 1 to 2 million units q6h

NOTE: Use erythromycin or cephalosporin in patients allergic to penicillin.

Facial erysipelas (include coverage for *Staphylococcus aureus*):
- PO dicloxacillin 500 mg q6h
- IV nafcillin or oxacillin 2 g q4h

DISPOSITION

Prognosis is good with antibiotic treatment but recurrence is common.

REFERRAL

For surgical debridement for patients with necrotizing fasciitis or for drainage of abscess

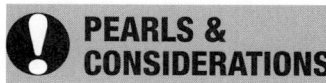 **PEARLS & CONSIDERATIONS**

Consider early surgical referral when necrotizing fasciitis suspected. Consider skin biopsy when not responding to appropriate antibiotics.

SUGGESTED READING
available at www.expertconsult.com

AUTHORS: **GAIL M. O'BRIEN, M.D.**, and **MARK J. FAGAN, M.D.**

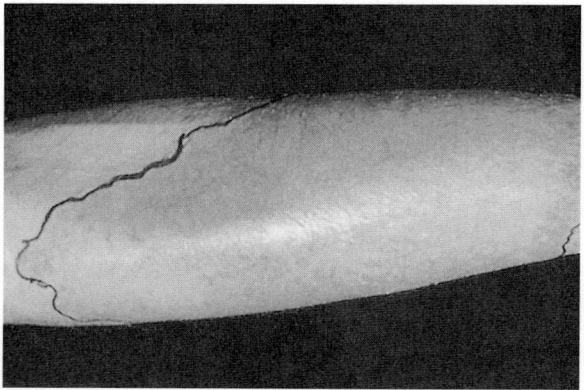

FIGURE 1-146 Erysipelas. Note well-demarcated erythematous plaque on arm. (From Goldstein B [ed]: *Practical dermatology,* ed 2, St Louis, 1997, Mosby. Courtesy Department of Dermatology, University of North Carolina at Chapel Hill.)

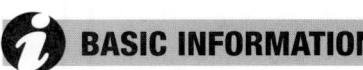

BASIC INFORMATION

DEFINITION

Erythema multiforme is an inflammatory disease characterized by eruption of annular, maculopapular lesions with dark raised, erythematous, or vesiculobullus center surrounded by a pale zone. It is believed to be caused by immune complex formation and subsequent deposition in the skin and mucous membranes. It is considered a hypersensitivity reaction to infection or drugs.

SYNONYMS

EM

ICD-9CM CODES

695.1 Erythema multiforme

EPIDEMIOLOGY & DEMOGRAPHICS

PREDOMINANT AGE: 20 to 40 yr
RISK FACTORS: Often associated with herpes simplex and other infectious agents, drugs, or connective tissue diseases.

PHYSICAL FINDINGS & CLINICAL PRESENTATION

- Prodromal symptoms are mild or absent. Itching or burning at the site of eruption may occur.
- Symmetric skin lesions with a classic "target" appearance (caused by the centrifugal spread of red maculopapules to circumference of 1 to 3 cm with a purpuric, cyanotic, or vesicular center) are present (Fig. 1-147). The papules may enlarge into plaques measuring a few centimeters in diameter with a dark or red central portion. Target lesions may not be apparent for several days.

- Lesions are most common in the back of the hands and feet and extensor aspect of the forearms and legs. Trunk involvement can occur in severe cases.
- Urticarial papules, vesicles, and bullae may also be present and generally indicate a more severe form of the disease.
- Individual lesions heal in 1 to 2 wk without scarring.
- Bullae and erosions may also be present in the oral cavity.

ETIOLOGY

- Immune complex formation and subsequent deposition in the cutaneous microvasculature may play a role in the pathogenesis of erythema multiforme.
- The majority of cases follow outbreaks of herpes simplex virus 1 and 2.
- Mycoplasma pneumoniae, fungal infections, medications (bupropion, sulfonamides, penicillins, nonsteroidal anti-inflammatory drugs, barbiturates, phenothiazines, hydantoins).
- In >50% of patients no specific cause is identified.

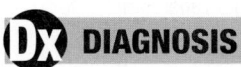

DIAGNOSIS

DIFFERENTIAL DIAGNOSIS

- Chronic urticaria
- Secondary syphilis
- Pityriasis rosea
- Contact dermatitis
- Pemphigus vulgaris
- Lichen planus
- Serum sickness
- Drug eruption
- Granuloma annulare
- Polymorphic light eruption
- Viral exanthem

WORKUP

- Medical history with emphasis on drug ingestion
- Laboratory evaluation in patients with suspected collagen-vascular diseases
- Skin biopsy when diagnosis is unclear

LABORATORY TESTS

- Complete blood count with differential
- Antinuclear antibody
- Serology for *Mycoplasma pneumoniae*, HSV-1, HSV-2
- Urinalysis

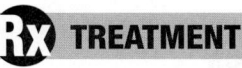

TREATMENT

NONPHARMACOLOGIC THERAPY

- Mild cases generally do not require treatment; lesions resolve spontaneously within 1 mo.
- Potential drug precipitants should be removed.

ACUTE GENERAL Rx

- Treatment of associated diseases (e.g., acyclovir for herpes simplex, erythromycin for *Mycoplasma* infection).
- Prednisone 40 to 80 mg/day for 1 to 3 wk may be tried in patients with many target lesions; however, the role of systemic steroids remains controversial.
- Levamisole, an immunomodulator, may be effective in the treatment of patients with chronic or recurrent oral lesions (dose is 150 mg/day for 3 consecutive days used alone or in combination with prednisone).
- IV immunoglobulins in severe cases.

DISPOSITION

The rash generally evolves over a 2-wk period and resolves within 3 to 4 wk without scarring. A severe bullous form can occur (see entry for Stevens-Johnson Syndrome).

REFERRAL

Hospital admission in patients with suspected Stevens-Johnson syndrome

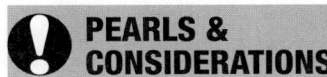

PEARLS & CONSIDERATIONS

COMMENTS

The risk of recurrence of erythema multiforme exceeds 30%. Recurrence may be treated with valacyclovir 500 to 1000 mg/day, famciclovir 125 to 250 mg/day, or acyclovir 400 mg bid. Dapsone, antimalarials, azathioprine, or cyclosporine use is reserved for cases resistant to antivirals.

SUGGESTED READINGS

available at www.expertconsult.com

AUTHOR: **FRED F. FERRI, M.D.**

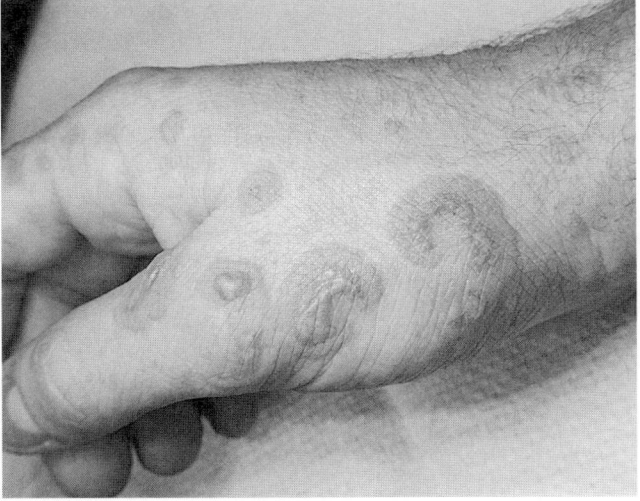

FIGURE 1-147 Iris and arcuate lesions of erythema multiforme. Note erythematous lesions with multiform configurations: target, arcuate, and vesicles. (From Noble J et al: *Textbook of primary care medicine,* ed 2, St Louis, 1995, Mosby.)

BASIC INFORMATION

DEFINITION
Erythema nodosum is an acute, tender, erythematous, nodular skin eruption resulting from inflammation of subcutaneous fat, often associated with bruising. It is the most common form of panniculitis.

ICD-9CM CODES
695.2 Erythema nodosum
017.10 Erythema nodosum, tuberculous, NOS

EPIDEMIOLOGY & DEMOGRAPHICS
INCIDENCE: Two to three cases/100,000 persons per yr
PREDOMINANT SEX: Female/male ratio of 3 to 4:1
PREDOMINANT AGE: 25 to 40 yr

PHYSICAL FINDINGS & CLINICAL PRESENTATION
- Acute onset of tender nodules typically located on the shins (Fig. 1-148) and occasionally seen on the thighs and forearms.
- The nodules are usually ⅛ to 1 inch in diameter but can be as large as 4 inches; they begin as light red lesions, then become darker and often ecchymotic. The nodules heal within 8 wk without ulceration.

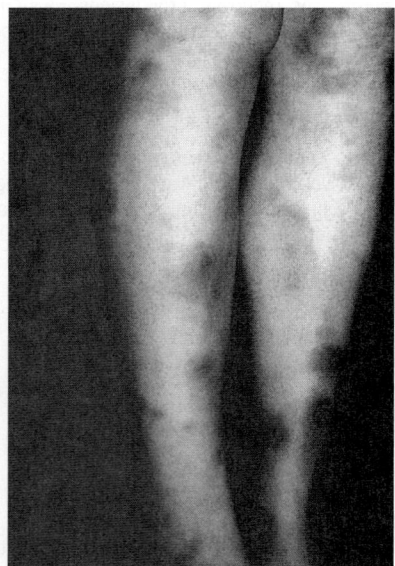

FIGURE 1-148 Erythema nodosum. (From Arndt KA et al: *Cutaneous medicine and surgery, vol 1,* Philadelphia, 1997, WB Saunders.)

- Associated findings:
  1. Fever
  2. Lymphadenopathy
  3. Arthralgia
  4. Signs of the underlying illness

ETIOLOGY
Cell-mediated hypersensitivity reaction is seen more frequently in persons with human leukocyte antigen (HLA) B8. The lesion results from an exaggerated interaction between an antigen and cell-mediated immune mechanisms leading to granuloma formation. Up to 55% of cases of erythema nodosum are idiopathic.
Infections:
- Bacteria
  - Streptococcal pharyngitis (28% to 48%)
  - *Salmonella* enteritis
  - *Yersinia* enteritis
  - Psittacosis
  - *Chlamydia pneumoniae* infection
  - *Mycoplasma* pneumonia
  - Meningococcal infection
  - Gonorrhea
  - Syphilis
  - Lymphogranuloma venereum
  - Tularemia
  - Cat-scratch disease
  - Leprosy
  - Tuberculosis
- Fungi
  - Histoplasmosis
  - Coccidioidomycosis
  - Blastomycosis
  - *Trichophyton verrucosum*
- Viruses
  - Cytomegalovirus
  - Hepatitis B
  - Epstein-Barr virus
- Drugs (3% to 10%)
  - Sulfonamides
  - Penicillins
  - Oral contraceptives
  - Gold salts
  - Prazosin
  - Aspirin
  - Bromides
- Sarcoidosis (11% to 25%)
- Cancer, usually lymphoma
- Ankylosing spondylosis and reactive arthropathies (e.g., associated with inflammatory bowel disease)

DIAGNOSIS

DIFFERENTIAL DIAGNOSIS
- Insect bites
- Posttraumatic ecchymoses
- Vasculitis

- Weber-Christian disease
- Fat necrosis associated with pancreatitis
- Necrobiosis lipoidica
- Scleroderma
- Lupus panniculitis
- Subcutaneous granuloma
- Alpha-1 antitrypsin deficiency

WORKUP
- Physical examination
- Diagnosis of underlying illness by history, physical examination, and laboratory tests as indicated

LABORATORY TESTS
- Erythrocyte sedimentation rate
- Throat culture and antistreptolysin O titer
- PPD
- Others depending on index of suspicion (e.g., stool culture and evaluation for ova and parasites in patients with diarrhea and gastrointestinal symptoms)
- Skin biopsy in doubtful cases:
  1. Early lesion: inflammation and hemorrhage in subcutaneous tissue
  2. Late lesion: giant cells and granulomata

IMAGING STUDIES
Chest radiograph to rule out sarcoidosis and tuberculosis

TREATMENT
- The disease is self-limited and treatment is symptomatic. Erythema nodosum nodules develop in pretibial locations and resolve spontaneously over several weeks without scarring or ulceration.
- Treatment of underlying disorders.
- Avoidance of contact irritation of affected areas.
- Nonsteroidal anti-inflammatory drugs for pain.
- Systemic steroids (prednisone 1 mg/kg of body weight/day, tapered over several days) may be useful in severe cases if underlying risk of sepsis and malignancy have been excluded.

PROGNOSIS
Typical case:
- Pain for 2 wk
- Resolution within 8 wk

SUGGESTED READING
available at www.expertconsult.com

AUTHOR: **FRED F. FERRI, M.D.**

BASIC INFORMATION

DEFINITION

Approximately 15% of esophageal tumors arise in the proximal esophagus, 50% in the middle third of the esophagus, and 35% in the lower third. Due to decreases in alcohol and tobacco use, rates of midesophagus squamous cell carcinoma are decreasing while rates of distal esophagus adenocarcinomas are increasing.

SYNONYMS

Neoplasm of the esophagus
Malignancy of the esophagus

ICD-10 CODES
C15.X Malignant neoplasm of the esophagus (X defines location)
D00.2 Carcinoma of esophagus, in situ

EPIDEMIOLOGY & DEMOGRAPHICS

Carcinomas of the esophageal epithelium, both squamous cell and adenocarcinoma, are by far the most common tumors of the esophagus (see Table 1-49). Barrett's esophagus from chronic gastric acid reflux is considered a precancerous lesion. Benign neoplasms are much less common (leiomyoma, papilloma, and fibrovascular polyps).

PREVALENCE: Varies widely worldwide. It is the eighth most common incident cancer and the sixth leading cause of cancer death. Rates are increasing every decade and are highest in the Asian esophageal cancer belt, extending from the Caspian Sea to northern China, with certain high-incidence pockets in Finland, Ireland, southeast Africa, and northwest France. In the United States, 16,500 new cases and 14,300 deaths are expected in 2008, making it the seventh leading cause of death by cancer among men. Incidence has increased sixfold since 1975. The majority are diagnosed at an advanced stage (unresectable or metastatic disease).

TABLE 1-49 Classification of Esophageal Cancer

Epithelial

Squamous cell
  Ordinary squamous cell
  Verrucous squamous cell
  Spindle cell (carcinosarcoma)
Adenocarcinoma
  Ordinary
  Adenoacanthoma
  Mucoepidermoid
  Adenoid cystic
Small cell
Melanoma
Choriocarcinoma

Metastatic Disease

Lymphoma
Sarcoma

Abeloff MD: *Clinical Oncology*, ed 3, Philadelphia, 2004, Elsevier.

RACE, AGE, & SEX PREDOMINANCE: Esophageal cancer is more common among blacks than whites and has a high male/female ratio of 3:1. It usually develops in the seventh and eighth decades and is associated with lower socioeconomic status.

GENETICS: Increasing evidence shows that genetics may play a role by increasing susceptibility to esophageal cancer, but it has had no impact on clinical practice.

CLINICAL PRESENTATION

Symptoms and signs:
- Dysphagia (74%): initially occurs with solid foods and gradually progresses to include semisolids and liquids; latter signs usually indicate incurable disease with tumor involving more than 60% of the esophageal circumference. May be felt as chest pain.
- Unintentional weight loss: usually of short duration. Losing >10% of body mass predicts poor outcome.
- Hoarseness: suggests recurrent laryngeal nerve involvement.
- Odynophagia and halitosis: unusual symptoms.
- Cervical adenopathy: usually involving supraclavicular lymph nodes.
- Dry cough: suggests tracheal involvement.
- Aspiration pneumonia: caused by development of a fistula between the esophagus and trachea.
- Massive hemoptysis or hematemesis: results from the invasion of vascular structures.
- Advanced disease spreads to lymph nodes, liver, lungs, peritoneum, and pleura.
- Hypercalcemia: associated with squamous cell carcinoma from secretion of a parathyroid-like tumor peptide.

ETIOLOGY

Pathogenesis of esophageal cancers is attributable to chronic recurrent oxidative damage from any of the following etiologic agents, which cause inflammation, and esophagitis, increased cell turnover, and, ultimately, initiation of the carcinogenic process.

ETIOLOGIC AGENTS:
- Excess alcohol consumption accounts for 80% to 90% of esophageal cancer in the United States; whiskey is associated with a higher incidence than wine or beer.
- Tobacco and alcohol use combined increases risk substantially for squamous cell cancer.
- Obesity, hiatal hernia, and low-vitamin, high-fat diet.
- Other ingested carcinogens:
  - Nitrates (converted to nitrites): South Asia, China
  - Smoked opiates: Northern Iran
  - Fungal toxins in pickled vegetables
  - Betel nut chewing
- Mucosal damage:
  - Long-term exposure to extremely hot tea (>70° C)
  - Lye ingestion
- Radiation-induced strictures

- Chronic achalasia: incidence of esophageal cancer is seven times greater in this population
- Host susceptibility as a result of precancerous lesions:
  - Plummer-Vinson syndrome (Paterson-Kelly): glossitis with iron deficiency
  - Congenital hyperkeratosis and pitting of palms and soles
- Chronic GERD leading to Barrett's metaplasia and adenocarcinoma (whites are affected more than blacks). The annual rate of transformation from Barrett's to adenocarcinoma is 0.5%. Zollinger-Ellison syndrome increases risk due to increased gastric acid production.
- Possible association with celiac sprue or dietary deficiencies of molybdenum, zinc, vitamin A.
- Questionable relationship with prolonged bisphosphonate use (≥10 prescriptions, or use >3 yr).

DIAGNOSIS

DIFFERENTIAL DIAGNOSIS
- Achalasia
- Scleroderma of the esophagus
- Diffuse esophageal spasm
- Esophageal rings and webs

LABORATORY TESTS

Complete blood cell count, blood chemistry, liver enzymes. No biomarkers are available currently to diagnose, monitor, or predict outcomes.

IMAGING STUDIES
- Double-contrast esophagogram effectively identifies large esophageal lesions (Fig. 1-149).
  - In contrast to benign esophageal leiomyomata, which cause narrowing with preservation of normal mucosal pattern, esophageal carcinomas cause ragged ulcerating mucosal changes in association with deeper infiltration.
- Esophagoscopy may be performed initially if suspicion is high, to visualize smaller tumors missed by esophagogram, and to allow histopathologic confirmation. In conjunction, an endoscopic sonogram is often performed to determine the depth of tumor invasion.
  - Endoscopic inspection of the larynx, trachea, and bronchi may identify concomitant cancers of head, neck, and lung.
  - Endoscopic biopsies fail to recover malignant tissue one third of the time; thus cytologic examination of tumor brushings should be routinely performed.
  - Examination of the fundus of the stomach by retroflexion of the endoscope is imperative.
- Chest and abdominal CT and/or integrated CT-PET scans can determine tumor spread for preoperative staging.
- Staging laparoscopy may alter treatment plans in 20% to 30% of cases.

TREATMENT

ACUTE GENERAL Rx

SURGICAL RESECTION:
- Surgical resection of squamous cell carcinoma and adenocarcinoma of the lower third of the esophagus is indicated if no widespread metastasis is detected by CT-PET. Stomach or colon typically is used for esophageal replacement.
- Endoscopic resection may replace radical surgical resection in early tumors with no lymph node involvement, but a recent Cochrane review found no studies comparing endoscopic treatment vs. surgery.
- Complications of surgery:
  - Anatomic fistula (usually with colon interposition, subphrenic abscesses)
  - Respiratory complications
  - Cardiovascular complications are most common, including MI, CVA, and PE

RADIATION THERAPY:
- Squamous cell carcinomas are more radiosensitive than adenocarcinoma. Radiation achieves good local control and is an excellent palliative modality for obstructive symptoms but is rarely curative. It is best used for upper esophageal tumors.
- Approximately 40% of tumors cannot be destroyed even after 6000 rads.
- Palliative radiation therapy for bone metastasis is also effective.
- Complications of radiation therapy:
  - Esophageal stricture, radiation-induced pulmonary fibrosis, and transverse myelitis are the most feared.
  - Radiation-induced cardiomyopathy and skin changes are rare.

COMBINATION CHEMOTHERAPY, RADIATION Rx, & SURGICAL Rx:
- Single-agent chemotherapy resulted in significant tumor regression in 15% to 25% of patients.
- Most beneficial chemotherapy appeared to be a cisplatin/5-fluorouracil–based combination.
- Combination chemotherapy including cisplatin achieved significant tumor reduction in 30% to 60% of patients.
- Capecitabine and oxaliplatin are as effective as fluorouracil and cisplatin, respectively, in patients with previously untreated esophagogastric cancer
- Complications of chemotherapy include mucositis, GI toxicity, myelosuppression, nephrotoxicity; ototoxicity and neurotoxicity occur with cisplatin.
- 2-yr survival is improved with chemoradiotherapy (30%) vs. radiotherapy alone (10%).
- Preoperative chemoradiotherapy plus surgery significantly reduced the 3-yr mortality rate compared with surgery alone in patients with resectable esophageal cancer. Trimodal therapy is the standard of care for most esophageal cancers, whether performed preoperatively, perioperatively, or postoperatively.

CHRONIC Rx

Palliative procedures such as repeated endoscopic dilation, surgical placement of feeding tube, or polyvinyl prosthesis to bypass tumors have been used for unresectable patients.

DISPOSITION
- Overall 5-yr survival is 13%
- Surgery: 5-yr survival rate is 48% in stages I and II, 20% in advanced stages
- Radiation therapy: 5-yr survival rate of 6%-20%
- Chemotherapy: Single-agent response rate of 15% to 38%; combination response rate 80%
- Combined trimodality: 18% response rate
- Patients with stage IV disease receive palliative chemotherapy with a median survival of less than 1 year

REFERRAL
- To gastroenterologist or general surgeon for endoscopy for patients with chronic dysphagia, odynophagia, or unexplained weight loss
- To medical oncologist for evaluation of preoperative chemotherapy
- To radiation oncologist for palliative therapy if tumor is unresectable or obstruction is present
- To hospice if appropriate

PEARLS & CONSIDERATIONS

COMMENTS
More than 50% of patients with esophageal cancer are diagnosed when the disease is metastatic or unresectable.

PREVENTION
- A diet high in fruits and vegetables is associated with lower risk of esophageal cancer.
- Avoid tobacco and excessive alcohol use.
- Avoid ingested toxins known to cause esophageal cancers.
- There is no evidence that vitamins, Chinese herbal regimens, or green tea prevent esophageal cancer.
- Although screening the general population is not recommended, endoscopic evaluation of persons with chronic dysphagia or GERD symptoms is indicated. If Barrett's esophagus is detected, regularly scheduled surveillance endoscopies are necessary with consideration for radiofrequency ablation therapy.

PATIENT/FAMILY EDUCATION
Provide education and support about the likely prognosis because most esophageal cancers are diagnosed at an advanced stage.

EVIDENCE

available at www.expertconsult.com

SUGGESTED READINGS
available at www.expertconsult.com

AUTHOR: **LYNN MCNICOLL, M.D., F.R.C.P.C.**

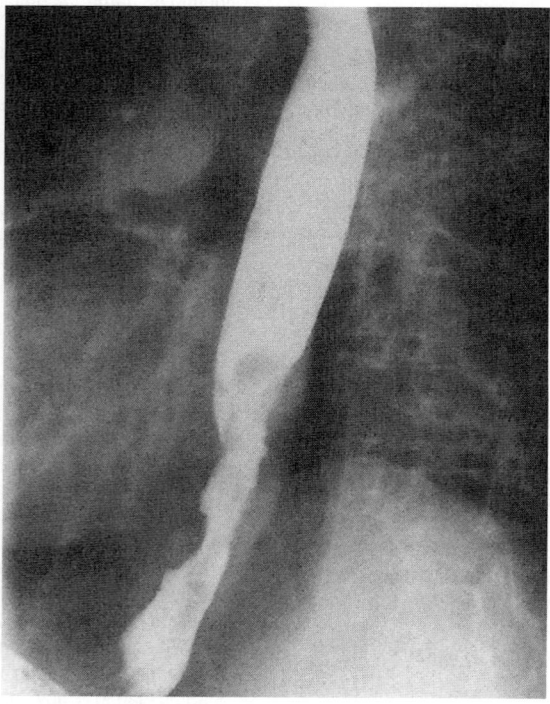

FIGURE 1-149 Barium swallow demonstrating the classic findings in cancer of the distal third of the esophagus. (Reprinted from Noble J [ed]: *Primary care medicine*, ed 2, St Louis, 1996, Mosby.)

BASIC INFORMATION

DEFINITION

A predominantly postural and action tremor that is bilateral and tends to progress slowly over the years in the absence of other neurological abnormalities.

SYNONYMS

Benign essential tremor
Familial tremor

ICD-9CM CODES
333.1 Essential tremor

EPIDEMIOLOGY & DEMOGRAPHICS

PREDOMINANT AGE: Can begin at any age, but incidence increases after age 40 yr. Prevalence is 6% to 9% for those >60 yr.
GENETICS: No gender or racial predominance.

PHYSICAL FINDINGS & CLINICAL PRESENTATION

- Patients complain of tremor that is most bothersome when writing or holding something such as a newspaper or trying to drink from a cup. Worsens under emotional distress.
- Tremor, 4 to 12 Hz, bilateral postural and action tremor of the upper extremities. May also affect the head, voice, trunk, and legs. Typically it is the same amplitude throughout the action, such as bringing a cup to the mouth. No other neurologic abnormalities on examination except difficulty with tandem gait. Patients often note improvement with intake of small amounts of alcohol.

ETIOLOGY

Often an inherited disease, autosomal dominant; sporadic cases without a family history are frequently encountered

DIAGNOSIS

DIFFERENTIAL DIAGNOSIS
(see Table 1-50)

- Parkinson's disease—tremor is usually asymmetric, especially early on in the disease, and is predominantly a resting tremor. Patients with Parkinson's disease will often also have increased tone, decreased facial expression, slowness of movement, and shuffling gait.
- Cerebellar tremor—an intention tremor that increases at the end of a goal-directed movement (such as finger to nose testing). Other associated neurologic abnormalities include ataxia, dysarthria, and difficulty with tandem gait.
- Drug-induced—there are many drugs that enhance normal, physiologic tremor. These include caffeine, nicotine, lithium, levothyroxine, β-adrenergic bronchodilators, amiodarone, valproate, and SSRIs.
- Wilson's disease—wing-beating tremor that is most pronounced with shoulders abducted, elbows flexed, and fingers pointing towards each other. Usually there are other neurologic abnormalities including dysarthria, dystonia, and Keyser Fleischer rings on ophthalmologic examination.
- Physiologic tremor.

WORKUP

- All imaging studies normal (MRI, CT) and are usually unnecessary unless there are other associated neurologic abnormalities
- Check TSH
- In patients younger than 40 yrs with other neurologic abnormalities, send ceruloplasmin, serum Cu, 24-hr urine Cu to rule out Wilson's disease

TREATMENT

Treat essential tremor when it is functionally impairing. Treatments are up to 75% effective.

NONPHARMACOLOGIC THERAPY

Reduction of stress. Minimize use of caffeine. Small quantities of alcohol at social functions may be beneficial.

ACUTE GENERAL Rx

Can take a dose of propranolol (20 to 40 mg) in preparation for specific event.

CHRONIC Rx

First-line agents:
- Propranolol/Propranolol LA: Usual starting dose is 30 mg. The usual therapeutic dose is 160 to 320 mg. Although not contraindicated, they must be used with caution in those with asthma, depression, cardiac disease, and diabetes.
- Primidone: Usual starting dose is 12.5 to 25 mg qhs. Usual therapeutic dose is between 62.5 and 750 mg daily (assuming side effects are tolerated). Sedation and nausea when first begin medication are biggest side effects.
- Topiramate: 25 mg qhs, may titrate up to about 400 mg

Other agents:
- Gabapentin: 400 mg qhs, usual therapeutic dose is 1200 to 3600 mg
- Alprazolam: 0.75 to 2.75 mg
- Botulinum toxin injected focally may decrease tremor

SURGICAL Rx

Thalamic deep brain stimulation (or possibly thalamotomy) contralateral to side of tremor

DISPOSITION

Patients should be reassured that the condition is not associated with other neurologic disabilities; however, it can become quite functionally disabling over time.

REFERRAL

This is a condition that usually can be treated by the primary care physician; however, if patient fails first-line therapies then patient should be referred to specialists for other drug trials and other possible surgical options.

PEARLS & CONSIDERATIONS

Essential tremor is the most common of all movement disorders.

EVIDENCE

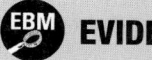

available at www.expertconsult.com

SUGGESTED READINGS
available at www.expertconsult.com

AUTHOR: **CINDY ZADIKOFF, M.D.**

TABLE 1-50 Overlapping Features of Various Types of Tremor

Feature	Parkinson's Syndrome	Cerebellar Tremor	Essential Tremor
Present at rest	Yes	No	Yes
Increased tone	Yes	No	No
Decreased tone	No	Yes	No
Postural abnormality	Yes	Yes	No
Head involvement	Yes	Yes	Yes
Intentional component	No	Yes	Yes
Incoordination	No	Yes	No

Remmel KS, Bunyan R, Brumback RA, Gascon GA, Olson WH: *Handbook of symptom-oriented neurology*, ed 3, St Louis, 2002, Mosby.

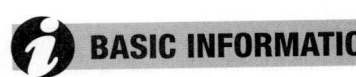 **BASIC INFORMATION**

DEFINITION

Factitious physical disorder occurs when an individual intentionally strives to create signs or symptoms of disease. The individual may create signs or symptoms by (1) lying, (2) simulating (e.g., putting drops of blood into a urine sample), or (3) actually creating disease (e.g., injecting bacteria or medications). The primary aim is to achieve the patient role, and the individual may seek invasive diagnostic testing, surgery, or treatment. Munchausen's syndrome is the most severe variant of factitious physical disorder and is characterized by exaggerated lying (pseudologia fantastica), sociopathy, geographic wandering from hospital to hospital, and a continuous life of patienthood.

SYNONYMS

Factitious disorder
Munchausen's syndrome (the most severe variant of factitious disorder)
Munchausen by proxy (factitious disorder created in another person, usually a child)
Deliberate disability
Hospital addiction syndrome
Artifactual illness
Peregrinating problem patients
Dermatitis artefacta
Surreptitious illness

ICD-9CM CODES
300.19 Factitious disorder

EPIDEMIOLOGY & DEMOGRAPHICS

INCIDENCE (IN U.S.): Unknown
PEAK INCIDENCE: 30 to 40 yr
PREVALENCE (IN U.S.): Unknown but considerable in specific illnesses. For example, 3.3% of patients with fever of unknown origin have a factitious disorder.
PREDOMINANT SEX: Male/female ratio of 2:1 for Munchausen's syndrome but 1:2 for individuals with non-Munchausen type of factitious physical disorder.
PREDOMINANT AGE: 30 to 40 yr
GENETICS: No genetic predisposition known

PHYSICAL FINDINGS & CLINICAL PRESENTATION

- False complaints or self-inflicted injury or symptoms without clear secondary gain. The intentional aspect of the disorder is often evident, such as injecting bacteria to produce infection or taking medication to produce an abnormality.
- Presentation may be acute and dramatic, but the condition can be a chronic, recurring problem.
- Workup is usually negative for naturally occurring organic etiology.
- Clinical picture is atypical for the natural history of disease (e.g., an infection that does not respond to multiple courses of appropriate antibiotics).

ETIOLOGY

- A history of significant childhood illness; physical or sexual abuse are thought to predispose.
- Personality disorders and psychodynamic factors often play a significant role.

 DIAGNOSIS

The diagnosis can be made by (1) direct observation of fabrication, (2) the presence of signs or symptoms that contradict laboratory testing, (3) nonphysiologic response to treatment, (4) the presence of physical evidence of fabrication (e.g., syringes), and (5) recurrent patterns of illness exacerbation (e.g., just before discharge) or failure to follow the natural history of disease (e.g., a wound that does not heal for no apparent reason).

DIFFERENTIAL DIAGNOSIS

- Malingering: falsifying an illness for a clear secondary gain (e.g., financial gain or avoidance of unwanted duties).
- Somatoform disorders or hypochondriasis: these disorders are produced unconsciously and are not intentionally produced.
- Self-injurious behavior is common in many other psychiatric conditions; in those conditions the patients confess the intentional self-harm and describe motivating factors. The main intent is the self-harm and not to attain the patient role, as occurs in factitious disorder.
- May also present as Munchausen by proxy, in which a mother (86% of time) or other caregiver induces illness in a child (52% between ages of 3 and 13 yr) for the purpose of obtaining medical attention or some other psychological need. Mothers often have a history of somatoform, factitious, or personality disorder themselves.

WORKUP

- Dictated by the presenting complaints.
- No specific tests for Munchausen's syndrome.
- Diagnosis may be made when the patient is caught in the act of lying or inducing an injury. The diagnosis often rests on organic workup failing to reveal a plausible natural organic disease. The failure of usual, or even extensive, treatment to ameliorate a condition is an important clue.

LABORATORY TESTS

- Laboratory testing often reveals inconsistencies.
- Other laboratory abnormalities may reflect the underlying factitious behavior (e.g., hypokalemia in an individual surreptitiously taking furosemide).

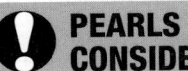 **TREATMENT**

NONPHARMACOLOGIC THERAPY

Two major approaches:
- Nonpunitive confrontation. Primary physician and psychiatrist conjointly meet with patient and say, "You must be in a lot of distress to be harming yourself as we believe you have been. We would like to help you deal with your distress more adaptively and get you into psychiatric treatment."
- Avoid overt confrontation with patient but provide him or her with a face-saving way to recover. For example, a therapeutic double bind would involve saying, "There are two possibilities here, one is that you have a medical problem that should respond to the next intervention we do, or two, you have a factitious disorder. The outcome will give us the answer."
- Munchausen's syndrome is the most severe variant and may be virtually impossible to treat except to avoid further invasive and iatrogenic disease.

ACUTE GENERAL Rx

Treatment of comorbid psychiatric disorders may be helpful. Treatment with antidepressants or psychotherapy may ameliorate the factitious behavior. Multidisciplinary staff meetings are useful to ventilate feelings and develop cohesive treatment plans.

DISPOSITION

- After being confronted with their behavior, patients may cease factitious behavior, but they more commonly seek other physicians or hospitals, as in the Munchausen variant. Other factitious disorder patients may enter psychotherapy, particularly when they have been given a face-saving approach with an avoidance of a humiliating confrontation.
- Extensive medical workups and exploratory surgery are frequent.

REFERRAL

Always obtain psychiatric referral. Risk management attorneys and hospital ethicists may contribute to challenging decision making in these patients.

! **PEARLS & CONSIDERATIONS**

Think of factitious disorders whenever there is an unexplained medical course that continues to repeat despite appropriate treatment, particularly in patients associated with the health care field. There is current consideration of whether factitious disorders should be classified in the upcoming DSM-V as a subset of somatoform disorders. This possibility is related to the challenge of discriminating whether an illness state is being consciously (factitious) or unconsciously (somatoform) produced. Future research will investigate the utility of this possible change in classification.

SUGGESTED READINGS
available at www.expertconsult.com

AUTHOR: **STUART J. EISENDRATH, M.D.**

BASIC INFORMATION

DEFINITION

A fall is an "event which results in a person coming to rest inadvertently on the ground and other than a consequence of the following: loss of consciousness, sudden onset of paralysis, or epileptic seizure" (Kellogg International Work Group, *Danish Medical Bulletin,* 34, 1-24).

SYNONYMS

Syncope
Collapse

ICD-9CM CODES

Accidental fall (E880-E888.9)

EPIDEMIOLOGY & DEMOGRAPHICS

INCIDENCE:

- Falls are the leading cause of accidental death among older adults.
- The incidence of falls among community-dwelling older adults is 35% to 40%.
- The incidence of falls for nursing home and hospitalized older adults is three times the rate of community-dwelling older adults.
- 20% to 30% of older adults who fall suffer significant injury leading to immobility and dependence.

PREDOMINANT SEX & AGE:

- Fall-related mortality is highest among older white men followed by white women, black men, and black women.
- The incidence rates of falls increase with advancing age.
- Older adults aged 85 years and over are 10 to 15 times more likely to have a fracture compared with those aged 60 to 65 years.

RISK FACTORS: Three groups of risk factors for falls have been identified (Table 1-51):
1. Intrinsic factors inherent in the older adult who falls
2. Extrinsic factors circumstantial to the older adult who falls
3. Situational or the activity in which the older adult is engaged in when a fall occurs

CLINICAL PRESENTATION

- Older adults who fall may present with minor soft tissue injuries, such as lacerations or bruising, hip fracture or head trauma; however, most falls are not reported unless an injury has occurred.
- A detailed history of events and circumstances surrounding fall, risk factors, medications, chronic illnesses, and a review of systems for acute medical illnesses, cognitive status, and functional status should be obtained.

- Physical examination should focus on the identified risk factors and include:
  - Cardiovascular examination: heart rate and rhythm, orthostatics, carotid pulses
  - Neurologic examination: mental status, visual screen, lower extremity assessment of strength, tone, proprioception, sensation, reflexes and testing of cortical and cerebellar function
  - Gait and balance assessment: "Get up and go test"

ETIOLOGY

- Falls are a multifactorial syndrome resulting from the cumulative effects of impaired gait and balance, aging, polypharmacy, depression, cognitive impairment, acute medical illness, or environmental factors (Fig. 1-150).
- Most falls among community-dwelling older adults are due to environmental factors, whereas falls among nursing home residents are a result of confusion, gait impairment, or postural hypotension.

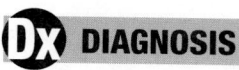 **DIAGNOSIS**

DIFFERENTIAL DIAGNOSIS

Falls are often a nonspecific symptom of an acute illness (such as a UTI, acute anemia, or pneumonia) or an exacerbation of a chronic disease (CHF or COPD).

WORKUP

- Older adults presenting with a noninjurious fall need a detailed history and physical exam to identify acute medical illnesses and potential modifiable risk factors. Laboratory and neuroimaging studies may be necessary if the history and physical exam indicate a specific problem. ECG and Holter monitoring may be considered if cardiac arrhythmia is suspected.
- See Fig. 1-150.

LABORATORY TESTS

CBC, chemistries, thyroid function, drug levels, and urinalysis depending on physical/historical findings

IMAGING STUDIES

- CT or MRI of the brain or cervical spine films in the presence of neurologic or gait impairment.
- Consider ECG, echocardiography, or Holter monitor if suspicious for structural cardiac abnormality or syncope.

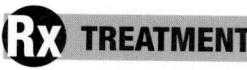 **TREATMENT**

NONPHARMACOLOGIC THERAPY

- Assisted devices such as a cane, walker to improve mobility
- Fall prevention equipment including bed alarms, low beds, and hip protectors
- Physical therapy evaluation for gait and balance training and home safety assessment

---

TABLE 1-51 Risk Factors for Falls in the Elderly

Intrinsic

Aging
Age-related decline in vestibular function might lead to increased sway, dizziness, and falls. Aging of the vision system may result in decreased visual acuity, inability to discriminate dark/light, and decreased spatial perception.

Cardiac
Cardiac arrhythmias, carotid sinus hypersensitivity

Neurologic
Parkinson's disease, normal pressure hydrocephalus (NPH), sensory neuropathy, dementia/impaired cognition, cervical myelopathy, senile gait disorder, prior stroke

Musculoskeletal
Lower extremity weakness, deconditioning, arthritis, foot abnormalities (such as bunions, calluses, or nail abnormalities)

Vascular
Vertebrobasilar insufficiency, postural hypotension, postprandial hypotension

Metabolic
Hypoglycemia, hypothyroidism, hyponatremia

Psychiatric
Depression

Extrinsic

Medications
Use of more than four medications may be associated with an increased risk of falls. Medications that may increase fall risk include benzodiazepines, sleeping medications, neuroleptics, antidepressants, anticonvulsants, class I antiarrhythmics, and antihypertensives (Rao, 2005).

Environmental
Inadequate lighting, ill-fitting shoes, slippery floor surfaces, loose rugs, uneven steps

Situational

Tripping over obstacles, carrying heavy items, descending/ascending stairs, rapid turning, reaching overhead, climbing ladders

- Discontinuation of certain medications associated with falls
- Exercise program to improve strength and balance
- Evaluation of proper footwear, hard sole, and low heel height

ACUTE GENERAL Rx

Hospitalization may be necessary for treatment of hip fracture, subdural hematoma, lacerations, or trauma as well as the treatment of underlying cause of the fall such as infection, metabolic disturbances, cardiovascular or neurologic abnormality.

CHRONIC Rx

- Screen and treat for osteoporosis as low bone density increases the risk of hip or other fractures.
- Optimize treatment of chronic illnesses such as CHF, COPD, OA, Parkinson's disease, dementia, and visual problems.

COMPLEMENTARY & ALTERNATIVE MEDICINE

T'ai chi has been shown to reduce the risk of falls in community-dwelling study participants.

DISPOSITION

Falls increase the older adult's risk of hospitalization, institutionalization, and mortality.

REFERRAL

- Referral may be appropriate to cardiologist, ophthalmologist, neurologist, or podiatrist depending on the presence of a specific condition.
- Consider referral to physical therapist for gait and balance training, evaluation for assisted device, or strengthening program.

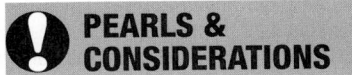

PEARLS & CONSIDERATIONS

COMMENTS

- Fear of falling may lead to restriction of activities, social isolation, and dependence.
- Older adults with four or more risk factors have a 78% chance of falling.

PREVENTION

The USPSTF does recommend counseling elderly patients about fall prevention during routine visits as well as arranging individualized multifactorial home interventions for high-risk elders (USPSTF Guidelines, 1996).

PATIENT/FAMILY EDUCATION

Counseling patient and family about reducing the risks of falling

SUGGESTED READINGS
available at www.expertconsult.com

AUTHORS: **SEAN H. UITERWYK, M.D.,** and **ALICIA J. CURTIN, PH.D., G.N.P.**

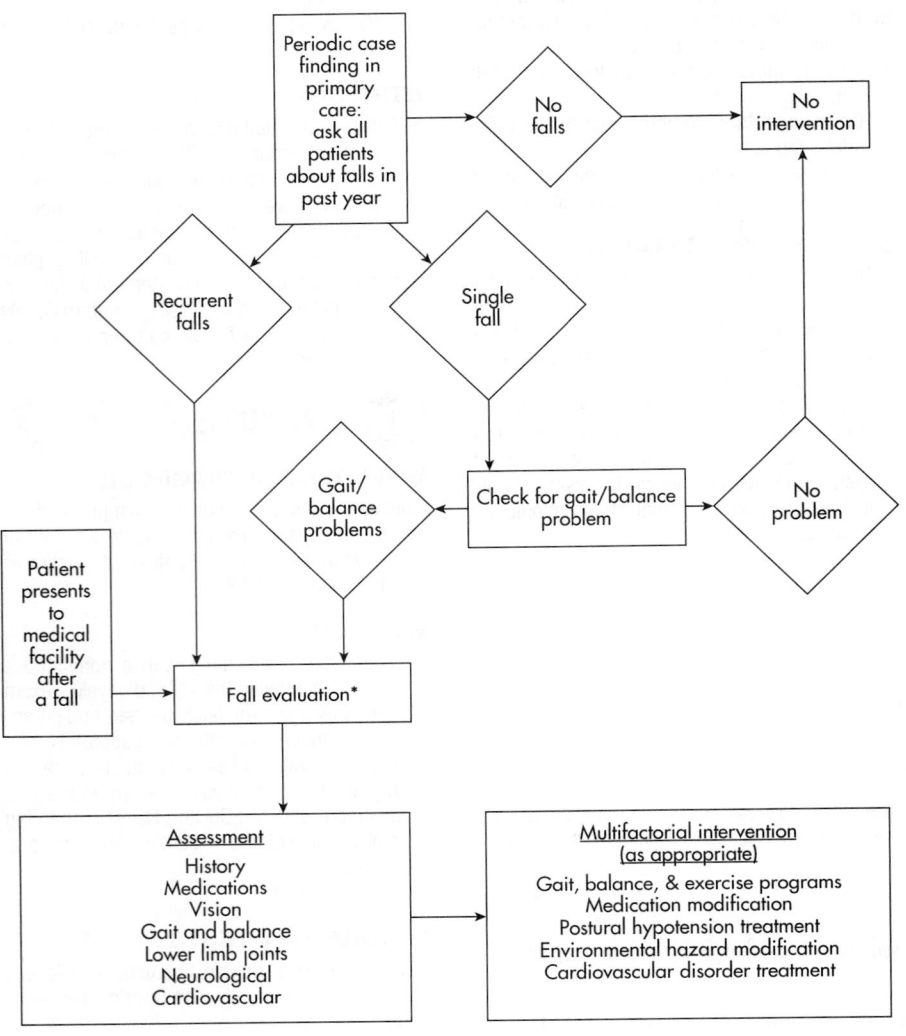

*See text for details

FIGURE 1-150 Guideline for the prevention of falls in older persons. Algorithm summarizing the assessment and management of falls. (From American Geriatrics Society, British Society, and American Academy of Orthopaedic Surgeons Panel on Falls Prevention.)

BASIC INFORMATION

DEFINITION

Acute fatty liver of pregnancy (AFLP) is characterized histologically by microvesicular fatty cytoplasmic infiltration of hepatocytes with minimal hepatocellular necrosis.

SYNONYMS

Acute fatty metamorphosis
Acute yellow atrophy

ICD-9CM CODES
646.7 Liver disorders in pregnancy

EPIDEMIOLOGY & DEMOGRAPHICS

INCIDENCE:
- Approximately one in 10,000 pregnancies
- Equal frequencies in all races and at all maternal ages

AVERAGE GESTATIONAL AGE: 37 wk (range 28 to 42 wk)

RISK FACTORS:
- Primiparity
- Multiple gestation
- Male fetus

GENETICS: Some with a familial deficiency of long-chain 3-hydroxyacyl-coenzyme A dehydrogenase (LCHAD)

PHYSICAL FINDINGS & CLINICAL PRESENTATION

- Initial manifestations:
  1. Nausea and vomiting (70%)
  2. Pain in right upper quadrant or epigastrium (50% to 80%)
  3. Malaise and anorexia
- Jaundice often in 1 to 2 wk
- Late manifestations:
  1. Fulminant hepatic failure
  2. Encephalopathy
  3. Renal failure
  4. Pancreatitis
  5. Gastrointestinal and uterine bleeding
  6. Disseminated intravascular coagulation
  7. Seizures
  8. Coma
- Liver:
  1. Usually small
  2. Normal or enlarged in preeclampsia, eclampsia, HELLP syndrome (hemolysis, elevated liver enzymes, and low platelets), and acute hepatitis
  3. Coexistent preeclampsia in up to 46% of patients

ETIOLOGY

- Postulated that inhibition of mitochondrial oxidation of fatty acids may lead to microvesicular fatty infiltration of liver
- Fatty metamorphosis of preeclamptic liver disease believed to be of different etiology

DIAGNOSIS

DIFFERENTIAL DIAGNOSIS

- Acute gastroenteritis
- Preeclampsia or eclampsia with liver involvement
- HELLP syndrome
- Acute viral hepatitis
- Fulminant hepatitis
- Drug-induced hepatitis caused by halothane, phenytoin, methyldopa, isoniazid, hydrochlorothiazide, or tetracycline
- Intrahepatic cholestasis of pregnancy
- Gallbladder disease
- Reye's syndrome
- Hemolytic-uremic syndrome
- Budd-Chiari syndrome
- Systemic lupus erythematosus

WORKUP

- A clinical diagnosis is based predominantly on physical and laboratory findings.
- Most definitive diagnosis is through liver biopsy with oil red O staining and electron microscopy.
- Liver biopsy is reserved for atypical cases only and only after any existing coagulopathy corrected with fresh frozen plasma.

LABORATORY TESTS

Tests to determine the following:
- Hypoglycemia (often profound <60 mg/dl)
- Hyperammonemia
- Elevated aminotransferases (usually <500 U/ml)
- Thrombocytopenia
- Leucocytosis (white blood cell count >15,000)
- Hyperbilirubinemia (usually <10 mg/dl)
- Low albumin
- Hypofibrinogenemia (<300 mg/dl)
- Disseminated intravascular coagulation (DIC) (in 75%)

IMAGING STUDIES

- Ultrasound: best used to rule out other diseases in the differential diagnosis such as gallbladder disease
- CT scan: plays minimal role because of a high false-negative rate

TREATMENT

NONPHARMACOLOGIC THERAPY

- Patient is admitted to intensive care unit for stabilization.
- Fetus is delivered; spontaneous resolution usually follows delivery.
- Mode of delivery is based on obstetric indications and clinical assessment of disease severity.

ACUTE GENERAL Rx

- Decrease in endogenous ammonia through dietary protein restriction; neomycin 6 to 12 g/day PO to decrease presence of ammonia-producing bacteria; magnesium citrate 30 to 50 ml PO or enema to evacuate nitrogenous wastes from colon
- Administration of IV fluids with glucose to keep glucose levels >60 mg/dl
- Coagulopathy corrected with fresh frozen plasma
- Avoidance of drugs metabolized by liver
- Aggressive avoidance and treatment for nosocomial infections; consideration of prophylactic antibiotics
- Monitor closely for development of complications such as hepatic encephalopathy, pulmonary edema, DIC, and respiratory arrest

CHRONIC Rx

Orthotopic liver transplantation is the only treatment for irreversible liver failure.

DISPOSITION

- Before 1980, both maternal and fetal mortality rates were approximately 85%
- Since 1980, both maternal and fetal mortality rates are less than 20%
- Usually rapid return of liver function to normal after delivery
- Minimal risk of recurrence with future pregnancies

REFERRAL

- To tertiary health care facility as soon as diagnosis is suspected.
- Infants of mothers with AFLP should be evaluated for LCHAD deficiency.

SUGGESTED READINGS
available at www.expertconsult.com

AUTHORS: **ARUNDATHI G. PRASAD, M.D.,** and **RUBEN ALVERO, M.D.**

F

Diseases and Disorders

I

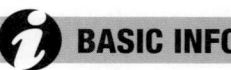

BASIC INFORMATION

DEFINITION

Felty's syndrome (FS) is defined as the triad of rheumatoid arthritis (RA), splenomegaly, and neutropenia. The hallmark of FS is a persistent, idiopathic neutropenia, which is defined as a neutrophil count $<2000/mm^3$. Splenomegaly is extremely variable in its extent and no longer required as an absolute diagnostic requirement. It is an extraarticular manifestation of seropositive RA in which recurrent local and systemic infections are the major source of morbidity and mortality.

ICD-9CM CODES
714.1 Felty's syndrome

EPIDEMIOLOGY & DEMOGRAPHICS

- The lifetime risk of FS for a patient initially diagnosed with RA is estimated to be 1% to 3%.
- 60% to 80% are women.
- Recognized in patients in their late 40s or early 50s who have had RA for 10 yr or more.
- Patients with FS are more likely to have a family history of RA and HLA-DRB1*0401.
- Rare in African Americans (low frequency of HLA-DRB1*0401).

CLINICAL PRESENTATION

- Rarely, splenomegaly and neutropenia are present before the arthritis.
- Articular involvement is usually more severe in patients with FS compared with other patients with RA; however, one third may have relatively inactive synovitis with elevated erythrocyte sedimentation rate (ESR).
- Degree of splenomegaly varies and may be detectable only by imaging studies; degree of splenomegaly has no correlation with the degree of neutropenia.
- Patients with FS have a greater frequency of extraarticular manifestations (rheumatoid nodules, vasculitis, skin lesions, pleuropericarditis, etc.) than other patients with RA.
- Mild hepatomegaly is common (up to 68%).
- Patients with FS have a twentyfold increased frequency of bacterial infections compared with other RA patients.

ETIOLOGY

The pathogenesis of FS is probably multifactorial, and no clear explanation has been elucidated.

DIAGNOSIS

DIFFERENTIAL DIAGNOSIS

- Systemic lupus erythematosus
- Large granular lymphocytic (LGL) leukemia
- Drug reaction
- Myeloproliferative disorders
- Lymphoma/reticuloendothelial malignances
- Cirrhosis with portal hypertension
- Sarcoidosis
- Tuberculosis
- Amyloidosis
- HIV infection

LABORATORY TESTS

- There is no single diagnostic test for FS.
- Complete blood count with differential to detect neutropenia, mild to moderate anemia, and mild to moderate thrombocytopenia.
- High ESR, C-reactive protein (CRP).
- Rheumatoid factor: positive in 98%, usually high titer.
- Antinuclear antibody (ANA): positive in 67%.
- Antihistone antibody: positive in 83%.
- Antineutrophil cytoplasmic antibodies (ANCA): positive in 77%.
- HLA-DRB1*0401: positive in 98%.
- Immunoglobulins: level may be higher than in RA patients.
- Complement level may be lower than in RA patients.
- Bone marrow examination is often necessary to exclude other cause of neutropenia. It usually shows myeloid hyperplasia with maturation arrest.
- Clonal cytogenetic abnormalities or clonal *TCR* gene recombination in patients with characteristic lymphocyte phenotypes suggests LGL leukemia.

IMAGING STUDIES

Ultrasonography or CT scan may be useful in diagnosing splenomegaly.

TREATMENT

ACUTE GENERAL Rx

- Splenectomy
  - It was the principal treatment therapy for FS but has now been replaced by drug therapy.
  - Usually reserved for patients with profound neutropenia ($<1000/mm^3$) and severe recurrent infections.
  - Acutely reverses hematologic abnormalities.
  - 25% to 30% will have recurrent neutropenia, but the granulocyte count usually remains above the presplenectomy level.
  - Improvement in frequency of recurrent infection is variable and not correlated with degree of hematologic improvement.

- Antirheumatic drugs: second-line drugs for RA may improve the neutropenia in FS.
  - Gold salt injections: good hematologic response in 60%, partial response in 20%. The recovery of neutrophil count is usually slow.
  - Methotrexate: series of studies with small numbers of patients suggest the efficacy in FS. Follow-up durations are still short. Granulocyte count may begin to rise within several weeks in responders.
  - Penicillamine, sulfasalazine: limited experience; not first choice for FS.
- Corticosteroids
  - Overwhelming infection is the main barrier to the use of corticosteroids.
  - Prednisone 30 mg/day or more can elevate the neutrophil count, but this effect is often not sustained when the dose is reduced.
  - Pulse dosing is a potential alternative for short-term elevation of neutrophils.
- Others
  - Limited experience with cyclophosphamide, cyclosporine, azathioprine, leflunomide, anti–tumor necrosis factor-alpha antibody, rituximab, lithium, and testosterone.
- Recombinant granulocyte colony-stimulating factor/granulocyte-macrophage colony-stimulating factor
  - Improves neutrophil count but not arthritis and anemia of FS.
  - May be useful as adjunctive therapy during serious infection or in preparation for surgery.

DISPOSITION

- Poor prognosis with recurrent infections because of neutropenia.
- Articular involvement can be severe in FS.

REFERRAL

- To hematologist for treatment of neutropenia
- To rheumatologist for treatment of RA

PEARLS & CONSIDERATIONS

COMMENTS

- Recurrent infections are the major cause of death.
- Neutropenia of FS can be effectively treated with disease-modifying antirheumatic drugs, the widest experience being with methotrexate.

SUGGESTED READINGS
available at www.expertconsult.com

AUTHOR: ETSUKO AOKI, M.D., PH.D.

BASIC INFORMATION

DEFINITION

A femoral neck fracture occurs within the capsule of the hip joint between the base of the head and the intertrochanteric line.

SYNONYMS

Hip fracture
Intracapsular fracture
Subcapital fracture

ICD-9CM CODES

820.8 Femoral neck fracture

EPIDEMIOLOGY & DEMOGRAPHICS

PREVALENCE: Lifetime risk in women ~16%
PREDOMINANT SEX: Female/male ratio of 3:1
PREDOMINANT AGE: 90% >60 yr

PHYSICAL FINDINGS & CLINICAL PRESENTATION

- Hip or groin pain
- Affected limb usually shortened and externally rotated in displaced fractures
- Impacted fractures: possibly no deformity and only mild pain with hip motion
- Mild external bruising

ETIOLOGY

- Trauma
- Age-related bone weakness, usually caused by osteoporosis
- Increased risk of fractures in elderly (decline in muscle function, use of psychotropic medication, etc.)

DIAGNOSIS

DIFFERENTIAL DIAGNOSIS

- Osteoarthritis of hip
- Pathologic fracture
- Lumbar disc syndrome with radicular pain
- Insufficiency fracture of pelvis

WORKUP

Diagnosis is usually obvious based on clinical and radiographic findings.

IMAGING STUDIES

- Standard roentgenograms consisting of an anteroposterior view of the pelvis and a cross-table lateral view of the hip to confirm the diagnosis (Fig. 1-151).
- If initial roentgenograms are negative and diagnosis of an occult femoral neck fracture is suspected, hospital admission and further radiographic assessment with either bone scanning or MRI are recommended.
- Bone scanning is sensitive after 48 to 72 hr.

TREATMENT

- Orthopedic consultation
- Surgery indicated in most cases, usually within 24 hr
- Deep vein thrombosis prophylaxis

DISPOSITION

- Older adults have a five- to eightfold increased risk for all-cause mortality during the first 3 mo after hip fracture. Mortality rate within 1 yr in elderly patients is 25% to 30%. Excess annual mortality persists over time for both women and men, but at any given age, excess annual mortality after hip fracture is higher in men than in women.
- Dementia is a particularly poor prognostic sign.

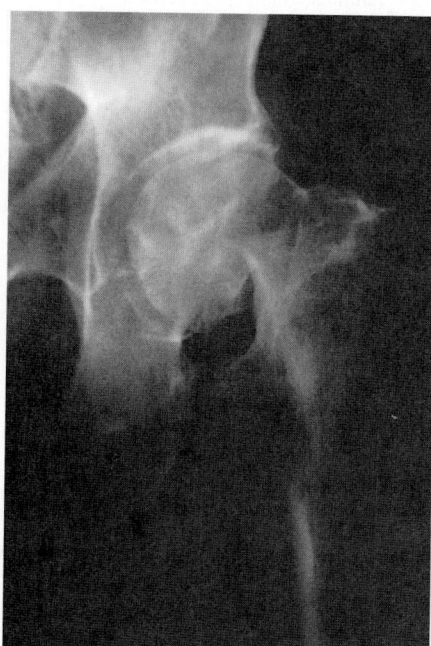

FIGURE 1-151 Femoral neck fracture. (From Scudieri G [ed]: *Sports medicine: principles of primary care,* St Louis, 1997, Mosby.)

REFERRAL

For surgical consideration when the diagnosis is made

PEARLS & CONSIDERATIONS

COMMENTS

- Complications: nonunion and avascular necrosis
- Intracapsular fractures: occasionally occur in nonambulatory patients
  1. Usually treated nonsurgically, especially in the patient with dementia and limited pain perception
  2. Early bed-to-chair mobilization and vigilant nursing care to avoid skin breakdown
  3. Fracture usually pain free in a short time even if solid bony healing does not occur
- As a result of the increasing life span of the female population, femoral neck fractures are becoming more common. The initial physical examination and roentgenographic studies may be completely negative. Groin pain, sometimes quite severe, may be the only early clue to the diagnosis.
- The rate of hip fracture could be reduced by:
  1. Elimination of environmental hazards (poor lighting, loose rugs)
  2. Regular exercise for balance and strength
  3. Patient education about fall prevention
  4. Medication review to minimize side effects
  5. Prevention and treatment of osteoporosis
- In the U.S., hip fracture rates and subsequent mortality among persons aged 65 yr and older are declining, and comorbidities among patients with hip fractures have increased. Hip fractures are also very expensive ($40,000 in the first year following hip fracture for direct medical costs and $5,000 in subsequent years).

EVIDENCE

available at www.expertconsult.com

SUGGESTED READINGS

available at www.expertconsult.com

AUTHOR: **LONNIE R. MERCIER, M.D.**

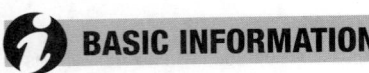 **BASIC INFORMATION**

DEFINITION

- The adverse effects of alcohol on the developing human represent a spectrum of structural anomalies and behavioral and neurocognitive disabilities, most accurately termed fetal alcohol spectrum disorder (FASD) (Table 1-52).
- Children at the severe end of the spectrum have been defined as having the fetal alcohol syndrome (FAS).

ICD-9CM CODES
760.71 Fetal alcohol syndrome

EPIDEMIOLOGY & DEMOGRAPHICS

- Alcohol is considered to be the most common major teratogen to which the fetus is liable to be exposed.
- 10% report drinking alcohol during pregnancy and 2% to 4% admit to binge drinking.
- FAS represent the most common form of mental retardation in U.S.
- Its prevalence is 1 to 2 per 1000 live births across United States.
- Each year 40,000 babies are born with fetal alcohol spectrum disorder.

RISK FACTORS

- Advance maternal age (>30 yr)
- High parity
- African-American, Alaskan Natives, and Native Indian race
- Binge drinking (more than four drinks per occasion)
- History of prior affected child
- Genetic susceptibility
- Undernutrition
- Low socioeconomic group

PHYSICAL FINDINGS & CLINICAL PRESENTATION

Typical features:
- Growth retardation
  - Prenatal or postnatal
  - Height and/or weight <10%
- Facial dysmorphia
  - Smooth philtrum
  - Thin vermilion border
  - Small palpebral fissure (<10%)
  - Others: epicanthic folds, ptosis of eyelids, flat nasal bridge and midface, upturned nose, railroad track ears, and so forth
- CNS abnormalities
  - Structural
    - Head circumference, 10%
    - Clinically significant brain abnormalities observable through imaging
  - Neurologic
    - Neurologic problems not due to a postnatal insult or fever
  - Functional
    - Intellectual deficit
    - Cognitive or developmental deficits
    - Executive function deficits
    - Motor function delays
    - Problem with attention and hyperactivity
    - Social skills
    - Other problems such as sensory, pragmatic language, and memory

Rare birth defects:
- Cardiac
  - Ventricular septal defect (VSD)
  - Atrial septal defect (ASD)
  - Tetralogy of Fallot
  - Aberrant great vessels
- Skeletal
  - Radioulnar synostosis
  - Hypoplastic nails
  - Clinodactyly
  - Shortened fifth digit
  - Pectus excavatum and carinatum
  - Klippel-Feil syndrome
  - Hemivertebrae
  - Camptodactyly
  - Scoliosis
- Renal
  - Aplastic kidneys
  - Dysplastic kidneys
  - Ureteral duplication
  - Hypoplastic kidneys
  - Hydronephrosis
  - Horseshoe kidneys
- Ocular
  - Strabismus
  - Refractive problems
  - Retinal vascular abnormalities
- Auditory
  - Conductive hearing loss
  - Neurosensory hearing loss
- Others
  - Hockey stick–like palmar crease

ETIOLOGY

- Prenatal damage as a result of chronic alcoholism comes about primarily because of direct action of ethanol or its metabolites (e.g., acetaldehyde) on the fetus.
- The exact damaging mechanism is not clear.
- Although the damaging effect of alcohol is different in the various phases of pregnancy, it is by no means limited to first trimester.
- There is no exact dose-response relationship between the amount of alcohol consumed during the prenatal period and the extent of damage inflicted on the infant.
- An occasional drink during pregnancy carries no risk to the fetus, but no level of drinking is known to be safe during pregnancy.
- The least significant effect recognized at two drinks per day has been slightly smaller birth weight (160 g smaller than average).
- It is not until four to six drinks per day are consumed that additional subtle clinical features are evident.
- Most of the children believed to have FAS have been born to frankly alcoholic mothers whose intake is eight to ten drinks or more per day, and those who engage in binge drinking.
- The risk of serious problem in the offspring of a chronically alcoholic woman has been estimated to be 30% to 50%, the greatest risk being varying degree of mental retardation.

SECONDARY DISABILITIES

- Mental health problems
- Dependent living
- Employment problems
- Disruptive school problems
- Trouble with law
- Confinement
- Inappropriate sexual behavior
- Alcohol or drug problems

DX DIAGNOSIS

- It is a diagnosis of exclusion.
- Diagnosis is difficult both prenatally and at birth. Unfortunately, most cases are not diagnosed until school age.
- As the characteristic facial features tend to become decreasingly recognizable as the child reaches adolescence, the diagnosis becomes increasingly difficult with advancing age.
- Prenatal exposure to alcohol is not sufficient to warrant a diagnosis. According to the Centers for Disease Control and Prevention the diagnosis of FAS requires three specific findings along with the history of prenatal alcohol exposure:
  - Growth restriction (intrauterine or postnatal)
  - Central nervous system involvement

TABLE 1-52 The Institute of Medicine's Diagnostic Criteria for Fetal Alcohol-Related Abnormalities	
Category 1 FAS with confirmed maternal alcohol exposure	Presence of classic triad of growth retardation, characteristic facial dysmorphology and neurodevelopmental abnormalities. This is often defined as full-blown FAS
Category 2 FAS without confirmed maternal alcohol exposure	Triad in category 1 is present without confirmed maternal drinking
Category 3 Partial FAS with confirmed maternal alcohol exposure	Presence of some of the characteristic facial anomalies plus growth retardation or central nervous system neurodevelopmental abnormalities or behavioral/cognitive abnormalities
Category 4 FAS with confirmed maternal alcohol exposure and alcohol-related birth defects	These patients will have some congenital anomalies as a result of alcohol toxicity
Category 5 FAS with confirmed maternal alcohol exposure and alcohol-related neurodevelopmental disorder	There is evidence of CNS neurodevelopmental abnormalities or a complex patter of behavioral/cognitive abnormalities or both, but not necessarily any obvious physical changes

○ Documentation of all three facial abnormalities (smooth philtrum, thin vermilion border, and short palpebral fissure)
- Imaging recommendation during pregnancy with alcohol exposure:
  ○ High-risk anatomy scan
  ○ Serial growth scan
  ○ Fetal echocardiogram at 22 to 24 weeks' intrauterine pregnancy
- Measurement of the ethyl esters of fatty acids in the meconium and hair of the newborn can substantiate maternal alcohol exposure.
- In school-aged children, the diagnostic process should include a through psychologic evaluation that assesses multiple domains. Also, supplement the observation by obtaining standardized testing through early intervention programs, public schools, and psychologists in private practice.

DIFFERENTIAL DIAGNOSIS

- Other causes of symmetrical growth retardation including intrauterine infection and aneuploidy
- Aneuploidy (T21, T18, T13)
- Syndromes with overlapping features of FAS:
  ○ Fetal anticonvulsant syndrome
  ○ Maternal phenylketonuria
  ○ Toluene embryopathy
  ○ Velocardiofacial syndrome (deletion 22q11)
  ○ William syndrome
  ○ Dubowitz syndrome
  ○ Cornelia de Lange syndrome

℞ TREATMENT

- As there is no cure for FAS, we need to emphasize prevention.
- For those women who are planning pregnancy or who have the potential to become pregnant, the U.S. Surgeon General has recommended that the safest course is to avoid alcohol entirely during pregnancy.
- Women of childbearing age who are not pregnant should drink no more than seven alcoholic drinks per week and no more than three drinks on any one occasion.
- Preconception counseling should be offered to women of childbearing age who are at risk for an alcohol-exposed pregnancy.
- Screen all pregnant women for alcohol use.
- The National Institute on Alcohol Abuse and Alcoholism recommend that any woman who reports drinking more than seven drinks per week or more than three drinks on any given day be further assessed for alcohol-related problems.
- The following two questionnaires are used to identify women drinking sufficiently to potentially damage the fetus. The CAGE questionnaire is less sensitive for screening pregnant women:
  ○ T-ACE (Table 1-53)
  ○ TWEAK (Table 1-54)
- Effective treatment alternatives for women who screen positive for hazardous alcohol use include brief interventions to promote reductions in alcohol use and that facilitate referral to specialized treatment programs.

- Discontinuation or reduction of alcohol consumption at any point in pregnancy may be beneficial.
- The use of alcohol-containing tonics and medications with an alcohol base should be avoided. This applies to medications with an alcohol base, at least when the concentration exceeds 10%.
- Alcoholism is one of the few situations in which pregnancy interruption may be discussed with the patient as it may result in FAS.
- Early diagnosis and appropriate treatment may decrease secondary disabilities and recurrence in future pregnancies.
- A child should be referred for full FAS evaluation when substantial prenatal alcohol use by the mother has been confirmed (more than seven drinks per week, or more than three drinks on multiple occasions, or both).
- If substantial prenatal exposure is known, in the absence of any other positive criteria, the physician should document this exposure and closely monitor the child's ongoing growth and development.
- When information about prenatal exposure is unknown, a child should be referred for full FAS if any of the following conditions are present: (1) all three dysmorphic facial features (smooth philtrum, thin vermilion border, and small palpebral fissure), (2) one or more of these facial features with growth deficit, (3) one or more facial features with one or more CNS abnormalities, (4) one or more dysmorphic facial features with growth deficit and one or more CNS abnormalities, or (5) any report of concern by a caregiver or parent that a child has or may have FAS.
- Infants and children who are diagnosed with FAS should be evaluated by a physician who is knowledgeable and competent in the evaluation of neurodevelopment and psychosocial problems associated with the diagnosis.
- A multidisciplinary team including a clinical geneticist, developmental pediatrician, mental health professional, social worker, and education specialist is often necessary for management.
- Treatment options include:
  ○ Medications to help with symptoms
  ○ Behavior and education therapy
    Friendship training
    Specialized math training

Executive function training
Parent-child interaction training
Parenting and behavior management training
- Parenting training
  Concentrate on child's strengths and talents
  Accept child's limitations
  Be consistent with everything
  Use concrete language and examples
  Use stable routine that does not change daily
  Keep everything simple
  Be specific (i.e., say exactly what you mean)
  Structure your child's world to provide a foundation for daily living
  Use visualized aids, music, and hands-on activities to help your child learn
  Use positive reinforcement often
  Supervise
  Repeat, repeat, and repeat
- Emphasis on the following protective factors helps reduce the effects and also assists people with this condition to reach their full potential:
  Diagnosing before 6 yr
  Living in stable nurturing home environment in school years
  Absence of violence
  Involvement in special education and social services
- Alternative approaches such as biofeedback, auditory training, relaxation therapy, visual imagery, yoga/exercise, acupuncture/acupressure, massage, Reiki, energy healing, animal-assisted therapy, and so forth may play a role.

TABLE 1-53 T-ACE Questions*

T (tolerance)	How many drinks does it take to make you feel high? (3 or more drinks = 2 points)
A (annoyed)	Have people annoyed you by criticizing your drinking? (Yes = 1 point)
C (cut down)	Have you felt you ought to cut down on your drinking? (Yes = 1 point)
E (eye opener)	Have you ever had to drink first thing in the morning to steady your nerves or to get rid of a hangover? (Yes = 1 point)

*A score of 2 or more indicates heavy or problem drinker. Its sensitivity is 70% and specificity is 85%.

TABLE 1-54 TWEAK*

T (tolerance)	How many drinks does it take before you begin to feel the first effects of alcohol? (3 or more drinks = 2 points)
W (worried)	Have close friends or relatives worried about your drinking in the past year? (Yes = 2 points)
E (eye opener)	Do you sometimes take a drink in the morning when you first get up? (Yes = 1 point)
A (amnesia)	Has a friend or family member ever told you about things you said or did while you were drinking that you could not remember? (Yes = 1 point)
K (kut down)	Do you sometimes feel the need to cut down on your drinking? (Yes = 1 point)

*A total of 3 or more points indicates the woman is likely to be a heavy or problem drinker. Its sensitivity is 79% and specificity is 83%.

SUGGESTED READINGS
available at www.expertconsult.com

AUTHOR: **HEMANT SATPATHY, M.D.**

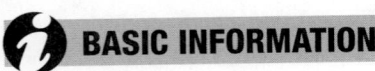

BASIC INFORMATION

DEFINITION

Fever of undetermined origin (FUO) was defined by Petersdorf and Beeson in 1961 as an illness characterized by temperatures >101° F on several occasions for >3 wk with no known cause despite extensive workup.

- Persistence for >2 wk separates an FUO from an insignificant viral illness.
- Traditionally, diagnosis was made only after a 1-wk inpatient workup. In contemporary practice, much of the workup is performed as an outpatient.

SYNONYMS

Fever of unknown origin

ICD-9CM CODES

780.6 Pyrexia of undetermined origin

EPIDEMIOLOGY & DEMOGRAPHICS

- The incidence of undiagnosed FUO dropped to <10% in the 1950s but has steadily increased since then.
- True FUOs are uncommon.

CLINICAL PRESENTATION

Fever (101° F or more) >3 wk.

ETIOLOGY

(Most common etiologies italicized)
- Infection (16%)
  - *Abscess: abdominal, pelvic*
  - *Tuberculosis*
  - HIV infection
  - Nosocomial (febrile for 3 days in hospital): urinary tract infection, pneumonia, line-related bacteremia, *Clostridium difficile* diarrhea, sinusitis
  - Bacterial endocarditis (especially caused by difficult-to-isolate organisms)
  - Biliary tract infection
  - Osteomyelitis, vertebral and mandibular
  - Less common infections: Q fever, leptospirosis, psittacosis, tularemia, secondary syphilis, gonococcemia, chronic meningococcemia, Whipple's disease, yersiniosis, fungal infections
- Malignancy (7%): *lymphoma* (especially non-Hodgkin's lymphoma) and *leukemia,* renal cell carcinoma, hepatocellular carcinomas, other tumors metastatic to liver
- Noninfectious inflammatory disease (22%)
  - Juvenile rheumatoid arthritis (younger patients)
  - Temporal arteritis (elderly patients)
  - Other vasculitis: polyarteritis nodosa, Takayasu's arteritis, Wegener's granuloma-

tosis, mixed cryoglobulinemia, adult Still's disease
- Other (4%)
  - Drug-induced fever
  - Inflammatory bowel disease
  - Sarcoidosis
  - Granulomatous hepatitis
  - Deep venous thrombosis
  - Alcoholic hepatitis
- No diagnosis (51%)

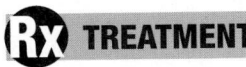

DIAGNOSIS

DIFFERENTIAL DIAGNOSIS

Factitious fever

WORKUP

- Accurate history and careful physical examination are essential.
- Laboratory tests and imaging dependent on medical history clues and physical findings.
- When in doubt, perform another complete history and physical examination.

MEDICAL HISTORY CLUES

- Fever duration, tempo; inciting factors
- Rash, myalgia, weight loss, pain
- Sick contacts
- Past medical history: tuberculosis, HIV, malignancies, surgeries
- Medications
- Family history: tuberculosis, malignancies, familial Mediterranean fever
- Social history: daily routine, rural versus urban, pets and animal contacts, arthropod bites, recent and remote travel, socioeconomic status, occupation, military service, sexual history

PHYSICAL FINDINGS

- HEENT (head, ears, eyes, nose, throat): sinus tenderness, dental abscesses, funduscopic lesions
- Neck: adenopathy, palpable thyroid
- Lungs: auscultate for rales
- Heart: murmur
- Abdomen: organomegaly
- Rectal: prostate tenderness
- Pelvic: cervical motion tenderness, fundal or adnexal masses or pain; inguinal adenopathy
- Extremities: clubbing, splinter hemorrhages; tenderness or fluctuance at IV access site
- Musculoskeletal: joint effusions
- Skin: rashes, wounds

LABORATORY TESTS

- Most FUO workups include:
  - Blood cultures
  - Complete blood count with differential
  - Erythrocyte sedimentation rate or C-reactive protein

  - Urinalysis
  - Transaminases
  - Serum lactate dehydrogenase
  - PPD testing
- Consider
  - HIV antibody testing
  - Creatinine phosphokinase
  - Rheumatoid factor
  - Serum protein electrophoresis
  - Lumbar puncture
  - Thyroid function testing
  - Stool culture and *C. difficile* assay
  - Bone marrow biopsy
  - Skin biopsy
  - Antinuclear antibody testing

May need to repeat tests at regular intervals until diagnosis is established.

IMAGING STUDIES

- Most workups eventually include chest radiograph and abdominal CT scan.
- Further imaging is based on medical history clues and physical findings.

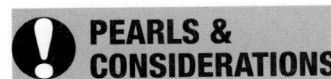

TREATMENT

ACUTE GENERAL Rx

Antibiotics and other treatment indicated only after definitive or highly probable diagnosis is established unless patient is severely ill or septic.

DISPOSITION

Diagnoses are found in majority of cases of FUO. In some cases a diagnosis is not made for years. At 5-yr follow-up, mortality rate among patients with undiagnosed FUO was only 3.2% in one study.

REFERRAL

To an infectious disease specialist, hematologist, or rheumatologist if no diagnosis after thoughtful workup

PEARLS & CONSIDERATIONS

COMMENTS

Because of improvements in imaging and laboratory tests, fewer cases of FUO are attributed to infectious causes and more are diagnosed as attributable to tumors and collagen-vascular diseases.

SUGGESTED READINGS

available at www.expertconsult.com

AUTHOR: ETSUKO AOKI, M.D., PH.D.

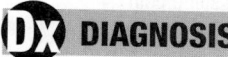 **BASIC INFORMATION**

DEFINITION

Fibrocystic breast disease (FCD) is a "nondisease" that includes nonmalignant breast lesions such as microcystic and macrocystic changes, fibrosis, ductal or lobular hyperplasia, adenosis, apocrine metaplasia, fibroadenoma, papilloma, papillomatosis, and other changes. Atypical ductal or lobular hyperplasia is associated with a moderate increase in breast cancer risk.

SYNONYMS

Cystic changes
Chronic cystic mastitis
Mammary dysplasia

ICD-9CM CODES
610.0 Solitary cyst of the breast
610.1 Fibrocystic disease of the breast

EPIDEMIOLOGY & DEMOGRAPHICS

- Ubiquitous in premenopausal women after 20 yr of age
- Palpable nodular changes in the breast termed FCD clinically; such changes observable in more than half of adult women aged 20 to 50 yr

PHYSICAL FINDINGS & CLINICAL PRESENTATION

- Tender breasts
- Nodular areas
- Dominant mass
- Thickening
- Nipple discharge
- Can vary with menstrual cycle

ETIOLOGY

- Although it is frequently seen and diagnosed, mechanism of development is not understood.

- Because it is found in the majority of healthy breasts, it is regarded as a nonpathologic process.
- With hormone replacement therapy, the condition may be carried into menopause.

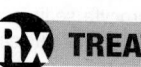 **DIAGNOSIS**

DIFFERENTIAL DIAGNOSIS

- If presenting as dominant mass or masses, exclude possible carcinoma.
- Carcinoma: detection is difficult with FCD, particularly among premenopausal women.
- If presenting with nipple discharge, differentiate from discharge of possible malignant origin.

WORKUP

- Exclude breast carcinoma if breast mass, thickening, discharge, and/or pain are present.
- Perform biopsy of suspected area for histologic confirmation.

IMAGING STUDIES

Mammography and ultrasound studies required:
- For mammographic changes (suspicious densities, microcalcifications, architectural distortion): careful evaluation, including possibly biopsy to exclude breast cancer
- Ultrasound study: to establish cystic nature of clinical or mammographic mass lesion

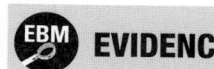 **TREATMENT**

NONPHARMACOLOGIC THERAPY

- Not considered a "disease" and does not require treatment
- Surgical intervention diagnostic to eliminate possibility of breast cancer
- Periodic physician examination to monitor patients with FCD who have pronounced nodular features

- Aspiration for palpable cysts (NOTE: Cysts often recur; repeat aspiration is not always required unless pain is a problem.)

ACUTE GENERAL Rx

The majority of women require no treatment.

CHRONIC Rx

For breast pain:
- Danocrine (Danazol): limited success reported
- Bromocriptine or tamoxifen: used less frequently
- Limited caffeine intake: not as successful in controlling pain or nodularity as originally suggested

DISPOSITION

- Careful evaluation to exclude suspicious changes for breast cancer, then reassurance and periodic reevaluation as required
- Regular self-examination, annual physician examination, and annual mammograms for women with atypical ductal or lobular hyperplasia

REFERRAL

- For further evaluation and/or biopsy if there are suspicious changes that may be associated with FCD (including changing of dominant mass or thickening, persistent or spontaneous discharge, suspicious mammographic changes or lesions)
- To alleviate anxiety associated with breast symptoms or changes

EBM **EVIDENCE**

available at www.expertconsult.com

AUTHORS: **TAKUMA NEMOTO, M.D.,** and **RUBEN ALVERO, M.D.**

F

Diseases and Disorders

I

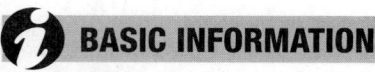 **BASIC INFORMATION**

DEFINITION

Fibromyalgia is a poorly defined disorder characterized by multiple trigger points and referred pain.

SYNONYMS

Myofascial pain syndrome
Fibrositis
Psychogenic rheumatism
Nonarticular rheumatism
Fibromyalgia syndrome (FS)

ICD-9CM CODES
729.0 Rheumatism, unspecified and fibrositis
729.1 Myalgia and myositis, unspecified

EPIDEMIOLOGY & DEMOGRAPHICS

PREVALENCE: 1% to 2% of the general population
PREDOMINANT SEX: Female/male ratio of 9:1
PREDOMINANT AGE: 30 to 50 yr

PHYSICAL FINDINGS

Tender "nodules" and tender points (Fig. 1-152)

ETIOLOGY

• Unknown. Genetic, environmental, and psychosocial factors appear to influence its expression.
• Pain magnification may play a role

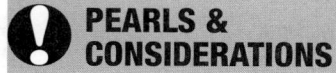 **DIAGNOSIS**

DIFFERENTIAL DIAGNOSIS

• Polymyalgia rheumatica
• Referred discogenic spine pain
• Rheumatoid arthritis
• Localized tendinitis
• Connective tissue disease
• Osteoarthritis
• Thyroid disease
• Spondyloarthropathies

WORKUP

• Subsets of this disorder are often described:
  1. If symptoms develop in conjunction with other conditions (rheumatoid disease or acute stress)
  2. If findings are more regionally distributed, such as those in the neck after motor vehicle accidents
• The primary condition is often suggested by the following criteria from the American College of Rheumatology:
  1. History of widespread pain
  2. Pain in 11 of 18 selected tender spots on digital palpation (mainly in the spine, elbows, and knees)

LABORATORY TESTS

There are no abnormalities in fibromyalgia, but laboratory assessment may be required to rule out other conditions and may include:
• Complete blood count, erythrocyte sedimentation rate, rheumatoid factor, antinuclear antibody
• Creatine phosphokinase, T_4

TREATMENT

ACUTE GENERAL Rx

• Self-management
• Explanation, reassurance
• Aerobic and stretching exercise, particularly swimming
• Mild analgesics; avoidance of chronic narcotic use
• Pregabalin 120 mg/day may be effective in symptom control (Lyrica), a GABA analog (75 mg bid), duloxetine (Cymbalta), an SNRI (60-120 mg/day), and milnacipam (Savella), an SNRI (50 mg bid), may be effective in symptom control
• Low-dose tricyclic antidepressants for sleep disturbance (amitriptyline 10 to 25 mg)
• Tricyclic antidepressants for sleep disturbance (amitriptyline 10 to 25 mg)
• Trigger point injections
• Physical therapy
• Tai chi: several trials have shown that tai chi offers a therapeutic benefit in patients with fibromyalgia

DISPOSITION

• Prognosis is uncertain.
• Symptoms come and go for years despite an aggressive, multifaceted approach to treatment.

REFERRAL

Consultation with rheumatology, psychiatry, and physical medicine may all be helpful.

PEARLS & CONSIDERATIONS

Some investigators consider myofascial pain syndrome to be a separate condition, perhaps with a better prognosis.

COMMENTS

• Before making this diagnosis, all other more likely disorders should be ruled out.
• The term "fibrositis" is often used, but no inflammation has ever been found.
• The number of trigger points needed to establish the diagnosis is debated.

SUGGESTED READINGS
available at www.expertconsult.com

AUTHOR: **LONNIE R. MERCIER, M.D.**

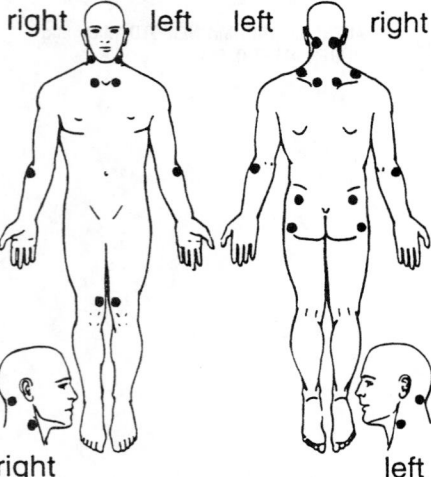

1. Occiput
2. Low cervical
3. Trapezius
4. Supraspinatus
5. Second rib
6. Lateral epicondyle
7. Gluteal
8. Greater trochanter
9. Knees

FIGURE 1-152 The sites of the 18 tender points of the 1990 American College of Rheumatology criteria for the classification of fibromyalgia. (From Conn R: *Current diagnosis,* ed 9, Philadelphia, 1997, WB Saunders.)

BASIC INFORMATION

DEFINITION

Parvovirus B-19 is a nonenveloped DNA virus that causes a spectrum of human disease. Classically, it has been associated with "fifth disease," also known as "erythema infectiosum")—viral exanthem of school-aged children historically considered to be the "fifth" in a series of viral exanthems. There is a growing awareness that parvovirus B-19 also causes a spectrum of disease in adults, specifically in immunocompromised populations.

SYNONYMS

Erythema infectiosum

ICD-9CM CODES
057.0 Fifth disease (eruptive)

EPIDEMIOLOGY & DEMOGRAPHICS

PEAK INCIDENCE: Late winter and spring, especially April and May
PREDOMINANT AGE: 5 to 18 yr
GENETICS: 50% to 60% of adults have demonstrated protective antibodies to parvovirus B-19.

PHYSICAL FINDINGS & CLINICAL PRESENTATION

- Typical bright red, nontender maxillary rash with circumoral pallor over cheeks, producing the classic "slapped cheek" appearance (Fig. 1-153).
- In adults, 90% with erythematous rash, 25% with classic reticular lacy, erythematous, maculopapular rash over trunk and extremities lasting for up to several weeks after the acute episode. May be worsened by heat or

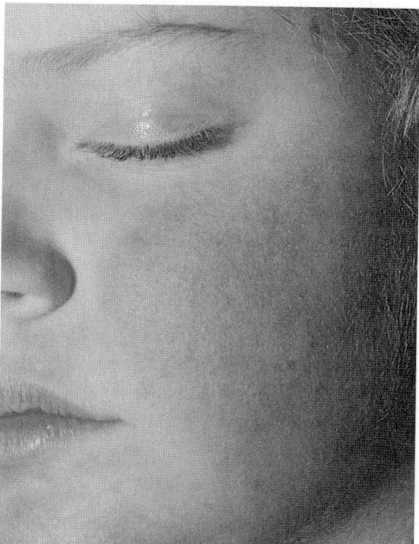

FIGURE 1-153 Fifth disease (erythema infectiosum). Facial erythema "slapped cheek." The red plaque covers the cheek and spares the nasolabial and the circumoral region. (From Habif TP: *Clinical dermatology: a color guide to diagnosis and therapy,* ed 3, St Louis, 1996, Mosby.)

sunlight. 60% report pruritus, primarily in lower extremities.
- Polyarthritis and arthralgias are commonly seen in older patients and less commonly in children. Arthritis involves small joints of the extremities in symmetric fashion and typically occurs one week after the initial symptoms (5.5 ± 3.2 days).
- Mild fever is seen in up to one third of children, whereas 70% of adults report a fever.

ETIOLOGY

Syndrome caused by parvovirus B-19, a single-stranded DNA virus, which has been reclassified in the new genus *Erythrovirus.* Transmission is primarily through droplet exposure to the respiratory tract. As it is heat stable and nonenveloped, parvovirus transmission has been demonstrated through exposure to blood products, although recent studies have failed to demonstrate transmission in a large surgical cohort (references).

DIAGNOSIS

DIFFERENTIAL DIAGNOSIS

- Juvenile rheumatoid arthritis (Still's disease)
- Rubella, measles (rubeola), and other childhood viral exanthems
- Mononucleosis
- Lyme disease
- Acute HIV infection
- Drug eruption

WORKUP

Diagnosis made by typical clinical presentation; laboratory tests can support diagnosis (see next).

LABORATORY TESTS

- Parvovirus B-19 IgM
  - An antibody seen in 90% of patients with acute illness. Usually not necessary, as clinical presentation and typical rash are sufficient to establish diagnosis.
  - Complete blood count (in specific populations at risk for marrow toxicity). Transient aplastic crisis is a syndrome distinct from fifth disease, which may be seen in patients with chronic hematologic illness (described with sickle cell disease, spherocytosis, and other hemolytic processes) or AIDS who are infected with parvovirus B-19. There have been recent case reports of patients treated with rituximab who developed aplastic crisis in the setting of parvovirus infection.
    a. Usually self-limited and associated with prodrome of fever and malaise. Lasts for 1 to 2 wk, followed by marrow recovery.
    b. Rash is usually absent.
    c. These patients are highly infective.
- Human chorionic gonadotropin (in women of childbearing age)
  - Infection during early pregnancy may result in fetal death (10%) or severe anemia but is usually asymptomatic and not associated with congenital malformations.

- Quantitative polymerase chain reaction.
- Used for early, rapid diagnosis in immunocompromised patients and to screen plasma products.

TREATMENT

ACUTE GENERAL Rx

- Treatment is supportive only
- Nonsteroidal anti-inflammatory drugs for arthralgias and arthritis
- IV immunoglobulin and transfusion support has anecdotal success reported in patients with immunocompromised state with red cell aplasia.
- Consider immunoglobulin treatment or prophylaxis in pregnancy
- Bone marrow transplantation has been used in individuals with nonresolving aplastic crisis.

DISPOSITION & PROGNOSIS

- Typically self-limited illness lasting 1 to 2 wk.
- Arthritis lasts for weeks. In some patients it may be chronic and develop into rheumatoid arthritis as adults.
- Pregnant women should avoid contact with patients who have marrow suppression. Maternal parvovirus infection in pregnancy may have a wide range of fetal effects, including hydrops fetalis, and warrants close monitoring of fetal development and health.
- Patients with transient aplastic crisis or chronic parvovirus B-19 infection pose a risk for nosocomial spread and, when hospitalized, should be isolated with contact and respiratory precautions.
- Children with fifth disease are not contagious and may attend school and day care.
- A vaccine is under development.
- Some infected individuals develop aplastic anemia and require bone marrow transplantation.

REFERRAL

- To hematologist for signs of marrow suppression
- To rheumatologist for signs of severe or erosive arthritis

PEARLS & CONSIDERATIONS

- Self-limited disease lasting 1 to 2 wk
- Symmetric arthritis involving small joints is common in adults, whereas facial rash is common in children
- Can cause aplastic anemia in patients with an underlying hematologic disorder such as sickle cell disease, in an immunocompromised state, and after transplantation.

SUGGESTED READINGS

available at www.expertconsult.com

AUTHORS: **WILLIAM HAHN, M.D.,** and **DOMINICK TAMMARO, M.D.**

F

Diseases and Disorders

I

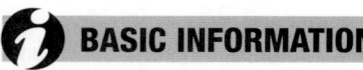

DEFINITION

Filariasis is a general term for an infection caused by subcutaneous nematodes (roundworms) of the genera *Wuchereria* and *Brugia*, found in the tropical and subtropical regions of the world. The disease is variably characterized by acute lymphatic inflammation or chronic lymphatic obstruction associated with intermittent fevers or recurrent episodes of dyspnea and bronchospasm.

SYNONYMS

Lymphatic filariasis
Elephantiasis

ICD-9CM CODES
125.0 Bancroftian
125.1 Brugian
125.9 Filariasis

EPIDEMIOLOGY & DEMOGRAPHICS

INCIDENCE (IN U.S.): Unknown
PEAK INCIDENCE: Unknown
PREDOMINANT SEX: Male
PREDOMINANT AGE: For both males and females, risk is greatest between the ages of 15 and 35 yr.

PHYSICAL FINDINGS & CLINICAL PRESENTATION

- Clinical manifestations result from acute lymphatic inflammation or chronic lymphatic obstruction.

- Many patients are asymptomatic despite the presence of microfilaremia.
- Episodes of lymphangitis and lymphadenitis are associated with fever, headache, and back pain.
- Acute funiculitis and epididymitis or orchitis may also be present; all usually resolve within days to weeks but tend to recur.
- Chronic infections may be associated with lymphedema, most commonly manifested by hydrocele.
- It is a progressive disease, leading to nonpitting edema and brawny changes that may involve a whole limb (Fig. 1-154).
- Elephantiasis occurs in about 10% of patients, with skin of the scrotum or leg becoming thickened and fissured; patient is thereafter plagued by recurrent ulceration and infection.
- Chyluria, a condition that develops when lymphatic vessels rupture into the urinary tract, may occur.

ETIOLOGY

Caused by one of three types of nematode parasite, all of which are transmitted to humans by *Culex* spp. mosquitoes.

- *W. bancrofti:* distributed in Africa, areas of Central and South America, the Pacific Islands, and the Caribbean Basin
- *B. malayi:* restricted to Southeast Asia
- *B. timori:* confined to the Indonesian archipelago

After bite of an infected mosquito:

- Filarial larvae move into lymphatic vessels and nodes, settling and maturing over 3 to 15 mo into adult male and female worms (Fig. 1-55).

- After fertilization, the female nematode produces large numbers of larvae or microfilariae that enter into the bloodstream via the lymphatics.
- Nocturnal periodicity, characteristic of *B. malayi*, is an increased presence of microfilariae in the circulation during the night.
- Microfilariae of *W. bancrofti* are maximal during late afternoon.
- Most microfilariae remain in the body as immature forms for 6 mo to 2 yr.
- Infected larvae are ingested by mosquitoes, then transmitted to humans, where the microfilariae mature into new adult worms.

Acute and chronic inflammatory and granulomatous changes in the lymphatic channels:

- Result from complex interaction of adult worms and host's immune systems
- Eventually lead to fibrosis and obstruction
- Most likely to develop into obstructive lymphatic disease with recurrent exposure over many years

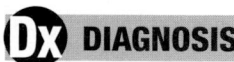
DIAGNOSIS

DIFFERENTIAL DIAGNOSIS

Elephantiasis is distinguished from other causes of chronic lymphedema, including Milroy's disease, postoperative scarring, and lymphedema of malignancy.

WORKUP

Diagnosis is suspected in individuals who have resided in endemic areas for at least 3 to 6 mo or more and complain of recurrent episodes of lymphangitis, lymphadenitis, scrotal edema, or thrombophlebitis, with or without fever.

LABORATORY TESTS

- Demonstration of microfilariae on a blood smear for definitive diagnosis
- For patients from southeastern Asia: blood sample drawn at night, especially between midnight and 2 A.M.
- Occasionally, microfilaremia in chylous urine or hydrocele fluid
- Prominent eosinophilia only during periods of acute lymphangitis or lymphadenitis
- Serologic tests for antibody, including enzyme-linked immunosorbent assay and indirect fluorescent antibody (often unable to distinguish among the various forms of filariasis or between acute and remote infection)
- Immunoassays (such as circulating filaria antigen [CFA]): more successful in antigen detection in patients who are microfilaremic than in those who are amicrofilaremic

IMAGING STUDIES

- Chest radiograph: reticular nodular infiltrates (tropical pulmonary eosinophilia syndrome)
- In men proven to be microfilaremic, scrotal ultrasonography to aid in the detection of adult worms
- Compared with adults, children with FS have more sleep disturbances, fewer tender points, and a better prognosis

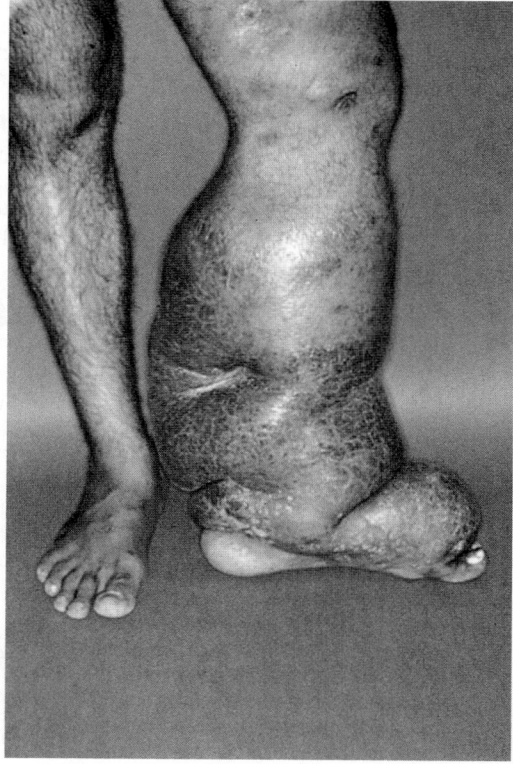

FIGURE 1-154 Filariasis that eventually leads to elephantiasis. Note massive swelling of the extremity. (From Goldstein B [ed]: *Practical dermatology,* ed 2, St Louis, 1997, Mosby.)

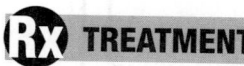

TREATMENT

NONPHARMACOLOGIC THERAPY

- Standard of care for elephantiasis:
  1. Elevation of the affected limb
  2. Use of elastic stockings
  3. Local foot care
- General wound care for chronic ulcers and prevention of secondary infection

ACUTE GENERAL Rx

- Diethylcarbamazine citrate (DEC) to reduce microfilaremia by 90%
  1. Effect on adult worms, especially those of the *Wuchereria* species, less certain
  2. Given in an oral dose of 6 mg/kg qd for 12 to 14 days
- Ivermectin alone or in combination with diethylcarbamazine citrate to decrease microfilaremia
- Both drugs are similar in efficacy and tolerability; advantage of ivermectin: administration in a single oral dose of 200 to 400 μg/kg. Side effects of these drugs include severe hypotensive reactions with dizziness, headache, fever, and vomiting, especially in patients with high microfilarial loads.
- World Health Organization (WHO) recommendation: DEC given as a single dose, alone or (preferably) in combination with ivermectin as treatment in endemic areas
- Antibacterial agents (a penicillin or cephalosporin) may be indicated to treat coexisting bacterial soft tissue infection (cellulitis or lymphangiitis), which frequently complicates filariasis of the lower extremities.

CHRONIC Rx

- Surgical drainage of hydroceles
- No satisfactory therapy for those patients with chyluria

DISPOSITION

Rarely fatal, but the psychologic impact of limb and scrotal deformities associated with elephantiasis is substantial.

REFERRAL

To a surgeon for management of hydrocele

PEARLS & CONSIDERATIONS

- Studies in endemic areas suggest that filarial-specific IgG1 is associated with amicrofilaremic states highest in children, regardless of sex.
- Levels of IgE and IgG4 increase with age and are associated with increased levels of microfilaremia.

COMMENTS

Individuals who intend to travel or reside in endemic areas should be advised to institute preventive measures such as the use of netting and insect repellents containing DEET, especially at night.

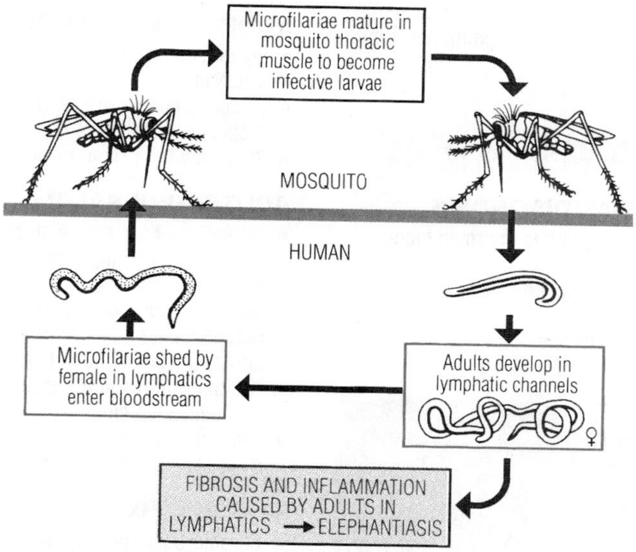

FIGURE 1-155 Lifecycle of lymphatic filariasis. (From Souhami RL, Moxham J: *Textbook of medicine,* ed 4, London, Churchill Livingstone, 2002.)

SUGGESTED READINGS

available at www.expertconsult.com

AUTHORS: **GLENN G. FORT, M.D., M.P.H.,** and **DENNIS J. MIKOLICH, M.D.**

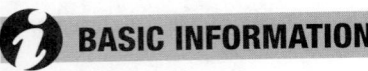

BASIC INFORMATION

DEFINITION

Folliculitis is inflammation of the hair follicle as a result of infection, physical injury, or chemical irritation.

SYNONYMS

Sycosis barbae

ICD-9CM CODES
704.8 Other specified diseases of hair and hair follicles

EPIDEMIOLOGY & DEMOGRAPHICS

PREVALENCE: Staphylococcal folliculitis is the most common form of infectious folliculitis; it occurs most commonly in persons with diabetes.
PREDOMINANT SEX: Sycosis barbae occurs most frequently in men who have commenced shaving.

PHYSICAL FINDINGS & CLINICAL PRESENTATION

- The lesions generally consist of painful yellow pustules surrounded by erythema; a central hair is present in the pustules.
- Patients with sycosis barbae may initially present with small follicular papules or pustules that increase in size with continued shaving; deep follicular pustules may occur surrounded by erythema and swelling; the upper lip is frequently involved (Fig. 1-156).
- "Hot tub" folliculitis occurs within 1 to 4 days after the use of a hot tub with poor chlorination. It is characterized by pustules with surrounding erythema generally affecting the torso, buttocks, and limbs.

ETIOLOGY

- *Staphylococcus* infection (e.g., sycosis barbae), *Pseudomonas aeruginosa* ("hot tub" folliculitis)
- Gram-negative folliculitis *(Klebsiella, Enterobacter, Proteus)* associated with antibiotic treatment of acne
- Chronic irritation of the hair follicle (use of cocoa butter or coconut oil, chronic irritation from workplace)
- Initial use of systemic corticosteroid therapy (steroid acne), eosinophilic folliculitis (AIDS patients), *Candida albicans* (immunocompromised patients)
- *Pityrosporum orbiculare*

DIAGNOSIS
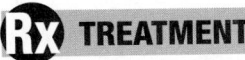

DIFFERENTIAL DIAGNOSIS

- Pseudofolliculitis barbae (ingrown hairs)
- Acne vulgaris
- Dermatophyte fungal infections
- Keratosis biliaris
- Cutaneous candidiasis

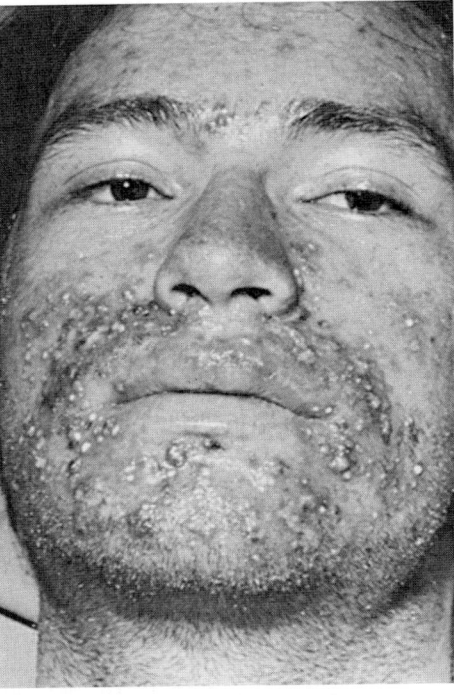

FIGURE 1-156 Folliculitis. Note the pustular eruption with small abscess formation in the hair-bearing areas of the face. General symptoms are usually absent. (From Mandell GL: *Mandell, Douglas, and Bennett's principles and practice of infectious diseases,* ed 6, New York, 2004, Churchill Livingstone.)

- Superficial fungal infections
- Miliaris

WORKUP

Physical examination and medical history (e.g., use of hot tub: "hot tub" folliculitis; adolescent patients who have started shaving: sycosis barbae; use of occlusive topical steroid therapy: *Staphylococcus* folliculitis).

LABORATORY TESTS

- Generally not necessary.
- Gram stain is useful to identify the infective organisms in infectious folliculitis and to differentiate infectious folliculitis from noninfectious.

TREATMENT
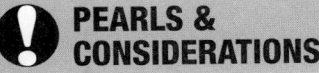

NONPHARMACOLOGIC THERAPY

- Prevention of chemical or mechanical skin irritation
- Glycemic control in diabetics
- Proper chlorination of hot tubs and spas
- Shaving with a clean razor

ACUTE GENERAL Rx

- Cleansing of the area with chlorhexidine and application of saline compresses to involved area
- Application of 2% mupirocin ointment or 1% Retapamulin ointment for bacterial folliculitis affecting a limited area (e.g., sycosis barbae)
- Treatment of severe cases of *Pseudomonas* folliculitis with ciprofloxacin
- Treatment of *S. aureus* folliculitis with dicloxacillin 250 mg qd for 10 days

CHRONIC Rx

- Chronic nasal or perineal *S. aureus* carriers with frequent folliculitis can be treated with rifampin 300 mg bid for 5 days.
- Mupirocin or Retapamulin ointment applied to nares bid is also effective for nasal carriers.

DISPOSITION

- Most cases of bacterial folliculitis resolve completely with proper treatment.
- Steroid folliculitis responds to discontinuation of steroids.

PEARLS & CONSIDERATIONS

COMMENTS

Patients should be instructed in good personal hygiene and avoidance of sharing razors, towels, and washcloths.

AUTHOR: **FRED F. FERRI, M.D.**

BASIC INFORMATION

DEFINITION

Food allergy is an adverse immune response to food proteins. Food allergies are categorized into IgE-mediated or non–IgE-mediated processes.

EPIDEMIOLOGY & DEMOGRAPHICS

INCIDENCE: Food allergies have a cumulative incidence of 6% to 8% for the first 3 yr of life.
PREVALENCE:
- Food allergies affect 5% to 7% of children and 1% to 2% of adults. 30% of food allergies are self-reported.
- Cow's milk allergy is found in 2.5% infants. IgE-mediated allergy occurs in 1% of children and non–IgE-mediated allergy occurs in 1.5 % of children.
- Egg allergy occurs in 1.5% to 3.2% children and 1% to 6% of infants have soy allergy.
- There is no predilection for race.

PREDOMINANT SEX: Males are more affected than females among children and among adults females are more frequently affected.
GENETICS: Children with parents or close relatives with allergies may have a tendency to become allergic to foods.

PHYSICAL FINDINGS & CLINICAL PRESENTATION

- IgE-mediated reactions: (immediate) pruritus, urticaria or angioedema, atopic dermatitis, GI symptoms, conjunctival injection, sneezing, nasal congestion, rhinorrhea, bronchospasm, and anaphylaxis
- Non–IgE-mediated reactions: food-induced enterocolitis, celiac disease, Crohn's disease, dermatitis herpetiformis, and pulmonary reactions such as Heiner syndrome
- Assess overall nutritional status, growth parameters, and signs of other allergic diseases such as atopic dermatitis, allergic rhinitis, or asthma
- Skin: eczema (dermatitis), angioedema, urticaria
- HEENT: nasal congestion, boggy mucous membranes, lymphoid tissue hypertrophy, postnasal mucous discharge, conjunctival injection
- Oropharyngeal: cobblestoning
- Lungs: stridor or wheezing
- Tachycardia or hypotension may indicate anaphylactic shock

ETIOLOGY

There is insufficient evidence to support the hypothesis that early exposure to food allergens may cause an immature immune system to produce IgE. Eight common foods have been found to be responsible for >90% of food allergies. Foods allergies with the greatest likelihood of spontaneous resolution are those involving milk, soy, egg, and wheat. Allergies least likely to resolve spontaneously are peanut, tree nuts, fish, and shellfish.

DIAGNOSIS

- Thorough history and physical exam should be performed.
- Differential diagnosis should include toxic reactions (food poisoning), psychologic reactions (strongly held beliefs), and carbohydrate malabsorption.
- Skin testing: simple, inexpensive, with excellent sensitivity and negative predictive value. A wheal of 3 mm or greater is considered a positive test. Skin testing if negative can reliably exclude food allergies, but as it has variable specificity and positive predictive value, it does not confirm food allergies when the test is positive. In such cases a food challenge is often necessary.
- In vitro testing: RAST testing: Historically it is less sensitive than skin testing, but sensitivity has improved with cut off points indicating a positive predictive value of 95% for allergies to eggs, milk, peanuts, wheat, and fish.
- Atopy patch test: used in conjunction with RAST and skin testing in multiallergic children to plan widen the elimination diet.
- Double-blind, placebo-controlled food challenges are the gold standard test for determining food allergies. These need to be done in a supervised and controlled setting.
- In summary, if the history and lab tests are suggestive of specific food allergy, that food should be eliminated from the diet. If reaction involves various food allergens then positive skin tests or specific IgE measurements should be confirmed by double-blind, placebo-controlled food challenge.

DIFFERENTIAL DIAGNOSIS

- Gastrointestinal disorders
- Irritable bowel syndrome
- Carcinoid syndrome
- Giardiasis
- Structural abnormalities like hiatal hernia, pyloric stenosis, Hirschsprung's disease, tracheoesophageal fistula
- Disaccharidase deficiencies: lactase, sucrase-isomaltase complex, glucose-galactose complex
- Pancreatic insufficiency: cystic fibrosis
- Gallbladder disease
- Peptic ulcer disease
- Malignancy
- Metabolic disorders
- Galactosemia
- Phenylketonuria
- Pharmacologic-related conditions
- Gustatory rhinitis
- Auriculotemporal syndrome (facial flush from tart food)

TREATMENT

NONPHARMACOLOGICAL THERAPY

- Elimination diet should be used.
- Formula-fed infants: brief trial of hydrolyzed milk formula as most children with milk allergy induced skin symptoms will respond to the change of formula. Nonresponders may require amino acid–based formula.
- In older children: elimination of one to two suspected foods are appropriate for 2 wk or longer and then reintroducing the foods to determine if symptoms recur.
- Epinephrine and antihistamines should be readily available during food challenges should anaphylactic reactions occur.

ACUTE GENERAL Rx

Antihistamines (both H_1 and H_2 antihistamines), albuterol if wheezing, epinephrine and glucocorticoids in patients with anaphylaxis.

NEW TREATMENTS FOR FOOD ALLERGIES

- Oral and sublingual immunotherapy may play a role in management of food allergies, but this is currently under investigation.
- Recombinant vaccines and other immunomodulatory strategies are under development, although monoclonal anti-IgE antibody has shown benefit in adults with peanut allergy.

PEARLS & CONSIDERATIONS

- Eczema that develops in first 6 to 12 mo of life is usually the first manifestation of atopy.
- Egg allergy or sensitization is the strongest recognized predictor of respiratory allergies in children and asthma in adults.
- Consultation with trained dietitian is critical to avoid potentially adverse nutritional consequences in children with multiple food allergies.
- Skin testing is the preferred method for identifying food-specific IgE. RAST is useful if there is chance of severe food reaction causing risk to the patient.
- American Academy of Pediatrics recommends avoiding influenza vaccine in patients with severe systemic allergic reactions to egg. Skin prick testing using influenza vaccine containing egg is recommended before vaccination in children with egg allergy and asthma. Skin prick testing not required before MMR vaccine in children with egg allergy.

COMMENTS

- Milk allergy usually resolves by age 5. Risk factors for persistence are early cutaneous manifestations following milk ingestion, development of other atopic conditions, and persistence of milk-specific high IgE titers. Soy milk is recommended for these children, keeping in mind that about 15% risk of these children can develop soy allergy.
- Egg allergy has been thought to resolve in 66% of children by 5 yr of age and in 75% of children by 7 yr of age.
- Wheat allergy found to resolve by 5 yr of age and soybean allergy by 2 yr of age.

PREVENTION

- There is conflicting evidence regarding the protective effect of breastfeeding on food allergies.
- There is no evidence to suggest that exclusive breastfeeding for 6 mo or more is superior to exclusive breastfeeding for 4 to 6 mo in terms of developing food allergies.
- In high-risk infants that are not exclusively breast fed, there is limited evidence to suggest that feeding with hydrolyzed formula compared to cow's milk formula reduces allergies.
- Currently, there is no evidence to support the use of prebiotics, probiotics, or synbiotics for the prevention of allergic diseases.
- No current evidence exists to support delaying the introduction of solid foods beyond 4 to 6 mo.

PATIENT/FAMILY EDUCATION

Information can be found on American Academy of Allergy Asthma and Immunology (www.aaaai.org), the Food Allergy and Anaphylaxis Network (www.foodallergy.org), and the Anaphylaxis Campaign (www.anaphylaxis.org.uk).

SUGGESTED READINGS
available at www.expertconsult.com

AUTHOR: **DIVJOT SOOCH, M.D.**

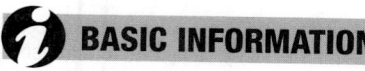

BASIC INFORMATION

DEFINITION

Food poisoning is an illness caused by ingestion of food contaminated by bacteria and/or bacterial toxins. Table 1-55 describes pathogenic mechanisms in bacterial foodborne disease.

SYNONYMS

Enterotoxin-poisoning
Epidemic vomiting disease

ICD-9CM CODES

See specific illness.

EPIDEMIOLOGY & DEMOGRAPHICS

INCIDENCE (IN U.S.):
- Estimated range of 6 to 8 million cases/yr
- Majority of identifiable causes are bacterial, although more than 250 known diseases can be transmitted through food

PEAK INCIDENCE: Varies with specific organism
- Summer: *Staphylococcus aureus, Salmonella, Shigella* spp.
- Summer and fall: *Clostridium botulinum, Vibrio parahaemolyticus*
- Spring and fall: *Campylobacter jejuni*
- Winter: *Clostridium perfringens, Yersinia enterocolitica*

PREDOMINANT AGE: Varies with specific agent
NEONATAL INFECTION: Rare but severe with *Shigella* and *Salmonella* spp.

PHYSICAL FINDINGS & CLINICAL PRESENTATION

- Any combination of GI symptoms and fever
- Specific organisms suspected on the basis of the incubation period and predominant symptoms, although a great deal of overlap exists
1. Short incubation period (1 to 6 hr): involve the ingestion of preformed toxin; noninvasive
   a. *S. aureus:* nausea, profuse vomiting, and abdominal cramps common; diarrhea possible, but fever uncommon; usually resolves within 24 hr; foods implicated in outbreaks include meats, mayonnaise, and cream pastries
   b. *B. cereus:* two forms, a short incubation (emetic) form (characterized by vomiting and abdominal cramps in virtually all patients, diarrhea in one third of patients, fever uncommon) and a long incubation (diarrheal) form; illness usually mild, resolves within 12 hr; unrefrigerated rice most often implicated as vehicle
2. Moderate incubation period (8 to 16 hr): involves the in vivo production of toxin; noninvasive
   a. *C. perfringens:* severe crampy abdominal pain and watery diarrhea common; fever and vomiting unlikely; symptoms usually resolving within 24 hr; outbreaks invariably related to cooked meat or poultry that is allowed to cool without refrigeration; most cases in the fall and winter months
   b. *B. cereus:* diarrheal (or long incubation) form most commonly beginning with diarrhea, abdominal cramps, and occasionally vomiting; fever uncommon; usually resolves within 24 hr; the responsible food is usually fried rice
3. Long incubation period (>16 hr): some toxin-mediated, some invasive
   a. Toxin-producing organisms include:
      (1) *C. botulinum:* should be considered when a diarrheal illness coincides with or precedes paralysis; severity of illness related to the quantity of toxin ingested; characteristic cranial nerve palsies progressing to a descending paralysis; fever usually absent; usually associated with home-canned foods
      (2) Enterotoxigenic *E. coli* (ETEC): most common cause of travelers' diarrhea; after 1- to 2-day incubation period, abdominal cramps and copious diarrhea occur; vomiting and fever uncommon; usually resolves after 3 to 4 days; vehicle usually unbottled water or contaminated salad or ice
      (3) Enterohemorrhagic *E. coli* (EHEC): can cause severe abdominal cramps and watery diarrhea, which may eventually become bloody; bacteria (strain 0157:H7) are noninvasive; no fever; illness may be complicated by hemolytic-uremic syndrome; associated with contaminated beef
      (4) *V. cholerae:* varies from a mild, self-limited illness to life-threatening cholera; diarrhea, nausea, and vomiting, abdominal cramps, and muscle cramps; no fever; severe cases may progress to shock and death within hours of onset; survivors usually have resolution of symptoms in 1 wk; U.S. cases are either imported or result from ingestion of imported food
   b. Invasive organisms include:
      (1) *Salmonella:* associated most often with nontyphoidal strains; incubation period generally 12 to 48 hr; nausea, vomiting, diarrhea, and abdominal cramps typical; fever possible; outbreaks of gastroenteritis related to contaminated poultry, meat, and dairy products
      (2) *Shigella:* asymptomatic infection possible, but some with fever and watery diarrhea that may progress to bloody diarrhea and dysentery; with mild illness, usually self-limited, resolves in a few days; with severe illness, may develop complications; transmission usually from person to person but can occur via contaminated food or water
      (3) *C. jejuni:* the most common foodborne bacterial pathogen; incubation period is about 1 day, then a prodrome of fever, headache, and myalgias; intestinal phase marked by diarrhea associated with fever, malaise, and abdominal pain; diarrhea mild to profuse and bloody; usually resolves in about 7 days, but relapse is possible; associated with undercooked meats and poultry, unpasteurized dairy products, and drinking from freshwater streams
      (4) *Y. enterocolitica* and *Y. pseudotuberculosis:* infrequent causes of enteritis in U.S.; children affected more often than adults; fever, diarrhea, and abdominal pain lasting 1 to 3 wk; some with mesenteric adenitis that mimics acute appendicitis; contaminated food or water is usually responsible
      (5) *V. parahaemolyticus:* In U.S., most outbreaks in coastal states or on

Preformed Toxin	Toxin Production in Vivo	Tissue Invasion	Toxin Production and/or Tissue Invasion
Staphylococcus aureus *Bacillus cereus* (short incubation) *Clostridium botulinum*	*Clostridium perfringens* *B. cereus* (long incubation) *C. botulinum* (infant botulism) Enterotoxigenic *Escherichia coli* *Vibrio cholerae* 01 or 0139 *V. cholerae* non-01 Shiga toxin–producing *E. coli*	*Campylobacter jejuni* *Salmonella* *Shigella* Invasive *E. coli*	*Vibrio parahaemolyticus* *Yersinia enterocolitica*

TABLE 1-55 Pathogenic Mechanisms in Bacterial Foodborne Disease

Mandell GL, Bennett JE, Dolin R: *Principles and practice of infectious diseases,* ed 6, Philadelphia, 2005, Elsevier.

F

Diseases and Disorders

I

cruise ships during the summer months; incubation period usually <1 day, followed by explosive watery diarrhea in the majority of cases; nausea, vomiting, abdominal cramps, and headache also common; fever less common; usually resolves by 1 wk; related to ingestion of seafood

(6) Enteroinvasive *E. coli* (EIEC): a rare cause of disease in the U.S.; high incidence of fever and bloody diarrhea; may resemble bacillary dysentery

(7) *V. vulnificus:* may cause serious, often fatal illness in persons with chronic liver disease; GI symptoms usually absent, but fever, chills, hypotension, and hemorrhagic skin lesions possible; patients with liver disease or at increased risk of developing liver disease should avoid eating raw oysters

ETIOLOGY

Classically categorized as either inflammatory (invasive) or noninflammatory:

- Noninflammatory: *B. cereus, S. aureus, C. botulinum, C. perfringens, V. cholerae,* enterotoxigenic *E. coli* (ETEC), and enterohemorrhagic *E. coli* (EHEC); toxin-producing organisms that are noninvasive; fecal leukocytes are not seen.
- Inflammatory: *Campylobacter,* enteroinvasive *E. coli* (EIEC), *Salmonella, Shigella, V. parahaemolyticus,* and *Yersinia;* cause disease by invasion of intestinal tissue; fecal leukocytes are seen.

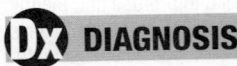 DIAGNOSIS

DIFFERENTIAL DIAGNOSIS

Gastroenteritis caused by viruses (Norwalk, Noro, or rotavirus), parasites *(Amoeba histolytica, Giardia lamblia),* or toxins (ciguatoxins, mushrooms, heavy metals)

LABORATORY TESTS

- Test stool for fecal leukocytes to help narrow the differential diagnosis:
  1. Send stool for culture and for ova and parasites.

2. Send stool for *C. difficile* toxin in patients with current or recent antibiotic use.
3. NOTE: Some pathogens are not identified on routine stool culture; laboratory should be advised if *Yersinia, C. botulinum, Vibrio,* or enterohemorrhagic *E. coli* (O157:H7) are suspected.
4. Finding *B. cereus, C. perfringens,* or *E. coli* in stool is of little value, because these may be part of the normal bowel flora.

- If botulism suspected, send food, serum, and stool for toxin assay.
- Blood cultures are needed for all febrile patients.

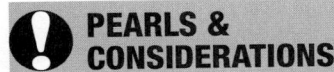 TREATMENT

NONPHARMACOLOGIC THERAPY

Adequate rehydration is the mainstay of therapy.

ACUTE GENERAL Rx

- Gastroenteritis caused by the following organisms requires no antimicrobial treatment: *B. cereus, S. aureus, C. perfringens, V. parahaemolyticus, Yersinia,* and enterohemorrhagic and enteroinvasive *E. coli.*
- The usual cause of traveler's diarrhea is enterotoxigenic *E. coli.* Although usually a self-limited illness, antibiotics can shorten the course.
  1. SMX/TMP one DS tab bid for 3 days
  2. Ciprofloxacin 500 mg PO bid for 3 days
- The mainstay of therapy for cholera is fluid replacement. Antibiotics should be given to decrease shedding and duration of illness.
  1. Doxycycline 100 mg PO bid for 3 days
  2. SMX/TMP one DS tab bid for 3 days
- Treatment is not indicated for *Salmonella* gastroenteritis. Patients who are at high risk of developing bacteremia may be treated for 48 to 72 hr (see "Salmonellosis").
- Although shigellosis tends to be a self-limited illness, antibiotics shorten the course of illness and may limit transmission of the illness (see "Shigellosis").

- Those with moderate or severe *Campylobacter* diarrhea may benefit from treatment.
  1. Erythromycin 500 mg PO qid for 5 days
  2. Ciprofloxacin 500 mg PO bid for 5 days
- *V. vulnificus* sepsis should be treated with:
  1. Doxycycline 100 mg IV bid for 2 wk
  2. Ceftazidime 2 g IV q8h for 2 wk
- For suspected botulism, antitoxin should be administered early (see "Botulism").

CHRONIC Rx

Patients with *Salmonella* infections may become carriers and may require treatment (see "Salmonellosis").

DISPOSITION

- Most infections are self-limited and do not require therapy.
- In immunocompromised host or patient with underlying disease, serious complications are possible.
- Postinfectious syndromes are important with some infections:
  1. Reiter's syndrome: *Salmonella, Shigella, Campylobacter, Yersinia* spp.; more common in genetically susceptible host (HLA-B27+)
  2. Guillain-Barré syndrome: *Campylobacter* spp.

REFERRAL

If more than a mild illness

❗ PEARLS & CONSIDERATIONS

COMMENTS

- Grossly underreported and undiagnosed
- All cases to be reported to the local health department

SUGGESTED READINGS

available at www.expertconsult.com

AUTHORS: **DENNIS J. MIKOLICH, M.D.,** and **GLENN G. FORT, M.D., M.P.H.**

BASIC INFORMATION

DEFINITION

Friedreich's ataxia is the most common neurodegenerative hereditary ataxic disorder, caused by degeneration of dorsal root ganglions, posterior columns, spinocerebellar and corticospinal tracts, and large sensory peripheral neurons.

ICD-9CM CODES
334.0 Friedreich's ataxia

EPIDEMIOLOGY & DEMOGRAPHICS

INCIDENCE (IN U.S.): Estimated at one in 30,000 whites
PEAK INCIDENCE: 8 to 15 yr
PREVALENCE (IN U.S.): Two to four per 100,000. Carrier rate 1:120 to 1:160. Lower prevalence in Asians and people of African descent.
PREDOMINANT SEX: Males and females affected equally
GENETICS: Autosomal recessive; 96% of affected patients are homozygous and 4% are compound heterozygous (two different mutations). Trinucleotide repeat expansion accounts for 94% to 98% of cases, whereas point mutations account for 2% to 6% of cases.

PHYSICAL FINDINGS & CLINICAL PRESENTATION

- Onset of progressive appendicular and gait ataxia, with absent muscle stretch reflexes in the lower extremities.
- With disease progression (within 5 yr): dysarthria, distal loss of position and vibration sense, pyramidal leg weakness, areflexia in all four limbs, and extensor plantar responses.
- Common findings: progressive scoliosis, distal atrophy, pes cavus, and cardiomyopathy (symmetric concentric hypertrophic form in most cases).
- Insulin-requiring diabetes mellitus may occur in 10% of patients, with glucose intolerance occurring in an additional 10% to 20%.

ETIOLOGY

- Genetic: frataxin gene is localized to the centromeric region of chromosome 9q13.
- Normal sequence has six to 27 repeats; abnormal sequence has 120 to 1700 GAA repeats.
- Frataxin deficiency leads to impaired mitochondrial iron homeostasis.

DIAGNOSIS

DIFFERENTIAL DIAGNOSIS

- Charcot-Marie-Tooth disease type 2
- Abetalipoproteinemia
- Severe vitamin E deficiency with malabsorption
- Early-onset cerebellar ataxia with retained reflexes

- Autosomal-dominant cerebellar ataxia (spinocerebellar ataxia)

WORKUP

- Diagnostic criteria include electrophysiologic evidence for a generalized axonal sensory or sensorimotor neuropathy.
- ECG may show widespread T-wave inversion and evidence of left ventricular hypertrophy. ECG abnormalities are present in 65% of patients.
- Sural nerve biopsy shows loss of large myelinated fibers.
- Specific gene testing for the expanded GAA trinucleotide repeat.

LABORATORY TESTS

- Electromyography or nerve conduction study
- ECG and echocardiogram
- Peripheral blood smear for acanthocytes
- Lipid profile
- Two-hour glucose tolerance test
- Vitamin E levels (if necessary)

IMAGING STUDIES

MRI of the spinal cord may demonstrate spinal cord atrophy with essentially normal cerebrum, brainstem, and cerebellum (Fig. 1-157).

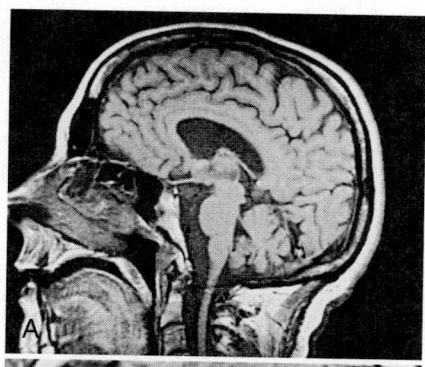
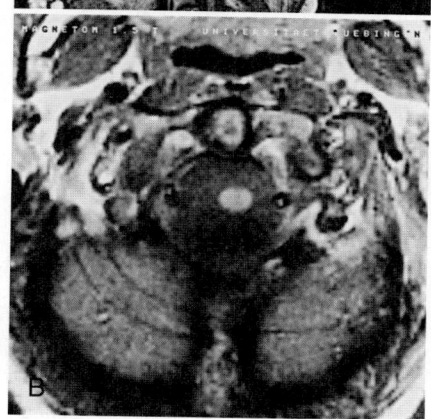

FIGURE 1-157 T1 MRI of the brain (midsagittal section) and spinal cord (axial slice at level of the dens) showing severe shrinkage of the cervical cord, but the cerebellum and brain stem are of normal size. (From Goetz CG: *Textbook of clinical neurology,* Philadelphia, 1999, WB Saunders.)

TREATMENT

NONPHARMACOLOGIC THERAPY

- Surgical correction of scoliosis and foot deformities in selected patients
- Prosthetic devices as required (e.g., ankle-foot orthosis for foot drop)
- Physical therapy
- Communication devices for patients with severe dysarthria

ACUTE GENERAL Rx

None established.
- An antioxidant, idebenone (short-chain analogue of coenzyme Q10), administered orally at 5 to 10 mg/kg/day with or without vitamin E may improve outcomes in patients with cardiomyopathy without clinical deterioration. This treatment is experimental, and research may be reviewed at http://www.idebenone.org.
- Further research with various antioxidants and iron chelators is ongoing. An open-label pilot study of antioxidants (coenzyme Q10, 400 mg/day, and vitamin E, 2100 U/day) suggested slowing in progression in generalized ataxia and kinetic function and significant improvement in cardiac function with unaltered deterioration in posture, gait, and hand dexterity.

CHRONIC Rx

Chronic management of congestive heart failure is required. Cardiac arrhythmias will warrant pacemaker implantation.

DISPOSITION

- Loss of ambulation typically occurs within 15 yr of symptom onset, and 95% are wheelchair bound by age 45 yr.
- Life expectancy is reduced, particularly if heart disease with or without diabetes mellitus is present.

REFERRAL

- If uncertain about diagnosis
- For genetic counseling (recommended if available)

PEARLS & CONSIDERATIONS

Friedreich's ataxia should be considered in all preadolescent and adolescent children presenting with progressive ataxia. Early recognition of cardiac failure and arrhythmias and institution of appropriate therapy helps prolong survival.

SUGGESTED READING
available at www.expertconsult.com

AUTHOR: **EROBOGHENE E. UBOGU, M.D.**

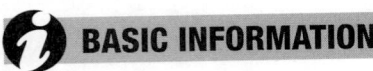

BASIC INFORMATION

DEFINITION

Frostbite represents tissue injury (or death) from freezing and vasoconstriction induced by severe environmental cold exposure.

SYNONYMS

Cold-induced tissue injury

ICD-9CM CODES
991.3 Frostbite

EPIDEMIOLOGY & DEMOGRAPHICS

- Environmental factors include wind chill factor, temperature, duration of exposure, altitude, and degree of wetness. Hands and feet account for 90% of injuries; earlobes, nose, and male genitalia are also more susceptible.
- Host factors include older age, psychiatric illness, neuroleptic and sedative drugs (especially alcohol), immobility, previous frostbite, skin damage, malnutrition, tobacco use, peripheral neuropathy, peripheral vascular disease, hypothyroidism, fatigue, and constricting clothing and footwear.

PHYSICAL FINDINGS & CLINICAL PRESENTATION

- Frostbite may be classified into grades I to IV of injury severity or, more practically, into *superficial* and *deep* groups. This can only be accurately determined after rewarming as initially most frostbite injuries appear similar.
- *Superficial* frostbite involves the skin and subcutaneous tissue. The frozen part is waxy, white (or mottled), and firm but soft and resilient below the surface when gently depressed. After rewarming, there is an initial hyperemia that may be followed by swelling and formation of superficial blisters with clear or milky fluid within 6 to 24 hr (Fig. 1-158). There is no ultimate tissue loss.
- *Deep* frostbite also involves muscles, nerves, tendons, or bones. The skin may be hard or wooden, without tissue resilience. Non-blanching cyanosis, hemorrhagic blisters (after 3 to 7 days), tissue necrosis, and gan-

grene may develop. Affected tissue has a poor prognosis and debridement or amputation is generally required.
- Patients initially feel numbness, prickling, and itching. More severe injury can produce paresthesias and stiffness, with burning or throbbing pain on thawing.

ETIOLOGY

Two mechanisms of tissue injury:
1. Cellular death occurring at time of exposure from intracellular water crystallization and temperature-induced protein changes.
2. Subsequent vascular impairment from vasoconstriction and endothelial injury result from tissue thawing and associated edema. On a cellular level, Prostaglandin F and Thromboxane AZ are involved in platelet aggregation and thrombosis leading to ischemia. Hemorrhage, necrosis, and gangrene may develop. Most frostbite injury occurs in this phase.

DIAGNOSIS

DIFFERENTIAL DIAGNOSIS

- Frostnip: transient tingling and numbness without associated permanent tissue damage
- Pernio (chilblains): self-limited, cold-induced vasculitis associated with purple plaques or nodules, often affecting dorsum of hands and feet; seen with prolonged cold exposure to above-freezing temperatures
- Cold immersion (trench foot): caused by ischemic injury resulting from sustained, severe vasoconstriction in appendages exposed to wet cold at temperatures above freezing

WORKUP

- Laboratory work is not indicated unless the patient has systemic hypothermia.
- No reliable predictors of tissue viability. Small series show MRI/MRA and triple-phase bone scanning (with technetium) to be the most promising modalities. (Some centers have reduced amputation rates by imaging within 24 hr of injury and giving thrombolytics to those with impaired blood flow.)

TREATMENT (3 PHASES)

1. FIELD MANAGEMENT

- Remove constricting or wet clothing. Gently insulate, splint, and elevate affected area.
- Avoid thawing if there is any risk of refreezing.
- Never rub or massage the affected area. Avoid dry heat (e.g., fires and heaters) and exercising the affected area.
- If hypothermic (core body temperature <32° C), initiate active core rewarming (e.g., pleural and peritoneal irrigation, hemodialysis or cardiopulmonary bypass) and adjunctive treatment with warmed, humidified oxygen, heated IV saline (45° C), and warming blankets before thawing frostbitten extremities.

2. REWARMING

- Rapid rewarming is the key objective.
- Immerse affected area in circulating warm water bath with a mild antibacterial agent (e.g., chlorhexidene or povidone-iodine) maintained at 40 to 42° C for 15 to 30 min. Repeat until capillary refill returns and tissue is supple and flushed. Active motion during rewarming is advisable; massage is not.
- IV narcotics for pain during thawing.
- Tetanus prophylaxis and topical antibiotics if potentially contaminated skin wound.
- Streptococcal prophylaxis for 48 to 72 hr with IV penicillin for severe cases.
- Thrombolytic therapy followed by short-term anticoagulation appears to considerably improve reperfusion and reduce subsequent digit amputations.
- Dextran, heparin, vasodilators, and hyperbaric oxygen are of potential but unproven benefit.

3. POST-THAW Rx

- Daily dressing changes with dry, sterile, noncompressive, and nonadherent dressings. Splint and elevate hands and feet to reduce edema and separate digits with cotton gauze. Avoid even slightest abrasion to limit risk of infection.
- Whirlpool hydrotherapy with warm water (38° C) and an antiseptic for 20 to 30 min bid to tid for several weeks.
- Debride broken clear vesicles and avoid disrupting intact blisters (especially hemorrhagic ones) unless they interfere with mobility.
- Topical aloe vera q6h and ibuprofen 400 to 600 mg tid for 1 wk may be beneficial as thromboxane inhibitors.
- Gentle, progressive physical therapy after edema resolves.
- Avoid all vasoconstrictors, including nicotine.

DISPOSITION

A majority of patients have long-term residual symptoms, including neuropathic pain, sensory deficits, hyperhidrosis, secondary Raynaud's disease, edema, hair or nail deformities, and (rarely) arthritis. Treatment with antiadrenergics or calcium channel blockers and careful protection from further cold exposure are often helpful.

REFERRAL

- Hospitalize for hypothermia or deep frostbite; a burn unit is best.
- Surgical decisions regarding amputation should be deferred until demarcation of viable tissue is clear (1 to 3 mo) unless refractory pain, sepsis, or gangrene occurs.

SUGGESTED READINGS
available at www.expertconsult.com

AUTHOR: **MICHAEL P. JOHNSON, M.D.**

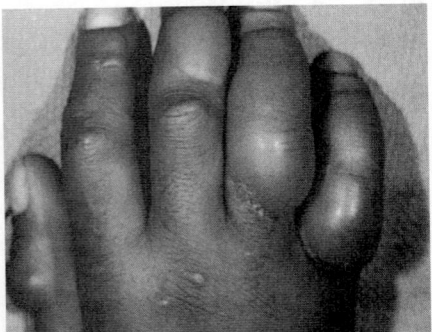

FIGURE 1-158 Large, clear frostbite blisters on the right hand. (From Rosen P [ed]: *Emergency medicine,* ed 4, St Louis, 1998, Mosby.)

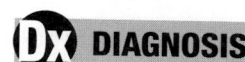

BASIC INFORMATION

DEFINITION

Frozen shoulder is a condition that describes a stiffened glenohumoral joint characterized by pain and restricted passive and active range of motion (Fig. 1-159). Its natural history occurs in three phases that usually includes full resolution of pain and return of function.

SYNONYMS

Adhesive capsulitis
Periarthritis
Pericapsulitis
Check-rein shoulder

ICD-9CM CODES
726.0 Adhesive shoulder capsulitis

EPIDEMIOLOGY & DEMOGRAPHICS

Its prevalence is 2% to 5%.
PREDOMINANT SEX: Females are affected more often than males
PREDOMINANT AGE: 40 to 60 yr

PHYSICAL FINDINGS & CLINICAL PRESENTATION

- Arm held protectively at the side with apprehension caused by pain
- Varying degrees of deltoid and spinatus atrophy
- Generalized shoulder tenderness
- Varying degrees of restricted active and passive shoulder motion. Internal and external rotation are most severely affected.

ETIOLOGY

- Primary or idiopathic and secondary as a result of an underlying disorder.
- Common predisposing factors include: (1) rotator cuff tendinopathy, (2) acute subacromial bursitis, (3) paralytic stroke, and (4) fractures about the humeral head and neck.
- Fig. 1-159 illustrates the sequence of events terminating in frozen shoulder.

DIAGNOSIS

DIFFERENTIAL DIAGNOSIS

- Secondary causes of shoulder stiffness (prolonged immobilization after trauma or surgery)
- Posterior shoulder dislocation
- Ruptured rotator cuff
- Glenohumeral osteoarthritis
- Rotator cuff tendonopathy
- Superior sulcus tumor
- Cervical disk disease
- Brachial neuritis

WORKUP

Laboratory studies are generally normal.

Radiographic evaluation may be normal, although nonspecific findings may also include calcification of the tendons of the rotator cuff.

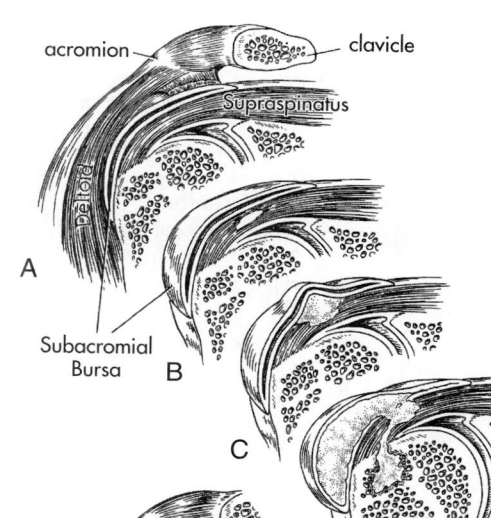

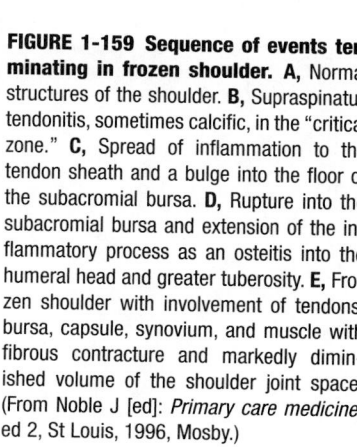

FIGURE 1-159 Sequence of events terminating in frozen shoulder. **A,** Normal structures of the shoulder. **B,** Supraspinatus tendonitis, sometimes calcific, in the "critical zone." **C,** Spread of inflammation to the tendon sheath and a bulge into the floor of the subacromial bursa. **D,** Rupture into the subacromial bursa and extension of the inflammatory process as an osteitis into the humeral head and greater tuberosity. **E,** Frozen shoulder with involvement of tendons, bursa, capsule, synovium, and muscle with fibrous contracture and markedly diminished volume of the shoulder joint space. (From Noble J [ed]: *Primary care medicine*, ed 2, St Louis, 1996, Mosby.)

TREATMENT

NONPHARMACOLOGIC THERAPY

Prevention is important. Shoulder motion should be maintained when the patient may be inactive as a result of illness or injury.

ACUTE GENERAL Rx

- Initial conservative therapy with heat, analgesics generally with nonsteroidal anti-inflammatory medications, and gentle stretching.
- A local steroid/lidocaine injection into the subacromial space (see "Epicondylitis" entry for guidelines to common steroid injections).
- Home exercise program including passive stretching and range of motion exercises. This should be performed regularly during the early stages of treatment. Physical therapy may be needed.
- Manipulation of shoulder under anesthesia (rarely needed).

DISPOSITION

- The initial stage of pain followed by stiffness may last several months; recovery phase may also last several months; complete recovery is typical.
- Recurrence in the same shoulder is rare, although the opposite limb may develop the same symptoms.
- Some patients have mild residual loss of movement but without any significant functional impairment.

REFERRAL

Orthopedic consultation in patients with resistant disease who fail to respond to conservative treatment after 6 mo.

PEARLS & CONSIDERATIONS

COMMENTS

- "Capsulitis" with an inflammatory infiltrate is not consistently found pathologically.
- Frozen shoulder is more common in patients with diabetes, thyroid disease, and recent cardiopulmonary conditions.
- Some cases have findings of reflex sympathetic dystrophy.

SUGGESTED READINGS

available at www.expertconsult.com

AUTHORS: **ANISHKA ROLLE, M.D.**, and **LONNIE R. MERCIER, M.D.**

F

Diseases and Disorders

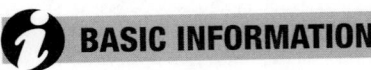

BASIC INFORMATION

DEFINITION

Galactorrhea can be defined as inappropriate lactation (in the absence of pregnancy or post-partum state) as a result of nonphysiologic augmentation of prolactin release.

ICD-9CM CODES
611.6 Galactorrhea

PHYSICAL FINDINGS & CLINICAL PRESENTATION

- Milky discharge from nipples usually occurring bilaterally
- Evidence of chest wall irritation from ill-fitting clothing, herpes zoster, or atopic dermatitis may be present
- Visual field defects may be present with prolactinomas
- Evidence of acromegaly, Cushing's disease, or hypothyroidism when galactorrhea is caused by these disorders

ETIOLOGY

- Medications (phenothiazines, metoclopramide, selective serotonin reuptake inhibitors, anxiolytics, buspirone, atenolol, valproic acid, conjugated estrogen and medroxyprogesterone, methyldopa, verapamil, H_2 receptor blockers, octreotide, danazol, tricyclic antidepressants, isoniazid, amphetamine, reserpine, opiates, sumatriptan, rimantadine, oral contraceptive formulations); after infancy, galactorrhea is usually medication induced
- Breast stimulation (prolonged suckling), sexual intercourse
- Pituitary tumors (prolactinomas, craniopharyngiomas)
- Chest wall irritation from ill-fitting clothing, herpes zoster, atopic dermatitis, burns
- Hypothyroidism (diminished feedback inhibition increases thyroid-releasing hormone [TRH], which increases prolactin)
- Increased stress, major trauma
- Chronic renal failure (decreased prolactin clearance)

- Cushing's disease
- Herbs (e.g., fennel, red clover, anise, red raspberry, marshmallow)
- Cannabis
- Spinal cord surgery or injury, or tumors
- Severe gastroesophageal reflux disease, esophagitis (stimulation of thoracic nerves by the cervical and thoracic ganglia)
- Breast surgery
- Idiopathic
- Neonatal ("witch's milk" produced by 2% to 5% of neonates because of precipitous drop in maternal estrogen and progesterone post-delivery)
- Lymphomas, Hodgkin's disease, bronchogenic carcinoma, renal adenocarcinomas
- Sarcoidosis and other infiltrative disorders
- Tuberculosis affecting pituitary gland
- Pituitary stalk resection
- Multiple sclerosis
- Empty sella syndrome
- Acromegaly

DIAGNOSIS

DIFFERENTIAL DIAGNOSIS

- Intraductal papilloma
- Breast cancer
- Paget's disease of breast
- Breast abscess

WORKUP

- Complete history focusing on menstrual irregularity, infertility, previous pregnancies, duration of galactorrhea, medications, visual complaints, fatigue. Age of onset is also significant (e.g., prolactinoma most common between ages 20 and 35 yr; neonatal galactorrhea is usually secondary to transplacental transfer of maternal estrogen)
- Physical examination: hirsutism, acne, obesity, visual field defects, goiter
- Breast examination for presence of nodules, evaluation of discharge (milky versus serosanguineous versus purulent)
- Laboratory testing and imaging studies (see "Laboratory Tests")

LABORATORY TESTS

- Prolactin level (elevated, often >200 ng/ml in prolactinoma)
- Human chorionic gonadotropin level (positive in pregnancy)
- TSH, TRH (both elevated in hypothyroidism)
- Blood urea nitrogen, creatinine (elevated in renal failure), glucose (elevated in Cushing's syndrome)
- Urinalysis (hematuria in renal cell carcinoma)
- Microscopic examination of nipple discharge (scant cellular material, numerous fat globules)

IMAGING STUDIES

- MRI of brain if prolactin level is elevated, amenorrhea is present, or visual field defects are detected on physical examination.
- High-resolution CT of brain with special coronal cuts through the pituitary region may be helpful in patients with contraindications to MRI; however, it may miss small lesions.

TREATMENT

- Discontinuation of potential offending agents.
- Avoidance of excessive breast stimulation.
- Galactorrhea resulting from prolactinoma can be managed medically or with careful surveillance depending on size and growth of tumor, associated symptoms, and prolactin level. Surgical treatment of prolactinomas is usually reserved for medication failures. Please refer to "Prolactinoma" in Section I for additional information.

REFERRAL

Endocrine and surgical consultation if prolactinoma is detected

SUGGESTED READINGS
available at www.expertconsult.com

AUTHOR: **FRED F. FERRI, M.D.**

BASIC INFORMATION

DEFINITION

A fluid-filled sac (cyst) overlying a tendon sheath or joint

SYNONYMS Ganglion

ICD-9CM CODES
727.43 Ganglion

EPIDEMIOLOGY & DEMOGRAPHICS

- Ganglia are more common in women than men (3:1)
- Can occur at any age, but usually between second and fourth decades of life
- Most common soft tissue tumor of the hand and wrist

PHYSICAL FINDINGS & CLINICAL PRESENTATION

- Most ganglia occur on the dorsum of the wrist (50% to 70%) (Fig. 1-160).
- The volar wrist (18% to 20%) is the next most common site.
- Can also involve the proximal digital flexor tendons and the distal interphalangeal joints.
- Left and right hands are equally affected.
- Ganglia are usually solitary, firm, smooth, round, and fluctuant.
- Pain from mass effect or compression against nearby structure may be present (e.g., median nerve and radial nerve).
- Hand numbness may be present.
- Patient may have hand muscle weakness.
- Ganglia usually develop over a period of months but may arise suddenly.

ETIOLOGY

Ganglia are believed to derive from synovial herniation or expansion from the joint capsule or tendon sheath. Repetitive movement as an eti-

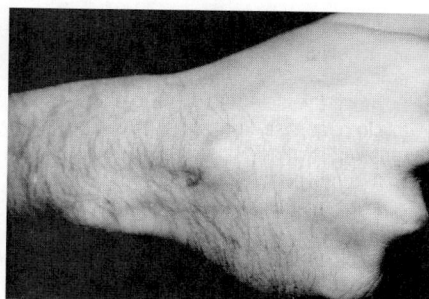

FIGURE 1-160 Round and firm ganglion cyst bulging from the dorsal aspect of the hand. (From Kelly WN: *Textbook of rheumatology,* ed 5, Philadelphia, 1997, WB Saunders.)

ology is uncertain, although it may cause enlargement of the lesion or worsen symptoms.

DIAGNOSIS

Direct inspection and localization of the cyst often is enough to make the diagnosis of ganglia. Transillumination is an easy method of differentiating ganglia from solid tumors; ganglia transilluminate while solid tumors do not.

DIFFERENTIAL DIAGNOSIS

- Lipoma
- Fibroma
- Epidermoid inclusion cyst
- Osteochondroma
- Hemangioma
- Infection (tuberculosis, fungi, and secondary syphilis)
- Gout
- Rheumatoid nodule
- Radial artery aneurysm

WORKUP

The workup of ganglia usually consists of history, physical examination, and x-ray imaging.

LABORATORY TESTS

Blood tests are not specific in the diagnosis of ganglia.

IMAGING STUDIES

- Radiographs of the hand and wrist are taken to rule out other bone or joint abnormalities.
- Ultrasound studies are helpful in the diagnosis of ganglia by demonstrating smooth cystic walls that may be septated.
- CT scan can be done if the ultrasound is equivocal.
- MRI helps differentiate malignant bone lesions from cystic structures.
- Arthrography may demonstrate a communication between the joint and ganglia (not commonly done).

TREATMENT

Expectant treatment is appropriate if the mass is not painful or interfering with motor function.

NONPHARMACOLOGIC THERAPY

- Attempts to rupture the cyst by sharp blows with a book or with finger compression are not recommended.
- Aspiration, heat, and sclerotherapy have been tried but have met with high recurrence rates (60%).

ACUTE GENERAL Rx

- Aspiration at the base with a large-bore needle (18-gauge) followed by injection of 20 to 40 mg of triamcinolone acetonide can be tried.
- This may be repeated if the ganglia recurs (35% to 40%).

CHRONIC Rx

Total ganglionectomy and repair of the defect after tracing its connection to the tendon sheath is effective and the surgical procedure of choice.

DISPOSITION

- Ganglia spontaneously resolve in approximately 40% to 50% of cases.
- Aspiration with steroid injection is successful in approximately 65% of cases.
- Surgery provides cure in 85% to 95% of the cases.
- Complications of ganglia include:
  1. Carpal tunnel syndrome with pain and muscle atrophy
  2. Radial nerve impingement
  3. Radial artery compression
- Complications of ganglion surgery include:
  1. Infection
  2. Recurrence (5% to 15%), usually from inadequate excision
  3. Reflex sympathetic dystrophy
  4. Scar formation

REFERRAL

It is best to refer patients with symptomatic ganglia to a hand surgeon.

PEARLS & CONSIDERATIONS

- Dorsal ganglia usually originate from the scapholunate ligament.
- Volar ganglia typically originate between the tendons of the flexor carpi radialis and brachioradialis.

COMMENTS

A ganglion's synovial membrane maintains its secretory function. Aspiration of ganglia often demonstrates a viscous, mucinous, clear fluid containing albumin, globulin, and hyaluronic acid.

EVIDENCE

available at www.expertconsult.com

SUGGESTED READINGS
available at www.expertconsult.com

AUTHORS: **RYAN W. ZUZEK, M.D.,** and **IMMAD SADIQ, M.D.**

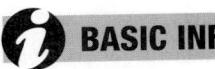

BASIC INFORMATION

DEFINITION

Gardner's syndrome is a variant of familial adenomatous polyposis (FAP), with prominent extraintestinal manifestations. It is a highly penetrant autosomal-dominant condition characterized by the following:
- Adenomatous intestinal polyps
- Soft tissue tumors
- Osteomas

SYNONYMS

Familial adenomatous polyposis

ICD-9CM CODES

211.3 Familial adenomatous polyposis

EPIDEMIOLOGY & DEMOGRAPHICS

- FAP occurs in approximately 1 in 10,000 births.
- FAP accounts for about 1% of all colorectal cancers.
- Individuals develop hundreds to thousands of adenomatous colorectal polyps.
- Polyps usually present in adolescence.
- 100% lifetime risk for colorectal cancer; most diagnosed by 40 yr of age.
- Gastric, duodenal, periampullary, and small bowel polyps occur but have lower malignant potential.
- Increased risk for other tumors: desmoid (15%), duodenal/periampullary (7%), thyroid (2%), brain (1%), childhood hepatoblastoma (1%), nasopharyngeal angiofibroma, pancreatic (2%), adrenal, adenoma, and gastric (1%).

PHYSICAL FINDINGS & CLINICAL PRESENTATION

Phenotypic variability is seen in individuals and families with the same mutation. Soft tissue and bone abnormalities may precede intestinal disease.
- Congenital hypertrophy of the retinal pigment epithelium (CHRPE): benign fundus lesions, usually present at birth
- Dental abnormalities: supernumerary or unerupted teeth
- Soft tissue lesions: epidermal or sebaceous cysts, fibromas, lipomas, desmoid tumors (benign, locally invasive, connective tissue tumors)
- Osteomas (benign bone growths): skull, mandible, long bone
- Anemia, occult blood in stool, bowel obstruction, weight loss

ETIOLOGY

- Caused by mutations of the tumor suppressor gene adenomatous polyposis coli (APC) on chromosome 5q21-q22; more than 700 diseases causing mutations identified. The site of the mutation may explain the prominent extraintestinal lesions found in Gardner's syndrome.
- De novo mutations are responsible for approximately 20% of FAP cases. A subset of these patients have somatic cell mosaicism, which is seen when a new mutation occurs in the APC gene post-fertilization and is present in only a subset of cell types or tissues.

DIAGNOSIS

In individuals with a family history, more than 100 adenomatous colorectal polyps, CHRPE lesions, or genetic testing confirms diagnosis. In those without a family history, more than 100 adenomatous colorectal polyps suggest the diagnosis and genetic testing confirms it.

DIFFERENTIAL DIAGNOSIS

- Turcot's syndrome
- Attenuated familial adenomatous polyposis
- MYH-associated polyposis
- Peutz-Jeghers syndrome
- Juvenile polyposis syndrome
- Hereditary mixed polyposis syndrome
- Hyperplastic polyposis

WORKUP

History, physical examination, laboratory tests, imaging studies

DIAGNOSTIC SCREENING OPTIONS

GENETIC TESTING

- Should be offered to first-degree relatives of affected individuals (with an identified mutation) at age 10 to 12 yr and clinically suspected individuals.
- Able to identify a mutation in approximately 80% of families. To ensure that the family has a detectable mutation, test an affected family member first.
- If positive in the affected individual, the test can differentiate with 100% accuracy affected and unaffected family members. If negative in the affected individual, screening family members will not be useful in determining disease status.
- If no known family history exists, screening the clinically suspected individual is reasonable. A positive test rules in FAP but a negative test does not rule it out.
- Numerous testing techniques available; may require multiple tests to identify the mutation.

NOTE: Genetic counseling should be performed and written informed consent obtained before testing.

SIGMOIDOSCOPY

- Individuals with a positive genetic test: annual flexible sigmoidoscopy beginning at 10 to 12 yr of age.
- Untested at-risk family members or patients from families with an unidentified APC mutation: annual flexible sigmoidoscopy beginning at 10 to 12 yr until 25 yr of age, then decreasing frequency until age 50 yr, when age-appropriate guidelines may be followed.
- Once adenomatous polyps are detected, patients should undergo colonoscopy and evaluation for colectomy.
- Negative genetic test in patients from families with an identified mutation: average risk screening.

CHRPE: Lesions occur in approximately 80% of families and are a reliable indicator of affected status in these families.

TREATMENT

- Prophylactic colectomy or proctocolectomy: timing determined by polyp number, size, and degree of dysplasia.
- Consider celecoxib therapy to reduce polyposis.
- Screening of remaining GI tract and screening for extraintestinal manifestations must continue after colectomy.
  - Annual physical examination: history, examination (including thyroid), and blood tests
  - Upper endoscopy to screen for duodenal polyps: baseline at age 20 yr and repeated every 1 to 5 yr based on findings
  - Some recommend annual thyroid ultrasound
  - Other possible cancer sites imaged if symptoms occur or if these cancers have occurred in relatives
- Treat soft tissue lesions and osteomas for symptoms or cosmetic concerns. Treat desmoid tumors if they pose a risk to adjacent structures.

DISPOSITION

- 100% chance of colorectal cancer in untreated individuals. Many other neoplasms occur at higher rates.
- Metastatic colorectal cancer is the leading cause of death (58%), followed by desmoid tumors (11%) and duodenal/periampullary adenocarcinoma (8%).

REFERRAL

- Patients should be managed at centers with expertise in FAP, including a gastroenterologist, medical geneticist, and surgeon.
- Genetic counseling and testing sites can be found at GeneTests (www.ncbi.nlm.nih.gov/sites/GeneTests).

PEARLS & CONSIDERATIONS

- Management should be individualized based on genotype, phenotype, and individual preferences.
- Sulindac (nonselective NSAID) and celecoxib (cyclooxygenase-2 inhibitor) cause polyp regression in individuals with FAP. Celecoxib is FDA approved for this indication. Cancer risk remains; neither replaces colon resection for cancer prevention.
- Desmoid tumors frequently occur in the abdomen and are difficult to treat with high rates of recurrence. Growth is stimulated by surgery and pregnancy.
- Screen children of affected parents yearly (from infancy to age 10 yr) with alpha-fetoprotein level and liver ultrasound to rule out hepatoblastoma.
- Preimplantation genetic diagnosis and prenatal diagnosis are available.

SUGGESTED READINGS

available at www.expertconsult.com

AUTHOR: **SUDEEP KAUR AULAKH, M.D.**

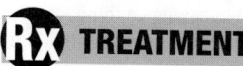

BASIC INFORMATION

DEFINITION

Gastric cancer is an adenocarcinoma arising from the stomach.

SYNONYMS

Stomach cancer
Linitis plastica

ICD-9CM CODES
451 Malignant neoplasm of stomach

EPIDEMIOLOGY & DEMOGRAPHICS

- Annual incidence of gastric cancer in the U.S. is seven cases per 100,000 persons. The incidence is much higher in Japan, with rates as high as 80 cases per 100,000 persons.
- Most gastric cancers arise in the antrum (35%).
- The incidence of distal stomach tumors has greatly declined, whereas that of proximal tumors of the cardia and fundus is on the rise.
- Gastric cancer occurs most commonly in male patients >65 yr (70% of patients are >50 yr).
- Incidence of gastric cancer has been declining over the past 30 yr.
- Male/female ratio is 3:2.
- Familial diffuse gastric cancer is a disease with autosomal-dominant inheritance in which gastric cancer develops at a young age. Germline truncating mutations in the E-cadherin gene (CDH1) are found in these families.

PHYSICAL FINDINGS & CLINICAL PRESENTATION

- Medical history may reveal complaints of postprandial fullness with significant weight loss (70% to 80%), nausea/emesis (20% to 40%), dysphagia (20%), and dyspepsia, usually unrelieved by antacids; epigastric discomfort, usually lessened by fasting and exacerbated by food intake, is also common.
- Epigastric or abdominal mass (30% to 50%), epigastric pain.
- Skin pallor from anemia.
- Hard, nodular liver: generally indicates metastatic disease to the liver.
- Hemoccult-positive stools.
- Ascites, lymphadenopathy, or pleural effusions: may indicate metastasis.

ETIOLOGY

Risk factors:
- Chronic *Helicobacter pylori* gastritis. Gastric cancer develops in persons infected with *H. pylori* but not in uninfected persons. Those with histologic findings of severe gastric atrophy, corpus-predominant gastritis, or intestinal metaplasia are at increased risk. Persons with *H. pylori* infection and duodenal ulcer are not at risk, whereas those with gastric ulcers, nonulcer dyspepsia, and gastric hyperplastic polyps are. Eradication of *H. pylori* reduces gastric cancer risk.
- Tobacco abuse, alcohol consumption.
- Food additives (nitrosamines), smoked foods, occupational exposure to heavy metals, rubber, asbestos.

- Chronic atrophic gastritis with intestinal metaplasia, hypertrophic gastritis, and pernicious anemia.

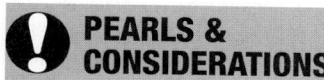

DIAGNOSIS

DIFFERENTIAL DIAGNOSIS

- Gastric lymphoma (5% of gastric malignancies)
- Hypertrophic gastritis
- Peptic ulcer
- Reflux esophagitis

WORKUP

Upper endoscopy with biopsy will confirm diagnosis. Endoscopic ultrasonography in combination with CT scanning and operative lymph node dissection can be used in staging of the tumor. Table 1-56 describes staging systems for gastric carcinoma.

LABORATORY TESTS

- Microcytic anemia
- Hemoccult-positive stools
- Hypoalbuminemia
- Abnormal liver enzymes in patients with metastasis to the liver
- Mutation-specific predictive genetic testing by polymerase chain reaction amplification followed by restriction: enzyme digestion and DNA sequencing for truncating mutations in CDH1 is recommended in families of patients with familiar diffuse cancer because gastric cancer develops in three of every four carriers of a mutant CDH1 gene.

IMAGING STUDIES

Abdominal CT scan to evaluate for metastasis (70% accurate for regional node metastases)

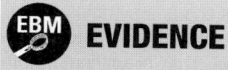

TREATMENT

ACUTE GENERAL Rx

- Gastrectomy with regional lymphadenectomy is performed in patients with curative potential (<30% of patients at time of diagnosis). In patients with operable gastric cancer, a perioperative regimen of epirubicin, cisplatin, and infused fluorouracil (ECF) decreases tumor size and stage and significantly improves progression-free and overall survival. Postoperative adjuvant chemoradiation therapy using 5-fluorouracil and leucovorin is now the standard of care for resected patients able to tolerate such treatment. Postoperative chemotherapy and radiotherapy, compared with surgical resection alone, can extend the survival rate of patients with gastric cancer in those who are able to complete adjuvant therapy.
- When surgical cure is not possible, palliative resection may prolong duration and quality of life.
- Chemotherapy (FAM: 5-fluorouracil, Adriamycin, and mitomycin C) may provide some palliation; however, it generally does not prolong survival. Chemotherapy with docetaxel, cisplatin, and 5-fluorouracil can be used for chemotherapy-naive patients with metastatic or locally recurrent gastric cancer.

DISPOSITION

- 5-yr survival rate of gastric carcinoma is 12% overall.
- 5-yr survival for early gastric cancers (usually detected incidentally with endoscopy in populations where screening is recommended) is >35%.

PEARLS & CONSIDERATIONS

COMMENTS

- Gastrectomy patients will need vitamin B_{12} replacement. They are also at risk for dumping syndrome and should be advised to ingest frequent, small meals.
- Prophylactic gastrectomy should be considered in young, asymptomatic carriers of germ-line truncating *CDH1* mutations who belong to families with highly penetrant heredity diffuse gastric cancer.

EBM EVIDENCE

available at www.expertconsult.com

SUGGESTED READING

available at www.expertconsult.com

AUTHOR: **FRED F. FERRI, M.D.**

TABLE 1-56 Staging Systems for Gastric Carcinoma*

Modified Astler-Coller	TNM	Characteristics
A	TisN0	Nodes negative; lesion limited to mucosa
B1	T1–2N0	Nodes negative; extension of lesion beyond mucosa but still within gastric wall
B2	T3N0	Nodes negative; extension beyond the entire wall (including serosa if present) without adherence to or invasion of surrounding organs or structures
B3	T4N0	Nodes negative; beyond wall with adherence to or invasion of surrounding organs or structures
C1	Tis–2N1–3	Nodes positive; lesion limited to wall
C2	T3N1–3	Nodes positive; extension of lesion through the entire wall (including serosa)
C3	T4N1–3	Nodes positive; beyond wall with adherence to or invasion of surrounding organs or structures

*Comparison of TNM system with a modification of the Astler-Coller rectal system by Gunderson and Sosin.
Abeloff MD: *Clinical oncology,* ed 3, Philadelphia, 2004, Elsevier.

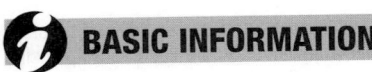

DEFINITION

Histologically, gastritis refers to inflammation in the stomach. Endoscopically, gastritis refers to a number of abnormal features such as erythema, erosions, and subepithelial hemorrhages. Gastritis can also be subdivided into erosive, nonerosive, and specific types of gastritis with distinctive features both endoscopically and histologically.

SYNONYMS

Erosive gastritis
Hemorrhagic gastritis
Helicobacter pylori gastritis

ICD-9CM CODES
535.5 Gastritis (unless otherwise specified)
535.0 Gastritis, acute
535.3 Alcoholic gastritis
535.1 Atrophic (chronic) gastritis
535.4 Erosive gastritis
535.2 Hypertrophic gastritis

EPIDEMIOLOGY & DEMOGRAPHICS

- Erosive and hemorrhagic gastritis is most commonly seen in patients taking nonsteroidal anti-inflammatory drugs (NSAIDs), alcoholics, and critically ill patients (usually on ventilator support).
- *H. pylori* infection with gastritis is believed to be present in 30% to 50% of the population; however, the majority are asymptomatic.
- The prevalence of *H. pylori* infection increases with age from <10% in whites <40 yr to >50% in patients >50 yr.

PHYSICAL FINDINGS & CLINICAL PRESENTATION

- Patients with gastritis generally present with nonspecific clinical signs and symptoms (e.g., epigastric pain, abdominal tenderness, bloating, anorexia, nausea [with or without vomiting]). Symptoms may be aggravated by eating.
- Epigastric tenderness in acute alcoholic gastritis (may be absent in chronic gastritis).
- Foul-smelling breath.
- Hematemesis ("coffee grounds" emesis).

ETIOLOGY

- Alcohol, NSAIDs, stress (critically ill patients usually on mechanical respiration), hepatic or renal failure, multiorgan failure
- Infection (bacterial, viral)
- Bile reflux, pancreatic enzyme reflux
- Gastric mucosal atrophy, portal hypertension gastropathy
- Irradiation

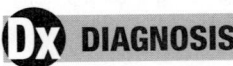 **DIAGNOSIS**

DIFFERENTIAL DIAGNOSIS

- Peptic ulcer disease
- Gastroesophageal reflux disease
- Nonulcer dyspepsia
- Gastric lymphoma or carcinoma
- Pancreatitis
- Gastroparesis

WORKUP

Diagnostic workup includes a comprehensive history and endoscopy with biopsy.

LABORATORY TESTS

- *H. pylori* testing by urea breath test, stool antigen test (*H. pylori* stool antigen), endoscopic biopsy, or specific antibody test is recommended.
  1. The urea breath test documents active infection (sensitivity and specificity >90%). A new card test for ^{14}C urea has recently been developed, providing a testing option in primary care settings. It uses a flat breath card read by a small analyzer.
  2. The stool antigen test is an enzymatic immunoassay (ELISA) that identifies *H. pylori* antigen in a stool specimen with a polyclonal anti–*H. pylori* antibody. It is as accurate as the urea breath test for diagnosis of active infection and follow-up evaluation of patients treated for *H. pylori*. A negative result on the stool antigen test 8 wk after completion of therapy identifies patients in whom eradication of *H. pylori* was unsuccessful.
  3. Histologic evaluation of endoscopic biopsy samples is considered by many the gold standard for accurate diagnosis of *H. pylori* infection. However, detection of *H. pylori* depends on the site and number of biopsy samples, the method of staining, and experience of the pathologist.
  4. Serologic testing for antibodies to *H. pylori* is easy and inexpensive; however, the presence of antibodies demonstrates previous but not necessarily current infection. Antibodies to *H. pylori* can remain elevated for months to years after infection has cleared; therefore antibody levels must be interpreted in light of patient's symptoms and other test results (e.g., peptic ulcer disease (PUD) seen on upper gastrointestinal series).
- Vitamin B_{12} level in patients with atrophic gastritis.
- Hematocrit (low if significant bleeding has occurred).

Rx TREATMENT

NONPHARMACOLOGIC THERAPY

- Avoidance of mucosal irritants such as alcohol and NSAIDs
- Lifestyle modifications with avoidance of tobacco and foods that trigger symptoms

ACUTE GENERAL Rx

Eradication of *H. pylori,* when present, can be accomplished with various regimens:
1. Proton pump inhibitor (PPI) bid *plus* amoxicillin 500 mg bid *plus* metronidazole 500 mg for 10 days.
2. PPI bid *plus* clarithromycin 500 mg bid *and* metronidazole 500 mg bid for 10 days. This regimen is useful in those with penicillin allergy.
3. A 1-day quadruple-therapy regimen may be as effective as a 7-day triple-therapy regimen. The 1-day quadruple-therapy regimen consists of two tablets of 262 mg bismuth subsalicylate qd, one 500-mg metronidazole tablet qd, 2 g of amoxicillin suspension qd, and two capsules of 30 mg of lansoprazole.
4. A 5-day treatment with three antibiotics (amoxicillin 1 g bid, clarithromycin 250 mg bid, and metronidazole 400 mg bid) plus either lansoprazole 30 mg bid or ranitidine 300 mg bid is an efficacious, cost-saving option for patients >55 yr with no history of PUD.
5. A combination of levofloxacin 250 mg bid, amoxicillin 1000 mg bid, and a PPI bid for 10 to 14 days can be used as salvage therapy after unsuccessful attempts to eradicate *H. pylori* using other regimens.
   - A 10-day sequential therapy has been reported to be superior to standard triple therapy for eradication of *H. pylori*. It consists of 5 days of treatment with a PPI and one antibiotic (usually amoxicillin) followed by 5-day treatment with the PPI and two other antibiotics (usually clarithromycin and metronidazole).
6. Prophylaxis and treatment of stress gastritis with sucralfate suspension 1 g orally q4-6h, H_2-receptor antagonists, or PPIs in patients on ventilator support.

CHRONIC Rx

- Omeprazole 20 mg/qd in patients receiving long-term NSAIDs
- Avoidance of alcohol, tobacco, and prolonged NSAID or corticosteroid use

DISPOSITION

- Undetectable stool antigen 4 wk after therapy accurately confirms cure of *H. pylori* infection in initially seropositive healthy subjects with reasonable sensitivity.
- Surveillance gastroscopy in patients with atrophic gastritis (increased risk of gastric cancer).

AUTHOR: **FRED F. FERRI, M.D.**

ⓘ BASIC INFORMATION

DEFINITION

Gastroesophageal reflux disease (GERD) is a motility disorder characterized primarily by heartburn and caused by the reflux of gastric contents into the esophagus. A current definition is a condition that develops when the reflux of stomach contents causes at least two heartburn episodes per week and/or complications.

SYNONYMS

Peptic esophagitis
Reflux esophagitis
GERD

ICD-9CM CODES
530.81 Gastroesophageal reflux disease
530.1 Esophagitis
787.1 Heartburn

EPIDEMIOLOGY & DEMOGRAPHICS

- GERD is one of the most prevalent gastrointestinal disorders. It is the most common GI diagnosis recorded during visits to outpatient clinics. From 14% to 20% of adults are affected.
- Nearly 7% of persons in the U.S. have heartburn daily, 20% have it monthly, and 60% have it intermittently. Incidence in pregnant women exceeds 80%.
- Nearly 20% of adults use antacids or over-the-counter H_2 blockers at least once a week for relief of heartburn.

PHYSICAL FINDINGS & CLINICAL PRESENTATION

- Physical examination: generally unremarkable

- Clinical signs and symptoms: heartburn, dysphagia, sour taste, regurgitation of gastric contents into the mouth
- Chronic cough and bronchospasm
- Chest pain, laryngitis, early satiety, abdominal fullness, and bloating with belching
- Dental erosions in children

ETIOLOGY

- Incompetent lower esophageal sphincter (LES) (see Fig. 1-161)
- Medications that lower LES pressure (calcium channel blockers, alpha-adrenergic antagonists, nitrates, theophylline, anticholinergics, sedatives, prostaglandins)
- Foods that lower LES pressure (chocolate, yellow onions, peppermint)
- Tobacco abuse, alcohol, coffee
- Pregnancy
- Gastric acid hypersecretion
- Hiatal hernia (controversial) present in >70% of patients with GERD; however, most patients with hiatal hernia are asymptomatic
- Obesity is associated with a statistically significant increase in the risk for GERD symptoms, erosive esophagitis, and esophageal carcinoma

ⒹⓍ DIAGNOSIS

DIFFERENTIAL DIAGNOSIS

- Peptic ulcer disease
- Unstable angina
- Esophagitis (from infections such as herpes, *Candida*), medication induced (doxycycline, potassium chloride)
- Esophageal spasm (nutcracker esophagus)
- Cancer of esophagus

WORKUP

- Aimed at eliminating the conditions noted in the differential diagnosis and documenting the type and extent of tissue damage. Generally, when symptoms of GERD are typical and the patient responds to therapy, there is no need for further diagnostic tests to verify the diagnosis.
- Upper GI endoscopy is useful to document the type and extent of tissue damage in persistent GERD and to exclude potentially malignant conditions such as Barrett's esophagus. The American College of Gastroenterology recommends endoscopy to screen for Barrett's esophagus in patients who have chronic GERD symptoms. The data demonstrating the cost-effectiveness of endoscopic screening remain controversial. Also, there is imperfect correspondence between symptoms attributed to the condition and endoscopic features of the disease.

LABORATORY TESTS

- 24-hr esophageal pH monitoring and Bernstein test are sensitive diagnostic tests; however, they are not practical and generally not done. They are useful in patients with atypical manifestations of GERD, such as chest pain or chronic cough.
- Esophageal manometry is indicated in patients with refractory reflux in whom surgical therapy is planned.

IMAGING STUDIES

An upper GI series is useful in patients unwilling to have endoscopy or with medical contraindications to the procedure. It can identify ulcerations and strictures; however, it may miss mucosal abnormalities. Only one third of patients with GERD have radiographic signs of esophagitis on an upper GI series.

ⓇⓍ TREATMENT

NONPHARMACOLOGIC THERAPY

- Lifestyle modifications with avoidance of foods (e.g., citrus- and tomato-based products, onions, spicy foods, carbonated beverages, mint, chocolate, fried foods) and drugs that exacerbate reflux (e.g., caffeine, β-blockers, calcium channel blockers, α-adrenergic agonists, theophylline)
- Avoidance of tobacco and alcohol use
- Elevation of head of bed (4 to 8 in) with blocks
- Avoidance of lying down directly after late or large evening meals, consumption of smaller and more frequent meals
- Weight reduction to BMI <25, decreased fat intake
- Avoidance of clothing that is tight around the waist

GENERAL Rx

- Proton pump inhibitors (PPIs) (esomeprazole 40 mg qd, omeprazole 20 mg qd, lansoprazole 30 mg qd, rabeprazole 20 mg qd, or pantoprazole 40 mg qd, or dexlansoprazole

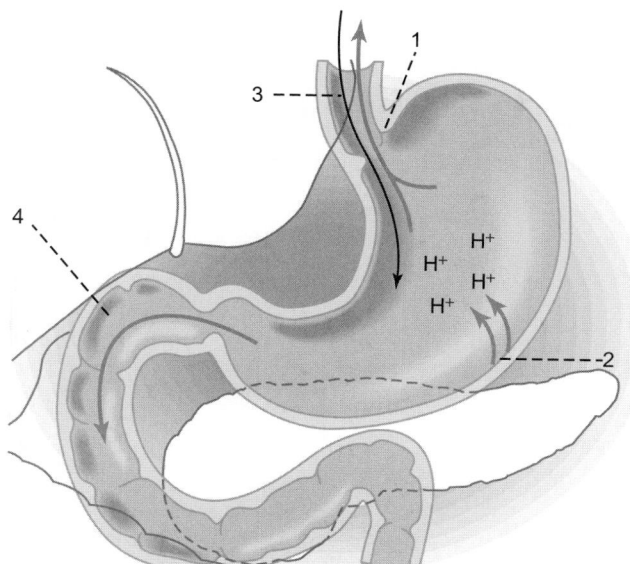

FIGURE 1-161 Pathogenesis of gastroesophageal reflux disease: (1) impaired lower esophageal sphincter-low pressures or frequent transient lower esophageal sphincter relaxation; (2) hypersection of acid; (3) decreased acid clearance resulting from impaired peristalsis or abnormal saliva production; (4) delayed gastric emptying or duodengastric reflux of bile salts and pancreatic enzymes. (From Andreoli TE, Benjamin IJ, Griggs RC, Wing EJ: *Andreoli and Carpenter's cecil essentials of medicine,* ed 8, Philadelphia, 2010, Saunders.)

- 30 mg) are safe, tolerated, and highly effective in most patients.
- H₂ blockers (nizatidine 300 mg qhs, famotidine 40 mg qhs, ranitidine 300 mg qhs, or cimetidine 800 mg qhs) can be used but are generally much less effective than PPIs.
- Antacids (may be useful for relief of mild symptoms; however, they are generally ineffective in severe cases of reflux).
- Prokinetic agents (metoclopramide) are indicated only when PPIs are not fully effective. They can be used in combination therapy; however, side effects limit their use.
- For refractory cases: surgery with Nissen fundoplication. Potential surgical candidates should have reflux esophagitis documented by esophagogastroduodenoscopy and normal esophageal motility as evaluated by manometry. Surgery generally consists of reduction of hiatal hernia when present and placement of a gastric wrap around the gastroesophageal (GE) junction (fundoplication). Although laparoscopic fundoplication is now widely used, surgery should not be advised with the expectation that patients with GERD will no longer need to take antisecretory medications or that the procedure will prevent esophageal cancer among those with GERD and Barrett's esophagus.

- Endoscopic radiofrequency heating of the GE junction (Stretta procedure) is a newer treatment modality for GERD patients unresponsive to traditional therapy. Its mechanism of action remains unclear. Endoscopy gastroplasty (EndoCinch procedure) is also aimed at treating GERD. Initial results appear encouraging; however, long-term studies are needed before recommending these procedures.
- Lifestyle modification must be followed for life because this is generally an irreversible condition.

DISPOSITION
- Recurrence of reflux is common if treatment is discontinued.
- The majority of patients respond well to therapy. In patients with chronic GERD, long-term outcomes are similar between medical therapy with PPIs and anti-reflux surgery.
- Postsurgical complications occur in nearly 20% of patients (dysphagia, gas, bloating, diarrhea, nausea). Long-term follow-up studies also reveal that within 3 to 5 yr, 52% of patients who had undergone antireflux surgery are taking antireflux medications again.

REFERRAL
- There is a strong and probably causal relation between symptomatic prolonged and un-treated GERD, Barrett's esophagus, and esophageal adenocarcinoma. GI referral for upper endoscopy is needed when there are concerns about associated peptic ulcer disease, Barrett's esophagus, or esophageal cancer.
- Patients with Barrett's esophagus should undergo surveillance endoscopy with mucosal biopsy every 2 yr or less because the risk of developing adenocarcinoma of esophagus is at least 30 times greater than that of the general population.
- Testing and treating for *Helicobacter pylori* in patients with GERD has not been shown to improve symptoms.
- All children with dental erosions should be evaluated for GERD.

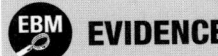

EVIDENCE

available at www.expertconsult.com

SUGGESTED READINGS

available at www.expertconsult.com

AUTHOR: **FRED F. FERRI, M.D.**

BASIC INFORMATION

DEFINITION

Glucose intolerance that begins, or is first recognized, during pregnancy. Women are first screened with a 1-hr, nonfasting glucose tolerance test. If the result is >130 mg/dl, a 3-hr glucose tolerance test is ordered. The diagnosis is made if two or more of the glucose values are met or exceeded:

Fasting: 95 mg/dl
1-hr: 180 mg/dl
2-hr: 155 mg/dl
3-hr: 140 mg/dl

Pregnant women with diabetes mellitus (DM) (gestational or preexisting) are classified according to White's classification (Table 1-57).

SYNONYMS

Gestational diabetes
Sugar of pregnancy
Diet-controlled gestational diabetes (A1)
Insulin-treated gestational diabetes (A2)

ICD-9CM CODES
648.8; if using insulin to treat, add V58.67

EPIDEMIOLOGY & DEMOGRAPHICS

INCIDENCE: Approximately 7% of all pregnancies (may range from 1% to 14% in the U.S. depending on the population studied and the diagnostic tests used)
PREDOMINANT SEX AND AGE: Women of childbearing age
GENETICS: Higher rate in women with family history of gestational DM (GDM) or type 2 diabetes; specific HLA alleles (DR3 or DR4) predispose to the development of DM type 1 after delivery

RISK FACTORS

- Obesity
- Family history of GDM or type 2 diabetes
- Glycosuria at first prenatal visit
- Polycystic ovarian syndrome
- Twin gestation
- Hypertension
- Chronic systemic steroid use
- Maternal birth weight >9 lb or <6 lb
- Age >25 y
- Previous infant weighing >9 lb or with shoulder dystocia
- Unexplained perinatal loss or malformation
- Personal history of abnormal glucose tolerance or GDM
- Latin American, Native American, African American, or Asian ethnicity

POTENTIAL RISK FACTORS

- Mixing or applying agricultural pesticides in the first trimester
- Limited physical activity the year before pregnancy
- Prepregnancy diet low in fiber and high in glycemic load

PHYSICAL FINDINGS & CLINICAL PRESENTATION

Suspect GDM if:
- Fetal size greater than dates
- Macrosomia on ultrasound
- Marked maternal obesity or weight gain

ETIOLOGY

- During normal pregnancy there is increased insulin resistance because of placental secretion of diabetogenic hormones in the late second and third trimesters. Pancreatic beta-cell secretion increases to compensate for the increased insulin resistance. GDM occurs when this need cannot be met.
- Insulin resistance is also exacerbated by an increase in maternal adipose deposition, decreased exercise, and increased caloric intake.

Dx DIAGNOSIS

DIFFERENTIAL DIAGNOSIS

Preexisting type 1 or 2 DM not previously diagnosed

WORKUP

- History with focus on personal medical history, prior pregnancy history, and family history
- Routine prenatal examination
- Laboratory evaluation

LABORATORY TESTS

- Screening with 1-hr glucose tolerance test (Nonfasting; 50-g oral glucose load)
  - For screening without risk factors, order at 24 to 28 wk
  - For screening with risk factors, order at first prenatal visit, then repeat at 24 to 28 wk if initial screen was normal. If abnormal at intake, consider possibility of undiagnosed preexisting DM and check hemoglobin A1c.
- If 1-hr test result is abnormal (>130 mg/dl), order 3-hr glucose tolerance test
  - Performed after 3 days of unrestricted diet (carbohydrate load is probably not necessary)
  - Fasting
  - 100-g oral glucose load
- If one fourth of values on 3-hr glucose tolerance test is abnormal, repeat in 1 month and consider beginning a diabetic diet
- The U.S. Preventive Services Task Force (USPSTF) concludes that the evidence is insufficient to recommend for or against routine screening for gestational diabetes. The current evidence is insufficient to assess the balance between the benefits and harms of screening women for GDM either before or after 24 weeks' gestation. Harms of screening include short-term anxiety in some women with positive screening results and inconvenience to many women and medical practices because most positive screening tests are likely false-positives. Until there is better evidence, clinicians should discuss screening for GDM with their patients and make case-by-case decisions. The discussion should include information about the uncertain benefits and harms as well as the frequency and uncertain meaning of a positive screening test result.

IMAGING STUDIES

Ultrasound for fetal size at least once at 36 to 37 wk; more frequently if macrosomia suspected

Rx TREATMENT

NONPHARMACOLOGIC THERAPY

- Glucose monitoring:
  - Four times daily: fasting and 2-hr postprandial
  - Goals: fasting <95 to 105 mg/dl; 2-hr postprandial <110 to 120 mg/dl
  - Can also use 1-hr postprandial goal of <130 to 140 mg/dl
- Dietary modifications aimed at glycemic control:
  - Follow a low-fat, high-fiber diet; avoid sugar and concentrated sweets; and eat small, frequent meals.
  - Nutrition counseling for diet that adequately meets the needs of pregnancy but restricts carbohydrates to 35% to 40% of daily calories.

TABLE 1-57   White's Classification for Pregnant Women with Diabetes (Gestational or Preexisting)

Class	Description
A1	DM diagnosed during pregnancy and controlled by diet
A2	DM diagnosed during pregnancy and requiring medication
B	Insulin-requiring DM diagnosed before pregnancy, age >20 yr, lasting <10 yr
C	Insulin-requiring DM, onset at age 10 to 19 yr, with a duration 10 to 19 yr
D	Onset >10 yr or duration >20 yr, or associated with hypertension or background retinopathy
F	DM with renal disease
H	DM with coronary artery disease
R	DM with proliferative retinopathy
T	DM with renal transplant

- ○ For women with a body mass index >30, restrict calories to 25 kcal/kg actual weight per day.
- Regular moderate exercise

PHARMACOLOGIC Rx

Begin if >20% of glucose values are elevated after trial of diet control:

- Oral hypoglycemics:
  - ○ Glyburide: begin at 2.5 mg qd and titrate up to a maximum of 20 mg qd (10 mg bid). Increase dose as needed by 2.5 to 5 mg/wk.
  - ○ Metformin use in pregnancy remains controversial because it crosses the placenta.
- Insulin:
  1. One commonly used regimen:
     - ○ Insulin 0.7 U/kg/day SQ, with two thirds of the total daily dose given in the morning and one third of the total daily dose given in the evening
     - ○ One third of each dose is given as short-acting insulin and the remaining two thirds as NPH insulin
  2. Another option:
     - ○ If fasting values are elevated, use NPH at bedtime with initial dose of 0.2 U/kg
     - ○ If postprandial values are elevated, use rapid-acting insulin before meals with initial dose 1.5 U/10 g carbohydrate at breakfast and 1 U/10 g carbohydrate at lunch and dinner
  3. Long-acting insulin such as Lantus does not have sufficient data to determine whether it crosses the placenta; it may be continued in persons with preexisting diabetes who are well controlled but is not recommended in patients with newly diagnosed GDM
  4. Glyburide and insulin have overall similar rates of clinical effectiveness and fetal safety

ANTENATAL TESTING

Routine blood pressure and urine protein monitoring:

- Class A1: NST/AFI at 40 wk
- Class A2: weekly NST/AFI beginning at 32 wk or when insulin is started
- Poorly controlled diabetes, vascular complications, or hypertension: biweekly NST/AFI beginning at 28 wk and consider admission for initial glycemic control

TIMING AND ROUTE OF DELIVERY

- Class A1 (well controlled): deliver by 41 wk
- Class A2: deliver by 40 wk
- Offer elective cesarean section at 38 wk if estimated fetal weight >4500 g
- Consider delivery by 37 wk if poor control or intrauterine growth retardation after confirmed fetal lung maturity by amniocentesis

INTRAPARTUM MANAGEMENT

- Goal is normoglycemia (80 to 110 mg/dl) using insulin and D5 lactated Ringer's IV fluid
- Monitor glucose hourly
- Preparation for shoulder dystocia
- If on glyburide, discontinue in labor or 12 hr before a scheduled induction

NEONATAL MANAGEMENT

- Check 30- and 60-min glucose
- Watch for signs of hypoglycemia, hypocalcemia, hyperbilirubinemia, and polycythemia

POSTPARTUM MANAGEMENT

- Class A2: check fasting level before discharge; if abnormal, continue checking at home and early follow up with primary care physician to confirm diagnosis of DM
- 6-wk postpartum visit: screen for diabetes with 2-hr glucose tolerance test or two fasting values
- If no evidence of DM, screen annually for DM and counsel on risk factor modification

REFERRAL

- Nutritionist
- High-risk obstetrician
- Maternal-fetal medicine
- Diabetes educator

COMPLICATIONS

- Maternal: preeclampsia, future type 2 DM or GDM, operative delivery
- Fetal: polyhydramnios, macrosomia, shoulder dystocia, birth trauma, congenital malformations
- Neonatal: hypoglycemia, hypocalcemia, hyperbilirubinemia, polycythemia, perinatal death, future obesity and DM, impaired fine and gross motor functions; increased rates of inattention and hyperactivity

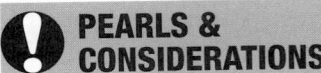

PEARLS & CONSIDERATIONS

Trials have shown that although treatment of mild gestational DM did not significantly reduce the frequency of a composite outcome that included stillbirth or perinatal death and several neonatal complications, it did reduce the risks of fetal overgrowth, shoulder dystocia, cesarean delivery, and hypertensive disorders.

PREVENTION

Regular exercise, maintenance of ideal body weight, and high-fiber low-glycemic diet

PATIENT & FAMILY EDUCATION

Gestational Diabetes Patient Information
American Academy of Family Physicians
http://www.aafp.org/afp/20031101/1775ph.html

American Dietetic Association
Consumer Nutrition Information and Referrals
http://www.eatright.org
Telephone: 800-366-1655

American Diabetes Association: Gestational Diabetes
http://www.diabetes.org
800-DIABETES (800-342-2383)

NOAH: New York Online Access to Health
http://www.noah-health.org

National Institute of Child Health and Human Development
Managing Gestational Diabetes: A Patient's Guide to a Healthy Pregnancy
http://www.nichd.nih.gov/publications/pubs/gest_diabetes/
800-370-2943

Food and Nutrition Information Center
Food Guide Pyramid
http://www.nal.usda.gov.

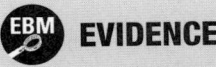 **EVIDENCE**

available at www.expertconsult.com

SUGGESTED READINGS

available at www.expertconsult.com

AUTHORS: **JORDAN WHITE, M.D.,**
NIRALI BORA, M.D.,
HEIDI H. PETERSON, M.D., and
SUSANNA R. MAGEE, M.D., M.P.H.

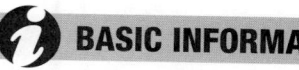

BASIC INFORMATION

DEFINITION

Giant cell arteritis (GCA) is a segmental systemic granulomatous arteritis affecting medium and large arteries in individuals >50 yr. Peak incidence is in patients aged 60 to 80 yr. Inflammation primarily targets extracranial blood vessels, and although the carotid system is usually affected, pathology in the posterior cerebral artery has been reported.

SYNONYMS

Temporal arteritis
Cranial arteritis
GCA

ICD-9CM CODES
446.5 Temporal arteritis

EPIDEMIOLOGY & DEMOGRAPHICS

INCIDENCE: 17 to 23.3 new cases per 100,000 persons >50 yr
PREVALENCE: 200 cases per 100,000 persons; female/male predominance of twofold to fourfold

PHYSICAL FINDINGS & CLINICAL PRESENTATION

GCA can present with the following clinical manifestations:
- Headache, often associated with marked scalp tenderness

TABLE 1-58 Atypical Manifestations of Giant Cell Arteritis (GCA)

Fever of unknown origin
Respiratory symptoms (especially cough)
Otolaryngeal manifestations
  Glossitis
  Lingual infarction
  Throat pain
  Hearing loss
Large-artery disease
  Aortic aneurysm
  Aortic dissection
  Limb claudication
  Raynaud's phenomenon
Neurologic manifestations
  Peripheral neuropathy
  Transient ischemic attack (TIA) or stroke
  Dementia
  Delerium
Myocardial infarction
Tumorlike lesions
  Breast mass
  Ovarian and uterine mass
Syndrome of inappropriate antidiuretic hormone
  secretion (SIADH)
Microangiopathic hemolytic anemia

Harris ED, Budd RC, Genovese MC, Firestein GS, Sargent JS, Sledge JS, Rubby S: *Kelly's textbook of rheumatology,* ed 7, Philadelphia, 2005, Saunders.

- Constitutional symptoms (fever, weight loss, anorexia, fatigue)
- Polymyalgia syndrome (aching and stiffness of the trunk and proximal muscle groups)
- Visual disturbances (transient or permanent monocular visual loss)
- Intermittent claudication of jaw and tongue on mastication
- Table 1-58 describes atypical manifestations of giant cell arteritis

Important physical findings in GCA:
- Vascular examination: tenderness, decreased pulsation, and nodulation of temporal arteries; diminished or absent pulses in upper extremities

ETIOLOGY

Vasculitis of unknown etiology

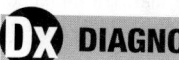

DIAGNOSIS

Clinical history and vascular examination are cornerstones of diagnosis.
- Age of onset >50 yr
- New-onset or new type of headache
- Temporal artery tenderness or decreased pulsation
- Westergren erythrocyte sedimentation rate (ESR) elevated (typically >50 mm/hr)
- Jaw claudication
- Temporal artery biopsy with vasculitis and mononuclear cell infiltrate or granulomatous changes

DIFFERENTIAL DIAGNOSIS

- Other vasculitic syndromes
- Nonarteritic anterior ischemic optic neuropathy (AION)
- Primary amyloidosis
- Transient ischemic attack, stroke
- Infections
- Occult neoplasm, multiple myeloma

LABORATORY TESTS

- ESR elevated; up to 22.5% patients with GCA have normal ESR before treatment.
- C-reactive protein is typically included in laboratory investigation; it may have greater sensitivity than ESR.
- Mild to moderate normochromic normocytic anemia, elevated platelet count.

IMAGING STUDIES

- Reliability of color duplex ultrasonography of temporal artery is controversial because it is believed to not improve diagnostic accuracy over careful physical examination.
- Fluorescein angiogram of ophthalmic vessels may be warranted to differentiate between arteritic AION (i.e., GCA) and nonarteritic AION.

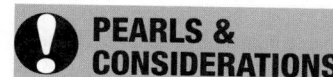

TREATMENT

ACUTE GENERAL Rx

- IV methylprednisolone (250 to 1000 mg qd for 3 to 5 days) is indicated in those with significant clinical manifestations (e.g., visual loss).
- Oral prednisone (1 mg/kg/day). High-dose oral regimen should be continued at least until symptoms resolve and ESR returns to normal. Prednisone treatment may last up to 2 yr and is tapered over several weeks to months.
- Other immunosuppressive agents may be used when steroids are contraindicated.

DISPOSITION

If steroid therapy is initiated early, GCA has excellent prognosis; however, once there is visual loss, improvement is dismal. In one study only 4% of eyes improved in both visual acuity and central visual field.

REFERRAL

- Surgical referral for biopsy of temporal artery
- Ophthalmology referral in patients with visual disturbances and after initiation of corticosteroid therapy
- Rheumatology referral for patients in whom steroids are contraindicated

PEARLS & CONSIDERATIONS

The diagnostic utility of temporal artery biopsy is not compromised if performed within days of starting steroid therapy.

COMMENTS

- The relation between polymyalgia rheumatica and GCA is unclear, but the two frequently coexist.
- Clinical picture rather than ESR should be the prime yardstick for continuing prednisone therapy. A rising ESR in a clinically asymptomatic patient with normal hematocrit should raise suspicion for alternate explanations (e.g., infections, neoplasms).
- GCA is associated with a markedly increased risk for the development of aortic aneurysm, which is often a late complication and may cause death. Annual chest radiograph in chronic CGA patients has been suggested, as well as emergent chest CT or MRI for clinical suspicion.

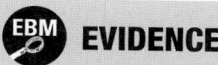

EVIDENCE

available at www.expertconsult.com

SUGGESTED READINGS

available at www.expertconsult.com

AUTHOR: **U. SHIVRAJ SOHUR, M.D., PH.D.**

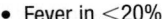

DEFINITION

Giardiasis is an intestinal and/or biliary tract infection caused by the protozoal parasite *Giardia lamblia*. The organism is a widespread zoonotic parasite and frequently contaminates fresh water sources worldwide.

SYNONYMS

Giardiasis
Giardia duodenalis
Giardia intestinalis

ICD-9CM CODES
007.1 Giardiasis

EPIDEMIOLOGY & DEMOGRAPHICS

INCIDENCE (IN U.S.):
- Exact incidence unknown
- Frequently occurs as water-borne outbreaks

PREVALENCE (IN U.S.): 4%
PREDOMINANT SEX: Male = female
PREDOMINANT AGE:
- Preschool children, especially if in day care
- 20 to 40 yr of age, especially among sexually active homosexual men

PEAK INCIDENCE:
- Varies with risk factors, outbreaks, but peak onset from early summer through early fall
- All age groups affected

GENETICS: Familial disposition: Patients with common variable immunodeficiency or X-linked agammaglobulinemia are at increased risk of infection.

PHYSICAL FINDINGS & CLINICAL PRESENTATION

- More than 70% with one or more intestinal symptoms (diarrhea, flatulence, cramps, bloating, nausea)

- Fever in <20%
- Chronic diarrhea, malabsorption, and weight loss
- GI bleeding is unusual
- Continuous or intermittent symptoms, lasting for weeks
- Of infected patients, 20% to 25% are asymptomatic

ETIOLOGY

Infection is acquired by ingestion of viable cysts of the organism, typically in contaminated water or by fecal-oral contact.

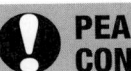 **DIAGNOSIS**

DIFFERENTIAL DIAGNOSIS

- Other agents of infective diarrhea (amebae, *Salmonella* sp., *Shigella* sp., *Staphylococcus aureus*, *Cryptosporidium*, etc.)
- Noninfectious causes of malabsorption

WORKUP

- Stool specimen (three specimens yield 90% sensitivity) or duodenal aspirate for microscopic examination to establish diagnosis and exclude other pathogens (Fig. 1-162)
- Immunoassays for *Giardia* sp. Antigens in stool samples are now routinely used in most clinical laboratories. These assays are 85% to 98% sensitive and 90% to 100% specific.

LABORATORY TESTS

Serum albumin, vitamin B_{12} levels, and stool fat test to exclude malabsorption

IMAGING STUDIES

- Not necessary unless biliary obstruction is suspected
- In detection of organism, possible interference by barium in stool from radiographic studies

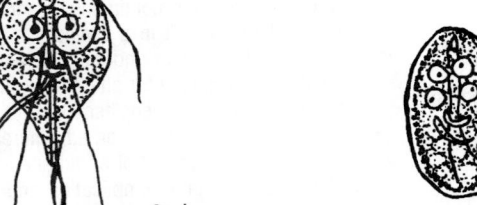

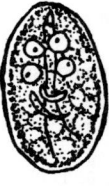

Scale:
0 ⊢————⊣ 12 μ

FIGURE 1-162 *Giardia* **organisms.** The trophozoite *(left)* is 12 to 15 μm long and has four pairs of flagella. This form is not commonly seen in stools. Cysts *(right)* are 9 to 19 μm long and may have two to four nuclei. (From Hoekelman R [ed]: *Primary pediatric care,* ed 3, St Louis, 1997, Mosby.)

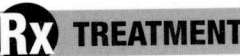 **TREATMENT**

NONPHARMACOLOGIC THERAPY

Avoidance of milk products to reduce symptoms of transient lactase deficiency that occur in many patients

ACUTE GENERAL Rx

Adult and pediatric:
- Metronidazole 250 mg PO three times daily for 5 to 7 days is considered the drug of choice in the United States. Pediatric dose: 5 mg/kg tid × 7 days (metronidazole should be avoided in pregnancy).
- Tinidazole: 2 g single dose, (50 mg/kg in children) is a congener of metronidazole
- Nitazoxanide: aged 12 to 47 mo: 100 mg bid × 3 days. Age 4 to 11 yr: 200 mg bid × 3 days
- Paromomycin 25 to 30 mg/kg/day in three doses for 5 to 10 days
- Other alternatives include furazolidone (100 mg qid × 7 to 10 days in adults, 2 mg/kg qid × 10 days in children and albendazole: 400 mg qid × 5 days in adults, 15 mg/kg/day × 5 to 7 days (max. 400 mg)

CHRONIC Rx

May require retreatment.

DISPOSITION

Reinfection is possible.

REFERRAL

For evaluation by gastroenterologist if malabsorption and persistent weight loss

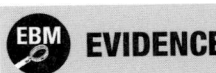 **PEARLS & CONSIDERATIONS**

COMMENTS

Travelers to endemic areas (developing world, wilderness areas) should be cautioned to boil drinking water or use water purification tablets.

EBM EVIDENCE

available at www.expertconsult.com

SUGGESTED READINGS

available at www.expertconsult.com

AUTHORS: **GLENN G. FORT, M.D., M.P.H.,** and **DENNIS J. MIKOLICH, M.D.**

BASIC INFORMATION

DEFINITION

Gilbert's disease is an autosomal-dominant disease characterized by indirect hyperbilirubinemia caused by impaired glucuronyl transferase activity.

SYNONYMS

Gilbert's syndrome

ICD-9CM CODES
277.4 Gilbert's syndrome

EPIDEMIOLOGY & DEMOGRAPHICS

INCIDENCE (IN U.S.): Probable autosomal-dominant disease affecting >5% of the U.S. population
PREDOMINANT SEX: Male/female ratio of 3:1
GENETICS: Most common hereditary hyperbilirubinemia (genotypic prevalence 12%)

PHYSICAL FINDINGS & CLINICAL PRESENTATION

- No abnormalities on physical examination other than mild jaundice when bilirubin exceeds 3 mg/dl.
- A family history of unconjugated hyperbilirubinemia may be present.

ETIOLOGY

- Decreased elimination of bilirubin in bile is caused by inadequate conjugation of bilirubin.
- Alcohol consumption and starvation diet can increase bilirubin level.
- The pathogenesis of Gilbert's syndrome has been linked to a reduction in the bilirubin UGT-1 gene *(HUG-Brl)* transcription, resulting from a mutation in the promoter region.

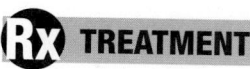 **DIAGNOSIS**

DIFFERENTIAL DIAGNOSIS

- Hemolytic anemia
- Liver disease (chronic hepatitis, cirrhosis)
- Crigler-Najjar syndrome

WORKUP

- Most patients are diagnosed during or after adolescence, when isolated hyperbilirubinemia is detected as an incidental finding on routine biochemical testing.
- Laboratory evaluation to exclude hemolysis and liver diseases as a cause of the elevated bilirubin level (Table 1-59).

LABORATORY TESTS

Elevated indirect (unconjugated) bilirubin (rarely exceeds 5 mg/dl)

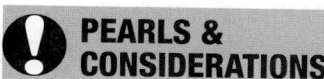 **TREATMENT**

ACUTE GENERAL Rx

Treatment is generally unnecessary. Phenobarbital (if clinical jaundice is present) can rapidly decrease serum indirect bilirubin level.

DISPOSITION

Prognosis is excellent. Treatment is generally unnecessary.

REFERRAL

Referral is generally not necessary.

❗ PEARLS & CONSIDERATIONS

COMMENTS

- Patients should be reassured about the benign nature of their condition.
- Fasting for 2 days or significant dehydration may raise the bilirubin level and result in the clinical recognition of jaundice.

AUTHOR: **FRED F. FERRI, M.D.**

G

Diseases and Disorders

I

TABLE 1-59 Characteristic Patterns of Liver Function Tests

Disorder	Bilirubin	Alkaline Phosphatase	AST	ALT	Prothrombin Time	Albumin
Gilbert's syndrome (abnormal bilirubin metabolism)	↑	NL	NL	NL	NL	NL
Bile duct obstruction (pancreatic cancer)	↑↑↑	↑↑↑	↑	↑	↑-↑↑	NL
Acute hepatocellular damage (toxic, viral hepatitis)	↑-↑↑↑	↑-↑↑	↑↑↑	↑↑↑	NL-↑↑↑	NL-↓↓
Cirrhosis	NL-↑	NL-↑	NL-↑	NL-↑	NL-↑↑	NL-↓↓

From Andreoli TE (ed): *Cecil essentials of medicine*, ed 6, Philadelphia, 2005, WB Saunders.
ALT, Alanine aminotransferase; *AST*, aspartate aminotransferase; *NL*, normal; ↑, increase; ↓, decrease (arrows indicate extent of change: ↑-↑↑↑, slight to large).

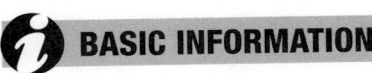

BASIC INFORMATION

DEFINITION

Inflammation of the gums covering the maxilla and mandible

SYNONYMS

None

ICD-9CM CODES
523.1   Chronic gingivitis
523.01 Acute gingivitis

EPIDEMIOLOGY & DEMOGRAPHICS

Gingivitis generally occurs in adults.

PHYSICAL FINDINGS & CLINICAL PRESENTATION

- Inflammation is usually painless.
- Bleeding may occur with minor trauma such as brushing teeth.
- A bluish discoloration of the gums and halitosis are sometimes present.
- Subgingival plaque may be seen on close examination, and in time, there is detachment of soft tissue from the tooth surface.
- Longstanding infection may lead to destructive periodontal disease, which may involve teeth and bones.
- A dramatic form of gingivitis called acute ulcerative necrotizing gingivitis (ANUG or "trench mouth") can occur. This is manifested by acute, painful inflammation of the gingivae, with bleeding, ulceration, and halitosis. At times this is accompanied by fever and lymphadenopathy.
- Linear gingival erythema ("HIV Gingivitis") presents as a brightly inflamed band of marginal gingiva. It may be painful, with easy bleeding and rapid destruction.
- Severe periodontitis can occur in patients with diabetes mellitus or HIV infection and in primary HIV infection (acute retroviral syndrome).

- Pregnancy may be associated with an acute form of gingivitis. Gingivae become inflamed and hypertrophic; this is likely the result of hormonal shifts.

ETIOLOGY

- A variety of organisms may be found in the environment of plaque. Anaerobes play a predominant role in periodontal disease.
- Improper hygiene and poorly fitting dentures may contribute to the development of gingivitis.
- Excessive use of tobacco and alcohol may predispose individuals to gingival disease.
- In patients with HIV infection, gram-negative anaerobes, enteric organisms, and yeast predominate.
- Appropriate oral hygiene, such as flossing and tooth brushing, can prevent the accumulation of bacterial plaque; once dense plaque is present, adequate hygiene becomes more difficult.

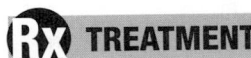 DIAGNOSIS

DIFFERENTIAL DIAGNOSIS

Gingival hyperplasia, which may be caused by long-term use of phenytoin or nifedipine

WORKUP

Oral examination

LABORATORY TESTS

Elevated serum glucose in diabetics

IMAGING STUDIES

Radiographs of the teeth and facial bones may reveal extension of infection to these structures.

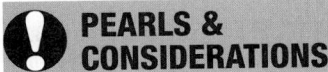 TREATMENT

NONPHARMACOLOGIC THERAPY

Removal of plaque, and at times, debridement of soft tissue

ACUTE GENERAL Rx

- Penicillin VK, 500 mg PO qid for 1 to 2 wk or
- Clindamycin, 300 mg PO qid for 1 to 2 wk
- For linear gingival erythema, chlorhexidine gluconate rinses and nystatin rinses or troches may be used

CHRONIC Rx

Extensive or recurrent infection may require periodic evaluation and debridement.

DISPOSITION

Continued inflammation can eventually lead to destruction of teeth and bone.

REFERRAL

Patients should be referred to a dentist or periodontist.

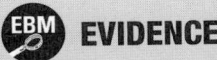

PEARLS & CONSIDERATIONS

COMMENTS

- Presence of periodontal disease is associated with an increased incidence of anaerobic pleuropulmonary infections.
- Existing data support the recommendation to change a toothbrush every 3 mo. Worn brushes seem to be less effective in plaque reduction.

EBM EVIDENCE

available at www.expertconsult.com

SUGGESTED READINGS

available at www.expertconsult.com

AUTHORS: **GLENN G. FORT, M.D., M.P.H.,** and **DENNIS J. MIKOLICH, M.D.**

BASIC INFORMATION

DESCRIPTION

Necrotizing ulcerative gingivitis (NUG) is a distinct painful infectious disease primarily of the interdental and marginal gingiva. It is characterized by a symptom triad that includes gingival pain, ulcer, and bleeding.

SYNONYMS

Trench mouth
Acute necrotizing ulcerative gingivitis (ANUG)
Vincent's stomatitis
Fusospirochetal gingivitis
Acute ulcerative gingivitis

ICD-9CM CODES

101 Acute necrotizing ulcerative gingivitis

EPIDEMIOLOGY

- Unlike in the developing world, NUG is seen rarely in developed countries.
- Occurs in the 2nd and 3rd decades of life in the developed world.
- In contrast, it affects young children more often in developing countries.
- Slightly more prevalent in males than in females because the latter group tend to have a better oral hygiene.

RISK FACTORS

- Poor oral hygiene
- Smoking/chewing tobacco
- Alcohol use
- Drug addiction
- Poor socioeconomic status
- Psychological stress
- Preexisting gingivitis
- Lack of sleep
- Malnutrition
- Overcrowding
- Living near livestock
- History of prior NUG
- Recent illness
- Underlying systemic diseases
- Acatalasia
- Various infections such as measles, malaria, and infestation with intestinal parasites
- Trauma
- Immunosuppression
  - Dermatomyositis (DM)
  - Steroid use
  - HIV/AIDS
  - Use of chemotherapeutic drugs
  - Leukemia and other malignancies

ETIOLOGY

- Polymicrobial
- Often caused by both Fusobacterium and spirochetes

PATHOGENESIS

- Unknown
- For the most part it appears to result from an opportunistic infection in a host with lowered resistance.

CLINICAL FEATURES

- Onset of the disease is usually sudden
- Severe gingival pain
- Gingival tissue is inflamed, edematous, friable, and necrotic; the normal pointed interdental papillae are blunted, but there is no loss of attachment
- Gingival bleeding with little or no provocation
- Punched out ulcerations are seen along the interdental papillae around the anterior incisors and posterior molars. A grayish-white pseudomembrane often covers these ulcers. These punched out ulcers along the pseudomembrane are pathognomonic of NUG.
- Other features include
  - Halitosis
  - Alteration in taste, such as a metallic flavor
  - Wooden teeth feeling
  - Odynophagia
  - Fever and fatigue
  - Cervical lymphadenopathy

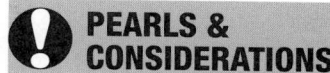 DIAGNOSIS

- Based on the clinical features
- WBC may be elevated
- Gram stain and aerobic/anaerobic culture
- Dental x-ray or x-ray of face to check on the extent of the disease
- HIV testing is recommended for patients refractory to antibiotic therapy

DIFFERENTIAL DIAGNOSIS

- Gingivitis
- Acute herpetic gingivostomatitis
- Aphthous stomatitis
- Chronic periodontal disease
- Desquamative gingivitis
- Gonococcal and streptococcal gingivostomatitis
- Oral candidiasis
- Ludwig's angina
- HIV-associated idiopathic ulcerations

TREATMENT

- Improve oral hygiene by flushing and brushing at least twice a day.
- Improve nutrition and hydrations.
- Eliminate contributing factors such as smoking, alcohol, carbonated beverages, spicy/hot foods, poor nutrition, stress, and so on.
- Antibiotics coverage for 5 to 10 days. Most recommend oral penicillin V 250 to 500 mg orally every 6 to 8 hr and metronidazole 250 to 500 mg orally every 8 hr. Tetracycline is given instead of penicillin in patients allergic to the latter. As an alternative one could give only clindamycin instead of the drug combination of penicillin and metronidazole.
- Rinsing the mouth at least twice a day with warm saline (1/2 teaspoon of salt in 1 cup of water), 0.12% chlorhexidine, or dilute 3% hydrogen peroxide (mixed half and half with water).
- Pain is controlled with oral pain medications and topical application of 2% viscous lidocaine (15 ml oral rinse every 6 to 8 hr as needed) to the inflamed gum.
- Surgical debridement is needed in severe cases.
- Scaling and root planning following the resolution of infection and the acute inflammation.
- At times reconstructive surgery may be needed.

COMPLICATIONS

- Cancrum oris (noma) results when NUG involves the deeper tissue
- Vincent's angina from the involvement of tonsils and pharynx
- Necrotizing ulcerative periodontitis
- Loss of teeth
- Periodontal abscess
- Alveolar bone destruction
- Disfigurement
- Cellulitis
- Dehydration/malnutrition

PROGNOSIS

- Dramatic relief of symptoms within 24 hr of initiating antibiotics and supportive treatment is characteristic.
- Risk of recurrence is high.

PEARLS & CONSIDERATIONS

PREVENTION

- Good oral hygiene
- Use of power toothbrush is better than a manual brush
- Good general health including proper nutrition, sleep, and exercise
- Routine dental checks
- Avoidance of smoking and alcohol
- Stress management

PATIENT EDUCATION

Not a communicable disease

SUGGESTED READING

available at www.expertconsult.com

AUTHOR: **HEMANT K. SATPATHY, M.D.**

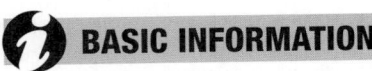

BASIC INFORMATION

DEFINITION

Primary angle-closure glaucoma (PACG) occurs when elevated intraocular pressure is associated with closure of the filtration angle or obstruction in the circulating pathway of the aqueous humor.

SYNONYMS

Acute glaucoma, angle-closure glaucoma (ACG)
Pupillary block glaucoma
Narrow-angle glaucoma

ICD-9CM CODES
365.2 Primary angle-closure glaucoma (PACG)

EPIDEMIOLOGY & DEMOGRAPHICS

INCIDENCE (IN U.S.):
- 2% to 8% of all patients with glaucoma
- Higher incidence among those with hyperopia, small eyes, dense cataracts, shallow anterior chambers

PEAK INCIDENCE: Greater >50 yr; high association with hypopia, cataracts, and eye trauma
PREDOMINANT SEX: Females are affected more often than males
PREDOMINANT AGE: 50 to 60 yr
GENETICS: High family history

PHYSICAL FINDINGS & CLINICAL PRESENTATION

- Hazy cornea (Fig. 1-163)
- Narrow angle
- Red eyes
- Pain
- Injection of conjunctiva
- Shallow anterior chamber
- Thick cataract
- Old trauma
- Chronic eye infections

ETIOLOGY

- Narrow angles with acute closure: blockage of circulatory path of the aqueous humor causing increase in interior ocular pressure. ACG occurs more commonly in eyes with shorter axial length, shallower anterior chamber, and a relatively larger lens
- Secondary angle-closure glaucoma (SACG) resulting from neovascularization of iris, iris tumors, pharmacology, lens induced, iris scarring, trauma, chronic inflammation with scarring, malignant glaucoma with aqueous misdirection

DIAGNOSIS

DIFFERENTIAL DIAGNOSIS

- High pressure
- Optic nerve cupping
- Field loss
- Shallow chamber
- Open-angle glaucoma
- Conjunctivitis
- Corneal disease, keratitis
- Uveitis
- Scleritis
- Allergies
- Contact lens wearing with irritation

WORKUP

- Intraocular pressure
- Gonioscopy
- Slit lamp examination
- Visual field examination
- GDx examination (laser scan of nerve fiber layer), OCT
- Optic nerve evaluation
- Anterior chamber depth
- Cataract evaluation
- High hyperopia
- Dilantin provocative testing

LABORATORY TESTS

- Blood sugar and complete blood count (if diabetes or inflammatory disease is suspected)
- Visual field
- GDx nerve fiber analysis, OCT, Heidelberg retinal tomography

IMAGING STUDIES

- Fundus photography
- Fluorescein angiography for neurovascular disease

TREATMENT

The goal of treatment is to acutely lower pressure on the eye and keep it down.

NONPHARMACOLOGIC THERAPY

Laser iridotomy early in disease process

ACUTE GENERAL Rx

- IV mannitol
- Pilocarpine
- β-blockers
- Diamox
- Laser iridotomy
- Anterior chamber paracentesis (as emergency treatment)

CHRONIC Rx

- Iridotomy
- Trabeculectomy
- Filter valves
- Other laser procedures

DISPOSITION

Refer to ophthalmologist immediately.

REFERRAL

This is an emergency; refer immediately to an ophthalmologist.

PEARLS & CONSIDERATIONS

COMMENTS

- Do not use antihistamines or vasodilators with narrow-angle glaucoma.
- After iridotomy, the majority of patients will be totally cured and will need no further medication and have no visual loss.
- Lower socioeconomic status and higher levels of social deprivation are risk factors for delayed detection and probable worse outcomes in glaucoma.

EVIDENCE

available at www.expertconsult.com

SUGGESTED READINGS
available at www.expertconsult.com

AUTHOR: **MELVYN KOBY, M.D.**

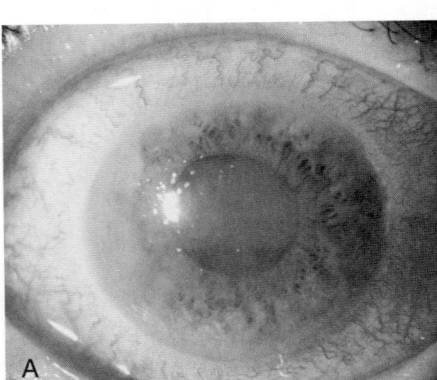
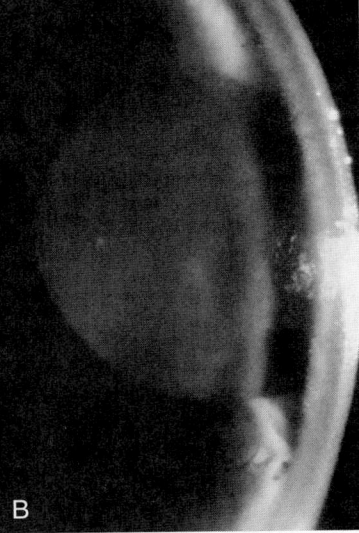

FIGURE 1-163 Acute angle-closure glaucoma. A, Acutely elevated pressure produces an inflamed eye with corneal edema (note fragmented light reflex) and a mid-dilated pupil. **B,** Slit lamp examination shows a very shallow central anterior chamber (space between cornea and iris) and no peripheral chamber. (From Palay D [ed]: *Ophthalmology for the primary care physician,* St Louis, 1997, Mosby.)

BASIC INFORMATION

DEFINITION

Glenohumeral dislocation (Fig. 1-164) is complete separation or displacement of the humeral head from the glenoid surface (partial separation is termed *subluxation*). Most often the cause is traumatic, and the humeral head dislocates anteriorly and inferiorly. This may cause a tear of the glenoid labrum (the Bankart lesion). Less commonly the head dislocates posteriorly.

Rarely, multidirectional instability may be present in which dislocation or subluxation, often bilateral, may occur in multiple directions, usually the result of excessive joint laxity and generally without trauma.

ICD-9CM CODES
831.01 Anterior
831.02 Posterior
831.03 Inferior
718.31 Recurrent
718.81 Instability

PHYSICAL FINDINGS & CLINICAL PRESENTATION

Traumatic:
- The arm is held in external rotation with anterior dislocation and internal rotation with posterior dislocation.
- Little movement is possible without pain.
- The acromion may appear more prominent, and there is absence of the normal "fullness" beneath the acromion.
- The status of the axillary nerve must always be checked (sensation to the mid-deltoid should be assessed).

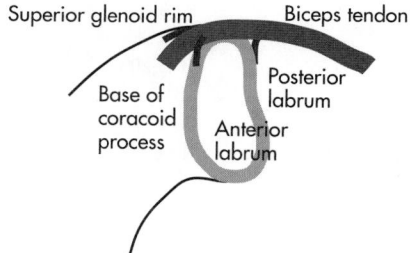

FIGURE 1-164 Glenohumeral dislocation. (From Weisslederer R, Wittenberg J, Harisinghani MG, Chen JW: *Primer of diagnostic imaging*, St Louis, 2007, Mosby.)

- The apprehension test may become positive if anterior instability persists (pain and apprehension that the shoulder will dislocate when the relaxed arm is manually placed in the "throwing position" of external rotation and abduction).
- Recurrent episodes of anterior dislocation may occur with minor movement, such as putting on a coat or turning off a light.

Multidirectional:
- Often difficult to diagnose, especially if only subluxation occurs.
- Recurrent episodes of giving out and weakness, often bilateral and without trauma.
- Sulcus sign is often positive (the arms are pulled downward with the patient standing; a sulcus [indentation] will form between the acromion and humeral head, indicating excessive inferior movement of the head).
- Other signs of generalized joint laxity may be present, such as joint hyperextensibility and the ability of the patient to touch the thumb against the flexor aspect of the forearm.

ETIOLOGY
- Trauma
- Generalized joint laxity (multidirectional)
- Seizures (posterior dislocations)

DIAGNOSIS

DIFFERENTIAL DIAGNOSIS
- Rotator cuff rupture
- Frozen shoulder (posterior dislocation)
- Suprascapular nerve paralysis
- Anterior instability

IMAGING STUDIES
- Acute shoulder injury: true anteroposterior roentgenogram plus lateral view of the glenohumeral joint, either transaxillary or transcapular
- MRI: to determine soft tissue status, especially the presence of Bankart lesion or rotator cuff tear; may be indicated after a second episode of dislocation

TREATMENT

- Reduction of the acute dislocation by gentle straight traction in the relaxed patient followed by light immobilization

- Gentle limited range-of-motion exercises as pain subsides followed by strengthening exercises at 2 wk

DISPOSITION
- Recurrence of anterior dislocation is common in the young; these patients may have to avoid the arm position associated with dislocation (external rotation with abduction).
- Primary dislocations in patients >40 yr are not generally complicated by recurrence but may result in shoulder stiffness and associated rotator cuff injuries.
- There is an almost 100% recurrence after the third dislocation.

REFERRAL

Surgical reconstruction may be required in the recurrent dislocator.

PEARLS & CONSIDERATIONS

COMMENTS
- It is important to know if there was an injury involved in the first episode and if a radiograph was taken to determine direction of the dislocation.
- Up to 50% of posterior dislocations are missed by the first examiner, usually the result of an inadequate lateral radiograph of the glenohumeral joint.
- "Voluntary" posterior dislocators should always be treated nonsurgically.
- Sports activities may be resumed when there is pain-free full flexibility and normal strength.
- Multidirectional instabilities are usually treated nonsurgically with strengthening exercises.
- Dislocations in either direction are occasionally overlooked. If the injury is over 2 to 4 weeks old, enough tissue healing will have occurred to make closed reduction fail. Open reduction or arthroplasty will then be needed in the young. Older patients may improve with therapeutic exercises, and the resultant disability is often acceptable.

SUGGESTED READINGS
available at www.expertconsult.com

AUTHOR: **LONNIE R. MERCIER, M.D.**

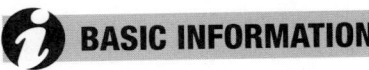

BASIC INFORMATION

DEFINITION

Acute glomerulonephritis is an immunologically mediated inflammation primarily involving the glomerulus that can result in damage to the basement membrane, mesangium, or capillary endothelium. Table 1-60 summarizes primary renal diseases that present as acute glomerulonephritis.

SYNONYMS

Postinfectious glomerulonephritis
Acute nephritic syndrome

ICD-9CM CODES
583.9 Glomerulonephritis, acute

EPIDEMIOLOGY & DEMOGRAPHICS

- More than 50% of cases involve children <13 yr.
- Glomerulonephritis is the most common cause of chronic renal failure (25%).
- Immunoglobulin A (IgA) nephropathy glomerulonephritis (Berger's disease) is the most common glomerulonephritis worldwide.

PHYSICAL FINDINGS & CLINICAL PRESENTATION

- Edema (peripheral, periorbital, or pulmonary)
- Joint pains, oral ulcers, malar rash (frequently seen with lupus nephritis)
- Dark urine
- Hypertension
- Findings of palpable purpura in patients with Henoch-Schönlein purpura
- Heart murmurs may indicate endocarditis
- Impetigo, skin pallor, tenderness in the abdomen and/or back, pharyngeal erythema may be present

ETIOLOGY

Acute glomerulonephritis may be caused by primary renal disease or a systemic disease. A number of pathogenic processes (e.g., antibody deposition, cell-mediated immune mechanisms, complement activation, hemodynamic alterations) have been implicated in the pathogenesis of glomerular inflammation. Medical disorders generally associated with glomerulonephritis are:

- Group A beta-hemolytic *Streptococcus* infection (other infectious etiologies including endocarditis and visceral abscess)
- Collagen-vascular diseases (systemic lupus erythematosus [SLE])
- Vasculitis (Wegener's granulomatosis, polyarteritis nodosa)
- Idiopathic glomerulonephritis (membranoproliferative, idiopathic, crescentic, IgA nephropathy)
- Goodpasture's syndrome
- Other cryoglobulinemia (Henoch-Schönlein purpura)
- Drug-induced (gold, penicillamine)

Table 1-60 summarizes primary renal diseases that present as acute glomerulonephritis.

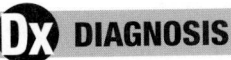

DIAGNOSIS

DIFFERENTIAL DIAGNOSIS

- Cirrhosis with edema and ascites
- Congestive heart failure
- Acute interstitial nephritis
- Severe hypertension
- Hemolytic-uremic syndrome
- SLE, diabetes mellitus, amyloidosis, preeclampsia, sclerodermal renal crisis

WORKUP

Initial evaluation of suspected glomerulonephritis consists of laboratory testing.

LABORATORY TESTS

- Urinalysis (hematuria [dysmorphic erythrocytes and red cell casts], proteinuria)
- Serum creatinine (to estimate glomerular filtration rate [GFR]), blood urea nitrogen
- 24-hr urine for protein excretion and creatinine clearance (to document degree of renal dysfunction and amount of proteinuria). Proteinuria in acute glomerulonephritis typically ranges from 500 mg/day to 3 g/day, but nephrotic-range proteinuria (>3.5 g/day) may be present.
- Streptococcal tests (Streptozyme), antistreptolysin O (ASO) quantitative titer (highest in 3 to 5 wk); ASO titer, however, is not related to severity of renal disease, duration, or prognosis.

TABLE 1-60 Summary of Primary Renal Diseases that Present as Acute Glomerulonephritis

Diseases	PSGN	IgA Nephropathy	Membranoproliferative Glomerulonephritis	Idiopathic RPGN
Clinical manifestations	All ages; mean, 7 yr, 2:1 male	15-35 yr; 2:1 male	15-30 yr; 6:1 male	Mean, 58 yr; 2:1 male
Age and sex	90%	50%	90%	90%
Acute nephritic syndrome	Occasionally	50%	Rare	Rare
Asymptomatic hematuria	10%-20%	Rare	Rare	10%-20%
Nephrotic syndrome	70%	30%-50%	Rare	25%
Hypertension	50% (transient)	Very rare	50%	60%
Acute renal failure	Latent period of 1-3 wk	Follows viral syndromes	Pulmonary hemorrhage; iron-deficiency anemia	None
Other				
Laboratory findings	↑ ASO titers (70%) Positive streptozyme (95%) ↓ C3-C9; Normal C1, C4	↑ Serum IgA (50%) IgA in dermal capillaries	Positive anti-GBM antibody	Positive ANCA
Immunogenetics	HLA-B12, D "EN" (9)*	HLA-Bw 35, DR4 (4)*	HLA-DR2 (16)*	None established
Renal Pathology				
Light microscopy	Diffuse proliferation	Focal proliferation	Focal → diffuse proliferation with crescents	Crescentic GN
Immunofluorescence	Granular IgG, C3	Diffuse mesangial IgA	Linear IgG, C3	No immune deposits
Electron microscopy	Subepithelial humps	Mesangial deposits	No deposits	No deposits
Prognosis	95% resolve spontaneously 5% RPGN or slowly progressive	Slow progression in 25%-50%	75% stabilize or improve if treated early	75% stabilize or improve if treated early
Treatment	Supportive	None established	Plasma exchange, steroids, cyclophosphamide	Steroid pulse therapy

Modified from Goldman L, Ausiello D (eds): *Cecil textbook of medicine,* ed 22, Philadelphia, 2004, WB Saunders.
ANCA, Antineutrophil cytoplasm antibody; *ASO,* antistreptolysin O; *GBM,* glomerular basement membrane; *GN,* glomerulonephritis; *HLA,* human leukocyte antigen; *Ig,* immunoglobulin; *PSGN,* post-streptococcal glomerulonephritis; *RPGN,* rapidly progressive glomerulonephritis.
*Relative risk.

- Additional useful tests depending on the history: anti-DNA antibodies (rule out SLE), CH_{50} level (if elevated, obtain C_3, C_4 levels), triglycerides, cryoglobulins, hepatitis B and C serologies, antineutrophil cytoplasmic antibody (ANCA), c-ANCA (in suspected cases of Wegener's granulomatosis), p-ANCA found in pauciimmune (lack of immune deposits) idiopathic rapidly progressive glomerulonephritis with or without systemic vasculitis, and antiglomerular basement membrane (type alpha[3] IV collagen) antibodies.
- Hematocrit (decrease in glomerulonephritis) and platelet count (thrombocytopenia in cases of lupus nephritis).
- Anti–glomerular basement membrane antibody (in Goodpasture's syndrome).
- Blood cultures are indicated in all febrile patients.

IMAGING STUDIES
- Chest x-ray: pulmonary congestion, Wegener's granulomatosis, and Goodpasture's syndrome.
- Renal ultrasound if GFR is depressed to evaluate renal size and determine extent of fibrosis. A kidney size of <9 cm is suggestive of extensive scarring and low likelihood of reversibility.
- Echocardiogram in patients with new cardiac murmurs or positive blood cultures to rule out endocarditis and pericardial effusion.
- Renal biopsy and light (Fig. 1-165), electron, and immunofluorescent microscopy to confirm diagnosis.
- Kidney biopsy: generally reveals a granular pattern in poststreptococcal glomerulonephritis and a linear pattern in Goodpasture's syndrome; absence of immune deposits suggests vasculitis. Renal biopsy, although helpful to define the etiology of glomerulonephritis, is not usually essential. It is useful to determine the degree of inflammation and fibrosis. It is also especially important for patients with rapidly progressive glomerulonephritis, in whom prompt diagnosis and treatment are essential.
- Immunofluorescence: generally reveals C_3. Negative immunofluorescence suggests Wegener's granulomatosis, idiopathic crescentic glomerulonephritis, or polyarteritis nodosa.
- Angiography or biopsy of other affected organs if systemic vasculitis is suspected.

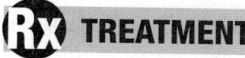 **TREATMENT**

NONPHARMACOLOGIC THERAPY
- Avoidance of salt if edema or hypertension is present
- Low-protein intake (approximately 0.5 g/kg/day) in patients with renal failure
- Fluid restriction in patients with significant edema
- Avoidance of high-potassium foods

ACUTE GENERAL Rx
- Correction of electrolyte abnormalities (hypocalcemia, hyperkalemia) and acidosis (if present)
- Treatment of streptococcal infection with penicillin (or erythromycin in penicillin-allergic patients)
- Furosemide in patients with significant hypertension and/or edema; hydralazine or nifedipine in patients with hypertension
- Immunosuppressive treatment in patients with heavy proteinuria or rapidly decreasing GFR (high-dose steroids, cyclosporin A, cyclophosphamide); corticosteroids generally not useful in poststreptococcal glomerulonephritis
- Fish oil (n-3 fatty acids) 12 g/day; may prevent or slow loss of renal function in patients with IgA nephropathy
- Plasma exchange therapy and immunosuppressive drugs (prednisone and cyclophosphamide); effective in Goodpasture's syndrome

- Short-term therapy with IV cyclophosphamide followed by maintenance therapy with mycophenolate mofetil or azathioprine is more efficacious and safer than long-term therapy with IV cyclophosphamide in patients with proliferative lupus nephritis

CHRONIC Rx
- Frequent monitoring of urinalysis, serum creatinine, and blood pressure in the initial 12 mo
- Monitoring for onset of hypertensive retinopathy, encephalopathy
- Aggressive treatment of infections, particularly streptococcal infections
- Dosage adjustment of all renally excreted medications

DISPOSITION
- Prognosis is generally related to histology, with excellent prognosis in patients with minimal change in glomerulonephritis and focal segmental proliferative glomerulonephritis. Between 25% and 30% of patients with mesangial IgA disease and membranous glomerulonephritis generally progress to chronic renal failure; >70% of patients with mesangial capillary glomerulonephritis will develop chronic renal failure.
- In general, prognosis is worse in patients with heavy proteinuria, severe hypertension, and significant elevations of creatinine.
- Recovery of renal function occurs within 8 to 12 wk in 95% of patients with poststreptococcal glomerulonephritis.

REFERRAL
- Nephrology consultation. The urgency for referral depends on the GFR. Urgent consultation is recommended if GFR is significantly abnormal or rapidly deteriorating or if the patient has systemic symptoms.
- Surgical referral for biopsy in selected cases.

(!) PEARLS & CONSIDERATIONS

COMMENTS
- Anticoagulation to prevent deep vein thrombosis should be considered in patients with a low level of physical activity.
- Monitoring of lipids and aggressive treatment of hyperlipidemias are recommended.
- Close monitoring of side effects of immunosuppressive drugs and complications of corticosteroids is necessary.

SUGGESTED READINGS
available at www.expertconsult.com

AUTHOR: **FRED F. FERRI, M.D.**

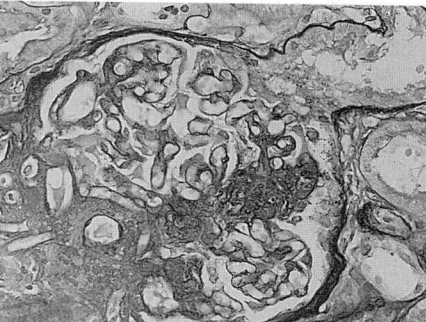
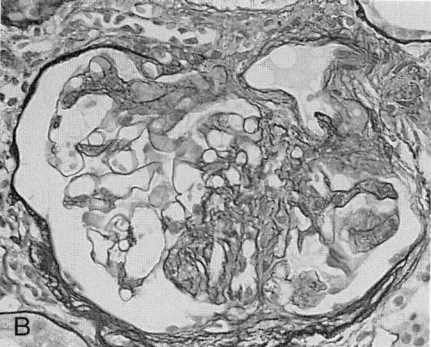

FIGURE 1-165 Light microscopic appearances in focal segmental glomerulosclerosis. Segmental scars with capsular adhesions in otherwise normal glomeruli. A, Periodic acid-Schiff, ×300. **B,** Methenamine silver stain, ×300. (Courtesy Dr. D. Davies. From Johnson RJ, Feehally J: *Comprehensive clinical nephrology,* ed 2, St Louis, 2000, Mosby.)

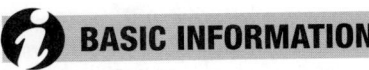

BASIC INFORMATION

DEFINITION

Glossitis is an inflammation of the tongue that can lead to loss of filiform papillae.

ICD-9CM CODES
529.0 Glossitis

EPIDEMIOLOGY & DEMOGRAPHICS

Glossitis is seen more frequently in patients of lower socioeconomic status, malnourished patients, alcoholics, smokers, elderly patients, immunocompromised patients, and patients with dentures.

PHYSICAL FINDINGS & CLINICAL PRESENTATION

- The appearance of the tongue varies depending on the etiology of the glossitis. Loss of filiform papillae results in a red, smooth-surfaced tongue (Fig. 1-166).
- The tongue may appear pale in patients with significant anemia.

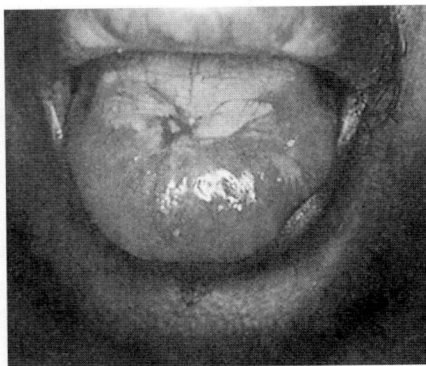

FIGURE 1-166 Glossitis. (From Seidel HM [ed]: *Mosby's guide to physical examination*, ed 4, St Louis, 1999, Mosby.)

- Pain and swelling of the tongue may be present when glossitis is associated with infections, trauma, or lichen planus.
- Ulcerations may be present in patients with herpetic glossitis, pemphigus, or streptococcal infection.
- Excessive use of mouthwash may result in a "hairy" appearance of the tongue.

ETIOLOGY

- Nutritional deficiencies (vitamin E, riboflavin, niacin, vitamin B_{12}, iron)
- Infections (viral, candidiasis, tuberculosis, syphilis)
- Trauma (generally caused by poorly fitting dentures)
- Irritation of the tongue from toothpaste, medications, alcohol, tobacco, citrus
- Lichen planus, pemphigus vulgaris, erythema multiforme
- Neoplasms

DIAGNOSIS

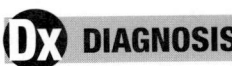

DIFFERENTIAL DIAGNOSIS

- Infections
- Use of chemical irritants
- Neoplasms
- Skin disorders (e.g., Behçet's syndrome, erythema multiforme)

WORKUP

- Laboratory evaluation to exclude infectious processes, vitamin deficiencies, and systemic disorders
- Biopsy of lesion only when there is no response to treatment

LABORATORY TESTS

- Complete blood count: decreased hemoglobin and hematocrit, low mean corpuscular volume (MCV) (iron-deficiency anemia), elevated MCV (vitamin B_{12} deficiency)
- Vitamin B_{12} level
- 10% KOH scrapings in patients with white patches suspect for candidiasis

TREATMENT

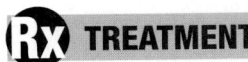

NONPHARMACOLOGIC THERAPY

Avoidance of primary irritants such as hot foods, spices, tobacco, and alcohol

ACUTE GENERAL Rx

Treatment varies with the etiology of the glossitis.

- Malnutrition with avitaminosis: multivitamins
- Candidiasis: fluconazole 200 mg on day 1, then 100 mg/day for at least 2 wk or nystatin 400,000 U suspension qid for 10 days or 200,000 pastilles dissolved slowly in the mouth four to five times qd for 10 to 14 days
- Painful oral lesions: rinsing of the mouth with 2% lidocaine viscous, 1 to 2 tablespoons q4h prn; triamcinolone 0.1% applied to painful ulcers prn for symptomatic relief

CHRONIC Rx

- Lifestyle changes with elimination of tobacco, alcohol, and other primary irritants
- Dental evaluation for correction of ill-fitting dentures
- Correction of associated metabolic abnormalities such as hyperglycemia from diabetes mellitus

DISPOSITION

Most patients experience prompt improvement with identification and treatment of the cause of the glossitis.

REFERRAL

Surgical referral for biopsy of solitary lesions unresponsive to treatment to rule out neoplasm

PEARLS & CONSIDERATIONS

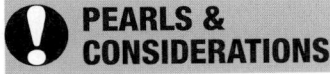

COMMENTS

If the primary cause of glossitis is not identified or cannot be corrected, enteric nutritional replacement therapy should be considered in malnourished patients.

AUTHOR: **FRED F. FERRI, M.D.**

BASIC INFORMATION

DEFINITION

Gonorrhea is a sexually transmitted bacterial infection with a predilection for columnar and transitional epithelial cells. It commonly manifests as urethritis, cervicitis, or salpingitis. Infection may be asymptomatic. It differs between males and females in course, severity, and ease of recognition.

SYNONYMS

Gonococcal urethritis
Gonococcal vulvovaginitis
Gonococcal cervicitis
Gonococcal bartholinitis
Clap; GC

ICD-9CM CODES
098 Gonococcal infections

EPIDEMIOLOGY & DEMOGRAPHICS

- The disease is common worldwide, affects both sexes and all ages, especially younger adults; highest incidence is in inner-city areas, with an estimated 700,000 new cases annually.
- Asymptomatic anterior urethral carriage may occur in 12% to 50% of cases in men.
- Asymptomatic in 50% to 80% of cases in women. Most common dissemination by mucosal passage to fallopian tubes, resulting in pelvic inflammatory disease (PID) in 10% to 15% of infected women. Hematogenous spread may result in septic arthritis and skin lesions. Conjunctivitis rarely occurs but may result in blindness if not rapidly treated. Infection can occur in both men and women in oropharynx and anorectally.
- 700,000 new infections per year (second most commonly reported bacterial STD).

PHYSICAL FINDINGS & CLINICAL PRESENTATION

- Males: purulent discharge from anterior urethra (Fig. 1-167) with dysuria appearing 2 to 7 days after infecting exposure. May have rectal infection causing pruritus, tenesmus, and discharge or may be asymptomatic.

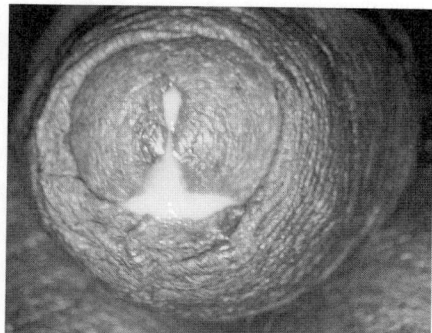

FIGURE 1-167 Purulent urethral discharge from a man with gonococcal urethritis. (From Mandell GL et al: *Principles and practice of infections diseases,* ed 6, Philadelphia, 2005, Elsevier.)

- Females: initial urethritis or cervicitis may occur a few days after exposure, frequently mild. In approximately 20% of cases uterine invasion occurs after menstrual period with signs and symptoms of endometritis, salpingitis, or pelvic peritonitis. The patient may have purulent discharge or inflamed Skene's or Bartholin's glands.
- Classic presentation of acute gonococcal PID is fever, abdominal and adnexal tenderness, and often absence of purulent discharge. Physical examination may be normal if asymptomatic.

ETIOLOGY

Neisseria gonorrhoeae is the gonococcus. Plasmids coding for β-lactamase render some strains resistant to penicillin or tetracycline. There is an increasing frequency of chromosomally mediated resistance to penicillin, tetracycline, fluoroquinolones, and cefoxitin. In the Far East, high-level resistance to spectinomycin is endemic.

There are a rising number of cases of quinolone-resistant *N. gonorrhoeae* worldwide, with the expected number to rise in the U.S. from importation.

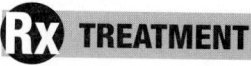

DIAGNOSIS

DIFFERENTIAL DIAGNOSIS

- Nongonococcal urethritis (NGU)
- Nongonococcal mucopurulent cervicitis
- *Chlamydia* trachomatis

WORKUP

- Diagnosis depends on bacteriologic investigation.
- Gram-negative intracellular diplococci are diagnostic in male urethral smears. There is a false-negative rate of 60% to 70% in female cervical or urethral smears. Culture, nucleic acid hybridization tests, and nucleic acid amplification tests (NAATs) are available for the detection of genitourinary infection with *N. gonorrhoeae.* Culture and nucleic acid hybridization tests require female endocervical or male urethral swab specimen. NAATs allow testing of the widest variety of specimen types including endocervical swabs, vaginal swabs, urethral swabs (men), and urine (from both men and women).

LABORATORY TESTS

- Gonorrhea culture on Thayer-Martin medium (organism is fastidious; requires aerobic conditions with increased carbon dioxide atmosphere; incubate ASAP). Culture has a sensitivity of 95% or more for urethral specimens from men with symptomatic urethritis and 80% to 90% for endocervical infection in women.
- NAATs: These tests have largely replaced culture in many settings where persons are screened for asymptomatic genital infection. They are not more sensitive than culture for detecting *N. gonorrhoeae* in cervical or urethral specimen; however, they have specificities >99% and retain sensitivity when used to test voided urine or self-collected vaginal swabs.
- Nonamplified DNA probe tests are less sensitive than culture or NAATs and are not useful in the diagnosis of rectal or pharyngeal infection or for testing urine; however, they are inexpensive, readily available and offered in many laboratories in combination assays for *C. trachomatis.*
- Concomitant serologic testing for syphilis on all patients
- Concomitant *Chlamydia* testing on all patients
- Offer of HIV counseling and testing to all patients

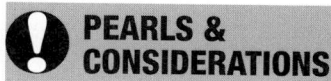

TREATMENT

ACUTE GENERAL Rx

Uncomplicated infections of the cervix, urethra, and rectum:
- Ceftriaxone 250 mg IM × 1 dose or
- Cefixime 400 mg po × 1 dose
Alternatives:
- Single-dose injectable cephalosporin (ceftizoxime 500 mg IM, cefotaxime 500 mg IM, or cefoxitin 2 g IM plus probenecid 1 g PO) plus azithromycin 1 g orally single dose or doxycycline 100 mg bid × 7 days

DISPOSITION

- Pregnant patients require test of cure (as do those treated with regimens other than ceftriaxone/doxycycline); reculture 4 to 7 days after treatment.
- Treatment failure in nonpregnant patients is rare, and test of cure is not required. Rescreening in 1 to 2 mo detects treatment failures and reinfections.
- All sexual partners should be identified, examined, tested, and receive presumptive treatment.

REFERRAL

PID requiring hospitalization, disseminated gonococcal infection

PEARLS & CONSIDERATIONS

COMMENTS

- This is a reportable disease.
- The proportion of gonorrhea cases in heterosexual men who are fluoroquinolone resistant (QRNG) has reached 6.7%, an elevenfold increase from 0.6% in 2001. Fluoroquinolone antibiotics are no longer recommended to treat gonorrhea in the U.S.

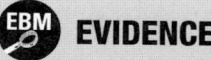

EVIDENCE

available at www.expertconsult.com

AUTHORS: **MARIA A. CORIGLIANO, M.D.,** and **RUBEN ALVERO, M.D.**

BASIC INFORMATION

DEFINITION

Goodpasture's syndrome is characterized by idiopathic recurrence of alveolar hemorrhage and rapidly progressive glomerulonephritis. It can also be defined by the triad of glomerulonephritis, pulmonary hemorrhage, and antibody to basement membrane antigens.

ICD-9CM CODES
446.2 Goodpasture's syndrome

EPIDEMIOLOGY & DEMOGRAPHICS

- Goodpasture's syndrome affects predominantly young, white, male smokers.
- Male/female ratio is 6:1.
- Goodpasture's syndrome accounts for 5% of all cases of rapidly progressive glomerulonephritis.
- 80% of patients are HLA-BR2 positive.

PHYSICAL FINDINGS & CLINICAL PRESENTATION

- Dyspnea, cough, hemoptysis
- Skin pallor, fever, arthralgias (may be mild or absent at the time of initial presentation)

ETIOLOGY

Presence of glomerular basement membranes (GBM) antibody deposition in kidneys and lungs with subsequent pulmonary hemorrhage and glomerulonephritis. In the kidneys circulating antibodies bind to the non-collagenous-1 (NC1) domain of type IV collagen in the GBM.

DIAGNOSIS

DIFFERENTIAL DIAGNOSIS

- Wegener's granulomatosis
- Systemic lupus erythematosus
- Systemic necrotizing vasculitis
- Idiopathic rapidly progressive glomerulonephritis
- Drug-induced renal pulmonary disease (e.g., penicillamine)

WORKUP

Laboratory evaluation, diagnostic imaging, immunofluorescence studies of renal biopsy

LABORATORY TESTS

- Presence of circulating serum anti-GBM antibodies
- Absence of circulating immunocomplexes, antineutrophils, cytoplasmic antibodies, and cryoglobulins
- Urinalysis revealing microscopic hematuria and proteinuria
- Elevated blood urea nitrogen and creatinine from rapidly progressive glomerulonephritis
- Immunofluorescence studies of renal biopsy material: linear deposits of anti-GBM antibody, often accompanied by C3 deposition
- Anemia from iron deficiency (from blood loss and iron sequestration in the lungs)

IMAGING STUDIES

Chest radiograph: fluffy alveolar infiltrates, evidence of pulmonary hemorrhage (Fig. 1-168)

TREATMENT

ACUTE GENERAL Rx

- Plasma exchange therapy
- Immunosuppressive therapy with prednisone (1 mg/kg/day) and cyclophosphamide (2 mg/kg/day)
- Dialysis support in patients with renal failure

DISPOSITION

Life-threatening pulmonary hemorrhage and irreversible glomerular damage are the major causes of death.

REFERRAL

- Referral for renal biopsy to guide the management
- Referral of patients with renal failure to dialysis center
- Consideration for renal transplantation in patients with end-stage renal failure

SUGGESTED READINGS
available at www.expertconsult.com

AUTHOR: **FRED F. FERRI, M.D.**

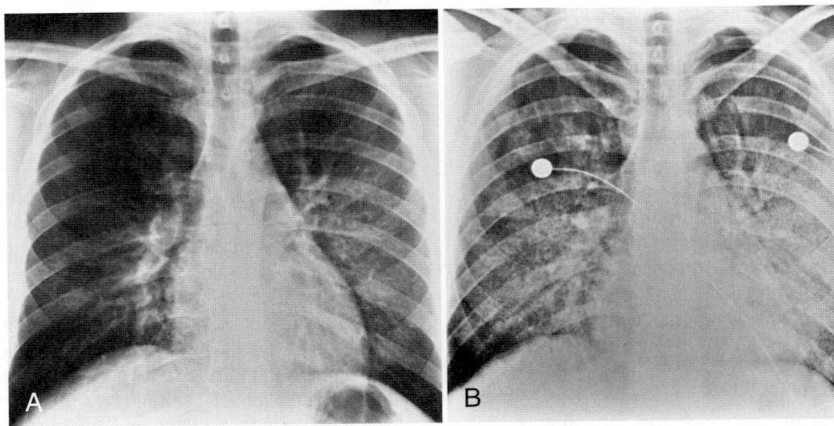

FIGURE 1-168 Goodpasture's syndrome. Posteroanterior chest radiographs several days apart demonstrate consolidation in the left lung **(A),** which progressed to diffuse alveolar disease (consolidation) **(B).** (From McLoud TC [ed]: *Thoracic radiology: the requisites,* St Louis, 1998, Mosby.)

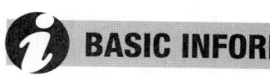 **BASIC INFORMATION**

DEFINITION

Gout is a disease caused by tissue deposition of monosodium urate due to prolonged hyperuricemia. Clinical manifestations of gout include acute arthritis, soft tissue inflammation, chronic tophus formation, gouty nephropathy, and nephrolithiasis. Untreated hyperuricemia in patients with gout may lead to chronic destructive deforming arthritis

ICD-9CM CODES
274.00 Gouty arthritis
274.01 Acute gout
274.02 Chronic gout
274.03 Gout with tophus

EPIDEMIOLOGY & DEMOGRAPHICS

PREVALENCE: 5 cases per 1000 persons in the United States. Incidence is rising.
PREDOMINANT SEX: Male:female ratio ~4:1
PREDOMINANT AGE: 30 to 50 yr in men. Older than 60 yr in women

ETIOLOGY

- Hyperuricemia and gout develop from excessive uric acid production, a decrease in the renal excretion of uric acid, or both.
- Primary hyperuricemia results from an inborn error of metabolism and may be attributed to several biochemical defects.
- Secondary hyperuricemia may develop as a complication of acquired disorders (e.g., leukemia) or as a result of the use of certain drugs (e.g., diuretics).
- Individuals with hyperuricemia who are predisposed with genetic factors develop clinical gout.

PHYSICAL FINDINGS & CLINICAL PRESENTATION
ACUTE GOUT:
- Rapid onset of pain and swelling and erythema of a distal joint and/or periarticular soft tissue
- May present as monoarthritis of any joint
- 10% to 15% of attacks are polyarticular
- Spontaneous resolution occurs over days to weeks

CHRONIC TOPHACEOUS GOUT (Fig. 1-169)
- Insidious onset of painless arthritis and soft tissue swelling
- Distal small joints characteristic
- May be confused with nodal osteoarthritis

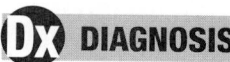 **DIAGNOSIS**

DIFFERENTIAL DIAGNOSIS OF ACUTE GOUT
- Infectious arthritis
- Cellulitis
- Pseudogout

DIFFERENTIAL DIAGNOSIS OF CHRONIC GOUT
- Osteoarthritis (especially nodal OA in women)
- Rheumatoid arthritis
- Psoriatic arthritis
Section II describes the differential diagnosis of acute monoarticular and oligoarticular arthritis.

WORKUP
Arthrocentesis and examination of synovial fluid

LABORATORY TESTS
- Uric acid: All patients with gout are hyperuricemic at some time, but during an acute attack the serum uric acid may be normal or low.
- Synovial aspirate: usually cloudy and markedly inflammatory in nature. Urate crystals in fluid are needle-shaped and strongly positively birefringent under polarized microscopy.
- CBC: mild leukocytosis often present
- Inflammatory markers: ESR and CRP often elevated

IMAGING STUDIES
- Plain radiography for diagnosis and evaluation.
- No typical findings in early gouty arthritis but late disease is associated with characteristic punched-out marginal erosions and overhanging edges

Rx **TREATMENT OPTIONS FOR ACUTE GOUT**

- Nonsteroidal anti-inflammatory medication (see Table 1-61)
  ○ Indomethacin 75 mg bid
  ○ Ibuprofen 800 tid
  ○ Naproxen 500 bid
- Low-dose colchicine (less toxic and as effective as traditional high-dose colchicine): 1.2 mg colchicine po, followed by 0.6 mg PO 1 hr later.

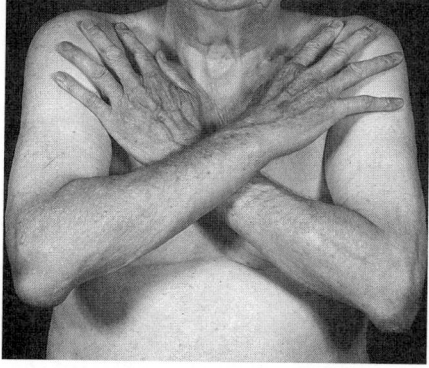

FIGURE 1-169 Tophi on the elbows in a patient with chronic polyarthritis affecting the fingers. The patient was thought to have nodular rheumatoid arthritis and was treated with sodium aurothiomalate injections despite a negative test for rheumatoid factor. (From Hochberg MC et al [eds]: *Rheumatology*, ed 3, St Louis, 2003, Mosby.)

- Intra-articular corticosteroid injection (treatment of choice for monoarticular large joint attack): Triamcinolone hexacetomide 40 mg or equivalent for knee
- Systemic corticosteroid therapy: Prednisone 40 mg PO for 3 days, then taper over 10 days (effective and safe, but evidence is lacking)

NONPHARMACOLOGIC THERAPY
Lifestyle and dietary modification may be effective in highly motivated patients. Should be attempted only inpatients with modestly elevated uric acid, as dietary modification can only lower uric acid 1 mg%. Discontinuation of diuretic therapy may help.

PHARMACOLOGIC TREATMENT OF SYMPTOMATIC HYPERURICEMIA
ALLOPURINOL: Allopurinol is very effective and safe when used properly. Correct dosing and patient compliance are essential elements in the prevention of erosive and tophaceous gout. Patients with renal insufficiency are at increased risk for allopurinol hypersensitivity, which is manifest as fever, rash, and hepatitis occurring most commonly in the first 3 mo of therapy. The rash may progress to life-threatening toxic epidermal necrolysis if not recognized early.

Therapy with allopurinol should be initiated several weeks after the acute attack has resolved. The initial dose should be low (≤100 mg/day depending on creatinine clearance) in patients with renal insufficiency and those with very high uric acid levels. The serum uric acid should be reevaluated after 4-6 wk of therapy, and the allopurinol dose adjusted to reduce the serum uric acid to less than 6 mg%. The most common therapeutic dosage of allopurinol is 300 mg/day, but dose may be increased as needed to achieve the target serum uric acid level. Some authors have reported using doses as high as 800 mg daily without excess toxicity.
BENEMID SULFINPYRAZONE: These uricosuric agents may only be used in patients with good renal function and urinary uric acid less than 600 mg in a 24-hr collection. Compliance is reduced due to necessity of taking drugs more often than once daily
FEBUXOSTAT: Novel xanthine oxidase inhibitor that has been shown to be more potent than allopurinol 300 mg daily for reducing serum uric acid. The chemical structure of febuxostat is different from allopurinol, making cross-reactive allergy unlikely. The metabolism of febuxostat is primarily hepatic, which obviates the need for dose adjustments due to renal insufficiency. Some cases of hepatic toxicity have been reported, and it is recommended that liver function tests be monitored periodically. Febuxostat has not been tested in patients with severe renal failure.

The primary indication for febuxostat is previous allergy to allopurinol.
PEGLOTICASE: Pegylated uricase approved by the FDA in 2010 for treatment of severe refractory tophaceous gout. Use will be limited by high cost and significant side effect profile.

PATIENT/FAMILY EDUCATION

It is essential that patients, families, physicians, and other members of the health care team appreciate the importance of compliance with a daily allopurinol regime if recurrent flares and progression to chronic arthritis and tophi are to be avoided. Allopurinol should be discontinued only for symptoms suggesting the hypersensitivity syndrome. It should be continued during flares, medical illnesses, and surgical procedures.

REFERRAL

- Rheumatologist if diagnosis is not clear or therapy is complicated
- Podiatrist for management of pedal complications

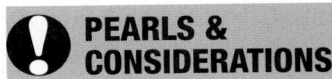

Do not stop allopurinol during hospitalizations, surgery, or acute attacks unless there is evidence of drug allergy.

SUGGESTED READINGS
available at www.expertconsult.com

AUTHOR: **BERNARD ZIMMERMANN, M.D.**

TABLE 1-61 Treatment of Gout

Acute Gout	Interval Gout	Treatment of Hyperuricemia
NSAIDs (preferred): Indomethacin 50 mg qid or ibuprofen 800 mg tid (or other NSAID in full doses). Contraindicated in patients with renal insufficiency and gastrointestinal disorders *Or* **Colchicine, oral:** 1.2 mg followed by a second dose of 0.6 mg 1 hr later. Contraindicated in patients with renal insufficiency and gastrointestinal disorders *Or* **Intra-articular steroids** (Treatment of choice for large joint monoarthritis): Triamcinolone 40 mg or equivalent for knee *Or* Systemic steroid therapy (for patients in whom NSAIDs and colchicine are contraindicated) Prednisone 30-50 mg PO daily or in divided doses. May use lower dose in diabetic or postsurgical patients	**Colchicine, oral:** 0.6-1.2 mg/day as prophylaxis against recurrent attacks. **NSAIDs may also be used for prophylaxis.** **Hypouricemic agent:** Indicated for patients with recurrent attacks despite prophylaxis, severe hyperuricemia, presence of tophi, urolithiasis, or gouty arthritis **Other:** Weight loss, reduce alcohol (especially beer), diet low in seafood, red meat, organ meat, and fructose	**Colchicine, oral:** 0.6-1.2 mg/day for 4-6 wk before initiating hypouricemic therapy and for several months afterward to prevent recurrent attacks during initiation of hypouricemic therapy. *And* **Allopurinol:** Initial dose 100 mg/day in patients with renal insufficiency or very high uric acid levels. Increase dose as needed to attain uric acid less than 6 mg/dl *Or* **Uricosuric agent** (Use only in patients with good renal function and <600 mg uric acid in a 24-hr collection): probenecid, 0.5-1 g bid, or sulfinpyrazone 100 mg tid or qid **Other:** Consider febuxostat for patients allergic to allopurinol. Pegloticase may be useful for selected patients with severe tophaceous gout.

NSAIDs, Nonsteroidal anti-inflammatory drugs.

BASIC INFORMATION

DEFINITION

Granuloma annulare (GA) is a chronic, usually self-limited, inflammatory disorder of the dermis that classically presents as arciform to annular plaques located on the extremities.

SYNONYMS

Pseudorheumatoid nodule—subcutaneous granuloma annulare
GA

ICD-9CM CODES
695.89 Granuloma annulare

EPIDEMIOLOGY & DEMOGRAPHICS

- Most common in children and young adults; most cases of localized granuloma annulare are diagnosed in patients <30 yr
- Female predominance (2:1)
- Disseminated form associated with diabetes mellitus
- Recurrent in 40% of affected individuals
- A generalized form of GA can occur in up to 15% of patients

PHYSICAL FINDINGS & CLINICAL PRESENTATION

- The four main clinical variants of granuloma annulare are localized (75%), disseminated (>10 lesions), subcutaneous (occurring primarily in children aged 2 to 5 yr), and perforating (rare form manifesting with 1- to 4-mm papules with a central crust).
- Localized granuloma annulare starts as a small ring of colored skin or pale erythematous papules.
- Lesions coalesce and evolve into annular plaques over several weeks.
- Plaques undergo central involution and increase in diameter over several months (0.5 to 5 cm) (Fig. 1-170).
- Most frequently found on the lateral and dorsal surfaces of the hands and feet.
- Most lesions resolve spontaneously after several months.
- The generalized form of GA is characterized by hundreds to thousands of small, flesh-colored papules in a symmetric distribution on the trunk and extremities.
- Deep dermal (subcutaneous GA) presents as large, painless, skin-colored nodules that are frequently mistaken for rheumatoid nodules.

ETIOLOGY

Unknown, but may be related to vasculitis, trauma, monocyte activation, or delayed hypersensitivity.

DIAGNOSIS

DIFFERENTIAL DIAGNOSIS

- Tinea corporis
- Lichen planus
- Necrobiosis lipoidica diabeticorum
- Sarcoidosis
- Rheumatoid nodules
- Late secondary or tertiary syphilis
- Arcuate and annular plaques of mycosis fungoides
- Papular GA can simulate insect bites, secondary syphilis, xanthoma
- Annular elastolytic giant cell granuloma

WORKUP

- Diagnosis based on clinical appearance and presentation
- Biopsy when diagnosis is unclear

LABORATORY TESTS

- No laboratory tests will help confirm the diagnosis.

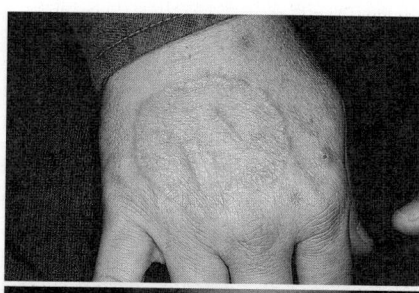
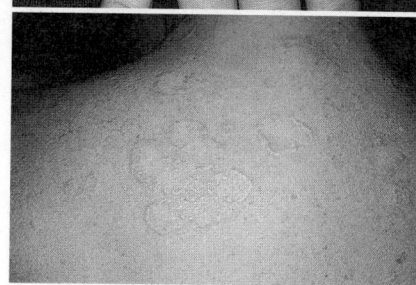

FIGURE 1-170 Granuloma annulare. (From Callen JP [ed]: *Color atlas of dermatology,* ed 2, Philadelphia, 2000, WB Saunders.)

- Biopsy shows focal degeneration of collagen and elastic fibers, mucin deposition, and perivascular and interstitial lymphohistiocytic infiltrate in the upper and middle dermis.

TREATMENT

NONPHARMACOLOGIC THERAPY

Reassurance, given the self-limited and benign nature of GA

CHRONIC Rx

High-potency topical corticosteroids with or without occlusion and intralesional steroid injection into elevated border with triamcinolone 2.5 to 10 mg/ml are useful first-line local therapies.

- Cryosurgery, psoralen ultraviolet-A (UVA) range or UVA-1 therapy, and carbon dioxide laser treatment can also be used.
- Systemic agents (e.g., niacinamide, hydroxychloroquine, chloroquine, cyclosporine, dapsone) are generally reserved for severe cases. Recent case reports indicate positive outcomes with tacrolimus and pimecrolimus and the tumor necrosis factor infliximab.

DISPOSITION

Most lesions resolve spontaneously within 2 yr.

REFERRAL

Dermatology referral recommended for symptomatic, disseminated disease

PEARLS & CONSIDERATIONS

COMMENTS

GA has been described as a paraneoplastic granulomatous reaction to Hodgkin's disease, non-Hodgkin's lymphoma, solid organ tumors, and mycosis fungoides.

SUGGESTED READING
available at www.expertconsult.com

AUTHOR: **FRED F. FERRI, M.D.**

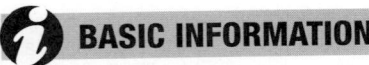

DEFINITION

Granuloma inguinale is a genital ulcerative disease caused by a gram-negative bacterium, *Calymmatobacterium granulomatis,* which may be sexually transmitted, possibly by anal intercourse. It can also be spread through close, long-term, nonsexual contact.

SYNONYMS

Donovanosis

ICD-9CM CODES
099.2 Granuloma inguinale

EPIDEMIOLOGY & DEMOGRAPHICS

INCIDENCE: Rare in the U.S. (<100 cases reported annually) and other developed countries
PREVALENCE: Endemic in Australia, India, Caribbean, and Africa; incubation period is variable (1 to 2 wk)
PREDOMINANT SEX: Can affect both males and females

PHYSICAL FINDINGS & CLINICAL PRESENTATION

- Clinically, the disease is commonly characterized as painless, slowly progressive ulcerative lesions on the genitals or perineum without regional lymphadenopathy; subcutaneous granulomas (pseudobobes) might also occur. The lesions are highly vascular (i.e., beefy red appearance [Fig. 1-171]) and bleed easily on contact.
- Pathogenic features:
  1. Large, infected mononuclear cell containing many Donovan bodies
  2. Intracytoplasmic location

ETIOLOGY

C. granulomatis is a gram-negative bacillus that reproduces within polymorphonuclear cells, plasma cells, and histiocytes, causing the infected cells to rupture 20 to 30 organisms.

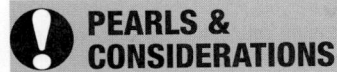 DIAGNOSIS

DIFFERENTIAL DIAGNOSIS

- Carcinoma
- Secondary syphilis: condylomata lata
- Amebiasis: necrotic ulceration
- Concurrent infections
- Lymphogranuloma venereum
- Chancroid
- Genital herpes

WORKUP

- Check for clinical manifestations.
  1. Lesions bleed easily.
  2. Lesions sharply defined and painless.
  3. Secondary infection may ensue.
  4. Inguinal involvement may cause pseudobuboes.
  5. Elephantiasis can result from obstruction of lymphatics.
  6. Suppuration and sinus formation are rare in female patients.
- Screen for other sexually transmitted diseases.
- Exclude other causes of lesions.
- Obtain stained, crushed prep from lesion.

A clinical algorithm for evaluation of genital ulcer disease is described in Section III.

Section II describes the differential diagnosis of genital sores.

LABORATORY TESTS

- The causative organism is difficult to culture, and diagnosis requires visualization of dark staining Donovan bodies with Wright stain (observation of Donovan bodies [intracellular bacteria]; organisms in vacuoles within macrophages)
- HIV testing of all patients

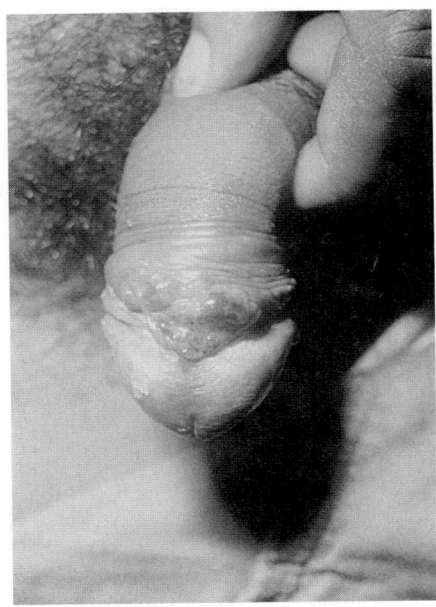

FIGURE 1-171 Involvement of the penis, with a beefy red, granulomatous ulceration in a patient with granuloma inguinale. (From Goldstein B [ed]: *Practical dermatology,* ed 2, St Louis, 1997, Mosby.)

TREATMENT

ACUTE GENERAL Rx

Recommended regimen:
- Doxycycline 100 mg orally bid × 3 wk minimum

Alternative regimens:
- Azithromycin 1 g PO/wk × 3 wk
- Ciprofloxacin 750 mg PO bid × 3 wk
- Erythromycin base 500 mg PO daily × 3 wk
- Trimethoprim/sulfamethoxazole, one double-strength tablet PO bid × 3 wk minimum
- All gentamicin 1 mg/kg IV q8h if no improvement within the first few days of therapy

CHRONIC Rx

If there is a poor initial response, extend treatment. Treatment of relapses is often necessary. Patients should be counseled to avoid risky sex practices and not resume having sex until infection is cleared.

DISPOSITION

Follow up clinically until signs and symptoms have resolved, then routine annual or semiannual visits

REFERRAL

If response is poor, consider referral to infectious disease specialist.

PEARLS & CONSIDERATIONS

COMMENTS

- Sexual partners within 60 days before onset of patient's symptoms should be examined and offered therapy.
- Pregnant women should be treated with erythromycin regimen.
- Patient education material can be obtained from local and state health clinics and also from American College of Obstetricians and Gynecologists.

SUGGESTED READING

available at www.expertconsult.com

AUTHORS: **GEORGE T. DANAKAS, M.D.,** and **RUBEN ALVERO, M.D.**

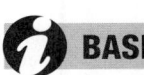

BASIC INFORMATION

DEFINITION

Graves' disease is a hypermetabolic state caused by circulating immunoglobulin (Ig) G antibodies that bind to and activate the G-protein–coupled thyrotropin receptor. This activation stimulates follicular hypertrophy and hyperplasia, causing thyroid enlargement as well as increases in thyroid hormone production. It is characterized by thyrotoxicosis, diffuse goiter, and infiltrative ophthalmopathy (edema and inflammation of the extraocular muscles and an increase in orbital connective tissue and fat); infiltrative dermopathy characterized by lymphocytic infiltration of the dermis; accumulation of glycosaminoglycans; and occasionally edema.

SYNONYMS

Thyrotoxicosis

ICD-9CM CODES
242.0 Toxic diffuse goiter

EPIDEMIOLOGY & DEMOGRAPHICS

INCIDENCE/PREVALENCE: Hyperthyroidism affects 2% of women and 0.2% of men in their lifetimes. More than 80% of these cases are caused by Graves' disease.
PREDOMINANT AGE: Peak incidence is between 40 and 60 yr.
GENETICS: Increased prevalence of HLA-B8 and HLA-DR3 in whites with Graves' disease. Concordance rate is 20% among monozygotic twins.

PHYSICAL FINDINGS & CLINICAL PRESENTATION

- Tachycardia, palpitations, tremor, hyperreflexia
- Goiter, exophthalmos (50% of patients), lid retraction, lid lag
- Nervousness, weight loss, heat intolerance, atrial fibrillation
- Increased sweating, brittle nails, clubbing of fingers
- Localized dermopathy (1% to 2% of patients) is most frequent over the anterolateral aspects of the skin but can be found at other sites (especially after trauma)
- Men may have gynecomastia, reduced libido, and erectile dysfunction. Women often have irregular menses

ETIOLOGY

Autoimmune etiology: the activity of the thyroid gland is stimulated by the action of T cells, which induce specific B cells to synthesize antibodies against thyroid-stimulating hormone (TSH) receptors in the follicular cell membrane.

DIAGNOSIS

DIFFERENTIAL DIAGNOSIS

- Anxiety disorder
- Premenopausal state
- Thyroiditis
- Other causes of hyperthyroidism (e.g., toxic multinodular goiter, toxic adenoma)
- Other: metastatic neoplasm, diabetes mellitus, pheochromocytoma

WORKUP

The diagnostic workup includes a detailed medical history followed by laboratory and imaging studies and ECG. Patients often present with anxiety, heat intolerance, menstrual dysfunction, increased appetite, and weight loss. Elderly patients can have an atypical presentation (apathetic hyperparathyroidism). For additional information, refer to the topic "Hyperthyroidism."

LABORATORY TESTS

- Increased free thyroxine (T_4) and free triiodothyronine (T_3)
- Decreased TSH
- Presence of thyroid-stimulating immunoglobulin or thyrotropin-receptor antibodies (useful in selected patients to differentiate Graves' disease from toxic nodular goiter)

IMAGING STUDIES

- 24-hr radioactive iodine uptake (RAIU): increased homogeneous uptake
- CT or MRI of the orbits is useful if there is uncertainty about the cause of ophthalmopathy

TREATMENT

NONPHARMACOLOGIC THERAPY

- Patient education and discussion of therapeutic options
- Smoking cessation: smoking is associated with an increased risk of progression of Graves' ophthalmopathy.

ACUTE GENERAL Rx

- Antithyroid drugs (ATDs) to inhibit thyroid hormone synthesis or peripheral conversion of T_4 to T_3:
  1. Methimazole or propylthiouracil (PTU) are available. Methimazole is generally preferred because it has a longer half-life, allowing for once-daily dosing. PTU is preferred during pregnancy.
  2. Side effects: skin rash (3% to 5%), arthralgias, myalgias, granulocytopenia (0.5%); rare side effects: aplastic anemia, hepatic necrosis (PTU), cholestatic jaundice.
- Radioactive iodine (RAI):
  1. Treatment of choice for patients >21 yr and younger patients who have not achieved remission after 1 yr of ATD therapy

  2. Contraindicated during pregnancy and lactation
- Surgery: near-total thyroidectomy is rarely performed. Indications: obstructing goiters despite RAI and ATD therapy, patients who refuse RAI and cannot be adequately managed with ATDs, and pregnant women inadequately managed with ATDs.
- Adjunctive therapy: Beta-adrenergic receptor blockers (e.g. atenolol 25 to 100 mg/day) to alleviate the β-adrenergic symptoms of hyperthyroidism (tachycardia, tremor); contraindicated in patients with bronchospasm.
- Graves' ophthalmopathy: methylcellulose eye drops to protect against excessive dryness, sunglasses to decrease photophobia, intraocular and systemic high-dose corticosteroids for severe exophthalmos. Worsening of ophthalmopathy after RAI therapy is often transient and can be prevented by the administration of prednisone. Other treatment options include antiinflammatory and immunosuppressive agents, radiation, and corrective surgical procedures.

CHRONIC Rx

Patients undergoing treatment with ATDs should be seen every 1 to 3 mo until euthyroidism is achieved and every 3 to 4 mo while they are receiving ATDs.

DISPOSITION

- ATDs induce sustained remission in <60% of cases.
- The incidence of hypothyroidism after RAI is >50% within the first year and 2% per year thereafter.
- Complications of surgery include hypothyroidism (28% to 43% after 10 yr), hypoparathyroidism, and vocal cord paralysis (1%).
- Successful treatment of hyperthyroidism requires lifelong monitoring for the onset of hypothyroidism or the recurrence of thyrotoxicosis.
- RAI therapy is followed by the appearance or worsening of ophthalmopathy more often than is therapy with methimazole, particularly in patients who are cigarette smokers. It can be prevented with the administration of prednisone 0.5 mg/kg body weight per day starting 2 to 3 days after RAI, continued for 1 mo, then tapered off over 2 mo.
- Mild to moderate ophthalmopathy often improves spontaneously. Severe cases can be treated with high-dose glucocorticoids, orbital irradiation, or both. Orbital decompression may be used in patients with optic neuropathy and exophthalmos (see "Hyperthyroidism").

SUGGESTED READINGS
available at www.expertconsult.com

AUTHOR: **FRED F. FERRI, M.D.**

BASIC INFORMATION

DEFINITION
Guillain-Barré syndrome (GBS) is an acute immune-mediated polyradiculoneuropathy (affects nerve roots and peripheral nerves), with predominant motor involvement. It is the most common cause of acute flaccid paralysis in the Western hemisphere and probably worldwide. By definition, maximal clinical weakness occurs within 4 wk of disease onset.

SYNONYMS
AIDP (acute inflammatory demyelinating polyradiculoneuropathy)
Acute polyneuropathy
Ascending paralysis
Postinfectious polyneuritis

ICD-9CM CODES
357.0 Guillain-Barré

EPIDEMIOLOGY & DEMOGRAPHICS
INCIDENCE:
- 0.6 to 1.9 cases/100,000 persons annually without geographic variation. Incidence increases with age. A slight peak in incidence occurs between late adolescence and early adulthood. A slight male preponderance (1.25:1) also exists.
- GBS consists of several clinical variants based on the pattern of clinical involvement and electrophysiologic findings. These include:
  - AIDP (most common form in Europe and North America)
  - Acute motor axonal neuropathy (AMAN; most prevalent form in China and Japan)
  - Acute motor and sensory axonal neuropathy (AMSAN; has more severe sensory involvement and is associated with more severe clinical course and poorer prognosis)
  - Miller Fisher syndrome (MFS; triad of ophthalmoplegia, ataxia, and areflexia)
  - Acute pandysautonomia (rapid onset of parasympathetic and sympathetic failure without motor or sensory involvement)
  - Regional variants (e.g., pharyngeal-cervical-brachial GBS, pure ataxic GBS)

PREDISPOSING FACTORS: Viral (HIV, CMV, EBV, influenza) and bacterial *(Campylobacter jejuni, Mycoplasma pneumonia)* infections; systemic illness (Hodgkin's lymphoma, immunizations)

PHYSICAL FINDINGS & CLINICAL PRESENTATION
- Symmetric weakness, most commonly involving proximal muscles initially, subsequently involving both proximal and distal muscles; difficulty in ambulating, getting up from a chair, or climbing stairs.
- Depressed or absent reflexes bilaterally.
- Minimal to moderate glove and stocking paresthesias/dysesthesia/anesthesia or back pain.
- Pain (caused by involvement of posterior nerve roots) may be prominent.
- Autonomic abnormalities (brady- or tachyarrhythmias, hypo- or hypertension).
- Respiratory insufficiency (caused by weakness of bulbar/intercostal muscles).
- Facial paresis, ophthalmoparesis, dysphagia (secondary to cranial nerve involvement).

ETIOLOGY
- Unknown
- Preceding infectious illness 1 to 4 wk before disease onset in 66% of patients
- Humoral and cell-mediated immune attack of peripheral nerve myelin, Schwann cells; sometimes with primary axonal involvement

DIAGNOSIS

DIFFERENTIAL DIAGNOSIS
- Toxic peripheral neuropathies: heavy metal poisoning (lead, thallium, arsenic), medications (vincristine, disulfiram), organophosphate poisoning, hexacarbon (glue sniffer's neuropathy)
- Nontoxic peripheral neuropathies: acute intermittent porphyria, fulminant vasculitic polyneuropathy, infectious (poliomyelitis, diphtheria, Lyme disease, West Nile virus); tick paralysis
- Neuromuscular junction disorders: myasthenia gravis, botulism, snake envenomations
- Myopathies such as polymyositis, acute necrotizing myopathies caused by drugs
- Metabolic derangements such as hypermagnesemia, hypokalemia, hypophosphatemia
- Acute CNS disorders such as basilar artery thrombosis with brain stem infarction, brain stem encephalomyelitis, transverse myelitis, or spinal cord compression
- Hysterical paralysis or malingering

WORKUP
1. Exclude other causes based on clinical history, examination, and laboratory tests.
2. Lumbar puncture (may be normal in the first 1 to 2 wk of the illness).
   Typical findings include elevated CSF protein with few mononuclear leukocytes (albuminocytologic dissociation) in 80% to 90% of patients. Elevated CSF cell counts is an expected feature in cases associated with HIV seroconversion.
3. EMG/NCS: may be normal in the first 10 to 14 days of the disease. The earliest electrodiagnostic abnormality is prolongation or absence of H-reflexes. EMG/NCS evidence of demyelination (prolonged distal latency, conduction velocity slowing, conduction block, temporal dispersion, and prolonged F-waves) in two or more motor nerves confirms diagnosis of AIDP in the appropriate clinical context.

LABORATORY TESTS
- CBC may reveal early leukocytosis with left shift. Electrolytes are tested to exclude metabolic causes.
- Heavy metal testing, urine porphyria screen, creatine kinase, HIV titers, neuroimaging of the brain and spinal cord if diagnosis uncertain. Nerve root enhancement may be seen on MRI of the lumbosacral spine.
- Antibodies against ganglioside GQ1b may be present in up to 90% of patients with MFS. IgG antibodies against ganglioside GM1 may be associated with AMAN. There are no antiganglioside antibodies commonly associated with AIDP.
- In equivocal cases (especially if peripheral nerve vasculitis is a concern), nerve biopsy may aid in confirming a diagnosis of GBS. Sensory nerve biopsy demonstrates segmental demyelination with infiltration of monocytes and T cells into the endoneurium. Axonal loss is commonly seen in sensory nerve biopsy specimens in GBS.

TREATMENT

NONPHARMACOLOGIC THERAPY
- Close monitoring of respiratory function (frequent measurements of vital capacity, negative inspiratory force, and pulmonary toilet), because respiratory failure is the major complication in GBS
- Frequent repositioning of patient to minimize formation of pressure sores
- Prevention of thromboembolism with antithrombotic stockings and SC heparin (5000 U q12h) in nonambulatory patients
- Emotional support and social counseling

ACUTE GENERAL Rx
- Infusion of IV immunoglobulins (IVIG; 0.4 g/kg/day for 5 days). Always check serum IgA levels before infusion to prevent anaphylaxis in deficient patients.
- Early therapeutic plasma exchange (TPE or plasmapheresis: 200 to 250 ml/kg over five sessions every other day), started within 7 days of onset of symptoms, is beneficial in reducing the need for mechanical ventilation in patients with rapidly progressive disease and results in improved rate of recovery. It is contraindicated in patients with cardiovascular disease (recent MI, unstable angina), active sepsis, and autonomic dysfunction.
- There is no proven benefit from combining IVIG and plasma exchange.
- Mechanical ventilation may be needed if FVC is <12 to 15 ml/kg, vital capacity is rapidly decreasing or is <1000 ml, negative inspiratory force <20 cm H$_2$O, PaO$_2$ is <70, the patient is having significant difficulty clearing secretions or is aspirating.

CHRONIC Rx
- Ventilatory support: may be necessary in 10% to 20% of patients. Adequate fluid/electrolyte support and nutrition are necessary, especially in patients with dysautonomia or bulbar dysfunction.
- Aggressive nursing care to prevent decubitus, infections, fecal impactions, and pressure nerve palsies.
- Monitoring and treatment of autonomic dysfunction (bradyarrhythmias or tachyarrhyth-

mias, orthostatic hypotension, systemic hypertension, altered sweating).

- Treatment of back pain and dysesthesia with low-dose tricyclics, gabapentin, and so on. Opiate narcotics can be used cautiously in the short term but may compound dysautonomia.
- Stress ulcer prevention in patients receiving ventilator support.
- Physical and occupational therapy rehabilitation, including supportive devices.

DISPOSITION

- Mortality is approximately 5% to 10% worldwide. Causes of death include cardiac arrest, pulmonary embolism, and fulminant infections. A recent study showed 62% complete motor recovery, 14% mild weakness, 9% moderate weakness, 4% bed-bound or ventilated, and 8% dead at 1 yr. Another study suggested that about 33% of patients were free from sensory symptoms at 1 yr, with residual sensory loss present in the lower extremities in 67% and 36% in the upper extremities. About 32% had to change their

work, 30% were unable to function at home as well as they could before the disease, and 52% had to alter their leisure activities 1 yr after GBS onset. Excessive fatigue is a common complaint in patients during the recovery phase of GBS. This may be treated with exercise therapy (e.g., bicycle exercise training).

- Predictors for poor recovery (inability to walk independently at 1 yr): age >60 yr, preceding diarrheal illness, recent CMV infection, fulminant or rapidly progressing course, ventilatory dependence, reduced motor amplitudes (<20% normal), or inexcitable nerves on NCS. Outcomes may also be influenced by complications of medical therapy.
- GBS is typically a monophasic illness. Recurrence may occur in <5% of patients following full recovery.

REFERRAL

Tracheostomy may be necessary in patients with prolonged ventilatory support. Percutaneous endoscopic gastrostomy may be temporarily required.

 PEARLS & CONSIDERATIONS

- GBS is the most common cause of acute flaccid paralysis.
- Close monitoring of ventilatory function with respiratory mechanics (FVC and NIF) is of paramount importance in all patients with suspected GBS.

COMMENTS

Patient education information may be obtained from the Guillain-Barré Foundation International, The Holly Building, 104 1/2 Forrest Avenue, Narberth, PA 19072; phone: (610) 667-0131; fax: (610) 667-7036; toll-free: (866) 224-3301; E-mail: info@gbs-cidp.org

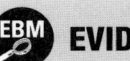 **EVIDENCE**

available at www.expertconsult.com

SUGGESTED READINGS

available at www.expertconsult.com

AUTHOR: **EROBOGHENE E. UBOGU, M.D.**

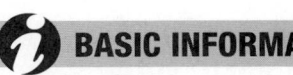 BASIC INFORMATION

DEFINITION
Gynecomastia is a benign enlargement of male breast, resulting from proliferation of glandular breast tissue.

ICD-9CM CODES
611.1 Gynecomastia

EPIDEMIOLOGY
- Most common reason for male breast evaluation.
- Seen in patients of all age groups.
- 60% to 90% of infants have transient gynecomastia due to high estrogenic state of pregnancy.
- Prevalence during adolescence ranges from 4% to 69%. It results from transient increase of estradiol concentration at the onset of puberty.
- Higher incidence in body builders due to use of anabolic steroids.
- 24% to 65% of older men have gynecomastia. It is secondary to decrease testosterone production with advanced age, increased peripheral conversion of testosterone to estrogen, and at times from side effects of medications.

PATHOPHYSIOLOGY
Altered estrogen-androgen balance, in favor of estrogen.

ETIOLOGY
Physiological
  Infancy
  Puberty
  Persistent pubertal gynecomastia seen in 25% of cases
  Elderly
Pathological
  Idiopathic (25%)
  Increased estrogen production or action
    Testicular tumors (3%)
    Chronic liver disease
    Malnutrition
    Hyperthyroidism
    Adrenal tumors
    Familial gynecomastia
  Decreased testosterone production or action (10%)
    Testicular trauma
    Testicular torsion
    Viral orchitis
    Congenital anorchia
    Renal failure (1%)
    Hyperthyroidism (1.5%)
    Malnutrition
    Androgen insensitivity syndrome
    Five-alpha reductase deficiency
    Pituitary tumors
    Kallmann syndrome
    Klinefelter's syndrome
  Medications (10% to 25%)
    Estrogen, gonadotropins, clomiphene, phenytoin, ketoconazole, metronidazole, metoclopramide, alkylating agents, busulfan, methotrexate, cisplatin, cimetidine, ranitidine, omeprazole, flutamide, finasteride, etomidate, HAART therapy, INH, tricyclic antidepressants, phenothiazines, diazepam, haloperidol, calcium channel blocker, ACE inhibitors, spironolactone, digoxin, amiodarone, methyldopa, alcohol, marijuana, heroin, methadone, amphetamine, anabolic steroids

CLINICAL FEATURES
- Although gynecomastia is usually bilateral, it could be unilateral.
- Characterized by concentric rubbery to firm disk of tissue, which is often mobile and located directly beneath the areola.
- Pain is usually not severe. Varying degree of tenderness and nipple sensitivity are more common than pain, usually in the first 6 mo.

Dx DIAGNOSIS

- Good history and physical examination including review of all medications the patient is taking is helpful.
- Mammogram is recommended for suspected breast cancer.
- Serum concentration of hCG, LH, testosterone, and estradiol should be measured, preferably in the morning, unless the cause is clearly apparent. There is no uniformity of opinion regarding what biochemical evaluation, if any, should be performed in patients with asymptomatic gynecomastia (see Fig. 1-172).

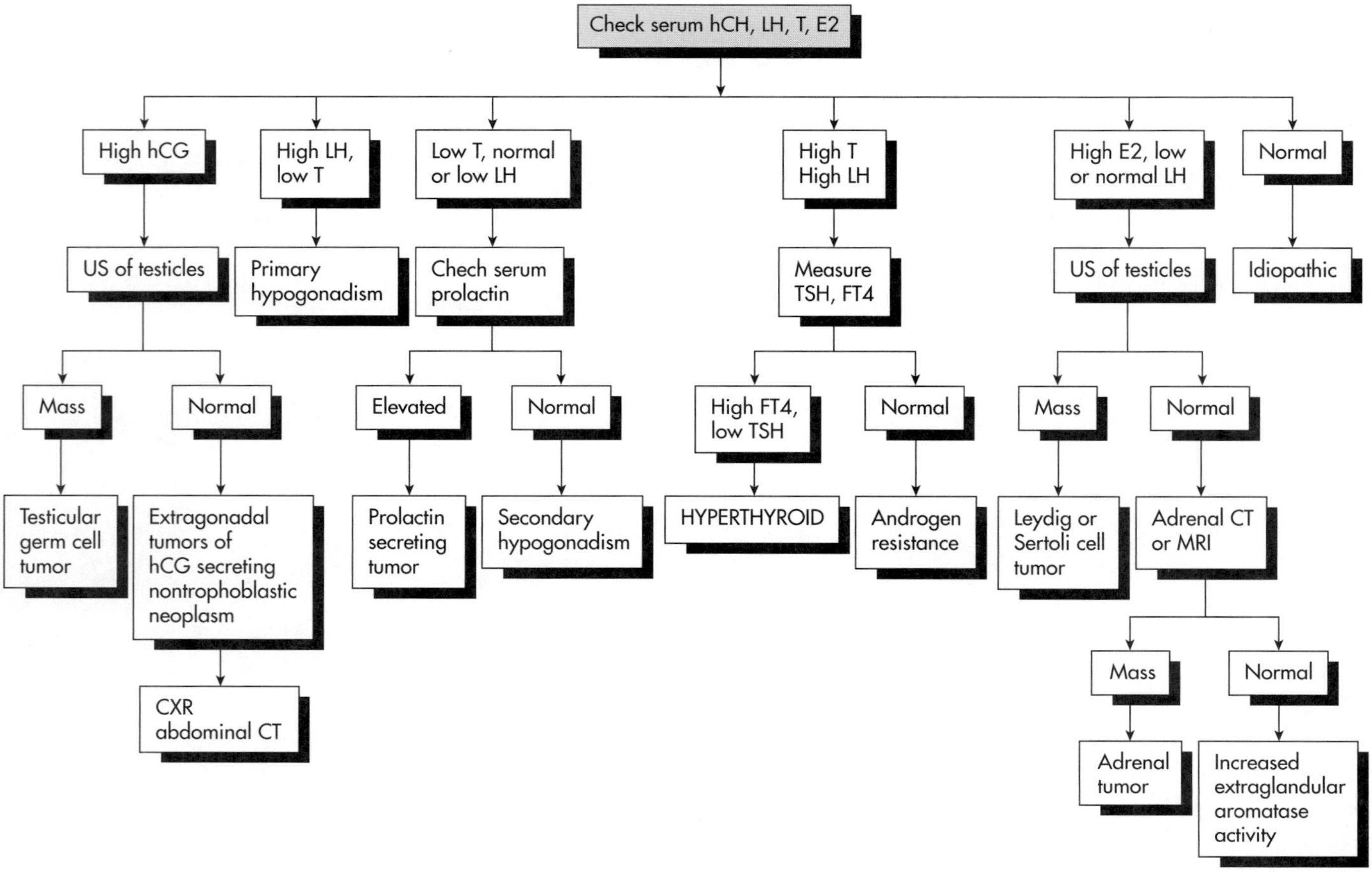

Check serum hCH, LH, T, E2

| High hCG | High LH, low T | Low T, normal or low LH | High T High LH | High E2, low or normal LH | Normal |

US of testicles — Primary hypogonadism — Chech serum prolactin — Measure TSH, FT4 — US of testicles — Idiopathic

Mass — Normal — Elevated — Normal — High FT4, low TSH — Normal — Mass — Normal

Testicular germ cell tumor — Extragonadal tumors of hCG secreting nontrophoblastic neoplasm — Prolactin secreting tumor — Secondary hypogonadism — HYPERTHYROID — Androgen resistance — Leydig or Sertoli cell tumor — Adrenal CT or MRI

CXR abdominal CT

Mass — Normal

Adrenal tumor — Increased extraglandular aromatase activity

FIGURE 1-172 Gynecomastia algorithm

DIFFERENTIAL DIAGNOSIS

- Breast cancer
  - Mass is usually firm to hard
  - Unilateral
  - Eccentric in location
  - Could be associated with nipple discharge and retraction, lymphadenopathy, and skin dimpling
- Pseudogynecomastia or lipomastia
  - Characterized by fat deposition without glandular proliferation
  - Seen in obese men
  - Bilateral
  - Remain unchanged over time

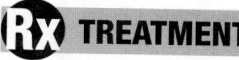 **TREATMENT**

- Observation is recommended for most patients with physiological gynecomastia. They often regress spontaneously. Reassurance and follow-up examination in 3 to 6 mo usually suffice.
- Treat the underlying cause, and stop the offending medications.
- Treatment is most effective in the early stages (first 6 mo). Medical therapy often fails when given for longstanding (>12 mo) cases because of the presence of fibrosis.
- Potential indications of early therapy include severe breast enlargement, pain, tenderness, and psychological embarrassment. Consider giving tamoxifen 10 mg orally twice a day to these patients for up to 3 mo. It is not FDA-approved for this purpose. It results in regression of gynecomastia in approximately 80% of patients and, of which, only 60% had complete regression. As far as breast symptoms, such as pain and tenderness, some improvement is usually seen within a month of therapy.
- Surgery is offered for symptomatic gynecomastia that does not respond to medical therapy. However, for adolescents, surgery is deferred until puberty is completed. The different surgical options include subcutaneous mastectomy, ultrasound-guided liposuction, and suction-assisted lipectomy.
- For prevention of gynecomastia in patients with prostate cancer using antiandrogen therapy, one could offer tamoxifen or radiotherapy.

SUGGESTED READINGS

available at www.expertconsult.com

AUTHOR: **HEMANT K. SATPATHY, M.D.**

G

Diseases and Disorders

I

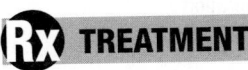
BASIC INFORMATION

DEFINITION

Hand-foot-mouth (HFM) disease is a viral illness characterized by superficial lesions of the oral mucosa and skin of the extremities. HFM is transmitted primarily by respiratory droplet contact in developed areas and feco-oral contact in developing countries. Although children are predominantly affected, adults are also at risk. This disease is usually self-limited and benign, although outbreaks in the Asia Pacific Region have been increasingly complicated by neurological and cardiopulmonary sequelae.

SYNONYMS

Vesicular stomatitis with exanthem
Coxsackievirus infection

ICD-9CM CODES
074.0 Hand-foot-mouth disease

EPIDEMIOLOGY & DEMOGRAPHICS

- Children <5 yr are at the highest risk and have the most severe cases.
- HFM is usually found in children <10 yr.
- HFM is contagious. Close contacts of affected children, including family members and health care workers, are the most commonly affected adults.
- Infection is spread from person to person by direct contact with nasal discharge or stool.
- A person is most contagious during the first week of illness.
- Outbreaks tend to occur during the summer.
- Infection leads to immunity, but a second episode may occur after infection with a different agent.

PHYSICAL FINDINGS & CLINICAL PRESENTATION

Symptoms:
- After a 4- to 6-day incubation period, patients may report odynophagia, sore throat, malaise, and fever (38.3° to 40° C).
- 1 to 2 days later the characteristic oral lesions appear.
- In 75% of cases skin lesions on the extremities accompany these oral manifestations.
- 11% of adults have cutaneous findings.
- Lesions appear over the course of 1 or 2 days.

Physical findings:
- Oral lesions, usually between five and ten, are commonly found on the tongue, buccal mucosa, gingivae, and hard palate.
- Oral lesions initially start as 1- to 3-mm erythematous macules and evolve into gray vesicles on an erythematous base.
- Vesicles are frequently broken by the time of presentation and appear as superficial gray ulcers with surrounding erythema.
- Skin lesions of the hands and feet start as linear erythematous papules (3 to 10 mm in diameter) that evolve into gray vesicles that may be mildly painful (Fig. 1-173). These vesicles are usually intact at presentation and remain so until they desquamate within 2 wk.
- Involvement of the buttocks and perineum is present in 31% of cases.
- In rare cases, encephalitis, meningitis, myocarditis, poliomyelitis-like paralysis, and pulmonary edema may develop. Sporadic acute paralysis and long term neurologic sequelae have been reported with Enterovirus 71.
- Although information is limited, there is no clear evidence that pregnancy outcomes are affected.

ETIOLOGY

- Coxsackievirus group A, type 16, was the first and is the most common viral agent isolated.
- Coxsackie viruses A5, A7, A9, A10, B1, B2, B3, B5, and Enterovirus 71 have also been implicated.
- Enterovirus 71 infection rates have been rising in the Asian Pacific region. This virus may lead to more severe cases of the disease including CNS involvement.

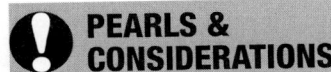
DIAGNOSIS

DIFFERENTIAL DIAGNOSIS

- Aphthous stomatitis
- Herpes simplex infection
- Herpangina
- Behçet's disease
- Erythema multiforme
- Pemphigus
- Gonorrhea
- Acute leukemia
- Lymphoma
- Allergic contact dermatitis

WORKUP

The diagnosis is usually made on the basis of history and characteristic physical examination.

LABORATORY TESTS

- Not indicated unless the diagnosis is in doubt.
- Throat culture or stool specimen may be obtained for viral testing but may take from 2 to 4 wk for results.

TREATMENT

ACUTE GENERAL Rx

- Palliative therapy is given for this usually self-limited disease.
- Limited data suggest acyclovir may have a role in treatment of certain cases.

DISPOSITION

Prognosis is excellent except in rare cases of central nervous system or cardiac involvement. Most are managed as outpatients.

REFERRAL

Not usually needed

PEARLS & CONSIDERATIONS

- Frequent handwashing, disinfection of contaminated surfaces, and washing of soiled articles of clothing can help reduce transmission.
- HFM has no relation to hoof and mouth disease in cattle.

SUGGESTED READINGS
available at www.expertconsult.com

AUTHORS: **JAMES J. NG, M.D.,** and **JENNIFER JEREMIAH, M.D.**

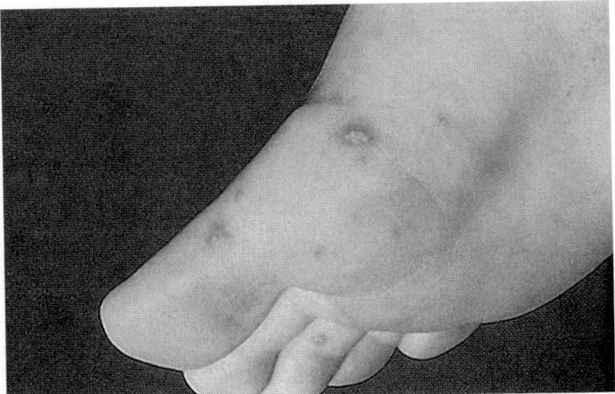

FIGURE 1-173 Hand-foot-mouth disease. Note oval lesions on an erythematous base. (From Goldstein B [ed]: *Practical dermatology,* ed 2, St Louis, 1997, Mosby.)

BASIC INFORMATION

DEFINITION

Hantavirus pulmonary syndrome (HPS) is a severe infectious cardiopulmonary illness usually caused by the Sin Nombre virus (SNV), whose main vector is the deer mouse.

SYNONYMS

Four Corners disease
Hantavirus cardiopulmonary syndrome

ICD-9CM CODES
079.81

EPIDEMIOLOGY & DEMOGRAPHICS

- First identified in the U.S. in 1993, Hantavirus has been found throughout the Continental U.S. and the Americas.
- As of 2005, 396 cases have been identified in 31 states with a mortality rate of 37%.
- The peak incidence to date was in June and July 1993 in the Four Corners region of the U.S.
- HPS is more common in the spring and summer.
- HPS is more prevalent among males, most likely because of increased environmental exposure.
- Mean age is 38 yr.
- HPS has not been found at the extremes of age.
- Risk factors include exposure to rodent populations, rural locales, occupations with increased exposure to rodents, and entering infrequently opened structures.

CLINICAL PRESENTATION

- The most common symptoms are fever, headache, nausea, vomiting, cough, shortness of breath, and myalgia. It is not associated with rhinorrhea or nasal congestion.
- The most common signs on physical examination include fever, hypoxemia, and tachypnea. Rash, mucosal bleeding, or peripheral edema is not found with HPS.
- There are two phases of HPS, the prodromal phase and the cardiopulmonary phase. The prodromal phase is characterized by:
  - Fever, chills, headache, and myalgias, especially in the legs and back
  - Cough, nausea, vomiting, and general malaise
  - Tachypnea, tachycardia, hypoxemia

- The cardiopulmonary phase has the following characteristics:
  - Cough and dyspnea
  - Acute pulmonary edema
  - Hypotension
  - Decreased cardiac output

ETIOLOGY

- HPS is most often caused by the Sin Nombre virus.
- The main vector is the deer mouse.
- It is transmitted by inhalation of aerosolized feces, urine, or saliva from infected rodents.
- No cases of person-to-person transmission have been reported.

DIAGNOSIS

DIFFERENTIAL DIAGNOSIS

- Acute respiratory distress syndrome
- Pneumonia
- Congestive heart failure
- Pulmonary edema
- Acute bacterial endocarditis
- Gastroenteritis
- Plague
- Tularemia ("rabbit fever")
- Histoplasmosis
- Coccidioidomycosis
- Cardiogenic shock
- HIV/AIDS
- Myocardial infarction
- Goodpasture's syndrome—an autoimmune pulmonary disease

WORKUP

- Complete blood count q8h.
  1. All patients manifest thrombocytopenia, and its progression is the most consistent indicator heralding the cardiopulmonary phase of HPS.
  2. Differential usually reveals a left shift. White blood cell counts are an unreliable indicator of severity of infection.
- Lactate level >4 mg/dl is associated with a high mortality rate.
- Rapid immunoblot strip assay for SNV antibodies.
- Diagnosis is confirmed by identification of immunoglobulin M and G antibodies to SNV.

IMAGING STUDIES

Chest radiograph: pulmonary edema

TREATMENT

NONPHARMACOLOGIC THERAPY

- Intensive care unit admission in tertiary care center
- Mechanical ventilation with high pulmonary end-expiratory pressure and high Fio_2
- Pulmonary artery catheterization
- Extracorporeal membrane oxygenation (ECMO)

ACUTE GENERAL Rx

- Supportive measures
- Supplemental oxygen
- Intubation when indicated
- Fluid resuscitation
- Hemodynamic monitoring
- Initial broad-spectrum antibiotics
- Pressors
- No medication is effective against SNV

DISPOSITION

- Patients who survive cardiopulmonary phase of HPS have rapid clinical improvement.
- There are no serious sequelae.

REFERRAL

University of New Mexico Hospital is the only facility with experience in ECMO for treatment of HPS. This modality is only for hemodynamically unstable, critically ill patients who do not respond to conventional therapies.

PEARLS & CONSIDERATIONS

COMMENTS

- Although rare, HPS should be a consideration in those with acute respiratory illness and a history suggestive of HPS exposure. The combination of thrombocytopenia, left shift, circulating immunoblasts, and hemoconcentration is rare in other viral illnesses.
- Testing for hantavirus should always be considered in cases of thrombocytopenia and fever of unknown origin, especially in areas endemic for the infection.

PREVENTION

Rodent control is the primary way to prevent Hantavirus infection.

SUGGESTED READINGS
available at www.expertconsult.com

AUTHOR: **CATHERINE SHAFTS, D.O.**

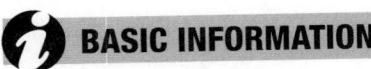

BASIC INFORMATION

DEFINITION

The term *cluster headache* refers to attacks of severe, unilateral pain that is orbital, supraorbital, temporal, or any combination of these sites, lasting 15 to 180 minutes, and occurring from once every other day to eight times a day. The attacks are associated with one or more of the following, all of which are ipsilateral: conjunctival injection, lacrimation, nasal congestion, rhinorrhea, forehead and facial sweating, miosis, ptosis, and eyelid edema. Most patients are restless or agitated during an attack.

SYNONYMS

Ciliary neuralgia
Erythromelalgia of the head
Erythroprosopalgia of Bing
Horton's headache

ICD-9CM CODES
346.2 Variants of migraine

EPIDEMIOLOGY & DEMOGRAPHICS

INCIDENCE: Estimated to occur in 0.05% to 1% of the population
PREDOMINANT SEX: Occurs in males at least five times more commonly than in females
PREDOMINANT AGE: Peak age of onset between 20 and 40 yr
GENETICS: May be inherited (autosomal dominant) in approximately 5% of cases

PHYSICAL FINDINGS & CLINICAL PRESENTATION

- During attack: ipsilateral conjunctival injection, lacrimation, nasal congestion, rhinorrhea, facial sweating, Horner's syndrome.
- In contrast to migraine sufferers, patients are agitated and active during an attack.
- Permanent partial Horner's syndrome in 5% of patients; otherwise examination is normal.

ETIOLOGY

Activation of the posterior hypothalamic grey matter resulting in trigeminal activation coupled with parasympathetic activation. The pathophysiology remains controversial.

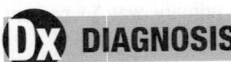

DIAGNOSIS

- Severe or very severe unilateral orbital, supraorbital, and/or temporal pain lasting 15 to 180 minutes.

- Frequency of every other day to eight per day; they may cluster seasonally or at a certain time in a patient's life.
- Headache is accompanied by at least one of the following (ipsilateral):
  1. Conjunctival injection and/or lacrimation
  2. Nasal congestion and/or rhinorrhea
  3. Eyelid edema
  4. Forehead and facial sweating
  5. Miosis and/or ptosis
  6. Restlessness or agitation

DIFFERENTIAL DIAGNOSIS

- Migraine
- Trigeminal neuralgia
- Temporal arteritis
- Postherpetic neuralgia
- Venous sinus thrombosis
- Carotid-cavernous fistula or other cavernous sinus lesions
- Other trigeminal autonomic cephalalgias
- Section II describes the differential diagnosis of headaches

WORKUP

Diagnosis is usually established by characteristic history.

IMAGING STUDIES

None, unless history or examination suggests focal neurologic deficit or headaches change in character or are of new onset.

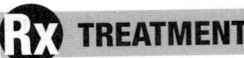

TREATMENT

NONPHARMACOLOGIC THERAPY

Avoidance of alcohol, histamine, nitroglycerine, and tobacco during clusters

ABORTIVE Rx

- Inhalation of 100% oxygen by face mask for 15 min often aborts an attack.
- About 75% of users of triptans (sumatriptan, zolmatriptan) will be pain free within 20 minutes.
- Cafergot, octreotide, intranasal lidocaine, or dihydroergotamine may abort an attack or prevent one if given just before a predictable episode. Acute episode is typically resolved before oral analgesics become effective, although indomethacin and other NSAIDs may also be effective in prolonged attacks.

- Acute episode is typically resolved before oral analgesics become effective, although indomethacin and other NSAIDs may also be effective in prolonged attacks.

PROPHYLAXIS Rx

Various medications have been tried without great success, although good responses may be obtained in up to 50% of cases. Examples include:

- Valproic acid: start at 500 mg/day
- Topiramate: up to 50 mg bid
- Verapamil: up to 480 mg/day as tolerated
- Lithium: 200 mg tid with frequent monitoring and adjustment to maintain therapeutic serum level of 0.4 to 1 mEq/L. Equally effective as verapamil, but with more side effects
- Methysergide: 1 to 2 mg tid; requires familiarity with the potential adverse effects and use of "drug holidays" to decrease risk of fibrosis
- Ergotamine tartrate: 3 to 4 mg/day during clusters
- Prednisone: 60 mg PO qd for 1 wk followed by taper; headaches can return during taper

DISPOSITION

Headache-free periods tend to increase with increasing age.

REFERRAL

Refractory cluster headaches may require referral to a headache specialist.

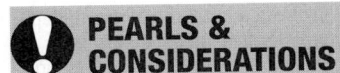

PEARLS & CONSIDERATIONS

COMMENTS

- Cluster headaches are divided into episodic (attacks lasting up to 1 yr with more than 1 mo pain-free periods) and chronic (>1 yr without remission).
- Home oxygen therapy is reasonable for cluster headache sufferers.

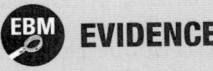

EVIDENCE

available at www.expertconsult.com

SUGGESTED READINGS
available at www.expertconsult.com

AUTHOR: **CHUN LIM, M.D., PH.D.**

BASIC INFORMATION

DEFINITION

Migraine headaches are recurrent headaches preceded by a focal neurologic symptom (migraine with aura), occur independently (migraine without aura), or have atypical presentations (migraine variants). The migraine aura typically is characterized by visual or sensory symptoms that develop over a period of 5 to 20 min. In both migraine with and without aura the headache is typically unilateral, pulsatile, and associated with nausea and vomiting, photophobia, and phonophobia.

ICD-9CM CODES
346 Migraine

EPIDEMIOLOGY & DEMOGRAPHICS

INCIDENCE: Increases from infancy, peaks during the third decade of life, then decreases
PREVALENCE (IN U.S.): Females: 18%; males: 6%. More than 50% of persons affected by migraine headaches report reduced work or school productivity.
PREDOMINANT SEX: Female/male ratio of 3:1
GENETICS:
- Familial predisposition, with more than 50% of migraine sufferers having an affected family member
- Autosomal-dominant transmission for some rare migraine variants (familial hemiplegic migraine; cerebral autosomal-dominant arteriopathy with subcortical infarcts and leukoencephalopathy [CADASIL])

PHYSICAL FINDINGS & CLINICAL PRESENTATION
- Normal between episodes.
- Normal for migraine without aura. Focal motor or sensory abnormalities possible with migraine with aura or migraine variants.
- Common aura types include scintillating scotomata, bright zigzags, homonymous visual disturbance such as paresthesias, speech disturbances, or hemiparesis (familial or sporadic hemiplegic migraine).

ETIOLOGY

The pathophysiology of migraines is not clearly understood. It is believed that a primary neuronal event results in a trigeminovascular reflex causing neurogenic inflammation. Serotonin, substance P, nitric oxide, and calcitonin-gene-related peptide also play a role, but the exact mechanism is unknown. Cortical spreading depression is probably responsible for the aura.

DIAGNOSIS

Migraine without aura:
- Five attacks fulfilling criteria
- Headache attacks lasting 4 to 72 hr
- Headache has at least two of the following characteristics:
  1. Unilateral location
  2. Pulsating quality
  3. Moderate or severe pain intensity
  4. Aggravation or causing avoidance of routine physical activity
- During headache at least one of the following:
  1. Nausea and/or vomiting
  2. Photophobia and phonophobia

Migraine with aura:
- At least two attacks
- Aura consisting of at least one of the following, but no motor weakness:
  1. Fully reversible visual symptoms, including positive features and/or negative features
  2. Fully reversible sensory symptoms, including positive and/or negative features
- At least two of the following:
  1. Homonymous visual symptoms and/or unilateral sensory symptoms
  2. At least one aura symptom develops gradually over >5 min and/or different aura symptoms occur in succession over >5 min
- A migraine occurring during or within 60 min of the aura

DIFFERENTIAL DIAGNOSIS
- Subarachnoid hemorrhage
- Cluster headache
- Chronic daily headaches
- Arteriovenous malformation
- Vasculitis
- Intracranial mass lesion
- Section II describes the differential diagnosis of headaches

WORKUP
- In general, no additional investigation is needed with recurrent, typical attacks with usual age of onset, family history, and a normal physical examination.
- If there is an unusual presentation and/or unexpected findings on examination, investigation for other causes is required.

LABORATORY TESTS

Lumbar puncture for history of abrupt-onset headaches and uncertain diagnosis of migraine

IMAGING STUDIES
- Imaging should be done in patients with headaches and an unexplained abnormal finding on the neurologic examination.
- Imaging should be considered in patients with rapidly increasing headache frequency, history of dizziness or incoordination, headache causing wakening from sleep, or headaches worsening with Valsalva maneuver.

TREATMENT

Consider the use of a headache log/diary to identify triggers of headaches, record efficacy of treatments, and track history of the headaches.

NONPHARMACOLOGIC THERAPY
- Avoid any identifiable provoking factors: caffeine, tobacco, and alcohol may trigger attacks, as may dietary or other environmental precipitants (less common)
- Avoid stressors in life and minimize variations in daily routine with regular sleep, meals, and exercise
- Relaxation training, behavioral therapy, and biofeedback

ACUTE ANALGESIC Rx
- Many oral agents are ineffective because of poor absorption from migraine-induced gastric stasis. Non-oral route of administration should be selected in patients with severe nausea or vomiting.
- Acetaminophen, NSAIDS, combination analgesics, benzodiazepines, opioids, barbiturates.

ACUTE ABORTIVE Rx
- IV antiemetics (prochlorperazine, metoclopramide, domperidone). Acute dystonic reactions and akathisia are rare side effects. These are generally not used as monotherapy.
- Ergotamine and ergotamine combinations (PO/PR) and dihydroergotamine (DHE 45) (SC, IV, IM, intranasal) have well-documented efficacy against migraines. DHE is usually administered in combination with an antiemetic drug (Table 1-62).
- Triptans (SC, PO, and intranasal) are now considered the drug class of choice for abortive therapy. Meta-analysis suggests that 10 mg rizatriptan, 80 mg eletriptan, and 12.5 mg almotriptan are most effective.
- Early administration improves effectiveness.

PROPHYLAXIS Rx
- Prophylactic treatment is generally indicated when headaches occur more than once a week or when symptomatic treatments are contraindicated or not effective. They are most effective when initiated during a headache-free period. All prophylaxis should be maintained for at least 3 mo before deeming the medication a failure.
- Well-established options for prophylactic treatment include β-blockers (propranolol, timolol, atenolol, metoprolol), tricyclic antidepressants (amitriptyline), and the antiepileptic drug valproic acid.
- Less-established options include calcium channel blockers, selective serotonin reuptake inhibitors, and the antiepileptic drugs gabapentin and topiramate.
- The FDA has recently approved injection of onabotulinum toxin A (Botox) for prevention of headaches in adult patients with chronic migraines (≥15 headache days/mo for ≥3 mo). The recommended total dose is 155 total units administered intramuscularly every 12 wk divided among 31 sites in head and neck area (frontalis, corrugator, procerus, occipitalis, temporalis, trapezius, cervical paraspinal muscle group).

TABLE 1-62 Abortive and Analgesic Therapy for Migraine*

Drug	Route	Dose
Triptans (Serotonin Agonists)		
Sumatriptan	Subcutaneous	6 mg, repeat in 2 hr (max 2 doses/day)
Sumatriptan	Oral	25 mg, 50 mg, repeat in 2 hr (max 200 mg/day)
Sumatriptan	Nasal spray	5 mg, 20 mg, repeat in 2 hr (max 40 mg/day)
Zolmitriptan	Oral	1.25, 2.5, 5 mg, repeat in 2 hr (max 10 mg/day)
Zolmitriptan	Nasal spray	5 mg, repeat in 2 hr (max 10 mg/day)
Zolmitriptan	Orally disintegrating tab	2.5, 5 mg, repeat in 2 hr (max 10 mg/day)
Naratriptan	Oral	1 mg, 2.5 mg, repeat in 4 hr (max 5 mg/day)
Rizatriptan	Oral	5 mg, 10 mg, repeat in 2 hr (max 30 mg/day)
Almotriptan	Oral	6.25 mg, 12.5 mg, may repeat in 2 hr (max 25 mg/day)
Eletriptan	Oral	20 mg, 40 mg, may repeat in 2 hr (max 80 mg/day)
Frovatriptan	Oral	2.5 mg, may repeat in 2 hr (max 7.5 mg/day)
Ergotamine Preparations		
Ergotamine and caffeine	Oral	2 tablets, may repeat 1 tab q30 min (max 6/day)
Ergotamine and caffeine	Rectal	1 suppository, repeat in 1 hr (max 2/day)
Ergotamine	Sublingual	1 tablet, repeat in 1 hr (max 2/day)
Dihydroergotamine	Intramuscular Subcutaneous Intravenous Nasal spray	0.5-1.0 mg, repeat twice at 1-hr intervals (max 3 mg/attack)
Sympathomimetics (with or without Barbiturates or Codeine)		
Isometheptene + dichloralphenazone + acetaminophen	Oral	1 to 2 capsules, repeat in 4 hr (max 8/day)
Nonsteroidal Anti-inflammatory Drugs		
Acetaminophen +	Oral	2 tablets, repeat in 6 hr (max 8/day aspirin + caffeine)
Naproxen	Oral	550-750 mg, repeat in 1 hr (max 3 times/wk)
Meclofenamate	Oral	100-200 mg, repeat in 1 hr (max 3 times/wk)
Flurbiprofen	Oral	50-100 mg, repeat in 1 hr (max 3 times/wk)
Ibuprofen	Oral	200-300 mg, repeat in 1 hr (max 3 times/wk)
Antiemetics		
Promethazine	Oral Intramuscular	50-125 mg
Prochlorperazine	Oral Rectal Intramuscular	1-25 mg 2.5-25 mg (suppository) 5-10 mg
Chlorpromazine	Oral Rectal Intravenous	10-25 mg 50-100 mg (suppository) Up to 35 mg
Trimethobenzamide	Oral Rectal	250 mg 200 mg
Metoclopramide	Oral Intramuscular Intravenous	5-10 mg 10 mg 5-10 mg
Dimenhydrinate	Oral	50 mg

Modified from Wiederholt WC: *Neurology for non-neurologists*, ed 4, Philadelphia, 2000, WB Saunders.
*For side effects and contraindications consult the manufacturer's drug insert before prescribing any of these drugs.

DISPOSITION
After age 30 yr, 40% of patients are migraine free.

REFERRAL
If uncertain about diagnosis or treatment not effective

 PEARLS & CONSIDERATIONS

- Avoid overuse of narcotics, barbiturates, caffeine, and benzodiazepines because they are habit-forming.
- Long-term use of analgesic medications can result in drug-induced or rebound headaches.

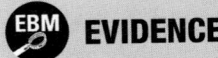 **EVIDENCE**

available at www.expertconsult.com

SUGGESTED READINGS
available at www.expertconsult.com

AUTHOR: **CHUN LIM, M.D., PH.D.**

BASIC INFORMATION

DEFINITION

Tension-type headaches (TTH) are recurrent headaches lasting 30 min to 7 days without nausea or vomiting and with at least two of the following characteristics: pressing or tightening quality (nonthrobbing), mild or moderate intensity, bilateral, and not aggravated by routine physical activity.

SYNONYMS

Muscle contraction headache
Tension headache
Stress headache
Essential headache

ICD-9CM CODES
307.81 Tension headache

EPIDEMIOLOGY & DEMOGRAPHICS

INCIDENCE (IN U.S.): Most common type of headache; as high as 70% of all headaches presenting to primary care physician
PEAK INCIDENCE: Occurs at all ages
PREVALENCE (IN U.S.): Males: 63%/yr; females: 86%/yr
PREDOMINANT SEX: Females are affected more often than males

PHYSICAL FINDINGS & CLINICAL PRESENTATION

Pressure or "bandlike" tightness all around the head; may be worse at the vertex. Cervical, paracervical, and trapezius muscle spasm and/or tenderness on palpation may be present. Scalp tenderness or hypersensitivity to pain also occurs. Symptoms suggestive of migraine are usually not present (e.g., throbbing pain, nausea/vomiting, visual complaints, aura). Either one symptom of photo or phonophobia does not exclude the diagnosis of TTH.

ETIOLOGY

- Unclear; little data to support postulated muscle contraction component. More recently has been thought of as a multifactorial disorder with several possible concurrent pathophysiologic mechanisms.

- No recent data to support the longstanding belief that these headaches arise from stress or other psychological factors. However, components of stress, sleep deprivation, hunger, and eyestrain may exacerbate symptoms.

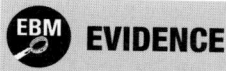

DIAGNOSIS

DIFFERENTIAL DIAGNOSIS

- Migraine (would expect associated symptoms; see entry "Headache, Migraine")
- Cervical spine disease
- Intracranial mass (may present with focal neurologic signs, seizures, or headache awakening patient from sleep)
- Idiopathic intracranial hypertension (found more often in obese women of child-bearing age, may have papilledema, visual loss, or diplopia)
- Rebound headache from overuse of analgesics
- Secondary headache (e.g., temporomandibular joint syndrome, thyrotoxicosis, polycythemia, drug side effects)
- Migraine and TTH may often coexist and may be difficult to differentiate (suggest headache calendar)
- Section II describes the differential diagnosis of headaches

WORKUP

- Thorough history and physical examination for any new-onset headache.
- Neuroimaging should be performed when unexplained neurologic findings are present on examination or in cases of atypical new-onset sudden and severe headaches.

LABORATORY TESTS

- No routine tests
- Erythrocyte sedimentation rate in elderly patients suspected of having cranial arteritis

IMAGING STUDIES

CT scan and/or MRI may be used to exclude intracranial pathology. MRI is better for imaging the posterior fossa. Contrast should be used if mass lesion is suspected.

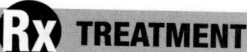 TREATMENT

NONPHARMACOLOGIC THERAPY

- Relaxation and cognitive behavioral therapy (especially in adolescents and children), Schultz-type autogenic training (relaxation technique based on passive concentration and body awareness of specific sensations), transcutaneous electrical nerve stimulation, heat
- Physical therapy, including stretching exercises, massage, and ultrasound

ACUTE GENERAL Rx

Nonnarcotic analgesics with limited frequency to prevent drug-induced and/or rebound headache

CHRONIC Rx

- Tricyclic antidepressants (e.g., amitriptyline 10 to 150 mg hs) and SSRIs
- Avoid narcotics, limit NSAIDs, consider indomethacin; if related to cervical muscle spasm, may consider trial of muscle relaxants (e.g., Skelaxin 400 to 800 mg tid)

DISPOSITION

May not respond fully to treatment

REFERRAL

If uncertain about diagnosis or unexplained focal neurologic findings on examination

PEARLS & CONSIDERATIONS

It is imperative to avoid overuse of caffeine- and barbiturate-containing medications because of the risk of rebound headaches.

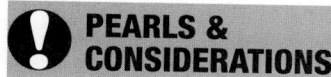 EVIDENCE

available at www.expertconsult.com

SUGGESTED READINGS

available at www.expertconsult.com

AUTHOR: **RICHARD S. ISAACSON, M.D.**

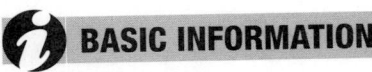

BASIC INFORMATION

DEFINITION

HAIs are infections associated with health care, generally occurring more than 48 hr after admission to a hospital. Classification criteria are established by the National Healthcare Safety Network (NHSN).

SYNONYMS

Nosocomial infections

ICD-9CM CODES

008.45 *Clostridium difficile*
041.12 MRSA
482.42 MRSA pneumonia
038.12 MRSA septicemia
998.59 Other postoperative infection
999.31 Infection due to central venous catheter
997.31 Ventilator-assisted pneumonia
996.31 Due to urethral [indwelling] catheter

EPIDEMIOLOGY & DEMOGRAPHICS

INCIDENCE (IN U.S.):
- Develop in at least 5% of hospitalized patients.
- In 2002, HAIs accounted for more than 98,000 deaths.
- In 2002, the annual cost of HAIs in the U.S. was estimated as >$5 billion to $10 billion; adjusts to >$35 billion in 2007 values.
- At least one third of hospital-acquired infections are preventable.

PREVALENCE (IN U.S.): 2 million to 4 million cases/yr

PREDOMINANT SEX:
- Overall, approximately equal
- Elderly women: predominantly nosocomial urinary tract infections

PREDOMINANT AGE: Newborns and elderly patients (>60 yr) at highest risk

PEAK INCIDENCE: Varies widely with infection site

RISK FACTORS: Patients with the following conditions can develop HAIs at any age:
- In ICU
- Intubation
- Chronic lung disease
- Renal disease
- Comatose
- Chronic urethral or vascular catheterization
- Malnutrition
- Postoperative state
- Diabetic

PHYSICAL FINDINGS & CLINICAL PRESENTATION

Vary with specific HAIs

ETIOLOGY

- Bacteria (gram-negative bacteria are responsible for >30% of HAIs)
- Fungi
- Viruses

SOURCES AND MODES OF TRANSMISSION:

- Patient's own flora
  - Comprises resistant organisms associated with hospitalization
  - Frequently maintained thereafter by persistent GI colonization
- Unwashed hands of staff
  - Physicians
  - Nurses
- Invasion of protective defenses (intact skin, respiratory cilia, urinary sphincters, and mucosa)
  - IV lines/central lines
  - Catheters
  - Respiratory equipment
  - Surgical wounds
  - Scopes and other imaging devices
- Failure to provide adequate negative pressure, high-volume air flow chambers for airborne infection isolation of patients with TB or disseminated herpes zoster/chickenpox
- Failure to rapidly identify and provide appropriate care (with isolation or precautions) for patients with communicable diseases
- Inanimate environment
- Food
- Fomites

RISKS AMPLIFIED:

- Use of broad-spectrum antibiotics
  - Select highly resistant bacteria
  - Establish highly resistant bacteria as endemic flora in microenvironments within the hospital
- Highly vulnerable patients with specific risk factors
  - Immunosuppression (as a result of therapy, transplantation, AIDS)
  - Old age
  - Postsurgery
  - Prolonged surgery
  - Chronic lung disease
  - Ventilator dependence
  - Antacid therapy
  - Vascular lines
  - Hyperalimentation
  - ICU stay
  - Recent antibiotic therapy
- Clustering of seriously ill patients
  - Often with wounds or drainage of contaminated materials
  - Intensifying probability of cross-infection

PREVENTION STRATEGIES: Handwashing/hand hygiene between all patient contacts is the single most important method of decreasing HAI:
- Regular soap and water for at least 15 sec
- Chlorhexidine (particularly good for gram-positive organisms like methicillin-resistant *Staphylococcus aureus* [MRSA]), alcohol hand-rub or other antiseptic for resistant organisms
- Purpose of soap and water handwash
  - Degrease hand surfaces
  - Wash away oils and associated bacteria, removal of visible dirt or body fluids
- Procedure
  - Lukewarm water
  - Must include all surfaces

- Special attention to areas between fingers and to the dirtier dominant hand (most people reflexively wash the cleaner, nondominant hand more vigorously)
- The widespread availability of alcohol-based hand hygiene solutions throughout hospital settings has been shown to improve handwashing frequency (less drying to hands, faster, and no need for wash basin and towels for drying) and to significantly reduce hospital-associated infections; now recommended in essentially all routine health-care settings

METHICILLIN-RESISTANT *STAPHYLOCOCCUS AUREUS* (MRSA)

- Invasive HAIs caused by MRSA decreased 9.4% per year from 2005 through 2008 in the United States.
- Health-care–associated MRSA strains are typically resistant to many antibiotics, remaining susceptible to vancomycin and trimethoprim/sulfamethoxazole.
- High-risk factors include dialysis, recent stay in acute or long-term care facilities.
- Control measures include hand hygiene, disinfection of equipment, protective attire for isolation, and standard precautions.
- Community-acquired (CA-MRSA) associated with soft tissue, presenting as boils, rash, or so-called spider bite, and typically occurs in patients who have no recent health-care or hospital interaction.
- CA-MRSA often not found in nares.

VANCOMYCIN-RESISTANT *ENTEROCOCCUS FAECIUM* (VREF):

- The percentage of HAIs caused by VREF increased more than twentyfold between 1989 and 1993, rising from 0% to 3% to 7% to 9%. By 2005, VREF, vancomycin-resistant *E. faecalis,* and other vancomycin-resistant species of enterococci had become common and endemic nosocomial pathogens accounting for 15% to 40% of all enterococci isolated in the hospital setting.
- A high percentage of VREF isolated, 80%, are also ampicillin resistant.
- Factors predisposing to VREF colonization or infection include a high percentage of hospital days receiving antibiotic therapy, use of IV, underlying disease, immunosuppression, and abdominal surgery.
- Evidence suggests that the vehicle is the hands of medical personnel.
- Control measures:
  - Aggressive isolation of colonized or infected patients
  - Restraint in using broad-spectrum antibiotics
  - Compliance with hand-hygiene best practices

CLOSTRIDIUM DIFFICILE:

- Causes diarrhea as a result of pseudomembranous colitis.
- Can be transmitted among hospitalized patients.
- Warrants contact precautions and bleach for disinfection.

- Alcohol-based hand rub may not eliminate spores of this organism, so can use soap and water to wash hands at sink.
- Spores can be dispersed in the air or room environment surrounding patients.
- Treatment is tiered based on severity.
- Rising incidence of *C. difficile* infection with emerging strains that have up to twenty-threefold more toxin production.
- Can present in healthy patients with no known risk factors.

NOROVIRUS:
- Patients present with sudden onset of nausea, vomiting, and/or diarrhea.
- Now considered year-round rather than seasonal.
- Disinfection with bleach.
- Often need to isolate exposed persons for average incubation period, such as 3 days, to prevent outbreak.

SURVEILLANCE
- Crucial for early identification of infections:
  - Enables immediate intervention
  - Education
- Prospective, concurrent, hospital surveillance:
  - Electronic data mining provides accurate review
  - Feasible with sophisticated computerized data collection and analysis
- Targeted surveillance address high-risk procedures and patient populations
- Routine rate calculations and statistical analyses:
  - Uses device-specific days or patient-days as denominators
  - Enhances early recognition of microclusters of infections by body site and by organism
  - Facilitates proper early control of potential outbreaks
- Active surveillance cultures for multi-drug resistant organisms (MDROs); for example, high-risk populations for MRSA

ⓓ DIAGNOSIS

MOST COMMON HAI:
- Urinary tract infections (UTIs) (32%)
- Surgical wound and other soft tissue infections (22%)
- Pneumonia (15%)
- Bloodstream infections (14%)

HEALTH-CARE–ASSOCIATED UTIs:
- General associations:
  - Foley catheters
  - Inappropriate catheter care (including opening catheter junctions)
  - Female sex
  - Absence of systemic antibiotics
- Physical findings:
  - Fever
  - Dysuria
  - Leukocytosis
  - Pyuria
  - Flank or costovertebral angle tenderness

- Usual organisms:
  - *E. coli*
  - *Candida*
  - *Enterococcus*
  - *Pseudomonas*
  - *Klebsiella*
  - *Enterobacter*
- Sepsis in 1% to 3% of hospital-associated UTIs
- Prevention:
  - Meticulous technique during insertion and daily perineal care
  - Never open the catheter-collection tubing junction
  - Obtain all specimens using sterile syringe
  - Substitute intermittent catheterization for Foley catheters

HEALTH-CARE–ASSOCIATED BLOODSTREAM INFECTIONS:
- General associations:
  - IV lines
  - Arterial lines
  - CVP lines: leads to catheter-associated bloodstream infection (CLABSI)
  - Phlebitis
  - Hyperalimentation
- Fever possibly only presenting sign
- Exit site of all vascular lines carefully evaluated for:
  - Erythema
  - Induration
  - Tenderness
  - Purulent drainage
- Usual organism for device-associated bacteremia
  - *S. aureus* (including MRSA)
  - *Staphylococcus epidermidis* for long-term IV lines
  - *Enterobacter*
  - *Klebsiella*
  - *Candida* spp.
  - *Pseudomonas aeruginosa* may come from a water source or reflect cutaneous bacteria
- Phlebitis in 1.3 million patients yearly
- Approximately 10,000 annual deaths from IV sepsis
- Prevention:
  - Meticulous sterile technique during IV insertion.
  - Emphasis should be placed on attention to detail, including handwashing, adherence to guidelines for catheter insertion and maintenance, appropriate use of antiseptic solutions such as chlorhexidine (CHG) for CVPs or chlorhexidine or iodine to prepare the skin around the catheter insertion site, and use of sterile technique for central catheter insertion.
  - Modified catheter may reduce risk for endoluminal colonization and catheter-related sepsis in subclavian lines.
  - Decrease use of routine IVs and encourage PO intake
  - Avoid using a femoral insertion site. Subclavian site is associated with lower infection rate than jugular.

  - Use of bundle to prevent central line associated bloodstream infections (CLABSIs) to include hand hygiene, chlorhexidine skin prep for insertion of central lines, full barrier protection for insertion of central lines, removal of unnecessary lines.

HEALTH-CARE–ASSOCIATED PNEUMONIAS:
- More common in ICUs
- General associations:
  - Aspiration
  - Intubation: leads to ventilator-associated pneumonia (VAP)
  - Altered consciousness
  - Old age
  - Chronic lung disease
  - Postsurgery
  - Antacids
  - Head of bed not elevated
- Signs of pneumonia common among patients on general wards:
  - Cough
  - Sputum
  - Fever
  - Leukocytosis
  - New infiltrate on chest x-ray examination
- Signs more subtle in ICUs, because many patients have purulent sputum because of chronic intubation
  - Change in sputum character or volume
  - Small changes on chest x-ray examination
- Usual organisms:
  - *S. aureus* (including MRSA)
  - *Pseudomonas aeruginosa*
  - *Enterobacter*
  - *Acinetobacter*
  - *Klebsiella*
- Less common organisms:
  - *Stenotrophomonas* spp.
  - *Legionella, Flavobacterium*
  - Respiratory syncytial virus (infants)
  - Adenovirus
- 1% of hospitalized patients affected
- Mortality rate high (40%)
- Prevention:
  - Use meticulous sterile technique during suctioning and handling airway.
  - Do not routinely change ventilator breathing circuits and components. For heat and moisture exchangers, no more frequently than every 48 hr.
  - Drain respirator tubing without allowing fluid to return to respirator.
  - Wash hands routinely to prevent colonization of patients and transfer of organisms among patients.
  - Use of a bundle to prevent ventilator-associated pneumonias (VAPs) to include: elevate the head of bed, provide deep vein thrombosis (DVT) prophylaxis, provide peptic ulcer disease (PUD) prophylaxis, hold sedation, test for ability to extubate, control glucose, gastric decontamination.

SURGICAL AND HEALTH-CARE–ASSOCIATED SOFT TISSUE INFECTIONS:
- Associations:
  - Decubitus ulcers
  - Surgical site risks: contaminated or dirty/infected, the American Society of Anesthe-

siologists' (ASA) physical status classification of ASA 3 or 4, duration of surgery over national average, usually 3 hr
- ○ Abdominal surgery
- ○ Presence of drain
- ○ Preoperative length of stay
- ○ Surgeon
- ○ Presence of other infection
- Physical findings:
  - ○ Decubitus ulcer with fluctuance at margin or under firm eschar
  - ○ Erythema extending >2 cm beyond margin of surgical wound
  - ○ Tenderness
  - ○ Induration
  - ○ Erythema
  - ○ Fluctuance
  - ○ Purulent drainage
  - ○ Dehiscence of sutures
- Usual organisms:
  - ○ S. aureus (including MRSA)
  - ○ Enterococcus
  - ○ Enterobacter
  - ○ Acinetobacter
  - ○ E. coli
- Prevention:
  - ○ Use careful skin care and frequent, proper positioning of patient to prevent decubitus ulcer.
  - ○ Use meticulous sterile surgical technique.
  - ○ Wash hands to decrease colonization when handling postoperative wound.
  - ○ Limit prophylactic antibiotics to 24 hr perioperatively.
  - ○ Double-wrap contaminated dressings (hold in gloved hand and evert gloves over dressings) before disposal.
  - ○ Surgical Care Improvement Project (SCIP) bundle to include antibiotic prophylaxis selection, receipt of antibiotic within 1 hr prior to surgery, discontinuation of antibiotic within 24 hr after surgery, clip rather than shave prep, postoperative normothermia for colorectal surgery patients.
  - ○ Preadmission nares MRSA screening often beneficial for open heart and orthopedic implants when time is allowed for decolonization, chlorhexidine showers, and appropriate antibiotic prophylaxis selection.

LABORATORY TESTS
- Appropriate to specific HAI and specific patient's condition
- Cultures generally indicated for proper confirmation of responsible pathogens:
  - ○ Urine
  - ○ Blood
  - ○ Sputum
  - ○ Soft tissue
- Molecular analysis of nosocomial epidemics:
  - ○ Plasmid fingerprinting
  - ○ Restriction endonuclease digestion (plasmid and genomic DNA)
  - ○ Peptide analysis
  - ○ Immunoblotting
  - ○ Ribosomal RNA (rRNA) typing
  - ○ DNA probes
  - ○ Multilocus enzyme electrophoresis

- ○ Restriction fragment length polymorphism (RFLP)
- ○ Polymerase chain reaction (PCR)
- ○ Provide confirmation of point-source or common strains and corroboration of hypotheses reached utilizing classic epidemiology

IMAGING STUDIES
Rarely needed for diagnosis of HAI

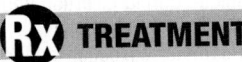
TREATMENT

ACUTE GENERAL Rx
- Appropriate to etiologic organism:
  - ○ Antibiotic
  - ○ Antifungal
  - ○ Antiviral
- Specific therapy determined after careful consideration of resident flora within the microenvironment in which the patient was hospitalized
  - ○ Empiric therapy
    Frequently difficult to fashion accurately
    Often undesirable, unless the patient's clinical condition requires urgent treatment
- Consultation for expert advice regarding antibiotic selection in view of known epidemiologic risks within the hospital
  Infection preventionist
  Hospital epidemiologist
- Avoid unnecessary treatment for organisms that are colonizing but not infecting patients
- Prevention of spread of communicable diseases, often requiring isolation or precautions
  - ○ Classic schema (strict, respiratory isolation and contact [skin and wound] precautions) being replaced by more streamlined revised guidelines (airborne, droplet, contact isolation precautions, and combinations thereof)
  - ○ Less careful response to some diseases (e.g., hemorrhagic fevers) inadvertently induced by removal of strict isolation category
  - ○ Universal/standard precautions and body substance isolation continue within a new standard isolation precautions guideline
  - ○ Tracking patients of roommates with communicable disease, such as Norovirus, influenza
- Universal/standard precautions used for all patients during all anticipated contacts with blood, body fluids, or secretions
  - ○ Gloves
  - ○ Goggles/eye shield
  - ○ Impermeable gowns if aerosol or splash is likely
- Consider aggressive isolation to restrict spread of resistant organisms and their plasmids
  - ○ MRSA
  - ○ VREF
  - ○ Highly resistant gram-negative organisms, including extended spectrum β-lactamases (ESBL) gram-negative rods

and carbapenem-resistant Enterobacteriaceae (CRE), some Acinetobacter baumanni
- ○ New Delhi metallo-β-lactamase 1 (NDM-1): these are gram-negative Enterobacteriaceae with a new type of carbapenem-resistance gene.

DISPOSITION
The infection prevention and control service and/or hospital epidemiologist should be notified when infectious complications occur in the hospital setting; most, but not all, HAIs are potentially avoidable, and every effort should be taken to minimize the risk of infections associated with health care.

REFERRAL
- To infection preventionist
- To hospital epidemiologist

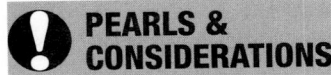
PEARLS & CONSIDERATIONS

COMMENTS
- Sharp and splash injuries to staff are relatively rare, but nearly all are preventable.
  - ○ Nurses incur most injuries.
  - ○ Usual causes:
    1. Needle sticks
    2. Scalpel and surgical needle injuries
    3. Blood splashes
  - ○ Prevention:
    1. Never recap needles.
    2. Dispose of needles only in rigid, impermeable plastic containers.
    3. Clearly announce instrument passes in the operating room or during procedures and use passing trays.
    4. Use needleless systems for vascular access and connectors whenever possible to limit health-care workers' use of sharp medical devices.
    5. Use gloves, mask, and goggles/eye shield if aerosol or splash is likely.
    6. Never leave needles or other sharp items in beds.
    7. Never dispose of sharp items in regular trash bags.
  - ○ Infection prevention and control or employee health staff should be consulted immediately after exposure to determine need for prophylaxis for hepatitis B or HIV.
  - ○ All clinical staff should be immune to hepatitis B (natural or vaccine).
- Fungi previously considered to be contaminants are now risks for patients with cancer and organ transplantation.
  - ○ Candida spp.
    1. C. guilliermondii
    2. C. krusei
    3. C. parapsilosis
    4. C. tropicalis
  - ○ Aspergillus spp.
  - ○ Curvularia spp.
  - ○ Bipolaris spp.
  - ○ Exserohilum spp.

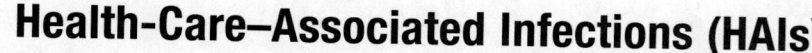

- ○ *Alternaria* spp.
- ○ *Fusarium* spp.
- ○ *Scopulariopsis* spp.
- ○ *Pseudallescheria boydii*
- ○ *Trichosporon beigelii*
- ○ *Malassezia furfur*
- ○ *Hansenula* spp.
- ○ *Microsporum canis*
- Focused, committed efforts by the entire health-care staff continuously directed toward prevention:
  - ○ Each HAI addressed as an opportunity to improve the organization and delivery of care

- ○ Essential that individual staff members understand that small risks applied to large populations result in a large number of total events (i.e., HAIs)
- The Centers for Medicare & Medicaid Services (CMS) denies inpatient payments for certain HAIs.
- The number of surgical-site *S. aureus* infections acquired in the hospital can be reduced by rapid screening and decolonizing of nasal carriers of *S. aureus* on admission.

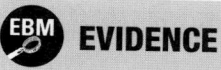 **EVIDENCE**

available at www.expertconsult.com

SUGGESTED READINGS

available at www.expertconsult.com

AUTHORS: **MARLENE FISHMAN, M.P.H., C.I.C.,** and **GLENN G. FORT, M.D., M.P.H.**

H

Diseases and Disorders

I

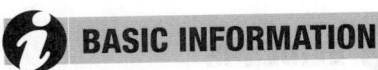

BASIC INFORMATION

DEFINITION

Complete heart block (CHB) is the absence of electrical impulse transmission from the atria to the ventricles.

SYNONYMS

Third-degree AV block

ICD-9CM CODES
426.0 Complete heart block

EPIDEMIOLOGY & DEMOGRAPHICS

- The prevalence of CHB is 0.04%.
- The prevalence of CHB increases with age.

PHYSICAL FINDINGS & CLINICAL PRESENTATION

Physical examination may be normal. Patients may present with the following clinical manifestations:

- Dizziness, palpitations
- Syncope or presyncope
- Fatigue, impaired exercise tolerance
- Mental status changes
- Congestive heart failure
- Angina pectoris
- Some patients may be asymptomatic (e.g., congenital CHB)

ETIOLOGY

- Fibrosis or sclerosis of the conduction system
- Acute myocardial infarction (may be seen in inferior or anterior wall MI)
- Drug effect (digitalis, calcium channel blockers, beta-blockers, amiodarone)
- Cardiomyopathy and myocarditis
- Infiltrative processes of the myocardium (amyloidosis, sarcoidosis, tumor)
- Metabolic abnormalities (hyperkalemia, hypoxia, hypothyroidism)
- Lyme carditis
- Neuromuscular disorders (Becker muscular dystrophy, myotonic muscular dystrophy)
- Congenital (birth from mothers with systemic lupus)
- Iatrogenic (cardiac surgery, catheter ablation of arrhythmias, percutaneous coronary intervention)

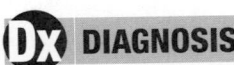

DIAGNOSIS

DIFFERENTIAL DIAGNOSIS

The differential diagnosis includes lesser degree of atrioventricular (AV) block, junctional rhythms, and nonconducted premature atrial contractions.

WORKUP

- Workup such as routine labs, cardiac biomarkers, and cardiac imaging should be dictated by the clinical circumstances.
- ECG: diagnostic of the disease (Fig. 1-174):
  - P waves are present with a regular atrial rate that is faster than the ventricular rate.
  - P waves are not related to the QRS complexes. The PR intervals are variable.
  - RR intervals are regular.
  - QRS complexes may be of normal width or abnormally wide, depending on the location of the block in the conduction system.

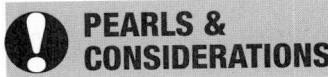

TREATMENT

ACUTE GENERAL Rx

- Initial treatment should focus on the hemodynamic stability and symptoms of the patient.
- Consider temporary pacemaker insertion if ventricular escape rate is slow (<40 beats per minute [bpm]) and associated with symptoms or hemodynamic compromise.
- Withdraw AV-nodal blocking agents if any.
- Atropine may be used to increase the rate of the escape rhythm.
- Isoproterenol may be used as a bridge to pacer insertion.
- Symptomatic CHB in the absence of a condition that is likely to resolve is an ACC/AHA/HRS Class I indication for permanent pacemaker placement.
- Class 1 indications for permanent pacing in asymptomatic patients according to the ACC/AHA guidelines include:
  - Patients in sinus rhythm, with documented asystolic pauses greater than or equal to 3.0 seconds or an escape rate less than 40 bpm, or with an escape rhythm that is below the AV node
  - Patients with atrial fibrillation and bradycardia with one or more pauses of at least 5 seconds or longer
  - After catheter ablation of the AV junction
  - If cardiomegaly or LV dysfunction is present or if the site of CHB is below the AV node
  - CHB after cardiac surgery block that is not expected to resolve
  - When it is associated with neuromuscular diseases, such as: Erb dystrophy (limb-girdle muscular dystrophy), Kearns-Sayre syndrome, myotonic muscular dystrophy, and peroneal muscular atrophy
  - CHB present during exercise in the absence of myocardial ischemia
- Therapy is directed toward the underlying etiology if there is a reversible source.

CHRONIC Rx

Patients with permanent pacemakers need regular follow-up and pacemaker monitoring to ensure proper device functioning.

DISPOSITION

- Prognosis is favorable after insertion of pacemaker and related to the underlying etiology of complete AV block (e.g., myocardial infarction, cardiomyopathy).
- Nonrandomized studies have shown that permanent pacemaker insertion improves survival in patients with CHB.

REFERRAL

All patients with CHB should be referred to a cardiologist for consideration of temporary and/or permanent pacemaker implantation.

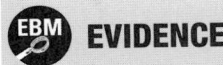

PEARLS & CONSIDERATIONS

COMMENTS

- Patients should be instructed to avoid activities that may damage the pacemaker (e.g., contact sports).
- Pacemaker manufacturers do not recommend any special restrictions regarding proximity to typical household items.
- The presence of a permanent pacemaker is a strong relative contraindication to MRI.

EBM EVIDENCE

available at www.expertconsult.com

SUGGESTED READINGS

available at www.expertconsult.com

AUTHORS: **THOMAS J. EARL, M.D.,**
JOSHUA SILVERSTEIN, M.D.,
FRED F. FERRI, M.D., and
WEN-CHIH WU, M.D.

THIRD-DEGREE (COMPLETE) AV BLOCK

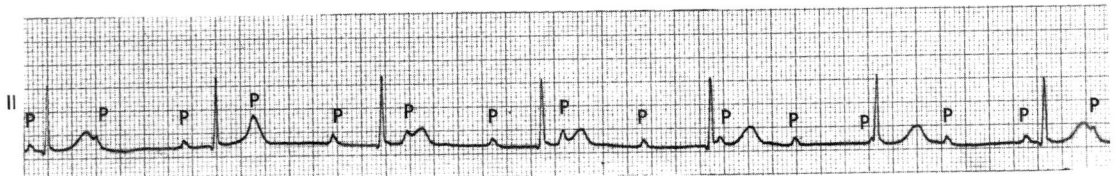

FIGURE 1-174 Third-degree complete atrioventricular heart block is characterized by independent atrial (P) and ventricular (QRS) activity. The atrial rate is always faster than the ventricular rate. The PR intervals are completely variable. Some P waves fall on the T wave, distorting its shape. Others may fall in the QRS complex and be "lost." Notice that the QRS complexes are of normal width, indicating that the ventricles are being paced from the atrioventricular junction. (From Goldberger AL [ed]: *Clinical electrocardiography,* ed 5, St Louis, 1994, Mosby.)

BASIC INFORMATION

DEFINITION

Second-degree heart block is the blockage of some impulses from the atria to the ventricles. There are three types of second-degree atrioventricular (AV) block:
- Mobitz type I (Wenckebach):
  - There is a progressive prolongation of the PR interval before an impulse is completely blocked; the cycle may repeat periodically, leading to "grouped beating."
  - Site of block is usually AV node (proximal to the bundle of His).
- Mobitz type II:
  - There is a sudden interruption of AV conduction without prior prolongation of the PR interval.
  - Site of block is usually infranodal.
- Advanced or high-grade second-degree block is the term used to describe the block of two or more consecutive P waves with some beats conducted (in contrast to third degree or complete heart block), indicating some preservation of AV conduction.

SYNONYMS

Wenckebach block (Mobitz type I block)
Mobitz type II block

ICD-9CM CODES
426.13 Mobitz type I
426.12 Mobitz type II

EPIDEMIOLOGY & DEMOGRAPHICS

Mobitz type I block is more common and may occur in individuals with heightened vagal tone or as a side effect of some medications, such as β-blockers or calcium channel blockers.

PHYSICAL FINDINGS & CLINICAL PRESENTATION

- Patients with Mobitz type I are usually asymptomatic.
- Sudden loss of consciousness without warning (Adams-Stokes attack) can occur in patients with Mobitz type II; however, it is much more common in patients with complete heart block.
- Irregular pulse with dropped beats is present (Mobitz type I).
- Irregular pulse with occasional dropped beats is present (Mobitz type II).

ETIOLOGY

- High vagal tone (young patients, athletes at rest)
- Degenerative changes in the AV conduction system
- Ischemia at the AV nodes (particularly in inferior wall myocardial infarction [MI])
- Drugs (digitalis, quinidine, procainamide, adenosine, calcium channel blockers, β-blockers)
- Cardiomyopathies
- Myocarditis (infectious, e.g., Lyme disease, and noninfectious, e.g., systemic lupus erythematosus, Chagas disease)
- Hyperkalemia
- Hypothyroidism
- Prior cardiac valve surgery
- Catheter ablation for arrhythmias

DIAGNOSIS

DIFFERENTIAL DIAGNOSIS

The ECG will distinguish between Mobitz type I and Mobitz type II block and other conduction abnormalities.

WORKUP

ECG, 24-hr Holter monitor (selected patients)
- Mobitz type I (Fig. 1-175) ECG shows:
  1. Gradual prolongation of PR interval leading to a blocked beat
  2. Shortened PR interval after dropped beat
  3. The R-R interval will often shorten prior to each dropped beat.
  4. Usually see "grouped beating" pattern.
- Mobitz type II ECG shows:
  1. Fixed duration of PR interval
  2. Sudden appearance of blocked beats
- In 2:1 AV block, it cannot be determined based on the 12-lead EKG whether there is Mobitz type I or type II AV block, although a wide QRS complex is suggestive of Mobitz type II.

TREATMENT

NONPHARMACOLOGIC THERAPY

Elimination of drugs that may induce AV block

ACUTE GENERAL Rx

Mobitz type I:
- Treatment is usually not necessary unless the resting heart rate is less than 40 beats per min while awake.
- If symptomatic (e.g., dizziness), atropine 1 mg (may repeat once after 5 min) may be tried to increase AV conduction; if no response, trial of dobutamine or isoproterenol may be helpful prior to insertion of temporary pacemaker.
- If block is the result of drugs (e.g., digitalis), discontinue the drug.
- If associated with anterior wall MI and wide QRS escape rhythm, consider insertion of a temporary pacemaker.
- Permanent pacemaker implantation is indicated for second-degree AV block with symptomatic bradycardia regardless of the site of the block.

Mobitz type II:
- Pacemaker insertion is usually needed if the patient is symptomatic or if the resting heart rate is less than 40 beats per min while awake because this type of block is usually permanent and often progresses to complete AV block.

DISPOSITION

Prognosis is good with insertion of a pacemaker.

REFERRAL

Referral for pacemaker insertion (see "Acute General Rx")

PEARLS & CONSIDERATIONS

COMMENTS

Patients with Mobitz type I should be followed up routinely for potential development of high-grade AV block.

SUGGESTED READINGS

available at www.expertconsult.com

AUTHORS: **JOSHUA SILVERSTEIN, M.D., FRED F. FERRI, M.D.,** and **WEN-CHIH WU, M.D.**

WENCKEBACH (MOBITZ TYPE I) SECOND-DEGREE AV BLOCK

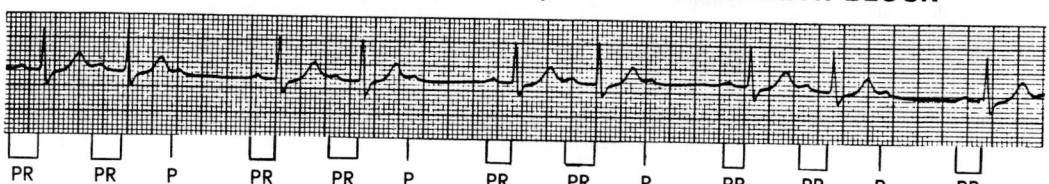

PR PR P PR PR P PR PR P PR PR P PR

FIGURE 1-175 Wenckebach (Mobitz type I) second-degree atrioventricular block. Notice the progressive increase in PR intervals, with the third P wave in each sequence not followed by a QRS. Wenckebach block produces a characteristically syncopated rhythm with grouping of the QRS complexes (group beating). (From Goldberger AL [ed]: *Clinical electrocardiography*, ed 5, St Louis, 1994, Mosby.)

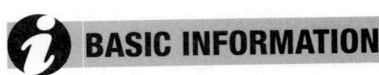

BASIC INFORMATION

DEFINITION

Heart failure (HF) is a complex clinical syndrome characterized by impaired myocardial performance, resulting in the heart's inability to deliver sufficient oxygenated blood to meet the metabolic demands of peripheral tissues. It can result from any structural or functional cardiac disorder that impairs the ability of the ventricle to fill with or eject blood at normal filling pressures and is associated with progressive activation of the neuroendocrine system leading to volume overload and circulatory insufficiency. The term "congestive heart failure" (CHF) usually denotes a volume-overloaded status as a result of HF. Given that not all patients have volume overload at the time of the evaluation, "congestive heart failure" should be distinguished from the broader term "heart failure."

CLASSIFICATION: The American College of Cardiology/American Heart Association (ACC/AHA) describe the following four stages of heart failure, emphasizing the evolution and progression of HF over a continuum and the preventability of HF in at-risk patients:

Stage A: Patients at high risk (e.g., patients with hypertension) for HF but without structural heart disease or symptoms of HF

Stage B: Patients with structural heart disease (e.g., left ventricular [LV] dysfunction) but without symptoms of HF

Stage C: Patients with structural heart disease with prior or current symptoms of HF

Stage D: Patients with refractory HF requiring specialized interventions

The New York Heart Association (NYHA) defines the following functional classes, commonly used to categorize signs and symptoms. This classification may often be modified by therapy:

I. Asymptomatic
II. Symptomatic with moderate exertion (2 city blocks or 1 flight of stairs in a faster than usual pace)
III. Symptomatic with minimal exertion (less than 2 city blocks or 1 flight of stairs)
IV. Symptomatic at rest

TERMINOLOGY

HF has been traditionally dichotomized as systolic versus diastolic (see Table 1-63), right-sided versus left-sided, and high-output versus low-output. Systolic HF is defined by the presence of impaired contractility of the left ventricle, as measured by ejection fraction (EF); while a consensus definition of diastolic heart failure is lacking, it usually involves signs or symptoms of HF, normal LV systolic function, and evidence of diastolic dysfunction. The term "heart failure with preserved EF" is preferred over the term "diastolic heart failure" given that many of the physiologic derangements in this subset of HF are not solely restricted to diastole. Right-sided HF denotes peripheral signs and symptoms of HF without evidence of pulmonary congestion, as opposed to left HF, which typically manifests with pulmonary congestion and subsequent signs and symptoms of right-sided HF. High-output HF involves signs and symptoms of HF but features an elevated cardiac output unable to meet the abnormally high metabolic demands of peripheral tissues, the result of myriad systemic disorders. The term "acute decompensated congestive HF" (ADCHF) refers to worsening of signs or symptoms of HF due to a wide range of causes.

SYNONYMS

Congestive heart failure
Cardiac failure
Heart failure
Cardiogenic pulmonary edema
CHF

ICD-9CM CODES
428.0 Congestive heart failure

EPIDEMIOLOGY & DEMOGRAPHICS

- There is marked variability in the reported demographics of HF due to the absence of reliable, population-based studies to elucidate epidemiologic data and heterogeneous definitions and classifications of HF.
- Congestive HF is the most common inpatient diagnosis in the U.S. for patients aged >65 yr and is the discharge diagnosis in >3.5 million hospitalizations annually.
- HF occurs in ~5.2 million persons in the U.S. and an estimated 23 million persons worldwide, and more commonly afflicts African Americans than whites. The prevalence of HF is rising, especially in the elderly, particularly due to aging of the population and improved survival from other conditions (e.g., valvular and coronary disease).
- There are 100 to 400 new cases of HF per 100,000 persons per year, and incidence is higher in the elderly, approaching 1000 or more new cases per 100,000 persons aged >65 yr per year. Before age 75, the incidence of HF is higher in males but both sexes are equally affected after this age cutoff.

PHYSICAL FINDINGS & CLINICAL PRESENTATION

Clinical and physical exam findings with HF vary depending on the severity of disease, precipitant factor, comorbid conditions, and whether the failure symptoms are predominantly right-sided or left-sided.

- Common clinical manifestations are:
  - Dyspnea on exertion, progressively worsening to dyspnea at rest, and caused by

TABLE 1-63 Systolic Versus Diastolic Heart Failure*

Parameters	Systolic	Diastolic
History		
Coronary artery disease	+++†	++
Hypertension	++	++++
Diabetes	++	++
Valvular heart disease	++++	+
Paroxysmal dyspnea	++	+++
Physical Examination		
Cardiomegaly	+++	+
Soft heart sounds	++++	+
S_3 gallop	+++	+
S_4 gallop	+	+++
Hypertension	++	++++
Mitral regurgitation	+++	+
Rales	++	+
Edema	+++	+
Jugular venous distention	+++	+
Chest Radiograph		
Cardiomegaly	+++	+
Pulmonary congestion	+++	+++
Electrocardiogram		
Left ventricular hypertrophy	++	++++
Q waves	++	+
Low voltage	+++	−
Echocardiogram		
Left ventricular hypertrophy	++	++++
Left ventricular dilation	++	−
Left atrial enlargement	++	++
Reduced ejection fraction	++++	−

From Zipes DP et al (eds): *Braunwauld's heart disease*, ed 7, Philadelphia, 2005, Elsevier.
*Certain aspects of the history and physical examination, along with clinical measurements, may help to distinguish diastolic from systolic heart failure. For example, patients with hypertensive heart disease and severe left ventricular hypertrophy often experience heart failure because of diastolic dysfunction.
†*Plus signs* indicate "suggestive" (the number reflects relative weight). *Minus signs* indicate "not very suggestive."

increasing pulmonary vascular congestion due to inadequate forward flow and subsequent increased pulmonary venous pressure
- Orthopnea, caused by increased venous return in the recumbent position and further elevated pulmonary venous pressure
- Paroxysmal nocturnal dyspnea (PND) resulting from multiple factors including increased venous return in the recumbent position, decreased Pao_2 and decreased adrenergic stimulation of myocardial function during sleep
- Nocturnal angina resulting from increased myocardial oxygen demand (secondary to increased venous return in the recumbent position causing increased preload) in patients with concomitant coronary artery disease (CAD)
- Cheyne-Stokes respiration (alternating phases of apnea and hyperventilation) caused by prolonged circulation time from lungs to brain as a result of impaired cardiac output
- Fatigue, lethargy, and decreased functional capacity resulting from low cardiac output and hypoperfusion of peripheral tissues
- Physical examination: fine pulmonary crackles, wheezes, tachypnea, hypoxia (due to elevated pulmonary pressures); tachycardia and narrowed pulse pressure (due to increased sympathetic tone); S_3 gallop, paradoxical splitting of S_2, jugular venous distention, peripheral edema in dependent tissues, congestive hepatomegaly, ascites, and hepatojugular reflux (due to volume overload); and perioral and peripheral cyanosis, decreased capillary refill, pulsus alternans, and cool extremities (due to decreased cardiac output)
- Acute precipitants of HF exacerbations are: noncompliance with salt restriction or medications, infection, arrhythmias, new medications (e.g., calcium channel blockers/antiarrhythmic agents), nonsteroidal anti-inflammatory drugs (NSAIDs), renal dysfunction, uncontrolled hypertension, toxins, ischemia, infarction, or valvular catastrophe.

ETIOLOGY

LEFT VENTRICULAR FAILURE: The dichotomy of whether HF occurs in the setting of preserved or abnormal LV systolic function plays an important role in treatment strategies, as patients with HF with preserved EF may have significant abnormalities in active relaxation and passive stiffness of the LV, renal function, or arterial vasoreactivity.
- Abnormal LV systolic function
  - CAD (acute or chronic ischemia, myocardial infarction [MI], LV aneurysm)
  - Pressure overload (severe hypertension, aortic stenosis)
  - Volume overload (mitral regurgitation, aortic regurgitation)
  - Cardiomyopathy (dilated cardiomyopathy, dilated phase of hypertrophic cardiomyopathy, ischemic cardiomyopathy)
  - Infectious (Chagas, myocarditis)

- Infiltrative (amyloidosis, sarcoidosis, hemochromatosis)
  - Toxins (ethanol, cocaine, anthracyclines)
  - Tachycardia induced
- Preserved LV systolic function
  - Impaired relaxation: (myocardial ischemia, diabetes mellitus, metabolic syndrome)
  - Tachyarrhythmia (featuring reduced diastolic filling)
  - Restrictive cardiomyopathy (myocardial stiffness, such as hypereosinophilic syndrome, amyloidosis, hemochromatosis)
  - High cardiac output (thiamine deficiency, anemia, thyrotoxicosis, arteriovenous malformations)
  - Increased afterload (aortic stenosis, hypertrophic obstructive cardiomyopathy, hypertensive crisis)
  - Hypervolemia (oliguric renal failure, iatrogenic)

RIGHT VENTRICULAR FAILURE:
- Pulmonary embolism
- Valvular heart disease (mitral stenosis or regurgitation)
- Primary pulmonary hypertension
- Chronic hypoxemic pulmonary disease
- Right-to-left shunts that cause systemic hypoxemia (e.g., large patent foramen ovale)
- Left-to-right shunts that cause volume overload (e.g., atrial septal defect, severe tricuspid regurgitation)
- Bacterial endocarditis (right-sided)
- Right ventricular infarction

Dx DIAGNOSIS

DIFFERENTIAL DIAGNOSIS
- Cirrhosis
- Nephrotic syndrome
- Venous occlusive disease
- COPD, asthma
- Pulmonary embolism
- ARDS (adult respiratory distress syndrome)
- Heroin overdose
- Pneumonia

WORKUP
- Blood work (to diagnose potentially reversible causes, identify comorbidities, and assess disease severity)
  - CBC (to evaluate for anemia, infections), blood urea nitrogen (BUN), creatinine, electrolytes, liver enzymes, thyroid function (especially in the elderly or patients with comorbid atrial fibrillation or known thyroid disease)
  - B-type natriuretic peptide (BNP) is a cardiac neurohormone secreted from the atria in response to elevated LV end-diastolic pressure. The sensitivity is low in asymptomatic patients (but elevated BNP levels have been shown to have a negative predictive value up to 90% in symptomatic patients), and BNP elevation generally correlates with severity of disease and parallels closely morbidity and mortality outcome measures.

- Cardiac biomarkers may be elevated if ischemia is the precipitant factor. In patients with ADCHF, a positive cardiac troponin test is associated with higher in-hospital mortality
  - Routine screening for dyslipidemia and glucose intolerance, given that CAD remains the predominant cause of HF
- Electrocardiogram (ECG)
  - Look for signs of prior MI, chamber enlargement, hypertrophy, heart block, arrhythmia, and evidence of pericardial effusion
  - More than 25% of patients with CHF have some form of intraventricular conduction abnormality that is manifest as an increased QRS duration. The most common pattern seen is left bundle-branch block
- Chest radiography
  - Evaluate for pulmonary venous congestion, pulmonary edema, pleural effusion, cardiomegaly, chamber dilation, and Kerley B lines
- Doppler echocardiography
  - Plays a critical diagnostic role in patients with HF and is useful in assessment of systolic, diastolic, and valvular structure and function
- Exercise stress testing
  - May be useful in evaluating concomitant CAD and assessment of degree of disability
- Cardiac catheterization
  Useful in select patients to evaluate intracardiac filling pressures, estimates of valvular areas, presence of intracardiac shunts, coronary artery anatomy, and calculation of hemodynamic properties such as cardiac output, systemic vascular resistance, and pulmonary artery wedge pressure to further guide management

Rx TREATMENT

NONPHARMACOLOGIC GENERAL MEASURES
- Assess the etiology and severity of disease
- Identify and correct precipitating factors (e.g., anemia, thyrotoxicosis, infections, increased sodium load, medication noncompliance, etc.) and address lifestyle modification (e.g., smoking and alcohol cessation, weight reduction etc.)
- Restrict sodium intake to <2 g/day
- Restriction of fluid intake to <2 L/day in patients with hyponatremia
- Caloric supplementation should be provided to patients with advanced HF with weight loss and muscle wasting due to cardiac cachexia
- For patients with coexisting obstructive sleep apnea, continuous positive airway pressure (CPAP) is often recommended after polysomnography, thereby reducing systolic blood pressure and improving LV function.

TREATMENT OF ADCHF
- Main goals are short-term hemodynamic stabilization, support of oxygenation and ventilation, symptom relief, optimization of tissue perfusion, and recognition of more immedi-

ately life-threatening conditions (arrhythmias, valvular catastrophe, MI, cardiac tamponade, etc.), followed by optimization of chronic oral therapy. Much of the initial therapy of ADCHF is similar regardless of whether a patient exhibits primarily systolic or diastolic dysfunction. An effort should be made to identify patients who may benefit from coronary revascularization

- Maximize oxygenation via upright positioning to reduce work of breathing, administering supplemental oxygenation and considering noninvasive positive pressure ventilation (which has been showed to decrease the need for intubation and is particularly beneficial in patients with hypercapnia) or mechanical ventilation if indicated
- Vasodilators (may be used in patients with ADCHF who are not in cardiogenic shock and do not have comorbid severe aortic stenosis, in an effort to reduce preload and/or afterload)
  - Nitroglycerin (0.4 to 0.8 mg sublingually every 3 to 5 min, or by intravenous infusion starting at 0.2 to 0.4 mcg/kg/min with subsequent titration) may be administered in the emergency setting until relative hypotension ensues. Nitrates are contraindicated after use of phosphodiesterase inhibitors such as sildenafil due to risk of hypotension.
  - Sodium nitroprusside (0.1 to 0.2 mcg/kg/min as an intravenous infusion) is a potent vasodilator with balanced venous and arteriolar effects that usually requires hemodynamic monitoring with an arterial line and may precipitate coronary steal and thiocyanate toxicity.
- Diuretics (have an immediate vasodilator effect, in addition to gradually decreasing intravascular volume)
  - Furosemide (20 to 80 mg intravenous) produces prompt venodilation and diuresis. Intravenous therapy may cause more effective diuresis than oral therapy, and when changing from IV to PO furosemide, doubling the dose is usually necessary for a similar therapeutic effect. Administration of smaller doses of short-acting loop diuretics multiple times daily is preferable to a single large dose, and monitoring of urine output, renal function, and electrolytes is recommended. The addition of metolazone to furosemide often enhances diuresis. Diuretics should be used with caution in patients with aortic stenosis and are contraindicated in patients with severe hypotension or cardiogenic shock.
- Inotropic agents (should be considered when signs and symptoms of ADCHF persist despite vasodilators and diuretics in patients with systolic failure). Inotropic therapy is used for temporary hemodynamic support, but has not been shown to improve survival
  - Dobutamine (starting at 2.5 to 5 mcg/kg/min) can be used for inotropic support but is associated with increased oxygen demand and cardiac arrhythmias and may

result in hypotension from decreased systemic vascular resistance.
  - Milrinone (37.5 to 75 mcg/kg loading dose, followed by 0.375 to 0.75 mcg/kg/min) can be used as a vasodilator and inotropic agent, but is associated with increased oxygen demand and cardiac arrhythmias, and may result in hypotension from decreased systemic vascular resistance.
- Hemodialysis (can be used as an alternative to pharmacologic diuresis in ADCHF when renal function is significantly compromised)
- ACE inhibitors or angiotensin receptor blockers (ARBs), if part of a patient's chronic medication regimen, should be continued in the absence of hypotension, acute renal failure, or hyperkalemia. Beta-blockers, if part of a patient's chronic medication regimen, may be continued or reduced in dosage in mild exacerbations of HF but should be discontinued in patients with hypotension or those requiring inotropic support. Beta-blockers should not be initiated to patients who are not on chronic beta-blocker therapy until the patient is judged to be euvolemic
- Morphine sulfate may be used to reduce patient work of breathing and anxiety and for modest venodilation, but recent retrospective studies have suggested increased incidence of mechanical ventilation and in-hospital mortality in patients who are administered morphine
- If ADCHF with preserved EF is suspected, therapy is usually aimed at symptom control and correction of the inciting factor (e.g., tachycardia, hypertension). Treatment generally involves diuretics to reduce pulmonary congestion with caution not to overdiuresis given the need for elevated filling pressures in these patients to ensure adequate stroke volume and cardiac output. Nitrates may be useful in providing symptomatic relief but may precipitate hypotension. Ventricular rate should be controlled in the presence of atrial fibrillation, which, at rapid rates, is poorly tolerated in patients with impaired diastolic filling. Beta-blockers and calcium channel blockers can be used with caution

CHRONIC TREATMENT OF HF SECONDARY TO SYSTOLIC DYSFUNCTION:

- ACE inhibitors
  - Reduce morbidity and mortality
  - Produce both venous and arterial vasodilation acutely, thereby reducing both preload and afterload
  - Potential mechanism of long-term benefit is attenuation of renin-angiotensin-aldosterone system (RAAS) activation
  - Used as first-line therapy for asymptomatic LV dysfunction (LVEF <40%) and symptomatic systolic HF (ACC/AHA grades A–D)
  - Therapy should be initiated at low doses to prevent hypotension and rapidly titrated to higher doses as tolerated
  - Contraindications to the use of ACE inhibitors are renal insufficiency (creatinine clearance <30 ml/min), bilaterally renal

artery stenosis, hyperkalemia, hypotension, or adverse reactions (e.g., angioedema)
- ARBs
  - Receptor antagonists to the angiotensin II type 1 receptor, inhibiting the effects of angiotensin II
  - Clinical trials have not shown any superiority compared to ACE inhibitors in patients with systolic HF (LVEF <40%)
  - Reserved for patients who are ACE inhibitor intolerant
  - There are conflictive data on the utility of combination therapy with ARBs and ACE inhibitors in addition to beta-blockers for patients who remain symptomatic in the absence of renal dysfunction, hyperkalemia, and outside the post-MI period
  - Have a similar contraindication profile to ACE inhibitors
- Combination of isosorbide dinitrate and hydralazine
  - Function in venous (nitrates) and arteriolar (hydralazine) vasodilation resulting in decreased preload and afterload
  - Combination therapy has been shown to confer morbidity and mortality benefit in African American patients with NYHA class III-IV systolic HF (LVEF <35%) already medicated with ACE inhibitors or ARBs; also indicated in patients unable to tolerate ACE inhibitors or ARBs
  - Adverse effects of nitrates include hypotension, headaches, and tolerance, and reflex tachycardia and lupuslike syndrome for hydralazine
- Beta-adrenergic blockers (beta-blockers)
  - Benefit is thought to be conferred by blockade of sympathetic effects of neurohormonal stimulation due to HF; they have been shown to reduce hospitalizations, sudden death, and overall mortality in CHF
  - Are considered first-line therapy for symptomatic patients with systolic HF (NYHA class ≥II and LVEF <35%)
  - Only carvedilol, bisoprolol, and metoprolol succinate have been approved for the medical treatment of chronic HF; these agents are generally started in patients judged to be euvolemic and dosage is to be slowly uptitrated as tolerated
  - Adverse effects include worsening HF (due to negative inotropic effects), dizziness, bradycardia, hypotension, and bronchospasm
- Aldosterone receptor antagonists
  - Indicated in patients with NYHA class III-IV HF, with LVEF <35%, already treated with ACE inhibitors and beta-blockers without significant renal insufficiency or hyperkalemia
  - Spironolactone may cause gynecomastia, galactorrhea, and hyperkalemia (especially in patients with baseline renal insufficiency or type 4 renal tubular acidosis). Eplerenone is associated with less endocrine side effects
- Diuretics
  - Are used to maintain euvolemia and to improve symptoms

- Loop diuretics such as furosemide are commonly used initially, with subsequent addition of thiazide diuretics such as metolazone or hydrochlorothiazine as needed. Loop diuretics with better bioavailability such as torsemide and bumetanide may be used in diuretic-resistant patients but are generally more expensive
- Digoxin
  - Positive inotropic and negative chronotropic drug that works by inhibition of the sodium-potassium transmembrane exchange pump
  - Commonly used in patients with concomitant atrial fibrillation
  - Has been shown to reduce HF-related hospitalizations but does not confer any mortality benefit
  - Caution must be used in patients with abnormal renal function to avoid digoxin toxicity and life-threatening arrhythmia
- Cardiac resynchronization therapy (CRT)
  - The presence of a bundle-branch block or other intraventricular conduction delay (IVCD) can cause ventricular dyssynchrony, which induces regional loading disparities and reduces the efficiency of ventricular contraction, thereby further impairing the systolic function of a failing ventricle.
  - CRT is recommended in patients with advanced HF (NYHA class III-IV despite optimal medical therapy), severe systolic dysfunction (LVEF <35%), and IVCD (QRS duration >120 msec). CRT is NOT indicated in patients whose functional status and life expectancy are limited predominantly by chronic noncardiac conditions.
  - In the appropriate subset of patients, CRT in addition to optimal medical therapy has been shown in numerous clinical trials to improve symptoms by at least one NYHA class, improve 6-min walk distance and quality of life, reduce rate of HF-related

hospitalization, and reduce rate of all-cause and cardiovascular mortality.
- Implantable cardioverter-defibrillators (ICDs)
  - Sudden cardiac death (SCD) is a common cause of death in patients with HF. Ventricular tachycardia (VT) degenerating into ventricular fibrillation (VF) is the culprit in the majority of patients with SCD, although bradyarrhythmias do also occur with less frequency.
  - In patients with nonischemic cardiomyopathy, primary prevention of SCD with an ICD is appropriate in patients with LVEF <35% and NYHA class II-III HF (and NYHA class IV HF if likelihood of survival is >1 yr). In patients with LVEF <35%, class III-IV HF, and QRS duration >120 msec, a combined biventricular pacemaker and ICD device is indicated. For patients with a history of prior MI and LVEF <30% (>40 days post MI and 3 mo post CABG or PCI), regardless of NYHA classification, an ICD is indicated. In patients who do not meet the above criteria who experience nonsustained VT, the appropriateness of ICD placement is based on electrophysiologic studies.
  - Patients with HF who survive an episode of sudden cardiac arrest or experience sustained VT in the presence of LVEF <35% are at high risk for future arrhythmic events and SCD and obtain a mortality benefit from ICD placement for secondary prevention, with or without adjunctive therapies such as antiarrhythmic drugs, radiofrequency ablation, surgery, or transplant.
- The routine use of anticoagulation is not suggested in patients with HF without history of atrial fibrillation or systemic embolism
- Antiplatelet agents are recommended for patients with concomitant CAD
- Percutaneous coronary intervention (PCI) or surgical revascularization should be consid-

ered in patients with HF and significant CAD who are revascularization candidates

CHRONIC
TREATMENT OF HF WITH PRESERVED SYSTOLIC FUNCTION
- To date, there is a relative dearth of clinical trials examining effective chronic treatment strategies in this subset of patients with HF.
- Therapy centers on relief of volume overload with judicious diuretic use, treatment of ischemia via coronary revascularization, heart rate and blood pressure control to prevent acute decompensation, and sodium and fluid restriction to prevent volume overload.
- Surgical options for contributing critical aortic stenosis, constrictive pericarditis, and hypertrophic cardiomyopathy (HCM) should be entertained in appropriate patients.

DISPOSITION
- Annual mortality of systolic HF ranges from 10% in stable patients with mild symptoms to 50% in patients with NYHA class IV disease (a mortality rate rivaling some malignancies).
- Cardiac transplantation has a 5-yr survival rate of ~70% and represents a viable option in selected patients.
- The use of an LV assist device in patients with advanced HF can result in a clinically meaningful survival benefit and improve quality of life in patients who are not candidates for cardiac transplantation.

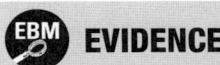

EVIDENCE

available at www.expertconsult.com

SUGGESTED READINGS
available at www.expertconsult.com

AUTHORS: **MAHIM KAPOOR, M.D.,**
FRED F. FERRI, M.D., and **WEN-CHIH WU, M.D.**

BASIC INFORMATION

DEFINITION

Heat exhaustion and heat stroke are part of a continuum of heat-related illness, and unless factors leading to heat exhaustion are corrected swiftly, affected patients can progress to heat stroke.

- Heat exhaustion: an illness resulting from prolonged, heavy activity in a hot environment with subsequent dehydration, electrolyte depletion, and rectal temperature >37.8° C but ≤40° C.
- Heat stroke: a life-threatening heat illness characterized by extreme hyperthermia, dehydration, and neurologic manifestations (core temperature >40° C).

SYNONYMS

Heat illness
Hyperthermia

ICD-9CM CODES
992.0 Heat stroke
992.5 Heat exhaustion

EPIDEMIOLOGY & DEMOGRAPHICS

INCIDENCE (IN U.S.): Incidence of heat stroke is approximately 20 cases/100,000 population.
PREDOMINANT AGE: Heat exhaustion and stroke occur more frequently in elderly patients, especially those taking diuretics or medications that impair heat dissipation (e.g., phenothiazines, anticholinergics, antihistamines, beta-blockers).

PHYSICAL FINDINGS & CLINICAL PRESENTATION

Heat exhaustion:
- Generalized malaise, weakness, headache, muscle and abdominal cramps, nausea, vomiting, hypotension, tachycardia
- Rectal temperature is usually normal
- Sweating is usually present
Heat stroke:
- Neurologic manifestations (seizures, tremor, hemiplegia, coma, psychosis, other bizarre behavior)
- Evidence of dehydration (poor skin turgor, sunken eyeballs)
- Tachycardia, hyperventilation
- Skin is hot, red, and flushed
- Sweating is often (not always) absent, particularly in elderly patients

ETIOLOGY

- Exogenous heat gain (increased ambient temperature)
- Increased heat production (exercise, infection, hyperthyroidism, drugs)
- Impaired heat dissipation (high humidity, heavy clothing, neonatal or elderly patients, drugs [phenothiazines, anticholinergics, antihistamines, butyrophenones, amphetamines, cocaine, alcohol, β-blockers])
- Diuretics, laxatives

Dx **DIAGNOSIS**

DIFFERENTIAL DIAGNOSIS

- Infections (meningitis, encephalitis, sepsis)
- Head trauma
- Epilepsy
- Thyroid storm
- Acute cocaine intoxication
- Malignant hyperthermia
- Heat exhaustion can be differentiated from heat stroke by the following:
  1. Essentially intact mental function and lack of significant fever in heat exhaustion
  2. Mild or absent increases in creatine phosphokinase (CPK), aspartate aminotransferase (AST), lactate dehydrogenase (LDH), and alanine aminotransferase (ALT) in heat exhaustion

WORKUP

- Heat stroke: comprehensive history, physical examination, and laboratory evaluation
- Heat exhaustion: in most cases, laboratory tests are not necessary for diagnosis

LABORATORY TESTS

Laboratory abnormalities may include the following:
- Elevated blood urea nitrogen, creatinine, hematocrit
- Hyponatremia or hypernatremia, hyperkalemia or hypokalemia
- Elevated LDH, AST, ALT, CPK, bilirubin
- Lactic acidosis, respiratory alkalosis (from hyperventilation)
- Myoglobinuria, hypofibrinogenemia, fibrinolysis, hypocalcemia

Rx **TREATMENT**

- Treatment of heat exhaustion consists primarily of placing the patient in a cool, shaded area and providing rapid hydration and salt replacement.
  1. Fluid intake should be at least 2 L q4h in patients without history of CHF.
  2. Salt replacement can be accomplished by using one-quarter teaspoon of salt or two 10-grain salt tablets dissolved in 1 L of water.
  3. If IV fluid replacement is necessary, young athletes can be given normal saline IV (3 to 4 L over 6 to 8 hr); in elderly patients, consider using D5½NS IV with the rate titrated to cardiovascular status.
- Patients with heat stroke should undergo rapid cooling.
  1. Remove the patient's clothes and place the patient in a cool and well-ventilated room.
  2. If patient is unconscious, position on his or her side and clear the airway. Protect airway and augment oxygenation (e.g., nasal O_2 at 4 L/min to keep oxygen saturation >90%).

3. Monitor body temperature every 5 min. Measurement of the patient's core temperature with a rectal probe is recommended. The goal is to reduce the body temperature to 39° C (102.2° F) in 30 to 60 min.
4. Spray the patient with a cool mist and use fans to enhance airflow over the body (rapid evaporation method).
5. Immersion of the patient in ice water, stomach lavage with iced saline solution, intravenous administration of cooled fluids, and inhalation of cold air are advisable only when the means for rapid evaporation are not available. Immersion in tepid water (15° C, 59° F) is preferred over ice water immersion to minimize risk of shivering.
6. Use of ice packs on axillae, neck, and groin is controversial because they increase peripheral vasoconstriction and may induce shivering.
7. Antipyretics are ineffective because the hypothalamic set point during heat stroke is normal despite the increased body temperature.
8. Intubate a comatose patient, insert a Foley catheter, and start nasal O_2. Continuous ECG monitoring is recommended.
9. Insert at least two large-bore IV lines and begin IV hydration with NS or Ringer's lactate.
10. Draw initial laboratory studies: electrolytes, complete blood count, blood urea nitrogen, creatinine, AST, ALT, CPK, LDH, glucose, PT (INR), PTT, platelet count, Ca^{2+}, lactic acid, and arterial blood gases.
11. Treat complications as follows:
    a. Hypotension: vigorous hydration with normal saline or Ringer's lactate.
    b. Convulsions: diazepam 5 to 10 mg IV (slowly).
    c. Shivering: chlorpromazine 10 to 50 mg IV.
    d. Acidosis: use bicarbonate judiciously (only in severe acidosis).
12. Observe for evidence of rhabdomyolysis and hepatic, renal, or cardiac failure and treat accordingly.

DISPOSITION

Most patients recover completely within 48 hr. Central nervous system injury is permanent in 20% of cases. Mortality rate can exceed 30% in patients with prolonged and severe hyperthermia.

SUGGESTED READING

available at www.expertconsult.com

AUTHOR: **FRED F. FERRI, M.D.**

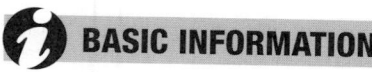

BASIC INFORMATION

DEFINITION

Infection of the human gastric mucosa with the organism *Helicobacter pylori,* a spiral-shaped gram-negative organism with unique features that allow it to survive in the hostile gastric environment.

SYNONYMS

Previously known as *Campylobacter pylori*

ICD-9CM CODES
041.86 *Helicobacter pylori (H. pylori)*

EPIDEMIOLOGY & DEMOGRAPHICS

H. pylori is the most common chronic bacterial infection in human beings, probably affecting 50% of the earth's population in all age groups and probably 30% to 40% of the U.S. population. Infection is acquired at an earlier age and occurs more frequently in developing nations.

CLINICAL PRESENTATION

- *H. pylori* causes histologic gastritis in all affected individuals. The majority of cases are asymptomatic and unlikely to proceed to serious consequences.
- *H. pylori* is a causative agent in peptic ulcer disease (PUD), gastric adenocarcinoma, and gastric mucosa-associated lymphoid tissue lymphoma, and may be a risk factor for iron-deficiency anemia and chronic idiopathic thrombocytopenic purpura. It may present with the signs and symptoms of these disorders, including abdominal pain, bloating, anorexia, and early satiety. Fig. 1-176 describes association of *H. pylori* infection and disease states.
- "Alarm symptoms" that should prompt more immediate and aggressive workup include weight loss, dysphagia, protracted nausea or vomiting, anemia, melena, and palpable abdominal mass.

ETIOLOGY

- Route of acquisition is unknown but is presumed to be person to person by oral–oral or fecal–oral exposure.
- The majority of cases are acquired in childhood. Socioeconomic status and living conditions in childhood affect risk of acquisition of infection. These factors include housing density, number of siblings, overcrowding, sharing a bed, and lack of running water.
- *H. pylori* does not invade gastroduodenal tissue, but disrupts the mucous layer, causing the underlying mucosa to be more vulnerable to acid peptic damage.
- What differentiates the subset of patients with *H. pylori* who go on to develop ulcers or cancer remains unclear.

DIAGNOSIS

DIFFERENTIAL DIAGNOSIS

- Infection with *H. pylori* should be considered in the face of PUD, gastric cancer, gastritis, and gastric MALT lymphoma.
- Upper gastrointestinal (GI) tract disease, including non-ulcer dyspepsia, reflux esophagitis, biliary tract disease, gastroparesis, pancreatitis, and ischemic bowel, may be considered in the differential diagnosis of *H. pylori.*

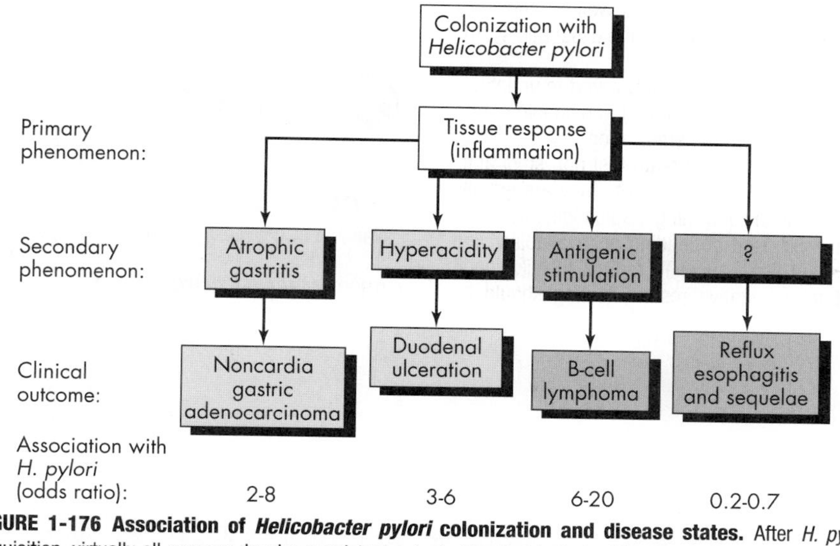

FIGURE 1-176 Association of *Helicobacter pylori* colonization and disease states. After *H. pylori* acquisition, virtually all persons develop persistent colonization that lasts for life. Colonization induces tissue responses termed *chronic gastritis*. This process affects gastric physiology, including glandular structure, acid secretion, and antigen processing, which in turn affect disease risk. Colonization with *H. pylori* increases the risk for certain diseases (duodenal ulcer, gastric ulcer, noncardia gastric adenocarcinoma, and B-cell lymphomas) but appears to decrease the risk for gastroesophageal reflux disease and its complications, including Barrett's esophagus, and adenocarcinoma of the esophagus or gastric cardia. (Mandell GL et al: *Principles and practice of infectious diseases,* ed 7, Philadelphia, 2010, Elsevier.)

WORKUP

- Workup is indicated in patients with active PUD, a past history of documented peptic ulcer, or gastric MALT lymphoma. The role of routine screening in high-risk population is not clear. However, numerous studies suggest that *H. pylori* eradication is protective against progression of premalignant lesions. Consider a test-and-treat approach in asymptomatic first-degree relatives of gastric cancer patients.
- Routine identification and treatment of *H. pylori* in cases of non-ulcer dyspepsia, gastroesophageal reflux disease (GERD), nonsteroidal anti-inflammatory drug (NSAID) use, and in asymptomatic individuals in populations at high risk for gastric cancer are considered controversial, although it may be indicated in specific cases. A test-and-treat strategy may be used in patients aged <55 yr with uncomplicated dyspepsia who have no alarm symptoms.
- Efficacy of testing is related to the individual patient's likelihood of *H. pylori* infection based on demographic risk factors. In the U.S. population, increased probability of infection exists in African Americans, Hispanics/Latinos, immigrants from developing nations, patients with poor socioeconomic status, Native Americans from Alaska, and persons >50 yr.
- Routine screening for *H. pylori* is not indicated in asymptomatic patients who are at low risk of infection.
- There is no evidence that *H. pylori* causes symptoms of nonulcer dyspepsia.

LABORATORY TESTS

- Testing may be invasive or noninvasive depending on the need for endoscopy. There is no indication for endoscopy solely to diagnose *H. pylori.*
- Tests for *H. pylori* are differentiated as active or passive. Active tests provide direct evidence that *H. pylori* infection is currently present and include urea breath testing and stool antigen testing. Passive testing, which includes all serologic testing for *H. pylori,* gives indirect evidence of its presence by detecting the presence of antibodies to the organism. Serologic testing is limited by its inability to distinguish between current, active infection and prior infection that has resolved.
- Tests that use urease as a marker (urea breath and stool antigen tests and biopsy for urease activity) may result in false-negative results in patients taking antibiotics, bismuth, or antisecretory therapy, as well as those with active ulcer bleeding. Patients should be off antibiotics for 4 wk and off protein pump inhibitors for 2 wk before urea breath or stool antigen testing.
- When diagnostic endoscopy is indicated (for suspicion or follow-up of PUD or gastric MALT), antral biopsy should be tested for urease activity. If urease testing is likely to show a false-negative result because of re-

cent proton pump inhibitor (PPI), bismuth, or antibiotic use or active ulcer bleeding, the sample should undergo histologic examination.

- In cases in which biopsy is not indicated, urea breath testing or stool antigen testing are indicated to evaluate for active infection. The sensitivities and specificities of these two tests are similar (>90%). Urea breath testing is slightly more expensive than stool antigen testing, but both costs are in the modest range. Choice can be made based on patient preference and availability.
- Serologic testing may be useful in cases in whom the pretest probability of infection is high or when it is impractical or contraindicated to stop antisecretory therapy for the required duration. It cannot be used to document eradication of infection.

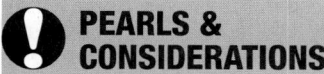 **TREATMENT**

ACUTE GENERAL Rx

- Test only patients whom you intend to treat if positive (see "Workup" above). At this time, the value of eradicating *H. pylori* infection is proven in patients with PUD or gastric MALT lymphoma.
- The optimal antibiotic regimen has not been defined. In addition to efficacy, side effects, cost, and ease of administration must be considered.
- The following regimens are effective in 85% of patients:
  ○ PPI twice daily, with twice-daily clarithromycin (500 mg) and amoxicillin (1 g).
  ○ In cases of penicillin allergy, metronidazole (500 mg bid) may be substituted for amoxicillin. This may reduce effectiveness of treatment because metronidazole resistance has increased.
  ○ PPI twice daily, combined with bismuth four times daily, as well as tetracycline (500 mg qid) and metronidazole (250 mg) four times daily.
- Available data suggest that extending triple therapy beyond 7 days is unlikely to be a clinically useful strategy.
- Prior exposure to a macrolide or metronidazole, for any reason, is associated with increased resistance. A preferable regimen

would include medications to which the patient has not been previously exposed.
- Diarrhea and abdominal cramping are commonly observed with many of the regimens. Other side effects may include a metallic taste with metronidazole or clarithromycin, neuropathy, seizures, and disulfiram-like reaction with metronidazole, diarrhea with amoxicillin, photosensitivity with tetracycline, and *Clostridium difficile* infection with any antibiotic exposure. Bismuth may cause black stool and constipation. Tetracycline is contraindicated in pregnant patients.
- 20% of patients may not respond to initial therapy. Optimal retreatment regimens are under investigation. Use either an alternative regimen with a different combination of medications or quadruple therapy consisting of twice-daily PPI and bismuth-based triple therapy. Levofloxacin-based triple therapy for persistent infections appears effective in international studies but has not been evaluated in U.S. studies. It is important to reinforce compliance.
- A 10-day sequential therapy has been reported to be superior to standard triple therapy for eradication of *H. pylori*. It consists of 5 days of treatment with a PPI and one antibiotic (usually amoxicillin) followed by 5-day treatment with the PPI and two other antibiotics (usually clarithromycin and metronidazole).

CHRONIC Rx

- Data do not support routine testing for cure. Accepted indications for testing to prove eradication include *H. pylori*–associated ulcers, MALT lymphoma, and early gastric cancer. It may be considered in those with persistent dyspepsia despite a test-and-treat management strategy (as well as consideration of other causes for the dyspeptic symptoms).
- Serology does not reliably revert to undetectable levels after treatment and should not be used to determine eradication.
- Active tests (urea breath test and stool antigen testing) are preferable. They are equally accurate in confirming eradication, and either may be used depending on availability and patient preference. To reduce the likelihood of false-negative results, testing should be

performed 4 wk after eradication therapy with PPI and antibiotics or 2 wk after the cessation of PPI therapy.

DISPOSITION

Consider further evaluation in patients with recurrent symptoms after appropriate treatment.

REFERRAL

- Patients with gastric MALT lymphoma should be followed by a gastroenterologist and oncologist with expertise in the care of lymphoid neoplasms.
- Patients with dyspepsia who have tested positive for *H. pylori* and been treated without resolution should be referred for endoscopy.
- Consider referral for biopsy for culture and sensitivity in patients who have not responded to two attempts at treatment.

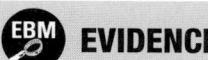 **PEARLS & CONSIDERATIONS**

- Whether *H. pylori* eradication reduces the risk of gastric cancer is unclear.
- Outcomes in PUD and gastric MALT lymphoma are improved with treatment of associated *H. pylori* infection.
- Tests that provide direct evidence of active *H. pylori* infection (urea breath and stool antigen testing) are preferred but may result in false-negative results in patients taking antibiotics, bismuth, or antisecretory agents.
- Serologic testing does not differentiate active from prior infection. It may be useful when active tests are not indicated, particularly in high-risk patients.
- Be aware of high-risk populations in low-prevalence settings, including immigrants from Mexico, South America, Southeast Asia, and Eastern Europe.

EBM **EVIDENCE**

available at www.expertconsult.com

SUGGESTED READINGS

available at www.expertconsult.com

AUTHOR: **MARGARET TRYFOROS, M.D.**

BASIC INFORMATION

DEFINITION

The HELLP syndrome is a serious variant of preeclampsia. HELLP is an acronym for **h**emolysis, **e**levated **l**iver function, and **l**ow **p**latelet count. It is the most frequently encountered microangiopathy of pregnancy. There are three classes of the syndrome based on the degree of maternal thrombocytopenia as a primary indicator of disease severity:

Class 1:   Platelets 50,000/mm^3
Class 2:   Platelets >50,000/mm^3 to 100,000/mm^3
Class 3:   Platelets >100,000/mm^3

ICD-9CM CODES
642.50 HELLP, episode of care
642.51 HELLP, delivered
642.52 HELLP, delivered with postpartum complications
642.53 HELLP, antepartum complications
642.54 HELLP, postpartum complications

EPIDEMIOLOGY & DEMOGRAPHICS

- Among women with severe preeclampsia, 6% will manifest with one abnormality suggestive of HELLP syndrome, 12% will develop two abnormalities, and approximately 10% will develop all three.
- The HELLP syndrome, like preeclampsia, is rare before 20 wk of gestation.
- One third of all cases occur postpartum; of these, only 80% are typically diagnosed with preeclampsia before delivery.

RISK FACTORS: Women >35 yr, white, multiparity
RECURRENCE RATE: 3% to 25%

PHYSICAL FINDINGS & CLINICAL PRESENTATION

- Definitive laboratory criteria remain to be validated prospectively.
- Most commonly used criteria include hemolysis defined by the presence of an abnormal peripheral smear with schistocytes, lactate dehydrogenase (LDH) >600 U/L, and total bilirubin >1.2 mg/dl; elevated liver enzymes as serum aspartate aminotransferase (AST) >70 U/L and LDH >600 U/L; low platelet count as less than 100,000/mm^3.
- Although many women with HELLP syndrome are asymptomatic, 80% report right upper quadrant pain and 50% to 60% present with excessive weight gain and worsening edema.

ETIOLOGY

As with other microangiopathies, endothelial dysfunction, with resultant activation of the intravascular coagulation cascade, has been proposed as the central pathogenesis of HELLP syndrome.

DIAGNOSIS

DIFFERENTIAL DIAGNOSIS

- Appendicitis
- Gallbladder disease
- Peptic ulcer disease
- Enteritis
- Hepatitis
- Pyelonephritis
- Systemic lupus erythematosus
- Thrombotic thrombocytopenic purpura/hemolytic-uremic syndrome
- Acute fatty liver of pregnancy

WORKUP

Because HELLP syndrome is a disease entity based on laboratory values, initial assessment is detailed below.

LABORATORY TESTS

- Initial assessment of suspected HELLP syndrome should include a complete blood count to evaluate platelets, urinalysis, serum creatinine, LDH, uric acid, indirect and total bilirubin levels, and AST/alanine aminotransferase (ALT).
- Tests of prothrombin time, partial thromboplastin time, fibrinogen, and fibrin split products are reserved for women with a platelet count well below 100,000/mm^3.

IMAGING STUDIES

No imaging modalities aid in diagnosis.

TREATMENT

Treatment depends on gestational age of the fetus, severity of condition, and maternal status. Stabilization of the mother is the first priority.

ACUTE GENERAL Rx

- Assess gestational age thoroughly. Fetal status should be monitored with nonstress tests, contraction stress tests, and/or biophysical profile

- Maternal status should be evaluated by history, physical examination, and laboratory testing
- Magnesium sulfate is administered for seizure prophylaxis regardless of blood pressure
- Blood pressure control is achieved with agents such as hydralazine or labetalol
- Indwelling Foley catheter to monitor maternal volume status and urine output

CHRONIC Rx

- In pregnancies of 34 wk or with class 1 HELLP syndrome, delivery, either vaginal or abdominal, within 24 hr is the goal.
- In the preterm fetus corticosteroid therapy to enhance fetal lung maturation is indicated.
- Some reports have shown temporary amelioration of HELLP severity with the administration of high-dose steroids measured by increased urine output, improvement in platelet count, and liver function test.
- Judicious use of blood products, especially in those requiring surgery.
- The patient requires intensive observation for 48 hr postpartum; laboratory levels should begin to improve during this time.

DISPOSITION

The natural history of this disorder is a rapidly deteriorating condition requiring close monitoring of maternal and fetal well-being.

REFERRAL

Preterm patients with HELLP syndrome should be stabilized hemodynamically and transferred to a tertiary care center. Term patients can be treated at a local hospital depending on the availability of obstetric, neonatal, and blood banking services.

PEARLS & CONSIDERATIONS

- Not all women with HELLP have hypertension or proteinuria.
- Life-threatening hemorrhage is a rare event in HELLP Syndrome. Identifiable risk factors predictative of a major hemorrhage are thrombocytopenia (<100,000/mm^3), AST >70 IU/L, and previous gestations.

SUGGESTED READINGS
available at www.expertconsult.com

AUTHORS: **SONYA S. ABDEL-RAZEQ, M.D.**, and **RUBEN ALVERO, M.D.**

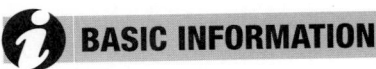

BASIC INFORMATION

DEFINITION

Hemochromatosis is an autosomal-recessive disorder characterized by increased accumulation of iron in various organs (adrenals, liver, pancreas, heart, testes, kidneys, pituitary) and eventual dysfunction of these organs if not treated appropriately.

SYNONYMS

Bronze diabetes

ICD-9CM CODES
275.0 Hemochromatosis

EPIDEMIOLOGY & DEMOGRAPHICS

INCIDENCE: In whites, approximately 1 in 385 persons.

PREDOMINANT SEX AND AGE:

Generally diagnosed in males in their fifth decade. Diagnosis in females is generally not made until 10 to 20 yr after menopause.

GENETICS:

Most common genetic disorder in North European ancestry. Homozygosity for the *C282Y* mutation is now found in approximately 5 of every 1000 persons of European descent.

PHYSICAL FINDINGS & CLINICAL PRESENTATION

- In earlier stages patients completely asymptomatic and diagnosed due to abnormal laboratory tests
- Hepatic dysfunction leading to hepatomegaly, fibrosis, and eventually cirrhosis
- Arthritis
- Gonadal insufficiency leading to loss of libido and testicular atrophy
- Diabetes mellitus: risk greater in patients with family history
- Iron-induced cardiac disease resulting in cardiomyopathy, heart failure, and arrhythmias
- Skin pigmentation

ETIOLOGY

- The majority of the patients diagnosed with hemochromatosis have mutation in the *HFE* gene and are either homozygous for the *C282Y* mutation (*C282Y/C282Y*) or compound heterozygote for the *C282Y* mutation and either the mutation *H63D* (*C282Y/H63D*) or less commonly the *S65C* (*C282Y/S65C*).
- The remainder of the patients are classified as non–*HFE*-associated hemochromatosis.

DIAGNOSIS

DIFFERENTIAL DIAGNOSIS

- Hereditary anemias with defect of erythropoiesis
- Cirrhosis, chronic liver disease, Porphyria cutanea tarda
- Repeated blood transfusions
- African dietary iron overload

WORKUP

Medical history, physical examination, and laboratory evaluation should be focused on affected organ systems (see "Physical Findings & Clinical Presentation"). Liver biopsy is the gold standard for diagnosis; it reveals iron deposition in hepatocytes, bile ducts, and supporting tissues.

LABORATORY TESTS

- Transferrin saturation is the best screening test. Values >45% are an indication for further testing.
- Elevated serum ferritin is good evidence of iron overload, but other causes like chronic inflammatory conditions, malignancy, and so forth needs to be ruled out as ferritin is also an acute phase reactant.
- Genotypical screening for *C282Y* and *H63D* mutation in *HFE* gene should be done in patients with high transferring saturation, elevated ferritin, or both.
- Liver biopsy is the gold standard but is not needed in somebody who has a persistently elevated transferring saturation, elevated ferritin, or both.
- Hepatic iron index can help differentiate between various causes of iron overload.
- Elevated aspartate aminotransferase, alanine aminotransferase, and alkaline phosphatase are seen.
- Hyperglycemia is found.
- Endocrine abnormalities (decreased testosterone, luteinizing hormone, follicle-stimulating hormone) are noted.

IMAGING STUDIES

Routine radiologic imaging is not needed.

TREATMENT

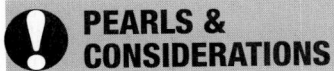

The goal of therapy is the removal of excess iron and maintaining it at a normal or near normal level.

NONPHARMACOLOGIC THERAPY

Phlebotomy is the treatment of choice.

ACUTE GENERAL Rx

- The timing and frequency of phlebotomy needs to be individualized for each patient.
- For patients with heavy iron overload twice weekly phlebotomies should be started.

- The effectiveness of treatment is monitored by periodic ferritin measurement. The goal is to bring ferritin level below 50 μg.
- Patients with iron overload due to transfusion dependent anemias may not tolerate phlebotomy. For these patients iron chelation may be needed.
- The chelating agent deferoxamine has to be given daily as a 9 to 12 hr IV or SC infusion and compliance is difficult.
- An oral chelating agent deferasirox (Exjade) was approved by the FDA in 2005.

CHRONIC Rx

After the ferritin has been brought to less than 50 μg, phlebotomy is needed on an as needed basis to keep the ferritin at that level.

DISPOSITION

Prognosis is good if phlebotomy is started early (before onset of cirrhosis or diabetes mellitus); women can have the full phenotypic expression of the disease, including cirrhosis, and should also be aggressively treated.

REFERRAL

For liver biopsy if diagnosis is uncertain

PEARLS & CONSIDERATIONS

COMMENTS

- Patients with hemochromatosis and serum ferritin levels <1000 μg/L are unlikely to have cirrhosis. Liver biopsy to screen for cirrhosis may be unnecessary in such patients.
- Cirrhotic patients must be periodically monitored (ultrasound or CT scan) because of their increased risk of hepatocellular carcinoma.
- *HFE* gene testing for *C282Y* mutation is a cost-effective method of screening relatives of patients with hereditary hemochromatosis. The American College of Gastroenterology recommends genotyping persons who have abnormal iron screening tests and first-degree relatives of those identified with *C282Y* homozygosity.
- Established cirrhosis, hypogonadism, destructive arthritis, and insulin-dependent diabetes mellitus secondary to hemochromatosis cannot be reversed with repeated phlebotomy, but their progress can be slowed.
- In patients who are heterozygotes for *C282Y* or *H63D* mutation, clinically meaningful iron overload does not develop.

SUGGESTED READINGS
available at www.expertconsult.com

AUTHORS: **BILAL H. NAQVI M.D.**, and **FRED F. FERRI, M.D.**

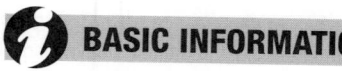

BASIC INFORMATION

DEFINITION

Hemolytic-uremic syndrome (HUS) refers to an acute syndrome characterized by microangiopathic hemolytic anemia, thrombocytopenia, and severe renal failure.

SYNONYMS

HUS

ICD-9CM CODES

283.11 Hemolytic-uremic syndrome

EPIDEMIOLOGY & DEMOGRAPHICS

- HUS affects mainly children younger than 5 yr with incidence rate of 6.1 cases/100,000.
- Overall incidence is 1 to 2 cases/100,000.
- May be epidemic, most commonly occurring during the summer months in rural populations.
- Most common cause of acute renal failure in children.
- In the U.S., 300 to 700 new cases occur each year.

PHYSICAL FINDINGS & CLINICAL PRESENTATION

- HUS usually preceded by diarrhea in 90% of cases, bloody in 75%
- Abdominal pain, vomiting, and fever
- Neurologic symptoms principally seizure and somnolence were observed in 20% to 25% of cases. Stroke or coma: may occur and associated with significant mortality
- Hypertension
- Hepatomegaly and abnormality in liver function tests
- Anuria or oliguria
- Glucose intolerance and transient diabetes (10%)

ETIOLOGY

Pathologically, it is thought that thrombin generation (probably the result of accelerated thrombogenesis) and inhibition of fibrinolysis leads to renal arteriolar and capillary microthrombi preceding renal injury.
In children:
- *Escherichia coli* serotype O157:H7 is the leading cause of HUS.
- The infection is acquired by eating undercooked red meat, nonpasteurized milk or milk products, water, fruits, or vegetables.
- Other causes of HUS in children and adults are:
  - Drugs (cyclosporine, mitomycin, tacrolimus, ticlopidine, clopidogrel, cisplatin, quinine, penicillin, penicillamine, oral contraceptives, and quinine used to treat muscle cramps) and toxins
  - Infection (*Salmonella, Shigella, Yersinia,* Group A streptococci, *Clostridium difficile, Campylobacter,* coxsackievirus, rubella, influenza virus, Epstein-Barr virus)
  - HIV-associated thrombotic microangiopathy
  - Pneumococcal infection
- Complement disorders involving factors H, I, and membrane cofactors protein have been associated with cases of nondiarrhea-associated HUS (atypical HUS).
- Mutations that impair the function of thrombomodulin occur in about 5% of patients with atypical HUS.

DIAGNOSIS

The triad of thrombocytopenia, acute renal failure, and microangiopathic hemolytic anemia establishes the diagnosis of HUS.

DIFFERENTIAL DIAGNOSIS

The differential is vast, including all causes of bloody and nonbloody diarrhea because the GI symptoms usually precede the triad of HUS:
- Thrombotic thrombocytopenic purpura
- Disseminated intravascular coagulation
- Prosthetic valve hemolysis
- Malignant hypertension
- Vasculitis
- Catastrophic antiphospholipid syndrome
- Postpartum acute renal failure
- Scleroderma renal crisis

WORKUP

The workup for suspected HUS patients includes blood tests and stool cultures.

LABORATORY TESTS

- Anemia (hemoglobin <8 g/dl) with peripheral smear shows the hallmark microangiopathic hemolytic anemia with schistocytes, burr cells, and helmet cells
- Thrombocytopenia (platelet counts usually <60,000/mm³)
- Reticulocyte count high
- LDH level elevated
- Haptoglobin low
- Indirect bilirubin elevated
- Negative Coombs test
- BUN and creatinine elevated
- Urinalysis: proteinuria, microscopic hematuria, and pyuria
- Stool cultures for *E. coli* O157:H7 are positive in more than 90% of cases if obtained during the first week of illness. After the first week only one third positive

IMAGING STUDIES

Imaging studies are not very helpful in the diagnosis of HUS.

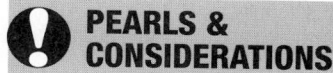

TREATMENT

The treatment of HUS is primarily supportive.

NONPHARMACOLOGIC THERAPY

- Blood transfusions are used for severe anemia.
- Antibiotics and antimotility should be avoided and are not indicated for the treatment of *E. coli* O157:H7.
- Correction of electrolyte abnormalities and fluid management should be performed.
- Platelet transfusion is preserved only for patients with HUS who have significant bleed or invasive procedure is required.
- Although unproven in patients with HUS, plasma exchange has been used in patients with severe CNS involvement.
- Tissue-type plasminogen activator (PAI-1) may have a role in improving renal function in recent studies.

ACUTE GENERAL Rx

Hypertension and seizure control

CHRONIC Rx

For anuric or oliguric renal failure, dialysis may be required.

DISPOSITION

- Adults presenting with HUS have a worse prognosis than do children with HUS.
- Mortality rate is less than 5%.
- Morbidity includes:
  - Proteinuria (31%)
  - Renal insufficiency (31%)
  - Hypertension (6%)

REFERRAL

- The local health department should be notified if the bacteria *E. coli* O157:H7 has been isolated; large food-borne outbreaks have occurred with commercial beef products and asparagus.
- Consultation with hematology and nephrology specialist is recommended in patients with HUS.

PEARLS & CONSIDERATIONS

COMMENTS

- Children testing positive for the *E. coli* O157:H7 serotype should not return to school or day care facilities until two consecutive stools test negative for the microorganism.
- *E. coli* O157:H7 can be transmitted from person to person; therefore universal precautions and hand washing are recommended in preventing the spread of the infection.
- *E. coli* O111 can also be associated with HUS. In 2008 the largest known U.S. serotype 1 *E. coli* O111 occurred in Oklahoma, causing 341 illnesses. The HUS attack rate in this *E. coli* O111 outbreak was comparable to that for *E. coli* O157-related illness, but most cases occurred among adults.

SUGGESTED READINGS

available at www.expertconsult.com

AUTHORS: **MONZR M. AL MALKI, M.D.,** **GLENN G. FORT, M.D., M.P.H.,** and **DENNIS J. MIKOLICH, M.D.**

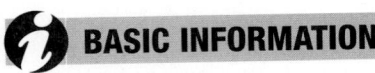

BASIC INFORMATION

DEFINITION

Hemophilia is a hereditary bleeding disorder caused by low factor VIII coagulant activity (hemophilia A) or low levels of factor IX coagulant activity (hemophilia B).

SYNONYMS

Hemophilia A: Classic hemophilia, factor VIII deficiency hemophilia
Hemophilia B: Christmas disease, factor IX hemophilia

ICD-9CM CODES
286.0 Hemophilia A
286.1 Hemophilia B

EPIDEMIOLOGY & DEMOGRAPHICS

INCIDENCE/PREVALENCE (IN U.S.): Hemophilia A: 100 cases per 1 million males; hemophilia B: 20 cases per 1 million males. Approximately 400,000 patients have severe hemophilia worldwide.
GENETIC: Both hemophilias have an X-linked recessive pattern of inheritance with only males affected.

PHYSICAL FINDINGS & CLINICAL PRESENTATION

- The clinical features of hemophilia A and B are generally indistinguishable from each other.
- Bleeding is most commonly seen in joints (knees, ankles, elbows), resulting in hot, swollen, painful joints and subsequent crippling joint deformity.
- Bleeding can also occur into the muscles and the gastrointestinal tract.
- Compartment syndrome can occur from large hematomas.
- Hematuria may be present.

ETIOLOGY

- Hemophilia A: low factor VIII coagulant (VIII:C) activity; can be classified as mild if factor VIII:C levels are >5%, moderate if levels are 1% to 5%, and severe if levels are <1%.
- Hemophilia B: low levels of factor IX coagulant activity.
- Both disorders are congenital.
- Spontaneous acquisition of factor VIII inhibitors (acquired hemophilia) is rare.

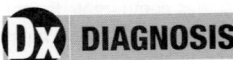 DIAGNOSIS

DIFFERENTIAL DIAGNOSIS

- Other clotting factor deficiencies
- Platelet function disorders
- Vitamin K deficiency

WORKUP

Patients with mild hemophilia bleed only in response to major trauma or surgery and may not be diagnosed until young adulthood. Diagnostic workup includes laboratory evaluation (see "Laboratory Tests").

LABORATORY TESTS

- Partial thromboplastin time (PTT) is prolonged.
- Reduced factor VIII:C level distinguishes hemophilia A from other causes of prolonged PTT.
- Factor VIII antigen, prothrombin time, fibrinogen level, and bleeding time are normal.
- Factor IX coagulant activity levels are reduced in patients with hemophilia B.
- Coagulation factor activity measurement is useful to correlate with disease severity. Normal range is 50 to 150 U/dl; 5 to 20 U/dl indicates mild disease, 2 to 5 U/dl indicates moderate disease, and <2 U/dl indicates severe disease with spontaneous bleeding episodes.

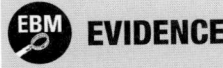 TREATMENT

NONPHARMACOLOGIC THERAPY

- Avoidance of contact sports
- Patient education regarding the disease; promotion of exercises such as swimming
- Avoidance of aspirin or other NSAIDs
- Orthopedic evaluation and physical therapy evaluation in patients with joint involvement
- Hepatitis vaccination

ACUTE GENERAL Rx

Hemophilia A:
- Reversal and prevention of acute bleeding in hemophilia A and B are based on adequate replacement of deficient or missing factor protein.
- The choice of the product for replacement therapy is guided by availability, capacity, concerns, and cost. Recombinant factors cost two to three times as much as plasma-derived factors, and the limited capacity to produce recombinant factors often results in periods of shortage. In the U.S., 60% of patients with severe hemophilia use recombinant products.
- Factor VIII concentrates are effective in controlling spontaneous and traumatic hemorrhage in severe hemophilia. The new recombinant factor VIII is stable without added human serum albumin (decreased risk of transmission of infectious agents).
- Recombinant activated factor VII is useful to stop spontaneous hemorrhages and prevent excessive bleeding during surgery in 75% of patients with inhibitors. Recommended dose

is 90 μg/mg of body weight every 2 to 3 hr for treatment of life-threatening hemorrhage. It is, however, very expensive ($1 per μg).
- Desmopressin acetate 0.3 μg/kg q24h (causes release of factor VIII:C) may be used in preparation for minor surgical procedures in mild hemophiliacs.
- Aminocaproic acid (EACA, Amicar) 4 g PO q4h can be given for persistent bleeding that is unresponsive to factor VIII concentrate or desmopressin.

Hemophilia B:
- Infuse factor IX concentrates. It is important to remember that factor IX concentrates contain other proteins that may increase the risk of thrombosis with recurrent use. Therefore factor IX concentrates must be used only when clearly indicated.
- Daily administration of oral cyclophosphamide and prednisone without empirical factor VIII therapy is an effective and well-tolerated treatment for acquired hemophilia.

CHRONIC Rx

- The aim of chronic treatment is to prevent spontaneous bleeding and excessive bleeding during any surgical intervention.
- Prophylaxis with recombinant factor VIII can prevent joint damage and decrease the frequency of joint and other hemorrhages in young boys with severe hemophilia A. The estimated annual cost for treatment of one patient with recombinant factor VIII is $300,000.
- Implantation of genetically altered fibroblasts that produce factor VIII is safe and well tolerated. This form is feasible in patients with severe hemophilia. Hemophilia will likely be the first common, severe genetic disease to be cured by gene therapy.

DISPOSITION

- Despite the advent of virally safe blood products and blood treatment programs, nearly 70% of hemophiliacs are HIV seropositive. Survival is of normal expectancy in HIV-negative patients with mild disease.
- Intracranial bleeds are the second most common cause of death in hemophiliacs after AIDS. They are fatal in 30% of patients, occur in 10% of patients, and are generally the result of trauma.

EVIDENCE

available at www.expertconsult.com

SUGGESTED READING
available at www.expertconsult.com

AUTHOR: **FRED F. FERRI, M.D.**

BASIC INFORMATION

DEFINITION

Coughing up of blood originating from the lower respiratory tract, ranging from blood-streaked sputum to gross blood. If greater than 100 to 600 ml in 24 hours, considered massive hemoptysis

ICD-9CM CODES
786.3 Hemoptysis

EPIDEMIOLOGY & DEMOGRAPHICS

INCIDENCE: Unknown, varies based on underlying pathology
RISK FACTORS: Tobacco smoking predisposes to lung cancer, a common cause of hemoptysis. Free-base ("crack") cocaine has been associated with diffuse alveolar hemorrhage. Anticoagulation can worsen bleeding.

PHYSICAL FINDINGS & CLINICAL PRESENTATION

- Presentation of hemoptysis is variable and can range from minimal blood-tinged sputum to more than 500 ml of gross blood in 24 hr. Other symptoms depend on the underlying etiology and can include cough, sputum production, fever, shortness of breath, weight loss, night sweats, wheezing, and chest pain.
- There are no specific exam findings, but clues to the etiology may be present, for example, focal wheezing, rhonchi or rales on pulmonary exam, murmur of mitral stenosis on cardiac exam.

ETIOLOGY

- There are many potential causes of hemoptysis including airway disease (bronchitis, bronchiectasis, lung neoplasm), infection (necrotizing pneumonia, lung abscess, tuberculosis, fungal infection), inflammatory diseases (Wegener's granulomatosis, Goodpasture's syndrome, lupus), cardiac disease (mitral stenosis after rheumatic heart disease, congenital heart diseases), and others (pulmonary embolism, cocaine use, foreign body, airway trauma, iatrogenic and cryptogenic).

- In one study of 208 patients, the most common causes of hemoptysis were bronchiectasis, lung cancer, bronchitis, and pneumonia, respectively.

DIAGNOSIS

DIFFERENTIAL DIAGNOSIS

- Various potential causes of lower respiratory tract bleeding
  - Airway disease (bronchitis, bronchiectasis, lung neoplasm)
  - Infection (necrotizing pneumonia, lung abscess, tuberculosis, fungal infection)
  - Inflammatory diseases (Wegener's granulomatosis, Goodpasture's syndrome, lupus)
  - Cardiac disease (mitral stenosis after rheumatic heart disease, congenital heart diseases)
  - Pulmonary embolism
  - Cocaine use
  - Foreign body
  - Airway trauma
- Bleeding from upper respiratory tract
- Hematemesis
- Coagulopathy

WORKUP

Complete history and physical exam may suggest a particular etiology, important to ask about duration and quantity of hemoptysis and smoking history.

LABORATORY TESTS

- Complete blood count
- Coagulation profile
- Serum chemistries including creatinine, urinalysis (these latter studies if pulmonary-renal syndromes are in the differential)
- Arterial blood gas to assess oxygenation
- Sputum for cultures and cytologic studies

IMAGING STUDIES

- Chest x-ray: all patients with hemoptysis should have a chest x-ray but will likely need additional studies to localize site of bleeding.
- Chest CT: chest CT scan combined with flexible bronchoscopy has the highest yield for localizing the site of bleeding.

TREATMENT

Varies based on underlying etiology and non-massive versus massive hemoptysis

NONPHARMACOLOGIC THERAPY

Massive hemoptysis:
- Arteriographic embolization of bronchial arteries and/or collateral systemic vessels
- Surgical resection of affected lung

ACUTE GENERAL Rx

Massive hemoptysis:
- Stabilize hemodynamic status and oxygenation.
- Reverse any coagulopathy.
- If site of bleeding is known, place patient with bleeding lung in dependent position to prevent blood from spilling into nonaffected lung.
- Bronchoscopic lavage with iced saline or topical application of epinephrine can be tried as a temporizing measure.
- Bronchoscopic balloon tamponade of bleeding site can be used as temporizing measure.
- Early consultation with interventional radiology and thoracic surgery for definitive intervention is recommended.

Nonmassive hemoptysis:
For nonmassive hemoptysis, identify and treat underlying condition. Referral to pulmonologist or hematologist if indicated.

CHRONIC Rx

For patients requiring anticoagulation or antiplatelet therapy for another disorder, consider risks/benefits of continued anticoagulation or antiplatelet therapy.

DISPOSITION

Generally, patients have a good prognosis after an episode of hemoptysis, but those with massive bleeding and/or malignancy tend to have a poorer prognosis.

SUGGESTED READINGS
available at www.expertconsult.com

AUTHOR: **SARAH TAPYRIK, M.D.**

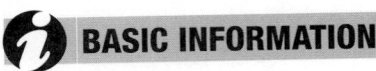

BASIC INFORMATION

DEFINITION

A hemorrhoid is a varicose dilation of a vein of the superior or inferior hemorrhoidal plexus, resulting from a persistent increase in venous pressure. External hemorrhoids are below the pectinate line (inferior plexus). Internal hemorrhoids are above the pectinate line (superior plexus) (Fig. 1-177).

SYNONYMS

Piles

ICD-9CM CODES
455.6 Hemorrhoids

EPIDEMIOLOGY & DEMOGRAPHICS

Potential for development of symptomatic hemorrhoids in all adults
PREVALENCE: Estimated 50% of the adult population in the United States.
PREDOMINANT SEX: Males and females affected equally

PHYSICAL FINDINGS & CLINICAL PRESENTATION

- Painless bleeding with defecation; bleeding is bright red and staining on toilet paper
- Perianal irritation
- Mucofecal staining of underclothes
- Acute external hemorrhoids: painful, swollen, and often thrombosed
- Pain on sitting, standing, or defecating (thrombosed hemorrhoid)
- Prolapse
- Constipation

ETIOLOGY

- Low-fiber, high-fat diet
- Chronic constipation and straining with defecation
- High resting anal sphincter pressures
- Pregnancy
- Obesity
- Rectal surgery (i.e., episiotomy)
- Prolonged sitting
- Anal intercourse

DIAGNOSIS

DIFFERENTIAL DIAGNOSIS

- Fissure
- Abscess
- Anal fistula
- Condylomata acuminata
- Hypertrophied anal papillae
- Rectal prolapse
- Rectal polyp
- Neoplasm

WORKUP

- Inspection
- Digital rectal examination
- Anoscopy
- Sigmoidoscopy

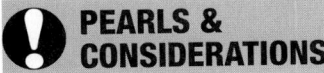

TREATMENT

NONPHARMACOLOGIC THERAPY

- Avoidance of constipation and straining with defecation
- Avoidance of prolonged sitting on toilet
- High-fiber diet (20 to 30 g/day)
- Increased fluid intake (six to eight glasses of water per day)
- Cleaning with mild soap and water after defecation
- Warm soaks or ice to soothe
- Sitz baths

ACUTE GENERAL Rx

- Fiber supplements to provide bulk (psyllium extracts or mucilloids)
- Medicated compresses with witch hazel
- Topical hydrocortisone (1% to 3% cream or ointment)
- Topical anesthetic spray
- Glycerin suppositories
- Stool softeners
- Surgically remove during first 72 hr after onset

CHRONIC Rx

- Rubber-band ligation
- Injection sclerotherapy
- Photocoagulation
- Cryodestruction
- Hemorrhoidectomy

- Anal dilation
- Laser or cautery hemorrhoidectomy
- Observance for complications: thrombosis, bleeding, infection, anal stenosis or weakness

DISPOSITION

Should resolve, but there is a high rate of recurrence

REFERRAL

To colorectal or general surgeon for any hemorrhoid that does not respond to conservative therapy

PEARLS & CONSIDERATIONS

COMMENTS

- Patients need to understand the importance of a healthy diet, regular exercise, and rectal hygiene.
- Stress the importance of avoiding prolonged sitting and straining on the toilet.
- Stress the need not to defer the urge to defecate.

EVIDENCE

available at www.expertconsult.com

SUGGESTED READING

available at www.expertconsult.com

AUTHORS: **MARIA A. CORIGLIANO, M.D.,** and **RUBEN ALVERO, M.D.**

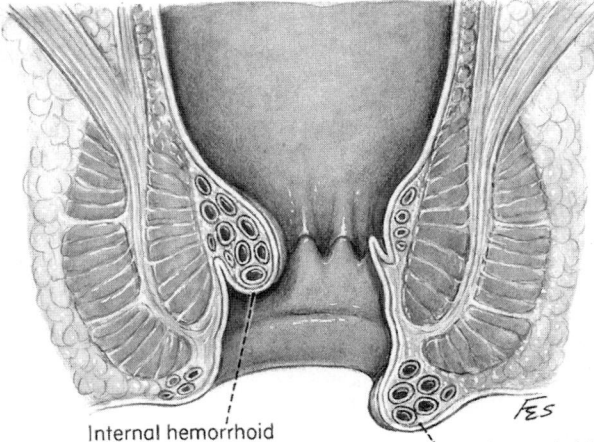

FIGURE 1-177 Anatomy of internal and external hemorrhoids. (From Noble J [ed]: *Textbook of primary care medicine,* ed 2, St Louis, 1996, Mosby.)

Internal hemorrhoid

External hemorrhoid

BASIC INFORMATION

DEFINITION

Henoch-Schönlein purpura (HSP) is a systemic, small-vessel, IgA immune complex–mediated leukocytoclastic vasculitis characterized by a triad of palpable purpura, abdominal pain, and arthritis. It may also present with gastrointestinal (GI) bleeding, arthralgias, and renal involvement.

SYNONYMS

Anaphylactoid purpura
Allergic purpura

EPIDEMIOLOGY & DEMOGRAPHICS

INCIDENCE: Annual incidence of 20 cases/100,000 population
PEAK INCIDENCE: Majority in spring, rarely in summer
PREVALENCE: Most common vasculitis seen in children and younger age groups; whites and Asians more common than black patients
PREDOMINANT SEX: 2:1 male/female ratio
PREDOMINANT AGE: Seen mostly from ages 4 to 15, although can be seen in older adolescents and young adults

PHYSICAL FINDINGS & CLINICAL PRESENTATION

- Palpable purpura of dependent areas, especially lower extremities (Fig. 1-178) and areas subjected to pressure, such as the beltline in adults or buttocks in toddlers.
- Subcutaneous edema.
- Arthralgias and arthritis in 80%. Typically oligoarticular, affecting lower extremity and large joints. Periarticular swelling and tenderness also noted.
- GI symptoms are seen in approximately one third of patients. Common findings are nausea, vomiting, diarrhea, cramping, abdominal pain, hematochezia, and melena. Complications include GI bleeding (20% to 30%), bowel ischemia, intussusception, and bowel perforation.

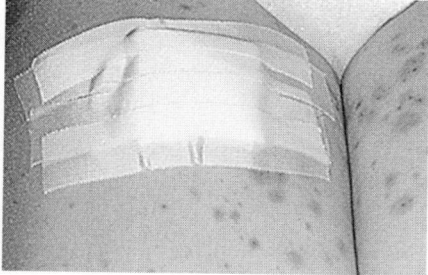

FIGURE 1-178 Henoch-Schönlein purpura on the lower extremities of a child. (Courtesy Medical College of Georgia, Division of Dermatology. From Goldstein B [ed]: *Practical dermatology,* ed 2, St Louis, 1997, Mosby.)

- Anecdotally may follow upper respiratory infection.
- Renal involvement is seen in as many as 80% of older children, usually within the first month of illness. Fewer than 5% progress to end-stage renal failure, a major cause of morbidity. Renal manifestations may range from isolated hematuria or proteinuria to acute nephropathy with renal insufficiency.

ETIOLOGY

- Presumptive etiology is exposure to a trigger antigen that causes antibody formation.
- Antigen-antibody (immune) complex deposition then occurs in arteriole and capillary walls of skin, renal mesangium, and GI tract. Immunoglobulin (Ig) A deposition is most common.
- Antigen triggers postulated include drugs, foods, immunization, and upper respiratory and other viral illnesses. Group A streptococcal infection is the most common precipitant in children, seen in up to one third of cases. A recent adult case triggered by pantoprazole has also been reported.
- Serologic and pathologic evidence suggests an association between Parvovirus B19 and HSP, which may explain observed cases of HSP that do not respond to corticosteroids or other immunosuppressive therapy.
- Case reports describing development of HSP after treatment with immunosuppressive agents (e.g., etanercept) have been published.
- Recent studies suggest an association with the "Mediterranean fever" (MEFV) gene.

DIAGNOSIS

- Diagnosis is clinical.
- Skin manifestations are most common.
- Palpable purpura is seen in 70% of adult patients, whereas GI symptoms are more common in children.
- Skin biopsy shows leukocytoclastic vasculitis. Renal biopsy shows mesangial IgA deposition.
- The presence of two of the following four American College of Rheumatology criteria yields a diagnostic sensitivity of 87.1% and specificity of 87.7%:
  - Palpable purpura unrelated to thrombocytopenia
  - Age <20 yr at onset of first symptoms
  - Bowel angina or ischemia
  - Granulocytic infiltration of arteriole or venule walls on biopsy

DIFFERENTIAL DIAGNOSIS

- Polyarteritis nodosa
- Meningococcemia
- Thrombocytopenic purpura
- Hypersensitivity vasculitis
- Microscopic polyangitis
- Wegener granulomatosis

WORKUP

History, physical examination, laboratory testing, skin or renal biopsy

LABORATORY TESTS

- Electrolytes, blood urea nitrogen, and creatinine
- Urinalysis
- Complete blood count
- Prothrombin time, fibrinogen, and fibrin degradation products
- Blood cultures

Laboratory abnormalities are not specific for HSP. Leukocytosis and eosinophilia may be seen. IgA levels are elevated in approximately 50% of patients. Glomerulonephritis may be present (microscopic hematuria, proteinuria, and red blood cell casts).

IMAGING STUDIES

Imaging studies are generally not useful in the diagnosis of HSP. Arteriography or magnetic resonance angiography may be helpful in distinguishing from polyarteritis nodosa. Abdominal ultrasound can be used to detect intussusception.

TREATMENT

- Nonsteroidal antiinflammatory drugs for arthritis and arthralgias.
- Prednisone 1 mg/kg PO is given if renal or severe GI disease, although clear benefits in renal disease have not been demonstrated according to a recent Cochrane Systematic review.
- A recent double-blind, randomized, controlled trial found that early treatment with prednisone reduced abdominal pain and joint symptoms but did not prevent development of renal disease. It was effective in the treatment of renal disease once it was established.
- Corticosteroids and azathioprine may be beneficial if rapidly progressive glomerulonephritis is present. Pulse methylprednisolone therapy has also been proposed in patients with glomerulonephritis, mesenteric vasculitis, or pulmonary involvement. A recent report described improvement in rapidly progressive glomerulonephritis after treatment with mycophenolate mofetil.
- Hospitalization for significant GI or Renal involvement.

NONPHARMACOLOGIC THERAPY

Supportive care with pain management, adequate hydration, and nutrition

DISPOSITION & PROGNOSIS

- Prognosis excellent, with spontaneous recovery of most patients within 4 wk.
- End-stage renal disease occurs in 1% to 5% of patients. Chronic renal insufficiency is the most common long-term morbidity.
- GI complications (mesenteric infarction, perforation, and intussusception).
- Recurrences in up to one third of patients, especially within first 4 to 6 mo after initial episode and most commonly in patients with renal involvement. Recurrences less severe than initial episode.

REFERRAL

Nephrologist or gastroenterologist

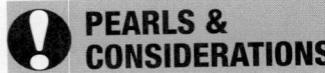

PEARLS & CONSIDERATIONS

- HSP is an IgA-related vasculitis.
- Organ systems involved are skin, joints, GI tract, and kidneys.
- Palpable purpura more common in adults; GI symptoms more common in children.
- Most with spontaneous recovery within 4 wk of onset of symptoms.
- End-stage renal disease occurs in only 5% of patients.
- Steroids and immunosuppressive agents may offer some benefit.

SUGGESTED READINGS

available at www.expertconsult.com

AUTHORS: **NIDA CHAUDHARY, M.D.,** and **DOMINICK TAMMARO, M.D.**

BASIC INFORMATION

DEFINITION

There are two forms of heparin-induced thrombocytopenia (HIT). Type 1 HIT is a mild, transient decrease in platelet count that occurs during the first few days of heparin exposure due to platelet agglutination. This form is benign, and the platelet count will return to normal while heparin is continued. This section will refer to Type 2 HIT, an antibody-mediated thrombocytopenia that is associated with a high risk of developing thrombosis.

SYNONYMS

Type II heparin-induced thrombocytopenia
Heparin-induced thrombocytopenia and thrombosis (HITT)
White clot syndrome
Heparin-associated immune thrombocytopenia

ICD-9CM CODES
289.84

EPIDEMIOLOGY & DEMOGRAPHICS

INCIDENCE: Occurs in 1% to 5% of patients exposed to heparin. Unfractionated heparin is associated with a 10 times higher risk of HIT compared to low-molecular-weight heparin.
PREDOMINANT SEX AND AGE: Females are at slightly higher risk than males. More common in adults but may also occur in children.
RISK FACTORS: Longer duration of exposure to heparin, type of heparin (unfractionated heparin has a greater risk), type of patient (surgical patients, especially cardiac and orthopedic surgery, at higher risk than medical patients).

PHYSICAL FINDINGS & CLINICAL PRESENTATION

Suspect in a patient with:
- Exposure to heparin for 4 to 14 days OR who was exposed to heparin in the prior 3 mo
- Unexplained platelet count decrease to 50% below pretreatment baseline
- Onset of thrombocytopenia 5 to 10 days after heparin initiation
- Evidence of acute venous or arterial thrombosis
- Skin lesions/necrosis at heparin injection sites
- Acute anaphylactoid reaction during administration of heparin bolus

ETIOLOGY

Occurs due to the formation of antibodies, directed against heparin in complex with platelet factor 4, which bind to and activate platelets. Activated platelets release platelet factor 4 (leading to more antibody production) and undergo aggregation and premature removal from the circulation (resulting in thrombocytopenia). This platelet activation and antibody formation also can lead to thrombosis.

DIAGNOSIS

DIFFERENTIAL DIAGNOSIS

Thrombocytopenia due to other causes including:
- Sepsis
- Disseminated intravascular coagulation
- Thrombocytopenic thrombotic purpura
- Hemolytic uremic syndrome
- Drug-induced thrombocytopenia (other than heparin)
- Antiphospholipid antibody syndrome.

WORKUP

HIT is a clinical diagnosis. See Table 1-64 for workup based on pretest probability. If the patient has a low pretest probability score, heparin can be safely continued, and there is no need to send for further testing for HIT. If the patient has a moderate pretest probability, HIT testing and imaging studies for lower extremity deep venous thrombosis should be performed (also consider imaging of upper extremities if swelling is present or venous catheters are in place). If the patient has a high pretest probability, no further testing is required and the patient should be treated for HIT. Imaging for the presence of deep venous thrombosis may help determine length of treatment needed.

LABORATORY TESTS

In the appropriate clinical setting, testing for HIT antibodies with an enzyme-linked immunosor-

TABLE 1-64 A Diagnostic and Treatment Approach to Heparin-Induced Thrombocytopenia

Suspicion of HIT based upon the "4 T's"	Score	Pre-test Probability Score Criteria		
		2	1	0
Thrombocytopenia	☐	nadir 20-100, or >50% platelet fall	nadir 10-19, or 30-50% platelet fall	nadir <10, or <30% platelet fall
Timing of onset of platelet fall	☐	day 5-10, or ≤day 1 with recent heparin*	>day 10 or timing unclear (but fits with HIT)	≤day 1 (no recent heparin)
Thrombosis or other sequelae	☐	proven thrombosis, skin necrosis, or ASR†	progressive, recurrent, or silent thrombosis; erythematous skin lesions possible	none
OTher cause of platelet fall	☐	none evident		definite
Total Pre-test Probability Score	☐	periodic reassessment as new information can change pre-test probability (e.g., positive blood cultures)		

Total Pre-test Probability Score				
High		Moderate	Low	
8	7	6	5	4	3	2	1	0
Stop heparin‡, give alternative non-heparin anticoagulant argatroban¶ or lepirudin# or danaparoid** (or bivalirudin†† or fondaparinux‡‡)		Physician judgment	Continue (LMW) heparin	

Positive test for HIT antibodies ← **HIT Test** → **Negative** test for HIT antibodies
Continue non-heparin anticoagulant until platelet count recovery | Consider continuing or switching back to (LMW) heparin ##

Thrombosis*** ← **Imaging studies for lower-limb DVT †††** → **No Thrombosis**
If HIT, continue non-heparin anticoagulant until platelet count recovery, then **cautious coumarin overlap¶¶** | If HIT, consider anticoagulating until platelet count recovery, even if no thrombosis apparent (± coumarin ¶¶)

* recent heparin indicates exposure within the past 30 days (2 points) or past 30-100 days (1 point)
† ASR, acute systemic reaction following i.v. heparin bolus (see Table 4)
‡ stop all heparin, including catheter "flushes" and, possibly, heparin-coated catheters
¶ argatroban: approved (U.S., Canada) for isolated HIT and HIT complicated by thrombosis (2 μg/kg/min i.v., adjusted to 1.5-3.0X patient's baseline aPTT or the mean of the laboratory normal range); reduce dose for hepatobiliary compromise: may increase INR more than the other direct thrombin inhibitors, thus requiring care in managing coumarin overlap (see ¶¶ below)
# lepirudin: approved (U.S., Canada, E.U., elsewhere) for treatment of thrombosis complicating HIT (±0.4 mg/kg i.v. bolus, then 0.15 mg/kg adjusted to 1.5-2.5X patient's baseline aPTT or mean of the laboratory normal range); used (off-label) also to treat isolated HIT (0.1 mg/kg/h, adjusted by aPTT); to avoid overdosing and anaphylaxis, it may be preferable to omit the bolus, and begin as i.v. infusion (except when facing life- or limb-threatening thrombosis); reduce dose for renal insufficiency
** danaparoid: usual i.v. bolus, 2,250 U (body weight 60-75 kg) followed by infusion (400 U/hr for 4 h, then 300 U/h for 4 h, then 200 U/h, adjusted by anti-factor Xa levels); this therapeutic-dose regimen is appropriate both for isolated HIT and for HIT complicated by thrombosis (though higher than approved dose in some jurisdictions); withdrawn from U.S. market (2002)
†† bivalirudin: no bolus, i.v. infusion 0.15 mg/kg/h adjusted by aPTT; limited experience (off-label)
‡‡ fondaparinux: dosing for HIT not established; limited experience (off-label)
¶¶ delay coumarin pending substantial platelet count recovery (at least >100, preferably >150); begin coumarin in low doses, with at least 4-5 day overlap, stopping alternative anticoagulant when INR therapeutic for 2 days and platelets recovered
depending on physician confidence in the laboratory's ability to rule out HIT antibodies (usually, negative PF4-dependent enzyme-immunoassay and/or washed platelet activation assay performed by an experienced laboratory)
*** some thrombi may require special treatment, e.g., thrombectomy for large limb artery thrombosis
††† routine ultrasound of lower-limb veins recommended, since many HIT patients have subclinical deep-vein thrombosis (DVT)

From Warkentin TE et al: Platelet-endothelial interactions: sepsis, HIT, and antiphospholipid syndrome, *Hematol (Am Soc Hematol Educ Prog* 506-507, 2003.

bent assay, or ELISA, can be useful. This test is very sensitive, but not specific. The majority of patients with positive testing for HIT antibodies will not develop clinical HIT. Thus, HIT antibody testing is more effective for ruling out the diagnosis than confirming the diagnosis of HIT. A more specific test is the serotonin release assay (^{14}C-SRA). Donor platelets are incubated with radiolabeled serotonin. The platelets internalize the serotonin and are then exposed to the patient's serum and heparin at a therapeutic concentration. The platelets undergo a release reaction if antibodies to the platelet factor 4–heparin complex are present in the patient's serum and the released radioactive serotonin is then measured. Unfortunately, results of this test are usually not available for about 2 wk and thus are not clinically helpful in most situations.

IMAGING STUDIES

Doppler sonography of the extremities in the correct clinical setting

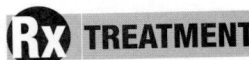

- For patients with a high pretest probability, or a moderate pretest probability with evidence of thrombosis and/or positive HIT antibody testing, DISCONTINUE ALL HEPARIN EXPOSURE. Even if the patient does not have a clinically evident thrombosis, they are at a 50% risk of developing a clot within the subsequent 30 days. Thus, the patient must be started on an alternate anticoagulant.
- Three agents, all direct thrombin inhibitors, are approved for this indication:
  - argatroban (avoid in liver dysfunction)
  - lepirudin (avoid in renal dysfunction)
  - bivalirudin (bivalirudin is approved only for patients with HIT or at risk of HIT who are undergoing PCI).
- These drugs should be continued as a single agent until the platelet count returns to baseline (or at least to a platelet count of 150 × 10^9/L), then warfarin can be added at a maximum dose of 5 mg/day. This overlap therapy should continue until the platelet count has reached a stable plateau, the INR has reached the intended target (remember that argatroban artificially elevates the INR), and after a minimum overlap of 5 days of both the direct thrombin inhibitor and warfarin. The length of treatment is controversial, but most clinicians agree that one month of alternate anticoagulation is sufficient in the absence of thrombosis, while three months of treatment is required in the presence of thrombosis.

NONPHARMACOLOGIC THERAPY

All non-pharm therapies including surgical procedures.

REFERRAL

Consider hematology consult

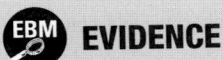
PEARLS & CONSIDERATIONS

COMMENTS

HIT paradoxically causes thrombocytopenia and CLOTTING, not bleeding.

PREVENTION

Consider the use of low-molecular-weight heparin (as opposed to unfractionated heparin) as DVT prophylaxis

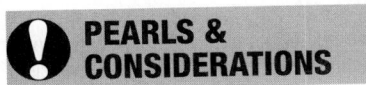 **EVIDENCE**

available at www.expertconsult.com

SUGGESTED READINGS

available at www.expertconsult.com

AUTHOR: **ANGELA PLETTE, M.D.**

BASIC INFORMATION

DEFINITION

Hepatic encephalopathy (HE) is a neuropsychiatric syndrome occurring in patients with severe impairment of liver function and consequent accumulation of toxic products not metabolized by the liver. It is characterized by gradual impairment of the ability to perform mental tasks and to react to external stimuli.

SYNONYMS Hepatic coma

ICD-9CM CODES
572.2 Hepatic encephalopathy

EPIDEMIOLOGY & DEMOGRAPHICS

INCIDENCE/PREVALENCE: Hepatic encephalopathy occurs in >50% of all cases of cirrhosis.

PHYSICAL FINDINGS & CLINICAL PRESENTATION

Hepatic encephalopathy can be classified in stages or grades 1 to 4:
- Grades 1 and 2: mild obtundation
- Grades 3 and 4: stupor to deep coma, with or without decerebrate posturing

The physical examination in hepatic encephalopathy varies with the stage and may reveal the following abnormalities:
- Skin: jaundice, palmar erythema, spider angiomata, ecchymosis, dilated superficial periumbilical veins (caput medusae) in patients with cirrhosis
- Eyes: scleral icterus, Kayser-Fleischer rings (Wilson's disease)
- Breath: fetor hepaticus
- Chest: gynecomastia in men with chronic liver disease
- Abdomen: ascites, small nodular liver (cirrhosis), tender hepatomegaly (congestive hepatomegaly)
- Rectal examination: hemorrhoids (portal hypertension), guaiac-positive stool (alcoholic gastritis, bleeding esophageal varices, peptic ulcer disease, bleeding hemorrhoids)
- Genitalia: testicular atrophy in males with chronic liver disease
- Extremities: pedal edema from hypoalbuminemia
- Neurologic: flapping tremor (asterixis), obtundation, coma with or without decerebrate posturing

ETIOLOGY
- Precipitating factors in patients with underlying cirrhosis (upper gastrointestinal bleeding, hypokalemia, hypomagnesemia, analgesic and sedative drugs, sepsis, alkalosis, increased dietary protein)
- Acute fulminant viral hepatitis
- Drugs and toxins (e.g., isoniazid, acetaminophen, diclofenac and other NSAIDs, statins, methyldopa, loratadine, propylthiouracil, lisinopril, labetalol, halothane, carbon tetrachloride, erythromycin, nitrofurantoin, troglitazone)
- Reye's syndrome
- Shock and/or sepsis
- Fatty liver of pregnancy

- Metastatic carcinoma, hepatocellular carcinoma
- Other: autoimmune hepatitis, ischemic veno-occlusive disease, sclerosing cholangitis, heat stroke, amebic abscesses

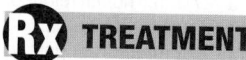

DIAGNOSIS

DIFFERENTIAL DIAGNOSIS
- Delirium caused by medications or illicit drugs
- Cerebrovascular accident, subdural hematoma
- Meningitis, encephalitis
- Hypoglycemia
- Uremia
- Cerebral anoxia
- Hypercalcemia
- Metastatic neoplasm to brain
- Alcohol withdrawal syndrome

WORKUP

Exclude other etiologies with comprehensive history (obtained from patient, relatives, and others), physical examination, and laboratory and imaging studies. A pertinent history should include exposure to hepatitis, ethanol intake, drug history, exposure to toxins, IV drug abuse, measles or influenza with aspirin use (Reye's syndrome), and history of carcinoma (primary or metastatic).

LABORATORY TESTS
- Alanine aminotransferase, aspartate aminotransferase, bilirubin, alkaline phosphatase glucose, calcium, electrolytes, blood urea nitrogen, creatinine, albumin
- Complete blood count, platelet count, prothrombin time, partial thromboplastin time
- Serum and urine toxicology screen in suspected medication or illegal drug use
- Blood and urine cultures, urinalysis
- Venous ammonia level
- Arterial blood gases

IMAGING STUDIES

CT scan of the head may be useful in selected patients to exclude other etiologies.

TREATMENT

NONPHARMACOLOGIC THERAPY
- Identification and treatment of precipitating factors
- Restriction of protein intake (30 to 40 g/day) to reduce toxic protein metabolites

ACUTE GENERAL Rx

Reduction of colonic ammonia production:
- Lactulose 30 ml of 50% solution qid initially; dose is subsequently adjusted depending on clinical response. Ornithine aspartate 9 g tid is also effective. Lactulose may improve hepatic encephalopathy but may be less effective than antibiotics.
- Neomycin 1 g PO q4 to 6h or given as a 1% retention enema solution (1 g in 100 ml of isotonic saline solution); neomycin should be used with caution in patients with renal insufficiency. Metronidazole 250 mg qid may be as effective as neomycin and is not nephrotoxic; however, long-term use can be associated with neurotoxicity.

- A combination of lactulose and neomycin can be used when either agent is ineffective alone.
- The oral antibiotic rifaximin (550 mg PO bid) is effective in reducing the risk of recurrent hepatic encephalopathy in patients with cirrhosis. It can be taken with lactulose. It is well tolerated but expensive.
- Rifamycin is a newer minimally absorbed nonaminoglycoside antibacterial agent effective in reducing ammonia-producing intestinal bacteria. Dose is 550 mg PO bid.

Treatment of cerebral edema:
- Cerebral edema is often present in patients with acute liver failure, and it accounts for nearly 50% of deaths. Monitoring intracranial pressure by epidural, intraparenchymal, or subdural transducers and treatment of cerebral edema with mannitol (100 to 200 ml of 20% solution [0.3 to 0.4 g/kg of body weight]) given by rapid IV infusion are helpful in selected patients (e.g., potential transplantation patients).
- Dexamethasone and hyperventilation (useful in head injury) are of little value in treating cerebral edema from liver failure.

CHRONIC Rx
- Avoidance of any precipitating factors (e.g., high-protein diet, medications)
- Consideration of liver transplantation in selected patients with progressive or recurrent encephalopathy. Liver transplantation remains the only curative therapeutic option.

DISPOSITION

Prognosis varies with the underlying etiology of the liver failure and the grade of encephalopathy (generally good for grades 1 or 2; poor for grades 3 or 4).

REFERRAL

The early stages of hepatic encephalopathy can be managed in the outpatient setting, whereas stages 3 or 4 require hospital admission.

PEARLS & CONSIDERATIONS

COMMENTS
- Patients not responding to supportive therapy should be evaluated for liver transplantation.
- Not all patients with cirrhosis develop hepatic encephalopathy. It has been shown that 40% of persons with cirrhosis and minimal hepatic encephalopathy do not develop overt hepatic encephalopathy in long-term follow-up. There are genetic factors associated with development of hepatic encephalopathy in patients with cirrhosis. Genetic analyses have shown that glutaminase TACC and CACC haplotypes are linked to the risk for overt hepatic encephalopathy.

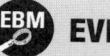 EVIDENCE

available at www.expertconsult.com

SUGGESTED READING
available at www.expertconsult.com

AUTHOR: FRED F. FERRI, M.D.

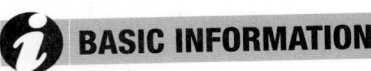

DEFINITION

Hepatitis A is generally an acute self-limiting infection of the liver by an enterically transmitted picornavirus, hepatitis A virus (HAV). Infection may range from asymptomatic to fulminant hepatitis.

SYNONYMS

Infectious hepatitis
Short incubation hepatitis
Type A hepatitis
HAV (hepatitis A virus)

ICD-9CM CODES
070.1 Hepatitis A

EPIDIMIOLOGY & DEMOGRAPHICS

INCIDENCE:
- Hepatitis A occurs worldwide, affecting 1.4 million people annually and accounting for 20% to 40% of cases of viral hepatitis in the United States.
- The seroprevalence increases with age, ranging from 10% in individuals aged <5 yr to 74% in those aged >50 yr.
- In the United States, average disease rate was ~15 cases/100,000 persons/yr prior to routine vaccination of all children in certain states. The incidence after 2005 is about 1 case/100,000.
- The incidence is relatively higher in some regions in the United States, including Arizona, Alaska, California, Idaho, Nevada, New Mexico, Oklahoma, Oregon, South Dakota, and Washington.
- At-risk groups include:
  1. Residents and staff of group homes
  2. Children and employees of day care centers
  3. People who engage in oral–anal contact, regardless of sexual orientation
  4. IV drug abusers
  5. Travel to endemic areas
  6. Areas of overcrowding, poor sanitation, inadequate sewage treatment

PREVALENCE:
- Approximately three fourths of the U.S. population has serologic evidence of prior infection.
- Anti-HAV prevalence has an inverse relation to income and household size.

PREDOMINANT SEX: None, except higher infection rates seen in homosexual males who engage in oral–anal contact.

PREDOMINANT AGE/PEAK INCIDENCE:
- In areas of high rates of hepatitis A, virtually all children are infected while younger than 10 yr, but disease is rare.
- In areas of moderate rates of hepatitis A, disease occurs in late childhood and young adults.
- In areas of low rates of hepatitis A, most cases occur in young adults.

INCUBATION PERIOD: Averages 30 days (15 to 50)

PHYSICAL FINDINGS & CLINICAL PRESENTATION

- Infection with HAV may have acute or sub-acute presentation, icteric or anicteric. Severity of illness seems to increase with age (90% of infection in children aged <5 yr may be subclinical).
- A preicteric, prodromal phase of approximately 1 to 14 days. 15% no apparent prodrome. Symptoms are usually abrupt in onset and may include anorexia, malaise, nausea, vomiting, fever, headache, and abdominal pain.
- Less common symptoms are chills, myalgias, arthralgias, upper respiratory symptoms, constipation, diarrhea, pruritus, urticaria.
- Jaundice occurs in >70% of patients.
- The icteric phase is preceded by dark urine.
- Bilirubinuria is typically followed a few days later by clay-colored stools and icterus.

PHYSICAL EXAMINATION

- Jaundice
- Hepatomegaly
- Splenomegaly
- Cervical lymphadenopathy
- Evanescent rash
- Petechiae
- Cardiac arrhythmias

COMPLICATIONS

- Cholestasis
- Fulminant hepatitis
- Arthritis
- Myocarditis
- Optic neuritis
- Transverse myelitis
- Thrombocytopenic purpura
- Aplastic anemia
- Red cell aplasia
- Henoch-Schönlein purpura
- IgA dominant glomerulonephritis

ETIOLOGY

- Caused by HAV, a 27-nm, nonenveloped, icosahedral, positive-stranded RNA virus.
- Transmission is fecal-oral route, from person to person. Transmission occurs with close contact or with food- or water-borne outbreaks with inadequately purified water or cooked foods. Recent outbreaks have involved green onions and tomatoes.
- Parenteral transmission is considered rare.
- Vertical transmission has also been reported.

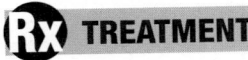
DIAGNOSIS

DIFFERENTIAL DIAGNOSIS

- Other hepatitis virus (B, C, D, E)
- Infectious mononucleosis
- Cytomegalovirus infection
- Herpes simplex virus infection
- Leptospirosis
- Brucellosis
- Drug-induced liver disease
- Ischemic hepatitis
- Autoimmune hepatitis

WORKUP

- IgM antibody specific for HAV
- Liver function tests; ALT and AST elevations are sensitive for liver damage but not specific for HAV
- Elevated ESR
- CBC; may find mild lymphocytosis

LABORATORY TESTS

- DIAGNOSIS confirmed by IgM anti HAV; it is detectable in almost all infected patients at presentation and remains positive for 3 to 6 mo.
- A fourfold rise in titer of total antibody (IgM and IgG) to HAV confirms acute infection.
- HAV detection in stool and body fluids by electron microscopy.
- HAV RNA detection in stool, body fluids, serum, and liver tissue.
- ALT and AST usually more than 8 times normal in acute infection.
- Bilirubin usually 5 to 15 times normal.
- Alkaline phosphatase minimally elevated but higher level in cholestasis.
- Albumin and prothrombin time are generally normal; if elevated, they may herald hepatic necrosis.
- Fig. 1-179 Illustrates the typical course of hepatis A.

IMAGING STUDIES

- Rarely useful
- Sonogram (fulminant hepatitis)

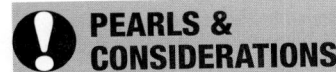
TREATMENT

- Usually self-limited
- Supportive care
- Those with fulminant hepatitis may require hospitalization and treatment of associated complications
- Activity as tolerated
- Advise to avoid alcohol and hepatotoxic drugs
- Patients with fulminant hepatitis should be assessed for liver transplantation

CHRONIC Rx

No chronic HAV and no chronic carrier state

DISPOSITION

Follow-up as outpatient

REFERRAL

- To a hepatologist if severe, fulminant hepatitis develops
- To a transplant surgeon if liver transplant becomes a consideration for fulminant hepatitis and liver failure

PEARLS & CONSIDERATIONS

- All cases of hepatitis A should be reported to the public heath authorities because food-borne or water-borne outbreaks may occur, and public health efforts (mass vaccination or

immunoglobulin therapy) may prevent secondary cases.
- Hepatitis A is a common illness in internationally traveled and developing countries. Pretravel vaccination is strongly recommended for travelers who are HAV susceptible.

PREVENTION
- Improvement in hygiene and sanitation
- Heating food
- Avoidance of water and foods from endemic area

PASSIVE IMMUNIZATION
- Immunoglobulin provides protection against HAV through passive transfer of antibody.
- Preexposure prophylaxis indicated for people traveling to endemic areas (Ig 0.02 or 0.06 ml/kg given IM). The lower dose is effective for up to 3 mo, and the higher dose is effective for up to 5 mo.
- Postexposure prophylaxis (Ig 0.02 ml/kg given IM) is indicated for people with recent exposure (within 2 wk) to HAV and who have not been previously vaccinated. In high-risk patients, vaccine may be administered with immunoglobulin.

ACTIVE IMMUNIZATION
- There are several inactivated and attenuated hepatitis vaccines; only the inactivated vaccines are currently available for use and they have been found to be safe and highly immunogenic: HAVRIX or VAQTA. These can be used in adults and children older than 12 mo. They are given as a two-dose regimen 6 mo to 1 yr apart. A combined hepatitis A and hepatitis B vaccine called TWINRX is also available.
- Protective antibody levels were reached in 94% to 100% of adults 1 mo after the first dose, similar results have been found for children and adolescents.
- Theoretic analyses of antibody levels estimate duration of immunity to be 10 to 20 yr.
- Vaccine should be considered for persons who are at risk: those traveling to or working in endemic areas, homosexual men, illegal drug users, persons with chronic liver disease, children in areas with high rates of hepatitis A infection.
- Beginning in May 2006, the Advisory Committee on Immunization Practices recommended routine hepatitis A vaccination for all children beginning at 12 to 23 mo of age.

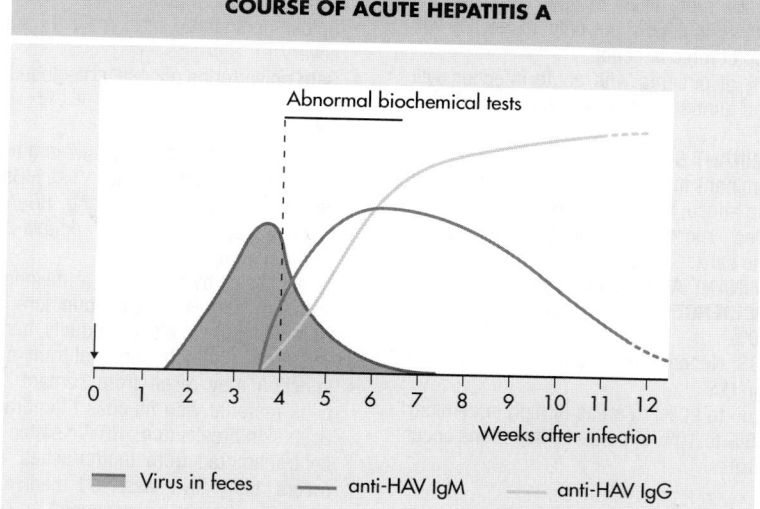

COURSE OF ACUTE HEPATITIS A

Abnormal biochemical tests

Weeks after infection

Virus in feces   anti-HAV IgM   anti-HAV IgG

FIGURE 1-179 Course of acute hepatitis A. (From Cohen J, Powderly WG: *Infectious diseases,* ed 2, St Louis, 2004, Mosby.)

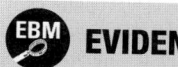 **EVIDENCE**

available at www.expertconsult.com

SUGGESTED READINGS

available at www.expertconsult.com

AUTHORS: **GLENN G. FORT, M.D., M.P.H.,** and **DENNIS J. MIKOLICH, M.D.**

Diseases and Disorders

H

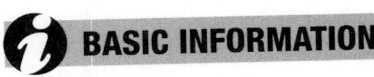

DEFINITION

Hepatitis B is an acute infection of the liver parenchymal cells caused by the hepatitis B virus (HBV).

SYNONYMS

Serum hepatitis
Long incubation (30 to 180 days) hepatitis

ICD-9CM CODES
070.3 Hepatitis B

EPIDEMIOLOGY & DEMOGRAPHICS

INCIDENCE (IN U.S.):

- ~200,000 to 300,000 infections annually in the United States.
- Much higher incidence in Europe (~1 million new cases annually) and in areas of high endemicity.
- In U.S., transmission is mainly horizontal (percutaneous and mucous membrane exposure to infectious blood and other body fluids [e.g., sexual transmission, either homosexual or heterosexual]); also from needle sharing among drug abusers; occupational exposure to contaminated blood and blood products; persons receiving transfusions of blood and blood products; and hemodialysis patients.

NOTE: Improved screening of blood and blood products has greatly reduced, although not eliminated, the risk of posttransfusion HBV infection.

- In areas of high endemicity, transmission is largely vertical (perinatal): HBV exists in the blood and body fluids. Perinatal transmission from HBsAg-positive mothers is as high as 90% unless immunoprophylaxis is given.

PREVALENCE (IN U.S.):

- North America, Western Europe, and Australia are areas of low prevalence, <2%.
- Africa, Asia, and the Western Pacific region are areas of high prevalence, ≥8%.
- Southern and Eastern Europe have intermediate rates, 2% to 7%.
- Chronically infected persons, those with positive HBsAg for >6 mo, represent the major source of infection.
- As many as 95% of infants and children aged <5, who typically have subclinical acute infection, will become chronic HBV carriers.
- Adults are more likely to have clinically evident acute infection, but only 1% to 5% will develop chronic infection.
- ~0.1% of patients with acute infection will develop fulminant acute hepatitis resulting in death.

PREDOMINANT SEX:

- Predominant in males because of increased IV drug abuse, homosexuality
- Females more commonly terminate in chronic carrier state

PREDOMINANT AGE: 20 to 45 yr
PEAK INCIDENCE: 30 to 45 yr of age, at rates of 5% to 20%
GENETICS: Neonatal infection:

- Rare in U.S.
- High (up to 90%) in areas of high endemicity (only 5% to 10% of perinatal infections occur in utero)

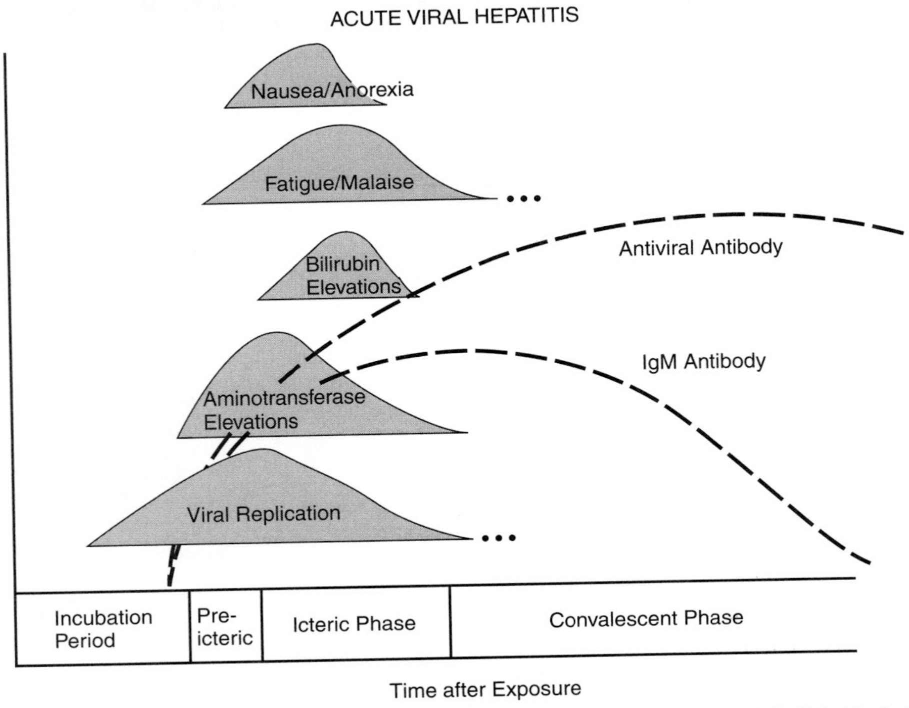

PHYSICAL FINDINGS & CLINICAL PRESENTATION (Fig. 1-180)

- Often nonspecific symptoms
- Profound malaise
- Many asymptomatic cases
- Prodrome:
  1. 15% to 20% serum sickness (urticaria, rash, arthralgia) during early HBsAg
  2. HBsAg-Ab complex disease (polyarteritis nodosa–arthritis, arteritis, glomerulonephritis)
- Hepatomegaly (87%) with right upper quadrant (RUQ) tenderness
  1. Hepatic punch tenderness
  2. Splenomegaly: rare (10% to 15%)
- Jaundice, dark urine, with occasional pruritus
- Variable fever (when present, generally precedes jaundice and rapidly declines following onset of icteric phase)
- Spider angiomata: rare; resolves during recovery
- Rare polyarteritis nodosa, cryoglobulinemia

ETIOLOGY

- Caused by hepatitis B virus (42-nm hepadnavirus with an outer surface coat [HBsAg], inner nucleocapsid core [HBcAg; HBeAg]; DNA polymerase; and partially double-stranded DNA genome).
- Transmission by parenteral route (needle use, tattooing, ear piercing, acupuncture, transfusion of blood and blood products, hemodialysis, sexual contact), perinatal transmission.
- Infection may result from contact of infectious material with mucous membranes and open skin breaks (e.g., HBV is stable and can be transmitted from toothbrushes, utensils, razors, baby toys, assorted medical equipment [respirators, endoscopes]).
- Oral intake of infectious material may result in infection through breaks in the oral mucosa.
- Food or water are virtually never found to be sources of HBV infection.
- Infection occurs primarily in liver, where necrosis probably results from cytotoxic T-cell response, direct cytopathic effect of HBcAg (core antigen), high-level HBsAg (surface antigen) expression, or coinfection with delta (D) hepatitis virus (RNA delta core within HBsAg envelope).
- Recovery (>90%):
  - Fulminant hepatitis occurring in <1% (especially if coinfected with hepatitis D); 80% fatal
  - Unusual (5%) prolonged acute disease for 4 to 12 mo, with recovery
  - Overall fatality increases with age and viral inoculation (e.g., transfusions)
- Chronic infection (1% to 2%):
  - Persistent carrier state without hepatitis (HBsAg positive)
  - Chronic persistent hepatitis (CPH) (clinically well), or chronic active hepatitis (CAH) (HBsAg positive and HBeAg positive)
  - Cirrhosis
  - Hepatocellular carcinoma (especially after neonatal infection)

ACUTE VIRAL HEPATITIS

Nausea/Anorexia

Fatigue/Malaise

Bilirubin Elevations

Antiviral Antibody

IgM Antibody

Aminotransferase Elevations

Viral Replication

| Incubation Period | Pre-icteric | Icteric Phase | Convalescent Phase |

Time after Exposure

FIGURE 1-180 The typical course of acute viral hepatitis. (From Goldman L, Ausiello D [eds]: *Cecil textbook of medicine*, ed 22, Philadelphia, 2004, WB Saunders.)

○ Chronic infection: more common following low-dose exposure and mild acute hepatitis, with earlier age of infection, in males, and in immunosuppressed patients
○ One third to one quarter of chronically infected will develop progressive liver disease (cirrhosis, hepatocellular carcinoma)

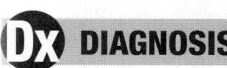 **DIAGNOSIS**

DIFFERENTIAL DIAGNOSIS

- Acute disease confused with other viral hepatitis infections (A, C, D, E)
- Any viral illness producing systemic disease and hepatitis (e.g., yellow fever, EBV, CMV, HIV, rubella, rubeola, coxsackie B, adenovirus, herpes simplex or zoster)
- Nonviral causes of hepatitis (e.g., leptospirosis, toxoplasmosis, alcoholic hepatitis, drug-induced [e.g., acetaminophen, INH], toxic hepatitis [carbon tetrachloride, benzene])

WORKUP

- Acute serum specimen for hepatitis B serology (HBsAg, HBsAb, HBcAb, HBeAg, HBeAb), HBDNA
- LFTs
- CBC
- Liver biopsy: rarely indicated for diagnosis of fulminant viral hepatitis, chronic hepatitis, cirrhosis, carcinoma

LABORATORY TESTS

- Diagnosis of acute HBV infection is best confirmed by IgM HBcAb in acute or early convalescent serum or by HBDNA.
  ○ Generally, IgM present during onset of jaundice
  ○ Coexisting HBsAg
- HBsAg and IgG-HBcAb during acute jaundice are strongly suggestive of remote HBV infection and another cause for current illness (Fig. 1-181).

- HBsAb alone is suggestive of immunization response.
- With recovery, HBeAg is rapidly replaced by HBeAb in 2 to 3 mo, and HBsAg is replaced by HBsAb in 5 to 6 mo.
- In chronic HBV hepatitis, HBsAg and HBeAg are persistent without corresponding Ab.
- In chronic carrier state, HBsAg is persistent, but HBeAg is replaced by HBeAb.
- HBcAb develops in all outcomes.
- HBeAg correlation with highest infectivity; appearance of HBeAb heralds recovery.
- LFTs:
  ○ ALT and AST: usually more than eight times normal (often 1000 U/L) at onset of jaundice (minimal acute ALT/AST rises often followed by chronic hepatitis or hepatocellular carcinoma)
  ○ Bilirubin: variably elevated in icteric viral hepatitis
  ○ Alkaline phosphatase: minimally elevated (one to three times normal) acutely
- Albumin and prothrombin time:
  ○ Generally normal
  ○ If abnormal, possible harbinger of impending hepatic necrosis (fulminant hepatitis)
- WBC and ESR: generally normal

IMAGING STUDIES

- Rarely useful
- Sonogram to document rapid reduction in liver size during fulminant hepatitis or mass in hepatocellular carcinoma

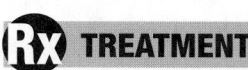 **TREATMENT**

NONPHARMACOLOGIC THERAPY

- Symptomatic treatment as necessary
- Activity as tolerated
- High-calorie diet preferred; often best tolerated in morning

ACUTE GENERAL Rx

- In most cases of acute HBV infection no treatment necessary; >90% of adults will spontaneously clear infection
- Hospitalization advisable for any patient in danger from dehydration caused by poor oral intake, whose PT is prolonged, who has rising bilirubin level >15 to 20 μg/dl, or who has any clinical evidence of hepatic failure
- IV therapy needed (rarely) for hydration during severe vomiting
- Avoid hepatically metabolized drugs
- No therapeutic measures are beneficial
- Steroids not shown helpful

CHRONIC Rx

- The aim of therapy in chronic HBV infection is to eradicate the virus.
- The two modalities of therapy available to achieve this goal have been immune modulators (interferon alfa) and antiviral agents in the form of nucleoside analogues (e.g., lamivudine).
- Pegylated interferon alpha (IFN-α) given as a once-a-week SQ injection for 48 wk is a mainstay of therapy and has largely replaced interferon alpha without pegylation, which required daily or thrice weekly injections. Its mechanism of action is to stimulate the immune system to attack HBV-infected hepatocytes, thus inhibiting viral protein synthesis.
- A 12-mo course of treatment results in a 30% to 40% response with significant reduction of serum HBV DNA, normalization of ALT, and loss of HBeAg. Seroconversion from HBeAg to HBeAb occurs in 15% to 20%.
- Factors that increase the likelihood of response to IFN-α therapy include:
  ○ Adult onset of infection
  ○ High baseline ALT
  ○ Low baseline HBV DNA
  ○ Absence of cirrhosis
  ○ Female
  ○ HBeAg positive

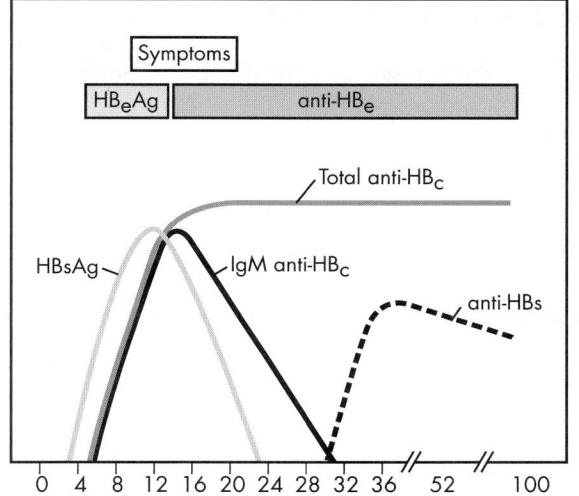

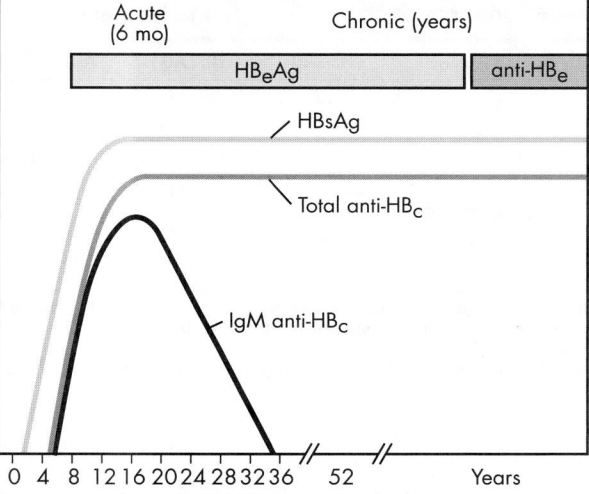

FIGURE 1-181 Typical course of hepatitis B. Left, Typical course of acute hepatitis B. **Right,** Chronic hepatitis B. *HBc,* Hepatitis B core; *HBe,* hepatitis B early; *HBsAg,* hepatitis B surface antigen; *IgM,* immunoglobulin M. (From Mandell GL et al: *Principles and practice of infectious diseases,* ed 7, Philadelphia, 2010, Elsevier.)

- Infrequent relapse after successful completion of therapy.
- 80% of patients who lose HBeAg during therapy lose HBsAg in the decade after therapy.
- >50% of patients who do not seroconvert after initial therapy develop a delayed HBeAg seroconversion months to years after therapy.
- Overall incidence of cirrhosis and hepatocellular carcinoma is decreased in those treated with IFN-α.
- IFN-α is successful only in patients with an active immune response; therefore it is not effective in patients with HIV infection and organ transplant patients.
- Asians respond poorly to IFN-α.
- Treatment with IFN-α in general is not well tolerated: side effects include flulike symptoms, injection-site reactions, rash, weight loss, anxiety, depression, alopecia, thrombocytopenia, granulocytopenia, and thyroid dysfunction.
- Nucleoside analogues block viral replication by inhibiting HBV polymerase.
- Lamivudine was the first nucleoside analogue approved for treatment of chronic HBV infection; it has been shown to rapidly reduce HBV replication and suppress HBV DNA to undetectable levels after a few wk of treatment, and treatment for 1 yr is as effective as IFN-α with respect to loss of HBeAg seroconversion to HBeAb and loss of HBV DNA. Emergence of resistant HBV strains while on therapy has limited the use of lamivudine (YMDD variants [tyrosine-methionine-aspartate-aspartate]).
- Adefovir dipivoxil is a nucleotide reverse transcriptase inhibitor that also has antiviral activity against HBV. It is a prodrug that is converted to the active drug adefovir. It is highly active against HBV and may be useful as a first-line agent or as salvage therapy for patients who are refractory or intolerant to lamivudine. (Nephrotoxicity is a potential side effect, but emergence of resistant strains is less than with lamivudine.)

- Entecavir is a potent nucleoside agent approved for the treatment of hepatitis B, and it appears to be more effective and to present fewer concerns than lamivudine or adefovir regarding the emergence of resistant strains.
- Telbivudine, a thymidine nucleosidase analogue, has demonstrated greater and more consistent HBV DNA suppression than lamivudine or adefovir after 24 wk of treatment but selects for the same resistant strains as lamivudine.
- Tenofovir: more potent than adefovir and suppresses lamivudine resistant strains.
- Emtricitabine: nucleoside analogue similar to lamivudine but with more potent activity.
- Combination therapy with two or three nucleoside analogues or combination therapy with IFN-α are currently under investigation.
- Liver transplantation (should be considered for fulminant hepatitis).

DISPOSITION

- Follow-up as outpatient
- Acute disease: usually <6 wk
- Rare fatalities (fulminant hepatitis)
- Possible chronic carrier state, cirrhosis, hepatocellular carcinoma

REFERRAL

To infectious disease specialist and gastroenterologist for consultation regarding fulminant hepatitis or prolonged cholestasis, for cases of uncertain etiology, or for treatment of CAH

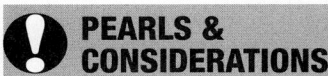

! PEARLS & CONSIDERATIONS

COMMENTS

- Virus and HBsAg in high titers in blood for 1 to 7 wk before jaundice and for a variable time thereafter.
- Transmission is possible during entire period of HBsAg (and especially during HBeAg) in serum.

- Universal precautions should be followed for all contacts with blood or secretions/excretions contaminated with blood.
- Preventing before exposure:
  ○ Lifestyle changes
  ○ Meticulous testing of blood supply (although some chronically infected, infectious donors are HBsAg negative)
  ○ Sterilization via steam or hypochlorite
  ○ Hepatitis B vaccine for high-risk groups given IM in deltoid to induce HBsAb (response should be confirmed) is protective (>90% effective)
  ○ Recommendation for universal childhood immunization with doses at birth, 1 mo, and 6 mo
- Prevention after exposure:
  ○ HBV hyperimmune globulin (HBIG) given immediately after needlestick, within 14 days of sexual exposure, or at birth, followed by HBV vaccination
  ○ Standard immune globulin: nearly as effective as HBIG
- Preventive therapy with lamivudine for patients who test positive for HBsAg and are undergoing chemotherapy may reduce the risk for HBV reactivation and HBV-associated morbidity and mortality,
- Hepatitis B prophylaxis is described in Section V
- Table 1-65 summarizes interpretation of serologic markers and serum DNA in hepatitis B

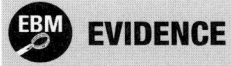

EBM **EVIDENCE**

available at www.expertconsult.com

SUGGESTED READINGS

available at www.expertconsult.com

AUTHORS: **GLENN G. FORT, M.D., M.P.H.**, and **DENNIS J. MIKOLICH, M.D.**

TABLE 1-65 Interpretation of Serologic Markers and Serum DNA in Hepatitis B

	HBsAg	HBeAg	Anti-HBc IgM	Anti-HBc IgG	Anti-HBs	Anti-HBe	HBV DNA*
Acute hepatitis	+	+/−	+				+
Acute hepatitis, window period			+				
Recovery from acute hepatitis			+	+	+	+/−	
Chronic hepatitis	+	+					+
Chronic hepatitis (precore mutant)	+					+	+
Inactive carrier	+					+/−	
Vaccinated					+		

HBsAg, Hepatitis B surface antigen; *HBeAg*, hepatitis Be antigen; *anti-HBc IgM*, hepatitis B core antibody (IgM type); *anti-HBc IgG*, hepatitis B core antibody (IgG type); *anti-HBs*, hepatitis B surface antibody; *anti-HBe*, hepatitis Be antibody; *HBV DNA*, hepatitis B viral DNA.
*HBV DNA > 10⁵ copies/mL.
Andreoli TE et al: *Andreoli and Carpenter's Cecil essentials of medicine,* ed 8, Philadelphia, 2010, Saunders/Elsevier.

BASIC INFORMATION

DEFINITION

Hepatitis C is an acute liver parenchymal infection caused by hepatitis C virus (HCV).

SYNONYMS

Transfusion-related non-A, non-B hepatitis (incubation period averages 6 wk, intermediate between hepatitis A and B)

ICD-9CM CODES
070.51 Other viral hepatitis

EPIDEMIOLOGY & DEMOGRAPHICS

Hepatitis C infection is the most common chronic blood-borne infection in the U.S.
INCIDENCE (IN U.S.):
- 150,000 new cases/yr (37,500 symptomatic; 93,000 later chronic liver disease; 30,700 cirrhosis). The incidence of acute HCV has declined substantially over the past 30 yr
- ~9000 of these ultimately die of HCV infection; most common (40%) cause of nonalcoholic liver disease in the United States

PREVALENCE (IN U.S.):
- Overall prevalence of anti-HCV antibody is 1.8% (an estimated 3.9 million persons nationwide)
- Highest prevalence in hemophiliacs transfused before 1987 and users of injection drugs, 72% to 90%
- Among low-risk groups, prevalence 0.6%

PREDOMINANT SEX: Slight male predominance
PREDOMINANT AGE: Highest prevalence in 30- to 49-yr age group (65%)
PEAK INCIDENCE:
- 20 to 39 yr of age
- African Americans and whites have similar incidence of acute disease; Hispanics have higher rates
- Prevalence is substantially higher among non-Hispanic blacks than among non-Hispanic whites

GENETICS: Neonatal infection is rare; increased risk with maternal HIV-1 coinfection

PHYSICAL FINDINGS & CLINICAL PRESENTATION

- Symptoms usually develop 7 to 8 wk after infection (range of 2 to 26 wk), but 70% to 80% of cases are subclinical.
- 10% to 20% report acute illness with jaundice and nonspecific symptoms (abdominal pain, anorexia, malaise).
- Fulminant hepatitis may rarely occur during this period.
- After acute infection, 15% to 25% have complete resolution (absence of HCV RNA in serum, normal ALT).
- Progression to chronic infection is common, 50% to 84%. 74% to 86% have persistent viremia; spontaneous clearance of viremia in chronic infection is rare. 60% to 70% of patients will have persistent or fluctuating ALT levels; 30% to 40% with chronic infection have normal ALT levels.
- 15% to 20% of those with chronic HCV will develop cirrhosis over a period of 20 to 30 yr; in most others, chronic infection leads to hepatitis and varying degrees of fibrosis.
- 0.4% to 2.5% of patients with chronic infection develop hepatocellular carcinoma.
- 25% of patients with chronic infection continue to have an asymptomatic course with normal LFTs and benign histology.
- In chronic HCV infection, extrahepatic sequelae include a variety of immunologic and lymphoproliferative disorders (e.g., cryoglobulinemia, membranoproliferative glomerulonephritis, and possibly Sjögren's syndrome, autoimmune thyroiditis, polyarteritis nodosa, aplastic anemia, lichen planus, porphyria cutanea tarda, B-cell lymphoma, others).

ETIOLOGY

- Caused by HCV (single-stranded RNA flavivirus).
- Most HCV transmission is parenteral.
- In the United States, advances in screening of blood and blood products in 1990 and 1992 have made transfusion-related HCV infection rare (the risk is estimated to be 0.001% per unit transfused).
- Injecting-drug use accounts for most HCV transmission in the United States (60% of newly acquired cases, 20% to 50% of chronically infected persons).
- Occupational needlestick exposure from an HCV-positive source has a seroconversion rate of 1.8% (range 0% to 7%).
- Nosocomial transmission rates (from surgery and procedures such as colonoscopy and hemodialysis) are extremely low.
- Sexual transmission and maternal-fetal transmission are infrequent (estimated at 5%).
- No identifiable risk in 40% to 50% of community-acquired hepatitis C, but snorting of cocaine by shared use of straw or rolled-up paper has been identified as a risk factor because it causes microscopic bleeding of nasal mucosa.
- HCV infection may stimulate production of cytotoxic T lymphocytes and cytokines (INF-γ), which probably mediate hepatic necrosis.

DIAGNOSIS

DIFFERENTIAL DIAGNOSIS

- Other hepatitis viruses (A, B, D, E)
- Other viral illnesses producing systemic disease (e.g., yellow fever, EBV, CMV, HIV, rubella, rubeola, coxsackie B, adenovirus, HSV, HZV)
- Nonviral hepatitis (e.g., leptospirosis, toxoplasmosis, alcoholic hepatitis, drug-induced hepatitis [acetaminophen, INH], toxic hepatitis)

WORKUP

- Acute hepatitis C antibody
- LFTs; CBC
NOTE: ALT is an easy and inexpensive test to monitor infection and efficacy of therapy. However, ALT levels may fluctuate or even be normal in active or chronic infection and even with cirrhosis, and ALT may remain elevated even after clearance of viremia.

- Liver biopsy with histologic staging is the gold standard for assessing the degree of disease activity and the likelihood of disease progression, and also to help rule out other causes of liver disease

LABORATORY TESTS

- Diagnosis is often by exclusion, because it takes 6 wk to 12 mo to develop anti-HCV antibody (70% positive by 6 wk, 90% positive by 6 mo).
- Diagnostic tests include serologic assays for antibodies and molecular tests for viral particles.
  - Enzyme immunoassay is the test for anti-HCV antibody:
    The current version can detect antibody within 4 to 10 wk after infection.
    False-negative rate in low-risk populations is 0.5% to 1%.
    False-negatives also occur in immune-compromised persons, HIV-1, renal failure, HCV-associated essential mixed cryoglobulinemia.
    False positives in autoimmune hepatitis, paraproteinemia, and persons with no risk factors.
  - Recombinant immunoblot is used to confirm positive enzyme immunoassays:
    Recommended only in low-risk settings.
  - Qualitative and quantitative HCV RNA tests using PCR:
    Lower limit of detection is <43 IU/ml
    Used to confirm viremia and to assess response to treatment.
    Qualitative polymerase chain reaction (PCR) useful in patients with negative enzyme immunoassay in whom infection is suspected.
    Quantitative tests use either branched-chain DNA or reverse transcription PCR; the latter is more sensitive.
  - Viral genotyping can distinguish among genotypes 1, 2, 3, and 4, which is helpful in choosing therapy; most of these tests use PCR (genotypes 1, 2, 3, and 4 predominate in the U.S. and Europe [1 is especially common in North America]).
  - LFTs:
    ALT and AST may be elevated to more than eight times normal in acute infection; in chronic infection ALT may be normal or fluctuate.
    Bilirubin may be five to 10 times normal.
    Albumin and prothrombin time generally normal; if abnormal, may be harbinger of impending hepatic necrosis.
  - WBC and erythrocyte sedimentation rate (ESR) are generally normal.

IMAGING STUDIES

Sonogram: rapid liver size reduction during fulminant hepatitis or mass in hepatocellular carcinoma

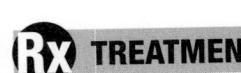

TREATMENT

NONPHARMACOLOGIC THERAPY
Activity and diet as tolerated

ACUTE GENERAL Rx
- Supportive care.
- Avoid hepatically metabolized drugs.
- Specific Rx for acute HCV infection.
- Recent studies demonstrate that early treatment with interferon-alpha-2b during acute HCV infection prevents chronic infection. The aim is to decrease viral load early in infection and allow the patient's immune system to control viral replication, thus preventing progression to chronic infection. The primary end point was sustained virologic response, with absence of HCV RNA in serum 24 wk after completion of therapy.
- Further investigations are in progress.

CHRONIC Rx
- Response to therapy is influenced by HCV genotype. Patients with genotype 1 and genotype 4 have sustained virologic response and cure rates much lower than patients with genotypes 2 and 3. Cure rates for genotypes 1 and 4 are about 45% to 50%, whereas cure rates for genotypes 2 and 3 are as high as 75% to 80%.
- Mainstay of therapy currently is with a pegylated interferon-alpha as a weekly SC injection and oral weight-based ribavirin. For genotypes 1 and 4, the therapy is for 48 wk. For genotypes 2 or 3, the length of therapy is 24 wk.
- Pegylated interferons are interferon-alpha with an attached polyethylene glycol (PEG) molecule. The PEG molecule confers a longer half-life and extended therapeutic activity compared with interferon-alpha and reduced dosing to once a week. A third type of interferon, known as consensus interferon, is also available for treatment of hepatitis C, but it is not a long-acting form like the pegylated interferons.
- Two formulations of PEG interferon are available. Peginterferon alpha-2b (PEG INTRON) uses a weight-based dosage in a once-a-week SC Redipen injection. Peginterferon alpha-2a (Pegasys) uses a fixed dosage in a once-a-week premixed syringe, also SC.
- Both PEG interferon-alpha and ribavirin have numerous contraindications (absolute and relative) to use and may cause a variety of side effects. Interferon-alpha can cause flu-like symptoms, thrombocytopenia, granulocytopenia, rash, alopecia, anorexia, psychiatric disturbances, and other side effects. Ribavirin can cause hemolysis, nausea, anemia, nasal congestion, and pruritus. Ribavirin is contraindicated in pregnancy and patients should not get pregnant while on therapy and for 6 mo after therapy.
- In patients who fail to respond to interferon-alpha and ribavirin, <10% will respond to retreatment.
- Treatment trials have shown that pegylated interferon alone achieves higher hepatitis C–specific T-helper-1 response and clinical response rates than does interferon-alpha alone in patients with chronic hepatitis C without cirrhosis, and in patients with chronic hepatitis C with cirrhosis or bridging fibrosis.
- Liver transplantation:
  - Hepatitis C is the main indication for liver transplantation in the United States.
  - It is the only option for patients with deteriorating HCV-related cirrhosis and for some patients with hepatocellular carcinoma.
  - Recurrent infection occurs in almost all patients with progressive fibrosis and cirrhosis; as many as 20% progress to cirrhosis within 5-yr posttransplant.
- Coinfection with HIV:
  - These patients have a poor response to pegylated interferon-alpha and ribavirin if the immune system is depleted, with a low CD4 count as seen in the AIDS category. It is, however, important to treat patients coinfected with HIV and hepatitis C with HAART (highly active antiretroviral therapy). Many coinfected patients are stable from their HIV disease, but have significant morbidity and mortality from their hepatitis C.
  - Newer agents that are proteases inhibitors such as telaprevir and boceprevir expected to become available in 2011 that may dramatically improve the cure rates for genotypes 1 and 4 and only require 24 wk of therapy. They would be used in a cocktail with a pegylated interferon plus ribavirin.

DISPOSITION
- Follow-up as outpatient
- Monitor ALT levels as a clue for chronic disease
- Chronic carrier state, cirrhosis, hepatic carcinoma more common than with hepatitis A and B
- Periodic abdominal ultrasonography and measurement of alpha-fetoprotein for hepatocellular carcinoma screening

REFERRAL
- To a hepatologist or infectious disease specialist for treatment for hepatitis C
- To an oncologist if hepatocellular carcinoma (HCC) develops. HCC is the fastest rising cause of cancer-related deaths in the United States. This increase is most attributable to an increase in HCV-related HCC.
- To a transplant surgeon for consideration of liver transplant if indicated

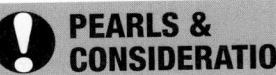

PEARLS & CONSIDERATIONS

- More rapid progression of disease in persons who drink alcohol regularly, persons of advanced age at time of infection, and those coinfected with other viruses (HIV, hepatitis B).
- No preventive vaccine available; postexposure Ig provides minimal protection.
- Preventive measures include use of universal precautions, careful screening of blood and blood products, lifestyle changes.
- Side effects of interferon include neutropenia that may require use Neupogen. Ribavirin may cause sufficient anemia that may require use Epogen or Procrit or even blood transfusions.
- Eltrombopag is an orally active thrombopoietin-receptor agonist that stimulates thrombopoiesis. It has been reported effective in increasing platelet counts in patients with thrombocytopenia caused by HCV-related cirrhosis.
- Regression of cirrhosis has been demonstrated after antiviral therapy in some patients with chronic hepatitis C. Regression is associated with decreased disease-related morbidity and improved survival.

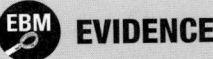 **EVIDENCE**

available at www.expertconsult.com

SUGGESTED READINGS
available at www.expertconsult.com

AUTHORS: **GLENN G. FORT, M.D., M.P.H.,** and **DENNIS J. MIKOLICH, M.D.**

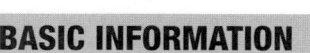 **BASIC INFORMATION**

DEFINITION

Autoimmune hepatitis is a chronic inflammatory condition of the liver characterized by elevated serum globulin levels and the presence of circulating autoantibodies. Two types have been described:

- Type 1, or "classic," autoimmune hepatitis is the most predominant form in the U.S. and worldwide (80%); patients are positive for antinuclear antibodies (ANA) and/or anti-smooth muscle antibodies (ASMA). Occurs across all age ranges and may be underdiagnosed in the elderly.
- Type 2 is rare in the U.S. and primarily affects young children. Type 2 is characterized by the presence of antibodies to liver/kidney microsomes (anti-LKM-1) or liver cytosol 1.

SYNONYMS

Autoimmune chronic active hepatitis
Chronic active hepatitis
Lupoid hepatitis

ICD-9CM CODES
571.49 Chronic hepatitis

EPIDEMIOLOGY & DEMOGRAPHICS

- Annual incidence (estimated): 1.9 cases per 100,000
- Point prevalence (estimated): 16.9 per 100,000
- Type 1: all age groups; type 2: more common in teenagers and young adults
- Female/male ratio is 3.6:1
- Approximately 100,000 to 200,000 persons affected in the U.S.
- Accounts for 5.9% of liver transplants in U.S.
- Associated with HLA DRB1*0301 and HLA DRB1*0401

CLINICAL PRESENTATION

- Varies from asymptomatic elevations of liver enzymes to fulminant hepatitis to advanced cirrhosis.
- Symptoms may include fatigue, anorexia, nausea, abdominal pain, pruritus, and arthralgia.
- Jaundice.
- Hepatomegaly/splenomegaly.
- Autoimmune findings may include arthritis, xerostomia, keratoconjunctivitis, cutaneous vasculitis, and erythema nodosum.
- Patients with advanced disease show ascites, edema, abnormal bleeding, and jaundice.

ETIOLOGY

- Exact etiology is unknown; liver histology demonstrates cell-mediated immune attack against hepatocytes.
- Presence of a variety of autoantibodies suggests an autoimmune mechanism.
- Strong genetic predisposition.
- Potential triggering agents such as virus (hepatitis A) or drugs (minocycline, nitrofurantoin).

(Dx) DIAGNOSIS

A simplified diagnostic criteria for routine clinical practice has been developed by the International Autoimmune Hepatitis Group (see Table 1-66).

DIFFERENTIAL DIAGNOSIS

- Acute viral hepatitis (A, B, C, D, E, cytomegalovirus, Epstein-Barr, herpes)
- Chronic viral hepatitis (B, C)
- Toxic hepatitis (alcohol, drugs)
- Primary biliary cirrhosis
- Primary sclerosing cholangitis
- Hemochromatosis
- Nonalcoholic steatohepatitis
- SLE
- Wilson's disease
- Alpha-1 antitrypsin deficiency

WORKUP

- History and physical examination with attention to the presence of autoimmune abnormalities such as thyroiditis, Graves' disease, ulcerative colitis, and rheumatoid arthritis
- Liver function tests and serum gamma-globulins
- Tests for autoantibodies
- Liver biopsy for establishing diagnosis and disease severity

LABORATORY TESTS

- Aminotransferases generally elevated, may fluctuate
- Bilirubin and alkaline phosphatase moderately elevated or normal
- Elevation of gamma globulin and immunoglobulin G
- Circulating autoantibodies often present:
  1. Rheumatoid factor
  2. ANAs
     a. Present in two thirds of patients
     b. Typical pattern is homogeneous or speckled
     c. Titer does not correlate with the stage, activity, or prognosis
  3. ASMAs
     a. Present in 87% of patients
     b. Titer does not correlate with course or prognosis

4. Anti-LKM antibodies
   a. Typically found in patients who are ANA negative and ASMA negative
   b. Found in <$\frac{1}{25}$ of patients in U.S.
   c. Present in pediatric population and up to 20% of adults in Europe; also present in patients with drug-induced hepatitis
5. Autoantibodies against soluble liver antigen and liver-pancreas antigen (anti-SLA/LP)
   a. Present in 10% to 30% of patients
   b. Associated with higher rate of relapse after corticosteroid therapy
   c. Several studies suggest that patients with anti-SLA/LP have a more severe course
- Hypoalbuminemia and prolonged prothrombin time with advanced disease
- There is a well-described overlap syndrome with primary biliary cirrhosis (7%), primary sclerosing cholangitis (6%), and autoimmune cholangitis (11%)

IMAGING STUDIES

Ultrasound of liver and biliary tree to rule out obstruction or hepatic mass

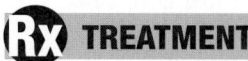 TREATMENT

NONPHARMACOLOGIC THERAPY

- Avoid alcohol and hepatotoxic medications.
- Liver transplantation is an option for end-stage disease or fulminant hepatic failure.

PHARMACOLOGIC THERAPY

- Initial treatment:
  1. Prednisone 60 mg/day PO or combination treatment with prednisone 30 mg/day PO plus azathioprine 50 mg/day PO. A combination of oral budesonide (6 to 9 mg/day) and azathioprine (1 to 2 mg/kg/day) can be used to induce and maintain remission in patients with non-cirrhotic AIH, with a lower rate of steroid-specific side effects.
  2. Combination therapy allows lower prednisone doses and fewer steroid side effects.
  3. Goal of therapy is remission (normalization of gamma-globulin and bilirubin, reduction of aminotransferases to less than twice the upper limit of normal).

TABLE 1-66 Diagnostic Criteria for Autoimmune Hepatitis

Variable	Cutoff	Points	Cutoff	Points
ANA or SMA	≥1:40	1	≥1:80	2
LKM			≥1:40	2
SLA			Positive	2
IgG	≥ULN	1	≥1.1 × ULN	2
Histology	Compatible with AIH	1	Typical of AIH	2
Absence of viral hepatitis			Yes	2

Maximum number of points for all antibodies = 2, total = 8.
Probable AIH ≥6 points, definite AIH ≥7 points.
AIH, Autoimmune hepatitis; *ANA,* antinuclear antibody; *IgG,* immunoglobulin G; *LKM,* liver/kidney microsomes; *SLA,* soluble liver antigen; *SMA,* smooth muscle antibody; *ULN,* upper limit of normal.

- Indications for treatment:
  1. Serum aminotransferase >10 times the upper limit of normal
  2. Serum aminotransferase more than five times the upper limit of normal, with serum gamma-globulin level twice the upper limit of normal
  3. Histologic features of bridging necrosis or multiacinar necrosis
  4. Incapacitating symptoms such as fatigue and arthralgia
- Evaluation of treatment response:
  1. Goal is the absence of symptoms, resolution of liver function test abnormalities, and histologic improvement.
  2. Patients whose transaminase levels normalize may continue to have ongoing active hepatitis involving inflammation and fibrosis. 5% to 10% of patients with normal transaminase levels progress to cirrhosis.
  3. Histologic improvement may lag behind clinical and laboratory improvement by as much as 6 mo.
  4. Repeat liver biopsy should be considered after normalization of transaminase levels.
  5. Complete normalization on biopsy is associated with a 15% to 20% risk of relapse.
  6. Persistent interface hepatitis is associated with a 90% risk of relapse.

DISPOSITION

- Follow up as outpatient.
- Long-term treatment may be necessary for sustained remission.
- Sixty-five percent of patients achieve remission by 18 mo; 80% achieve remission by 3 yr.
- Approximately 10% of patients do not improve with therapy.
- Patients in whom end-stage liver develops are candidates for liver transplantation. Recurrent disease may occur after liver transplantation.

REFERRAL

Patients with advanced cirrhosis or who progress to end-stage liver disease are candidates for liver transplantation and should be referred to appropriate medical centers that provide liver transplantation services.

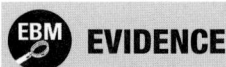

PEARLS & CONSIDERATIONS

COMMENTS

- A variety of autoimmune conditions can be seen in association with autoimmune hepatitis, including thyroiditis, Graves' disease, ulcerative colitis, rheumatoid arthritis, uveitis, pernicious anemia, Sjögren's syndrome, mixed connective tissue disease, CREST syndrome, and vitiligo.
- Variant forms of autoimmune hepatitis (overlap syndrome) have clinical and serologic findings of autoimmune hepatitis plus features of other forms of chronic liver disease such as primary biliary cirrhosis (PBC) or primary sclerosing cholangitis (PSC).

PREVENTION

None

PATIENT & FAMILY EDUCATION

- American Liver Foundation (ALF) Phone: 800-GO-LIVER (465-4837) E-mail: Internet: www.liverfoundation.org
- National Digestive Diseases Information clearinghouse: http://digestive.niddk.nih.gov/ddiseases/pubs/autoimmunehep

EVIDENCE

available at www.expertconsult.com

SUGGESTED READINGS
available at www.expertconsult.com

AUTHOR: **KITTICHAI PROMRAT, M.D.**

BASIC INFORMATION

DEFINITION

Hepatocellular carcinoma (HCC) is a malignant tumor of the hepatocytes.

SYNONYMS

Hepatoma
HCC

ICD-9CM CODES
155.0 Hepatocellular carcinoma

EPIDEMIOLOGY & DEMOGRAPHICS

Fifth most common cancer worldwide and third most common cause of cancer deaths. Incidence varies worldwide:

- Areas with high rates of hepatitis B and C (Asia, sub-Saharan Africa) have high rates of HCC.
- Males more affected than females, with ratios between 2:1 and 4:1.
- Peak incidence: fifth and sixth decades in Western countries, earlier in areas with perinatal transmission of hepatitis B.
- Incidence rapidly growing in U.S. secondary to hepatitis C infection.
  - Incidence: increased more than twofold in the past 20 years; 3.3/100,000 per year between 1999 and 2001
  - Mean age of diagnosis approximately 65 yr
  - HCC is the fastest rising cause of cancer-related deaths in the United States
- Risk factors:
  - Hepatitis B infection
  - Chronic hepatitis C infection
  - Cirrhosis from causes other than viral hepatitis: alcoholic liver disease, nonalcoholic steatohepatitis, primary biliary cirrhosis, hemochromatosis, α-1-antitrypsin deficiency, and autoimmune hepatitis
  - Hepatotoxins: alcohol and aflatoxin B1
  - Systemic diseases affecting the liver such as tyrosinemia
  - Obesity and diabetes mellitus

PHYSICAL FINDINGS & CLINICAL PRESENTATION

- One third of patients are asymptomatic. Abdominal pain may be the initial presentation.
- Signs of underlying cirrhosis and portal hypertension are often present.
- Previously compensated cirrhosis with new ascites, encephalopathy, jaundice, or bleeding.
- Paraneoplastic syndromes (hypoglycemia, erythrocytosis, hypercalcemia, severe diarrhea) may be present.

DIAGNOSIS

DIFFERENTIAL DIAGNOSIS

- Metastatic tumor to liver
- Benign liver tumors such as adenomas, focal nodular hyperplasia, and hemangiomas
- Focal fatty infiltration

WORKUP

- History regarding risk factors
- Physical examination with attention to signs of chronic liver disease
- Laboratory evaluation and imaging studies

LABORATORY TESTS

- Liver function tests
- Elevated α-fetoprotein in 70% of patients (sensitivity, 40% to 65%; specificity, 80% to 94%).
- Paraneoplastic syndromes associated with HCC may cause hypercalcemia, hypoglycemia, and polycythemia
- Elevated serum HBV DNA level (≥10,000 copies/ml) is a strong risk predictor of HCC independent of HBeAg, serum aminotransferase level, and liver cirrhosis

IMAGING STUDIES

Ultrasound (US), CT scan (Fig. 1-182), or MRI. Ultrasound is most commonly used as a screening test for HCC in high-risk patients. Multiphasic CT and MR scans are usually performed when a focal lesion is present on US or strong clinical suspicion of HCC.

BIOPSY: Percutaneous biopsy under ultrasound or CT scan usually is diagnostic. Tissue diagnosis is the gold standard. However, HCC can be reliably diagnosed when:

- Mass >2 cm that shows characteristics typical of HCC (hypervascular in the arterial phase with washout in the portal venous or delayed phase) seen on two imaging modalities, or
- Single positive imaging method with AFP >200 μg/ml

SCREENING: Screening high-risk patients with US every 6 mo is currently recommended to identify HCC at an early stage. The use of AFP alone should be discouraged due to limited sensitivity and specificity. Newer tumor markers (lectin-bound AFP [AFP-L3%] and Des-gamma carboxy-prothrombin [DCP]) have not been

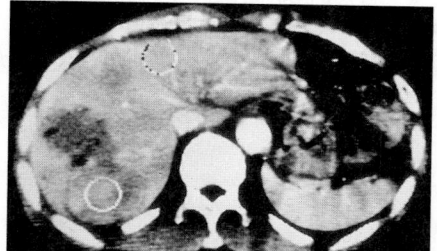

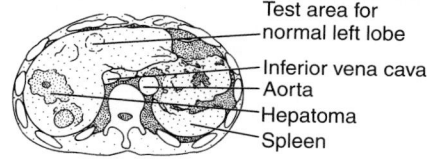

Test area for
normal left lobe

Inferior vena cava
Aorta
Hepatoma
Spleen

FIGURE 1-182 Hepatoma. CT scan shows a diffuse lesion in the right lobe of an otherwise normal liver. (From Skarin AT: *Atlas of diagnostic oncology*, ed 3, St Louis, 2003, Mosby.)

shown to be more sensitive than AFP, thus they have very limited clinical utility. Patients on transplant waiting lists should be regularly screened for HCC because in the U.S. the development of HCC gives increased priority for liver transplantation. Screening for HCC is recommended in the following groups:

- Hepatitis B carriers (HBsAg positive): Asian males >40 yr, Asian females >50 yr, all cirrhotic hepatitis B carriers, family history of HCC and Africans older than age 20 yr
- Cirrhosis (nonhepatitis B): hepatitis C, alcoholic cirrhosis, hemochromatosis, primary biliary cirrhosis, and possibly α1-antitrypsin deficiency, autoimmune hepatitis, and nonalcoholic steatohepatitis

STAGING: According to the Barcelona Clinic Liver Cancer (BCLC) staging classification, treatment is determined according to stage:

- Early stage (A): asymptomatic single tumor 5 cm or 3 nodules, each ≤3 cm (known as Milan criteria)
- Intermediate stage (B): patients with tumors that exceed early criteria but do not yet show cancer-related symptoms, vascular invasion, or metastases
- Advanced stage (C): patients with mild cancer-related symptoms and/or vascular invasion or extrahepatic spread
- End-stage (D): patients with advanced, symptomatic disease

TREATMENT

- Early stage: curative treatment (surgical resection or liver transplantation). Patients who have a single lesion can be offered surgical resection if they are noncirrhotic or have cirrhosis but still have well-preserved liver function, normal bilirubin, and no significant portal hypertension. Liver transplantation is an effective option for patients with HCC corresponding to the Milan criteria. Living donor transplantation can be offered for HCC if the waiting time is expected to be long. Local ablation is safe and effective therapy for patients who cannot undergo resection or as a bridge to transplantation. With these options, survival at 5 yr ranges from 50% to 70%.
- Intermediate stage: Transarterial chemoembolization (TACE) is recommended as first-line noncurative therapy for nonsurgical patients with large/multifocal HCC who do not have vascular invasion or extrahepatic spread. Median survival with this option exceeds 2 yr.
- Advanced stage: sorafenib, an oral multikinase inhibitor of the vascular endothelial growth factor receptor (VEGF), the platelet-derived growth factor receptor (PDGF), and Raf, a serine-threonine kinase, has been shown to improve survival and delay disease progression. The SHARP trial included patients with advanced HCC in Child-Pugh A cirrhosis and showed increased median survival from 7.9 to 10.7 mo.
- End stage: palliative care.

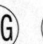

DISPOSITION

For unresectable tumors, prognosis is poor; 5-yr survival after surgical resection ranges from 30% to 50%.

REFERRAL

To gastroenterologist for treatment planning

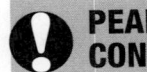

PEARLS & CONSIDERATIONS

PREVENTION

- Universal hepatitis B vaccination in children in endemic areas has been shown to decrease the incidence of HCC.
- Treatment of patients with chronic hepatitis B–associated cirrhosis with lamivudine reduces the incidence of HCC.

- HCC screening is recommended in high-risk patients because curative therapies are available for small and early HCC.
- The expression patterns of microRNAs in liver tissue in patients with HCC differ between men and women. The miR-26 expression status of such patients is associated with survival and response to adjuvant therapy with interferon alfa.
- Several observational studies have suggested that radiofrequency ablation (RFA) may have survival benefits similar to hepatic resection (HR) in cirrhotic patients affected by HCC who are not candidates for liver transplantation.
- Recent trials have shown that among patients with advanced HCC, treatment with sorafenib

plus doxorubicin monotherapy resulted in greater median time to progression-free survival. The degree in which this improvement may represent synergism between sorafenib and doxorubicin remains to be defined.

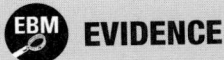 **EVIDENCE**

available at www.expertconsult.com

SUGGESTED READINGS

available at www.expertconsult.com

AUTHOR: **KITTICHAI PROMRAT, M.D.**

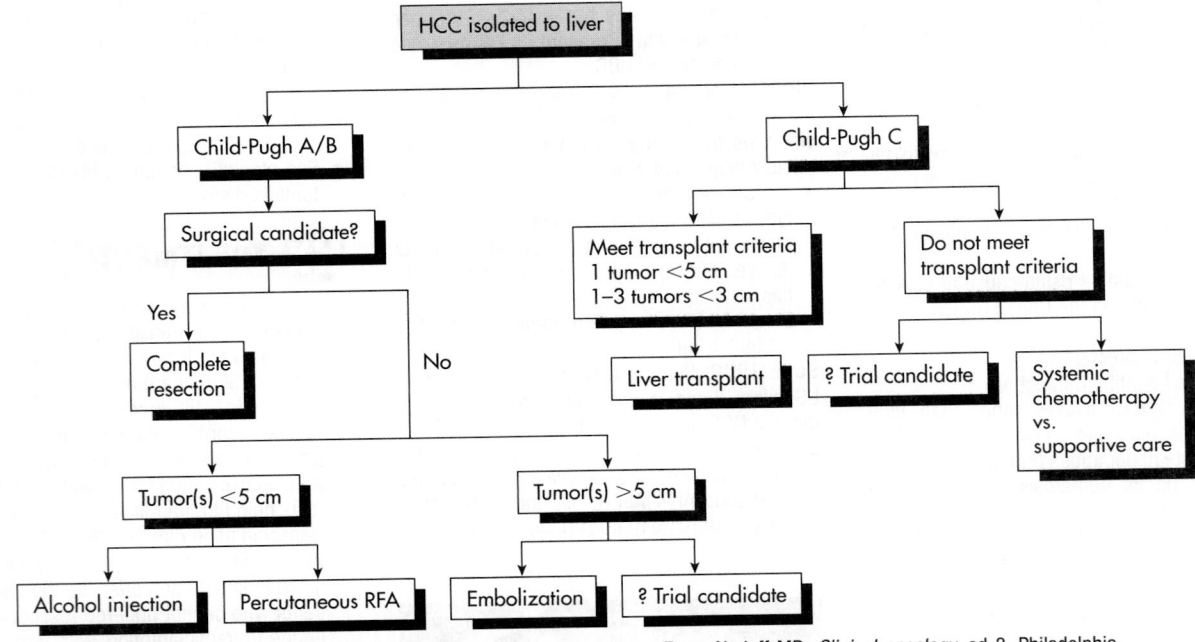

FIGURE 1-183 Treatment algorithm for hepatocellular carcinoma. (From Abeloff MD: *Clinical oncology,* ed 3, Philadelphia, 2004, Elsevier.)

BASIC INFORMATION

DEFINITION
Hepatopulmonary syndrome is characterized by intrapulmonary vascular dilatation in the setting of liver disease causing an increased alveolar-arterial (A-a) gradient.

SYNONYMS
None

ICD-9CM CODES
417.9 Unspecified disease of pulmonary circulation

EPIDEMIOLOGY & DEMOGRAPHICS
PREVALENCE: Between 4% and 47% of patients with liver disease; wide range due to lack of diagnostic criteria
PREDOMINANT SEX AND AGE: There are no data on gender or age prevalence.
RISK FACTORS: Can occur with any degree or etiology of liver disease but is more common in patients with established cirrhosis and portal hypertension. There is no clear relationship between severity of hepatic dysfunction and level of hypoxemia.
GENETICS: There are new data suggesting that genes involved in the regulation of angiogenesis are associated with the risk of hepatopulmonary syndrome.

PHYSICAL FINDINGS & CLINICAL PRESENTATION
- Dyspnea
- Platypnea: worsened dyspnea when sitting upright compared to supine position due to further ventilation-perfusion mismatch
- Orthodeoxia: decreased PaO_2 when the patient is sitting upright compared to supine position due to ventilation-perfusion mismatch
- Spider angiomata seen in high number
- Signs of severe hypoxemia (e.g., cyanosis and clubbing of the digits)

ETIOLOGY
Dilation of intrapulmonary arterioles and dilated vascular channels between pulmonary arteries and veins leading to a ventilation-perfusion match and right-to-left shunting (Fig. 1-184). Research shows that nitric oxide plays a role in vasodilation. The relationship of vasodilation to liver disease is unclear. New areas of research include endothelin-1 receptors, pulmonary angiogenesis, and opiate receptors influence on NO production.

DIAGNOSIS

DIFFERENTIAL DIAGNOSIS
- Portopulmonary hypertension
- Cavo-pulmonary anastomosis
- Hereditary hemorrhagic telangiectasia (Rendu-Osler-Weber syndrome)
- Chronic lung disease (i.e., COPD or pulmonary fibrosis) with coexisting liver disease

WORKUP
Workup includes lab testing and imaging studies (see following), but diagnosis is based on clinical findings.

LABORATORY TESTS
- Arterial blood gas at rest, both supine and erect; Pao_2 <80 mm Hg
- Pulmonary function tests will show nonspecific reduction in DL_{CO}

IMAGING STUDIES
- Chest x-ray may show nonspecific bibasilar interstitial pattern.
- Transthoracic echocardiogram with bubble study to rule out right-to-left cardiac shunt; microbubble opacification in left atrium shows vasodilation of pulmonary vascular bed.
- Scintigraphic perfusion scanning: technetium-99m–labeled albumin found in brain or spleen indicates dilated pulmonary vasculature or cardiac right-to-left shunt.
- Pulmonary angiography rarely used unless there is potential to embolize arteriovenous malformation.

TREATMENT

Ideal treatment would be targeted against pulmonary vasodilation but no effective medications yet exist. Liver transplantation is the only successful treatment, however severe hypoxemia with Pao_2 <50 has been associated with a high posttransplant mortality. Some studies have shown benefit of transjugular portosystemic shunting although it is not currently established treatment. Coil embolization in the setting of pulmonary arteriovenous malformations (AVMs) is another possible area of treatment.

NONPHARMACOLOGIC THERAPY
Oxygen to correct hypoxemia; Pao_2 will partially correct with administration of supplemental O_2.

ACUTE GENERAL Rx
Correct hypoxemia with supplemental O_2.

CHRONIC Rx
Liver transplantation is only successful treatment.

COMPLEMENTARY AND ALTERNATIVE MEDICINE
One study suggested that garlic supplements might decrease A-a gradient in patients with hepatopulmonary syndrome. Studies of diets containing low amount of L-arginine have not shown benefit.

DISPOSITION
The diagnosis of hepatopulmonary syndrome confers a poor prognosis. Patients with hepatopulmonary syndrome have high mortality and shorter median survival than other patients with liver disease, even after adjusting for severity of liver disease. According to one natural history study, compared with patients with similar severity of liver disease and comorbidities whose 5-yr survival was estimated at 63%, those patients with the diagnosis of hepatopulmonary syndrome had a 5-yr survival rate of 23%.

REFERRAL
- Referral to pulmonologist to help in establishing diagnosis
- Referral to a liver transplant center should be considered for patients who would be eligible

PEARLS & CONSIDERATIONS

COMMENTS
Consider the diagnosis of hepatopulmonary syndrome in patients with cirrhosis who present with dyspnea without signs of pulmonary edema from fluid overload.

SUGGESTED READINGS
available at www.expertconsult.com

AUTHOR: **BEVIN KENNEY, M.D.**

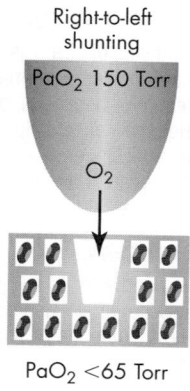

FIGURE 1-184 Pathophysiology of hypoxemia in hepatopulmonary syndrome. Abnormal intrapulmonary vascular dilatation in combination with increased pulmonary blood flow leads to diffusion-perfusion disturbance and arterial hypoxemia, correctable by oxygen supplementation. Most severe intrapulmonary vascular dilatation or formation of arteriovenous malformations causes right-to-left shunting only partially correctable by oxygen administration. (From Hoeper MM et al: Portopulmonary hypertension and hepatopulmonary syndrome, *Lancet* 363:1461, 2004.)

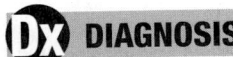 **BASIC INFORMATION**

DEFINITION

Hepatorenal syndrome (HRS) is a condition of intense renal vasoconstriction resulting from loss of renal autoregulation occurring as a complication of severe liver disease. Criteria for hepatorenal syndrome are:

1. Serum creatinine concentration >1.5 mg/dl or 24-hr creatinine clearance <40 ml/min
2. Absence of shock, ongoing infection, and fluid loss and no current treatment with nephrotoxic drugs
3. Absence of sustained improvement in renal function (decrease in serum creatinine to <1.5 mg/dl after discontinuation of diuretics and a trial of plasma expansion)
4. Absence of proteinuria (<500 mg/day) or hematuria (<50 red blood cells/high power field)
5. Absence of ultrasonographic evidence of obstructive uropathy or parenchymal renal disease
6. Urinary sodium concentration <10 mmol/L

There are two types of hepatorenal syndrome:

1. Type 1: progressive impairment in renal function as defined by a doubling of initial serum creatinine >2.5 mg/dl in <2 wk
2. Type 2: stable or slowly progressive impairment of renal function not meeting the above criteria

SYNONYMS

Hepatic nephropathy
Oliguric renal failure of cirrhosis
HRS

ICD-9CM CODES
572.4 Hepatorenal syndrome

EPIDEMIOLOGY & DEMOGRAPHICS

The probability of HRS in patients with cirrhosis is 18% at 1 yr and 39% at 5 yr.

PHYSICAL FINDINGS & CLINICAL PRESENTATION

- Evidence of cirrhosis is usually present: jaundice, spider angiomas, splenomegaly, ascites, fetor hepaticus, pedal edema
- Hepatic encephalopathy: flapping tremor (asterixis), coma
- Tachycardia and bounding pulse
- Oliguria

ETIOLOGY

An exacerbation of end-stage liver disease, HRS may occur after significant reduction of effective blood volume (e.g., paracentesis, GI bleeding, diuretics) or in the absence of any precipitating factors.

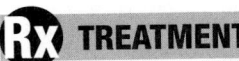 **DIAGNOSIS**

DIFFERENTIAL DIAGNOSIS

- Prerenal azotemia: response to sustained plasma expansion is good (prompt diuresis with volume expansion). Volume challenge (to increase mean arterial pressure) followed by large-volume paracentesis (to increase cardiac output and decrease renal venous pressure) may be useful to distinguish HRS from prerenal azotemia in patients with FENa <1%. In patients with prerenal azotemia, the increase in renal perfusion pressure and renal blood flow will result in prompt diuresis; the volume challenge can be accomplished by giving a solution of 100 g of albumin in 500 ml of isotonic saline.
- Acute tubular necrosis: urinary sodium >30 mEq/L, fractional excretion of sodium (FENa) >1.5%, urinary/plasma creatinine ratio <30, urine/plasma osmolality ratio = 1, urine sediment reveals casts and cellular debris, no significant response to sustained plasma expansion.

WORKUP

Patients with acute azotemia and oliguria in the setting of liver disease should undergo laboratory evaluation to differentiate HRS from acute tubular necrosis and volume challenge to differentiate HRS from prerenal azotemia if FENa <1%.

LABORATORY TESTS

- Obtain serum electrolytes, blood urea nitrogen, creatinine, osmolality, urinalysis, urinary sodium, urinary creatinine, urine osmolality
- Calculate FENa
- In HRS: urinary sodium <10 mEq/L, FENa <1%, urinary plasma creatinine ratio >30, urinary plasma osmolality ratio >1.5, urine sediment unremarkable

IMAGING STUDIES

Renal ultrasound may be indicated if renal obstruction is suspected.

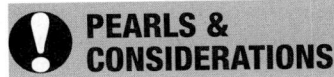 **TREATMENT**

NONPHARMACOLOGIC THERAPY

- Avoidance of precipitating factors.
- Transjugular intrahepatic portosystemic shunts may be effective in selected patients, but data are limited.
- Dialysis with molecular adsorbent recirculating systems remains investigational until more data are available.

ACUTE GENERAL Rx

- The only effective treatment of HRS is liver transplantation; ornipressin is used in some liver units to avoid further deterioration of renal function in patients awaiting liver transplantation. In general, dopamine and prostaglandins are ineffective in treating patients with hepatorenal syndrome.
- The best approach to the management of HRS based on its pathogenesis is the administration of vasoconstrictor drugs (terlipressin, norepinephrine, midodrine). Terlipressin may improve renal perfusion by reversing splanchnic vasodilation, which is the hallmark of HRS. Encouraging results were found in a recent study using continuous IV noradrenalin in combination with albumin and furosemide. In this study, reversal of HRS was achieved in 10 of 12 patients.
- Treatment of hepatorenal syndrome with vasoconstrictors for 5 to 15 days in attempt to reduce serum creatinine to <1.5 mg/dl is as follows:
  1. Administration of one of the following drugs or drug combinations:
     a. Norepinephrine (0.5 to 3.0 mg/hr IV)
     b. Midodrine (7.5 mg PO tid, increased to 12.5 mg tid if needed) in combination with octreotide (100 micrograms SC tid, increased to tid prn)
     c. Terlipressin (0.2 to 2.0 mg IV q4 to 12h)
  2. Concomitant administration of albumin (1 g/kg IV on day 1, followed by 20 to 40 g daily)

DISPOSITION

Mortality rate exceeds 80%; liver transplantation is the only curative treatment.

REFERRAL

Referral for liver transplantation when indicated (see "Comments")

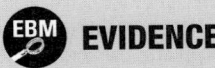 **PEARLS & CONSIDERATIONS**

COMMENTS

Liver transplantation may be indicated in otherwise healthy patients (age preferably <65 yr) with sclerosing cholangitis, chronic hepatitis with cirrhosis, or primary biliary cirrhosis. Contraindications to liver transplantation are AIDS, most metastatic malignancies, active substance abuse, uncontrolled sepsis, and uncontrolled cardiac or pulmonary disease.

EBM EVIDENCE

available at www.expertconsult.com

SUGGESTED READINGS
available at www.expertconsult.com

AUTHOR: **FRED F. FERRI, M.D.**

Diseases and Disorders

I

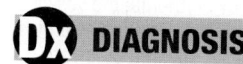

BASIC INFORMATION

DEFINITION

Herpangina is a self-limited upper respiratory tract infection associated with a characteristic vesicular rash on the soft palate.

SYNONYMS

Vesicular stomatitis
Acute lymphonodular pharyngitis

ICD-9CM CODES
074.0 Herpangina

EPIDEMIOLOGY & DEMOGRAPHICS

INCIDENCE (IN U.S.): Unknown
PEAK INCIDENCE: Summer outbreaks common
PREVALENCE (IN U.S.): Unknown
PREDOMINANT SEX: Male = female
PREDOMINANT AGE: 3 to 10 yr

PHYSICAL FINDINGS & CLINICAL PRESENTATION

- Characterized by ulcerating lesions typically located on the soft palate (Fig. 1-185)
- Usually fewer than six lesions that evolve rapidly from a diffuse pharyngitis to erythematous macules and subsequently to vesicles that are moderately painful
- Fever, vomiting, and headache in the first few days of illness but subsiding spontaneously
- Pharyngeal lesions typical for several more days

ETIOLOGY

- Most cases caused by coxsackie A viruses (A2, A4, A5, A6, A10)
- Occasional cases caused by other enteroviruses (Echovirus and Enterovirus 71)

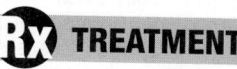

DIAGNOSIS

DIFFERENTIAL DIAGNOSIS

- Herpes simplex
- Bacterial pharyngitis
- Tonsillitis
- Aphthous stomatitis
- Hand-foot-mouth disease

WORKUP

Diagnosis is typically based on characteristic lesions on the soft palate.

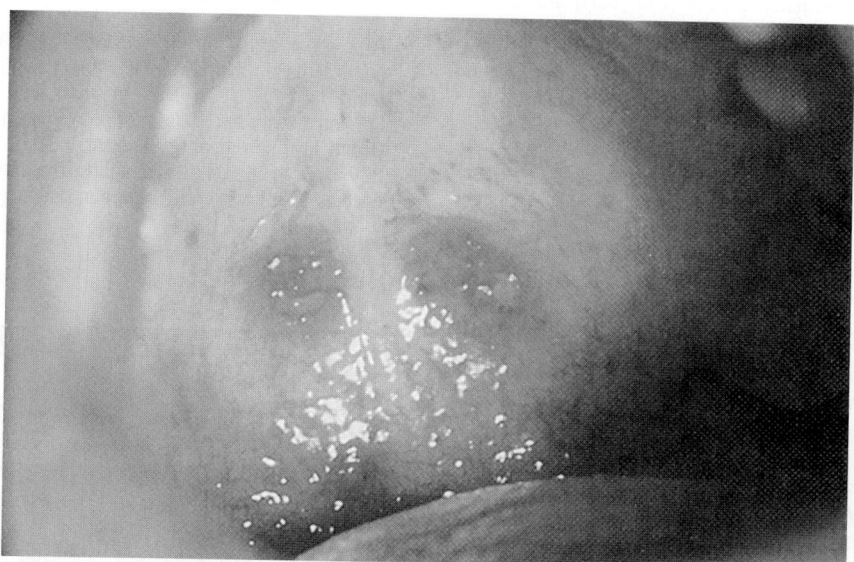

FIGURE 1-185 Herpangina with shallow ulcers in the roof of the mouth. (Courtesy Marshall Guill, M.D. From Goldstein B [ed]: *Practical dermatology*, ed 2, St Louis, 1997, Mosby.)

LABORATORY TESTS

Viral and bacterial cultures of the pharynx to exclude herpes simplex infection and streptococcal pharyngitis if the diagnosis is in doubt

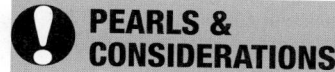

TREATMENT

- Give symptomatic treatment for sore throat: saline gargles and analgesics, and encourage oral fluids.
- No antiviral therapy indicated; avoid antibacterial agents because they are ineffective, increase cost, might result in side effects, and promote antibiotic resistance.

NONPHARMACOLOGIC THERAPY

Analgesic throat lozenges are helpful in some cases.

ACUTE GENERAL Rx

Antipyretics when indicated

CHRONIC Rx

Self-limited infection

DISPOSITION

- Generally, resolution of symptoms within 1 wk
- Persistence of fever or mouth lesions beyond 1 wk suggestive of an alternative diagnosis (see "Differential Diagnosis")

REFERRAL

For consultation with otolaryngologist or infectious disease specialist if the diagnosis is in doubt

PEARLS & CONSIDERATIONS

COMMENTS

Household outbreaks may occur, especially during the summer months.

SUGGESTED READINGS
available at www.expertconsult.com

AUTHORS: **GLENN G. FORT, M.D., M.P.H.,** and **DENNIS J. MIKOLICH, M.D.**

DEFINITION

Herpes simplex is a viral infection caused by the herpes simplex virus (HSV). HSV-1 is associated primarily with oral infections, and HSV-2 causes mainly genital infections. However, either type can infect any site. After the primary infection, the virus enters the nerve endings in the skin directly below the lesions and ascends to the dorsal root ganglia, where it remains in a latent stage until it is reactivated.

SYNONYMS

Genital herpes
Herpes labialis
Herpes gladiatorum
Herpes digitalis

ICD-9CM CODES
054.10 Genital herpes
054.9   Herpes labialis

EPIDEMIOLOGY & DEMOGRAPHICS

- More than 85% of adults have serologic evidence of HSV-1 infection. The seroprevalence of adults with HSV-2 in the U.S. is 25%; however, only approximately 20% of these persons recall having symptoms of HSV infection.
- Most cases of eye or digital herpetic infections are caused by HSV-1.
- Frequency of recurrence of HSV-2 genital herpes is higher than HSV-1 oral labial infection.
- The frequency of recurrence is lowest for oral labial HSV-2 infections.
- The incidence of complications from herpes simplex (e.g., herpes encephalitis) is highest in immunocompromised hosts.
- Male circumcision significantly reduces the incidence of HSV-2.

PHYSICAL FINDINGS & CLINICAL PRESENTATION

Primary infection:
- Symptoms occur from 3 to 7 days after contact (respiratory droplets, direct contact).
- Constitutional symptoms include low-grade fever, headache and myalgias, regional lymphadenopathy, and localized pain.
- Pain, burning, itching, and tingling last several hours.
- Grouped vesicles (Fig. 1-186), usually with surrounding erythema, appear and generally ulcerate or crust within 48 hr.
- The vesicles are uniform in size (differentiating it from herpes zoster vesicles, which vary in size).
- During the acute eruption the patient is uncomfortable; involvement of lips and inside of mouth may make it unpleasant for the patient

to eat; urinary retention may complicate involvement of the genital area.
- Lesions generally last from 2 to 6 wk and heal without scarring.

Recurrent infection:
- Generally caused by alteration in the immune system; fatigue, stress, menses, local skin trauma, and exposure to sunlight are contributing factors.
- The prodromal symptoms (fatigue, burning and tingling of the affected area) last 12 to 24 hr.
- A cluster of lesions generally evolves within 24 hr from a macule to a papule and then vesicles surrounded by erythema; the vesicles coalesce and subsequently rupture within 4 days, revealing erosions covered by crusts.
- The crusts are generally shed within 7 to 10 days, revealing a pink surface.
- The most frequent location of the lesions is on the vermilion border of the lips (HSV-1), the penile shaft or glans penis and the labia (HSV-2), buttocks (seen more frequently in women), fingertips (herpetic whitlow), and trunk (may be confused with herpes zoster).
- Rapid onset of diffuse cutaneous herpes simplex (eczema herpeticum) may occur in certain atopic infants and adults. It is a medical emergency, especially in young infants, and should be promptly treated with acyclovir.
- Herpes encephalitis, meningitis, and ocular herpes can occur in patients with immunocompromised status and occasionally in normal hosts.

ETIOLOGY

HSV-1 and HSV-2 are both DNA viruses.

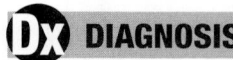

DIFFERENTIAL DIAGNOSIS

- Impetigo
- Behçet's syndrome
- Coxsackie virus infection
- Syphilis
- Stevens-Johnson syndrome
- Herpangina
- Aphthous stomatitis
- Varicella
- Herpes zoster

WORKUP

Diagnosis is based on clinical presentation. Laboratory evaluation confirms diagnosis.

LABORATORY TESTS

- Direct immunofluorescent antibody slide tests provide a rapid diagnosis.
- Viral culture is the most definitive method for diagnosis; results are generally available in 1 or 2 days. The lesions should be sampled during the vesicular or early ulcerative stage; cervical samples should be taken from the endocervix with a swab.
- Tzanck smear is a readily available test that will demonstrate multinucleated giant cells. However, it is not a highly sensitive test.
- Pap smear will detect HSV-infected cells in cervical tissue from women without symptoms.
- Serologic tests for HSV: immunoglobulin (Ig) G and IgM serum antibodies. Antibodies to HSV occur in 50% to 90% of adults. The presence of IgM or a fourfold or greater rise in IgG

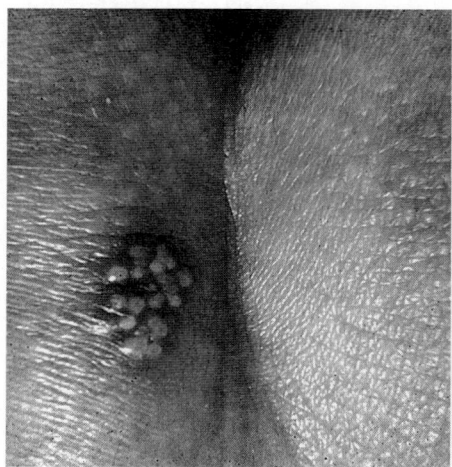 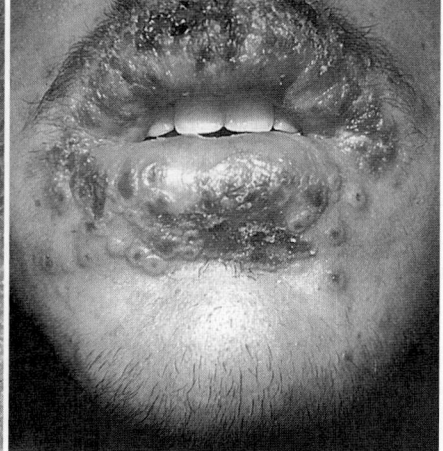

FIGURE 1-186 Herpes simplex. (From Scuderi G [ed]: *Sports medicine: principles of primary care,* St Louis, 1997, Mosby.)

titers indicates a recent infection (convalescent sample should be drawn 2 to 3 wk after the acute specimen is drawn).

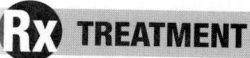 **TREATMENT**

- Table 1-67 summarizes antiviral chemotherapy for herpes simplex virus infection.
- Topical acyclovir, penciclovir, and docosanol are optional treatments for recurrent herpes labialis, but they are less effective than oral treatments.

DISPOSITION

Most patients recover from the initial episode or recurrences without complications; immunocompromised hosts are at risk for complications (e.g., disseminated herpes simplex infection, herpes encephalitis).

REFERRAL

- Hospital admission in patients with herpes encephalitis or herpes meningitis and in immunocompromised hosts with diffuse herpes simplex infection
- Ophthalmology referral in patients with suspected ocular herpes

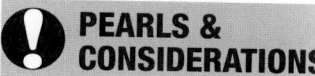 **PEARLS & CONSIDERATIONS**

COMMENTS

- Provide patient education regarding transmission of HSV.
- Condom use offers significant protection against HSV-1 infection in susceptive women.
- Patients should be instructed on the use of condoms for sexual intercourse and on avoiding kissing or sexual intercourse until lesions are crusted.
- Patients should also avoid contact with immunocompromised hosts or neonates while lesions are present.

- Proper handwashing techniques should be explained.
- Patients with herpes gladiatorum (cutaneous herpes in athletes involved in contact sports) should be excluded from participation in active sports until lesions have resolved.
- Many new HSV-2 infections are asymptomatic, but new symptoms may result from old infections.

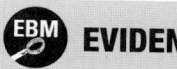 **EVIDENCE**

available at www.expertconsult.com

SUGGESTED READINGS

available at www.expertconsult.com

AUTHOR: **FRED F. FERRI, M.D.**

TABLE 1-67 Antiviral Chemotherapy for Herpes Simplex Virus Infection

Mucocutaneous HSV Infections
Infections in Immunosuppressed Patients
Acute symptomatic first or recurrent episodes: IV acyclovir (5 mg/kg q8h) and oral acyclovir (400 mg qid), famciclovir (500 mg PO tid), or valacyclovir (500 mg PO bid) for 7-10 days are effective. Treatment duration may vary from 7-14 days.
Suppression of reactivation disease: IV acyclovir (5 mg/kg q8h), valacyclovir (500 mg PO bid), or oral acyclovir (400-800 mg three to five times per day) prevents recurrences during the immediate 30-day post-transplantation period. Longer term suppression is often used for persons with continued immunosuppression. In bone marrow and renal transplant recipients, valacyclovir 2 g four times daily is also effective in preventing CMV infection. Valacyclovir 4 g four times daily has been associated with TTP after extended use in HIV-positive persons. In HIV-infected persons, oral famciclovir (500 mg bid) is effective in reducing clinical and subclinical reactivations of HSV-1 and -2.
Genital Herpes
First episodes: Oral acyclovir (200 mg five times per day or 400 mg tid), oral valacyclovir (1000 mg bid), or famciclovir (250 mg bid) for 10-14 days is effective. IV acyclovir (5 mg/kg q8h for 5 days) is given for severe disease or neurologic complications such as aseptic meningitis.
Symptomatic recurrent genital herpes: Oral acyclovir (200 mg five times per day for 5 days, 800 mg PO tid for 2 days) valacyclovir (500 mg bid for 3 or 5 days), or famciclovir (125 mg bid for 5 days). All these therapies are effective in shortening lesion duration.
Suppression of recurrent genital herpes: Oral acyclovir (200-mg capsules bid or tid, 400 mg bid, or 800 mg qd), famciclovir (250 mg bid), or valacyclovir (500 mg or 1000 mg qd or 500 mg bid) prevents symptomatic reactivation. Persons with frequent reactivation (<9 episodes/year) can take 500 mg daily; those with >9 episodes/year should take 1000 mg/daily or 500 mg bid.
Oral-Labial HSV Infections
First episode: Oral acyclovir (200 mg) is given four or five times per day. Famciclovir (250 mg bid) or valacyclovir (1000 mg bid) has been used clinically.
Recurrent episodes: Valacyclovir 1000 mg bid for 1 day or 500 mg bid for 3 days is effective in reducing pain and speeding healing. Self-initiated therapy with six times daily topical 1% penciclovir cream is effective in speeding the healing of oral-labial HSV; topical acyclovir cream has also been shown to speed healing.
Suppression of reactivation of oral-labial HSV: Oral acyclovir (400 mg bid), if started before exposure and continued for the duration of exposure (usually 5-10 days), prevents reactivation of recurrent oral-labial HSV infection associated with severe sun exposure.

Herpetic Whitlow
Oral acyclovir (200 mg) five times daily for 7-10 days.
HSV Proctitis
Oral acyclovir (400 mg five times per day) is useful in shortening the course of infection. In immunosuppressed patients or in patients with severe infection, IV acyclovir (5 mg/kg q8h) may be useful.
Herpetic Eye Infections
In acute keratitis, topical trifluorothymidine, vidarabine, idoxuridine, acyclovir, penciclovir, and interferon are all beneficial. Debridement may be required; topical steroids may worsen disease.
CNS HSV Infections
HSV encephalitis: Intravenous acyclovir (10 mg/kg q8h; 30 mg/kg per day) for 14-21 days is preferred.
HSV aseptic meningitis: No studies of systemic antiviral chemotherapy exist. If therapy is to be given, IV acyclovir (15-30 mg/kg/day) should be used.
Autonomic radiculopathy: No studies are available.
Neonatal HSV infections: Acyclovir (60 mg/kg/day, divided into three doses) is given. The recommended duration of treatment is 21 days. Monitoring for relapse should be undertaken, and some authorities recommend continued suppression with oral acyclovir suspension for 3 to 4 mo.
Visceral HSV Infections
HSV esophagitis: IV acyclovir (15 mg/kg per day). In some patients with milder forms of immunosuppression, oral therapy with valacyclovir or famciclovir is effective.
HSV pneumonitis: No controlled studies exist. IV acyclovir (15 mg/kg per day) should be considered.
Disseminated HSV infections: No controlled studies exist. Intravenous acyclovir (10 mg/kg q8h) nevertheless should be tried. No definite evidence indicates that therapy decreases the risk of death.
Erythema multiforme-associated HSV: Anecdotal observations suggest that oral acyclovir (400 mg bid or tid) or valacyclovir (500 mg bid) suppresses erythema multiforme.
Surgical prophylaxis: Several surgical procedures such as laser skin resurfacing, trigeminal nerve root decompression, and lumbar disk surgery have been associated with HSV reactivation. Intravenous acyclovir (3 mg/kg) and oral acyclovir 800 bid, valacyclovir 500 bid, or famciclovir 250 bid is effective in reducing reactivation. Therapy should be initiated 48 hours before surgery and continued for 3 to 7 days.
Infections with acyclovir-resistant HSV: Foscarnet (40 mg/kg IV q8h) should be given until lesions heal. The optimal duration of therapy and the usefulness of its continuation to suppress lesions are unclear. Some patients may benefit from cutaneous application of trifluorothymidine or 5% cidofovir gel.

CMV, Cytomegalovirus; *CNS,* central nervous system; *HIV,* human immunodeficiency virus; *HSV,* herpes simplex virus; *TTP,* thrombotic thrombocytopenic purpura.
Mandell GI, Bennett JE, Dolin R: *Principles and practice of infectious diseases,* ed 6, Philadelphia, Elsevier, 2005.

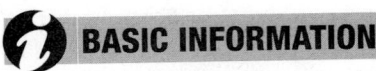

BASIC INFORMATION

DEFINITION

Herpes zoster is a disease caused by reactivation of the varicella-zoster virus (VZV). After the primary infection (chickenpox), the virus becomes latent in the dorsal root ganglia and re-emerges when there is a weakening of the immune system (as a result of disease or advanced age).

SYNONYMS

Shingles

ICD-9CM CODES
053.9 Herpes zoster

EPIDEMIOLOGY & DEMOGRAPHICS

- Herpes zoster occurs during the lifetime of 10% to 20% of the population.
- There is an increased incidence in immunocompromised patients (AIDS, malignancy), the elderly, and children who acquired chickenpox when younger than 2 mo.

PHYSICAL FINDINGS & CLINICAL PRESENTATION

- Pain generally precedes skin manifestation by 3 to 5 days and is generally localized to the dermatome that will be affected by the skin lesions.
- Constitutional symptoms are often present (malaise, fever, headache).
- The initial rash consists of erythematous maculopapules generally affecting one dermatome (thoracic region in majority of cases). Typically the rash does not cross the midline. Some patients (<30%) may have scattered vesicles outside the affected dermatome.
- The initial maculopapules evolve into vesicles and pustules by the third or the fourth day.
- The vesicles have an erythematous base, are cloudy, and have various sizes (a distinguishing characteristic from herpes simplex, in which the vesicles are of uniform size).
- The vesicles subsequently become umbilicated and then form crusts that generally fall off within 3 wk; scarring may occur.
- Pain during and after the rash is generally significant.
- Secondary bacterial infection with *Staphylococcus aureus* or *Streptococcus pyogenes* may occur.
- Regional lymphadenopathy may occur.
- Herpes zoster may involve the trigeminal nerve (most frequent cranial nerve involved); involvement of the geniculate ganglion can cause facial palsy and a painful ear, with the presence of vesicles on the pinna and external auditory canal (Ramsay Hunt syndrome).

ETIOLOGY

Reactivation of varicella virus (human herpes virus III)

DIAGNOSIS

DIFFERENTIAL DIAGNOSIS

- Rash: herpes simplex and other viral infections
- Pain from herpes zoster: may be confused with acute myocardial infarction, pulmonary embolism, pleuritis, pericarditis, renal colic

LABORATORY TESTS

Laboratory tests are generally not necessary (viral cultures and Tzanck smear will confirm diagnosis in patients with atypical presentation).

TREATMENT

NONPHARMACOLOGIC THERAPY

- Wet compresses (using Burow's solution or cool tap water) applied for 15 to 30 min five to 10 times a day are useful to break vesicles and remove serum and crust.
- Care must be taken to prevent any secondary bacterial infection.

ACUTE GENERAL Rx

- Gabapentin 100 to 600 mg tid is effective in the treatment of pain and sleep interference associated with postherpetic neuralgia. Other effective agents are pregabalin, duloxetine, and tricyclic antidepressants.
- Lidocaine patch 5% (Lidoderm) is also effective in relieving postherpetic neuralgia. Patches are applied to intact skin after resolution of blisters and crusts to cover the most painful area for up to 12 hr within a 24-hr period.
- Oral antiviral agents can decrease acute pain, inflammation, and vesicle formation when treatment is begun within 48 hr of onset of rash. Treatment options are:
  1. Acyclovir (Zovirax) 800 mg 5 times daily for 7 to 10 days
  2. Valacyclovir (Valtrex) 1000 mg tid for 7 days
  3. Famciclovir (Famvir) 500 mg tid for 7 days
- Immunocompromised patients should be treated with IV acyclovir 500 mg/m^2 or 10 mg/kg q8h in 1-hr infusions for 7 days, with close monitoring of renal function and adequate hydration; vidarabine (continuous 12-hr infusion of 10 mg/kg/day for 7 days) is also effective for treatment of disseminated herpes zoster in immunocompromised hosts.
- Patients with AIDS and transplant recipients may develop acyclovir-resistant varicella-zoster; these patients can be treated with foscarnet (40 mg/kg IV q8h) continued for at least 10 days or until lesions are completely healed.
- Capsaicin cream (Zostrix) can be useful for treatment of postherpetic neuralgia. It is generally applied 3 to 5 times daily for several weeks after the crusts have fallen off.

- Sympathetic blocks (stellate ganglion or epidural) with 0.25% bupivacaine and rhizotomy are reserved for severe cases unresponsive to conservative treatment.
- Corticosteroids should be considered in older patients within 72 hr of clinical presentation or if new lesions are still appearing if there are no contraindications. Initial dose is prednisone 40 mg/day decreased by 5 mg/day until finished. When used there is a decrease in the use of analgesics and time to resumption of usual activities, but there is no effect on the incidence and duration of postherpetic neuralgia.

DISPOSITION

- The incidence of postherpetic neuralgia (defined as pain that persists more than 30 days after onset of rash) increases with age (30% by age 40 yr, >70% by age 70 yr); antivirals reduce the risk of postherpetic neuralgia.
- Incidence of disseminated herpes zoster is increased in immunocompromised hosts (e.g., 15% to 50% of patients with active Hodgkin's disease).
- Immunocompromised hosts are also more prone to neurologic complications (encephalitis, myelitis, cranial and peripheral nerve palsies, acute retinal necrosis). The mortality rate is 10% to 20% in immunocompromised hosts with disseminated zoster.
- Motor neuropathies occur in 5% of all cases of zoster; complete recovery occurs in >70% of patients.

REFERRAL

- Hospitalization for IV acyclovir in patients with disseminated herpes zoster.
- Patients with herpes zoster ophthalmicus should be referred to an ophthalmologist.
- Vaccination: immunocompetent adults ≥60 yr are appropriate candidates for a single dose of varicella-zoster vaccine (VZV) whether or not they have had a previous episode of herpes zoster. Immunization with VZV (Zostavax) boosts waning immunity in older adults and reduces the severity and duration of pain caused by herpes zoster by 61%. Adults who are VZV seronegative (never had varicella) should be immunized against varicella with two doses of varicella vaccine (Varivax). Despite its efficacy and safety, use of this vaccine remains low (<8% of potential recipients).

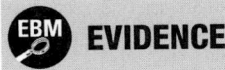 **EVIDENCE**

available at www.expertconsult.com

SUGGESTED READINGS

available at www.expertconsult.com

AUTHOR: **FRED F. FERRI, M.D.**

BASIC INFORMATION

DEFINITION

A hiatal hernia is the protrusion of a portion of the stomach into the thoracic cavity through the diaphragmatic esophageal hiatus.

SYNONYMS

Hiatus hernia
Diaphragmatic hernia

ICD-9CM CODES

553.3 Diaphragmatic hernia without obstruction or gangrene
750.6 Congenital hiatal hernia
756.6 Congenital diaphragmatic hernia

EPIDEMIOLOGY & DEMOGRAPHICS

- Found in 50% of patients older than 50.
- Prevalence increases with age.
- More prevalent in Western countries than in Africa and Asia.
- Paraesophageal hiatal hernias are more common in women than in men (4:1).
- Associated with diverticulosis (25%), esophagitis (25%), duodenal ulcers (20%), and gallstones (18%).
- More than 90% of patients with endoscopic documentation of esophagitis have hiatal hernias.

PHYSICAL FINDINGS & CLINICAL PRESENTATION

Most patients are asymptomatic. If symptoms are present, they resemble those of gastroesophageal reflux disease (GERD).

- Heartburn
- Dysphagia
- Regurgitation of gastric contents
- Chest pain
- Postprandial fullness
- GI bleed
- Dyspnea
- Hoarseness
- Wheezing with bowel sounds heard over the left lung base

ETIOLOGY

- The repetitive stretching of the gastroesophageal (GE) junction with swallowing and actions (e.g., vomiting) or states (e.g., obesity, pregnancy) that increase intraabdominal pressure may cause widening of the hiatus, rupture of the phrenoesophageal ligament, and onset of the hernia.
- Hiatal hernias are classified as:
  1. Type I: Sliding (Fig. 1-187, A), axial, or concentric hiatal hernia (most common type, 99%). Only the GE junction protrudes into the thoracic cavity and the phrenoesophageal ligament remains intact.
  2. Type II: Paraesophageal or rolling hernia (Fig. 1-187, B) (1%). The GE junction stays at the level of the diaphragm, but part of the stomach bulges into the thoracic cavity through a defect in the phrenoesophageal ligament.
  3. Type III: Mixed (rare), a combination of type I and type II.
  4. Type IV: Large defect in hiatus that allows other intraabdominal organs to enter the hernia sac.

DIAGNOSIS

DIFFERENTIAL DIAGNOSIS

- Peptic ulcer disease
- Unstable angina
- Esophagitis (caused by *Candida*, herpes, NSAIDs, etc.)
- Esophageal spasm
- Barrett's esophagus
- Schatzki's ring
- Achalasia
- Zenker's diverticulum
- Esophageal cancer

WORKUP

- Exclude conditions noted in the differential diagnosis and document the presence of a hiatal hernia. Upper endoscopy may also be needed to exclude abnormal metaplasia, dysplasia, or neoplasia.
- A clinical algorithm for evaluation of heartburn is described in Section III.

LABORATORY TESTS

- Blood tests are not specific.
- Esophageal manometry, although not commonly done, can be used in establishing a diagnosis (low sensitivity, but high specificity when compared with endoscopy).

IMAGING STUDIES

- Upper gastrointestinal (UGI) barium contrast swallow series: best defines the anatomic abnormality. Demonstration that the gastric cardia is herniated 2 cm above the hiatus is diagnostic. UGI may also reveal a tortuous esophagus (Fig. 1-188). If endoscopy is performed preoperatively, a barium swallow is generally not necessary.
- UGI endoscopy: documents the presence of a hiatal hernia and also excludes common associated findings of esophagitis and Barrett's esophagus (recommended at least once during the workup). Greater than 2 cm of gastric rugal fold seen above the margins of the diaphragmatic crura is diagnostic.
- Abdominal ultrasonography: simple, well tolerated. A transdiaphragmatic esophageal diameter of more than or equal to 18 mm is highly suggestive of the presence of a sliding hiatal hernia.

TREATMENT

NONPHARMACOLOGIC THERAPY

- Lifestyle modifications: avoid foods and drugs that decrease lower-esophageal pressure (e.g., caffeine, chocolate, mint, calcium channel blockers, and anticholinergics)
- Weight loss
- Avoid large quantities of food with meals
- Sleep with the head of the bed elevated 6 inches

ACUTE GENERAL Rx

- Antacids may be useful to relieve mild symptoms.
- H_2 antagonists (e.g., cimetidine 400 mg bid, ranitidine 150 mg bid, or famotidine 20 mg bid).
- If significant GERD is present with documented esophagitis, proton pump inhibitors (e.g., omeprazole 20 mg qd or lansoprazole 30 mg qd) are used. Refractory symptoms may require higher doses (e.g., bid dosing).
- Prokinetic agents (e.g., metoclopramide 10 mg taken 30 min before each meal) can be added to an H_2 antagonist or proton pump inhibitor.

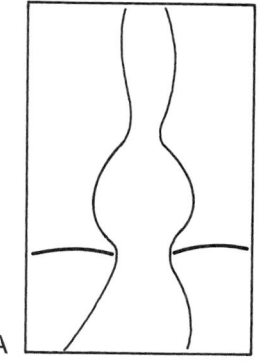
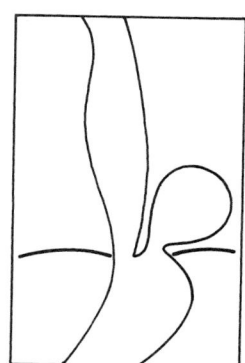

FIGURE 1-187 Types of esophageal hiatal hernia. A, Sliding hiatal hernia, the most common type. **B,** Paraesophageal hiatal hernia. (From Behrman RE: *Nelson textbook of pediatrics,* ed 17, Philadelphia, 2004, WB Saunders.)

A   B

CHRONIC Rx

- When indicated, surgery (laparoscopic or open) can be done in patients with refractory symptoms impairing quality of life, or causing intestinal (e.g., recurrent GI bleeds) or extraintestinal complications (e.g., aspiration pneumonia, asthma, or ear-nose-throat complications).
- Prophylactic surgery is a consideration in all paraesophageal hernias because they have a higher incidence of strangulation.

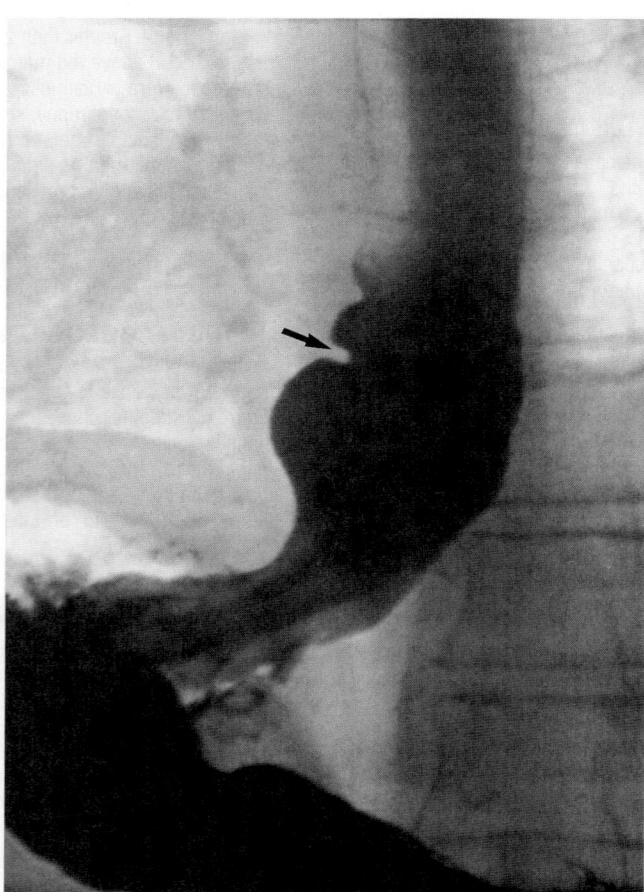

FIGURE 1-188 A sliding hiatal hernia confirmed by the presence of an incisural notch *(arrow)* on the greater curve aspect. (From Grainger RG et al [eds]: *Grainger & Allison's diagnostic radiology,* ed 4, Philadelphia, 2001, Churchill Livingstone.)

DISPOSITION

- More than 90% of patients having GERD symptoms respond well to medical therapy.
- Complications of hiatal hernias are similar to complications occurring in patients with GERD:
  1. Erosive esophagitis
  2. Ulcerative esophagitis
  3. Barrett's esophagus
  4. Peptic stricture
  5. GI hemorrhage
  6. Extraintestinal complications
  7. Lung collapse or heart failure (severe cases)

REFERRAL

Gastroenterologist: for symptoms refractory to conventional therapy (H$_2$ antagonists, antacids, and proton pump inhibitors) or having complications previously mentioned.

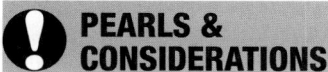

PEARLS & CONSIDERATIONS

COMMENTS

- Gastric ulceration and erosions (Cameron's lesion) can occur in the paraesophageal hernia pouch and are an uncommon cause of UGI bleeding.
- May cause iron deficiency anemia.
- Gastric volvulus or torsion can also occur and presents as dysphagia and postprandial pain.
- High incidence of esophagitis even after the eradication of *Helicobacter pylori.*
- The appearance of hiatal hernia may resemble a left atrial mass by echocardiography.

SUGGESTED READINGS

available at www.expertconsult.com

AUTHOR: **MARK F. BRADY, M.D., M.P.H., M.M.S.**

BASIC INFORMATION

DEFINITION

Hidradenitis suppurativa is a chronic, relapsing suppurative cutaneous disease manifested by abscesses, fistulating sinus tracts and chronic infection leading to scarring.

SYNONYMS

Acne inversa
Apocrinitis
Verneuil's disease
Pyoderma fistulas significa

ICD-9CM CODES
705.83 Hidradenitis

EPIDEMIOLOGY & DEMOGRAPHICS

- Onset is postpubertal, with an average age of onset of 23 yr
- An increased frequency is seen in people of African American descent, possibly due to due to a greater density of apocrine glands; however, this has not been fully studied.

PREVALENCE: Overall prevalence in the United States is ~1% to 2%.

PREDOMINANT SEX: Female to male ratio is 4:1.

RISK FACTORS:
- Hyperandrogenism
- Obesity
- Family history
- Shorter menstrual cycles and longer duration of menses
- Personal or family history of acne or pilonidal cysts
- Cigarette smoking

PHYSICAL FINDINGS & CLINICAL PRESENTATION

The diagnosis is primarily clinical based on the development of typical lesions in a characteristic distribution, with a relapsing nature.

- Early symptoms include pain, itching, burning, erythema, and hyperhidrosis.
- Typical lesions include:
  - Painful and/or tender erythematous papules and nodules
  - Painful or tender abscesses and inflamed papules or nodules with foul smelling discharge
  - Dermal contractures and ropelike elevation of the skin
  - Comedones in the apocrine, gland-bearing skin
- The axilla is the most common site (Fig. 1-189).
- Less common sites include inguinal and perineal region, the areola of the breast, and the submammary folds.
- There is a strong tendency toward relapse and recurrence.
- Other characteristics of the disease are:
  - Poor response to conventional antibiotics
  - Often no pathogens from routine cultures of pus from boils

ETIOLOGY

- Keratinous materials plug apocrine glands in hair follicles leading to stasis and dilatation in glands.
- Bacteria are trapped and multiply leading to gland rupture with surrounding inflammation and local bacterial infection causing skin and tissue damage and scarring.
- Infectious agents such as *Streptococcus, Staphylococcus,* and *Escherichia coli,* and enteric flora have been identified in cultures, but are likely a secondary cause of the disease.
- There is likely some correlation with androgen levels and a genetic component to the disease.
- HS has been associated with other endocrine disorders such as diabetes, Cushing's disease, and acromegaly.

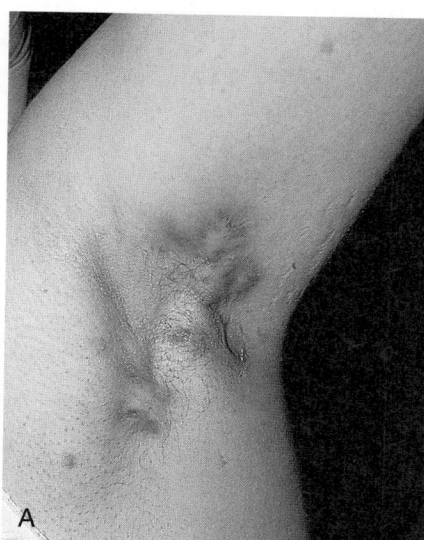

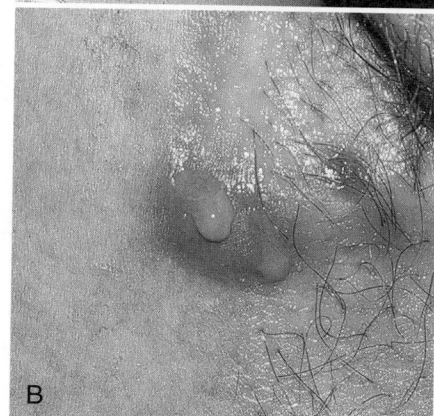

FIGURE 1-189 Hidradenitis suppurativa (HS). A, HS of the axilla. This is the classic appearance with inflammatory nodules and scarred areas. This condition is commonly misdiagnosed as a bacterial infection. **B,** HS of the axilla; a close-up view of the draining pus. When intact, the lesions represent sterile abscesses. Once open, they may become secondarily infected. (From White GM, Cox NH [eds]: *Diseases of the skin: a color atlas and text,* ed 2, St Louis, 2006, Mosby.)

DIAGNOSIS

DIFFERENTIAL DIAGNOSIS

- Follicular pyodermas such as folliculitis, furuncles, carbuncles, and pilonidal cysts
- Granuloma inguinale
- Perianal and vulvar manifestations of Crohn's disease
- Actinomycosis
- Lymphogranuloma venereum
- Dermoid, epidermoid, or Bartholin's cysts
- Tuberculous inflammation of the skin
- Lymphadenitis
- Cat scratch disease
- Tularemia
- Erysipelas

WORKUP

Primarily a clinical diagnosis based on typical lesion (see "Physical Findings & Clinical Presentation")

LABORATORY TESTS

- Patients with acute lesions may have an elevated erythrocyte sedimentation rate or WBC.
- Febrile and toxic appearing patients should have complete blood count, chemistries, and blood cultures.
- Any pus should be sampled for bacterial culture and sensitivity.

TREATMENT

There is no definitive cure for hidradenitis.

NONPHARMALOGIC THERAPY

- Avoidance of shaving, depilatory creams, deodorants
- Warm compresses
- Weight loss
- Smoking cessation
- Avoiding tight, synthetic clothing and hot humid climates
- Stress management to reduce flare-ups
- Hydrotherapy
- Incision and drainage of nonpurulent lesions not recommended
- Early wide excision recommended by some surgeons before significant progression
- Radiotherapy and cryotherapy currently under study

ACUTE AND CHRONIC Rx

- NSAIDs for inflammation and pain.
- Topical anesthetics and antibacterial soap.
- Antibiotics never proven to be effective; however, are mainstay of treatment.
  - Clindamycin is the only topical antibiotic proven to be effective in randomized controlled trial.
  - For oral therapy: cephalosporins, dicloxacillin, clindamycin, erythromycin, minocycline, tetracycline.

- Tailor therapy based on location of lesions (antistaphylococcal for axilla, broad spectrum for perineal lesions).
  - Severe, recurrent disease can require >2 mo of antibiotics.
- Oral contraceptives with low androgenic progesterone for women show mixed effectiveness.
- Isotretinoin (Accutane) has been used with mixed effectiveness.
- Corticosteroids and other immune suppressants such as cyclosporin, infliximab, and etanercept are under study currently.

COMPLICATIONS

- Dermal contraction
- Local and systemic infection
- Arthritis secondary to inflammatory injury
- Squamous cell carcinoma
- Scarring and restricted limb mobility

- Lymphedema caused by scarring of lymphatics
- Rectal or urethral fistulas

REFERRAL

- Referral to dermatology for patients who fail initial medical therapy.
- Referral to a surgeon is indicated with progression to multiple abscesses, sinus tract formation, and scarring.

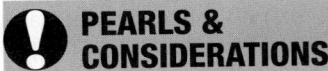

PEARLS & CONSIDERATIONS

COMMENTS

- Patients with hidradenitis are at risk for severe depression, social isolation, and negatively impacted sexuality as a result of their disease.

- It is important to maximize nonmedical treatment, start medical treatment, and refer to a surgeon early in the disease course to ensure the best quality of life for patients.
- The only definitive treatment for hidradenitis is wide excision of the involved skin.

PATIENT & FAMILY EDUCATION

Handout included in: Shah N: Hidradenitis suppurativa: a treatment challenge, *Am Fam Physician* 72:1547-1552, 1554, 2005.

SUGGESTED READINGS

available at www.expertconsult.com

AUTHOR: **MARY BETH SUTTER, M.D.**

BASIC INFORMATION

DEFINITION

The development of stiff, pigmented (terminal) facial and body hair (male distribution) in women as a result of excess androgen production.

SYNONYMS

Excessive hair growth

ICD-9CM CODES
704.1 Hirsutism

EPIDEMIOLOGY & DEMOGRAPHICS

- Overall prevalence unknown, estimated 5% to 10% in reproductive age women.
- Race and genetics should be considered. Some distinct ethnic populations have minimal body hair and others (Mediterranean, Middle Eastern, South Asian) have moderate to large amounts of body hair while serum androgen levels are similar.
- Social norms and culture also determine how much body hair is cosmetically acceptable.
- Half of all cases of mild hirsutism do not have hyperandrogenemia.
- Incidence and presentation of hirsutism is dependent on underlying cause of androgen excess (see "Differential Diagnosis").

PHYSICAL FINDINGS & CLINICAL PRESENTATION

- Timing of symptoms: abrupt onset, short duration, rapid progression, progressive worsening, more severe signs of virilization, or later age of onset suggest androgen-producing tumor, late-onset congenital adrenal hyperplasia, or Cushing's syndrome. Weight increases may produce increased androgen production.

- Menstrual history: menarche, cycle regularity and symptoms of ovulation, fertility, and contraception use. Anovulatory cycles are the most common underlying cause of androgen excess.
- Medication use history: some drugs cause hirsutism or produce androgenic effects (danazol, phenytoin, valproic acid, androgenic progestins (e.g., norgestrel), cyclosporin, minoxidil, metoclopramide, phenothiazines, methyldopa, diazoxide, penicillamine).
- Family history: known or suspected family history of hirsutism, congenital adrenal hyperplasia, insulin resistance, polycystic ovary syndrome (PCOS), infertility, obesity, menstrual irregularity may be found.
- Physical exam reveals deepening voice, body habitus, increased muscle mass, galactorrhea, abdominal and pelvic exam.
- Associated cutaneous manifestations (Fig. 1-190) are acne, acanthosis nigricans, striae, hair distribution, location and quantity, frontotemporal balding, muscle mass, clitoromegaly.

ETIOLOGY

- Presence of hirsutism indicates androgen excess. Total testosterone may be normal, but free testosterone is elevated.
- Androgens induce vellus hair follicles in sex-specific areas to develop into thicker, more heavily pigmented terminal hairs.
- Anovulatory ovaries are usual source of excess androgens through thecal cell steroidogenesis and conversion of androstenedione to testosterone.
- Conditions that decrease hepatic production of sex hormone binding globulin (SHBG) decrease protein-bound testosterone and increase free testosterone fraction (e.g., low estrogen, high androgen, and hyperinsulinemic states).

- Late-onset, congenital adrenal hyperplasia enzyme deficiency (most commonly 21-hydroxylase deficiency) produces excess 17 hydroxy-progesterone (17-OHP) and over-production of androstenedione.
- Rare ovarian tumors primarily derived from Sertoli-Leydig cells, granulosa theca cells, or hilus cells produce excess androgens.
- Rare adrenal tumors produce excess androgens.
- Rare pituitary or hypothalamic tumors produce excess prolactin and can lead to anovulation.

DIAGNOSIS

DIFFERENTIAL DIAGNOSIS

- Androgen-independent vellus hair: soft, unpigmented hair that covers entire body
- Hypertrichosis: diffusely increased total body hair (vellus or lanugo-type) not restricted to androgen-dependent areas often an adverse response to a medication or systemic illness
- PCOS 75%
- Idiopathic 5% to 15%
- Congenital adrenal hyperplasia 1% to 8%
- Insulin resistance syndrome 3% to 4%
- Cushing's syndrome <1%
- Drug induced <1%
- Ovarian tumor <1%
- Adrenal tumor <1%
- Hyperthecosis <1%
- Hyperprolactinemia <1%

WORKUP

- Hirsutism is a clinical diagnosis.
- Management of hirsutism is largely independent of the etiology.
- Workup in selected hirsute women is directed to determine underlying cause of androgen excess.
- Check androgen levels in women with moderate or severe hirsutism, sudden onset, rapid progression, or associated menstrual dysfunction, central obesity, clitoromegaly, or acanthosis nigricans.
- See specific conditions for more detailed workup of individual diagnoses.

LABORATORY TESTS

Total plasma testosterone or free testosterone: early morning on day 4 to 10 of menstrual cycle to screen for testosterone secreting tumors. If markedly elevated may image adrenals and ovaries.

Other laboratory test considerations if appropriate:

- Dehydroepiandrosterone sulfate (DHEA-S): screen for adrenal androgen production as almost entirely produced by adrenals
- Prolactin: moderately elevated values should prompt imaging of pituitary-hypothalamic region
- 17-OHP (17 α-hydroxyprogesterone): screen for adrenal enzyme deficiencies

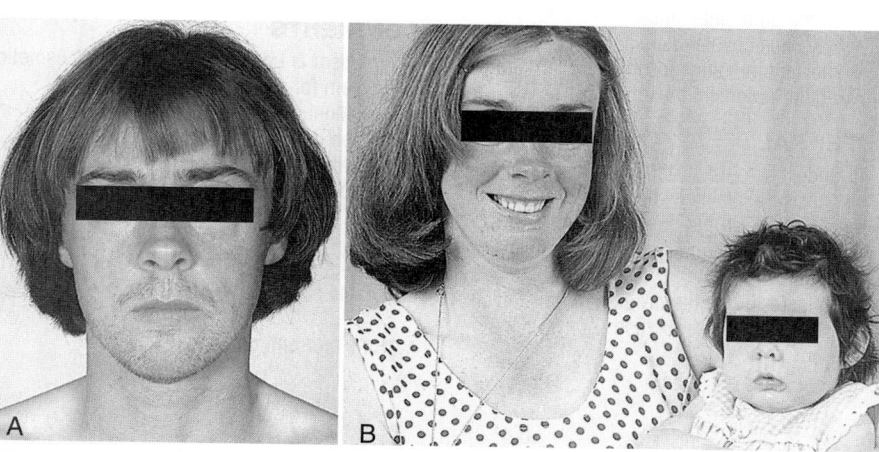

FIGURE 1-190 A patient with an arrhenoblastoma with associated polycystic ovaries before and after treatment. **A,** Before treatment, the patient had marked facial hirsutism. **B,** The patient is shown successfully treated. The tumor was resected and ovulation ensued with clomiphene and human chorionic gonadotropin therapy. (From Besser CM, Thorner MO: *Comprehensive clinical endocrinology,* ed 3, St Louis, 2002, Mosby.)

Other laboratory test considerations if appropriate:
- Follicle-stimulating hormone: (FSH): rule out hypoestrogen state (perimenopausal)
- Luteinizing hormone: (LH): typically elevated in PCOS with low or normal FSH
- Thyroid-stimulating hormone (TSH): rule out hypothyroidism
- 24-hour urinary free cortisol: rule out Cushing's syndrome and overproduction of cortisol
- Overnight single-dose dexamethasone suppression test: rule out Cushing's syndrome and adrenal hyperfunction
- Fasting blood sugar (FBS), 2-hr 75-g oral glucose tolerance test, fasting insulin levels: rule out insulin resistance syndrome

IMAGING STUDIES

Imaging study considerations if appropriate:
- Pelvic ultrasound (high resolution, transvaginal): rule out ovarian tumor
- Abdominal CT/MRI: rule out adrenal tumor
- Pituitary-hypothalamic region CT/MRI: rule out pituitary tumor
- Laparoscopy/laparotomy: rule out small ovarian tumor in cases of elevated testosterone levels without radiologic evidence of adrenal or ovarian pathology

Rx TREATMENT

NONPHARMACOLOGIC THERAPY

- Weight reduction: can reduce androgen production indirectly by reducing insulin-stimulated theca cell androgen production and improve menstrual function, and slow hair growth in obese women.
- Cosmetic: temporary.
  - Shaving: does not stimulate hair growth; lasts days, leaves stubble.
  - Epilation: electronic plucking.
  - Bleaching: removes hair pigment. May cause skin irritation.
  - Mechanical waxing/plucking.
  - Depilatories: gels, lotions, or creams that chemically disrupt sulfide bonds of hair causing dissolution of hair shaft. No stubble.
  - Photoepilation (laser and intense pulsed light [IPL]): hair follicles destroyed by wavelengths of light absorbed by melanin. Good for pigmented hair; laser treatment is more effective than shaving, waxing, and electrolysis. It lasts 3 to 6 mo as vellus follicles remain and can be converted to terminal pigmented hair under excess androgens.
- Cosmetic: permanent. Electrolysis: destroys individual hair follicles. May be expensive and time consuming.

ACUTE GENERAL Rx
See "Pharmacologic Therapy."

CHRONIC Rx
See "Pharmacologic Therapy."

PHARMACOLOGIC THERAPY

- Usually second-line treatment following non-pharmacologic, physical methods of hair control, and in consideration of patient's co-morbidities and risk factors, patient preferences, area of excess hair amenable to treatment, and access and affordability of treatments.
- Pharmacologic treatments categorized as topical, oral contraceptive pills (OCPs), anti-androgens, other treatments directed at underlying etiology.
- Topical: Eflornithine topical cream 13.9%: temporary cosmetic treatment for facial hair. Applied directly to unwanted facial hair bid with at least 8 hr spaced applications. Does not remove hair, rather slows growth. Slow response over 4 to 8 wk. Hair growth returns upon discontinuation of treatment.
- OCPs: Suppress ovarian steroidogenesis and LH through low-dose estrogen and low androgenic progestational agents. Slow response to treatment. Suppresses new hair growth. Established hair unaffected. Low-dose OCPs with low androgenic progestational agents, for example, norethindrone, desogestrel, norgestimate, drospirenone, cyproterone acetate (not available in U.S.). Avoid norgestrel and levonorgestrel (higher androgenic progestational agents).
- Antiandrogens: Spironolactone: when OCPs unacceptable or may be added for disappointing results after 6 mo of OCP treatment.
  - Aldosterone-antagonist diuretic inhibits adrenal and ovarian biosynthesis of androgens. May get ovulation.
  - Slow response usually 6 mo or more.
  - 200 mg PO qd, then decrease to 25 to 50 mg qd maintenance.
  - May cause hyperkalemia.
  - Anovulatory, unopposed estrogen states require progestin management.

REFERRAL

- To endocrinologist if difficulty in determining diagnosis, achieving therapeutic goals, or resistant to first-line therapies
- Consider referral or consultation for following therapies:
  1. Finasteride: antiandrogen, in hair follicle blocks 5 α–reductase conversion of testosterone to intranuclearly active 5 α–dihydrotestosterone (DHT)
     - Use only with reliable contraception because DHT necessary for normal male fetus urogenital development
     - Not FDA approved for treatment of hirsutism
     - 1 to 5 mg PO qd
  2. Flutamide: inhibits androgen uptake and receptor binding
     - Not recommended by Endocrine Society Clinical Practice Guidelines and not FDA approved for treatment of hirsutism, but used by some European endocrinologists
     - Use only with reliable contraception
     - Reserved for women with severe, resistant hirsutism because of risk of hepatic dysfunction
     - 250 mg PO bid
- Other treatments directed at underlying etiology:
  - Metformin/thiazolidinediones: therapy reserved for documented insulin resistant states.
  - GnRH agonists: recommended only in women with severe hyperandrogenemia (e.g., ovarian hyperthecosis) with suboptimal response to combination low-dose estrogen/progestin pills and antiandrogen treatment. Inhibits gonadotropin and consequently ovarian androgen and estrogen secretion.
  - Dexamethasone: adrenal glucocorticoid suppression is reserved for diagnosis of adrenal enzyme deficiency.
  - Total abdominal hysterectomy/bilateral salpingo-oopherectomy reserved for recalcitrant hirsutism in older female with hyperthecosis and undesired fertility.

(!) PEARLS & CONSIDERATIONS

COMMENTS

- Hirsutism is both an endocrine and cosmetic problem for patients.
- Ovulation induction therapy is indicated in women desiring pregnancy.
- Evaluation of incidental adrenal mass is warranted.

SUGGESTED READINGS
available at www.expertconsult.com

AUTHOR: **RICHARD LONG, M.D.**

BASIC INFORMATION

DEFINITION

Histiocytosis X, now known as Langerhans cell histiocytosis (LCH), is a rare disorder characterized by the abnormal proliferation of pathologic Langerhans cells. These dendritic cells form characteristic infiltrates with eosinophils, lymphocytes, and other histiocytes found in various organs.

SYNONYMS

Eosinophilic granuloma
Hand-Schüller-Christian disease
Letterer-Siwe disease
Langerhans cell histiocytosis
Langerhans cell granulomatosis
Diffuse reticuloendotheliosis

ICD-9CM CODES	
202.5	Acute Histiocytosis X
277.89	Chronic Histiocytosis X

EPIDEMIOLOGY & DEMOGRAPHICS

- LCH is mainly a childhood disorder with a peak incidence from age 1 to 4 yr.
- The annual incidence in the pediatric population is 2 to 5 per million.
- LCH affects males more often than females, 2:1.
- Pulmonary LCH (a localized form more commonly found in adults) has an equal male:female incidence, if not female predominance, probably because of increased prevalence of smoking in women.
- Usually more common in Caucasians.
- Disseminated LCH usually occurs before 2 yr of age.

PHYSICAL FINDINGS & CLINICAL PRESENTATION

- Clinical presentation is variable, and ranges from:
  - A benign isolated bony lesion (eosinophilic granuloma), most often found in children younger than 15 yr of age.
  - Multiple bone lesions with soft tissue gingival and oral mucosal involvement (Hand-Schüller-Christian disease); generally occurs in children younger than 10 yr of age.
  - An aggressive disseminated disease infiltrating organs and causing organ dysfunction (Letterer-Siwe disease). It is the rarest form of LCH, affecting mostly children younger than 2 yr.
- Bone lesions (80% to 100%).
  - May be isolated or multiple
  - Painful, often worse at night
  - Skull most often involved, followed by long bones; lesions rarely seen in small bones of hands and feet
  - Proptosis
  - Mastoiditis
  - Loose teeth
  - Gingival hypertrophy

- Skin is involved in >80% of patients with disseminated disease and in 30% of patients with less extensive disease.
  - Seborrhea-like scaling of scalp, petechial and purpuric lesions, ulcers, and bronzing of the skin may occur.
  - Common sites: scalp, neck, trunk, groin, and extremities.
- Lymphadenopathy (10%): cervical and inguinal.
- Pulmonary disease is very frequent in adults (usually as isolated disease), but can be seen in 23% to 50% of children as well. Lung involvement always occurs as part of the disseminated disease in children.
- Pulmonary involvement may manifest with cough, tachypnea, cyanosis, inspiratory crackles, pleural effusions, or pneumothorax. Diffuse emphysema associated with pulmonary fibrosis is the end stage of a mixed restrictive and obstructive pattern of disease.
- Liver involvement manifesting as hepatomegaly with or without jaundice (50% to 60%).
- Involvement of the biliary tree may be seen as biliary fibrosis or sclerosing cholangitis.
- Splenomegaly (5%).
- CNS involvement occurs in 25% to 35% of patients, most often in those with disseminated disease. The most common cerebral site affected is the hypothalamic-neurohypophyseal region, where infiltration and destruction usually result in diabetes insipidus with insatiable thirst and urination. The second most common site of involvement is the cerebellum.
- Involvement of the thymus, parotid glands, and GI tract has been reported in rare cases.

ETIOLOGY

- The etiology of LCH is unknown, though multiple theories have been proposed.
- Some degree of genetic predisposition has been proposed and recent evidence suggests LCH as a monoclonal proliferative neoplastic disorder in children.
- In adults, pulmonary LCH appears to be primarily an immune-mediated reactive process and has been linked to cigarette smoking. Cigarette smoke had not been observed as a causative factor in other forms of LCH.

DIAGNOSIS

Tissue biopsy of organ lesions reveals pathological Langerhans cells characterized by the presence of multiple surface nucleoproteins including CD1a, the presence of which establishes definitively histological diagnosis of LCH. The infiltration by eosinophils forming pseudo-abscesses is characteristic.

DIFFERENTIAL DIAGNOSIS

The differential diagnosis is extensive, including all causes of diabetes insipidus, lytic bone lesions, dermatitis, hepatomegaly, and lymphadenopathy.

WORKUP

Baseline evaluation should include bone scan, chest x-ray, skeletal x-ray, abdominal ultrasound, and routine laboratory to assess the extent of disease involvement.

LABORATORY TESTS

- CBC is not specific but may reveal cytopenias in patients with bone marrow involvement.
- Electrolytes, BUN, creatinine, urinalysis, and urine and serum osmolality are helpful in the diagnosis of diabetes insipidus during fluid deprivation testing.
- Liver function tests (LFTs) may be elevated in patients with liver involvement.
- Bronchoalveolar lavage may show increased numbers of CD1a-positive histiocytes or Langerhans cells in patients with pulmonary LCH.

IMAGING STUDIES

- Radiograph studies of affected areas show lytic lesions with or without sclerotic margins.
- Radiograph bone survey is done searching for other lesions.
- Bone scan complements the bone survey studies.
- Panoramic dental view of the mandible and maxilla for children with oral involvement.
- Chest radiograph can show interstitial reticulonodular infiltrates. This pattern typically progresses toward frank honeycombing fibrosis later in the course of the disease (Fig. 1-191).

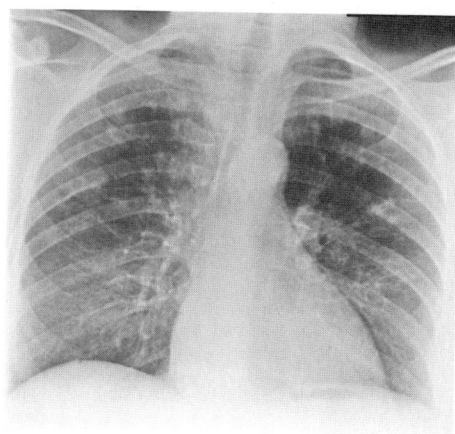

FIGURE 1-191 Langerhans cell histiocytosis (LCH; histiocytosis X). There is a reticular nodular pattern in the upper lobes. The lung volumes are preserved. (From McLoud TC [ed]: *Thoracic radiology, the requisites,* St Louis, 1998, Mosby.)

- High-resolution CT scan of the chest confirms interstitial lung scarring, nodules, and cysts, and represents an excellent noninvasive means for diagnosis and follow-up of pulmonary LCH. Pulmonary cysts are bilateral and symmetric, showing slight upper-lobe predominance with relative sparing of the costophrenic angles.
- CT scans of the temporal bone searching for mastoid, and inner and middle ear involvement.
- Ultrasound of the abdomen may show hepatosplenomegaly.
- Conventional cholangiography or MRI cholangiopancreatography can confirm the presence of disease in patients suspected to have biliary involvement.
- MRI of the brain to visualize the hypothalamic-hypophyseal region in patients suspected of having diabetes insipidus.

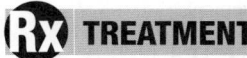 **TREATMENT**

Treatment is still evolving and is based on organ involvement and the extent of disease.

ACUTE GENERAL Rx

Isolated bone lesions can be treated by:
- Curettage of affected site and implantation of allograft bone chips or polymethylmethacrylate
- Intralesional prednisone or prednisone and vinblastine
- Bisphosphonates
- NSAIDs
- Radiation therapy is useful only for bone lesions of the vertebrae or femoral neck at risk of collapse

Single skin lesions are treated with:
- Topical steroid (e.g., triamcinolone acetonide) applied bid
- Nitrogen mustard in 20% solution
- Surgery
- Intralesional interferon
- Isotretinoin

Treatment of solitary lymph node involvement:
- Excision at the time of diagnosis
- Systemic oral prednisone

Treatment for multiple bone lesions, skull base lesions, or multisystem disease includes:
- Vinblastine 6 mg/m^2 IV bolus every wk for 6 mo or etoposide 150 mg/m^2 IV for 3 days every 3 wk for 6 mo and oral prednisone for 6 mo

CHRONIC Rx

- For severe, high-risk, disseminated cases not responding within 6 wk of initial treatment, salvage therapy, including high dose of the purine analog cladribine along with high-dose cytosine arabinoside followed by allogeneic blood stem cell transplantation, should be considered. Additionally, liver or lung transplantation might be the treatment of choice for terminal liver and lung failure patients.
- Diabetes insipidus is treated with DDAVP 0.1 to 0.8 mg PO or 1 spray bid to tid.
- Adults with isolated pulmonary LCH do not require aggressive treatment, and will benefit from smoking cessation.
- Empirical use of steroids, in either short pulses or longer exposures, has also been suggested in the treatment of pulmonary disease; however, data regarding effectiveness are still limited.
- Lung transplantation has been tried in both children and adults with advanced pulmonary disease and limited lung function, but failure rates are high because of local recurrence after transplantation.

DISPOSITION

- Patients with disease localized to only one organ system have a good prognosis and appear to need minimal, if any, treatment. For patients with isolated pulmonary LCH, the 5-yr survival rate is around 80%.
- Patients with disseminated disease have an increased risk for poor outcome, with a reported mortality rate of 10% to 20%, and 50% risk of life-impairing morbidity. A poor prognostic feature is the failure to respond to therapy in the first 6 wk.
- In patients with disseminated LCH and <2 yr of age, the mortality rate is 30%.

REFERRAL

Multidisciplinary approach: pediatric oncologist, radiation oncologists, oral maxillary surgeons, ear-nose-throat specialists, audiology, dermatology, endocrinology, and family counseling

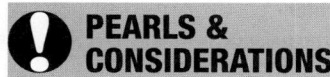 **PEARLS & CONSIDERATIONS**

COMMENTS

- The course of LCH is often unpredictable and varies from spontaneous resolution to rapid progression and death, or multiple recurrences and regressions with risk for permanent sequelae.
- The association of LCH with other malignancies (e.g., acute lymphocytic leukemia, acute nonlymphoblastic leukemia, and solid tumors) has been cited.

PREVENTION

Effective antismoking measures may prevent pulmonary LCH.

PATIENT/FAMILY EDUCATION

- Instruct patients to promptly report the development of hemoptysis. This symptom may indicate malignancy or superimposed bacterial/fungal infection, such as *Aspergillus* species infection.
- Educate about the likely etiologic role of cigarette smoking.

SUGGESTED READINGS
available at www.expertconsult.com

AUTHOR: **MARK F. BRADY, M.D., M.P.H., M.M.S.**

BASIC INFORMATION

DEFINITION

Histoplasmosis is caused by the fungus *Histoplasma capsulatum* and characterized by a primary pulmonary focus with occasional progression to chronic pulmonary histoplasmosis (CPH) or various forms of dissemination. Progressive disseminated histoplasmosis (PDH) may present with a diverse clinical spectrum, including adrenal necrosis, pulmonary and mediastinal fibrosis, and ulcerations of the oropharynx and GI tract. In those patients coinfected with HIV, it is a defining disease for AIDS.

SYNONYMS

North American histoplasmosis
Ohio Valley fever
Vanderbilt disease

ICD-9CM CODES
115.90 Histoplasmosis
115.94 Histoplasmosis with endocarditis
115.91 Histoplasmosis with meningitis
115.93 Histoplasmosis with pericarditis
115.95 Histoplasmosis with pneumonia
115.92 Histoplasmosis with retinitis

EPIDEMIOLOGY & DEMOGRAPHICS

INCIDENCE (IN U.S.):
- Unknown for acute pulmonary disease
- For CPH, estimated at 1/100,000 cases in endemic areas
- For PDH in immunocompetent adults, estimated at 1/2000 cases of histoplasmosis

PREVALENCE: Unknown

PREDOMINANT SEX: Clinically evident disease is most common in males; male:female ratio of 4:1

PREDOMINANT AGE:
- CPH is most often seen in males >50 yr old with an associated history of COPD.
- Presumed ocular histoplasmosis syndrome (POHS) is seen between ages of 20 and 40 yr.

PEAK INCIDENCE: Unknown

PHYSICAL FINDINGS & CLINICAL PRESENTATION

- Conidia are deposited in alveoli then converted to yeast forms where they spread to regional lymph nodes and other organs, especially liver and spleen.
- 1 to 2 wk later, a granulomatous inflammatory response begins to contain the yeast in the form of discrete granulomas.
- Delayed-type hypersensitivity to *Histoplasma* antigens occurs 3 to 6 wk after exposure.
- Clinical disease manifests in various forms, depending on host cellular immunity and inoculum size:
  1. Acute primary pulmonary histoplasmosis
     a. An overwhelming number of patients are asymptomatic.
     b. Most clinically apparent infections manifest by complaints of fever, headache, malaise, pleuritic chest pain, nonproductive cough, and weight loss.

c. Less than 10%, mainly women, complain of arthralgias, myalgias, and skin manifestations such as erythema multiforme or erythema nodosum.
     d. Acute pericarditis presents in a smaller percentage of patients.
     e. Hepatosplenomegaly is most commonly observed in children.
     f. With particularly heavy exposure, there is severe dyspnea, marked hypoxemia, impending respiratory failure.
     g. Most patients are asymptomatic within 6 wk.
  2. CPH
     a. Presents insidiously with low-grade fever, malaise, weight loss, cough, sometimes with blood-streaked sputum or frank hemoptysis.
     b. Most patients with cavitary lesions present with associated COPD or chronic bronchitis, masking underlying fungal disease.
     c. Tends to worsen preexisting pulmonary disease and further contribute to eventual respiratory insufficiency.
  3. PDH
     a. In both acute and subacute forms, constitutional symptoms of fever, fatigue, malaise, and weight loss are common.
     b. Acute form (seen in infants and children) presents with respiratory symptoms, fever ≥101° F (38.3° C), generalized lymphadenopathy, marked hepatosplenomegaly, and fulminant course resembling septic shock associated with a high fatality rate.
     c. Subacute form is more common in adults and associated with lower temperatures, hepatosplenomegaly, oropharyngeal ulceration, focal organ involvement (including adrenal destruction, endocarditis, chronic meningitis, and intracerebral mass lesions).
     d. Course of subacute form is relentless, with untreated patients dying within 2 yr.
     e. Chronic PDH is found in adults and marked by gradual symptoms of weight loss, weakness, easy fatigability; low-grade fever when present; oropharyngeal ulcerations and hepatomegaly and/or splenomegaly in one third of patients.
     f. Less clinical evidence of focal organ involvement in chronic form than in subacute form.
     g. Natural history of chronic form is protracted and intermittent, spanning months to years.
- Histoplasmoma
  1. A healed area of caseation necrosis surrounded by a fibrous capsule
  2. Usually asymptomatic
- Mediastinal fibrosis
  1. A rare consequence of a fibroblastic process that encases caseating mediastinal lymph nodes producing severe retraction,

compression, and distortion of mediastinal structures
  2. Constriction of the bronchi resulting in bronchiectasis, also esophageal stenosis associated with dysphagia, and superior vena cava syndrome
- POHS
  1. Diagnosis characterized by distinct clinical features, including atrophic choroidal scars and maculopathy in patients with histories suggestive of exposure to the fungus (e.g., residence in an endemic area)
  2. Patient complains of distortion or loss of central vision without pain, redness, or photophobia
  3. Usually no evidence of infection except for a positive skin reaction to histoplasmin
- In patients with AIDS
  1. Possible presentation as overwhelming infection similar to acute PDH seen in children
  2. Constitutional symptoms: fever, weight loss, malaise, cough, dyspnea
  3. About 10% with cutaneous maculopapular, erythematous eruptions or purpuric lesions on face, trunk, and extremities
  4. Up to 20% with CNS involvement, manifesting as intracerebral mass lesions, chronic meningitis, or encephalopathy

ETIOLOGY

- *H. capsulatum* is a dimorphic fungus present in temperate zones and river valleys worldwide.
- In the U.S., it is highly endemic in southeastern, mid-Atlantic, and central states.
- Exists as mold at ambient temperature and favors soils enriched with bird or bat droppings.

Dx **DIAGNOSIS**

DIFFERENTIAL DIAGNOSIS

- Acute pulmonary histoplasmosis
  1. *Mycobacterium tuberculosis*
  2. Community-acquired pneumonias caused by *Mycoplasma* and *Chlamydia*
  3. Other fungal diseases, such as *Blastomyces dermatitidis* and *Coccidioides immitis*
- Chronic cavitary pulmonary histoplasmosis: *M. tuberculosis*
- Histoplasmomas: true neoplasms

WORKUP

- Suspect diagnosis in patients who present with a history of residence or travel in an endemic area, especially if engaged in occupations (e.g., outside construction or street cleaning) or hobbies (e.g., cave exploring) that increase the likelihood of exposure to fungal spores.
- Suspect diagnosis in immunosuppressed patients with remote history of exposure, especially if associated with characteristic calcifications on chest x-ray.

LABORATORY TESTS

- Demonstration of organism on culture from body fluid or tissues to make definitive diagnosis
  1. Especially high yield in patients with AIDS
  2. Characteristic oval yeast cells in neutrophils with Giemsa stain from peripheral smear
  3. Preparations of infected tissue with Gomori's silver methenamine for revealing yeast forms, especially in areas of caseation necrosis
- Serologic tests, including complement-fixing (CF) antibodies and immunodiffusion assays
- Detection of *Histoplasma* antigen in urine: may be influenced by infections with *Blastomyces* and *Coccidioides*
- In PDH
  1. Pancytopenia
  2. Marked elevations in alkaline phosphatase and alanine aminotransferase (ALT) common
- In chronic meningitis (majority of cases)
  1. CSF pleocytosis with either lymphocytes or neutrophils predominating
  2. Elevated CSF protein levels
  3. Hypoglycorrhachia

IMAGING STUDIES

- Chest radiograph examination in acute pulmonary histoplasmosis
  1. Singular or multiple patchy infiltrates, especially in the lower lung fields
  2. Hilar or mediastinal lymphadenopathy with or without pneumonitis
  3. Diffuse nodular or confluent bilateral miliary infiltrates characteristic of heavier exposure
  4. Infrequent pleural effusions, except when associated with pericarditis
- Chest radiograph examination in histoplasmoma: coin lesion displaying central calcification, ranging from 1 to 4 cm in diameter, predominantly located in the subpleural regions
- Chest radiograph examination in CPH:
  1. Upper lobe disease frequently associated with cavities
  2. Preexisting calcifications in the hilum associated with peribronchial streaking extending to the parenchyma
- Chest radiograph examination in acute PDH: hilar adenopathy and/or diffuse nodular infiltrates

- CT scan of adrenals to reveal bilateral enlargement and low-attenuation centers

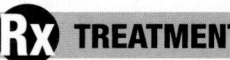 **TREATMENT**

NONPHARMACOLOGIC THERAPY

For life-threatening disease seen in acute disseminated disease or infection in patients with AIDS: supportive therapy with IV fluids

ACUTE GENERAL Rx

- No drug therapy is required for asymptomatic pulmonary disease.
- A course of therapy with ketoconazole 400 mg/day or itraconazole 200 mg/day PO for 3 to 6 wk may be beneficial in some patients with acute pulmonary distress. Avoid fluconazole because it is not as active.
- Same therapy appropriate for immunocompetent, mild to moderately symptomatic patients with CPH and subacute and chronic forms of PDH, but duration for 6 to 12 mo.
- Use amphotericin B 0.7 to 1 mg/kg IV for 6 to 12 mo in patients hypersensitive to or intolerant of azole therapy.
- Give amphotericin B for life-threatening disease or continued illness as a result of primary failure or relapse of adequate azole therapy. A lipid formulation of amphotericin B can be used to avoid nephrotoxicity.
  1. For acute pulmonary histoplasmosis associated with acute respiratory distress syndrome (ARDS), acute PDH, and histoplasma meningitis: dose of 0.7 to 1 mg/kg IV q24h
  2. End point of therapy for patient with complicated acute pulmonary disease: total dose of 500 mg
  3. End point for patient with acute PDH: total dose 35 mg/kg or 2.5 g total
  4. Prednisone 60 to 80 mg/day beneficial for severe fungal hypersensitivity complicating acute pulmonary disease
- Endocarditis: surgical treatment with excision of infected valve or graft combined with amphotericin for a total dose of 35 mg/kg or 2.5 g.
- For pericardial disease:
  1. Antifungal therapy: no apparent benefit
  2. Best managed with NSAIDs
- For POHS:
  1. Antifungal therapy: no apparent benefit
  2. May respond to laser therapy

CHRONIC Rx

In patients with AIDS: lifelong suppressive therapy with either itraconazole, given 200 mg PO qid, or IV amphotericin B at a dose of 50 mg once weekly; a triazole compound posaconazole (400 mg PO bid) may be useful in refractory cases, but clinical experience is limited at this point.

DISPOSITION

For those with chronic or progressive disease, especially if immunocompromised, prognosis is dependent on prompt recognition and timely administration of appropriate antifungal drugs.

REFERRAL

- To an infectious disease specialist in suspected cases of disseminated disease, especially if immunocompromised
- To a pulmonologist for patients with CPH form because of progressive respiratory compromise
- To a thoracic surgeon for decompression procedures for progressive mediastinal fibrosis

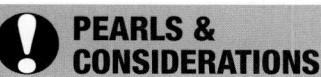 **PEARLS & CONSIDERATIONS**

- *H. capsulatum,* variety *duboisii,* also known as African histoplasmosis, is restricted to Senegal, Nigeria, Zaire, and Uganda.
- Unlike *H. capsulatum,* pulmonary forms of *duboisii* are not seen, and the disease is limited to the skin, soft tissues, and bone.

COMMENTS

- Patients living in endemic areas, especially if immunocompromised, should take appropriate respiratory precautions when disposing of bird waste from rooftop or home aviaries.
- Appropriate respiratory precautions should also be taken when leisure traveling to areas that act as a natural haven for the fungus, such as bat caves.

SUGGESTED READINGS
available at www.expertconsult.com

AUTHORS: **GLENN G. FORT, M.D., M.P.H.,** and **DENNIS J. MIKOLICH, M.D.**

BASIC INFORMATION

DEFINITION

Patients with histrionic personality disorder present with a pervasive pattern of excessive emotionality and attention-seeking behavior that generally begins in early adulthood.

SYNONYMS

Hysterical personality disorder
Psycho-infantile personality disorder
Personality disorder (nonspecific)

ICD-9CM CODES

301.5 Histrionic personality disorder (ICD-9 and DSM IV code)

EPIDEMIOLOGY & DEMOGRAPHICS

PREVALENCE (IN U.S.):

- Diagnosed more often in women; rarely found in men
- Prevalence: 1% to 2%

PREDOMINANT SEX: Female. Cultural factors (e.g., attention-seeking behavior not as acceptable in men) may lead to more common diagnosis in women.

PREDOMINANT AGE: Generally begins in early childhood

PHYSICAL FINDINGS & CLINICAL PRESENTATION

Features include five or more of the following:
1. Is uncomfortable in situations where he or she is not the center of attention.
2. Interaction with others is often characterized by inappropriate sexually seductive or provocative behavior.
3. Displays rapidly shifting and shallow expression of emotions.
4. Consistently uses physical appearance to draw attention to self.
5. Has a style of speech that is excessively impressionistic and lacking in detail.
6. Shows self-dramatization, theatricality, and exaggerated expression of emotion.
7. Is suggestible (i.e., easily influenced by others or circumstances).
8. Considers relationships to be more intimate than they actually are.

ETIOLOGY

- Unknown
- Hypothesized that childhood events, psychosocial adversity, and genetics are contributory

DIAGNOSIS

DIFFERENTIAL DIAGNOSIS

- Other personality disorders (e.g., borderline personality disorder, antisocial personality disorder, narcissistic personality disorder)
- Personality change attributable to general medical condition
- Symptoms in association with chronic substance abuse

WORKUP

There is no formal test to establish diagnosis.

TREATMENT

NONPHARMACOLOGIC THERAPY

- Long-term individual psychotherapy is treatment of choice.
- No controlled psychotherapy studies.
- Unlike other people who have personality disorders, these individuals often seek treatment and exaggerate their symptoms and difficulties in functioning.
- Patients tend to be more emotionally needy and are often reluctant to terminate therapy.

ACUTE GENERAL Rx

- No placebo-controlled trials.
- Care should be given when prescribing medications because of the potential for self-destructive or otherwise harmful behaviors.

DISPOSITION

Therapeutic approaches should not focus on the long-term personality change, but rather short-term alleviation of difficulties within the person's life.

REFERRAL

Primarily treated by mental health professionals

PEARLS & CONSIDERATIONS

- This disorder is difficult to treat.
- Like most personality disorders, patients present for treatment only when stress or other situational factor within their lives has made their ability to function and cope effectively impossible.
- Suicidality should be assessed on a regular basis, and suicidal threats and self-mutilation should not be ignored or dismissed.

PATIENT & FAMILY EDUCATION

Group and family therapy approaches are generally not recommended because individuals with this disorder often try to draw attention to themselves and exaggerate every action and reaction.

SUGGESTED READINGS

available at www.expertconsult.com

AUTHORS: **MITCHELL D. FELDMAN, M.D., M.PHIL.,** and **MARK ZIMMERMAN, M.D.**

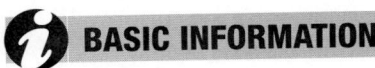

DEFINITION

Hodgkin's lymphoma is a malignant disorder of lymphoreticular origin, characterized histologically by the presence of multinucleated giant cells (Reed-Sternberg cells) usually originating from B lymphocytes in germinal centers of lymphoid tissue.

ICD-9CM CODES
201.9 Hodgkin's lymphoma, unspecified
201.4 Hodgkin's lymphoma, lymphocyte predominance
201.5 Hodgkin's lymphoma, nodular sclerosis
201.6 Hodgkin's lymphoma, mixed cellularity
201.7 Hodgkin's lymphoma, lymphocyte depletion

EPIDEMIOLOGY & DEMOGRAPHICS

- There is a bimodal age distribution (15 to 34 yr and >50 yr).
- Concordance for Hodgkin's lymphoma in identical twins suggests that a genetic susceptibility underlies Hodgkin's lymphoma in young adulthood.
- The disease is more common in males (in childhood Hodgkin's lymphoma, >80% occur in males), whites, and higher socioeconomic groups.
- Overall incidence of Hodgkin's lymphoma in the United States is ~4 per 100,000. There are >8000 new cases of Hodgkin's lymphoma diagnosed annually in the United States.

PHYSICAL FINDINGS & CLINICAL PRESENTATION

- Palpable lymphadenopathy that is generally painless is the most common presenting symptom
- Most common site of involvement: neck region
- Fever and night sweats: fever in a cyclical pattern (days or weeks of fever alternating with afebrile periods) is known as Pel-Epstein fever
- Weight loss, generalized malaise
- Persistent, nonproductive cough
- Pain associated with alcohol ingestion often because of heavy eosinophil infiltration of the tumor sites is relatively uncommon
- Pruritus
- Other: superior vena cava syndrome, spinal cord compression (rare), erythema nodosum, ichthyosis

ETIOLOGY

Unknown; evidence implicating Epstein-Barr virus remains controversial.

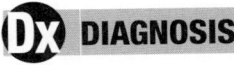 DIAGNOSIS

DIFFERENTIAL DIAGNOSIS

- Non-Hodgkin's lymphoma
- Sarcoidosis

- Infections (e.g., cytomegalovirus, Epstein-Barr virus, toxoplasmosis, HIV)
- Drug reaction

WORKUP

Diagnosis is confirmed by lymph node biopsy. The World Health Organization classifies Hodgkin's lymphoma into two groups: classical Hodgkin's lymphoma (92% to 97%) and nodular lymphocyte-predominant Hodgkin's lymphoma (3% to 8%). Classic Hodgkin's lymphoma has four main histologic subtypes based on the number of lymphocytes, Reed-Sternberg cells (Fig. 1-192), and the presence of fibrous tissue:
1. Nodular sclerosis (60% to 80%)
2. Mixed cellularity (15% to 30%)
3. Lymphocyte predominance (2% to 7%)
4. Lymphocyte depletion (1% to 6%)

Nodular sclerosis occurs mainly in young adulthood, whereas the mixed cellularity type is more prevalent after age 50 yr.

Staging for Hodgkin's disease follows the Ann Arbor staging classification:
- Stage I: Involvement of a single lymph node region
- Stage II: Two or more lymph node regions on the same side of the diaphragm
- Stage III: Lymph node involvement on both sides of diaphragm, including spleen
- Stage IV: Diffuse involvement of external sites

- Suffix A: No systemic symptoms
- Suffix B: Presence of fever, night sweats, or unexplained weight loss of ≥10% body weight over 6 mo
- Suffix X: Indicates bulky disease more than one third of the widening of the mediastinum or >10 cm maximum dimension of nodal mass on a chest film

Proper staging requires the following:
- Detailed history (with documentation of "B symptoms" and physical examination)
- Surgical biopsy
- Laboratory evaluation (complete blood count, erythrocyte sedimentation rate, blood urea nitrogen, creatinine, alkaline phosphatase, liver function tests, albumin, lactate dehydrogenase, uric acid), immunophenotypic markers (see Table 1-68). Gene-expression profiling for tumor-associated macrophages is a new biomarker for risk stratification
- Chest x-ray (posteroanterior and lateral)
- CT scan of chest, abdomen, pelvis, neck
- Positron emission tomography scan
- Bilateral bone marrow biopsy (selected patients)
- Exploratory laparotomy and splenectomy (now rarely performed):
  1. Decision to perform staging laparotomy depends on the therapeutic plan; it is generally not indicated in patients who

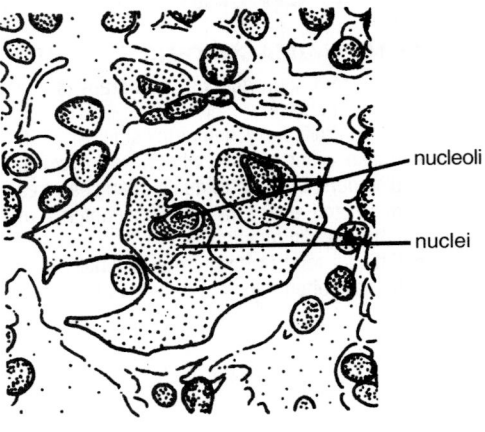

nucleoli

nuclei

FIGURE 1-192 Hodgkin's disease. High-power photomicrograph demonstrates a binucleate Reed-Sternberg cell exhibiting prominent inclusion-like eosinophilic nucleoli, giving it an "owl's eye" appearance. (From Skarin AT: *Atlas of diagnostic oncology,* ed 3, St Louis, 2003, Mosby.)

TABLE 1-68 Selected Immunophenotypic Markers and Histologic Characteristics of Use in the Differential Diagnosis of Hodgkin's Lymphoma and Other Lymphoid Neoplasms

Marker	Classical HL	Nodular Lymphocyte Predominant HL	TCRBCL	ALCL
CD30	+	−	−	+
CD15	+	−	−	−
CD20	−/+*	+	+	−
CD45	−	+	+	+/−
CD79a	−	+	+	−
ALK	−	−	−	+/−
EMA	−	+	+	+
Nodular growth protein	+/−†	+	−	−

+, >90% of cases positive; +/−, majority of cases positive; −/+, minority of cases positive; −, <10% of cases positive; ALCL, anaplastic large cell lymphoma; HL, Hodgkin's lymphoma; TCRBCL, T-cell rich B-cell lymphoma.
*CD20 positivity in classical Hodgkin's lymphoma is quite heterogeneous, with a wide range in brightness of staining.
†In classical Hodgkin's lymphoma, a nodular growth pattern is confined to the nodular sclerosing subtype.
From Abeloff MD: *Clinical oncology,* ed 3, Philadelphia, 2004, Elsevier.

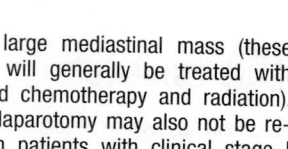

have a large mediastinal mass (these patients will generally be treated with combined chemotherapy and radiation). Staging laparotomy may also not be required in patients with clinical stage I disease or those who are unlikely to have abdominal disease (e.g., females with supradiaphragmatic disease).

2. Exploratory laparotomy and splenectomy may be used for selected patients with clinical stage I to IIA or IIB.
3. It is useful in identifying patients who can be treated with irradiation alone with curative intent.
4. Polyvalent pneumococcal vaccine should be given prophylactically to all patients before splenectomy (increased risk of sepsis from encapsulated organisms in splenectomized patients).

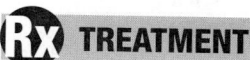 **TREATMENT**

ACUTE GENERAL Rx

The main therapeutic modalities are radiotherapy and chemotherapy; the indication for which one varies with pathologic stage and other factors. In general, chemotherapy plus involved-field radiotherapy can be used as standard

---

TABLE 1-69 Characteristics of the ABVD Regimen

Agents: doxorubicin, bleomycin, vinblastine, dacarbazine
All intravenous, total compliance
80% complete response rate
10% primary refractory disease
60%-65% overall disease-free survival
Most relapses occur within the first 4 yr; however, about 10% of all relapses occur beyond 5 yr
Major side effects are nausea, phlebitis, myelosuppression, less cumulative myelotoxicity than MOPP
No infertility
No leukemia

From Abeloff MD: *Clinical oncology*, ed 3, Philadelphia, 2004, Elsevier.

---

treatment for Hodgkin's lymphoma in early stages with favorable prognostic features. In patients with unfavorable features, four courses of chemotherapy plus involved-field radiotherapy should be the standard treatment. Commonly used therapeutic modalities are:

- Stage I and II: radiation therapy alone (involved-field radiotherapy [35 Gy]) unless a large mediastinal mass is present (mediastinal to thoracic ratio ≥1.3); in the latter case, a combination of chemotherapy and radiation therapy is indicated.
- Stage IB or IIB: total nodal irradiation is often used, although chemotherapy is performed in many centers.
- Stage IIIA: treatment is controversial. It varies with the anatomic substage after splenectomy.
  1. III₁A and minimum splenic involvement: radiation therapy alone may be adequate.
  2. III₂ or III₁A with extensive splenic involvement: there is disagreement whether chemotherapy alone or a combination of chemotherapy and radiation therapy is the preferred treatment modality.
  3. IIIB and IVB: the treatment of choice is chemotherapy with or without adjuvant radiotherapy.

Various regimens can be used for combination of chemotherapy. Most oncologists prefer the combination of doxorubicin plus bleomycin plus vincristine plus dacarbazine (ABVD). Table 1-69 describes characteristics of the ABVD regimen. Recent trials have shown that in patients with early-stage Hodgkins's lymphoma and favorable prognosis, treatment with two cycles of ABVD followed by 20 Gy of involved-field radiation therapy may be as effective as, and less toxic than four cycles of ABVD followed by 30 Gy of involved-field radiation therapy. Long-term effects of this approach need to be fully assessed before it becomes standard of care.

- Definitions of treatment groups are described in Table 1-70.
- Recommendations for the primary treatment of Hodgkin's lymphoma outside of clinical trials are described in Table 1-71.

DISPOSITION

- The overall survival at 10 yr is ~60%.
- Cure rates as high as 75% to 80% are now possible with appropriate initial therapy.
- Poor prognostic features (Table 1-72) include presence of B symptoms, advanced age, advanced stage at initial presentation, mixed cellularity and lymphocyte depletion histology, and increased number of tumor-associated macrophages.
- Chemotherapy significantly increases the risk of leukemia.
- The peak in risk of leukemia is seen approximately 5 yr after the initiation of chemotherapy.
- The risk of leukemia is greater for those who undergo splenectomy and patients with advanced stages of Hodgkin's disease; the risk is unaffected by concomitant radiotherapy.
- Involved-field radiotherapy does not improve the outcome in patients with advanced-stage Hodgkin's lymphoma who have a complete remission after MOPP (mechlorethamine, vincristine, procarbazine, and prednisone)–ABV chemotherapy. Radiotherapy may benefit patients with a partial response after chemotherapy.
- Mediastinal irradiation increases the risk of subsequent death from heart disease caused by sclerosis of the coronary artery from irradiation. Risk increases with high mediastinal doses, minimal protective cardiac blocking, young age at irradiation, and increased duration of follow-up.
- Both chemotherapy and radiation therapy increase the risk of developing secondary solid tumors (Table 1-73).
- Table 1-74 describes potential late complications of Hodgkin's lymphoma treatment and appropriate clinical responses and preventive strategies.

REFERRAL

- To surgery for lymph node biopsy
- Hematology/oncology

H

Diseases and Disorders

I

TABLE 1-70 Definition of Treatment Groups According to the EORTC/GELA and GHSG

Treatment Group	EORTC/GELA	GHSG	NCIC/ECOG
Early-stage favorable	CS I-II without risk factors (supradiaphragmatic)	CS I-II without risk factors	Standard risk group: favorable CSD I-II (without risk factors)
Early-stage unfavorable (intermediate)	CS I-II with ≥1 risk factors (supradiaphragmatic)	CS I, CSIIA ≥1 risk factors; CS IIB with C/D but without A/B	Standard risk group: unfavorable CS I-II (at least one risk factor)
Advanced stage	CS III-IV	CS IIB with A/B; CS III-IV	High risk group: CS I or II with bulky disease; intraabdominal disease; CS III, IV
Risk factors (RF)	A large mediastinal mass B age ≥50 yr C elevated ESR* D ≥4 involved regions	A large mediastinal mass B extranodal disease C elevated ESR* D ≥3 involved areas	A ≥ 40 years B not NLPHL or NS histology C ESR ≥ 50 mm/h D ≥ 4 involved nodal regions

*erythrocyte sedimentation rate (≥50 mm/h without or ≥30 mm/h with B-symptoms).
ECOG, Eastern Cooperative Oncology Group; *EORTC*, European Organization for Research and treatment of Cancer; *GELA*, Groupe d'Etude des Lymphomes de l'Adulte; *GHSG*, German Hodgkin Study Group; *NCIC*, National Cancer Institute of Canada.
From Hoffman R et al: *Hematology, basic principles and practice*, ed 5, New York, 2009, Churchill Livingstone.

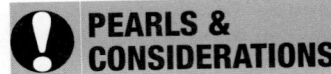

COMMENTS

- Young male patients should consider sperm banking before the initiation of therapy.

- Chemotherapy plus involved-field radiotherapy should be the standard treatment for Hodgkin's disease with favorable prognostic features. In patients with unfavorable features, four courses of chemotherapy plus involved-field radiotherapy should be the standard of treatment.

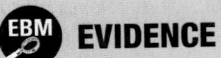

available at www.expertconsult.com

SUGGESTED READINGS

available at www.expertconsult.com

AUTHOR: **FRED F. FERRI, M.D.**

TABLE 1-71 Recommendations for the Primary Treatment of Hodgkin's Lymphoma Outside of Clinical Trials

Group	Stage	Recommendation
Early stages (favorable)	CS I-II A/B, no RFs*	2 cycles ABVD; 6 cycles EBVP; or VBM ± IF RT, (20-30 Gy)
	Early stages (unfavorable, intermediate)	4-6 cycles ABVD; BEACOPP-baseline, Stanford V; or
	CS I-II A/B + RFs	MOPP/ABV ± IF RT, 20-30Gy
Advanced stages	CS IIB + RFs, CS III A/B, CS IV A/B	6-8 cycles ABVD; MOPP/ABV; ChIVPP/EVA; BEACOPP-escalated or BEACOPP-14 ± RT, 20-30 Gy for residual tumor (PET positive) and/or bulk disease

*RF, Risk factors
ABVD regimen, doxorubicin, vinblastine, bleomycin, and dacarbazine; BEACOPP-baseline regimen, bleomycin, etoposide, doxorubicin (Adriamycin), cyclophosphamide, vincristine (Oncovin), procarbazine, and prednisone; BEACOPP-escalated regimen, bleomycin, etoposide, doxorubicin (Adriamycin), cyclophosphamide, vincristine (Oncovin), procarbazine, prednisone, and G-CSF; BEACOPP-14 regimen, bleomycin, etoposide, doxorubicin (Adriamycin), cyclophosphamide, vincristine (Oncovin), procarbazine, prednisone, and G-CSF; ChIVPP/EVA regimen, chlorambucil, vinblastine, procarbazine, prednisolone, etoposide, vincristine, Adriamycin (doxorubicin); CS, clinical stage; EBVP regimen, epirubicin, bleomycin, vinblastine, and prednisone; IF, involved field; MOPP regimen, mechlorethamine, vincristine (Oncovin), procarbazine, and prednisone; PET, positron emission tomography; RT, radiation therapy; Stanford V regimen, nitrogen mustard, doxorubicin, vinblastine, bleomycin, vincristine, etoposide, and prednisone; VBM regimen, vinblastine, methotrexate, and bleomycin.
From Hoffman R et al: Hematology, basic principles and practice, ed 5, New York, 2009, Churchill Livingstone.

TABLE 1-72 Prognostic Factors of Importance in Advanced Hodgkin's Lymphoma*

Gender	male
Age	>45 yr
Stage	IV
Hemoglobin	<105 g/L
White blood cell count	>15 × 10⁹/L
Lymphocyte count	<0.6 × 10⁹/L or <8% of the white cell differential
Serum albumin	<40 g/L

*Identified by the International Prognostic Factors Project on Advanced Hodgkin's Disease.
From Abeloff MD: Clinical oncology, ed 3, Philadelphia, 2004, Elsevier.

TABLE 1-73 Second Neoplasms Seen with Increased Frequency after Successful Hodgkin's Lymphoma Treatment

Acute myelogenous leukemia/myelodysplasia
Non-Hodgkin's lymphoma
Melanoma
Soft tissue sarcoma
Adenocarcinoma
 Breast
 Thyroid
 Lung
 Stomach and esophagus
Squamous cell carcinoma
 Skin
 Uterine cervix
 Head and neck

From Abeloff MD: Clinical oncology, ed 3, Philadelphia, 2004, Elsevier.

TABLE 1-74 Potential Late Complications Hodgkin's Lymphoma Treatment and Appropriate Clinical Responses and Preventive Strategies

Risk/Problem	Incidence/Response
Dental caries	Neck or oropharyngeal irradiation can cause decreased salivation. Patients should have careful dental care follow-up and should make their dentist aware of the previous irradiation.
Hypothyroidism	After external beam irradiation that encompasses the thyroid with doses sufficient to cure Hodgkin's lymphoma, at least 50% of patients will eventually become hypothyroid. All patients whose TSH level becomes elevated should be treated with lifelong thyroxine replacement in doses sufficient to suppress thyroid-stimulating hormone (TSH) levels to low normal. This is also necessary to assure that the radiation-damaged thyroid is not subjected to long-term stimulation by thyroid-stimulating hormone, which can increase the risk of thyroid neoplasm.
Infertility	ABVD is not known to cause any permanent gonadal toxicity, although oligospermia for 1 to 2 years after treatment is common. Direct or scatter radiation to gonadal tissue can cause infertility, amenorrhea, or premature menopause, but this seldom occurs with the current fields used for the treatment of Hodgkin's lymphoma. Thus, with the current chemotherapy regimens and radiation fields used, most patients will not develop these problems. In general, after treatment, women who continue menstruating are fertile, but men require semen analysis to provide a specific answer. High-dose chemoradiotherapy and hematopoietic stem cell transplantation almost always cause permanent infertility in both genders, although some young women occasionally recover fertility.
Impaired immunity to infections	Hodgkin's lymphoma and its treatment can lead to lifelong impairment of full immunity to infection. All patients should be given annual influenza immunization and pneumococcal immunization every five years. Patients whose spleen has been irradiated or removed should also be immunized against meningococcal types A and C and Hemophilus influenza type B. As for all adults, diptheria and tetanus immunizations should be kept up-to-date.
Secondary neoplasms	Although uncommon, certain secondary neoplasms occur with increased frequency in patients who have been treated for Hodgkin's lymphoma. These include acute myelogenous leukemia, thyroid, breast, lung, and upper gastrointestinal carcinoma and melanoma and cervical carcinoma in situ. It is appropriate to screen for these neoplasms for the rest of the patient's life because they might have lengthy induction periods.

From Abeloff MD: Clinical oncology, ed 3, Philadelphia, 2004, Elsevier.

BASIC INFORMATION

DEFINITION

Hookworm is a parasitic infection of the intestine caused by helminths.

SYNONYMS

Ground itch
Ancylostoma duodenale infection
Necator americanus infection

ICD-9CM CODES

126.35 Hookworm

EPIDEMIOLOGY & DEMOGRAPHICS

INCIDENCE (IN U.S.):

- Varies greatly in different areas of the U.S.
- Most common in rural areas of southeastern U.S.
- Poor sanitation and increased rainfall increase incidence

PREVALENCE (IN U.S.): Varies from 10% to 90% in regions where it is found

PREDOMINANT AGE: Schoolchildren

PHYSICAL FINDINGS & CLINICAL PRESENTATION

- Nonspecific abdominal complaints
- Because these organisms consume host RBCs, symptoms related to iron-deficiency anemia, depending on the amount of iron in the diet and the worm burden
- Fatigue, tachycardia, dyspnea, and high-output failure
- Hypoproteinemia and edema from loss of proteins into the intestinal tract
- Unusual for pulmonary manifestations to occur when the larvae migrate through the lungs
- Skin rash at sites of larval penetration in some individuals without prior exposure

ETIOLOGY

Two species can cause this disease: *N. americanus* and *A. duodenale*. *N. americanus* is the predominant cause of hookworm in the U.S. They are soil nematodes (Geohelminthic infections) that are acquired by skin contact (i.e., bare feet) with contaminated soils in moist, warm climate.

- Infection occurs via penetration of the skin by the larval form, with subsequent migration via the bloodstream to the alveoli, up the respiratory tract, then into the GI tract (Fig. 1-193)
- *Ancylostoma* spp. infection can also occur via the oral route through ingestion of contaminated water supplies
- Sharp mouth parts allow for attachment to intestinal mucosa
- *Ancylostoma* spp. are more likely to cause iron deficiency anemia because they are larger and remove more blood daily from the bowel wall than the other hookworm species, *N. americanus*

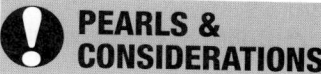

DIAGNOSIS

DIFFERENTIAL DIAGNOSIS

- Strongyloidiasis
- Ascariasis
- Other causes of iron deficiency anemia and malabsorption

WORKUP

Examine stool for hookworm eggs.

LABORATORY TESTS

CBC to show hypochromic, microcytic anemia; possible mild eosinophilia and hypoalbuminemia

IMAGING STUDIES

Chest x-ray examination: occasionally shows opacities

TREATMENT

NONPHARMACOLOGIC THERAPY

- Prevention of disease by not walking barefoot and by improving sanitary conditions
- Vaccines are in development

ACUTE GENERAL Rx

- Mebendazole 100 mg PO bid for 3 days or as a 500-mg single dose.
- Albendazole 400 mg once PO has become preferred treatment.
- Iron supplementation may be helpful in patients with iron deficiency.

DISPOSITION

Easily treated

REFERRAL

If diagnosis uncertain

PEARLS & CONSIDERATIONS

COMMENTS

- Appropriate disposal of human wastes is important in controlling the disease in areas with a high prevalence of hookworm infestation.
- Wearing shoes will avoid contact with contaminated soils, and the provision of safe water and sanitation for disposing human excreta is important in control of hookworm.

SUGGESTED READINGS

available at www.expertconsult.com

AUTHORS: **GLENN G. FORT, M.D., M.P.H.** and **DENNIS J. MIKOLICH, M.D.**

FIGURE 1-193 Life cycle of intestinal nematodes with a migratory phase through the lungs. Eggs are passed with stools in *Ascaris lumbricoides* (A.l.), *Necator americanus,* or *Ancylostoma duodenale* (A.d.), or they hatch on their way out in *Strongyloides stercoralis* (S.s.). Ascaris eggs mature in soil, and humans are infected upon ingestion of these eggs. With hookworm and strongyloidiasis, humans are infected via skin penetration by filariform larvae. In all three infections, larvae pass through a migratory phase via the lungs before reaching maturity at their final habitat in the small intestine. (Mandell GL et al: *Principles and practice of infectious diseases,* ed 7, Philadelphia, 2010, Elsevier.)

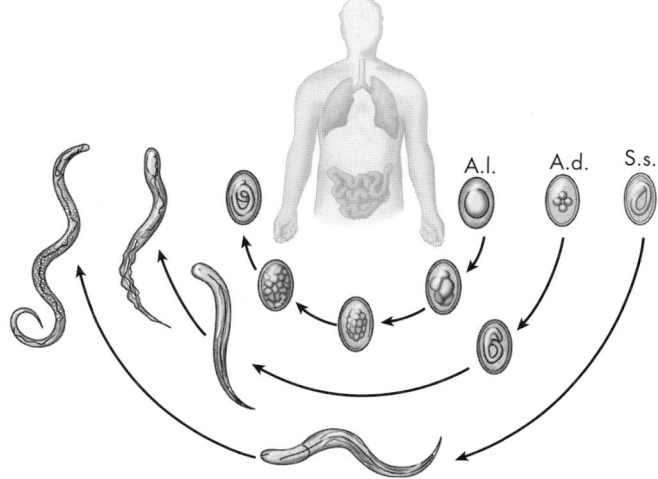

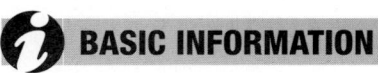

BASIC INFORMATION

DEFINITION

A hordeolum is an acute inflammatory process affecting the eyelid and arising from the meibomian (posterior) or Zeis (anterior) glands. It is most often infectious and usually caused by *Staphylococcus aureus*.

SYNONYMS

Stye

ICD-9CM CODES

373.11 External hordeolum
373.12 Internal hordeolum

EPIDEMIOLOGY & DEMOGRAPHICS

INCIDENCE (IN U.S.): Unknown
PREVALENCE (IN U.S.): Unknown
PREDOMINANT SEX: No gender predilection
PREDOMINANT AGE: May occur at any age
NEONATAL INFECTION: Rare in the neonatal period
PEAK INCIDENCE: May occur at any age

PHYSICAL FINDINGS & CLINICAL PRESENTATION

- Abrupt onset with pain and erythema of the eyelid
- Localized, tender mass in the eyelid (Fig. 1-194)
- May be associated with blepharitis
- External hordeolum: points toward the skin surface of the lid and may spontaneously drain
- Internal hordeolum: can point toward the conjunctival side of the lid and may cause conjunctival inflammation

ETIOLOGY

- 75% to 95% of cases are caused by *S. aureus.*
- Occasional cases are caused by *Streptococcus pneumoniae*, other streptococci, gram-negative enteric organisms, or mixed bacterial flora.

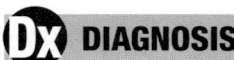

DIAGNOSIS

DIFFERENTIAL DIAGNOSIS

- Eyelid abscess
- Chalazion
- Allergy or contact dermatitis with conjunctival edema
- Acute dacryocystitis
- Herpes simplex infection
- Cellulitis of the eyelid

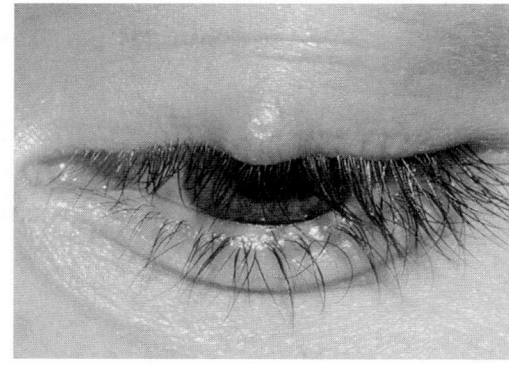

FIGURE 1-194 External stye. (From Palay D [ed]: *Ophthalmology for the primary care physician,* St Louis, 1997, Mosby.)

LABORATORY TESTS

- Generally, none are necessary.
- If incision and drainage are performed, specimens should be sent for bacterial culture.

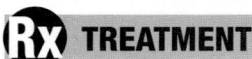

TREATMENT

NONPHARMACOLOGIC THERAPY

Usually responds to warm compresses

ACUTE GENERAL Rx

- Systemic antibiotics generally not necessary
- In refractory cases, an oral antistaphylococcal agent (e.g., dicloxacillin 500 mg PO qid) possibly helpful
- Topical erythromycin ophthalmic ointment applied to the lid margins two to four times daily until resolution
- Incision and drainage: rarely needed but should be considered for progressive infections

DISPOSITION

- Usually sporadic occurrence
- Possible relapse if resolution is not complete

REFERRAL

- For evaluation by an ophthalmologist if visual acuity or ocular movement is affected or if the diagnosis is in doubt
- For surgical drainage if necessary

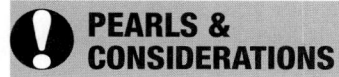

PEARLS & CONSIDERATIONS

COMMENTS

Seborrheic dermatitis may coexist with hordeolum.

SUGGESTED READINGS

available at www.expertconsult.com

AUTHORS: **GLENN G. FORT, M.D., M.P.H.,** and **DENNIS J. MIKOLICH, M.D.**

BASIC INFORMATION

DEFINITION

Horner's syndrome is the clinical triad of ipsilateral ptosis, miosis, and sometimes facial anhidrosis. Disruption of any of the three neurons in the oculosympathetic pathway (central, preganglionic, or postganglionic) can cause Horner's syndrome.

SYNONYMS

Oculosympathetic paresis

Raeder's paratrigeminal syndrome: Horner's syndrome of the postganglionic neuron associated with pain in the trigeminal nerve distribution

ICD-9CM CODES
337.9 Horner's syndrome

EPIDEMIOLOGY & DEMOGRAPHICS

Congenital or acquired

PHYSICAL FINDINGS & CLINICAL PRESENTATION

- Ptosis is usually mild. It results from loss of sympathetic tone to Müller's muscle, which contributes approximately 2 mm of upper eyelid elevation. Weakness of the corresponding muscle in the lower eyelid causes it to elevate slightly. This combination causes narrowing of the palpebral fissure. Levator function of the eyelid is preserved.
- Miosis results from loss of sympathetic innervation to the iris dilator muscle (Fig. 1-195). The affected pupil reacts normally to bright light and accommodation. Anisocoria is greater in dim light.
  - Dilation lag: Horner's pupil dilates more slowly than the normal pupil when lights are dimmed (20 vs. 5 sec) because it dilates passively as a result of relaxation of the iris sphincter.
- Presence of facial anhidrosis is variable and depends on the site of injury. It occurs with lesions affecting central or preganglionic neurons.
- Congenital Horner's syndrome may result in heterochromia. The affected eye has a lighter colored iris.
- Acute cases may also present with conjunctival injection from the loss of sympathetic vasoconstriction.

ETIOLOGY

Lesions affecting any neuron in the oculosympathetic pathway. Central lesions are least common but are usually caused by pathology in the hypothalamus, brainstem, or cervicothoracic spinal cord. Preganglionic lesions are often caused by disease involving the spinal cord, lung apex, or anterior neck. Postganglionic lesions are usually seen with disease in the internal carotid artery, skull base, cavernous sinus, or orbital apex. Location is often suggested by the presence of associated findings. Vascular disease and neoplasms must be considered.

Mechanical:
- Syringomyelia
- Trauma
- Tumors: benign, malignant (thyroid, Pancoast, mediastinal, metastatic)
- Lymphadenopathy
- Neurofibromatosis
- Cervical rib
- Cervical spondylosis

Vascular (ischemia, hemorrhage or arteriovenous malformation):
- Brain stem lesion: commonly occlusion of the posterior inferior cerebellar artery but other arteries may be responsible (vertebral; superior, middle or inferior lateral medullary arteries; superior or anterior inferior cerebellar arteries)
- Carotid artery aneurysm or dissection. Can also be from injury to other major vessels (internal carotid artery, subclavian artery, ascending aorta)
- Cavernous sinus thrombosis
- Cluster headache, migraine

Miscellaneous:
- Idiopathic
- Congenital
- Demyelination (multiple sclerosis)
- Infection (apical tuberculosis, herpes zoster, Lyme's disease)
- Pneumothorax
- Iatrogenic (angiography, internal jugular/subclavian catheter, chest tube, neck or upper thoracic surgery, epidural spinal anesthesia)

DIAGNOSIS

DIFFERENTIAL DIAGNOSIS

Causes of anisocoria (unequal pupils):
- Normal variant
- Mydriatic use
- Prosthetic eye
- Prior eye surgery
- Unilateral cataract
- Iritis

Causes of ptosis are described in Section II.

WORKUP

History, physical examination, imaging

IMAGING STUDIES

Accompanying signs and symptoms may guide imaging:
- MRI brain: brain stem (diplopia, vertigo, ataxia); cavernous sinus (eye movement abnormalities, sixth nerve palsy)
- MRI cervical and upper thoracic spinal cord: weakness of extremities, bowel/bladder dysfunction
- MR angiography (or ultrasound, CT angiography): carotid artery dissection (acute Horner's syndrome with face or neck pain)
- CT chest and neck: evaluate lung apex, perivertebral areas, mediastinum if symptoms do not localize to the central nervous system; brachial plexus lesion (arm/hand pain or weakness)

TREATMENT

- Treatment depends on underlying cause.
- Ptosis can be surgically corrected or treated with medication (phenylephrine drops).

DISPOSITION

- Prognosis depends on underlying cause.
- Horner's syndrome is an uncommon presentation for malignancy.
- In one study, 40% of cases were idiopathic.

REFERRAL

- Ophthalmologist to confirm diagnosis and localize lesion.
- Topical cocaine test: confirms sympathetic denervation (drops dilate normal pupil but not Horner's pupil).
- Topical apraclonidine test: confirms diagnosis (drops reverse anisocoria by causing dilatation of Horner's pupil and constriction of normal pupil).
- Topical hydroxyamphetamine test: distinguishes central and preganglionic from postganglionic sympathetic lesions (drops dilate normal pupil and central or preganglionic Horner's pupil, but not postganglionic Horner's pupil).

PEARLS & CONSIDERATIONS

- May be the presentation of a life-threatening condition.
- Anisocoria greater in bright light is likely caused by a defect in parasympathetic innervation, and anisocoria greater in dim light is likely caused by a sympathetic defect.
- Normal variant anisocoria:
  - Occurs in 20% of people
  - Usually <1-mm difference between pupils; more apparent in darkness
  - Pupils are round and display a normal, brisk constriction and dilation response to light

SUGGESTED READINGS
available at www.expertconsult.com

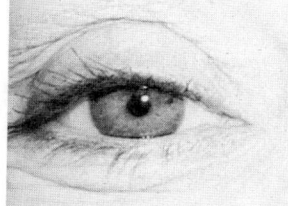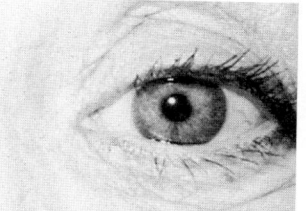

FIGURE 1-195 Horner's syndrome. The mild ptosis (1 to 2 mm) and the smaller pupil (in room light) can be seen on the affected right side. (From Palay D [ed]: *Ophthalmology for the primary care physician*, St Louis, 1997, Mosby.)

AUTHOR: SUDEEP KAUR AULAKH, M.D.

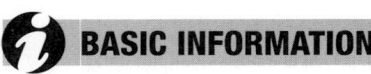

BASIC INFORMATION

DEFINITION

Sudden onset of intense warmth that begins in the neck or face, or in the chest and progresses to the neck and face; often associated with profuse sweating, anxiety, and palpitations.

ICD-9CM CODES
627.2 Hot flashes

EPIDEMIOLOGY & DEMOGRAPHICS

- Hot flashes affect 75% of postmenopausal women.
- Most hot flashes begin 1 to 2 yr before menopause and resolve after 2 yr.
- 15% of women report duration of hot flashes >15 yr.

PHYSICAL FINDINGS & CLINICAL PRESENTATION

- Profuse sweating and red blotching of skin may be noted during the vasomotor event.
- Palpitations and hyperreflexia may be present during the hot flash.
- Hot flashes typically last 1 to 5 min.
- Each hot flash is associated with increase in temperature, increased pulse rate, and increased blood flow into the hands and face.
- Hot flashes during sleep are common and are referred to as *night sweats.*
- There is considerable variation in the frequency of hot flashes. One third of women report more than 10 flashes per day.

ETIOLOGY

- Dysfunction of central thermoregulatory centers caused by changes in estrogen level at the time of menopause
- Tamoxifen use
- Chemotherapy-induced ovarian failure
- Androgen ablation therapy for prostate carcinoma

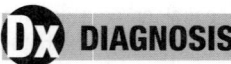

DIAGNOSIS

DIFFERENTIAL DIAGNOSIS

- Carcinoid syndrome
- Anxiety disorder
- Idiopathic flushing
- Lymphoma (night sweats)

- Hyperthyroidism
- Hyperhidrosis

WORKUP

Evaluation of hot flashes is aimed at excluding the conditions listed in the differential diagnosis.

LABORATORY TESTS

- Follicle-stimulating hormone (FSH), luteinizing hormone, estradiol level. The serum FSH levels rather than estradiol levels are associated with greater severity of hot flashes in older postmenopausal women, suggesting that nonestrogen feedback systems may be important in modulating the severity of hot flashes. It is not necessary to obtain an FSH to make the diagnosis of menopausal status, however. An amenorrheic woman over age 50 with vasomotor symptoms is assumed to have made the menopausal transition and serum markers of menopause are not required to complete the diagnosis.
- Thyroid-stimulating hormone.

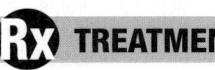

TREATMENT

NONPHARMACOLOGIC THERAPY

- Behavioral interventions such as relaxation training and paced respiration have been reported effective in reducing symptoms in some women.
- Avoidance of caffeine, alcohol, tobacco, and spicy foods may be beneficial.

GENERAL Rx

- Estrogen replacement therapy reduces hot flashes by 80% to 90%. Estrogen therapy, however, is contraindicated in many women, and others are fearful of its use. Potential risks and side effects should be considered before using estrogen in any patient. When using estrogen, it is best to use low-dose (e.g., Prempro [conjugated equine estrogen 0.45 mg or 0.3 mg plus medroxyprogesterone 1.5 mg]). Femring is an intravaginal ring that is changed every 3 mo and approved to treat vasomotor symptoms in women who have had a hysterectomy. It provides both local and systemic estrogen.
- Megestrol acetate, a progestational agent, is a safer alternative to estrogen in women with a history of breast or uterine cancer and in

men receiving androgen ablation therapy for prostate cancer. Usual dose is 20 mg bid.
- The antidepressant venlafaxine has been reported to be 60% effective in reducing hot flashes and represents an alternative treatment modality in women unable or unwilling to use estrogens. Starting dose is 37.5 mg qd, increased as tolerated up to a maximum of 300 mg/day. Other antidepressants such as desvenlafaxine and escitalopram have also been shown to be effective in reducing the number and severity of menopausal hot flashes. A recent trial showed that paroxetine is an effective agent for diminishing hot flashes in men receiving androgen ablation therapy.
- The anticonvulsant gabapentin (300 to 1200 mg/day) represents another nonhormonal alternative in the treatment of hot flashes and can be used alone or in combination with venlafaxine.
- The antihypertensive clonidine is also somewhat effective in reducing the frequency of hot flashes in mild cases. Adverse effects include dry mouth, sedation, and dizziness.
- Vitamin E (800 IU/day) may be effective in patients with mild symptoms that do not interfere with sleep or daily function.
- Soy protein (use of soy extracts that contain plant-derived estrogens [phytoestrogens]) is often used; however, clinical trials have not shown clear efficacy.
- Several classes of herbal remedies are available to patients and are commonly used, generally without significant benefit. Frequently used agents are *Cimicifuga racemosa* (black cohosh, snakeroot, bugbane), *Angelica sinensis,* and evening primrose (evening star). Recent trials using the isopropanolic extract of black cohosh rootstock (Remefemin) did show some improvement in controlling menopausal symptoms.

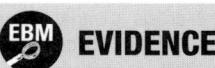

EVIDENCE

available at www.expertconsult.com

SUGGESTED READINGS
available at www.expertconsult.com

AUTHOR: **FRED F. FERRI, M.D.**

BASIC INFORMATION

DEFINITION

Human granulocytic ehrlichiosis (HGE [also known as HGA]) is a zoonotic infection of granulocytes, caused by *Anaplasma phagocytophilum*, an *Ehrlichia* species closely related to *Ehrlichia chaffeensis* and *E. ewingii*, with multisystem manifestations.

SYNONYMS

Ehrlichiosis
Ehrlichia phagocytophila
Anaplasma phagocytophilum

ICD-9CM CODES
082-8   Other tick-borne rickettsiosis

EPIDEMIOLOGY & DEMOGRAPHICS

INCIDENCE (IN U.S.): Highest overall incidence in Rhode Island (36.5 per 1 million), New York, New Jersey, Connecticut, Wisconsin, Minnesota, and northern California; >3000 cases identified in the United States since 2006.
PREDOMINANT SEX: Males outnumber females by 2 to 1.
PREDOMINANT AGE: Most severe disease 50 to 70 yr
PEAK INCIDENCE: Occurs throughout the year, with peak incidence between May and July and again in November.

PHYSICAL FINDINGS & CLINICAL PRESENTATION

- Most common initial symptoms
  1. Fever
  2. Chills, rigor
  3. Headache
  4. Myalgia
- Subsequent symptoms
  1. Anorexia, nausea
  2. Arthralgia
  3. Cough
  4. Confusion
  5. Abdominal pain
  6. Rash (erythematous to pustular) rare (<11%)
- Complications
  1. Hepatitis
  2. Interstitial pneumonitis; acute respiratory distress syndrome
  3. Renal and respiratory failure
  4. Demyelinating polyneuropathy
  5. Toxic shock–like syndrome
  6. Life-threatening opportunistic infections

ETIOLOGY

- Obligate intracellular gram-negative bacterium (family Rickettsiaceae, genus *Ehrlichia*), now renamed *Anaplasma phagocytophilum*

- Vector
  1. Almost certainly tick-borne, recently confirmed to be rarely transmitted by infected blood (including nosocomial infection).
  2. Transmitted by *Ixodes scapularis* in the northeastern and upper midwestern states and *Ixodes pacificus* in the Pacific western states.
  3. Tick exposure reported in >90% of patients, with ~60% reporting tick bite.
- Mammalian host: deer, horses, dogs, white-footed mice, cattle, sheep, goats, bison
- Host inflammatory and immune responses define final spectrum of disease beyond granulocytes, including hepatitis, interstitial pneumonitis, and nephritis with mild azotemia
- Between 6% and 21% of patients with HGE also have serologic evidence of other *Ixodes* spp. tick-borne diseases: Lyme disease or babesiosis
- Recovery is usual outcome; fatality rate of HGE is <1%
- ICU care required: 7%

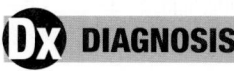 **DIAGNOSIS**

DIFFERENTIAL DIAGNOSIS

- Human monocytic ehrlichiosis (HME)
  1. Caused by *E. chaffeensis* (vector: tick *Amblyomma americanum*)
  2. Rash more common, sometimes petechial
  3. Morulae in monocytes
- Rocky Mountain spotted fever, Colorado tick fever, Q fever, relapsing fever
- Babesiosis
- Leptospirosis
- Lyme disease
- Tularemia
- Typhoid fever, paratyphoid fever
- Brucellosis
- Viral hepatitis
- Meningococcemia
- Infectious mononucleosis
- Hematologic malignancy

WORKUP

- Acute blood samples for Giemsa-stained smears
- CBC, liver function, BUN/creatinine
- Acute serum samples for serology
- Chest radiograph examination
- Bone marrow rarely needed

LABORATORY TESTS

- Giemsa-stained smear demonstrating morulae of the organism within granulocytes (sensitivity 20% to 75%)
- CBC progressive leukopenia and thrombocytopenia with nadir near day 7
- C reactive protein concentration is generally elevated

- Liver function tests (LFTs): increase in hepatic transaminases, lactate dehydrogenase, and alkaline phosphatase
- Elevated plasma creatinine concentration may be seen
- Serologic titer (IFA) >80 or fourfold increase in titer to *E. equi* antigen
- Polymerase chain reaction (PCR) to facilitate early diagnosis
- Culture on the first 7 days of illness; not readily available in most clinical laboratories

IMAGING STUDIES

- Chest radiograph examination to show interstitial pneumonitis (unusual)
- MRI of the brain

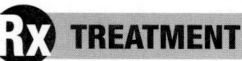 **TREATMENT**

ACUTE GENERAL Rx

- Immediate therapy to limit extent of acute illness and complication
- Doxycycline: 100 mg twice a day for 10 days is therapy of choice for adults and children >8 yr (4 mg/kg/day in 2 divided doses)
- Rifampin: 300 mg twice a day for 7 to 10 days can be used in pregnancy and for children <8 yr at 10 mg/kg twice per day
- Most patients defervesce within 24 to 48 hr given appropriate treatment

PROGNOSIS

Poor prognostic indicators include:
- Advanced age
- Concomitant chronic illness (such as diabetes mellitus, collagen-vascular disease)
- Lack of diagnosis recognition
- Delayed onset of specific antibiotic therapy
- Concomitant HIV or organ transplant status

DISPOSITION

Repeat CBC every 2 to 4 wk until normal

REFERRAL

For consultation with infectious diseases specialist and hematologist in suspected cases

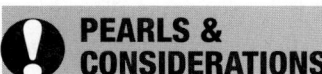 **PEARLS & CONSIDERATIONS**

COMMENTS

Duration of time tick must be attached to produce illness as few as 4 hr.

SUGGESTED READINGS
available at www.expertconsult.com

AUTHOR: **PATRICIA CRISTOFARO, M.D.**

BASIC INFORMATION

DEFINITION

The human immunodeficiency virus, type 1 (HIV) causes a chronic infection that culminates, usually after 5 to 10 yr, in AIDS.

SYNONYMS

AIDS: when a patient with HIV infection meets specific diagnostic criteria (See "Acquired Immunodeficiency Syndrome" in Section I.)

ICD-9CM CODES
044.9 HIV, unspecified

EPIDEMIOLOGY & DEMOGRAPHICS

INCIDENCE (IN U.S.):
- In 2006, there were an estimated 56,300 new HIV infections
- Greatest incidence is in metropolitan areas with population >500,000.

PREVALENCE (IN U.S.): Estimated at 1 million to 2 million cases at the end of 2003.

PREDOMINANT SEX:
- Adults: Males accounted for 73% of new infections in 2006.
- Children: male = female

RACIAL DATA:
- In 2006, the rate of HIV diagnosis for black males was eight times the rate for whites.
- Black females are disproportionately affected by HIV: the rate of HIV diagnosis for black females is 19 times the rate for white females.
- The rate for Hispanic women is five times that for white females.

PEAK INCIDENCE: More than half of new infections in 2006 were in patients ages 25 to 44.

GENETICS:

Familial Disposition:
Although there is no proven genetic predisposition, individuals with deletions in the CCR5 gene are immune from infection with macrophage tropic virus (the predominant virus in sexual transmission).

Congenital Infection:
- 80% of childhood cases are caused by peripartum infection, which may occur in utero, during delivery, or after delivery via breastfeeding.
- No specific congenital abnormalities are associated with HIV infection, although risk of spontaneous abortion and low birth weight is greater.

Neonatal Infection:
- May occur during delivery or via breastfeeding
- Typically asymptomatic

PHYSICAL FINDINGS & CLINICAL PRESENTATION

- Signs and symptoms are variable with stage of disease.
- In acute infection:
  1. May cause a self-limited mononucleosis-like illness characterized by fever, sore throat, lymphadenopathy, headache, and a rash resembling roseola

  2. In a minority of acute cases: frank aseptic meningitis, Bell's palsy, or peripheral neuropathy
  3. Rarely, opportunistic infections such as thrush or *Pneumocystis jiroveci* pneumonia (PJP) may occur.
- Later in the course of infection, after a prolonged asymptomatic phase: nonspecific symptoms of lymphadenopathy, weight loss, diarrhea, and skin changes including seborrheic dermatitis, localized herpes zoster, or fungal infection.
- Advanced disease: characterized by the infections and malignancies associated with AIDS (see specific disorders).
- Some studies suggest that HIV infection in women is associated with lower levels of viral load at comparable degrees of immunosuppression when compared with men. Furthermore, women may, on average, have higher CD4 lymphocyte counts at the time of AIDS diagnosis.
- Another special consideration in women infected with HIV is the high incidence of human papillomavirus (HPV) coinfection and the risk for cervical neoplasm that this presents. Even women with normal Pap smears should have this test repeated after 6 mo and annually thereafter.
- Coinfection with HIV and hepatitis C is common because of common transmission risk. Patients with HIV and hepatitis C progress faster to cirrhosis. Patients may already have signs of advanced liver disease at the time of diagnosis.

ETIOLOGY

- RNA retrovirus (Fig. 1-196) HIV-1 was probably derived from transmission of a simian immunodeficiency virus (SIV) from chimpanzees in Central Africa; a related virus HIV-2 was derived from an SIV found in sooty mangabey monkeys from West Africa.
- HIV-1 is the predominant pathogenic retrovirus in human populations; HIV-2 has limited distribution (primarily in West Africa) and tends to be less rapidly immunosuppressive than HIV-1.

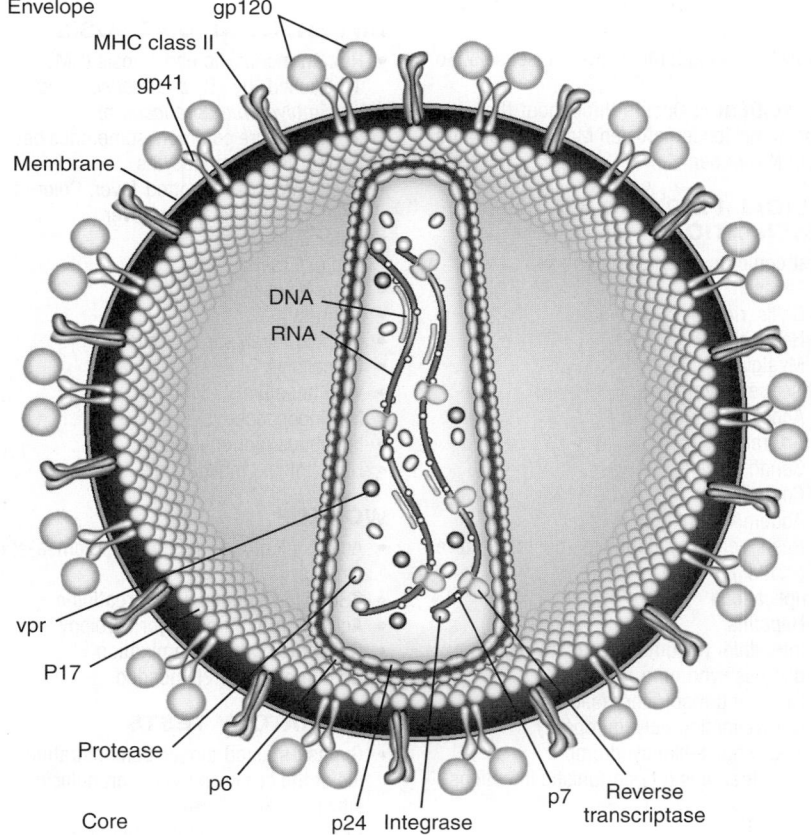

FIGURE 1-196 Structure of the HIV-1 virion. The viral envelop is formed from the host cell membrane, into which the HIV-1 envelop proteins gp41 and gp120 have been inserted and may include several host cell proteins, most significantly the major histocompatibility complex class II proteins. The matrix between the envelop and the core is formed predominantly from Gag protein p17. The core contains the viral RNA, closely associated with Gag protein p7, in addition to RT and integrase. It has also been proven that virions contain complementary DNA, as shown, synthesized by the RT. The major structural proteins of the core are Gag proteins p24 and p6. Also present within the virion are the protease and two cleavage products from the Gag precursor protein (p1 and p2, not shown) of undetermined position within the virion is also package in the virion and is thought to be localized within the core, as shown. (From Mandell GL et al: *Principles and practice of infectious diseases,* ed 7, Philadelphia, 2010, Elsevier.)

- Transmitted by sexual contact, shared needles, blood transfusion, or from mother to child during pregnancy, delivery, or breastfeeding.
- Primary target of infection: CD4 lymphocyte.
- Direct CNS involvement: manifested as encephalopathy, myelopathy, or neuropathy in advanced cases.
- Renal failure, rheumatologic disorders, thrombocytopenia, or cardiac abnormalities may be seen in association with HIV.

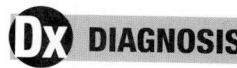 **DIAGNOSIS**

DIFFERENTIAL DIAGNOSIS
- Acute infection: mononucleosis or other respiratory viral infections
- Late symptoms: similar to those produced by other wasting illnesses such as neoplasms, TB, disseminated fungal infection, malabsorption, or depression
- HIV-related encephalopathy: confused with Alzheimer's disease or other causes of chronic dementia (cognitive impairment in HIV infection is described in Section II); myelopathy and neuropathy possibly resembling other demyelinating diseases such as multiple sclerosis

WORKUP
Since the debut of HIV/AIDS in the 1980s, diagnosis has been established by voluntary testing for antibody to the virus. The CDC is now recommending routine testing for patients in all health care settings unless the patient declines (opt-out screening). This includes routine testing of pregnant women. It is also recommended that separate written consent should no longer be required, although by law this is being addressed on a state-by-state basis.

LABORATORY TESTS
HIV antibody detected by a two-step technique:
- ELISA as a sensitive screening test.
- Confirmation of positive ELISA tests with the more specific Western blot technique.

- The CD4 count and HIV RNA polymerase chain reaction (PCR) should be measured in all patients.
- The CD4 count is a marker of current immune status.
The HIV RNA PCR (viral load) is predictive of disease progression.
- Rapid serologic tests have been increasingly used and are useful in specific settings: occupational exposures, pregnant women in labor without previous testing, and patients in high seroprevalence areas (for immediate results). Specimens are either blood or saliva and results are given within 20 min. Although sensitivity is high (99.1% to 99.7%), false-positive tests are more common in low seroprevalence populations. Thus, all positive results must be confirmed with standard serology, including western blot.
Fig. 1-197 describes the immunologic response to HIV infection.

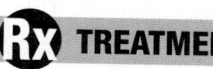 **TREATMENT**

NONPHARMACOLOGIC THERAPY
Maintenance of adequate nutrition

ACUTE GENERAL Rx
- Acute management of opportunistic infections and malignancies (see AIDS-associated disorders, "*Pneumocystis carinii* (now *P. jirovecii*) Pneumonia," "Cryptococcosis," "Tuberculosis," "Toxoplasmosis" elsewhere in this text.)
Acute HIV syndrome:
- No definitive evidence supports routine initiation of antiretroviral therapy in primary HIV infection.

CHRONIC Rx
Naïve, chronically infected patients should be considered for therapy based on their current CD4 counts, likelihood for disease progression (viral loads), and ability to remain adherent with combination antiretroviral therapy. Please see current HIV treatment guidelines of the Depart-

ment of Health and Human Services (www.aidsinfo.nih.gov/guidelines).
1. Therapy is recommended for all patients with symptomatic established HIV disease. Symptomatic HIV disease is defined as the presence of any of the following: thrush, vaginal candidiasis, herpes zoster, peripheral neuropathy, bacillary angiomatosis, cervical dysplasia in situ, constitutional symptoms such as fever or diarrhea for more than 1 mo, ITP, PID, or listeriosis.
2. In asymptomatic individuals, therapy should be initiated before the CD4 count declines below 350 cells/mm³.
3. For all patients with CD4 count >350, there is insufficient evidence showing clear benefit. Decisions to start treatment above this threshold should be based on several factors: presence of comorbidities or risk factors for cardiovascular and other non-AIDS diseases that favor earlier therapy, rapid decline in CD4 count (>100/yr), or HIV-1 RNA level of >100,000.
4. Antiretroviral therapy using combinations of nucleoside/nucleotide reverse transcriptase inhibitor (NRTI) agents: zidovudine (AZT), lamivudine (3TC), emtricitabine (FTC), tenofovir, abacavir, stavudine (D4T), or didanosine (DDI); in addition to boosted (with ritonavir) protease inhibitors (PI) such as lopinavir/ritonavir, atazanavir, fosamprenavir, darunavir, saquinavir, indinavir, or nonnucleoside reverse transcriptase inhibitors (NNRTI), such as nevirapine or efavirenz. The PI ritonavir is often used, in low dose, in combination with other PIs to obtain more sustained drug levels. Adding a fourth drug to the three-drug regimen does not improve viral suppression or outcome and is not recommended. Treatment interruptions based upon CD4 responses appear harmful in recent comparative studies versus standard continuous treatment protocols and should be avoided.
5. Usual initial dosing regimen consists of two nucleoside/nucleotide reverse transcriptase inhibitors (nRTIs) and a nonnucleoside reverse transcriptase inhibitor (NNRTI) or a PI. Data support inclusion of lamivudine or emtricitabine as one of the two nRTIs.
Standard nRTIs include:
- Truvada (tenofovir/emtricitabine) 1 tablet once daily.
  - Tenofovir: individuals with underlying renal dysfunction or requiring other nephrotoxic agents may be at increased risk of renal toxicity.
  - Epzicom (abacavir/lamivudine) 1 tablet once daily
- Abacavir: association with increased risk of myocardial infarction. Use with caution in patients with cardiovascular risk.
  - Combivir (Zidovudine/lamivudine) 1 tablet twice daily
  - Zidovudine: associated with lipoatrophy and anemia. GI and CNS side effects.

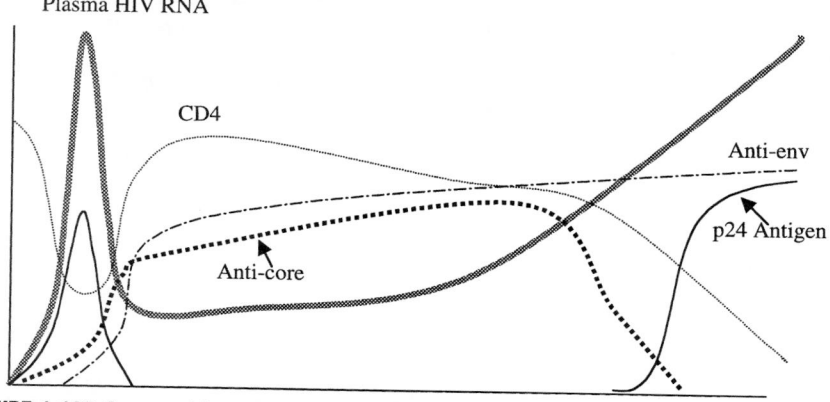
FIGURE 1-197 Course of human immunodeficiency virus infection. (From Mandell GL [ed]: *Mandell, Douglas, and Bennett's principles and practice of infectious diseases,* ed 6, New York, 2005, Churchill Livingstone.)

Standard Backbone Regimens include:

- NNRTI
  - Efavirenz 600 mg daily: not recommended for women in the first trimester or those who are contemplating pregnancy
  - Nevirapine 200 mg two times a day: avoid with CD4 count >250 in men and >350 in women because of the risk of hepatitis
- PIs (ritonavir boosted)
  - Lopinavir/ritonavir (200 mg/50 mg) 2 tablets twice a day (or 4 tablets once a day): most likely to cause diarrhea and has the greatest negative effect on triglyceride levels.
  - Atazanavir and ritonavir (300 mg and 100 mg) 2 tablets a day: lower pill burden, but use with caution with acid reducing agents—can alter absorption.
  - Fosamprenavir and ritonavir (700 mg and 100 mg) 2 tablets twice a day (or 4 tablets once a day): cannot take fosamprenavir with sulfa allergy
  - Saquinavir and ritonavir
  - Darunavir and ritonavir: Used more in treatment of experienced patients with multidrug-resistant virus
- All these drugs have their own unique, as well as class-specific, side effects and require careful follow-up to achieve optimal antiviral effects. Compliance with the drug regimen and tolerance of common side effects are critically important to maintain drug efficacy. Antiviral response should be monitored by baseline HIV viral load and CD4 count and repeat measurement at 2 and 4 wk into treatment and then periodically (every 3 mo) to ensure viral suppression.
- All patients should have genotypic resistance testing on entry into medical care.
- Later, an antiretroviral regimen should be constructed based on past antiretroviral experience and the results of genotypic or phenotypic testing.
- Patients with CD4 lymphocyte count <200/mm^3 should be given preventive therapy for *Pneumocystis jirovecii* pneumonia (PJP) (see "*Pneumocystis jirovecii [P. carinii]* Pneumonia").
- Evaluation of chronic diarrhea in patients with HIV is described in Section III, "HIV-Infected Patient, Acutely Ill."
- Criteria for discontinuing and restarting opportunistic prophylaxis for adults with HIV

infection is described in Section I, "Acquired Immunodeficiency Syndrome."

- HIV infection in a pregnant woman poses special challenges and considerations. Appropriate and timely antiretroviral therapy given to mother and newborn has been shown to dramatically reduce the risk of perinatal transmission of HIV. The goal of therapy is to achieve an undetectable viral load. For HIV-infected pregnant women who are already receiving ART: (1) Continue therapy if suppressing viral replication, but avoid use of efavirenz in the first trimester (substitution is recommended in the first trimester); (2) If viremia on therapy, genotypic testing is recommended; (3) Nevirapine should be continued, regardless of CD4 count, if there is viral suppression. For HIV-infected pregnant women who have never received ART: (1) Women who require ART for their own health should start on ART in the first trimester. Most antiretrovirals are safe in pregnancy, however, Sustiva should be avoided because of tetrogenicity (Class D), DDI and D4T should be avoided (potential of lactic acidosis), and some protease inhibitors may be dose-altered in pregnancy. Nevirapine should not be initiated in an antiretroviral naive pregnant patient with CD4 counts >250 because of the risk of hepatotoxicity. (2) Women who do not need ART for their own health should also initiate three-drug therapy, but may do so at the end of the first trimester. (3) Zidovudine (AZT) is recommended as a component of antiretroviral therapy.
- Therapy should continue through the baby's birth. Zidovudine is given intravenously at the time of labor, regardless of whether it is an existing component of her three-drug regimen. In women with viral loads persistently >1000 copies/ml despite appropriate ARV, cesarean section may further lower risk of transmission. Zidovudine (AZT) should also be given to the newborn for the first 6 wk of life, and mothers should completely avoid nursing.

DISPOSITION

- Ongoing care consisting of frequent medical evaluations and T-lymphocyte subset analysis along with the plasma HIV load
- Long-term care focused on providing up-to-date antiretroviral therapy and prophylaxis of

PJP and other opportunistic infections, as well as early detection of complications (see Section III.)
- Ongoing assessment for cardiovascular risk
- Screening and treatment for Hepatitis B and C
- Yearly screening for STIs (Chlamydia, gonorrhea, syphilis)
- Consideration of AIDS (lymphomas, HPV) and non-AIDS related (screening for general population, age specific cancers)

REFERRAL

To a physician knowledgeable and experienced in the management of HIV infection and its complications

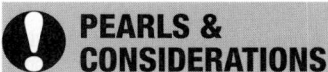

COMMENTS

- HIV chemoprophylaxis after occupational exposure is described in Section V.
- A recent analysis of the impact of the highly active anti-retroviral therapy (HAART) era indicates that antiretroviral therapy has saved at least 3 million years of life since the introduction of HAART into medicine more than 10 yr ago.
- In persons with HIV infection, screening for TB needs to include questions about combination of symptoms rather than only inquiring about chronic cough.
- Trials involving antiretroviral chemoprophylaxis before exposure for the prevention of HIV acquisition in men who have sex with men have shown that oral tenofovir disoproxil fumarate (FTC-TDF) provides protection against acquisition of HIV infection. Detected blood levels strongly correlated with the prophylactic effect.

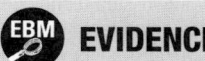 **EVIDENCE**

available at www.expertconsult.com

SUGGESTED READINGS
available at www.expertconsult.com

AUTHOR: **DENNIS J. MIKOLICH, M.D.**

BASIC INFORMATION

DEFINITION

Huntington's disease is an inherited neurodegenerative disorder characterized by involuntary movements, psychiatric disturbance, and cognitive decline.

SYNONYMS

Huntington's chorea

ICD-9CM CODES
333.4 Huntington's chorea

EPIDEMIOLOGY & DEMOGRAPHICS

PEAK INCIDENCE: Late 30s and 40s, with onsets from ages 2 to 70 yr
PREVALENCE (IN U.S.): 4.1 to 8.4 cases/100,000 persons
PREDOMINANT SEX: Female = male
PREDOMINANT AGE: Adulthood
GENETICS: Autosomal dominant

PHYSICAL FINDINGS & CLINICAL PRESENTATION

- Chorea (irregular, rapid, flowing, nonstereotyped involuntary movements). When there is a writhing quality, it is referred to as choreoathetosis. Chorea is present early on and tends to decrease in end stages of disease.
- Dancelike, lurching gait, often caused by chorea.
- Westphal variant: cognitive dysfunction, bradykinesia, and rigidity. This variant is more commonly seen in juvenile-onset Huntington's.
- Oculomotor abnormalities are common early on and include increased latency of response and insuppressible eye blinking.
- Psychiatric disorders (can be present early on): depression is commonly seen as well as obsessive-compulsive behaviors and aggression associated with impaired impulse control.

ETIOLOGY

- Trinucleotide repeat disorder.
- The responsible gene is the Huntington gene located on chromosome 4. Its function is not known.

DIAGNOSIS

DIFFERENTIAL DIAGNOSIS

- Drug-induced chorea: dopamine, stimulants, anticonvulsants, antidepressants, and oral contraceptives have all been known to cause chorea.
- Sydenham's chorea: decreased incidence with decline of rheumatic fever.
- Benign hereditary chorea: autosomal dominant with onset in childhood. There is no progression of symptoms and no associated dementia or behavioral problems.
- Senile chorea: possibly vascular in origin.
- Wilson's disease: autosomal recessive; tremor, dysarthria, and dystonia are more common presentations than chorea. A total of 95% of patients with neurologic manifestations will have Keyser-Fleischer rings.
- Postinfectious.
- Systemic lupus erythematosus: can be the presenting feature of lupus (rare).
- Chorea gravidarum: presents during first 4 to 5 mo of pregnancy and resolves after delivery.
- Paraneoplastic: seen most commonly in small-cell lung cancer and lymphoma.

WORKUP

Onset of symptoms in an individual with an established family history requires no additional investigation.

LABORATORY TESTS

- Genetic testing.
- If normal, obtain complete blood count with smear, erythrocyte sedimentation rate, electrolytes, serum ceruloplasmin, 24-hr urinary copper excretion, TFTs, antinuclear antibody, liver function tests, HIV, and ASO titer. Consider paraneoplastic markers.

IMAGING STUDIES

CT scan or MRI scan will show atrophy, most notably in the caudate and putamen. The cortex is involved to a lesser extent. A normal scan does not exclude the diagnosis.

TREATMENT

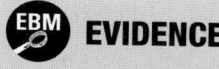

NONPHARMACOLOGIC THERAPY

- Supportive counseling
- Physical and occupational therapy
- Home health care
- Genetic counseling

CHRONIC Rx

- Chorea does not need to be treated unless it is disabling.
- Tetrabenazine (TBZ), now available in the United States, was recently approved by the FDA for the treatment of chorea associated with Huntington's disease. It is a reversible inhibitor of the vesicle monoamine transporter type 2 (VMAT-2). It inhibits primarily dopamine and to a lesser degree serotonin and norepinephrine. Side effects include parkinsonism and depression.
- Neuroleptics at low doses (e.g., haloperidol 1 to 10 mg/day).
- Amantadine (up to 300 to 400 mg divided tid).
- Depression with suicidal ideation is common; may improve with tricyclic antidepressants or SSRI

DISPOSITION

Relentless course of variable duration leading to progressive disability and death

REFERRAL

- Should refer to psychiatry and neurology for treatment of mood disorders and movement disorders
- Genetic counseling

PEARLS & CONSIDERATIONS

- Suicide rate is fivefold that of the general population.
- The number of repeats does correlate with age of onset but does not clearly correlate with disease severity. Interpretation of number of repeats is still difficult at this time; therefore it is debatable whether to disclose this information to patients.

EVIDENCE

available at www.expertconsult.com

SUGGESTED READINGS

available at www.expertconsult.com

AUTHOR: **CINDY ZADIKOFF, M.D.**

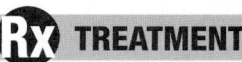

BASIC INFORMATION

DEFINITION

A hydrocele is a fluid collection in a serous scrotal space, usually between the layers of the tunica vaginalis (Figs. 1-198 and 1-199). A hydrocele that fills with fluid from the peritoneum is termed *communicating*. This is distinguished from a *noncommunicating* hydrocele by history of variation in size throughout the day and palpation of a thickened cord above the testicle on the affected side. A communicating hydrocele is a small inguinal hernia in which fluid, but not peritoneal structures, traverses the processus vaginalis.

ICD-9CM CODES
603.9 Hydrocele

PHYSICAL FINDINGS & CLINICAL PRESENTATION

Symptoms:
- Scrotal enlargement
- Scrotal heaviness or discomfort radiating to the inguinal area
- Back pain

Physical findings:
- Scrotal distention (testicle may be impossible to palpate)
- Transillumination

ETIOLOGY

Hydroceles may occur as a congenital abnormality in which the processus vaginalis fails to close. In this case an inguinal hernia is virtually always associated with the malformation. Congenital hydroceles are most common in infants and children. In adults, hydroceles are more frequently caused by infection, tumor, or trauma. Infection of the epididymis often results in the development of a secondary hydrocele. Tropical infections such as filariasis may produce hydroceles.

DIAGNOSIS

DIFFERENTIAL DIAGNOSIS
- Spermatocele
- Inguinoscrotal hernia
- Testicular tumor
- Varicocele
- Epididymitis

IMAGING STUDIES

Scrotal ultrasound (useful to rule out a testicular tumor as the cause of the hydrocele). The acute development of a hydrocele might be associated with the onset of epididymitis, testicular tumor, trauma, and torsion of a testicular appendage. An ultrasound of the scrotum may provide important diagnostic information.

TREATMENT

- No treatment if asymptomatic and testicle is believed to be normal.
- Surgical repair. Communicating hydroceles should be repaired in the same manner as an indirect hernia. The indications for repair of a noncommunicating hydrocele include failure to resolve and increase in size to one that is large and tense.

AUTHOR: **FRED F. FERRI, M.D.**

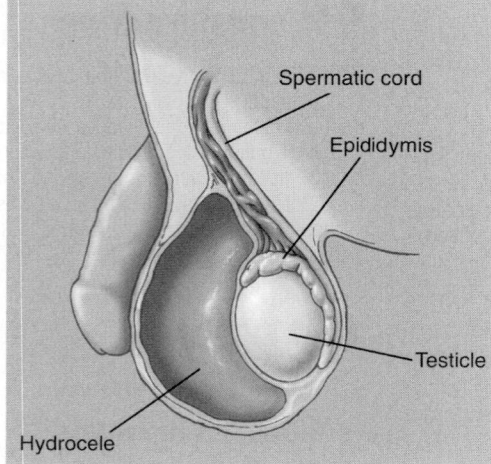

FIGURE 1-198 Schematic representation of the testicle, epididymis, spermatic cord, and a hydrocele. (Lipshultz LI, Khera M, Atwal DT: *Urology and the primary care practitioner,* ed 3, Philadelphia, 2008, Elsevier.)

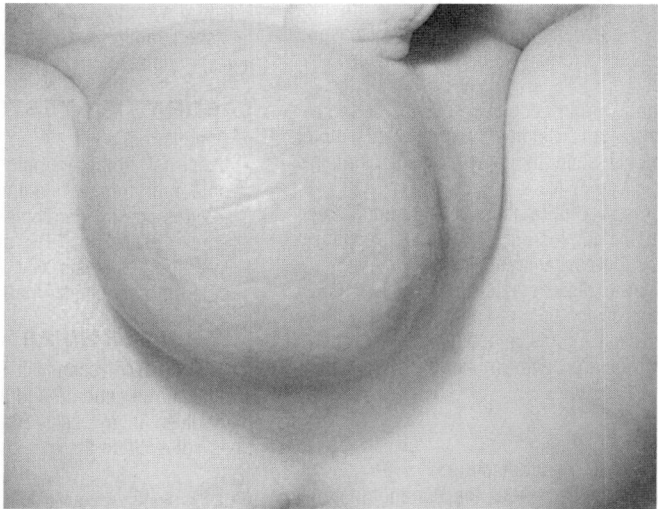

FIGURE 1-199 Newborn with large right hydrocele. (From Behrman RE: *Nelson textbook of pediatrics,* ed 16, Philadelphia, 2000, WB Saunders.)

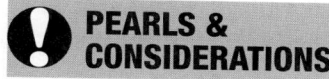

BASIC INFORMATION

DEFINITION

Normal pressure hydrocephalus (NPH) is a syndrome of symptomatic hydrocephalus in the setting of normal cerebrospinal fluid (CSF) pressure. The classic clinical triad of NPH includes gait disturbance, cognitive decline, and incontinence.

SYNONYMS

Occult hydrocephalus
Extraventricular obstructive hydrocephalus
Chronic hydrocephalus

ICD-9CM CODES
331.3 Communicating hydrocephalus

EPIDEMIOLOGY & DEMOGRAPHICS

INCIDENCE: The exact incidence is not known. It may account for up to 5% of dementia in the U.S. Hospital discharge data suggest approximately 11,500 new cases diagnosed annually (may be overestimated).
PREDOMINANT SEX: Males = females
PREDOMINANT AGE: NPH is more common with increasing age.

PHYSICAL FINDINGS & CLINICAL PRESENTATION

- Gait difficulty: patients often have difficulty initiating ambulation, and the gait may be broad based and shuffling, with the appearance that the feet are stuck to the floor ("magnetic gait" or "frontal gait disorder").
- Cognitive decline: mental slowing, forgetfulness and inattention typically without agnosia, aphasia, or other cortical disturbances.
- Incontinence: initially may have urinary urgency; incontinence later develops. Fecal incontinence also occasionally occurs.
- Gegenhalten (paratonia) or other frontal lobe signs may be seen.

ETIOLOGY

- Approximately 50% of cases are idiopathic; the remaining cases have a variety of causes, including prior subarachnoid hemorrhage, meningitis, trauma, or intracranial surgery.
- Symptoms are presumed to result from stretching of sacral motor and limbic fibers that lie near the ventricles as dilation occurs.

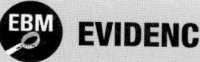

DIAGNOSIS

DIFFERENTIAL DIAGNOSIS

- Alzheimer's disease with extrapyramidal features

- Cognitive impairment in the setting of Parkinson's disease or parkinsonism-plus syndromes
- Diffuse Lewy body disease
- Frontotemporal dementia
- Cervical spondylosis with cord compromise in the setting of degenerative dementia
- Multiinfarct dementia
- HIV dementia

WORKUP

- Large-volume lumbar puncture:
  1. Mental status testing and time to walk a prespecified distance (usually 25 feet) are measured, followed by removal of 40 to 50 ml of CSF.
  2. Retest of mental status and timed walking are done later (sometimes at 1 and 4 hr). Patients who have significant improvement in gait or mental status may have a better surgical outcome; those with mild or negative response can have variable outcomes.
  3. Opening and closing pressure are measured; if pressure is elevated, alternative causes must be considered. Higher *normal* pressure may predict a good outcome from CSF shunting.
- Measurement of CSF outflow resistance by an infusion test, CSF pressure monitoring, and prolonged external lumbar drainage are sometimes used to help predict surgical outcome.

LABORATORY TESTS

CSF should be sent for routine fluid analysis to exclude other pathologies.

IMAGING STUDIES

- CT scan or MRI can be used to document ventriculomegaly. The distinguishing feature of NPH is ventricular enlargement out of proportion to sulcal atrophy.
- MRI has advantages over CT, including better ability to visualize structures in the posterior fossa, visualize transependymal CSF flow, and document extent of white matter lesions. On MRI a flow void in the aqueduct and third ventricle ("jet sign") may be seen.
- Isotope cisternography and dynamic MRI studies have not been shown to be superior in predicting shunt outcome.

TREATMENT

There is no evidence that NPH can be effectively treated with medications.

NONPHARMACOLOGIC THERAPY

Response to ventriculoperitoneal shunting is variable. Some patients (variable depending on

series reported) show significant improvement from shunting.
  Factors that may predict positive outcome with surgery:
- NPH caused by prior trauma, subarachnoid hemorrhage, or meningitis
- History of mild impairment in cognition <2 yr duration
- Onset of gait abnormality before cognitive decline
- Imaging demonstrates hydrocephalus without sulcal enlargement
- Transependymal CSF flow visualized on MRI
- Large-volume tap produces dramatic but temporary relief of symptoms
- High *normal* opening pressure
Factors that may predict negative outcome with surgery:
- Extensive white matter lesions or diffuse cerebral atrophy on MRI
- Moderate to severe cognitive impairment
- Onset of cognitive impairment before gait disorder
- History of alcohol abuse

ACUTE GENERAL Rx

Shunting in selected patients

DISPOSITION

Symptoms of NPH may progress over time. Prompt diagnosis may improve chances for treatment success.

REFERRAL

To neurologist for initial evaluation, including lumbar puncture, followed by neurosurgeon for shunting in appropriate patients

PEARLS & CONSIDERATIONS

Each of the cardinal symptoms of NPH is commonly seen in the elderly and occurs in multiple disease processes; therefore differential diagnoses should always be considered carefully.

CAUTION

Shunt complications, including subdural or intracerebral hematoma, may occur in 30% to 40% of patients.

EVIDENCE

available at www.expertconsult.com

SUGGESTED READINGS
available at www.expertconsult.com

AUTHOR: **TAMARA G. FONG, M.D., Ph.D.**

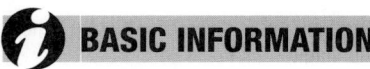

BASIC INFORMATION

DEFINITION

Hydronephrosis is dilation of the renal pyelocalyceal system, most often as a result of impairment of urinary flow.

SYNONYMS

Hydroureter (dilation of ureter, often seen with hydronephrosis when obstruction is in lower urinary tract)
Urinary tract obstruction

ICD-9CM CODES
591   Acquired hydronephrosis
753.2   Congenital hydronephrosis

EPIDEMIOLOGY & DEMOGRAPHICS

Children usually have congenital malformations, whereas adults tend to have acquired defects as etiologies.

CLINICAL PRESENTATION

HISTORY:

- Pain is caused by distention of collecting system or renal capsule and is more related to the rate of onset than the degree of obstruction. It can vary in location from flank to the lower abdomen to the testes/labia. Pain in the flank occurring only on micturition is highly suggestive of vesicoureteral reflux.
- Anuria can occur with total obstruction of urinary flow (bilateral hydronephrosis, or unilateral if only one kidney is present).
- Polyuria or nocturia can occur with chronic (incomplete) obstruction because of deleterious effects on renal concentrating ability (nephrogenic diabetes insipidus).
- Urinary frequency, hesitancy, poor stream, and postvoid dribbling are all symptoms that can occur with obstruction at or below the bladder (e.g., prostatic hyperplasia).
- Chronic urinary infections can either result from chronic urinary obstruction (organisms favoring growth with stasis of urine) or lead to conditions (e.g., urine pH changes) that favor stone formation and subsequent obstruction.

PHYSICAL EXAMINATION:

- Hypertension can be caused by increased renin release in acute or subacute obstruction.
- Fever or costovertebral angle (CVA) tenderness can suggest urinary tract infection.
- Palpate bladder to detect if distention is present.
- Rectal examination to evaluate prostate for size and nodularity and also to check rectal sphincter tone.
- Pelvic examination to assess for vaginal anatomy, pelvic mass, or pelvic inflammatory disease.
- Penile examination to rule out meatal stenosis or phimosis.
- Bladder catheterization to assess postvoid residual volume if urinary tract obstruction is considered. Should rule out postrenal obstruction in unexplained acute renal failure.

ETIOLOGY

MECHANICAL IMPAIRMENTS:

Congenital:
- Ureteropelvic junction narrowing
- Ureterovesical junction narrowing
- Ureterocele
- Retrocaval ureter
- Bladder neck obstruction
- Urethral valve
- Urethral stricture
- Meatal stenosis

Acquired:
- Intrinsic to urinary tract:
  - Calculi
  - Inflammation
  - Trauma
  - Sloughed papillae
  - Ureteral tumor
  - Blood clots
  - Prostatic hypertrophy or cancer
  - Bladder cancer
  - Urethral stricture
  - Phimosis
- Extrinsic to urinary tract:
  - Gravid uterus
  - Retroperitoneal fibrosis or tumor (e.g., lymphoma)
  - Aortic aneurysm
  - Uterine fibroids
  - Trauma (surgical or nonsurgical)
  - Pelvic inflammatory disease
  - Pelvic malignancies (e.g., prostate, colorectal, cervical, uterine, bladder)

FUNCTIONAL IMPAIRMENTS:

- Neurogenic bladder (often with adynamic ureter) can occur with spinal cord disease or diabetic neuropathy.
- Pharmacologic agents such as alpha-adrenergic antagonists and anticholinergic drugs can inhibit bladder emptying.
- Vesicoureteral reflux may occur.
- Pregnancy can cause hydroureter and hydronephrosis (on the right more often than left) as early as the second month. Hormonal effects on ureteral tone combine with mechanical factors.

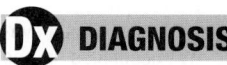

DIAGNOSIS

DIFFERENTIAL DIAGNOSIS

- Urinary stones
- Neoplastic disease
- Prostatic hypertrophy
- Neurologic disease
- Urinary reflux
- Urinary tract infection
- Medication effects
- Trauma
- Congenital abnormality of urinary tract

LABORATORY TESTS

- Serum blood urea nitrogen and creatinine to assess for renal insufficiency (usually implies bilateral obstruction or unilateral obstruction of a solitary kidney).
- Electrolytes may reveal hypernatremia (if nephrogenic diabetes insipidus), hyperkalemia (from renal failure and effects on tubular function), or distal renal tubular acidosis.
- Urinalysis and examination of sediment may reveal white blood cells, red blood cells, or bacteria in the appropriate setting (e.g., infection, stones), but often the sediment is normal in obstructive renal disease.

IMAGING STUDIES

- Assess kidney and bladder size with ultrasound as well as contour of collecting system and ureters. Ultrasound is >90% sensitive and specific for hydronephrosis and is noninvasive; therefore it will not worsen preexisting renal insufficiency.
- Abdominal CT scan without IV contrast provides excellent localization of the site of obstruction (Fig. 1-200).

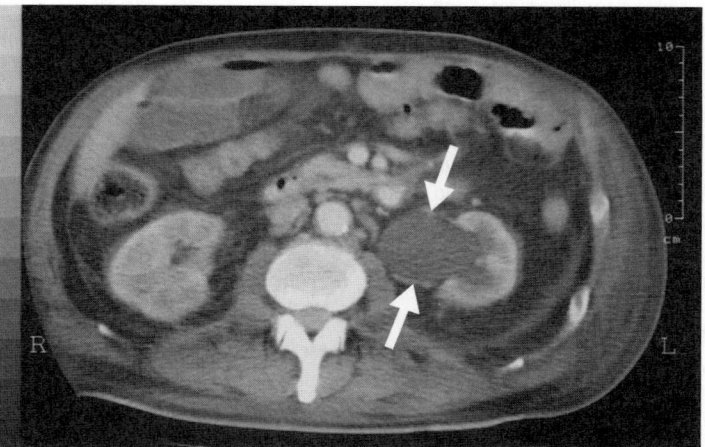

FIGURE 1-200 CT scan of the abdomen showing a grossly hydronephrotic kidney on the left. *Arrows* mark dilated renal pelvis. Dilated loops of small bowel are seen in the right hypochondrium. Sequential sections demonstrated that the ureter was dilated along its length and that there was a pelvic mass, which was responsible for both bowel and left ureteric obstruction. The mass was subsequently shown to be arising from a carcinoma of the colon. (From Johnson RJ, Feehally J: *Comprehensive clinical nephrology,* ed 2, St Louis, 2000, Mosby.)

H

Diseases and Disorders

I

- Once diagnosed, antegrade or retrograde ureterograms can further delineate the point of obstruction.
- Voiding cystourethrogram is helpful in diagnosing vesicoureteral reflux and obstructions of the bladder neck or urethra.

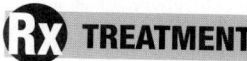 **TREATMENT**

NONPHARMACOLOGIC THERAPY

- Urgent treatment is required if urinary tract obstruction is associated with urinary tract infection, acute renal failure, or uncontrollable pain.
- Conservative management of calculi with IV fluids, IV antibiotics (if evidence of infection), and aggressive analgesia may be enough to treat acute unilateral urinary tract obstruction depending on the size (90% of stones <5 mm will pass spontaneously).
- Urethral catheter is adequate to relieve most obstructions at or distal to the bladder, but occasionally a suprapubic catheter will be required (e.g., impassable urethral stricture or urethral injury). Neurogenic bladder may require intermittent clean catheterization if frequent voiding and pharmacologic treatments are ineffective.
- Nephrostomy tube can be placed percutaneously to facilitate urinary drainage.
- Extracorporeal shock wave lithotripsy (ESWL) is used to fragment large stones to facilitate

spontaneous passage or subsequent extraction. (Note: ESWL is contraindicated in pregnancy.)
- Nephroscopy is performed for extraction of proximal stones under direct visualization.
- Cystoscopy with ureteroscopy is used to remove distal ureteral stones with a loop or basket with or without fragmentation by ultrasonic or laser lithotripsy.
- Ureteral stents can be used for extrinsic and some intrinsic ureteral obstructions.
- Urethral dilation or internal urethrotomy can be used for urethral strictures.
- Nephrectomy or ureteral diversion may be required in severe cases (e.g., malignancy).
- Ureterovesical reimplantation can be used for reflux disease.
- Transurethral retrograde prostatectomy is used for severe obstruction from benign prostatic hypertrophy.
- IV fluid and electrolyte replacement are needed; the patient must be monitored closely during the postobstructive diuresis (usually lasting several days to a week).

ACUTE GENERAL Rx

Antibiotics if indicated

DISPOSITION

Aggressive treatment of infections and early relief of obstruction can usually prevent progressive loss of renal function; however, chronic

bilateral obstruction (often from benign prostatic hypertrophy) can lead to chronic renal failure.

REFERRAL

- Urologist consultation early for diagnostic or therapeutic procedures
- Oncologist if a neoplasm is diagnosed
- Gynecologist if pregnancy or female pelvic anatomy is involved

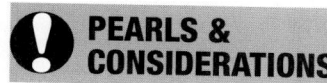 **PEARLS & CONSIDERATIONS**

COMMENTS

- Not a primary disorder: an underlying etiology should be sought.

PREVENTION

May be achieved through prevention of an underlying potential etiology (e.g., medical or surgical management of benign prostatic hypertrophy before obstruction occurring or medical treatment to avoid formation of renal stones).

SUGGESTED READINGS
available at www.expertconsult.com

AUTHORS: **SHEENAGH M. BODKIN, M.D.,** and **PAUL A. PIRRAGLIA, M.D., M.P.H.**

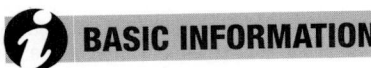

BASIC INFORMATION

DEFINITION

Primary hyperaldosteronism is a clinical syndrome characterized by hypokalemia, hypertension, low plasma renin activity (PRA), and excessive aldosterone secretion.

SYNONYMS

Hyperaldosteronism
Aldosteronism
Primary aldosteronism
Conn's syndrome

ICD-9CM CODES

255.1 Primary aldosteronism

EPIDEMIOLOGY & DEMOGRAPHICS

INCIDENCE: 1% to 2% of patients with hypertension
PREVALENCE: More common in females

PHYSICAL FINDINGS & CLINICAL PRESENTATION

- Generally asymptomatic
- If significant hypokalemia is present, possible muscle cramping, weakness, paresthesias
- Hypertension
- Polyuria, polydipsia

ETIOLOGY

- Aldosterone-producing adenoma (>60%)
- Idiopathic hyperaldosteronism (>30%)
- Glucocorticoid-suppressible hyperaldosteronism (<1%)
- Aldosterone-producing carcinoma (<1%)

DIAGNOSIS

DIFFERENTIAL DIAGNOSIS

- Diuretic use
- Hypokalemia from vomiting, diarrhea
- Renovascular hypertension
- Other endocrine neoplasm (pheochromocytoma, deoxycorticosterone-producing tumor, renin-secreting tumor)

WORKUP

CT, MRI, and adrenal vein sampling (AVS) are used to distinguish unilateral from bilateral increased aldosterone secretion. This distinction will dictate treatment options since unilateral primary aldosteronism is treated surgically rather than medically. In patients with hypokalemia and a low PRA, confirming tests for primary hyperaldosteronism include the following:

- 24-hr urine test for aldosterone and potassium levels (potassium >40 mEq and aldosterone >15 mcg).
- Captopril test: administer 25 to 50 mg of captopril (an angiotensin-converting enzyme [ACE] inhibitor) and measure plasma renin and aldosterone levels 1 to 2 hr later. A plasma aldosterone level >15 ng/dl confirms the diagnosis of primary aldosteronism. This test is more expensive and is best reserved for situations in which the 24-hr urine test for aldosterone is ambiguous.
- 24-hr urinary tetrahydroaldosterone (<65 mcg/24 hr) and saline infusion test (plasma aldosterone >10 ng/dl) can also be used in ambiguous cases.
- The renin-aldosterone stimulation test (posture test) is helpful in differentiating idiopathic hyperaldosteronism (IHA) from aldosterone-producing adenoma (APA). Patients with APA have a decrease in aldosterone levels at 4 hr, whereas patients with IHA have an increase in aldosterone levels.
- As a screening test for primary aldosteronism, an elevated plasma aldosterone-renin ratio (ARR), drawn randomly from patients taking hypertensive drugs, is predictive of primary aldosteronism (positive predictive value 100% in a recent study). ARR is calculated by dividing plasma aldosterone (mg/dl) by PRA (mg/ml/hr). ARR >100 is considered elevated.
- Bilateral AVS may be done to localize APA when adrenal CT scan is equivocal. In APA, ipsilateral/contralateral aldosterone level is >10:1, and ipsilateral venous aldosterone concentration is very high (>1000 ng/dl).
- A diagnostic evaluation of hypertensive patients with suspected aldosteronism is described in the online version of Section III.

LABORATORY TESTS

Routine laboratory tests can be suggestive but are not diagnostic of primary aldosteronism. Common abnormalities are:

- Spontaneous hypokalemia or moderately severe hypokalemia while receiving conventional doses of diuretics
- Possible alkalosis and hypernatremia

IMAGING STUDIES

- Adrenal CT scans (with 3-mm cuts) or MRI may be used to localize neoplasm.
- Adrenal scanning with iodocholesterol (NP-59) or 6-beta-iodomethyl-19-norcholesterol after dexamethasone suppression. The uptake of tracer is increased in those with aldosteronoma and absent in those with IHA and adrenal carcinoma.

TREATMENT

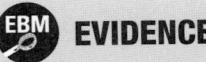

NONPHARMACOLOGIC THERAPY

- Regular monitoring and control of blood pressure
- Low-sodium diet, tobacco avoidance, maintenance of ideal body weight, and regular exercise

ACUTE GENERAL Rx

- Control of blood pressure and hypokalemia with spironolactone, amiloride, or ACE inhibitors
- Surgery (unilateral adrenalectomy) for APA

CHRONIC Rx

Chronic medical therapy with spironolactone, amiloride, or ACE inhibitors to control blood pressure and hypokalemia is necessary in all patients with bilateral IHA.

DISPOSITION

- Unilateral adrenalectomy normalizes hypertension and hypokalemia in 70% of patients with APA after 1 yr. After 5 yr, 50% of patients remain normotensive.
- Experimental animal studies have suggested that long-term exposure to increased aldosterone levels in untreated aldosteronism may result in renal structural damage. However, clinical trials have shown that primary aldosteronism is characterized by partially reversible renal dysfunction in which elevated albuminuria is a marker of a dynamic rather than structural renal defect.

REFERRAL

Surgical referral for unilateral adrenalectomy after confirmation of unilateral APA or carcinoma

PEARLS & CONSIDERATIONS

- Frequent monitoring of blood pressure and electrolytes postoperatively is necessary because normotension after unilateral adrenalectomy may take up to 4 mo.
- Recent investigations regarding serum aldosterone and the incidence of hypertension in nonhypertensive persons indicate that increased aldosterone levels within the physiologic range predispose to the development of hypertension.

EVIDENCE

available at www.expertconsult.com

SUGGESTED READINGS

available at www.expertconsult.com

AUTHOR: **FRED F. FERRI, M.D.**

BASIC INFORMATION

DEFINITION

Hypercholesterolemia refers to a blood cholesterol measurement >200 mg/dl. A cholesterol level of 200 to 239 mg/dl is considered borderline high, and a level of >240 mg/dl is considered high.

SYNONYMS

Hypercholesteremia
Dyslipidemia
Type II familial hyperlipoproteinemia

ICD-9CM CODES
272.0 Pure hypercholesterolemia

EPIDEMIOLOGY & DEMOGRAPHICS

- More than half of all U.S. adults have dyslipidemia: 50.4% of men and 50.9% of women.
- Only ~12% of people with high cholesterol are being treated.
- Elevated cholesterol requires drug therapy in ~60 million Americans.
- Incidence of heterozygous familial hypercholesterolemia: ~1:500.
- Incidence of homozygous familial hypercholesterolemia: ~1:1 million.
- Prevalence of hypercholesterolemia increases with increasing age.
- Familial hypercholesterolemia: autosomal-dominant disorder.
- Familial combined hyperlipidemia: possibly an autosomal-dominant disorder.
- Multifactorial predilection: apparent in majority of affected individuals.

PHYSICAL FINDINGS & CLINICAL PRESENTATION

- A detailed medication history should be performed because some medications may affect lipid levels (e.g., thiazides, corticosteroids, beta-blockers, and estrogens).
- The physical examination should include measurements of BMI and BP, thyroid and liver assessments, and examining peripheral pulses including carotids for bruits.
- Physical findings, particularly in the familial forms may include
  1. Tendon xanthomas
  2. Xanthelasma
  3. Arcus corneae
  4. Arterial bruits (young adulthood)

ETIOLOGY

Primary:
- Genetics
- Obesity
- Dietary intake

Secondary:
- Hypothyroidism
- Diabetes mellitus
- Nephrotic syndrome
- Obstructive liver disease: Hepatoma, extrahepatic biliary obstruction, primary biliary cirrhosis
- Alcohol or tobacco use
- Drugs: Oral contraceptives, progesterone, corticosteroids, thiazide diuretics, b-blockers, androgenic steroids, retinoic acid derivatives

DIAGNOSIS

DIFFERENTIAL DIAGNOSIS

- Always consider underlying secondary causes for the elevated cholesterol.
- Patients with very high LDL cholesterol usually have genetic forms of hypercholesterolemia (see hyperlipoproteinemias). Early detection of these cases and family testing to identify similarly affected relatives is important.
- Metabolic syndrome:
  1. A constellation of lipid and nonlipid risk factors of a metabolic origin
  2. Diagnosed when three or more of the following are present: abdominal obesity (waist circumference >40 in in men and >35 in in women); triglycerides >150 mg/dl; HDL <40 mg/dl in males and <50 mg/dl in females; systolic BP >130 mmHg and diastolic BP >85 mmHg; fasting glucose >110 mg/dl

WHO SHOULD BE SCREENED:
- The National Cholesterol Education Program Adult Treatment Panel III (NCEP-ATP III) recommends screening of all adults at age 20 yr with fasting lipid profile measurement every 5 yr, regardless of their CHD risk profile.
- The USPSTF supports routine screening for men aged >35 yr and women aged >45 yr by measurement of nonfasting total and HDL cholesterol alone.
- Clinicians should also screen younger adults (men aged 20 to 35 or women aged 20 to 45) who have other risk factors for CVD, family history of premature CHD, or familial lipid disorder or who have evidence of hyperlipidemia on physical examination.
- In 2010, the USPSTF recommended routine screening for overweight and obesity in persons aged <20 yr.

LABORATORY TESTS
- Risk assessment to modify LDL goals (Table 1-75)
- Evaluate for CHD* and CHD equivalents (Table 1-76).

TREATMENT

NONPHARMACOLOGIC THERAPY
- First line of treatment: dietary therapy (use of NCEP-ATP III Therapeutic Lifestyle Change TLC Diet can result in 5% to 15% reduction in LDL cholesterol level).
- Composition of the TLC diet:
  1. Total fat 25% to 30% of total calories
  2. Polyunsaturated fat up to 10% of total calories

---

*CHD includes history of MI, unstable angina, stable angina, coronary procedures (angioplasty or bypass surgery),

  3. Monounsaturated fat up to 20% of total calories
  4. Saturated fats <7% of total calories
  5. Carbohydrate 50% to 60% of total calories
  6. Protein 15% of total calories
  7. No more than 200 mg/day of cholesterol
  8. Fiber 20 to 30 g/day
- Increased physical activity: encourage 20 to 30 min of aerobic exercise three or four times a week
- Weight reduction
- Smoking cessation
- Counseling on CAD risk factors
- Plant-based diets (including stanol-containing margarines, oat bran, and nuts) have shown effectiveness in controlling lipids.

ACUTE GENERAL Rx
No acute treatment needed

CHRONIC Rx
- Elevated LDL cholesterol is the primary target of cholesterol-lowering therapy.
- Risk assessment should be made based on the presence of risk factors (see Table 1-75), CHD and CHD risk equivalents (see Table 1-76) and 10-yr CHD risk using Framingham risk calculator (Table 1-77).
- Drug therapy should be instituted in patients with:
  - LDL >190 and 0-1 risk factor
  - LDL >160 and ≥2 risk factors and <10% 10-yr risk
  - LDL >130 and ≥2 risk factors and 10% to 20% 10-yr risk
  - LDL >100 with CHD, CHD risk equivalents, and >20% 10-yr risk
- Optional goal of LDL cholesterol <70 mg/dl is favored for "very high risk" patients, which

---

TABLE 1-75 Risk Factors That Modify LDL Goals

1. Cigarette smoking
2. Hypertension (BP ≤140/90 mm Hg or on medications)
3. Low HDL cholesterol (<40 mg/dl)*
4. Family history of premature CHD (<55 yr in first-degree male relative or <65 yr in first-degree female relative)
5. Age (men ≥45 yr, women ≥55 yr)

*HDL cholesterol >60 mg/dl counts as a negative risk factor; its presence removes one risk factor from the total count.

TABLE 1-76 Coronary Heart Disease Equivalents

1. Diabetes mellitus
2. Aortic aneurysm
3. Peripheral vascular disease (ABI <0.9)
4. Symptomatic carotid artery disease (stroke, transient ischemic attack)
5. 10-yr risk for coronary artery disease >20% using Framingham risk equation

includes the presence of established CVD plus multiple major risk factors (especially diabetes), severe and poorly controlled risk factors (especially continued cigarette smoking), multiple risk factors of the metabolic syndrome, and in patients with acute coronary syndromes.

- Non–HDL cholesterol should be secondary target of therapy in patients with elevated triglycerides (>200 mg/dl). The non–HDL cholesterol goal is 30 mg/dl higher than the LDL cholesterol goal.
- Medications that can be used (Table 1-78):
  1. Bile acid sequestrants
  2. Niacin
  3. HMG-CoA reductase inhibitors (statins)
  4. Fibric acids
  5. Ezetimibe
  6. Omega-3 fatty acids

- Bile acid sequestrants are the first-line drugs to lower cholesterol in children and in pregnant women.
- The management of metabolic syndrome includes weight reduction and increased physical activity and treatment of hypertension, elevated triglycerides, and low HDL cholesterol.

DISPOSITION AND FOLLOW-UP

- The NCEP-ATP III recommends that a 3- to 6-mo trial of lifestyle changes and TLC diet should be completed before initiating treatment.
- It also recommends that 6 weekly reassessments with fasting lipid profiles should be performed once lipid lowering therapy is initiated and further intensification of therapy be considered until goal LDL cholesterol is achieved.

- The ACP guideline does not recommend routine liver function tests in patients treated with statins.
- Counseling about behavioral lifestyle changes and risk factors for CHD should be provided at every follow-up visit.

REFERRAL

Patients with rare lipid disorders, hyperlipoproteinemias, patients resistant to treatment, on complex regimens, and with evidence of disease progression despite treatment should be referred to a lipid specialist.

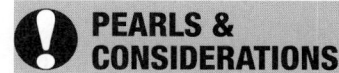

COMMENTS

- Nonoptimal levels of LDL and HDL cholesterol during young adulthood are independently associated with coronary atherosclerosis 2 decades later.
- The American Academy of Pediatrics (AAP) guideline (*Pediatrics* 122:198, 2008) recommends consideration towards pharmacologic treatment for children with LDL >190 mg/dl or >160 mg/dl if other risk factors are present
- See "Hyperlipoproteinemia" topic for additional information on hypercholesterolemia.

SUGGESTED READINGS

available at www.expertconsult.com

AUTHOR: **PRIYA BANSAL, M.D., M.P.H.**

TABLE 1-77 Framingham Risk Calculator

Risk Group	Goal LDL Cholesterol (mg/dl)	Initiate Therapeutic Lifestyle Changes	Consider Drug Therapy
High Risk CHD or CHD equivalents (>20% 10-yr risk)	<100 (optional goal <70)	>100	>130 (optional if <100)
Moderately High Risk >2 risk factors (10%-20% 10-yr risk)	<130 (optional goal <100)	>130	>130 (optional if 100-129)
Moderate Risk >2 risk factors (<10% 10-yr risk)	<130	>130	>160
Lower Risk 0-1 risk factor	<160	>160	>190 (optional if 160-189)

TABLE 1-78 Drugs Affecting Lipoprotein Metabolism

Drug Class	Agents and Daily Doses	Lipid/Lipoprotein Effects	Side Effects	Contraindications
HMG-CoA reductase inhibitors (statins)	Lovastatin (10-40 mg) Pravastatin (10-80 mg) Simvastatin (5-80 mg) Fluvastatin (20-40 mg) Atorvastatin (10-80 mg) Rosuvastatin (5-40 mg) Pitavastatin (2-4 mg)	LDL ↓ 20%-60% HDL ↑ 5%-15% TG ↓ 7%-30%	Myalgias, myositis increased liver enzymes	Active or chronic liver disease Pregnancy Concomitant use of certain drugs*
Bile acid sequestrants	Colestipol (5-20 g) Colesevelam (2.6-3.8 g) Cholestyramine (4-16 g)	LDL ↓ 15%-30% HDL ↑ 3%-5% TG No change or increase	Gastrointestinal distress, constipation, drug interaction, hypertriglyceridemia	TG >300 mg/dl GI motility disorder
Omega-3 fatty acids	Fish oils (4-6 g)	TG ↓ 45% HDL ↑ 13%	Increase bleeding time nausea	Caution with anticoagulant therapy
Nicotinic acid	Immediate release (niacin) (1.5-3 g) Extended-release (Niaspan) (1-2 g)	LDL ↓ 5%-25% HDL ↑ 15%-35% TG ↓ 20%-50%	Flushing hyperglycemia hyperuricemia (or gout) upper GI distress hepatotoxicity	Chronic liver disease Severe gout Diabetes Peptic ulcer disease Pregnancy/lactation
Fibric acids	Gemfibrozil (600 mg bid) Fenofibrate (45-145 mg)	LDL ↓ 5%-20% HDL ↑ 10%-20% TG ↓ 20%-50%	Dyspepsia gallstones myopathy	Severe renal disease Severe hepatic disease Caution with statins Can worsen LDL cholesterol
Ezetimibe (cholesterol absorption inhibitor)	Ezetimibe (10 mg)	LDL ↓ 18% HDL ↑ 1% TG ↓ 8%	Abdominal pain; myalgias	Liver disease Avoid with resins and fibrates

Modified from The National Cholesterol Education Program, *JAMA* 285:2486, 2001.
*Cyclosporine, macrolide antibiotics, various antifungal agents, and cytochrome P-450 inhibitors (fibrates and niacin should be used with appropriate caution).

BASIC INFORMATION

DEFINITION

An inherited or acquired condition associated with an increased risk of thrombosis

SYNONYMS

Thrombophilia

ICD-9CM CODES
289.8 Hypercoagulable state

EPIDEMIOLOGY & DEMOGRAPHICS

See Table 1-79.

- Risk of thrombosis increases with age and with multiple risk factors.
- Most people with a genetic defect will not have thrombotic disease. When thrombosis occurs, it is often associated with an acquired risk factor (e.g., surgery, pregnancy, oral contraceptive [OC] use). Annual risk of thrombosis is <1%.
- Low risk of recurrent thrombosis in patients with a single genetic defect.
- Multiple genetic defects are not uncommon (1% to 2% prevalence in patients with idiopathic venous thromboembolism [VTE]); strong synergistic effect when multiple defects are present.
- Approximately half of patients with unprovoked thrombosis have an identifiable inherited thrombophilia.
- Significant variations in the prevalence rates and thrombotic risks for thrombophilia are reported. This may reflect geographic variation in the prevalence of genetic defects, different populations, or the presence of other unidentified thrombophilic risk factors.

HISTORY

A hypercoagulable state is strongly suggested by the following:

- Age <50 yr at first episode of unprovoked thrombosis
- Family history: first-degree relative with thrombosis at age <50 yr
- Recurrent thrombotic events
- Thrombosis in unusual anatomic location (i.e., portal, hepatic, mesenteric, or cerebral vein)

- Thrombosis associated with pregnancy or OC use
- Warfarin-induced skin necrosis
- Adverse pregnancy outcomes may be associated with thrombophilia: recurrent pregnancy loss, preeclampsia, placental abruption, intrauterine growth restriction. Association is weak for inherited thrombophilias but strong for antiphospholipid antibodies

PHYSICAL FINDINGS & CLINICAL PRESENTATION

- Inherited thrombophilia is usually associated with VTE, most commonly deep vein thrombosis (DVT)
- Some acquired thrombophilias are associated with arterial thrombosis
- Pregnancy complications
- Medical conditions associated with increased risk of thrombosis

ETIOLOGY

See Table 1-79. The differential diagnosis of the patient presenting with thrombosis or thrombotic diathesis is described in Section II.

- Often a multifactorial process with genetic, environmental, and acquired factors.
- Thrombotic risk increases with use of OCs or hormone replacement therapy (HRT) and during the pregnancy/postpartum period.
- Adverse pregnancy outcomes may be caused by thrombosis of the uteroplacental circulation.

INHERITED:

Factor V Leiden (FVL) mutation:

- Autosomal-dominant mutation with low penetrance.
- Causes activated protein C resistance (APCR); 90% of APCR is caused by FVL mutation.
- Most common inherited thrombophilia; accounts for 40% to 50% of cases.
- OC use in heterozygous carriers is associated with an eightfold increased risk of VTE compared with noncarriers and a thirty-fivefold increased risk of VTE compared with noncarriers not using OCs.
- May be associated with cardiovascular disease in select high-risk subgroups.

Prothrombin G20210A mutation:

- Autosomal-dominant mutation with low penetrance.
- OC use in heterozygous carriers is associated with a sixteenfold increased risk of VTE compared with noncarriers not using OCs.

- May be associated with cardiovascular disease in select high-risk subgroups and young patients with ischemic stroke.

Protein C, protein S, antithrombin (AT) deficiency:

- Autosomal-dominant inheritance; many mutations identified for each of these conditions.
- Decreased level (type I deficiency) or abnormal function (type II deficiency).
- First episode of thrombosis is usually in young adults.

Protein C and protein S:

- Homozygous condition is very rare; usually associated with lethal thrombosis in infancy.
- Associated with warfarin-induced skin necrosis, which occurs secondary to depletion of vitamin K–dependent anticoagulant factors sooner than procoagulant factors in the first few days of therapy.

AT deficiency:

- Most thrombogenic of the inherited thrombophilias; 50% lifetime risk of thrombosis.
- Homozygous condition is very rare, probably not compatible with normal fetal development.
- Arterial thrombosis can occur rarely.
- Can cause heparin resistance.

Elevated factor VIII level:

- May be an important risk factor for thrombosis in African-American population.
- Increased risk of recurrent thrombosis.
- Genetic etiology is suspected but not yet identified.

Other possible causes: Non-O blood group, dysfibrinogenemia, elevated thrombin-activatable fibrinolysis inhibitor, elevated factor IX and factor XI levels

ACQUIRED:

Antiphospholipid antibody syndrome (APS):

- Most common cause of acquired thrombophilia.
- Can present as arterial or venous thrombosis, recurrent pregnancy loss, and adverse pregnancy outcomes.
- Thromboembolic events occur in up to 30% of population; high risk of recurrent thrombosis (up to 70% reported).
- See "Antiphospholipid Antibody Syndrome" for more information.

Hyperhomocysteinemia:

- Can be inherited (most commonly an autosomal recessive mutation in methylene tetrahydrofolate reductase gene) but more fre-

TABLE 1-79   Hypercoagulable Conditions

	Prevalence in General Population (%)	Prevalence in Population with Thrombosis (%)	A/V Events	Relative Risk of Thrombosis
FVL mutation	5% of whites; rare in nonwhites	12%-40%	V	Heterozygous: 3-7; homozygous: 80
Prothrombin G20210A mutation	3% of whites; rare in nonwhites	6%-18%	V	3
AT deficiency	0.02%	1%-3%	V	20-50
PC deficiency	0.2%-0.4%	3%-5%	V	7-15
PS deficiency	0.03%-0.1%	1%-5%	V	5-11
Antiphospholipid antibody syndrome	1%-2%	5%-21%	V + A	2-11
Hyperhomocysteinemia	5%-7%	10%	V + A	3
Elevated factor VIII level	11%	25%	V + A	5

A, Arterial; AT, antithrombin; FVL, factor V Leiden; PC, protein C; PS, protein S; V, venous.

quently acquired; folate, vitamin B_6, or vitamin B_{12} deficiency account for two thirds of cases. Other acquired causes include renal disease, hypothyroidism, malignancy, smoking, and certain medications.

- Acquired causes may be associated with VTE and atherosclerotic disease (cardiovascular, cerebrovascular, and peripheral vascular). Inherited causes may be associated with atherosclerotic disease and adverse pregnancy outcomes.

Conditions associated with increased risk of thrombosis:

- Prior thrombosis
- Trauma
- Medical illness: heart failure, respiratory failure, infection, diabetes mellitus, obesity, nephrotic syndrome, inflammatory bowel disease, paroxysmal nocturnal hemoglobinuria, sickle cell anemia
- Pregnancy (sixfold increased risk of VTE), postpartum, OC use (fourfold increased risk, higher risk with third-generation OCs), transdermal contraceptive patch, HRT (twofold increased risk), tamoxifen, raloxifene
- Immobilization, travel
- Surgery (especially orthopedic), central venous catheters
- Hyperviscosity syndromes
- Myeloproliferative disorders
- Malignancy: disease or treatment related
- Heparin-induced thrombocytopenia and thrombosis
- Smoking

Dx DIAGNOSIS

WORKUP

- History (presence of conditions or use of medications predisposing to thrombosis, family history of thrombosis), physical examination, laboratory tests, imaging studies.
- Age-appropriate cancer screening.
- No consensus exists regarding screening for thrombophilia; little cost-effectiveness or outcomes data are available. Thrombophilia screening is probably overused, as results usually don't change management.
- Thrombophilia screening is not recommended for primary prevention of VTE; some advocate testing prior to OC use or pregnancy in women with a strong family history of thrombosis or thrombophilia.
- Screening not recommended if VTE was associated with an identified risk factor. A possible exception is thrombosis associated with pregnancy, the postpartum period or with OC use.
- Unprovoked VTE:
  - Screen individuals for APCR, prothrombin G20210A mutation, protein C, protein S, AT deficiency, and APS if any of the following are present: <50 yr of age at first episode of thrombosis, family history of thrombosis, recurrent thrombosis, thrombosis in unusual anatomic location, life-threatening thrombotic event, warfarin-induced skin necrosis, thrombosis in

pregnancy/postpartum /with OC use, or characteristic pregnancy complications.
  - Screen all Caucasians <50 yr of age and all women on HRT for APCR, prothrombin G20210A mutation, and APS.
  - Screen all others for APS.
- Arterial thrombosis: Screen for APS.
- Note: Routine screening for factor VIII level or hyperhomocysteinemia is not recommended.

TIMING OF WORKUP:

- Ideally >3 wk after discontinuation of anticoagulation (except for APS, which requires prolonged anticoagulation).
- Note: Acute thrombosis, anticoagulation, pregnancy, and many medical conditions can affect the results and must be considered in the timing and interpretation of the workup.

LABORATORY TESTS

- CBC with peripheral smear, electrolytes, calcium, renal and liver function tests, prothrombin time/partial thromboplastin time, prostate-specific antigen (in men aged >50 yr), urinalysis
- Note: Genetic counseling and written informed consent should be obtained before genetic testing. Abnormal nongenetic tests should be repeated after 6 wk to decrease false-positive results.
- APCR: APC-resistance assay (using factor V–deficient plasma) and if positive confirm with genetic test for FVL mutation; use genetic test if lupus anticoagulant present.
- Prothrombin G20210A mutation test.
- AT, protein C, and protein S deficiency: functional assays; if decreased perform antigenic assay to determine type of deficiency. Antigenic assays for protein S should measure free and total levels. In protein C and protein S deficiency, the functional assay may be falsely low in the presence of APCR or elevated factor VIII level and falsely high if lupus anticoagulant is present.
- APS: any of the following found on two occasions at least 12 wk apart: lupus anticoagulant or anticardiolipin antibodies or anti–B_2-glycoprotein-I antibodies.
- Hyperhomocysteinemia: fasting plasma homocysteine level (if normal but suspicion is high, can proceed with methionine loading test and genotyping for methylene tetrahydrofolate reductase).
- Factor VIII level functional assay.

IMAGING STUDIES

Chest radiograph and other tests as appropriate to diagnose thrombosis and rule out associated conditions

Rx TREATMENT

NONPHARMACOLOGIC THERAPY

OC/HRT use and smoking should be avoided.

PROPHYLAXIS

- Prophylactic anticoagulation in high-risk situations.

- Patients with AT deficiency may benefit from antithrombin concentrates in high-risk situations.
- Although homocysteine levels can be lowered with folic acid, vitamin B_6, and vitamin B_{12} supplements, correcting hyperhomocysteinemia does not decrease risk of thrombosis and routine supplementation is not indicated.
- Vitamin E supplements may decrease risk of VTE in women.
- Pregnancy prophylaxis: timing and intensity of therapy is based on the patient's risk (genetic or acquired defect and clinical history). Women with thrombophilia and recurrent adverse pregnancy outcomes may benefit from prophylaxis with heparin and low-dose aspirin.

ACUTE GENERAL Rx

Initial therapy is the same as for individuals without thrombophilia (exceptions for protein C and AT deficiency).

Venous thrombosis:

- Begin low-molecular-weight heparin (LMWH) and warfarin simultaneously. Continue heparin for at least 5 days and until international normalized ratio (INR) is therapeutic for 2 consecutive days; continue warfarin for at least 3 mo. Aim for INR of 2 to 3. Unfractionated heparin (UH) or Fondaparinux (factor Xa inhibitor) may be used as alternatives to LMWH. LMWH is preferred over UH (except in patients with massive pulmonary embolism, increased risk of bleeding or renal failure) because of equivalent or superior effectiveness and a better safety profile.
- Thrombophilia is not associated with a higher risk of recurrent VTE during warfarin therapy, with the exception of cancer patients in whom LMWH for 3 to 6 mo is associated with lower rates of recurrence than warfarin therapy.
- In pregnancy, anticoagulate with heparin throughout pregnancy and for at least 6 wk postpartum. Minimum duration of anticoagulation should be 6 mo. LMWH is preferred over UH. Warfarin may be used postpartum.
- Consider thrombolysis or thrombectomy in patients with massive pulmonary embolism or large proximal lower extremity DVT.

Protein C deficiency:

- Warfarin-induced skin necrosis: Discontinue warfarin, give vitamin K, and start heparin anticoagulation. Consider protein C replacement with protein C concentrate or fresh frozen plasma. Warfarin may be restarted at a low dose (2 mg qd for 3 days and increase by 2 to 3 mg qd until target INR is reached). Continue heparin for at least 5 days and until warfarin-induced anticoagulation is achieved.

AT deficiency:

- AT concentrates may be used if difficulty achieving anticoagulation (heparin resistance), severe thrombosis, or recurrent thrombosis despite adequate anticoagulation.

Arterial thrombosis:

- Anticoagulation and evaluation for thrombolysis or surgery.

Duration of therapy:
- Optimal duration of anticoagulation remains unknown. Length of therapy may be individualized by assessing the risk of recurrence. Residual thrombosis (on ultrasonography) or elevated D-dimer levels after completion of anticoagulation are associated with an increased risk of recurrence. With these findings, consider prolonging anticoagulation.
- Must consider risk and benefit; risk of major bleeding 2% to 3% annually in general population on anticoagulation but higher in the elderly (7% to 9% per year). Long-term anticoagulation is usually not indicated given the low risk of recurrent thrombosis for most conditions and the bleeding risk associated with anticoagulation.
- Indefinite anticoagulation considered if ≥2 spontaneous thromboses or spontaneous thrombosis associated with any of the following:
  1. Life-threatening thrombosis or thrombosis at an unusual site
  2. More than a single genetic defect
  3. Presence of AT deficiency or APS
- Patients with active cancer may benefit from indefinite anticoagulation.

DISPOSITION
Depends on underlying condition

REFERRAL
Hematology, maternal-fetal medicine, obstetric medicine

 PEARLS & CONSIDERATIONS

- Warfarin therapy effectively reduces the risk of recurrent VTE; when therapy is discontinued VTE risk increases.
- Previous episode of VTE is a major risk factor for recurrence regardless of the presence of thrombophilia. Risk is greatest in the first 2 yr after thrombosis. ~20% of all patients with unprovoked VTE have recurrence within 5 yr.
- Risk of post thrombotic syndrome decreases if compression stockings are worn for at least 1 year, starting in the first month after the DVT.
- Genetic risk factors for thrombosis in nonwhites remain largely unknown.
- Interpreting workup: many medical conditions cause acquired abnormalities.
  - Acute thrombosis may be associated with lupus anticoagulant, increased anticardiolipin antibodies, and elevated factor VIII levels
  - Heparin therapy: antithrombin levels decrease by up to 30%; can affect lupus anticoagulant testing
  - Warfarin therapy: cannot measure protein C and protein S (levels and function decrease); antithrombin levels may increase; can affect lupus anticoagulant testing
  - Protein C, protein S, and antithrombin levels decrease with acute thrombosis (<2 wk), surgery, liver disease, disseminated intravascular coagulation and chemotherapy. Protein C level also decreases with severe infection but levels increase with age and hyperlipidemia. Protein S and Antithrombin levels also decrease with nephrotic syndrome, pregnancy and estrogen therapy (HRT, OC)
  - APCR is increased with pregnancy, estrogen therapy (HRT, OCs), and certain cancers; elevated factor VIII level and antiphospholipid antibodies can cause APCR

SUGGESTED READINGS
available at www.expertconsult.com

AUTHOR: **SUDEEP KAUR AULAKH, M.D.**

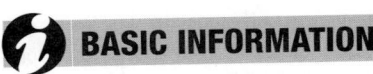

BASIC INFORMATION

DEFINITION

Hyperemesis gravidarum is persistent nausea and vomiting with onset in the first trimester of pregnancy, resulting in weight loss and fluid and electrolyte and acid–base imbalances.

ICD-9CM CODES
643.1 Hyperemesis gravidarum

EPIDEMIOLOGY & DEMOGRAPHICS

INCIDENCE: 0.5 to 10 cases per 1000 pregnancies
GENETICS: No genetic disposition
RISK FACTORS:
- Multiple pregnancy
- Molar pregnancy
- Previous history of unsuccessful pregnancy
- Nulliparity
- Hyperemesis gravidarum in a prior pregnancy
- No correlation with race, socioeconomic status, or marital status

PEAK ONSET: 8 to 12 wk of gestation

PHYSICAL FINDINGS & CLINICAL PRESENTATION

- Weight loss
- Rapid heart rate
- Fall in blood pressure
- Dry mucous membranes
- Loss of skin elasticity
- Ketotic odor
- In severe cases, Wernicke's encephalopathy as a result of thiamine deficiency

ETIOLOGY

Specific etiology is unknown.

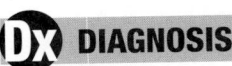

DIAGNOSIS

DIFFERENTIAL DIAGNOSIS

- Pancreatitis
- Cholecystitis
- Hepatitis
- Pyelonephritis

WORKUP

Hyperemesis gravidarum is a diagnosis of exclusion. A detailed history and physical examination along with laboratory tests to rule out other causes of vomiting in early pregnancy are indicated (see Box 1-6).

LABORATORY TESTS

- Urinalysis to document ketonuria and proteinuria
- Urine culture and sensitivity to rule out pyelonephritis
- Serum electrolytes to rule out electrolyte and acid–base imbalance
- Serum concentration of aminotransferases and bilirubin to rule out hepatitis
- Serum amylase to rule out pancreatitis
- Free T_4 and thyroid-stimulating hormone (TSH). (Elevated T_4 with suppressed TSH levels present in as many as 60% of patients with hyperemesis gravidarum. This biochemical hyperthyroidism usually spontaneously resolves after 18 wk.)

IMAGING STUDIES

- Pelvic ultrasound examination to rule out multiple gestation and molar pregnancy
- Ultrasound of the gallbladder to rule out cholecystitis

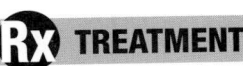

TREATMENT

NONPHARMACOLOGIC THERAPY

- Reassurance
- Psychologic support
- Avoidance of foods that trigger nausea
- Frequent small meals once oral intake has resumed
- Acupressure with the use of a wrist band
- Ginger has been studied as a promising herbal remedy, but data are relatively sparse

ACUTE GENERAL Rx

- Nothing by mouth order.
- Fluid and electrolyte replacement.
- Parenteral vitamin supplementation.
- Daily supplementation of thiamine 100 mg IM or IV to prevent Wernicke's encephalopathy.
- Pyridoxine (vitamin B_6) 30 mg daily may reduce nausea.
- Antiemetics, such as promethazine (Phenergan) or droperidol (Inapsine), have not been found to be associated with fetal malformations when given in early pregnancy. Promethazine given as a low-dose continuous infusion of 25 mg in each liter of IV fluid has been shown to be effective in controlling nausea and vomiting.
- The combination of doxylamine and vitamin B_6 has been used effectively in the past. A series of lawsuits alleging neonatal abnormalities prevented its use despite the fact the FDA and others found no association with fetal defects.
- Recently, the use of ondansetron (Zofran) has been found to be very effective in this disorder although the cost is somewhat limiting.
- Restart oral intake gradually no less than 48 hr after vomiting has ceased.

CHRONIC Rx

If the previous acute therapy does not resolve vomiting and oral intake is not feasible, parenteral hyperalimentation may be necessary.

DISPOSITION

- Untreated hyperemesis gravidarum can result in maternal renal and hepatic damage or death from fluid and electrolyte imbalance.
- Hyperemesis gravidarum with severe weight loss has been associated with lower average birth weight and central nervous system malformations in neonates.

REFERRAL

For parenteral hyperalimentation if required

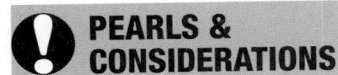

PEARLS & CONSIDERATIONS

COMMENTS

Although the specific etiology of hyperemesis gravidarum is not known, psychogenic causes proposed in older literature have been largely discredited. "Behavioral therapies" for hyperemesis gravidarum are inappropriate.

SUGGESTED READING
available at www.expertconsult.com

AUTHORS: **LAUREL M. WHITE, M.D.,** and **RUBEN ALVERO, M.D.**

BOX 1-6   Diagnostic Evaluation of the Expected Hyperemetic Patient

History: Young primigravida, single parent, ambivalent about pregnancy, Caucasian, high socioeconomic class, dependent personality
Physical: Postural vital signs, dry mucous membranes, poor skin turgor, in severe cases hepatocellular jaundice, generally clear lungs, nontender abdomen and no costovertebral angle tenderness, normal uterine size for gestational age but may be enlarged secondary to multiple gestation or molar pregnancy
Laboratory: Serum-positive pregnancy test (b-hCG), hypokalemia, hyponatremia, hypochloremia, metabolic alkalosis, elevated blood urea nitrogen (BUN) and creatinine, urine ketosis and elevated specific gravity of urine
Other differential diagnoses:
    Medical conditions: gallbladder disease, hepatitis, pancreatitis, gastroenteritis, appendicitis, pyelonephritis
    Pregnancy conditions: molar pregnancy, twin gestation

From Carl KJ et al: *Primary care of women,* ed 2, St Louis, 2002, Mosby.

BASIC INFORMATION

DEFINITION

Hypereosinophilic syndrome (HES) refers to a group of disorders of unknown cause characterized by sustained overproduction of eosinophils, in which eosinophilic infiltration and mediators release cause organ dysfunction.

SYNONYMS

Idiopathic hypereosinophilic syndrome (IHES)

ICD-9CM CODES
288.3 Hypereosinophilic syndrome

EPIDEMIOLOGY & DEMOGRAPHICS

PREDOMINANT SEX: Occurs in men more often than women (9:1)
PREDOMINANT AGE: Usually occurs between the ages of 20 and 50 yr

PHYSICAL FINDINGS & CLINICAL PRESENTATION

- Clinical presentation of HES may vary from an incidental finding of eosinophilia to sudden onset of cardiac or neurologic symptoms.
- Early presentation includes fatigue, cough, breathlessness, muscle pain, angioedema, rash, and fever.
- Cardiac manifestations (58%) include dyspnea, orthopnea, and signs and symptoms of congestive heart failure. Including three stages: Acute necrotic stage secondary to endocardial infiltration of eosinophils, Thrombus formation and fibrotic stage. This may result in a restrictive or dilated cardiomyopathy and/or valvular heart disease.
- Neurologic manifestations (54%) may be of three types:
  1. Thromboembolic (e.g., cardiac emboli or local vascular thrombosis)
  2. CNS dysfunction: confusion, loss of memory, ataxia, upper motor neuron signs, seizures, and behavior changes
  3. Peripheral neuropathy (most common) may be symmetric or asymmetric, sensory or mixed sensory and motor deficits
- Pulmonary manifestations (40%) include a chronic persistent nonproductive cough, shortness of breath, and dyspnea on exertion. Diffuse or focal infiltrate may present in 20% of cases. Complications may include pulmonary fibrosis, congestive heart failure (CHF), or pulmonary embolus (PE).
- Cutaneous manifestations (56%) usually include eczema, lichenifications, urticaria, angioedema, or erythematous pruritic papules and nodules.
- GI manifestations (23%) include diarrhea, but findings of gastritis, colitis, pancreatitis, cholangitis, and hepatitis can occur.
- Ocular manifestations (23%) are thought to be the result of retinal microemboli.
- Vascular manifestations include venous or arterial thrombosis of unknown mechanism such as femoral artery occlusion, intracranial sinus thrombosis, and digital gangrene.

ETIOLOGY

- The etiology of HES is unknown and is thought of as a composite of many diseases.
- In some cases, a fusion event generating an abnormal and oncogenic tyrosine kinase (FIP1L1-PDGFRA) appears to be causative especially in males.

DIAGNOSIS

Criteria for the diagnosis of idiopathic HES include:
- Persistent eosinophilia of >1500 eosinophils/mm^3 for more than 6 mo
- Exclusion of other conditions causing eosinophilia (e.g., parasites, allergies)
- Signs and symptoms of organ system dysfunction (e.g., heart, liver, lung)

DIFFERENTIAL DIAGNOSIS

The differential includes all causes of peripheral blood eosinophilia. Parasitic infections, coccidioidomycosis, cat-scratch disease, asthma, Churg-Strauss syndrome, allergic rhinitis, atopic dermatitis, drug-induced eosinophilia, aspergillosis, eosinophilic pneumonia, hypersensitivity pneumonitis, HIV, eosinophilic gastroenteritis, inflammatory bowel disease, leukemias (CML and CMML), systemic mastocytosis with eosinophilia.

WORKUP

The workup of a patient who is suspected of having HES should exclude other causes mentioned in the "Differential Diagnosis" section leading to peripheral eosinophilia.

LABORATORY TESTS

- CBC with differential; often the total WBC ranges from 10,000 to 30,000/mm^3 with eosinophilia of 30% to 70%, anemia is present in 50% of the cases, and either thrombocytopenia or thrombocytosis may be noted
- Erythrocyte sedimentation rate (ESR) and rheumatoid factor
- Liver function tests (LFTs), electrolytes, urinalysis, BUN, and creatinine
- HIV assay
- Stools for ova and parasites ×3
- Serologic blood tests for parasitic infections (e.g., Strongyloides)
- Total IgE level
- Bone marrow aspirate and biopsy
- Duodenal aspirate
- ECG
- Tissue biopsies as indicated
- Serum levels of vitamin B$_{12}$
- Serum levels of tryptase

IMAGING STUDIES

- Chest radiograph may be clear or show infiltrates, effusions, or fibrotic scarring
- CT scan of chest, abdomen, and pelvis
- Echocardiogram (or cardiac MRI for early cardiac involvement) can assess for ventricular function and valvular pathology including regurgitation and thrombi formation

TREATMENT

Treatment is initiated only if there is evidence of organ involvement.

NONPHARMACOLOGIC THERAPY

In patients with hypereosinophilia without organ involvement, serial echocardiograms, blood chemistries, and pulmonary function tests are recommended at 6-mo intervals.

ACUTE GENERAL Rx

- In patients with organ involvement without FIP1L1-PDGFRA fusion, initial therapy is with prednisone 1 mg/kg/day or 60 mg/day in adults.
- Patient's symptoms and peripheral eosinophil counts are monitored.
- Doses may be tapered to alternate-day prednisone use in patients whose eosinophil counts have been suppressed.

CHRONIC Rx

- Patients not responding to corticosteroids, hydroxyurea 1 to 2 g/day may be tried.
- Patient with FIP1L1-PDGFRA fusion with or without organ involvement should be started on tyrosine kinase imatinib or dasatinib for resistant cases.
- If the disease continues to progress, vincristine, etoposide, interferon-α, cyclosporine, and leukapheresis are alternative choices.
- Anticoagulation and/or antiplatelet agents are often used in patients with HES.
- If all else fails, bone marrow transplantation may be considered.

DISPOSITION

- Before the use of cardiac imaging (echo) and cardiac surgeries (valve replacement), patients with HES had a poor prognosis with a mean survival of 9 mo and a 3-yr survival of 12%.
- Deaths usually result from congestive heart failure, endocarditis, and systemic emboli.
- 5-yr and 15-yr survival rates are 80% and 42%, respectively.

REFERRAL

HES is a rare and complicated disorder requiring a multidisciplinary approach.

PEARLS & CONSIDERATIONS

COMMENTS

There is still much to be learned about HES. The etiology and exact mechanism of organ damage caused by eosinophils remains unknown.

SUGGESTED READINGS

available at www.expertconsult.com

AUTHORS: **MONZR M. AL MALKI, M.D.**, **DENNIS J. MIKOLICH, M.D.**, and **GLENN G. FORT, M.D., M.P.H.**

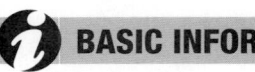

BASIC INFORMATION

DEFINITION

- Primary hyperlipoproteinemia is a group of genetic disorders of the lipid transport proteins in the blood that manifests as abnormally elevated levels of cholesterol, triglycerides, or both in the serum of affected patients.
- Usually defined as total cholesterol, LDL, triglycerides or lipoprotein A levels above 90th percentile or HDL or apo A-1 levels below the 10th percentile for the general population. Table 1-80 describes the ATP classification for cholesterol.

SYNONYMS

Hyperlipidemia

ICD-9CM CODES
272.4 Hyperlipoproteinemia
272.3 Fredrickson type I
272.0 Fredrickson type IIa
272.2 Fredrickson type IIb, III
272.1 Fredrickson type IV
272.3 Fredrickson type V

EPIDEMIOLOGY & DEMOGRAPHICS

INCIDENCE: The most common types are lipoprotein A excess, hypertriglyceridemia, and combined hyperlipidemia.
GENETICS:
- Familial lipoprotein lipase deficiency: autosomal recessive, resulting in an elevation in the plasma chylomicrons and triglycerides
- Familial apoprotein CII deficiency: autosomal recessive, resulting in increased serum chylomicrons, very-low-density lipoprotein (VLDL), and hypertriglyceridemia
- Familial type 3 hyperlipoproteinemia: single-gene defect requiring contributory factors to manifest
- Familial hypercholesterolemia: autosomal-dominant defect of the LDL receptor, resulting in an elevated serum cholesterol level and normal triglycerides
- Familial hypertriglyceridemia: common, autosomal-dominant defect resulting in elevated VLDL and triglycerides
- Multiple lipoprotein–type hyperlipidemia: autosomal dominant, manifesting as isolated hypercholesterolemia, isolated hypertriglyceridemia, or hyperlipidemia
- Polygenic hypercholesterolemia: multifactorial
- Polygenic hyperalphalipoproteinemia: autosomal dominant or polygenic, causing an elevated high-density lipoprotein

PHYSICAL FINDINGS & CLINICAL PRESENTATION

- Familial lipoprotein lipase deficiency: recurrent bouts of abdominal pain in infancy, eruptive xanthomas, hepatomegaly, splenomegaly, lipemia retinalis
- Familial apoprotein CII deficiency: occasional eruptive xanthomas

- Familial type 3 hyperlipoproteinemia: xanthoma striata palmaris or tuberoeruptive xanthomas, xanthelasmas, arterial bruits at a young age, gangrene of the lower extremities at a young age
- Familial hypercholesterolemia: tendon xanthomas, arcus corneae, xanthelasma
- Familial hypertriglyceridemia: associated obesity; eruptive xanthomas can develop with exacerbations

ETIOLOGY

- Genetic defects causing lipid abnormalities
- Environmental influences including diet, drugs, and alcohol intake

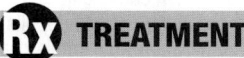

DIAGNOSIS

DIFFERENTIAL DIAGNOSIS

Secondary causes of hyperlipoproteinemias:
- Hypothyroidism
- Diabetes mellitus
- Pancreatitis
- Autoimmune hyperlipoproteinemia
- Nephrotic syndrome
- Biliary obstruction

WORKUP

- Family history for premature cardiac disease
- Personal history of recurrent pancreatitis
- Detailed physical examination

LABORATORY TESTS

- Standard lipid profile
- If normal, further testing with measurement of lipoprotein A, apo B, and apo A-1

TABLE 1-80 ATP III Classification of LDL, Total, and HDL Cholesterol (mg/dl)

LDL cholesterol

<100	Optimal
100-129	Near or above optimal
130-159	Borderline high
160-189	High
≥190	Very high

Total cholesterol

<200	Desirable
200-239	Borderline high
>240	High

HDL cholesterol

<40	Low
>60	High

From National Cholesterol Education Program Expert Panel on Detection, Evaluation, and Treatment of High Blood Cholesterol in Adults (Adult Treatment Panel III), National Institutes of Health, *JAMA* 285:2486, 2001.
ATP, Adult treatment panel; *HDL,* high-density lipoprotein; *LDL,* low-density lipoprotein.

- Lipoprotein electrophoresis and ultracentrifugation (for phenotypic classification)
- Workup for secondary causes: TSH, fasting glucose, liver function, renal function, urinary protein

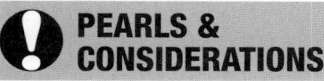

TREATMENT

NONPHARMACOLOGIC THERAPY

- Cornerstone of treatment: dietary therapy
  - TLC diet (**t**herapeutic **l**ifestyle **c**hanges): see "hyperlipidemias" section
- Risk factor reduction includes smoking cessation, treatment of hypertension, exercise
- Familial lipoprotein lipase deficiency and familial apoprotein CII deficiency: fat-free diet
- Remainder of cases, except those with polygenic hyperalphalipoproteinemia: fat- and cholesterol-restricted diets
- Interventions to improve adherence are described in Table 1-81

ACUTE GENERAL Rx

No acute treatment needed

CHRONIC Rx

- Familial lipoprotein lipase deficiency, polygenic hyperalphalipoproteinemia, or familial apoprotein CII deficiency: no chronic drug therapy
- Familial type 3 hyperlipoproteinemia: usually responds well to secondary causes being treated and diet therapy; if not, fibric acids may be tried
- Familial hypercholesterolemia: bile acid sequestrants, HMG-CoA reductase inhibitors, or niacin
- Familial hypertriglyceridemia: fibric acids
- Multiple lipoprotein–type hyperlipidemia: drug therapy aimed at the predominant lipid abnormality noted
- Recent data suggest in patients with lipoprotein abnormalities that treatment goals should be based on non-HDL cholesterol rather than LDL cholesterol

DISPOSITION

- Those with polygenic hyperalphalipoproteinemia: excellent prognosis for longevity
- Those with familial hypercholesterolemia, familial type 3 hypercholesterolemia, or multiple lipoprotein–type hyperlipidemia: even with aggressive treatment, at high risk for accelerated atherosclerosis and coronary artery disease

PEARLS & CONSIDERATIONS

COMMENTS

- Patient information is available through the American Heart Association.
- Lipid-lowering drug therapy is recommended for children ≥10 yr whose LDL-C levels re-

TABLE 1-81 Interventions to Improve Adherence

Focus on the Patient

Simplify medication regimens.

Provide explicit patient instruction and use good counseling techniques to teach the patient how to follow the prescribed treatment.

Encourage the use of prompts to help patients remember treatment regimens.

Use systems to reinforce adherence and maintain contact with the patient.

Encourage the support of family and friends.

Reinforce and reward adherence.

Increase visits for patients unable to achieve treatment goal.

Increase the convenience and access to care.

Involve patients in their care through self-monitoring.

Focus on the Physician and Medical Office

Teach physicians to implement lipid treatment guidelines.

Use reminders to prompt physicians to attend to lipid management.

Identify a patient advocate in the office to help deliver or prompt care.

Use patients to prompt preventive care.

Develop a standardized treatment plan to structure care.

Use feedback from past performance to foster change in future care.

Remind patients of appointments and follow up missed appointments.

Focus on the Health Delivery System

Provide lipid management through a lipid clinic.

Utilize case management by nurses.

Deploy telemedicine.

Utilize the collaborative care of pharmacists.

Execute critical care pathways in hospitals.

From National Cholesterol Education Program Expert Panel on Detection, Evaluation, and Treatment of High Blood Cholesterol in Adults (Adult Treatment Panel III), National Institutes of Health, *JAMA* 285:2486, 2001.

main extremely elevated after 6 mo to 1 yr of dietary modification. Drug therapy also can be considered for children with LDL-C levels of ≥190 mg/dl. Children who may also require treatment are those whose levels are >160 mg/dl and who have ≥2 risk factors for CVD or a family history of premature CVD.

- Refer "hyperlipidemias" section for NCEP-ATP III guidelines for management.

SUGGESTED READINGS

available at www.expertconsult.com

AUTHOR: **PRIYA BANSAL, M.D., M.P.H.**

TABLE 1-82 Classification of Lipoprotein Disorders by Phenotypes, Genotypes, and Corresponding Clinical Manifestations

Phenotype (Frederickson Type)	Genotype	Elevated Cholesterol Type	Genetic Defect	Xanthomas	Other Clinical Manifestations
I (rare)	Familial hyperchylomicronemia	Elevated chylomicrons	Familial lipoprotein lipase deficiency, Apo C-II deficiency	Eruptive skin xanthomas	Recurrent abdominal pain, hepatosplenomegaly
IIA	Familial hypercholesterolemia	Elevated LDL	FHC, LDL receptor deficiency	Tendon xanthomas, xanthelasma, tuberous; planar palmar (homozygous)	Premature CAD, arcus corneae, arthritic symptoms
IIB	Familial combined hypercholesterolemia	Elevated LDL and VLDL	Reduced LDL receptor and increased apo B		
III (rare)	Familial dysbetalipoproteinemia	Elevated IDL	Defective apo E2 synthesis	Tuberous, Planar (palmar)	Premature CAD and peripheral vascular disease, male > female, obesity, abnormal glucose tolerance, hyperuricemia, aggravated by hypothyroiditis, good response to therapy
IV	Familial hyperlipemia	Elevated VLDL	Increased VLDL production	None	CAD and peripheral vascular disease, obesity, abnormal glucose tolerance, hyperuricemia, arthritic
V (rare)	Endogenous hypertriglyceridemia	Elevated VLDL, chylomicrons	Increased VLDL production and reduced LPL	Eruptive	

Modified from Graber MA: *The family practice handbook,* ed 4, St Louis, 2001, Mosby.

Apo, Apolipoprotein; *CAD,* coronary artery disease; *FHC,* familial hypercholesterolemia.

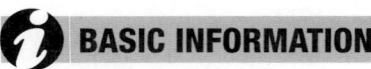

BASIC INFORMATION

DEFINITION

Hyperosmolar hyperglycemic syndrome (HHS) is a state of extreme hyperglycemia, marked dehydration, serum hyperosmolarity, altered mental status, and absence of ketoacidosis.

SYNONYMS

HHS
Hyperosmolar coma
Nonketotic hyperosmolar syndrome
Hyperosmolar nonketotic state

ICD-9CM CODES
250.2 Hyperosmolar coma

PHYSICAL FINDINGS & CLINICAL PRESENTATION

- Evidence of extreme dehydration (poor skin turgor, sunken eyeballs, dry mucous membranes)
- Neurologic defects (reversible hemiplegia, focal seizures)
- Orthostatic hypotension, tachycardia
- Evidence of precipitating factors (pneumonia, infected skin ulcer)
- Coma (25% of patients), delirium

ETIOLOGY

- Infections, 20% to 25% (e.g., pneumonia, urinary tract infection, sepsis)
- New or previously unrecognized diabetes (30% to 50%)
- Reduction or recent discontinuation of diabetic medication
- Stress (myocardial infarction, cerebrovascular accident)
- Drugs: diuretics (dehydration), phenytoin, diazoxide (impaired insulin secretion), glucocorticoids, chemotherapeutic agents, calcium channel blockers, total parenteral nutrition, substance abuse (alcohol, cocaine)

DIAGNOSIS

DIFFERENTIAL DIAGNOSIS

- Diabetic ketoacidosis
- The differential diagnosis of coma is described in Section II

LABORATORY TESTS

- Hyperglycemia: serum glucose usually >600 mg/dl, serum/urine ketones absent or "small."
- Hyperosmolarity: serum osmolarity usually >320 mOsm/L.
- Serum sodium: may be low, normal, or high; if normal or high, the patient is severely dehydrated because an elevated glucose draws fluid from intracellular space, decreasing the serum sodium. The corrected sodium can be obtained by increasing the serum sodium concentration by 1.6 mEq/dl for every 100 mg/dl increase in the serum glucose level over normal.

- Serum potassium: may be low, normal, or high; regardless of the initial serum level, the total body deficit is approximately 5 to 15 mEq/kg.
- Serum bicarbonate: usually >15 mEq/L (average 17 mEq/L).
- Arterial pH: usually >7.3; both serum bicarbonate and arterial pH may be lower if lactic acidosis is present.
- Blood urea nitrogen: azotemia (prerenal) is usually present (generally ranges from 60 to 90 mg/dl).
- Phosphorus: hypophosphatemia (average deficit is 70 to 140 mmol).
- Calcium: hypocalcemia (average deficit is 50 to 100 mEq).
- Magnesium: hypomagnesemia (average deficit is 50 to 100 mEq).
- Complete blood count with differential, urinalysis, and blood and urine cultures should be performed to rule out infectious etiology.
- ECG to rule out a concomitant myocardial infarction.

IMAGING STUDIES

Chest radiograph is useful to rule out infectious process. The initial radiograph may be negative if the patient has significant dehydration. Repeat chest x-ray after 24 hr of hydration if pulmonary infection is suspected.

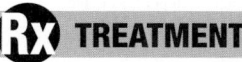

TREATMENT

NONPHARMACOLOGIC THERAPY

- Monitor mental status, vital signs, urine output hourly until improved, then monitor q2-4h.
- Monitor electrolytes, renal function, and glucose level (see "Acute General Rx").

ACUTE GENERAL Rx

- Vigorous fluid replacement: the volume and rate of fluid replacement are determined by renal and cardiac function. Typically, infuse 1000 to 1500 ml/hr for the initial 1 to 2 L; then decrease the rate of infusion to 500 ml/hr and monitor urinary output, blood chemistries, and blood pressure. Use 0.9% NS (isotonic solution) if the patient is hypotensive or serum osmolarity is <320 mOsm/L; otherwise use 0.45% NS solution. Slower infusion rate may be used initially in patients with compromised cardiovascular or renal status. When serum glucose reaches 300 mg/dl, change to 5% dextrose with 0.45% NS.
- Replace electrolytes and monitor serum levels frequently (e.g., serum sodium and potassium q2h for the first 12 hr). KCl replacement in patients with normal renal function and adequate urinary output when the serum potassium level is <5.2 mEq/L (e.g., 10 mEq KCl/hr if potassium level is 4 to 5.2 mEq/L). Continuous telemetry monitoring and hourly measurement of urinary output are recommended. In patients with severe hypokalemia (potassium <3.3 mEq/L), give 40 mEq of potassium/hr until potassium is >3.3 mEq/L.

- Correct hyperglycemia. The goal is for plasma glucose to decline by at least 50 to 100 mg/dl/hr.
  1. Vigorous IV hydration will decrease the serum glucose level in most patients by 80 mg/dl/hr; a regular insulin IV bolus (0.15 U/kg of body weight) is often not necessary. Insulin should not be administered until serum potassium is >3.3 mEq/L to prevent life-threatening hypokalemia.
  2. Low-dose insulin infusion at 0.1 U/kg/hr (e.g., 25 U of regular insulin in 250 ml of 0.9% saline solution at 20 ml/hr) until the serum glucose level approaches 300 mg/dl; then the patient is started on regular SC insulin with sliding scale coverage. If the plasma glucose level does not decrease over 2 to 4 hr despite adequate fluid administration and urine output, consider doubling the hourly insulin dose.
  3. Glucose should be monitored q1 to 2h in the initial 12 hr.
- In the absence of renal failure, phosphate can be administered at a rate of 0.1 mmol/kg/hr (5 to 10 mmol/hr) to a maximum of 80 to 120 mmol in 24 hr. Magnesium replacement, in the absence of renal failure, can be administered IM (0.05 to 0.10 ml/kg of 20% magnesium sulfate) or as IV infusion (4 to 8 ml of 20% magnesium sulfate [0.08 to 0.16 mEq/kg]). Repeat magnesium, phosphate, and calcium levels should be obtained after 12 to 24 hr.
- On day 2 begin or resume feeding if patient is able and glucose is under control (<200 mg/dl). Begin or resume SC insulin. For patients with type 2 diabetes, a mixture of NPH plus a short acting (such as Lispro, Aspart) insulin is preferred, timing the injection with a planned meal. Total daily dose (TDD) can be 0.5 U/kg. Insulin proportions are typically 60% in the AM and 40% in the PM.
- Individual patients may be appropriate for a trial of oral agents.

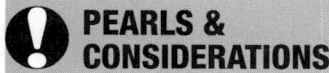

PEARLS & CONSIDERATIONS

COMMENTS

The typical patient is an elderly or bed-confined diabetic with impaired ability to communicate thirst who is evaluated after an interval of 1 to 2 wk of prolonged osmotic diuresis.

SUGGESTED READINGS
available at www.expertconsult.com

AUTHORS: **ANTHONY GEMIGNANI, M.D.**, **FRED F. FERRI, M.D.**, and **WEN-CHIH WU, M.D.**

BASIC INFORMATION

DEFINITION

Hyperparathyroidism is an endocrine disorder caused by excessive secretion of parathyroid hormone (PTH) from the parathyroid glands. Autonomous production of PTH resulting in hypercalcemia defines primary hyperparathyroidism. Secondary hyperparathyroidism occurs when the parathyroid glands appropriately increase PTH production in response to low calcium states. Primary hyperparathyroidism is the focus of this section.

ICD-9CM CODES
252.00 Hyperparathyroidism, unspecified
252.01 Hyperparathyroidism, primary
252.02 Hyperparathyroidism, secondary (non-renal)
588.81 Hyperparathyroidism, secondary (renal)

EPIDEMIOLOGY & DEMOGRAPHICS

INCIDENCE: 2 cases/100,000 person-yr
PREVALENCE: 1 case/1000 persons
PREDOMINANT SEX AND AGE: Women:men 2:1, peaks 50 to 60 yr

PHYSICAL FINDINGS & CLINICAL PRESENTATION

The majority of patients with primary hyperparathyroidism are asymptomatic. The development of symptoms varies with severity and rapidity of disease progression and reflects both the hypercalcemic and hyperparathyroid components of the disease process.

- Cardiovascular: hypertension, shortened QT interval, arrhythmia, valvular calcification
- GI: anorexia, nausea, vomiting, constipation, abdominal pain, peptic ulcer disease, pancreatitis
- GU: nephrolithiasis, nephrocalcinosis, renal insufficiency, polyuria, nocturia, nephrogenic diabetes insipidus, renal tubular acidosis
- Musculoskeletal: weakness, myopathy, bone pain, osteoporosis, gout, pseudogout, chondrocalcinosis, osteitis fibrosa cystica
- CNS: confusion, anxiety, fatigue, obtundation, depression, coma
- Other: hypomagnesemia, hypophosphatemia, pruritus, metastatic calcifications, band keratopathy

ETIOLOGY

Most cases of primary hyperparathyroidism are sporadic but it can be associated with rare genetic conditions such as multiple endocrine neoplasia (MEN)-1 and MEN-2. Pathologic characteristics include adenoma (89%), hyperplasia (10%), or carcinomas (<1%).

Dx DIAGNOSIS

DIFFERENTIAL DIAGNOSIS

- Other causes of hyperparathyroidism (i.e., secondary hyperparathyroidism) include:
  - Medication: loop diuretics
  - Calcium or vitamin D deficiency
  - Chronic kidney disease
  - Pseudohypoparathyroidism (PTH resistance)
- Other causes of hypercalcemia include:
  - Medications: thiazide diuretics, lithium therapy
  - Vitamin D intoxication, milk-alkali syndrome
  - Familial hypocalciuric hypercalcemia (FHH)
  - Renal failure (tertiary hyperparathyroidism)
  - Granulomatous disorders (e.g., sarcoidosis)
  - Malignancy (e.g., lung cancer, lymphoma, myeloma, bone metastasis)
  - Prolonged immobilization

WORKUP

- Primary hyperparathyroidism is confirmed with an elevated serum calcium and PTH level.
  - Two measurements of serum calcium are required for the confirmation of hypercalcemia. Total calcium should be corrected for low albumin utilizing the formula: Corrected Calcium = $(0.8 \times [4 - \text{serum albumin}]) + \text{serum calcium}$. If a reliable laboratory is available, an ionized calcium should be considered especially in condition associated with acid-base disturbances or low albumin states.
  - The serum intact PTH (iPTH) level is the single best test to evaluate the etiology of hypercalcemia. PTH is elevated in hyperparathyroidism and decreased in most other conditions associated with elevated calcium.
- Rule out other causes of hypercalcemia. These are typically associated with low PTH levels. Exceptions include lithium use and FHH.
  - Review medication history to determine lithium, thiazide, vitamin D or calcium intake
  - Check 24-hr urine calcium:creatinine to rule out FHH. Urine calcium is usually low in FHH and high in hyperparathyroidism. PTH can be low, normal, or high in FHH.
  - Consider parathyroid hormone–related peptide (PTHrP) to evaluate hypercalcemia related to malignancies and vitamin D 1,25 to assess hypercalcemia secondary to glaucomatous diseases or lymphomas. Multiple myeloma and bone metastasis can also result in a high calcium state and therefore must be appropriately evaluated.
- Rule out other causes of elevated PTH (i.e., secondary hyperparathyroidism). Serum calcium is typically low or low-normal in secondary hyperparathyroidism.
  - Check calcium and 25 OH-vitamin D to rule out deficiency states.
  - Assess renal function to evaluate for chronic renal failures.

LABORATORY TESTS

- Elevated serum calcium (ionized or corrected calcium)
- Low or low-normal serum phosphorus
- Elevated PTH

- 24-hr urine calcium to evaluate risk for renal stones and to rule out FHH
- Rule out other etiologies for hypercalcemia by checking PTHrp and 1,25 OH-vitamin D levels.
- Evaluation of 25 OH-vitamin D is recommended in all patients with hyperparathyroidism. Vitamin D deficiency can decrease calcium and increase PTH levels. Due to the clinical impact of vitamin D deficiency, normalization is required prior to making any diagnostic and therapeutic decisions.
- ECG may reveal shortening of the QT interval secondary to severe hypercalcemia (>12 mg/dl)

IMAGING STUDIES

- Parathyroid localization with technetium-99m sestamibi can identify potential adenomas.
- Bone mineral density of the spine, hip, and forearm is recommended for all patients with hyperparathyroidism in order to assess the risk for osteoporosis and fragility fractures. Cortical bone loss (i.e., forearm or hip) is greater in hyperparathyroidism.
- Renal ultrasound can be considered to assess asymptomatic renal stones.
- Plain x-rays may reveal high bone turnover (Fig. 1-201).

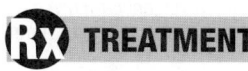

Rx TREATMENT

NONPHARMACOLOGIC THERAPY

- Surgery is the only definitive treatment for symptomatic primary hyperparathyroidism.

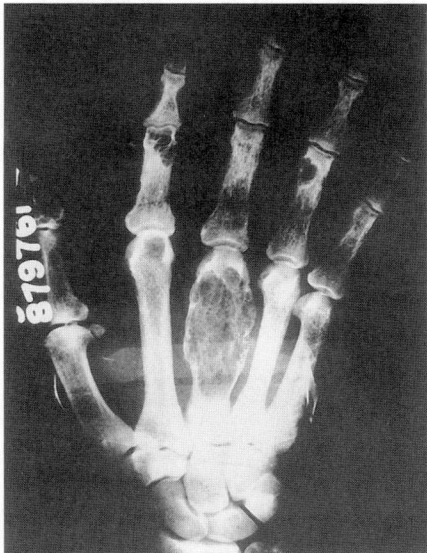

FIGURE 1-201 Radiograph of hand from a patient with severe primary hyperparathyroidism. Note the dramatic remodeling associated with the intense region of high bone turnover in the third metacarpal, in addition to widespread evidence of subperiosteal and trabecular resorption. (Courtesy Fuller Albright Collection, Massachusetts General Hospital. From Larsen PR et al [eds]: *Williams textbook of endocrinology,* ed 10, Philadelphia, 2003, WB Saunders.)

Surgery can normalize calcium levels, decrease the risk for kidney stones, increase bone mineral density, and improve quality of life measures.

○ Indications for parathyroidectomy
1. All patients younger than 50 yr
2. Hypercalcemia (Ca >1 mg/dl above upper limit normal)
3. Creatinine clearance <60 ml/min
4. Osteoporosis (T-score <−2.5 or fragility fracture)
5. Symptomatic hyperparathyroidism such as nephrolithiasis

○ Surgical approaches include:
1. The conventional surgical approach is bilateral neck exploration under general anesthesia. An experienced endocrine surgeon cures >95% of patients undergoing bilateral neck exploration and incurs <1% perioperative mortality.
2. Minimally invasive parathyroidectomy under local anesthesia with intraoperative monitoring of PTH before and after removal is becoming more popular.

• Medical monitoring is recommended for asymptomatic primary hyperparathyroidism. Majority of patients do not manifest disease progression during observation.

○ Indications for medical monitoring
1. Clinically asymptomatic
2. Serum calcium level only mildly elevated (<1 mg/dl above upper limit normal)
3. GFR >60 ml/min and no nephrolithiasis or nephrocalcinosis
4. No evidence of osteoporosis

• ~25% of asymptomatic patients will require surgery over a 10-yr follow-up period. Therefore patients will require regular monitoring of symptoms and assessment of serum calcium and creatinine levels yearly. Bone mineral density can be monitored every 2 yr.

• Medical management
1. Avoid medications that precipitate hypercalcemia (e.g., thiazide or lithium)

2. Since inadequate calcium and vitamin D status stimulates PTH, calcium and vitamin D intake should be the same as for patients without hyperparathyroidism (i.e., 1000 mg of elemental calcium and 600 to 800 IU of vitamin D daily).
3. Encourage physical activity since immobilization increases bone resorption.
4. Recommend adequate hydration (at least 2 L) to minimize the risk of nephrolithiasis.

PHARMACOLOGIC THERAPY

For patients who are not surgical candidates, pharmacologic options are available. Indications include symptomatic hyperparathyroidism or osteopenia associated with an increased fracture risk.

• Agents that inhibit bone resorption such as bisphosphonates (e.g., alendronate, pamidronate, zoledronate), estrogens, and selective estrogen receptor modulators (e.g., Raloxifene) have been shown to improve bone mineral density and decrease calcium levels in patients with hyperparathyroidism.
• Cinacalcet (Sensipar) is an oral calcimimetic agent that activates the calcium sensing receptor in the parathyroid gland. It decreases PTH production and subsequently serum calcium levels. Its role in the management of primary hyperparathyroidism is under evaluation. However, it is indicated for the treatment of secondary hyperparathyroidism associated with chronic kidney disease and hypercalcemia associated with parathyroid carcinoma.

ACUTE GENERAL Rx

Severe and/or symptomatic hypercalcemia may require hospitalization especially if serum calcium >12 mg/dl. Acute management of hypercalcemia includes:

• Vigorous hydration with IV normal saline (2 to 4 L/day). Fluid status must be monitored in

patients with cardiac or renal insufficiency in order to avoid fluid overload.
• Bisphosphonates can effectively decrease calcium levels. Zoledronate (4 mg IV over 15 min) or pamidronate (60-90 mg IV over 4 hr) are both effective. Onset of action after 24 to 48 hr.
• Calcitonin (4 units/kg IM/SC every 12 hr) may be used with bisphosphonates to achieve a more rapid reduction of calcium levels. Onset of action is within hours.

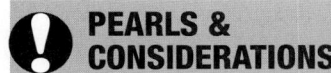 **PEARLS & CONSIDERATIONS**

COMMENTS
• Parathyroidectomy should be considered for all patients with symptomatic hyperparathyroidism.
• Asymptomatic patients can be monitored with serial creatinine, calcium and bone mineral density measurements. Disease progression may result in surgery. Most patients can be managed medically by limiting factors that result in hypercalcemia (i.e., dehydration, immobilization, thiazide diuretics etc.) and maintaining normal calcium and vitamin D intake. Patients with osteopenia and high fracture risk may require antiresorptive therapy such as bisphosphonates.

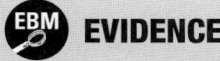 **EVIDENCE**
available at www.expertconsult.com

SUGGESTED READINGS
available at www.expertconsult.com

AUTHORS: **ALLISON D. GRAZIADEI, M.D.,** and **GEETHA GOPALAKRISHNAN, M.D.**

BASIC INFORMATION

DEFINITION

Hypersensitivity pneumonitis (HP) is a group of immunologically mediated pulmonary diseases provoked by recurrent exposure to various environmental agents.

SYNONYMS

Extrinsic allergic alveolitis (EAA)
Some specific examples:
- Bird fancier's lung
- Farmer's lung
- Chemical worker's lung
- Humidifier lung
- Hot tub lung
- Sauna taker's lung

ICD-9CM CODES
495.9 Pneumonitis, hypersensitivity

EPIDEMIOLOGY & DEMOGRAPHICS

- Prevalence and incidence of HP vary considerably.
- Depend on definition and methods to establish diagnosis, intensity of exposure, environmental conditions, and genetic risk factors that remain poorly understood.
- More than 300 causative agents have been identified, and the number continues to grow.
- Causative agents in residential and occupational exposures include birds, mold, humidifiers, wind instruments (e.g., trombone, saxophone), and organic and inorganic chemicals, including metalworking fluids. Likely several genes are involved that cause an exaggerated lung response to an offending agent. The major histocompatibility complex is the most studied thus far.
- A viral connection has been implicated that may enhance clinical exposure to an offending agent.

PHYSICAL FINDINGS & CLINICAL PRESENTATION

Vary depending on frequency and intensity of antigen exposure.
- Acute: fever, cough, malaise, and dyspnea 4 to 6 hr after an intense exposure, lasting 18 to 24 hr
- Subacute: insidious onset of productive cough, dyspnea on exertion, anorexia, and weight loss, usually from a heavy, sustained exposure
- Chronic: gradually progressive cough, dyspnea, malaise, and weight loss, usually from low-grade or recurrent exposure
- Physical examination: cyanosis and crepitant rales, possible fever

ETIOLOGY

- Numerous environmental agents, often encountered in occupational settings
- Common sources of antigens: "moldy" hay, silage, grain, or vegetables; bird droppings or feathers; low-molecular-weight chemicals (e.g., isocyanates); pharmaceutical products

DIAGNOSIS

- Accurate diagnosis is important for differentiating HP from other interstitial disorders because the prognosis and treatment may differ.
- There is no gold standard for diagnosis.
- The clinical syndrome is indistinguishable from an acute respiratory infection without a history of illness occurring within hours of exposure to an antigen.
- Need high index of suspicion.
- Detailed occupational and home exposure history is required.
- Lung biopsy is often necessary for diagnosis.

DIFFERENTIAL DIAGNOSIS

Acute Stages	Chronic Stages
Acute bronchopulmonary aspergillosis	Idiopathic pulmonary fibrosis (IPF)
Pulmonary embolism	Bronchiectasis
Asthma	Chronic bronchitis
Aspiration pneumonia	Nonspecific interstitial pneumonia (NSIP)
Recurrent pneumonia	Connective tissue–related lung disease
Bronchiolitis obliterans–organizing pneumonia	
Sarcoidosis	
Churg-Strauss syndrome	
Wegener granulomatosis	

WORKUP

No single radiologic, physiologic, or immunologic test is specific for the diagnosis of HP. HP must be suspected in any patient presenting with cough, dyspnea, fever, and malaise. A thorough history focusing on potential exposures is essential.

Environmental and occupational history questions should ask about grain dusts; animal handling; food processing; cooling towers; fountains; metalworking fluids; symptom improvement away from exposure; pets (particularly birds); hobbies involving chemicals, feathers, or fur; organic dusts; presence of humidifiers, dehumidifiers, or hot tubs/saunas; leaking or flooding indoors; visible fungal growth in living or working environment; feather pillows or bedding.

Major criteria:
- History of symptoms compatible with HP that appear to worsen within hours after antigen exposure
- Confirmation of exposure to the offending agent by history, investigation of the environment, serum precipitin test, or bronchoalveolar lavage (BAL) antibody
- Compatible changes on chest radiograph or high-resolution CT (HRCT) of the chest
- BAL fluid lymphocytosis (if performed)
- Compatible histologic changes by lung biopsy (if performed): bronchiolocentric interstitial pneumonia, nonspecific interstitial pneumonia (NSIP)

- Positive natural challenge (reproduction of symptoms and laboratory abnormalities after exposure to the suspected environment) or controlled inhalation challenge
Minor criteria:
- Basilar crackles
- Decreased diffusion capacity
- Arterial hypoxemia (either at rest or with exercise)

LABORATORY TESTS

- Routine laboratory tests do not make the diagnosis, but typically the erythrocyte sedimentation rate, C-reactive protein, lactate dehydrogenase, and leukocyte count are increased; elevated immunoglobulins IgG and IgM are nonspecific; rheumatoid factor (RF) and immune complexes are often positive; peripheral eosinophil count and serum IgE are generally normal.
- Lactate dehydrogenase is increased and tends to decrease with improvement.
- Pulmonary function tests: restrictive ventilatory patterns are typically seen. Decreased FEV_1, decreased forced vital capacity, decreased total lung capacity, decreased diffusing capacity, and decreased static compliance.
- Arterial blood gases show mild hypoxemia (worsens with exercise).
- A-a gradient shows slight increase.
- Serum precipitin test IgG antibody against offending antigen detected in serum. It is sensitive but not specific for HP (asymptomatic patients may have IgG antibodies in serum).
- Skin testing: unclear if helpful. However, some believe it to be a safe, effective, and rapid procedure in the diagnosis and follow-up of patients with HP. Sensitivity is similar to that of the precipitin test but the specificity is higher.

IMAGING STUDIES

Chest radiograph: nonspecific; may be normal in early stage.
- Acute/subacute: bilateral interstitial and alveolar nodular infiltrates (Fig. 1-202) in a patchy or homogeneous distribution. Apices are often spared.
- Chronic: diffuse reticulonodular infiltrates and fibrosis.
High-resolution chest CT scan: no pathognomonic features but demonstrates airspace and interstitial patterns in the acute and subacute stage. The chronic stage reveals honeycombing and bronchiectasis.

TREATMENT

NONPHARMACOLOGIC THERAPY

Early recognition and avoidance of the causative antigen

ACUTE GENERAL Rx

- Glucocorticoids accelerate initial lung recovery but may have no effect long term (from a controlled study in farmer's lung). No prospective, randomized, placebo-controlled trials for other types of HP or subacute and chronic stages.

- Prednisone 0.5 to 1 mg/kg usually over 1 to 2 wk then tapered over 4 wk. Some patients, particularly those with subacute or chronic presentation, may require a longer course of therapy.

DISPOSITION/PROGNOSIS

Prognosis is generally better in patients with acute or subacute HP, and with the finding of NSIP pathologically. Prognosis is worse in those with older age, desaturation during exercise, and findings of severe fibrosis by lung biopsy.

Acute: 4 to 48 hr
- Clinical: fever, chills, cough, hypoxia, malaise
- HRCT: ground-glass infiltrates
- Immunopathology: poorly formed, noncaseating granulomas or mononuclear cell infiltration in a peribronchial distribution, frequently with giant cells
- Prognosis: good

Subacute: weeks to 4 mo
- Clinical: dyspnea, cough, episodic flares
- HRCT: micronodules, air trapping
- Immunopathology: more well-formed noncaseating granulomas, bronchiolitis, organizing pneumonia and interstitial fibrosis
- Prognosis: good

Chronic: 4 mo to years
- Clinical: dyspnea, cough, fatigue, weight loss
- HRCT: fibrosis (possible), honeycombing, emphysema
- Immunopathology: granulomatous pneumonitides may be seen in addition to bronchiolitis obliterans (with or without organizing pneumonia) and honeycombing and fibrosis, lymphocytic infiltration, centrilobular and bridging fibrosis, neutrophil-mediated air space destruction, giant cells

REFERRAL

- Bronchoscopy: BAL provides useful supportive data in the diagnosis of HP. Usually reveals intense lymphocytosis (typically T cells >50%) of predominantly CD8+ suppressor cells. In the acute stage neutrophils predominate, but as the disease progresses to chronic form the ratio of CD4+ to CD8+ cells increase. When fibrosis is present the number of neutrophils increases.
- Lung biopsy: the histopathologic features of HP are distinctive but not pathognomonic. Bronchiolitis and interstitial pneumonitis with granuloma formation typically is seen. Variable degrees of interstitial fibrosis are seen in the chronic form. Chronic hypersensitivity pneumonitis may be difficult to distinguish from IPF or NSIP pathologically.
- Laboratory inhalation challenge: testing to prove a direct relation between a suspected antigen and disease; extract of antigen is inhaled by nebulizer.

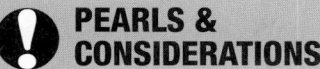

PEARLS & CONSIDERATIONS

A clinical prediction rule using six features has high specificity and sensitivity for the diagnosis of acute and subacute HP:
- Exposure to a known offending agent
- Positive specific precipitating antibody
- Recurrent episodes of symptoms
- Inspiratory crackles
- Symptoms occurring 4 to 8 hr after exposure
- Weight loss

No diagnostic gold standards; requires combination of clinical, environmental, radiologic, physiologic, and pathologic findings that represent a diagnostic challenge.

HP occurs more frequently in smokers than nonsmokers (likely from an immunosuppressive effect).

SUGGESTED READINGS

available at www.expertconsult.com

AUTHORS: **CAROLYN J. O'CONNOR, M.D.,** and **KRISTINA KRAMER, M.D.**

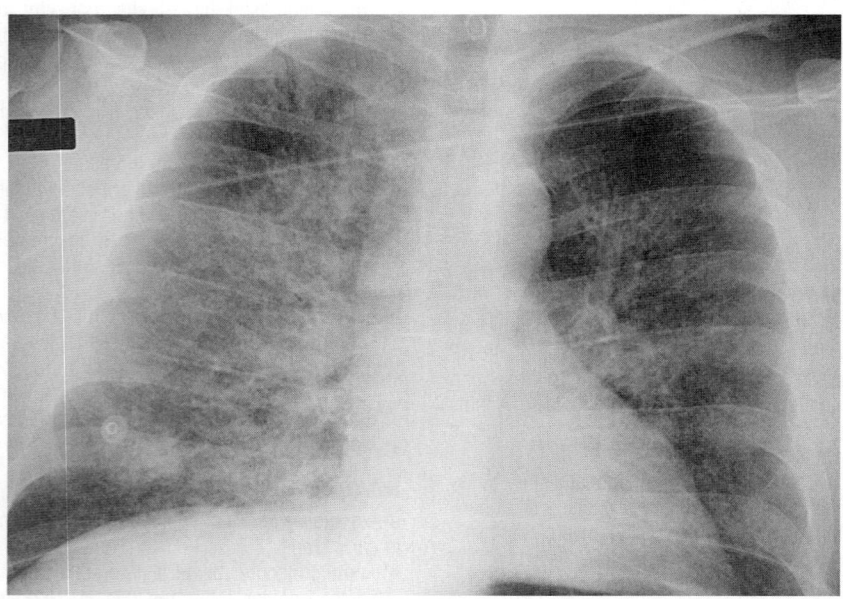

FIGURE 1-202 Chest radiograph of a patient with acute hypersensitivity pneumonitis. Bilateral interstitial infiltrates are evident, more on the right side than the left. Note the absence of pleural effusion, hilar adenopathy, and hyperinflation. (From Altman LV [ed]: *Allergy in primary care,* Philadelphia, 2000, WB Saunders.)

BASIC INFORMATION

DEFINITION

Hypersplenism is a syndrome characterized by splenomegaly, cytopenia (one or more of the following: anemia, thrombocytopenia, or leukopenia), and compensatory hyperplastic bone marrow. The cytopenias are correctable with splenectomy.

ICD-9CM CODES
289.4 Hypersplenism

EPIDEMIOLOGY & DEMOGRAPHICS

Most often seen in patients with liver disease, hematologic malignancy, and infection

PHYSICAL FINDINGS & CLINICAL PRESENTATION

- Symptoms depend on the size of the spleen, rate of growth, and underlying disease.
- History: early satiety, abdominal discomfort or fullness, left upper quadrant pleuritic pain (abscess, infarction), episodes of acute left upper quadrant pain (sequestration crisis), referred pain to left shoulder
- Physical examination: splenomegaly (normal spleen not palpable), presence of a rub in left upper quadrant (suggestive of a splenic infarct), stigmata of cytopenias

ETIOLOGY

The spleen is an important component of cellular and humoral immunity: antigen recognition, antibody production, and clearance of antibody-coated particles and microorganisms from circulation. It is also responsible for the modification (removal of particles and parasites) and clearance of damaged or old red blood cells (RBCs) from the circulation. The spleen is a platelet reservoir, storing 30% of platelet mass. It can become the site of hematopoiesis in certain disease states. The spleen's normal activities are augmented when enlarged.
- Splenomegaly increases the proportion of blood channeled through the red pulp, causing inappropriate splenic pooling of both normal and abnormal blood cells. The size of the spleen determines the amount of cell sequestration. Up to 90% of platelets may be pooled in an enlarged spleen.
- Splenomegaly leads to increased destruction of RBCs. Platelets and white blood cells (WBCs) have about normal survival time even when sequestered and may be available if needed.
- Splenomegaly causes plasma volume expansion, exacerbating cytopenias by dilution.

DIAGNOSIS

DIFFERENTIAL DIAGNOSIS

Hypersplenism can be caused by splenomegaly of almost any cause.
- Splenic congestion: cirrhosis (portal hypertension); congestive heart failure; portal, splenic, or hepatic vein thrombosis

- Hematologic causes: hemolytic anemia, sickle cell anemia, thalassemia, spherocytosis, elliptocytosis, extramedullary hematopoiesis, following use of granulocyte colony-stimulating factor
- Infections: viral (hepatitis, infectious mononucleosis, cytomegalovirus, HIV), bacterial (abscess, endocarditis, tuberculosis, salmonella, brucella, Lyme's disease), parasitic (babesiosis, malaria, leishmaniasis, schistosomiasis, toxoplasmosis), fungal
- Malignancy: acute or chronic leukemia, lymphoma, myeloproliferative diseases (polycythemia vera, essential thrombocythemia, myelofibrosis), metastatic tumors
- Inflammatory diseases: rheumatic fever, rheumatoid arthritis (Felty's syndrome), systemic lupus erythematosus, sarcoid, serum sickness
- Infiltrative diseases: amyloidosis, Gaucher's disease, Niemann-Pick disease, glycogen storage disease
- Anatomic abnormalities: cyst, pseudocyst, hemangioma, hamartoma

WORKUP

History (including travel), physical examination, laboratory tests, imaging studies

LABORATORY TESTS

- CBC with differential: cytopenia, neutrophilia (infection)
- Peripheral smear: RBC and WBC morphology (abnormal cells may suggest infection, malignancy, bone marrow disease, rheumatologic disease), organisms (bacteria, malaria, babesiosis)
- Bone marrow biopsy: hyperplasia of cytopenic cell lines; hematologic, infiltrative, or infectious disorders
- Tests to diagnose suspected cause of splenomegaly: liver function, hepatitis serology, HIV, rheumatoid factor, antinuclear antibody, tissue biopsy
- Note: red cell mass (^{51}Cr assay) may be used to assess severity of anemia. RBC mass measurement will differentiate true anemia (decrease in RBCs) from dilutional anemia (plasma volume expansion).

IMAGING STUDIES

- Ultrasound: splenic size, presence of cyst or abscess
- CT: estimate volume, obtain structural information: cyst, abscess, tumor, infarct
- MRI: most useful for assessing vascular lesions and infections
- Liver-spleen scan: assess anatomy and function; may suggest presence of portal hypertension
- Consider other studies as suggested by history and examination: chest radiograph, echocardiogram

TREATMENT

ACUTE GENERAL Rx

- Treat underlying disease
- Splenectomy is considered if:
  1. Indicated for the management of the underlying cause
  2. Persistent symptomatic disease (severe cytopenia) not responding to therapy
  3. Necessary for diagnosis

Risks:
- Infections (especially encapsulated organisms): risk greatest in the first 2 yr after splenectomy. Mortality rate from sepsis is fiftyfold greater in asplenic patients. Attempts to decrease risk include:
  ○ Immunization with pneumococcal, meningococcal, and haemophilus influenzae vaccines 3 wk before splenectomy. Revaccination for pneumococcal in 5 yr. Annual influenza vaccination.
  ○ Prophylactic antibiotics after splenectomy in highest risk patients.
  ○ Patient education regarding the importance of rapid initiation of antibiotics at the first sign of infection.
- Rapid increase in platelet count may cause thromboembolic complications.
- Possible increased risk of atherosclerotic heart disease.
- Splenectomy should not be performed if the spleen is the main site of hematopoiesis as a result of bone marrow failure (e.g., myelofibrosis).
- Other options include partial splenectomy, partial splenic embolization, portosystemic shunting (for congestive splenomegaly).

DISPOSITION

- Cytopenias are usually correctable with splenectomy; cell counts return to normal within a few weeks.
- Splenectomy may alleviate portal hypertension.
- Prognosis depends on the underlying disease.

REFERRAL

Hematology

PEARLS & CONSIDERATIONS

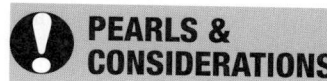

- Thrombocytopenia in hypersplenism is usually moderately severe ($>50 \times 10^9$ /L) and asymptomatic; severe thrombocytopenia ($<20 \times 10^9$/L) suggests another diagnosis.
- Neutropenia of hypersplenism is rarely symptomatic.

SUGGESTED READING
available at www.expertconsult.com

AUTHOR: **SUDEEP KAUR AULAKH, M.D.**

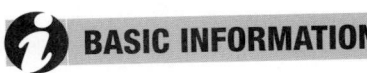

BASIC INFORMATION

DEFINITION

The Joint National Committee on Prevention, Detection, Evaluation, and Treatment of High Blood Pressure (JNC 7) classifies normal blood pressure (BP) in adults as <120 mm Hg systolic and <80 mm Hg diastolic. *Prehypertension* is defined as systolic BP from 120 to 139 mm Hg or diastolic BP from 80 to 89 mm Hg. *Stage 1 hypertension* (HTN) is systolic BP from 140 to 159 mm Hg or diastolic BP from 90 to 99 mm Hg. *Stage 2 hypertension* is systolic BP ≥160 mm Hg or diastolic BP ≥100 mm Hg.

SYNONYMS

Essential hypertension
Idiopathic hypertension
High BP

ICD-9CM CODES
401.1 Essential hypertension (HTN)
401.0-9 with 5th digit 1 Renovascular hypertension
405 Secondary hypertension
642 Hypertension complicating pregnancy
437.2 Hypertensive encephalopathy

EPIDEMIOLOGY & DEMOGRAPHICS

PREVALENCE: 25% to 30% of adult population, 65 million individuals in the United States and ~1 billion individuals worldwide meet the criteria for diagnosis of HTN. In the United States, as many as 15 million may have undiagnosed hypertension.
PEAK PREVALENCE: Males and the elderly

PHYSICAL FINDINGS & CLINICAL PRESENTATION

Physical examination may be entirely within normal limits except for the presence of HTN. A proper initial physical examination on a hypertensive patient should include the following:

- The BP should be measured with an appropriately sized cuff (bladder of the cuff should cover at least two thirds of the circumference of the arm) and in both arms (the higher of the readings being used).
- Postural BP change is best assessed by going from the lying to the standing position and should include notation of the change in heart rate with position change.
- A diagnosis of HTN may be established if the BP is markedly elevated (>180/110 mm Hg); otherwise such a diagnosis should wait until BP is found elevated on at least two occasions where white coat HTN is highly unlikely.
- Measure heart rate, height and weight, body mass index, and waist circumference.
- Evaluate skin for the presence of café-au-lait spots (neurofibromatosis), uremic appearance (renal failure), striae (Cushing's syndrome).
- Perform careful funduscopic examination; check for papilledema, retinal exudates, hemorrhages, arterial narrowing, arteriovenous compression.
- Examine the neck for carotid bruits, distended neck veins, or enlarged thyroid gland.

- Perform extensive cardiopulmonary examination: check for loud aortic component of S_2, S_4, ventricular lift, murmurs, and arrhythmias.
- Check abdomen for masses (pheochromocytoma, polycystic kidneys), and frank bruit (renal artery stenosis), as well as pulsatile periumbilical mass suggestive of dilation of the aorta.
- Obtain two or more BP measurements separated by 2 min with the patient either supine or seated and after standing for at least 2 min. Measure BP in both upper extremities (if values differ, use the higher value).
- Examine arterial pulses (dilated or absent femoral pulses and BP greater in upper extremities than lower extremities suggest aortic coarctation).
- Note the presence of truncal obesity (Cushing's syndrome) and pedal edema (congestive heart failure [CHF]).
- The clinical evaluation should help to determine if the patient has primary or secondary (possibly reversible) HTN, if there is target organ disease present, and whether additional cardiovascular risk factors are present.

ETIOLOGY

- Essential (primary) HTN (85%)
- Drug induced or drug related (5%)
  1. NSAIDs
  2. Oral contraceptives
  3. Corticosteroids
- Renal HTN (5%)
  1. Renal parenchymal disease (3%)
  2. Renovascular hypertension (RVH) (<2%)
- Endocrine (<2%)
  1. Primary aldosteronism (0.5%)
  2. Pheochromocytoma (0.2%)
  3. Cushing's syndrome and long-term steroid therapy (0.2%)
  4. Hyperparathyroidism or thyroid disease (0.2%)
- Coarctation of the aorta (0.2%)

DIAGNOSIS

WORKUP

- The objective for the initial evaluation of HTN is to establish the diagnosis and stage of HTN.
- By gathering office and nonoffice BP readings, assessing presence of target organ damage (TOD), assessing the level of global cardiovascular disease risk and to produce a plan for individualized monitoring and therapy.
- ECG, CXR, renal imaging, and tests for plasma aldosterone/plasma rennin activity are not routinely recommended at the initial evaluation stage of the patient with newly diagnosed HTN.
- Patient counseling and education should be prominent features of the initial evaluation.
Pertinent history:
- Age of onset of HTN, previous antihypertensive therapy
- Family history of HTN, stroke, cardiovascular disease

- Diet, salt intake, alcohol, drugs (e.g., oral contraceptives, NSAIDs, decongestants, steroids)
- Occupation, lifestyle, socioeconomic status, psychologic factors
- Other cardiovascular risk factors: hyperlipidemia, obesity, diabetes mellitus
- Symptoms of secondary HTN:
  1. Headache, palpitations, excessive perspiration (possible pheochromocytoma)
  2. Weakness, polyuria (consider hyperaldosteronism)
  3. Claudication of lower extremities (seen with coarctation of aorta)

An algorithm for investigation of suspected endocrine HTN is described in Section III.

LABORATORY TESTS

- Urinalysis with microscopic evaluation, blood urea nitrogen and creatinine, and an albumin/creatinine ratio; for evidence of renal disease. High-serum creatinine is a predictor of cardiovascular risk in essential HTN.
- Nonoffice (home, workplace, 24-hr ambulatory BP determination to establish the pattern of HTN (sustained, "white coat," or "masked" HTN).
- Serum electrolyte levels: low potassium is suggestive of primary aldosteronism or diuretic use.
- Screening for coexisting diseases that may adversely affect prognosis:
  1. Fasting serum glucose
  2. Serum lipid panel, uric acid, calcium
  3. If pheochromocytoma is suspected: 24-hr urine for VMA and metanephrines

IMAGING STUDIES

- ECG: check for presence of left ventricular hypertrophy (LVH) with strain pattern.
- Magnetic resonance angiography of the renal arteries in suspected renovascular hypertension (renal artery stenosis).

TREATMENT

NONPHARMACOLOGIC THERAPY

Lifestyle modifications:
- Weight loss if overweight (target BMI <25).
- Limit alcohol intake to 1 oz of ethanol per day (<2 drinks/day) in men or 0.5 oz (<1 drink/day) in women.
- Regular aerobic exercise (at least 30 min/day on most days).
- Reduce sodium intake to <100 mmol/day (<1.5 g of sodium/day).
- Maintain adequate dietary potassium (>3500 mg/day) intake in patients with normal kidney function.
- Stop smoking.
- The BP reduction seen ranges from 2 to 20 mm Hg, most significant with substantial weight loss and the implementation of the Dietary Approaches to Stop Hypertension (DASH) eating plan, which relies on a diet high in fruits and vegetables, moderate in low-fat dairy products, and low in animal protein but with substantial amount of plant protein from legumes and nuts.

ACUTE GENERAL Rx

According to the JNC 7:

For patients with prehypertension and no other complications, recommend lifestyle modifications to prevent progression to sustained HTN.

For patients with prehypertension and diabetes or chronic kidney disease, aggressive pharmacologic treatment should be undertaken to reduce BP to <130/80 mm Hg.

Antihypertensive drug therapy should be initiated in patients with stage 1 HTN. Thiazide diuretics are preferred for initial therapy unless there are compelling indications to use other agents for initial therapy. Chlorthalidone has been shown to be more effective than an ACE inhibitor in lowering blood pressure and at least as effective as a calcium blocker or an ACE inhibitor in prevention of cardiovascular events.

Compelling indications for individual drug classes:

Congestive heart failure (CHF) due to systolic dysfunction: ACE inhibitors, angiotensin-receptor blockers (ARBs), beta-blockers, diuretics, aldosterone antagonists

Post MI: beta-blockers, ACE inhibitors, aldosterone antagonists

High cardiovascular risk: beta-blockers, ACE inhibitors, calcium channel blockers (CCBs), diuretics

Diabetes: ACE inhibitors, ARBs, CCBs, beta-blockers, diuretics

Chronic kidney disease: ACE inhibitors, ARBs

Recurrent stroke prevention: ACE inhibitors, diuretics

A two-drug combination is necessary for most patients with stage 2 HTN. The combination of a diuretic with another agent is preferred unless there is a compelling indication to use other agents.

When selecting drugs, also consider the cost of the medication, metabolic and subjective side effects, and drug-drug interactions.

The major advantages and limitations of each class of drugs are described as follows:

1. Diuretics:
   a. Advantages: inexpensive, once-daily dosing. Useful in edematous states, CHF, chronic renal disease, elderly patients (decreased incidence of hip fractures in elderly patients)
   b. Disadvantages: significant adverse metabolic effects, increased risk of cardiac arrhythmias, sexual dysfunction, possible adverse effects on lipids and glucose levels
2. Beta-blockers:
   a. Advantages: ideal in hypertensive patients with ischemic heart disease or status post MI. Favored in hyperkinetic, young patients (resting tachycardia, wide pulse pressure, hyperdynamic heart) and stable CHF patients
   b. Disadvantages: adverse effect on quality of life (increased incidence of fatigue, depression, impotence, bronchospasm, hypoglycemia, peripheral vascular disease, adverse effects on lipids, masking of signs and symptoms of hypoglycemia in diabetics)

3. Calcium antagonists:
   a. Advantages: helpful in hypertensive patients with ischemic heart disease. Generally favorable effect on quality of life; can be used in patients with bronchospastic disorders, renal disease, peripheral vascular disease, metabolic disorders, and salt sensitivity. CCBs BP-lowering effect is independent of Na^+ intake.
   b. Disadvantages: diltiazem and verapamil should be avoided in patients with CHF due to systolic dysfunction because of their negative inotropic effects; pedal edema may occur with nifedipine and amlodipine; constipation can be severe in elderly patients receiving verapamil. CCB-related edema is positional in nature, it improves with lying position, additional strategies include; switching CCB classes; reducing dosage; giving the medication later in the day; and adding a venodilator (nitrates, an ACE, or an ARB); diuretics may improve edema, but at the expense of a reduction in plasma volume.
4. ACE inhibitors:
   a. Advantages: well tolerated, favorable impact on quality of life; useful in HTN complicated by CHF; helpful in prevention of diabetic renal disease; effective in decreasing left ventricular hypertrophy (LVH).
   b. Disadvantages: cough is a frequent side effect (5% to 20% of patients); hyperkalemia may occur in patients with diabetes or severe renal insufficiency; hypotension may occur in volume-depleted patients.
5. ARBs:
   a. Advantages: well tolerated, favorable impact on quality of life; useful in patients unable to tolerate ACE inhibitors because of persistent cough and in CHF and diabetic patients; single daily dose. An episode of renal insufficiency with ACE inhibitors does not rule out future therapy with an ARB unless high-grade bilateral renal artery stenosis exists.
   b. Disadvantages: excessive cost; hypotension may occur in volume-depleted patients; contraindicated in pregnancy.
6. Renin inhibitors: newest class of antihypertensives (Aliskiren, Tekturna):
   a. Advantages: generally well tolerated; once-daily dosing; can be used alone or in combination with other antihypertensive agents.
   b. Disadvantages: contraindicated in pregnancy; should not be used in patients with impaired renal function, excessive cost, paucity of cardiovascular outcomes data showing benefit.
7. Alpha-adrenergic blockers:
   a. Advantages: no adverse effect on blood lipids or insulin sensitivity; helpful in benign prostatic hypertrophy.
   b. Disadvantages: postural hypotension, sedation; syncope can be avoided by giving an initial low dose at bedtime.
8. Central alpha-antagonists:
   a. Oral clonidine mainstay of therapy for hypertensive urgencies because of the ease of administration and relative safety.

   b. Transdermal clonidine; useful in management of labile HTN, the hospitalized patient who cannot take medications by mouth, and patients subject to early morning BP surges. At equivalent doses, transdermal clonidine is more apt to precipitate salt and water retention than is the case with oral clonidine.
   c. Dose beyond 0.4 mg causes fatigue, sedation and dry mouth, salt and water retention, and rebound HTN upon abrupt termination of the medication.
9. Combined alpha- and beta-adrenergic receptor blockers:
   a. Labetalol, nebivolol, and carvedilol: Use is reserved to treat complicated hypertensive patient when an antihypertensive effect beyond beta-blockade is sought. IV labetalol is used for hypertensive emergencies. Carvedilol is shown to have less adverse effect on glycemic control than metoprolol and to reduce urinary protein excretion in hypertensive diabetic patients.

TREATMENT OF RENOVASCULAR HYPERTENSION: The therapeutic approach varies with the cause of the RVH (refer to "Renal Artery Stenosis" for additional information).

1. Young patients with fibromuscular dysplasia refractory to medical therapy can be treated with percutaneous transluminal renal angioplasty (PTRA).
2. Medical therapy is advisable in elderly patients with atheromatous RVH; useful agents are:
   a. Beta-blockers: highly effective in patients with elevated plasma renin
   b. ACE inhibitors: highly effective; however, should be avoided in patients with bilateral renal artery stenosis or with a solitary kidney and renal stenosis
   c. Diuretics: often used in combination with ACE inhibitors
3. Surgical revascularization is generally reserved for atheromatous RVH in patients responding poorly to medical therapy (uncontrolled HTN, deteriorating renal function).

HTN DURING PREGNANCY:

1. HTN complicates 5% to 12% of all pregnancies.
2. The American Obstetrical Committee defines BP of 130/80 mm Hg as the upper limit of normal at any time during pregnancy.
3. A rise of 30 mm Hg systolic or 15 mm Hg diastolic is also considered abnormal regardless of the absolute values obtained.
4. Chronic HTN (occurring before pregnancy) must be distinguished from preeclampsia because the risk to mother and fetus is much greater in the latter.
5. Treatment of chronic HTN during pregnancy is as follows:
   a. Initial treatment with conservative measures (proper nutrition, limited physical activity).
   b. When drug therapy is necessary, initiation of methyldopa, hydralazine, labetalol, or atenolol is preferred.
   c. ACE inhibitors can cause fetal and neonatal complications; their use should be avoided in pregnancy.
   d. The safety of CCBs remains unclear.

e. Diuretics should be used only if there is a specific reason for initiating and maintaining their use (e.g., HTN associated with severe fluid overload or left ventricular dysfunction).

MALIGNANT HTN, HYPERTENSIVE EMERGENCIES, AND HYPERTENSIVE URGENCIES:

Definitions:

1. Malignant HTN is a potentially life-threatening situation caused by elevated BP.
   a. The rate of BP rise is a critical factor.
   b. The clinical manifestations are grade IV hypertensive retinopathy (exudates, hemorrhages, and papilledema), cardiovascular or renal compromise, and encephalopathy.
   c. Requires immediate BP reduction (not necessarily into normal ranges) to prevent or limit target organ disease.
2. Hypertensive emergencies require rapid (within 1 hr) lowering of BP to prevent end-organ damage.
3. Hypertensive urgencies are significant BP elevations that should be corrected within 24 hr of presentation.

Therapy: The choice of therapeutic agents varies with the cause.

1. Nitroprusside is the drug of choice in hypertensive encephalopathy, HTN and intracranial bleeding, malignant HTN, HTN and heart failure, dissecting aortic aneurysm (used in combination with propranolol); its onset of action is immediate.
2. Fenoldopam is a vasodilator agent useful for the short-term (up to 48 hr) management of severe HTN when rapid but quickly reversible reduction of BP is required.
3. Other commonly used agents are the IV CCBs nicardipine and clevidipine (useful for urgent treatment of HTN in the intensive care unit or operating room), the beta-blocker esmolol (useful in aortic dissection or postoperative HTN), labetalol (combined β-adrenergic and α-blocker useful in patients with coronary disease), phentolamine (useful for catecholamine-related emergencies), IV nitroglycerin (used in patients with cardiac ischemia and hypertensive crisis), and hydralazine (used for hypertensive emergencies in pregnancy).

4. Table 1-83 describes parenteral agents for management of hypertensive emergencies. *The following are important points to remember when treating hypertensive emergencies:*
   a. Introduce a plan for long-term therapy at the time of the initial emergency treatment.
   b. Agents that reduce arterial pressure can cause the kidney to retain sodium and water; therefore the judicious administration of diuretics should accompany their use.
   c. The initial goal of antihypertensive therapy is not to achieve a normal BP, but rather to gradually reduce the BP; cerebral hypoperfusion may occur if the mean BP is lowered >40% in the initial 24 hr.

PEARLS & CONSIDERATIONS

COMMENTS

- For patients with prehypertension, every 20/10 mm Hg increase in BP doubles the risk of cardiovascular events.
- Most patients will require at least two medications for BP control.
- Guidelines now suggest that, if BP is greater than 20/10 mm Hg above goal, therapy should be initiated with two drugs.
- A practical approach to multidrug therapy is use of fixed-dose antihypertensive combinations as an alternative to the sequenced addition of two or three drugs.
- Resistant HTN: HTN is considered resistant if the BP cannot be reduced below target levels in patients who are compliant with an optimal triple-drug regimen that includes a diuretic. Terms *refractory* and *resistant* are used interchangeably. Causes include pseudohypertension, measurement artifact, medication nonadherence, volume overload, and secondary HTN.
  - Pseudohypertension in elderly: hardened and sclerotic artery is not compressible hence falsely elevates BP measurement artifact
  - Measurement artifact: BP taken with a small cuff in people with large arm diameter. BP should be taken with the patient in the seated position and the arm supported at heart level, the bladder within the cuff should encircle at least 80% of the arm diameter.
- Section III describes an algorithm for patients with resistant HTN.
- Barriers to BP control: system issues, provider issues; patients issues and behavior issues. The rate at which physicians adopt recommended changes based on evidence based findings can be quite slow and has been properly described as "clinical inertia."
- ACE-ARB combination therapy has gained popularity in the primary care setting, but this practice should be discouraged. Recent studies assessing dual renin-angiotensin-aldosterone system blockade with ACE-ARB combination have not supported the use of this combination.

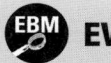 **EVIDENCE**

available at www.expertconsult.com

SUGGESTED READINGS

available at www.expertconsult.com

AUTHORS: **ANTHONY GEMIGNANI, M.D., FRED F. FERRI, M.D.,** and **WEN-CHIH WU, M.D.**

TABLE 1-83 Parenteral Agents for Management of Hypertensive Emergencies

Agent	Dose	Onset of Action	Precautions
Parenteral Vasodilators			
Sodium nitroprusside	0.25-10 mcg/kg/min IV infusion	Immediate	Thiocyanate toxicity with prolonged use
Nitroglycerin	5-100 mcg/min IV infusion	2-5 min	Headache, tachycardia, tolerance
Nicardipine	5-15 mg/hr IV infusion	1-5 min	Protracted hypotension after prolonged use
Fenoldopam mesylate	0.1-0.3 mcg/kg/min IV infusion	1-5 min	Headache, tachycardia, increased intraocular pressure
Hydralazine	5-10 mg as IV bolus or 10-40 mg IM; repeat every 4-6 hr	10 min IV 20 min IM	Unpredictable and excessive falls in blood pressure; tachycardia, angina exacerbation
Enalaprilat	0.625-1.25 mg every 6 hr IV bolus	15-60 min	Unpredictable and excessive falls in blood pressure; acute renal failure in patients with bilateral renal artery stenosis
Parenteral Adrenergic Inhibitors			
Labetalol	20-80 mg as slow IV injection every 10 min, or 0.5-2.0 mg/min IV as infusion	5-10 min	Bronchospasm, heart block, orthostatic hypotension
Metoprolol	5 mg IV every 10 min for three doses	5-10 min	Bronchospasm, heart block, heart failure, exacerbation of cocaine-induced myocardial ischemia
Esmolol	500 mcg/kg IV over 3 min; then 25-100 mg/kg/min as IV infusion	1-5 min	Bronchospasm, heart block, heart failure
Phentolamine	5-10 mg IV bolus every 5-15 min	1-2 min	Tachycardia, orthostatic hypotension

IM, Intramuscular; *IV,* intravenous.
From Andreoli TE et al: *Andreoli and Carpenter's Cecil essentials of medicine,* ed 8, Philadelphia, 2010, Saunders.

BASIC INFORMATION

DEFINITION

Hyperthyroidism is a hypermetabolic state resulting from excess thyroid hormone.

SYNONYMS

Thyrotoxicosis

ICD-9CM CODES
242.9 Hyperthyroidism
242.0 Hyperthyroidism with goiter
242.2 Hyperthyroidism, multinodular
242.3 Hyperthyroidism, uninodular

EPIDEMIOLOGY & DEMOGRAPHICS

INCIDENCE/PREVALENCE:
- Hyperthyroidism affects 2% of women and 0.2% of men in their lifetimes.
- Toxic multinodular goiter usually occurs in women >55 yr and is more common than Graves' disease in the elderly.

PHYSICAL FINDINGS & CLINICAL PRESENTATION

- Patients with hyperthyroidism generally present with tachycardia, tremor, hyperreflexia, anxiety, irritability, emotional lability, panic attacks, heat intolerance, sweating, increased appetite, diarrhea, weight loss, menstrual dysfunction (oligomenorrhea, amenorrhea). Presentation may be different in elderly patients (see below).
- Patients with Graves' disease may present with exophthalmos, lid retraction, and lid lag (Graves' ophthalmopathy). The following signs and symptoms of ophthalmopathy may be present: blurring of vision, photophobia, increased lacrimation, double vision, and deep orbital pressure. Clubbing of fingers associated with periosteal new bone formation in other skeletal areas (Graves' acropachy) and pretibial myxedema may also be noted.
- Clinical signs of hyperthyroidism in the elderly may be masked by manifestations of coexisting disease (e.g., new-onset atrial fibrillation, exacerbation of congestive heart failure).

ETIOLOGY

- Graves' disease (diffuse toxic goiter): 80% to 90% of all cases of hyperthyroidism
- Toxic multinodular goiter (Plummer's disease)
- Toxic adenoma
- Iatrogenic and factitious
- Transient hyperthyroidism (subacute thyroiditis, Hashimoto's thyroiditis)
- Rare causes: hypersecretion of thyroid-stimulating hormone (TSH) (e.g., pituitary neoplasms), struma ovarii, ingestion of large amount of iodine in a patient with preexisting thyroid hyperplasia or adenoma (Jod-Basedow phenomenon), hydatidiform mole, carcinoma of thyroid, amiodarone therapy

DIAGNOSIS

DIFFERENTIAL DIAGNOSIS

- Anxiety disorder
- Pheochromocytoma
- Metastatic neoplasm
- Diabetes mellitus
- Premenopausal state

WORKUP

Suspected hyperthyroidism requires laboratory confirmation and identification of its etiology because treatment varies with cause. A detailed medical history will often provide clues to the diagnosis and etiology of the hyperthyroidism.

LABORATORY TESTS

- Elevated free thyroxine (T_4)
- Elevated free triiodothyronine (T_3): generally not necessary for diagnosis
- Low TSH (unless hyperthyroidism is a result of the rare hypersecretion of TSH from a pituitary adenoma)
- Thyroid autoantibodies useful in selected cases to differentiate Graves' disease from toxic multinodular goiter (absent thyroid antibodies)

IMAGING STUDIES

- 24-hr radioactive iodine uptake (RAIU) is useful to distinguish hyperthyroidism from iatrogenic thyroid hormone synthesis (thyrotoxicosis factitia) and from thyroiditis.
- An overactive thyroid shows increased uptake, whereas a normal underactive thyroid (iatrogenic thyroid ingestion, painless or subacute thyroiditis) shows normal or decreased uptake.
- The RAIU results also vary with the etiology of the hyperthyroidism:
  - Graves' disease: increased homogeneous uptake
  - Multinodular goiter: increased heterogeneous uptake
  - Hot nodule: single focus of increased uptake
- RAIU is also generally performed before the therapeutic administration of radioactive iodine to determine the appropriate dose.

TREATMENT

NONPHARMACOLOGIC THERAPY

Patient education regarding thyroid disease and discussion of the therapeutic options. Patients should be informed that radioiodine, antithyroid drugs, and surgery are all reasonable treatment options for hyperthyroidism. It is crucial for the physician to have a detailed discussion with the patient about the benefits and risks relative to lifestyle, patients' values, and coexisting conditions.

ACUTE GENERAL Rx

ANTITHYROID DRUGS (THIONAMIDES): Propylthiouracil (PTU) and methimazole inhibit thyroid hormone synthesis by blocking production of thyroid peroxidase (PTU and methimazole) or inhibit peripheral conversion of T_4 to T_3 (PTU). Methimazole is favored by most endocrinologists. PTU is preferred in pregnant women because methimazole has been associated with aplasia cutis and with choanal and esophageal atresia. Complete blood count and differential should be obtained before their use.

1. Dosage: methimazole 15 to 30 mg/day given as a single dose; PTU 50 to 100 mg PO q8h.
2. Antithyroid drugs can be used as the primary form of treatment or as adjunctive therapy before radioactive therapy or surgery or afterward if the hyperthyroidism recurs.
3. Side effects: skin rash (3% to 5% of patients), arthralgias, myalgias, granulocytopenia (0.5%). Rare side effects are aplastic anemia, hepatic necrosis from PTU, cholestatic jaundice from methimazole.
4. When antithyroid drugs are used as primary therapy, they are usually given for 6 to 18 mo; prolonged therapy may cause hypothyroidism. Monitor thyroid function every 2 mo for 6 mo, then less frequently.
5. The use of antithyroid drugs before radioiodine therapy is best reserved for patients in whom exacerbation of hyperthyroidism after radioactive iodine therapy is hazardous (e.g., elderly patients with coronary artery disease or significant coexisting morbidity). In these patients the antithyroid drug can be stopped 2 days before radioactive iodine therapy, resumed 2 days later, and continued for 4 to 6 wk.

RADIOIODINE THERAPY (RADIOACTIVE IODINE [RAI; ^{131}I]):
1. RAI is the treatment of choice for patients aged >21 yr and younger patients who have not achieved remission after 1 yr of antithyroid drug therapy. RAI is also used in hyperthyroidism caused by toxic adenoma or toxic multinodular goiter.
2. Contraindicated during pregnancy (can cause fetal hypothyroidism) and lactation. Pregnancy should be excluded in women of childbearing age before RAI is administered.
3. A single dose of RAI is effective in inducing a euthyroid state in nearly 80% of patients.
4. There is a high incidence of post-RAI hypothyroidism (>50% within first year and 2%/yr thereafter); these patients should be frequently evaluated for the onset of hypothyroidism (see "Chronic Rx").

SURGICAL THERAPY (SUBTOTAL THYROIDECTOMY):
1. Indicated in obstructing goiters, in any patient who refuses RAI and cannot be adequately managed with antithyroid medications (e.g., patients with toxic adenoma or toxic multinodular goiter), and in pregnant patients who cannot be adequately managed with antithyroid medication or develop side effects to them.
2. Patients should be rendered euthyroid with antithyroid drugs before surgery.
3. Complications of surgery include hypothyroidism (28% to 43% after 10 yr), hypoparathyroidism, and vocal cord paralysis (1%).
4. Hyperthyroidism recurs after surgery in 10% to 15% of patients.

ADJUNCTIVE THERAPY: Propranolol alleviates the beta-adrenergic symptoms of hyperthyroidism; initial dose is 20 to 40 mg PO q6h; dosage is gradually increased until symptoms are controlled. Major contraindications to propranolol are congestive heart failure and bronchospasm. Diagnosis and treatment of thyrotoxic storm is also discussed in Section I.

CHRONIC Rx

- Patients undergoing treatment with antithyroid drugs should be seen every 1 to 3 mo until euthyroidism is achieved and every 3 to 4 mo while they remain on antithyroid therapy. After treatment is stopped, periodic monitoring of thyroid function tests with TSH is recommended every 3 mo for 1 yr, then every 6 mo for 1 yr, then annually.
- Orbital decompression surgery can be used to correct Graves' orbitopathy (Fig. 1-203).

DISPOSITION

Successful treatment of hyperthyroidism requires lifelong monitoring for the onset of hypothyroidism or the recurrence of thyrotoxicosis.

REFERRAL

- Endocrinology referral is recommended at the time of initial diagnosis and during treatment.
- Surgical referral in selected patients (see "Surgical Therapy").
- Hospitalization of all patients with thyroid storm.

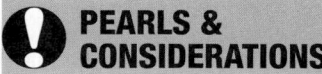

PEARLS & CONSIDERATIONS

COMMENTS

- Elderly hyperthyroid patients may have only subtle signs (weight loss, tachycardia, fine skin, brittle nails). This form is known as *apathetic hyperthyroidism* and manifests with lethargy rather than hyperkinetic activity. An enlarged thyroid gland may be absent. Coexisting medical disorders (most commonly cardiac disease) may also mask the symptoms. These patients often have unexplained congestive heart failure, worsening of angina, or new-onset atrial fibrillation resistant to treatment. See the entry on Graves' disease for additional information on diagnosis and treatment.
- Subclinical hyperthyroidism is defined as a normal serum-free thyroxine and free triiodothyronine levels with a TSH level suppressed below the normal range and usually undetectable. These patients usually do not present with signs or symptoms of overt hyperthyroidism. Treatment options include observation or a therapeutic trial of low-dose antithyroid agents for 6 mo to attempt to induce remission.
- *Thyrotoxic periodic paralysis (TPP)* is a hyperthyroidism-related hypokalemia and muscle-weakening condition resulting from a sudden shift of potassium into cells. Many patients do not have other symptoms of hyperthyroidism. Typical presentation involves an Asian adult male with acute fatigue and muscle weakness initially presenting in the lower extremities. Physical examination reveals decreased deep tendon reflexes, hypertension, and tachycardia. ECG often reveals U waves, high QRS voltage, and first-degree atrioventricular block. Additional laboratory testing reveals normal acid-base state, hypokalemia with low urinary potassium excretion (spot urinary potassium concentration <20 mEq/L from potassium shift into cells), hypophosphatemia, hypophostaturia, and hypercalciuria. Electromyography during attacks shows low-amplitude compound muscle action potential of the tested muscle. Therapy consists of cautious potassium supplementation (increased risk of rebound hyperkalemia). Use of nonselective beta-blockers (e.g., propranolol) to counteract hyperadrenergic activity, which may be causing TPP, may also be useful.

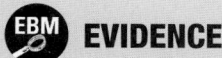

EVIDENCE

available at www.expertconsult.com

SUGGESTED READINGS

available at www.expertconsult.com

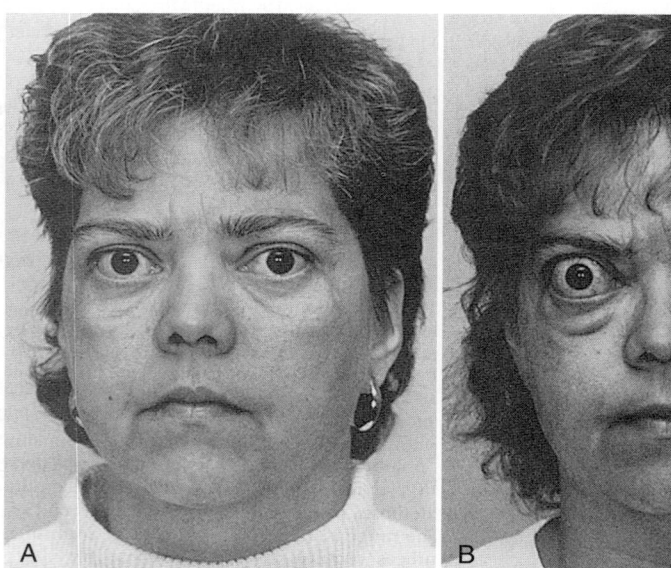

FIGURE 1-203 Characteristic signs of Graves' orbitopathy. A, Subsequently corrected by orbital decompression surgery. **B,** Note the thyroid stare, asymmetry, proptosis, and periorbital edema before correction. (Courtesy Dr. Jack Rootman, University of British Columbia, Vancouver, Canada. From Larsen PR et al [eds]: *Williams textbook of endocrinology,* ed 10, Philadelphia, 2003, Saunders.)

AUTHOR: **FRED F. FERRI, M.D.**

BASIC INFORMATION

DEFINITION

Hypertrophic osteoarthropathy (HOA) is a syndrome of clubbing of the digits, periostitis of long bones, skin changes, and arthritis. HOA may be primary or secondary to other underlying disease processes.

SYNONYMS

- Primary hypertrophic osteoarthropathy:
  1. Pachydermoperiostosis
  2. Idiopathic clubbing
  3. Touraine-Solente-Golé syndrome
- Secondary hypertrophic osteoarthropathy

ICD-9CM CODES
731.2 Hypertrophic osteoarthropathy

EPIDEMIOLOGY & DEMOGRAPHICS

- Primary HOA is a familial autosomal-dominant disease affecting the age group between 1 and 20 yr and is rare.
- Secondary HOA is more common, typically occurs in adults, and is associated with other illnesses, including:
  1. Pulmonary: bronchogenic carcinoma, lung abscesses, bronchiectasis, cystic fibrosis, pulmonary fibrosis, mesothelioma, sarcoidosis
  2. Gastrointestinal: esophageal carcinoma, colon cancer, inflammatory bowel disease (Crohn's disease, ulcerative colitis), hepatocellular carcinoma, liver cirrhosis, amebiasis
  3. Cardiac: infective endocarditis, right-to-left cardiac shunts, aortic aneurysms
  4. Thymoma
  5. Lymphoma
  6. Connective tissue diseases
  7. Thyroid acropachy

PHYSICAL FINDINGS & CLINICAL PRESENTATION

- Primary HOA typically presents with the insidious onset of clubbing of the hands and feet, described as "spadelike." Other signs and symptoms include:
  1. Joint pain and swelling
  2. Decreased use of the fingers and hands
  3. Facial changes, coarse facial skin grooves
  4. Thickening of the arms and legs
  5. Oily skin, diaphoresis, gynecomastia, and acne
- Secondary HOA patients may present with clinical symptoms before the underlying disorder can be detected. Signs and symptoms are similar to the above in addition to findings related to the underlying disease (e.g., bronchogenic carcinoma, infective endocarditis).

ETIOLOGY

The pathogenesis of HOA is not fully understood; current knowledge suggests that HOA results from the activation of one or more growth factors, such as vascular endothelial growth factor (VEGF) and platelet-derived growth factor, that are normally inactivated in the lungs and systemic circulation.

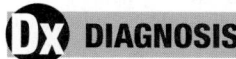 **DIAGNOSIS**

Diagnosis is primarily clinical; radiographs and bone scans can help confirm the diagnosis.

DIFFERENTIAL DIAGNOSIS

Other causes of HOA include Paget's disease, Reiter's syndrome, psoriasis, syphilis, osteoarthritis, rheumatoid arthritis, and osteomyelitis.

WORKUP

HOA warrants an investigation into any associated illnesses.

LABORATORY TESTS

- Routine laboratory studies such as blood count, electrolytes, and urine studies are typically normal in primary and secondary HOA.
- Erythrocyte sedimentation rate is elevated in secondary HOA.
- Liver function tests may be abnormal in patients with secondary HOA from gastrointestinal pathology.
- Alkaline phosphatase may be elevated as a result of periostitis of long bones.
- Analysis of the synovial fluid from joint effusions reveals a low white blood cell count with normal viscosity, color, and complement levels.

IMAGING STUDIES

- Radiographs of the long bones show periosteal new bone formation.
- A chest radiograph should be obtained to rule out underlying lung cancer.
- Bone scan with technetium-99m reveals uptake along the long bones, phalanges, and periarticular joint spaces.

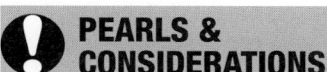 **TREATMENT**

ACUTE GENERAL Rx

- Treatment of primary HOA is symptomatic. Nonsteroidal antiinflammatory medications such as aspirin, salicylate, ibuprofen, naproxen, or indomethacin can be used.
- Treatment of secondary HOA is to eradicate the underlying disease (e.g., antibiotics for infective endocarditis, surgery for bronchogenic carcinoma). Correction of heart malfor-

mation or removal of an underlying tumor is rapidly followed by regression of HOA.

CHRONIC Rx

In patients with secondary HOA refractory to NSAIDs and aspirin, vagotomy has been tried with some success. However, the definitive treatment is to treat the underlying disease.

DISPOSITION

- Patients with primary HOA typically have symptoms of joint pain and swelling for the early part of their life. However, the disease becomes quiescent thereafter.
- Prognosis and disease course in patients with secondary HOA will depend on the underlying cause. The insidious development of clubbing suggests an infectious process, whereas the rapid progression of clubbing may suggest underlying malignancy.

REFERRAL

Referral should be made to rheumatology when the diagnosis of HOA is suspected and the cause remains unclear.

PEARLS & CONSIDERATIONS

Promidronate is a promising agent to relieve intractable pains associated with periosteal proliferation. Some bisphosphonates, including pamidronate, inhibit VEGF expression.

COMMENTS

- Infections and intrathoracic malignancies are the most common causes of secondary HOA.
- Some cases of primary HOA may later be found to be associated with a underlying disease such as patent ductus arteriosus, Crohn's disease, or myelofibrosis, in which case they become secondary.
- The periostosis and the extent of involvement do not depend on the form of the disease (primary or secondary), but rather on its duration.
- HOA secondary to infection of an arterial graft has been reported.
- Primary HOA and polyneuropathy, organomegaly, endocrinopathy, M-protein, and skin changes (POEMS) syndrome share important clinical features.

SUGGESTED READINGS
available at www.expertconsult.com

AUTHOR: **SHAHNAZ PUNJANI, M.D.**

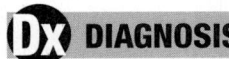

BASIC INFORMATION

DEFINITION

Hyperuricemia may be defined as serum uric acid >7.0 mg/dl in males or >6.0 mg/dl in females. Some individuals who are normouricemic by this definition will have levels of uric acid that exceed the limit of solubility of uric acid in tissue. Most people with hyperuricemia are asymptomatic; 20% of those with serum uric acid >9 mg/dl will develop gout in 5 yr. Hyperuricemia is associated with gout, obesity, diabetes, and cardiovascular disease.

ASYMTOMATIC HYPERURICEMIA

Definition: Laboratory evidence of elevated serum uric acid without clinical disease known to be caused by hyperuricemia

ETIOLOGY

Overproduction of uric acid accounts for a minority of cases of hyperuricemia. Most cases are due to decreased renal clearance of uric acid and high dietary purine consumption.

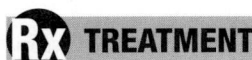

DIAGNOSIS

EVALUATION

The finding of hyperuricemia should prompt a thorough evaluation of potential causes and related diseases. If there is no clinical evidence of gout, nephrolithiasis, or acute kidney injury, the patient may be said to have asymptomatic hyperuricemia. Patient with hyperuricemia should be evaluated for potential causes of elevated uric acid including malignancy, renal insufficiency, toxins, and dietary indiscretion.

LABORATORY TESTS

- CBC with differential
- BUN/creatinine
- Urinalysis
- Lipid profile

TREATMENT

No specific therapy is indicated for most patients with asymptomatic hyperuricemia. Lifestyle and dietary modification are often advisable.

NONPHARMACOLOGIC THERAPY

- Weight loss
- Reduce alcohol intake, especially beer
- Reduce consumption of foods known to be high in purines such as red meat, organ meat, and high-fructose soft drinks.

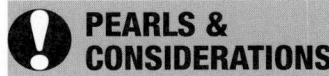

PEARLS & CONSIDERATIONS

- Research in progress suggest there may be a causal relationship between hyperuricemia and early hypertension.
- Very high levels of serum uric acid may warrant treatment even if asymptomatic.
- Patient with hyperuricemia and a family history of gout should be followed closely for the development of gouty arthritis.
- Hyperuricemia in patients with gout should almost always be treated with urate lowering medication (see chapter on gout).

SUGGESTED READINGS

available at www.expertconsult.com

AUTHOR: **BERNARD ZIMMERMANN, M.D.**

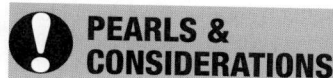 BASIC INFORMATION

DEFINITION

Hypoaldosteronism is defined as an aldosterone deficiency or impaired aldosterone function.

ICD-9CM CODES
255.4 Hypoadrenalism

EPIDEMIOLOGY & DEMOGRAPHICS

Selective hypoaldosteronism accounts for as many as 10% of cases of unexplained hyperkalemia.

PHYSICAL FINDINGS & CLINICAL PRESENTATION

- Physical examination may be entirely within normal limits.
- Hypertension may be present in some patients.
- Profound muscle weakness and cardiac arrhythmias may be present.

ETIOLOGY

- Hyporeninemic hypoaldosteronism (renin-angiotensin dependent): decreased aldosterone production as a result of decreased renin production; the typical patient has renal disease attributable to various factors (e.g., diabetes mellitus, interstitial nephritis, multiple myeloma).
- Hyperreninemic hypoaldosteronism (renin-angiotensin independent): renin production by the kidneys is intact; the defect is in aldosterone biosynthesis or in the action of angiotensin II. Common causes of this form of hypoaldosteronism are medications (ACE inhibitors, heparin), lead poisoning, aldosterone enzyme defects, and severe illness.

DIAGNOSIS

DIFFERENTIAL DIAGNOSIS

Pseudohypoaldosteronism: renal unresponsiveness to aldosterone. In this condition both renin and aldosterone levels are elevated. Pseudohypoaldosteronism can be caused by medications (spironolactone), chronic interstitial nephritis, systemic disorders (systemic lupus erythematosus, amyloidosis), or primary mineralocorticoid resistance.

WORKUP

Measurement of plasma renin activity after 4 hr of upright posture can differentiate hyporeninemic from hyperreninemic causes. Renin levels in the normal or low range identify cases that are renin-angiotensin dependent, whereas high renin levels identify cases that are renin-angiotensin independent. The diagnosis and etiology of hypoaldosteronism can be confirmed with the renin-aldosterone stimulation test:

- Hyporeninemic hypoaldosteronism: low stimulated renin and aldosterone levels
- End-organ refractoriness to aldosterone action: high stimulated renin and aldosterone levels
- Adrenal gland abnormality: high stimulated renin and low aldosterone levels

LABORATORY TESTS

- Increased potassium, normal or decreased sodium
- Hyperchloremic metabolic acidosis (caused by the absence of hydrogen-secreting action of aldosterone)
- Increased BUN and creatinine (secondary to renal disease)
- Hyperglycemia (diabetes mellitus is common in these patients)

TREATMENT

NONPHARMACOLOGIC THERAPY

- Low-potassium diet with liberal sodium intake (at least 4 g of sodium chloride per day)
- Avoidance of ACE inhibitors and potassium-sparing diuretics

ACUTE GENERAL Rx

- Judicious use of fludrocortisone (0.05 to 0.1 mg PO every morning) in patients with aldosterone deficiency associated with deficiency of adrenal glucocorticoid hormones
- Furosemide 20 to 40 mg qd to correct hyperkalemia of hyporeninemic hypoaldosteronism

DISPOSITION

Prognosis varies with the etiology of hypoaldosteronism and presence of associated disorders.

REFERRAL

Endocrinology referral for renin-aldosterone stimulation test

⚠ PEARLS & CONSIDERATIONS

COMMENTS

Treatment of pseudohypoaldosteronism is the same as for hypoaldosteronism; however, effect is limited because of impaired renal sensitivity.

AUTHOR: **FRED F. FERRI, M.D.**

BASIC INFORMATION

DEFINITION

Hypochondriasis is the preoccupation with the fear of having, or the idea that one has, a serious disease. The fear is usually based on a misinterpretation of bodily signs or symptoms and persists despite medical reassurance, although the belief does not have the intensity of a delusion. The preoccupation causes clinically significant distress or impairment in social, occupational, or other important areas of functioning and lasts for at least 6 mo.

ICD-9CM CODES
300.7 Hypochondriasis

EPIDEMIOLOGY & DEMOGRAPHICS

PREVALENCE: 1% to 5%, but thought to be higher in primary care outpatient settings, where estimates range from 3% to 10%.
PREDOMINANT SEX: Equal frequency in men and women.
PREDOMINANT AGE: Onset at any age, but most commonly between ages 20 and 30 yr
GENETICS/RISK: No genetic component identified, and neither socioeconomic nor educational factors appear to predispose to this disorder. Patients with hypochondriasis are more likely than the general population to have Axis I disorders, such as generalized anxiety, obsessive-compulsive disorder, and depression, and Axis II personality disorders. Serious childhood illnesses common in past medical history.

PHYSICAL FINDINGS & CLINICAL PRESENTATION

- Patient presents with a complaint of a physical symptom or sign (e.g., dizziness, pain) and remains preoccupied with the concern, despite evidence to the contrary, that it represents a serious disease.
- Associated distress and impairment last at least 6 mo.
- Variable degree of insight (i.e., recognition that the concern about serious illness is excessive or unreasonable).
- Hypochondriacal symptoms often correlated with psychosocial stressors.
- No specific physical examination findings.

ETIOLOGY

Unknown etiology, but psychological theories include disturbance of perception (amplification of normal somatic sensations), cognition (tendency to attribute sensations to a pathologic process), or interpersonal relationships (learning and then reinforcement of the sick role); or variant of another psychiatric condition such as depression.

DIAGNOSIS

DIFFERENTIAL DIAGNOSIS

- Underlying medical condition, such as multiple sclerosis, hypothyroidism, or systemic lupus erythematosus
- Somatization disorder
- Body dysmorphic disorder (restricted to a circumscribed concern about appearance)
- Factitious disorder or malingering
- Generalized anxiety disorder with health concerns as one worry among many others
- Major depressive disorder with health concerns occurring only during depressive episodes
- Psychosis, as may occur with depression and schizophrenia

WORKUP

- History, physical examination, and laboratory and imaging tests, as appropriate, to exclude underlying medical condition.
- Symptom measures (e.g., Health Anxiety Inventory, Whiteley Index of Hypochondriasis) may be used for detection and monitoring of severity over time.
- Evaluation for other psychiatric disorders associated with hypochondriasis such as depression and anxiety.

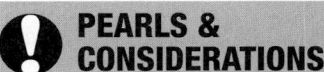
TREATMENT

NONPHARMACOLOGIC THERAPY

- Reassurance and education, including linking the diagnosis to psychologic stressors
- Individual or group therapy, including problem-solving (focusing on understanding and coping with symptoms) or cognitive-behavioral (with techniques to alter or restructure maladaptive thinking) approaches

- Brief and regularly scheduled appointments with the primary care physician
- Avoidance of laboratory tests, imaging studies, and diagnostic and surgical procedures unless otherwise indicated
- Elimination of sources of secondary gain
- Limit on reading medical texts or websites
- Benign interventions (e.g., exercise, massage)

CHRONIC Rx

- Antidepressants may be helpful even in patients without features of depression: placebo-controlled trials of fluoxetine and paroxetine suggest benefit; imipramine and fluvoxamine have been studied in small, open-label trials.
- Treatment of comorbid psychiatric conditions, if present.

DISPOSITION

Waxing and waning course over decades; recovery rates between 30% and 50%. Positive prognostic factors include acute onset, absence of secondary gain, lack of comorbid psychiatric disorder, and high socioeconomic status.

REFERRAL

Referral to a therapist and/or psychiatrist may be helpful; however, some patients may resist referral given the belief that symptoms are due to an undiagnosed medical illness.

PEARLS & CONSIDERATIONS

- Psychotherapy and pharmacotherapy may be helpful treatment modalities for patients open to treatment not directed at the perceived illness.
- The onset of physical symptoms late in life is almost always the result of a medical disorder.

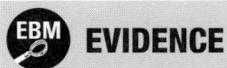
EVIDENCE

available at www.expertconsult.com

SUGGESTED READINGS
available at www.expertconsult.com

AUTHOR: **LUCY KALANITHI, M.D.**

BASIC INFORMATION

DEFINITION

A decrease in parathyroid hormone (PTH) secretion or function results in hypoparathyroidism. In primary hypoparathyroidism, absence or dysfunction of the parathyroid gland results in inadequate PTH secreation and subsequent hypocalcemia and hyperphosphatemia. Impaired function of PTH (i.e., PTH resistance or pseudohypoparathyroidism) can also cause hypocalcemia and hyperphosphatemia but the measured PTH level is elevated in this circumstance. Secondary hypoparathyroidism, a condition in which PTH levels are low in response to hypercalcemic states, is discussed in "Hypercalcemia." The focus of this section is primary hypoparathyroidism.

ICD-9CM CODES
252.1 Hypoparathyroidism

EPIDEMIOLOGY & DEMOGRAPHICS

The incidence and prevalence of primary hypoparathyroidism depends on the etiology of the condition. Postoperative hypoparathyroidism is the most common etiology and has an incidence as high as 3.8% in patients undergoing total or near-total thyroidectomy. Autoimmune disorders are more common in women (female:male ratio of 1.4:1.0). Autoimmune polyglandular syndrome type I is reported to have an incidence of 1:100,000 and prevalence of 1:25,000. Typically, patients with this syndrome present in childhood. Other etiologies of primary hypoparathyroidism are very rare.

PHYSICAL FINDINGS & CLINICAL PRESENTATION

The symptoms of primary hypoparathyroidism are primarily related to hypocalcemia. The presentation of symptoms varies with the severity and duration of illness.
- Cardiovascular: prolonged QT intervals, QRS and ST segment changes, ventricular arrhythmias
- Musculoskeletal: muscle cramps, laryngospasm, osteomalacia (adults), rickets (children), weakened tooth enamel, osteosclerosis
- CNS: tetany (Chvostek's sign and Trousseau's sign), seizures, paresthesias, visual impairment from cataract formation, altered mental status, papilledema, and basal ganglia calcifications with longstanding disease
- GI: abdominal pain
- Renal: hypercalciuria and nephrolithiasis
- Other: dry scaly skin, brittle nails, dry hair

ETIOLOGY

There are several etiologies of primary hypoparathyroidism.
- Genetic disorders
  - Branchial dysembryogenesis (DiGeorge's syndrome)
  - Congenital absence of parathyroids
  - Activating mutation of the calcium sensing receptor alters the set point of the receptor and decreases PTH secretion
- Autoimmune
  - Autoimmune polyglandular syndrome type 1 presents in early childhood and is defined by a classic triad of mucocutaneous candidiasis, autoimmune hypoparathyroidism, and Addison's disease.
  - Activating antibodies to calcium sensing receptor alters the set point of the receptor and decreases PTH secretion.
- Postsurgical (most common etiology)—can be transient or permanent
  - Parathyroidectomy
  - Complication of neck surgery such as thyroidectomy
- Radiation to the neck
- Infiltration
  - Metastatic carcinoma
  - Wilson's disease
  - Hemochromatosis
  - Granulomas
- Other
  - Hypermagnesemia and hypomagnesemia
  - Severe burns and sepsis

DIAGNOSIS

DIFFERENTIAL DIAGNOSIS

- Other causes of hypoparathyroidism (i.e., secondary hypoparathyroidism as a result of hypercalcemia) include:
  - Medications: thiazide diuretics
  - Vitamin D intoxication, milk-alkali syndrome
  - Granulomatous disorders (e.g., sarcoidosis)
  - Malignancy (e.g., lung cancer, lymphoma, myeloma, bone metastasis)
  - Prolonged immobilization
- Other causes of hypocalcemia (i.e., secondary hyperparathyroidism) include:
  - PTH resistance (i.e., target organs unresponsive to PTH action)
    1. Pseudohypoparathyroidism (see Table 1-84): heterogeneous disorder presenting in childhood characterized by hypocalcemia, hyperphosphatemia and elevated PTH levels
    2. Hypomagnesemia

- Vitamin D deficiency or resistance
- Hyperphosphatemia (i.e., renal failure, rhabdomyolysis, tumor lysis)
- Osteoblastic metastasis
- Acute pancreatitis
- Drugs: calcium chelators, bisphosphonates, foscarnet, cisplatin

WORKUP

- Primary hypoparathyroidism: serum calcium is usually low and phosphorus is elevated in primary hypoparathyroidism.
  - Two measurements of serum calcium are required for the confirmation of hypocalcemia. Total calcium should be corrected for low albumin utilizing the formula: Corrected Calcium = measured calcium-albumin + 4. If a reliable laboratory is available, an ionized calcium should be considered especially in conditions associated with acid-base disturbances or low albumin states.
  - The serum intact PTH (iPTH) level is the single best test to evaluate the etiology of hypocalcemia. PTH is decreased in primary hypoparathyroidism and elevated in most other conditions associated with low calcium levels.
  - Serum phosphorus is usually high normal or elevated in primary hypoparathyroidism.
- Rule out other causes of hypoparathyroidism (i.e., secondary hypoparathyroidism). These conditions are associated with hypercalcemia and subsequent PTH suppression.
- Rule out other causes of hypocalcemia. These conditions are typically associated with elevated PTH levels.

LABORATORY TESTS

- Total and ionized calcium: low in primary hypoparathyroidism and high in secondary hypoparathyroidism
- PTH: low in primary and secondary hypoparathyroidism and high in PTH resistance states like pseudohypoparathyroidism
- Phosphorus: high-normal or high in primary hypoparathyroidism
- Magnesium: both hypomagnesemia and hypermagnesemia can cause hypoparathyroidism
- ECG should be considered in both hypercalcemic and hypocalcemic states. Hypocalcemia associated with prolonged QT interval, rarely ST-segment elevations
- 24-hr urine for calcium to evaluate the risk for renal stones
- Other tests to consider includes vitamin D 25, vitamin D 1,25, creatinine, PTHrp, SPEP/UPEP, and amylase. These tests evaluate for conditions discussed in the differential diagnosis.

TREATMENT

NONPHARMACOLOGIC THERAPY

Parathyroid autotransplantation:
Hypoparathyroidism and subsequent hypocalcemia are common problems after neck exploration for total or near-total thyroidectomy or parathyroidectomy. In cases where there is con-

TABLE 1-84 Types of Hypoparathyroidism

Type	Calcium	PO$_4$	PTH	Comments
Hypoparathyroidism	↓	↑	↓	Surgical removal (most common cause)
Pseudohypoparathyroidism	↓	↑	Ø↑	End-organ resistance to PTH (hereditary)
Pseudo-pseudohypoparathyroidism	Ø	Ø	Ø	Only skeletal abnormalities (Albright's hereditary osteodystrophy)

Ø, No change.
From Weisslederer R et al: *Primer of diagnostic imaging*, St Louis, 2007, Mosby.

cern for postoperative hypoparathyroidism, parathyroid autotransplantation of one or two parathyroid glands into the forearm or sternocleidomastoid muscle should be performed to prevent postoperative hypoparathyroidism.

PHARMACOLOGIC THERAPY

The mainstay of treatment for primary hypoparathyroidism is through pharmacologic therapy with calcium and vitamin D supplementation. The goals of therapy are to control symptoms and minimize complications of therapy. The aim should be to obtain low-normal serum calcium, 24-hr urinary calcium <300 mg/day, and a calcium-phosphorus product <55.

- Vitamin D:
  - There are several vitamin D preparations available on the market but the treatment of choice for patients with primary hypoparathyroidism is calcitriol. It is an active metabolite that does not require hydroxylation in the liver or kidney and therefore bypasses the PTH-mediated 1-α hydroxylation defect that occurs with hypoparathyroidism.
  - Dose of 0.25 to 1 μg once or twice daily is usually required to correct hypocalcemia and improves symptoms. Its maximal effect is seen after 10 hr and it lasts for 2 to 3 days.
- Calcium:
  - Calcium carbonate or calcium citrates are common oral agents used to treatment hypocalcemia associated with hypoparathyroidism. Calcium carbonate requires an acidic environment for effective absorption, and as a result, it must be taken with food. Its effectiveness is decreased with concomitant use of H$_2$ blockers or proton pump inhibitors. However, calcium carbonate is cheaper in cost than other calcium supplements and therefore it is first line in the management of hypocalcemia for some patients. The advantage of calcium citrate is that it does not require an acidic environment for effective absorption.
  - Start with a dose of 500 to 1000 mg of elemental calcium TID and adjust the dose for a desired calcium in the low-normal range.
- Magnesium: hypocalcemia is difficult to correct without normalizing magnesium levels. Magnesium sulfate IV 2 g over 20 min followed by 1 g/hr infusion can be considered in severe deficiency states. Milder deficiencies can be managed with oral magnesium 100 mg tid.
- Thiazide diuretics: thiazides diuretics decrease urine calcium excretion and decrease kidney stones. They should be considered in individuals with urine calcium >250 mg/day.
- PTH replacement:
  - Preliminary studies involving injectable synthetic human PTH(1-34) have been performed with results showing a decrease in urinary calcium excretion and maintenance of serum calcium in the normal range.
  - It is not FDA approved for use in hypoparathyroidism.

ACUTE GENERAL RX

Severe and/or symptomatic hypocalcemia requires hospitalization. Acute management of hypocalcemia includes:
- Telemetry monitoring for arrhythmias associated with severe hypocalcemia
- IV infusion of calcium gluconate 10 ml of 10% solution to receive a bolus of 90 mg of elemental calcium followed by an infusion of 0.5 to 2 mg/kg/hr until ionized calcium levels are $\geq$4 mg/dl.

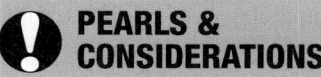

COMMENTS
- The mainstay of treatment for primary hypoparathyroidism is calcitriol and calcium supplementation to maintain a goal serum calcium level in the low-normal range. IV calcium should be considered if calcium <7.0 mg/dl. Magnesium levels should be assessed and appropriately replaced in all patients with hypocalcemia. Clinical trials are under way to evaluate the role of recombinant PTH for the treatment of primary hypoparathyroidism.
- In patients undergoing neck exploration, consideration should be given to the parathyroids and autotransplantation of one or more parathyroid glands should be considered when appropriate to prevent postoperative hypoparathyroidism.

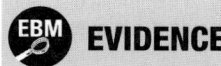

available at www.expertconsult.com

SUGGESTED READINGS
available at www.expertconsult.com

AUTHORS: **JENNIFER MIRANDA, M.D.,** and **GEETHA GOPALAKRISHNAN, M.D.**

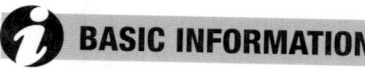 **BASIC INFORMATION**

DEFINITION

Hypopituitarism (from the Latin *pituita,* meaning phlegm) is the deficiency of one or more of the hormones of the anterior or posterior pituitary gland resulting from diseases of the hypothalamus or pituitary gland. Panhypopituitarism indicates the loss of all the pituitary hormones but is often used in clinical practice to describe patients deficient in growth hormone (GH), gonadotropins, corticotrophin, or thyrotropin in whom posterior pituitary function remains intact.

SYNONYMS

Panhypopituitarism
Pituitary insufficiency

ICD-9CM CODES
253.2 Panhypopituitarism

EPIDEMIOLOGY & DEMOGRAPHICS

Incidence of 4.2 cases per 100,000 persons

PHYSICAL FINDINGS & CLINICAL PRESENTATION

Symptoms depend on type of onset, number and severity of hormone deficiencies, their target organs, and age of onset.
- Mass effect of a pituitary tumor can cause headaches and visual disturbances (typically as bitemporal hemianopsia).
- Rhinorrhea.
- Corticotropin deficiency:
  ○ Fatigue and weakness, no appetite, abdominal pain, nausea, vomiting, failure to thrive in children, and hyponatremia. If the onset is abrupt, hypotension and shock
- Thyrotropin deficiency:
  ○ Fatigue and weakness, weight gain, cold intolerance, anemia, constipation
  ○ Bradycardia, hung-up reflexes, pretibial edema, change in voice, and hair loss
- Gonadotropin deficiency:
  ○ Loss of libido, erectile dysfunction, amenorrhea, hot flashes, dyspareunia, infertility, gynecomastia, decreased muscle mass, and anemia
- GH deficiency:
  ○ Growth retardation in children
  ○ Easy fatigue, hypoglycemia
  ○ Lean mass is reduced and fat mass is increased, leading to obesity
  ○ Decreased bone mineral density, increased low density lipoprotein cholesterol, obesity, increased inflammatory cardiovascular markers (interleukin-6 and C-reactive protein)
- Hyperprolactinemia:
  ○ Galactorrhea, hypogonadism, inability to lactate after delivery
  ○ Posterior pituitary (vasopressin; antidiuretic hormone [ADH] deficiency): diabetes insipidus with polyuria, polydipsia, nocturia, hypotension, and dehydration

ETIOLOGY

It can be congenital or acquired:
- Congenital: mutations in transcription factors produce multiple hormonal deficiencies. Mutations in genes produce single hormonal deficiency.
- Acquired: the result of destruction of pituitary cells caused by:
  1. Pituitary apoplexy: hemorrhage or infarction of the pituitary gland. Predisposing factors include diabetes mellitus, anticoagulation therapy, head trauma, and radiation therapy. Sheehan's syndrome: postpartum necrosis, a rare complication after pregnancy.
  2. Infiltrative disease, including sarcoidosis, hemachromatosis, histiocytosis X, Wegener's granulomatosis, lymphocytic hypophysitis, and infection of the pituitary (tuberculosis, mycosis, syphilis).
  3. Primary empty sella syndrome: flattening of the pituitary gland caused by extension of the subarachnoid space and filling of cerebrospinal fluid into the sella turcica.
  4. Pituitary tumors: classified by size (microadenomas, <10 mm; macroadenomas, >10 mm) and function. Prolactin-secreting tumors and nonfunctioning tumors account for the majority of pituitary adenomas.
  5. Suprasellar tumors: craniopharyngiomas are the most common.

DX DIAGNOSIS

The diagnosis of hypopituitarism is suspected by clinical history and physical findings and is established by blood tests to confirm the presence of hormone deficiency.

DIFFERENTIAL DIAGNOSIS

The differential diagnosis is as outlined under "Etiology."

WORKUP

Includes baseline determination of each anterior pituitary hormone followed by dynamic provocative stimulation tests, radiograph imaging, and formal visual field testing.

LABORATORY TESTS

- Corticotropin deficiency:
  1. The presence of a 9:00 AM cortisol level >20 mcg/dl or <4 mcg/dl usually confirms sufficiency or deficiency, respectively.
  2. Corticotropin stimulation test using 250 mcg of corticotropin given IV and measuring serum cortisol before and 30 and 60 min after administration. A normal response is an increase in serum cortisol level >20 mcg/dl.
  3. With pituitary disease these test results may be indeterminate, and more dynamic testing such as an insulin-tolerance or metyrapone test may be necessary.
- Thyrotropin deficiency:
  1. Thyroid-stimulating hormone (TSH) and free T_4 measurements

2. Primary hypothyroidism shows elevated TSH with low free T_4. Secondary hypothyroidism shows normal or low TSH with low free T_4 and low T_3 resin uptake.
- Gonadotropin deficiency:
  1. Follicle-stimulating hormone (FSH), luteinizing hormone (LH), estrogen, and testosterone measurements.
  2. In men, hypogonadotropic hypogonadism is seen with low testosterone levels and normal or low FSH and LH levels (ideally measured at 9:00 AM because of diurnal rhythm). Check free testosterone if patient is obese.
  3. In premenopausal women with amenorrhea, low estrogen with normal or low FSH and LH levels is typically seen.
- GH deficiency:
  1. Insulin-induced hypoglycemia stimulation test using 0.1 to 0.15 unit/kg regular insulin given IV and measuring growth hormone 30, 60, and 120 min after administration. A normal response is a growth hormone level >3 mcg/dl. This test is contraindicated in seizure disorder or ischemic heart disease.
  2. Combination of GH-releasing hormone plus arginine is an alternative test, with a diagnostic threshold of 9 mcg/L.
  3. Because the relation between serum insulinlike growth factor (IGF)-1 and GH levels blurs with age, a normal serum IGF-1 does not exclude the diagnosis in older adults.
- Hyperprolactinemia: prolactin levels may be elevated in prolactin-secreting pituitary adenomas.
- Vasopressin deficiency:
  1. Urinalysis shows low specific gravity.
  2. Urine osmolality is low.
  3. Serum osmolality is high.
  4. Fluid deprivation test over 18 hr with inability to concentrate the urine.
  5. Serum vasopressin level is low.
  6. Electrolytes may show hyponatremia and exclude hyperglycemia.

IMAGING STUDIES

- Imaging is the first step in identifying an underlying cause.
- MRI is more sensitive than CT in visualizing the pituitary fossa, sella turcica, optic chiasm, pituitary stalk, and cavernous sinuses. It is also more sensitive in detecting pituitary microadenomas. CT with contrast can be used if MRI is not available.
- Surveillance scan at baseline and 12 mo thereafter depending on protocol and clinical symptoms.

RX TREATMENT

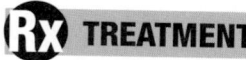

Threefold: removing underlying cause (surgery or radiation), treating hormonal deficiencies, and addressing any other repercussions from deficiency.

NONPHARMACOLOGIC THERAPY

- IV fluid resuscitation, correction of electrolyte and metabolic abnormalities with potassium bicarbonate, and oxygen therapy.
- Transsphenoidal surgery for tumors causing specific symptoms.
- Radiation or stereotactic radiosurgery ("gamma knife") for medically unresponsive, surgically unresectable tumors and tumors for which other modalities are contraindicated. It is both safe and effective for recurrent or residual pituitary adenomas.

ACUTE GENERAL Rx

Acute situations such as adrenal crisis or myxedema coma can occur in untreated hypopituitarism and should be treated accordingly with IV corticosteroids (e.g., hydrocortisone 100 to 250 mg bolus followed by hydrocortisone 100 mg IV q6h for 24 hr) and levothyroxine (e.g., 5 to 8 mcg/kg IV over 15 min, then 100 mcg IV q24h).

CHRONIC Rx

Treatment is lifelong:
- Adrenocorticotropic hormone (ACTH) deficiency: hydrocortisone 10 mg PO every morning and 5 mg PO every evening or prednisone 5 mg PO every morning and 2.5 mg PO every evening. Dexamethasone or prednisone is often preferred because of longer duration of action.
- LH and FSH deficiency:
  - In men, testosterone enanthate or propionate 200 to 300 mg IM every 2 to 3 wk, or transdermal testosterone scrotal patches can be tried.
  - In women who are not interested in fertility, conjugated estrogen 0.3 to 1.25 mg/day and held the last 5 to 7 days of each month with the addition of medroxyprogesterone 10 mg/day given during days 15 to 25 of the normal menstrual cycle. In those who have secondary hypogonadism and wish to become pregnant, pulsatile gonadotropic-releasing hormone may be of benefit.
- TSH deficiency: levothyroxine 0.05 to 0.15 mg/day.
- GH deficiency:
  - GH replacement in children is universally accepted.
  - GH replacement in adults is not generally recommended and requires careful consideration of each individual case. It may have effects on quality of life, body composition, bone density, and cardiovascular risk factors.
  - Side effects of replacement includes peripheral edema, arthralgia, and headaches.
  - Usual GH dose is between 0.2 and 0.4 mg, determined by the age and gender of a patient and increments of 0.1 mg every 2 to 4 wk until serum IGF-1 is in the upper part of the normal range. Young adults and women taking estrogen require a higher dose.
- ADH deficiency:
  - Desmopressin (DDAVP) 10 to 20 mcg by intranasal spray or 0.05 to 0.1 mg PO bid is used in patients with diabetes insipidus.
  - Vasopressin: 5-10 U given IM or SC q6h.

DISPOSITION

- Hormone replacement therapy is adjusted according to serum hormone monitoring.
- If untreated can lead to adrenal crisis, severe hyponatremia and hypothyroidism, metabolic abnormalities, and death.
- Complications: visual deficit, adrenal crisis, susceptibility to infection and other stressors.
- Prognosis: stable patients have a favorable prognosis with replacement hormone therapy. Patients with acute decompensation are in critical condition with a high mortality rate.

REFERRAL

Consultation with an endocrinologist and neurosurgeon for surgical treatment

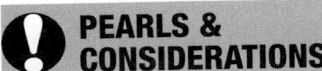 **PEARLS & CONSIDERATIONS**

- All patients sustaining moderate to severe head injury should undergo assessment of anterior pituitary function during the acute phase and at 6 mo.
- IGF-1 can be used as a marker of GH deficiency.
- All tests of GH secretion are more likely to give false-positive results in obese patients.

- The GH axis is the most vulnerable to the effects of radiotherapy; doses as low as 18 Gy in children have caused GH deficiency.
- Sequence of hormonal disruption: GH secretion then gonadotropin secretion. TSH and adrenocorticotropic hormone secretion are somewhat resistant.
- Thyroxine supplementation increases the rate of cortisol metabolism and can lead to adrenal crisis, so corticosteroids should be replaced first.
- All patients receiving glucocorticoid replacement therapy should wear proper identification stating the need for this therapy.
- Stress doses of corticosteroids are indicated before surgery or for any medical emergency (e.g., sepsis, acute myocardial infarction).
- Antidiuretic hormone deficiency may be masked if there is ACTH deficiency with symptoms only appearing when cortisol has been replaced.

COMMENTS

- Mineralocorticoid replacement is not necessary in secondary adrenal insufficiency because the renin-angiotensin-aldosterone system is unaffected by pituitary failure.
- Patients with adult-acquired GH deficiency must meet at least two criteria before replacement therapy: a poor GH response to at least two standard stimuli and hypopituitarism from pituitary or hypothalamic damage. The criteria are different in children in whom GH is required for normal growth.
- Prevention of acute decompensation can be accomplished by reminding patients to increase the dose of hydrocortisone in response to stress.
- Medical therapy should precede surgical therapy.

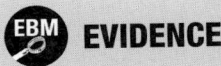 **EVIDENCE**

available at www.expertconsult.com

SUGGESTED READINGS
available at www.expertconsult.com

AUTHOR: **SHAHNAZ PUNJANI, M.D.**

BASIC INFORMATION

DEFINITION

Hypospadias is a developmental abnormality of the penis characterized by:
- Abnormal ventral opening of the urethral meatus anywhere from the ventral aspect of the glans penis to the perineum
- Ventral curvature of the penis (chordee)
- Dorsal foreskin hood

ICD-9CM CODES
752.61
Congenital chordee: 752.63

EPIDEMIOLOGY & DEMOGRAPHICS

PREVALENCE: One male in 250
GENETICS:
- Pertinent familial aspects of hypospadias include the finding of hypospadias in 6.8% of fathers of affected boys and in 14% of male siblings.
- An 8.5-fold higher rate of hypospadias is reported in monozygotic twins, suggesting insufficient production of human chorionic gonadotropin (hCG) by the single placenta.

PHYSICAL FINDINGS & CLINICAL PRESENTATION
- Genetics: normal karyotypes are seen with glandular hypospadias; abnormal karyotypes are noted in more severe forms of hypospadias
- Cryptorchidism: 8% to 9% occurrence
- Inguinal hernia: 9% to 10% occurrence
- Hydrocele: 9% to 16% occurrence

PENILE CURVATURE (CHORDEE): Three theories:
1. Abnormal development of the urethral plate
2. Abnormal fibrotic mesenchymal tissue at the urethral meatus
3. Corporal disproportion

ETIOLOGY

Multifactorial:
- Endocrine factors:
  1. Abnormal androgen production
  2. Limited androgen sensitivity in the target tissues
  3. Premature cessation of androgenic stimulation as a result of Leydig cell dysfunction
  4. Insufficient testosterone-dihydrotestosterone synthesis as a result of deficient 5-alpha reductase enzyme activity
- Arrested development

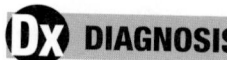

DIAGNOSIS

WORKUP

Made by observation and examination

LABORATORY TESTS

Intersex evaluation should be undertaken if there is associated cryptorchidism. The evaluation should include ultrasound; genitographic studies; and chromosomal, gonadal, biochemical, and molecular studies.

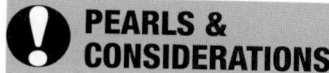

TREATMENT

ACUTE GENERAL Rx
DESIGNATION/CLASSIFICATION:
- Anterior: 33%
- Middle: 25%
- Posterior: 41%

SPECIAL CONSIDERATIONS:
- The only reason for operating on any patient with hypospadias is to correct deformities that interfere with the function of urination and procreation.
- Another reason for intervention is cosmetic concern.
- The American Academy of Pediatrics recommends the best time for surgical intervention to be 6 to 12 mo.

HORMONAL MANIPULATION:
- Controversial.
- hCG administration is given before repair of proximal hypospadias.
- The effect of hCG administration is decreased hypospadias and chordee severity in all patients, increased vascularity and thickness of the proximal corpus spongiosum.
- Application of topical testosterone increases mean penile circumference and length without any lasting side effects.
- Prepubertal exogenous testosterone does not adversely effect ultimate penile growth.

CHRONIC Rx
SURGICAL PROCEDURES:
- Orthoplasty (correcting penile curvature)
- Urethroplasty
- Meatoplasty
- Glanuloplasty
- Skin coverage

There is no single universally acceptable applicable technique for hypospadias repair.

TYPES OF REPAIR:
- Anterior hypospadias: MAGPI, Thiersch-Duplay urethroplasty, glans approximation procedure, tubularized incised plate (TIP) urethroplasty, Mathieu perimeatal flap, Mustarde technique, megameatus intact prepuce, pyramid procedure
- Midlevel hypospadias: TIP, Mathieu flap, onlay island flap (OIF), King procedure
- Posterior hypospadias:
  1. One-stage repair: OIF, double-onlay preputial flap, pedicled preputial flap, transverse preputial island flap
  2. Two-stage repair: orthoplasty to correct chordee followed 6 mo later or longer by Thiersch-Duplay, bladder and/or buccal mucosal hypospadias repair

COMPLICATIONS OF REPAIR: Hematoma, meatal stenosis, fistula, urethral stricture, urethral diverticulum, wound infection, impaired healing, balanitis xerotica obliterans, penile curvature

PEARLS & CONSIDERATIONS

- Apparent simple isolated hypospadias may be the only visible indication of an underlying abnormality.
- The dorsal hood of redundant foreskin is used in the repair of hypospadias, so the patient with hypospadias and a dorsal hood should not be circumcised.

SUGGESTED READINGS
available at www.expertconsult.com

AUTHORS: **PHILIP J. ALIOTTA, M.D., M.S.H.A.,** and **RUBEN ALVERO, M.D.**

H

Diseases and Disorders

I

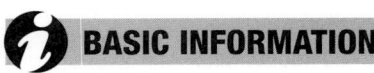

BASIC INFORMATION

DEFINITION

Hypothermia is a rectal temperature <35° C (95.8° F). Accidental hypothermia is an unintentionally induced decrease in core temperature in the absence of preoptic anterior hypothalamic conditions.

ICD-9CM CODES
991.6 Accidental hypothermia
780.9 Hypothermia not associated with low environmental temperature

EPIDEMIOLOGY & DEMOGRAPHICS

- Hypothermia occurs most frequently in the following groups: alcoholics; learning-impaired; patients with cardiovascular, cerebrovascular, or pituitary disorders; those using sedatives or tranquilizers; and elderly patients.
- ~700 persons in the United States die from hypothermia annually.

PHYSICAL FINDINGS & CLINICAL PRESENTATION

The clinical presentation varies with the severity of hypothermia. Shivering may be absent if body temperature is <33.3° C (92° F) or in patients taking phenothiazines.

Hypothermia may masquerade as cerebrovascular accident, ataxia, or slurred speech, or the patient may appear comatose or clinically dead.

Physiologic stages of hypothermia:
1. Mild hypothermia (32.2° to 35° C [90° to 95° F]): arrhythmias, ataxia
2. Moderate hypothermia (28° to 32.2° C [82.4° to 90° F]):
   a. Progressive decrease of level of consciousness, pulse, cardiac output, and respiration
   b. Fibrillation, dysrhythmias (increased susceptibility to ventricular tachy-cardia)
   c. Elimination of shivering mechanism for thermogenesis
3. Severe hypothermia (≤28° C [82.4° F]):
   a. Absence of reflexes or response to pain
   b. Decreased cerebral blood flow, decreased CO_2
   c. Increased risk of ventricular fibrillation or asystole

ETIOLOGY

Exposure to cold temperatures for a prolonged period. Contributing factors include:
1. Drugs: ethanol, phenothiazines, sedative-hypnotics
2. Skin disorders: extensive burns, severe psoriasis, exfoliative dermatitis
3. Metabolic disorders: hypopituitarism, hypothyroidism, hypoadrenalism
4. Neurologic abnormalities: stroke, head trauma, acute spinal cord transaction, impaired shivering
5. Other: lack of acclimatization, aggressive fluid resuscitation, sepsis, heat stroke treatment

DIAGNOSIS

DIFFERENTIAL DIAGNOSIS

- Cerebrovascular accident
- Myxedema coma
- Drug intoxication
- Hypoglycemia

LABORATORY TESTS

1. Metabolic and respiratory acidosis are usually present.
   a. When blood cools, the arterial pH increases, oxygen tension (Po_2) increases, and the Pco_2 falls:
      (1) pH increases 0.008 U/° F (or 0.015 U/° C), causing a decrease in temperature.
      (2) Pao_2 increases 3.3%/° F, causing a decrease in temperature. Oxygenation considerations during hypothermia are described in Box 1-7.
      (3) $Paco_2$ decreases 2.4%/° F, causing a decrease in temperature.
   b. Blood gas analyzers warm the blood to 37° C, increasing the partial pressure of dissolved gases, resulting in higher oxygen and carbon dioxide levels and a lower pH than the patient's actual values. Correction of arterial blood gases for temperature is unnecessary as a guide to therapy. The use of uncorrected values also permits reference to the standard acid–base nomograms.
2. A decrease in K^+ initially, then an increase K^+ with increasing hypothermia; extreme hyperkalemia indicates a poor prognosis.
3. Hematocrit increases (caused by hemoconcentration), decreasing leukocytes and platelets (caused by splenic sequestration).
4. Blood viscosity, increased clotting time

IMAGING STUDIES

- Chest x-ray: generally not helpful; may reveal evidence of aspiration (e.g., intoxicated patient with aspiration pneumonia)
- ECG: prolonged PR, QT, and QRS segments, depressed ST segments, inverted T waves, atrioventricular block, and hypothermic J

waves (Osborne waves) may appear at 25° to 30° C; characterized by notching of the junction of the QRS complex and ST segments (Fig. 1-204).

TREATMENT

NONPHARMACOLOGIC THERAPY

- Treatment of hypothermia varies with the following:
  1. Degree of hypothermia
  2. Existence of concomitant diseases (e.g., cardiovascular insufficiency)
  3. Patient's age and medical condition (e.g., elderly, debilitated patients vs. young, healthy patients)
- General measures:
  1. Secure an airway before warming all unconscious patients; precede endotracheal intubation with oxygenation (if possible) to minimize the risk of arrhythmias during the procedure.
  2. Peripheral vasoconstriction may impede placement of a peripheral intravenous catheter; consider femoral venous access as an alternative to the jugular or subclavian sites to avoid ventricular stimulation.
  3. A Foley catheter should be inserted, and urinary output should be monitored and maintained >0.5 to 1 ml/kg/hr with intravascular volume replacement.
  4. Box 1-8 summarizes measures for preparing hypothermic patients for transport.

ACUTE GENERAL Rx

Continuous ECG monitoring of patients is recommended. Ventricular arrhythmias can be treated with bretylium; lidocaine is generally ineffective, and procainamide is associated with an increased incidence of ventricular fibrillation in hypothermic patients.

Correct severe acidosis and electrolyte abnormalities.

Hypothyroidism, if present, should be promptly treated (see "Myxedema Coma").

If clinical evidence suggests adrenal insufficiency, administer IV methylprednisolone.

BOX 1-7 Oxygenation Considerations During Hypothermia

Detrimental Factors
Oxygen consumption increases with rise in temperature; caution if rapid rewarming; shivering also increases demand
Decreased temperature shifts oxyhemoglobin dissociation curve to the left
Ventilation-perfusion mismatch; atelectasis; decreased respiratory minute volume; bronchorrhea; decreased protective airway reflexes
Decreased tissue perfusion from vascoconstriction; increased viscocity
"Functional hemoglobin" concept: capability of hemoglobin to unload oxygen is lowered
Decreased thoracic elasticity and pulmonary compliance

Protective Factors
Reduction of oxygen consumption: 50% at 28° C (82.4° F); 75% at 22° C (71.6° F); 92% at 10° C (50° F)
Increased oxygen solubility in plasma
Decreased pH and increased $Paco_2$ shift oxyhemoglobin dissociation curve to right

From Auerbach P: *Wilderness medicine,* ed 4, St. Louis, 2001, Mosby.

In patients unresponsive to verbal or noxious stimuli or with altered mental status, 100 mg of thiamine, 0.4 mg of naloxone, and 1 ampule of 50% dextrose may be given.

Warm (104° to 113° F [40° to 45° C]), humidified oxygen should also be given if available.

Specific treatment:

1. Mild hypothermia (rectal temperature <32.3° C [90° F]): passive external rewarming is indicated. Place the patient in a warm room (temperature >21° C [69.8° F]), and cover with insulating material after gently removing wet clothing; recommended rewarming rates vary between 0.5° and 20° C/hr but should not exceed 0.55° C/hr in elderly persons.
2. Moderate to severe hypothermia:
   a. Active core rewarming
      (1) Delivery of heat by way of fluids: warm gastrointestinal irrigation (with saline enemas and by nasogastric tube); IV fluids (usually D₅NS without potassium) warmed to 104° to 107.6° F (40° to 42° C), peritoneal dialysis with dialysate heated to 40.5° to 42.5° C.
      (2) Inhalation of heated, humidified oxygen (warmed to 40° C [104° F]) increases core temperature by 1° C (1.8° F) per hr and decreases evaporative heat loss from respiration.
   b. Active external rewarming: immersion in a bath of warm water (40° to 41° C); active external rewarming may produce shock because of excessive peripheral vasodilation. Ideal candidates are previously healthy, young patients with acute immersion hypothermia.
   c. Extracorporeal blood warming with cardiopulmonary bypass appears to be an efficacious rewarming technique in young, otherwise healthy persons.

(EBM) **EVIDENCE**

available at www.expertconsult.com

SUGGESTED READING

available at www.expertconsult.com

AUTHOR: **FRED F. FERRI, M.D.**

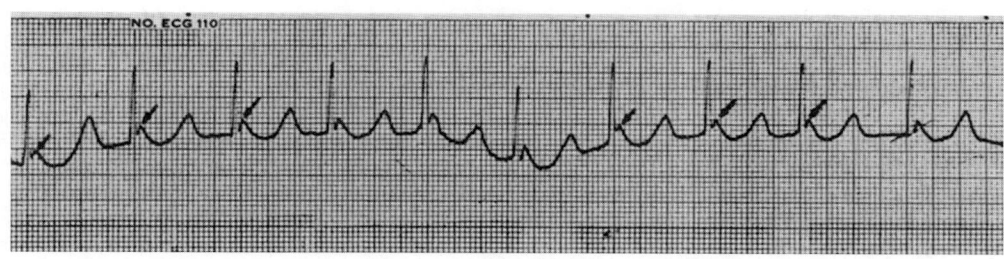

FIGURE 1-204 Hypothermic J waves (Osborne waves) *(arrows)* **in an 80-year-old man with core temperature of 86° F (30° C).** These waves disappeared with rewarming. (From Morse CD, Rial WY: Emergency medicine. In Rakel RE [ed]: *Textbook of family practice,* ed 4, Philadelphia, 1990, WB Saunders.)

BOX 1-8 Preparing Hypothermic Patients for Transport

1. The patient must be dry. Gently remove or cut off wet clothing and replace it with dry clothing or a dry insulation system. Keep the patient horizontal, and do not allow exertion or massage of the extremities.
2. Stabilize injuries (i.e., the spine; place fractures in the correct anatomic position). Open wounds should be covered before packaging.
3. Initiate intravenous infusions (IVs) if feasible; bags can be placed under the patient's buttocks or in a compressor system. Administer a fluid challenge.
4. Active rewarming should be limited to heated inhalation and truncal heat. Insulate hot water bottles in stockings or mittens and then place them in the patient's axillae and groin.
5. The patient should be wrapped. The wrap starts with a large plastic sheet, on which is placed an insulated sleeping pad. A layer of blankets, a sleeping bag, or bubble wrap insulating material is laid over the sleeping bag; the patient is placed on the insulation; the heating bottles are put in place along with IVs, and the entire package is wrapped layer over layer. The plastic is the final closure. The face should be partially covered, but a tunnel should be created to allow access for breathing and monitoring of the patient.

From Auerbach P: *Wilderness medicine,* ed 4, St. Louis, 2001, Mosby.

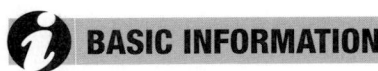 **BASIC INFORMATION**

DEFINITION

Hypothyroidism is a disorder caused by the inadequate secretion of thyroid hormone.

SYNONYMS

Myxedema

ICD-9CM CODES
244 Acquired hypothyroidism
243 Congenital hypothyroidism
244.1 Surgical hypothyroidism
244.3 Iatrogenic hypothyroidism
244.8 Pituitary hypothyroidism
246.1 Sporadic goitrous hypothyroidism

EPIDEMIOLOGY & DEMOGRAPHICS

INCIDENCE/PREVALENCE: 1.5% to 2% of women and 0.2% of men
PREDOMINANT AGE: Incidence of hypothyroidism increases with age; among persons older than 60 yr, 6% of women and 2.5% of men have laboratory evidence of hypothyroidism (thyroid-stimulating hormone [TSH] more than twice normal level).

PHYSICAL FINDINGS & CLINICAL PRESENTATION

- Hypothyroid patients generally present with the following signs and symptoms: fatigue, lethargy, weakness, constipation, weight gain, cold intolerance, muscle weakness, slow speech, slow cerebration with poor memory.
- Skin: dry, coarse, thick, cool, sallow (yellow color caused by carotenemia); nonpitting edema in skin of eyelids and hands (myxedema) secondary to infiltration of subcutaneous tissues by a hydrophilic mucopolysaccharide substance.
- Hair: brittle and coarse; loss of outer third of eyebrows.
- Facies: dulled expression, thickened tongue, thick and slow-moving lips.
- Thyroid gland: may or may not be palpable (depending on the cause of the hypothyroidism).
- Heart sounds: distant, possible pericardial effusion.
- Pulse: bradycardia.
- Neurologic: delayed relaxation phase of the deep tendon reflexes, cerebellar ataxia, hearing impairment, poor memory, peripheral neuropathies with paresthesia.
- Musculoskeletal: carpal tunnel syndrome, muscular stiffness, weakness.

ETIOLOGY

1. Primary hypothyroidism (thyroid gland dysfunction): the cause of >90% of the cases of hypothyroidism
   - Hashimoto's thyroiditis is the most common cause of hypothyroidism after age 8 yr
   - Idiopathic myxedema (nongoitrous form of Hashimoto's thyroiditis)
   - Previous treatment of hyperthyroidism (radioiodine therapy, subtotal thyroidectomy)
   - Subacute thyroiditis
   - Radiation therapy to the neck (usually for malignant disease)
   - Iodine deficiency or excess
   - Drugs (lithium, para-aminosalicylate, sulfonamides, phenylbutazone, amiodarone, thiourea)
   - Congenital (approximately one case per 4000 live births)
   - Prolonged treatment with iodides
2. Secondary hypothyroidism: pituitary dysfunction, postpartum necrosis, neoplasm, infiltrative disease causing deficiency of TSH
3. Tertiary hypothyroidism: hypothalamic disease (granuloma, neoplasm, or irradiation causing deficiency of TRH)
4. Tissue resistance to thyroid hormone: rare

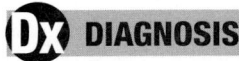 **DIAGNOSIS**

DIFFERENTIAL DIAGNOSIS

- Depression
- Dementia from other causes
- Systemic disorders (e.g., nephrotic syndrome, congestive heart failure, amyloidosis)

LABORATORY TESTS

- Increased TSH: TSH may be normal if patient has secondary or tertiary hypothyroidism, is receiving dopamine or corticosteroids, or the level is obtained after severe illness
- Decreased free T_4
- Other common laboratory abnormalities: hyperlipidemia, hyponatremia, and anemia
- Increased antimicrosomal and antithyroglobulin antibody titers: useful when autoimmune thyroiditis is suspected as the cause of the hypothyroidism

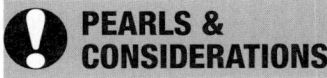 **TREATMENT**

NONPHARMACOLOGIC THERAPY

Patients should be educated regarding hypothyroidism and its possible complications. Patients should also be instructed about the need for lifelong treatment and monitoring of their thyroid abnormality.

ACUTE GENERAL Rx

Start replacement therapy with levothyroxine (L-thyroxine) 25 to 100 μg/day, depending on the patient's age and the severity of the disease. Physiologic combinations of L-thyroxine plus liothyronine do not offer any objective advantage over L-thyroxine alone. The levothyroxine dose may be increased every 6 to 8 wk, depending on the clinical response and serum TSH level. Elderly patients and patients with coronary artery disease should be started with 12.5 to 25 μg/day (higher doses may precipitate angina). The average maintenance dose of levothyroxine is 1.7 μg/kg/day (100 to 150 μg/day in adults). The elderly may require <1 μg/kg/day, whereas children generally require higher doses (up to 3 to 4 μg/kg/day). Pregnant patients also have increased requirements. Estrogen therapy may also increase the need for thyroxine. Women with hypothyroidism should increase their levothyroxine dose by approximately 30% as soon as pregnancy is confirmed. Close monitoring of serum thyrotropin levels and adjustment of levothyroxine dose is recommended throughout pregnancy.

CHRONIC Rx

- Periodic monitoring of TSH level is an essential part of treatment. Patients should be evaluated initially with office visit and TSH levels every 6 to 8 wk until the patient is clinically euthyroid and the TSH level is normalized. The frequency of subsequent visits and TSH measurement can then be decreased to every 6 to 12 mo. Pregnant patients should be checked every trimester.
- For monitoring therapy in patients with central hypothyroidism, measurement of serum free thyroxine (free T_4 level) is appropriate and should be maintained in the upper half of the normal range.

REFERRAL

Admission to the hospital intensive care unit is recommended in all patients with myxedema coma. Additional information on the diagnosis and treatment of this life-threatening complication of hypothyroidism is available under "Myxedema Coma" in Section I.

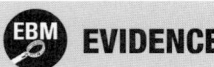 **PEARLS & CONSIDERATIONS**

COMMENTS

Subclinical hypothyroidism occurs in as many as 15% of elderly patients and is characterized by an elevated serum TSH and a normal free T_4 level. Subclinical hypothyroidism is associated with an increased risk of coronary heart disease events and mortality, particularly in those with a TSH concentration of 10 mU/L or greater. Treatment is individualized. In general, replacement therapy is recommended for all patients with serum TSH >10 mU/L and with presence of goiter or thyroid autoantibodies.

(EBM) EVIDENCE

available at www.expertconsult.com

SUGGESTED READINGS
available at www.expertconsult.com

AUTHOR: **FRED F. FERRI, M.D.**

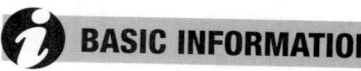

BASIC INFORMATION

DESCRIPTION
The term refers to an acute dermatitis developing at cutaneous sites distant from a primary inflammatory focus and is not explained by the inciting primary inflammation.

SYNONYMS
Autoeczematization

ICD-9CM CODES
692.89 Contact dermatitis and other eczema

EPIDEMIOLOGY
- Exact prevalence in U.S. is unknown.
- Seen in all ages
- Males and females are equally affected
- No particular race or ethnicity is more vulnerable

ETIOLOGY
- Infection with dermatophytes, mycobacterium, histoplasma, viruses, bacteria, or parasites (e.g., lice)
- Dermatitis such as contact, stasis, or eczematous
- Other causes include retained sutures, ionizing radiation, blunt trauma

PATHOGENESIS
- Unknown, but possible explanations include:
  1. Abnormal immune recognition of autologous skin antigens
  2. Stimulation of normal T cells by altered skin constituents
  3. Lowering of the threshold for skin irritation
  4. Dissemination of infectious antigen resulting in a secondary response
  5. Hematogenous dissemination of cytokines from the primary site of inflammation

CLINICAL FEATURES
- Usually associated with exacerbation of primary dermatitis
- Characteristics of the rash in ID reaction include:
  - Sudden onset of rash appearing within a week or two of primary inflammation
  - The rash could not be identified as a common dermatosis
  - Lesions are most commonly seen in the side of the fingers. But, it could be generalized. Particularly in patients with stasis dermatitis, it appears in forearms, thighs, legs, trunk, face, hands, neck, and feet in descending order of frequency.
  - Extremely pruritic
  - Often symmetrical in distribution
  - Most of the time it is vesicular.
- It resolves upon treatment of primary inflammation

DIAGNOSIS

- It is a clinical diagnosis
- Fungus when suspected could be isolated only from the primary site by using potassium hydroxide or by using fungal culture
- At times skin biopsy is done. The biopsy findings are not pathognomonic for ID reaction. These include spongiotic epidermal vesicles associated with superficial perivascular lymphocytic infiltration of dermis, which may also contain scattered eosinophils. Most of the lymphocytes in the epidermis are CD3 and CD8 T cells, whereas those in the dermis are primarily CD4 cells.
- Patch testing may be considered to exclude primary or secondary allergic contact dermatitis.

DIFFERENTIAL DIAGNOSIS
- Atopic dermatitis
- Contact dermatitis
- Drug eruptions
- Dyshidrotic eczema
- Folliculitis
- Scabies
- Dermatophytic infection
- Viral exanthema

TREATMENT

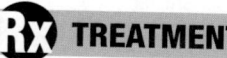

- The treatment is best directed toward the inciting cause.
- Medications used for symptomatic treatment of ID reaction include:
  1. Local or systemic steroids
  2. Local or systemic antihistamines
  3. Topical or systemic antibiotics for secondary bacterial infection
  4. Aluminum sulfate or calcium acetate for weeping skin lesions
  5. Rarely, local or systemic macrolactams (e.g. cyclosporine)

COMPLICATIONS
- Secondary bacterial infection

PROGNOSIS
- It almost always resolves within days when the primary dermatitis is adequately treated.

PATIENT EDUCATION
Treat primary dermatitis promptly.

AUTHOR: **HEMANT K. SATPATHY, M.D.**

BASIC INFORMATION

DEFINITION

Idiopathic intracranial hypertension (IIH) (pseudotumor cerebri) is a syndrome of increased intracranial pressure without underlying hydrocephalus or mass lesion and with normal cerebrospinal fluid analysis.

SYNONYMS

Pseudotumor cerebri
IIH
Benign intracranial hypertension

ICD-9CM CODES
348.2 Pseudotumor cerebri

EPIDEMIOLOGY & DEMOGRAPHICS

- One case per 100,000 women
- 19 cases per 100,000 women aged 20 to 44 yr and >20% of ideal body weight
- 0.3 to 1.5 cases per 100,000 men
- Female/male ratio from 4.3:1 to 8:1
- More than 90% of IIH patients are obese
- Mean age at diagnosis is 30 yr

PHYSICAL FINDINGS & CLINICAL PRESENTATION

Symptoms:
- Headaches: generalized, throbbing, slowly progressive, worse with straining maneuvers, worse in the morning.
- Transient visual obscurations as a brief blurring of vision or scotomata lasting <30 sec. Occur frequently with Valsalva maneuver and may be monocular.
- Double vision: most often in the horizontal plane (because of pseudo–sixth nerve palsy).
- Pulsatile tinnitus: may be initial symptom.
- Photopsia: lights, sparkles in the eyes.
- Pain: mainly retro-orbital. Pain may also be located in the shoulders or neck. Could be present without a headache. May be associated with Lhermitte's sign.

Signs:
- Papilledema: in virtually all cases; bilateral but may be asymmetric
- Sixth nerve palsy: in approximately 10% to 20% of patients
- Visual field defects: enlarged physiologic blind spot, constricted visual fields
- Loss of vision: end result of longstanding and untreated IIH

ETIOLOGY

IIH may be explained on the basis of decreased cerebrospinal fluid (CSF) absorption and increased intracerebral blood volume.

- Decreased CSF absorption from increased venous sinus pressure: this hypothesis is supported by direct retrograde venography studies and would explain higher incidence of IIH in patients with CHF, hypertension, and obesity.
- Increase in cerebral blood volume: supported by MRI and positron emission tomography, as well as the presence of edema on microscopic evaluation.

DIAGNOSIS

DIFFERENTIAL DIAGNOSIS

- The symptoms and signs of IIH are essentially those of raised intracranial pressure (ICP), and the differential diagnosis includes any condition that may be associated with raised ICP. Here we consider only those disease processes in which elevated ICP occurs in the context of normal CSF analysis and normal MRI. (Of note, venous sinus thrombosis [VST] is on this list despite associated MRI findings. VST should be excluded in all individuals with suspected IIH.)
- Medications: vitamin A and retinoids, steroids (both use and withdrawal), oral contraceptives
- Autoimmune disorders: systemic lupus erythematosus, Behçet's disease
- Vascular disease: venous sinus thrombosis
- Other conditions: hypertension, CHF, pregnancy, obesity, uremia, obstructive sleep apnea

LABORATORY TESTS

- CSF analysis
  1. Shows elevated opening pressure
  2. Shows normal protein, glucose, and cell count
- Hypercoagulability workup if suspicion for VST

IMAGING STUDIES

- MRI of the brain to rule out underlying structural lesions
  1. Empty sella sign often associated with IIH but is not pathognomonic
- Cerebral venography to evaluate venous flow
  1. Magnetic venography
  2. CT venography
  3. Conventional contrast venography
- CT
  1. Slitlike ventricles

TREATMENT

NONPHARMACOLOGIC THERAPY

- Weight loss in obese patients
- Continuous positive airway pressure if obstructive sleep apnea is suspected

ACUTE GENERAL Rx

- Acetazolamide 250 mg to 4 g per day: reduces CSF production by inhibition of carbonic anhydrase, occasionally causing anorexia and resultant weight loss.
- Furosemide 40 to 120 mg/day in divided doses: apparent mechanism of action is by reduced sodium transport, leading to decreased total CSF volume.
- Topiramate 100 to 400 mg/day: antiepileptic medication, recently reported to be effective in treatment of IIH. Weak carbonic anhydrase inhibitor with weight loss as one of its primary side effects.
- Serial lumbar punctures: attempted in patients with severe headaches resistant to medical therapy. Goal is to reduce spinal fluid pressure, allowing immediate reduction in headache severity. This treatment should be reserved only for the most resistant cases and should be used as a conduit to future surgical intervention.

CHRONIC Rx

Surgical intervention is indicated in cases of treatment failure and progressive visual loss.
- Optic nerve fenestration: preferred for patients with visual loss and easily controlled headaches. Proposed mechanism is decompression of the optic nerve. Highly effective; however, has been associated with significant number of failure rates.
- CSF shunting: neurosurgical procedure. Performed in patients with significant visual deterioration and difficult-to-control headaches. Provides rapid improvement in symptoms; however, reported to have significant rates of shunt revisions because of shunt malfunction.

DISPOSITION

- IIH is a self-limiting disease with occasional periods of relapses. Each episode may last from 1 to several years.
- All patients with IIH should undergo MR or CT venography to rule out the possibility of VST.
- The major complication of IIH is visual loss, and treatment should be directed toward reducing ICP to prevent visual loss.

REFERRAL

- Neuro-ophthalmologist for serial evaluation of visual fields and fundus photographs
- Nutritionist for weight loss
- General neurologist for the initial workup and eventual treatment of raised ICP

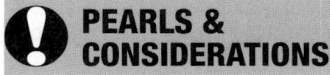

PEARLS & CONSIDERATIONS

COMMENTS

- IIH is a diagnosis of exclusion.
- IIH is a disease of young obese women.
- Ongoing treatment is essential to avoid progressive visual loss, which is the most significant complication of this disorder.

PREVENTION

Maintenance of ideal body weight is one of the best preventative mechanisms for avoidance of IIH. However, it does occur in patients with normal body weight. In these cases there are no known preventable risk factors.

PATIENT & FAMILY EDUCATION

The combination of weight loss and medical therapy is highly effective in treatment of IIH. Given that most patients with IIH are young and otherwise healthy, high success rates can be accomplished. Because IIH is a self-limiting condition, patients with IIH may expect to become both symptom and medication free after intracranial hypertension resolves.

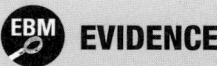 **EVIDENCE**

available at www.expertconsult.com

SUGGESTED READINGS

available at www.expertconsult.com

AUTHOR: GENNA GEKHT, M.D.

BASIC INFORMATION

DEFINITION

Idiopathic pulmonary fibrosis (IPF) is a specific form of chronic fibrosing interstitial pneumonia with histopathologic characteristics of usual interstitial pneumonia (UIP). Disease characterized by progressive parenchymal scarring and loss of pulmonary function.

SYNONYMS

Cryptogenic fibrosing alveolitis
Usual interstitial pneumonia
Pulmonary fibrosis

ICD-9CM CODES

516.3 Idiopathic pulmonary fibrosis

EPIDEMIOLOGY & DEMOGRAPHICS

- Incidence: 7 to 16 cases/100,000 persons worldwide
- Most commonly presents in fifth and sixth decades
- More common in men than women
- Familial forms account for 3% to 25% of cases. Genetic variants: include mutations in surfactant protein C and abnormal telomere shortening
- No distinct geographic distribution; no clear racial predilection

PHYSICAL FINDINGS & CLINICAL PRESENTATION

- Most present with gradual onset (>6 mo) of exertional dyspnea and nonproductive cough. Progressive dyspnea is usually the most prominent symptom.
- Fine bibasilar inspiratory crackles in >80% of patients, with progression upward as the disease advances.
- Clubbing is found in 25% to 50% of patients.
- Cyanosis and right heart failure (cor pulmonale) may occur late in the disease course.
- Extrapulmonary involvement rarely occurs. Fever and wheezing are rare and suggest alternative diagnosis.

ETIOLOGY

- Unknown.
- There are numerous hypotheses, including environmental insults such as metal and wood dust, infectious causes, chronic aspiration, or exposure to certain drugs (antidepressants).
- New research suggests important role of aberrant tissue repair and fibrosis and downplays the importance of generalized inflammation.

DX DIAGNOSIS

DIFFERENTIAL DIAGNOSIS

- Sarcoidosis
- Drug-induced interstitial lung disease
- Pulmonary manifestations of collagen vascular diseases (e.g., rheumatoid arthritis [RA], systemic sclerosis)
- Hypersensitivity pneumonitis
- Occupational exposures (e.g., asbestos, silica) may cause pneumoconiosis that mimics IPF
- Other idiopathic interstitial pneumonias:
  o Desquamative interstitial pneumonia
  o Respiratory bronchitis interstitial lung disease
  o Acute interstitial pneumonia
  o Nonspecific interstitial pneumonia
  o Cryptogenic organizing pneumonia

WORKUP

- Almost all patients have abnormal chest radiograph at presentation, with bilateral reticular opacities most prominent in the periphery and lower lobes. Peripheral honeycombing may be seen.
- High-resolution CT scan shows patchy peripheral reticular abnormalities with intralobular linear opacities, irregular septal thickening, subpleural honeycombing, and ground-glass appearance.
- Pulmonary function tests show restrictive pattern and reduced carbon monoxide diffusion into the lung.
- Six-min walk test may show reduced exercise tolerance and/or exertional hypoxia.
- Laboratory abnormalities (nondiagnostic): mild anemia; increases in erythrocyte sedimentation rate, lactate dehydrogenase, C-reactive protein; low titer antinuclear antibody seen in up to 30% of patients.
- There is a limited role for bronchioalveolar lavage either in diagnosis or monitoring IPF.
- Gold standard for diagnosis is lung biopsy (open thoracotomy or video-assisted thoracoscopy). Hallmark features: heterogeneous distribution of parenchymal fibrosis against background of mild inflammation (UIP).
- Lung biopsy is critical to distinguish IPF from diseases with better prognosis and treatment options, especially in patients with any atypical features.
- In absence of or contraindication to lung biopsy, the combination of clinical and radiographic features is often enough to establish the diagnosis.

Rx TREATMENT

- No proven treatment for IPF and little evidence to support the routine use of any specific therapy. With the lack of evidence supporting specific therapies in IPF, evaluation for participation in clinical trials of new therapies may be warranted.
- In patients with mild-moderate disease who desire treatment, conventional treatment includes a trial of corticosteroids combined with azathioprine for 3 to 6 mo; 10% to 30% of patients may respond. The addition of N-acetylcysteine may help to slow the deterioration of lung function but has not been shown to impact survival.
- Treatment is continued for up to 24 mo if the patient improves or is stable. Long-term treatment only with objective evidence of continued improvement or stabilization.
- In patients with severe disease, treatment options include supportive care (pulmonary rehabilitation, supplemental oxygen, influenza and pneumococcal vaccination) and potential lung transplantation.
- Lung transplantation is the only therapy shown to prolong survival in IPF. Posttransplant 5-yr survival for IPF patients is approximately 40%. Median survival time is longer after bilateral lung transplantation than single lung transplantation but is associated with more complications during the first year.
- Treatment agents designed to target the fibrotic process include pirfenidone, bosentan, Coumadin, and etanercept. Clinical trials are ongoing, but results, to date, have been variable.
- Acute exacerbation of IPF, defined as worsening dyspnea (<1 mo), the presence of new opacities on radiograph, and the lack of evidence of infection, has an incidence of 10% to 57%. Progressive respiratory failure may require mechanical ventilation. Treatment often includes high dose corticosteroids and broad-spectrum antibiotics.

DISPOSITION

- Spontaneous remissions do not occur.
- Natural history includes progressive loss of pulmonary function.
- There is an 8 to 14× increased risk of lung cancer.
- Mean survival after the diagnosis of biopsy-confirmed IPF is 3 to 5 yr.
- Respiratory failure is the most common cause of death.

REFERRAL

To pulmonologist for review of abnormal chest imaging and establishing diagnosis

PEARLS & CONSIDERATIONS

- The course is progressive, with a high mortality rate.
- Critical to differentiate IPF from other interstitial lung diseases because prognosis and response to treatment differ.
- There is no proven treatment for IPF. Novel therapeutic agents targeting aberrant epithelial cell activation and repair may prove beneficial.
- Consider early referral for lung transplant.

SUGGESTED READINGS

available at www.expertconsult.com

AUTHORS: **LYNN BOWLBY, M.D.**, and **MICHAEL BLUNDIN, M.D.**

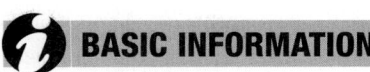

BASIC INFORMATION

DEFINITION

Immunoglobulin A (IgA) nephropathy is a proliferative glomerulonephritis associated with predominant deposition of IgA in the mesangium.

SYNONYMS

Berger's disease

ICD-9CM CODES
583.81 IgA Nephropathy

EPIDEMIOLOGY & DEMOGRAPHICS

INCIDENCE: It is the most common type of glomerulonephropathy worldwide.

PREVALENCE: Prevalence rate is lower in the U.S. (10% to 15%) compared with Asian countries. Lower rates could be explained by a conservative approach by nephrologists in the U.S., who are reluctant to do renal biopsy in asymptomatic patients with minimal renal abnormalities. In most reports prevalence rates are expressed as a percentage of cases of primary glomerulonephritis or as a percentage of total series of renal biopsies.

PREDOMINANT SEX AND AGE: It is most prevalent in the second and third decades of life with a male/female ratio of 6:1 in the U.S.

GENETICS: Although it is considered a sporadic disease, genetic linkage to locus called *IgAN1* on 6q22 and 6q23 has been shown.

RISK FACTORS: It has a higher association with Asians, whites, and Native Americans and is rarely seen in African Americans.

PHYSICAL FINDINGS & CLINICAL PRESENTATION

- Two common presentations include (1) recurrent macroscopic hematuria often associated with upper respiratory infection and (2) persistent microscopic hematuria.
- Loin pain may be associated with macroscopic hematuria.
- Physical findings are usually unremarkable, except hypertension seen in 20% to 30% of patients with chronic disease and edema in 5% of patients with nephrotic range proteinuria.
- Mild proteinuria is common.
- Rarely, IgA nephropathy presents as acute renal failure in 5% of patients and chronic renal failure in 10% to 20% of patients.

ETIOLOGY

- Most cases are idiopathic/primary.
- Secondary causes of IgA nephropathy include Henoch-Schönlein purpura; hepatitis B; alcoholic cirrhosis; celiac disease; inflammatory bowel disease; psoriasis; sarcoidosis; cystic fibrosis; cancer of the lungs, larynx, or pancreas; HIV infection; systemic lupus erythematosus; rheumatoid arthritis; diabetic nephropathy; Sjögren's syndrome; and Reiter's syndrome.
- Fig. 1-205 illustrates the pathogenesis of IgA nephropathy.

DIAGNOSIS

DIFFERENTIAL DIAGNOSIS

- Henoch-Schönlein purpura
- Hereditary nephritis
- Thin glomerular basement membrane disease
- Lupus nephritis
- Poststreptococcal nephritis
- Secondary causes associated with IgA nephropathy mentioned above

WORKUP

- The diagnosis is suspected on the basis of clinical history and laboratory data but is confirmed by renal biopsy showing IgA deposits in the mesangium.
- Renal biopsy is restricted to patients with sustained proteinuria >1 g/day or worsening renal function.

LABORATORY TESTS

- Urine analysis showing protein, red blood cells and casts, and white blood cells.
- Serum creatinine may be elevated.
- 24-hour urine assay for quantifying proteinuria and to check creatinine clearance.
- Serum IgA is elevated in only 50% of patients and has no clinical utility.

TREATMENT

Although initially considered a benign disease, IgA nephropathy is now recognized as a common cause of renal failure. Currently there is no cure.

NONPHARMACOLOGIC THERAPY

- Moderate dietary protein restriction
- Discourage smoking

ACUTE AND CHRONIC GENERAL Rx

- Aggressive therapy for hypertension, preferably with angiotensin-converting enzyme (ACE) inhibitors. Goal blood pressure is <125/75 mm Hg in the presence of proteinuria >1 g/day.
- Patients with recurrent gross hematuria or isolated microscopic hematuria, no or minimal proteinuria (<1 g/day), normal blood pressure, and normal kidney function should only be monitored every 6 to 12 mo to assess disease progression.
- If bouts of recurrent macroscopic hematuria are associated with tonsillitis, tonsillectomy may benefit these patients.
- Patients with persistent proteinuria >1 g/day with or without hypertension are treated with ACE inhibitors and/or angiotensin receptor blockers (ARBs). Steroids are reserved for patients with persistent proteinuria >1 g/day despite ACE and/or ARB administration.
- Patients with nephrotic syndrome, preserved kidney function, and minimal change in disease are treated with steroids for 6 mo.
- Patients with severe renal disease or crescentic, rapidly progressive glomerulonephritis in the absence of changes of chronic kidney disease in biopsy are treated with steroid and cyclophosphamide combination for the first 2 mo, followed by steroids and azathioprine for 2 yr for maintenance treatment.

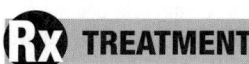
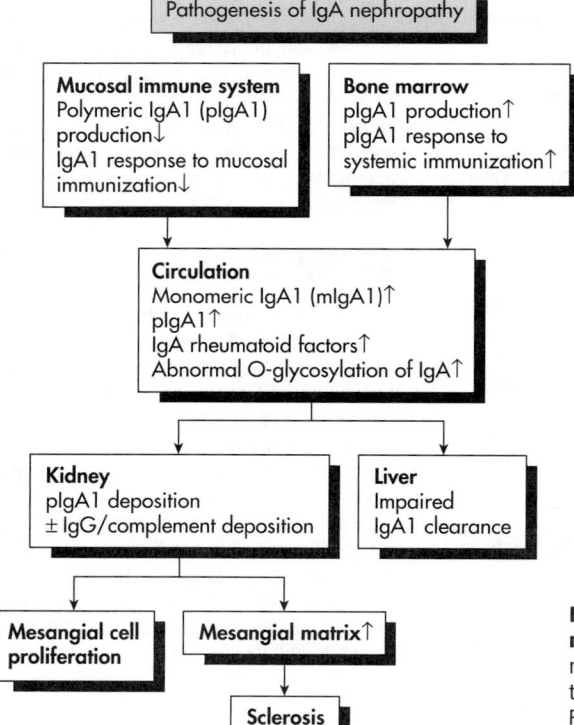

FIGURE 1-205 Pathogenesis of IgA nephropathy. Abnormalities in IgA immunity leading to mesangial IgA deposition and injury. (Modified from Johnson RJ, Feehally J: *Comprehensive clinical nephrology,* ed 2, St Louis, 2000, Mosby.)

- Patients with acute renal failure need renal biopsy to rule out acute tubular necrosis, which needs only supportive therapy, from crescentic IgA nephropathy, which needs aggressive medical management.
- Kidney transplantation is the treatment of choice for end-stage kidney disease. There is no difference in survival in living versus cadaver donors. At present, kidneys with IgA deposits are not used for transplantation.
- Statins are indicated for all IgA nephropathy patients with dyslipidemia, hypertension, and other cardiovascular risks.

- Role of mycophenolate and plasmapheresis is controversial.

COMPLEMENTARY & ALTERNATIVE MEDICINE

Role of fish oil is controversial

DISPOSITION

- Complete remission occurs in <10% of patients.
- End-stage renal failure develops in 15% to 20% of patients within 10 yr of onset and in 30% to 35% of patients within 20 yr. Prognostic markers at presentation in IgA nephropathy are described in Box 1-9.
- Poor prognostic indicators include (1) male gender, (2) older age, (3) young age at the onset of the disease, (4) absence of episodes of recurrent macroscopic hematuria, (5) hypertension, (6) extent of renal insufficiency, (7) extent of proteinuria, (8) elevated serum uric acid, and (9) certain histologic changes seen in renal biopsy, such as crescents, glomerulosclerosis, and tubulointerstitial fibrosis or atrophy.

REFERRAL

Patients with IgA nephropathy are commonly referred to nephrologists.

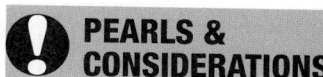 PEARLS & CONSIDERATIONS

COMMENTS

- IgA nephropathy seems to be a kidney-restricted form of Henoch-Schönlein purpura.
- IgA nephropathy is not an entirely benign condition, even when microhematuria is the only clinical presentation.

SUGGESTED READINGS

available at www.expertconsult.com

AUTHOR: **HEMANT K. SATPATHY, M.D.**

BOX 1-9 Prognostic Markers at Presentation in IgA Nephropathy

Clinical	Histopathologic
Poor prognosis	**Poor prognosis**
Increasing age	Glomerular sclerosis
Duration of preceding symptoms	Tubular atrophy
Severity of proteinuria	Interstitial fibrosis
Hyperuricemia	Vascular wall thickening
Hypertension	Capillary-loop IgA deposits
Renal impairment	
Good prognosis	
Recurrent macroscopic hematuria	
No impact on prognosis	**No impact on prognosis**
Gender	Intensity of IgA deposits
Serum IgA level	

None of the clinical or histopathologic adverse features, except capillary-loop IgA deposits, are specific to IgAN.
From Johnson RJ, Feehaly J: *Comprehensive clinical nephrology,* ed 2, St Louis, 2000, Mosby.

Diseases and Disorders

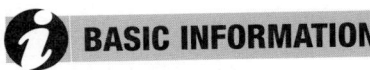

BASIC INFORMATION

DEFINITION

Immune thrombocytopenic purpura (ITP) is an autoimmune disorder in which antibody-coated or immune complex–coated platelets are destroyed prematurely by the reticuloendothelial system, resulting in peripheral thrombocytopenia.

ICD-9CM CODES
287.3 Idiopathic thrombocytopenic purpura (ITP)

EPIDEMIOLOGY & DEMOGRAPHICS

INCIDENCE: 100 cases per 1 million persons annually
PREVALENCE: Five to 10 cases per 100,000 persons
PREDOMINANT SEX: 72% of patients >10 yr are female; in children, males and females are affected equally
PREDOMINANT AGE: Children ages 2 to 4 yr and young women (70% are <40 yr)

PHYSICAL FINDINGS & CLINICAL PRESENTATION

The presentation of ITP is different in children and adults:

- Children generally present with sudden onset of bruising and petechiae from severe thrombocytopenia.
- In adults the presentation is insidious; a history of prolonged purpura may be present; many patients are diagnosed incidentally on the basis of automated laboratory tests that now routinely include platelet counts.
- The physical examination may be entirely normal.
- Patients with severe thrombocytopenia may have petechiae, purpura, epistaxis, or heme-positive stool from gastrointestinal bleeding.
- Splenomegaly is unusual; its presence should alert to the possibility of other etiologies of thrombocytopenia.
- The presence of dysmorphic features (skeletal anomalies, auditory abnormalities) may indicate a congenital disorder as the cause of the thrombocytopenia.

ETIOLOGY

Increased platelet destruction caused by autoantibodies to platelet-membrane antigens. Hundreds of medications can cause thrombocytopenia. Drugs commonly implicated are quinidine, heparin, antibiotics (linezolid, vancomycin, sulfonamides, rifampin), platelet inhibitors (tirofiban, abciximab, eptifibatide), cimetidine, NSAIDs, thiazide diuretics, antirheumatic agents (gold salts, penicillamine), acetaminophen, and chemotherapeutic agents (cyclosporine, fludarabine, oxaliplatin).

Dx DIAGNOSIS

DIFFERENTIAL DIAGNOSIS

- Falsely low platelet count (resulting from EDTA-dependent or cold-dependent agglutinins)
- Viral infections (e.g., HIV, mononucleosis, rubella)
- Drug-induced (e.g., heparin, quinidine, sulfonamides)
- Hypersplenism resulting from liver disease
- Myelodysplastic and lymphoproliferative disorders
- Pregnancy, hypothyroidism
- SLE, TTP, hemolytic-uremic syndrome
- Congenital thrombocytopenia (e.g., Fanconi's syndrome, May-Hegglin anomaly, Bernard-Soulier syndrome)

LABORATORY TESTS

- Complete blood count, platelet count, and peripheral smear: platelets are decreased but are normal in size or may appear larger than normal. Red blood cells and white blood cells have a normal morphology.
- Additional tests may be ordered to exclude other causes of the thrombocytopenia when clinically indicated (e.g., HIV, ANA, TSH, liver enzymes, bone marrow examination).
- The direct assay for the measurement of platelet-bound antibodies has an estimated positive predictive value of 80% to 83%. A negative test cannot be used to rule out the diagnosis.

IMAGING STUDIES

CT scan of abdomen/pelvis in patients with splenomegaly to exclude other disorders causing thrombocytopenia

Rx TREATMENT

NONPHARMACOLOGIC THERAPY

- Minimize activity to prevent injury or bruising (e.g., contact sports should be avoided).
- Stop any potentially offending drugs (see "Etiology"). Avoid medications that increase the risk of bleeding (e.g., aspirin and other NSAIDs).

ACUTE GENERAL Rx

- Treatment varies with the platelet count, patient's age, and bleeding status.
- Observation and frequent monitoring of platelet count are needed in asymptomatic patients with platelet counts >30,000/mm^3.
- Methylprednisolone 30 mg/kg/day IV infused over a period of 20 to 30 min (maximum dose of 1 g/day for 2 or 3 days) plus IV immunoglobulin (1 g/kg/day for 2 or 3 days) and infusion of platelets should be given to patients with neurologic symptoms, internal bleeding, or those undergoing emergency surgery.
- Prednisone 1 to 2 mg/kg qd, continued until the platelet count is normalized then slowly tapered off, is indicated in adults with platelet counts <20,000/mm^3 and those who have counts <50,000/mm^3 and significant mucous membrane bleeding. Response rates

range from 50% to 75%, and most responses occur within the first 3 wk. Oral dexamethasone at a dosage of 40 mg/day for 4 consecutive days has also been reported to induce a high response rate (85%).
- Splenectomy should be considered in adults with platelet count <30,000/mm^3 after 6 wk of medical treatment or after 6 mo if more than 10 to 20 mg of prednisone per day is required to maintain a platelet count >30,000/mm^3. In children, splenectomy is generally reserved for persistent thrombocytopenia (>1 yr) and clinically significant bleeding. Appropriate immunizations (pneumococcal vaccine in adults and children, *Haemophilus influenzae* vaccine, meningococcal vaccine in children) should be administered before splenectomy.
- Romiplostim, a recombinant fusion protein, and the oral thrombopoietin-receptor agonist eltrombopag are effective in increasing platelet count in patients with chronic ITP refractory to corticosteroids and/or splenectomy. Recent trials have shown that patients treated with romiplostim had a higher rate of a platelet response, lower incidence of treatment failure and splenectomy, less bleeding and fewer blood transfusions, and a higher quality of life than patients treated with the standard of care (glucocorticoids). However, it is an expensive treatment required indefinitely.
- Platelet transfusion is needed only in case of life-threatening hemorrhage.
- High-dose immunoglobulins (IgG 0.4 g/kg/day IV, infused on 3 to 5 consecutive days) or high-dose parenteral glucocorticoids (methylprednisolone 30 mg/kg/day) can be used in children with a platelet count <20,000/mm^3 and significant bleeding or adults with severe thrombocytopenia or bleeding. However, responses are generally transient, lasting no longer than 4 wk.
- Use of danazol, an attenuated androgen, and chemotherapy with cyclophosphamide, vincristine, and prednisone (CVP) has been partially effective in chronic ITP.
- Rituximab, a monoclonal antibody directed against the CD$_{20}$ antigen, has been reported useful for patients with ITP who are resistant to conventional treatment; it may help prevent serious or fatal bleeding. Encouraging results have also been shown in trials involving AMG 531, a thrombopoiesis-stimulating protein in patients with chronic ITP.

DISPOSITION

- More than 80% of children have a complete remission within 8 wk.
- In adults, the course of the disease is chronic; only 5% of adults have spontaneous remission.
- The principal cause of death from ITP is intracranial hemorrhage (1% of children, 5% of adults).

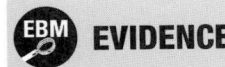 **EVIDENCE**

available at www.expertconsult.com

AUTHOR: FRED F. FERRI, M.D.

BASIC INFORMATION

DEFINITION

Impetigo is a superficial skin infection generally caused by *Staphylococcus aureus* and/or *Streptococcus* spp.

Common presentations are bullous impetigo (generally caused by staphylococcal disease) and nonbullous impetigo (from streptococcal infection and possible staphylococcal infection); the bullous form is caused by an epidermolytic toxin produced at the site of infection.

SYNONYMS

Impetigo vulgaris
Pyoderma

ICD-9CM CODES
684 Impetigo

EPIDEMIOLOGY & DEMOGRAPHICS

- Bullous impetigo is most common in infants and children. The nonbullous form is most common in children ages 2 to 5 yr with poor hygiene in warm climates.
- The overall incidence of acute nephritis with impetigo varies between 2% and 5%.

PHYSICAL FINDINGS & CLINICAL PRESENTATION

- Nonbullous impetigo begins as a single red macule or papule that quickly becomes a vesicle. Rupture of the vesicle produces an erosion of which the contents dry to form honey-colored crusts. Multiple lesions with golden yellow crusts and weeping areas are often found on the skin around the nose, mouth, and limbs (Fig. 1-206).

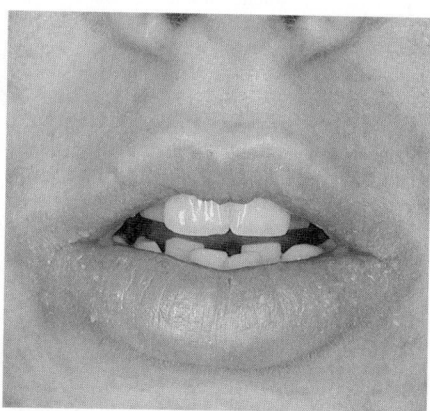

FIGURE 1-206 Impetigo. Serum and crust at the angle of the mouth is a common presentation for impetigo. (From Habif TB: *Clinical dermatology: a color guide to diagnosis and therapy,* ed 4, St Louis, 2000, Mosby.)

- Bullous impetigo is manifested by the presence of vesicles that enlarge rapidly to form bullae with contents that vary from clear to cloudy. There is subsequent collapse of the center of the bullae; the peripheral areas may retain fluid, and a honey-colored crust may appear in the center. As the lesions enlarge and become contiguous with the others, a scaling border replaces the fluid-filled rim; there is minimal erythema surrounding the lesions.
- Regional lymphadenopathy is most common with nonbullous impetigo.
- Constitutional symptoms are generally absent.

ETIOLOGY

- *S. aureus* coagulase positive is the dominant microorganism.
- *S. pyogenes* (group A β-hemolytic streptococci): M-T serotypes of this organism associated with acute nephritis are 2, 49, 55, 57, and 60.

DIAGNOSIS

DIFFERENTIAL DIAGNOSIS

- Atopic dermatitis
- Herpes simplex infection
- Ecthyma
- Folliculitis
- Eczema
- Insect bites
- Scabies
- Tinea corporis
- Pemphigus vulgaris and bullous pemphigoid
- Chickenpox

WORKUP

Diagnosis is clinical.

LABORATORY TESTS

- Generally not necessary
- Gram stain and culture and sensitivity to confirm the diagnosis when the clinical presentation is unclear
- Sedimentation rate parallel to activity of the disease
- Increased anti-DNAse B and antihyaluronidase
- Urinalysis revealing hematuria with erythrocyte casts and proteinuria in patients with acute nephritis (most frequently occurring in children between ages 2 and 4 yr in the southern part of the U.S.)

TREATMENT

NONPHARMACOLOGIC THERAPY

Remove crusts by soaking with wet cloth compresses (crusts block the penetration of antibacterial creams).

GENERAL Rx

- Application of 2% mupirocin ointment tid for 10 days or retapamulin 1% applied bid for 5 days to the affected area or until all lesions have cleared.
- Oral antibiotics are used in severe cases: commonly used agents are dicloxacillin 250 mg qid for 7 to 10 days, cephalexin 250 mg qid for 7 to 10 days, azithromycin 500 mg on day 1, 250 mg on days 2 through 5, amoxicillin/clavulanate 500 mg q8h.
- Impetigo can be prevented by prompt application of mupirocin or triple-antibiotic ointment (bacitracin, Polysporin, and neomycin) to sites of skin trauma.
- Patients who are carriers of *S. aureus* in their nares should be treated with mupirocin ointment applied to their nares bid for 5 days.
- Fingernails should be kept short, and patients should be advised not to scratch any lesions to avoid spread of infection.

DISPOSITION

Most cases of impetigo resolve promptly with appropriate treatment. Both bullous and nonbullous forms of impetigo heal without scarring.

REFERRAL

Nephrology referral in patients with acute nephritis

PEARLS & CONSIDERATIONS

COMMENTS

- Patients should be instructed on use of antibacterial soaps and avoidance of sharing of towels and washcloths because impetigo is extremely contagious.
- Children attending day care should be removed until 48 to 72 hr after initiation of antibiotic treatment.

EVIDENCE

available at www.expertconsult.com

AUTHOR: **FRED F. FERRI, M.D.**

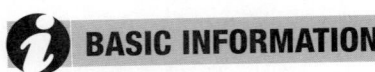

BASIC INFORMATION

DEFINITION

Inclusion body myositis (IBM) is the most common myopathy with onset after the age of 50 yr. Although classified among the inflammatory myopathies, its underlying pathophysiology has not yet been delineated.

SYNONYMS

None

ICD-9CM CODES
359.71 Inclusion body myositis

EPIDEMIOLOGY & DEMOGRAPHIC S

INCIDENCE: 0.22 to 0.79 cases/100,000 persons
PREVALENCE: 0.5 to 7.1 cases/100,000 persons
PREDOMINANT SEX: Male:female ratio 1.2-3:1
PREDOMINANT AGE: 87% older than 50 yr
PEAK INCIDENCE: Seventh decade
RISK FACTORS: None known
GENETICS: Less than 10% of cases familial

PHYSICAL FINDINGS & CLINICAL PRESENTATION

- Insidious onset of slowly progressive proximal leg and distal arm weakness.
- Time to diagnosis from symptom onset often lags by years to a decade.
- Functional loss of strength in the legs most often precedes arm weakness.
- The cardinal clinical features include early weakness and atrophy of quadriceps muscles (difficulty climbing stairs, arising from chairs, and getting out of cars) along with wrist and finger flexor muscles (difficulty grasping, opening jars and turning doorknobs). Ankle dorsiflexion weakness may also be prominent leading to foot drop and tripping.
- When examining strength, side to side asymmetries are seen in one or more muscle groups in the majority of patients. This stands in contrast to the symmetrical, proximal involvement of polymyositis and most muscular dystrophies.
- Dysphagia and/or mild facial weakness are present in over half of cases.
- Although sensory symptoms are usually lacking, one third will have evidence for peripheral neuropathy on physical examination and electrodiagnostic testing.
- 10% to 15% of patients have concomitant autoimmune disorders such as systemic lupus erythematosus, Sjögren's syndrome, scleroderma, sarcoidosis, or thrombocytopenia. However, different from polymyositis and dermatomyositis, IBM does not portend an increased risk of heart or lung disease nor cancer.

ETIOLOGY

The pathogenesis of IBM is not known. Inflammatory, degenerative, viral and prion etiologies have been postulated, but none substantiated.

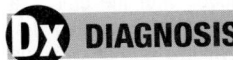

DIAGNOSIS

DIFFERENTIAL DIAGNOSIS

- Polymyositis
- Amyotrophic lateral sclerosis
- Late-onset muscular dystrophies
- Acid maltase deficiency

WORKUP

- Thorough neurologic examination with emphasis on the motor exam is important.
- Nerve conduction studies should be performed to exclude other causes and EMG to document a myopathy.
- The diagnosis of definite IBM requires the following features on muscle biopsy: (1) inflammation, (2) inflammatory cells invading healthy muscle fibers, (3) vacuoles, and (4) either amyloid deposits by Congo red staining or tubulofilaments on electron microscopy.

LABORATORY TESTS

Creatine kinase level (labs for collagen vascular diseases may be obtained after the diagnosis). A complete blood count and coagulation studies should be drawn in anticipation of the muscle biopsy.

IMAGING STUDIES

MRI of the forearms to document atrophy and signal abnormalities in volar forearm muscle groups may be performed to increase clinical certainty.

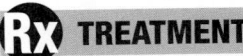

TREATMENT

NONPHARMACOLOGIC THERAPY

- Assistive devices for mobility such as canes, walkers, and wheelchairs are the mainstay of therapy.
- Occasionally knee orthoses or ankle-foot orthoses may improve and prolong ambulation.

ACUTE GENERAL Rx

None

CHRONIC Rx

- Experts have not found clinically significant improvement in functional strength with any pharmacologic therapy. Clinical trials of corticosteroids, methotrexate, intravenous immunoglobulin, anti-T lymphocyte globulin, etanercept, interferon β-1a, and oxandrolone have all failed to demonstrate functional improvements in limb strength.
- A short, small trial of a home exercise program demonstrated mild improvements in strength.
- IBM is generally refractory to therapy.

COMPLEMENTARY & ALTERNATIVE MEDICINE

Some patients choose to self-treat with creatine supplementation, coenzyme Q10, or lithium. There is no evidence supporting these treatments.

REFERRAL

- Patients with suspected IBM should be referred to a neurologist with subspecialty expertise in neuromuscular medicine.
- Physical therapy and occupational therapy consultations help the patient optimize ambulation and fine motor tasks, respectively.
- Speech therapy consultations can assist with symptomatic dysphagia.

PROGNOSIS

Life expectancy is not significantly altered in this late-onset, slowly progressive disorder. Some patients require wheelchair use 10 to 20 yr after disease onset.

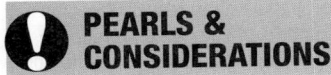

PEARLS & CONSIDERATIONS

COMMENTS

The key to diagnosis rests in finding weakness of finger or wrist flexors on examination (evident in over 95% of patients at initial presentation).

PREVENTION

None known

PATIENT/FAMILY EDUCATION

Patient information and support groups can be found at: www.ninds.nih.gov/disorders/inclusion_body_myositis and http://www.myositis.org.

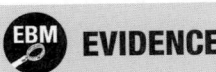

EVIDENCE

available at www.expertconsult.com

SUGGESTED READINGS

available at www.expertconsult.com

AUTHOR: **MATTHEW P. WICKLUND, M.D.**

BASIC INFORMATION

DEFINITION

Fecal incontinence is defined as the loss of voluntary bowel control, leading to the inability to hold gas or feces in the rectum.

SYNONYMS

Fecal Incontinence
Anal Incontinence

ICD-9CM CODES
787.6 Incontinence of feces
307.7 Encopresis of non-organic origin

EPIDEMIOLOGY & DEMOGRAPHICS

INCIDENCE: It affects 0.5% to 1.5% of the population younger than age 65 yr but >10% older than age 65. Also more common in institutionalized patients.
PREVALENCE: 2.2% in general population and 21% in older adults. Prevalence increases with age and body mass index (BMI) in women.
PREDOMINANT SEX AND AGE: More common in females as compared to males
RISK FACTORS:
- History of urinary incontinence (present in 50% of the cases)
- Demented or cognitively impaired individuals
- Age >70 yr
- Presence of neurologic or psychiatric disease
- Poor mobility
- Fecal impaction from chronic constipation

PHYSICAL FINDINGS & CLINICAL PRESENTATION

- On inspection and by performing a digital rectal exam to ascertain the presence of fecal material, prolapsed hemorrhoid, dermatitis, scars, absence of perianal creases, or a gaping anus.
- Also assess for anocutaneous reflex. This can be done by stroking skin in each perianal quadrant (normal response is brisk anal wink).
- Assess the length of the anal sphincter.
- Assess resting and squeezing anal tone.
- Assess for rectal prolapsed or excessive perianal descent when patient strains.

ETIOLOGY

- Often multifactorial
- Radiation-induced inflammation and fibrosis

- Rectal inflammation secondary to ulcerative colitis or Crohn's disease
- Neurological disorders:
  - Status post stroke
  - Dementia
  - Multiple sclerosis
  - Dorsal and spinal cord lesions
- Surgery
  - Anorectal surgery for hemorrhoids, fistula, and fissures
- Medicines
  - Narcotics
  - Antidepressants
  - Antipsychotics
  - Calcium channel blockers
- Number of births and episiotomies in females
- Childhood abuse and adult sexual abuse

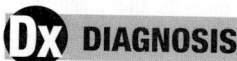 **DIAGNOSIS**

DIFFERENTIAL DIAGNOSIS

- Fecal encopresis

WORKUP

- Detailed history taking that includes the onset and precipitating events, duration and severity, stool consistency and urgency, and the presence of coexisting problems including urinary incontinence, surgery, or back injury is important.
- Diagnostic workup includes anal manometry, anorectal ultrasound, proctosigmoidoscopy, and anal electromyography (EMG)

IMAGING STUDIES

- Anal endosonography (most widely used and least expensive)
- MRI

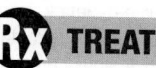 **TREATMENT**

Loperamide hydrochloride, diphenoxylate/atropine sulphate (mainstay of treatment), estrogen replacement therapy in postmenopausal women (uncontrolled trials)

NONPHARMACOLOGIC THERAPY

- Supportive therapy
  - Education/counseling/habit training
  - Diet (increase fiber, lactulose, and fructose)

- Biofeedback therapy:
  - Anal sphincter muscle strengthening
  - Rectal sensory conditioning
  - Rectoanal coordination training
- Modified Kegel exercises
- Surgery:
  - Sphincteroplasty
  - Anterior repair
  - Artificial bowel sphincter
  - Sacral nerve stimulation
  - Colostomy

REFERRAL

Refer to colorectal surgeon

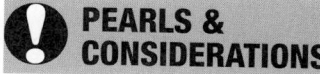 **PEARLS & CONSIDERATIONS**

COMMENTS

- The shame, embarrassment, and stigma associated with fecal and urinary incontinence pose significant barriers to seeking professional treatment, resulting in many people who suffer from these conditions without help.

PREVENTION

- Endoanal ultrasound to detect and repair anal sphincter tears in women with second-degree perineal tears may reduce severe fecal incontinence (mid-level evidence).
- Routine episiotomy is the most easily preventable risk factor for fecal incontinence in females.

PATIENT/FAMILY EDUCATION

Website: www.familydoctor.org/online/famdoc en/home/seniors/common-older/067.html digestive.niddk.nih.gov/ddiseases/pubs/fecal incontinence

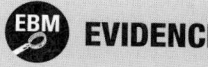 **EVIDENCE**

available at www.expertconsult.com

SUGGESTED READINGS
available at www.expertconsult.com

AUTHOR: **NADIA MUJAHID, M.D.**

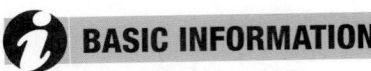

BASIC INFORMATION

DEFINITION

Incontinence is the involuntary loss of urine. The International Continence Society defines overactive bladder as "urinary urgency, usually accompanied by frequency and no uturia, with or without urgency urinary incontinence, in the absence of urinary tract infection or other obvious pathology" and urgency urinary incontinence as "involuntary loss of urine associated with urgency."

ICD-9CM CODES
788.3   Incontinence
625.6   Stress incontinence
788.33 Mixed stress and urge incontinence
788.32 Male incontinence
788.39 Neurogenic incontinence
307.6   Nonorganic origin

EPIDEMIOLOGY & DEMOGRAPHICS

INCIDENCE/PREVALENCE: In the general population between the ages of 15 and 64 yr, 1.5% to 5% of men and 10% to 25% of women have incontinence. In the nursing home population, 50% of the population has some degree of incontinence. Nearly 20% of children through the mid-teenage years have episodes of urinary incontinence.

CLINICAL, PSYCHOLOGIC, & SOCIAL IMPACT

Fewer than 50% of the individuals with incontinence living in the community consult health care providers, preferring to "suffer silently," turning to home remedies, commercially available absorbent materials, and supportive aids. As their condition worsens, they become depressed, sacrifice their independence, suffer from recurrent urinary tract infection and its sequelae, limit social interaction, refrain from sexual intimacy, and become homebound. In terms of costs, for all ages living in the community, it is estimated that $7 billion is spent for incontinence annually.

MAJOR TYPES OF INCONTINENCE

- **Transient incontinence:** Incontinence occurring as a result or reaction to an acute medical problem affecting the lower urinary tract. Many of these problems can be reversed with treatment of the underlying problem.
- **Urge incontinence:** Involuntary loss of urine associated with an abrupt and strong desire to void. It is usually associated with involuntary detrusor contractions on urodynamic investigation. In neurologically impaired patients, the involuntary detrusor contraction is referred to as *detrusor hyperreflexia*. In neurologically normal patients the involuntary contraction is called *detrusor instability*.
- **Stress incontinence** (Fig. 1-207): The involuntary loss of urine with physical activities that increase abdominal pressure in the absence of a detrusor contraction or an overdistended bladder. Classification of stress incontinence:
  1. Type 0: Report of incontinence without demonstration of leakage.
  2. Type I: Incontinence in response to stress but with little descent of the bladder neck and urethra.
  3. Type II: Incontinence in response to stress with >2 cm descent of the bladder neck and urethra.
  4. Type III: Bladder neck and urethra wide open without bladder contraction; intrinsic sphincter deficiency; denervation of the urethra. The most common causes include urethral hypermobility and displacement of the bladder neck with exertion, intrinsic sphincter deficiency from failed antiincontinence surgery, prostatectomy, radiation, cord lesions, epispadias, and myelomeningocele.
- **Overflow incontinence:** Loss of urine resulting from overdistention of the bladder with resultant overflow or spilling of the urine.

Causes include hypotonic-to-atonic bladder resulting from drug effect, fecal impaction, or neurologic conditions such as diabetes, spinal cord injury, surgery, or vitamin B_{12} deficiency. It is also caused by obstruction at the bladder neck and urethra. In this situation prostatism, prostatic cancer, urethral stenosis, antiincontinence surgery, pelvic prolapse, and detrusor-sphincter dyssynergia cause the incontinence.
- **Functional incontinence:** Involuntary loss of urine resulting from chronic impairments of physical and/or cognitive functioning. This is a diagnosis of exclusion. The condition can sometimes be improved or cured by improving the patient's functional status, treating comorbidities, changing medications, and reducing environmental barriers.
- **Mixed stress and urge incontinence.** (Fig. 1-207)
- **Sensory urgency incontinence:** Involuntary loss of urine as a result of decreased bladder compliance and increased intravesical pressures accompanied by severe urgency and bladder hypersensitivity without detrusor overactivity. This is seen with radiation cystitis, interstitial cystitis, eosinophilic cystitis, myelomeningocele, and radical pelvic surgery. Nephropathy can occur as a complication of this vesicoureteral reflux.
- **Sphincteric incontinence:**
  1. *Urethral hypermobility:* The basic abnormality is a weakness of pelvic floor support. Because of this weakness, during increases in abdominal pressure there is rotational descent of the vesical neck and proximal urethra. If the urethra opens concomitantly, stress urinary incontinence ensues. Urethral hypermobility is often present in women who are not incontinent. Its mere presence is not sufficient evidence to make the diagnosis of sphincteric abnormality unless incontinence is shown.
  2. *Intrinsic sphincter deficiency:* There is an intrinsic malfunction of the sphincter itself. It is characterized by an open vesical neck at rest and a low leak point pressure (<65 cm water). Urethral hypermobility and intrinsic sphincter deficiency may coexist in the same patient. Causes of intrinsic sphincter deficiency are previous pelvic surgery, antiincontinence surgery, urethral diverticulectomy, radical hysterectomy, abdominoperineal resection of the rectum, urethrotomy, Y-V plasty of the vesical neck, myelodysplasia, anterior spinal artery syndrome, lumbosacral disease, aging, and hyperestrogenism.

DIAGNOSIS

HISTORY

- History of present illness, psychosocial factors, congenital disorders, access issues for the physically challenged, neurologic disorders, and disorders pertinent to the urologic tract
- Review of prescription and nonprescription medications

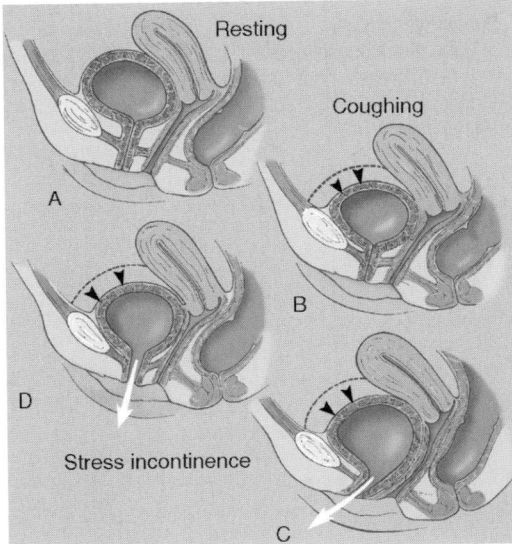

FIGURE 1-207 A, Bladder and urethra in normal position. **B,** Intra-abdominal pressure transmitted to the bladder. **C,** Bladder and urethra in abnormal position with loss of support (hypermobile). **D,** Loss of urethral closure. (From Lipshultz LI et al: *Urology and the primary care practitioner,* ed 3, Philadelphia, 2008, Elsevier.)

- Voiding diary to assess total voided volume, frequency of micturition, mean volume voided, largest single volume, diurnal distribution, nature and severity of incontinence

WORKUP

- Physical examination including general examination, gait of the patient (neuromuscular deficits), estrogen status, vaginal examination to include the periurethral region, evaluation for cystocele, rectocele, and enterocele
- Pelvic floor strength assessment
- Rectal examination to assess sphincter tone and bulbocavernosus reflex
- Neurologic examination
- Postvoid residual check with bladder scan or catheter

LABORATORY TESTS

Urinalysis, urine culture, urine cytology, blood urea nitrogen, creatinine

IMAGING STUDIES

- Radiographs of the kidney, ureter, and bladder to assess bony skeleton
- Intravenous pyelography to rule out upper tract abnormalities, developmental anomalies, bladder configuration, and fistula
- Renal ultrasound if dye study is contraindicated

SPECIALIZED STUDIES

Simple cystometrogram, complex urodynamics for leak point pressures and uroflowmetry, endoscopic evaluation, cystogram

Rx TREATMENT

- Transient incontinence: Treatment of underlying medical conditions and behavioral therapy to include habit training and timed voiding
- Urge incontinence: Bladder relaxants (tolterodine, oxybutynin, imipramine), trospium chloride, estrogen, biofeedback, Kegel exercises, and surgical removal of obstructing or other pathologic lesions. Recent trials reveal promising results with direct intravesical instillation of a botulinum type A toxin/dimethyl sulfoxide (DMSO) solution for the treatment of idiopathic detrusor overactivity in women.
- Stress incontinence: Pelvic floor exercises, Kegel exercises, α-adrenergic agonists (e.g., ephedrine), estrogen, biofeedback
  - Cystourethropexy (see Table 1-85): Marshall-Marchetti-Krantz procedure, Burch procedure, Raz procedure, Stamey-Raz procedure, Gittes procedure, in situ transvaginal sling, pubovaginal sling with autologous or cadaver graft, laparoscopic Burch procedure, laparoscopic sling, tension-free vaginal tape
  - For intrinsic sphincter deficiency: bulking agents (e.g., collagen), sling, and artificial sphincter
- Overflow incontinence: surgical removal of any obstructing lesions, clean intermittent catheterization, indwelling catheter
- Functional incontinence: behavioral training to include habit training and timed voiding, incontinence undergarments and pads, external collecting devices, environmental manipulation

TABLE 1-85 Surgical Treatment of Stress Incontinence

Anterior Colporrhaphy
Transvaginal Needle Suspension
Pereyra
Stamey
Gittes
Raz
Abdominal Retropubic Urethropexy (Suspension)
Marshall-Marchetti-Krantz
Burch operation
Paravaginal repair
Lapides procedure
Sling Procedure
Pubovaginal (bladder neck) sling
Autologous
Rectus abdominus fascia
Tensor fascia lata
Anterior vagina wall sling
Allograft (cadaveric fascia lata fascia)
Xenograft
Porcine dermis
Small intestinal submucosa
Synthetic mesh (polypropylene)
Tension-free midurethral sling (polypropylene)
TVT
TVT-O
TOT
SPARC
Urethral Bulking Agent
Bovine collagen
Carbon-coated zirconium beads
Ethylene vinyl alcohol copolymer
Calcium hydroxyapatite
Artificial Urinary Sphincter

SPARC, Suprapubic arc sling system; *TOT,* trans-obturator tape; *TVT,* tension-free vaginal tape; *TVT-O,* TVT-obturator.
From Lipshultz LI et al: *Urology and the primary care practitioner,* ed 3, Philadelphia, 2008, Elsevier.

- Mixed urgency and stress incontinence: use of measures recommended in the management of stress and urge incontinence
- Sensory urgency: bladder relaxants (e.g., anticholinergics, muscle relaxants, and tricyclic antidepressants), behavior therapy to include habit training and timed voiding, cystoscopy and hydrodilation
- Sphincteric deficiency: urethral bulking agents, sling procedure, artificial sphincter, mechanical clamp, external collection devices

PEARLS & CONSIDERATIONS

COMMENTS

Overweight and obese women with urinary incontinence have a high prevalence of monthly fecal incontinence (16% found to be associated with low dietary fiber intake after adjustment for other known risk factors for fecal incontinence

Other forms of incontinence:

- Nocturnal enuresis: (ICD-9CM Code: 788.3) Can be caused by sphincter abnormalities and detrusor overactivity; can occur as idiopathic, neurogenic, and with outlet obstruction
- Postvoid dribble: (ICD-9CM Code: 599.2) A postsphincteric collection of urine seen with urethral diverticulum; can be idiopathic
- Extraurethral incontinence: Enterovesical (ICD-9CM Codes: 596.1 and 596.2), urethral (ICD-9CM Code: 599.1); also known as *fistula*

Conditions that predispose to surgical failure: Advanced age, postmenopausal state, hysterectomy, prior failed incontinence surgery, concurrent detrusor instability, abnormal perineal electromyography, pelvic radiation

EBM EVIDENCE

available at www.expertconsult.com

SUGGESTED READINGS

available at www.expertconsult.com

AUTHORS: **PHILIP J. ALIOTTA, M.D., M.S.H.A.,** and **RUBEN ALVERO, M.D.**

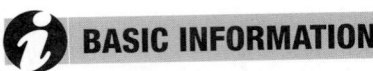
DEFINITION

Hypotonia typically describes the inability to move or maintain posture against forces that stretch the body, mainly gravity. The cause can be at any level in the neuroaxis, so the differential is extensive. A detailed history and physical exam are the key tools to localizing the lesion.

SYNONYMS Floppy infant

ICD-9CM CODES
343.8 Infantile cerebral palsy

EPIDEMIOLOGY & DEMOGRAPHICS

Central causes for hypotonia outweigh peripheral causes 3:1

PHYSICAL FINDINGS & CLINICAL PRESENTATION

To assess tone, first observe the fully awake child looking for movement, position, and signs of decreased fetal movement (hip dislocation, arthrogryposis, plagiocephaly, pectus excavatum). When supine, infants with low tone will lay with their extremities extended and abducted, termed the *frog-leg position*. The head needs to be straight to avoid inducing the tonic neck reflex, which can make tone falsely appear to be asymmetric. When pulled gently by the hands toward the sitting position, normal infants will have a *traction response* that involves flexion at the hips, knees, and ankles with the head rising off the bed. Infants with hypotonia will have significant head lag and very little resistance to the examiner. Keep in mind, however, that this response is not present until after 33 wk gestational age. When held under the arms by the axilla in *vertical suspension*, hypotonic infants will start to slip through the examiner's hands, while infants with normal tone will have the same flexion reflex as with the traction response. If held prone with support under the torso in *horizontal suspension*, normal infants will keep their back straight, have flexion at the hips, knees, and ankles, and keep their head up. They will also make efforts to maintain this position, whereas a hypotonic infant will fall limply into an "inverted U" position.

Look for other signs that the hypotonia may have central origin (Table 1-86), for example abnormal head shape or size, decreased level of consciousness, dysmorphic features, other organs with malformations, seizures, apnea, or abnormal sleep-wake cycles. Reflexes should be brisk, but may be decreased acutely after an injury. Infants with peripheral hypotonia (i.e., a lesion in the motor unit) are typically alert and profoundly weak. Reflexes are reduced or absent and muscles may be atrophic. With anterior horn cell disease, the tongue may have fasciculations and the child may have an intention tremor, as well. The rest of the neurologic and general exams can provide pertinent clues to specific diagnoses. Cardiac murmurs, skin lesions, hepatosplenomegaly, and so forth help narrow down the differential.

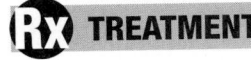 **DIAGNOSIS**

DIFFERENTIAL DIAGNOSIS

Common central causes
- Acquired brain insult
  - Infection
  - Hypoxic encephalopathy
  - Intracranial hemorrhage
- Brain anomalies: neuromigrational disorders
- Genetic disorders
  - Kabuki syndrome
  - Williams syndrome
  - MECP2 duplication syndrome
  - Down syndrome
  - Fragile X syndrome
  - Prader-Willi syndrome
- Congenital syndromes: benign congenital hypotonia

Peripheral causes of hypotonia in infants
- Anterior horn cell disease
  - Spinal muscular atrophy
  - Hypoxic injury
  - Neurogenic arthrogryposis
- Polyneuropathies (motor or sensory)
  - Hereditary motor-sensory neuropathy
  - Charcot-Marie-Tooth disease
  - Guillain-Barré syndrome
  - Congenital hypomyelinating disorder
- Neuromuscular junction disorders
  - Infantile botulism
  - Congenital myasthenia gravis
  - Transient neonatal myasthenia

- Congenital myopathies
  - Central core disease
  - Nemaline rod myopathy
  - Fiber-type disproportion myopathy
  - Multi-Minicore disease
  - Myotubular myopathy
- Muscular dystrophies
  - Congenital dystrophinopathy
  - Congenital muscular dystrophy
  - Congenital myotonic dystrophy
- Metabolic disorders
  - Acid maltase deficiency (Pompe's disease)
  - Cerebrohepatorenal syndrome (Zellweger)
  - Cytochrome-c oxidase deficiency
  - Mitochondrial myopathies
  - Neonatal adrenoleukodystrophy

LABORATORY TESTS
- Evaluate neonate for sepsis
- Electrolytes including glucose, creatinine, calcium
- Liver function tests
- Ammonia level
- Creatinine kinase level
- Lactate
- Consider TORCH titers
- Karyotype or specific genetic testing
- Serum amino acids
- Urine organic acids
- Acylcarnitine/carnitine panel
- Very long chain fatty acids
- EMG/nerve conduction velocity (NCV)
- Muscle biopsy

IMAGING STUDIES
MRI with spectroscopy

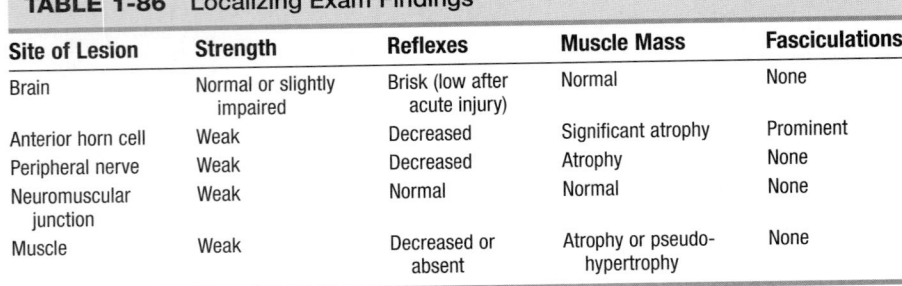 **TREATMENT**

Most of these disorders have no specific treatment.

CHRONIC Rx
- Physical therapy, occupational therapy, and other therapies tailored to the patient's specific needs can provide significant improvement in quality of life and ability to function.
- Respiratory illnesses are common in these children, so vaccinations should be kept up to date

DISPOSITION
- Long-term outcome varies greatly among different diseases.
- As a general rule, a hypotonic infant that requires mechanical ventilation cannot survive extubation (unless the cause is neonatal myasthenia).

EBM EVIDENCE

available at www.expertconsult.com

SUGGESTED READINGS
available at www.expertconsult.com

AUTHOR: **KIMBERLY JONES, M.D.**

TABLE 1-86 Localizing Exam Findings

Site of Lesion	Strength	Reflexes	Muscle Mass	Fasciculations
Brain	Normal or slightly impaired	Brisk (low after acute injury)	Normal	None
Anterior horn cell	Weak	Decreased	Significant atrophy	Prominent
Peripheral nerve	Weak	Decreased	Atrophy	None
Neuromuscular junction	Weak	Normal	Normal	None
Muscle	Weak	Decreased or absent	Atrophy or pseudo-hypertrophy	None

BASIC INFORMATION

DEFINITION

Infertility in a reproductive age couple is the inability to conceive after adequate coital attempts have been made for ≥1 yr. In couples where the female partner is >35 yr of age, an evaluation is justified after 6 mo without successful pregnancy.

SYNONYMS

Sterility

ICD-9CM CODES
628.0 Infertility, female, associated with anovulation
628.2 Infertility, female, of tubal origin
628.9 Infertility, of unspecified origin

EPIDEMIOLOGY & DEMOGRAPHICS

PEAK INCIDENCE: The incidence of infertility increases with increasing age. Subtle decreases in female fertility start as early as age 30. The rate of infertility increases dramatically after age 37 and spontaneous pregnancies become extremely uncommon as women reach the mid-40s. There is also a more subtle but still detectable decrease in male fertility that can also start as early as age 30.

PREVALENCE: One in eight reproductive age couples experience infertility. This prevalence is consistent in all developed countries and there is evidence that it is historically stable.

PREDOMINANT SEX AND AGE: By definition this is a diagnosis of reproductive age couples. Infertility increases with aging in both males and females but more dramatically in women. Male factor is responsible in ~40% of couples and the female factor is responsible in ~40% of couples. The remainder of the cases are either combined male and female or unexplained infertility, meaning a clear cause in not identified.

RISK FACTORS: Aging is among the most common of risk factors, predominantly among females. Women are increasingly deferring pregnancy as a result of careers, which is likely associated with the increasing prevalence in certain sectors of the population. Sexually transmitted disease with *Chlamydia* and gonorrhea is associated with pelvic inflammatory disease, which frequently results in tubal factor infertility. Extremes of weight, especially overweight, are associated with ovulatory dysfunction. Male factor infertility is most commonly idiopathic, although trauma, infection, varicocele, and exposure to environmental toxins may be associated with compromise of semen parameters. Smoking is the most common lifestyle choice that impairs fertility.

PHYSICAL FINDINGS & CLINICAL PRESENTATION

- Age (both partners)
- Previous fertility, particularly if no pregnancy has occurred in another relationship despite absence of contraception (both partners)
- Absence of secondary sexual characteristics (both partners)
- Irregular or absent menstruation (female)
- Hirsutism, acne and alopecia suggestive of hyperandrogenism (female)
- Pelvic exam suggestive of uterine abnormality such as fibroids (female)
- Trauma or torsion of the testes (male)
- Small, firm testes (male)

ETIOLOGY

- Advanced age, especially female
- Pelvic inflammatory disease (results in tubal factor infertility)
- Endometriosis (results in tubal factor infertility)
- Female anatomic (uterine fibroids, polyps, intrauterine adhesions)
- Oligoovulation, most frequently due to polycystic ovarian syndrome (PCOS)
- Idiopathic, both male and female

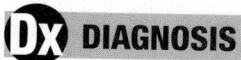

DIAGNOSIS

DIFFERENTIAL DIAGNOSIS

- Recurrent spontaneous abortion
- Ineffective attempts at natural conception
- Sterility due to previous permanent sterilization procedure

WORKUP

- The components of evaluation depend greatly on whether the female patient is reliably ovulating based on history (regular menses, premenstrual molimina such as breast tenderness) and laboratory testing (midluteal progesterone, basal body temperature testing, urinary LH predictor kits, mid-cycle ovulatory pain [Mittelschmerz], cervical mucus testing)
- Where the menstrual cycle is important in testing, the first day is defined as the first day of full menstrual flow
- If the female patient does not appear to be ovulating, testing should consist of:
  - TSH
  - Prolactin
  - Total testosterone/free testosterone (to assess for PCOS)
  - Transvaginal pelvic ultrasound to assess for polycystic appearing ovaries
  - 17-Hydroxyprogesterone (to assess for cryptic congenital adrenal hyperplasia)
  - 2-hr glucose tolerance testing (if the patient has PCOS)
  - FSH/LH
  - Lipid panel (if the patient has PCOS, secondary to overlap with metabolic syndrome)
  - Liver function test (if the patient has PCOS, in case treatment with insulin-sensitizing agents indicated)
  - BUN/creatinine (if the patient has PCOS, in case treatment with insulin-sensitizing agents indicated)
  - Semen analysis in the male partner
  - Hysterosalpingogram (if the history suggests previous pelvic infection)

- If the female patient appears to be ovulating, testing should consist of:
  - Semen analysis in the male partner
  - Hysterosalpingogram
  - Mid-luteal progesterone, urinary LH predictor kits (to assess for ovulation)
  - FSH, estradiol, anti-mullerian hormone on day 2 to 3 of menstrual cycle (ovarian reserve testing)
  - Transvaginal pelvic ultrasound to assess for uterine anomalies and antral follicle count as a measure of ovarian reserve

LABORATORY TESTS

- Semen analysis, using Kruger strict morphology after 2 to 3 days of abstinence (male)
- Day 2 or 3 FSH, estradiol, and anti-mullerian hormone as a measure of ovarian reserve (female)
- Mid-luteal progesterone (ideally 7 days after ovulatory surge)
- Urinary LH ovulatory kits
- See "Workup" for evaluation of couples where the female partner is oligo- or anovulatory

IMAGING STUDIES

- Hysterosalpingogram (between days 6 and 12 of the menstrual cycle)
- Day 2 or 3 transvaginal pelvic ultrasound to assess uterine abnormalities and to count the number of small antral follicles (2 to 9 mm) as a measure of ovarian reserve. If oligo- or anovulatory, to assess for polycystic appearing ovary

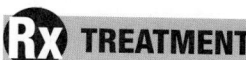

TREATMENT

Once the patient presents for evaluation, testing should be completed as quickly as possible, ideally within one menstrual cycle. The couple should follow up with the evaluating provider once all testing is completed and treatment initiated as abnormalities are found.

ACUTE GENERAL Rx

- Mild male factor infertility may be treated with intrauterine insemination but more severe forms will usually require assisted reproductive technologies (ART) with intracytoplasmic sperm injection (ICSI), where sperm is injected directly into the oocyte.
- Tubal factor infertility may be treated surgically if mild and if the female patient is young and can afford the time to attempt pregnancy over multiple menstrual cycles. If the patient is older or if the tubal pathology moderate to severe, then the patient should use in vitro fertilization (IVF) to achieve pregnancy.
- Oligo- or anovulation should be treated with ovulation induction agents. Women with euestrogenic ovulatory dysfunction can be treated with clomiphene citrate as a first-line agent, using 50 mg in the first cycle attempt and increasing the dose by 50 mg up to a maximum dose of 200 mg if the patient fails to ovulate. Far less commonly, ovulatory dysfunction is the result of hypothalamic dys-

function. In these patients, once hypothalamic or pituitary abnormalities are excluded with MRI, ovulation can be achieved using injected gonadotropins.

- Uterine anatomic abnormalities such as submucous fibroids, polyps, or intrauterine adhesions should be corrected if they are identified. Fibroids that do not impact the uterine cavity probably do not interfere with fertility. Removal of intramural or subserosal fibroids is reserved for situations in which these cause excessive vaginal bleeding, pain, or pressure.
- Unexplained infertility can be treated empirically using superovulation with clomiphene citrate or gonadotropins combined with intrauterine insemination with partner's sperm. Most providers recommend using clomiphene citrate with insemination as a first-line superovulatory agent since it is inexpensive. After 3 to 4 such cycles, few pregnancies occur and the couple should be advised to become more aggressive. Controversy exists as to whether gonadotropins with insemination or IFV should be used after clomiphene citrate superovulation induction. There is evidence suggesting that moving to IVF in a "fast-track" fashion shortens the time interval to achieving pregnancy.

COMPLEMENTARY AND ALTERNATIVE MEDICINE

Acupuncture is widely used by women being treated for infertility. Limited data suggest some benefit, with possible mechanisms of action including increasing blood flow to the uterus. Patients may additionally benefit from the stress relief that acupuncture provides.

DISPOSITION

- Most couples will achieve a pregnancy, provided that they are willing to use aggressive techniques, including ART such as IVF and gamete donation.
- Adoption can also be used but patients should be aware that this can also be difficult because of limited availability of adoptable children and because of the expense and bureaucratic hurdles.

REFERRAL

Couples should be referred to a Reproductive Endocrinologist once the complexity of treatment exceeds the comfort level of the provider, whether a Family Physician, Internist or general Gynecologist. Complex ovulation and superovulation induction and ART are usually managed by a board certified Reproductive Endocrinologist.

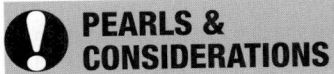

PEARLS & CONSIDERATIONS

COMMENTS

- ~1% of all live births in the United States currently are the result of IVF.

- The incidence of heterotopic pregnancy in patients who have undergone IVF is ~1%; identification of a patient with ultrasound-proved intrauterine pregnancy who used ART to conceive should NOT necessarily exclude the possibility of an ectopic gestation.

PREVENTION

- Techniques that reduce the incidence of pelvic inflammatory disease, such as condom use, can reduce pelvic adhesions that are associated with tubal factor infertility.
- Women can be made aware of the fact that delaying pregnancy into the later reproductive years can reduce the chances for successful pregnancy.

PATIENT/FAMILY EDUCATION

Patient support groups such as *Resolve* (www.resolve.org) are available to help couples during evaluation and treatment of infertility, which can be extraordinarily stressful.

SUGGESTED READINGS

available at www.expertconsult.com

AUTHOR: **RUBEN ALVERO, M.D.**

BASIC INFORMATION

DEFINITION

Influenza is an acute febrile illness caused by infection with influenza type A or B virus. Seasonal influenza can include the H1N1 virus. Severe acute respiratory syndrome (SARS) is a similar respiratory illness caused by a coronavirus called SARS-associated coronavirus (SARS-CoV). See Table 1-87 at end of chapter.

SYNONYMS

Flu
Influenza-like illness (ILI)

ICD-9CM CODES
487.1 Influenza

EPIDEMIOLOGY & DEMOGRAPHICS

PEAK INCIDENCE: Winter outbreaks lasting 5 to 6 wk
PREDOMINANT SEX: Male = female
PREDOMINANT AGE: Attack rates are higher among children than adults, although children are less prone to develop pulmonary complications.
INCIDENCE (IN U.S.): Annual incidence of influenza-related deaths is ~36,000 deaths/yr

PANDEMICS

DEFINITION: Widespread human community-level outbreaks in ≥two countries in one World Health Organization (WHO) region.
HISTORICAL:
- In the twentieth century, pandemics occurred from H1N1 resulting in 40 to 100 million deaths worldwide in 1918, 70,000 deaths in the United States in 1957 from H2N2, and 36,000 deaths in the United States in 1968 from H3N2.
- H5N1 emerged in Hong Kong in 1997, quickly infecting poultry and birds. More than 400 humans were infected with Avian flu (H5N1) by 2009, but transmission from human to human was not efficient.
Novel influenza A (H1N1) virus:
- WHO declared the H1N1 outbreaks a public health emergency in April 2009, and announced a global pandemic in June 2009. The U.S. emergency ended in June 2010, and the WHO declared an end to the global pandemic in August 2010.
- H1N1 is predicted to continue circulation as a seasonal virus for years to come.
- The 2009 H1N1 virus affected more young adults than the elderly.
- In 2009 in the United States, it is estimated that there were 43 million to 88 million cases, 192,000 to 398,000 hospitalizations, and as many as 18,000 deaths from H1N1.

PHYSICAL FINDINGS & CLINICAL PRESENTATION

- "Classic flu" is characterized by abrupt onset of fever, headache, myalgias, anorexia, and malaise after a 1- to 2-day incubation period.

- Clinical syndromes are similar to those produced by other respiratory viruses, including pharyngitis, common colds, tracheobronchitis, bronchiolitis, and croup.
- Respiratory symptoms such as cough, sore throat, and nasal discharge are usually present at the onset of illness, but systemic symptoms predominate.
- Elderly patients may experience fever, weakness, and confusion without any respiratory complaints.
- Acute deterioration to status asthmaticus may occur in patients with asthma.
- Influenza pneumonia: rapidly progressive cough, dyspnea, and cyanosis may occur after typical flu onset. This may be caused by primary influenza pneumonia or secondary bacterial pneumonia (often pneumococcal or staphylococcal infection).

ETIOLOGY

- Variation in the surface antigens of the influenza virus, hemagglutinin (HA) and neuraminidase (NA), leading to infection with variants to which resistance is inadequate in the population at risk
- Transmitted by small-particle aerosols and deposited on the respiratory tract epithelium

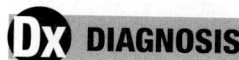 **DIAGNOSIS**

DIFFERENTIAL DIAGNOSIS

- Respiratory syncytial virus, adenovirus, parainfluenza virus infection
- Secondary bacterial pneumonia or mixed bacterial-viral pneumonia

WORKUP

- Virus isolation from nasal or throat swab or sputum specimens is the most rapid diagnostic method in the setting of acute illness.
- Specimens are placed into virus transport medium and processed by a reference laboratory.
- For serologic diagnosis:
  1. Paired serum specimens, acute and convalescent, the latter obtained 10 to 20 days later
  2. Fourfold rises or falls in the titer of antibodies (various techniques) considered diagnostic of recent infection

LABORATORY TESTS

Septic syndrome presentation: CBC, ABG analysis, blood cultures

IMAGING STUDIES

- Chest x-ray examination to demonstrate findings of viral pneumonia: peribronchial and patchy interstitial infiltrates in multiple lobes with atelectasis
- Possible progression to diffuse interstitial pneumonitis

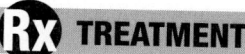 **TREATMENT**

NONPHARMACOLOGIC THERAPY

- Bed rest
- Hydration

ACUTE GENERAL Rx

- Supportive care: antipyretics; avoid use of aspirin in children because of the association with Reye's syndrome
- Antibiotics if bacterial pneumonia is proven or suspected
- Amantadine (100 mg PO twice daily for children >10 yr and adults <65 yr; once daily in patients >65 yr) or rimantadine (same dose schedule as amantadine)
  1. Further dose adjustments needed with renal insufficiency
  2. Fewer CNS side effects with rimantadine
  3. There are clinical limitations to their use due to resistance. See Table 1-87.
- Neuraminidase inhibitors block release of virions from infected cells, resulting in shortened duration of symptoms and decrease in complications; effective against both influenza A and B
  1. Zanamivir, administered via inhaler:
     For treatment, 10 mg (2 inhalations of 5 mg each) twice daily for 5 days
     For prevention in households, 10 mg (2 inhalations of 5 mg each) once daily for 10 days
  2. Oseltamivir, administered orally:
     For treatment, 75 mg PO twice daily for 5 days
     For prevention, 75 mg PO once daily for a minimum of 2 wk in an outbreak setting
  3. Emergency use authorization by the Centers for Disease Control and Prevention (CDC) for intravenous peramivir during the H1N1 pandemic was terminated in June 2010. Intravenous peramivir is still available as an experimental drug.
- Placebo-controlled studies have suggested that antiviral therapy with any of the previously mentioned agents must be initiated within 1 to 2 days of the onset of symptoms and reduces the duration of illness by ~1 day.
- Oseltamivir resistance developed on therapy in individuals with avian flu (H5N1) in Asia, and this is associated with poor outcome.
- Amantadine and rimantadine resistance are documented for novel (H1N1) influenza and H3N2 influenza virus.

DISPOSITION

Patients are hospitalized if signs of pneumonia are present.

REFERRAL

Infectious disease and/or pulmonary consultation when influenza pneumonia is suspected

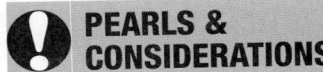

COMMENTS

- Prevention of influenza in patients at high risk is an important goal of primary care.
- Vaccines reduce the risk of infection and the severity of illness.
  1. Antigenic composition of the vaccine is updated annually. The 2010 to 2011 season vaccine includes one influenza A (H3N2) virus, one influenza A (H1N1) virus, and one influenza B virus.
  2. Vaccination should be given at the start of the flu season (September-October) for all persons aged ≥6 mo. Vaccination is particularly important for persons who are at increased risk for severe complications from influenza. When vaccine supply is limited, vaccination efforts should focus on the following groups:
     a. All children aged 6 mo to 4 yr (59 mo).
     b. Adults and children with chronic cardiac or pulmonary disease, including asthma
     c. Adults and children with illness requiring frequent follow-up (e.g., hemoglobinopathies, diabetes mellitus)
     d. Children aged 6 mo to 18 yr who are receiving long-term aspirin therapy
     e. Immunocompromised patients (including HIV-infected persons)
     f. Residents of nursing homes and other long-term care facilities
     g. American Indians/Alaska Natives
     h. Persons who are morbidly obese (BMI ≥40).
     i. Health care workers
     j. Women who are or will be pregnant during the influenza season
     k. Household contacts and caregivers of persons in the previous groups
  3. Contraindication to vaccination is anaphylactic hypersensitivity to eggs or to other components of the influenza vaccine unless the recipient has been desensitized.
  4. Vaccination should be delayed for persons with moderate to severe acute febrile illness. Precautions include:
     Guillain-Barré syndrome within 6 wk following a previous dose of influenza vaccine
     Moderate or severe acute illness with or without fever (for trivalent inactivated influenza vaccine).
  5. Special efforts should be made to vaccinate high-risk patients <65 yr, only 10% to 15% of whom are vaccinated each year.
- Chemoprophylaxis:
  1. Table 1-87 describes antiviral agents for influenza. Amantadine and rimantadine approved for prophylaxis against influenza A; they are ineffective against influenza B and H1N1.
  2. Consider (after the current circulating strain of influenza has been shown to be sensitive):
     a. For high-risk patients in whom vaccination is contraindicated
     b. When the available vaccine is known not to include the circulating strain
     c. To provide added protection to immunosuppressed patients likely to have a diminished response to vaccination
     d. In the setting of an outbreak, when immediate protection of unvaccinated or recently vaccinated patients is desired
  3. Give for 2 wk in the case of late vaccination and for the duration of the flu season in all other patients
- Other prevention strategies:
  1. Hand hygiene, cough etiquette (cover your cough), respiratory hygiene (use of tissues, facemasks for the ill and proper disposal)
  2. Personal protective equipment (PPE)—wear gloves and gowns as for universal/standard precautions. Per Centers for Disease Control and Prevention, wear facemask, adhering to Droplet Precautions for 7 days after illness onset or until 24 hr after fever and respiratory symptoms are resolved, whichever is longer. Patient placement in a negative pressure room and N95 respirator for health care workers are recommended when procedures are conducted that generate respiratory aerosols.
  3. Management of ill health care workers—exclude from work until at least 24 hr after they no longer have a fever (without the use of fever-reducing medication). Extended exclusion time period when caring for severely immunocompromised patients.
  4. Standard cleaning and disinfection procedures.

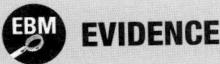 **EVIDENCE**

available at www.expertconsult.com

SUGGESTED READINGS

available at www.expertconsult.com

AUTHORS: **MARLENE FISHMAN, M.P.H., C.I.C.,** and **GLENN G. FORT, M.D., M.P.H.**

TABLE 1-87 Antiviral Agents for Influenza

	Amantadine	Rimantadine	Zanamivir	Oseltamivir
Protein target	M2	M2	Neuraminidase	Neuraminidase
Activity	A only (H1N1 and H3N2 are resistant)	A only (H1N1 and H3N2 are resistant)	A and B	A and B
Side effects	CNS (13%)	GI (6%)	? Bronchospasm	GI (9%)
	GI (3%)	GI (3%)		
Metabolism	None	Multiple (hepatic)	None	Hepatic
Excretion	Renal	Renal, + others	Renal	Renal (tubular secretion)
Drug interactions	Antihistamines, anticholinergics	None	None	Probenecid (increased levels of oseltamivir)
Dose adjustments needed	≥65 yr old	≥65 yr old	None	CrCl <30 ml/min
	CrCl <50 ml/min	CrCl <10 ml/min		Severe liver dysfunction
Contraindications	Acute-angle glaucoma	Severe liver dysfunction	Underlying airway disease, asthma	

FDA-Approved Indications

	Amantadine	Rimantadine	Zanamivir	Oseltamivir
Therapy	Adults and children ≥1 yr old	Adults only	Adults and children ≥7 yr old	Adults and children ≥1 yr old*
Prophylaxis	Yes	Yes	Adults and children >5 yr old	Adults and children ≥13 yr old†

CrCl, Creatinine clearance; *FDA,* U.S. Food and Drug Administration; *GI,* gastrointestinal.
*FDA has authorized treatment of S-OIV (novel H1N1) virus with oseltamivir in children ≥3 mo of age.
†FDA has authorized prophylaxis for S-OIV (novel H1N1) virus with oseltamivir in children ≥1 yr of age.
(From Mandell GL et al: *Principles and practice of infectious diseases,* ed 7, Philadelphia, 2010, Elsevier.)

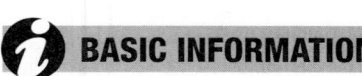

BASIC INFORMATION

DEFINITION
Avian influenza is a virus originating in birds that has the capacity to infect humans. The prior influenza pandemics of the twentieth century (from the devastating 1918 pandemic, in which 40 to 100 million people died, to the lesser pandemics of 1957 and 1968, of 1 to 6 million deaths) were caused by highly virulent, efficiently transmitted influenzas that evolved from avian strains. The highly pathogenic avian influenza A (H5N1), which is capable of only incidentally infecting humans but with a near 60% mortality rate, threatens to bring another pandemic flu. H5N1 avian influenza emerged in 1997 in Hong Kong, and by September 2010 had infected more than 500 humans as it spread via migrating waterfowl from Asia to Europe and Africa.

SYNONYMS
Bird flu
Pandemic flu

ICD-9CM CODES
488 Avian influenza

EPIDEMIOLOGY & DEMOGRAPHICS
Avian influenza A H5N1 is an influenza virus related to those that bring our yearly influenzas, against which populations are routinely vaccinated. Influenza viruses are enveloped RNA viruses with segmented genomes and great antigenic diversity. They are categorized by their core proteins (A, B, C), species of origin (avian, swine, human), geographic site of isolation, serial number, and influenza subtypes based on the major antigenic surface glycoproteins, hemagglutinin (HA), and neuraminidase (NA).

Often human and avian viruses meet and resort in a pig respiratory system. Southeast Asia is often the birthplace of new flu strains because birds, pigs, and people live in close proximity. It is where avian influenza A H5N1 emerged, first infecting domestic poultry, then wild birds that migrated across Eurasia. It is transmitted directly from birds to their keepers. Antigenic drift or shift may allow avian influenza A H5N1 to gain the ability to be easily transmissible from human to human, transforming it from a highly virulent influenza strain to a pandemic flu.

PREDOMINANT SEX AND AGE: Children and young adults

RISK FACTORS: Poultry work, possibly swine work (in case of reassortment), travel to affected areas

PHYSICAL FINDINGS & CLINICAL PRESENTATION
- Presenting features include fever of at least 100.4° F (38° C) with leukopenia or lymphopenia nearly always followed by viral pneumonia with escalating respiratory distress.
- Ventilatory support is often required within 48 hr of hospitalization for acute respiratory distress syndrome (ARDS).
- Symptom onset is 2 to 5 days after exposure, longer than with human influenza.
- Respiratory symptoms may also be accompanied by watery diarrhea.
- Complications include respiratory failure, renal dysfunction, cardiac compromise, pulmonary hemorrhage, pneumothorax, and multiorgan failure. A common cause of death is superinfection with bacterial pneumonias.

ETIOLOGY
H5N1 resists host antiviral cytokines, inducing excessive host pro-inflammatory responses. It may cause death by "cytokine storm" rather than by inherent pathogenicity. It attaches to sialic acid molecules via an α2-3 galactose receptor (common in birds) also found in human alveoli, leading to heavy damage to lower lungs. It causes severe pulmonary injury with diffuse alveolar damage. In the bone marrow, there is a reactive histiocytosis with hemophagocytosis that may lead to pancytopenia.

DIAGNOSIS

DIFFERENTIAL DIAGNOSIS
Atypical pneumonia, typical respiratory virus infections (e.g., influenza, respiratory syncytial virus), severe acute respiratory syndrome, upper respiratory infection with conjunctivitis (e.g., adenovirus). Clinical symptoms indistinguishable from other illnesses

WORKUP
Comprehensive travel, occupational and epidemiologic history

LABORATORY TESTS
- Aspartate aminotransferase, alanine aminotransferase, blood urea nitrogen, creatinine, complete blood count should be performed.
- Throat swab within 3 days of onset of symptoms to be sent for viral culture and polymerase chain reaction assay for avian influenza A (H5N1) RNA with appropriate biosafety precautions. The throat swab is more effective than nasal swabs since avian influenza preferentially infects the throat and lower respiratory tract. In the U.S. the FDA has approved the release of influenza H/A5 (Asian lineage) Virus Real-Time Reverse Transcription-PCR Primer and Probe Set for more than 140 labs in 50 states, which will return preliminary results in 4 hr.
- High-risk patients who must be tested include those with history of travel within 10 days of symptom onset to a country with documented H5N1 avian flu as well as patients with radiographically confirmed pneumonia, ARDS, or severe respiratory illness without alternate etiology.
- Low-risk patients are those who have contact with domestic poultry, or contact with people who have traveled to a country with documented H5N1 avian flu, who have fever >38° C and cough, sore throat, shortness of breath.

IMAGING STUDIES
- Chest x-rays detect infiltrates a median of 7 days after onset of fever. They may be diffuse, multifocal/patchy infiltrates, or interstitial infiltrates, or segmental/lobular consolidation. Progression to respiratory failure is indicated by diffuse bilateral ground-glass infiltrates.
- See ARDS imaging studies.

TREATMENT

Vaccines and antivirals are the usual means for preventing and treating flu, but there are limited supplies worldwide. The traditional means of vaccine production using embryonated hens' eggs has been limited because the bird flu kills the eggs. Promising new vaccine production methods are advancing through the experimental stages, including adenovirus vectors that have the possibility of allowing rapid large-scale production of vaccines.

NONPHARMACOLOGIC THERAPY
- N95 particulate masks should help prevent person-to-person transmission of H5N1. Surgical masks prevent only large-droplet transmission.
- In preparation for pandemic flu: increase worldwide surveillance and disease reporting, kill infected birds, increase the numbers of available intensive care unit beds with mechanical ventilators and increase emergency capacity, educate medical personnel and the public, produce vaccines.
- In response, use influenza surveillance, social distancing (school closures), travel restrictions, quarantine, respirator masks, communications networking, and international teamwork to cordon off affected areas.

ACUTE GENERAL Rx
- The neuraminidase inhibitor oseltamivir can reduce the severity and duration of symptoms if treatment is initiated in the first 48 hr after symptom onset.
  - TREATMENT: adults 75 mg PO twice daily for 5 days
  - Postexposure prophylaxis: 75 mg PO daily for 7 to 10 days
- H5N1 demonstrates amantadine and rimantadine resistance.

PEARLS & CONSIDERATIONS

As of September 2010, the World Health Organization level of alert for avian influenza was phase 3, pandemic preparedness. Health-care workers should stay abreast of developments in terms of epidemiology, preventive measures, and treatments.

PREVENTION
See "Nonpharmacologic Therapy."

PATIENT & FAMILY EDUCATION
The American Council on Science and Health: Avian influenza: what you need to know. Available at http://acsh.org/publications/pubid.1294/pub_detail.asp

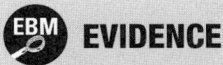 **EVIDENCE**

available at www.expertconsult.com

SUGGESTED READINGS
available at www.expertconsult.com

AUTHOR: **KOHAR JONES, M.D.**

Diseases and Disorders

I

BASIC INFORMATION

DEFINITION

Insomnia is a disturbance of initiating or maintaining sleep. Restless, nonrestorative sleep may also be described as insomnia. The disturbance occurs despite adequate circumstances and opportunity for sleep and is accompanied by significant distress or impairment in daytime functioning.

SYNONYMS

Sleeplessness
Sleep disorder, sleep disturbance, dyssomnia (NOTE: The terms *sleep disorder, sleep disturbance,* and *dyssomnia* are generic and can refer to disorders of wakefulness [hypersomnia] or sleep-related behavior disorders [parasomnias]).

ICD-9CM CODES
780.52 Insomnia
780.51 Insomnia with sleep apnea
307.41 Insomnia, nonorganic origin
307.42 Insomnia, persistent (primary)
307.41 Insomnia, transient
307.49 Subjective complaint

DSM IV-TR CODES
307.42 Primary insomnia
307.45 Circadian rhythm disorders
780.52 Insomnia due to a general medical condition
291.89, 292.89 Substance-induced insomnia

EPIDEMIOLOGY & DEMOGRAPHICS

INCIDENCE (IN U.S.): 30% to 45% of adults experience insomnia per year.
PREVALENCE (IN U.S.): 1% to 15% of all adults and 25% of older adults develop persistent insomnia.
PREDOMINANT SEX: More common in women.
PREDOMINANT AGE: Transient insomnia can occur at any age; persistent insomnia is more common after age 60 yr.
GENETICS: Can run in families and may be genetically influenced. Circadian rhythm disorders and narcolepsy have been traced to specific genes.

PHYSICAL FINDINGS & CLINICAL PRESENTATION

- Difficulty falling asleep, difficulty staying asleep, early morning awakening, restless or nonrestorative sleep, or difficulty sleeping at desired times.
- Significant distress or impairment in daytime functioning such as fatigue or low energy, sleepiness, cognitive impairments, mood disturbances, or behavioral problems.
- Difficulty occurs despite adequate opportunity for sleep.
- Symptoms may be acute and self-limited, chronic but intermittent, or chronic and frequent.

ETIOLOGY

- Transient insomnia:
  1. Stress
  2. Illness
  3. Travel (across time zones)
  4. Environmental disruptions (noise, heat, cold, poor bedding, unfamiliar surroundings, etc.)
- Persistent insomnia:
  1. Mood and anxiety disorders (depression, hypomania/mania, PTSD)
  2. Primary or psychophysiologic insomnia (with or without poor sleep hygiene)
  3. Sleep-related breathing disorders (e.g., obstructive apnea and hypopnea, increased upper airway resistance)
  4. Chronobiologic (also known as circadian rhythm) disorder (delayed sleep phase, advanced sleep phase, shift work, free-running rhythm secondary to blindness)
  5. Drug and alcohol abuse
  6. Restless legs syndrome and periodic leg movements
  7. Neurodegenerative (Alzheimer's disease, Parkinson's disease, etc.)
  8. Medical (pain, GERD, nocturia, orthopnea, medications, etc.)

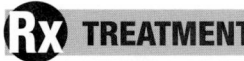 **DIAGNOSIS**

DIFFERENTIAL DIAGNOSIS

Primary or psychophysiologic insomnia is diagnosed when other etiologies (see "Etiology") are ruled out. However, it can be precipitated by a "primary" medical or mental health disorder and continue even after the "primary disorder" has been treated.

WORKUP

- History (with bed partner interview, if possible)
- Sleep diary for 2 wk (sample sleep diary available at http://www.sleepfoundation.org)
- Validated sleep-quality rating scale (optional)
  1. Pittsburgh Sleep Quality Index or Insomnia Severity Index
  2. Epworth Sleepiness Scale (see Daytime Sleepiness Test at http://www.sleep foundation.org)

LABORATORY TESTS

- Evaluate for anemia, uremia (for restless legs), thyroid function (if other signs present).
- Polysomnography (in home or in sleep laboratory) should be reserved for patients whose history suggests specific sleep-related breathing or movement disorders of breathing. It is indicated for symptoms suggesting of: daytime sleepiness (obstructive sleep apnea, narcolepsy), nonrestorative sleep (periodic leg movements), or sleep behavior suggesting parasomnia (somnambulism, REM sleep behavior).

IMAGING STUDIES

- Not generally helpful for insomnia
- Brain CT or MRI for severe daytime sleepiness or acute onset

Rx **TREATMENT**

NONPHARMACOLOGIC THERAPY

- Sleep hygiene measures (Box 1-10) as a monotherapy is not very effective. More useful combined with procedures described next.
- Cognitive-behavioral therapy for insomnia (CBT-I) addresses insomnia-perpetuating behaviors and conditioned arousal and anxiety. CBT-I has been shown to reduce time to fall asleep and time awake during the night and can reduce reliance on sleep medications.
- The cognitive component of CBT-I involves education to address concerns that increase anxiety about sleeplessness. The behavioral component attempts to change habits that may perpetuate insomnia. The four components are relaxation techniques, control of stimuli that create arousal when attempting to sleep, restricting time in bed to increase sleep drive; and improving sleep hygiene practices (e.g., exercise, avoiding heavy meals at night, and avoiding or eliminating caffeine, nicotine, and alcohol intake). Increased daytime activity improves total sleep duration, sleep-onset latency, and global sleep quality.
- Insomnia attributable to circadian rhythm disturbances, such as in shift workers, many blind individuals who lack light–dark cycle to synchronize body clock, adolescents and

---

BOX 1-10 Sleep Habits (Sleep Hygiene Measures) That May Improve Sleep

1. Reduce caffeine, alcohol, or tobacco late in the day or evening.
2. Avoid heavy meals at night.
3. Increase daytime activity.
4. Increase daytime exposure to natural light.
5. Take warm bath as part of bedtime ritual.
6. Restrict bed to sleep and sex.
7. Get out of bed if not asleep after 30 minutes and return when drowsy.
8. Repeat above if awakened during the night.
9. Maintain regular sleep and wake times.
10. Go to bed with calm mind; resolve arguments or deal with problems earlier in day.

young adults with delayed sleep phase syndrome, and jet lag can be treated with chronobiologic therapies such as bright light exposure, melatonin, or melatonin agonists.

ACUTE GENERAL Rx

- Benzodiazepine receptor agonists zolpidem 5 to 10 mg and zaleplon 5 to 10 mg for sleep-onset insomnia, and zolpidem continuous-release formulation 6.25 to 12.5 mg and eszopiclone 1 to 3 mg for maintenance insomnia.
- Benzodiazepine sedative-hypnotics (e.g., temazepam 7.5 to 30 mg, triazolam 0.125 to 0.25 mg).
- In critical care: lorazepam 0.25 to 0.5 mg PO, SL, or IV as needed for sleep. In patients with acute delirium, haloperidol 0.25 to 0.5 mg IV as needed up to 2 mg/day may be less likely to worsen confusion.
- Melatonin agonist ramelteon 8 mg for sleep-onset insomnia when a mild agent without benzodiazepine side effects is desired.
- Avoid antihistamines except for occasional use.
- Optimize treatment of medical symptoms, especially pain.
- Most prescription and over-the-counter medications carry significant risk of adverse events and drug interactions, especially in the geriatric patient. Preferred pharmacotherapeutic agents in the elderly are zolpidem, zalepton, eszopiclone, and ramelteon.

CHRONIC Rx

- Considerable research supports the efficacy of CBT-I, with acute treatment outcomes equivalent to pharmacotherapy, with better long-term outcomes and maintenance of treatment gains. Three sedative-hypnotics—zolpidem continuous release, eszopiclone, and ramelteon—FDA approved for long-term use.

- Some evidence shows that benzodiazepines and benzodiazepine receptor agonists can be used for chronic insomnia on either intermittent or nightly use with moderate risk of tolerance and dependence but low risk of addiction.
- Sedating antidepressants (e.g., trazodone 25 to 150 mg, mirtazapine 7.5 to 30 mg, amitriptyline 25 to 50 mg) are in widespread use, with limited data on safety and efficacy. Amitriptyline should be avoided in older adults.
- Sedating antipsychotics (e.g., quetiapine 25 to 200 mg, olanzapine 2.5 to 10 mg at night) considered for severe mood or psychotic disorders associated with insomnia.

COMPLEMENTARY & ALTERNATIVE MEDICINE

Melatonin may shorten sleep-onset latency in some individuals. It may have more use in the treatment of circadian rhythm disorders.

DISPOSITION

- Transient insomnia: usually self-limited. May require follow-up if stress-related or illness-related because of risk of depression or persistence.
- Persistent insomnia: Studies has shown that patients who respond well to CBT-I often continue to maintain gains at 1- and 2-yr follow-ups. Insomnia patients may need periodic follow-up to reinforce good sleep hygiene and stimulus control and for reevaluation of pharmacologic therapies. Evidence is growing that insomnia is associated with significant negative mental and health effects over time.

REFERRAL

- A referral to a behavioral medicine specialist may be required for CBT-I for circadian rhythmn disturbances

- Excessive daytime sleepiness not obviously caused by insomnia (e.g., narcolepsy, sleep-related breathing disorder)
- Nighttime behavior suggestive of a parasomnia (e.g., somnambulism, REM behavior disorder)
- Severe insomnia not responsive to basic interventions

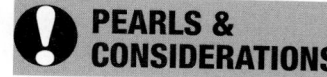

COMMENTS

Treatment should focus on reducing daytime sleepiness and improving daytime function rather than on trying to achieve the elusive goal of uninterrupted nighttime sleep. CBT-I often results in worse sleep and more fatigue in the short run. Patients often respond to initial worsening of symptoms as a sign of failure.

PREVENTION

Effective treatment of transient insomnia may reduce the risk of developing persistent insomnia.

PATIENT/FAMILY EDUCATION

The National Sleep Foundation (http://www.sleepfoundation.org) is a comprehensive resource for health care providers and patients.

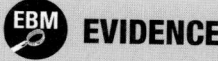 **EVIDENCE**

available at www.expertconsult.com

SUGGESTED READINGS

available at www.expertconsult.com

AUTHORS: **DONN POSNER, PH.D., C.B.S.M.,** and **MITCHELL D. FELDMAN, M.D., M.PHIL.**

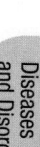
Diseases and Disorders

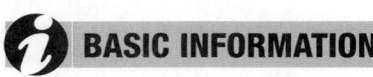

BASIC INFORMATION

DEFINITION

Insulinoma is a pancreatic insulin-secreting tumor that causes symptoms associated with hypoglycemia.

ICD-9CM CODES
M8151/0 Insulinoma

EPIDEMIOLOGY & DEMOGRAPHICS

INCIDENCE: One case per 250,000 persons annually. Ninety percent of insulinomas are benign.
PREDOMINANT SEX AND AGE: Insulinomas occur in both sexes (approximately 60% in women) and at all ages. In a Mayo Clinic series, the median age at diagnosis was 50 yr in sporadic cases but 23 yr in patients with multiple endocrine neoplasia, type 1 (MEN-1).

PHYSICAL FINDINGS & CLINICAL PRESENTATION

Symptoms typically occur in the morning before breakfast (i.e., fasting hypoglycemia as opposed to reactive hypoglycemia, which is not commonly associated with insulinoma)

Neuroglycopenic Symptoms	%
Various combinations of diplopia, blurred vision, sweating, palpitations, or weakness	85
Confusion or abnormal behavior	80
Unconsciousness or amnesia	53
Grand mal seizures	12
Adrenergic Symptoms	%
Sweating	43
Tremulousness	23
Hunger, nausea	12
Palpitations	10

ETIOLOGY, PATHOLOGY, PATHOPHYSIOLOGY

- Insulinomas are almost always solitary. Malignant insulinomas account for 5% of the total; they tend to be larger (6 cm). Metastases are usually to the liver (47%), regional lymph nodes (30%), or both.

- Insulinomas are evenly distributed in the head, body, and tail of the pancreas; ectopic insulinomas are rare (1% to 3%). Tumor size: 5% are ≤0.5 cm, 34% are 0.5 to 1 cm, 53% are 1 to 5 cm, and 8% are >5 cm.
- Histologic classification includes insulinoma in 86% of patients, adenomatosis in 5% to 15%, nesidioblastosis in 4%, and hyperplasia in 1%. Adenomatosis consists of multiple macroadenomas or microadenomas and occurs especially in patients with MEN-1. Nesidioblastosis is also a diffuse lesion in which islet cells form as buds on ductular structures.

DIAGNOSIS

DIFFERENTIAL DIAGNOSIS (OF FASTING HYPOGLYCEMIA)

Hyperinsulinism:
- Insulinoma
- Nonpancreatic tumors
- Severe congestive heart failure
- Severe renal insufficiency in non-insulin-dependent diabetes

Hepatic enzyme deficiencies or decreased hepatic glucose output (primarily in infants and children):
- Glycogen storage diseases
- Endocrine hypofunction
- Hypopituitarism
- Addison's disease
- Liver failure
- Alcohol abuse
- Malnutrition

Exogenous agents:
- Sulfonylureas, biguanides
- Insulin
- Other drugs (aspirin, pentamidine)

Functional fasting hypoglycemia:
- Autoantibodies to insulin receptor or insulin

LABORATORY TESTS

- An overnight fasting blood sugar level combined with a simultaneous plasma insulin, proinsulin, and/or C peptide level will establish the existence of fasting organic hypoglycemia in 60% of patients. Table 1-88 describes biochemical patterns in patients with

various causes of hyperinsulinemic hypoglycemia.
- If single overnight fasting glucose and insulin levels are nondiagnostic, a 72-hr fast is usually done with blood glucose and insulin levels determined at 2- to 4-hr intervals. A total of 75% of patients with insulinoma develop symptoms and a blood sugar level of <40 mg/dl by 24 hr, 92% to 98% develop these by 48 hr, and virtually all patients develop them by 72 hr. The test is considered positive for insulinoma if the plasma insulin/glucose ratio is more than 0.3. If at any point the patient becomes symptomatic, plasma insulin and glucose values should be obtained and IV glucose should be administered.
- Plasma proinsulin, C-peptide, antibodies to insulin, and plasma sulfonylurea levels may be used to rule out factitious use of insulin or hypoglycemic agents or autoantibodies against the insulin receptor or insulin.
- See Section III, "Hypoglycemia," for a description of the diagnostic approach to patients with documented hypoglycemia and elevated insulin.

IMAGING STUDIES

- Abdominal CT scan or MRI detects half to two thirds of insulinomas (abdominal ultrasound is not effective); should be done only after laboratory tests for insulinoma have confirmed the diagnosis
- Intraoperative ultrasound
- Arteriography
- Octreotide scan

TREATMENT

NONPHARMACOLOGIC THERAPY

- Enucleation of single insulinoma
- Partial pancreatectomy for multiple adenomas

ACUTE GENERAL Rx

- Carbohydrate administration
- Diazoxide directly inhibits insulin release and has an extrapancreatic, hyperglycemic effect that enhances glycogenolysis
- Lanreotide and octreotide (somatostatin analogs)
- Streptozotocin

REFERRAL

At some point in the workup the patient will probably be referred to an endocrinologist and then a surgeon. A combination of fasting hypoglycemia and elevated insulin level is probably a good point at which to refer.

SUGGESTED READING
available at www.expertconsult.com

AUTHOR: **FRED F. FERRI, M.D.**

TABLE 1-88 Biochemical Patterns in Patients with Various Causes of Hyperinsulinemic Hypoglycemia

Insulin	C Peptide	Proinsulin	Sulfonylurea	Insulin Antibody	Diagnosis
↑	↓	↓	−	−	Exogenous insulin
↑	↑	↑*	−	−	Insulinoma, CHI[†]
↑	↑	↑	+	−	Sulfonylurea
↑	↑‡	↑‡	−	+	Insulin autoimmune
±↑	↓	↓	−	−	Insulin receptor autoimmune[§]

*> 20% of insulin value.
[†]Congenital hyperinsulinism.
‡Free C peptide and proinsulin ↓.
[§]Insulin receptor antibody +.

Larsen PR, Kronenberg HM, Melmed S, Polonsky KS: *Williams textbook of endocrinology*, ed 10, Philadelphia, Saunders, 2003.

BASIC INFORMATION

DEFINITION

The International Continence Society defines interstitial cystitis (IC), otherwise known as painful bladder syndrome, as a clinical syndrome consisting of suprapubic pain related to bladder filling and accompanied by other symptoms such as increased daytime and nighttime frequency in the absence of proven infection or other obvious pathology.

SYNONYMS

Painful bladder syndrome
Tic douloureux of bladder

ICD-9CM CODES
595.1

EPIDEMIOLOGY & DEMOGRAPHICS

INCIDENCE: 21 cases per 100,000 women and four cases per 100,000 men annually
PREVALENCE:
- 197 per 100,000 women and 41 per 100,000 men in the U.S.
- Because the disease is substantially underdiagnosed, it may actually affect one in five women and one in 20 men.
- More than 81% of women diagnosed with chronic pelvic pain and up to 84% of men initially diagnosed with chronic prostatitis actually have IC.
- More than 90% of patients diagnosed with overactive bladder who do not respond to anticholinergics are subsequently diagnosed with IC.

PREDOMINANT SEX AND AGE:
- White women constitute 95% of patients with IC.
- Female/male ratio of 5 to 10:1.
- Most prevalent in fourth and fifth decades of life.

PHYSICAL FINDINGS & CLINICAL PRESENTATION

- Urinary urgency, frequency (>8 in daytime), nocturia (>2 at night), and suprapubic pain are the most common symptoms.
- Suprapubic pain is worse with bladder filling or urinating and relieved after emptying.
- Dyspareunia.
- Symptoms lasting longer than 6 mo.
- Intensity of symptoms waxes and wanes.
- Insidious onset and worsens to the final stage within 5 to 15 yr.
- Exercise, stress, sexual activity, ejaculation, certain foods with high potassium and acids (beer, spices, bananas, tomatoes, chocolate, strawberries, artificial sweeteners, oranges, cranberries, caffeine), menstruation, prolonged sitting, and activation of allergies exacerbate the symptoms.
- Often associated with irritable bowel syndrome, migraine, endometriosis, skin sensitivities, multiple drug allergies, other allergies, vulvodynia, fibromyalgia, chronic fatigue

syndrome, systemic lupus erythematosus, and mood disorders.
- Dysphoric mood.
- Lower abdominal tenderness.
- Tender prostate in digital rectal examination.
- Levator ani tenderness in female.
- Tenderness of anterior vaginal wall/bladder neck in female.

ETIOLOGY

Unknown

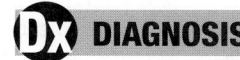 **DIAGNOSIS**

DIFFERENTIAL DIAGNOSIS

- Chronic pelvic pain
- Overactive bladder
- Recurrent urinary tract infection
- Endometriosis
- Pelvic adhesions
- Vulvar vestibulitis
- Vulvodynia
- Urethral pain syndrome
- Chronic nonbacterial prostatitis
- Frequent vaginitis
- Benign prostatic hyperplasia

WORKUP

- Interstitial cystitis can be considered a diagnosis of exclusion when no known cause of painful bladder can be identified.
- There is no definite diagnostic test.
- Validated questionnaires such as Pelvic Pain and Urgency/Frequency scale (PUF), O'Leary-Sant symptoms and problem index, and Wisconsin IC scale. PUF is the most commonly used.
- Voiding diary shows low volume (<100 ml) and high-frequency voiding pattern.
- National Institute of Diabetes and Diseases of the Kidney diagnostic criteria misses 60% of IC patients and is not clinically used any more.
- Anesthetic bladder challenge: with this test the symptoms dissipate on instillation of an anesthetic cocktail into the bladder.
- Cystoscopy and hydrodistension under general anesthesia may show terminal hematuria, glomerulation, Hunner's ulcers, and small bladder capacity of less than 350 ml.
- Bladder biopsy is not essential for diagnosis of IC.
- Parson's potassium sensitivity test (PST).
- Urodynamics are unnecessary in diagnosis of IC.

LABORATORY TESTS

- Urine analysis and culture.
- Urine cytology should be performed if microscopic or gross hematuria is present, or with other risk factors such as smoking, age >40 yr, and other bladder cancer risk factors.
- Culture of sexually transmitted diseases if clinically indicated. Nonbacteriuric patients with pyuria should be screened for *Chlamydia*.

- Urine biomarkers (e.g., antiproliferative factor) are promising but not ready for clinical use.

IMAGING STUDIES

CT or ultrasound of abdomen and pelvis may be considered to rule out other pathology.

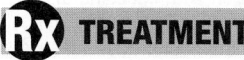 **TREATMENT**

- There is no consensus for optimal management.
- There is no cure for this disease.

NONPHARMACOLOGIC THERAPY

- Avoidance of activities associated with flare-ups
- Avoidance of smoking
- Dietary restriction
- Physical therapy
- Exercise
- Behavioral therapy
- Bladder retraining
- Biofeedback
- Warm sitz bath, ice, heating pad
- Thiele massage (transrectal and transvaginal manual therapy of pelvic floor muscle) in presence of pelvic floor muscle tenderness and spasm
- Hydrodistension only gives temporary relief, so it is not commonly used anymore

ACUTE AND CHRONIC Rx

- A course of empiric antibiotics if not tried yet.
- Oral therapy is tried first.
- Pentosan polysulfate sodium (Elmiron) is the only FDA approved and most effective oral therapy.
- Most treatment takes 3 to 6 mo before maximum benefit is seen.
- Adjunct oral therapy includes tricyclic antidepressants (amitriptyline), antihistaminics (hydroxyzine, montelukast), neuroleptics (gabapentin, topiramate), analgesics (NSAIDS, opioid analgesics), and occasionally antimuscarinics.
- Oral therapies can be used in combination.
- Antihistaminics are preferred for patients with an allergy history or those who show mast cells in bladder biopsy.
- Oral prednisone is used in presence of Hunner's ulcers.
- Other drugs rarely used for IC are cyclosporin A, interleukin-10, imatinib, methotrexate, suplatast, misoprostol, and quercetin.
- Growth factor inhibitors, gene therapy, RDP 58, and vitamin B_3 analogue (BXL 628) may represent future therapies.
- Intravesical treatment is used when oral medications fail, for acute flare-ups, or before the oral medications take full effect.
- Dimethyl sulfoxide (DMSO), heparin, lidocaine, hyaluronic acid, bacille Calmette-Guérin, capsaicin, resiniferatoxin, botulinum toxin A, chondroitin sulfate, steroids, and Elmiron are drugs used for intravesical treatment.

- DMSO is the only FDA-approved intravesical treatment.
- DMSO is used less often now because of its side effects, specifically a garlic-like odor or taste on breath or skin that lasts 72 hr after treatment.
- Intravesical therapy typically involves mixture of heparin or Elmiron with lidocaine and sodium bicarbonate.
- Silver nitrate and Clorpactin have fallen out of favor.

SURGERY

- Major surgical intervention is not the mainstay of treatment.
- Patients whose condition is extreme and who are miserable may consider surgery if medications fail.
- Sacral neuromodulation (InterStim) is the current preferred surgical intervention.
- Laser ablation, fulguration, or resection is offered when Hunner's ulcers are seen in cystoscopy.
- Augmentation cystoplasty is not recommended.
- Cystourethrectomy with urinary diversion is rarely done.

COMPLEMENTARY & ALTERNATIVE MEDICINE

- Transcutaneous electric nerve stimulation
- Intravaginal electric nerve stimulation
- Acupuncture
- Urinary chelating agents such as Polycitra-K crystals, Urocit-K
- Prelief, an over-the-counter food additive
- Herbal remedies such as Algnot Plus, Cysto-Protek, Cysta-Q, aloe vera

DISPOSITION

- Close follow-up every month for 3 mo and every 3 mo thereafter.
- Voiding diary and symptom questionnaire are helpful to monitor response to treatment.

REFERRAL

- Urologist
- Pain specialist
- Physical therapist

⚠ PEARLS & CONSIDERATIONS

COMMENTS

- On average these patients see five physicians and endure irritating voiding symptoms for 5 yr before the disease is identified.

- Besides symptom questionnaire and urine analysis, all other diagnostic tests are optional.
- PST is well tolerated.
- Negative cystoscopy does not rule out IC.

PREVENTION

Early identification and timely intervention improve patient outcome.

PATIENT & FAMILY EDUCATION

- IC support groups
- Interstitial Cystitis Association
- Interstitial Cystitis Network

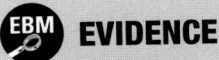 **EVIDENCE**

available at www.expertconsult.com

SUGGESTED READINGS
available at www.expertconsult.com

AUTHOR: **HEMANT K. SATPATHY, M.D.**

BASIC INFORMATION

DEFINITION

Diffuse interstitial lung disease (ILD) includes a large group of nonmalignant disorders, which are characterized by diffuse damage to the lung parenchyma via inflammation and fibrosis, and/or granulomatous reaction in interstitial or vascular areas.

SYNONYMS

Interstitial lung disease
ILD

ICD-9CM CODES
136.3 Acute interstitial lung disease
515   Chronic interstitial lung disease

EPIDEMIOLOGY & DEMOGRAPHICS

PREVALENCE: Varies with type of ILD. The most common type of ILD is idiopathic interstitial fibrosis, with a prevalence of 20 cases/100,000 people in the general population, increasing with age to 175 cases/100,000 people aged 75 yr or older.
PREDOMINANT SEX & AGE: Some ILDs are more common in women, such as those resulting from connective tissue disorders. One exception is rheumatoid arthritis, which is more common in men. Lymphangiomyomatosis occurs exclusively in postmenopausal women. ILD caused by occupational exposures are more common in men. Generally, ILD occurs in people >50 yr.
RISK FACTORS: History of tobacco abuse; environmental exposures such as to silicone, asbestos, or beryllium; reactions to drugs such as amiodarone, methotrexate, or bleomycin; history of connective tissue disease such as rheumatoid arthritis or systemic lupus erythematosus.

PHYSICAL FINDINGS & CLINICAL PRESENTATION

- Dyspnea
- Tachypnea
- Bibasilar end inspiratory dry crackles
- Pulmonary hypertension
- Cyanosis, clubbing

ETIOLOGY

- The hallmark of ILD is restriction caused by decreased lung compliance. The decreased compliance can be the result of a number of factors depending on the type of ILD. Different types of ILD are characterized by three distinct patterns in the alveolar walls:
  1. Inflammatory changes, which are early and potentially reversible
  2. Fibrotic changes
  3. Lung destruction
- Specific changes may be seen:
  - Granulomatous: accumulation of T lymphocytes, macrophages, and epithelioid cells into granulomas in lung parenchyma
  - Inflammation and fibrosis: injury to epithelium causes inflammation; if chronic, inflammation spreads to interstitium and vascular areas
  - Occupational exposure: pneumoconiosis, asbestosis, silicosis, organic dust
  - Drug induced
  - Connective tissue disorder: systemic lupus erythematosus, rheumatoid arthritis, dermatomyositis, interstitial pneumonitis

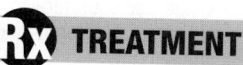

DIAGNOSIS

DIFFERENTIAL DIAGNOSIS

- Congestive heart failure
- Chronic renal failure

WORKUP

- Well-defined patterns in pulmonary function tests are usually consistent with restrictive defect (decreased FRC, RV, and TLC) owing to decreased lung compliance caused by alveolar wall thickening as a result of inflammation and fibrosis. Diffusing capacity is usually reduced also because of inflammation and thickening of alveolar walls, though nonspecific. FEV1/FVC is usually normal or increased because lung stiffness keeps small airways open, although some conditions (e.g., sarcoidosis) may reduce air flow.
- Bronchoscopy and BAL may help identify type of ILD. However, their role in defining stage of disease and response to therapy is controversial.
- Biopsy is the most effective method for confirming diagnosis and assessing disease activity.

LABORATORY TESTS

- ABGs may be normal or show respiratory alkalosis.
- Antinuclear antibodies, anti-immunoglobulin antibodies (rheumatoid factors), LDH.
- Serum precipitins confirm exposure if hypersensitivity pneumonitis is suspected.
- Antineutrophil cytoplasmic antibodies or anti-basement membrane antibodies if vasculitis is suspected.
- Elevation in angiotensin-converting enzyme level in sarcoidosis.
- ECG and echocardiogram will check for evidence of pulmonary hypertension.

IMAGING STUDIES

- A chest x-ray may be normal but commonly shows a bibasilar reticular pattern.
- A high-resolution CT is superior to chest x-ray; it is also useful for determining potential biopsy sights.

TREATMENT

NONPHARMACOLOGIC THERAPY

Avoidance of tobacco and occupational exposures

ACUTE GENERAL Rx

- Supplemental oxygen in patients with hypoxemia.
- Glucocorticoids are the mainstay of therapy, but success rate is low. Common starting dose is prednisone 0.5 to 1 mg/kg once daily for 4 to 12 wk. Patients should be reevaluated after this initial course of treatment. If they are stable, steroids may be tapered. If not, the same course may be maintained for another 4 to 12 wk. If patient's condition continues to decline, may consider adding second agent (cyclophosphamide, azathioprine).

REFERRAL

- Surgical referral for biopsy
- Pulmonary referral for bronchoscopy or BAL

SUGGESTED READINGS
available at www.expertconsult.com

AUTHORS: **GRACE SHIH, M.D.,** and **CINDY GLEIT, M.D.**

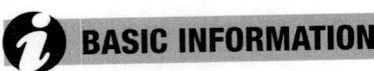

BASIC INFORMATION

DEFINITION

Falls into two broad categories: acute and chronic:

Acute: Defined as a decrease in renal function resulting from immune-mediated injury characterized histopathologically with edema and inflammation of the renal interstitium, classically sparing the glomeruli and blood vessels. Most often induced by drugs.

Chronic: Represents a large and diverse group of disorders characterized by interstitial fibrosis with mononuclear leukocyte infiltration and tubular atrophy. It is a final common pathway of many chronic kidney diseases including chronic bacterial infections, obstruction, and high-grade vesicoureteral reflux. Histopathologically seen as atrophy and fibrosis of the renal interstitium.

SYNONYMS

Acute tubulointerstitial nephritis, contracted kidney, cirrhosis of the kidney, granular kidney, gouty kidney, renal sclerosis, chronic productive nephritis without exudation

ICD-9CM CODES

583   Nephritis and nephropathy not specified as acute or chronic
583.7   Nephritis and nephropathy, not specific as acute or chronic, with lesion of renal medullary necrosis
583.8   Nephritis and nephropathy, not specific as acute or chronic, with other specified pathological lesion in kidney
583.9   With unspecified pathological lesions in the kidney

EPIDEMIOLOGY & DEMOGRAPHICS

PREVALENCE: 2% to 3% of all renal biopsies; in cases of acute renal failure, the incidence of acute interstitial nephritis is 7% to 15%.
PREDOMINANT SEX AND AGE: Older patients generally at higher risk given reduced glomerular filtration rates.
PEAK INCIDENCE: Median age at presentation is 65 yr.
GENETICS: Risk of acute interstitial nephritis due to drugs (e.g., NSAIDs, penicillins, sulfa drugs, etc.) increases with volume depletion, underlying kidney disease, age >65 yr, congestive heart failure, and diabetes. Some autoimmune disorders are also risk factors.

PHYSICAL FINDINGS & CLINICAL PRESENTATION

Nonspecific but acutely can present with renal failure, oliguria, hematuria, malaise, mental status changes, rash, nausea, and vomiting. Classic triad of low-grade fever, rash, and arthralgias is present in only 5% of cases of AIN. Chronic interstitial nephritis can be asymptomatic with elevations in BUN or creatinine or the appearance of abnormal urinary sediment.

ETIOLOGY

- Drug induced (71%) usually hypersensitivity reaction occurring about 15 days after exposure to the drug: antibiotics (penicillins, cephalosporins sulfonamides), NSAIDs, diuretics, proton pump inhibitors, anticonvulsants
- Infection associated (15%) can be either primary renal infection (acute bacterial pyelonephritis, renal tuberculosis, and fungal nephritis) or complication of systemic infections
  - Bacterial: *Corynebacterium diphtheriae, Legionella,* staphylococci, streptococci, *Yersinia*
  - Viral: Cytomegalovirus, Epstein-Barr virus, hantaviruses, hepatitis C, herpes simplex virus, human immunodeficiency virus, mumps, polyomavirus
  - Other: *Mycobacterium, Mycoplasma, Rickettsia,* syphilis, toxoplasmosis
- Immune disorders: systemic lupus erythematosus, Sjogren's and Wegener)
- Neoplastic disorders (multiple myeloma)
- Metabolic diseases (urate nephropathy, hypercalcemic nephropathy, hypokalemic nephropathy, oxalate nephropathy)
- Heavy metals (chronic form)
- Chronic urinary tract obstruction

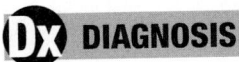

DIAGNOSIS

DIFFERENTIAL DIAGNOSIS

Any other causes of acute renal failure including acute tubular necrosis, glomerulonephritis, hypertensive nephrosclerosis, prerenal azotemia, obstructive nephropathy, renal vascular disease, and various electrolyte abnormalities

WORKUP

Medical history with focus on recent infection illness or new medication in the presence of acute to chronic onset of kidney failure; evaluation for underlying infection or insult

LABORATORY TESTS

- Urinalysis, urine microscopy (especially eosinophiluria), serum chemistry profile, complete blood count with differential (eosinophilia occurs in 50% of AIN patients), liver function tests, 24-hr urine specimen collection, consider serum IgE levels
- Renal biopsy is the gold standard for diagnosis but is indicated only when diagnosis is unclear, removal of offending agent does not result in improvement, and there are no contraindications to the procedure

IMAGING STUDIES

Neither ultrasound nor gallium 67 scan is diagnostic but may be useful for ruling out AIN

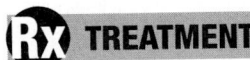

TREATMENT

NONPHARMACOLOGIC THERAPY

Largely supportive, removal of offending agent will resolve 60% of all cases.

ACUTE GENERAL Rx

- Correct fluid and electrolyte imbalances, maintain adequate hydration and urine output but avoid volume overload.
- Identify and treat infection as indicated.
- Remove offending drug, substitute as appropriate.
- Avoid medications that impair renal blood flow.
- Initiation of steroids is controversial, but retrospective studies have shown that early steroid treatment may reduce need for chronic dialysis in patients with drug-induced AIN. A reasonable choice is prednisone 1 mg/kg/d for 2 to 3 wk.
- Consider treatment with cyclophosphamide (Cytoxan) if patients fail to respond to corticosteroids.

CHRONIC Rx

- Limit exposure to known nephrotoxic agents.
- Renally adjust medications as indicated by glomerular filtration rate.
- Tight control of blood pressure, diabetes, and cholesterol to preserve kidney function as needed

DISPOSITION

With acute interstitial nephritis, 40% of patients will improve in time. Relapse is common with reexposure to offending agents.

REFERRAL

Refer to nephrology with question in diagnosis, multiple comorbidities, with failure to respond to supportive care, or with decision to evaluate for biopsy.

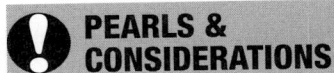

PEARLS & CONSIDERATIONS

COMMENTS

Once known mainly as a complication of streptococcal infection, today acute interstitial nephritis is most often due to drugs; 88% of the time, the drug was started in the past 30 days. Significant fibrosis of the tubules seen in biopsy is the best predictor of transition to chronic interstitial nephritis.

PREVENTION

Use known offending agents with care, especially in the elderly and those with known underlying kidney disease.

SUGGESTED READINGS

available at www.expertconsult.com

AUTHOR: **ELIZABETH BROWN, M.D.**

BASIC INFORMATION

DEFINITION

Irritable bowel syndrome (IBS) is a chronic functional disorder manifested by alteration in bowel habits and recurrent abdominal pain and bloating. IBS is a symptom complex influenced by a variety of physiologic determinants from gut to brain and back. The ROME III criteria for diagnosis of IBS are:

- Recurrent abdominal pain or discomfort at least 3 days per month in the past 3 mo associated with ≥two of the following:
  - Pain is relieved or improved with defecation.
  - Its onset is associated with a change in the frequency of bowel movement.
  - Its onset is associated with a change in the form or appearance of the stool.
- The criteria must be fulfilled for at least the past 3 mo with symptom onset at least 6 mo before the diagnosis.

SYNONYMS

Irritable colon
Spastic colon
IBS

ICD-9CM CODES
564.1 Irritable bowel syndrome

EPIDEMIOLOGY & DEMOGRAPHICS

- IBS is the most common functional bowel disorder. An estimated 15 million people in the United States have IBS.
- IBS occurs in 20% of the population of industrialized countries and is responsible for >50% of gastrointestinal (GI) referrals. Worldwide adult prevalence is 12%. Incidence increases during adolescence and peaks in third and fourth decades of life.
- Female:male ratio is 2:1.
- Nearly 50% of patients have psychiatric abnormalities, with anxiety disorders being most common.

PHYSICAL FINDINGS & CLINICAL PRESENTATION

- The clinical presentation of IBS consists of abdominal pain and abnormalities of defecation, which may include loose stools, usually after meals and in the morning, alternating with episodes of constipation.
- Physical examination is generally normal.
- Nonspecific abdominal tenderness and distention may be present.

ETIOLOGY

- Unknown
- Associated pathophysiology includes altered GI motility, alteration in gut flora, and increased gut sensitivity
- Risk factors: anxiety, depression, personality disorders, history of childhood sexual abuse, and domestic abuse in women

DIAGNOSIS

DIFFERENTIAL DIAGNOSIS

- Inflammatory bowel disease (IBD)
- Diverticulitis
- Colon malignancy
- Endometriosis
- Peptic ulcer disease
- Biliary liver disease
- Chronic pancreatitis
- Constipation caused by medications (opiates, calcium channel blockers, anticholinergics)
- Diarrhea caused by medications (metformin, colchicine, proton pump inhibitors, antacids, antibiotics)
- Small-bowel overgrowth
- Celiac disease
- Parasites
- Lymphoma of GI tract

WORKUP

Diagnostic workup is aimed primarily at excluding the conditions listed in the differential diagnoses. It is important to identify red flags of other diseases, such as weight loss, rectal bleeding, onset in patients >50 yr, fever, nocturnal pain, and family history of malignancy or IBD. Additional red flags include abnormal examination (e.g., mass, enlarged lymph nodes, stool positive for occult blood, muscle wasting) and abnormal laboratory values (anemia, leukocytosis, abnormal chemistry).

Common clinical criteria for diagnosis of IBS are >3 mo of symptoms, including abdominal pain that is relieved by a bowel movement, or pain accompanied by a change in bowel pattern, and abnormality in bowel movement 25% of the time, characterized by two of the following features:

- Abdominal distention
- Abnormal consistency
- Abnormal defecation (e.g., straining, sense of incomplete evacuation)
- Abnormal frequency
- Mucus with bowel movement

LABORATORY TESTS

- Blood work is generally normal. CBC is reasonable to evaluate for anemia. The presence of anemia should alert to the possibility of a colonic malignancy or IBD.
- Testing of stool for ova and parasites should be considered only in patients with chronic diarrhea. Evaluation of stool for *Clostridium difficile* may be helpful in patients with predominant diarrhea symptoms who have recently taken antibiotics.

IMAGING STUDIES

Imaging studies (e.g., flat and upright abdominal radiograph, small-bowel series, sonogram or CT of abdomen and pelvis) are normal and not necessary for diagnosis.

Lower endoscopy is generally normal except for the presence of some spasms. Colonoscopic imaging should be performed only in persons who have alarm features to rule out organic disease and in persons older than 50 yr to screen for colorectal cancer.

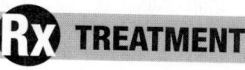

TREATMENT

NONPHARMACOLOGIC THERAPY

- The patient should be encouraged to maintain an adequate fiber intake and to eliminate foods that aggravate symptoms. Avoidance of caffeine, dairy products, fatty foods, and dietary excesses is also helpful.
- Cognitive-behavioral therapy is also recommended, particularly in younger patients because psychosocial stressors are important triggers of IBS. Reassurance and education about trigger avoidance and stress management are important.
- Importance of regular exercise and adequate fluid intake should be stressed.

GENERAL Rx

- The mainstay of treatment of IBS is a high-fiber diet. Fiber is helpful for relief of constipation but not for relief of pain. Because symptoms are chronic, the use of laxatives should generally be avoided.
- Soluble fiber (psyllium) is more effective in symptom relief than insoluble fiber (bran). Fiber supplementation with psyllium 1 tbsp bid or calcium polycarbophil (FiberCon) 2 tablets one to four times daily followed by 8 oz of water may be necessary in some patients.
- Patients should be instructed that there might be some increased bloating on initiation of fiber supplementation, which should resolve within 2 to 3 wk. It is important that patients take these fiber products on a regular basis and not only as needed. Fiber is not effective in patients with diarrhea-predominant IBS and may worsen symptoms in these patients.
- Patients who appear anxious can benefit from use of sedatives or selective serotonin reuptake inhibitors (SSRIs). Tricyclic antidepressants in low doses are also effective in some patients with IBS.
- C-2 chloride channel activators: Lubiprostone (Amitiza) is a chloride channel activator that stimulates chloride-rich intestinal fluid secretion and accelerates small intestine and colonic transit time. It may be effective in chronic constipation-predominant IBS unresponsive to conventional treatment. Usual dose is 8 to 24 mcg bid with food. Side effects include headache and nausea.
- Loperamide is effective for diarrhea. Alosetron, a serotonin type-3 receptor antagonist previously withdrawn because of severe constipation and ischemic colitis, has been reintroduced with limited availability. It is indicated only for women with severe chronic diarrhea-predominant IBS unresponsive to conventional therapy and not caused by anatomic or metabolic abnormality. Starting dose is 1 mg qd.

- Alterations in gut flora have been identified as potentially contributing to IBS (84% of IBS patients have an abnormal lactulose breath test, suggesting small-intestinal bacterial overgrowth). Rifaximin, a gut-selective antibiotic, has been used in recent trials to eradicate bacterial overgrowth (70% eradication rate). A dose of 400 mg tid for 10 days was reported effective in improving IBS symptoms up to 10 wk after discontinuation of therapy. Until additional evidence is available, use of rifaximin or other antibiotics in IBS should be reserved for patients with proven bacterial overgrowth.
- Antispasmodics-anticholinergics (e.g., dicyclomine, hyoscyamine) are often used, but efficacy data from clinical trials are inconclusive.
- Probiotics: Bifidobacteria and some combinations of probiotics have shown some limited efficacy. Lactobacilli do not appear to be effective for the treatment of IBS. Additional data showing efficacy is needed before probiotics can be endorsed for treatment of IBS

- Antidepressants: SSRIs are more effective than placebo for relief of global IBS symptoms.

DISPOSITION

More than 60% of patients respond successfully to treatment over the initial 12 mo; however, IBS is a chronic, relapsing condition and requires prolonged therapy.

REFERRAL

GI referral is recommended in patients with rectal bleeding, fever, nocturnal diarrhea, anemia, weight loss, or onset of symptoms >40 yr. Consultation is also necessary if specialized diagnostic procedures such as endoscopy are necessary.

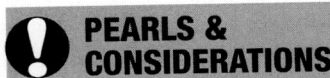

COMMENTS

- Patients should be educated regarding maintenance of a high-fiber diet and elimination of

stressors, which can precipitate attacks of IBS. They should be reassured that their condition does not lead to cancer.
- Recent drug efforts (alosetron, tegaserod) are aimed at serotonergic receptors in the gut because most of the serotonin in the body is found in the GI tract and is believed to be involved in the mediation of visceral sensation and motility.
- Cognitive-behavioral therapy is effective in the treatment of patients with IBS and should be considered as part of the armamentarium against this disorder.

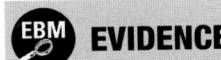

available at www.expertconsult.com

SUGGESTED READINGS
available at www.expertconsult.com

AUTHOR: **FRED F. FERRI, M.D.**

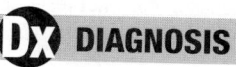

BASIC INFORMATION

DEFINITION

Jaundice is a yellowish discoloration of the sclera, skin, and mucous membranes caused by an excessive amount of bilirubin in the bloodstream. Clinically detectable jaundice in adults is a serum bilirubin of 2.5 to 3 mg/dl.

SYNONYMS

Icterus

ICD-9CM CODES
782.4 Jaundice
283.9 Hemolytic jaundice
576.8 Obstructive jaundice

EPIDEMIOLOGY & DEMOGRAPHICS

The major causes of jaundice by age and sex:
- Young adults: viral hepatitis
- Women over 30: choledocholithiasis
- Middle adulthood (both sexes): drug induced and cirrhosis
- Middle-aged and older men: alcoholic liver disease, pancreatic cancer, hepatoma, primary hemochromatosis
- Women: primary biliary cirrhosis, chronic active hepatitis, choledocholithiasis, carcinoma of the gallbladder

CLINICAL PRESENTATION

Presentation can vary from asymptomatic to acute and life threatening. History and physical examination give important clues to the underlying condition.
Key history:
- Duration of jaundice
- Previous episodes
- Pain
- Color of urine and stool
- Systemic symptoms (fever, chills)

- Alcohol use
- Medications, herbal products
- Injection of illicit drugs
- Blood transfusions
- Hepatitis exposure (e.g., other jaundiced people)
- Shellfish ingestion
- Travel
- Occupation/exposure to toxins
- Anorexia/weight loss
- Prior abdominal/biliary surgery

Key physical: vital signs
- Fever, signs of chronic liver disease (palmar erythema, spider angiomas, bruising, gynecomastia, testicular atrophy), size of liver, abdominal tenderness (and location), abdominal mass, splenomegaly, ascites, edema, weight loss, Kayser-Fleischer rings (Wilson's disease)

ETIOLOGY

Disruption in any of the three phases of bilirubin metabolism can lead to jaundice:
- Prehepatic phase: bilirubin is produced from the metabolism of heme—80% from red blood cell catabolism, 20% from ineffective erythropoiesis and breakdown of muscle myoglobin and cytochromes—and transported to the liver for conjugation and excretion.
- Intrahepatic phase: unconjugated (indirect) bilirubin, which is fat soluble but water insoluble, is conjugated within the hepatocyte to the water-soluble, conjugated (direct) bilirubin.
- Posthepatic phase: conjugated bilirubin dissolves in the bile and travels through the biliary system to the gallbladder, where it is stored, or passes into the duodenum through the ampulla of Vater. Some bilirubin is excreted in the stool and the rest is converted to urobilinogens by the gut flora and reabsorbed. Most of the urobilinogen is excreted

by the kidney. A small amount is reabsorbed by the gut and re-excreted into the bile.

DIAGNOSIS

DIFFERENTIAL DIAGNOSIS

Prehepatic causes:
- Unconjugated hyperbilirubinemia: excessive heme metabolism from hemolysis (e.g., sickle cell disease, spherocytosis, G6PD, immune hemolysis), ineffective erythropoiesis (e.g., thalassemia, folate, severe iron deficiency), or large hematoma reabsorption.

Intrahepatic causes:
- Unconjugated hyperbilirubinemia: disorders of enzyme metabolism such as Gilbert's disease (common, benign), Crigler-Najjar syndrome (rare, severe), or drugs such as rifampin and probenecid
- Conjugated hyperbilirubinemia: intrahepatic cholestasis
  1. Viruses: hepatitis A, B, and C; Epstein-Barr
  2. Alcohol: alcoholic hepatitis, alcoholic cirrhosis
  3. Autoimmune: primary biliary cirrhosis, primary sclerosing cholangitis
  4. Drug induced: acetaminophen, penicillins, oral contraceptives, chlorpromazine (Thorazine), steroids (estrogenic or anabolic), some herbals
  5. Hereditary metabolic: hemochromatosis, Wilson's disease, Dubin-Johnson and Rotor's syndromes, alpha-antitrypsin deficiency
  6. Systemic disease: sarcoidosis, amyloidosis, glycogen storage diseases, celiac disease, tuberculosis, *Mycobacterium avium intracellulare*
  7. Other: sepsis, total parenteral nutrition, pregnancy, graft-versus-host disease, environmental toxins

Posthepatic causes:
- Conjugated hyperbilirubinemia: intrinsic or extrinsic obstruction of the biliary system
  1. Intrinsic blockage: gallstones, cholangitis, strictures, infection (e.g., cytomegalovirus, cryptosporidium in AIDS patients, parasites, cholangiocarcinoma, gallbladder cancer)
  2. Extrinsic blockage: pancreatitis, pancreatic carcinoma, pancreatic pseudocyst

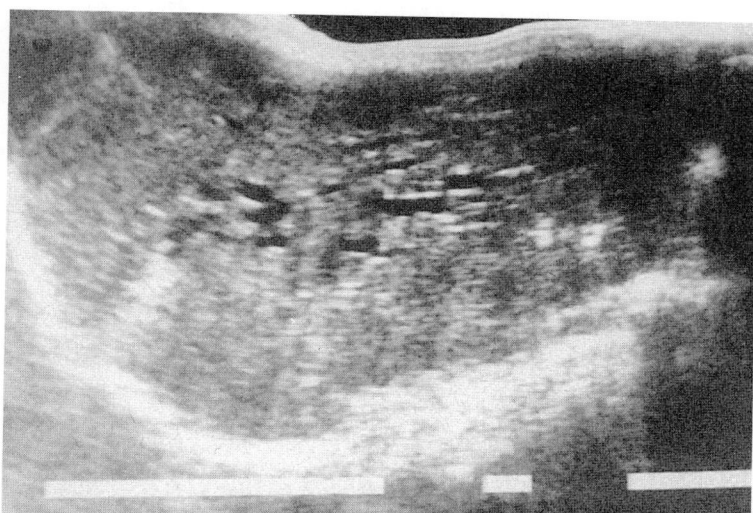

FIGURE 1-208 Ultrasound showing a large calculus in the extrahepatic biliary tree. Dilated bile ducts can be seen to the left. (Courtesy of Dr. M.C. Collins. Forbes A, Misiewicz JJ, Compton CC, Levine MS, Quraishy MS, Rubesin SE, Thuluvath PJ [eds]: *Atlas of clinical gastroenterology,* ed 3, Mosby, 2005.)

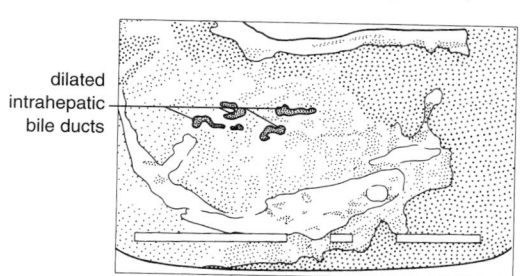

dilated intrahepatic bile ducts

FIGURE 1-209 Schematic representation of ultrasound abnormality seen on Figure 1-208. (Forbes A, Misiewicz JJ, Compton CC, Levine MS, Quraishy MS, Rubesin SE, Thuluvath PJ [eds]: *Atlas of clinical gastroenterology,* ed 3, Mosby, 2005.)

- Pseudojaundice: caused by an excessive ingestion of foods containing beta-carotene (carrots, melons, squash); does *not* result in hyperbilirubinemia or scleral icterus

WORKUP

History and physical examination as above are key to diagnosis.

LABORATORY TESTS

First-line tests:
- Serum total and direct bilirubin
- Urinalysis
- If first-line tests are normal, consider pseudojaundice

If urine is positive for bilirubin and serum has elevated total and direct bilirubin (conjugated hyperbilirubinemia):
- Initial evaluation: liver function tests (AST, ALT, GGTP, alk phos), CBC, liver synthetic function (albumin, PT, PTT), pancreatic function (amylase, lipase).
- Additional tests if diagnosis unclear:
  1. Screen for hepatitis A, B, and C; if still unclear then consider options 2 to 6 below
  2. Other viruses (Epstein-Barr virus, cytomegalovirus)
  3. Autoimmune disorders: antimitochondrial antibody, immunoglobulin (Ig) M (elevated in primary biliary cirrhosis); smooth muscle antibody, antinuclear antibody, IgG (autoimmune chronic active hepatitis); antinuclear cytoplasmic antibody (primary sclerosing cholangitis)
  4. Ceruloplasmin (Wilson's disease)
  5. Alpha-1 antitrypsin deficiency (cirrhosis and emphysema)
  6. Ferritin, Fe saturation (elevated in hemochromatosis)

If urine is negative for bilirubin, increased t. bili and normal d. bili (unconjugated hyperbilirubinemia):
- Hemolysis? (complete blood count, smear for abnormal red blood cell types)
- Genetic syndrome? (e.g., Gilbert's)
- Hematoma?

Liver biopsy: essential in diagnosis of chronic hepatitis. Can be used for diagnosis of liver masses but carries a substantial risk.

IMAGING STUDIES

- Abdominal ultrasound: first-line study (Figs. 1-208, 1-209). Most sensitive for biliary tract stones and extrahepatic biliary obstruction.
- Abdominal CT: more information on liver, pancreas, and biliary system.
- Endoscopic retrograde cholangiopancreatography: best for lower duct obstruction.
- Percutaneous transhepatic cholangiography: best for hilar obstructions.
- Magnetic resonance cholangiopancreatography: noninvasive visualization of bile and pancreatic ducts; becoming more available.

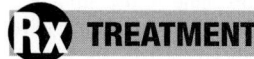 **TREATMENT**

NONPHARMACOLOGIC THERAPY

Depends on underlying cause of the jaundice, rapidity of onset, and clinical stability of the patient. Generally, obstructive causes require surgical treatment and nonobstructive causes require medical treatment.

ACUTE GENERAL Rx

Acute, life-threatening illness such as acute cholecystitis or ascending cholangitis requires prompt diagnosis and emergent surgical or endoscopic intervention in conjunction with medical management.

CHRONIC Rx

Chronic causes may require such treatment as stopping certain medications; stopping alcohol; antihistamines for pruritus; cholestyramine to bind bilirubin and decrease pruritus; interferon for hepatitis B or C; penicillamine for Wilson's disease; phlebotomy for hemochromatosis; surgical resection for liver for pancreatic cancer; liver transplant for eligible patients with end-stage cirrhosis; and N-acetylcysteine for acetaminophen overdose.

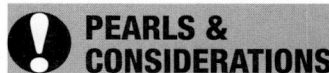 **PEARLS & CONSIDERATIONS**

COMMENTS

- The key to the management of the jaundiced adult is accurate diagnosis of the underlying cause.
- Prompt diagnosis and treatment of life-threatening illness is essential.
- Careful history and physical examination followed by selective laboratory and imaging studies will lead to accurate diagnosis.
- Collaboration with surgical and gastroenterology colleagues is helpful in complex patient care scenarios.

SUGGESTED READINGS

available at www.expertconsult.com

AUTHOR: **GOWRI ANANDARAJAH, M.D.**

BASIC INFORMATION

DEFINITION
Juvenile idiopathic arthritis (JIA), previously referred to as juvenile rheumatoid arthritis (JRA), is a diverse spectrum of arthritides presenting before 16 yr of age. The arthritis symptoms must be persistent and objective in ≥one joints for at least 6 wk with the exclusion of any other known cause.

SYNONYMS
Still's disease
JIA

ICD-9CM CODES
714.3 Polyarticular juvenile rheumatoid arthritis, chronic or unspecified

EPIDEMIOLOGY & DEMOGRAPHICS
PREVALENCE (IN U.S.): 57 to 220 per 100,000 children

PHYSICAL FINDINGS & CLINICAL PRESENTATION
JIA is subdivided into seven categories based on the 2001 International League of Associations for Rheumatology (ILAR) classification criteria (subtype characterisits are summarized in Table 1-89)
Systemic onset JIA
Arthritis in ≥one joints with or preceded by fever of at least 2 wk duration that is quotidian (once daily) for at least 3 days and associated with at least one of the following: (1) evanescent erythematous rash, (2) generalized lymph node enlargement, (3) hepatomegaly, splenomegaly, or both, and (4) serositis such as pleuritis, pericarditis, or peritonitis.
Oligoarticular JIA
Arthritis in one to four joints during a 6-mo period of time. There are two subtypes:
Persistent: ≤four joints throughout the disease course
Extended: ≤four joints during the first 6 mo extending to >four joints after 6 mo.
Polyarthritis, rheumatoid factor (RF) negative
Arthritis involves >six joints during first 6 mo of the disease with negative RF.
Polyarthritis, RF positive
Arthritis involves >six joints during first 6 mo of the disease with positive RF on at least two tests run 3 mo apart.
Anti–cyclic citrullinated (CCP) antibodies may also be present
Psoriatic arthritis
Psoriasis and arthritis or psoriasis and ≥two of the following:
Dactylitis, nail pitting, onycholysis, and psoriasis in a first-degree relative
Enthesitis-related arthritis
Arthritis and enthesitis or arthritis or enthesitis and ≥two of the following:
Presence of or a history of SI joint pain, positive HLA-B27, boy aged >6 yr, acute anterior uveitis, or history of ankylosing spondylitis, reactive arthritis, sacroiliitis with inflammatory bowel disease or acute anterior uveitis in a first-degree relative

ETIOLOGY
Idiopathic: Both genetic and environmental triggers thought to play a role.

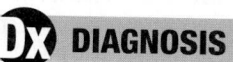

DIAGNOSIS

DIFFERENTIAL DIAGNOSIS
- Infection: viral or rheumatic fever
- Systemic lupus erythematosus
- Malignancy
- Serum sickness
- Lyme arthritis

LABORATORY TESTS
- Increased erythrocyte sedimentation rate and CRP
- Low-grade anemia
- Leukocytosis
- Rheumatoid factor: rarely demonstrable in the serum of children
- Antinuclear antibodies: often found in children with ocular complications
- If macrophage activation syndrome suspected in patients with systemic JIA: decreased platelets, WBC, and fibrinogen with high ferritin and liver function tests. Bone marrow biopsy is needed to confirm diagnosis.

IMAGING STUDIES
- Roentgenographic findings are similar to those in adult, with soft tissue swelling and periarticular osteopenia early in the disease.
- Joint destruction is less frequent.
- Bony erosion and cyst formation may be present as a result of synovial hypertrophy.

TABLE 1-89 Overview of the Main Features of the Subtypes of Juvenile Idiopathic Arthritis (JIA)

ILAR Subtype	Peak Age of Onset (yr)	Female: Male; % of All JIA	Arthritis Pattern	Extra-articular Features	Investigations	Notes on Therapy
Systemic arthritis	2-4	1:1; ~10% of JIA cases	Polyarticular, often knees, wrists, and ankles; also fingers, neck, and hips	Daily fever; evanescent rash; pericarditis; pleuritis	Anemia; WBC ↑↑; ESR ↑↑; CRP ↑↑; ferritin ↑; platelets ↑↑ (normal or ↓ in MAS)	Less responsive to standard treatment with MTX and anti-TNF agents; consider IL-1Ra in resistant cases
Oligoarthritis	<6	4:1; 50%-60% of JIA (but ethnic variation)	Knees + +; ankles, fingers +	Uveitis in ~30%	ANA positive in ;60%; other tests usually normal; may have mildly ↑ ESR/CRP	NSAIDs and intra-articular steroids; occasionally require MTX
Polyarthritis, RF negative	6-7	3:1; 30% of JIA cases	Symmetric or asymmetric; small and large joints; cervical spine; TMJ	Uveitis in ~10%	ANA positive in 40%; RF negative; ESR ↑ or ↑↑; CRP ↑/normal; mild anemia	Standard therapy with MTX and NSAIDs, then if non-responsive, anti-TNF agents or other biologics
Polyarthritis, RF positive	9-12	9:1; <10% of JIA cases	Aggressive symmetric polyarthritis	Rheumatoid nodules in 10%; low-grade fever	RF positive; ESR ↑↑; CRP ↑/normal; mild anemia	Long-term remission unlikely; early aggressive therapy is warranted
Psoriatic arthritis	7-10	2:1; <10% of JIA cases	Asymmetric arthritis of small or medium sized joints	Uveitis in 10%; psoriasis in 50%	ANA positive in 50%; ESR ↑; CRP ↑/normal; mild anemia	NSAIDS and intra-articular steroids; second-line agents less commonly
Enthesitis-related arthritis	9-12	1:7; 10% of JIA cases	Predominantly lower limb joints affected; sometimes axial skeleton (but less than adult AS)	Acute anterior uveitis; association with reactive arthritis and IBD	80% HLA-B27+	NSAIDS and intra-articular steroids; consider sulfasalazine as alternative to MTX

ANA, Antinuclear antibody; *AS*, ankylosing spondylitis; *CRP*, C-reactive protein; *ESR*, erythrocyte sedimentation rate; *IBD*, inflammatory bowel disease; *ILAR*, International League of Associations for Rheumatology; *IL-1Ra*, interleukin-1 receptor antagonist; *MAS*, macrophage activation syndrome; *MTX*, methotrexate; *NSAID*, nonsteroidal anti-inflammatory drug; *RF*, rheumatoid factor; *TMJ*, temporomandibular joint; *TNF*, tumor necrosis factor; *WBC*, white blood cell count.
From Firestein G et al: *Kelley's textbook of rheumatology*, ed 8, Philadelphia, 2008, Elsevier, p. 1659, Table 97-2.

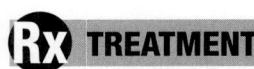

NONPHARMACOLOGIC THERAPY

Proper management requires close cooperation among primary physician, physical and occupational therapists, pediatric rheumatologist, social workers, and orthopedist.

- Rest
- Physical and occupational therapy
- Patient and family education
- Proper diet and weight maintenance

ACUTE GENERAL Rx

- NSAIDs
- DMARDs: methotrexate, leflunomide, sulfasalazine
- Biologics:
  - Tumor necrosis factor blockers such as etanercept and adalimumab
  - T-cell modulator CTLA-4 fusion protein, abatacept
  - IL-6 (tocilizumab) and IL-1 inhibitors (anakinra) particularly in systemic JIA
- Intra-articular steroids
- Systemic corticosteroids

DISPOSITION

- Complete remission occurs in the majority of patients and may occur at any age.
- 70% to 85% of children regain normal function.
- Mortality is three- to fourteenfold greater than the general population of the same age. Macrophage activation syndrome is a life-threatening complication in systemic JIA.
- Oligoarticular JIA patients with positive ANA are at the highest risk for blindness due to chronic iridocyclitis and require frequent ophthamologic monitoring.
- Systemic and localized growth disturbance can lead to generalized growth failure and leg length discrepancies.
- Arthritis of the temporomandibular joint can lead to jaw malformation.

REFERRAL

- Early rheumatology consultation
- Ophthalmology consultation at diagnosis and regularly thereafter particularly in ANA+, oligoarticular JIA
- Orthopedic consultation for corrective surgery

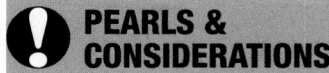

COMMENTS

The spontaneous adverse event reports (SERS) in the FDA surveillance system has recently reported a warning for risk of malignancy related to anti-TNF agents in the pediatric population. However, baseline risk of malignancy in children with JIA is unknown and the SERS reporting system has limitations including incomplete adverse event reporting. Initiation of anti-TNF therapy should be a decision made between families and pediatric rheumatologists.

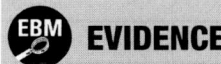

available at www.expertconsult.com

SUGGESTED READINGS
available at www.expertconsult.com

AUTHOR: **ELISABETH B. MATSON, D.O.**

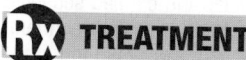

BASIC INFORMATION

DEFINITION

Kaposi's sarcoma (KS) is a vascular neoplasm most frequently occurring in AIDS patients. It can be divided into the following four subsets:
1. Classic Kaposi's sarcoma: most frequently found in elderly Eastern European and Mediterranean males. It consists initially of violaceous macules and papules with subsequent development of plaques and red-purple nodules. Growth is slow, and most of the patients die of unrelated causes.
2. Epidemic or AIDS-related Kaposi's sarcoma: most frequently occurs in homosexual men. Lesions are generally multifocal and widespread. Lymphadenopathy may be associated.
3. Endemic Kaposi's sarcoma: usually affects African children and adults. An aggressive lymphadenopathic form affects African children in particular.
4. Immunosuppression-associated, or transplantation-associated, Kaposi's sarcoma: usually associated with chemotherapy.

SYNONYMS

KS

ICD-9CM CODES
173.9 Malignant neoplasm of the skin

EPIDEMIOLOGY & DEMOGRAPHICS

- AIDS-related KS affects >35% of AIDS cases.
- Highest incidence is in homosexual men.

PHYSICAL FINDINGS & CLINICAL PRESENTATION

- AIDS-related KS: multifocal and widespread red-purple or dark plaques and/or nodules on cutaneous or mucosal surfaces (Fig. 1-210).
- Generalized lymphadenopathy at the time of diagnosis is present in >50% of patients with AIDS-related KS; the initial lesions have a rust-colored appearance; subsequent progression to red or purple nodules or plaques occurs.
- Most frequently affected areas are the face, trunk, oral cavity, and upper and lower extremities.

ETIOLOGY

A herpesvirus (HHV-8, Kaposi's sarcoma–associated herpesvirus KSHV) has been isolated from patients with most forms of KS and is believed to be the causative agent. It can be transmitted sexually (homosexual or heterosexual activities) and by other forms of nonsexual contact such as maternal-infant transmission (common in African countries).

DIAGNOSIS

DIFFERENTIAL DIAGNOSIS

- Stasis dermatitis
- Pyogenic granuloma
- Capillary hemangiomas
- Granulation tissue
- Postinflammatory hyperpigmentation
- Cutaneous lymphoma
- Melanoma
- Dermatofibroma
- Hematoma
- Prurigo nodularis

The differential diagnosis of cutaneous lesions in patients with HIV infection is described in Section III.

WORKUP

Diagnosis can generally be made on clinical appearance; tissue biopsy will confirm diagnosis.

LABORATORY TESTS

HIV in patients suspected of AIDS

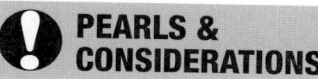

TREATMENT

NONPHARMACOLOGIC THERAPY

Observation is a reasonable option in patients with slowly progressive disease.

GENERAL Rx

- Excisional biopsy often provides adequate treatment for single lesions and resected recurrences in classic Kaposi's sarcoma.
- Liquid nitrogen cryotherapy can result in complete response in 80% of lesions.
- Interlesional chemotherapy with vinblastine is useful for nodular lesions >1 cm in diameter. Intralesional injection of interferon alfa-2b has also been reported as effective and well tolerated.

- Radiation therapy is effective in non-AIDS KS and for large tumor masses that interfere with normal function.
- Systemic therapy with interferon is also effective in AIDS-related KS and is often used in combination with zidovudine.
- Systemic chemotherapy (vinblastine, bleomycin, doxorubicin, and dacarbazine) can be used for rapidly progressive disease and for classic and African endemic KS.
- Sirolimus (rapamycin), an immunosuppressive drug, is effective in inhibiting the progression of dermal Kaposi's sarcoma in kidney transplant recipients.
- Oral etoposide is also effective and has less myelosuppression than vinblastine.
- Paclitaxel is also effective in patients with advanced KS and represents an excellent second-line therapy.
- Thalidomide, retinoids.

DISPOSITION

- Prognosis is poor in AIDS-related KS. Death is often a result of other AIDS-defining illnesses.
- Prognosis is better in African cutaneous KS and classic sarcoma (patients usually die of unrelated causes).

PEARLS & CONSIDERATIONS

COMMENTS

Immunosuppression-associated KS usually regresses with the cessation, reduction, or modification of immunosuppression therapy in most patients. Similarly, in HIV patients KS responds concurrently with the decrease in serum HIV RNA and increase in the CD4 count.

SUGGESTED READING

available at www.expertconsult.com

AUTHOR: **FRED F. FERRI, M.D.**

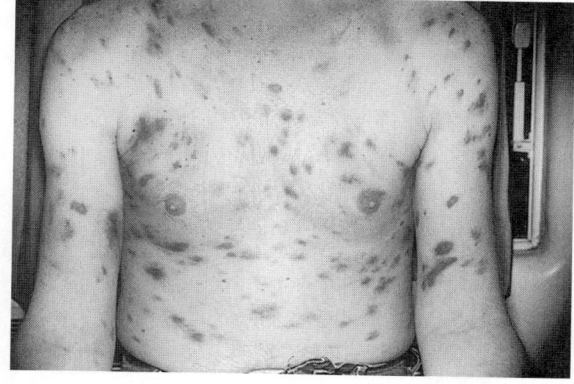

FIGURE 1-210 Kaposi's sarcoma. More advanced lesions. Note widespread hemorrhagic plaques and nodules. (From Noble J [ed]: *Textbook of primary care medicine,* ed 2, St Louis, 1995, Mosby.)

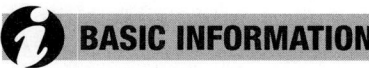

BASIC INFORMATION

DEFINITION

Kawasaki disease (KD) is an acute, febrile, vasculitis that predominantly affects children.

SYNONYMS

Kawasaki syndrome
Mucocutaneous lymph node syndrome
Infantile polyarteritis

ICD-9CM CODES
446.1 Kawasaki disease

EPIDEMIOLOGY & DEMOGRAPHICS

- KD is the leading cause of acquired heart disease in children in developing countries.
- Commonly occurs in children <5 yr (80%); peak incidence is in infants aged 9 to 11 mo to 24 mo.
- More prevalent in boys than girls (1.5:1).
- The highest incidence is found in Japan (~174 cases/100,000 children).
- Temporal clustering and seasonality have been observed in KD cases in Japan, supporting an environmental or infectious etiology.
- Incidence of KD in the U.S. is 17 to 18 cases/ 100,000 children <5 yr.
- Children of Asian descent have the highest incidence of KD compared with those of European or African descent.
- ~4200 new cases are diagnosed each year in the United States.
- In the United States, KD has now surpassed acute rheumatic fever as the leading cause of acquired heart disease in children.

PHYSICAL FINDINGS & CLINICAL PRESENTATION

- Diagnosis of KD is based on characteristic clinical signs and symptoms and includes fever persisting for >5 days and the presence of at least four of the following five principal features:
  1. Bilateral, painless bulbar conjunctival injection without exudate
  2. Oral mucosal changes: erythema and fissured lips, strawberry tongue (Fig. 1-211, B), diffuse injection of the oropharyngeal mucosae
  3. Polymorphous exanthema (usually in truncal region) (Fig. 1-212, A and B)
  4. Extremity changes: (a) acute: erythema and edema of hands and feet (Fig. 1-153, A); (b) convalescent: membranous desquamation of fingertips
  5. Cervical lymphadenopathy (<1.5 cm in diameter, predominantly unilateral and anterior)
- The fever of KD is usually higher than 102.2° F (39° C) and often >104.0° F (40° C); if untreated, it lasts for an average of 12 days.
- Coronary artery aneurysms can develop in as many as 25% to 30% of untreated children. This subset of patients can over time develop ischemic heart disease, myocardial infarction, congestive heart failure, and, occasionally, death.
- Morbidity and mortality rates are highest if aneurysm diameter is >8 mm.
- Children with KD who are <1 yr or >6 yr are more likely to develop the cardiac sequelae and are most likely to not respond treatment.
- Patients with fever and fewer than four principal symptoms but evidence of coronary artery disease are diagnosed as having atypical KD (10%).
- Cervical lymphadenopathy is the most common physical manifestation absent in atypical KD, followed by exanthema and then extremity changes.
- Oral mucosal changes are the most common manifestations of KD (either typical or atypical).
- On rare occasions aneurysms of peripheral arteries (e.g., axillary) may be seen.
- Beau's lines (transverse grooves of the nails), diarrhea, dyspnea, arthralgia, and myalgia may also been seen.

ETIOLOGY

The cause of KD is not known, although evidence substantiates an infectious etiology precipitating an immune-mediated reaction in genetically susceptible individuals.

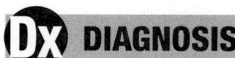

DIAGNOSIS

Diagnosis of KD is made on the basis of clinical features (see "Physical Findings & Clinical Presentation"). The illness begins with the abrupt onset of fever. Typically, the clinical signs appear over the course of several days. Laboratory evaluation may be helpful in making the diagnosis in atypical KD.

DIFFERENTIAL DIAGNOSIS

- Scarlet fever
- Stevens-Johnson syndrome
- Drug eruption
- Henoch-Schönlein purpura
- Toxic shock syndrome
- Measles
- Rocky Mountain spotted fever
- Infectious mononucleosis
- Juvenile rheumatoid arthritis
- Mercury hypersensitivity

WORKUP

Clinical findings in addition to laboratory and imaging studies are useful in searching for multiorgan system involvement and complications (e.g., cardiac, lung, liver).

LABORATORY TESTS

Inflammatory markers will be increased in kawasaki disease.

Clinical and laboratory findings observed in patients with this disease are frequently helpful in diagnosis:
- Complete blood count commonly shows a normochromic normocytic anemia, elevated platelet count, and elevated white blood cell count with neutrophil predominance.
- Abnormal liver function tests are found: elevated transaminases (hepatic congestion), elevated bilirubin (gallbladder hydrops), low albumin.
- Elevated erythrocyte sedimentation rate is found (often >40 mm/hr and not uncommonly elevated to levels of >100 mm/hr).
- Elevated C-reactive protein (levels of >3 mg/ dl) is identified.
- Urinalysis may show sterile pyuria.

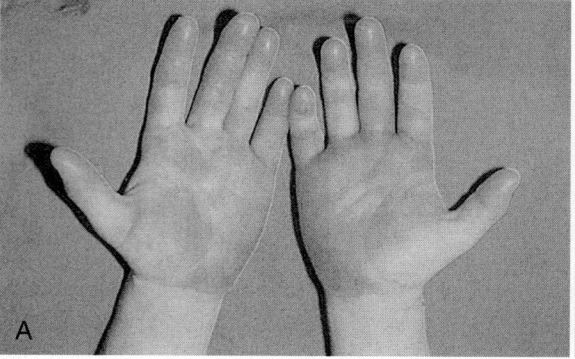
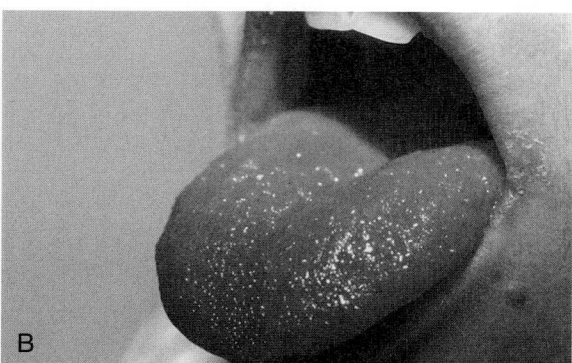

FIGURE 1-211 A, Erythema of the hands, to be followed by desquamation. **B,** Strawberry tongue in a patient with Kawasaki disease. **(A** Courtesy Department of Dermatology, University of North Carolina at Chapel Hill. In Goldstein B [ed]: *Practical dermatology,* ed 2, St Louis, 1997, Mosby. **B** Courtesy Marshall Guill, M.D. In Goldstein B [ed]: *Practical dermatology,* ed 2, St Louis, 1997, Mosby.)

IMAGING STUDIES

- Chest radiograph may reveal pulmonary infiltrates; cardiomegaly may also be present.
- Echocardiogram is recommended at the time of illness, and repeat in 6 wk and 6 mo. Echocardiogram should include careful assessment of the coronary arteries for size and aneurysms, mural or intraluminal thrombi, effusions, valve function, and myocardial function.
- Coronary angiogram, computed tomography angiography, and magnetic resonance angiography can be used to visualize the arterial system and the presence of coronary artery aneurysms. Echocardiography may be able to visualize these aneurysms in infants.
- Intravascular ultrasound can assess for luminal irregularities of the coronary arteries.
- Exercise testing with myocardial perfusion studies can be done to assess for coronary blood flow and the presence of myocardial ischemia.
- ECG changes (arrhythmias, abnormal Q waves, prolonged PR and/or QT intervals, occasionally low voltage, or ST-T wave changes) can be seen.

Rx TREATMENT

Treatment of KD in the acute phase is directed at reducing inflammation in the systemic and coronary arteries and preventing arterial thrombosis. Long-term therapy in individuals who develop coronary aneurysms is aimed at preventing myocardial ischemia or infarction.

NONPHARMACOLOGIC THERAPY

- Oxygen in selected patients
- Salt restriction in patients with congestive heart failure
- Emollient creams for peeling skin and balms for fissured lips

ACUTE GENERAL Rx

- IV immunoglobulin (IVIG) 2 g/kg over 8 to 12 hr is the treatment of choice in children diagnosed with KD and ideally should be given within the first 10 days of the illness.
- Aspirin 80 to 100 mg/kg/day (anti-inflammatory dosing) given in four divided doses until the patient is no longer febrile for 48 hr. Thereafter, aspirin 3 to 5 mg/kg/day (antiplatelet dosing) is continued until laboratory studies (e.g., platelet count, sedimentation rate) return to normal, generally within 6 to 8 wk.
- In patients who do not defervesce within 48 hr or have recrudescent fever after initial IVIG treatment, a second dose of IVIG 2 g/kg IV over 8 to 12 hr should be considered.
- NSAIDs are not effective in the treatment of KD.
- The effect of corticosteroids on coronary artery aneurysms is unclear. Therefore most experts recommend withholding steroids unless fever persists after at least two courses of IVIG.
- Other therapies, including pentoxifylline, infliximab (monoclonal antibody against tumor necrosis factor-α), plasma exchange, abciximab (platelet glycoprotein IIb/IIIa receptor

inhibitor), and immunosuppressive agents (methotrexate, cyclosporine, tacrolimus, antithymocyte globulin, cyclophosphamide) have been used, but data are limited on their success.
- Acute management of patients with coronary artery abnormalities depends on the severity of the lesion.
- Most patients with large or giant coronary artery aneurysms (diameter >8 mm) are maintained on aspirin (or clopidogrel) and warfarin to prevent thrombosis within the aneurysm and myocardial infarction.

CHRONIC Rx

Interventional and surgical procedures can be tried in children who have developed cardiac complications of KD:

- Percutaneous transluminal coronary angioplasty with or without stenting may be performed.
- Coronary bypass graft surgery using the internal mammary artery or the gastroepiploic artery has met with greater patency success than saphenous vein grafts. Patency rates for internal thoracic artery grafts have been shown to be 87% at 20 yr, and patency rates for vein grafts at 1, 10, and 25 yr after surgery have been shown to be 84%, 57%, and 51%, respectively.
- Cardiac transplantation is an option and is indicated in patients with:
  - Severe left ventricular failure
  - Malignant arrhythmias
  - Multivessel coronary artery disease

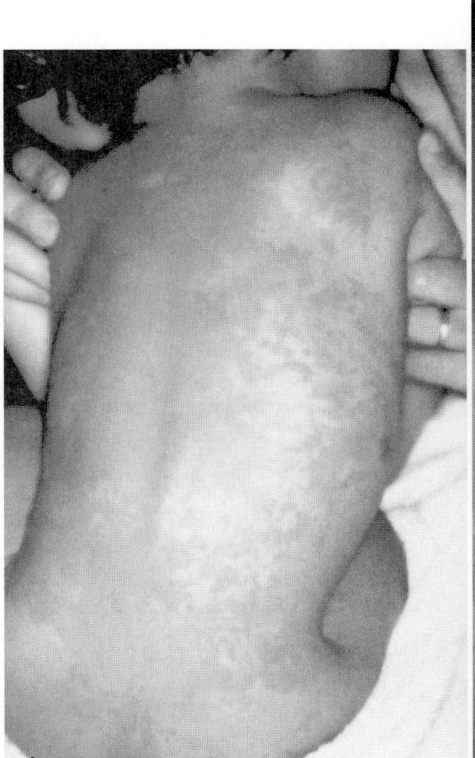 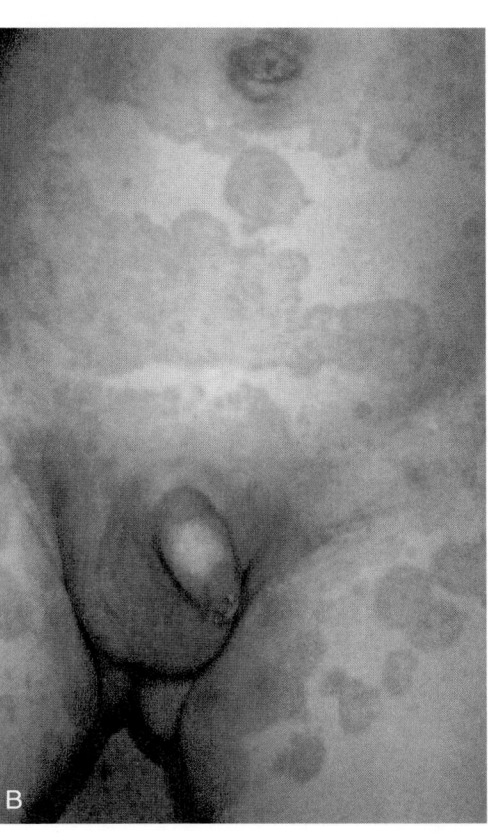

FIGURE 1-212 Clinical manifestations of Kawasaki disease. Polymorphous exanthema **(A, B).**

A

B

For patients with persistent giant (≥8 mm) aneurysms, anticoagulation with warfarin for a goal international normalized ratio of 2.0 to 2.5 should be considered.

DISPOSITION

- Mortality rate of children with KD is 0.5% to 2.8%, usually from coronary aneurysm thrombosis and myocardial infarction.
- Death usually occurs in the third to fourth week of the illness.
- Before the use of IVIG, ~20% of all patients with KD developed coronary artery aneurysms.
- Treatment with IVIG has reduced the incidence of coronary aneurysms by 80%.
- IVIG has also been shown to improve left ventricular function during the acute stages of the disease.
- Risk factors for the development of coronary aneurysms or giant coronary aneurysms 8 mm or greater are:
  ○ Fever lasting >10 days
  ○ Age <1 yr or >6 yr
  ○ Male
  ○ Recurrence of fever
- 1% to 2% of patients have recurrences of KD.

REFERRAL

Multiple specialists may be consulted to assist in the diagnosis of KD, including dermatology, rheumatology, and infectious disease. Cardiology consultation is recommended in any patient with cardiac involvement and in the long-term follow-up of patients with KD.

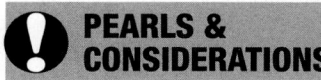

COMMENTS

- KD was first described by Dr. Tomisaku Kawasaki in 1967 and published in the *Journal of Allergology.*
- KD is not transmitted from person to person.
- Atypical or incomplete KD can be detected using clinical plus laboratory criteria along with typical findings on echocardiography.
- The mechanism of action of IVIG therapy for KD remains unknown.
- Failure of corticosteroids suggests that the inflammatory response is different compared with other vasculitic conditions.

PREVENTION

- Without a known etiologic agent for KD, primary prevention is not possible.
- Low-dose aspirin (3 to 5 mg/kg/day, given as a single dose) should be continued until 6 to 8 wk after disease onset if there are no coronary artery abnormalities or indefinitely if abnormalities are present.

- Thrombosis leading to myocardial infarction in a stenotic or aneurysmal coronary artery is the leading cause of death in these children and occurs most often in the first year after illness onset. Therefore serial imaging and stress tests are necessary in patients with significant coronary artery abnormalities (by coronary angiography).

PATIENT & FAMILY EDUCATION

- The Kawasaki Disease Foundation, a non-profit organization dedicated to KD issues (http://www.kdfoundation.org).
- The American Heart Association has developed guidelines for the diagnosis of KD (http://www.americanheart.org).

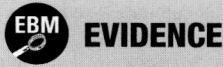 **EVIDENCE**

available at www.expertconsult.com

SUGGESTED READINGS

available at www.expertconsult.com

AUTHORS: **ABDULRAHMAN ABDULBAKI, MD.,** and **WEN-CHIH WU, M.D.**

BASIC INFORMATION

DESCRIPTION

Keloid may be defined as a benign growth of dense fibrous tissue developing from an abnormal healing response to cutaneous injury, extending beyond the original borders of the wound or inflammatory response (Fig. 1-213).

In 1806, Alibert used the term *cheloide*, derived from the Greek *chele*, or crab's claw, to describe lateral growth of tissue into unaffected skin.

ICD-9CM CODES
701.4 Keloid scar

EPIDEMIOLOGY

- Keloid is seen 5 to 15 times more often in pigmented ethnic groups than in whites.
- Its prevalence is 16% in blacks and Hispanics.
- The highest incidence is seen in the second decade.
- It affects both sexes equally.
- Combined incidence of keloid and hypertrophic scar ranges from 40% to 70% following surgery to up to 91% following burns.

ETIOLOGY

- Wounds from trauma, surgery, or body piercing
- Burn
- Other injuries such as insect bites, vaccination, folliculitis, acne, and so on
- Rarely can be spontaneous without obvious injury
- Familial predisposition seen in some patients

RISK FACTORS

- Family history of keloids
- Personal history of keloids

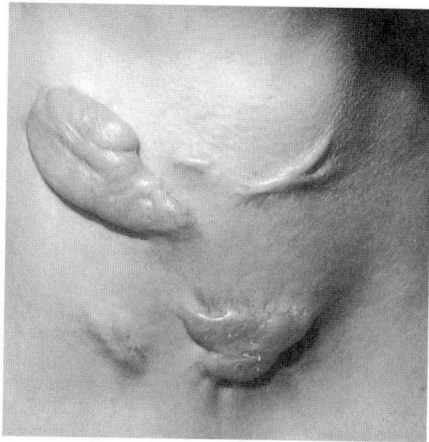

FIGURE 1-213 Keloids. An abnormal reparative reaction to skin injury, keloids are characterized by proliferation of fibroblasts and collagen that extends beyond the margins of the original wound. (From Zitelli BJ, Davis HW: *Atlas of pediatric physical diagnosis*, ed 5, Philadelphia, 2007, Mosby.)

- Blacks, Hispanics, and Asians
- Pregnancy
- Puberty
- Patients with blood group A
- Injury over bones

PATHOGENESIS

- Pathophysiology of keloid is not completely understood
- Caused by benign dermal fibroproliferation because of disorder in the regulation of cellularity during the wound healing process

CLINICAL FEATURES

- Keloids usually appear within a few months of the injury, in contrast to the hypertrophic scars, which develop within a few weeks. At times it could take up to a year to appear because the growth is slow.
- Keloids are often symptomatic in the early stages. Common complaints are pruritus, burning, pain, and tenderness.
- Keloids are commonly seen on the shoulders, sternum, upper back, nape of neck, ear lobes, mandibular border, and cheek. Hands and feet are often spared.
- Skin lesions vary from papules to nodules to large tuberous lesions. They have the normal skin color most of the time with well-defined borders. Early on they can appear erythematous, whereas older lesions may be hypo- or hyperpigmented. They can be firm to hard in consistency with smooth surface and are tender to touch. Hair follicles are absent in these keloids.
- Unlike with hypertrophic scar, in keloids the scar extends beyond the margin of the initial wound.

DIAGNOSIS

- Workup is usually not necessary because it is a clinical diagnosis.
- Biopsy is usually avoided because it may increase the keloid size. When biopsy is done, the histology shows randomly organized large collagen fibers in a dense connective tissue matrix. In fact, both major components of extracellular matrix, collagen and glycosaminoglycans, are increased.

DIFFERENTIAL DIAGNOSIS

- Hypertrophic scar
- Dermatofibroma
- Dermatofibrosarcoma protuberance
- Desmoid tumor
- Foreign body granuloma
- Scar with sarcoidosis
- Lobomycosis

TREATMENT

- There is no universally accepted treatment protocol. Prevention is the best strategy.
- Combination treatment is most effective.
- Surgical excision using cold knife followed by intralesional steroids is the preferred method.

- Treatment outcome is the best when it is initiated shortly after the keloid formation.
- Different treatment options include:
  1. Unlike with hypertrophic scars, **surgery** alone is associated with a 55% to 100% recurrence rate in patients with keloids. Results are significantly better when it is followed by intralesional steroids, radiotherapy, pressure therapy, or silicon application. Both complete and near total excision has been advocated. Few recommend core extirpation. Use of Z-plasties or any wound lengthening techniques is strongly discouraged.
  2. **Intralesional steroid** every 2 to 4 wk is administered either alone or following surgery. Duration of treatment depends on the treatment response. Triamcinolone is the most studied steroid and is used at a concentration of 10 to 40 mg/ml. Higher concentration is used for denser, more calcitrant lesions, and those located in trunks or extremities. It could be used in combination with lidocaine to reduce the discomfort. A 27- to 30-gauge needle is used for its administration. To distribute the suspension evenly, it should be injected while continuously advancing the needle. No more than 20 to 30 mg of the drug is used during each treatment. Liquid nitrogen is applied to the injection briefly for 2 to 4 seconds about 10 to 15 min prior to steroid injection for better dispersal of the steroid and to minimize deposition into surrounding normal tissue. Hypopigmentation, skin atrophy, ulceration, and telangiectasia are the side effects associated with this treatment.
  3. **Cryotherapy** has been used for smaller lesions. When this treatment is chosen, the entire lesion is treated with 2 to 3 freeze-thaw cycles of 30 seconds' duration each. Most lesions need 2 to 10 treatment sessions at 4-wk intervals. Pain and hypopigmentation are the main adverse events.
  4. **Silicone gel sheeting or cushioning** can prevent keloids from recurring after surgery. These are applied as soon as re-epithelialization is achieved and are worn for at least 12 hr/day for 2 to 4 mo.
  5. **Application of pressure** by compression devices has been advocated in the treatment of keloids. These compression treatments include button compression, pressure ear rings, pressure gradient garments, ACE bandages, elastic adhesive bandages, compression wraps, Spandex or Elastane bandages, and support bandages. About 24 to 40 mm Hg pressure must be maintained. It must be instituted for long periods (>23 hr/day for 6 to 12 mo) before significant effect can be achieved. Unfortunately many parts of the body are not amenable to this pressure. Patient discomfort frequently reduces compliance.

6. **Radiation** following surgery can also reduce the recurrence rate. X-rays of 700 to 1500 cGy in fractions over 5 to 6 treatments is the most frequently used treatment. It is usually initiated within 10 days, preferably within 24 hr of surgery. It is avoided in pediatric and pregnant patients. At times brachytherapy is used using interstitial iridium 192. Most physicians use radiation only for keloids over the extremities. The reported risk of radiation-induced malignancy is theoretical.

7. **5-Fluorouracil** can be used as an individual agent, following surgery, or in combination with intralesional steroids. Weekly injection of 0.5 to 2 ml at a 50 mg/ml concentration of 5-fluorouracil for 12 wk is the recommended dose.

8. Superiority of **laser** use to simple excision currently has not been demonstrated.

9. Topical 5% **imiquimod** cream has some role when used following surgery locally every night for a minimum of 2 mo.

10. Other treatments include Cordran tape, bleomycin, interferon, vitamin A, nitrogen mustard, antihistamines, zinc, tacrolimus, sirolimus, allantoin, botulinum toxin, colchicine, salicylic acid, calcipotriol, NSAIDs, d-penicillamine, relaxin, quercetin, dinoprostone, doxorubicin, ACE inhibitors, hyaluronidase, pentoxifylline, tranilast, mitomycin-C, tamoxifen, silver sulfadiazine, onion extract, vitamin E, intralesional verapamil.

FOLLOW-UP

Because of the high risk of recurrence, a follow-up of at least 12 mo is necessary to fully evaluate the effectiveness of therapy.

PREVENTION

- Avoid nonessential surgery such as body piercing, which carry a high risk for keloid formation.
- LASIK eye surgery and CO_2 laser resurfacing should be avoided in patients with a tendency for keloids.
- Use a laparoscopic approach when surgery is needed.
- Avoid making incisions over joint spaces or over midchest, and ensure that they follow skin creases.
- Handle tissue gently during surgery.
- Ensure good hemostasis intraoperatively.
- Use tension-free primary wound closure.
- Use monofilament, synthetic permanent sutures.
- Use adhesives instead of sutures when possible for closure of wounds.
- Compressive pressure dressing is preferred in high risk patients following surgery.
- Avoid of wound infection.
- Avoid tattoos.
- Aggressively treat inflammatory acnes.

COMPLICATIONS

- Psychological effects secondary to disfigurement.
- Contracture from keloids may result in loss of function if overlying a joint.

PROGNOSIS

- Unlike with hypertrophic scars, keloids do not regress with time. However, they may continue to expand in size for decades.
- Regardless of the type of treatment there is a high recurrence rate.
- Keloids never become malignant.

SUGGESTED READINGS

available at www.expertconsult.com

AUTHOR: **HEMANT K. SAPATHY, M.D.**

BASIC INFORMATION

DEFINITION

Klinefelter's syndrome is a congenital disorder in which a 47,XXY chromosome complement is associated with hypogonadism and infertility.

SYNONYMS

47,XXY Hypogonadism

ICD-9CM CODES
758.7 Klinefelter's syndrome

EPIDEMIOLOGY & DEMOGRAPHICS

INCIDENCE: One in 500 men (most common sex chromosome disorder)
GENETICS: The most common mosaic complement is 46,XY/47,XXY. 47,XXY karyotype 48,XXYY, 48,XXXY, or 49,XXXXY have been reported. The manifestations vary in severity by patient (see Table 1-90). This sex chromosome mosaicism is believed to account for the variable presentation. Fertility, although very rare, has been reported in men with Klinefelter's syndrome.

TABLE 1-90 Clinical Features of Klinefelter's Syndrome

Karyotype	47,XXY
Inheritance	Sporadic; associated with advanced maternal age; nondisjunction during first or second meiotic division in either parent (67% maternal, 33% paternal); mitotic nondisjunction
Genitalia	Male
Wolffian duct derivatives	Normal
Müllerian duct derivatives	Absent
Gonads	Small, firm testes; seminiferous tubule dysgenesis; azoospermia; Leydig cell hyperplasia
Habitus	Poor to normal virilization at puberty: gynecomastia; disproportionately long legs
Hormone profile	Testosterone levels variable but usually decreased; increased levels of plasma LH and FSH postpubertally

FSH, Follicle-stimulating hormone; *LH,* luteinizing hormone.
Larsen PR, Kronenberg HM, Melmed S, Polonsky KS: *Williams textbook of endocrinology,* ed 10, Philadelphia, Saunders, 2003.

PHYSICAL FINDINGS & CLINICAL PRESENTATION

- Classic triad: Small firm testes, azoospermia, and gynecomastia.
- Prepubertal: Small testes; gonadal volume <1.5 ml is a result of loss of germ cells before puberty.
- Postpubertal: Gynecomastia (periductal fat growth) with small, firm testes. Exaggerated growth of the lower extremities results in a decreased crown-to-pubis/pubis-to-floor ratio. There is diminished strength, diminished ability to grow a full beard or mustache, and infertility. Decreased intellectual development and antisocial behavior are believed to occur with high frequency.

ETIOLOGY

- Several postulated mechanisms: nondisjunction during meiosis and mitosis and anaphase lag during mitosis or meiosis
- Reason: maternal age
  1. The incidence of Klinefelter's syndrome rises from 0.6% when the maternal age is ≤35 yr to 5.4% when the maternal age is >45 yr.
  2. Of note, the extra X chromosome has a paternal origin as often as a maternal origin.

DIAGNOSIS

- Markedly elevated follicle-stimulating hormone levels.
- Total plasma testosterone levels are decreased in 50% to 60% of patients.
- Free testosterone levels are decreased.
- Plasma estradiol is increased, stimulating the increase in levels of testosterone-binding globulin with resultant decrease in the testosterone/estradiol ratio, which is believed to be the cause of gynecomastia.

LABORATORY TESTS

- Normal to low serum testosterone.
- Increased sex hormone–binding globulin (acts to further suppress any available free testosterone).
- Normal to increased estradiol (a result of augmented peripheral conversion of testosterone to estradiol).
- Testis biopsy shows azoospermia, Leydig cell hyperplasia, hyalinization, and fibrosis of the seminiferous tubules. Mosaics may have focal areas of spermatogenesis and, on rare occasions, a sperm may appear in the ejaculate. The extra X chromosome is the pivotal factor controlling spermatogenesis and also affects neuronal function directly, leading to the behavioral abnormalities related to decreased IQ.

- Buccal smear: one sex chromatin body.
- Prepubertal male: gonadotropin levels are normal.
- Postpubertal male: Gonadotropin levels are elevated even when the testosterone level is normal.
- Disease associations:
  - Malignancies: breast cancer (20 times greater than XY men and 20% the rate of occurrence in women), nonlymphocytic leukemia, lymphomas, marrow dysplastic syndromes, extragonadal germ cell neoplasms
  - Autoimmune disorders: chronic lymphocytic thyroiditis, Takayasu arteritis, taurodontism (enlarged molar teeth), mitral valve prolapse, varicose veins, asthma, bronchitis, osteoporosis, abnormal glucose tolerance testing, diabetes, varicose veins

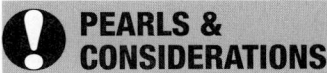 TREATMENT

- Revolves around three facets of Klinefelter's syndrome:
  1. Hypogonadism: androgen replacement in the form of testosterone
  2. Gynecomastia: cosmetic surgery
  3. Psychosocial problems: androgen therapy and educational support
- After extensive genetic counseling, intracytoplasmic sperm insertion has been used to treat infertility with limited success in mosaic men

PEARLS & CONSIDERATIONS

COMMENTS

- Androgen therapy should not be used in the case of severe mental retardation.
- Rule out breast and prostate cancer before initiating or continuing androgen therapy.
- Androgen therapy will not improve fertility; it may suppress any spermatogenesis that is taking place within the testes.
- Other causes of primary hypogonadism:
  1. Myotonic muscular dystrophy
  2. Sertoli cell–only syndrome
  3. Kartagener's syndrome
  4. Anorchia
  5. Acquired hypogonadism

SUGGESTED READINGS
available at www.expertconsult.com

AUTHORS: **PHILIP J. ALIOTTA, M.D., M.S.H.A.,** and **RUBEN ALVERO, M.D.**

Diseases and Disorders

I

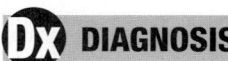

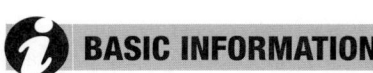 **BASIC INFORMATION**

DEFINITION

Korsakoff's psychosis is a disorder of learning and memory, out of proportion to other cognitive functions, associated with thiamine deficiency. It is classically seen with chronic alcohol abuse and may follow the presentation of Wernicke's encephalopathy (see relevant entry).

SYNONYMS

Korsakoff's syndrome
Wernicke-Korsakoff syndrome
Alcoholic polyneuritic psychosis

ICD-9CM CODES

291.1 Alcohol amnestic syndrome

EPIDEMIOLOGY & DEMOGRAPHICS

- Formerly seen commonly in chronic alcohol users, but declining in recent years as a result of better nutrition and awareness by health professionals.
- Slightly more common in males.
- Age of onset evenly distributed between ages 30 and 70.

PHYSICAL FINDINGS & CLINICAL PRESENTATION

- Impairment of ability to remember new material.
- Remote memory is relatively better preserved but is commonly impaired on neuropsychologic testing.
- Confabulation (the fabrication of false memories to fill memory gaps) is common.

ETIOLOGY

Thiamine deficiency is the underlying cause. This is most commonly seen in alcoholics and other malnourished populations, although it may be iatrogenic from prolonged infusion of dextrose-containing fluids without thiamine repletion.

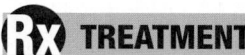 **DIAGNOSIS**

DIFFERENTIAL DIAGNOSIS

- Stroke, trauma, or tumor affecting the temporal lobes or hippocampus
- Cerebral anoxia
- Transient global amnesia
- Dementia of multiple causes

WORKUP

A high index of suspicion should be maintained in all alcoholics and others in malnourished states.

LABORATORY TESTS

- CBC
- Serum chemistries
- Serum pyruvate is elevated
- Whole-blood or erythrocyte transketolase are decreased; rapid resolution to normal in 24 hr with thiamine repletion

IMAGING STUDIES

MRI may show T_2 hyperintense diencephalic and mesencephalic lesions acutely, but there is no definitive radiologic study for diagnosis.

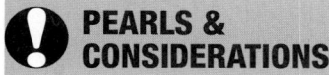 **TREATMENT**

NONPHARMACOLOGIC THERAPY

A supervised environment may be required.

ACUTE GENERAL Rx

- Thiamine 100 mg IV or IM should be given immediately.
- Thiamine given acutely during Wernicke's phase (disorders of extraocular movements, confusion, and ataxia) may prevent the development of Korsakoff's psychosis.

CHRONIC Rx

- It is impossible to predict acutely the degree of recovery of an individual patient, although the vast majority will have lasting deficits. Decisions regarding long-term institutionalization should therefore be made cautiously.
- Chronic treatment with thiamine.

DISPOSITION

Patient often must live in a protected environment for the rest of his or her life.

REFERRAL

- Neurology to confirm the diagnosis.
- Neuropsychologic testing may be helpful.

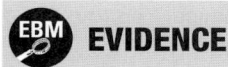 **PEARLS & CONSIDERATIONS**

COMMENTS

- This disease may be underdiagnosed, and memory problems may persist, even in "recovered" patients.
- Replace thiamine in patients at risk, even if clinical symptoms are not evident.
- A preventable cause is prolonged use of dextrose-containing IV fluids without supplemental thiamine.

EBM **EVIDENCE**

available at www.expertconsult.com

SUGGESTED READINGS
available at www.expertconsult.com

AUTHOR: **DANIEL T. MATTSON, M.S., M.SC. (MED.)**

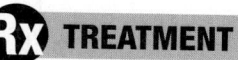

BASIC INFORMATION

DEFINITION

Labyrinthitis is a peripheral vestibulopathy characterized by acute onset of vertigo usually associated with nausea and vomiting. It may be associated with hearing loss. It may be either serous or purulent.

SYNONYMS

Acute labyrinthitis
Acute vestibular neuronopathy
Vestibular neuronitis
Viral neurolabyrinthitis

ICD-9CM CODES

386.12 Vestibular neuronitis (active and recurrent)
386.3 Labyrinthitis

EPIDEMIOLOGY & DEMOGRAPHICS

INCIDENCE (IN U.S.): Most common cause of prolonged spontaneous vertigo associated with nausea at any age
PREDOMINANT AGE: Any

CLINICAL PRESENTATION

- Vertigo, nausea, and vomiting with onset over several hr.
- Symptoms usually peak within 24 hr, then resolve gradually over several wk.
- During the first day, the patient usually has difficulty focusing the eyes because of spontaneous nystagmus.
- Usually has benign course, with complete recovery within 1 to 3 mo, although older patients may have intractable dizziness that persists for many mo.

PHYSICAL FINDINGS

- Nystagmus
- Nausea
- Vomiting
- Vertigo worsening with head movement
- Abnormal caloric ENG tests
- Possible hearing loss in the affected ear
- Normal otoscopic exam typically
- Otherwise normal neurologic exam, except may possibly have signs of vestibular loss, such as a positive head thrust test

ETIOLOGY

Often preceded for 1 to 2 wk by a viral-like illness. It may be either bacterial or viral, and be either tympanogenic (i.e., resulting from spread of infection into the inner ear from the middle ear, antrum, or petrous apex), meningogenic, or hematogenic from encephalitis or brain abscess. The round window membrane is considered the most likely pathway of inflammatory mediators from the middle to the inner ear that subsequently give rise to labyrinthitis.

DIAGNOSIS

DIFFERENTIAL DIAGNOSIS

- Acute labyrinthine ischemia (vascular insufficiency)
- Other forms of labyrinthitis (bacterial and syphilitic)
- Labyrinthine fistula
- Benign positional vertigo
- Meniere's syndrome
- Cholesteatoma
- Drug induced
- Eighth nerve tumor
- Head trauma
- Vertebrobasilar stroke

WORKUP

- Otoscopic examination
- Neurologic examination, with close attention to cranial nerves
- Bedside test of vestibular function, that is, head thrust or head heave test
- Audiogram if symptoms accompanied by hearing loss
- Caloric test if presentation is atypical

LABORATORY TESTS

- Routine laboratory tests are generally not helpful.
- If there is a history of significant emesis, check electrolytes, BUN, and creatinine.

IMAGING STUDIES

Usually not necessary, but enhancement of bony labyrinth may be seen by MRI after injection of contrast material. Do a head CT with fine cuts through temporal bones if there is a history of trauma or suspicion of cholesteatoma. Use an MRI of the brain with and without contrast with fine cuts through the internal auditory canal if there is an abnormal cranial nerve exam or suspicion of eighth nerve tumor.

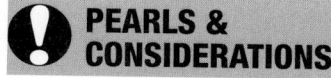

TREATMENT

NONPHARMACOLOGIC THERAPY

- Reassurance.
- Initial bed rest, then encourage increase in activity as tolerated.

ACUTE GENERAL Rx

- Phenergan or other antiemetics are typically effective.
- Vestibular suppressant: meclizine 12.5 to 25 mg qid is often used. Scopolamine patch is also effective.
- Methylprednisolone 100 mg per day for 3 days, with slow taper over 3 wk.
- Valacyclovir has not been shown to be helpful.

CHRONIC Rx

No specific chronic therapy

DISPOSITION

Usually does not require hospital admission unless the patient is unable to tolerate oral intake of liquids.

REFERRAL

- Refer if symptoms persist or neurologic abnormalities are present.
- Consider vestibular rehabilitation, particularly in the elderly.

PEARLS & CONSIDERATIONS

COMMENTS

Labyrinthitis is a term that usually implies peripheral vestibulopathy associated with hearing loss. The term vestibular neuronitis is typically used when hearing is not affected. Despite this technical distinction, many physicians use these terms interchangeably.

SUGGESTED READINGS

available at www.expertconsult.com

AUTHOR: **SHARON S. HARTMAN POLENSEK, M.D., PH.D.**

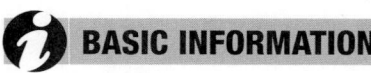

BASIC INFORMATION

DEFINITION

Lactose intolerance is the insufficient concentration of lactase enzyme, leading to fermentation of malabsorbed lactose by intestinal bacteria with subsequent production of intestinal gas and various organic acids, manifesting clinically with diarrhea, abdominal pain, flatulence, or bloating after lactose intolerance. *Lactose malabsorption* occurs when a substantial amount of lactose is not absorbed in the intestine. *Lactase deficiency* is defined as brush-border lactase activity that is markedly reduced relative to the activity observed in infants.

SYNONYMS

Lactase deficiency
Milk intolerance

ICD-9CM CODES
271.3 Lactose intolerance

EPIDEMIOLOGY & DEMOGRAPHICS

Nearly 50 million people in the United States have partial or complete lactose intolerance. There are racial differences, with <25% of white adults being lactose intolerant but >85% of Asian Americans and >60% of African Americans having some form of lactose intolerance.

PHYSICAL FINDINGS & CLINICAL PRESENTATION

- Abdominal tenderness and cramping, bloating, flatulence
- Diarrhea
- Symptoms are directly related to the osmotic pressure of substrate in the colon and occur approximately 2 hr after ingestion of lactose
- Physical examination: may be entirely within normal limits

ETIOLOGY

- Congenital lactase deficiency: common in premature infants; rare in term infants and generally inherited as a chromosomal recessive trait
- Secondary lactose intolerance: usually a result of injury of the intestinal mucosa (Crohn's disease, viral gastroenteritis, AIDS enteropathy, cryptosporidiosis, Whipple's disease, sprue)

DIAGNOSIS

DIFFERENTIAL DIAGNOSIS

- IBD
- IBS
- Pancreatic insufficiency
- Nontropical and tropical sprue
- Cystic fibrosis
- Diverticular disease
- Bowel neoplasm
- Laxative abuse
- Celiac disease
- Parasitic disease (e.g., giardiasis)
- Viral or bacterial infections

WORKUP

- The diagnosis can usually be made on the basis of the history and improvement with dietary manipulation.
- Diagnostic workup may include confirming the diagnosis with hydrogen breath test and excluding other conditions listed in the differential diagnosis that may also coexist with lactase deficiency.

LABORATORY TESTS

- Lactose breath hydrogen test: a rise in breath hydrogen >20 ppm within 90 min of ingestion of 50 g of lactose is positive for lactase deficiency. This test is positive in 90% of patients with lactose malabsorption. Common causes of false-negative results are recent use of oral antibiotics or recent high colonic enema.
- The lactose tolerance test is an older and less accurate testing modality (20% rate of false-positive and false-negative results). The patient is administered an oral dose of 1 to 1.5 g of lactose/kg body weight. Serial measurement of blood glucose level on an hourly basis for 3 hr is then performed. The test is considered positive if the patient develops intestinal symptoms and the blood glucose level rises <20 mg/dl above the fasting baseline level.
- Diarrhea associated with lactase deficiency is osmotic in nature with an osmotic gap and a pH <6.5.

IMAGING STUDIES

Imaging studies are generally not indicated. A small bowel series may be useful in patients with significant malabsorption.

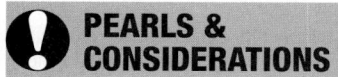 TREATMENT

NONPHARMACOLOGIC THERAPY

Management consists of reducing lactose exposure by avoiding milk and milk-containing products or using milk in which the lactose has been prehydrolized with lactase. A lactose-free diet generally results in prompt resolution of symptoms. Lactose is primarily found in dairy products but may be present as an ingredient or component of common foods and beverages. Possible sources of lactose include breads, candies, cold cuts, dessert mixes, cream soups, bologna, commercial sauces and gravies, chocolate, drink mixes, salad dressings, and medications. Labels should be read carefully to identify sources of lactose.

ACUTE GENERAL Rx

- Addition of lactase enzyme supplement (Lactaid tablets, Dairy Ease) before the ingestion of milk products may prevent symptoms in some patients. However, it is not effective for all lactose-intolerant patients.
- Lactose-intolerant patients must ensure adequate calcium intake. Calcium supplementation is recommended to prevent osteoporosis.

CHRONIC Rx

Patient education regarding foods high in lactose, such as milk, cottage cheese, or ice cream, is recommended.

DISPOSITION

Clinical improvement with restriction or elimination of milk products

REFERRAL

GI referral for endoscopic procedures if concomitant GI disorders are suspected

PEARLS & CONSIDERATIONS

COMMENTS

- There is great variability in signs and symptoms in patients with lactose intolerance depending on the degree of lactase deficiency. Most individuals with presumed lactose malabsorption can tolerate 12 to 15 g of lactose or up to 12 oz of milk daily without symptoms.
- Nondairy synthetic drinks (e.g., Coffee-Mate) and use of rice milk are well tolerated.

SUGGESTED READINGS
available at www.expertconsult.com

AUTHOR: **FRED F. FERRI, M.D.**

 **BASIC INFORMATION**

DEFINITION

Lambert-Eaton myasthenic syndrome (LEMS) is a disorder of neuromuscular transmission caused by antibodies directed against presynaptic voltage-gated P/Q calcium channels on motor and autonomic nerve terminals. There are two forms: paraneoplastic (most common) and nonparaneoplastic (autoimmune).

SYNONYMS

Eaton-Lambert syndrome

ICD-9CM CODES
199.1 Malignant neoplasm without specification of site, other

EPIDEMIOLOGY & DEMOGRAPHICS

INCIDENCE (IN U.S.): Uncertain; estimated at five cases per 1 million persons annually
PEAK INCIDENCE: Sixth decade
PREVALENCE (IN U.S.): Uncertain; estimated at one per 100,000. Up to 3% of small-cell lung cancer (SCLC) patients are estimated to develop LEMS.
PREDOMINANT SEX: Male:female ratio of 2:1.

PHYSICAL FINDINGS & CLINICAL PRESENTATION

- Weakness with diminished or absent muscle stretch reflexes
- Proximal lower extremity muscles affected most
- Ocular and bulbar muscles less commonly affected
- Transient strength improvement with brief exercise
- Reflexes may be facilitated by repeatedly tapping the tendon
- Autonomic dysfunction common (dry mouth in 75%, sexual dysfunction, blurred vision, constipation, orthostasis, etc.)

ETIOLOGY

- Antibodies directed against presynaptic voltage-gated P/Q calcium channels are present in most patients. The reduction in calcium influx causes a reduction in acetylcholine release at motor and autonomic nerve terminals.
- Paraneoplastic forms, usually associated with SCLC, are present in 50% to 70% of patients.
- Autoimmune forms, usually in patients with other autoimmune diseases, occur in 10% to 30%.

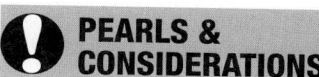 **DIAGNOSIS**

DIFFERENTIAL DIAGNOSIS

- Myasthenia gravis
- Polymyositis
- Primary myopathies
- Carcinomatous myopathies
- Polymyalgia rheumatica
- Botulism
- Guillain-Barré syndrome

Section II describes the differential diagnosis of muscle weakness.

WORKUP

Confirm diagnosis by characteristic electrodiagnostic (EMG/NCS) findings: reduced motor amplitudes with normal sensory studies; >10% decrement in motor amplitudes on slow repetitive nerve stimulation (RNS) at 2 to 3 Hz, with >100% increment on fast RNS (20 to 30 Hz) or immediately after 10 sec of maximum exercise (postexercise facilitation).

LABORATORY TESTS

Check P/Q calcium channel antibody titers (commercially available).

IMAGING STUDIES

Screen for an underlying malignancy. Presentation with LEMS may precede diagnosis of SCLC by up to 5 yr. Chest radiograph or CT of the chest may be required every 6 to 12 mo for SCLC.

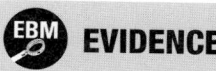 **TREATMENT**

NONPHARMACOLOGIC THERAPY

Symptomatic treatment for autonomic dysfunction.

ACUTE GENERAL Rx

- Anticholinesterase agents (pyridostigmine 30 to 60 mg q4-6h) may yield some improvement.
- Guanidine hydrochloride: start 5 to 10 mg/kg/day up to 30 mg/kg/day in 3-day intervals.
- Plasma exchange (200 to 250 ml/kg over 10 to 14 days) or IV immunoglobulins (2 g/kg over 2 to 5 days) often produce significant, temporary improvement.
- Prednisone 1.0 to 1.5 mg/kg/day can be gradually tapered over months to minimal effective dose.
- Azathioprine can be given alone or in combination with prednisone. Give up to 2.5 mg/kg/

day. If patient is intolerant, can administer cyclosporine up to 3 mg/kg/day instead.
- 3,4-diaminopyridine (3,4-DAP) 10 to 20 mg PO qid (maximum of 100 mg/day) may improve muscle strength and reduce autonomic symptoms in up to 85% of patients in uncontrolled series. It is available in Europe and may be available in the U.S. on a compassionate use basis.

CHRONIC Rx

Treat underlying malignancy if present.

DISPOSITION

- Gradually progressive weakness leading to impaired mobility if untreated
- Clinical remission may occur with chronic immunosuppressive therapy in 43% of cases
- Possible substantial improvement with successful treatment of underlying malignancy

REFERRAL

To a neurologist (recommended) because of the infrequency of this disease and risks associated with some treatments. Referral to specialist centers for 3,4-DAP therapy may be warranted in the U.S. Surgical referral for tumor debulking in paraneoplastic forms necessary.

⚠ PEARLS & CONSIDERATIONS

COMMENTS

- Prominent autonomic symptoms (dry eyes, dry mouth, impotence, orthostasis) are often the clue to the diagnosis in the appropriate clinical context.
- Many drugs may worsen weakness and should be used only if absolutely necessary. Included are succinylcholine, d-tubocurarine, quinine, quinidine, procainamide, aminoglycoside antibiotics, β-blockers, and calcium channel blockers.

EBM EVIDENCE

available at www.expertconsult.com

SUGGESTED READINGS
available at www.expertconsult.com

AUTHOR: **EROBOGHENE E. UBOGU, M.D.**

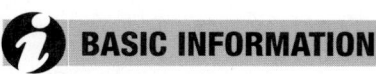

DEFINITION

Cancer of the larynx, including the vocal cords (glottis), supraglottis, and subglottis.

SYNONYMS

Laryngeal cancer

Head and neck cancer (subsite); other sites include oral cavity, pharynx, paranasal sinus, and salivary glands

ICD-9CM CODES
231.0 Carcinoma of larynx

EPIDEMIOLOGY & DEMOGRAPHICS

INCIDENCE: 12,000 new cases per year in the U.S.

PEAK INCIDENCE: Sixth decade

PREDOMINANT SEX: 80% male predominance (current, with past and projected increase in female rates as a result of changing smoking habits)

PHYSICAL FINDINGS & CLINICAL PRESENTATION

Glottis:
- Early diagnosis possible because of voice change (hoarseness). Any voice change of more than 2-wk duration should prompt a laryngeal examination.
- Supraglottis:
  1. No early symptom
  2. Cervical lymphadenopathy
  3. Neck pain or ear pain
  4. Discomfort during swallowing
  5. Odynophagia
  6. Later: hoarseness, dysphagia, airway obstruction
- Subglottis: Even more subtle than supraglottic lesion; the same signs occur, only later in the course.

ETIOLOGY

- Smoking (cigarette, cigar, or pipe)
- Alcohol intake/abuse
- Diet and nutritional deficiencies
- Gastroesophageal reflux
- Voice abuse
- Chronic laryngitis
- Exposure to wood dust
- Asbestosis
- Exposure to radiation
- Possible role of human papilloma virus

DIAGNOSIS

DIFFERENTIAL DIAGNOSIS

- Laryngitis
- Allergic and nonallergic rhinosinusitis
- Gastroesophageal reflux
- Voice abuse leading to hoarseness
- Laryngeal papilloma
- Vocal cord paralysis attributable to a neurologic condition or entrapment of the recurrent laryngeal nerve caused by mediastinal compression
- Tracheomalacia

STAGING:

Supraglottic:
- T_1: Tumor limited to one subsite with normal cord mobility
- T_2: Tumor invades mucosa of more than one subsite (e.g., base of tongue, vallecula, pyriform sinus) without fixation of larynx
- T_3: Tumor limited to larynx with vocal cord fixation or invasion of postcricoid area or preepiglottis
- T_4: Tumor invades thyroid cartilage or extends into soft tissue of the neck, thyroid, or esophagus

Glottic:
- T_1: Tumor limited to vocal cord with normal mobility
- T_{1a}: Tumor limited to one vocal cord
- T_{1b}: Tumor involves both vocal cords
- T_2: Tumor extends to supra or subglottis or impairs cord mobility
- T_3: Tumor limited to larynx with cord fixation
- T_4: Tumor invades through cartilage or other tissues beyond larynx

Stage grouping:
- Stage I: T_1, N0, M0
- Stage II: T_2, N0, M0
- Stage III: T_3, N0, M0
- T_1, T_2, T_3, N1, M0
- Stage IV: T_4, N0, N1, M0
- Any T, N2, N3, M0
- Any T, any N or M >0

WORKUP

- Laboratory: none
- Endoscopic laryngeal inspection
- After (and only after) diagnosis of the malignancy, imaging with CT or MRI should be undertaken to stage the disease

HISTOLOGIC CLASSIFICATION

Epithelial cancers:
- Squamous cell carcinoma in situ
- Superficially invasive cancer
- Verrucous carcinoma
- Pseudosarcoma
- Anaplastic cancer
- Transitional cell carcinoma
- Lymphoepithelial cancer
- Adenocarcinoma
- Neuroendocrine tumors, including small cell and carcinoid

Sarcomas:
- Metastatic malignancies

TREATMENT

ACUTE GENERAL Rx

- Early stage (T or T_2) has two options:
  1. Conservative surgery (partial laryngectomy) with neck dissection
  2. Primary radiation
- Intermediate stage has four options:
  1. Primary radiation alone
  2. Supraglottic laryngectomy with neck dissection
  3. Supraglottic laryngectomy with postoperative radiation
  4. Chemotherapy with radiation
- Advanced stage:
  1. Chemotherapy and radiation with total laryngectomy reserved for treatment failure

Glottis:
- Carcinoma in situ
  1. Microexcision
  2. Laser vaporization
  3. Radiation
- Early stage (T or T_2) has two options:
  1. Voice conservation surgery
  2. Radiation
- Intermediate stage (T_3)
  1. Combined radiation and chemotherapy (cisplatin and 5-fluorouracil)
  2. Total laryngectomy for treatment failure
- Advanced stage (T_4)
  1. Combined radiation and chemotherapy
  2. Total laryngectomy and neck dissection followed by postoperative radiation in unfavorable lesion or treatment failure

Subglottis:
- Total laryngectomy and approximate neck surgery to excise the tumor, followed by radiation

Unresected cancers:
- Induction chemotherapy and radiation followed by neck dissection in chemosensitive tumors, or by laryngectomy and neck dissection in chemoresistant tumors
- If hypopharyngeal involvement exists: laryngopharyngectomy, neck dissection, and postoperative radiation

DISPOSITION

Supraglottis 5-yr control:
- T_1 95% to 100%
- T_2 80% to 90%
- T_3 65% to 85%
- T_4 40% to 55%

Glottis 5-yr control:
- T_1 95% to 100%
- T_2 50% to 85%
- T_3 35% to 85%
- T_4 20% to 65%

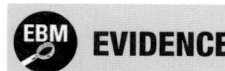 EVIDENCE

available at www.expertconsult.com

AUTHOR: **FRED F. FERRI, M.D.**

BASIC INFORMATION

DEFINITION

Laryngitis is an acute or chronic inflammation of the laryngeal mucous membranes.

SYNONYMS

Lower respiratory tract infection

ICD-9CM CODES
464.0 Acute laryngitis
476.0 Chronic laryngitis

EPIDEMIOLOGY & DEMOGRAPHICS

It is a common illness in both genders and all age groups, but the diagnosis is imprecise and, therefore, statistics are not readily available with respect to incidence and prevalence.

PHYSICAL FINDINGS & CLINICAL PRESENTATION

ACUTE LARYNGITIS:

- Clinical syndrome characterized by the onset of hoarseness, voice breaks, or episodes of aphonia; may also have accompanying sore throat, cough, nasal congestion, and rhinorrhea
- Usually associated with viral upper respiratory infection
- Larynx with diffuse erythema, edema, and vascular engorgement of the vocal folds, and occasionally mucosal ulceration
- In young children subglottis is often affected, resulting in airway narrowing with marked hoarseness, inspiratory stridor, dyspnea, and restlessness
- Respiratory compromise rare in adults

CHRONIC LARYNGITIS: Characterized by hoarseness or dysphonia persisting for longer than 2 wk

ETIOLOGY

ACUTE LARYNGITIS:

- Most often caused by viruses so treatment consists of supportive measures as outlined in "Nonpharmacologic Therapy" section.
- Studies evaluating the use of antibiotics (erythromycin, penicillin) in acute laryngitis failed to show objective clinical benefit over placebo so they are not routinely recommended. Antibiotics and other antimicrobials may be indicated in cases in which specific treatable pathogens are identified.
- Avoid decongestants because of their drying effect.
- Guaifenesin may be a useful adjunct as a mucolytic agent.

- In GERD-associated laryngitis use acid-suppressive therapy (H_2 blockers, proton pump inhibitors) and nocturnal antireflux precautions.

CHRONIC LARYNGITIS:

- Results from any of the following: tuberculosis, usually through bronchogenic spread; leprosy, from nasopharyngeal or oropharyngeal spread; syphilis, in secondary and tertiary stages; rhinoscleroma, extending from the nose and nasopharynx; actinomycosis; cryptococcosis histoplasmosis; blastomycosis; paracoccidiomycosis; coccidiosis; candidiasis; aspergillosis; sporotrichosis; rhinosporidiosis; parasitic infections including leishmaniasis and Clinostomum infection following raw fresh-water fish ingestion.
- Noninfectious causes of both acute and chronic laryngitis include malignancy, voice abuse (singers), GERD, and chemical or environmental irritants such as cigarettes and allergens. Other causes of inflammatory or granulomatous lesions of the larynx include relapsing polychondritis, Wegener's granulomatosis, and sarcoidosis.

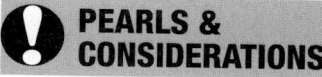

DIAGNOSIS

DIFFERENTIAL DIAGNOSIS

- Young children with signs of airway obstruction:
  - Supraglottitis (epiglottitis)
  - Laryngotracheobronchitis
  - Tracheitis
  - Foreign body aspiration
- Adults with persistent hoarseness, consider noninfectious causes of laryngitis as listed previously

WORKUP

- History and physical examination: diagnosis is usually apparent.
- Laryngoscopy for severe or persistent cases.
- Laryngeal cultures should be performed if a cause other than acute viral infection is suspected.
- Imaging not indicated unless there is evidence of airway compromise. Obtain plain radiographs of neck, anteroposterior and lateral views, to differentiate laryngitis from acute laryngotracheobronchitis or supraglottitis.

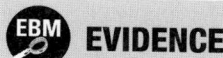

TREATMENT

NONPHARMACOLOGIC THERAPY

- Rest the voice.
- Use an air humidifier.

- Ensure adequate hydration. Avoid alcohol and caffeine because of diuretic effect.

ACUTE GENERAL Rx

- Antibiotics and other antimicrobials: indicated only when a specific pathogen is isolated; commonly employed antibacterial agents are macrolides; clarithromycin 500 mg by mouth bid for 5 to 7 days or azithromycin 500 mg followed by 250 mg once daily for 4 to 5 days if the cause of laryngitis is found to be *Mycoplasma pneumoniae* or *Chlamydiophila pneumoniae* (the new name for what was formerly known as *Chlamydia pneumoniae*).
- Avoid decongestants because of their drying effect.
- Guaifenesin may be a useful adjunct as a mucolytic agent.
- In GERD-associated laryngitis use acid-suppressive therapy (H_2 blockers, proton pump inhibitors) and nocturnal antireflux precautions.

DISPOSITION

Uncomplicated laryngitis is usually benign, with gradual resolution of symptoms.

REFERRAL

- If symptoms persist for >2 wk, refer to otolaryngologist for laryngoscopy.
- Consider referral to gastroenterologist if GERD is suspected.

PEARLS & CONSIDERATIONS

- Most cases of uncomplicated acute laryngitis are viral in origin, and antibacterial agents should not be routinely administered.
- A recent Cochrane analysis found no evidence for the use of empiric antibiotics in adults with laryngitis.
- The most difficult clinical challenge is often convincing patients with acute laryngitis that they do not need and will not benefit from antibacterial agents.

EVIDENCE

available at www.expertconsult.com

SUGGESTED READINGS

available at www.expertconsult.com

AUTHORS: **GLENN G. FORT, M.D., M.P.H.,** and **DENNIS J. MIKOLICH, M.D.**

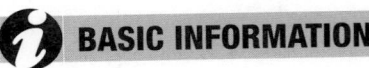 **BASIC INFORMATION**

DEFINITION

Acute laryngotracheobronchitis is a viral infection of the upper and lower respiratory tract leading to erythema and edema of the tracheal walls and narrowing of the subglottic region.

SYNONYMS

Croup

ICD-9CM CODES
464.4 Croup

EPIDEMIOLOGY & DEMOGRAPHICS

- Croup is primarily a disease of children occurring between the ages of 1 and 6 yr.
- The peak incidence of croup is the second yr of life (50 cases/1000 children).
- Most cases occur in the fall and represent parainfluenza type 1 viral infection.
- Winter outbreaks usually represent infection by influenza A and B viruses.
- Croup accounts for 10% to 15% of lower respiratory tract infections in young children.
- Boys are affected more often than girls.

PHYSICAL FINDINGS & CLINICAL PRESENTATION

Most children with croup present with symptoms of an upper respiratory infection for several days.

- Rhinorrhea
- Cough
- Low-grade fever
- Barking cough that usually occurs at night and awakes the child
- Sore throat
- Stridor
- Apprehension
- Use of accessory muscles of respiration
- Tachypnea
- Tachycardia
- Wheezing

ETIOLOGY

- Parainfluenza viruses (types 1, 2, and 3) are the most common causes of croup in the U.S.
- Influenza A and B, although not common causes of croup, do lead to more severe cases of the disease.
- Adenovirus.
- Respiratory syncytial virus.
- *Mycoplasma pneumoniae* (rare).

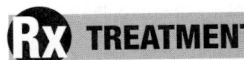 **DIAGNOSIS**

The diagnosis of croup is usually based on the characteristic clinical presentation of a young child between the ages of 1 and 6 yr waking up with a barking cough ("seal's bark") and stridor.

DIFFERENTIAL DIAGNOSIS

- Spasmodic croup
- Epiglottitis
- Bacterial tracheitis
- Angioneurotic edema
- Diphtheria
- Peritonsillar abscess
- Retropharyngeal abscess
- Smoke inhalation
- Foreign body

WORKUP

- The workup of a child with croup is to differentiate viral laryngotracheobronchitis from noninfectious causes of stridor and epiglottitis caused by *H. influenzae.*
- The clinical presentation and plain films of the soft tissues of the neck assist in differentiating viral from nonviral and noninfectious causes.

LABORATORY TESTS

- Laboratory tests are not often used to make the diagnosis of viral tracheobronchitis.
- CBC, viral serology, and tissue cultures can be ordered and may detect the infecting agent in up to 65% of cases.
- Pulse oximetry and ABG determination for patients with tachypnea and respiratory distress.

IMAGING STUDIES

- Plain (AP and lateral) films of the soft tissues of the neck may show the classic radiographic finding of subglottic stenosis or "steeple" sign.
- CT scan of the soft tissues of the neck may be performed in cases in which the differentiation between croup, epiglottitis, and noninfectious is more difficult.
- Direct visualization via laryngoscopy may be useful in some situations under a controlled setting.

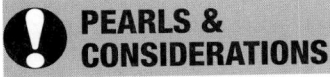 **TREATMENT**

Treatment of croup focuses on airway management.

NONPHARMACOLOGIC THERAPY

- Oxygen
- Cool mist
- Hot steam

ACUTE GENERAL Rx

- 0.25 to 0.75 ml of 2.25% racemic epinephrine every 20 min is used in children with severe respiratory symptoms, rest stridor, and impending intubation.
- Corticosteroids (e.g., dexamethasone 0.6 mg/kg IV or PO, prednisone 2 mg/kg/day) have been shown to be effective.
- Budesonide, a nebulized corticosteroid given at 4 mg, has been shown to improve symptoms in patients with moderate to severe croup.

DISPOSITION

- Croup is usually benign and self-limited, resolving within 3 to 4 days.
- Complications include:
  1. Airway obstruction
  2. Otitis media
  3. Pneumonia
  4. Dehydration

REFERRAL

If intubation is needed (rarely), an emergency consultation with ENT and/or anesthesiology is recommended.

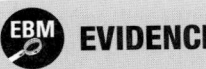 **PEARLS & CONSIDERATIONS**

COMMENTS

- Most patients with croup can be managed at home (e.g., patients without stridor and in no respiratory distress).
- Hospitalization and observation is required for children with moderate to severe croup (e.g., rest stridor, respiratory distress refractory to the previously mentioned acute treatments).

EBM EVIDENCE

available at www.expertconsult.com

SUGGESTED READING
available at www.expertconsult.com

AUTHORS: **GLENN G. FORT, M.D., M.P.H.,** and **DENNIS J. MIKOLICH, M.D.**

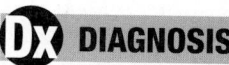

BASIC INFORMATION

DEFINITION

Lead is a potent, pervasive neurotoxicant. Lead poisoning refers to multisystem abnormalities resulting from excessive lead exposure.

SYNONYMS

Plumbism

ICD-9CM CODES
984.0 Lead poisoning

EPIDEMIOLOGY & DEMOGRAPHICS

- Lead poisoning is most common in children ages 1 to 5 yr (17,000 cases/100,000 persons). The highest rates are among blacks, those with low income, and urban children.
- In 1991 the Centers for Disease Control and Prevention (CDC) lowered the definition of a safe blood lead level to <10 μg/dl of whole blood (a blood lead level of 25 μg/dl was considered acceptable before 1991).
- It is estimated that >15% of preschoolers in the U.S. have a blood lead level >15 μg/dl.

PHYSICAL FINDINGS & CLINICAL PRESENTATION

- Findings vary with the degree of toxicity. Examination may be normal in patients with mild toxicity.
- Myalgias, irritability, headache, and general fatigue may be present initially.
- Abdominal cramping, constipation, weight loss, tremor, paresthesias and peripheral neuritis, seizures, and coma may occur with severe toxicity.
- Motor neuropathy is common in children with lead poisoning; learning disorders are also frequent.

ETIOLOGY

Chronic, repeated exposure to paint containing lead, plumbing, storage of batteries, pottery, or lead soldering. Concentration of lead is generally highest in lead-based paint on exterior surfaces. Among interior surfaces, windows are most likely to have the highest lead content.

DIAGNOSIS

DIFFERENTIAL DIAGNOSIS

- Polyneuropathies from other sources
- Anxiety disorder, attention deficit disorder
- Malabsorption, acute abdomen
- Iron-deficiency anemia

WORKUP

Laboratory screening: all U.S. children should be considered to be at risk for lead poisoning and should be screened routinely starting at age 1 yr for low-risk children and age 6 mo for high-risk children.

LABORATORY TESTS

- Venous blood lead level: normal level, <10 μg/dl; levels of 50 to 70 μg/dl, indicative of moderate toxicity; levels >70 μg/dl, associated with severe poisoning
- Mild anemia with basophilic stippling on peripheral smear
- Elevated zinc protoporphyrin levels or free erythrocyte protoporphyrin level
- An increased body burden of lead with previous high-level exposure in patients with occupational lead poisoning can be demonstrated by measuring the excretion of lead in urine after premedication with calcium ethylenediamine tetraacetic acid (EDTA) or another chelating agent

IMAGING STUDIES

- Imaging studies are generally not necessary.
- A plain abdominal film can visualize lead particles in the gut.
- "Lead lines" may be noted on x-ray films of long bones.

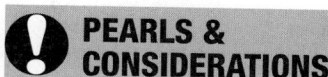 TREATMENT

NONPHARMACOLOGIC THERAPY

- Provide adequate amounts of calcium, iron, zinc, and protein in patient's diet
- Family education on sources of lead exposure and potential adverse health effects

ACUTE GENERAL Rx

- For children with blood levels of 10 to 19 mcg/dl, the CDC recommends nonpharmacologic interventions (see "Nonpharmacologic Therapy").
- For children with blood levels between 20 and 44 μg/dl, the CDC recommendations include case management by a qualified social worker, clinical management, environmental assessment, and lead hazard control. Chelation therapy should be considered in children with refractory blood lead levels.

Chelation therapy is indicated in children with blood lead levels >45 μg/dl:
- Succimer (DMSA) 10 mg/kg PO q8h for 5 days then q12h for 2 wk can be used in patients with levels between 45 and 70 μg/dl.
- Edetate calcium disodium (EDTA) and dimercaprol (BAL) are effective in patients with severe toxicity.

- Use of both EDTA and DMSA is indicated in children with blood levels >70 μg/dl.
- d-Penicillamine (Cuprimine) can also be used for lead poisoning, but it is not FDA approved for this condition.

CHRONIC Rx

- Reduce exposure, remove any potential lead sources.
- Correct iron deficiency and any other nutritional deficiencies.
- Recheck blood lead level 7 to 21 days after chelation therapy.

DISPOSITION

Patients with mild to moderate toxicity generally improve without any residual deficits. The presence of encephalopathy at diagnosis is a poor prognostic sign. Residual neurologic deficits may persist in these patients. Chelation therapy seems to slow the progression of renal insufficiency in patients with mildly elevated body lead burden.

REFERRAL

If exposure to lead is work related, it should be reported to the Office of the United States Occupational Safety and Health Administration (OSHA). Follow-up testing is mandatory in all patients after an abnormal screening blood lead level.

PEARLS & CONSIDERATIONS

COMMENTS

- Even blood lead concentrations <10 mcg/dl are inversely associated with children's IQ scores at age 3 and 5 yr.
- Screening of household members of affected individuals is recommended.
- In children with blood lead levels of >45 mg/dl, treatment with succimer does not improve scores on tests of cognition, behavior, or neuropsychological function.
- Lead toxicity may delay growth and pubertal development in girls.
- Low-level environmental lead exposure may accelerate progressive renal insufficiency in patients without diabetes who have chronic renal disease. Repeated chelation therapy may improve renal function and slow the progression of renal failure.

SUGGESTED READINGS

available at www.expertconsult.com

AUTHOR: **FRED F. FERRI, M.D.**

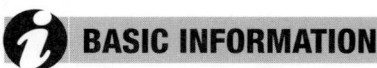

BASIC INFORMATION

DEFINITION

Legg-Calvé-Perthes disease is a self-limited disorder of unknown etiology caused by ischemia of the immature femoral head that leads to bone necrosis and variable amounts of collapse during the reparative process.

SYNONYMS

Coxa plana
Capital femoral osteochondrosis

ICD-9CM CODES
732.1 Perthes' disease

EPIDEMIOLOGY & DEMOGRAPHICS

PREVALENCE: One case in 1300 children
PREDOMINANT SEX: Male:female ratio of 4:1
PREDOMINANT AGE: 3 to 10 yr

PHYSICAL FINDINGS & CLINICAL PRESENTATION

- Initial symptom: usually a mildly painful limp
- Pain referred down the inner aspect of the thigh to the knee
- Moderate restriction of motion resulting from hip synovitis (abduction and internal rotation are especially limited)
- Pain at the extremes of movement and tenderness over anterior hip joint

ETIOLOGY

Unknown

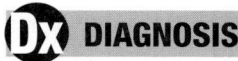

DIAGNOSIS

DIFFERENTIAL DIAGNOSIS

- Transient synovitis
- Low-grade septic arthritis
- Juvenile rheumatoid arthritis

WORKUP

Diagnosis is usually based on the physical findings and eventual radiographic findings.

IMAGING STUDIES

- Plain roentgenography to establish the diagnosis (Fig. 1-214)
- AP and frog-leg lateral radiographs
- Technetium bone scanning to help confirm the diagnosis in early cases

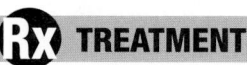

TREATMENT

ACUTE GENERAL Rx

- A brief period of bed rest (1 to 3 days) followed by bracing (except in mild cases)
- Bracing possibly required for 2 to 3 yr in small percent of patients

DISPOSITION

- Prognosis depends on age of patient and degree of involvement of the femoral head at onset.
- Young patients (<6 yr) with minimal involvement do well.
- Older patients (>8 yr) often do poorly.
- A few patients eventually develop degenerative arthritis.

REFERRAL

For orthopedic consultation when diagnosis is suspected

PEARLS & CONSIDERATIONS

Both the etiology and treatment of Legg-Calvé-Perthes disease remain controversial. Treatment recommendations vary widely and continue to evolve.

COMMENTS

There is great uncertainty regarding treatment and its effect on outcome. Bracing may have no effect whatsoever on the end result.

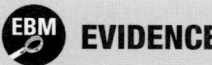

EVIDENCE

available at www.expertconsult.com

SUGGESTED READINGS

available at www.expertconsult.com

AUTHOR: **LONNIE R. MERCIER, M.D.**

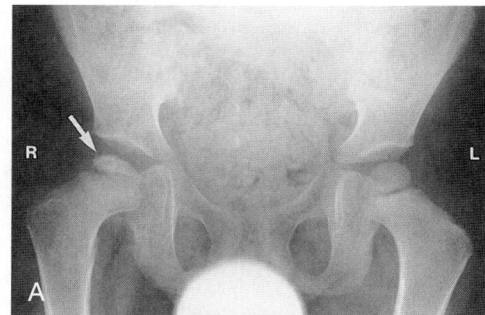

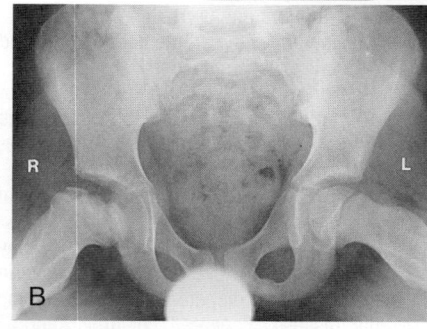

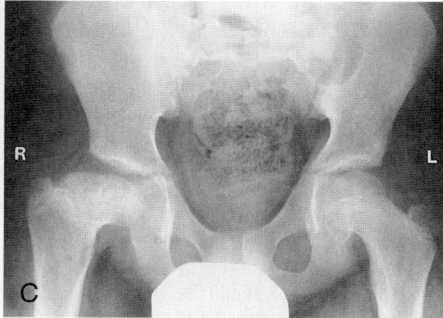

FIGURE 1-214 Legg-Calvé-Perthes disease. A, An anteroposterior view of the pelvis demonstrates fragmentation and sclerosis of the right femoral epiphysis *(arrow)* in this 6-year-old boy. **B,** A follow-up film obtained 8 years later shows continuing deformity resulting from the osteonecrosis. The patient developed significant degenerative arthritis **(C)** by the age of 12 years. (From Mettler FA [ed]: *Primary care radiology,* Philadelphia, 2000, WB Saunders.)

BASIC INFORMATION

DEFINITION

Leishmaniasis is an infectious disease caused by a heterogeneous group of protozoan parasites belonging to the genus *Leishmania* and resulting in a variety of different clinical syndromes.

SYNONYMS

Kala azar
Old world leishmaniasis
New world leishmaniasis

ICD-9CM CODES
085.9 Leishmaniasis

EPIDEMIOLOGY & DEMOGRAPHICS

INCIDENCE: ~2 million total new cases and 500,000 visceral cases occur each year with almost 400 million people at risk for the disease.
- Can be classified geographically into new world versus old world disease.
- Infection can be divided into cutaneous, mucocutaneous, visceral disease.
- Incubation period: from 1 wk to many mo for cutaneous and mucosal leishmaniasis; 2 to 6 mo (range is 10 days to years) for visceral leishmaniasis.
- Mode of transmission: by the female sandfly vector; can also be spread via shared needles, blood transfusions, organ transplants, vertically from the mother to fetus, or sexually.
- Cutaneous leishmaniasis has been reported in U.S. military personnel in Iraq (more than 500 cases from 2002 to 2004).
- Travelers to endemic areas have become infected after <1 week exposure.

PHYSICAL FINDINGS & CLINICAL PRESENTATION

Cutaneous syndrome
- Localized cutaneous leishmaniasis
- Mucosal leishmaniasis
- Leishmania recidivans
- Diffuse cutaneous leishmaniasis
Visceral syndrome
- Viscerotrophic leishmaniasis: fever, chronic fatigue, malaise, cough, intermittent diarrhea, and abdominal pain. Signs include adenopathy, hepatosplenomegaly, hyperpigmentation of skin, petechiae, jaundice, edema, and ascites
- Post–kala-azar dermal leishmaniasis: generalized cutaneous rash that is often papular or nodular; severe forms with desquamation of skin and mucosa

ETIOLOGY
- Old-world parasite: *Leishmania tropica, L. major, L. aethiopica, L. donovani, L. infantum*
- New-world parasite: *L. braziliensis* and *L. mexicana complex, L. chagasi, L. b. guyanensis, L. b. panamensis*

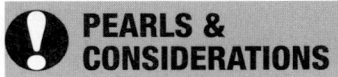 **DIAGNOSIS**

DIFFERENTIAL DIAGNOSIS
- Malaria
- African trypanosomiasis
- Brucellosis
- Enteric fever
- Bacterial endocarditis
- Generalized histoplasmosis
- Chronic myelocytic leukemia
- Hodgkin's disease and other lymphomas
- Sarcoidosis
- Hepatic cirrhosis
- Tuberculosis

WORKUP
- CBC
- LFTs
- Renal panel
- Serology
- Biopsy for histology and culture
- PCR
- Bone marrow bx for visceral disease
- Splenic aspirate often done in resource-poor settings.

LABORATORY TESTS
- CBC: anemia, neutropenia, thrombocytopenia, and eosinopenia
- LFTs: hypergammaglobulinemia, hypoalbuminemia, and hyperbilirubinemia
- Elevated BUN and creatinine
- Specific diagnosis confirmed by intracellular amastigote in Giemsa-stained impression smears or sectioned tissue or culture performed in NMN (Novy, MacNeal, Nicolle) or Schneider's medium
- Serologic diagnosis: ELISA, direct agglutination tests, K39 ELISA, PCR, and monoclonal antibody staining of tissue smears; ELISA and DAT on urine specimens
- Montenegro skin test

Rx **TREATMENT**

Nonspecific or supportive care
1. Nutritional diet
2. Antimicrobial agents for concurrent infections
3. Blood transfusions
4. Iron and vitamins
Specific antileishmanial therapy
1. Miltefosine (2.5 mg/kg/day orally in two divided doses for 28 days) is an optional choice for visceral disease.
2. Pentavalent antimonials: sodium stibogluconate and sodium antimony gluconate may be used, but resistance has emerged in some geographic areas (e.g., in Asia).
3. Liposomal amphotericin B in various regimens is the preferred drug for visceral leishmaniasis.
4. Fluconazole 200 mg PO daily for 6 wk probably effective for cutaneous disease, but not a first-line drug.
5. Pentamidine 2 to 4 mg/kg/day for 15 doses IV. Extreme toxicity. Often used as salvage therapy.
6. Other agents: paromomycin (combined with other regimens).
7. Immunotherapy: IFN-γ.
8. Local or tropical treatments and physical therapy, including thermal treatments.
9. Plastic surgery.

DISPOSITION

Follow-up examination is important for the early detection and treatment relapse.

REFERRAL

To infectious disease experts for accurate diagnosis and management

PEARLS & CONSIDERATIONS

COMMENTS
- Prevention by reservoir control: destruction of animal reservoir hosts, mass treatment of humans in kala-azar–prevalent areas.
- Prevention by vector control: insecticide spraying in domestic and peridomestic areas.
- Vaccines are in various stages of development and clinical trials. None are licensed or commercially available at this time.
- Co-infection with HIV requires more intense therapy as well as HAART.

SUGGESTED READINGS
available at www.expertconsult.com

AUTHOR: **PATRICIA CRISTOFARO, M.D.**

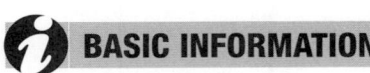

ℹ️ BASIC INFORMATION

DEFINITION
Leprosy is a chronic granulomatous infection of humans that primarily affects the skin and peripheral nerves.

SYNONYMS
Hansen's disease

ICD-9CM CODES
030.9 Leprosy

EPIDEMIOLOGY & DEMOGRAPHICS
- The number of cases worldwide has fallen from more than 5 million cases in 1985 to about 612,000 cases in 2002 according to the WHO.
- Nearly 75% of the cases of leprosy are found in India, Brazil, Nepal, Mozambique, Madagascar, and Myanmar (see Fig. 1-216).
- More than 85% of the cases diagnosed in the U.S. are found among immigrants.
- Annual incidence in the United States is between 100 and 200 new cases per year.
- Leprosy is more common in men than women (2:1).
- Leprosy can occur at any age but usually is found in young children.

PHYSICAL FINDINGS & CLINICAL PRESENTATION
- A skin lesion: most common initial presentation
- Sensory loss
- Anhidrosis
- Neuritic pain
- Palpable peripheral nerves
- Nerve damage (most commonly affected nerves are ulnar, median, common peroneal, posterior tibial, radial cutaneous nerve of the wrist, facial, and posterior auricular)
- Muscle atrophy and weakness
- Foot drop
- Claw hand and claw toes
- Lagophthalmos, nasal septal perforation, collapse of bridge of nose (Fig. 1-215A), loss of eyebrows resulting in "leonine" facies
- Leprosy can present along a spectrum from simple cutaneous skin lesions with minimal sensory loss (Fig. 1-215B) to severe extensive skin involvement, painful neuritis, muscle wasting and contractures, and multiple peripheral nerve damage.

ETIOLOGY
- Leprosy is caused by *Mycobacterium leprae,* an obligate intracellular acid-fast rod.
- The mode of transmission remains elusive. Spread in humans is thought to occur via the respiratory route or entry through broken skin in patients with multibacillary disease or extensive paucibacillary disease.
- Zoonotic transmission from armadillos has been shown in only a few case reports.
- The majority of people exposed to patients with leprosy do not develop the disease because of their natural immunity. Variants of genes in the *NOD2*-mediated signaling pathway (which regulates the innate immune response) are associated with susceptibility to infection with *M. leprae.*
- Incubation period is 3 to 5 yr.

℞ DIAGNOSIS

- The diagnosis of leprosy relies on a detailed history and physical examination and is established by the demonstration of acid-fast bacilli in skin smears or skin biopsies of the affected sites.
- Leprosy has been classified according to the WHO system into:
  1. Paucibacillary leprosy is defined as <five skin lesions with no bacilli on skin smear.
  2. Multibacillary leprosy is defined as >five skin lesions and may be skin-smear positive.
- Leprosy has also been classified by the Ridley-Jopling system based on the type of skin lesions, sensory and motor deficits, and biopsy into:
  1. Indeterminate leprosy
  2. Tuberculoid leprosy (paucibacillary [few organisms], intense inflammatory reaction; few, well-demarcated skin lesions)
  3. Borderline tuberculoid leprosy
  4. Borderline lepromatous leprosy
  5. Lepromatous leprosy (multibacillary [numerous organisms], inadequate host response; diffuse, poorly organized skin lesions)

DIFFERENTIAL DIAGNOSIS
The differential diagnosis of leprosy includes: sarcoidosis, rheumatoid arthritis, systemic lupus erythematosus, lymphomatoid granulomatosis, carpal tunnel syndrome, cutaneous leishmaniasis, fungal infections and other causes of hypopigmented, hyperpigmented, and erythematous skin lesions.

WORKUP
Any patient who presents with skin lesions and a sensory or muscle deficit should have a workup for leprosy.

LABORATORY TESTS
- *Mycobacterium leprae* cannot be cultured on artificial media. The bacteria proliferate when

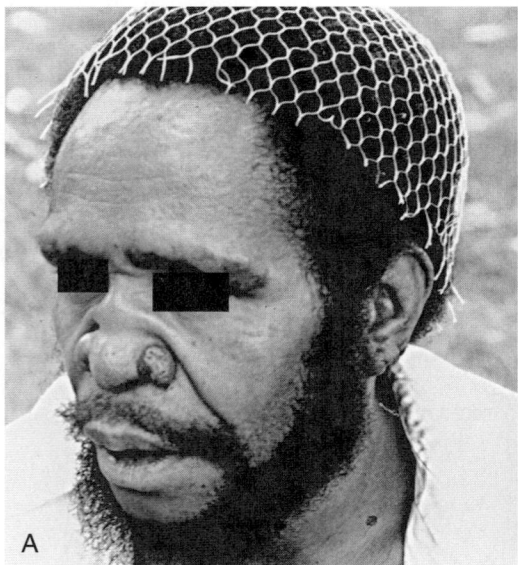
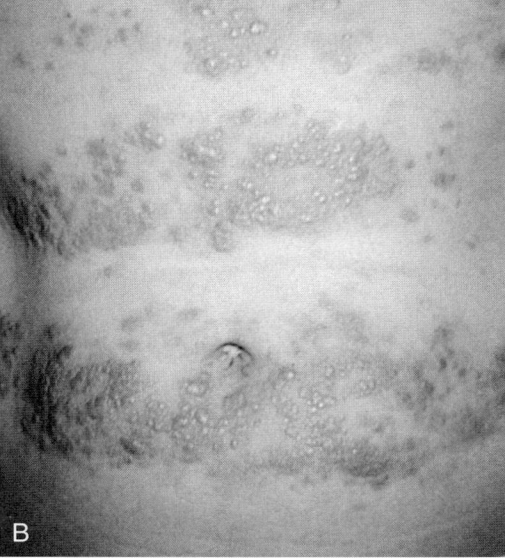

FIGURE 1-215 A, Advanced lepromatous leprosy with collapse of the nasal septum. **B,** Lepromatous leprosy characterized by extensive papule formation over abdomen. Minimal or no sensory loss is present in the affected areas. (**A,** From Gorbach SL: *Infectious diseases,* ed 2, Philadelphia, 1998, WB Saunders; **B,** From Mandell GL: *Mandell, Douglas, and Bennett's principles and practice of infectious diseases,* ed 5, New York, 2000, Churchill Livingstone.)

injected into the footpads of mice or armadillos and can be used for drug-sensitivity testing.
- Serologic tests, including the antibody to phenolic glycolipid 1 (PGL-1) and bacilli detection in tissue using PCR, are available and used for diagnostic confirmation and research epidemiologic studies.
- Lepromin intradermal skin test is not diagnostic and not for commercial use.
- Skin smears are taken from active sites or most commonly from the earlobe, elbows, or knees and are stained for acid-fast bacilli.
- Skin biopsies of active sites are stained for acid-fast bacilli.
- Peripheral nerve biopsy can be done in patients with sensory loss and no skin lesions. Common nerves biopsied are the radial cutaneous nerve of the wrist and the sural nerve of the ankle.

IMAGING STUDIES

Radiograph studies are usually of no benefit in the diagnosis or treatment of leprosy.

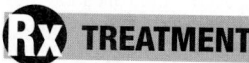 **TREATMENT**

NONPHARMACOLOGIC THERAPY
- Physical therapy for patients with upper and lower extremity deformities
- Proper foot care and footwear to prevent ulcer formation

ACUTE GENERAL Rx
CURRENT STANDARD US REGIMENS:
For paucibacillary leprosy:
- Dapsone 100 mg PO q day plus rifampin 600 mg PO q day for 6 mo, followed by dapsone monotherapy for 3 yr for indeterminate and tuberculoid leprosy and 5 yr for borderline tuberculoid leprosy.

For multibacillary leprosy:
- Dapsone 100 mg PO q day plus rifampin 600 mg PO q day for 3 yr, followed by dapsone montherapy for 10 yr for borderline and indefinitely for borderline lepromatous or lepromatous.
- If dapsone resitance suspected, clofazimine 50 mg daily should be added.

CHRONIC Rx
- If relapse occurs, the patient is treated with the same medical regimen; drug resistance is low.
- If relapse is from paucibacillary to multibacillary, the medical regimen for multibacillary should be used for therapy.

DISPOSITION
- Relapse is <1% for multibacillary and just over 1% in paucibacillary cases.
- Patients are initially followed up monthly and, when treatment is completed, every 3 to 6 mo for the next 5 to 10 yr.
- Some patients develop reactions known as erythema nodosum leprosum and reversal reaction, usually during treatment.
  1. Erythema nodosum leprosum results in tender nodules and is treated with thalidomide 100 mg qid then tapered with response. Cases not responsive to thalidomide are treated with prednisone 60 to 80 mg q day.
  2. Reactive reaction results in the development of new skin lesions with swelling and erythema of existing lesions. Treatment is with prednisone 60 to 80 mg a day then a taper dose. Clofazimine aqnd dapsone are options. Do not use thalidomide.
  3. Other agents used in the treatment of leprosy include ofloxacin, moxifloxacin, minocycline and clarithromycin.

REFERRAL
- National Hansen's Disease Programs (NHDP) Center in Baton Rouge, Louisiana, and 15 outpatient clinics in the United States offer consultations and treatment. Telephone: 1-800-642-2477.
- Directly observed therapy (DOT), much like DOT for tuberculosis, is highly desirable and should be used if feasible, at least in the first 6 to 12 mo of therapy.
- Any suspected case of leprosy merits an infectious disease consultation. Consultation with orthopedic, podiatry, ophthalmology, physical therapy, plastic surgery, and psychology are all in order for any of the potential sequelae of the disease.

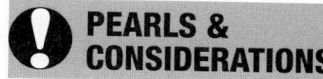 **PEARLS & CONSIDERATIONS**

COMMENTS
- The risk of transmission is low in patients with leprosy, and therefore no infection control precautions of hospitalized patients is needed.
- Family members and close contacts need to be examined frequently for the development of lesions.
- Dapsone or rifampin prophylaxis is not recommended in the prevention of leprosy.
- BCG vaccination has a 50% efficacy in the prevention of leprosy and may be considered.

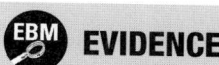 **EVIDENCE**

available at www.expertconsult.com

SUGGESTED READINGS
available at www.expertconsult.com

AUTHORS: **GLENN G. FORT, M.D., M.P.H.,** and **DENNIS J. MIKOLICH, M.D.**

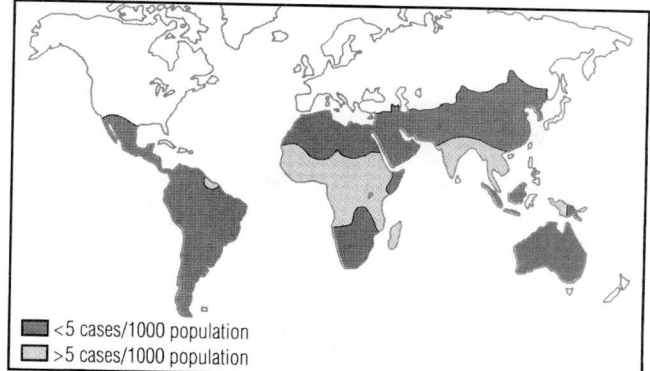

■ <5 cases/1000 population
□ >5 cases/1000 population

FIGURE 1-216 Geographical distribution of leprosy. (From Souhami RL, Moxham J: *Textbook of medicine,* ed 4, London, 2002, Churchill Livingstone.)

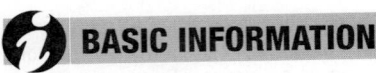

BASIC INFORMATION

DEFINITION

Leptospirosis is a zoonosis caused by the spirochete *Leptospira interrogans.*

SYNONYMS

Weil's disease

ICD-9CM CODES
100.9 Leptospirosis

EPIDEMIOLOGY & DEMOGRAPHICS

INCIDENCE (IN U.S.):

- 0.05 cases/100,000 persons
- Significant underestimation because of underreporting
- Hawaii consistently has the highest reported annual incidence rate in U.S.

PEAK INCIDENCE: Summer months, into the fall
PREDOMINANT SEX: Male (4:1)
PREDOMINANT AGE: Teenagers and young adults
GENETICS: Neonatal infection can occur

PHYSICAL FINDINGS & CLINICAL PRESENTATION (see Table 1-91)

ANICTERIC FORM:

- Milder and more common presentation of disease
- A self-limited systemic illness with two stages:
  1. Septicemic stage: presents abruptly with fevers, headache, severe myalgias, rigors, prostration, and sometimes circulatory collapse; conjunctival suffusion is common; skin rash, pharyngitis, lymphadenopathy, hepatomegaly, splenomegaly.
  2. Immune stage: occurs a few days after first stage with similar symptoms; hallmark is aseptic meningitis.

ICTERIC LEPTOSPIROSIS (WEIL'S SYNDROME):

1. Denotes severe cases, with symptoms of hepatic, renal, and vascular dysfunction
2. Biphasic course: persistence of fever, jaundice, and azotemia
3. Complications: oliguria or anuria, hemorrhage, hypotension, vascular collapse

ETIOLOGY

Caused by a spirochete, *L. interrogans*
- Infects a variety of animals, including most mammals
- Specific serotypes associated with different hosts—*pomona* in livestock, *canicola* in dogs, and *icterohaemorrhagiae* in rodents
- Organism penetrates skin or mucous membranes through exposure to animal urine or infected water

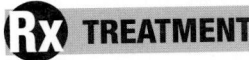

DIAGNOSIS

DIFFERENTIAL DIAGNOSIS

- Bacterial meningitis
- Viral hepatitis
- Influenza
- Legionnaire's disease

WORKUP

Culture of blood, CSF, and urine:
- Organism can be isolated from blood or CSF during first 10 days of illness.
- Urine should be cultured after first wk and for up to 30 days after onset of illness.

LABORATORY TESTS

- Normal or elevated WBCs, at times with leukemoid reactions up to 70,000/mm^3
- Elevated transaminases or bilirubin
- Anemia, azotemia, hypoprothrombinemia in those with icteric illness
- Elevated CK in first phase
- Meningitis in both phases, but aseptic in second phase

IMAGING STUDIES

Chest radiographs to show interstitial nonlobar infiltrates

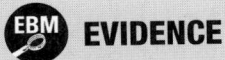

TREATMENT

NONPHARMACOLOGIC THERAPY

- Supportive
- Observation for dehydration, hypotension, renal failure, hemorrhage

ACUTE GENERAL Rx

- IV penicillin G 1 million U q4h
- Doxycycline 100 mg PO bid for 7 days
- Vitamin K administration if hypoprothrombinemia present
- Possible Jarisch-Herxheimer reaction when treated with penicillin

DISPOSITION

- In anicteric leptospirosis, antibiotics can decrease severity and duration of symptoms.
- Icteric leptospirosis, even with supportive therapy, may have a mortality as high as 10%.

REFERRAL

- If more than mild disease
- If no response to treatment

EBM EVIDENCE

available at www.expertconsult.com

SUGGESTED READINGS

available at www.expertconsult.com

AUTHORS: **DENNIS J. MIKOLICH, M.D.,** and **GLENN G. FORT, M.D.**

TABLE 1-91 Signs and Symptoms of Admission in Patients with Leptospirosis in Large Case Series

	Puerto Rico, 1963 n = 208	China, 1965 n = 168	Vietnam, 1973 n = 150	Korea, 1987 n = 93	Barbados, 1990 n = 88	Seychelles, 1998 n = 75	Brazil, 1999 n = 193	Hawaii, 2001 n = 353	India, 2002 n = 74
Percent with:									
Jaundice	49	0	1.5	16	95	27	93	39	34
Anorexia	—	46	—	80	85	—	—	82	—
Headache	91	90	98	70	76	80	75	89	92
Conjunctival suffusion	99	57	42	58	54	—	28.5	73	35
Vomiting	69	18	33	32	50	40	—	91	—
Myalgia	97	64	79	40	49	63	94	59	68
Arthralgia	—	36	—	—	—	31	—	51	12
Abdominal pain	—	26	28	40	43	41	—	77	—
Nausea	75	29	41	46	37	—	—	—	—
Dehydration	—	—	—	—	37	—	—	—	—
Cough	24	57	20	45	32	39	—	—	—
Hemoptysis	9	51	—	40	—	13	20	16	35
Hepatomegaly	69	28	15	17	27	—	—	—	15
Lymphadenopathy	24	49	21	—	21	—	—	53	—
Diarrhea	27	20	29	36	14	11	—	8	12
Rash	6	—	7	—	2	—	—	—	—

Mandell GL, Bennett JE, Dolin R: *Principles and practice of infectious diseases,* ed 7, Philadelphia, 2010, Elsevier.

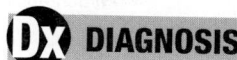 BASIC INFORMATION

DEFINITION

Acute lymphoblastic leukemia (ALL) is characterized by uncontrolled proliferation of abnormal, immature lymphocytes and their progenitors, ultimately replacing normal bone marrow elements.

SYNONYMS

Lymphoid leukemia
ALL

ICD-9CM CODES
204.0 Acute lymphoblastic leukemia

EPIDEMIOLOGY & DEMOGRAPHICS

- ALL is primarily a disease of children (peak incidence from ages 2 to 10 yr).
- It is diagnosed in 3000 to 4000 persons in the U.S. each year; two thirds are children.

PHYSICAL FINDINGS & CLINICAL PRESENTATION

- Skin pallor, purpura, or easy bruising
- Lymphadenopathy or hepatosplenomegaly
- Fever, bone pain, oliguria, weakness, weight loss, mental status changes

ETIOLOGY

- Unknown; increased risk in patients with a previous use of antineoplastic agents (e.g., chemotherapy of non-Hodgkin's lymphoma, Hodgkin's disease, ovarian cancer, myeloma)
- Environmental factors (e.g., ionizing radiation), toxins (e.g., benzene)

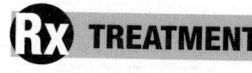 DIAGNOSIS

DIFFERENTIAL DIAGNOSIS

- Acute myeloid leukemia (AML): the distinction between ALL and AML (see Table 1-92) and the classification of the various subtypes are based on the following factors:
  1. Cell morphology
     - Lymphoblasts: a high nucleus/cytoplasmic ratio; cytoplasmic granules are usually not present.
     - Myeloblasts: abundant cytoplasm; cytoplasmic granules (Auer rods) are often present.
  2. Histochemical stains
     - Peroxidase and Sudan black stains: negative in ALL; useful to distinguish nonlymphoid from lymphoid cells.
     - Chloracetate esterase: a pink cytoplasmic reaction identifies granulocytes; useful to distinguish granulocytes from monocytes in patients with AML.
- Lymphoblastic lymphoma
- Aplastic anemia
- Infectious mononucleosis
- Leukemoid reaction to infection
- Multiple myeloma

WORKUP

- Laboratory evaluation
- Bone marrow examination (with biopsy, cytochemistry, immunophenotyping, and cytogenetics)
- Lumbar puncture and imaging studies

LABORATORY TESTS

- Complete blood count reveals normochromic, normocytic anemia, thrombocytopenia.
- Peripheral smear will reveal lymphoblasts.
- Initial blood work should also include blood urea nitrogen, creatinine, serum electrolytes, uric acid, and lactate dehydrogenase.
- Special diagnostic tests include immunophenotyping, cytogenetics, and cytochemistry.
- The French, American, British (FAB) Cooperative Study Group has classified ALL into three groups (L1 to L3) on the basis of cell size, cytoplasmic appearance, nucleus shape, and chromatin pattern. The most common form is the L2 type.
- Immunologic classification is made on the basis of expression of surface antigens by blast cells: T lineage and B lineage.

IMAGING STUDIES

- Chest x-ray to evaluate for the presence of mediastinal mass
- CT scan or ultrasound of abdomen/pelvis to assess splenomegaly or leukemic infiltration of abdominal organs

TREATMENT

ACUTE GENERAL Rx
Table 1-93 summarizes the preferred approach to the treatment of adult ALL patients.

DISPOSITION

- Prognosis is generally poorer in adult disease compared with childhood disease (40% adult cure rate versus 80% cure rate in children).
- Five-year leukemia-free survival is <40%.
- The different clinical outcomes associated with the various subtypes of ALL can be attributed primarily to drug sensitivity or resistance of leukemic blasts harboring specific genetic abnormalities. For example, cases of ALL expressing the TEL-AML1 fusion protein are very responsive to intensive chemotherapy with asparaginase, whereas the presence of Philadelphia chromosome (Ph{ΣY}+ {/ΣY}), monosomy 5 and 7, and abnormalities of 11q23 are bad prognostic signs in ALL.
- Genetic alteration (deletion) of IKZF1 is associated with a very poor outcome in B-cell-progenitor ALL.
- Outcome of adult ALL patients according to subgroups is summarized in Table 1-94.

REFERRAL

Referral to a hematologist is indicated in all cases of ALL.

TABLE 1-92 Morphologic, Cytochemical, and Biochemical Characteristics Helpful in Distinguishing Acute Lymphoblastic Leukemia from Acute Myelocytic Leukemia

Morphologic Features	ALL	AML
Nuclear/cytoplasmic ratio	High	Low
Nuclear chromatin	Clumped	Spongy
Nucleoli	0-2	2-5
Granules	−	+
Auer rods	−	+/−
Cytoplasm	Blue	Blue-gray
Cytochemical Reaction		
Peroxidase	−	+
Sudan Black B	−	+
Periodic Acid-Schiff	+/−	−
Naphthyl AS-D chloroacetate esterase	−	+/−
α-Naphthyl acetate esterase	−	+/−
α-Naphthyl butyrate esterase	−	−
Terminal deoxynucleotidyl transferase	+*	−

Table provides information on characteristics that may be useful in differentiating acute lymphoblastic leukemia (ALL) from acute myelocytic leukemia (AML) (see text for details). Wide variation in morphology is encountered in both disease categories. Diagnostic evaluation should include more refined classification of disease according to FAB subtype.
*Terminal deoxynucleotidyl transferase is usually negative in FAB L3 ALL.
Hoffman R, Benz EJ, Shattil SJ, Furie B, Silberstein LE, McGlave P, Heslop H: *Hematology, basic principles, and practice*, ed 5, Churchill Livingstone, 2009.

TABLE 1-93 Preferred Approach to the Treatment of Adult Acute Lymphocytic Leukemia Patients

	Low-Risk ALL	High-Risk ALL	Very High-Risk ALL	Mature B-ALL
Definition	*B-lineage* WBC <30,000/μl Time to CR <4 wk No Pro-B/ t(4;11) *T-lineage* Thy ALL Molecular CR	*B-lineage* WBC >30,000/μl Time to CR >4 wk Pro-B/ t(4;11) *T-lineage* Early T, mature T No molecular CR	Ph/BCR-ABL positive	
Multidrug-induction	Yes	Yes	Yes + imatinib	Short intensive cycles including HDM, fractionated C, HDAC and other drugs Rituximab
CNS prophylaxis*	Yes	Yes	Yes	Yes
Consolidation (also other combinations)	Alternating cycles, e.g., HDM, HDAC, Asparaginase reinduction	One cycle	One cycle + imatinib	6 cycles
SCT in CR1	None	Allogeneic SCT (if matched related or unrelated donor) Autologous SCT After additional (if no donor and negative MRD, consolidation)		None
Maintenance	6-MP/M + intensification for 2-2½ yr		imatinib	None

AC, Cytosine arabinoside; *ALL,* acute lymphocytic leukemia; *CR,* complete remission; *HDM,* high-dose methotrexate; *SCT,* stem cell transplantation; *MRD,* minimal residual disease; *Thy ALL,* thymic ALL.
*Intrathecal therapy with M or triple combination (M, AC, steroid) continued during maintenance therapy; additional CNS irradiation and/or high-dose chemotherapy according to subgroup.
Hoffman R, Benz EJ, Shattil SJ, Furie B, Silberstein LE, McGlave P, Heslop H: *Hematology, basic principles, and practice,* ed 5, Churchill Livingstone, 2009.

TABLE 1-94 Outcome of Adult Lymphocytic Leukemia Patients According to Subgroup*

Subgroup	No. of Patients	CR Rate	No. of Patients	LFS
Age				
<30	669	88%	510	42%-60%[‡]
30-59	610	79%	412	33%
≥60	215	58%	141	15%
Subtype				
T-ALL[†]	976	88%	850	40%-60%[‡]
B-Precursor ALL	2366	82%	2036	40%-60%
Pro-B-ALL	987	75%	107	37%-60%[§]
Cytogenetics				
Ph/bcr-abl + (without imatinib)	633	72%	633	21%
Ph/bcr-abl + (with imatinib + Chemo)		90%		50%
WBC				
<30,000/μl	698	81%	746	40%
>30,000/μl	387	75%	409	28%
Time to CR				
<4 wk			1433	44%
>4 wk			253	36%

CR, Complete remission; *LFS,* leukemia-free survival; *MRD,* median remission duration.
*Pooled data from published studies.
[†]Depends on T-ALL subtype.
[‡]Depending on protocol and subtype.
[§]Including allogeneic SCT.
Hoffman R, Benz EJ, Shattil SJ, Furie B, Silberstein LE, McGlave P, Heslop H: *Hematology, basic principles, and practice,* ed 5, Churchill Livingstone, 2009.

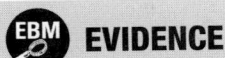

EVIDENCE

available at www.expertconsult.com

SUGGESTED READINGS

available at www.expertconsult.com

AUTHOR: **FRED F. FERRI, M.D.**

BASIC INFORMATION

DEFINITION

Acute myelogenous leukemia (AML) is a disorder characterized by uncontrolled proliferation of primitive myeloid cells (blasts), ultimately replacing normal bone marrow elements and frequently resulting in hematopoietic insufficiency (granulocytopenia, thrombocytopenia, or anemia) with or without leukocytosis.

SYNONYMS

Acute nonlymphoblastic leukemia (ANLL)
Acute nonlymphocytic leukemia
Acute myeloid leukemia (AML)

ICD-9CM CODES
205.0 Acute myelogenous leukemia

EPIDEMIOLOGY & DEMOGRAPHICS

- AML usually affects adults (most patients are 30 to 60 yr; median age at presentation is 50 yr).
- Annual incidence is 2 to 4 cases/100,000 persons.

PHYSICAL FINDINGS & CLINICAL PRESENTATION

Patients generally come to medical attention because of the effects of the cytopenias:
- Anemia manifests with weakness or fatigue.
- Thrombocytopenia can manifest with bleeding, petechiae, and ecchymosis.
- Neutropenia can result in infections and fever.
- Physical examination may reveal skin pallor, bruises, petechiae; abdominal examination may reveal hepatosplenomegaly; peripheral lymphadenopathy may also be present.
- Hyperleukocytosis can lead to symptoms of leukostasis, such as ocular and cerebrovascular dysfunction or bleeding.

ETIOLOGY

Risk factors are previous use of antineoplastic agents, chromosomal abnormalities, ionizing radiation, toxins, immunodeficiency states, and chronic myeloproliferative disorders. Congenital disorders or acquired factors predisposing to AML are described in Table 1-95.

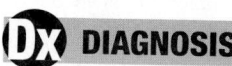

DIAGNOSIS

DIFFERENTIAL DIAGNOSIS

- Acute lymphocytic leukemia
- Leukemoid reaction
- Myelodysplastic syndrome
- Infiltrative diseases of the bone marrow
- Epstein-Barr virus, other viral infection

LABORATORY TESTS

- Complete blood count reveals anemia and thrombocytopenia. Peripheral white blood cell count varies from <5000/mm³ to >100,000/mm³.

- Additional laboratory findings may include elevated lactate dehydrogenase and uric acid levels, decreased fibrinogen, and increased fibrin degradation product as a result of disseminated intravascular coagulation (DIC).
- Cytogenetic abnormalities are common (chromosome 8 is most frequently involved in AML). Table 1-96 describes gene mutations in patients with AML. DNMT3A mutations are highly recurrent in patients with de novo AML with an intermediate-risk cytogenetic profile and are independently associated with a poor outcome.
- The distinction between acute lymphoblastic leukemia (ALL) and AML and the classification of the various subtypes are based on the following factors:
  1. Cell morphology: myeloblasts reveal abundant cytoplasm; cytoplasmic granules are often present (Auer rods).
  2. Histochemical stains:
     - Peroxidase and Sudan black stains are negative in ALL.
     - Chloracetate esterase: a pink cytoplasmic reaction identifies granulocytes;

TABLE 1-95 Congenital Disorders or Acquired Factors Predisposing to Acute Myeloid Leukemia

Genetic Factors

Down syndrome
Fanconi anemia
Bloom syndrome
Neurofibromatosis type I
Klinefelter syndrome
Turner syndrome

Congenital Bone Marrow Failure Syndromes

Kostmann syndrome
Diamond-Blackfan anemia

Drugs

Benzene
Alkylating agents
Epipodophyllotoxins
Ionizing radiation
Myelodysplastic syndromes

From Hoffmann R et al: *Hematology: basic principles and practice,* ed 5, Philadelphia, 2009, Churchill Livingstone.

TABLE 1-96 Gene Mutations in Patients with Acute Myelogenous Leukemia, and Normal Karyotype

Gene Mutation	Frequency (%)	Prognosis
NPM	45-63	Favorable
FLT3	23-33	Adverse
MLL	5-30	Adverse
C/EBP	8-19	Favorable

From Hoffmann R et al: *Hematology: basic principles and practice,* ed 5, Philadelphia, 2009, Churchill Livingstone.

useful to distinguish granulocytes from monocytes in patients with AML.
- AML is diagnosed by the presence of at least 30% blast cells and positive peroxidase or Sudan black histochemical stain in the bone marrow aspirate.
- The French, American, British (FAB) Cooperative Study Group has classified AML into seven categories (M1 to M7) based on the type and percentage of immature cells. The WHO classification of AML is described in Table 1-97.
- A stepwise algorithm for diagnosis and classification of AML using cytomorphology, cytochemistry, immunophenotyping, cytogenetics, and molecular genetics is described in Box 1-11 and in the online version of Section III. Cytogenetic risk categories in AML are described in Table 1-98.

IMAGING STUDIES

- Chest x-ray is useful to evaluate for the presence of mediastinal masses.
- CT scan of the abdomen may reveal hepatosplenomegaly or leukemic involvement of other organs.

TREATMENT

ACUTE GENERAL Rx

- Emergency treatment consisting of one or more of the following is indicated in patients with intracerebral leukostasis:
  1. Cranial irradiation
  2. Leukapheresis
  3. Oral hydroxyurea
- Urate nephropathy can be prevented by vigorous hydration and lowering uric acid level with allopurinol and urine alkalinization with acetazolamide.
- Infections must be aggressively treated with broad-spectrum antibiotics.
- Correct significant thrombocytopenia with platelet transfusions.
- Bleeding from DIC is treated with heparin and replacement of clotting factors.
- Intensive induction chemotherapy to destroy a significant number of leukemic cells and achieve remission usually consists of cytarabine and daunorubicin. It is a 7 + 3 regimen consisting of 7 days of continuous IV infusion of cytarabine and 3 days of daunorubicin. With this regimen, the chance of obtaining a complete remission is 65% to 70% with significantly lower rates in older patients (>56 yr old). All-trans retinoic acid is effective for the induction of remission of AML M3 subtype (acute promyelocytic leukemia).
- High-dose cytarabine (ARA-C) (HiDAC) can be used in patients with refractory or relapsed AML. It usually takes 28 to 32 days from the start of therapy to achieve remission. The duration of remission is variable; the median duration of remission in an adult with AML is 1 yr.
- Post remission therapy following complete remission with induction chemotherapy may include either allogeneic bone marrow trans-

plant (younger patients with donor match) or consolidation chemotherapy.

- Consolidation therapy consists of an aggressive course of chemotherapy with or without radiation shortly after complete remission has been obtained; its purpose is to prolong the remission period or cure. Complications of consolidation therapy are usually attributable to severe bone marrow suppression (anemia, thrombocytopenia, granulocytopenia).
- Goal of therapy is to maintain a state of remission. A postinduction course of high-dose cytarabine can provide equivalent disease-free survival and somewhat better overall survival than autologous marrow transplantation in adults.
- Autologous bone marrow transplantation is indicated in patients <55 yr without a sibling donor. Allogeneic bone marrow transplantation is generally available to <20% of patients; it is usually performed only in patients <40 yr because of higher incidence of graft-versus-host disease with advancing age.

DISPOSITION

- Remission can be achieved in nearly 80% of patients <55 yr. Remission rates are highest in children. Patient characteristics relating to duration of remission are described in Table 1-99.
- Allogeneic stem cell transplantation (SCT) after myoablative conditioning is a curative option in younger patients with AML in first complete remission (CR1). However, concerns related to toxicity limit its use. Cure for allogeneic bone marrow transplantation approaches 60%; cure rates with autologous transplantation are lower. Compared with nonallogeneic SCT therapies, allogeneic SCT has significant relapse-free survival (RFS) and overall survival benefit for intermediate- and poor-risk AML but not for good-risk AML in first complete remission.
- Favorable cytogenics are inv (16) (p13;q22) and t(8;21), t(15;17).
- High expression of an LSC (leukemic stem cell) gene signature is independently associated with adverse outcomes with AML.

TABLE 1-97 WHO Classification of Acute Myeloid Leukemia

Acute myeloid leukemia with recurrent genetic abnormalities

Acute myeloid leukemia with t(8;21)(q22;q22), (AML1/ETO)

Acute myeloid leukemia with abnormal bone marrow eosinophils and inv(16)(p13;q22) or t(16;16) (p13;q22), (CBFβ/MYH11)

Acute promyelocytic leukemia with t(15;17)(q22;q12), (PML/RARα) and variants

Acute myeloid leukemia with 11q23 (MLL) abnormalities

Acute myeloid leukemia with multilineage dysplasia

Following MDS or MDS/MPD

Without antecedent MDS or MDS/MPD, but with dysplasia in at least 50% of cells in two or more myeloid lineages

Acute myeloid leukemia and myelodysplastic syndromes, therapy related

Alkylating agent/radiation-related type

Topoisomerase II inhibitor-related type (some may be lymphoid)

Others

Acute myeloid leukemia, not otherwise categorized

Classify as:

Acute myeloid leukemia, minimally differentiated

Acute myeloid leukemia without maturation

Acute myeloid leukemia with maturation

Acute myelomonocytic leukemia

Acute monoblastic/acute monocytic leukemia

Acute erythroid leukemia (erythroid/myeloid and pure erythroleukemia)

Acute megakaryoblastic leukemia

Acute basophilic leukemia

Acute panmyelosis with myelofibrosis

Myeloid sarcoma

From Hoffmann R et al: *Hematology: basic principles and practice*, ed 5, Philadelphia, 2009, Churchill Livingstone.

BOX 1-11 Stepwise Algorithm for Diagnosis and Classification of Acute Myelogenous Leukemia Using Cytomorphology, Cytochemistry, Immunophenotyping, Cytogenetics, and Molecular Cytogenetics

The criteria are based on Wright-Giemsa–stained blood and marrow smears and biopsy. The percentage of blast cells separates acute myeloid leukemia (AML) from myelodysplastic syndrome (MDS). The World Health Organization (WHO) classification defines AML as greater than 20% blasts in the marrow or blood. The next step is to define the blast population by immunophenotyping and/or immunohistochemistry. The initial evaluation separates AML from ALL. A history of exposure to prior cytoxic chemotherapy or agents associated with AML defines the leukemia as *therapy-related acute myeloid leukemia* (t-AML). The WHO recognizes the unique clinical and biologic features of the therapy-related leukemias (t-AML). This subtype results from prior exposure to cytotoxic chemotherapy and/or radiation therapy. A majority of patients will have clonal cytogenetic abnormalities and now account for more than 40% of all patients with AML. The WHO recognizes two types of t-AML based on the type of prior exposure or treatment: alkylating agent–related AML and topoisomerase II inhibitor–related AML. The WHO classification defines major subgroups of AML that manifest recurring cytogenetic abnormalities. As a group, these AMLs have chromosomal translocations that result in the production of chimeric proteins, which are pivotal in the leukemogenic process. The genetic abnormalities define a specific biology, clinical course, and prognosis and therefore are important to classify them separately. In this group of patients, the diagnosis is defined by the cytogenetic abnormality independent of the percentage of blasts. There are four recurrent translocations in this group. The diagnosis is defined by the cytogenetic abnormalities and is not dependent on the number of blasts: (a) AML with t(8;21)(q22;q22), (AML1/ETO) (RUNX/CBFA2T1); (b) AML with abnormal bone marrow eosinophils and inv[16](p13;q22) or t(16;16)(p13;q22), (CBFB/MYH11); (c) acute promyelocytic leukemia: AML with t(15;17)(q22;q21) (PML/RARA) or t(11;17)(q23;q12) (PLZF/RARA) or t(5;17)(q23;q12)(NPM/RARA), or t(11;17)(q13;q12) (NuMA/RARA); and (d) AML with 11q23 (MLL) abnormalities. If multilineage dysplasia is present, then the leukemia is classified as *acute leukemia with multilineage dysplasia*.

AML with multilineage dysplasia is characterized by the presence of 20% or more blasts in the marrow and dysplasia in at least 50% of the cells of at least two of the three main hemopoietic lines. The leukemia may occur de novo or after a preceding myelodysplastic, myeloproliferative, or overlap myelodysplastic/myeloproliferative syndrome unrelated to prior exposure to chemotherapy. If such a syndrome preceded the development of acute leukemia, the AML is best designated as AML "evolving from a myelodysplastic syndrome." When a leukemia fails to satisfy the cytogenetic, morphologic, or clinical criteria for the newly defined subgroups, it is classified as AML not otherwise categorized. The *not otherwise categorized* designation essentially applies the original FAB classification with some modifications, namely, acute promyelocytic leukemia (M3) is no longer included; a pure erythroleukemia has been distinguished from erythroleukemia, acute erythroid/myeloid type; and acute basophilic leukemia (very rare) has been added, as is a rare entity termed acute panmyelosis with myelofibrosis and the solid tumor myeloid sarcoma.

(From Hoffmann R et al: *Hematology, basic principles and practice*, ed 5, Philadelphia, 2009, Churchill Livingstone.)

CD, Cluster designation; *MPO*, myeloperoxidase; *NEC*, nonerythroid cells; *NSE*, nonspecific esterase; *PAS*, periodic acid–Schiff; *SBB*, Sudan black B; *TdT*, terminal deoxynucleotidyl transferase; *TNC*, total nucleated cells.

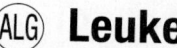 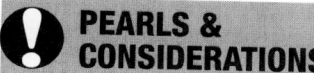

TABLE 1-98 Cytogenetic Risk Categories in Acute Myelogenous Leukemia

Category	Abnormality
Favorable	t(8;21),* t(15;17), inv(16) with or without other abnormalities
Intermediate	Normal, +6, +8, +21, +22 −Y, del(9q)
Unfavorable	−5/del(5q), −7/Del(7q), abn(3q) t(9;22),t(6;9), abn(11q), 20q or 21q, abn(17p), complex karyotype

*Without deletion 9q or complex karyotype.
From Hoffmann R et al: *Hematology: basic principles and practice*, ed 5, Philadelphia, 2009, Churchill Livingstone.

TABLE 1-99 Patient Characteristics Relating to Duration of Remission

Characteristics	Favorable Value
Cytogenetics	t(15;17), t(8;21), inv(16)
Leukocyte count	<100,000 μL^{-1}
Secondary acute myeloid leukemia	Not present
FAB subtype	M1 or M2 with Auer rods, M3 and M4eo
FLT3	Wild-type
Courses to complete remission	1

From Hoffmann R et al: *Hematology: basic principles and practice*, ed 5, Philadelphia, 2009, Churchill Livingstone.

PEARLS & CONSIDERATIONS

- The major complication of chemotherapy is profound marrow depression with pancytopenia lasting 3 to 4 wk. Treatment is aimed at red blood cell and platelet replacement and aggressive monitoring and treatment of suspected infections.
- Low doses of arsenic trioxide can induce complete remission in patients with acute promyelocytic leukemia.

SUGGESTED READINGS
available at www.expertconsult.com

AUTHOR: **FRED F. FERRI, M.D.**

Diseases and Disorders

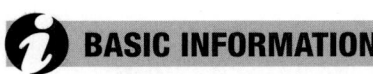

BASIC INFORMATION

DEFINITION

Chronic lymphocytic leukemia (CLL) is a lympho-proliferative disorder characterized by proliferation and accumulation of mature-appearing neoplastic lymphocytes.

SYNONYMS

CLL

ICD-9CM CODES

204.1 Leukemia, chronic lymphocytic

EPIDEMIOLOGY & DEMOGRAPHICS

- Most frequent form of leukemia in Western countries (10,000 new cases annually in the United States)
- Generally occurs in middle-aged and elderly patients (median age 65 yr)
- Male:female ratio of 2:1

PHYSICAL FINDINGS & CLINICAL PRESENTATION

- Lymphadenopathy, splenomegaly, and hepatomegaly in the majority of patients
- Variable clinical presentation according to stage of the disease
- Abnormal complete blood count: many cases are diagnosed on the basis of laboratory results obtained after routine physical examination

- Some patients come to medical attention because of weakness and fatigue (as a result of anemia) or lymphadenopathy

ETIOLOGY

CLL is a disease derived from antigen-experienced B lymphocytes that differ in the level of immunoglobulin V-gene mutations.

DIAGNOSIS

- Identification of cells bearing the phenotype of CLL in peripheral blood (CD5-positive/CD19-positive)
- Absolute B lymphocyte count in the peripheral blood $\geq 5000/\mu l$ for >3 mo with a preponderant population of morphologically mature-appearing small lymphocytes
- Demonstration of clonality of circulating B lymphocytes by flow cytometry of peripheral blood
- Table 1-100 describes the evaluation of CLL patients at diagnosis

DIFFERENTIAL DIAGNOSIS

- Hairy cell leukemia
- Adult T-cell lymphoma
- Prolymphocytic leukemia
- Viral infections
- Waldenström's macroglobulinemia

LABORATORY TESTS

- Proliferative lymphocytosis ($\geq 15,000/dl$) of well-differentiated lymphocytes is the hall-

mark of CLL. B-cell clones are early markers for CLL and can be detected in peripheral blood >6 yr before a CLL diagnosis.

- There is monotonous replacement of the bone marrow by small lymphocytes (marrow contains $\geq 30\%$ of well-differentiated lymphocytes).
- Hypogammaglobulinemia and elevated lactate dehydrogenase may be present at the time of diagnosis.
- Anemia or thrombocytopenia, if present, indicates poor prognosis.
- Trisomy-12 is the most common chromosomal abnormality, followed by 14 q+, 13 q, and 11 q; these all indicate a poor prognosis.
- New laboratory techniques (CD 38, fluorescence in situ hybridization) can identify patients with early-stage CLL at higher risk of rapid disease progression. Staining of mononuclear cells by a two-color (fluorescein isothiocyanate/phycoerythrin) flow cytometric assay using antibodies to the chemokine receptors (CXCR1, CXCR2, etc.) can help in the staging and prognosis of patients. Increase in expression of chemokine receptors CXCR4 and CCR7 correlates with advanced Rai stage (stage IV). The presence of V-gene mutations, CD38+, or ZAP-70+ cells also has prognostic relevance. Patients with clones having few or no V-gene mutations or many CD38+ or ZAP-70+ B cells are associated with an aggressive, usually fatal course.
- The percentage of smudge cells (CLL cells ruptured during smear preparation) is associated with mutated IgVH gene status, a favorable prognostic factor. A high percentage of smudge cells on peripheral smear indicates a longer time to treatment from initial diagnosis and better overall survival in patients with early stage CLL.

STAGING:

Rai et al. divided CLL into five clinical stages:

- Stage 0: Characterized by lymphocytosis only ($>15,000/mm^3$ on peripheral smear, bone marrow aspirate $\geq 40\%$ lymphocytes). The coexistence of lymphocytosis and other factors increases the clinical stage.
- Stage 1: Lymphadenopathy
- Stage 2: Lymphadenopathy/hepatomegaly
- Stage 3: Anemia (hemoglobin [Hgb] <11 g/mm^3)
- Stage 4: Thrombocytopenia (platelets <100,000/mm^3)

Another well-known staging system developed by Binet divides CLL into three stages:

- Stage A: Hgb >10 g/dl, platelets >100,000/mm^3, and fewer than three areas involved (the cervical, axillary, and inguinal lymph nodes [whether unilaterally or bilaterally]; the spleen; and the liver)
- Stage B: Hgb >10 g/dl, platelets >100,000/mm^3, and three or more areas involved
- Stage C: Hgb <10 g/dl, low platelets (<100,000/mm^3), or both (independent of the areas involved)

TABLE 1-100 Evaluation of Chronic Lymphocytic Leukemia (CLL) Patients at Diagnosis

History

B-symptom and fatigue assessment
Infectious history assessment
Occupational assessment for chemical exposure
Familial history of CLL and lymphoproliferative disorders
Preventive interventions for infections and secondary cancers

Physical Exam

Laboratory Assessment

Complete blood count with differential
Morphology assessment of lymphocytes
Chemistry, LFT enzymes, LDH
Flow cytometry assessment to confirm immunophenotype of CLL
Serum immunoglobulins
Serum β_2M levels
Interphase cytogenetics for del(17p13.1), del(11q22.3), del(13q14), del(6q21), and trisomy 12
IgV$_H$ mutational analysis
Stimulated metaphase karyotype (if available)

Selected Tests Under Certain Circumstances

Direct antiglobulin test (DAT), haptoglobin, reticulocyte count if anemia present
CT Scan if unexplained abdominal pain or enlargement present
PET Scan and/or biopsy if large nodal mass present
Bone marrow aspirate and biopsy if cytopenias present
Familial counseling if first-degree relative with CLL

Teaching

Varicella zoster identification instruction
Skin cancer identification
Disease education (Leukemia and Lymphoma Society, CLL Topics, ACOR)

From Hoffmann R et al: *Hematology: basic principles and practice*, ed 5, Philadelphia, 2009, Churchill Livingstone.

IMAGING STUDIES

CT scans at diagnosis for assessment of end-organ involvement is not recommended in diagnostic guidelines. However, CT scan of abdomen may be done to evaluate for hepatomegaly and splenomegaly in patients with poor prognostic features.

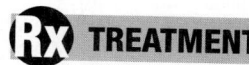 **TREATMENT**

NONPHARMACOLOGIC THERAPY

- Treatment goals are relief of symptoms and prolongation of life.
- Observation is appropriate for patients in Rai stage 0 or Binet stage A.

ACUTE GENERAL Rx

- Symptomatic patients in Rai stage I or II or Binet stage B: chlorambucil; local irradiation for isolated symptomatic lymphadenopathy and lymph nodes that interfere with vital organs.
- Fludarabine is an effective treatment for CLL that does not respond to initial treatment with chlorambucil. Recent reports indicate that when used as the initial treatment for CLL, fludarabine yields higher response rates and a longer duration of remission and progression-free survival than chlorambucil; overall survival, however, is not enhanced.
- Rai stages III or IV, Binet stage C: chlorambucil chemotherapy with or without prednisone:
  1. Fludarabine, CAP (**c**yclophosphamide, **A**driamycin, **p**rednisone), or cyclophosphamide, doxorubicin, vincristine, and prednisone (mini-CHOP) can be used in patients who respond poorly to chlorambucil.
  2. The human anti-CD20 monoclonal antibodies rituximab and ofatumumab have received FDA approval for treatment of patients with CLL refractory to fludarabine.
  3. Splenic irradiation can be used in selected patients with advanced disease.
- An algorithm to treatment approach to first relapsed CLL is described in Fig. 1-217.

CHRONIC Rx

Treatment of systemic complications:

- Hypogammaglobulinemia is frequent in CLL and is the chief cause of infections. Immune globulin (250 mg/kg IV every 4 wk) may prevent infections but has no effect on survival rate. Infections should be treated with broad-spectrum antibiotics. Patients should be monitored for opportunistic infections.
- Recombinant hematopoietic cofactors (e.g., granulocyte-macrophage colony stimulating factor and granulocyte colony stimulating factor) may be useful to overcome neutropenia related to treatment.
- Erythropoietin may be useful to treat anemia that is unresponsive to other measures.

DISPOSITION

The patient's prognosis is generally directly related to the clinical stage (e.g., the average survival in patients in Rai stage 0 or Binet stage A is >120 mo, whereas for RAI stage 4 or Binet stage C it is approximately 30 mo). Overall 5-yr survival is 60%. Measurement of ZAP-70 intracellular protein (where available) is also a useful indicator of prognosis.

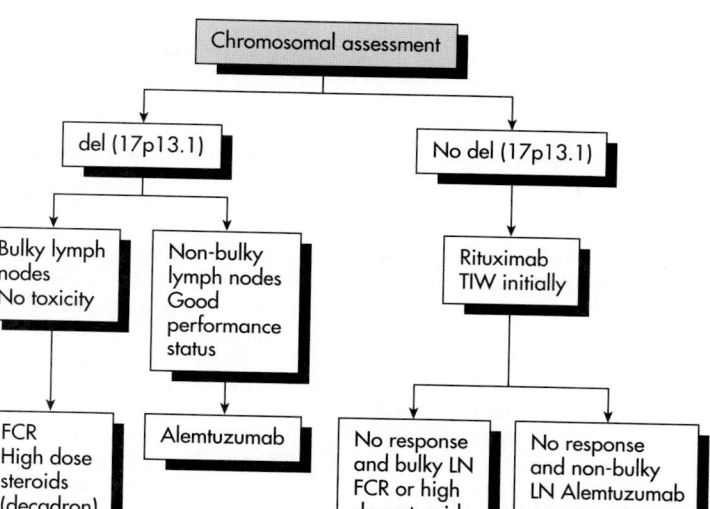

FIGURE 1-217 Algorithm to treatment approach to first relapsed chronic lymphocytic leukemia. (Modified from Hoffmann R et al: *Hematology: basic principles and practice*, ed 5, Philadelphia, 2009, Churchill Livingstone.)

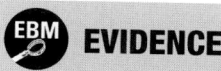 **EVIDENCE**

available at www.expertconsult.com

SUGGESTED READINGS

available at www.expertconsult.com

AUTHOR: **FRED F. FERRI, M.D.**

BASIC INFORMATION

DEFINITION

Chronic myelogenous leukemia (CML) is a malignant clonal stem disease caused by an acquired somatic mutation that fuses, through chromosomal translocation, the *ABL* and *BCR* genes on chromosomes 9 and 22 and is characterized by abnormal proliferation and accumulation of immature granulocytes. CML manifests with a chronic phase (CP-CML) lasting months to years, followed by an advanced phase (AP-CML) characterized by poor response to therapy, worsening anemia, or decreased platelet count; the second phase then evolves into a terminal phase (acute transformation) that degenerates into acute leukemia (mostly myeloid and approximately 20% lymphoid subtype), characterized by elevated number of blast cells and numerous complications (e.g., sepsis, bleeding).

SYNONYMS

CML
Chronic granulocytic leukemia
Chronic myeloid leukemia

ICD-9CM CODES
201.1 Chronic myelogenous leukemia

EPIDEMIOLOGY & DEMOGRAPHICS

- CML usually affects elderly patients (median age at presentation is 65 yr) and accounts for 15% of adult cases of leukemia
- Incidence is one to two cases per 100,000 people annually

PHYSICAL FINDINGS & CLINICAL PRESENTATION

- The chronic phase usually reveals splenomegaly; hepatomegaly is not infrequent, but lymphadenopathy is highly unusual and generally indicates the accelerated proliferative phase of the disease.
- Common symptoms at the time of diagnosis are weakness or discomfort from an enlarged spleen (abdominal discomfort or pain). Splenomegaly is present in up to 40% of patients at time of diagnosis.
- 40% of patients are asymptomatic, and diagnosis is based solely on an abnormal blood count.

ETIOLOGY

Current evidence strongly implicates the chromosome translocation t (9;22) (q34;q11.2) as the cause of chronic granulocytic leukemia. This translocation is present in >95% of patients. The remaining patients have a complex or variant translocation involving additional chromosomes that have the same end result (fusion of the *BCR* [break point cluster region] gene on chromosome 22 to *ABL* [Ableson leukemia virus] gene on chromosome 9).

DIAGNOSIS

DIFFERENTIAL DIAGNOSIS

- Splenic lymphoma
- Chronic lymphocytic leukemia
- Myelodysplastic syndrome

LABORATORY TESTS

- Elevated white blood cell count (generally >100,000/mm^3) with broad spectrum of granulocytic forms.
- Bone marrow demonstrates hypercellularity with granulocytic hyperplasia, increased ratio of myeloid cells to erythroid cells, and increased number of megakaryocytes. Blasts and promyelocytes constitute <10% of all cells.
- Philadelphia chromosome (which results from the reciprocal translocation between the long arms of chromosomes 9 and 22) is present in >95% of patients with CML; its presence (Ph^1) is a major prognostic factor because survival rate of patients with Philadelphia chromosome is approximately eight times better than that of those without it. Some believe that Ph^1(+) defines CML and that those who are Ph^1(−) have another disease.
- Leukocyte alkaline phosphatase is markedly decreased (used to distinguish CML from other myeloproliferative disorders).
- Anemia and thrombocytosis are often present.
- Additional laboratory results are elevated vitamin B$_{12}$ levels (caused by increased transcobalamin 1 from granulocytes) and elevated blood histamine levels (because of increased basophils).

IMAGING STUDIES

Chest radiograph and CT scan of abdomen/pelvis

TREATMENT

ACUTE GENERAL Rx

Treatment with a potential to either cure CML or prolong survival should be used during the chronic phase of the disease because it is often futile when administered during the advanced phase. Imatinib mesylate, an oral tyrosine kinase inhibitor, is effective and indicated as first-line treatment for CML myeloid blast crisis, accelerated phase, or CML in its chronic phase. More than 75% of patients have major cytogenetic response (<35% Philadelphia chromosome-positive cells in the marrow), and more than 80% have progression-free survival after 24 mo. Complete hematologic response usually occurs in <1 mo. Nilotinib and dasatinib are newer, more effective agents that also inhibit the activity of the BCR-ABL fusion protein by binding to a particular site and can be used after failure of imatinib and eventually may become first line agents.

- Symptomatic hyperleukocytosis (e.g., central nervous system symptoms) can be treated with leukapheresis and hydroxyurea; allopurinol should be started to prevent urate nephropathy after the rapid lysis of the leukemia cells.
- Allogeneic stem-cell transplantation (SCT) is the only curative treatment for CML in the chronic phase unresponsive to imatinib. In general only 20% of patients are candidates for SCT given the limitations of age or lack of HLA-matched related donors.
  1. It should be considered in "young" patients (increased survival in patients <55 yr) with compatible siblings.
  2. Early transplantation is also important for patient's survival.
- Interferon-alfa is an acceptable alternative in the early chronic phase for patients who do not tolerate tyrosine kinase inhibitors.
- Recent trials have shown that as compared with other treatments, the addition of peginterferon alfa-2a to imatinib therapy resulted in significantly higher rates of molecular response in patients with chronic-phase CML.
- Transplantation of marrow from an HLA-matched, unrelated donor is also now recognized as safe and effective therapy for selected patients with chronic myelogenous leukemia.

SUGGESTED READINGS
available at www.expertconsult.com

AUTHOR: **FRED F. FERRI, M.D.**

BASIC INFORMATION

DEFINITION

Hairy cell leukemia is a lymphoid neoplasm characterized by the proliferation of mature B cells with prominent cytoplasmic projections (hairs).

SYNONYMS

Leukemic reticuloendotheliosis

ICD-9CM CODES
202.4 Hairy cell leukemia

EPIDEMIOLOGY & DEMOGRAPHICS

PREVALENCE: Occurs predominantly in men between ages 40 and 60 yr. Approximately 2% of leukemia cases are of the hairy cell type.
PREDOMINANT SEX: Male:female ratio of 4:1

PHYSICAL FINDINGS & CLINICAL PRESENTATION

- Usually, splenomegaly (present in >90% of cases) caused by tumor cell infiltration
- Pallor, ecchymosis, and evidence of infection if the pancytopenia is severe
- Weakness, lethargy, and fatigue
- Infections (resulting from impaired resistance caused by neutropenia) and easy bruising (caused by thrombocytopenia) also common

ETIOLOGY

Neoplastic disease of the lymphoreticular system of unknown etiology

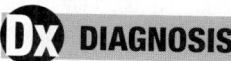

DIAGNOSIS

DIFFERENTIAL DIAGNOSIS

- Other forms of leukemia
- Lymphoma
- Viral syndrome

WORKUP

Comprehensive history, physical examination, and laboratory evaluation to confirm the diagnosis

LABORATORY TESTS

- Pancytopenia involving erythrocytes, neutrophils, and platelets is common; anemia is usually present and varies from minimal to severe.
- Hairy cells (Fig. 1-218) can account for 5% to 80% of cells in the peripheral blood. The cytoplasmic projections on the cells are redundant plasma membranes.
- Leukemic cells stain positively for tartrate-resistant acid phosphatase stain.
- Bone marrow may result in a "dry tap" (because of increased marrow reticulin).

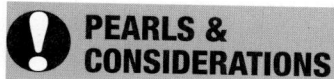

TREATMENT

NONPHARMACOLOGIC THERAPY

Approximately 8% to 10% of patients are asymptomatic and have minimal splenomegaly and minor cytopenia. They are usually detected on routine laboratory evaluation and do not require initial therapy. They should, however, be frequently monitored for progression of disease.

ACUTE GENERAL Rx

- Drugs of choice are the purine analogues 2-chloro-2 deoxyadenosine (Cladribine) or 2-deoxycoformycin (DCF, Pentostatin). They induce complete remissions in up to 85% of patients and partial responses in 5% to 25%.

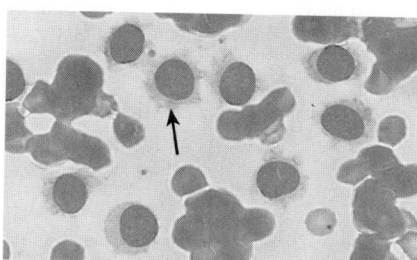

FIGURE 1-218 Hairy cell leukemia. Note the lymphocytes with hairlike cytoplasmic projections surrounding the nucleus. (From Rodak BF: *Diagnostic hematology,* Philadelphia, 1995, WB Saunders.)

- 2-Chloro-2 deoxyadenosine (CdA) 0.14 mg/kg qd for 7 days has minimal toxicity and is able to induce complete durable responses with a single course of therapy.
- Interferon-α produces a partial remission in 30% to 70% of patients and complete remission, often of short duration, in 5% to 10% of patients.
- The anti-CD 22 recombinant immunotoxin BL 22 can induce complete remission in patients with hairy cell leukemia resistant to treatment with purine analogues.

CHRONIC Rx

Patients should be monitored with periodic examination and laboratory tests for progression of disease.

DISPOSITION

Prognosis has become increasingly favorable with the newer agents. Approximately 90% of patients who are treated have a complete or partial response.

REFERRAL

Hematology consultation is recommended in all patients.

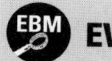

PEARLS & CONSIDERATIONS

COMMENTS

The diagnosis of hairy cell leukemia is occasionally missed and subsequently made by the histopathologist after removal of the spleen for diagnostic purposes.

EBM EVIDENCE

available at www.expertconsult.com

SUGGESTED READING

available at www.expertconsult.com

AUTHOR: **FRED F. FERRI, M.D.**

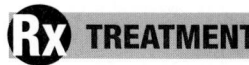
DEFINITION
Oral hairy leukoplakia (OHL) is a painless, white, nonremovable, plaquelike lesion typically located on the lateral aspect of the tongue.

ICD-9CM CODES
528.6 Oral hairy leukoplakia

EPIDEMIOLOGY & DEMOGRAPHICS
INCIDENCE AND PREVALENCE: Epstein-Barr virus (EBV) seroprevalence occurs in high incidence in individuals who are HIV seropositive. However, OHL occurs in only 25% of these cases.
RISK FACTORS: OHL is usually found in HIV-seropositive individuals (median CD4 count is 468/μl) but may also be identified in other immunocompromised patients such as transplant recipients (particularly renal) and patients taking steroids. Diagnosing OHL is an indication to institute a workup to evaluate and manage HIV disease.

PHYSICAL FINDINGS & CLINICAL PRESENTATION
- Varying morphology and appearance.
- May be unilateral or bilateral.
- White and can be small with fine, vertical corrugations on the lateral margin of the tongue (Fig. 1-219).
- Irregular surface; may have prominent folds or projection, occasionally markedly resembling hairs.
- May spread to cover the entire dorsal surface or spread onto the ventral surface of the tongue where the lesions usually appear flat.
- Rarely, lesions can manifest on the soft palate, buccal mucosa, or posterior oropharynx.

- Usually asymptomatic, but some patients have mouth pain, soreness, or a burning sensation; impaired taste; or difficulty eating; others complain of its unsightly appearance.
- OHL may progress to oral squamous cell carcinoma, which has a poor prognosis.

ETIOLOGY
EBV is implicated in its etiology, and OHL is a result of replication EBV in the epithelium of keratinized cells. OHL differs from most EBV-related diseases in that infection is predominantly lytic rather than latent.

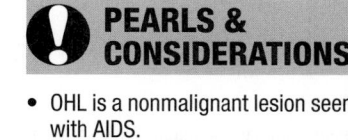
DIAGNOSIS

DIFFERENTIAL DIAGNOSIS
- *Candida albicans*
- Lichen planus
- Idiopathic leukoplakia
- White sponge nevus
- Dysplasia
- Squamous cell carcinoma

WORKUP
Requires physical examination and evaluation of HIV disease

LABORATORY TESTS
The *provisional* diagnosis is clinical and based on:
- Visual inspection
- Inability to scrape the lesion off the tongue with a blade
- Failure to respond to antifungal therapy
The *presumptive* diagnosis requires biopsy and histologic demonstration of:
- Epithelial hyperplasia with hairs
- Absence of inflammatory cell infiltrate

The *definitive* diagnosis requires:
- In situ hybridization of histologic or cytologic specimens revealing EBV DNA *or*
- Electron microscopy of specimens revealing herpes-like particles
- Measurement of the DNA content in cells of oral leukoplakia may be used to predict the risk of oral carcinoma
NOTE: Specimens obtained from lesions may demonstrate hyphae of *Candida albicans,* which may coexist and potentiate EBV-induced OHL.

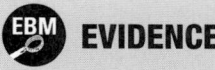
TREATMENT

NONPHARMACOLOGIC THERAPY
OHL is usually asymptomatic and requires no specific therapy. It may resolve spontaneously and has no known premalignant potential.

ACUTE GENERAL Rx
- Highly active antiretroviral therapy (HAART) has considerably changed the frequency of oral lesions caused by opportunistic infections in HIV-seropositive individuals.
- Topical retinoids (0.1% vitamin A) may improve the appearance of OHL-affected oral surfaces through their dekeratinizing and immunomodulation effects; however, they are expensive and prolonged use may result in a burning sensation over the treated area.
- Topical podophyllin resin 25% solution has been reported to induce resolution.
- Surgical excision and cryotherapy may help, but the lesions may recur.
- High-dose acyclovir 800 mg five times per day, valacyclovir 1000 mg tid, famciclovir 500 mg tid, ganciclovir 1000 mg tid, or foscarnet 40 mg/kg IV tid will cause lesions to resolve but only temporarily.

PEARLS & CONSIDERATIONS

- OHL is a nonmalignant lesion seen in patients with AIDS.
- The incidence has decreased significantly in the era of HAART.

EBM EVIDENCE

available at www.expertconsult.com

SUGGESTED READING
available at www.expertconsult.com

AUTHOR: **SAJEEV HANDA, M.D.**

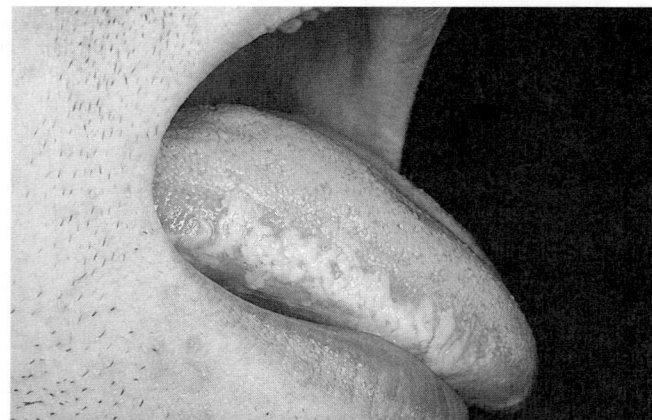
FIGURE 1-219 Oral hairy leukoplakia. Note white verrucoid plaques on the lateral border of the tongue. (From Noble J: *Primary care medicine,* ed 3, St Louis, 2001, Mosby.)

BASIC INFORMATION

DEFINITION

Lichen planus refers to a papular skin eruption characteristically found over the flexor surfaces of the extremities, genitalia, and mucous membranes.

SYNONYMS

Lichen
Lichen planus et atrophicus

ICD-9CM CODES
697.0 Lichen planus

EPIDEMIOLOGY & DEMOGRAPHICS

INCIDENCE: One in every 100 new patients seen in dermatology clinics in the U.S. is diagnosed with lichen planus
PREVALENCE: 440 cases/100,000 persons
PREDOMINANT SEX: Found equally between males and females (1:1)
PREDOMINANT AGE: Usually found in people between the ages of 30 and 60 yr
PREDISPOSING FACTORS:
1. Associated with other autoimmune disorders (e.g., primary biliary cirrhosis, myasthenia gravis, ulcerative colitis, diabetes)
2. Associated with hepatitis C infection
3. Drug-induced form affects any area of the body surface (e.g., beta-blocker, methyldopa, penicillamine, quinidine, nonsteroidal anti-inflammatory drugs, angiotensin-converting enzyme inhibitors, sulfonylurea agents)

PHYSICAL FINDINGS & CLINICAL PRESENTATION

History:
- Usually starts on an extremity and may remain localized or spread to involve other areas over a 1- to 4-mo period
- Pruritic

Physical findings:
- Anatomic distribution:
  1. Flexor surface of wrists, forearms, shins, and upper thighs
  2. Neck and back area
  3. Nails
  4. Scalp (lichen planopilaris)
  5. Oral mucosa, buccal mucosa, tongue, gingiva, and lips
  6. Vulva, penis

Genital mucosa:
- Lesion configuration:
  1. Linear
  2. Annular (more common)
  3. Reticular pattern noted on oral mucosa and genital area

- Lesion morphology:
  1. Papules most common presentation (flat, smooth, shiny)
  2. Hypertrophic
  3. Follicular
  4. Vesicular
- Color:
  1. Dark red, bluish red, purplish-violaceous color is noted in cutaneous lichen planus.
  2. Individual lesions characteristically have white lines visible (Wickham's striae).
  3. Oral and genital lichen planus has a reticular network of white lines that may be raised or annular in appearance.
- Scalp lesions may result in alopecia.

ETIOLOGY

The cause of lichen planus is unknown.

DIAGNOSIS

- Clinical history and physical findings usually establish the diagnosis of lichen planus.
- Skin biopsy (deep shave or punch biopsy of the most developed lesion) can be performed to confirm the diagnosis.

DIFFERENTIAL DIAGNOSIS

Drug eruption, psoriasis, Bowen's disease, leukoplakia, candidiasis, lupus rash, secondary syphilis, seborrheic dermatitis, chronic graft vs. host disease

WORKUP

If the diagnosis is questionable, a skin biopsy is performed.

LABORATORY TESTS

Laboratory tests are not specific for the diagnosis of lichen planus.

IMAGING STUDIES

Imaging studies are not helpful in diagnosing lichen planus.

TREATMENT

NONPHARMACOLOGIC THERAPY
- Avoid scratching.
- Use mild soaps and emollients after bathing to prevent dryness.

ACUTE GENERAL Rx

For cutaneous lichen planus:
- Topical steroids (e.g., triamcinolone acetonide 0.1%, fluocinonide 0.05%, clobetasol propionate 0.05% cream or ointment) with occlusion used twice daily.

- Acitretin 30 mg/day PO for 8 wk.
- Systemic prednisone 30 to 60 mg/day as a starting dose and tapered to 15 to 20 mg/day maintenance for 6 wk.
- Intradermal steroid triamcinolone acetonide 5 mg/ml can be tried for thick hyperkeratotic lesions.
- Hydroxyzine 25 mg PO q6h can be used for pruritus.

For oral lichen planus:
- Topical steroid fluocinonide in an adhesive base used six times/day for 9 wk.
- Topical calcineurin in steroid unresponsive cases.
- Topical or systemic retinoids 0.1% retinoic acid in an adhesive base or gel.
- Etretinate 75 mg/day for 2 mo.

CHRONIC Rx

Refer to acute general treatment

DISPOSITION
- Spontaneous remissions of cutaneous lichen planus occur in more than 65% of cases within the first year.
- Spontaneous remission of oral lichen planus usually occurs by 5 yr.
- Approximately 10% to 20% of patients will have recurrence.

REFERRAL

Dermatology

PEARLS & CONSIDERATIONS

COMMENTS
- Lichen planus can be remembered as purple, planar, pruritic, polygonal, papules, and plaques (six P's).
- Lesions can develop at the site of prior skin injury (Koebner's phenomenon).
- Although transformation to skin cancer has been seen in patients with lichen planus, it remains unclear if there is a true correlation.

EVIDENCE

available at www.expertconsult.com

SUGGESTED READINGS
available at www.expertconsult.com

AUTHOR: **TANYA ALI, M.D.**

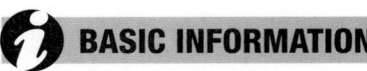

BASIC INFORMATION

DEFINITION

Chronic inflammatory condition of the skin usually affecting the vulva, perianal area, and groin

ICD-9CM CODES
701.0 Lichen sclerosus

EPIDEMIOLOGY & DEMOGRAPHICS

- Most common in postmenopausal women and men between ages 40 and 60 yr
- More common in females
- Can occur in children (usually prepubertal girls with involvement of the vulva and perineum)

PHYSICAL FINDINGS & CLINICAL PRESENTATION

- Erythema may be the only initial sign. A characteristic finding is the presence of ivory-white atrophic lesions on the involved area.
- Close inspection of the affected area will reveal the presence of white-to-brown follicular plugs on the surface (dells).
- When the genitals are involved, the white, parchment-like skin assumes an hourglass configuration around the introital and perianal area ("keyhole" distribution; Fig. 1-220). Inflammation, subepithelial hemorrhages, and chronic ulceration may develop.

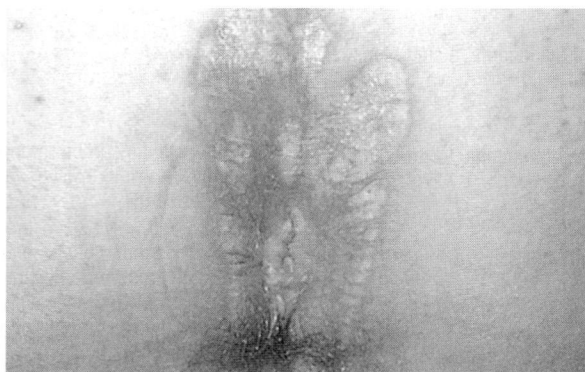

FIGURE 1-220 Lichen sclerosus. Perianal area is thinned and chalk white (keyhole distribution). (Courtesy Department of Dermatology, University of North Carolina at Chapel Hill. From Goldstein BG, Goldstein AO: *Practical dermatology,* ed 2, St Louis, 1997, Mosby.)

- Dyspareunia, genital bleeding, and anal bleeding are common.

ETIOLOGY

Unknown. There may be an autoimmune association and a genetic familial component.

DIAGNOSIS

DIFFERENTIAL DIAGNOSIS

- Localized scleroderma (morphea)
- Cutaneous discoid lupus erythematosus
- Atrophic lichen planus
- Psoriasis

WORKUP

Diagnosis is based on close examination of the lesions for the presence of ivory-white atrophic lesions and typical location.

LABORATORY TESTS

Punch or deep shave biopsy can be used to confirm the diagnosis.

TREATMENT

NONPHARMACOLOGIC THERAPY

Attention to hygiene and elimination of irritants or excessive bathing with harsh soaps

GENERAL Rx

- Application of clobetasol propionate 0.05% topically bid for up to 4 wk is usually effective. Repeat courses of corticosteroids may be necessary because of the chronic nature of this disorder. Continual application of topical steroids may lead to atrophy of the vulva.
- Use of topical testosterone (2%) has been found to be less effective than topical corticosteroids.
- Lubricants (e.g., Nutraplus cream) are useful to soothe dry tissues.
- Hydroxyzine 25 mg at bedtime is effective in decreasing nocturnal itching.
- Use of intralesional steroids, etretinate, and surgical management are usually reserved for refractory cases.

DISPOSITION

- The disease persists in approximately one third of patients.
- Most prepubertal girls improve spontaneously at menarche.
- Squamous cell carcinoma can develop within the lesions in 3% to 10% of older patients; therefore periodic examination and biopsy of suspicious areas are indicated.

PEARLS & CONSIDERATIONS

COMMENTS

- Prepubertal lichen sclerosus may be confused with sexual abuse in prepubertal girls and may lead to false accusations and investigations.
- Lichen sclerosus of the vulva (kraurosis vulvae) usually occurs after menopause and is generally chronic. It can be painful and interfere with sexual activity.
- Lichen sclerosus of the penis (balanitis xerotica obliterans) is seen more commonly in uncircumcised males. It affects the glans and prepuce and may lead to stricture if it encroaches into the urinary meatus.

AUTHOR: **FRED F. FERRI, M.D.**

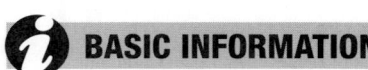

BASIC INFORMATION

DEFINITION

Listeriosis is a systemic infection caused by the gram-positive aerobic bacterium *Listeria monocytogenes*.

SYNONYMS

Listerial infection
Granulomatosis infantisepticum

ICD-9CM CODES
027.0 Listeriosis
771.2 Congenital listeriosis
771.2 Fetal listeriosis
665.4 Suspected fetal damage affecting management of pregnancy

EPIDEMIOLOGY & DEMOGRAPHICS

INCIDENCE (IN U.S.):
- Listeria meningitis: about 0.7 cases/100,000 persons (fourth most common cause of community-acquired bacterial meningitis in adults)
- Perinatal listeriosis: 8.6 cases/100,000 persons
- Nonperinatal listeriosis: 3 cases/1 million persons

PREDOMINANT SEX: Pregnant women are more susceptible to listeria bacteremia, accounting for up to one third of reported cases.

PREDOMINANT AGE:
- Pregnant women
- Immunocompromised patients of any age
- Elderly patients are susceptible even in the absence of recognized immunocompromised states

GENETICS:
Congenital infection:
- With transplacental transmission, syndrome termed *granulomatosis infantisepticum* in neonate
- Characterized by disseminated abscesses in multiple organs, skin lesions, and conjunctivitis
- Mortality: 33% to 100%

Neonatal infection:
- Infant becoming ill after 3 days of age; mother invariably asymptomatic
- Clinical picture of sepsis of unknown origin

PHYSICAL FINDINGS & CLINICAL PRESENTATION

Infections in pregnancy
1. More common in third trimester
2. Usually present with fever and chills without localizing symptoms or signs of infection

Meningoencephalitis
1. More common in neonates and immunocompromised patients, but up to 30% of adults have no underlying condition
2. In neonates: poor appetite with or without fever possibly the only presenting signs
3. In adults: presentation often subacute, with low-grade fever and personality change as only signs
4. Focal neurologic signs seen without demonstrable brain abscess on CT scan

Cerebritis/rhombencephalitis:
1. Headache and fever may be only presenting complaints
2. Progressive cranial nerve palsies, hemiparesis, seizures, depressed level of consciousness, cerebellar signs, respiratory insufficiency may also be seen

Focal infections
1. Ocular infections (purulent conjunctivitis) and skin lesions (granulomatosis infantisepticum) as a result of inadvertent inoculation by laboratory and veterinary personnel
2. Others: arthritis, prosthetic joint infections, peritonitis, osteomyelitis, organ abscesses, cholecystitis

ETIOLOGY

- Direct invasion of skin and eye has been documented, but mechanism of GI entry is unclear.
- Organism's intracellular life cycle explanatory of:
  1. Importance of cell-mediated immunity in host defense
  2. Increased infection in neonates, pregnant women, and immunocompromised hosts

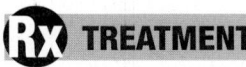

DIAGNOSIS

DIFFERENTIAL DIAGNOSIS

- Meningitis caused by other bacteria, mycobacteria, or fungi
- CNS sarcoidosis
- Brain neoplasm or abscess
- Tuberculous and fungal (especially cryptococcal) meningitis
- Cerebral toxoplasmosis
- Lyme disease
- Sarcoidosis

WORKUP

Dictated by age, end-organ involvement, and immune status

LABORATORY TESTS

- Cultures of blood and other appropriate body fluids
- Variable CSF findings, but neutrophils usually predominate

- Organisms uncommonly seen on Gram stain and may be difficult to identify morphologically
- Monoclonal antibodies, polymerase chain reaction, and DNA probe techniques to detect *Listeria* in foods

IMAGING STUDIES

- If focal cerebral involvement suspected: CT scan or MRI
- MRI most sensitive for evaluation of brainstem and cerebellum

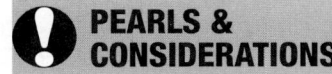

TREATMENT

Empiric therapy should be administered when diagnosis is suspected because overall mortality is 23%.

ACUTE GENERAL Rx

- Drugs of choice:
  1. IV ampicillin 8 to 12 g/day in divided doses
  2. IV penicillin 12 to 24 million U/day in divided doses
- Continuation of therapy for 2 wk
- Alternative (if penicillin allergic): trimethoprim/sulfamethoxazole or vancomycin
- Gentamicin added to provide synergy in meningitis or endocarditis

CHRONIC Rx

Relapses reported, especially in immunocompromised hosts, after 2 wk of therapy.

DISPOSITION

Long-term follow-up of immunodeficiency state

REFERRAL

Infectious disease consultation for all patients

PEARLS & CONSIDERATIONS

COMMENTS

- Foodborne cases have been linked to various products: coleslaw, soft cheeses, unpasteurized milk and milk products, vegetables, undercooked chicken, hot dogs, luncheon meats, refrigerated smoked seafood, and so on.
- Complete decontamination of food products is difficult because *Listeria* is resistant to pasteurization and refrigeration.

SUGGESTED READINGS
available at www.expertconsult.com

AUTHORS: **GLENN G. FORT, M.D., M.P.H.,** and **DENNIS J. MIKOLICH, M.D.**

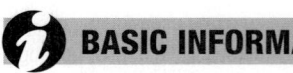

BASIC INFORMATION

DEFINITION
Long QT syndrome is a disorder of myocardial repolarization characterized by a prolonged QT interval on the ECG associated with an increased risk of developing life-threatening ventricular arrhythmias, most commonly torsades de pointes (a specific type of polymorphic ventricular tachycardia).

SYNONYMS
LQTS
Congenital forms:
Jervell and Lange-Nielsen syndrome (associated with deafness)
Romano-Ward syndrome (associated with normal hearing)

ICD-9CM CODES
427.9 Unspecified cardiac dysrhythmia

EPIDEMIOLOGY & DEMOGRAPHICS
- Congenital long QT syndrome is thought to account for more than 3000 deaths per year in the United States.
- Incidence of long QT syndrome is thought to be between 1:2500 and 1:10,000 in the general population, although it has been difficult to estimate due to incomplete penetrance.
- The congenital form associated with deafness is autosomal recessive (Jervell and Lange Nielsen syndrome) and is less common than the autosomal dominant form.
- The congenital form associated with normal hearing (Romano-Ward syndrome) is autosomal dominant. Although inheritance of long QT syndrome is autosomal dominant, female predominance has often been observed and has been attributed to an increased susceptibility to cardiac arrhythmias in women.
- More than 10 subtypes of congenital LQTS have been identified.
- Long QT syndrome is more common in women than in men.
- Genetic mutations in the congenital long QT syndrome are described in Table 1-101.

PHYSICAL FINDINGS & CLINICAL PRESENTATION
- Palpitations, presyncope
- Syncope caused by ventricular tachycardia
- Sudden cardiac death (SCD)
- Seizure
- Family history of long QT syndrome, but a family history of SCD has not been proven to be a risk factor for SCD in patients with long QT syndrome
- Abnormal ECG (prolonged QT) in asymptomatic relatives of known case
- Prolonged QTc interval on ECG (QTc should be <440 ms in women and <420 ms in men)

ETIOLOGY
- Cardiac repolarization abnormality
- Congenital cause (hundreds of mutations on more than 10 genes have been identified)

- Most of the gene mutations affect function of ion channels leading to prolonged repolarization (i.e., sodium and potassium channels)
- Acquired causes:
  - Drugs: dofetilide, ibutilide, bepridil, quinidine, procainamide, sotalol, amiodarone, ranolazine, disopyramide, phenothiazines and antiemetic agents (droperidol, domperidone), tricyclic antidepressants, quinolones, astemizole or cisapride given with ketoconazole or erythromycin, clarithromycin, and antimalarials, particularly among patients with asthma or those using potassium-lowering medications; also common in patients receiving methadone
  - Hypokalemia, hypomagnesemia, hypocalcemia (especially in patients with malabsorption syndrome)
  - Liquid protein diet
  - Central nervous system lesions
  - Mitral valve prolapse
  - Hypothyroidism

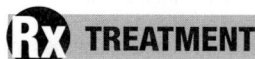

DIAGNOSIS

DIFFERENTIAL DIAGNOSIS
See "Syncope."
Diagnostic criteria for the congenital long QT syndrome:

ECG Criteria
Corrected QT >480 ms	3 points
Corrected QT 460-480 ms	2 points
Corrected QT 450-460 ms (males)	1 point
Torsades de pointes	2 points
T-wave alternans	1 point
Notched T wave in 3 leads	1 point
Bradycardia	0.5 point
History	
Syncope with stress	2 points
Syncope without stress	1 point
Congenital deafness	0.5 point
Definite family history of long QT	1 point
Unexplained cardiac death in first-degree relative <30 yr	0.5 point

Total score = 4: definite long QT syndrome; total score = 2 to 3: intermediate probability; total score = 1: low probability.

WORKUP
Cardiology referral is recommended for all cases.
Genetic analysis is useful for risk stratification of patients with congenital prolonged QT and is important for identification of potential mutation carriers within the proband family.
In relatives of known patients with long QT syndrome or in young patients with syncope:
- Stress test may prolong the QT interval or cause T-wave alternans
- Valsalva maneuver: may prolong the QT interval or cause T-wave alternans
- Prolonged ECG monitoring with various stimulations aimed at increasing catecholamines and assess for QT prolongation (perform in a setting that can provide resuscitation)
- Epinephrine-induced prolongation of the QT interval (epinephrine infusion QT stress test)
- Genetic analysis
  - LQT1 locus of KCNQ1 potassium channel gene
  - LQT2 locus of KCNH2 potassium channel gene
  - LQT3 locus of SCN5A sodium channel gene
- Risk stratification: QT interval duration was the strongest predictor of risk for cardiac events (syncope, SCD); a QTc exceeding 500 ms identifies patients with the highest risk of becoming symptomatic by age 40; patients with the Jervell Lange-Nielsen and other homozygous syndromes and patients with long QT associated with syndactyly are at higher risk
  - High risk (>50% of cardiac event): QTc >500 ms and LQT1 and LQT2 or male with LQT3
  - Moderate risk (30% to 50%): QTc <500 ms in male with LQT3 or in female with LQT2, and female with LQT3
  - Low risk (<30%): QTc <500 ms and LQT1 or male LQT2

TREATMENT

NONPHARMACOLOGIC
- Swimming should be avoided or performed under supervision in patients with LQT1.

TABLE 1-101 Genetic Mutations in the Congenital Long QT Syndrome

		Location	Gene	Current	Effect
Romano-Ward syndrome (autosomal-dominant inheritance)	LQT1	11p15.5	KvLQT1 (K⁺ channel)	I_{Ks}	↓ Function ↓ Repolarization
	LQT2	7q35-36	HERG (K⁺ channel)	I_{Kr}	↓ Function ↓ Repolarization
	LQT3	3q21-24	SCN5A (Na⁺ channel)	I_{Na}	↑ Function ↑ Depolarization
	LQT4	4q25-27	Unknown	Unknown	Unknown
	LQT5	21q22	KCNE1 (K⁺ channel, subunit minK)	I_{Ks}	↓ Function ↓ Repolarization
Jervell and Lange-Nielsen syndrome (autosomal-recessive inheritance)		11p15.5	KvLQT1 (K⁺ channel)	I_{Ks}	↓ Function ↓ Repolarization
		21q22	KCNE 1 (K⁺ channel, subunit minK)	I_{Ks}	↓ Function ↓ Repolarization

From Crawford MH et al (eds): *Cardiology*, ed 2, St Louis, 2004, Mosby.

- Patients with *LQT2* patients should avoid sudden or excessive acoustic stimuli, especially during sleep (e.g., avoid telephone and/or alarm clock in the proximity).
- Avoid competitive sports.
- Implantable defibrillator is recommended according to the ACC/AHA guidelines for patients with a good functional status for more than 1 yr and the following conditions:
  ○ Survivors of cardiac arrest (class 1)
  ○ Patients with syncope or ventricular tachycardia while receiving β-blockers (class 2a)
  ○ Primary prevention in patients with characteristics that suggest high risk, such as *LQT2* and *LQT3* (class 2b)

PHARMACOLOGIC

- β-blocker at maximum tolerated dose
- Avoidance of medications that may further prolong the QT interval or deplete magnesium or potassium
- Table 1-102 summarizes management of patients with long QT syndrome

PROGNOSIS

The timing and frequency of syncope, QTc prolongation, and gender are predictive of risk for aborted cardiac arrest and sudden cardiac death during adolescence. Higher risk is present in those with one or two or more episodes of syncope in the last 10 yr compared with those with no syncopal episodes, those with QTc >530 ms, and males ages 10 to 12.

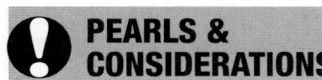

COMMENTS

Family history should be assessed for a history of sudden death and other deaths that may have occurred as manifestations of long QT syndrome (e.g., sudden infant death, drowning, loss of consciousness while driving).

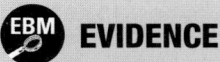

available at www.expertconsult.com

SUGGESTED READINGS
available at www.expertconsult.com

AUTHORS: **JOSHUA R. SILVERSTEIN, M.D., FRED F. FERRI, M.D.,** and **WEN-CHIH WU, M.D.**

TABLE 1-102 Management of Patients With Long QT Syndrome

Type of Syndrome	Management	Indication
Congenital	Beta blockers	Asymptomatic patients, symptomatic patients (who do not have broncospasm)
	Cervicothoracic sympathectomy	Refractory symptoms, especially in pediatric patients
	Cardiac pacing	Refractory symptoms associated with bradycardia, pauses
	Implantable cardioverter–defibrillator	Cardiac arrest, refractory syncope
Acquired	Elimination of causative drug or condition	All patients
	Magnesium sulfate	Nonsustained ventricular tachycardia, torsades de pointes (even with a normal serum magnesium concentration)
	Administration of potassium (to keep serum K^+ >4.5mEq/l)	Serum K^+ <4.5 mEq/l
	Maneuvers to increase heart rate (cardiac pacing, isoproterenol)	Bradycardia, arrhythmias refractory to magnesium sulfate

K^+, Potassium.
From Crawford MH et al (eds): *Cardiology,* ed 2, St Louis, 2004, Mosby.

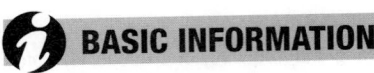

BASIC INFORMATION

DEFINITION

Lumbar disk syndrome includes diseases resulting from disk disorder, either herniation or degenerative change (spondylosis). Massive disk protrusion may rarely lead to paralysis in the lower extremity, a condition termed *cauda equina syndrome*. Gradual narrowing of the spinal canal (lumbar stenosis), usually from spondylosis, may also cause lower extremity symptoms.

SYNONYMS

Lumbago
Sciatica

ICD-9CM CODES
722.10 Lumbar disk displacement
724.02 Lumbar stenosis
344.60 Cauda equina syndrome
721.3 Lumbar spondylosis

EPIDEMIOLOGY & DEMOGRAPHICS

PREVALENCE:
- Variable
- At least one episode in 80% of adults

PREDOMINANT SEX: Approximately equal
PREDOMINANT AGE:
- Herniation: 20 to 40 yr
- Stenosis: >40 to 50 yr
- Disk symptoms: rare <20 yr

PHYSICAL FINDINGS & CLINICAL PRESENTATION

- Overlapping clinical syndromes that may result:
  1. Mild herniation without nerve root compression
  2. Herniation with nerve root compression
  3. Cauda equina syndrome
  4. Chronic degenerative disease with or without leg symptoms
  5. Spinal stenosis
- Low back pain, often worsened by activity or coughing and sneezing
- Local lumbar or lumbosacral tenderness
- Paresthesias, usually unilateral
- Restricted low back motion
- Increased pain on bending toward affected side
- Weakness and reflex changes (L4—knee jerk and quadriceps, L5—extensor hallucis longus, S1—ankle jerk and toe walking)
- Sensory examination usually not helpful
- Lumbar stenosis that possibly produces symptoms (pseudoclaudication), which are often misinterpreted as being vascular (Pseudoclaudication usually recovers quickly with sitting or spine flexion. Vascular disease is unaffected by spine position and is typically associated with atrophic skin changes and diminished pulses.)
- Positive straight leg raising test if nerve root compression is present

ETIOLOGY
Unknown

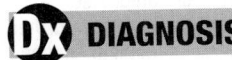

DIAGNOSIS

DIFFERENTIAL DIAGNOSIS
- Soft tissue strain or sprain
- Tumor
- Degenerative arthritis of hip
- Insufficiency fracture of hip or pelvis
  Section II describes the differential diagnosis of common low back pain syndromes.

WORKUP
In most cases the diagnosis can be established on a clinical basis alone.

IMAGING STUDIES
- Plain roentgenograms may be indicated within the first few weeks; they are usually normal in soft disk herniation, but with chronic degenerative disk disease loss of height of the disk space and osteophyte formation can occur.
- Myelography, CT scanning, and MRI (Fig. 1-221) may be indicated in patients whose symptoms do not resolve or when other spinal pathology may be suspected.
- Electrodiagnostic studies may confirm the diagnosis or rule out peripheral nerve disorders.

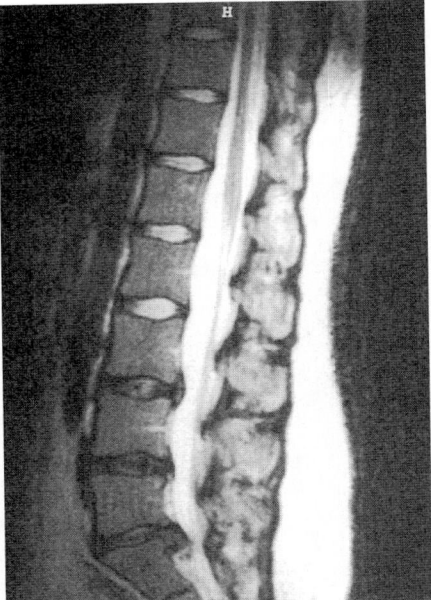

FIGURE 1-221 MRI showing a prolapsed L5/S1 disc. (From Carr A, Hamilton W: *Orthopedics in primary care*, ed 2, Philadelphia, 2005, Elsevier.)

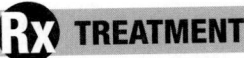

TREATMENT

NONPHARMACOLOGIC THERAPY
- Short course (3 to 5 days) of bed rest for acute disk herniation with leg pain
- Physical therapy for modalities plus a careful gradual exercise program
- Lumbosacral corset brace during rehabilitation process in conjunction with exercise program
- Percutaneous electrical nerve stimulation may be beneficial in selected patients with chronic back pain

ACUTE GENERAL Rx
- NSAIDs
- Muscle relaxants for sedative effect
- Analgesics
- Epidural steroid injection for leg symptoms in selected patients

DISPOSITION
- Almost all lumbar disk syndromes improve with time.
- Recurrent episodes usually respond to medical management.
- Recovery from the rare paralytic event is often incomplete.

REFERRAL
- For orthopedic or neurosurgical consultation for intractable pain or significant neurologic deficit
- Emergency referral for cauda equina syndrome

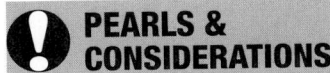

PEARLS & CONSIDERATIONS

Red flags suggesting a more serious condition as a cause of the back pain include:
1. Fever
2. History of malignancy
3. Pain at rest
4. Incontinence
5. Sudden worsening in level of pain
6. Weight loss
7. Significant motor loss, especially if associated with saddle anesthesia

COMMENTS
- Surgery is most consistently helpful when leg pain (not back pain) predominates.
- A clinical algorithm for evaluation of back pain is described in Section III.

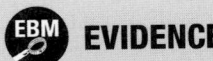

EVIDENCE
available at www.expertconsult.com

SUGGESTED READINGS
available at www.expertconsult.com

AUTHOR: **LONNIE R. MERCIER, M.D.**

BASIC INFORMATION

DEFINITION

A primary lung neoplasm is a malignancy arising from lung tissue. The World Health Organization distinguishes 12 types of pulmonary neoplasms. The major types are squamous cell carcinoma, adenocarcinoma, small cell carcinoma, and large cell carcinoma. However, the crucial difference in the diagnosis of lung cancer is between small cell and non–small cell types because the prognosis and therapeutic approach are different.

ADENOCARCINOMA: Represents 35% to 40% of lung carcinomas; frequently located in mid-lung and periphery; initial metastases are to lymphatics; frequently associated with peripheral scars

SQUAMOUS CELL (EPIDERMOID): 20% to 30% of lung cancers; central location; metastasis by local invasion; frequent cavitation and obstructive phenomena

SMALL CELL (OAT CELL): 20% of lung carcinomas; central location; metastasis through lymphatics; associated with lesion of the short arm of chromosome 3; high cavitation rate

LARGE CELL: 10% to 15% of lung carcinomas; frequently located in the periphery; metastasis to central nervous system and mediastinum; rapid growth rate with early metastasis

BRONCHOALVEOLAR: 5% of lung carcinomas; frequently located in the periphery; may be bilateral; initial metastasis through lymphatic, hematogenous, and local invasion; no correlation with cigarette smoking; cavitation rare

SYNONYMS

Lung cancer

ICD-9CM CODES
162.9 Malignant neoplasm of bronchus and lung, unspecified

EPIDEMIOLOGY & DEMOGRAPHICS

- Lung cancer is responsible for >30% of cancer deaths in males and >25% of cancer deaths in females. It has been the most common cancer in the world since 1985 and is the leading cause of cancer-related death.
- Tobacco smoking is implicated in 85% of cases; second-hand smoke is responsible for approximately 20% of cases.
- There are >200,000 new cases of lung cancer yearly in the U.S., most occurring at age >50 yr (<4% in patients <40 yr).
- Among women there has been a 600% increase in incidence of lung cancer during the past 80 years. The rates of death among women with lung cancer in the U.S. are the highest in the world.

PHYSICAL FINDINGS & CLINICAL PRESENTATION

- Weight loss, fatigue, fever, anorexia, dysphagia
- Cough, hemoptysis, dyspnea, wheezing
- Chest, shoulder, and bone pain
- Paraneoplastic syndromes (see Table 1-103):
  - Lambert-Eaton syndrome: myopathy involving proximal muscle groups
  - Endocrine manifestations: hypercalcemia, ectopic adrenocorticotropic hormone, syndrome of inappropriate excretion of adrenocorticotropic hormone
  - Neurologic: subacute cerebellar degeneration, peripheral neuropathy, cortical degeneration
  - Musculoskeletal: polymyositis, clubbing, hypertrophic pulmonary osteoarthropathy
  - Hematologic or vascular: migratory thrombophlebitis, marantic thrombosis, anemia, thrombocytosis, or thrombocytopenia
  - Cutaneous: acanthosis nigricans, dermatomyositis
- Pleural effusion (10% of patients), recurrent pneumonias (from obstruction), localized wheezing
- Superior vena cava syndrome:
  - Obstruction of venous return of the superior vena cava is most commonly caused by bronchogenic carcinoma or metastasis to paratracheal nodes.
  - The patient usually reports headache, nausea, dizziness, visual changes, syncope, and respiratory distress.
  - Physical examination reveals distention of thoracic and neck veins, edema of face and upper extremities, facial plethora, and cyanosis.
- Horner's syndrome: constricted pupil, ptosis, facial anhidrosis caused by spinal cord damage between C8 and T1 as a result of a superior sulcus tumor (bronchogenic carcinoma of the extreme lung apex); Pancoast tumor: a superior sulcus tumor associated with ipsilateral Horner's syndrome and shoulder pain

ETIOLOGY

- Tobacco abuse
- Environmental agents (e.g., radon) and industrial agents (e.g., ionizing radiation, asbestos, nickel, uranium, vinyl chloride, chromium, arsenic, coal dust)
- Lung cancer susceptibility and risk increased in inherited cancer syndromes caused by germ-line mutations in p53, retinoblastoma, and germ-line mutation in the epidermal growth factor receptor (EGFR) gene; also an association between single-nucleotide polymorphism variation at 15q24-15q25.1 and susceptibility to lung cancer

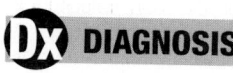

DIAGNOSIS

DIFFERENTIAL DIAGNOSIS

- Pneumonia
- Tuberculosis (TB)
- Metastatic carcinoma to the lung
- Lung abscess
- Granulomatous disease
- Carcinoid tumor
- Mycobacterial and fungal diseases
- Sarcoidosis
- Viral pneumonitis
- Benign lesions that simulate thoracic malignancy:
  - Lobar atelectasis: pneumonia, TB, chronic inflammatory disease, allergic bronchopulmonary aspergillosis
  - Multiple pulmonary nodules: septic emboli, Wegener's granulomatosis, sarcoidosis, rheumatoid nodules, fungal disease, multiple pulmonary atrioventricular fistulas
  - Mediastinal adenopathy: sarcoidosis, lymphoma, primary TB, fungal disease, silicosis, pneumoconiosis, drug-induced (e.g., phenytoin, trimethadione)
  - Pleural effusion: congestive heart failure, pneumonia with parapneumonic effusion,

TABLE 1-103 Paraneoplastic Syndromes Associated With Bronchogenic Carcinoma

Syndrome	Cell Type	Mechanism
Hypertrophic pulmonary osteoarthropathy and clubbing	All except small cell	Unknown
Hyponatremia	Small cell most common; may be any type	SIADH, ectopic antidiuretic hormone production by tumor
Hypercalcemia	Usually squamous cell	Bone metastases, osteoclast-activating factor, parathyroid hormone–like hormone, prostaglandins
Cushing's syndrome	Usually small cell	Ectopic ACTH production
Eaton-Lambert myasthenic syndrome	Usually small cell	Voltage-sensitive calcium channel antibodies in >75%; affects presynaptic neuronal calcium channel activity
Other neuromyopathic disorders	Small cell most common; may be any type	Antineuronal nuclear antibodies, also known as anti-Hu; others unknown
Thrombophlebitis	All types	Unknown

ACTH, Adrenocorticotropic hormone; *SIADH,* syndrome of inappropriate secretion of antidiuretic hormone.
From Andreoli TE et al: *Andreoli and Carpenter's Cecil essentials of medicine,* ed 8, Philadelphia, 2010, Saunders.

TB, viral pneumonitis, ascites, pancreatitis, collagen-vascular disease

WORKUP
Workup generally includes chest radiograph, CT scan of chest, positron-emission tomographic (PET) scan, and tissue biopsy.

LABORATORY TESTS
Obtain tissue diagnosis. Various modalities are available:
- Biopsy of any suspicious lymph nodes (e.g., supraclavicular node)
- Flexible fiberoptic bronchoscopy: brush and biopsy specimens are obtained from any visualized endobronchial lesions
- Transbronchial needle aspiration: done with a special needle passed through the bronchoscope; this technique is useful to sample mediastinal masses or paratracheal lymph nodes
- Transthoracic fine-needle aspiration biopsy with fluoroscopic or CT scan guidance to evaluate peripheral pulmonary nodules
- Mediastinoscopy and anteromedial sternotomy in suspected tumor involvement of the mediastinum
- Pleural biopsy in patients with pleural effusion
- Thoracentesis of pleural effusion and cytologic evaluation of the obtained fluid: may confirm diagnosis

IMAGING STUDIES
- Chest radiograph (Fig. 1-222): The radiographic presentation often varies with the cell type. Pleural effusion, lobar atelectasis, and mediastinal adenopathy can accompany any cell types.
- CT scan of chest is performed to evaluate mediastinal and pleural extension of suspected lung neoplasms.
- PET with ^{18}F-fluorodeoxyglucose (^{18}FDG-PET), a metabolic marker of malignant tissue, is superior to CT scan in detecting mediastinal

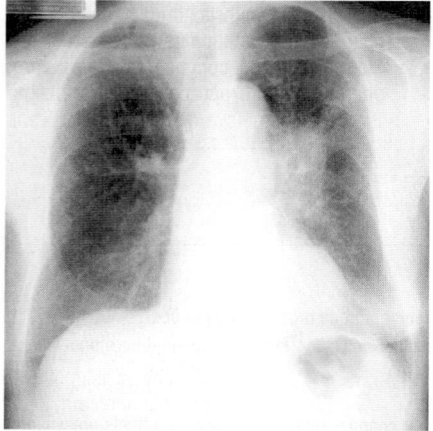

FIGURE 1-222 Chest radiograph shows small cell carcinoma of lung manifesting as left hilar mass. (From Weinberg SE, Cockrill BA, Mandel J: *Principles of pulmonary medicine*, ed 5, Philadelphia, 2008, Saunders.)

and distant metastases in non–small cell lung cancer (NSLC). It is useful for preoperative staging of NSLC.
- The use of PET-CT for preoperative staging of NSLC reduces both the total number of thoracotomies and the number of futile thoracotomies but does not affect overall mortality.
- The combination of endoluminal ultrasound (EUS) and endobronchial ultrasound (EBUS) with fine-needle aspiration has been reported to have a 93% sensitivity and 97% specificity for establishing the presence of mediastinal disease in lung cancer patients.

STAGING
After confirmation of diagnosis, patients should undergo staging:
1. The international staging system is the most widely accepted staging system for NSLC. In this system, stage I (N0 [no lymph node involvement]) and stage II (N1 [spread to ipsilateral bronchopulmonary or hilar lymph nodes]) include localized tumors for which surgical resection is the preferred treatment. Stage III is subdivided into IIIA (potentially resectable) and IIIB. The surgical management of stage IIIA disease (N2 [involvement of ipsilateral mediastinal nodes]) is controversial. Only 20% of N2 disease is considered minimal disease (involvement of only one node) and technically resectable. Stage IV indicates metastatic disease. The pathologic staging system uses a tumor/nodal involvement/metastasis system.
2. In patients with small cell lung cancer, a more practical accepted staging system is the one developed by the Veterans Administration Lung Cancer Study Group. This system contains two stages:
   a. Limited-stage disease: confined to the regional lymph nodes and to one hemithorax (excluding pleural surfaces)
   b. Extensive-stage disease: spread beyond the confines of limited-stage disease
3. Pretreatment staging procedures for lung cancer patients, in addition to complete history and physical examination, generally include the following tests:
   a. Chest radiograph (posteroanterior and lateral), ECG
   b. Laboratory evaluation: complete blood count, complete metabolic panel, arterial blood gases, pulse oximetry. The identification of molecular signatures of lung cancer to predict prognosis with data from microarray and/or reverse-transcription polymerase chain reaction analysis has been validated in recent trials. A five-gene signature (*DUSP6, MMD, STAT1, ERBB3,* and *LCK*) is closely associated with relapse-free and overall survival among patients with NSLC. Detection of mutations in epidermal growth factor receptor (EGFR) in circulating tumor cells from the blood of patients with lung cancer offers the possibility of monitoring changes in epithelial tumor genotypes during the course of treatment
   c. Pulmonary function studies

   d. CT scan of chest and PET scan: a recent Dutch trial revealed a 51% relative reduction in futile thoracotomies for patients with suspected NSLC who underwent preoperative assessment with PET with the tracer 18FDG-PET in addition to conventional workup
   e. Mediastinoscopy or anterior mediastinotomy in patients being considered for possible curative lung resection
   f. Biopsy of any accessible suspect lesions
   g. CT scan of liver and brain; radionuclide scans of bone in all patients with small cell carcinoma of the lung and patients with NSLC neoplasms suspected of involving these organs
   h. Bone marrow aspiration and biopsy only in selected patients with small cell carcinoma of the lung. In the absence of an increased lactate dehydrogenase or cytopenia, routine bone marrow examination not recommended
   i. Newer technologies in preoperative staging include endoscopic bronchial ultrasonography and esophageal ultrasonography to guide biopsies; however, cervical mediastinoscopy is criterion standard in preoperative nodal staging (sensitivity >93%, specificity >95%)

Rx TREATMENT

NONPHARMACOLOGIC THERAPY
- Nutritional support
- Avoidance of tobacco and other substances toxic to the lungs
- Supplemental O_2 prn

ACUTE GENERAL Rx
NON–SMALL CELL CARCINOMA:
- Surgical resection is the best hope for cure in patients with operable NSLC.
  1. Surgical resection is indicated in patients with limited disease (not involving mediastinal nodes, ribs, pleura, or distant sites). This represents approximately 15% to 30% of diagnosed cases.
  2. Preoperative evaluation includes review of cardiac status (e.g., recent myocardial infarction, major arrhythmias) and evaluation of pulmonary function (to determine if the patient can tolerate any loss of lung tissue). Pneumonectomy is possible if the patient has a preoperative $FEV_1 = 2$ L or if the maximal voluntary ventilation is >50% of predicted capacity. Individuals with FEV_1 >1.5 L are suitable for lobectomy without further evaluation unless there is evidence of interstitial lung disease or undue dyspnea on exertion. In that case, carbon dioxide diffusion in the lung (DLCO) should be measured. If the DLCO is <80% predicted normal, the individual is not clearly operable.
  3. Preoperative chemotherapy should be considered in patients with more advanced disease (stage IIIA) who are being considered for surgery because it in-

creases the median survival time in patients with NSLC compared with the use of surgery alone. Gene expression profiles that predict the risk of recurrence in patients with early stage (IA) NSLC have been identified. These patients are at high risk of recurrence and may also benefit from adjuvant chemotherapy.

4. Postoperative adjuvant chemotherapy (chemotherapy given after surgical resection of an apparently localized tumor to eradicate occult metastases) with vinorelbine plus cisplatin significantly increases 5-yr survival (69% vs. 54%) in patients with completely resected stage IB or stage II NSLC and good performance status. Adjuvant chemotherapy is generally indicated for patients with resected stages IIA through IIIA.

- Treatment of unresectable NSLC:
1. Radiotherapy can be used alone or in combination with chemotherapy; it is used primarily for treatment of central nervous system and skeletal metastases, superior vena cava syndrome, and obstructive atelectasis. Although thoracic radiotherapy is generally considered standard therapy for stage 3 disease, it has limited effect on survival. Palliative radiotherapy should be delayed until symptoms occur because immediate therapy offers no advantage over delayed therapy and results in more adverse events from the radiotherapy. Conventional radiotherapy fails to durably control the primary lung tumor in nealy 70% of patients and 2-yr survival is less than 40%. Stereotactic body radiation (SBRT) uses several highly focused radiation beams to deliver high doses in 15 treatments and appears to be more effective than conventional radiotherapy, with a survival rate of 55.8% at 3 yr for inoperable early stage lung cancer.

2. Chemotherapy: various combination regimens are available. Current drugs of choice are paclitaxel plus either carboplatin or cisplatin, cisplatin plus vinorelbine, gemcitabine plus cisplatin, and carboplatin or cisplatin plus docetaxel. The overall results are disappointing, and none of the standard regimens for NSLC is clearly superior to the others. The addition of bevacizumab to paclitaxel plus carboplatin results in significant survival benefit but carries an increased risk of treatment-related death. Gefitinib and erlotinib are oral inhibitors of *EGFR* tyrosine kinase. Activating mutations in the *EGFR* gene confer hypersensitivity to these medications. Both agents are currently approved only for patients who have not responded to at least one prior chemotherapy regimen. Sensitivity of lung neoplasms to these agents is seen primarily in tumors with somatic mutations in the tyrosine kinase domain (more common in adenocarcinomas found in patients who never smoked and in Asian patients). Recent trials revealed that gefitinib is superior to carboplatin-paclitaxel as an initial treatment for pulmonary adenocarcinoma among nonsmokers or former smokers in East Asia. In these patients the presence in the tumor of a mutation of the *EGFR* gene was a strong predictor of a better outcome with gefitinib. Oncogenic fusion genes consisting of EML4 and anaplastic lymphoma kinase (ALK) are present in a subgroup of non–small-cell lung cancers, representing 2% to 7% of such tumors. The inhibition of ALK in lung tumors with crizotinib, an orally available small-molecule inhibitor of the ALK tyrosine kinase has resulted in tumor shrinkage or stable patients in preliminary trials.

3. The addition of chemotherapy to radiotherapy improves survival in patients with locally advanced, unresectable NSLC. The absolute benefit is relatively small, however, and should be balanced against the increased toxicity associated with the addition of chemotherapy.

SMALL CELL LUNG CANCER:
- Limited-stage disease: standard treatments include thoracic radiotherapy and chemotherapy (cisplatin and etoposide)
- Extensive-stage disease: standard treatments include combination chemotherapy (cisplatin or carboplatin plus etoposide or combination of irinotecan and cisplatin)
- Prophylactic cranial irradiation for patients in complete remission to decrease the risk of central nervous system metastasis

DISPOSITION
- The 5-yr survival of patients with NSLC when the disease is resectable is approximately 30%.
- Median survival time in patients with limited-stage disease and small cell lung cancer is 15 mo; in patients with extensive stage disease, it is 9 mo. Among patients with metastatic non–small cell lung cancer, early palliative care results in longer survival and significant improvements in both quality of life and mood.
- Methylation of the promoter region of certain genes (*P16, CDH13, APC,* and *RASSF1A*) in a resected NSLC specimen is associated with recurrence of the tumor.

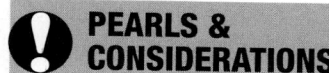

PEARLS & CONSIDERATIONS

COMMENTS
CT screening for detection of lung cancer among persons with a heavy history of smoking increases the percentage of lung cancer cases that are diagnosed in stage 1. However, randomized trials to assess whether such screening reduces mortality rates have not shown a significant benefit for CT screening. Current data do not support screening for lung cancer with any method.

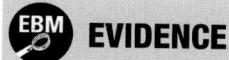

EVIDENCE
available at www.expertconsult.com

SUGGESTED READINGS
available at www.expertconsult.com

AUTHOR: **FRED F. FERRI, M.D.**

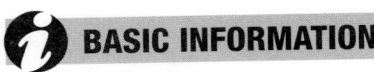

BASIC INFORMATION

DEFINITION

Lyme disease is a multisystem inflammatory disorder caused by the transmission of a spirochete, *Borrelia burgdorferi*. Lyme disease is spread by the bite of infected *Ixodes* ticks, taking 36 to 48 hr for a tick to feed and transmit the infecting organism *B. burgdorferi* to the host.

SYNONYMS

Bannworth's syndrome (Europe)
Acrodermatitis chronica atrophicans

ICD-9CM CODES
088.8 Lyme disease

EPIDEMIOLOGY & DEMOGRAPHICS

INCIDENCE (IN U.S.): 4.4 cases/100,000 persons; 90% of cases in the U.S. are found in: Massachusetts, Connecticut, Rhode Island, New York, New Jersey, Pennsylvania, Minnesota, Wisconsin, and California.
PEAK INCIDENCE: May to November
PREDOMINANT SEX: Male = female
PREDOMINANT AGE: Median age of 28 yr

PHYSICAL FINDINGS & CLINICAL PRESENTATION

Lyme disease may present in the following stages:
- *Early localized:* early Lyme disease, erythema migrans (EM); skin rash, often at site of tick bite; possible fever, myalgias 3 to 32 days after tick bite
- *Early disseminated:* days to weeks later; multiorgan system involvement, including CNS, joints, cardiac; related to dissemination of spirochete
- *Late persistent:* mo to yr after tick exposure; affects central and peripheral nervous system, cardiac, joints

Common presenting signs and symptoms include:
- EM (Fig. 1-223).
- Lymphadenopathy, neck pains, pharyngeal erythema, myalgias, hepatosplenomegaly.

- Patients will complain of malaise, fatigue, lethargy, headache, fever/chills, neck pain, myalgias, back pain.

ETIOLOGY

B. burgdorferi transmitted from bite of an *Ixodes* tick

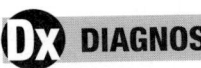

DIAGNOSIS

Clinical presentation, exposure to ticks in endemic area, and diagnostic testing for antibody response to *B. burgdorferi*

DIFFERENTIAL DIAGNOSIS

- Chronic fatigue/fibromyalgia
- Acute viral illnesses
- Babesiosis
- Ehrlichiosis

WORKUP

- ELISA testing-Western blot IgM and IgG
- Immunofluorescent assay
- Early disease often difficult to diagnose serologically secondary to slow immune response
- Culturing of skin lesions (EM) and polymerase chain reaction (PCR) of skin biopsy and blood to give definitive diagnosis (available only in reference laboratories)

IMAGING STUDIES

- Echocardiogram if conduction abnormalities are present with cardiac involvement
- CT scan, MRI of head for CNS involvement

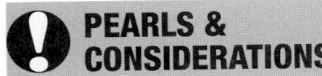

TREATMENT

- Early Lyme disease.
- Doxycycline 100 mg bid or amoxicillin 500 mg tid for 14 days (doxycycline should be avoided in children and pregnant females).
- Alternative treatments: cefuroxime axetil 500 mg bid for 14 to 21 days, azithromycin 500 mg PO for 7 to 10 days but should not be used as a first-line agent.
- Early disseminated and late persistent infection: 28 days of treatment necessary; doxycycline and ceftriaxone appear equally effective for acute disseminated Lyme disease.
- Arthritis: 28 days of doxycycline or amoxicillin plus probenecid.
- Neurologic involvement requires parenteral antibiotics. Those who fail to respond should be treated with IV ceftriaxone or cefotaxime.
- Ceftriaxone 2 g/day for 21 to 28 days; alternative: cefotaxime 2 g q8h; alternative: penicillin G 5 million U qid.
- Cardiac involvement: IV ceftriaxone or penicillin plus cardiac monitoring.
- Prolonged treatment with IV or PO antibiotic therapy for up to 90 days did not improve symptoms more than placebo.

DISPOSITION

The patient often needs careful follow-up and supportive care for the arthralgia-neuritis symptoms.

REFERRAL

- To a neurologist if significant neurologic complications (meningitis, myelitis, ophthalmoplegia, Bell's palsy)
- To a cardiologist if the patient develops evidence of cardiac conduction disturbances or pericarditis

PEARLS & CONSIDERATIONS

- The Lyme disease vaccine was taken off the U.S. market in 2002 because of concerns about possible side effects (arthralgia, arthritis) and its infrequent use.
- A physician diagnosis of classic erythema migrans in an endemic region of Lyme disease is sufficient to make a definitive diagnosis.
- In some patients with Lyme disease, nonspecific complaints such as headache, fatigue, and arthralgia may persist for months after appropriate (and ultimately successful) antibiotic treatment.
- There is no evidence of current or previous Borrelia burgdorferi infection in most patients evaluated at university-based Lyme disease referral centers. Psychiatric comorbidity and other psychological factors are prominent in the presentation and outcome of some patients who inaccurately ascribe longstanding symptoms to "chronic Lyme disease."
- A single dose of 200 mg doxycycline given within 72 hr of *Ixodes* tick bite can prevent development of Lyme disease.

SUGGESTED READINGS
available at www.expertconsult.com

AUTHORS: **GLENN G. FORT, M.D., M.P.H.,** and **DENNIS J. MIKOLICH, M.D.**

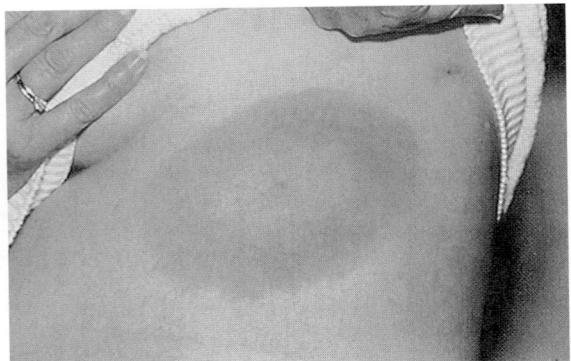

FIGURE 1-223 Erythema migrans. Note expanding erythematous lesion with central clearing on trunk. (Courtesy John Cook, M.D. From Goldstein B [ed]: *Practical dermatology*, ed 2, St Louis, 1997, Mosby.)

BASIC INFORMATION

DEFINITION

Lymphangitis refers to the inflammation of lymphatic vessels.

SYNONYMS

Nodular lymphangitis
Sporotrichoid lymphangitis

ICD-9CM CODES
457.2 Lymphangitis

EPIDEMIOLOGY & DEMOGRAPHICS

INCIDENCE (IN U.S.): Several hundred cases/yr of sporotrichoid lymphangitis

PHYSICAL FINDINGS & CLINICAL PRESENTATION

ACUTE LYMPHANGITIS:
- Commonly associated with a bacterial cellulitis
- May or may not recognize site of skin trauma (i.e., laceration, puncture, ulcer)
- In hours to days, distal appearance of erythema, edema, and tenderness, with linear erythematous streaks extending proximally to regional lymph nodes
- Possible lymphadenitis and fever
- Predisposition to group A streptococcal infection of the skin in those with chronic lymphedema and superficial fungal infections (e.g., tinea pedis)

SPOROTRICHOID OR NODULAR LYMPHANGITIS:
- Includes subcutaneous nodules that develop along the path of involved lymphatics
- Most commonly results from inoculation of the skin of the hand
- Usually preceded by well-defined episode of cutaneous inoculation or trauma
- Lesions apparent from one to several wk after inoculation
- Initially, nodular or papular lesion; may ulcerate
- May have frank pus or a serosanguineous discharge
- Systemic complaints uncommon, but infection with certain microorganisms associated with fever, chills, myalgias, and headache

ETIOLOGY

- Acute lymphangitis: usually associated with *Streptococcus pyogenes* (group A streptococcus), but staphylococcal organisms are increasingly recognized as a cause of severe soft tissue infections such as lymphangitis, including community-acquired methicillin-resistant *S. aureus* (CA-MRSA)
- Nodular lymphangitis caused by one of several organisms
  1. *Sporothrix schenckii*
     a. Most common recognized cause in the U.S., usually in the Midwest
     b. Found in soil and plant debris
  2. *Nocardia brasiliensis:* found in soil
  3. *Mycobacterium marinum:* associated with trauma related to water (e.g., aquariums, swimming pools, fish)
  4. *Leishmania brasiliensis*
     a. Protozoal parasite transmitted to humans by sandflies, mostly to travelers in endemic areas
     b. Small endemic focus in Texas
  5. *Francisella tularensis*
     a. Most often in Midwestern states
     b. Associated with contact with infected mammals (e.g., rabbits) or tick bites

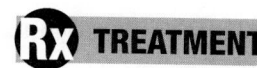 DIAGNOSIS

DIFFERENTIAL DIAGNOSIS

- Nodular lymphangitis
- Insect or snake bites
- Filariasis

WORKUP

- Acute lymphangitis: blood cultures
- Nodular lymphangitis: various stains and cultures of drainage or biopsy specimens of inoculation sites to make definitive diagnosis

LABORATORY TESTS

- WBCs possibly elevated with cellulitis
- Eosinophilia common with helminthic infections

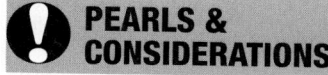 TREATMENT

NONPHARMACOLOGIC THERAPY

Limb elevation

ACUTE GENERAL Rx

- Penicillin possibly sufficient, but 1 wk of dicloxacillin or cephalexin 500 mg PO qid commonly used to ensure antistaphylococcal coverage; if CA-MRSA suspected, then use oral Bactrim DS: one PO bid is the best oral agent and with vancomycin 1 g IV every 12 hr being reserved for patients requiring IV therapy.
- If allergic to penicillin:
  1. Clindamycin 300 mg PO qid for 7 days *or*
  2. Erythromycin 500 mg PO qid for 7 days
- Nodular lymphangitis: specific therapy directed at etiologic agent.
- For superficial fungal infections: treatment may prevent recurrence of acute lymphangitis.

DISPOSITION

- Acute lymphangitis: usually resolves with therapy
- Recurrent attacks: may lead to chronic lymphedema of limb, rarely resulting in elephantiasis nostras (nonfilarial elephantiasis)
- Nodular lymphangitis: usually responds to appropriate therapy

REFERRAL

- If acute lymphangitis is more than a mild disease or involves the face
- If nodular lymphangitis or filariasis is suspected

! PEARLS & CONSIDERATIONS

COMMENTS

- Outside of the U.S., initial episodes of filariasis caused by *Brugia malayi* resemble acute lymphangitis.
- Chronic lymphedema or elephantiasis results from recurrent episodes.

SUGGESTED READINGS
available at www.expertconsult.com

AUTHORS: **GLENN G. FORT, M.D., M.P.H.,** and **DENNIS J. MIKOLICH, M.D.**

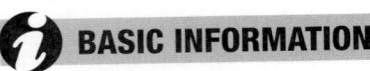
DEFINITION

Lymphedema refers to excessive accumulation of interstitial protein-rich fluid typically resulting from impaired regional lymphatic drainage.

SYNONYMS

Elephantiasis

ICD-9CM CODES
457.1 Lymphedema: acquired (chronic), praecox, secondary
457.1 Elephantiasis (nonfilarial)

EPIDEMIOLOGY & DEMOGRAPHICS

PRIMARY LYMPHEDEMA:
- Found in 1.1/100,000 people aged <20 yr
- Females outnumber males 3.5:1.
- Incidence peaks between ages 12 and 16

SECONDARY LYMPHEDEMA: See specific etiology (e.g., filariasis, breast cancer, prostate cancer)

PHYSICAL FINDINGS & CLINICAL PRESENTATION

Edema:
- Painless and progressive
  1. Initially the edema is pitting and smooth (Fig. 1-224); however, with advanced cases, the edema becomes nonpitting (this depends on the extent of fibrosis that has occurred).
  2. Elevation of the leg resolves the swelling in the early stages but not in the advanced stages.
- More often unilateral, but can be bilateral depending on the etiology

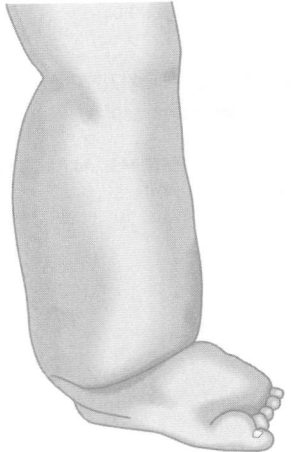

FIGURE 1-224 Lymphedema with characteristic loss of the normal perimalleolar shape resulting in a "tree trunk" pattern. Dorsum of the foot is characteristically swollen, resulting in the appearance of the "buffalo hump." (From Townsend CM, Beauchamp RD, Evers BM, Mattox KL [eds]: *Sabiston textbook of surgery,* ed 17, Philadelphia, 2004, Saunders.)

- Not always restricted to the lower extremities; may involve the genitals, face, or upper extremities (e.g., arm swelling after mastectomy)
- Stemmer's sign (squaring of the toes caused by edema in the digits)
- "Buffalo hump" appearance of the dorsum of the foot
- Loss of the ankle contour, giving a "tree trunk" appearance of the leg

Skin:
- Hard, thick, leathery skin caused by fibrosis induced by chronic stasis
- Occasional drainage of lymph
- Infections (cellulitis, lymphangitis, onychomycosis)

ETIOLOGY

Lymphedema is caused by a reduction in lymphatic transport and is classified into primary and secondary forms.

Primary idiopathic lymphedema is believed to result from developmental abnormalities such as lymphatic hypoplasia and functional insufficiency or absence of lymphatic valves. Subclasses of this type of lymphedema include:
- Congenital lymphedema:
  1. Detected at birth or recognized within first 2 yr of life
  2. Involves one or both extremities, usually the entire leg
  3. May be familial (Milroy's disease)
- Lymphedema praecox:
  1. Onset in teenage years
  2. Usually unilateral
  3. Most common form of primary lymphedema (up to 94% of cases)
  4. More common in females (10:1), suggesting estrogen has a role in pathogenesis
  5. May be familial (Meige's disease)
- Lymphedema tarda:
  1. Usually occurs after age 30 yr
  2. Uncommon, accounting for <10% of cases of primary lymphedema

Secondary lymphedema develops after disruption or obstruction of the lymphatic system as a consequence of:
- Surgery for malignant tumors (e.g., breast, prostate, lymphoma)
- Edema of the arm after axillary lymph node dissection is the most common cause of lymphedema in the United States
- Incidence of lymphedema is approximately 14% in patients after mastectomy with adjuvant radiation treatment
- Inflammation (streptococci, filariasis)
- Filariasis is the most common cause of lymphedema in the world
- Trauma
- Radiation with lymph node removal

DX DIAGNOSIS

- Lymphedema is primarily a clinical diagnosis made on the basis of physical features that distinguish it from other causes of chronic edema of the extremities, such as the presence of cutaneous and subcutaneous fibrosis (peau d'orange) and the Stemmer sign.
- When physical examination is inconclusive, other available imaging tests can help make the diagnosis: isotopic lymphoscintigraphy, indirect and direct lymphography, lymphatic capillaroscopy, MRI, CT, or ultrasound.

DIFFERENTIAL DIAGNOSIS

Exclude other causes of edema (e.g., cirrhosis, nephrosis, congestive heart failure, myxedema, hypoalbuminemia, chronic venous stasis, reflex sympathetic dystrophy, obstruction from abdominal or pelvic malignancy).

WORKUP

A detailed history and physical examination should help exclude most of the differential diagnoses.

LABORATORY TESTS

- Blood urea nitrogen, creatinine, liver function tests, albumin, urine analysis, and thyroid function tests are obtained to exclude possible systemic causes of edema.
- Noninvasive venous studies help exclude venous insufficiency.
- Genetic testing may be practical in defining a specific hereditary syndrome with a discrete gene mutation such as lymphedema-distichiasis *(FOXC2)* and some forms of Milroy disease *(VEGFR-3).*

IMAGING STUDIES

- Lymphoscintigraphy:
  1. Diagnostic image of choice
  2. Sensitivity and specificity of 100% in diagnosing lymphedema
  3. Currently considered the gold standard for diagnosis of lymphedema
- CT scan: to exclude malignancy leading to obstruction.
- Duplex ultrasound to rule out venous obstruction as a cause for edema.
- Lymphangiography: lymphoscintigraphy is preferred over lymphangiography. Lymphangiography is contraindicated in malignancy.

Rx TREATMENT

NONPHARMACOLOGIC THERAPY

Complex decongestive therapy (CDT) is backed by longstanding experience as the primary treatment of choice for lymphedema in both children and adults. It involves a two-stage treatment program:
1. Reduce leg swelling and size:
   - Leg elevation
   - Limb massage
   - Pneumatic leg compression
2. Maintain edema-free state:
   - Elastic support stockings that are properly fitted according to compression pressure and length are essential to prevent edema from returning.
   - Compression pressures are graduated; most of the pressure is distal with

L

decreasing pressure from the stockings moving proximally.

- Compression pressures range from 20 to 30 mm Hg, 30 to 40 mm Hg, 40 to 50 mm Hg, and 50 to 60 mm Hg. Most prefer 40 to 50 mm Hg for lymphedema.
- The length should cover the edematous site. Choices include below the knee, thigh-high, and pantyhose lengths.

ACUTE GENERAL Rx

- No drugs have been shown to be beneficial. Diuretics, in particular, should not be used because they may promote the development of volume depletion.
- Infections such as lymphangitis (usually caused by group A streptococci) should be treated promptly.
- In secondary lymphedema, treating the underlying cause is indicated (e.g., prostate cancer, breast cancer). If the etiology is filariasis caused by the parasites *Wuchereria bancrofti* or *Brugia malayi,* treatment is diethylcarbamazine citrate 5 mg/kg in divided doses for 3 wk.
- Mesotherapy (hyaluronidase), immunological therapy (autologous lymphocyte injection), and fluid restriction all have uncertain benefit in the treatment of lymphedema.
- In children with chylous reflux syndromes, a diet low in long-chain triglycerides and high in short- and medium-chain triglycerides has been shown to be of benefit in treatment.

CHRONIC Rx

Surgery for chronic lymphedema should act as an adjunct to CDT or as an alternative if CDT has proven unsuccessful. Operative treatment is considered with:

- Continued increase in leg size despite medical treatment
- Impaired leg function
- Recurrent infections
- Emotional lability as a result of the cosmetic appearance

Surgical procedures are divided into two types:
- Those performed to improve lymph node drainage (e.g., anastomoses of the lymph system with the venous system)
- Those performed to excise the subcutaneous tissue (e.g., Charles' procedure, Thompson's procedure, and the modified Homans' procedure)
- Liposuction in combination with long-term CDT has been shown to be more effective in reducing edema than long-term CDT alone

DISPOSITION

- Lymphedema is a slowly progressive disorder that can lead to significant disfigurement of the extremities or other body parts.
- The extent of fibrotic change to the skin of the affected limb increases with the chronicity of lymphatic stasis.
- In many patients the maximum girth of the affected limb is reached within the first year after onset, unless complications such as recurrent cellulitis supervene.
- Patients with lymphedema commonly manifest psychiatric comorbidities as a result of their disease, such as anxiety, depression, adjustment problems, and difficulty in vocational, domestic, or social domains.

- Chronic lymphedema can be complicated by cellulitis or, in rare cases, development of lymphangiosarcomata or other cutaneous malignancies.

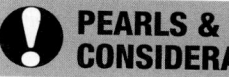 **PEARLS & CONSIDERATIONS**

- Lymphedema is a chronic, generally incurable ailment that requires lifelong care and attention along with psychosocial support.
- It is important to remember that surgery is not a cure.
- Children and adolescents (along with parents and adults) should be encouraged to pursue a normal life, participating in school activities and sports (preferably noncontact, such as swimming).
- It should also be remembered that cases of lymphangiosarcomas have been associated, although rarely, with postmastectomy lymphedema.
- Gene therapy to develop new lymphangioles in the affected limbs is a potential clinical remedy in the future.

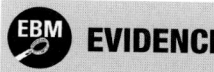 **EVIDENCE**

available at www.expertconsult.com

SUGGESTED READINGS
available at www.expertconsult.com

AUTHOR: **TANYA ALI, M.D.**

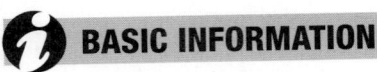

BASIC INFORMATION

DEFINITION

Lymphogranuloma venereum (LGV) is a sexually transmitted, systemic disease caused by *Chlamydia trachomatis,* serovars L_1, L_2, or L_3.

SYNONYMS

Tropical bubo
Poradenitis inguinalis
LGV

ICD-9CM CODES
099.1 Lymphogranuloma venereum

EPIDEMIOLOGY & DEMOGRAPHICS

INCIDENCE (IN U.S.): Rare; 285 cases reported in 1993
PREVALENCE: Endemic in Africa, India, parts of Southeast Asia, South America, and the Caribbean
PREDOMINANT SEX: Male:female ratio is 5:1

PHYSICAL FINDINGS & CLINICAL PRESENTATION

Primary stage:
- Primary lesion caused by multiplication of organism at site of infection
- Papule, shallow ulcer
- Herpetiform lesion at site of inoculation (most common)
- Incubation period of 3 to 21 days
- Most common site of lesion in women: posterior wall, fourchette, or vulva
- Spontaneous healing without scarring

Second stage:
- Inguinal syndrome: characteristic inguinal adenopathy
- Begins 1 to 4 wk after primary lesion
- Syndrome is the most frequent clinical sign of the disease
- Unilateral inguinal adenopathy in 70% of cases
- Symptoms: painful, extensive adenitis (bubo) and suppuration may occur with numerous sinus tracts
- "Groove sign" signaling femoral and inguinal node involvement (20%); most often seen in men
- Involvement of deep iliac and retroperitoneal lymph nodes in women may present as a pelvic mass

Third stage (anogenital syndrome):
- Subacute: proctocolitis
- Late: tissue destruction or scarring, sinuses, abscesses, fistulas, strictures of perineum, elephantiasis

ETIOLOGY

Chlamydia trachomatis is the causative agent. There are three serotypes: L1, L2, and L3.

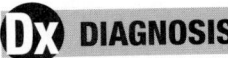

DIAGNOSIS

DIFFERENTIAL DIAGNOSIS

- Inguinal adenitis, suppurative adenitis, retroperitoneal adenitis, proctitis, schistosomiasis.
- Section II describes the differential diagnosis of genital sores.

WORKUP

- Diagnosis is based on clinical suspicion, epidemiologic information, and the exclusion of other etiologies for proctocolitis, inguinal lymphadenopathy, or genital or rectal ulcers.
- Screening for other STDs.
- A clinical algorithm for evaluation of genital ulcer disease is described in Section III, "Genital Lesions."

LABORATORY TESTS

- Genital and lymph node specimens (i.e., lesion swab or bubo aspirate) can be tested for *C. trachomatis* by culture, direct immunofluorescence, or nucleic acid detection.
- Positive Frei test:
  1. Intradermal chlamydial antigen
  2. Nonspecific for all *Chlamydia*
  3. No longer available (historical significance only)
- Complement fixation test:
  1. Titer >1:64 in active infection
  2. Convalescent titers no difference
- Cell culture of *Chlamydia* aspiration of fluctuant node yields highest rates of recovery
- Complete blood count: mild leukocytosis with lymphocytosis or monocytosis
- Elevated sedimentation rate
- VDRL and HIV screening to rule out other sexually transmitted diseases

IMAGING STUDIES

- CT scan for suspected retroperitoneal adenitis

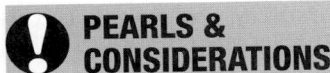

TREATMENT

NONPHARMACOLOGIC THERAPY

- Avoid milk and milk products while taking medication.
- Practice sexual abstinence.
- Treat sexual partners. Persons who have had sexual contact with a patient who has LGV within 60 days before onset of the patient's symptoms should be examined, tested for urethral or cervical chlamydial infection, and treated with a chlamydia regimen (azithromycin 1 g orally single dose or doxycycline 100 mg orally twice a day for 7 days.

ACUTE GENERAL Rx

- Doxycycline 100 mg PO bid × 21 days
- Erythromycin base 500 mg PO qid × 21 days
- Azithromycin 1 g orally once weekly for 3 wk is probably effective
- Surgical:
  1. Aspirate fluctuant nodes
  2. Incise and drain abscesses

CHRONIC Rx

- Longer course of therapy will be needed for chronic or relapsing cases, which may be caused by reinfection and/or inadequate treatment.
- A rectal stricture requires a colostomy.
- Surgery should be considered only after antibiotic treatment.

DISPOSITION

Good prognosis with early treatment, usually resulting in complete resolution of symptoms.

REFERRAL

Surgical consultation if patient develops obstruction, fistula, or rectal stricture. May need referral to plastic surgeon if patient has lymphatic obstruction.

PEARLS & CONSIDERATIONS

COMMENTS

- Pregnant and lactating women should be treated with erythromycin regimen.
- Congenital transmission does not occur, but infection may be acquired through an infected birth canal.
- Patient education materials may be obtained through local and state health clinics.

SUGGESTED READING
available at www.expertconsult.com

AUTHORS: **GEORGE T. DANAKAS, M.D.,** and **RUBEN ALVERO, M.D.**

BASIC INFORMATION

DEFINITION

Non-Hodgkin lymphoma (NHL) is a heterogeneous group of malignancies of the lymphoreticular system.

SYNONYMS

NHL

ICD-9CM CODES
201.9 Lymphoma, non-Hodgkin

EPIDEMIOLOGY & DEMOGRAPHICS

INCIDENCE (IN U.S.): Sixth most common neoplasm (56,000 new cases annually). Incidence increases with age. In patients with HIV, NHL is the second most common tumor (after Kaposi's sarcoma).
PREDOMINANT AGE: Median age at time of diagnosis is 50 yr.

PHYSICAL FINDINGS & CLINICAL PRESENTATION

- Patients often present with asymptomatic lymphadenopathy.
- Approximately one third of NHLs originate extranodally. Involvement of extranodal sites can result in unusual presentations (e.g., gastrointestinal tract involvement can simulate peptic ulcer disease).
- NHL cases associated with HIV occur predominantly in the brain.
- Pruritus, fever, night sweats, and weight loss are less common than in Hodgkin's disease.
- Hepatomegaly and splenomegaly may be present.

DIAGNOSIS

DIFFERENTIAL DIAGNOSIS

- Hodgkin's disease
- Viral infections
- Metastatic carcinoma

A clinical algorithm for evaluation of lymphadenopathy is described in Section III. The differential diagnosis of lymphadenopathy is described in Section II.

WORKUP

Initial laboratory evaluation may reveal only mild anemia and elevated lactate dehydrogenase (LDH) and erythrocyte sedimentation rate (ESR). Proper staging of NHL requires the following:

- A thorough history, physical examination, and adequate biopsy. Laparoscopic lymph node biopsy can be used on an outpatient basis for most patients with intraabdominal lymphoma.
- Routine laboratory evaluation (complete blood count, ESR, urinalysis, LDH, blood urea nitrogen, creatinine, serum calcium, uric acid, liver function tests, serum protein electrophoresis).
- Chest x-ray (posteroanterior and lateral).
- Bone marrow evaluation (aspirate and full bone core biopsy).

- CT scan of abdomen and pelvis; CT scan of chest if chest x-ray films abnormal.
- Bone scan (particularly in patients with histiocytic lymphoma).
- Depending on the histopathology, the results of the above studies and the planned therapy, some other tests may be performed (e.g., positron-emission tomographic scan).
- β-2 microglobulin levels should be obtained initially (prognostic value) and serially in patients with low-grade lymphomas (useful to monitor therapeutic response of the tumor).
- Serum interleukin levels have prognostic value in diffuse large cell lymphoma.

CLASSIFICATION: The working formulation of NHL for clinical use subdivides lymphomas into low grade, intermediate grade, high grade, and miscellaneous (Table 1-104).
STAGING: The Ann Arbor staging system with Cotswold modification is described in Table 1-105. Histopathology has greater therapeutic implications in NHL than in Hodgkin's disease. The frequency of indolent lymphomas among all lymphomas is described in Table 1-106. The classification of aggressive lymphomas is described in Table 1-107.

TREATMENT

ACUTE GENERAL Rx

The therapeutic regimen varies with the histologic type and pathologic stage. Following are the commonly used therapeutic modalities:
LOW-GRADE NHL (e.g., NODULAR, POORLY DIFFERENTIATED):

1. Local radiotherapy for symptomatic obstructive adenopathy.
2. Deferment of therapy and careful observation in asymptomatic patients.
3. Single-agent chemotherapy with cyclophosphamide or chlorambucil and glucocorticoids
4. Combination chemotherapy alone or with radiotherapy: generally indicated only when the lymphoma becomes more invasive, with poor response to less aggressive treatment.
5. Monoclonal antibodies directed against B-cell surface antigens can also be used to treat follicular lymphomas resistant to conventional therapy. The anti-CD20 monoclonal antibody rituximab is effective against low-grade NHL in patients who have not received previous treatment.
6. The addition of rituximab to CHOP is generally well tolerated; however, additional studies may be necessary to clarify the role of CHOP plus rituximab in patients with indolent NHL.
7. Ibritumomab tiuxetan (Zevalin), an immunoconjugate that combines the linker-chelator tiuxetan with the monoclonal antibody ibritumomab, can be used as part of a two-step regimen for treatment of patients with relapsed or refractory low-grade, follicular, or transformed B-cell NHL refractory to rituximab.

8. New purine analogs (FLAMP, 2CDA) can be used in salvage treatment of refractory lymphomas. They all have activity in follicular lymphomas.
9. Table 1-108 summarizes treatment strategies for indolent lymphomas.

INTERMEDIATE- AND HIGH-GRADE LYMPHOMAS (E.G., DIFFUSE HISTIOCYTIC LYMPHOMA): Combination chemotherapy regimens (e.g., CHOP, PRO-MACE-CYTABOM, MACOP-B, M-BACOD). An anthracycline-containing regimen (such as CHOP) given in standard doses and schedule is generally best for treatment of older patients with advanced stage, aggressive-histology lymphoma who do not have significant comorbid illness.

1. High-dose sequential therapy is superior to standard-dose MACOP-B for patients with diffuse large-cell lymphoma of the B-cell type.
2. Dose-modified chemotherapy should be considered for most HIV-infected patients with lymphoma.
   - Three cycles of CHOP followed by involved-field radiotherapy may be superior to eight cycles of CHOP alone in patients with localized intermediate- and high-grade NHL.
   - High-dose chemotherapy with autologous stem-cell support has been reported to be superior to CHOP in adults with disseminated aggressive lymphoma.
   - The addition of rituximab against CD20 B-cell lymphoma to the CHOP regimen increases the complete response rate and prolongs event-free and overall survival in elderly patients with diffuse large B-cell lymphoma without a clinically significant increase in toxicity. Bexxar, a combination of the mononuclear antibody tositumomab and radiolabeled iodine-131, can be used for a single treatment of relapsed follicular NHL in patients who are refractory to rituximab.
   - In patients <61 yr, chemotherapy with three cycles of ACVBP (doxorubicin, cyclophosphamide, vindesine, bleomycin, and prednisone) followed by sequential consolidation has been reported to be superior to three cycles of CHOP plus radiotherapy for treatment of newly diagnosed aggressive lymphoma (diffuse mixed, diffuse large cell, or immunoblastic according to the working formulation).
   - Granulocyte-colony stimulating factor: may be effective in reducing the risk of infection in patients with aggressive lymphoma undergoing chemotherapy.
   - Radioimmunotherapy with (^{131}I) anti-B1 antibody therapy for NHL either by itself or in combination with other treatments represents a new modality in the armamentarium against lymphomas.
   - Treatment with high-dose chemotherapy and autologous bone marrow transplant: compared with conventional chemotherapy, increases event-free and overall survival in patients with chemotherapy-sensitive NHL in relapse.

TABLE 1-104 Classification Systems for Grading Lymphomas

Kiel Classification	Working Formulation	Revised European-American Classification

Low-grade malignancy
  Lymphocytic, CLL
  Lymphocytic, other
  Lymphoplasmacytoid
  Centrocytic
	Low grade
	  A. Malignant lymphoma, small lymphocytic
	     Consistent with CLL
	
	  B. Malignant lymphoma, follicular, predominantly small
	     cleaved cell
		B-cell lymphomas
		
		  B-CLL/SLL
		  Lymphoplasmacytoid lymphoma
		  Follicle center lymphomas

Centroblastic/centrocytic
    Follicular without sclerosis
    Follicular with sclerosis
    Follicular and diffuse, without sclerosis
	Diffuse areas
	  Sclerosis
	  C. Malignant lymphoma, follicular mixed, small cleaved
	     and large cell
		Marginal zone lymphomas (MALT)
		  Mantle cell lymphoma

Follicular and diffuse, with sclerosis
    Diffuse
  Low-grade malignant lymphoma, unclassified
High-grade malignancy
  Centroblastic
  Lymphoblastic, Burkitt's type
  Lymphoblastic, convoluted cell type
  Lymphoblastic, other (unclassified) immunoblastic
  High-grade malignant lymphoma, unclassified
	Diffuse areas
	  Sclerosis
	Intermediate grade
	  D. Malignant lymphoma, follicular
	    Diffuse areas
	  E. Malignant lymphoma, diffuse small cleaved cell
		Diffuse large B-cell lymphoma
		  Primary mediastinal large B-cell lymphoma
		  Burkitt's lymphoma
		T-cell lymphomas
		
		  T-CLL
		  Mycosis fungoides/Sézary syndrome

Malignant lymphoma unclassified (unable to specify high
  grade or low grade)
Composite lymphoma
	F. Malignant lymphoma, diffuse mixed, small and large
	     cell sclerosis
	  G. Malignant lymphoma diffuse
	
	  Large cell
	  Cleaved cell
	  Noncleaved cell
	  Sclerosis
	  High grade
	  H. Malignant lymphoma large cell, immunoblastic
	  Plasmacytoid
	  Clear cell
	  Polymorphous
	  Epithelioid cell component
	  I. Malignant lymphoma lymphoblastic
	  Convoluted cell
	  Nonconvoluted cell
	  J. Malignant lymphoma small noncleaved cell
	  Burkitt's
	  Follicular areas
		Peripheral T-cell lymphoma, unspecified
		
		  Angioimmunoblastic T-cell lymphoma
		  Angiocentric lymphoma
		  Intestinal T-cell lymphoma
		  Adult T-cell lymphoma/leukemia
		  Anaplastic large cell lymphoma
		  Precursor T-lymphoid lymphoma/leukemia

B-CLL, B-cell chronic lymphoid leukemia; *CLL,* chronic lymphocytic leukemia; *MALT,* mucosa-associated lymphoid tumor; *SLL,* lymphoid leukemia; *T-CLL,* T-cell CLL.
From Abeloff MD: *Clinical oncology,* ed 3, New York, 2004, Churchill Livingstone.

TABLE 1-105 Ann Arbor Staging System for Lymphomas

Stage*	Cotswold Modification of Ann Arbor Classification
I	Involvement of a single lymph node region or lymphoid structure
II	Involvement of two or more lymph node regions on the same side of the diaphragm (the mediastinum is considered a single site, whereas the hilar lymph nodes are considered bilaterally); the number of anatomic sites should be indicated by a subscript (e.g., II_3)
III	Involvement of lymph node regions on both sides of the diaphragm: III_1 (with or without involvement of splenic hilar, celiac, or portal nodes) and III_2 (with involvement of para-aortic, iliac, and mesenteric nodes)
IV	Involvement of one or more extranodal sites in addition to a site for which the designation E has been used

*All cases are subclassified to indicate the absence (A) or presence (B) of the systemic symptoms of significant fever (>38.0° C [100.4° F]), night sweats, and unexplained weight loss exceeding 10% of normal body weight within the previous 6 months. The clinical stage (CS) denotes the stage as determined by all diagnostic examinations and a single diagnostic biopsy only. In the Ann Arbor classification, the term pathologic stage (PS) is used if a second biopsy of any kind has been obtained, whether negative or positive. In the Cotswold modification, the PS is determined by laparotomy; X designates bulky disease (widening of the mediastinum by more than one third or the presence of a nodal mass >10 cm), and E designates involvement of a single extranodal site that is contiguous or proximal to the known nodal site.
From Hoffmann R et al: *Hematology: basic principles and practice,* ed 5, Philadelphia, 2009, Churchill Livingstone.

TABLE 1-106 Frequency of Indolent Lymphomas Among All Lymphomas in the WHO Classification

Follicular lymphoma	22.1%
Extranodal marginal zone lymphoma of mucosa-associated lymphoid tissue type	7.6%
Small lymphocytic lymphoma/chronic lymphocytic leukemia	6.7%
Mantle cell	6.0%
Splenic marginal zone lymphoma	1.8%
Lymphoplasmacytic lymphoma	1.2%
Nodal marginal zone B-cell lymphoma (±monocytoid B cells)	1.0%

From Hoffmann R et al: *Hematology: basic principles and practice,* ed 5, Philadelphia, 2009, Churchill Livingstone.

TABLE 1-107 Classification of Aggressive Lymphomas

B Cell Neoplasms

Precursor B-cell lymphoma
Precursor B lymphoblastic leukemia/lymphoma
Mature B-cell lymphoma
Mantle cell lymphoma
Diffuse large B-cell lymphoma
Mediastinal (thymic) large B-cell lymphoma
Intravascular large B-cell lymphoma
Primary effusion lymphoma
Burkitt lymphoma/leukemia
B-cell proliferations of uncertain malignant potential
Lymphomatoid granulomatosis
Posttransplant lymphoproliferative disorder, polymorphic

T-cell and NK-cell Neoplasms

Precursor T-cell
Precursor T lymphoblastic leukemia/lymphoma
Blastic NK cell lymphoma
Mature T-cell and NK-cell lymphoma
Adult T-cell leukemia/lymphoma
Extranodal NK/T cell lymphoma, nasal type
Hepatosplenic T-cell lymphoma
Peripheral T-cell lymphoma, unspecified
Angioimmunoblastic T-cell lymphoma
Anaplastic large cell lymphoma

From Hoffmann R et al: *Hematology: basic principles and practice*, ed 5, Philadelphia, 2009, Churchill Livingstone.

TABLE 1-108 Treatment Strategies for Indolent Lymphomas

Advanced Stage Disease

"Watchful waiting"
Alkylating agents
Purine analogs
Combination chemotherapy
Monoclonal antibodies
   Unconjugated
   Conjugated — radioimmunoconjugates and immunotoxins
Chemotherapy + monoclonal antibodies (chemoimmunotherapy)
High dose chemotherapy plus autologous/allogeneic hematopoietic cell transplantation
Reduced intensity conditioning allogeneic transplantation
Palliative radiotherapy

Localized Disease

Radiotherapy
"Watchful waiting"

From Hoffmann R et al: *Hematology: basic principles and practice*, ed 5, Philadelphia, 2009, Churchill Livingstone.

- An algorithm for the management of non-Hodgkin lymphoma in pediatric patients is described in the online version of Section III.

DISPOSITION

- Patients with low-grade lymphoma, despite their long-term survival (6 to 10 yr average), are rarely cured, and the great majority (if not all) eventually die of the lymphoma, whereas patients with a high-grade lymphoma may achieve a cure with aggressive chemotherapy.
- Complete remission occurs in 35% to 50% of patients with intermediate- and high-grade lymphoma. Prognostic factors include the histologic subtype, age of patient, and bulk of disease. Table 1-109 describes the International Prognostic Index for aggressive lymphomas.
- Patients who present with AIDS-related NHL and a low CD4 cell count have a poor prognosis (median duration of survival is 15 to 34 mo).

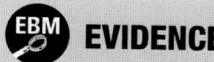 **EVIDENCE**

available at www.expertconsult.com

SUGGESTED READINGS
available at www.expertconsult.com

AUTHOR: **FRED F. FERRI, M.D.**

TABLE 1-109 International Prognostic Index for Aggressive Lymphomas*

Risk Group	IPI Score	CR Rate (%)	5 year overall survival (%)
Low	0, 1	87	73
Low intermediate	2	67	51
High intermediate	3	55	43
High	4, 5	44	26

*One point is given for the presence of each of the following characteristics: age >60 years, elevated serum LDH level, ECOG performance status ≥ 2, Ann Arbor stage III or IV, and more than two extranodal sites.
CR, Complete response; *ECOG*, Eastern Cooperative Oncology Group; *IPI*, International Prognostic Index; *LDH*, lactate dehydrogenase.
From Hoffmann R et al: *Hematology: basic principles and practice*, ed 5, Philadelphia, 2009, Churchill Livingstone.

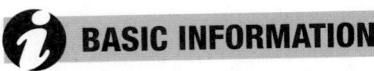

BASIC INFORMATION

DEFINITION

Lynch syndrome is a hereditary predisposition to malignancy of the colon that is explained by a germline mutation in a DNA mismatch repair gene.

SYNONYMS

Hereditary nonpolyposis colorectal cancer
Hereditary site-specific colon cancer

ICD-9CM CODES
1539 Lynch syndrome

EPIDEMIOLOGY & DEMOGRAPHICS

The lifetime risk for developing colon cancer in the U.S. is approximately 6%. Of these cases, 2% to 3% may be attributable to Lynch syndrome. The incidence of Lynch syndrome is estimated to be between 1:660 and 1:2000. The average age of diagnosis for Lynch syndrome is 48 yr, although diagnosis can occur as early as the 20s or as late as the 70s.

RISK FACTORS: Family history of colon cancer or other hereditary nonpolyposis colorectal cancer (HNPCC)-related cancers such as endometrial (up to 40% of women with Lynch syndrome may develop endometrial cancer), biliary tract, ovarian, stomach, or brain.

GENETICS: Autosomal-dominant inheritance pattern

ETIOLOGY

Lynch syndrome is thought to be secondary to germline mutations in DNA mismatch repair genes. The predominant genes involved are *MSH2* and *MLH1,* which are tumor suppressor genes, although other genes have documented involvement *(PMS1, PMS2, MSH6, MLH3).* Mutations in these genes prevent repair of DNA mismatches during DNA replication. This is most prevalent in regions of DNA called microsatellites causing DNA microsatellite instability and leading to an increased risk for malignancy, especially colon cancer.

PHYSICAL FINDINGS & CLINICAL PRESENTATION

- Changes in bowel habits (prolonged constipation)
- Melena
- Hematochezia
- Abdominal pain
- Unexplained weight loss
- Decreased appetite

DIAGNOSIS

DIFFERENTIAL DIAGNOSIS

- Familial adenomatosis polyposis
- Peutz-Jeghers syndrome
- Juvenile polyposis
- Nonhereditary colorectal cancer
- Gardner syndrome

WORKUP

If an individual presents with numerous adenomatous polyps or has multiple relatives with cancer at a young age, a family history complete with pedigree must be obtained. Clinical diagnosis of the Lynch syndrome can be made with the Amsterdam criteria or, if these are not met, the Bethesda criteria, which are more sensitive (see following list).

- Amsterdam criteria (must meet all criteria):
  1. Colorectal carcinoma and/or endometrial carcinoma or transitional cell carcinoma of the ureter or carcinoma of the small bowel in at least three individuals in the family
  2. One of the patients is a first-degree family member of two other patients
  3. Involved patients occur in at least two successive generations
  4. At least one of the diagnoses was made before age 50
  5. The diagnoses are histologically confirmed
  6. Familial adenomatous polyposis is excluded
- Bethesda criteria (must meet all criteria):
  1. Colorectal cancer before age 50
  2. Multiple colorectal cancers or other HNPCC-related cancers such as biliary tract, endometrial, stomach, or ovary
  3. Colorectal cancer with microsatellite instability histology <60 yr of age
  4. Colorectal cancer or HNPCC-related cancer in first-degree relative <50 yr of age
  5. Colorectal cancer or HNPCC-related cancer in at least two first- or second-degree relatives, any age
- If criteria for the Lynch syndrome are not met, no further analysis is necessary (although a genetic syndrome cannot be definitively excluded and genetic referral may be warranted).

LABORATORY TESTS

- If a patient meets criteria for Lynch syndrome, immunohistochemistry can be performed for the presence or absence of mismatch repair genes *MLH1, MSH2, MSH6,* and *PMS2.*
- Microsatellite instability analysis should also be performed if criteria for Lynch syndrome are met.

TREATMENT

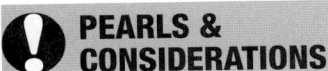

- If the mutation has been identified in a family member, screening for this mutation can be performed via genetic testing. Informed consent must be obtained after a thorough explanation has been provided to each individual.
- Surveillance using colonoscopy can be performed in individuals who screen positive, while those who screen negative can be discharged. The mismatch repair gene that is mutated guides screening.
- According to the Netherlands Surveillance Protocol, for example, individuals with mutations in *MLH1, MSH2,* or *MSH6* should have colonoscopies every 1 to 2 yr starting at age 20 to 25 yr; urine cytology every 1 to 2 yr starting at age 30 to 35 yr; gastroscopy every 1 to 2 yr starting at age 30 to 35 yr; and, in females, ultrasound of endometrium and CA-125 every 1 to 2 yr starting at age 30 to 35 yr.

REFERRALS

- To gastroenterology for surveillance colonoscopies
- To genetic counselor if patient satisfies Bethesda criteria
- To psychologist as necessary for psychologic support

PEARLS & CONSIDERATIONS

- Prior to genetic testing being instituted, informed consent must be obtained because consequences of this testing include the necessity of lifelong screenings such as colonoscopies.
- The risk of pancreatic cancer is increased in families with Lynch syndrome compared with the U.S. population.

PATIENT & FAMILY EDUCATION

- For information on local genetic counselors, visit the National Society of Genetic Counselors Web site at www.nsgc.org.
- For information on Lynch syndrome, visit www.mayoclinic.com/health/lynch-syndrome/DS00669.

SUGGESTED READINGS
available at www.expertconsult.com

AUTHORS: **PAUL F. GEORGE, M.D.,** and **JOANNE M. SILVIA, M.D.**

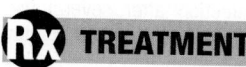

BASIC INFORMATION

DEFINITION

Macular degeneration refers to a group of diseases associated with loss of central vision and damage to the macula. Degenerative changes occur in the pigment, neural, and vascular layers of the macula. Dry macular degeneration is usually ischemic in etiology, and wet macular degeneration is associated with leakage of fluid from blood vessels, usually referred to as *age-related macular degeneration* (AMD).

ICD-9CM CODES
362.5 Degeneration of macula and posterior pole

EPIDEMIOLOGY & DEMOGRAPHICS

INCIDENCE (IN U.S.):
- Leading cause of irreversible blindness in people ≥50 yr in the developed world.
- Increases with age.
- More than 8 million Americans have AMD. The overall prevalence is projected to increase by >50% by 2020.

PEAK INCIDENCE:
- Ages 75 to 80 yr
- Dramatically increases in incidence and prevalence with age until ~80% of people ≥75 yr have senile macular degeneration

PREVALENCE (IN U.S.): Varies, but ~5% of people >50 yr have some signs of macular degeneration

PREDOMINANT SEX: Males and females are affected equally (15% of white women >80 yr have severe AMD)

PREDOMINANT AGE: >50 yr

RISK FACTORS:
- Advancing age
- Genetic factors
- Complement factor H, Tyr402His variant
- *LOC387715/ARMS2*, Ala69Ser variant
- History of smoking within past 20 yr
- Dietary factors (low intake of antioxidants and zinc, high fat intake)
- Obesity
- White race

PHYSICAL FINDINGS & CLINICAL PRESENTATION

- Decreased central vision
- Macular hemorrhage, pigmentation, edema, atrophy
- The most common abnormality seen in AMD is the presence of drusen, or yellowish deposits deep to the retina; this may be early in the course of disease
- Choroidal neovascular membrane (CNVM) develops with rapid change in vision

ETIOLOGY

- Subretinal neovascular membrane early
- Pigmentary and vascular changes with exudate, edema, and scar tissue development
- Dry-type atrophy of macular pigment epithelium

DIAGNOSIS

DIFFERENTIAL DIAGNOSIS

- Diabetic retinopathy (with neovascularization, can mimic CNVM)
- Hypertension
- Histoplasmosis (less common cause of CNVM)
- Trauma with scar

WORKUP

- Complete eye examination, including visual field and fluorescein angiography
- Optical coherence tomography (OCT)

LABORATORY TESTS

Evaluate for diabetes and other metabolic problems as well as vascular diseases

IMAGING STUDIES

- OCT
- Fluorescein angiography

TREATMENT

NONPHARMACOLOGIC THERAPY

- Laser treatment to stop progression of disease; photodynamic treatment with verteporfin IV
- Laser (Argon) for certain classic membranes (CNVM)
- A high dietary intake of antioxidants, vitamins C and E, and zinc has been reported to substantially reduce the risk of AMD in elderly persons

ACUTE GENERAL Rx

- The introduction of therapies blocking vascular endothelial growth factor (VEGF) dramatically changed the management of AMD and it is now standard practice for clinicians to offer intravitreal injections of anti-VEGF agents (ranibizumab, bevacizumab) as first-line treatment for neovascular AMD. Intravitreal administration of ranibizumab, a monoclonal antibody Fab that neutralizes all active forms of VEGF A, has shown to be effective in preventing vision loss and improving mean visual acuity in patients with AMD. It has also been reported to be superior to photodynamic therapy with verteporfin in the treatment of predominantly classic neovascular AMD. Bevacizumab, a monoclonal antibody to

BEGF, is also often used off-label as intravitreal therapy. Its cost per intravitreal dose is significantly lower than that of ranibizumab. A major concern regarding anti-VEGF treatment is the potential increased risk of stroke and cardiovascular disease.
- Intravitreal steroids; photodynamic treatment with laser.
- Intravitreous injections of pegaptanib (Macugen), an anti-VEGF, have been reported as effective therapy in slowing vision loss in neovascular AMD. Pegaptanib is administered once every 6 wk by intravitreous injection into one eye.

CHRONIC Rx

- Repeated laser treatments
- Antioxidants and zinc may slow progression of AMD

DISPOSITION

- Follow closely by ophthalmologist, retinal specialist.
- Most bevacizumab or ranibizumab treatment failures are due to missed follow-up visits. Patients should be reminded repeatedly to call if their vision worsens. There should also be a system in place for calling patients who have been lost to follow-up due to the high risk of recurrent neurovascularization and vision loss in these patients.

REFERRAL

- To ophthalmologist early in the course of the disease if vision is to be saved
- Immediate referral if any change in vision

PEARLS & CONSIDERATIONS

COMMENTS

- Sildenafil has no significant effect on macular degeneration.
- Statistically, the vision of only 1 of 10 affected persons can be saved, but the disease is so devastating that vigorous therapy should be considered in all patients.
- Statins plus aspirin may slow progression.
- Vitamins with zinc and antioxidants may slow progression of AMD.

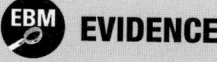 **EVIDENCE**

available at www.expertconsult.com

SUGGESTED READINGS
available at www.expertconsult.com

AUTHOR: **MELVYN KOBY, M.D.**

M

Diseases and Disorders

I

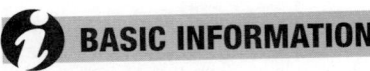

BASIC INFORMATION

DEFINITION

Malaria is a protozoan disease caused by the genus *Plasmodium* and transmitted by female *Anopheles* spp. mosquitoes. It is endemic throughout most of the tropics and is characterized by hectic fever and often presents with classic malarial paroxysm. Four species of genus plasmodium usually infect humans:

- *P. falciparum*
- *P. vivax*
- *P. malariae*
- *P. ovale*

SYNONYMS

Periodic fever
Tertian malaria
Quartan malaria
Tropical splenomegaly

ICD-9CM CODES

084.6 Malaria

EPIDEMIOLOGY & DEMOGRAPHICS

Global:
- ~300 million cases a year in more than 100 countries
- Around 900,000 deaths per year, with more than 80% of the deaths ocurring in children of sub-Saharan Africa
- 3 billion people live in malaria endemic areas

U.S.:
- ~1500 cases reported to the CDC in the United States each year.
- More than 50% of the reported cases in the U.S. are *P. falciparum*. On average, there are six deaths per year in the United States.
- Most infections limited to:
  1. Immigrant population
  2. Returned travelers or troops from endemic area
- Occasionally, transmission through exposure to infected blood product or shared intravenous needles by users of injection drugs.
- Congenital transmission is possible.
- Local mosquito-borne transmission has been reported.
- Competent mosquito vectors are present.
  1. *A. albimanus* in eastern United States
  2. *A. freeborni* in western United States

Geographic distribution:
- *P. falciparum:* Sub-Saharan Africa, Papua New Guinea, Solomon Islands, Haiti, Indian subcontinent
- *P. vivax:* Central America, South America, North Africa, Middle East, Indian subcontinent
- *P. ovale:* West Africa
- *P. malariae:* worldwide

Parasite life cycle (Fig. 1-225):
- Human infection begins when a female anopheline mosquito bites (only female anopheline mosquito takes blood meal) and inoculates plasmodial sporozoites into bloodstream. The bite usually occurs between dusk and dawn.
- The sporozoites then travel to liver and invade hepatocytes.

- In the hepatocytes, the sporozoites mature to tissue schizont or become dormant hypnozoites.
- The tissue schizonts amplify the infection by producing large number of merozoites (10,000 to 30,000).
- Each merozoite is capable of invading an RBC and can establish the asexual cycle of replication in RBCs.
- Asexual cycles produce and release 24 to 32 merozoites at the end of 48- or 72-hr (*P. malariae*) cycles.
- The hypnozoites are only found in relapsing malaria *P. vivax* or *P. ovale* and may remain dormant for up to 5 yr.
- Eventually some intraerythrocytic parasites develop into gametocytes. Male and female gametocytes are taken up by a female anopheline mosquito with a blood meal where they fertilize in the mosquito gut to produce a diploid zygote that matures to an ookinete; haploid sporozoites are generated that migrate to the salivary gland of the mosquito to infect another human.

PHYSICAL FINDINGS & CLINICAL PRESENTATION

- Fever is the hallmark of malaria, known as malarial paroxysm, initially daily until synchronization of infection after several wk, when fever may occur every other day (tertian) in *P. vivax, P. ovale,* or *P. falciparum* malaria or every third day (quartan) in *P. malariae* malaria.
- Classic malarial paroxysm characterized by
  1. Cold stage: abrupt onset of cold feeling associated with rigors, shakes
  2. Hot stage: high fever (~40° C) associated with restlessness
  3. Sweating stage: patient defervesces
- Nonspecific symptoms are
  1. Headache
  2. Cough
  3. Myalgia
  4. Vomiting
  5. Diarrhea
  6. Jaundice
- *P. falciparum*:
  ○ Most pathogenic of the four species.
  ○ Rapidly progresses to high-level parasitemia.
  ○ Important cause of the fatal malaria.
  ○ Classic malarial paroxysm is usually absent.
  ○ Incubation period after exposure is 12 days (range: 9 to 60 days).
  ○ Cytoadherence and resetting of RBCs play central role in pathogenesis.
  ○ The sequestration of RBCs in vital organs leads to fatal complications.
  ○ Cerebral malaria is a feared complication.

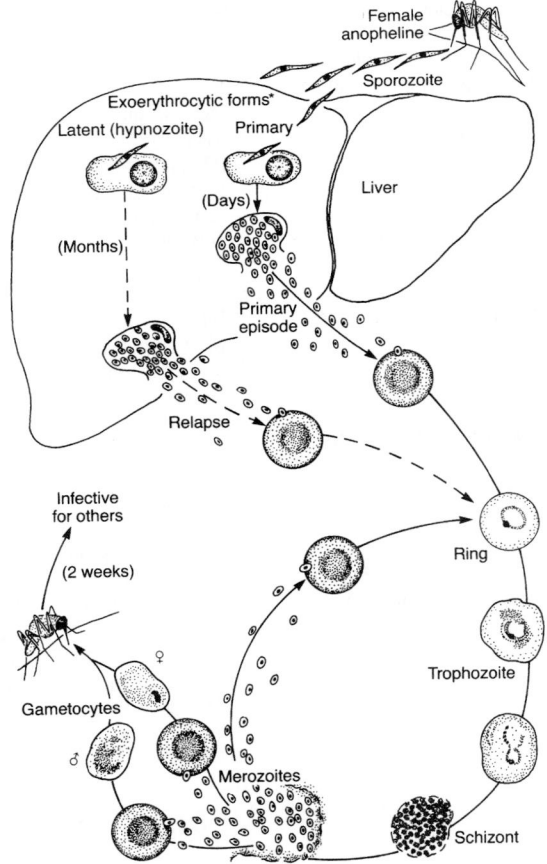

FIGURE 1-225 Life cycle of plasmodia in humans. Exoerythrocytic forms are also called schizonts. (From Gorbach SL: *Infectious diseases*, ed 2, Philadelphia, 1998, WB Saunders.)

- Invades erythrocytes of all ages.
- Lacks hypnozoites (intrahepatic stage), does not relapse.
- Blood smear usually shows ring form only.
- Pigment color is black.
- Banana-shaped gametocytes; if seen in blood, smear is diagnostic.
- Chloroquine resistance is widely present.

• *P. vivax:*
  - Known as tertian malaria: fever occurs every other day.
  - Duffy blood-group antigen FYA- or FYB-related receptor is needed for attachment to RBC.
  - FyFy phenotype (most West African) individuals are resistant to *P. vivax* malaria.
  - Incubation period after exposure is 14 days (range: 8 to 27 days).
  - Hypnozoites may cause relapse of infection after years.
  - Infects mainly reticulocytes.
  - Irregularly shaped large rings and trophozoites, enlarged RBCs, and Schüffner's dot are seen in peripheral blood smear (Fig. 1-226).
  - Pigment color is yellow-brown.
  - *P. vivax* from Papua New Guinea have reduced sensitivity to chloroquine.
  - Primaquine is needed to eradicate the hypnozoites.

• *P. ovale:*
  - Also known as tertian malaria; fever occurs every other day.
  - Occurs mainly in tropical Africa.
  - Incubation period after exposure is 14 days (range: 8 to 27 days).
  - Hypnozoites may cause relapse of infection.
  - Infects mainly reticulocytes.
  - Infected RBC are seen as enlarged, oval shape containing large ring or trophozoites with Schüffner's dot.
  - Pigment color is dark brown.
  - Primaquine needed to eradicate the hypnozoites.
  - No chloroquine resistance has been encountered.

• *P. malariae:*
  - Known as quartan malaria; fever occurs every third day.
  - Common cause of chronic malarial infection.
  - May persist for 20 to 30 yr after leaving the endemic area.
  - Worldwide distribution.
  - Incubation period after exposure is 30 days (range: 16 to 60 days).
  - Lacks hypnozoites (intrahepatic stage).
  - May persist in blood for many years if treated inadequately.
  - Chronic infection may cause soluble immune-complex, resulting in nephritic syndrome.
  - Infects mainly mature RBCs.
  - Band or rectangular forms of trophozoites are commonly seen in peripheral blood smear.
  - Pigment color is brown-black.

• Cerebral malaria:
  - Feared complication of *P. falciparum* infection.
  - Mortality is ~20%.
  - Pathogenesis is poorly understood.
  - Ischemia as a result of sequestration of parasites or cytokines induced by parasite toxin(s) is the key debate.
  - Seizure and altered mental status leading to coma are cardinal manifestation.
  - Hypoglycemia, lactic acidosis, and elevated circulating TNF-α may be present.
  - CSF studies: no increase of WBC count or protein, raised lactate concentrate, and increased opening pressure, especially in children, may be present.

Dx DIAGNOSIS

DIFFERENTIAL DIAGNOSIS

- Typhoid fever
- Dengue fever
- Yellow fever
- Viral hepatitis
- Influenza
- Brucellosis
- UTI
- Leishmaniasis
- Trypanosomiasis
- Rickettsial diseases
- Leptospirosis

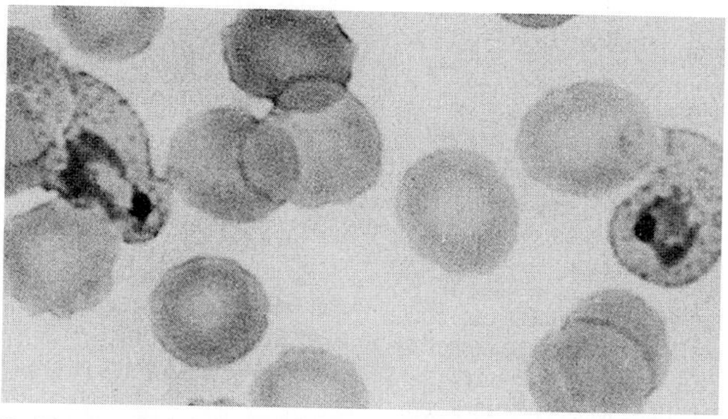

FIGURE 1-226 Giemsa-stained blood smear in *Plasmodium vivax* malaria. Asexual parasites. Note that the parasites are large and ameboid; the infected erythrocytes are the largest cells in the field (because they are reticulocytes), and the erythrocytes contain numerous pink dots (Schüffner's dots) (×2000). (From Klippel JH et al (eds): *Internal medicine,* ed 5, St Louis, 1998, Mosby.)

WORKUP

- Clinical diagnosis is notoriously inaccurate.
- Demonstration of malarial parasites in blood smear is essential.
- Newer molecular diagnostic techniques are promising.

LABORATORY TESTS

- The thick and thin blood film is required to identify malarial parasites.
- The thick smears are more sensitive and primarily used to detect the presence of parasites.
- The thin smears are used for species differentiation and parasite density estimation.
- A patient who is suspected of having malaria but who has no parasite seen in blood smears should have blood smears repeated every 12 to 24 hr for 3 consecutive days.

PREPARATION OF BLOOD SMEAR:

- Must be prepared from fresh blood obtained by pricking the fingers.
- The thin smear is fixed in methanol before staining.
- The thick smear is stained unfixed.
- The smear should be stained with a 3% Giemsa solution (pH of 7.2) for 30 to 45 min.
- The parasite density should be estimated by counting the percentage of RBCs infected, not the number of parasites, under an oil immersion lens on thin film.

COMMON ERRORS IN READING MALARIAL SMEARS:

- Platelets overlying an RBC
- Misreading artifacts as parasites
- Concern about missing a positive slide

MOLECULAR DIAGNOSIS OF MALARIA:

- Rapid diagnostic tests (RDT)
  1. Employ immunochromatographic lateral flow technology for antigen detection.
  2. Thus far only one RDT has been FDA approved: BinaxNOW Malaria test kit.
  3. This kit is based on antigens HRP-2 and aldolase.
  4. For *P. flaciparum*: sensitivity 95% and specificity 94%.
  5. For *P. vivax*: sensitivity 69% and specificity 100%.
- Limitations of the BinaxNOW Malaria test:
  1. Not approved for mixed infections
  2. Should not be used for *P. malariae* and *P. ovale* as data are limited
  3. Negative results require confirmation by thick and thin smears
  4. This test cannot be used to monitor therapy as antigen persists after the elimination of the parasite causing false positives
- Other diagnostic tests available include:
  1. Tagged monoclonal antibodies for malaria antigen detection
  2. Nucleic acid amplification and detection: PCR can detect parasites down to a level of 1 to 5 parasites per microliter of blood. PCR can detect mixed species infection
  3. Fluorescence microscopy with acridine orange or other staining
  4. Dark field microscopy

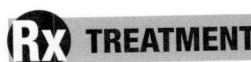 **TREATMENT**

NONPHARMACOLOGIC THERAPY

ANTIMOSQUITO MEASURES:
1. Eradication of mosquito breeding places by chemical spray
2. Use of mosquito nets properly in the endemic areas
3. Use of protective clothing
4. Use of insect spray (permethrin), mosquito coils, or repellents such as diethyltoluamide (DEET). For adults, DEET (30% to 50%) is generally protective for at least 4 hr. For smaller children, use DEET at ≤20% concentration.

ACUTE GENERAL Rx

A definitive diagnosis of malaria is essential for specific antimalarial chemotherapy.

NON-*FALCIPARUM* MALARIA:
- Chloroquine 600 mg base (1000 mg chloroquine phosphate) PO loading dose, 6 hr later 300 mg base (500 mg salt), then 300 mg base (500 mg salt) daily for 2 days.
- In the case of *P. vivax* and *P. ovale,* treatment with primaquine 15 mg daily for 14 days is needed to eradicate the exoerythrocytic forms, especially the hypnozoites responsible for relapses.
- G6PD should be measured before primaquine is given.
- Chloroquine-resistant *P. vivax* has been documented; in that case, quinine is given.

FALCIPARUM MALARIA:
- Chloroquine can be used cautiously for *falciparum* malaria acquired in chloroquine-sensitive areas (chloroquine is more rapidly effective than quinine)
- Mainstay of treatment is oral quinine sulfate 10 mg (salt)/kg (usually 650 mg) q8h for 3 to 7 days + doxycycline 100 mg PO BID both for 7 days for adults. Pediatrics: quinine sulfate: 10 mg/kg PO tid plus clindamycin: 20 mg/kg per day divided in tid dose both for 7 days.
- Atovaquone-proguanil (Malarone): 250 mg atovaquone/100 mg proguanil): 4 adult tabs PO once a day for 3 days with food in adults or for pediatrics: pediatric tablets (62.5 mg atovaquone/25 mg proguanil) are used based on weight:
  - 5 to 8 kg: 2 pediatric tab PO once daily for 3 days
  - 9 to 10 kg: 3 pediatric tabs PO once daily for 3 days
  - 11 to 20 kg: 1 adult tab PO once daily for 3 days
  - 21 to 30 kg: 2 adult tabs PO once daily for 3 days
  - 31 to 40 kg: 3 adult tabs PO once daily for 3 days
  - >40 kg: 4 adult tabs PO once daily for 3 days artemether-lumefantrine (Coartem) tablets: 4 tabs PO (at time zero and 8 hr later) then bid × 2 days for a total of six doses. For pediatrics:
    - 5 to <15 kg: 1 tablet per dose
    - 15 to <25 kg: 2 tablets per dose

- 25 to <35 kg: 3 tablets per dose
- >35 kg: 4 tablets per dose. The child should receive initial dose based on weight, then followed by second dose 8 hr later, then 1 dose PO bid for following 2 days

ALTERNATIVES:
- Quinine sulfate plus clindamycin 900 mg tid for 7 days in adults, or
- Mefloquine 750 mg PO then 500 mg PO 6 to 12 hr later in adults

NOTE: Parasitemia may paradoxically rise in the first 24 to 36 hr and is not an indication of treatment failure.

SEVERE *FALCIPARUM* MALARIA:
- It is a medical emergency; intensive care is preferred.
- Measurement of blood glucose, lactate, ABG is important.
- IV quinidine gluconate 10 mg salt/kg loading dose (maximum 600 mg) in NS; infuse slowly over 1 to 2 hr, followed by continuous infusion of 0.02 mg/kg/min until patient can swallow.
- Need to monitor ECG for observation of QT interval as can prolong. Also need to monitor blood pressure and glucose to avoid hypoglycemia.
- Alternatively, IV artesunate: 2.4 mg/kg IV first dose then at 12 and 24 hr followed by 2.4 mg/kg once daily.
- Plasmapheresis is an option for parasitemia >30% or in pregnant woman and in elderly with severe malaria.

NOTE: WHO recommends IV artesunate as the treatment of choice for severe malaria in adults and children in area of low transmission. Data on children in high-transmission regions are limited, and WHO recommends treatment with artesunate, artemether, or quinine.

MULTIDRUG-RESISTANT MALARIA:
- Mefloquine 1250 mg as a single dose, or
- Halofantrine 500 mg every 6 hr for 3 doses, repeat same course after 1 wk
- Combination therapy usually preferred

DISPOSITION

RISK FACTORS FOR FATAL MALARIA:
- Failure to take chemoprophylaxis
- Delay in seeking medical care
- Misdiagnosis

COMPLICATIONS OF MALARIA:
- Anemia
- Acidosis
- Hypoglycemia
- Respiratory distress
- DIC
- Blackwater fever
- Renal failure
- Shock

REFERRAL
- To an infectious disease specialist or travel medicine expert for severe malaria complications
- To an intensive care specialist if severe cerebral malaria or other major organ failure develops

PEARLS & CONSIDERATIONS

HOST RESPONSE:
- The specific immune response to malaria confers protection from high-level parasitemia and disease, but not from infection.
- Asymptomatic parasitemia without illness (premunition) is common among adults in endemic areas.
- Immunity is specific for both the species and the strain of infecting malarial parasites.
- Immunity to all strains is never achieved.
- Normal spleen function is an important host factor because of immunologic as well as filtering functions of the spleen.
- Both humoral and cellular immunity are necessary for protection.
- Polyclonal increase in serum level of IgG, IgM, and IgA occur in immune individuals.
- Antibody to antigenically variant protein PfEMP1 is important for protection in case of *P. falciparum* malaria.
- Passively transferred IgG from immune individuals has been shown protective.
- Maternal antibody confers relative protection of infants from severe disease.
- Genetic disorders (sickle cell disease, thalassemia, and G6PD deficiency) confer protection from death because parasites are unable to grow efficiently in low-oxygen tensions, thus preventing high-level parasitemias. Individuals deficient of Duffy factor in RBCs are resistant to infection by *P. vivax.*
- Nonspecific defense mechanisms, such as cytokines (TNF-α, IL-1, -6, -8), also play an important role in protection, causing fever (temperatures of 40° C damage mature parasites) and other pathologic effects.

PREVENTION OF MALARIA: Medications are available for the prophylaxis of malaria and will vary depending on level of chloroquine resistence in a given area.

Areas free of chloroquine-resistant Falciparum malaria:
Chloroquine 300 mg base (500 mg chloroquine phosphate) PO/wk. Start 1 wk prior to arrival in malaria area, then weekly while there and for 4 wk on leaving malaria area. Pediatric dose: 8.3 mg/kg (5 mg/kg base). Alternatives for adults include atovaquone-proguanil (Malarone): 1 adult tablet per day starting 1 to 2 days prior to arriving in malaria area, then daily while there and then for 7 days daily on leaving malaria area. For children, atovaquone-proguanil pediatric tablets based on weight:
  - 11 to 20 kg 1 pediatric tablet
  - 21 to 30 kg 2 pediatric tablets
  - 31 to 40 kg 3 pediatric tablets
  - >40 kg 1 adult tablet

Areas with chloroquine-resistant Falciparum malaria:
- Atovaquone-proguanil (Malarone): dosing as above
- Mefloquine 250 mg (228 mg base) PO/wk, starting 1 wk before arriving in malaria area, weekly while there and then weekly for 4 wk

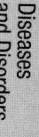

on return. In children, mefloquine dose is based on weight:
<15 kg 5 mg/kg
15 to 19 kg ¼ adult dose
20 to 30 kg ½ adult dose
31 to 45 kg ¾ adult dose
>45 kg adult dose

- Doxycycline 100 mg PO/day for adults and children aged >8. Start 1 to 2 days before travel, daily while in malaria area and then daily for 4 wk on return.

SPECIAL CONSIDERATIONS:
- Long-term visitors or travelers
- Children aged <12 yr
- Immunocompromised host

- Pregnant women: chloroquine and mefloquine are safe in pregnancy but not atovaquone-proguanil. Avoid doxycycline and primaquine.

VACCINATION:
- No effective and safe vaccine available yet
- A live, attenuated, whole sporozoite vaccine shown to work
- A synthetic peptide (SPf66) vaccine proved ineffective
- New DNA-based vaccines are in development

MALARIA INFORMATION:
- CDC Travelers' Health Hotline (877) 394–8747; CDC Travelers' Health Fax (888) 232–3299

- CDC Malaria Epidemiology (770) 488–7788; internet: www.cdc.gov

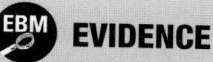 **EVIDENCE**

available at www.expertconsult.com

SUGGESTED READINGS
available at www.expertconsult.com

AUTHORS: **GLENN G. FORT, M.D., M.P.H.,** and **DENNIS J. MIKOLICH, M.D.**

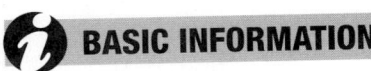

BASIC INFORMATION

DEFINITION

In the setting of recently administered anesthetic agents, most commonly halogenated inhalation agents (halothane) or depolarizing muscle relaxants (succinylcholine), patients with malignant hyperthermia (MH) quickly develop muscle rigidity and elevated temperature.

SYNONYMS

Malignant hyperthermia of anesthesia
Malignant hyperpyrexia

ICD-9CM CODES
995.86 Malignant hyperthermia of anesthesia

EPIDEMIOLOGY & DEMOGRAPHICS

INCIDENCE: Between 1/200 and 1/250,000. A study by Larach et al demonstrates a mortality rate of 1.4%.
PEAK INCIDENCE: Children, but any age may be affected
PREVALENCE: Difficult to determine because of great variations in both penetrance of gene and severity of illness
PREDOMINANT SEX AND AGE: Children and either sex may be affected
GENETICS: MH may be considered a pharmaco-genetic disorder that is triggered by exposure to anesthetics or depolarizing muscle relaxants in predisposed individuals. Half of cases are autosomal dominant, mostly involving a mutation of the rynodine receptor. Others unknown.
RISK FACTORS: Known family history of malignant hyperthermia or significant problems with general anesthesia. Muscular build increases risk of dying fourteenfold and the risk of cardiac arrest nineteenfold. Northern Europeans seem more affected. Also associated with history of anesthesia-associated masseter spasm.

PHYSICAL FINDINGS & CLINICAL PRESENTATION

- Within minutes to hours after anesthetic is given, patient develops muscle rigidity (especially masseter spasm), hyperthermia (up to 45° C), tachycardia that may progress to other dysrhythmias, and hypotension. Skin initially reddens but then becomes cyanotic and mottled. There is also increased carbon dioxide production.
- Rhabdomyolysis, acute renal failure, and disseminated intravascular coagulation may soon follow.

ETIOLOGY

- In contrast to fever, in which elevated core temperature is related to hypothalamus set point adjustment by cytokines, malignant hyperthermia results from overproduction of heat via skeletal muscle metabolism in the context of a normal hypothalamic set point.
- In genetically susceptible individuals, administration of anesthetic agents results in release of calcium from the sarcoplasmic reticulum of skeletal muscles, causing muscle rigidity and hypermetabolism. This results in significant heat production that overwhelms the body's normal ability to dissipate heat.

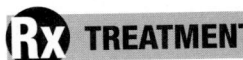 DIAGNOSIS

DIFFERENTIAL DIAGNOSIS

- Neuroleptic malignant syndrome
- Fever
- Heat stroke
- Thyrotoxicosis
- Pheochromocytoma
- Central nervous system infection or space-occupying lesion
- MDMA (Ecstasy), cocaine, alcohol withdrawal, or amphetamine use
- Serotonin syndrome
- Adverse reaction to monoamine oxidase inhibitor or anticholinergic drug
- Strychnine poisoning

WORKUP

Based on history, it is usually easy to distinguish malignant hyperthermia from other causes of hyperthermia. A thorough history, especially including medications and any illicit substances, is important. Consider lumbar puncture to rule out infection.

LABORATORY TESTS

- If the cause of hyperthermia is uncertain, a complete blood count, thyroid function studies, toxicology screen, and urine vanillylmandelic acid (VMA) may be useful.
- Once diagnosis is established, it is important to follow electrolytes (especially potassium, calcium, and phosphorus), creatinine, blood urea nitrogen, liver transaminases, and creatinine kinase.
- Prothrombin time and partial thromboplastin time should be followed to evaluate for disseminated intravascular coagulation.

IMAGING STUDIES

CT scan to assess for space-occupying lesion if diagnosis is uncertain

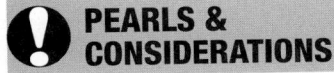 TREATMENT

The most important measures for treatment include stopping the anesthetic agents, starting dantrolene, physical cooling, and preventing sequelae. Antipyretics are not useful because the hypothalamic set point is not altered by cytokines.

NONPHARMACOLOGIC THERAPY

- Cooling by ice bath, ice packs in the groin and axillae, cool spray with fans, or cooling blankets. In severe instances extracorporeal partial bypass or iced peritoneal lavage may be used. Stop cooling when core temperature reaches 38° C to prevent overcooling.
- Careful monitoring of cardiovascular and respiratory status with constant core temperature measurements.

ACUTE GENERAL Rx

- Dantrolene is the mainstay of treatment, starting with a bolus of 5 mg/kg IV, which should be repeated every 5 min until symptoms abate or a maximum of 10 to 20 mg/kg is reached. Then 24 hr of 10 mg/kg/day IV should be given.
- Beta-blockers or lidocaine may be useful for dysrhythmias, but verapamil should be avoided as its use with dantrolene has been shown to depress cardiac function.
- Sodium bicarbonate may be necessary to reverse acidosis.
- Aggressive hydration with forced diuresis and urine alkalinization should be instituted as treatment for rhabdomyolysis.

CHRONIC Rx

This is an acute illness.

COMPLEMENTARY & ALTERNATIVE MEDICINE

None

DISPOSITION

Patient will likely need intensive monitoring, necessitating an intensive care unit bed.

REFERRAL

Anesthesia consultants will likely already be involved. Consider cardiac, renal, or hematologic consult if sequelae are significant.

PEARLS & CONSIDERATIONS

COMMENTS

Malignant hyperthermia is a life-threatening condition that requires prompt recognition of the signs and symptoms to minimize illness and end-organ damage.

PREVENTION

- Careful family and personal history of significant adverse effects with general anesthesia are important tip-offs.
- Prophylactic dantrolene therapy is no longer recommended in susceptible individuals.

PATIENT & FAMILY EDUCATION

Because family history is so important in this illness, it is important for patients and families to be aware of a history of problems with general anesthesia.

SUGGESTED READINGS
available at www.expertconsult.com

AUTHOR: **CRISTINA ANTONIO PACHECO, M.D.**

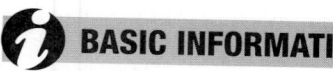 BASIC INFORMATION

DEFINITION

A Mallory-Weiss tear (MWT) is a longitudinal mucosal laceration in the region of the gastro-esophageal junction.

SYNONYMS

Mallory-Weiss syndrome

ICD-9CM CODES
530.7   Gastroesophageal laceration-hemorrhage syndrome
530.82 Esophageal hemorrhage

EPIDEMIOLOGY & DEMOGRAPHICS

- Accounts for 5% to 15% of cases of upper gastrointestinal (GI) bleeding
- Reported from early childhood to old age; the majority of patients are age 40 yr to 60 yr
- More common in males
- Alcohol use is present in 30% to 60%

PHYSICAL FINDINGS & CLINICAL PRESENTATION

- Vomiting, retching, or vigorous coughing will often, but not always, precede hematemesis.
- Patients may be clinically stable or present with tachycardia, hypotension, melena, or hematochezia.
- Bleeding may be self-limited or severe.
- Tears may be seen in association with other upper GI tract lesions, including hiatus hernia (present in as many as 90% of patients), ulcers, and esophageal varices, particularly in alcoholics.

ETIOLOGY

- An acute increase in intraabdominal pressure is transmitted to the esophagus, resulting in mucosal laceration.
- Vomiting may be associated with alcohol use, ketoacidosis, ulcer disease, uremia, pancreatitis, cholecystitis, pregnancy (in particular associated with hyperemesis gravidarum), myocardial infarction, or the postoperative period.
- Tears may be iatrogenic, related to endoscopy (especially in struggling or retching patients), esophageal dilation, lower esophageal pneumatic disruption therapy for achalasia, transesophageal echocardiography, or in association with polyethylene glycol electrolyte colonic lavage preparation.

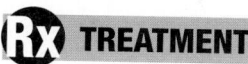 DIAGNOSIS

DIFFERENTIAL DIAGNOSIS

- Esophageal or gastric varices
- Esophagitis or esophageal ulcers (peptic or pill-induced)
- Gastric erosions
- Gastric or duodenal ulcer
- Dieulafoy lesion
- Arteriovenous malformations
- Neoplasms (usually gastric)
- Boerhaave's syndrome

WORKUP

Endoscopy is the diagnostic method of choice.

LABORATORY TESTS

- Complete blood count, prothrombin time, partial thromboplastin time
- Electrolytes, blood urea nitrogen, creatinine, liver function tests, pregnancy test, tests to evaluate for predisposing conditions

IMAGING STUDIES

Upper GI series is usually not sensitive. Patients with concurrent chest pain, dyspnea, shock, or physical examination findings of crepitus or pleural effusion should have a chest radiograph or CT to exclude Boerhaave's syndrome.

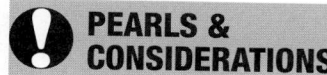 TREATMENT

NONPHARMACOLOGIC THERAPY

- Supportive care
- Avoidance of aspirin, nonsteroidal anti-inflammatory drugs, and anticoagulants

ACUTE GENERAL Rx

- Patients with active bleeding or hemodynamic instability require large-bore IVs, fluid resuscitation, and transfusion of blood products (red blood cells, fresh frozen plasma, and platelets) as appropriate.
- Nasogastric decompression and antiemetics may be considered.
- Endoscopic therapy for patients with active or ongoing hemorrhage. Therapeutic modalities include electrocoagulation, injection (e.g., 1:10,000 epinephrine, polidocanol), sclerotherapy (for bleeding associated with esophageal varices), band ligation, or endoscopic hemoclips (therapies may be used alone or in combination).
- Arterial embolization in patients with active bleeding who are poor surgical candidates.
- Laparotomy, with gastrotomy and oversewing of the tear, is required in a small percentage of patients with uncontrolled bleeding.

CHRONIC Rx

- Healing will usually occur without specific therapy.
- H_2 blockers or proton pump inhibitors may be given to help facilitate healing but should not be used long term unless appropriate indications are present.

DISPOSITION

- Prognosis is good, with spontaneous cessation of bleeding in upwards of 90% of patients. Endoscopic features can guide treatment.
- Delayed rebleeding is described in patients with high-risk stigmata (shock at initial presentation, spurting or oozing at initial endoscopy).
- Death has been reported in 3% to 12%, often with severe bleeding and underlying comorbid conditions such as coagulopathy, thrombocytopenia, alcohol use, and multisystem organ failure.

REFERRAL

- Gastrointestinal referral for endoscopy
- Surgical referral for bleeding unresponsive to endoscopic treatment or in the setting of co-existent perforation

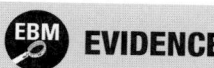 PEARLS & CONSIDERATIONS

Conditions predisposing to retching or vomiting should be identified and treated at presentation.

EBM EVIDENCE

available at www.expertconsult.com

SUGGESTED READINGS
available at www.expertconsult.com

AUTHOR: **HARLAN G. RICH, M.D.**

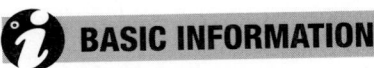

BASIC INFORMATION

DEFINITION

Marfan's syndrome is an inherited disorder of connective tissue involving the skeleton, cardiovascular system, eyes, lungs, and central nervous system.

ICD-9CM CODES
759.82 Marfan's syndrome

EPIDEMIOLOGY & DEMOGRAPHICS

PREVALENCE:
- One case per 10,000 persons.
- Both sexes are affected equally by this autosomal-dominant syndrome.
- Approximately 30% of cases are a new mutation.

PHYSICAL FINDINGS & CLINICAL PRESENTATION

Diagnostic criteria for Marfan's syndrome (Fig. 1-227):
- Skeleton: joint hypermobility, tall stature, pectus excavatum, reduced thoracic kyphosis, scoliosis, arachnodactyly, dolichostenomelia, pectus carinatum, and erosion of the lumbosacral vertebrae from dural ectasia*

- Eye: myopia, retinal detachment, elongated globe, ectopia lentis*
- Cardiovascular: mitral valve prolapse, endocarditis, arrhythmia, dilated mitral annulus, mitral regurgitation, tricuspid valve prolapse, aortic regurgitation, aortic dissection,* dilation of the aortic root*
- Pulmonary: apical blebs, spontaneous pneumothorax
- Skin and integument: inguinal hernias, incisional hernias, striae atrophicae
- Central nervous system: attention deficit disorder, hyperactivity, verbal-performance discrepancy, dural ectasia, anterior pelvic meningocele*

If the family history is positive for a close relative clearly affected by Marfan's syndrome, manifestations should be present in the skeleton and one of the other organ systems and the diagnosis confirmed by linkage analysis or mutation detection.

If the family history is negative or unknown, the patient should have manifestations in the skeleton, the cardiovascular system, and one other system and at least one of the manifestations indicated by an asterisk in the above lists.

Manifestations are listed within each organ system in increasing specificity for Marfan's syndrome; although none is completely specific, those indicated by an asterisk are the most specific.

ETIOLOGY

Mutations in the gene that encodes fibrillin-1, the major constituent of microfibrils, which form the frame for elastic fibers. All the manifestations of Marfan's syndrome can be explained by the defective microfibrils.

DIAGNOSIS

DIFFERENTIAL DIAGNOSIS

Each of the clinical manifestations of the syndrome may have other causes; however, if the diagnostic criteria are met, the diagnosis is made.

WORKUP

- Echocardiography to establish:
  1. Mitral valve prolapse
  2. Mitral regurgitation
  3. Tricuspid valve prolapse
  4. Aortic regurgitation
  5. Dilation of the aortic root
- Chest radiograph
- Transesophageal echocardiography, chest CT scan, chest MRI, or aortography for suspected aortic dissection
- Chest radiograph for pulmonary apical bullae
- Ophthalmologic examination by ophthalmologist

TREATMENT

- Regular cardiac and aorta monitoring by physical examination and echocardiography.
- Endocarditis prophylaxis.
- Restriction of contact sports, weight lifting, and overexertion.
- Beta-blockers are commonly prescribed to slow the rate of aortic root dilation in children; recent trials, however, have shown that this approach is not effective. Recent reports indicate that use of angiotensin receptor blockers significantly slowed the rate of progressive aortic root dilation.
- Early use of angiotensin-converting enzyme inhibitors in young patients with Marfan's syndrome and valvular regurgitation may lessen the need for mitral valve surgery.
- Genetic counseling.
- Monitor aorta during pregnancy because of the increased risk of dissection.

SUGGESTED READINGS

available at www.expertconsult.com

AUTHOR: FRED F. FERRI, M.D.

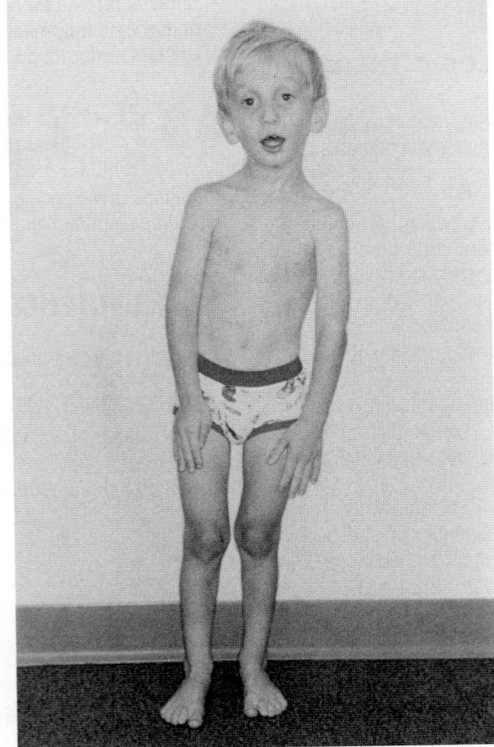

FIGURE 1-227 Marfan's syndrome. Note the elongated facies, droopy lids, apparent dolichostenomelia, and mild scoliosis. (From Behrman RE: *Nelson's textbook of pediatrics*, Philadelphia, 2004, WB Saunders.)

BASIC INFORMATION

DEFINITION

Local painful inflammation of the breast, which may or may not be accompanied by infection, flulike symptoms, and abscess formation.

ICD-9CM CODES
611.0 Inflammatory disease of the breast
675.1 Postpartum abscess of the breast
675.2 Postpartum nonpurulent mastitis

EPIDEMIOLOGY & DEMOGRAPHICS

- In lactating mothers, mastitis typically occurs in the first 3 mo postpartum (74% to 95% cases)
- When severe, mastitis can lead to a breast abscess (5% to 11%) or septicemia
- In nonlactating women of childbearing age it often presents as granulomatous mastitis (GM)
- In older nonlactating women it is called peri-ductal mastitis (PM) and is caused by in-flamed milk ducts near the nipple
- Mastitis can also occur in early infancy, when breast hypertrophy from maternal hormonal stimulation can lead to infection

PREVALENCE: 9.5% to 33% depending on defi-nition and postpartum timeline
PREDOMINANT SEX: Females
RISK FACTORS:
- Previous mastitis
- Cracked, fissured, or sore nipples
- Primiparity and infant attachment difficulties
- Cleft lip or palate or short frenulum in infant
- Milk stasis and missed feedings
- Poor maternal nutrition
- Using antifungal nipple cream (presumably for nipple thrush) in the same week
- Tight clothing or bras
- Use of manual breast pump
- Diabetes
- Use of steroids
- Lumpectomy with radiation
- Breast implants
- Nipple piercings

PHYSICAL FINDINGS & CLINICAL PRESENTATION

- Warmth, redness, tenderness in breast
- Unilateral or bilateral
- Malaise, myalgias, fevers, chills
- Pain with nursing
- Decreased milk output
- Area of breast is hard, wedge shaped, and swollen
- In PM, breast mass near nipple with retrac-tion or discharge
- In GM, enlarged axillary lymph nodes or sinus tract formation

ETIOLOGY

- Milk stasis and irritation of the milk ducts due to local immune response to milk proteins.
- Bacterial infection of subcutaneous tissue due to breaks in skin.
- The most common organism is *S. aureus* and, less commonly, group A beta-hemolytic *streptococci, S. pneumoniae, E. coli, Candida albicans,* and *M. tuberculosis.*
- GM from inflammation with epithelioid histio-cytes and multinucleated giant cells can be caused by etiologies like tuberculosis, sar-coidosis, foreign body reaction, parasitic and mycotic infections, or idiopathic (IGM).
- Mastitis in neonates is caused by infections with *S. aureus* or gram-negative enteric bac-teria.

DIAGNOSIS

DIFFERENTIAL DIAGNOSIS

- Engorgement, plugged duct (see Table 1-110)
- Breast abscess
- Inflammatory or other breast cancer (3% women diagnosed with breast cancer are lactating)
- Mastitis as a symptom of hyperprolactinemia or galactorrhea
- GM can be a manifestation of systemic dis-ease including sarcoidosis, Wegener granulo-matosis, giant cell arteritis, polyarteritis no-dosa, TB, syphilis

WORKUP

- History of signs and symptoms and clinical exam including thorough breast exam with assessment for axillary nodes and nipple discharge are sufficient to make diagnosis
- Recurrent mastitis should include workup for underlying breast disease

LABORATORY TESTS

- Simple mastitis requires no milk culture or laboratory studies
- Obtain midstream sample of milk for culture for antibiotic sensitivities in refractory masti-tis or in MRSA-suspected cases
- CBC and blood cultures in toxic-appearing patients
- In abscess formation, culture of drainage or aspirate fluid
- Gram stain and culture indicated in infant mastitis

IMAGING STUDIES

- Not necessary unless refractory mastitis or abscess suspected
- Consider ultrasound to evaluate for abscess or mammogram in appropriate patients to exclude carcinoma
- In GM, use of mammogram and ultrasound guided FNA are standard studies

TREATMENT

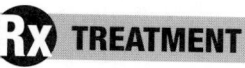

NONPHARMACOLOGIC THERAPY

- Mainstay of therapy is effective milk removal through continued breastfeeding
- Consider referral to a certified lactation con-sultant
- Warm compresses, increased fluid intake, good nutrition, and rest
- In abscess formation, surgical drainage or needle aspiration is necessary, followed by antibiotic therapy based on sensitivities of culture

ACUTE GENERAL Rx

- NSAIDs and analgesics (e.g., acetaminophen, ibuprofen)
- There are no randomized controlled trials examining the effectiveness, type, or duration of antibiotic therapy. Common regimens in-clude:
  - Amoxicillin/clavulanate (Augmentin) 875 mg twice daily for 10 to 14 days
  - Cephalexin (Keflex) 500 mg four times a day for 10 to 14 days
  - Clindamycin (Cleocin) 300 mg four times daily for 10 to 14 days (for penicillin al-lergy, MRSA coverage)
  - Dicloxacillin 500 mg four times daily for 10 to 14 days
  - Trimethoprim/sulfamethoxazole (Bactim) 160 mg/800 mg twice daily for 10 to 14 days (MRSA coverage, but should not be used in healthy infants aged <2 mo or compromised infants)
- Oxytocin nasal spray if letdown reflex dis-turbed
- Mastitis in early infancy should be treated with parenteral antibiotics based on results of gram stain

CHRONIC Rx

Systemic corticosteroids or wide surgical resec-tion in GM.

COMPLEMENTARY AND ALTERNATIVE MEDICINE

- Complementary therapies have not been as-sessed in prospective studies: *Belladonna, Phytolacca, Chamomilla,* sulfur, and *Bellis perenis*

TABLE 1-110 Comparison of Findings of Engorgement, Plugged Duct, and Mastitis

Characteristics	Engorgement	Plugged Duct	Mastitis
Onset	Gradual, immediately	Gradual, after feedings	Sudden, after 10 days post-partum
Site	Bilateral	Unilateral	Usually unilateral
Swelling and heat	Generalized	May shift/little or not heat	Localized red hot, and swollen
Body temperature	<38.4° C	<38.4° C	>38.4° C
Systemic symptoms	Feels well	Feels well	Flulike symptoms

From Lawrence RA, Lawrence RM: *Breastfeeding: a guide for the medical profession,* ed 5, St Louis, 1999, Mosby.

- Several strains of lactobacilli have shown promise as probiotic agents that might be useful in treating mastitis. *L. formentum* and *L. salivarius* have been found to be an effective alternative to antibiotics in recent trials on treatment of infectious mastitis during lactation. These intriguing results should be replicated before this approach is adopted widely.

REFERRAL

Referral to a surgeon for severe PM or significant abscess that does not resolve with conservative measures

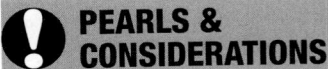

PEARLS & CONSIDERATIONS

COMMENTS

- One quarter of breastfeeding mothers with one episode of mastitis will stop breastfeeding.
- Increasing incidence of MRSA mastitis.
- In reassessing refractory mastitis, the most important consideration is the possibility of cancer.
- Mastitis can be a manifestation of systemic disease.
- Mastitis is a risk factor for vertical transmission of infections including increased transmission of retroviruses (especially HIV-1), CMV, measles, hepatitis B and C.
- GM mimics breast cancer both clinically and radiologically (>50% of reported cases are initially mistaken for carcinoma). This includes fine needle aspiration, which is sometimes interpreted as malignant.
- All infants with diagnosis of mastitis should receive parenteral antibiotics.

PATIENT & FAMILY EDUCATION

La Leche League International (web site: http://www.llli.org),
International Lactation Consultant Association (web site: http://www.ilca.org)

SUGGESTED READINGS

available at www.expertconsult.com

AUTHORS: **MARY BETH SUTTER, M.D., JEFFREY M. BORKAN, M.D., Ph.D.,** and **ANDREI LEVCHENKO, M.D.**

BASIC INFORMATION

DEFINITION

- Pain in the breast
- Usually cyclical condition but may be noncyclic or extramammary

SYNONYMS

Mastalgia

ICD-9CM CODES
611.71 Mastodynia

EPIDEMIOLOGY & DEMOGRAPHICS

- Mastodynia affects up to 70% of women at some time in their reproductive lives.
- Severe cyclical mastodynia lasting more than 5 days/mo and of sufficient intensity to interfere with sexual, physical, social, and work-related activities is reported among 30% of premenopausal women.
- Underlying fear of breast cancer is the reason most of these women seek medical consultation.
- One tenth of women with mastodynia require pain-relieving therapy.

PHYSICAL FINDINGS & CLINICAL PRESENTATION

- Usually the breasts are normal bilaterally
- Full, tender breasts
- Generalized breast nodularity without discrete lumps
- Chest wall tenderness: extramammary breast pain
- Distinguishing mammary from extramammary pain can be difficult
- With the patient lying on her side so that the breast tissue falls away from the chest wall, tenderness can then be reproduced by direct pressure over the offending site
- Cyclical mastodynia presents in the luteal phase of the menstrual cycle
- Women with cyclical mastodynia tend to have abdominal bloating, leg swelling, and other symptoms of premenstrual syndrome
- Noncyclic mastodynia, on the other hand, is unrelated to the menstrual cycle
- Extramammary breast pain simulates noncyclic mastodynia

ETIOLOGY

- Hormonal imbalance
- Abnormal lipid metabolism
- Premenstrual syndrome (20%)
- Fibrocystic breast disease
- Emotional abuse and anxiety
- Excessive caffeine intake
- Breast cancer (10%)
- Tietze syndrome (idiopathic costochondritis)

DIAGNOSIS

DIFFERENTIAL DIAGNOSIS

- See "Etiology."
- The majority of women with mastodynia have no underlying abnormality.

- Breast fullness and tenderness associated with hormonal changes fluctuate with the menstrual cycle.
- Similarly, breast nodularity, which may or may not be the result of fibrocystic breast disease, also fluctuates with the menstrual cycle.
- Discrete breast lumps need full evaluation to rule out malignancy.
- Tietze syndrome is usually unilateral and may be associated with chest wall swelling.

WORKUP

- Complete history and thorough clinical examination.
- Pain analogue cards may be helpful in establishing the pattern of symptomatology. In patients >35 yr, mammography should be performed as part of the baseline investigation.
- Most women presenting with severe mastodynia are <35 yr. This group has a lower risk of subclinical breast cancer, and their breasts have increased density. In this younger group, radiologic investigations are of limited value unless a discrete breast lump is palpated.

LABORATORY TESTS

Although hormonal imbalance and abnormal lipid metabolism have been implicated in the etiopathogenesis of mastodynia, there is no good evidence to support any consistent pattern of serum hormonal or lipid profile in women with mastodynia. These tests are therefore not recommended.

IMAGING STUDIES

- Mammography should be part of the baseline investigation if the woman is >35 yr.
- Ultrasound can be performed as needed; it is particularly helpful in the assessment of cystic breast lesions.
- In women <35 yr, imaging investigations are not helpful unless a lump has been palpated clinically.
- There are no radiologic features associated with mastodynia: rather, radiologic investigations are performed to exclude the rare presence of a subclinical carcinoma.

TREATMENT

NONPHARMACOLOGIC THERAPY

- 85% of the women with mastodynia can be reassured after full clinical evaluation.
- The remaining 15% require some form of therapy in addition to reassurance.
- A firm, supportive brassiere designed for postpartum use is particularly helpful if mastodynia is associated with breast swelling.
- Follow a low-fat, high-carbohydrate diet.
- Reduce caffeine intake.

ACUTE GENERAL Rx

- Evening primrose oil, which contains gamma-linolenic acid, has been shown to have some effectiveness and is an acceptable treatment for mastodynia.

- Topical NSAID preparations may confer some benefit and can be prescribed for these women.
- Hormonal therapy is the mainstay of treatment.
- Danazol is the only drug approved by the FDA for the treatment of mastodynia. Danazol has some androgenic and peripheral antiestrogenic effects. Its efficacy is well established, with significant relief of mastodynia in 70% to 93% of cases.
- Widespread use of danazol is limited because of its adverse side effects. These include menstrual irregularities, depression, acne, hirsutism and, in severe cases, voice deepening. Women taking danazol should be advised to use effective nonhormonal contraception because of the drug's potential adverse effects on the fetus.
- The side effects of danazol can be significantly reduced by using a low dose (100 mg daily) and confining treatment to 2 wk preceding menstruation.
- Tamoxifen, a synthetic antiestrogen, has also been shown to be effective in the treatment of mastodynia. Although effective in relieving symptoms, its use is extremely limited because of side effects. When used, it should be at a low dosage of 10 mg/day and duration should be limited to 6 mo at a time. In the U.S. this agent is not approved for use in women with mastodynia.
- Bromocriptine is a dopamine-receptor agonist whose primary action is inhibition of prolactin release. It has been used extensively in the treatment of severe cyclical mastodynia and is effective. Again, side effects such as headache and lightheadedness have limited its use.
- Lisuride maleate was recently found to be effective by one study.
- Other hormonal agents that have been reported to be effective in small studies cannot be recommended. They either have unacceptable side effect profiles or their efficacy is not established. These agents include gestrinone, gonadotropin-releasing hormone analogues, progesterone, and hormone replacement therapy.

CHRONIC Rx

- Longstanding cases of mastodynia can be managed with intermittent low-dose danazol therapy to limit side effects. In between these courses of hormone, nonpharmacologic and nonhormonal therapy can be used.
- Severe, unremitting mastodynia that does not respond to medical treatment may require mastectomy; this is rare.

DISPOSITION

- Cyclical mastodynia resolves spontaneously in 20% to 30% of women.
- Up to 60% of women may develop recurrent symptoms 2 yr after treatment.
- Noncyclic mastodynia responds poorly to treatment but may resolve spontaneously in up to 50% of women.

REFERRAL

- Detection of a breast lump or any other findings suggestive of neoplasm should be fully investigated with an immediate referral.
- Women with chronic, unremitting mastodynia that does not respond to pharmacologic therapy should be referred for possible mastectomy; this is rare.

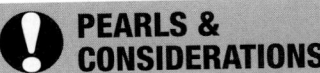

PEARLS & CONSIDERATIONS

COMMENTS

- There is no good evidence to support the use of vitamin B_6, diuretics, and vitamin E. Mastodynia may represent a presenting symptom of another, more generalized disorder (e.g., premenstrual syndrome, psychologic disturbance).

- In these cases treating mastodynia in isolation will not work; the underlying conditions must be appropriately addressed.

SUGGESTED READINGS

available at www.expertconsult.com

AUTHORS: **ALEXANDER B. OLAWAIYE, M.D.,** and **RUBEN ALVERO, M.D.**

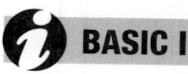 **BASIC INFORMATION**

DEFINITION

Mastoiditis is inflammation of the mastoid process and air cells, a complication of otitis media.

SYNONYMS

Mastoid abscess

ICD-9CM CODES
383.00 Mastoiditis, acute or subacute
383.1 Mastoiditis, chronic

EPIDEMIOLOGY & DEMOGRAPHICS

INCIDENCE (IN U.S.): Since the introduction of antibiotic therapy and use of broad-spectrum antibiotics, there has been a marked decline in the incidence of acute mastoiditis.
PREDOMINANT SEX: More common in males
PREDOMINANT AGE: 2 mo to 18 yr
PEAK INCIDENCE: Early childhood

PHYSICAL FINDINGS & CLINICAL PRESENTATION

- Acute mastoiditis is usually a complication of acute otitis media.
- Most common presenting symptom is pain and tenderness in the postauricular region.
- Other signs or symptoms include:
  1. Fever
  2. Postauricular erythema and edema
  3. Protrusion of the pinna inferiorly and anteriorly
  4. Tympanic membrane usually intact with signs of acute otitis media
- Complications of acute mastoiditis include:
  1. Subperiosteal abscess (most common complication)
  2. Hearing loss
  3. Facial nerve palsy
  4. Labyrinthitis
  5. Intracranial complications such as hydrocephalus, meningitis, encephalitis, intracranial abscess, and lateral sinus thrombosis
- Chronic mastoiditis is characterized by chronic otorrhea and chronic tympanic membrane perforation.

ETIOLOGY

- Continuity exists between the middle air space and the mastoid cavity.
- Initial hyperemia and edema of the mucosal lining of the air cells results in accumulation of purulent exudate.
- Dissolution of calcium from bony septae and osteoclastic activity in the inflamed periosteum lead to bone necrosis and coalescence of air cells.
- Most common bacterial isolates are:
  1. *Streptococcus pneumoniae*
  2. *Streptococcus pyogenes*
  3. *Haemophilus influenzae*
  4. *Moraxella catarrhalis*
  5. *Staphylococcus aureus*
- Often, there are multiple organisms in chronic mastoiditis, with predominance of anaerobes and gram-negative bacteria.
- *Mycobacterium tuberculosis,* nontuberculous mycobacteria, *Aspergillus* and *Rhodococcus equi* have been reported in cases of mastoiditis in severely immunocompromised individuals.

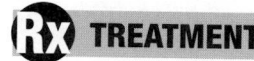 **DIAGNOSIS**

DIFFERENTIAL DIAGNOSIS

- Children
  1. Rhabdomyosarcoma
  2. Histiocytosis X
  3. Leukemia
  4. Kawasaki syndrome
- Adults
  1. Fulminant otitis externa
  2. Histiocytosis X
  3. Metastatic disease

WORKUP

A thorough history and physical examination are important in establishing diagnosis.

LABORATORY TESTS

- Fluid for Gram stain and culture may be obtained by myringotomy.
- If there is a perforation in the tympanic membrane with drainage, cultures of this may be taken after carefully cleaning the external canal.

IMAGING STUDIES

- Plain x-rays of the mastoid region may demonstrate clouding or opacification in areas of pneumatization.
- CT scan can demonstrate early involvement of bone (mastoiditis with bone destruction).
- MRI is more sensitive than CT scan in evaluating soft-tissue involvement and is useful in conjunction with CT scan to investigate other complications of mastoiditis.

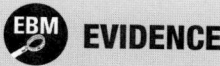 **TREATMENT**

NONPHARMACOLOGIC THERAPY

Myringotomy, if the ear is not already draining

ACUTE GENERAL Rx

- Initiated with IV antibiotics directed against the common organisms *S. pneumoniae* and *H. influenzae*. If the disease in the mastoid has had a prolonged course, coverage for *Staphylococcus aureus* with gram-negative enteric bacilli may be considered for initial therapy until results of cultures become available.
- Continued until all signs of mastoiditis have resolved
- Directed against enteric gram-negative organisms and anaerobes in chronic mastoiditis
- Indications for mastoidectomy:
  1. Failure to improve after 72 hr of therapy
  2. Persistent fever
  3. Imminent or overt signs of intracranial complications
  4. Evidence of a subperiosteal abscess in the mastoid bone

DISPOSITION

Proceed with mastoidectomy when medical therapy fails.

REFERRAL

- To otorhinolaryngologist:
  1. If diagnosis is in doubt
  2. If aural complications present
  3. To evaluate for surgical intervention
- To neurosurgeon if intratemporal or intracranial extension of infection suspected
  1. Aural complications: bone destruction, subperiosteal abscess, petrositis, facial paralysis, labyrinthitis
  2. Intracranial complications: extradural abscess, lateral sinus thrombophlebitis or thrombosis, subdural abscess, meningitis, brain abscess, otitic hydrocephalus

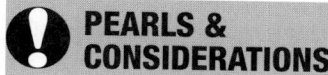 **PEARLS & CONSIDERATIONS**

Mastoiditis is particularly difficult to eradicate because the mastoid air cells are poorly vascularized and difficult to drain.

EBM EVIDENCE

available at www.expertconsult.com

SUGGESTED READINGS

available at www.expertconsult.com

AUTHORS: **GLENN G. FORT, M.D., M.P.H.,** and **DENNIS J. MIKOLICH, M.D.**

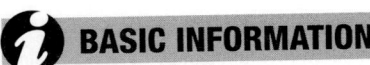

BASIC INFORMATION

DEFINITION

Measles is a childhood exanthem caused by an RNA virus called *Morbillivirus,* belonging to the family *Paramyxoviridae.*

SYNONYMS

Rubeola

ICD-9CM CODES
055.9 Measles
055.0 Encephalitis
055.1 Pneumonia
V04.2 Vaccination

EPIDEMIOLOGY & DEMOGRAPHICS

- Before the introduction of an effective vaccine in 1963, measles was one of the most common childhood illnesses. In developing countries, where it mostly strikes children <5 yr, it remains a leading cause of childhood death.
- 30 million cases occur worldwide each year.
- In developed countries, measles outbreaks occasionally occur in adolescents and young adults who have not been immunized (incidence up to 10 per 100,000 person-years).

PHYSICAL FINDINGS & CLINICAL PRESENTATION

- Incubation: 10 to 14 days (up to 3 wk in adults)
- Prodrome: 2 to 4 days; malaise, fever, rhinorrhea, conjunctivitis, cough
- Exanthem phase: 7 to 10 days
- The fever increases and peaks at 104° to 105° F together with the rash; it persists for 5 or 6 days. The patient's fever decreases over 24 hr.
- Rash: erythematous maculopapular eruption begins behind the ears, progresses to the forehead and neck (Fig. 1-228), then spreads to face, trunk, upper extremities, buttocks, and lower extremities, in that order. After 3 days the rash fades in the same sequence by becoming copper brown and then desquamating.
- Enanthem: *Koplik spots* are white papules 1 to 2 mm in diameter on an erythematous base. They first appear on the buccal mucosa opposite the lower molar 2 days before the rash and spread over 24 hr to involve most of the buccal and lower labial mucosa. They fade after 3 days.
- Other symptoms and signs: malaise, anorexia, vomiting, diarrhea, abdominal pain, pharyngitis, lymphadenopathy, and occasional splenomegaly.

Atypical measles (in vaccinated persons):
- Incubation: 10 to 14 days
- Prodrome: 1 to 3 days; high fever and headache
- Rash: maculopapular, urticarial, or petechial rash that begins peripherally and progresses centrally
- Modified measles applies to patients who have received immune serum globulin and develop a milder illness
- Complications (30% of all cases):
  ○ Otitis media
  ○ Laryngitis, tracheitis
  ○ Pneumonia (accounts for 90% of measles deaths)
  ○ Encephalitis with lethargy, irritability, and seizures; 60% recover completely, 25% have neurologic sequelae (mental retardation, hemiplegia, paraplegia, epilepsy, deafness), and 15% die
  ○ Myocarditis, pericarditis, hepatitis
  ○ Complications more common in immunocompromised hosts and persons with AIDS

ETIOLOGY & PATHOGENESIS

- The measles virus is transmitted through the respiratory tract by airborne droplets.
- It initially infects the respiratory epithelium; the patient becomes viremic during the prodromal phase and the virus is disseminated to the skin, respiratory tract, and other organs.
- Viral clearance is achieved by cellular immunity.

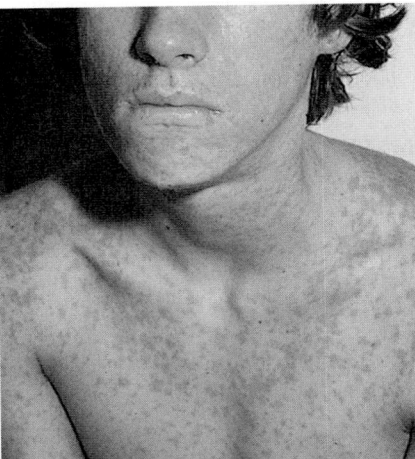

FIGURE 1-228 Rubeola. (From Zitelli BJ, Davis HW: *Atlas of pediatric physical diagnosis,* ed 5, St Louis, 2005, Mosby.)

DIAGNOSIS

DIFFERENTIAL DIAGNOSIS

- Other viral infections by enteroviruses, adenoviruses, human parvovirus B-19, rubella
- Scarlet fever
- Allergic reaction
- Kawasaki disease

WORKUP

Knowledge of outbreak, history and physical findings (Koplik spots are diagnostic), laboratory tests

LABORATORY TESTS

- Complete blood count: leukopenia
- Enzyme-linked immunosorbent assay for measles antibodies, which appear shortly after the onset of the rash and peak 3 to 4 wk later
- Cerebrospinal fluid analysis in encephalitis may reveal pleocytosis (lymphocytes) and an elevated protein

IMAGING STUDIES

Chest radiograph if pneumonia is suspected

TREATMENT

- Supportive
- Vitamin A
- Ribavirin for severe measles pneumonitis

PEARLS & CONSIDERATIONS

PREVENTION

- Passive immunization: human immunoglobulin 0.25 ml/kg IM within 6 days of exposure. Double the dose for immunocompromised persons.
- Active immunization (see Section V).

EVIDENCE

available at www.expertconsult.com

SUGGESTED READING

available at www.expertconsult.com

AUTHOR: **FRED F. FERRI, M.D.**

BASIC INFORMATION

DEFINITION

Meckel diverticulum is an ileal diverticulum located 100 cm proximal to the cecum. It results from failure of the omphalomesenteric duct to obliterate completely (as it should by the eighth week of gestation).

SYNONYMS

MD

ICD-9CM CODES
751.0 Meckel diverticulum

EPIDEMIOLOGY & DEMOGRAPHICS

- Meckel diverticulum, based on autopsy studies and intraoperative evidence, occurs in 0.3% to 4% of the population and is the most prevalent congenital anomaly of the gastrointestinal (GI) tract. Complications occur more frequently in males.
- Most patients who develop symptoms are <10 yr.
- The lifetime risk of complications developing in a case of Meckel diverticulum is 4%.
- In adults, complications (small bowel obstruction [25% to 40%], diverticulitis [20%]) are usually attributable to factors other than heterotopic mucosa.
- Tumors have rarely been reported in symptomatic Meckel diverticulum, with carcinoid being the most common type.

PHYSICAL FINDINGS & CLINICAL PRESENTATION

- Painless lower GI bleeding (4%)
- Intestinal obstruction caused by intussusception, volvulus, herniation, or entrapment of a loop of bowel through a defect in the diverticular mesentery (6%)
- Meckel's diverticulitis mimics acute appendicitis (5%)
- Rare primary tumor arising from diverticulum (carcinoid, sarcoma, leiomyoma, adenocarcinoma)
- Asymptomatic (80% to 95%)

ETIOLOGY & PATHOGENESIS

- As a remnant of the omphalomesenteric duct, Meckel diverticulum contains all layers of the intestinal wall and has its own mesentery and blood supply (branch of the superior mesenteric artery).
- The majority of complicated cases of Meckel diverticulum contain ectopic mucosa (75%

gastric, 15% pancreatic). It causes ulceration and bleeding of ileal mucosa adjacent to the acidic ectopic gastric secretions. Alkaline secretions of ectopic pancreatic tissue can also cause ulcerations.

DIAGNOSIS

DIFFERENTIAL DIAGNOSIS

- Appendicitis
- Crohn's disease
- All causes of lower GI bleeding (polyp, colon cancer, arteriovenous malformation, diverticulosis, hemorrhoids)

WORKUP

- Diagnosis is often made intraoperatively when the preoperative diagnosis is appendicitis.
- Preoperative detection of symptomatic Meckel diverticulum requires a high index of suspicion.
- In the case of GI bleeding of unknown source, a technetium scan will identify Meckel diverticulum (sensitivity: 85% in children, 62% in adults; specificity: 95% in children, 9% in adults) (Fig. 1-229).
- In patients with suspected small-bowel obstruction, intussusception, or diverticulitis, a CT scan of the abdomen and pelvis is helpful.

TREATMENT

- Surgical resection in symptomatic patients.
- There is controversy regarding the need to remove an incidentally found diverticulum, with most surgeons arguing in favor of resection.

SUGGESTED READINGS

available at www.expertconsult.com

AUTHOR: **FRED F. FERRI, M.D.**

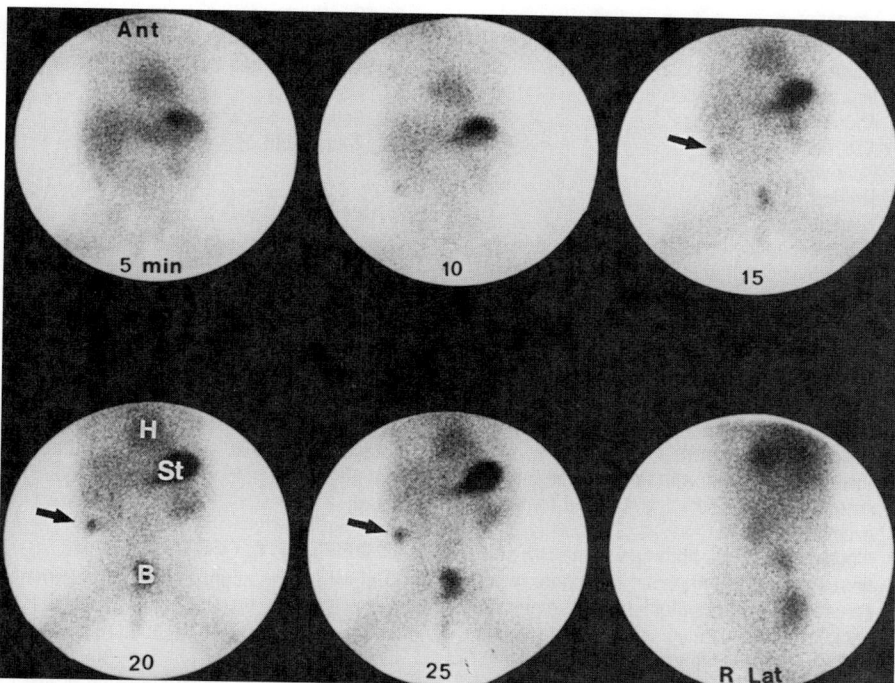

FIGURE 1-229 Meckel diverticulum. In this 2-year-old child who had unexplained rectal bleeding, a nuclear medicine study was performed with radioactive material that concentrates in gastric mucosa (technetium-99m pertechnetate). Sequential 5-min images of the abdomen are obtained. On the 20-min image, the heart *(H)*, stomach *(St)*, and bladder *(B)* are clearly seen in addition to an ectopic focus of activity *(arrow)* representing a Meckel diverticulum. (From Mettler FA [ed]: *Primary care radiology*, Philadelphia, 2000, WB Saunders.)

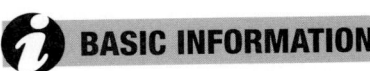

DEFINITION

Meigs' syndrome is characterized by the presence of a benign solid ovarian tumor associated with ascites and predominantly right hydrothorax that disappear after tumor removal.

ICD-9CM CODES
620.2 Ovarian mass (unspecified)
220.0 Benign ovarian lesion
789.5 Ascites
511.9 Pleural effusion

EPIDEMIOLOGY & DEMOGRAPHICS

- Occurs in <1% of ovarian fibromas (associated with approximately 0.004% of ovarian tumors)
- Most frequently encountered during middle age (average age, approximately 48 yr)

PHYSICAL FINDINGS & CLINICAL PRESENTATION

- Asymptomatic pelvic mass on bimanual examination
- Intermittent pelvic pain (intermittent torsion)
- Acute pelvic tenderness
- Acute abdominal tenderness
- Abdominal pelvic mass
- Abdominal bloating
- Fluid wave
- Shifting dullness
- "Puddle sign"
- Hyperresonance or flatness to chest percussion, absence of tactile and vocal fremitus
- Absent or loud bronchial breath sounds, rales, mediastinal displacement, tracheal shift
- Weight loss and emaciation

ETIOLOGY

- Not specifically known
- Usually associated with "edematous" fibromas (or other benign ovarian solid tumor) in excess of 10 cm
- Plausible that large fibroma with narrow stalk has inadequate lymphatic drainage; when coupled with intermittent torsion, results in backflow transudation into the peritoneal cavity; accumulated peritoneal ascites then pass to the right pleural cavity by the lymphatics (overloaded thoracic duct) or abdominal pleural commutation (i.e., foramen of Bochdalek)

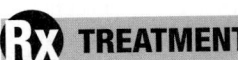

DIFFERENTIAL DIAGNOSIS

- Abdominal ovarian malignancy
- Various gynecologic disorders:
  1. Uterus; endometrial tumor, sarcoma, leiomyoma ("pseudo-Meigs' syndrome")
  2. Fallopian tube: hydrosalpinx, granulomatous salpingitis, fallopian tube malignancy
  3. Ovary: benign, serous, mucinous, endometrioid, clear cell, Brenner tumor, granulosa, stromal, dysgerminoma, fibroma, metastatic tumor
- Nongynecologic (gastrointestinal tract or genitourinary tract tumor or pathology) causes of pelvic mass
  1. Ascites
  2. Portal vein obstruction
  3. Inferior vena cava obstruction
  4. Hypoproteinemia
  5. Thoracic duct obstruction
  6. Tuberculosis
  7. Amyloidosis
  8. Pancreatitis
  9. Neoplasm
  10. Ovarian hyperstimulation
  11. Pleural effusion
  12. Congestive heart failure
  13. Malignancy
  14. Collagen-vascular disease
  15. Pancreatitis
  16. Cirrhosis

WORKUP

- Clinical condition characterized by ovarian mass, ascites, and predominantly right-sided pleural effusion (the pleural effusion can also be left-sided in a small number of cases)
- Ovarian malignancy and the other causes (see "Differential Diagnosis") of pelvic mass, ascites, and pleural effusion to be considered
- History of early satiety, weight loss with increased abdominal girth, bloating, intermittent abdominal pain, dyspnea, nonproductive cough

LABORATORY TESTS

- Complete blood count to rule out inflammatory process
- Tumor markers (CA-125, hCG, AFP, CEA) to evaluate malignancy
- Chemical and liver function testing profile to evaluate metabolic or hepatic involvement

IMAGING STUDIES

- Pelvic sonography (color-flow Doppler evaluation of adnexal mass) to evaluate pelvic pathology (CT scan or MRI if etiology indeterminate)
- Chest x-ray examination
- Arterial blood gases if respiratory compromise

Rx TREATMENT

NONPHARMACOLOGIC THERAPY

- Informed consent and proper preparation of patient for possible staging laparotomy (total abdominal hysterectomy and bilateral salpingo-oophorectomy, omentectomy, possible bowel resection, pelvic/periaortic lymphadenectomy)
- Bowel prep if considering pelvic malignancy

ACUTE GENERAL Rx

Depending on clinical presentation, size of pelvic mass, amount of ascites, and pleural effusion:
- If pelvic mass <10 cm with minimal ascites/pleural effusion: consider diagnostic open laparoscopy (possible exploratory laparotomy) and salpingo-oophorectomy with removal of ovarian fibroma (tumor).
- If pelvic mass >10 cm with moderate/large amount ascites/pleural effusion: consider pleurocentesis if respiratory compromise (cytology: AFB) and exploratory laparotomy with salpingo-oophorectomy and removal of ovarian fibroma (tumor).
- Treat pelvic malignancy, gastrointestinal or genitourinary tumor as indicated.

CHRONIC Rx

- Resolution of ascites and right-sided pleural effusion after removal of ovarian fibroma
- No long-term follow-up for benign ovarian fibroma

DISPOSITION

Excellent progress and complete survival are expected.

REFERRAL

To gynecologist or gynecologic oncologist for evaluation and treatment, especially if malignancy considered or encountered

SUGGESTED READINGS
available at www.expertconsult.com

AUTHORS: **DENNIS M. WEPPNER, M.D.,** and **RUBEN ALVERO, M.D.**

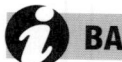

BASIC INFORMATION

DEFINITION

Melanoma is a skin neoplasm arising from the malignant degeneration of melanocytes. It is classically subdivided in four types:
1. Superficial spreading melanoma (70%) (Fig. 1-230, *A*)
2. Nodular melanoma (15% to 20%) (Fig. 1-230, *B*)
3. Lentigo maligna melanoma (5% to 10%)
4. Acral lentiginous melanoma (7% to 10%)

SYNONYMS

Malignant melanoma

ICD-9CM CODES
172.9 Melanoma of the skin, site unspecified

EPIDEMIOLOGY & DEMOGRAPHICS

- Annual incidence of melanoma is 13 cases per 100,000 persons.
- Melanoma has doubled to tripled in incidence over the past 25 yr.
- Melanoma is the most common cancer among women ages 20 to 29 yr.
- Melanoma is much more common in whites (17.2/100,000 white men) than in African Americans (1 in 100,000 African American men).
- Lifetime risk of cutaneous melanoma for white Americans is 1 in 90.
- Melanoma is the leading cause of death from skin disease.
- Median age at diagnosis is 53 yr.
- Superficial spreading melanoma occurs most often in young adults on sun-exposed areas.
- Acral lentiginous melanoma is most often found in Asian Americans and African Americans and is not related to sun exposure.
- Death rate for white men with melanoma is 3 per 100,000.
- 8% to 10% of melanomas arise in people with a family history of the disease.

PHYSICAL FINDINGS & CLINICAL PRESENTATION

Variable depending on the subtype of melanoma:

- Superficial spreading melanoma is most often found on the lower legs, arms, and upper back. It may have a combination of many colors or may be uniformly brown or black.
- Nodular melanoma can be found anywhere on the body, but it most frequently occurs on the trunk on sun-exposed areas. It has a dark-brown or red-brown appearance and can be dome shaped or pedunculated. Lesions are frequently misdiagnosed because they may resemble a blood blister or hemangioma and may also be amelanotic.
- Lentigo maligna melanoma is generally found in older adults in areas continually exposed to the sun and frequently arising from lentigo maligna (Hutchinson's freckle) or melanoma in situ. It might have a complex pattern and variable shape; color is more uniform than in superficial spreading melanoma.
- Acral lentiginous melanoma frequently occurs on soles, subungual mucous membranes, and palms (sole of the foot is the most prevalent site). Unlike other types of melanoma, it has a similar incidence in all ethnic groups.
- The warning signs that the lesion may be a melanoma can be summarized with the ABCD mnemonic:
  - **A:** Asymmetry (e.g., lesion is bisected and halves are not identical)
  - **B:** Border irregularity (uneven, ragged border)
  - **C:** Color variegation (presence of various shades of pigmentation)
  - **D:** Diameter enlargement (>6 mm)
  Recent data regarding small-diameter melanoma suggest that the ABCD criteria for gross inspection of pigmented skin lesions and early diagnosis of cutaneous melanoma should be expanded to ABCDE to include *e*volving (i.e., lesions that have changed over time).

ETIOLOGY

- Ultraviolet light is the most important cause of malignant melanoma.
- There is a modest increase in melanoma risk in patients with small nondysplastic nevi and a much greater risk in those with dysplastic lesions.
- The *CDKN2A* gene, residing at the *9p21* locus, is often deleted in people with familial melanoma.

- A mutated signal transduction molecule v-raf murine sarcoma viral oncogene homolog B₁ (BRAF) has been identified in about 50% of patients with metastatic melanoma.

DIAGNOSIS

DIFFERENTIAL DIAGNOSIS

- Dysplastic nevi
- Solar lentigo
- Vascular lesions
- Blue nevus
- Basal cell carcinoma
- Seborrheic keratosis

WORKUP

- Perform excisional biopsy with elliptical excision that includes 1 to 2 mm of normal skin surrounding the lesion and extends to the subcutaneous tissue; incisional punch biopsy is sometimes necessary in surgically sensitive areas (e.g., digits, nose).
- Sentinel lymph node dissection should be considered in patients with intermediate (1 to 4 mm) melanomas or high-risk skin tumors to obtain information regarding a patient's subclinical lymph node status with minimal morbidity. It involves the use of radiologic lymphoscintigraphy to map lymphatic drainage from the site of the primary melanoma to the first sentinel lymph node in the region. When properly performed, if the sentinel node is negative the remaining lymph nodes in the region will not have metastases in more than 98% of cases. The staging of intermediate thickness (1.2 to 3.5 mm) primary melanomas, according to the results of sentinel node biopsy, provides important prognostic information and identifies patients with nodal metastases whose survival can be prolonged by immediate lymphadenectomy.
- The staging system for melanoma adapted by the American Joint Committee on Cancer (AJCC) is as follows:

T*	Thickness of primary tumor
Tis	In situ
T1	≤1.0 mm
T2	1.01-2.0 mm
T3	2.01-4.0 mm
T4	>4.0 mm
N†	Number of positive lymph nodes

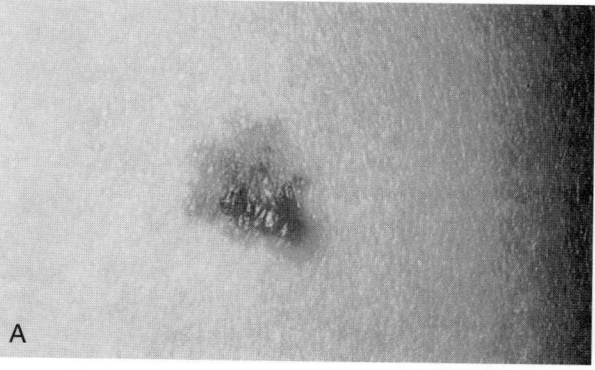
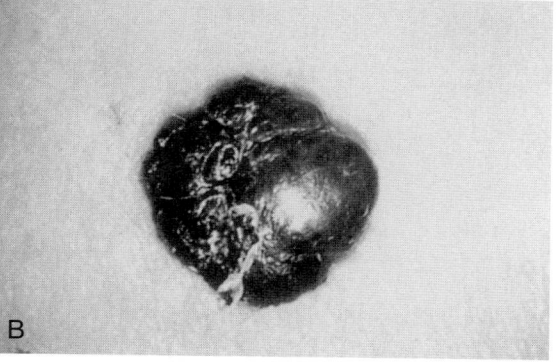

FIGURE 1-230 A, Superficial spreading melanoma. **B,** Nodular melanoma. (From Abeloff MD [ed]: *Clinical oncology,* ed 3, New York, 2004, Churchill Livingstone.)

N0	0
N1	1
N2	2 or 3
N3	≥4 (or combination of in-transit metastases, satellite lesions, or an ulcerated primary lesion with any number of nodes)
M	Metastases
M0	0
M1	Distant subcutaneous or lymph node metastases
M2	Lung metastases
M3	All other visceral or any distant metastases or an elevated lactate dehydrogenase level not attributable to another cause

Clinical Stage

0	(T0N0M0)
IA	(T1aN0M0)
IB	(T1bN0M0) (T2aN0M0)
IIA	(T2bN0M0) (T3aN0M0)
IIB	(T3bN0M0) (T4aN0M0)
IIC	(T4bN0M0)
IIIA	(T1-T4aN1bM0)
IIIB	(T1-T4aN2bM0)
IIIC	(AnyT, N2c, M0) (Any T, N3, M0)
IV	(Any T, Any N, >M1)

*a, Without ulceration; b, with ulceration.

†a, Micrometastasis; b, macrometastases; c, in-transit metastases with metastatic lymph nodes.

LABORATORY TESTS

The pathology report should indicate the following:

- Tumor thickness (Breslow microstage).
- Tumor depth (Clark level): the depth of invasion is the most important histologic prognostic parameter in evaluating the primary tumor.
- Mitotic rate: tabulated as mitoses per square millimeter in the dermal part of the tumor in which most mitoses are identified.
- Radial growth rates versus vertical growth rate: radial growth phase describes the growth of melanoma within the epidermis and along the dermal-epidermal junction.
- Tumor infiltrating lymphocytes have a strong predictive value in vertical growth phase melanomas and are defined as brisk, nonbrisk, or absent.
- Histologic regression: characterized by the absence of melanoma in the epidermis and

dermis flanked on one or both sides by melanoma.
- Reverse-transcription polymerase chain reaction assay for tyrosine messenger RNA is a useful marker for the presence of melanoma cells. It is performed on sentinel lymph node biopsy and is useful for detection of submicroscopic metastases.
- Identification of somatic mutations in the gene encoding the serine-threonine protein kinase B-RAF (*BRAF*) may be useful for treatment options (see later).

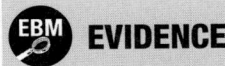

TREATMENT

- Initial excision of the melanoma
- Reexcision of the involved area after histologic diagnosis:
  1. The margins of reexcision depend on the thickness of the tumor.
  2. Low-risk or intermediate-risk tumors require excision of 1 to 3 cm.
  3. Melanomas of moderate thickness (0.9 to 2.0 mm) can be excised safely with 2-cm margins.
  4. A 1-cm margin of excision for melanoma with a poor prognosis (as defined by a tumor thickness ≥2 mm) is associated with a significantly greater risk of regional recurrence than is a 3-cm margin, but with a similar overall survival rate.
- Lymph node dissection: recommended in all patients with enlarged lymph nodes. Lymph node evaluation is important in patients with melanoma 1 mm in depth because it determines the overall prognosis and need for therapeutic lymph node dissection or adjuvant treatment.
  1. Elective lymph node dissection remains controversial.
  2. It is indicated with positive sentinel node. It may be considered in those with a primary melanoma between 1 and 4 mm thick (especially in patients <60 yr).
- Adjuvant therapy with interferon alfa-2b (intron A) in patients with metastatic melanoma is approved by the FDA for AJCC stages IIb and III melanoma; however, its statistical benefit remains unclear.
- Dacarbazine and interleukin-2 can be used in metastatic melanoma. Results are generally poor, with median survival time in patients

with distant metastatic melanoma approximately 6 mo.
- Recent attention has focused on combinations of dacarbazine and cisplatin with interleukin-2 and interferon-alfa (biochemotherapy).
- Novel therapeutics involve cancer vaccines and use of granulocyte-macrophage colony-stimulating factor and angiogenesis inhibitors. Trials with ipilimumab, an agent that blocks cytotoxic T-lymphocyte–associated antigen 4 to potentiate an antitumor T-cell response, have shown improved overall survival in patients with previously treated metastatic melanoma. In patients that carry the V600E *BRAF* mutation, trials involving treatment with PLX4032 (also known as RG7204), an oral inhibitor of mutated *BRAF*, have shown complete or partial tumor regression in the majority of patients with metastatic melanoma.
- Patients with a history of melanoma should be followed up with skin examinations every 6 mo or sooner if patient detects any new lesions; the assessments usually consist of medical history, physical examination, laboratory values, and chest radiograph.

DISPOSITION

- Prognosis varies with the stage of the melanoma. The 5-yr survival related to thickness is as follows: <0.76 mm, 99% survival; 0.6 to 1.49 mm, 85%; 1.5 to 2.49 mm, 84%; 2.5 to 3.9 mm, 70%; >4 mm, 44%.
- The 5-yr survival in patients with distant metastasis is <10%.
- Treatment of advanced disease consists (in addition to surgical excision and lymph node dissection) of chemotherapy, immunotherapy, and radiation therapy.

EBM EVIDENCE

available at www.expertconsult.com

SUGGESTED READINGS
available at www.expertconsult.com

AUTHOR: **FRED F. FERRI, M.D.**

BASIC INFORMATION

DEFINITION

Meniere's disease is a syndrome characterized by recurrent vertigo with fluctuating hearing loss, tinnitus, and fullness in the ear.

SYNONYMS

Endolymphatic hydrops
Lermoyez's syndrome

ICD-9CM CODES
386.01 Meniere's disease, cochleovestibular (active)

EPIDEMIOLOGY & DEMOGRAPHICS

INCIDENCE (IN U.S.): 100 cases/100,000 persons
PREVALENCE (IN U.S.): 15 cases/100,000 persons
PREDOMINANT SEX: Male = female
PEAK INCIDENCE: 20 to 50 yr

PHYSICAL FINDINGS & CLINICAL PRESENTATION

- Hearing may be unilaterally decreased.
- Pallor, sweating, and nausea may occur during a severe attack.
- Usually the patient develops a sensation of fullness and pressure along with decreased hearing and tinnitus in a single ear.
- The patient typically experiences severe vertigo, which peaks within min, then slowly subsides over hr.
- May see spontaneous nystagmus on examination.
- Persistent sense of disequilibrium for days is typical after an acute episode
- May have vestibulopathy demonstrable with a positive head thrust test.

ETIOLOGY

- Unknown; viral and autoimmune causes have been suggested.
- Associated with endolymphatic hydrops.

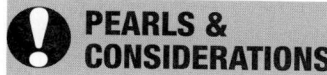 DIAGNOSIS

Proposed criteria by the American Academy of Otolaryngology-Head and Neck Surgery (AAO-HNS) for diagnosis of Meniere's disease include the following four features, of which (1) and at least one of (2), (3), or (4) must be present:
1. Two spontaneous episodes of vertigo lasting 20 min or longer without loss of consciousness
2. Hearing loss that is usually, but not always, fluctuating
3. Tinnitus in the ear, which may fluctuate
4. Aural fullness in the ear, which may fluctuate

DIFFERENTIAL DIAGNOSIS

- Acoustic neuroma
- Migrainous vertigo
- Multiple sclerosis
- Autoimmune inner ear syndrome
- Otitis media
- Vertebrobasilar disease
- Labyrinthitis

WORKUP

- Electronystagmography may show peripheral vestibular deficit.
- Electrocochleography and glycerol test used by some otoneurologists and ENT specialists.

LABORATORY TESTS

Audiogram may show sensorineural hearing loss, with lower frequencies primarily affected.

IMAGING STUDIES

MRI to rule out acoustic neuroma, especially if cerebellar or CNS dysfunction is present

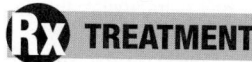 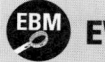 TREATMENT

NONPHARMACOLOGIC THERAPY

Limit activity during attacks

ACUTE GENERAL Rx

- Prochlorperazine 5 to 10 mg PO q6h or 25 mg PO bid
- Promethazine 12.5 to 25 mg PO q4 to 6h
- Diazepam 5 to 10 mg IV/PO for acute attack
- Meclizine 25 mg q6h
- Scopolamine patch

CHRONIC Rx

- Diuretics such as hydrochlorothiazide or acetazolamide, salt restriction, and avoidance of caffeine are traditional.
- For refractory cases, surgical interventions.

DISPOSITION

- Patients are usually followed by an otoneurologist or ENT specialist.
- Usual course of disease consists of alternating attacks and remissions.
- Majority of patients can be managed medically. Of patients, 10% to 30% will undergo surgical intervention for persistent incapacitating vertigo.

REFERRAL

To an otolaryngologist for surgical intervention if attacks persist despite medical therapy

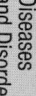 PEARLS & CONSIDERATIONS

COMMENTS

- There are many variations of the classical clinical picture. The essential features for diagnosis are episodic vertigo and sensorineural hearing loss audiometrically documented on at least one occasion.
- In one third of patients, both ears are eventually involved.
- There is some evidence that Meniere's disease and migraines may be pathophysiologically linked.

EBM EVIDENCE

available at www.expertconsult.com

SUGGESTED READINGS
available at www.expertconsult.com

AUTHOR: **SHARON S. HARTMAN POLENSEK, M.D., PH.D.**

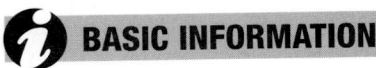

BASIC INFORMATION

DEFINITION

Meningiomas are generally slow-growing tumors arising from arachnoid cells of the arachnoid villi; 90% are benign.

ICD-9CM CODES
225.2 Cerebral meninges

EPIDEMIOLOGY & DEMOGRAPHICS

INCIDENCE: 6/100,000 persons/yr; accounts for about one third of primary intracranial tumors and are the second most common brain tumor in adults; often underreported.

PREDOMINANT SEX AND AGE: Female:male ratio of almost 3:1 in the brain and up to 6:1 in the spinal cord; male > female in childhood and male = female among African Americans

PEAK INCIDENCE: Males: sixth decade, females: seventh decade, incidence increases with age; rare in childhood

RISK FACTORS: Ionizing radiation results in increased incidence and a shorter latency period

GENETICS: Meningiomas may be isolated or found in association with other genetic diseases, such as neurofibromatosis type 2 and familial meningioma. Approximately half of meningiomas have allelic losses involving of the NF2 and DAL-1 genes. Allelic losses of chromosomes 1p, 2p, 6q, 9q, 10q, 14q, 17p, and 18q may be associated with histologic progression.

PHYSICAL FINDINGS & CLINICAL PRESENTATION

- Neurologic symptoms vary with location and size (see Table 1-111); meningiomas can arise from the dura at any site, although most commonly occur over the cerebral convexities, often associated with the falx. Other common locations include the sphenoid wing, olfactory groove and optic nerve sheath. Focal symptoms depend on the site of origin.
- Most common presentation is with a focal or generalized seizure or gradually worsening

TABLE 1-111 Locations and Presentations of Meningiomas

Location	Presenting Manifestation
Parasagittal	Urinary incontinence, dementia, gradual paraparesis, seizures
Lateral convexity	Variable depending on structures compressed, including slow hemiparesis, speech abnormalities
Olfactory groove	Anosmia, visual disturbance, dementia, Foster–Kennedy syndrome
Suprasellar	Hormonal failure, bitemporal hemianopia, optic atrophy
Sphenoid ridge	Extraocular nerve paresis, exostoses, proptosis, seizures

Goetz CG, Pappert EJ: *Textbook of clinical neurology,* Philadelphia, 1999, Saunders.

neurologic deficit. Seizures are present preoperatively in 30% to 40%.
- Typically are slow growing and asymptomatic; discovered incidentally on a neuroimaging study or at autopsy.

ETIOLOGY

- Meningiomas are thought to arise from a multistep progression of genetic changes.
- Mutations of the NF2 gene on chromosome 22 are found in patients with neurofibromatosis type 2 and >50% of sporadic meningiomas. This gene is thought to act as a tumor suppressor gene; the protein product, merlin, is also involved in cytoskeletal organization.
- DAL-1 is another tumor suppressor gene, located on chromosome 18p, that has been identified in a subset of the approximately 40% of sporadic meningiomas with neither the NF2 gene mutations nor allelic loss of chromosome 22q.
- Cranial radiation may be responsible for some cases following an appropriate latency period from 10 to 20 yr. Meningiomas that result from radiation are generally more aggressive.
- The link with steroid hormones and their receptors is suggested by the increase in growth rate and/or development of meningiomas during pregnancy and increased incidence in women who use postmenopausal hormones or in association with breast carcinomas.

DIAGNOSIS

DIFFERENTIAL DIAGNOSIS

Other well-circumscribed intracranial tumors that involve the dura or subdural space.
- Acoustic schwannoma (typically at the pontocerebellar junction)

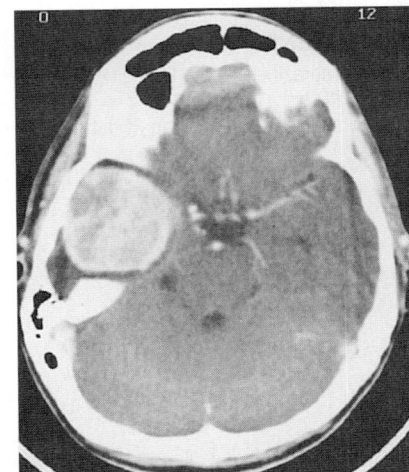

FIGURE 1-231 Contrast-enhanced CT scan demonstrates a large contrast-enhancing right sphenoid wing meningioma. (From Specht N [ed]: *Practical guide to diagnostic imaging,* St Louis, 1998, Mosby.)

- Ependymoma, lipoma, and metastases within the spinal cord
- Metastatic disease from lymphoma/adenocarcinoma, inflammatory disease, or infections such as tuberculosis

WORKUP

Imaging studies with CT or MRI, followed by surgical removal with histologic confirmation

LABORATORY TESTS

According to the World Health Organization (WHO) classification, there are nine benign histologic variants (account for 90% of all meningiomas) and four variants associated with increased recurrence and rates of metastasis. Ninety percent of meningiomas are classified as benign meningiomas or WHO grade I.

IMAGING STUDIES

- Cranial CT scanning or MRI can detect and determine the extent of meningiomas (Fig. 1-231). CT can show hyperostosis and/or intratumoral calcifications. MRI (Fig. 1-232) is preferable to show the dural origin of the tumor in most cases, with the characteristic "tail" sign.
- On nonenhanced scans, meningiomas typically are isodense to slightly hyperdense to brain and are homogeneous in appearance. Meningiomas show homogeneous enhancement; gadolinium can facilitate imaging of smaller additional lesions that are missed on unenhanced images.
- Indistinct margins, marked edema, mushroomlike projections from tumor, brain parenchymal infiltration and heterogeneous enhancement are suggestive of more aggressive behavior.

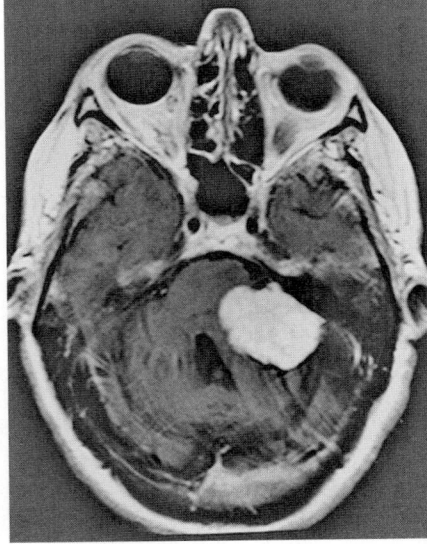

FIGURE 1-232 MRI picture of a posterior fossa meningioma, demonstrated an extra-axial homogeneously contrast-enhanced mass arising from the tentorium and compressing the cerebellar hemisphere. (Goetz CG, Pappert EJ: *Textbook of clinical neurology,* Philadelphia, 1999, Saunders.)

M

Diseases and Disorders

I

- PET scan may help in predicting the aggressiveness of the tumor and the potential for recurrence.

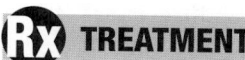 **TREATMENT**

Primary management depends on signs or symptoms, age of patient, and location and size of tumor. Observation may be appropriate if tumors are discovered incidentally and/or if growth is indolent and unlikely to cause symptoms.

NONPHARMACOLOGIC THERAPY

- The mainstay of treatment for meningiomas remains surgical removal. Complete resection is usually attempted, when feasible. After total excision, recurrence rates of 0% to 20% have been observed, while 20% to 50% of patients recur within 5 yr of a subtotal resection.
- Active surveillance to monitor for tumor recurrence is important.
- Radiation therapy is the only validated form of adjuvant therapy and may be beneficial in patients with incomplete resections or inoperable tumors. Stereotactic radiosurgery can provide local control with more limited toxicity.

ACUTE GENERAL Rx

- For lesions that cause significant mass effect, steroids are sometimes used to decrease brain edema.
- Anticonvulsants to control seizures. The use of prophylactic anticonvulsants is controversial without a clear history of seizures.

CHRONIC Rx

- Prophylactic use of anticonvulsants is not recommended in patients without a history of seizures.
- There is limited data on the efficacy of traditional chemotherapy and the evidence is largely anecdotal. The most extensively evaluated agents are hydroxyurea, mifepristone (RU486), and interferon alfa-2b. Recently, somatostatin analogs have been evaluated in multicenter clinical trials.

DISPOSITION

- Estimated surgical mortality is 7%. Significant morbidity and mortality can be observed in meningiomas with otherwise favorable pathology secondary to unfavorable location (e.g., skull base).
- Long-term outcome varies, based on pathology, tumor grade, location, and completeness of resection.
- Most incidentally discovered meningiomas remain asymptomatic and experience a slow rate of growth. Calcified tumors may be less likely to progress than noncalcified ones.
- Meningiomas may recur after surgical resection. In addition, some tumors show histologic progression to a higher grade. Features suggesting increased rate of recurrence include multiple allelic chromosomal losses, local brain invasion, high rate of mitosis and highly anaplastic features.

REFERRAL

- Neurosurgical consultation for all cases
- Neurology, radiation oncology, and oncology depending on presence of other sequelae and in setting of recurrence

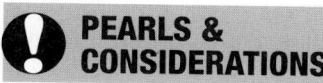 **PEARLS & CONSIDERATIONS**

COMMENTS

- Many meningiomas are discovered incidentally; most are benign and remain asymptomatic.
- "Dural tail" is classic finding on neuroimaging studies.
- Individuals with neurofibromatosis type 2 are at high risk to develop meningiomas.

PATIENT/FAMILY EDUCATION

Meningioma mommas: www.meningiomamommas.org
Meningioma Support and Patient Information Group
Meningioma Online Support Group: http://www.brainstrust.org/meningioma.htm

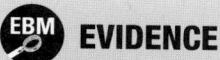 **EVIDENCE**

available at www.expertconsult.com

SUGGESTED READINGS

available at www.expertconsult.com

AUTHOR: **NICOLE J. ULLRICH, M.D., PH.D.**

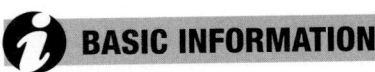

DEFINITION

Bacterial meningitis is an inflammation of meninges with increased intracranial pressure, and pleocytosis or increased WBCs in cerebrospinal fluid (CSF) secondary to bacteria in the pia-subarachnoid space and ventricles, leading to neurologic sequelae and abnormalities.

SYNONYMS

Spinal meningitis

ICD-9CM CODES
320 Bacterial meningitis

EPIDEMIOLOGY & DEMOGRAPHICS

INCIDENCE (IN U.S.): 3 cases/100,000 persons; 1.2 million cases per year in the world; 135,000 deaths annually worldwide
PREDOMINANT SEX: Male = female
PREDOMINANT AGE: All ages, neonate to geriatric

PHYSICAL FINDINGS & CLINICAL PRESENTATION

- Fever
- Headache
- Neck stiffness, nuchal rigidity, meningismus
- Altered mental state, lethargy
- Vomiting, nausea
- Photophobia
- Seizures
- Coma; lethargy, stupor
- Rash: petechial associated with meningococcal infection (Fig. 1-233)
- Myalgia
- Cranial nerve abnormality (unilateral)
- Papilledema
- Dilated, nonreactive pupil(s)
- Posturing: decorticate/decerebrate
- Physical examination findings of Kernig's sign and Brudzinski's sign in adults with meningitis are often not helpful in determining meningeal inflammation

ETIOLOGY

Neisseria meningitidis is now more common than *Haemophilus influenzae* as a cause of bacterial meningitis in children as well as adults. *H. influenzae* is the cause of >30% of cases of meningitis (usually in infants and children <6 yr of age). It is associated with sinusitis, otitis media.

- Neonates: group B streptococci, *Escherichia coli*, *Listeria monocytogenes*, *Klebsiella* sp.
- Infants: 1 to 23 mo
  1. *S. pnemoniae*
  2. *N. meningitidis*
  3. *S. agalactiae* (group B streptococci)
  4. *Haemophilus influenzae*
  5. *E. coli*
- Ages 2 to 50 yr
  1. *N. meningitidis*
  2. *S. pneumoniae*
- >50 yr of age
  1. *S. pneumoniae*
  2. *N. meningitidis*
  3. *L. monocytogenes*
  4. Aerobic gram-negative bacilli

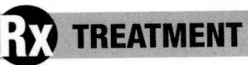 DIAGNOSIS

Diagnostic approach is based on patient presentation and physical examination. Key elements to diagnosis are CSF evaluation and CT scan or MRI if the patient is in a coma or has focal neurologic deficits, pupillary abnormalities, or papilledema.

DIFFERENTIAL DIAGNOSIS

- Endocarditis, bacteremia
- Intracranial tumor
- Lyme disease
- Brain abscess
- Partially treated bacterial meningitis
- Medications
- SLE
- Seizures
- Acute mononucleosis
- Other infectious meningitides
- Neuroleptic malignant syndrome
- Subdural empyema
- Rocky Mountain spotted fever

WORKUP

CSF examination:
- Opening pressure >100 to 200 mm Hg
- WBC <5 to >100 mm^3
- Neutrophilic predominance: >80%
- Gram stain of CSF: positive in 60% to 90% of patients
- CSF protein: >50 mg/dl
- CSF glucose: <40 mg/dl
- Culture: positive in 65% to 90% of cases
- CSF bacterial antigen: 50% to 100% sensitivity
- E-test for susceptibility of pneumococcal isolates

LABORATORY TESTS

Blood culturing, WBC with differential, and CSF examination (see "Workup")

IMAGING STUDIES

- CT scan or MRI of head: necessary with increased intracranial pressure, coma, neurologic deficits
- Sinus CT: if sinusitis suspected

(Rx) TREATMENT

Empiric therapy is necessary with IV antibiotic treatment if patient has purulent CSF fluid at time of lumbar puncture, is asplenic, or has signs of DIC/sepsis pending Gram stain and culture results. Therapy after Gram stain pending cultures is recommended for the following:

1. Neonates: ampicillin plus cefotaxime
2. Infants/children: ampicillin or third-generation cephalosporin (plus chloramphenicol if purulent or patient compromised)
3. Adults (18 to 50 yr): third-generation cephalosporin (e.g., Ceftriaxone: 2 g IV q12hr)
4. Older adults (>50 yr): ampicillin plus third-generation cephalosporin
   - Penicillin-resistant pneumococcus: because of an increasing incidence of this organism, empiric treatment with ceftriaxone or cefotaxime plus vancomycin (30 to 60 mg/kg/day) has been recommended.
   - Table 1-112 describes common pathogens of bacterial meningitis and their empiric treatment based on age.
   - Table 1-113 describes specific antibiotic treatments for known pathogens.
   - Steroids: dexamethasone 0.15 mg/kg q6h for first 4 days of therapy should be used in adults with bacterial meningitis and mental status changes or acute neurologic phenomenon. Decreased mortality and neurologic sequelae are seen with adjunct therapy.
   - Dexamethasone also benefits children with Hib or pneumococcal meningitis and should be given within the first 2 days of illness.

DISPOSITION

Bacterial meningitis is a reportable disease that needs to be reported to local health authorities. Droplet precautions should be used for first 24 hr of therapy for suspected or confirmed *N. meningitidis* infection.

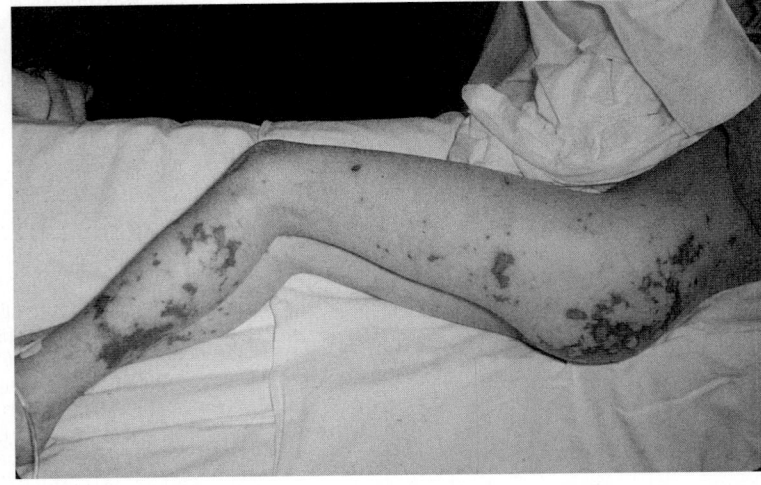

FIGURE 1-233 Fully developed, almost pathognomonic hemorrhagic rash of meningococcal sepsis. (From Cohen J, Powderly WG: *Infectious diseases*, ed 2, St Louis, 2004, Mosby.)

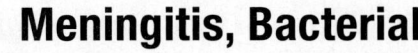
Diseases and Disorders

I

REFERRAL

- To a neurologist if persistent neurologic sequelae develop after bacterial meningitis
- To an infectious disease consultant if a patient has recurrent bacterial meningitis; such patients deserve a workup for an anatomic (CSF dural leak) or immunologic defect (complement defect, hyposplenism, immunoglobulin deficiency)

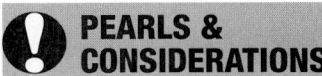
PEARLS & CONSIDERATIONS

COMMENTS

- Nosocomial bacterial meningitis may result from invasive procedures (e.g., placement of ventricular catheters, lumbar puncture, craniotomy, spinal anesthesia). Treatment of this different spectrum of microorganisms requires empirical antimicrobial therapy with vancomycin plus cefepime, ceftazidime, or meropenem. In cases of basilar skull fracture, effective empirical antimicrobial therapy consists of vancomycin plus a third-generation cephalosporin.
- Prevention of meningitis can be achieved through chemoprophylaxis of close contacts (household members and anyone exposed to oral secretions).
- Effective medications are rifampin 10 mg/kg PO bid for 2 days or ceftriaxone 250 mg IM single dose in patients older than age 12; 125 mg IM if age 12 or younger.

- Ciprofloxacin 500 mg for prevention of *Neisseria* meningitis can be given to patients older than 18 yr who cannot tolerate rifampin to eradicate pharyngeal colonization.
- Menactra: a protein-conjugate vaccine against serogroup A, C, Y, W-135 capsular polysaccharides is available for adults (up to 55 yr) and children older than 2 yr.

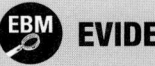 **EVIDENCE**

available at www.expertconsult.com

SUGGESTED READINGS

available at www.expertconsult.com

AUTHORS: **GLENN G. FORT, M.D., M.P.H.,** and **DENNIS J. MIKOLICH, M.D.**

TABLE 1-112 Common Pathogens of Bacterial Meningitis and Their Empiric Treatment Based on Age

Age	Common Pathogens	Treatment*	Duration (days)
0-1 mo	Group B streptococci *Listeria monocytogenes* *Escherichia coli*	Ampicillin and third-generation cephalosporin[†] or ampicillin and aminoglycoside	14-21 14-21 21
1-3 mo	*Streptococcus pneumoniae* Group B streptococci, *E. coli*, *L. monocytogenes* *S. pneumoniae* *Neisseria meningitidis*, *Haemophilus influenzae*	Ampicillin and third-generation cephalosporin[†]	10-14 14-21 14-21 10-14 7-10
3 mo-18 yr	*H. influenzae*, *H. meningitidis*, *S. pneumoniae*	Third-generation cephalosporin[†] or meropenem or chloramphenicol	7-10 (*N. influenzae* and *N. meningitidis*) 10-14 (*S. pneumoniae*)
18-50 yr	*H. influenzae*, *N. meningitidis*, *S. pneumoniae*	Third-generation cephalosporin[†] or meropenem or ampicillin and chloramphenicol	Same as above
>50 yr	*S. pneumoniae*, *L. monocytogenes*, gram-negative bacilli	Ampicillin and third-generation cephalosporin[†] or ampicillin and fluoroquinolone[‡] or meropenem	10-14 (*S. pneumoniae*) 14-21 (*L. monocytogenes*) 21 Gram-negative bacilli other than *H. influenzae*

From Rakel RE (ed): *Principles of family practice*, ed 6, Philadelphia, 2002, WB Saunders.
*Add vancomycin in areas where there is greater than 2% incidence of highly drug-resistant *S. pneumoniae*.
[†]Ceftriaxone or cefotaxime.
[‡]Ciprofloxacin or levofloxacin.

TABLE 1-113 Specific Antibiotic Treatments for Known Pathogens

Pathogen	Primary Therapy	Alternative*
Group B streptococci	Penicillin G or ampicillin	Vancomycin or third-generation cephalosporin[†]
Streptococcus pneumoniae (MIC < 0.1)	Third-generation cephalosporin[†]	Meropenem, penicillin
S. pneumoniae (MIC > 0.1)	Vancomycin and third-generation cephalosporin*	Substitute rifampin for vancomycin; or meropenem; or vancomycin as monotherapy if highly allergic to other alternatives
Haemophilus influenzae (β-lactamase-negative)	Ampicillin	Third-generation cephalosporin[†] or chloramphenicol or aztreonam
H. influenzae (β-lactamase-positive)	Third-generation cephalosporin[†]	Chloramphenicol or aztreonam or fluoroquinolones[‡]
Listeria monocytogenes	Ampicillin and gentamicin	Trimethoprim-sulfamethoxazole
Neisseria meningitidis	Penicillin G or ampicillin	Third-generation cephalosporin[†]
Enterobacteriaceae	Third-generation cephalosporin[†] and aminoglycoside	Trimethoprim-sulfamethoxazole or aztreonam or fluoroquinolones or antipseudomonal penicillin (or ampicillin) and aminoglycoside
Pseudomonas aeruginosa	Ceftazidime and aminoglycoside	Aminoglycoside and aztreonam or aminoglycoside and antipseudomonal penicillin[§]
Staphylococcus aureus (methicillin-sensitive)	Antistaphylococcal penicillin[¶] and rifampin	Vancomycin and rifampin or trimethoprim-sulfamethoxazole and rifampin
S. aureus (methicillin-resistant)	Vancomycin and rifampin	
Staphylococcus epidermidis	Vancomycin and rifampin	

From Rakel RE (ed): *Principles of family practice*, ed 6, Philadelphia, 2002, WB Saunders.
MIC, Minimum inhibitory concentration.
*If patient is highly allergic or intolerant of primary therapy.
[†]Ceftriaxone or cefotaxime.
[‡]Ciprofloxacin or levofloxacin.
[§]Piperacillin, mezlocillin, or ticarcillin.
[¶]Nafcillin, oxacillin, or methicillin.

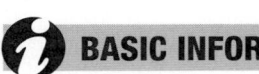

BASIC INFORMATION

DEFINITION
Viral meningitis is an acute febrile illness with signs and symptoms of meningeal irritation, usually with a lymphocytic pleocytosis of the cerebrospinal fluid (CSF) and negative CSF bacterial stains and cultures.

SYNONYMS
Aseptic meningitis

ICD-9CM CODES
047.8 Meningitis, aseptic

EPIDEMIOLOGY & DEMOGRAPHICS (Table 1-114)
INCIDENCE (IN U.S.): 11 cases/100,000 persons
PREDOMINANT SEX: Male = female
GENETICS: Those with abnormal humoral immunity and agammaglobulinemia have associated difficulty with viral clearance.

PHYSICAL FINDINGS & CLINICAL PRESENTATION
- Fever
- Headache
- Nuchal rigidity
- Photophobia
- Myalgias
- Vomiting
- Rash

ETIOLOGY
- Enterovirus: 85% to 95% of all cases
- Parechoviruses
- Mumps virus
- Measles
- Arboviruses from mosquitoes: EEE, West Nile, St Louis
- Herpes: HSV-1, HSV-2, VZV, HHV-6, and HHV-7
- Acute HIV
- Lymphocytic choriomeningitis virus
- Adenovirus
- CMV and EBV
- Other arthropod-borne viruses: Powassan virus
- Influenza A and B virus

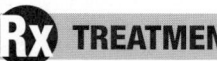

DIAGNOSIS

The diagnostic approach is similar to that for bacterial meningitis (see "Meningitis, Bacterial"); the foremost need is to rule out bacterial meningitis with CSF evaluation. Presentation may be similar to that of meningitis with bacterial involvement.

DIFFERENTIAL DIAGNOSIS
- Bacterial meningitis
- Meningitis secondary to Lyme disease, TB, syphilis, amebiasis, leptospirosis
- Rickettsial illnesses: Rocky Mountain spotted fever
- Migraine headache
- Medications
- SLE
- Acute mononucleosis/Epstein-Barr virus
- Seizures
- Carcinomatous meningitis

WORKUP
CSF examination:
- Usually shows pleocytosis
- Lymphocytic predominance (neutrophils in early stages)
- Opening pressure: 200 to 250 mm Hg
- WBC: 100 to 1000 mm^3
- Increased CSF protein
- Decreased or normal CSF glucose
- Negative Gram stain, cultures, CIE, latex agglutination
- Viral cultures or serologic testing may be diagnostic
- Polymerase chain reaction for HSV, West Nile, or enterovirus (which could shorten duration of antibiotic treatment and hospitalization if bacterial meningitis was suspected)

LABORATORY TESTS
CBC with differential, blood culturing, and CSF examination (see "Workup")

IMAGING STUDIES
CT scan or MRI: if cerebral edema, focal neurologic findings develop

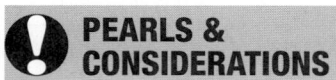

TREATMENT

No specific antiviral therapy for most viruses. Treatment is supportive unless HSV is detected, which would be treated with IV acyclovir: 10 mg/kg q8hr in adults. Up to 20 mg/kg q8hr in children <12 yr.

DISPOSITION
Viral meningitis is almost always an uncomplicated illness that will resolve; however, relapsing headache, myalgia, and weakness may occur for 2 to 3 wk after onset of symptoms.

PEARLS & CONSIDERATIONS

- Enteroviruses are the most common cause of viral meningitis and are transmitted by fecal-oral and less commonly by the respiratory route.
- Herpes simplex type 2 (HSV-2) causes both primary and recurrent lymphocytic meningitis. HSV-2 meningitis presents most often without a history of genital herpes, recurrent meningitis, or genital symptoms.

SUGGESTED READINGS
available at www.expertconsult.com

AUTHORS: **GLENN G. FORT, M.D., M.P.H.,** and **DENNIS J. MIKOLICH, M.D.**

TABLE 1-114 Epidemiology of Acute Viral Meningitis

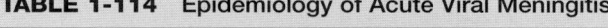

		EPIDEMIOLOGIC FACTORS*		
Season	Patient's Age (yr)	Patient's Sex	Risk Factor	Suggested Viral Agent
Summer-fall	Infant	—	Infected mother	Coxsackievirus B
	1-15	—	Swimming pools, closed communities	Enteroviruses
			Geographic area: California, southeastern United States	California serogroup virus
Winter	1-15	—	School exposure	Varicella virus, measles virus
		Male/female 3:1		Mumps virus
	16-21	—	College exposure	Measles virus
		Male/female 3:1		Mumps virus
		—		Epstein-Barr virus (mononucleosis)
	Any	—	Mice, rats, hamsters	Lymphocytic choriomeningitis virus
	Adults	—	Varicella-zoster	Varicella-zoster virus
Any	Any	—	Immunocompromise	Adenovirus
		—	Acquired immunodeficiency syndrome	Human immunodeficiency virus

From Gorbach SI: *Infectious diseases,* ed 2, Philadelphia, 1998, WB Saunders.
*Epidemiologic factors are suggestive but should not be used to exclude diagnoses in individual cases.

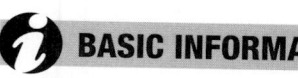

BASIC INFORMATION

DEFINITION

Meningomyelocele is the most common type of spina bifida and is characterized by herniation of the spinal cord, nerves, or both through a bony defect of the spine.

SYNONYMS

Myelomeningocele
Spina bifida cystica

ICD-9CM CODES
741.9 Spina bifida without mention of hydrocephalus
741.9 Meningomyelocele

EPIDEMIOLOGY & DEMOGRAPHICS

INCIDENCE (IN U.S.): 4.6/10,000 births
PREDOMINANT SEX: Male = female
PEAK INCIDENCE: Newborn
GENETICS: Environmental and genetic factors have a joint role.

PHYSICAL FINDINGS & CLINICAL PRESENTATION

- Evident at birth—a sac protruding in the lumbar region (Fig. 1-234)
- Severity of neurologic deficits depends on the location of the lesion along the neuroaxis
- Motor dysfunction in the legs
- Lack of bladder or bowel control
- Often associated with Chiari II malformation and resulting obstructive hydrocephalus

ETIOLOGY

- Failure of neural tube to close completely at about 4 wk gestation
- Associated with maternal valproate use
- A small proportion of cases are associated with chromosomal or single-gene disorders

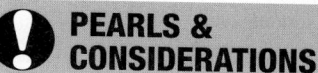

DIAGNOSIS

- Prenatal diagnosis through ultrasound and MRI is being made more frequently
- Coexisting hydrocephalus detected by measurement of head size, ultrasonography, CT, or MRI

DIFFERENTIAL DIAGNOSIS

- Teratoma
- Meningocele

WORKUP

- Evaluate for hydrocephalus
- Evaluate for other congenital abnormalities, such as congenital heart disease, hydronephrosis, intestinal malformation, club foot, and skeletal deformities

LABORATORY TESTS

Prenatal testing often reveals elevated alpha-fetoprotein in amniotic fluid or maternal serum.

IMAGING STUDIES

- MRI of spine
- X-ray studies of skull exhibit craniolacuna, a honeycombed pattern associated with hydrocephalus
- CT or MRI of head: may reveal hydrocephalus

TREATMENT

- Surgical closure of myelomeningocele is performed soon after birth
- Control of hydrocephalus (shunt)
- Management of urinary incontinence (bladder catheterization)

ACUTE GENERAL Rx

- Immediate goal after delivery is to close defect and prevent infection; surgery usually performed within 24 hr of birth

- Shunt placement for obstructive hydrocephalus
- Treatment of seizures, if present

CHRONIC Rx

- Follow closely for development of hydrocephalus
- Bladder catheterization
- Avoid use of latex-containing products to prevent development of latex allergy

DISPOSITION

Followed by a team of specialists including neurosurgeons, urologists, orthopedists, and myelodysplasia nurses

PEARLS & CONSIDERATIONS

All mothers of children with neural tube defects should be instructed on nutritional supplementation with folate for future pregnancies.

COMMENTS

- Intrauterine repair of meningomyelocele decreases the incidence of hindbrain herniation and shunt-dependent hydrocephalus in infants, but increases the incidence of premature delivery.
- U.S. Public Health Service recommends 400 μg of folate intake per day for all women capable of becoming pregnant for primary prevention of neural tube defects.

SUGGESTED READINGS
available at www.expertconsult.com

AUTHOR: **MAITREYI MAZUMDAR, M.D., M.P.H.**

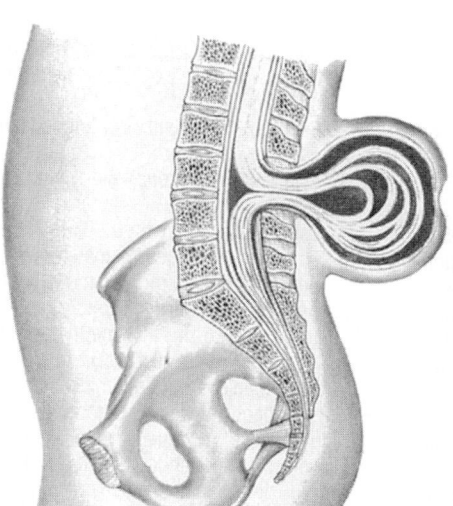
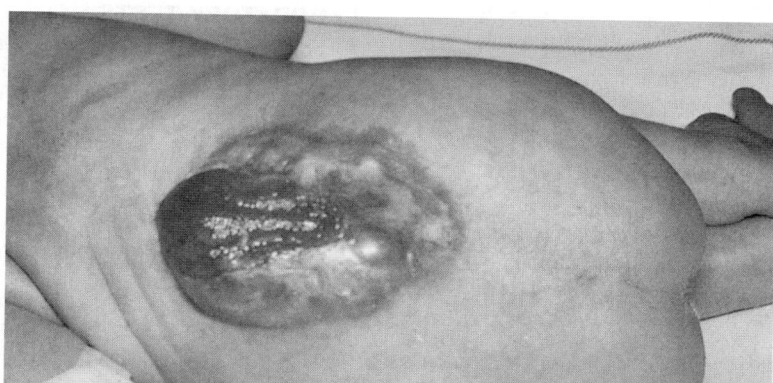

FIGURE 1-234 Meningomyelocele. (From Wong DL: *Whaley's and Wong's nursing care of infants and children,* ed 5, St Louis, 1995, Mosby.)

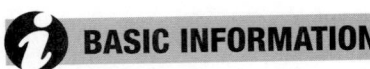

BASIC INFORMATION

DEFINITION

Menopause is the permanent cessation of menstrual periods for 1 yr after age 40 yr or permanent cessation of ovulation after lost ovarian activity. It is a climacteric reproductive stage of life marked by waxing and waning estrogen levels followed by decreasing ovarian function. Premature ovarian failure and no menstrual periods may also occur because of depletion of ovarian follicles before the age of 40 yr.

SYNONYMS

Change of life
Climacteric ovarian failure

ICD-9CM CODES
627   Premenopausal menorrhagia
627.2 Menopausal or female climacteric states
627.4 States associated with artificial menopause
716.3 Climacteric arthritis

EPIDEMIOLOGY & DEMOGRAPHICS

- Average age of menopause in the United States is 51 yr.
- Age at which menopause occurs is genetically determined.
- Smokers experience menopause an average of 1.5 yr earlier than nonsmokers.
- More than one third of a woman's life will be spent after menopause.
- Onset of perimenopause is usually in a woman's mid- to late-40s.
- ~4000 women each day begin menopause.

PHYSICAL FINDINGS & CLINICAL PRESENTATION

- Atrophic vaginitis, which can cause burning, itching, bleeding, dyspareunia
- Either complete cessation of menses or a period of irregular cycles and diminished or heavier bleeding
- Osteoporosis
- Psychologic dysfunction:
  1. Anxiety
  2. Depression
  3. Insomnia
  4. Nervousness
  5. Irritability
  6. Inability to concentrate
- Sexual changes, decreased libido, dyspareunia
- Urinary incontinence
- Vasomotor symptoms (hot flashes, flushes), night sweats, cardiovascular disease, coronary artery disease, atherosclerosis, headaches, tiredness, and lethargy

ETIOLOGY

- The most common etiology: physiologic, caused by depleted granulosa and theca cells that fail to react to endogenous gonadotropins, producing less estrogen; decreased negative feedback in the hypothalamic pituitary access, increased follicle-stimulating hormone (FSH), and increased luteinizing hormone (LH), which leads to stromal cells that continue to produce androgens as a result of the LH stimulation
- Surgical castration
- Family history of early menopause, cigarette smoking, blindness, abnormal chromosomal karyotype (Turner's syndrome, gonadal dysgenesis), precocious puberty, and left-handedness

DIAGNOSIS

DIFFERENTIAL DIAGNOSIS

- Asherman's syndrome
- Hypothalamic dysfunction
- Hypothyroidism
- Pituitary tumors
- Adrenal abnormalities
- Ovarian abnormalities
- Polycystic ovarian syndrome
- Pregnancy
- Ovarian neoplasm
- Tuberculosis of the endometrium

WORKUP

- If the clinical picture is highly suggestive of menopause, estrogen can be prescribed. If all symptoms resolve, then diagnosis has essentially been made. Before estrogen is prescribed, a complete history and physical examination are needed. If a patient has estrogen-dependent malignancy, unexplained abnormal uterine bleeding, history of thrombophlebitis, or acute liver disease, estrogen therapy is contraindicated.
- Progesterone challenge test: medroxyprogesterone 10 to 20 mg PO or progesterone 100 mg IM to induce withdrawal bleeding. If no withdrawal bleeding is obtained, a hypoestrogenic state is assumed to be present.
- Physical examination, height, weight, blood pressure, breast examination, and pelvic examination are needed.
- Assess risk for coronary artery disease, osteoporosis, cigarette smoking, personal history, history of breast cancer, liver disease, active coagulation disorder, or any unexplained vaginal bleeding.

LABORATORY TESTS

- FSH, LH, and estrogen levels: markedly elevated FSH and markedly depressed estrogen level constitute laboratory diagnosis of ovarian failure; LH only if polycystic ovarian disease is to be ruled out in a younger patient. It is not necessary to obtain an FSH if the patient fulfills the clinical criteria for menopause. Similarly, since estradiol levels vary during the menstrual cycle, estradiol levels are rarely necessary or informative
- TSH to rule out thyroid dysfunction and prolactin level if patient has symptoms of galactorrhea and if suspicion of pituitary adenoma exists
- A general chemistry profile to check for any systemic diseases
- Pap smear, endometrial biopsy, or dilation and curettage in patients who have had irregular periods or intermenstrual or postmenopausal bleeding
- Mammogram

IMAGING STUDIES

- CT scan or MRI of sella if pituitary tumor is suspected
- Bone density studies if high-risk condition for osteoporosis exists
- Pelvic ultrasound to check endometrial stripe

TREATMENT

NONPHARMACOLOGIC THERAPY

- A balanced diet: low in fat, with total fat intake being <30% of calories; total calories sufficient to maintain body weight or produce weight loss if that is needed
- Avoidance of smoking and excessive alcohol or caffeine intake
- Exercise: weight-bearing exercise for osteoporosis prevention
- Kegel exercises for strengthening the pelvic floor
- Adequate calcium intake: 1500 mg qd is necessary to maintain zero calcium balance in postmenopausal women
- Change in the ambient temperature (may ameliorate hot flashes and reduce night sweats)
- Vitamin E
- Avoidance of caffeine, alcohol, and spicy foods if they trigger hot flashes
- Vaginal lubricants to help with the dyspareunia attributable to vaginal dryness (e.g., Replens, K-Y Jelly, or Gyne-Moistrin cream)

ACUTE GENERAL Rx

Estrogen replacement in symptomatic patients can be done in a variety of forms, including oral estrogen and transdermal estrogen patch. The lowest effective dose should be prescribed.

- Examples of oral estrogen include:
  1. Conjugated estrogens: start with 0.3 mg qd and increase to 1.25 mg qd depending on symptoms.
  2. Estradiol: start with 0.5 mg qd and increase to 2 mg qd.
  3. Esterified estrogens: start with 0.3 to 1.25 mg qd.
  4. Estropipate: start with 0.625 to 2.5 mg qd.
  5. Esterified estrogen/testosterone combination: give 1.25 mg and methyltestosterone 2.5 mg (Estratest) and esterified estrogen 0.625 mg and methyltestosterone 1.25 mg (Estratest HS). May improve sexual enjoyment and libido.
- If the patient has had a hysterectomy for benign disease, estrogen alone is sufficient. However, if she still has her uterus, progestin should be added for its protective effect against endometrial cancer. Progestins can be prescribed as continual daily dose or cyclic fashion. Most commonly prescribed progestins include medroxyprogesterone acetate 2.5 mg, 5 mg, and 10 mg; Prometrium

100 mg, 200 mg, and 400 mg; and Aygestin 5 mg. Continuous hormone replacement therapy is preferred because after time the patient should be amenorrheic. Patients should be counseled that they may experience some irregular spotting for the first 6 to 9 mo after starting the hormone replacement therapy. Cyclic therapy will cause withdrawal bleeding.

- Combination oral preparations Femhrt, Prefest, Prempro, Activella, Premphase.
- Transdermal patches can be either estradiol (Estraderm, Vivelle, FemPatch) 0.025 to 0.1 mg applied twice weekly or Climara 0.025 to 0.1 mg used once a week. With these preparations, progesterone should be used in a similar fashion. Apply CombiPatch twice weekly (combination estrogen and progesterone) or Climara Pro once per week (one patch).
- Vaginal creams can be used; these should be reserved for local therapy of atrophic vaginitis. Systemic absorption does occur; however, blood levels are unpredictable. Usual dose 0.5 to 2 g intravaginally daily, cyclically 3 wk on 1 wk off. When symptoms improve, once to twice weekly is adequate maintenance.
- Vagifem estradiol vaginal tablets. Initial dosage: one Vagifem tablet, inserted vaginally, qd for 2 wk. Maintenance dose: one Vagifem tablet, inserted vaginally, twice weekly.
- Femring vaginal ring delivering the equivalent of 0.5 mg/day inserted every 3 mo or Estring 0.0075 mg/day.
- EstroGel 0.06% (estradiol gel) One Pump (1.25 g/day) applied to one arm from wrist to shoulder.
- For women in whom estrogen is contraindicated or for those who do not wish to take estrogen, the following regimens can be used:
  1. Serotonin reuptake inhibitors
  2. Depo-Provera 150 mg IM every month (may be helpful in alleviating hot flashes)
  3. Clonidine 0.05 to 0.15 mg qd (questionable efficacy)
  4. Bellergal-S (questionable efficacy)
- Tibolone significantly improves vasomotor symptoms, libido, and vaginal lubrication.

CHRONIC Rx

Hormone replacement therapy should be used only for the short term unless benefits outweigh the risks of long-term use. As a result of the results of the Women's Health Initiative, the FDA has instituted a "black box" warning on postmenopausal hormone replacement products suggesting that the lowest dose should be used for the shortest period of time. This necessitates a considered and nuanced counseling session with patients contemplating hormone replacement prior to the initiation of therapy and then on a periodic basis after that, usually at least a yearly basis.

DISPOSITION

If treated, the patient should have resolution of her symptoms and reduced incidence of osteoporosis. Lifelong medical supervision is necessary to monitor adequacy of treatment and prevention of complications. This should include annual Pap smears, pelvic examinations, breast examinations, mammography, and endometrial sampling of any type of abnormal bleeding. If untreated, the vasomotor symptoms will eventually disappear; however, this may take several years in a small percentage of women. Some women who are in their 80s have experienced hot flashes. Urogenital atrophy will continue to worsen. Osteoporosis and coronary artery disease risks will increase with every passing year. Women using estrogen replacement therapy for >10 yr may have increased risk of developing ovarian cancer.

REFERRAL

Most menopausal women are managed by their gynecologists. However, this condition can be managed adequately by the patient's primary care physician who has an interest in treating menopausal women.

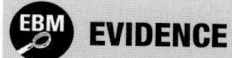 **PEARLS & CONSIDERATIONS**

COMMENTS

- Short-term risks of hormone replacement therapy (HRT) include an eighteenfold increased rise for cholecystitis, three-and-a-half-fold risk of a thrombocardiac event in the first year, and probably increased risk of stroke and myocardial infarction.
- Results of the WHI study found that for every 10,000 women taking HRT for 1 yr (10,000 person-yr), seven more would have coronary events, eight would have more strokes, eight would have more pulmonary emboli, and eight would have earlier breast cancer than would 10,000 women taking placebo. Benefits of HRT were six fewer cases of colorectal cancer and five fewer hip fractures per 10,000 women.
- HRT should not be initiated or continued for the primary or secondary prevention of coronary heart disease.
- Estrogen-replacement therapy or HRT should only be prescribed for patients with sufficient menopausal symptoms that impact the patient's quality of life.

EBM EVIDENCE

available at www.expertconsult.com

SUGGESTED READINGS

available at www.expertconsult.com

AUTHORS: **GEORGE T. DANAKAS, M.D.,** and **RUBEN ALVERO, M.D.**

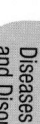

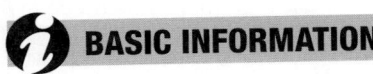

BASIC INFORMATION

DEFINITION

Acute mesenteric lymphadenitis is a syndrome of acute right lower quadrant abdominal pain associated with mesenteric lymph node enlargement and a normal appendix.

ICD-9CM CODES
289.2 Mesenteric adenitis

EPIDEMIOLOGY & DEMOGRAPHICS

- Incidence unknown
- Affects mostly children (<18 yr) with no sex preference
- When *Yersinia* enterocolitis is the cause, boys are more frequently involved

PHYSICAL FINDINGS & CLINICAL PRESENTATION

- Abdominal pain of variable severity (mild ache to severe colic) beginning in upper abdomen or right lower quadrant; eventually localizes in the right side but not in a precise location (unlike appendicitis)
- In *Yersinia* infection outbreaks (see Table 1-115), symptoms include abdominal pain (84%), diarrhea (78%), fever (43%), anorexia (22%), nausea (13%), and vomiting (8%)

- Physical findings:
  - Other lymphadenopathy (20% of cases)
  - Right lower quadrant tenderness (site of maximal tenderness may vary from one examination to the next)
  - Guarding (rare)
  - Mild fever

ETIOLOGY & PATHOGENESIS

- Reactive hyperplasia of lymph nodes that drain the ileocecal region, similar to that seen in inflammatory or allergic conditions. One study reported that approximately two thirds of cases are secondary (reactive) and one third are primary (no demonstrable associated inflammatory process).
- *Yersinia enterocolitica, Y. pseudotuberculosis, Salmonella* species, *Escherichia coli,* and streptococci have been implicated in mesenteric adenitis. Clinical manifestations of yersiniosis are described in Table 1-116.

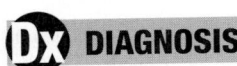

DIAGNOSIS

In general, the diagnosis is made on exploration of the abdomen of a patient suspected of having acute appendicitis. On examination the appendix appears normal, and enlarged mesenteric lymph nodes are noted. Excision of an enlarged lymph node with culture and nodal histology may provide information regarding the etiology but is not routinely used.

DIFFERENTIAL DIAGNOSIS

- Acute appendicitis (5% to 10% of patients admitted to hospitals with a diagnosis of appendicitis are discharged with a diagnosis of mesenteric adenitis)
- Crohn's disease
  Section II describes the differential diagnosis of right lower quadrant abdominal pain.

LABORATORY TESTS

- Complete blood count may show leukocytosis
- Abdominal sonography and helical appendiceal CT scan may be useful
- Laparotomy if appendicitis is suspected

PROGNOSIS

Recurrent bouts are common; therefore if laparotomy is performed and a normal appendix is found, it should be removed.

SUGGESTED READING

available at www.expertconsult.com

AUTHOR: **FRED F. FERRI, M.D.**

TABLE 1-115 Symptoms in Four Outbreaks of Mesenteric Adenitis Caused by *Yersinia* Enterocolitis

Location	Japan (110)	Japan (111)	Japan (111)	United States (112)
Serotype	03	03	03	08
Number ill	198	188	544	38
Percentage with				
Abdominal pain	76	86	64	97
Fever	61	76	50	100
Diarrhea	36	60	32	74
Vomiting	12	4	11	—
Percentage undergoing appendectomy	2	—	—	42

Mandell GL, Bennett JE, Dolin R: *Principles and practice of infectious diseases,* ed 7, Philadelphia, Elsevier, 2010.

TABLE 1-116 Clinical Manifestations of Yersiniosis

Yersinia enterocolitica	*Yersinia pseudotuberculosis*
Gastroenteritis	Mesenteric lymphadenitis
Mesenteric lymphadenitis	Ulcerative ileitis
Ulcerative ileitis	Septicemia
Septicemia	Erythema nodosum
Hepatic or splenic abscesses	
Reactive polyarthritis (HLA-B27)	
Reiter's syndrome	
Erythema nodosum	
Meningitis	
Exudative pharyngitis	

Cohen J, Powderly WG: *Infectious diseases,* ed 2, St Louis, Mosby, 2004.

BASIC INFORMATION

DEFINITION

Acute mesenteric ischemia (AMI) is the sudden onset of intestinal hypoperfusion caused by emboli, arterial or venous thrombosis (Fig. 1-235), or vasoconstriction from low-flow states.

ICD-9CM CODES
ICD-557.1 Mesenteric vascular insufficiency

EPIDEMIOLOGY & DEMOGRAPHICS

INCIDENCE:
- AMI accounts for 0.1% of hospital admissions.
- The incidence appears to be increasing, likely due to increased awareness among clinicians and aging of the population.
- Improved intensive care, and longer survival of sicker patients, has allowed mesenteric ischemia to occur more frequently as a complication of the initial illnesses.

PREDOMINANT SEX AND AGE:
- AMI caused by arterial embolism or thrombosis occurs more frequently in the elderly.
- AMI from mesenteric venous thrombosis often presents in younger age groups.

GENETICS: No specific genetic predisposition but may be related to underlying factors such as cardiac disease, atherosclerosis, and hypercoagulable states.

RISK FACTORS:
- Advanced age, atherosclerosis, low cardiac output (especially atrial fibrillation), severe cardiac valvular disease, intraabdominal malignancy.
- In the subgroup of cases caused by venous thrombosis, risk factors include hypercoagulable states, portal hypertension, abdominal infection, blunt trauma, pancreatitis, and portal malignancy.

- Additional risk factors for AMI caused by non-occlusive mesenteric ischemia include recent cardiac surgery, dialysis, and cocaine use.
- AMI may occur rarely in patients with no identifiable risk factors.

PHYSICAL FINDINGS & CLINICAL PRESENTATION
- The classic presentation is rapid onset of severe periumbilical pain out of proportion to physical examination findings.
- Nausea and vomiting are commonly associated.
- Initial abdominal examination may be normal, with no rebound or guarding, or may include minimal distension or stool positive for occult blood.
- Later in the course the patient may present with gross distension, absence of bowel sounds, and peritoneal signs. In the elderly, mental status changes may occur.

ETIOLOGY
The pathophysiologic mechanisms that cause AMI include:
- Mesenteric arterial embolism: typically from the left atrium, left ventricle, or cardiac valves. The superior mesenteric artery is most commonly affected.
- Mesenteric arterial thrombosis: often in patients with prior progressive atherosclerotic stenoses, with superimposed abdominal trauma or infection.
- Mesenteric venous thrombosis may occur in the setting of hypercoagulable states (acquired or inherited), blunt trauma, abdominal infection, portal hypertension, pancreatitis, and portal malignancy.
- Nonocclusive mesenteric ischemia is caused by reduced intestinal perfusion, such as may be seen in a patient with an acute cardiovascular disease process being treated with drugs that reduce intestinal perfusion, or with use of ergot, cocaine, or amphetamines.

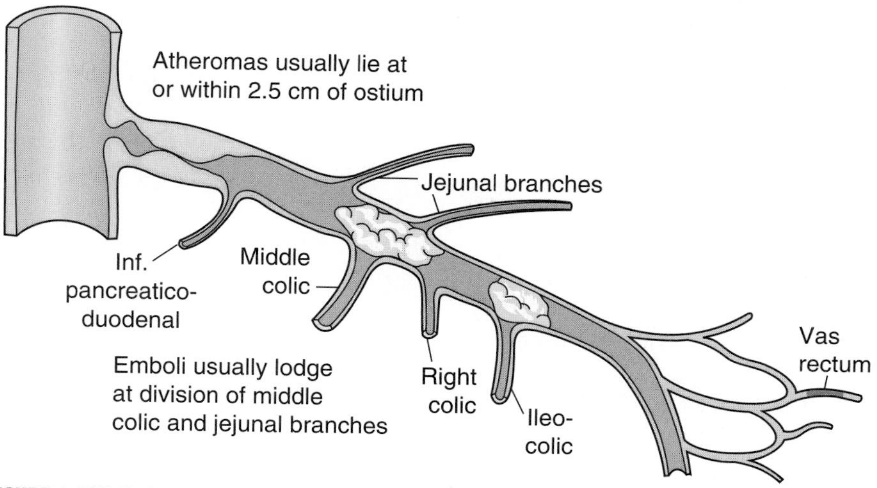

DIAGNOSIS

DIFFERENTIAL DIAGNOSIS
Initially include other causes of abdominal pain of acute onset, including perforated peptic ulcer and early appendicitis. Ultimately, the varied causes of peritonitis.

WORKUP
- Early diagnosis is key. Treatment success is related to the duration of symptoms before diagnosis.
- Consider early laparotomy for diagnosis in cases with a high index of suspicion when angiography is not available.

LABORATORY TESTS
- Laboratory test results are nonspecific, especially early in the course. Later they can include leukocytosis, acidosis, and elevated hematocrit from hemoconcentration. Most abnormalities occur after progression to bowel necrosis.
- When a hypercoagulable state is suspected, workup may include proteins C and S, antithrombin III, and factor V Leiden. This will likely not affect the diagnosis of AMI but may help guide long-term therapy.
- D-dimer testing has been reported to be useful for the early diagnosis of AMI.

IMAGING STUDIES
- The gold standard is mesenteric angiography; however, in practice, this is being replaced by CT angiography, which is noninvasive, more readily available, and similarly sensitive.
- With strong clinical suspicion, workup should proceed directly to angiography without delay for CT scan or other testing. If angiography cannot be done emergently, diagnositic laparotomy should not be delayed.
- Plain films are normal 25% of the time in the early stages. Suggestive findings may include ileus, bowel wall thickening, or intramural gas. Intraluminal barium should not be used as it is rarely helpful in making a positive diagnosis and will interfere with angiographic studies.
- Doppler ultrasound evaluation of intestinal blood flow is often limited by the presence of air-filled loops of bowel and is not an appropriate part of the diagnostic workup if AMI is the leading working diagnosis.
- CT findings also are commonly nonspecific and more often found late in the course. Portal venous gas or intramural gas may be seen after the development of gangrene; in many cases, even at that advanced stage CT findings remain nonspecific. The use of IV contrast material may affect interpretation of subsequent angiography.
- CT scanning has been found to be more useful in cases of mesenteric vein thrombosis causing AMI, with sensitivity approaching 90%. It has also been found useful in monitoring the progress of patients with superior

---

Atheromas usually lie at or within 2.5 cm of ostium

Jejunal branches

Inf. pancreatico-duodenal

Middle colic

Emboli usually lodge at division of middle colic and jejunal branches

Right colic

Ileo-colic

Vas rectum

FIGURE 1-235 Typical location of superior mesenteric artery obstruction in patients with embolic and thrombotic occlusion. (From Donaldson MC: Mesenteric vascular disease. In Braunwald S, Creager MA [eds]: *Atlas of heart diseases*, St Louis, 1996, Mosby, pp. 5-6.)

mesenteric venous thrombosis who are treated nonsurgically.

- Recent studies suggest that multidetector CT angiography may be a useful diagnostic modality.

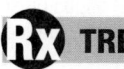 **TREATMENT**

- The goal of treatment is to restore blood flow as rapidly as possible to ischemic bowel before the occurrence of infarction.
- Treatment varies depending on etiology.

ACUTE GENERAL Rx

- Initial management should include hemodynamic monitoring and support, correction of acidosis, administration of broad-spectrum antibiotics, and gastric decompression by nasogastric tube.
- Vasoconstricting agents should be avoided.
- Systemic anticoagulation may be started. Optimal timing of initiation is unclear.

NONPHARMACOLOGIC THERAPY

- Signs of peritonitis mandate early laparotomy and resection of infarcted bowel.
- When workup is positive for major superior mesenteric artery (SMA) embolus, embolectomy is considered standard treatment in the absence of peritoneal signs. Depending on the location and degree of occlusion of the embolus, surgical revascularization, intraarterial infusion of thrombolytics or vasodilators, or systemic anticoagulation may be considered.
- In cases of SMA thrombosis, emergency surgical revascularization is the treatment of choice; stent placement may be a viable alternative.

- Angiography is needed to diagnose nonocclusive mesenteric ischemia before infarct and should be followed up by intraarterial vasodilator infusion. This approach has been shown to significantly reduce mortality rate in this situation.
- In patients with mesenteric vein thrombosis, treatment depends on the presence or absence of peritoneal signs. Laparotomy and resection of infarcted bowel is indicated in more advanced cases. If there are no peritoneal signs, immediate anticoagulant therapy with heparin, and ultimately warfarin, may be adequate treatment.
- Percutaneous treatment with lytic therapy, balloon angioplasty, or stenting may be limited by the frequent presence of nonviable bowel, which would require laparotomy despite success with the percutaneous treatment.

CHRONIC Rx

In the subgroup of patients with mesenteric venous thrombosis, prevention of further thrombosis is indicated. The optimal duration of anticoagulation is unclear.

DISPOSITION

- Prognosis is best in AMI due to mesenteric venous thrombosis and after surgical treatment for acute arterial embolism. It remains poor in cases of arterial thrombosis and nonocclusive ischemia.
- With delayed diagnosis, intestinal infarction—resulting in perforation or gangrenous bowel, sepsis, shock, and death—is typical.

REFERRAL

- Early surgical consultation should be considered. There should be no delay with peritoneal signs.
- If diagnostic angiography is unavailable, surgery may be warranted for diagnostic purposes.

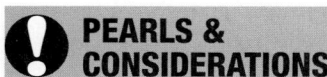 **PEARLS & CONSIDERATIONS**

COMMENTS

- The diagnosis of AMI should be considered in any patient with acute onset of abdominal pain out of proportion to physical findings, particularly in at-risk patients.
- Early diagnosis, before intestinal infarction occurs, is critical and correlates with improved survival rates.
- In a recent case series, the primary location of the ischemic colitis was in the right, transverse, left, and distal colon in 25%, 10%, 33%, and 25% of cases, respectively; 7% were pancolonic.

PREVENTION

Prevention of the underlying factors, most notably atherosclerotic disease

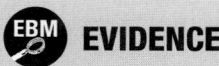 **EVIDENCE**

available at www.expertconsult.com

SUGGESTED READINGS

available at www.expertconsult.com

AUTHOR: **MARGARET TRYFOROS, M.D.**

BASIC INFORMATION

DEFINITION

Mesenteric venous thrombosis (MVT) is a thrombotic occlusion of the mesenteric venous system involving major trunks or smaller branches and leading to intestinal infarction in its acute form.

ICD-9CM CODES
557.0 Mesenteric venous thrombosis

EPIDEMIOLOGY & DEMOGRAPHICS

Between 5% and 15% of patients with acute mesenteric infarction have MVT. MVT is slightly more common in men than women. The typical age of occurrence is 50 to 60 yr.

PHYSICAL FINDINGS & CLINICAL PRESENTATION

Acute MVT:
- Symptoms: abdominal pain in 90% of patients, typically out of proportion to the physical findings. Nausea and vomiting occur in 50% and gastrointestinal (GI) bleeding occurs in 50% (occult) and 15% (gross).
- Physical findings:
  o Early: abdominal tenderness, decreased bowel sounds, abdominal distention
  o Later: guarding and rebound tenderness, fever, septic shock

Subacute MVT:
- Symptoms: nonspecific abdominal pain for weeks or months
- Physical findings: none

Chronic MVT:
- Symptoms: upper GI hemorrhage from bleeding varices
- Physical findings: none other than signs of blood loss if significant

ETIOLOGY & PATHOGENESIS

Hypercoagulable states:
- Peripheral deep venous thrombosis
- Neoplasms
- Antithrombin III, protein C, protein S deficiencies
- Lupus anticoagulant (antiphospholipid antibody)
- Oral contraceptive use, pregnancy
- Polycythemia vera
- Thrombocytosis
- Paroxysmal nocturnal hemoglobinuria

Portal hypertension:
- Cirrhosis

Inflammation:
- Pancreatitis
- Peritonitis (e.g., appendicitis, diverticulitis, perforated viscus)
- Inflammatory bowel disease
- Pelvic or intraabdominal abscess
- Intraabdominal cancer

Postoperative state or trauma:
- Blunt abdominal trauma
- Postoperative states (abdominal surgery)

Thrombosis may begin in small mesenteric branches (e.g., in hypercoagulable states) and propagate to the major venous mesenteric trunks or begin in large veins (e.g., in cirrhosis, intraabdominal cancer, surgery) and extend distally. If collateral drainage is inadequate the intestine becomes congested, edematous, cyanotic, and hemorrhagic and eventually may infarct.

DIAGNOSIS

DIFFERENTIAL DIAGNOSIS

All other causes of abdominal pain (e.g., peritonitis, intestinal obstruction, pancreatitis, peptic ulcer disease, gastritis, inflammatory bowel disease, perforated viscus). Also to be considered in the differential diagnosis of GI hemorrhage.

WORKUP

Laboratory tests and imaging studies

LABORATORY TESTS
- Complete blood count: leukocytosis
- Electrolytes: metabolic acidosis (lactic) indicates bowel infarction
- Elevated amylase
- Tests for hypercoagulable status

IMAGING STUDIES
- Abdominal plain radiograph: ileus, ascites, bowel dilation, bowel wall thickening, loop separation, thumbprinting
- Abdominal CT scan (diagnostic in 90%): bowel wall thickening, venous dilation, venous thrombus
- Arteriography if CT scan is not diagnostic
- Diagnosis occasionally made by laparotomy

TREATMENT

- Anticoagulation or thrombolytic therapy
- Laparotomy if intestinal infarction is suspected
- Short ischemic segment: resection
- Long ischemic segment:
  1. Nonviable: resection or close
  2. Viable: intraarterial papaverine and/or thrombectomy followed by "second look" intervention
- Treatment of chronic MVT is the same as for portal hypertension

PROGNOSIS
- Mortality rate of acute mesenteric venous thrombosis: 20% to 50%
- Recurrence rate: 15% to 25%

SUGGESTED READINGS
available at www.expertconsult.com

AUTHOR: **FRED F. FERRI, M.D.**

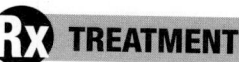

Diseases and Disorders

M

I

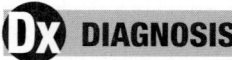

BASIC INFORMATION

DEFINITION

Malignant mesothelioma is a rare neoplastic lesion associated with asbestos exposure. There are three major histologic subtypes: epithelial (most common), sarcomatous, and mixed (epithelial/sarcomatous).

ICD-9CM CODES
199.1 Malignant mesothelioma, site NOS

EPIDEMIOLOGY & DEMOGRAPHICS

- Associated with asbestos exposure (all fiber types)
- More than 3000 new cases diagnosed in the United States annually
- More common in men as a result of asbestos exposure in the workplace
- Right-sided involvement is more common
- Incidence of mesothelioma increases with age; median age at presentation is >60 yr
- More than 8 million persons in the United States are currently at risk for mesothelioma because of prior asbestos exposure

PHYSICAL FINDINGS & CLINICAL PRESENTATION

- Dyspnea
- Nonpleuritic chest pain
- Fever, weight loss, sweats, fatigue, loss of appetite
- Dysphagia, superior vena cava syndrome, Horner's syndrome in advanced stages
- Auscultation may reveal unilateral loss of breath sounds
- Dullness on percussion may be present

ETIOLOGY

- Asbestos exposure
- Other reported potentially causal factors include prior radiation therapy and extravasated Thorotrast, zeolite, and erionite fibers

DIAGNOSIS

DIFFERENTIAL DIAGNOSIS

Metastatic adenocarcinomas (from lung, breast, ovary, kidney, stomach, prostate)

WORKUP

- Staging evaluation includes complete history (including occupational history), physical examination, and testing to determine potential operability (CT, bone scan, pulmonary function tests [PFTs])
- Thoracoscopy, pleuroscopy, and open-lung biopsy are useful in obtaining adequate tissue samples for diagnosis
- Pulmonary function tests
- Staging: the International Union Against Cancer (UICC) staging uses the TNM categories to organize mesothelioma in stages I to IV in a manner similar to that used for non–small cell lung cancer

LABORATORY TESTS

- Diagnostic thoracentesis is generally insufficient for diagnosis because pleural effusions may only reveal atypical mesothelial cells.
- Immunohistochemistry is useful to distinguish adenocarcinoma from epithelial malignant mesothelioma (mesotheliomas are generally carcinoembryonic antigen negative and cytokeratin positive).
- Thrombocytosis and anemia may be found on initial laboratory evaluation.
- Serum osteopontin levels (when available) can be used to distinguish persons with exposure to asbestos who do not have cancer from those with exposure to asbestos who have pleural mesothelioma.

IMAGING STUDIES

- Chest radiographs may reveal pleural plaques (Fig. 1-236) or calcifications in the diaphragm.
- CT scans of the chest and abdomen and bone scan are used to assess the extent of disease.

TREATMENT

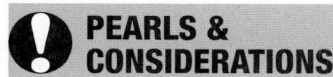

GENERAL Rx

- Operable patient (epithelial type, no positive nodes, confined to pleura, adequate PFTs): the two surgical techniques for therapeutic intervention are decortication (pleurectomy) and extrapleural pneumonectomy. Postoperative chemotherapy with cisplatin, doxorubicin, and cyclophosphamide and subsequent

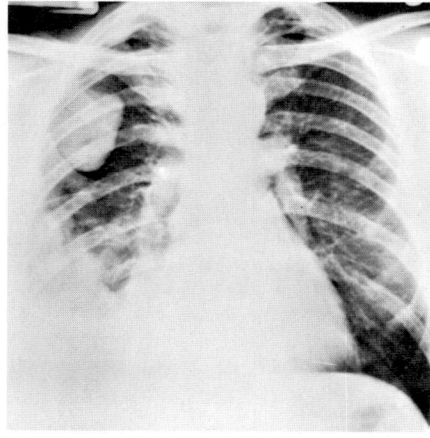

FIGURE 1-236 Chest radiograph of patient with mesothelioma. Note several lobulated, pleural-based masses in right hemithorax accompanied by right pleural effusion. (From Weinberg SE, Cockrill BA, Mandel J: *Principles of pulmonary medicine,* ed 5, Philadelphia, 2008, Saunders.)

external-beam radiation are used in some centers with limited success.
- Inoperable patient (disease too extensive, sarcomatous or mixed histology type, poor PFTs): supportive care with or without radiation therapy for symptoms or supportive care plus chemotherapy. Combined modality therapies (surgery, radiation therapy, chemotherapy, and biologics) have also been used to reduce both local and distant recurrences. The combination of pemetrexed (an antimetabolite that inhibits enzymes involved in folate metabolism) and cisplatin is used for chemotherapy of unresectable malignant pleural mesothelioma.
- Intrapleural instillation of cisplatin or biologics (e.g., interferons, interleukin-2) is generally limited to very early disease because it can only penetrate a very limited depth of the tumor and there is a propensity of the pleural space to become progressively obliterated with advancing disease.
- The role of radiation therapy in the treatment of mesotheliomas remains uncertain. It is often used for palliation of local pain despite lack of trials to prove its utility.
- Obliteration of the pleural space (pleurodesis) with instillation of tetracycline, bleomycin, or biologic substances such as *Cryptosporidium parvum* into the pleural cavity is often attempted in the treatment of recurrent symptomatic pleural effusions.

DISPOSITION

Median survival is from 6.7 to 21 mo for patients undergoing pleurectomy ranges and from 4 to 21 mo for extrapleural pneumonectomy. Survival is better for patients with the epithelial form.

PEARLS & CONSIDERATIONS

COMMENTS

- Patients with early disease should be referred to treatment centers specializing in mesothelioma treatment before attempts are made to obliterate the pleural space with pleurodesis.
- An approach to the evaluation and treatment of mesothelioma is described in Section III, online version.

EVIDENCE

available at www.expertconsult.com

SUGGESTED READINGS
available at www.expertconsult.com

AUTHOR: FRED F. FERRI, M.D.

BASIC INFORMATION

DEFINITION

Hyperglycemia, dyslipidemia, abdominal obesity, and hypertension are critical components of metabolic syndrome. Over the years, many definitions of the syndrome have been proposed and debated. In 2009, a consensus statement from several organizations including the International Diabetes Federation (IDF) and American Heart Association defined "metabolic syndrome" as the presence of any three of the following criteria:

- Abdominal waist circumference >94 cm (37 in) in men and >80 cm (31 in) in women (the use of population- and country-specific definitions are suggested; however, until better data are available, IDF recommends using these cutoffs)
- Serum hypertriglyceridemia ≥150 mg/dl (1.7 mmol/L) or drug treatment for elevated triglycerides
- Serum high-density lipoprotein (HDL) cholesterol <40 mg/dl (1 mmol/L) in men and <50 mg/dl (1.3 mmol/L) in women or drug treatment for low HDL-C
- Blood pressure ≥130/85 mm Hg or drug treatment for elevated blood pressure
- Fasting glucose ≥100 mg/dl (5.6 mmol/L) or drug treatment for elevated blood glucose

SYNONYMS

Syndrome X
Insulin resistance syndrome
Obesity dyslipidemia syndrome

ICD-9CM CODES
277.7 Metabolic syndrome

EPIDEMIOLOGY & DEMOGRAPHICS

- Affects 22% of U.S. adults.
- Prevalence increases with age, affecting more than 40% of individuals >60 yr.
- Increasing prevalence among women especially in the African American and Mexican American populations.
- Weight or body mass index is a major risk factor (5% of normal weight, 22% of overweight, and 60% of obese individuals have the metabolic syndrome).
- Genetic factors account for up to 50% of the variation noted in the development of metabolic syndrome. Other risk factors include low socioeconomic status, lack of physical activity, high carbohydrate diet, no alcohol intake, smoking, and postmenopausal status.

CLINICAL PRESENTATION

- Obesity, hypertension, dyslipidemia, and hyperglycemia as defined.
  - Blood pressure: ≥130/85 mm Hg
  - Abdominal obesity with waist circumference: >94 cm (37 in) in men and >80 cm (31 in) in women
  - Triglycerides: ≥150 mg/dl (1.7 mmol/L)
  - HDL: <40 mg/dl (1 mmol/L) in men and <50 mg/dl (1.3 mmol/L) in women

- High fasting glucose: ≥100 mg/dl (5.6 mmol/L)
- Patients with the metabolic syndrome are at twice the risk of developing cardiovascular disease and have a fivefold increase in risk for type 2 diabetes compared to patients without the syndrome. Other complications include cognitive decline, fatty liver disease, polycystic ovary syndrome, obstructive sleep apnea, and chronic kidney disease.
- Focus history on symptoms of diabetes and its complications, obesity and its complications, coronary artery disease (angina), and polycystic ovary syndrome.
- Complete physical examination, including height, weight, waist circumference, and blood pressure.

ETIOLOGY

- Genetic predisposition and environmental factors associated with obesity lead to the development of metabolic syndrome.
- Abdominal obesity is associated with insulin resistance and hyperinsulinemia.
- Insulin resistance results in ineffective glucose and fatty acid utilization leading to type 2 diabetes mellitus.
- Elevations in inflammatory markers and cytokines (i.e., plasminogen activator inhibitor [PAI]-1, interleukin-6, and C-reactive protein) have been associated with insulin resistance.
- Hyperinsulinemia and cytokines play an important role in development of abnormal lipid profile, hypertension, and vascular endothelial dysfunction, which can lead to the development of atherosclerotic cardiovascular disease.
- Accumulating evidence suggests that the cardiovascular and renal abnormalities associated with insulin resistance are mediated in part by aldosterone acting on the mineralocorticoid receptor.

DIAGNOSIS

DIFFERENTIAL DIAGNOSIS

- Other causes of weight gain or obesity (Cushing's syndrome, hypothyroidism)
- Other causes of hyperlipidemia (familial hyperlipidemia, hypothyroidism)
- Other causes of hypertension (Cushing's syndrome, hyperaldosteronism)
- Other forms of diabetes (type 1)

LABORATORY TESTS

- Fasting lipid profile (total cholesterol, low-density lipoprotein [LDL] cholesterol, HDL cholesterol, and triglyceride)
- Fasting glucose

TREATMENT

NONPHARMACOLOGIC THERAPY

- Lifestyle modification:
  - Dietary modifications aimed at weight loss
  - Physical activity of moderate intensity (i.e., brisk walking): 30 min daily
  - Smoking cessation

- Consider bariatric surgery in the management of obesity:
  - Body mass index (BMI) ≥40 kg/m² in patients who have not responded to diet and exercise (with or without drug therapy).
  - Individuals with BMI >35 kg/m² and comorbidities (hypertension, impaired glucose tolerance, diabetes mellitus, dyslipidemia, sleep apnea) are also potential surgical candidates.

ACUTE GENERAL Rx

- Treat obesity (see "Obesity"): Pharmacologic treatment: consider sibutramine, orlistat, phentermine, and diethylpropion in individuals who have not responded to diet and exercise if BMI >30 kg/m² or a BMI of 27 to 30 kg/m² with comorbid conditions.
- Treat hypertension (see "Hypertension"): Systolic blood pressures >130/80 mm Hg: consider angiotensin-converting enzyme inhibitors or angiotensin II receptor blocker as first-line therapy.
- Treat hyperlipidemia:
  - Serum LDL cholesterol of <100 mg/dl (2.6 mmol/L) is recommended for secondary prevention (i.e., coronary artery disease [CAD] or CAD equivalent such as diabetes); however, recent studies suggest greater benefit with a more aggressive goal of <80 mg/dl (2.1 mmol/L). For primary prevention, an LDL goal <130 mg/dl (3.4 mmol/L) is recommended for individuals with more than two coronary heart disease risk factors. HMG-CoA reductase inhibitors (statins) are commonly used as first-line agents.
  - Patients with high triglycerides (>200 mg/dl) may benefit from fibric acid derivatives to achieve secondary non-HDL cholesterol target (LDL goal + 30).
- Treat diabetes:
  - Goal fasting blood glucose <100 mg/dl
  - Metformin as first-line therapy to improve insulin sensitivity
- Treat cardiovascular risk factors:
  - Consider aspirin.
  - Risk can be lowered with weight loss, exercise, smoking cessation, blood pressure control, diabetes management, and treatment of hyperlipidemia.

CHRONIC Rx

- Encourage lifestyle modification as above.
- Pharmacologic and surgical management to maintain therapeutic goals described above.

DISPOSITION

Weight loss can prevent disease progression. Appropriate treatment of obesity, hypertension, hyperlipidemia, and diabetes can improve morbidity and mortality rates.

REFERRAL

- To nutritionist for diet counseling
- To weight loss and exercise programs
- To endocrinologist if difficulty reaching therapeutic goals

- To bariatric surgeon if meets surgical criteria (as noted previously)

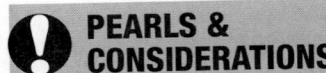

PEARLS & CONSIDERATIONS

PREVENTION

- Weight loss is essential for the prevention and treatment of metabolic syndrome.
- Recommend dietary modifications and moderate physical activity.

- Consider pharmacologic and surgical options in select individuals (as above).

PATIENT & FAMILY EDUCATION

- Weight reduction programs, including Weight Watchers, Curves, etc.
- American Diabetes Association: http://www.diabetes.org
- Polycystic Ovarian Syndrome Association: http://www.pcosupport.org
- The Hormone Foundation: http://www.hormone.org

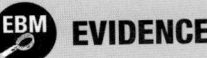 **EVIDENCE**

available at www.expertconsult.com

SUGGESTED READINGS

available at www.expertconsult.com

AUTHORS: **MICHAEL SCHAEFER, M.D.,** and **GEETHA GOPALAKRISHNAN, M.D.**

BASIC INFORMATION

DEFINITION

The diagnosis of metatarsalgia includes multiple etiologies of pain involving the plantar aspect of the lesser metatarsals or metatarsophalangeal joints (Fig. 1-237).

ICD-9CM CODES
726.7 Metatarsalgia

PHYSICAL FINDINGS & CLINICAL PRESENTATION

- Pain beneath any or all of metatarsal heads 2, 3, 4, and 5
- Pain on metatarsophalangeal joint range of motion
- Often associated with hammertoe deformity
- May include predislocation syndrome
- Common with bunion deformity
- Often obesity, recent weight gain, or increased activity

ETIOLOGY

- Primary structural/functional factors: cavus foot, ankle equinus, and pseudoequinus, all yielding increased pressure on the plantar forefoot
- Transferred pressure from hypermobile first or fifth rays
- Friction resulting from compensation to structural/biomechanical factors
- Decreased shock absorption to hammertoe deformity, predislocation syndrome, translocation of the plantar fat pad
- Relative fixed dorsiflexion or plantarflexion of adjacent joints causing increased pressure or joint instability
- Elongated lesser metatarsal(s), exceeding the optimal metatarsal parabola
- Trauma: Rupture of plantar plate, MTPJ capsule, or tendon
- Degenerative joint diseases (OA, RA, psoriatic arthritis, etc.)

DIAGNOSIS

DIFFERENTIAL DIAGNOSIS

- Interdigital neuroma, most commonly third interspace (Morton's)
- Metatarsal traumatic fracture or stress fracture
- Foreign body, infection, gout
- Freiberg's infraction, usually of the second metatarsal head, frequently in teenage females
- Ganglion cyst, bone tumor, rheumatoid nodules
- Skin: Verrucous plantaris, intractable plantar keratoma, tinea pedis, etc.
- Neuropathy or peripheral vascular disease

LABORATORY TESTS

As necessary if suspicion of a systemic cause of joint arthritis/destruction

IMAGING STUDIES

- X-rays: Rule out fracture, tumor, avascular necrosis, arthritic process/joint disease.
- MRI: Will reveal any plantar plate injury, capsular injury, tendon rupture, or neuroma if present. Provides closer look at degenerative processes.

TREATMENT

- Silicone sleeve padding for acute pain, providing pressure and friction relief.
- Moleskin or padding will reduce friction forces.
- Custom orthotics with proximal metatarsal pad or submetatarsal cutout to offload.
- Heel lift or shoes with short heel are especially effective when equinus is etiology.
- Rocker-bottom to prevent motion in severe or high-risk diabetic patients.
- Nonsteroidal anti-inflammatory drugs.
- Intraarticular injection if indicated, based on underlying etiology. Caution with injection: plantar plate ruptures are common in this area!

DISPOSITION

Varies depending on etiology.

REFERRAL

To podiatric or foot/ankle orthopedic surgeon for biomechanical exam/orthotic management and surgical management as needed (not common).

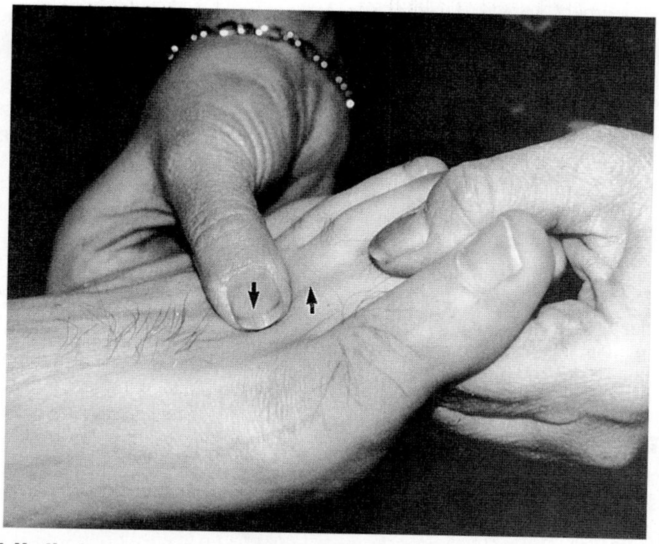

FIGURE 1-237 Vertical stress test for metatarsophalangeal stability. One of the examiner's hands stabilizes the metatarsal head while the other grasps the proximal phalanx. Examiner attempts to displace the proximal phalanx dorsally. A positive test result is the ability to displace dorsally while reproducing symptoms. (From Scuderi G [ed]: *Sports medicine: principles of primary care,* St Louis, 1997, Mosby.)

SUGGESTED READINGS
available at www.expertconsult.com

AUTHOR: **BROOKE E. KEELEY, D.P.M.**

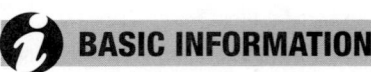

BASIC INFORMATION

DEFINITION

Significant cognitive impairment in the absence of dementia with preserved activities of daily living (ADLs). Mild cognitive impairment (MCI) can also be thought of as an intermediate state between normal cognitive function and dementia.

SYNONYMS

Minimal dementia; isolated short term memory loss; cognitive impairment not dementia (CIND); predementia; dementia prodrome

ICD-9CM CODES
331.83 Mild cognitive impairment, so stated

ICD-10CM CODES
F06.7

EPIDEMIOLOGY & DEMOGRAPHICS

INCIDENCE:
- 12 to 15 cases per 1000 person-yr age ≥65
- 51 to 77 cases per 1000 person-yr age ≥75

PEAK INCIDENCE: In the elderly

PREVALENCE: 15% to 25% in those older than age 70.

PREDOMINANT SEX AND AGE: Male, age ≥75

GENETICS: A*POE4* genotype
- Various pathways result in amyloid accumulation and deposition.

RISK FACTORS: Male sex, age, lower socioeconomic status, lower educational level

CLINICAL PRESENTATION

- Subjective memory problems, preferably corroborated by another person.
- Preserved functional status (ADLs).
- Normal general thinking and reasoning skills.
- Subtypes of MCI include amnestic vs. non-amnestic with involvement of single domain vs. multiple domains.
- Domains affected in MCI include memory, visuospatial skills, language, attention, and executive function.

ETIOLOGY

Neurodegenerative, vascular, traumatic, depression, or due to underlying medical condition

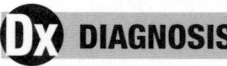 DIAGNOSIS

DIFFERENTIAL DIAGNOSIS

- Delirium
- Dementia
- Depression
- "Reversible" cognitive impairment:
  ○ Medication related (anticholinergics)
  ○ Hypothyroidism
  ○ Vitamin B₁₂ deficiency
- Reversible CNS conditions
  ○ Subdural hematoma
  ○ Normal pressure hydrocephalus
  ○ Metastatic disease

WORKUP

History
- Focus on cognitive deficits and impairment.
- Review all medications that may impact cognition (i.e., anticholinergics).
- Rule out depression and delirium.
- Perform functional assessment.

Physical exam
- Check blood pressure
- Neurologic exam to rule out reversible CNS causes of cognitive impairment

Cognitive function testing:
Brief mental status testing using MMSE (Mini-Mental Status Exam), MOCA (Montreal Cognitive Assessment), or SLUMS (Saint Louis University Mental Status) for office screening followed by neuropsychological testing if appropriate for specific deficits in cognitive domains.

LABORATORY TESTS

- Complete blood count
- Comprehensive metabolic profile
- TSH
- Vitamin B₁₂
- Lipids
- Vitamin D level

IMAGING STUDIES

- CT imaging can detect most reversible CNS conditions leading to cognitive impairment.
- MRI further evaluates vascular, infectious, neoplastic, and inflammatory conditions.

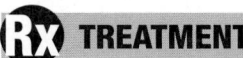 TREATMENT

- There is insufficient evidence to recommend use of Cholinesterase inhibitors (Table 1-117) for MCI.
- Consider treatment with these medications only if memory complaints appear to be affecting day-to-day quality of life in individual patients or in amnestic subtypes of MCI.

NONPHARMACOLOGIC THERAPY

- Role of cognitive rehabilitation to target specific deficits
- Caregiver education and counseling
- Physical and mental exercises to maintain cognition should be recommended

COMPLEMENTARY & ALTERNATIVE MEDICINE

No clear indications for antioxidants, and studies in humans are inconclusive.

DISPOSITION

- Progression to Alzheimer's at the rate of 5% to 15% per year
  ○ Risk factors for progression to dementia include presence of vascular risk factors, significant cognitive impairment, depression, and presence of extrapyramidal signs.
- Mortality of those with MCI is twice that of those without MCI.
- Two- to threefold increase in risk of nursing home placement in those with MCI.

REFERRAL

Consider referral to a memory specialist if more than just memory is involved or for further evaluation of specific deficits.

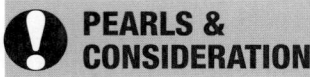 PEARLS & CONSIDERATIONS

COMMENTS

Patients with MCI usually report short-term memory concerns such as misplacing things, not remembering names of people, word-finding difficulties, forgetting day-to-day tasks, not being able to read a book, or not being able to follow a conversation.

MCI becomes clinically relevant when quality of life is affected such as problems making financial decisions and problems with personal day-to-day interactions.

Depression should be ruled out prior to making a diagnosis of MCI since it is highly prevalent in the elderly.

Anticholinergic medication use should be evaluated carefully prior to making a diagnosis of MCI.

PREVENTION

Patients with MCI should be counseled on strategies to prevent progression to dementia. They should remain physically and mentally active, have a well-balanced diet, continue activities that are socially engaging, reduce stress in their lives, and aggressively pursue treatment of vascular risk factors.

PATIENT/FAMILY EDUCATION

Patients with MCI typically have poor retention and rapid loss of newly learned information.

For additional information for patients, families, and clinicians: Alzheimer's Association (www.alzheimers.org)

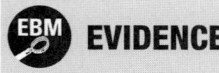 EVIDENCE

available at www.expertconsult.com

SUGGESTED READINGS

available at www.expertconsult.com

AUTHORS: **BIRJU B. PATEL, M.D., F.A.C.P.,** and **N. WILSON HOLLAND, M.D., F.A.C.P.**

TABLE 1-117 Characteristics and Properties of Cholinesterase Inhibitors

Drug Name	Starting Dose	Maintenance Dose	Serum Half-life	Taken with Food?	Elimination
Donepezil	5 mg	10 mg	70 hr	+/−	Hepatic
Rivastigmine pill	1.5 mg bid	6 mg bid	2-8 hr	+	Hepatic
Rivastigmine patch	4.6 mg/24 hr	9.5 mg/24 hr	N/A	N/A	Hepatic
Galantamine	4 mg bid or 8 mg SA daily	12 mg bid or 24 mg SA daily	6-8 hr	+	Hepatic and renal

Adapted from *Physicians' desk reference*, ed 62, Montvale, New Jersey, 2008, Thomson PDR.

Milk-Alkali Syndrome

BASIC INFORMATION

DEFINITION

Milk-alkali syndrome is the consumption of large amounts of calcium and alkali, resulting in the triad of hypercalcemia, metabolic alkalosis, and renal insufficiency.

SYNONYMS

Burnett's syndrome (acute form)
Cope's syndrome (subacute form)

ICD-9CM CODES
275.42 Milk-alkali syndrome

EPIDEMIOLOGY & DEMOGRAPHICS

In the early 20th century the milk-alkali syndrome was associated with an antacid regimen created by F.W. Sippy that included large amounts of calcium and bicarbonate. With the development of more effective and less toxic treatments, the syndrome virtually disappeared. Since the 1980s, however, there has been a small resurgence of hypercalcemia associated with use of calcium-containing products for the prevention of osteoporosis and the use of calcium bicarbonate rather than aluminum bicarbonate in patients with chronic renal failure. The term milk-alkali syndrome has been used for these more modern cases. The milk-alkali syndrome was the third leading cause of hypercalcemia (12%) in a review of hypercalcemia in hospitalized patients from 1990 to 1993.

PHYSICAL FINDINGS & CLINICAL PRESENTATION

- Asymptomatic hypercalcemia:
  - Less than half of cases are detected by an incidental finding of hypercalcemia and occasionally renal failure.
- Symptomatic hypercalcemia:
  - Symptoms: nausea, vomiting, anorexia, fatigue, vague abdominal pain, nephrolithiasis- and pancreatitis-related pain, constipation, myalgia, confusion, and psychosis. In more chronic cases polyuria and polydipsia may be reported.
  - Physical examination and further testing: mental status changes such as anxiety, depression, and cognitive dysfunction; shortened QT interval.

ETIOLOGY

Overconsumption of supplemental calcium bicarbonate with reported ranges of 2.5 to 20 g/day, particularly when associated with volume depletion, renal insufficiency, or use of hydrochlorothiazide or calcium-containing substances.

Betel nut chewing, a practice in Asia and the South Pacific, has been associated with a milk-alkali syndrome. Betel nuts are prepared with a compound that can be converted to calcium carbonate.

DIAGNOSIS

DIFFERENTIAL DIAGNOSIS

Hypercalcemia secondary to hyperparathyroidism or malignancy

LABORATORY TESTS

- Elevated plasma calcium (wide variation reported).
- Renal insufficiency.
- Elevated plasma bicarbonate and arterial pH, metabolic alkalosis.
- Parathyroid hormone, which is usually suppressed with milk-alkali syndrome, may be elevated, particularly if checked after treatment has begun.
- Phosphate level is variable.

TREATMENT

NONPHARMACOLOGIC THERAPY

Hemodialysis has been indicated for some patients with significant renal failure.

ACUTE GENERAL Rx

- Discontinuation of calcium bicarbonate supplements.
- Aggressive hydration and furosemide if symptomatic hypercalcemia.
- Monitor for rebound hypocalcemia as a result of elevation of parathyroid hormone with treatment.
- Patient education regarding appropriate calcium supplementation. Standard over-the-counter calcium supplements and some antacids contain calcium carbonate.

PROGNOSIS

Hypercalcemia and symptoms resolve with withdrawal of excess calcium supplementation and treatment of hypercalcemia. Acute cases typically resolve in 1 to 2 days while chronic cases will take longer. Patients initially presenting with renal failure may have residual renal insufficiency.

DISPOSITION

Treatment is determined by degree of hypercalcemia and symptoms. Hospital admission is required for patients who require IV hydration and other intensive treatments for hypercalcemia.

REFERRAL

Differentiation from hyperparathyroidism can be difficult and may require the assistance of an endocrinologist. Referral to a nutritionist is generally not required because the excess calcium is from nutritional supplements rather than dietary factors.

PEARLS & CONSIDERATIONS

COMMENTS

Detailed history of dietary supplements and over-the-counter medications (see Table 1-118) can provide the most important clues. Many patients do not list dietary supplements as a medication.

SUGGESTED READINGS
available at www.expertconsult.com

AUTHOR: **MICHELLE STOZEK ANVAR, M.D.**

TABLE 1-118 Potential Sources of Alkali

Alkali/Alkali Precursor	Source
Bicarbonate	NaHCO₃: pills, intravenous solutions Proprietary brands, e.g., Alka Seltzer Baking soda KHCO₃: pills, oral solutions
Lactate	Ringer's solution, peritoneal dialysis solutions
Acetate Glutamate Propionate	Parenteral nutrition
Citrate	Blood products, plasma exchange, K⁺ supplements, alkalinizing agents
Calcium compounds (alkalinizing effect minimal when given by mouth) Acetate Citrate Carbonate	Calcium supplements, phosphate binders

Johnson RJ, Feehally J: *Comprehensive clinical nephrology*, ed 2, St Louis, Mosby, 2000.

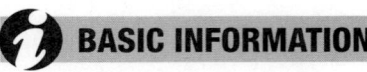

BASIC INFORMATION

DEFINITION
Mitral regurgitation (MR) is retrograde blood flow into the left atrium resulting from an incompetent mitral valve. This condition can lead to left ventricular (LV) failure as well as increased left atrial and pulmonary pressures, with consequent right heart failure.

SYNONYMS
Mitral insufficiency
MR

ICD-9CM CODES
424.0 Mitral regurgitation

EPIDEMIOLOGY & DEMOGRAPHICS
The incidence of MR has increased over the past 30 yr; however, this may be due to increasing availability of echocardiography and MR diagnosis rather than any real increase in the prevalence of this condition.

PHYSICAL FINDINGS & CLINICAL PRESENTATION
- Many patients with mild to moderate MR will remain asymptomatic and without evidence of hemodynamic compromise for years.
- Symptomatic patients with MR generally present with the following:
  - Symptoms suggestive of heart failure (fatigue, dyspnea, orthopnea, paroxysmal nocturnal dyspnea, edema)
  - Hemoptysis (caused by pulmonary hypertension)
  - Atrial fibrillation
- Hyperdynamic apex, sometimes with palpable LV lift and apical thrill.
- Holosystolic, high-pitched, "blowing" murmur at apex with radiation to base, left axilla, or back; there is a poor correlation between the intensity of the systolic murmur and the degree of regurgitation. However, an early diastolic to mid-diastolic rumble (pseudomitral stenosis) suggests severe MR.
- The murmur of acute MR (e.g., from papillary muscle rupture) can be very soft or inaudible.

ETIOLOGY
- Idiopathic myxomatous degeneration of the mitral valve, mitral valve prolapse (most common cause of MR in industrialized countries)
- Papillary muscle dysfunction or rupture (typically as a result of an inferior wall myocardial infarction)
- Ruptured chordae tendineae
- Infective endocarditis
- Calcified mitral valve annulus
- LV dilation (e.g., secondary to dilated cardiomyopathy)
- Rheumatic valvulitis (may be combined with mitral stenosis; common in Third World countries)
- Hypertrophic cardiomyopathy

- Systemic lupus erythematosus (Libman-Sacks endocarditis)
- Fenfluramine, dexfenfluramine, pergolide, cabergoline

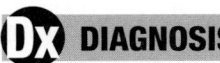

DIAGNOSIS

DIFFERENTIAL DIAGNOSIS
- Hypertrophic cardiomyopathy
- Tricuspid regurgitation
- Aortic stenosis
- Aortic sclerosis
- Ventricular septal defect
- Atrial septal defect

WORKUP
- Diagnostic workup consists of echocardiography, ECG, and chest radiograph; cardiac catheterization sometimes needed to confirm severity of the disease.
- There are data suggesting that in patients with severe asymptomatic MR and normal LV function, elevations of brain natriuretic peptide (BNP) levels (beyond 105 pg/ml) have an independent and additive prognostic value that may identify patients at high risk and aid in the selection of patients for early surgery.

IMAGING STUDIES
- Echocardiography: dilated left atrium, hyperdynamic left ventricle (erratic motion of the leaflet is seen in patients with ruptured chordae tendineae); color flow Doppler will show evidence of MR. The most important aspect of the echocardiographic examination is the quantification of the severity of MR, LV systolic performance, and estimated right ventricular (RV) systolic pressure.
- Chest x-ray:
  - Left atrial enlargement LV enlargement
  - Possible pulmonary congestion, though most often normal
- ECG:
  - Left atrial enlargement
  - LV hypertrophy
  - Atrial fibrillation
- Cardiac catheterization: to confirm severity of MR, or to rule out presence of coronary artery disease in patients being evaluated for surgical replacement

TREATMENT

NONPHARMACOLOGIC THERAPY
Salt restriction

ACUTE GENERAL Rx
- Medical: medical therapy is primarily directed toward treatment of the source or its complications (e.g., atrial fibrillation, ischemic heart disease, infective endocarditis and heart failure).
  - The utility of afterload reduction (to decrease the regurgitant fraction and to increase cardiac output) depends upon the etiology of MR and the administration of afterload reducers. In acute MR, intrave-

nous nitroprusside has shown some utility. Long-term use of oral afterload reducers (e.g., ACE inhibitors or angiotensin receptor blockers [ARBs]) has shown mixed results in small studies but may be given if another indication for their use exists (hypertension, LV dysfunction, diabetes).
  - Control ventricular response only if atrial fibrillation with rapid ventricular response is present.
  - Anticoagulants if atrial fibrillation occurs.
- Surgery: surgery is the only definitive treatment for MR. Transesophageal echocardiography allows accurate assessment of the feasibility of valve repair and is indicated before surgical intervention. The timing of surgical repair varies. In general surgery is indicated (Class I recommendation) in:
  - Acute severe MR
  - Symptomatic patients with severe MR despite optimal medical therapy
  - Asymptomatic patients with severe MR but with evidence of declining LV function (EF <60%) or progressive dilatation (LV at end-systole >40 mm)
  - In addition, surgery is reasonable (Class IIa recommendation) in:
  - Severe MR with new onset atrial fibrillation, even if asymptomatic
  - Asymptomatic severe MR with pulmonary hypertension (≥50 mm Hg at rest or ≥60 mm Hg during exercise)
  - Symptomatic severe MR with severe LV dysfunction or dilatation (LVEF <30% or LV at end-systole >55 mm, respectively) in whom mitral valve repair is likely and the LV dysfunction is not the primary cause for the MR (as opposed to the other way around)
  - Asymptomatic severe MR with preserved LV EF (>60%) and size (<40 mm in end-systole) in whom the likelihood of successful repair without residual MR is >90%
  - Note that the last two criteria above apply to mitral valve repair only, in which the subvalvular apparatus is conserved, as opposed to valve replacement done otherwise
  - Quantitative grading of MR is a powerful predictor of the clinical outcome of asymptomatic MR. In general, patients with regurgitant orifice areas of >40 mm² should be considered for prompt surgery, whereas those with orifices between 20 and 39 mm² can be followed closely

DISPOSITION
Prognosis is generally good unless there is significant impairment of left ventricle or significantly elevated pulmonary artery pressures. Most patients remain asymptomatic for many years (average interval from diagnosis to onset of symptoms is 16 yr).

REFERRAL
Surgical referral in selected patients (see "Acute General Rx"). Emergency surgery is usually necessary in patients with acute MR caused by

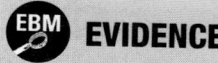

ruptured papillary muscle or chordae tendineae after myocardial infarction.

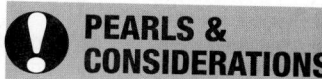

PEARLS & CONSIDERATIONS

COMMENTS

Patients should be counseled regarding weight reduction (if obese), avoidance of tobacco, and maintenance of normal (nonstrenuous) activities.

In 2007, the AHA guidelines for prevention of infectious endocarditis were revised and routine antibiotic prophylaxis to undergo dental or other invasive procedures is no longer recommended, unless the patient has prior endocarditis.

EBM EVIDENCE

available at www.expertconsult.com

SUGGESTED READINGS

available at www.expertconsult.com

AUTHORS: **GABRIEL A. DELGADO, M.D., FRED F. FERRI, M.D.,** and **DAVID J. FORTUNATO, M.D., F.A.C.C.**

M

Diseases and Disorders

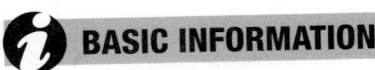

DEFINITION

Mitral stenosis is a narrowing of the mitral valve orifice that prevents proper opening during diastole. The cross-section of a normal orifice measures 4 to 6 cm^2. Symptoms usually develop with exercise when the orifice measures <2.5 cm^2, and symptoms may develop at rest when the orifice is <1.5 cm^2.

SYNONYMS

MS

ICD-9CM CODES
394.0 Mitral stenosis

EPIDEMIOLOGY & DEMOGRAPHICS

- The predominant cause of mitral stenosis is rheumatic heart disease; however, the occurrence of mitral valve stenosis has decreased worldwide over the past 30 yr (particularly in developed countries) as a result of declining incidence of rheumatic fever.
- The incidence of MS is higher in women (2:1 female-to-male ratio).

PHYSICAL FINDINGS & CLINICAL PRESENTATION

- Dyspnea is the most common symptom along with fatigue and decreased exercise capacity. These occur secondary to an inability to increase cardiac output and elevated pulmonary capillary pressures.
- Paroxysmal nocturnal dyspnea (PND) and orthopnea secondary to elevated left atrial pressure may occur.
- Acute pulmonary edema may occur after an increase in flow across the mitral valve secondary to an increase in cardiac output or heart rate (exertion, tachyarrhythmias, fever).
- Pulmonary hypertension can lead to right ventricular (RV) dysfunction and signs and symptoms of right heart failure (hepatomegaly, pulsatile liver, peripheral edema, ascites).
- Hemoptysis can be present secondary to pulmonary capillary vessel rupture or pulmonary vascular congestion.
- Systemic embolic events are caused by left atrial thrombi. These are associated with atrial fibrillation 80% of the time.
- Chest pain can be caused by RV pressure overload and/or concomitant coronary artery disease in up to 15% of patients.
- Irregularly irregular pulse caused by atrial fibrillation.
- Signs of left and subsequently right heart failure.
- Loud first heart sound (S$_1$) caused by delayed valve closure and rapid rising left ventricular (LV) pressure.
- A low pitched, rumbling diastolic murmur heard best at the apex. The intensity of the murmur is not related to the severity of the stenosis, but the duration is holodiastolic in severe MS.
- An opening snap (OS) caused by tensing of the valve leaflets after the cusps have opened completely. The OS follows S$_2$ by 0.03 to 0.14 sec and the shorter the S$_2$-OS interval, the more severe the MS, due to higher left atrial pressures.
- Prominent A wave on the venous pulse of patients in normal sinus rhythm.
- A diastolic thrill may be palpable at the apex, especially with the patient in the left lateral recumbent position.
- An RV lift may be palpable at the left sternal border secondary RV hypertrophy and pulmonary hypertension.
- An accentuated P$_2$ and/or a soft, early diastolic decrescendo murmur (Graham Steell murmur) caused by pulmonary regurgitation may be present in patients with pulmonary hypertension.

ETIOLOGY

- Rheumatic fever (RF) is the predominant cause of MS. RF causes thickening of the leaflet edges, commissure fusion, and chordal shortening and fusion.
- Congenital defect (parachute valve) has the usual two mitral leaflets, but the chordae, instead of diverging to insert into two papillary muscles, converge into one major papillary muscle, which allows little mobility of the leaflets.
- Rare causes are severe mitral annular calcification, endomyocardial fibroelastosis, malignant carcinoid syndrome, systemic lupus erythematosus, Whipple disease, and Fabry disease.

DIFFERENTIAL DIAGNOSIS

- Left atrial myxoma
- Ball valve thrombus
- Other valvular abnormalities (e.g., tricuspid stenosis, mitral regurgitation)
- Atrial septal defect

WORKUP

Physical examination and echocardiography

IMAGING STUDIES

- Echocardiography:
  - Two-dimensional echocardiogram can measure valve area by direct planimetry or calculate it by the Doppler pressure half-time method (this may be inaccurate in patients with concomitant diastolic dysfunction or aortic insufficiency) or the continuity equation. The transmitral gradient can also be calculated.
  - Echocardiography will also show a markedly diminished E-to-F slope of the anterior mitral valve leaflet during diastole; there is also fusion of the commissures, resulting in "doming" of the leaflets during diastole.
  - Grading of leaflet thickness, mobility, calcification and chordal involvement with a score of 0 to 4 for each characteristic can

predict hemodynamic results and outcome of balloon mitral valvuloplasty (a low score of less than 8 is favorable for angioplasty and a high score is unfavorable).
  - Doppler echocardiography can be used to assess for pulmonary hypertension and to give an estimate of the pulmonary artery pressure.
- Chest radiograph:
  - Straightening of the left cardiac border caused by dilated left atrium
  - Left atrial enlargement on lateral chest radiograph
  - Prominence of pulmonary arteries
  - Possible pulmonary congestion and edema (Kerley B lines)
- ECG:
  - RV hypertrophy; right axis deviation caused by pulmonary hypertension
  - Left atrial enlargement (broad, notched P waves)
  - Atrial fibrillation
- Cardiac catheterization:
  - Allows the measurement of pulmonary artery pressure and transmitral pressure gradients at rest or with exercise (supine biking or raising weights with arms while lying supine).
  - Allows the measurement of transmitral flow and calculation of the valve area.
  - Is not routinely recommended for the evaluation of MS but is useful when the echocardiographic findings are nondiagnostic or discrepant with the clinical scenario.

NONPHARMACOLOGIC THERAPY

Decrease level of activity in symptomatic patients and salt restriction if pulmonary congestion is present.

ACUTE GENERAL Rx

- Medical:
  - Antibiotic prophylaxis to prevent recurrent rheumatic fever is usually not indicated unless presence of high-risk features such as prior endocarditis, prosthetic heart valves, valvulopathy of the transplanted heart, and certain cases of cyanotic congenital heart disease.
  - Anticoagulation for the prevention of systemic embolic events in patients with MS and:
    1. Atrial fibrillation
    2. Prior embolic event
    3. Documented left atrial thrombus
    4. Severe left atrial enlargement and spontaneous echo contrast indicating stagnant blood flow (class 2b indication)
  - Ventricular rate control (to increase diastolic filling period) with beta blockers, calcium channel blockers or digitalis and aggressive treatment of tachyarrhythmias.
  - Treat congestive heart failure with diuretics and sodium restriction.

- Table 1-119 summarizes approaches to mechanical relief of mitral stenosis.
- Percutaneous balloon mitral valvotomy (BMV) is the therapy of choice for symptomatic patients with moderate to severe MS (valve area ≤1.5 cm²) with a favorable valve score, minimal or no mitral regurgitation and no left atrial thrombus. Balloon valvotomy is also indicated in asymptomatic patients with moderate to severe MS that has resulted in pulmonary artery pressures of 50 mm Hg at rest or 60 mm Hg with exercise. Percutaneous BMV is also considered the procedure of choice in pregnant women with rheumatic MS and in NYHA class 3 to 4 and/or unresponsive to adequate medical treatment. In addition, it is a reasonable option for patients who are at high risk for surgery even when their valve morphology is not ideal (class 2a indication).
- Surgical intervention is indicated for patients with moderate to severe symptomatic MS when BMV is not available, contraindicated or the valve is calcified and the surgical risk is acceptable. The surgical approaches include closed mitral valvotomy, open valvotomy and repair (preferred) and mitral valve replacement.

DISPOSITION

- Prognosis is generally good except in patients with chronic pulmonary hypertension.

- Operative mortality rates for mitral valve replacement are 1% to 5% at most institutions.

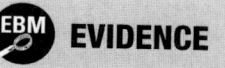 **EVIDENCE**

available at www.expertconsult.com

AUTHORS: **SCOTT COHEN, M.D.,
FRED F. FERRI, M.D.,** and
GAURAV CHOUDHARY, M.D.

M

Diseases
and Disorders

I

TABLE 1-119 Approaches to Mechanical Relief of Mitral Stenosis

Approach	Advantages	Disadvantages
Closed surgical valvotomy	Inexpensive Relatively simple Good hemodynamic results in selected patients Good long-term outcome	No direct visualization of valve Only feasible with flexible, noncalcified valves Contraindicated if MR >2+ Surgical procedure with general anesthesia
Open surgical valvotomy	Visualization of valve allows directed valvotomy Concurrent annuloplasty for MR is feasible	Best results with flexible, noncalcified valves Surgical procedure with general anesthesia
Valve replacement	Feasible in all patients regardless of extent of valve calcification or severity of MR	Surgical procedure with general anesthesia Effect of loss of annular-papillary muscle continuity on LV function Prosthetic valve Chronic anticoagulation
Balloon mitral valvotomy	Percutaneous approach Local anesthesia Good hemodynamic results in selected patients Good long-term outcome	No direct visualization of valve Only feasible with flexible, noncalcified valves Contraindicated if MR >2+

From Otto CM: *Valvular heart disease*, ed 2, Philadelphia, 2004, WB Saunders, p. 296.
LV, Left ventricular; *MR,* mitral regurgitation.

 **BASIC INFORMATION**

DEFINITION

Mitral valve prolapse (MVP) is the bulging of one or both of the mitral valve leaflets into the left atrium during systole. MVP syndrome refers to a constellation of MVP and associated symptoms (e.g., autonomic dysfunction, palpitations) or other physical abnormalities (e.g., pectus excavatum).

SYNONYMS

MVP
Mitral click murmur syndrome
Barlow's syndrome

ICD-9CM CODES
424.0 Mitral valve disorders
394.9 Other and unspecified mitral valve diseases

EPIDEMIOLOGY & DEMOGRAPHICS

- MVP can be found by two-dimensional echocardiogram in 1% to 4% of the general population (females more often than males).
- Increased incidence is seen with autoimmune thyroid disorders, Ehlers-Danlos syndrome, Marfan's syndrome, pseudoxanthoma elasticum, pectus excavatum, anorexia nervosa, and bulimia.
- Compared to men, women with MVP have less posterior prolapse (22% vs. 31%), less flail (2% vs. 8%), more leaflet thickening (32% vs. 28%), and less frequent severe regurgitation (10% vs. 23%).
- Although MVP is more common in women than men, men more often develop severe regurgitation requiring surgical intervention.

PHYSICAL FINDINGS & CLINICAL PRESENTATION

- Usually, young female patient with narrow anteroposterior chest diameter, low body weight, low blood pressure
- Mid to late systolic click, heard best at the apex
- Crescendo mid to late systolic murmur, may have a "honking" quality
- Timing of click within the cardiac cycle varies with loading conditions within the left ventricle (i.e., may occur earlier with standing or Valsalva and later with squatting or expiration)
- Most patients with MVP are asymptomatic; symptoms (if present) consist primarily of chest pain and palpitations
- Neurologic abnormalities (e.g., transient ischemic attack [TIA] or stroke) rare
- Patients may also complain of anxiety, fatigue, and dyspnea

ETIOLOGY

- Myxomatous degeneration of connective tissue within mitral valve
- Congenital deformity of mitral valve and supportive structures
- Secondary to other disorders of connective tissue such as Ehlers-Danlos, Marfan, or pseudoxanthoma elasticum; association with other connective tissue disorders suggests MVP result of defective embryogenesis in cells of mesenchymal origin

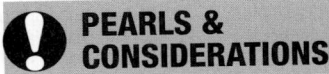 **DIAGNOSIS**

DIFFERENTIAL DIAGNOSIS

- Other valvular abnormalities (especially mitral regurgitation [MR])
- Anxiety/panic disorders
- Pulmonary embolism
- Atypical chest pain

WORKUP

- Medical history and physical examination, with increased suspicion in patients with other findings of connective tissue disorder.
- Workup consists primarily of echocardiography in patients with a systolic click or murmur on careful auscultation.
- ECG is most often normal but may show nonspecific ST-T wave changes, prolonged QT interval or prominent Q waves.

IMAGING STUDIES

Echocardiography shows one or more leaflet prolapsing at least 2 mm into the left atrium during systole. Mitral leaflets may be thickened (>5 mm). MR may or may not be present, and sometimes it is only present during exertion. If moderate or severe MR is present, findings of dilated left atrium, LV dilation and/or dysfunction, and elevated estimated RV systolic pressures may also be present. There is an increased incidence of secundum-type atrial septal defects (ASDs) in patients with MVP, which may also be identified with echocardiography.

Rx **TREATMENT**

NONPHARMACOLOGIC THERAPY

Avoidance of stimulants (e.g., caffeine, nicotine) in patients with palpitations

ACUTE GENERAL Rx

β-blockers may be tried in symptomatic patients (e.g., palpitations, chest pain); they decrease the heart rate and contractility, thus potentially decreasing the stretch on the prolapsing valve leaflets.

CHRONIC Rx

Monitoring for complications:
- Bacterial endocarditis (risk is three to eight times that of the general population)
- TIA or stroke caused by embolic phenomena (from fibrin and platelet thrombi) in patients with thickened leaflets; risk in young patients is <0.05% per year, if present aspirin (75-325 mg) is indicated for secondary prevention
- Cardiac arrhythmias (the vast majority are supraventricular and benign)
- Sudden death (rare occurrence, most often caused by ventricular arrhythmias associated with other structural heart disease)
- MR (most common complication of MVP, on rare occasion may occur acutely due to rupture of chordae tendineae)

DISPOSITION

The incidence of complications of MVP is very low (<1% per year) and generally associated with an increase in mitral leaflet thickness to >5 mm; young patients (age <45 yr) with absence of mitral systolic murmur or MR on Doppler echocardiography are at low risk for any complications.

REFERRAL

Surgical referral may be necessary in patients who develop progressive MR with surgical indications as per guidelines for valvular heart disease (see chapter on MR).

! **PEARLS & CONSIDERATIONS**

COMMENTS

- Recent studies suggest that the prevalence of MVP and its propensity to cause symptoms and serious complications have been overestimated in the past.
- Asymptomatic patients with MVP and mild or no MR can be evaluated clinically every 3 to 5 yr. High-risk patients (those with symptoms, arrhythmias, or significant regurgitation) should undergo a follow-up examination once a year.
- Among patients with severe regurgitation, women have higher mortality and lower surgery rates than men.
- In 2007, the AHA guidelines for prevention of infectious endocarditis were revised and prophylactic antibiotics are no longer recommended for patients with MVP without previous endocarditis.

SUGGESTED READINGS
available at www.expertconsult.com

AUTHORS: **DAVID J. FORTUNATO, M.D., F.A.C.C.,** and **FRED F. FERRI, M.D.**

BASIC INFORMATION

DEFINITION

An overlap syndrome with clinical features seen in systemic lupus erythematous (SLE), polymyositis (PM) and systemic sclerosis (Scl) in association with high titer of anti U1-RNP antibodies, especially to the 70-kD epitope. Not all clinical features are present initially, and it usually takes several years before enough overlapping features are present to be confident that mixed connective tissue disease (MCTD) is the most likely diagnosis. Because of the nonspecific signs and symptoms at presentation, most of the patients may be initially classified as undifferentiated connective tissue disease.

ICD-9CM CODES

710.9 Diffuse connective tissue disease NOS

EPIDEMIOLOGY & DEMOGRAPHICS

PREVALENCE: Variable by population.
PREDOMINANT SEX: Female/male ratio of 15:1
PREDOMINANT AGE: 4 to 80 yr

PHYSICAL FINDINGS & CLINICAL PRESENTATION

- General: malaise, fatigue, fever
- Joints: arthralgias are early symptom that can evolve to arthritis resembling RA but without severe erosions.
- Skin and mucosas: Raynaud's phenomenon is an early finding. Malar rash, discoid plaques, oral or genital ulcers, sicca symptoms, subcutaneous nodules, abnormal nail fold capillaries can be seen.

- Muscle: myalgias, inflammatory myopathy
- Lung: interstitial lung disease leading to pulmonary fibrosis
- Heart: pulmonary hypertension, pericarditis
- Hematopoetic: anemia of chronic disease, lymphopenia, thrombocytopenia
- Gastrointestinal tract: altered motility, mesenteric vasculitis, pancreatitis, hepatitis
- Kidney: membranous glomerulonephritis, diffuse proliferative glomerulonephritis
- Nervous system: trigeminal neuropathy, headache, aseptic meningitis

ETIOLOGY

Autoimmune disorder

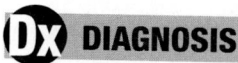

DIAGNOSIS

DIFFERENTIAL DIAGNOSIS

Other connective tissue disorders (SLE, progressive systemic sclerosis, polymyositis)

WORKUP (Table 1-120)

Alarcon-Segovia: Serologic criterion accompanied by three or more clinical criteria, one of which must be synovitis or myositis (sensitivity 81.3%, specificity 86.2%).
Kahn: Serologic criterion accompanied by Raynaud's phenomenon and at least two of the three remaining clinical criteria.

LABORATORY TESTS

- Positive Antinuclear antibody (ANA) speckled pattern >1:1000 to 1:10,000.
- U1-RNP antibodies especially to the 70-kD antigen (high titers).

- Antibodies to double-stranded DNA, Sm, Ro, and La (transient).
- Rheumatoid factor positive (50% to 70%).

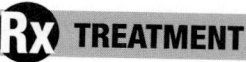

TREATMENT

- Considered to be a steroid-responsive disease
- Aimed at the specific features of the overlap syndrome
- Arthralgias, arthritis, fatigue, myalgias usually respond to NSAIDs, antimalarials, and/or steroids. Immunosuppressive medications such as methotrexate and azathioprine can also be used
- Keeping warm, avoiding beta blockers, stop smoking and dyhydropiridine calcium channel blockers can be used for Raynaud's
- Pulmonary hypertension: Therapies include steroids, cyclophosphamide, low-dose aspirin, anticoagulation, ACE inhibitors, endothelin receptor antagonist, IV prostacyclin, sildenafil

DISPOSITION

- Patients with high titers of U1-RNP antibodies have low prevalence of serious renal disease and life-threatening neurologic disorders.
- Disease-related mortality is usually related to pulmonary hypertension and its cardiac sequelae.

REFERRAL

Rheumatology consultation for clarification and assistance in treatment

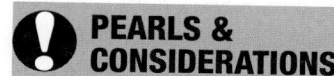

PEARLS & CONSIDERATIONS

COMMENTS

A clinical algorithm for evaluation of a positive ANA titer is described in Section III, "Antinuclear Antibody Testing."

SUGGESTED READINGS

available at www.expertconsult.com

AUTHOR: **DANIEL E. MENDEZ-ALLWOOD, M.D.**

TABLE 1-120 Diagnostic Criteria by Alarcon-Segovia and Kahn

	Alarcon-Segovia Criteria	Kahn Criteria
Serology	Anti-RNP at hemagglutination titer of ≥1:1600	High-titer anti-RNP corresponding to a speckled ANA of ≥1:1200
Clinical	Swollen hands Synovitis Myositis Raynaud's phenomenon Acrosclerosis	Swollen fingers Synovitis Myositis Raynaud's phenomenon

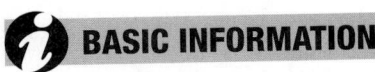

BASIC INFORMATION

DEFINITION

Molar pregnancy is a premalignant gestational disorder. Molar pregnancies are classified as complete or partial based on morphologic and pathologic examination. Both complete and partial molar pregnancies have an abnormal placenta with enlargement and swelling of the chorionic villi and hyperplasia of the villous trophoblastic cells. Most molar pregnancies are complete and are characterized by generalized hydropic villous changes with no fetal tissue. Partial moles are characterized by a mixture of large hydropic villi and normal placental tissue and often have fetal tissue present. The risk of malignant sequelae (gestational trophoblastic neoplasia) for a complete mole is 18% to 29% and for a partial mole is 0% to 11%.

SYNONYMS

Hydatidiform mole
Gestational trophoblastic disease

ICD-9-CM CODES
630 Hydatidiform mole

EPIDEMIOLOGY & DEMOGRAPHICS

INCIDENCE: 0.57 to 2/1000 pregnancies with wide regional variation
PREDOMINANT SEX AND AGE: Females of reproductive age, highest rates at extremes of reproductive ages
RISK FACTORS: Extremes of reproductive age (<21 and >40 yr), previous molar pregnancy, history of spontaneous abortion

PHYSICAL FINDINGS & CLINICAL PRESENTATION

Complete molar pregnancy:
- 80% to 90% present with vaginal bleeding at 6 to 16 wk gestational age
- 28% with uterine enlargement greater than expected for gestational age
- 8% with hyperemesis gravidarum
- 1% with gestational hypertension in the first or second trimester
- 15% with bilateral theca lutein cysts
- 15% will have a beta hCG >100,000

Partial molar pregnancy
- 90% present with an incomplete or missed abortion
- 75% present with vaginal bleeding
- <10% will have a beta hCG of >100,000

ETIOLOGY

Complete molar pregnancy
- Fertilization of an oocyte with absent or inactive maternal chromosomes and duplication of paternal chromosomes (90% are 46, XX) or fertilization of an empty oocyte with 2 sperm (46, XY or XX)
- Uniform villous enlargement and no development of a fetus

Partial molar pregnancy
- Fertilization of a normal oocyte with 2 sperm (usually 69, XXY)
- Focal villous edema with identifiable fetus

DIAGNOSIS

DIFFERENTIAL DIAGNOSIS

Complete mole, partial mole, ectopic pregnancy, abortion (incomplete or spontaneous), normal intrauterine pregnancy

WORKUP

- Pelvic exam to evaluate for uterine size and bleeding
- Blood pressure to assess for gestational hypertension or preeclampsia (systolic blood pressure >140 or diastolic blood pressure >90)

LABORATORY TESTS

- Quantitative beta human chorionic growth hormone (beta hCG), significantly elevated levels >100,000 will raise suspicion for molar pregnancy
- Complete blood count (CBC) to assess for acute anemia from vaginal bleeding
- Comprehensive metabolic panel to evaluate for renal or liver disease
- TSH to evaluate for hyperthyroidism
- Urinalysis for proteinuria to evaluate for preeclampsia
- Type and screen to evaluate Rh and to prepare for surgery

IMAGING STUDIES

- Pelvic ultrasound
  - Complete molar pregnancy will show diffuse vesicular changes with no evidence of fetal tissue and may show theca lutein cysts
  - Partial molar pregnancy will show focal cystic changes in the placenta and fetal tissue may be present
- Baseline chest x-ray to use for comparison if malignant trophoblastic disease develops

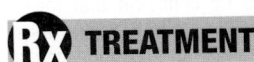 TREATMENT

NONPHARMACOLOGIC THERAPY

Surgical uterine evacuation with dilation and curettage (D&C)

ACUTE GENERAL Rx

D&C, Rh immune globulin if Rh negative

CHRONIC Rx and Disposition

If pathology results are consistent with complete or partial mole, patients must be followed to evaluate for trophoblastic neoplasia. 15% to 20% of complete moles and 1% to 5% of partial moles will develop into trophoblastic neoplasia. Quantitative beta hCG should be followed weekly until three consecutive results show normal levels. After that, check quantitative beta hCG every 3 mo for a total of 6 mo. Patients should remain on reliable contraception during this time to prevent confusion from a rising beta hCG in the case of a new pregnancy.

REFERRAL

- If there is concern for a molar pregnancy, the patient should be managed by a gynecologist for uterine evacuation and follow-up.
- If there is a plateau or rise of the beta hCG during follow-up, the patient should be referred to a gynecologic oncologist for treatment with chemotherapy.

SUGGESTED READINGS
available at www.expertconsult.com

AUTHOR: **LAUREN ROTH, M.D.**

BASIC INFORMATION

DEFINITION

Viral infection characterized by discrete skin lesions with central umbilication (Fig. 1-238).

ICD-9CM CODES
078.0 Molluscum contagiosum

EPIDEMIOLOGY & DEMOGRAPHICS

- Molluscum contagiosum spreads by autoinoculation, scratching, or touching a lesion.
- It usually occurs in young children. It is also common in sexually active adults and patients with HIV infection.
- Incubation period varies between 4 and 8 wk.
- Spontaneous resolution in immunocompetent patients can occur after several months.

PHYSICAL FINDINGS & CLINICAL PRESENTATION

- The individual lesion appears initially as a flesh-colored, firm, smooth-surfaced papule with subsequent central umbilication. Lesions are frequently grouped. The size of each lesion generally varies from 2 to 6 mm in diameter.
- Typical distribution in children involves the face, extremities, and trunk. Mucous membranes are spared.
- Distribution in adults generally involves pubic and genital areas.

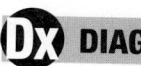

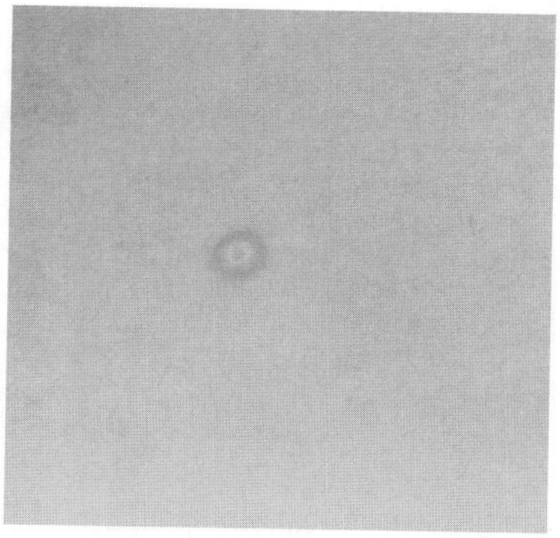

FIGURE 1-238 Molluscum contagiosum. (From Rakel RE: *Textbook of family practice,* ed 6, Philadelphia, 2002, WB Saunders.)

- Erythema and scaling at the periphery of the lesions may be present as a result of scratching or hypersensitivity reaction.
- Lesions are not present on the palms and soles.

ETIOLOGY

Viral infection of epithelial cells caused by a pox virus

DIAGNOSIS

Diagnosis is usually established by the clinical appearance of the lesions (distribution and central umbilication). A magnifying lens can be used to observe the central umbilication. If necessary, the diagnosis can be confirmed by removing a typical lesion with a curette and examining the content on a slide after adding potassium hydroxide and gentle heating. Staining with toluidine blue will identify viral inclusions.

DIFFERENTIAL DIAGNOSIS

- Verruca plana (flat warts): no central umbilication, not dome shaped, irregular surface, can involve palms and soles
- Herpes simplex: lesions become rapidly umbilicated
- Varicella: blisters and vesicles are present
- Folliculitis: no central umbilication, presence of hair piercing the pustule or papule
- Cutaneous cryptococcosis in AIDS patients: budding yeasts will be present on cytologic examination of the lesions
- Basal cell carcinoma: multiple lesions are absent

WORKUP

Careful examination of the papules

LABORATORY TESTS

Generally not indicated in children. Screening for other sexually transmitted diseases is recommended in all cases of genital molluscum contagiosum.

TREATMENT

GENERAL THERAPY

- Therapy is individualized depending on number of lesions, immune status, and patient's age and preference.
- Observation for spontaneous resolution is reasonable in patients with few, small, nonir-

ritated, and nonspreading lesions. Genital lesions should be treated in all sexually active patients.
- Liquid nitrogen cryotherapy.
- Carbon dioxide laser.
- Curettage after pretreatment of the area with combination prilocaine 2.5% with lidocaine 2.5% cream (EMLA) for anesthesia is useful for treatment of a few lesions. Curettage should be avoided in cosmetically sensitive areas because scarring may develop.
- Treatments with liquid nitrogen therapy in combination with curettage are effective in older patients who do not object to some discomfort.
- Application of cantharidin 0.7% to individual lesions covered with clear tape will result in blistering over 24 hr and possible clearing without scarring. This medication should be avoided on facial lesions.
- Other treatment measures include use of imiquimod cream or tretinoin 0.025% gel or 0.1% cream at bedtime, daily use of salicylic acid (Occlusal) at bedtime, and use of laser therapy.
- Trichloroacetic acid peel generally repeated every 2 wk for several weeks is useful in immunocompromised patients with extensive lesions.

DISPOSITION

Most patients respond well to the therapeutic modalities listed previously. Spontaneous resolution can occur after 6 to 9 mo in some immunocompetent patients.

REFERRAL

To dermatology when diagnosis is in doubt or in patients with extensive lesions

PEARLS & CONSIDERATIONS

COMMENTS

Genital molluscum contagiosum in children may be indicative of sexual abuse.

EVIDENCE

available at www.expertconsult.com

AUTHOR: FRED F. FERRI, M.D.

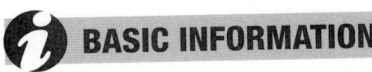

BASIC INFORMATION

DEFINITION

Mononucleosis is a symptomatic infection caused by Epstein-Barr virus (EBV) characterized by fever, tonsillar pharyngitis, and lymphadenopathy.

SYNONYMS

Infectious mononucleosis (IM)

ICD-9CM CODES
075 Infectious mononucleosis

EPIDEMIOLOGY & DEMOGRAPHICS

INCIDENCE (IN U.S.): 500 cases/100,000 persons/yr
PREDOMINANT SEX: Incidence is the same, but occurs earlier in females.
PREDOMINANT AGE: Most common between the ages of 15 and 24 yr.

PHYSICAL FINDINGS & CLINICAL PRESENTATION

- Following an incubation period of 1 to 2 mo, a prodrome may occur, with fever, chills, malaise, and anorexia for several days. This is followed by the classic triad, which includes pharyngitis, fever, and adenopathy. Although fatigue and malaise may be prominent, pharyngitis is usually the most severe symptom. Exudates are common.
- Lymphadenopathy is most prominent in the cervical region but may be diffuse.
- Splenomegaly may occur, most commonly during the second wk of illness.
- Rash is uncommon but will occur in nearly all patients who receive ampicillin.
- At times, IM can present as fever and adenopathy without pharyngitis. Although complications may be severe, they are uncommon and tend to resolve completely. Involvement of the hematologic, pulmonary, cardiac, or nervous system may occur; splenic rupture is rare. IM is usually a self-limited illness, but symptoms of malaise and fatigue may last months before resolving.

ETIOLOGY

The cause of IM is primary infection with EBV. Primary infection during childhood causes few or no symptoms. Infection during childhood is more common in lower socioeconomic groups. The frequency of IM in late adolescence is attributed to the onset of social contact between the sexes.

Close personal contact is usually necessary for transmission. Transfer via saliva while kissing may be responsible for many cases. Virus can persist in oropharynx of patients with IM for up to 18 mo. Transmission may also occur sexually as EBV can be isolated in cervical epithelial cells and male seminal fluid and can also be transmitted by blood transfusion.

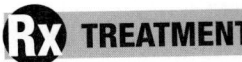

DIAGNOSIS

DIFFERENTIAL DIAGNOSIS

- Heterophile-negative infectious mononucleosis caused by cytomegalovirus (CMV); although clinical presentation may be similar, CMV more frequently follows transfusion
- Bacterial and viral causes of pharyngitis
- Toxoplasmosis
- Acute retroviral syndrome of HIV, lymphoma

WORKUP

Heterophile antibody (monospot) and CBC should be sent.

LABORATORY TESTS

- Increased WBC is common, with a relative lymphocytosis and neutropenia. Atypical lymphocytes are the hallmark of IM, but are not pathognomonic. Mild thrombocytopenia is common. A falling hematocrit may signal splenic rupture or severe immune-mediated hemolytic anemia. Elevated hepatocellular enzymes and cryoglobulins occur in most cases. Heterophile antibody, as measured by the Monospot test, may be positive at presentation, or may appear later in the course of illness. A negative test should be repeated if clinical suspicion is high. If this test remains negative for 8 wk, other causes of IM are likely. The monospot usually remains positive for 3 to 6 mo, but can last for 1 yr.
- A positive test has been reported with primary HIV infection.
- In addition to the heterophile antibody, virus-specific antibodies may result in response to IM. Determination of these EBV-specific antibodies is rarely necessary to diagnose IM, although early diagnosis in monospot negative cases may be made by isolating IgM to the viral capsid antigen (VCA), which is usually positive during the acute illness.

IMAGING STUDIES

Chest radiograph may rarely show infiltrates. An elevated left hemidiaphragm may occur in cases of splenic rupture.

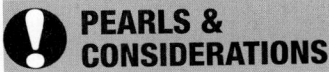

TREATMENT

NONPHARMACOLOGIC THERAPY

- Supportive rest is advocated by some, but effect on outcome is not clear
- Splenectomy if rupture occurs; transfusions for severe anemia or thrombocytopenia

ACUTE GENERAL Rx

- Pharmacologic therapy is not indicated in uncomplicated illness.
- The use of steroids is suggested in patients who have severe thrombocytopenia or hemolytic anemia, or impending airway obstruction as a result of enlarged tonsils. Prednisone, 60 to 80 mg PO qid for 3 days, then tapered over 1 to 2 wk. There is no role for antiviral agents such as acyclovir in the management of IM.

CHRONIC Rx

A rare, chronic form of IM with persistent organ infection and inflammation has been described. This should not be confused with chronic fatigue syndrome, which is unrelated to EBV.

DISPOSITION

Eventual resolution of all symptoms is the rule.

REFERRAL

More than mild illness

PEARLS & CONSIDERATIONS

COMMENTS

- Contact sports should be avoided during the first mo of illness, because splenic rupture can occur, even in the absence of clinically detectable splenomegaly.
- A total of 30% to 75% of college freshmen are seronegative for EBV. Each year nearly 20% of susceptible persons becomes infected and up to 50% of these persons develops infectious mononucleosis.

SUGGESTED READINGS
available at www.expertconsult.com

AUTHORS: **GLENN G. FORT, M.D., M.P.H.,** and **DENNIS J. MIKOLICH, M.D.**

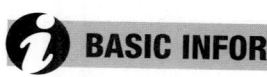 **BASIC INFORMATION**

DEFINITION

Morton's neuroma refers to an inflammatory fibrosing process of the plantar digital nerve characterized by pain in the sole of the foot. Morton's neuroma is also described as an interdigital plantar neuropathy with or without plantar neuroma.

SYNONYMS

Morton metatarsalgia
Morton toe
Interdigital neuroma

ICD-9CM CODES
355.6 Morton's neuroma

EPIDEMIOLOGY & DEMOGRAPHICS

- Morton's neuroma most commonly involves the plantar digital nerve between the heads of the third and fourth metatarsals.
- May also involve the second and third metatarsal and can involve both simultaneously.
- Commonly occurs in people wearing tight-fitting shoes in toe region and high heels.
- Morton's neuroma is usually unilateral.
- Morton's neuroma is found more often in women than in men.
- Morton's neuroma can occur in both young and old.

PHYSICAL FINDINGS & CLINICAL PRESENTATION

- Pain is usually located in a specific region, usually in the sole of the foot between the third and fourth metatarsal area, and is unilateral in the majority of cases.
- Numbness may occur.
- Pain is exacerbated with exercise and relieved with rest and may radiate to the toes and to the ankle.
- Point tenderness is noted on examination, and palpation reveals fullness at the site of discomfort.
- An audible, painful click called *Murder's click* is noted in patients with Morton's neuroma after compressing and releasing the forefoot.
- Patients may have neuroma but silent lesions without symptoms.

ETIOLOGY

- Morton's neuroma is thought to be caused by nerve thickening from repeated injury.
- The typical finding is swelling of the plantar digital nerve that pathologically resembles

other nerve entrapment syndromes (e.g., median nerve compression in carpal tunnel syndrome).

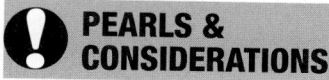 **DIAGNOSIS**

The diagnosis of Morton's neuroma is strictly made on clinical grounds alone because there are no laboratory tests or x-ray imaging studies that are specific for this disorder.

DIFFERENTIAL DIAGNOSIS

- Diabetic neuropathy
- Alcoholic neuropathy
- Nutritional neuropathy
- Toxic neuropathy
- Osteoarthritis
- Trauma (e.g., fracture)
- Gouty arthritis
- Rheumatoid arthritis

WORKUP

Exclude other causes as mentioned in the "Differential Diagnosis" section.

LABORATORY TESTS

- Laboratory studies are not specific for the diagnosis of Morton's neuroma.
- CBC and ESR are usually normal.
- Blood glucose.
- B_{12} and folic acid level.

IMAGING STUDIES

- X-ray imaging is primarily done to exclude other causes of foot pain (e.g., fractures, osteoarthritis, or gouty arthritis).
- MRI can detect and localize a neuroma but is rarely needed to make the diagnosis. An MRI can also be performed in patients with recurrent pain after surgical excision of a Morton's neuroma.
- Ultrasound imaging is also being used to locate Morton's neuroma but is rarely needed to make the diagnosis.

TREATMENT

NONPHARMACOLOGIC THERAPY

- Changing the type of footwear is the first line of treatment.
- Use open footwear and custom shoe inserts and avoid weight-bearing activities.
- A metatarsal pad with arch support is helpful.
- Participate in ultrasound therapy.

ACUTE GENERAL Rx

- If conservative measures are unsuccessful, injection of the intermetatarsal bursa with hydrocortisone may help. Ultrasound–guided injections of ethyl alcohol plus bupivaine have also been reported effective for Morton's neuroma
- Nonsteroidal anti-inflammatory agents (e.g., ibuprofen 400 to 800 mg PO tid or naproxen 250 to 500 mg bid)

CHRONIC Rx

- If nonpharmacologic and acute treatments do not give sufficient relief, surgical excision of the nerve has been successful in 95% of the cases.
- Surgery can be performed in the physician's office using local anesthesia.
- Numbness in the area where the nerve was excised is a common postoperative finding.

DISPOSITION

- Postoperative patients return to their normal activities in 3 to 6 wk.
- In cases in which pain persists after surgery a "stump neuroma" may be present.
- Approximately 80% of patients who fail to have relief with the initial surgery do find relief with a second procedure.

REFERRAL

If surgery is being considered, a consultation with either a podiatrist or an orthopedic surgeon is indicated.

PEARLS & CONSIDERATIONS

COMMENTS

- Dr. Thomas G. Morton is given credit for describing this disorder in 1876.
- Morton's neuroma occurs just before the nerve bifurcates at the metatarsal area to innervate sides of two adjacent toes.
- A recent Cochrane analysis of treatment options for Morton's neuroma found insufficient evidence to support any treatment other than surgical excision for refractory cases.

SUGGESTED READINGS
available at www.expertconsult.com

AUTHORS: **GLENN G. FORT, M.D., M.P.H.,** and **DENNIS J. MIKOLICH, M.D.**

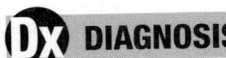 **BASIC INFORMATION**

DEFINITION

Clinical syndrome associated with motion or perception of motion. Patients with motion sickness suffer perspiration, nausea, vomiting, increased salivation, and generalized malaise in response to movement.

SYNONYMS

Physiologic vertigo

ICD-9CM CODES
994.6 Motion sickness

EPIDEMIOLOGY & DEMOGRAPHICS

INCIDENCE (IN U.S.): Common
PEAK INCIDENCE: Any age
PREVALENCE (IN U.S.): Common
PREDOMINANT SEX: Male = female
PREDOMINANT AGE: Any age
GENETICS: Not known to be genetic

PHYSICAL FINDINGS & CLINICAL PRESENTATION

- Vomiting
- Sweating
- Pallor

ETIOLOGY

- Motion (e.g., amusement rides, rides in automobiles or planes)
- Exacerbated by anxiety, fumes (e.g., industrial pollutants), visual stimuli

 DIAGNOSIS

DIFFERENTIAL DIAGNOSIS

- Acute labyrinthitis
- Gastroenteritis
- Metabolic disorders
- Viral syndrome

WORKUP

None necessary in routine case

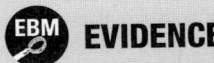 **TREATMENT**

NONPHARMACOLOGIC THERAPY

- Fixate on far object
- Cease motion
- Avoid reading
- Avoid alcohol

ACUTE GENERAL Rx

- Scopolamine patch is most effective. It should be applied to a hairless area behind the ear every 3 days prn. It should be applied >4 hr before antiemetic effect is required.
- Over-the-counter oral preparations (e.g., Dramamine) are less effective.
- Meclizine 12.5 to 25 mg q6h may be effective.

CHRONIC Rx

- Rarely chronic
- Symptoms generally resolve completely with cessation of motion exposure

DISPOSITION

Follow-up is not needed.

REFERRAL

If another diagnosis is suspected (e.g., purulent ear, fever, cranial nerve abnormalities)

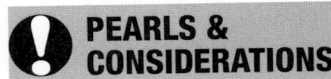 **PEARLS & CONSIDERATIONS**

COMMENTS

- Many patients with migraine report having severe motion sickness as a child.
- Improved ventilation, avoidance of large meals before travel, semirecumbent sitting, and avoidance of reading while in motion will minimize the risk of motion sickness.

EBM EVIDENCE

available at www.expertconsult.com

SUGGESTED READINGS
available at www.expertconsult.com

AUTHOR: **FRED F. FERRI, M.D.**

BASIC INFORMATION

DEFINITION

Mucormycosis is a fungal infection by *Zygomycetes fungi* and includes species in the order Mucorales (*Rhizopus* sp., *Rhizomucor, Cunninghamella, Apophysomyces, Saksenaea, Asbsidia, Syncephalastrum, Cokeromyces, Mortierella*) and in the order Entomophthorales (*Conidiobolus* and *Basidiobolus*).

ICD-9CM CODES
117.7 Mucormycosis

EPIDEMIOLOGY & DEMOGRAPHICS

- These fungi are ubiquitous in nature and can be found in soil and decaying vegetation. Infection is seen in association with underlying conditions, including diabetes mellitus especially with ketoacidosis, hematologic malignancies, stem cell or solid organ transplants, severe burns or trauma, treatment with deferoxamine or iron overload states, steroid treatment, immunodeficiency states (e.g., AIDS), injection drug use, and malnutrition. Immunocompetent hosts may become infected in tropical climates.
- The fungus gains entry to the body most commonly through the respiratory tract. The spores are deposited in the nasal turbinates and may be inhaled into the pulmonary alveoli. In cases of cutaneous mucormycosis, the spores are introduced directly into the skin lesion.

PHYSICAL FINDINGS & CLINICAL PRESENTATION

- Rhinocerebral-rhinoorbital-paranasal syndrome may present with fever, facial and orbital pain, headache, diplopia, loss of vision, facial or orbital cellulitis, facial anesthesia, cranial nerve dysfunction, black nasal discharge, epistaxis, and seizure. Physical findings in this situation include proptosis; chemosis; nasal, palatal, or pharyngeal necrotic ulcerations; and retinal infarction. Thrombosis of the cavernous sinus or internal carotid artery may occur. This form of mucormycosis is found most commonly in diabetics, primarily in the presence of acidosis, and in patients with leukemia and neutropenia.
- Pulmonary mucormycosis can present with pneumonia, lung abscess, pulmonary infarction, pleurisy, pleural effusion, hemoptysis, chills, and fever. This form of mucormycosis is found most commonly in immunocompromised neutropenic hosts after chemotherapy for hematologic malignancies.
- Gastrointestinal zygomycosis presents with abdominal pain, diarrhea, gastrointestinal hemorrhage, ulcers, peritonitis, and bowel infarction. This form of mucormycosis is found most commonly in patients with extreme malnutrition and is believed to arise from ingestion of spores of the fungi.
- Cutaneous zygomycosis presents as nodular lesions (hematogenous seeding) or a wound infection. It primarily involves the epidermis and dermis after use of occlusive dressings that have not been properly sterilized.
- Cardiac mucormycosis is a form of endocarditis.
- Septic arthritis and osteomyelitis.
- Brain abscess occurs most often from extension of the fungus from the nose or paranasal sinuses through adjacent bones in severely debilitated patients.
- Disseminated zygomycosis (rare but uniformly fatal).
- Physical findings depend on the location of the infection.

ETIOLOGY & PATHOGENESIS

The cause of mucormycosis is infection by a fungus of the *Zygomycetes* class (see "Definition"). Normal host defenses include leukocytes and pulmonary macrophages. Quantitative (e.g., neutropenia) or qualitative (e.g., diabetes mellitus or steroid treatment) disruption in the host defenses predisposes the patient to infection.

DIAGNOSIS

The hallmark of mucormycosis is infarction and necrosis of host tissues that result from invasion of the vasculature by the fungal elements. Black eschars and discharges should be closely evaluated. Diagnosis depends on the demonstration of the organism in the tissue of a biopsy specimen.

DIFFERENTIAL DIAGNOSIS

- Infection of the sites described previously by other organisms (bacterial [including tuberculosis and leprosy], viral, fungal, or protozoan)
- Noninfectious tissue necrosis (e.g., neoplasia, vasculitis, degenerative) of the sites described previously

WORKUP

- Biopsy of infected tissue with direct-light microscopy examination establishes the diagnosis within minutes of the biopsy in the case of nasopharyngeal infection. Fungal hyphae are broad (5- to 15-micron diameter) and irregularly branched and have rare septations, in contrast to molds such as *Aspergillus,* which are narrower, have regular branching, and have many septations.
- Bronchoalveolar lavage or bronchoscopy with biopsy for smear, culture, and histologic examination.
- Radiographs and other imaging studies such as CT of symptomatic sites may be required before infection is suspected and tissue specimens are obtained.

TREATMENT

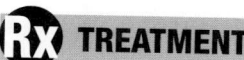

Aggressive correction of underlying disease (e.g., hyperglycemia, high steroid doses, use of immunosuppressive drugs) should be undertaken.

Standard therapy for invasive mucormycosis is treatment with amphotericin B given IV at a daily dose of 1.0 to 1.5 mg/kg infused over 2 to 4 hr for a total of 1 to 4 g. Adverse reactions may be managed as follows:

- Fever, chills, headache, myalgias, nausea, and vomiting: premedicate with aspirin (650 mg PO), acetaminophen (650 mg PO), diphenhydramine (25 to 50 mg IV), hydrocortisone (25 to 100 mg IV), or meperidine (25 to 50 mg IV).
- Hypokalemia and hypomagnesemia are treated with potassium and magnesium replacement.
- Nephrotoxicity and renal tubular acidosis can be mitigated to some extent with 500 ml of NS infusion 30 min before and after each dose of amphotericin. Amphotericin dose reduction may also be necessary.
- Renal function and electrolytes should be monitored twice a week during the entire course of amphotericin.
- Lipid preparations of amphotericin B are now used by many clinicians as they are less toxic (e.g., amphotericin B lipid complex (Abelcet), and liposomal amphotericin B (AmBisome) at a dose of 5 mg/kg daily). Higher doses up to 10 mg/kg have also been used.
- Other antifungals do not appear to be effective except possibly posaconazole, which may serve as step down therapy after amphotericin B and caspofungin, which may be beneficial in combination therapy with amphotericin B.
- Surgical debridement or radical resection of necrotic tissue is required.
- The role of colony-stimulating factors remains unclear, beyond that of increasing the neutrophil count in patients with neutropenia.

PROGNOSIS

- Sinus infection with no underlying disease: 75% survival.
- Sinus infection with diabetes: 60% survival.
- Sinus infection with renal disease: 25% survival.
- Surgery may increase survival by 5% to 20%.
- Early diagnosis improves survival as well as control of the underlying condition.

SUGGESTED READINGS

available at www.expertconsult.com

AUTHORS: **GLENN G. FORT, M.D., M.P.H.,** and **DENNIS J. MIKOLICH, M.D.**

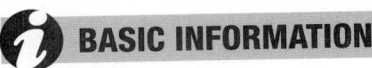

BASIC INFORMATION

DEFINITION

Multifocal atrial tachycardia (MAT) is a supraventricular, moderately rapid arrhythmia (rate 100 to 140 beats/min) with P waves having at least three or more different morphologies and irregular P-P intervals. An isoelectric baseline further differentiates MAT from atrial fibrillation or atrial flutter.

SYNONYMS

Chaotic atrial rhythm
The term *wandering pacemaker* is used for a similar arrhythmia associated with a normal or slow heart rate.

ICD-9CM CODES
427.89 Multifocal atrial tachycardia

EPIDEMIOLOGY & DEMOGRAPHICS

Estimated prevalence in hospitalized patients of 0.05% to 0.32%. Average age is 70s. Usually associated with underlying pulmonary disease. COPD is present in approximately 55% of patients with MAT.

PHYSICAL FINDINGS & CLINICAL PRESENTATION

Symptoms:
- Palpitation
- Lightheadedness
- Syncope
- Symptoms of the underlying pulmonary disease
- Physical findings associated with the underlying pulmonary disease

ETIOLOGY

- Exact mechanism unknown
- Associated abnormalities include pulmonary disease, cardiac disease, hypoxia, hypercarbia, acidosis, electrolyte disturbances, digitalis toxicity

DIAGNOSIS

DIFFERENTIAL DIAGNOSIS

- Atrial fibrillation
- Atrial flutter
- Sinus tachycardia
- Paroxysmal atrial tachycardia
- Extrasystole

WORKUP

- ECG (Fig. 1-239)
- Chest x-ray
- Pulmonary function tests
- Electrolytes
- Arterial blood gases
- Digoxin level (if patient on digoxin)

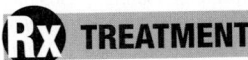

TREATMENT

- Improve the pulmonary or metabolic dysfunction if possible
- Electrolyte repletion, especially magnesium and potassium
- Calcium channel blockers
- β-blockers if not contraindicated by obstructive lung disease or acute heart failure
- If the arrhythmia is asymptomatic, it can be left untreated
- Direct current cardioversion is ineffective

SUGGESTED READINGS
available at www.expertconsult.com

AUTHORS: **ALEXANDER G. TRUESDELL, M.D., FRED F. FERRI, M.D.,** and **WEN-CHIH WU, M.D.**

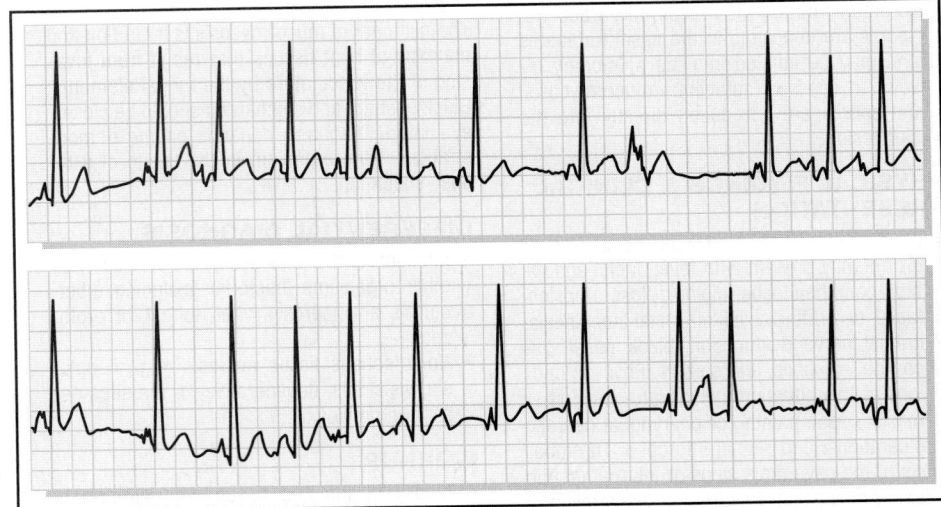

FIGURE 1-239 Chaotic (multifocal) atrial tachycardia. Premature atrial complexes occur at varying cycle lengths and with differing contours. (Zipes DP, Libby P, Bonow RO, Braunwald E (eds): *Braunwald's heart disease,* ed 7, Philadelphia, 2005, Elsevier.)

BASIC INFORMATION

DEFINITION

Multiple myeloma is a malignancy of plasma cells characterized by overproduction of intact monoclonal immunoglobulin or free monoclonal kappa or lambda chains. Diagnostic criteria require the following:
1. Presence of ≥10% plasma cells on examination of the bone marrow (or biopsy of a tissue with monoclonal plasma cells).
2. Monoclonal protein in the serum or urine. Occasional patients without detectable monoclonal protein are considered to have nonsecretory myeloma.
3. Evidence of end-organ damage (*c*alcium elevation, *r*enal insufficiency, *a*nemia, or *b*one lesions [CRAB]).

ICD-9CM CODES
203.0 Multiple myeloma

EPIDEMIOLOGY & DEMOGRAPHICS

ANNUAL INCIDENCE: Five cases/100,000 persons (blacks affected twice as frequently as whites, males more than females); multiple myeloma accounts for 10% of all hematologic cancers. It is the most common primary bone malignancy. There are 16,000 new cases diagnosed annually in the United States.
PREDOMINANT AGE: Peak incidence is in the seventh decade at a median age of 69 yr.

PHYSICAL FINDINGS & CLINICAL PRESENTATION

The patient usually comes to medical attention because of one or more of the following:
- Bone pain (58%) (back, thorax) or pathologic fractures (30%) caused by osteolytic lesions
- Fatigue (32%) or weakness because of anemia from bone marrow infiltration with plasma cells
- Recurrent infections as a result of impaired neutrophil function and deficiency of normal immunoglobulins
- Nausea and vomiting caused by constipation and uremia
- Delirium resulting from hypercalcemia
- Neurologic complications, such as spinal cord or nerve root compression, blurred vision from hyperviscosity
- Pallor and generalized weakness from anemia
- Purpura, epistaxis from thrombocytopenia
- Evidence of infections from impaired immune system
- Paresthesias (5%), weight loss (24%)
- Swelling on ribs, vertebrae, and other bones

DIAGNOSIS

DIFFERENTIAL DIAGNOSIS

- Metastatic carcinoma
- Lymphoma (B-cell NHL)
- Bone neoplasms (e.g., sarcoma)
- Monoclonal gammopathy of undetermined significance
- Primary amyloidosis
- Chronic lymphocytic leukemia
- Waldenström's macroglobulinemia

LABORATORY TESTS

- Normochromic, normocytic anemia; rouleaux formation on peripheral smear.
- Hypercalcemia is present in 15% of patients at diagnosis.
- Elevated blood urea nitrogen, creatinine, uric acid, and total protein.
- Proteinuria from overproduction and secretion of free monoclonal kappa or lambda chains (Bence Jones protein).
- Tall homogeneous monoclonal spike (M spike) on protein immunoelectrophoresis in approximately 75% of patients (Fig. 1-240); decreased levels of normal immunoglobulins (Ig).
  1. The increased immunoglobulins are generally IgG (75%) and IgA (15%).
  2. Approximately 17% of patients have a flat level of immunoglobulins but increased light chains in the urine by electrophoresis.
  3. A small percentage (<2%) of patients have nonsecreting myeloma (no increase in immunoglobulins and no light chains in the urine) but have other evidence of the disease (e.g., positive bone marrow examination).
- Reduced ion gap from the positive charge of the M proteins and the frequent presence of hyponatremia in myeloma patients.
- Hyponatremia, serum hyperviscosity (more common with production of IgA).
- Bone marrow examination: usually demonstrates nests or sheets of plasma cells, which comprise >30% of the bone marrow; ≥10% are immature.
- Serum beta-2 microglobulin has little diagnostic value; it is useful for prognosis because levels >8 mg/L indicate high tumor mass and aggressive disease.

- Elevated serum levels of lactate dehydrogenase at the time of diagnosis define a subgroup of myeloma patients with very poor prognosis.
- Increased interleukin-6 in serum during active stage of myeloma.
- The production of DKK1, an inhibitor of osteoblast differentiation, by myeloma cells is associated with the presence of lytic bone lesions in patients with multiple myeloma.
- Nearly all patients with myeloma present with abnormal chromosomes identified by fluorescence in situ hybridization (FISH). The Mayo Clinic Stratification of Myeloma, for purposes of therapy, identifies high-risk patients (<25% of patients at diagnosis) as those who have any of the following: FISH deletion 17p, FISH translocation 4;14, FISH translocation 14;16, cytogenetic deletion 13q, cytogenetic hypodiploidy, or plasma cell labeling index ≥3%.

IMAGING STUDIES

Radiograph films of painful areas may demonstrate punched-out lytic lesions or osteoporosis (Fig. 1-240). MRI is the preferred technique for suspected spinal compression or soft tissue plasmacytomas. Bone scans are not useful because lesions are not blastic. PET and CT scans are emerging as useful tools.

STAGING

Table 1-121 describes a multiple myeloma staging system

TREATMENT

NONPHARMACOLOGIC THERAPY

Prevention of renal failure with adequate hydration and avoidance of nephrotoxic agents and dye contrast studies

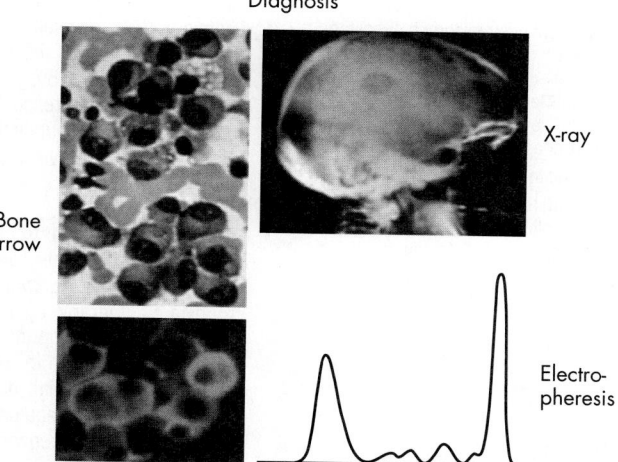

Diagnosis

Bone marrow

X-ray

Electrophoresis

FIGURE 1-240 Common diagnostic features in multiple myeloma. Light chain-restricted plasma cells in a bone marrow aspirate; multiple lytic lesions in a skull radiograph; large monoclonal spike in the γ-globulin area in serum electrophoresis. (From Hoffmann R et al: *Hematology, basic principles and practice,* ed 5, Philadelphia, 2009, Churchill Livingstone.)

ACUTE GENERAL Rx

- Newly diagnosed patients with good performance status are best treated with autologous stem cell transplantation.
  1. Autologous transplantation is recommended for patients with stage II or III myeloma and good performance status.
  2. Induction therapy before stem cell harvest is administered in four cycles. It includes dexamethasone alone or thalidomide-dexamethasone (Thal-Dex).
  3. High-dose chemotherapy (HDCT) with vincristine, melphalan, cyclophosphamide, and prednisone (VMCP) alternating with vincristine, carmustine, doxorubicin, and prednisone (BVAP) combined with bone marrow transplantation improves the response rate, event-free survival, and overall survival in patients with myeloma. Current HDCT regimen with autologous stem cell support achieves complete response in approximately 20% to 30% of patients, with the best results seen in good-risk patients, defined as young patients (<50 yr) with good performance status and a low tumor burden (beta-2 microglobulin ≤2.5 mg/L).
- Induction therapy in patients ineligible for transplantation (old age, coexisting conditions, poor physical conditions) includes the following chemotherapeutic agents:
  1. Thalidomide in combination with melphalan and prednisone.
  2. Melphalan and prednisone: the rates of response to this treatment range from 40% to 60%. Adding continuous low-dose inter-

feron to standard melphalan-prednisone therapy does not improve response rate or survival; however, response duration and plateau phase duration are prolonged by maintenance therapy with interferon.
  3. Vincristine, doxorubicin, and dexamethasone (VAD) can be used in patients not responding or relapsing after treatment with melphalan and prednisone; methylprednisolone is substituted for dexamethasone (VAMP) in some centers.

- Therapy for relapsed and refractory myeloma:
  1. If the relapse occurs more than 6 mo after conventional therapy is stopped, the initial chemotherapy regimen can be reinstituted.
  2. Consider autologous stem cell transplantation as salvage therapy in patients who had stem cells cryopreserved early in the course of the disease.
  3. Chemotherapy with vincristine, doxorubicin, and dexamethasone.
  4. Thalidomide, an agent with antiangiogenic properties, is also useful to induce responses in patients with multiple myeloma refractory to chemotherapy. Lenalidomide (CC-5013) is an active analogue of thalidomide developed to overcome the toxic effects of thalidomide.
  5. Bortezomib is a protease inhibitor that is cytotoxic for multiple myeloma. It is indicated for treatment of refractory multiple myeloma. It is superior to high-dose dexamethasone for treatment of patients who have had relapse. Bortezomib plus melphalan-prednisone has also been reported to be superior to melphalan plus prednisone alone as initial therapy for patients with myeloma who are not candidates for hematopoietic stem cell transplantation.

- ~15% of patients with newly diagnosed multiple myeloma are recognized incidentally and present without significant symptoms (smoldering myeloma). The rate of progression of smoldering myeloma to symptomatic disease is 10% per year for the initial 5 yr, decreasing to 5% for the next 5 yr, and decreasing further to 1.5% per year thereafter. Observation alone is reasonable in these patients because no survival advantage has been demonstrated by treating them.

CHRONIC Rx

- Promptly diagnose and treat infections. Common bacterial agents are *Streptococcus pneumoniae* and *Haemophilus influenzae*. Prophylactic therapy against *Pneumocystis jirovecii* with trimethoprim sulfamethoxazole must be considered in patients receiving chemotherapy and high-dose corticosteroid regimens. Vaccinate against *S. pneumoniae*, influenza, and *H. influenzae*.

- Control hypercalcemia with IV fluids and corticosteroids. Monthly infusions of the bisphosphonate pamidronate provide significant protection against skeletal complications and improve the quality of life of patients with advanced multiple myeloma. Zoledronic acid (Zometa) at doses of 2 mg and 4 mg in patients with osteolytic lesions has been shown to be as effective as pamidronate in terms of reducing the need for radiation to bone, increasing bone mineral density, and decreasing bone resorption. It can be infused over 15 min for treatment of hypercalcemia of malignancy. Bisphosphonates (pamidronate, zoledronate, and ibandronate) also appear to have an antitumor effect.
- Control pain with analgesics; radiation therapy to treat painful bone lesions or cord compression. Surgical stabilization of pathologic fractures. Consider vertebroplasty or kyphoplasty for selected vertebral lesions.
- Treat anemia with erythropoietin.
- Aggressive treatment of reversible causes of renal failure such as dehydration, hypercalcemia, and hyperuricemia.

DISPOSITION

- The median length of survival after diagnosis is 3 yr. Prognosis is better in asymptomatic patients with indolent or smoldering myeloma. Median survival time is approximately 10 yr in persons with no lytic bone lesions and a serum myeloma protein concentration <3 g/dl. Adverse outcome is associated with increased levels of beta-2 microglobulin, low levels of serum albumin, circulating plasma cells, plasmablastic features in bone marrow, increased plasma cell labeling index, complete deletion of chromosome 13 or its long arm, t (4;14) or t (14;16) translocation, and increased density of bone marrow microvessels.
- Compared with a single autologous stem cell transplantation, double transplantation (two successive autologous stem cell transplantations) improves survival among patients with myeloma, especially those who do not have a very good partial response after undergoing one transplantation.
- Recent trials reveal that among patients with newly diagnosed myeloma, survival in recipients of a hematopoietic stem cell autograft followed by a stem cell allograft from an HLA-identical sibling is superior to that in recipients of tandem stem cell autografts.

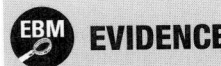

EBM EVIDENCE

available at www.expertconsult.com

SUGGESTED READINGS

available at www.expertconsult.com

AUTHOR: **FRED F. FERRI, M.D.**

Stage	Criteria

I	All of the following:
	1. Hemoglobin >10 g/dL
	2. Serum calcium <12 mg/dL
	3. Normal bone radiograph or solitary lesion
	4. Low M-component production
	  a. IgG level <5 g/dL
	  b. IgA level <3 g/dL
	  c. Urine light chain <4 g/24 hr

II	Fitting neither I nor III

III	One or more of the following:
	1. Hemoglobin <8.5 g/dL
	2. Serum calcium >12 mg/dL
	3. Advanced lytic bone lesions
	4. High M-component production
	  a. IgG level >7 g/dL
	  b. IgA level >5 g/dL
	  c. Urine light chains >12 g/24 hr

TABLE 1-121 Myeloma Staging System

Subclassification:
  A Serum creatinine <2 mg/dl.
  B Serum creatinine <2 mg/dl.

BASIC INFORMATION

DEFINITION

Multiple sclerosis (MS) is a chronic autoimmune demyelinating disease of the central nervous system (CNS) characterized by clinical attacks correlated with lesions separated in time and space. A clinical attack or relapse is the sub-acute onset of neurologic dysfunction that lasts for a minimum of 24 hr.

Subtypes include:
- Relapsing-remitting MS (RRMS) (most common): relapses followed by complete or near-complete recovery, 50% to 85% of which later transition to secondary progressive MS
- Secondary progressive MS (SPMS): progression of disability with few or no relapses
- Primary progressive MS (PPMS) (<5%): progression from the onset
- Progressive relapsing MS (PRMS): seen in 10% to 15%

Rare MS variants include:
- Neuromyelitis optica (NMO; Devic's disease): Recurrent relapses limited to optic nerves and spinal cord.
- Marburg's disease (malignant MS): MRI reveals a tumorlike lesion with significant edema in one cerebral hemisphere. Pathology shows severe inflammation with necrosis. Typically acute onset with a fulminant course, leading to coma or death.
- Balo's concentric sclerosis: Neuroimaging and pathology show alternating rings of myelination and demyelination. Typically more fulminant progression than classic MS.
- Schilder's diffuse sclerosis: Childhood onset with one to two large symmetric lesions.
- Relapsing optic neuritis.

SYNONYMS

MS
Disseminated sclerosis

ICD-9CM CODES
340 Multiple sclerosis

EPIDEMIOLOGY & DEMOGRAPHICS

PEAK INCIDENCE: 20 to 40 yr in two thirds of patients; remaining cases of MS usually before age 20 yr (0.3% to 0.4% occur in first decade). Overall mean age of onset is 37.5 yr

PREVALENCE: MS is more common in people raised in northern latitudes and in certain genetic clusters. Prevalence per 10^5 varies from 6 to 14 in southern United States and southern Europe to 30 to 80 in Canada, northern United States and northern Europe; 16 to 30 in Middle Eastern Arabs and 30 to 38 in Israeli Jews; and less than 10 in Asia, Central America, and most of Africa.

PREDOMINANT SEX & AGE: Female/male ratio is 2 to 3:1. MS is most commonly a disease of young adults.

GENETICS: Frequency of MS in dizygotic twins and siblings is 3% to 5% and 20% to 40% in monozygotic twins. Most common associations include human leukocyte antigen classes I and II (DRB1*1501, DQA1*0102, DQB1*0602), (DRB1*0405-DQA1*0301-DQB1*0302 in Mediterranean population), T-cell receptor-beta, CTLA4, and ICAM1.

PHYSICAL FINDINGS & CLINICAL PRESENTATION

- Common: both vague and nonspecific complaints such as fatigue, blurred vision, diplopia, vertigo, falls, hemiparesis, paraparesis, monoparesis, numbness, paresthesias, ataxia, cognitive deficits, depression, sexual dysfunction, and urinary dysfunction
- Visual abnormalities: horizontal nystagmus, visual field defects, Marcus Gunn pupil (i.e., relative afferent papillary defect—normal direct and consensual light reflexes; however, when swinging flashlight from one eye to the other, direct light causes dilatation of pupil of affected eye), internuclear ophthalmoplegia (paresis of the adducting eye on conjugate lateral gaze with horizontal nystagmus of the abducting eye)
- Corticospinal tract(s) involvement: leads to upper motor neuron signs such as spasticity, hyperreflexia, clonus, extensor plantar responses, and UMN pattern of weakness (shoulder abduction, elbow, hand and finger extension, hip and knee flexion, foot dorsiflexion)
- Sensory loss: numbness, and tingling may or may not follow anatomic distribution, dermatomal loss of pain and temperature, loss of vibration (common) and position sense, and a thoracic band of sensory loss
- Ataxia: intention tremor, heel-to-shin ataxia, inability to tandem gait
- Bladder dysfunction: detrusor hyperreflexia (urge incontinence), flaccidity (neurogenic bladder), and dyssynergia (bladder contracts against a closed sphincter)
- Lhermitte's sign: flexion of the neck elicits an electrical sensation extending down the spine and occasionally into the extremities
- Uhthoff's phenomenon: transient worsening of preexisting symptoms with small increases in body temperature

ETIOLOGY

The precise etiology of MS is uncertain. There is evidence that autoimmunity (autoreactive T and B cells) plays an important role. It is believed that an interaction between multiple genes influencing the immune system and environmental factors [such as certain viruses (e.g., Epstein-Barr virus and human herpes virus 6), low vitamin D level, smoking, and sun exposure] are important factors.

DX DIAGNOSIS

- MS: based on revised 2005 McDonald criteria (Table 1-122)
- RRMS: at least two relapses—two clinical lesions distinctly separated in space and time or one clinical lesion plus paraclinical testing (Table 1-122)
- PPMS: insidious progression of disability with a positive CSF and either dissemination in both space and time or ongoing progression for at least 1 yr

DIFFERENTIAL DIAGNOSIS

- Autoimmune: acute disseminated encephalomyelitis (ADEM), postvaccination encephalomyelitis
- Degenerative: subacute combined degeneration of the cord (B_{12} deficiency), amyotrophic lateral sclerosis
- Infections: Lyme's disease, neurosyphilis, HIV, tropical spastic paraparesis, progressive multifocal leukoencephalopathy, Whipple's disease
- Inflammatory: systemic lupus erythematosus, vasculitis, sarcoidosis, Sjögren's disease, Behçet's disease, celiac disease
- Inherited metabolic disorders: leukodystrophies
- Mitochondrial: Leber's hereditary optic neuropathy, mitochondrial encephalopathy lactic acidosis and strokelike episodes (MELAS)
- Neoplasms: CNS lymphoma, metastases
- Vascular: subcortical infarcts, Binswanger's disease

TABLE 1-122 Summary of Revised 2005 McDonald Criteria for Diagnosis of MS

Clinical Attacks	Clinical Lesions	Paraclinical Testing Needed
2	2	None
2	1	MRI dissemination in space or two lesions on MRI consistent with MS plus positive CSF
1	2	MRI dissemination in time
1	1	MRI dissemination in space or two MRI lesions consistent with MS and positive CSF, and MRI dissemination in time

Evidence of clinical lesions by physical examination or evoked potentials.
CSF, Cerebrospinal fluid; MRI, magnetic resonance imaging; MRI dissemination in space, at least three of the following: (1) one enhancing lesion or nine T2 hyperintense lesions, (2) one infratentorial lesion, (3) one juxtacortical lesion, and (4) three periventricular lesions. Note: One spinal cord lesion may be substituted for one brain lesion; MRI dissemination in time, a new enhancing at least 3 mo or a new nonenhancing lesion at least 6 mo after the initial attack; MS, multiple sclerosis; positive CSF, positive oligoclonal bands or elevated immunoglobulin G index.
Modified from Degenhardt A: Ferri's clinical advisor, ed 11, St Louis, 2011, Elsevier, p. 700.

WORKUP

- Lumbar puncture for all first-time relapses and all cases in which the diagnosis of MS is not definite. Typical CSF abnormalities include increased protein (less than 100 mg/dl), mild elevation of mononuclear white blood cells and increased Ig G synthesis rate. An elevated CSF immunoglobulin (Ig) G index and positive oligoclonal bands are seen in 70% and 90%, respectively, of clinically definite MS. (Serum MS profile needs to be sent to lab simultaneously with CSF MS profile.) False-positive results with IgG index and rarely with positive OCBs (at least two CSF OCBs with polyclonal or negative serum) can be seen in CNS infections (SSPE, neurosyphilis), inflammation (vasculitis), and CNS lymphoma. CSF myelin basic protein is typically elevated following an acute exacerbation.
- Serum: complete blood count (CBC), erythrocyte sedimentation rate, CHEM 7, liver function tests (LFTs), antinuclear antibody, vitamin B_{12}.
- Consider: anti–SS-A antibody, anti–SS-B antibody, neuromyelitis optica IgG antibody, Lyme titer, angiotensin-converting enzyme, TSH, free T_4, anti–thyroglobulin antibody, very-long-chain fatty acids, arylsulfatase A, and possibly heavy metal screen (urine) in select cases.
- Consider evoked potentials (visual, somatosensory and brainstem auditory evoked response). Demyelination causes slow conduction velocities. Visual evoked potentials reveal prolongation of P100.

IMAGING STUDIES

Head imaging (CT or MRI) is strongly recommended. MRI of the head with gadolinium is the most sensitive (Fig. 1-241). MRI of the cervical spine can be helpful. MRI helps to assess disease load, acute lesions, and atrophy.

A normal MRI of the brain does not conclusively exclude MS.

Rx TREATMENT

NONPHARMACOLOGIC THERAPY

Patient education regarding disease characteristics, treatment options, and prognosis. Advise patient to schedule intermittent rest periods on a daily basis and avoid exposure to heat as much as possible. Provide encouragement regarding improved quality of life with new disease modifying drug options.

Recommend physical therapy for spasticity/disability.

ACUTE GENERAL Rx

Relapses: high-dose IV methylprednisolone (3 to 5 days of 1 g/day; alternative dose is 15 mg/kg/day), often followed by a 7- to 10-day prednisone taper. There is no evidence to suggest that high dose corticosteroids alter the long term course of disease.

If marked acute disability and acute corticosteroid therapy has failed, plasma exchange (5 to 7 exchanges on alternate days) have shown benefit.

CHRONIC Rx

- *Disease-modifying therapy:* includes interferon beta-1a (IM Avonex, SC Rebif), interferon beta-1b (SC Betaseron), and glatiramer acetate (SC Copaxone). Interferons require routine CBC and LFT checks (initially in 1 mo, q3mo thereafter), occasionally thyroid-stimulating hormone. None needed with glatiramer acetate. Interferons can frequently cause flu-like symptoms.
- Fingolimod, a sphingosine-1-phosphate receptor modulator, was recently approved as the first oral disease modifying agent. Com-

mon side effects: liver toxicity, bradycardia with first dose only, pancytopenia.
- Dalfampridine (Ampyra) is a potassium channel blocker recently approved to improve walking speed in patients with MS.
- Cytotoxic: methotrexate or azathioprine is occasionally used in RRMS or PPMS. Consider cyclophosphamide or mitoxantrone (causes dose-dependent cardiotoxicity) for frequent relapses with significant disability progression and for early secondary progressive MS.
- Monoclonal antibodies: natalizumab (Tysabri) is approved for treatment of RRMS in the form of monthly infusions. It has been associated with an increased risk of developing progressive multifocal leukoencephalopathy (rare and fatal brain infection). Patients taking natalizumab must enter into a registry for monitoring.
- Spasticity: onabotulinom toxin type A injection is FDA approved as first-line therapy for upper limb spasticity. Baclofen, tizanidine, dantrolene diazepam, lorazepam, and intrathecal baclofen are other alternatives.
- Pain: carbamazepine, gabapentin, or amitriptyline.
- Spastic bladder: oxybutynin, tolterodine, or propantheline. Prazosin for spastic sphincter.
- Fatigue: consider amantadine 100 mg bid, modafinil (most effective for somnolence), or fluoxetine.
- Tremor: clonazepam, carbamazepine, propranolol, or gabapentin. Wrist splints may be helpful.
- Depression: selective serotonin receptor inhibitors or tricyclic antidepressants.

DISPOSITION

Most patients have complete or near-complete recovery weeks to months after a relapse. Typically, two flares occur in RRMS patient per year (75% will have at least one flare). Although the rate of disease progression is highly variable, 50% to 75% of patients progress from RRMS to SPMS.

REFERRAL

- Referral to neurology on diagnosis is recommended.
- Consider referrals for physical therapy and occupational therapy to prevent/minimize disability. Consider referral to urology if post-void residual by bladder scan is more than 100 ml.
- Referral to MS specialist should be strongly considered in case of poor response to therapy, possibility of cytotoxic treatment, and/or concern regarding accuracy of diagnosis.

PEARLS & CONSIDERATIONS

- Clinically isolated syndrome (CIS): when there is chronic CNS inflammatory syndrome with no prior history of neurologic symptoms. If brain MRI is completely normal, 20% to 25% chance of subsequent MS. If there are two or more T2 hyperintensities on neu-

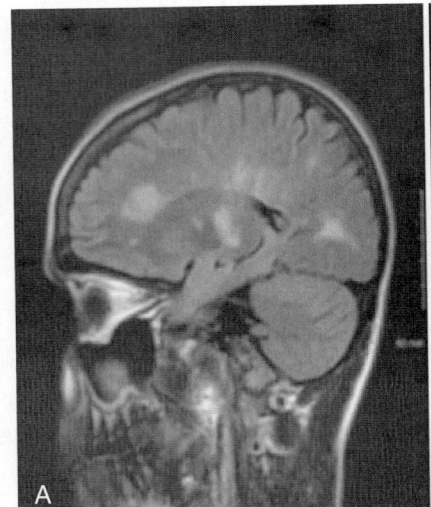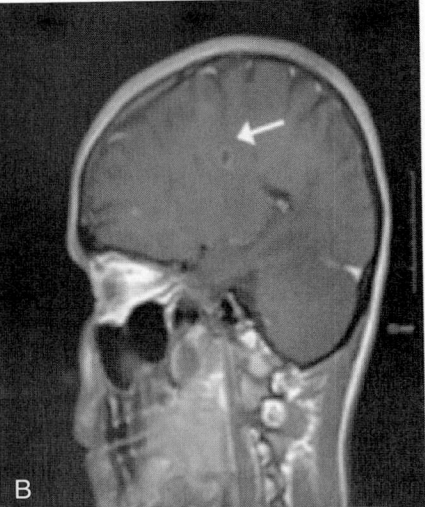

FIGURE 1-241 Multiple sclerosis. (A) Sagittal FLAIR image magnetic resonance scan shows multiple lesions in corpus callosum (periventricular and perpendicular to corpus callosum, known as "Dawson's fingers") along with lesions in right frontal, occipital lobes. (B) Gadolinium-enhanced scan shows one enhancing lesion (arrow).

roimaging, there is a 70% to 90% chance of subsequent MS.
- Pseudorelapses may occur with heat, fever, or infections (urinary tract infections common in patients with MS).
- Preliminary trials have shown that cladribine (a drug that provides immunomodulation through selective targeting of lymphocyte subtypes) significantly reduce relapse rates, the risk of disability progression, and MRI measures of disease activity at 96 wk. Ongoing phase III trials for alemtuzumab, laquinimod, and trifluoride. Results anticipated in late 2012 and 2013, respectively.

- It is important to rule out neuromyelitis optica (NMO) as the prognosis is poorer than with MS and typical disease-modifying drugs for MS (interferons, glatiramer acetate) are not efficacious in NMO. First-line treatment for NMPO includes mycophenolate mofetil, azathioprine, and rituximab.
- In an African American patient with clinical suspicion for MS, strongly consider possibility of neurosarcoidosis and order CXR, CSF angiotensin-converting enzyme level, and perhaps noncontrast chest CT.

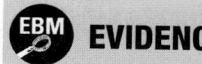

EVIDENCE
available at www.expertconsult.com
SUGGESTED READINGS
available at www.expertconsult.com

AUTHOR: **DIVYA SINGHAL, M.D.**

Diseases and Disorders

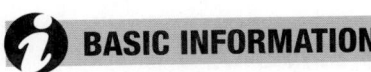

BASIC INFORMATION

DEFINITION

Mumps is an acute generalized viral infection that is usually characterized by nonsuppurative swelling and tenderness of one or both parotid glands. It is caused by mumps virus, a paramyxovirus and member of the paramyxoviridae family.

SYNONYMS

Viral parotitis
Parotitis

ICD-9CM CODES
072.9 Mumps

EPIDEMIOLOGY & DEMOGRAPHICS

INCIDENCE (IN U.S.):
- About 1600 infections/yr. Sporadic outbreaks occur
- More than 150,000 cases/yr before licensure of mumps vaccine in 1967

PREDOMINANT SEX: Males = females
PREDOMINANT AGE: 75% of disease in teenage year
PEAK INCIDENCE: Late winter and early spring months
GENETICS:
Congenital infection:
- First-trimester infection is associated with excessive fetal deaths.
- Second- and third-trimester infection is not associated with increased fetal mortality.
Neonatal infection:
- Uncommon
- Uncommon in infants <1 yr because of passive immunity conferred by placental transfer of maternal antibody

PHYSICAL FINDINGS & CLINICAL PRESENTATION

- Prodromal period: includes low-grade fever, malaise, anorexia, and headache
- Parotid swelling and tenderness are often the first signs of infection.
  1. Progresses over 2 to 3 days, then opposite side may become involved
  2. Unilateral parotitis in 25% of cases
  3. Considerable pain with parotid swelling, causing trismus and difficulty with mastication and pronunciation
  4. Pain exacerbated by eating or drinking citrus and other acidic foods
  5. Possible fever with parotid swelling, ranging up to 40° C
  6. Parotid swelling, usually resolving within 1 wk
- CNS involvement:
  1. May occur from 1 wk before to 2 wk after the onset of parotitis or even in its absence
  2. Meningitis:
     a. Occurs in 1% to 10% of patients with mumps parotitis
     b. Occurs three times more often in males than females
     c. Symptoms: headache, fever, nuchal rigidity, and vomiting
     d. Full recovery with no sequelae
  3. Encephalitis:
     a. May develop early, as a result of direct viral invasion of neurons, or late, around the second wk after onset of parotitis, and is a postinfectious demyelinating process.
     b. Mumps accounted for only 0.5% of viral meningitis.
     c. Symptoms: fever, alterations in the level of consciousness, possible seizures, paresis or paralysis, and aphasia. Fever can be quite high (40° to 41° C).
     d. Cerebellitis and hydrocephalus are serious complications of mumps encephalitis.
     e. May result in permanent sequelae or death.
  4. Other rare neurologic complications: include cerebellar ataxia, transverse myelitis, Guillain-Barré syndrome and facial palsy.
- Epididymoorchitis:
  1. Most common extra salivary gland complication of mumps in adult men
  2. Occurs in 38% of postpubertal males who have mumps
  3. Most often unilateral but is bilateral in 30% of males who develop this complication
  4. May precede development of parotitis and may be only manifestation of mumps
  5. Two thirds of cases develop during first week of parotitis
  6. Symptoms
     a. Severe pain, swelling, and tenderness of the testes and scrotal erythema
     b. Fever and chills
  7. Some degree of testicular atrophy in 50% of cases, mo to yr later
  8. Sterility from bilateral orchitis is rare
- Involvement of pancreas and ovaries:
  1. Pancreas: abdominal pain, fever, and vomiting
  2. Ovaries: oophoritis
     a. Occurs in 5% of postpubertal women with mumps
     b. Symptoms include fever, nausea, vomiting, and lower abdominal pain
     c. May rarely result in decreased fertility and premature menopause
- Transient renal impairment: common and manifested by hematura and polyuia
- Joint involvement:
  1. Migratory polyarthritis is most frequent
  2. Infrequently affects adults with mumps
  3. Occurs rarely in children
  4. Self-limited, with complete resolution
- Deafness:
  1. Most often unilateral, involving high frequencies; may rarely cause bilateral involvement
  2. Most patients recover
  3. Permanent unilateral deafness reported in 1 in 20,000 cases
  4. Labyrinthitis and end lymphatic hydrops also reported
- Myocardial involvement:
  1. Uncommon
  2. Rarely causes progressive and culminant fatal myocarditis with dilated cardiomyopathy
  3. Refractory arrhythmia and congestive heart failure
  4. Coronary artery involvement
- Eye involvement:
  1. Corneal endothelitis following mumps parotitis

ETIOLOGY

- Virus is spread via direct contact, droplet nuclei, fomites, or oral or nasal secretions.
- Patients are contagious from 48 hr before to 9 days after parotid swelling.

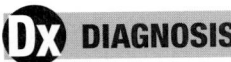 DIAGNOSIS

DIFFERENTIAL DIAGNOSIS

- Other viruses that may cause acute parotitis:
  1. Parainfluenza types 1 and 3
  2. Coxsackie viruses
  3. Influenza A
  4. Cytomegalovirus
- Suppurative parotitis:
  1. Most often caused by *Staphylococcus aureus*
  2. May be differentiated from mumps
     a. Extreme indurations, tenderness and erythema overlying the gland
     b. Ability to express pus from Stensen's duct or massage of parotid
- Other conditions that may occur with parotid enlargement or swelling:
  1. Sjögren's syndrome
  2. Leukemia
  3. Diabetes mellitus
  4. Uremia
  5. Malnutrition
  6. Cirrhosis
- Drugs that cause parotid swelling:
  1. Phenothiazines
  2. Phenylbutazone
  3. Thiouracil
  4. Iodides
- Conditions that cause unilateral swelling:
  1. Tumors
  2. Cysts
  3. Stones causing obstruction
  4. Strictures causing obstruction

WORKUP

- Diagnosis based on history of exposure and physical finding of parotid tenderness with mild to moderate constitutional symptoms.
- Diagnosis is confirmed by a variety of serologic tests or isolation of the virus.

LABORATORY TESTS

- Diagnosis is confirmed by a positive IgM mumps antibody or by fourfold rise between acute and convalescent sera by CF, ELISA, or neutralization tests. A polymerase chain reaction (PCR) assay is also available.

- Virus can be isolated from the saliva, usually from 2 to 3 days before to 4 to 5 days after the onset of parotitis.
- Virus can be cultured from CSF in patients with meningitis during the first 3 days of meningeal findings. More rapid confirmation of mumps in the CSF is IgM antibody capture immunoassay and nested PCR assay.
- Virus can be detected in urine during the first 2 wk of infection.
- WBC:
  1. May be normal or possible mild leucopenia with a relative lymphocytosis
  2. Leucocytosis with left shift with extra salivary gland involvement, such as meningitis, orchitis, or pancreatitis
- Serum amylase:
  1. Elevated in the presence of parotitis
  2. May remain elevated for 2 to 3 wk
  3. May be differentiated from mumps and parotids by isoenzyme analysis or serum pancreatic lipase
- Mumps meningitis:
  1. CSF WBCs from 10 to 2000 WBC/mm³ with a predominance of lymphocytes
  2. In 20% to 25% of patients, predominance of polymorphonuclear cells
  3. CSF protein normal or mildly elevated
  4. CSF glucose low, <40 mg/dl, in 6% to 30% of patients

TREATMENT

NONPHARMACOLOGIC THERAPY
- Supportive treatment
- Adequate hydration and nutrition

ACUTE GENERAL Rx
- Analgesics and antipyretics to relieve pain and fever
- Narcotic analgesics, along with bed rest, ice packs, and a testicular bridge, to relieve pain associated with mumps orchitis
- IV fluids for patients with frequent vomiting associated with mumps pancreatitis or meningitis

DISPOSITION
Most patients recover without incident.

REFERRAL
- To a neurologist if significant neurologic complications develop during or following mumps (myelitis, encephalitis, cranial nerve involvement, cerebellar ataxia, etc.)
- To a cardiologist if viral perimyocarditis develops
- To a urologist if orchitis develops

PEARLS & CONSIDERATIONS

COMMENTS
Prevention:
- Attenuated live mumps virus vaccine has been available since 1967.
  1. Usually given in combination with measles and rubella vaccines
  2. Should be given at 15 mo of age, and again at 5 to 12 yr
  3. Seroconversion in about 100% of infants given the vaccine
  4. Contraindicated in pregnant women and immunocompromised patients
  5. Patients with asymptomatic HIV infection and patients with symptomatic HIV infection, in the absence of severe immunosuppression, can safely receive mumps, measles, and rubella (MMR) vaccine
  6. Adverse events of vaccination include local pain, indurations, thrombocytopenic purpura, Guillain-Barré syndrome, and cerebellar ataxia
- The CDC and American Academy of Pediatrics (AAP) recommends that patients with mumps stay home from work or school for 5 days after onset of clinical symptoms.
- Because virus may be shed before the onset of parotid swelling, isolation possibly not of great value in limiting spread of infection. Use droplet precautions as per CDC and AAP.

EVIDENCE
available at www.expertconsult.com

SUGGESTED READINGS
available at www.expertconsult.com

AUTHORS: **GLENN G. FORT, M.D., M.P.H.,** and **DENNIS J. MIKOLICH, M.D.**

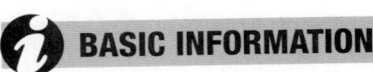

DEFINITION

Muscular dystrophy (MD) refers to a heterogeneous group of inherited disorders resulting in characteristic patterns of muscle weakness, some with cardiac involvement. Only disorders with childhood or adult onset are considered here (i.e., excluding congenital myopathies).

ICD-9CM CODES

| 359 | Muscular dystrophies and other myopathies |
| 359.1 | Hereditary progressive muscular dystrophy |

EPIDEMIOLOGY & DEMOGRAPHICS

INCIDENCE:

- Most common childhood MD is Duchenne's muscular dystrophy (DMD) with an incidence of 1/3500 male births
- Most common adult MD is myotonic dystrophy with an incidence as high as 1/8000

GENETICS:

- **Dystrophinopathies:** X-linked recessive defect in dystrophin gene resulting in either absence (DMD) or reduced/defective (Becker's MD [BMD]) dystrophin.
- **Myotonic Dystrophy:** Autosomal dominant (AD) CTG trinucleotide repeat.
- **Limb-Girdle Muscular Dystrophy:** Autosomal recessive, also autosomal dominant forms with deficiency identified in multiple proteins (sarcoglycan, calpain, dysferlin, telethonin, lamin A/C, myotilin, and caveolin-3).
- **Emery-Dreifuss Muscular Dystrophy:** X-linked recessive defect in nuclear protein emerin or AR defect in inner nuclear lamina proteins lamin A/C.
- **Facioscapulohumeral Muscular Dystrophy:** AD; genetic mutation causes deletion of 3.3 kb repeat.
- **Oculopharyngeal Muscular Dystrophy:** AD GCG trinucleotide repeat resulting in deficient mRNA transfer from nucleus.

PHYSICAL FINDINGS & CLINICAL PRESENTATION

- **Dystrophinopathies:** Proximal arm and leg weakness with hypertrophic calf muscles, delayed motor milestones, cognitive impairment, cardiac involvement, progressive course resulting in respiratory complications and respiratory failure
  - DMD (Fig. 1-242) onset at 2 to 3 yr old, typically wheelchair-bound by 12 yr
  - BMD onset at 5 to 15 yr old, ambulatory beyond age 15
- **Myotonic Dystrophy:** Variable age of onset and severity manifesting as predominately distal weakness with long face, percussion and grip myotonia, temporalis and masseter wasting, ptosis, hypersomnolence, cognitive impairment, and cardiac conduction defects. May be associated with frontal balding, cataracts, impaired glucose tolerance, and male infertility.
- **Limb-Girdle MD:** Phenotypically and genetically heterogenous characterized by proximal hip and shoulder girdle weakness, some genotypes featuring cardiac involvement.
- **Emery-Dreifuss MD:** Early adulthood onset with predominately humeroperoneal weakness, early contractures, and cardiac dysfunction.
- **Facioscapulohumeral MD:** Onset typically in late childhood or adolescence with weakness mostly in face and shoulder girdle musculature and possible later, mild involvement of lower extremities.
- **Oculopharyngeal MD:** Symptom onset typically in mid-adult life with ptosis, dysphagia, dysarthria, and proximal muscle weakness.

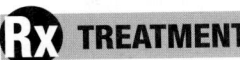

DIAGNOSIS

DIFFERENTIAL DIAGNOSIS

Myasthenia gravis, inflammatory myopathy, metabolic myopathy, endocrine myopathy, toxic myopathy, mitochondrial myopathy

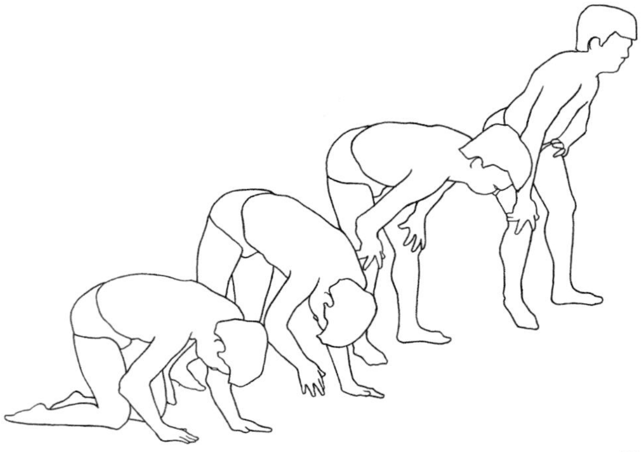

WORKUP

- CK
- ECG, Holter monitor, echocardiography
- EMG
- Muscle biopsy with immunohistochemistry useful for diagnosis of dystrophinopathies and limb-girdle MD
- DNA analysis helpful if clinical suspicion is for myotonic, Emery-Dreifuss, facioscapulohumeral, and oculopharyngeal MDs
- Assessment of respiratory parameters, including forced vital capacity (FVC)

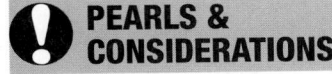

TREATMENT

NONPHARMACOLOGIC THERAPY

- Genetic counseling
- Physical, occupational, respiratory, speech therapy as symptoms dictate
- Screening for sleep-disordered breathing with overnight polysomnogram (PSG) if clinically indicated
- Pacemaker placement may be necessary if cardiac conduction defect present

ACUTE GENERAL Rx

- Prednisone may modestly prolong ambulation in DMD.

CHRONIC Rx

- Vigilance to avoid cardiac and respiratory complications, joint contractures

DISPOSITION

Variable course, because severity of phenotype is contingent upon both diagnosis and genotype

REFERRAL

- Surgical referral for correction of scoliosis or contractures may be necessary.
- Assessment and follow-up in a muscular dystrophy specialty clinic.

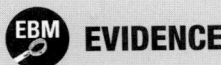

PEARLS & CONSIDERATIONS

Formal evaluation by anesthetist recommended before any operation with general anesthesia in patients with dystrophinopathy

EVIDENCE

available at www.expertconsult.com

SUGGESTED READINGS

available at www.expertconsult.com

AUTHOR: **TAYLOR HARRISON, M.D.**

FIGURE 1-242 In Duchenne's muscular dystrophy, the patient will get up from the floor with Gower's maneuver. The boy will "walk up" his body with his hands as he arises. (Remmel KS, Bunyan R, Brumback RA, Gascon GA, Olson WH: *Handbook of symptom-oriented neurology,* ed 3, St Louis, 2002, Mosby.)

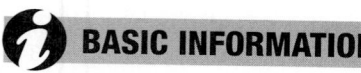

BASIC INFORMATION

DEFINITION

Mushroom poisoning is intoxication resulting from ingestion of poisonous mushrooms.

ICD-9CM CODES
988.1 Mushroom poisoning

EPIDEMIOLOGY & DEMOGRAPHICS

- 5% of all mushrooms are poisonous. Distinction between poisonous and edible mushrooms may be difficult even by experienced persons.

- Common poisonous species include *Amanita*, *Russula*, *Gyromitra*, and *Omphalotus*.

PHYSICAL FINDINGS & CLINICAL PRESENTATION (Table 1-123)

- *Russula* causes confusion, delirium, visual disturbance, tachycardia, and diarrhea within a few hours of ingestion. Prognosis: spontaneous recovery (mortality rate <1%).
- *Amanita* (Fig. 1-243) and *Gyromitra* intoxication begins with symptoms of gastroenteritis (nausea, vomiting, diarrhea, abdominal cramps) approximately 10 hr after ingestion. *Amanita* then causes cardiomyopathy and hepatic and renal failure. *Gyromitra* produces jaundice and seizures. Both mushrooms are associated with a 50% mortality rate.
- *Omphalotus* causes symptoms of gastroenteritis that subside spontaneously within 24 hr.

ETIOLOGY

- *Amanita* contains cytotoxic substances and isoxazoles that are gamma-aminobutyric acid neurotransmitter analogs.
- *Gyromitra* contains a pyridoxine antagonist that disrupts the gastrointestinal mucosa and causes hemolysis.
- *Russula* contains a cholinergic substance.

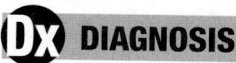

DIAGNOSIS

DIFFERENTIAL DIAGNOSIS

- Food poisoning
- Overdose of prescription or illegal drug
- Other intoxications
- See topic on specific organ failure (e.g., renal or hepatic failure) for differential diagnosis of those conditions

WORKUP

- History
- Inspection and identification of suspected mushrooms
- Mushroom or gastric content analysis (by thin-layer chromatography or radioimmunoassay)

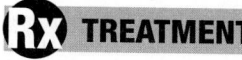

TREATMENT

- Gastric lavage
- Repeated administration of activated charcoal
- Supportive care as needed (may require respiratory assistance, hemodialysis, or emergency liver transplantation)

AUTHOR: **FRED F. FERRI, M.D.**

TABLE 1-123   Mushroom Poisoning Syndromes

Syndrome	Incubation Period (hr)	Species	Toxin
Confusion, restlessness, visual disturbances, lethargy	2	*Amanita muscaria* *Amanita pantherina*	Ibotenic acid, muscimol
Parasympathetic activity	2	*Inocybe* spp. *Clitocybe* spp.	Muscarine
Hallucinations	2	*Psilocybe* spp. *Panacolus* spp.	Psilocybin Psilocin
Disulfiram	2	*Coprinus atramentarius*	Disulfiram-like substances
Gastroenteritis	2	Many	Unknown
Hepatorenal failure	6-24	*Amanita phalloides* *Amanita virosa* *Amanita verna* *Galerina autumnalis* *Galerina marginata* *Galerina venenata*	Amatoxins Phallotoxins
Hepatic failure	6-24	*Gyromitra* spp.	Gyromitrin

From Gorbach SL: *Infectious diseases*, ed 2, Philadelphia, 1998, WB Saunders.

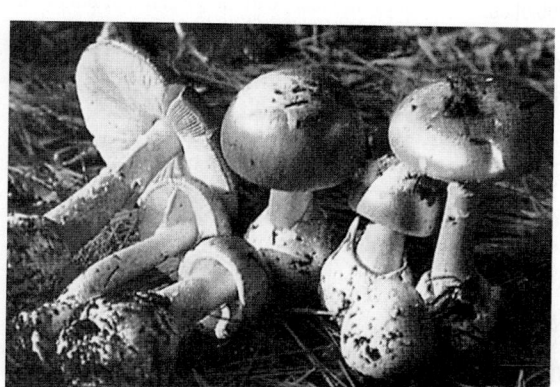

FIGURE 1-243 Death cap (*Amanita phalloides*). (Auerbach P: *Wilderness medicine*, ed 4, St Louis, Mosby.)

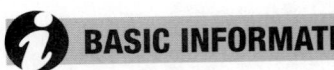

BASIC INFORMATION

DEFINITION

Myasthenia gravis (MG) is an autoimmune disorder of postsynaptic neuromuscular transmission classically directed against the nicotinic acetylcholine receptor (AChR) of the neuromuscular junction, resulting in a decrease in functional postsynaptic ACh receptors and consequent weakness.

ICD-9CM CODES
358.0 Myasthenia gravis

EPIDEMIOLOGY & DEMOGRAPHICS

INCIDENCE (IN U.S.): Two to five cases annually per 1 million persons
PEAK INCIDENCE: Female, second to third decades; male, sixth to seventh decades
PREVALENCE (IN U.S.): One per 20,000 persons
PREDOMINANT SEX: Females are affected more often than males (3:2) in adults; they are equally affected in the elderly
GENETICS: Increased frequency of HLA-B8, DR3

PHYSICAL FINDINGS & CLINICAL PRESENTATION

- The hallmark of MG is fluctuating weakness worsened with exercise and improved with rest.
- Generalized weakness involving proximal muscles, diaphragm, and neck extensors is common.
- Weakness is confined to eyelids and extraocular muscles in approximately 15% of patients.
- Bulbar symptoms of ptosis, diplopia, dysarthria, and dysphagia are common.
- Reflexes, sensation, and coordination are normal.

ETIOLOGY

Antibody-mediated decrease in nicotinic AChR in the postsynaptic neuromuscular junction resulting in defective neuromuscular transmission and subsequent muscle weakness and fatigue

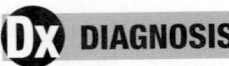

DIAGNOSIS

DIFFERENTIAL DIAGNOSIS

Lambert-Eaton myasthenic syndrome, botulism, medication-induced myasthenia, chronic progressive external ophthalmoplegia, congenital myasthenic syndromes, thyroid disease, basilar meningitis, intracranial mass lesion with cranial neuropathy, Miller-Fisher variant of Guillain-Barré syndrome

WORKUP

- Tensilon test: useful in MG patients with ocular symptoms. Cardiac monitoring and atropine ready at the bedside are essential.
- Repetitive nerve stimulation: successive stimulation shows decrement of muscle action potential in clinically weak muscle; may be negative in up to 50%.
- Single-fiber electromyography: highly sensitive; abnormal in up to 95% of patients.
- Serum AChR antibodies found in up to 80% of patients.
- A subset of patients with seronegative MG may have muscle-specific tyrosine kinase (MUSK) antibodies.

ADDITIONAL TESTS

- Spirometry to document pulmonary function
- CT scan of anterior chest to look for thymoma or residual thymic tissue
- Thyroid-stimulating hormone, free T_4 to rule out thyroid disease

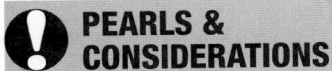

TREATMENT

NONPHARMACOLOGIC THERAPY

- Patient education to facilitate recognition of worsening symptoms and impress need for medical evaluation at onset of clinical deterioration
- Avoidance of selected drugs known to provoke exacerbations of MG (beta-blockers, aminoglycoside and quinolone antibiotics, class I antiarrhythmics)
- Prompt treatment of infections, diet modification, and speech evaluation with dysphagia

ACUTE GENERAL Rx

- Symptomatic treatment with acetylcholinesterase inhibitors:
  1. Pyridostigmine 30 to 60 mg PO q4 to 6h initially; onset of effects is 30 min, duration 4 hr
- Immunosuppressive treatment with corticosteroids, azathioprine, cyclosporine for long-term disease-modifying therapy
  1. Prednisone initiated at 15 to 20 mg qd titrate by 5-mg increments to effect or dose of 1 mg/kg/day with improvement in 2 to 4 wk and maximal response by 3 to 6 mo
  2. Azathioprine initiated at 50 mg qd titrated to 2 to 3 mg/kg/day with clinical effect in 6 to 12 mo
  3. Cyclosporine initiated at 5 mg/kg/day with clinical effect within 1 to 2 mo
- Plasmapheresis and IV immunoglobulin are short-term options for immunotherapy, including during an exacerbation.
- Mechanical ventilation is lifesaving in setting of a myasthenic crisis. Consider elective intubation if forced vital capacity <15 ml/kg, maximal expiratory pressure <40 cm H_2O, or negative inspiratory pressure <25 cm H_2O.

SURGICAL Rx

- In thymomatous MG, thymectomy is indicated in all patients.
- For nonthymomatous autoimmune MG, thymectomy is an option in select patients, typically <40 yr.

DISPOSITION

Course of disease is highly variable.

REFERRAL

Surgical referral for thymectomy in selected cases (see "Surgical Rx")

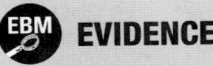

PEARLS & CONSIDERATIONS

- Sustained upward or lateral gaze and arm abduction for 120 sec may be necessary to elicit subtle signs on examination.
- Myasthenic patients can worsen rapidly and warrant close, careful observation during an exacerbation.

EVIDENCE

available at www.expertconsult.com

SUGGESTED READINGS
available at www.expertconsult.com

AUTHOR: **TAYLOR HARRISON, M.D.**

BASIC INFORMATION

DEFINITION

Mycosis fungoides refers to a T-cell lymphoproliferative disorder with characteristic cutaneous skin lesions and the potential to disseminate into lymph nodes and viscera.

SYNONYMS

Cutaneous T-cell lymphoma

ICD-9CM CODES
202.1 Mycosis fungoides

EPIDEMIOLOGY & DEMOGRAPHICS

- Incidence of mycosis fungoides is four cases per 1 million persons.
- ~1000 new cases are diagnosed annually in the United States.
- More commonly affects males than females (2:1).
- Affects blacks more often than whites (2:1).
- Usually found in males ages 40 to 60.

PHYSICAL FINDINGS & CLINICAL PRESENTATION

Mycosis fungoides characteristically progresses through three phases:

- A *premycotic phase* featuring scaly, erythematous patches that can last from months to years. During this stage the diagnosis can only be suspected because the histopathologic features are not definitive for mycosis fungoides. Lesions are pruritic and can appear anywhere but are usually found in sun-shielded areas. Parapsoriasis in plaques, poikilodermatous parapsoriasis, parapsoria-

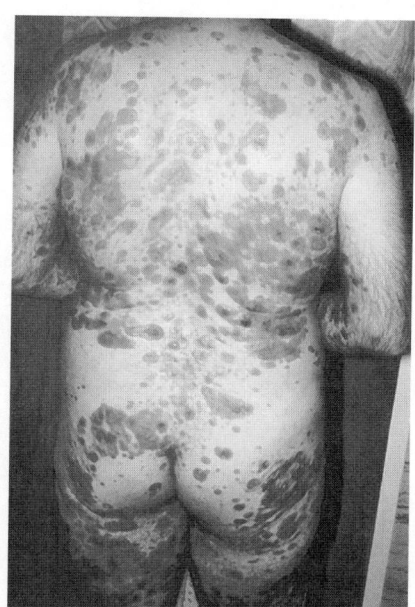

FIGURE 1-244 Cutaneous T-cell lymphoma (mycosis fungoides). Note patch, plaque, and tumor stages. (From Noble J [ed]: *Textbook of primary care medicine,* ed 2, St Louis, 1996, Mosby.)

sis lichenoides, and variegata are skin lesions suspicious of representing premycotic cutaneous T-cell lymphoma.

- The *infiltrative plaque phase* features raised, indurated erythematous palpable plaques that are pruritic and may be associated with alopecia.
  - Stage IA disease is defined as a patch or plaque skin disease involving <10% of the skin surface area and with absence of blood involvement or with low blood tumor burden (<5% of atypical T cells [Sézary cells] in the peripheral blood).
  - Stage IB disease (Fig. 1-244) is defined as a patch or plaque skin disease involving ≥10% of the skin surface area with absence of blood involvement or low blood tumor burden (<5% Sézary cells).
- The *tumor phase* is characterized by large, lumpy nodules arising from a premycotic patch, plaque, or unaffected skin and represents systemic infiltration and spreading. The tumors can be pruritic and large (>10 cm) and ulceration can occur.
  - Stage IIA and stage IIB diseases are defined by the presence of tumors with or without clinically abnormal peripheral lymph nodes with absence of blood involvement or low blood tumor burden. In approximately 5% of cases of mycosis fungoides, the presentation may be a diffuse, painful, pruritive erythroderma with Sézary cells in the peripheral blood (known as Sézary syndrome).
  - Stage III disease is defined by the presence of generalized erythroderma from the spread of cancer cells through the skin but not yet to the lymph nodes.
- Lymphadenopathy can occur during the plaque or tumor stages and may be regional or diffuse.
  - Stage IVA disease is defined by a lymph node biopsy showing large clusters of atypical cells, more than six cells, or total effacement by atypical cells.
- Infiltration of the liver, spleen, lungs, bone marrow, kidney, stomach, and brain can occur.
  - Stage IVB disease is defined by the presence of visceral involvement.

ETIOLOGY

The specific cause of mycosis fungoides is not known. Infection with the retrovirus HTLV-1 has been suspected, given the association of individuals infected with HTLV-1 and those with T-cell leukemia. Other considerations listed but unsubstantiated include environmental toxins (e.g., tobacco, pesticides, herbicides, and solvents) and genetic predisposition.

DIAGNOSIS

The diagnosis of mycosis fungoides is established by skin biopsy. This may be difficult to differentiate from other skin lesions in the early phases of the disease (e.g., premycotic patch or early plaque lesions); therefore the diagnosis can only be suspected.

DIFFERENTIAL DIAGNOSIS

- Contact dermatitis
- Atopic dermatitis
- Nummular dermatitis
- Parapsoriases
- Superficial fungal infections
- Drug eruptions
- Psoriasis
- Photodermatitis
- Alopecia mucinosa
- Lymphomatoid papulosis

WORKUP

Any patient who is suspected of having mycosis fungoides should have a staging workup. Prognosis in patients with mycosis fungoides depends on the type of skin lesions and the extent of disease. The workup should focus on:

1. Complete physical examination:
   - The type of skin lesion and the extent of skin involvement of the body (e.g., skin involvement is >10% or <10% of the skin surface)
   - Identification of palpable lymph node (especially those >1.5 cm in largest diameter)
   - Identification of organomegaly (e.g., lungs, liver)
2. Skin biopsy:
   - Biopsy of the most indurated area
   - Immunophenotyping
   - Evaluation for clonality
3. Blood test:
   - Complete blood count with differential, liver function tests, lactate dehydrogenase, chemistry
   - T-cell receptor gene rearrangement
   - Determination of Sézary cell count and/or flow cytometry
4. Radiologic tests
   - Depending on the stage of the disease, chest radiograph; ultrasound; and CT scan of the chest, abdomen, and pelvis alone, with or without fluorodeoxyglucose positron emission tomography scan
5. Lymph node biopsy
   - Excisional biopsy
   - Biopsy of the largest lymph node
   - If multiple nodes enlarged, order of preference is cervical, axillary, and inguinal areas
   - Histopathology, flow cytometry, T-cell receptor gene rearrangement

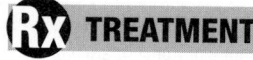 TREATMENT

Treatment is guided according to the stage of disease. A treatment algorithm is described in the online version of Section III.

NONPHARMACOLOGIC THERAPY

- For dry, cracking skin, emollients (e.g., lanolin and petrolatum) are applied bid.
- Moisturizing lotion (e.g., ammonium lactate) applied bid.
- Topical antibiotics (e.g., bacitracin) are used on ulcerative tumors.

ACUTE GENERAL Rx

- Treatment of patients with stage IA limited patch or plaque phase include:
  - Topical nitrogen mustard 10 to 20 mg per 100 ml in water or ointment base applied to affected areas daily until cleared (usually 1 to 2 mo).
  - Psoralen ultraviolet A (PUVA) light therapy where 0.6 mg/kg of 8-methoxypsoralen is ingested 1 to 2 hr before exposure of the skin to UVA light (320 to 400 nm). This is done three times per wk and tapered to twice per wk until all the lesions have cleared. This is typically continued for 6 mo with a 90% complete remission rate.
- Treatment of patients with stage IB and IIA disease is similar to stage IA, with topical nitrogen mustard or PUVA.
  - Total skin electron beam therapy is considered in patients with thick plaques.
  - Interferon-alpha 5 million units SQ three times weekly can be considered in patients with stage IB or IIA disease.
  - Retinoids in combination with PUVA are used in refractory cases. Isotretinoin 1 mg/kg per day or acitretin 25 to 50 mg per day is the standard dosing.
- Treatment of patients with stage IIB disease with generalized tumor and plaque disease includes:
  - Total skin electron beam therapy in doses of 3000 to 3600 cGy given over 8 to 10 wk followed by adjuvant therapy with topical mustard can be used.

CHRONIC Rx

- In patients developing diffuse erythroderma, stage III disease (e.g., Sézary syndrome, extracorporeal photophoresis), 8-methoxypsoralen is ingested and peripheral blood is exposed to UVA through a membrane filter.
- In stage IV disease, interferon and other systemic chemotherapeutic agents (e.g., methotrexate, cyclophosphamide, doxorubicin, vincristine, prednisone) are considered.

DISPOSITION

- The patients with limited patch or plaque disease have excellent prognosis with long-term life expectancy that is similar to an age-, sex-, and race-matched control population.

- The patients with generalized patch or plaque without evidence of extracutaneous involvement have a median survival of greater than 11 yr.
- The patients with cutaneous tumor and generalized erythroderma without extracutaneous involvement have a median survival of 3 to 4.6 yr.
- The patients with extracutaneous disease at presentation involving either lymphnode or a viscera have median survival of 13 mo.

REFERRAL

Any patient with suspected mycosis fungoides should be referred to a dermatologist for definitive diagnosis and initial therapy. Oncology consultation is also indicated in patients with more advanced disease.

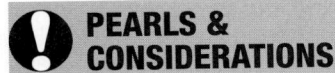 PEARLS & CONSIDERATIONS

A TNM staging classification of mycosis fungoides has been in use for guiding therapy since 1979. The International Society for Cutaneous Lymphomas (ISCL) and the Cutaneous Lymphoma Task Force of the European Organization of Research and Treatment of Cancer (EORTC) recommended revisions to the TNM classification and staging system of cutaneous T-cell lymphoma in 2007. Table 1-124 compares EORTC and WHO classifications of primary cutaneous lymphoma.

COMMENTS

Mycosis fungoides is thought to represent one class of the spectrum of cutaneous T-cell lymphomas.

SUGGESTED READINGS
available at www.expertconsult.com

AUTHOR: **TANYA ALI, M.D.**

TABLE 1-124 Comparison of EORTC and WHO Classifications of Primary Cutaneous Lymphoma

EORTC Classification	WHO Classification
Cutaneous T-Cell Lymphoma	
Indolent clinical behavior	Mycosis fungoides
Mycosis fungoides variants	Mycosis fungoides variants
Follicular mycosis fungoides	Follicular mycosis fungoides
Pagetoid reticulosis	Pagetoid reticulosis
CTCL, large cell, CD30+	Primary cutaneous CD30+ ALCA (CD30+ lymphoproliferative disease, including lymphomatoid papulosis)
Lymphomatoid papulosis	
Aggressive clinical behavior	Sézary syndrome
Sézary syndrome	Peripheral T-cell lymphoma, unspecified (most); extranodal NK/T-cell lymphoma, nasal type
CTCL, large cell, CD-30-negative	
Provisional entities	
CTCL, pleomorphic, small/medium sized	
Subcutaneous panniculitis-like T-cell lymphoma	Subcutaneous panniculitis-like T-cell lymphoma
Cutaneous B-Cell Lymphoma	
Indolent clinical behavior	Extranodal marginal zone B-cell lymphoma
Primary cutaneous immunocytoma (marginal zone B-cell lymphoma)	
Follicle Center Cell Lymphoma (any grade)	
Intermediate clinical behavior	
Primary cutaneous large B-cell	
Lymphoma of the leg	
Provisional Entities	
Primary cutaneous plasmacytoma	Plasmacytoma
Intravascular large B-cell lymphoma	Diffuse large B-cell lymphoma (intravascular)

ALCL, Anaplastic large cell lymphoma; *CTCL,* cutaneous T-cell lymphoma; *EORTC,* European Organization for the Research and Treatment of Cancer; *NK,* natural killer; *WHO,* World Health Organization.
From Hoffman R et al: *Hematology: basic principles and practice,* ed 5, Philadelphia, 2009, Churchill Livingstone.

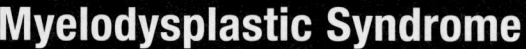
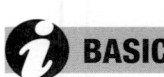 BASIC INFORMATION

DEFINITION

Myelodysplastic syndrome (MDS) is a group of acquired clonal disorders affecting the hemopoietic stem cells and characterized by cytopenias with hypercellular bone marrow and various morphologic abnormalities in the hemopoietic cell lines. MDS shows abnormal (dysplastic) hemopoietic maturation. Marrow cellularity is increased, reflecting an effective hematopoiesis, but inadequate maturation results in peripheral cytopenias.

CLASSIFICATION

- Myelodysplasia encompasses several heterogenous syndromes. The French-American-British (FAB) classification of MDSs is based on the proportion of immature blast cells in the blood and marrow and on the presence or absence of ringed sideroblasts or peripheral monocytosis (Table 1-125). It includes refractory anemia, refractory anemia with ringed sideroblasts, refractory anemia with excess blasts, chronic myelomonocytic leukemia, and refractory anemia with excess blasts in transformation.
- In 1999 the World Health Organization modified the FAB by incorporating newer morphologic insights and cytogenetic findings. It includes the disease subtypes refractory anemia, refractory anemia with ringed sideroblasts, refractory cytopenia with multilineage dysplasia, refractory cytopenia with multilineage dysplasia and ringed sideroblasts, refractory anemia with excessive blasts (1, 2), unclassified MDS, and MDS associated with isolated del(5q).

SYNONYMS

MDS
Preleukemia
Dysmyelopoietic syndrome

ICD-9CM CODES
238.7 Myelodysplastic syndrome

EPIDEMIOLOGY & DEMOGRAPHICS

INCIDENCE (IN U.S.): Approximately 82 cases/100,000 persons per yr. An estimated 7000 to 12,000 new cases are diagnosed annually in the U.S.
PREDOMINANT AGE: More common in elderly patients; median age, >65 yr

PHYSICAL FINDINGS & CLINICAL PRESENTATION

- Splenomegaly, skin pallor, mucosal bleeding, and ecchymosis may be present.
- Patients often present with fatigue.
- Fever, infection, and dyspnea are common.

ETIOLOGY

Unknown. However, exposure to radiation, chemotherapeutic agents, benzene, or other organic compounds is associated with myelodysplasia. Table 1-126 describes predisposing factors and epidemiologic associations of patients with myelodysplastic syndrome.

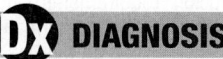 DIAGNOSIS

DIFFERENTIAL DIAGNOSIS

- Hereditary dysplasias (e.g., Fanconi's anemia, Diamond-Blackfan syndrome)
- Vitamin B_{12}/folate deficiency
- Exposure to toxins (drugs, alcohol, chemotherapy)
- Renal failure

- Irradiation
- Autoimmune disease
- Infections (tuberculosis, viral infections)
- Paroxysmal nocturnal hemoglobinuria

WORKUP

Diagnostic workup includes laboratory evaluation and bone marrow examination. Cytogenetic analysis by conventional metaphase karyotyping should be performed in patients with MDS. Physical examination, medical history, and laboratory tests aiding in diagnosis of myelodysplastic syndrome are described in Table 1-127.

TABLE 1-125   French-American-British Classification Criteria

Subtype	Abbreviation	Peripheral Blood	Bone Marrow
Refractory anemia	RA	Blasts <1%	Blasts <5%
Refractory anemia with ringed sideroblasts	RARS	Blasts <1%	Blasts <5%, and >15% ringed sideroblasts
Refractory anemia with excess blasts	RAEB	Blasts <5%	Blasts 5%-20%
Refractory anemia with excess blasts in transformation	RAEB-T	Blasts >5%	Blasts 20%-30% or Auer rods
Chronic myelomonocytic leukemia	CMML	Monocytes $>1 \times 10^9$/L	Any of the above
Acute myelogenous leukemia	AML	Blasts >30%	

From Hoffmann R et al: *Hematology, basic principles and practice*, ed 5, Philadelphia, 2009, Churchill Livingstone.

TABLE 1-126   Predisposing Factors and Epidemiologic Associations of Patients with Myelodysplastic Syndrome

Heritable

Constitutional Genetic Disorders

Trisomy 8 mosaicism
Familial monosomy 7
Down syndrome (trisomy 21)
Neurofibromatosis 1
Germ cell tumors [embryonal dysgenesis del(12p)]

Congenital Neutropenia

Kostmann syndrome
Shwachman-Diamond syndrome

DNA Repair Deficiencies

Fanconi anemia
Ataxia-telangiectasia
Bloom syndrome
Xeroderma pigmentosum
Pharmacogenomic polymorphisms (GSTq1-null)

Acquired

Senescence

Mutagen Exposure

Alkylator therapy (chlorambucil, cyclophosphamide, melphalan, N-mustards)
Topoisomerase II inhibitors (anthracyclines)
β Emitters (32P)
Autologous stem cell transplantation
Environmental/occupational (benzene)
Tobacco
Aplastic anemia
Paroxysmal nocturnal hemoglobinuria

Hoffmann R et al: *Hematology, basic principles and practice*, ed 5, Philadelphia, 2009, Churchill Livingstone.

Rx TREATMENT

NONPHARMACOLOGIC THERAPY
Red blood cell transfusions in patients with severe symptomatic anemia

ACUTE GENERAL Rx
- Erythropoietin (10,000 to 40,000 U/wk) in patient with symptomatic anemia.
- DNA methyltransferase inhibitors: Azacitidine (Vidaza), a pyrimidine nucleoside analog of cytidine, has been shown to improve the quality of life for patients with MDS and probably prolong survival. Decitabine (Dacogen), another nucleoside analog, has also been FDA approved for patients with MDS. These agents may also be useful in preventing the transition of MDS to AML.
- Immunomodulators: Lenalidomide (Revlimid), a novel analogue of thalidomide, has demonstrated hematologic activity in patients with low-rise MDS who have no response to erythropoietin or who are unlikely to benefit from conventional therapy. Lenalidomide can also reduce transfusion requirements and reverse cytologic and cytogenetic abnormalities in patients who have MDS with the 5q31 deletion.
- Allogeneic stem cell transplantation should be considered in patients ≤60 yr because this is the established procedure with cure potential.
- Results of chemotherapy are generally disappointing. Combination chemotherapy regimens (e.g., cytarabine plus doxorubicin) generally induce a complete response in only a minority of patients, and the average duration of response is <1 yr.
- The role of myeloid growth factors (granulocyte colony-stimulating factor (G-CSF), granulocyte-macrophage CSF) and immunotherapy is undefined. In a recent trial, 34% of patients treated with antithymocyte globulin (40 mg/kg for 4 days) became transfusion independent. Response was also associated with a statistically significantly longer survival.

CHRONIC Rx
Monitor for infections, bleeding, and complications of anemia. Supportive measures include blood transfusions and erythropoietin for anemia and antibiotics to treat opportunistic infections. Iron overload from frequent transfusions may require iron chelation therapy.

DISPOSITION
- Cure rates in young patients with allogeneic bone marrow transplantation approach 30% to 50%.
- The risk of transformation to acute myelogenous leukemia varies with the percentage of blasts in the bone marrow.
- Advanced age, male sex, and deletion of chromosomes 5 and 7 are associated with a poor prognosis.
- The 1997 International Prognostic Scoring System uses the following three elements for staging: (1) the proportion of myeloblasts in the patient's marrow, (2) the number of blood cell lineage deficits, and (3) the type of chromosomal abnormality present (e.g., poor risk includes abnormalities of chromosome 7; good risk includes clonal loss of the Y chromosome). According to the International Myelodysplastic Syndrome Risk Analysis Workshop, the most important variables in disease outcome are the specific cytogenetic abnormalities, the percentage of blasts in the bone marrow, and the number of hematopoietic lineages involved in the cytopenias.

REFERRAL
Hematology referral in all patients with MDS

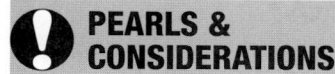

PEARLS & CONSIDERATIONS

COMMENTS
- Patients with cytogenetic abnormalities associated with poor prognosis should be considered for aggressive treatment with high-dose chemotherapy and stem cell transplantation.
- Many younger patients who respond to immunosuppressive therapy with drugs such as antithymocyte globulin and cyclosporine have clonal expansions of cytotoxic $CD8^+$ T cells that suppress normal hematopoiesis, as well as expansion of $CD4^+$ helper T-cell subsets that promote and sustain autoimmunity.
- Nearly 50% of the deaths that result from MDS are the result of cytopenia associated with bone marrow failure.

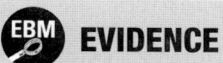 **EVIDENCE**

available at www.expertconsult.com

SUGGESTED READINGS

available at www.expertconsult.com

TABLE 1-127 Physical Examination, Medical History, and Laboratory Tests Aiding in Diagnosis of Myelodysplastic Syndrome

Medical History

Duration of symptoms
History of blood disease
History of exposure to occupational toxins or cytotoxic agents
Medication history
Alcohol intake
Comorbid conditions

Physical Examination

Pallor
Petechiae
Purpura
Bruising
Tachypnea
Signs of infection
Splenomegaly

Laboratory Testing

Complete blood count with a manual differential
Reticulocyte count
Vitamin B_{12} and folate levels
Consider methylmalonic acid and red blood cell folate levels
Iron, total iron-binding capacity, and ferritin level
Thyroid-stimulating hormone level
Lactate dehydrogenase
Antinuclear antibody
Coombs test and haptoglobin
Serum erythropoietin level
Human leukocyte antigen (histocompatibility antigens) typing in appropriate patients
Paroxysmal nocturnal hemoglobinuria screen

Bone Marrow Testing

Hematopathology
 Percentage of blasts on 200 cell aspirate differential
 Presence or absence of Auer rods
 Percentage of cellularity of bone marrow biopsy
 Iron stain on aspirate (ringed sideroblasts)
 Iron stain on biopsy (storage)
 Dysplastic features (% and number of dysplastic lineages)
Cytogenetics (karyotype of 20 metaphase cells)
Fluorescent in situ hybridization
Flow cytometry (not useful for quantitation)

From Hoffmann R et al: *Hematology, basic principles and practice,* ed 5, Philadelphia, 2009, Churchill Livingstone.

AUTHOR: **FRED F. FERRI, M.D.**

BASIC INFORMATION

DEFINITION

- Myocardial infarction (MI) is characterized by myocardial necrosis resulting from an insufficient supply of oxygenated blood to an area of the heart. According to the European Society of Cardiology/American College of Cardiology, either one of the following criteria for acute evolving or recent MI satisfies the diagnosis:
  a. Typical rise and gradual fall (troponin) or more rapid rise and fall (creatine kinase–MB fraction [CK-MB]) of biochemical markers of myocardial necrosis with at least one of the following:
     i. Ischemic symptoms
     ii. Development of pathologic Q waves on ECG
     iii. ECG changes indicative of ischemia (ST-segment elevation or depression)
     iv. Coronary artery intervention (e.g., coronary angioplasty)
  b. Pathologic findings of acute MI
  Myocardial infarction may be classified as ST-elevation segment elevation MI (STEMI) and non–ST-segment elevation myocardial infarction [NSTEMI]) depending on the ECG findings on MI presentation.
- The *European Heart Journal* and the *Journal of the American College of Cardiology* published a new definition of acute MI (see later) to account for advances in diagnosis and management. It includes subtypes of acute MI, imaging tests supporting the diagnosis, and biomarker thresholds after percutaneous coronary intervention (PCI) or coronary artery bypass grafting (CABG).
  - Type 1: Spontaneous MI related to ischemia due to a primary coronary event such as plaque erosion and/or rupture, fissuring, or dissection
  - Type 2: MI secondary to ischemia due to either increased oxygen demand or decreased supply (e.g., coronary artery spasm, coronary embolism, anemia, arrhythmias, hypertension, or hypotension)
  - Type 3: Sudden unexpected cardiac death, including cardiac arrest, often with symptoms suggestive of myocardial ischemia, accompanied by presumably new ST elevation, new left bundle branch block, or evidence of fresh thrombus in a coronary artery by angiography and/or at autopsy, but death occurring before blood samples could be obtained or at a time before the appearance of cardiac biomarkers in the blood
  - Type 4a: MI associated with percutaneous coronary intervention
  - Type 4b: MI associated with stent thrombosis as documented by angiography or at autopsy
  - Type 5: MI associated with coronary artery bypass grafting

SYNONYMS

MI
Myocardial infarction
Non–ST elevation MI
ST-elevation MI
Heart attack
Coronary thrombosis
Coronary occlusion

ICD-9CM CODES

410.9 Acute myocardial infarction, unspecified site

EPIDEMIOLOGY & DEMOGRAPHICS

INCIDENCE/PREVALENCE (IN U.S.):
- >500 cases/100,000 persons.
- >500,000 MIs in the United States annually.
- More prominent in males between the ages of 40 and 65 yr; no predominant sex after age 65 yr.
- Women experience more lethal and severe first acute MIs than men regardless of comorbidity, previous angina, or age.
- At least one fourth of all myocardial infarctions are clinically unrecognized.

PHYSICAL FINDINGS & CLINICAL PRESENTATION

Clinical presentation:
- Crushing substernal chest pain usually lasts longer than 30 min.
- Pain is unrelieved by rest or sublingual nitroglycerin or is rapidly recurring.
- Pain radiates to the left or right arm, neck, jaw, back, shoulders, or abdomen and is not pleuritic in character.
- Pain may be associated with dyspnea, diaphoresis, nausea, or vomiting.
- There is no pain in ~20% of infarctions (usually in diabetic or elderly patients).
Physical findings:
- Skin may be diaphoretic, with pallor (because of decreased oxygen).
- Rales may be present at the bases of lungs (indicative of congestive heart failure [CHF]).
- Cardiac auscultation may reveal an apical systolic murmur caused by mitral regurgitation from papillary muscle dysfunction; S_3 or S_4 may also be present.
- Physical examination may be completely normal.

ETIOLOGY

- Coronary atherosclerosis and plaque rupture.
- Coronary artery spasm.
- Coronary embolism (caused by infective endocarditis, rheumatic heart disease, intracavitary thrombus).
- Periarteritis and other coronary artery inflammatory diseases.
- Dissection into coronary arteries (aneurysmal or iatrogenic).
- Metabolic derangements such as hypoxemia, anemia, sepsis, hypotension, or hyperthyroidism leading to ischemic necrosis due to supply-demand mismatch.

- MI with normal coronaries: more frequent in younger patients and cocaine addicts. The risk of acute MI is increased by a factor of 24 during the 60 min after the use of cocaine in persons who are otherwise at relatively low risk. Most patients with cocaine-related MI are young, nonwhite, male cigarette smokers without other risk factors for arteriosclerotic heart disease who have a history of repeated cocaine use. Blood and urine toxicology screen for cocaine is recommended in all young patients who present with acute MI.
- Hypercoagulable states, increased blood viscosity (polycythemia vera).

DIAGNOSIS

DIFFERENTIAL DIAGNOSIS

The various causes of myocardial ischemia are described in Section II along with the differential diagnosis of chest pain.

LABORATORY TESTS

- Cardiac troponin levels: cardiac-specific troponin T (cTnT) and cardiac-specific troponin I (cTnI) are generally indicative of myocardial injury. Increases in serum levels of cTnT and cTnI >99th percentile of normal reference population. Detection of a rise and/or fall pattern of the measurements is essential to the diagnosis of acute MI. The rise may occur relatively early after muscle damage (3 to 12 hr), peak within 24 hr, and may be present for several days after MI (up to 7 days for cTnI and up to 10 to 14 days for cTnT). cTnT or cTnI tests can be falsely positive in patients with renal failure.
- CK-MB isoenzyme is also a useful marker for MI if troponin levels are not available. It is released in the circulation in amounts that correlate with the size of the infarct. An increased CK-MB value for the diagnosis of MI is defined as a measurement above the 99th percentile of the upper reference limit.
- Neither CK-MB nor troponin consistently appear in the blood within 6 hr after an ischemic event; therefore serial testing (e.g., on presentation and after 6 to 9 hr) is necessary to definitely rule out MI.
- ECG: common ECG findings suggestive of acute myocardial ischemia include inverted T waves ≥1 mm deep and/or ST-segment depression ≥0.5 mm in two contiguous leads. The presence of pathologic Q waves (Fig. 1-245) indicates an area of infarction (usually develops after 3 to 6 hr) of continuous ischemia. STEMI is considered to be present when there is ST segment elevation in two contiguous leads, ≥0.20 mV for men and ≥0.15 mV for women measured at the J point in leads V2 and V3 or ≥0.10 mV in other leads.

IMAGING STUDIES

- Chest radiograph is useful to evaluate for pulmonary congestion and exclude other causes of chest pain.

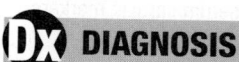

M

- Echocardiography can evaluate wall motion abnormalities and identify mural thrombus or mitral regurgitation, which can occur acutely after MI.

RISK ASSESSMENT

Several risk assessment models are available. The Thrombolysis in Myocardial Infarction risk score uses the seven following variables: age ≥65 yr, at least three conventional risk factors for coronary artery disease, prior coronary stenosis ≥50%, ST-segment deviation on ECG at presentation, two or more anginal events in the preceding 24 hr, use of aspirin in the prior 7 days, and elevated serum cardiac markers.

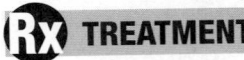 **TREATMENT**

NONPHARMACOLOGIC THERAPY

- Limit patient's activity: bed rest for the initial 12 to 24 hr; if the patient remains stable, gradually increase activity.
- Diet: nothing by mouth until stable, then no added salt and a low-cholesterol diet.
- Patient education to decrease the risk of subsequent cardiac events (proper diet, cessation of smoking, regular exercise) should be initiated when the patient is medically stable.

ACUTE GENERAL Rx

- Any patient with suspected acute MI should immediately receive the following:
  ○ Antiplatelet therapy: aspirin, 160 to 325 mg PO unless true aspirin allergy is suspected. If the first dose is chewed, a blood level is achieved more rapidly than if it is swallowed. Clopidogrel 75 mg qd may be substituted if true allergy is present or given in addition to aspirin.
  ○ Nitrates: increase the supply of oxygen by reducing coronary vasospasm and de-

creasing consumption of oxygen by reducing ventricular preload. Sublingual nitroglycerin (0.4 mg) can be administered immediately on suspicion of MI (unless systolic blood pressure is <90 mm Hg or ≤30 mm Hg below baseline or heart rate is <50 beats/min or >100 beats/min); IV nitroglycerin can be subsequently used. Nitroglycerin should be used with great caution in patients with inferior wall MI; nitrate use can result in hypotension because these patients are sensitive to change in preload. It should also be avoided in patients suspected of having right ventricular infarction (increased risk of preload reduction) and if a patient has used sildenafil or vardenafil within the previous 24 hr or tadalafil in the previous 48 hr.
  ○ Adequate analgesia: morphine sulfate 2 to 4 mg IV initially with increments of 2 to 8 mg IV at 5 to 15 min intervals can be given for severe pain unrelieved by nitroglycerin. Hypotension from morphine can be treated with careful IV hydration with saline solution. If sinus bradycardia accompanies hypotension, use atropine (0.5 to 1.0 mg IV every 5 min prn to a total dose of 2.5 mg). Respiratory depression caused by morphine can be reversed with naloxone 0.8 mg.
  ○ Nasal oxygen: administer at 2 to 4 L/min.
- Prompt myocardial reperfusion in STEMI can be accomplished with PCI, fibrinolytic therapy, or CABG surgery. If readily available without delay, PCI is superior to thrombolytic therapy. It is effective and generally results in more favorable outcomes than thrombolytic therapy. If PCI is planned, use of parenteral anticoagulation is recommended with either unfractionated heparin, enoxaparin, fondaparinux, or bivalirudin. In patients at high risk of bleeding, use of bivalirudin, is

reasonable. Aspirin and a thienopyridine (e.g., clopidogrel) should be loaded before PCI and continued for at least 12 mo in patients who receive a stent. Continuation beyond 15 mo may be considered in patients who receive a drug-eluting stent. Thienopyridines can be discontinued early if there is a high risk for bleeding. If coronary artery bypass grafting is planned, the drug should be withheld for at least 5 days unless the urgency of revascularization outweighs the risk of bleeding. Neither facilitation of PCI with reteplase plus abciximab nor facilitation with abciximab alone significantly improves the clinical outcomes compared with abciximab given at the time of PCI in patients with STEMI. Coronary stents after PCI are useful to decrease ischemia, improve long-term patency, and lower the rate of restenosis of the infarct-related artery. In patients with acute MI, treatment with drug-eluting stents is associated with decreased 2-yr mortality rates and a reduction in the need for repeat revascularization procedures compared with treatment with bare-metal stents.
- Thrombolytic therapy (Table 1-128): in STEMI, if the duration of pain has been <12 hr and primary angioplasty is not readily available, recanalization of the occluded arteries should be attempted with thrombolytic agents. Because the effectiveness of thrombolytics is time dependent, these agents should ideally be administered either in the field or within 30 min of the patient's arrival in the emergency department. When tissue plasminogen activator (tPA) or reteplase is used, heparin is given to increase the likelihood of patency in the infarct-related artery for 24 to 48 hr. In patients receiving fibrinolysis for STEMI, treatment with enoxaparin is superior to treatment with unfractionated heparin for 48 hr, but is associated with an increase in major bleeding episodes. In patients receiving streptokinase

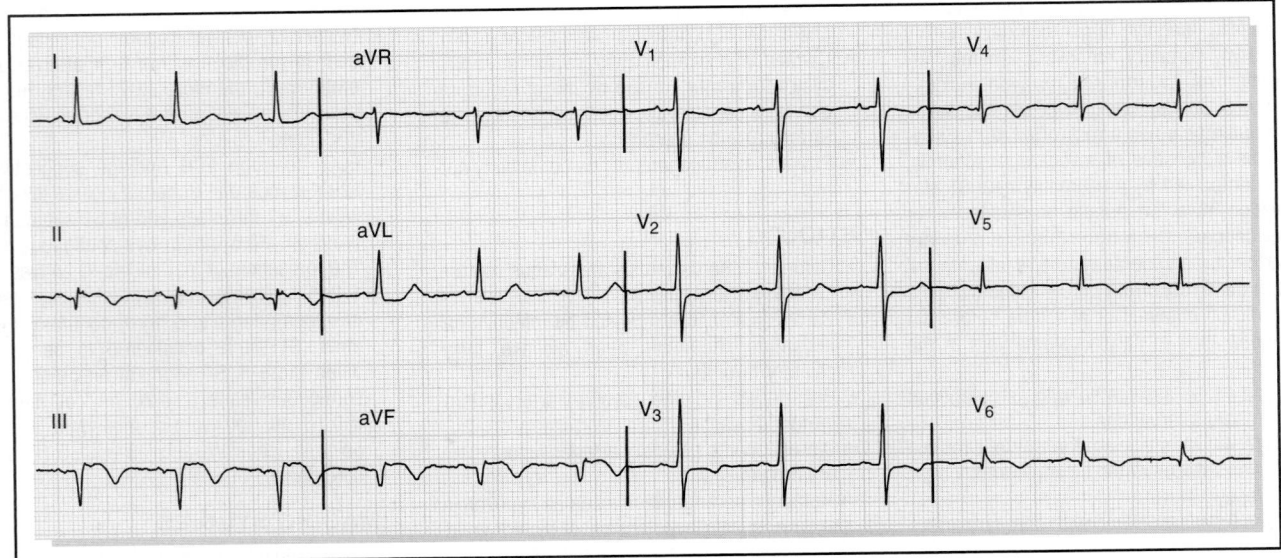

FIGURE 1-245 Evolving inferoposterolateral infarction. Note the prominent Q waves in leads II, III, and aV1, along with ST elevation and T-wave inversion in these leads, as well as V3 through V6. ST depression in I, aV1, V1, and V2 is consistent with a reciprocal change. Relatively tall R waves are also present in V1 and V2. (From Zipes DP et al [eds]: *Braunwald's heart disease*, ed 7, Philadelphia, 2005, Elsevier.)

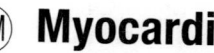

or APSAC, heparin after thrombolysis is not indicated because it does not offer any additional benefit and can result in increased bleeding complications. Tenecteplase and reteplase are comparable with accelerated infusion recombinant tPA in terms of efficacy and safety, but are more convenient because they are administered by bolus injection. Lanoplase and heparin bolus plus infusion are as effective as tPA with regard to mortality rate, but the rate of intracranial hemorrhage is significantly higher. Absolute contraindications to thrombolytic therapy (Table 1-129) include active internal bleeding, intracranial neoplasm or arteriovenous malformation, intracranial surgery in past 6 mo, stroke in past year, head trauma with loss of consciousness in past 6 mo, surgery in noncompressible location in past 6 wk, alteration in mental status, and infectious endocarditis.

- Beta-adrenergic blocking agents should generally be given to all patients with evolving acute MI. Before using beta-blockers, some of the contraindications and side effects (i.e., exacerbation of asthma, central nervous system effects, hypotension, bradycardia) must be carefully assessed. Beta-blockers are useful to reduce myocardial oxygen consumption and prevent tachyarrhythmias. Early IV beta-blockage (in the initial 24 hr) followed by institution of an oral maintenance regimen is also effective in reducing recurrent infarction and ischemia. Frequently used agents are:
  ○ Metoprolol: IV 5 mg q2min for three doses, then PO 25 to 50 mg q6h, given 15 min after last IV dose, continued for 48 hr; maintenance dosage is 50 to 100 mg bid.
  ○ Atenolol: IV 5 mg over 5 min, repeat in 10 min if initial dose is well tolerated, then start PO dose 10 min after the last IV dose; PO 50 mg qd, increasing to 100 mg as tolerated.
- Angiotensin-converting enzyme inhibitors (ACEIs) reduce left ventricular dysfunction and dilation and slow the progression of CHF during and after acute MI. They should be initiated within hours of hospitalization, provided the patient does not have hypotension or a contraindication (bilateral renal stenosis, renal failure, or history of angioedema caused by previous treatment with ACEIs). Angioten-sin receptor blockers offer no advantage over ACEIs and should be considered only in patients who have a contraindication to the use of ACEIs or cannot tolerate them.
  ○ Commonly used ACEIs are ramipril 2.5 mg qd, captopril 12.5 mg PO bid, enalapril 2.5 mg bid, or lisinopril 2.5 to 5 mg qd initially, with subsequent titration as needed. Ramipril is associated with lower mortality rate than most ACEIs.
  ○ ACEIs may be stopped in patients without complications and no evidence of left ventricular dysfunction after 6 to 8 wk.
  ○ ACEIs should be continued indefinitely in patients with impaired left ventricular function (ejection fraction <40%) or clinical CHF.
- Glycoprotein IIb receptor inhibitors (tirofiban, eptifibatide), when administered with heparin and aspirin, further reduce the incidence of ischemic events in high-risk patients with NSTEMI. The use of IV glycoprotein IIb/IIIa inhibitors (e.g., abciximab) during PCI also reduces the risk of target vessel closure after angioplasty. However, the usefulness of initiating therapy for PCI prior to arrival to the cardiac catheterization laboratory is uncertain.
- Assess fasting lipid profile preferably within 24 hr of MI, and initiate statin therapy before hospital discharge to keep low-density lipoprotein cholesterol <70 mg/dl. Consider addition of fenofibrate or niacin if triglycerides are significantly elevated or high-density lipoprotein cholesterol is very low.
- Long-term aldosterone blockade should be prescribed for post-STEMI patients without significant renal dysfunction (Cr ≤2.5 mg/dl in men and ≤2.0 mg/dl in women) or hyperkalemia who are already taking an ACEI and have left ventricular ejection fraction <0.40, and have symptomatic heart failure or diabetes.
- Patients with STEMI who are not undergoing reperfusion therapy and do not have a contraindication to anticoagulation may be treated with IV or SC unfractionated heparin or with SC low-molecular-weight heparin for at least 48 hr. In the patient with prolonged bed rest or limited activity, treatment should continue until the patient is ambulatory.

CHRONIC Rx

- Discharge medications in all patients with MI (unless contraindicated) should include antiischemic medications (e.g., nitroglycerin, beta-blocker), lipid-lowering agents, and aspirin (81 to 325 mg/day). Clopidogrel 75 mg/day can be given in addition to aspirin for up to 12 mo or in place of aspirin in those who cannot tolerate aspirin. If CABG is planned, clopidogrel should be withheld 5 to 7 days before the procedure.
- The addition of ACEIs is also recommended in all patients with diabetes, CHF, and in those with ejection fraction <40%.
- Evaluation of post-MI patients:
  ○ Submaximal exercise (low level) treadmill test (can be done 1 to 3 wk after MI) in

TABLE 1-128 Dosing Regimens of Commonly Used Thrombolytic Agents

Thrombolytic Agents	Dosing Regimen
t-PA (alteplase)	15 mg bolus IV, followed by 0.75 mg/kg body weight (not to exceed 50 mg) over 30 min, followed by 0.5 mg/kg (not to exceed 35 mg) over 60 min
r-PA (reteplase)	Two 10U IV boluses, given 30 min apart
TNK-tPA (tenecteplase)	Single bolus IV 0.5 mg/kg (dose rounded to the nearest 5 mg, ranging from 30 to 50 mg)
Streptokinase	1.5 million U IV over 60 min

IV, Intravenous; *PA*, plasminogen activator; *r-PA*, reteplase plasminogen activator; *TNK-tPA*, tenecteplase tissue plasminogen activator; *U*, units.
From Andreoli TE et al: *Andreoli and Carpenter's Cecil essential of medicine*, ed 8, Philadelphia, 2010, Saunders.

TABLE 1-129 Contraindications to Thrombolytic Therapy in Acute Myocardial Infarction

Absolute

Suspected aortic dissection
Active bleeding*
Any prior cerebral hemorrhage
Intracranial neoplasm
Cerebral aneurysm or arteriovenous malformation
Ischemic cerebrovascular accident within 3 months

Relative

Bleeding diathesis, coagulopathy, or anticoagulant use
Major surgery within 3 wk
Puncture of a noncompressible vessel, internal bleeding, or head or major body trauma within previous 2 wk
Nonhemorrhagic stroke or gastrointestinal hemorrhage within 6 mo
Proliferative retinopathy
Active peptic ulcer disease
History of chronic, severe, poorly controlled hypertension
Severe uncontrolled hypertension on presentation (systolic blood pressure >180 mm Hg or diastolic blood pressure >110 mm Hg)
Traumatic or prolonged (>10 min) cardiopulmonary resuscitation
Pregnancy

*Does not include menstrual bleeding.
From Andreoli TE et al: *Andreoli and Carpenter's Cecil essential of medicine*, ed 8, Philadelphia, 2010, Saunders.

stable patients who did not undergo cardiac catheterization.

1. Useful to assess the patient's functional capacity and formulate an at-home exercise program
2. Helpful to determine the patient's prognosis

○ Radionuclide angiography or two-dimensional echocardiography:

1. To evaluate patient's left ventricular ejection fraction
2. To evaluate ventricular size and segmental wall motion
3. Echocardiography to rule out presence of mural thrombi in patients suspected of having an extensive infarction; contrast echocardiography is added if mural thrombosis is suspected

○ Primary prevention of sudden cardiac death: Forty days after MI, patients with left ventricular ejection fraction <40% and nonsustained ventricular tachycardia may be candidates for programmed electrical stimulation studies and implanted defibrillator, depending on the results of these studies. Patients with left ventricular ejection fraction <35% and class 2 or 3 heart failure, or left ventricular ejection fraction ≤30% with or without heart failure should be considered for implanted defibrillator if the life expectancy is >1 yr.

DISPOSITION

The prognosis after MI depends on multiple factors:

- Use of beta-blockers: the mortality rate of patients on a regular regimen of beta-blockers is significantly decreased compared with that of control groups. Discharge medication in patients with UA/NSTEMI should include a beta-blocker in all patients without contraindications.
- In patients ≤75 yr who have STEMI and receive aspirin and a standard fibrinolytic regimen, the addition of clopidogrel improves the patency rate of the infarct-related artery and reduces ischemic complications.
- Presence of arrhythmias, frequent ventricular ectopy (≥10/hr), or repetitive forms of ventricular ectopic beats (couplets, triplets) indicates an increased risk (two to three times greater) of sudden cardiac death. New bundle branch block, Mobitz II second-degree block, and third-degree heart block also adversely affect outcome.

- Size of infarct: the larger it is, the higher the post-MI mortality rate. Significant myocardial stunning with subsequent improvement of ventricular function occurs in most patients after anterior MI. A lower level of creatine kinase, an estimate of the extent of necrosis, is independently predictive of recovery of function.
- Site of infarct: inferior wall MI carries a better prognosis than anterior wall MI; however, patients with inferior wall MI and right ventricular involvement have a high risk for arrhythmic complications and cardiac shock.
- Ejection fraction after MI: the lower the left ventricular ejection fraction, the higher the mortality rate after MI. The risk of death is highest in the first 30 days after MI among patients with left ventricular dysfunction, heart failure, or both.
- Presence of post-MI angina indicates a high mortality rate.
- Performance on low-level exercise test: the presence of ST-segment changes during the test is a predictor of high mortality rate during the first year.
- Presence of pericarditis during the acute phase of MI increases mortality rate at 1 yr.
- Type A behavior (competitive drive, ambitiousness, hostility) is associated with a lower mortality rate after symptomatic MI.
- The Killip classification is an independent predictor of all-cause mortality in patients with non–ST elevation acute coronary syndromes.
- Self-reported moderate alcohol consumption in the year before acute MI is associated with reduced 1-yr mortality rate.
- Discharge medication in patients with MI should include lipid-lowering agents. Statins may also lower vascular inflammation and damage by mechanisms other than reduction of low-density lipoprotein cholesterol. Early initiation of statin treatment in patients with acute MI is associated with reduced 1-yr mortality rate.
- Additional poor prognostic factors include cigarette smoking, history of hypertension or prior MI, presence of ST-segment depression in acute MI, increasing age, diabetes mellitus, and female sex (especially women >50 yr).
- Renal disease, even mild, as assessed by the estimated glomerular filtration rate, is a major risk factor for cardiovascular complications after MI.
- Although black patients with MI have worse outcomes than white patients, these differences did not persist after adjustment for patient factors and site of care.

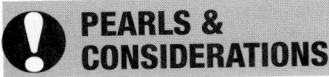

PEARLS & CONSIDERATIONS

COMMENTS

- A recent trial (ICTUS) comparing early invasive and selectively invasive management for acute coronary syndromes failed to show that, given optimized medical therapy, an early invasive strategy is superior to a selective invasive strategy in patients with NSTEMI. All 1200 patients in this trial received aggressive medical therapy, including aspirin, clopidogrel, enoxaparin for 48 hr, abciximab during PCI, and intensive lipid-lowering therapy. The mortality rate was the same in the two groups (2.5%).
- Approximately 1.5 million patients undergo PCI in the United States each year. Depending on local practices and the diagnostic criteria used, 5% to 30% of these patients have evidence of a periprocedural myocardial infarction.
- The 12-lead ECG has low sensitivity for the detection of MI if the culprit lesion is in the left circumflex artery (LCA). If the initial 12 lead ECG is not diagnostic and high clinical suspicion for acute coronary syndrome exists, it is reasonable to obtain additional posterior chest leads (V7-V9) to detect LCA occlusion.

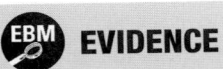 **EVIDENCE**

available at www.expertconsult.com

SUGGESTED READINGS
available at www.expertconsult.com

AUTHORS: **WEN-CHIH WU, M.D.,** and **FRED F. FERRI, M.D.**

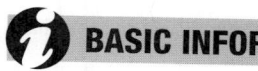

BASIC INFORMATION

DEFINITION

Myocarditis is an inflammatory condition of the myocardium.

ICD-9CM CODES
429.0	Myocarditis, nonspecific
391.2	Myocarditis, rheumatic
422.91	Myocarditis, viral (except Coxsackie)
074.23	Myocarditis, Coxsackie
422.92	Myocarditis, bacterial

EPIDEMIOLOGY & DEMOGRAPHICS

- The incidence of focal myocarditis reported at autopsy is 1% to 7% in asymptomatic patients and ≥50% in patients infected with HIV.
- Myocarditis is a major cause of sudden unexpected death (15% to 20% of cases) in adults <40 yr.

PHYSICAL FINDINGS & CLINICAL PRESENTATION

- Persistent tachycardia out of proportion to fever
- Faint S_1, S_4 sound on auscultation
- Murmur of mitral regurgitation
- Pericardial friction rub if associated with pericarditis
- Signs of biventricular failure (hypotension, hepatomegaly, peripheral edema, distention of neck veins, S_3)
- Patients may present with a history of recent flulike syndrome (fever, arthralgias, malaise); children often have a more fulminant presentation. Difficulty breathing is the most common presentation of pediatric myocarditis
- Most common presentations are dyspnea (72% of patients), chest pain (32%), arrhythmias (18%)
- Sudden cardiac death

ETIOLOGY

- Infection
  1. Viral (Coxsackie B virus, cytomegalovirus, echovirus, polio virus, adenovirus, mumps, HIV, Epstein-Barr virus)
  2. Bacterial (*Staphylococcus aureus, Clostridium perfringens,* diphtheria, and any severe bacterial infection)
  3. Mycoplasma
  4. Mycotic (*Candida, Mucor, Aspergillus*)
  5. Parasitic (*Trypanosoma cruzi—most common worldwide, Trichinella, Echinococcus,* amoeba, *Toxoplasma*)
  6. *Rickettsia rickettsii*
  7. Spirochetal (*Borrelia burgdorferi*–Lyme carditis)
- Rheumatic fever
- Drugs (e.g., cocaine, emetine, doxorubicin, sulfonamides, isoniazid, methyldopa, amphotericin B, tetracycline, phenylbutazone, lithium, 5-fluoruracil, phenothiazines, interferon-alfa, tricyclic antidepressants, cyclophosphamides)
- Toxins (carbon monoxide, ethanol, diphtheria toxin, lead, arsenicals)
- Systemic and collagen-vascular disease (systemic lupus erythematosus, scleroderma, sarcoidosis, and Kawasaki syndrome)
- Radiation
- Postpartum status

DIAGNOSIS

DIFFERENTIAL DIAGNOSIS

- Cardiomyopathy
- Acute myocardial infarction
- Valvulopathies

The differential diagnosis of chest pain is described in Section II.

WORKUP

- Medical history: the clinical presentation of myocarditis is nonspecific and can consist of fatigue, palpitations, dyspnea, precordial discomfort, and myalgias.
- Diagnostic workup includes chest x-ray examination, ECG, laboratory evaluation, echocardiogram, cardiac catheterization, and endomyocardial biopsy (in selected patients on the basis of the likelihood of finding specific treatable disorders such as giant cell myocarditis).

LABORATORY TESTS

- Elevated cardiac troponin T is suggestive of myocarditis in patients with clinically suspected myocarditis. Troponin I specificity is 89%; sensitivity is 34%. A normal level does not rule out the diagnosis.
- Increased creatine kinase (with elevated MB fraction, lactate dehydrogenase), and aspartate aminotransferase from myocardial necrosis.
- Increased erythrocyte sedimentation rate (nonspecific but may be of value in following the progress of the disease and the response to therapy).
- Increased white blood cell count (increased eosinophils if parasitic infection).
- Viral titers (acute and convalescent).
- Cold agglutinin titer, antistreptolysin O titer, blood cultures.
- Lyme disease antibody titer.

IMAGING STUDIES

- Chest radiograph: enlargement of cardiac silhouette
- ECG: sinus tachycardia with nonspecific ST-T wave changes; interventricular conduction defects and bundle branch block may be present
  1. Lyme disease and diphtheria cause all degrees of heart block.
  2. Changes of acute myocardial infarction can occur with focal necrosis.
- Echocardiogram:
  1. Dilated and hypokinetic chambers
  2. Segmental wall motion abnormalities
- Cardiac catheterization and angiography:
  1. To rule out coronary artery disease and valvular disease.
  2. A right ventricular endomyocardial biopsy can confirm the diagnosis, although a negative biopsy result does not exclude myocarditis. Recent studies have shown that myocardial biopsy may be unnecessary because immunosuppression therapy based on biopsy results is generally ineffective.

- Cardiac MRI is a newer promising modality in suspected myocarditis. Regions of myocarditis are reported to correlate closely with regions of abnormal signal on cardiac MRI.

TREATMENT

NONPHARMACOLOGIC THERAPY

- Supportive care is the first line of therapy for patients with myocarditis.
- Restrict physical activity (to decrease cardiac work). Bed rest is advisable during viremia.

ACUTE GENERAL Rx

- Treat underlying cause (e.g., use specific antibiotics for bacterial infection).
- Treat congestive heart failure (CHF) with diuretics, angiotensin-converting enzyme inhibitors, and salt restriction. A beta-blocker may be added once clinical stability has been achieved. Digoxin should be used with caution and only at low doses.
- Antiarrhythmics if needed for ventricular arrhythmias.
- Provide anticoagulation to prevent thromboembolism in severe left ventricular dysfunction or if atrial fibrillation occurs.
- Ionotropes or mechanical assist devices if severe heart failure or cardiovascular collapse is present.
- Corticosteroid use is contraindicated in early infectious myocarditis; it may be justified in only selected patients with intractable CHF, severe systemic toxicity, and severe life-threatening arrhythmias.
- Immunosuppressive drugs (prednisone with cyclosporine or azathioprine) do not have any significant effect on the prognosis of myocarditis and should not be used in the routine treatment of patients with myocarditis. Immunosuppression may have a role in the treatment of myocarditis from systemic autoimmune disease (e.g., lupus, scleroderma) and in patients with idiopathic giant cell myocarditis.

DISPOSITION

Nearly 50% of patients with myocarditis will die within 5 yr of diagnosis. Prognosis is best for patients with fulminant lymphocytic myocarditis (severe hemodynamic compromise, rapid onset of symptoms, or high fever). These patients tend to have complete recovery with total resolution of myocarditis on repeat biopsy.

REFERRAL

Consider heart transplant if patient develops intractable CHF.

EVIDENCE

available at www.expertconsult.com

SUGGESTED READINGS

available at www.expertconsult.com

AUTHORS: **SCOTT COHEN, M.D.,**
FRED F. FERRI, M.D., and
GAURAV CHOUDHARY, M.D.

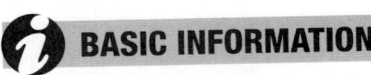

BASIC INFORMATION

DEFINITION

Myoclonus is defined as sudden, brief, jerky, "shocklike" involuntary movements that can involve the muscles of the extremities, face, or trunk. Positive myoclonus is caused by muscle contraction, whereas negative myoclonus is caused by inhibition of active (such as postural) muscles. Myoclonus is a symptom that can be seen in a number of different neurologic disorders.

ICD-9CM CODES
333.2 Myoclonus

EPIDEMIOLOGY & DEMOGRAPHICS

INCIDENCE: 1.3/100,000 persons
PREVALENCE: 8.6/100,000 persons
PREDOMINANT SEX AND AGE: No gender preference; age of onset varies by the etiology of the myoclonus.
GENETICS: Varies by etiology, can be hereditary or sporadic

PHYSICAL FINDINGS & CLINICAL PRESENTATION

- Clinically, myoclonus can be classified by its distribution: focal (only one body part involved), multifocal, segmental (spread to adjacent body parts), axial (muscles innervated by one or several spinal levels), or generalized. It can be stimulus-induced or occur at rest.
- Myoclonus can be seen with involvement or lesions of the cerebral cortex, brainstem, spinal cord, or peripheral nerve. The location of the lesion may not always influence the characteristics of the myoclonus.
- Negative myoclonus is typically seen in postural muscles of the legs, causing a "bobbing" while walking. Asterixis is another form of negative myoclonus.

ETIOLOGY

- The causes of myoclonus are numerous and can be grouped into the categories of physiologic, essential, epileptic, and symptomatic.
- Physiologic myoclonus ranges from sleep (hypnic) jerks to exercise-induced myoclonus and can be seen in normal subjects.
- Essential myoclonus occurs in the absence of other neurologic symptoms and is usually autosomal dominant. When dystonia is present it is called myoclonus-dystonia. The my-

oclonus is often responsive to alcohol in this condition.
- In epileptic myoclonus, seizures dominate the clinical picture. Syndromes include infantile spasms and juvenile myoclonic epilepsy among others.
- Symptomatic or secondary myoclonus comprises myoclonus in the setting of an underlying neurologic disorder or other precipitant. The number of secondary causes prevents giving a full list, but common etiologies include neurodegenerative diseases (Alzheimer's, atypical forms of parkinsonism), CNS infections (Creutzfeldt-Jakob disease, viral encephalitis), metabolic derangements (uremia, hepatic failure), drug-induced (selective serotonin reuptake inhibitors [SSRIs], tricyclics, lithium), and posthypoxic etiologies.

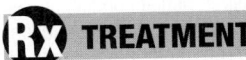

DIAGNOSIS

DIFFERENTIAL DIAGNOSIS

- Tremor: a rhythmic oscillation around a point; slower than myoclonus
- Tic: complex patterned movements that can be suppressed voluntarily for a short time unlike myoclonus, which is simple jerks that are persistent
- Dystonia: patterned contractions of agonist/antagonist muscles causing twisting or pulling; slower than myoclonus
- Chorea: typically slower, writhing, patterned movements
- Psychogenic myoclonus: variable in duration and location, distractible, or entrainable

LABORATORY TESTS

- Evaluate for metabolic precipitants (renal and hepatic function, Mg, Ca, thyroid studies)
- Toxicology screen
- Lumbar puncture if encephalitis is suspected
- Electroencephalography (EEG) to evaluate for epileptic myoclonus

IMAGING STUDIES

MRI of the brain can evaluate for a seizure focus if the myoclonus is epileptic. Creutzfeldt-Jakob disease can show diffusion weighted abnormalities in the striatum and cortex.

TREATMENT

NONPHARMACOLOGIC THERAPY

- Treatment should be directed toward correcting the underlying cause if it is reversible (e.g. hepatic or renal failure).

- Carefully remove or decrease potentially causative medications.

ACUTE GENERAL Rx

For acute treatment of epileptic myoclonus, antiepileptic drugs such as valproic acid, levetiracetam, or clonazepam are helpful.

CHRONIC Rx

- Clonazepam, valproic acid, levetiracetam are typically used for all forms of myoclonus, and often combinations of several medications seem to be more effective.
- If dystonia is present (myoclonus-dystonia), a trial of levodopa is worthwhile although only rarely responsive. Anticholinergics may also help dystonia. Botulinum toxin injections are used for focal dystonias.
- Peripheral focal myoclonus can also be helped by botulinum toxin injections.

DISPOSITION

The ultimate prognosis depends on the etiology of the myoclonus.

REFERRAL

Referral to a general neurologist or movement disorders center is appropriate.

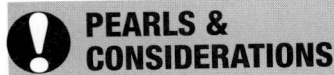

PEARLS & CONSIDERATIONS

COMMENTS

- When myoclonus is seen with parkinsonism, atypical forms of parkinsonism should be high on the differential such as dementia with Lewy bodies, corticobasal degeneration, and multiple system atrophy. Myoclonus is only rarely seen in idiopathic Parkinson's disease.
- Symptomatic palatal myoclonus is a specific syndrome that is often associated with a focal brainstem lesion. In essential palatal myoclonus (no lesion), ear "clicking" is an additional symptom, which is not seen in the symptomatic form.

SUGGESTED READINGS
available at www.expertconsult.com

AUTHOR: **ANDREW DUKER, M.D.**

BASIC INFORMATION

DEFINITION

Inflammatory myopathies are idiopathic diseases of muscle characterized clinically by muscle weakness and pathologically by inflammation and muscle fiber breakdown. The three most common are dermatomyositis (DM), polymyositis (PM), and inclusion body myositis (IBM). See separate topic on "Inclusion Body Myositis" for details regarding the latter.

SYNONYMS

Idiopathic inflammatory myopathies
Myositis syndromes
Polymyositis
Dermatomyositis

ICD-9CM CODES
710.3 Dermatomyositis
710.4 Polymyositis

EPIDEMIOLOGY & DEMOGRAPHICS

DM:

- Occurs in children and in adults (bimodal age peak)
- Average age at diagnosis is 40 in adults. Age range in children: 5 to 14 yr
- More common in females than in males (2:1)
- Incidence 1:100,000
- Prevalence 1 to 10 cases/million in adults and 1 to 3.2 cases/million in children
- Up to one third of patients older than 50 with DM have an associated malignancy

PM:

- Occurs mostly in adults, very rare in children
- Average age at diagnosis >20 yr
- More common in females
- Least common inflammatory myopathy
- Exact incidence unknown

PHYSICAL FINDINGS & CLINICAL PRESENTATION

DM and PM:

- Most patients have a subacute onset over weeks to months.
- Pattern is typically symmetric proximal muscle weakness involving the proximal limbs (shoulder and pelvic girdles).
- Weakness of neck flexion and extension is common.
- Difficulty getting up from a chair, climbing stairs, reaching for objects above head, or combing hair.
- Distal muscle and ocular involvement is uncommon.
- Sensation is preserved.
- Reflexes may be preserved or diminished.
- Dysphagia and dysphonia result from involvement of striated muscle of the pharynx and proximal esophagus.
- Esophageal dysmotility is common in DM.
- Respiratory failure from associated pulmonary fibrosis.
- Cardiac conduction abnormalities can be seen with DM.

- Systemic autoimmune disease occurs frequently in PM, and rarely in DM.
- Skin findings in DM:
  - Heliotrope rash on the upper eyelids (Fig. 1-246)
  - Erythematous rash on the face (see Fig. 1-246)
  - May also involve the back and shoulders (shawl sign), neck and chest (V-shape), knees, and elbows
  - Photosensitivity
  - Gottron's papules (violaceous papules overlying dorsal interphalangeal or metacarpophalangeal areas, elbow or knee joints—Fig. 1-247)
  - Nail cracking, thickening, and irregularity with periungual telangiectasia (see Fig. 1-247)
  - Mechanic's hand: fissured, hyperpigmented, scaly, and hyperkeratotic; also associated with increased risk of interstitial lung disease

ETIOLOGY

DM: complex, immune-mediated microangiopathy. Adaptive immune response via humorally mediated complement attack
PM: unknown

- Cell-mediated immune major histocompatibility-I (MHC-1) process directed against muscle fibers is likely, given biopsy features.
- A viral etiology has been proposed secondary to the presence of autoantibodies to histidyl transferase, anti-Jo-1, and signal recognition particle.

DIAGNOSIS

- Myopathic pattern of muscle weakness
- Characteristic rash in DM
- EMG shows myopathic (small-amplitude, short-duration, polyphasic) motor potentials with early recruitment

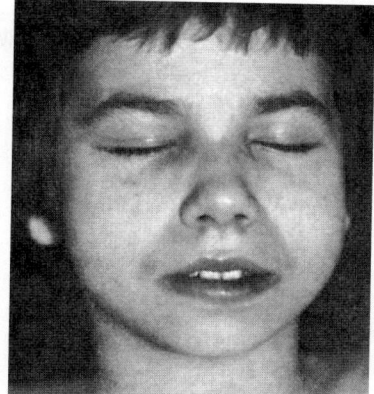

FIGURE 1-246 The facial rash of juvenile dermatomyositis. There is erythema over the bridge of the nose and malar areas, with violaceous (heliotropic) discoloration of the upper eyelids. (From Behrman RE: *Nelson textbook of pediatrics,* ed 17, Philadelphia, 2004, WB Saunders.)

- Majority of patients have "irritable" features (fibrillations and positive sharp waves) on EMG
- See "Laboratory Tests."
- Biopsy is required for diagnosis and should confirm inflammation before treatment is started: myopathic features (variation in fiber size, fiber splitting, fatty replacement of muscle tissue, and increased endomysial connective tissue) should be seen in addition to the following:
  - DM: perifascicular atrophy, MAC deposition along capillaries
  - PM: endomysial infiltrates composed of CD8+ T cells and macrophages invading nonnecrotic muscle fibers that express MHC-I antigen

DIFFERENTIAL DIAGNOSIS

- IBM
- Muscular dystrophies
- Amyloid myoneuropathy
- Amyotrophic lateral sclerosis
- Myasthenia gravis
- Eaton-Lambert syndrome
- Drug-induced myopathies (e.g., quinidine, NSAIDs, penicillamine, HMG CoA-reductase inhibitors)
- Diabetic amyotrophy
- Guillain-Barré syndrome
- Hyperthyroidism or hypothyroidism
- Lichen planus
- Amyopathic DM (rash without weakness)
- Dermatomyositis siné rash (weakness with characteristic biopsy, but no rash)
- Systemic lupus erythematosus (SLE)
- Contact atopic or seborrheic dermatitis
- Psoriasis

LABORATORY TESTS

- Creatine kinase (CK) is the most sensitive muscle enzyme test for muscle breakdown. It should be checked at onset, and serially monitored several times during treatment.
- CK is typically elevated (5-50x normal) in active PM.

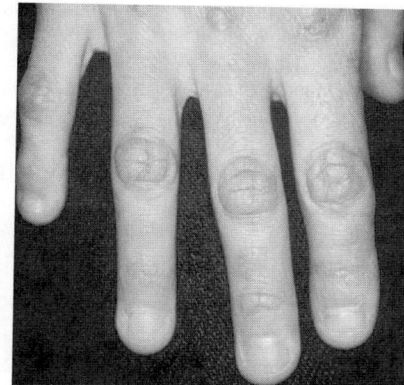

FIGURE 1-247 Dermatomyositis (Gottron's papules). Note erythematous papules over joints and periungual telangiectasias. (From Noble J [ed]: *Textbook of primary care medicine,* ed 2, St Louis, 1996, Mosby.)

- CK may be normal or only slightly elevated in DM.
- Aldolase, AST, ALT, alkaline phosphatase, and LDH may be elevated.
- Anti-Jo-1 antibodies are seen in myositis with associated interstitial lung disease but are not specific for either DM or PM.
- Electrolytes, thyroid-stimulating hormone (TSH), Ca, and Mg should be evaluated to exclude other causes of weakness.
- Check ECG for cardiac involvement.

IMAGING STUDIES

- Chest x-ray is used to rule out pulmonary involvement. If suspicious for pulmonary interstitial disease, a high-resolution CT scan of the chest may be helpful.
- Video fluoroscopy or barium swallow study to look for upper esophageal dysfunction in patients with dysphagia and DM.

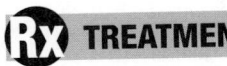 **TREATMENT**

Goal: maintain function, minimize disease/iatrogenic sequelae

NONPHARMACOLOGIC THERAPY

- Sun-blocking agents with SPF 15 or greater for skin protection in patients with DM
- Physical therapy beneficial for gait training and increasing muscle tone and strength
- Occupational therapy assists with activities of daily living
- Speech therapy to monitor patients with swallowing dysfunction

ACUTE GENERAL Rx

- Corticosteroids are the mainstay of therapy. Start prednisone 1 to 2 mg/kg per day, up to a maximum dose of 100 mg/day. Continue until muscle strength improves or muscle enzymes have normalized for at least 4 wk. Begin tapering by 10 mg/mo until 60 mg/day, then slowly taper by 5 mg/mo. Consider every-other-day prednisone treatment at same dose (may decrease side effects).
- Consider IV immunoglobulin (IVIG) if patient fails to improve on prednisone, or muscle enzymes begin rising when tapering off prednisone. See "Chronic Rx" for specific dosage.
- Hydroxychloroquine can be used to treat the cutaneous lesions of DM.

CHRONIC Rx

- Chronic prednisone therapy may be needed for years, but other immunosuppressive ("steroid-sparing") agents may be added early to decrease long-term steroid side effects.
- Azathioprine 2 to 3 mg/kg per day tapered to 1 mg/kg per day once steroid is tapered to 15 mg/day. Reduce dosage monthly by 25-mg intervals. Maintenance dosage is 50 mg/day.
- Methotrexate 7.5 to 10 mg PO/wk, increased by 2.5 mg/wk to total of 25 mg/wk; consider IM dosing if PO is ineffective.
- IV immunoglobulin 2 g/kg total dose over 2 to 5 days.
- IV cyclophosphamide 1 g/M^2 monthly for 6 mo is preferred to oral dosing for refractory cases. However, oral dosing of cyclophosphamide is 1 to 3 mg/kg per day PO or 2 to 4 mg/kg per day in conjunction with prednisone.
- Cyclosporin A: initial dose 2.0 to 2.5 mg/kg bid; long-term maintenance is lowest effective dose.
- Mycophenolate mofetil 500 mg PO bid, titrate to 1500 mg PO bid over 1 to 2 mo.
- Hydroxychloroquine 200 mg PO daily; monitor for visual changes.

DISPOSITION

- 30% to 40% of patients achieve clinical remission with treatment.
- In patients with residual weakness, deficits typically remain stable over long-term follow-up.
- 10% experience recurrent disease.
- Serum CK often returns to normal before symptoms improve.
- During exacerbations, enzymes may rise before clinical symptoms appear.
- Poor prognostic indicators include delay in diagnosis, older age, recalcitrant disease, malignancy, interstitial pulmonary fibrosis, dysphagia, leukocytosis, fever, and anorexia.
- Infection, malignancy, and cardiac and pulmonary dysfunction are the most common causes of death.
- With early treatment, 5- and 8-yr survival rates of 80% and 73%, respectively, have been reported.

REFERRAL

Neurology or rheumatology referral should be made to help establish the diagnosis and implement treatment.

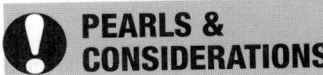 **PEARLS & CONSIDERATIONS**

- Do not implement treatment before muscle biopsy.
- When assessing response to treatment, clinical muscle strength is more important than muscle enzyme tests.
- The concern for malignancies (ovary, lung, breast, GI) associated with DM is legitimate and merits screening in patients older than age 40 at time of diagnosis and every 2 to 3 yr thereafter.
- There does not appear to be any association between juvenile DM and malignancy.
- Overlap syndrome refers to patients with DM who also meet criteria for a connective tissue disorder (e.g., rheumatoid arthritis, scleroderma, SLE).
- In any patient taking steroids, closely monitor for:
  - Diabetes or glucose intolerance (2-hour oral glucose tolerance test)
  - Osteopenia/osteoporosis (DEXA scan q6mo)
  - Cataracts (yearly ophthalmologic appointment)
  - Hypertension
  - Psychiatric side effects including depression or psychosis
  - Poor sleep
  - Peptic ulcer disease (prescribe H+ antagonist or proton pump inhibitor)
- Clinical and immune response features can be used for categorizing heterogeneous myositis syndromes and mutually exclusive and stable phenotypes and are useful for predicting clinical signs and symptoms, associated environmental and genetic risk factors, and responses to therapy and prognosis.

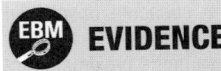 **EVIDENCE**

available at www.expertconsult.com

AUTHOR: **GAVIN BROWN, M.D.**

BASIC INFORMATION

DEFINITION

Myotonia is a type of muscular dystrophy in which relaxation of a muscle after contraction is delayed or prolonged. The most common type of muscular dystrophy with myotonia is myotonic dystrophy.

SYNONYMS

Myotonic dystrophy

ICD-9CM CODES
359.2   Myotonic disorders
728.85 Muscle spasm

EPIDEMIOLOGY & DEMOGRAPHICS

- Three to five cases/100,000 persons.
- Genetic disorder inherited as an autosomal-dominant illness.
- Symptoms usually manifest during adolescence or early adulthood. Cases of infantile myotonic dystrophy have been described.

PHYSICAL FINDINGS & CLINICAL PRESENTATION

- Usual first symptom is distal extremity weakness sometimes associated with muscle stiffness, cramps, or difficulty relaxing grasp.
- Weakness spreads to eventually involve all muscle groups. Flexor neck muscle weakness and masseter and temporal wasting are often prominent features, as is dysarthria.
- Percussion of a muscle produces a slow contraction followed by prolonged relaxation. The myotonic reflex is best tested by percussing the thenar muscles and observing a slow flexion followed by slow relaxation of the thumb.
- As the disease progresses, generalized weakness becomes more pronounced and myotonia becomes less evident.
- Extramuscular involvement:
  - Mental retardation of variable severity (may be absent)
  - Frontal baldness (Fig. 1-248)
  - Cataracts
  - Diabetes mellitus
  - Hypogonadism
  - Adrenal failure
  - Cardiomyopathy
- Infantile myotonic dystrophy presents as neonatal extreme hypotonia with "shark mouth" deformity (upper lip forming an inverted V).

ETIOLOGY & PATHOGENESIS

Genetic disorder encoded on chromosome 19 leading to sustained firing of the muscle membrane, causing prolonged muscle contraction. Myotonic dystrophy 1 (the more common form) is caused by an expanded CTG repeat within the noncoding 3′ untranslated region of the myotonic dystrophy protein kinase *(DMPK)* gene. The less common form (myotonic dystrophy 2) is caused by an expanded CCTG repeat in the first intron of the zinc finger protein 9 *(ZNF9)* gene.

DIAGNOSIS

DIFFERENTIAL DIAGNOSIS

The disease is limited to muscles and causes hypertrophy and stiffness after rest. Muscle function normalizes with exercise. There is no weakness. Symptoms are exacerbated by exposure to cold.

- Myotonia congenita (Thomsen's disease)
- May be autosomal dominant or recessive (two distinct varieties)
- Paramyotonia congenita (autosomal-dominant disease): weakness and stiffness of facial muscles and distal upper extremities, especially or exclusively on cold exposure
- Muscular dystrophies
- Inflammatory myopathies (polymyositis)
- Metabolic muscle diseases
- Myasthenic syndromes
- Motor neuron disease

WORKUP

- History and physical examination usually sufficient

- Muscle enzymes usually abnormal (creatine phosphokinase, aldolase, aspartate aminotransferase)
- Electromyography: typical myotonic "dive bomber" bursts
- Muscle biopsy: type I fiber atrophy, ring fibers, increased central nucleation

TREATMENT

- Phenytoin
- Quinine
- Quinidine
- Procainamide
- Acetazolamide
- Genetic counseling
- Assistive devices, orthotics

DISPOSITION

In myotonic dystrophy, death is usually caused by the wasting of skeletal muscle and defects in cardiac function.

REFERRAL

To neurologist

SUGGESTED READINGS
available at www.expertconsult.com

AUTHOR: **FRED F. FERRI, M.D.**

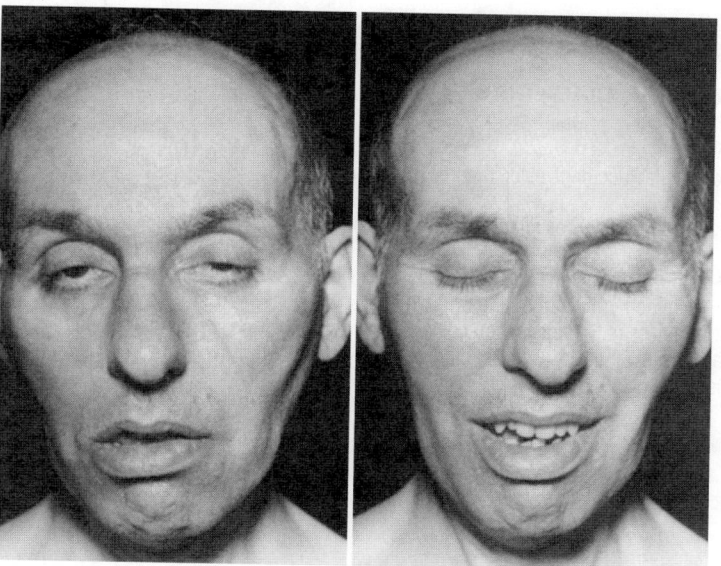

FIGURE 1-248 Myotonic dystrophy with typical myopathic facies, frontal balding, and sunken cheeks. (From Dubowitz V: *Muscle disorders in childhood,* London, 1995, WB Saunders.)

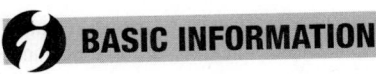

BASIC INFORMATION

DEFINITION

Myxedema coma is a life-threatening complication of hypothyroidism characterized by profound lethargy or coma and usually accompanied by hypothermia.

ICD-9CM CODES
244.8 Myxedema, pituitary
244.1 Myxedema, primary

PHYSICAL FINDINGS & CLINICAL PRESENTATION

- Profound lethargy or coma
- Hypothermia (rectal temperature <35° C [95° F]); often missed by using ordinary thermometers graduated only to 34.5° C or because the mercury is not shaken below 36° C
- Bradycardia, hypotension (attributable to circulatory collapse)
- Delayed relaxation phase of deep tendon reflexes, areflexia
- Myxedema facies (Fig. 1-249)
- Alopecia, macroglossia, ptosis, periorbital edema, nonpitting edema, doughy skin
- Bladder dystonia and distention

ETIOLOGY

Decompensation of hypothyroidism from:
- Sepsis
- Exposure to cold weather
- Central nervous system depressants (sedatives, narcotics, antidepressants)
- Trauma, surgery

DIAGNOSIS

DIFFERENTIAL DIAGNOSIS

- Severe depression, primary psychosis
- Drug overdose
- Cerebrovascular accident, liver failure, renal failure
- Hypoglycemia, CO_2 narcosis, encephalitis

WORKUP

Diagnosis of hypothyroidism and exclusion of contributing factors (e.g., sepsis, cerebrovascular accident) with laboratory and radiographic studies (see "Laboratory Tests")

LABORATORY TESTS

- Markedly increased thyroid-stimulating hormone (if primary hypothyroidism), decreased serum free T_4
- Complete blood count with differential, urine and blood cultures to rule out infectious process
- Electrolytes, blood urea nitrogen, creatinine, liver function tests, calcium, glucose
- Arterial blood gases to rule out hypoxemia and carbon dioxide retention
- Cortisol level to rule out adrenal insufficiency
- Elevated CPK
- Hyperlipidemia

IMAGING STUDIES

- CT scan of head in suspected cerebrovascular accident
- Chest radiograph to rule out infectious process

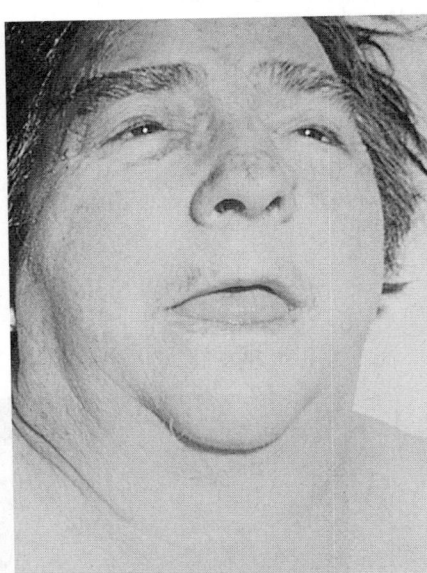

FIGURE 1-249 Myxedema facies. Note dull, puffy, yellowed skin; coarse, sparse hair; temporal loss of eyebrows; periorbital edema; prominent tongue. (Courtesy Paul W. Ladenson, M.D., The Johns Hopkins University and Hospital, Baltimore. In Seidel HM [ed]: *Mosby's guide to physical examination,* ed 5, St Louis, 2004, Mosby.)

TREATMENT

NONPHARMACOLOGIC THERAPY

- Prevent further heat loss; cover the patient but avoid external rewarming because it may produce vascular collapse.
- Support respiratory function; intubation and mechanical ventilation may be required.
- Monitor patients in the intensive care unit.

ACUTE GENERAL Rx

- Give levothyroxine 5 to 8 mcg/kg (300 to 500 mcg) IV infused over 15 min, then 100 mcg IV q24h.
- Glucocorticoids should also be administered until coexistent adrenal insufficiency can be ruled out. Hydrocortisone hemisuccinate 100 mg IV bolus is initially given, followed by 50 mg IV q12h or 25 mg IV q6h until initial plasma cortisol level is confirmed normal.
- IV hydration with D_5NS is used to correct hypotension and hypoglycemia (if present); avoid overhydration and possible water intoxication because clearance of free water is impaired in these patients.
- Rule out and treat precipitating factors (e.g., antibiotics in suspected sepsis).

CHRONIC Rx

Refer to "Hypothyroidism" in Section I.

DISPOSITION

Mortality rate in myxedema coma is 20% to 50%.

REFERRAL

Endocrinology consultation

PEARLS & CONSIDERATIONS

COMMENTS

If the diagnosis is suspected, initiate treatment immediately without waiting for confirming laboratory results.

AUTHOR: **FRED F. FERRI, M.D.**

BASIC INFORMATION

DEFINITION

Narcissistic personality disorder (NPD) is characterized by a pattern of grandiosity, need for admiration, and lack of empathy that begins by early adulthood and causes significant distress or impairment in multiple domains of functioning. The individual must meet five or more of the following criteria:

1. Grandiose sense of self-importance. For example, the person may exaggerate achievements and talents or expect recognition as superior without commensurate achievements.
2. Preoccupied with fantasies of unlimited success, power, brilliance, beauty, or ideal love.
3. Views self as "special" and unique and should only associate with other special or highly regarded people and institutions.
4. Requires excessive admiration.
5. Sense of entitlement. For example, unreasonable expectations of especially favorable treatment or automatic compliance with his or her expectations.
6. Interpersonally exploitative.
7. Lacks empathy—unwilling to recognize or identify with the feelings or needs of others.
8. Often envious of others or believes others envious of him or her.
9. Shows arrogant or haughty behaviors.

SYNONYMS

None

ICD-9CM CODES

301.81

EPIDEMIOLOGY & DEMOGRAPHICS

PREVALENCE: Less than 1% of the general population; estimates range from 2% to 16% in the clinical population
PREDOMINANT SEX: More commonly diagnosed in males (up to 3:1)
PREDOMINANT AGE: 20s and 30s

CLINICAL PRESENTATION

- Patients have an underlying sense of inferiority and inadequacy.
- May be related to the failure of parents or parental surrogates to impart a sense of self-worth.
- To avoid these beliefs and their associated painful effects, patients seek to convince self and others that they are special, the best, or unusually talented.
- Astutely aware of status, pecking order.
- Vulnerability in self-esteem makes these patients exquisitely sensitive to criticism, defeat, or perceived weakness, which in turn can lead to feeling humiliated, degraded, and empty.

- These patients react to perceived slights with either more intense grandiosity and admiration seeking or with disdain and rage. Either approach seeks to bolster their sense of self often by devaluing or criticizing the other person.
- Experiences of self-deflation lead to social withdrawal or depressed mood or to feigned humility that protects grandiosity.
- Interpersonal relationships are typically shallow and limited.
- Although ambition and confidence may lead to high achievement, vocational functioning may be disrupted by intolerance for criticism.

ETIOLOGY

- Limited knowledge about role of genetic loading and neurobiologic vulnerability.
- Prevailing hypotheses focus on impaired development of self as "worthy" because of insufficient affirmation and warmth from parents.

DIAGNOSIS

DIFFERENTIAL DIAGNOSIS

- Mania and hypomania
- Dysthymia and major depressive episode
- Substance-induced euphoria, especially cocaine abuse
- Histrionic, borderline, antisocial, and paranoid personality disorders share common features and are often comorbid
- Personality changes from a general medical condition, including central nervous system processes in the frontal-temporal regions of the brain

WORKUP

- History: collateral information essential to establishing presence of longstanding interpersonal pattern in multiple domains of the patient's life
- Physical examination
- Mental status examination

LABORATORY TESTS

Tests necessary to rule out medical causes of personality changes

IMAGING STUDIES

Those necessary to rule out medical causes of personality changes

TREATMENT

NONPHARMACOLOGIC THERAPY

- Cognitive-behavioral therapy to help patients control rage, manage perceived criticism, and develop social skills

- Psychodynamic psychotherapy to help develop improved self-concept, affect tolerance, and interpersonal functioning

ACUTE GENERAL Rx

Benzodiazepines or low-dose antipsychotics to control rage

CHRONIC Rx

- Selective serotonin reuptake inhibitors for impulsivity or comorbid depression
- Mood stabilizers if comorbid bipolar or to improve impulse control

DISPOSITION

- Severity is variable and course is chronic. The majority of patients obtain greater functioning in fifth decade and beyond when pessimism replaces grandiosity. Often lifelong difficulty maintaining intimate relationships.
- At increased risk for major depressive disorder and substance abuse or dependence (especially cocaine).

REFERRAL

If pharmacotherapy is contemplated

PEARLS & CONSIDERATIONS

COMMENTS

- Illness threatens these patients' image of superiority.
- To defend against this threat, patients may minimize symptoms or deny presence of illness.
- Patients will commonly demand special treatment from senior and well-known physicians.
- Patients may devalue, criticize, or question the behavior or credentials of the treating physician.
- Management guidelines:
  1. Be respectful and nonconfrontational.
  2. Help patient use self-perceived talents in service of treatment.
  3. Do not personalize patient's devaluation, but understand their criticalness as an attempt to manage their own intense insecurity.
  4. Appeal to the patient's narcissism. In other words, agree with the patient that he or she is "entitled" to appropriate care.

SUGGESTED READINGS

available at www.expertconsult.com

AUTHOR: **JOHN Q. YOUNG, M.D., M.P.P.**

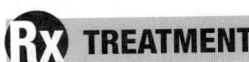

BASIC INFORMATION

DEFINITION

Narcolepsy is a chronic neurologic sleep disorder characterized by excessive daytime sleepiness and dysregulation of rapid eye movement (REM) sleep. It is the second most common cause of disabling daytime sleepiness after obstructive sleep apnea. Symptoms of REM sleep dysregulation include cataplexy, sleep paralysis, and hallucinations during transition between wake and sleep.

SYNONYMS

Hypersomnia of central origin
Narcolepsy with cataplexy
Narcolepsy-cataplexy syndrome
Narcolepsy with hypocretin deficiency
Gelineau syndrome

ICD-9CM CODES

347.00 Narcolepsy without cataplexy
347.01 Narcolepsy with cataplexy

EPIDEMIOLOGY & DEMOGRAPHICS

INCIDENCE: 0.74/100,000 person/yr
PREVALENCE: 5 to 50/100,000 people
PREDOMINANT SEX: Males and females are equally affected.
AGE OF ONSET: Peak 15 to 30 yr (range, 10-55 yr)
GENETICS:
- Associated with specific human leukocyte antigen (HLA) subtypes (e.g., *DQB1*0602*)
- Risk of narcolepsy increases 20 to 40 times if a family member is affected.
- Monozygotic concordance rate is 17% to 36%, thus indicating an incomplete penetrance and suggesting an environmental factor in the disease process.

PHYSICAL FINDINGS & CLINICAL PRESENTATION

- Overwhelming urge to sleep with chronic hypersomnia may occur during the day.
- Cataplexy occurs in 60% to 100% of patients with narcolepsy and is reported as a partial or complete loss of voluntary muscle control with preserved consciousness that is precipitated by a strong emotion, more commonly with laughter. This is the most specific symptom and is considered pathognomonic for narcolepsy.
- Hypnagogic (wake to sleep) or hypnopompic (sleep to wake) hallucinations have been reported in 60% to 80% of patients with narcolepsy.
- Sleep paralysis, defined as loss of muscle tone during the transition between sleep and wakefulness, occurs in 60% to 80% of patients with narcolepsy. It may occur with hallucinations and can be interrupted by sensory stimuli.
- Fragmented sleep is seen in 60% to 80% of narcolepsy patients and can often be mistaken for insomnia or other intrinsic sleep disorder.

- Other symptoms that have been reported in narcolepsy include automatic behavior or semipurposeful movements in 40% of patients and memory disturbance in 50% of patients.

ETIOLOGY

The loss of hypocretin/orexin signaling, genetic factors, and rare brain lesions are presently identified factors in the development of narcolepsy.

HYPOCRETIN/OREXIN:
- Loss of hypocretin-1 and hypocretin-2 (also known as orexin-A and orexin-B) producing neurons in the lateral hypothalamus.
- Human cerebrospinal fluid (CSF) levels of hypocretin-1 are low to undetectable in narcoleptics with cataplexy.
- Narcolepsy without cataplexy may have a different cause because CSF hypocretin levels are usually normal in these patients, so there may be a completely separate mechanism in these patients, or it may result from less extensive loss of hypocretin neurons or impaired signaling.

SECONDARY ETIOLOGIES:
- Tumors, vascular malformations, and strokes have all been reported to cause secondary narcolepsy.
- Direct injury to the hypocretin neurons or their projections is the most likely cause of secondary narcolepsy due to central nervous system lesions.
- Narcolepsy has been reported in genetic syndromes, including Prader-Willi syndrome and Niemann-Pick disease type C, as well as paraneoplastic syndromes.

DIAGNOSIS

DIFFERENTIAL DIAGNOSIS

Excessive daytime somnolence:
- Autism
- Autosomal dominant cerebellar ataxia, deafness, and narcolepsy
- Behaviorally induced insufficient sleep syndrome
- Central or obstructive sleep apnea (sleep-disordered breathing)
- Circadian rhythm disorder
- Depression
- Diencephalic lesions
- Drug or alcohol abuse
- Hypothyroidism
- Idiopathic hypersomnia with long or short sleep time
- Inadequate sleep hygiene
- Increased intracranial pressure
- Insomnia
- Kleine-Levin syndrome
- Medication effect
- Menstrual-related hypersomnia
- Posttraumatic narcolepsy
- Seizures
- Sleep fragmentation (multiple causes)

Cataplexy:
- Seizures
- Periodic paralysis
- Cardiovascular insufficiency
- Psychogenic (multiple causes)

WORKUP

- Narcolepsy is often diagnosed by clinical history. The Epworth Sleepiness Scale is very useful in determining the degree of excessive daytime sleepiness.
- The diagnosis of narcolepsy can be made if there is a clear history of cataplexy in the setting of excessive daytime somnolence, without need for further diagnostic testing. Sleep laboratory testing or possibly laboratory testing is required if these symptoms do not exist.
- The medical history should include questions regarding severity of daytime hypersomnia while also evaluating for sleep-disordered breathing, transient muscle weakness triggered by emotion, hallucinations while falling asleep or upon awakening, and inability to move after awakening. The clinical evaluation should also address symptoms of seizures and paraneoplastic disorders while also asking about previous stroke or genetic disorders. A detailed family history is imperative. Hypothalamic dysfunction such as unexplained weight gain, endocrine abnormalities, circadian dysrhythmias, and autonomic nervous system problems may provide useful insight.
- A thorough examination including a detailed neurological examination should be performed.
- Nocturnal polysomnography followed by a multiple sleep latency test remains to be the gold standard for the diagnosis of narcolepsy. A drug screen should also be performed to rule our pharmacological modulations of sleep.

LABORATORY TESTS

HLA subtyping and CSF hypocretin/orexin levels may be attempted in suspected cases of narcolepsy. CSF hypocretin/orexin analysis is primarily a research tool. CSF hypocretin levels below 110 pg/ml are indicative of narcolepsy, but high CSF hypocretin levels do not exclude the diagnosis.

TREATMENT

NONPHARMACOLOGIC THERAPY

Avoidance of over-the-counter drugs and illicit drugs, optimal sleep hygiene and scheduled daily naps, and psychosocial support can be used for symptoms of excessive daytime somnolence. However, nonpharmacologic therapy is typically not sufficient for treatment of narcolepsy alone but is often used as adjunct therapy with medications.

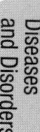

PHARMACOLOGIC THERAPY

For excessive daytime somnolence:
- Sodium oxybate (Xyrem): a central nervous system depressant that can be used for the treatment cataplexy and REM-related symptoms
- Modafinil (Provigil) 200 to 600 mg PO every morning or divided bid
- Armodafinil (Nuvigil) 150 or 250 mg PO as a single dose in the morning
- Methylphenidate (Ritalin) 5 to 15 mg PO bid to tid
- Methylphenidate SR (Concerta) 18 to 54 mg PO every morning or divided bid
- Dextroamphetamine (Dexedrine) 10 to 60 mg PO qd
- Eldepryl (Selegiline HCl) 5 mg PO bid

For cataplexy:
- Sodium oxybate (Xyrem): a central nervous system depressant that can be used for the treatment of cataplexy and REM-related symptoms
- Fluoxetine (Prozac) 20 mg PO qd initially
- Sertraline (Zoloft) 25 mg PO qd initially
- Venlafaxine (Effexor) 25 mg PO qd initially
- Clomipramine (Anafranil) 25 mg/day initially
- Protriptyline (Vivactil) 5 mg tid initially
- Imipramine (Tofranil) 25 to 50 mg/day initially
- Desipramine (Norpramin) 10 mg bid initially

DISPOSITION

This is a chronic sleep disorder that may worsen for the first few years and then persist for life.

REFERRAL

Because of the complexity of this disorder and its ever-changing management and treatment, patients should be referred to centers or programs with highly trained sleep specialists with expertise caring for these patients, especially if sodium oxybate (Xyrem) therapy is needed.

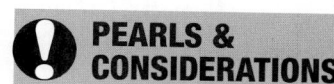

PEARLS & CONSIDERATIONS

Many narcoleptics report the onset of symptoms beginning in childhood to early adulthood with a long delay of actual diagnosis on the order of 10 to 15 yr. Typically, excessive daytime sleepiness is the initial symptom followed by REM dysregulation (e.g., cataplexy, sleep paralysis, hypnagogic hallucinations). Patients with narcolepsy also have higher than expected incidence of other sleep disorders, including obstructive sleep apnea, periodic limb movements of sleep, and REM sleep behavior disorder.

COMMENTS

Narcolepsy is a rare disorder that is underdiagnosed. Cataplexy is specific for narcolepsy, but other symptoms of REM dysregulation, including sleep paralysis and hypnagogic or hypnopompic hallucinations can occur even in normal patients. Sleep-onset REM or REM periods on a MSLT study may occur as a result of sleep deprivation or withdrawal from REM suppressing drugs.

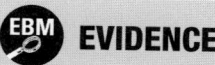 **EVIDENCE**

available at www.expertconsult.com

SUGGESTED READINGS

available at www.expertconsult.com

AUTHOR: **DON HAYES, JR., M.D.**

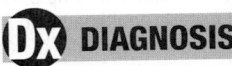

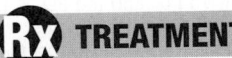 BASIC INFORMATION

DEFINITION

Necrotizing fasciitis is a rapidly spreading bacterial infection with associated inflammation involving deep fascia, leading to necrosis of subcutaneous tissue planes associated with trauma, surgical wounds, or spontaneous or idiopathic.

SYNONYMS

Soft tissue gangrene
Flesh eating bacteria
Fournier's gangrene

ICD-9CM CODES
728.86 Necrotizing fasciitis

EPIDEMIOLOGY & DEMOGRAPHICS

PREDOMINANT SEX: Male > female
PREDOMINANT AGE: 6 to 50 yr of age; rare in children

PHYSICAL FINDINGS & CLINICAL PRESENTATION

- Minor skin trauma, toxic appearing patient
- Open skin wound
- Severe pain at injury or surgical site
- Fever, confusion, weakness, diarrhea
- Early skin erythema, quickly spread hours to days
- Skin redness changes to purple discoloration
- Gangrenous skin changes may develop
- Loosening of skin and subcutaneous skin association with deep fascial necrosis
- Muscle involvement, thrombosis of blood vessels, and myonecrosis may develop
- Bullae and gas formation at site

ETIOLOGY

- Polymicrobal
- Group A streptococci *(S. pyogenes)*
- *S. aureus*
- *C. perfringens*
- *Bacteroides fragilis*
- *Vibrio vulnificus*
- MRSA

DIAGNOSIS

DIFFERENTIAL DIAGNOSIS

- Cellulitis
- Vasculitis
- Gas gangrene

WORKUP

- Labs
  - CBC differential
  - Cultures of skin, soft tissue, or debrided tissue
- Imagining
  - X-rays: subcutaneous gas in fascial planes
  - CT/MRI: may be helpful

TREATMENT

- Aggressive surgical debridement of involved necrotic tissues
- Fasciotomies may be necessary of extremities
- Hyperbaric oxygen (HBO) evaluation
- Empiric antibiotic treatment:
  - Penicillin or extended spectrum penicillins
  - Clindamycin
  - Metronidazole
  - Ceftriaxone, gentamicin

SUGGESTED READINGS
available at www.expertconsult.com

AUTHOR: **DENNIS J. MIKOLICH, M.D.**

BASIC INFORMATION

DEFINITION

Malignant renal tumor derived from primitive metanephric blastoma. Most tumors are unicentric, but some are multifocal in one or both kidneys. Associated anomalies may be present.

SYNONYMS

Wilms' tumor

ICD-9CM CODES
189.0 Nephroblastoma

EPIDEMIOLOGY & DEMOGRAPHICS

- Pediatric malignancy mean presentation is at 41.5 mo in boys and 46.9 mo in girls
- Slightly more frequent in girls
- Incidence rate is 7.9 cases per year per 1 million white children <15 yr (a little over 500 new cases annually in the U.S.); the incidence is double in black children
- Associated syndromes:
  1. Cryptorchidism
  2. Hypospadias
  3. Hemihypertrophy with or without the Beckwith-Wiedemann syndrome, aniridia
  4. Denys-Drash syndrome (nephroblastoma, pseudohermaphrodism, glomerulonephritis)
  5. WAGR syndrome (**W**ilms' tumor, **a**niridia, **g**enitourinary malformations, and mental **r**etardation)
- Familial nephroblastoma occurs in 1.5% (with younger age at diagnosis and more frequent multifocal tumors)

PHYSICAL FINDINGS & CLINICAL PRESENTATION

- Nephroblastoma often is discovered when a parent notices a mass while bathing or dressing a child, most commonly a child who is approximately age 3 yr, or during a routine physical examination. The mass is unilateral, firm, and nontender and below the costal margin.
- Abdominal swelling and/or pain
- Nausea
- Vomiting
- Constipation
- Loss of appetite
- Fever of unknown origin
- Night sweats
- Hematuria (less common than in adult renal malignancies)
- Malaise
- High blood pressure that is triggered when the tumor obstructs the renal artery
- Varicocele
- Signs of associated syndromes

ETIOLOGY & PATHOGENESIS

- Three cell types: blastomal, stromal, and epithelial may be present. Structural diversity is characteristic.
- Anaplasia is evidenced by the presence of gigantic polyploid nuclei. The term *focal anaplasia* is used to describe such findings when it is confined within the primary tumor in the kidney.
- Staging:
  Stage I: Tumor limited to the kidney whose capsule is intact. The tumor is completely excised.
  Stage II: Tumor extends beyond the kidney but is completely excised. No peritoneal involvement.
  Stage III: Residual tumor confined to the abdomen after surgery. No hematogenous metastases.
  Stage IV: Hematogenous metastases present.
  Stage V: Bilateral renal involvement at time of initial diagnosis.

DIAGNOSIS

DIFFERENTIAL DIAGNOSIS

- Other renal malignancies
  1. Hypernephroma
  2. Transitional cell carcinoma
  3. Lymphoma
  4. Clear cell sarcoma
  5. Rhabdoid tumor of the kidney
- Renal cyst
- Other intraabdominal or retroperitoneal tumors

LABORATORY TESTS

- Complete blood count
- Transaminases (alanine aminotransferase, aspartate aminotransferase)
- Alkaline phosphatase
- Blood urea nitrogen and creatinine
- Serum calcium
- Urinalysis

IMAGING STUDIES

- Renal ultrasound to confirm existence of a solid mass in a kidney
- Abdominal CT scan with contrast (Fig. 1-250)
- Chest radiograph or CT scan

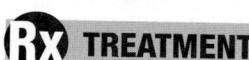 TREATMENT

- Surgical resection and surgical staging:
  1. Stages I and II: surgery followed by chemotherapy
  2. Stages III and IV: surgery followed by radiation and chemotherapy
- Chemotherapeutic agents used in the treatment of nephroblastoma include vincristine, dactinomycin, and doxorubicin

PROGNOSIS

- Stage I: 95% survival
- Stage II: 91% survival
- Stage III: 91% survival
- Stage IV: 81% survival
- Prognosis is better for patients <2 yr

AUTHOR: **FRED F. FERRI, M.D.**

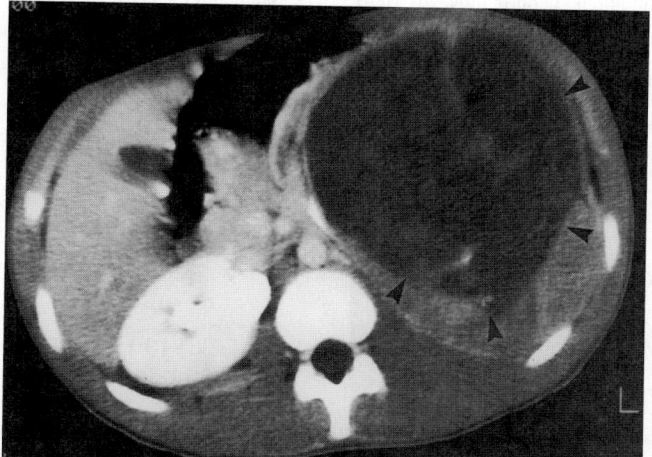

FIGURE 1-250 Transverse computed tomographic image of a nephroblastoma (Wilms' tumor) shows a large intrarenal mass. (From Abeloff MD [ed]: *Clinical oncology*, ed 3, Philadelphia, 2004, Elsevier.)

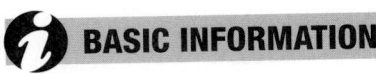

BASIC INFORMATION

DEFINITION

Nephrotic syndrome is characterized by high urine protein excretion (>3.5 g/1.73 m^3/24 hr), peripheral edema, and metabolic abnormalities (hypoalbuminemia, hypercholesterolemia).

ICD-9CM CODES
581.9 Nephrotic syndrome

EPIDEMIOLOGY & DEMOGRAPHICS

- Nephrotic syndrome occurs predominantly in children ages 2 to 6 yr (2 new cases/100,000 persons/yr) and in adults of all ages (3 to 4 new cases/100,000 persons/yr).
- Membranous glomerulonephritis is the most common cause of nephrotic syndrome.

PHYSICAL FINDINGS & CLINICAL PRESENTATION

- Peripheral edema, eyelid edema (Fig. 1-251)
- Ascites, anasarca
- Hypertension
- Pleural effusion
- Typically patients present with severe peripheral edema, exertional dyspnea, and abdominal fullness secondary to ascites. There is a significant amount of weight gain in most patients

ETIOLOGY

- Idiopathic (may be secondary to the following glomerular diseases: minimal change disease [nil disease, lipoid nephrosis], focal segmental glomerular sclerosis, membranous nephropathy, membranoproliferative glomerular nephropathy) PLA 2 R is a major antigen in the majority of patients with idiopathic membranous nephropathy. An HLA-DQA$_1$ allele on chromosome 6p21 is most closely associated with idiopathic membranous nephropathy in persons of white ancestry. This allele may facilitate an autoimmune response against targets such as variants of PLA 2 R1
- Associated with systemic diseases (diabetes mellitus, SLE, amyloidosis). Amyloidosis and dysproteinemias should be considered in patients older than 40 yr
- Majority of children with nephrotic syndrome have minimal change disease (this form also associated with allergy, nonsteroidals, and Hodgkin's disease)
- Focal glomerular disease: can be associated with HIV infection, heroin abuse. A more severe form of nephrotic syndrome associated with rapid progression to end-stage renal failure within months can also occur in HIV seropositive patients and is known as "collapsing glomerulopathy"
- Membranous nephropathy: can occur with Hodgkin's lymphoma, carcinomas, SLE, gold therapy
- Membranoproliferative glomerulonephropathy: often associated with upper respiratory infections

DIAGNOSIS

DIFFERENTIAL DIAGNOSIS

- Other edema states (CHF, cirrhosis)
- Primary renal disease (e.g., focal glomerulonephritis, membranoproliferative glomerulonephritis). The differentiation between nephrotic syndrome and nephritic syndrome is described in Table 1-130. Table 1-131 summarizes primary renal diseases that present as idiopathic nephrotic syndrome
- Carcinoma, infections
- Malignant hypertension
- Polyarteritis nodosa
- Serum sickness
- Toxemia of pregnancy

WORKUP

Diagnostic workup consists of family history and history of drug use or toxin exposure and laboratory evaluation. Renal biopsy is generally performed in individuals with persistent proteinuria in whom the etiology of the proteinuria is unclear.

LABORATORY TESTS

- Urinalysis reveals proteinuria. The presence of hematuria, cellular casts, and pyuria is suggestive of nephritic syndrome. Oval fat bodies (tubular epithelial cells with cholesterol esters) are also found in the urine in patients with nephrotic syndrome.
- 24-hr urine protein excretion is >3.5 g/ 1.73 m^3/24 hr.
- Abnormalities of blood chemistries include serum albumin <3 g/dl, decreased total protein, elevated serum cholesterol, glucose, azotemia.
- Additional tests in patients with nephrotic syndromes depending on the history and physical examination are ANA, serum and urine immunoelectrophoresis, C3, C4, CH-50, LDH, liver enzymes, alkaline phosphatase, hepatitis B and C screening, and HIV.

IMAGING STUDIES

- Ultrasound of kidneys
- Chest radiograph

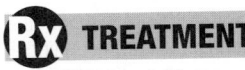 TREATMENT

NONPHARMACOLOGIC THERAPY

- Bed rest as tolerated, avoidance of nephrotoxic drugs, low-fat diet, fluid restriction in hyponatremic patients; normal protein intake unless urinary protein loss exceeds 10 g/24 hr (some patients may require additional dietary protein to prevent negative nitrogen balance and significant protein malnutrition)
- Improved urinary protein excretion and serum lipid changes have been observed with a low-fat soy protein diet providing 0.7 g of protein/kg/day. However, because of increased risk of malnutrition, many nephrologists recommend normal protein intake
- Strict sodium restriction to help manage peripheral edema
- Close monitoring of patients for development of peripheral venous thrombosis and renal vein thrombosis because of hypercoagulable state secondary to loss of antithrombin III and other proteins involved in the clotting mechanism

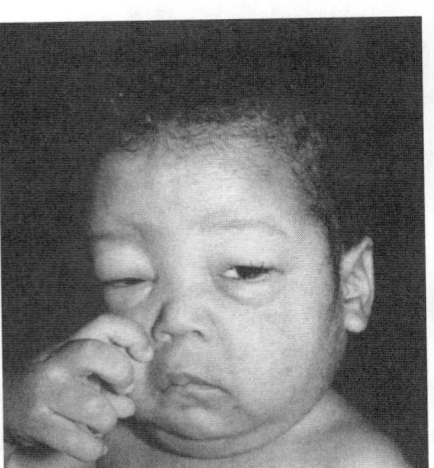

FIGURE 1-251 Marked eyelid edema in a 2-year-old boy with minimal change disease and nephrotic syndrome. Eyelid edema in any child should prompt the performance of urinalysis rather than the presumption of allergy. (From Zitelli BJ, Davis HW: *Atlas of pediatric physical diagnosis*, ed 5, Philadelphia, 2007, Mosby.)

TABLE 1-130 Differentiation between Nephrotic Syndrome and Nephritic Syndrome

Typical Features	Nephrotic	Nephritic
Onset	Insidious	Abrupt
Edema	++++	++
Blood pressure	Normal	Raised
Jugular venous pressure	Normal/low	Raised
Proteinuria	++++	++
Hematuria	May/may not occur	+++
Red-cell casts	Absent	Present
Serum albumin	Low	Normal/slightly reduced

Johnson RJ, Feehally J: *Comprehensive clinical nephrology*, ed 2, St Louis, 2000, Mosby.

ACUTE GENERAL Rx

- Furosemide is useful for severe edema.
- Use of ACE inhibitors to reduce proteinuria is generally indicated even in normotensive patients.
- Anticoagulant therapy should be administered as long as patients have nephrotic proteinuria, an albumin level <20 g/L, or both.

The mainstay of therapy is treatment of the underlying disorder:

- Minimal change disease generally responds to prednisone 1 mg/kg/day. Relapses can occur when steroids are discontinued. In these individuals, cyclophosphamide and chlorambucil may be useful.
- Focal and segmental glomerulosclerosis: steroid therapy is also recommended. However, response rate is approximately 35% to 40%, and most patients progress to end-stage renal disease within 3 yr.
- Membranous glomerulonephritis: prednisone 2 mg/kg/day may be useful in inducing remission. Cytotoxic agents can be added if there is poor response to prednisone.
- Membranoproliferative glomerulonephritis: most patients are treated with steroid therapy and antiplatelet drugs. Despite treatment, the majority of patients will progress to end-stage renal disease within 5 yr.

CHRONIC Rx

- Patients should be monitored for azotemia and should be aggressively treated for hypertension and hyperlipidemia. Furosemide is useful for severe edema. Anticoagulants may be necessary for thromboembolic events. Prophylactic anticoagulation should be considered in patients with membranous glomerulonephritis.
- Oral vitamin D is useful in the treatment of hypocalcemia (because of vitamin D loss).

REFERRAL

Nephrology consultation is recommended in all cases of nephrotic syndrome.

SUGGESTED READING

available at www.expertconsult.com

AUTHOR: **FRED F. FERRI, M.D.**

TABLE 1-131 Summary of Primary Renal Diseases That Present as Idiopathic Nephrotic Syndrome

	Minimal-Change Nephropathy Syndrome (MCNS)	Focal Segmental Sclerosis	Membranous Nephrotic	MEMBRANOPROLIFERATIVE GLOMERULONEPHRITIS (MPGN)	
				Type I	Type II
Frequency*					
Children	75%	10%	<5%	10%	10%
Adults	15%	15%	50%	10%	10%
Clinical Manifestations					
Age (yr)	2-6	2-10	40-50	5-15	5-15
Sex	2:1	1.3:1	2:1 male	Male-female	Male-female
Nephrotic syndrome	100%	90%	80%	60%	60%
Asymptomatic proteinuria	0	10%	20%	40%	40%
Hematuria	10%-20%	60%-80%	60%	80%	80%
Hypertension	10%	20% early	Infrequent	35%	35%
Rate of progression to renal failure	Does not progress	10 years	50% in 10-20 yr	10-20 yr	5-15 yr
Associated conditions	Allergy? Hodgkin's disease, usually none	None			
Laboratory Findings	Manifestations of nephrotic syndrome	Manifestations of nephrotic syndrome	Renal vein thrombosis, cancer, SLE, hepatitis B	None	Partial lipodystrophy
	↑ BUN in 15%-30%	↑ BUN in 20%-40%	Manifestations of nephrotic syndrome	Low C1, C4, C3–C9	Normal C1, C4, low C3–C9
Immunogenetics	HLA-B8, B12 (3.5)†	Not established	HLA-DRW3 (12–32)†	Not established	C3 nephritic factor
Renal Pathology					Not established
Light microscopy	Normal	Focal	Thickened	Thickened	Lobulation
Immunofluorescence	Negative	IgM	Fine	Granular	C3 only
Electron microscopy	Foot process fusion	Foot	Subepithelial	Mesangial	Dense deposits
Response of Steroids	90%	15%-20%	May slow progression	Not established	Not established

Modified from Goldman L, Ausiello D (eds): *Cecil textbook of medicine,* ed 22, Philadelphia, 2004, WB Saunders.
*Approximate frequency as a cause of idiopathic nephrotic syndrome. About 10% of adult nephrotic syndrome is due to various diseases that usually present with acute glomerulonephritis.
†Relative risk.
↑, Elevated; *BUN,* blood urea nitrogen; *C,* complement; *GBM,* glomerular basement membrane; *hepatitis B,* hepatitis B virus; *HLA,* human leukocyte antigen; *Ig,* immunoglobulin; *SLE,* systemic lupus erythematosus.

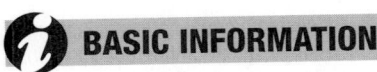

BASIC INFORMATION

DEFINITION

Neuroblastomas are tumors of postganglionic sympathetic neurons that typically originate in the adrenal medulla or the sympathetic chain/ganglion. Often present at birth, but not diagnosed until later, when the child shows symptoms of the disease. They are almost exclusively a disease of childhood.

ICD-9CM CODES
194.0 Neuroblastoma, unspecified site

EPIDEMIOLOGY & DEMOGRAPHICS

INCIDENCE (IN U.S.): 8%-10% of all solid tumors of childhood (third most common childhood cancer, after leukemia and brain tumors); 1/10,000 children <15 yr.

PREDOMINANT SEX: Male:female ratio of 1:1.3

PEAK AGE: Early childhood. Mean age of onset is 18 mo; 33% onset by 1 year; 75% onset by 5 year; 97% by 10 year. In rare cases, neuroblastoma can be discovered by fetal ultrasound.

GENETICS: Chromosomal deletions (loss of heterozygosity) found in nearly half of tumors, most commonly localized to chromosomes 1p, 11q, and 14q. Deletion of 1p36 (leading to amplification and overexpression of *N-MYC* protooncogene) associated with poor prognosis. There is a small subset with an autosomal dominant pattern of inheritance.

PHYSICAL FINDINGS & CLINICAL PRESENTATION

- Mass in abdomen, neck, or chest. Approximately two thirds of tumors arise in the abdomen; of these, two thirds arise in the adrenal glands. 70% to 80% of children have regional lymph node involvement or distant metastases at time of presentation.
- Spinal cord/paraspinal: can present with back pain, signs of compression—paraplegia, stool/urine retention.
- Horner's syndrome (ptosis, miosis, anhidrosis).
- Thoracic: difficulty breathing, dysphagia, infections, chronic cough.
- Secondary symptoms referable to metastatic disease: fatigue, chronic pain (typically bony pain), pancytopenia, periorbital ecchymosis, proptosis, anorexia, weight loss, unexplained fever, multiple subcutaneous bluish nodules, irritability.
- Paraneoplastic syndromes: opsoclonus-myoclonus syndrome is described as "dancing eyes, dancing feet," which manifest as myoclonic jerks and chaotic eye movements in all directions. This may be initial presentation before tumor diagnosis; present in 1% to 3% of patients with neuroblastoma; of all patients with opsoclonus-myoclonus, 20% to 50% have an underlying neuroblastoma. Patients who present with this syndrome often

have neuroblastomas with more favorable biologic features.
- Progressive cerebellar ataxia.
- Abnormal secretion of vasoactive intestinal peptide by the tumor, leading to distention of the abdomen and secretory diarrhea.

DIAGNOSIS

WORKUP
- Careful general physical examination
- Biopsy and resection of tumor when possible

LABORATORY TESTS
- Complete blood count, coagulation studies, erythrocyte sedimentation rate.
- 24-hour urine for catecholamines: homovanillic acid (HVA) and vanillylmandelic acid (VMA) are secreted by up to 90% of tumors.
- Nonspecific serum markers such as neuron-specific enolase, lactate dehydrogenase, and ferritin.
- Bone marrow biopsy and aspirate: karyotype, DNA index, *N-MYC* copy number.
- Minimum criteria for diagnosis is based on one of the following: (1) unequivocal pathologic diagnosis made from tumor tissue or (2) combination of bone marrow aspirate with unequivocal tumor cells and increased levels of serum or urinary catecholamine metabolites, as described above.
- Genetic/biologic variables have been studied in children with neuroblastoma, in particular the histology, aneuploidy of tumor DNA, and amplification of the *N-MYC* oncogene within tumor tissue, because treatment decisions may be based on these factors.
  - Hyperdiploid DNA is associated with favorable prognosis, especially in infants.
  - *N-MYC* amplification is associated with poor prognosis, regardless of patient age, likely due to association with deletion of chromosome 1p and gain of chromosome 17q.
  - Other biologic factors studied include profile of GABAergic receptors, expression of neurotrophin receptors, level of telomerase RNA and serum ferritin and lactate dehydrogenase.

IMAGING STUDIES
- Chest radiograph, abdominal radiograph, skeletal survey, abdominal ultrasound
- Renal/bladder ultrasound
- CT scan or MRI of the chest and abdomen to provide information about regional lymph nodes, vessel invasion, and distant metastases (Fig. 1-252)
- Body scan with ^{131}I-MIBG (meta-iodobenzylguanidine), which is taken up by neuroblasts and is sensitive to metastases in the bone and soft tissue
- Bone scan with Tc-99 MDP to visualize lytic bone lesions and metastases

- STAGING (International Neuroblastoma Staging System)
  - I. Confined to single organ
  - IIA. Localized tumor with incomplete gross resection; lymph nodes negative
  - IIB. Localized tumor with incomplete gross resection; ipsilateral lymph nodes positive
  - III. Extension across midline, with or without lymph node involvement
  - IV. Distant metastases to lymph nodes, bone, bone marrow, liver, skin
  - IVs. Localized primary tumor with dissemination limited to skin, liver, or bone marrow; limited to infants

DIFFERENTIAL DIAGNOSIS
- Other small, round, blue-cell childhood tumors, such as lymphoma, rhabdomyosarcoma, soft tissue sarcoma, and primitive neuroectodermal tumors (PNETs)
- Wilms' tumor
- Hepatoblastoma

TREATMENT

- Assure patient and family that there is hope for recovery with aggressive treatment.
- Overall, treatment will be determined by several factors, including age at diagnosis, stage of disease, site of primary tumor and metastases, and tumor histology.

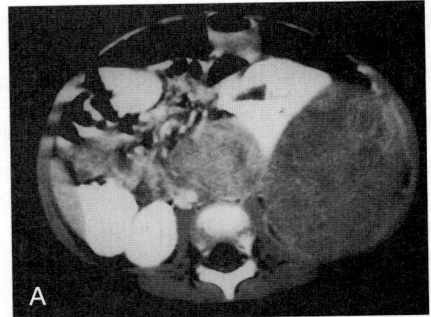
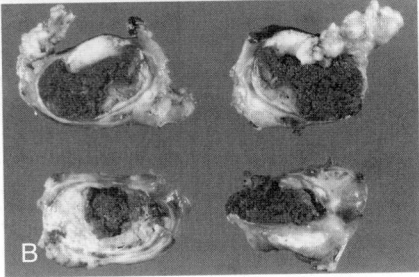

FIGURE 1-252 Computed tomographic scan **(A)** shows adrenal neuroblastoma at diagnosis. Serial sections through adrenal neuroblastoma **(B)** show tumor with large areas of diffuse hemorrhage and calcification. (From Abeloff MD [ed]: *Clinical oncology,* ed 3, Philadelphia, 2004, Elsevier.)

- Surgery, particularly for low-risk tumors.
- Radiation therapy may be tried for unresectable tumors or tumors that are not responsive to chemotherapy.
- Multiagent chemotherapy is mainstay of treatment (e.g., cisplatinum, etoposide, Adriamycin, cyclophosphamide, carboplatin).
- Autologous bone marrow transplantation following aggressive chemotherapy for stage IV disease or patients who are at highest risk based on presence of disseminated disease or unfavorable markers such as *N-MYC* amplification.
- Novel therapies include immunotherapy using monoclonal antibodies and vaccines that attempt to initiate an immune reaction against the disease and targeting of tumor cells with drugs that induce apoptosis or have antiangiogenic effect. Immunotherapy with ch14.18, a monoclonal antibody against the tumor-associated disialoganglioside GD2 has activity against neuroblastoma. Recent trials have shown that immunotherapy with ch14.18, GM-CSF, and interleukin-2 is associated with a significantly improved outcome as compared with standard therapy in patients with high-risk neuroblastoma.
- Adrenocorticotropic hormone (ACTH) treatment is thought to be effective for patients with opsoclonus/myoclonus syndrome.

DISPOSITION

- Overall survival is >40%. Children under the age of 1 yr have a cure rate as high as 90%.
- Approximately 70% of patients with neuroblastoma have metastases at diagnoses.
- Prognosis is related to age at time of diagnosis, clinical stage, and regional lymph node involvement. Children with localized disease and infants <1 year at diagnosis and favorable disease characteristics have better prognosis whereas poorer prognosis is noted in older children with stage IV disease (20% survival compared with >95% in stage I), age >1 year at diagnosis, increased number of *N-MYC* copies, adrenal tumor, and chronic 1p deletion.
- Children treated for neuroblastoma may be at risk for second malignancies, including renal cell carcinoma.

REFERRAL

Multidisciplinary oncology team with experience in treating cancers of childhood and adolescence.

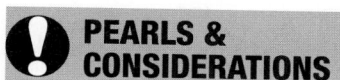

PEARLS & CONSIDERATIONS

- Predominantly a tumor of early childhood that originates in the sites where the sympathetic nervous system tissue is present.

- Most common symptoms due to tumor mass or bone pain from metastases.
- Children can present with classic paraneoplastic neurologic symptoms including cerebellar ataxia and opsoclonus/myoclonus.
- Recent trials have shown a very high rate of survival among patients with intermediate-risk neuroblastoma with biologically based treatment assignment involving a substantially reduced duration of chemotherapy and reduced doses of chemotherapeutic agents as compared with regimens used in earlier trials. These data provide support for further reduction in chemotherapy with more refined risk stratifications.
- Despite recent advances, 50% to 60% of patients with high-risk neuroblastoma have a relapse and currently there are no salvage treatment regimens known to be curative.

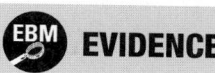 **EVIDENCE**

available at www.expertconsult.com

SUGGESTED READINGS
available at www.expertconsult.com

AUTHOR: **NICOLE J. ULLRICH, M.D., PH.D.**

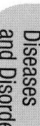

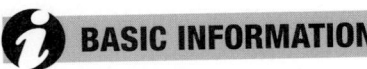

BASIC INFORMATION

DEFINITION

Neurofibromatosis (NF) is an autosomal-dominant disorder affecting bone, the nervous system, soft tissue, and skin. There are three major subtypes of neurofibromatosis disorders: NF type 1 (NF1), NF type 2 (NF2), and schwannomatosis. Schwannomatosis has only recently been recognized as a distinct disorder; currently very little is known about it.

SYNONYMS

NF1: von Recklinghausen disease, peripheral NF
NF2: bilateral acoustic neurofibromatosis, central NF

ICD-9CM CODES
237.70 Neurofibromatosis, unspecified
237.71 Type 1, von Recklinghausen's
237.72 Type 2, acoustic

EPIDEMIOLOGY & DEMOGRAPHICS

- Incidence of NF1 (one case/3000 live births), NF2 (one case/25,000 live births).
- Prevalence of NF1 (one case/5000 persons), NF2 (one case/210,000 persons).
- NF1 and NF2 are autosomal dominant; approximately 50% of cases have no family history.
- The two disorders affect approximately 100,000 people in the U.S.
- Affects males and females equally.
- NF1 may be associated with optic gliomas, astrocytomas, spinal neurofibromas, pheochromocytomas, and chronic myeloid leukemia.
- NF2 may be associated with meningiomas, spinal schwannomas, and cataracts.
- For schwannomatosis, the incidence is one per 30,000 persons, and the disease is mostly sporadic in nature.

PHYSICAL FINDINGS & CLINICAL PRESENTATION

- Common features of NF1 include:
  1. Café-au-lait macules (100% of children by age 2 yr)
     a. Hyperpigmented skin lesions occurring anywhere on the body except the face, palms, and soles
     b. Appear early in life and increase in size and number during puberty
     c. Are focal or diffuse
  2. Axillary and inguinal freckling (70%).
  3. Multiple neurofibromas (Figs. 1-253 and 1-254) can be soft or firm; three subtypes:
     a. Cutaneous: circumscribed, not specific for NF1
     b. Subcutaneous: circumscribed, not specific for NF1
     c. Plexiform: noncircumscribed, thick and irregular; can cause disfigurement of supportive structures and specific for NF1

  4. Lisch nodule (small hamartoma of the iris) found in >90% of adult cases.
  5. Visual defects possibly related to optic gliomas (2% to 5%).
  6. Neurodevelopment problems such as learning disability and mental retardation (30% to 40%).
  7. Skeletal disorders, including long bone dysplasia, pseudoarthrosis, scoliosis, short stature, and decreased bone mineral density.
- Common features of NF2 include:
  1. Hearing loss and tinnitus related to bilateral acoustic neuromas (>90% of adults)
  2. Cataracts (81%)
  3. Headache
  4. Unsteady gait
  5. Cutaneous and subcutaneous neurofibromas, but less than NF1
  6. Café-au-lait macules (1%)
- Common features of schwannomatosis include painful multiple schwannomas of the spinal, peripheral, or cranial nerves *except* the vestibular nerve.

ETIOLOGY

- NF1 is caused by DNA mutations located on the long arm of chromosome 17 responsible for encoding the protein neurofibromin.
- NF2 is caused by DNA mutations located in the middle of the long arm of chromosome 22 responsible for encoding the protein merlin, which is a potent inhibitor of glioma growth.
- Both proteins are speculated to act as tumor suppressors.

- The etiology of schwannomatosis remains unclear; however, biallelic NF2 mutations are found in the schwannomas but nowhere else, suggesting that they are secondary mutations.

DIAGNOSIS

- NF1 is diagnosed if the person has two or more of the following features:
  1. Six or more café-au-lait macules >5 mm in prepubertal patients and >15 mm in postpubertal patients
  2. Two or more neurofibromas of any type or one plexiform neurofibroma
  3. Axillary or inguinal freckling
  4. Optic glioma
  5. Two or more Lisch nodules (iris hamartomas)
  6. Sphenoid wing dysplasia or cortical thinning of long bones, with or without pseudoarthrosis
  7. A first-degree relative (parent, sibling, or child) with NF1 based on the previous criteria
- NF2 is diagnosed if the person has either of the following two criteria:
  1. Bilateral eighth nerve masses seen by appropriate imaging studies (e.g., CT, MRI)
  2. A first-degree relative with NF2 and either a unilateral eighth nerve mass or two of the following: neurofibroma, meningioma, glioma, schwannoma, or juvenile posterior subcapsular lenticular opacity

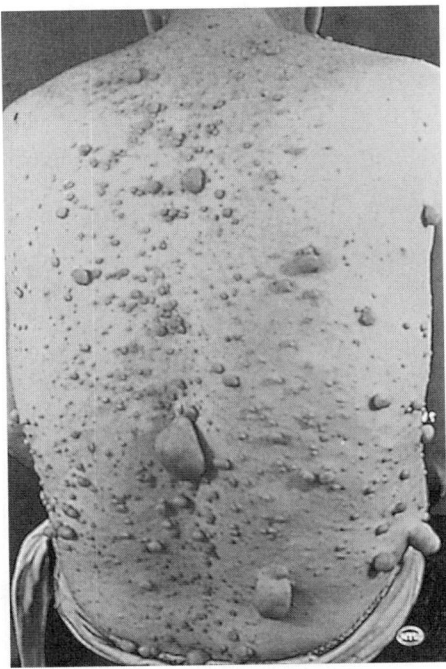

FIGURE 1-253 Nodules. Solid, large (>1 cm), deep-seated mass in dermal or subcutaneous tissues. These nodules are neurofibromas in a patient with neurofibromatosis. (From Goldman L, Ausiello D [eds]: *Cecil textbook of medicine,* ed 22, Philadelphia, 2004, WB Saunders.)

- Schwannomatosis is diagnosed in an individual >30 yr having either of the following two criteria:
  1. Two nonintradermal schwannomas, no vestibular tumor found on MRI scan, no NF2 mutation
  2. One nonvestibular schwannoma and a first-degree relative fitting the above criteria

DIFFERENTIAL DIAGNOSIS

- Abdominal neurofibromatosis
- Myxoid lipoma
- Nodular fasciitis
- Fibrous histiocytoma
- Segmental NF

WORKUP

The diagnosis of NF is usually self-evident. Workup is dictated by clinical symptoms in NF1 and usually includes MRI evaluation of the head and spine in NF2 and schwannomatosis. In fact, if NF2 is suspected but no vestibular nerve schwannomas are found, the diagnosis points to schwannomatosis.

LABORATORY TESTS

- Genetic testing is possible in individuals who desire prenatal diagnosis for NF1. There is no single standard test and multiple tests are required. Results can only tell if an individual is affected but cannot predict the severity of the disease due to variable expression.
- In NF2, linkage analysis testing provides a >99% certainty the individual has NF2.

IMAGING STUDIES

- MRI with gadolinium is the imaging study of choice in both NF1 and NF2 patients. MRI increases detection of optic gliomas, tumors of the spine, acoustic neuromas, and "bright spots" believed to represent hamartomas.
- MRI of the spine is recommended in all patients diagnosed with NF2 to exclude intramedullary tumors.

OTHER TESTS

- Wood lamp examination may be useful in patients with very pale skin for visualizing café-au-lait spots.
- Slit-lamp examination is recommended for children >6 yr to confirm the presence of Lisch nodules and subcapsular opacity.

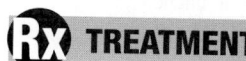 **TREATMENT**

Treatment is directed primarily at symptoms and complications of NF1 and NF2. As for schwannomatosis, resection should be reserved for tumors that are symptomatic or threaten to cause spinal cord compression.

NONPHARMACOLOGIC THERAPY

- Counseling addressing prognosis and genetic, psychological, and social issues
- Hearing testing and speech pathology evaluation

ACUTE GENERAL Rx

- Surgery is usually not done on skin tumors unless cosmetically requested or if suspicion of malignant transformation exists.
- Surgery may be indicated for spinal or cranial neurofibromas, gliomas, or meningiomas.
- Acoustic neuromas can be treated by surgical excision.

CHRONIC Rx

- Radiation may be indicated in optic nerve gliomas and patients whose central nervous system tumors show image progression.
- Stereotactic radiosurgery with a gamma knife may be an alternative approach to surgery for acoustic neuromas.

DISPOSITION

- Prognosis varies according to the severity of involvement.
- There is no cure for neurofibromatosis.

REFERRAL

A multidisciplinary team of consultants is needed in patients with neurofibromatosis, including neurosurgeon, otolaryngologist, dermatologist, neurologist, audiologist, speech pathologist, geneticist, and neuropsychologist.

(!) PEARLS & CONSIDERATIONS

- Friedrich Daniel von Recklinghausen first reported his cases in 1882, although there had been similar accounts dating back to the 1600s.
- The first report in the literature of NF2 was by Wishart in 1822.
- A high SPRED1 mutation detection rate has been identified in NF1 mutation-negative families with an autosomal dominant phenotype of CALMs with or without freckling and no other NF1 features.

COMMENTS

For additional information and patient resources, refer to the National Neurofibromatosis Foundation (www.nf.org) or Neurofibromatosis Inc. (www.nfinc.org).

SUGGESTED READINGS

available at www.expertconsult.com

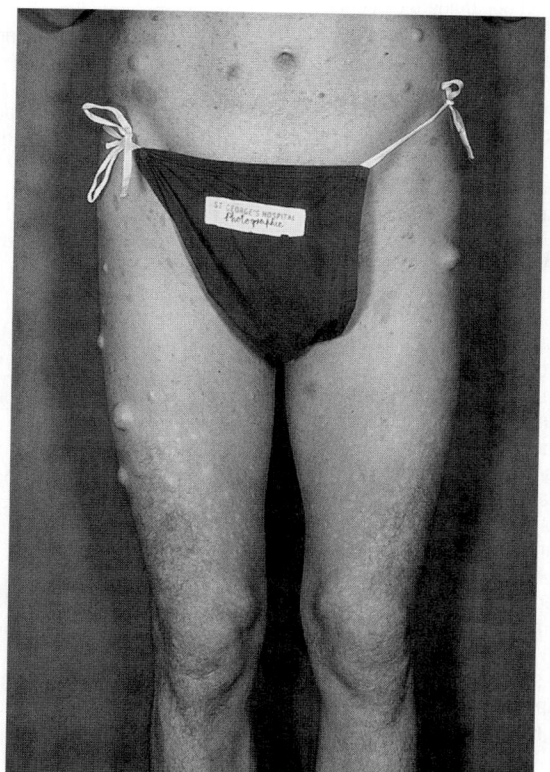

FIGURE 1-254 Type 1 neurofibromatosis: widespread cutaneous neurofibromata are a prominent feature of the classical variant. Courtesy of R.A. Marsden, M.D., St George's Hospital, London. (From McKee PH, Calonje E, Granter SR [eds]: *Pathology of the skin with clinical correlations,* ed 3, St Louis, 2005, Mosby.)

AUTHORS: **MARK F. BRADY, M.D., M.P.H.,** and **WEN Y. WU-CHEN, M.D.**

Diseases and Disorders

I

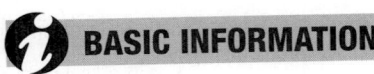

DEFINITION

Neuroleptic malignant syndrome (NMS) is a disorder characterized by hyperthermia, muscular rigidity, autonomic dysfunction, and depressed/fluctuating levels of arousal that evolve over 24 to 72 hr. This occurs as an idiosyncratic adverse reaction most commonly to dopamine-receptor antagonists (especially the D2/4 receptor) or sudden withdrawal from a dopaminergic agent or agonist, such as antiparkinsonian medications.

SYNONYMS

None

ICD-9CM CODES
333.92 Neuroleptic malignant syndrome

EPIDEMIOLOGY & DEMOGRAPHICS

INCIDENCE (IN U.S.): 0.07% to 0.15% annual incidence in psychiatric population.
PREDOMINANT SEX: More than two thirds of patients are male.
PREDOMINANT AGE: Young and middle-aged adults
PREDISPOSING FACTORS:
- High-potency dopamine antagonists
- Long-acting depot preparations or multiple agents

PHYSICAL FINDINGS & CLINICAL PRESENTATION

- Muscle rigidity (hypertonia, cogwheeling, or "lead pipe" rigidity)
- Hyperthermia (38.6° to 42.3° C, usually <40° C)
- Autonomic symptoms: diaphoresis, sialorrhea, skin pallor, urinary incontinence
- Tachycardia, tachypnea
- Labile blood pressure (hypertension or postural hypotension)
- Agitation, catatonia, fluctuating consciousness, obtundation

ETIOLOGY

- Unknown. Impaired thermoregulation in hypothalamus and limbic cortex may occur as a result of relative lack of dopamine activity (central dopamine-blockade hypothesis: most accepted).
- Neuroleptic drugs have different potencies for inducing NMS:
  1. Typical neuroleptics: high potency, haloperidol; medium potency, chlorpromazine, fluphenazine; low potency, levomepromazine, loxapine
  2. Atypical neuroleptics: low potency, risperidone, olanzapine, clozapine, quetiapine

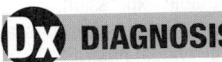
DIAGNOSIS

DIFFERENTIAL DIAGNOSIS

- Heatstroke, drug-induced states and overdose (ecstasy abuse, phencyclidine), thyrotoxicosis, pheochromocytoma, serotonin syndrome
- Malignant hyperthermia, catatonia, acute psychosis with agitation
- CNS or systemic infections, including sepsis

WORKUP

Careful drug history

LABORATORY TESTS

- Elevated creatine phosphokinase (CPK) (sensitivity 0.71)
- Urinary myoglobin
- Leukocytosis, usually 10,000 to 40,000/mm^3
- Electrolytes and renal function
- Blood gases
- Drug levels

TREATMENT

NONPHARMACOLOGIC THERAPY

- Stop all neuroleptic agents and reinstitute any recently discontinued dopaminergic agents.
- Respiratory support; nutritional support in cases with dysphagia or comatose.
- Careful fluid balance monitoring with adequate hydration (intravenous in severe cases).
- Active cooling (cooling blanket and antipyretics).
- Skilled nursing care is necessary to prevent decubitus ulcers in bed-confined patients.

ACUTE GENERAL Rx

- IV benzodiazepines (e.g., diazepam 2 to 10 mg, with total daily dose of 10 to 60 mg) to relax muscles and control agitation.
- Bromocriptine, a dopamine receptor agonist, is the mainstay of therapy for patients with neuroleptic malignant syndrome. Initial doses of 2.5 to 10 mg are given IV q8h and are increased by 5 mg/day until clinical improvement is seen. The drug should be continued for at least 10 days after the syndrome has been controlled and then tapered slowly.
- Amantadine, an NMDA receptor antagonist with possible dopaminergic properties, administered orally at doses of 100 to 200 mg PO bid, has been shown to reduce mortality in comparison to supportive therapy alone.
- Dantrolene therapy is also effective. Initially, patients can be given 0.25 mg/kg IV q6-12h, followed by a maintenance dose up to 3 mg/kg/day. After 2 to 3 days, patients may be given the drug orally (25 to 600 mg/day in divided doses). Oral dantrolene therapy (50 to 600 mg/day) may be continued for several days afterward.
- Electroconvulsive therapy with neuromuscular blockage in pharmacologically refractory cases. Succinylcholine should not be used because it may cause hyperkalemia and cardiac arrhythmias in patients with rhabdomyolysis or dysautonomia.

CHRONIC Rx

- Respiratory care, nutritional support, and physical therapy may be required in more severe cases.
- Appropriate therapy would be required in patients with persistent neuropsychiatric sequelae of NMS (e.g., antidepressants for depression, cognitive behavioral therapy for cognitive deficits, rehabilitation for contractures).

DISPOSITION

- Mortality rate is currently 5% to 10% despite therapeutic measures. Serious sequelae may occur in a further 20%. Complete recovery occurs in >70% of patients. Causes of death include cardiac arrhythmias, myocardial infarction, renal failure secondary to rhabdomyolysis, seizures, pulmonary edema, and bronchopneumonia.
- Factors adversely affecting mortality are development of renal failure and core temperature >104°F (40° C).
- Late neuropsychiatric sequelae.
- Monitor closely for future complications of pharmacologic therapy.

REFERRAL

If the patient's condition is critical, it is preferable to treat the patient in a medical/neurologic ICU.

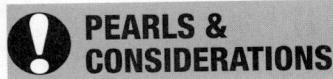
PEARLS & CONSIDERATIONS

COMMENTS

Early detection and diagnosis lead to a more favorable outcome. Treatment is a medical emergency.

SUGGESTED READINGS
available at www.expertconsult.com

AUTHOR: **EROBOGHENE E. UBOGU, M.D.**

BASIC INFORMATION

DEFINITION

Neuropathic pain is not itself a disease, but rather a symptom that is associated with multiple different diseases. Thus it is not enough to define its presence without searching for a cause. It is defined as the sensation derived from the abnormal discharges of impaired or injured neural structures in either the peripheral or central nervous system. Descriptors include:

- Hyperesthesia: heightened sensitivity to non-painful stimuli (e.g., light touch)
- Hyperalgesia: heightened sensitivity to painful stimuli (e.g., pinprick), or reduced threshold to feel pain
- Allodynia: pain provoked by a stimulus that is not normally painful

SYNONYMS

Neuralgia

ICD-9CM CODES
782.0 Numbness, paresthesias
729.1 Myositis/myalgia, not otherwise specified
729.2 Neuralgia, neuritis, or radiculitis, not otherwise specified

EPIDEMIOLOGY & DEMOGRAPHICS

- Estimates of the prevalence of neuropathic pain in the general population range from 1.6% to 8.2%.
- Demographics vary widely depending on etiology, for example:
  - Postherpetic neuralgia: affects elderly, pain seen in almost 100% of cases
  - AIDS: 30% of patients affected
  - Diabetes mellitus: 20% to 24% affected (prevalence rates vary, increasing with longer disease duration)
  - Fabry disease: affects mostly children, pain in 81% to 90% of patients

PHYSICAL FINDINGS & CLINICAL PRESENATION

- History: localize the disease with questions
  - Quality (description) of neuropathic pain: burning, hot or cold, "icy hot," "pins and needles," stinging, lancinating, sharp, shooting
  - Distribution of symptoms may aid in localization (i.e., "stocking-glove" symptoms in generalized neuropathy, numbness in a peripheral nerve territory in focal neuropathy)
  - Generalized small fiber neuropathy: dysesthesias without numbness common, but many etiologies (e.g., diabetes) cause both small and large fiber dysfunction
  - Large fiber neuropathy (LFPN): coexisting numbness, hyporeflexia, or weakness may be seen, usually worse distally
  - Nerve root: coexisting neck or low back pain that radiates along a specific dermatome; most common cause is structural compression

  - Spinal cord symptoms: coexisting spasticity, bowel or bladder involvement, sensory level
  - Prior history of thalamic stroke in central thalamic pain syndrome (Dejerine-Roussy syndrome)
  - Family history may suggest a genetic cause
- Examination: see Table 1-132 and Section III, "Neuropathic Pain."

ETIOLOGY & LABORATORY EVALUATION (Table 1-133)

- Metabolic: diabetes mellitus; malnutrition and alcoholism; vitamin B_{12} deficiency; thiamine deficiency; porphyria; Fabry's disease
- Inflammatory: immune vasculitides (lupus, Sjögren's syndrome, polyarteritis nodosa, etc.), acute inflammatory demyelinating polyneuropathy (classically presents with ascending weakness and numbness, though pain is also a common feature), chronic inflammatory demyelinating polyneuropathy, sarcoid, multiple sclerosis
- Infiltrative: amyloidosis, paraproteinemias (e.g., monoclonal gammopathy of uncertain significance [MGUS])
- Infectious: postviral (brachial neuritis), HIV/AIDS, HSV, varicella-zoster virus (VZV; postherpetic neuralgia), Lyme disease, leprosy (thickened nerves and skin lesions), syphilis
- Neoplastic and paraneoplastic-carcinomatous infiltration of nerve/nerve root, anti-Hu
- Drugs/toxins: history of exposure to alcohol, chemotherapeutic agents (paclitaxel, vincristine), isoniazid, metronidazole, or heavy metals (thallium, arsenic)

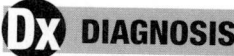 **DIAGNOSIS**

LABORATORY TESTS

- Fasting blood glucose (FBG)
- 2-hour oral glucose tolerance test (OGTT)
- Vitamin B_1 level
- If B_{12} level normal: serum methylmalonic acid and homocysteine levels
- Serum erythrocyte sedimentation rate (ESR), ANA, SS-A and SS-B, c-ANCA, p-ANCA
- RPR or FTA-ABS
- Serum ACE level (sarcoid)
- HIV antibody
- SPEP, UPEP, immunofixation
- Urine and stool protoporphyrins, if porphyria is suspected clinically
- Hu antibody: can be seen in both small cell and non–small cell lung cancers, may be positive without evidence of lung cancer
- Lumbar puncture: protein elevation, oligoclonal bands, CSF/serum IgG index, herpes simplex virus (HSV), VZV, Lyme polymerase chain reaction (PCR), VDRL

ELECTROPHYSIOLOGY STUDIES

- Electrophysiologic testing (electromyography with nerve conduction studies): may be normal in small fiber neuropathies or CNS lesion, but often abnormal in large fiber neuropathies
- Quantitative sensory testing: abnormal in small and large fiber neuropathy
- Evoked potentials (only if suspicion for spinal cord lesion)

TABLE 1-132 Examination

Exam Finding	Localization
Pinprick/temperature loss alone	Small fibers only
Pinprick/temperature loss + vibratory/proprioceptive loss	Small and large fibers
Sensory loss and motor dysfunction worse distally than proximal	Large fiber neuropathy
Sensory loss and motor dysfunction along single nerve distribution	Single nerve
Sensory loss and motor dysfunction along multiple single nerves	Multiple mononeuropathies (i.e., mononeuropathy multiplex)
Motor and sensory loss involving multiple nerves belonging to specific region of brachial or lumbar plexus	Plexopathy
Sensory loss along dermatome with multiple myotomal muscles affected	Nerve root lesion
Asymmetric sensory loss without weakness and pseudoathetosis	Dorsal root ganglion
Vibratory/proprioceptive loss without pinprick/temperature loss	Dorsal column dysfunction (from compressive lesion, B_{12} deficiency, or tabes dorsalis from neurosyphilis)
Sensory level with weakness below the level of lesion and long tract signs (spasticity/Babinski's sign)	Spinal cord lesion
Hemisensory hyperalgesia	Contralateral thalamus

PATHOLOGY STUDIES

- Nerve biopsy is occasionally useful in selected cases, particularly when vasculitis, sarcoid, or amyloid neuropathy are in the differential.
- Skin biopsy for intraepidermal nerve fiber (IENF) density may be useful for small fiber neuropathy when other studies are normal.
- Rectal or abdominal fat pad biopsy may show amyloid deposition in systemic amyloidosis.

IMAGING STUDIES

- MRI (with and without contrast):
  - Of the brain to exclude thalamic pathology if symptoms and signs are consistent with thalamic lesion
  - Of the spinal cord and nerve roots to exclude structural, inflammatory, neoplastic, or infectious causes
  - Of the lumbar spine to evaluate for arachnoiditis
- If MRI cannot be performed, consider:
  - CT of the brain for thalamic pathology
  - CT myelography of the spinal cord to evaluate for structural/neoplastic disease, but only if clinical signs of spinal or nerve root compromise are present

℞ TREATMENT

NONPHARMACOLOGIC THERAPY

- Counseling should be initiated at the beginning of therapy to address psychologic issues exacerbating physiologic pain
- Physical therapy: especially in cases of chronic neck and low back pain

ACUTE GENERAL Rx

- Antidepressants:
  - Tricyclic antidepressants (TCAs): nortriptyline preferred over amitriptyline (fewer anticholinergic side effects with nortriptyline). Begin 25 mg PO qd in adults, or 10 mg qd in elderly. Increase dose by 25 mg every week as tolerated until usual maximal effective dose of 150 mg/day.
  - Paroxetine: begin 10 mg PO qd, increase by 10 mg/wk to a max dose of 60 mg qd.
  - Duloxetine: begin 30 mg daily, increase to 60 to 120 mg daily, qd or bid.
- Antiepileptics:
  - Gabapentin: begin 300 mg PO qd, advance to 300 mg PO tid by the end of the first week. Effective dose: higher than 1600 mg/day. Max dose: 1500 mg PO tid.
  - Carbamazepine: for trigeminal neuralgia. Begin 400 mg PO bid, increase to tid if necessary. Side effects and drug levels help to determine optimal dosing. Risk of aplastic anemia and hyponatremia (monitor CBC and chemistries).
  - Oxcarbazepine: better tolerated than carbamazepine. Start 150 mg PO bid and gradually increase to a maximal dose of 600 mg bid.
  - Lamotrigine: begin 25 mg PO bid, increase slowly (by 100 mg biweekly) until maximum effective dose of 200 to 300 mg PO bid. Risk: Stevens-Johnson syndrome.
  - Pregabalin: begin 50 mg PO tid, increase slowly to 100 to 200 mg PO tid.
- Analgesics:
  - Tramadol: 150 mg/day (50 mg tid), increase by 50 mg/wk, max 200 to 400 mg/day.
  - Morphine (oral): 15 to 30 mg q8h, max 90 to 360 mg/day.
  - Oxycodone: 20 mg q12h, increase by 10 mg/wk, max 40 to 160 mg/day.
  - Fentanyl patch: 25 to 100 mcg transdermally q3 days.
- Topical anesthetics:
  - 5% lidocaine patch, apply to area of pain, max three patches every 12 hr.

TABLE 1-133 Clinical Presentation and Laboratory Findings

Neuropathy Type	Predisposition	Examination Findings	EMG/NCS	Laboratory Analysis
Idiopathic small fiber PN	Age >50	Strength: normal Reflexes: normal Pos/Vib: normal Pain/Temp: decreased distally	Normal	Serum studies: normal Skin biopsy: abnormal Sudomotor studies: abnormal
Diabetic PN	Longstanding disease Family history	Strength normal to reduced, sensation reduced distally	Abnormal	Abnormal glucose tolerance High fasting glucose
Inherited PN	Family history	Pes cavus, hammer toes, reduced reflexes, sensation reduced distally	Abnormal	Genetic studies may be abnormal, other studies normal
Familial amyloid PN	Family history	Pain/temp loss Reduced reflexes Orthostasis	Abnormal if large fibers affected; also carpal tunnel syndrome	Transthyretin genetic study
Acquired amyloid PN	Monoclonal gammopathy	Pain/temp loss Reduced reflexes Orthostasis	Abnormal if large fibers affected; also carpal tunnel syndrome	SPEP, UPEP, immunofixation abnormal
Fabry's disease	Age Renal failure Strokes	Normal; possible reduced pain/temp sensation	Normal	α-galactosidase levels in cultured fibroblasts
PN + mixed connective tissue disease	History of lupus, rheumatoid arthritis, Sjögren's syndrome	Reduced reflexes and distal sensation	Abnormal	ANA, RF, SS-A/SS-B may be abnormal
Peripheral nerve vasculitis	Asymmetric disease	Multiple peripheral nerves involved	Abnormal	ANA, RF, SS-A/SS-B, ANCA, cryoglobulins may be abnormal
Paraneoplastic neuropathy	Lung cancer risk factors, chemical exposures	Asymmetric sensory loss, pseudoathetosis, relatively preserved strength	Abnormal	Anti-Hu
Sarcoidosis	Pulmonary sarcoid	Multiple mononeuropathies	Abnormal	Abnormal biopsy, elevated serum ACE, CXR abnormal
Arsenic	Pesticides, copper smelting	Reduced reflexes and distal sensation	Abnormal	Elevated arsenic in plasma, urine, and hair
HIV	Promiscuity, unprotected sex, IV drug abuse, blood transfusion	Variable, but most often reduced reflexes and distal sensation	Abnormal if large fibers involved	HIV antibody

ACE, Angiotensin-converting enzyme; *ANA*, antibody to nuclear antigens; *ANCA*, antineutrophil cytoplasmic antibodies; *CXR*, chest x-ray; *EMG*, electromyography; *HbA1C*, glycosylated hemoglobin; *HIV*, human immunodeficiency virus; *IV*, intravenous; *NCS*, nerve conduction studies; *PN*, polyneuropathy; *Pos*, position sensation; *RF*, rheumatoid factor; *SPEP*, serum protein electrophoresis; *SS-A*, Sjögren syndrome A; *SS-B*, Sjögren syndrome B; *Temp*, temperature sensation; *UPEP*, urine protein electrophoresis; *Vib*, vibration sensation.
Adapted from Mendell JR, Sahenk Z: Painful sensory neuropathy, *N Engl J Med* 348(13):1243, 2003.

- ○ Capsaicin is inconsistent in its ability to relieve pain and may exacerbate it. Use not recommended.
- Procedural/surgical: this option is considered mostly when the patient suffers from pain secondary to spinal cord or cauda equina injury. Studies are limited and benefit is not completely established. Procedures should be considered only when all other therapeutic modalities have failed. In addition, the patient should be cautioned that surgical procedures may not result in pain relief and may be associated with significant morbidity and even mortality.
  - ○ Dorsal root rhizotomy
  - ○ Nerve blocks
  - ○ Spinal cord stimulator

DISPOSITION
Prognosis depends on multiple factors including:
- Etiology of pain
- Treatment of any underlying condition

- Initiation of appropriate (often multiple) therapeutic modalities
- Patient compliance with prescribed regimen
Most care is accomplished in the outpatient setting, except when surgery is required.

REFERRAL
- Pain clinic
- Neurology
- Psychiatry
- Psychology
- Physiatry
- Anesthesiology (nerve blocks)
- Neurosurgery if considering surgical management

⚠ PEARLS & CONSIDERATIONS

- Factitious disorder and malingering frequently manifest with pain complaints. These are diagnoses of exclusion, and require negative evaluation for organic etiologies before diagnosis is made.
- Peripheral neuropathy in diabetics increases the risk of foot ulceration by sevenfold. Abnormal results in monofilament testing and vibratory perception (alone or in combination with the appearance of the feet, ulceration, and ankle reflexes) are the most helpful sign for the detection of LFPN.

EBM EVIDENCE
available at www.expertconsult.com

SUGGESTED READINGS
available at www.expertconsult.com

AUTHOR: **GAVIN BROWN, M.D.**

N

Diseases and Disorders

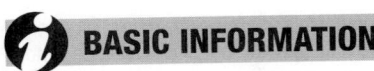

DEFINITION

Any disorder affecting the peripheral nervous system, including nerve roots, plexuses, and individual peripheral nerves, that has a genetic basis of inheritance and has been or is capable of being transmitted along generations.

There are many different types of hereditary peripheral neuropathies, including Dejerine-Sottas disease, inherited metabolic neuropathies, hereditary sensory and autonomic neuropathies (HSANs), and hereditary motor neuropathies such as spinal muscular atrophy (SMA). Most disorders are diagnosed in infancy or childhood; as such, adult clinicians rarely see these patients. For this reason, this chapter discusses only the hereditary motor and sensory neuropathies that an adult clinician might encounter.

SYNONYMS

Charcot-Marie-Tooth (CMT) disease, a.k.a. hereditary motor-sensory neuropathy (HMSN)
Hereditary neuropathy with liability to pressure-sensitive palsies (HNPP)

ICD-9CM CODES
CMT: 356.1
HNPP: 689

EPIDEMIOLOGY & DEMOGRAPHICS

All CMT: approximately 30 per 100,000
- CMT type 1 (demyelinating pathophysiology): 1 in 2500
- CMT type 2 (axonal pathophysiology): 7 in 1000
- CMT type 4 and CMT-X: rare (either axonal or demyelinating pathophysiology)
HNPP: 2 to 5 per 100,000

PHYSICAL FINDINGS & CLINICAL PRESENATION

CMT: Highly variable
- Age at onset earlier for CMT-1 than CMT-2, but both may present from childhood to old age.
- Severely affected patients have severe distal weakness and muscle atrophy with hand (prominently affecting interossei) and foot deformities (pes cavus, high arched feet, hammer toes).
- Mildly affected patients may have only foot deformity (pes cavus) with little or no weakness/sensory loss.
- Legs can be affected greater than arms, and patients will complain of gait abnormalities (steppage), which cause them to trip and fall.
- Sensory complaints (paresthesias, numbness, dysesthesia) are uncommon despite physical findings of impaired sensation.
- Decreased or absent reflexes.
- Some patients may have postural tremor of the upper limbs.

HNPP (a.k.a. tomaculous neuropathy):
- Age at onset is commonly adolescence.
- Disorder is characterized by recurrent entrapment of peripheral nerves with accompanying signs and symptoms (paresthesias and/or weakness in anatomical distributions). Most common are:
  1. Median nerve at the wrist (carpal tunnel syndrome)
  2. Ulnar nerve at the elbow (cubital tunnel syndrome)
  3. Painless brachial plexopathies
  4. Lateral femoral cutaneous nerve (meralgia paresthetica)
  5. Peroneal nerve at the fibular head
- May be associated with a generalized polyneuropathy.

ETIOLOGY

CMT: more than 30 subgroups have been identified and have various chromosomal abnormalities.
- Most common mutation is PMP-22 duplication, giving rise to CMT 1A demyelinating phenotype.
- Other mutations include P0 (demyelinating) and neurofilament light chain mutations (demyelinating or axonal phenotype)—see the following.
- Updated information may be available at http://www.neuro.wustl.edu/neuromuscular.
HNPP: deletion of chromosome 17p11.2–12.

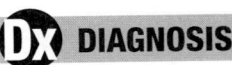 DIAGNOSIS

DIFFERENTIAL DIAGNOSIS

CMT: other genetic, metabolic, and multisystem disorders including:
- Spinocerebellar ataxias
- Friedreich's ataxia
- Leukodystrophies
- Refsum's disease (elevated serum phytanic acid)
- Distal spinal muscular atrophies and distal myopathies, which can present with pes cavus and other foot deformities
- Chronic inflammatory demyelinating polyneuropathy (CIDP)
HNPP:
- Hereditary neuralgic amyotrophy (HNA), which typically is painful rather than painless. In addition, in HNA, there is no evidence of generalized polyneuropathy.
- Multifocal motor neuropathy with conduction block (MMNCB)—autoimmune-mediated pure motor neuropathy
- Neuropathy associated with renal failure
- Lead neuropathy
- Neuropathy relating to paraproteinemia (demyelinating pathophysiology)

EVALUATION

CMT
- History of gradual onset symptoms is important to distinguish CMT from other forms of neuropathy.

- Detailed family history with *pedigree* is essential. Consider examination of multiple family members.
- History should evaluate for potential heavy metal exposure.
- History of dysesthesias is uncommon and should prompt search for acquired neuropathy or other inherited neuropathies (e.g., Fabry's disease).
HNPP: genetic testing after identification of multiple entrapment neuropathies on EMG and nerve conduction studies

LABORATORY TESTS

- Neurophysiology: electromyography (EMG) and nerve conduction studies (NCSs) must be done first to determine type of pathophysiology: demyelinating or axonal. This will guide genetic testing.
- NCSs in CMT-1 will reveal demyelinating physiology characterized by very slow conduction velocities (around 15 to 30 m/s) with prolonged distal latencies. Inherited demyelinating disorders can be distinguished from acquired demyelinating disorders (e.g., chronic inflammatory demyelinating polyneuropathy or CIDP) by the presence of conduction block in the latter.
- In HNPP, diffusely prolonged distal latencies with superimposed entrapment neuropathies at common sites will be seen on NCSs.
- EMG will reveal reinnervation characterized by long-duration, large-amplitude, polyphasic motor unit potentials (MUPs) with decreased MUP recruitment.
- Genetic tests are available for some CMT subtypes:
  1. CMT-1A: chromosome 17p11-PMP-22 duplication
  2. CMT-1B: chromosome 1q22-P0 mutation
  3. CMT-2E: chromosome 8p21-neurofilament light chain (NF-L) point mutation
  4. CMT-X: connexin 32 mutations
  5. HNPP: chromosome 17p11 deletion, which includes the PMP-22 gene
- Serum and 24-hour urine levels of heavy metals (arsenic, lead, etc.)
- SPEP, UPEP, immunofixation (for paraprotein).
- Anti-GM1 antibody (positive in ~50% of patients with MMNCB).
- Lumbar puncture may reveal elevated CSF protein in CIDP.
- Peripheral nerve biopsy:
  1. Demyelination with "onion bulb formation." Tomaculae, or focal thickening of myelin sheaths, seen in HNPP
  2. Generally not indicated unless diagnosis is uncertain

IMAGING STUDIES

- Spine plain films: for evaluation of scoliosis.
- MRI: indicated if dissociative sensory loss (dorsal column dysfunction with intact spinothalamic tract function) or if upper motor neuron findings (spasticity, Babinski's sign, clonus, increased tendon reflexes) are present.

- Exclusion of involvement of brain or spinal cord compressive lesions causing arm or leg weakness.
- Some inherited peripheral demyelinating disorders (i.e., CMT-X) are associated with intracerebral white matter abnormalities on MRI.
- Exclusion of structural, infectious, or inflammatory nerve root pathology.

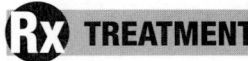

There is no known cure for any of these disorders. Management is supportive.

NONPHARMACOLOGIC THERAPY

- Physical therapy (PT) and occupational therapy (OT) to provide assistance with gait and coordination.
- PT and OT might provide walking aid such as ankle foot orthosis (AFO), cane, walker, or wheelchair depending on the severity of the neuropathy.
- Wrist splints for superimposed carpal tunnel syndrome.
- Elbow pads (Heelbo Pads) to cushion the ulnar nerve at the elbow.
- Heel-cord strengthening.
- Stretching exercises.
- Analgesics for pain associated with foot deformity.
- Surgical correction of foot deformities by orthopedic surgeons if indicated.

Vincristine may worsen existing neuropathy (important for oncologist to know if patient develops cancer requiring chemotherapy).

SURGICAL TREATMENT

- Patients with HNPP should probably not undergo surgical decompression of the median nerve at the wrist or the ulnar nerve at the elbow; these nerves are sensitive to manipulation. Poor results have been reported with ulnar nerve transposition.
- Anesthesiologists should be aware of HNPP diagnosis in patients undergoing surgery to prevent compression neuropathies from occurring during surgical procedures.

GENETIC COUNSELING

Must be routinely done for patient and family when diagnosis is established. Many aspects of the patient and family's life are affected including:

- Future progeny of patient and/or patient's parents or children
- Psychosocial aspects including social functioning, marriage, employment
- Financial needs
- Medical and life insurability

PROGNOSIS

- CMT: slowly progressive, and patients often remain ambulatory until late in life. Life expectancy is normal. Patients with respiratory

involvement (i.e., phrenic nerve involvement with diaphragm paresis) may have shorter life expectancy.
- HNPP: benign prognosis.

DISPOSITION

Outpatient care. Routine follow-up appointments should be done initially every 6 mo, and then every 1 to 2 yr.

REFERRAL

- Neurology and/or neuromuscular disease specialist
- Podiatry for recurrent foot problems, including appropriate arches

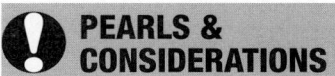

PATIENT & FAMILY EDUCATION

Patients can benefit from use of Muscular Dystrophy Association (MDA) resources.

SUGGESTED READINGS

available at www.expertconsult.com

AUTHOR: **GAVIN BROWN, M.D.**

N

Diseases
and Disorders

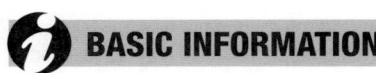

BASIC INFORMATION

DEFINITION

Nocardiosis is an infection caused by aerobic actinomycetes found in soil and characterized by lung, soft tissue, or central nervous system (CNS) involvement.

SYNONYMS

Mycetoma
Nocardia

ICD-9CM CODES
039   Actinomycotic infections
039.9 Nocardiosis NOS, of unspecified site

EPIDEMIOLOGY & DEMOGRAPHICS

- *Nocardia* species are found worldwide in the soil.
- Nocardiosis is found most commonly in patients who are immunocompromised (e.g., those receiving steroids or immunosuppressive therapy; those with lymphoma, leukemia, or lung cancer; transplant recipients; and those with pulmonary infections).
- Other underlying conditions associated with nocardiosis are pemphigus vulgaris, Whipple's disease, Goodpasture's syndrome, Cushing's disease, cirrhosis, ulcerative colitis, and rheumatoid arthritis.
- Use of steroids is an independent risk factor for developing nocardiosis.
- Between 500 and 1000 new cases are diagnosed each year in the U.S.
- Approximately 2% of patients with AIDS develop nocardiosis.
- Occurs more commonly in men than in women (2:1).
- Adults are affected more often than children.

PHYSICAL FINDINGS & CLINICAL PRESENTATION

- Inhalation of *Nocardia* organisms is the most common mode of entry, and pneumonia is the most common presentation, with 75% manifesting with fever, chills, dyspnea, and a productive cough (Fig. 1-255).
  1. Presentation can be acute, subacute, or chronic.
  2. Nocardiosis should be suspected if soft tissue abscesses or CNS tumors or abscesses form in conjunction with the pulmonary infection.
  3. Pulmonary infection may spread into the pericardium, mediastinum, and superior vena cava.
- Cutaneous disease usually occurs by direct inoculation of the organism as a result of skin puncture by a thorn or splinter, surgery, IV catheter use, or animal scratches or bites manifesting in:
  1. Cellulitis
  2. Lymphocutaneous nodules appearing along lymphatic sites draining the infected puncture wound
  3. Mycetoma (Madura foot), a chronic deep nodular infection usually involving the

hands or feet that can cause skin breakdown or fistula formation and that spreads along the fascial planes to infect surrounding skin, subcutaneous tissue, and bone
- The CNS system is infected in approximately one third of all cases. Brain abscess is the most common pathologic finding.
- Dissemination of nocardiosis may infect other tissues and organs, including the kidney, heart, skin, and bone.

ETIOLOGY

- The most common *Nocardia* species leading to infection in human beings are:
  1. *N. asteroides* (causing more than 80% of the cases of pulmonary nocardiosis)
  2. *N. brasiliensis* (most common cause of mycetoma)
  3. *N. otitidiscaviarum*
- *N. asteroides* has two subgroups:
  1. *N. farcinica*
  2. *N. nova*

DIAGNOSIS

The diagnosis of nocardiosis requires a high index of suspicion in the proper clinical setting and is confirmed by bacteriologic staining and growth of the organism in culture.

DIFFERENTIAL DIAGNOSIS

There are no pathognomonic findings separating nocardiosis pneumonia from other infectious etiologies of the lung. Diagnoses presenting in a similar manner and often confused for nocardiosis include:
1. Tuberculosis
2. Lung abscess
3. Lung tumor
4. Other causes of pneumonia
5. Actinomycosis
6. Mycosis
7. Cellulitis
8. Coccidioidomycosis
9. Histoplasmosis
10. Aspergillosis
11. Kaposi's sarcoma

WORKUP

All patients with suspected nocardiosis need laboratory identification of the microorganism by obtaining sputum in the case of pneumonia, cultures of the infected skin lesions in mycetoma or lymphocutaneous disease, or the sampling of any purulent material (e.g., brain abscess, lung abscess, or pleural effusion).

LABORATORY TESTS

- Blood tests are not very sensitive in the diagnosis of nocardiosis.
- Gram stain shows gram-positive beaded filaments with multiple branches (Fig.1-256).
- Gomori methenamine silver staining may detect the organism.
- *Nocardia* species are acid-fast on a modified Ziehl-Neelsen stain.
- *Nocardia* are slow-growing organisms; colony growth in cultures may take up to 2 to 3 wk.

IMAGING STUDIES

- Chest radiograph may demonstrate infiltrates, densities, nodules, cavitary masses, or multiple abscesses.
- CT scan of the brain is indicated in the appropriate clinical setting to exclude CNS brain abscesses.

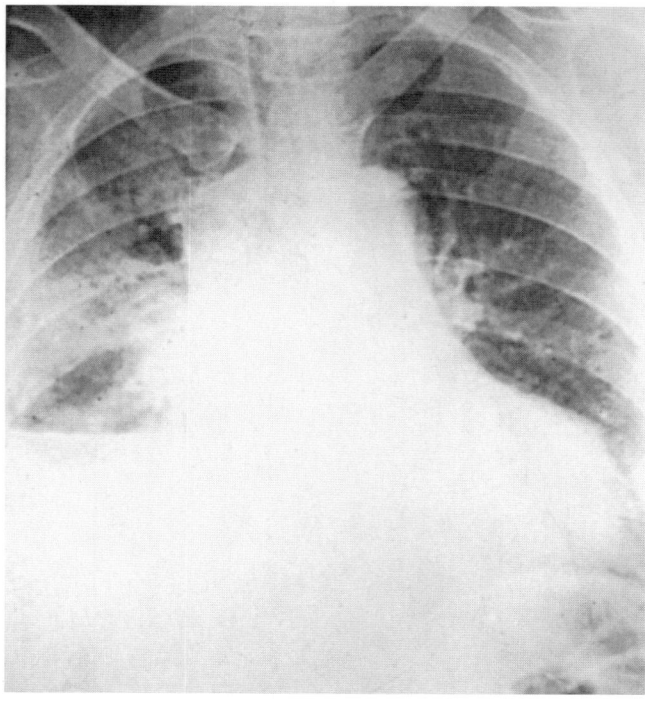

FIGURE 1-255 Right lower lobe *Nocardia* pneumonia in a kidney transplant recipient. (From Gorbach SL: *Infectious diseases,* ed 2, Philadelphia, 1998, WB Saunders.)

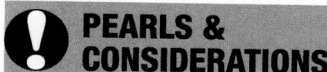 **Nocardiosis** 703

N

Diseases and Disorders

Rx TREATMENT

NONPHARMACOLOGIC THERAPY
- Supportive therapy with oxygen in patients with pneumonia
- Chest physiotherapy
- For any abscess formation, surgical drainage is indicated (e.g., skin, lung, or brain)

ACUTE GENERAL Rx
- There are no prospective, randomized trials to date highlighting the most effective treatment of nocardiosis. Nevertheless, sulfonamides are considered the treatment of choice. Sulfadiazine 6 to 10 g is given in 4 to 6 divided oral doses.
- For cutaneous infection, trimethoprim-sulfamethoxazole (TMX-SMX) 5 mg/kg of the trimethoprim component divided in 2 doses
- Severe infection: life-threatening pulmonary or disseminated disease; immunocompromised patients with severe disease should receive two-drug therapy: TMP-SMX 15 mg/kg IV of the trimethoprim component divided into two to four doses and amikacin 7.5 mg/kg IV q12h.

- In patients with CNS disease, ceftriaxone 2 g IV q12h or cefotaxime 2 g IV q8h or imipenem 500 mg IV q6h is substituted for amikacin.
- Sulfonamide-resistant disease: any of the following two-drug regimens: amikacin plus one of the following: ampicillin/sulbactam, imipenem, meropenem, ceftriaxone, or cefotaxime.
- Alternative drug treatment includes:
  1. Imipenem
  2. Third-generation cephalosporin
  3. Minocycline 100 to 200 mg bid
  4. Extended-spectrum fluoroquinolones (moxifloxacin)
  5. Linezolid (use of linezolid >4 wk is associated with hematologic toxicity)

CHRONIC Rx
- Although the optimal duration of therapy has not been determined, long-term therapy is generally recommended for all infections caused by *Nocardia*.
- Patients with cellulitis and lymphocutaneous syndrome are treated for 2 to 4 mo depending on whether there is bone involvement.

- Mycetomas are best treated with antibiotics for 6 to 12 mo but may require surgical drainage.
- Pulmonary and systemic nocardiosis excluding the CNS is treated for 6 to 12 mo.
- CNS involvement is treated with drainage and antibiotics for 12 mo.
- All immunosuppressed patients should receive 12 mo of antibiotic therapy.

DISPOSITION
- Patients with pulmonary nocardiosis have a mortality rate of 15% to 30%.
- CNS involvement carries a >40% mortality rate.
- Isolated skin lesions have a low mortality rate.

REFERRAL
Whenever the diagnosis of nocardiosis is suspected, consultation with infectious disease is indicated. Pulmonary evaluation and assistance may be needed in pulmonary nocardiosis. Neurosurgery consultation is indicated in patients with single or multiple brain abscesses.

! PEARLS & CONSIDERATIONS

- Nocardiosis does not spread from animal to animal.
- Nocardiosis is not transmitted from person to person.
- Nocardiosis is distinguished by its ability to disseminate to any organ and its tendency to relapse despite appropriate antibiotic therapy.

COMMENTS
Tuberculosis and nocardiosis may coexist in the same patient.

SUGGESTED READINGS
available at www.expertconsult.com

AUTHOR: **TANYA ALI, M.D.**

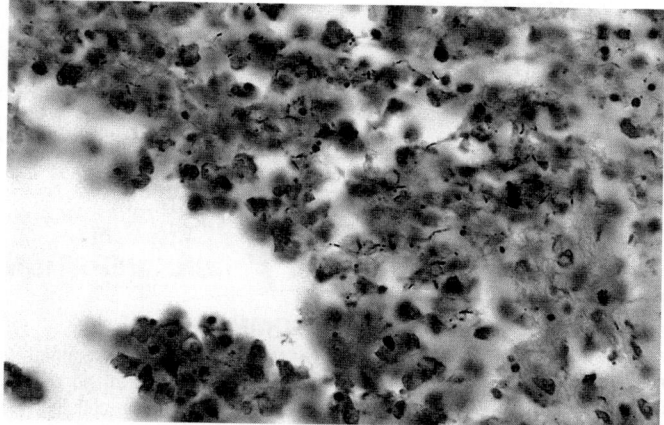

FIGURE 1-256 *Nocardia* **pneumonia.** Thin, branching, irregularly staining Gram-positive bacilli course through necrotic pulmonary tissue (Brown-Hopps Gram, ×1000). (From Silverberg SG et al [eds]: *Silverberg's principles and practice of surgical pathology and cytopathology,* ed 4, Philadelphia, 2006, Churchill Livingstone.)

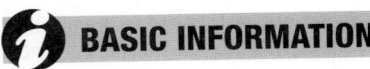

BASIC INFORMATION

DEFINITION

Spectrum of diseases based on histiopathologic findings and representing a morphologic rather than a clinical diagnosis. It is liver disease occurring in patients who do not abuse alcohol and manifesting histologically by mononuclear cells and/or polymorphonuclear cells, hepatocyte ballooning, and spotty necrosis. A diagnosis of nonalcoholic fatty liver disease is contingent on the following factors:

1. Alcohol consumption in amounts less than those considered hepatotoxic
2. Absence of serologic evidence of other hepatic diseases or disorders
3. Liver biopsy showing predominant macrovesicular steatosis or steatohepatitis

SYNONYMS

Nonalcoholic steatohepatitis (NASH)
NAFLD
Fatty liver hepatitis
Diabetes hepatitis
Alcohol-like liver disease
Laënnec's disease

ICD-9CM CODES
571.8 Fatty liver

EPIDEMIOLOGY & DEMOGRAPHICS

- Nonalcoholic fatty liver disease (NAFLD) affects 10% to 24% of the general population
- Increased prevalence in obese persons (57% to 74%), type 2 diabetes mellitus, and hyperlipidemia (primarily hypertriglyceridemia)
- Most common cause of abnormal liver test results in adults in the United States (accounts for up to 90% of cases of asymptomatic ALT elevations)
- 30 million obese adults have steatosis, 8.6 million may have steatohepatitis
- There is a 3:1 female-to-male predominance

PHYSICAL FINDINGS & CLINICAL PRESENTATION

- Most patients are asymptomatic
- Patients may report a sensation of fullness or discomfort on the right side of the upper abdomen
- Nonspecific complaints of fatigue or malaise may be reported
- Hepatomegaly is generally the only positive finding on physical examination
- Acanthosis nigricans may be found in children

ETIOLOGY

- Insulin resistance is the most reproducible factor in the development of nonalcoholic fatty liver disease. High baseline and continuously increasing fasting insulin levels are independent determinants for future development of NFLD
- Risk factors are obesity (especially truncal obesity), diabetes mellitus, hyperlipidemia

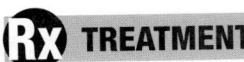

DIAGNOSIS

DIFFERENTIAL DIAGNOSIS

- Alcohol-induced liver disease (a daily alcohol intake of 20 g in females and 30 g in males [three 12-oz beers or 12 oz of wine] may be enough to cause alcohol-induced liver disease)
- Viral hepatitis
- Autoimmune hepatitis
- Toxin- or drug-induced liver disease

WORKUP

Diagnosis is usually suspected on the basis of hepatomegaly, asymptomatic elevations of transaminases, or "fatty liver" on sonogram of abdomen in obese patients with little or no alcohol use. Liver biopsy will confirm diagnosis and provide prognostic information. It should be considered in patients with suspected advanced liver fibrosis (presence of obesity or type 2 diabetes, AST/ALT ratio 1, age 45 yr).

LABORATORY TESTS

- Elevated ALT, AST: AST/ALT ratio is usually <1, but can increase as fibrosis advances
- Negative serology for infectious hepatitis; generally normal GGTP and serum alkaline phosphatase
- Hyperlipidemia (primarily hypertriglyceridemia) may be present
- Elevated glucose levels may be present
- Prolonged prothrombin time, hypoalbuminuria, and elevated bilirubin may be present in advanced stages
- Elevated serum ferritin and increased transferrin saturation may be found in up to 10% of patients; however, hepatic iron index and hepatic iron level are normal
- Liver biopsy may show a wide spectrum of liver damage, ranging from simple steatosis to advanced fibrosis and cirrhosis

IMAGING STUDIES

- Ultrasound generally reveals diffuse increase in echogenicity as compared with that of the kidneys; CT scan reveals diffuse low-density hepatic parenchyma.
- Occasionally patients may have focal rather than diffuse steatosis, which may be misinterpreted as a liver mass on ultrasound or CT; use of MRI in these cases will identify focal fatty infiltration.

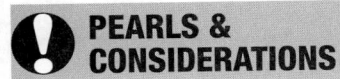

TREATMENT

NONPHARMACOLOGIC THERAPY

- Weight reduction in all obese patients (500 g per week in children and 1600 g per week in adults is preferred)
- Increase physical activity
- Alcohol has a deleterious effect on NAFLD and should be avoided

GENERAL Rx

- No medications have been proved to directly improve liver damage from nonalcoholic fatty liver disease.
- Medications to control hyperlipidemia (e.g., fenofibrates for elevated triglycerides) and hyperglycemia (e.g., metformin) can lead to improvement in abnormal liver test results.
- Pioglitazone therapy (30 mg/day) and vitamin E (800 IU/day) provide modest benefits in non-alcoholic steatohepatitis

DISPOSITION

- Patients with pure steatosis on liver biopsy generally have a relatively benign course.
- The presence of steatohepatitis or advanced fibrosis on liver biopsy is associated with a worse prognosis.

REFERRAL

- Liver transplantation should be considered in patients with decompensated, end-stage disease; however, in these patients there may be a recurrence of NAFLD post transplantation.

PEARLS & CONSIDERATIONS

COMMENTS

- NAFLD is closely associated with metabolic disorders, even in nonobese, nondiabetic subjects. It can be considered an early predictor of metabolic disorders, particularly in the normal-weight population. The presence of metabolic syndrome is a strong predictor of NAFLD.
- NAFLD is associated with an increased risk of incident cardiovascular disease that is independent of the risk conferred by traditional risk factors and components of the metabolic syndrome.

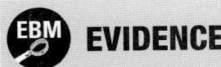 EVIDENCE

available at www.expertconsult.com

SUGGESTED READINGS
available at www.expertconsult.com

AUTHOR: **FRED F. FERRI, M.D.**

BASIC INFORMATION

DEFINITION

Obesity refers to having an excess amount of body fat in relation to lean body mass, or a body mass index (BMI) of $\geq$30 kg/m². Overweight is defined as BMI of 25 to 29.9 kg/m² and morbid obesity refers to adults with a BMI $\geq$40 kg/m². BMI is used as a surrogate measure of obesity. These conditions result from an imbalance between energy intake and expenditure.

SYNONYMS

Overweight

ICD-9CM CODES
278.0 Obesity

EPIDEMIOLOGY & DEMOGRAPHICS

- The World Health Organization first recognized obesity as a worldwide epidemic in 1997. As of 2005, 1.6 billion adults worldwide were classified as overweight, 400 million of whom were obese. It is predicted that the combination of overweight and obesity will soon eclipse more traditional public health issues like malnutrition and infectious diseases as the most significant cause of poor health.
- Based on data from the 2003 to 2004 U.S. National Health and Nutrition Examination Survey (NHANES), ~66 million American adults (30 million men and 36 million women) are obese and an additional 74 million (42 million men and 32 million women) are overweight. By 2015, it is estimated that two in every five adults and one in every four children in the U.S. will be obese.
- The present cost of obesity in the U.S. population is estimated at $100 billion annually.
- The prevalence of individuals who are overweight and obese increases with advancing age until the sixth decade, after which it begins to decline.
- For persons with a BMI $\geq$30 kg/m², all-cause mortality is increased by 50% to 100% above that of persons with BMI in the range of 20 to 25 kg/m².
- Obesity is an independent risk factor for cardiovascular disease (CVD) and CVD risks associated with obesity have also been documented in children.
- Obese individuals are at increased risk of morbidity and death from type 2 diabetes, hypertension, coronary heart disease (CHD), cancer (particularly colon, prostate, and breast cancer), sleep apnea, degenerative joint disease, thromboembolic disorders, digestive tract diseases (gallstones), and dermatologic disorders.
- Significant morbidity and risk of death are projected to begin in young adulthood, resulting in more than 100,000 excess cases of CHD by 2035, even with the most modest projection of future obesity.
- Obesity in adolescence is significantly associated with increased risk of incident severe obesity in adulthood, with variations by sex and race/ethnicity.
- Obesity is a major preventable cause of death and disability in the United States (the other is tobacco).
- Extensive data indicate that weight loss can reverse or arrest the harmful effects of obesity.

PHYSICAL FINDINGS & CLINICAL PRESENTATION

- Physical examination should assess the degree and distribution of body fat and signs of secondary causes of obesity.
- Increased waist circumference is apparent. Excess abdominal fat is clinically defined as a waist circumference >40 inches (>102 cm) in men and >35 inches (>88 cm) in women (in Asian men and women, >36 inches and >33 inches, respectively).
- Symptoms associated with hypertension, coronary artery disease (CAD), and diabetes (e.g., polyuria, polydipsia, retinopathy, and neuropathy) may be present.
- Obesity is associated with cardiac hypertrophy, diastolic dysfunction, and increased aortic stiffness, which are independent predictors of cardiovascular risk.
- Joint pain and swelling are associated with degenerative joint disease secondary to obesity.
- The physical exam and ECG often underestimate the presence and extent of cardiac dysfunction in obese patient. Jugular venous distention and hepatojugular reflux may not be seen and heart sounds are frequently distant. Obesity is associated with changes in the ECG such as a reduction in voltage and nonspecific ST-T changes that may affect the diagnosis of left ventricular hypertrophy (LVH) or CAD.
- A large quantity of fluid is present in the interstitial space of adipose tissue, as the interstitial space is ~10% of the tissue wet weight. Excess fluid in this compartment may have important repercussions in obese individuals with heart failure if this extra volume is redistributed into the circulation. Obese individuals have higher cardiac output and a lower total peripheral resistance than do lean individuals and obesity is associated with persistence of elevated cardiac filling pressure during exercise.
- Obesity predisposes to heart failure through several different mechanisms: increased total blood volume, increased cardiac output, LVH, left ventricular diastolic dysfunction, and adipositas cordis (excessive epicardial fat and fatty infiltration of the myocardium).

ETIOLOGY

- The pathophysiology of obesity is complex and poorly understood, but includes social, nutritional, physiologic, psychological, and genetic factors.
- Environmental factors such as a sedentary lifestyle and chronic ingestion of excess calories can cause obesity.
- Obesity may be related to genetic factors, which are thought to be polygenic. Genetic studies with adopted children have demonstrated that they have similar BMIs to their biologic parents but not their adoptive parents. Twin studies also demonstrate a genetic influence on BMI.

 DIAGNOSIS

- BMI will establish the diagnosis of obesity. BMI is a measure of an adult's weight in relation to his or her height—more specifically, the adult's weight in kilograms divided by the square of his or her height—and is closely correlated with total body fat content.
- BMI values can categorize patients into three classes of obesity:
  - Class I (mild): BMI of 30.0 to 34.9 kg/m²
  - Class II (moderate): BMI of 35.0 to 39.9 kg/m²
  - Class III (severe): BMI of $\geq$40 kg/m²
- Although BMI is commonly used to define obesity, it is not a highly accurate indicator of body fat composition in children, who are undergoing rapid changes in height, or in bodybuilders or athletes who have large amounts of muscle tissue.
- Waist circumference or waist-hip ratio is indicative of visceral adipose tissue, or intraabdominal fat, which may be more deleterious than overall overweight or obesity.

DIFFERENTIAL DIAGNOSIS

It is important to rule out specific causative medical disorders in obese patients. Hypothalamic disorders, hypothyroidism, Cushing's syndrome, insulinoma, depression, and drugs (corticosteroids, antidepressants, second generation antipsychotics, and HIV protease inhibitors) can cause obesity.

WORKUP

History should be obtained regarding weight change, family history of obesity, social circles, and eating and exercise behavior. Assessment for eating disorders and depression should be made. Attention should be directed to the use of nutritional supplements, over-the-counter medications, hormones, diuretics, and laxatives. The workup of an obese patient typically requires laboratory work to assess for risks and complications as well as to rule out underlying causative medical conditions.

LABORATORY TESTS

- Obese patients should be assessed for medical consequences of their obesity by screening for metabolic syndrome (measure high density lipoprotein, triglycerides, blood pressure, fasting glucose, and waist circumference).
- In the proper clinical setting, thyroid function studies, dexamethasone suppression testing, morning cortisol level, and insulin level with C-peptide measurements will exclude hypothyroidism, Cushing's syndrome, and insulinoma as underlying causes of obesity.

IMAGING STUDIES

- Several methods are available for determining or calculating total body fat but offer no

significant advantage over the BMI. These include measurement of total body water, total body potassium, bioelectrical impedance, and dual-energy x-ray absorptiometry.
- Buoyancy testing is an accurate method for determining total body fat composition.

(Rx) TREATMENT

The National Heart, Lung, and Blood Institute (NHLBI) developed guidelines for selecting treatment strategies for overweight and obese patients based on BMI and comorbidities. They recommend a combination of dietary management, physical activity management, and behavior therapy for anyone with a BMI ≥25. Pharmacotherapy should also be considered for patients with a BMI between 27 and 29.9 with comorbidities and for any patient with a BMI ≥30.

Surgery is indicated for patients with a BMI between 35 and 39.9 with comorbidities and for any patient with a BMI ≥40 (Table 1-134).

NONPHARMACOLOGIC THERAPY

- The cornerstones for weight management and reduction are calorie restriction, exercise, and behavioral modification.
- The NHLBI guidelines recommend an initial diet to produce a calorie deficit of 500 to 1000 kcal/day. This has been shown to reduce total body weight by an average of 8% over 3 to 12 mo.
- These guidelines recommend the use of a food diary to focus on dietary substitutes.
- Thirty minutes of moderate-intensity activity on 5 or more days of the week results in health benefits for obese individuals. Moreover, several studies indicate that 60 to 80 min of moderate to vigorous physical activity may provide additional benefit.
- Increased physical activity without caloric restriction (minimal or no weight loss) can reduce abdominal (visceral) adipose tissue and improve insulin resistance.
- The key features of the standard behavioral-modification program include goal setting, self-monitoring, stimulus control (modification of one's environment to enhance behaviors that will support weight management), cognitive restructuring (increased awareness of perceptions of oneself and one's weight), and prevention of relapse (weight regain).
- Mammalian sleep is closely integrated with the regulation of energy balance. Trials have shown that the amount of human sleep contributes to the maintenance of fat-free body mass at times of decreased energy intake. Lack of sufficient sleep may compromise the efficacy of typical dietary interventions for weight loss and related metabolic risk reduction.

ACUTE GENERAL Rx

- According to the NHLBI *Guidelines on the Identification, Evaluation, and Treatment of Overweight and Obesity in Adults* and the U.S. Food and Drug Administration (FDA), pharmacotherapy is indicated for:
  - Obese patients with a BMI ≥30 *or*
  - Overweight patients with a BMI of ≥27 and concomitant obesity-related risk factors or diseases, such as hypertension, diabetes, or dyslipidemia
- Two general classes of medications are currently approved by the FDA for treating obesity:
  - Gastrointestinal lipase inhibitors: orlistat (Xenical) blocks the digestion and absorption of ingested dietary fat. It is a reversible inhibitor of pancreatic, gastric, and carboxyl ester lipases and phospholipase A2, which are required for the hydrolysis of dietary fat in the gastrointestinal tract.
  - Sympathomimetic medications approved for short-term use: phentermine is an am-

phetamine derivative that increases the amount of norepinephrine in the neuronal cleft, resulting in appetite suppression. Similar drugs include diethylpropion, benzphetamine, and phendimetrazine. In 1997 both dexfenfluramine and fenfluramine were withdrawn from the market because of side effects of valvular heart lesions and pulmonary hypertension.
- Other medications in clinical trials include bupropion (Wellbutrin), topiramate (Topamax), and metformin (Glucophage).

CHRONIC Rx

- According to the NHLBI guidelines, surgical intervention is an option for selected patients with clinically severe obesity (a BMI ≥40 or a BMI ≥35 with comorbid conditions), when patients are at high risk for obesity-associated morbidity or death, and when less invasive methods of weight loss have failed.
- Bariatric surgery for weight loss falls into one of two categories:
  - Restrictive surgeries that limit the amount of food the stomach can hold and slow the rate of gastric emptying. These include vertical banded gastroplasty and laparoscopic adjustable silicone gastric banding (lap banding).
  - Restrictive malabsorptive bypass procedures combine the elements of gastric restriction and selective malabsorption. These include Roux-en-Y gastric bypass (considered the gold standard because of its high level of effectiveness and durability) and biliopancreatic diversion.
- A study on bariatric surgery patients demonstrated a significant reduction in long-term cardiovascular events. Ten-year follow-up estimated relative risk reductions ranging from 18% to 79% according to the Framingham risk score and 8% to 62% with the PROCAM risk score.

DISPOSITION

- The incidence of venous thromboembolism in the upper tertile of BMI was 2.42 times that of the lowest BMI tertile. Obese patients have a higher incidence of postoperative thromboembolic events when undergoing noncardiac surgery.
- Venous insufficiency: in the absence of right heart failure, surgically-induced weight loss is effective in correcting the venous stasis disease in the large majority of the patients.
- Perioperative obesity (>140% ideal body weight) may increase morbidity and mortality rates after heart transplantation.
- Weight stable obese subjects have an increased risk of arrhythmias and sudden death even in the absence of cardiac dysfunction.
- Obesity and the cardiac autonomic nervous system are intrinsically related. A 10% increase in body weight is associated with a decline in parasympathetic tone accompanied by a rise in mean heart rate, and conversely, heart rate declines during weight reduction.

TABLE 1-134 Weight-Loss Treatment Guidelines from the National Heart, Lung, and Blood Institute*

Treatment	BMI				
	25.0-26.9	27.0-29.9	30.0-34.9	35.0-39.9	>40.0
Diet, physical activity, behavioral therapy, or all three	Yes	Yes	Yes	Yes	Yes
Pharmacotherapy†		In patients with obesity-related diseases	Yes	Yes	Yes
Surgery‡				In patients with obesity-related diseases	Yes

*Data are from www.nhlbi.nih.gov/guidelines/obesity/ob_home.htm. These guidelines are generally consistent with those from the American Heart Association, the American Medical Association, the American Diabetic Association, the Obesity Society (Practical Guide), the American Diabetes Association, the American Academy of Family Physicians, the American College of Sports Medicine, and the American Cancer Society. BMI denotes body mass index, calculated as the weight in kilograms divided by the square of the height in meters.
†Pharmacotherapy should be considered only in patients who are not able to achieve adequate weight loss with available conventional lifestyle modifications and who have no absolute contraindications for drug therapy.
‡Bariatric surgery should be considered only in patients who are unable to lose weight with available conventional therapy and who have no absolute contraindications for surgery.

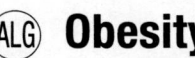
- A 10% weight loss in severely obese patients is associated with significant improvement in autonomic nervous system cardiac modulation. This translates into decreased heart rate and increased heart rate variability (HRV); decreased HRV is associated with increased cardiac mortality, independent of ejection fraction.
- Postmortem Determinants of Atherosclerosis in Youth (PDAY) study data provided convincing evidence that obesity in adolescents and young adults accelerates the progression of atherosclerosis decades before the appearance of clinical manifestations.
- Obesity accelerates the progression of native coronary atherosclerosis and after coronary artery bypass grafting.
- In older adults, obesity is associated with protection against hip fracture, but this protective effect on bone status does not offset the extensive array of potential adverse effects on conditions common in the older population.

REFERRAL

- Obesity is commonly seen in the primary care setting. If pharmacologic therapy is considered, consultation with physicians specializing in obesity and experienced with the use of the drug is recommended. In addition, consultation with nutritionists and behavioral therapists is also helpful. A consultation with general surgery is indicated in patients being considered for surgical intervention.
- Recent trials have shown that among adolescents, use of gastric banding compared with lifestyle intervention results in a greater percentage achieving a loss of 50% of excess weight corrected for age. There were associated benefits to health and quality of life.

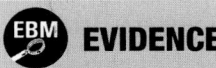
PEARLS & CONSIDERATIONS

COMMENTS

- The NHLBI launched the Obesity Education Initiative in January 1991. The overall purpose of the initiative is to help reduce the prevalence of overweight along with the prevalence of physical inactivity to reduce the risk of CHD and overall morbidity and mortality rates from CHD.
- The American Medical Association, in association with the Robert Wood Johnson Foundation and the U.S. Department of Health and Human Services, produced a primer for the assessment and management of adult obesity. The primer consists of 10 booklets that offer practical recommendations for addressing adult obesity in the primary care setting and is available for free at: http://www.ama-assn.org/ama1/pub/upload/mm/433/booklet1.pdf.
- Recent research indicates that brown adipose tissue represents a natural target for the modulation of energy expenditure. The presence of brown adipose tissue in humans may be quantified with the use of ^{18}F-FDG PET-CT. The amount of brown adipose tissue is inversely correlated with body mass index, suggesting a potential role of brown adipose tissue in adult human metabolism.
- Obesity, glucose intolerance, and hypertension in childhood are strongly associated with increased rates of premature death from endogenous causes in this population.
- Sibutramine (Meridia) is no longer FDA approved for treatment of obesity. Trials have shown that subjects with pre-existing cardiovascular conditions who were receiving long-term sibutramine treatment had an increased risk of non-fatal myocardial infarction and non-fatal stroke.

PREVENTION

- Prevention of overweight and obesity involves both increasing physical activity and dietary modification to reduce caloric intake.
- There is compelling evidence that prevention of weight regain in formerly obese individuals requires 60 to 90 min of moderate intensity activity or lesser amounts of vigorous intensity activity.
- Moderate intensity activity of approximately 45 to 60 min per day, or 1.7 physical activity level (PAL) is required to prevent the transition to overweight or obesity. For children, even more activity time is recommended.
- Clinicians can help guide patients to develop personalized eating plans and help them recognize the contributions of fat, concentrated carbohydrates, and large portion sizes.
- Clinicians must work with patients to modify other risk factors such as tobacco use, high glycemic intake, and elevated blood pressure to prevent the long-term chronic disease sequelae of obesity.
- Regular screening of body weight and BMI measurements at routine office visits can help identify early weight gain.

PATIENT & FAMILY EDUCATION

Information can be obtained on the American Obesity Association website (http://www.obesity.org) and the American Medical Association website (http://www.ama-assn.org).

EBM EVIDENCE

available at www.expertconsult.com

SUGGESTED READINGS

available at www.expertconsult.com

AUTHORS: **ANTHONY GEMIGNANI, M.D., FRED F. FERRI, M.D.,** and **WEN-CHIH WU, M.D.**

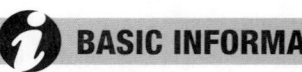

BASIC INFORMATION

DEFINITION

Obsessive-compulsive disorder (OCD) involves recurrent obsessions (intrusive and unwanted thoughts, urges, or images) and/or compulsions (behaviors or mental acts performed in response to obsessions, or according to rules that must be applied rigidly) that are time-consuming (e.g., >1 hr/day) or cause marked impairment or distress. The symptoms are usually perceived as excessive and unreasonable.

SYNONYMS

Compulsive hoarding, washing, list-making
Intrusive thoughts with ritualized and repetitive behaviors

ICD-9CM CODES
F42.8 Obsessive-compulsive disorder
(DSM-IV 300.3)

EPIDEMIOLOGY & DEMOGRAPHICS

PEAK INCIDENCE: Mean age at onset is 19.6 yr.
LIFETIME PREVALENCE (IN U.S.): 2.5% of adults
PREDOMINANT SEX: Approximately equal distribution between sexes
PREDOMINANT AGE:
- Modal age of onset for females is between 20 and 29 yr.
- Modal age of onset for males is between 6 and 15 yr.

DISEASE COURSE:
- Condition is chronic with waxing and waning pattern.
- Symptoms typically worsen with stress.
- 15% show progressive deterioration, whereas 5% show an episodic course with little impairment between episodes.

GENETICS:
- There is no clear genetic pattern.
- Rate of concordance is higher in monozygotic (33%) compared with dizygotic (7%) twins.
- Rate of disorder is also higher in first-degree relatives of individuals with OCD and Tourette's disorder than in the general population.

PHYSICAL FINDINGS & CLINICAL PRESENTATION

- Persistent and recurrent intrusive and ego-dystonic obsessive ideas, thoughts, urges, or images that are perceived as alien and beyond one's control.
- Frequent experiencing of obsessions related to contamination (e.g., when using the telephone), excessive doubt (e.g., was the door locked?), organization (the need for a particular order), violent impulses (e.g., to yell obscenities in church), or intrusive sexual imagery.
- Obsessions possibly leading to compulsive behaviors meant to temporarily ameliorate the anxiety caused by obsessions (e.g., repeated hand washing, checking, rearranging), or mental tasks (e.g., counting, repeating phrases).
- Obsessions and compulsions almost always accompanied by high anxiety and subjective distress. Both are usually seen as excessive and unreasonable.

ETIOLOGY

- Strong evidence of neurobiologic etiology.
- OCD may have onset after infectious illness of central nervous system (e.g., Von Economo's encephalitis, Sydenham's chorea).
- OCD may follow head trauma or other premorbid neurologic condition, including birth hypoxia and Tourette's syndrome.
- Serotonergic pathways believed important in some ritualistic instinctual behaviors, with dysfunction of these pathways possibly giving rise to OCD.

DIAGNOSIS

DIFFERENTIAL DIAGNOSIS

- Obsessive-compulsive personality disorder (OCPD) is a maladaptive personality style defined by excessive rigidity, need for order and control, preoccupation with details, and excessive perfectionism. Unlike OCD, OCPD is ego-syntonic.
- Other psychiatric disorders in which obsessive or intrusive thoughts occur (e.g., body dysmorphic disorder, eating disorders, hypochondriasis, phobias, posttraumatic stress disorder).
- Impulse control disorders (e.g., trichotillomania, pathologic gambling, compulsive shopping, kleptomania, paraphilias/sexual compulsions).
- Neurologic disorders with repetitive behaviors (e.g., Tourette's syndrome, Sydenham's chorea, torticollis, autism).
- Delusions or psychosis, which may be mistaken for obsessive thoughts; unlike OCD, these individuals do not believe their obsessions are unreal and may likely meet criteria for another psychotic spectrum disorder that fully accounts for the obsessions (e.g., schizophrenia).

WORKUP

- Careful history leading to diagnosis.
- Typically long delay between symptom onset and treatment.
- Neurologic examination to rule out concomitant Tourette's or other tic disorder.
- In adolescents and children: psychological testing to reveal learning disabilities.

LABORATORY TESTS

No specific tests are indicated.

IMAGING STUDIES

No specific studies are indicated.

TREATMENT

NONPHARMACOLOGIC THERAPY

- Treatment will help approximately 50% of patients achieve partial remission within the first 6 mo.
- Cognitive-behavioral therapy (especially exposure with response prevention) is successful in up to 70% of patients, but nearly 25% drop out of treatment because of the initial anxiety the exposures create. Best results are found for contamination obsessions and washing compulsions.

ACUTE GENERAL Rx

Clonazepam may be helpful in patients with extreme anxiety or those with a history of seizure disorder.

CHRONIC Rx

- Antidepressants with serotonergic reuptake blockade, including clomipramine, fluvoxamine, fluoxetine, paroxetine, sertraline, citalopram and escitalopram, venlafaxine, and duloxetine; optimal dosages are typically at the high end of the prescription range.
- Most improve with treatment, but few become symptom-free. No response in 15% of patients.
- Likely indefinite treatment. Relapse is common if medications are discontinued.
- Recent studies suggest that combination cognitive-behavioral therapy and pharmacotherapy yields superior outcomes. More severe symptoms warrant combination therapy.
- Patients who do not respond to first-line treatments and those with comorbid psychosis and/or tic disorders may benefit from augmentation with a first- or second-generation antipsychotic medication (e.g., haloperidol, olanzapine, risperidone).
- Surgical intervention (e.g., cingulotomy, deep brain stimulation) is an option for the most extreme, refractory cases.

DISPOSITION

- Most mild to moderate cases can be managed on a regular outpatient basis. Treatment should typically start with selective serotonin reuptake inhibitor (SSRI) monotherapy with regular follow-up to assess treatment response and side-effect management. Dose should be increased to maximum tolerated.
- Patient and family education may help improve medical adherence and support.

REFERRAL

- If distinction from other psychiatric conditions, particularly delusional disorder, is not clear.
- If patient is refractory to drug treatment and/or requests cognitive-behavioral therapy.

PEARLS & CONSIDERATIONS

Patients with OCD typically have insight regarding the irrationality of their obsessions and compulsions but lack the ability to control them. This may cause intense shame and avoidance of medical care unless patient education and support are provided. Screen for OCD, especially among patients who present with "depression" or "anxiety."

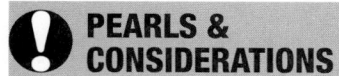 **EVIDENCE**

available at www.expertconsult.com

SUGGESTED READINGS
available at www.expertconsult.com

AUTHORS: **AUGUSTIN G. YIP, M.D., PH.D.,**
JASON M. SATTERFIELD, PH.D., and
MITCHELL D. FELDMAN, M.D., M.PHIL.

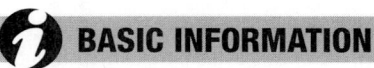

BASIC INFORMATION

DEFINITION
The term *ocular foreign body* refers to a foreign body on the surface of the corneal epithelium.

ICD-9CM CODES
930 Foreign body in external eye

EPIDEMIOLOGY & DEMOGRAPHICS
INCIDENCE (IN U.S.): Universal, with a predominance in active people
PEAK INCIDENCE: Childhood through active adult years
PREDOMINANT SEX: Perhaps slightly more common in men
PREDOMINANT AGE: Childhood through active adult years

PHYSICAL FINDINGS & CLINICAL PRESENTATION
- Pain is most common symptom.
- Causes of most common foreign bodies:
  - Grinding (Fig. 1-257)
  - Drilling
  - Auto repair
  - Working beneath cars
  - Airborne particles, such as blown by fans

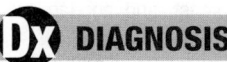

DIAGNOSIS

DIFFERENTIAL DIAGNOSIS
- History of corneal foreign body seen
- Hemorrhage, loss of vision
- Distorted anterior chamber, soft eye
- Corneal abrasion
- Corneal ulceration or laceration
- Glaucoma
- Herpes ulcers
- Infection
- Other keratitis
- Intraocular foreign body

WORKUP
- Fluorescein stain, slit-lamp examination if no foreign body is found
- Ultrasound examination
- Plain radiographs

LABORATORY TESTS
Intraocular pressure to make certain that eye has not been penetrated

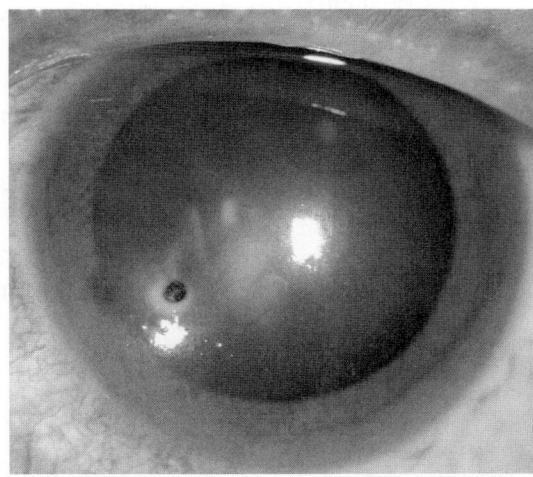

FIGURE 1-257 A small iron foreign body may be seen on external examination. (Courtesy Department of Dermatology, University of North Carolina at Chapel Hill. In Goldstein GB, Goldstein AO: *Practical dermatology,* ed 2, St Louis, 1997, Mosby.)

IMAGING STUDIES
Occasionally, MRI of the orbits to identify foreign bodies not found by other means. Do not perform MRI if suspect metallic foreign body. Plain radiographs and ultrasound are sufficient.

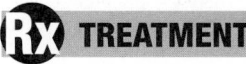

TREATMENT

NONPHARMACOLOGIC THERAPY
- Remove foreign body
- Treat infection
- Repair eye if ruptured
- Treat corneal abrasion or injury

ACUTE GENERAL Rx
- Saline irrigation
- Removal of foreign body with moist cotton-tipped applicator after instillation of topical anesthetic drops
- Use Burr or more aggressive treatment if needed
- Cycloplegics, antibiotics, and pressure dressing after removal of foreign body
- Repair corneal laceration or damaged eye

DISPOSITION
If symptoms persist 24 hr after examination, refer to an ophthalmologist.

REFERRAL
To ophthalmology within 24 hr if patient not completely comfortable

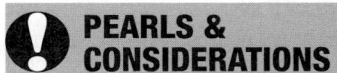

PEARLS & CONSIDERATIONS

COMMENTS
- Make sure foreign body is not intraocular (inside eye).
- Alkaline or acidic chemical foreign bodies can be dangerous; pH test must be performed if either of these is suspected (for all chemical foreign bodies).

SUGGESTED READINGS
available at www.expertconsult.com

AUTHOR: **MELVYN KOBY, M.D.**

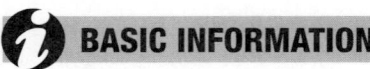

DEFINITION

Onychomycosis is defined as a persistent fungal infection affecting the toenails and fingernails.

SYNONYMS

Tinea unguium
Ringworm of the nails

ICD-9CM CODES
110.1 Onychomycosis

EPIDEMIOLOGY & DEMOGRAPHICS

- Onychomycosis is most commonly found in people between the ages of 40 and 60 yr.
- Onychomycosis rarely occurs before puberty.
- Incidence: 20 to 100 cases/1000 population.
- Toenail infection is 4 to 6 times more common than fingernail infection.
- Onychomycosis affects men more often than women.
- Occurs more frequently in patients with diabetes, peripheral vascular disease, and any conditions resulting in the suppression of the immune system.
- Occlusive footwear, physical exercise followed by communal showering, and incompletely drying the feet predisposes the individual to developing onychomycosis.

PHYSICAL FINDINGS & CLINICAL PRESENTATION

- Onychomycosis causes nails to become thick, brittle, hard, distorted, and discolored (yellow to brown color). Eventually, the nail may loosen, separate from the nail bed, and fall off (Fig. 1-258).
- Onychomycosis is frequently associated with tinea pedis (athlete's foot).

ETIOLOGY

- The most common causes of onychomycosis are dermatophyte, yeast, and nondermatophyte molds.
- The dermatophyte *Trichophyton rubrum* accounts for 80% of all nail infections caused by fungus.
- *Trichophyton interdigitale* and *Trichophyton mentagrophytes* are other fungi causing onychomycosis.
- The yeast *Candida albicans* is responsible for 5% of the cases of onychomycosis.
- Nondermatophyte molds *Scopulariopsis brevicaulis* and *Aspergillus niger,* although rare, can also cause onychomycosis.
- Onychomycosis is classified according to the clinical pattern of nail bed involvement. The main types are:
  1. Distal and lateral subungual onychomycosis (DLSO)
  2. Superficial onychomycosis
  3. Proximal subungual onychomycosis
  4. Endonyx onychomycosis
  5. Total dystrophic onychomycosis

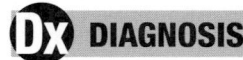

DIAGNOSIS

The diagnosis of onychomycosis is based on the clinical nail findings and confirmed by direct microscopy and culture.

DIFFERENTIAL DIAGNOSIS

- Psoriasis
- Contact dermatitis
- Lichen planus
- Subungual keratosis
- Paronychia
- Infection (e.g., *Pseudomonas*)
- Trauma
- Peripheral vascular disease
- Yellow nail syndrome

WORKUP

The workup of suspected onychomycosis is directed at confirming the diagnosis of onychomycosis by visualizing hyphae under the microscope by KOH prep or by culturing the organism. Although the standard for the diagnosis of fungal nail disease is a positive result on microscopical examination and culture of nail clippings with subungal debris or from surface debris in superficial white onychomycosis, treatment is often prescribed in absence of confirmatory findings.

LABORATORY TESTS

- KOH prep: specificity is high but sensitivity is variable
- Fungal cultures on Sabouraud medium: culture may take 4 to 6 wk
- Dermatophyte test medium (DTM): an alternative to Sabaoraud's, which takes only 3 to 7 days and can be done in office setting. A color change indicates dermatophyte growth.
- Nail plate biopsy with periodic acid–Schiff (PAS) stain
- Blood tests are not specific in the diagnosis of onychomycosis and therefore not useful

IMAGING STUDIES

- Imaging studies are not very specific in making the diagnosis of onychomycosis and not useful.
- If an infection is present and osteomyelitis is a consideration, an x-ray of the specific area and a bone scan may help establish the diagnosis.

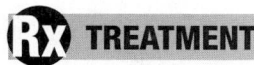

TREATMENT

NONPHARMACOLOGIC THERAPY

- Surgical removal of the nail plate is a treatment option; however, the relapse rate is high.
- Prevention of reinfection by wearing properly fitted shoes, avoiding public showers, and keeping feet and nails clean and dry.

ACUTE GENERAL Rx

- Topical antifungal creams are used for early superficial nail infections.
  1. Miconazole 2% cream applied over the nail plate bid
  2. Clotrimazole 1% cream bid
  3. Ciclopirox: topical antifungal nail lacquer can be used for moderate onychomycosis that spares the lunula. Success rate <10%
  4. Amorolfine: nail lacquer for infecton that spares lunula but not available in the U.S.
- Oral agents.
  1. Terbinafine
     a. For toenails: 250 mg/day for 3 mo
     b. For fingernails: 250 mg/day for 6 wk
  2. Itraconazole
     a. For toenails: 200 mg PO daily for 3 mo
     b. For fingernails: 200 mg PO daily for 6 wk
  3. Fluconazole: not as effective as terbinafine or itraconazol

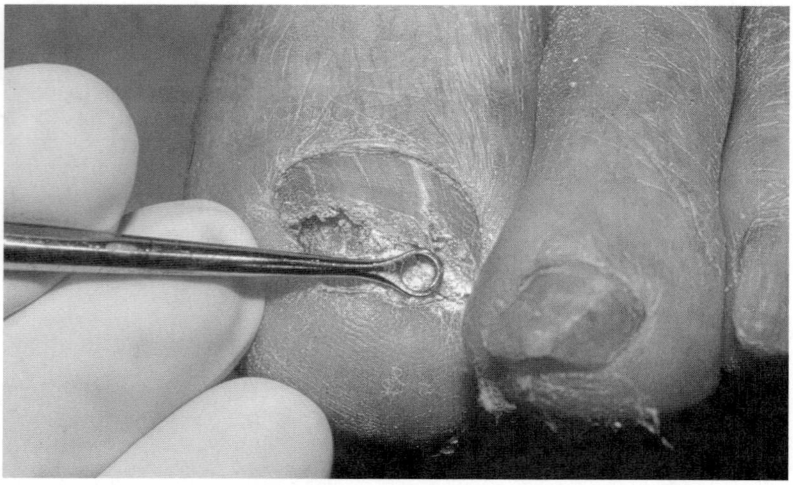

FIGURE 1-258 Collection of nail for culture. The subungual debris is the most valuable material for culture. After cutting back the nail, a curette may be used. Clippings of the nail may be added to the culture. (From White GM, Cox NH [eds]: *Diseases of the skin, a color atlas and text,* ed 2, St Louis, 2006, Mosby.)

a. For toenails: 150 to 300 mg once weekly for 18 to 26 wk
b. For fingernails: 150 to 300 mg once weekly for 12 to 16 wk

- All oral agents used for onychomycosis require periodic monitoring of liver function blood tests. Patients should be advised to watch for symptoms of drug-induced hepatitis (anorexia, fatigue, nausea, right upper quadrant pain) while taking these oral antifungal agents. They should stop their medication and contact their physician immediately if symptoms occur.
- Itraconazole is contraindicated in patients taking cisapride, astemizole, triazolam, midazolam, and terfenadine. Statins should be discontinued during itraconazole therapy. Itraconazole requires gastric acidity for absorption; patients should be advised not to take oral antacids, H_2 blockers, or proton pump inhibitors while taking itraconazole.
- Fluconazole is contraindicated in patients taking cisapride and terfenadine.

- Oral antifungal agents should not be initiated during pregnancy.
- Near-infrared laser therapy, ultraviolet light therapy, and photodynamic therapy are currently being evaluated.

DISPOSITION

- Spontaneous remission of onychomycosis is rare.
- A disease-free toenail is reported to occur in approximately 25% to 50% of patients treated with the oral antifungal agents mentioned previously.

REFERRAL

- Podiatry consultation is indicated in diabetic patients for proper instruction in foot care, footwear, and nail debridement or surgical removal of the toenail.
- Dermatology consultation is indicated in patients refractory to treatment or if another diagnosis is considered (e.g., psoriasis).

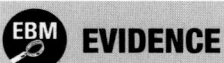 **PEARLS & CONSIDERATIONS**

COMMENTS

- The growth of fungus on an infected nail typically begins at the end of the nail and spreads under the nail plate to infect the nail bed as well.
- Carefully consider the informational insert regarding drug-drug interactions and contraindications before initiating oral antifungal agents.

EBM **EVIDENCE**

available at www.expertconsult.com

SUGGESTED READINGS

available at www.expertconsult.com

AUTHORS: **GLENN G. FORT, M.D., M.P.H.,** and **DENNIS J. MIKOLICH, M.D.**

Diseases and Disorders

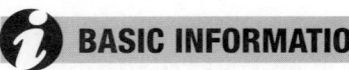

BASIC INFORMATION

DEFINITION

- Opioid addiction/dependence is defined as a cluster of cognitive, behavioral, and physiologic symptoms in which the individual continues use of opiates despite significant opiate-induced problems. Opiate dependence is a chronic, relapsing disorder characterized by repeated self-administration that usually results in opiate tolerance, withdrawal, and compulsive drug use. Dependence may occur with or without the physiologic symptoms of tolerance and withdrawal.
- There are four stages of addiction:
  1. Stage I, acute drug effects: rewarding effects of drug result from neurobiologic changes in response to the acute drug use. Duration varies from hours to days.
  2. Stage II, transformation to addiction: associated with changes in neuronal function that accumulate with repeated administration and diminish over days or weeks after discontinuation of drug use.
  3. Stage III, relapse after extended periods of abstinence: precipitated by an incubation of cue-induced craving (people, places, and things as triggers) and priming (relapse precipitated by drug exposure).
  4. Stage IV, end-stage addiction: vulnerability to relapse endures for years and results from prolonged changes at the cellular level.
- Pseudoaddiction: undertreatment of pain resulting in "opiate-seeking" behaviors such as "doctor shopping" and multiple emergency department visits. These behaviors disappear with adequate treatment of pain.

SYNONYMS

Opiate addiction
Opiate abuse
Narcotic addiction
Narcotic abuse

ICD-9CM CODES
304.7X/304.8X Opioid dependence

EPIDEMIOLOGY & DEMOGRAPHICS

INCIDENCE: There are 980,000 opiate addicts in the U.S.; less than one third are in treatment.

PREVALENCE:
- Approximately 6 million persons age ≥12 yr used psychotherapeutic drugs for nonmedical purposes in 2004, which represents 2.5% of the population. Most of them reported abusing opiate pain relievers.
- In 2004, 2.4 million persons age ≥12 yr initiated nonmedical use of prescription pain relievers, surpassing for the first time those who initiated abuse of marijuana (2.1 million).
- Opiate addiction is becoming an adolescent disease. Among twelfth-graders, in 2005, 9.5% reported past-year nonmedical use of oxycodone (Vicodin) and 5.5% reported past-

year nonmedical use of oxycodone slow-release tablets (OxyContin).
- The percentage of eighth-, tenth-, and twelfth-graders who have used heroin has more than doubled since the late 1990s. This increase has largely been attributed to decreased price and increased purity in the last decade.

PREDOMINANT SEX: Males abuse opiates more commonly than females, with a male/female ratio of 3:1 for heroin and 1.5:1 for prescription opiates.

PEAK INCIDENCE: The majority of new abusers of opiates are <26 yr.

RISK FACTORS:
- Family history
- Prior history of addiction
- Psychiatric disorders

GENETICS:
- Genetic epidemiologic studies suggest a high degree of heritable vulnerability for opiate dependence.
- Gene polymorphism for dopamine receptor/transporters, opioid receptors, serotonin receptors/transporters, proenkephalin, and catechol-o-methyltransferase all appear to be associated with vulnerability to opiate dependence. Future interventions for opiate dependence may include medications identified through genetic research.

PHYSICAL FINDINGS & CLINICAL PRESENTATION

- Physical examination is often noncontributory.
- Small-sized pupils may be the only observable sign of use because only mild tolerance develops for miosis.
- Scars or tracks from chronic IV use may be visible over the veins of the arms, hands, ankles, neck, and breasts.
- Inflamed nasal mucosa or respiratory wheezing may be apparent in patients who are snorting heroin or OxyContin.
- Patients in withdrawal may have more dramatic findings such as tachycardia, hypertension, fever, piloerection (goose flesh), mydriasis, lacrimation, central nervous system (CNS) arousal, irritability, and repeated yawning. In patients with sympathetic overactivity and panic attacks, use of CNS stimulants, such as amphetamines or cocaine, should also be ruled out.
- Although gastrointestinal symptoms of nausea, vomiting, and abdominal pain are common in opiate withdrawal, other causes such as gastroenteritis, pancreatitis, peptic ulcer disease, and intestinal obstruction need to be ruled out.
- The history may provide relevant information in making the diagnosis. Significant findings may include:
  1. A long history of opiate self-administration, typically by the IV or intranasal route but sometimes through smoking as well.
  2. Polysubstance use. Intoxication by drugs other than narcotics (e.g., benzodiazepines, barbiturates) should be ruled out in unconscious patients.

3. A high incidence of non-opiate-related psychiatric disorders (>80%).
4. History of problems at work, school, or relationships associated with drug use.
5. History of legal problems associated with drug use, such as arrest for possession, robbery, or prostitution.
6. History of interpersonal violence (as perpetrator or victim).
7. History of physical problems such as skin infections, phlebitis, endocarditis, or liver diseases attributable to acetaminophen toxicity (Vicodin/Percocet) or viral hepatitis. Hepatitis C is the most prevalent blood-borne pathogen. It is present in approximately 90% of opiate-dependent people and is often spread by sharing IV drug paraphernalia or snorting devices. There is also a higher incidence of HIV infection.

ETIOLOGY

Opioid dependence is a biopsychosocial disorder. Pharmacologic, social, genetic, and psychodynamic factors interact to influence abusive behaviors. Pharmacologic factors are especially prominent in opiate addiction because these drugs are strong reinforcing agents because of their euphoric effects and their ability to reduce anxiety and increase self-esteem and the patient's subjective feelings of improved ability to cope with daily challenges.

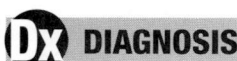 DIAGNOSIS

DIFFERENTIAL DIAGNOSIS

- Psychiatric disorders (e.g., anxiety, depression, bipolar disorder).
- Acute medical illness (e.g., hypoglycemia, seizure disorder, sepsis, renal or hepatic insufficiency) may mimic opiate withdrawal symptoms.

WORKUP

- The history is the most important part of the workup.
- Observation of opiate withdrawal is indicative of opiate addiction.
- Observation of purposeful behaviors such as complaints and manipulations directed at getting more drugs and anxiety during withdrawal is suggestive of opiate addiction.
- Screen blood and urine for opiate metabolites.
- Screen for communicable diseases: HIV, hepatitis B and hepatitis C, tuberculosis.
- Screen for endocarditis in patients with newly diagnosed murmurs.

LABORATORY TESTS

- Urine and serum toxicology screen
- Complete blood count
- Chemistries (alanine aminotransferase, aspartate aminotransferase, serum creatinine): elevated liver function test (LFT) results may be from viral hepatitis or acetaminophen toxicity

- Hepatitis screen: if hepatitis C antibody positive, follow up with hepatitis C polymerase chain reaction (viral load) even in patients with normal LFTs
- HIV
- PPD

IMAGING STUDIES

Generally not helpful in routine diagnosis and treatment. Consider echocardiography in patients with heart murmurs and liver sonography or CT scan in patients with elevated LFTs or who are positive for hepatitis C or B (increased risk of hepatocellular carcinoma).

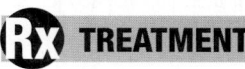 **TREATMENT**

NONPHARMACOLOGIC THERAPY

- Brief counseling interventions during a visit with their primary care physician or OB/GYN have proven efficacious in motivating patients for treatment.
- Therapeutic communities (residential).
- 12-step or other self-help groups (e.g., Alcoholics Anonymous, Narcotics Anonymous).
- Relapse prevention (counseling).

ACUTE Rx

- Medical withdrawal (not overdosed).
- Short- (30 days) or long-term (30 to 180 days) protocols.
- Buprenorphine (opioid partial agonist) or methadone (opioid agonist) is initiated in tapering doses.
- Clonidine 0.1 mg bid to tid can be used to minimize autonomic symptoms (sweating) and craving.
- Nonsteroidal antiinflammatory drugs for body and muscle aches.
- The anticholinergic dicyclomine can be used to minimize gastrointestinal hyperactivity.
- Nonbenzodiazepine hypnotics, low-dose atypical antipsychotics (e.g., Quetiapine), or low-dose tricyclic antidepressants are effective for promoting adequate sleep.

CHRONIC Rx

Opioid antagonist treatment:
- Naltrexone: does not stabilize neuronal circuitry like partial or full opioid agonists and generally results in poor outcomes, much like Antabuse for alcohol.
- Opioid partial agonist therapy: buprenorphine.
- Opioid agonist therapy: methadone.

NOTE: Buprenorphine and methadone are both metabolized by the cytochrome P450 3a4 and 2d6 I isoenzyme pathways. Prescribers should be aware of multiple possible drug interactions.

PATIENT SELECTION FOR BUPRENORPHINE OR METHADONE

- Appropriate patients for buprenorphine office-based treatment:
  - Patients interested (highly motivated) in treatment
  - Have no major contraindications (see following)
  - Can be expected to be reasonably compliant with treatment
  - Understand the benefits and risks of buprenorphine treatment
  - Willing to follow safety precautions
- Less likely to be appropriate for office-based treatment:
  - Have comorbid dependence on benzodiazepines or other CNS depressants (including ethylene alcohol)
  - Have significant untreated psychiatric comorbidities
  - Have active or chronic suicidal or homicidal ideation or attempts
  - Have multiple previous treatments with frequent relapses
  - Have poor response to previous treatment with buprenorphine
  - Have significant medical complications (e.g., hepatic insufficiency, bacterial endocarditis, active tuberculosis)
- Methadone maintenance: narcotic treatment program (clinic setting) indications
- Evidence of opiate addiction >1 yr
- Two failed previous treatment attempts
- Patients not appropriate for office-based treatment
- Eligible without active "use" if prior methadone maintenance patient within previous 2 mo
- Pregnancy

DISPOSITION

- Opioid addiction is a chronic, relapsing disease.
- High rate of relapse after "detox."
- Relapse potential after medically supervised withdrawal from methadone:
  - 90% after 1 yr stable in treatment
  - 80% after 3 yr stable in treatment
  - 70% after 5 yr stable in treatment

REFERRAL

Refer to addiction medicine specialist or narcotic treatment program when the neurobiologic disease of opioid addiction is identified.

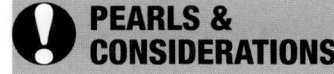 **PEARLS & CONSIDERATIONS**

COMMENTS

- Methadone maintenance is the gold standard for the pregnant opiate-addicted patient re-

gardless of the duration of the addiction or prior treatment attempts. Detoxification is contraindicated during pregnancy.
- Breastfeeding is encouraged in mothers on methadone maintenance. The American Academy of Pediatrics statement regarding "Transfer of Drugs and Other Chemicals into Human Milk" has placed methadone into the "usually compatible with breastfeeding" group based on the assumption that maternal urine is monitored to detect use of illicit drugs. The U.S. Department of Health and Human Services also recommends that mothers on methadone be encouraged to breastfeed.
- When a physician identifies a patient as a "drug seeker," it is imperative that the physician avoids abruptly stopping the opiate prescription because this will often result in the patient buying the drugs illegally. These patients should be counseled and referred for treatment.
- Patients on methadone or buprenorphine who have pain resulting from an acute injury will need pain medication in addition to their daily dose of methadone or buprenorphine. They will require higher than usual doses of pain medications because of opiate receptor blockade attributable to their methadone or buprenorphine use.
- Opiate-dependent patients have a lower pain threshold resulting from hyperalgesia caused by the long-term use of opiates.

PREVENTION

Education is the hallmark of prevention.
- School drug prevention education programs.
- Educate children about their family medical history, including diseases of addiction.
- Address childhood psychiatric disorders to prevent self-medicating.

PATIENT & FAMILY EDUCATION

- Stigma of addictions and treatment often interferes with good treatment.
- Family needs to be educated so they can support the patient's efforts.
- Encourage family meeting with addiction specialist, counselor.
- Recommend support groups for family members.

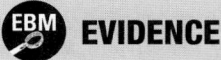 **EVIDENCE**

available at www.expertconsult.com

SUGGESTED READINGS
available at www.expertconsult.com

AUTHOR: **STEVEN PELIGIAN, D.O.**

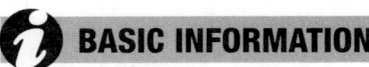

DEFINITION

- Optic atrophy refers to the degeneration of the axons of the optic nerve.
- It is a symptom rather than a disease.

SYNONYMS

Unilateral/bilateral optic atrophy

ICD-9CM CODES
377.10 Atrophy, optic nerve

EPIDEMIOLOGY & DEMOGRAPHICS

PREDOMINANT SEX: Unilateral optic atrophy in women is most commonly multiple sclerosis (MS); may also occur after head injury (more commonly in men)
PREDOMINANT AGE: 21 to 40 yr
PEAK INCIDENCE: Varies depending on cause

PHYSICAL FINDINGS & CLINICAL PRESENTATION

- Asymmetry of disc color is often first subtle finding.
- Temporal part of optic disc is pale initially (Fig. 1-259); later the entire disc becomes pale/white.
- Optic disc pallor occurs 4 to 6 wk after optic nerve injury.

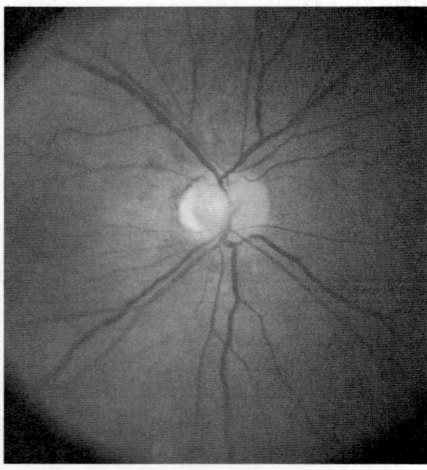

FIGURE 1-259 Optic atrophy. Patient's right eye shows atrophy. (Courtesy John W. Payne, M.D., The Wilmer Ophthalmological Institute, The Johns Hopkins University and Hospital, Baltimore. From Seidel HM [ed]: *Mosby's guide to physical examination,* ed 4, St Louis, 1999, Mosby.)

- Unilateral lesion produces a relative afferent pupillary defect (RAPD): swing flashlight eye to eye; abnormal pupil dilates to direct light.
- Decreased visual acuity, blurred vision, visual field deficits (e.g., central scotoma), abnormal color vision (e.g., red desaturation).

ETIOLOGY

- Optic neuritis—MS, sarcoidosis, infections (syphilis, CMV, HIV, Lyme disease)
- Vascular—ischemic optic neuropathy, central retinal artery occlusion, temporal arteritis
- Compression—glaucoma, pituitary tumor, meningioma, thyroid eye disease
- Hereditary—Leber's hereditary optic neuropathy
- Nutritional, toxic, and metabolic—Amiodarone, Isoniazid, B_{12} deficiency, tobacco, alcohol
- Trauma

DIAGNOSIS

DIFFERENTIAL DIAGNOSIS

- Nutritional, toxic, and hereditary causes are usually bilateral.
- Unilateral optic atrophy in a young person is more commonly MS.
- Postviral atrophy may be seen in childhood.

WORKUP

- Depends on suspected cause/clinical presentation. History including age of onset, risk factors, acuity of onset of symptoms, trauma, presence of pain, family history, toxic/nutritional factors, and other associated neurologic findings should be considered.
- Visual field testing may help identify cause (e.g., centrocecal field defects may occur with nutritional/toxic causes), but specificity is low.
- To differentiate between optic nerve and macular disease an Amsler chart and/or visual evoked responses may be helpful.
- If high clinical suspicion for MS, consider MRI of brain with contrast, evoked potentials, and LP with oligoclonal bands.
- Measure intraocular pressure (glaucoma).

LABORATORY TESTS

- Depends on suspected cause: none for trauma, tumor, or MS
- Serum B_{12}
- Autoimmune diseases: ESR, ANA, ACE

IMAGING STUDIES

- MRI of the brain with contrast, fat suppression and special (thin) cuts through orbits are necessary to identify compressive lesions in all patients with unexplained optic atrophy; especially important in patients with positive predictive factors for abnormal imaging (e.g., young age, progression, bilateral findings).
- If sarcoid is suspected, order chest x-ray.

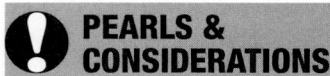
TREATMENT

ACUTE GENERAL Rx

Treat the underlying cause—discontinue identifiable toxins, use B_{12} replacement, neurosurgical intervention is necessary if tumor is found; consider IV steroids if there is evidence for active demyelinating disease.

CHRONIC Rx

The optic nerve does not regenerate, although symptoms often improve.

DISPOSITION

- Visual loss usually occurs over weeks to months.
- Appointment with neurologist or ophthalmologist.

REFERRAL

If tumor or demyelinating lesions are found or if etiology is unknown

PEARLS & CONSIDERATIONS

COMMENTS

- An experienced clinician should be able to identify pale optic discs and a relative afferent pupillary defect.
- Pupillary dilation with mydriatic agents (e.g., Pilocarpine) may be necessary to optimize funduscopic examination.
- Patient education material can be obtained from the National Eye Institute, Department of Health and Human Services, 9000 Rockville Pike, Bethesda, MD 20892.

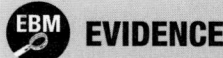
EVIDENCE

available at www.expertconsult.com

SUGGESTED READINGS
available at www.expertconsult.com

AUTHOR: **RICHARD S. ISAACSON, M.D.**

BASIC INFORMATION

DEFINITION

Optic neuritis is an inflammation of the optic nerve resulting in impaired visual function.

SYNONYMS

Optic papillitis
Retrobulbar neuritis

ICD-9CM CODES
377.3 Optic neuritis

EPIDEMIOLOGY & DEMOGRAPHICS

INCIDENCE (IN U.S.): 1 to 5/100,000 person(s) per year; rates vary according to incidence of multiple sclerosis (MS).
PREVALENCE (IN U.S.): Common in patients with MS.
PREDOMINANT SEX: Female/male ratio: 1.8:1
PEAK INCIDENCE: 20 to 49 yr, mean 30.
GENETICS: MS is more common in patients with certain HLA blood types and in monozygotic twins of affected siblings. See topic "Multiple Sclerosis."

PHYSICAL FINDINGS & CLINICAL PRESENTATION

- Presents with acute or subacute (days) visual loss and most often tenderness with movement of affected eye.
- Marcus Gunn pupil (relative afferent pupillary defect [RAPD]): direct and consensual response is normal; however, when swinging flashlight from eye to eye, the affected eye's pupil dilates to direct light.
- Decreased visual acuity.
- Unilateral visual field abnormalities—often a central scotoma.
- Color desaturation, red is most often affected.
- Normal orbit and fundus; occasionally there is disc edema acutely (Fig. 1-260), uveitis, or periphlebitis.

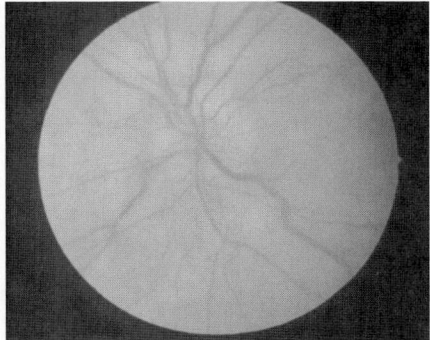

FIGURE 1-260 A case of optic neuritis. The optic disc edema seen here is often not present. Note the otherwise normal fundus. (Courtesy of J. Barton, M.D., Beth Israel Deaconess Medical Center, Boston.)

- May have movement or light-induced phosphenes (flashes of light lasting 1 to 2 sec).
- Uhthoff's phenomenon (benign exercise- or heat-induced deterioration of vision) is seen in some. Vision may also worsen in bright sunlight.
- Over time the optic disc may atrophy and become pale.

ETIOLOGY

An inflammatory response associated with an infection, autoimmune disease (such as MS), or, rarely, a mitochondrial disorder.

DIAGNOSIS

Consistent clinical presentation and exclusion of alternate ocular pathology, infection, and CNS mass lesions. Classic triad includes loss of vision, pain, and dyschromatopsia. 70% unilateral and 30% bilateral.

DIFFERENTIAL DIAGNOSIS

- Inflammatory: MS, neuromyelitis optica, sarcoidosis, lupus, Sjögren's, Behçet's, postinfectious, postvaccination
- Infectious: syphilis, TB, Lyme disease, *Bartonella*, HIV, CMV, herpes
- Ischemic: giant cell arteritis, anterior and posterior ischemic optic neuropathies, diabetic papillopathy, branch or central retinal artery or vein occlusion
- Mitochondrial: Leber's hereditary optic neuropathy
- Mass lesion: pituitary tumor, aneurysm, meningioma, glioma, metastases, sinus mucocele
- Ocular: optic drusen, retinal detachment, vitreous hemorrhage, uveitis, posterior scleritis, neuroretinitis, maculopathies and retinopathies
- Toxic: B_{12} deficiency, tobacco-ethanol amblyopia, methanol or ethambutol intoxication (painless, most bilateral, typically slowly progressive)
- Other: acute papilledema, retinal migraine, factitious visual loss

WORKUP

A thorough neurologic examination; recommend dilated ophthalmoscopy.

LABORATORY TESTS

- Recommend CBC, ANA, ESR.
- Consider HIV Ab, Lyme titer, ACE, RPR, LHON mtDNA mutations.

IMAGING STUDIES

MRI of the brain and orbits (thin section fat-suppressed T_2-weighted) with gadolinium is needed to look for compressive and infiltrative causes. Often enhancement of the optic nerve is seen. The risk to develop MS can also be assessed.

TREATMENT

NONPHARMACOLOGIC THERAPY

Assure patient that in most cases there is near complete recovery of vision.

ACUTE GENERAL Rx

Not all ophthalmologists and neurologists recommend treatment, but treat if the visual loss is severe or if there is an abnormal MRI (higher risk of MS). Consider methylprednisolone (MP) 250 mg IV every 6 hr for 3 days followed by an oral prednisone taper of 11 days. MP 1 g IV every day for 3 days followed by a prednisone taper is an alternative.

CHRONIC Rx

None, unless at high risk to develop MS. See topic "Multiple Sclerosis."

DISPOSITION

Most often vision is worst at the end of week 1, followed by recovery over several months. In the Optic Neuritis Treatment Trial (ONTT), 90% had 20/40 or better vision at 1 yr and 3% had 20/200 or worse. Of initial 20/200 or worse cases, only 5% remained in that group at 6 mo.

REFERRAL

- To neurologist if patient has other neurologic signs; urgently needed if proptosis or ophthalmoplegia present.
- To ophthalmologist when atypical features or slowly progressive, and urgently when other ocular pathology is present.
- To ophthalmologist if vision worsens or does not improve after several wk, severe or persistent pain, or deteriorates as steroids are tapered.

PEARLS & CONSIDERATIONS

- Bilateral optic neuritis, especially with poor recovery, suggests possible Leber's hereditary optic neuropathy or toxic optic neuropathies.
- Acute bilateral loss with a severe headache or diplopia should raise concern for pituitary apoplexy.

EVIDENCE

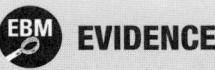

available at www.expertconsult.com

SUGGESTED READINGS

available at www.expertconsult.com

AUTHOR: **ALEXANDRA DEGENHARDT, M.D.**

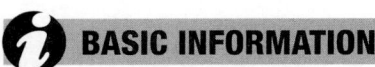 **BASIC INFORMATION**

DEFINITION

Orchitis is an inflammatory process (usually infectious) involving the testicles. Infection may be viral or bacterial and can be associated with infection of other male sex organs (prostate, epididymis, or bladder) or lower urogenital tract or sexually transmitted diseases often via hematogenous spread. Common causes are:

- Viral: Mumps—20% postpubertal; coxsackie B virus
- Bacterial: Pyogenic via spread from involving epididymis; bacteria include *Escherichia coli, Klebsiella pneumoniae, P. aeruginosa, Staphylococcus, Streptococcus* or *Rickettsia, Brucella* spp
- Other:
  - Viral—HIV-associated, CMV
  - Fungi
    1. Cryptococcosis
    2. Histoplasmosis
    3. *Candida*
    4. Blastomycosis
  - *Mycobacterium tuberculosis* and *M. leprae*
  - Parasitic causes: toxoplasmosis, filiariasis, schistosomiasis

SYNONYMS

Epididymoorchitis
Testicular infection
Testicular inflammation

ICD-9CM CODES
0.72	Mumps
098.13	Acute gonococcal orchitis
095.8	Syphilitic orchitis
016.50	Tuberculous orchitis, unspecified

EPIDEMIOLOGY & DEMOGRAPHICS

PREDOMINANT SEX: Male
PREDOMINANT ORGANISM: The leading cause of viral orchitis is mumps. The mumps virus rarely causes orchitis in prepubertal males but involves one or both testicles in nearly 30% of postpubertal males.

PHYSICAL FINDINGS & CLINICAL PRESENTATION

- Testicular pain, unilateral or bilateral swelling
- May have associated epididymitis, prostatitis, fever, scrotal edema, erythema cellulitis
- Inguinal lymphadenopathy
- Acute hydrocele (bacterial)
- Rare development: abscess formation, pyocele of scrotum, testicular infarction
- Spermatic cord tenderness may be present

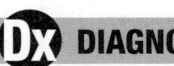 **DIAGNOSIS**

Clinical presentation as described previously with possible history of acute viral illness or concomitant epididymitis. Table 1-135 describes a classification of epididymitis and orchitis based on etiology.

DIFFERENTIAL DIAGNOSIS

- Epididymoorchitis-gonococcal
- Autoimmune disease
- Vasculitis
- Epididymyosis
- Mumps, with or without parotitis
- Neoplasm
- Hematoma
- Spermatic cord torsion

LABORATORY TESTS

- CBC with differential
- Urinalysis
- Viral titer—mumps
- Urine culture
- Ultrasound of testicle to rule out abscess

IMAGING STUDIES

Ultrasound if abscess suspected

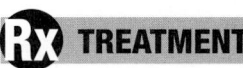 **TREATMENT**

- Dependent on cause
- Viral (mumps): observation; bed rest, ice packs, analgesics, and a scrotal sling for support may provide some relief of discomfort that accompanies mumps orchitis
- Bacterial: empiric antibiotic treatment with parenteral antibiotic treatment until pathogen identified: ceftriaxone (250 mg IM once) plus doxycycline (100 mg PO bid for 10 days), ofloxacin (300 mg PO bid for 10 days), ciprofloxacin (500 mg PO bid or 400 mg IV bid)
- Surgery for abscess, pyogenic process

DISPOSITION

Follow-up for evidence of recurrence, hypogonadism, and infertility may be needed with bilateral orchitis.

REFERRAL

- To a urologist if surgical drainage is needed
- To an endocrinologist if hypogonadism develops
- To a fertility specialist if infertility develops

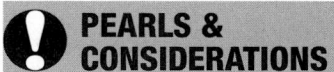 **PEARLS & CONSIDERATIONS**

Consider tuberculous orchitis if symptoms fail to respond to standard antibacterial therapy, even in the absence of chest radiographic evidence of pulmonary tuberculosis.

SUGGESTED READINGS
available at www.expertconsult.com

AUTHORS: **DENNIS J. MIKOLICH, M.D.** and **GLENN G. FORT, M.D., M.P.H.**

TABLE 1-135 Classification of Epididymitis and Orchitis

Acute Epididymitis or Epididymo-orchitis	Granulomatous Epididymitis or Orchitis	Viral Orchitis
Neisseria gonorrhoeae	*Mycobacterium tuberculosis*	Mumps
Chlamydia trachomatis	*Treponema pallidum*	Enteroviruses
Escherichia coli		
Streptococcus pneumoniae	*Brucella* spp.	
Klebsiella spp.	Sarcoid	
Salmonella spp.	Fungal	
Other urinary tract pathogens	Parasitic	
Idiopathic	Idiopathic	

Cohen J, Powderly WG: *Infectious diseases*, ed 2, St Louis, 2004, Mosby.

BASIC INFORMATION

DEFINITION

Orthostatic hypotension (OH) is defined as the presence of at least one of the following: a decrease in systolic blood pressure by $\geq$20 mm Hg or a decrease in diastolic blood pressure by $\geq$10 mm Hg within 3 min of standing. It is a physical sign that requires further investigation to discern its underlying etiology.

SYNONYMS

Postural hypotension

ICD-9CM CODES
458.0 Orthostatic hypotension

EPIDEMIOLOGY & DEMOGRAPHICS

- The incidence of OH is increased in older people.
- OH may cause up to 30% of all syncopal events in the elderly, and OH is associated with an increased risk of cardiovascular disease and all-cause mortality among those aged 55 yr and older.

PHYSICAL FINDINGS & CLINICAL PRESENTATION

- Symptoms may include dizziness, lightheadedness, syncope, visual and auditory disturbances, weakness, diaphoresis, pallor, and nausea. OH may also be asymptomatic, especially in older hypertensive patients.
- Associated with increased autonomic activity during meals (from increased splanchnic blood flow), exercise, and hot weather.
- Supine and nocturnal hypertension in patients with OH may indicate an underlying autonomic dysfunction.

ETIOLOGY

- The assumption of an upright posture results in the pooling of approximately 500 ml of blood in the lower extremities due to gravity and leads to decreased venous return, decreased cardiac output, and decreased arterial pressure. The consequent increase in sympathetic tone due to increased carotid baroreceptor activity causes arterial and venous constriction as well as positive inotropic and chronotropic effects, thereby limiting the fall in blood pressure in the upright position. Peripheral vasoconstriction is also mediated by increased activity of the renin-angiotensin system and decreased activity of atrial natriuretic factor.
- Impairment of the baroreceptor reflex, as in central or peripheral autonomic dysfunction and aging, may cause OH because decreased blood pressure cannot be counteracted by the aforementioned regulatory mechanisms.

DIAGNOSIS

DIFFERENTIAL DIAGNOSIS

Common:
- Medications: antihypertensives, antidepressants (tricyclics), antipsychotics (phenothiazines), alcohol, narcotics, barbiturates, insulin, nitrates, PDE-5 inhibitors, alpha-adrenergic antagonists
- Reduced intravascular volume (hemorrhage, dehydration, hyperglycemia, hypoalbuminemia)
- Postprandial effect (especially in the elderly)
- Vasovagal syncope
- Deconditioning
- Central autonomic dysfunction (Parkinson's disease)
- Peripheral autonomic dysfunction (diabetes mellitus, Guillain-Barré syndrome)

Uncommon:
- Central autonomic dysfunction (Shy-Drager syndrome)
- Postganglionic autonomic dysfunction: impaired norepinephrine release
- Autoimmune autonomic dysfunction: nicotinic acetylcholine receptor autoantibodies
- Paraneoplastic autonomic dysfunction: anti-Hu antibodies (in small–cell lung cancer)
- Postural tachycardia syndrome (POTS): usually occurs in young women; an abnormally large increase in heart rate is observed in the upright position caused by increased venous pooling from autonomic dysfunction of the lower extremities, but blood pressure is not affected because of an excess of plasma norepinephrine
- Impaired cardiac output (myocardial infarction, aortic stenosis, arrhythmias)
- Cerebrovascular accident
- Adrenal insufficiency
- Deconditioning
- Carotid sinus hypersensitivity
- Anxiety, panic attacks
- Seizures
- Sepsis
- Idiopathic

WORKUP

- Measure supine blood pressure after the patient has been resting comfortably to ensure stability of the supine blood pressure measurement, stand for 3 min, then measure upright blood pressure. The blood pressure cuff must be held at the level of the right atrium; holding the cuff below this level will result in a 5 to 10 mm Hg underestimation of blood pressure.
- Thorough neurologic examination should be performed.
- Rule out treatable causes (e.g., medications, volume depletion).

LABORATORY TESTS

- Hemoglobin and hematocrit
- Consider when treatable causes of OH have been ruled out:
  - Blood pressure and heart rate monitoring with a tilt table test
  - Plasma norepinephrine measurements (to distinguish postganglionic autonomic dysfunction from preganglionic autonomic dysfunction)
  - Other methods, which use the Valsalva maneuver or measure sweating as indirect means of evaluating the autonomic nervous system

IMAGING STUDIES

None

TREATMENT

NONPHARMACOLOGIC THERAPY

- Patient education (leg crossing, prolonged sitting before first standing in the morning, avoid excessive straining and hot baths)
- High-salt diet (e.g., bouillon cubes); caution if history of heart failure
- Liberal fluid intake
- Take needed antihypertensive medications at different times of the day
- Raise the head of the bed at night
- Compression stockings (to include splanchnic circulation)
- Multiple low-carbohydrate meals to avoid postprandial orthostatic hypotension
- Avoid large carbohydrate loads and excess alcohol consumption

ACUTE GENERAL Rx

- Correction of volume status
- Review medication list and attempt to eliminate medications potentially contributing to OH

CHRONIC Rx

- Fludrocortisone: 0.1 mg/day (may combine with an alpha-1 agonist to lower the dose of each); monitor for electrolyte disturbances and supine hypertension
- Midodrine (alpha-1 agonist): 10 mg three times a day; monitor for supine hypertension
- Erythropoietin (consider if anemic)
- Caffeine (for postprandial hypotension)

OTHER TREATMENTS

- Pyridostigmine (enhances renal sodium reabsorption): 0.2 to 0.6 mg/day (not FDA approved for this indication)
- Octreotide: 300 to 600 mg/day (not FDA-approved for this indication)
- Indomethacin (prostaglandin inhibitor)
- DDAVP (experimental)

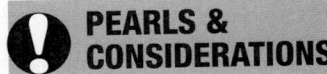

PEARLS & CONSIDERATIONS

COMMENTS

- The presence of OH should always trigger a search for an underlying etiology.
- OH is diagnosed by observing changes in blood pressure, not by observing changes in heart rate.
- Volume depletion should cause an increased heart rate on standing; a lack of heart rate response in this setting suggests autonomic dysfunction.
- Pharmacotherapy with mineralocorticoids may require concomitant potassium replenishment and monitoring for hypertension.
- The etiology of OH is often multifactorial in older patients, but increased susceptibility to volume depletion due to decreased baroreceptor reflexes frequently contributes.
- The physical examination of patients with dizziness, gait disturbance, and/or falls should include an assessment for OH.
- Because OH may be asymptomatic, physical examination of those at risk must include assessment of blood pressure in both the supine and upright positions.

SUGGESTED READINGS

available at www.expertconsult.com

AUTHOR: **TIMOTHY W. FARRELL, M.D.**

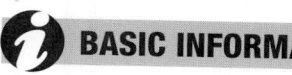

BASIC INFORMATION

DEFINITION

Osgood-Schlatter disease is a painful swelling of the tibial tuberosity that occurs in adolescence.

ICD-9CM CODES

732.4 Osgood-Schlatter disease

EPIDEMIOLOGY & DEMOGRAPHICS

PREVALENCE: 4 cases/100 adolescents
PREDOMINANT SEX: Male/female ratio of 3:1
PREDOMINANT AGE: 11 to 15 yr (bilateral in 20%)

PHYSICAL FINDINGS & CLINICAL PRESENTATION

- Pain at the tibial tubercle aggravated by activity, especially stair-walking and squatting
- Tender swelling and enlargement of the tibial tubercle
- Increased pain with knee extension against resistance

ETIOLOGY

- Unknown
- May be traumatically induced inflammation

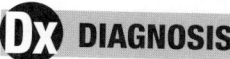

DIAGNOSIS

DIFFERENTIAL DIAGNOSIS

- Referred hip pain (any child with hip pain should have a thorough clinical hip examination)
- Patellar tendinitis

WORKUP

In most cases, the diagnosis is obvious on a clinical basis.

IMAGING STUDIES

- Lateral roentgenogram of the upper portion of the tibia with the leg slightly internally rotated may reveal variable degrees of separation and fragmentation of the upper tibial epiphysis (Fig. 1-261).
- Fragmented area occasionally fails to unite to the tibia and persists into adulthood.

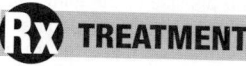

TREATMENT

ACUTE GENERAL Rx

- Ice, especially after exercise
- Nonsteroidal antiinflammatory drugs
- Gentle hamstring and quadriceps stretching exercises
- Abstinence from physical activity
- Temporary immobilization in a knee splint for 2 to 4 wk in resistant cases

DISPOSITION

- Prognosis for complete restoration of function and relief from pain is excellent.
- Condition usually heals when the epiphysis closes.
- Complications are rare.
- Symptoms in the adult:
  1. Although unusual, prominence of the tibial tubercle is usually permanent
  2. May be more susceptible to local irritation, especially when kneeling
  3. Rarely, nonunion of the epiphyseal fragment, but it is usually asymptomatic
  4. Surgery rarely required

REFERRAL

For orthopedic consultation when diagnosis is uncertain or when symptoms persist.

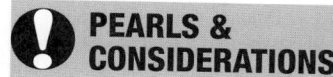

PEARLS & CONSIDERATIONS

COMMENTS

Larsen-Johansson disease is a similar disorder that can develop where either the quadriceps or patellar tendon inserts into the patella. Treatment and prognosis are the same as with Osgood-Schlatter disease.

SUGGESTED READINGS

available at www.expertconsult.com

AUTHOR: **LONNIE R. MERCIER, M.D.**

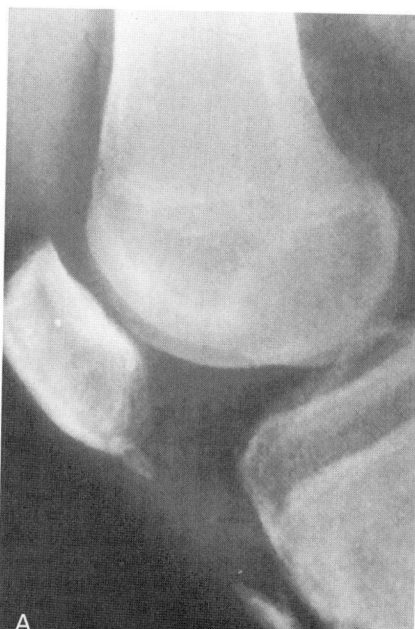
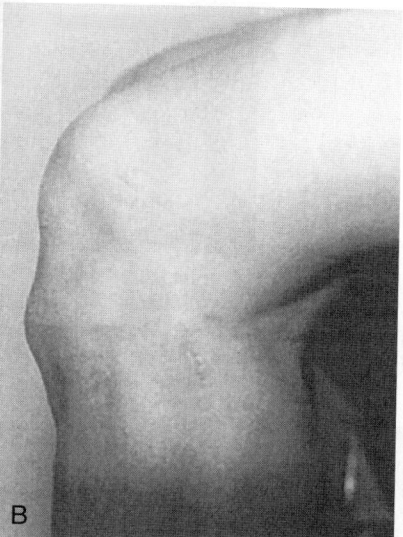

FIGURE 1-261 **A,** Radiograph of Osgood-Schlatter disease demonstrating thickening of patella tendon, fragmentation of the tibial tubercle, and soft tissue swelling. **B,** Clinical picture of bony prominence anteriorly at the tibial tubercle. (From Scuderi G [ed]: *Sports medicine: principles of primary care,* St Louis, 1997, Mosby.)

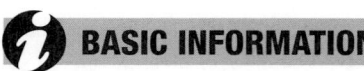

DEFINITION

Osteoarthritis (OA) is a disease of the joint with different etiologies but with similar morphologic, biologic, and clinical outcomes. It is a failure of the whole joint, which considers not only the subchondral bone and cartilage but also ligaments, joint capsule, synovium, as well as periarticular muscles. Because of its heterogeneity, it is aptly defined in epidemiologic studies as radiographic evidence of OA with pain on most days of the month within the past year.

SYNONYMS

Degenerative joint disease
Osteoarthrosis
Arthrosis

ICD-9CM CODES
715.0 Osteoarthrosis and allied disorders

EPIDEMIOLOGY & DEMOGRAPHICS

PREVALENCE: 2% to 6% of general population
PREDOMINANT SEX: Females slightly more than males in a 2:1 ratio
PREDOMINANT AGE: >50 yr
GENETICS: 39% to 65% heritability rate in twin studies of women who have generalized OA, concordance rate of 0.64 in monozygotic twins.
RISK FACTORS: Nonmodifiable are age, gender, hormonal status, geographic, genetic, and presence of congenital or developmental conditions. Modifiable risk factors such as obesity, high bone density, nutritional deficiencies such as vitamin D deficiency and presence of crystal arthropathies such as gout. Local factors are trauma during physical activities, type of occupation, muscle strength, anatomic malalignment of the lower extremities, as well as biomechanical factors such as knee laxity, leg length discrepancy, and proprioceptive deficits.

PHYSICAL FINDINGS & CLINICAL PRESENTATION

- Similar symptoms in most forms: stiffness, pain, crepitus
- Joint tenderness, swelling
- Decreased range of motion
- Crepitus with motion
- Bouchard's nodes: bony enlargement on the proximal interphalangeal (PIP) joints of the hand
- Heberden's nodes: bony enlargement of the distal interphalangeal (DIP) joints of the hand (Fig. 1-262)
- Pain with range of motion

ETIOLOGY

Primary or idiopathic OA can be mono-, oligo-, or polyarticular.

Secondary OA is due to an identifiable condition such as trauma, type of occupation, developmental, mechanical, metabolic, and inflammatory conditions.

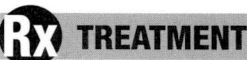 **DIAGNOSIS**

DIFFERENTIAL DIAGNOSIS

- Bursitis, tendinitis
- Inflammatory arthritides
- Infectious arthritis
- Crystal arthropathies such as gout and pseudogout

WORKUP

- No diagnostic test exists for degenerative joint disease.
- Laboratory evaluation is normal.
- Rheumatoid factor, erythrocyte sedimentation rate, complete blood count, and antinuclear antibody tests may be required if inflammatory component is suggested by history.
- Arthrocentecis of swollen joints: synovial fluid examination is generally normal or noninflammatory in character.

IMAGING STUDIES

- Plain x-ray of the involved joints is the first step and usually of high diagnostic value.
- Roentgenographic evaluation (Fig. 1-263) reveals:
  1. Joint space narrowing
  2. Subchondral sclerosis
  3. New bone formation in the form of osteophytes
- MRI can detect other sources of pain such as synovial thickening, effusions, bone marrow edema, bony attrition, and periarticular lesions.

Rx TREATMENT

- Optimal use of both pharmacologic and non-pharmacologic measures
- Education and reassurance

NONPHARMACOLOGIC THERAPY

- Assisted strength conditioning
- Regular nonvigorous exercise
- Assistive devices such as cane or walkers
- Braces, proper footwear, wedged insoles

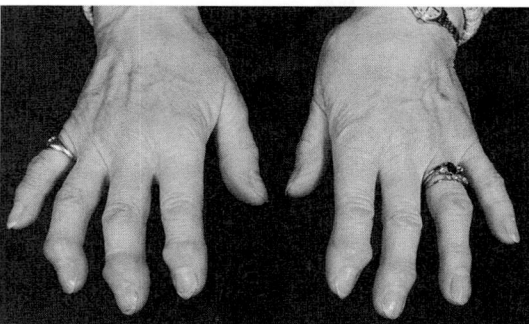

FIGURE 1-262 Osteoarthritis of the distal interphalangeal (DIP) joints. This patient has the typical clinical findings of advanced osteoarthritis of the DIP joints, including large, firm swellings (Heberden's nodes), some of which are tender and red because of associated inflammation of the periarticular tissues and the joint. (From Klippel J et al [eds]: *Primary care rheumatology,* London, 1999, Mosby.)

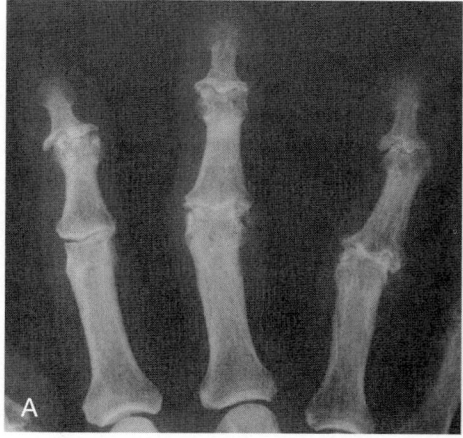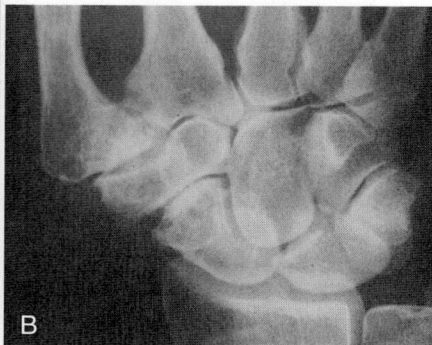

FIGURE 1-263 Osteoarthritis (degenerative joint disease). A, Primary osteoarthritis of the fingers with characteristic cartilage loss, deviations, and spurs of the proximal (Bouchard's nodes) and distal (Heberden's nodes) interphalangeal joints. **B,** Primary osteoarthritis of the carpus showing characteristic involvement of the radial side with cartilage loss, subchondral sclerosis, and small spur formation from the base of the first metacarpal to the distal articular surface of the scaphoid. (From Grainger RG, Allison D: *Grainger & Allison's diagnostic radiology, a textbook of medical imaging,* ed 4, 2001, Churchill Livingstone.)

ACUTE GENERAL Rx

- Rest and ice
- Acetaminophen recommended for mild to moderate pain
- NSAIDs effectively proven in placebo-controlled trials but not first line
- May add weak opioids such as tramadol
- Topical NSAIDs available, less effective but low toxicity
- Arthrocentecis of the acutely swollen joint followed by intra-articular steroid injection
- Chronic Physical therapy for gentle assisted strengthening exercises
- Weight control on obese patients
- If considering NSAID as long term, evaluate for risk factors such as age, GI bleed, cardiovascular (CV) risks

- If with risk for GI bleed (age >60 yr), may add PPI or use COX-2 inhibitors
- If with CV risks, consider using naproxen
- Viscosupplementation (injection of hyaluronic acid products into the degenerative joint) is of uncertain benefit
- Nutritional supplements (glucosamine and chondroitin) are unproven

DISPOSITION

Progression is not always inevitable, and the prognosis is variable depending on the site and extent of the disease.

REFERRAL

Surgical consultation for patients not responding to medical management

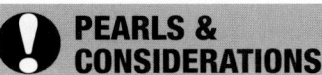

COMMENTS

Surgical intervention is generally helpful in degenerative joint disease. Arthroplasty, arthrodesis, and realignment osteotomy are the most common procedures performed. Arthroscopic debridement (of the knee) appears to be of questionable value.

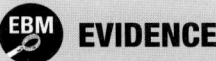

available at www.expertconsult.com

SUGGESTED READINGS
available at www.expertconsult.com

AUTHOR: **CRISOSTOMO R. BALIOG, JR, M.D.**

Diseases and Disorders

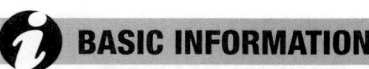

BASIC INFORMATION

DEFINITION
Osteochondritis dissecans is a disorder in which a portion of cartilage and underlying subchondral bone separates from a joint surface and may even become detached.

SYNONYMS
Osteochondrosis
Talar dome fracture: commonly used in describing the lesion of the talus
Panner's disease (capitellum)

ICD-9CM CODES
732.7 Osteochondritis dissecans

EPIDEMIOLOGY & DEMOGRAPHICS
PREVALENCE: 0.3 cases/1000 persons
PREDOMINANT SEX: Male/female ratio of 3:1
PREDOMINANT AGE: Onset at 10 to 30 yr
The most common joint affected is the knee, with the lateral surface of the medial femoral condyle the most frequent area involved. The capitellum of the humerus, dome of the talus, shoulder, and hip may also be affected.

PHYSICAL FINDINGS & CLINICAL PRESENTATION
- Pain, stiffness, and swelling
- Intermittent locking if the fragment becomes detached
- Occasionally palpable loose body
- Tenderness at the site of the lesion
- When the knee is involved, positive Wilson's sign (pain with knee extension and internal rotation)
- Some asymptomatic cases

ETIOLOGY
Unknown

DIAGNOSIS

DIFFERENTIAL DIAGNOSIS
- Acute fracture
- Neoplasm

IMAGING STUDIES
- Plain roentgenography to confirm the diagnosis (Fig. 1-264)
- "Tunnel view" helpful in knee cases
- Typical finding: radiolucent, semilunar line outlining the oval fragment of bone (but findings variable depending on the amount of healing and stability)
- MRI or bone scanning usually not necessary in establishing diagnosis but helpful in determining prognosis and management, especially regarding stability of the lesion

TREATMENT

ACUTE GENERAL Rx
- Observation every 4 to 6 mo for patients in whom the lesion is asymptomatic

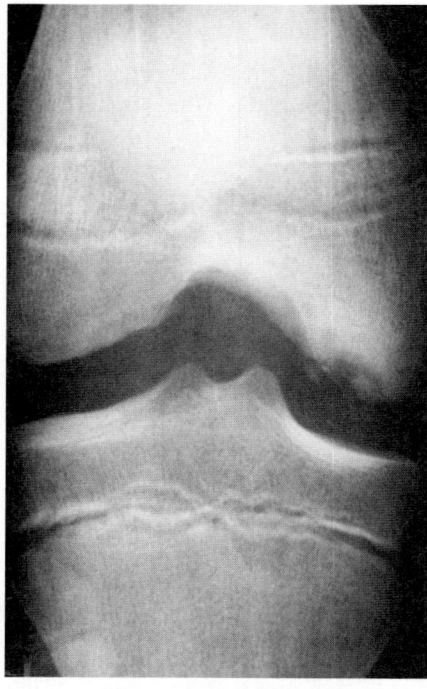

FIGURE 1-264 Osteochondritis dissecans of the knee. The "tunnel" view is often helpful in visualizing the defect. This fragment may become detached and form a loose body. This area should not be confused with the normal irregularity of the distal femoral epiphysis in young children.

- Symptomatic patients who are skeletally immature:
  1. Observation with an initial period of non–weight bearing for 6 to 8 wk (in knee cases)
  2. When symptoms subside, gradual resumption of activities

DISPOSITION
- Juvenile cases with open epiphyses have a favorable prognosis.
- Cases developing after skeletal maturity are more likely to develop osteoarthritis.
- Large fragments, especially those in weight-bearing areas, have a more unfavorable prognosis, especially if they involve the lateral femoral condyle.
- Loose body formation and degenerative joint disease are more common when condition develops after age 20 yr.

REFERRAL
For orthopedic consultation:
- For most adults with unstable lesions
- If a loose body is present
- If symptomatic care has failed

PEARLS & CONSIDERATIONS

COMMENTS
- Although inflammation is suggested by the name, it has not been shown to be of significance in this disorder. *Osteochondral lesion* or *osteochondrosis dissecans* may be more appropriate terms to describe these disorders.
- Repetitive trauma with ischemic necrosis is the most likely cause.
- The condition is often bilateral, especially in the knee, which could suggest the possibility of an endocrine or genetic basis.
- This condition should always be considered in the patient whose "sprained ankle" does not improve over the usual course of treatment.

SUGGESTED READINGS
available at www.expertconsult.com

AUTHOR: **LONNIE R. MERCIER, M.D.**

BASIC INFORMATION

DEFINITION

Osteomyelitis is an acute or chronic infection of the bone secondary to the hematogenous or contiguous source of infection or direct traumatic inoculation, which is usually bacterial.

SYNONYMS

Bone infection

ICD-9CM CODES
730.1 Chronic osteomyelitis
730.2 Acute or subacute osteomyelitis

EPIDEMIOLOGY & DEMOGRAPHICS

PREDOMINANT SEX: Male > female
PREDOMINANT AGE: All ages

PHYSICAL FINDINGS & CLINICAL PRESENTATION

HEMATOGENOUS OSTEOMYELITIS:
- Usually occurs in tibia/fibula (children)
- Localized inflammation: often secondary to trauma with accompanying hematoma or cellulitis
- Abrupt fever
- Lethargy
- Irritability
- Pain in involved bone

VERTEBRAL OSTEOMYELITIS:
- Usually hematogenous
- Fever: 50%
- Localized pain/tenderness. Back pain is the most common initial symptom (86% of cases)
- Neurologic defects: motor/sensory (sensory loss, weakness, radiculopathy)

CONTIGUOUS OSTEOMYELITIS:
- Direct inoculation
- Associated with trauma, fractures, surgical fixation
- Chronic infection of skin/soft tissue
- Fever, drainage from surgical site

CHRONIC OSTEOMYELITIS:
- Bone pain
- Sinus tract drainage, nonhealing ulcer
- Chronic low-grade fever
- Chronic localized pain

ETIOLOGY
- *Staphylococcus aureus*
- *S. aureus* (methicillin-resistant)
- *Pseudomonas aeruginosa*
- *Enterobacteriaceae*
- *Streptococcus pyogenes*
- *Enterococcus*
- *Mycobacteria*
- Fungi
- Coagulase-negative staphylococci
- *Salmonella* (in sickle cell disease)

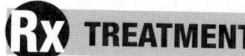

DIAGNOSIS

DIFFERENTIAL DIAGNOSIS
- Gaucher's disease
- Bone infarction
- Charcot's joint
- Fracture

WORKUP
- ESR, C-reactive protein
- Blood culturing
- Bone culture. A culture of a biopsy specimen has a significantly higher overall diagnostic yield than does a blood culture. Bone samples should be cultured for aerobic and anaerobic bacteria and for fungi
- Pathologic evaluation of bone biopsy for acute/chronic changes consistent with necrosis or acute inflammation
- PCR analysis of specimens obtained by means of biopsy or puncture may be useful for organisms that are difficult to identify (anaerobic bacteria, *Bartonella* sp., *Kingella kingae*); however, broad-range PCR has suboptimal sensitivity and specificity due to contamination and may not provide sufficient information on the the susceptibility of the microorganisms to antibiotics

IMAGING STUDIES
- Bone radiograph examination: initial study but not sensitive in early osteomyelitis
- MRI (Fig. 1-266): most accurate imaging study. CT only if patient has contraindication to MRI
- Triple-phase technetium-99m bone scan (Fig. 1-265). Typically positive within a few days after onset of symptoms but accuracy is lower than that of MRI
- Gallium scan (Ga-67) scintigraphy with single-photon emission CT (SPECT) has higher accuracy than bone scan but is less sensitive for detection of epidural abscess in vertebral osteomyelitis
- Indium-111–labeled leukocyte scintigraphy scan; low sensitivity (<20%) for vertebral osteomyelitis
- Positron-emission tomography (PET) scanning with ^{18}F-fluorodeoxyglucose has high accuracy (similar to MRI) and is useful in patients with metallic implants

TREATMENT
- Surgical debridement in biopsy-positive cases will guide direction for antibiotic therapy. This will vary with type of osteomyelitis. Duration of therapy is usually 6 wk for acute osteomyelitis; chronic osteomyelitis may need a longer course of medication
- *S. aureus*: cefazolin IV, nafcillin IV, vancomycin IV (in patient allergic to penicillin)
- *S. aureus* (methicillin resistant): vancomycin IV, linezolid, daptomycin, or tigecycline
- *Streptococcus* spp.: ceftriaxone, IV penicillin G in sensitive species
- *P. aeruginosa*: piperacillin plus aminoglycoside or cefepime plus aminoglycoside
- Enterobacteriaceae quinolone-susceptible: fluoroquinolone or ceftriaxone
- Enterobacteriaceae quinolone-resistant: carbapenem (imipenem)

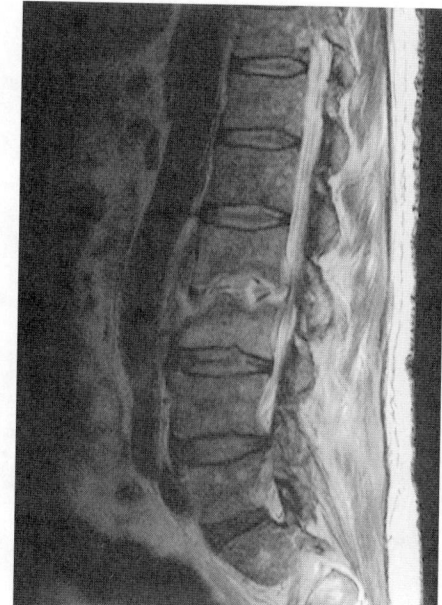

Figure 1-266 T1-weighted magnetic resinance images show an abnormal signal in the disk between L2 & L3 with associated vertebral osteomyelitis. A fluid collection is located in the posterior part of L2 and L3 resulting in the evaluation of the posterior ligament. A computed tomography-guided aspirate grew *Staphylococcus aureus*. (From Mandell GL et al: *Principles and practice of infectious diseases*, ed 7, Philadelphia, 2010, Elsevier.)

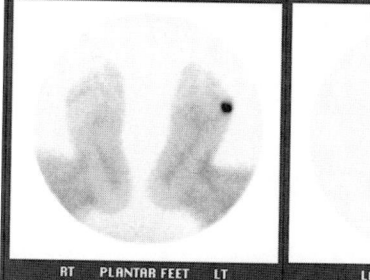
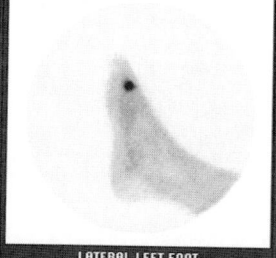

RT   PLANTAR FEET   LT   LATERAL LEFT FOOT

FIGURE 1-265 Osteomyelitis. Intense accumulation of Tc-99m WBC in proximal phalanx of fifth digit of left foot at 4 hr after injection (From Specht N [ed]: *Practical guide to diagnostic imaging*, St Louis, 1998, Mosby.)

- Anaerobes: clindamycin
- Hyperbaric oxygen therapy: may be useful in chronic osteomyelitis
- Surgical debridement of all devitalized bone and tissue
- Immobilization of affected bone (plaster, traction) if bone is unstable

DISPOSITION

Acute hematogenous osteomyelitis usually resolves without recurrence or long-term complications, but contiguous focus osteomyelitis, bone infections from open fractures, or osteomyelitis frequently recur.

REFERRAL

- To an orthopedic surgeon if chronic osteomyelitis with need for bone debridement, bone grafting, or stabilization of infected tissue adjacent to a bone fracture
- To an infectious disease specialist for appropriate treatment for difficult-to-treat or recalcitrant infections
- To an hyperbaric oxygen chamber service for nonhealing, chronic osteomyelitis

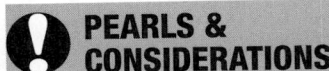 **PEARLS & CONSIDERATIONS**

Chronic osteomyelitis is one of the most challenging infections to treat; the high failure rate is a consequence of poor vascular supply, nondistensible bone tissue, and limited penetration of bone tissue.

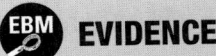 **EVIDENCE**

available at www.expertconsult.com

SUGGESTED READINGS

available at www.expertconsult.com

AUTHORS: **GLENN G. FORT, M.D., M.P.H.,** and **DENNIS J. MIKOLICH, M.D.**

BASIC INFORMATION

DEFINITION

Osteoporosis is characterized by a progressive decrease in bone mass that results in increased bone fragility and a higher fracture risk. The various types are as follows:

PRIMARY OSTEOPOROSIS: Affects 80% of women and 60% of men with osteoporosis.

- Idiopathic osteoporosis: unknown pathogenesis; may occur in children and young adults
- Type I osteoporosis: may occur in postmenopausal women (ages 51 to 75); characterized by accelerated and disproportionate trabecular bone loss and associated with vertebral body and distal forearm fractures (estrogen withdrawal effect)
- Type II osteoporosis (involutional): occurs in both men and women aged >70 yr; characterized by both trabecular and cortical bone loss and associated with fractures of the proximal humerus and tibia, femoral neck, and pelvis

SECONDARY OSTEOPOROSIS: Affects 20% of women and 40% of men with osteoporosis; osteoporosis that exists as a common feature of another disease process, heritable disorder of connective tissue, or drug side effect (see "Differential Diagnosis")

ICD-9CM CODES
733.0 Osteoporosis

EPIDEMIOLOGY & DEMOGRAPHICS

PREVALENCE (IN U.S.):
- ~25 million men and women
- Twice as common in women
- Results in 1.5 million fractures annually (70% women)
- Osteoporosis-related fractures in 50% women and 20% men aged >65 yr
- Results: institutionalization, death, and costs in excess of $10 billion annually

RISK FACTORS:
- Age: each decade after 40 yr associated with a fivefold increase risk
- Genetics:
  1. Ethnicity (white/Asian are affected more often than blacks, with Polynesians affected the least)
  2. Gender (females affected more often than males)
  3. Family history
- Environmental factors: poor nutrition, calcium deficiency, physical inactivity, medication (steroids/heparin), tobacco use, ethylene alcohol use, traumatic injury
- Chronic disease states: estrogen deficiency, androgen deficiency, hyperthyroidism, inflammatory bowel disease, hypercortisolism, cirrhosis, gastrectomy

PHYSICAL FINDINGS & CLINICAL PRESENTATION

- Most commonly silent with no signs and symptoms

- Insidious and progressive development of dorsal kyphosis (dowager's hump), loss of height, and skeletal pain typically associated with fracture; other physical findings related to other conditions with associated increased risk for osteoporosis (see "Risk Factors")

ETIOLOGY

- Primary osteoporosis: multifactorial, resulting from a combination of factors including nutrition, peak bone mass, genetics, level of physical activity, age of menopause (spontaneous vs. surgical), and estrogen status
- Secondary osteoporosis: associated decrease in bone mass resulting from an identified cause, including endocrinopathies, hypogonadism, hyperthyroidism, hyperparathyroidism, Cushing's syndrome, hyperprolactinemia, acromegaly, diabetes mellitus, gastrointestinal disease, malabsorption, primary biliary cirrhosis, gastrectomy, malnutrition (including anorexia nervosa), and medications (corticosteroids, PPIs, rosiglitazone, pioglitazone)

DX DIAGNOSIS

DIFFERENTIAL DIAGNOSIS

- Malignancy (multiple myeloma, lymphoma, leukemia, metastatic carcinoma)
- Primary hyperparathyroidism
- Osteomalacia
- Paget's disease
- Osteogenesis imperfecta: types I, III, and IV (see also "Epidemiology and Demographics" and "Etiology")

WORKUP

- History and physical examination (20% of women with type I osteoporosis have associated secondary cause), with appropriate evaluation for identified risk factors and secondary causes
- Diagnosis of osteoporosis made by bone mineral density (BMD) determination (BMD should ideally evaluate the hip, spine, and wrist):
  1. Dual-energy x-ray absorptiometry
  2. Single-energy x-ray
  3. Peripheral dual-energy x-ray
  4. Single-photon absorptiometry
  5. Dual-photon absorptiometry
  6. Quantitative CT scan
  7. Radiographic absorptiometry

LABORATORY TESTS

- Biochemical profile to evaluate renal and hepatic function, primary hyperparathyroidism, and malnutrition
- Complete blood count for nutritional status and myeloma
- Thyroid-stimulating hormone to rule out the presence of hyperthyroidism
- Consideration of 24-hr urine collection for calcium (excess skeletal loss, vitamin D malabsorption/deficiency), creatinine, sodium, and free cortisol (to detect occult Cushing's disease); no need to measure calci-

tropic hormones (parathyroid hormone, calcitriol, calcitonin) unless specifically indicated
- Biochemical markers of bone remodeling; may be useful to predict rate of bone loss and/or follow therapy response; specific biochemical markers followed (e.g., 3-mo interval) to document normalization as a response to therapy
  1. High-turnover osteoporosis: high levels of resorption markers (lysyl pyridinoline, deoxy lysyl pyridinoline, n-telopeptide of collagen cross-links, C-telopeptide of collagen cross-links) and formation markers (osteocalcin, bone-specific alkaline phosphatase, carboxy-terminal extension peptide of type I procollagen); accelerated bone loss responding best to antiresorptive therapy
  2. Low-normal-turnover osteoporosis: normal or low levels of the markers of resorption and formation (see "high turnover osteoporosis" listed previously); no accelerated bone loss; responds best to drugs that enhance bone formation

IMAGING STUDIES

- BMD determination (see "Workup") should be performed on all women with determined risk factors and/or associated secondary causes; accepted screening criteria are currently being investigated
  1. Normal: BMD <1 SD of the young adult reference mean
  2. Osteopenia: BMD 1 to 2.5 SD below the young adult reference mean
  3. Osteoporosis: BMD >2.5 SD below the young adult reference mean
- For patient undergoing treatment: annual BMD to follow response to therapy
- X-ray examination of appropriate part of skeleton to evaluate clinical osteoporotic fracture only (Fig. 1-267)

RX TREATMENT

NONPHARMACOLOGIC THERAPY

Prevention:
- Identification and minimization of risk factors
- Appropriate diagnosis and treatment of secondary causes
- Behavioral modification: proper nutrition (dietary calcium >800 mg/day, vitamin D 400 to 800 U/day), physical activity, fracture prevention strategies

ACUTE GENERAL Rx

- Vitamin D supplement: 400 U/day.
- Calcium supplement: 1000 to 1500 mg/day.
- Ibandronate 150 mg once monthly, swallow whole with 8 oz water on empty stomach, with no oral intake for at least 60 min. Do not lie down for 60 min after dose.
- Alendronate 70 mg once weekly on awakening, with 8 oz water on empty stomach, with no oral intake for at least 30 min. Use 70-mg dose for treatment of postmenopausal osteo-

porosis and a 35-mg tablet for the prevention of osteoporosis in postmenopausal women.

- Risedronate: 35 mg once weekly or 75 mg taken on 2 consecutive days per month on awakening, with 8 oz water on empty stomach, with no oral intake for at least 30 min.
- Synthetic salmon calcitonin: 100 U/day SC or 200 U/day intranasally.
- Raloxifene: 60 mg qd.
- Zoledronic acid: a bisphosphonate given by IV infusion over at least 15 min, 5 mg once/year.
- Teriparatide is a recombinant human parathyroid hormone used for postmenopausal women with osteoporosis who are at high risk for fracture. It is also used in men with primary or hypogonadal osteoporosis who are at high risk of fracture. It is administered by injection 20 mcg qd SQ into the thigh or abdominal wall. Use for >2 yr not recommended. It reduces the risk of fracture but may increase the risk of stroke in older women with osteoporosis.
- Denosumab is an osteoclast inhibitor approved for use in postmenopausal women with osteoporosis at high risk of fracture or patients who have failed or are intolerant to other therapy. It is a human IgG_2 monoclonal antibody that binds to human receptor activator of nuclear factor kappaB ligand (RANKL). It prevents RANKL from interacting with its receptors on the surface of osteoclasts and their precursors, thereby inhibiting osteoclast formation, function, and survival.
- Other FDA-approved drugs (without osteoporosis indication) used to treat osteoporosis:
  1. Calcitriol
  2. Etidronate
  3. Thiazide

- Estrogen (conjugated equine estrogen or equivalent): 0.3 to 0.625 mg/day.
- Progestin: continuous (e.g., 2.5 mg medroxyprogesterone acetate/day or equivalent) or cyclic (e.g., 10 mg medroxyprogesterone acetate days 16 to 25 each mo or equivalent) co-administered in nonhysterectomized women.
- Combination estrogen/alendronate or estrogen-progestin/alendronate may be considered in individualized patients on hormone replacement therapy with identified osteoporosis. BMD baseline obtained before onset of therapy and at 1 yr; decrease of 2% or greater results in dosage adjustment or medication change.
- A recent trial on the effects of lasofoxifene on the risk of fractures showed that in postmenopausal women with osteoporosis, lasofoxifene (0.5 mg/day) decreased risk of vertebral and non-vertebral fractures. It also lowered the risk of ER-positive breast cancer, coronary heart disease, and stroke but it increased the risk of venous thromboembolic events.
- Baseline biochemical markers of remodeling baseline considered; identified high-turnover osteoporosis patients rescreened at 3 mo to document marker return to normal.

CHRONIC Rx

- Lifelong disorder requiring lifelong attention to behavior modification issues (nutrition, physical activity, fracture prevention strategies) and compliance with pharmacologic intervention

- Continuing need to eliminate high-risk factors when possible and to diagnose and optimally manage secondary causes of osteoporosis

DISPOSITION

Goal for diagnosis and treatment: identification of women at risk; initiation of preventive measures for all women lifelong; institution of treatment modalities that will result in a decrease in fracture risk; and reduction of morbidity, mortality, and unnecessary institutionalization, thereby improving quality of independent life and productivity.

REFERRAL

- To reproductive endocrinologist, endocrinologist, gynecologist, or rheumatologist if unfamiliar with diagnosis and management of osteoporosis
- If multidisciplinary management is required, to other specialties depending on presence of acute fracture and/or secondary associated disorders

❗ PEARLS & CONSIDERATIONS

COMMENTS

- Osteonecrosis of the jaw is a known complication of high-dose IV biphosphonate therapy for cancer, however there is considerable debate on whether low-dose biphosphonates used for osteoporosis can also cause this disorder. Evidence for this is inconclusive.
- Long-term use (>10 yr) of biphosphonates has been reported to increase risk of atypical subtrochanteric or femoral shaft fractures in several uncontrolled case series. A prodrome of thigh pain, lack of trauma prior to the procedure, and specific radiological characteristics have been reported. The evidence remains inconclusive. Patients can be reassured that short or intermediate use of biphosphonates does not increase the risk of atypical femoral fractures. Current stragies should include considering a 12-mo interruption in therapy after 5 yr in patients who are clinically stable and considering teriparatide treatment in individuals who experience an atypical fracture while receiving biphosphonate therapy.

EBM EVIDENCE

available at www.expertconsult.com

SUGGESTED READINGS

available at www.expertconsult.com

AUTHORS: **DENNIS M. WEPPNER, M.D.,** and **RUBEN ALVERO, M.D.**

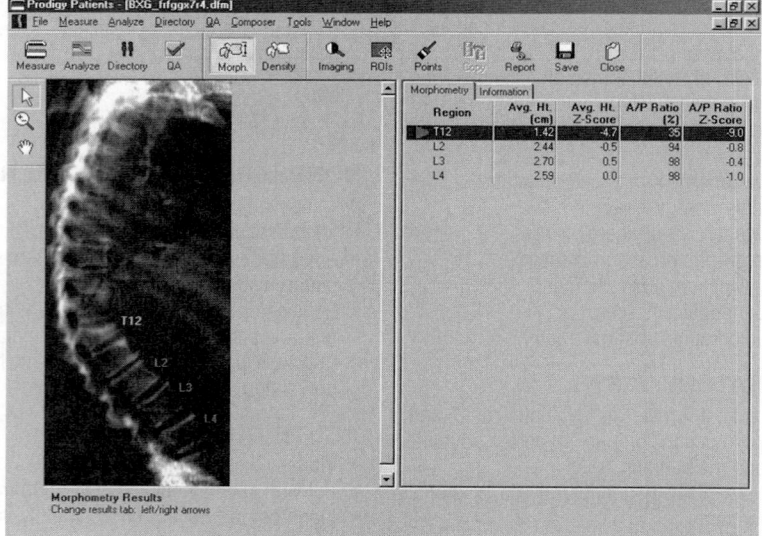

FIGURE 1-267 Vertebral fracture assessment from a dual x-ray absorptiometry image of the spine. Use of dual energy images facilitates the visualization of the lumbar and thoracic spine in a single image. In this example, a fracture has been identified at T12. (From Hochberg MC et al [eds]: *Rheumatology,* ed 3, St Louis, 2003, Mosby.)

BASIC INFORMATION

DEFINITION

Otitis externa is a term encompassing a variety of conditions causing inflammation and/or infection of the external auditory canal (and/or auricle and tympanic membrane). There are six subgroups of otitis externa:
1. Acute localized otitis externa (furunculosis)
2. Acute diffuse bacterial otitis externa (swimmer's ear)
3. Chronic otitis externa
4. Eczematous otitis externa
5. Fungal otitis externa (otomycosis)
6. Invasive or necrotizing (malignant) otitis externa (Fig. 1-268)

SYNONYMS

See "Definition."

ICD-9CM CODES
38.10 Otitis externa

EPIDEMIOLOGY & DEMOGRAPHICS

INCIDENCE (IN U.S.):
- Among the most common disorders
- Affects 3% to 10% of patients seeking otologic care

PREVALENCE (IN U.S.):
- Diffuse otitis externa (swimmer's ear) is most often seen in swimmers and in hot, humid climates, conditions that lead to water retention in the ear canal.
- Necrotizing otitis externa is more common in elderly, diabetics, and immunocompromised patients.

PREDOMINANT SEX: None

PREDOMINANT AGE:
- Occurs at all ages
- Necrotizing otitis externa: typically occurs in elderly: mean age >65 yr

PHYSICAL FINDINGS & CLINICAL PRESENTATION

The two most common symptoms are otalgia, ranging from pruritus to severe pain exacerbated by motion (e.g., chewing), and otorrhea. Patients may also experience aural fullness and hearing loss as a result of swelling with occlusion of the canal. More intense symptoms may occur with bacterial otitis externa, with or without fever, and lymphadenopathy (anterior to tragus). There are also findings unique to the various forms of the infection:
- Acute localized otitis externa (furunculosis):
  1. Occurs from infected hair follicles, usually in the outer third of the ear canal, forming pustules and furuncles
  2. Furuncles are superficial and pointing or deep and diffuse
- Impetigo:
  1. In contrast to furunculosis, this is a superficial spreading infection of the ear canal that may also involve the concha and the auricle
  2. Begins as a small blister that ruptures, releasing straw-colored fluid that dries as a golden crust
- Erysipelas:
  1. Caused by group A streptococcus
  2. May involve the concha and canal
  3. May involve the dermis and deeper tissues
  4. Area of cellulitis, often with severe pain
  5. Fever, chills, malaise
  6. Regional adenopathy
- Eczematous otitis externa:
  1. Stems from a variety of dermatologic problems that can involve the external auditory canal
  2. Severe itching, erythema, scaling, crusting, and fissuring possible
- Acute diffuse otitis externa (swimmer's ear):
  1. Begins with itching and a feeling of pressure and fullness in the ear that becomes increasingly tender and painful
  2. Mild erythema and edema of the external auditory canal, which may cause narrowing and occlusion of the canal, leading to hearing loss
  3. Minimal serous secretions, which may become profuse and purulent
  4. Tympanic membrane may appear dull and infected
  5. Usually absence of systemic symptoms such as fever, chills
- Otomycosis:
  1. Chronic superficial infection of the ear canal and tympanic membrane
  2. In primary fungal infection, major symptom is intense itching
  3. In secondary infection (fungal infection superimposed on bacterial infection), major symptom is pain
  4. Fungal growth of variety of colors
- Chronic otitis externa:
  1. Dry and atrophic canal
  2. Typically lack of cerumen
  3. Itching, often severe, and mild discomfort rather than pain
  4. Occasionally mucopurulent discharge
  5. With time, thickening of the walls of the canal, causing narrowing of the lumen
- Necrotizing otitis externa (also known as malignant otitis externa). Typically seen in older patients with diabetes or in patients who are immunocompromised.
  1. Redness, swelling, and tenderness of the ear canal
  2. Classic finding of granulation tissue on the floor of the canal and the bone–cartilage junction
  3. Small ulceration of necrotic soft tissue at bone–cartilage junction
  4. Most common symptoms: pain (often severe) and otorrhea
  5. Lessening of purulent drainage as infection advances
  6. Facial nerve palsy often the first and only cranial nerve defect
  7. Possible involvement of other cranial nerves

ETIOLOGY

- Acute localized otitis externa: *Staphylococcus aureus*
- Impetigo:
  1. *S. aureus*
  2. *Streptococcus pyogenes*
- Erysipelas: *S. pyogenes*
- Eczematous otitis externa:
  1. Seborrheic dermatitis
  2. Atopic dermatitis
  3. Psoriasis
  4. Neurodermatitis
  5. Lupus erythematosus
- Acute diffuse otitis externa:
  1. Swimming
  2. Hot, humid climates
  3. Tightly fitting hearing aids
  4. Use of ear plugs
  5. *Pseudomonas aeruginosa*
  6. *S. aureus*
- Otomycosis:
  1. Prolonged use of topical antibiotics and steroid preparations

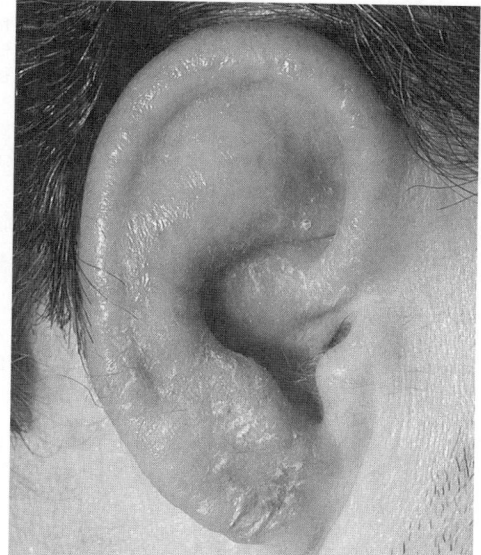

FIGURE 1-268 Malignant external otitis. Severe infection of the ear has occurred after months of chronic inflammation of the pinna. (From Habif TP: *Clinical dermatology: a color guide to diagnosis and therapy,* ed 3, St Louis, 1996, Mosby.)

2. *Aspergillus* (80% to 90%)
3. *Candida*
- Chronic otitis externa: persistent low-grade infection and inflammation
- Necrotizing otitis externa (NOE):
  1. Complication of persistent otitis externa
  2. Extends through Santorini's fissures, small apertures at the bone–cartilage junction of the canal, into the mastoid and along the base of the skull
  3. *P. aeruginosa*

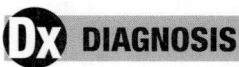

DIAGNOSIS

DIFFERENTIAL DIAGNOSIS
- Acute otitis media
- Bullous myringitis
- Mastoiditis
- Foreign bodies
- Neoplasms

WORKUP
Thorough history and physical examination

LABORATORY TESTS
- Cultures from the canal are usually not necessary unless the condition does not respond to treatment.
- Leukocyte count normal or mildly elevated.
- Erythrocyte sedimentation rate is often quite elevated in malignant otitis externa.

IMAGING STUDIES
- CT scan is the best technique for defining bone involvement and extent of disease in malignant otitis externa.
- MRI is slightly more sensitive in evaluation of soft tissue changes.
- Gallium scans are more specific than bone scans in diagnosing NOE.
- Follow-up scans are helpful in determining efficacy of treatment.

NOTE: Expert opinion supports history and physical examination as the best means of diagnosis. Persistent pain that is constant and severe should raise the question of NOE (particularly in the elderly, diabetics, and immunocompromised patients).

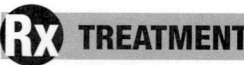

TREATMENT

NONPHARMACOLOGIC THERAPY
- Cleansing and debridement of the ear canal with cotton swabs and hydrogen peroxide or other antiseptic solution allows a more thorough examination of the ear.
- If the canal lumen is edematous and too narrow to allow adequate cleansing, a cotton wick or gauze strip inserted into the canal serves as a conduit for topical medications to be drawn into the canal. Usually remove wick after 2 days.
- Local heat is useful in treating deep furunculosis.
- Incision and drainage is indicated in treatment of superficial pointing furunculosis.

ACUTE GENERAL Rx
Topical medications:
- An acidifying agent, such as 2% acetic acid, inhibits growth of bacteria and fungi
- Topical antibiotics (in the form of otic or ophthalmic solutions) or antifungals, often in combination with an acidifying agent and a steroid preparation
- The following are some of the available preparations:
  1. Neomycin otic solutions and suspensions:
     a. With polymyxin-B-hydrocortisone (Corticosporin)
     b. With hydrocortisone-thonzonium (Coly-Mycin S)
  2. Polymyxin-B-hydrocortisone (Otobiotic)
  3. Quinolone otic solutions:
     a. Ofloxacin 0.3% solution (Floxin Otic)
     b. Ciprofloxacin 0.3% with hydrocortisone (Cipro HC)
  4. Quinolone ophthalmic solutions:
     a. Ofloxacin 0.3% (Ocuflox)
     b. Ciprofloxacin 0.3% (Ciloxan)
  5. Aminoglycoside ophthalmic solutions:
     a. Gentamicin sulfate 0.3% (Garamycin)
     b. Tobramycin sulfate 0.3% (Tobrex)
     c. Tobramycin 0.3% and dexamethasone 0.1% (TobraDex)
  6. Chloramphenicol 0.5% otic solution or 0.25% ophthalmic solution (Chloromycetin)
  7. Gentian violet (methylrosaniline chloride 1%, 2%)
  8. Antifungals:
     a. Amphotericin B 3% (Fungizone lotion)
     b. Clotrimazole 1% solution (Lotrimin)
     c. Tolnaftate 1% (Tinactin)
- Topical preparations should be applied qid (bid for quinolones, antifungals), generally for 3 days after cessation of symptoms (average 10 to 14 days total)

Systemic antibiotics:
- Reserved for severe cases, most often infections with *P. aeruginosa* or *S. aureus*
- Treatment usually for 10 days with ciprofloxacin 750 mg q12h or ofloxacin 400 mg q12h, or with antistaphylococcal agent (e.g., dicloxacillin or cephalexin 500 mg q6h)

Treatment for NOE:
- Requires prolonged therapy up to 3 mo; whether to use oral parenteral therapy based on clinical judgment
- Oral quinolones, ciprofloxacin 750 mg q12h or ofloxacin 400 mg q12h may be appropriate initial therapy or used to shorten the course of IV therapy
- Intravenous antipseudomonals with or without aminoglycosides are also appropriate
- Local debridement

Pain control:
- May require NSAIDs or opioids
- Topical corticosteroids to reduce swelling and inflammation

CHRONIC Rx
- Patients prone to recurrent infections should try to identify and avoid precipitants to infection.
- Swimmers should try tight-fitting ear plugs or tight-fitting bathing caps and remove all excess water from the ears after swimming.
- Treat underlying systemic diseases and dermatologic conditions that predispose to infection.

DISPOSITION
Inadequate treatment of otitis externa may lead to NOE and mastoiditis.

REFERRAL
To an otolaryngologist:
- NOE
- Treatment failure
- Severe pain

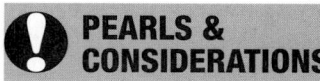

PEARLS & CONSIDERATIONS

Otitis externa varies in severity from a mild irritation of the external acoustic canal (swimmer's ear) that resolves spontaneously by simply removing the offending agent (stay out of fresh water or wear ear plugs) to a life-threatening infection with the risk of intracranial extension, gram-negative bacterial meningitis, and severe neurologic impairment with multiple cranial neuropathy. Do not miss severe malignant otitis externa in patients who are diabetic or immunocompromised.

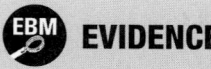

EVIDENCE

available at www.expertconsult.com

SUGGESTED READINGS
available at www.expertconsult.com

AUTHORS: **GLENN G. FORT, M.D., M.P.H.,** and **DENNIS J. MIKOLICH, M.D.**

BASIC INFORMATION

DEFINITION

Otitis media is the presence of fluid in the middle ear accompanied by signs and symptoms of infection.

SYNONYMS

Acute suppurative otitis media
Purulent otitis media
Acute otitis media
AOM

ICD-9CM CODES

382.9 Acute or chronic otitis media
382.10 381.00 Otitis media with effusion

EPIDEMIOLOGY & DEMOGRAPHICS

INCIDENCE (IN U.S.):

- Affects patients of all ages but is largely a disease of infants and young children
- Occurs once in approximately 75% of all children
- Occurs three or more times in one third of all children by age 3 yr
- The diagnosis of acute otitis media increased from 9.9 million in 1975 to 25.5 million in 1990
- From 1975 to 1990, office visits for acute otitis media increased threefold for children <2 yr, doubled for children ages 2 to 5 yr, and almost doubled for children ages 6 to 10 yr

PEAK INCIDENCE:

- Between 6 and 36 mo
- Second peak between ages 4 and 6 yr
- Fall, winter, early spring

PREDOMINANT SEX: Males

PREDOMINANT AGE:

- 47% to 60% of all children have their first episode of otitis media during their first year of life and 60% to 70% by their fourth birthday
- Incidence of infection declines with age; seen infrequently in adults

GENETICS:

Familial disposition:

- Native Americans
- Eskimos
- Australian aborigines
- Those with a strong family history

Congenital infection: high incidence in children born with cleft palates and other craniofacial abnormalities

PHYSICAL FINDINGS & CLINICAL PRESENTATION

- Fluid in the middle ear along with signs and symptoms of local inflammation (Figs. 1-269 and 1-270).
  1. Erythema with diminished light reflex
- Erythema of the tympanic membrane without other abnormalities is not a diagnostic criterion for acute otitis media because it may occur with any inflammation of the upper respiratory tract, crying, or nose blowing.

- As infection progresses, middle ear exudation occurs (exudative phase); the exudate rapidly changes from serous to purulent (suppurative phase).
  1. Retraction and poor motility of the tympanic membrane, which then becomes bulging and convex
- At any time during the suppurative phase the tympanic membrane may rupture, releasing the middle ear contents.
- Symptoms:
  1. Otalgia, ranging from slight discomfort to severe, spreading to the temporal region
  2. Ear stuffiness and hearing loss may precede or follow otalgia
  3. Otorrhea
  4. Vertigo, nystagmus, tinnitus, fever, lethargy, irritability, nausea, vomiting, anorexia
- After an episode of acute otitis media:
  1. Persistence of effusion for weeks or months (called secretory, serous, or non-suppurative otitis media)
  2. Fever and otalgia usually absent
  3. Hearing loss possible (10 to 50 dB, with predominant involvement of the low frequencies)

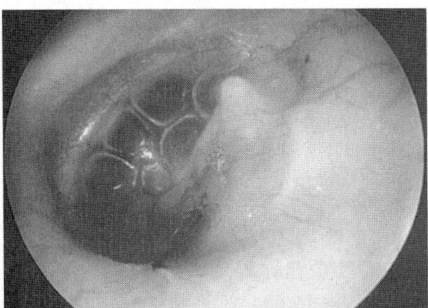

FIGURE 1-269 Otitis media with effusion of left ear. Retracted eardrum, prominent short process of malleus, and air bubbles seen anteriorly through the tympanic membrane. (From Behrman RE: *Nelson textbook of pediatrics,* ed 16, Philadelphia, 1996, WB Saunders.)

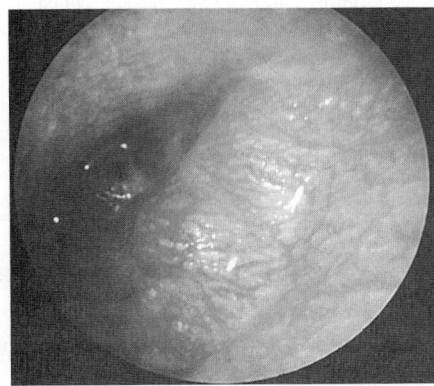

FIGURE 1-270 Acute left otitis media. (From Behrman RE: *Nelson textbook of pediatrics,* ed 16, Philadelphia, 1996, WB Saunders.)

ETIOLOGY

- Most common etiologic factor is an upper respiratory tract infection (often viral), which causes inflammation and obstruction of the eustachian tube. Bacterial colonization of the nasopharynx in conjunction with eustachian tube dysfunction leads to infection.
- May occasionally develop as a result of hematogenous spread or by direct invasion from the nasopharynx.
- Most common bacterial pathogens:
  1. *Streptococcus pneumoniae* causes 40% to 50% of cases and is the least likely of the major pathogens to resolve without treatment
  2. *Haemophilus influenzae* causes 20% to 30% of cases
  3. *Moraxella catarrhalis* causes 10% to 15% of cases
  4. Of increasing importance, infection caused by penicillin-nonsusceptible *S. pneumoniae* (MIC >0.1 μg/ml), ranging from 8% to 34%. About 50% of PNSSP isolates are penicillin-intermediate (MIC 0.1 to 2.0 μg/ml)
- Viral pathogens:
  1. Respiratory syncytial virus
  2. Rhinovirus
  3. Adenovirus
  4. Influenza
- Others:
  1. *Mycoplasma pneumoniae*
  2. *Chlamydia trachomatis*

DIAGNOSIS

DIFFERENTIAL DIAGNOSIS

- Otitis externa
- Referred pain
  1. Mouth
  2. Nasopharynx
  3. Tonsils
  4. Other parts of the upper respiratory tract
- Section II describes the differential diagnosis of earache

WORKUP

Thorough otoscopic examination. Adequate visualization of the tympanic membrane requires removal of cerumen and debris.

- Tympanometry
  1. Measures compliance of the tympanic membrane and middle ear pressure
  2. Detects the presence of fluid
- Acoustic reflectometry
  1. Measures sound waves reflected from the middle ear
  2. Useful in infants >3 mo
  3. Increased reflected sound correlated with the presence of effusion

LABORATORY TESTS

- Tympanocentesis
  1. Not necessary in most cases because the microbiology of middle ear effusions has been shown to be quite consistent

2. May be indicated in:
    a. Highly toxic patients
    b. Patients who do not respond to treatment in 48 to 72 hr
    c. Immunocompromised patients
- Cultures of the nasopharynx: sensitive but not specific
- Blood counts: usually show a leukocytosis with polymorphonuclear elevation
- Plain mastoid radiographs: generally not indicated; will reveal haziness in the periantral cells that may extend to entire mastoid
- CT or MRI may be indicated if serious complications suspected (meningitis, brain abscess)

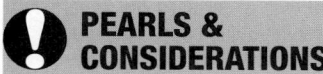

TREATMENT

ACUTE GENERAL Rx

Hydration, avoidance of irritants (e.g., tobacco smoke), nasal systemic decongestants, cool mist humidifier
Antimicrobials:

NOTE: Most uncomplicated cases of acute otitis media resolve spontaneously, without complications. Studies have demonstrated limited therapeutic benefit from antibiotic therapy. However, when opting to use antibiotic therapy:

- Amoxicillin remains the drug of choice for first-line treatment of uncomplicated acute otitis media despite increasing prevalence of drug-resistant *S. pneumoniae.*
- Treatment failure is defined by lack of clinical improvement of signs or symptoms after 3 days of therapy.
- With treatment failure, in the absence of an identified etiologic pathogen, therapy should be redirected to cover:
    1. Drug-resistant *S. pneumoniae*
    2. β-lactamase–producing strains of *H. influenzae* and *M. catarrhalis*
- Agents fulfilling these criteria include amoxicillin/clavulanate, second-generation cephalosporins (e.g., cefuroxime axetil, cefaclor), and ceftriaxone (given IM). Cefaclor, cefixime, loracarbef, and ceftibuten are active against *H. influenzae* and *M. catarrhalis* but less active against pneumococci, especially drug-resistant strains, than the agents listed previously.
- TMP/SMX and macrolides have been used as first- and second-line agents, but pneumo-

coccal resistance to these agents is rising (up to 25% resistance to TMP/SMX and up to 10% resistance to erythromycin).
- Cross-resistance between these drugs and the β-lactams exists; therefore patients who do not respond to amoxicillin are more likely to have infections resistant to TMP/SMX and macrolides.
- Newer fluoroquinolones (grepafloxacin, levofloxacin, moxifloxacin) have enhanced activity against pneumococci compared with older agents (ciprofloxacin, ofloxacin).
- Treatment should be modified according to cultures and sensitivities.
- Generally treatment course is 10 to 14 days.
- Follow up approximately 4 wk after discontinuation of therapy to verify resolution of all symptoms, return to normal otoscopic findings, and restoration of normal hearing.

NOTE: Effusions may persist for 2 to 6 wk or longer in many cases of adequately treated otitis media.

SURGICAL Rx

- No evidence to support the routine of myringotomy, but in severe cases it provides prompt pain relief and accelerates resolution of infection.
- Purulent secretions retained in the middle ear lead to increased pressure that may lead to spread of infection to contiguous areas. Myringotomy to decompress the middle ear is necessary to avoid complications.
- Complications include mastoiditis, facial nerve paralysis, labyrinthitis, meningitis, and brain abscess.
- Other procedures used for drainage of the middle ear include insertion of a ventilation tube and/or simple mastoidectomy.

CHRONIC Rx

- Myringotomy and tympanostomy tube placement for persistent middle ear effusion unresponsive to medical therapy for ≥3 mo if bilateral or ≥6 mo if unilateral.
- Adenoidectomy, with or without tonsillectomy, often advocated for treatment of recurrent otitis media, although indications for this procedure are controversial.
- Long-term complications include tympanic membrane perforations, cholesteatoma, tympanosclerosis, ossicular necrosis, toxic or

suppurative labyrinthitis, and intracranial suppuration.

DISPOSITION

Patients can be treated at home as outpatients with the rare exception of patients with evidence of local suppurative complications (e.g., meningitis, acute mastoiditis, brain abscess, cavernous sinus, or lateral vein thrombosis).

REFERRAL

- To otorhinolaryngologist if:
    1. Medical treatment failure
    2. Diagnosis uncertain: adults with one or more episodes of otitis media should be referred for ear-nose-throat evaluation to rule out underlying process (e.g., malignancy)
    3. Any of the above-mentioned acute and chronic complications

PEARLS & CONSIDERATIONS

COMMENTS

- Utoscopic findings are critical to accurate acute otitis media (AOM) diagnosis. AOM microbiology has changed with use of pneumococcal conjugate vaccine (PCV7). Antibiotics are modestly more effective than no treatment but cause adverse effects in 4% to 10% of children. Most antibiotics have comparable clinical success.
Prevention:
- Multiple component conjugate vaccines hold promise for decreasing recurrent episodes of acute otitis media
- Breastfeed and bottle-feed infants in an upright position
- Avoidance of irritants (e.g., tobacco smoke)

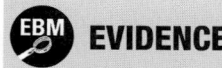 **EVIDENCE**

available at www.expertconsult.com

SUGGESTED READINGS

available at www.expertconsult.com

AUTHORS: **GLENN G. FORT, M.D., M.P.H.,** and **DENNIS J. MIKOLICH, M.D.**

BASIC INFORMATION

DEFINITION

Otosclerosis is conductive hearing loss caused by fixation of the stapes, resulting in gradual hearing loss. Approximately 15% of cases affect only one ear.

ICD-9CM CODES
387.9 Otosclerosis

EPIDEMIOLOGY & DEMOGRAPHICS

INCIDENCE (IN U.S.): Most common cause of hearing loss in young adults
PEAK INCIDENCE: Middle age
PREVALENCE (IN U.S.): Five cases per 1000 persons
PREDOMINANT SEX: Male/female ratio of 2:1
PREDOMINANT AGE: Symptoms start between ages 15 and 30 yr, with slowly progressive hearing loss.
GENETICS: Half of cases are dominantly inherited.

PHYSICAL FINDINGS & CLINICAL PRESENTATION

- Tympanic membrane is normal in most cases (tested with tuning fork).
- Bone conduction is greater than air conduction.
- Weber test localizes to affected ear.

ETIOLOGY

- A disease in which a vascular type of spongy bone is laid down
- Unknown

 DIAGNOSIS

DIFFERENTIAL DIAGNOSIS

- Hearing loss from any cause: cochlear otosclerosis, polyps, granulomas, tumors, osteogenesis imperfecta, chronic ear infections, trauma.
- A clinical algorithm for evaluation of hearing loss is described in Section III.
- Table 1-136 describes common types of conductive and sensorineural hearing loss.

WORKUP

Audiometry

LABORATORY TESTS

None, unless infection suspected

IMAGING STUDIES

MRI or CT with specific cuts through inner ear (Fig. 1-271)

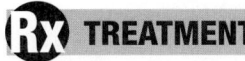 **TREATMENT**

NONPHARMACOLOGIC THERAPY

Hearing aid only of temporary use

CHRONIC Rx

Progresses to deafness without surgical intervention

DISPOSITION

Referral to ear-nose-throat (ENT) specialist

REFERRAL

To ENT specialist for surgery if moderate hearing loss suspected

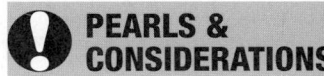 **PEARLS & CONSIDERATIONS**

COMMENTS

A full ENT evaluation in a young or middle-aged person with hearing loss is mandatory unless the cause is obvious (such as trauma or repeated infection).

SUGGESTED READING
available at www.expertconsult.com

AUTHOR: **FRED F. FERRI, M.D.**

TABLE 1-136 Common Types of Conductive and Sensorineural Hearing Loss

Conductive Hearing Loss	Sensorineural Hearing Loss
Otitis media with effusion	Presbycusis (hearing loss with aging)
TM perforation	Ototoxicity
Tympanosclerosis	Ménière's disease
Retracted TM (eustachian tube dysfunction)	Idiopathic loss
Ossicular problems	Noise-induced loss
Otosclerosis	Perilymphatic fistula
Foreign body in ear canal	Hereditary (congenital) loss
Cerumen impaction	Multiple sclerosis
Tumor of the ear canal or middle ear	Diabetes
Cholesteatoma	Syphilis, acoustic neuroma

From Rakel RE (ed): *Principles of family practice,* ed 6, Philadelphia, 2002, WB Saunders.
TM, Tympanic membrane.

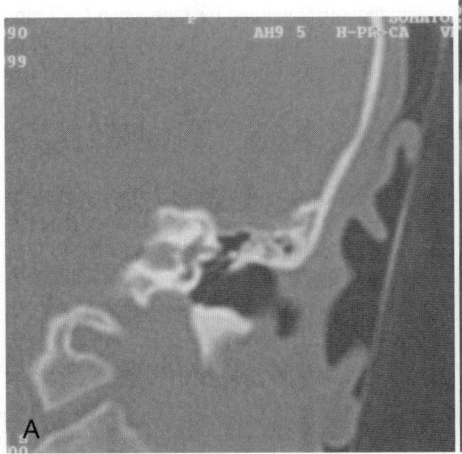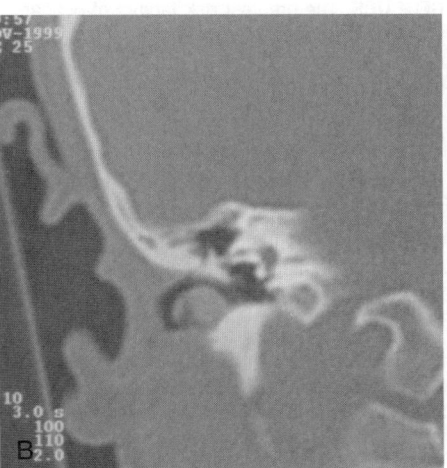

FIGURE 1-271 A patient with conductive hearing loss. By comparing the normal **(A)** and abnormal **(B)** sides on CT scan, the narrowing of the oval window can be clearly appreciated. This results in fixation of the stapes footplate and conductive hearing loss. (From Grainger RG et al [eds]: *Grainger & Allison's diagnostic radiology,* ed 4, Philadelphia, 2001, Churchill Livingstone.)

Diseases and Disorders

Ovarian Cancer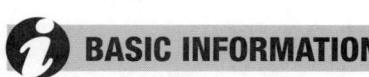

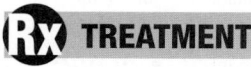 BASIC INFORMATION

DEFINITION

Ovarian tumors can be benign, requiring operative intervention but not recurring or metastasizing; malignant, recurring, metastasizing, and having decreased survival; or borderline, having a small risk of recurrence or metastases but generally having a good prognosis.

SYNONYMS

Epithelial ovarian cancer
Germ cell tumor
Sex cord stromal tumor
Ovarian tumor of low malignant potential

ICD-9CM CODES

183.0 Malignant neoplasm of ovary

EPIDEMIOLOGY & DEMOGRAPHICS

INCIDENCE: 12.9 to 15.1 cases/100,000 persons; ~25,000 new cases annually
PREVALENCE: Median age of 61 yr; peaks at age 75 to 79 yr (54/100,000)
RISK FACTORS: Low parity, delayed childbearing, use of talc on the perineum (unlikely), high-fat diet, fertility drugs (unlikely), Lynch II syndrome (nonpolyposis colon cancer, endometrial cancer, breast cancer, and ovarian cancer clusters in first- and second-degree relatives), breast-ovarian familial cancer syndrome, site-specific familial ovarian cancer. Hormone therapy is associated with an increased risk of ovarian cancer regardless of the duration of use, the formulation, estrogen dose, regimen, progestin type, and route of administration.
GENETICS: The greatest risk factors of ovarian cancer are a family history and associated genetic syndromes. Familial susceptibility has been shown with the *BRCA1* gene located on 17q12 to 21. This correlates with breast-ovarian cancer syndrome.

PHYSICAL FINDINGS & CLINICAL PRESENTATION

- 60% present with advanced disease
- Abdominal fullness, early satiety, dyspepsia
- Pelvic pain, back pain, constipation
- Pelvic or abdominal mass
- Lymphadenopathy (inguinal)
- Sister Mary Joseph nodule (umbilical mass)

ETIOLOGY

- Can be inherited as site-specific familial ovarian cancer (two or more first-degree relatives have ovarian cancer)
- Breast-ovarian cancer syndrome (clusters of breast and ovarian cancer among first- and second-degree relatives)
- Lynch syndrome
- No family history and unknown etiology in the majority of ovarian cancer cases

DIAGNOSIS

DIFFERENTIAL DIAGNOSIS

- Primary peritoneal cancer mesothelioma
- Benign ovarian tumor
- Functional ovarian cyst
- Endometriosis
- Ovarian torsion
- Pelvic kidney
- Pedunculated uterine fibroid
- Primary cancer from breast, gastrointestinal tract, or other pelvic organ metastasized to the ovary

WORKUP

- Definitive diagnosis made at laparotomy; epithelial ovarian cancer most common type of ovarian cancer
- Careful physical and history, including family history
- Exclusion of nongynecologic etiologies
- Observation of small cystic masses in premenopausal women for regression for 2 mo
- FIGO classification of ovarian carcinoma is described in Table 1-137

LABORATORY TESTS

- Complete blood count.
- Chemistry profile.
- CA-125 or lysophosphatidic acid level. Only about 50% of early-stage ovarian cancers will be associated with elevated CA-125. Additionally, false elevations may occur with uterine leiomyoma, endometriosis, pregnancy, and intra-abdominal infections.
- Consider: human chorionic gonadotropin, inhibin, alpha-fetoprotein, neuron-specific enolase, and lactate dehydrogenase in patients at risk for germ cell tumors.
- A panel of 3 serum biomarkers (apolipoprotein A-1 [ApoA-1], transthyretin [TTR], and transferrin [TF] has been reported useful in distinguishing normal samples from early-stage ovarian cancer with a sensitivity of 84% and normal samples from late-stage ovarian cancer with a sensitivity of 97%.

IMAGING STUDIES

- Ultrasound
- Chest x-ray examination
- Mammogram
- CT scan to help evaluate extent of disease (Fig. 1-272)
- Other studies (barium enema, MRI, intravenous pyelogram, etc.) as clinically indicated

TREATMENT

NONPHARMACOLOGIC THERAPY

Virtually all cases of ovarian cancer involve surgical exploration. This includes:
- Abdominal cytology
- Total abdominal hysterectomy and bilateral salpingo-oophorectomy (except in early stages in which fertility is an issue)
- Omentectomy
- Diaphragm sampling
- Selective lymphadenectomy (pelvis and para-aortic)
- Primary cytoreduction with a goal of residual tumor diameter <2 cm
- Bowel surgery, splenectomy if needed to obtain optimal (<2 cm) cytoreduction
- Conventional treatment includes surgical debulking followed by chemotherapy

ACUTE GENERAL Rx

- Optimal cytoreduction is generally followed by chemotherapy (except in some early-stage disease).

TABLE 1-137	FIGO Classification of Ovarian Carcinoma	
Stage I	Growth limited to the ovaries:	
	Stage IA:	Growth limited to one ovary, no ascites and no tumour present on the external surface; capsule intact
	Stage IB:	Growth limited to both ovaries, no ascites and no tumour present on the external surface; capsule intact
	Stage IC:	Stage 1A or 1B where there is tumor on the surface of either ovary; or with ruptured capsules or with ascites containing malignant cells or positive peritoneal washings
Stage II	Growth involving one or both ovaries with pelvic extension:	
	Stage IIA:	Extension and/or metastases to the uterus and tubes
	Stage IIB:	Extension to other pelvic tissues
	Stage IIC:	Stage IIA or IIB with tumour on the surface of either ovary or positive peritoneal washings or malignant ascites
Stage III	Growth involving one or both ovaries with peritoneal implants outside the pelvis or positive retroperitoneal or inguinal lymph nodes:	
	Stage IIIA:	Microscopic seeding of abdominal peritoneal surfaces
	Stage IIIB:	Macroscopic disease outside the pelvis less than 2 cm in diameter
	Stage IIIC:	Abdominal implants greater than 2 cm and/or positive nodes
Stage IV	Growth involving one or both ovaries with distant metastases including parenchymal (but not superficial) liver metastases and pleural effusions containing malignant cells	

From Symonds EM, Symonds IM: *Essential obstetrics and gynaecology*, ed 4, London, 2004, Churchill Livingstone.

- Cisplatin-based combination chemotherapy is used for stage II or greater, 6-mo treatment. Compared with IV paclitaxel plus cisplatin, IV paclitaxel plus intraperitoneal cisplatin and paclitaxel improves survival rates in patients with optimally debulked stage III ovarian cancer.
- Chemotherapy regimens continue to change as research continues.
- Consider second-look surgery when chemotherapy is complete.

- Recent trials have shown that neoadjuvant chemotherapy followed by interval debulking surgery is not inferior to debulking surgery followed by chemotherapy as a treatment option for patients with bulky stage IIIC or IV ovarian carcinoma. Complete resection of all macroscopic disease, whether performed as primary treatment or after neoadjuvant chemotherapy, remains the objective whenever cytoreductive surgery is performed.

CHRONIC Rx

- If CA-125 elevated, may have recurrent disease
- Physical and pelvic examinations every 3 mo for 2 yr, every 4 mo during third year, then every 6 mo
- CA-125 every visit
- Yearly Pap smear

DISPOSITION

- Overall 5-yr survival rates remain low because of the preponderance of late-stage disease:
  - Stage I and II: 80% to 100%
  - Stage III: 15% to 20%
  - Stage IV: 5%
- Younger patients (<50 yr) in all stages have a considerably better 5-yr survival than older patients (40% vs. 15%).

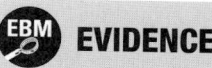 **EVIDENCE**

available at www.expertconsult.com

SUGGESTED READINGS

available at www.expertconsult.com

AUTHORS: **GIL M. FARKASH, M.D.,** and **RUBEN ALVERO, M.D.**

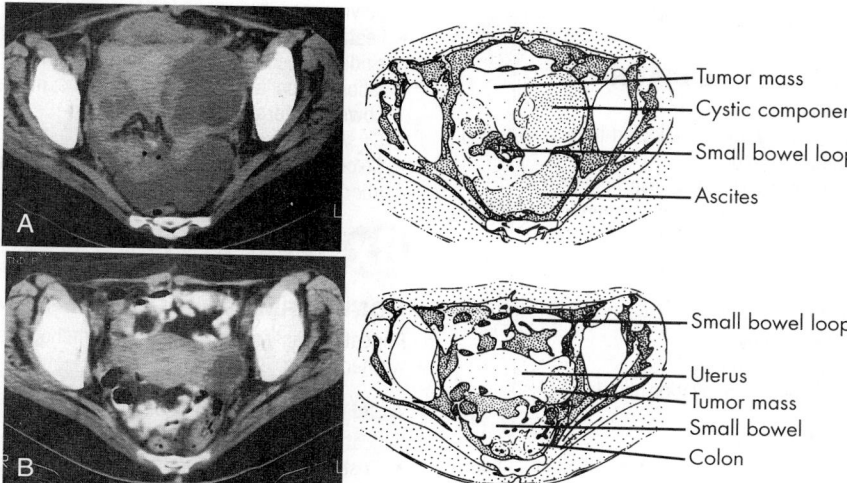

FIGURE 1-272 labels:
- Tumor mass
- Cystic component
- Small bowel loop
- Ascites
- Small bowel loop
- Uterus
- Tumor mass
- Small bowel
- Colon

FIGURE 1-272 Response to chemotherapy. A 51-year-old woman presented with a rapid increase in abdominal girth. **A,** On CT scan, she was found to have a 12 × 8 cm ovarian mass with a cystic component; peritoneal involvement was extensive and 6 L of ascites were removed. Pathologic examination showed a poorly differentiated tumor. The tumor was not resectable, and she was treated with combination chemotherapy. After one cycle of therapy, her abdomen returned to normal size. **B,** A CT scan reveals only a small residual ovarian mass. Surgery after four cycles of chemotherapy showed no gross or microscopic tumor. She received four more cycles of chemotherapy but relapsed 1 year later with abdominal metastases. (From Skarin AT: *Atlas of diagnostic oncology,* ed 3, St Louis, 2003, Mosby.)

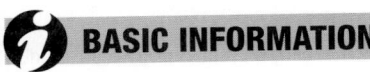

DEFINITION

Benign ovarian neoplasms are often clinically indistinguishable from their malignant counterparts. Therefore all persistent adnexal masses must be considered malignant until proven otherwise. Nonneoplastic tumors include:
- Germinal inclusion cyst
- Follicle cyst
- Corpus luteum cyst
- Pregnancy luteoma
- Theca lutein cysts
- Sclerocystic ovaries
- Endometrioma

Neoplastic tumors derived from coelomic epithelium include:
- Cystic tumors: serous cystoma, mucinous cystoma, mixed forms
- Tumors with stromal overgrowth: fibroma, adenofibroma, Brenner tumor

Tumors derived from germ cells are dermoids (benign cystic teratomas).

ICD-9CM CODES
220 Benign neoplasm of ovary

EPIDEMIOLOGY & DEMOGRAPHICS

- Reproductive years:
  1. Most common benign ovarian neoplasms: serous cystadenoma and benign cystic teratoma
  2. Most common adnexal mass: functional cyst
- Risk of malignancy increases after age 40 yr.
- Infants: adnexal masses are usually follicular cysts attributable to maternal hormone stimulation that regress during first few months of life.
- Childhood:
  1. Adnexal masses are rare
  2. 8% malignant
  3. Almost always dysgerminomas or teratomas (germ cell origin)
  4. Frequency of malignancy inversely correlated with age
- Adolescence:
  1. Most common adnexal mass is a functional cyst.
  2. Most common neoplastic ovarian tumor is a benign cystic teratoma.
  3. Solid/cystic adnexal tumors are rare and almost always dysgerminomas or malignant teratomas.

PHYSICAL FINDINGS & CLINICAL PRESENTATION

- Usually asymptomatic
- Pelvic pain or pressure
- Dyspareunia
- Abdominal pain ranging from mild to severe peritoneal irritation
- Increasing abdominal girth or distention
- Adnexal mass of pelvic examination
- Children: abdominal or rectal mass

ETIOLOGY

- Physiologic
- Endometriosis
- Unknown

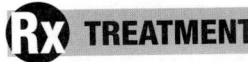 DIAGNOSIS

DIFFERENTIAL DIAGNOSIS

- Ovarian torsion
- Malignancy: ovary, fallopian tube, colon
- Uterine fibroid
- Diverticular abscess, diverticulitis
- Appendiceal abscess, appendicitis (especially in children)
- Tubo-ovarian abscess
- Paraovarian cyst
- Distended bladder
- Pelvic kidney
- Ectopic pregnancy
- Retroperitoneal cyst or neoplasm

WORKUP

- Complete history and physical examination
- Pelvic or rectovaginal examination to reveal firm, irregular, mobile mass
- Laparoscopy or laparotomy to establish diagnosis

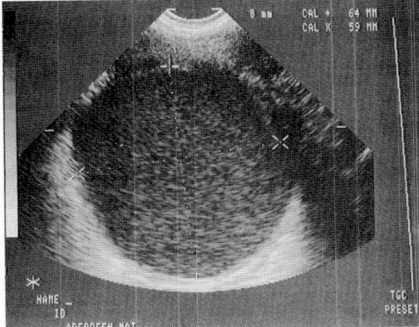

FIGURE 1-273 Ultrasonogram, which reveals a cyst 6.5 cm across, which was found at laparotomy to be an endometrioma, full of altered blood: the so-called chocolate cyst. This may cause cyclical or chronic pelvic pain. Greer IA, Cameron IT, Kitchner HC, Prentice A: *A Mosby's color atlas and text of obstetrics and gynecology*, London, 2001, Harcourt.

LABORATORY TESTS

- Pregnancy test
- Serum tumor markers:
  1. Cancer antigen 125 (CA 125)
  2. Alpha-fetoprotein (endodermal sinus tumor, immature teratoma)
  3. Beta-human chorionic gonadotropin
  4. Lactate dehydrogenase (dysgerminoma)

IMAGING STUDIES

Ultrasound (Fig. 1-273):
- May differentiate adnexal mass from other pelvic masses
- Features that increase risk of malignancy include solid component, papillae, multiple septations or solitary thick septa, ascites, matted bowel, bilaterality, irregular borders
- CT scan with contrast
- Colonoscopy or barium enema, if symptomatic

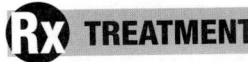 TREATMENT

NONPHARMACOLOGIC THERAPY

Repeat pelvic examination for premenopausal women in 4 to 6 wk

ACUTE GENERAL Rx

Indications for surgery:
- Postmenopausal or premenarcheal palpable adnexal mass
- Adnexal mass with suspicious ultrasound features
- Premenopausal woman with persistent cyst >5 cm
- Any adnexal mass >10 cm
- Suspected torsion or rupture

CHRONIC Rx

- Depends on diagnosis
- Possible suppression of formation of new cysts by oral contraceptives

DISPOSITION

Depends on diagnosis

REFERRAL

- If malignancy suspected
- If surgery required

SUGGESTED READINGS
available at www.expertconsult.com

AUTHORS: **GEORGE T. DANAKAS, M.D.,** and **RUBEN ALVERO, M.D.**

BASIC INFORMATION

DEFINITION

Paget's disease of the bone is a focal disorder of chaotic bone remodeling with increased osteoblastic and osteoclastic activity that results in disorganized woven and lamellar bone in one or more skeletal sites. The end result is bone of poor quality that is enlarged, hypervascular, and susceptible to deformation and fracture.

SYNONYMS

Osteitis deformans

ICD-9CM CODES
731.0 Paget's disease (osteitis deformans)

EPIDEMIOLOGY & DEMOGRAPHICS

Epidemiologic data suggest an origin of Paget's disease in Great Britain spreading to other areas by English colonists beginning in the seventeenth century. Highest prevalence occurs in Eastern and Western Europe and in those who have emigrated to New Zealand, Australia, South Africa, and North America. Rarely seen in Japanese, Chinese, Asian Indians, sub-Saharan Africans, and middle eastern Arabs.

Most commonly diagnosed in those aged >50 yr and rare before 40 yr.

Prevalence estimates of up to 3% of population aged > 50 yr and up to 10% in those aged >90 yr.

PREDOMINANT SEX: Variable preponderance of males.

PREDOMINANT AGE: Middle or advanced years.

FAMILIAL INCIDENCE: Common, family history positive in up to 40% of cases.

PHYSICAL FINDINGS & CLINICAL PRESENTATION

- Most common sites of involvement: pelvis, spine, sacrum, femora, skull, tibiae, humeri, scapulae.
- Uncommon: hands, feet, fibulae.
- Lesions in one (monostotic) or more bones (polyostotic).
- Gradual progression of disease in affected bone(s) with rare appearance at new site(s).
- Many patients are asymptomatic.
- Symptoms and signs include bone and articular pain often related to secondary arthritis, bone deformities and enlargement, increased warmth over pagetic bone, skull enlargement and nerve entrapment or compression syndromes, cranial nerve deficits especially deafness, spinal cord compression and vascular steal syndromes, fissure fractures, fractures, and neoplastic degeneration.

ETIOLOGY

Etiology remains unknown.

Extensive epidemiologic and laboratory data are in keeping with potential role of paramyxo-

viral infection of osteoclasts in a genetically susceptible individual with or without documented genetic mutations.

DIAGNOSIS

DIFFERENTIAL DIAGNOSIS

- Osteosclerosis
- Hyperphosphatasia
- Familial expansile osteolysis
- Fibrous dysplasia
- Skeletal neoplasm (primary or metastatic)
- Osteomalacia with secondary hyperparathyroidism

LABORATORY TESTS

- Increased serum alkaline phosphatase (SAP)
- Increase in urine NTx/creatinine ratio or plasma CTx
- Bone biopsy may be necessary to rule out sarcomatous degeneration or metastases

IMAGING STUDIES

Bone scintigraphy is the most sensitive test for delineating the extent and site of pagetic lesions but nonspecific in that areas of uptake may be related to arthritis or metastatic lesions. Radiographs (Fig. 1-274) will further delineate characteristic pagetic changes.

TREATMENT

Indications for therapy include extensive or symptomatic disease; neurologic complications; involvement of weight-bearing bones, skull, vertebrae, and other areas of critical involvement, for example, in proximity to joints; and preven-

tion of excess bleeding from orthopedic procedures on pagetic bone.

NONPHARMACOLOGIC THERAPY

Optimization of calcium and vitamin D intake and appropriate guidance regarding ambulatory needs.

SPECIFIC THERAPY

Bisphosphonates are the mainstay of therapy and include oral alendronate or risedronate, and intravenous pamidronate or zoledronic acid.

- SC salmon calcitonin when bisphosphonates are not tolerated or contraindicated as in those with GFR of <35 ml/min
- Acetaminophen, aspirin, and nonsteroidal drugs for relief of pain

DISPOSITION

- Without treatment, progression of disease is common
- With treatment, remissions of varying duration in most patients
- Careful and regular clinical and biochemical followup at 3- to 6-mo intervals with necessity of retreatment in patients with continued pagetic activity or reactivation
- With first ever intravenous dose of pamidronate or zoledronic acid, patients may experience a flu-like syndrome for several days that may be prevented with acetaminophen

SUGGESTED READINGS

available at www.expertconsult.com

AUTHOR: **JOSEPH R. TUCCI, M.D.**

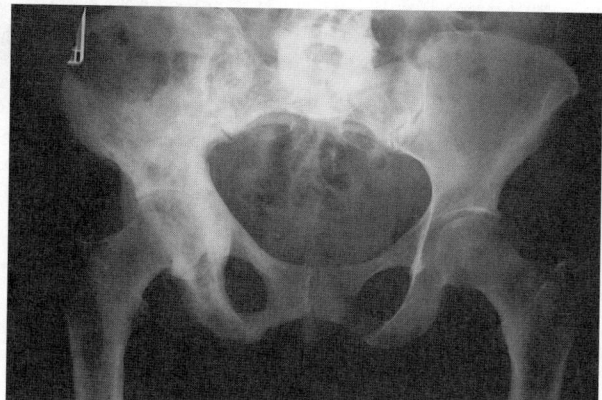

FIGURE 1-274 Frontal radiograph of the pelvis shows marked prominence to the trabeculae in the right ilium, ischium, and pubic bones, with small lytic areas identified as compatible with the later stages of Paget's disease. (From Specht N [ed]: *Practical guide to diagnostic imaging*, St Louis, 1998, Mosby.)

BASIC INFORMATION

DEFINITION

Paget's disease of the breast is a malignant disease that presents itself as a scaly, sore, eroding, bleeding ulcer of the nipple. Microscopically, typical large clear cells (Paget's cells) with pale and abundant cytoplasm and hyperchromatic nuclei with prominent nucleoli are found in the epidermal layer. Paget's disease is more often associated with primary invasive or in situ carcinoma of the breast.

ICD-9CM CODES
174.0 Malignant neoplasm of female breast, nipple, and areola

EPIDEMIOLOGY & DEMOGRAPHICS
- Not common
- Found in one in 100 to 200 breast cancer patients

PHYSICAL FINDINGS & CLINICAL PRESENTATION
- Variable
- Itching or burning nipple and/or reported lump
- Very minimal scaly lesion that may bleed when scales are lifted
- Typical ulcer located on nipple with serous fluid weeping or small amount of bleeding coming from it (Fig. 1-275)
- Palpable carcinoma in the breast of some patients

ETIOLOGY
- Exact origin unknown
- Possibly migration of either in situ or invasive carcinoma cells in breast to nipple skin to produce Paget's disease

DIAGNOSIS

DIFFERENTIAL DIAGNOSIS
- Chronic dermatitis
- Florid papillomatosis of the nipple or nipple adenoma
- Eczema

WORKUP
- Clinically apparent
- Careful breast examination with diagnosis in mind
- Palpable mass or mammographic lesions in 60% to 70% of patients

A clinical algorithm for the evaluation of nipple discharge is described in Section III, "Breast, Nipple Discharge Evaluation."

LABORATORY TESTS
Biopsy of nipple lesion

IMAGING STUDIES
Mammograms to search for possible primary carcinoma

TREATMENT

NONPHARMACOLOGIC THERAPY
- Fewer patients:
  1. Paget's disease of nipple only finding when mammographically negative breast
  2. Consideration of wide excision of nipple with or without radiation
- Other patients: additional invasive or in situ carcinoma recognized
- Either modified mastectomy or breast conservation treatment
- Presence of underlying in situ or invasive carcinoma in mastectomy specimen of majority of patients

ACUTE GENERAL Rx
Systemic adjuvant therapy depending on extent of invasive carcinoma found

DISPOSITION
- Parallel prognosis to that of breast cancer patient without Paget's disease
- Regular follow-up as in other invasive or in situ carcinoma patients

REFERRAL
At outset, all suspicious nipple lesions should be referred for evaluation and treatment.

SUGGESTED READINGS
available at www.expertconsult.com

AUTHORS: **TAKUMA NEMOTO, M.D.,** and **RUBEN ALVERO, M.D.**

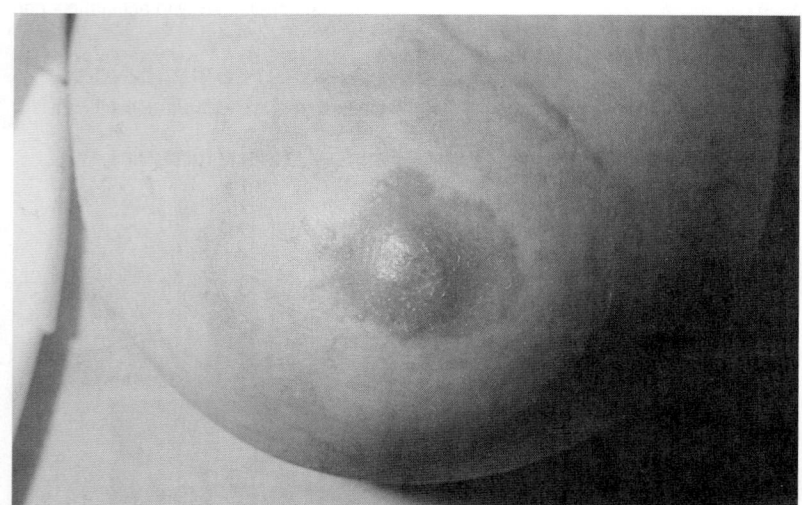

FIGURE 1-275 Paget's disease of the breast. The lesion has insidiously spread for 1 year to infiltrate the areola and surrounding skin. (From Habif TP: *Clinical dermatology: a color guide to diagnosis and therapy,* ed 3, St Louis, 1996, Mosby.)

BASIC INFORMATION

DEFINITION

Pancreatic cancer is an adenocarcinoma derived from the epithelium of the pancreatic duct.

ICD-9CM CODES
157.9 Pancreatic cancer
157.0 (head)
157.1 (body)
157.2 (tail)
157.3 (duct)
230.9 (in situ)

EPIDEMIOLOGY & DEMOGRAPHICS

INCIDENCE: One case in 10,000 persons annually. In the U.S. there are >35,000 patients diagnosed with pancreatic cancer and >30,000 deaths yearly. Less than 20% of patients present with localized, potentially respectable tumors.
PREDOMINANT SEX: Male/female ratio of 2:1
PREDOMINANT AGE: Seventh and eighth decades of life

PHYSICAL FINDINGS & CLINICAL PRESENTATION

Presenting symptoms:
- Jaundice
- Abdominal pain: generally dull upper abdominal pain or vague abdominal discomfort
- Weight loss
- Anorexia/change in taste, aesthenia
- Nausea
- Uncommonly: depression, gastrointestinal bleeding, acute pancreatitis (from obstruction of the pancreatic duct), back pain

Physical findings:
- Icterus
- Cachexia, temporal wasting
- Ascites, peripheral lymphadenopathy, hepatomegaly
- Excoriations from scratching pruritic skin

ETIOLOGY

Unknown, but several conditions have been associated with pancreatic cancer:
- Smoking
- Alcoholism
- Genetics: 5% to 10% of patients have a family history of the disease
- Gallstones
- Diabetes mellitus
- Chronic pancreatitis
- Diet rich in animal fat
- Occupational exposures: oil refining, paper manufacturing, chemical industry
- Overweight or obesity during early adulthood is associated with a greater risk of pancreatic cancer and a younger age of disease onset. Obesity at an older age is associated with a lower overall survival in patients with pancreatic cancer.

DIAGNOSIS

DIFFERENTIAL DIAGNOSIS

- Common duct cholelithiasis
- Cholangiocarcinoma
- Common duct stricture
- Sclerosing cholangitis
- Primary biliary cirrhosis
- Autoimmune pancreatitis
- Drug-induced cholestasis (e.g., phenothiazines)
- Chronic hepatitis
- Sarcoidosis
- Other pancreatic tumors (islet cell tumor, cystadenocarcinoma, epidermoid carcinoma, sarcomas, lymphomas)

WORKUP

Routine Laboratory Tests	% Abnormal
Alkaline phosphatase	80
Bilirubin	55
Total protein	15
Amylase	15
Hematocrit	60

Ca 19-9: Not useful as a screening tool because it may be elevated in other conditions, such as cholestasis, but is useful for therapeutic monitoring and early detection of recurrent disease after treatment

IMAGING STUDIES

Multidetector helical CT with IV administration of contrast is the imaging procedure of choice for initial evaluation. Endoscopic ultrasonography is useful when there is no identifiable mass on CT and diagnosis is strongly suspected and in obtaining tissue for diagnostic purposes. Fine-needle aspiration biopsy combined with endoscopic ultrasonography is the preferred modality for evaluation of cystic or mass lesions to determine malignancy. Endoscopic retrograde cholangiopancreatography (ERCP) is useful in patients with jaundice needing an endoscopic stent to relieve obstruction.

Noninvasive Imaging	% Abnormal
Abdominal ultrasonography	60
Abdominal CT scan (with contrast) (Fig. 1-276)	90
Abdominal MRI scan	90
Invasive Imaging	
ERCP	90
CT scan or ultrasonography-guided needle aspiration cytology	90-95

STAGING FOR PANCREATIC CANCER

PRIMARY TUMOR (T):
TX	Primary tumor cannot be assessed
T0	No evidence of primary tumor
T1	Tumor <2 cm
T2	Tumor >2 cm, confined to the pancreas
T3	Tumor extends locally beyond the pancreas
T4	Tumor involves celiac or superior mesenteric arteries

LYMPH NODES (N):
NX	Regional lymph nodes cannot be assessed
N0	No regional lymph node metastasis
N1	Regional lymph node metastasis

DISTANT METASTASES (M):
MX	Presence of distant metastasis cannot be assessed
M0	No distant metastasis
M1	Distant metastasis

STAGING GROUP:
IA	T1, N0, M0
IB	T2, N0, M0
IIA	T3, N0, M0
IIB	T1-3, N1, M0
III	T4, N0-1, M0
IV	T1-4, N0-1, M1

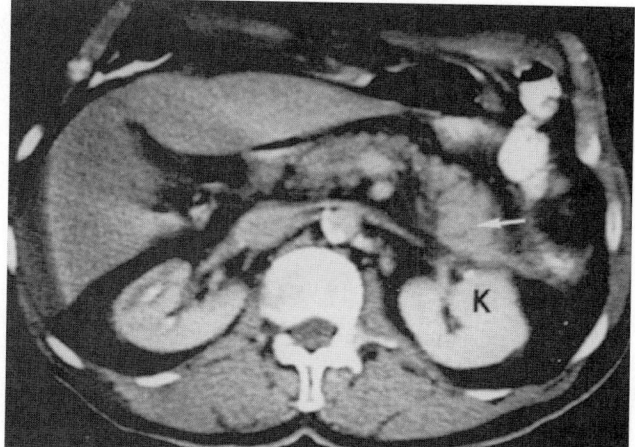

FIGURE 1-276 CT scan of a patient with adenocarcinoma of the body and tail of the pancreas. The tumor *(arrow)* is seen anterior and adjacent to the left kidney *(K)*. At operation, the tumor was invading Gerota's fascia. (From Sabiston D: *Textbook of surgery,* ed 17, Philadelphia, 2005, WB Saunders.)

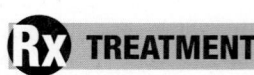

SURGERY

Curative cephalic pancreatoduodenectomy (Whipple's procedure) is appropriate for only 10% to 20% of patients whose lesion is <5 cm, solitary, and without metastases. Surgical mortality rate is 5%. Adjuvant chemotherapy may improve postoperative survival. The addition of gemcitabine to adjuvant fluorouracil and leucovorin chemotherapy has been reported to have a survival benefit for patients with resected pancreatic cancer. An emerging strategy is the use of neoadjuvant preoperative treatment in patients with respectable pancreatic cancer

PALLIATIVE SURGERY (FOR BILIARY DECOMPRESSION/ DIVERSION)

Palliative therapeutic ERCP with stents

CHEMOTHERAPY

In patients with advanced disease an accepted approach is the administration of gemcitabine given alone or combined with a platinum agent, erlotinib, or fluoropyrimidine.

RADIATION

- External-beam radiation for palliation of pain.
- Combined chemotherapy and radiation provides a median survival of 11 mo.
- Celiac plexus block by an experienced anesthesiologist provides pain relief in 80% to 90% of cases.

DISPOSITION

- Adjunct chemotherapy has a significant survival benefit in patients with resected pancreatic cancer.
- Recent trials have shown that adjuvant postoperative chemotherapy with gemcitabine significantly delays the development of recurrent disease after complete resection of pancreatic cancer.

PEARLS & CONSIDERATIONS

COMMENTS

- The U.S. Preventive Services Task Force (USPSTF) recommends against routine screening for pancreatic cancer in asymptomatic adults by abdominal palpation, ultrasonography, or serologic markers. The USPSTF found no evidence that screening for pancreatic cancer is effective in reducing mortality rates. There is potential for significant harm because of the low prevalence of pancreatic cancer, limited accuracy of available screening tests, invasive nature of diagnostic tests, and poor outcome of treatment. As a result, the USPSTF concluded that the harms of screening for pancreatic cancer exceed any potential benefits.
- Recent trials indicate that pancreatic cancer may have a distinct microRNA (miRNA) expression pattern that may differentiate it from normal pancreas and chronic pancreatitis. Current research is aimed at using miRNA expression patterns to distinguish between long- and short-term survivors.

EVIDENCE

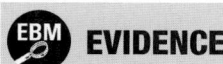

available at www.expertconsult.com

SUGGESTED READINGS
available at www.expertconsult.com

AUTHOR: **FRED F. FERRI, M.D.**

BASIC INFORMATION

DEFINITION

- Acute pancreatitis is an inflammatory process of the pancreas with intrapancreatic activation of enzymes that may also involve peripancreatic tissue and/or remote organ systems.
- Severe acute pancreatitis (SAP) is diagnosed by the presence of any of the following four criteria:
  1. Organ failure with one or more of the following: shock (systolic blood pressure <90 mm Hg), pulmonary insufficiency (Pao$_2$ ≤60 mm Hg), renal failure (serum creatinine >2 mg/dl after rehydration), and gastrointestinal bleeding (>500 ml/24 hr)
  2. Local complications such as necrosis, pseudocyst, or abscess
  3. At least three of Ranson's criteria (see below) or
  4. At least eight of the Acute Physiology and Chronic Health Evaluation II (APACHE II) criteria

ICD-9CM CODES
577.0 Acute pancreatitis

EPIDEMIOLOGY & DEMOGRAPHICS

- Acute pancreatitis is most often secondary to biliary tract disease and alcohol.
- Incidence in urban areas is twice that of rural areas (20/100,000 persons in urban areas).
- 20% of patients have necrotizing pancreatitis; the remainder have interstitial, or edematous, pancreatitis.
- Acute pancreatitis accounts for >220,000 hospital admissions in the U.S. each year.

PHYSICAL FINDINGS & CLINICAL PRESENTATION

- Epigastric tenderness and guarding, often radiating to the back; pain usually developing suddenly, reaching peak intensity within 10 to 30 min, severe and lasting several hours without relief
- Hypoactive bowel sounds (from ileus)
- Tachycardia, shock (from decreased intravascular volume)
- Confusion (from metabolic disturbances)
- Fever
- Tachycardia, decreased breath sounds (atelectasis, pleural effusions, acute respiratory distress syndrome [ARDS])
- Jaundice (from obstruction or compression of biliary tract)
- Ascites (from tear in pancreatic duct, leaking pseudocyst)
- Palpable abdominal mass (pseudocyst, phlegmon, abscess, carcinoma)
- Evidence of hypocalcemia (Chvostek's sign, Trousseau's sign)
- Evidence of intraabdominal bleeding (hemorrhagic pancreatitis):
  1. Gray-blue discoloration around the umbilicus (Cullen's sign)
  2. Bluish discoloration involving the flanks (Grey Turner's sign)
- Tender subcutaneous nodules (caused by subcutaneous fat necrosis)

ETIOLOGY

- In >90% of cases: biliary tract disease (calculi or sludge) or alcohol, most common after 5-10 yr of heavy drinking
- Drugs (e.g., thiazides, furosemide, corticosteroids, tetracycline, estrogens, valproic acid, metronidazole, azathioprine, methyldopa, pentamidine, ethacrynic acid, procainamide, sulindac, nitrofurantoin, angiotensin-converting enzyme inhibitors, danazol, cimetidine, piroxicam, gold, ranitidine, sulfasalazine, isoniazid, acetaminophen, cisplatin, opiates, erythromycin, metformin, sitagliptin)
- Abdominal trauma
- Surgery
- Endoscopic retrograde cholangiopancreatography (ERCP)
- Infections (predominantly viral infections)
- Peptic ulcer (penetrating duodenal ulcer)
- Pancreas divisum (congenital failure to fuse of dorsal or ventral pancreas)
- Idiopathic
- Pregnancy
- Vascular (vasculitis, ischemic)
- Hypolipoproteinemia (types I, IV, and V)
- Hypercalcemia
- Pancreatic carcinoma (primary or metastatic)
- Renal failure
- Hereditary pancreatitis
- Occupational exposure to chemicals: methanol, cobalt, zinc, mercuric chloride, creosol, lead, organophosphates, chlorinated naphthalenes
- Others: scorpion bite, obstruction at ampulla region (neoplasm, duodenal diverticula, Crohn's disease), hypotensive shock, autoimmune pancreatitis

DIAGNOSIS

DIFFERENTIAL DIAGNOSIS

- PUD
- Acute cholangitis, biliary colic
- High intestinal obstruction
- Early acute appendicitis
- Mesenteric vascular obstruction
- DKA
- Pneumonia (basilar)
- Myocardial infarction (inferior wall)
- Renal colic
- Ruptured or dissecting aortic aneurysm
- Mesenteric ischemia

LABORATORY TESTS

Pancreatic enzymes:

- Amylase is increased, usually elevated in the initial 3 to 5 days of acute pancreatitis. Isoamylase determinations (separation of pancreatic cell isoenzyme components of amylase) are useful in excluding occasional cases of salivary hyperamylasemia. The use of isoamylase rather than total serum amylase reduces the risk of erroneously diagnosing pancreatitis and is preferred by some as initial biochemical test in patients suspected of having acute pancreatitis.
- Urinary amylase determinations are useful to diagnose acute pancreatitis in patients with lipemic serum, to rule out elevated serum amylase caused by macroamylasemia, and to diagnose acute pancreatitis in patients whose serum amylase is normal.
- Serum lipase levels are elevated in acute pancreatitis; the elevation is less transient than serum amylase; concomitant evaluation of serum amylase and lipase increases diagnostic accuracy of acute pancreatitis. An elevated lipase/amylase ratio is suggestive of alcoholic pancreatitis.
- Elevated serum trypsin levels are diagnostic of pancreatitis (in absence of renal failure).
- Serum C-reactive protein at 48 hr is an excellent laboratory marker of severity.
- Rapid measurement of urinary trypsinogen-2 (if available) is useful in the emergency department as a screening test for acute pancreatitis in patients with abdominal pain; a negative dipstick test for urinary trypsinogen-2 rules out acute pancreatitis with a high degree of probability, whereas a positive test indicates need for further evaluation.

Additional tests:

- Complete blood count: reveals leukocytosis; hematocrit (Hct) may be initially increased as a result of hemoconcentration; decreased Hct may indicate hemorrhage or hemolysis.
- Blood urea nitrogen (BUN) is increased because of dehydration. Serial BUN measurements are the most valuable lab test for predicting mortality during the initial 48 hr.
- Elevation of serum glucose in a previously normal patient correlates with the degree of pancreatic malfunction and may be related to increased release of glycogen, catecholamines, and glucocorticoid release and decreased insulin release.
- Liver profile: aspartate aminotransferase (AST) and lactate dehydrogenase (LDH) are increased as a result of tissue necrosis; bilirubin and alkaline phosphatase may be increased from common bile duct obstruction. A threefold or greater rise in serum alanine aminotransferase concentrations is an excellent indicator (95% probability) of biliary pancreatitis.
- Serum calcium is decreased as a result of saponification, precipitation, and decreased parathyroid hormone response.
- Arterial blood gases: Pao$_2$ may be decreased as a result of ARDS, pleural effusion(s); pH may be decreased as a result of lactic acidosis, respiratory acidosis, and renal insufficiency.
- Serum electrolytes: potassium may be increased from acidosis or renal insufficiency; sodium may be increased from dehydration.

IMAGING STUDIES

- Abdominal plain films are useful initially to distinguish other conditions that may mimic pancreatitis (perforated viscus). They may reveal localized ileus (sentinel loop), pancreatic calcifications (chronic pancreatitis), blur-

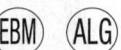
ring of left psoas shadow, dilation of transverse colon, calcified gallstones.

- Chest x-ray may reveal elevation of one or both diaphragms, pleural effusions, basilar infiltrates, or platelike atelectasis.
- Abdominal ultrasonography is useful in detecting gallstones (sensitivity of 60% to 70% for detecting stones associated with pancreatitis). It is also useful for detecting pancreatic pseudocysts. Its availability and noninvasive nature make it the initial imaging study of choice; its major limitation is the presence of distended bowel loops overlying the pancreas.
- CT scan is superior to ultrasonography in identifying pancreatitis and defining its extent, and it also plays a role in diagnosing pseudocysts (they appear as a well-defined area surrounded by a high-density capsule); gastrointestinal fistulation or infection of a pseudocyst can also be identified by the presence of gas within the pseudocyst. Sequential contrast-enhanced CT is useful for detection of pancreatic necrosis. The severity of pancreatitis can also be graded by CT scan. (A = normal pancreas, B = enlarged pancreas [1 point], C = pancreatic and/or peripancreatic inflammation [2 points], D = single peripancreatic collection [3 points], E = at least two peripancreatic collections and/or retroperitoneal air [4 points]. Percentage of pancreatic necrosis <30% [2 points], 30% to 50% [4 points], >50% [6 points]. The CT severity index is calculated by adding grade points to points assigned for percentage of necrosis.)
- Magnetic resonance cholangiopancreatography (MRCP) has >90% sensitivity for choledocholithiasis and can identify other anatomical abnormalities.
- Endoscopic ultrasonography (EUS) is useful to identify anatomical abnormalities of the pancreas and has good sensitivity and specificity for small gallstones (≤5 mm).
- ERCP indications: useful to perform biliary sphincterotomy and stone removal in the presence of a retained bile duct stone seen on imaging.

℞ TREATMENT

NONPHARMACOLOGIC THERAPY

- Bowel rest with avoidance of liquids or solids during the acute illness
- Avoidance of alcohol and any drugs associated with pancreatitis

ACUTE GENERAL Rx

General measures:
- Maintain adequate intravascular volume with vigorous IV hydration. Aggressive fluid resuscitation is critical in managing acute pancreatitis.
- Patient should remain NPO until clinically improved, stable, and hungry. Enteral feedings are preferred over total parenteral nutrition. Enteral nutrition reduces mortality, mul-

tiple organ failure, systemic infections, and operative interventions more than total parenteral nutrition does in patients with acute pancreatitis. Parenteral nutrition may be necessary in patients who do not tolerate enteral feeding or in whom an adequate infusion rate cannot be reached within 2 to 4 days.
- Nasogastric suction is useful only in severe pancreatitis to decompress the abdomen in patients with ileus.
- Control pain: IV morphine or fentanyl. Meperidine or hydromorphine are also commonly used narcotics for pain control.
- Correct metabolic abnormalities (e.g., replace calcium and magnesium as necessary).

Specific measures:
- Pancreatic or peripancreatic infection develops in 40% to 70% of patients with pancreatic necrosis. However, IV antibiotics should not be used prophylactically for all cases of pancreatitis; their use is justified if the patient has evidence of septicemia, pancreatic abscess, or pancreatitis caused by biliary calculi. Their use should generally be limited to 5 to 7 days to prevent development of fungal superinfection. Appropriate empiric antibiotic therapy should cover:
  - *Bacteroides fragilis* and other anaerobes (cefotetan, cefoxitin, metronidazole, or clindamycin plus aminoglycoside)
  - *Enterococcus* (ampicillin)
- Surgical therapy has a limited role in acute pancreatitis; it is indicated in the following:
  - Gallstone-induced pancreatitis: cholecystectomy when acute pancreatitis subsides.
  - Perforated peptic ulcer.
  - Necrotizing pancreatitis with infected necrotic tissue is associated with an elevated rate of complications and increased risk of death. Traditional treatment has been open necrosectomy; however, recent trials have shown that a step-up approach consisting of percutaneous drainage followed, if necessary, by minimally invasive retroperitoneal necrosectomy may have a lower rate of complications and death.
- Identification and treatment of complications:
  - Pseudocyst: round or spheroid collection of fluid, tissue, pancreatic enzymes, and blood.
    - Diagnosed by CT scan or sonography
    - Treatment: CT scan or ultrasound-guided percutaneous drainage (with a pigtail catheter left in place for continuous drainage) can be used, but the recurrence rate is high; the conservative approach is to reevaluate the pseudocyst (with CT scan or sonography) after 6 to 7 wk and surgically drain it if the pseudocyst has not decreased in size. Generally, pseudocysts <5 cm in diameter are reabsorbed without intervention, whereas those >5 cm require surgical intervention after the wall has matured.

  - Phlegmon: represents pancreatic edema. It can be diagnosed by CT scan or sonography. Treatment is supportive because it usually resolves spontaneously.
  - Pancreatic abscess: diagnosed by CT scan (presence of bubbles in the retroperitoneum); Gram staining and cultures of fluid obtained from guided percutaneous aspiration usually identify bacterial organism. Therapy is surgical (or catheter) drainage and IV antibiotics (imipenem-cilastatin is the drug of choice).
  - Pancreatic ascites: usually caused by leaking of pseudocyst or tear in pancreatic duct. Paracentesis reveals very high amylase and lipase levels in the pancreatic fluid; ERCP may demonstrate the lesion. Treatment is surgical correction if exudative ascites from severe pancreatitis does not resolve spontaneously.
  - Gastrointestinal bleeding: caused by alcoholic gastritis, bleeding varices, stress ulceration, or disseminated intravascular coagulation (DIC).
  - Renal failure: caused by hypovolemia, resulting in oliguria or anuria, cortical or tubular necrosis (shock, DIC), or thrombosis of renal artery or vein.
  - Hypoxia: caused by ARDS, pleural effusion, or atelectasis.

DISPOSITION

Prognosis varies with the severity of pancreatitis; overall mortality rate in acute pancreatitis is 5% to 10%; poor prognostic signs according to the Ranson criteria are as follows:
- Age >55 yr
- Fluid sequestration >6000 ml
- Laboratory abnormalities on admission: white blood cell count >16,000, blood glucose >200 mg/dl, serum LDH >350 IU/L, AST >250 IU/L
- Laboratory abnormalities during the initial 48 hr: decreased Hct >10% with hydration or Hct <30%, BUN rise >5 mg/dl, serum calcium <8 mg/dl, arterial Po_2 <60 mm Hg, and base deficit >4 mEq/L

REFERRAL

- Hospitalization is indicated in moderate to severe cases of pancreatitis.
- Surgical consultation is needed in suspected gallstone pancreatitis, perforated peptic ulcer, or presence of necrotic or infected foci.
- Gastroenterology consultation in severe pancreatitis, recurrent pancreatitis, or when the cause of pancreatitis is unclear.

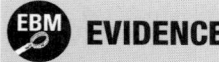 **EVIDENCE**

available at www.expertconsult.com

SUGGESTED READINGS

available at www.expertconsult.com

AUTHOR: **FRED F. FERRI, M.D.**

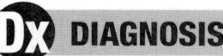 **BASIC INFORMATION**

DEFINITION
Chronic pancreatitis is a recurrent or persistent inflammatory process of the pancreas characterized by chronic pain and by pancreatic exocrine and/or endocrine insufficiency.

ICD-9CM CODES
577.1 Chronic pancreatitis

EPIDEMIOLOGY & DEMOGRAPHICS
- Chronic pancreatitis occurs in approximately five to 10 per 100,000 persons in industrialized countries.
- Average age at diagnosis is 35 to 55 yr; male/female ratio is 5:1.

PHYSICAL FINDINGS & CLINICAL PRESENTATION
- Persistent or recurrent epigastric and left upper quadrant pain that may radiate to the back
- Tenderness over the pancreas, muscle guarding
- Significant weight loss
- Bulky, foul-smelling stools, greasy in appearance
- Epigastric mass (10% of patients)
- Jaundice (5% to 10% of patients)

ETIOLOGY
- Chronic alcoholism.
- Obstruction (ampullary stenosis, tumor, trauma, pancreas divisum, annular pancreas).
- Hereditary pancreatitis.
- Severe malnutrition.
- Idiopathic.
- Untreated hyperparathyroidism (hypercalcemia).
- Mutations of the cystic fibrosis transmembrane conductance regulator *(CFTR)* gene and the TF genotype.
- Autoimmune pancreatitis (5% of chronic pancreatitis cases): presents clinically with jaundice (63% of patients) and abdominal pain (35%). CT may reveal diffusely enlarged pancreas, enhanced peripheral rim of hypoattenuation "halo," and low-attenuation mass in head of pancreas. Laboratory values reveal elevated serum immunoglobulin (Ig) G4, elevated serum Ig or gamma-globulin level, presence of antilactoferrin antibody (ALA), anticarbonic anhydrase (ACA) II level, antismooth-muscle antibody (ASMA), or antinuclear antibody (ANA).
- Sclerosing pancreatitis: a form of chronic pancreatitis characterized by infrequent attacks of abdominal pain, irregular narrowing of the pancreatic duct, and swelling of the pancreatic parenchyma; patients have high levels of serum immunoglobulins (IgG4).

Chronic sclerosing pancreatitis is also known as *autoimmune pancreatitis.*

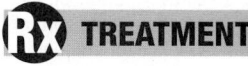 **DIAGNOSIS**

DIFFERENTIAL DIAGNOSIS
- Pancreatic cancer
- Peptic ulcer disease
- Cholelithiasis with biliary obstruction
- Malabsorption from other etiologies
- Recurrent acute pancreatitis
- Renal insufficiency
- Intestinal ischemia or infarction
- Other: Crohn's disease, gastroparesis, inflammatory bowel disease

WORKUP
Medical history with focus on alcohol use, laboratory tests, diagnostic imaging

LABORATORY TESTS
- Serum amylase and lipase may be elevated (normal amylase levels, however, do not exclude the diagnosis).
- Hyperglycemia, glycosuria, hyperbilirubinemia, and elevated serum alkaline phosphatase may also be present.
- 72-hr fecal fat determination (rarely performed) reveals excess fecal fat. Fecal elastase test requires only 20 g of stool.
- Secretin stimulation test is the best test for diagnosing pancreatic exocrine insufficiency.
- Lipid panel: significantly elevated triglycerides can cause pancreatitis.
- Serum calcium: hyperparathyroidism is a rare cause of chronic pancreatitis.
- Elevated levels of serum IgG4 are found in sclerosing pancreatitis and autoimmune pancreatitis.
- Elevated serum Ig or gamma globulin level, presence of ALA, ACA II level, ASMA, or ANA in autoimmune pancreatitis.

IMAGING STUDIES
- Plain abdominal radiographs may reveal pancreatic calcifications (95% specific for chronic pancreatitis).
- Ultrasound of abdomen may reveal duct dilation, pseudocyst, calcification, and presence of ascites.
- Contrast-enhanced CT scan of abdomen is the initial modality of choice. It is useful to detect calcifications, evaluate for ductal dilation, and rule out pancreatic cancer.
- Endoscopic retrograde cholangiopancreatography (ERCP) has been traditionally used to evaluate for the presence of dilated ducts, strictures, pseudocysts, and intraductal stones. However, for the evaluation of pancreatic parenchyma and duct system newer, less invasive modalities such as magnetic resonance cholangiopancreatography (MRCP) and endoscopic ultrasonography (EUS) may be preferred. EUS has a sensitivity of 97% and a specificity of 60% for chronic pancreatitis and

a very low complication rate. Fine-needle aspiration biopsy (FNAB) combined with EUS is the preferred modality for evaluation of cystic or mass lesions to determine malignancy.

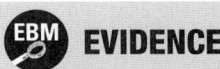 **TREATMENT**

NONPHARMACOLOGIC THERAPY
- Avoidance of alcohol and tobacco
- Frequent, small-volume, low-fat meals

ACUTE GENERAL Rx
- Avoidance of narcotics if possible (simple analgesics or nonsteroidal anti-inflammatory drugs can be used).
- Treatment of steatorrhea with pancreatic supplements (e.g., Pancrease, Creon, Pancrelipase titrated prn based on the amount of steatorrhea and patient's weight loss). Proton pump inhibitors and H₂ blockers reduce inactivation of the enzymes from gastric acid.
- Treatment of complications (e.g., type 1 diabetes mellitus).
- Glucocorticoid therapy in patients with autoimmune pancreatitis and sclerosing pancreatitis can induce clinical remission and significantly decrease serum concentrations of IgG4, immune complexes, and the IgG4 subclass of immune complexes.

CHRONIC Rx
- Surgical intervention may be necessary to eliminate biliary tract disease and improve flow of bile into the duodenum by eliminating obstruction of pancreatic duct.
- ERCP with endoscopic sphincterectomy and stone extraction is useful in selected patients.
- Transduodenal sphincteroplasty or pancreaticojejunostomy in selected patients. Surgery should also be considered in patients with intractable pain.

DISPOSITION
- Long-term survival is poor (50% of patients die within 10 yr from chronic pancreatitis or malignancy).
- Prognosis is best in patients with recurrent acute pancreatitis resulting from cholelithiasis, hyperparathyroidism, or stenosis of the sphincter of Oddi.

REFERRAL
Gastrointestinal referral for ERCP, surgical referral in selected patients (see "Chronic Rx").

EBM EVIDENCE
available at www.expertconsult.com

SUGGESTED READINGS
available at www.expertconsult.com

AUTHOR: **FRED F. FERRI, M.D.**

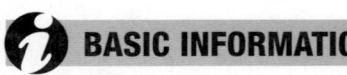 **BASIC INFORMATION**

DEFINITION

- A panic attack is a relatively brief, sudden episode of intense fear or apprehension, often associated with a sense of impending doom and various uncomfortable and disquieting physical symptoms. Panic attacks may be uncued ("out of the blue") or cued (i.e., triggered by a particular object or situation). Panic attacks may be present in a variety of different anxiety-related disorders (e.g., phobias, social anxiety, obsessive-compulsive disorder).
- Panic disorder is diagnosed after two uncued panic attacks have occurred followed by at least 1 mo (or more) of significant concern about future attacks, worry about their implications, or a major change in behavior related to these attacks. Agoraphobia is anxiety about, and avoidance of, places or situations in which the ability to escape is limited or embarrassing or in which help might not be available in the event of having a panic attack.

SYNONYMS

Anxiety attacks
Fear attacks
Ataque de nervios

ICD-9CM CODES
F41.0   Panic disorder without agoraphobia (DSM-IV 300.01)
F40.01 Panic disorder with agoraphobia (DSM-IV 300.21)

EPIDEMIOLOGY & DEMOGRAPHICS

INCIDENCE (IN U.S.): 1% 1-mo incidence of panic attacks.
PREVALENCE (IN U.S.):
- 15% to 20% lifetime prevalence of one or more panic attacks.
- Panic disorder much more uncommon, with a lifetime prevalence of 1.5% to 3.5%; chronicity of condition reflected by a similar 1-yr prevalence rate of 1% to 2%.
- Agoraphobia relatively rare; 0.3% to 1% lifetime prevalence; 30% to 50% of patients diagnosed with panic disorder also have agoraphobia.
PEAK INCIDENCE:
- Chronic condition with a waxing and waning course.
- Bimodal incidence peaks noted, with the first peak between ages 15 and 24 yr and second peak between ages 35 and 44 yr.
PREDOMINANT SEX:
- Women more commonly affected (>85% of clinical population).
- Panic disorder twice as common in women.
- Panic disorder with agoraphobia three times as common in women.
PREDOMINANT AGE:
- Age of onset is typically late adolescence to mid-30s. Onset earlier in males (24 yr) than females (28 yr).

- Onset after age 45 yr is rare and should raise suspicion of different etiology.
GENETICS:
- Risk of developing panic disorder in first-degree relatives of individuals with panic disorder is four to seven times that of general population.
- Findings in twin studies: approximately 60% of contributing factors to panic are genetic.

PHYSICAL FINDINGS & CLINICAL PRESENTATION

Panic disorder:
- Present either with a panic attack or with fear and anxiety related to anticipation of a future panic attack or its implications.
- Typical presentation: unexpected, untriggered periods of intense anxiety and fear with associated physiologic changes (e.g., palpitations, sweating, tremulousness, shortness of breath, chest pain, gastrointestinal distress, faintness, derealization, paresthesia). This is accompanied by associated fears of dying, heart attack, stroke, passing out, losing control, or losing one's mind. Panic attacks are often described as "the most terrifying" episode an individual has experienced.
- Emergency or physician visits often occasioned by physical symptoms such as chest pain, dizziness, or difficulty breathing.
Agoraphobia:
- Rare complaints to physician. May manifest in missed office visits or tardiness. Patients may request home visits or telephone care.
- Activities usually self-limited by avoiding public situations where the patient might experience a panic attack and would be unable to exit readily, such as the following:
  1. Crowded public areas (stores, public transportation, flying, church)
  2. Individual interactions (hairdresser, neighborhood meetings)
  3. Driving (especially if alone, over bridges, through tunnels, or on isolated roads)
- On exposure to or anticipation of exposure to such situations, significant anxiety occurs. Anxiety may generate somatic symptoms that trigger a full-blown panic attack, further reinforcing avoidance of such situations.

ETIOLOGY

Hypotheses (NOTE: There are sufficient data to support each model. Models are not mutually exclusive.)
1. Central dyscontrol of autonomic arousal (typically localized to the locus ceruleus); similar symptoms may be chemically induced with yohimbine, caffeine, or cholecystokinin.
2. Cognitive overreaction (i.e., "catastrophic misinterpretation") to relatively mild or benign physiologic cues that then triggers a genuine autonomic cascade and further misinterpretations.
3. Dysfunction of a central suffocation alarm mechanism; some signs of compensated respiratory alkalosis. Can be experimentally induced with sodium lactate or carbon dioxide.

Dx DIAGNOSIS

DIFFERENTIAL DIAGNOSIS

Medical conditions:
- Endocrinopathies:
  1. Hyperthyroidism
  2. Hyperparathyroidism
  3. Pheochromocytoma
  4. Carcinoid tumor
- Cardiac and respiratory diseases:
  1. Arrhythmias
  2. Myocardial infarction
  3. Chronic obstructive pulmonary disease
  4. Asthma
  5. Mitral valve prolapse
- Metabolic:
  1. Hypoglycemia
  2. Electrolyte imbalances
  3. Porphyria
- Seizure disorders
- Psychiatric disorders (NOTE: Panic attacks are common in a variety of psychiatric disorders. Panic disorder could be conceptualized as a phobia of the somatic sensations or situations that have become paired with panic attacks.)
  1. Phobias (e.g., specific phobia or social phobia). Note that fear of going on a plane because of crashing would be a specific phobia, whereas fear of going on a plane because one is then trapped and worries about panic is more suggestive of panic disorder with agoraphobia.
  2. Obsessive-compulsive disorder (cued by exposure to the object of the obsession)
  3. Posttraumatic stress disorder (cued by recall of a stressor)
- Therapeutic (theophylline, steroids) and recreational (cocaine, amphetamine, caffeine, diet pills) drugs and drug withdrawal (alcohol, barbiturates, benzodiazepines)

WORKUP

- Emergency presentation: cardiac, respiratory, or neurologic symptoms
- History and physical examination to rule out a concomitant medical or substance-related condition
NOTE: Panic disorder and agoraphobia are not diagnoses of exclusion, but exclusion of other conditions is usually required.

LABORATORY TESTS

- Thyroid profile
- Electrolyte measures, including calcium
- Toxicology screen
- ECG
- Acute cases: possible monitoring and cardiac enzymes to rule out arrhythmia or ischemia

IMAGING STUDIES

- For temporal lobe dysfunction (e.g., temporal lesions or as ictal or interictal manifestation of temporal lobe seizures): brain CT scan or MRI or an electroencephalogram in some patients
- Holter monitor to rule out occult or episodic arrhythmias

- Chest x-ray examination, arterial blood gases, or pulmonary function tests if respiratory compromise suspected

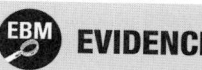 **TREATMENT**

NONPHARMACOLOGIC THERAPY

Cognitive-behavioral therapy (CBT) is generally very effective, with strongest results for cognitive restructuring (i.e., challenging catastrophic misinterpretations of somatic symptoms), in vivo or imaginal exposures (i.e., exposure to feared situations that are likely to produce panic and are carried out in a hierarchical fashion from least to most difficult), and interoceptive exposures (i.e., repeated recreation and management of feared somatic sensations via activities such as chair spinning, straw breathing, and hyperventilation). CBT effect sizes are equal to or larger than for pharmacotherapy, attrition rates are lower, and relapse rates are lower. Treatment may take several sessions spread over weeks and may require referral to a behavioral specialist.

ACUTE GENERAL Rx

- Benzodiazepines, particularly alprazolam: highly effective in the acute setting.
- Low-dose alprazolam for patients with rare panic attacks and asymptomatic periods (0.25 to 0.5 mg PO or sublingually prn).
- Start patient on selective serotonin reuptake inhibitor (SSRI) or similar agent and taper patient off of benzodiazepine by wk 2 to 3.

CHRONIC Rx

- Preferred pharmacologic agents: antidepressants with a significant serotonin reuptake inhibitory action. Generally start at low dose and titrate upward. Minimum treatment duration is 6 to 8 mo, but many patients need to take medications indefinitely.
  1. SSRIs: paroxetine (10 to 60 mg/day), sertraline (50 to 200 mg/day), citalopram (20 to 60 mg/day), escitalopram (5 to 30 mg/day), and fluoxetine (5 to 60 mg/day)
  2. Imipramine (100 to 300 mg/day)
  3. Venlafaxine (75 to 225 mg/day)
- Combination CBT plus SSRI has shown good long-term effects and is somewhat better than antidepressants or CBT alone. Combination CBT plus benzodiazepine does not provide any added benefit and may undermine CBT (interoceptive and in-vivo exposures may be less effective if patient is taking a benzodiazepine).

DISPOSITION

- Typical course is chronic but with significant waxing and waning (common to have long periods of remission).
- Presence of agoraphobia associated with a more chronic course.
- Findings with long-term follow-up studies: 6 to 10 yr after treatment some 30% are in remission, 40% to 50% have improved with residual symptoms, and the remainder either are unchanged or worse.

REFERRAL

- If patients do not respond to an SSRI.
- Cognitive-behavioral therapy is the preferred treatment.

PEARLS & CONSIDERATIONS

- Patient and family education is an important first step in the management of panic disorder. Education provides more adaptive explanations for the benign somatic sensations paired with panic. Presentation of genetic information and explanation of the benign nature of the physiology of each of the symptoms the patient experiences serve as a good start to allay fears and reduce stigma.
- Resumption of avoided activities or situations is a positive prognostic sign and may promote further therapeutic gains.

EBM EVIDENCE

available at www.expertconsult.com

SUGGESTED READINGS

available at www.expertconsult.com

AUTHORS: **DONN POSNER, PH.D,** **JASON M. SATTERFIELD, PH.D.,** and **MITCHELL D. FELDMAN, M.D., M.PHIL.**

P

Diseases and Disorders

I

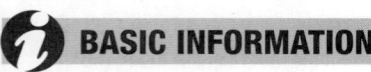

DEFINITION

Paranoid personality disorder (PPD) is characterized by a pattern of pervasive distrust and suspiciousness of others that leads the person to assign malevolence to the motives of others. PPD begins by early adulthood and causes significant distress or impairment in multiple domains of functioning. Individuals must meet four or more of the following criteria:

1. Suspect, without justification, that others are exploiting, harming, or deceiving them.
2. Preoccupied with unwarranted doubts about the loyalty or trustworthiness of friends or associates.
3. Reluctant to confide in others because of unjustified fear that the information will be used against them in a malicious fashion.
4. Infer demeaning or threatening statements from benign remarks or events.
5. Bear grudges for extended periods. For example, PPD patients are unforgiving of perceived or real insults and slights.
6. Perceive attacks on their character that are not apparent to others. Quick to react angrily or to counterattack.
7. Recurrent suspicions, without justification, regarding fidelity of spouse or partner.

SYNONYMS

None

ICD-9CM CODES

301.0

EPIDEMIOLOGY & DEMOGRAPHICS

PREVALENCE: From 0.5% to 4.4% in the general population, 10% to 30% in inpatient psychiatric settings, and 2% to 10% in outpatient mental health clinics.
PREDOMINANT SEX: More commonly diagnosed in males in clinical samples.
GENETICS: Increased prevalence of PPD in relatives of probands with schizophrenia and delusional disorder, paranoid type.

CLINICAL PRESENTATION

- Signs of PPD in childhood include solitariness, poor peer relationships, social anxiety, underachievement in school, hypersensitivity, peculiar thoughts and language, and idiosyncratic fantasies.
- As children, these patients may have appeared "odd" or "eccentric" and attracted teasing.
- Their excessive suspiciousness often leads to either overt argumentativeness and recurrent complaining or quiet, hostile aloofness.
- These patients maintain interpersonal distance and may refuse to answer personal questions, saying the information is "nobody's business."
- Misinterpret benign actions by others as malicious assaults. PPD patients may, for example, interpret an honest mistake as a deliberate attempt to harm, a casual humorous remark as a serious character attack, a compliment as a veiled criticism, and an offer of help as a judgment of failure.
- Close relationships are impaired by hypervigilance for threats and associated guardedness. May appear as "cold." Suspiciousness can lead to pathologic jealousy where they gather circumstantial evidence to support contention of betrayal.
- To protect themselves from the perceived malice of others, these patients often maintain a high degree of control of relationships and interactions, constantly questioning the whereabouts, intentions, or actions of the other.
- Often rigid and critical of others but have great difficulty accepting criticism themselves.
- Given their lack of trust of others, PPD patients have an excessive need for self-sufficiency and autonomy.
- Quick to counterattack and may be litigious.
- May join "cults" or groups that share their paranoid belief system.
- In response to stress, may experience very brief psychotic episodes (minutes to hours).

ETIOLOGY

- At this point, limited knowledge about role of genetic loading and neurobiologic vulnerability.
- However, increased prevalence in families of probands with schizophrenia and delusional disorder, paranoid type, suggests possible genetic role.

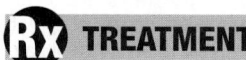

DIFFERENTIAL DIAGNOSIS

- Schizophrenia, paranoid type, delusional disorder, paranoid type, and mood disorder with psychotic symptoms: require presence of persistent positive psychotic symptoms such as delusions and hallucinations. To give an additional diagnosis of PPD, the personality disorder must be present before the onset of psychotic symptoms and must persist when the psychotic symptoms are in remission.
- Substance-induced paranoia, especially in the context of cocaine, PCP, or methamphetamine abuse or dependence.
- Personality changes caused by a general medical condition that affects the central nervous system.
- Paranoid traits associated with a sensory disability; for example, hearing impairment.
- Increased risk for major depressive disorder, obsessive-compulsive disorder, agoraphobia, and substance abuse or dependence.
- The most common co-occurring personality disorders are schizotypal, schizoid, narcissistic, avoidant, and borderline:
  1. Schizotypal personality disorder includes magical thinking and unusual perceptual experiences.
  2. Schizoid and borderline personality disorders do not have prominent paranoid ideation.
  3. Avoidant personality disorder includes fear of embarrassment.
  4. Narcissistic personality disorder includes the fear that hidden "flaws" or "inferiority" may be revealed.

WORKUP

- History: collateral information is essential to establishing the presence of longstanding interpersonal pattern in multiple domains of the patient's life.
- Physical examination.
- Mental status examination.

LABORATORY TESTS

Those necessary to rule out medical causes of personality changes

IMAGING STUDIES

Those necessary to rule out medical causes of personality changes

TREATMENT

NONPHARMACOLOGIC THERAPY

- Cognitive-behavioral therapy to help patients control rage, manage perceived criticism, and develop social skills.
- Psychodynamic psychotherapy to help patient develop capacity to trust and improved interpersonal functioning.

ACUTE GENERAL Rx

Benzodiazepines or low-dose antipsychotics to control hostility and paranoia

CHRONIC Rx

- Low-dose antipsychotic medication. Increase dose in small increments to minimize risk of side effects.
- Selective serotonin reuptake inhibitors if comorbid depression, obsessive-compulsive disorder, or agoraphobia.
- Substance abuse treatment if comorbid dependence.

COMPLEMENTARY & ALTERNATIVE MEDICINE

No evidence of efficacy in PPD.

DISPOSITION

- Severity is variable and course is chronic. Often lifelong difficulty maintaining intimate relationships.
- At increased risk for major depressive disorder, obsessive-compulsive disorder, agoraphobia, and substance abuse or dependence.
- In some cases, PPD is a prepsychotic antecedent of delusional disorder, paranoid type.

REFERRAL

- If pharmacotherapy or psychotherapy is contemplated
- If patient's social or occupational functioning is impaired

PEARLS & CONSIDERATIONS

COMMENTS

- Illness exacerbates these patients' sense of vulnerability.
- Communicating personal information to the physician challenges the guarded, self-protective approach to others and will often heighten PPD patients' fear that the physician will harm them.
- The encounter with the physician intensifies hypervigilance. As a result, innocuous or even overtly helpful behaviors by the physician may be perceived as manipulating or threatening.
- With the perceived threat, these patients will often confront and challenge the physician on their motives and their rationale for diagnosis and treatment. Conflict and argument are not uncommon.
- Thus establishing an alliance with the patient can be challenging.
- Faced with such a patient, physicians may understandably react defensively to unfounded suspicion or distance and not respond to the patient's concerns. Both responses increase the patient's anxiety and paranoia.
- Management guidelines:
  1. Convey intent "to do no harm."
  2. Address the patient's fears and concerns, no matter how irrational, in a clear, direct, and detailed manner.
  3. Remember that behind the patient's hostility lie fears that are real to him or her.
  4. Maintain a professional and neutral stance.
  5. Responding with too much warmth and friendliness will intensify paranoia.
  6. Give patient detailed and factual information about treatment plan.
  7. Give patient as much control as possible, including maximum participation at each decision node.
  8. Do not personalize patient's hostility and suspicion, but understand his or her distrust as an attempt to manage intense fear.
  9. Validate patient's concerns about the diagnosis or treatment plan.

SUGGESTED READINGS
available at www.expertconsult.com

AUTHOR: **JOHN Q. YOUNG, M.D., M.P.P.**

DEFINITION

Idiopathic Parkinson's disease (PD) is a progressive neurodegenerative disorder characterized clinically by rigidity, tremor, postural instability, and bradykinesia.

SYNONYMS

Paralysis agitans

ICD-9CM CODES
332.0 Idiopathic Parkinson's disease, primary
332.1 Parkinson's disease, secondary

EPIDEMIOLOGY & DEMOGRAPHICS

PREVALENCE:
- Affects more than 1 million people in North America.
- In age group <40 yr, <5/100,000 are affected.
- In those aged >70 yr, 700/100,000 are affected.
- Highest incidence in whites, lowest incidence in Asians and African Americans.

PHYSICAL FINDINGS & CLINICAL PRESENTATION

- Tremor (Fig. 1-277)—typically a resting tremor with a frequency of 4 to 6 Hz that is often first noted in the hand as a pill-rolling tremor (thumb and forefinger). Can also involve the leg and lip. Tremor improves with purposeful movement. Usually starts asymmetrically.
- Rigidity—increased muscle tone that persists throughout the range of passive movement of a joint. This, too, is usually asymmetric at onset.
- Akinesia/bradykinesia—slowness in initiating movement.

- Postural instability—tested by "pull test." Ask patient to stand in place with back to examiner. Examiner pulls patient back by the shoulders, and proper response would be to take no steps back or very few steps back without falling. Retropulsion is a positive test as is falling straight back. This is not usually severe early on. If falls and postural reflexes are greatly impaired early on, then consider other disorders.
- Masked facies—face seems expressionless, giving the appearance of depression. Decreased blink; often there is excess drooling.
- Gait disturbance.
- Stooped posture, decreased arm swing.
- Difficulty initiating the first step; small shuffling steps that increase in speed (festinating gait). Steps become progressively faster and shorter while the trunk inclines further forward.
- Other complaints and findings early on include micrographia—handwriting becomes smaller, and hypophonia—voice becomes softer and often "gruffer."

ETIOLOGY

- Unknown.
- Most cases are sporadic, with age being the most common risk factor, although there is probably a combination of both environmental and genetic factors contributing to disease expression. There are rare familial forms with at least seven different genes identified; these include the parkin gene, which is a significant cause of early-onset autosomal recessive PD and LRRK2, which is the most common cause of familial and sporadic parkinsonism.

![Dx] **DIAGNOSIS**

A clinical diagnosis can be made based on a comprehensive history and physical examina-

tion. The four cardinal signs used to diagnose Parkinson's disease are (mnemonic = TRAP):
1. **T**remor (resting, typically 4-6Hz)
2. **R**igidity, of the Cogwheel type
3. Bradykinesia/**a**kinesia—slowness of movement
4. **P**ostural instability—failure of postural "righting" reflexes leading to poor balance and falls

One need not show all four cardinal signs to make a presumptive diagnosis of PD and begin treatment.

DIFFERENTIAL DIAGNOSIS

- Multiple system atrophy—distinguishing features include autonomic dysfunction (including urinary incontinence, orthostatic hypotension, and erectile dysfunction), parkinsonism, cerebellar signs, and normal cognition.
- Diffuse Lewy body disease—parkinsonism with concomitant dementia. Patients often have early hallucinations and fluctuations in level of alertness and mental status.
- Corticobasal degeneration—often begins asymmetrically with apraxia, cortical sensory loss in one limb, and sometimes alien limb phenomenon.
- Progressive supranuclear palsy—tends to have axial rigidity greater than appendicular (limb) rigidity. These patients have early and severe postural instability. Hallmark is supranuclear gaze palsy that usually involves vertical gaze (especially downward) before horizontal.
- Essential tremor—bilateral postural and action tremor.
- Secondary (acquired) parkinsonism.
  1. Iatrogenic—any of the neuroleptics and antipsychotics. The high-potency D_2-blocker neuroleptics are most likely to cause parkinsonism. Quetiapine is an atypical antipsychotic with lower risk of causing parkinsonism. Metoclopramide can also cause parkinsonism.
  2. Postinfectious parkinsonism—von Economo's encephalitis.
  3. Parkinson's pugilistica—after repeated head trauma.
  4. Toxins (e.g., MPTP, manganese, carbon monoxide).
  5. Cerebrovascular disease "vascular parkinsonism" (basal ganglia infarcts); often lower limbs (especially gait) affected more than upper extremities.

WORKUP

Identification of clinical signs and symptoms associated with PD (see "Physical Findings") and elimination of conditions that may mimic it with a comprehensive history and physical examination.

Routine genetic testing is not recommended.

IMAGING STUDIES

Computed tomographic (CT) scan has almost no role in investigations. Magnetic resonance imaging (MRI) of the head may sometimes distinguish between idiopathic PD and other condi-

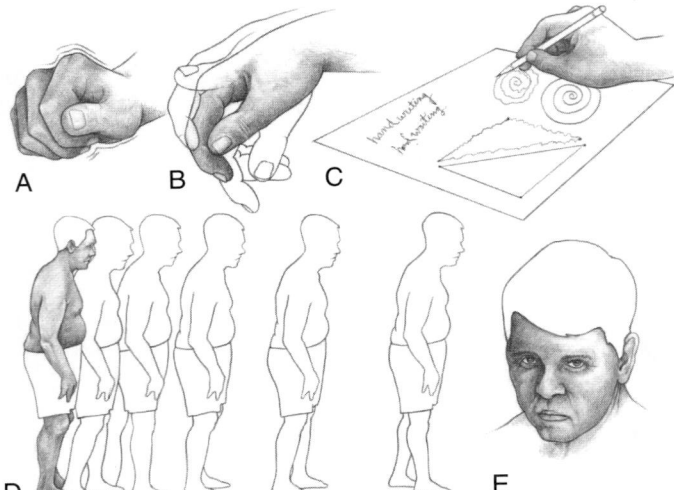

FIGURE 1-277 The parkinsonian syndrome. A, The "pill-rolling" tremor. **B,** Tremor that can worsen with emotional stress. **C,** Handwriting abnormalities, which include micrographia. **D,** Typical posture and gait, which becomes faster (festination). **E,** Lack of facial expression as well as "stare" from decreased blinking. (From Remmel KS, Bunyan R, Brumback RA, Gascon GA, Olson WH: *Handbook of symptom oriented neurology,* ed 3, St Louis, 2002, Mosby.)

tions that present with signs of parkinsonism (see "Differential Diagnosis").

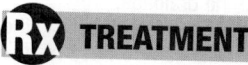 **TREATMENT**

NONPHARMACOLOGIC THERAPY

- Physical therapy, patient education and reassurance, treatment of associated conditions (e.g., depression)
- Avoidance of drugs that can induce or worsen parkinsonism: neuroleptics (especially high potency), certain antiemetics (prochlorperazine, trimethobenzamide), metoclopramide, nonselective MAO inhibitors (may induce hypertensive crisis), reserpine, methyldopa

ACUTE GENERAL Rx

- There is persistent controversy whether levodopa or dopamine agonists should be the initial treatment. In younger patients, agonists are usually the drug of choice; in patients >70 yrs, levodopa is typically the drug of choice.
- It is appropriate to initiate pharmacotherapy when required by symptoms; prior practice of waiting for limitation of ADLs is now outdated.
- Motor complications do develop during the course of the disease and likely reflect the combination of disease progression together with the side effects of dopaminergic medications.

CHRONIC Rx

- Levodopa therapy
  1. Cornerstone of symptomatic therapy—should be used with a peripheral dopa decarboxylase inhibitor (carbidopa) to minimize side effects (nausea, light-headedness, postural hypotension). The combination of the two drugs is marketed under the trade name Sinemet. Levodopa therapy has been found to reduce morbidity and mortality in PD patients.
  2. Usual starting dose is 25/100 mg (carbidopa/levodopa) tid 1 hr before meals.
  3. Controlled-release preparations (Sinemet CR) are available, but their use should be deferred to a neurologist.
  4. Stalevo (combination Sinemet and entacapone, a COMT inhibitor). Useful for patients with motor fluctuations (wearing off). Has no role in treating early patients with PD.
- Dopamine receptor agonists (Ropinirole and Pramipexole) are not as potent as levodopa, but they are often used as initial treatment in

younger patients to attempt to delay the onset of complications (dyskinesias, motor fluctuations) associated with levodopa therapy. These medications are more expensive than levodopa. In general they cause more side effects than levodopa, including nausea, vomiting, light-headedness, peripheral edema, confusion, and somnolence. They can also cause impulse control behaviors such as hypersexuality, binge eating, and compulsive shopping and gambling. Presence of these must be assessed at each visit.
  1. Ropinirole (Requip): initial dose is 0.25 mg tid
  2. Pramipexole (Mirapex): initial dose is 0.125 mg tid
- MAO-B inhibitors can be used as monotherapy early in the disease or as adjunctive therapy in later stages. Milder symptomatic benefit than dopamine agonists or levodopa. Well tolerated and easy to titrate. Concurrent use of stimulants and sympathomimetics should be avoided. Certain food restrictions may apply.
  1. Rasagiline (Azilect): initial dose is 0.5 mg qd, then 1 mg daily. A recent study, ADAGIO, suggests that 1 mg Rasagiline may have disease-modifying benefits, but results must be interpreted with caution.
  2. Selegiline: Usual dose, 5 mg bid with breakfast and lunch. Has amphetamine byproduct so has mild stimulant-like effects, which can be beneficial in some patients.
  3. Amantadine (Symmetrel) can be used alone early in the disease. It is especially useful in the treatment of dyskinesias. Dosage is 100 mg tid (titrate q week from 100 mg qd). Must adjust for elderly and renal impairment. The most notable side effect, especially in the elderly, is confusion.
- Anticholinergic agents are only helpful in treating tremor and drooling in patients with PD. Potential side effects include constipation, urinary retention, memory impairment, and hallucinations. They should be avoided in the elderly.
  1. Trihexyphenidyl (Artane): initial dose, 1 mg PO tid
  2. Benztropine (Cogentin): usual dose, 0.5 to 1 mg qd or bid

SURGICAL OPTIONS

- Pallidal (globus pallidus interna) and subthalamic deep-brain stimulation (subthalamic nucleus) are currently the surgical options of

choice for patients with advanced Parkinson's disease; Similar improvement in motor function and adverse effects have been reported after either procedure. Thalamic DBS may be useful for refractory tremor.
- Surgery is limited to patients with disabling, medically refractory problems, and patients must still have a good response to L-dopa to undergo surgery. DBS results in decreased dyskinesias, fluctuations, rigidity, and tremor.

DISPOSITION

Parkinson's disease usually follows a slowly progressive course leading to disability over the course of several years. However, every patient will progress individually, and patients should be reassured that this diagnosis does not, by definition, result in being either wheelchair- or bedbound.

REFERRAL

- Neurology consultation is recommended on initial diagnosis of PD.
- Exercise is important for all patients with PD.
- Participation in outpatient physical therapy program is recommended for patients with moderate to advanced disease.

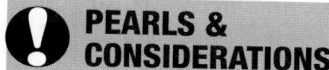 **PEARLS & CONSIDERATIONS**

- Asymmetry of symptoms at onset is very useful in distinguishing PD from other causes of parkinsonism.
- Although resting tremor is a common presenting symptom, up to 25% of patients with idiopathic PD do not have classic resting tremor.

COMMENTS

Additional patient information on PD can be obtained from the Internet at www.parkinson. org and from the National Parkinson Foundation, Inc., 1501 Ninth Avenue NW, Miami, FL 33136; phone: (800) 327-4545.

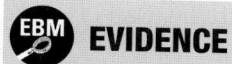 **EVIDENCE**

available at www.expertconsult.com

SUGGESTED READINGS

available at www.expertconsult.com

AUTHOR: **CINDY ZADIKOFF, M.D.**

P

Diseases and Disorders

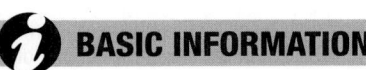

BASIC INFORMATION

DEFINITION

Paronychia is a localized superficial infection or abscess of the lateral and proximal nail fold. Paronychia may be acute or chronic.

SYNONYMS

Nail bed infection
Nail bed abscess

ICD-9CM CODES

681.9 Paronychia

EPIDEMIOLOGY & DEMOGRAPHICS

- Acute paronychia affects males and females equally.
- Chronic paronychia is more common in females than males (9:1).
- Acute paronychia most often occurs in children.
- Chronic paronychia usually presents in the fifth or sixth decade of life.
- Paronychia is the most common infection of the hand.

PHYSICAL FINDINGS & CLINICAL PRESENTATION

- Acute paronychia usually presents with the sudden onset of redness, swelling, and pain with abscess or cellulitis formation in the nail fold. Fluid with purulence is often present.
- Chronic paronychia is insidious, presenting with mild swelling and erythema of the nail folds.
- Acute paronychia usually involves only one finger.
- Chronic paronychia may involve more than one finger.
- Acute paronychia usually involves the thumb.
- Chronic paronychia commonly involves the middle finger.

ETIOLOGY

- Any disruption of the seal between the proximal nail fold and the nail plate can cause paronychial infections.
- Acute paronychia is almost always bacterial in origin (e.g., *Staphylococcus aureus* [most common], *Streptococcus pyogenes*, *Enterococcus faecalis*, *Proteus* and *Pseudomonas* species, and anaerobes).

- Chronic paronychia is commonly caused by *Candida albicans* (70%), with bacterial organisms accounting for the remaining 30%.
- Trauma, nail biting, hangnails, diabetes, and long-term exposure to water are common predisposing features of paronychia.

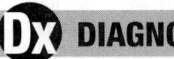

DIAGNOSIS

The diagnosis of paronychia is self-evident on physical examination.

DIFFERENTIAL DIAGNOSIS

- Herpetic whitlow
- Pyogenic granuloma
- Viral warts
- Ganglions
- Squamous cell carcinoma

WORKUP

A workup is usually not pursued unless there is treatment failure.

LABORATORY TESTS

- Gram stain and culture any purulent drainage.
- Potassium hydroxide mount may show pseudohyphae.

IMAGING STUDIES

Radiographs of the digit if concerned about osteomyelitis.

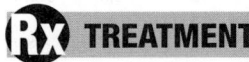

TREATMENT

NONPHARMACOLOGIC THERAPY

- For acute paronychia without purulent drainage, warm soaks tid or qid are helpful. If pus is present, surgical drainage is required.
- For chronic paronychia, avoid frequent immersion in water or exposure to moisture.

ACUTE GENERAL Rx

- First-generation cephalosporin (e.g., cephalexin 250 to 500 mg qid) or penicillinase-resistant penicillin (e.g., dicloxacillin 250 to 500 mg qid) are usually the antibiotics of choice for acute paronychia.
- Alternative antibiotic choices include clindamycin and amoxicillin-clavulanate potassium.
- Surgical drainage is indicated if purulent discharge is noted.

- A No. 11 blade scalpel is used to lift the lateral perionychium and proximal eponychium off the nail, facilitating drainage.
- If the pus is located beneath the nail, the lateral edge of the nail can be lifted off the nail bed and excised.

CHRONIC Rx

- If no fungal organism is found, tincture of iodine (2 drops bid) helps keep the nail and skin dry.
- Chronic paronychia caused by *Candida albicans* is treated with topical antifungal agents (e.g., miconazole or ketoconazole applied tid).
- Unresponsive cases may be treated with itraconazole or fluconazole but should be done in consultation with dermatology and/or infectious disease.
- Surgery may be needed in refractory cases.

DISPOSITION

- Most acute paronychias with appropriate treatment resolve within 7 to 10 days.
- Osteomyelitis is a potential complication of paronychia.
- Untreated chronic paronychia leads to thickening and discoloration with eventual nail loss.

REFERRAL

Chronic paronychia refractory to topical medical therapy is best referred to dermatology and/or infectious disease. A hand surgeon is consulted if abscess drainage or surgery is being considered.

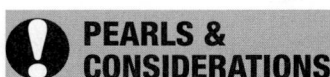

PEARLS & CONSIDERATIONS

COMMENTS

The gastrointestinal tract, including the mouth and bowel, and the genitourinary tract in women are the usual sources of *C. albicans* in chronic paronychia.

SUGGESTED READINGS

available at www.expertconsult.com

AUTHORS: **GLENN G. FORT, M.D., M.P.H.,** and **DENNIS J. MIKOLICH, M.D.**

BASIC INFORMATION

DEFINITION

Paroxysmal cold hemoglobinuria (PCH) is the first, albeit rarest, auto-immune hemolytic anemia to be identified. It is characterized by transient or episodic massive intravascular hemolysis after exposure to cold temperatures. It was first described in patients with secondary or tertiary syphilis, and was classified as acute transient, chronic syphilitic, and chronic non-syphilitic. In modern times, chronic PCH is very rare, usually occurs in the elderly, and is associated with a malignancy. Most cases are of the acute transient type, which is usually idiopathic in adults and secondary to a viral syndrome or immunization in children.

SYNONYMS

PCH
Donath-Landsteiner hemoglobinuria

ICD-9CM CODES

283.2 Hemoglobinuria caused by hemolysis from external causes

EPIDEMIOLOGY & DEMOGRAPHICS

- No race predilection, but mild male sex predilection with reported male-to-female ratio of 2:1 to 5:1.
- Accounts for up to 5% of adult cases of auto-immune hemolytic anemia
- Accounts for nearly 30% of childhood cases of autoimmune hemolytic anemia

PHYSICAL FINDINGS & CLINICAL PRESENTATION

- Within minutes to a few hours after cold exposure, there is a sudden onset of fever, rigors, and chills followed by red to brown urination.
- Associated symptoms include back, leg, and abdominal pain.
- Headaches, nausea, vomiting, diarrhea, and esophageal spasm are common.
- Oliguria and anuria can develop following renal dysfunction.
- May be associated with Raynaud's phenomenon.
- Associated with cold urticaria.
- Transient splenomegaly and hepatomegaly with jaundice may occur.
- Symptoms and gross hemoglobinuria usually resolve within hours.
- Symptoms believed to be mediated by smooth muscle dysfunction as a result of nitric oxide toxicity associated with hemoglobinemia.

ETIOLOGY & PATHOGENESIS

- The Donath-Landsteiner antibody is a biphasic, usually polyclonal, immunoglobulin (Ig) G. It is known to bind to various antigens such as I-, i-, p-, Pr-, which are normally present on the red blood cell (RBC) surface; yet, the glycosphingolipid P antigen is considered its primary target. It sensitizes RBCs in the cold, and as blood warms to 37° C, complement-mediated hemolysis ensues.
- In children, the appearance of the antibody usually follows the onset of a viral respiratory illness by 1 to 3 wk. Symptoms may persist for several weeks.
- PCH has been associated with multiple infectious pathogens, including syphilis, *Haemophilus influenzae,* Epstein-Barr virus (EBV), cytomegalovirus (CMV), influenza A, varicella, measles, mumps, adenovirus, parvovirus B19, coxsackie A9, Mycoplasma pneumonia, and Klebsiella pneumonia.

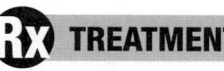 DIAGNOSIS

DIFFERENTIAL DIAGNOSIS

- Cold agglutinin disease, paroxysmal nocturnal hemoglobinuria, and malaria.
- Other causes of acute massive intravascular hemolysis and myoglobinuria secondary to rhabdomyolysis.
- Table 1-138 differentiates various types of autoimmune hemolytic anemias.

LABORATORY TESTS

- The presence of IgG that reacts with the RBC at reduced temperatures but not at body temperature. In the Donath-Landsteiner test, a patient's serum is incubated with papain-ized pooled donated RBCs and complement at 4° C then warmed to 37° C. Lysis is observed in a positive test.
- A more sensitive test involves using radiolabelled monoclonal anti-IgG. This is incubated at 4° C with the patient's serum and donor RBCs. The degree of radioactivity on the separated RBCs will be elevated in PCH compared with a control run at 37° C.
- Elevated bilirubin and lactate dehydrogenase, low haptoglobin, free plasma hemoglobin, low complement (C2, C3, C4).
- Abnormal RBC forms on the peripheral blood smear such as poikilocytosis, spherocytosis, anisocytosis and nucleated RBCs.

- Erythrophagocytosis by neutrophils and monocytes may be seen.

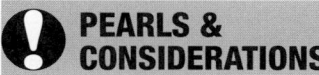 TREATMENT

NONPHARMACOLOGIC THERAPY

The mainstay of treatment is the avoidance of exposure to cold and presence of supportive care.

ACUTE GENERAL Rx

- In children in particular, transfusion may be necessary because the anemia may become life threatening and hemolysis may be ongoing for several weeks.
- Testing and treatment for underlying secondary condition.
- Hydration and alkalinization of the urine may be necessary to prevent renal failure.
- Steroids, although commonly used, were not shown to be beneficial.
- Plasma exchange therapy with 5% albumin fluid replacement has been successfully employed.
- Splenectomy is not indicated.
- Treatment with rituximab has resulted in termination of hemolysis in a case report.
- Azathioprine has also been suggested in case reports.

DISPOSITION

- Postinfectious varieties are self-limited.
- Adult idiopathic form is generally manageable by avoiding environmental exposure.

REFERRAL

To hematologist to aid in diagnosis

PEARLS & CONSIDERATIONS

- PCH is associated with brown or red discoloration of urine after cold exposure in adults or after a viral infection in children.
- PCH can be associated with viral or bacterial infections, including syphilis, *H. influenzae,* EBV, CMV, influenza A, varicella, measles, mumps, and adenovirus, or malignancy, especially in adults.
- PCH can cause life-threatening hemolysis in children.

SUGGESTED READINGS

available at www.expertconsult.com

AUTHORS: **LARA KFOURY, M.D.,** and **SUSIE L. HU, M.D.**

TABLE 1-138 Characteristics of Autoimmune Hemolytic Anemia

Characteristic	TYPE OF AUTOIMMUNE HEMOLYTIC ANEMIA		
	Warm Autoimmune Hemolytic Anemia	Cold Agglutinin Disease	Paroxysmal Cold Hemoglobinuria
Antibody isotope	IgG, rare IgA, IgM	IgM	IgG
Direct antiglobulin test (DAT) result	IgG and/or C3	C3	C3
Antigen specificity	Multiple, primarily Rh	i/I, Pr	P
Hemolysis	Primarily extravascular	Primarily extravascular	Intravascular
Common disease associations	B-cell neoplasia/lymphoproliferative, collagen-vascular	Viral, neoplasia	Syphilis, viral

Hoffman R et al: *Hematology basic principles and practice,* ed 5, Philadelphia, 2009, Churchill Livingstone.

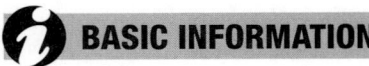

BASIC INFORMATION

DEFINITION

Paroxysmal nocturnal hemoglobinuria (PNH) is a rare disease characterized by episodes of intravascular hemolysis and hemoglobinuria usually occurring at night. Thrombocytopenia, leukopenia, and recurrent venous thrombosis are also associated with PNH.

SYNONYMS

PNH

ICD-9CM CODES
283.2 Paroxysmal nocturnal hemoglobinuria

EPIDEMIOLOGY & DEMOGRAPHICS

- Affects patients of any age (reported spectrum 6 to 82 yr) but most common in patients aged 30 to 50 yr
- Affects both sexes (slight female predominance) and all races

PHYSICAL FINDINGS & CLINICAL PRESENTATION

1. Initial manifestations
   - Anemia symptoms (35%)
   - Hemoglobinuria (25%)
   - Bleeding (20%)
   - Aplastic anemia (15%)
   - Gastrointestinal symptoms (10%)
   - Hemolytic anemia (10%)
   - Iron-deficiency anemia (5%)
   - Venous thrombosis (5%)
   - Infections (5%)
   - Neurologic symptoms
2. Hemoglobinuria
   - Typically the first morning void reveals dark urine with progressive clearing during the day. The cause for the circadian rhythm is unknown.
3. Hemolysis
   - In addition to the circadian hemolysis and resulting hemoglobinuria, episodes of hemolytic exacerbations can accompany infections, menstruation, transfusion, surgery, iron therapy, and vaccinations. Symptoms of severe hemolysis include chest, back, or abdominal pain, headache, fever, malaise, and fatigue.
4. Aplastic anemia
   - Aplastic anemia may be the presenting manifestation of PNH (therefore PNH must be in the differential diagnosis of aplastic anemia) or may develop as a later complication of PNH.
5. Thrombosis (leading cause of death in PNH; occurs in 40% of patients)
   - Lower extremity deep vein thrombosis (DVT)
   - Subclavian thrombosis
   - Portal or mesenteric vein thrombosis
   - Hepatic vein thrombosis (Budd-Chiari syndrome)
   - Cerebrovascular thromboses
6. Renal failure
   - Acute renal failure associated with massive hemoglobinuria (acute tubular necrosis)
   - Progressive renal failure associated with thrombosis within renal small veins
7. Dysphagia
8. Infections (associated with leukopenia or steroid treatment)
9. Physical findings include:
   - Pallor (anemia)
   - Jaundice (hemolysis)
   - Splenomegaly
   - Unilateral extremity swelling (DVT)
   - Ascites (Budd-Chiari syndrome)

ETIOLOGY & PATHOGENESIS

- Complement-mediated hemolysis; the erythrocytes are abnormally sensitive to acidified serum.
- Patients have two populations of red blood cells (RBCs): some sensitive to hemolysis (PNH III cells) and others not (PNH I cells), in variable proportions (10% to 75% PNH III cells). Approximately 20% PNH III are required for hemoglobinuria to be detectable.
- The RBC defects in PNH are in the membrane proteins as follows:
  - Decay-accelerating factor deficiency
  - Membrane inhibitor of reactive lysis deficiency
  - C-8 binding protein deficiency
- These protein deficiencies are the result of an acquired mutation located in the X chromosome, which regulates glycosyl phosphatidyl inositol (GPI). GPI anchors the above-mentioned proteins in the RBC membrane; GPI-deficient RBCs proliferate as an abnormal clone. Because women are affected at least as frequently as men are, the mutation must be expressed as dominant gene. The mechanism by which the mutant stem cells can dominate hematopoiesis in PNH is unknown.
- The pathophysiology of the relation of PNH and aplastic anemia is unknown.

DIAGNOSIS

Clinical situations:
- Intravascular hemolysis
- Hemoglobinuria
- Pancytopenia associated with hemolysis
- Iron deficiency associated with hemolysis
- Recurrent venous thrombosis
- Recurrent episodes of abdominal pain, headache, or back pain associated with hemolysis

DIFFERENTIAL DIAGNOSIS

- See "Hemolytic Anemia" in Section I.
- See "Aplastic Anemia" in Section I.
- See "Anemia" algorithm in Section III.

LABORATORY TESTS

- Complete blood count: anemia, leukopenia, thrombocytopenia
- Reticulocytosis
- RBC smear: spherocytes
- Negative Coombs test
- Low leukocyte alkaline phosphatase
- Elevated lactate dehydrogenase
- Low serum haptoglobin
- Low serum iron saturation, low ferritin
- Elevated urine hemoglobin, urine urobilinogen, urine hemosiderin
- Positive Ham test (acidified serum RBC lysis)
- Normoblastic hyperplasia on bone marrow aspirate or biopsy
- Identification of GPI-anchored protein deficiency on hematopoietic cells by using monoclonal antibodies or flow cytometry; flow cytometric analysis of granulocytes is the best way to diagnose PNH
- Cytogenetic studies are not diagnostic

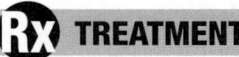 TREATMENT

- Prednisone (15 to 40 mg qod) helpful, but prolonged use should be avoided
- Eculizumab, a humanized antibody that inhibits the activation of terminal complement components, is an effective therapy for PNH; it reduces intravascular hemolysis, hemoglobinuria, and need for transfusion in patients with PNH. It is very expensive and requires lifelong administration.
- Iron replacement, folic acid supplementation
- Transfusions
- Treatment and prevention of thrombosis (heparin, Coumadin)
- Avoidance of oral contraceptives
- Bone marrow transplantation

REFERRAL

To hematologist

PROGNOSIS

- 50% survival to 10 to 15 yr
- 25% survival to 25 yr
- If thrombosis at presentation, only 40% survival to 4 yr
- 1% incidence of leukemia
- 5% incidence of myelodysplastic syndrome

SUGGESTED READINGS
available at www.expertconsult.com

AUTHOR: **FRED F. FERRI, M.D.**

BASIC INFORMATION

DEFINITION

Paroxysmal supraventricular tachycardia (SVT) is a group of tachyarrhythmias that originate from within or above the atrioventricular (AV) node and are characterized by sudden onset and abrupt termination. The most common types include AV nodal reentrant tachycardia (AVNRT), AV reentrant tachycardia (AVRT), and paroxysmal atrial tachycardia (PAT).

SYNONYMS

PAT (old terminology for SVT)
PSVT
Supraventricular tachycardia

ICD-9CM CODES
427.0 Paroxysmal atrial tachycardia

PHYSICAL FINDINGS & CLINICAL PRESENTATION

- Patient is usually asymptomatic.
- Patient may be aware of "fast" heartbeat (palpitations) or have presyncope, syncope, or chest pain.
- Hemodynamic status during arrhythmia may vary and can depend on the patient's comorbidities and presence of underlying structural heart disease.

ETIOLOGY

- AVNRT—Dual electrical pathways within or near the AV node
- AVRT—Accessory pathway (concealed [not evident on ECG], only retrograde ventriculoatrial conduction without antegrade atrioventricular conduction)
- Pre-excitation [Wolff-Parkinson-White] syndrome, evident on ECG as described below
- Paroxysmal atrial tachycardia—abnormal automaticity of atrial tissue or triggered activity

DIAGNOSIS

WORKUP

- Regular rhythm at rate of >100 beats/min is present.
- P waves may or may not be seen (the presence of P waves depends on the relation of atrial to ventricular depolarization).
- Wide QRS complex (>0.12 sec) with initial slurring (delta wave) during sinus rhythm and short PR (<0.12 sec) is characteristic of WPW syndrome.
- QRS complex during supraventricular tachycardia is usually narrow; however, may be widened because of intrinsic conduction disease, myocardial disease, or rate-related bundle branch block. It may also be widened if the patient has pre-excitation syndrome.
- Echocardiography is appropriate to assess for the presence of underlying structural heart disease.

TREATMENT

NONPHARMACOLOGIC THERAPY

- Valsalva maneuver in the supine position is the most effective way to terminate SVT; carotid sinus massage (after excluding occlusive carotid disease) is also commonly used to elicit vagal efferent impulses.
- Synchronized DC shock is used if patient shows signs of hemodynamic instability.
- Table 1-139 describes useful features to differentiate ventricular tachycardia from SVT with aberrancy.

ACUTE GENERAL Rx

- Adenosine is useful for treatment of AVRT and AVNRT, and can uncover the underlying rhythm in paroxysmal atrial tachycardia; it is the first choice of therapy for treatment of almost all episodes of SVT unresponsive to vagal maneuvers. The dose is 6 mg given as a rapid IV bolus; tachycardia is usually terminated within a few seconds. If necessary, may repeat with 12-mg IV bolus. Contraindications are second- or third-degree atrioventricular block, sick sinus syndrome, and atrial fibrillation. Adenosine may cause bronchospasm in asthmatics.
- Verapamil 5 to 10 mg IV is given over 5 min; if no effect, may repeat in 30 min.
  1. Verapamil should be used cautiously in patients with SVT associated with hypotension.
  2. Slow injection of calcium chloride (10 ml of a 10% solution given over 5 to 8 min before verapamil administration) decreases the hypotensive effect without compromising its antiarrhythmic effect.
- Repeat carotid massage after IV verapamil if SVT persists.
- Metoprolol (IV 5 mg/2 min up to 15 mg) or esmolol (500 µg/kg IV bolus, then 50 µg/kg/min) may be effective in the treatment of SVT.
- IV digitalization (0.75 to 1 mg slow IV loading) if other agents are not effective.
  1. Repeat carotid massage 30 min later; if not successful, give additional 0.25 mg IV digoxin and repeat carotid sinus massage 1 hr later.
  2. Digoxin, beta-blockers, and calcium-channel blockers should be avoided in patients with pre-excitation syndrome to avoid increased conduction through the accessory pathway.

DISPOSITION

Most patients respond well with resolution of the paroxysmal atrial tachycardia upon treatment (see "Acute General Rx"). Some patients may need chronic AV blocking agents for recurrence.

REFERRAL

Radiofrequency ablation (RFA) is the procedure of choice in symptomatic patients who are refractory to medical therapy. RFA has high efficacy rates (single procedure success is 93.2%), low all-cause mortality (0.1%), and low adverse events (2.9%). Despite high reported success rates, RFA appears to be underused in clinical practice.

PEARLS & CONSIDERATIONS

COMMENTS

Accessory pathways occur in 0.1% to 0.3% of the general population.

SUGGESTED READINGS

available at www.expertconsult.com

AUTHORS: **ALEXANDER G. TRUESDELL, M.D., FRED F. FERRI, M.D.,** and **WEN-CHIH WU, M.D.**

TABLE 1-139 Features that May Differentiate Ventricular Tachycardia from Supraventricular Tachycardia with Aberrancy

Helpful Features	Implications
Positive QRS concordance	Diagnostic of VT
Presence of AV dissociation, capture beats, or fusion beats	Diagnostic of VT
Atypical RBBB (monophasic R, QR, RS, or triphasic QRS in V_1; R:S ratio < 1, QS or QR, monophasic R in V_6)	Suggests VT
Atypical LBBB (R >30 min or R to S [nadir or notch] > 60 min in V_1 or V_2; R:S ratio < 1, QS or QR in V_6)	Suggests VT
Shift of axis from baseline	Suggests VT
History of CAD	Suggests VT
QRS during tachycardia identical to QRS during sinus rhythm	Suggests SVT
Termination with adenosine	Suggests SVT

AV, Atrioventricular; *CAD,* coronary artery disease; *LBBB,* left bundle branch block; *RBBB,* right bundle branch block; *SVT,* supraventricular tachycardia; *VT,* ventricular tachycardia.
Andreoli TG, Benjamin IJ, Griggs RC, Wing EJ: *Andreoli and Carpenter's Cecil essentials of medicine,* ed 8, Philadelphia, 2010, Saunders.

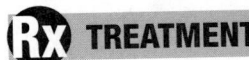

BASIC INFORMATION

DEFINITION

Overuse or overload of the patellofemoral region leading to anterior knee pain

SYNONYMS

PFPS
Retropatellar pain syndrome
Runner's knee
Lateral facet compression syndrome
Idiopathic anterior knee pain

ICD-9CM CODES

719.46 Patellofemoral pain syndrome

EPIDEMIOLOGY & DEMOGRAPHICS

PREVALENCE: Estimated >20% of adolescents. PFPS is the most common diagnosis in outpatients presenting with knee pain. PFPS also constitutes 16% to 25% of all injuries to runners.
PREDOMINANT SEX AND AGE: Nearly 2:1 female predominance; disproportionately affects active adolescents and adults in the second and third decades of life
RISK FACTORS: Increase in physical activity intensity or duration, overuse, joint overload, trauma, anatomic abnormalities, malalignment, patellar hypermobility, quadriceps weakness

PHYSICAL FINDINGS & CLINICAL PRESENTATION

- Gradual or acute onset of anterior knee pain
- Sometimes localized under or around the patella
- Also described as a catching sensation under the patella
- Worsened pain with squatting, running, prolonged sitting, or ascending or descending steps
- Effusion implies intraarticular pathology not explained by PFPS
- Pain may be elicited by compression of the patella into the trochlear groove while the leg is extended

ETIOLOGY

No clear consensus; likely multifactorial, including muscle overuse or joint overload with malalignment and/or trauma potentially contributing resulting in imbalances in the forces controlling patellar tracking during knee flexion and extension

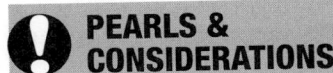

DIAGNOSIS

DIFFERENTIAL DIAGNOSIS

- Patellofemoral arthritis
- Patellar instability
- Patellar stress fracture
- Osgood-Schlatter disease
- Articular cartilage injury
- Prepatellar bursitis
- Pes anserine bursitis
- Iliotibial band syndrome
- Plica synovitis
- Chondromalacia
- Bony abnormalities
- Bone tumors
- Patellar tendinopathy
- Other: Referred pain from lumbar spine or hip joint pathology, loose bodies, osteochondritis dissecans, Sinding-Larse-Johansson syndrome, symptomatic bipartite patella

WORKUP

- PFPS is a clinical diagnosis of exclusion; evaluate and rule out other possibilities on the differential. Dynamic patellar tracking can be assessed by having the patient perform a single leg squat and stand. Physical exam should also include patellar mobility testing (displacement >3 quadrants is considered hypermobile), patellar grind (or inhibition) test (positive test if pain is produced), and patellar tilt test to assess for tightness of the lateral structures.
- Physical exam findings consistent with PFPS include eliciting pain by compression of the patella into the trochlear groove while the leg is extended.

IMAGING STUDIES

- No imaging is necessary in the initial workup.
- Consider plain films if symptoms do not improve after 1 to 2 mo of therapy.

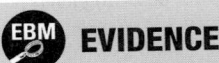

TREATMENT

There is a general lack of consensus. Management should focus on the implementation of a comprehensive rehabilitation program.

NONPHARMACOLOGIC THERAPY

Physical therapy; quadriceps, hamstring, iliotibial band, and calf-stretching exercises; quadriceps and hip abductor strengthening

ACUTE GENERAL Rx

Short-term (2 to 3 wk) NSAIDs for pain relief; activity modification; ice for 10 to 20 min after activity

CHRONIC Rx

- Physical therapy; strengthening and flexibility exercises; consider arch supports or evaluation for custom orthotics.
- Spontaneous resolution may occur in some cases.

DISPOSITION

Outpatient management

REFERRAL

Consider referral to orthopedics for surgical evaluation as a last resort if conservative therapies fail. Surgical options include release of the lateral retinaculum; articular cartilage procedures; and proximal realignment, usually with anteromedialization of the tibial tubercle.

PEARLS & CONSIDERATIONS

COMMENTS

Treatment is most successful when the patient has a disciplined approach.

PATIENT/FAMILY EDUCATION

The American Academy of Family Practice website www.familydoctor.org contains frequently asked questions, patient information, and example stretching and strengthening exercises.

EVIDENCE

available at www.expertconsult.com

SUGGESTED READING

available at www.expertconsult.com

AUTHOR: **KATE MAVRICH, M.D.**

BASIC INFORMATION

DEFINITION

- Patent foramen ovale (PFO) is a vestige of the fetal circulation, and results from failure of the primum and secundum septa to fuse postnatally. Persistence of the one-way flap valve overlying this foramen ovale allows right to left blood flow when right atrial pressure exceeds that of the left.
- Foramen ovale remains open during intrauterine life, in a valve-like manner, to allow highly oxygenated blood to reach the left atrium from the inferior vena cava. High right atrial pressure in the fetus keeps it open.
- Soon after birth, as the pulmonary circulation fills, the left atrial pressure rises higher than that of the right atrium. This pushes the septum primum against septum secondum, closing the right-to-left pathway through the foramen ovale.

ICD-9CM CODES
745.5 Patent foramen ovale

EPIDEMIOLOGY & DEMOGRAPHICS

- PFO fails to close in as many as a fourth of the population.
- PFO has similar frequency among males and females.

PHYSICAL FINDINGS & CLINICAL PRESENTATION

- Most patients with isolated PFO are asymptomatic.
- It cannot be detected on clinical examination.

COMPLICATIONS
- Cryptogenic stroke (particularly <55 yr).
- The proposed mechanism of stroke with PFO includes paradoxical embolization, in situ thrombosis within the canal of the PFO, associated atrial arrhythmia and concomitant hypercoagulable state.
- Migraine with aura.
- Decompression sickness and air embolism.
- Increases risk of hypoxemia during sleep in patients with obstructive sleep apnea.
- Platypnea-orthodeoxia syndrome (characterized by both dyspnea and arterial desaturation in the upright position with improvement in supine position).
- Increased risk of postoperative atrial fibrillation and hypoxemia, in off-pump coronary artery bypass surgery.

ETIOLOGY
- Unknown

DIAGNOSIS

- Testing for PFO is primarily performed in patients with a cerebral ischemic event of uncertain origin.
- A variety of echocardiography modalities have been used to diagnose PFO. These include:
  1. Transthoracic echocardiography (TTE)
  2. Transesophageal echocardiogram (TEE) (Fig. 1-278)

3. Transmitral Doppler (TMD)
4. Transcranial Doppler (TCD) of middle cerebral artery after injection of agitated saline peripherally
- TEE, especially when performed with contrast injected during a cough or valsalva, is the most sensitive and preferred test for diagnosing PFO.
- Essentially, a PFO is suggested by the presence of echo dropout in the atrial septum visualized in more than one plane during echocardiography. The appearance of microbubbles in the left atrium within three to five cardiac cycles after injection of agitated saline peripherally is considered diagnostic of PFO with associated with right-to-left shunt (RLS).
- The diagnosis of PFO is enhanced with multiple intravenous contrast injections with maneuvers that cause transient elevations of right atrial pressure (cough or valsalva) to enhance RLS.
- TCD has the advantage of being noninvasive and easy to perform at bedside. But it can only detect a right-to-left shunt, not the location of the shunt or other cardiac structural anomalies.

TREATMENT

- Management guidelines from professional societies are shown in Table 1-140.
- Most patients with a PFO as an isolated finding receive no special treatment. This is because the yearly risk of cryptogenic stroke in healthy persons with PFO may be as low as 0.1%.
- As it is not associated with increased risk for endocarditis, antibiotic prophylaxis is not indicated.

PHARMACOLOGICAL TREATMENT

When PFO is associated with an otherwise unexplained neurological event, traditional treatment has been antiplatelet treatment (e.g., aspirin) therapy alone in low-risk patients and combined with therapeutic anticoagulants (e.g., warfarin) in high-risk patients.

Risk factors associated with a higher risk of complications, particularly stroke include:
- Coexisting atrial septal aneurysm
- Large PFO
- Spontaneous right-to-left shunting
- Major shunt (>50 bubbles)
- Valsalva provoking activity preceding the onset of stroke
- Presence of Chiari network (a congenital remnant of the right valve of the sinus venosus)
- Eustachian valves
- Younger age (<55 yr)
- Multiple clinical events or infarcts
- Pulmonary hypertension
- Failure or contraindications to anticoagulants
- High risk for recurrent deep venous thrombosis
- Pulmonary embolism at time of initial event
- Hypercoagulable state

PERCUTANEOUS TRANSCATHETER CLOSURE OF PFO

Percutaneous method of closure is usually preferred over open surgical closure because of invasiveness, procedure time, and patient convenience.
- Indications:
  1. Recurrent cryptogenic stroke due to presumed paradoxical embolism through PFO while on adequate medical treatment with antiplatelets or anticoagulants
  2. In presence of contraindications to anticoagulants

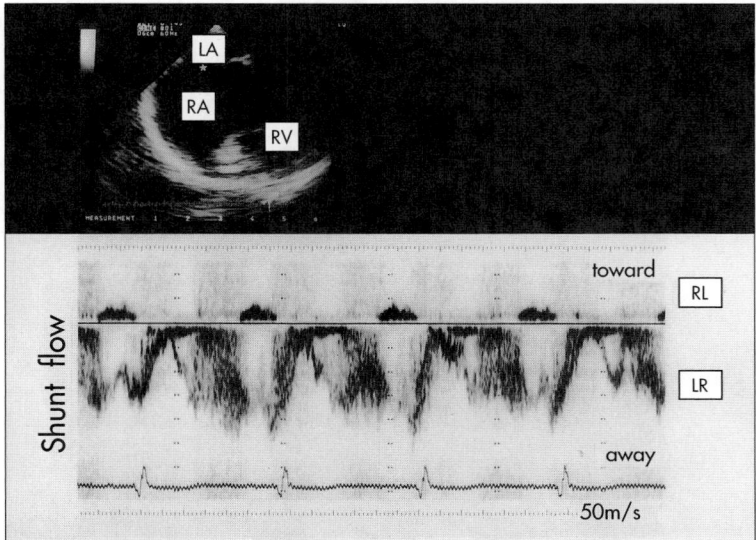

FIGURE 1-278 Transesophageal echocardiography of an internal defects and pulsed Doppler flow signal. Pulsed Doppler echocardiographic signal is consistent with left-to-right level. *LA,* Left atrium; *RA,* right atrium; *RV,* right ventricle; *LR,* left-to-right shunt signal; *RL,* right-to-left shunt signal. (From Crawford, MH, DiMaxcro JP, Paulus WJ [eds]: *Cardiology,* ed 2, St Louis, 2004, Mosby.

- Contraindications:
  1. Presence of thrombus on the implant site or in the venous system used for access
  2. Active endocarditis or bacteremia
  3. Inadequate size of femoral vein for access
  4. Atrial septal anatomy without an adequate rim to hold the device
  5. Atrial septal anatomy that may result in the occlude obstructing an intracardiac structure

  6. Known hypercoagulable state
  7. Presence of an intracardiac mass or vegetation
- The Food and Drug Administration (FDA) has approved CardioSEAL Septal Occlusion System and Amplatzer PFO Occluder devices for percutaneous PFO closure.
- Requires SBE prophylaxis and antiplatelets (aspirin and clopidogrel for first 3 mo, followed by aspirin for another 3 mo) for 6 mo

postprocedure. During this period of endothelialization, the risk of recurrent stroke is highest.
- The 1-yr rate of recurrent neurological events ranged from 0% to 5% with percutaneous closure group vs. 4% to 12% with medical therapy group.
- MRI or metal detectors do not affect these implants, as they are not metallic in nature.

SURGICAL CLOSURE (OPEN THORACOTOMY)

- Indications:
  1. PFO >25 mm in size
  2. Inadequate rim of tissue around the defect
  3. Percutaneous device failure
  4. In presence of other indication for open heart surgery

TABLE 1-140	Management Guidelines from Professional Societies	
	American Academy of Neurology	**American College of Chest Physicians**
PFO	1. Evidence is insufficient to determine whether warfarin or aspirin is superior in preventing recurrent strokes or death, but minor bleeding is more frequent with warfarin. 2. There is insufficient evidence to evaluate the efficacy of surgical or endovascular closure.	
PFO alone		1. Antiplatelet therapy recommended over no therapy 2. Antiplatelet therapy suggested over warfarin
PFO with other risk factors		Inadequate data available to allow recommendation of optimal medical therapy vs. endovascular or surgical closure
PFO with concomitant deep vein thrombosis or pulmonary embolism	At least 3 mo of anticoagulation	Anticoagulation recommended

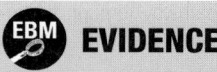 **EVIDENCE**

available at www.expertconsult.com

SUGGESTED READINGS

available at www.expertconsult.com

AUTHOR: **HEMANT K. SATPATHY, M.D.**

BASIC INFORMATION

DEFINITION

Medication errors represent failure of intended prescription, dispensation, or administration of desired drug therapy. Medication errors may result in inappropriate medication use or an adverse drug event (ADE) (i.e., direct harm or injury to the patient).

SYNONYMS

Dosing errors or mistakes. Medication errors are not synonymous with ADEs because not all cause harm (a requirement of ADEs).

ICD-9CM CODES
Not applicable

EPIDEMIOLOGY & DEMOGRAPHICS

INCIDENCE:
- 15% of pediatric outpatient prescriptions are either underdosed (7%) or overdosed (8%).
- Nearly 6% of medication orders for a hospitalized child contain an error. One percent of medication orders for a child will result in a potential ADE (i.e., an error that would have caused harm but was intercepted before reaching the patient). Less than 1% of medication orders for a child will contain an error that ultimately results in harm or injury.

PEAK INCIDENCE: Among outpatient prescriptions, medication errors occur more frequently in children <4 yr compared with older children (20% vs. 13%)

PREVALENCE: Not applicable

PREDOMINANT SEX AND AGE: Children <4 yr

GENETICS: Not applicable

RISK FACTORS:
- Patient aged <4 yr, particularly with prescriptions for asthma and allergy medications or antibiotics
- Off-label (non-FDA approved) medication use
- Prescriptions for analgesics (most commonly written for potential overdose)
- Lack of computerized prescriber order entry (CPOE), standardized order sets, or alert systems
- Prescriptions for antiseizure medications (most commonly written for potential underdose)
- Infants or children with multiple health care needs or those in intensive care

PHYSICAL FINDINGS & CLINICAL PRESENTATION

- Signs and symptoms of toxicity specific to the current drug regimen
- Lack of clinical efficacy of the current drug regimen

ETIOLOGY

Common sources of pediatric medication errors include:
- Prescribing errors: lack of knowledge of medication; lack of recognition of the impact growth and development may have on the pharmacokinetics of a specific drug; use of

medical abbreviations within the prescription or medication order
- Calculation errors: mg/kg/*dose* versus mg/kg/*day* dosing recommendations; "tenfold" decimal mistakes such as the use of trailing zeros (1 vs. 1.0) and naked decimals (0.1 vs. 1); patient weight in pounds versus kilograms
- Administration errors: incomplete education provided to patient or caregiver; lack of appropriate drug administration tools such as graduated oral syringes or medication spoons; deviation from the "five rights," (i.e., the *right* drug at the *right* dose for the *right* patient by the *right* route at the *right* time)
- Dispensing errors: inappropriate formulation recommended, prescribed, or dispensed; use of adult formulations for children

 DIAGNOSIS

DIFFERENTIAL DIAGNOSIS

- Iatrogenic adverse drug reaction (unpreventable ADEs)
- Patient nonadherence (may be considered a medication error if appropriate instructions and/or education is not provided to the patient or caregiver)

WORKUP

Alert from CPOE systems, deviation from standardized order set, or detection on review of prescription or medication order by pharmacist or nurse:
- Immediately discontinue medication order or prescription
- Determine if suspected error has reached the patient
- Assess harm to patient and intervene if necessary (if ADE has occurred)
- Determine source of error if possible
- Resume correct drug therapy with appropriate monitoring of efficacy and toxicity
- Report error to institution or facility for tracking and quality improvement purposes
- Report sentinel events (an adverse event that led to death, serious physical or psychologic injury, or the risk of such injury) to the Joint Commission

LABORATORY TESTS

Supratherapeutic or subtherapeutic serum drug concentrations (if applicable)

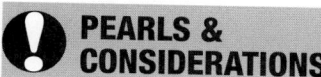 **TREATMENT**

Management of a medication error resulting in harm to the patient may include acute treatment of a toxic ADE or long-term management of a suboptimally treated condition. It should always include the workup described above.

ACUTE GENERAL Rx

If the medication error has reached the patient and resulted in an ADE, immediate intervention may be required. Disclosure to the patient or caregiver of an error resulting in harm to the patient is necessary.

CHRONIC Rx

Long-term management of injury or harm resulting from a medication error may be necessary.

DISPOSITION

- Prescribers may need to reestablish trust with the patient or caregiver after an error that resulted in harm to ensure optimal care in the future.
- The reporting of medication errors should be nonpunitive in nature and intent on individual education and correction of health systems–related flaws.

REFERRAL

Consultation with a pharmacist trained in pediatric pharmacotherapy may improve individual drug therapy and ensure age-specific drug dosing. Interpreters may be necessary to ensure drug information is accurately relayed to non-English-speaking patients or caregivers.

 PEARLS & CONSIDERATIONS

COMMENTS

- 20% of ADEs occurring in hospitalized children are preventable.
- The most common tenfold dosing errors in children ≤12 mo in age involve histamine H_2 antagonist medications (e.g., ranitidine) and metoclopramide. For children >12 mo of age, tenfold dosing errors most commonly involve antibiotics or antihistamine-decongestant combination products.
- Medication errors must be reported for health systems–related flaws to be identified and corrected.
- Careful attention must always be focused on the impact growth and development has on the pharmacokinetic characteristics of drugs used in children. From birth through adolescence, the absorption, distribution, metabolism, and elimination of a particular drug must not be assumed constant, and age-specific dosing recommendations should be used. A child's dose should not exceed that of an adult. Equations that calculate proportionate doses based on body weight or body surface area do not take into consideration these age-related changes.

PREVENTION

- Health systems management: double-checking of calculations and verification of medication orders by pharmacists and nurses reduce preventable ADEs. Eliminate the use of medical abbreviations within medication orders and prescriptions. The use of CPOE, standardized order sets, and electronic prescription filing can provide a prompt at the time of prescribing or ordering and will reduce medication errors resulting from illegible handwriting.
- Communication: open lines of communication between the prescriber, nurse, and phar-

macist will help ensure medication errors do not occur. Drug information must be presented and reinforced at a level and in a language understandable to patients or caregivers.

- Education: health care professionals must remain knowledgeable of current standards of care as well as new drug therapy options.
- Review of drug therapy: reassessment of prescriptions for accurate age-appropriate dosing and the indication for drug therapy, monitoring of efficacy and toxicity, and reconfirming a patient or caregiver's understanding of the drug regimen will limit medication errors and potential harm in chronic medication use.

PATIENT & FAMILY EDUCATION

- Caregivers should always remind a child's doctor of any drug allergies or side effects the child has had in the past.
- Do not use over-the-counter cough and cold medicines for children less than 4 yr.
- A list of all the medicines a child uses should be kept and shared with all the doctors the child sees. Remember to include over-the-counter medicines such as cough medicine and analgesics.
- Caregivers should ask a child's doctor or pharmacist as many questions as needed so that they understand how to correctly use the child's medicine.

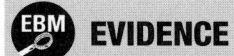

EVIDENCE

available at www.expertconsult.com

SUGGESTED READINGS

available at www.expertconsult.com

AUTHOR: **BRIAN J. COWLES, PHARM.D.**

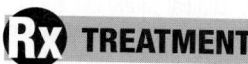 BASIC INFORMATION

DEFINITION

Pediculosis is lice infestation. Human beings can be infested with three kinds of lice: *Pediculus capitis* (head louse [Fig. 1-279]), *Pediculus corporis* (body louse), and *Phthirus pubis* (pubic, or crab, louse). Lice feed on human blood and deposit their eggs (nits) on the hair shafts (head lice and pubic lice) and along the seams of clothing (body lice). Nits generally hatch within 7 to 10 days. Lice are obligate human parasites and cannot survive away from their hosts for longer than 7 to 10 days.

SYNONYMS

Lice

ICD-9CM CODES
132.9 Pediculosis

EPIDEMIOLOGY & DEMOGRAPHICS

- There are 6 million to 12 million cases of head lice in the U.S. yearly.
- Lice infestation of the scalp is most common in children (girls affected more often than boys).
- Infestation of the eyelashes is most frequently seen in children and may indicate sexual abuse.
- The chance of acquiring pubic lice from one sexual exposure with an infested partner is >90% (most contagious STD known).
- Body lice is most common in conditions of poor hygiene.

PHYSICAL FINDINGS & CLINICAL PRESENTATION

- Pruritus with excoriation may be caused by hypersensitivity reaction, inflammation from saliva, and fecal material from the lice.
- Nits can be identified by examining hair shafts.
- The presence of nits on clothes is indicative of body lice.
- Lymphadenopathy may be present (cervical adenopathy with head lice, inguinal lymphadenopathy with pubic lice).

- Head lice is most frequently found in the back of the head and neck, behind the ears.
- Scratching can result in pustules and crusting.
- Pubic lice may affect the hair around the anus.

ETIOLOGY

Lice are transmitted by close personal contact or use of contaminated objects (e.g., combs, clothing, bed linen, hats).

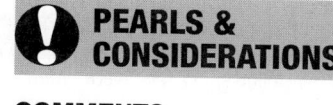 DIAGNOSIS

DIFFERENTIAL DIAGNOSIS

- Seborrheic dermatitis
- Scabies
- Eczema
- Other: pilar casts, trichonodosis (knotted hair), monilethrix

WORKUP

Diagnosis is made by seeing the lice or their nits. Combing hair with a fine-toothed comb is recommended because visual inspection of the hair and scalp may miss more than 50% of infestations.

LABORATORY TESTS

Wood's light examination is useful to screen a large number of children: live nits fluoresce, empty nits have a gray fluorescence, nits with unborn louse reveal white fluorescence.

TREATMENT

NONPHARMACOLOGIC THERAPY

- Patients with body lice should discard infested clothes and improve their hygiene.
- Combing out nits is a widely recommended but unproven adjunctive therapy.
- Personal items such as combs and brushes should be soaked in hot water for 15 to 30 min.
- Close contacts and household members should also be examined for the presence of lice.

ACUTE GENERAL Rx

The following products are available for treatment of lice:

- Benzyl alcohol lotion, 5% (Ulesfia) can be used for treatment of head lice in patients >6 mo old. The lotion is applied to dry hair and left on for 10 min. Treatment must be repeated after 7 days because the drug is not ovicidal.
- Permethrin: available over the counter (1% permethrin [Nix]) or by prescription (5% permethrin [Elimite]); should be applied to the hair and scalp and rinsed out after 10 min. A repeat application is generally not necessary in patients with head lice. It can be applied to clean, dry hair and left on overnight (8 to 14 hours) under a shower cap.
- Eyelash infestation can be treated with the application of petroleum jelly rubbed into the eyelashes three times a day for 5 to 7 days. The application of baby shampoo to the eyelashes and brows three or four times a day for 5 days is also effective. The use of fluorescein drops applied to the lids and eyelashes is also toxic to lice.
- In patients who have previously not responded to treatment or in whom resistance with 1% permethrin cream rinse occurs, a 10-day course of trimethoprim-sulfamethoxazole (TMP-SMX) 8 mg/kg/day in divided doses is an effective treatment for head lice infestation, especially for eyelash infestations with *Phthirus pubis*.
- Ivermectin, an antiparasitic drug, given as an oral dose of 400 mcg/kg of body weight on days 1 and 8 is effective for head lice resistant to other treatments (currently not FDA approved for pediculosis).
- Malathion, an organophosphate, is effective in head lice. It is available by prescription. Use should be avoided in children ≤2 yr. It is not commonly used because of its objectionable odor, fear of flammability, and prolonged application time (8 to 12 hr).

PEARLS & CONSIDERATIONS

COMMENTS

- Patients with pubic lice should notify their sexual contacts. Sex partners within the last month should be treated.
- Parents of patients should also be educated that head lice infestation (unlike body lice) does not indicate poor hygiene.

SUGGESTED READINGS

available at www.expertconsult.com

AUTHOR: **FRED F. FERRI, M.D.**

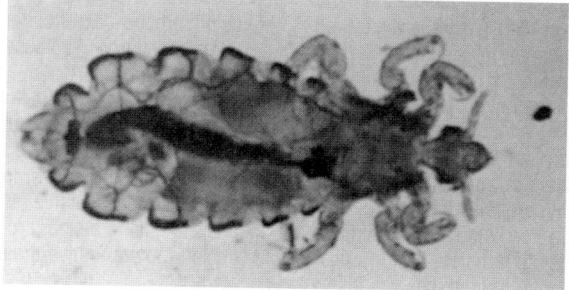

FIGURE 1-279 *Pediculus humanus* var. *capitis* (head louse). (From Mandell GL [ed]: *Mandell, Douglas, and Bennett's principles and practice of infectious diseases,* ed 6, New York, 2005, Churchill Livingstone.)

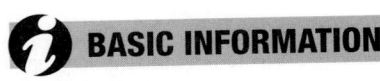

DEFINITION

According to the DSM-IV-R, pedophilia is one of nine possible paraphilias. A paraphilia is an enduring sexual preference that is highly unusual or illegal and results in distress or impairment. The sexual preference of a pedophile is for young children. The pedophile must experience at least 6 mo of intense sexual urges, fantasies, or behaviors involving *prepubescent* children. The pedophile must experience distress or impairment. According to the DSM-IV-R, if the individual acts upon his/her sexual urge with a child, or if the sexual urge puts them at odds with society or with the law, the functional impairment criterion has been met. The pedophile must be older than 16 yr and at least 5 yr older than the object of their longings. DSM-IV-TR subtypes pedophiles into categories based on his/her victim gender preference (boys, girls or both), on the exclusivity of his/her sexual urges toward children (children only or affinity for adults and children), and based upon his/her relationship with the victim (family or extrafamilial).

ICD-10 CODES
F65.4/302.2

EPIDEMIOLOGY & DEMOGRAPHICS

PREVALENCE (IN U.S.): Prevalence rates are largely based on self-reports of convicted child molesters, who are not necessarily pedophiles. According to this data, 3% to 9% of men self-report sexual contact or sexual fantasy with prepubescent children. Convenience samples suggest an upper limit of 5% for pedophilia.

ONSET & PREDOMINANT AGE: Pedophilia has an early onset and a chronic course. A study of 4007 self-admitted child molesters (2429 pedophiles) found that 40% of pedophiles molest before age 15 and the majority molest before age 20. Dickey et al reviewed charts of 174 sex offenders, 68 of whom were pedophiles. The pedophiles were distributed across the three age groups as follows: 17.6% were young adults, 38.2% were adults, and 44.1% were older adults, aged 40 to 70 yr old.

PREDOMINANT SEX: The significant majority of pedophiles are men (females comprise 1% to 6% of child molesters).

PHYSICAL FINDINGS & CLINICAL PRESENTATION

According to Abel and Harlow's study of 4007 child molesters:

- Child molesters match the general population with regards to education, marital status, and religion.
- 93% of child molesters reported some sexual interest in adults.
- 51% of men who abuse boys reported being exclusively heterosexual. 8% reported being exclusively homosexual.
- 60% have other paraphilias.

Sex offenders have higher rates of *general* crime recidivism than *sexual* crime recidivism. When known child molesters are rearrested, ~40% of their rearrests are for sexual offenses.

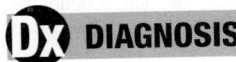

DIFFERENTIAL DIAGNOSIS

Pedophilia is often confused with terms such as child molester, sex offender, and hebephile. Not all child molesters are pedophiles. For example, individuals with Antisocial Personality Disorder may have an exclusive sexual preference for adults but may take a child's presence as an opportunity to gratify their sexual impulses. An individual who is hypersexual, indiscriminate, disinhibited, and who has very little opportunity for sexual gratification with their preferred age group may molest a child. A hebephile is one who has a sexual affinity for pubescent adolescents, rather than prepubescent youth. The term "sexual offender" represents a broad group of individuals who sexually offend against a variety of populations, including adult women.

WORKUP

Requires comprehensive data from multiple sources, including self-report, past sexual offense convictions, past and present partner report, psychophysiological assessments, forensic computer analysis, and/or scales. Deviant sexual preferences and lifestyle instability/criminality are strongly associated with general sexual recidivism. Therefore, clinical interview should explore sexual preferences (sex drive, paraphilic interests, victim characteristics), past sexual behaviors (including inquiry into the use of child pornography), and a history of rule violation, substance abuse, and risk taking. It is also important to explore opportunities that the individual has to be around children as well as exploring an individual's strengths and protective factors (lifestyle stability).

Investigation into comorbid disorders should include substance abuse, antisocial personality disorder, other paraphilias, personality disorders, and affective and anxiety disorders.

SCALES AND LABORATORY TESTS

- Phallometric/Plethysmographic Testing: The penile volume or circumference is measured in response to a variety of sexual materials. The result is thought to be a predictor of sexual recidivism among sex offenders. However, ~20% to 30% of individuals tested are considered low or nonresponders. Further, in the U.S., possession of the viewing material (child pornography) presents a legal dilemma for researchers. Other limitations include its lack of applicability to females, lack of applicability to males with impotence, and ability of individuals to try to suppress sexual feelings via distraction. This form of testing is not currently admissible in court for the purpose of determining guilt.
- Viewing Time: Viewing time is correlated with self-reported sexual interest and phallomet-

ric sexual arousal to children. No studies report that this measure predicts recidivism.
- Scales: For the prediction of general sexual recidivism, the most accurate approach appears to be the use of certain actuarial and mechanical measures. Some of the measures include the Static 99, MnSOST-R, Risk Matrix-2000 sex and the SVR 20. An individual's likelihood to recidivate is estimated based on the average risk of a group of individual's with similar characteristics.

NONPHARMACOLOGIC THERAPY

- Many models of sex offender treatment include identification of the offender's "sexual assault cycle." A response prevention intervention is devised. Triggers and relapse cues are identified, high-risk factors are avoided, and skills are taught to interrupt an offending response. An individuals's life skills are enhanced via training in anger management, self-regulation, intimacy and relationships, and general coping. Comorbidity such as substance abuse and mania should be treated. Treatment of pedophilia focuses on diminishing the pedophile's likelihood of acting on their urges rather than on changing the core sexual orientation. Scales have been developed in order to monitor progress in sex offender treatment.
- Hanson and Morton-Bourgon reported that recidivism rates over 5 to 6 yr for general sexual offenders vary from 13% (sexual recidivism) to 36% (any type of recidivism). Other sources range from 10% to 50% for pedophiles. There is no clear and consistent support for the efficacy of current treatment for sexual offenders. A 2009 Cochrane Collaboration Review on Management for people with disorders of sexual preference and for convicted sexual offenders concluded that the area lacked a strong evidence base.
- Treatment should develop positive life competencies, such as skills and beliefs, that will enhance the likelihood of a prosocial life and that are incompatible with offending behaviors.
- Community interventions might include the education of parents (re: high-risk situations, neighborhood sex offenders) and the education of children (re: assertiveness training, etc).
- Behavioral treatments are controversial interventions that are not the standard of care. They were devised to decrease sexual arousal to children. Examples include the introduction of aversive stimuli, habituation, and increasing sexual arousal to adults. It is unclear how effective these treatments are.

ACUTE GENERAL Rx & CHRONIC Rx

- Cyproterone acetate (CPA), medroxyprogesterone, and leuprolide acetate interfere with testosterone. These agents may reduce the frequency or intensity of sexual urges and arousal. There are no large well-controlled studies. They require close monitoring. Long-term consequences are unknown. Hormone therapy is expensive.

- SSRIs are supported by open label trials and case reports. They may decrease urges and lessen sexual preoccupation.
- Surgical castration involves removal of the testes. A significant minority of surgically castrated individuals continue to be able to have erections and to achieve ejaculation. Testosterone may be purchased by the sex offender in order to circumvent the function of their surgical castration.

REFERRAL

Refer to specialty mental health.

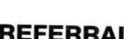

PEARLS & CONSIDERATIONS

- Pedophiles with no known risk of prior sexual contacts with children are at unknown risk to offend.
- Physicians should be aware of reporting requirements in their jurisdiction.

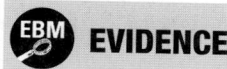

EVIDENCE

available at www.expertconsult.com

SUGGESTED READINGS

available at www.expertconsult.com

AUTHOR: **SARAH L. XAVIER, D.O.**

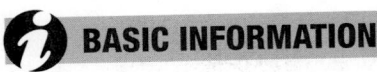

DEFINITION

Pelvic inflammatory disease (PID) is a spectrum of inflammatory disorders of the upper genital tract, including a combination of any of the following:
- Endometritis, salpingitis, tubo-ovarian abscess, or pelvic peritonitis
- Resulting from an ascending lower genital tract infection
- Not related to obstetric or surgical intervention

SYNONYMS

Adnexitis
Pyosalpinx
Salpingitis
Tubo-ovarian abscess

ICD-9CM CODES
614.9 Unspecified inflammatory disease of female pelvic organs and tissue

EPIDEMIOLOGY & DEMOGRAPHICS

INCIDENCE/PREVALENCE:
- Estimated 600,000 to 1 million cases annually (U.S.)
- Diagnosed in 2% to 5% of women seen in sexually transmitted disease clinics
- Most common cause of female infertility and ectopic pregnancy

RISK FACTORS:
- Adolescent sexually active females <20 yr (1:8)
- Previous episode of gonococcal PID
- Multiple sexual partners
- Vaginal douching

PHYSICAL FINDINGS & CLINICAL PRESENTATION
- Lower abdominal pain
- Abnormal vaginal discharge
- Abnormal uterine bleeding
- Dysuria
- Dyspareunia
- Nausea and vomiting (suggestive of peritonitis)
- Fever
- Right upper quadrant tenderness (perihepatitis): 5% of PID cases
- Cervical motion tenderness and adnexal tenderness
- Adnexal mass

ETIOLOGY
- *Chlamydia trachomatis*
- *Neisseria gonorrhoeae*
- Polymicrobial infection: *Bacteroides fragilis, Escherichia coli, Gardnerella vaginalis, Haemophilus influenzae, Mycoplasma hominis, Ureaplasma urealyticum*
- *Mycobacterium tuberculosis* (an important cause in developing countries)
- Cytomegalovirus (CMV)

DIAGNOSIS

DIFFERENTIAL DIAGNOSIS
- Ectopic pregnancy
- Appendicitis
- Ruptured ovarian cyst
- Endometriosis
- Urinary tract infection (cystitis or pyelonephritis)
- Renal calculus
- Adnexal torsion
- Proctocolitis

WORKUP
Diagnostic considerations:
- Clinical diagnosis is difficult and imprecise. A clinical algorithm for the evaluation of pelvic pain is described in Section III, "Pelvic Pain, Reproductive-Age Woman"; evaluation of vaginal discharge is described in Section III, "Vaginal Discharge."
- Clinical diagnosis of symptomatic PID has a positive predictive value of 65% to 90% compared with laparoscopy as the standard.
- No single historical, physical, or laboratory finding is both sensitive and specific for the diagnosis of PID.
- Empiric treatment for PID should be initiated in sexually active young women and other women at risk for STDs if they are experiencing pelvic or lower abdominal pain, if no cause for the illness other than PID can be identified, and if one or more of the following minimum criteria are present on pelvic examination:
  - Uterine tenderness
  - Adnexal tenderness
  - Cervical motion tenderness
- The requirement that all three minimum criteria be present before the initiation of empiric treatment could result in insufficient sensitivity for the diagnosis of PID. The presence of signs of lower genital tract inflammation (predominance of leukocytes in vaginal secretions, in addition to one of the three minimum criteria, increases the specificity of the diagnosis.
- Additional criteria to increase the specificity of the diagnosis of PID in women with severe clinical signs:
  - Oral temperature >38.3° C (101° F)
  - Abnormal cervical or vaginal discharge
  - Elevated erythrocyte sedimentation rate (ESR)
  - Elevated C-reactive protein
  - Laboratory documentation of cervical infection with *N. gonorrhoeae* or *C. trachomatis*
- Presence of abundant numbers of WBC on saline microscopy of vaginal fluid.
- Definitive criteria for diagnosing PID warranted in selected cases:
  - Laparoscopic abnormalities consistent with PID
  - Histopathologic evidence of endometritis on biopsy. Endometrial biopsy is warranted in women undergoing laparoscopy who do not have visual evidence of salpingitis because endometritis is the only sign of PID in some women
  - Transvaginal sonography or other imaging techniques showing thickened fluid-filled tubes with or without free pelvic fluid or tubo-ovarian complex

LABORATORY TESTS
- Leukocytosis
- Elevated acute phase reactants: ESR >15 mm/hr, C-reactive protein
- Gram stain of endocervical exudate: >30 polymorphonuclear cells per high-power field correlates with chlamydial or gonococcal infection
- Endocervical cultures for *N. gonorrhoeae* and *C. trachomatis*
- Fallopian tube aspirate or peritoneal exudate culture if laparoscopy performed
- Human chorionic gonadotropin to rule out ectopic pregnancy

IMAGING STUDIES
- Transvaginal ultrasound to look for adnexal mass has sensitivity for PID of 81%, specificity of 78%, and accuracy of 80%.
- MRI has sensitivity for PID of 95%, specificity of 89%, and accuracy of 93%. It is useful for establishing the diagnosis of PID and detecting other processes responsible for the symptoms. Disadvantages are its higher cost and unavailability in certain areas.

TREATMENT

NONPHARMACOLOGIC THERAPY
- Most patients are treated as outpatients.
- Criteria for hospitalization (CDC, 2006) as follows:
  - Surgical emergencies such as appendicitis cannot be excluded
  - Tubo-ovarian abscess
  - Pregnant patient
  - Patient is immunodeficient
  - Severe illness, nausea, or vomiting precluding outpatient management
  - Patient unable to follow or tolerate outpatient regimens
  - No clinical response to outpatient therapy

ACUTE GENERAL Rx

Regimens for treatment of PID should also be effective against *N. gonorrhoeae* and *C. trachomatis* because endocervical screening for these organisms does not rule out upper reproductive tract infections.

Recommended parenteral regimen A
- Cefotetan 2 g IV q12h
  OR
- Cefoxitin 2 g IV q6h
  PLUS
- Doxycycline 100 mg PO or IV q12h

Recommended parental regimen B
- Clindamycin 900 mg IV q8h
  PLUS
- Gentamicin loading dose IV or IM (2 mg/kg of body weight), followed by a maintenance dose (1.5 mg/kg) q8h. Single daily dosing (3 to 5 mg/kg) can be substituted.

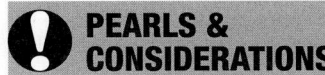

Alternative parenteral regimens
- Ampicillin/sulbactam 3 g IV q6h
  PLUS
- Doxycycline 100 mg PO or IV q12h

OUTPATIENT ORAL TREATMENT:
Recommended regimen
- Ceftriaxone 250 mg IM in a single dose
  PLUS
- Doxycycline 100 mg PO bid for 14 days
  WITH or WITHOUT
- Metronidazole 500 mg PO bid for 14 days
  OR
- Cefoxitin 2 g IM in a single dose and Proben-ecid, 1 g PO administered concurrently in a single dose
  PLUS
- Doxycycline 100 mg PO bid for 14 days
  WITH or WITHOUT
- Metronidazole 500 mg PO bid for 14 days
  OR
- Other parenteral third-generation cephalo-sporin (e.g., ceftizoxime or cefotaxime)
  PLUS

- Doxycycline 100 mg PO bid for 14 days
  WITH or WITHOUT
- Metronidazole 500 mg PO bid for 14 days

CHRONIC Rx

Hospitalized patients receiving IV therapy:
1. Significant clinical improvement is char-acterized by defervescence, decreased abdominal tenderness, and decreased uterine, adnexal, and cervical motion ten-derness within 3 to 5 days.
2. If no clinical improvement occurs, further diagnostic workup is necessary, including possible surgical intervention.

DISPOSITION
- Long-term sequelae of PID: recurrent PID, chronic pelvic pain, ectopic pregnancy, infer-tility, Fitz-Hugh-Curtis syndrome (Fig. 1-280)
- Risk of tubal infertility related to episodes of PID: first episode, 8%; second episode, 20%; third episode, 40%

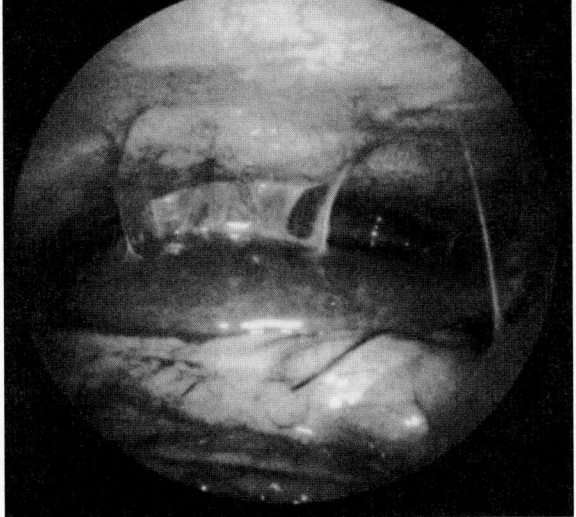

FIGURE 1-280 "Violin string" adhesions are visualized in this patient with Fitz-Hugh-Curtis syndrome. (From Copeland LJ: *Textbook of gynecology,* ed 2, Philadelphia, 2000, WB Saunders.)

- Essential to evaluate and treat male sex part-ners

REFERRAL

If there is no clinical improvement with outpa-tient therapy observed within 72 hr, patient should be hospitalized and gynecology consult requested.

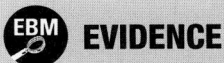
PEARLS & CONSIDERATIONS

COMMENTS
- Maintain a low threshold for the diagnosis of PID.
- Women with documented chlamydial or gonococcal infections have a high rate of re-infection within 6 mo of treatment. Repeat testing of all women who have been diag-nosed with chlamydia or gonorrhea is recom-mended 3 to 6 mo after treatment, regardless of whether their sex partners were treated.
- All women diagnosed with acute PID should be offered HIV testing.
- Male sex partners of women with PID should be examined and treated if they had sexual contact with the patient during 60 days pre-ceding the patient's onset of symptoms. If a patient's last sexual intercourse was >60 days before onset of symptoms or diagnosis, the patient's most recent sex partner should be treated.
- Patients should be instructed to abstain from sexual intercourse until therapy is completed and until they and their sex partners no lon-ger have symptoms.

EBM EVIDENCE

available at www.expertconsult.com

SUGGESTED READING

available at www.expertconsult.com

AUTHORS: **GEORGE T. DANAKAS, M.D.,** and **RUBEN ALVERO, M.D.**

P

Diseases and Disorders

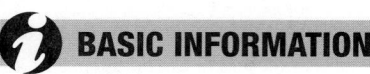

DEFINITION

Pelvic organ prolapse or uterine prolapse refers to the protrusion of the uterus into or out of the vaginal canal. In a first-degree uterine prolapse, the cervix is visible when the perineum is depressed. In a second-degree uterine prolapse, the uterine cervix has prolapsed through the vaginal introitus, with the fundus remaining within the pelvis proper. In a third-degree uterine prolapse (i.e., complete uterine prolapse, uterine procidentia), the entire uterus is outside the introitus. Table 1-141 compares the various types of prolapse.

SYNONYMS

Genital prolapse
Uterine descensus
Uterine prolapse
POP

ICD-9CM CODES
618.8 Genital prolapse
618.1 Uterine descensus
618.8 Pelvic organ prolapse

EPIDEMIOLOGY & DEMOGRAPHICS

PREVALENCE: Most prevalent in postmenopausal multiparous women.
RISK FACTORS:
- Pregnancy, especially POP symptoms during pregnancy
- Labor
- Vaginal childbirth
- Obesity
- Chronic coughing
- Constipation
- Pelvic tumors
- Ascites
- Strenuous physical exertion, especially during pregnancy
- Maternal history of prolapse
- Caucasian race
GENETICS: Increased incidence in women with spina bifida occulta.

PHYSICAL FINDINGS & CLINICAL PRESENTATION

- Pelvic pressure
- Bearing-down sensation
- Bilateral groin pain
- Sacral backache
- Coital difficulty
- Protrusion from vagina
- Spotting
- Ulceration
- Bleeding
- Examination of patient in lithotomy, sitting, and standing positions and before, during, and after a maximum Valsalva effort
- Erosion or ulceration of the cervix possible in the most dependent area of the protrusion

ETIOLOGY

- Vaginal childbirth and chronic increases in intraabdominal pressure leading to detach-ments, lacerations, and denervations of the vaginal support system
- Further weakening of pelvic support system by hypoestrogenic atrophy
- Direct injury to the levator ani, neurologic injury from stretching of the pudendal nerves
- Some cases from congenital or inherited weaknesses within the pelvic support system
- Neonatal uterine prolapse mostly coexistent with congenital spinal defects

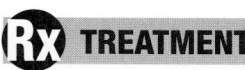 **DIAGNOSIS**

DIFFERENTIAL DIAGNOSIS

- Occasionally, elongated cervix; body of the uterus remains undescended.
- Diagnosis is based on history and physical examination. Currently there is only one genital tract prolapse classification system that has attained international acceptance and recognition: the patient pelvic organ prolapse quantification (POP-Q) (Boxes 1-12 and 1-13).

WORKUP

- If erosion or ulceration of the cervix is present, a Pap smear followed by a cervical biopsy should be performed if indicated.
- If urinary symptoms are significant, further urodynamic workup is indicated, looking for concurrent cystourethrocele, cystocele, enterocele, or rectocele.

LABORATORY TESTS

Urine culture

IMAGING STUDIES

Ultrasound if concurrent fibroids need further evaluation

TREATMENT

NONPHARMACOLOGIC THERAPY
- Prophylactic measures
  1. Diagnosis and treatment of chronic respiratory and metabolic disorders

---

TABLE 1-141   Types of Genital Prolapse

Original Position of Organs	Prolapse	Symptoms (in addition to the general symptoms of discomfort, dragging, the feeling of a 'lump' and, rarely, coital problems)
Anterior	Urethrocele Cystocele	Urinary symptoms (stress incontinence, urinary frequency)
Central	Cervix/uterus: 1st, 2nd, and 3rd degree Procidentia	Bleeding and/or discharge from ulceration in association with procidentia
Posterior	Rectocele Enterocele	Bowel symptoms, particularly the feeling of incomplete evacuation and sometimes having to press the posterior wall backwards to pass stool

From Drife J, Magowan B: *Clinical obstetrics and gynaecology,* Philadelphia, 2004, Saunders.

BOX 1-12   Staging of Pelvic Organ Prolapse Based on POP-Q Examination

Stage 0	No prolapse.
Stage I	Most distal prolapse >1 cm above hymenal ring.
Stage II	Most distal point is ≤1 cm above hymenal ring.
Stage III	Most distal point is >1 cm below the hymenal ring but not farther than 2 cm less than the total vaginal length (TVL) (i.e., ≥1 cm but ≤ (TVL − 2) cm.
Stage IV	Complete vaginal eversion.

From Pemberton J (ed): *The pelvic floor,* Philadelphia, 2002, WB Saunders.

BOX 1-13   Points of Reference for POP-Q

Point A: 3 cm above the hymen on anterior vaginal wall (Aa) or posterior vaginal wall (Ap). Point Aa roughly corresponds with the urethrovesical junction. These points can range from −3 cm (no prolapse) to +3 cm (maximal prolapse).
Point B: The lowest extent of the segment of vagina between point A and the apex of the vagina. Unlike point A, it is not fixed but will be the same as A if point A is the most protruding point. In maximal prolapse it will be the same as point C.
Point C: The most distal part of the cervix or vaginal vault.
Point D: The posterior fornix, which is omitted in women with prior hysterectomy.
Genital hiatus: From midline external urethral meatus to inferior hymenal ring.
Perineal body: From inferior hymenal ring to middle of anal orifice.
Vaginal length: This should be measured without undue stretching of the vagina.

From Pemberton J (ed): *The pelvic floor,* Philadelphia, 2002, WB Saunders.

2. Correction of constipation
3. Weight control, nutrition, and smoking cessation counseling
4. Teaching of pelvic muscle exercises
- Supportive pessary therapy
  1. Ring-type pessary useful for first- or second-degree prolapse
  2. Gellhorn pessary preferred for more advanced prolapse
  3. Use of pessaries in conjunction with continuous hormone replacement therapy, unless contraindicated
  4. Perineorrhaphy under local anesthesia possibly needed to support the pessary if the vaginal outlet is very relaxed

ACUTE GENERAL Rx

- Patients who are only infrequently symptomatic: insertion of a tampon or diaphragm for temporary relief when prolonged standing is anticipated
- Neonatal uterine prolapse: simple digital reduction or the use of a small pessary

CHRONIC Rx

- Hormone replacement therapy at the time of menopause helps preserve tissue strength, maintain elasticity of the vagina, and promote the durability of surgical repairs.
- Gold standard for therapy is vaginal hysterectomy.
- Vaginal apex should be well suspended, but a prophylactic sacrospinous ligament fixation is not routinely required.
- If occult enterocele present, McCall culdoplasty is performed.
- If vaginal approach to hysterectomy is contraindicated, abdominal hysterectomy is performed; vaginal apex likewise well supported.
- Colpocleisis is considered for the elderly patient who is sexually inactive and is a high-risk patient from a surgical point of view; can be done rapidly under local anesthesia with mild sedation if necessary.
- For symptomatic women who desire childbearing: management with pessaries or pelvic muscle exercises is recommended; if surgical correction is required, transvaginal sacrospinous fixation is the preferred method.
- Other surgical options are sling operations and sacral cervicopexy.

DISPOSITION

If untreated, uterine prolapse progressively worsens.

REFERRAL

To a gynecologist/urologist if pessary fitting or surgical intervention is needed

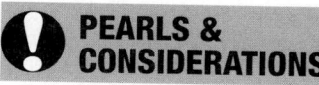

PEARLS & CONSIDERATIONS

COMMENTS

Surgery contraindicated in mild or asymptomatic uterine prolapse because the patient will seldom benefit from the operation although exposed to its risks.

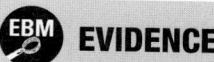

EVIDENCE

available at www.expertconsult.com

SUGGESTED READINGS

available at www.expertconsult.com

AUTHORS: **ARUNDATHI G. PRASAD, M.D.,** and **RUBEN ALVERO, M.D.**

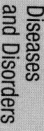

Diseases and Disorders

P

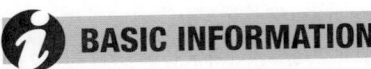
BASIC INFORMATION

DEFINITION

- Pemphigus refers to a group of rare, potentially fatal, chronic, autoimmune blistering diseases of the skin and mucous membranes
- Pemphigus has four main subtypes:
  1. Pemphigus vulgaris (PV) (most common) (Fig. 1-281)
     - Pemphigus vegetans, a rare clinical variant of PV
  2. Pemphigus foliaceus (PF)
     - Pemphigus erythematosus, a variant of PF
  3. Paraneoplastic pemphigus
  4. Immunoglobulin (Ig) A pemphigus

SYNONYMS

Pemphigus
Fogo selvagem: endemic pemphigus foliaceus
Senear-Usher syndrome: pemphigus erythematosus

ICD-9CM CODES
694.4 Pemphigus

EPIDEMIOLOGY & DEMOGRAPHICS

- Incidence is approximately one case per 100,000 persons and varies substantially by geographic region.
- More common in Ashkenazi Jews and people of Middle Eastern descent.
- Typically occurs in the fourth and fifth decades of life, though range of ages affected is broad and may occur in the very young or elderly.
- No gender predilection.

PHYSICAL FINDINGS & CLINICAL PRESENTATION

- History:
  1. Multiple oropharyngeal ulcerations and erosions typically occur first, which can then be followed by a more generalized bullous eruption involving the skin within several weeks or months
  2. Blisters are fragile and rupture easily, leaving painful erosions and ulcerations that may be the predominant clinical finding
  3. Pain associated with oral mucosal blistering often results in dysphagia and hoarseness
  4. Not commonly pruritic
- Physical findings:
  1. Anatomic distribution
     a. Oral mucosa
     b. Can also involve the pharynx, larynx, vagina, penis, anus, and conjunctival mucosa
     c. Generalized cutaneous involvement (Figs. 1-282 and 1-283)
  2. Lesion configuration
     a. Any stratified squamous epithelial surfaces can become involved
  3. Lesion morphology
     a. Flaccid bullae and vesicles
     b. Erosion with crusting commonly occurs

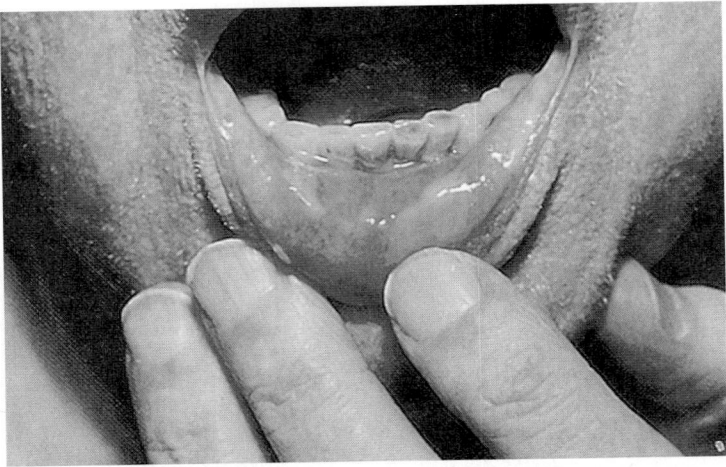

FIGURE 1-281 Pemphigus vulgaris with oral lesions and no intact bullae. (Courtesy Department of Dermatology, University of North Carolina at Chapel Hill. From Goldstein BG, Goldstein AO: *Practical dermatology,* ed 2, St Louis, 1997, Mosby.)

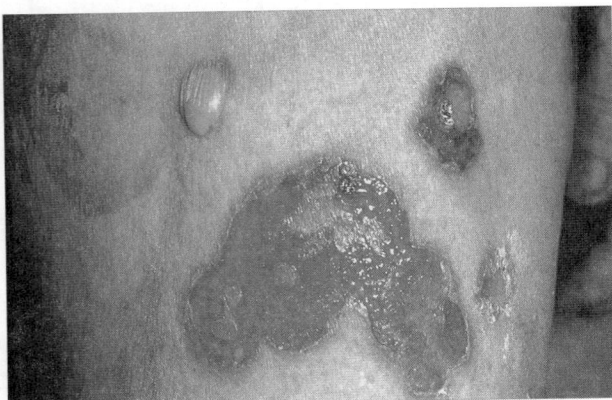

FIGURE 1-282 Pemphigus vulgaris; extensive erosions and blisters are present on the shin. (Courtesy R. A. Marsden, M.D., St. George's Hospital, London. From McKee PH et al [eds]: *Pathology of the skin with clinical correlations,* ed 3, St Louis, 2005, Mosby.)

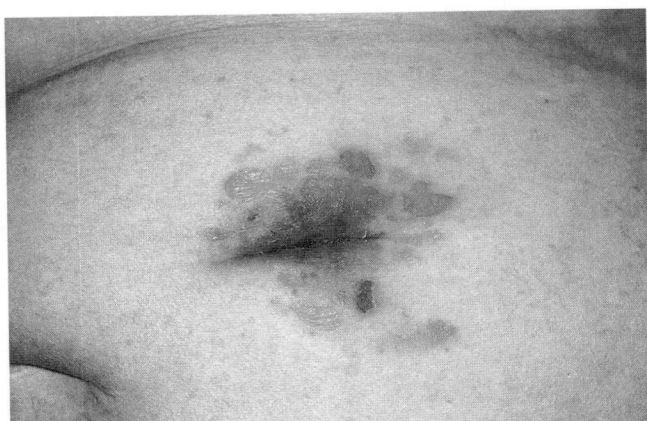

FIGURE 1-283 Pemphigus vulgaris: umbilical lesions showing intact blisters as well as raw erosions. (Courtesy R. A. Marsden, M.D., St. George's Hospital, London. From McKee PH et al [eds]: *Pathology of the skin with clinical correlations,* ed 3, St Louis, 2005, Mosby.)

4. Positive Nikolsky sign: when the clinician applies lateral pressure to normal-appearing skin at the periphery of active lesions, separation of the superficial epidermis occurs

ETIOLOGY

Autoimmune disease caused by autoantibodies against the cell surface of keratinocytes. The predominant antibody in PV is directed against desmoglein 3; in PF it is directed against desmoglein 1.

DIAGNOSIS

The diagnosis of pemphigus vulgaris should be suspected in patients with painful oral erosions and flaccid bullae or erosions on the skin.

DIFFERENTIAL DIAGNOSIS

- Bullous pemphigoid (Table 1-142)
- Cicatricial pemphigoid
- Behçet's syndrome
- Erythema multiforme
- Hailey-Hailey disease
- Aphthous stomatitis
- Bullous lupus erythematosus
- Drug eruptions

WORKUP

Skin biopsy is diagnostic; specimens should be sent for routine histochemical staining and direct immunofluorescence. Certain laboratory values may also be useful in establishing the diagnosis of pemphigus.

LABORATORY TESTS

- Skin biopsy reveals intraepidermal vesicles, also called *acantholysis* (loss of cell adhesion between the epidermal cells).

- Indirect immunofluorescence may detect circulating autoantibodies.
- Direct immunofluorescence studies of perilesional skin demonstrate IgG directed against keratinocyte surfaces in the epidermis.

Rx TREATMENT

NONPHARMACOLOGIC THERAPY

- Mild soaps and emollients to skin
- Burow's solution may be useful for weeping erosions
- Soft diet and viscous lidocaine can be used in patients with oral lesions

ACUTE GENERAL Rx

- For localized disease, topical steroids may be effective
- For generalized disease, systemic corticosteroids (prednisone) are the mainstay of therapy and often work rapidly to halt blistering
  - Initial dose of prednisone is usually 1 mg/kg/day, then tapered over weeks as blistering decreases
  - Steroid-sparing immunosuppressive therapies are often initiated simultaneously with prednisone to minimize the side effects of prolonged corticosteroid therapy

CHRONIC Rx

- Adjuvant therapy such as immunosuppressants, anti-inflammatories, chemotherapeutic agents, and biologics are useful for disease control and to shorten the length of treatment with oral steroids; treatment duration and dosing are determined by clinical response:
  1. Azathioprine 50 to 100 mg/day
  2. Cyclophosphamide 1 to 3 mg/kg/day
  3. Mycophenolate mofetil 500 mg to 2 g daily

- Refractory disease:
  1. IV Ig
  2. Rituximab (anti-CD20 monoclonal antibody)
  3. Plasmapheresis

DISPOSITION

- Before the use of oral corticosteroids, pemphigus was usually a fatal disease with most patients dying within 5 yr of diagnosis
- Combined corticosteroids and adjuvant therapy has decreased mortality rates to <10%
- Death generally occurs from sepsis or complications related to medical therapy

REFERRAL

Dermatology
Otolaryngology

PEARLS & CONSIDERATIONS

COMMENTS

- PV, unlike bullous pemphigoid, is a disease of middle-aged persons
- Early diagnosis of pemphigus is important to initiate prompt treatment
- Oral corticosteroids have many substantial side effects, and patients should be monitored for osteoporosis, hypertension, and diabetes

SUGGESTED READINGS
available at www.expertconsult.com

AUTHORS: **JESSICA RISSER, M.D., M.P.H.,** and **KACHIU LEE, B.A.**

TABLE 1-142	Differentiation of Pemphigus Vulgaris and Bullous Pemphigoid	
Characteristics	**Pemphigus Vulgaris**	**Bullous Pemphigoid**
Age	Usually occurs in middle aged persons	>60 yr
Site	Oral mucosa, face, chest, groin	Flexural areas, groin, axilla; less often involving mucosal surfaces
Findings	Flaccid bullae and erosions, intraepidermal blisters, IgG autoantibodies against keratinocyte surfaces	Intact bullae, subepidermal blisters, IgG autoantibodies against hemidesmosomal antigens
Treatment	Prednisone 1 mg/kg/day with adjuvant immunosuppressant agents; refractory disease may require IV Ig, plasmapheresis or rituximab	Prednisone 1 mg/kg/day with adjuvant immunosuppressant therapy; localized disease may be controlled with topical steroids
Prognosis	>90% respond; steroid side effects significant	>90% respond; remissions and recurrences common

Ig, Immunoglobulin; *IV,* intravenous.

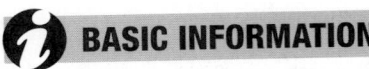

BASIC INFORMATION

DEFINITION

Peptic ulcer disease (PUD) is an ulceration in the stomach or duodenum resulting from an imbalance between mucosal protective factors and various mucosal damaging mechanisms (see "Etiology").

SYNONYMS

PUD
Duodenal ulcer (DU)
Gastric ulcer (GU)

ICD-9CM CODES
536.8 Peptic ulcer disease
531.3 Peptic ulcer, stomach, acute
531.7 Peptic ulcer, stomach, chronic
532.3 Peptic ulcer, duodenum, acute
532.7 Peptic ulcer, duodenum, chronic

EPIDEMIOLOGY & DEMOGRAPHICS

- Incidence: 250,000 to 500,000 (200,000 to 400,000 duodenal; 50,000 to 100,000 gastric) annually; duodenal ulcer/gastric ulcer ratio is 4:1.
- Anatomic location: >90% of duodenal ulcers occur in the first portion of the duodenum; gastric ulcers occur most frequently in the lesser curvature near the incisura angularis.

PHYSICAL FINDINGS & CLINICAL PRESENTATION

- Physical examination is often unremarkable.
- Patient may have epigastric tenderness, tachycardia, pallor, hypotension (from acute or chronic blood loss), nausea and vomiting (if pyloric channel is obstructed), boardlike abdomen and rebound tenderness (if perforated), and hematemesis or melena (with a bleeding ulcer).

ETIOLOGY

Often multifactorial. The following are common mucosal damaging factors:

- *Helicobacter pylori* infection. *H. pylori* is the major cause of peptic ulcer disease. It is found in more than 70% of patients with duodenal ulcers and gastric ulcers in the U.S. Rates are much higher (>90%) in other parts of the world. Eradication of *H. pylori* markedly reduces peptic ulcer recurrence.
- Medications (nonsteroidal anti-inflammatory drugs [NSAIDs], glucocorticoids). Risk factors for development of NSAID-related ulcers are described in Table 1-143
- Incompetent pylorus or lower esophageal sphincter
- Bile acids
- Impaired proximal duodenal bicarbonate secretion
- Decreased blood flow to gastric mucosa
- Acid secreted by parietal cells and pepsin secreted as pepsinogen by chief cells
- Cigarette smoking
- Alcohol

DIAGNOSIS

DIFFERENTIAL DIAGNOSIS

- Gastroesophageal reflux disease
- Cholelithiasis syndrome
- Pancreatitis
- Gastritis
- Nonulcer dyspepsia
- Neoplasm (gastric carcinoma, lymphoma, pancreatic carcinoma)
- Angina pectoris, myocardial infarction, pericarditis
- Dissecting aneurysm
- Other: high small-bowel obstruction, pneumonia, subphrenic abscess, early appendicitis

WORKUP

Comprehensive history and physical examination to exclude other diagnoses. Diagnostic modalities include endoscopy or upper gastrointestinal (GI) series. Endoscopy is preferred.

LABORATORY TESTS

- Routine laboratory evaluation is usually unremarkable.
- Anemia may be present in patients with significant GI bleeding.
- *H. pylori* testing by endoscopic biopsy, urea breath test, stool antigen test (*H. pylori* stool antigen), or specific antibody test is recommended:
  1. Serologic testing for antibodies to *H. pylori* is easy and inexpensive; however, the presence of antibodies demonstrates previous but not necessarily current infection. Antibodies to *H. pylori* can remain elevated for months to years after infection has cleared; therefore antibody levels must be interpreted in light of the patient's symptoms and other test results (e.g., PUD seen on upper GI series).
  2. The urea breath test documents active infection (sensitivity and specificity >90%). The patient ingests a small amount of urea labeled with carbon 13 or carbon 14. If urease is present (produced

---

TABLE 1-143 Risk Factors for Development of NSAID-Related Ulcers

Definite

Advanced age
History of ulcer
Concomitant corticosteroid therapy
Concomitant anticoagulation therapy
High doses of NSAIDs
Serious systemic disorders

Possible

Concomitant infection with *Helicobacter pylori*
Cigarette smoking
Consumption of alcohol

NSAIDs, Nonsteroidal anti-inflammatory drugs.
Andreoli, TE et al: *Andreoli and Carpenter's Cecil essentials of medicine*, ed 8, Philadelphia, 2010, Saunders.

---

by the organism), the urea is hydrolyzed and the patient exhales labeled carbon dioxide that is then collected and measured. This test is more expensive and not as readily available. Use of proton pump inhibitors (PPI) within 2 wk of the urea breath test may interfere with test results. Recently a new card test for ^{14}C urea has been developed, providing a testing option in primary care settings. It uses a flat breath card that is read by a small analyzer.

3. Histologic evaluation of endoscopic biopsy samples is considered by many the gold standard for accurate diagnosis of *H. pylori* infection. However, detection of *H. pylori* depends on the site and number of biopsy samples, the method of staining, and experience of the pathologist.

4. Stool antigen test is an enzyme-linked immunosorbent assay (ELISA) that identifies *H. pylori* antigen in a stool specimen through a polyclonal anti–*H. pylori* antibody. It is as accurate as the urea breath test for diagnosis of active infection and follow-up evaluation of patients treated for *H. pylori*. A negative result on the stool antigen test 8 wk after completion of therapy identifies patients in whom eradication of *H. pylori* was unsuccessful.

- Additional laboratory evaluation is indicated only in specific cases (e.g., amylase level in suspected pancreatitis, serum gastrin level in suspected Zollinger-Ellison [ZE] syndrome).

IMAGING STUDIES

Conventional upper GI barium studies identify approximately 70% to 80% of PUD; accuracy can be increased to approximately 90% by using double contrast.

TREATMENT

NONPHARMACOLOGIC THERAPY

- Stop smoking; smoking increases the risk of PUD, decreases the healing rate, and increases the frequency of recurrence.
- Avoid NSAIDs and alcohol.
- Special diets have been proved unrelated to ulcer development and healing; however, avoid foods that cause symptoms.

ACUTE GENERAL Rx

Eradication of *H. pylori,* when present, can be accomplished with various regimens:

1. PPI (e.g., omeprazole 20 mg bid or lansoprazole 30 mg bid, esomeprazole 40 mg qd) *plus* clarithromycin 500 mg bid *and* amoxicillin 1000 mg bid for 10 days. This regimen achieves an eradication rate of 80% to 90% and can be used as first-line therapy for patients not allergic to penicillin.
2. PPI bid *plus* amoxicillin 500 mg bid *plus* metronidazole 500 mg bid for 10 days.
3. PPI bid *plus* clarithromycin 500 mg bid *and* metronidazole 500 mg bid for 10 days. This regimen is useful in those with penicillin allergy.

4. A 1-day quadruple therapy may be as effective as a 7-day triple-therapy regimen. The 1-day quadruple-therapy regimen consists of 2 tablets of 262-mg bismuth subsalicylate qid, 1 500-mg metronidazole tablet qid, 2 g of amoxicillin suspension qid, and 2 capsules of 30 mg of lansoprazole.
5. Bismuth compound qid *plus* tetracycline 500 mg qid *and* metronidazole 500 mg qid for 14 days.
6. A combination of levofloxacin 250 mg bid, amoxicillin 1000 mg bid, and a PPI bid for 10 to 14 days can be used as salvage therapy after unsuccessful attempts to eradicate *H. pylori* using other regimens.

A 10-day sequential therapy has been reported to be superior to standard triple therapy for eradication of *H. pylori*. It consists of 5 days of treatment with a PPI and one antibiotic (usually amoxicillin) followed by 5-day treatment with the PPI and two other antibiotics (usually clarithromycin and metronidazole).

PUD patients testing negative for *H. pylori* should be treated with antisecretory agents:
- H_2 receptor antagonists (H_2RAs): cimetidine, ranitidine, famotidine, and nizatidine are all effective; they are usually given in split dose or at nighttime.
- PPIs: can also induce rapid healing; they are usually given 30 min before meals.

Antacids and sucralfate are also effective agents for the treatment and prevention of PUD.

CHRONIC Rx

Maintenance therapy in duodenal ulcer patients is indicated in the following situations:
- Persistent smokers
- Recurrent ulcerations
- Long-term treatment with NSAIDs, glucocorticoids
- Elderly or debilitated patients
- Aggressive or complicated ulcer disease (e.g., perforation, hemorrhage)
- Asymptomatic bleeders

Misoprostol therapy (100 μg qid with food, increased to 200 μg qid if well tolerated) is useful for the prevention of NSAID-induced gastric ulcers in all patients on long-term NSAID therapy; it is contraindicated in women of childbearing age because of its abortifacient properties. PPIs are at least as effective as misoprostol and more effective than H2 receptor antagonists at healing ulcers and maintaining remission in patients on long-term NSAIDs.

DISPOSITION

- The recurrence rate for untreated PUD is ~60% (>70% in smokers). Treatment decreases the recurrence rate by nearly 30%.
- Patients with recurrent ulcers should be retreated for an additional 8 wk and then placed on maintenance therapy with H_2RAs, PPIs, sucralfate, or antacids.
- An ulcer is considered refractory to treatment if healing is not evident after 8 wk for duodenal ulcers and 12 wk for gastric ulcers. In these patients maximum acid inhibition (e.g., esomeprazole 40 mg bid) is preferred over continued therapy with standard antiulcer therapy.
- Eradication of *H. pylori* (when present) is indicated in all patients. A negative stool antigen test for *H. pylori* 6 wk after treatment accurately confirms cure of *H. pylori* infection with reasonable sensitivity in initially seropositive healthy subjects.
- Screening for ZE syndrome should also be considered in patients with multiple recurrent ulcers; in patients with ZE, the serum gastrin level is >1000 pg/ml and the basal acid output is usually >15 mEq/hr.
- Surgery for refractory ulcers is now only rarely performed; it consists of highly selective vagotomy for duodenal ulcers or ulcer removal with antrectomy or hemigastrectomy without vagotomy for gastric ulcers.

REFERRAL
- GI referral for patients requiring endoscopy
- Surgical referral for patients with nonhealing ulcers despite appropriate medical therapy

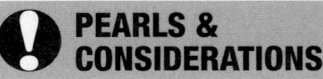 **PEARLS & CONSIDERATIONS**

COMMENTS
- Patients with gastric ulcers should have repeat endoscopy after 4 to 6 wk of therapy to document healing and test exfoliative cytology for gastric carcinoma.
- After endoscopic treatment of bleeding peptic ulcers, bleeding recurs in up to 20% of patients. PPI administration intravenously by continuous infusion substantially reduces the risk of recurrent bleeding. High-dose IV esomeprazole (80 mg IV bolus followed by 8 mg/hr infusion over 72 hr) given after successful endoscopic therapy to patients with high-risk peptic ulcer bleeding has been reported to reduce recurrent bleeding at 72 hr and to maintain sustained clinical benefits for up to 30 days.
- Among low-dose aspirin recipients who had peptic ulcer bleeding, continuous aspirin therapy may increase the risk for recurrent bleeding; however, mortality was reported higher among those who stopped aspirin therapy and were at risk for cardiovascular events

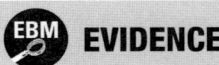 **EVIDENCE**

available at www.expertconsult.com

SUGGESTED READINGS
available at www.expertconsult.com

AUTHOR: **FRED F. FERRI, M.D.**

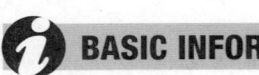

BASIC INFORMATION

DEFINITION

Pericarditis is the inflammation (or infiltration) of the pericardium associated with a wide variety of causes (see "Etiology").

ICD-9CM CODES
420.91 Pericarditis

EPIDEMIOLOGY & DEMOGRAPHICS

- The incidence of acute pericarditis is 2% to 6%.
- Increased incidence found in male and in adults compared with children.
- The use of thrombolytic agents and early revascularization have greatly reduced the incidence of both early postinfarction pericarditis and Dressler's syndrome.

PHYSICAL FINDINGS & CLINICAL PRESENTATION

- Severe, constant pain that localizes over the anterior chest and may radiate to arms and back; it can be differentiated from myocardial ischemia because in pericarditis the pain intensifies with inspiration and is relieved by sitting up and leaning forward (the pain of myocardial ischemia is typically neither pleuritic nor positional).
- A pericardial friction rub is a classic finding, although not present in all patients. It is best heard with the patient sitting up and leaning forward and by pressing the diaphragm of the stethoscope firmly against the chest at the lower left sternal border during inspiration. It is often confused with the pleural rub. The pericardial friction rub corresponds temporally to movement of the heart within the pericardial sac. Typically the rub is a high-pitched scratchy or squeaky sound heard best at the left sternal border at end expiration. It consists classically of three short, scratchy sounds:
  1. Systolic component
  2. Diastolic component
  3. Late diastolic component (associated with atrial contraction)
  However, in reality, the rub is reported to be triphasic in approximately half of patients, biphasic in a third, and monophasic in the remainder.
- Small pericardial effusions are common. Cardiac tamponade may occur as a complication of large or rapidly accumulating effusions. Classic tamponade findings include: hypotension, jugular venous distention, and muffled heart sounds (Beck's triad). In addition, tachycardia and pulsus paradoxus are usually present.

ETIOLOGY

- Most common cause (>40%) of pericarditis is idiopathic
- Infectious (viral, bacterial [1% to 2%], tuberculous [4%], fungal, amebic, toxoplasmosis)
- Collagen-vascular disease (systemic lupus erythematosus, rheumatoid arthritis, scleroderma, vasculitis, dermatomyositis): 3% to 5% of cases
- Drug-induced lupus syndrome (procainamide, hydralazine, phenytoin, isoniazid, rifampin, doxorubicin, mesalamine)
- Acute myocardial infarction (MI) (usually transmural MIs)
- Trauma or posttraumatic
- After MI (Dressler's syndrome. Usually 2 wk post MI)
- After pericardiotomy
- After mediastinal radiation (e.g., patients with Hodgkin's disease)
- Uremia
- Sarcoidosis
- Neoplasm (primary or metastatic [breast, lung, leukemia, lymphoma]): 7% of cases
- Leakage of aortic aneurysm into pericardial sac
- Familial Mediterranean fever
- Rheumatic fever
- Other: anticoagulants, amyloidosis, idiopathic thrombocytopenia purpura

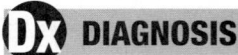

DIAGNOSIS

DIFFERENTIAL DIAGNOSIS
- Angina pectoris
- Pulmonary infarction
- Dissecting aneurysm
- Gastrointestinal abnormalities (e.g., hiatal hernia, esophageal rupture)
- Pneumothorax
- Hepatitis
- Cholecystitis
- Pneumonia with pleurisy

WORKUP

Diagnosis is clinical, based on history and physical examination. ECG may help confirm the diagnosis if typical changes are found. Laboratory tests may help on elucidating the potential cause, and an ECG may assist in ruling out significant pericardial effusion.

LABORATORY TESTS

Laboratory tests are generally not clinically helpful, and the clinical presentation should guide any ordering. Initial blood work should be limited to the following tests:
- Complete blood count with differential
- Erythrocyte sedimentation rate (not specific but may be of value in following the course of the disease and the response to therapy)
- Blood urea nitrogen, creatinine
- Troponin I (plasma troponins are elevated in 35% to 50% of patients with pericarditis, and indicate involvement of the myocardium, i.e., myopericarditis)
The following tests may be useful in the absence of an obvious cause:
- Viral titers (acute and convalescent)
- Antinuclear antibody, rheumatoid factor
- Purified protein derivative (PPD), antistreptolysin O titers
- Blood cultures

- Pericardiocentesis is indicated in patients with pericardial tamponade, in those with purulent pericarditis, or when a neoplastic origin is suspected. The fluid should be analyzed for red and white blood cell counts, cytology, glucose, lactate dehydrogenase, protein, pH, triglyceride level, and cultured. Polymerase chain reaction assays or elevated levels of adenosine deaminase activity (>30 U/L) are useful when suspecting tuberculous pericarditis.
- Pericardial biopsy may be helpful in recurrent pericardial effusion if the diagnosis remains elusive.

IMAGING STUDIES

- Echocardiogram to detect and determine amount of pericardial effusion; absence of effusion does not rule out the diagnosis of pericarditis. Variation in atrioventricular valve inflow with respiration is present in cardiac tamponade and constrictive pericarditis.
- ECG: the changes vary with the evolutionary stage of pericarditis:
  1. Acute phase: PR-segment depression and diffuse ST-segment elevations (particularly evident in the precordial leads), which can be distinguished from acute MI by:
     a. Absence of reciprocal ST-segment depression in oppositely oriented leads. Elevated ST segments concave upward
     b. Absence of Q waves
     c. Reciprocal PR elevation may be seen in aVR and V1
  2. Intermediate phase: return of PR and ST segments to baseline, and T-wave inversion in leads previously showing ST-segment elevation (Fig. 1-284)
  3. Late phase: resolution of the T-wave changes
- Chest radiograph: done primarily to rule out abnormalities of the mediastinum or lung fields that may be responsible for the pericarditis
  1. Cardiac silhouette appears enlarged if more than 250 ml of fluid has accumulated.
  2. Calcifications around the heart may be seen with constrictive pericarditis.

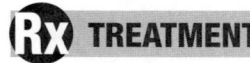

TREATMENT

NONPHARMACOLOGIC THERAPY
- Limitation of activity until the pain abates
- Patient education regarding potential complications (e.g., cardiac tamponade, constrictive pericarditis)

ACUTE GENERAL Rx
- NSAID therapy (e.g., ibuprofen 800 mg tid, naproxen 500 mg bid). NSAIDS are contraindicated and aspirin is preferred in patients with recent MI.
- Colchicine 0.6 mg bid may be used in combination or as an alternative to NSAIDs. There is evidence of colchicine being effective in both reducing symptoms and the rates of recur-

rent pericarditis. Its use is recommended for first episodes and recurrent disease.

- Use of corticosteroids is controversial. There is evidence of their use being associated with increased recurrence, side effects, and hospitalizations. The 2004 European Society of Cardiology guidelines recommend that systemic steroid therapy be restricted to patients with acute pericarditis caused by connective tissue disease, autoimmune-mediated pericarditis, and uremic pericarditis. One study found that using a lower dose (0.2 to 0.5 mg/kg per day) maintained for 4 weeks, and followed by a slow taper had same efficacy and fewer adverse effects.
- Close observation of patients when there is suspicion for cardiac tamponade.
- Avoidance of anticoagulants (increased risk of hemopericardium).

TREATMENT OF UNDERLYING CAUSE:
- Bacterial pericarditis: systemic antibiotics and surgical drainage of pericardium
- Collagen vascular disease and idiopathic: NSAIDs, prednisone
- Uremic: dialysis

POTENTIAL COMPLICATIONS FROM PERICARDITIS:
1. *Pericardial effusion:* the time required for pericardial effusion to develop is of critical importance. If the rate of accumulation is slow, the pericardium can gradually stretch and accommodate a large effusion (>1000 ml), whereas rapid accumulation can cause tamponade with as little as 200 ml of fluid.
2. Chronic constrictive pericarditis:
   a. Physical examination reveals jugular venous distention, Kussmaul's sign (increase in jugular venous distention during inspiration as a result of increased venous pressure), pericardial knock (early diastolic filling sound heard 0.06 to 0.1 sec after S2), clear lungs, tender hepatomegaly, pedal edema, ascites, scrotal edema, and possible anasarca.

b. Chest radiograph: clear lung fields, normal or slightly enlarged heart, pericardial calcification.
   c. ECG: low-voltage QRS complex.
   d. Echocardiography: may show respiratory inflow variation over the mitral and tricuspid valves (due to variations in the diastolic ventricular pressure gradients with respiration), pericardial thickening or may be normal.
   e. Cardiac catheterization to confirm elevation of right-sided filling pressures: shows a prominent y descent in the right atrial tracing, a "dip and plateau" tracing of the right ventricular pressure and discordance of right ventricular and left ventricular systolic pressures during respiration.
   f. Therapy: surgical stripping or removal of both layers of the constricting pericardium.
3. *Cardiac tamponade:* occurs in 15% of patients with idiopathic pericarditis but in nearly 60% of those with neoplastic, tuberculous, or purulent pericarditis.
   a. Signs and symptoms: dyspnea, orthopnea, interscapular pain.
   b. Physical examination: distended neck veins, distant heart sounds, decreased apical impulse, diaphoresis, tachypnea, tachycardia, Ewart's sign (an area of dullness at the angle of the left scapula caused by compression of the lungs by the pericardial effusion), pulsus paradoxus (decrease in systolic blood pressure >10 mm Hg during inspiration), hypotension, narrowed pulse pressure. Of all the clinical signs, a pulsus paradoxus >10 mm Hg in patients with pericardial effusion is the most specific for tamponade.
   c. Chest radiograph: cardiomegaly ("water-bottle" configuration of the cardiac silhouette may be seen) with clear lungs; the chest x-ray film may be normal when

acute tamponade occurs rapidly in the absence of prior pericardial effusion.
   d. ECG reveals decreased amplitude of the QRS complex, variation of the R-wave amplitude from beat to beat (electrical alternans). This results from the heart's oscillating motion in the pericardial sac from beat to beat and frequently occurs with neoplastic effusions.
   e. Echocardiography: may show diastolic collapse of the right ventricle and/or the right atrium, respiratory inflow variation over the mitral valve and tricuspid valve (due to transmission of respiratory changes in intrathoracic pressure to the ventricles), and a paradoxic wall motion may also be seen.
   f. Cardiac catheterization: equalization of pressures within chambers of the heart, elevation of right atrial pressure with a prominent x but no significant y descent.
   g. MRI can also be used to diagnose pericardial effusions.
   h. Therapy for pericardial tamponade consists of immediate pericardiocentesis, preferably by needle paracentesis with the use of echocardiography, fluoroscopy, or CT; in patients with recurrent effusions (e.g., neoplasms), placement of a percutaneous drainage catheter or pericardial window draining in the pleural cavity may be necessary.
4. Effusive-constrictive pericarditis:
   a. Uncommon pericardial syndrome characterized by concomitant tamponade caused by tense pericardial effusion and constriction caused by the visceral pericardium.
   b. Extensive epicardiectomy is the procedure of choice in symptomatic patients.

DISPOSITION
- Complete resolution of pain and other signs and symptoms during the initial 3 wk of therapy.
- Recurrence in 10% to 15% of patients within the initial 12 mo.
- Recurrent pericarditis in 28% of patients.
- Recurrence of large effusion after pericardiocentesis is common in patients with idiopathic chronic pericardial effusion. Pericardiectomy should be considered in these patients.
- Most cases of pericarditis can be treated in the outpatient setting. Indications for hospitalization are fever >38° C, immunosuppressed state, history of trauma, subacute onset, oral anticoagulant therapy, presence of myocarditis, large pericardial effusion, or tamponade.
- In patients with pericardial effusion after cardiac surgery, use of NSAIDs is not recommended because they have not been shown to reduce the size of the effusions or prevent late cardiac tamponade.

SUGGESTED READINGS
available at www.expertconsult.com

PERICARDITIS, EVOLVING PATTERN

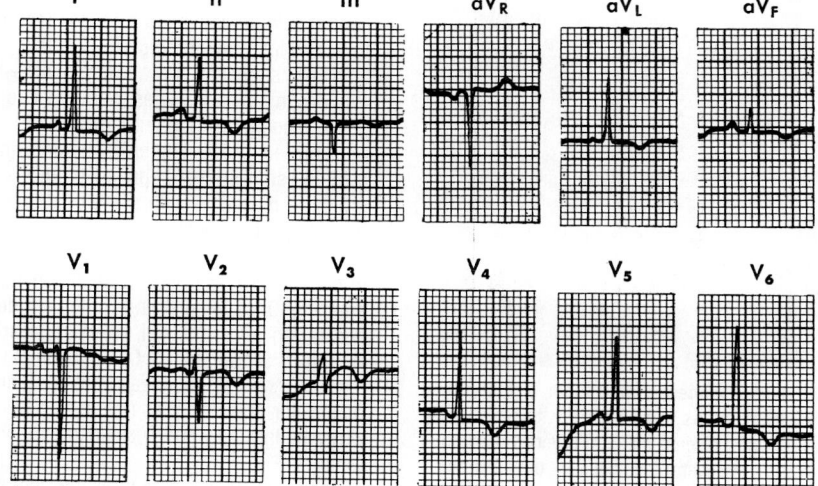

FIGURE 1-284 Note the diffuse T-wave inversions in leads I, II, III, aVL, aVF, and V2 to V6. (From Goldberg AL [ed]: *Clinical electrocardiography,* ed 5, St Louis, 1994, Mosby.)

AUTHORS: **GABRIEL A. DELGADO, M.D.,**
FRED F. FERRI, M.D., and
DAVID J. FORTUNATO, M.D., F.A.C.C.

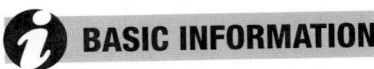

DEFINITION

Peripheral arterial disease (PAD) refers to atherosclerotic, occlusive, and aneurysmal diseases involving the abdominal aorta and its branch arteries. The following chapter focuses on PAD with an emphasis on infrainguinal disease, which is defined by atherosclerotic obstruction of the infrainguinal arteries of the legs, which reduce arterial blood flow during activity or rest.

SYNONYMS

Peripheral vascular disease (PVD)
Arteriosclerosis obliterans
Atherosclerotic occlusive disease
Atherosclerosis of the extremities
Peripheral arterial stenosis
Vaso-occlusive disease of the legs
Chronic critical limb ischemia

ICD-9CM CODES
443.9 Peripheral vascular disease

EPIDEMIOLOGY & DEMOGRAPHICS

- ~12% of the adult population has PAD, and the prevalence is equal in men and women. The prevalence of PAD increases with age: 2.5% in those aged 40 to 59 yr, 8.3% in those aged 60 to 69 yr, and 18.8% in those aged 70 to 79 yr.
- A prevalence of PAD up to 29% has been shown in those patients aged 50 to 69 yr who use tobacco or have diabetes. Cigarette smoking and diabetes mellitus are the strongest risk factors.
- Risk factors associated with PAD are similar to coronary artery disease, including tobacco use, diabetes, hyperlipidemia, hypertension, and advanced age.
- Nontraditional risk factors associated with increased prevalence of PAD include race and ethnicity (African Americans and those of Hispanic origin are at higher risk), chronic kidney disease, and the metabolic syndrome.
- Patients with newly diagnosed PAD are six times more likely to die within the next 10 yr when compared with patients without PAD.
- An inverse relationship has been suggested between PAD and alcohol consumption.
- In 2006, the American College of Cardiology/American Heart Association (ACC/AHA) suggested that the following individuals would be at risk from lower-extremity PAD:
  - Age <50 yr, with diabetes and one other atherosclerosis risk factor (smoking, dyslipidemia, hypertension, or hyperhomocysteinemia)
  - Ages 50 to 69 yr and history of smoking or diabetes
  - Age 70 yr or older
  - Symptoms with exertion involving the lower extremities (suggestive of claudication) or ischemic rest pain
  - Abnormal lower extremity pulse examination
  - Known atherosclerotic coronary, carotid, or renal artery disease

PHYSICAL FINDINGS & CLINICAL PRESENTATION

PAD is a largely under-diagnosed and untreated condition given that nearly 50% of patients with PAD are asymptomatic. Approximately one third of patients with PAD present with intermittent claudication, described as an aching, pain, cramping, or numbness in the calf and, less likely, in the lower thigh or arch of the foot. Symptoms are brought on by exertion and relieved by rest. However, patients often present with atypical symptoms of claudication involving the calf, thigh, or buttock making diagnosis difficult.

Individuals who present with symptoms associated with PAD often present with one or more of the following complaints or findings:
- Painful cramping in buttocks, hip, or leg that occurs while walking but goes away while resting
- Diminished pedal pulses
- Bruits heard over the distal aorta, iliac, or femoral arteries
- Changes in skin color, especially on feet (rubor with prolonged capillary refill on dependency or delayed pallor)
- Cool skin temperature
- Trophic changes of hair loss, brittle nails, and muscle atrophy
- Nonhealing ulcers (Fig. 1-285), necrotic tissue, and gangrene
- Weakness, numbness, or a feeling of heaviness in legs
- Aching or burning in toes and feet during rest and especially while lying flat, which may be a sign of ischemia and more serious PAD

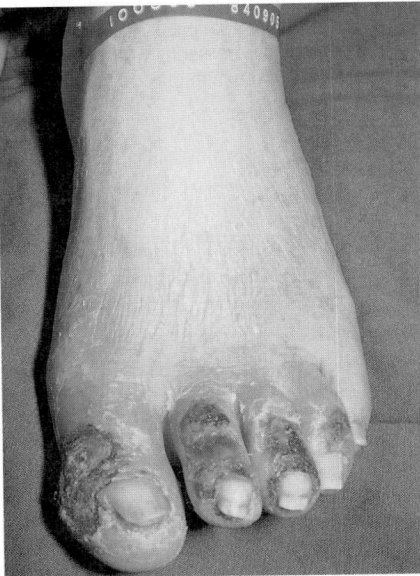

FIGURE 1-285 Ischemic skin ulcer induced by trauma from shoes. This patient with peripheral arterial occlusive disease suffered severe superficial skin necrosis of several toes because of shoes that were too tight. (From Crawford MH et al [eds]: *Cardiology,* ed 2, St Louis, 2004, Mosby.)

ETIOLOGY

PAD is primarily the result of an atherosclerotic process with formation of atherosclerotic plaques. The atheroma, or plaque, consists of a lipid core of cholesterol and inflammatory mediators with a fibrous intravascular covering. The disease typically is segmental, with significant variation, and may gradually progress to complete occlusion. Symptoms of claudication are a product of physiologically significant luminal stenoses of the peripheral vessels, limiting blood flow to limb muscles.

DIAGNOSIS

DIFFERENTIAL DIAGNOSIS

- Spinal stenosis
- Musculoskeletal disorder
- Lumbar spinal stenosis or nerve root compression (neurogenic or pseudoclaudication)
- Peripheral neuropathy
- Reflex sympathetic dystrophy
- Raynaud's disease
- Compartment syndrome

WORKUP

A thorough history and physical examination are critical for evaluating and diagnosing the etiology of lower-extremity pain. Since the differential of lower-extremity pain is relatively broad, careful questioning of symptom onset, duration, and intensity is critical to obtaining an accurate diagnosis. Physical examination for identification of PAD should include assessment of all the major arterial trees in each extremity:
- Measurement of blood pressure in both arms and notation of asymmetry.
- Palpation and recording of carotid pulses, upstroke, amplitude, and presence of bruits.
- Auscultation and palpation of abdomen for bruits, aortic pulsation, and diameter.
- Palpation of brachial, radial, ulnar, femoral, popliteal, dorsalis pedis, and posterior tibial pulses. Pulse intensity should be recorded as follows: 0, absent; 1+, diminished; 2+, normal; 3+, bounding.
- Auscultation of femoral arteries for the presence of bruits.
- Feet should be inspected for color, temperature, and integrity of the skin.
- Findings suggestive of severe PAD—hair loss, trophic skin changes, and hypertrophic nails—should be sought and recorded.
- Measurement of resting ankle-brachial index (ABI) to establish the diagnosis of PAD is appropriate in people with symptoms of exertional leg pain or nonhealing wounds who are aged 70 yr or older; or in people aged 50 yr or older with a history of diabetes mellitus or smoking. Once the presence of PAD is identified by an abnormal ABI, exercise treadmill testing is recommended. Comparison of resting and exercise ABI measurements can be helpful for objectively characterizing the severity of the individual's claudication symptoms.
- ABI also subjectively measures the severity of functional limitations related to the claudica-

tion. Postexercise ABI measurements can be especially useful in individuals with symptoms of intermittent claudication who have a normal resting ABI.

- Individuals with asymptomatic lower extremity PAD should be identified by examination and/or measurement of the ABI so that therapeutic interventions known to diminish their risk of cardiovascular disease, myocardial infarction, or stroke may be initiated.
- The ABI is calculated by dividing the highest ankle systolic pressure using either the dorsalis pedis or posterior tibial artery (in each leg) by the highest brachial systolic pressure from either arm. A normal ABI is 0.90 to 1.30.
- A diagnosis of PAD is based on the presence of limb symptoms or a low ABI.
- The lower the ABI the worse the prognosis.
- The severity of PAD is based on the ABI at rest and during treadmill exercise (1 to 2 mph, 5 min, or symptom limited). It is classified as follows:
  - Mild: ABI at rest 0.71 to 0.90 or ABI during exercise 0.50 to 0.90
  - Moderate: ABI at rest 0.41 to 0.70 or ABI during exercise 0.20 to 0.50
  - Severe: ABI at rest <0.40 or ABI during exercise <0.20
- An ABI >1.30 is an indication of vessel calcification. If the ABI is >1, then obtain a toe brachial index since there is no medial calci-

fication of the digital vessels. If the toe brachial index is <0.7, then this is an indication of PAD.
- Calculation of the ABI does not define the level of obstructive disease but does correlate with the severity of the perfusion abnormality.

LABORATORY TESTS

Currently there is no laboratory test that can diagnose PAD; however, measurement of lipid profile, hemoglobin A1C, homocysteine levels, fibrinogen, D-dimer, and CRP can be useful in the initiation of treatment for systemic atherosclerotic disease.

IMAGING STUDIES

- The diagnosis of PAD can be confirmed by measuring the ABI or toe-brachial index (determined according to the return of pulsatile flow on deflation of a small blood pressure cuff on the great or second toe with a plethysmographic device).
- Rest or exercise pulse volume recordings (PVR) and segmental limb pressures are also useful. PVR measure volume of limb flow per pulse in different segments of the limb (e.g., thigh, calf, ankle, metatarsal, and toes). They help to assess the location and severity of the lesion.

- Duplex ultrasonagraphy after an abnormal ABI can accurately determine the severity and location of stenosis and differentiate stenosis from occlusion. It is also an appropriate modality for surveillance evaluation after femoral popliteal or femoral tibial or pedal surgical bypass with a venous graft.
- Magnetic resonance angiography (MRA) can be used as a noninvasive approach to visualize the aorta and peripheral arterial vasculature. MRA has virtually replaced diagnostic angiography in determining what type of intervention is feasible. Contrast-enhanced MRA has high accuracy for identifying or excluding clinically relevant arterial steno-occlusions in adults with PAD symptoms.
- Computed tomographic angiography (CTA) high-resolution image acquisition can be performed quickly and has several advantages over conventional angiography besides being less invasive with fewer complications. The arterial anatomy can be defined from multiple angles and in multiple planes after a single acquisition.
- Duplex ultrasonagraphy, CTA, and MRA have largely replaced catheter-based angiography in the initial diagnostic evaluation; however, the advantage of catheter-based angiography is its ability to selectively evaluate individual vessels and provide physiologic information such as pressure gradients prior to percutaneous intervention. Contrast angiography (Fig. 1-286) is now reserved for pa-

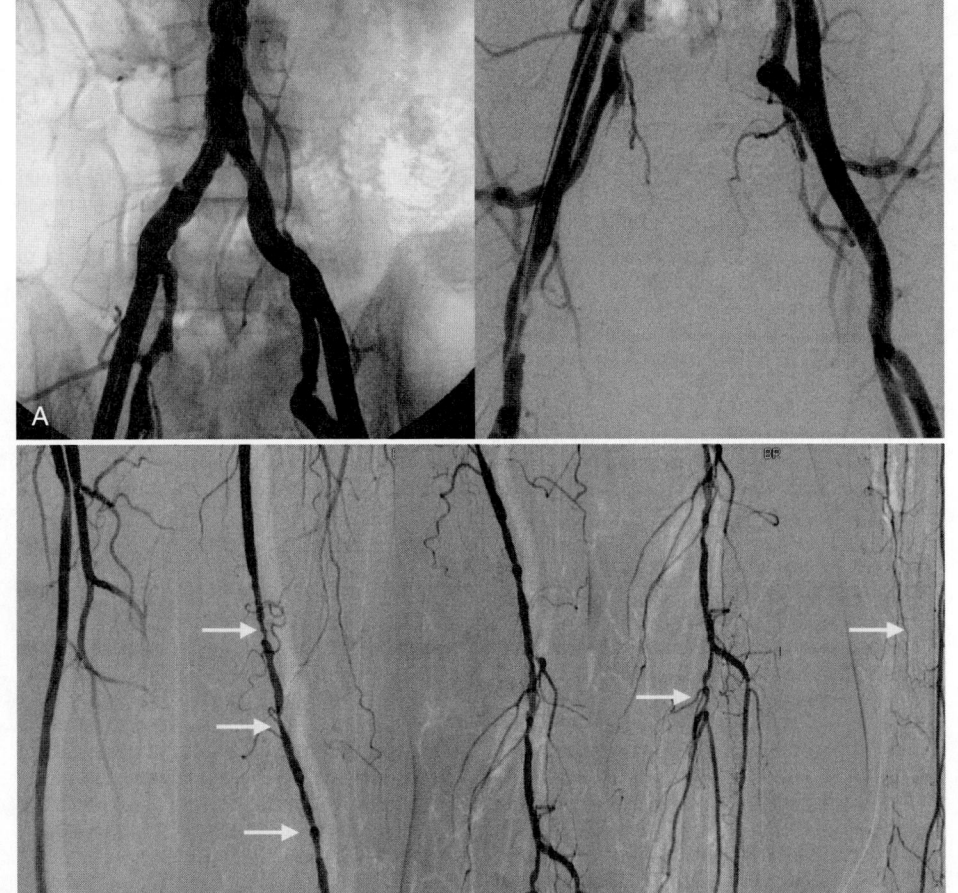

FIGURE 1-286 Angiogram of a patient with disabling left calf claudication. A, The aorta and bilateral common iliac arteries are patent. **B,** The left superficial femoral artery has multiple stenotic lesions *(arrows)*. There is a significant stenosis of the left tibioperoneal trunk and left posterior tibial artery *(arrows)*. From Zipes DP et al [eds]: *Braunwauld's heart disease,* ed 7, Philadelphia, 2005, Elsevier.

tients with PAD who are being considered for endovascular revascularization.

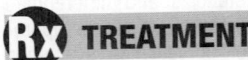 **TREATMENT**

The treatment goal in patients with PAD is to focus on cardiovascular risk-factor reduction to decrease morbidity and mortality as well as to improve limb-related symptoms. There are also medical and surgical approaches to management of limb-related symptoms that are discussed.

CHRONIC MEDICAL Rx

LOWERING CARDIOVASCULAR MORBIDITY AND MORTALITY:

- Smoking cessation should be emphasized in patients with PAD because decreased rates of PAD progression have been seen in patients who successfully stop smoking. A combined pharmacologic and support group approach is recommended to increase compliance with cessation.
- Lipid management should be implemented with a goal of LDL cholesterol of <100 mg/dl and <70 mg/dl in very high-risk patients. Alternatively, aim for reduction of LDL-cholesterol levels by 50% in patients with high-baseline LDL cholesterol if levels <70 mg/dl could not be achieved. If triglycerides are >200 mg/dl, non-HDL cholesterol should be lowered to <130 mg/dl.
- Emphasize management of hypertension with a goal of <140/90 mm Hg or <130/80 mm Hg if the patient has diabetes or chronic renal disease. Achieving goal blood pressure control is more important than the specific antihypertensive agent; however angiotensin-converting enzyme (ACE) inhibitors are often recommended as first line given their cardiovascular benefits.
- Antiplatelet therapy with aspirin 75 to 162 mg is recommended for secondary prevention in patients with PAD to reduce vascular events. The thienopyridines (Clopidogrel) may be considered as alternatives to aspirin, particularly in patients who cannot tolerate aspirin.
- No clear benefit has been observed with combination aspirin and Clopidogrel therapy, despite the common use of combined therapy in patients undergoing infrainguinal angioplasty and stenting. A combination of antiplatelet therapy and Warfarin has also shown no advantage over antiplatelet therapy alone.
- Weight management is important; the goal body mass index is 18.5 to 24.9 kg/m². Ideal waist circumference for men is <40 in and <35 in for women.
- Tight glycemic control (A1C <7%) in diabetic patients with PAD results in prevention of microvascular complications.

TREATMENT OF CLAUDICATION:

- Exercise therapy: A supervised training program is recommended in patients with PAD and has been shown to be an effective method of treating patients with claudication. Supervised training should be performed for a minimum of 30 to 45 min, in sessions performed at least three times per week for a minimum of 12 wk. Studies have shown that a rigorous exercise-training program may be as beneficial as lower-extremity bypass surgery in symptomatic improvement. Supervised treadmill training and resistance training improve functional performance measured by treadmill walking and quality of life evaluation.
- Pharmacologic therapy should be used as an adjunct to a supervised training program. Cilostazol (Pletal) 100 mg bid has been shown to increase pain-free and maximal walking distance by 40% to 60% in symptomatic patients with infrainguinal PAD after 12 to 24 wk of therapy.
- Cilostazol has also been shown to be superior to Pentoxifylline. The beneficial response of Pentoxifylline has been small in most patients, and the overall data are insufficient to support its use as first-line therapy. However, Pentoxifylline should be reserved for patients who cannot take Cilostazol or have not responded appropriately to therapy. Of note, Cilostazol is contraindicated in patients with congestive heart failure with an ejection fraction of less than 40% and long-term use in this patient population is associated with increased mortality.

SURGICAL Rx

Most individuals will respond fairly well to medical management with risk-factor modification, supervised exercise training, and pharmacologic therapy. The ACC/AHA guidelines on PAD have suggested that the following factors be considered prior to revascularization with either percutaneous or surgical methods:

- The patient has had inadequate response to a supervised exercise training program and pharmacologic therapy.
- Symptoms of claudication have resulted in significant disability resulting in an inability to perform normal work or other activities.
- The characteristics of the lesion allow for intervention at a low risk with a high likelihood of success.
- The patient has more urgent limb-threatening ischemia as manifested by ischemic rest pain, ischemic ulcers, or gangrene.

Advancements in catheter, guide wire, and balloon design, and the development of intravascular stents have resulted in a significant increase in the number of percutaneous procedures performed for PAD. Studies have shown no significant difference in outcome between percutaneous transluminal angioplasty (PTA) and bypass surgery for iliac or femoro-popliteal disease; however, although surgery is associated with a higher morbidity, PTA has a higher reintervention rate.

The site and length of the lesion determine the success of PTA. Features that may favor a surgical strategy include long segments; multifocal segments; long segment occlusions; and eccentric, calcified stenoses.

The ACC/AHA has suggested the following guidelines for revascularization therapy:

- A revascularization procedure is indicated in fewer than 10% of people with PAD.
- Endovascular intervention is recommended for TransAtlantic Inter-Society Consensus type A iliac and femoro-popliteal arterial lesions.
- Endovascular therapy is preferred in patients aged 50 yr or younger, because they have a higher risk of graft failure after surgical therapy than older patients.
- Endovascular intervention is not indicated as prophylactic therapy in an asymptomatic patient with lower-extremity PAD, or if there is no significant pressure gradient across a stenosis even after augmentation of flow with vasodilators.
- Primary stent placement is not recommended in the femoral, popliteal, or tibial arteries.
- Surgical intervention is not indicated to prevent progression to limb-threatening ischemia in patients with intermittent claudication.
- Prior to any surgical therapy, patients should have a preoperative cardiovascular risk evaluation.

DISPOSITION

Risk factors for atherosclerosis should be assessed, and appropriate modification instituted. Focus should be placed on smoking cessation, dietary adjustment, and pharmacotherapy for dyslipidemia, hyperglycemia, and hypertension. All patients with PAD should receive aspirin therapy unless contraindicated. Revascularization is performed if the symptoms of PAD do not improve with conservative therapy.

REFERRAL

Consultation with vascular medicine, vascular surgery, or other physicians with expertise in PAD is recommended in patients with rest pain, functional disability from pain, ABI <0.50 at rest, or any physical signs of limb ischemia or gangrene.

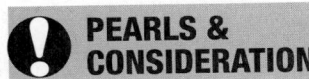 **PEARLS & CONSIDERATIONS**

COMMENTS

- Although the prevalence of PAD in Europe and North America is estimated at ~27 million people, PAD remains under diagnosed and undertreated.
- Studies of the natural history of claudication show the relative safety of initial conservative treatment of PAD in the absence of critical limb ischemia.
- When PAD limits a patient's ability to walk and exercise, percutaneous revascularization can be considered. Data reveal excellent outcomes with angioplasty and stenting in selected patients. Outcomes will likely be better as peripheral interventional technology and skills improve.

- In patients with peripheral arterial disease, the combination of an oral anticoagulant and antiplatelet therapy was not more effective than antiplatelet therapy alone in preventing major cardiovascular complications and was associated with an increase in life-threatening bleeding.
- Increasing levels of D-dimer and inflammatory biomarkers (CRP) are independently associated with higher mortality in persons with PAD.

PREVENTION

Cardiovascular disease is the major cause of death in patients with intermittent claudication. Therefore, the treatment of claudication is directed not only at improving walking distance but also at reducing cardiovascular risk.

PATIENT & FAMILY EDUCATION

The following organizations offer more information about PAD:

- American College of Cardiology (http://www.acc.org)
- Vascular Disease Foundation (http://www.vdf.org)

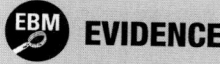 **EVIDENCE**

available at www.expertconsult.com

SUGGESTED READINGS

available at www.expertconsult.com

AUTHORS: **AHMAD EDRIS, M.D.,** and **PRANAV M. PATEL, M.D.**

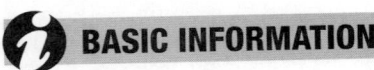 **BASIC INFORMATION**

DEFINITION

Peritonitis refers to the acute onset of severe abdominal pain caused by peritoneal inflammation.

Secondary peritonitis is a localized (abscess) or diffuse peritonitis originating from a defect in abdominal viscus.

SYNONYMS

Acute abdomen
Surgical abdomen

ICD-9CM CODES
567.2 Peritonitis

EPIDEMIOLOGY & DEMOGRAPHICS

Common presentation as a result of diverse etiologies; for example, 5% to 10% of the population has acute appendicitis at some point in their lives.

PHYSICAL FINDINGS & CLINICAL PRESENTATION

- Acute abdominal pain
- Abdominal distention and ascites
- Abdominal rigidity, rebound, and guarding
- Fever, chills
- Exacerbation with movement
- Anorexia, nausea, and vomiting
- Constipation
- Decreased bowel sounds
- Hypotension and tachycardia
- Tachypnea, dyspnea

ETIOLOGY

- Microbiology: most common is gram-negative bacteria (*Escherichia coli, Enterobacter, Klebsiella, Proteus*), gram-positive bacteria (enterococci, streptococci, staphylococci), anaerobic bacteria (*Bacteroides, Clostridium*), and fungi
- Acute perforation peritonitis: gastrointestinal perforation, intestinal ischemia, pelvic peritonitis and other forms
- Postoperative peritonitis: anastomotic leak, accidental perforation, and devascularization
- Posttraumatic peritonitis: after blunt or penetrating abdominal trauma

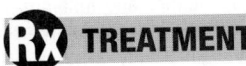 **DIAGNOSIS**

DIFFERENTIAL DIAGNOSIS

- Postoperative: abscess, sepsis, bowel obstruction, injury to internal organs
- Gastrointestinal: perforated viscus, appendicitis, inflammatory bowel disease, infectious colitis, diverticulitis, acute cholecystitis, peptic ulcer perforation, pancreatitis, bowel obstruction
- Gynecologic: ruptured ectopic pregnancy, pelvic inflammatory disease, ruptured hemorrhagic ovarian cyst, ovarian torsion, degenerating leiomyoma
- Urologic: nephrolithiasis, interstitial cystitis
- Miscellaneous: abdominal trauma, penetrating wounds, infections caused by intraperitoneal dialysis

WORKUP

- Acute peritonitis is mainly a clinical diagnosis based on patient history and physical examination.
- Laboratory and imaging studies (see "Laboratory Tests") assist in determining the need for and type of intervention.
- If patient is hemodynamically unstable, immediate diagnostic laparotomy should be performed in lieu of adjuvant diagnostic studies.

LABORATORY TESTS

- Complete blood count: leukocytosis, left shift, anemia
- SMA7: electrolyte imbalances, kidney dysfunction
- Liver function tests: ascites from liver disease, cholelithiasis
- Amylase: pancreatitis
- Blood cultures: bacteremia, sepsis
- Peritoneal cultures: infectious etiology
- Blood gas: respiratory versus metabolic acidosis
- Ascitic fluid analysis: exudate versus transudate
- Urinalysis and culture: urinary tract infection
- Cervical cultures for gonorrhea and *Chlamydia*
- Urine/serum human chorionic gonadotropin

IMAGING STUDIES

- Abdominal series: free air from perforation, small or large bowel dilation from obstruction, identification of fecalith

- Chest x-ray examination: elevated diaphragm, pneumonia
- Pelvic/abdominal ultrasound: abscess formation, abdominal mass, intrauterine versus ectopic pregnancy, identify free fluid suggestive of hemorrhage or ascites
- CT: mass, ascites

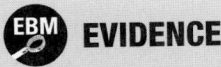 **TREATMENT**

NONPHARMACOLOGIC THERAPY

- IV hydration to correct dehydration, hypovolemia
- Blood transfusion to correct anemia from hemorrhage
- Nasogastric decompression, especially if obstruction is present
- Oxygen: intubation if necessary
- Bed rest

ACUTE GENERAL Rx

- Surgery to correct underlying pathology, such as controlling hemorrhage, correcting perforation, draining abscess
- Broad-spectrum antibiotics:
  1. Single agent: ceftriaxone 1 to 2 g IV q24h, cefotaxime 1 to 2 g IV q4 to 6h
  2. Multiple agents:
     a. Ampicillin 2 g IV q4 to 6h; gentamicin 1.5 mg/kg/day; clindamycin 600 to 900 mg IV q8h
     b. Ampicillin 2 g IV q4 to 6h; gentamicin 1.5 mg/kg/day; metronidazole 500 mg IV q6 to 8h
- Pain control: morphine or meperidine as needed (hold until diagnosis confirmed)

DISPOSITION

Depends on etiology of peritonitis, age of patient, coexisting medical disease, and duration of process before presentation

REFERRAL

Surgical consultation is required in all cases of acute peritonitis.

EBM **EVIDENCE**

available at www.expertconsult.com

SUGGESTED READINGS
available at www.expertconsult.com

AUTHORS: **ARUNDATHI G. PRASAD, M.D.,** and **RUBEN ALVERO, M.D.**

BASIC INFORMATION

DEFINITION

Spontaneous bacterial peritonitis (SBP) is an inflammatory reaction of the peritoneum secondary to the presence of bacteria or other microorganisms. More specifically, SBP is defined as an ascitic fluid infection without an evident intra-abdominal surgically treatable source occurring primarily in patients with advanced cirrhosis of the liver.

SYNONYMS

Primary peritonitis
SBP

ICD-9CM CODES
567.2 Peritonitis

EPIDEMIOLOGY & DEMOGRAPHICS

PREDOMINANT SEX: Males affected more often than females

PHYSICAL FINDINGS & CLINICAL PRESENTATION

- Acute fever with accompanying abdominal pain/ascites, nausea, vomiting, diarrhea
- In cirrhotic patients, presentation may be subtle with a low-grade temperature (100° F) with or without abdominal abnormalities
- In patients with ascites, a heightened degree of awareness is necessary for detection
- Jaundice and encephalopathy
- Deterioration of mental status and/or renal function

ETIOLOGY

- *Escherichia coli*
- *Klebsiella pneumoniae*
- *Streptococcus pneumoniae*
- *Streptococcus* and *Enterococcus* spp.
- *Staphylococcus aureus*
- Anaerobic pathogens: *Bacteroides, Clostridium* organisms
- Other: fungal, mycobacterial, viral

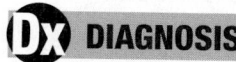 **DIAGNOSIS**

The diagnosis of SBP is established by a positive ascitic fluid bacterial culture and an elevated ascitic fluid absolute polymorphonuclear leukocyte count (≥250 cells/mm³).

DIFFERENTIAL DIAGNOSIS

- Appendicitis (in children)
- Perforated peptic ulcer
- Secondary peritonitis
- Peritoneal abscess
- Splenic, hepatic, or pancreatic abscess
- Cholecystitis
- Cholangitis

WORKUP

Paracentesis and ascitic fluid analysis will confirm diagnosis (see "Laboratory Tests").

LABORATORY TESTS

Ascitic fluid analysis reveals the following:
- Polymorphonuclear cell count >250/mm³
- Presence of bacteria on Gram stain
- pH <7.31
- Lactic acid >32 mg/dl
- Protein <1 g/dl
- Glucose >50 mg/dl
- Lactate dehydrogenase <225 mU/ml
- Positive culture of peritoneal fluid
- Measurement of the serum/ascites/albumin gradient: The serum/ascites/albumin gradient indirectly measures portal pressure. The albumin concentration of ascitic fluid and serum must be obtained on the same day. The ascitic fluid value is subtracted from the serum value to obtain the gradient. If the difference (not a ratio) is >1.1 g/dl, the patient has portal hypertension, with 97% accuracy. If the difference is <1.1 g/dl, portal hypertension is not present. The majority of patients with SBP have portal hypertension as a result of cirrhosis.

IMAGING STUDIES

- Abdominal ultrasound: if there is clinical difficulty in performing paracentesis
- CT scan: to rule out secondary peritonitis (if indicated) and to exclude abscess, mass

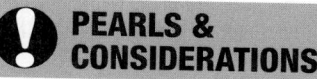 **TREATMENT**

ACUTE GENERAL Rx

Cefotaxime 1 to 2 g IV q8h or ceftriaxone 2 g IV q24h in patients with normal renal function; duration of treatment is generally 7 to 10 days. Oral quinolone therapy (ofloxacin 400 to 800 mg/day) or ciprofloxacin may be an acceptable alternative in selected patients.

PROPHYLAXIS

Give double-strength trimethoprim/sulfamethoxazole qd 5 days/wk or ciprofloxacin 750 mg/wk PO. Both have been shown to decrease occurrence of SBP in patients with cirrhosis.

DISPOSITION

- If possible, the initial management of SBP should be undertaken in the hospital setting; this permits careful follow-up for treatment-related complications, management of underlying portal hypertension, and workup for concomitant diseases.
- Once the diagnosis is confirmed and the patient is stabilized, oral antibiotic therapy can be continued in an outpatient setting if careful follow-up of the patient is ensured.

REFERRAL

- To a gastroenterologist for management of ascites and prevention of recurrent SBP
- To an infectious disease specialist for management of difficult-to-treat infections, antibiotic-resistant bacterial infections, or antibiotic drug intolerance

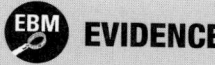 **PEARLS & CONSIDERATIONS**

COMMENTS

- Renal failure is a major cause of morbidity in cirrhotic patients with SBP. The use of IV albumin (1.5 g/kg at the time of diagnosis and 1 g/kg on day 3) may lower the rate of renal failure and mortality in patients with SBP.
- The criteria for the diagnosis of SBP require that abdominal paracentesis be performed and ascitic fluid be analyzed before a diagnosis of SBP can be made.
- Culturing ascitic fluid as if it were blood (with bedside inoculation of ascitic fluid into blood culture bottles) has been shown to significantly increase the culture positivity of the ascitic fluid.
- Laparotomy may be life threatening in end-stage cirrhosis.
- Positive blood cultures in an individual with ascites require exclusion of a peritoneal source by paracentesis.

EBM EVIDENCE

available at www.expertconsult.com

SUGGESTED READINGS
available at www.expertconsult.com

AUTHORS: **GLENN G. FORT, M.D., M.P.H.,** and **DENNIS J. MIKOLICH, M.D.**

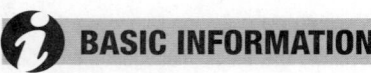

BASIC INFORMATION

DEFINITION

Peritonsillar abscess is an acute infection located between the capsule of the palatine tonsil and the superior constrictor muscle of the pharynx.

SYNONYMS

Quinsy

ICD-9CM CODES

475.0 Peritonsillar abscess

EPIDEMIOLOGY & DEMOGRAPHICS

INCIDENCE (IN U.S.): 30:100,000/yr. It is the most common deep infection of the head and neck
FREQUENCY: There is a bimodal frequency during the year, with highest occurrence from November to December and April to May.
PREDOMINANT SEX: Male = female
PREDOMINANT AGE: Common during adolescence and 20s. Young children may be affected if immunocompromised.

CLINICAL PRESENTATION

- Sore throat, which may be severe
- Dysphagia and odynophagia
- Otalgia
- Foul-smelling breath
- Facial swelling
- Drooling
- Headache
- Fever
- Trismus
- Hoarseness, muffled voice (also called "hot potato voice")
- Tender submandibular and anterior cervical lymph nodes
- Tonsillar hypertrophy
- Contralateral deflection of the uvula
- Stridor

ETIOLOGY

- Peritonsillar abscess is a complication of tonsillitis.
- Group A β-hemolytic Streptococcus is the most common bacterial cause, accounting for 15% to 30% of cases in children and 5% to 10% of cases in adults.

- Less common aerobic causes are *Staphylococcus aureus*, *Haemophilus influenzae*, *Neisseria* species.
- The most common anaerobic organism is *Fusobacterium*.

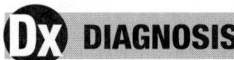

DIAGNOSIS

DIFFERENTIAL DIAGNOSIS

- Tonsillitis
- Infectious mononucleosis
- Peritonsillar cellulitis
- Retropharyngeal abscess
- Epiglottitis
- Dental abscess
- Lymphoma

WORKUP

Thorough history and physical exam

LABORATORY TESTS

- Rapid strep antigen detecting testing and throat swab culture and sensitivity
- Aspiration of the abscess for culture and sensitivity

IMAGING STUDIES

Ultrasound and CT scan can be considered to help differentiate mass from abscess, but the gold standard still remains a culture of the abscess.

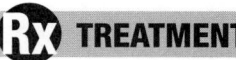

TREATMENT

NONPHARMACOLOGIC THERAPY

- Surgical drainage of the abscess by needle aspiration or by incision and drainage
- Possible subsequent surgery for tonsillectomy

ACUTE GENERAL Rx

- Several methods of initial surgical drainage are equally effective.
- Appropriate selection of antibiotic guided by culture and sensitivity of the organism. After performing aspiration or drainage, appropriate antibiotic therapy, possibly including penicillin, clindamycin, cephalosporins, or metronidazole, must be started.

CHRONIC Rx

- Tonsillectomy usually occurs 3 to 6 mo after diagnosis of abscess or recurrent tonsillitis.
- Though rare, in adults and children with peritonsillar abscess and a history of recurrent pharyngitis or previous peritonsillar abscess, the specialist may proceed with removal of the tonsils directly after placing the patient on IV antibiotics. This is known as a quinsy or hot tonsillectomy.

REFERRAL

Patients may be able to be treated as outpatients, but emergently consider hospitalization or consultation with an otolaryngologist if the patient's airway has the potential to become obstructed or if stridor is appreciated.

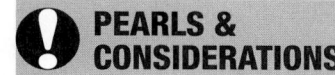

PEARLS & CONSIDERATIONS

COMMENTS

- Any person who has had a peritonsillar abscess is at risk for a recurrence, both immediately (within 4 days) and long term (2 to 3 yr).
- Most recurrences occur shortly after the initial presentation, suggesting continued infection rather than recurrence.
- Regardless of treatment modality, the overall recurrence rate is from 6% to 36%.

PREVENTION

- Strongly encourage completion of the full course of antibiotic treatment for acute pharyngitis (10 to 14 days) to prevent incomplete treatment of infection leading to abscess formation.
- Tonsillectomy is recommended in the event of recurrent peritonsillar abscess or tonsillitis in both children and adults.

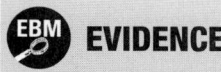

EVIDENCE

available at www.expertconsult.com

SUGGESTED READINGS

available at www.expertconsult.com

AUTHOR: **CHRISTINE HEALY, D.O.**

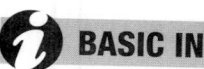 **BASIC INFORMATION**

DEFINITION

Pertussis is a prolonged bacterial infection of the upper respiratory tract characterized by paroxysms of an intense cough.

SYNONYMS

Whooping cough

ICD-9CM CODES
033.9 Pertussis

EPIDEMIOLOGY

INCIDENCE (IN U.S.): Approximately 5000 new cases annually (Fig. 1-287)
PEAK INCIDENCE:
- Childhood
- Usually affects children aged <1 yr
PREDOMINANT AGE:
- 50% in children aged <1 yr
- 20% in children aged >15 yr

PHYSICAL FINDINGS & CLINICAL PRESENTATION

- Usually begins with a 1- to 2-wk prodrome that resembles a common cold
- After this initial phase, increased production of mucus is noted
- Increased mucus production is followed by an intense, paroxysmal cough, ending with gasps and an inspiratory whoop
- In some children, cyanosis and anoxia are noted
- When prolonged, frank exhaustion and even apnea occur
- Pertussis is characterized by the finding of intense cough with a marked lymphocytosis; posttussive gagging and vomiting are characteristic of pertussis

ETIOLOGY

Gram-negative rod *Bordetella pertussis,* which adheres to human cilia

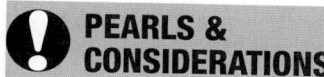 **DIAGNOSIS**

DIFFERENTIAL DIAGNOSIS

- Croup
- Epiglottitis
- Foreign body aspiration
- Bacterial pneumonia

WORKUP

Pertussis is often overlooked as a cause of chronic cough, especially in adolescents and adults. The presence or absence of posttussive emesis or inspiratory whoop increase the likelihood of pertussis but only modestly. Therefore, clinicians must use their overall impression in pursuing the diagnosis.
- Blood cultures in hospitalized patients
- Chest radiograph examination
- Culture of bacteria, usually from nasopharynx
- Immunofluorescent staining of nasopharyngeal secretions
- Enzyme-linked immunosorbent assay for detection of antibody to pertussis

LABORATORY TESTS

Complete blood count, which usually demonstrates marked lymphocytosis:
- Up to 18,000 white blood cells
- 70% to 80% lymphocytes

IMAGING STUDIES

Chest x-ray examination is of value if secondary bacterial pneumonia is suspected.

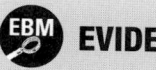 **TREATMENT**

ACUTE GENERAL Rx

- Intensive supportive care:
  1. Adequate hydration
  2. Control of secretions
  3. Maintenance of airway

- Antibiotics are indicated even though their ability to alter the course of the disease is controversial.
  1. Erythromycin 50 mg/kg/day for 14 days. Recent literature reports indicate that a 7-day treatment regimen may be as effective as a 14-day course of erythromycin. Azithromycin 500 mg on day 1, followed by 250 mg for days 2 to 5. TMP/SMX 320/1600 mg per day in divided doses can be used in patients with allergy or intolerance to macrolides.
  2. Although unproved, dexamethasone 1 mg/kg/day in four doses for severe, life-threatening paroxysms.
  3. Ceftriaxone 75 mg/kg/day in two doses for broad coverage of secondary bacterial pneumonias.
- Vaccination is successful in preventing the disease: universal vaccination is advised for all children aged <7 yr.
- Erythromycin is recommended for all close contacts in the household: TMP/SMX in two oral doses per day for those intolerant to erythromycin.

DISPOSITION

Close attention to accepted vaccination schedules is the best prevention.

REFERRAL

To intensive care setting for life-threatening infections:
- Pulmonologist
- Infectious disease specialist

PEARLS & CONSIDERATIONS

- The diagnosis of pertussis in a young child is easily recognized, but in adults pertussis can be a subtle diagnosis and is often missed. The tip-off is often a persistent, hacking, and productive cough with minor or no fever in a previously healthy person that lasts >2 wk.
- Approximately 11% of pertussis cases in the pediatric population are attributable to vaccine refusal, dispelling the myth that herd immunity protects children whose parents refuse pertussis vaccine.

EBM EVIDENCE

available at www.expertconsult.com

SUGGESTED READINGS

available at www.expertconsult.com

AUTHORS: **DENNIS J. MIKOLICH, M.D.,** and **GLENN G. FORT, M.D., M.P.H.**

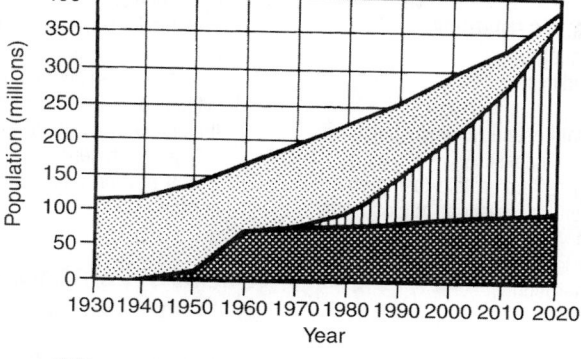

Pertussis post disease immune

Adult pertussis susceptibles

Pertussis vaccine immune (1 to 20 years old)

FIGURE 1-287 Pertussis epidemiology in the United States projected through the year 2020 with continued use of present-day whole-cell pertussis vaccines. (Modified from Bass JW, Stephenson SR: The return of pertussis, *Pediatr Infect Dis J* 6:141, 1987.)

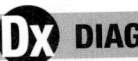

BASIC INFORMATION

DEFINITION

- A hamartomatous polyp is a benign intestinal growth that may contain all components of the intestinal mucosa. In gastrointestinal polyposis, multiple such polyps coexist within the intestinal tract, and associated manifestations are usually also present.
- Juvenile polyps are benign polyps composed of cystic dilatations of glandular structures within the fibroblastic stroma of the lamina propria. They may cause bleeding or intussusception.
- Commonly recognized syndromes are Peutz-Jeghers syndrome, juvenile polyposis syndrome, Cowden's disease, Bannagan-Ruvalcaba-Riley syndrome, and Cronkhite-Canada syndrome. Other lesser known inherited hamartomatous polyposis syndromes are hereditary mixed polyposis syndrome, intestinal ganglioneuromatosis and neurofibromatosis (variant of von Recklinghausen's syndrome), Devon family syndrome, basal cell nevus syndrome, and tuberous sclerosis (may involve gastrointestinal tract).

ICD-9CM CODES
759.6 (Peutz-Jeghers syndrome)
211.3 (Cronkhite-Canada syndrome)

EPIDEMIOLOGY

- Colonic adenomas, the precursors of nearly all colorectal cancers, are found in nearly 40% of patients by age 60 yr.
- 25% of men and 15% of women who undergo colonoscopy are found to have one or more adenomas.
- Detection of any adenoma in patients <60 yr confers an increased risk of colorectal cancer (by a factor of 2.6) in their first-degree relatives.

PHYSICAL FINDINGS & CLINICAL PRESENTATION

PEUTZ-JEGHERS SYNDROME:
- Transmission: autosomal dominant with incomplete penetrance
- Disease expression:
  - Stomach, small and large intestinal hamartomas with bands of smooth muscle in the lamina propria
  - Pigmented lesions around mouth (lips and buccal mucosa), nose, hands, feet, genital, and perineal areas
  - Ovarian tumors
  - Sertoli cell testicular tumors
  - Airway polyps
  - Pancreatic cancer
  - Breast cancer
  - Urinary tract polyps
- Cumulative lifetime cancer risk
  - Colon cancer: 39%
  - Stomach cancer: 29%

- Small intestine cancer: 13%
- Pancreatic cancer: 36%
- Breast cancer: 54%
- Ovarian cancer: 10%
- Sertoli cell tumor: 9%
- Overall cancer risk: 93%
- Clinical manifestation:
  - Gastrointestinal, small-bowel obstruction, intussusception, gastrointestinal bleeding
  - See chapters on relevant malignancies for their signs and symptoms

JUVENILE POLYPOSIS SYNDROME:
- Transmission: autosomal dominant
- Disease expression
  - Solitary juvenile polyps numbering 10 or more in the rectum or throughout the gastrointestinal tract; the polyps are smooth and covered with normal epithelium
  - Various congenital abnormalities coexist in 20%
- Cumulative cancer risk is increased (may be as high as 50%)
- Clinical manifestation
  - Intestinal obstruction
  - Intussusception
  - Gastrointestinal bleeding

COWDEN'S DISEASE:
- Transmission: autosomal dominant, rare
- Disease expression
  - Juvenile intestinal polyposis
  - Orocutaneous hamartomas
  - Fibrocystic breast disease and breast cancer
  - Goiter and thyroid cancer
  - Facial tricholemmomas (papules) in 83%
- Cumulative cancer risk
  - Gastrointestinal: same as general population
  - Thyroid: 3% to 10%
  - Breast: 25% to 50%

BANNAGAN-RUVALCABA-RILEY SYNDROME:
- Transmission: autosomal dominant, rare
- Disease expression
  - Juvenile intestinal polyposis
  - Macrocephaly
  - Developmental delay
  - Penile pigmented spots
  - Cumulative cancer risk unknown

CRONKHITE-CANADA SYNDROME:
- Transmission: acquired
- Age of onset: midlife
- Disease expression
  - Diffuse gastrointestinal juvenile polyposis (50% to 95% of cases)
  - Chronic diarrhea and protein-losing enteropathy (the entire intestinal mucosa may be inflamed), which leads to abdominal pain, weight loss, and various complications of malnutrition
  - Dystrophic nails
  - Alopecia
  - Hyperpigmentation

- Cumulative cancer risk: same as the average population

DIAGNOSIS

Diagnosis is suggested in many cases by family history and confirmed by colonoscopy and physical findings described previously.

TREATMENT

GENERAL Rx

Peutz-Jeghers syndrome:
- Colonoscopies with polypectomies
- Screening for breast cancer, testicular cancer, possibly ovarian cancer

Juvenile polyposis syndrome:
- Colonoscopies with polypectomies if few colon polyps
- Total colectomy if numerous polyps
- Esophagogastroscopies and polypectomies

Cowden's disease:
- Rigorous breast cancer screening or prophylactic simple bilateral mastectomy with reconstruction.

Cronkhite-Canada syndrome:
- Progressive malabsorption syndrome is the hallmark of this syndrome, and no specific treatment exists. Enteral or parenteral feeding is the cornerstone of management and can result in remission.

DISPOSITION

- The screening of first-degree relatives of patients with colonic adenomas detected before 60 yr of age is controversial. Some recommend beginning colonoscopic screening at age 40 yr or 10 yr younger than the age at diagnosis of the youngest person in the family with an adenoma.
- Recommended interval between colonoscopies from the U.S. Consensus Guidelines for Colonoscopic Surveillance after Polypectomy are as follows:
  - 10 yr for small, rectal hyperplastic polyps
  - 5 to 10 yr for one to two low-risk adenomas (tubular adenomas <1 cm)
  - 3 yr for low-risk adenomas or any high-risk adenoma (large [≥1 cm] or histologically advanced adenomas [tubulovillous or villous adenomas or villous adenomas and those with high-grade dysplasia])
  - <3 yr for presence of >10 adenomas
  - 2 to 6 mo for inadequately removed adenomas

SUGGESTED READING
available at www.expertconsult.com

AUTHOR: **FRED F. FERRI, M.D.**

BASIC INFORMATION

DEFINITION

Peyronie's disease is an abnormal curvature and shortening of the penis during an erection. This is caused by scarring of the tunica albuginea of the corpora cavernosa.

SYNONYMS

Plastic induration of the penis
Penile fibromatosis

ICD-9CM CODES

607.89 Peyronie's disease

EPIDEMIOLOGY & DEMOGRAPHICS

- Peyronie's disease occurs in approximately 1% of men.
- It is commonly seen between the ages of 45 and 60 yr.
- A genetic predisposition has been suggested.
- There are no incidence and prevalence data available in the literature.

PHYSICAL FINDINGS & CLINICAL PRESENTATION

- Painful erections
- Tenderness over the scar tissue area
- Erectile dysfunction
- Curvature of the erected penis interfering with penetration
- Dupuytren's contracture is a commonly associated finding in patients with Peyronie's disease

ETIOLOGY

- Specific cause is unknown. It is believed that scar tissue forms on either the dorsal or ventral midline surface of the penile shaft. The scar restricts expansion at the involved site, causing the penis to bend or curve in one direction.
- The precipitating factor appears to be trauma either from repetitive microvascular injury caused by vigorous sexual intercourse, accidents, or prior surgeries (e.g., transurethral or radical prostatectomy, cystoscopy).

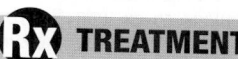

DIAGNOSIS

Diagnosis is based on the clinical findings.

DIFFERENTIAL DIAGNOSIS

- The history differentiates congenital from acquired curvatures of the penis.
- Other causes of erectile dysfunction must be excluded, including metabolic, diabetic, thyroid, and renal causes, in addition to hypogonadism and hyperprolactinemia.

WORKUP

History and physical examination alone will usually establish the diagnosis of Peyronie's disease.

LABORATORY TESTS

There are no specific blood tests to diagnose Peyronie's disease. Electrolytes, blood urea nitrogen, creatinine, glucose, thyroid function tests (thyroid-stimulating hormone, T_3U, T_4), testosterone, and prolactin levels are blood tests to exclude other medical causes of erectile dysfunction.

IMAGING STUDIES

Imaging studies are not specific.

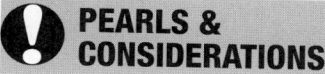

TREATMENT

NONPHARMACOLOGIC THERAPY

A conservative approach of reassurance and observation is taken at first because the disease process may be self-limiting.

ACUTE GENERAL Rx

Although not substantiated by direct randomized, controlled clinical trials, the following treatment modalities have been tried:
- Vitamin E 400 mg bid.
- Paraaminobenzoic acid 12 g/day.
- Colchicine 0.6 mg bid for 2 to 3 wk.
- Fexofenadine 60 mg bid for 3 mo.
- Steroid injection into the scar tissue.
- Collagenase injection into the scar tissue.
- Radiation to the scar tissue area.
- Extracorporeal shockwave therapy (ESWT): Current evidence on the safety, but not the efficacy, of ESWT appears adequate. From comparative studies, the main benefits of ESWT were the alleviation of pain and reduction of angulation of the penis. In one comparative study, 10 of 20 patients receiving ESWT had a decrease in the curvature of at least 30%. Case series evidence also suggested some improvement of sexual performance.
- Other medications that can be helpful include verapamil, tamoxifen, and interferon.

CHRONIC Rx

In patients who have progressed to intractable pain with erection or erectile dysfunction, surgical treatment with excision of the plaque and skin grafting may be indicated.

DISPOSITION

Peyronie's disease evolves slowly and in some cases can resolve on its own. Waiting for 1 yr before proceeding with surgical attempts is recommended.

REFERRAL

A urologic consultation is recommended in patients with progressive symptoms and erectile dysfunction.

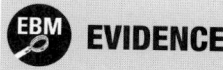

PEARLS & CONSIDERATIONS

COMMENTS

- Peyronie's disease is not commonly seen in younger patients because they are able to sustain intracorporeal pressures high enough to stretch the scar tissue, preventing it from deforming the penis during erection.
- Trauma from buckling of the erected penis is thought to be the precipitant cause of scar formation and Peyronie's disease. It is found more often in men who are sexually very active and vigorous, having sexual intercourse daily or almost daily.
- Sexual positions with the women being on top or thrusting the penis into the anterior vaginal wall is thought to increase the chances of developing Peyronie's disease.

EVIDENCE

available at www.expertconsult.com

SUGGESTED READINGS

available at www.expertconsult.com

AUTHOR: **TANYA ALI, M.D.**

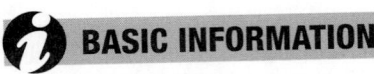

BASIC INFORMATION

DEFINITION

Pharyngitis/tonsillitis is inflammation of the pharynx or tonsils.

SYNONYMS   Sore throat

ICD-9CM CODES
462 Pharyngitis

EPIDEMIOLOGY & DEMOGRAPHICS

Acute pharyngitis accounts for 1.3% of outpatient visits to health care providers in the U.S.
PEAK INCIDENCE: Late winter/early spring (group A streptococcal infections)
PREDOMINANT SEX: Females and males affected equally
PREDOMINANT AGE:
- All ages affected
- Streptococcal pharyngitis most common among school-age children (5 to 15 yr of age). Group A strep is responsible for 5% to 15% of cases of pharyngitis in adults and 20% to 30% of cases in children
GENETICS: Neonatal infection: pharyngitis at age <3 yr is almost always of viral etiology.

PHYSICAL FINDINGS & CLINICAL PRESENTATION

- Pharynx:
  1. May appear normal to severely erythematous
  2. Tonsillar hypertrophy and exudates commonly seen but do not indicate etiology
- Viral infection:
  1. Rhinorrhea
  2. Conjunctivitis
  3. Cough
- Bacterial infection, especially group A streptococci:
  1. High fever
  2. Systemic signs of infection
- Herpes simplex or enterovirus infection: vesicles
- Streptococcal infection:
  1. Rare complications:
     a. Scarlet fever
     b. Rheumatic fever
     c. Acute glomerulonephritis
  2. Extension of infection: tonsillar, parapharyngeal, or retropharyngeal abscess presenting with severe pain, high fever, trismus
- Streptococcal tonsillitis is manifested as acute onset of fever, headache, neck pain, odynophagia, sore throat, otalgia, red tongue with enlargement of papillae, sore throat, red swollen uvula, and tender anterior cervical adenitis.
- Peritonsillar abscess (accumulation of pus between the tonsil and its capsule) is the most common complication of acute tonsillitis. Clinical signs include deformed posterior pharynx, medial displacement of the uvula, trismus, and muffled voice (hot-potato voice).
- Table 1-144 describes seven danger signs in patients with sore throat.

ETIOLOGY

- Viruses:
  1. Respiratory syncytial virus
  2. Influenza A and B
  3. Epstein-Barr virus
  4. Adenovirus
  5. Herpes simplex
- Bacteria:
  1. *Streptococcus pyogenes*
  2. *Neisseria gonorrhoeae*
  3. *Arcanobacterium haemolyticum*
- Other organisms:
  1. *Mycoplasma pneumoniae*
  2. *Chlamydophila pneumoniae*

DIAGNOSIS

DIFFERENTIAL DIAGNOSIS

- Sore throat associated with granulocytopenia, thyroiditis.
- Tonsillar hypertrophy associated with lymphoma.
- Section II describes the differential diagnosis of sore throat.

WORKUP

- Rapid streptococcal antigen test (culture should be performed if rapid test negative)
- Throat swab for culture to exclude *S. pyogenes*, *N. gonorrhoeae* (requires specific transport medium)
- Monospot if diagnosis is unclear

LABORATORY TESTS

- Complete blood count with differential
  1. May help support diagnosis of bacterial infection
  2. Streptococcal infection suggested by leukocytosis >15,000/mm^3
- Viral cultures, serologic studies rarely needed

IMAGING STUDIES

Seldom indicated. If necessary to distinguish between tonsillitis and peritonsillar abscess, CT or MRI imaging of the neck can be done.

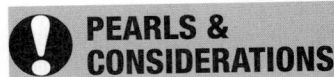 TREATMENT

NONPHARMACOLOGIC THERAPY

- Fluids
- Salt water gargles

TABLE 1-144   Seven Danger Signs in Patients with Sore Throat

1. Persistence of symptoms longer than 1 wk without improvement
2. Respiratory difficulty, particularly stridor
3. Difficulty in handling secretions
4. Difficulty in swallowing
5. Severe pain in the absence of erythema
6. A palpable mass
7. Blood, even in small amounts, in the pharynx or ear

Andreoli TE et al: *Andreoli and Carpenter's Cecil essentials of medicine,* ed 8, Philadelphia, 2010, Saunders.

ACUTE GENERAL Rx

- Aspirin (acetaminophen culture)
- If streptococcal infection proven or suspected:
  1. Penicillin V 500 mg PO bid for 10 days or benzathine penicillin 1.2 million U IM once (adults)
  2. Erythromycin 500 mg PO bid or 250 mg qid for 10 days if penicillin allergic
- If gonococcal infection proven or suspected: ceftriaxone 125 mg IM once
- Amoxicillin 500 mg tid for 10 days is the primary antibiotic treatment of streptococcal tonsillitis. Macrolides or clindamycin can be used in penicillin-allergic patients.
- Treatment of peritonsillar abscess is drainage through needle or incision.

CHRONIC Rx

- Recurrent streptococcal infections are common and may represent reinfection from other household.
- There is no conclusive evidence from randomized clinical trials that tonsillectomy is superior to antibiotic therapy for recurrent tonsillitis in adults.
- Tonsillopharyngitis is generally managed in an outpatient setting with follow-up arranged in 1 to 2 wk. Admission to the hospital is indicated for local suppurative complications (peritonsillar abscess; lateral pharyngeal or posterior pharyngeal abscess; impending airway closure; or inability to swallow food, medications, or water).

REFERRAL

- To otolaryngologist:
  1. If peritonsillar or other abscess is suspected
  2. If tonsillar hypertrophy persists
- To infectious disease expert if unusual pathogen is suspected

PEARLS & CONSIDERATIONS

COMMENTS

- Antibiotic therapy should be avoided unless bacterial etiology is suspected or proven, especially in adults.
- Beta hemolytic Group A streptococci is the most common cause of acute tonsillitis
- The major problem in the diagnosis and treatment of pharyngitis is not which guideline to follow to avoid testing and antibiotic prescribing to patients at low risk for streptococcal pharyngitis but that most physicians fail to follow any guidelines.

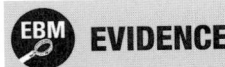 EVIDENCE

available at www.expertconsult.com

SUGGESTED READINGS
available at www.expertconsult.com

AUTHORS: **GLENN G. FORT, M.D., M.P.H.,** and **DENNIS J. MIKOLICH, M.D.**

BASIC INFORMATION

DEFINITION

Pheochromocytomas are catecholamine-producing tumors that originate from chromaffin cells of the adrenergic system. They generally secrete both norepinephrine and epinephrine, but norepinephrine is usually the predominant amine.

SYNONYMS

Paraganglioma

ICD-9CM CODES
194.0 Pheochromocytoma
255.6 Medulloadrenal hyperfunction

EPIDEMIOLOGY & DEMOGRAPHICS

- Incidence: 0.05% of population; peak incidence in 30s and 40s.
- "Rough" rule of 10: 10% are extraadrenal, 10% are malignant, 10% are familial, 10% occur in children, 10% involve both adrenals, 10% are multiple (other than bilateral adrenal).
- Approximately 25% of patients with apparently sporadic pheochromocytoma may be carriers of mutations.
- Pheochromocytoma is a feature of two disorders with autosomal-dominant pattern of inheritance:
  1. Multiple endocrine neoplasia (MEN) type 2
  2. Von Hippel-Lindau disease: angioma of the retina, hemangioblastoma of the central nervous system, renal cell carcinoma, pancreatic cysts, and epididymal cystoadenoma
- Pheochromocytomas occur in 5% of patients with neurofibromatosis type 1.

PHYSICAL FINDINGS & CLINICAL PRESENTATION

- Hypertension: can be sustained (55%) or paroxysmal (45%).
- Headache (80%): usually paroxysmal in nature and described as "pounding" and severe.
- Palpitations (70%): can be present with or without tachycardia.
- Hyperhidrosis (60%): most evident during paroxysmal attacks of hypertension.
- Physical examination may be entirely normal if done in a symptom-free interval; during a paroxysm the patient may demonstrate marked increase in both systolic and diastolic pressure, profuse sweating, visual disturbances (caused by hypertensive retinopathy), dilated pupils (from catecholamine excess), paresthesias in the lower extremities (caused by severe vasoconstriction), tremor, tachycardia.

ETIOLOGY

- Catecholamine-producing tumors that are usually located in the adrenal medulla.
- Specific mutations of the RET protooncogene cause familial predisposition to pheochromocytoma in MEN 2.
- Mutations in the von Hippel-Lindau tumor suppressor gene (*VHL* gene) cause familial disposition to pheochromocytoma in von Hippel-Lindau disease.
- Recently identified genes for succinate dehydrogenase subunit D (*SDHD*) and succinate dehydrogenase subunit B (*SDHB*) predispose carriers to pheochromocytoma and globus tumors.

DIAGNOSIS

DIFFERENTIAL DIAGNOSIS

- Anxiety disorder
- Thyrotoxicosis
- Amphetamine or cocaine abuse
- Carcinoid
- Essential hypertension

WORKUP

Laboratory evaluation and imaging studies to locate the neoplasm. Misdiagnosis of pheochromocytoma is not uncommon. Correct interpretation of biochemical tests and imaging is crucial to a correct diagnosis.

LABORATORY TESTS

- Although there is no consensus on the best test, plasma-free metanephrines have been suggested as the test of first choice for excluding or confirming the tumor. Plasma concentrations of normetanephrines >2.5 pmol/ml or metanephrine levels >1.4 pmol/ml indicate a pheochromocytoma with 100% specificity.
- 24-hr urine collection for metanephrines (up to 100% sensitive) will also show increased metanephrines; the accuracy of the 24-hr urinary levels for metanephrines can be improved by indexing urinary metanephrine levels by urine creatinine levels.
- The clonidine suppression test is useful for distinguishing between high levels of plasma norepinephrine from sympathetic nerves and those from a pheochromocytoma. A decrease <50% in plasma norepinephrine levels after clonidine administration is normal, whereas persistent elevations are indicative of pheochromocytoma.

IMAGING STUDIES

- Abdominal CT scan (88% sensitivity) is useful in locating pheochromocytomas >0.5 inch in diameter (90% to 95% accurate). There have been concerns that IV contrast may induce a hypertensive crisis. However, studies have shown that IV low-osmolar, contrast-enhanced CT can safely be used in patients with pheochromocytoma who are not receiving alpha or beta blockers.
- MRI: pheochromocytomas demonstrate a distinctive MRI appearance (up to 100% sensitivity); MRI may become the diagnostic imaging modality of choice.
- Scintigraphy with 131 or 1-123 I-MIBG (up to 100% sensitivity): this norepinephrine analog localizes in adrenergic tissue; it is particularly useful in locating extraadrenal pheochromocytomas.
- 6 [^{18}F] Fluorodopamine positron emission tomography is reserved for cases in which clinical symptoms and signs suggest pheochromocytoma and results of biochemical tests are positive but conventional imaging studies cannot locate the tumor. An alternative approach is to use vena caval sampling for plasma catecholamines and metanephrines.

TREATMENT

GENERAL Rx

Laparoscopic removal of the tumor (surgical resection for both benign and malignant disease):
1. Preoperative stabilization with combination of phenoxybenzamine, beta-blocker, metyrosine, and liberal fluid and salt intake starting 10 to 14 days before surgery.
2. Hypertensive crisis preoperatively and intraoperatively can be controlled with phentolamine (Regitine) 2 to 5 mg IV q1 to 2h prn or nitroprusside used in combination with beta-adrenergic blockers.

PEARLS & CONSIDERATIONS

COMMENTS

- Obtaining a detailed family history is important because 10% of pheochromocytomas are familial.
- Screening for pheochromocytoma should be considered in patients with any of the following:
  1. Malignant hypertension
  2. Poor response to antihypertensive therapy
  3. Paradoxical hypertensive response
  4. Hypertension during induction of anesthesia, parturition, surgery, or thyrotropin-releasing hormone testing
  5. Hypertension associated with imipramine or desipramine
  6. Neurofibromatosis (increased incidence of pheochromocytoma)
- All patients with pheochromocytoma should be screened for MEN-2 and von Hippel-Lindau disease with pentagastrin test, serum parathyroid hormone, ophthalmoscopy, MRI of the brain, CT scan of the kidneys and pancreas, and ultrasonography of the testes.
- In patients with pheochromocytoma, routine analysis for mutations of *RET, VHL, SDHD,* and *SDHB* is indicated to identify pheochromocytoma-associated syndromes.

EVIDENCE

available at www.expertconsult.com

SUGGESTED READINGS

available at www.expertconsult.com

AUTHORS: **MARK F. BRADY,** and **FRED F. FERRI, M.D.**

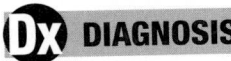

DEFINITION

Specific phobias are anxiety disorders characterized by an excessive, persistent fear elicited by a specific object or situation that is then avoided or tolerated with intense distress. The provoking stimulus may be a specific object, such as an animal or insect; natural environments, such as heights or water; or a specific situation, such as the sight of blood, the receiving of an injection, or being in a tunnel or on a bridge. Social phobia is a specific disorder characterized by a fear of being in social or performance situations. Also, those with panic disorder may also have agoraphobia, characterized by an intense anxiety about being in a place or situation from which they would not be able to escape in the event of a panic attack.

SYNONYMS

Simple phobia (obsolete name for specific phobia)
Phobias named for the provoking stimulus, such as arachnophobia (fear of spiders) and acrophobia (fear of heights)
Social anxiety disorder (social phobia)

ICD-9CM CODES
F40.2 Specific phobia (DSM-IV: 300.29)
F40.1 Social phobia (DSM-IV: 300.23), Agoraphobia (DSM-IV: 300.21 [with panic disorder], 300.22 [without panic disorder])

EPIDEMIOLOGY & DEMOGRAPHICS

PEAK INCIDENCE: Specific phobias are often lifelong conditions; some of those with childhood onset (e.g., some animal phobias) tend to remit spontaneously.
PREVALENCE (IN U.S.):
- Specific phobias are prevalent in 5% to 10% of the general population.
- Social phobia is prevalent in approximately 13% of the general population.
PREDOMINANT SEX AND AGE:
- Females with specific phobias outnumber males, though rates vary by phobia.
- More women than men (16% vs. 11%) are affected with social phobia.
- Agoraphobia is more prevalent in women.
- Most specific phobias have childhood onset.
- Situational phobias have two peaks—in childhood and the mid-20s.
- Onset of social phobia usually occurs in the mid-teens, with onset after age 25 being unusual; this disorder is generally lifelong.
GENETICS: Specific and social phobias more common in first-degree relatives.

PHYSICAL FINDINGS & CLINICAL PRESENTATION

- When approaching the phobic stimulus, the experience of extreme anxiety is often accompanied by autonomic symptoms such as tachycardia, tremor, and diaphoresis; depersonalization may occur. In blood or injection phobias, symptoms are often followed by a parasympathetic response that can cause vasovagal syncope.
- Specific phobias frequently occur with other anxiety disorders.
- Social phobias are distinguished from specific phobias in that what is feared is humiliation or embarrassment rather than a specific object or environment.

ETIOLOGY

There is no clear etiology.

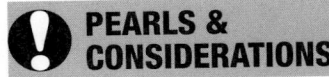 **DIAGNOSIS**

DIFFERENTIAL DIAGNOSIS

- Panic attacks (with or without agoraphobia): anxiety symptoms seen in specific phobia may resemble symptoms of panic attacks, but the stimulus in the specific or social phobia is clear, whereas panic attacks do not have a clearly associated provoking stimulus.
- Posttraumatic stress disorder (PTSD): anxiety and physiological arousal associated with specific cues from the traumatic event defining the PTSD may resemble the symptoms induced by a phobia.
- Generalized anxiety disorder (GAD): may be difficult to distinguish from social phobia, but in social phobia the focus is fear of embarrassment or humiliation from other people, whereas GAD has no specific focus for the worry.
- Avoidant personality disorder is often comorbid with social phobia.
- Psychotic disorders can present with a fear of being in public that arises from delusions.

WORKUP

- History: usually diagnostic. This should include information about other medical disorders, medications, any history of past trauma, and substance abuse.
- Physical examination: to confirm absence of cardiovascular abnormalities (e.g., a chronic sinus arrhythmia).

LABORATORY TESTS

No specific laboratory tests are indicated.

IMAGING STUDIES

No specific imaging studies are recommended.

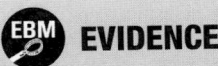 **TREATMENT**

NONPHARMACOLOGIC THERAPY

- Cognitive-behavioral therapy (CBT) and exposure-based treatments have been effective for treating social phobia in controlled trials.
- Behavioral treatments can involve relaxation training, often paired with visualization and progressive desensitization.

- Success rates in treating specific phobias are higher when the phobia is not complicated by other anxiety disorders.

ACUTE GENERAL Rx

- Benzodiazepines provide rapid relief of anxiety associated with exposure to provoking stimuli.
- Lorazepam or alprazolam can be administered sublingually to increase the rate of absorption.
- Beta-blockers (e.g., propranolol) have been used to decrease autonomic hyperarousal and tremor associated with performance situations (e.g., before public speaking).

CHRONIC Rx

- If the phobic stimulus is rarely encountered, benzodiazepines on an as-needed basis can be an appropriate long-term treatment.
- Selective serotonin reuptake inhibitors are the most effective pharmacologic treatment in reducing symptoms and improving function for people with social phobia.
- Monoamine oxidase inhibitors are also effective for treatment of social phobia.

COMPLEMENTARY & ALTERNATIVE MEDICINE

No definitive evidence supports complementary or alternative medicines in the treatment of phobic disorders.

DISPOSITION

Phobic disorders generally present for life, though outpatient-based treatment may effectively reduce symptoms.

REFERRAL

Recommended for confirmation of diagnosis and for evaluation for psychotherapy and other treatment modalities.

PEARLS & CONSIDERATIONS

People with social phobia often have low self-esteem and fear being scrutinized by others such that they avoid or are fearful of any situation in which others may assess or evaluate them directly or indirectly. More than half are concurrently affected by another anxiety disorder, and alcohol and other substance dependence is common because these patients often use substances to mask their anxiety.

EVIDENCE

available at www.expertconsult.com

SUGGESTED READINGS
available at www.expertconsult.com

AUTHOR: **ILJIE KIM FITZGERALD, M.D., M.S.**

BASIC INFORMATION

DEFINITION

From the Latin words *pilus,* meaning hair, and *nidus,* meaning nest.

A *pilonidal sinus* is a short tract that extends from the skin surface and most likely represents a distended hair follicle. It is most commonly found in the intergluteal fold sacrococcygeal region, but it can also occur in the interdigital area, umbilicus, chest wall, and scalp. An *acute pilonidal abscess,* which consists of pus and a wall of edematous fat, results from rupture of an infected follicle into fat. A *chronic pilonidal abscess* results when an infected follicle ruptures directly into surrounding tissues; the wall of a chronic pilonidal abscess consists of fibrous tissue. A *pilonidal cyst* develops from a chronic abscess of long duration as a thin and flat lining of epithelium grows into the cavity from the skin surface.

SYNONYMS

Jeep disease

ICD-9CM CODES
685.1 Pilonidal cyst

EPIDEMIOLOGY & DEMOGRAPHICS

INCIDENCE: 26 cases per 100,000 persons
PREDOMINANT SEX: Males are more commonly affected than females (2.2:1)
AVERAGE AGE OF PRESENTATION: 21 yr
RISK FACTORS:
- Male sex
- Caucasian race
- Family predisposition
- Obesity
- Sedentary lifestyle
- Occupation requiring prolonged sitting
- Local hirsutism
- Poor hygiene
- Increased sweat activity

PHYSICAL FINDINGS & CLINICAL PRESENTATION

- May manifest as asymptomatic pits or pores in the natal cleft
- Tenderness after physical activity or prolonged sitting
- Acute pilonidal abscess in 20% of patients with pilonidal disease
- Presents as a hot, tender, fluctuant swelling just lateral to the midline over the sacrum that may exude pus through the midline pit
- Chronic pilonidal abscess in 80% of patients with pilonidal disease
- Acute suppuration, tenderness, swelling, and heat
- Infrequently, systemic reaction: occasionally fever, leukocytosis, and malaise

ETIOLOGY

- Currently believed to be acquired rather than congenital.
- Drilling of hair shed from the perineum or the head into sebaceous or hair follicles in the natal cleft.
- Drilling is facilitated by the friction of the natal cleft.
- Subsequent infection by skin organisms leads to pilonidal abscess.

DIAGNOSIS

DIFFERENTIAL DIAGNOSIS

- Perianal abscess arising from the posterior midline crypt
- Hidradenitis suppurativa
- Carbuncle
- Furuncle
- Osteomyelitis
- Anal fistula
- Coccygeal sinus

WORKUP

- Diagnosis is based on history and physical examination.
- Midline pits present behind the anus overlying the sacrum and coccyx.
- Broken hairs are often seen extruding from the midline pits.
- Insert probe in pilonidal sinus in path away from the anus.
- Complicated anal fistula may be angulating posteriorly before passing into a retrorectal abscess, but thorough examination of the anal cavity usually discloses point of origin.

LABORATORY TESTS

Complete blood count

IMAGING STUDIES

CT scan in advanced, recurrent cases

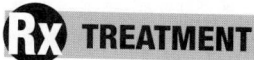 TREATMENT

NONPHARMACOLOGIC THERAPY

Prevention of exacerbations:
1. Local hygiene
2. Avoidance of prolonged sitting position
3. Weight reduction

ACUTE GENERAL Rx

- Procedure of choice for first-episode acute abscess: simple incision and drainage in an outpatient setting
- Cure rate of 76% after 18 mo
- Antibiotics: generally not indicated unless the patient has a medical condition such as rheumatic heart disease or is immunosuppressed

CHRONIC Rx

Elective treatment of pilonidal disease:
1. Minimal surgery:
   a. Remove hair from midline pits and shave buttocks.
   b. May use a fine wire brush with local anesthesia to clear the pits and any lateral openings of granulation tissue and hair.
   c. Keep area clean.
2. Fistulotomy and curettage:
   a. Used when minimal surgery does not control episodes of suppuration
   b. Pass probe to outline the pilonidal sinus and open tract surgically
   c. Curette granulation tissue at the base of the sinus and excise edges of the skin
   d. Keep open granulating wound meticulously clean and allow to heal
   e. If complete healing does not take place, use a skin graft or advancement flap to close the defect
3. Marsupialization:
   a. This is the treatment of choice for chronic pilonidal disease.
   b. Wide excision of the pilonidal area is performed, including all affected skin and subcutaneous tissues down to the presacral fascia.
   c. Wound is left open, allowed to marsupialize, or closed as a primary procedure.
   d. Give antibiotics for 24 hr (particularly those directed against *Staphylococcus* and *Bacteroides* species).
4. Other procedures:
   a. Excision and closure
   b. Excision and skin grafting
   c. Bascom procedure (follicle removal and lateral drainage)
   d. Flaps: *Z*-plasty, V-Y advancement flap, rhomboid flap, gluteus maximus myocutaneous flap

DISPOSITION

- Recurrence rate for excision (most definitive procedure): 1% to 6%
- Incidence of squamous cell carcinoma in a chronic, recurrent pilonidal sinus is rare <1%

REFERRAL

- Emergency department for incision and drainage for an acute abscess
- To a surgeon for elective treatment or management of chronic or recurrent disease

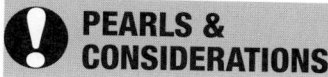 PEARLS & CONSIDERATIONS

COMMENTS

Because of significant associated morbidity, the elective surgical procedures outlined are performed only after the potential risks versus benefits are carefully weighed.

SUGGESTED READINGS
available at www.expertconsult.com

AUTHORS: **ARUNDATHI G. PRASAD, M.D.,** and **RUBEN ALVERO, M.D.**

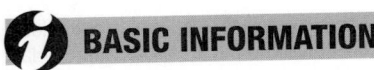

BASIC INFORMATION

DEFINITION

Pinworms are a noninvasive infestation of the intestinal tract by *Enterobius vermicularis*, a helminth of the nematode family.

SYNONYMS

Enterobiasis

ICD-9CM CODES
127.4 Enterobiasis

EPIDEMIOLOGY & DEMOGRAPHICS

- Most common intestinal nematode; approximately 30,000 cases annually in the U.S.
- Worldwide distribution, but most common in temperate climates.
- The prevalence of pinworm infection is lowest in infants and reaches highest infection rate in school-age children (ages 5 to 14 yr).
- Eggs are infective within 6 hr of oviposition and may remain so for 20 days.
- Clusters are found in families, institutionalized persons, and homosexual men.

PHYSICAL FINDINGS & CLINICAL PRESENTATION

- Most infested persons are asymptomatic.
- Perianal itching is the most common reported symptom, with scratching leading to excoriation and sometimes secondary infection.
- Rarely insomnia, irritability, anorexia, and weight loss are described.
- Granulomas have been described in various organs resulting from worms wandering outside the intestines and dying there.

ETIOLOGY & PATHOGENESIS

- *E. vermicularis* is highly prevalent throughout the world, particularly in countries of the temperate zone. Human beings are the only host for this worm. Infestation is by fecal–oral route; ingested eggs hatch in the stomach and the larvae migrate to the colon, where they mature. Gravid female worms containing an average of 10,000 ova migrate to the perianal skin at night, lay their eggs there, and die. The eggs embryonate within 6 hr and cause itching; scratching causes egg deposition under fingernails, from which they can contaminate food or lead to autoreinfection.
- *E. vermicularis* may be transmitted between sexual partners, especially those engaging in oral–anal sex.

DIAGNOSIS

DIFFERENTIAL DIAGNOSIS

- Perianal itching related to poor hygiene
- Hemorrhoidal disease and anal fissures
- Perineal yeast/fungal infections

Section II describes the causes of pruritus ani.

WORKUP

Identification of adult worms or eggs. *E. vermicularis* ova are ovoid but flattened on one side and measure approximately 56 × 27 micrometers (Fig. 1-288). The eggs can be identified on transparent tape placed on the perianal skin on awakening. (NOTE: Five consecutive negative tests rule out the diagnosis.) A single examination detects 50% of infections, three examinations detect 90%, and five examinations detect 99%.

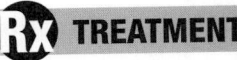

TREATMENT

- Single dose of mebendazole (100 mg) with a repeat dose given after 2 wk.
- Single dose of albendazole (400 mg) with a second dose given 2 wk later is also highly effective.
- Pyrantel pamoate (11 mg/kg up to 1 g) can prevent against *E. vermicularis*. It is available as a suspension and has minimal toxicity (mild transient gastrointestinal symptoms, headache, drowsiness). A repeat dose after 2 wk is recommended because of the frequency of reinfection and autoinfection.
- Other infected family members, classmates, or residents of long-term care facilities should be treated at the same time as the index case.

SUGGESTED READING

available at www.expertconsult.com

AUTHOR: **FRED F. FERRI, M.D.**

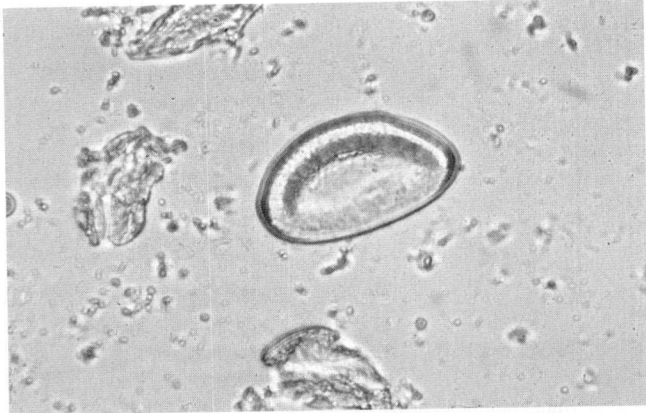

FIGURE 1-288 Enterobius vermicularis embryonated egg. Note larva inside (40 × 10 μm). (From Gorbach SL et al [eds]: *Infectious diseases,* ed 2, Philadelphia, 1998, WB Saunders.)

DEFINITION

Pituitary adenoma is a benign neoplasm of the anterior lobe of the pituitary that causes symptoms, either by excess secretion of hormones or by a local mass effect as the tumor impinges on other, nearby structures (e.g., optic chiasm, hypothalamus, pituitary stalk). Pituitary adenomas are classified by their size, function, and features that characterize their appearance. Microadenomas are <10 mm in size, and macroadenomas are ≥10 mm in size.

- *Acromegaly* is the disease state characterized by a pituitary adenoma that secretes growth hormone (GH).
- A *prolactinoma* secretes prolactin (PRL).
- *Cushing's disease* is a disease state of hypersecretion of adrenocorticotropic hormone (ACTH).
- *Thyrotropin-secreting pituitary adenomas* secrete primarily thyroid-stimulating hormone (TSH).
- *Nonsecretory pituitary adenomas* are those in which the neoplasm is a space-occupying lesion whose secretory products do not cause a specific disease state.

ICD-9CM CODES
253   Pituitary adenoma
253.0 Acromegaly
253.1 Prolactinoma

EPIDEMIOLOGY & DEMOGRAPHICS

CLASSIFICATION (BY HORMONE SECRETED):
- PRL only: 35%
- No hormone: 30%
- GH only: 20%
- PRL and GH: 7%
- ACTH: 7%
- Luteinizing hormone (LH), follicle-stimulating hormone (FSH), TSH: 1%

PREVALENCE/INCIDENCE:
- Pituitary adenomas: up to 10% to 15% of all intracranial neoplasms; 3% to 27% at autopsy series
- Prolactinomas: up to 20% in women with unexplained primary or secondary amenorrhea
- GH-secreting pituitary adenoma: 50 to 60 cases per 1 million persons
- Thyrotropin-secreting pituitary adenoma: 2.8% of pituitary adenomas with a slight female/male predominance of 1.7:1
- Corticotropin-secreting pituitary adenomas: female/male predominance of 8:1

PHYSICAL FINDINGS & CLINICAL PRESENTATION

PROLACTINOMAS:
- Females:
  1. Galactorrhea
  2. Amenorrhea
  3. Oligomenorrhea with anovulation
  4. Infertility
  5. Estrogen deficiency leading to hirsutism
  6. Decreased vaginal lubrication
  7. Osteopenia
- Males:
  1. Large tumors more common as a result of delayed diagnosis
  2. Possible impotence, decreased libido, or hypogonadism
  3. Galactorrhea rare because males lack the estrogen-dependent breast growth and differentiation

GH-SECRETING PITUITARY ADENOMA: ACROMEGALY
- Coarse facial features
- Oily skin
- Prognathism
- Carpal tunnel syndrome
- Osteoarthritis
- History of increased hat, glove, or shoe size
- Decreased exercise capacity
- Visual field deficits
- Diabetes mellitus

CORTICOTROPIN-SECRETING PITUITARY ADENOMA: CUSHING'S DISEASE
- Usually present when the tumor is small (1 to 2 mm)
- 50% of the tumors <5 mm
- Other symptoms:
  1. Truncal obesity
  2. Round facies (moon face)
  3. Dorsocervical fat accumulation (buffalo hump)
  4. Hirsutism
  5. Acne
  6. Menstrual disorders
  7. Hypertension
  8. Striae
  9. Bruising
  10. Thin skin
  11. Hyperglycemia

THYROTROPIN-SECRETING PITUITARY ADENOMA:
- In males, larger, more invasive, and more rapidly growing tumors that present later in life
- Other symptoms: thyrotoxicosis, goiter, visual impairment

NONSECRETORY PITUITARY ADENOMAS (ENDOCRINE INACTIVE PITUITARY ADENOMA):
- Usually large at the time of diagnosis
- Symptoms:
  1. Bitemporal hemianopsia as a result of compression of the optic chiasm
  2. Hypopituitarism from compression of the pituitary gland
  3. Hypogonadism in men and in premenopausal women
  4. Cranial nerve deficits caused by extension into the cavernous sinus
  5. Hydrocephalus from extension into the third ventricle, compressing the foramen of Monro
  6. Diabetes insipidus resulting from compression of the hypothalamus or pituitary stalk (a rare complication)

ETIOLOGY

Benign neoplasms of epithelial origin

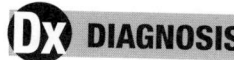

DIFFERENTIAL DIAGNOSIS

PROLACTINOMA:
- Pregnancy
- Postpartum puerperium
- Primary hypothyroidism
- Breast disease
- Breast stimulation
- Drug ingestion (especially phenothiazines, antidepressants, haloperidol, methyldopa, reserpine, opiates, amphetamines, and cimetidine)
- Chronic renal failure
- Liver disease
- Polycystic ovarian disease
- Chest wall disorders
- Spinal cord lesions
- Previous cranial irradiation

ACROMEGALY: Ectopic production of GH-releasing hormone from a carcinoid or other neuroendocrine tumor

CUSHING'S DISEASE:
- Diseases that cause ectopic sources of ACTH overproduction (including small-cell carcinoma of the lung, bronchial carcinoid, intestinal carcinoid, pancreatic islet cell tumor, medullary thyroid carcinoma, or pheochromocytoma)
- Adrenal adenomas, adrenal carcinoma
- Nelson's syndrome

THYROTROPIN-SECRETNG PITUITARY ADENOMAS: Primary hypothyroidism

NONSECRETORY PITUITARY ADENOMA: Non-neoplastic mass lesions of various etiologies (e.g., infectious, granulomatous)

WORKUP

See Section III, "Pituitary Tumor."

PROLACTINOMA:
First step: measurement of basal PRL levels (practitioners should be aware of discriminatory values in their own institutions)
- Elevated PRL levels are correlated with tumor size.
- Level >200 ng/ml is diagnostic, with levels of 100 to 200 ng/ml being equivocal.
- Basal PRL levels between 20 and 100 suggest a microadenoma as well as other conditions such as psychotropic drug ingestion, recent breast examination, and even a recent meal.
- Basal level <20 ng/ml is usually considered normal.
- Prolactin normative data should be developed by each institution for its population.
- Threshold level for obtaining imaging such as MRI should be developed by individual providers depending on the level of specificity and sensitivity desired.

ACROMEGALY:
- First screening tests are the measurement of the serum insulin-like growth factor I level, postprandial serum GH, and TRH stimulation test.
- Follow with an oral glucose tolerance test.
- Failure to suppress serum GH to <2 ng/ml with an oral load of 100 g glucose is considered conclusive.

- A GH-releasing hormone level >300 ng/ml is indicative of an ectopic source of GH.

CUSHING'S DISEASE:
- Normal or slightly elevated corticotropin levels ranging from 20 to 200 pg/ml; normal is 10 to 50 pg/ml (normative data should be developed by each institution for its population).
- Level <10 pg/ml usually indicates an autonomously secreting adrenal tumor.
- Level >200 pg/ml suggests an ectopic corticotropin-secreting neoplasm.
- Cushing's disease can be assessed by absence of cortisol suppression with the low-dose dexamethasone test but with the presence of cortisol suppression after the high-dose test. As a method to distinguish Cushing's disease from an ectopic source of ACTH, this test is robust.
- 24-hr urine collection should demonstrate an increased level of cortisol excretion.

THYROTROPIN-SECRETING PITUITARY ADENOMA:
- Highly sensitive thyrotropin assays, which evaluate the presence of thyrotoxicosis, are one way to detect a thyrotropin-secreting tumor.
- Free alpha subunit is secreted by >80% of tumors, with the ratio of the alpha subunit to thyrotropin <1.
- With central resistance to thyroid hormone, ratio is <1 and the sella is normal.
- Laboratory tests show elevated serum levels of both T_3 and T_4.

NONSECRETORY PITUITARY ADENOMA:
- Visual field testing
- Assessment of the pituitary and organ function to determine if there is hypopituitarism or hypersecretion of hormones (even if the effects of hypersecretion are subclinical)
- TRH to provoke secretion of FSH, LH, and LH-beta-subunit; will not elicit response in normal persons
- Exclusion of Klinefelter's syndrome in patient with longstanding primary hypogonadism, elevated gonadotropin levels, and enlargement of the sella

IMAGING STUDIES

Study of choice: MRI of the pituitary and hypothalamus
- When evaluating Cushing's disease, small size at the onset of symptoms noted
- MRI, in this case, only 60% sensitive at best and may yield false-positive results

- CT scan only when MRI is unavailable or is otherwise contraindicated

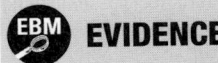

TREATMENT

NONPHARMACOLOGIC THERAPY
SURGERY:
- Selective transsphenoidal resection of the adenoma is the treatment of choice for acromegaly, Cushing's disease, and thyrotropin-secreting pituitary adenomas, all of which tend to be microadenomas at the time of onset of symptoms.
- Macroadenomas, such as the nonsecretory pituitary adenoma, may also be surgically removed, but risk of recurrence is greater with these tumors and adjunctive therapy such as irradiation may also be necessary.
- Radiotherapy is reserved for patients who have not responded to surgical treatment and who still have symptoms of the adenoma.
- Bilateral adrenalectomy has been performed in patients with Cushing's disease after failure of other therapies; complications requiring lifelong hormone replacement or Nelson's syndrome may occur.

RADIOTHERAPY:
- Generally reserved for patients who have not responded to surgical treatment
- Used with varying degrees of success in all the different pituitary adenomas

ACUTE GENERAL Rx
PROLACTINOMA:
- Bromocriptine, a dopamine analog, is generally given orally in divided doses of 1.5 to 10 mg.
- Side effects include orthostatic hypotension, nausea, and dizziness; avoided by beginning with low-dose therapy.
- Other compounds include pergolide mesylate, a long-acting ergot derivative with dopaminergic properties, as well as other nonergot derivatives.

ACROMEGALY:
- Octreotide, a somatostatin analog, 100 mcg SC, is the medical therapy of choice but is limited by side effects such as biliary sludge and gallstones, nausea, cramps, steatorrhea, and its parenteral administration.
- Bromocriptine 10 to 20 mg PO tid to qid is less effective than octreotide but has the advantage of oral administration.

CUSHING'S DISEASE:
- Ketoconazole, which inhibits the cytochrome P-450 enzymes involved in steroid biosynthesis, is effective in managing mild to moderate disease in daily oral doses of 600 to 1200 mg.
- Metyrapone and aminoglutethimide can be used to control hypersecretion of cortisol but are generally used when preparing a patient for surgery or while waiting for a response to radiotherapy.

THYROTROPIN-SECRETING PITUITARY ADENOMA:
- Ablative therapy with either radioactive iodide or surgery is indicated.
- Treatment directed to the thyroid alone may accelerate growth of the pituitary adenoma.
- Octreotide has been shown to be effective in doses similar to those used for acromegaly.

NONSECRETORY PITUITARY ADENOMA:
- There is no role for medical therapy at this time.
- Surgery and radiotherapy are indicated.

CHRONIC Rx

For all pituitary adenomas:
- Careful follow-up is important. Patients undergoing transsphenoidal microsurgical resection should be seen in 4 to 6 wk to ensure that the adenoma has been completely removed and that the endocrine hypersecretion is resolved.
- If there is good clinical response, patient should be monitored yearly for recurrence and to follow the level of the hypersecreted hormone.
- Patients who have undergone irradiation should have close follow-up with backup medical therapy because response to radiotherapy may be delayed; incidence of hypopituitarism also increases with time.

EBM EVIDENCE

available at www.expertconsult.com

SUGGESTED READINGS
available at www.expertconsult.com

AUTHORS: **BETH J. WUTZ, M.D.**, and **RUBEN ALVERO, M.D.**

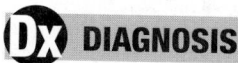

BASIC INFORMATION

DEFINITION

Pityriasis is a common self-limiting skin eruption of unknown etiology.

ICD-9CM CODES
696.3 Pityriasis rosea

EPIDEMIOLOGY & DEMOGRAPHICS

- Most cases of pityriasis rosea occur between ages 10 and 35 yr; mean age is 23 yr.
- The incidence of disease is highest in the fall and spring.
- Female/male ratio is 1.5:1.

PHYSICAL FINDINGS & CLINICAL PRESENTATION

- Initial lesion (herald patch) precedes the eruption by approximately 1 to 2 wk; typically measures 3 to 6 cm; it is round to oval in appearance and most frequently located on the trunk.
- Eruptive phase follows within 2 wk and peaks after 7 to 14 days.
- Lesions are most frequently located in the lower abdominal area. They have a salmon-pink appearance in whites and a hyperpigmented appearance in blacks.

- Most lesions are 4 to 5 mm in diameter; center has a "cigarette paper" appearance; border has a characteristic ring of scale (collarette).
- Lesions occur in a symmetric distribution and follow the cleavage lines of the trunk (Christmas tree pattern [Fig. 1-289]).
- The number of lesions varies from a few to hundreds.
- Most patients are asymptomatic; pruritus is the most common symptom.
- History of recent fatigue, headache, sore throat, and low-grade fever is present in approximately 25% of cases.

ETIOLOGY

Unknown, possibly viral (picornavirus)

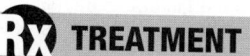

DIAGNOSIS

DIFFERENTIAL DIAGNOSIS

- Tinea corporis (can be ruled out by potassium hydroxide examination)
- Secondary syphilis (absence of herald patch, positive serologic test for syphilis)
- Psoriasis
- Nummular eczema
- Drug eruption: medications that may cause rashes similar to pityriasis rosea include clonidine, captopril, interferon, bismuth, bar-

biturates, gold, hepatitis B vaccine, and imatinib mesylate
- Viral exanthem
- Eczema
- Lichen planus
- Tinea versicolor (the lesions are more brown and the borders are not as ovoid)

WORKUP

Presence of herald lesion and characteristic rash are diagnostic. Skin biopsy is generally reserved for atypical cases.

LABORATORY TESTS

Generally not necessary; serologic test for syphilis if clinically indicated

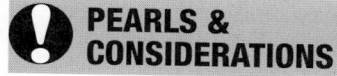

TREATMENT

NONPHARMACOLOGIC THERAPY

The disease is self-limited and generally does not require any therapeutic intervention.

ACUTE GENERAL Rx

- Use calamine lotion or oral antihistamines in patients with significant pruritus.
- Use prednisone tapered over 2 wk in patients with severe pruritus.
- Direct sun exposure or use of ultraviolet light within the first week of eruption is beneficial in decreasing the severity of disease.

DISPOSITION

- Spontaneous complete resolution of the rash within 4 to 8 wk
- Recurrence rare (<2% of cases)

PEARLS & CONSIDERATIONS

COMMENTS

Reassure patient that the disease is not contagious and its course is benign.

SUGGESTED READING
available at www.expertconsult.com

AUTHOR: **FRED F. FERRI, M.D.**

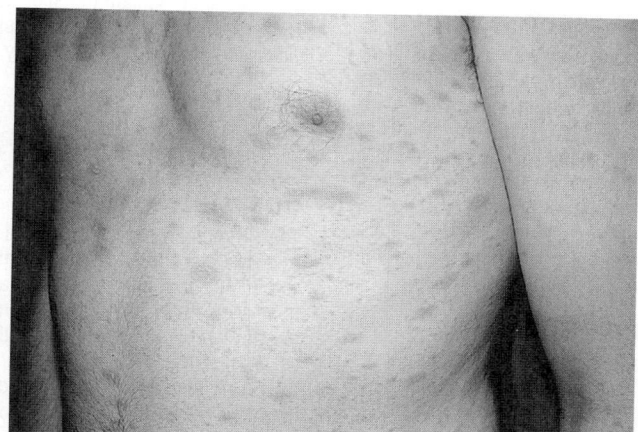

FIGURE 1-289 Scale (pityriasis rosea). Shows example of how unique scaling (collarette of fine scale within several lesions), distribution and shape of lesions (oval lesions with long axis paralleling natural skin cleavage lines), and color (salmon-pink) help in diagnosing skin disease. (From Noble J [ed]: *Textbook of primary care medicine,* ed 3, St Louis, 2001, Mosby.)

BASIC INFORMATION

DEFINITION

Placenta previa is the implantation of the placenta over the internal os. Four degrees of this abnormality (Fig. 1-290) have been traditionally defined, however, the accurate localization of the placental edge in relation to the discrete point of the internal os with transvaginal sonography makes the following terms outmoded:

1. Total placenta previa: the internal os is covered completely.
2. Partial placenta previa: the internal os is partially covered.
3. Marginal placenta previa: the edge of the placenta is at the margin of the internal os.
4. Low-lying placenta: the placenta is implanted in the lower uterine segment and, although its edge does not reach the internal os, is in close proximity to it.

ICD-9CM CODES
641.1 Placenta previa

EPIDEMIOLOGY & DEMOGRAPHICS

INCIDENCE: 0.26% to 0.7% of pregnancies
RISK FACTORS:
- Previous cesarean delivery (after one cesarean delivery, the risk is 1% to 4%; after four or more, the risk approaches 10%).
- Multiparity has also been associated with placenta previa.

PHYSICAL FINDINGS & CLINICAL PRESENTATION

The classic presentation of placenta previa is painless vaginal bleeding, usually in the second or third trimester. Uterine contractions may or may not be present. On physical examination, the uterus is soft and pain free. The fetus is often in breech, transverse lie, or high. Fetal distress is usually not present.

DIAGNOSIS

DIFFERENTIAL DIAGNOSIS

- Placenta accreta
- Placenta percreta
- Placenta increta
- Vasa previa
- Abruptio placentae
- Vaginal or cervical trauma
- Labor
- Local malignancy

WORKUP

- Do *not* perform a digital vaginal examination.
- The diagnosis of placenta previa can seldom be firmly established by physical examination alone. A speculum examination in a hospital setting to exclude any local bleeding may be performed.

- This diagnosis should not be dismissed until thorough evaluation, including sonography, has completely excluded its presence.

LABORATORY TESTS

- A complete blood count can be used to monitor hemoglobin and hematocrit
- A Kleihauer-Betke preparation of maternal blood in all Rh-negative women and Rh-immune globulin when indicated

IMAGING STUDIES

- The simplest and safest method of placental localization is transabdominal sonography with confirmatory imaging by transvaginal ultrasonography (TVS). Transabdominal ultrasound alone is inaccurate in the diagnosis of placenta previa and should be used only as a screening tool. TVS has become the gold standard for the diagnosis of placent previa. It is safe even in the presence of active bleeding. A distance of ≤20 mm from placental edge to interior cervical os is becoming a new criterion for performing term cesarean delivery in women with placenta previa.
- MRI has also been effective in detecting placenta previa, although sonography remains the preferred method.

TREATMENT

NONPHARMACOLOGIC THERAPY

- In preterm pregnancies with no active bleeding, close observation and expectant management are indicated. In those with active bleeding, conservative management, including blood transfusions for severe bleeds, is appropriate. The woman should stay in the hospital for at least 48 hr after the bleeding has stopped.
- Bed rest, preferably in a hospital setting, should be prescribed.

ACUTE GENERAL Rx

- Initial assessment for signs of maternal hemodynamic compromise or hemorrhagic

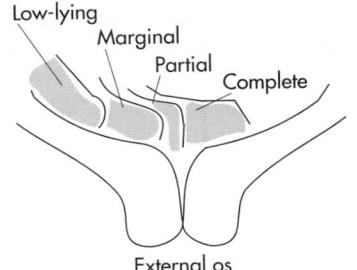

FIGURE 1-290 Depiction of degrees of placenta previa. (From Weisslederer R et al: *Primer of diagnostic imaging,* St Louis, 2007, Mosby.)

shock; large-bore IV access with crystalloid fluid resuscitation
- Assess fetal status and gestational age by sonogram and continuous fetal heart rate monitoring
- Cross-matched blood should be made available during bleeding episodes; if the hemorrhage is severe, cesarean delivery is indicated despite fetal immaturity
- Tocolytic therapy may be considered in those women in preterm labor, as well as the administration of corticosteroids to enhance fetal lung maturity

CHRONIC Rx

- Cesarean delivery is necessary in nearly all cases of placenta previa.
- Uncontrollable hemorrhage after placental removal should be anticipated as a result of the poorly contractile nature of the lower uterine segment. The need for hysterectomy to control bleeding should be discussed with the patient before delivery, if possible.

DISPOSITION

Because of the unpredictable nature of placenta previa, not all women with placenta previa can be treated expectantly.

REFERRAL

Affected women and their families should be aware of all signs and symptoms that would necessitate immediate transport to the hospital. The possibility of hysterectomy should also be discussed early during pregnancy.

PEARLS & CONSIDERATIONS

COMMENTS

Third-trimester measurement of the distance from the placental edge to the internal cervical os by TVS commonly is used to gauge the likelihood of need for cesarean section. The decision to offer women with a placenta that is situated 11 to 20 mm away a trial of labor remains controversial. Recent reports by Vergani et al indicate that more than two-thirds of women with a placental edge to cervical os distance of >10 mm fewer than 28 days before delivery can deliver vaginally without increased risk of hemorrhage

SUGGESTED READINGS
available at www.expertconsult.com

AUTHORS: **SONYA S. ABDEL-RAZEQ, M.D.,** and **RUBEN ALVERO, M.D.**

BASIC INFORMATION

DEFINITION

The plantar fascia arises from the calcaneal tuberosity and has various attachments as it travels longitudinally, ending at the digital level. It acts as a tension band supporting the medial longitudinal arch of the foot. Plantar fasciitis describes the local inflammation and subsequent pain occurring at the insertion at the medial calcaneal tuberosity or along the course of the fascial band.

SYNONYMS

Heel pain syndrome

ICD-9CM CODES
728.71 Plantar fasciitis
726.73 Calcaneal spur

EPIDEMIOLOGY & DEMOGRAPHICS

PREDOMINANT SEX: Females slightly greater than males, studies vary.
PREDOMINANT AGE: Commonly middle aged; any age group possible.
RISK FACTORS: Weight gain, obesity, increased activity, prolonged standing, trauma, certain activities (see etiology).

PHYSICAL FINDINGS & CLINICAL PRESENTATION

- Pain localized to the heel or along the course of the plantar fascia.
- Pain greatest upon the first steps in the morning and upon standing after rest.
- Symptoms may improve throughout the day or with ambulation, but may persist or increase with prolonged standing.
- Pain may be elicited with ankle dorsiflexion and simultaneous subtalar eversion.
- Often exquisitely tender upon palpation of the medial calcaneal tuberosity
- May have localized or medial heel edema.

ETIOLOGY

- Any factor that increases the tension at the insertion of the fascia on the medial calcaneal tuberosity, creating local inflammation. Evidence suggests that plantar spurs are secondary rather than an etiology; these are an incidental finding in about 30% of asymptomatic patients.
- Achilles/ankle equinus or pseudoequinus.
- Active STJ/rearfoot pronation, such as with calcaneal or forefoot varus.
- A strain of the fascia or dorsiflexory force of the forefoot on the midfoot or vice versa. Example: jumping from a height, sprinting from starting blocks.

DIAGNOSIS

DIFFERENTIAL DIAGNOSIS

- Calcaneal fracture, including traumatic or stress fracture, or bone bruise.
- Tarsal tunnel syndrome.
- Calcaneal osteomyelitis.
- Bone cyst or bone tumor.
- Posterior tibial tendon dysfunction.
- Plantar fascial fibromatosis (thickening/soft tissue mass along the plantar fascial band).
- Systemic cause: Gout, Psoriasis, Reiter's Syndrome, etc.

STUDIES

- Initial x-ray to rule out tumor or trauma. Lateral, oblique, calcaneal axial views.
- MRI/bone scan to rule out stress fracture (takes 2 wk to show on x-ray)
- MRI or ultrasound if suspected plantar fascial fibromatosis.
- May need to rule out tarsal tunnel syndrome with nerve studies.

TREATMENT

- Supportive lace-up sneakers with firm, cushioned sole.
- Ice, stretching exercises, NSAIDs, limit activity.
- Low-dye strapping/taping.
- Steroid/local anesthetic injections (Fig. 1-291) via several techniques.
- Custom orthotics will limit subtalar joint overpronation and other faulty biomechanics.
- Add heel cushion to orthotics if acute pain/inflammation.
- Heel lifts if the etiology is Achilles equinus or pseudoequinus.
- Night splints maintain ankle dorsiflexion overnight.

- Severe cases may require a cast or cast walker for 4 to 6 wk
- Recalcitrant cases may require surgical endoscopic or open fasciotomy.

DISPOSITION

Cases that are treated sooner and acute cases with sudden onset have a higher likelihood of resolving completely. Chronic, recalcitrant cases may require surgery.

REFERRAL

- For biomechanical exam or surgical consult (podiatric/orthopedic foot/ankle surgeon).
- Physical therapy is often beneficial when first-line therapy fails.

PEARLS & CONSIDERATIONS

COMMENTS

Caution: Common, seemingly simple diagnosis. Do not overlook differential diagnosis.

PREVENTION

- Avoid shoes with bendable/flexible soles and shoes without laces/straps.
- Maintain foot/ankle flexibility with stretching exercises.
- Seek treatment at first signs of pain.

SUGGESTED READINGS
available at www.expertconsult.com

AUTHOR: **BROOKE E. KEELEY, DPM**

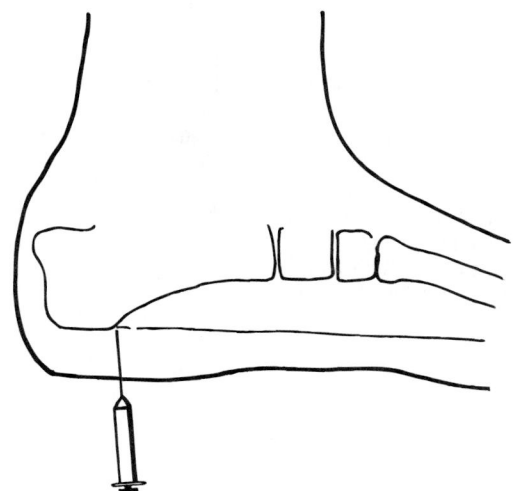

FIGURE 1-291 Injection site for plantar fasciitis. Injection should be through the sole into the area of maximum tenderness. A 25- or 27-gauge needle should be used and the medication injected slowly because some pain may occur. The total volume should be no greater than 1.5 ml. (From Mercier L: *Practical orthopedics*, ed 5, St Louis, 2002, Mosby.)

BASIC INFORMATION

DEFINITION

Pleurisy refers to the inflammation of the parietal pleural. This inflammation results in pleuritic chest pain that is characteristically worsened with respiration or movement.

SYNONYMS

Pleuritis

ICD-9CM CODES
511.0 Pleurisy

EPIDEMIOLOGY & DEMOGRAPHICS

INCIDENCE: One of the most common causes of pleuritic chest pain is viral pleurisy. However, there are a variety of disorders that may result in pleurisy. Infectious diseases, rheumatologic disorders, thromboembolic events, and trauma may all lead to pleural inflammation. Therefore, the incidence of pleurisy varies in accordance with the underlying etiology.

PHYSICAL FINDINGS & CLINICAL PRESENTATION

- The defining characteristic of pleurisy is chest pain that worsens with respiration, coughing, or sneezing.
- Pleuritic chest pain is typically described as sharp or stabbing. However, pleuritic chest pain may also be described as dull pain, burning pain, or a "catch" while breathing.
- Movements of the trunk or chest wall may exacerbate pain. Patients with pleurisy may locate the position of minimal discomfort and remain still in that position.
- Dyspnea may be associated with pleurisy.
- Physical exam may be remarkable for a pleural friction rub.
- Decreased breath sounds, rales, or egophony may be appreciated if pneumonia is the underlying etiology of the patient's pleurisy.

ETIOLOGY

- Pleurisy is caused by inflammation of the parietal pleura. The visceral pleura is not innervated by nociceptors. However, injury or inflammation at the periphery of the lung parenchyma often results in inflammation of the overlying parietal pleura. The parietal pleura, which lines the rib cage and the lateral portion of each hemidiaphragm, is innervated by intercostal nerves; therefore pain is localized to the cutaneous distribution of those nerves (over the chest wall). The parietal pleural of the central diaphragm is innervated by fibers that travel with the phrenic nerve; therefore pain associated with inflammation in this area is referred to the ipsilateral shoulder or neck.
- Various underlying etiologies may result in pleurisy, including:
  1. Thromboembolism (pulmonary embolism)
  2. Viral infection (coxsackie viruses, RSV, CMV, adenovirus, EBV, parainfluenza, influenza)
  3. Bacterial infection (pneumonia or tuberculous pleuritis)
  4. Fungal infection (coccidioidomycosis, histoplasmosis)
  5. Rheumatologic disease (rheumatoid arthritis, SLE)
  6. Medications (drug-induced lupus)
  7. Malignancy of the lung or pleura
  8. Trauma (rib fracture)
  9. Hereditary (familial Mediterranean fever, sickle cell disease)

DIAGNOSIS

DIFFERENTIAL DIAGNOSIS

- Cardiac: myocardial infarction, ischemia, pericarditis.
- Intraabdominal process: pancreatitis, cholecystitis.
- Thromboembolic: pulmonary embolism, infarction of lung parenchyma.
- Traumatic/mechanical: rib fracture or pneumothorax.
- Viral infection: viral infections may lead to epidemic pleurodynia (also known as Bornholm's disease). Implicated viruses include coxsackie viruses, RSV, CMV, adenovirus, EBV, parainfluenza, influenza. Of note, viral pleurisy is a diagnosis of exclusion.
- Bacterial infection: pneumonia or tuberculous pleurisy.
- Fungal infection: coccidioidomycosis, histoplasmosis.
- Rheumatologic disease: rheumatoid arthritis, SLE.
- Medications: drug-induced lupus.
- Hereditary causes: familial Mediterranean fever, sickle cell disease.
- Malignancy: malignancy affecting the lung or pleura.
- Uremia.

WORKUP

- A thorough history and physical exam of all patients presenting with pleuritic chest pain should be taken. The time course of the patient's symptoms can provide valuable diagnostic clues. Acute onset of symptoms is suggestive of traumatic injuries, spontaneous pneumothorax, pulmonary embolism, or myocardial infarction. Subacute onset of symptoms suggests a potential infectious, rheumatologic, or medication-induced cause. Viral pleurisy is often associated with prodromal symptoms of upper respiratory infection. Chronic or recurrent symptoms suggest a potential malignant, tuberculous, or hereditary cause.
- Chest x-ray to evaluate for pneumonia, pneumothorax, or pleural effusion.
- EKG to evaluate for infarction, ischemia, or pericarditis.
- Evaluation for pulmonary embolism should be undertaken if clinical suspicion exists.

LABORATORY TESTS

- Laboratory testing varies based on suspected underlying etiology.
- If a pleural effusion is present, diagnostic thoracentesis may provide valuable diagnostic clues to the underlying etiology.

IMAGING STUDIES

- Chest x-ray
- EKG

TREATMENT

- Treatment of pleurisy consists of pain control as well as treating the underlying condition.
- NSAIDs are the preferred first-line agent to control pain associated with pleurisy. Human studies have been limited to trials using indomethacin for pain control, although an NSAID class effect is presumed.
- Indomethacin 50 mg orally up to three times a day has been found to be effective in relieving pain and is associated with an improvement in mechanical lung function.

SUGGESTED READINGS

available at www.expertconsult.com

AUTHOR: **MARISA VAN POZNAK, M.D.**

BASIC INFORMATION

DEFINITION

Aspiration pneumonia is a vague term that refers to pulmonary abnormalities following abnormal entry of endogenous or exogenous substances in the lower airways. It is generally classified as:

- Aspiration (chemical pneumonitis)
- Primary bacterial aspiration pneumonia
- Secondary bacterial infection of chemical pneumonitis

ICD-9CM CODES
507.0 Aspiration pneumonia

EPIDEMIOLOGY & DEMOGRAPHICS

INCIDENCE (IN U.S.):
- Few reliable data
- 20% to 35% of all pneumonias
- 5% to 15% of all community acquired pneumonias

PEAK INCIDENCE: Elderly patients in hospitals or nursing homes

PREVALENCE (IN U.S.): Unknown (unreliable data)

PREDOMINANT SEX: Males and females affected equally

PREDOMINANT AGE: Elderly

PHYSICAL FINDINGS & CLINICAL PRESENTATION

- Shortness of breath, tachypnea, cough, sputum, fever after vomiting, or difficulty swallowing
- Rales, rhonchi, often diffusely throughout lung

ETIOLOGY

Complex interaction of etiologies, ranging from chemical (often acid) pneumonitis after aspiration of sterile gastric contents (generally not requiring antibiotic treatment) to bacterial aspiration

COMMUNITY-ACQUIRED ASPIRATION PNEUMONIA:

- Generally results from predominantly anaerobic mouth bacteria (anaerobic and microaerophilic streptococci, fusobacteria, gram-positive anaerobic non–spore-forming rods), *Bacteroides* species *(melaninogenicus, intermedius, oralis, ureolyticus)*, *Haemophilus influenzae*, and *Streptococcus pneumoniae*
- Rarely caused by *Bacteroides fragilis* (of uncertain validity in published studies) or *Eikenella corrodens*
- High-risk groups: the elderly; alcoholics; IV drug users; patients who are obtunded; stroke victims; and those with esophageal disorders, seizures, poor dentition, or recent dental manipulations.

HOSPITAL-ACQUIRED ASPIRATION PNEUMONIA:

- Often occurs among elderly patients and others with diminished gag reflex; those with nasogastric tubes, intestinal obstruction, or ventilator support; and especially those ex-

posed to contaminated nebulizers or unsterile suctioning.

- High-risk groups: seriously ill hospitalized patients (especially patients with coma, acidosis, alcoholism, uremia, diabetes mellitus, nasogastric intubation, or recent antimicrobial therapy, who are frequently colonized with aerobic gram-negative rods); patients undergoing anesthesia; those with strokes, dementia, or swallowing disorders; the elderly; and those receiving antacids or H_2 blockers (but not sucralfate).
- Hypoxic patients receiving concentrated O_2 have diminished ciliary activity, encouraging aspiration.
- Causative organisms:
  1. Anaerobes listed above, although in many studies gram-negative aerobes (60%) and gram-positive aerobes (20%) predominate.
  2. *E. coli, P. aeruginosa, S. aureus* including MRSA, *Klebsiella, Enterobacter, Serratia, Proteus* spp. *H. influenzae, S. pneumoniae, Legionella,* and *Acinetobacter* spp. (sporadic pneumonias) in two thirds of cases.
  3. Fungi, including *Candida albicans,* in fewer than 1%.

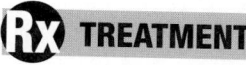

DIAGNOSIS

DIFFERENTIAL DIAGNOSIS

- Other necrotizing or cavitary pneumonias (especially tuberculosis, gram-negative pneumonias)
- See "Pulmonary Tuberculosis"

WORKUP

- Chest x-ray examination
- Complete blood count (CBC), blood cultures
- Sputum Gram stain and culture
- Consideration of tracheal aspirate

LABORATORY TESTS

- CBC: leukocytosis often present
- Sputum Gram stain
  1. Often useful when carefully prepared immediately after obtaining suctioned or expectorated specimen, examined by experienced observer.
  2. Only specimens with multiple white blood cells and rare or absent epithelial cells should be examined.
  3. Unlike nonaspiration pneumonias (e.g., pneumococcal), multiple organisms may be present.
  4. Long, slender rods suggest anaerobes.
  5. Sputum from pneumonia caused by acid aspiration may be devoid of organisms.
  6. Cultures should be interpreted in light of morphology of visualized organisms.

IMAGING STUDIES

- Chest x-ray often reveals bilateral, diffuse, patchy infiltrates and posterior segment upper lobes. Chemical pneumonitis typically affects the most dependent regions of the lungs.

- Aspiration pneumonia of several days' or longer duration may reveal necrosis (especially community-acquired anaerobic pneumonias) and even cavitation with air-fluid levels, indicating lung abscess.

TREATMENT

NONPHARMACOLOGIC THERAPY

- Airway management to prevent repeated aspiration
- Ventilatory support if necessary

ACUTE GENERAL Rx

Acute aspiration of acidic gastric contents without bacteria may not require antibiotic therapy; consult infectious disease or pulmonary expert.

- Community-acquired anaerobic aspiration pneumonia: clindamycin (600 mg IV twice daily followed by 300 mg q6h orally). Intravenous Peniucillion G (1 to 2 million U q4 to 6h) can also still be used. Alternative oral agents include: amoxacillin-clavulanate (875 mg orally twice daily), amoxicillin plus metronidazole or oral moxifloxacin (400 mg orally once daily).
- Nursing home aspirations: levofloxacin 500-750 mg qd or piperacillin-tazobactam 3.375 g q6h or ceftazidime 2 g q8h +/− Vancomycin if MRSA suspected or known
- Hospital-acquired aspiration pneumonia:
  ○ Piperacillin-tazobactam 3.375 g IV q6h, or cefoxitin 2 g IV q8h +/− Vancomycin IV to cover MRSA.
  ○ Knowledge of resident flora in the microenvironment of the aspiration within the hospital is crucial to intelligent antibiotic selection; consult infection control nurses or hospital epidemiologist.
  ○ Confirmed *Pseudomonas* pneumonia should be treated with antipseudomonal beta-lactam agent plus an aminoglycoside until antimicrobial sensitivities confirm that less toxic agents may replace the aminoglycoside.
  ○ Do not use metronidazole alone for anaerobes.

DISPOSITION

Repeat chest x-ray examination in 6 to 8 wk.

REFERRAL

For consultation with infectious disease and/or pulmonary experts for patients with respiratory distress, hypoxia, ventilatory support, pneumonia in more than one lobe, or necrosis or cavitation on x-ray examination or for those not responding to antibiotic therapy within 2 to 3 days.

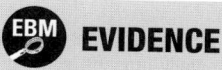
EVIDENCE

available at www.expertconsult.com

SUGGESTED READINGS

available at www.expertconsult.com

AUTHORS: **GLENN G. FORT, M.D., M.P.H.,** and **DENNIS J. MIKOLICH, M.D.**

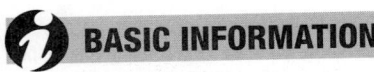

DEFINITION

Bacterial pneumonia is an infection involving the lung parenchyma.

ICD-9CM CODES
486.0 Pneumonia, acute
507.0 Pneumonia, aspiration
482.9 Pneumonia, bacterial
481 Pneumonia, pneumococcal
482.1 Pneumonia, Pseudomonas
482.4 Pneumonia, staphylococcal
482.0 Pneumonia, Klebsiella
482.2 Pneumonia, Haemophilus influenzae

EPIDEMIOLOGY & DEMOGRAPHICS

- The incidence of community-acquired pneumonia (CAP) is 1 in 100 persons.
- The incidence of health care facility–acquired pneumonia (HCAP) is 8 cases per 1000 persons annually.
- Primary care physicians see an average of 10 cases of pneumonia annually.
- Hospitalization rate for pneumonia is 15% to 20%.
- Most cases of pneumonia occur in the winter and in elderly patients.

PHYSICAL FINDINGS & CLINICAL PRESENTATION

- Fever, tachypnea, chills, tachycardia, cough
- Presentation varies with the cause of pneumonia, the patient's age, and the clinical situation:
  - Patients with streptococcal pneumonia usually present with high fever, shaking chills, pleuritic chest pain, cough, and copious production of rusty-appearing purulent sputum. Pleurisy and parapneumonic effusions are also common. Potential complications include bacteremia, empyema, and distant infections (e.g., meningitis).
  - *Mycoplasma pneumoniae:* insidious onset; headache; dry, paroxysmal cough that is worse at night; myalgias; malaise; sore throat; extrapulmonary manifestations (e.g., erythema multiforme, aseptic meningitis, urticaria, erythema nodosum) may be present.
  - *Chlamydia pneumoniae:* persistent, nonproductive cough, low-grade fever, headache, sore throat.
  - *Legionella pneumophila:* high fever, mild cough, mental status change, myalgias, diarrhea, respiratory failure.
  - MRSA pneumonia: often preceded by influenza, may present with shock and respiratory failure.
  - Elderly or immunocompromised hosts with pneumonia may initially present with only minimal symptoms (e.g., low-grade fever, confusion); respiratory and nonrespiratory symptoms are less commonly reported by older patients with pneumonia.
  - In general, auscultation of patients with pneumonia reveals crackles and diminished breath sounds.
  - Percussion dullness is present if the patient has pleural effusion.
  - The clinical impression of pneumonia has an overall sensitivity of 70% to 90%; specificity ranges from 40% to 70%.

ETIOLOGY

- *Streptococcus pneumoniae* (20% to 60% of CAP cases)
- *Haemophilus influenzae* (3% to 10% of CAP cases)
- *L. pneumophila* (1% to 5% of adult pneumonias) (2% to 8% of CAP cases)
- *Klebsiella, Pseudomonas, Escherichia coli*
- *Staphylococcus aureus* (3% to 5% of CAP cases)
- Atypical organisms such as *M. pneumoniae, C. pneumoniae,* and *L. pneumophila* implicated in up to 40% of cases of community-acquired pneumonia
- Pneumococcal infection responsible for 50% to 75% of community-acquired pneumonias. Influenza infection is one of the important predisposing factors to *S. pneumoniae* and *S. aureus* pneumonia; gram-negative organisms cause >80% of nosocomial pneumonias
- Predisposing factors:
  1. Chronic obstructive pulmonary disease: *H. influenzae, S. pneumoniae, Legionella*
  2. Seizures: aspiration pneumonia
  3. Compromised hosts: *Legionella,* gram-negative organisms
  4. Alcoholism: *Klebsiella, S. pneumoniae, H. influenzae*
  5. HIV: *S. pneumoniae*
  6. IV drug addicts with right-sided bacterial endocarditis: *S. aureus*
  7. Older patient with comorbid diseases: *C. pneumoniae*

Dx DIAGNOSIS

DIFFERENTIAL DIAGNOSIS

- Exacerbation of chronic bronchitis
- Pulmonary embolism or infarction
- Lung neoplasm
- Bronchiolitis
- Sarcoidosis
- Hypersensitivity pneumonitis
- Pulmonary edema
- Drug-induced lung injury
- Viral pneumonias
- Fungal pneumonias
- Parasitic pneumonias
- Atypical pneumonia
- Tuberculosis

WORKUP

Laboratory evaluation and chest x-ray. Useful tools for assessing severity of illness are the *CURB-65* (see following) and *Pneumonia Severity Index.* Poor prognostic indicators are: hypotension (SBP <90 or DBP <60), respiratory rate >30/min, hyperpyrexia (>40° C), or hypothermia (<35° C). None of these indices are as valuable as clinical judgement of the physician.

LABORATORY TESTS

- Complete blood count with differential; white blood cell count is elevated, usually with left shift.
- Blood cultures (hospitalized patients only): positive in approximately 20% of cases of pneumococcal pneumonia.
- Pneumococcal urinary antigen test can be used to detect the C-polysaccharide antigen of *S. pneumoniae.* It is a useful tool in the treatment of hospitalized adult patients with CAP.
- Direct immunofluorescent examination of sputum when suspecting *Legionella* (e.g., direct fluorescent antibody stain is a highly specific and rapid test for detecting legionellae in clinical specimen) or urine *Legionella* antigen test.
- Serologic testing for HIV in selected patients.
- Serum electrolytes (hyponatremia in suspected *Legionella* pneumonia), BUN, creatinine.
- Pulse oximetry or arterial blood gases: hypoxemia with partial pressure of oxygen <60 mm Hg while the patient is breathing room air, a standard criterion for hospital admission.

IMAGING STUDIES

Chest x-ray: findings vary with the stage and type of pneumonia and the hydration of the patient (Fig. 1-292).

- Classically, pneumococcal pneumonia presents with a segmental lobe infiltrate.
- Diffuse infiltrates on chest radiograph can be seen with *L. pneumophila, M. pneumoniae,* viral pneumonias, *P. jirovecii (carinii),* miliary tuberculosis, aspiration, aspergillosis.
- An initial chest radiograph is also useful to rule out the presence of any complications (pneumothorax, empyema, abscesses).

Rx TREATMENT

NONPHARMACOLOGIC THERAPY

- Avoidance of tobacco use
- Oxygen to maintain partial oxygen pressure in arterial blood >60 mm Hg
- IV hydration, correction of dehydration
- Assisted ventilation in patients with significant respiratory failure

ACUTE GENERAL Rx

- Initial antibiotic therapy should be based on clinical, radiographic, and laboratory evaluation.
- Macrolides (azithromycin or clarithromycin) or levofloxacin is recommended for empirical outpatient treatment of community-acquired pneumonia. Cefotaxime or a beta-lactam/beta-lactamase inhibitor can be added in

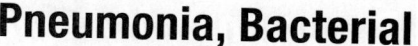
patients with more severe presentation who insist on outpatient therapy. Duration of treatment ranges from 7 to 14 days. The treatment of choice in suspected *Legionella* pneumonia is either a quinolone (e.g. moxifloxaxin) or a macrolide (e.g., azithromycin) antibiotic.

- In the hospital setting, patients admitted to the general ward can be treated empirically with a second- or third-generation cephalosporin (ceftriaxone, ceftizoxime, cefotaxime, or cefuroxime) plus a macrolide (azithromycin or clarithromycin) or doxycycline. An antipseudomonal quinolone (levofloxacin or moxifloxacin) can be substituted in place of the macrolide or doxycycline.

- Empiric therapy in ICU patients: IV beta-lactam (ceftriaxone, cefotaxime, ampicillin-sulbactam) plus an IV quinolone (levofloxacin, moxifloxacin) or IV azithromycin.

- In hospitalized patients at risk for *P. aeruginosa* infection, empirical treatment should consist of an antipseudomonal beta-lactam (Meropenem, Doripenem, Imipenem, or piperacillin-tazobactam) plus an aminoglycoside plus an antipseudomonal quinolone.

- In patients with suspected methicillin-resistant *S. aureus,* vancomycin or linezolid is effective.

CHRONIC Rx

Parapneumonic effusion empyema can be managed with chest tube placement for drainage. Instillation of fibrinolytic agents (streptokinase, urokinase) by chest tube may be necessary in resistant cases.

DISPOSITION

- Most patients respond well to antibiotic therapy.
- Indications for hospital admission are:
  1. Hypoxemia (oxygen saturation <90% while patient is breathing room air)
  2. Hemodynamic instability
  3. Inability to tolerate medications
  4. Active coexisting condition requiring hospitalization

A criterion often used to determine hospital admission is known as the "CURB-65": **C**onfusion, B**U**N >19.6 mg/dl, **R**espiratory rate >30 breaths/min, Systolic **B**P <90 mg Hg, and diastolic BP ≤60 mm Hg, age ≥**65**. Patients are generally admitted to the hospital if they fulfill 2 or more criteria and to the ICU if they have 3 or more criteria.

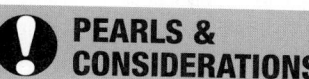

PEARLS & CONSIDERATIONS

COMMENTS

- Use of gastric acid suppressive therapy (H$_2$ receptor antagonists, proton pump inhibitors [PPIs]) has been associated with an increased risk of community-acquired pneumonia. It appears that PPI therapy started within the previous 30 days is associated with an increased risk for community-

acquired pneumonia, whereas longer-term current use is not.

- Causes of slowly resolving or nonresolving pneumonia:
  1. Difficult to treat infections: viral pneumonia, *Legionella*, pneumococci or staphylococci with impaired host response, tuberculosis, fungi
  2. Neoplasm: lung, lymphoma, metastasis
  3. Congestive heart failure
  4. Pulmonary embolism
  5. Immunologic or idiopathic: Wegener granulomatosis, pulmonary eosinophilic syndromes, systemic lupus erythematosus
  6. Drug toxicity (e.g., amiodarone)

- In patients with pneumonia, repeat films should be taken promptly in those who are not doing well. In those with complete clinical recovery, it is reasonable to wait 6 to 8 wk before repeating the radiograph to document clearing of the infiltrate.

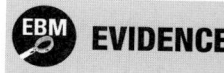 **EVIDENCE**

available at www.expertconsult.com

SUGGESTED READINGS
available at www.expertconsult.com

AUTHOR: **FRED F. FERRI, M.D.**

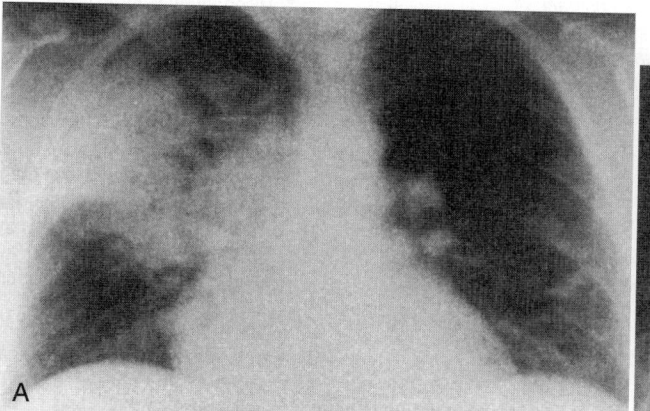 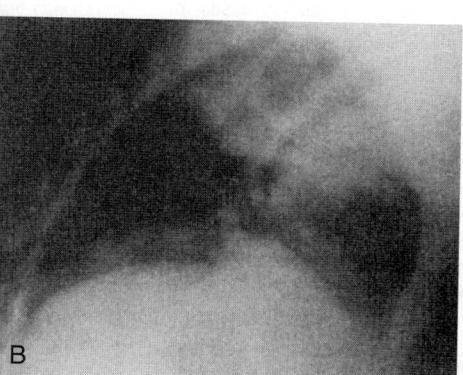

FIGURE 1-292 A, PA and, **B,** lateral chest radiographs reveal right upper-lobe pneumonia and patchy left lower-lobe infiltrate. A variety of organisms can produce this pattern, including *S. pneumoniae* and *H. influenzae.* (From Marx J [ed]: *Rosen's emergency medicine,* ed 5, St Louis, 2003, Mosby.)

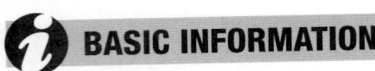

BASIC INFORMATION

DEFINITION

Mycoplasma pneumonia is an infection of the lung parenchyma caused by *Mycoplasma pneumoniae*.

SYNONYMS

Primary atypical pneumonia
Eaton's pneumonia
Walking pneumonia

ICD-9CM CODES

483 *Mycoplasma* pneumonia

EPIDEMIOLOGY & DEMOGRAPHICS

INCIDENCE (IN U.S.):

- Hard to determine incidence precisely because of difficulty in making the diagnosis, but it is a frequent cause of community-acquired pneumonia.
- Many cases probably resolve without coming to medical attention.
- Incidence is estimated at one case per 1000 persons annually.
- Incidence is estimated to at least triple every (approximately) 5 yr during epidemics.

PEAK INCIDENCE:

- Some increased incidence in fall to early winter
- Seems more prevalent in temperate climates

PREVALENCE (IN U.S.):

- Estimated to be present in one in every five patients hospitalized for pneumonia (generally a self-limited disease, so its true prevalence is unknown)
- Estimated to cause 7% of all cases of pneumonia and approximately half the cases in those aged 5 to 20 yr

PREDOMINANT SEX: Equal distribution

PREDOMINANT AGE:

- Most commonly affected: school-age children and young adults (ages 5 to 20 yr)
- Occurs in older adults as well, especially with household exposure to a young child
- More severe infections in affected elderly patients

GENETICS: Familial disposition:

- None known
- May be more severe in patients with sickle cell anemia

Neonatal infection: severe respiratory distress, sometimes requiring intubation, attributed to this disease in infants.

PHYSICAL FINDINGS & CLINICAL PRESENTATION

- Nonexudative pharyngitis (common)
- Headache, otalgia common
- Fever may be mild or not present
- Rhonchi or rales without evidence of consolidation (common) in lower lung zones
- Associated with bullous myringitis (nonspecific finding; perhaps no more frequently than in other pneumonias)
- Skin rashes in up to one fourth of patients
  1. Morbilliform
  2. Urticaria
  3. Erythema nodosum (unusual)
  4. Erythema multiforme (unusual)
  5. Stevens-Johnson syndrome (rare)
- Muscle tenderness (<50% of the patients)
- On examination (and confirmed with testing):
  1. Mononeuritis or polyneuritis
  2. Transverse myelitis
  3. Cranial nerve palsies
  4. Meningoencephalitis
- Lymphadenopathy and splenomegaly
- Conjunctivitis
- Table 1-145 summarizes the clinical manifestations of *Mycoplasma pneumoniae*

ETIOLOGY

Infection is spread by droplet infection from respiratory tract secretions.

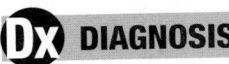

DIAGNOSIS

DIFFERENTIAL DIAGNOSIS

- *Chlamydia* (now known as *Chlamydophila*) pneumoniae
- *Chlamydophila psittaci*
- *Legionella* spp.
- *Coxiella burnetii*
- Several viral agents
- Q fever
- *Streptococcus pneumoniae*
- Pulmonary embolism or infarction

WORKUP

- Chest x-ray
- Thorough history and physical examination
- Laboratory tests
- Evaluation guided by symptoms and findings

LABORATORY TESTS

- White blood cells (WBC):
  1. WBC count >10,000/mm^3 in approximately one fourth of patients

  2. Differential count nonspecific
  3. Leukopenia rare
- Cold agglutinins:
  1. Detected in approximately half of the patients
  2. Also may be found in:
     a. Lymphoproliferative diseases
     b. Influenza
     c. Mononucleosis
     d. Adenovirus infections
     e. Occasionally, Legionnaires' disease
  3. Titers typically >1:64
     a. May be detectable with bedside testing
     b. Appear between days 5 and 10 of the illness (so may be demonstrable when patient is first examined) and disappear within 1 mo
- Complement fixation testing or other immunoassays specific for mycoplasm antigens of paired sera (fourfold rise) in patients with pneumonia and a compatible history:
  1. Considered diagnostic in the appropriate clinical setting
- Culture of the organism from specimens
  1. Only truly specific test for infection
  2. Technically difficult and done reliably by few laboratories
  3. May require weeks to get results
- Sputum
  1. Often no sputum produced for laboratory testing
  2. When present, gram-stained specimens show polymorphonuclear cells without organisms
- Infection occasionally complicated by pancreatitis or glomerulitis
- Disseminated intravascular coagulation is a rare complication
- Electrocardiographic evidence of pericarditis or myocarditis may be present

IMAGING STUDIES

- Predilection for lower lobe involvement (upper lobes involved in less than a fourth), with radiographic abnormalities frequently out of proportion to those on physical examination (Fig. 1-293)
- Small pleural effusions in approximately 30% of patients
- Large effusions: rare
- Infiltrates: patchy, unilateral, and with a segmental distribution, although multilobar involvement may be seen
- Evidence of hilar adenopathy on chest radiographs in 20% to 25%
- Rare cases reported:
  1. Associated lung abscess
  2. Residual pneumatoceles
  3. Lobar collapse
  4. Hyperlucent lung syndrome

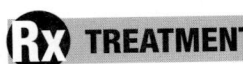

TREATMENT

ACUTE GENERAL Rx

- Therapy, or azithromycin (500 mg initially, then 250 mg daily for 4 days), clarithromycin (500 mg bid) (10 to 14 days) with erythromycin (500 mg qid) is preferred to tetracycline,

---

TABLE 1-145 Clinical Manifestations of *Mycoplasma Pneumoniae* Infection

Respiratory tract	Pharyngitis, laryngitis, acute bronchitis, bronchopneumonia
Skin and mucosa	Maculopapular and vesicular exanthema, urticaria, purpura, erythema nodosum, erythema multiforme, Stevens-Johnson syndrome
Central nervous system	Meningitis, meningoencephalitis, acute psychosis, cerebellitis, Guillain-Barré syndrome?
Parenchymatous organs	Pancreatitis, diabetes mellitus, non-specific reactive hepatitis, subacute thyroiditis?
Miscellaneous	Hemorrhagic bullous myringitis, hemolytic anemia, pericarditis, thromboembolism?

Some association remains uncertain.
Cohen J, Powderly WG: *Infectious diseases,* ed 2, St. Louis, 2004, Mosby.

especially in young children or women of childbearing age. Respiratory fluoroquinolones such as Levaquin or moxifloxacin are alternative agents for treatment but should not be used in young children.

- Therapy shortens the duration and severity of symptoms and may hasten radiographic clearing, but the disease is self-limiting.

CHRONIC Rx

- Effective antimicrobial therapy does not eliminate the organism from the respiratory secretions, which may be positive for weeks.
- Serum antibody response does not necessarily provide lifelong immunity.

- Chronic symptoms do not occur, although clinical relapses may occur 7 to 10 days after the initial response and may be associated with new areas of infiltration.

DISPOSITION

- Clinical improvement is almost universal within 10 days.
- Infiltrates generally clear within 5 to 8 wk.
- Rare deaths are likely attributable to underlying medical diseases.
- Person-to-person spread can be minimized by avoiding open coughing, especially in enclosed areas.

REFERRAL

- Not responding to treatment
- Severe infection
- Severe extrapulmonary manifestations
- Multilobe involvement accompanied by respiratory embarrassment (very rare)

⚠ PEARLS & CONSIDERATIONS

COMMENTS

X-ray resolution complete by 8 wk in approximately 90% of patients.

(EBM) EVIDENCE

available at www.expertconsult.com

SUGGESTED READINGS

available at www.expertconsult.com

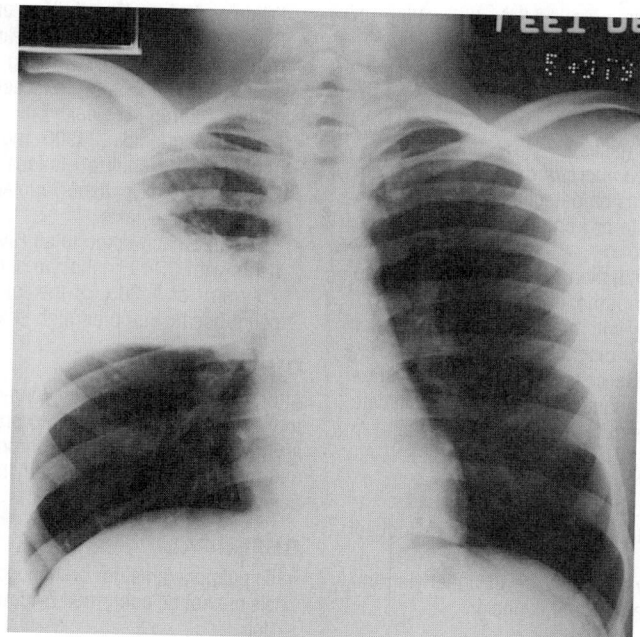

FIGURE 1-293 Localized airspace opacification resulting from *Mycoplasma pneumoniae.* (From Specht N [ed]: *Practical guide to diagnostic imaging,* St Louis, 1998, Mosby.)

AUTHORS: **GLENN G. FORT, M.D., M.P.H.,** and **DENNIS J. MIKOLICH, M.D.**

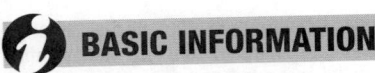
DEFINITION

Pneumocystis jirovecii pneumonia (PJP) is a serious respiratory infection caused by the fungal or protozoal organism *P. jirovecii* (formerly known as *P. carinii*).

SYNONYMS

PCP
PJP

ICD-9CM CODES
136.3 *Pneumocystis jirovecii* (*P. carinii*)
pneumonia

EPIDEMIOLOGY & DEMOGRAPHICS

INCIDENCE (IN U.S.):
- Seen primarily in the setting of AIDS
- Approximately 11 cases per 100 patient-years among HIV-infected patients with CD4 lymphocyte counts <100/mm^3
- Also seen in other immunocompromised patients with severe cell-mediated immune deficiency (congenital T-cell deficiency, acute leukemia, lymphoma, bone marrow or organ transplant deficiency)

PEAK INCIDENCE: Age 20 to 40 yr (parallel to AIDS epidemic)
PREDOMINANT SEX: Equal incidence when corrected for HIV status
PREDOMINANT AGE:
- <2 yr
- 20 to 40 yr

GENETICS: Neonatal infection:
- Most frequent opportunistic infection among HIV-infected children, occurring in approximately 30%
- Neonatal occurrence unusual

PHYSICAL FINDINGS & CLINICAL PRESENTATION

- Fever, cough, shortness of breath present in almost all cases
- Lungs frequently clear to auscultation, although rales occasionally present
- Cyanosis and pronounced tachypnea in severe cases
- Hemoptysis unusual
- Spontaneous pneumothorax

ETIOLOGY

- *P. jirovecii* (formerly *P. carinii*) recently reclassified as a fungal organism
- Reactivation of dormant infection
- Extrapulmonary involvement rare

DIFFERENTIAL DIAGNOSIS

- Other opportunistic respiratory infections:
  1. Tuberculosis
  2. Histoplasmosis
  3. Cryptococcosis
- Nonopportunistic infections:
  1. Bacterial pneumonia
  2. Viral pneumonia
  3. Mycoplasmal pneumonia
  4. Legionellosis
- Occurs virtually exclusively in the setting of profound depression of cellular immunity

WORKUP

- Chest x-ray.
- Arterial blood gases.
- Because *Pneumocystis* cannot be cultured, diagnosis relies on detection of the organism by colorimetric or immunofluorescent stains or PCR.
- Sputum examination for cysts of PJP and to exclude other pathogens.
- Bronchoscopy with bronchoalveolar lavage or lung biopsy for diagnosis if sputum examination is negative or equivocal. Stains such as Gomori methenamine silver stain or toluidine blue O are used to identify the organism.

LABORATORY TESTS

- Arterial blood gas monitoring
- Elevated lactate dehydrogenase in majority of cases
- HIV antibody test if cause of underlying immune deficiency state is unclear

IMAGING STUDIES

Diffuse uptake on gallium scanning of the lungs is suggestive but not diagnostic.

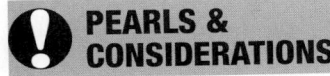
NONPHARMACOLOGIC THERAPY

- Supplemental oxygen
- Ventilatory support if needed
- Prompt thoracotomy if pneumothorax develops

ACUTE GENERAL Rx

For confirmed or suspected PJP:
- Trimethoprim-sulfamethoxazole (15 to 20 mg/kg trimethoprim and 75 to 100 mg/kg sulfamethoxazole qd) PO or IV per day divided and given q6 to 8h
- Pentamidine (4 mg/kg IV qd)
- Either regimen with prednisone (40 mg PO bid):
  1. If arterial oxygen pressure <70 mm Hg
  2. If arterial-alveolar oxygen pressure difference >35 mm Hg

3. Dose tapered to 20 mg bid after 5 days and 20 mg qd after 10 days
- Therapy continued for 3 wk
- Alternative therapies available for patients unable to tolerate conventional therapy:
  1. Dapsone/trimethoprim
  2. Clindamycin/primaquine
  3. Atovaquone

CHRONIC Rx

- After completion of therapy, lifelong prophylaxis should be maintained with trimethoprim-sulfamethoxazole (one single-strength tablet PO qd or double-strength three times weekly).
- Patients intolerant of this therapy should be treated with dapsone (50 mg PO qd) plus pyrimethamine (50 mg PO weekly) plus leucovorin (25 mg PO weekly).
- Inhaled pentamidine (300 mg monthly by standardized nebulizer) is less effective and is reserved for patients intolerant to other forms of prophylaxis.
- Same approach taken to all HIV-infected patients with CD4 lymphocyte counts <200 to 250/mm^3 or <20% of the total lymphocyte count because of their high risk of PJP.

DISPOSITION

After completion of therapy, long-term ambulatory follow-up is mandatory to provide secondary prevention of PJP (see "Chronic Rx" above) and management of the underlying immunodeficiency syndrome.

REFERRAL

- To pulmonologist for bronchoscopy if diagnosis cannot be confirmed by sputum examination
- To an infectious disease specialist if case is severe or difficult to manage

COMMENTS

All patients, especially those with severe infection or intolerant of conventional therapy, should be followed by a physician experienced in the management of PJP and, if appropriate, in the long-term management of HIV infection or other underlying disease.

Severe and life-threatening hypoglycemia may occur after 1 or 2 wk after start of IV pentamidine. Monitor closely and advise the patient of symptoms of hypoglycemia.

SUGGESTED READINGS
available at www.expertconsult.com

AUTHORS: **GLENN G. FORT, M.D., M.P.H.,** and **DENNIS J. MIKOLICH, M.D.**

BASIC INFORMATION

DEFINITION

Viral pneumonia is infection of the pulmonary parenchyma caused by any of a large number of viral agents. The most important viruses are discussed.

SYNONYMS

Nonbacterial pneumonia
Atypical pneumonia

ICD-9CM CODES

480.9 Viral pneumonia

EPIDEMIOLOGY & DEMOGRAPHICS

INCIDENCE (IN U.S.):

- Influenza virus:
  1. 10% to 20% of population in temperate zones infected during 1- to 2-mo epidemics occurring yearly during winter months.
  2. Up to 50% infected during pandemics.
  3. Pneumonia develops in small percentage of infected persons.
- Incidence of other important viral pneumonias is not known precisely.

PEAK INCIDENCE:

1. Influenza:
   - Winter months for influenza A
   - Year round for influenza B
   - Peak of pneumonia seen weeks into the outbreak of infection
2. Respiratory syncytial virus (RSV) and parainfluenza virus:
   - Winter and spring
3. Adenovirus:
   - Endemic (military)
4. Varicella:
   - Spring in temperate zones
5. Measles:
   - Year round
6. Cytomegalovirus (CMV):
   - Year round

PREVALENCE (IN U.S.):

- Often related to immune status of the population or presence of an epidemic
- Normal hosts (estimates):
  1. 86% of cases of pneumonia resulting in hospitalization in American adults
  2. 16% of pediatric pneumonias managed as outpatients
  3. 49% of hospitalized infants with pneumonia
- Important problem in hosts with impaired immunity

PREDOMINANT SEX:

- None generally
- Male sex may predispose to more severe respiratory disease in RSV infection

PREDOMINANT AGE:

1. Influenza:
   - Overall incidence greatest at age 5 yr
   - Falls with increasing age
   - The most serious sequelae in those with chronic medical illnesses, especially cardiopulmonary disease

- Hospitalizations greatest in infants and adults aged >64 yr
2. RSV and parainfluenza virus:
   - Young children (as the major cause of pneumonia)
   - Occurs throughout life
3. Adenoviruses:
   - Young children
   - Adults, primarily military recruits
4. Varicella:
   - Approximately 16% of adults (not infected in childhood) who contract chickenpox
   - Acute varicella during pregnancy more likely to be complicated by severe pneumonia
   - 90% of reported varicella pneumonia cases are in adults (highest incidence ages 20 to 60 yr)
5. Measles:
   - Young adults and older children who received a single vaccination (5% failure rate)
   - Measles during pregnancy more likely to be complicated by pneumonia
   - Underlying cardiopulmonary diseases and immunosuppression predispose to serious pneumonia complicating measles
   - Before availability of measles vaccine, 90% of pneumonias in those <10 yr
   - Currently more than one third of U.S. patients >14 yr
   - 3% to 50% of measles cases are complicated by pneumonia
6. CMV:
   - Neonatal through adult
   - Immunosuppression is key predisposing factor

GENETICS:

Familial disposition:
- Close contact, not genetics, is important in acquisition
- Congenital anomalies and immunosuppression worsen course of RSV pneumonia

Congenital infection:
- CMV is the most common intrauterine infection in the U.S.
- Pneumonia occurs occasionally in infants with symptomatic congenital infection.

Neonatal infection:
- Severe RSV pneumonia
- Adenovirus pneumonia
  1. 5% to 20% mortality rate
  2. Can lead to residual restrictive or obstructive functional abnormalities
- "Varicella neonatorum"
  1. Disseminated visceral disease including pneumonia
  2. May develop in neonates whose mothers develop peripartum chickenpox
- CMV pneumonia
  1. Generally fatal
  2. Associated with severe cerebral damage in this population

PHYSICAL FINDINGS & CLINICAL PRESENTATION

1. Influenza:
   - Fever
   - Uncomfortable or lethargic appearance

- Prominent dry cough (rarely hemoptysis)
- Flushed integument and erythematous mucous membranes
- Rales or rhonchi
2. RSV and parainfluenza:
   - Fever
   - Tachypnea
   - Prolonged expiration
   - Wheezes and rales
3. Adenoviruses:
   - Hoarseness
   - Pharyngitis
   - Tachypnea
   - Cervical adenitis
4. Measles:
   - Conjunctivitis
   - Rhinorrhea
   - Koplik's spots
   - Exanthem
   - Pneumonitis
     a. May occur as a complication in 3% to 4% of adolescents and young adults
     b. Coincident with rash
     c. May also develop after apparent recovery from measles
   - Fever
   - Dry cough
5. Varicella:
   - Fever
   - Maculopapular or vesicular rash
     a. Becomes encrusted
     b. Pneumonia typical 1 to 6 days after rash appears
     c. Pneumonia accompanied by cough and occasionally hemoptysis
   - Few auscultatory abnormalities noted on examination of the lungs
6. CMV:
   - Fever
   - Paroxysmal cough
   - Occasional hemoptysis
   - Diffuse adenopathy when pneumonia occurs after transfusion

ETIOLOGY

Viral infection can lead to pneumonia in both immunocompetent and immunocompromised hosts.

DIAGNOSIS

DIFFERENTIAL DIAGNOSIS

- Bacterial pneumonia, which frequently complicates (i.e., can follow or be simultaneous with) viral (especially influenza) pneumonia
- Other causes of atypical pneumonia:
  1. *Mycoplasma* spp.
  2. *Chlamydia* spp.
  3. *Coxiella* spp.
  4. Legionnaires' disease
- Acute respiratory distress syndrome (ARDS)
- Physical findings and associated hypoxemia confused with pulmonary emboli

WORKUP

- Information about the current prevalent strain of influenza virus can be obtained from local health departments or from the Centers for Disease Control and Prevention.

- Viral diagnostic tests are usually not necessary once an outbreak has been defined.
- Influenza and other viruses can be cultured from respiratory secretions during the initial few days of the illness (special media and techniques necessary).
- Paired sera antibody titers are also useful.
- Monoclonal antibody tests are available for influenza and other respiratory viruses.
- Measles and adenovirus pneumonia are usually diagnosed clinically.
- Polymerase chain reaction may be able to rapidly detect and identify viral nucleic acid.
- Open lung biopsy is required for definite diagnosis of CMV pneumonia.

LABORATORY TESTS

- Sputum Gram stain (usually produced in scanty amounts) typically shows few polymorphonuclear leukocytes and few bacteria.
- White blood cell count may vary from leukopenic to modest elevation, usually without a leftward shift.
- Disseminated intravascular coagulation occasionally complicates adenovirus type 7 pneumonia.
- Multinucleated giant cells on Tzanck preparation of an unroofed vesicular lesion are useful in diagnosing varicella in a patient with an infiltrate (also found in herpes simplex).
- Severe immunosuppression is associated with symptomatic CMV pneumonia (usually reactivation of latent infection or in previously seronegative recipients from the donor).
- Hypoxemia may be profound.
- Cultures may be helpful in identifying superinfecting bacterial pathogens.
- When they occur, parapneumonic pleural effusions are exudative.

IMAGING STUDIES

- Chest x-ray may demonstrate a spectrum of findings from ill-defined, patchy, or generalized interstitial infiltrates, which can be associated with ARDS.
- A localized dense alveolar infiltrate suggests a superimposed bacterial pneumonia.
- Small calcified nodules may develop as a radiographic residual of varicella pneumonia.

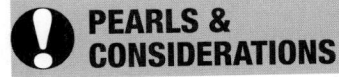 TREATMENT

NONPHARMACOLOGIC THERAPY

General:
- Measures to diminish person-to-person transmission
- Modified bed rest
- Maintenance of adequate hydration
- Possible ventilatory support for severe pneumonia or ARDS

Influenza:
- Yearly prophylactic strain-specific influenza vaccination (only subvirion vaccine should be used in children <13 yr) can be given to prevent infection.

- Live, attenuated influenza vaccines administered by nose drops as effective as injected inactivated viral vaccines.

RSV:
- Isolation techniques are important in limiting spread of RSV infections.
- Immunoglobulins with a high RSV-neutralizing antibody titer are beneficial in treatment.

Adenoviruses:
- Intestinal inoculation of respiratory adenoviruses has been used to successfully immunize military recruits.
- Although they produce no disease in recipients, the viruses may be shed chronically and may infect others at a later date.
- These vaccines are not available for civilian populations.

Varicella:
- Live, attenuated varicella vaccine has been successfully used in clinical trials.
- Varicella-zoster immune globulin should be administered within 4 days of exposure to prevent or modify the disease in susceptible persons.
- Nonimmunized persons exposed to varicella are potentially infectious between 10 and 21 days after exposure.

Measles:
- Effective measles vaccine is available:
  ○ The vaccine should be administered at age 15 mo.
  ○ A second dose should be administered at the time of school entry.
- Live, attenuated vaccine or gamma-globulin can prevent measles in unvaccinated persons if administered early after exposure.
- Vitamin A given PO for 2 days reduces morbidity and mortality rates from measles in exposed children.

Severe acute respiratory syndrome (SARS) = associated coronaviruses:
- No vaccine currently available.
- Supportive care: ribavirin ineffective, use of steroids or interferon-alpha of unclear value.

ACUTE GENERAL Rx

- **General:** Administer appropriate antibiotics for bacterial superinfections.
- **Influenza:**
  ○ Amantadine and rimantadine for influenza A (not active against influenza B). Early use can speed recovery from small airways dysfunction, but whether it influences the development or course of pneumonia is uncertain.
  ○ The neuraminidase inhibitors oseltamivir and zanamivir are effective if given in the first 48 hours of symptoms of influenza; their efficacy in established influenza pneumonia is unclear.
  ○ Aerosolized ribavirin or amantadine may have a role in severe influenza pneumonia but have not been approved for this indication.
- **RSV and parainfluenza:**
  ○ Ribavirin aerosol is effective for severe RSV pneumonia.
  ○ There is no approved antiviral therapy for parainfluenza virus pneumonia.

- **Adenoviruses:** no effective agent; some case reports of cidofovir use but unproved.
- **Varicella:**
  ○ Varicella pneumonia can be treated with IV acyclovir.
  ○ Adults who develop chickenpox should be considered for acyclovir treatment, which may prevent the development of pneumonia.
- **Measles:** no effective antimeasles agent.
- **CMV:**
  ○ Acyclovir can prevent CMV infection in renal transplant recipients.
  ○ Ganciclovir and foscarnet, with or without CMV hyperimmune globulin, show promise in the treatment of serious CMV infection, including pneumonia, in compromised hosts.

DISPOSITION

- Supportive therapy is useful.
- Death arise possible during acute illness.
- Residual functional abnormalities may be persistent, develop into, or predispose to chronic respiratory diseases in later life.
- Morbidity and mortality rates after most viral pneumonias are increased by bacterial superinfection.

REFERRAL

- Uncertainty about the diagnosis in a compromised host
- Symptoms or findings progressive
- Severe respiratory compromise, diffuse infiltrates, or the development of ARDS

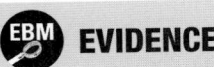 PEARLS & CONSIDERATIONS

COMMENTS

- Influenza spreads by close contact and by small droplets transmitted by cough.
- RSV is effectively transmitted by fomites and by direct contact (little by aerosol).
- Varicella is transmitted by direct contact or by aerosol.
- Of the three major forms of parainfluenza viruses (types 1 to 3), type 3 is the most common cause of viral pneumonia; types 1 and 2 primarily cause laryngotracheitis.
- Recent evidence indicates that a newly discovered virus known as metapneumovirus is a common cause of upper respiratory infections worldwide; this virus can cause pneumonia.

EBM EVIDENCE

available at www.expertconsult.com

SUGGESTED READINGS

available at www.expertconsult.com

AUTHORS: **DENNIS J. MIKOLICH, M.D.,** and **GLENN G. FORT, M.D., M.P.H.**

BASIC INFORMATION

DEFINITION

A spontaneous pneumothorax (SP) is defined as the accumulation of air into the pleural space, collapsing the lung. This can be primary SP (without any obvious underlying lung disease) or secondary SP (with underlying lung disease).

SYNONYMS

Primary spontaneous pneumothorax
Secondary spontaneous pneumothorax

ICD-9CM CODES

512.0S Spontaneous tension pneumothorax
512.8   Other spontaneous pneumothorax

EPIDEMIOLOGY & DEMOGRAPHICS

- Approximately 20,000 new cases of SP occur each year in the U.S.
- SP is more common in men than women (6:1).
- Incidence of primary SP is 7.4 per 100,000 in men and 1.2 per 100,000 in women.
- Incidence of secondary SP is 6.3 per 100,000 in men and 2.0 per 100,000 in women.
- SP is commonly seen in tall, thin young men aged 20 to 40 yr.
- Tobacco use increases the risk of SP.

PHYSICAL FINDINGS & CLINICAL PRESENTATION

- Sudden onset of pleuritic chest pain (90%), which often becomes dull after a few hours
- Pain is usually unilateral and can be sharp and agonizing and associated with considerable apprehension
- Dyspnea (80%), which often resolves within 24 hr, despite persistence of pneumothorax
- Cough (10%)
- Asymptomatic (5%); may take up to 7 days to come to medical attention
- Tachycardia
- Diminished breath sounds
- Subcutaneous emphysema may be present
- Hyperresonance on percussion

ETIOLOGY

- In primary SP, rupture of small blebs, usually located near the apex of the upper lobes, is a common cause. The check-valve mechanism is uncommon in this case; therefore, tension pneumothorax rarely occurs.
- In secondary SP, chronic obstructive pulmonary disease is the most common cause, but it can also be associated with pneumonia, bronchogenic carcinoma, mesothelioma, sarcoidosis, tuberculosis, cystic fibrosis, and many other lung diseases (Fig. 1-294).

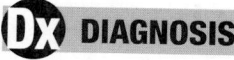 DIAGNOSIS

Established by the chest radiograph (CXR) or CT

DIFFERENTIAL DIAGNOSIS

- Pleurisy
- Pulmonary embolism
- Myocardial infarction
- Pericarditis
- Asthma
- Pneumonia

WORKUP

Includes CXR and, in some cases, CT scan of the chest

LABORATORY TESTS

Arterial blood gases may show hypoxemia and hypocapnia as a result of hyperventilation.

IMAGING STUDIES

- Spontaneous pneumothorax is usually confirmed by upright CXR:
  1. A white visceral pleural line. The absence of vessel markings peripheral to this line helps differentiate from mimicking conditions such as an overlying skin fold. A lateral width of 1 cm corresponds to 10% pneumothorax.
  2. The left lateral decubitus position is the most sensitive and supine position the least sensitive. The increased sensitivity of expiratory films in detecting pneumothorax has never been demonstrated in studies.
  3. As little as 50 ml of air can be detected on upright film.
- Tension pneumothorax is a medical emergency and should be suspected when the patient is hemodynamically unstable or with contralateral tracheal and mediastinal deviation and ipsilateral flattening or inversion of the diaphragm on the CXR.

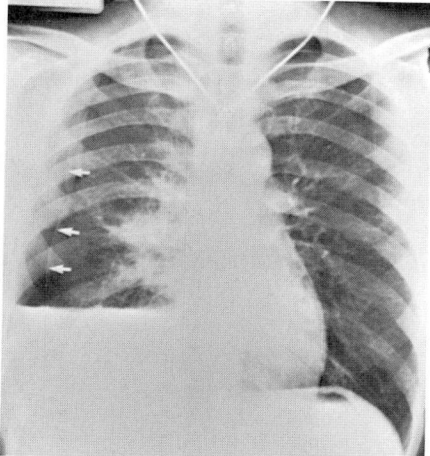

FIGURE 1-294 Chest radiograph shows right hydropneumothorax. Horizontal line in lower right hemithorax is interface between air and liquid in pleural space. *Arrows* point to visceral pleura above level of effusion. There is air in pleural space between visceral pleura and chest wall. (From Weinberg SE et al: *Principles of pulmonary medicine,* ed 5, Philadelphia, 2008, Saunders.)

- CT scan can be done in suspected but difficult-to-visualize pneumothoraces, to differentiate from large subpleural bullae or to evaluate for underlying lung pathology, especially in patients with secondary pneumothorax.

TREATMENT

NONPHARMACOLOGIC THERAPY

- 100% oxygen administration reduces the partial pressure of nitrogen in pleural capillaries, consequently quadrupling the rate of pneumothorax absorption, and should be administered to all patients with pneumothorax.
- Observation alone is acceptable in the asymptomatic patient with a small (<3 cm between lung and chest wall on CXR) pneumothorax. However, a repeat CXR is necessary to demonstrate the stability of the condition, which requires close monitoring.

ACUTE GENERAL Rx

- Initial management is directed at removing air from the pleural space, with subsequent management directed at preventing recurrence.
- Needle aspiration is performed emergently in unstable patients with a tension pneumothorax as a bridge to allow adequate time for chest tube placement.
- Needle aspiration technique or chest tube placement should be considered for stable patients with large primary spontaneous pneumothorax (>3 cm between the lung and chest wall on a CXR).
- There is no firm conclusion on the initial optimal treatment (simple aspiration versus chest tube insertion) for a first episode of primary SP. Studies suggest that shorter hospital stay can be achieved with the aspiration technique, but there is a potential risk of lung laceration.
- Needle aspiration can be done at the bedside using a large-bore angiocatheter needle or commercially available needle thoracotomy kit. The needle is introduced in the second intercostal space midclavicular line. The catheter is left in place and attached to a three-way stopcock and a large syringe. Air is aspirated until resistance is met or the patient experiences significant coughing. Repeat CXR is done immediately after aspiration and again in 4 to 24 hr to document reexpansion of the lung. If the pneumothorax fails to resolve with aspiration, a chest tube should be placed.
- If there is improvement but not complete resolution of pneumothorax after the aspiration, the catheter can be attached to a Heimlich (one-way) valve to allow further lung expansion. Some stable patients can be discharged home with this device in place if close follow-up monitoring can be obtained.
- Chest tube insertion has been recommended for patients with primary SP who do not respond to simple aspiration and for all patients

with secondary SP, recurrent pneumothorax, or tension pneumothorax.

PREVENTION

- Multiple techniques have been used to prevent recurrence, including pleurectomy, laser abrasion of parietal pleural, intrapleural instillation of sclerosing agents, and pleural abrasion with dry gauze. The overall recurrence rate is estimated at <5%.
- The current recommended approach is the use of video-assisted thoracoscopy (VATS) with an aim to excise the associated bullae or perform guided pleurodesis or treatment. Most pulmonologists recommend definitive management after the first recurrence. However, high-risk occupations such as divers or pilots should be considered for surgery after their first pneumothorax. Similarly, complex conditions such as patients with persistent bronchopleural fistula suggested by a persistent air leak from the chest tube should also be considered for VATS and early surgical intervention.
- The recurrence rates for the instillation of sclerosing agents (minocycline 5 mg/kg in 50 ml of normal saline or doxycycline 500 mg in 50 ml of normal saline) are higher than VATS-guided therapy. Therefore this mode of therapy should be reserved for patients who are poor surgical candidates.
- Talc has also been used as a sclerosing agent; however, there are case reports of acute respiratory distress syndrome and pleural calcification occurring after use.
- Open thoracotomy is performed in patients who do not respond to VATS or when VATS is not available.

DISPOSITION

- Approximately 25% of patients with primary SP will have recurrence within 2 yr.
- Smoking cessation should be advised.
- The rates of recurrence after the second and third episode of SP are 60% and 80%, respectively, with the majority of recurrences occurring on the same side as the first pneumothorax.
- Death from primary SP is uncommon. In patients with secondary SP and chronic obstructive pulmonary disease, mortality rates range from 1% to 16%.

REFERRAL

A pulmonary specialist and surgical consultation are recommended.

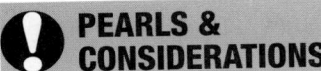

PEARLS & CONSIDERATIONS

- The rate of pleural air absorption is approximately 1.25% of the volume of the hemithorax per day. Therefore the interval for complete resolution of pneumothorax with observation can be estimated.
- Catamenial pneumothorax is a rare condition characterized by recurrent spontaneous pneumothorax coinciding with the onset of menses. It usually affects the right lung and is believed to be caused by endometriosis with involvement of the diaphragm and/or pleura. It is believed to be hormonally related, and treatment is aimed at endometrial suppression.

COMMENTS

- Patients with AIDS and *Pneumocystis carinii* infection have a high incidence of SP. Treatment typically requires chest tube placement and either thoracoscopy or open thoracotomy.

SUGGESTED READINGS

available at www.expertconsult.com

AUTHORS: **RICHARD REGNANTE, M.D.,** and **KENNETH KORR, M.D.**

BASIC INFORMATION

DEFINITION

Contact dermatitis caused by exposure to urushiol, the oil of plants of the genus *Toxicodendron*, which includes poison ivy, poison oak, and poison sumac.

SYNONYMS

Rhus dermatitis
Toxicodendron dermatitis

ICD-9CM CODES
ICD 692.6

EPIDEMIOLOGY & DEMOGRAPHICS

INCIDENCE: Affects 10 million to 40 million Americans annually
PEAK INCIDENCE: More frequent in months when outdoor activity is more common.
PREVALENCE: From 50% to 75% of the adult population is clinically sensitive to these plants. Sensitivity rates are lower in urban areas. (Tolerance is found in 10% to 15% of the population.)
PREDOMINANT SEX AND AGE: Sensitization occurs most commonly between ages 8 and 14 yr. Sensitivity wanes with age, especially with limited exposure and prior mild reactions.
GENETICS: There is believed to be a genetic susceptibility to sensitivity; however, the rash occurs in all ethnicities and skin types.
RISK FACTORS: Firefighters, forestry workers, farmers, and outdoor workers in general as well as those who participate in outdoor recreation. These plants are indigenous to the United States, Canada, and Mexico, and cases are most common in these areas.

PHYSICAL FINDINGS & CLINICAL PRESENTATION

- Patients typically present with intense pruritus and rash. The patient may not be aware of exposure to the plant.
- Symptoms typically peak from 1 to 14 days after exposure depending on the degree of exposure and thickness of affected skin.
- Dermatitis may initially present as erythema and may develop into papules, vesicles, and bullae.
- Lesions may be found in the classic linear configuration, typically in exposed areas likely to have been in contact with plants. Atypical appearance or location of dermatitis is more common with secondary exposure, such as through pets or infected tools or clothing.
- Face and genital involvement may present with significant edema.
- Inhalation of urushiol aerosolized by fire can cause significant respiratory tract inflammation. This can be a particular occupational hazard of forest firefighters.
- Post-inflammatory hyperpigmentation may occur, more commonly in dark skin types. This usually resolves with treatment.

ETIOLOGY

- Initial contact with oil of plants in this genus, which is released with damage to plant parts, causes a classic T-lymphocyte–mediated delayed-type allergic reaction.
- Subsequent exposures cause a cell-mediated cytotoxic immune response.

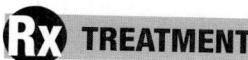

DIAGNOSIS

DIFFERENTIAL DIAGNOSIS

- Allergic contact dermatitis from other plants or nonplant substances
- Irritant contact dermatitis
- Nummular dermatitis
- Arthropod reactions, including scabies and bedbug bites

WORKUP

- Typically not needed. Diagnosis is based on characteristic rash and possibly history of exposure.

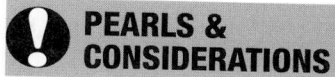

TREATMENT

Prevention is the most effective treatment.

NONPHARMACOLOGIC THERAPY

- After known exposure, patients should remove contaminated clothing and wash the skin gently with soap and water. Washing after appearance of dermatitis does not prevent further lesions.
- Calamine lotion, cool compresses, baking soda, or colloidal oatmeal baths may provide symptomatic relief.
- Keep nails short and clean to help prevent secondary bacterial infection.
- Exposed clothing, as well as tools, pets, and equipment, should be washed with soap and water to prevent secondary exposure.

ACUTE GENERAL Rx

- Topical steroids generally should be avoided. They may be effective in mild, early cases with erythema and pruritus but no vesiculation.
- Topical antibiotics should be avoided.
- Use of antihistamines for associated pruritus may be effective, but this has not been extensively studied.
- Systemic corticosteroids offer significant relief in moderate to severe rhus dermatitis, including generalized rash or severe facial or genital involvement.

- Effective dosing of oral prednisone is 1 mg/kg/day over 7 to 10 days (maximum 60 mg initial dose), with tapering over an additional 7 to 10 days.
- Inadequate doses or too-rapid tapering of systemic steroids may cause symptom rebound.
- IM treatment with long-acting triamcinolone suspension may be considered for patients intolerant of oral therapy.

CHRONIC Rx

- Recurrence may be caused by repeated exposure to fomites, including contaminated clothing, equipment, or pets.
- Secondary bacterial infection of the skin is the most common complication of rhus dermatitis. Staph and strep are the most common pathogens, but MRSA must be considered.

DISPOSITION

Untreated rhus dermatitis will resolve in 1 to 3 weeks.

REFERRAL

To dermatology if there is diagnostic confusion

PEARLS & CONSIDERATIONS

PREVENTION

- Patients should be educated regarding identification and avoidance as well as washing to remove the oil after known exposure.
- Total avoidance of the plants may not be practical.
- The use of barrier creams applied before exposure to prevent dermatitis may be of some benefit, particularly in potential occupational (therefore predictable) exposure.
- Products available for postexposure prophylaxis are effective; however, equal efficacy may be obtained from less expensive liquid dishwashing soap.
- Desensitization has not been found to be effective.

PATIENT & FAMILY EDUCATION

- "Leaves of three, let it be," is a helpful reminder for patients.
- Patient education material, including access to photographs of the leaves of these plants in a variety of seasons and conditions, may be useful.

SUGGESTED READINGS
available at www.expertconsult.com

AUTHOR: **MARGARET TRYFOROS, M.D.**

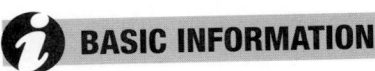

BASIC INFORMATION

DEFINITION

Poliomyelitis is a symptomatic infection caused by poliovirus, which (on rare occasions) may result in paralysis.

SYNONYMS

Polio
Infantile paralysis

ICD-9CM CODES
045.9 Poliomyelitis

EPIDEMIOLOGY & DEMOGRAPHICS

INCIDENCE (IN U.S.):
- Approximately 8 cases/yr.
- All cases in the U.S. and Western Hemisphere are now vaccine associated (because of oral polio vaccine [OPV]).

PREDOMINANT AGE: Almost always infants or young children
GENETICS:
Neonatal Infection: Most cases occur in otherwise healthy infants who receive OPV, or their contacts.

PHYSICAL FINDINGS & CLINICAL PRESENTATION

- Exposure of a nonimmune host to poliovirus usually results in asymptomatic infection.
- A small percentage of individuals may have one of three presentations:
  1. Abortive poliomyelitis: a flulike illness
     a. Fever
     b. Malaise
     c. Headache
     d. Sore throat
  2. Nonparalytic poliomyelitis: an aseptic meningitis that correlates with invasion of the CNS
     a. Headache
     b. Neck stiffness
     c. Change in mental status
  3. Paralytic poliomyelitis
     a. Most commonly affects the lumbar or bulbar regions
     b. Following paralysis, a period of variable degrees of recovery, the majority of which occurs in 2 to 6 mo
     c. Paralysis from involvement of motor neurons in the spinal cord
     d. Flaccid paralysis without sensory defects
     e. Postpolio syndrome late sequela, which may occur many years after the acute illness
     f. Functional deterioration of muscle groups that had recovered from initial paralysis thought to result from failure of reinnervation, which initially was able to restore function to weakened or paralyzed areas

ETIOLOGY

- Virus of genus *Enterovirus* (3 serotypes of polio virus [types 1 to 3])
- Classic endemic and epidemic disease caused by wild-type poliovirus
- All cases in the U.S. currently caused by a live, attenuated virus in the OPV
  1. Extremely rare complication that occurs in vaccine recipients or their contacts
  2. Paralysis from lower motor neuron damage caused by viral infection

DIAGNOSIS

DIFFERENTIAL DIAGNOSIS

- Guillain-Barré syndrome
- CVA
- Botulism food poisoning
- Spinal cord compression
- Other enteroviruses:
  1. Aseptic meningitis
  2. Paralysis (rare)

WORKUP

- Isolation of virus:
  1. Stool or a rectal swab
  2. Throat swabs
  3. Rarely CSF
- Paired sera for antibody titer determinations

LABORATORY TESTS

CSF:
- Aseptic meningitis
- Elevated WBCs
- Elevated protein
- Normal glucose

IMAGING STUDIES

MRI may show involvement of anterior horn of the spinal cord.

TREATMENT

NONPHARMACOLOGIC THERAPY

- Maintenance of respiration and hydration
- Early mobilization and exercise once fever subsides

ACUTE GENERAL Rx

- Aimed at reduction of pain and muscle spasm
- No agent to alter the course of disease

CHRONIC Rx

Physical therapy

DISPOSITION

- In the abortive and nonparalytic forms, complete recovery
- Paralytic disease:
  1. Variable degrees of recovery
  2. 80% usually in the first 6 mo following illness

REFERRAL

Always refer to an infectious disease consultant. Cases should be reported to public health agencies.

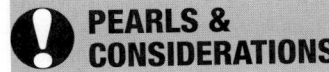

PEARLS & CONSIDERATIONS

COMMENTS

- Risk of disease in recipients of OPV is approximately 1 in 2.5 million.
- Use of inactivated polio vaccine (IPV) is not associated with disease:
  1. Does not confer local (mucosal) immunity
  2. Will not immunize nonvaccinated contacts
  3. Requires boosters
  4. Is given by injection
- To decrease the incidence of vaccine-associated polio, the routine childhood vaccination schedule has been changed. A recent recommendation for use of a sequential IPV-OPV schedule has again been modified. Exclusive use of IPV is now recommended. OPV use is limited to unvaccinated persons with plans for imminent (<4 wk) travel to polio-endemic areas.

SUGGESTED READINGS
available at www.expertconsult.com

AUTHORS: **DENNIS J. MIKOLICH, M.D.,** and **GLENN G. FORT, M.D., M.P.H.**

BASIC INFORMATION

DEFINITION

Polyarteritis nodosa is a vasculitic syndrome involving medium-sized to small arteries, characterized histologically by necrotizing inflammation of the arterial media and inflammatory cell infiltration.

SYNONYMS

Periarteritis nodosa
PAN
Necrotizing arteritis

ICD-9CM CODES
446.0 Polyarteritis nodosa

EPIDEMIOLOGY & DEMOGRAPHICS

INCIDENCE: One per 100,000 persons annually. Increased incidence in patients with hepatitis B surface antigen or hepatitis C virus.
PREDOMINANT SEX: Male/female ratio is 2:1.

PHYSICAL FINDINGS & CLINICAL PRESENTATION

- Typical presentation is subacute, with the onset of constitutional symptoms over weeks to months
- Weight loss, nausea, vomiting
- Testicular pain or tenderness
- Myalgias, weakness, or leg tenderness
- Neuropathy (mononeuritis multiplex), foot drop
- Livedo reticularis, ulceration of digits, abdominal pain after meals, hematemesis, hematochezia, hypertension, asymmetric polyarthritis (tending to involve large joints of lower extremities); true synovitis occurs only in a minority of patients
- Fever may be present (polyarteritis nodosa is often a cause of fever of unknown origin) and can range from intermittent, low-grade fevers to high fevers with chills
- Tachycardia is common and often striking

ETIOLOGY

- Unknown.
- Hepatitis B virus–associated polyarteritis nodosa appears to be an immune complex–mediated disease.

DIAGNOSIS

DIFFERENTIAL DIAGNOSIS

Cryoglobulinemia, systemic lupus erythematosus, infections (e.g., subacute bacterial endocarditis, trichinosis, *Rickettsia*), lymphoma

WORKUP

- Laboratory evaluation, arteriography, and biopsy of small or medium-sized arteries can confirm diagnosis. Clinical manifestations are variable and depend on the arteries involved and the organs affected (e.g., kidney involvement occurs in >80% of cases).
- The presence of any three of the following 10 items allows the diagnosis of polyarteritis nodosa with a sensitivity of 82% and a specificity of 86%:
  1. Weight loss >4 kg
  2. Livedo reticularis
  3. Testicular pain or tenderness
  4. Myalgias, weakness, or leg tenderness
  5. Neuropathy
  6. Diastolic blood pressure >90 mm Hg
  7. Elevated blood urea nitrogen (BUN) or creatinine
  8. Positive test for hepatitis B virus
  9. Arteriography revealing small or large aneurysms and focal constrictions between dilated segments
  10. Biopsy of small or medium-sized artery containing white blood cells

LABORATORY TESTS

- Elevated BUN or creatinine, positive test for hepatitis B virus or hepatitis C.
- Elevated erythrocyte sedimentation rate and C-reactive protein, anemia, elevated platelets, eosinophilia, proteinuria, hematuria.
- Biopsy of small or medium-sized artery of symptomatic sites (muscle, nerve) is >90% specific. Biopsy of the gastrocnemius muscle and sural nerve are commonly performed.
- Assays for antinuclear antibody and rheumatoid factor are negative; however, low, nonspecific titers may be detected.

IMAGING STUDIES

Arteriography can be done in patients with negative biopsies or if there are no symptomatic sites. Visceral angiography will reveal aneurysmal dilation of the renal, mesenteric (Fig. 1-295), or hepatic arteries.

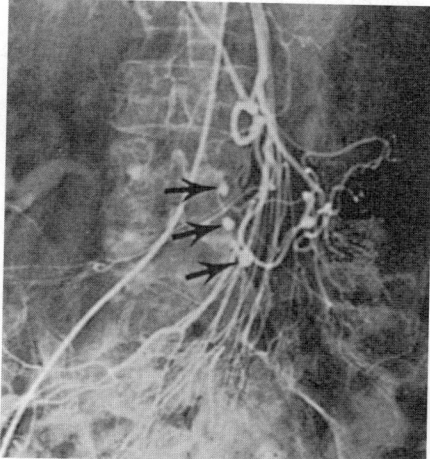

FIGURE 1-295 Superior mesenteric arteriogram in patients with polyarteritis. Several small aneurysms *(arrows)* are present in branches of superior mesenteric artery. (Courtesy of Dr. A.W. Stanson.) (Harris ED, Budd RC, Genovese MC, Firestein GS, Sargent JS, Sledge CB, Ruddy S: *Kelley's textbook of rheumatology,* ed 7, 2005, Saunders.)

TREATMENT

NONPHARMACOLOGIC THERAPY

Low-sodium diet in hypertensive patients

ACUTE GENERAL Rx

Prednisone 1 to 2 mg/kg/day; cyclophosphamide in refractory cases

CHRONIC Rx

Monitoring for infections and potential complications such as thrombosis, infarction, or organ necrosis

DISPOSITION

The 5-yr survival is <20% in untreated patients. Treatment with corticosteroids increases survival to approximately 50%. Use of both corticosteroids and immunosuppressive drugs may increase 5-yr survival to >80%. Poor prognostic signs are severe renal or gastrointestinal involvement.

REFERRAL

Surgical referral for biopsy

SUGGESTED READING
available at www.expertconsult.com

AUTHOR: **FRED F. FERRI, M.D.**

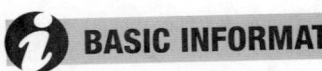

DEFINITION

Polycystic kidney disease (PKD) refers to a systemic hereditary disorder characterized by the formation of cysts in the cortex and medulla of both kidneys (Figs. 1-296 and 1-297).

SYNONYMS

Autosomal-dominant polycystic kidney disease (ADPKD)

ICD-9CM CODES	
753.1	Polycystic kidney, unspecified type
753.13	Polycystic kidney, autosomal dominant

EPIDEMIOLOGY & DEMOGRAPHICS

- The most common Mendelian disorder of the kidneys
- Affects all racial groups worldwide
- Results in kidney failure in the majority of individuals by the fifth to sixth decade
- PKD occurs in one in 700 to 1000 persons
- Usually presents in the third to fourth decades of life

PHYSICAL FINDINGS & CLINICAL PRESENTATION

- Characterized by focal development of renal and extrarenal cysts in an age-dependent manner, resulting in a slow, gradual, and massive kidney enlargement.

Symptoms:
- Pain (60%): acute pain can be associated renal hemorrhage, passage of stones (20% patients; usually uric acid or calcium oxalate), and urinary tract infections
- Palpable flank mass
- Hypertension: >60% of patients; usually develops before the loss of renal function
- Headache
- Nocturia, hematuria

Renal manifestations:
- Kidney and cyst volumes and renal blood flow (or vascular resistance) are the strongest predictors of renal function decline. Kidney function does not decline in individuals with PKD until kidney size is at least five times greater than normal.
- Morphometric analysis of sequential CT was shown to be sufficiently accurate to monitor rates of renal enlargement in PKD, and MRI-based methods have been developed. Two general groups of kidney volume increase: those with rapid rates (>5% increase in total kidney volume per year) and those with rates of progression <5% per year. Intervals between measurements as short as 6 mo may be adequate to determine an effect of treatment that reduces the rates of volume progression >50% in those with rapidly progressive disease.
- All cysts develop from preexisting renal tubule segments, and only a small portion of the nephrons (1%) undergoes cystic formation.
- Renal failure: in most patients renal function is maintained within normal range, despite relentless growth of cysts, until the fourth to sixth decades of life.
- Nephrolithiasis (20%)
- Urinary tract infection

Extrarenal manifestations:
- Associated with liver cysts (50% to 70%), pancreatic cysts (10%), splenic cysts (5%), central nervous system arachnoid cysts (5%), and cerebral aneurysms (20%)
- Polycystic liver disease: most common extrarenal manifestation-associated with both *PKD1* and non-*PKD1* genotypes
- Vascular manifestations: intracranial aneurysms (occur in approximately 6% of patients with a negative family history of aneurysms and 16% of those with a positive history), thoracic aortic and cervicocephalic artery dissection, and coronary artery aneurysms
- Increased incidence of diverticular disease and mitral valve prolapse

ETIOLOGY

- Dominantly inherited heterogenic systemic disease: mutations in *PKD1* (chromosome region 16p13.3; 85% of cases) or *PKD2* (4q21; approximately 15% of cases).
- Polycystin 1 and polycystin 2 are the protein products of PKD1 and PKD2, which interact and coassemble and seem to function together to regulate the morphologic configuration of epithelial cells. Although individuals with PKD1 are clinically indistinguishable from individuals with PKD2, patients with PKD2 have a less severe course of disease with a later mean age of diagnosis, hypertension, and end-stage renal disease (ESRD).
- Disease penetrance is 100%.

Sonographic imaging or CT scan:
1. In an individual with a family history for the disease, including:
   - Age <30 yr: at least two unilateral or bilateral cysts
   - 30 to 59 yr: two cysts in each kidney
   - ≥60 yr: four cysts in each kidney
2. In the absence of a family history: bilateral renal enlargement or cysts or the presence of multiple bilateral cysts with hepatic cysts together and in the absence of other manifestations suggesting a different renal cyst disease
   - Genetic testing can be used when the imaging results are equivocal and when a definitive diagnosis is required in a younger individual, such as a potential living related kidney donor.

DIFFERENTIAL DIAGNOSIS

- Simple cysts
- Autosomal-recessive polycystic kidney disease in children
- Tuberous sclerosis
- von Hippel Lindau syndrome
- Acquired cystic kidney disease

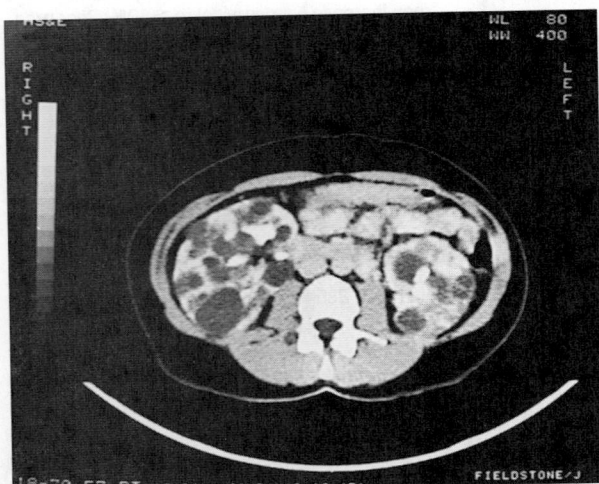

FIGURE 1-296 Tomogram of autosomal-dominant polycystic kidney disease. Kidney cysts. (From Stein JH [ed]: *Internal medicine,* ed 5, St Louis, 1998, Mosby.)

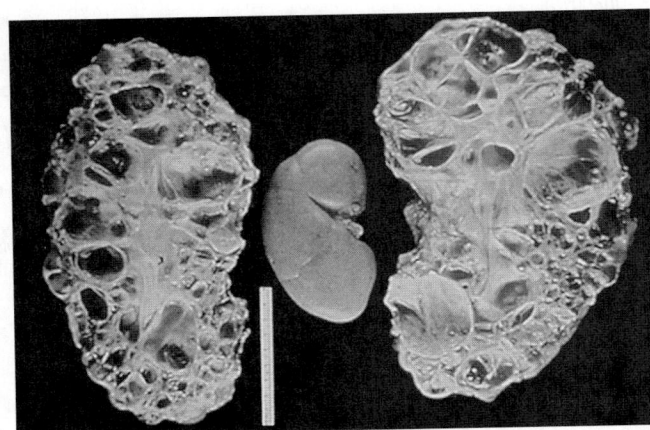

FIGURE 1-297 Markedly enlarged polycystic kidneys from a patient with autosomal-dominant polycystic kidney disease compared with a normal kidney *(middle)*. (From Johnson RJ, Feehally J: *Comprehensive clinical nephrology,* ed 2, St Louis, 2000, Mosby.)

LABORATORY TESTS

- Hemoglobin and hematocrit are elevated because of increased secretion of erythropoietin from functioning renal cysts.
- Electrolyte abnormalities commonly seen in any patients with renal insufficiency.
- Blood urea nitrogen and creatinine can be elevated.
- Urinalysis can show microscopic hematuria and proteinuria (seldom >1 g/24 hr). Proteinuria >2 g/day is unusual and suggests the presence of another kidney disease.

IMAGING STUDIES

- A cyst is considered to be present if it measures >2 mm in diameter.
- Abdominal renal ultrasound is the easiest and more cost-efficient test for renal cysts. Renal ultrasound can detect cysts from 1 to 1.5 cm.
- Abdominal CT scan is more sensitive than ultrasound and can detect cysts as small as 0.5 cm.
- Both studies can detect associated hepatic, splenic, and pancreatic cysts.
- MRI is more sensitive than ultrasound and may help distinguish renal cell carcinomas from simple cysts.

 TREATMENT

NONPHARMACOLOGIC THERAPY

- Treatment consists of the standard therapies for chronic renal disease, including good blood pressure control and control of hyperlipidemia.
- When conservative measures fail to control the pain, infection, or bleeding, surgical interventions such as cystic decompression by aspiration under ultrasound or CT guidance or laparoscopic or surgical cyst fenestration through lumbotomy or flank incision may be of benefit.
- When above measures fail, nephrectomy should be undertaken in ESRD.
- Combined percutaneous cyst drainage and antibiotic treatment provide the best treatment results for hepatic cyst infection.

ACUTE GENERAL Rx

- Kidney infections should be treated with antibiotics known to penetrate the cyst (e.g., trimethoprim-sulfamethoxazole 1 tablet PO bid or ciprofloxacin 250 mg PO bid).
- Early detection and treatment of hypertension is important because cardiovascular disease is the main cause of death.

CHRONIC Rx

- Dialysis for end-stage renal failure.
- Pretransplant nephrectomy is reserved for patients with a history of infected cyst or frequent bleeding.
- Renal transplantation is the treatment of choice for ESRD.
- Cyst infections are often difficult to treat. Lipophilic agents penetrate the cysts consistently. If fever persists after 1 to 2 wk of appropriate antimicrobial treatment, percutaneous or surgical drainage of the cysts may be needed. Several months of antibiotic treatment may be needed to eradicate the infection.
- Most cases of polycystic liver disease do not need treatment; patients should avoid estrogens and compounds that promote cyclic adenosine monophosphate accumulation (e.g., caffeine).

DISPOSITION

- Most patients with PKD will progress to renal failure.
- Gross hematuria is usually self-limited.

REFERRAL

- Nephrology consultation.
- Urology can also be consulted in patients with nephrolithiasis, for recurrent episodes of gross hematuria, or for consideration for nephrectomy before transplantation.
- Counseling should be done before PKD genetic testing. Benefits include certainty of diagnosis that could affect family planning, early detection and treatment of disease complications, and selection of genetically unaffected family members for living related donor transplantation. Potential discrimination in terms of insurability and employment associated with a positive diagnosis should be discussed.

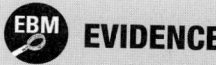 **PEARLS & CONSIDERATIONS**

- ESRD patients with PKD do better on dialysis than do patients with other causes of ESRD.
- There is no difference in patient survival after transplantation between patients with PKD and other ESRD populations.
- Widespread screening is not indicated. Indications for screening include family history of aneurysm, subarachnoid hemorrhage, previous aneurysm rupture, preparation for major elective surgery, high-risk occupations (airplane pilots), and patient anxiety despite adequate information.
- Kidney and cyst volumes are the strongest predictors of renal function decline.

COMMENTS

- Conservative management is recommended for patients with a small (<7 mm) cerebral aneurysm, particularly in the anterior circulation. Rescreening of patients with a family history of intracranial aneurysm after 5 to 10 yr seems reasonable.
- Trials with treatment protocols involving vasopressin antagonists, somatostatin, and rapamycin are underway to slow the progression of PKD. Results with the rapamycin (mTOR) inhibitors evarilus and sirolimus have been disappointing.

EBM EVIDENCE

available at www.expertconsult.com

SUGGESTED READINGS
available at www.expertconsult.com

AUTHOR: **SHAHNAZ PUNJANI, M.D.**

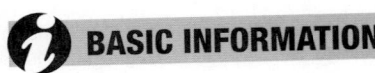

BASIC INFORMATION

DEFINITION

Polycystic ovary syndrome (PCOS) is characterized by an accumulation of incompletely developed follicles in the ovaries due to anovulation and associated with ovarian androgen production. In its complete form, it associates polycystic ovaries, amenorrhea, hirsutism, and obesity.

SYNONYMS

Stein-Leventhal syndrome
PCOS

ICD-9CM CODES

256.4 Polycystic ovary syndrome

EPIDEMIOLOGY & DEMOGRAPHICS

- 5% to 15% of reproductive-age women (most common endocrine disorder in this population).
- Symptoms usually begin around the time of menarche, and the diagnosis is often made during adolescence or young adulthood.
- Increased risk of endometrial and ovarian cancers.
- PCOS is the most common cause of anovulatory infertility

PHYSICAL FINDINGS & CLINICAL PRESENTATION

- Oligomenorrhea or amenorrhea
- Dysfunctional uterine bleeding
- Infertility
- Hirsutism
- Acne, alopecia, acanthosis nigricans
- Obesity (40% only), predominantly abdominal obesity
- Insulin resistance (type 2 diabetes mellitus)
- Hypertension

ETIOLOGY & PATHOGENESIS

Elevated serum luteinizing hormone (LH) concentrations and an increased serum LH/follicle-stimulating hormone (FSH) ratio result either from an increased gonadotropin-releasing hormone hypothalamic secretion or less likely from a primary pituitary abnormality. This results in dysregulation of androgen secretion and increased intraovarian androgen, the effect of which in the ovary is follicular atresia, maturation arrest, polycystic ovaries, and anovulation. Hyperinsulinemia is a contributing factor to ovarian hyperandrogenism, independent of LH excess. A role for insulin growth factor (IGF) receptors has been postulated for the association of PCOS and diabetes.

DIAGNOSIS

The diagnosis of PCOS excludes secondary causes (androgen-producing neoplasm, hyperprolactinemia, adult-onset congenital adrenal hyperplasia).
Clinical:
- The symptoms, signs, and biochemical features of PCOS vary greatly among women and may change over time.
- PCOS is the most common cause of chronic anovulation with estrogen present. A positive progesterone withdrawal test establishes the presence of estrogen. Medroxyprogesterone

(Provera) 10 mg qd is administered for 5 days and bleeding occurs if estrogen is present.
- The presence of oligomenorrhea, hirsutism, obesity, and documented polycystic ovaries establishes the diagnosis.

DIFFERENTIAL DIAGNOSIS

Causes of amenorrhea:
- Primary (unusual in PCOS)
  1. Genetic disorder (Turner's syndrome)
  2. Anatomic abnormality (e.g., imperforate hymen)
- Secondary
  1. Pregnancy
  2. Functional (cause unknown, anorexia nervosa, stress, excessive exercise, hyperthyroidism, less commonly hypothyroidism, adrenal dysfunction, pituitary dysfunction, severe systemic illness, drugs such as oral contraceptives, estrogens, or dopamine agonists)
  3. Abnormalities of the genital tract (uterine tumor, endometrial scarring, ovarian tumor)

LABORATORY TESTS

- Glucose tolerance test at the initial presentation and every 2 yr thereafter (rule out diabetes mellitus). Impaired glucose tolerance is very common, occurring in approximately 30% of women with PCOS
- Fasting lipid panel (rule out dyslipidemia), alanine aminotransferase, aspartate aminotransferase (rule out hepatic steatosis)
- Elevated LH/FSH ratio >2.5
- Prolactin level elevation in 25%
- Elevated androgens (testosterone [free and total levels], DHEA-S) (rule out androgen-secreting tumor)
- Other: thyroid-stimulating hormone (rule out hypothyroidism), 17-hydroxyprogesterone (rule out congenital adrenal hyperplasia), 24-h urine for cortisol and creatinine (rule out Cushing's syndrome)

IMAGING STUDIES

Pelvic ultrasound (or CT scan) reveals the presence of twofold to fivefold ovarian enlargement with a thickened tunica albuginea, thecal hyperplasia, and 20 or more subcapsular follicles

from 1 to 15 mm in diameter (Fig. 1-298). It is important to note that having polycystic ovaries alone does not make the diagnosis of PCOS because 20% of women with polycystic ovaries have no symptoms.

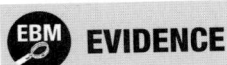

TREATMENT

The goal is to interrupt the self-perpetuating abnormal hormone cycle:
- Reduction of ovarian androgen secretion by laparoscopic ovarian wedge resection. Laparoscopic ovarian surgery (laparoscopic ovarian drilling [LOD]) is a useful alternative that does not trigger ovarian hyperstimulation
- Reduction of ovarian androgen secretion by using oral contraceptives or LH-releasing hormone (LHRH) analogs
- Weight reduction for all obese women with PCOS. Loss of abdominal fat seems to be crucial to restore ovulation
- FSH stimulation with clomiphene HMG or pulsatile LHRH
- Urofollitropin (pure FSH) administration
- Metformin improves ovulation, insulin sensitivity, and possibly hyperandrogenemia
Choice of treatment:
- The management of hirsutism without risking pregnancy includes oral contraceptives, glucocorticoids, LHRH analogs, or spironolactone (an antiandrogen). Finasteride and flutamide may be similarly effective in reducing hirsutism as spironolactone.
- Pregnancy can be achieved with clomiphene (alone or with glucocorticoids, human chorionic gonadotropin, or bromocriptine), HMG, urofollitropin, pulsatile LHRH, or ovarian wedge resection. (Metformin may induce ovulation.)

EVIDENCE

available at www.expertconsult.com

SUGGESTED READINGS

available at www.expertconsult.com

AUTHOR: FRED F. FERRI, M.D.

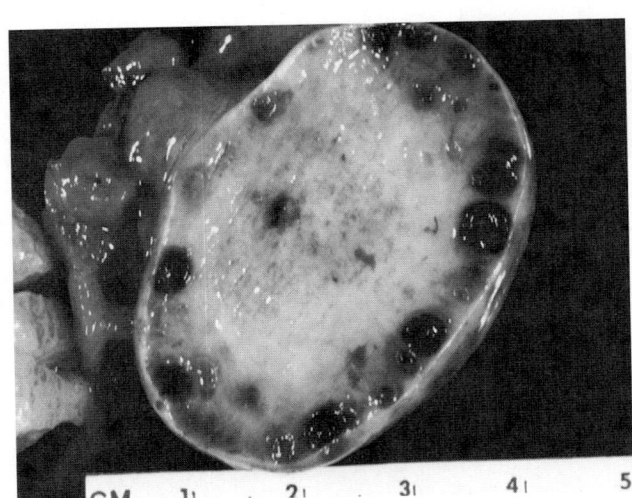

FIGURE 1-298 Sagittal section of a polycystic ovary illustrating large number of follicular cysts and thickened stroma. (From Mishell DR: *Comprehensive gynecology*, ed 3, St Louis, 1997, Mosby.)

BASIC INFORMATION

DEFINITION

Polycythemia vera is a chronic myeloproliferative disorder characterized mainly by erythrocytosis (increase in red blood cell [RBC] mass).

SYNONYMS

Primary polycythemia
Vaquez disease

EPIDEMIOLOGY & DEMOGRAPHICS

Incidence of 0.5 cases per 100,000 persons; mean age at onset is 60 yr; men are affected more often than are women.

PHYSICAL FINDINGS & CLINICAL PRESENTATION

The patient generally comes to medical attention because of symptoms associated with increased blood volume and viscosity or impaired platelet function:

- Impaired cerebral circulation resulting in headache, vertigo, blurred vision, dizziness, transient ischemic attack, cerebrovascular accident
- Fatigue, poor exercise tolerance
- Pruritus, particularly after bathing (caused by overproduction of histamine)
- Bleeding: epistaxis, upper gastrointestinal bleeding (increased incidence of peptic ulcer disease)
- Abdominal discomfort from splenomegaly; hepatomegaly may be present
- Hyperuricemia may result in nephrolithiasis and gouty arthritis

The physical examination may reveal:

- Facial plethora, congestion of oral mucosa, ruddy complexion
- Enlargement and tortuosity of retinal veins
- Splenomegaly (found in >75% of patients)

DIAGNOSIS

DIFFERENTIAL DIAGNOSIS

Smoking:

- Polycythemia is caused by increased carboxyhemoglobin, resulting in left shift in the hemoglobin (Hgb) dissociation curve.
- Laboratory evaluation shows increased hematocrit (Hct), RBC mass, erythropoietin level, and carboxyhemoglobin.
- Splenomegaly is not present on physical examination.

Hypoxemia (secondary polycythemia):

- Living for prolonged periods at high altitudes, pulmonary fibrosis, congenital cardiac lesions with right-to-left shunts.
- Laboratory evaluation shows decreased arterial oxygen saturation and elevated erythropoietin level.
- Splenomegaly is not present on physical examination.

Erythropoietin-producing states:

- Renal cell carcinoma, hepatoma, cerebral hemangioma, uterine fibroids, polycystic kidneys.
- The erythropoietin level is elevated in these patients, and the arterial oxygen saturation is normal.
- Splenomegaly may be present with metastatic neoplasms.

Stress polycythemia (Gaisböck's syndrome, relative polycythemia):

- Laboratory evaluation demonstrates normal RBC mass, arterial oxygen saturation, and erythropoietin level; plasma volume is decreased.
- Splenomegaly is not present on physical examination.

Hemoglobinopathies associated with high oxygen affinity:

- An abnormal oxyhemoglobin-dissociation curve (P50) is present.

WORKUP

Recent developments in molecular biology have identified a single, acquired point mutation in the Janus kinase 2 (JAK2) gene in the majority of patients with polycythemia vera and other pH-negative myeloproliferative disorders. The JAK2 mutation is found in >95% of patients with polycythemia vera and can be used for diagnostic purposes. Testing for the JAK2 V617F mutation with polymerase chain reaction assay is now available. In patients with high hematocrit (>52% in men or >48% in women) and in the absence of coexisting secondary erythrocytosis, the presence of the JAK2 mutation is sufficient for the diagnosis of polycythemia vera.

The WHO diagnostic criteria for P. Vera is described in Table 1-146.

A diagnostic algorithm for polycythemia is described in Section III.

LABORATORY TESTS

- Elevated RBC count (>6 million/mm^3), elevated Hgb (>18 g/dl in men, >16 g/dl in women), elevated Hct (>54% in men, >49% in women)
- Increased white blood cell count (often with basophilia); thrombocytosis in the majority of patients
- Elevated leukocyte alkaline phosphatase, serum vitamin B_{12}, and uric acid levels
- Low serum erythropoietin level
- Bone marrow aspiration revealing RBC hyperplasia and absent iron stores

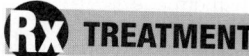

TREATMENT

NONPHARMACOLOGIC THERAPY

Phlebotomy to keep Hct <45% in men and <42% in women is the mainstay of therapy.

ACUTE GENERAL Rx

- Hydroxyurea can be used in conjunction with phlebotomy to decrease the incidence of thrombotic events.
- Interferon-alpha-2b is also effective in controlling RBC values without significant side effects.
- Myelosuppressive therapy with chlorambucil is effective but not routinely used because of its leukemogenic potential.
- Box 1-14 describes an algorithm for management of patients with PV.

CHRONIC Rx

- Patient education regarding need for lifelong monitoring and treatment.
- Adjunctive therapy: treatment of pruritus with antihistamines, control of significant hyperuricemia with allopurinol, reduction of gastric hyperacidity with antacids of H_2 blockers, low-dose aspirin to treat vasomotor symptoms in patients without bleeding diathesis. Low-dose aspirin can safely prevent thrombotic complications in patients with polycythemia vera.

DISPOSITION

- The median survival time without treatment is 6 to 18 mo after diagnosis; phlebotomy extends the average survival time to 12 yr.
- Prognosis is worse in patients >60 yr and those with a history of thrombosis.

TABLE 1-146 World Health Organization 2008 Diagnostic Criteria for Polycythemia Vera

Major Criteria

1. Hemoglobin (Hgb) >18.5 g/dl (men), >16.5 (women); or Hgb or hematocrit (Hct) >99% reference range for age, sex, or altitude of residence; or Hgb >17 g/dl (men), >15 g/dl (women) if associated with a sustained increase of ≥ 2g/dl from baseline that cannot be attributed to correction of iron deficiency; or elevated red cell mass (>25% above mean normal predicted value)
2. Presence of JAK2 V617F or similar mutation

Minor Criteria

1. Bone marrow trilineage myeloproliferation
2. Subnormal serum erythropoietin level
3. Endogenous erythroid colony formation in vitro

Either both major criteria and one minor criterion or the first major criterion and two minor criteria must be met for diagnosis of polycythemia vera.

Andreoli TE, Benjamin IJ, Griggs RC, Wing EJ: Andreoli and Carpenter's Cecil essentials of medicine, ed 8, Philadelphia, 2010, Saunders.

BOX 1-14 Algorithm for Management of Patients with PV

Low-risk young patients (<60 yr) and no prior history of thrombosis, platelet count <1.5×10^6 mm^{-3}

Phlebotomy + low-dose aspirin (81 mg/d) to maintain Hct <45% in males and <42% in females. Aspirin should not be used in patients with histories of hemorrhagic episode or with extreme thrombocytosis (>1.5×10^6 mm^{-3}) or acquired von Willebrand syndrome.

↓

Thrombosis or hemorrhage
Systemic symptoms
Severe pruritus refractory to histamine antagonists
Painful splenomegaly

↓

Pegylated interferon 90 to 180 μg/wk or interferon α (3×10^6 units three times/wk; alter dose depending on response and toxicity). Consider the use of pegylated interferon, which can be administered once/wk.

↓

If platelet control is inadequate or patient cannot tolerate interferon, one option could be the use of anagrelide. However, the use of this drug is controversial. In this case, supplemental phlebotomy is required to maintain Hct <45% in males and <42% in females, and the use of hydroxyurea should be considered, especially if patient continues to have thrombotic episodes.

↓

If the patient has increasing splenomegaly, systemic symptoms, or repeated thromboses in spite of adequate dose of hydroxyurea (2 to 3 g/d) start busulphan 4 to 6 mg/d PO for 4 to 8 wk. It should be mentioned that the sequential use of hydroxyurea and busulphan may be associated with an increased risk of leukemia. Supplemental phlebotomy may be required.

↓

Painful splenomegaly
Splenectomy + continued systemic therapy
High-risk patients (>60 yr), previous thrombosis, platelet count >1.5×10^6 mm^{-3}
Phlebotomy to Hct <42% in females and <45% in males
Aspirin (81 mg/d) to be given only in patients with platelet counts <1.5×10^6 mm^{-2}
Myelosuppressive therapy with hydroxyurea 30 mg/kg PO for 1 wk

↓

Then 15 to 20 mg/kg
If patient continues to have thrombotic episodes and has extreme thrombocytosis or cannot tolerate hydroxyurea, consider pegylated interferon 90 to 180 μg/wk or add busulphan 4 to 6 mg/d PO for 4 to 8 wk.

Stop when blood counts are normalized or platelet count is <300,000 mm^{-3}.

Occasional supplemental phlebotomy if Hct is >42% in females and >45% in males; when patient relapses (patient is symptomatic), initiate busulphan therapy again at same dose.

↓

If patient is poorly compliant, consider ^{32}P: 2.3 mCi/m^2 IV every 12 wk as needed (limit 5 mCi per dose).

Increase dose by 25% if no response
Patient age >70 yr
Phlebotomy + low-dose aspirin + hydroxyurea

↓

No response or poor compliance
Busulphan 4 to 6 mg/d PO for 4 to 8 wk. Stop when blood counts are normalized or platelet count is >300,000 mm^{-3}.

↓

No response ^{32}P

(From Hoffmann R et al: *Hematology: basic principles and practice,* ed 5, Philadelphia, 2009, Churchill Livingstone.)

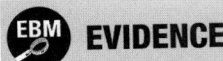

EVIDENCE
available at www.expertconsult.com

SUGGESTED READINGS
available at www.expertconsult.com

AUTHOR: **FRED F. FERRI, M.D.**

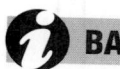

BASIC INFORMATION

DEFINITION

Polymyalgia rheumatica (PMR) is an inflammatory condition characterized by shoulder and pelvic girdle muscle pain and stiffness.

SYNONYMS

Anarthritic rheumatoid syndrome
PMR

ICD-9CM CODES

725.0 Polymyalgia rheumatica

EPIDEMIOLOGY & DEMOGRAPHICS

PREVALENCE: Some geographic variation with rates of 59 per 100,000 in Minnesota; 84 per 100,000 in UK; rare in African Americans
PREDOMINANT SEX: Female/male ratio of 2:1
PREDOMINANT AGE: Age >50 years with greater incidence as age increases.

PHYSICAL FINDINGS & CLINICAL PRESENTATION

- In majority of patients, sudden onset of muscle pain and stiffness.
- Neck, shoulders, and arms are most often affected. Pelvic girdle and thigh muscles also involved.
- Patients often note severe pain and stiffness.
- Constitutional symptoms of fatigue, malaise, and loss of appetite may accompany pain and stiffness.
- Physical exam is fairly benign; passive range of motion is typically preserved; may find minimal joint swelling, and strength testing is normal.
- Presence of fever, chills, night sweats, visual disturbances, headaches, or jaw claudication need to trigger a vasculitis workup; giant cell arteritis in particular must be ruled out.

ETIOLOGY

Appears to be related to the presence of HLA-D4 haplotypes which confer susceptibility to activation of the innate immune system leading to inflammation.

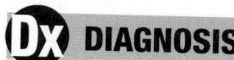

DIAGNOSIS

DIFFERENTIAL DIAGNOSIS

See Box 1-15

WORKUP

- Elderly patients with PMR symptoms should have initial laboratory evaluation with ESR, CBC, CPK
- ESR >40 is seen in majority of patients
- May have a normocytic, normochromic anemia and thrombocytosis
- Table 1-147 describes diagnostic criteria for PMR

BOX 1-15   Disease Entities with Polymyalgias

Rheumatoid arthritis
Rotator cuff syndrome
Osteoarthritis of shoulder and hip joints
Fibromyalgia
Polymyositis/dermatomyositis
Spondyloarthritis
Systemic lupus erythematosus
Vasculitides
Paraneoplastic myalgias
Infection-associated myalgias
RS3PE (remitting seronegative symmetrical synovitis and pitting edema)
Parkinson's disease
Hypothyroidism

From Hochberg M: *Rheumatology,* ed 4, 2007, Philadelphia, Mosby (Box 145-1).

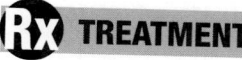

TREATMENT

ACUTE GENERAL Rx

- Prednisone 10 to 20 mg/day with dramatic improvement in symptoms typically noted in 24 to 48 hr.
- Initial dose of prednisone maintained for 2 to 4 wk with steroid dose reduced by 10% every 4 wk as long as patient remains symptom free.
- It is prudent to start a proton-pump inhibitor at initiation of therapy given the need for gastric protection in an elderly age group at high risk for GI toxicity.
- Attention should be paid to bone health given most patients are on steroids for 1 to 2 yr. Calcium and vitamin D supplementation should be started early on with possible bisphosphanate use if indicated by bone density measurement.

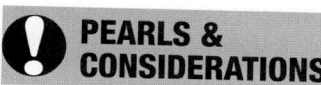

PEARLS & CONSIDERATIONS

Patients with PMR should be monitored carefully for the development of giant cell arteritis. Patients that have incomplete response to treatment with prednisone or have an evolving pattern of pain and swelling should be reevaluated for the possibility of a different diagnosis.

SUGGESTED READINGS

available at www.expertconsult.com

AUTHOR: **NUHA R. SAID, M.D.**

TABLE 1-147   Polymyalgia Rheumatica: Diagnostic Criteria

Chuang et al 1982	Healey 1984
<ul><li>Age of onset = 50 yr or older</li><li>Erythrocyte sedimentation rate >40 mm/h</li><li>Bilateral aching and stiffness for =1 mo and involving two of the following areas: neck or torso, shoulders or proximal regions of the arms, and hips or proximal aspects of the thighs</li><li>Exclusion of all other diagnoses causing PMR-like symptoms</li></ul>	<ul><li>Age of onset = 50 yr or older</li><li>Erythrocyte sedimentation rate >40 mm/h</li><li>Pain persisting for =1 mo and involving two of the following areas: neck, shoulders and pelvic girdle</li><li>Absence of other diseases capable of causing the musculoskeletal symptoms</li><li>Morning stiffness lasting more than 1 hr</li><li>Rapid response to prednisone (=20 mg/day)</li></ul>

From Hochberg M: *Rheumatology,* ed 4, 2007, Philadelphia, Mosby (Table 145-1).

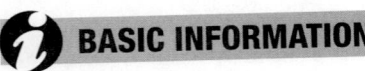

BASIC INFORMATION

DEFINITION

Polypharmacy is the concomitant use of more drugs than are clinically necessary. Older definitions have emphasized specific numbers of medications, commonly five or more drugs per day. The primary issue is that the drugs are inappropriate and potentially may increase the risk of medication errors, adverse drug reactions, drug interactions, hospitalizations, and/or cost without a clear benefit to the patient.

SYNONYMS

Potentially inappropriate medications (PIMs)

ICD-9CM CODES
Not applicable

EPIDEMIOLOGY & DEMOGRAPHICS

PEAK INCIDENCE: Estimates vary, but incidence appears to increase between age 70 and 84 yr.
PREVALENCE: One in five Americans receives potentially inappropriate drug therapy, although prevalence may be substantially higher in specific clinical settings.
PREDOMINANT SEX AND AGE:
- Adults aged 65 and older
- Women
RISK FACTORS:
- Multiple chronic diseases
- Frequent hospitalizations with incomplete medication reconciliation at care transitions
- Multiple providers such as primary care physician and specialists with inadequate communication
- Multiple pharmacies such as one pharmacy for inexpensive generics, one for free antibiotics, mail order for 90-day supply

PHYSICAL FINDINGS & CLINICAL PRESENTATION

- Presence of one or more drugs without a clearly defined purpose
- Presence of therapeutic duplication such as multiple proton pump inhibitors
- Presence of prescriptions for both generic and brand-name versions of the same drug
- Unexpected response to drug therapy ranging from lack of efficacy to exaggerated responses
- Expanding list of new medications for a patient late in life or at the end of life
- Decreased patient adherence
- Common unnecessary drugs in polypharmacy such as gastrointestinal and CNS agents
- Presence of a "geriatric syndrome" such as falling, excessive sedation and confusion, urinary retention or incontinence, reduced oral intake, and general failure to thrive

ETIOLOGY

- Inadequate communication between physicians, pharmacists, patients, and their caregivers
- Lack of coordination of medical care
- Extensive use of self-care with OTC drugs by patients
- Prescribing cascade (not recognizing new problem as a drug side effect and prescribing a second drug)
- Increasing number of available medications and intensive marketing to physicians and patients

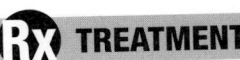

DIAGNOSIS

DIFFERENTIAL DIAGNOSIS

- Misuse, overuse, or underuse of drug therapy

WORKUP

- Obtain a thorough medication history including prescription and OTC drugs and dietary supplements.
- "Brown bag" approach: visually verify all medication bottles for actual ingredients.
- Although the presence of many drugs does not necessarily identify inappropriate prescribing, the likelihood of at least one or more problem drugs being present increases if at least seven drugs are prescribed.
- Use standard tools to evaluate drug regimens:
  1. Beers criteria drugs to recognize potentially dangerous or ineffective drugs
     Some of these drugs include propoxyphene, pentazocine, meperidine, indomethacin, ketorolac, amitriptyline, and imipramine (in antidepressant dosages); long-acting benzodiazepines, muscle relaxants, and antispasmodic agents; short-acting dipyridamole, ticlopidine, disopyramide, chlorpropamide, and drugs with strong anticholinergic properties.
  2. Zhan Criteria: Potentially inappropriate medication use in the community-dwelling elderly
  3. Classification by Expert Panel of 1997 Beers Criteria medications into three categories: always avoid, rarely appropriate, and appropriate for some indications.
  4. Medication Appropriateness Index evaluates key elements of appropriate prescribing
     ○ Is there an indication for the drug?
     ○ Is the medication effective for the condition?
     ○ Are the directions correct?
     ○ Are the directions practical?
     ○ Are there clinically significant drug–drug interactions?
     ○ Are there clinically significant drug–disease interactions?
     ○ Is there unnecessary duplication with other drugs?
     ○ Is the duration of therapy appropriate?
     ○ Is this drug the least expensive alternative compared with others of equal utility?
  5. The NCQA Healthcare Effectiveness Data and Information Set (HEDIS) 2009 measures include potentially harmful drug–disease interactions in the elderly and use of high-risk medications in the elderly.

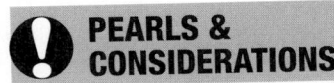

TREATMENT

The most important consideration in "treating" polypharmacy is to establish which conditions have the greatest priority for drug treatment, especially from the patient's perspective.

NONPHARMACOLOGIC THERAPY

As drugs are identified to be discontinued, ask patient about his or her interest in non-drug therapies.

ACUTE GENERAL Rx

If acute drug-related problems are identified, establish priorities for safely withdrawing/tapering the offending drugs (as appropriate for the specific agents).

CHRONIC Rx

- A key issue is whether the individual is likely to receive a benefit from a specific medication, especially if multiple comorbid conditions exist and/or their life expectancy is limited.
- Consideration should be given to the incremental benefit from each drug added to a complex drug regimen. For example, what would be the risk to benefit ratio to a 90 year-old individual from the addition of spironolactone to a regimen consisting of lisinopril, candesartan, and carvedilol for heart failure?
- The goal of therapy for each new medication should be clearly listed by the prescriber.

DISPOSITION

Safe discontinuation of inappropriate medications from a regimen may take at least several months depending on the specific drugs.

REFERRAL

Referral to a clinical pharmacist for a comprehensive drug regimen review and potentially to a geriatrician, especially for frail older adults.

PEARLS & CONSIDERATIONS

COMMENTS

The prevention and/or identification of polypharmacy should focus on the appropriateness of the medications for the *individual* person and not simply the number of medications. The decision regarding what is "appropriate" for an individual should first consider the patient's own priorities and expected risk and benefit to that individual before focusing on clinical practice guidelines that may or may not be applicable to a specific patient.

PREVENTION

- Polypharmacy is prevented by considering whether a drug is needed for a new symptom and whether a new symptom is actually an unrecognized adverse drug reaction.
- Use of electronic health records in which the medication history is updated regularly

against what the patient is actually taking may help to prevent polypharmacy.

- OTC drugs and dietary supplements should always be identified when taking a medication history. Certain points in the continuum of care are high risk for polypharmacy and inappropriate prescribing. Discharge from the hospital to home is a common point when patients may become confused about the intended drug regimen.
- Consistent use of generic drug names can decrease the risk of polypharmacy. Duplicate prescriptions for the same drug (furosemide and Lasix) commonly occur.
- Medication reconciliation: perform a complete review of medications for the appropriateness of their continued use at least every 6 mo (for older adults), after discharge from the hospital, and whenever new drugs are added.
- Regular evaluation of how frequently "as needed" medications are being used by the patient. For example, the "Rule of 2" for short-acting beta-agonists may identify a need for a change in maintenance therapy.

- Drug–drug interaction alerts in institutional record systems.
- Geriatric Evaluation and Management (GEM) Program: specialized program of services for both inpatient and outpatient settings. GEM uses an interdisciplinary approach to treatment, rehabilitation, health promotion and social service interventions in older adults. It aims to optimize drug prescribing and reduce unnecessary drug use.
- Use of positive Beers criteria for preferred CNS drugs in older adults can help prescribers select medications preferred for dementia, depression, Parkinson's disease, and psychosis, based on efficacy and safety.

PATIENT/FAMILY EDUCATION

- An up-to-date list of all drugs taken on a regular or as needed basis must be maintained. The list should include all prescription and OTC drugs including eye drops, inhalers, and skin creams. Dietary supplements such as vitamins and herbals should also be on the list. The National Transitions of Care Coalition's "My Medicine List" is an excellent tool

for patients (http://www.ntocc.org/Portals/0/My_Medicine_List.pdf), as well as My Medication Action Plan (MAP) from the American Pharmacists Association. Patient should ask physician or pharmacist to review all drugs at least once a year.
- After being discharged from the hospital, compare newly prescribed drugs to your existing drugs. Ask which drugs should be continued and which should be stopped.
- If enrolled in Medicare Part D, determine eligibility for Medication Therapy Management Programs (MTMP). MTMP may be available for beneficiaries who have multiple chronic diseases and Part D drugs, and who are likely to incur significant costs.

SUGGESTED READINGS
available at www.expertconsult.com

AUTHORS: **ANNE L. HUME, PHARM.D.,** and **CHRISTINE EISENHOWER, PHARM.D.**

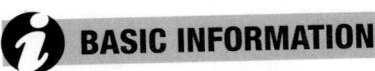

BASIC INFORMATION

DEFINITION

Clinically significant portal hypertension is defined as a portal vein pressure >10 mm Hg, most commonly attributable to liver disease.

SYNONYMS

None

> **ICD-9CM CODES**
> 572.3 Portal hypertension

EPIDEMIOLOGY & DEMOGRAPHICS

- Incidence of portal hypertension is not known.
- Cirrhosis is the most common cause of portal hypertension in the U.S.
- More than 90% of patients with cirrhosis develop portal hypertension.
- Alcoholic and viral liver diseases are the most common causes of cirrhosis and portal hypertension in the U.S.
- Schistosomiasis is the main cause of portal hypertension outside the U.S.
- Esophageal varices may appear when portal vein pressure rises to >10 mm Hg.
- Variceal hemorrhage is the most serious complication of portal hypertension and may occur when portal pressures rise >12 mm Hg.

PHYSICAL FINDINGS & CLINICAL PRESENTATION

- Jaundice
- Ascites (Figs. 1-299 and 1-300)
- Spider angiomata
- Testicular atrophy
- Gynecomastia
- Palmar erythema
- Dupuytren's contracture
- Asterixis (with advanced liver failure)
- Irritability, encephalopathy
- Splenomegaly
- Dilated veins in the anterior abdominal wall
- Venous pattern on the flanks
- Caput medusae (tortuous collateral veins around the umbilicus)
- Hemorrhoids
- Hematemesis
- Melena
- Pruritus

ETIOLOGY

Pathophysiologically caused by:
1. Conditions resulting in an increased resistance to flow
   - Prehepatic (e.g., portal vein thrombosis, splenic vein thrombosis, congenital stenosis)
   - Hepatic (e.g., cirrhosis, alcoholic liver disease, primary biliary cirrhosis, schistosomiasis)
   - Posthepatic (e.g., Budd-Chiari syndrome, constrictive pericarditis, inferior vena cava obstruction, cor pulmonale, tricuspid regurgitation)
2. Conditions leading to increase in portal blood flow
   - Splanchnic arterial vasodilation accompanying portal hypertension, mediated by local release of nitric oxide
   - Arterial-portal venous fistulae

DIAGNOSIS

- The diagnosis of portal hypertension is made on clinical grounds after a comprehensive history and physical examination.

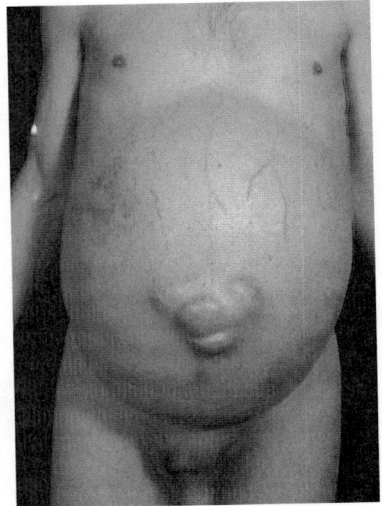

FIGURE 1-300 Ascites in a patient with alcoholic cirrhosis showing distended abdomen; dilated superficial collateral veins; hemorrhagic scratch marks due to pruritus and coagulopathy; umbilical varices; plaster in left iliac fossa indicating diagnostic paracentesis. (From Forbes A, Misiewicz JJ, Crompton CC, Levine M et al [eds]: *Atlas of clinical gastroenterology,* ed 3, Oxford, 2005, Mosby.)

- Noninvasive and invasive procedures confirm diagnosis and determine the severity of portal hypertension.

DIFFERENTIAL DIAGNOSIS

- Ascites from infection, neoplasm, or other inflammatory processes
- Obesity
- Abdominal organomegaly

WORKUP

The workup of portal hypertension includes blood tests and noninvasive imaging studies to determine if the cause of portal hypertension is prehepatic, hepatic, or posthepatic. Ascitic fluid analysis is a key part of the diagnosis.

LABORATORY TESTS

- Complete blood count with platelets
- Liver function tests with serum albumin
- Prothrombin and partial thromboplastin times
- Hepatitis B surface antigen and antibody
- Hepatitis C antibody
- In selected cases: iron, total iron-binding capacity, and ferritin; antinuclear antibody, anti–smooth muscle antibodies, antimitochondrial antibody, ceruloplasmin, alpha-1 antitrypsin.
- Ascitic fluid analysis: a serum-ascites albumin gradient ≥1.1 mg/dl suggests portal hypertension. Polymorphonuclear cells ≥250 cells/ml or positive Gram stain or culture suggest complicating spontaneous bacterial peritonitis (SBP).

IMAGING STUDIES

- Duplex-Doppler ultrasound is effective in screening for portal hypertension.
- Less commonly, CT/MRI/MRA scanning (Fig. 1-301) or liver-spleen nuclear medicine scanning can be used if the results from ultrasound are equivocal.
- Upper endoscopy is the most reliable test documenting the presence of esophageal varices.

TREATMENT

The treatment of portal hypertension is complex and involves measures to reduce the hypertension directly, minimize volume overload, correct underlying disorders, and prevent complications (most notably SBP and variceal bleeding).

NONPHARMACOLOGIC THERAPY

Dietary sodium restriction to generally 2000 mg/day forms the basis of therapy to limit fluid overload.

ACUTE GENERAL Rx

- For tense ascites, serial large volume paracentesis (LVP) is generally recommended. The use of albumin infusion (8 to 10 g/L of ascites fluid removed) during LVP >5 L has been shown to reduce the incidence of postparacentesis circulatory dysfunction, although its use remains somewhat controversial.

FIGURE 1-299 Ascites secondary to portal hypertension. Note the dilated collateral vein running up the right side of the abdomen. (From Forbes A, Misiewicz JJ, Crompton CC, Levine M et al [eds]: *Atlas of clinical gastroenterology,* ed 3, Oxford, 2005, Mosby.)

- IV diuretics, typically furosemide and spironolactone, are used to achieve natriuresis and net negative salt and water balance. Renal function and serum electrolytes are monitored frequently, with transition to an oral regimen for long-term therapy.
- SBP is treated with IV antibiotics directed against enteric bacteria.
- Acute variceal hemorrhage is treated with crystalloid and blood product resuscitation, IV octreotide, terlipressin/vasopressin or somatostatin, and urgent upper endoscopy, often with sclerotherapy or band ligation. Patients with acute variceal hemorrhage should receive antibiotic prophylaxis against SBP.
- Traditionally, a transjugular intrahepatic portosystemic shunt (TIPS) or surgical shunt placement may be considered in patients not responding to above measures. However, recent data show early TIPS placement improved outcomes in acute variceal hemorrhage.

CHRONIC Rx

- Dietary sodium restriction in combination with diuretics: the typical ratio of furosemide 40 mg to spironolactone 100 mg retains normal serum potassium levels in most patients.

- Nonselective beta-blockers (propranolol and nadolol) in dosages sufficient to reduce the resting heart rate by 25% have been shown to be effective in primary prophylaxis for first-time variceal bleeding and for preventing recurrent variceal bleeding. Dosages are usually given bid and decreased if heart rate falls to <55 beats/min or systolic blood pressure drops to <90 mm Hg. The addition of a long-acting nitrate (e.g., isosorbide-5-mononitrate) has been shown to improve portal hemodynamics. Findings of a prospective trial of beta-blockers to prevent the formation of varices were negative. The combination of beta-blockade plus endoscopic esophageal variceal banding is superior to either intervention alone.
- Intermittent LVP may be needed in "diuretic resistant" patients.
- Patients with prior SBP merit lifelong antibiotics for secondary prevention.
- Abstinence from alcohol or treatment for hepatitis B or hepatitis C. Vaccination for hepatitis A and B as appropriate.
- Hepatic transplantation is an option in selected patients.

DISPOSITION

- The most common complication associated with portal hypertension is variceal bleeding.

The risk of bleeding from varices is approximately 15% at 1 yr.
- Development of the hepatorenal syndrome (HRS) is associated with high near-term mortality. In particular, HRS may complicate SBP, which emphasizes the importance of making the diagnosis of SBP and instituting appropriate prophylaxis.

REFERRAL

Consultation with a gastroenterologist is recommended in all patients with portal hypertension to screen for esophageal varices.

⚠ PEARLS & CONSIDERATIONS

Splanchnic arterial vasodilation is increasingly recognized as an important component of the pathophysiology of portal hypertension and ascites. There may be vasodilation in other capillary beds as well; of note, pulmonary arteriolar vasodilation can create a significant shunt fraction and resultant hypoxemia in the absence of chest radiograph or CT chest evidence of parenchymal disease. The diagnosis is suspected when otherwise unexplained hypoxia arises in a patient with cirrhosis, along with platypnea (dyspnea worse when sitting upright) and orthodeoxia (desaturation with upright posture). The diagnosis is confirmed by echocardiography with agitated saline, in which there is delayed appearance of bubbles in the left heart after injection into a peripheral vein.

COMMENTS

Portal hypertension and its complications carry significant morbidity and mortality rates. Emphasize ethanol abstinence, provide vaccinations and prophylactic therapy where indicated, and consider early referral to a specialist for assistance with management and consideration for hepatic transplantation.

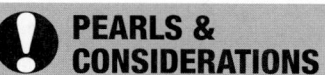

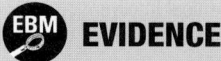 **EVIDENCE**

available at www.expertconsult.com

SUGGESTED READINGS

available at www.expertconsult.com

AUTHOR: **MEL L. ANDERSON, M.D.**

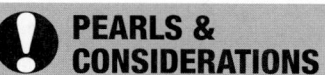

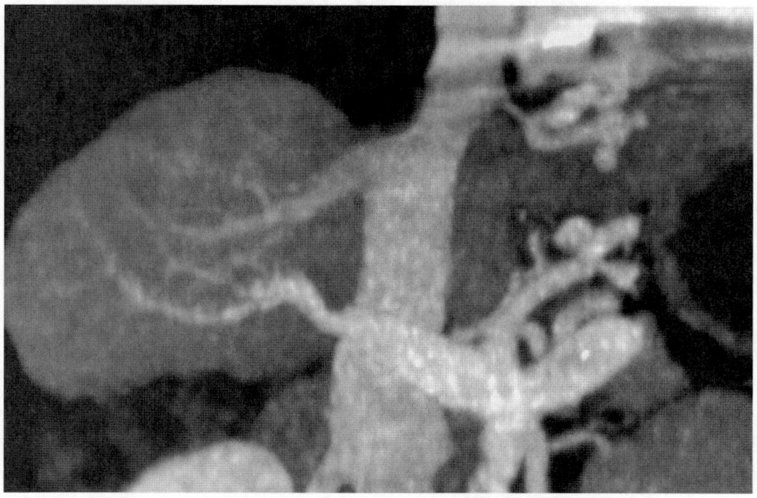

FIGURE 1-301 MR angiography showing portal hypertension with collaterals. The shrunken liver and collateral is obvious. (Forbes A, Misiewicz JJ, Compton CC, Levine MS, Quraishy MS, Rubesin SE, Thuluvath PJ [eds]: *Atlas of clinical gastroenterology*, ed 3, St Louis, 2005, Mosby.)

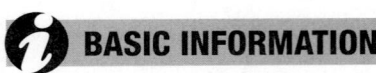

BASIC INFORMATION

DEFINITION
Portal vein thrombosis is thrombotic occlusion of the portal vein.

SYNONYMS
Pylethrombosis

ICD-9CM CODES
452   Portal vein thrombosis
572.1 Septic portal vein thrombosis

EPIDEMIOLOGY & DEMOGRAPHICS
Occurs with equal frequency in children (peak age: 6 yr) and adults (peak age: 40 yr)

PHYSICAL FINDINGS & CLINICAL PRESENTATION
Upper gastrointestinal hemorrhage (hematemesis and/or melena) caused by esophageal varices. If abdominal pain is present, mesenteric venous thrombosis should be suspected (see Mesenteric Venous Thrombosis in Section I).

ETIOLOGY & PATHOPHYSIOLOGY
In children: umbilical sepsis (pathophysiology unknown) In adults:
1. Hypercoagulable states
   - Antiphospholipid syndrome
   - Neoplasm (common cause)
   - Paroxysmal nocturnal hemoglobinuria
   - Myeloproliferative diseases
   - Oral contraceptives
   - Polycythemia vera
   - Pregnancy
   - Protein S or C deficiency
   - Sickle cell disease
   - Thrombocytosis
2. Inflammatory diseases
   - Crohn's disease
   - Pancreatitis
   - Ulcerative colitis
3. Complications of medical intervention
   - Ambulatory dialysis
   - Chemoembolization
   - Liver transplantation
   - Partial hepatectomy
   - Sclerotherapy
   - Splenectomy
   - Transjugular intrahepatic portosystemic shunt
4. Infections
   - Appendicitis
   - Diverticulitis
   - Cholecystitis
5. Miscellaneous
   - Cirrhosis (common cause)
   - Bladder cancer

Pathophysiology: portal vein thrombosis results in portal hypertension, leading to esophageal and gastrointestinal varices. The liver sustained by the hepatic artery maintains normal function.

DIAGNOSIS

DIFFERENTIAL DIAGNOSIS
Causes of upper gastrointestinal hemorrhage are covered in Section II.

WORKUP
- Determination of underlying cirrhosis of the liver should be the foremost step.
- Esophagogastroscopy shows esophageal varices.
- Abdominal ultrasound (Fig. 1-302) or MRI may show the portal vein thrombosis. Abdominal ultrasound color Doppler imaging has a 98% negative predictive value and is considered the imaging modality of choice in diagnosing portal vein thrombosis.

TREATMENT

- Oral anticoagulation if risks of bleeding are low. In patients with concomitant cirrhosis, long-term anticoagulation generally not recommended
- Variceal sclerotherapy or banding
- Surgical mesocaval or splenorenal shunt
- The roles of thrombolysis and transjugular intrahepatic portosystemic shunt continuing to evolve

REFERRAL
To gastroenterologist, surgeon, or both

SUGGESTED READING
available at www.expertconsult.com

AUTHOR: **FRED F. FERRI, M.D.**

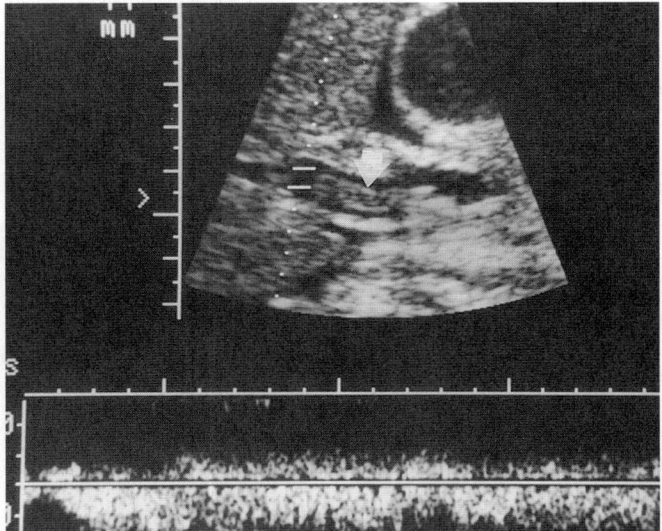

FIGURE 1-302 Thrombus in portal vein evident on pulsed Doppler ultrasonography. An echogenic thrombus *(arrow)* is within the lumen of the portal vein. Doppler tracing indicates flow within portal vein. (From Sabiston D: *Textbook of surgery,* ed 17, Philadelphia, 2005, WB Saunders.)

BASIC INFORMATION

DEFINITION

Postconcussive syndrome (PCS) refers to persistent neurologic symptoms that result from traumatic brain injury (TBI). PCS can also follow moderate and severe brain injury, although it is more commonly associated with mild brain injury or concussion. Concussion is an acute trauma-induced alteration of mental function lasting <24 hr, with or without preceding loss of consciousness.

SYNONYMS

Posttraumatic nervous instability or brain injury
Postcontusion syndrome or encephalopathy status post comotio cerebri

ICD-9CM CODES
310.2 Postconcussion syndrome

EPIDEMIOLOGY & DEMOGRAPHICS

- Incidence is approximately 27 cases per 100,000 persons/year.
- From 30% to 80% of patients with mild to moderate brain injury will experience some symptoms of PCS.
- Female gender and increasing age are risk factors for PCS.
- Usually seen in the young, ages 20 to 30 yr.

PHYSICAL FINDINGS & CLINICAL PRESENTATION

- Usually present without focal neurologic deficits on examination.
- Symptoms start within a few days after the head injury and usually persist after 3 mo.
- Can be divided into early and late or persistent (>6 mo).
- 15% of patients will have persistent symptoms 1 yr later.
- Symptoms include (at least three of the following after traumatic brain injury to meet ICD-10 criteria):
  1. Headache (usually of fronto-occipital location and showing characteristics of tension or migraine headache). The International Headache Society suggests that coding and attribution of headaches with characteristics of primary headaches but in the setting of an inticing event should be attributed to the event, unless there was a known history of the headache and the inticing event was seen as aggravating/initiating the preexisting migraine/tension headache.
  2. Fatigue
  3. Dizziness and/or vertigo
  4. Impaired memory
  5. Difficulty in concentrating
  6. Insomnia
  7. Irritability
  8. Lowered tolerance of stress, emotion, or alcohol
- Other associated symptoms: noise sensitivity, neck pain, non-dermatomal paresthesias, interference with social role functioning.

ETIOLOGY

- Caused by TBI from events such as falls, motor vehicle accidents, contact sports.
- Postmortem findings reveal diffuse axonal injury as the primary pathologic finding along with small petechial hemorrhages and local edema.
- Diffuse axon injury is believed to lead to altered neurotransmission and possibly to clinical manifestations.
- A psychogenic origin has been suggested by a number of empiric and clinical observations; however, limitations in methodology and differing definitions preclude firm conclusions.

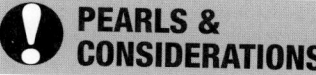 **DIAGNOSIS**

A careful history, a nonfocal neurologic examination, and a normal neurologic test will usually establish the diagnosis.

DIFFERENTIAL DIAGNOSIS

- Headache (dissection of the vertebral artery, occipital neuralgia)
- Epidural hematoma
- Subdural hematoma
- Skull fracture
- Cervical spine disk disease
- Whiplash
- Cerebrovascular accident
- Depression
- Anxiety

WORKUP

To exclude other causes of neurologic symptoms after TBI:
- Electroencephalography is normal.
- Evoked potentials are normal.
- Neuropsychologic testing is useful because it reveals difficulties in concentration, memory, language, and executive function.

LABORATORY TESTS

Blood tests are not specific.

IMAGING STUDIES

- 10% of CT scans of the head following mild TBI are abnormal, showing mild subarachnoid hemorrhage, subdural hemorrhage, or contusions.
- MRI of the head is abnormal in 30% of patients with normal CT scans and may show irregular brain contours or old cerebral contusions.

Rx TREATMENT

Must be recognized as a physiologic and psychologic problem and treated accordingly.

GENERAL Rx

- Must be individualized to the patient's particular symptoms.
- Simple reassurance is often the major treatment.
- Supportive care may include the use of non-narcotic analgesics and antiemetics.
- Pain management.
- Amitriptyline has been widely used for posttraumatic tension-type headaches as well as

for nonspecific symptoms such as irritability, dizziness, insomnia, and depression.
- Posttraumatic migraine-type headaches can be treated with a trial of propranolol or amitriptyline alone or in combination.
- Depression can be treated with selective serotonin reuptake inhibitors but may not respond as well when compared with patients without PCS who have depression.
- Some patients may be admitted for severe symptoms; most can be managed as an outpatient.

NONPHARMACOLOGIC THERAPY

- Early psychological intervention and cognitive rehabilitation are key for full recovery.
- Physical and occupational therapy.
- Avoidance of alcohol, narcotics, and sleep deprivation.
- Explanation of symptoms and expectations, combined with early follow-up with reassurance, may hasten resolution of symptoms.

DISPOSITION

- Most patients improve after mild TBI without any residual deficits within 3 months.
- Predictors for the development of persistent PCS include:
  - Female sex
  - Ongoing litigation (conflicting studies)
  - Low socioeconomic status
  - Prior headaches
  - Prior TBI
  - Prior psychiatric illnesses

REFERRAL

Early consultations with psychologists, psychiatrists, neurologists, and rehabilitation specialists in an outpatient setting would be beneficial.

PEARLS & CONSIDERATIONS

- PCS starts within a few days after the injury.
- Recognizing depression and treating pain symptoms early in the course may help prevent the development of persistent PCS (>1 yr).
- The severity of the trauma does not clearly predict the risk of PCS.
- The severity of the brain injury is usually documented by the initial Glasgow coma scale, the length of unconsciousness, and the duration of amnesia; however, the field may be moving towards more subtle tests of function, such as neuropsychological testing.

COMMENTS

- Attempts to determine how much of a role psychological and/or neurologic factors play in the PCS are important but very difficult.
- No medication at hospital discharge has been proven to change the natural course of the disease.

SUGGESTED READINGS
available at www.expertconsult.com

AUTHORS: **WEN Y. WU-CHEN, M.D.,** and **MARK F. BRADY, M.D., M.P.H.**

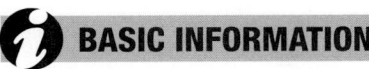

BASIC INFORMATION

DEFINITION

Postpoliomyelitis syndrome (PPS) is a disorder typically characterized by the gradual onset and slow progression of new weakness, fatigue, and pain in survivors of paralytic poliomyelitis after a period of partial or complete recovery and many years of neurological stability. The symptoms are persistent and cannot be explained by the presence of other neurologic, medical, or orthopedic conditions.

SYNONYMS

Postpolio syndrome
Progressive postpoliomyelitis muscular atrophy

ICD-9CM CODES
138 Late effects of acute poliomyelitis

EPIDEMIOLOGY & DEMOGRAPHICS

INCIDENCE: Estimates vary from 22% to 85% of individuals who survive acute poliomyelitis
PEAK INCIDENCE: Appears to be about 30 to 36 yr following acute poliomyelitis, although cases have been reported between 8 and 71 yr.
RISK FACTORS:
- Increasing age and greater length of time since the episode of acute poliomyelitis
- Acute poliomyelitis at an older age
- Greater severity of the acute poliomyelitis or chronic deficits after recovery

PHYSICAL FINDINGS & CLINICAL PRESENTATION

- The most common clinical features are new weakness (20% to 60%), fatigue (59% to 89%), and pain (38% to 86%).
- The symptoms typically have an insidious onset with gradual progression.
- The new weakness is typically, but not exclusively, in muscles that were previously affected by the acute poliomyelitis.
- Fatigue may be described as general or muscular in nature and is often the most disabling symptom.
- Pain is usually described as severe aching, cramping, or burning localized to the muscles or joints, particularly in areas previously affected by acute poliomyelitis
- Respiratory weakness and sleep-disordered breathing with nocturnal hypoventilation occur less frequently
- Other less common features include fasciculations, dysphagia, dysarthria, and cold intolerance
- Neurological examination reveals evidence of asymmetric, lower motor neuron weakness

ETIOLOGY

The pathophysiologic basis of PPS remains unclear, although there are several proposed mechanisms. The most popular hypothesis is that the reduced population of enlarged motor units present after acute poliomyelitis is subject to increased stress and overuse over the course of years. This is proposed to lead to the eventual distal degeneration of these motor units, which in turn results in ongoing denervation that in turn leads to the clinical symptoms.

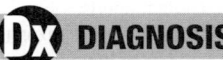

DIAGNOSIS

DIFFERENTIAL DIAGNOSIS

Postpoliomyelitis syndrome is a diagnosis of exclusion. A particular individual's symptoms will determine the differential, but some commonly considered entities:
- Amyotrophic lateral sclerosis
- Cervical or lumbosacral radiculopathy
- Acquired demyelinating polyneuropathies
- Myasthenia gravis
- Fibromyalgia
- Chronic fatigue syndrome
- Anemia
- Hypothyroidism
- Arthritis
- Depression
- Normal aging

WORKUP

- A detailed history to confirm the presence of a previous acute poliomyelitis with a period of stability prior to the emergence of the new symptoms
- A neurological exam to confirm weakness is consistent with a lower motor neuron disorder
- Nerve conduction studies and electromyography are helpful in confirming the presence of denervation and excluding other potential causes of weakness
- A sleep study should be strongly considered to evaluate for the presence of sleep-disordered breathing.
- Pulmonary function tests should be strongly considered to evaluate for evidence of respiratory weakness.
- A swallow study should be performed in patients with difficulty swallowing.

LABORATORY TESTS

Complete blood count, electrolytes, and thyroid function tests to exclude other causes of fatigue

IMAGING STUDIES

Magnetic resonance imaging of the brain and spine be helpful in excluding other potential causes of weakness

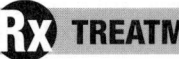

TREATMENT

There is no specific therapy for postpoliomyelitis syndrome. However, a multidisciplinary management program tailored to the patient's presentation can be very helpful in the management of symptoms, resulting in improved functionality and quality of life.
- Most individuals will benefit from physical activity regimens designed by a physical therapist to focus on energy conservation and pacing.
- Orthoses and assistive devices may facilitate ambulation and other activities of daily living as well as reduce the risk of falls.
- Pain can often be controlled with conservative measures such as activity and lifestyle modifications, but analgesic medications may be necessary in some cases.
- Several studies evaluating the use of pyridostigmine for the treatment of weakness and fatigue in postpoliomyelitis syndrome have had conflicting results.
- Studies evaluating amantadine, modafinil, prednisone, and human growth hormone have failed to show any definitive benefit.
- There have been promising initial results with limited studies of lamotrigine and intravenous immunoglobulin, but further trials are needed.

DISPOSITION

- The symptoms of postpoliomyelitis syndrome tend to be slowly progressive and may stabilize over the course of years.
- The weakness, fatigue, and pain may result in disability.
- Rarely fatal, but individuals with respiratory weakness and dysphagia are at increased risk.

REFERRAL

- A neuromuscular specialist can assist in diagnosis and management.
- Physiatry, physical therapy, and occupational therapy referrals can provide guidance for rehabilitation and assistive devices.
- A speech therapy referral is useful in patients with dysarthria or dysphagia.
- A pulmonary consult should be obtained for patients with symptoms or signs of respiratory weakness.
- An orthopedic consult may be necessary for patients requiring surgical correction of joint deformities.
- A mental health professional can assist with management of depression and other psychosocial issues

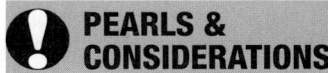

PEARLS & CONSIDERATIONS

COMMENTS

- A diagnosis of PPS should only be made after a thorough evaluation for other potential causes of the patient's symptoms has been completed.
- Due to the high incidence of PPS among the large number of poliomyelitis survivors, PPS is the most common motor neuron disease worldwide.

PATIENT/FAMILY EDUCATION

Website: http://www.mayoclinic.com/health/post-polio-syndrome/DS00494

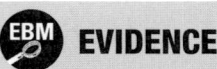

EVIDENCE

available at www.expertconsult.com

SUGGESTED READINGS

available at www.expertconsult.com

AUTHOR: **JEFFREY C. MCCLEAN II, M.D.**

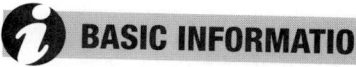

BASIC INFORMATION

DEFINITION

Posttraumatic stress disorder (PTSD) is an anxiety disorder that may arise when an individual has witnessed or experienced a potentially fatal or serious injury during which he or she felt helpless or horrified. The individual continues to experience the event in the form of flashbacks (reliving the trauma), intrusive recollections, dreams, or physiologic reactivity. These responses are associated with persistent hyperarousal (e.g., hypervigilance, exaggerated startle response, sleep disturbance, irritability, and difficulty concentrating) and avoidance (both physically and cognitively) of stimuli associated with the traumatic event. In children, the horror may be expressed by disorganized or agitated behavior.

SYNONYMS

Soldier's heart
Effort syndrome
Shell shock
Irritable heart
Traumatic necrosis
Survivor syndrome
Concentration camp syndrome
Gross stress reaction (DSM-I, published in 1952)
Developmental trauma disorder (for children)

ICD-9CM CODES
309.81 Posttraumatic stress syndrome

EPIDEMIOLOGY & DEMOGRAPHICS

INCIDENCE: Fewer than 10% of individuals who have experienced a traumatic event will develop PTSD.

PREVALENCE (IN U.S.):
- One of the most common psychiatric disorders; estimated lifetime prevalence 7.8% to 12.3%
- Prevalence among high-risk populations (e.g., combat veterans or victims of violent crimes) up to 58%
- ~80% have a comorbid psychiatric disorder (depression, anxiety disorder, or substance use)
- Factors most associated with development are subsequent life stress and perceived lack of social support

PREDOMINANT SEX: Twice as many women as men are affected with (prevalence 10% to 14% for women and 5% to 6% for men). More than 50% of cases in women are related to sexual assault.

PREDOMINANT AGE: No predisposing age factors

GENETICS: Twin studies have demonstrated genetic vulnerability related to combat.

PHYSICAL FINDINGS & CLINICAL PRESENTATION

- A life-threatening event evoking intense fear or horror (criterion A).

- Reexperiencing of traumatic events in the form of dreams, flashbacks, and intrusive memories (criterion B).
- Depersonalization, detachment, emotional numbing, and dissociation, with avoidance of physical or cognitive reminders of the event (criterion C).
- Hyperarousal, hypervigilance and exaggerated startle response, irritability, anxiety, and difficulty concentrating (criterion D).
- To meet DSM-IV criteria for PTSD, one must meet criterion A plus symptoms from each of the three symptoms clusters A, B, C, and D. A fifth criterion concerns duration of symptoms (>1 mo) and a sixth assesses function (must be impaired).
- Mneumonic: TRAUMA
  *T*raumatic event (criterion A)
  *R*e-experiencing (criterion B)
  *A*voidance (criterion C)
  *U*nable to function (criterion F)
  *M*onth at least (criterion E)
  *A*rousal (criterion D)

ETIOLOGY

- Interpersonal violence is more likely to give rise to PTSD than events such as motor vehicle accidents or natural disasters.
- Severity of physical injury is a weaker predictor of PTSD than the psychological distress; stress duration is the most important factor.
- Proposed mechanisms include excessive release of norepinephrine in the amygdala, exaggerated negative feedback inhibition of the HPA axis by glucocorticoids, and enhanced postsynaptic alpha-1 response to norepinephrine.
- Hippocampal volumes in adults with PTSD are smaller than normal. Whether this is a result of PTSD or a predisposing factor is unknown.

DIAGNOSIS

DIFFERENTIAL DIAGNOSIS

- In adjustment disorders, precipitating stress is less catastrophic and psychological reaction is less specific.
- Acute stress disorder, if symptoms last between 48 hr and 4 wk after trauma.
- Acute PTSD: duration of symptoms is <3 mo
- Chronic PTSD: symptoms last 3 mo or longer
- PTSD with delayed onset: symptoms develop >6 mo after the event.

WORKUP

- Among self-report questionnaires and structured diagnostic instruments, the best validated is the Posttraumatic Diagnostic Scale.
- Laboratory and imaging are not clinically useful. Medical conditions that can exacerbate symptoms should be ruled out.
- Primary care PTSD (PC-PTSD) screen recommended by the Veterans Administration. 3 "yes" answers is a positive screen.

In your life, have you ever had any experience that was so frightening, horrible, or upsetting that, in the past month, you:
1. Have had nightmares about it or thought about it when you did not want to? YES NO
2. Tried hard not to think about it or went out of your way to avoid situations that reminded you of it? YES NO
3. Were constantly on guard, watchful, or easily startled? YES NO
4. Felt numb or detached from others, activities, or your surroundings? YES NO

TREATMENT

NONPHARMACOLOGIC THERAPY

- Gold standard treatment is cognitive-behavioral therapy (CBT) with a trauma focus (may include mental imagery and other forms of exposure). Prolonged exposure (PE), a type of CBT that includes education on stress response, breathing training, and prolonged mental recounting of the event to decrease the emotional response, was found to be more effective than standard CBT in female veterans. There is some controversy regarding long-term efficacy of brief therapies and the potential role for long-term psychotherapy.
- Group therapy is helpful, particularly combat veterans.
- Eye movement desensitization reprocessing (EMDR) has shown efficacy in controlled trials.

ACUTE GENERAL Rx

- Immediate postincident debriefing may worsen outcome.
- A brief course of benzodiazepines may be helpful acutely but has not been shown to decrease development of core symptoms.
- Beta-adrenergic blockers may be helpful if given within hours after the trauma to disrupt the physiologic stress response.
- Sedating antidepressants or sleep aids may be helpful for initial insomnia.

CHRONIC Rx

- SSRIs are agents of choice.
- TCAs are also helpful in reducing symptoms.
- Guanfacine may be helpful in treating arousal symptoms.
- Prazosin may decrease distressing dreams and improve sleep quality.
- Mood stabilizers and antipsychotics may be needed for severe symptoms such as paranoia, extreme anxiety, or angry outbursts.

COMPLEMENTARY & ALTERNATIVE APPROACHES

Acupuncture has been shown to be as effective as CBT in decreasing symptoms of PTSD.

DISPOSITION

- Recovery rates are highest in the first 12 mo after onset.

- Average duration of symptoms is 36 mo for those who undergo treatment and 64 mo for those never treated.
- 50% chance of remission at 2 yr; 50% have chronic symptoms.
- Predictors of chronic course include previous trauma, premorbid psychiatric function, panic reaction at time of event, prolonged terror, or dissociation at time of event.

REFERRAL

Because early intervention improves outcome, refer to psychiatry as soon as diagnosis made.

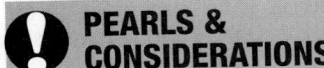

PEARLS & CONSIDERATIONS

- Screen for comorbid substance abuse.
- Treatment can be effective even if it begins years after the traumatic event occurred.
- PTSD is increasingly being conceived of as a stress-induced fear-circuitry disorder of the limbic system.

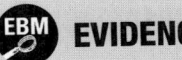

EVIDENCE

available at www.expertconsult.com

SUGGESTED READINGS
available at www.expertconsult.com

AUTHORS: **RADHIKA A. RAMANAN, M.D., M.P.H.,**
ALISON C. MAY, M.D., and
KAILA COMPTON, M.D., Ph.D.

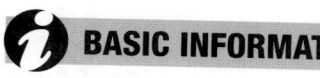

BASIC INFORMATION

DEFINITION

Precocious puberty is defined as sexual development occurring before age 8 yr in females and 9 yr in males.

SYNONYMS

Pubertas praecox

ICD-9CM CODES
259.1 Precocious puberty

EPIDEMIOLOGY & DEMOGRAPHICS

INCIDENCE: Estimated to be between one in 5000 to 10,000.
PREDOMINANT SEX: Females are affected more often than males for the idiopathic variant; for other causes, dependent on the underlying etiology.
GENETICS: The genetics for some of the etiologies of precocious puberty are known.

PHYSICAL FINDINGS & CLINICAL PRESENTATION

- In females: breast development, pubic hair development, accelerated growth, menarche
- In males: increase in testicular volume and penile length, pubic hair development, accelerated growth, muscular development, acne, change in voice, penile erections

ETIOLOGY

- Idiopathic or true: diagnosis of exclusion
- Central nervous system (CNS) pathology: tumors, hydrocephalus, ventricular cysts, benign lesions
- Severe hypothyroidism
- Posttraumatic head injury
- Genetic disorders: neurofibromatosis, tuberous sclerosis, McCune-Albright syndrome, congenital adrenal hyperplasia
- Gonadal tumors
- Nongonadal tumors: hepatoblastoma
- Exposure to exogenous sex steroids

DIAGNOSIS

DIFFERENTIAL DIAGNOSIS

- Most common diagnoses to consider: premature thelarche and premature adrenarche
- Gonadotropin hormone-releasing hormone (GnRH)-dependent precocious puberty: idiopathic, CNS tumors, hypothalamic hamartomas, neurofibromatosis, tuberous sclerosis, hydrocephalus, status after acute head injury, ventricular cysts, status after CNS infection
- GnRH-independent precocious puberty: congenital adrenal hyperplasia, adrenocortical tumors (males), McCune-Albright syndrome (females), gonadal tumors, ectopic human chorionic gonadotropin (hCG)-secreting tumors (chorioblastoma, hepatoblastoma), exposure to exogenous sex steroids, severe hypothyroidism

WORKUP

Thorough history and physical examination are essential to determine if the patient has true precocious puberty. Particular attention should be paid to growth, development, order of appearance of the secondary sexual characteristics, pubertal development in family members, medications, neurologic symptoms, Tanner staging, abdominal and neurologic examination. Section III, "Puberty, Precocious" describes a clinical approach to precocious puberty.

LABORATORY TESTS

- GnRH testing will help determine if dependent or independent cause
- Sex hormone studies: luteinizing hormone, follicle-stimulating hormone, hCG, testosterone (males), estrogen (females). Levels of sex steroids should be determined in the morning, with use of assays that have detection limits adapted to pediatric values. In girls, serum estradiol levels are highly variable and have a rather low sensitivity for the diagnosis of precocious puberty.
- T_4, thyroid-stimulating hormone

IMAGING STUDIES

- CT scan or MRI of the brain to evaluate for CNS pathology
- Consideration of pelvic ultrasound in female patients to evaluate for cysts or tumors
- Abdominal imaging with CT scan if intra-abdominal pathology suspected

TREATMENT

NONPHARMACOLOGIC THERAPY

- Good communication with the parents is essential to care.
- Psychologic support for the child may be needed with regard to self-image and problems with peer acceptance.

ACUTE GENERAL Rx

There is no acute therapy for precocious puberty.

CHRONIC Rx

Therapy depends on the etiology of precocious puberty. For the treatment of central or gonadotropin-dependent precocious puberty depot GnRH agonists (leuprorelin, leuprolide, triptorelin, goserelin, histrelin, buserelin) are effective.

- Leuprolide is given 0.25 to 0.3 mg/kg with a 7.5 mg minimum IM every 4 wk. Local side effects include pain, erythema, and inflammatory reactions. Other side effects include headaches and menopausal-like symptoms (asthenia, hot flashes).
- For other CNS lesions and extragonadal tumors, therapy is dependent on the type of lesion, location of the lesion, and the overall prognosis of the underlying problem.
- For severe hypothyroidism, treatment with thyroid hormone will result in regression of the sexual development. The child will subsequently undergo appropriate pubertal development later in life.
- For familial male gonadotropin-independent precocious puberty, the androgen-synthesis inhibitor ketoconazole can be used at doses of 600 mg/day divided tid, or a combination of the aromatase inhibitor testolactone and spironolactone can be used.

DISPOSITION

- For true precocious puberty and some CNS lesions, long-term outcome is usually very good. When drug therapy is instituted, it is continued until a time when further pubertal development is appropriate. It is then discontinued, allowing the child to progress through puberty.
- For other cases, long-term outcomes depend on the prognosis of the underlying cause.

REFERRAL

- Initial workup can be instituted by the primary care provider.
- Referral to an endocrinologist is indicated for most children because they will need long-term management, monitoring, and treatment.
- Attention to the emotional needs of the child is important.

SUGGESTED READING
available at www.expertconsult.com

AUTHORS: **BETH J. WUTZ, M.D.,** and **RUBEN ALVERO, M.D.**

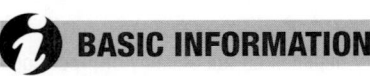

BASIC INFORMATION

DEFINITION

Preeclampsia involves the triad of hypertension, proteinuria, and edema that develops after the twentieth week of gestation. Mild preeclampsia is defined as a blood pressure of <140/90 mm Hg. Severe preeclampsia is associated with a blood pressure >160/110 mm Hg, proteinuria >5 g in a 24-hr urine collection, oliguria (<400 ml/24 hr), cerebral or visual disturbances, epigastric pain, pulmonary edema, thrombocytopenia, hepatic dysfunction, or severe intrauterine growth restriction.

SYNONYMS

Pregnancy-induced hypertension
Toxemia of pregnancy

ICD-9CM CODES
642.6 Preeclampsia

EPIDEMIOLOGY & DEMOGRAPHICS

INCIDENCE: 0% to 14% in primigravidas, 5.7% to 7.3% in multigravidas
RISK FACTORS: Increased incidence and severity with multiple gestations or renal or collagen-vascular diseases. Extremes of reproductive age, <20 or >35 yr, obesity, African American race, thrombophilia, previous preeclampsia.
GENETICS: Positive correlation with maternal and paternal family history.

PHYSICAL FINDINGS & CLINICAL PRESENTATION

- Generalized swelling or nondependent edema, possibly manifested by rapid weight gain (>4 lb/wk) even in the absence of edema
- Auscultation of pulmonary rales
- Right upper quadrant pain (HELLP syndrome [hemolysis, elevated liver enzymes, and low platelet count] or subcapsular liver hematoma)
- Hyperreflexia or clonus
- Vaginal bleeding (placental abruption)
- Acute or chronic fetal compromise manifested by intrauterine growth restriction or fetal tachycardia with late decelerations, respectively
- Wide range of symptoms attributable to multiorgan system dysfunction, involving hepatic, hematologic, renal, pulmonary, and central nervous systems
- Possibility of severe disease despite "normal" blood pressure readings, so a high index of suspicion must be maintained in high-risk situations

ETIOLOGY

- Exact etiology or toxic substance is unknown
- Theories:
  - Imbalance between thromboxane A_2 (vasoconstrictor and platelet aggregator) and prostacyclin (vasodilator)
  - Abnormal trophoblastic invasion of spiral arteries
  - Increased sensitivity to angiotensin II by the muscular walls of the arteries
  - Excess circulating soluble fms-like tyrosine kinase 1 (SFIT-1), which binds placental growth factor (PlGF) and vascular endothelial growth factor (VEGF), may have a pathogenic role
- Potential secondary effects of the metabolic, inflammatory endothelial alternatives in preeclampsia are described in Table 1-148

DIAGNOSIS

DIFFERENTIAL DIAGNOSIS

- Acute fatty liver of pregnancy
- Appendicitis
- Diabetic ketoacidosis
- Gallbladder disease
- Gastroenteritis
- Glomerulonephritis
- Hemolytic-uremic syndrome
- Hepatic encephalopathy
- Hyperemesis gravidarum
- Idiopathic thrombocytopenia
- Thrombotic thrombocytopenic purpura
- Nephrolithiasis
- Pyelonephritis
- Peptic ulcer disease
- Systemic lupus erythematosus
- Viral hepatitis

WORKUP

- Two blood pressure measurements with the patient in lateral recumbent position 6 hr apart, with an absolute pressure >140/90 mm Hg or an increase of 30 mm Hg systolic or 15 mm Hg diastolic from baseline, an increase in the mean arterial pressure (MAP) of 20 mm Hg, or an absolute MAP >105 mm Hg
- Evaluation for proteinuria as defined by >0.1 g/L on urine dipstick or >300 mg protein on a 24-hr urine collection
- Evaluation of fetal status for evidence of intrauterine growth restriction, oligohydramnios, alteration in umbilical or uterine artery Doppler flow, or acute compromise, such as abruption

- Because of the insidious nature of the disease with potential for multiple organ involvement, complete evaluation for preeclampsia in any pregnant patient presenting with central nervous system derangement or gastrointestinal symptoms after 20 wk of gestation
- Evaluation for associated conditions such as disseminated intravascular coagulation, hepatic dysfunction, or subcapsular hematoma

LABORATORY TESTS

- High-risk patients: baseline assessment of renal function (24-hr urine collection for protein and creatinine clearance), platelets, blood urea nitrogen, creatinine, liver function tests (LFTs), and uric acid should be obtained at the first prenatal visit.
- Complete blood count (hemoglobin, hematocrit, platelets) may show signs of volume contraction or HELLP syndrome.
- LFTs (aspartate aminotransferase, alanine aminotransferase, lactate dehydrogenase) are useful in evaluation for HELLP syndrome or to exclude important differentials.
- Hyperuricemia or increased creatinine may indicate decreasing renal function.
- Prothrombin time, partial thromboplastin time, and fibrinogen should be checked to rule out disseminated intravascular coagulation.
- Peripheral smear may demonstrate microangiopathic hemolytic anemia.
- Complement levels can be used to differentiate from an acute exacerbation of a collagen-vascular disease.
- Increased levels of SFIT-1 and reduced levels of PlGF predict subsequent development of preeclampsia.

IMAGING STUDIES

- CT scan of head if atypical presentation of eclampsia, possibility of intracerebral bleed, or prolonged postictal state
- Sonogram of fetus to evaluate for intrauterine growth restriction (Fig. 1-303), amniotic fluid, placenta
- Sonogram of maternal liver if suspect subcapsular hematoma

TABLE 1-148 Potential Secondary Effects of the Metabolic, Inflammatory Endothelial Alternatives in Preeclampsia

CVS	Increased peripheral resistance leading to hypertension Increased vascular permeability and reduced maternal plasma volume
Lungs	Laryngeal and pulmonary edema
Renal	Glomerular damage leading to proteinuria, hypoproteinemia, and reduced oncotic pressure which further exacerbates the hypovolemia. May develop acute renal failure ± cortical necrosis
Clotting	Hypercoagulability, with increased fibrin formation and increased fibrinolysis, i.e., disseminated intravascular coagulation
Liver	HELLP syndrome Hepatic rupture
CNS	Thrombosis and fibrinoid necrosis of the cerebral arterioles Eclampsia (convulsions), cerebral hemorrhage and cerebral edema
Fetus	Impaired uteroplacental circulation, potentially leading to FGR, hypoxemia, and intrauterine death

Drife J, Magowan B: *Clinical obstetrics and gynecology,* Philadelphia, 2004, Saunders.

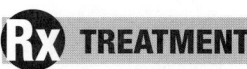

TREATMENT

NONPHARMACOLOGIC THERAPY
Bed rest in left lateral decubitus position

ACUTE GENERAL Rx
Delivery is the treatment of choice and the only cure for the disease. This must be taken in the context of the gestational age of the fetus, severity of the preeclampsia, and the likelihood of a successful induction and reliability of patient.
- Administer magnesium sulfate 6 g IV loading dose, with 2 to 3 g maintenance or phenytoin at 10 to 15 mg/kg loading dose, then 200 mg IV q8h starting 12 hr after loading dose.
- Hydralazine 10 mg IV, labetalol hydrochloride 20 to 40 mg IV, nifedipine 20 mg SL can be used for acute blood pressure control.

- Continuous fetal monitoring is needed.
- Epidural is anesthesia of choice for pain management in labor or cesarean section.
- All patients undergoing induction of labor should receive antiseizure medications regardless of severity of disease.

CHRONIC Rx
- Mild preeclampsia <37 wk: close observation for worsening maternal or fetal condition, with delivery at >37 wk with favorable cervix or at 40 wk regardless of cervical status.
- Severe preeclampsia: delivery in the presence of maternal or fetal compromise, labor, or >34 wk; at 28 to 34 wk consider steroids with close monitoring, and at <24 wk consider termination of pregnancy.
- Methyldopa is drug of choice for long-term blood pressure control during pregnancy.

DISPOSITION
Preeclampsia is a progressive and unpredictable disease process; a course of expectancy should be managed with caution. Up to 20% of patients who have seizures are normotensive.

REFERRAL
Obstetric management is indicated because of the insidious nature of the disease, with transfer of all cases <34 wk to a facility with a level three nursery.

PEARLS & CONSIDERATIONS

COMMENTS
- Low-dose aspirin 81 mg qd and calcium supplementation 1500 mg qd can be considered in high-risk patients to decrease the risk of recurrence.
- Begin after first trimester.
- Although the absolute risk of ESRD in women who have had preeclampsia is low, preeclampsia is a marker for an increased risk of subsequent ESRD.
- The development of preeclampsia may be one of the earliest identifiable risk markers for potential future cardiovascular disease in women. It has been shown that women who develop preeclampsia have a higher incidence of cardiovascular risk factors including components of the metabolic syndrome within 1 yr of delivery.

EBM EVIDENCE

available at www.expertconsult.com

SUGGESTED READINGS
available at www.expertconsult.com

AUTHORS: **SCOTT J. ZUCCALA, D.O.,** and **RUBEN ALVERO, M.D.**

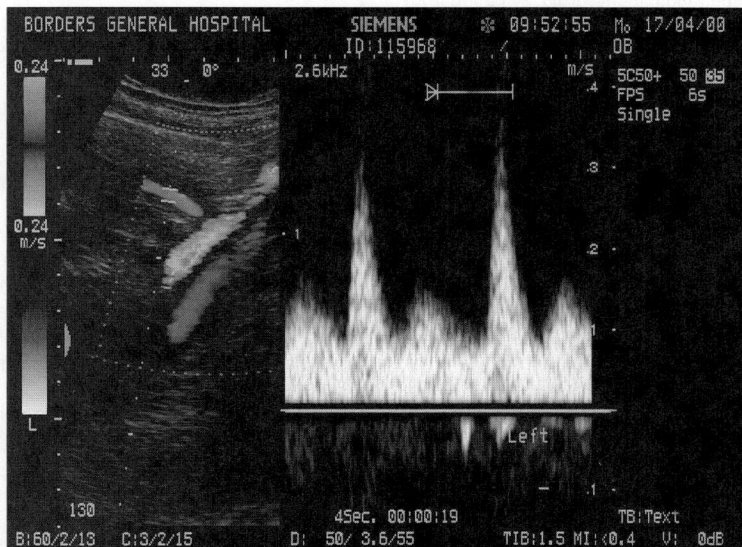
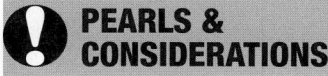
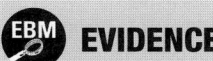

FIGURE 1-303 Uterine artery Doppler notching at 24 wk is predictive of preeclampsia and intrauterine growth restriction in high-risk mothers. (From Drife J, Magowan B: *Clinical obstetrics and gynecology,* Philadelphia, 2004, Saunders.)

Diseases and Disorders

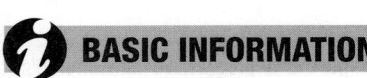 **BASIC INFORMATION**

DEFINITION

The *Diagnostic and Statistical Manual of Mental Disorders,* 4th edition, classifies premenstrual dysphoric disorder (PMDD) as a "depressive disorder not otherwise specified" and requires as criteria for definition the presence of five or more of the following symptoms in most menstrual cycles for the past year.

- The symptoms should be present most of the time during the last week of the luteal phase, with remission beginning within a few days after the onset of the follicular phase, and absent during the week after menses, with at least one of the symptoms being either 1, 2, 3, or 4:
  1. Marked depressed mood, feeling of hopelessness, or self-deprecating thoughts
  2. Marked anxiety, tension, feeling of being "keyed up" or "on edge"
  3. Marked affective lability (e.g., feeling suddenly sad or tearful or increased sensitivity to rejection)
  4. Persistent and marked anger or irritability or increased interpersonal conflicts
  5. Decreased interest in usual activities (e.g., work, school, friends, hobbies)
  6. Subjective sense of difficulty in concentrating
  7. Lethargy, easy fatigability, or marked lack of energy
  8. Marked change in appetite, overeating, or specific food cravings
  9. Hypersomnia or insomnia
  10. A subjective sense of being overwhelmed or out of control
  11. Other physical symptoms, such as breast tenderness or swelling, headaches, joint or muscle pain, a sensation of "bloating," or weight gain
- The disturbance markedly interferes with work or school or with usual social activities and relationships with others (e.g., avoidance of social activities, decreased production and efficiency at work or school).
- The disturbance is not merely an exacerbation of the symptoms of another disorder, such as major depressive disorder, panic disorder, dysthymic disorder, or a personality disorder (although it may be superimposed on any of these disorders).
- The first three criteria must be confirmed by prospective daily ratings during at least two consecutive symptomatic cycles (diagnosis may be made provisionally before such confirmation).

NOTE: In menstruating women, the luteal phase corresponds to the period between ovulation and the onset of menses, and the follicular phase begins with menses. In nonmenstruating women (e.g., women who have had a hysterectomy), determination of the timing of the luteal and follicular phases may require measurement of circulating reproductive hormones.

ICD-9CM CODES
625.4 Premenstrual dysphoric syndrome

EPIDEMIOLOGY & DEMOGRAPHICS

- PMDD affects 3% to 10% of women of reproductive age.
- Genetic factors play a significant role (increased incidence in monozygotic twins and in women whose mothers had PMDD).
- 30% to 76% of women with PMDD have a lifetime history of depression.

PHYSICAL FINDINGS & CLINICAL PRESENTATION

- Physical examination may be completely normal.
- Depressed mood, tachycardia, sweating from comorbid disorders (e.g., panic disorder, major depression) may be present.
- Symptoms occur during the last half of the menstrual cycle (the luteal phase) and are absent from the first day of menstruation until ovulation (follicular phase).

ETIOLOGY

- Unknown. Serotonin deficiency and altered sensitivity in serotoninergic system in response to phasic hormone fluctuations in the menstrual cycle are believed to play a role.
- Progesterone appears to be the main precipitating factor in PMDD symptoms, but estrogen may also provoke symptoms.

Dx **DIAGNOSIS**

DIFFERENTIAL DIAGNOSIS

- Premenstrual syndrome
- Dysthymic syndrome
- Personality disorder
- Panic disorder
- Major depressive disorder
- Hyperthyroidism
- Polycystic ovarian syndrome
- Drug or alcohol abuse
- Irritable bowel syndrome
- Endometriosis

WORKUP

- Diagnosis is based on obtaining a detailed history and ruling out the presence of physical or psychiatric disorders. No objective diagnostic tests exist.
- The diagnosis should be confirmed by using a symptom checklist prospectively for two consecutive menstrual cycles. Commonly used diagnostic instruments include the Calendar of Premenstrual Experiences and the Premenstrual Syndrome Diary.

LABORATORY TESTS

- None are usually necessary.
- A serum thyroid-stimulating hormone test to exclude thyroid problems, complete blood count to rule out anemia, and a chemistry profile to assess electrolytes may be ordered if diagnosis is unclear.

Rx **TREATMENT**

NONPHARMACOLOGIC THERAPY

- Reduction in intake of caffeine, refined sugars, or sodium may be helpful in some patients.
- Increased aerobic exercise, smoking cessation, alcohol restriction, and regular sleep are often beneficial.
- Stress reduction and management will decrease severity of symptoms.

GENERAL Rx

- Selective serotonin reuptake inhibitors are useful for the treatment of PMDD. Commonly used agents and initial doses are fluoxetine 10 mg qd, sertraline 50 mg qd, paroxetine 10 mg qd, and citalopram 20 mg qd. Many patients will require titration to significantly higher doses to achieve therapeutic benefit. These medications can be administered continuously during the menstrual cycle or only when the patients experience symptoms. Luteal phase or intermittent administration involves initiating medication at the time of ovulation and stopping it at the beginning of menses.
- Other useful agents are benzodiazepines (alprazolam 0.25 mg tid prn) and the tricyclic antidepressant clomipramine (25 mg qd as starting dose).
- Gonadotropin-releasing hormone (GmRH) agonists are effective in treating patients with PMDD. The accelerated bone loss and vasomotor symptoms associated with long-term use of a GmRH agonist will require add-back therapy. Hormonal intervention with monthly intramuscular injections of leuprolide has been reported effective in some patients; however, it should be reserved only for patients unresponsive to first- and second-line agents.
- Nutritional supplementation (vitamin B_6 up to 100 mg/day, vitamin E up to 600 IU/day, calcium carbonate up to 1200 mg/day, and magnesium up to 500 mg/day) are also commonly used and effective in symptom reduction in some patients.
- Ovariectomy may be considered in severe refractory cases.

SUGGESTED READING
available at www.expertconsult.com

AUTHOR: **FRED F. FERRI, M.D.**

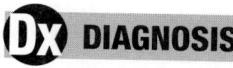

BASIC INFORMATION

DEFINITION

Premenstrual syndrome (PMS) is a cyclic recurrence during the luteal phase of the menstrual cycle of somatic, affective, and behavioral disturbances that are of sufficient severity to affect interpersonal relationships adversely or interfere with normal activities.

SYNONYMS

PMS
PMDD

ICD-9CM CODES
625.4 Premenstrual tension syndromes

EPIDEMIOLOGY & DEMOGRAPHICS

- PMS is believed to be extremely prevalent, intermittently affecting approximately one third of all premenopausal women.
- Severe cases occur in approximately 2% to 10% of women with PMS.
- Those seeking treatment for PMS are usually in their 30s or 40s.
- The natural history of PMS has not been clearly elucidated.

PHYSICAL FINDINGS & CLINICAL PRESENTATION

- Diverse and potentially disabling symptoms
- Associated with >150 psychological, physical, and behavioral symptoms
- Most frequent reason for seeking treatment: emotional symptoms
- Most common emotional symptoms: depression, irritability, anxiety, labile moods, anger, crying easily, sadness, extreme sensitivity, nervous tension
- Most common physical symptoms: headache, bloating, cramps, breast tenderness, migraines, fatigue, weight gain, aches and pains, palpitations
- Most common behavior symptom: food cravings
- Other behavioral symptoms: increased appetite, increased alcohol intake, decreased motivation, decreased efficiency, avoidance of activities, staying home, sleep changes, libido changes, forgetfulness, decreased concentration

ETIOLOGY

- Etiology remains obscure.
- Because of the multifactorial, multiorgan nature of PMS, a single etiologic cause is unlikely.

DIAGNOSIS

DIFFERENTIAL DIAGNOSIS

- A diagnosis of exclusion, so other medical or psychologic disorders should be ruled out.

- Most common disorders: depression or anxiety, thyroid disease.

WORKUP

- History
- Physical examination
- Laboratory studies to rule out alternative diagnosis
- If no alternative diagnosis confirms diagnosis of PMS, basal body temperature charting is used to determine if the patient is ovulating:
  1. If she is not ovulating, it is not PMS.
  2. If she is ovulating, symptoms should be charted for at least two cycles to determine if the symptoms occur in the luteal phase.
  3. If symptoms are not occurring in the luteal phase, it is not PMS and further investigation is needed.
     a. If symptoms occur in the follicular phase, patient has premenstrual exacerbation of another condition.
     b. If symptoms do not occur in the follicular phase, diagnosis of PMS is confirmed.

LABORATORY TESTS

- None available to specifically confirm the diagnosis of PMS
- Thyroid function tests to rule out thyroid disease

TREATMENT

NONPHARMACOLOGIC THERAPY

- Individualization of the treatment plan to maximize therapeutic response
- Psychosocial intervention:
  o Education
  o Stress management
  o Environmental changes
  o Adequate rest and sleep
  o Regular exercise
- Nutritional recommendations:
  o Regularly eaten, well-balanced meals
  o Adequate amounts of protein, fiber, and complex carbohydrates; low fat
  o Avoidance of foods that are high in salt and simple sugars; may promote water retention, weight gain, and physical discomfort
  o Avoidance of caffeine-containing beverages; stimulant effects of caffeine may worsen tension, irritability, and insomnia
  o Avoidance of alcohol and illicit drugs; may worsen emotional lability
  o Calcium supplementation (1000 mg/day for women 19 to 50 yr, 1300 mg/day for girls 14 to 18 yr) to reduce the physical and emotional symptoms
  o Magnesium (360 mg/day) to reduce water retention and the negative effect associated with PMS
  o Pyridoxine (vitamin B_6) 50 mg bid to improve depression, fatigue, irritability, and

natural diuretic ability; neurotoxicity observed at higher dosages

ACUTE GENERAL Rx

Suppression of ovulation:
- Oral contraceptives: one pill per day
- Progestin-only oral contraceptive: one pill per day
- Oral micronized progesterone: 100 mg every morning and 200 mg every evening on days 17 through 28 of menstrual cycle
- Progestin suppository: 200 to 400 mg bid on days 17 through 28 of menstrual cycle
- Oral contraceptive containing drosperinone/ethinyl estradiol: very effective in decreasing physical symptoms
- Medroxyprogesterone: 150 mg IM q3mo
- Levonorgestrel implants: surgical insertion every 5 yr
- Transdermal estradiol: one or two 100-μg patches every 3 days
- Danazol: 100 to 200 mg/day (ovulation not suppressed at this dose)
- Gonadotropin-releasing hormone (GnRH) agonists: daily by intranasal spray or monthly by depot injection

Suppression of physical symptoms:
- Spironolactone: 25 to 50 mg bid on days 14 through 28 of menstrual cycle
- Mefenamic acid
  o For fluid retention: 250 mg tid on days 24 through 28 of cycle
  o For pain: 500 mg tid on days 19 through 28 of cycle
- Bromocriptine: 5 mg/day on days 10 through 26 of cycle
- Danazol: 200 mg/day on days 19 through 28 of cycle
- Naproxen: 550 mg bid on days 17 through 28 of cycle, Naprosyn-500 mg bid on days 17 through 28 of cycle

Suppression of psychological symptoms:
- Nortriptyline: 50 to 125 mg/day
- Fluoxetine: 20 mg/day or 90 mg weekly (this medication has indications for premenstrual dysphoric disorder)
- Buspirone: 10 mg bid or tid on days 16 through 28 of cycle, then taper drug
- Alprazolam: 25 mg tid on days 16 through 28 of cycle, then taper drug
- Clonidine: 0.1 mg bid
- Naltrexone: 0.25 mg/day on days 9 through 18 of cycle
- Atenolol: 50 mg/day
- Paroxetine: 20 mg/day
- Sertraline: 50 to 100 mg/day
- Nefazodone: initial dosage 100 mg bid; after 1 wk increase to 150 mg bid
- Propranolol: 20 to 40 mg bid
- Verapamil: 100 to 320 mg qd

CHRONIC Rx

- Therapy is largely trial and error, with the goal of providing effective treatment with the safest and most simple therapy.

- For severe intractable PMS: hysterectomy with bilateral oophorectomy; give trial of GnRH therapy or danazol before surgery (hysterectomy and bilateral oophorectomy should be exceedingly rare).
- Estrogen replacement therapy recommended postoperatively to reduce the risk of osteoporosis, heart disease, and genitourinary atrophy.

DISPOSITION

Improved symptoms in 90% of women over time.

REFERRAL

- For counseling with a psychologist or psychiatrist if underlying psychiatric disorder is discovered (cognitive-behavioral therapy)
- To a gynecologist if surgical therapy is contemplated

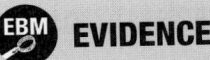

EVIDENCE

available at www.expertconsult.com

SUGGESTED READINGS

available at www.expertconsult.com

AUTHORS: **GEORGE T. DANAKAS, M.D.,** and **RUBEN ALVERO, M.D.**

BASIC INFORMATION

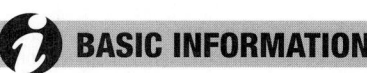

DEFINITION

Preoperative evaluation is the clinical risk evaluation for patients undergoing surgery. The goal of the assessment is to identify and treat unrecognized disease and risk factors that may increase the risk of surgery above baseline.

SYNONYMS

Preoperative evaluation and risk reduction; Risk reduction in patients undergoing invasive procedures.

ICD-9CM CODES
ICD-V72.84

EPIDEMIOLOGY & DEMOGRAPHICS

In the United States, the number of surgical procedures is increasing, although the percentage that occurs in inpatient facilities is decreasing. The scope of the issue is enormous: more than 46 million surgical procedures were performed in 2006 on hospital inpatients (National Health Services Statistics Report, July 30, 2008).

Some studies have shown the benefits of preoperative testing while others that have shown no added benefit. Lack of added benefit has been particularly true for otherwise healthy individuals: the prevalence of significant unrecognized disease and the predictive value of tests are both low for this population–leading to an excess of false positive tests.

Certain risk factors do exist that may be helpful: The nature and extent of surgery appears to play a role, as does increasing age, exercise capacity, and certain medications. Box 1-16 describes stratification of risk of common noncardiac surgical procedures.

There may be other reasons to perform preoperative evaluations: In the United States, individuals undergo an increasing number of surgical procedures of all kinds and seeing patients during the preoperative period may be a good opportunity to reach out to patients about other preventative, screening, and routine health care issues. The primary care physician is uniquely poised to provide an accurate assessment and risk stratification of patients and to develop care plans for follow-up. This information can then be used to help surgeons counsel patients and guide patients' decision making.

PEAK INCIDENCE: When there are adverse consequences from surgery, cardiovascular complications account for the majority of the morbidity and mortality in patients. Perioperative MIs (PMI) is one of the most important predictors of short- and long-term morbidity and mortality associated surgery. The highest incidence of PMI is in the first 3 to 5 days after surgery.

PHYSICAL FINDINGS & CLINICAL PRESENTATION

The history, physical and other studies need to assess the risks for myocardial infarction, arrhythmias, heart failure, endocarditis, stroke, pulmonary insufficiency, venous thrombosis and pulmonary embolism, hemorrhage, diabetic acidosis, renal or hepatic failure, and infection.

WORKUP
HISTORY

- Assess the urgency of the surgical procedure. A conversation with the surgical team is helpful for urgent and emergent procedures.
- Age is important to consider because age is often associated with an increasing number of comorbidities, which are in turn associated with an increase in perioperative risk.
- All patients should be asked about their exercise capacity before surgery. One way to assess functional capacity is in metabolic equivalents (METS). (Circulation, 2009). The ability to walk two blocks on level ground or carry two bags of groceries up stairs without symptoms are simple questions that that can give a approximate assessment of patient risk. One MET is defined as the energy expenditure for sitting quietly. For the average adult, this is equivalent to an oxygen consumption of 3.5 ml/kg body weight per minute. Studies have shown that those who have a low exercise capacity have twice as much risk for postoperative complications compared to those have high exercise capacity.
  - Can take care of self such as eat, dress or use toilet = 1 MET
  - Can walk up a flight of steps or hill = 4 METS
  - Can do heavy work around the house = 4 to 10 METS
  - Can participate in strenuous sports such as swimming, tennis, football and skiing = > 10 METS
- Assess other relevant risk factors by addressing the following questions:
  - What is patient's BMI?
  - Does the patient experience shortness of breath when lying flat?
  - Does the patient have any of the following cardiac conditions: heart disease, heart attack within the past 6 mo, angina, irregular heartbeat, heart failure?
  - Has the patient ever had any rheumatologic conditions, kidney disease, liver disease, diabetes?
  - Has the patient or any member of the patient's family had any adverse reactions to anesthesia?
  - Any family history of deep venous thrombosis or pulmonary embolism, bleeding problems, diabetes mellitus, elevated cholesterol, hypertension or heart disease?
  - For female patients, is it possible the patient is pregnant? What was the date of the patient's last menstrual period?
  - Is patient on any medications? Is the patient on any anticoagulants, antiplatelet drugs, or other medications which can increase bleeding risk? Can these medications be safely stopped for surgery?
- Consider further testing based on above risk factors.

PHYSICAL EXAM

- Vital signs: blood pressure, heart rate and rhythm, rate and ease of respirations, and temperature.
- Cardiovascular exam. Auscultate heart to check for heart murmurs, pathologic heart sounds, and ventricular systolic or diastolic dysfunction.
- Respiratory exam. Auscultate lungs for crackles, wheezes, decreased breath sounds.
- Vascular exam. Examine for carotid, abdominal and femoral bruits.
- Integumentary exam. Check for evidence of venous stasis in lower extremities, petechiae and unusual bruises.
- Mental Status. Conduct a mini-mental exam.

LABORATORY TESTS & IMAGING STUDIES

- Determine the patient's age, height, weight.
- EKG: Although it has often been routine to perform an EKG in patients older than age 55 (except those undergoing low risk procedures like endoscopy) and those patients with pre-existing cardiac conditions, a more nuanced approach is suggested by the 2007 Guidelines published by the American College of Cardiology (ACC) and the American Health Association which use Assessment of Risk for CAD and Assessment of Functional Capacity: Recommendations for Preoperative Resting 12-Lead ECG
  Class I
  1 Preoperative resting 12-lead ECG is recommended for patients with at least 1 clinical risk factor who are undergoing vascular surgical procedures. (Level of Evidence: B)

BOX 1-16 Stratification of Risk of Common Noncardiac Surgical Procedures

Higher Risk	Emergent and urgent major operations, especially in the elderly
	Aortic and noncarotid major vascular surgery
	Surgery associated with large fluid status change or blood loss
Intermediate Risk	Head and neck surgery
	Carotid endarterectomy surgery
	Major thoracic surgery
	Major abdominal surgery
	Orthopedic surgery
	Prostate surgery
Lower Risk	Eye and skin surgery
	Endoscopy

2 Preoperative resting 12-lead ECG is recommended for patients with known CHD, peripheral arterial disease, or cerebrovascular disease who are undergoing intermediate-risk surgical procedures. (Level of Evidence: C)

Class IIa

1 Preoperative resting 12-lead ECG is reasonable in persons with no clinical risk factors who are undergoing vascular surgical procedures. (Level of Evidence: B)

Class IIb

1 Preoperative resting 12-lead ECG may be reasonable in patients with at least 1 clinical risk factor who are undergoing intermediate-risk operative procedures. (Level of Evidence: B)

Class III

1 Preoperative and postoperative resting 12-lead ECGs are not indicated in asymptomatic persons undergoing low-risk surgical procedures. (Level of Evidence: B)

- Routine laboratory studies are not necessary unless there is a specific medical indication. (Anesthesiology, 2002). Testing need not be repeated if results are recently available, unless there has been a change in clinical status.
  - Low-risk procedures do not require routine basic metabolic panel, blood glucose, liver function, hemostasis evaluation or a urine analysis.
  - For intermediate and high-risk procedures as well as in the setting of diabetes, cardiac, or renal disease, obtain a complete blood count.
  - A CBC is recommended for all patients older than age 65 undergoing major surgery as well as any one undergoing a surgery with expected large amounts of blood loss.
  - Coagulation studies are only needed for patients with personal or family history of bleeding or thrombophilia.
- Chest x-ray is indicated for all patients with new respiratory symptoms, suspected congestive heart failure, valvular heart disease, or cardiac compromise. Clinicians should not order routine preoperative chest x-rays or pulmonary function tests.

MEDICATIONS

Most medications can be continued through the perioperative period with the exception of aspirin, clopidogrel, ticlopidine, warfarin, and non-steroidal anti-inflammatory drugs. If the patient is going to be NPO during the procedure, then hypoglycemia inducing agents should be reduced to half-dose the night before surgery and held the morning of surgery.

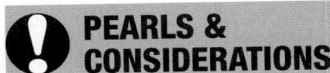

PEARLS & CONSIDERATIONS

COMMENTS

Although most individuals will not require any significant preoperative testing, certain conditions will require further workup.

- Ischemic heart disease
  - If patient has angina, determine frequency, precipitating factors, response to rest and nitroglycerin
  - If patient has had prior cardiac catheterizations or coronary revascularizations, obtain previous records
- Dysrhythmias & pacemakers
  - Examine current and prior EKGs for high grade atrioventricular block, symptomatic ventricular arrhythmias, supraventricular tachycardias at uncontrolled rates.
  - If patient has a pacemaker, establish the type and mode, date of implantation and when it was last interrogated.
- Valvular & congenital heart disease
  - Look for signs of severe valvular heart disease on last echo-cardiographic evaluations.
- Cerebrovascular disease
  - Inquire about prior carotid artery ultrasounds
- Venous thromboembolism
  - Determine results of studies for thrombophilia (factor V Leiden mutation, lupus anticoagulant, anti-thrombin III, protein C or S).

PATIENT/FAMILY EDUCATION

Advise patients that their preoperative evaluation visit with their PCP is another opportunity for them to bring up concerns or get questions answered about their upcoming procedure.

SUGGESTED READINGS

available at www.expertconsult.com

AUTHOR: **PRIYA SARIN GUPTA, M.D.**

BASIC INFORMATION

DEFINITION

Priapism is the persistent, usually painful erection associated or unassociated with sexual stimulation. There are two major forms: low-flow (veno-occlusive) priapism and high-flow priapism (associated with increased arterial inflow without increased venous outflow resistance).

ICD-9CM CODES
607.3 Priapism

EPIDEMIOLOGY & DEMOGRAPHICS

- Peak incidence is seen from ages 5 to 10 yr and 20 to 50 yr.
- In the younger group, priapism is often associated with sickle cell disease or neoplasm. In the older group it is often caused by pharmacologic agents.
- Low-flow (veno-occlusive priapism [type I]) is much more common than high-flow (type II).

PHYSICAL FINDINGS & CLINICAL PRESENTATION

- In idiopathic priapism the initial erection is associated with prolonged sexual excitement. Previous transient episodes are frequently reported. The erection involves the corpora cavernosa alone. Detumescence does not occur spontaneously.
- In secondary priapism, sexual excitement need not be involved. Otherwise the clinical picture is the same as in idiopathic priapism.
- Table 1-149 compares normal erection and priapism.

ETIOLOGY

Idiopathic: prolonged sexual arousal
Secondary or associated causes:
- Sickle cell disease
- Diabetes
- Leukemia (especially chronic myelogenous leukemia)
- Solid tumor (malignant) penile infiltration
- Spinal cord injury
- Perineal or penile trauma
- Iatrogenic
- Total parenteral nutrition, which includes a fat emulsion
- Hyperosmolar IV contrast
- Spinal or general anesthesia
- Anticoagulant therapy
- Phenothiazines
- Trazodone
- Intracorporeal injection therapy for impotence
- Phosphodiesterase type 5 inhibitors (e.g., sildenafil [Viagra], tadalafil [Cialis], vardenafil [Levitra])

PATHOPHYSIOLOGY

- Low-flow priapism: prolonged erection leads to edema of the cavernosal trabeculae, resulting in a sequence of statis, thrombosis, venous occlusion, fibrosis, scarring, and possibly impotence.
- High-flow priapism: cavernosal artery rupture leading to an arteriocavernous fistula.

DIAGNOSIS

WORKUP

None if the associated underlying causes are known to be present. Otherwise they should be ruled out. Low-flow priapism can be distinguished from high-flow priapism by obtaining a corporeal blood gas value. A $P_{O_2} <30$ mm Hg, $P_{CO_2} >60$ mm Hg, and a pH <7.25 are consistent with low-flow priapism. High-flow priapism can be confirmed by a perineal Doppler ultrasound or arteriography (useful to identify arterial-lacunar fistula).

TREATMENT

Goal: achieve detumescence with preservation of potency.
1. Medical therapies:
   - Ice packs
   - Ice water enemas
   - Hot water enemas
   - Pressure dressing
   - Sedatives
   - Analgesics
   - Antispasmodic/anticholinergic drugs
   - Estrogens
   - Anticoagulants
   - Procaine
   - Amyl nitrite
   - Local or general anesthesia
   - Ketamine (1 mg/lb)
2. In the patient with sickle cell disease: intravenous hydration, alkalinization, transfusion or exchange transfusion, oxygen.
3. Corporeal irrigation with normal saline may be used for low-flow priapism. The midshaft of the penis can be injected with a small-gauge butterfly needle and irrigated with 10 to 20 ml of normal saline, followed by an intracorporeal injection of an alpha-adrenergic agonist every 5 min until detumescence. Commonly used intracavernous vasoconstrictor agents are epinephrine (10 to 20 mcg), phenylephrine (250 to 500 mcg), and ephedrine (50 to 100 mg). It is mandatory to monitor the patient's blood pressure and pulse when using alpha-adrenergic agonists.
4. Surgery:
   - Cavernospongiosum shunt
   - Glans-cavernosum shunt
   - Cavernosaphenous shunt
   - In the less common situation of high-flow priapism (diagnosed by the finding of bright red arterial blood on aspiration), arterial embolization or surgical ligation is recommended.

PROGNOSIS

Impotence is associated with the duration of priapism, with 36 hr being an important threshold.

REFERRAL

To urologist

AUTHOR: **FRED F. FERRI, M.D.**

TABLE 1-149 Comparison of Normal Erection and Priapism

Factor	Normal Erection	Priapism
Portion of penis involved	Corpora cavernosa and corpus spongiosum and glans	Corpora cavernosa
Cause	Vasodilatation of penile arteries	Obstruction of venous outflow Disturbance of neuroarterial mechanism (imbalance between it and adrenergic activity) Increased viscosity
Sexual desire	Present	Absent
Pain	Absent	Present
Duration	Minutes to hours	Hours to days

From Nseyo UO (ed): *Urology for primary care physicians,* Philadelphia, 1999, WB Saunders.

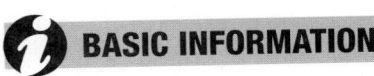

BASIC INFORMATION

DEFINITION

Glaucoma is a chronic degenerative optic neuropathy in which the neuro-retinal rim of the optic nerve becomes progressively thinner, thereby enlarging the optic-nerve cup. The classification of glaucomas is based on the appearance of the iridocorneal angle (open angle vs. closed angle) and is further subdivided into primary and secondary types. Primary open-angle glaucoma can occur with or without elevated intraocular pressure. Normal tension glaucoma refers to primary open-angle glaucoma without elevated intraocular pressure.

SYNONYMS

Chronic simple glaucoma
Chronic open-angle glaucoma (POAG)

ICD-9CM CODES
365.1 Open-angle glaucoma

EPIDEMIOLOGY & DEMOGRAPHICS

INCIDENCE (IN U.S.): Third most common cause of vision loss (75% to 95% of all forms of glaucoma are open angle)
PEAK INCIDENCE:
- Increases after age 40 yr
- Three million cases expected by 2020 because of the rapid increase in aging population

PREVALENCE (IN U.S.):
- Overall prevalence in U.S. population aged >40 yr is estimated to be 1.86%, with 1.57 million white and 398,000 black patients affected.
- 150,000 patients have bilateral blindness.
- Disease occurs in 2% of people >40 yr.
- Prevalence is higher in diabetics, those with high myopia, and older persons.
- More common in blacks (three times the age-adjusted prevalence than whites).

PREDOMINANT AGE:
- Persons >50 yr
- Can occur in 30s and 40s

GENETICS:
- Four to six times higher incidence in blacks than whites
- No clear-cut hereditary patterns but a strong hereditary tendency

PHYSICAL FINDINGS & CLINICAL PRESENTATION

- High intraocular pressures and large optic nerve cup (Ocular Hypertension Treatment Study results very important)
- Corneal edema causes vision loss and blurring
- Abnormal visual fields
- Open-angle gonioscopy
- Red eye
- Restricted vision and field

ETIOLOGY

- Uncertain hereditary tendency
- Topical steroids
- Trauma
- Inflammatory
- High-dose oral corticosteroids taken for prolonged periods

DIAGNOSIS

DIFFERENTIAL DIAGNOSIS

- Other optic neuropathies
- Secondary glaucoma from inflammation and steroid therapy
- Red eye differential
- Trauma
- Contact lens injury

WORKUP

- Intraocular pressure
- Slit lamp examination
- Visual fields
- Gonioscopy
- Nerve fiber analysis (e.g., GDx analyzer, Zeiss, Jena, Germany)
- Corneal thickness—very important in prognosis

LABORATORY TESTS

Blood sugar

IMAGING STUDIES

- Optic nerve photography—stereo photographs
- Visual field testing
- Laser scan of nerve fiber layer, OCT, HRT

TREATMENT

ACUTE GENERAL Rx

- β-blockers (e.g., Timolol) qd to bid depending on individual response to drug
- Diamox 250 mg qid or 500 mg bid
- Hyperosmotic agents (mannitol) in acute treatment (IV)
- Prostaglandins commonly used as first-line treatment
- Laser trabeculoplasty (SLT) as needed
- Pilocarpine qid

CHRONIC Rx

- At least biannual checks of intraocular pressure and adjustment of medication
- Poor control = frequent examinations; good control = drugs
- Trabeculectomy
- Filter valves

DISPOSITION

Must be followed by ophthalmologist

REFERRAL

Immediately to ophthalmologist

PEARLS & CONSIDERATIONS

COMMENTS

- Glaucoma is a serious blinding disease that must be monitored professionally by an ophthalmologist.
- Early diagnosis and treatment may minimize visual loss.
- Glaucoma is not solely caused by increased intraocular pressure because approximately 20% of patients with glaucoma have normal intraocular pressure. However, high pressure is definitely a risk factor to be considered. Potential sites of increased resistance to aqueous flow are described in Fig. 1-304.

EVIDENCE

available at www.expertconsult.com

SUGGESTED READINGS

available at www.expertconsult.com

AUTHOR: **MELVYN KOBY, M.D.**

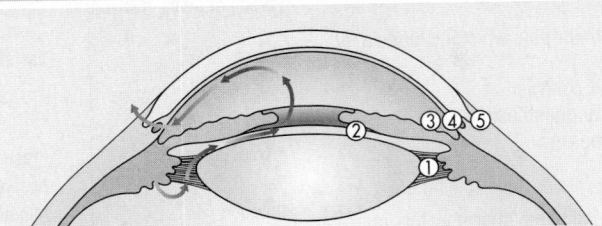

POTENTIAL SITES OF INCREASED RESISTANCE TO AQUEOUS FLOW

1 Ciliary body processes (when ciliary body swollen by congestion), fibrin debris, vitreous face against the lens equator
2 Pupillary block by anterior position of lens or swollen lens
3 Pretrabecular by neovascular or cellular membranes
4 Trabecular by abnormal accumulation of extracellular matrix
5 Post-trabecular by increased episcleral venous pressure

FIGURE 1-304 Potential sites of increased resistance to aqueous flow. (From Yanoff M, Duker JS: *Ophthalmology*, ed 2, St Louis, 2004, Mosby.)

BASIC INFORMATION

DEFINITION

- Woman younger than 40 yr of age with amenorrhea, oligomenorrhea, or dysfunctional uterine bleeding for 4 mo or more along with FSH levels in the menopausal range meet diagnostic criteria for primary ovarian insufficiency.
- Menopause younger than the age of 40 yr.

SYNONYMS

Hypergonadotropic hypogonadism
Premature ovarian failure
Premature menopause
Gonadal dysgenesis

ICD-9-CM CODES
256.31 Premature menopause

EPIDEMIOLOGY & DEMOGRAPHICS

INCIDENCE: Affects 1% to 4% of the female population in the U.S.
PREDOMINANT AGE: 1:250 incident cases by age 35 and 1:100 by age 40

PHYSICAL FINDINGS & CLINICAL PRESENTATION

- The most common presentation is disturbance in menstrual pattern due to intermittent ovarian function.
- Between 5% and 30% of affected women have another affected female relative.
- Between 10% and 30% of affected women already have a concurrent autoimmune condition, the most common of which is hypothyroidism.
- Symptoms of estrogen deficiency include hot flashes, night sweat, poor concentration, drying of the vagina and infertility.
- Physical exam may reveal stigmata of autoimmune condition such as vitiligo, thyroid enlargement or Turner's syndrome (webbed neck, short stature, and high-arched palate).

ETIOLOGY (see Table 1-150)
Idiopathic in 95% of cases

DIAGNOSIS

DIFFERENTIAL DIAGNOSIS

- Pregnancy
- Causes of secondary amenorrhea include polycystic ovarian disease, hypothalamic amenorrhea, hyperprolactinemia.

WORKUP

- After pregnancy is ruled out, the initial evaluation should include the measurement of serum prolactin, FSH, and thyrotropin (TSH) levels.
- If the FSH level is in the menopausal range, the test should be repeated in 1 month along with a serum estradiol measurement to confirm the diagnosis of Primary Ovarian Insufficiency.

LABORATORY TESTS

Once a diagnosis of premature ovarian failure is made, other evaluations include:
- Autoimmune disorders, adrenal insufficiency (seen in 3% of cases): serum anti-adrenal and anti-21 hydroxylase antibodies should be measured.
- Hypothyroidism: serum TSH, T4, and anti-TPO antibodies
- All cases should be screened for osteoporosis by DXA for bone mineral density.
- A karyotype analysis should be performed for all patients to look for chromosomal defects including Turner's variant or deletions of the X chromosome.
- Permutations for the Fragile X syndrome (FMR1 gene) should be checked for as well.

IMAGING STUDIES

Pelvic ultrasound has no proven benefit in the management of these patients.

TREATMENT

NONPHARMACOLOGIC THERAPY

Counseling or patient support group should be offered to all women with low self-esteem and depression due to the psychological scar left by the diagnosis.

ACUTE GENERAL Rx

- Physiologic estrogen and progestin replacement is reasonable in the cases of young women until they reach the age of natural menopause.
- A dose of 100 mcg of estradiol per day, administered by transdermal patch, achieves average estradiol level observed in normal menstruating women and effectively treats symptoms.
- Cyclic medroxyprogesterone at a dose of 10 mg per day for 12 days each month is the preferred progestin to provide protection against endometrial cancer.
- Pregnancy may occur while a woman is taking estrogen and progesterone therapy and the therapy should be stopped immediately if the pregnancy test is found to be positive.

CHRONIC Rx

- Intake of 1200 mg of elemental calcium and 800 units of vitamin D_3 per day should be encouraged to prevent bone loss. A serum 25-hydroxyvitamin D level of 30 ng per ml or higher should be maintained.
- Patients with positive tests for adrenal antibodies should be evaluated annually for adrenal insufficiency by corticotropin stimulation test.
- Patients who wish to avoid pregnancy should use a barrier method or an IUD.
- Options for parenthood include adoption, foster parenthood, egg donation, and embryo donation.

DISPOSITION

Women with the known diagnosis should be encouraged to maintain a lifestyle that optimizes bone and cardiovascular health, including regular weight-bearing exercises, adequate intake of calcium (1200 mg daily) and vitamin D (800 IU daily), healthy diet to prevent obesity, and screening for cardiovascular risk factors.

REFERRAL

Referral to gynecologist and reproductive endocrinologist may be helpful in patients who decide to pursue parenthood.

PEARLS & CONSIDERATIONS

COMMENTS

- Common etiologies should be ruled out, including chromosomal abnormalities, fragile X premutations and autoimmune causes.
- Management directed at symptom resolution and bone protection primarily, but should include psychosocial support for women facing this devastating diagnosis.

PREVENTION

Early diagnosis of primary ovarian insufficiency important for osteoporosis prevention and possibly prevention of coronary artery disease.

PATIENT/FAMILY EDUCATION

www.pofsupport.org

SUGGESTED READINGS
available at www.expertconsult.com

AUTHOR: **PRIYA BANSAL, M.D., M.P.H.**

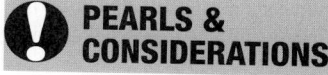

TABLE 1-150 Mechanisms and Causes of Primary Ovarian Insufficiency

Accelerated Follicular Depletion

Genetic: Turner's syndrome, Fragile X permutations, galactosemia
Toxic: Chemotherapy, radiation, infections such as mumps or CMV
Autoimmune: Polyglandular failure, hypothyroidism, Addison's disease, vitiligo, myasthenia gravis

Abnormal Follicular Stimulation

Gonadotropin receptor function: FSH/LH receptor mutation
Enzyme defects: Aromatase deficiency
Luteinized follicles

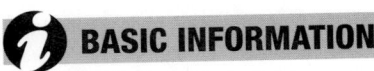

BASIC INFORMATION

DEFINITION

Primary sclerosing cholangitis (PSC) is a chronic progressive cholestatic liver disease characterized by segmental fibrosing and inflammation of intrahepatic and extrahepatic bile ducts complicated by recurrent cholangitis, cholangiocarcinoma, cirrhosis, and portal hypertension.

SYNONYMS

Chronic obliterative cholangitis
Fibrosing cholangitis
Stenosing cholangitis
PSC

ICD-9CM CODES
567.1 Cholangitis
698 Pruritus
780.7 Malaise and fatigue
782.4 Jaundice

EPIDEMIOLOGY & DEMOGRAPHICS

- The incidence and prevalence of PSC is 0.9 to 1.3 cases and 8.5 to 13.6 cases per 100,000 population, respectively.
- About 70% of patients with PSC are men with a M:F ratio of 3:1.
- Mean age of presentation is 40 yr old.
- 70% to 90% of patients with PSC also have inflammatory bowel disease (IBD), particularly with ulcerative colitis (UC). Patients with PSC and UC are at higher risk for developing colon cancer than patients with UC alone.
- PSC can coexist with other autoimmune liver disease. Autoimmune hepatitis and PSC overlap syndrome is mostly seen in young adults and children.
- The median survival from time of diagnosis is 10 to 15 yr without liver transplantation.

PHYSICAL FINDINGS & CLINICAL PRESENTATION

- Most patients are asymptomatic (15% to 40%) at the time of diagnosis with normal physical findings.
- More than 75% of asymptomatic patients develop symptoms, the most common being pruritis (70%) and fatigue (70%). Other complaints include abdominal discomfort, steatorrhea, jaundice, and weight loss, which are concerning for advance PSC, sepsis or mechanical obstruction (i.e., cholangitis) and malignancy (i.e., cholangiocarcinoma).
- Patients with advanced liver disease can present with decompensated cirrhosis (i.e., ascites, spontaneous bacterial peritonitis, hepatic encephalopathy, and variceal hemorrhage) and hepatic failure.
- Physical findings of symptomatic patients may reveal jaundice, skin excoriation and hyperpigmentation from scratching due to pruritis, hepatosplenomegaly, and xanthelasma. In patients with cirrhosis, physical findings may reveal a shrunken nodular liver and evidence of portal hypertension.

ETIOLOGY

- The cause of PSC is unknown but is thought to be multifactorial due to environmental, immunologic and genetic factors.
- Genetic and immunologic factors are supported by reports of familial occurrence of this disorder and increased frequency of HLA B8 and DR 3, which are known to be associated with several autoimmune disorders.
- Environment factor is implicated in PSC due to the close association of PSC with UC. This has led to the hypothesis that bacterial, viral, or toxic substances in the inflamed colonic mucosa might transmigrated to the biliary tree and cause chronic inflammation and fibrosis.

DIAGNOSIS

Diagnosis is based on characteristic cholangiographic findings in combination with clinical, biochemical and in some cases histologic features.

DIFFERENTIAL DIAGNOSIS

- Choledocholithiasis
- Surgical biliary trauma
- Recurrent pyogenic cholangitis
- Ischemic cholangitis
- Cholangiocarcinoma
- IgG4-associated cholangitis
- Intraarterial chemotherapy
- Diffuse intrahepatic metastasis
- Histiocytosis X

WORKUP

History, physical examination, laboratory evaluation, imaging studies +/− liver biopsy.

LABORATORY TESTS

- Serum biochemical tests usually indicate cholestasis with predominant elevation in the serum alkaline phosphatase (three to five times the upper limit of normal). Serum aminotransferase levels are elevated in the majority of patients (two to three times the upper limits of normal). Serum bilirubin is usually normal at the time of diagnosis unless patient has advanced liver disease.
- A wide range of autoantibodies can be detected in patients with PSC; however, they have no role in the routine diagnosis of PSC including the perinuclear antineutrophil cytoplasmic antibody (pANCA), which is nonspecific. However, autoantibodies such as antinuclear antigen (ANA) and/or smooth muscle antigen (ASMA) and/or serum IgG levels are useful in the diagnosis of PSC-autoimmune hepatitis(AIH) overlap syndrome.

IMAGING STUDIES

- Endoscopic retrograde cholangiography (ERC) is considered to be the "gold standard" for the diagnosis of PSC. Characteristic findings reveal segmental fibrosis of bile ducts with saccular dilatation of normal intervening areas resulting in a "beads-on-a-string" appearance (see Fig. 1-305).
- Magnetic resonance cholangiography (MRC) is the imaging modality of choice when PSC is suspected due to serious complications associated with ERC (i.e., pancreatitis and cholangititis) and high sensitivity and specificity of MRC.
- Liver biopsy is not necessary for the diagnosis of PSC in patients with typical cholangiographic findings. Liver biopsy is recommended for diagnosis in patients with suspected autoimmune hepatitis, PSC overlap syndrome or small duct PSC (normal cholangiogram) or for prognostication.

TREATMENT

- No medical therapy has been proven effective in halting the disease progression of PSC.
- Management of PSC patients are aimed at symptom relief and management of complications from PSC (i.e., obstruction/strictures, bacterial cholangitis, metabolic bone disease, portal hypertension, and malignancy).
- There has been mixed data on the use of ursodeoxycholic acid (UDCA) in adults with PSC. It is yet unclear if UDCA slows the progression of PSC-related liver disease and in high doses it has been shown to be harmful. Therefore UDCA is not recommended as medical therapy in patients with PSC.
- The use of corticosteroids and other immunosuppressive agents are not recommended in patients with PSC alone however it is recommended in patient with PSC and overlap syndrome.

ACUTE GENERAL Rx

- Bile acid sequestrants (i.e., cholestyramine 16 g/day) are the preferred chose for the initial management of pruritus. Alternative agents for pruritis refractory to bile acid sequestrants include rifampicin 150 to 300 mg

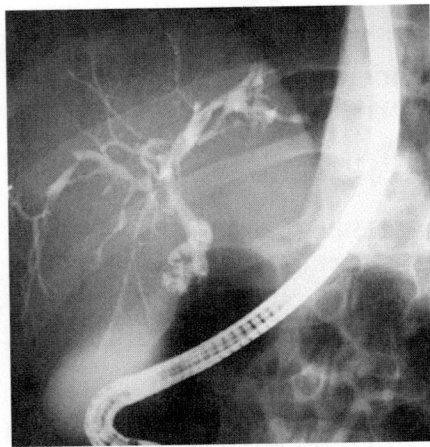

FIGURE 1-305 A 29-year-old male patient who was diagnosed with PSC for 5 years with both the intra- and extrahepatic bile ducts are involved at cholangiography. (From Parlak E et al: An endoscopic finding in patients with primary sclerosing cholangitis: retraction of the main duodenal papilla into the duodenum wall, *GIE* 65(3): 535, Figure 3B, 2007.)

twice daily, naltrexone 50 mg daily, and ser-traline 75 to 100 mg daily.
- Patients who present with increasing serum bilirubin and/or worsening pruritis, progressive bile duct dilatation on imaging studies and/or cholangitis needs to be evaluated for dominant strictures.
- ERC with balloon dilatation +/− stenting is recommended in patients with dominant strictures after the exclusion of malignancy. If ERC is unsuccessful percutaneous cholangiography +/− stenting should be considered.
- In non-cirrhotic patients with dominant strictures refractory to endoscopic and/or percutaneous management, surgery should be considered though this may complicate future liver transplantation surgery.
- Antibiotic usage is recommended in patients with dominant strictures/obstructions both acutely and for long-term prophylaxis in patients with recurrent cholangitis.

CHRONIC Rx

- Avoidance of alcohol advised to avoid further insults to the liver.
- All patients need to be vaccinated against Hepatitis A and B.
- Patients with PSC are at risk for metabolic bone disease. At time of diagnosis a DEXA scan is recommend to evaluate for osteopenia and osteoporosis. Calcium (1000 to 1500 g) and vitamin D 1,000 IU daily are recommended for patients with osteopenia and the addition of bisphosphonate is recommended in patients with osteoporosis.
- Patients with newly diagnosed PSC should have full a colonoscopy with biopsies to exclude concurrent IBD and for surveillance of colorectal cancer. In patients with established PSC and IBD continued surveillance colonoscopy with biopsies at 1 to 2 yr is recommended.
- Annual transabdominal ultrasound is recommended to screen for gallbladder mass due to risk of gallbladder malignancy and if detected cholecystectomy should be performed if underlying liver disease permits.
- Patients with cirrhosis are recommended to have gastroesophageal variceal and hepatocellular carcinoma (HCC) surveillance at regular intervals.
- All patients with deterioration in clinical performance status or liver biochemical parameters should be evaluated for development of cholangiocarcinoma and in patients with cirrhosis the development of hepatocellular carcinoma. Depending on underlying liver disease resection versus liver transplantation would be required.

DISPOSITION

Liver transplantation is the only effective treatment for patients with end-stage liver disease, portal hypertension, liver failure, and recurrent or intractable bacterial cholangitis.

REFERRAL

Gastroenterology and/or hepatology for treatment of PSC, management of its complications, surveillance of associated malignancy and evaluation for liver transplantation.

! PEARLS & CONSIDERATIONS

- Management of PSC targets symptom relief and complications of PSC and cirrhosis.
- Patients are at increase risk for the development of colorectal cancer, gallbladder cancer, and cholangiocarcinoma.
- In patient with cirrhosis surveillance for gastroesophageal varices and hepatocellular carcinoma are recommended.
- Liver transplant remain the only definitive therapy for complications of PSC.

SUGGESTED READINGS

available at www.expertconsult.com

AUTHORS: **CUI LI LIN, M.D.,** and **KITTICHAI PROMRAT, M.D.**

Diseases and Disorders

P

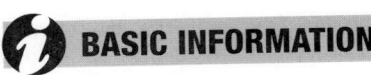

BASIC INFORMATION

DEFINITION

Progressive supranuclear palsy (PSP) is an atypical parkinsonian syndrome characterized by supranuclear gaze impairment, prominent and early postural instability with falls, axial greater than appendicular rigidity, and poor or absent response to levodopa.

SYNONYMS

Steele-Richardson-Olszewski syndrome
Progressive supranuclear ophthalmoplegia

ICD-9CM CODES
333.0 Other degenerative diseases of the basal ganglia

EPIDEMIOLOGY & DEMOGRAPHICS

INCIDENCE: 1.1 per 100,000 (5.3 per 100,000 over age 50)
PREVALENCE: 4.9 per 100,000 (6.4 per 100,000 age-adjusted)
PREDOMINANT SEX AND AGE: Slight male predominance; mean age onset 63 yr, very uncommon for onset <50 yr
GENETICS: Familial cases have been reported only rarely. The vast majority of cases are sporadic.

PHYSICAL FINDINGS & CLINICAL PRESENTATION

Tremorless parkinsonism is the general clinical presentation, and differentiation from idiopathic Parkinson's disease can be challenging early in the disease course. However, there are certain symptoms that can serve as "red flags" to consider PSP:

- Early postural instability and retropulsion leads to frequent falls; falls within the first year of onset of symptoms is typically the rule.
- Supranuclear gaze palsy is often preceded by slowing of vertical saccades; square wave jerks can be present; blepharospasm is common.
- Dystonia of the frontalis and procerus muscles gives the PSP patient a "surprised" or "frightened" expression as opposed to the hypomimia of Parkinson's disease (see Fig. 1-306).
- Speech is typically strained, spastic, hypernasal, with a low-pitched dysarthria.
- Pseudobulbar affect and "emotional incontinence" can be seen, with easy crying or laughter.
- Early cognitive impairment, most commonly with apathy, disinhibition, and anxiety.

ETIOLOGY

PSP is caused by neuronal degeneration of nuclei in the midbrain and basal ganglia, as a result of abnormal tau protein accumulation, most commonly in astrocyte inclusions and neurofibrillary tangles.

DIAGNOSIS

DIFFERENTIAL DIAGNOSIS

- Parkinson's disease: responds more robustly to levodopa, progression much slower, and lacks "red flag" symptoms above
- Corticobasal degeneration: also a tauopathy like PSP, but characterized by parkinsonism with prominent asymmetric dystonia, cortical sensory signs such as astereognosis, typically progressing to apraxia and sometimes an "alien hand" syndrome
- Multiple system atrophy: distinguished by autonomic involvement such as orthostatic hypotension, cerebellar ataxia, and inspiratory stridor
- Dementia with Lewy bodies: dementia coincident with parkinsonism, fluctuating mental status, visual hallucinations often preceding onset of dopaminergic treatment

WORKUP

- PSP is a clinical diagnosis, best made by a neurologist familiar with the disorder such as a movement disorders specialist.
- A robust response to a trial of levodopa may help to lead consideration away from PSP.
- MRI scan (see below) can be helpful.

LABORATORY TESTS

There are no diagnostic laboratory tests.

IMAGING STUDIES

- Dorsal midbrain atrophy is commonly seen on MRI.
- MRI regional apparent diffusion coefficients (rADC) in specific nuclei on diffusion-weighted imaging can reliably differentiate

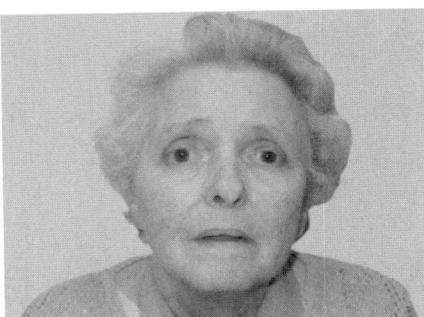

FIGURE 1-306 A patient with progressive supranuclear palsy with staring expression, frontalis overactivity, and retrocolitis. She is wearing a neck sling for a fractured wrist sustained in a fall. (From Burn D, Lees A: Progressive supranuclear palsy: where are we now? *Lancet Neurol* 1:359, 2002.)

PSP from Parkinson's disease, although not from multiple system atrophy.

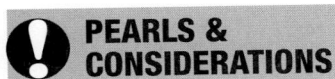

TREATMENT

NONPHARMACOLOGIC THERAPY

- Physical therapy, in particular focusing on fall prevention, is essential for avoiding the morbidity associated with frequent falls. Assistive devices such as a walker or wheelchair should be encouraged.
- Dysphagia is a common finding and should be monitored for closely in conjunction with a speech therapist.
- Prisms can be helpful in some patients for the eye movement abnormalities that can result in misalignment and diplopia.

CHRONIC Rx

- Although classically felt to be unresponsive to levodopa, there is often a transient response to this medication and it can be useful. The poor response to levodopa is most likely due to the loss of postsynaptic dopamine receptors.
- Anticholinergic medications should be avoided.
- Blepharospasm can be effectively treated with botulinum toxin injections.

DISPOSITION

- Median latency from symptom onset to wheelchair-bound state is 5 yr and to death is 7 yr.

REFERRAL

Referral to a general neurologist or movement disorders center is appropriate.

PEARLS & CONSIDERATIONS

COMMENTS

Consider PSP in a parkinsonian patient with the onset of falls within 1 yr of diagnosis, vertical eye movement abnormalities, early cognitive impairment, pseudobulbar affect, frontonasal dystonia, or poor response to levodopa.

PATIENT & FAMILY EDUCATION

Patient and caregiver information and resources can be found at www.wemove.org (a comprehensive movement disorders website) as well as the Society for Progressive Supranuclear Palsy at www.curepsp.org.

SUGGESTED READINGS
available at www.expertconsult.com

AUTHOR: **ANDREW DUKER, M.D.**

BASIC INFORMATION

DEFINITION

Prolactinomas are monoclonal tumors that secrete prolactin.

ICD-9CM CODES
253.1 Forbes-Albright syndrome

EPIDEMIOLOGY & DEMOGRAPHICS

INCIDENCE: Most common pituitary tumor; nearly 30% of all pituitary adenomas secrete enough prolactin to cause hyperprolactinemia.
PREDOMINANT SEX: Microadenomas are more common in women; macroadenomas are found more frequently in men.

PHYSICAL FINDINGS & CLINICAL PRESENTATION

- Men: decreased facial and body hair, infertility, small testicles; may also have decreased libido, erectile dysfunction,, and delayed puberty (caused by decreased testosterone as a result of inhibition of gonadotropin secretion).
- Women: physical examination may be normal; history may reveal amenorrhea, galactorrhea, oligomenorrhea, and anovulation.
- Both sexes: visual field defects and headache may occur depending on size of tumor and its expansion.

ETIOLOGY

Prolactin-secreting pituitary adenomas: microadenomas (<10 mm diameter) or macroadenomas (>10 mm diameter). No risk factors have been identified for sporadic prolactinomas. Rarely prolactinomas can be part of multiple endocrine neoplasia (MEN) type 1 syndrome.

DIAGNOSIS

DIFFERENTIAL DIAGNOSIS

Secretion of prolactin is under tonic inhibitory control by hypothalamic dopamine. Hyperprolactinemia may be caused by the following:
- Drugs: risperidone, phenothiazines, methyldopa, reserpine, monoamine oxidase inhibitors, androgens, progesterone, cimetidine, tricyclic antidepressants, haloperidol, meprobamate, chlordiazepoxide, estrogens, narcotics, metoclopramide, verapamil, amoxapine, cocaine, oral contraceptives
- Hepatic cirrhosis, renal failure, primary hypothyroidism
- Ectopic prolactin-secreting tumors (hypernephroma, bronchogenic carcinoma)
- Infiltrating diseases of the pituitary (sarcoidosis, histiocytosis)
- Head trauma, chest wall injury, spinal cord injury
- Polycystic ovary disease, pregnancy, nipple stimulation
- Idiopathic hyperprolactinemia, stress, exercise

WORKUP

- The diagnosis of prolactinoma is established by demonstration of an elevated serum prolactin level (after exclusion of other causes of hyperprolactinemia) and radiographic evidence of a pituitary adenoma.
  1. Normal mean prolactin levels are 8 ng/ml in women and 5 ng/ml in men.
  2. Levels >300 ng/ml are virtually diagnostic of prolactinomas.
  3. Prolactin levels can vary with time of day, stress, sleep cycle, and meals. More accurate measurements can be obtained 2 to 3 hr after awakening, preprandially, and when patient is not distressed.
  4. Serial measurements are recommended in patients with mild prolactin elevations.
- TSH, Free T4 , BUN, Creat, ALT, AST are useful tests. Pregnancy test in all women of childbearing age.
- All patients with prolactinomas should undergo visual field testing. Serial evaluation is recommended, particularly during pregnancy in patients with macroadenomas.

IMAGING STUDIES

- MRI with gadolinium enhancement is the procedure of choice in the radiographic evaluation of pituitary disease.
- In absence of MRI, a radiographic diagnosis is best accomplished with a high-resolution CT scanner and special coronal cuts through the pituitary region.

TREATMENT

NONPHARMACOLOGIC THERAPY

Pregnancy and breastfeeding should be avoided because they can encourage tumor growth.

ACUTE GENERAL Rx

- Management of prolactinomas depends on their size and encroachment on the optic chiasm and other vital structures, the presence or absence of gonadal dysfunction, and the patient's desires regarding fertility.
- Medical therapy is preferred when fertility is an important consideration.
  1. Bromocriptine: initial dose is 0.625 at bedtime for the first week. After 1 wk, add morning dose of 1.25 mg. Gradually increase dose by 1.25 mg/wk until dose of 5 to 10 mg/day is achieved. Bromocriptine decreases size of the tumor and generally lowers the prolactin level into the normal range when the initial serum prolactin is <500 ng/ml. Side effects of bromocriptine are nausea, constipation, dizziness, and nasal stuffiness. Bromocriptine appears to be safe during pregnancy.
  2. Cabergoline is a longer acting dopamine agonist that is more expensive but may be more effective and better tolerated than bromocriptine; initial dose is 0.25 mg twice weekly.
- Transsphenoidal resection: option in an infertile patient who cannot tolerate bromocriptine or cabergoline or when medical therapy is ineffective. The success rate depends on the location of the tumor (entirely intrasellar), experience of the neurosurgeon, and size of the tumor (<10 mm in diameter); the recurrence rate may reach 80% within 5 yr. Possible complications of transsphenoidal surgery vary with expeience and skill of the neurosurgeon and tumor anatomy and include transient diabetes insipidus, hypopituitarism, cerebrospinal fluid rhinorrhea, and infections (meningitis, wound infection).
- Pituitary irradiation is useful as adjunctive therapy of macroadenomas (>10 mm in diameter) and in patients with persistent hypersecretion after surgery. Potential complications include cranial nerve damage, radionecrosis, and cognitive abnormalities.
- Stereotactic radiosurgery (gamma knife) has become popular as a modality in the treatment of prolactinomas. A high dose of ionizing radiation is delivered to the tumor through multiple ports. Its advantage is minimal irradiation to surrounding tissues. Proximity of the tumor to the optic chiasm limits this therapeutic modality.

CHRONIC Rx

- Patients on medical therapy require periodic measurement of prolactin levels. An attempt to reduce the dose of bromocriptine or cabergoline can be made after the prolactin level has been normal for 2 yr. An MRI scan of the pituitary should be obtained to rule out tumor enlargement within 6 mo of initiation of tapering regimen.
- Evaluation and monitoring of pituitary function are recommended after transsphenoidal surgery.

DISPOSITION

- Transsphenoidal surgery will result in a cure in nearly 50% to 75% of patients with microadenomas and 10% to 20% of patients with macroadenomas.
- Nearly 20% of microprolactinomas resolve during long-term dopamine agonist treatment.

PEARLS & CONSIDERATIONS

COMMENTS

- Patients must be monitored for several years after surgery because up to 50% of microadenomas and nearly 90% of macroadenomas can recur.
- Pituitary microadenomas are found in 10.9% of autopsies, and 44% of these microadenomas are prolactinomas.

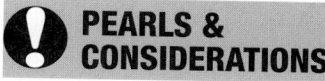

EVIDENCE

available at www.expertconsult.com

SUGGESTED READINGS
available at www.expertconsult.com

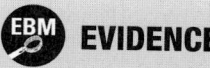

AUTHOR: **FRED F. FERRI, M.D.**

BASIC INFORMATION

DEFINITION
A form of compression neuropathy of the median nerve in the proximal forearm caused primarily by the pronator teres muscle (Fig. 1-307). Occasionally, only the anterior interosseus motor branch is affected, sometimes causing a specific separate clinical presentation.

SYNONYMS
Kiloh-Nevin syndrome (anterior interosseus syndrome)

ICD-9CM CODES
354.1 Median nerve entrapment
354.9 Mononeuritis of upper limb

EPIDEMIOLOGY & DEMOGRAPHICS
PREDOMINANT SEX: Males are affected more often than females.

INCIDENCE: Rare (comprises <1% of median nerve entrapment disorders); most common in dominant arm.

PHYSICAL FINDINGS & CLINICAL PRESENTATION
- Forearm discomfort and fatigue, often resulting from repetitive pronation.
- Insidious onset.
- Nocturnal paresthesias are not typical.
- Vague numbness in hand, primarily in thumb and index finger, may be present.
- Tenderness and enlargement of the pronator teres may be present.
- Tinel's sign may be positive at the site of compression.
- Although there are no reliable provocative tests, painful paresthesias may occasionally be elicited with forced pronation of the forearm against resistance.
- Motor impairment is rare.

Anterior interosseus nerve syndrome:
- Forearm pain and weakness.
- Patient may be unable to form a circle when trying to pinch the index finger and thumb because of the inability to flex distal phalanges of thumb and index finger.
- Sensation to the hand is not affected.

ETIOLOGY
- Localized anatomic compression
- Trauma
- Traumatic cut down or phlebotomy

DIAGNOSIS

DIFFERENTIAL DIAGNOSIS
- Carpal tunnel syndrome
- Cervical disc syndrome with radiculopathy
- Tendon rupture
- Tendinitis

WORKUP
- Electrodiagnostic studies may be helpful; they are indicated if symptoms persist >4 to 6 wk or if motor weakness is suspected
- Plain radiography to rule out bony abnormalities causing compression

TREATMENT

- Rest, bracing of forearm, sling
- Stretching exercises, physical therapy
- Nonsteroidal antiinflammatory drugs

DISPOSITION
Patients whose symptoms are mainly subjective often respond to nonsurgical management. Motor deficits may not be reversible despite surgery.

REFERRAL
Surgical referral in cases of failed medical management or when motor weakness is present

PEARLS & CONSIDERATIONS

COMMENTS
Prognosis for recovery is good. When indicated, surgical intervention is most effective if the diagnosis can be firmly established by objective testing.

SUGGESTED READINGS
available at www.expertconsult.com

AUTHOR: **LONNIE R. MERCIER, M.D.**

FOREARM ENTRAPMENT REGIONS

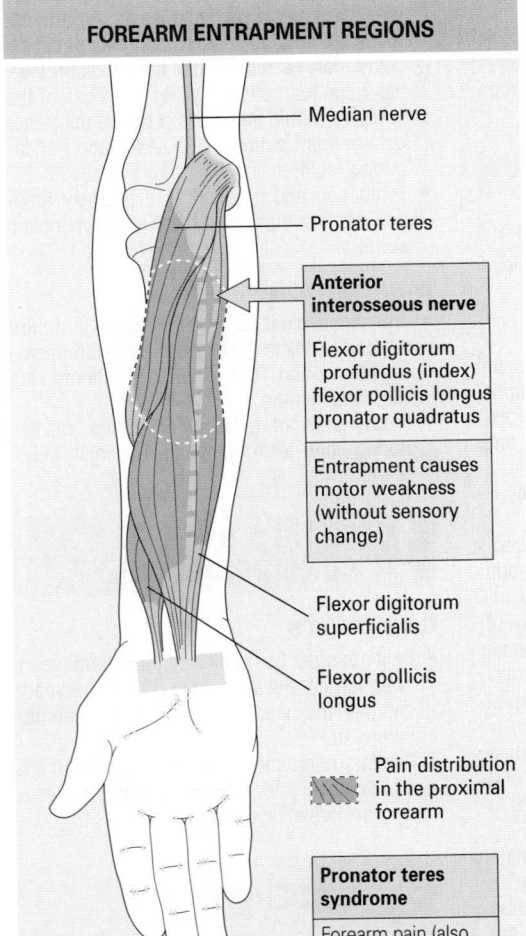

- Median nerve
- Pronator teres

Anterior interosseous nerve

Flexor digitorum profundus (index) flexor pollicis longus pronator quadratus

Entrapment causes motor weakness (without sensory change)

- Flexor digitorum superficialis
- Flexor pollicis longus

Pain distribution in the proximal forearm

Pronator teres syndrome

Forearm pain (also paresthesia in hand)

FIGURE 1-307 Forearm entrapment regions. The median nerve may be compressed at several locations in the forearm, most commonly as it traverses the pronator teres muscle. The anterior interosseous branch of the median nerve is solely motor, thus entrapment produces no sensory deficit. (From Hochberg MC et al [eds]: *Rheumatology,* 3rd ed, St Louis, 2003, Mosby.)

BASIC INFORMATION

DEFINITION & CLASSIFICATION

Prostate cancer is a neoplasm involving the prostate. Various classifications have been developed to evaluate malignancy potential and prognosis.

- The degree of malignancy varies with the stage:
  1. Stage A: Confined to the prostate, no nodule palpable
  2. Stage B: Palpable nodule confined to the gland
  3. Stage C: Local extension
  4. Stage D: Regional lymph nodes or distant metastases
- In the Gleason classification, two histologic patterns are independently assigned numbers 1 to 5 (best to least differentiated). These numbers are added to give a total tumor score between 2 and 10. Prognosis is best for highly differentiated tumors (e.g., Gleason score 2 to 4) compared with most poorly differentiated tumors (Gleason score 7 to 10).
- Another commonly used classification is the Tumor-Node-Metastasis (TNM) classification of prostate cancer.

ICD-9CM CODES
185 Malignant neoplasm of prostate

EPIDEMIOLOGY & DEMOGRAPHICS

- Prostate cancer has surpassed lung cancer as the most common nonskin cancer in men.
- In the U.S. more than 190,000 cases are diagnosed yearly, and nearly 30,000 males die from prostate cancer each year (second leading cause of death from cancer in U.S. men).
- Incidence of prostate cancer increases with age: uncommon <50 yr; 80% of new cases are diagnosed in patients aged ≥65 yr.
- Average age at time of diagnosis is 72 yr.
- Blacks in the U.S. have the highest incidence of prostate cancer in the world (one in every nine males).
- Incidence is low in Asians.
- Approximately 9% of all prostate cancers may be familial. Obesity is a risk factor for prostate cancer. High insulin levels may also increase the risk of prostate cancer.
- Mortality rates of prostate cancer have declined substantially in the past 15 yr from 34% in 1990 to <20% currently.

PHYSICAL FINDINGS & CLINICAL PRESENTATION

- Generally silent disease until it reaches advanced stages.
- Bone pain and pathologic fractures may be initial symptoms of prostate cancer.
- Local growth can cause symptoms of outflow obstruction.
- Digital rectal examination (DRE) may reveal an area of increased firmness; 10% of patients will have a negative DRE.
- Prostate may be hard, fixed, with extension of tumor to the seminal vesicles in advanced stages.

DIAGNOSIS

DIFFERENTIAL DIAGNOSIS

- Benign prostatic hypertrophy
- Prostatitis
- Prostate stones

LABORATORY TESTS

- Measurement of prostate-specific antigen (PSA) is controversial in early diagnosis of prostate cancer. PSA screening is associated with psychological harm, and its potential benefits remain uncertain. In asymptomatic men with no history of prostate cancer, screening using PSA does not reduce all-cause mortality or death from prostate cancer. Normal PSA is found in >20% of patients with prostate cancer, whereas only 20% of men with PSA levels between 4 ng/ml and 10 ng/ml have prostate cancer. The American Cancer Society recommends offering the PSA test and DRE yearly to men aged ≥50 yr who have a life expectancy of at least 10 yr. Earlier testing, starting at age 45 yr, is recommended for men at high risk (e.g., blacks, men with family history of prostate cancer). An isolated elevation in PSA level should be confirmed several weeks later before proceeding with further testing, including prostate biopsy. Screening for prostate cancer in men aged ≥75 yr is controversial and generally not recommended.
- Free PSA: the use of serum-free PSA for prostate screening has been proposed by some urologists as a means to decrease unwarranted biopsies without missing a significant number of prostate cancers. This approach is based on the higher free PSA in men with benign prostatic hyperplasia and the higher protein-bound PSA levels in men with prostate cancer. For example, in men with total PSA levels of 4 to 10 ng/ml, the cancer probability is 0.25, but if the percentage of free PSA is ≤17%, the probability of cancer increases to 0.45.
- PSA velocity: the rate of increase of serum PSA (PSA velocity) can aid in the diagnosis of prostate cancer. A yearly PSA velocity >0.75 ng/ml increases the likelihood of later malignancy when total PSA is still within normal range. Proper interpretation of PSA velocity requires at least three PSA measurements over an 18-month period because most PSA variations are physiologic.
- Age-adjusted PSA: there is evidence that the current threshold of 4.0 ng/ml is inadequate for younger men, because in a recent study 22% of men with PSA levels between 2.6 and 4.0 were found to have prostate cancer. The concept of age-related cutoffs remains controversial. Lowering the upper limit of normal for PSA would improve sensitivity but decrease specificity.
- Prostatic acid phosphatase can be used for evaluation of nonlocalized disease.
- Transrectal biopsy and fine-needle aspiration of prostate can confirm the diagnosis. Indications for biopsy include an abnormal PSA level, an abnormal DRE, or a previous biopsy specimen that showed prostatic intraepithelial neoplasia or prostatic atypia. The number of cores taken is patient specific, typically including a minimum of 10 cores. Prostate volume negatively affects cancer detection rate (23% in glands >50 cm³, 38% in glands <50 cm³).

IMAGING STUDIES

- Bone scan is useful to evaluate bone metastasis (present or eventually develops in almost 80% of patients). However, according to the American Urological Association (AUA), the routine use of bone scanning is not required for staging of prostate cancer in asymptomatic men with clinically localized cancer if the PSA level is ≤20 ng/ml.
- CT scan, MRI, and transrectal ultrasonography may be useful in selected patients to assess extent of prostate cancer. High-resolution MRI with magnetic nanoparticles has been used for the detection of small and otherwise undetectable lymph node metastases in patients with prostate cancer. However, according to the AUA, transrectal ultrasonography adds little to the combination of PSA and DRE. Similarly, CT and MRI imaging are generally not indicated for cancer staging in men with clinically localized cancer and PSA <25 ng/ml. With regard to pelvic lymph node dissection in staging, the AUA states that it may not be required in patients with PSA levels <10 ng/ml and when PSA level is <20 ng/ml and the Gleason score is <6.

TREATMENT

NONPHARMACOLOGIC THERAPY
Watchful waiting is reasonable in selected patients with early-stage (T-IA) and projected life expectancy <10 yr or in patients with focal and moderately differentiated carcinoma.

ACUTE GENERAL Rx
- Therapeutic approach varies with the following:
  1. Stage of the tumor
  2. Patient's life expectancy
  3. General medical condition
  4. Patient's treatment preference (e.g., patient may be opposed to orchiectomy)
- The optimal treatment of clinically localized prostate cancer is unclear.
  1. Radical prostatectomy is generally performed in patients with localized prostate cancer and life expectancy >10 yr. Radical prostatectomy reduces disease-specific mortality, overall mortality, and the risks of metastasis and local progression. The absolute reduction in the risk of death after 10 yr is small, but the reductions in

the risks of metastasis and local tumor progression are substantial. Postoperative complications of radical prostatectomy include urinary incontinence (10% to 20% depending on degree of neurovascular bundle and urethral preservation, patient age, and correct mucosal apposition) and erectile dysfunction (percentage exceeds 50% and varies with patient age, preoperative erectile dysfunction, stage of tumor at time of surgery, and preservation of neurovascular bundle). Lower complication rates occur in hospitals that perform a large number of prostatectomies. Fewer men will have postsurgical erectile dysfunction after unilateral or bilateral nerve-sparing surgery. Men undergoing minimally invasive prostatectomy (MIRP) experience shorter length of stay and fewer respiratory and miscellaneous surgical complications and strictures but experience more genitourinary complications, erectile dysfunction, and incontinence when compared with open retropubic radical prostatectomy (RPP).

2. Radiation therapy (external-beam irradiation or brachytherapy with implantation of radioactive pellets [iodine-125 or palladium-103 seeds] into the prostate gland) represents an alternative in patients with localized prostate cancer, especially poor surgical candidates or patients with a high-grade malignancy. The efficacy of brachytherapy is comparable to external radiation. In patients receiving external-beam radiation, a total dose of 79.2 Gy (high dose) compared with a total dose of 70.2 Gy (conventional dose) has been reported to lower the risk of recurrence without increased risk of morbidity and mortality. Patients with localized prostate cancer and high risk for extraprostatic disease and disease recurrence (e.g., Gleason score ≤7 with multiple positive biopsy cores and clinical stage T1b-T2b) may benefit (increased overall survival) with the addition of 6 mo of androgen suppression therapy to radiation therapy.

3. Watchful waiting is reasonable in patients who are too old or too ill to survive longer than 10 yr. If the cancer progresses to the point where it becomes symptomatic, palliation can be attempted with several methods. Conservative management is also reasonable for patients with Gleason score of 2 to 4 because these patients do not have a shortened life expectancy and treatment is associated with long-term side effects. Watchful waiting also appears to be safe in older men with less-aggressive disease. Individual preferences play a central role in the decision whether to treat or to pursue active surveillance.

- Patients with advanced disease and projected life expectancy <10 yr are candidates for radiation therapy and hormonal therapy (diethylstilbestrol, luteinizing hormone–releasing hormone analogs, antiandrogens, bilateral orchiectomy).

- Recommended treatment of patients with regional metastatic prostate cancer with projected life expectancy ≥10 yr includes radiation therapy and hormonal therapy.

- Androgen deprivation therapy (ADT) is the mainstay of treatment for metastatic prostate cancer. Adverse effects of ADT include decreased libido, impotence, hot flashes, osteopenia with increased fracture risk, metabolic alterations, and changes in mood and cognition. Adjuvant treatment with luteinizing hormone-releasing hormone (LHRH) agonists (goserelin leuprolide, or triptorelin) plus antiandrogens (flutamide, bicalutamide, or nilutamide), when started simultaneously with external-beam radiation, improves local control and survival in patients with locally advanced prostate cancer. Pamidronate inhibits osteoclast-mediated bone resorption and prevents bone loss in the hip and lumbar spine in men receiving treatment for prostate cancer. Gonadotropin-releasing hormone (GmRH) receptor antagonists can be used for rapid medical castration of men with advanced prostate cancer. Degarelix is an injectable GnRH agonist useful to suppress testosterone in patients with prostate cancer who are not good candidates for LHRH agonists and refuse surgical castration. Assessment of bone density and treatment with once-weekly oral alendronate can prevent and improve the bone loss that occurs in men receiving ADT for prostate cancer.

- Docetaxel plus prednisone or docetaxel plus estramustine can be used in metastatic hormone-refractory prostate cancer. Newer treatments for hormone-refractory prostate cancer (castration-resistant cancer) include immunotherapy with sipuleucel and cabazitaxel, a microtubule inhibitor that interferes with cell mitoxis and replication. Both agents can prolong survival but adverse effects can be severe and both agents are very expensive

CHRONIC Rx

- Patients should be monitored at 3- to 6-mo intervals with clinical examination and PSA for the first year, then every 6 mo for the second year, then yearly if stable. For patients who have undergone radical prostatectomy, a rising PSA level suggests evidence of residual or recurrent prostate cancer. Salvage radiotherapy may potentially cure patients with disease recurrence after radical prostatectomy.

- Chest radiography and bone scan should be performed yearly or sooner if patient develops symptoms.

DISPOSITION

- Prognosis varies with the stage of the disease and the Gleason classification (see "Definition"). For patients between ages 65 and 69 yr at diagnosis and a Gleason score of 2 to 4, the probability of dying from prostate cancer 15 yr after diagnosis is 0.06 and that of dying from other causes is 0.56. If the Gleason score is 7 to 10, the probability of dying from prostate cancer increases to 0.72 and from other causes varies from 0.25 to 0.36.

- The ploidy of the tumor also has prognostic value; prognosis is better with diploid tumor cells and worse with aneuploid tumor cells.

- For grade 1 tumors, the extended 10-yr, disease-specific survival is similar for patients with prostatectomy (94%), radiotherapy (90%), and conservative management (93%); survival rate is better with surgery than with radiotherapy or conservative management in patients with grade 2 or 3 localized prostate cancer.

- Expression of the gene *EZH2* has been identified as an important factor in the determination of the aggressiveness of prostate cancer. A recent study revealed that expression of the *EZH2* gene may be a better predictor of clinical failure than Gleason score, tumor stage, or surgical margin status. Testing for *EZH2* protein in prostate cancer tissue may be useful to determine prognosis and direct treatment.

- Preoperative PSA level and PSA velocity have prognostic significance. Men whose PSA level increases by >2.0 mcg/ml during the year before the diagnosis of cancer may have a relatively high risk of death from prostate cancer despite undergoing radical prostatectomy.

- Extraprostatic disease is detected at radical prostatectomy in 38% to 52% of patients and is associated with a risk of disease recurrence, progression, and death. In these patients, adjuvant radiotherapy results in significantly reduced risk of PSA relapse and disease recurrence; however, the improvements in metastases-free survival and overall survival are not statistically significant.

- The Prostate Cancer Prevention trial revealed that the use of 5-alpha-reductase inhibitors lowers the incidence of prostate cancer but also increases the incidence of high-grade tumors (Gleason score >7). It is possible that these agents delay diagnosis of prostate cancer by lowering PSA levels and decreasing prostate size.

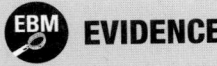 **EVIDENCE**

available at www.expertconsult.com

SUGGESTED READINGS
available at www.expertconsult.com

AUTHOR: **FRED F. FERRI, M.D.**

BASIC INFORMATION

DEFINITION

Benign prostatic hyperplasia (BPH) is the benign growth of the prostate, generally originating in the periureteral and transition zones, with subsequent obstructive and irritative voiding symptoms.

SYNONYMS

BPH
Prostatic hypertrophy

ICD-9CM CODES
600 Benign prostatic hyperplasia

EPIDEMIOLOGY & DEMOGRAPHICS

- 80% of men have evidence of BPH by age 80 yr.
- Medical and surgical intervention for problems caused by BPH is required in >20% of males by age 75 yr.
- Transurethral resection of the prostate (TURP) is the tenth most common operative procedure (>400,000/yr in U.S.).
- 10% to 30% of men with BPH have occult prostate cancer.

PHYSICAL FINDINGS & CLINICAL PRESENTATION

- Digital rectal examination (DRE) reveals enlargement of the prostate.
- Focal enlargement may be indicative of malignancy.
- There is poor correlation between size of prostate and symptoms (BPH may be asymptomatic if it does not encroach on the urethral lumen).
- Most patients with BPH report difficulty in initiating urination (hesitancy), decrease in caliber and force of stream, incomplete emptying of bladder often resulting in double voiding (need to urinate again a few minutes after voiding), postvoid "dribbling," and nocturia.

ETIOLOGY

Multifactorial; a functioning testicle is necessary for development of BPH (as evidenced by the absence in males who were castrated before puberty).

DIAGNOSIS

DIFFERENTIAL DIAGNOSIS

- Prostatitis
- Prostate cancer
- Strictures (urethral)
- Medications interfering with the muscle fibers in the prostate and also with bladder function
  - Opiates: impaired autonomic function
  - Decongestants: increased sphincter tone
  - Antihistamines: decreased parasympathetic tone
  - Tricyclic antidepressants: anticholinergic effects
- Neurogenic bladder
- Bladder cancer

WORKUP

Symptom assessment (use of American Urological Association [AUA] Symptom Index for BPH [Table 1-151]), laboratory tests, and imaging studies

LABORATORY TESTS

- Prostate-specific antigen (PSA): protease secreted by epithelial cells of the prostate; elevated in 30% to 50% of patients with BPH. Testing for PSA increases detection rate for prostate cancer and tends to detect cancer at an earlier stage. However, the PSA test does not discriminate well between patients with symptomatic BPH and those with prostate cancer, particularly if the cancer is pathologically localized and curable. The test may also trigger additional evaluation, including ultrasound biopsy of the prostate. Asymptomatic men with PSA levels <2 ng/ml do not need annual testing. According to the AUA, PSA testing and DRE should be offered to any asymptomatic man >50 yr with a life expectancy of 10 yr. PSA testing can also be offered at an earlier age in men at higher risk of prostatic cancer (e.g., first-degree relatives with prostate cancer; African American race).
- Measurement of "free" PSA is useful to assess the probability of prostate cancer in

TABLE 1-151 International Prostate Symptom Score (I-PSS)

Symptom	SCORE						Total Score
	Not at All	Less than 1 Time in 5	Less than Half the Time	About Half the Time	More than Half the Time	Almost Always	
Incomplete emptying: Over the past month, how often have you had a sensation of not emptying your bladder completely after you finished urinating?	0	1	2	3	4	5	
Frequency: Over the past month, how often have you had to urinate again <2 hr after you finished urinating?	0	1	2	3	4	5	
Intermittency: Over the past month, how often have you found you stopped and started again several times when you urinated?	0	1	2	3	4	5	
Urgency: Over the past month, how often have you found it difficult to postpone urination?	0	1	2	3	4	5	
Weak stream: Over the past month, how often have you had a weak urinary stream?	0	1	2	3	4	5	
Straining: Over the past month, how often have you had to push or strain to begin urination?	0	1	2	3	4	5	
	None	1 Time	2 Times	3 Times	4 Times	5 or More Times	
Nocturia: Over the past month, how many times did you most typically get up to urinate from the time you went to bed at night until the time you got up in the morning?	0	1	2	3	4	5	

Total I-PSS score =

patients with normal DRE and total PSA between 4 and 10 ng/ml. In these patients the global risk of prostate cancer is 25%. However, if the free PSA is >25%, the risk of prostate cancer decreases to 8%, whereas if the free PSA is <10%, the risk of cancer increases to 56%. Free PSA is also useful to evaluate the aggressiveness of prostate cancer. A low free PSA percentage generally indicates a high-grade cancer, whereas a high free PSA percentage is generally associated with a slower growing tumor.

- Urinalysis, urine culture, and sensitivity to rule out infection (if suspected).
- Blood urea nitrogen and creatinine to rule out postrenal insufficiency.

IMAGING STUDIES

- Transrectal ultrasound may be indicated in patients with palpable nodules or significant elevation of PSA. It is also useful to estimate prostate size. BPH may also be evident in suprapubic ultrasound and MRI.
- Uroflowmetry may be used to determine relative impact of obstruction on urine flow. Urethral pressure profile is useful to predict prostatic hypertrophy within the urethral lumen.
- Pressure flow studies, although invasive, are particularly helpful in patients whose history and/or examination suggest primary bladder dysfunction as a cause of symptoms of prostatism. They are also useful in patients for whom a distinction between prostatic obstruction and impaired detrusor contractility may affect the choice of therapy. However, pressure flow studies may not be useful in the workup of the usual patient with symptoms of prostatism.
- Postvoid residual urine measurement has not been proved useful in predicting the need for or response to treatment; it may be useful in monitoring the course of the disease in patients who elect nonsurgical treatment.
- Urethral cystoscopy is an option during later evaluation if invasive treatment is being planned.

Rx TREATMENT

NONPHARMACOLOGIC THERAPY

- Avoidance of caffeine or any other foods that may exacerbate symptoms
- Avoidance of medications that may exacerbate symptoms (e.g., most cold and allergy remedies)

GENERAL Rx

- Asymptomatic patients with prostate enlargement caused by BPH generally do not require treatment. Patients with mild to mod-

erate symptoms are candidates for pharmacologic treatment (see below). For patients who have specific complications from BPH, prostate surgery is usually the most appropriate form of treatment. However, surgery may result in significant complications (e.g., incontinence, infection).

- Alpha-blockers (e.g., tamsulosin, alfuzosin, doxazosin, prazosin, terazosin) relax smooth muscle of the bladder neck and prostate and can increase peak urinary flow rate. They have no effect on the size of the prostate. Alpha-1 blockers are useful in symptomatic patients to relieve symptoms of obstruction by causing relaxation of smooth muscle tone in the prostatic capsule, urethra, and bladder neck.
- Hormonal manipulation with finasteride, a 5-alpha-reductase inhibitor that blocks conversion of testosterone to dihydrotestosterone, can reduce the size of the prostate. Usual dose is 5 mg qd. Treatment requires ≥6 mo for maximal effect.
- Dutasteride is also a 5-alpha-reductase inhibitor useful to decrease prostate size and improve urinary flow. In addition to inhibiting the isoform of 5-alpha-reductase located in the prostate, the medication also inhibits a second isoform and reduces dihydrotestosterone formation in the skin and liver. Usual dose is 0.5 mg qd.
- The dietary supplement saw palmetto is commonly used for relief of symptoms of BPH. Recent trials using 160 mg of saw palmetto bid did not improve symptoms of BPH. This contrasts with the positive findings of many previous studies. Trials with higher dose-ranging protocols are currently in progress.
- TURP is the most commonly used surgical procedure for BPH. Transurethral incision of the prostate (TUIP), a procedure almost equivalent in efficacy, is limited to patients whose estimated resection tissue weight would be 30 g or less. TUIP can be performed in an ambulatory setting or during a 1-day hospitalization. Open prostatectomy is typically performed on patients with very large prostates.
- Laser therapy for BPH is a less invasive alternative to TURP; YAG laser enucleation has minimal effect on potency, libido, or patient satisfaction with his sex life and is associated with retrograde ejaculation. However, recent studies indicate that at least in the initial 7 mo after surgery, TURP is moderately more effective than laser therapy in relieving symptoms of BPH.
- Transurethral needle ablation with radiofrequency to remove periurethral prostate tissue is being increasingly used in patients with prostate volume <60 ml and moderate symptoms. It has a low morbidity rate, but

treatment failure is approximately 25% at 5 yr and >80% at 10 yr.
- Balloon dilation of the prostatic urethra is less effective than surgery for relieving symptoms but is associated with fewer complications. It is a reasonable treatment option for patients with smaller prostates and no middle lobe enlargement.
- Surgery need not be the treatment of last resort for most patients; that is, patients need not undergo other treatments for BPH before they can have surgery. However, recommending surgery on the grounds that a patient's surgical risk will "only increase with age" is generally inappropriate.

CHRONIC Rx

- Avoid medications and foods that exacerbate symptoms.
- Symptomatic improvement occurs in >70% of patients with proper treatment.

DISPOSITION

With appropriate therapy, symptoms improve or stabilize in >70% of patients with BPH.

REFERRAL

Urology referral for patients with severe or intolerable symptoms and for any patient suspected of having prostate cancer (10% to 30% of men with BPH).

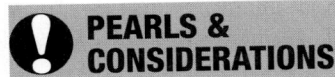 **PEARLS & CONSIDERATIONS**

COMMENTS

- Emerging technologies for treating BPH include lasers, coils, stents, thermal therapy, and hyperthermia. Laser prostatectomy appears promising; however, long-term effectiveness has not yet been demonstrated.
- The increase in the use of pharmacologic management has resulted in >30% reduction in the total number of TURP procedures.
- Combined drug therapy for BPH with an alpha-blocker and a 5-alpha-reductase inhibitor is superior to monotherapy with either agent.

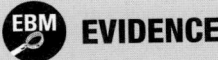 **EVIDENCE**

available at www.expertconsult.com

SUGGESTED READINGS
available at www.expertconsult.com

AUTHOR: **FRED F. FERRI, M.D.**

BASIC INFORMATION

DEFINITION

Prostatitis refers to inflammation of the prostate gland. There are four major categories:
1. Acute bacterial prostatitis (type I)
2. Chronic bacterial prostatitis (type II)
3. Chronic prostatitis/pelvic pain syndrome (CP/CPPS) (type III): subdivided in type IIIA (inflammatory) and IIIB (noninflammatory)
4. Asymptomatic inflammatory prostatitis (type IV)

ICD-9CM CODES
601.0   Prostatitis (acute)
601.1   Prostatitis (chronic)
099.54 Prostatitis (chlamydial)

EPIDEMIOLOGY & DEMOGRAPHICS

- 50% of men will have symptoms of prostatitis in their lifetime.
- Prostatitis accounts for >8% of visits to urologists and 1% of visits to primary care physicians.
- The prevalence of chronic bacterial prostatitis is 5% to 10%.
- CP/CPPS is the most common of the clinically defined prostatitis syndromes, with the prevalence of the syndrome ranging from 9% to 12% of men.

PHYSICAL FINDINGS & CLINICAL PRESENTATION

1. Acute bacterial prostatitis:
   - Sudden or rapidly progressive onset of:
     ○ Dysuria
     ○ Frequency
     ○ Urgency
     ○ Nocturia
     ○ Perineal pain that may radiate to the back, rectum, or penis
   - Hematuria or a purulent urethral discharge may occur.
   - Occasionally urinary retention complicates the course.
   - Fever, chills, and signs of sepsis can also be part of the clinical picture.
   - On rectal examination the prostate is typically tender.
2. Chronic bacterial prostatitis:
   - Characterized by positive culture of expressed prostatic secretions. May cause symptoms such as suprapubic, low back, or perineal pain; mild urgency, frequency, and dysuria with urination; and possibly recurrent urinary tract infections.
   - May be asymptomatic when the infection is confined to the prostate.
   - May present as an increase in severity of baseline symptoms of benign prostatic hypertrophy.
   - When cystitis is also present, urinary frequency, urgency, and burning may be reported.
   - Hematuria may be a presenting complaint.
   - In elderly men, new onset of urinary incontinence may be noted.

3. CP/CPPS:
   - Presents similarly with pain in the pelvic region lasting more than 3 mo. Symptoms also can include pain in the suprapubic region, low back, penis, testes, or scrotum.
   - The symptoms can be of variable severity and may include lower urinary tract symptoms, sexual dysfunction, and reduced quality of life.

ETIOLOGY

1. Acute bacterial prostatitis:
   - Acute, usually gram-negative infection of the prostate gland. *E. coli* is the most commonly isolated organism.
     ○ Generally associated with cystitis
     ○ Results from the ascent of bacteria into the urethra
   - Occasionally the route of infection is hematogenous or a lymphatogenous spread of rectal bacteria.
   - The condition is seen in young or middle-aged men.
2. Chronic bacterial prostatitis:
   - Often asymptomatic. *E. coli* is the most commonly isolated organism.
   - Exacerbation of symptoms of benign prostatic hypertrophy caused by the same mechanism as in acute bacterial prostatitis.
3. CP/CPPS:
   - Type IIIA: refers to symptoms of prostatic inflammation associated with the presence of white blood cells in prostatic secretions with no identifiable bacterial organism.
   - *Chlamydia* infection may be etiologically implicated in some cases.
   - Type IIIB: refers to symptoms of prostatic inflammation with no or few white blood cells in the prostatic secretion.
   - Its cause is unknown. Spasm in the bladder neck or urethra may be responsible for the symptoms.

DIAGNOSIS

DIFFERENTIAL DIAGNOSIS

- Benign prostatic hypertrophy with lower urinary tract symptoms
- Prostate cancer
- Also see differential diagnosis of "Hematuria" entry

WORKUP

- Rectal examination:
  1. Tender prostate most suggestive of acute bacterial prostatitis.
  2. Enlarged prostate common in chronic bacterial prostatitis.
  3. Normal prostate is consistent with chronic bacterial prostatitis and CP/CPPS.
- Expression of prostatic secretions by prostate massage is contraindicated in acute bacterial prostatitis but is appropriate in the other three situations.

LABORATORY TESTS

- Urinalysis.
- Urine culture and sensitivity.
- Bacterial localization studies can be performed but are cumbersome and impractical in most clinical settings.

- Cell count and culture of expressed prostatic secretions.
- The yield of a urine culture may be increased if the specimen is obtained after a prostatic massage.
- Prostate-specific antigen (PSA) is not used to diagnose prostatitis and is not recommended unless a nodule is present on digital examination. A rapid rise over baseline should raise the possibility of prostatitis even in the absence of symptoms. In such cases, a follow-up PSA after treatment of prostatitis is appropriate.
- Complete blood count and blood cultures if fever, chills, or signs of sepsis exist.
- If hematuria is present, a workup to rule out a urologic malignancy should be considered if the hematuria does not clear after treatment of prostatitis.

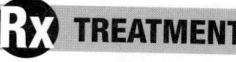

TREATMENT

1. Acute bacterial prostatitis:
   - Empiric therapy with quinolone at time of evaluation. Culture-guided antibiotic therapy for 4 wk (beginning with a few days of IV antibiotics if the infection is serious or if the patient is bacteremic)
2. Chronic bacterial prostatitis:
   - Trimethoprim-sulfamethoxazole (TMP-SMX) is first line choice for 4 wk if the organism is sensitive. Tissue penetration for TMP-SMX is not as good as quinolones and there is evidence of increasing uropathogenic resistance.
   - Second line choice for treatment failure or organisms resistant to TMP-SMX is with a quinolone (ciprofloxacin or levofloxacin).
   - Patient with refractory infection or with multiple relapses may be offered long-term suppressive therapy.
3. CP/CPPS:
   - No specific treatment. A brief course of nonsteroidal antiinflammatory drugs may be tried until urine localization cultures are completed. Alfzosin may reduce symptoms in men who have not received prior therapy with an alpha-blocker (*N Engl J Med* 359:2663, 2008).
   - Antibiotics are not generally effective and should be avoided in patients who are afebrile and have normal urinalysis results.
   - A trial of treatment with an alpha-adrenergic blocker (terazosin, doxazosin, or tamsulosin) may be considered, but recent trials failed to show a significant reduction in symptoms and the beneficial effects of alpha-blockers may be overestimated because of publication bias.
   - Contributing factors (e.g., stress, neuromuscular factors) should be addressed.
   - Any underlying bladder pathology should be ruled out by cystoscopy and treated if identified.

SUGGESTED READINGS
available at www.expertconsult.com

AUTHOR: **FRED F. FERRI, M.D.**

P

Diseases and Disorders

I

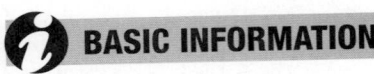

DEFINITION

Pruritus ani refers to an intense chronic itching of the anus and perianal skin.

ICD-9CM CODES
698.0 Pruritus ani

EPIDEMIOLOGY & DEMOGRAPHICS

- Any age can be affected.
- Occurs in 1% to 5% of the population.
- Male/female predominance of 4:1.

PHYSICAL FINDINGS & CLINICAL PRESENTATION

- Anal itching
- Anal fissures
- Hemorrhoids
- Excoriations
- Pinworms
- Fecal incontinence

ETIOLOGY

Anorectal diseases and fecal contamination:
- Diarrhea
- Anal incontinence
- Hemorrhoids
- Fissures
- Fistulae
- Rectal prolapse
- Malignancy: Bowen's disease, epidermoid cancer, perianal Paget's disease

Infections:
- Fungal: candidiasis, dermatophytes
- Parasitic: pinworms, scabies
- Bacterial: *Staphylococcus aureus,* erythrasma
- Lymphogranuloma venereum
- Granuloma inguinale
- Chancroid
- Molluscum contagiosa
- Trichomoniasis
- Venereal: herpes, gonococcal syphilis, human papillomavirus

Local irritants:
- Moisture, obesity, excessive perspiration
- Soaps, hygiene products
- Toilet paper: perfumed, dyed
- Underwear: irritating fabrics, detergents
- Anal creams, suppositories
- Dietary: coffee, beer, acidic foods
- Drugs: mineral oil, ascorbic acid, hydrocortisone sodium succinate, quinine, colchicine

Dermatologic diseases:
- Psoriasis
- Atopic dermatitis
- Seborrheic dermatitis

Section II also describes the various causes of pruritus ani.

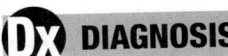 **DIAGNOSIS**

DIFFERENTIAL DIAGNOSIS

- Allergies
- Anxiety
- Dermatologic conditions
- Infections
- Parasites
- Diabetes mellitus
- Chronic liver disease
- Neoplasia
- Proctalgia fugax

WORKUP

- Detailed history regarding bowel habits, hygiene, use of perfumed products, and medical history
- Inspection of perianal area
- Possible biopsy to exclude neoplasia
- Microscopic inspection of scrapings
- Colposcopy of perineum

LABORATORY TESTS

- Chemistry profile
- Urinalysis
- Cultures
- Stool for ova and parasites
- Tape test
- Glucose tolerance test, if necessary

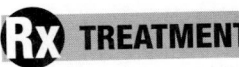 **TREATMENT**

NONPHARMACOLOGIC THERAPY

- Avoidance of tight, nonbreathable clothing and underclothing
- Discontinuation or curtailment of coffee, beer, citrus fruits, tomatoes, chocolate, and tea
- Cleansing of anal area after bowel movements with a premoistened pad or tissue and avoidance of perfumes and dyes present in toilet paper and soaps
- Avoidance of excessive perspiration
- Aggressive management of fecal leakage or incontinence to avoid soiling of perianal skin

ACUTE GENERAL Rx

- Minimization of frequent loose stools with antidiarrheals and fiber agents if appropriate
- Use of a 1% hydrocortisone cream sparingly bid during the acute phase of pruritus ani but not for >2 wk to avoid atrophy
- Treatment of predisposing factors, such as parasites, diabetes, liver disease, hemorrhoids, and other infections

CHRONIC Rx

- Possible complications: excoriation and secondary bacterial infection; must be treated aggressively
- Longstanding, intractable pruritus ani: good response to intracutaneous injections of methylene blue and other agents, steroid injection

DISPOSITION

- Usually good results with total resolution of symptoms
- In some, persistent and recurrent symptoms

REFERRAL

To colorectal specialist if conservative measures fail

SUGGESTED READING
available at www.expertconsult.com

AUTHORS: **MARIA A. CORIGLIANO, M.D.,** and **RUBEN ALVERO, M.D.**

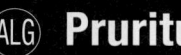

P

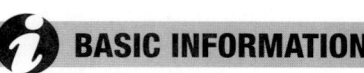 **BASIC INFORMATION**

DEFINITION

Pruritus vulvae refers to intense itching of the female external genitalia.

SYNONYMS

Vulvodynia

ICD-9CM CODES

698.1 Pruritus of genital organs

EPIDEMIOLOGY & DEMOGRAPHICS

- A female disorder that can affect women at any age
- Young girls: infection is usually causative
- Postmenopausal women: frequently affected because of hypoestrogenic state

PHYSICAL FINDINGS & CLINICAL PRESENTATION

Constant, intense itching or burning of the vulva

ETIOLOGY

- Approximately 50% are caused by monilial infection or trichomoniasis.
- Other infectious causes are herpes simplex, condylomata acuminata, and molluscum contagiosum.
- Other causes:
  1. Infestations with scabies, pediculosis pubis, and pinworms
  2. Dermatoses such as hypertrophic dystrophy, lichen sclerosus, lichen planus, and psoriasis
  3. Neoplasms such as Bowen's disease, Paget's disease, and squamous cell carcinoma
  4. Allergic or chemical dermatitis caused by dyes in clothing or toilet paper, detergents, contraceptive gels, vaginal medications, douches, or soaps
  5. Vulvar or vaginal atrophy
- Severe pruritus is probably caused by degeneration and inflammation of terminal nerve fibers.
- Most intense itching occurs with hyperplastic lesions.

- Children typically (75%) have nonspecific pruritus, lichen sclerosus, bacterial infections, yeast infection, or pinworm infestation.

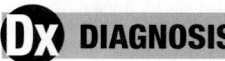 **DIAGNOSIS**

DIFFERENTIAL DIAGNOSIS

- Vulvitis
- Vaginitis
- Lichen sclerosus
- Squamous cell hyperplasia
- Pinworms
- Vulvar cancer
- Syringoma of the vulva

WORKUP

- Inspection of vulva, vagina, and perianal area for infection, fissures, ulcerations, induration, or thick plaques
- Must rule out trichomoniasis, candidiasis, bacterial vaginosis, allergy, vitamin deficiencies, diabetes

LABORATORY TESTS

- Wet prep of saline and potassium hydroxide of vaginal discharge
- Tape test to look for pinworms
- Vaginal cultures
- Biopsy when needed

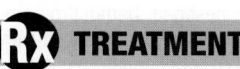 **TREATMENT**

NONPHARMACOLOGIC THERAPY

- Keep vulva clean and dry.
- Wear white cotton panties.
- Avoid perfumes and body creams over vulvar area because they can cause irritation.
- Reduce stress.
- Apply wet dressings with aluminum acetate (Burow's) solution frequently.
- Avoid coffee and caffeine-containing beverages, chocolate, and tomatoes.
- Sitz baths may be helpful.

ACUTE GENERAL Rx

Need to treat underlying problem:
- Yeast infection: any of the vaginal creams or Diflucan 150-mg one-time dose

- Trichomoniasis or *Gardnerella vaginalis:* Flagyl 500 mg or 375 mg PO bid for 7 days
- Urinary tract infection: treatment of specific organism
- Estrogen replacement therapy if atrophy is the cause of pruritus
- Pinworms: mebendazole (Vermox) 100 mg 1 tablet at diagnosis and repeated in 1 to 2 wk; also treat other members in family aged >2 yr
- Squamous cell hyperplasia: local application of corticosteroids
  1. One of the high- or medium-potency corticosteroids (0.025% or 0.01% fluocinolone acetonide or 0.01% triamcinolone acetonide) can be used to relieve itching.
  2. Rub into vulva bid or tid for 4 to 6 wk.
  3. Once itching is controlled, fluorinated steroid can be discontinued and patient can be switched to hydrocortisone preparation.
- Lichen sclerosus: topical 2% testosterone in petrolatum massaged into the vulvar tissue bid or tid; Temovate (clobetasol propionate gel 0.05%) cream tid for 5 days is effective
- Treatment with immune response modifiers

CHRONIC Rx

- If not relieved by topical measures: intradermal injection of triamcinolone (10 mg/ml diluted 2:1 saline); 0.1 ml of the suspension injected at 1-cm intervals and tissue gently massaged
- If symptoms still uncontrollable: SC injection of absolute alcohol 0.1 ml at 1-cm intervals

DISPOSITION

Usually controlled with conservative measures and topical steroids

REFERRAL

To a gynecologist for further workup if conservative measures do not give relief

SUGGESTED READINGS

available at www.expertconsult.com

AUTHORS: **MARIA A. CORIGLIANO, M.D.,** and **RUBEN ALVERO, M.D.**

BASIC INFORMATION

DEFINITION

The term "pseudogout" refers to an acute synovitis caused by calcium pyrophosphate dihydrate (CPPD) crystals. CPPD deposition diseases comprises a spectrum of clinical syndromes including pseudogout, chondrocalcinosis, and pyrophosphate arthropathy. Chondrocalcinosis (CC) refers to the presence of calcification in cartilage by radiograph and does not confirm the diagnosis of pseudogout as it can be present in other types of crystal deposition diseases or asymptomatic. Pyrophosphate arthropathy is the term used for a chronic structural arthropathy related to CPPD deposition.

SYNONYMS

Calcium pyrophosphate dihydrate crystal deposition disease (CPPD crystal deposition disease)
Chondrocalcinosis
Pyrophosphate arthropathy

ICD-9CM CODES
275.4 Chondrocalcinosis

EPIDEMIOLOGY & DEMOGRAPHICS

PREVALENCE:
- Uncertain
- Most linked with advancing age (average age of 70)

GENETICS:
- Associated with ANKH (ankylosis human) gene, which functions to transport inorganic pyrophosphate (PPi) out of cells. Familial mutations can increase extracellular PPi and lead to onset of CPPD disease in third or fourth decade of life

PHYSICAL FINDINGS & CLINICAL PRESENTATION

- Acute pseudogout: monoarticular attacks most commonly involve the knee but can be polyarticular. Patients, especially the elderly can have systemic manifestations such as fever and altered mental status.
- Asymptomatic CC
- Pyrophosphate arthropathy: chronic arthritis with osteoarthritic features
- "Pseudo-PMR": pain and stiffness in the neck and shoulder girdle mimicking polymyalgia rheumatica (PMR)
- "Pseudo-RA": symmetrical polyarthritis
- Crowned-dens syndrome caused by crystal deposition in the ligamentum flavum of the cervical spine either asymptomatic or causing acute neck pain.

ETIOLOGY
- Idiopathic
- Metabolic: Hyperparathyroidism, hypophosphatasia, hypomagnesemia, hemochromatosis, ochronosis, familial hypocalcuric hypercalcemia, x-linked hypophosphatemic rickets

DIAGNOSIS

DIFFERENTIAL DIAGNOSIS
- Gouty arthritis
- Septic arthritis
- Rheumatoid arthritis
- Polymyalgia rheumatica

Section II describes the differential diagnosis of acute monoarticular and oligoarticular arthritis and crystal-induced arthritides. An algorithm for evaluation of arthralgia is described in Section III, "Arthralgia Limited to One or Few Joints."

LABORATORY TESTS
- Arthrocentesis with presence of weakly positive birefringent rhomboid shaped crystals (yellow perpendicular and blue parallel to polarizer axis) (Fig. 1-308).
- Synovial fluid should always be analyzed for cell count with differential, crystals, gram stain, and culture because gout and septic arthritis can coexist with pseudogout.
- Evaluate for possible metabolic cause, especially in the younger patient aged <55 yr or the patient with florid polyarticular disease.
- Ca, TSH, Mg, Ferritin, **Alkaline Phosphatase, Liver Function Tests**

IMAGING STUDIES
- Plain radiographs often reveal CC located parallel to subchondral bone.
  - Classic locations for CC include knee menisci, wrist triangular fibrocartilage, and symphisis pubis (Fig. 1-309).

℞ TREATMENT

NONPHARMACOLOGIC THERAPY
General measures such as immobilization of inflamed joint

ACUTE GENERAL Rx
- Monoarticular pseudogout:
  - Aspiration with corticosteroid injection (often superior to systemic treatment in the elderly)
- Polyarticular pseudogout:
  - Oral corticosteroids or NSAIDs if not contraindicated

CHRONIC GENERAL Rx
- Prophylaxis: Daily low dose colchicine
  - "Pseudo" RA: Hydroxychloroquine
  - Treat underlying metabolic disease

DISPOSITION
Structural joint damage may occasionally occur, requiring arthroplasty in rare cases.

REFERRAL
Rheumatology

⚠ PEARLS & CONSIDERATIONS

COMMENTS
Acute pseudogout attacks have been reported to occur in the setting of surgical procedures, diuresis, bisphosphonate administration, and hyaluronate joint injections.

SUGGESTED READINGS
available at www.expertconsult.com

AUTHOR: **ELISABETH B. MATSON, D.O.**

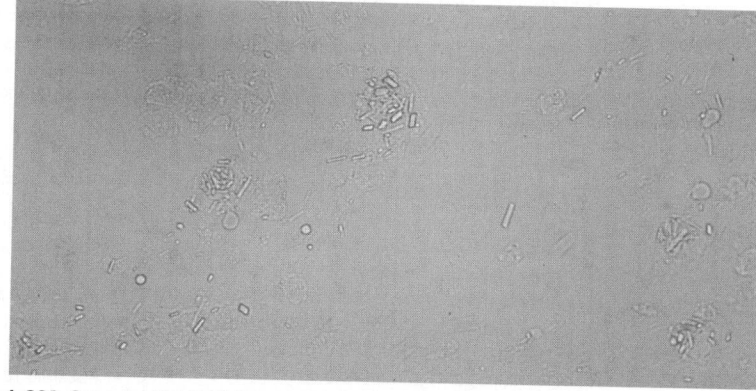

FIGURE 1-308 **Synovial fluid calcium pyrophosphate crystals.** (From Hochberg M et al: *Rheumatology*, Philadelphia, 2011, Mosby. Figure 186-6)

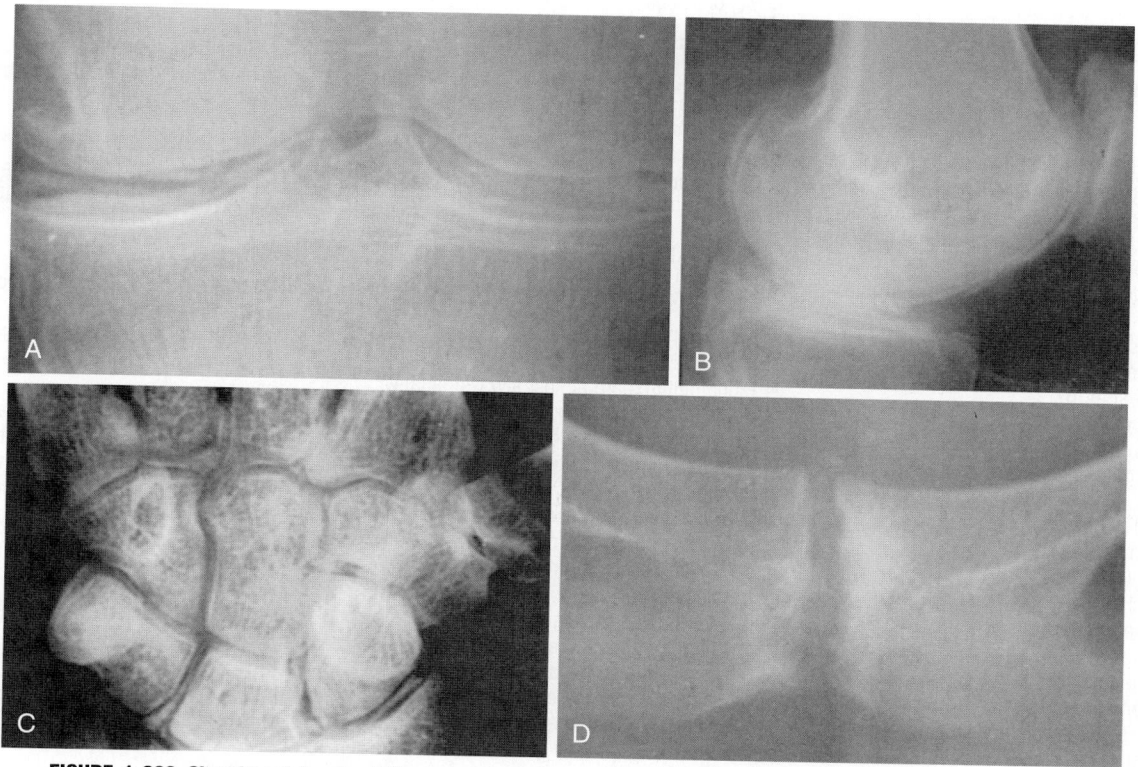

FIGURE 1-309 **Chondrocalcinosis of the most commonly affected joints in calcium pyrophosphate dehydrate deposition disease.** **A,** Lineal calcifications observed in knee menisci and fibrocartilage. **B,** Lateral view showing calcification of the articular cartilage as a line parallel to the femoral condyles. **C,** Calcification of intercarpal joints and triangular ligament. **D,** Calcification of the symphysis pubis fibrocartilage associated with subchondral bone erosions and subchondral increased bone density. (From Firestein G et al: *Kelley's textbook of rheumatology*, ed 8, Philadelphia, 2008, Elsevier. Figure 88-7)

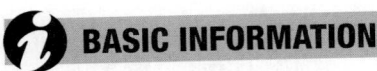

BASIC INFORMATION

DEFINITION

Psittacosis is a systemic infection caused by *Chlamydophila psittaci* (formerly known as *Chlamydia psittaci*).

SYNONYMS

Ornithosis
Parrot pneumonia

ICD-9CM CODES
073.9 Psittacosis

EPIDEMIOLOGY & DEMOGRAPHICS

INCIDENCE (IN U.S.):
- 21 cases reported in 2005
- True incidence possibly higher because infections may be subclinical
- Highest incidence among pet owners and people working with birds

PEAK INCIDENCE: Age 30 to 60 yr

PREVALENCE (IN U.S.):
- Low among human beings
- Organism carried by 5% to 8% of birds

PREDOMINANT SEX: Equal sex distribution

PREDOMINANT AGE: More common in adults

PHYSICAL FINDINGS & CLINICAL PRESENTATION

- Incubation period of 5 to 15 days
- Subclinical infection
- Onset abrupt or insidious
- Most common symptoms:
  1. Fever
  2. Myalgias
  3. Chills
  4. Cough
- Most common clinical syndrome: atypical pneumonia with fever, headache, dry cough, and a chest radiograph more dramatically abnormal than the physical examination
- Ranges from mild disease to respiratory failure and death, although this is extremely unusual
- Other clinical presentations:
  1. Mononucleosis-like syndrome
  2. Typhoidal form
- Most frequent physical findings:
  1. Fever
  2. Pharyngeal erythema
  3. Rales
  4. Hepatomegaly
- Less common findings:
  1. Somnolence
  2. Confusion
  3. Relative bradycardia
  4. Pleural rub
  5. Adenopathy
  6. Splenomegaly
  7. Horder's spots (pink blanching maculopapular rash)

- Besides the lungs, other specific end-organ involvement:
  1. Pericarditis
  2. Myocarditis
  3. Endocarditis
  4. Hepatitis
  5. Joints
  6. Kidneys (glomerulonephritis)
  7. Central nervous system

ETIOLOGY

- *C. psittaci* is an obligate intracellular bacterium.
- Infection is usually spread by the respiratory route from infected birds.
- There is a history of exposure to birds in 85% of patients.
- Strains from turkeys and psittacine birds are most virulent for human beings.
- Cows, goats, and sheep are occasionally implicated.

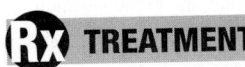

DIAGNOSIS

DIFFERENTIAL DIAGNOSIS

- Legionella
- Mycoplasma
- *Chlamydophila pneumoniae* (Taiwan acute respiratory strain)
- Viral respiratory infections
- Typhoid fever
- Viral hepatitis
- Aseptic meningitis
- Mononucleosis

WORKUP

- Complete blood count, renal and liver function tests
- *Chlamydophila* serology
- Chest x-ray examination
- Special immunostaining of respiratory secretions

LABORATORY TESTS

- White blood count is normal or slightly elevated.
- Mild liver function abnormalities are common (50%).
- Blood cultures are almost always negative.
- Studies on respiratory secretions:
  1. Direct immunofluorescent antibody of respiratory secretions with monoclonal antibodies to chlamydial antigens
  2. *Chlamydophila* lipopolysaccharide antigen by enzyme immunoassay
  3. Polymerase chain reaction
- Serologic studies:
  1. Complement-fixing antibodies
  2. Microimmunofluorescence
  3. Possible false-negative results and cross-reaction with other chlamydial species with both techniques

IMAGING STUDIES

- Chest x-ray examination is abnormal in 50% to 90% with a variety of patterns.
- Pleural effusions are common.

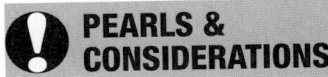

TREATMENT

NONPHARMACOLOGIC THERAPY

Oxygen supplementation as needed

ACUTE GENERAL Rx

- Tetracycline (500 mg PO qid) *or*
- Doxycycline (100 mg PO bid) *or*
- Erythromycin (500 mg PO qid): less effective

CHRONIC Rx

In the rare cases of endocarditis, combination of heart valve replacement and prolonged antibiotic course may be the treatment of choice.

DISPOSITION

- Mortality rate is low (0.7%)
- Poor prognostic factors:
  1. Advanced age
  2. Leukopenia
  3. Severe hypoxemia
  4. Renal failure
  5. Confusion
  6. Multilobe pulmonary involvement
- Possible reinfection

REFERRAL

- To infectious disease expert:
  1. Complicated atypical pneumonia or other end-organ involvement
  2. Suspicion of an outbreak
- To pulmonologist for diagnostic bronchoscopy

PEARLS & CONSIDERATIONS

COMMENTS

- Hospitalized patients do not require specific isolation precautions.
- Any confirmed or suspected case of psittacosis should be reported to public health authorities.
- Recent evidence indicates that *C. psittaci* may be associated with induction of a rare form of lymphoma found in the ocular adnexa; case reports have described regression of ocular lymphoma with antibiotic treatment for *C. psittaci*.

SUGGESTED READINGS
available at www.expertconsult.com

AUTHORS: **GLENN G. FORT, M.D., M.P.H.,** and **DENNIS J. MIKOLICH, M.D.**

BASIC INFORMATION

DEFINITION

Psoriasis is a chronic skin disorder characterized by excessive proliferation of keratinocytes, resulting in the formation of thickened scaly plaques, itching, and inflammatory changes of the epidermis and dermis. The various forms of psoriasis include guttate, pustular, and arthritis variants.

ICD-9CM CODES
696.0 Psoriasis, arthritis, arthropathic
696.1 Psoriasis, any type except arthropathic

EPIDEMIOLOGY & DEMOGRAPHICS

- Psoriasis affects 1% to 3% of the world's population. Most patients have limited psoriasis involving <5% of their body surface.
- There is a strong association between psoriasis and human leukocyte antigens (HLAs) B13, B17, and B27 (pustular psoriasis).
- Peak age of onset is bimodal (adolescents and at age 60 yr).
- Men and women are affected equally.

PHYSICAL FINDINGS & CLINICAL PRESENTATION

- The primary psoriatic lesion is an erythematous papule topped by a loosely adherent scale. Scraping the scale results in several bleeding points (Auspitz sign).
- Chronic plaque psoriasis generally manifests with symmetric, sharply demarcated, erythematous, silver-scaled patches affecting primarily the intergluteal folds, elbows, scalp, fingernails, toenails, and knees (Fig. 1-310, A). This form accounts for 80% of psoriasis cases.
- Psoriasis can also develop at the site of any physical trauma (sunburn, scratching). This is known as Koebner's phenomenon.
- Nail involvement is common (pitting of the nail plate), resulting in hyperkeratosis, onychodystrophy with onycholysis (Fig. 1-310, B).
- Pruritus is variable; soreness and bleeding may occur.
- Joint involvement can result in sacroiliitis and spondylitis.
- Guttate psoriasis is generally preceded by streptococcal pharyngitis and manifests with multiple droplike lesions on the extremities and the trunk (Fig. 1-310, C).
- Adverse effect on psychological and social functioning, with affected persons often feeling stigmatized.

ETIOLOGY

- Unknown, but there is a strong genetic component and high heritability. There are at least nine chromosomal loci with liinkage to psoriasis. These loci are called psoriasis susceptibility 1 through 9 (PSORS1-PSORS9). PSORS1 locus in the major histocompatibility complex (MHC) region on chromosome 6 is considered the most important susceptibility locus and is believed to account for 35% to 50% of the heritability of the disease.
- Familial clustering (genetic transmission with a dominant mode with variable penetrants).
- One third of persons affected have a positive family history.

DIAGNOSIS

DIFFERENTIAL DIAGNOSIS

- Contact dermatitis
- Atopic dermatitis
- Stasis dermatitis
- Tinea
- Nummular dermatitis
- Candidiasis
- Mycosis fungoides
- Cutaneous systemic lupus erythematosus
- Secondary and tertiary syphilis
- Drug eruption

WORKUP

- Diagnosis is clinical.
- Skin biopsy is rarely necessary.

LABORATORY TESTS

Generally not necessary for diagnosis

TREATMENT

NONPHARMACOLOGIC THERAPY

- Sunbathing generally leads to improvement.
- Eliminate triggering factors (e.g., stress, certain medications [e.g., lithium, beta-blockers, antimalarials]).
- Patients with psoriasis benefit from a daily bath in warm water followed by application of a cream or ointment moisturizer. Regular use or an emollient moisturizer limits evaporation of water from the skin and allows the stratum corneum to rehydrate itself.

GENERAL Rx

Therapeutic options vary according to the extent of disease. Approximately 70% to 80% of all patients can be treated adequately with topical therapy.

- Patients with limited disease (<20% of the body) can be treated with the following:
  1. Topical steroids: disadvantages are brief remissions, expense, and decreased effect with continued use. Salicylic acid can be compounded by pharmacist in concentrations of 2% to 10% and used in combination with a corticosteroid to decrease the amount of scale.
  2. Calcipotriene (Dovonex): a vitamin D analogue effective for moderate plaque psoriasis. Adults should comb the hair, apply solution to the lesions, and rub it in, avoiding uninvolved skin. Disadvantages include its cost and potential burning and skin irritation. It should not be used concurrently with salicylic acid because calcipotriene is inactivated by the acidic nature of salicylic acid. Taclonex ointment is a combination of calcipotriene and the high-potency corticosteroid betamethasone dipropionate. It is well tolerated and more effective than either agent used alone but also much more expensive.
  3. Tar products (Estar, LCD, psorigel) can be used overnight and are most effective when combined with ultraviolet B (UVB) light (Goeckerman regimen).
  4. Anthralin (Drithocreme): useful for chronic plaques; can result in purple-brown staining; best used with UVB light.
  5. Retinoids such as tazarotene 0.05%, 0.1% cream or gel, are effective in thinning plaques but are expensive and can cause irritation.
  6. Other useful measures include tape or occlusive dressing, UVB and lubricating agents, and interlesional steroids.
- Therapeutic options for persons with generalized disease (affecting >20% of the body) and for those with inadequate response to topical agents:
  1. UVB light exposure three times a week: this therapy does not require administration of a systemic drug (unlike psoralen plus ultraviolet A [PUVA]), but to be effective, it requires removal of scale with keratolytic agents and emollients.
  2. Oral PUVA administered two to three times weekly is effective for generalized disease. It is often considered in patients for whom narrow-band UVB therapy is ineffective. However, many PUVA treatments are required, necessitating frequent office visits, and it may be associated with phototoxicity, such as erythema and blistering, and increased risk of skin cancer.

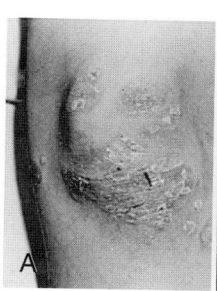 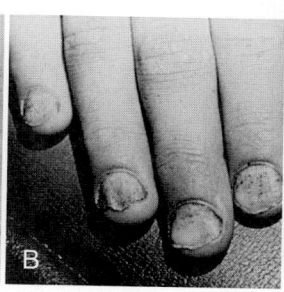 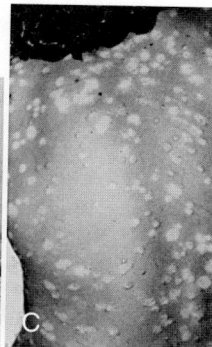

FIGURE 1-310 A, Chronic psoriatic plaques on the knee. **B,** Psoriatic nail changes of pitting and dystrophy. **C,** Guttate psoriasis in widespread distribution over the trunk. (From Behrman RE: *Nelson textbook of pediatrics,* ed 17, Philadelphia, 2004, WB Saunders.)

- Systemic treatments include methotrexate 25 mg/wk for severe psoriasis. Etretinate (Tegison) (a synthetic retinoid) is most effective for palmar-plantar pustular psoriasis. Dose is 0.5 to 1 mg/kg/day. It can cause liver enzyme and lipid abnormalities and is teratogenic.
- Cyclosporine is also effective in severe psoriasis; however, relapses are common.
- Chronic plaque psoriasis may be treated with alefacept, a recombinant protein that selectively targets T lymphocytes. Treatment with alefacept for 12 wk (0.025, 0.075, or 0.150 mg/kg of body weight IV weekly) may result in significant improvement. Some patients also demonstrate a sustained clinical response after the cessation of treatment. This medication is very expensive (a 12-wk course costs >$8000).
- TNF inhibitors: Treatment with etanercept, a tumor necrosis factor (TNF) antagonist, for 24 wk can also lead to a reduction in severity of plaque psoriasis. Efalizumab, a humanized monoclonal antibody that inhibits the activation of T cells, has also been reported to produce significant improvement in plaque psoriasis over a 24-wk treatment period. Adalimumab—a fully human, anti-TNF-alpha monoclonal antibody—has been reported to be effective for joint and skin manifestations of psoriasis.
- A newer biologic agent in patients with moderate to severe plaque psoriasis is ustekinumab (an interleukin-12 and interleukin-23 blocker). A recent trial showed that it was more effective than etanercept for the treatment of moderate-to-severe psoriasis.

DISPOSITION

The course of psoriasis is chronic, and the disease may be refractory to treatment.

REFERRAL

- Dermatology referral is recommended in all patients with generalized disease.
- Hospital admission may be necessary for severe diffuse or poorly responsive psoriasis. The Goeckerman regimen combines daily application of tar with UVB exposure and can result in prolonged remissions.

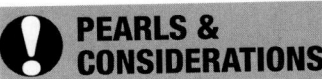

PEARLS & CONSIDERATIONS

COMMENTS

Psoriasis is more emotionally than physically disabling for most patients. Counseling may be indicated, particularly when it affects younger patients.

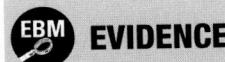 **EVIDENCE**

available at www.expertconsult.com

SUGGESTED READINGS
available at www.expertconsult.com

AUTHOR: **FRED F. FERRI, M.D.**

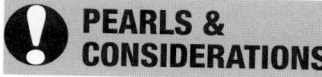 BASIC INFORMATION

DEFINITION

A state in which external reality is distorted by delusions and/or hallucinations (a delusion is a fixed false belief; a hallucination is a false auditory, visual, olfactory, tactile, or taste perception).

SYNONYMS

Psychosis is a key finding in many mental illnesses, such as brief psychotic disorder, delusional disorder, schizoaffective disorder, schizophrenia, schizophreniform disorder, or shared psychotic disorder.

EPIDEMIOLOGY & DEMOGRAPHICS

One-year prevalence: 4.5 per 1000. The demographics of psychosis depend on the underlying disorder.

PHYSICAL FINDINGS & CLINICAL PRESENTATION

History
- Past and current medical history important to identify potential medical etiologies
- Medication use
- Use of illicit substances
- Identification of functional and social impairment
- Behavior that is odd or unpredictable; patient may clearly be responding to internal stimuli
Examination:
- Examine for symptoms of:
  - Mood disorder: delusions or hallucinations are usually congruent with the mood (e.g., auditory hallucinations in a depressed patient may tell the patient what a terrible person he is).
  - Altered, or disorganized thought pattern: usually reflected in disorganized speech (including word salad, thought blocking, rhyming, clang).
  - Lack of insight into problems.
  - Signs of Parkinson's disease, dementia.

ETIOLOGY

- Involves an interaction among:
  1. Dopaminergic overactivity (particularly in the mesolimbic, nigrostriatal, and mesocortical systems)
  2. Environmental, social, or childhood factors
  3. Genetic predisposition

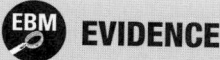 DIAGNOSIS

WORKUP

- Evaluate for potential confounding factors
- Underlying mental disorder: schizophrenia, major depression, brief psychotic disorder, delusional disorder, schizoaffective disorder, schizophreniform disorder, shared psychotic disorder
- Underlying personality disorder: borderline, paranoid, schizoid, schizotypal
- Underlying medical conditions: HIV/AIDS, Parkinson's disease, Huntington's disease, leprosy, malaria, sarcoidosis, systemic lupus erythematosus, prion disease, hypoglycemia, postpartum state, cerebrovascular event, temporal lobe epilepsy, brain neoplasm
- Medications: systemic steroids, anticonvulsants, antiparkinsonian medications, some chemotherapy, scopolamine
- Underlying dementia: Alzheimer's disease, Lewy body dementia
- Illicit drugs (usually with chronic use; can be caused by intoxication or withdrawal): LSD, PCP, cocaine, gamma-hydroxybutyrate (GHB; withdrawal), alcohol, amphetamines, marijuana
- Traumatic brain injury
- Intensive care unit stay: hypoxia, decreased cardiac output, infection, medications, sleep deprivation, alteration of diurnal cycle, sensory deprivation or overload, pain
- Emotional stress

LABORATORY TESTS

Consider checking chemistry panel (calcium), complete blood count, liver function tests, cortisol, HIV, rapid plasma reagin, thyroid-stimulating hormone, toxicology screen, lumbar puncture (LP).

IMAGING STUDIES

Consider chest x-ray examination (sarcoid), electroencephalography, head CT or MRI

Rx TREATMENT

NONPHARMACOLOGIC THERAPY

- Cognitive-behavioral therapy.
- Social and behavioral skills training.
- Training for self-management of disease.
- Aforementioned strategies favored over psychoanalytic techniques given the relative inability for abstract thought and lack of insight in psychotic patients.
- Family intervention, including education and strategies to reduce emotional expression.
- Counseling for substance abuse.

ACUTE GENERAL Rx

- Antipsychotics, such as haloperidol combined with promethazine, an antihistamine to reduce side effects; low doses should control first episode. Use with caution in elderly patients because adverse effects limit effectiveness.
- Benzodiazepines if agitation is severe.
- Discontinue offending medication if present.

CHRONIC Rx

Second-generation antipsychotics may reduce the incidence of tardive dyskinesia but may increase incidence of metabolic disorders compared with first-generation antipsychotics.

DISPOSITION

Prognosis varies according to etiology of psychosis. In general, the more severe and longer the psychotic episode, the worse the prognosis.

REFERRAL

Patient should be admitted for acute stabilization if actively psychotic to prevent harm to self and others as well as ensure administration of medications.

! PEARLS & CONSIDERATIONS

- Delusions and/or hallucinations are hallmarks of psychosis.
- Rule out medical or drug causes of psychosis.
- Antipsychotics are the mainstay of acute and chronic treatment.
- Consider alternatives to antipsychotics in elderly or intellectually disabled patients.

EBM EVIDENCE

available at www.expertconsult.com

SUGGESTED READINGS

available at www.expertconsult.com

AUTHOS: **MICHAEL K. ONG, M.D., PH.D.,** and **RICHARD J. GOLDBERG, M.D.**

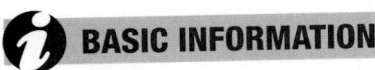 **BASIC INFORMATION**

DEFINITION
Pubertal delay refers to delayed development and maturation of the reproductive system. The diagnostic criterion is a delay of more than 2 standard deviations from the mean age of pubertal onset.

ICD-9CM CODES
259.0 Delay in sexual development and puberty, not elsewhere classified

EPIDEMIOLOGY & DEMOGRAPHICS
PREVALENCE: 2.5% of healthy adolescents have a diagnosis of pubertal delay using the statistical diagnostic criteria
GENETICS: Constitutional delay of puberty often runs in families. Pubertal delay occurs with some congenital syndromes, such as Prader-Willi syndrome and Noonan syndrome, and in patients with enzyme defects in sex steroid synthesis, as well as others.

PHYSICAL FINDINGS & CLINICAL PRESENTATION
Puberty is clinically delayed for girls if there is no evidence of breast development by 13 yr of age, absence of menarche by age 16 yr, or absence of menarche within 5 yr of pubertal onset. Puberty is clinically delayed for boys if there is no evidence of testicular enlargement by 14 yr of age, or >5 yr between start and completion of growth of genitalia.

ETIOLOGY
Puberty begins with increased pulsatile secretion of gonadotropin-releasing hormone (GnRH) from the hypothalamus, increased pituitary responsiveness to GnRH, secretion of gonadotropins, gonadal maturation, and increasing production of sex steroids. Increased concentration of sex steroids induces the development of secondary sexual characteristics, acceleration of growth, and fertility. Numerous causes can lead to pubertal delay, including chronic disease, normal variation, congenital syndromes, or other factors.

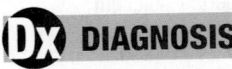 **DIAGNOSIS**

DIFFERENTIAL DIAGNOSIS
Normal or low serum gonadotropins
- Constitutional delay
- Hypothalamic dysfunction
  - Malnutrition or eating disorder
  - Strenuous exercise
  - Chronic illness
  - Severe obesity
  - Central nervous system tumors
- Hypopituitarism
  - Panhypopituitarism
  - Isolated gonadotropin deficiency
  - Kallman syndrome (associated with anosmia)
- Hypothyroidism
- Hyperprolactinemia
  - Pituitary adenoma
  - Drug-associated (cannabis, cocaine)

Increased serum gonadotropins
- Turner's syndrome (gonadal dysgenesis)
- Klinefelter syndrome
- Bilateral gonadal failure
  - Primary testicular failure
  - Anorchia
  - Premature ovarian failure
  - Resistant ovary syndrome
  - Irradiation, cytotoxic therapy
  - Trauma
  - Infections (e.g., mumps, orchitis)

Other conditions
- Prader-Willi syndrome
- Noonan syndrome
- Androgen resistance
- Steroidogenic enzyme defects

WORKUP
- Given the extensive differential diagnosis for pubertal delay, a systematic and focused approach is necessary. A careful history, including family history and social history, can identify eating and exercise habits, chronic illnesses, and parental history of pubertal delay.
- Growth measurement should include height and weight, a growth chart to assess rate of growth, and calculation of the sex-adjusted midparental height that represents the statistically most probable adult height for the child.
  - For boys, add 2.5 inches (6.5 cm) from the mean of the parents' heights. For girls, subtract 2.5 inches (6.5 cm) from the mean of the parents' heights.
  - Physical exam can reveal signs of sexual maturation, stigmata of congenital syndromes, and nutritional status. Include neurologic exam (visual fields, ophthalmologic), thyroid, chest, heart, abdomen, and Tanner staging.

LABORATORY TESTS
- Serum gonadotropin levels (luteinizing hormone, follicle-stimulating hormone) can help distinguish disorders of congenital or acquired gonadal failure from other causes. By bone age 10 to 12 yr gonadal failure produces elevated levels of serum gonadotropins. If levels are low or normal, constitutional delay is the most frequent diagnosis.
- Chromosomal analysis if there is a suspicion of gonadal dysgenesis or Klinefelter syndrome.
- Screening studies include complete blood count, erythrocyte sedimentation rate, serum prolactin, serum thyroid-stimulating hormone.
- Endocrinologist may do further studies such as IGF-1 to screen for growth hormone disorders and GnRH stimulation testing.

IMAGING STUDIES
Consider bone age (left hand and wrist film), which is delayed in constitutional delay and GnRH deficiency; MRI of the head to evaluate for tumors of pituitary or hypothalamus and absence of olfactory bulb and tract, which occurs in Kallman syndrome (absence of GnRH); and pelvic ultrasound, which can be helpful in detecting intraabdominal testes and to evaluate Mullerian anatomy.

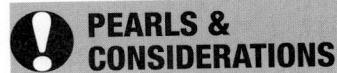 **TREATMENT**

- Treat underlying cause if it is identified.
- Constitutional delay can be managed with reassurance that the delay will have no effect on final adult height or development. Short-term hormonal therapy can be used to hasten puberty if the delay is causing severe psychosocial difficulties. Monthly testosterone injections are used for boys who have begun pubertal development.
- Gonadotropin deficiency or hypogonadism requires lifelong sex steroid replacement.
- Psychosocial evaluation, support, and treatment as needed.

REFERRAL
Pediatric endocrinology

! PEARLS & CONSIDERATIONS

COMMENTS
- Constitutional delay is the most common cause of pubertal delay and is often associated with a positive family history in parents and/or siblings, but other causes, such as Turner syndrome and systemic disorders, should be excluded.
- No studies reliably distinguish constitutional delay from gonadotropin deficiency.

PATIENT & FAMILY EDUCATION
- The Magic Foundation, a support group for patients and their families (http://www.magicfoundation.org)
- The American Academy of Family Physicians (http://www.aafp.org)
- American Academy of Pediatrics (http://www.aap.org)
- Pediatric Endocrine Society (http://www.lwpes.org)

SUGGESTED READINGS
available at www.expertconsult.com

AUTHOR: **NIRALI BORA, M.D.**

BASIC INFORMATION

DEFINITION

Acute cardiogenic pulmonary edema (ACPE) is a life-threatening condition that may occur if there is elevated left ventricular filling pressure related to systolic or diastolic dysfunction.

SYNONYMS

Cardiogenic pulmonary edema
Acute cardiogenic pulmonary edema
ACPE

ICD-9CM CODES

428.1 Acute pulmonary edema with heart disease

EPIDEMIOLOGY & DEMOGRAPHICS

- Leading cause of hospitalization (6.5 million hospital days in the U.S. each year)
- In-hospital mortality rate is 10% to 20%, particularly when associated with acute MI

PHYSICAL FINDINGS & CLINICAL PRESENTATION

- Dyspnea with rapid, shallow breathing
- Diaphoresis, perioral and peripheral cyanosis
- Pink, frothy sputum
- Moist, bilateral pulmonary rales
- Increased pulmonary second sound, S_3 gallop
- Hypertension (unless in cardiogenic shock and hypotensive)
- Tachycardia
- Bulging neck veins

ETIOLOGY

Increased pulmonary capillary pressure attributable to:

- Acute myocardial infarction
- Exacerbation of chronic congestive heart failure
- Valvular regurgitation (e.g., mitral regurgitation)
- Ventricular septal defect
- Severe myocardial ischemia
- Mitral stenosis
- Other: cardiac tamponade, endocarditis, myocarditis, arrhythmias, cardiomyopathy, hypertensive crisis

DIAGNOSIS

DIFFERENTIAL DIAGNOSIS

- Noncardiogenic pulmonary edema (see Fig. 1-311)
- Pulmonary embolism
- Exacerbation of asthma
- Exacerbation of chronic obstructive pulmonary disease
- Sarcoidosis
- Pulmonary fibrosis
- Viral pneumonitis and other pulmonary infections

LABORATORY TESTS

- Arterial blood gases (ABGs): respiratory and metabolic acidosis, decreased Pa_{O_2}, increased Pc_{O_2}, low pH. (NOTE: The patient may initially show respiratory alkalosis as a result of hyperventilation in attempts to maintain Pa_{O_2}.)
- Measurement of plasma brain natriuretic peptide (elevated).
- Cardiac biomarker: evaluate for possible acute myocardial infarction.
- Basic chemistries: hyponatremia is common in chronic heart failure; evaluate renal function.

IMAGING STUDIES

- ECG:
  1. May have evidence of ischemia, arrhythmias, or left ventricular hypertrophy (often seen in diastolic dysfunction)
- Chest radiograph:
  1. Pulmonary congestion with Kerley B lines; fluffy perihilar infiltrates in the early stages; bilateral interstitial alveolar infiltrates
  2. Pleural effusions
- Echocardiogram:
  1. Useful to evaluate valvular abnormalities, diastolic versus systolic dysfunction
  2. Can help differentiate cardiogenic versus noncardiogenic pulmonary edema
  3. Can also estimate pulmonary capillary wedge pressure and rule out presence of myxoma or atrial thrombus
- Right heart catheterization (selected patients): cardiac pressures and cardiogenic pulmonary edema reveal increased pulmonary artery diastolic pressure and pulmonary capillary wedge pressure (PCWP) ≥ 25 mm Hg

TREATMENT

ACUTE GENERAL Rx

All the following steps can be performed concomitantly:

- 100% oxygen by face mask. Noninvasive ventilation (continuous positive airway pressure [CPAP]) or noninvasive intermittent positive-pressure ventilation induces a more rapid improvement in respiratory distress and metabolic disturbance than does standard oxygen therapy but has no effect on short-term mortality rate. Both CPAP and bilevel PAP systems can improve oxygenation and lower carbon dioxide tensions. Monitor ABGs; if marked hypoxemia or severe respiratory acidosis, intubate the patient and place on a ventilator. Positive end-expiratory pressure increases functional capacity and improves oxygenation.
- Preload Reducers:
  1. Furosemide: 1 mg/kg IV bolus (typically 40 to 100 mg) to rapidly establish diuresis and decrease venous return through its venodilator action; may double the dose in 30 min if no effect.
  2. Nitrates: particularly useful if the patient has concomitant chest pain or hypertensive.
     a. Nitroglycerin: 150 to 600 mcg SL or nitroglycerin spray may be given immediately on arrival and repeated multiple times if the patient remains symptomatic and blood pressure remains stable.
     b. 2% nitroglycerin ointment: 1 to 3 inches out of the tube applied continuously; absorption may be erratic.

TYPES OF PULMONARY EDEMA

Signs	Cardiac	Renal	Lung Injury
Heart size	Enlarged	Normal	Normal
Blood flow	Inverted	Balanced	Normal
Kerley lines	Common	Common	Absent
Edema	Basilar	Central: butterfly	Diffuse
Air bronchograms	Not common	Not common	Very common
Pleural effusions	Very common	Common	Not common

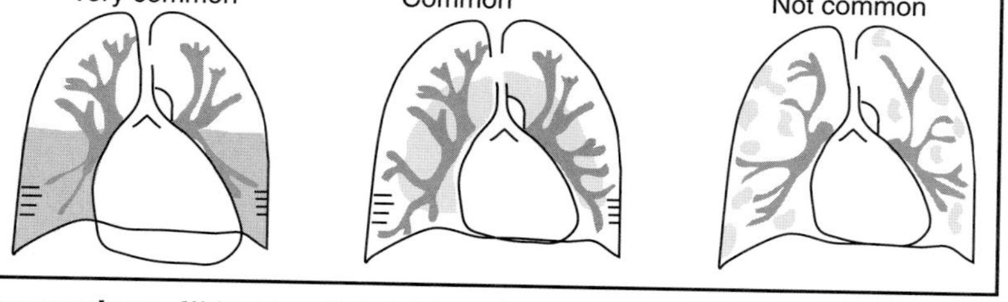

FIGURE 1-311 Types of pulmonary edema. (Weisslederer R et al: *Primer of diagnostic imaging*, St Louis, 2007, Mosby.)

c. IV nitroglycerin: 100 mg in 500 ml of D_5W solution; start at 6 mcg/min (2 ml/hr).
3. Morphine: 2 to 4 mg IV, SC, or IM; may repeat q15min prn. It decreases venous return, anxiety, and systemic vascular resistance (naloxone should be available at bedside to reverse the effects of morphine if respiratory depression occurs). Morphine may induce hypotension in volume-depleted patients.

• Vasodilator therapy:
1. Angiotensin-converting enzyme (ACE) inhibitors: Captopril 25 mg PO tablet can be used for SL administration (placing a drop or two of water on the tablet and placing it under the tongue helps dissolve it); onset of action is <10 min, peak effect can be reached in 30 min. ACE inhibitors can also be given IV (e.g., enalaprilat 1 mg IV given q2h prn).
2. Nitroprusside: useful for afterload reduction in hypertensive patients with decreased cardiac index (CI).
   a. Increases the CI and decreases left ventricular filling pressure.
   b. Nitroprusside use in patients with acute myocardial infarction is controversial because it may increase ischemia by decreasing blood flow to the myocardium.

• Ionotropes:
1. Dobutamine: parenteral inotropic agent of choice in severe cases of cardiogenic pulmonary edema. It can be administered at a dosage of 2.5 to 10 mcg/kg/min IV.
2. IV phosphodiesterase inhibitors (amrinone, milrinone) may be useful in refractory cases.

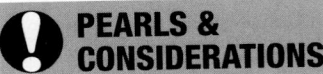

PEARLS & CONSIDERATIONS

COMMENTS

Although a recent large trial suggests that noninvasive ventillation may be less effective for ACPE and contradicts results from previous studies, the evidence in aggregate still favors the use of noninvasive ventillation in patients with ACPE

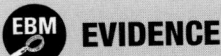 **EVIDENCE**

available at www.expertconsult.com

SUGGESTED READINGS

available at www.expertconsult.com

AUTHORS: **SCOTT COHEN, M.D.,**
FRED F. FERRI, M.D., and
GAURAV CHOUDHARY, M.D.

BASIC INFORMATION

DEFINITION

Pulmonary embolism (PE) refers to the lodging of a thrombus or other embolic material from a distant site in the pulmonary circulation.

SYNONYMS

Pulmonary thromboembolism
PE

ICD-9CM CODES
415.1 Pulmonary embolism and infarction

EPIDEMIOLOGY & DEMOGRAPHICS

- 650,000 cases of PE occur in the U.S. each year (increased incidence in women and with advanced age); annually, as many as 300,000 people in the U.S. die from acute PE, and the diagnosis is often not made until after autopsy. The incidence of PE is increasing with the increasing use of spiral CT scans, with a lower severity of illness and lower mortality, suggesting the increase is caused by earlier diagnosis.
- More than 90% of pulmonary emboli originate in the deep venous system of the lower extremities.
- Pulmonary thromboembolism is associated with >200,000 hospitalizations each yr in the U.S.
- 8% to 10% of victims of PE die within the first hr.

PHYSICAL FINDINGS & CLINICAL PRESENTATION

- Most common symptom: dyspnea (85%)
- Tachypnea (30%)
- Chest pain: may be nonpleuritic or pleuritic (infarction) (40%)
- Syncope (massive PE) (10%)
- Fever, diaphoresis, apprehension
- Hemoptysis (2%)
- Evidence of DVT may be present (e.g., swelling and tenderness of extremities)
- Cardiac examination: may reveal tachycardia (23%), increased pulmonic component of S_2, murmur of tricuspid insufficiency, right ventricular heave, right-sided S_3
- Pulmonary examination: may demonstrate rales, localized wheezing, friction rub

ETIOLOGY

- Thrombus, fat, or other foreign material
- Risk factors for PE:
  1. Prolonged immobilization, reduced mobility
  2. Postoperative state, major surgery
  3. Trauma to lower extremities, immobilizer or cast
  4. Estrogen-containing birth control pills, hormone replacement therapy
  5. Prior history of DVT or PE
  6. CHF
  7. Pregnancy and early puerperium
  8. Visceral cancer (lung, pancreas, alimentary and genitourinary tracts)
  9. Spinal cord injury
  10. Advanced age
  11. Obesity
  12. Hematologic disease (e.g., factor V Leiden mutation, antithrombin III deficiency, protein C deficiency, protein S deficiency, lupus anticoagulant, polycythemia vera, dysfibrinogenemia, paroxysmal nocturnal hemoglobinuria, acquired protein C resistance without factor V Leiden, G20210A prothrombin mutation)
  13. COPD, diabetes mellitus, acute medical illness
  14. Prolonged air travel
  15. Central venous catheterization

DIAGNOSIS

DIFFERENTIAL DIAGNOSIS

- Myocardial infarction
- Pericarditis
- Pneumonia
- Pneumothorax
- Chest wall pain
- GI abnormalities (e.g., peptic ulcer, esophageal rupture, gastritis)
- CHF
- Pleuritis
- Anxiety disorder with hyperventilation
- Pericardial tamponade
- Dissection of aorta
- Asthma

WORKUP

- Clinical assessment alone is insufficient to diagnose or rule out PE. It is also important to remember that no single noninvasive test has both high sensitivity and high specificity for PE. Consequently, in addition to clinical assessment, most patients would require an imaging test to diagnose PE. The Wells prediction rules can be used to estimate the probability of PE. Each of the following findings is assigned a score:
  1. Clinical signs/symptoms of deep vein thrombosis (score = 3.0)
  2. No alternate diagnosis likely or more likely than PE (score = 3.0)
  3. Heart rate >100/min (score = 1.5)
  4. Immobilization or surgery in last 4 weeks (score = 1.5)
  5. Previous history of DVT or PE (score = 1.5)
  6. Hemoptysis (score = 1.0)
  7. Cancer actively treated within last 6 months (score = 1.0)
- The probability of PE is high if total score is >6, moderate if 2-6; and low if <2.
- Spiral chest CT with contrast (see Fig. 1-313) is an excellent diagnostic modality.
- V/Q scan is reserved for patients with clinically significant contrast allergies or renal insufficiency.
- Pulmonary angiogram (when indicated) will confirm the diagnosis.
- Serial compressive duplex ultrasonography of lower extremities can be used in patients with "low-probability" lung scan and high clinical suspicion (see "Imaging Studies"). It is useful if positive, negative results do not exclude pulmonary embolism.
- A diagnostic approach to PE is described in Section III.

LABORATORY TESTS

- ABGs may reveal hypoxemia and respiratory alkalosis (decreased $PaCO_2$ and $PaCO_2$ and increased pH); normal results do not rule out PE.
- Alveolar-arteriolar (A-a) oxygen gradient, a measure of the difference in oxygen concentration between alveoli and arterial blood may be elevated. However, a normal A-a gradient does not rule out PE.
- Plasma D-dimer measurement: D-dimer assays by ELISA detect the presence of plasmin-mediated degradation products of fibrin that contain cross-linked D fragments in the whole blood or plasma. A normal plasma D-dimer level is useful to exclude PE in patients with a nondiagnostic lung scan and a low pretest probability of PE. However, it cannot be used to "rule in" the diagnosis because it increases with many other disorders (e.g., metastatic cancer, trauma, sepsis, postoperative state). Plasma D-dimer can also be used in conjunction with lower-extremity compression ultrasonography in patients with indeterminate V/Q and spiral CT scans. Absence of DVT and presence of a normal D-dimer level in these settings generally rules out clinically significant PE.
- Elevated cardiac troponin levels also occur in patients with PE because of right ventricular dilation and myocardial injury; therefore, PE should be considered in the differential diagnosis of all patients presenting with chest pain or dyspnea and elevated cardiac troponin levels.
- Elevated serum BNP levels in patients with acute PE may reflect RV overload.
- ECG is abnormal in 85% of patients with acute PE. Frequent abnormalities are sinus tachycardia; nonspecific ST-segment or T-wave changes; S-1, Q-3, T-3 pattern (10% of patients); S-1, S-2, S-3 pattern; T-wave inversion in V_1 to V_6; acute RBBB; new-onset atrial fibrillation; ST segment depression in lead II; right ventricular strain. A right ventricular strain pattern on ECG in patients with PG and normal blood pressure is associated with adverse short-term outcome and adds incremental prognostic value to echocardiographic evidence of right ventricular function.

IMAGING STUDIES

- Chest x-ray may be normal; suggestive findings include elevated diaphragm, pleural effusion, dilation of pulmonary artery, infiltrate or consolidation, abrupt vessel cut-off, oligemia distal to the PE (Westermark sign) or atelectasis. A wedge-shaped consolidation in the middle and lower lobes is suggestive of a pulmonary infarction and is known as "Hampton's hump."

- Lung scan (in patient with normal chest x-ray examination):
  1. A normal lung scan rules out PE.
  2. A ventilation-perfusion mismatch is suggestive of PE, and a lung scan interpretation of high probability is confirmatory (Fig. 1-312).
  3. If the clinical suspicion of PE is high and the lung scan is interpreted as low probability, moderate probability, or indeterminate, a pulmonary arteriogram is diagnostic; a positive arteriogram confirms diagnosis; a positive compressive duplex ultrasonography for DVT obviates the need for an arteriogram, because treatment with IV anticoagulants is indicated in these patients; the overall sensitivity of compressive ultrasonography for DVT in patients with PE is 29%, specificity 97%; adding ultrasonography in patients with a nondiagnostic lung scan prevents 9% of angiographies; however, this improvement in efficacy is achieved at the cost of unnecessary anticoagulant therapy in 26% of patients who have false-positive ultrasonography results.
- Angiography: pulmonary angiography is the gold standard; however, it is invasive, expensive, and not readily available in some clinical settings. False-positive pulmonary angiograms may result from mediastinal disorders such as radiation fibrosis and tumors.
- CT angiography is an accurate, noninvasive tool in the diagnosis of PE at the main, lobar, and segmental pulmonary artery levels. A major advantage of CT angiography over standard pulmonary angiography is its ability to diagnose intrathoracic disease other than PE that may account for the patient's clinical picture. It is also less invasive, less costly, and more widely available. Its major shortcoming is its poor sensitivity for subsegmental emboli. Gadolinium-enhanced magnetic resonance angiography (MRA) of the pulmonary arteries

has a moderate sensitivity and high specificity for the diagnosis of PE; MRA is best reserved for selected patients when CT scan and/or lung scan are inconclusive and the risk of pulmonary angiography is high.
- ECG: Useful for identifying patients with PE who may have poor prognosis. Moderate or severe hypokinesis, persistent pulmonary hypertension, patent foramen ovale, and free-floating right heart thrombus are markers for increased risk of death or recurrent thrombosis. Such patients should be considered for thrombolysis or embolectomy.

(Rx) TREATMENT

NONPHARMACOLOGIC THERAPY

Correction of risk factors (see "Etiology") to prevent future PE

ACUTE GENERAL Rx

- Unfractionated heparin (UFH) by continuous infusion for at least 5 days or low-molecular-weight heparin (LMWH); many experts recommend a larger initial IV heparin bolus (15,000 to 20,000 U) to block platelet aggregation and thrombi and subsequent release of vasoconstrictive substances.
- Thrombolytic agents (urokinase, tPA, streptokinase): provide rapid resolution of clots; thrombolytic agents are the treatment of choice in patients with massive PE who are hemodynamically unstable and with no contraindication to their use. The use of thrombolytic agents in the treatment of hemodynamically stable patients with acute submassive PE remains controversial. Use of the thrombolytic agents alteplase (100 mg IV over 2-hr period) in normotensive patients with moderate or severe right ventricular dysfunction identified by ECG has been advocated by some physicians. Use of alteplase in conjunction with heparin has been shown to

improve the clinical course of stable patients who have acute submassive PE without internal bleeding. Additional studies are needed to confirm these findings before recommending routine use of this therapeutic approach.
- Long-term treatment is generally carried out with warfarin therapy started on day 1 or 2 and given in a dose to maintain the INR at 2 to 3. Preliminary trials reveal that idraparinux, a long-acting inhibitor of activated factor X, given once weekly SC as a fixed dose for 3 or 6 mo has efficacy similar to that of heparin plus a vitamin-K antagonist in the treatment of DVT and causes less bleeding. However, in patients with PE, idraparinux was less efficacious than standard therapy.
- If thrombolytics and anticoagulants are contraindicated (e.g., GI bleeding, recent CNS surgery, recent trauma) or if the patient continues to have recurrent PE despite anticoagulation therapy, vena caval interruption is indicated by transvenous placement of a Greenfield vena caval filter.
- IVC filter may also be considered as an adjunct to anticoagulation in massive PE when thrombolytics cannot be used.
- Acute pulmonary artery embolectomy may be indicated in a patient with massive pulmonary emboli and refractory hypotension. It should also be considered for patients with right ventricular dysfunction that is an early sign of impending hemodynamic collapse.

CHRONIC Rx

Elimination of risk factors (see "Etiology") and monitoring of warfarin dose with INR on a routine basis

DISPOSITION

- Mortality can be reduced to <10% by rapid and effective treatment.
- Mortality from recurrent pulmonary emboli is 8% with effective treatment and >30% in patients with untreated pulmonary emboli.

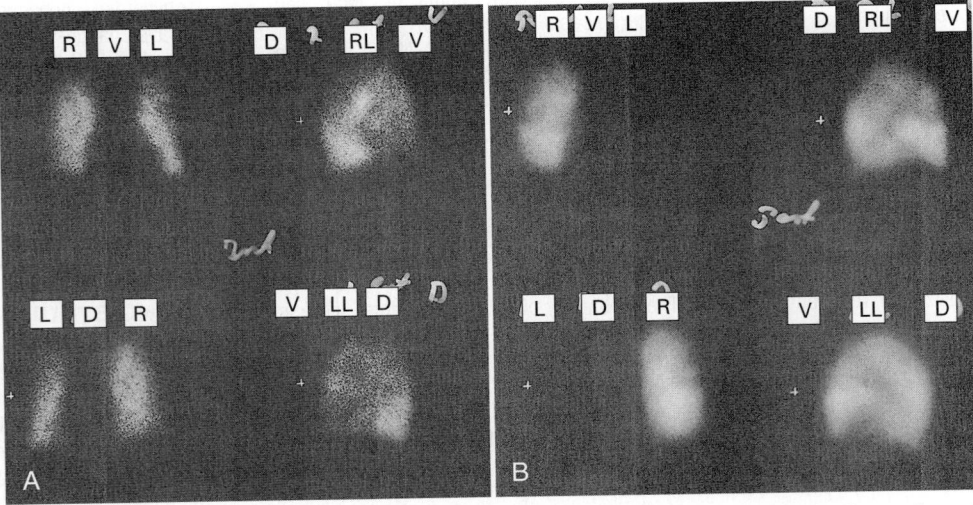

FIGURE 1-312 Ventilation-perfusion lung scan in massive pulmonary embolism. A, A normal pattern on the ventilation scan. **B,** The complete disappearance of the entire left lung from the perfusion scan indicates proximal occlusion of the left pulmonary artery. D, Dorsal; L, left; LL, left lobe; R, right; RL, right lobe; V, ventral. (From Crawford MH et al [eds]: *Cardiology,* ed 2, St Louis, 2004, Mosby.)

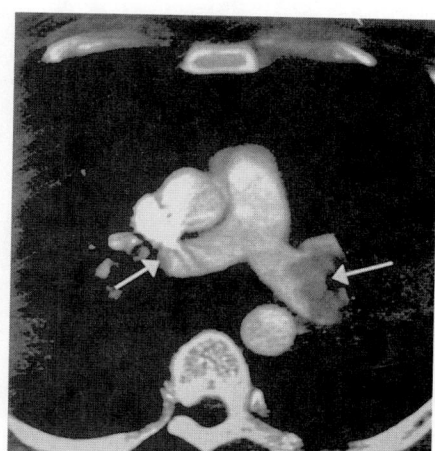

FIGURE 1-313 A 62-year-old physician suffered a massive pulmonary embolism 2 wk after prostatectomy. Spiral chest computed tomography with contrast provided a definitive diagnosis, with a large thrombus burden apparent in the right and left main pulmonary arteries *(arrows)*. (Zipes DP, Libby P, Bonow RO, Braunwald E [eds]: *Braunwald's heart disease,* ed 7, Philadelphia, 2005, Elsevier.)

PEARLS & CONSIDERATIONS

COMMENTS

- In hemodynamically stable patients with pulmonary embolism, initial treatment with once-daily SC administration of the synthetic antithrombotic agent fondaparinux without monitoring has been reported to be at least as safe and as effective as adjusted-dose IV UFH. Several other trials have also demonstrated fixed-dose LMWH to be as effective and safe as dose-adjusted IV UFH for the initial treatment of nonmassive PE.
- For cancer-related venous thromboembolism, LMWH is preferred.
- The duration of oral anticoagulant treatment is 6 mo in patients with reversible risk factors

and indefinitely in patients with persistence of risk factors that caused the initial PE.
- The risk for fatal PE is 0.19 to 0.49 events per 100 person-years for patients who have finished a course of anticoagulant therapy for a first episode of symptomatic venous thromboembolism. The case fatality rate for death from recurrent PE is 4% to 9%.

EVIDENCE

available at www.expertconsult.com

SUGGESTED READINGS

available at www.expertconsult.com

AUTHORS: **FREDERICK D. TRONCALES, M.D., FRED F. FERRI, M.D.,** and **GAURAV CHOUDHARY, M.D.**

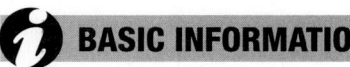

DEFINITION

Pulmonary hypertension (PH) is defined as mean pulmonary artery pressure (PAP) >25 mm Hg at rest or >30 mm Hg with exercise. Sustained elevation in PAP from increased pulmonary venous pressure, hypoxic pulmonary vasoconstriction, or increased flow is often referred to as *secondary pulmonary hypertension.*

SYNONYMS

Idiopathic pulmonary arterial hypertension (IPAH)
Secondary pulmonary hypertension

ICD-9CM CODES
416.0 Primary pulmonary hypertension
416.8 Secondary pulmonary hypertension

EPIDEMIOLOGY & DEMOGRAPHICS

- Idiopathic pulmonary arterial hypertension (IPAH) is rare, occurring in one to two cases per 1 million people per year, with an overall prevalence estimated at 1300 per 1 million.
- IPAH is more common in women than men (1.7:1), usually presenting in the third to fourth decades of life.
- Secondary pulmonary hypertension is more common than IPAH.
- Secondary pulmonary hypertension is the common pathophysiologic mechanism leading to cor pulmonale in patients with underlying pulmonary disease (e.g., chronic obstructive pulmonary disease [COPD], pulmonary embolism).

PHYSICAL FINDINGS & CLINICAL PRESENTATION

IPAH:
- Insidious, may go undetected for years
- Exertional dyspnea most common presenting symptom (60%)
- Fatigue and weakness
- Syncope, classically exertion related or after a warm shower with peripheral vasodilation
- Chest pain
- Hoarse voice from compression of recurrent laryngeal nerve by an enlarged pulmonary artery (Ortner's syndrome)
- Loud P2 component of the second heart sound and paradoxical splitting of second heart sound
- Right-sided S4
- Jugular venous distention
- Abdominal distention and ascites
- Prominent parasternal (right ventricular [RV]) impulse
- Holosystolic tricuspid regurgitation murmur heard best along the left fourth parasternal line that increases in intensity with inspiration
- Peripheral edema

SECONDARY PH: Similar to IPAH but from an underlying cause (e.g., left-sided congestive heart failure, mitral stenosis, COPD)

ETIOLOGY

- The etiology of IPAH is unknown. Most cases are sporadic, but there is a 6% to 12% familial incidence.
- PH is associated with several known risk factors: portal hypertension and liver cirrhosis, appetite-suppressant drugs (fenfluramine), hemoglobinopathies, and HIV disease. It is estimated that 10% of patients with hemoglobinopathies and 0.5% of patients with HIV infection develop moderate to severe pulmonary hypertension. Sickle cell disease and HIV disease may be the most common causes of pulmonary hypertension worldwide.
- Several genetic abnormalities have been associated with the familial form of IPAH, many of which are mutations in the genes that code for members of the tumor growth factor-beta family of receptors (BMPR-II, ALK-1) on chromosome 2q33.
- Familial pulmonary arterial hypertension (PAH) is an autosomal-dominant disease with variable penetrance, affecting only about 10% to 20% of carriers.
- Several factors play a role in the pathogenesis of PAH, including a genetic predisposition, endothelial cell dysfunction, abnormalities in vasomotor control, thrombotic obliteration of the vascular lumen, and vascular remodeling through cell proliferation and matrix production.
- New World Health Organization (WHO) grouping of PH (based on common clinical features)
  1. PAH
     ○ Idiopathic
     ○ Familial
     ○ Associated with collagen vascular diseases, congenital systemic to pulmonary shunts, HIV, portal hypertension, drugs, and toxins
     ○ Associated with significant venous or capillary involvement: pulmonary veno-occlusive disease, pulmonary capillary hemangiomatosis
     ○ Persistent PH of the newborn
  2. PH with left heart disease
     ○ Left-sided atrial, ventricular, or valvular heart disease
  3. PH associated with lung disease and/or hypoxemia
     ○ COPD, interstitial lung disease, sleep-disordered breathing, alveolar hypoventilation syndromes, long-term exposure to high altitude, neonatal lung disease, alveolar capillary dysplasia
  4. PH from chronic thrombotic and/or embolic disease
     ○ Pulmonary embolus (thrombus, tumor, parasites, foreign material)
  5. Miscellaneous: schistosomiasis, sarcoidosis, other

DX DIAGNOSIS

- PAH is a hemodynamic diagnosis involving the detection of elevated pressure in the pulmonary arteries; characterization of this abnormality determines its etiology.
- Right-sided heart catheterization must be performed in all patients suspected of having PAH to establish the diagnosis and to assess pulmonary hemodynamics and acute vasoreactivity response testing.
- Idiopathic PAH is a diagnosis of exclusion.

DIFFERENTIAL DIAGNOSIS

The differential diagnosis is as listed under "Etiology."

EVALUATION

- Consists of establishing the diagnosis and etiology.
- ECG with Doppler technique is a noninvasive measure of systolic PAP. Common findings include tricuspid regurgitation, right heart enlargement, abnormal movement of septum and, rarely, pericardial effusion.
- ECG shows RV enlargement, strain pattern, and right axis deviation.
- Chest radiograph (Fig. 1-314) shows enlarged central pulmonary arteries and right heart enlargement. Chest radiography is abnormal in 90% of patients at diagnosis. A normal chest radiograph does not rule out the diagnosis. High-resolution computed tomography (CT) can assist in the evaluation of thromboembolic disease (Fig. 1-315) or interstitial lung disease.
- Pulmonary function tests may show obstructive (airway disease) or restrictive disease (parenchymal disease) depending on etiology. Diffusion capacity of carbon monoxide in the lung is reduced, which suggests diffusion defect.
- Right heart catheterization is required to assess pulmonary hemodynamics, exclude shunts and left heart disease, and perform acute vasoreactivity response testing.
- Screening for the presence of PAH with Doppler echocardiography is warranted in individuals with a known predisposing genetic mutation or first-degree relative with IPAH, connective tissue diseases (especially scleroderma), congenital heart disease with left-to-right shunt, or portal hypertension undergoing evaluation for orthotopic liver transplantation.
- Determining the degree of functional impairment, as assessed by the WHO functional classification system (Classes I-IV) and the 6-min walk test (6MWT), is a useful way to monitor disease progression and assess response to treatment.

LABORATORY TESTS

- Complete blood count is usually normal in PAH but may show secondary polycythemia.
- Arterial blood gases show low PO_2 and oxygen saturation.
- Overnight oximetry and sleep study to rule out sleep apnea or hypopnea.
- Other blood tests: antinuclear antibody (ANA), antineutrophil cytoplasmic antibodies (ANCA), anti-Scl-70, anticentromere, ribonucleoprotein antibody levels, and rheumatoid factor

(RF) to screen for underlying connective tissue disease, HIV serology, liver function tests, and antiphospholipid antibodies.

- Ventilation perfusion lung scan has high sensitivity for chronic thromboembolic PAH. The diagnosis should be confirmed by pulmonary angiography, which has high specificity.

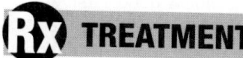 **TREATMENT**

- Most of the evidence in management of PAH is limited to IPAH. There is some evidence in treatment of PAH associated with connective tissue disease, especially scleroderma, and congenital heart disease. The recommendations for treating PAH associated with other causes are limited to case studies and expert opinions.
- There is some evidence for the use of advanced therapies for sarcoidosis-associated PH. The heterogeneity of sarcoid-associated PH complicates the interpretation.

NONPHARMACOLOGIC THERAPY

- Oxygen therapy to improve alveolar oxygen flow in both idiopathic and secondary PH.
- Avoidance of vigorous exercise and pregnancy.

GENERAL TREATMENT:

1. Diuretics (e.g., furosemide 40 to 80 mg qd) improve dyspnea by reducing afterload and peripheral edema.
2. Digoxin 0.25 mg qd has been used in patients with IPAH with inconclusive benefits.
3. Oral anticoagulation with warfarin B for IPAH, C for other PAH. Recommended INR is 1.5 to 2.5.

CHRONIC Rx

- Acute vasoreactivity response testing should be done in all patients at the time of right heart catheterization. Epoprostenol, adenosine, or nitric oxide is generally used to assess the response. A positive response is a

fall in mean PAP of >10 mm Hg to a value of <40 mm Hg, with increased or unchanged cardiac output. Fewer than 10% of patients are responders.

- The positive responders may benefit from treatment with calcium channel blockers (diltiazem, amlodipine, or nifedipine). Verapamil is not recommended because of its negative inotropic effects. All patients should be reassessed in 6 to 8 wk to demonstrate sustained benefit from the calcium channel blocker.
- Nonresponders or nonsustained responders are eligible for selective pulmonary vasodilators.
- Prostanoids (epoprostenol, treprostinil, iloprost, and beraprost) act as potent vasodilators of pulmonary arteries and inhibitors of platelet aggregation. Ideal for class IV patients.
  1. Epoprostenol: IV formulation with very short half-life. Requires long-term IV access with associated risks of infection and thrombosis. Rapid tachyphylaxis, and therefore dose escalation, is seen. Common side effects include jaw pain, abdominal cramping, and diarrhea. Limited evidence exists for use in secondary PAH patients.
  2. Treprostinil: IV and SQ formulation with longer half-life. Main disadvantage is pain at SQ pump site (no long-term evidence for IV formulation).
  3. Iloprost: aerosolized formulation with short half-life requiring 6 to 8 treatments/day.
  4. Beraprost: PO formulation. Not approved in U.S.
- Endothelin receptor antagonists:
  1. Bosentan (nonselective endothelin A and B receptor blocker): oral pulmonary vasodilator, requires monthly liver function tests, often response delay by weeks. Thus, it is not an ideal starting therapy for WHO class IV patients. They are effective in class II and III patients.

2. Sitaxsentan and ambrisentan (selective endothelin A receptor blockers).

- Phosphodiesterase inhibitors: (sildenafil and tadalafil): act by increasing concentration of nitric oxide. Sildenafil is administered as 20 mg PO tid up to 80 mg PO tid. Tadalafil dose is 40 mg once daily. Highly effective in WHO class II patients, both in IPAH and scleroderma-associated PAH.
- Combination therapies: considered when there is no improvement or deterioration on monotherapy.
- Bosentan + inhaled iloprost (STEP trial) showed some benefit over monotherapy.
- IV epoprostenol + oral bosentan (BREATH-2 trial) did not show much difference.
- IV epoprostenol + oral sildenafil (PACES trial) showed benefit over monotherapy.
- Lung transplantation and heart-lung transplantation are other options in patients with end-stage class IV disease. Atrial septostomy may be performed as a bridge to transplant. The defect can be closed at the time of transplantation.
- Atrial septostomy is recommended for individuals with a room air SaO_2 >90% who have severe right-sided heart failure (with refractory ascites) despite maximal diuretic therapy, or who have signs of impaired systemic blood flow (such as syncope) from reduced left heart filling.
- Lung transplant recipients with IPAH had survival rates of 73% at 1 yr, 55% at 3 yr, and 45% at 5 yr.

TREATMENT OF SECONDARY PAH:

- Directed toward cause. At present the guidelines for treatment of PAH do not differentiate between IPAH and secondary PAH. The level of difference varies. Some situations merit mention.
- PAH with congenital heart disease: Eisenmenger's syndrome. Medical treatment generally ineffective. Heart-lung transplantation required in most patients.
- PAH with lung disease or hypoxia: oxygen therapy, control of primary disease process.
- PAH with scleroderma: selective pulmonary vasodilators are effective.
- PAH with HIV: control of viral load by highly active antiretroviral therapy.

FOLLOW-UP

Regular follow-up at 3-mo intervals with clinical assessment: WHO class and 6MWT, 6- to 12-mo objective assessment of RV function by ECG and cardiac catheterization studies.

DISPOSITION

- The 6MWT is predictive of survival in patients with idiopathic PAH. Drop in O_2 saturation >10% during the test increases mortality risk 2.9 times over a median follow-up of 26 mo.
- WHO class II and III patients with PAH have a mean survival of 3.5 yr.
- WHO class IV patients have a mean survival of 6 mo.

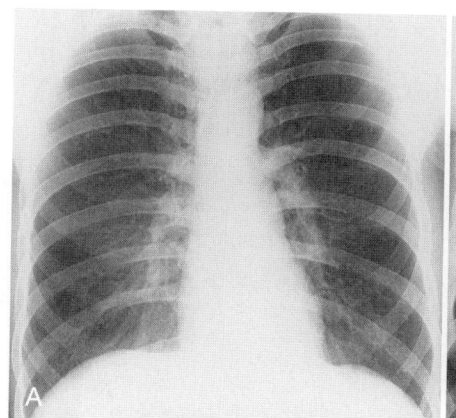 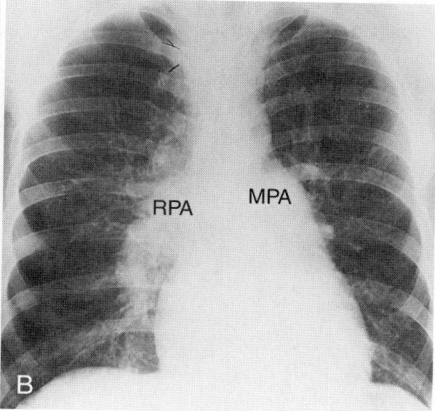

FIGURE 1-314 Progressive pulmonary arterial hypertension. This patient initially presented with a relatively normal chest radiograph **(A)**. However, several years later **(B)** there is increasing heart size and marked dilation of the main pulmonary artery (MPA) and right pulmonary artery (RPA). Rapid tapering of the arteries as they proceed peripherally is suggestive of pulmonary hypertension and is sometimes referred to as pruning. (From Mettler FA [ed]: *Primary care radiology,* Philadelphia, 2000, WB Saunders.)

REFERRAL

If the diagnosis of IPAH is suspected, a consultation with a pulmonary specialist is recommended. Secondary causes of PH may require disease-specific consultations.

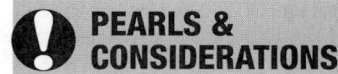

PEARLS & CONSIDERATIONS

- The exertional dyspnea of PAH is typically described by patients as being relentlessly progressive over several months to a year, often out of proportion to, or in the absence of, underlying heart or lung disease.

- Chest radiograph may reveal evidence of interstitial fluid within the lungs in cases of secondary PH. IPAH is not associated with infiltrates on chest radiograph.

COMMENTS

- RV systolic pressure (RVSP) as estimated by echocardiography is not a good indicator of the presence of PAH because RVSP increases with age and body mass index. Athletically conditioned men also have a higher resting RVSP. Thus, these measurements can be misleading.
- Abrupt development of pulmonary edema during acute vasodilator testing suggests pulmonary veno-occlusive disease or pulmonary capillary hemangiomatosis and is a contraindication to long-term vasodilator treatment.
- In advanced PAH, heart rate increase is the main compensatory mechanism and reflects increased sympathetic tone. A higher heart rate at rest is an important marker of prognosis and should be assessed at frequent intervals after initiation of treatment for PAH.

FUTURE TREATMENTS

- Serotonin receptor modulators, platelet-derived growth factor, Rho kinase inhibitors
- Potential of cardiac MRI in assessment of RV function

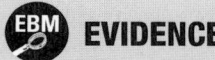 **EVIDENCE**

available at www.expertconsult.com

SUGGESTED READINGS

available at www.expertconsult.com

AUTHORS: **DOUGLAS W. MARTIN, M.D.**, and **GAURAV CHOUDHARY, M.D.**

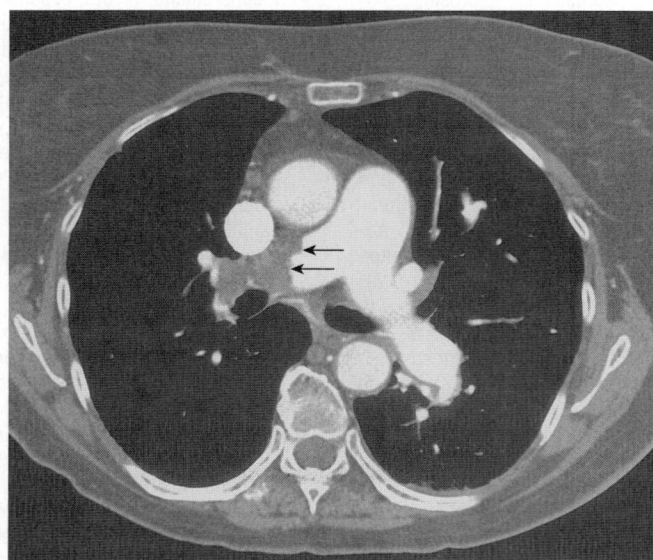

FIGURE 1-315 Chest computed tomographic (CT) scan of a 59-year-old woman with chronic thromboembolic pulmonary hypertensions. She has underlying antiphospholipid antibody syndrome. The chest CT scan demonstrated a large right pulmonary artery with an abrupt cut-off (arrows) in a jagged, irregular pattern due to chronic thromboembolism. (Zipes DP, Libby P, Bonow RO, Braunwald E [eds]: *Braunwald's heart disease,* ed 7, Philadelphia, 2005, Elsevier.)

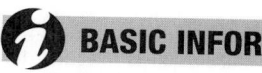

BASIC INFORMATION

DEFINITION

Pulseless electrical activity (PEA) is defined as the presence of organized electrical activity without a palpable pulse.

SYNONYMS

Electromechanical dissociation (EMD)

ICD-9CM CODES
427.5 Cardiac arrest

EPIDEMIOLOGY & DEMOGRAPHICS

- Accounts for about 30% of cardiac arrest cases
- Increasingly recognized as the cause of sudden cardiac death in patients with implantable cardioverter-defibrillators

PHYSICAL FINDINGS & CLINICAL PRESENTATION

PRIMARY PEA:
- Organized electrical activity (not VT/VF)
- No detectable pulse

SECONDARY PEA: As in primary PEA and may also have:
- Bradycardia: drug overdose
- Tachycardia: hypovolemia, massive PE
- Decreased jugular venous pressure (JVP): hypovolemia
- Elevated JVP and no pulse with CPR: cardiac tamponade, massive PE, tension pneumothorax
- Absent unilateral breath sounds and tracheal deviation: tension pneumothorax
- Cyanosis: hypoxia

ETIOLOGY

PRIMARY PEA: Myocardial electromechanical uncoupling secondary to advanced heart muscle disease

SECONDARY PEA: Because of changes in the loading conditions of the heart, ischemia, myocardial depressants
- Massive MI
- Massive PE
- Hypovolemia
- Cardiac tamponade
- Tension pneumothorax
- Hypothermia, hypoxia, acidosis
- Hyperkalemia/hypokalemia
- Hypomagnesemia
- Drug overdose: β-blockers, calcium channel blockers, digoxin, tricyclic antidepressants

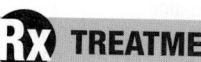

DIAGNOSIS

DIFFERENTIAL DIAGNOSIS

- EMD: no myocardial contractions
- Pseudo-EMD: myocardial contractions but no palpable pulse
- Idioventricular rhythm
- Postdefibrillation idioventricular rhythm

- Ventricular escape rhythm
- Bradyasystolic rhythm

WORKUP

- Stabilizing patient and workup to establish etiology should proceed simultaneously
- History, physical examination, laboratory tests, imaging studies

LABORATORY TESTS

- CBC
- Potassium, magnesium
- Arterial blood gas
- ECG (Fig. 1-316):
  Low voltage: tamponade
  Right heart strain: PE, pneumothorax
  Arrhythmias: MI, metabolic abnormalities, drug effects
  ST changes, Q waves: MI

IMAGING STUDIES

- Chest radiograph: rule out pneumothorax
- Chest CT/pulmonary arteriogram: rule out PE
- Echocardiogram: rule out pseudo-EMD, tamponade, valve dysfunction, and atrial myxoma
- Abdominal radiograph: rule out rupture of abdominal aortic aneurysm

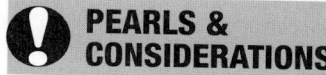

TREATMENT

Identifying and treating a reversible cause is critical.

NONPHARMACOLOGIC THERAPY

- Activate emergency medical service
- Begin CPR
- Intubate and ventilate
- Obtain IV access
- Fluid resuscitation
- Continuous cardiac monitor
- Confirm absence of blood flow with Doppler ultrasound, arterial line, or bedside echocardiogram

ACUTE GENERAL Rx

- Treat specific cause if known
- Epinephrine 1 mg IV push, q3 to 5min, or vasopressin 40 U IV given once may be used to replace the first or second dose of epinephrine

- If bradycardic: atropine 1 mg IV q3 to 5min to a maximum of 3 mg
- Normal saline (10 to 20 ml) should be given after the drug to improve distribution
- Alternate routes of medication delivery for epinephrine, vasopressin, and atropine. May take 2 min for medication to reach the heart via these routes:
  1. Intraosseous: safe and effective, use same dose
  2. Tracheal tube: least preferred as plasma concentrations are variable. Epinephrine and atropine given at 2 to 2.5 × the IV dose in 10 ml of sterile water

PROBABLY HELPFUL: Sodium bicarbonate 1 mEq/kg in:
- Severe hyperkalemia
- Tricyclic antidepressant overdose
- Severe preexisting metabolic acidosis

DISPOSITION

Of hospitalized patients who develop PEA, <15% survive to discharge. Survival rates much lower in patients with prehospital PEA. Survivors often have poor neurologic outcomes.

REFERRAL

As needed for underlying condition

PEARLS & CONSIDERATIONS

- Some support the use of vasopressin instead of or in addition to epinephrine during resuscitation. Randomized trials show no benefit of vasopressin over epinephrine in survival to hospital discharge and suggest it may worsen neurological outcomes.
- Therapeutic hypothermia (32° to 34° C for 12 to 24 hr) may improve neurological outcomes and reduce mortality in unconscious cardiac arrest survivors.
- Prognosis may be guided by median nerve somatosensory-evoked potentials (72 hr) or EEG (24 to 48 hr) after cardiac arrest.

SUGGESTED READINGS
available at www.expertconsult.com

AUTHOR: **SUDEEP KAUR AULAKH, M.D.**

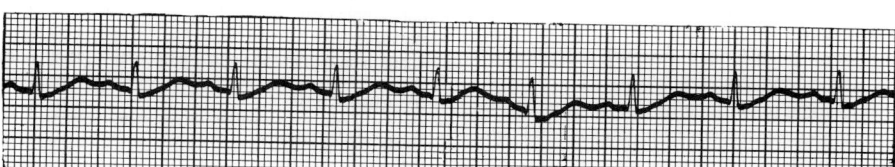

FIGURE 1-316 Sinus rhythm with pulseless electrical activity (PEA). Although the ECG showed sinus rhythm, the patient had no pulse or blood pressure. In this case the PEA was a result of depressed myocardial function after a cardiac arrest. (From Goldberg AL: *Clinical electrocardiography,* ed 5, St Louis, 1994, Mosby.)

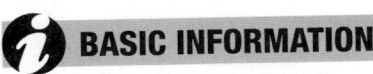

BASIC INFORMATION

DEFINITION

Pure red cell aplasia is characterized by a triad of severe anemia, reticulocytopenia and the absence of erythroid precursors in the bone marrow. All other cell lineages (namely, myeloid precursors and megakaryocytes) are normal.

SYNONYMS

Congenital hypoplastic anemia
Joseph-Blackfan-Diamond Syndrome
Acquired red cell aplasia

ICD-9-CM CODES
284.01 Constitutional red cell aplasia
284.81 Red cell aplasia (acquired) (adult) (with thymoma)

EPIDEMIOLOGY & DEMOGRAPHICS

- The frequency of this disease has been underestimated mainly due to self-limiting nature of most of the cases.
- Rare disease (WHO classification)

PREDOMINANT SEX AND AGE: The male to female ratio is 2:1 for pure red cell aplasia with thymoma. However, immune-mediated cases are seen more commonly in females.

GENETICS: Mutation in the gene RPS19 located at 19q13.2 has been seen in 25% of congenital hypoplastic anemia patients.

PHYSICAL FINDINGS & CLINICAL PRESENTATION

- Anemia is the primary problem in pure red cell aplasia.
- Patients with severe anemia can present with fatigue, pallor, tachycardia, and dyspnea.
- Congenital hypoplastic anemia is usually associated with physical findings of short stature, abnormal thumbs, and mental retardation.
- Other stigmata of underlying illnesses such as splenomegaly, enlarged parotid glands, lymphadenopathy, leg ulcers, and thymomas should be looked for.
- Physical findings related to complications from therapy including iron overload secondary to transfusion therapy; corticosteroid therapy and immunotherapy may be seen as well.

ETIOLOGY (see Table 1-152)

- Congenital: usually sporadic caused by injury to stem cells in utero
- Acquired:
  - acute, self-limited (usually secondary to drugs and viral infections)
  - chronic (with underlying thymomas, autoimmune disorders & immunocompromised states).

DIAGNOSIS

DIFFERENTIAL DIAGNOSIS

- Pure red cell aplasia:
  - Bone marrow findings: Normal cellularity except diminished RBC precursors

  - Peripheral blood: Anemia only
  - Cytogenetics: Negative
- Myelodysplastic syndrome
  - Bone marrow findings: Hypercellular
  - Peripheral blood: Pancytopenia with cellular dysplasia
  - Cytogenetics: Positive (5q deletion)
- Aplastic anemia
  - Bone marrow findings: Hypocellular
  - Peripheral blood: Pancytopenia
  - Cytogenetics: Negative

WORKUP

A search should always be made for the underlying condition.

LABORATORY TESTS

- CBC with peripheral smear: normocytic, normochromic anemia
- Reticulocyte count: diminished
- Bone marrow biopsy is essential to make this diagnosis and rule out other causes: normocellular marrow with normal myeloid precursors and megakaryocytes but absent erythroid precursors.
- Viral titers, if clinically indicated
- Antinuclear antibody testing
- Chest x-ray or chest CT should be ordered in all cases to rule out underlying thymoma.

TREATMENT

- Treatment of the underlying cause
- Red cell transfusions for symptomatic anemia

NONPHARMACOLOGIC THERAPY

- Treatment of underlying cause includes cessation of the offending drug. Viral infections usually resolve spontaneously in 2 to 3 wk.
- About 10% to 15% of patients have thymomas. Surgical resection results in amelioration of anemia in 30% of cases.

ACUTE GENERAL Rx

- Packed red cell transfusion is indicated for symptomatic anemia.
- A vast majority of patients have a protracted remitting and relapsing course, requiring long-term support of anemia with blood transfusions and long-term treatment with immunosuppressive agents.

CHRONIC Rx

- In refractory and relapsed cases, immunosuppressive therapy usually with prednisone or in combination with cyclosporine or cyclophosphamide or antithymocyte globulin (ATG) should be considered. This should always be done in consultation with a hematologist.
- Immunocompromised hosts with pure red cell aplasia secondary to parvovirus infection may not improve spontaneously and often benefit from high-dose intravenous immunoglobulin (IVIG) therapy.
- Certain cases of thymomas with pure red cell aplasia that do not respond to surgery may respond to somatostatin analogs (e.g., octreotide) in combination with prednisone.

DISPOSITION

- Acute self-limited pure red cell aplasia has an excellent prognosis.
- The mortality rate is low in most of the acquired chronic cases but may have significant morbidity related to the underlying condition and complication of therapy.
- Patients with congenital red cell aplasia undergo remission in 15% to 25% of cases and may not need treatment again, or may relapse after reaching adulthood.

REFERRAL

All patients should be referred to a hematologist for complete workup, diagnosis, to initiate appropriate treatments and monitor the response to therapy.

TABLE 1-152 Causes of Acquired Red Cell Aplasia

Drugs	Viruses
Procainamide	Parvovirus B19
Phenytoin	Mumps
Sulfonamides	Hepatitis
Zidovudine	Infectious Mononucleosis (EBV)
Azathioprine	Atypical mycoplasma
Chloramphenicol	
Isoniazid	
Recombinant erythropoietin therapy/anti-EPO antibodies	

Malignancies	Autoimmune Conditions
Thymomas (5%)	SLE
CLL	Rheumatoid disease
Hodgkin's disease	Autoimmune hemolytic anemia
LGL leukemia	

Immunocompromised states	Others
HIV	Pregnancy
HTLV-1	ABO incompatible hematopoietic cell transplantation
Idiopathic	

PEARLS & CONSIDERATIONS

COMMENTS
- Rare diagnosis
- Most cases self-limiting

PREVENTION
Medications implicated as the cause of pure red cell aplasia should be avoided.

PATIENT/FAMILY EDUCATION
- The consequences of iron overload and secondary hemosiderosis from repeated transfusion therapy should be explained to patients.
- The possibility of the transmission of infections with transfusions and immunotherapy should be discussed with the patients.
- Long-term use of corticosteroids, immunomodulators can result in significant adverse effects which should be explained to the patients.

SUGGESTED READINGS
available at www.expertconsult.com

AUTHOR: **PRIYA BANSAL, M.D., M.P.H.**

P

Diseases and Disorders

I

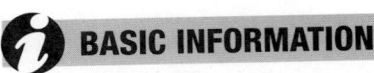

BASIC INFORMATION

DEFINITION
Pyelonephritis is an infection, usually bacterial in origin, of the upper urinary tract.

SYNONYMS
Acute pyelonephritis
Pyonephrosis
Renal carbuncle
Lobar nephronia
Acute bacterial nephritis

ICD-9CM CODES
590.81 Pyelonephritis
599.0 Urinary tract infection
595.9 Cystitis

EPIDEMIOLOGY & DEMOGRAPHICS
INCIDENCE (IN U.S.): Extremely common
PREDOMINANT SEX: Female
PREDOMINANT AGE:
- Sexually active years in women
- Usually age >50 yr in men

GENETICS: Congenital urologic structural disorders may predispose to infections at an early age.

PHYSICAL FINDINGS & CLINICAL PRESENTATION
- Fever, rigors, chills
- Flank pain
- Dysuria
- Polyuria
- Hematuria
- Toxic feeling and appearance
- Nausea and vomiting
- Headache
- Diarrhea
- Physical examination notable
  1. Costovertebral angle tenderness
  2. Exquisite flank pain

ETIOLOGY
- Gram-negative bacilli such as *Escherichia coli* and *Klebsiella* spp. in more than 95% of cases
- Other, more unusual gram-negative organisms, especially if instrumentation of the urinary system has occurred
- Resistant gram-negative organisms or even fungi in hospitalized patients with indwelling catheters
- Gram-positive organisms such as enterococci
- *Staphylococcus aureus:* presence in urine indicates hematogenous origin
- Viruses: rarely, but these are usually limited to the lower tract

DIAGNOSIS

DIFFERENTIAL DIAGNOSIS
- Nephrolithiasis
- Appendicitis
- Ovarian cyst torsion or rupture
- Acute glomerulonephritis
- Pelvic inflammatory disease
- Endometritis
- Other causes of acute abdomen
- Perinephric abscess
- Hydronephrosis

WORKUP
- No workup usually indicated in sexually active women
- Poorly responding infections, especially with azotemia and frank bacteremia
- Renal sonogram or CT scan to assess for underlying urologic pathology such as hydronephrosis
- Urologic imaging studies in all young men and boys
- Prostate assessment in older men

LABORATORY TESTS
- Complete blood count with differential
- Renal panel
- Blood cultures
- Gram stain of urine, urinalysis, and urine cultures
- Urgent renal sonography if obstruction or closed space infection suspected
- CT scans may better define the extent of collections of pus
- Helical CT scans excellent to detect calculi

TREATMENT

ACUTE GENERAL Rx
- Hospitalization for:
  1. Toxic patients
  2. Complicated infections
  3. Diabetes
  4. Suspected bacteremia
- Keep patients well hydrated.
- IV fluids are indicated for those unable to take adequate amounts of liquids.
- Give antipyretics such as acetaminophen when necessary.
- Antibiotic therapy should be initiated after cultures are obtained and guided by the results of culture and sensitivity testing.
  1. Oral TMP-SMX DS (bid for 10 days) or ciprofloxacin (500 mg PO bid for 10 days): adequate for stable patients who can tolerate oral medications with sensitive pathogens
  2. TMP-SMX or ciprofloxacin IV for more toxic patients
  3. Ceftazidime 1 g IV q6 to 8h
  4. Aminoglycosides such as gentamicin (2 mg/kg IV load followed by 1 mg/kg IV q8h adjusted for renal function) added, but nephrotoxicity possible, especially in diabetics with azotemia
  5. Vancomycin 1 g IV q12h or linezolid to cover gram-positive cocci such as enterococci or staphylococci
  6. Ampicillin 1 to 2 g IV q4 to 6h to cover enterococci with an aminoglycoside for synergy

7. Oral ampicillin or amoxicillin: no longer adequate for therapy of gram-negative infections because of resistance
- Prompt drainage with nephrostomy tube placement for obstruction.
- Surgical drainage of large collections of pus to control infection.
- Diabetic patients, as well as those with indwelling catheters, are especially prone to complicated infections and abscess formation.

CHRONIC Rx
- Repair underlying structural problems, especially when renal function is compromised.
  1. Reflux
  2. Obstruction
  3. Nephrolithiasis should be considered
- Patients with diabetes mellitus and indwelling urinary catheters are at particular risk of severe and complicated infections.
- When possible, remove catheters.

DISPOSITION
Most patients with uncomplicated pyelonephritis are now treated as outpatients or in short hospitalizations. Indications to admit a patient with pyelonephritis include pregnancy, suspected urinary obstruction, suspected renal abscess or perinephric abscess, bacterial sepsis, diabetes or other immunocompromised states, recurrent or refractory pyelonephritis, or infection with an unusual or antibiotic-resistant microorganism.

REFERRAL
- To a surgeon for correction of underlying urologic problems (e.g., reflux and hydronephrosis)
- To a pediatrician for detection of reflux to avoid recurrent urinary tract infection and loss of renal function
- To an internist for aggressive metabolic and urologic evaluation for patients with nephrolithiasis

PEARLS & CONSIDERATIONS

Pyelonephritis is a systemic illness and may be a source of bacteremia and sepsis, especially if accompanied by urinary obstruction. Workup for abscess, obstruction, papillary necrosis, and other local complications of pyelonephritis should be initiated if the patient is septic, if patient does not respond to antibiotic therapy after 72 hr of treatment, or if infection is accompanied by worsening renal function.

 EVIDENCE

available at www.expertconsult.com

SUGGESTED READINGS
available at www.expertconsult.com

AUTHORS: **GLENN G. FORT, M.D., M.P.H.,** and **DENNIS J. MIKOLICH, M.D.**

P

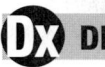 **BASIC INFORMATION**

DEFINITION

Pyoderma gangrenosum (PG) is a rare, non-infectious inflammatory skin disease that is characterized by a pustule that progresses to an ulcer or deep erosion with violaceous overhanging or undermined borders.

SYNONYMS

Classic pyoderma gangrenosum
Atypical pyoderma gangrenosum
Peristomal pyoderma gangrenosum

ICD-9CM CODES
686.01

EPIDEMIOLOGY & DEMOGRAPHICS

INCIDENCE: Unknown
PEAK INCIDENCE: Unknown
PREVALENCE: Between 3 and 10 per million cases or 1 in 100,000
PREDOMINANT AGE: Most common in ages 40 to 60 yr. Infants and adolescents are affected in 3% to 4% of cases.
PREDOMINANT SEX: Prevalence is roughly equal between the genders.
GENETICS: Unknown
RISK FACTORS: Autoimmune diseases particularly ulcerative colitis, Crohn's disease, and rheumatoid arthritis.

PHYSICAL FINDINGS & CLINICAL PRESENTATION

- Typically presents first as a pustule that rapidly and painfully progresses to an ulcer or erosion with tissue necrosis and enlargement of the area. The ulcer or erosion is surrounded by a violaceous or bluish border with erythema extending beyond that.
- Classic PG is commonly found on the legs. Atypical PG occurs more frequently in the upper extremities, head, and neck. Atypical PG lesions begin as pustules and become plaques that may be studded with pustules. Peristomal PG lesions appear similarly to classic PG lesions; however, they occur around surgically created stomas such as in Crohn's disease surgery.
- As many as 30% of lesions occur via pathergy. Pathergy is the development of skin lesions at the sites of injury, including minor injuries. Pathergy-induced PG lesions can be misdiagnosed as cellulitis. Surgery can also induce pathergy.
- Some patients only present with a single episode of PG, while others can have multiple episodes or a chronic relapsing course.
- Approximately 50% of PG sufferers have another underlying systemic disease, including inflammatory bowel disease, myeloproliferative diseases, or inflammatory arthritis.

ETIOLOGY

Exact etiology is unknown. However, neutrophilic infiltration causing cutaneous damage seems to be one part of the injury mechanism.

 DIAGNOSIS

DIFFERENTIAL DIAGNOSIS

- Wegener granulomatosis
- Cellulitis
- Fungal infection
- Brown recluse spider bite
- Systemic vasculitis such as polyarteritis nodosa
- Malignancies such as squamous cell carcinoma, cutaneous lymphoma, and metastatic carcinoma
- Sporotrichosis
- Antiphospholipid syndrome
- Erythema nodosum

WORKUP

PG is a diagnosis of exclusion. In particular, workup should include biopsy of lesions and evaluation for associated underlying illness such as inflammatory bowel disease, arthritis, or malignancy. History, particularly as to the timing and progression of the lesions and inciting injury, is particularly important, as well as the physical appearance of the lesions.

LABORATORY TESTS

Skin biopsy is not diagnostic in itself because the findings are nonspecific. However, it may be helpful in excluding other diseases. Histopathologic findings show sterile dermal neutrophilia with or without mixed inflammation or lymphocytic vasculitis. Other appropriate testing could include rheumatologic lab work or colonoscopy to evaluate for inflammatory arthritis or IBD. Tissue cultures should also be performed to rule out bacterial or fungal causes.

IMAGING STUDIES

Consider colonoscopy and/or CT to evaluate for IBD.

 TREATMENT

The major treatment modalities revolve around wound care for the ulcers themselves, as well as either topical or systemic therapy.

NONPHARMACOLOGIC THERAPY

Surgery or aggressive debridement should be avoided in PG lesions because the surgery can cause pathergy and worsen the lesions. When needed, grafting should be performed concurrently with systemic immune-modulating therapy to prevent worsening of the lesions.

ACUTE GENERAL Rx

Care may include one or more of the following:
- Topical wound care and moist healing
- Topical high potency steroids (e.g., clobetasone)
- Topical immune modulators (e.g., tacrolimus)
- Systemic glucocorticoids (e.g., prednisone)
- Systemic immune modulators (e.g., cyclosporine)
- Antibiotics—only in cases of super-infection and if used with one of above
- Infliximab in patients with Crohn's disease
- Thalidomide

CHRONIC Rx

Similar to above except for longer durations or in pulse therapy

COMPLEMENTARY & ALTERNATIVE MEDICINE

Not relevant

DISPOSITION

Can be treated in both inpatient and outpatient settings depending on severity and therapeutic modalities

REFERRAL

- Dermatology
- Rheumatology
- Gastroenterology, especially in cases of IBD-related PG

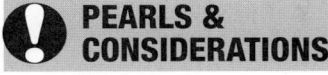 **PEARLS & CONSIDERATIONS**

COMMENTS

PG is a diagnosis of exclusion and should only be made after other diseases in the differential have been ruled out and the patient has been evaluated for the associated diseases seen in more than 50% of cases.

PATIENT/FAMILY EDUCATION

Support for PG can often be found in the support groups for associated diseases, particularly Crohn's disease, ulcerative colitis, and erythema nodosum.

EBM EVIDENCE

available at www.expertconsult.com

SUGGESTED READINGS
available at www.expertconsult.com

AUTHOR: **MICHAEL KLEIN, M.D.**

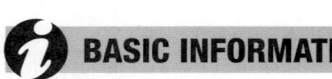

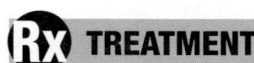 **BASIC INFORMATION**

DEFINITION

Pyogenic granuloma is a benign vascular lesion of the skin and mucous membranes. The lesions are caused by capillary proliferation, generally the result of trauma.

SYNONYMS

Granuloma pyogenicum
Tumor of pregnancy
Eruptive hemangioma
Lobular capillary hemangioma
Granulation tissue-type hemangioma

ICD-9CM CODES
686.1 Pyogenic granuloma

EPIDEMIOLOGY & DEMOGRAPHICS

- Common in children and young adults.
- Equally prevalent in males and females, with no racial or familial predisposition.
- Caused by trauma or surgery.
- Gingival lesions occur more frequently during pregnancy.

PHYSICAL FINDINGS & CLINICAL PRESENTATION

- Small (<1 cm), yellow to red, dome-shaped lesions (Fig. 1-317)
- May have surrounding scale at base
- Most commonly found on the head, neck, and extremities
- Often found on the gingiva during pregnancy (called *epulis*)
- Extremely friable, can easily ulcerate, and may bleed profusely with minor trauma

ETIOLOGY

Trauma causing focal capillary growth. These lesions are neither infectious in etiology nor granulomatous in histology.

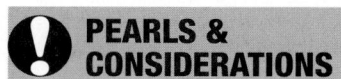 **DIAGNOSIS**

DIFFERENTIAL DIAGNOSIS

- Amelanotic melanoma
- Bacillary angiomatosis
- Glomus tumor
- Hemangioma
- Irritated nevus

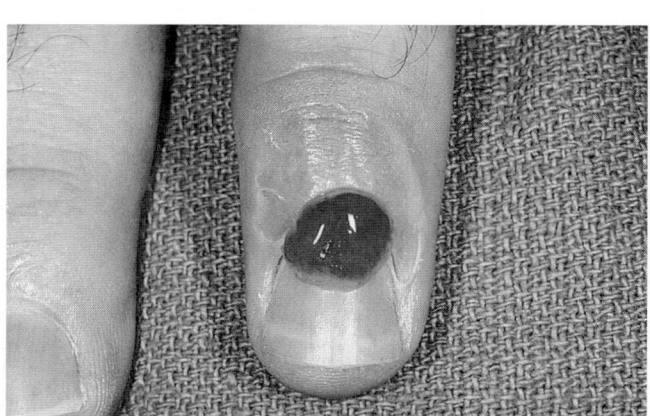

FIGURE 1-317 Pyogenic granuloma. Often the lesions have a collar or moat. (From Callen JP [ed]: *Color atlas of dermatology,* ed 2, Philadelphia, 2000, WB Saunders.)

- Wart
- Kaposi's sarcoma

WORKUP

Diagnosis is based on clinical history and appearance. Generally begins with trauma followed by the development of an erythematous papule. The lesion tends to bleed easily and develops over several days to weeks.

LABORATORY TESTS

Pathologic examination should be performed after excision to rule out melanoma.

Rx **TREATMENT**

ACUTE GENERAL Rx

- Excision: using 1% lidocaine for anesthesia, shave or curette at base and border. Follow with electrocauterization or cryotherapy.
- Pulsed-dye laser is also a safe and effective treatment modality.
- Pregnancy epulis generally resolve spontaneously after childbirth.

REFERRAL

Dermatology referral recommended if lesion recurs or multiple satellite lesions occur after excision.

! **PEARLS & CONSIDERATIONS**

COMMENTS

- Removal of entire lesion is essential because lesions may recur at the site of residual tissue.
- Patients and parents should be alerted to the possibility of recurrence after removal.
- Multiple satellite lesions occasionally develop near a primary pyogenic granuloma, usually after destruction of that lesion.

AUTHOR: **JENNIFER R. SOUTHER, M.D.**

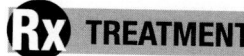

BASIC INFORMATION

DEFINITION

Q fever is a systemic febrile illness caused by *Coxiella burnetii* that may be acute or chronic.

SYNONYMS

C. burnetii infection

ICD-9CM CODES
083.0 Q fever

EPIDEMIOLOGY & DEMOGRAPHICS

- *C. burnetii* is found worldwide.
- Common animal reservoirs are cattle, sheep, and goats.
- Pets such as cats, rabbits, pigeons are also reservoirs (169 cases were reported in the U.S. in 2006).
- A parturient cat caused an outbreak in Nova Scotia just by delivering in the same room as a card game.
- Most cases are found in individuals who have direct contact with infected animals (e.g., farmers, veterinarians) or who are exposed to contaminated animal urine, feces, milk, or placental tissues.
- Q fever is seen more often in men than in women (ratio of 3:1).
- Its incidence in the U.S. is increasing, with more than 30 cases recently reported in U.S. military personnel recently deployed to Iraq and Afghanistan.
- *C. burnetii* is a CDC class B bioterrorism agent.

PHYSICAL FINDINGS & CLINICAL PRESENTATION

- Acute Q fever presentation:
  Fever
  Pneumonia
  Hepatitis
  Meningoencephalitis
- Chronic Q fever presentation:
  Endocarditis
  Hepatitis
- Most common clinical symptoms:
  Chills
  Sweats
  Nausea
  Vomiting
  Cough, nonproductive
  Headache
  Fatigue
- Most frequent physical findings:
  Fever
  Inspiratory rales
  Purpuric rash
  Hepatomegaly
  Splenomegaly

ETIOLOGY

- Q fever is caused by the proteobacterium *C. burnetii*.

- *C. burnetii* is a gram-negative coccobacillus transmitted from arthropods to animals to human beings.
- The disease is acquired most often by inhalation of aerosols. In the lungs, it proliferates in macrophages and then gains access to the bloodstream, producing a transient bacteremia. Thereafter it can invade many organs, most commonly the lungs and liver.
- There is an incubation period of 3 to 30 days before systemic symptoms manifest.
- Persons with abnormal heart valves, prosthetic valves, and endovascular grafts are at high risk of progression to chronic Q fever. This includes individuals with bicuspid aortic valves.

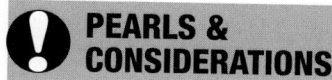

DIAGNOSIS

DIFFERENTIAL DIAGNOSIS

Q fever can have various presentations and must be in the differential diagnosis of fever, hepatitis, pneumonia, endocarditis, and meningitis.

WORKUP

- Complete blood count (CBC), erythrocyte sedimentation rate (ESR), and liver function tests
- Urinalysis
- Serology
- Chest radiograph

LABORATORY TESTS

In acute Q fever:
- CBC and white blood cell count are usually normal.
- Thrombocytopenia can occur (25%).
- Elevation of hepatic transaminases (two to three times the abnormal range) may be seen.
- Antibody detection by immunofluorescence assay is the most commonly used method because of its high sensitivity and specificity. Complement fixation (CF) shows a fourfold rise in titer between acute and convalescent samples.
- Polymerase chain reaction is a promising test for early detection of *C. burnetii* but test availability is limited to reference laboratories and research studies

In chronic Q fever (almost always endocarditis):
- ESR is elevated
- Anemia is present
- Microscopic hematuria
- Blood cultures are almost always negative
- MIF (microimmunofluorescence) titer of >1:800 to phase I antigen is diagnostic

IMAGING STUDIES

- Chest x-ray examination is abnormal, showing segmental lobe consolidation
- Pleural effusions (35%)

TREATMENT

NONPHARMACOLOGIC THERAPY

Oxygen as needed in patients with pneumonia

ACUTE GENERAL Rx

- Acute Q fever can be treated with doxycycline (100 mg bid) for 14 to 21 days *or*
- Erythromycin (500 mg qid) for 14 days now rarely used *(torsades)*; the newer macrolides have been shown to have potential
- Ofloxacin 200 mg PO q8h for 14 to 21 days
- Hydroxychloroquine plus doxycycline for endocarditis associated with Q fever
- Fluoroquinolones are recommended for suspected meningoencephalitis

CHRONIC Rx

- Chronic Q fever is treated with a combination of two antibiotics, doxycycline 100 mg bid and rifampin 300 mg qd *or*
- Doxycycline 100 mg bid and ofloxacin 200 mg PO q8h *or*
- Doxycycline 100 mg bid and hydroxychloroquine 200 mg PO tid
- Duration of treatment: 2 to 3 yr

DISPOSITION

- Patients with acute Q fever respond well with antibiotics, with deaths rarely reported.
- Mortality rate in chronic Q fever endocarditis is high (24%). Most patients will need valve replacement surgery.

REFERRAL

Referral to an infectious disease expert is recommended in any cases of suspected acute or chronic Q fever.

REPORTING

Q fever has been a reportable disease in the U.S. since 1999. The CDC must be notified of cases.

PEARLS & CONSIDERATIONS

COMMENTS

- An acellular (CMR) vaccine is available in the U.S. However, vaccines that are available in other countries such as Australia have been more thoroughly studied.
- Infected patients do not require specific isolation precautions.
- Q fever derived its name in 1935 from Derrick, who was suspicious of a new disease during a series of acute febrile illnesses in abattoir workers of Queensland, Australia, justifying the name of Q fever (for "query").

SUGGESTED READINGS
available at www.expertconsult.com

AUTHOR: **PATRICIA CRISTOFARO, M.D.**

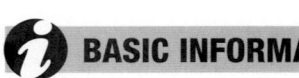 **BASIC INFORMATION**

DEFINITION
Rabies is a fatal illness caused by the rabies virus and transmitted to human beings by the bite of an infected animal.

SYNONYMS
Hydrophobia

ICD-9CM CODES
071 Rabies

EPIDEMIOLOGY & DEMOGRAPHICS
INCIDENCE (IN U.S.): Approximately two cases annually
PREDOMINANT SEX: Men are more commonly affected (70% of cases)
PREDOMINANT AGE: <16 yr and <55 yr

PHYSICAL FINDINGS & CLINICAL PRESENTATION
- Incubation period of 10 to 90 days
  1. Shorter with bites on the face
  2. Longer if extremities involved
- Prodrome
  1. Fever
  2. Headache
  3. Malaise
  4. Pain or anesthesia at exposure site
  5. Sore throat
  6. Gastrointestinal symptoms
  7. Psychiatric symptoms
- Acute neurologic period, with objective evidence of central nervous system involvement
  1. Extreme hyperactivity and bizarre behavior alternating with periods of relative calm
  2. Hallucinations, disorientation
  3. Seizures
  4. Paralysis
  5. Fear, pain, and spasm of the pharynx and larynx caused by drinking
  6. Coma, death

ETIOLOGY
- Rabies virus
- Cases in U.S. are associated with:
  1. Bats
  2. Raccoons
  3. Foxes
  4. Skunks
- In eight of the 32 cases occurring in the U.S. since 1980, there was a history of exposure to bats without a clinically evident bite or scratch.

- Imported cases are usually associated with dogs.
- Unusual acquisition:
  1. By organ transplantation
  2. By aerosol transmission in laboratory workers and spelunkers

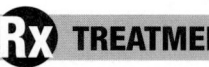 **DIAGNOSIS**

DIFFERENTIAL DIAGNOSIS
- Delirium tremens
- Tetanus
- Hysteria
- Psychiatric disorders
- Other viral encephalitides
- Guillain-Barré syndrome
- Poliomyelitis

WORKUP
- Rabies antibody
  1. Serum
  2. Cerebrospinal fluid (CSF)
- Viral isolation
  1. Saliva
  2. CSF
  3. Serum
- Rabies fluorescent antibody: skin biopsy from the hair-covered area of the neck
- Characteristic eosinophilic inclusions (Negri bodies) in infected neurons

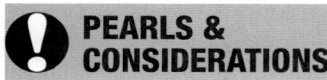 **TREATMENT**

NONPHARMACOLOGIC THERAPY
- Isolation of the patient to prevent transmission to others
- Supportive therapy

ACUTE GENERAL Rx
- No known beneficial therapy. A recent report describes a 15-yr-old girl who survived rabies and had been treated with a combination of ketamine, midazolam, ribavirin, and amantadine. This therapy is worth trying despite the fact this is a single case report.
- Emphasis is placed on prophylaxis of potentially exposed individuals after an exposure:
  1. Thorough wound cleansing and irrigation of the wound with soap and water as soon as possible. If available, a virucidal agent (e.g., povidine-iodine solution) should be used to irrigate the wounds.
  2. Active and passive immunization are most effective when used within 72 hr of exposure.
- Vaccinations: The CDC has recently recommended reducing the number of vaccine

doses for post-exposure prophylaxis. Current recommendations for rabies postexposure prophylaxis are as follows:
1. Human diploid cell vaccine (HDCV) or purified chick embryo cell vaccine (PCECV) 1 ml IM (deltoid area) 1 each on days 0, 3, 7, and 14 in patients not previously vaccinated. In patients previously vaccinated administer HDCV or PCECV 1 ml IM (deltoid area) 1 each on days 0 and 3. Human rabies hyperimmune globulin (RIG) 20 IU/kg body weight should be administered to persons not previously vaccinated. If anatomically feasible, the full dose should be infiltrated into the wound; any remaining volume should be given IM at a site separate from vaccine administration.
- Preexposure prophylaxis with HDCV or RVA (1 ml IM on days 0, 7, and 21 or 28) in individuals at high risk for acquisition:
  1. Veterinarians
  2. Laboratory workers working with rabies virus
  3. Spelunkers
  4. Visitors to endemic areas

DISPOSITION
Virtually always fatal

REFERRAL
- To infectious disease consultant
- To local health authorities

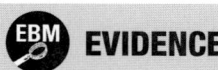 **PEARLS & CONSIDERATIONS**

COMMENTS
- Most cases in the U.S. are caused by:
  1. Bat bites, often after minimal contact and inapparent exposure to infected bat saliva
  2. Dog bites occurring outside the U.S.
- Rare cases can be transmitted by mucous membrane contact of aerosolized virus (caves, laboratory-acquired cases).

EBM **EVIDENCE**

available at www.expertconsult.com

SUGGESTED READINGS
available at www.expertconsult.com

AUTHORS: **GLENN G. FORT, M.D., M.P.H.,** and **DENNIS J. MIKOLICH, M.D.**

BASIC INFORMATION

DEFINITION

Radiation that has the potential for injury is called ionizing radiation. Ionizing radiation is a form of radiant energy strong enough to penetrate the body and eject electrons from atoms that form our tissues, creating ions. It consists of subatomic particles or electromagnetic waves that are energetic enough to detach electrons from atoms or molecules, thus ionizing them. The occurrence of ionization depends on the energy of the individual particles or waves, and not on their number. Examples of ionizing radiation include x-rays, gamma rays, and photons. The biological effects of ionizing radiation depend on the dose of exposure. These effects may produce direct cell damage and death, non-lethal changes in the DNA, which may result in neoplasm, and/or heritable DNA changes in reproductive cells.

TYPES OF RADIATION EXPOSURE:

- External irradiation: exposure to ionizing radiation from an external source.
- Internal irradiation: contamination with radioactive materials in the form of gases, liquids, or solids that are released into the environment and contaminate people through inhalation, ingestion, or skin exposure.
- Incorporation: uptake of radioactive materials by body cells, tissues, and target organs after contamination.

STOCHASTIC EFFECTS OF IONIZING RADIATION: Radiation can result in injury to the DNA or the cell itself. Stochastic effects result in direct DNA injury; These effects are related to the probability of a biologic effect caused by radiation and not its severity. The scientific community conservatively assumes that any amount of radiation may pose some risk for causing cancer and that the risk is higher for higher radiation exposures. A linear dose–response relationship is used to describe the relationship between radiation dose and the occurrence of cancer. Based on this assumption, any dose of ionizing radiation can alter DNA, causing mutations or carcinogenic changes that may take years to be expressed; hence, there is no safe dose per se and the risk is cumulative. This is mostly a concern with small, but prolonged or repetitive exposure to radiation, such as exposure from medical procedures.

DETERMINISTIC EFFECTS OF IONIZING RADIATION: Also known as non-stochastic effects, deterministic effects usually result in cellular injury. These effects are dose related, where there is no effect from the exposure below a certain threshold, but there is a dose-dependent effect above it. The higher the dose, the more severe the effects, such as cataracts, bone marrow suppression, organ atrophy, gonadal injury, skin erythema, desquamation, and necrosis. The deterministic effects of radiation are consequence of a large exposure, such as the explosion from an atomic bomb or nuclear reactor.

UNITS OF RADIATION:

- The measure of exposure is the roentgen (R). The roentgen is a unit of radiation exposure defined as the amount of ionization per mass of air due to gamma or x-rays, the most common form of human exposure. It indirectly measures a radiation field by its effect on air and is equal to 2.58×10^{-4} Coulombs/kg of air.
- Absorbed dose is the concentration of energy absorbed by a particular tissue. This unit is referred to as gray (Gy), where 1 Gy = 1 joule of energy concentrated in 1 kg of tissue. The older unit used was rad (radiation absorbed dose); 1 Gy = 100 rad.
- Equivalent dose is the estimate of the biologic potency a particular absorbed dose might have. It varies according to the type and energy of the ionizing radiation used. It is typically used for radiation protection purposes. This unit is the sievert (Sv). For x and gamma rays, 1 Sv = 1 Gy. The older unit was rem (radiation equivalent man); 1 Sv = 100 rem.
- Effective dose equivalent is a hypothetical uniform whole-body dose used to describe the risk of a non-uniform exposure. This allows for risk assessment and comparison between different exposures to particular areas of the body, based on an organ-specific weighting factor.

To put things in perspective, the average person in the United States receives an effective dose of 3.6 mSv per year from naturally occurring sources such as radon gas and cosmic radiation.

SYNONYMS

For large exposures (deterministic, or non-stochastic, effects of radiation):
Acute radiation syndrome
Radiation sickness

Chronic low-dose exposures produce stochastic effects. This has no common synonyms.

ICD-9CM CODES
990 Radiation exposure

PHYSICAL FINDINGS & CLINICAL PRESENTATION

Most of the data linking radiation to cancer comes from studies of the survivors of the atomic bombs. This data links sequela to a single, large exposure to radiation (>150 mSv). There is much less data on low exposures (<100 mSv) such as medical diagnostic imaging.

ACUTE RADIATION SYNDROME: This syndrome follows a large whole-body exposure of greater than 1 Gy in a very short period of time. The mean lethal dose of whole body radiation required to kill 50% of human beings at 60 days (lethal dose 50/60) is between 3.25 and 4 Gy in persons managed without supportive care, and 6 to 7 Gy when antibiotics and transfusion support are provided.

The sequence of events has four stages:
1. Stage 1 (prodromal phase): flulike syndrome with fatigue, anorexia, nausea, vomiting, and diarrhea usually occurring in the first 48 hr, but may develop in minutes up to 6 days after exposure. Onset of symptoms is dose dependent; however, symptom peak is usually at 6 to 8 hr.
2. Stage 2 (latent phase): a short period characterized by improvement in symptoms as the person appears to have recovered. Unfortunately this effect is transient, lasting for several days to 1 mo. The duration of this phase is inversely related to the dose of radiation received, and may be absent at the highest doses.
3. Stage 3 (manifest illness phase): occurs at the third to fifth week after exposure and is the most difficult to manage. This stage is characterized by recurrence of prodromal symptoms along with additional features such as intense immunosuppression. If the person survives this stage, recovery is likely. Signs and symptoms consist of abdominal pain, diarrhea, hair loss, bleeding, and infection. During this stage, several subsyndromes may coexist, overlap, or occur in sequence.
   - Cerebrovascular syndrome: fever, nervousness, hypotension, ataxia, apathy, lethargy, and seizures. These symptoms may be observed in those receiving more than 50 Gy of radiation. The prodromal phase is characterized by disorientation, confusion, and prostration. The physical examination may show papilledema, ataxia, decreased or absent deep tendon reflexes, and corneal reflexes. If death occurs during this phase, it is thought to be caused by cerebral edema from small vessel leakage and hemorrhage, and occurs within 3 days.
   - Cutaneous syndrome: caused by thermal or radiation burns and characterized by loss of epidermis, local edema, and increased risk for a compartmental syndrome.
   - Gastrointestinal syndrome: will usually occur with doses greater than 10 Gy. Radiation induces loss of intestinal crypts and breakdown of the mucosal barrier as a result of necrosis and mitotic arrest of mucosal stem cells. These changes result in abdominal pain, anorexia, nausea, vomiting, diarrhea, and dehydration, and predispose patients to super infection, electrolyte imbalance, and sepsis. Survival is unlikely with this syndrome, death occurs within 2 wk.
   - Hematopoietic syndrome: exposure range is 0.7 to 10 Gy; it can have a latency of 2 to 3 wk. Lymphopenia is common and occurs before the onset of other cytopenias. Pancytopenia with bleeding diathesis, and sepsis often follow possibly resulting in death. A predictable decline in lymphocytes occurs after irradiation. A potentially lethal exposure is characterized by a 50% decline in absolute lymphocyte count within the first 24 hr after exposure, followed by a further, more severe decline within 48 hr. The onset of cytopenias varies depending on the dose and dose rate. Granulocyte counts may transiently increase before decreasing in patients with exposure to <5 Gy. This transient increase before decline is known

as an *abortive rise* and may indicate a survivable exposure. The survival rate decreases with increasing dose.

4. Stage 4: recovery, lasting weeks to months. If patients survive, they will need lifelong follow up because of the potential for unusual infections, organ dysfunction, and carcinogenesis.

The prognosis of the patient depends on the dose absorbed by the body and the availability of medical care.

When expressed in grays:

- Exposure <1 Gy: almost certain survival, even without medical care
- Exposure 1 to 2 Gy: 90% survival with medical care
- Exposure 2 to 3.5 Gy: probable survival with medical care

  At a dose of <3 Sv received, a lymphocyte count >1200/mm^3 at 48 hr confers a favorable prognosis; if the count is <1200/mm^3, a fatal dose is possible and more aggressive medical management is warranted. A drop in the number of granulocytes or platelets also portends an increased risk of complications.

- Exposure 3.5 to 5.5 Gy: 50% survival with medical care
- Exposure 5.5 to 10 Gy: probable death
- Exposure >10 Gy: certain death

CHRONIC LOW-DOSE EXPOSURE: In controlled conditions, an excess of cancers has never been detected in animals or humans for exposures below 100 mSv. However, there is some epidemiologic data from the survivors of the atomic bomb, of a small but significant risk at low exposures (5-100 mSv). Although the evidence is scant, the National Academies' Biological Effects of Ionizing Radiation 7th Report (BEIR VII Phase 2) stated that cancer risk decreases with age and is the highest in children and young adults. This is because children have more years of life during which a potential cancer can be expressed and they are inherently more radiosensitive, since they have a larger proportion of dividing cells (more DNA material). There is usually a long latent period between the exposure and the appearance of a neoplasm, from 2 yr to several decades.

Radiation exposure to the eye can damage the cells covering the posterior surface of the crystalline lens. Symptoms range from cloudy vision to severe impairment, and can appear as soon as 1 to 2 yr after exposure. The exposure threshold is thought to be somewhere between 0 and 0.8 Gy[2].

(Dx) DIAGNOSIS

The key to making the diagnosis of acute radiation exposure and its associated injuries lies in obtaining a complete history including the timing of any radiation exposure, and, if possible, the dose to which the patient was subjected. If the dose is unknown physical dosimetry can provide an estimate of individual dose; however this process is very slow and time consuming.

Internal radiation dose can be estimated by ion chambers and spectroscopes. Biologic markers, such as time to onset of emesis, lymphocyte depletion kinetics, and chromosomal aberrations help to evaluate for radiation exposure.

For low-dose chronic exposures, it is currently impossible to determine whether a cancer is radiation induced. Cancers associated with high-dose exposure include leukemia, breast, bladder, colon, liver, lung, esophagus, ovarian, multiple myeloma, and stomach cancers. There is also a possible association between ionizing radiation exposure and prostate, nasal cavity/sinuses, pharyngeal, laryngeal, and pancreatic cancer The diagnosis of lens and skin lesions lesions will also rely on the history of exposure and the physical findings noted above.

ETIOLOGY

SOURCE OF RADIATION:
- Natural background radiation comes from four primary sources: cosmic radiation, solar radiation, external terrestrial sources, and radon.
  1. Natural internal radioisotopes.
     ○ Potassium-40.
     ○ Thorium and uranium.
  2. Cosmic origin: this cosmic radiation consists of positively-charged ions from protons to iron nuclei. This radiation interacts in the atmosphere to create secondary radiation that rains down, including x-rays, muons, protons, alpha particles, pions, electrons, and neutrons:
     ○ Galactic rays: originate outside our solar system.
     ○ Solar radiations: solar wind and flares from the sun.
  3. Terrestrial origin: radon (domestic and mining industry): radon-222 is produced by the decay of radium-226 which is present wherever uranium is found. Radon gas is emitted out of uranium-containing soils. It is often the single largest contributor to an individual's background radiation dose and could be the second largest cause of lung cancer in America, after smoking.
  4. Manmade radiation sources:
- Medical radiation: It is estimated that nearly 4 million Americans receive cumulative effective doses that exceed 20 mSv per year from imaging procedures (nuclear medicine and radiologic procedures). The most common source is CT scans followed by nuclear imaging. A chest x-ray usually provides an effective dose of 0.04 mSv; this is in contrast to 0.7 mSv from a mammogram, 2 to 10 mSv from computed tomography, 7.5 to 57 mSv from coronary angioplasty and 14 mSv from a PET scan. Physicians should use these procedures appropriately and adequately inform patients of the risks of exposure to radiation.
  ○ Consumer products (e.g., tobacco).
  ○ Occupational (e.g., nuclear energy).
  ○ Weapons and fallout.

(Rx) TREATMENT
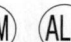

- For all accidental radiation contamination, the following decontamination steps are considered mandatory:
  1. Perform at site of exposure unless there is continued radiation exposure.
  2. Remove all clothing (and treat as radioactive waste). Providers should use strict isolation precautions, including donning of gown, mask, cap, double gloves, and shoe covers, when evaluating and treating contaminated patients.
  3. Wash patient with mild soap (neutral pH) and tepid water. Dispose of contaminated water as radioactive waste.
  4. Scrub any open wound.
  5. Depending on the situation, the regional emergency response system should be called for additional measures such as evacuation.
- Management of acute radiation syndrome:
  1. Establish IV access.
  2. Monitor physiologic signs.
  3. Manage the airway.
  4. Manage burns.
  5. Identify and treat other injuries.
  6. Provide analgesia.
  7. Give antiemetics (e.g., ondansetron).
  8. Manage bleeding and transfuse if necessary.
  9. Diagnose and treat sepsis. Administration of antibiotics reduces the mortality rate. In nonneutropenic patients, antibiotic therapy should be directed toward foci of infection and the most likely pathogens. Fluoroquinolones are useful for prophylaxis in neutropenic patients.
  10. Confirm initial dose estimate using chromosome aberration cytogenetic bioassay when possible.
  11. Consider colony-stimulating factors (CSFs). In any adult with whole-body or significant partial body exposure >3 Gy, treatment with CSFs should be rapidly initiated (e.g., G-CSF or filgrastim, 5 mcg/kg of body weight per day). CSFs may be withdrawn when the absolute neutrophil count reaches a level greater than 1.0×10^9 after recovery from the nadir.
  12. Consider stem cell transplantation in people with exposure dose of 7 to 10 Gy who do not have significant burns or other major organ toxicity and who have an appropriate donor.
  13. Provide counseling; 75% of individuals exposed to nuclear weapon denotations exhibit some form of psychological symptoms, ranging from insomnia to difficulty concentrating and social withdrawal.
- Chronic low-dose exposures: Treatment of radiation-induced organ damages would not differ significantly from non–radiation-induced cancers, cataracts, or skin lesions. Prevention of radiation-induced injuries is paramount, carefully assessing the risks and benefits of each medical imaging procedure, especially in

patients who have had these procedures repeatedly. Special attention should be placed in minimizing the dose of radiation utilized for each study.

! PEARLS & CONSIDERATIONS

COMMENTS

- The three most useful elements for calculating the acute exposure dose are time to onset of emesis, lymphocyte depletion kinetics, and the presence of chromosome aberrations, such as dicentrics or ring formation. The presence of chromosomal aberrations is the gold standard for biodosimetry.

- A radiation casualty management software program (biologic assessment tool) is available at the Armed Forces' Radiobiology Research Institute website (http://www.afrri.usuhs.mil).
- Complete blood count (CBC) analysis every 2 to 3 hr with special attendance to lymphocyte count if known or suspected exposure to large radiation dose. This should be done during the first 8 hr after exposure, every 4 to 6 hr the next 2 to 3 days, twice per day for the following 6 days, then weekly until a nadir in neutrophil count is obtained. If an unknown dose was received, consider a baseline CBC and chromosome analysis.
- The chromosome aberration cytogenetic bioassay should be obtained from a qualified radiation cytogenetic biodosimetry laboratory.

- Ionizing radiation from medical imaging procedures is not negligible. Since the early 1980s, the per capita dose of radiation from medical imaging has increased by a factor of nearly 6.

 EVIDENCE

available at www.expertconsult.com

SUGGESTED READINGS

available at www.expertconsult.com

AUTHORS: **AMANDA M. DONOHUE, D.O., FRED F. FERRI, M.D.,** and **PRANAV M. PATEL, M.D.**

R

Diseases and Disorders

I

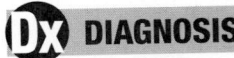

BASIC INFORMATION

DEFINITION

Ramsay Hunt syndrome is a localized herpes zoster infection involving the seventh nerve and geniculate ganglia, resulting in hearing loss, vertigo, and facial nerve palsy.

SYNONYMS

Herpes zoster oticus
Geniculate herpes
Herpetic geniculate ganglionitis

ICD-9CM CODES
053.11 Ramsay Hunt syndrome

EPIDEMIOLOGY & DEMOGRAPHICS

PREDOMINANT SEX: Equal sex distribution
PREDOMINANT AGE:
- Increasingly common with advancing age
- Rare in childhood

PHYSICAL FINDINGS & CLINICAL PRESENTATION

- Characteristic vesicles:
  1. On pinna
  2. In external auditory canal
  3. In distribution of the facial nerve and, occasionally, adjacent cranial nerves
- Facial paralysis on the involved side

ETIOLOGY

Reactivation of dormant infection with varicella-zoster virus after primary varicella

DIAGNOSIS

- Usually made by recognition of the clinical features detailed previously

- Viral culture and/or microscopic examination of specimens taken from active vesicles

DIFFERENTIAL DIAGNOSIS

- Herpes simplex
- External otitis
- Impetigo
- Enteroviral infection
- Bell's palsy of other etiologies
- Acoustic neuroma (before appearance of skin lesions)

The differential diagnosis of headache and facial pain is described in Section II.

WORKUP

If the diagnosis is in doubt, confirm varicella-zoster virus infection.

LABORATORY TESTS

- Viral culture of specimens of vesicular fluid and scrapings of the vesicle base
- Tzanck preparation, which may reveal multinucleated giant cells
- Direct immunofluorescent staining of scrapings

IMAGING STUDIES

MRI may demonstrate enhancement of the facial and vestibulocochlear nerves before appearance of vesicles.

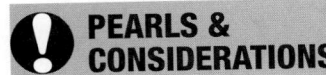 TREATMENT

ACUTE GENERAL Rx

- Prednisone (40 mg PO for 2 days, 30 mg for 7 days, followed by tapering course) is recommended by some authors.
- Acyclovir (800 mg PO five times qd for 10 days), famciclovir (500 mg tid for 7 days),

or valacyclovir (1 g q8h for 7 days) may hasten healing.
- Analgesics should be used as indicated.

CHRONIC Rx

- Amitriptyline is effective in some cases of postherpetic pain.
- Other agents for postherpetic pain include gabapentin (Neurontin) and pregabalin (Lyrica).
- Narcotic analgesics may occasionally be necessary.

DISPOSITION

Recurrences are unusual.

REFERRAL

To otolaryngologist: patients with persistent facial paralysis for potential surgical decompression of the facial nerve

PEARLS & CONSIDERATIONS

COMMENTS

Immunodeficiency states, particularly HIV infection, should be considered in:
- Younger patients
- Severe cases
- Patients with a history of specific risk behavior

SUGGESTED READINGS
available at www.expertconsult.com

AUTHORS: **GLENN G. FORT, M.D., M.P.H.,** and **DENNIS J. MIKOLICH, M.D.**

BASIC INFORMATION

DEFINITION

Raynaud's phenomenon (RP) is a vasospastic disorder that produces an exaggerated response to cold temperatures and/or emotional stress, resulting in episodic digital ischemia. It is characteristically manifest as a cold-induced, symmetric, sharply demarcated white or blue discoloration of the distal fingers or toes, followed by erythema at a variable time after rewarming.

SYNONYMS

Primary Raynaud's phenomenon or Raynaud's disease
Secondary Raynaud's phenomenon

ICD-9CM CODES
443.0 Raynaud's syndrome, Raynaud's disease, Raynaud's phenomenon (secondary)
785.4 If gangrene present

EPIDEMIOLOGY & DEMOGRAPHICS

- RP is classified clinically into primary or secondary forms and affects approximately 3% to 5% of the general population.
- Primary RP usually occurs between the ages of 15 and 25 yr. It is more likely to affect women than men (4:1) and appears to be more common in colder climates.
- 5% to 15% of patients with primary Raynaud's phenomenon develop a secondary cause later in the course of the disease (mostly a connective tissue disorder).
- Secondary RP tends to begin after age 35 to 40 yr.
- Secondary RP occurs in more than 90% of patients with scleroderma and in approximately 30% of patients with systemic lupus erythematosus or Sjögren's syndrome.
- There is also some suggestion that secondary RP may be associated with drugs (nicotine, caffeine, ergotamine, vinyl chloride) or trauma to the hands from vibrating tools such as jack hammers.

PHYSICAL FINDINGS & CLINICAL PRESENTATION

- The typical manifestation of RP is the biphasic color response of the digits to cold exposure and rewarming, which may or may not be accompanied by pain. RP most often affects the hand (Fig. 1-318).
  1. White (pallor) or blue (cyanotic) discoloration of the digit(s) resulting from vasospasm on cold or vibration exposure.
  2. Red (rubor) with or without pain and paresthesia when vasospasm resolves and blood returns to the digit.
- Color changes can sometimes be induced by placing the hand in an ice bath, although this is not recommended as a diagnostic maneuver because responses may be inconsistent even in patients with definite RP.

- Color changes are well delineated, symmetric, and usually bilateral, involving the fingers and toes. The index, middle, and ring fingers are commonly involved and the thumb is usually not.
- Fingertips are most often involved, but feet, ears, nose, tongue, and nipples can also be affected.
- During cold response, patients with RP may exhibit livedo reticularis; this is a violaceous or reticular pattern of skin of arms and legs, sometimes with regular, unbroken circles.
- Duration of attacks can range from seconds to hours and average 15 to 20 min.
- Chronic skin changes resulting from repeated attacks may include skin thickening and brittle nails. Ulcerations and, rarely, gangrene may occur.
- Physical examination should also include examination for symptoms associated with autoimmune disease, such as fever, rash, arthritis, dry eyes, dry mouth, myalgias, or cardiopulmonary abnormalities.

ETIOLOGY

- Primary RP can also be called idiopathic Raynaud's phenomenon, primary Raynaud's syndrome, or Raynaud's disease. It occurs in the absence of any associated disease.
- With primary RP, the possibility that another first-degree family member is affected is reported as approximately 25%.
- Secondary RP is associated with an underlying pathologic condition or disorder, use of certain drugs, or related occupation. Secondary RP is associated with:
  1. CREST syndrome (calcinosis, RP, esophageal involvement, sclerodactyly, and telangiectasia)
  2. Scleroderma, Sjögren's syndrome
  3. Mixed connective tissue disease, polymyositis, and dermatomyositis
  4. Systemic lupus erythematosus, arteritis
  5. Rheumatoid arthritis
  6. Thromboangiitis obliterans (Buerger's disease)
  7. Drugs (beta-blockers, ergotamine, methysergide, vinblastine, bleomycin, oral contraceptives, nicotine, clonidine, co-

caine, caffeine, vinyl chloride, tegafur, interferon alfa, interferon beta)
  8. Hematologic disorders (polycythemia, cryoglobulinemia, cold agglutinins, paraproteinemia)
  9. Carpal tunnel syndrome
  10. Use of tools that vibrate
  11. Endocrine disorders (hypothyroidism, carcinoid syndrome, pheochromocytoma, metabolic syndrome)
  12. Estrogen replacement therapy without progesterone
  13. Hypercoagulable states, protein C, protein S, antithrombin III deficiency, factor V Leiden deficiency, and anti-phospholipid syndrome
  14. Poliomyelitis is a rare cause
  15. Primary biliary cirrhosis
  16. Vasospastic disorders (migraines, prinzmetal angina)
  17. Malignancies (angiocentric lymphoma, ovarian cancer)
  18. Primary pulmonary hypertension
  19. Peripheral emboli

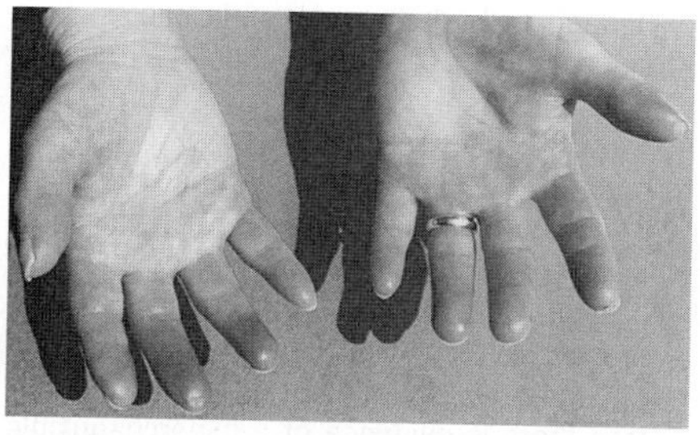

DIAGNOSIS

Clinical criteria:
- Definite RP: repeated episodes of biphasic color change on cold exposure
- Possible RP: Uniphasic color changes plus numbness or paresthesia on cold exposure
- No RP: No color change on cold exposure
The suggested criteria for primary RP are:
- Symmetric attacks
- Absence of tissue necrosis, ulceration, or gangrene
- Absence of a secondary cause on the basis of a patient's history and general physical examination
- Negative nailfold capillary examination
- Negative test for antinuclear antibody (ANA)
- Normal erythrocyte sedimentation rate (ESR)
Secondary RP is suggested by the following findings:
- Onset of symptoms after age 30 yr
- Male gender
- Episodes that are painful, asymmetric, or associated with ischemic skin lesions
- Clinical features suggestive of a connective-tissue disease
- Elevated specific autoantibody tests and ESR
- Evidence of microvascular disease on microscopy of nail-fold capillaries

DIFFERENTIAL DIAGNOSIS

- Neurogenic thoracic outlet syndrome or carpal tunnel syndrome
- Frostbite or cold weather injury
- Medication reaction (ergotamine, chemotherapeutic agents)
- Atherosclerosis, thromboembolic disease
- Buerger's disease, embolic disease
- Acrocyanosis
- Livedo reticularis
- Injury from repetitive motion

FIGURE 1-318 Raynaud's phenomenon. Sharply demarcated cyanosis of the fingers with proximal venular congestion (livedo reticularis) is seen. (From Klippel J et al [eds]: *Primary care rheumatology,* London, 1999, Mosby.)

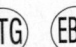
WORKUP

- Once the diagnosis of RP is established, differentiating primary from secondary is helpful in treatment and prognosis.
- Patients who are younger when their symptoms occur, have a normal history and physical examination and normal nail-fold capillaries, and have no history of digital ischemic lesions can be considered as having primary RP. These patients can be monitored clinically without any further testing.
- If a secondary cause of RP is suspected, appropriate laboratory testing is recommended (see "Laboratory Tests"). Secondary RP has associated abnormal nail-fold microscopy.

LABORATORY TESTS

- CBC, serum electrolytes, blood urea nitrogen, creatinine, ESR, ANAs, VDRL antibody test, rheumatoid factor, and urinalysis should be included in the initial evaluation.
- If the history, physical examination, and initial laboratory tests suggest a possible secondary cause, specific serologic testing (e.g., anti-centromere antibodies, anti-Scl 70, cryoglobulins, complement testing, and serum protein electrophoresis) may be indicated.
- Noninvasive vascular testing includes finger systolic blood pressures, segmental blood pressure measurements, cold recovery time (measure vasoconstrictor and vasodilator responses of finger to cold), fingertip thermography, and laser Doppler with thermal challenge (measures relative change in skin blood flow with ambient warming).

IMAGING STUDIES

- The diagnosis of RP should not be made on the basis of laboratory tests, and imaging studies should not replace a good history and physical examination.
- Duplex ultrasound can image the palmar arch and digital arteries for patency.
- Magnetic resonance angiography is useful for imaging larger arteries.
- Contrast angiography is the gold standard for arterial imaging.
- Nail-fold capillary microscopy can differentiate primary from secondary RP.

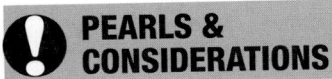 TREATMENT

NONPHARMACOLOGIC THERAPY

- Avoid drugs that may precipitate RP (see "Etiology").
- Avoid cold exposure. Use warm gloves, hats, and garments during the winter months or before going into cold environments (e.g., air-conditioned rooms). Sudden shifts in temperature are more likely to precipitate RP.
- Avoid stressful situations, and use relaxation techniques in preventing RP attacks.

ACUTE GENERAL Rx

- Acute measures to terminate an attack include rotating the arms in a windmill pattern, placing the hands under warm water or in a warm body fold such as the axilla, and the swing-arm maneuver. The swing-arm maneuver involves the patient raising both arms over the shoulders in one direction and forcefully swinging them across the body.
- Medications are indicated in the treatment of RP if there are signs of critical ischemia or if the quality of life of the patient is affected to the degree that activities of normal living are no longer possible and preventive techniques do not work.

CHRONIC Rx

- Dihydropyridine calcium channel blockers (e.g., nifedipine, amlodipine, felodipine, nisoldipine, isradipine) are the most effective pharmacologic treatment for RP and are the drugs of choice.
- Nifedipine is most often prescribed at a dose of 10 to 20 mg 30 min before cold exposure. If symptoms occur with long duration, nifedipine XL 30 to 180 mg PO qd is often effective.
- Patients who do not tolerate or do not respond to calcium channel blocker therapy can sometimes benefit from other drugs that directly or indirectly cause vasodilation, either alone or in combination, although data for these therapies are less robust. Some potential therapeutic options include direct vasodilators such as nitroprusside, hydralazine, papaverine, minoxidil, niacin, and griseofulvin. Topical 1% nitroglycerine or topical L-arginine, ethyl nicotinate, hexyl nicotinate, thurfyl salicylate may also be useful, particularly if low blood pressure is a concern.
- Phosphodiesterase inhibitors (cilostazol, pentoxifylline, and sildenafil), angiotensin 2 receptor antagonists (losartan), and selective serotonin reuptake inhibitors (Flouxetine) have been used with some limited success.
- Alpha receptor antagonists such as prazosin and phenoxybenzamine have shown some effectiveness in treating RP.
- The prostaglandins, including inhaled iloprost, IV epoprostenol, and alprostadil, may be promising in severe RP. However, additional experience and controlled studies are needed.
- Anticoagulation with IV unfractionated heparin or subcutaneous low-molecular-weight heparin and addition of aspirin can be considered during the acute phase of a severe ischemic event. Aspirin (81 mg/day) therapy can be considered in all patients with secondary RP with a history of ischemic ulcers or thrombotic events; however, caution should be exercised because aspirin can theoretically worsen vasospasm by the inhibition of prostacyclin. Long-term anticoagulation with heparin or warfarin is not recommended unless there is evidence of a hypercoagulable state.
- Bypass surgery can be performed for severe RP associated with reconstructible arterial occlusive disease.
- Sympathectomy is available for unreconstructible occlusive disease or pure vasospastic disease refractory to medical treatment.
- Microsurgical revascularization of the hand and digital reconstruction may improve digital vascular perfusion and heal digital ulcers when proximal arterial occlusion is associated by digital vasospasm.
- Ischemic digital lesions should be treated with topical antibiotics and daily cleansing with soap and water. Digits that progress to dry gangrene should be permitted to undergo autoamputation. Surgical amputation is limited for intractable pain or deep tissue infection.

DISPOSITION

The prognosis of patients with RP depends on the etiology.

- Primary RP is fairly benign, usually remaining stable and controlled with nonpharmacologic medical treatment.
- Patients with secondary RP, specifically those with scleroderma, CREST syndrome, or thromboangiitis obliterans, may develop severe ischemic digits with ulceration, gangrene, and autoamputation.

REFERRAL

- Rheumatology consult is indicated if secondary collagen vascular disease is diagnosed.
- Vascular surgery consult is indicated if ulcers, gangrene, or threatened digit loss is noted.

⚠ PEARLS & CONSIDERATIONS

- Most patients with RP can be managed by a primary care provider.
- It is important to differentiate primary from secondary forms. Secondary forms may become manifest as far out as 10 yr from the diagnosis of RP. It is important to take immediate action during an attack and patients are encouraged to:
  1. Keep warm
  2. Not use tobacco products
  3. Avoid aggravating medications
  4. Control stress
  5. Exercise
  6. Follow up with a physician

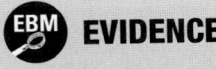 **EVIDENCE**

available at www.expertconsult.com

SUGGESTED READINGS
available at www.expertconsult.com

AUTHORS: **SYEDA M. SAYEED, M.D.**, and **FRED F. FERRI, M.D.**

BASIC INFORMATION

DEFINITION

Reiter's syndrome is one of the seronegative spondyloarthropathies, so called because serum rheumatoid factor is not present in these forms of inflammatory arthritis. There is an international consensus that the term *reactive arthritis* should replace the name "Reiter's syndrome" to describe this constellation of signs and symptoms. Unfortunately, the original name is still associated with the syndrome. Reiter's syndrome is an asymmetric polyarthritis that affects mainly the lower extremities and is associated with one or more of the following:
- Urethritis
- Cervicitis
- Dysentery
- Inflammatory eye disease
- Mucocutaneous lesions

SYNONYMS

Reiter's disease
Reactive arthritis
Seronegative spondyloarthropathy

ICD-9CM CODES
099.3 Reiter's syndrome

EPIDEMIOLOGY & DEMOGRAPHICS

INCIDENCE (IN U.S.): 0.0035% annually of men ≤50 yr
PEAK INCIDENCE: Most common in the third decade
PREDOMINANT SEX: Male
PREDOMINANT AGE: 20 to 40 yr
GENETICS: Familial disposition: strongly associated with HLA-B27 (63% to 96%)

PHYSICAL FINDINGS & CLINICAL PRESENTATION

- Polyarthritis
  1. Affecting the knee and ankle
  2. Commonly asymmetric
- Heel pain and Achilles tendinitis, especially at the insertion of the Achilles tendon
- Plantar fasciitis
- Large effusions
- Dactylitis, or "sausage toe"
- Urethritis
- Uveitis or conjunctivitis; uveitis can progress to blindness without treatment
- Keratoderma blennorrhagicum, circinate balanitis
  1. Hyperkeratotic lesions on soles of the feet, toes, penis, hands
  2. Closely resembles psoriasis
- Aortic regurgitation similar to that seen in ankylosing spondylitis

ETIOLOGY

- Epidemic Reiter's syndrome after outbreaks of dysentery has been well described.
- Genetically susceptible HLA-B27 individuals are at risk for developing Reiter's syndrome after infection with certain pathogens:
  - *Salmonella*
  - *Shigella*
  - *Yersinia enterocolitica*
  - *Chlamydia trachomatis*
- Symptom complex indistinguishable from Reiter's syndrome has been described in association with HIV infection.

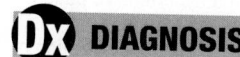

DIAGNOSIS

DIFFERENTIAL DIAGNOSIS

- Ankylosing spondylitis
- Psoriatic arthritis
- Rheumatoid arthritis
- Gonococcal arthritis-tenosynovitis
- Rheumatic fever

WORKUP

- X-ray examination of affected joints
- Synovial fluid examination and culture
- Careful examination of eyes and skin
- Cultures for gonococcus (urethral, cervical, stool)

LABORATORY TESTS

- Elevated but nonspecific erythrocyte sedimentation rate
- No specific laboratory tests to diagnose Reiter's syndrome

IMAGING STUDIES

Plain radiographs:
- Juxtaarticular osteopenia of affected joints
- Erosions and joint space narrowing in more advanced disease
- Periostitis and reactive new bone formation at the insertions of the Achilles tendon and the plantar fascia
- Sacroiliitis:
  1. Unilateral or bilateral
  2. Indistinguishable from ankylosing spondylitis
- Vertebral bridging osteophytes

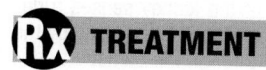

TREATMENT

NONPHARMACOLOGIC THERAPY

Physical therapy to maintain range of motion of the spine and other joints

ACUTE GENERAL Rx

- Flares treated with nonsteroidal anti-inflammatory drugs such as indomethacin (25 to 50 mg PO tid).

- Enteric or urethral infection should be treated with appropriate antibiotic coverage.
- Uveitis should be treated with steroid eye drops in consultation with an ophthalmologist.
- Achilles tendinitis and plantar fasciitis should be treated with injections of methylprednisolone (40 to 80 mg).
- Sulfasalazine (2 to 3 g PO tid) may be effective.
- Careful monitoring for the following is essential:
  - Gastrointestinal toxicity
  - Hypersensitivity
  - Bone marrow suppression
- Persistent and uncontrolled disease should be managed with cytotoxic drugs (methotrexate, azathioprine) in consultation with a rheumatologist.

CHRONIC Rx

Chronic disease is best managed by a team approach with the collaboration of a rheumatologist or other experienced physician and physical therapist.

DISPOSITION

- Recurrences are frequent, even with treatment.
- Long-term sequelae:
  - Persistent polyarthritis
  - Chronic back pain
  - Heel pain
  - Progressive iridocyclitis
  - Aortic regurgitation

REFERRAL

- To ophthalmologist if uveitis is suspected
- To rheumatologist if arthritis and tendinitis fail to improve rapidly after a course of nonsteroidal anti-inflammatory drugs

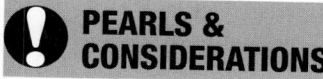

PEARLS & CONSIDERATIONS

COMMENTS

- Infection with HIV is associated with particularly severe cases of Reiter's syndrome.
- HIV testing is recommended, especially if risk factors such as unprotected sexual activity or IV drug use are identified.

SUGGESTED READINGS
available at www.expertconsult.com

AUTHORS: **GLENN G. FORT, M.D., M.P.H.,** and **DENNIS J. MIKOLICH, M.D.**

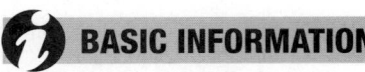

DEFINITION

Renal artery stenosis (RAS) is the progressive narrowing of the renal artery and may be acute or chronic. RAS may cause renovascular hypertension or ischemic nephropathy.

SYNONYMS

Acute:
  Renal artery thrombosis
  Renal artery embolism
Chronic:
  Renovascular hypertension

ICD-9CM CODES

593.81 Renal artery occlusion
440.1 Renal artery stenosis
405.01 Renovascular hypertension, secondary
447.9 Renal artery hyperplasia

EPIDEMIOLOGY & DEMOGRAPHICS

- Acute renal artery occlusion: epidemiology depends on the underlying cause (see "Etiology" and "Pathogenesis" below).
- Chronic renal artery stenosis:
  1. Atherosclerotic renovascular disease accounts for ~90% of chronic renal artery stenosis:
     a. In the general population >65 yr of age, the prevalence is 6.8% (5.5% of women, 9.1% of men, 6.7% of African Americans, and 6.9% of Caucasians)
     b. In patients with malignant hypertension, the prevalence is 43% in Caucasians and 7% in African Americans)
     c. In patients with peripheral artery disease, the prevalence is 22% to 59%
  2. Fibromuscular dysplasia accounts for approximately 10% of chronic renal artery stenosis. It is typically seen in women aged <30 yr

PHYSICAL FINDINGS & CLINICAL PRESENTATION

Acute renal artery occlusion:
- Flank or abdominal pain
- Fever
- Nausea or vomiting
- Leukocytosis
- Hematuria (microscopic or gross)
- Elevated aspartate aminotransferase, lactate dehydrogenase, and alkaline phosphatase
- Oliguric renal failure if occlusion is bilateral; normal or near-normal renal function in unilateral occlusion
- Cholesterol or septic emboli: depending on distribution of emboli, patients may have multisystem manifestations such as visual disturbance, painful distal extremities, abdominal pain, signs of organ or limb ischemia; laboratory findings include eosinophiluria, proteinuria, renal failure, elevated erythrocyte sedimentation rate

Progressive renal artery stenosis:
- Fibromuscular dysplasia: new onset hypertension at age <30, or hypertension in any patient without family history or risk factors
- Atherosclerotic renal artery disease: new onset hypertension at age >55 yr, with risk factors for or evidence of atherosclerotic disease
- Uncontrolled hypertension refractory to three or more medications
- Abdominal bruit (40% of cases)
- Renal failure
- Hypertensive retinopathy
- Pulmonary edema in a hypertensive patient
- Hypokalemia
- Acute renal failure after the administration of an ACE inhibitor (ACEI) has previously been considered a marker for bilateral RAS, but is neither sensitive nor specific

ETIOLOGY

Renal artery thrombosis:
- Atherosclerosis: risk factors for atherosclerosis include family history, smoking, diabetes, hypertension, and hyperlipidemia
- Fibromuscular dysplasia: etiology unknown. Classified into three categories based on the layer of arterial wall affected: medial (>90%), intimal (<10%), adventitial (<1%)
- Extrinsic compression (e.g., neoplasm)
- Neurofibromatosis and fibrous bands
- Vasculitides, including autoimmune (Takayasu's, antiphospholipid syndrome), infectious (syphilis)
- Renal artery aneurysm
- Hypercoagulable state
- Complication of renal transplantation (role of cyclosporine)
Renal artery embolism (cardiac conditions [90%]):
- Left ventricular thrombus (may be the result of myocardial infarction or other cardiomyopathy)
- Atrial fibrillation
- Endocarditis
- Paradoxical emboli from deep vein thrombosis in patient with atrio- or ventricular septal defect
- Atheromatous plaques (cholesterol emboli)

PATHOGENESIS

The macula densa of the kidney senses a decreased systemic blood pressure caused by the reduced blood flow through the stenotic artery. The decreased perfusion pressure leads to decreased blood flow (hypoperfusion) to the kidney and a decrease in the glomerular filtration rate. Renal hypoperfusion or ischemia produces an increase in plasma renin that stimulates the conversion of angiotensin I to angiotensin II, causing vasoconstriction and aldosterone secretion, sodium retention, and potassium wasting. Hypertension results and can be self-sustaining after some time, even in the case of unilateral RAS, because of hypertensive damage to the contralateral kidney.

Dx DIAGNOSIS

SCREENING

American College of Cardiology and American Heart Association (ACC/AHA) guidelines for identifying patients who should be screened for RAS
- Onset of hypertension at age <30 yr or severe hypertension at age >55 yr
- Malignant hypertension: hypertension with coexistent evidence of acute end-organ damage (acute renal failure, acute decompensated heart failure, new visual or neurologic disturbance, and/or retinopathy)
- Accelerated hypertension: sudden and persistent worsening
- Resistant hypertension: full doses of a three-drug regimen that includes a diuretic
- Sudden unexpected pulmonary edema
- New azotemia or acute renal failure after ACEI or angiotensin receptor blockers (ARBs)

LABORATORY TESTS

- Basic chemistry, including sodium, potassium, and creatinine
- Glomerular filtration rate
- Urinalysis

IMAGING STUDIES

- Duplex ultrasound, CT angiography, and magnetic resonance angiography (MRA) are effective diagnostic screening methods. The choice of imaging modality will depend on the availability of the diagnostic tool, the experience and local accuracy of each modality, and patient characteristics, including body size, renal function, contrast allergy, and presence of prior stents.
- Duplex ultrasound is safe and inexpensive. When compared with angiography, duplex ultrasound has a sensitivity of 84% to 98% and a specificity of 62% to 99% for detecting RAS. An end-diastolic velocity of >150 cm/sec predicts severe RAS. Duplex ultrasonography may be used to measure the renal dimensions and the renal resistive index. When ultrasound examination shows size discrepancy >1.5 cm, this suggests significant RAS involving the smaller kidney. Limitations include operator-dependent imaging, patient body habitus, and poor visualization of accessory renal arteries.
- MRA (Fig. 1-319) provides good visualization of both main and accessory renal arteries. Limitations include the associated risk of nephrogenic systemic fibrosis with gadolinium infusion, high cost, inability to image within a previously placed metallic stent, and lack of widespread availability.
- CT angiography is fast and effective but requires radiation exposure and infusion of potentially nephrotoxic iodinated contrast.
- IV digital subtraction catheter angiography (88% sensitivity, 90% specificity) is the reference standard for anatomic diagnosis of RAS. It is not a first-line screening tool but is rec-

ommended, if noninvasive tests are inconclusive but clinical suspicion is high. Renal fractional flow reserve (FFR) at the time of catheter angiography can be used to assess severity of RAS using maximal vasodilatation with papaverine. A FFR of <0.9 corresponds to an approximate systolic gradient of 25 mm Hg and is associated with a significant increase in renin production.

Rx TREATMENT

Acute renal artery thrombosis:
- Thrombolytic therapy.
- Anticoagulation.
- Revascularization (endovascular therapy or surgery). Endovascular renal artery stenting is favored over surgery, and has shown better clinical results when compared with balloon angioplasty (without stenting). Primary open revascularization can be considered selectively for nonatherosclerotic renal artery disease (NARAD) in some young patients or patients who need complex renal reconstructions.
- Blood pressure control.

Cholesterol emboli:
- Supportive care

Renovascular hypertension:
- Because of the activation of the renin-angiotensin-aldosterone system in renal artery stenosis, ACEI/ARBs are recommended for the treatment of renovascular hypertension. Renal function should be monitored carefully when initiating or titrating these medications, particularly in patients with bilateral RAS or unilateral stenosis with solitary kidney, so as to avoid precipitating acute renal failure.
- Beta-blockers are recommended for the treatment of hypertension in patients with RAS of all types.
- Angioplasty/stent or surgical revascularization should be reserved for patients whose blood pressure control with medication is difficult and for patients with progressive disease. The ACC/AHA guidelines for clinical indications of renal artery revascularization in the presence of significant stenosis include:
1. Accelerated, resistant, or malignant hypertension
2. Hypertension with unilateral small kidney
3. Hypertension with intolerance to medication
4. Treatment of cardiac destabilization syndromes such as unexplained heart failure exacerbations, episodes of flash pulmonary edema, and refractory or unstable angina
5. Progressive chronic kidney disease with bilateral RAS or RAS associated with a solitary functioning kidney

NATURAL HISTORY

- RAS caused by fibromuscular dysplasia generally does not progress. Fibromuscular dysplasia RAS responds well to angioplasty with long-term patency of the lesion typically observed.
- RAS associated with atherosclerosis is progressive. Of patients with >60% stenosis, 5% progress to total occlusion in 1 yr and 11% progress in 2 yr.
- An increased pulse pressure (PP), defined as systolic minus diastolic blood pressure, has been implicated in the development and progression of small-vessel disease and has been shown to reflect more advanced renal disease. It can help identify patients who are less likely to benefit from percutaneous interventions.

EBM EVIDENCE

available at www.expertconsult.com

SUGGESTED READINGS

available at www.expertconsult.com

AUTHORS: **JEANNETTE P. LIN, M.D.,** **FRED F. FERRI, M.D.,** and **PRANAV M. PATEL, M.D.**

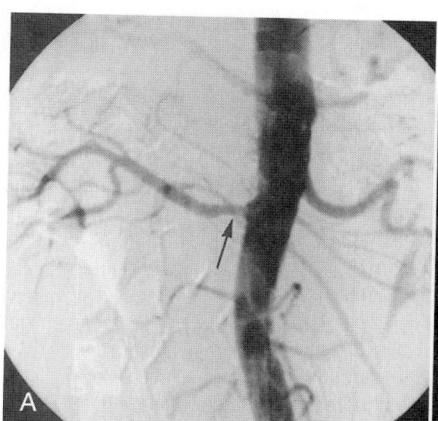 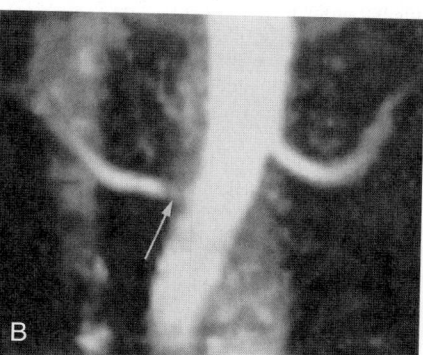

FIGURE 1-319 Renal arteriograms. A, Conventional renal digital subtraction (DSA) showing mild renal stenosis *(arrows)* on the right. **B,** Magnetic resonance angiogram (MRA) of the same patient. The stenosed segment *(arrows)* is clearly seen in this coronal projection. (Photograph provided by Dr. W. Gedroyc.) (From Souhami RL, Moxham J: *Textbook of medicine,* ed 4, London, 2002, Churchill Livingstone.)

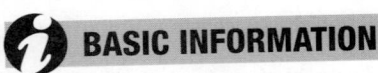

DEFINITION

Renal cell adenocarcinoma (RCA) is a primary adenocarcinoma originating in the renal parenchyma from the malignant transformation of proximal renal tubular epithelial cells.

SYNONYMS

Hypernephroma
Clear cell carcinoma of the kidney
Grawitz tumor

ICD-9CM CODES
189.0 Adenocarcinoma of kidney
189.1 (Renal pelvis)

EPIDEMIOLOGY & DEMOGRAPHICS

INCIDENCE: Approximately one in 10,000 persons annually (3% of all adult malignancies). In the U.S., renal cancer is the seventh leading malignant condition among men and twelfth among women. Two percent of cases of renal cancer are associated with inherited syndromes.
PREDOMINANT SEX: Male/female ratio of 2:1
PREDOMINANT AGE: Peaks at age 50 to 70 yr

PHYSICAL FINDINGS & CLINICAL PRESENTATION

The classic presentation of RCA includes the triad of flank pain, hematuria, and a palpable abdominal mass. This now represents an unusual presentation. Current presenting findings in RCA patients now include:

Hematuria	50% to 60%
Elevated erythrocyte sedimentation rate	50% to 60%
Abdominal mass	25% to 45%
Anemia	20% to 40%
Flank pain	35% to 40%
Hypertension	20% to 40%
Weight loss	30% to 35%
Fever	5% to 15%
Hepatic dysfunction	10% to 15%
Classic triad (hematuria, abdominal mass, flank pain)	5% to 10%
Hypercalcemia	3% to 6%
Erythrocytosis	3% to 4%
Varicocele	2% to 3%

ETIOLOGY

Hereditary forms:
- Familial renal carcinoma
- Renal carcinoma associated with von Hippel-Lindau disease
- Hereditary papillary renal cell carcinoma

Risk factors:
- Cigarette smoking
- Obesity
- Use of diuretics
- Phenacetin-containing analgesics
- Asbestos exposure
- Gasoline and other petroleum products
- Lead
- Cadmium
- Thorotrast
- Role of the *VHL* gene on chromosome 3

DIAGNOSIS

DIFFERENTIAL DIAGNOSIS
- Transitional cell carcinomas of the renal pelvis (8% of all renal cancers)
- Wilms' tumor
- Other rare primary renal carcinomas and sarcomas
- Renal cysts
- All causes of hematuria (see Section II)
- Retroperitoneal tumors

WORKUP
- Laboratory tests and imaging studies.
- Section III, "Renal Mass," describes patient evaluation.

LABORATORY TESTS
- Complete blood count: anemia or erythrocytosis
- Elevated sedimentation rate (nonspecific)
- Nonmetastatic hepatic dysfunction with elevated alkaline phosphatase, prolonged prothrombin time, and hypoalbuminemia
- Hypercalcemia (caused by parathyroid-related protein)
- Other: elevated ferritin, elevated insulin and glucagon levels, elevated alpha-fetoprotein, and elevated beta–human chorionic gonadotropin
- Recent reports indicate that urine AQP1 and ADFP concentrations quantified by Western blot appear to be sensitive and specific biomarkers of kidney cancers of proximal tubule origin and may be useful to diagnose an imaged renal mass and scree for kidney cancer at an early stage. Additional investigations are underway to determine if these tests should become standard tumor markers in the investigation of renal masses.

IMAGING STUDIES

Nearly 50% of renal cancers are now detected because a renal mass is incidentally detected on radiographic evaluation.
- Renal ultrasound
- Abdominal CT scan with contrast (Fig. 1-320)
- MRI
- Renal arteriogram
- Intravenous pyelography

STAGING
See Table 1-153.

COMMON SITES OF METASTASES

Lung	50% to 60%
Bone	30% to 40%
Regional nodes	15% to 30%
Main renal vein	15% to 20%
Perirenal fat	10% to 20%
Adrenal (ipsilateral)	10% to 15%
Vena cava	10% to 15%
Brain	10% to 15%
Adjacent organs (colon, pancreas)	10%
Kidney (contralateral)	2%

TREATMENT

- Surgery
  - Surgical nephrectomy is the only effective management for stages I, II, and some stage III tumors.
  - Various forms of partial nephrectomy may be available for patients with bilateral cancers or with a solitary kidney.
  - The role of nephrectomy in patients with metastatic renal cell carcinoma is controversial and should probably be reserved for patients who have a solitary metastasis amenable to surgical resection.
- Angioinfarction (for palliation)
- Radiotherapy (for palliation)
- Chemotherapy: inhibitors of vascular endothelial growth factor (VEGF) such as the anti-

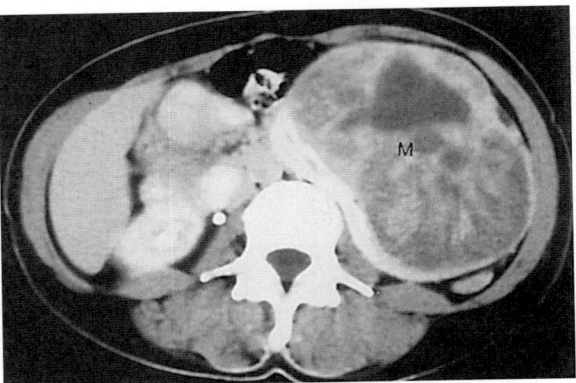

FIGURE 1-320 Large renal cell carcioma. Large mass *(M)* containing areas of high enhancement, low enhancement, and necrosis. (From Stein JH [ed]: *Internal medicine,* ed 5, St Louis, 1998, Mosby.)

vascular endothelial growth factor antibody Bevacizumab or mammalian target of rapamycin (mTOR) are often used. Inhibitors such as everolimus and temsirolimus are newer effective agents. Sunitinib, pazopanib, and sorafenib are oral multi- tyrosine kinase inhibitors useful for therapy of advanced renal cell carcinoma (as first-line therapy) or in patients not responding to or intolerant of cytokine therapy.

- Hormonal therapy (high-dose progesterone may achieve a 15% to 20% response rate)
- Immunotherapy (interleukin-2 may achieve a 15% to 30% response rate; alpha-, beta-, and gamma-interferons are somewhat less effective; for example, interferon alfa-2b increased postnephrectomy median survival by 30% in one recent trial)

PROGNOSIS

Prognosis of surgically treated patients:

TNM Stage	5-yr Survival (%)
I	95
II	88
III (renal vein or vena cava)	50 to 60
III (nodal involvement)	15 to 25
IV	5 to 20

REFERRAL

To urologist

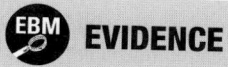

available at www.expertconsult.com

SUGGESTED READINGS
available at www.expertconsult.com

AUTHOR: **FRED F. FERRI, M.D.**

TABLE 1-153 Comparison of Conventional and TNM Staging Classification of RCAs

Robson Stage	T	N	M
I: Tumor confined by capsule	T_1 (tumor $\leq$2.5 cm) T_2 (tumor >2.5 cm, limited to kidney)		
II: Tumor extension to perirenal fat or ipsilateral adrenal but confined by Gerota's fascia	T_3a (tumor invades adrenal gland or perinephric fat but not beyond Gerota's fascia)		
IIIa: Renal vein or inferior vena caval involvement	T_3b (renal vein or caval involvement below diaphragm)	N_0 (nodes negative)	M_0 (no distant metastases)
IIIb: Lymphatic involvement	T_{1-4}	N_1 (single lymph node $\leq$2 cm) N_2 (single node 2 to 5 cm, or multiple N_3 (single or multiple nodes >5 cm)	T_3c (caval involvement above nodes <5 cm)
IIIc: Combination of IIIa and IIIb	$T_{3,4}$		
IVa: Spread to contiguous	T_4 (tumor extends beyond organs except ipsilateral adrenal Gerota's fascia)		
IVb: Distant metastases	T_{1-4}		M_1 (distant metastases)

RCC, Renal cell carcinoma.

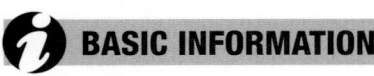

BASIC INFORMATION

DEFINITION
Acute renal failure (ARF) is the rapid impairment in renal function resulting in retention of products in the blood that are normally excreted by the kidneys.

SYNONYMS
ARF

ICD-9CM CODES
584.9 Acute renal failure, unspecified

EPIDEMIOLOGY & DEMOGRAPHICS
- ARF requiring dialysis develops in five in 100,000 persons annually.
- >10% of intensive care unit patients develop ARF.
- >40% of hospital ARF is iatrogenic.
- The most common cause of ARF in hospitalized patients is intrinsic renal failure caused by acute tubular necrosis.
- Acute renal failure occurs in 20% of patients with moderate sepsis and more than 50% of patients with septic shock and positive blood cultures.

PHYSICAL FINDINGS & CLINICAL PRESENTATION
- The physical examination should focus on volume status. The physical findings noted below vary with the duration and rapidity of onset of renal failure.
- Peripheral edema
- Skin pallor, ecchymoses
- Oliguria (however, patients can have nonoliguric renal failure), anuria
- Delirium, lethargy, myoclonus, seizures
- Back pain, fasciculations, muscle cramps
- Tachypnea, tachycardia
- Weakness, anorexia, generalized malaise, nausea

ETIOLOGY
- Prerenal: inadequate perfusion caused by hypovolemia, congestive heart failure, cirrhosis, sepsis. Sixty percent of community-acquired cases of ARF are from prerenal conditions.
- Postrenal: outlet obstruction from prostatic enlargement, ureteral obstruction (stones), bilateral renal vein occlusion. Postrenal causes account for 5% to 15% of community-acquired ARF.
- Intrinsic renal: glomerulonephritis, acute tubular necrosis, drug toxicity, contrast nephropathy. Contrast-induced nephropathy (increase in serum creatinine > 25% within 3 days of intravascular contrast administration in absence of an alternative cause) is the third most common cause of new ARF in hospitalized patients.
- Causes of acute renal failure are described in Section II.

DIAGNOSIS

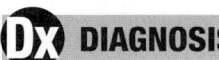

DIFFERENTIAL DIAGNOSIS
Refer to "Etiology."

LABORATORY TESTS
- Elevated serum creatinine: the rate of rise is approximately 1 mg/dl/day in complete renal failure.
- Elevated blood urea nitrogen (BUN): BUN/creatinine ratio is >20:1 in prerenal azotemia, postrenal azotemia, and acute glomerulonephritis; it is <20:1 in acute interstitial nephritis and acute tubular necrosis (Table 1-154).
- Electrolytes (potassium, phosphate) are elevated; bicarbonate level and calcium are decreased.
- Complete blood count may reveal anemia because of decreased erythropoietin production, hemoconcentration, or hemolysis.
- Urinalysis may reveal the presence of hematuria (glomerulonephritis), proteinuria (nephrotic syndrome), casts (e.g., granular casts in acute tubular necrosis, red blood cell casts in acute GN, white blood cell casts in acute interstitial nephritis), eosinophiluria (acute interstitial nephritis).
- Urinary sodium and urinary creatinine should also be obtained to calculate the fractional excretion of sodium (FE_{Na}) (FE_{Na} = Urine sodium/Plasma sodium × Plasma creatinine/Urine creatinine × 100). FE_{Na} is <1 in prerenal failure and >1 in intrinsic renal failure in patients with urine output <400 ml/day.
- Urinary osmolarity is 250 to 300 mOsm/kg in ATN, <400 mOsm/kg in postrenal azotemia, and >500 mOsm/kg in prerenal azotemia and acute glomerulonephritis (Table 1-155).
- Additional useful studies are blood cultures for patients suspected of sepsis, liver function tests, immunoglobulins, and protein electrophoresis in patients suspected of myeloma; and creatinine kinase in patients with suspected rhabdomyolysis.
- Renal biopsy may be indicated in patients with intrinsic renal failure when considering specific therapy; major uses of renal biopsy are differential diagnosis of nephrotic syndrome, separation of lupus vasculitis from other vasculitis and lupus membranous from idiopathic membranous, confirmation of hereditary nephropathies on the basis of the ultrastructure, diagnosis of rapidly progressing glomerulonephritis, separation of allergic interstitial nephritis from ATN, separation of primary glomerulonephritis syndromes. The biopsy may be performed percutaneously or by open method. The percutaneous approach is favored and generally yields adequate tissue in >90% of cases. Open biopsy is generally reserved for uncooperative patients, those with solitary kidney, and patients at risk for uncontrolled bleeding.

IMAGING STUDIES
- Chest x-ray is useful to evaluate for congestive heart failure and for pulmonary renal syndromes (Goodpasture's syndrome, Wegener's granulomatosis).
- Ultrasound of kidneys is used to evaluate kidney size (useful to distinguish acute from

TABLE 1-154 Serum and Radiographic Abnormalities in Renal Failure

	Prerenal	Postrenal (Acute)	Intrinsic Renal (Acute)	Intrinsic Renal (Chronic)
BUN	↑ 10:1 > Cr	↑ 20-40/day	↑ 20-40/day	Stable; ↑ varies with protein intake
Serum creatinine	N/moderate ↑	↑ 2-4/day	↑ 2-4/day	Stable ↑ (production equals excretion)
Serum potassium	N/moderate ↑	↑ varies with urinary volume	↑↑ (particularly when patient is oliguric)	Normal until end stage, unless tubular dysfunction (type 4 RTA)
			↑↑↑ with rhabdomyolysis	
Serum phosphorus	N/moderate ↑	Moderate ↑	↑	Becomes significantly elevated when serum creatinine surpasses 3 mg/dl
		↑↑ with rhabdomyolysis	Poor correlation with duration of renal disease	
Serum calcium	N	N/↓ with PO_4^{-3} retention	↓ (poor correlation with duration of renal failure)	Usually ↓
Renal size				
By ultrasonography	N/↑	↑ and dilated calyces	N/↑	↓ and with ↑ echogenicity
FE_{Na}*	<1	<1 → >1	>1†	>1

In Ferri FF (ed): *Practical guide to the care of the medical patient*, ed 8, St Louis, 2011, Mosby.
↑, Increase; ↓, decrease; ↑↑, large increase; ↑↑↑, very high increase; *BUN*, blood urea nitrogen; *Cr*, creatinine; *N*, normal; *Na*, sodium; *P*, plasma; *RTA*, renal tubular acidosis; *U*, urine.

$$*FE_{Na} = \left[\frac{U/P_{Na^+}}{U/P_{Cr}} \times 100 \right]$$ (useful only in oliguric patient).

†May be ≤1 in radiocontrast-induced myoglobinuric acute tubular necrosis and in early sepsis.

chronic renal failure), evaluate for the presence of obstruction, and evaluate renal vascular status (with Doppler evaluation).

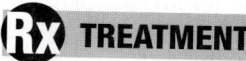 **TREATMENT**

NONPHARMACOLOGIC THERAPY
- Stop all nephrotoxic medications.
- Dietary modification to supply adequate calories while minimizing accumulation of toxins; appropriate control of fluid balance. Physicians should recommend a nutrition program with an energy prescription of 120 to 150 KJ/kg/day and restriction of potassium (60 mEq/day), sodium (90 mEq/day), and phosphorus (800 mg/day). Ideal protein supplementation ranges from 0.6 to 1.4 g/kg depending on whether dialysis is required.
- Daily weight.
- Modifications of dosage of renally excreted drugs.

ACUTE GENERAL Rx
Treatment is variable with etiology of ARF:
- Prerenal: IV volume expansion in hypovolemic patients.
- Intrinsic renal: discontinuation of any potential toxins and treatment of condition causing the renal failure.
  1. Low-dose dopamine is at times used to influence renal dysfunction and may offer transient improvement in renal physiology; however, there is lack of evidence that it

offers significant clinical benefits to patients with or at risk for acute renal failure.
  2. Fenoldopam, a dopamine alpha-1 receptor agonist currently approved for inpatient management of severe hypertension, has been reported to be beneficial in patients at risk for renal failure related to reduced renal blood flow.
  3. Although furosemide is used frequently to convert oliguric to nonoliguric renal failure in patients with early ARF, it has no effect on mortality rate, dialysis requirement, or proportion of patients with persistent oliguria. Its use in a high dose is also associated with increased risk of tinnitus and temporary deafness.
- Postrenal: removal of obstruction.

CHRONIC Rx
- Monitoring of renal function and electrolytes.
- Prevention of further insults to the kidneys with proper hydration, especially before contrast studies, and avoidance of nephrotoxic agents. Hydration with sodium bicarbonate (addition of 154 ml of 1000 mEq/L sodium bicarbonate to 846 ml of 5% dextrose in water) before contrast exposure is more effective than hydration with sodium chloride for prophylaxis of contrast-induced renal failure. Administration of *N*-acetylcysteine prophylaxis has been shown to reduce the risk of contrast-induced nephropathy.
- See "Chronic Renal Failure" entry for indications for initiation of dialysis. Daily hemodialysis is superior to every-other-day hemodi-

alysis in patients with acute tubular necrosis and ARF.

DISPOSITION
- General indications for initiation of dialysis are:
  1. Florid symptoms of uremia (encephalopathy, pericarditis)
  2. Severe volume overload
  3. Severe acid–base imbalance
  4. Significant derangement in electrolyte concentrations (e.g., hyperkalemia, hyponatremia)
- Intermittent hemodialysis and continuous renal replacement therapy have similar outcomes for patients with ARF.
- Renal function recovery (ability to discontinue dialysis) varies from 50% to 75% in survivors of ARF.
- Overall mortality rate in ARF is nearly 50%, varying from 60% in patients with ATN to 35% in patients with prerenal or postrenal ARF.
- The combination of ARF and sepsis is associated with a 70% mortality rate.

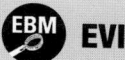 **EVIDENCE**

available at www.expertconsult.com

SUGGESTED READINGS
available at www.expertconsult.com

AUTHOR: **FRED F. FERRI, M.D.**

TABLE 1-155 Urinary Abnormalities in Renal Failure

	Prerenal	Postrenal (Acute)	Intrinsic Renal (Acute)	Intrinsic Renal (Chronic)
Urinary volume	↓	Absent-to-wide fluctuation	Oliguric or nonoliguric	1000 ml + until end stage
Urinary creatinine	↑ (U/P Cr ±40)	↓ (U/P Cr ±20)	↓ (U/P Cr <20)	↓ (U/P Cr <20)
Osmolarity	↑ (±400 mOsm/kg)	(<350 mOsm/kg)	(<350 mOsm/kg)	(<350 mOsm/kg)
Degree of proteinuria	Minimum	Absent	Varies with cause of renal failure: Modest with ATN Nephrotic range common with acute glomerulopathies, usually <2 g/24 hr with interstitial disease*	Varies with cause of renal disease (from 1-2 g/day to nephrotic range)
Urinary sediment	Negative, or occasional hyaline cast	Negative or hematuria with stones or papillary necrosis Pyuria with infectious prostatic disease	ATN: muddy brown casts Interstitial nephritis: lymphocytes, eosinophils (in stained preparations), and WBC casts RPGN: RBC casts Nephrosis: oval fat bodies	Broad casts with variable renal "residual" acute findings

In Ferri FF (ed): *Practical guide to the care of the medical patient,* ed 8, St Louis, 2011, Mosby.

↑, Increased; ↓, decreased; *ATN,* acute tubular necrosis; clearance $= \dfrac{\text{urinary concentration} \times \text{urinary volume}}{\text{plasma concentration}}$; *Cr,* creatinine; *RBC,* red blood cell; *RPGN,* rapidly progressive glomerulonephritis; *U/P,* urine/plasma; *WBC,* white blood cell.

*Except nonsteroidal anti-inflammatory drug-induced allergic interstitial nephritis with concomitant "nil disease."

BASIC INFORMATION

DEFINITION

Chronic renal failure (CRF) is a progressive decrease in renal function (glomerular filtration rate [GFR] <60 ml/min for >3 mo) with subsequent accumulation of waste products in the blood, electrolyte abnormalities, and anemia. The National Kidney Foundation Disease Outcomes Quality Initiative defines chronic kidney disease (CKD) as follows, regardless of clinical diagnosis: kidney damage (usually defined as an albumin-creatinine ratio [ACR] ≥30 mg/g) or a glomerular filtration rate (GFR) <60 ml/min per 1.73 m² (usually estimated from the serum creatinine level) for at least 3 mo.

SYNONYMS

CRF
Chronic kidney disease
CKD
End-stage renal disease

ICD-9CM CODES
585 Chronic renal failure

EPIDEMIOLOGY & DEMOGRAPHICS

- The prevalence of patients with chronic kidney disease in the U.S. is approximately 11%.
- The number of patients with end-stage renal disease (ESRD) is increasing at the rate of 7% to 9% per year in the U.S. Each year two in 10,000 persons develop end-stage CRF.
- In the U.S., >250,000 people per year receive dialysis treatment for ESRD.
- Although kidney transplantation is considered the best choice for renal replacement therapy, many patients are not eligible for transplantation and more than 100,000 patients start dialysis each year.

PHYSICAL FINDINGS & CLINICAL PRESENTATION

- Skin pallor, ecchymoses.
- Edema, leg cramps, restless legs, peripheral neuropathy.
- Hypertension.
- Emotional lability and depression, decreased mental acuity.
- The clinical presentation varies with the degree of renal failure and its underlying etiology. Common symptoms are generalized fatigue, nausea, anorexia, pruritus, sleep disturbances, smell and taste disturbances, hiccups, and seizures.

ETIOLOGY

- Diabetes (37%), hypertension (30%), chronic glomerulonephritis (12%)
- Polycystic kidney disease
- Tubular interstitial nephritis (e.g., drug hypersensitivity, analgesic nephropathy), obstructive nephropathies (e.g., nephrolithiasis, prostatic disease)
- Vascular diseases (renal artery stenosis, hypertensive nephrosclerosis)

DIAGNOSIS

- CRF is primarily distinguished from acute RF by the duration (progression over several months).
- Sonographic evaluation of the kidneys reveals smaller kidneys with increased echogenicity in CRF.

WORKUP

- Laboratory evaluation and imaging studies should be aimed at identifying reversible causes of acute decrements in GFR (e.g., volume depletion, urinary tract obstruction, congestive heart failure [CHF]) superimposed on chronic renal disease.
- Kidney biopsy: generally not performed in patients with small kidneys or with advanced disease.
- GFR is the best overall indicator of kidney function. It can be estimated by using prediction equations that take into account the serum creatinine level and some or all specific variables (body size, age, sex, race). GFR calculators are available on the National Kidney Foundation website (http://www.kidney.org/kls/professionals/gfr_calculator.cfm).

LABORATORY TESTS

- Elevated blood urea nitrogen (BUN), creatinine, creatinine clearance.

- Urinalysis: may reveal proteinuria, red blood cell casts.
- Serum chemistry: elevated BUN and creatinine, hyperkalemia, hyperuricemia, hypocalcemia, hyperphosphatemia, hyperglycemia, decreased bicarbonate. Fig. 1-321 Illustrates calcium and phosphate homeostasis in the setting of renal failure.
- Measure urinary protein excretion. The finding of a protein/creatinine ratio of >1000 mg/g suggests the presence of glomerular disease.
- Special studies: serum and urine immuno-electrophoresis (in suspected multiple myeloma), antinuclear antibody (in suspected systemic lupus erythematosus).
- Cystatin C is a cysteine proteinase inhibitor produced by all nucleated cells, freely filtered at the glomerulus but not secreted by tubular cells. Given these characteristics, it may be superior to creatinine concentration both in kidney disease and as a marker of acute kidney injury. It is a better index of kidney function in elderly patients and a better predictor of outcomes than creatinine. The association of cystatin C is stronger than the association of measured GFR with all-cause and cardiovascular mortality in patients with advanced chronic kidney disease.

IMAGING STUDIES

Ultrasound of kidneys to measure kidney size and rule out obstruction

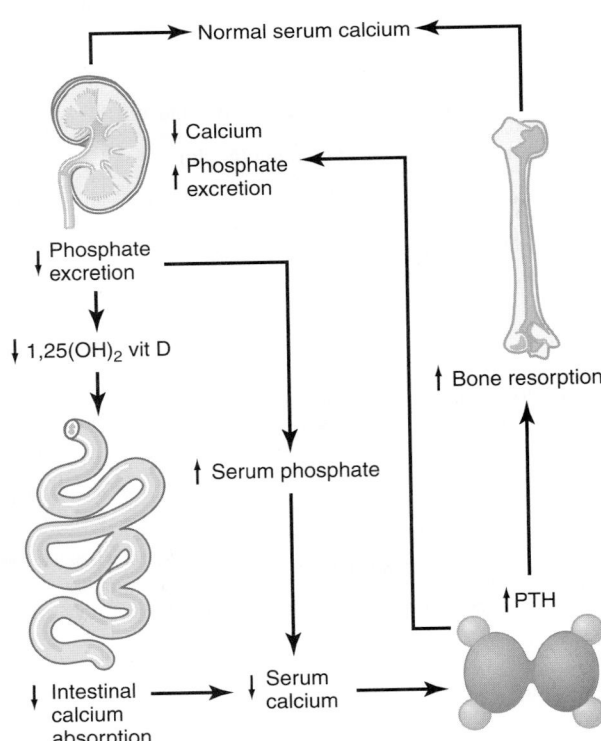

FIGURE 1-321 Calcium and phosphate homeostasis in the setting of renal failure. The decreased excretion of phosphate initiates the cycle directed at normalization of the serum calcium concentration. PTH, parathyroid hormone. (From Andreoli, TE et al: *Andreoli and Carpenter's Cecil essentials of medicine,* ed 8, Philadelphia, 2010, Saunders.)

Rx TREATMENT

NONPHARMACOLOGIC THERAPY

- Provide adequate nutrition and calories (147 to 168 kJ/kg/day in energy intake, chiefly from carbohydrate and polyunsaturated fats). Referral to a dietician for nutritional therapy for patients with GFR <50 ml/1.73 m² is recommended and is now a covered service by Medicare.
- Restrict sodium (approximately 100 mmol/day), potassium (≤60 mmol/day), and phosphate (<800 mg/day).
- Adjust drug doses to correct for prolonged half-lives.
- Restrict fluid if significant edema is present.
- Protein restriction (≤0.8 g/kg/day) may slow deterioration of renal function; however, recent studies have not confirmed this benefit. Table 1-156 describes traditional recommendations regarding intake of protein and energy in kidney failure; however, there is insufficient evidence to strongly recommend or advise against routine restriction of protein intake.
- Resistance exercise training can preserve lean body mass, nutritional status, and muscle function in patients with moderate chronic kidney disease.
- Avoid radiocontrast agents. Hydration with sodium bicarbonate before contrast exposure is more effective than hydration with sodium chloride for prophylaxis of contrast-induced renal failure.
- Smoking cessation.
- Initiate hemodialysis, usually performed in center three times per week, or peritoneal dialysis, usually done by the patient at home (see "Acute General Rx").
- Prompt referral to nephrologist is essential. Late evaluation of patients with chronic renal disease is associated with greater burden and severity of comorbid disease and shorter survival.
- Kidney transplantation in selected patients.

ACUTE GENERAL Rx

- Angiotensin-converting enzyme (ACE) inhibitors and angiotensin receptor blockers are useful in reducing proteinuria and slowing the progression of chronic renal disease, especially in hypertensive diabetic patients. The combination of ACEi and ARBs should be used with great caution in patients with chronic kidney disease due to increased risk of hyperkalemia, hypotension, and worsening renal failure. A systolic blood pressure between 110 and 129 mm Hg may be beneficial in patients with urine protein excretion >1.0 g/day. Systolic blood pressure <110 mm Hg may be associated with a higher risk for kidney disease progression.
- Initiation of dialysis:
  1. Urgent indications: uremic pericarditis, neuropathy, neuromuscular abnormalities, CHF, hyperkalemia, seizures.
  2. Judgmental indications: creatinine clearance 10 to 15 ml/min; progressive anorexia, weight loss, reversal of sleep pattern, pruritus, uncontrolled fluid gain with hypertension and signs of CHF.
- Erythropoiesis-stimulating agents epoetin-alpha and darbepoetin-alpha can be used to reduce the need for transfusions in patients with anemia. Anemia should not be fully corrected in patients with chronic kidney disease. Maintaining a target hemoglobin of 10 g/dl or hematocrit 30% to 33% is satisfactory. Targeting higher hemoglobin levels in CKD may increase risks for stroke, hypertension, and serious cardiovascular events.
- Diuretics for significant fluid overload (loop diuretics are preferred).
- Correction of hypertension to at least 130/85 mm Hg with ACE inhibitors (avoid in patients with significant hyperkalemia), ARBs, and/or nondihydropyridene calcium channel blockers (verapamil, diltiazem) can be used in patients intolerant to ACE inhibitors or when other agents are needed to control blood pressure.
- Correction of electrolyte abnormalities (e.g., calcium chloride, glucose, sodium polysty-

rene sulfonate for hyperkalemia), sodium bicarbonate in patients with severe metabolic acidosis.
- Lipid-lowering agents in patients with dyslipidemia; target low-density lipoprotein cholesterol is <100 mg/dl.
- Control of renal osteodystrophy with calcium supplementation and vitamin D. Starting dose of calcium carbonate is 0.5 g with each meal, increased until the serum phosphorus concentration is normalized (most patients require 5 to 10 g/day). Calcitriol 0.125 to 0.25 mcg/day PO is effective in increasing serum calcium concentration. Paricalcitol, a new vitamin D analogue, has been reported to be more effective than calcitriol in lessening the elevations in serum calcium and phosphorus levels.
- Dietary phosphate restriction effectively reduces serum phosphate levels and is recommended in all patiens with ESRD. For additional management of hyperphosphatemia, calcium-based agents are inexpensive, well tolerated, and should be the first-line phosphate binders for patients undergoing dialysis. Sevelamer and lanthanum are also effective ad phosphate binders, but are much more expensive.

DISPOSITION

- Prognosis is influenced by comorbidity of multisystem diseases. Late referral of patients to a nephrologist is associated with higher mortality and morbidity rates and higher costs. Despite recommendations for early referral, up to 64% of patients with CRF are still referred late.
- Lower predialysis serum sodium concentration is associated with an increased risk of death.
- Apolipoprotein E variation predicts chronic kidney disease progression, independent of diabetes, race, lipid, and nonlipid factors. The e2 allele moderately increases risk of kidney disease progression, whereas allele e4 decreases the risk.
- Kidney transplantation in selected patients improves survival. The 2-yr kidney graft survival rate for living related donor transplantations is >80%, whereas the 2-yr graft survival rate for cadaveric donor transplantation is approximately 70%.

EBM **EVIDENCE**

available at www.expertconsult.com

SUGGESTED READINGS

available at www.expertconsult.com

TABLE 1-156 Recommended Intake of Protein and Energy in Kidney Failure

Chronic Kidney Disease	Protein	Energy
Stage 1-3 (GFR > 30 ml/min)	No restriction	No restriction
Stage 4-5 (GFR < 30 ml/min)	0.60-0.75 g/kg/day*	35 kcal/kg/day†
Dialysis		
Hemodialysis	>1.2 g/kg/day	35 kcal/kg/day†
Peritoneal dialysis	>1.3 g/kg/day	35 kcal/kg/day†

Andreoli, TE, Benjamin, IJ, Griggs, RC, Wing, EJ: *Andreoli and Carpenter's Cecil essentials of medicine*, ed 8, Philadelphia, 2010, Saunders.

*With close supervision and frequent dietary counseling.
†30 kcal/kg/day for individuals 60 years or older.
GFR, Glomerular filtration rate.

AUTHOR: **FRED F. FERRI, M.D.**

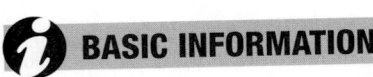

BASIC INFORMATION

DEFINITION

Renal tubular acidosis (RTA) is a disorder characterized by inability to excrete H^+ or inadequate generation of new HCO_3^-. Renal tubular acidosis syndromes are summarized in Table 1-157. There are four main types of renal tubular acidosis described in the medical literature:

- Type I (classic, distal RTA): abnormality in distal hydrogen secretion, resulting in hypokalemic hyperchloremic metabolic acidosis.
- Type II (proximal RTA): decreased proximal bicarbonate reabsorption, resulting in hypokalemic hyperchloremic metabolic acidosis.
- Type III (RTA of glomerular insufficiency): normokalemic hyperchloremic metabolic acidosis as a result of impaired ability to generate sufficient NH_3 in the setting of decreased glomerular filtration rate (<30 ml/min). This type of RTA is described in older textbooks and is considered by many not to be a distinct entity.
- Type IV (hyporeninemic hypoaldosteronemic RTA): aldosterone deficiency or antagonism, resulting in decreased distal acidification and decreased distal sodium reabsorption with subsequent hyperkalemic hyperchloremic acidosis.

SYNONYMS

RTA

ICD-9CM CODES
588.8 Renal tubular acidosis

EPIDEMIOLOGY & DEMOGRAPHICS

RTA type IV affects mostly adults, whereas RTA types I and II are more frequent in children.

PHYSICAL FINDINGS & CLINICAL PRESENTATION

- Examination may be normal.
- Poor skin turgor may be present from dehydration.
- Muscle weakness and muscle aches from hypokalemia may occur.
- Low back pain and bone pain may be present in patients with abnormalities of calcium metabolism (RTA II).
- There is failure to thrive in children (RTA II).

ETIOLOGY

- Type I RTA: autoimmune disorders, primary biliary cirrhosis and other liver diseases, medications (amphotericin, nonsteroidals), systemic lupus erythematosus, Sjögren's syndrome, genetic disorders (Ehlers-Danlos syndrome, Marfan syndrome, hereditary elliptocytosis), toxins (toluene), disorders with nephrocalcinosis (hyperparathyroidism, vitamin D intoxication, idiopathic hypercalciuria), tubulointerstitial disease (obstructive uropathy, renal transplantation)
- Type II RTA: Fanconi's syndrome, primary hyperparathyroidism, multiple myeloma, medications (acetazolamide)
- Type IV RTA: diabetes mellitus, sickle cell disease, Addison's disease, urinary obstruction

DIAGNOSIS

DIFFERENTIAL DIAGNOSIS

- Diarrhea with significant bicarbonate loss
- Other causes of metabolic acidosis
- Respiratory acidosis

WORKUP

Detection of hyperchloremic metabolic acidosis with arterial blood gases (ABGs) and serum electrolytes and evaluation of potential causes (see "Etiology")

LABORATORY TESTS

- ABGs reveal metabolic acidosis; serum potassium is low in RTA types I and II, normal in type III, and high in type IV.
- Minimal urine pH is >5.5 in RTA type I and <5.5 in types II, III, and IV.
- Urinary anion gap is 0 or positive in all types of RTA.
- Additional useful studies include serum calcium level and urine calcium.
- Anion gap is normal.
- Parathyroid hormone measurement is useful in patients suspected of primary hyperparathyroidism (may be associated with type II RTA).

IMAGING STUDIES

- Plain abdominal radiography is useful to evaluate for nephrocalcinosis.
- Renal sonogram can be used to evaluate renal size or presence of stones.
- Intravenous pyelogram in patients with nephrocalcinosis or nephrolithiasis.

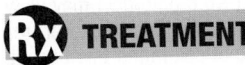 TREATMENT

ACUTE GENERAL Rx

- Types I and II are treated with oral sodium bicarbonate (1 to 2 mEq/kg/day in RTA I, 2 to 4 mEq/kg/day in RTA type II) titrated to correct acidosis.
- Potassium supplementation is needed in hypokalemic patients.
- Type IV RTA can be treated with furosemide to lower elevated potassium levels and sodium bicarbonate to correct significant acidosis. Fludrocortisone 100 to 300 μg/day can be used to correct mineralocorticoid deficiency.

CHRONIC Rx

- Frequent monitoring of potassium levels in RTA type IV
- Monitoring for bone disease in RTA type II
- Monitoring for nephrocalcinosis and nephrolithiasis in RTA type I

DISPOSITION

- Prognosis varies with the presence of associated conditions (see "Etiology").
- Untreated distal RTA may result in hypercalcemia, hyperphosphaturia, nephrolithiasis, and nephrocalcinosis.

PEARLS & CONSIDERATIONS

COMMENTS

Patient education material can be obtained from the National Kidney and Urologic Diseases Information Clearinghouse, Box NKUDIC, Bethesda, MD 20893.

AUTHOR: **FRED F. FERRI, M.D.**

TABLE 1-157 Renal Tubular Acidosis Syndromes

Type	Locus	Defect
Proximal	S_1-S_3	↓ HCO_3^- threshold
Hyperkalemic	CCD principal cell	↓ V_M (−) leading to ↓ H^+ secretion
Gradient limited	OMCD intercalated cells	Three specific defects in H^+ secretion

Andreoli TE, Benjamin IJ, Griggs RC, Wing EJ, *Andreoli and Carpenter's Cecil essentials of medicine*, ed 8, Philadelphia, 2010, Saunders.
CCD, Cortical collecting duct; *OMCD*, outer medullary collecting duct; *S*, segment; V_M (−), negative transepithelial voltage in the OMCD.

BASIC INFORMATION

DEFINITION

Renal vein thrombosis is the thrombotic occlusion of one or both renal veins.

ICD-9CM CODES

453.3 Renal vein thrombosis

EPIDEMIOLOGY & DEMOGRAPHICS

- Incidence unknown; probably an underdiagnosed condition
- May occur at any age with no gender preference
- Epidemiology tied to the underlying cause

PHYSICAL FINDINGS & CLINICAL PRESENTATION

Acute bilateral renal vein thrombosis:
- Back and bilateral flank pain
- Acute renal failure

Acute unilateral renal vein thrombosis:
- Flank pain
- Decline in renal function
- Hematuria
- Increase in the amount of proteinuria if associated with nephrotic syndrome

Chronic unilateral renal vein thrombosis:
- May be silent
- Pulmonary emboli and hemolysis
- Back pain
- Deep vein thrombosis in lower extremities
- Edema
- Glycosuria
- Hyperchloremic acidosis
- Left varicocele (if the left renal vein is thrombosed)
- Dilated abdominal veins

ETIOLOGY & PATHOGENESIS

- Extrinsic compression by a tumor or retroperitoneal mass
- Invasion of the renal vein or inferior vena cava by tumor (almost always renal cell cancer)
- Trauma
- Hypercoagulable states
- Dehydration
- Glomerulopathies (membranous glomerulonephritis, crescenting glomerulonephritis, systemic lupus erythematosus, amyloidosis) especially in the presence of nephrotic syndrome when the serum albumin is <2 g/dl
- NOTE: For unknown reasons, diabetic nephropathy is not commonly associated with renal vein thrombosis even if the nephrotic syndrome is present

A controversy has existed regarding whether the renal vein thrombosis association with nephrotic syndrome is a complication of nephrotic syndrome or whether renal vein thrombosis occurring in the setting of increased renal vein pressure (e.g., with congestive heart failure, constrictive pericarditis, or extrinsic compression) can independently cause proteinuria. Current evidence is that renal vein thrombosis does not cause nephrotic syndrome.

DIAGNOSIS

DIFFERENTIAL DIAGNOSIS

The diagnosis of renal vein thrombosis does not include any differential consideration. The differential diagnosis is that of proteinuria. Renal vein thrombosis should be considered if proteinuria worsens or if renal function worsens in a patient with glomerulonephritis. Renal vein thrombosis should also be considered in patients with pulmonary emboli and no lower-extremity deep vein thrombosis.

WORKUP

Clinical suspicion (see "Differential Diagnosis") and imaging studies

IMAGING STUDIES

- Abdominal ultrasound
- Abdominal MRI or CT with contrast (Fig. 1-322)
- Renal arteriography (delayed films during venous phase)
- Selective renal vein venography (inferior venacavogram images should be obtained before advancing the catheter in the vena cava because clots, if present, could be dislodged)
- Renal biopsy may be indicated if evidence of nephritis is present (e.g., active urinary sediment)

TREATMENT

- Anticoagulation in acute renal vein thrombosis to prevent pulmonary emboli and in attempt to improve renal function and decrease proteinuria
- Thrombolytic therapy or surgical thrombectomy has also been reported to be effective
- The value of anticoagulation in chronic renal vein thrombosis is dubious except in nephrotic patients with membranous glomerulonephritis with profound hypoalbuminemia where prolonged prophylactic anticoagulation may be of benefit even if renal vein thrombosis has not been documented

PROGNOSIS

Probable worsening of the underlying glomerulonephritis by acute renal vein thrombosis; the effect of chronic renal vein thrombosis is unclear.

AUTHOR: **FRED F. FERRI, M.D.**

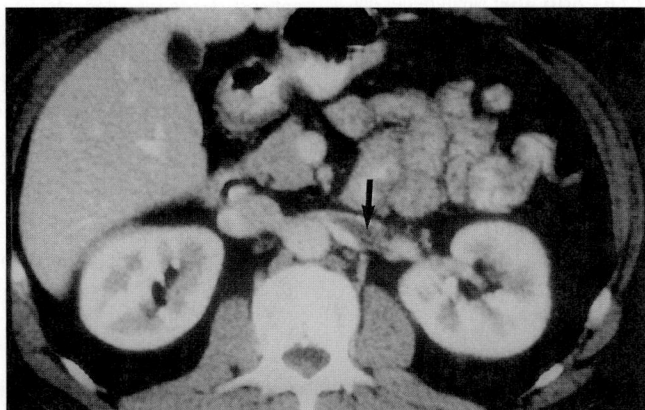

FIGURE 1-322 Renal vein thrombus in a patient with nephritic syndrome. Contrast medium–enhanced CT at the level of the renal vein shows thrombus in the left renal vein *(arrow)*. (From Grainger RG et al [eds]: *Grainger & Allison's diagnostic radiology,* ed 4, Philadelphia, 2001, Churchill Livingstone.)

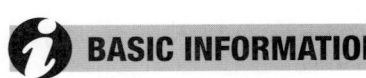
BASIC INFORMATION

DEFINITION
Respiratory syncytial virus (RSV) is an RNA virus that tends to form syncytia in tissue culture. RSV causes repeated acute respiratory tract infections in people of all ages. It is highly contagious and is the leading cause of severe lower respiratory tract infections in infants and young children, while it usually manifests as URIs, bronchiolitis, or tracheobronchitis in older children and adults.

SYNONYMS
RSV

ICD-9-CM CODES
ICD-079.6

EPIDEMIOLOGY & DEMOGRAPHICS
INCIDENCE: 64 million infections worldwide annually, resulting in 160,000 deaths; it is associated with 120,000 U.S. pediatric hospitalizations annually.
PEAK INCIDENCE: In nontropical areas of the northern hemisphere, seasonal outbreaks usually occur November to April, with a peak in January or February; in nontropical areas of the southern hemisphere, May to September, with a peak in May, June, or July. In the tropics, seasonal outbreaks usually occur during the rainy season. Incubation ranges from 2 to 8 days; though 4 to 6 days is most common.
PREVALENCE: Nearly everyone is infected by age 2, with reinfections occurring at all ages.
PREDOMINANT SEX AND AGE: None generally, but male sex may predispose to more severe respiratory disease in RSV infection.
GENETICS: Severe disease is associated with polymorphisms in various interleukins and CCR5.
RISK FACTORS: For children, risk factors include attending daycare or school and inpatient hospitalization. Severe disease is seen primarily in infants and young children (especially those born before 35 wk of gestation); the elderly; and in patients with cardiac, pulmonary, or immune system dysfunction.

PHYSICAL FINDINGS & CLINICAL PRESENTATION
Physical findings include fever, tachypnea, prolonged expiration, wheezes and rales, cough, rhinorrhea, coryza, conjunctivitis, and otitis media. Clinical presentation can include pneumonia and bronchiolitis.

ETIOLOGY
Humans are the only known reservoir. Transmission is by large respiratory droplets via close contact or contaminated surfaces, where it can survive for several hours. The CDC recommends handwashing, gowns and gloves to prevent nosocomial infection, which is especially common on pediatric wards. However, the CDC does not recommend excluding children with respiratory illnesses who are well enough to attend school or daycare, as RSV is often spread during early stages of illness.

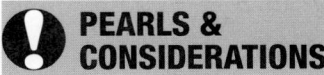
DIAGNOSIS

DIFFERENTIAL DIAGNOSIS
Influenza, parainfluenza, and adenovirus

WORKUP
- History with a focus on upper and lower respiratory symptoms, fever, and (in infants) apnea.
- Focused physical exam including temperature and pulse oximetry, as well as lung and HEENT exam.

LABORATORY TESTS
Nasopharyngeal specimens can be analyzed using rapid diagnostic assays, such as immunofluorescent and enzyme immunoassay techniques for detection of viral antigen and are generally reliable in infants and young children. Virus isolation is also possible, but requires 1 to 5 days and accuracy may vary. Serologic testing (serum antibodies) is less useful because it is unreliable in infants and is confounded in other patients due to repeated infections.

IMAGING STUDIES
Chest x-ray for suspected pneumonia, but not routinely in suspected bronchiolitis

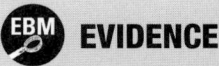
TREATMENT

NONPHARMACOLOGIC THERAPY
Early diagnosis and isolation techniques are important in limiting spread of RSV infections.

ACUTE GENERAL Rx
Primary treatment is supportive and may include hydration, careful clinical assessment of respiratory status, measurement of oxygen saturation, use of supplemental oxygen, suction of the upper airway, and, if necessary, intubation and mechanical ventilation.

- Mild disease: symptomatic treatment and supportive therapy
- Severe disease may require oxygen therapy, bronchodilators, corticosteroids, hospitalization, intubation, and mechanical ventilation.
- Ribavirin is not recommended for routine use but is specifically indicated for treatment of severe lower respiratory tract RSV infections in patients with additional underlying compromising conditions such as chronic lung conditions, prematurity, BPD congenital heart disease, immunodeficiency, immunosuppression, or organ transplantation. It may be used in selected patients with documented, potentially life-threatening RSV.

REFERRAL
To pulmonology for severe disease

PEARLS & CONSIDERATIONS

PREVENTION
Primary prevention is through avoidance of transmission through handwashing, proper procedures to avoid spread in healthcare facilitates, and diagnosis of suspected cases.

No benefit has been found from the use of RSV prophylaxis IGIV or RSV immune globulin (IG) monoclonal antibody and RSV-IGIV is no longer available. Palivizumab, a humanized mouse monoclonal antibody, is used for prevention of RSV lower respiratory tract disease in certain infants and children with chronic lung disease of prematurity, history of preterm birth (less than 35 wk gestation), or with congenital heart disease. Updated eligibility criteria for prophylaxis can be found in the American Academy of Pediatrics Red Book 2009 or in their online version.

PATIENT & FAMILY EDUCATION
Handwashing

EVIDENCE
available at www.expertconsult.com

SUGGESTED READINGS
available at www.expertconsult.com

AUTHORS: **STEVEN BUSSELEN, M.D.,** and **JEFFREY BORKAN, M.D., PH.D.**

BASIC INFORMATION

DEFINITION

Restless legs syndrome (RLS) is an awake phenomenon consisting of an urge to move legs, usually associated with feeling of discomfort in legs.

SYNONYMS Wittmaack-Ekbom's syndrome.

ICD-9CM CODES
333.94 Restless leg syndrome

EPIDEMIOLOGY & DEMOGRAPHICS

PREVALENCE: Average prevalence rate is 1% to 29%. Prevalence estimates in Europe are around 10%, and 0.1% to 12% in East Asian population.
PEAK PREVALENCE: 10% in persons aged 30 to 79 and 19% in persons aged 80 or above.
PREDOMINANT SEX: Early onset RLS is more common in females, with 2:1 female:male ratio.
PREDOMINANT AGE: Prevalence of RLS increases with age and is more commonly seen in elderly population.
GENETICS: Genetic basis of RLS has been reported, particularly in early onset RLS.
- Autosomal dominant disorder
- Common among first-degree relatives.
- Association between sequence in chromosome 6p,12q, 14q, 9p, 20p, 2p, 16p and RLS.
RISK FACTORS: Iron deficiency anemia, end-stage renal disease requiring hemodialysis, pregnancy, rheumatoid arthritis, Parkinson's disease, diabetes mellitus, neuropathy, and myelopathy.

CLASSIFICATION

- Primary RLS is without any obvious cause, with no associated disorder.
- Secondary RLS is associated with other medical conditions. The most frequently found associations are pregnancy, iron deficiency anemia, end-stage renal disease and parkinson disease.

PHYSICAL FINDINGS & CLINICAL PRESENTATION

- Wide spectrum of severity of clinical manifestations has been reported in RLS.
- Most common symptom is unpleasant sensations in legs, reported as discomfort or "creepy-crawling" sensations, mostly bilateral. Arms are occasionally involved.
- There is an extreme urge to move their legs and relief is sustained as long as the movement continues.
- Symptoms are worse at night or evening. Best sleep is usually early in the morning.

ETIOLOGY

The exact etiology of Restless leg syndrome is not clear. Pharmacologic, pathologic, physiologic and new imaging studies have implicated dopaminergic pathways, brain iron metabolism and endogenous opioid pathways.

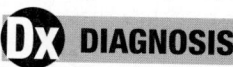

DIAGNOSIS

DIFFERENTIAL DIAGNOSIS

- Periodic limb movement disorder (PLMD)
- Nocturnal leg cramps
- Painful peripheral neuropathy
- Akathisias
- Positional discomfort
- Volitional movements, foot tapping, leg rocking

WORKUP

- Diagnosis of the RLS is based on clinical criteria and normal neurological examination.
- Other testing is done to determine possible cause of secondary RLS.
- Polysomnography to document periodic limb movements during sleep.
- Leg activity monitors to determine limb movements during sleep but they are unable to distinguish periodic limb movements from periodic movements associated with sleep apnea.
- Nerve conduction studies and electromyography for associated peripheral neuropathy.

LABORATORY TESTS

- Iron status: Serum ferritin, total iron binding capacity, percent saturation.
- Complete blood count for anemia, in case of iron deficiency.
- Metabolic panel: blood urea nitrogen and serum creatinine for renal insufficiency.

IMAGING STUDIES

No imaging studies are required for diagnosis for Restless leg syndrome.

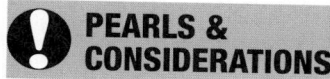

TREATMENT

Treatment options for RLS include:
- Dopaminergic agents, levodopa and dopamine agonists help to ameliorate RLS symptoms, decrease periodic limb movements and improve sleep. Augmentation, that is increase in severity and duration of symptoms, has been seen with levodopa but rarely with dopamine agonists. Dopamine agonists, pramipexole and ropinirole, are first line agents in the treatment of RLS.
- Anticonvulsants, Gabapentin is shown to be effective in multiple studies. Limited case reports reveal use of lamotrigine, gabatril and topiramate in patients who are intolerant to other agents.
- Opiates, mostly methadone, are generally reserved as last line of treatment.
- Iron replacement should be started in case of iron deficiency.

NONPHARMACOLOGIC THERAPY

- Avoidance of caffeine, alcohol, nicotine and medications that exacerbate RLS.
- Physical and mental activity.
- Good sleep hygiene.

ACUTE GENERAL Rx

Once the diagnosis of RLS is considered on the basis of clinical criteria as mentioned in Table 1-158, and causes impairment of quality of life, dopamine agonist should be started at low dose and then gradually tapered up depending on tolerance.

CHRONIC Rx

Dopamine agonists are given daily on chronic basis. Oral iron replacement is added to the regimen in case of iron deficiency.

DISPOSITION

It is usually a life-long disorder, presenting as relapses and remissions. Usually, medications are able to control symptoms and improve sleep quality.

REFERRAL

Refer to neurologist if diagnosis is uncertain or any underlying disorder is suspected.

PEARLS & CONSIDERATIONS

COMMENTS

RLS is diagnosed on the basis of patient's history and physical examination. Laboratory tests are done only to exclude secondary RLS. Neurological examination in idiopathic RLS is normal unless another neurological diagnosis is suspected with it. Pharmacological therapy should be limited to those individuals who meet the specific diagnosis criteria. Severity of the disease, subjective complaints, age and desire of the patient for treatment should be considered.

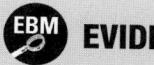 **EVIDENCE**

available at www.expertconsult.com

SUGGESTED READINGS
available at www.expertconsult.com

AUTHOR: **FARIHA ZAHEER, M.D.**

TABLE 1-158 Diagnostic Criteria for RLS

Minimal Criteria

1. Desire to move the legs usually associated with paraesthesias.
2. Motor restlessness, as characterized by floor pacing, leg rubbing, stretching, and flexing.
3. Worse at rest, with relief by activity.
4. Worse at night.

Additional Criteria

1. Sleep disturbances, as difficulty in sleep onset and maintaining sleep, daytime fatigue or somnolence.
2. Involuntary movements, as periodic limb or leg movements in sleep and periodic or aperiodic limb movements while awake.
3. Neurologic examination is normal in idiopathic RLS.
4. Clinical course may begin at any age but most severe in middle and older age.
5. Family history suggest autosomal dominant mode of inheritance in 1/3 of the cases.

Stiansy K, Oertel WH, Trenkwalder C: Clinical symptology and treatment of restless leg syndrome and periodic limb movement disorder, *Sleep medicine reviews* 6(4):253-265, 2002, Elsevier Inc.

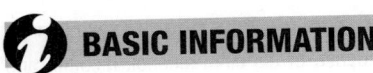

BASIC INFORMATION

DEFINITION

Retinal detachment is a retinal separation in which the inner or neural layer of the retina separates from the pigment epithelial layer. It results from numerous causes.

SYNONYMS

Inflammatory lesions of choroid
Uveitis
Tumor
Vascular lesions
Congenital disorders

ICD-9CM CODES
361 Retinal detachment and defects

EPIDEMIOLOGY & DEMOGRAPHICS

INCIDENCE (IN U.S.):
- 0.02% of the population
- Particularly common in patients with high myopia of 5 diopters or more

PEAK INCIDENCE: Incidence increases with increasing age or increasing myopia.

PREVALENCE (IN U.S.): Busy ophthalmologists may see one or two acute retinal detachments per month.

PREDOMINANT AGE:
- Congenital in younger patients
- Usually trauma in patients aged 30 to 40 yr and older
- High myopia a predisposition

PHYSICAL FINDINGS & CLINICAL PRESENTATION
- Elevation of retina and vessels associated with tears in the retina, fluid, and/or hemorrhage beneath the retina and changes in the vitreous (Fig. 1-323).
- Reports of flashing lights and floaters.

ETIOLOGY
- Trauma
- Tears in the retina
- Uveitis
- Fluid accumulation beneath the retina
- Tumors
- Scleritis
- Inflammatory disease
- Diabetes
- Collagen-vascular disease
- Vascular abnormalities

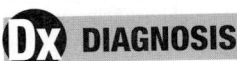 DIAGNOSIS

DIFFERENTIAL DIAGNOSIS
- Detachment
- Hemorrhage
- Tumors

WORKUP
- Full eye examination
- Fluorescein angiography
- Visual fields
- Ultrasonography to show the retinal detachment or tumors beneath it
- Medical workup only when inflammation or systemic disease considered

LABORATORY TESTS
Usually not necessary

IMAGING STUDIES
B scan of the eye

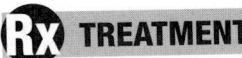 TREATMENT

NONPHARMACOLOGIC THERAPY
Immediate surgery. The three principal methods for reattachment of the retina in patients with primary retinal detachment are scleral buckling, vitrectomy, and pneumatic retinopexy. There is a paucity of randomized trials comparing these procedures and the choice remains subjective. Some data suggests that vitrectomy may be preferable for detachment in pseudophakic eyes, whereas primary detachment in phakic eyes with complexity exceeding the original indications for rheumatic retinopexy may be treated with scleral buckling or vitrectomy.

ACUTE GENERAL Rx
- Early surgery to repair the detachment
- Treatment of the underlying disorder

CHRONIC Rx
Occasionally, steroids or other treatment of underlying disease is indicated.

DISPOSITION
- Immediately refer to an ophthalmologist.
- Early intervention improves outcomes.

REFERRAL
Immediately

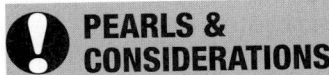 PEARLS & CONSIDERATIONS

COMMENTS
If treated early, most patients will recover a substantial portion of their vision.

SUGGESTED READINGS
available at www.expertconsult.com

AUTHOR: **MELVYN KOBY, M.D.**

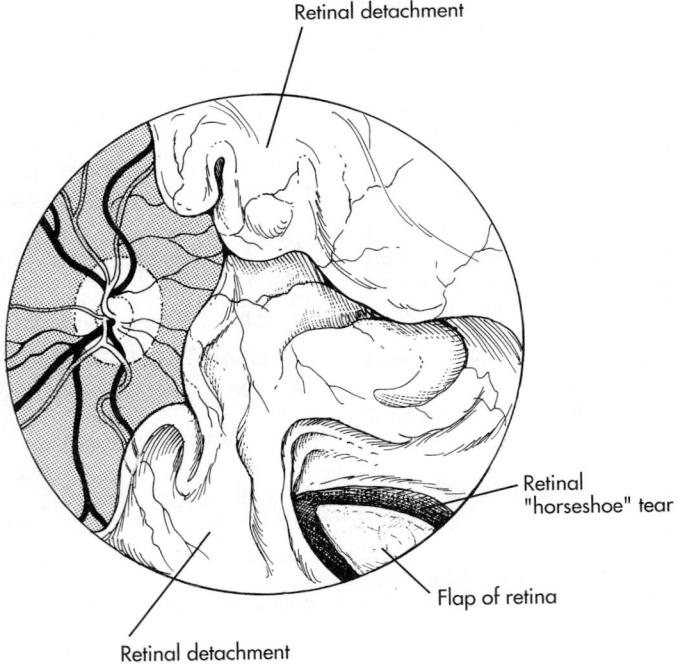

FIGURE 1-323 Retinal detachment. (From Scuderi G [ed]: *Sports medicine: principles of primary care,* St Louis, 1997, Mosby.)

BASIC INFORMATION
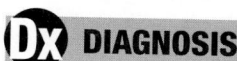

DEFINITION

In a retinal hemorrhage, blood accumulates in the retinal and subretinal areas as a result of multiple causes.

SYNONYMS

Pseudoxanthoma elasticum
Coats' disease
Retinal trauma
High-altitude retinopathy

ICD-9CM CODES
362.81 Retinal hemorrhage

EPIDEMIOLOGY & DEMOGRAPHICS

INCIDENCE (IN U.S.): Busy ophthalmologists see one or two cases a month.
PEAK INCIDENCE:
- In children: associated primarily with trauma and hematologic disorders (must consider shaken baby syndrome)
- Associated with trauma, diabetes, vascular disease, macular degeneration, altitude changes (mountain climbing)

PREDOMINANT AGE: Degenerative disease in older patients

PHYSICAL FINDINGS & CLINICAL PRESENTATION

- Hemorrhage within the retina or subretinal area (Fig. 1-324)
- Evidence of retinal tears, tumors, and inflammation; macular degeneration, drugs, diabetes

ETIOLOGY

- Diabetes
- Hypertension
- Trauma
- Inflammation
- Tumors
- Subretinal neovascularization
- Associated with diabetes and aging
- Rapid changes in altitude (mountain climbing or scuba diving)

DIAGNOSIS
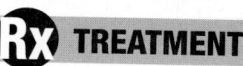

DIFFERENTIAL DIAGNOSIS

- Evaluate patients for local and systemic diseases.
- Trauma in children or adults.
- Venous or arterial occlusion associated with atherosclerotic or heart disease may cause retinal hemorrhage.
- Rule out malignant melanoma, trauma, hypertensive cardiovascular disease.

Section II describes the differential diagnosis of acute painless loss of vision.

WORKUP

Complete general physical examination, evaluate for trauma; look for systemic diseases and medication etiologies.

LABORATORY TESTS

- Minimum: complete blood count, erythrocyte sedimentation rate, complete blood chemistries
- Fluorescein
- Angiography
- Visual field testing

IMAGING STUDIES

- Usually not necessary
- Trauma: skull radiographs or head CT
- Ultrasound
- Fluorescein angiography

TREATMENT
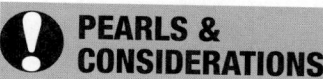

NONPHARMACOLOGIC THERAPY

- Laser or treatment of underlying disorder
- Treat medical problems (age-related macular degeneration, etc.)

ACUTE GENERAL Rx

- Laser treatment is often indicated.
- Steroids may be indicated with macular degeneration (intravitreal injection).
- Treat underlying disease.
- Repair any damage from trauma.

CHRONIC Rx

- Laser treatment if hemorrhage is recurrent
- Vitamin therapy: high in zinc and antioxidants

DISPOSITION

Consider this condition an emergency.

REFERRAL

Immediate referral to an ophthalmologist; early treatment significantly affects outcome

PEARLS & CONSIDERATIONS

COMMENTS

- Vision may return substantially.
- Complete recovery depends on amount of scar tissue formed.
- Chronic situations have poor prognosis.

SUGGESTED READINGS

available at www.expertconsult.com

AUTHOR: **MELVYN KOBY, M.D.**

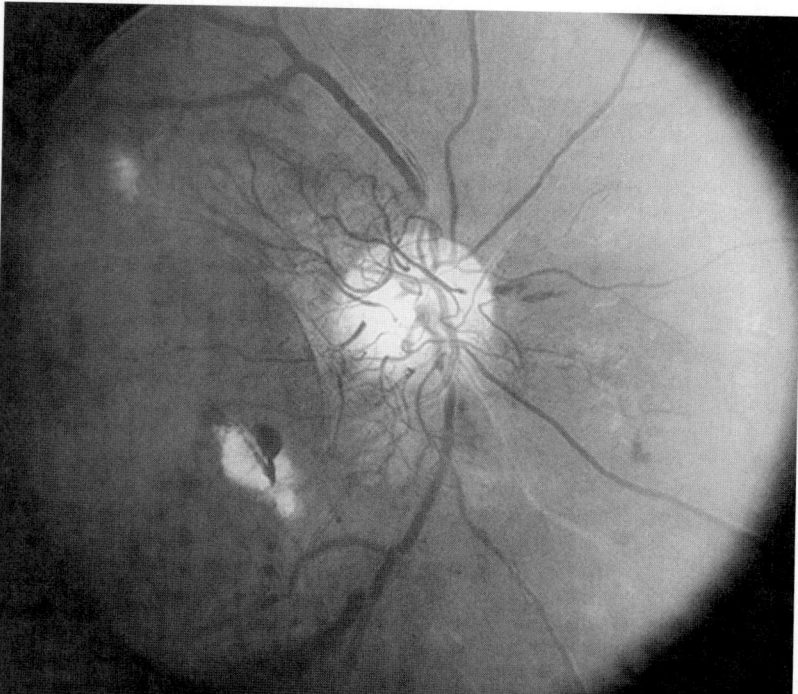

FIGURE 1-324 Fronds of neovascularization on the disc are present in this right eye. Temporally, two cotton-wool spots have adjacent intraretinal hemorrhage and preretinal hemorrhage. Native retinal arteries are narrowed and show evidence of sclerosis. (From Palay D [ed]: *Ophthalmology for the primary care physician*, St Louis, 1997, Mosby.)

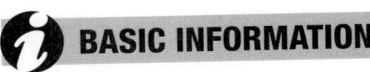

BASIC INFORMATION

DEFINITION

Retinitis pigmentosa is a generalized retinal pigment degeneration associated with a variety of inheritance patterns resulting in decreased vision. A simple recessive pattern is most severe. It may be associated with some rare neurologic syndromes.

ICD-9CM CODES
362.74 Retinitis pigmentosa, pigmentary retinal dystrophy

EPIDEMIOLOGY & DEMOGRAPHICS

PEAK INCIDENCE:
- Recessive incidence: in the 20s
- Dominant form: in the 40s

PREVALENCE (IN U.S.): One in 4000 persons
PREDOMINANT SEX: Depends on inheritance
PREDOMINANT AGE: 60 yr
GENETICS:
- 19% dominant
- 19% recessive
- 8% X-linked
- 46% not known to be genetically related (mutations)
- 8% undetermined cause

PHYSICAL FINDINGS & CLINICAL PRESENTATION

- Deposition of retinal pigment in midperiphery and centrally in the retina with a pale optic nerve and narrowing of blood vessels (Fig. 1-325)
- Possible cataracts and macular edema
- Decrease in night vision and peripheral vision. Patients typically lose night vision to a greater extent than they lose day vision, and they lose peripheral vision before losing central vision.

ETIOLOGY

Usually hereditary

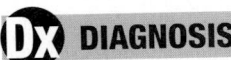

DIAGNOSIS

DIFFERENTIAL DIAGNOSIS

- Syphilis
- Old inflammatory scars
- Old hemorrhage
- Diabetes
- Toxic retinopathies (phenothiazines, chloroquine)

WORKUP

- Electrophysiologic studies
- Dark adaptation studies
- Visual fields

LABORATORY TESTS

- Usually not necessary
- VDRL (syphilis), glucose (selected patients)

IMAGING STUDIES

- Usually not necessary
- Rate of decline of vision for different groups cannot be accurately determined; decline rates are fastest with patients with mutations

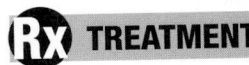

TREATMENT

CHRONIC Rx

- No proven effective therapy
- Correction of biochemical abnormalities. Some success has been reported with subretinal gene therapy in which patients with mutations in the gene encoding RPE65 were treated with delivery under the retina of a normal RPE65 gene by intraocular injection
- Nutritional supplements: sometimes vitamin E or vitamin A may be helpful
- In patients with advanced disease, treatment options may include attempts to regenerate photoreceptors by transplantation or genetic manipulation of nonphotoreceptor retinal cell types

DISPOSITION

Disease may be either mild or severe, but if the patient is expected to progress to total blindness, counseling and early education are important.

REFERRAL

To ophthalmologist to confirm diagnosis

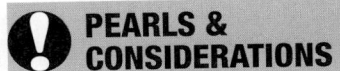

PEARLS & CONSIDERATIONS

COMMENTS

- The spider web–like appearance of macular degeneration should not be confused with the extra pigments sometimes seen in dark-skinned individuals.
- Patient education material can be obtained from the Retinitis Pigmentosa Foundation Fighting Blindness, 1401 Mt. Royal Avenue, 4th Floor, Baltimore, MD 21217.
- Research in fetal retinal pigment transplantation and computer chip implantation is ongoing.

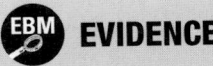

EVIDENCE

available at www.expertconsult.com

SUGGESTED READINGS

available at www.expertconsult.com

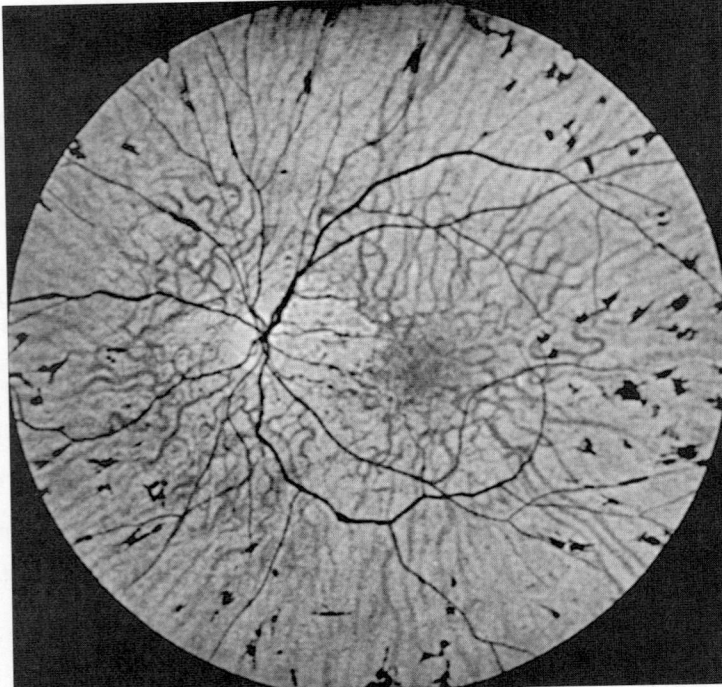

FIGURE 1-325 Retinitis pigmentosa. (From Behrman RE [ed]: *Nelson textbook of pediatrics*, Philadelphia, 2005, WB Saunders.)

AUTHOR: **MELVYN KOBY, M.D.**

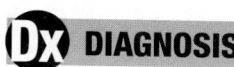 BASIC INFORMATION

DEFINITION

Retinoblastoma is an inherited, highly malignant congenital neoplasm arising from the neural layers of the retina.

ICD-9CM CODES
190.5 Retinoblastoma, malignant neoplasm of eyes, retina

EPIDEMIOLOGY & DEMOGRAPHICS

INCIDENCE (IN U.S.): Retinoblastoma affects 1 in 15,000 children, with ~300 children newly diagnosed each year in the United States. It is the most common primary intraocular malignancy of childhood.

PEAK INCIDENCE:
- 6 to 13 mo. Mean age at diagnosis is 12 mo for bilateral tumors and 24 mo for unilateral tumors.
- 72% diagnosed by age 3 yr
- 90% diagnosed by age 4 yr

PREDOMINANT AGE: 8 mo

GENETICS:
- Gene mutation or an autosomal-dominant gene with 80% to 95% penetration
- 5% mutations

PHYSICAL FINDINGS & CLINICAL PRESENTATION

- Leukokoria (white reflex or white pupil) (Fig. 1-326)
- White elevated retinal masses
- Strabismus
- Glaucoma
- Uveitis
- Vitreous masses and opacity

ETIOLOGY

The retinoblastoma gene is a tumor suppressor gene located on the long arm of chromosome 13 at region 14 that codes for the RB protein. ~60% of retinoblastomas are attributable to somatic, nonhereditary mutations.

DIAGNOSIS

DIFFERENTIAL DIAGNOSIS

Examination of eye
- Strabismus
- Retinal detachment
- Uveitis
- Other tumors
- Glaucoma
- Coats' disease (pathologic telangiectatic retinal vessels that leak and lead to accumulation of subretinal fluid and lipid)
- Endophthalmitis
- Cataract
- Infectious

WORKUP

Diagnosis is by ophthalmologic examination. An awake examination to determine if the patient can fixate and extent of eye mobility should be done. Examination should also include visual acuity, papillary examination, extraocular movements, slit-lamp examination for evidence of iris neovascularization, hyphema or hypopyon, and indirect ophthalmoscopy with 360 degrees of scleral depression, and fundus photographs documenting all lesions. Opthalmologic examination is followed by ultrasonography of the eye and MRI of the orbits and brain to exclude extraocular extension and trilateral retinoblastoma.

CLASSIFICATION

Retinoblastoma is separated into intraocular and extraocular disease. The Reese-Ellsworth classification system became outdated as chemoreduction strategies became widely used for salvage therapy and a new international classification system for intraocular retinoblastoma was formulated in 2003, which more accurately reflects response to standardized chemotherapy regimen used in conjunction with focal consolidative therapy. The international classification system is subdivided into group A (small), group B (medium), group C (confined, medium), group D (diffuse, large), and group E (enucleation, advanced)

IMAGING STUDIES

- MRI: may show calcifications in retina
- Ultrasonography: good delineation of mass

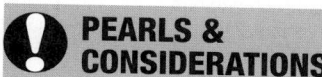 TREATMENT

Usually treated by a multidisciplinary team consisting of a pediatrician, an ophthalmologist, a pediatric oncologist, and pediatric radiation oncologist. Treatment depends on location and stage of tumor when diagnosed:
- Chemotherapy for larger tumors usually with carboplatin, etoposide, and vincristine. The goal of chemotherapy is to reduce the tumor volume for focal therapy with cryotherapy, laser, thermotherapy, or plaque bradytherapy.
- Radioactive plaque brachytherapy with iodine 125 or ruthenium 106 plaques and cryotherapy
- Surgical enucleation of the eye
- Radiation and chemotherapy

DISPOSITION

Overall there is a high cure rate (93% 5-yr survival in the United States) for retinoblastoma. Group A tumors generally have good visual and survival prognosis with focal consolidative therapy alone, groups B and C are treated with chemotherapy and focal therapy with good results (vision salvage rates up to 93%), group D patients often eventually require enucleation despite treatment.

REFERRAL

- To ophthalmologist, pediatric oncologist, and pediatric radiation oncologist
- Prospective parents with a family history of retinoblastoma should be referred for genetic counseling. Genetic testing should be carried out for most retinoblastoma patients unless it is declined.

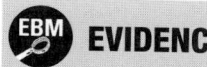 PEARLS & CONSIDERATIONS

COMMENTS

- High incidence of second tumor in survivors compared with general population.
- High incidence of lung cancer, bladder, and other epithelial cancers.

EBM EVIDENCE

available at www.expertconsult.com

SUGGESTED READINGS

available at www.expertconsult.com

AUTHORS: **MELVYN KOBY, M.D.,** and **FRED FERRI, M.D.**

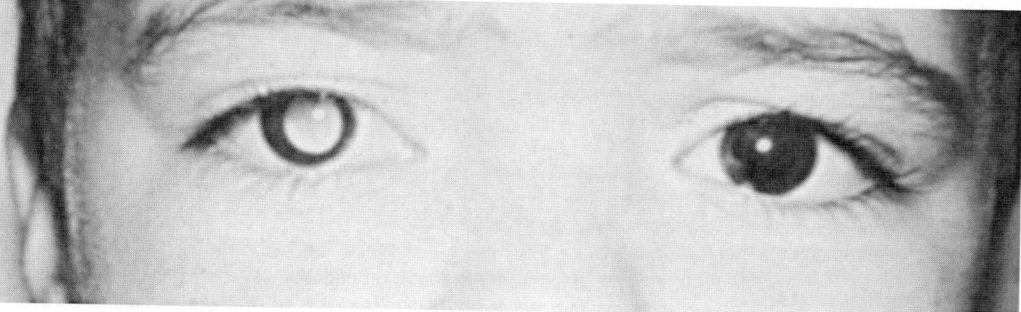

FIGURE 1-326 Leukocoria. White papillary reflex in a child with retinoblastoma. (From Behrman RE [ed]: *Nelson textbook of pediatrics,* Philadelphia, 2005, WB Saunders.)

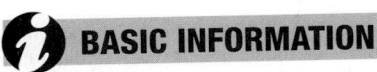

BASIC INFORMATION

DEFINITION

Diabetic retinopathy is an eye abnormality of the retina associated with diabetes and consisting of microaneurysms, punctate hemorrhages, white and yellow exudates, flame hemorrhages, and neovascular vessel growth and can ultimately end in blindness. Diabetic retinopathy can be classified into two stages: nonproliferative and proliferative (Fig. 1-327).

SYNONYMS

Nonproliferative diabetic retinopathy (NPDR)
Proliferative (advanced) diabetic retinopathy (PDR)
Diabetic retinopathy (DR)

ICD-9CM CODES
250.5   Diabetes with ophthalmic manifestations
362.1   Retinopathy, diabetic, background
362.02 Retinopathy, diabetic, proliferative

EPIDEMIOLOGY & DEMOGRAPHICS

INCIDENCE (IN U.S.):
- Affects 11 million persons
- A leading cause of blindness in people aged 20 to 70 yr
- 5000 new cases annually

PEAK INCIDENCE: Begins 10 yr after onset of diabetes

PREVALENCE (IN U.S.): Prevalence of retinopathy increases with duration of diabetes. Found in 18% of people diagnosed with diabetes for 3- to 4-yr duration and in up to 80% of diabetics with a diagnosis of ≥15 yr.

PREDOMINANT SEX: Males and females affected equally

PREDOMINANT AGE: ≥30 yr

GENETICS: Type 1 diabetes: 80% have retinopathy before 30 yr, with 30% having vision-threatening retinopathy.

PHYSICAL FINDINGS & CLINICAL PRESENTATION

- Microaneurysms
- Hemorrhages
- Exudates
- Macular edema
- Neovascularization
- Retinal detachment
- Hemorrhages in the vitreous
- In early cases, patient may not report a visual disturbance

ETIOLOGY

Vascular endothelial growth factor and erythropoietin have been identified as factors involved in angiogenesis in proliferative diabetic retinopathy. Risk factors for diabetic retinopathy are duration of diabetes, hyperglycemia/glycated hemoglobin value, hypertension, hyperlipidemia, pregnancy, and nephropathy or renal disease.

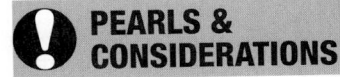

DIAGNOSIS

DIFFERENTIAL DIAGNOSIS

- Retinal examination: look for background retinopathy, microaneurysms, exudate, macular edema, retinal hemorrhage, proliferative neovascular growth on surface of retina
- Retinal inflammatory diseases
- Tumor
- Trauma
- Arteriosclerotic vascular disease
- Hypertension
- Vein or artery occlusion

WORKUP

- Fluorescein angiogram
- Frequent retinal examinations

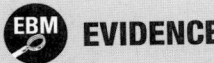

TREATMENT

NONPHARMACOLOGIC THERAPY

- Tight glycemic control remains the cornerstone in the primary prevention of diabetic retinopathy
- Laser treatment when indicated
- Laser treatment with proliferative disease or macular edema
- Photo coagulation of neovascular areas
- Exercise, diet, sugar and lipids control can slow progression of background retinopathy but have no effect on proliferative retinopathy. Trials have shown that glycemic control and combination treatment of dyslipidemia, but not intensive blood-pressure control, reduce the rate of diabetic retinopathy. Intensive glycemic therapy (vs. standard therapy) lowers the incidence of progressive retinopathy (7.3% vs. 10.4%) but not vision loss (16.3% vs. 16.7%) and can result in excess mortality (ACCORD trial)

ACUTE GENERAL Rx

- Laser therapy: pan-retinal and focal retinal laser photocoagulation reduces the risk of visual loss in patients with severe diabetic retinopathy and macular edema
- Vitrectomy
- Repair of retinal detachment
- Medical control of disease and complications and associated diseases (e.g., hypertension)

CHRONIC Rx

- Repeated laser treatments may be necessary
- Diet and exercise; good medical control of disease

DISPOSITION

- Retinal examination should be performed on all routine medical visits. Referral if abnormality seen.
- Routine annual eye examination in all patients with diabetes.
- Prognosis is improved with early diagnosis and treatment.

REFERRAL

Refer to ophthalmologist immediately on finding retinal abnormality to institute early treatment.

PEARLS & CONSIDERATIONS

COMMENTS

- Early laser treatment of severe, nonproliferative, and proliferative retinopathy may minimize complications and visual loss.
- Retinopathy is an independent risk marker for cardiovascular disease in patients with type 2 DM.

EVIDENCE

available at www.expertconsult.com

SUGGESTED READINGS

available at www.expertconsult.com

AUTHORS: **MELVYN KOBY, M.D.,** and **FRED F. FERRI, M.D.**

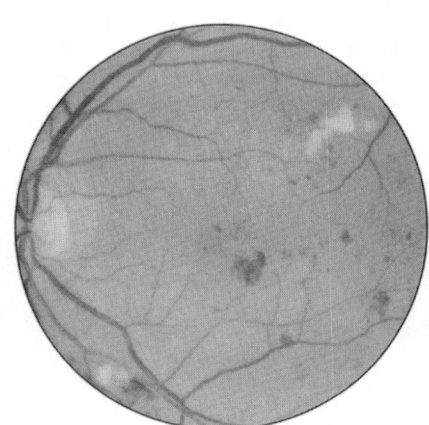
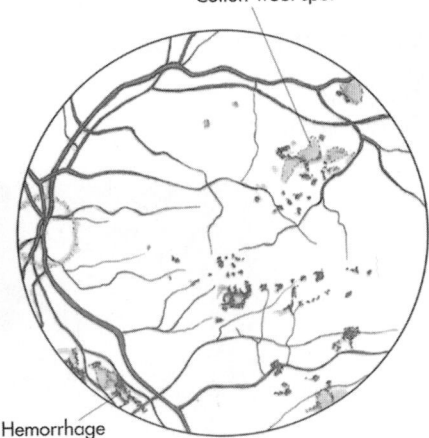

FIGURE 1-327 Background diabetic retinopathy. Note flame-shaped and dot-blot hemorrhages, cotton-wool spots, and microaneurysms. (From Barkaukas VH et al: *Health and physical assessment,* ed 2, St Louis, 1998, Mosby.)

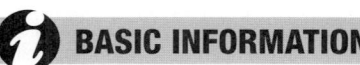

BASIC INFORMATION

DEFINITION

Retropharyngeal abscess is a soft tissue infection of the throat involving retropharyngeal space. The anatomic boundaries of the retropharyngeal space are the middle layer of the deep cervical fascia (abutting the posterior esophageal wall) anteriorly and the deep layer of the deep cervical fascia posteriorly (Fig. 1-328). These two fasciae fuse inferiorly at the level between the first and second thoracic vertebra.

ICD-9CM CODES
478.79

EPIDEMIOLOGY & DEMOGRAPHICS

Retropharyngeal abscess occurs most commonly in children between the ages of 2 and 4 yr, analogous to suppurative cervical adenitis. This represents the peak age group for numerous viral upper respiratory tract infections and their attendant complications, acute otitis media and sinusitis. Retropharyngeal space infection is less common in older children and adults because the lymph nodes atrophy by the age of 3 or 4 yr.

PHYSICAL FINDINGS & CLINICAL PRESENTATION

- The onset of a retropharyngeal infection may be insidious, with little more than fever, irritability, drooling, a muffled voice (dysphonia), or possibly nuchal rigidity.
- The acute symptoms relate to pressure and inflammation produced by the abscess on either the airway or the upper digestive tract and pharynx. The patient may have intense dysphagia, drooling, and odynophagia, or there may be some element of respiratory distress from edema and inflammation of the airway (stridor, tachypnea, or both).

- Unwillingness to move the neck because of discomfort is often a prominent presenting feature and should lead to consideration of retropharyngeal abscess if the child is febrile and irritable.
- Extension of the neck is usually affected more than flexion. This causes the patient to hold his or her neck stiffly or to present with torticollis.
- Trismus is unusual.
- On physical examination it may be possible to appreciate midline or unilateral swelling of the posterior pharyngeal wall. The mass may be fluctuant to the examining finger, and care must be taken to avoid rupture of the abscess into the upper airway.

Complications are numerous and could be fatal; these include airway obstruction, septicemia, thrombosis of the internal jugular vein, carotid artery rupture, and acute necrotizing mediastinitis. Aspiration with resultant pneumonia may complicate retropharyngeal abscess if rupture of the abscess occurs and empties into the airway. Infection can spread from one space in the neck to another.

The most dreaded complication is jugular vein suppurative thrombophlebitis (Lemierre's syndrome), in which the vessels of the carotid sheath become infected, leading to bacteremia and metastatic spread of infection to the lungs, brain, and mediastinum.

ETIOLOGY

- The retropharyngeal space comprises two chains of lymph nodes that drain the nasopharynx, adenoids, posterior paranasal sinuses, middle ear, and eustachian tube. Accordingly, suppurative infections in these areas may provide the seeds for infection for retropharyngeal abscess.
- The predominant bacterial species are *Streptococcus pyogenes* (group A *Streptococcus*), *Staphylococcus aureus*, and respiratory anaerobes (including *Fusobacteria*, *Prevotella*,

and *Veillonella* species). *Haemophilus* species are also occasionally found.
- In young children, infection usually reaches this space by lymphatic spread from a septic focus in the pharynx or sinuses.
- In adults, infection may reach the retropharyngeal space from either local or distant sites. Penetrating trauma (e.g., from chicken bones or after instrumentation) is the usual source of local spread. More distant sources of infection include odontogenic sepsis and peritonsillar abscess (now a rare cause).

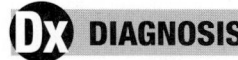

DIAGNOSIS

DIFFERENTIAL DIAGNOSIS
- Cervical osteomyelitis
- Pott's disease
- Meningitis
- Calcific tendonitis of the long muscle of the neck

IMAGING STUDIES
- A lateral neck film may be helpful in delineating the presence of a retropharyngeal abscess and may demonstrate cervical lordosis; the retropharyngeal space is considered widened and pathologic if it is greater than 7 mm at C2 or 14 mm at C6 (Fig. 1-329).
  - There must be attention to technical issues when performing the study, especially in children. The film should be a perfect lateral, and the child must keep the neck in extension during inspiration to avoid a false thickening of the retropharyngeal space. Crying, particularly in infants, may also cause false thickening of the retropharyngeal space.
- A CT scan of the neck is the best tool to identify abscesses in the retropharyngeal area, but it is not perfect. Both the sensitivity and specificity of the CT scan in predicting the presence of drainable purulent material

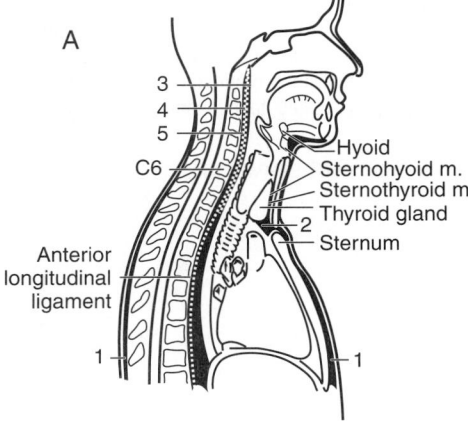

Layers of deep cervical fascia
Superficial ─────────
Middle ── ── ── ── ──
Deep ·················

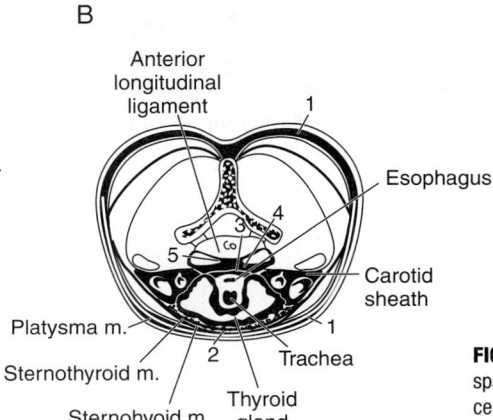

FIGURE 1-328 Relation of various cervical fascial spaces to the superficial and deep layers of the cervical fascia. **A,** Cross-section of the neck at the level of the thyroid isthmus. **B,** Coronal section in the suprahyoid region of the neck. *1,* Superficial space; *2,* pretracheal space; *3,* retropharyngeal space; *4,* "danger" space; *5,* prevertebral space.

are quite variable from study to study, ranging between 68% and 100%.

○ The CT scan provides more information than the plain radiograph because it can generally differentiate between retropharyngeal cellulitis and retropharyngeal abscess and can demonstrate extension of the retropharyngeal abscess to contiguous spaces in the neck. Findings on CT common to both cellulitis and abscess are a low-density core, soft tissue swelling, obliterated fat planes, and mass effect. The best differential finding on CT scan is "complete rim enhancement," which is indicative of abscess (Fig. 1-330). The abscess may be seen as a mass impinging on the posterior pharyngeal wall.

● MRI of the neck is more sensitive than CT, and technetium scanning can be helpful in detecting bone involvement. T2-weighted images may identify and localize areas of pus for drainage or aspiration. Gadolinium enhancement is important to accurately define the soft tissue component. Finally, MRI is useful for imaging vascular lesions, such as jugular thrombophlebitis.

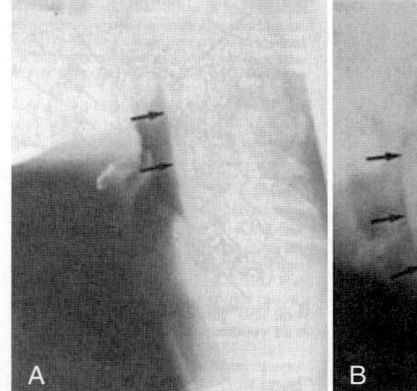 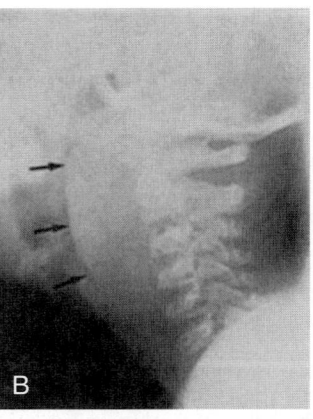

FIGURE 1-329 Lateral radiographs of the neck show normal lateral cervical view **(A)** and expansion of the prevertebral soft tissues by a retropharyngeal abscess **(B)**.

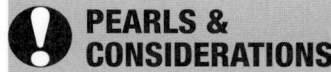 **TREATMENT**

ACUTE GENERAL & CHRONIC Rx

● High-dose penicillin (2 million to 4 million units IV q4h) plus metronidazole (500 mg IV q8h) or ampicillin-sulbactam (50 mg/kg/dose IV q6h) or clindamycin (13 mg/kg/dose IV q8h) are effective antimicrobial selections. Parenteral treatment is maintained until the patient is afebrile and clinically improved. Antibiotics should be adjusted as culture data become available, and oral therapy is continued to complete at least a 14-day course.

● Surgical intervention has historically played a prominent role in the management of retropharyngeal abscess in conjunction with antibiotic therapy. Drainage is indicated when there is a large hypodense area or when a patient has not responded to parenteral therapy alone.

● When the CT does not demonstrate a large hypodense area, a trial of antibiotic therapy without drainage is appropriate. Some investigators also support a trial of IV antibiotic therapy alone when small abscesses are identified by CT scans as long as there is no compromise of the airway.

PEARLS & CONSIDERATIONS

PREVENTION

The complications of deep neck infection in any space are numerous and potentially fatal. Early diagnosis, with prompt and appropriate management, is key to avoiding these complications.

AUTHOR: **RUBY SATPATHY, M.D.**

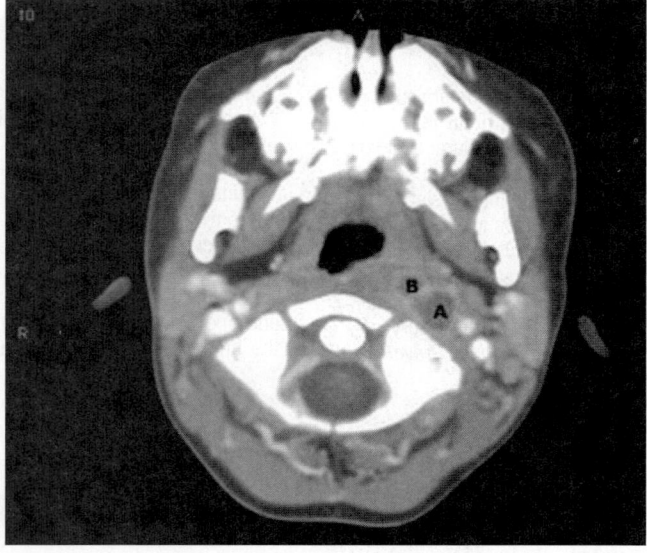

FIGURE 1-330 CT scan of a retropharyngeal abscess **(A** and **B)** demonstrates a low-density core, soft tissue swelling, obliterated fat planes, mass effect, and rim enhancement.

BASIC INFORMATION

DEFINITION

Reye's syndrome is a postinfectious triad consisting of encephalopathy, fatty liver degeneration, and transaminase elevation.

ICD-9CM CODES
331.81 Reye's syndrome

EPIDEMIOLOGY & DEMOGRAPHICS

- During the 1970s, 300 to 600 cases were being reported yearly in the U.S.
- Since the mid-1980s, after the understanding that aspirin is associated with Reye's syndrome, the yearly count has fallen to <20 cases
- Seasonal relation with influenza and varicella outbreaks
- Age: rare in persons aged >18 yr; peak age (in the U.S.) is 6 to 8 yr
- Case fatality rate: 25% to 50%

PHYSICAL FINDINGS & CLINICAL PRESENTATION

Shortly after recovery from a viral infection (flu or chickenpox), an afebrile child begins to vomit intractably. Hepatomegaly is often present. The vomiting can lead to dehydration. Occasionally, symptoms of hypoglycemia are present. After 2 days symptoms of encephalopathy dominate the clinical picture (lethargy, confusion, stupor, coma, seizures, decorticate or decerebrate posture) (Table 1-159).

ETIOLOGY

- Temporal association with influenza and varicella infection
- Epidemiologic association with aspirin or other salicylate use to treat the viral infection
- Possible association with aflatoxin and pesticides
- Pathology
- Liver: no inflammation; the striking finding is panlobular microvesicular hepatocyte infiltration on light microscopy and mitochondrial injury on electron microscopy
- Brain: no inflammation but cerebral edema and anoxic degeneration
- Pathogenesis: not fully understood but mitochondrial dysfunction is clearly center stage

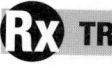 **DIAGNOSIS**

DIFFERENTIAL DIAGNOSIS

- Inborn errors of metabolism (e.g., carnitine deficiency, ornithine transcarbamylase deficiency)
- Salicylate or amiodarone intoxication
- Jamaican vomiting sickness
- Hepatic encephalopathy of any cause

WORKUP

According to the Centers for Disease Control case definition, the following conditions must be met for consideration as a Reye's syndrome case:
1. Acute noninflammatory encephalopathy documented by:
   - Alteration in the level of consciousness and, if available, a record of cerebrospinal fluid containing ≤8 leukocytes per mm³ or
   - Histologic specimen demonstrating cerebral edema without perivascular or meningeal inflammation
2. Hepatopathy documented either by a liver biopsy or autopsy considered to be diagnostic of Reye's syndrome or by a threefold or greater rise in the levels of serum aspartate aminotransferase, serum alanine aminotransferase, or serum ammonia and
3. No more reasonable explanation for the cerebral and hepatic abnormalities

LABORATORY TESTS

- Elevated transaminase (alanine aminotransferase and aspartate aminotransferase)
- Elevated ammonia level
- Occasional elevation of creatine phosphokinase, lactate dehydrogenase, and bilirubin and prolongation of prothrombin time
- Occasional hypoglycemia (in patients <4 yr)
- Cerebrospinal fluid is normal or contains <8 white blood cells per milliliter
- Rarely a liver biopsy is indicated (in infants or in recurrent cases)

Rx TREATMENT

- Supportive
- Mannitol, glycerol, or hyperventilation for cerebral edema if present
- Interferon-alfa (experimental)
- Prevention
  - Influenza vaccine
  - Varicella vaccine
  - Avoidance of aspirin in children, especially during influenza and varicella outbreaks

AUTHOR: **FRED F. FERRI, M.D.**

Grade	Symptoms at Time of Admission
I	Usually quiet, **lethargic** and sleepy, vomiting, laboratory evidence of liver dysfunction
II	Deep lethargy, **confusion,** delirium, combative, hyperventilation, hyperreflexic
III	Obtunded, **light coma,** seizures, decorticate rigidity, intact pupillary light reaction
IV	Seizures, deepening coma, **decerebrate rigidity,** loss of oculocephalic reflexes, fixed pupils
V	Coma, loss of deep tendon reflexes, respiratory arrest, fixed dilated pupils, **flaccidity/decerebrate** intermittent isoelectric electroencephalogram

TABLE 1-159   Clinical Staging of Reye's Syndrome

From Behrman RE: *Nelson textbook of pediatrics,* ed 17, Philadelphia, 2005, WB Saunders.

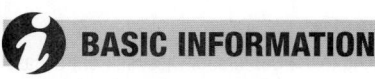

BASIC INFORMATION

DEFINITION

Rh incompatibility occurs when an absence of the D antigen on maternal red blood cells (RBCs) and its presence on fetal RBCs causes risk of isoimmunization.

ICD-9CM CODES
656.1 Rh incompatibility

EPIDEMIOLOGY & DEMOGRAPHICS

INCIDENCE:
- The absence of the D antigen (Rh− blood type) occurs in 15% of whites, 8% of blacks, and virtually no Asians or Native Americans. If the father's blood type is not known, the chance that an Rh− pregnant woman is bearing an Rh+ fetus is approximately 60%.
- Of those pregnancies complicated by Rh incompatibility, the risk of maternal isoimmunization to the D antigen is approximately 8% for each ABO-compatible pregnancy if no prophylaxis is given.
- Maternal-fetal ABO incompatibility is somewhat protective against Rh isoimmunization.

GENETICS: Five major loci determine Rh status: C, D, E, c, e. The presence of the D antigen results in an Rh+ individual. Its absence results in an Rh− individual. Of Rh+ fathers, 45% are homozygous, and 55% are heterozygotes. For homozygous Rh+ fathers, the probability of an Rh+ offspring is 100%. The probability for heterozygotes is approximately 50%.

RISK FACTORS:
- Antepartum: fetal-to-maternal transfusion
- Intrapartum: fetal-to-maternal transfusion, spontaneous abortion, ectopic pregnancy, abruptio placentae, abdominal trauma, chorionic villus sampling, amniocentesis, percutaneous umbilical blood sampling (PUBS), external cephalic version, manual removal of the placenta, therapeutic abortion, autologous blood product administration

ETIOLOGY

The initial response to D antigen exposure is production of immunoglobulin (Ig) M (molecular weight 900,000) that does not cross the placenta. With a repeated exposure, IgG (MW 160,000) is produced. IgG can cross the placenta and enter the fetal circulation, producing hemolysis in the fetus. This may produce erythroblastosis fetalis or hemolytic disease in the newborn, resulting in antepartum or neonatal death or neurologic damage to the fetus because of hyperbilirubinemia and kernicterus.

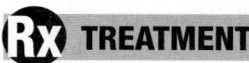

DIAGNOSIS

LABORATORY TESTS

ABO and Rh blood type and an antibody screen as part of the initial prenatal profile
- If antibody screen negative:
  1. Repeat antibody screen at 28 wk gestation.
  2. Obtain neonatal blood type after delivery.
  3. If Rh incompatibility is confirmed by the neonatal blood type, a Kleihauer-Betke or rosette test should be performed to determine the amount of fetomaternal transfusion in the following high-risk circumstances: abruptio placentae, placenta previa, cesarean delivery, intrauterine manipulation, manual removal of the placenta.
- If anti-D antibody screen is positive:
  1. Maternal indirect Coombs test is needed to determine antibody titer.
  2. Determine paternal Rh status and zygosity.
  3. If father is heterozygous, PUBS or amniotic fluid is needed to determine fetal Rh status.

IMAGING STUDIES

Ultrasound evaluation can diagnose hydrops fetalis, but it cannot predict it.

TREATMENT

PREVENTION OF D ISOIMMUNIZATION

- 50 mcg of D immunoglobulin: after spontaneous or induced abortion or ectopic pregnancy <13 wk gestation.
- 300 mcg of D immunoglobulin (protects against 30 ml of fetal blood):
  1. After spontaneous or induced abortion <13 wk gestation, amniocentesis, chorionic villous sampling, PUBS, external cephalic version, or other intrauterine manipulation.
  2. As antepartum prophylaxis at 28 wk gestation. Maternal anti-D prophylaxis does not cause hemolysis in the fetus or newborn.
  3. At delivery if the neonate is D- or Du-positive.
  4. If Kleihauer-Betke or rosette test confirms >30 ml of fetal red blood in maternal circulation, additional D immunoglobulin is indicated. Confirm adequacy of therapy by a maternal indirect Coombs test 48 to 72 hr after Rh immune globulin is given.

MANAGEMENT OF D ISOIMMUNIZED PREGNANCIES

- Serial amniocentesis for assessment of OD_{450} after 25 wk gestation with interpretation of the Delta OD450 according to criteria established by Liley
- PUBS if ultrasonographic evidence of hydrops, rising zone II Delta OD_{450} values on amniocentesis, or maternal history of a severely affected child
- Intrauterine exchange transfusion if severe anemia is documented remote from term
- Initiation of steroids for lung maturation at 28 wk in severely affected pregnancies with delivery at lung maturity
- Delivery as soon as lung maturation is achieved in mild to moderately affected pregnancies

DISPOSITION

Survival of nonhydropic infants is 90%. Of infants with hydrops, 82% survive.

REFERRAL

Refer all Rh isoimmunized pregnancies to a tertiary care center before 18 to 20 wk gestation.

SUGGESTED READING
available at www.expertconsult.com

AUTHOR: **LAUREL M. WHITE, M.D.**

BASIC INFORMATION

DEFINITION

Rhabdomyolysis is the dissolution or disintegration of muscle, which causes membrane lysis and leakage of muscle constituents, resulting in the excretion of myoglobin in the urine. Renal damage can occur as a result of tubular obstruction by myoglobin as well as hypovolemia.

ICD-9CM CODES
728.89 Rhabdomyolysis

EPIDEMIOLOGY & DEMOGRAPHICS

PREDOMINANT AGE: Rare in children. Increased risk in advanced age (>80 yr).
ONSET: The average length of time on statin therapy before rhabdomyolysis is 1 yr. Average time for onset of rhabdomyolysis after addition of fibrate to statin therapy is 32 days.

PHYSICAL FINDINGS & CLINICAL PRESENTATION

- Variable muscle tenderness. Rhabdomyolysis apart from statin use presents with muscle symptoms only 50% of the time.
- Weakness
- Muscular rigidity
- Fever
- Altered consciousness
- Muscle swelling
- Malaise, fatigue. In statin-induced rhabdomyolysis, fatigue (74%) is nearly as common as muscle pain (88%).
- Dark urine

ETIOLOGY

- Exertion (exercise-induced)
- Electrical injury
- Drug-induced (statins, combination of statins with fibrates, or erythromycin, simvastatin and amiodarone, amphetamines, haloperidol)
- Compartment syndrome
- Multiple trauma
- Malignant hyperthermia
- Limb ischemia
- Reperfusion after revascularization procedures for ischemia
- Extensive surgical (spinal) dissection, bariatric surgery
- Tourniquet ischemia
- Prolonged static positioning during surgery
- Infectious and inflammatory myositis
- Metabolic myopathies
- Hypovolemia and urinary acidification are important precipitating causes in the development of acute renal failure
- Sickle cell trait is a predisposing condition
- Hypothyroidism
- Alcoholism
- Seizures

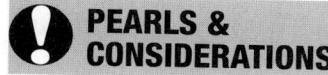 **DIAGNOSIS**

DIFFERENTIAL DIAGNOSIS

"Creatine Kinase Elevation" in Section III describes a clinical algorithm for the evaluation of creatine phosphokinase (CPK) elevation.

LABORATORY TESTS

- Screening for myoglobinuria with a simple urine dipstick test using orthotoluidine or benzidine
- Blood urea nitrogen, creatinine
- Increased CK (Fig. 1-331)
- Hyperkalemia
- Hypocalcemia
- Hyperphosphatemia
- Increased urinary myoglobin
- Pigmented granular casts
- Hyperuricemia

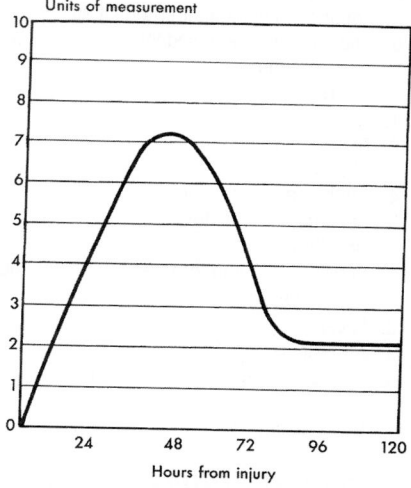

FIGURE 1-331 Typical creatine kinase elimination curve. (From Rosen P [ed]: *Emergency medicine*, ed 4, St Louis, 1998, Mosby.)

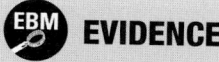 **TREATMENT**

ACUTE GENERAL Rx

- Early, aggressive, high-volume IV fluid replacement.
- Initiate volume repletion with normal saline at a rate of 200 to 1000 ml/hour depending on the setting and severity. Consider treatment with mannitol (up to 200 g/day and cumulative dose up to 800 g) to induce diuresis to prevent acute renal failure. Check for plasma osmolality and plasma osmolal gap. Discontinue mannitol if diuresis (>20 ml/hr) is not established. Maintain volume repletion until myoglobinuria is cleared (negative urine dipstick for blood).
- Monitor serum potassium frequently. Correct electrolyte imbalances. Correct hypocalcemia only if symptomatic or if severe hyperkalemia occurs.
- Treatment of electrolyte imbalances
- Alkalinization of urine is controversial but appears helpful in research models

DISPOSITION

The condition is easily treatable, but early diagnosis and management are necessary to avoid renal failure, which occurs in 30% of cases.

REFERRAL

Renal consultation

! PEARLS & CONSIDERATIONS

COMMENTS

- A clinical algorithm for the evaluation of muscle cramps and aches is described in Section III.
- Statin-induced rhabdomyolysis is 12× more frequent when statins are combined with fibrates compared with statin monotherapy.

EBM EVIDENCE

available at www.expertconsult.com

SUGGESTED READINGS

available at www.expertconsult.com

AUTHOR: **LONNIE R. MERCIER, M.D.**

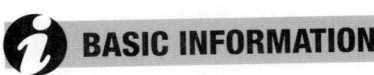

BASIC INFORMATION

DEFINITION

Rheumatic fever is a multisystem inflammatory disease that occurs in the genetically susceptible host after a pharyngeal infection with group A streptococci.

SYNONYMS

Acute rheumatic fever
Rheumatic carditis

ICD-9CM CODES
390; 716.9 Rheumatic fever

EPIDEMIOLOGY & DEMOGRAPHICS

INCIDENCE (IN U.S.):
- 0.1% to 3% in patients with untreated streptococcal pharyngitis
- Higher incidence of streptococcal pharyngitis with:
  1. Crowding
  2. Poverty
  3. Young age

PREDOMINANT AGE:
- Age 5 to 15 yr for first attack
- Possible relapses later

PEAK INCIDENCE: School-age children
GENETICS: Familial disposition: predisposition to the disease is likely to be genetically determined.

PHYSICAL FINDINGS & CLINICAL PRESENTATION

- Acute streptococcal pharyngitis, which may be subclinical and not reported by the patient
- After latent period of 1 to 5 wk (average, 19 days), acute rheumatic attack
- Patient is febrile, with a migratory polyarthritis of knees, ankles, wrists, elbows; typically severe for 1 wk, remits by 3 to 4 wk
- Carditis
  1. New heart murmur
     a. Mitral regurgitation
     b. Aortic insufficiency
     c. Diastolic mitral murmur
  2. Cardiomegaly
  3. CHF
  4. Pericardial friction rub or effusion
- Rarely, pancarditis is severe and fatal
- Subcutaneous nodules can be palpated over extensor tendon surfaces or bony prominences, such as the skull
- Chorea (Sydenham's chorea) is characterized by rapid involuntary movements affecting all muscles
  1. Muscular weakness
  2. Emotional lability
  3. Rarely seen after adolescence and almost never in adult males

- Erythema marginatum
  1. Evanescent, pink, well-demarcated spreading to trunk and proximal extremities
  2. Not specific
- Arthralgias (joint pain without swelling)
- Abdominal pain

ETIOLOGY

- Group A streptococci not recovered from tissue lesions.
- It does not occur in the absence of a streptococcal antibody response.
- Immunologic cross-reactivity between certain streptococcal antigens and human tissue antigens suggests an autoimmune cause.
- Both initial attacks and recurrences can be completely prevented by prompt treatment of streptococcal pharyngitis with penicillin.

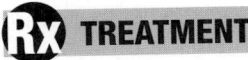

DIAGNOSIS

DIFFERENTIAL DIAGNOSIS

- Rheumatoid arthritis
- Juvenile rheumatoid arthritis (Still's disease)
- Bacterial endocarditis
- Systemic lupus
- Viral infections
- Serum sickness

WORKUP

- "Jones Criteria (revised) for Guidance in the Diagnosis of Rheumatic Fever"
- One major and two minor criteria if supported by evidence of an antecedent group A streptococcal infection
- Major criteria
  1. Carditis
  2. Migratory arthritis
  3. Chorea
  4. Erythema marginatum
  5. Subcutaneous nodules
- Minor criteria
  1. Previous rheumatic fever or rheumatic heart disease
  2. Fever
  3. Arthralgia
  4. Increased acute-phase reactants
     a. ESR
     b. C-reactive protein
     c. Leukocytosis
  5. Prolonged P-R interval

LABORATORY TESTS

- Throat cultures are usually negative.
- Streptococcal antibody tests are more useful in establishing the diagnosis.
  1. Peak at the beginning of the attack
  2. Can document a recent streptococcal infection

- ASO (antistreptolysin O) titers peak:
  1. 4 to 5 wk after a streptococcal throat infection
  2. During the second or third wk of illness
- Anti-DNase B (Streptozyme) is also commonly used but is less reliable.
- High-titer streptococcal antibodies:
  1. Are supportive of diagnosis, but not proof
  2. Should be interpreted in the context of clinical criteria

IMAGING STUDIES

- Chest x-ray to assess heart size
- Echocardiogram:
  1. To evaluate murmurs
  2. To rule out pericardial effusion

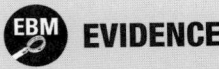

TREATMENT

ACUTE GENERAL Rx

- Course of penicillin to eradicate throat carriage of group A streptococci
- Arthralgia or arthritis without carditis: aspirin 40 mg/lb/day for 2 wk, followed by 20 mg/lb/day for 4 to 6 wk
- Carditis and heart failure:
  1. Prednisone 40 to 60 mg/day
  2. IV corticosteroids, such as methylprednisolone, 10 to 40 mg/day for severe carditis

CHRONIC Rx

Secondary prevention (prevention of recurrences):
- Monthly treatment with benzathine penicillin 1.2 million U IM
- Erythromycin in patients with penicillin allergy

DISPOSITION

- Damage of heart valves because of fibrosis
  1. Late sequela of recurrent attacks
  2. Frequent cause of valvular heart disease in developing countries
- May progress to heart failure

REFERRAL

To cardiologist for management of severe carditis

EVIDENCE

available at www.expertconsult.com

SUGGESTED READINGS

available at www.expertconsult.com

AUTHORS: **GLENN G. FORT, M.D., M.P.H.,** and **DENNIS J. MIKOLICH, M.D.**

BASIC INFORMATION

DEFINITION

Rheumatoid arthritis (RA) is a systemic disorder characterized by chronic joint inflammation that most commonly affects peripheral joints. This process results in the development of pannus, a destructive tissue that damages cartilage.

ICD-9CM CODES
714.0 Rheumatoid arthritis

EPIDEMIOLOGY & DEMOGRAPHICS

PREVALENCE: 5 to 10 cases/1000 adults. It is the most common autoimmune disease in the world.
PREDOMINANT SEX:
- Female/male ratio of 3:1
- After age 50 yr, sex difference less marked

PREDOMINANT AGE: 35 to 45 yr

PHYSICAL FINDINGS & CLINICAL PRESENTATION

- Usually gradual onset; common prodromal symptoms of weakness, fatigue, and anorexia
- Initial presentation: multiple symmetric joint involvement, most often in the hands and feet, usually metacarpophalangeal, metatarsophalangeal, and proximal interphalangeal joints (Fig. 1-332)
- Joint effusions, tenderness, and restricted motion usually present early in the disease
- Eventual characteristic deformities: subluxations, dislocations, joint contractures
- Extraarticular findings:
  1. Tendon sheaths and bursae frequently affected by chronic inflammation
  2. Possible tendon rupture
  3. Rheumatoid nodules over bony prominences such as the elbow and shaft of the ulna
  4. Splenomegaly, pericarditis, vasculitis
  5. Findings of carpal tunnel syndrome resulting from flexor tenosynovitis

ETIOLOGY

Unknown. There is increasing evidence that the inflammation and destruction of bone and cartilage that occur in many rheumatic diseases are the result of the activation by some unknown mechanism of proinflammatory cells that infiltrate the synovium. These cells, in turn, release various substances, such as cytokines and tumor necrosis factor (TNF)-alpha, which subsequently cause the pathologic changes typical of this group of diseases. Many of the newer therapeutic agents are directed at the suppression of these final mediators of inflammation.

Dx DIAGNOSIS

DIFFERENTIAL DIAGNOSIS

- Systemic lupus erythematosus
- Seronegative spondyloarthropathies
- Polymyalgia rheumatica
- Acute rheumatic fever
- Scleroderma

According to the American College of Rheumatology (ACR) previous criteria published in 1987, rheumatoid arthritis exists when four of seven criteria are present, with criteria 1 to 4 being present for at least 6 wk:
1. Morning stiffness >1 hr
2. Arthritis in three or more joints with swelling
3. Arthritis of hand joints with swelling
4. Symmetric arthritis
5. Rheumatoid nodules
6. Roentgenographic changes typical of RA
7. Positive serum rheumatoid factor

The ACR and the European League Against Rheumatism have developed a new classification criteria for RA. Four variables constitute the new criteria.
1. The number and size of involved joints (score 0-5)
2. Results of rheumatoid factor and anti-citrullinated protein antibody testing (score 0-3)
3. Abnormal sedimentation rate or elevated C-reactive protein (1 point)
4. Symptom duration >6 wk (1 point)

Scores ≥6 points are considered to have "definite RA." Maximum score is 10 points.

LABORATORY TESTS

- Increase in rheumatoid factor (RF) in 80% of cases (rheumatoid factor also present in the normal population). RF is an antibody directed against the Fc region of the IgG that has been used as a diagnostic marker for rheumatoid arthritis. Patients with rheumatoid arthritis also have autoantibodies against cyclic citrullinated peptide (CCP). Anti-CCp autoantibodies are more specific than RF for diagnosing rheumatoid arthritis and may better predict erosive disease. Sensitivity and specificity of the anti-CCP test for RA is 67% and 95% respectively.
- Possible mild anemia
- Usually, elevated acute phase reactants (erythrocyte sedimentation rate, C-reactive protein)
- Possible mild leukocytosis
- Usually, turbid joint fluid, which forms a poor mucin clot; elevated cell count, with an increase in polymorphonuclear leukocytes

IMAGING STUDIES

Plain radiography:
- Usually reveals soft tissue swelling and osteoporosis early (Fig. 1-333)
- Eventually, joint space narrowing, erosion, and deformity visible as a result of continued inflammation and cartilage destruction

Rx TREATMENT

NONPHARMACOLOGIC THERAPY

Proper management requires close cooperation among primary physician, therapist, rheumatologist, and orthopedist.
- Patient education is important.
- Rest with proper exercise and splinting can prevent or correct joint deformities.
- Maintain proper diet and control obesity.

CHRONIC Rx

- Nonsteroidal anti-inflammatory drugs (NSAIDs): commonly used as the initial treatment to relieve inflammation (drug of choice for most patients is aspirin, but other NSAIDs are also effective)
- Disease-modifying drugs (DMARDs): traditionally begun when NSAIDs are not effective; current recommendations favor early aggressive treatment with DMARDs, seeking to minimize long-term joint damage. Commonly used agents are methotrexate, cyclosporine, hydroxychloroquine, sulfasalazine, leflunomide, and infliximab. Most of these are associated with potential toxicity and require close monitoring. They are also usually slow-acting drugs that require >8 wk to become effective (Table 1-160)
- Oral prednisone
- Intrasynovial steroid injections

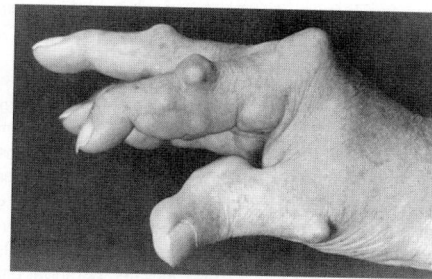

FIGURE 1-332 Rheumatoid arthritis. Hand of a 60-year-old man with seropositive rheumatoid arthritis. There are fixed deformities and gross rheumatoid nodules. (From Canoso JJ: *Rheumatology in primary care*, Philadelphia, 1997, WB Saunders.)

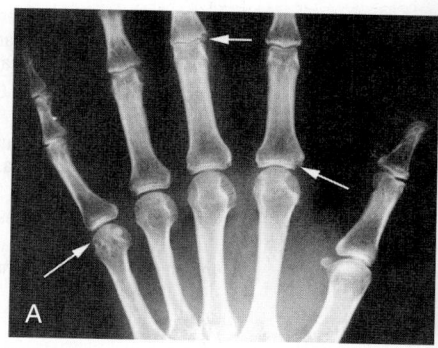
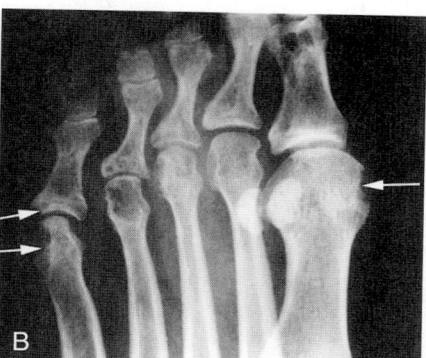

FIGURE 1-333 Rheumatoid arthritis. A, Periarticular osteopenia and marginal erosions in metacarpophalangeal joints and a proximal interphalangeal *(arrows)*. **B,** In the same patient, marginal erosions at metatarsal heads. (From Canoso JJ [ed]: *Rheumatology in primary care*, Philadelphia, 1997, WB Saunders.)

- Etanercept, a tumor necrosis factor (TNF) α-blocker, is useful in moderately to severely active RA in patients who respond inadequately to DMARDs. The combination of etanercept and methotrexate has been reported to be effective and promising in the treatment of RA
- New treatment agents include rituximab (anti-CD 20), abatacept (cytotoxic T-lymphocyte antigen 4 immunoglobulin), and tocilizumab (anti-interleukin 6 receptor). There is no solid evidence that any one TNF inhibitor is more effective than any other for treatment of rheumatoid arthritis.

DISPOSITION

- Remissions and exacerbations are common, but condition is chronically progressive in the majority of cases.

- Joint degeneration and deformity often lead to disability.
- Early diagnosis and treatment are important and can improve quality of life.

REFERRAL

- Early referral to rheumatologist
- Orthopedic consultation for corrective surgery

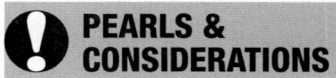

- RA often develops acutely in the postpartum patient, a common time for the onset of autoimmune diseases.

- Because of the poor outcomes associated with previous treatment protocols, a much more aggressive approach, often using IV therapies, is presently advocated by many rheumatologists.

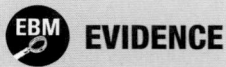 **EVIDENCE**

available at www.expertconsult.com

SUGGESTED READINGS

available at www.expertconsult.com

AUTHOR: **LONNIE R. MERCIER, M.D.**

TABLE 1-160 Selected Disease-Modifying Antirheumatic Drugs

Type Generic (Trade) Name	Recommended Dosages	Toxic Effects	Recommended Monitoring
Gold compounds (Myochrysine)	IM: 10 mg followed by 25 mg 1 wk later, then 25-50 mg/wk until there is toxicity, major clinical improvement, or cumulative dose ≥1 g. If effective, interval between doses is increased.	Pruritus, dermatitis (frequent in one third of patients), stomatitis, nephrotoxicity, blood dyscrasias, "nitritoid" reaction: flushing, weakness, nausea, dizziness 30 min after injection.	CBC, platelet count before every other injection
Aurothioglucose (Solganal)	IM: 10 mg; second and third doses 25 mg, fourth and subsequent doses 50 mg. Interval between doses: 1 wk. If improvement and no toxicity, decrease dose to 25 mg or increase interval between doses.	Dermatitis, stomatitis, nephrotoxicity, blood dyscrasias.	CBC, platelet count every 2 wk. Urinalysis before each dose.
Auranofin (Ridaura)	Oral: 3 mg bid or 6 mg qd; may increase to 3 mg tid after 6 mo.	Loose stools, diarrhea (up to 50%), dermatitis.	Baseline CBC, platelet count, U/A, renal, liver function, at onset then CBC with platelet count, U/A 9 mo.
Antimalarial Hydroxychloroquine (Plaquenil)	Oral: 400-600 mg qd with meals then 200-400 mg qd.	Retinopathy, dermatitis, muscle weakness, hypoactive DTRs, CNS.	Ophthalmologic examination every 3 mo (visual acuity, slit lamp, funduscopic, visual field tests), neuromuscular examination.
Penicillamine (Cuprimine, Depen)	Oral: 125-250 mg qd, then increasing at monthly intervals doses to max 750-1000 mg by 125-250 mg.	Pruritus, rash/mouth ulcers, bone marrow depression, proteinuria, hematuria, hypogeusia, myasthenia, myositis, GI distress, pulmonary toxicity, teratogenic.	CBC every 2 wk until dose stable, then every month.
Methotrexate (Rheumatrex)	Oral: 7.5-15 mg/wk.	Pulmonary toxicity, ulcerative stomatitis, leukopenia, thrombocytopenia, GI distress, malaise, fatigue, chills, fever, CNS, elevated LFTs/liver disease, lymphoma, infection.	U/A weekly until dose stable, then every month; hCG as needed.
Azathioprine (Imuran)	Oral: 50-100 mg qd, increase at 4-wk intervals by 0.5 mg/kg/day up to 2.5 mg/kg/day.	Leukopenia, thrombocytopenia, GI, neoplastic if previous Rx with alkylating agents.	CBC with platelet count, LFTs weekly for 6 wk then monthly LFTs, U/A periodically, hCG as needed.
Sulfasalazine (Azulfidine)	Oral: 500 mg/day then increase up to 3 g/day.	GI, skin rash, pruritus, blood dyscrasias, oligospermia.	CBC with platelet count, weekly × 1 mo, 2×/mo. × 2 mo, then monthly, HCG as needed.
Alkylating agents Cyclophosphamide (Cytoxan)	Oral: 50-100 mg/day up to 2.5 mg/kg/day.	Leukopenia, thrombocytopenia, hematuria, GI, alopecia, rash, bladder cancer, non-Hodgkin's lymphoma, infection.	CBC, U/A every 2 wk for 3 mo, then monthly for 9 mo, then every 6 mo.
Chlorambucil (Leukeran)	Oral: 0.1-0.2 mg/kg/day.	Bone marrow suppression, GI, CNS, infection.	CBC with platelet count regularly; hCG as needed.
Cyclosporine (Sandimmune)	Oral 2.5-5 mg/kg/day.	Nephrotoxicity, tremor, hirsutism, hypertension, gum hyperplasia.	CBC with platelet count every week. WBCs 3-4 days after each CBC during first 3-6 wk at therapy; hCG as needed.
Pyrimidine, synthesis inhibitors	Loading dose: 100 mg/day for 3 days.	Hepatotoxicity, carcinogenesis.	Renal function, liver function.
Leflunomide (Arava)	Maintenance therapy: 20 mg/day; if not tolerated, 10 mg/day.	Immunosuppression, long half-life.	LFTs every month, drug levels after discontinuation (after 1 mo therapy, remains in blood for 2 yr without use of cholestyramine).

From Rakel RE (ed): *Principles of family practice*, ed 6, Philadelphia, 2002, WB Saunders.
bid, Twice a day; *CBC,* complete blood count; *CNS,* central nervous system; *DTR,* deep tendon reflex; *GI,* gastrointestinal; *hCG,* human chorionic gonadotropin; *IM,* intramuscular; *LFT,* liver function test; *qd,* every day; *tid,* three times a day; *U/A,* urinalysis; *WBC,* white blood cell count.

BASIC INFORMATION

DEFINITION

Allergic rhinitis is an IgE-mediated hypersensitivity response to nasally inhaled allergens that causes sneezing, rhinorrhea, nasal pruritus, and congestion. It may be seasonal or perennial.

SYNONYMS

Hay fever
IgE-mediated rhinitis

ICD-9CM CODES
477.9 Allergic rhinitis

EPIDEMIOLOGY & DEMOGRAPHICS

- Allergic rhinitis affects approximately 10% to 20% of the U.S. population and 40% of children.
- Mean age of onset is 8 to 12 yr.
- The prevalence of allergic rhinitis in patients presenting to their primary care provider with nasal symptoms is estimated to be 30% to 60%.

PHYSICAL FINDINGS & CLINICAL PRESENTATION

- Pale or violaceous mucosa of the turbinates caused by venous engorgement (this can distinguish it from erythema present in viral rhinitis)
- Nasal polyps
- Lymphoid hyperplasia in the posterior oropharynx with cobblestone appearance
- Erythema of the throat, conjunctival and scleral injection
- Clear nasal discharge
- Clinical presentation: usually consists of sneezing, nasal congestion, cough, postnasal drip, loss of or alteration of smell, and sensation of plugged ears

ETIOLOGY

- Pollens in the springtime, ragweed in fall, grasses in the summer
- Dust, mites, animal allergens
- Smoke or any irritants
- Perfumes, detergents, soaps
- Emotion, changes in atmospheric pressure or temperature

DIAGNOSIS

DIFFERENTIAL DIAGNOSIS

- Infections (sinusitis; viral, bacterial, or fungal rhinitis)
- Rhinitis medicamentosa (cocaine, sympathomimetic nasal drops)
- Vasomotor rhinitis (e.g., secondary to air pollutants)
- Septal obstruction (e.g., deviated septum), nasal polyps, nasal neoplasms
- Systemic diseases (e.g., Wegener's granulomatosis, hypothyroidism [rare])

WORKUP

- The initial strategy should be to determine whether patients should undergo diagnostic testing or receive empirical treatment.
- Workup is often unnecessary if the diagnosis is apparent. A detailed medical history is useful in identifying the culprit allergen.
- Selected patients with allergic rhinitis that is not controlled with standard therapy may benefit from allergy testing to target allergen avoidance measures or guide immunotherapy. Allergy testing can be performed using skin testing or radioallergosorbent (RAST) testing. Immunoglobulin E (IgE) testing using newest generation assays is also an excellent tool for diagnosing the cause of symptoms related to rhinitis. Allergy testing should generally be reserved for ambiguous or complicated cases.
- Examination of nasal smears for the presence of neutrophils to rule out infectious causes and the presence of eosinophils (suggestive of allergy) may be useful in selected patients.
- Peripheral blood eosinophil counts are not useful in allergy diagnosis.

TREATMENT

NONPHARMACOLOGIC THERAPY

- Maintain allergen-free environment by covering mattresses and pillows with allergen-proof casings, eliminating carpeting, eliminating animal products, and removing dust-collecting fixtures.
- Use of air purifiers and dust filters is helpful.
- Maintain humidity in the environment below 50% to prevent dust mites and mold.
- Use air conditioners, especially in the bedroom.
- Remove pets from homes of patients with suspected sensitivity to animal allergens.

ACUTE GENERAL Rx

- Determine if the patient is troubled by swollen turbinates (best treated with decongestants) or blockages secondary to mucus (effectively treated by antihistamines).
- Topical nasal steroids are very effective and are preferred by many as first-line treatment for allergic rhinitis in adults. Patients should be instructed on proper use and informed that improvement might not occur for at least 1 wk after initiation of therapy. Commonly available inhalers follow.
  - Beclomethasone dipropionate: one to two sprays in each nostril bid
  - Fluticasone: initially two sprays in each nostril qd or one spray in each nostril bid, decreasing to one spray in each nostril qd based on response
  - Flunisolide: initially two sprays in each nostril bid
  - Budesonide: two sprays in each nostril bid or four sprays in each nostril qam
- Most first-generation antihistamines can cause considerable sedation and anticholinergic symptoms. The second-generation antihistamines (loratadine, fexofenadine, cetirizine, levocetirizine, desloratadine) are preferred because they do not have any significant anticholinergic or sedative effects.
- Montelukast (Singulair), a leukotriene receptor antagonist commonly used for asthma, is also effective for allergic rhinitis. Usual adult dose is 10 mg qd.
- Azelastine (Astelin) is an antihistamine nasal spray effective for seasonal allergic rhinitis. Olopatadine (Patanase) is an intranasal H1-antihistamine alternative to azestaline in mild to moderate seasonal allergic rhinitis.

CHRONIC Rx

- Cromolyn sodium : one spray to each nostril three to four times daily can be used for prophylaxis (mast cell stabilizer).
- Immunotherapy is generally reserved for patients responding poorly to the above treatments.

DISPOSITION

Most patients experience significant relief with avoidance of allergens and proper use of medications.

REFERRAL

Allergy testing in patients with severe symptoms who are unresponsive to therapy or when the diagnosis is uncertain

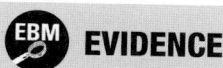

EVIDENCE

available at www.expertconsult.com

SUGGESTED READINGS
available at www.expertconsult.com

AUTHOR: **FRED F. FERRI, M.D.**

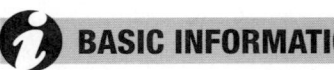

BASIC INFORMATION

DEFINITION

Rickets is a systemic disease of infancy and childhood in which mineralization of growing bone is deficient as a result of abnormal calcium, phosphorus, or vitamin D metabolism. Osteomalacia is the same condition in the adult. *Renal osteodystrophy* is a term used to describe a similar condition in patients with chronic kidney disease. Certain forms of the disorder may respond only to high doses of vitamin D and are referred to as vitamin D–resistant rickets (VDRR).

ICD-9CM CODES
268.0 Active rickets
275.3 Vitamin D–resistant rickets
588.0 Renal rickets (renal osteodystrophy)
268.2 Osteomalacia

PHYSICAL FINDINGS & CLINICAL PRESENTATION

The child with classic rickets usually develops a number of specific abnormalities:
- Softening of the skull bones (craniotabes) early in the disorder
- Enlargement of the ribs at the costochondral junctions, producing the "rachitic rosary"
- Limb deformities and epiphyseal swelling (Fig. 1-334)
- Height below normal range
- Irritability and easy fatigability
- Pigeon breast deformity and an indentation of the lower ribcage at the insertion of the diaphragm, sometimes referred to as *Harrison's groove;* possible decrease in thoracic volume, resulting in diminished pulmonary ventilation

Physical findings in the adult with osteomalacia are more subtle:
- Possible malaise and bone pain
- Many patients presumed to have osteoporosis but may also have osteomalacia

ETIOLOGY

- Deficiency states
  1. True classic VDRR is rare in Western society.
  2. Absorption of vitamin D, however, may be blocked in several gastrointestinal disorders.
  3. Similar disorders may also prevent absorption of calcium and phosphorus, but in the absence of these other diseases deficiencies of calcium and phosphorus are also rare.
- VDRR, type I results from abnormalities in the gene coding for 25 (OH)D3-1-alpha-hydroxylase, and type II results from defective vitamin D receptors.
- Acquired or inherited renal tubular abnormalities that cause resorptive defects and result in rickets and osteomalacia; syndromes include classical VDRR (probably the most common form of rickets seen in general practice). VDRR are familial hypophosphatemic rickets and hereditary hypophosphatemic rickets with hypercalciuria.

- Chronic renal failure:
  1. Can produce renal rickets or renal osteodystrophy
  2. Results in the retention of phosphate

DIAGNOSIS

DIFFERENTIAL DIAGNOSIS
- Osteoporosis
- Hyperparathyroidism
- Hyperthyroidism

LABORATORY TESTS
- Requires a high degree of interest because many of the conditions are so similar that only a complicated laboratory evaluation may establish the diagnosis
- Blood urea nitrogen, creatinine, alkaline phosphatase, calcium, and phosphorus levels in any patient suspected of having metabolic bone disease

IMAGING STUDIES
- In rickets:
  1. Characteristic radiographic changes in the ends of growing long bones caused by the lack of calcification of the cartilage matrix
  2. Widening and irregularity of the epiphyseal plate
- Radiographs in the adult with osteomalacia:
  1. More subtle and often confused with osteoporosis
  2. Possible pseudofractures (Looser's zones) where major arteries cross bone
  3. Insufficiency compression deformities in the vertebral bodies

TREATMENT

- VDRR, type I is treated with vitamin D. Various vitamin D (oral or intramuscular) are available. The earliest biochemical change after initiation of treatment is an increase in the level of phosphorus followed by a rise in calcium level. Serum calcium, phosphorus, alkaline phosphatase and calcidiol levels and urine calcium and phosphorus levels should be obtained within 2 wk of initiation of therapy and periodically. The treatment of type II is more complex and requires consultations with an endocrinologist and nephrologists.
- Familial hypophosphatemic rickets is treated with calcitriol and oral phosphorus.
- Oral phosphorus alone is the treatment of choice for hereditary hypophosphatemic rickets with hypercalciuria.

REFERRAL
- Because of the complex nature of many of these disorders, a qualified endocrinologist and nephrologist should be consulted for treatment.
- The need for orthopedic intervention is rare.
- Surgical care is indicated for slipped capital femoral epiphysis, which is fairly common in renal rickets.
- Deformity may require bracing.

SUGGESTED READINGS
available at www.expertconsult.com

AUTHOR: **LONNIE R. MERCIER, M.D.**

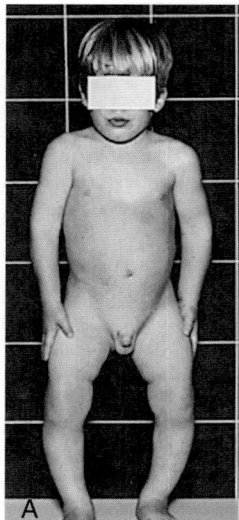
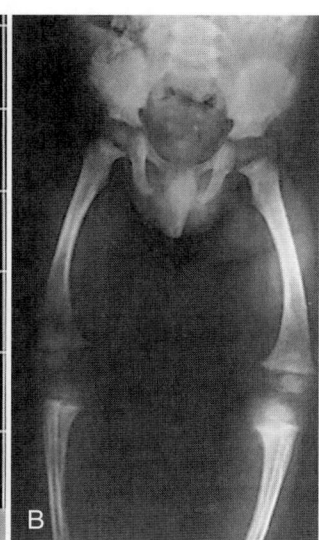

FIGURE 1-334 Clinical **(A)** and radiographic **(B)** appearance of a young boy with X-linked hypophosphatemic rickets. Note the striking bowing of the legs, apparent in both femora and tibiae, with flaring of the ends of the bones at the knee. (Courtesy Dr. Sara B. Arnaud. From Bikle DB: Osteomalacia and rickets. In Wyngaarden JB et al [eds]: *Cecil textbook of medicine,* ed 19, Philadelphia, 1992, WB Saunders.)

BASIC INFORMATION

DEFINITION

Rocky Mountain spotted fever (RMSF) is a life-threatening, tick-borne febrile illness caused by infection with *Rickettsia rickettsii*. The infection occurs when *R. rickettsii* in the salivary glands of a vector tick is transmitted into the dermis, spreading and replicating in the cytoplasm of endothelial cells and eliciting widespread vasculitis and end-organ damage.

ICD-9CM CODES

082.0 Rocky Mountain spotted fever

EPIDEMIOLOGY & DEMOGRAPHICS

INCIDENCE: 0.18 to 0.32 cases per 100,000 person-years

PREVALENCE: Most prevalent in the Southeast, followed by the South Central states, but seen anywhere. It has recently been reported in eastern Arizona, with common brown dog ticks (*Rhipicephalus sanguineus*) implicated as a vector of *R. rickettsii*.

PREDOMINANT SEX: Affects both genders equally

PREDOMINANT AGE: Occurs at any age, but more likely in children ages 5 to 14 yr

PHYSICAL FINDINGS & CLINICAL PRESENTATION

- Incubation: 3 to 12 days
- First symptoms: fever, headache, malaise, myalgias

Common History, Signs, or Symptoms	%
Tick bite	65
Fever	100
Rash	90
Rash on palms and soles	80
Headache	90
Myalgia	75
Nausea or vomiting	60
Abdominal pain	40
Conjunctivitis	30
Edema	20
Pneumonitis	15
Any severe neurologic complication (including stupor, delirium, seizures, ataxia, papilledema, focal neurologic deficits, and coma)	30

- Rash:
  - Appears during first 3 days in 50%; by day 5, 80% have it. No rash in 10%.
  - Initial appearance: blanching erythematous macules on wrists and ankles that then spread to trunk, palms, and soles.
  - Lesions may evolve into papules and eventually become nonblanching (petechiae or palpable purpura).
- Gastrointestinal symptoms:
  - Nausea, vomiting, and abdominal pain are common
  - Occasionally may mimic an "acute abdomen" (e.g., appendicitis, cholecystitis)
  - Mild hepatitis
- Cardiopulmonary involvement:
  - Interstitial pneumonitis
  - Myocarditis
- Renal problems:
  - Prerenal azotemia
  - Interstitial nephritis
  - Glomerulonephritis
- Neurologic involvement:
  - Encephalitis (confusion, lethargy, delirium)
  - Ataxia
  - Convulsion
  - Cranial nerve palsy
  - Speech impediment
  - Hemiparesis or paraparesis
  - Spasticity
- Fulminant Rocky Mountain spotted fever
  - Early, widespread vascular necrosis leading to multisystem illness and death

ETIOLOGY & PATHOGENESIS

- Infectious agent: *R. rickettsii* (an intracellular bacterium).
- Vector: dog tick and wood tick (vertical transmission exists in ticks, but horizontal transmission involving rodents represents an important reservoir for the agent). In the United States *R. rickettsii* is transmitted mainly by the American dog tick (*Dermacentor variabilis*) and the Rocky Mountain wood tick (*D. andersoni*).
- Pathogenesis: the spread of *R. rickettsii* is hematogenous with attachment to the vascular endothelium, causing a vasculitis. The manifestations of this illness are caused by increased vascular permeability.

DIAGNOSIS

DIFFERENTIAL DIAGNOSIS

Influenza A, enteroviral infection, typhoid fever, leptospirosis, infectious mononucleosis, viral hepatitis, sepsis, ehrlichiosis, gastroenteritis, acute abdomen, bronchitis, pneumonia, meningococcemia, disseminated gonococcal infection, secondary syphilis, bacterial endocarditis, toxic shock syndrome, scarlet fever, rheumatic fever, measles, rubella, typhus, rickettsialpox, Lyme disease, drug hypersensitivity reactions, idiopathic thrombocytopenic purpura, thrombotic thrombocytopenic purpura, Kawasaki disease, immune complex vasculitis, connective tissue disorders

WORKUP

Consider RMSF in any patient with an acute febrile illness with headache and myalgia, especially with an associated history of tick exposure. Absence of rash does not rule out the diagnosis.

LABORATORY TESTS

Routine Tests	%
White cell count	
<10,000/mm³	72
>10% bands	69
Platelet count	
<150,000/mm³	52
<99,000/mm³	32
Serum sodium value <132 mEq/L	56
Aspartate aminotransferase ≥2× normal	62
Alanine aminotransferase ≥2× normal	39
Bilirubin value >1.4 mg/dl	30
Cerebrospinal fluid	
Opening pressure ≥250 mm H₂O	14
Glucose value ≤50 mg/dl	8
Protein value ≥50 mg/dl	35
White cell count ≥5/mm³	38
Mononuclear cell predominance	46
Polymorphonuclear cell predominance	50

- Etiologic tests:
  - Antibody titers to *R. rickettsii* (by indirect fluorescent antibody test). The diagnosis of RMSF requires a fourfold increase 2 wk apart and thus is not helpful in the care of the patients despite a sensitivity and specificity of near 100%.
  - The only test that can provide a timely diagnosis is the immunohistologic demonstration of *R. rickettsii* in skin biopsy specimens.

TREATMENT

- Oral or IV doxycycline, 200 mg/day in 2 divided doses
- Oral tetracycline, 25 to 50 mg/kg/day in 4 divided doses
- Chloramphenicol, 50 to 75 mg/kg/day in 4 divided doses; chloramphenicol may be preferred during pregnancy because of the effects of tetracycline on fetal bones and teeth; therapy continued for at least 2 days after defervescence

PROGNOSIS

Fatality rate: 1% to 4% (five times greater if treatment is initiated after day 5 of illness, which is more likely in the absence of rash and during seasonal nonpeak tick activity). Long-term sequelae seen in patients who recover from severe RMSF: paraparesis, hearing loss; peripheral neuropathy; bladder and bowel incontinence; cerebellar, vestibular, and motor dysfunction; language disorders; limb amputation; and scrotal pain after cutaneous necrosis.

SUGGESTED READINGS

available at www.expertconsult.com

AUTHOR: **FRED F. FERRI, M.D.**

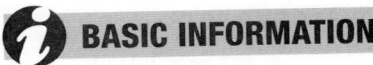

BASIC INFORMATION

DEFINITION

Rosacea is a chronic skin disorder characterized by papules and pustules affecting the face and often associated with flushing and erythema.

SYNONYMS

Acne rosacea

ICD-9CM CODES
695.3 Rosacea

EPIDEMIOLOGY & DEMOGRAPHICS

- Rosacea occurs in one in 20 Americans
- Onset often between ages 30 and 50 yr
- More common in people of Celtic origin; however, this disease may be overlooked in nonwhites because skin pigmentation results in atypical presentation
- Female/male ratio of 3:1

PHYSICAL FINDINGS & CLINICAL PRESENTATION

- Facial erythema, presence of papules, pustules, and telangiectasia.
- Excessive facial warmth and redness is the predominant presenting symptom.
- Itching is generally absent.
- Comedones are absent (unlike acne).
- Women are more likely to show symptoms on the chin and cheeks, whereas in men the nose is commonly involved.
- Ocular findings (mild dryness and irritation with blepharitis, conjunctival injection, burning, stinging, tearing, eyelid inflammation, swelling, and redness) are present in 50% of patients.

Rosacea can be classified into four major subtypes:
1. Erythematotelengiectatic: erythema in central part of face, telangiectasia, flushing
2. Papulopustular: presence of dome-shaped erythematous papules and small pustules, in addition to facial erythema, flushing, and telangiectasia
3. Phymatosis: presence of thickened skin with prominent pores that may affect the nose (rhinophyma), chin (gnathophyma), forehead (metophyma), eyelids (blepharophyma), and ears (otophyma)
4. Ocular: conjunctival injection, sensation of foreign body in the eye, telangiectasia and erythema of lid margins, scaling.

ETIOLOGY

- Unknown.
- Hot drinks, alcohol, and sun exposure may accentuate the erythema by causing vasodilation of the skin.

- Flare-ups may also result from reactions to medications (e.g., simvastatin, angiotensin-converting enzyme inhibitors, vasodilators, fluorinated corticosteroids), stress, extreme heat or cold, wind, humidity, strenuous exercise, spicy drinks, menstruation.

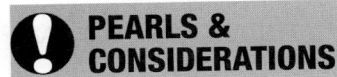

DIAGNOSIS

DIFFERENTIAL DIAGNOSIS

- Drug eruption
- Acne vulgaris
- Contact dermatitis
- Systemic lupus erythematosus
- Carcinoid flush
- Idiopathic facial flushing
- Seborrheic dermatitis
- Facial sarcoidosis
- Photodermatitis
- Mastocytosis
- Perioral dermatitis
- Granulomas of the skin

WORKUP

Diagnosis is based on clinical findings. Distinguishing features between acne and rosacea are the presence of telangiectasia and deep diffuse erythema and absence of comedones in rosacea.

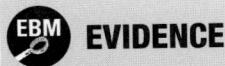

TREATMENT

NONPHARMACOLOGIC THERAPY

- Avoid alcohol, excessive sun exposure, and hot drinks of any type.
- Use of mild, nondrying soap is recommended; local skin irritants should be avoided.
- Reassure patient that rosacea is completely unrelated to poor hygiene.

GENERAL Rx

- Several classes of drugs are used in treatment of rosacea, including the metronidazole family, the tetracycline family, and azelaic acid.
- Topical therapy with metronidazole aqueous gel (MetroGel) applied bid is effective as initial therapy for mild cases or after the use of oral antibiotics. A new 1% formulation of metronidazole (Noritate) applied daily may improve patient compliance. Clindamycin lotion (Cleocin), sulfacetamide, or erythromycin 2% solution may also be effective.
- Systemic antibiotics: Doxycycline 100 mg qd tetracycline 250 mg qid until symptoms diminish, then taper off; doxycycline 100 mg bid is also effective.
- Minocycline 50 to 100 mg qd should be used only in resistant cases because this medication is expensive.

- Oral metronidazole (200 mg qd to bid) for 4 to 6 wk is also effective.
- Isotretinoin (Accutane) 0.5 to 1 mg/kg/day in two divided doses for 15 to 20 wk can be used for refractory papular and pustular rosacea; use of retinoids may, however, worsen erythema and telangiectasis.
- Laser treatment is an option for progressive telangiectasias or rhinophyma.
- Erythema and flushing may respond to low-dose clonidine (0.05 mg bid).
- Treatment of phymatous rosacea: oral tetracyclines, oral isotretinoin, ablative/pulsed dye laser therapy, electrosurgery.
- Treatment of ocular rosacea: topical or oral tetracyclines, artificial tears, and/or lid cleansing for eyelid hygiene.

DISPOSITION

- Rosacea is often resistant to initial treatment and recurrent. Periods of remission and relapse are common.
- The progression of rosacea is variable. Typical stages include:
  1. Facial flushing
  2. Erythema and/or edema and ocular symptoms
  3. Papules and pustules
  4. Rhinophyma

PEARLS & CONSIDERATIONS

COMMENTS

- The course of the disease is typically chronic, with remissions and relapses.
- Patients with resistant cases may have *Demodex folliculorum* mite infestation or tinea infection (diagnosis can be confirmed with potassium hydroxide examination); the role of *D. folliculorum* in rosacea is unclear. These mites can sometimes be found in large numbers in the lesions; however, their numbers do not generally decline with treatment.
- Rosacea can result in emotional and social stigmas, especially because many people associate rosacea and rhinophyma with alcohol abuse.
- Early consultation with an ophthalmologist is recommended in patients with suspected ocular involvement.

EVIDENCE

available at www.expertconsult.com

SUGGESTED READINGS
available at www.expertconsult.com

AUTHOR: **FRED F. FERRI, M.D.**

BASIC INFORMATION

DEFINITION

Roseola is a benign viral illness found in infants and characterized by high fevers, followed by a rash.

SYNONYMS

Exanthem subitum
Sixth disease
Roseola infantum

ICD-9CM CODES
057.8 Roseola

EPIDEMIOLOGY & DEMOGRAPHICS

- Nearly one third of all infants develop roseola before the age of 2 yr.
- More than 90% of children older than 2 yr of age are seropositive for the virus causing roseola.
- Roseola is spread from person to person. It is not known how it is spread, but it must be very efficiently spread and presumably via the respiratory tract.
- There is no predilection for gender or time of year.

PHYSICAL FINDINGS & CLINICAL PRESENTATION

- Typically the child develops a high fever, usually up to 104° F (40° C), that lasts for 3 to 5 days
- Fever may be associated with a runny nose, irritability, and fatigue
- A rash appears within 48 hr of defervescence, mainly on the face, neck, trunk, arms, and legs
- Faint pink maculopapular rash that blanches when palpated
- The rash usually fades away within 48 hr
- Anorexia
- Seizures
- Cervical adenopathy

ETIOLOGY

- Roseola is caused by human herpesvirus-6 (HHV-6).
- The incubation period is between 5 and 15 days.

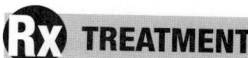 # DIAGNOSIS

The diagnosis of roseola is usually made by the clinical presentation as stated previously.

DIFFERENTIAL DIAGNOSIS

- Measles
- Rubella
- Fifth disease
- Drug eruption
- Mononucleosis
- All causes of fever (e.g., otitis media, pneumonia, and urinary tract infection)
- Meningitis

WORKUP

- If unsure of the diagnosis of roseola in a febrile infant, a fever workup is done to rule out other infectious causes.
- The decision to proceed with a fever workup is a clinical judgment call.

LABORATORY TESTS

- CBC with differential, erythrocyte sedimentation rate (ESR), blood cultures as indicated
- Urinalysis and urine cultures
- Stool cultures if diarrhea is present
- Lumbar puncture if needed to rule out meningitis
- Commercial assays can be used to detect HHV-6-specific IgG antibody responses but IgM assays are not always reliable for acute infection

IMAGING STUDIES

Chest x-ray to rule out pneumonia

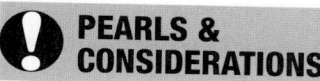 # TREATMENT

NONPHARMACOLOGIC THERAPY

- Supportive care
- Maintain hydration by drinking clear fluids: water, fruit juice, lemonade, and so forth
- Sponge bathe with lukewarm water if febrile

ACUTE GENERAL Rx

- Acetaminophen 10 to 15 mg/kg per dose at 4-hr intervals for fever
- Ibuprofen 5 to 10 mg/kg per dose at 6-hr intervals (maximal dose 600 mg)

CHRONIC Rx

Roseola is a viral disease that is short lasting; chronic treatment is usually not an issue.

DISPOSITION

- Roseola is generally a benign, self-limited disease that usually lasts approximately 1 wk.
- Complications, although rare, can occur and include:
  1. Febrile seizures
  2. Meningitis
  3. Encephalitis
  4. Pneumonitis
  5. Hepatitis

REFERRAL

Subspecialty consultation is made with the appropriate discipline if any of the previously mentioned complications occur (e.g., neurology for seizures).

! PEARLS & CONSIDERATIONS

COMMENTS

- A child with fever and rash should be excluded from day care.
- HHV-6 is named accordingly because it is the sixth herpesvirus discovered after herpes simplex 1 (HSV-1), HSV-2, cytomegalovirus (CMV), Epstein-Barr virus (EBV), and varicella-zoster virus (VZV).
- Roseola is called sixth disease because it represents the sixth childhood "exanthem"; the other five are measles, scarlet fever, rubella, Dukes disease, and erythema infectiosum.

SUGGESTED READINGS

available at www.expertconsult.com

AUTHORS: **GLENN G. FORT, M.D., M.P.H.,** and **DENNIS J. MIKOLICH, M.D.**

BASIC INFORMATION

DEFINITION

The rotator cuff comprises four muscle tendon units that stabilize the humeral head within the shoulder joint and aid in moving the upper extremity. Rotator cuff syndrome refers to a spectrum of afflictions involving the tendons of the rotator cuff (primarily the supraspinatus), ranging from simple strains and tendinitis to complete, massive rupture with cuff-tear arthropathy.

SYNONYMS

Impingement syndrome
Painful arc syndrome
Internal derangement of the subacromial joint
Supraspinatus syndrome
Bursitis of shoulder

ICD-9CM CODES
726.10 Rotator cuff syndrome
727.61 Rotator cuff rupture

EPIDEMIOLOGY & DEMOGRAPHICS

PREVALENCE: 5% to 10% of the general population
PREDOMINANT SEX: More common in males than females
PREDOMINANT AGE: Uncommon <20 yr of age

PHYSICAL FINDINGS & CLINICAL PRESENTATION

- Pain, often at night
- Rotator cuff tenderness
- Referred pain down deltoid, especially with abduction between 70 and 120 degrees ("the painful arc") (Fig. 1-335)
- Weakness in abduction or forward flexion
- Increased pain with overhead activities
- Atrophy in longstanding cases of complete tear
- Positive "drop-arm" test (weakness of abduction against downward pressure at 90 degrees)

ETIOLOGY

- Microtrauma from repetitive use
- Abnormally shaped acromion
- Shoulder instability
- Worsening of process by the overhead throwing motion
- Microcirculatory changes at the musculotendinous junction

DIAGNOSIS

DIFFERENTIAL DIAGNOSIS

- Shoulder instability
- Degenerative arthritis
- Cervical radiculopathy
- Avascular necrosis
- Suprascapular nerve entrapment

WORKUP

- In chronic tendinitis, clinical findings similar to those seen in partial rupture
- Even with complete rupture, may have full, active range of motion in shoulder

IMAGING STUDIES

- Plain radiography
- Ultrasonography may be useful but only in diagnosing moderately large tears
- MRI to evaluate full- or partial-thickness tears, chronic tendinitis, and other causes of shoulder pain
- Since MRI, arthrography is rarely used

TREATMENT

ACUTE GENERAL Rx

- Rest to avoid overhead activity
- Ice or heat for comfort
- Carefully supervised program of stretching and strengthening
- Medication: nonsteroidal antiinflammatory drugs, subacromial corticosteroid injection (once or twice at 2-wk intervals)

DISPOSITION

- All forms are likely to respond to nonsurgical management.
- Even many complete rotator cuff tears have minimal pain and little loss of function.

REFERRAL

For orthopedic consultation in patients who do not respond to medical management or in whom rotator cuff tear is suspected

PEARLS & CONSIDERATIONS

COMMENTS

- There is considerable disagreement regarding the likelihood of recovery once a significant rotator cuff rupture has developed.
- Indications for surgery vary among surgeons.
- Injection is contraindicated in the presence of local infection.
- As with other similar musculoskeletal disorders, the underlying pathology involved may be more degenerative (tendinopathy, tendinosis) than inflammatory.
- Once a separation ("tear") develops, there is no way to predict whether it will ever become worse or not.

SUGGESTED READINGS
available at www.expertconsult.com

AUTHOR: **LONNIE R. MERCIER, M.D.**

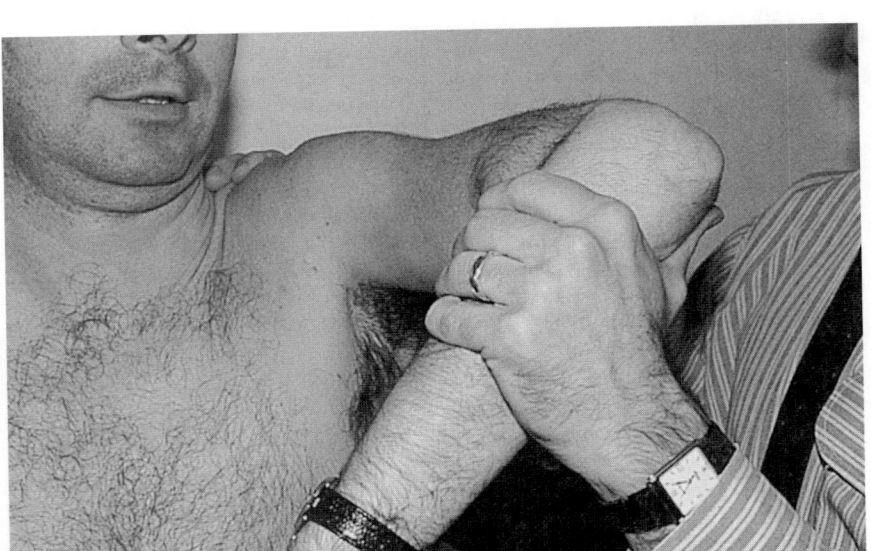

FIGURE 1-335 Rotator cuff lesions are often accompanied by painful impingement of the upwardly subluxating humerus onto the acromion. Evidence for this as a cause of pain is elicited by impingement tests—for example, by forced, passive, internal rotation, and abduction of the shoulder, as shown here. (From Klippel J et al [eds]: *Primary care rheumatology,* London, 1999, Mosby.)

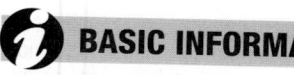

BASIC INFORMATION

DEFINITION

Rubella is a mild illness caused by the rubella virus that can cause severe congenital problems by in vitro transmission to a fetus when a pregnant woman becomes infected.

SYNONYMS

German measles

ICD-9CM CODES
056.9 Rubella
771.0 (Congenital)
V04.3 (Vaccination)

EPIDEMIOLOGY & DEMOGRAPHICS

- Before vaccination (i.e., before 1969):
  - 28 reported cases per 100,000 person-years, eight of which were in persons >15 yr
  - Four cases of congenital rubella syndrome per 100,000 live births
- After mass vaccination (i.e., after 1980) most cases have occurred in unimmunized people, with fewer than one case per 100,000 person-years (acquired and congenital).
- Currently, 10% to 20% of childbearing-age women are susceptible.
- The highest risk of developing long-term complications of congenital infection exists during the first trimester of gestation; both risk of congenital infection and long-term complications drop during the second trimester, and although the risk of congenital infection increases during the third trimester, there is no risk of long-term complication at that point.

PHYSICAL FINDINGS & CLINICAL PRESENTATION

1. Acquired infection:
   - Incubation: 14 to 21 days
   - Prodrome: 1 to 5 days; low-grade fever, headache, malaise, anorexia, mild conjunctivitis, coryza, pharyngitis, cough, and cervical, suboccipital, and postauricular lymphadenopathy
   - Rash: 1 to 5 days
2. Enanthema: palatal macules
3. Exanthema (rash): blotchy eruption beginning on face and neck and then spreading to trunk and limbs
   - Occasional splenomegaly and hepatitis (during rash)
   - Complications: arthritis (15%, mostly in adult women), thrombocytopenia, myo-

carditis, optic neuritis, encephalitis (all <0.1%)
4. Congenital infection:
   - Deafness: 85%
   - Intrauterine growth retardation: 70%
   - Cataracts: 35%
   - Retinopathy: 35%
   - Patent ductus arteriosus: 30%
   - Pulmonary artery hypoplasia: 25%
   - In utero death: 20%
   - Mental retardation: 10% to 20%
   - Meningoencephalitis: 10% to 20%
   - Behavior disorder: 10% to 20%
   - Hepatosplenomegaly: 10% to 20%
   - Bone radiolucencies: 10% to 20%
   - Diabetes mellitus (type 1): 10% to 20% by age 35 yr
   - Other congenital heart defects: 2% to 5%

ETIOLOGY & PATHOGENESIS

1. Acquired infection:
   - Viral portal of entry is upper respiratory tract.
   - Viral replication occurs in lymph nodes, then hematogenous dissemination occurs to many organs, including placenta if present.
   - Immune complexes may be cause of rash and arthritis.
2. Congenital infection:
   - Fetus is infected by the placenta during maternal acquired infection.
   - Cellular damage in the fetus results from cytolysis of fetal cells, mostly by fetal vasculitis or from immune-mediated inflammation and damage.

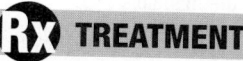

DIAGNOSIS

DIFFERENTIAL DIAGNOSIS

1. Acquired rubella syndrome:
   - Other viral infections by enteroviruses, adenoviruses, human parvovirus B-19, measles
   - Scarlet fever
   - Allergic reaction
   - Kawasaki disease
2. Congenital rubella syndrome:
   - Congenital syphilis, toxoplasmosis, herpes simplex, cytomegalovirus, and enterovirus can cause a similar set of problems.

WORKUP

1. Acquired infection:
   - Serologic test (hemagglutination inhibition, neutralization tests, complement

fixation tests, passive agglutination, enzyme immunoassay [EIA], enzyme-linked immunosorbent assay [ELISA])
   - Immunoglobulin (Ig) M antibodies (by EIA) are detected early: second to fourth week
   - IgG antibodies (by ELISA) can be measured as acute phase (7 days after rash onset) and convalescent phase (14 days later)
2. Congenital infection:
   - Viral culture (from nasopharynx)
   - Serologic studies: IgM antirubella virus detection by EIA is the method of choice (after the newborn is age 5 mo)

IMMUNIZATION

- Four existing vaccines provide persisting immunity in 92% of vaccines. Indications:
  - All children ≥12 mo (as part of the measles-mumps-rubella [MMR] vaccine)
  - Postpubertal women
- Vaccinate if not known to be immunized (advise not to become pregnant within 3 mo of vaccination)
- Premarital serologic screening for rubella immunity
- Prenatal or antepartum serologic screening for rubella
- Vaccinate susceptible women postpartum
- Serologic screening for female workers likely to be exposed to rubella (e.g., teachers, child care employees, health care workers)
Contraindications:
- Pregnancy
- Recent receipt of immune globulin or blood transfusion (2 wk before to 3 mo after)
- Immunodeficiency (except AIDS)
Adverse reactions:
- Fever, rash, or lymphadenopathy: 5% to 15%
- Arthralgias: 0.5% in children; 25% in adult women
- Transient peripheral neuropathy (rare)

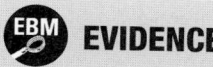

TREATMENT

- No known effective antiviral therapy
- Management of specific congenital problems as appropriate

EVIDENCE

available at www.expertconsult.com

SUGGESTED READINGS
available at www.expertconsult.com

AUTHOR: **FRED F. FERRI, M.D.**

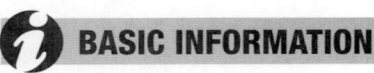

DEFINITION

Salivary gland neoplasms are benign or malignant tumors of a salivary gland (parotid, submandibular, or sublingual).

SYNONYMS

These tumors are often named according to their histologic type (see "Diagnosis").

ICD-9CM CODES
142.9 Salivary gland neoplasm
142.0 (Parotid)
142.1 (Submandibular)
142.2 (Sublingual)

EPIDEMIOLOGY & DEMOGRAPHICS

INCIDENCE: One to two cases per 100,000 person-years (1% of all head and neck tumors)
DISTRIBUTION:
- Parotid gland, 85% (80% are benign)
- Submandibular gland, 10% (55% are benign)
- Sublingual and minor glands, 5% (35% are benign)

PHYSICAL FINDINGS & CLINICAL PRESENTATION

- Parotid gland:
  1. Painless swelling overlying the masseter muscle (under the temporomandibular joint)
  2. Pain
  3. Facial nerve palsy
  4. Cervical lymph nodes
  5. Mass in oral cavity
- Submandibular gland: swelling under anterior portion of the mandible
- Sublingual gland: intraoral swelling under the tongue, medial to the mandible

Dx DIAGNOSIS

PATHOLOGY
HISTORY:
Benign Tumors:
- Mixed tumor (usually parotid)
- Adenolymphoma (Warthin's tumor)

- Pleomorphic adenoma
- Capillary hemangioma, lymphangioma (in children)
- Intraductal papilloma
- Other (e.g., myoepithelioma, canalicular adenoma, basal cell adenoma)

Malignant Tumors:
- Mucoepidermoid carcinoma (most common malignant tumor of the parotid gland)
- Adenoid cystic carcinoma
- Adenocarcinoma
- Malignant mixed tumor
- Squamous cell carcinoma
- Other

STAGE (TNM):
T_0 No evidence of primary tumor
T_1 Tumor <2 cm
T_2 Tumor 2 to 4 cm
T_3 Tumor 4 to 6 cm
T_4 Tumor >6 cm
All subdivided into
- Without local extension
- With local extension

N_0 No lymph node metastasis
N_1 Single ipsilateral node <3 cm
N_2 Ipsilateral, contralateral, or bilateral node <6 cm
N_3 Any node >6 cm
M_0 No distant metastasis
M_1 Distant metastasis
Stage I T_{1a} or $_{2a}N_0M_0$
Stage II $T_{1b,2b,3a}$ N_0M_0
Stage III $T_{3b,4a}$ N_0M_0 or any T except $_{4b}N_1M_0$
Stage IV T_{4b} any N any M or any T $N_{2,3}M_0$ or any T, any N_1M_1

WORKUP

- Fine-needle aspiration. The sensitivity, specificity, and accuracy of parotid gland aspirates is approximately 92%, 100%, and 98%, respectively
- Imaging by CT scan or MRI
- Open biopsy (rarely indicated)

Rx TREATMENT

Malignant tumors:
- Surgery is the mainstay of treatment; gland resection and neck dissection if lymph nodes are involved.

- A lateral lobectomy with preservation of facial nerve should be considered for tumors confined to the superficial lobe of the parotid gland. Gross tumor should not be left in situ, but if the facial nerve is able to be preserved by "peeling" tumor off the nerve, it should be attempted, followed by radiation therapy for microscopic disease.
- Postoperative radiation is indicated for high-grade malignancies demonstrating extraglandular disease, perineural invasion, direct invasion of surrounding tissues, or regional metastases.
- Chemotherapy.

Benign tumors: surgery for tumor resection

PROGNOSIS OF MALIGNANT TUMORS

Five-year survival rates:
- Mucoepidermoid carcinoma: 75% to 95%
- Adenoid cystic carcinoma: 40% to 80%
- Adenocarcinoma: 20% to 75%
- Malignant mixed tumor: 35% to 75%
- Squamous cell carcinoma: 25% to 60%

! PEARLS & CONSIDERATIONS

COMMENTS

Salivary gland neoplasms most often present as slow-growing, well-circumscribed masses. Pain, rapid growth, nerve weakness, fixation to skin or underlying muscle, and paresthesias usually are indicative of malignancy.

SUGGESTED READING
available at www.expertconsult.com

AUTHOR: **FRED F. FERRI, M.D.**

BASIC INFORMATION

DEFINITION

Salmonellosis is an infection caused by one of several serotypes of *Salmonella*.

SYNONYMS

Typhoid fever
Paratyphoid fever
Enteric fever

ICD-9CM CODES
003.0 Salmonellosis

EPIDEMIOLOGY & DEMOGRAPHICS

INCIDENCE (IN U.S.):
- Estimated 1 million cases/yr of nontyphoidal salmonellosis
- Approximately 500 cases of *Salmonella typhi* infection reported each yr
- Largest outbreak: 200,000 people who ingested contaminated milk

PEAK INCIDENCE: Summer and fall

PREDOMINANT AGE:
- <20 yr old
- >70 yr old
- Highest rates of infection in infants, especially neonates

GENETICS:
Neonatal infection:
- Highly susceptible to infection with nontyphoidal *Salmonella*

PHYSICAL FINDINGS & CLINICAL PRESENTATION

- Infections
  1. Localized to GI tract (gastroenteritis)
  2. Systemic (typhoid fever)
  3. Localized outside of GI tract
- Gastroenteritis
  1. Incubation period: 12 to 48 hr
  2. Nausea, vomiting
  3. Diarrhea, abdominal cramps
  4. Fever
  5. Bacteremia: Occurs mostly in the immunocompromised host or those with underlying conditions, including HIV infection
  6. Self-limited illness lasting 3 or 4 days
  7. Colonization of GI tract persistent for months, especially in those treated with antibiotics
- Typhoid fever
  1. Incubation period of few days to several wk
  2. Prolonged fever, often with a stepwise-increasing temperature pattern
  3. Myalgias
  4. Headache, cough, sore throat
  5. Malaise, anorexia
  6. Abdominal pain
  7. Hepatosplenomegaly
  8. Diarrhea or constipation early in the course of illness
  9. Rose spots (faint, maculopapular, blanching lesions) sometimes seen on chest or abdomen

- Untreated disease
  1. Fever lasting 1 to 2 mo
  2. Main complication: GI bleeding caused by perforation from ulceration of Peyer's patches in the ileum (Fig. 1-336)
  3. Rare complications:
     a. Mental status changes
     b. Shock
  4. Relapse rate of approximately 10%
- Infections outside GI tract
  1. Can occur in virtually any location
  2. Usually occur in patients with underlying diseases
  3. Endocarditis, endovascular infections are caused by seeding of atherosclerotic plaques or aneurysms
  4. Hepatic or splenic abscesses in patients with underlying disease in these organs
  5. Urinary tract infections in patients with renal TB or schistosomiasis
  6. Salmonellae are a frequent cause of gram-negative meningitis in neonates
  7. Osteomyelitis in children with hemoglobinopathies (particularly sickle cell disease)

ETIOLOGY

- More than 2000 serotypes of *Salmonella* exist, but only a few cause disease in humans.
- Raw produce is an increasingly recognized vehicle for salmonellosis. In 2008 there was a large outbreak of Salmonella Saintpaul involving 1500 persons, of which 21% were hospitalized and 2 died. It was due to contaminated jalapeno and serrano peppers.
- Some found only in humans are the cause of enteric fever.
  1. *S. typhi*
  2. *S. paratyphi*
- Some responsible for gastroenteritis and frequently isolated from raw meat and poultry and uncooked or undercooked eggs.
  1. *S. typhimurium*
  2. *S. enteritidis*
- *S. choleraesius* is a prototype organism that causes extraintestinal nontyphoidal disease.
- Transmission generally via ingestion of contaminated food or drink.
- Outbreaks of gastroenteritis related to contaminated poultry, meat, and dairy products are common.
- Typhoid fever is a systemic illness caused by serotypes exclusive to humans.
  1. Acquisition by ingestion of food or water contaminated by other humans
  2. Most cases in the U.S. are:
     a. Acquired during foreign travel
     b. Acquired by ingestion of food prepared by chronic carriers, many of whom have acquired the organism outside of the U.S.

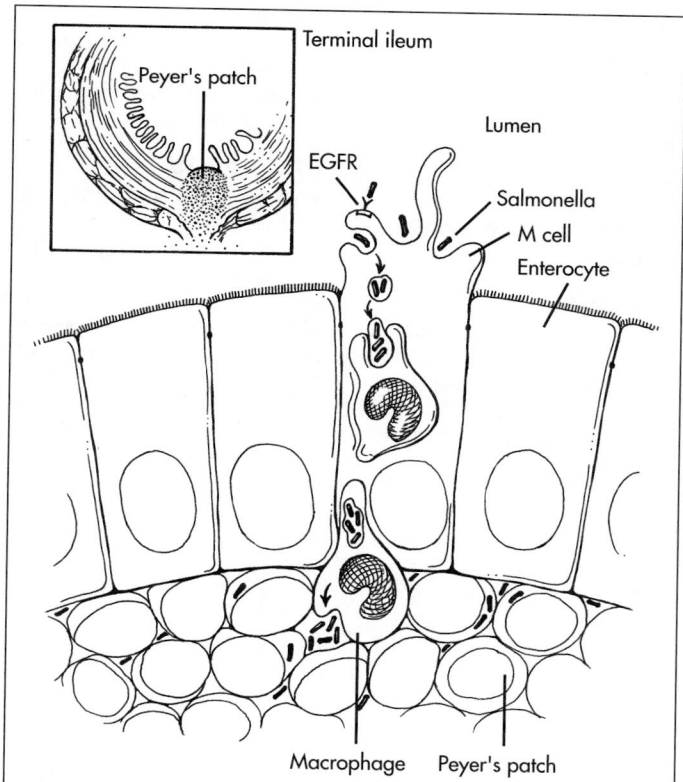

FIGURE 1-336 *Salmonella typhi* invade M cells through membrane ruffling and EGF receptor-dependent pathways. Macrophages originating from Peyer's patch take up *S. typhi* in close association with M cells. *S. typhi* replicate from Peyer's patches and then enter the lymphatic system, leading to bacteremia. Replication in Peyer's patches causes hypertrophy followed by necrosis, which can cause intestinal perforation. (From Stein JH [ed]: *Internal medicine*, ed 5, St Louis, 1998, Mosby.)

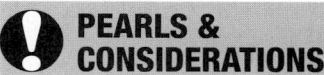 DIAGNOSIS

DIFFERENTIAL DIAGNOSIS

- Other causes of prolonged fever:
  1. Malaria
  2. TB
  3. Brucellosis
  4. Amebic liver abscess
- Other causes of gastroenteritis:
  1. Bacterial: *Shigella, Yersinia, Campylobacter* spp
  2. Viral: Norwalk virus, rotavirus
  3. Parasitic: *Entamoeba histolytica, Giardia lamblia*
  4. Toxic: enterotoxigenic *E. coli, Clostridium difficile*

WORKUP

- Typhoid fever
  1. Cultures of blood, stool, urine; repeat if initially negative.
  2. Blood cultures are more likely to be positive early in the course of illness.
  3. Stool and urine cultures are more commonly positive in the second and third wk of illness.
  4. Highest yield with bone marrow biopsy cultures: 90% positive.
  5. Serology using Widal's test is helpful in retrospect, showing a fourfold increase in convalescent titers.
- Gastroenteritis: stool cultures
- Extraintestinal localized infection:
  1. Blood cultures
  2. Cultures from the site of infection

LABORATORY TESTS

- Neutropenia is common
- Transaminitis is possible
- Culture to grow organism: blood, body fluids, biopsy specimens

IMAGING STUDIES

- Radiographs of bone may be suggestive of osteomyelitis (particularly in patients with sickle cell disease and bone infarctions).
- CT scan or sonogram of abdomen:
  1. May reveal hepatic or splenic abscesses or pleural involvement
  2. May reveal aortic aneurysm

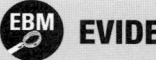 TREATMENT

NONPHARMACOLOGIC THERAPY

Adequate hydration and electrolyte replacement in people with diarrhea

ACUTE GENERAL Rx

- Typhoid fever:
  1. Ciprofloxacin 500 mg PO bid or 400 mg IV bid for 14 days
  2. Ceftriaxone 2 g IV qd for 14 days
  3. If sensitive, may switch therapy to TMP/SMX 1 to 2 DS tabs PO bid or amoxicillin 2 g PO q8h to complete 14 days
  4. Dexamethasone 3 mg IV initially, followed by 1 mg IV q6h for eight doses for patients with shock or mental status changes
- Gastroenteritis:
  1. Usually not indicated for gastroenteritis alone because this illness usually self-limited
  2. May prolong the carrier state
  3. Prophylactic treatment for patients who are at high risk of developing complications from bacteremia
     a. Neonates
     b. Patients with hemoglobinopathies
     c. Patients with atherosclerosis
     d. Patients with aneurysms
     e. Patients with prosthetic devices
     f. Immunocompromised patients
  4. Treatment can be oral or parenteral, with the same regimens used for typhoid, but only for 48 to 72 hr
- Intravascular infections require 6 wk of parenteral therapy.

CHRONIC Rx

- Carrier states are possible in those with typhoid fever.
- More common in people >60 yr of age and in people with gallstones.
- Usual site of colonization is the gallbladder.
- Treatment should be considered for those with persistently positive stool cultures and for food handlers.
- Suggested regimens for eradication of carrier state:
  1. Ciprofloxacin 500 mg PO bid for 4 wk

  2. SMX/TMP 1 to 2 DS tabs PO bid for 6 wk (if susceptible)
  3. Amoxicillin 2 g PO q8h for 6 wk (if susceptible)
- Cholecystectomy may be required in carriers with gallstones who fail medical therapy, but this is rarely indicated for nontyphoidal salmonellosis currently.
- Prolonged course of oral therapy or lifetime suppression for patients with AIDS who have chronic infection.

DISPOSITION

- Typhoid fever
  1. Treated patients usually respond to therapy; small percentage of chronic carriers.
  2. Untreated patients may have serious complications.
- Gastroenteritis
  1. Usually self-limited
  2. May be recurrent or persistent in AIDS patients

REFERRAL

- If gastroenteritis is persistent or recurrent
- If there is evidence of extraintestinal infection, typhoid fever, or chronic carriers

ⓘ PEARLS & CONSIDERATIONS

COMMENTS

- Quinolones should not be used in children or pregnant women.
- Infections should be reported to local health departments.
- Recent outbreaks in the U.S. have been traced back to raw tomatoes, peanut butter, and frozen pot pies.

EBM EVIDENCE

available at www.expertconsult.com

SUGGESTED READINGS
available at www.expertconsult.com

AUTHORS: **GLENN G. FORT, M.D., M.P.H.,** and **DENNIS J. MIKOLICH, M.D.**

BASIC INFORMATION

DEFINITION

Sarcoidosis is a chronic multisystem granulomatous disease characterized histologically by the presence of nonspecific, noncaseating granulomas.

SYNONYMS

Boeck's sarcoid

ICD-9CM CODES
135.0 Sarcoidosis

EPIDEMIOLOGY & DEMOGRAPHICS

INCIDENCE (IN U.S.): 11 in 100,000 whites and 35 in 100,000 blacks; presents most commonly in the winter and early spring
PREDOMINANT SEX: Increased incidence in females
PREDOMINANT AGE: 20 to 40 yr
GENETICS: Familial clustering has been described. Having a first-degree relative with sarcoidosis increases the risk for disease fivefold.

PHYSICAL FINDINGS & CLINICAL PRESENTATION

- Clinical manifestations often vary with the stage of the disease and degree of organ involvement. Patients may be asymptomatic, but a chest radiograph may demonstrate findings consistent with sarcoidosis (see "Imaging Studies" in next column). Nearly 50% of patients with sarcoidosis are diagnosed by incidental findings on chest radiograph. Thoracic involvement occurs in >90% of patients with sarcoidosis.
- Frequent manifestations:
  1. Pulmonary manifestations: dry, nonproductive cough; dyspnea; chest discomfort
  2. Constitutional symptoms: fatigue, weight loss, anorexia, malaise
  3. Visual disturbances: blurred vision, ocular discomfort, conjunctivitis, iritis, uveitis (65% of patients)
  4. Dermatologic manifestations (30% of patients): erythema nodosum (10% of patients), macules, papules, subcutaneous nodules, hyperpigmentation, lupus pernio (indurated violaceous lesions on the nose, lips, ears, and cheeks that can erode into underlying cartilage and bone)
  5. Myocardial disturbances, arrhythmias, cardiomyopathy. Cardiac sarcoidosis is much more common than clinically appreciated and is found in up to 25% of patients in the United States
  6. Splenomegaly, hepatomegaly
  7. Rheumatologic manifestations: arthralgias have been reported in up to 40% of patients
  8. Neurologic and other manifestations: cranial nerve palsies, diabetes insipidus, meningeal involvement, parotid enlargement, hypothalamic and pituitary lesions, peripheral adenopathy. Neurosarcoidosis is detected in up to 25% of patients and can occur in the absence of apparent disease elsewhere

ETIOLOGY

Unknown. A cardinal feature of sarcoidosis is the presence of CD4+ T cells that interact with antigen-presenting cells to initiate the formation and maintenance of granulomas. Multiple lines of evidence suggest that sarcoidosis may result from the interaction of multiple genes with environmental exposures or infection.

Dx DIAGNOSIS

DIFFERENTIAL DIAGNOSIS

- Tuberculosis
- Lymphoma
- Hodgkin's disease
- Metastases
- Pneumoconioses
- Enlarged pulmonary arteries
- Infectious mononucleosis
- Lymphangitic carcinomatosis
- Idiopathic hemosiderosis
- Alveolar cell carcinoma
- Pulmonary eosinophilia
- Hypersensitivity pneumonitis
- Fibrosing alveolitis
- Collagen disorders
- Parasitic infection

Section II describes the differential diagnosis of granulomatous lung disease and a classification of granulomatous disorders.

WORKUP

- No pathognomonic diagnostic test exists for sarcoidosis, so the diagnosis remains one of exclusion. Workup is aimed at excluding critical organ involvement, determining extent and severity of disease, and excluding other disease. A complete neurologic and ophthalmologic examination is mandatory. A complete occupational and environmental exposure history is recommended.
- Initial laboratory evaluation should include complete blood count, serum chemistries (alanine aminotransferase, aspartate aminotransferase, alkaline phosphatase, electrolytes, blood urea nitrogen, creatinine, serum calcium), urinalysis, and 24-hour urinary excretion of calcium.
- Chest radiograph and ECG should also be obtained in all patients with sarcoidosis.
- Pulmonary function testing; spirometry, diffusion capacity of carbon monoxide–single breath.
- Biopsy should be done on accessible tissues suspected of sarcoid involvement (conjunctiva, skin, lymph nodes); bronchoscopy with transbronchial biopsy (85% diagnostic yield) is the procedure of choice in patients without any readily accessible site. Endobronchial ultrasound-guided fine needle aspiration of intrathoracic lymph nodes also has high diagnostic yield and makes use of mediastinoscopy mostly unnecessary.

LABORATORY TESTS

Laboratory abnormalities:
- Hypergammaglobulinemia, anemia, leukopenia
- Liver function test abnormalities

- Hypercalcemia (11% of patients), hypercalciuria (40% of patients; attributable to increased gastrointestinal absorption, abnormal vitamin D metabolism, and increased calcitriol production by sarcoid granuloma)
- Angiotensin-converting enzyme: elevated in approximately 60% of patients with sarcoidosis; nonspecific and generally not useful as a diagnostic tool and in following the course of the disease

IMAGING STUDIES

- Chest radiograph (Fig. 1-337): adenopathy of the hilar and paratracheal nodes is a frequent finding. Parenchymal changes may also be present, depending on the stage of the disease (stage 0, normal radiograph; stage I, bilateral hilar adenopathy; stage II, stage I plus pulmonary infiltrate; stage III, pulmonary infiltrate without adenopathy; stage IV, advanced fibrosis with evidence of "honeycombing," hilar retraction, bullae, cysts, and emphysema).
- Pulmonary function tests (spirometry and diffusing capacity of the lung for carbon dioxide): may be normal or may reveal a restrictive pattern and/or obstructive pattern.
- For patients without apparent lung involvement, ^{18}F-fluorodeoxyglucose positron emission tomography (FDG-PET) is useful in identifying sites for diagnostic biopsy.
- CT imaging is generally unnecessary for most patients with sarcoidosis. It is indicated when the chest radiograph is atypical for sarcoidosis or if the patient has hemoptysis.
- FDG-PET and MRI with gadolinium are useful in patients with suspected cardiac and neurologic involvement.
- Gallium-67 scan: represents an older testing modality. It will localize in areas of granulomatous infiltrates; however, it is not specific and not necessary. The "panda" sign (localization in the lacrimal and salivary glands, giving a "panda" appearance to the face) is suggestive of sarcoidosis.

Rx TREATMENT

GENERAL Rx

- Many patients with sarcoidosis will not require any treatment. In general, treatment should be instituted when organ function is threatened. Corticosteroids (Table 1-161) are the mainstay of therapy when treatment is required (e.g., prednisone 40 mg qd for 8 to 12 wk with gradual tapering of the dose to 10 mg qod over 8 to 12 mo); corticosteroids should be considered in patients with severe symptoms (e.g., dyspnea, chest pain); hypercalcemia; ocular, central nervous system, or cardiac involvement; or progressive pulmonary disease. Patients with interstitial lung disease benefit from oral steroid therapy for 6 to 24 mo.
- Patients with progressive disease refractory to corticosteroids may be treated with methotrexate 7.5 to 15 mg once per week.
- Hydroxychloroquine is effective for chronic disfiguring skin lesions, hypercalcemia, and neurologic involvement.

- Nonsteroidal anti-inflammatory drugs are useful for musculoskeletal symptoms and erythema nodosum.
- Pulmonary rehabilitation in patients with significant respiratory insufficiency. Consider liver and lung transplantation in patients unresponsive to conventional treatment.

DISPOSITION

- The majority of patients with sarcoidosis have spontaneous remission within 2 yr and do not require treatment. Their course can be followed by periodic clinical evaluation, chest radiographs, and pulmonary function tests.
- Blacks have increased rates of pulmonary involvement, a worse long-term prognosis, and more frequent relapses.
- Up to one third of patients have unrelenting disease, leading to clinically significant organ impairment. Adverse prognostic factors in sarcoidosis include age of onset >40 yr, cardiac involvement, neurosarcoidosis, progressive pulmonary fibrosis, chronic hypercalcemia, chronic uveitis, involvement of nasal mucosa, nephrocalcinosis, and presence of cystic bone lesions and lupus pernio.

REFERRAL

Ophthalmologic examination is indicated in all patients with suspected sarcoidosis because ocular findings (iridocyclitis, uveitis, conjunctivitis, and keratopathy) are found in ≥25% of documented cases.

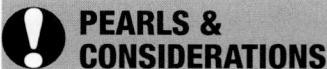

COMMENTS

- Approximately 15% to 20% of patients with lung involvement advance to irreversible lung impairment (bronchiectasis, cavitation, progressive fibrosis, pneumothorax, and respiratory failure). Death from pulmonary failure occurs in 5% to 7% of patients with sarcoidosis.
- Newer treatment approaches are aimed at targeting mechanisms involving CD$_4$ type 1 helper T cells.

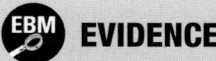

EVIDENCE
available at www.expertconsult.com

SUGGESTED READINGS
available at www.expertconsult.com

AUTHOR: **FRED F. FERRI, M.D.**

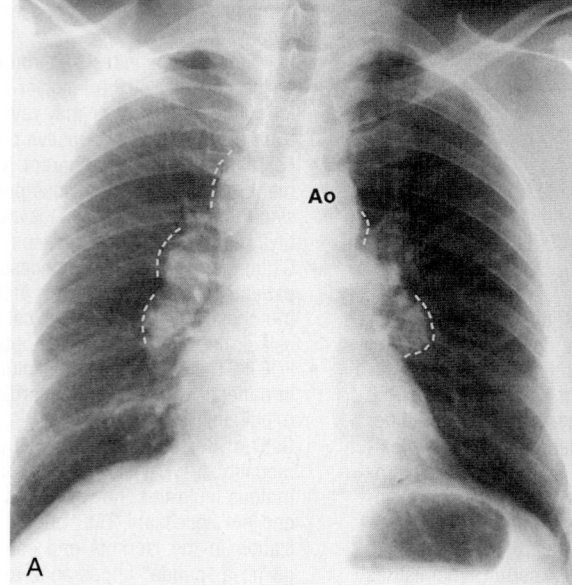
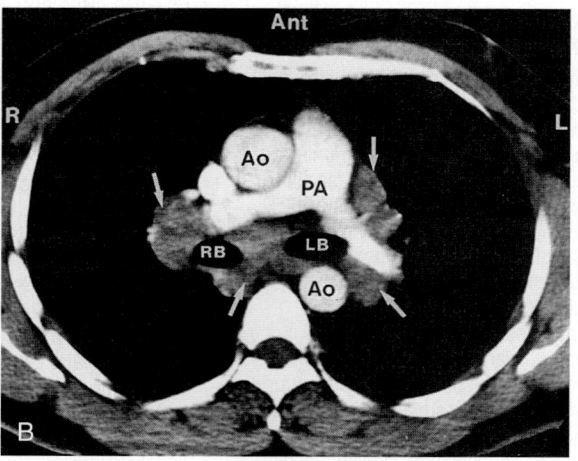

FIGURE 1-337 Sarcoid. Marked lymphadenopathy *(dotted lines)* is seen in the region of both hila in the right paratracheal region **(A).** The transverse contrast-enhanced CT scan of the upper chest **(B)** clearly shows the ascending and descending aorta *(Ao)* as well as the pulmonary artery *(PA)* and superior vena cava. The right and left mainstem bronchus area is also seen. The arrows indicate the extensive lymphadenopathy. *LB,* Left bronchus; *RB,* right bronchus. (From Mettler FA [ed]: *Primary care radiology,* Philadelphia, 2000, WB Saunders.)

TABLE 1-161 Indications for Use of Corticosteroids in Sarcoidosis

Disorder	Treatment
Iridocyclitis	Corticosteroid eye drops; local subconjunctival deposit of cortisone
Posterior uveitis	Oral prednisone
Pulmonary involvement	Steroids rarely recommended for stage I; typically used if infiltrate remains static or worsens over 3-mo period or the patient is symptomatic
Upper airway obstruction	Rare indication for intravenous steroids
Lupus pernio	Oral prednisone shrinks the disfiguring lesions
Hypercalcemia	Responds well to corticosteroids
Cardiac involvement	Corticosteroids usually recommended if patient has arrhythmias or conduction disturbances
CNS involvement	Response is best in patients with acute symptoms
Lacrimal/salivary gland involvement	Corticosteroids recommended for disordered function, not gland swelling
Bone cysts	Corticosteroids recommended if symptomatic

From Andreoli TE (ed): *Cecil essentials of medicine,* ed 8, Philadelphia, 2010, WB Saunders.
CNS, Central nervous system.

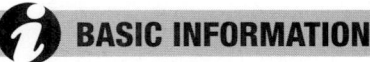

BASIC INFORMATION

DEFINITION

Scabies is a contagious disease caused by the mite *Sarcoptes scabiei*.

ICD-9CM CODES
133.0 Scabies

EPIDEMIOLOGY & DEMOGRAPHICS

- Scabies is generally acquired by sleeping with or in the bedding of infested individuals.
- It is generally associated with poor living conditions and is also common in hospitals and nursing homes.

PHYSICAL FINDINGS & CLINICAL PRESENTATION

- Primary lesions are caused when the female mite burrows within the stratum corneum, laying eggs within the tract she leaves behind; burrows (linear or serpiginous tracts) end with a minute papule or vesicle.
- Primary lesions are most commonly found in the web spaces of the hands, wrists, buttocks, scrotum, penis, breasts, axillae, and knees.
- Secondary lesions result from scratching or infection.
- Intense pruritus, especially nocturnal, is common; it is caused by an acquired sensitivity to the mite or fecal pellets and is usually noted 1 to 4 wk after the primary infestation.
- Examination of the skin may reveal burrows, tiny vesicles, excoriations, inflammatory papules.

- Widespread and crusted lesions (Norwegian or crusted scabies) may be seen in elderly and immunocompromised patients.

ETIOLOGY

Human scabies is caused by the mite *S. scabiei*, var. *hominis* (Fig. 1-338).

DIAGNOSIS

DIFFERENTIAL DIAGNOSIS

- Pediculosis
- Atopic dermatitis
- Flea bites
- Seborrheic dermatitis
- Dermatitis herpetiformis
- Contact dermatitis
- Nummular eczema
- Syphilis
- Other insect infestation

WORKUP

Diagnosis is made on the clinical presentation and on the demonstration of mites, eggs, or mite feces.

LABORATORY TESTS

- Microscopic demonstration of the organism, feces, or eggs: a drop of mineral oil may be placed over the suspected lesion before removal; the scrapings are transferred directly to a glass slide; a drop of potassium hydroxide is added and a cover slip is applied.
- Skin biopsy is rarely necessary to make the diagnosis.

TREATMENT

NONPHARMACOLOGIC THERAPY

Clothing, underwear, and towels used in the 48 hr before treatment must be laundered.

ACUTE GENERAL Rx

- Permethrin 5% cream (Elimite) is usually effective with one treatment; it should be massaged into the skin from head to soles of feet; remove 8 to 14 hr later by washing. If living mites are present after 14 days, treat again.
- A single dose (150 to 200 micrograms/kg in 6-mg tablets) of ivermectin, an antihelmintic agent, is also effective for the treatment of scabies. It is the best treatment for generalized crusted scabies.
- Pruritus generally abates 24 to 48 hr after treatment but can last up to 2 wk; oral antihistamines are effective in decreasing postscabietic pruritus.
- Topical corticosteroid creams may hasten the resolution of secondary eczematous dermatitis.
- If the patient is a resident of an extended care facility, it is important to educate the patients, staff, family, and frequent visitors about scabies and the need to have full cooperation in treatment. Scabicide should be applied to all patients, staff, and frequent visitors, whether symptomatic or not; symptomatic family members of staff and visitors should also receive treatment.

DISPOSITION

Refractory cases usually are seen with immunocompromised hosts or patients with underlying skin diseases.

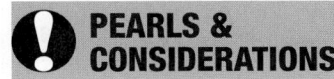

PEARLS & CONSIDERATIONS

COMMENTS

- Lindane is potentially neurotoxic and should not be used on infants or pregnant women (permethrin is safe and effective in these situations).
- Sexual partners should be notified and treated.

SUGGESTED READING
available at www.expertconsult.com

AUTHOR: **FRED F. FERRI, M.D.**

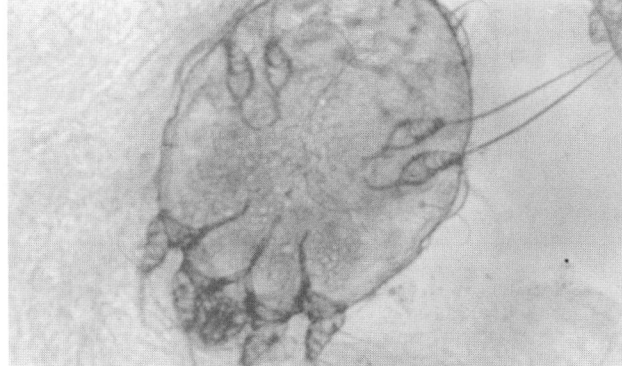

FIGURE 1-338 Scabies organism in a wet mount preparation. (From Mandell GL: *Mandell, Douglas, and Bennett's principles and practice of infectious diseases*, ed 5, New York, 2000, Churchill Livingstone.)

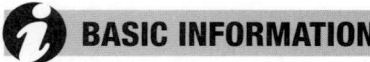

DEFINITION

Scarlet fever is a rash involving the skin and tongue and complicating streptococcal group A pharyngitis.

SYNONYMS

Scarlatina
SF

ICD-9CM CODES
034.1 Scarlet fever

EPIDEMIOLOGY & DEMOGRAPHICS

- Same as streptococcal pharyngitis; namely, children ages 5 to 15 yr. May also complicate impetigo.
- Most common in cooler climates during the late fall, winter, and early spring.
- Most cases follow tonsillitis or pharyngitis; however, it has also been reported after wounds ("surgical scarlet fever"), burns, and pelvic or puerperal infections.

PHYSICAL FINDINGS & CLINICAL PRESENTATION

- Diffuse erythema, beginning on face and spreading to neck, back, chest, rest of trunk, and extremities. Most intense on inner aspects of arms and thighs.
- Erythema blanches, but nonblanching petechiae may be present or produced by a tourniquet.
- Strawberry or raspberry tongue.
- Rash lasts approximately 1 wk and then desquamates.
- Febrile illness with headache, malaise, anorexia, and pharyngitis begins after a 2- to 4-day incubation period.
- Scarlatinal rash begins 1 or 2 days after the onset of pharyngitis (Fig. 1-339).

ETIOLOGY

Caused by group A beta-hemolytic *Streptococcus* infection, which produces one of three erythrogenic toxins (NOTE: *Some streptococcal species have the ability to cause both scarlet fever and rheumatic fever*).

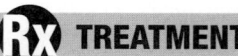

DIFFERENTIAL DIAGNOSIS

- Viral exanthems (covered in Section II)
- Kawasaki disease
- Toxic shock syndrome
- Drug rashes

See differential diagnosis of "Pharyngitis" in Section I.

WORKUP

- Identification of group A *Streptococcus* by throat culture
- Streptolysin O antibody titers

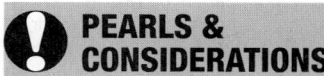

- Penicillin 250 mg PO qid for 10 days or erythromycin 250 mg PO qid for 10 days in penicillin-allergic patients. A clinical response can be expected in 24 to 48 hr.
- Benzathine penicillin 1 to 2 million U IM once; may be used for a patient who cannot swallow pills.

COMPLICATIONS (RARE)

- Peritonsillar abscess
- Mastoiditis
- Otitis media
- Pneumonia
- Sepsis and distant foci of infection
- Acute rheumatic fever
- Inability to swallow liquids or upper airway obstruction requiring hospitalization

NOTE: Failure to respond to penicillin should raise doubt about the diagnosis because *Streptococcus* may be carried in the pharynx without causing infection.

PEARLS & CONSIDERATIONS

COMMENTS

Patients with antibodies against the toxin are spared the rash but still develop other symptoms of the infection (e.g., sore throat).

AUTHOR: **FRED F. FERRI, M.D.**

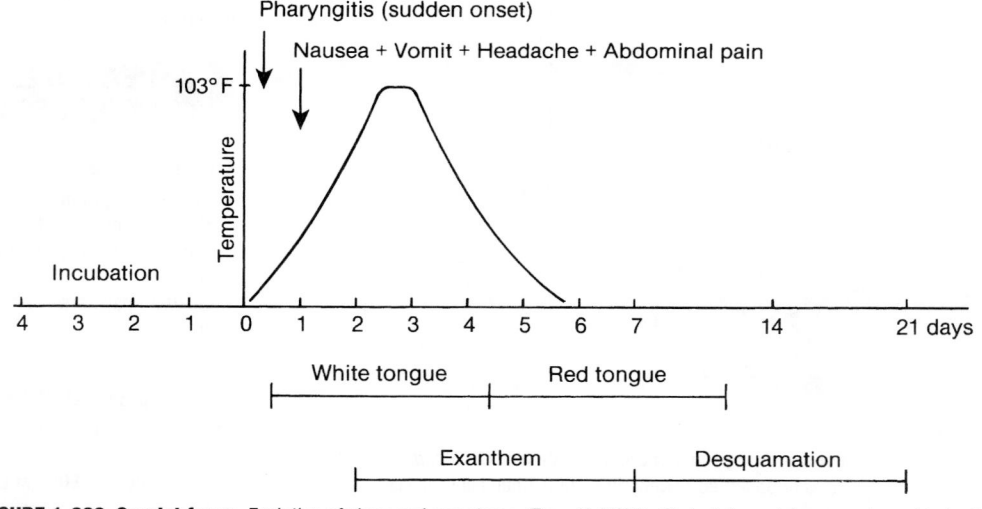

FIGURE 1-339 Scarlet fever. Evolution of signs and symptoms. (From Habif TP: *Clinical dermatology: a color guide to diagnosis and therapy*, ed 3, St Louis, 1996, Mosby.)

BASIC INFORMATION

DEFINITION

Schistosomiasis is caused by infection with parasite blood flukes known as schistosomes.

SYNONYMS

Bilharziasis
Urinary schistosomiasis
Hepatosplenic schistosomiasis
Swimmers itch
Katayama fever

ICD-9CM CODES

120.9 Schistosomiasis

EPIDEMIOLOGY & DEMOGRAPHICS

INCIDENCE:
- More than 200 million people worldwide and more than 200,000 deaths annually. In U.S., estimated to exceed 400,000 people.
- Geographic distribution of schistosomiasis is confined to an area between 36° north and 34° south latitude, where fresh water temperatures average 25° to 30° C.

PREVALENCE: The greatest cercarial exposure usually occurs in boys ages 5 to 10 yr

DISTRIBUTION:
- *S. mansoni* in tropical and subtropical areas of sub-Saharan Africa, the Middle East, South America, and the Caribbean
- *S. haematobium* in North Africa, sub-Saharan Africa, the Middle East, and India
- *S. japonicum* in Asia, particularly in China, the Philippines, Thailand, and Indonesia
- *S. intercalatum* in central and west Africa
- *S. mekongi* in Cambodia

ETIOLOGY & PATHOGENESIS

- Human infections are caused by *S. mansoni*, *S. haematobium*, *S. japonicum*, *S. mekongi*, and *S. intercalatum*.
- Acquisition of disease via contact with fresh water containing infectious free-living cercarial larvae.
- In U.S., most cases are acquired during foreign travel.
- Human disease is primarily associated with the host's granulomatous response to eggs retained in the tissue.

PHYSICAL FINDINGS & CLINICAL PRESENTATION

ACUTE SYMPTOMS:
- Swimmers itch
- Katayama fever

CHRONIC SYMPTOMS:
- Intestinal schistosomiasis
  1. Abdominal pain
  2. Bloody diarrhea
  3. Iron-deficiency anemia
  4. Intestinal polyp
  5. Bowel ulcer and strictures
- Hepatic schistosomiasis
  1. Hepatomegaly
  2. Splenomegaly
  3. Portal hypertension
  4. Esophageal varices
- Urinary schistosomiasis
  1. Hematuria
  2. Dysuria
  3. Urinary frequency
  4. Fibrosis of bladder and ureters
  5. Squamous cell ca of bladder
  6. Proteinuria
  7. Nephrotic syndrome

COMPLICATIONS:
- Neurologic complication
  1. Granuloma of spinal cord or brain
  2. Transverse myelitis
  3. Epilepsy or focal neurologic deficit
- Pulmonary complication
  1. Granulomatous pulmonary endarteritis
  2. Pulmonary hypertension
  3. Cor pulmonale
- Other complications include tubal obstruction and infertility
- Recurrent bacteremia and recurrent UTI

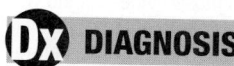 DIAGNOSIS

DIFFERENTIAL DIAGNOSIS

- Amebiasis
- Bacillary dysentery
- Bowel polyp
- Prostatic disease
- Genitourinary tract cancer
- Bacterial infections of the urinary tract

WORKUP

- Microscopy in urine or stool
- Tissue biopsy
- Serology
- CBC
- LFT
- US of abdomen
- CT scan of abdomen

LABORATORY TESTS

- CBC shows eosinophilia, anemia, thrombocytopenia
- LFT with mild increase in alkaline phosphatase and GGT
- Microscopy: stool and urine
- Serology: ELISA for detecting both schistosomal antibodies and antigen
- Rectal biopsy or bladder mucosal biopsy

IMAGING STUDIES

- X-ray of abdomen shows "fetal head" calcification.
- Sonography also documents a thickened bladder wall, hydronephrosis and hydroure-ter, and bladder polyps or calcification. It also demonstrates the thickened fibrosed portal tracts.
- Esophagoscopy documents esophageal varices.
- Liver biopsy may also demonstrate granuloma and clay pipestem fibrosis.

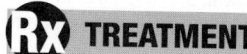 TREATMENT

- Praziquantel 40 mg/kg of body weight PO in one or two doses
- Oxamniquine 15 mg/kg PO once or 20 mg/kg PO daily for 3 days for recalcitrant infections
- Metrifonate 7.5 to 10 mg/kg of body weight given PO in three doses at 2-wk intervals

DISPOSITION

Treated patients usually respond to therapy. Definitive cure has occurred only when there is total disappearance of viable eggs from the excreta for a total of 6 mo after treatment.

REFERRAL

- To an infectious disease specialist knowledgeable in parasitology and geographic medicine for treatment and follow-up
- To a gastroenterologist for sclerotherapy of bleeding esophageal varices, if needed in advanced hepatosplenic schistosomiasis
- To a urologist for management and follow-up of urinary complications of *S. haematobium* infection of the genitourinary tract

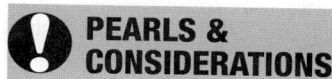 PEARLS & CONSIDERATIONS

COMMENTS

Prevention:
- Chemotherapy
  1. Mass
  2. Targeted population
- Snail control
  1. Mollusciciding
  2. Environmental modification
  3. Biologic control
- Reduction of water contact and contamination
  1. Provision of domestic water supplies
  2. Provision for sanitary disposal of excreta
- Vaccination
- Improved living standards

SUGGESTED READINGS

available at www.expertconsult.com

AUTHORS: **GLENN G. FORT, M.D., M.P.H.,** and **DENNIS J. MIKOLICH, M.D.**

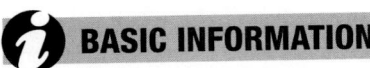

BASIC INFORMATION

DEFINITION

Schizophrenia is a disorder that causes significant distortions in thinking, perception, speech, and behavior. Characteristics include psychosis, apathy, social withdrawal, and cognitive impairment, which result in significant social impairment.

SYNONYMS

Dementia praecox

ICD-9CM CODES
295.9 Schizophrenia

EPIDEMIOLOGY & DEMOGRAPHICS

INCIDENCE: 0.2 per 1000
PREVALENCE: 0.5%; lifetime prevalence risk, 0.4%
PREDOMINANT SEX: Males have a more severe illness with earlier onset; however, distribution is probably equal.
PREDOMINANT AGE:
- Age of onset of psychotic symptoms is the early 20s for males and the late 20s for females.
- Age of onset of negative symptoms is usually earlier (i.e., the mid-teenage years).
PEAK INCIDENCE: Between ages of 16 and 30 yr
GENETICS:
- Genetics account for 70% of risk; the remaining 30% associated with other factors such as urban environments, migration, or cannabis use.
- First-degree relatives have a 10 times greater chance of becoming schizophrenic.
- Discordant rates among identical twins are higher than expected with the simple inheritance pattern.
- Associations with several chromosomes have been described, but none have been replicated.
- Evidence exists that triplet nucleotide repeat expansion (e.g., such as that seen with Huntington's disease) may play a role in the inheritance of the disease.

PHYSICAL FINDINGS & CLINICAL PRESENTATION

- Schizophrenia is best defined as a dementing illness that begins early in life and that progresses slowly throughout the lifetime.
- Frequent structural brain imaging findings include the enlargement of the ventricular system, a loss of brain volume and cortical gray matter, and an alteration of the white matter tracts.
- The initial "negative" symptoms of adolescence—cognitive decline, social withdrawal and awkwardness, loss of motivation and pleasure, and loss of emotional expressiveness—begin after a period of normal development.
- During early adulthood, positive symptoms of psychosis and thought disturbance occur; psychotic symptoms then wax and wane throughout life. Treatment ameliorates positive symptoms but generally does little for negative ones.
- The condition is also accompanied by cognitive impairment, including problems with attention and concentration, psychomotor speed, learning, memory, and executive functions (e.g., abstract thinking, problem solving).
- Social and occupational dysfunction can be profound.

ETIOLOGY

- The basic determination of whether this is a degenerative or developmental condition has not been made.
- The major hypothesis is that abnormality of the mesocortical pathways produces the hypofrontality and the negative symptoms. This occurs along with a compensatory hyperactivation of the mesolimbic pathways, which produces the positive symptoms of psychosis.

DIAGNOSIS

DIFFERENTIAL DIAGNOSIS

- Schizophrenia is diagnosed when an individual has experienced at least 1 mo of hallucinations, delusions, thought disorders, catatonia, or negative symptoms (e.g., avolition, anhedonia, social isolation, affective flattening).
- Any medical condition, medicine, or substance that can affect brain homeostasis can cause psychosis; this is distinguished from schizophrenia by a relatively brief course and an alteration in mental status that suggests an underlying delirium.
- Other neurologic conditions that have psychosis as the initial presentation (e.g., Huntington's disease) need to be ruled out.
- Mood disorders with psychosis: These are indistinguishable from schizophrenia cross-sectionally but have a longitudinal course that includes full recovery.
- Delusional disorder involves nonbizarre delusions and lacks the thought disturbance, hallucinations, and negative symptoms of schizophrenia.
- Autism in the adult has an early age of onset and lacks significant hallucinations or delusions.

WORKUP

- History and physical examination to help determine whether the psychosis is primary or secondary
- Neurologic examination to uncover the soft neurologic signs (e.g., clumsiness, cortical thumb, loss of fine motor movements) that are common with schizophrenia

LABORATORY TESTS

- No laboratory tests are specific.
- Laboratory examinations (e.g., chemistry profile, blood count, sedimentation rate, toxicology screen, urinalysis) are geared toward excluding a primary medical condition.

IMAGING STUDIES

- CT or MRI of the brain during the initial workup; repeated if the course of the illness varies from what is expected
- EEG may reveal slowing when psychosis is the result of an encephalopathy

TREATMENT

NONPHARMACOLOGIC THERAPY

- Significant social support is required by most schizophrenic patients, but available support services are grossly inadequate. Schizophrenic patients constitute nearly one third of all homeless individuals. They usually require help with basic social, occupational, and interactive skills.
- Family stress can precipitate relapse and rehospitalization. Family interventions can reduce morbidity.
- Cognitive behavioral therapy can reduce the severity of both psychotic and negative symptoms.
- Illness management training for patients can increase medication adherence and reduce symptom distress.
- Integrated treatment that includes assertive community treatment, family involvement programs, and social skills training reduces the severity of both psychotic and negative symptoms, reduces comorbid substance misuse, reduces hospital days, increases adherence to treatment, and increases satisfaction with treatment.

ACUTE GENERAL Rx

- Acute psychosis is usually adequately controlled with antipsychotic agents.
- Few differences in effectiveness exist between first-generation antipsychotics (e.g., haloperidol, perphenazine, fluphenazine, chlorpromazine) and second-generation antipsychotics (e.g., risperidone, olanzapine, quetiapine, ziprasidone, aripiprazole, clozapine, lurasidone) for nonrefractory patients. First-generation antipsychotics are slightly more likely than second-generation antipsychotics to cause a parkinsonian state and eventual tardive dyskinesia (rate of tardive dyskinesia, 15% to 30%). Antiparkinsonian drugs (e.g., benztropine, amantadine) are used to ameliorate the parkinsonism. Risperidone has been shown to be superior to haloperidol for the prevention of acute psychotic relapse.
- Sedatives (i.e., benzodiazepines and, to a lesser degree, barbiturates) can be used transiently if a patient is in an agitated state.

CHRONIC RX

- Relapse prevention is a major goal of treatment. Noncompliance is common and leads to high relapse rates. Antipsychotic agents usually must be continued at the same doses that controlled psychosis. For noncompliant patients, depot preparations given biweekly or monthly can be used.
- Most patients frequently switch among antipsychotics; there is considerable individual

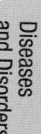

variability with regard to antipsychotic response and vulnerability to specific adverse effects.

- Clozapine is more effective than other agents for treatment-refractory patients. However, it requires monitoring to prevent life-threatening adverse effects. Olanzapine may also be more effective than less expensive first-generation drugs but has substantial adverse metabolic effects. Lurasidone is a newer second-generation antipsychotic that appears to be better tolerated, but longer-term studies are needed.
- Neurocognitive improvement associated with antipsychotic treatment among patients with schizophrenia is small and does not differ between first-generation and second-generation antipsychotics.
- Antiparkinsonian agents may also need to be continued for the long term.
- Tardive dyskinesia (i.e., choreoathetoid movements of the muscles of tongue and face and occasionally of other muscle groups) can occur in as many as 30% of patients with the long-term use of neuroleptics.
- The negative symptoms of schizophrenia can resemble depression. In addition, depressive disorders may occur in schizophrenic patients. Antidepressant treatment of the negative symptoms is usually not effective. However, antidepressants can improve the symptoms of a discrete comorbid depressive episode.
- Mood stabilizers (e.g., lithium, valproate, carbamazepine) are of little use unless the patient has a comorbid impulse control disorder.

- Substance abuse is a major problem for more than a third of schizophrenic patients. More than half of these patients smoke cigarettes. Unfortunately, these individuals do poorly in traditional substance abuse treatment programs. Specialized "dual-diagnosis" programs with highly structured aftercare are required.
- Specific antipsychotic medications have been associated with weight gain (i.e., olanzapine and clozapine) and QT prolongation. Hyperlipidemia and diabetes mellitus are associated with second-generation antipsychotics, and hyperprolactinemia is associated with first-generation antipsychotics. Clozapine is associated with agranulocytosis.

DISPOSITION

- The positive symptoms of as many as 20% to 30% of schizophrenic patients do not respond to available treatments. A much higher fraction of patients experience relapse as a result of poor compliance.
- Negative symptoms are responsible for the 50% to 70% of patients in whom deterioration in occupational and social function continues.
- Approximately 10% of schizophrenic patients will complete suicide.
- The course of the illness most strongly predicted by level of social development attained at the onset of psychosis.
- Schizophrenic patients die 12 to 15 yr sooner than the average population, mostly as a result of physical causes related to a lack of

access to health care or as a result of health risk factors (e.g., smoking, obesity).

REFERRAL

- If hospitalization is required
- If patient is noncompliant
- If patient is resistant to treatment

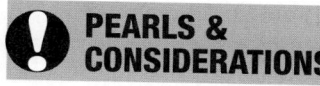

PEARLS & CONSIDERATIONS

- Rule out delirium caused by medical conditions, medications, or substance abuse before diagnosing an individual's psychotic behavior as schizophrenia.
- All antipsychotic medications have high discontinuation rates in chronic schizophrenia treatment. Olanzapine and clozapine may be more effective than other antipsychotics for chronic treatment, but they have significant side effects.
- Significant social support is required for most patients with schizophrenia. Nonpharmacologic therapy should be used in conjunction with pharmacotherapy.

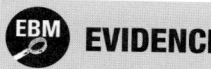

EVIDENCE

available at www.expertconsult.com

SUGGESTED READINGS

available at www.expertconsult.com

AUTHORS: **MICHAEL K. ONG, M.D., Ph.D.,** and **RICHARD J. GOLDBERG, M.D.**

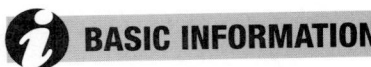

BASIC INFORMATION

DEFINITION
Scleritis is inflammation of the sclera.

SYNONYMS
Anterior scleritis
Diffuse nodular, necrotizing scleritis
Scleromalacia perforans
Scleral melt syndrome

ICD-9CM CODES
379.0 Scleritis and episcleritis

EPIDEMIOLOGY & DEMOGRAPHICS
PEAK INCIDENCE: Increases with increasing age
INCIDENCE (IN U.S.): Busy ophthalmologists may see one or two cases a year
PREVALENCE (IN U.S.): Relatively rare
PREDOMINANT SEX: 61% women
PREDOMINANT AGE: 52 yr

PHYSICAL FINDINGS & CLINICAL PRESENTATION
- Deep, boring eye pain
- Photophobia
- Tearing
- Conjunctival injection (Fig. 1-340)
- Thinning of the sclera

- More than 50% of patients have an underlying systemic autoimmune disease. Most common rheumatic problem is rheumatoid arthritis. Most patients with systemic disease are diagnosed before development of scleritis.

ETIOLOGY
- Inflammatory
- Allergic
- Toxic
- Infectious scleritis (herpes virus, bacteria, fungi) is uncommon, accounting for 4% to 18% of cases

DIAGNOSIS

DIFFERENTIAL DIAGNOSIS
- Most common causes are rheumatoid arthritis and other collagen-vascular diseases.
- Occasionally there are allergic, infectious, or traumatic causes.
- Conjunctivitis, iritis, and episcleritis should be considered in the differential diagnosis.

WORKUP
- Fluorescein angiography
- Eye examination
- Visual field examination
- Workup for autoimmune disease
- Workup for vasculitis
- Collagen vascular workup

LABORATORY TESTS
Rheumatoid factor, antinuclear antibody, erythrocyte sedimentation rate may be useful for underlying etiology

IMAGING STUDIES
Usually not necessary; CT scan of orbit may be useful in selected patients for collagen vascular disease or vasculitis

TREATMENT

NONPHARMACOLOGIC THERAPY
- Bandage lenses
- Surgery if thinning of the sclera is severe to prevent eye rupture

ACUTE GENERAL Rx
Immunotherapy (with steroids and Imuran, etc.):
- Steroids (topical, periocular, and systemic)
- Cycloplegic drops
- Nonsteroidal anti-inflammatory drugs (topical and systemic); systemic more effective than topical
- Other immunosuppressive drugs

CHRONIC Rx
- Systemic steroids can be given for the underlying disease.
- Local steroids may be helpful.
- Control underlying disease.

DISPOSITION
Urgent referral to ophthalmologist

REFERRAL
If not referred to an ophthalmologist early, patients may develop uveitis and other complications.

PEARLS & CONSIDERATIONS

COMMENTS
An ominous diagnosis because these patients often have other severe underlying debilitating disease processes.

SUGGESTED READINGS
available at www.expertconsult.com

AUTHOR: **MELVYN KOBY, M.D.**

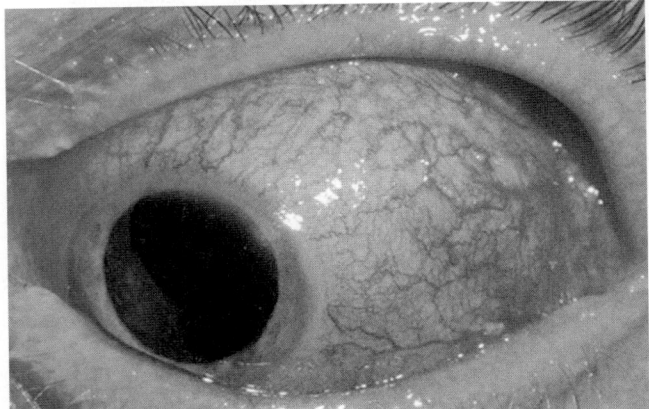

FIGURE 1-340 In diffuse anterior scleritis, widespread injection of the conjunctival and deep episcleral vessels occurs. (From Palay D [ed]: *Ophthalmology for the primary care physician,* St Louis, 1997, Mosby.)

BASIC INFORMATION

DEFINITION

Scleroderma (systemic sclerosis [SSc]) is a connective tissue disorder that is characterized by thickening and fibrosis of the skin and variably severe involvement of diverse internal organs. It can be subdivided into two major subgroups: (1) limited cutaneous SSc (lcSSc), which involves mainly the face, neck, arms, and hands; and (2) diffuse cutaneous SSc (dcSSc), which affects the skin in a more generalized distribution including the entire extremities, face, neck, and trunk. Both subgroups typically have characteristic internal organ involvement.

SYNONYMS

Systemic sclerosis
Morphea applies to localized scleroderma that affects only the skin
Scleredema is a disease of the skin that is distinct from scleroderma.

ICD-9CM CODES
710.1 Scleroderma
701.0 Morphea

EPIDEMIOLOGY & DEMOGRAPHICS

INCIDENCE: There are 2.3 to 22.8 cases per 1 million persons per yr, but many mild cases go unrecognized.
PREVALENCE: 50 to 300 cases per 1 million persons
PREDOMINANT SEX: Female/male ratio of 4:1
PREDOMINANT AGE: 30 to 50 yr
DISTRIBUTION: Worldwide

PHYSICAL FINDINGS & CLINICAL PRESENTATION

PHYSICAL FINDINGS:
1. Skin
   - Tightening of the skin begins on the hands and then progresses to the forearms, face, and neck; the skin is shiny, taut, and sometimes red, with a loss of creases and hair.
   - Later, skin tightening may limit movement by causing flexion contractures of the fingers, wrists, and elbows.
   - Pigmentary changes may occur.
   - Skin atrophy occurs during later stages.
2. Musculoskeletal
   - Joint pain and swelling
   - Symmetric inflammatory arthritis
   - Myopathy
3. Gastrointestinal involvement
   - Esophageal dysmotility with heartburn, dysphagia, and odynophagia
   - Delayed gastric emptying
   - Small-bowel dysmotility with abdominal cramps and diarrhea
   - Colon dysmotility with constipation
   - Primary biliary cirrhosis (see "Cirrhosis, Primary Biliary" in Section I)

4. Pulmonary manifestations
   - Pulmonary fibrosis with symptoms of dyspnea and nonproductive cough as well as fine inspiratory crackles on examination
   - Pulmonary hypertension
5. Cardiac involvement
   - Myocardial fibrosis that leads to congestive heart failure
6. Renal involvement
   - Malignant hypertension
   - Rapidly progressive renal failure
7. Other organ involvement
   - Hypothyroidism
   - Erectile dysfunction
   - Sjögren's syndrome
   - Entrapment neuropathies
8. CREST syndrome (term now replaced by limited cutaneous SSc)
   - Calcinosis, Raynaud's syndrome, Esophageal dysmotility, Sclerodactyly, Telangiectasias—with CREST syndrome, scleroderma is limited to the distal extremities. This acronym is now considered obsolete by many because it does not accurately reflect the burden of internal organ involvement.

CLINICAL PRESENTATION:
- Raynaud's phenomenon: initial complaint in 70% of patients (NOTE: The prevalence of Raynaud's phenomenon is 5% to 10% in the general population; most cases do not progress to scleroderma.)
- Finger or hand swelling that is sometimes associated with carpal tunnel syndrome
- Arthralgias/arthritis
- Internal organ involvement

ETIOLOGY

The etiology of this condition is unknown. Genetic profiles show clustering of different alleles acoording to the subtype of SSc. There is abnormal selection of fibroblasts and aberrant control of connective tissue synthesis by fibroblasts and other cells. Although there are characteristic autoantibodies detected, it is not clear that they directly participate in the pathogenesis of the disease.
- Extracellular connective tissue activation
- Frequent immunologic abnormalities including autoantibodies
- Inflammation in the early stages of disease
- Vasoconstriction

DIAGNOSIS

DIFFERENTIAL DIAGNOSIS
DERMATOLOGIC:
- Scleredema
- Amyloidosis
- Porphyria cutanea tarda
- Eosinophilic fasciitis
- Reflex sympathetic dystrophy
- Nephrogenic systemic fibrosis
SYSTEMIC:
- Idiopathic pulmonary fibrosis
- Primary pulmonary hypertension

- Primary biliary cirrhosis
- Cardiomyopathies
- Gastrointestinal dysmotility problems
- Systemic lupus erythematosus and overlap syndromes

WORKUP
Laboratory tests and imaging studies

LABORATORY TESTS
- Antinuclear antibodies (homogeneous, speckled, or nucleolar patterns)
- Negative antibody to native DNA
- Negative anti–smooth muscle antibody
- Autoantibodies against ribonucleoprotein positive in 20% of patients
- Rheumatoid factor positive in 20% of patients
- Anticentromere antibodies in one third of patients with lcSSc
- Positive extractable nuclear antibody to Scl-70 in 40% of patients with dcSSc
- Routine biochemistry tests may indicate specific organ involvement (e.g., liver, kidney, muscle)

IMAGING AND OTHER STUDIES
1. Arthritis: joint radiographs
2. Gastrointestinal
   - Endoscopy (diagnostic procedure of choice; may be therapeutic)
   - Cine-esophagography (in rare circumstances)
   - Barium swallow (occasionally indicated)
   - Esophageal manometry (almost never necessary)
3. Pulmonary
   - Chest x-ray
   - Pulmonary function tests (especially single-breath diffusion capacity for CO)
   - Chest computed tomography (CT) scan
   - Bronchoscopy with biopsy
   - Gallium lung scan
   - Bronchoalveolar lavage
4. Heart
   - ECG
   - Ambulatory (Holter) ECG monitoring
   - Echocardiography
   - Cardiac catheterization
5. Kidney: renal biopsy
6. Skin: skin biopsy

TREATMENT

1. No disease-modifying therapy available. Immunosuppressive agents used in individual patients. Prednisone should be used with extreme caution, especially in doses >20 mg/day
2. Raynaud's syndrome:
   - Calcium channel blockers (i.e., long-acting dihydropyridines)
   - Peripheral α_1-adrenergic blockers
   - Angiotensin II receptor blockers
   - Pentoxifylline
   - Phosphodiesterase inhibitors
   - Stellate ganglionic blockades
   - Digital sympathectomy

3. Arthralgias: nonsteroidal anti-inflammatory drugs
4. Skin: For extensive skin fibrosis, immuno-modulatory drugs have been used such as methotrexate mycophenolate, and cyclo-phosphamide but have not been proved to be beneficial
5. Esophageal reflux
   - H_2-receptor blockers
   - Proton pump inhibitors
6. Pulmonary hypertension and fibrosis
   - Oxygen
   - Diuretics (with caution)
   - Endothelin-1 receptor inhibitors (bosen-tan, ambrisentan)
   - Sildenafil, tadalafil
   - Prostacyclin analogues (epoprostenol, ilo-prost, treprostinil)
   - Lung transplantation
   - Cyclophosphamide chemotherapy for symptomatic scleroderma-related inter-stitial lung disease
7. Renal involvement
   - Angiotensin-converting enzyme inhibitors
   - Dialysis
   - Renal transplantation

REFERRAL
Rheumatology consultation

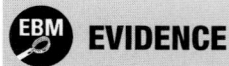 **EVIDENCE**

available at www.expertconsult.com

SUGGESTED READINGS
available at www.expertconsult.com

AUTHORS: **EDWARD V. LALLY, M.D.,** and **FRED F. FERRI, M.D.**

BASIC INFORMATION

DEFINITION

Scoliosis is a lateral curvature of the spine in the upright position, usually 10 degrees or greater. Scoliosis may be classified as either structural (fixed, nonflexible) or nonstructural (flexible, correctable).

ICD-9CM CODES
737.30 Idiopathic scoliosis
737.39 Paralytic scoliosis
754.2 Congenital scoliosis
724.3 Sciatic scoliosis
737.43 Associated with neurofibromatosis

EPIDEMIOLOGY & DEMOGRAPHICS (IDIOPATHIC FORM)

PREDOMINANT SEX: Females are affected more often than males (7:1)
PREVALENCE: Four cases per 1000 persons
PREDOMINANT AGE:
- Onset variable
- Most curves found in adolescents (age ≥11 yr)

PHYSICAL FINDINGS & CLINICAL PRESENTATION

- Record patient age (in years plus months) and height.
- Perform neurologic examination to rule out neuromuscular disease.
- Inspect the shoulders and iliac crests to determine if they are level.
- Palpate the spinous processes to determine their alignment.

- Have the patient bend forward symmetrically at the waist with the arms hanging free (Adams' position); observe from the back or front to detect abnormal spine rotation (Fig. 1-341).

ETIOLOGY

- 90% unknown, usually referred to as *idiopathic* (genetic)
- Congenital spine deformity
- Neuromuscular disease
- Leg-length inequality
- Local inflammation or infection
- Acute pain (disk disease)
- Chronic degenerative disk disease with asymmetric disk narrowing
  Curves of an idiopathic nature or those accompanying congenital deformity or neuromuscular disease are associated with structural changes. The nonstructural types (leg-length discrepancy, inflammation, or acute pain) disappear when the offending disorder is corrected.

DIAGNOSIS

WORKUP

- Curvatures associated with congenital spine abnormalities, neuromuscular disease, and other less common forms of scoliosis can usually be identified by history or associated radiographic or physical findings.
- Section III, "Scoliosis," describes an approach to scoliosis screening.

IMAGING STUDIES

- Diagnosis of idiopathic scoliosis is confirmed by a standing roentgenogram of the spine.

- Severity of the curve is measured in degrees, usually by the Cobb method.
- MRI is usually not indicated unless there is pain, a neurologic deficit, or a left thoracic curve (which is often associated with an underlying spinal disorder).

TREATMENT

ACUTE GENERAL Rx

- Treatment or correction of cause if curve is nonstructural
- Early detection is key in treating genetic curve
- Regular observation for curves <20 degrees
- Bracing for idiopathic curves of 20 to 40 degrees to prevent progression
- Surgery for idiopathic curves >40 to 50 degrees in immature patient

DISPOSITION

- The larger the curve at detection, the greater the chance of progression.
- Progression is more common in young children who are beginning their growth spurt.
- Curves in females are more likely to progress.
- Curves <20 degrees will improve spontaneously >50% of the time.
- Failure to diagnose and treat these curves may allow progressive deformity, pain, and cardiopulmonary compromise to develop.
- Spinal deformities >50 degrees in adults may progress and eventually become painful.
- There is no difference in the rate of back pain in the general population and patients with adolescent idiopathic scoliosis.

REFERRAL

For orthopedic consultation if structural curve is present

PEARLS & CONSIDERATIONS

COMMENTS

- Congenital scoliosis has a high incidence of cardiac and urinary tract abnormalities.
- Bracing is not intended to completely straighten the idiopathic curve. It may improve the curvature but is mainly used to stabilize and prevent progression.

SUGGESTED READINGS
available at www.expertconsult.com

AUTHORS: **LONNIE R. MERCIER, M.D.,** and **HAROLD HALL, M.D.**

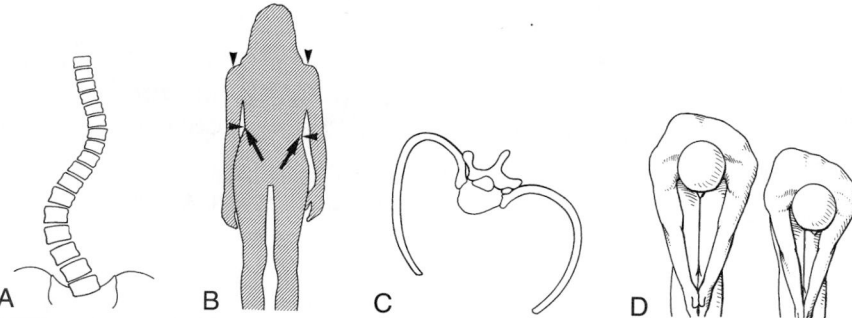

FIGURE 1-341 Structural changes in idiopathic scoliosis. A, As curvature increases, alterations in body configuration develop in both the primary and compensatory curve regions. **B,** Asymmetry of shoulder height, waistline, and the elbow-to-flank distance are common findings. **C,** Vertebral rotation and associated posterior displacement of the ribs on the convex side of the curve are responsible for the characteristic deformity of the chest wall in scoliosis patients. **D,** In the school screening examination for scoliosis, the patient bends forward at the waist. Rib asymmetry of even a small degree is obvious. (From Scoles PV: Spinal deformity in childhood and adolescence. In Behrman RE, Vaughn VC III [eds]: *Nelson textbook of pediatrics*, ed 5, Philadelphia, 1989, WB Saunders.)

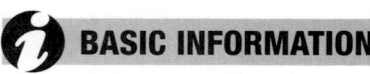

BASIC INFORMATION

DEFINITION

Recurrent depressive episodes during autumn and winter alternating with nondepressive episodes during spring and summer. Patients with seasonal affective disorder (SAD) have experienced two episodes of major depression in the past 2 yr that demonstrate the temporal seasonal relations and have had no nonseasonal episodes over this period.

SYNONYMS

Seasonal depression
Winter depression
Wintertime blues

ICD-9CM CODES

296.30 Seasonal affective disorder

EPIDEMIOLOGY & DEMOGRAPHICS

- Climate, genetic vulnerability, and sociocultural factors all play a role. The risk of seasonal mood swings is clearly associated with northern latitudes. The prevalence of SAD is estimated to be 0.5% to 1.5% in northern European populations, but up to 10% to 20% of these populations report milder, recurrent episodes consistent with subsyndromal SAD.
- As with other depressive disorders, women are affected disproportionately.

PHYSICAL FINDINGS & CLINICAL PRESENTATION

- The symptoms of SAD can be identical to those of other depressive episodes but tend to include features associated with atypical major depression, including low energy, irritability, weight gain, and overeating.
- Average duration is 5 mo, generally beginning in November.

ETIOLOGY

- Explanations focus on biologic models. Shorter photoperiod and decrease in sunlight are hypothesized to be the triggers.

- Several neurotransmitters implicated, including dopamine, serotonin, and norepinephrine.

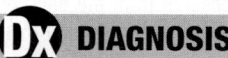

DIAGNOSIS

Diagnostic workup similar to that for major depression.

DIFFERENTIAL DIAGNOSIS

- Major depressive disorder
- Minor depression or adjustment disorder
- Bipolar affective disorder
- Evaluate for substance use (especially alcohol)
- Medical illness or medications that may contribute to depression (e.g., endocrine disorders, neurologic disease)

WORKUP

- As with major depression, consider medical etiologies and rule out as indicated by the presenting signs and symptoms. Consider endocrine evaluation, especially thyroid function; sleep studies and a toxicology screen might be considered.
- Structured Interview Guide for the Hamilton Depression Rating Scale–Seasonal Affective Disorders Version (SIGH-SAD) used in research settings.

LABORATORY TESTS

As directed by presenting symptoms

IMAGING STUDIES

Generally not indicated

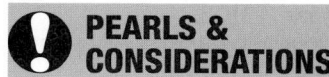

TREATMENT

NONPHARMACOLOGIC THERAPY

- Phototherapy presupposes that artificial light at a similar strength to natural sunlight will prevent the biologic changes that mediate SAD.
- Some trials of light treatment have found a benefit; others have been unable to demonstrate a benefit over placebo.

- Phototherapy tends to use 2500 to 10,000 lux delivered by a commercial light box or a portable head-mounted unit. Phototherapy is recommended to begin within 2 wk of the start of symptoms and continue through the winter months. Patients are instructed to sit ~18 in from the light box for 30 min up to several hours once or twice per day for a minimum of 1 wk.
- Some studies have found efficacy for high density negative ions, though negative studies also exist and more research is needed.

PHARMACOLOGIC THERAPY

Bupropion effective in preventing recurrence

ACUTE GENERAL Rx

Necessary if patient is suicidal.

CHRONIC Rx

No conclusive evidence to support use of SSRIs.

DISPOSITION

Psychiatric referral may be helpful to confirm diagnosis. Recommended for high-risk and suicidal patients.

REFERRAL

For active suicidal ideation, psychosis, symptoms suggestive of bipolar disorder

PEARLS & CONSIDERATIONS

Patients with SAD may present with a complaint of overeating, particularly food high in carbohydrates.

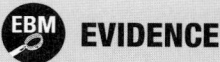 **EVIDENCE**

available at www.expertconsult.com

SUGGESTED READINGS

available at www.expertconsult.com

AUTHORS: **MARK ZIMMERMAN, M.D.,** and **MITCHELL D. FELDMAN, M.D., M.PHIL.**

BASIC INFORMATION

DEFINITION

Mild to severe rash characterized by scaling and erythema that occurs in areas of the skin rich in sebaceous glands.

SYNONYMS

Dandruff
Cradle cap
Sebopsoriasis
Seborrheic eczema
Pityriasis capitis

ICD-9CM CODES
690.10 Seborrheic dermatitis

EPIDEMIOLOGY & DEMOGRAPHICS

PREVALENCE: Affects between 1% and 3% of otherwise healthy adults.
PREDOMINANT SEX AND AGE: Can occur from infancy through old age, with peak incidence in adolescents and young adults and increasing again after age 50 yr. More common in men than women.
RISK FACTORS: More common in patients with HIV/AIDS, Parkinson's disease, other neurologic disorders, mood disorders, chronic alcoholic pancreatitis, hepatitis, cancer, and genetic disorders (e.g., Down syndrome). Occurs more often during winter season.

PHYSICAL FINDINGS & CLINICAL PRESENTATION

Mild, greasy scaling of the scalp and nasolabial folds, postauricular skin, beard area, eyebrows, trunk and sometimes the central face. Blepharitis, otitis externa and coexisting acne vulgaris or pityriasis may also be present. Itching and stinging of lesions can occur. Increased occurrence during times of stress or sleep deprivation.

ETIOLOGY

Actual etiology is unknown but has been linked to hormone levels, fungal infections, altered immune function, nutritional deficits, and neurogenic factors. Fungal infections of the *Malassezia* species have been associated with SD.

 DIAGNOSIS

DIFFERENTIAL DIAGNOSIS

- Atopic dermatitis
- Candidiasis
- Dermatophytosis
- Langerhans cell histiocytosis
- Psoriasis
- Rosacea
- Systemic lupus erythematosus
- Tinea infection

WORKUP

- Diagnosis usually based on clinical identification of lesions
- Skin biopsies can be performed, if warranted, to distinguish SD from similar disorders

LABORATORY TESTS

Microscopic examination with special stains can be used to determine if yeast cells are present in keratinocytes

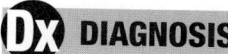 **TREATMENT**

NONPHARMACOLOGIC THERAPY

- Patient education that SD is a chronic condition and treatment is aimed at resolving lesions but does not prevent recurrence.
- General recommendations: wash skin regularly, soften and remove scales, and apply moisturizing emollients after washing.
- Scale removal can be accomplished through the application of mineral or olive oil and removed with a comb or brush after 1 hr.

ACUTE GENERAL Rx

- Topical steroids: can be in the form of shampoos, creams, or ointments
- Calcineurin inhibitors (e.g., tacrolimus ointment, pimecrolimus cream): good when face and ears are affected
- Keratolytics (e.g., tar, salicylic acid, zinc pyrithione)
- Antifungals (e.g., Nizoral, selenium sulfide, ketoconazole [the most evidence for effectiveness among antifungals], ciclopirox, fluconazole)
- Treatment of any secondary bacterial infection with oral antibiotics
- Reserve oral therapy for patients with widespread SD or SD that is refractory to topical therapy. Itraconazole 200 mg/day for 7 days is a sample oral regimen.

CHRONIC Rx

Recalcitrant seborrheic dermatitis: topical azole combined with desonide regimen (limit use to 2 wk)

COMPLEMENTARY AND ALTERNATIVE MEDICINE

Tea tree oil (Melaleuca oil)

REFERRAL

Consider referral to dermatology for recalcitrant cases or uncertain diagnosis

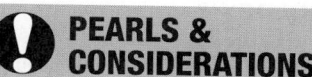 **PEARLS & CONSIDERATIONS**

- Use a combination of topical steroids and antifungal cream for severe SD
- Limit use of steroids to 2-wk course of treatment due to risk of cutaneous atrophy and telangiectasias
- SD of the scalp can be treated with an antifungal (e.g., 2% ketoconazole) or keratolytic shampoo. Limit use of antifungal shampoos to twice a week to prevent drying of the scalp. Alternate the use of antifungal shampoos with a moisturizing shampoo.
- In patients with widespread SD, consider testing for HIV infection

SUGGESTED READINGS

available at www.expertconsult.com

AUTHOR: **ANNGENE GIUSTOZZI, M.D., M.P.H., F.A.A.F.P.**

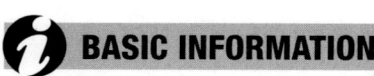

BASIC INFORMATION

DEFINITION

Absence seizures are a type of generalized seizures, characterized by brief episodes of staring with impairment of consciousness (absence). They usually last a few seconds up to 20 to 30 sec. The onset and the end of the seizures are sudden. Usually the patients are not aware of them and resume the activity they were doing prior to the seizure. The electroencephalogram signature of absence seizures consists of generalized 3-Hz spike and slow wave discharges.

SYNONYMS

Childhood absence epilepsy, previously known as petit mal.

ICD-9CM CODES
345.0 Generalized nonconvulsive epilepsy

EPIDEMIOLOGY & DEMOGRAPHICS

INCIDENCE: 1 to 10 cases per 100,000 population.
PEAK INCIDENCE: 6 to 7 yr
PREVALENCE: Represent up to 18% of all pediatric epilepsy syndromes
PREDOMINANT SEX AND AGE: More common in girls than in boys, absences typically begin between 4 and 8 yr

PHYSICAL FINDINGS & CLINICAL PRESENTATION

- Patients with absence seizures usually have normal physical and neurologic examinations.
- During the seizures, the patients are unresponsive and can have motor phenomena (automatisms, eye blinks, mouth and hand movements).
- Tonic-clonic seizures are not usually a feature of this syndrome. If this is the case, other etiologies should be investigated such as juvenile absence epilepsy, juvenile myoclonic epilepsy, etc.

ETIOLOGY

Genetic

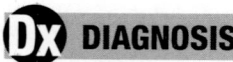 DIAGNOSIS

DIFFERENTIAL DIAGNOSIS

- Juvenile absence epilepsy
- Juvenile myoclonic epilepsy
- Complex partial seizures

WORKUP

- EEG with hyperventilation and photic stimulation is crucial in the diagnosis.
- Ambulatory EEG and video EEG are recommended for patients with diagnostic uncertainty.

LABORATORY TESTS

Routine blood workup (CBC, CMP, electrolytes)

IMAGING STUDIES

- MRI of the brain should be performed in all epilepsy patients, especially if the EEG does not show the typical characteristic of absence seizures (3-Hz spike and slow wave discharges).
- CT scans of the head should be avoided in children due to unnecessary exposure to radiation and the low yield of the test. CT scans of the head are reserved for neurologic emergencies and are adjusted for weight in children.

 TREATMENT

The medication of choice based on the best current data available is ethosuximide, followed by valproic acid and lamotrigine.

NONPHARMACOLOGIC THERAPY

Not applicable

GENERAL Rx

- Ethosuximide: Initial dose: 10 mg/kg/dat; then after 7 days, 20 mg/kg
- Valproic acid (Depakote): Initial dose: 5-10 mg/kg/day (divided bid), maximum dose 60 mg/kg/day
- Lamotrigine: Dose for patients on no other antiepileptic drugs. Wk 1 and 2: 0.3 mg/kg/day. Wk 3 and 4: 0.6 mg/kg/day. Wk 5 onward: Increase every 1 to 2 wk by 0.6 mg/kg/day. Maintenance: 4.5 to 7.5 mg/kg/day. Warning: Should be used with caution due to the potential for toxicity and Steven-Johnson syndrome. Patients on other antiepileptic drugs can also have severe adverse reactions.

CHRONIC Rx

- Children with recurrent seizures require chronic treatment.
- If children are seizure free for a period of 1 to 2 yr, a trial on no medications should be considered; children, unlike adults, can "outgrow" seizures.

COMPLEMENTARY AND ALTERNATIVE MEDICINE

Not applicable

DISPOSITION

- Response to treatment is excellent.
- Absence seizures tend to remit in teenage years.

REFERRAL

Patients with epilepsy and seizures should be referred for a consultation by a neurologist, preferably to one specializing in epilepsy.

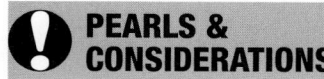 PEARLS & CONSIDERATIONS

COMMENTS

- Absence seizures can be present in other epilepsy syndromes.
- Valproic acid should be avoided in girls and women with childbearing potential due to the risk of teratogenicity.
- Carbamazepine and phenytoin should be avoided in the treatment of absence seizures, since these medications may worsen seizures and could provoke absence status epilepticus.
- All women of childbearing age taking antiepileptic drugs should take folic acid supplementation (1 to 4 mg/day) for the prevention of neural tube defects.

PREVENTION

Sleep deprivation and alcohol consumption should be avoided.

PATIENT/FAMILY EDUCATION

- Patients with epilepsy have normal lives.
- The goal of treatment is no seizures and no side effects to medications.
- Patient education and information can be obtained from the Epilepsy Foundation: www.epilepsyfoundation.org
- Pregnant women with epilepsy should visit the Antiepileptic Drug Pregnancy Registry website for information and assistance: www2.massgeneral.org/aed
- Patients with ongoing seizures are forbidden from driving; check your state regulations and laws regarding driving and epilepsy.

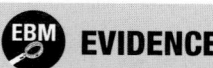 EVIDENCE

available at www.expertconsult.com

SUGGESTED READINGS
available at www.expertconsult.com

AUTHOR: **PATRICIO SEBASTIAN ESPINOSA, M.D., M.P.H.**

BASIC INFORMATION

DEFINITION

Febrile seizures are seizures that occur in febrile children between the ages of 6 and 60 mo who do not have an intracranial infection, metabolic disturbance, or history of a febrile seizure. Febrile seizures are subdivided into 2 categories: simple and complex. Simple febrile seizures last <15 min, are generalized (without a focal component), and occur once in a 24-hr period, whereas complex febrile seizures are prolonged (>15 min), show focal neurologic signs, or occur more than once in 24 hr.

SYNONYMS

Febrile convulsions

ICD-9CM CODES
780.6 Febrile seizures

EPIDEMIOLOGY & DEMOGRAPHICS

INCIDENCE: 2% to 5% of children will have a febrile seizure by age 60 mo.
PREDOMINANT SEX AND AGE: Slightly more common in boys than girls.
PEAK INCIDENCE: 6 to 60 mo
PREVALENCE: Represent up to 18% of all pediatric epilepsy syndromes

PHYSICAL FINDINGS & CLINICAL PRESENTATION

- Children with febrile seizures have normal physical and neurologic examinations.
- Viral illnesses are the predominant cause of febrile seizures.

ETIOLOGY

Genetic

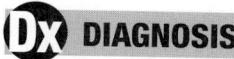

DIAGNOSIS

DIFFERENTIAL DIAGNOSIS

- CNS infection (ie, meningitis)
- Epilepsy

WORKUP

- It is important to first investigate whether an underlying infection exists.
- In patients with simple self-limited febrile seizures with rapid return to consciousness and a normal neurologic examination, further workup is not routinely recommended.
- In patients with complex febrile seizures, laboratory workup and brain imaging are recommended.
- EEG is not routinely recommended, but there is controversy in usefulness of this test in the setting of febrile seizures. In the opinion of the author, a screening EEG should be obtained as a baseline and for comparison in the future if needed.

LABORATORY TESTS

Routine blood workup (CBC, CMP, electrolytes), blood and urine cultures, chest x-ray, CSF (analysis if pertinent)

IMAGING STUDIES

- MRI of the brain is not required in patients with simple febrile seizures.
- Imaging of the brain should be considered in children with complex febrile seizures and in children with focal neurologic deficits.
- CT scans of the head should be avoided in children, if possible, due to exposure to radiation and the relative low yield of the test compared to MRI. CT scans of the head are reserved for neurologic emergencies and are adjusted for weight in children.

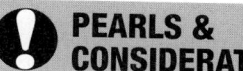

TREATMENT

Febrile seizures do not usually require antiepileptic drug treatment.

NONPHARMACOLOGIC THERAPY

Not applicable

GENERAL Rx

Treat the cause of the fever.

CHRONIC Rx

No chronic treatment for febrile seizures is recommended.

COMPLEMENTARY AND ALTERNATIVE MEDICINE

Not applicable

DISPOSITION

- Treatment is not recommended.
- Febrile seizures should stop by age 60 mo.

REFERRAL

Patients with recurrent febrile seizures need to be referred for a consultation by a pediatric neurologist.

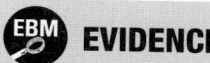

PEARLS & CONSIDERATIONS

COMMENTS

- It is crucial to find out the etiology of the fever and to treat it appropriately.
- Patient with seizures and fever after age 60 mo are not classified as febrile seizures.

PREVENTION

Antipyretics do not reduce the recurrence risk of febrile seizures. However, fever should be treated and worked up independently of the diagnosis of febrile seizures.

PATIENT/FAMILY EDUCATION

- Children with febrile seizures do not need antiepileptic drug treatment.
- Patient education and information can be obtained at the Epilepsy Foundation: www.epilepsyfoundation.org

EVIDENCE

available at www.expertconsult.com

SUGGESTED READINGS

available at www.expertconsult.com

AUTHOR: **PATRICIO SEBASTIAN ESPINOSA, M.D., M.P.H.**

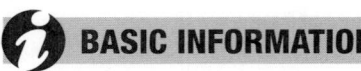

BASIC INFORMATION

DEFINITION

Tonic clonic seizures are characterized by sudden loss of consciousness, muscle contraction (tonic phase) followed by rhythmic jerking activity (clonic phase).

SYNONYMS

Convulsive seizures, previously known as grand mal

ICD-9CM CODES

345.1 Generalized convulsive epilepsy

EPIDEMIOLOGY & DEMOGRAPHICS

INCIDENCE: 30 to 50 cases per 100,000 person-yr (epilepsy incidence)
PEAK INCIDENCE: Not applicable
PREVALENCE: 5 to 8 cases per 1000 persons (epilepsy incidence)
PREDOMINANT SEX AND AGE: No gender preference

PHYSICAL FINDINGS & CLINICAL PRESENTATION

- Patients with tonic clonic seizures usually have normal physical and neurologic examinations (interictally).
- During the seizures, the patients are unresponsive and can have violent postures with severe repetitive muscle contractions.
- After the seizure, the patients are usually lethargic and confused.
- Tonic clonic seizures are associated with injuries, bladder incontinence, and tongue biting.
- Focal postictal weakness may point toward a focal neurologic lesion (Todd's paralysis).

ETIOLOGY

- Seizures are a cardinal sign of cortical neurologic injury.
- The etiology of seizures can be idiopathic (likely genetic), cryptogenic (possibly genetic), and symptomatic (due to a neurologic injury).

DIAGNOSIS

DIFFERENTIAL DIAGNOSIS

- Convulsive syncope
- Nonepileptic spells

WORKUP

- EEG
- Ambulatory EEG and/or video EEG recommended for patients with diagnostic uncertainty

LABORATORY TESTS

- Routine blood workup (CBC, CMP, glucose, electrolytes)
- Urine drug screen
- Lumbar puncture is recommended in patients with the suspicion of meningitis

IMAGING STUDIES

- In the acute setting, a CT scan of the head is high yield to rule out space-occupying lesions.
- MRI of the brain epilepsy protocol should be performed in all patients with recurrent seizures.
- CT scans of the head should be avoided in children due to unnecessary exposure to radiation and the low yield of the test. CT scans of the head are reserved for neurologic emergencies and are adjusted for weight in children.

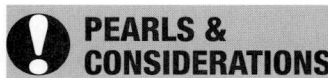

TREATMENT

- The treatment is based in the type and etiology of the seizures (i.e., metabolic disturbance, infectious, etc.).
- Levetiracetam is an effective and well-tolerated antiepileptic drug for treating generalized tonic clonic seizures.
- Valproic acid is better tolerated than topiramate and more efficacious than lamotrigine in patients with generalized and unclassified epilepsy types.
- Valproic acid should be avoided in girls and women with childbearing potential due to the risk of teratogenicity.

NONPHARMACOLOGIC THERAPY

Not applicable

GENERAL Rx

- First unprovoked seizure with normal imaging, EEG, and laboratory workup requires no treatment.
- Recurrent seizures and seizures with abnormal studies require treatment depending on the etiology.
- Valproic acid (Depakote): Initial dose: 10 to 15 mg/kg/day (divided bid), maximum dose 60 mg/kg/day.
- Levetiracetam (Keppra): Initial dose 250 to 500 bid, maximum dose 1500 mg bid.

CHRONIC Rx

Chronic treatment with antiepileptic drugs is indicated for ≥2 nonprovoked seizures or in patients with one seizure with abnormal workup.

COMPLEMENTARY AND ALTERNATIVE MEDICINE

Not applicable

DISPOSITION

- Response to treatment is excellent.
- No driving until seizure freedom in accordance with local laws and regulations.

REFERRAL

Patients with epilepsy and seizures should be referred for a consultation by a neurologist, preferably one with epilepsy training.

PEARLS & CONSIDERATIONS

COMMENTS

- It is crucial to understand that tonic clonic seizures can occur in variety of acute neurologic diseases.
- Successful treatment depends on the correct choice of antiepileptic drugs based on the type (partial vs. generalized in onset) and etiology of the seizures.
- Valproic acid should be avoided in girls and women with childbearing potential due to the risk of teratogenicity.
- All women of childbearing age taking antiepileptic drugs should take folic acid supplementation (1-4 mg/day) for the prevention of neural tube defects.

PREVENTION

Sleep deprivation and alcohol consumption should be avoided.

PATIENT/FAMILY EDUCATION

- Patients with epilepsy have normal lives.
- The goal of treatment is no seizures and no side effects to medications.
- Patient education and information can be obtained at the Epilepsy Foundation: www.epilepsyfoundation.org
- Pregnant women with epilepsy should visit the Antiepileptic Drug Pregnancy Registry website for information and assistance: www2.massgeneral.org/aed
- Patients with ongoing seizures are forbidden from driving; check your state regulations and laws regarding driving and epilepsy.

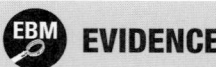 **EVIDENCE**

available at www.expertconsult.com

SUGGESTED READINGS
available at www.expertconsult.com

AUTHOR: **PATRICIO SEBASTIAN ESPINOSA, M.D., M.P.H.**

BASIC INFORMATION

DEFINITION

Partial seizures are characterized by focal cortical discharges that provoke seizure symptoms related to the area of the brain involved. Simple partial seizures do not cause impairment of consciousness.

SYNONYMS

Simple partial seizures
Focal seizures

ICD-9CM CODES

345.5 Localization-relate (focal) (partial) epilepsy and epileptic syndromes with simple partial seizures.

EPIDEMIOLOGY & DEMOGRAPHICS

INCIDENCE: 30 to 50 cases per 100,000 person-yr
PREVALENCE: 5 to 8 cases per 1000 persons
PREDOMINANT SEX AND AGE: No gender preference

PHYSICAL FINDINGS & CLINICAL PRESENTATION

- Patients with partial seizures usually have normal physical and neurologic examinations unless the focal seizures are due to a structural abnormality such as a stroke, wherein the patient will have a neurologic exam consistent with the area of CNS structural damage.
- During partial seizures the patients are conscious, unless there is spread of the epileptic focus causing secondary generalization and unresponsiveness. A focal seizure can evolve to a generalized tonic clonic seizure.
- Patients with partial seizures can experience postictal weakness/paralysis that usually resolves within 24 hr (Todd's paralysis). However, focal neurologic deficits may also be indicative of a structural brain lesion.

ETIOLOGY

- Seizures in general are a cardinal sign of cortical neurologic injury.
- The etiology of partial seizures can be idiopathic (likely genetic), cryptogenic (unknown, possibly genetic), and symptomatic (due to a neurologic injury).
- Frequent causes of partial seizures are tumor, stroke, CNS infections (cysticercosis, abscesses), arteriovenous malformations (AVMs), traumatic brain injury, cortical malformations, and others.

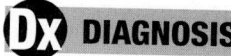 **DIAGNOSIS**

DIFFERENTIAL DIAGNOSIS

- TIA
- Movement disorders
- Nonepileptic spells

WORKUP

- EEG
- Ambulatory EEG and/or video EEG recommended for patients with diagnostic uncertainty

LABORATORY TESTS

Routine blood workup (CBC, CMP, glucose, electrolytes)

IMAGING STUDIES

- In the acute setting, a CT scan of the head is high yield to rule out space-occupying lesions.
- MRI of the brain with a defined epilepsy protocol should be performed in all patients with recurrent seizures.
- CT scans of the head should be avoided in children if possible, unless in an emergency setting.

 TREATMENT

- Carbamazepine traditionally has been the standard initial drug treatment for partial seizures.
- Lamotrigine and levetiracetam are effective and well-tolerated antiepileptic drugs for treating partial seizures.
- Other antiepileptic drugs may be used by an epilepsy specialist in specific cases.
- Surgical treatments (e.g., temporal lobectomy in mesial temporal sclerosis) may be indicated in refractory cases of partial seizures.

GENERAL Rx

- First unprovoked seizure with normal imaging, EEG, and laboratory workup generally requires no treatment.
- Recurrent seizures and seizures with abnormal studies require treatment.

DISPOSITION

- Response to treatment often depends on the etiology of the partial seizures.
- 47% of patients become seizure free with monotherapy and 67% with polytherapy.
- No driving until seizure freedom in accordance with local laws and regulations.

REFERRAL

Patients with epilepsy and seizures should be referred for a consultation by a neurologist, preferably to one with a special interest in epilepsy.

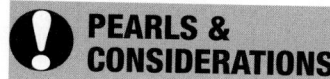 **PEARLS & CONSIDERATIONS**

COMMENTS

- It is crucial to understand that partial seizures can be due to a variety of neurologic diseases.
- Successful treatment depends on the correct choice of antiepileptic drugs based on patient's gender and comorbidities.
- Valproic acid should be avoided in girls and women with childbearing potential due to the risk of teratogenicity.
- All women in childbearing age taking antiepileptic drugs should take folic acid supplementation (1 to 4 mg/day) for the prevention of neural tube defects.

PREVENTION

- Sleep deprivation and alcohol consumption should be avoided.
- Drug compliance is compulsory to prevent seizure recurrence.

PATIENT/FAMILY EDUCATION

- People with epilepsy can lead normal lives.
- The goal of treatment is no seizures and no side effects to medications.
- Patient education and information can be obtained at the Epilepsy Foundation: www.epilepsyfoundation.org
- Pregnant women with epilepsy should visit the Antiepileptic Drug Pregnancy Registry website for information and assistance: www2.massgeneral.org/aed
- Patients with ongoing seizures are forbidden from driving; check your state regulations and laws regarding driving and epilepsy.
- Patients should be counseled on general seizure precautions such as swimming, bathing, and heights.

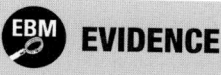 **EVIDENCE**

available at www.expertconsult.com

SUGGESTED READINGS

available at www.expertconsult.com

AUTHOR: **PATRICIO SEBASTIAN ESPINOSA, M.D., M.P.H.**

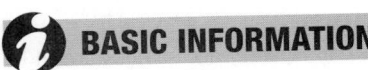

DEFINITION

Septicemia is a systemic illness caused by generalized bacterial or fungal infection and characterized by evidence of infection, fever or hypothermia, hypotension, and evidence of end-organ compromise.

SYNONYMS

Sepsis
Sepsis syndrome
Severe sepsis
Systemic inflammatory response syndrome
Septic shock

ICD-9CM CODES
038.9   Sepsis
038.40 Sepsis, gram-negative bacteremia
038.1   Sepsis, *Staphylococcus*

EPIDEMIOLOGY & DEMOGRAPHICS

INCIDENCE (IN U.S.):
- Exact incidence is unknown
- Approximately 750,000 cases of severe sepsis occur among hospitalized patients each year in the U.S.
- Complicates a minority of bacteremia cases and may occur in the absence of documented bacteremia

PREDOMINANT SEX: Males slightly more commonly affected than females

PREDOMINANT AGE:
- Neonatal period
- Patients >65 yr of age account for 60% of all cases of severe sepsis

GENETICS:
- Familial disposition: a great variety of congenital immunodeficiency states and other inherited disorders may predispose to septicemia.
- Neonatal infection: incidence is high in neonatal period.

PHYSICAL FINDINGS & CLINICAL PRESENTATION
- Fever or hypothermia
- Hypotension
- Tachycardia
- Tachypnea
- Altered mental status
- Bleeding diathesis
- Skin rashes
- Symptoms that reflect primary site of infection: urinary tract, GI tract, CNS, respiratory tract

ETIOLOGY
- Disseminated infection with a great variety of bacteria:
  A. Gram-negative bacteria
    1. *E. coli*
    2. *Klebsiella* spp.
    3. *Pseudomonas aeruginosa*
    4. *Proteus* spp.
    5. *Neisseria meningitidis*
  B. Gram-positive bacteria
    1. *Staphylococcus aureus*
    2. *Streptococcus* spp.
    3. *Enterococcus* spp.
- Less common infections:
  1. Fungal
  2. Viral
  3. Rickettsial
  4. Parasitic
- Activation of coagulation, inflammatory cytokines, complement, and kinin cascades with release of a variety of vasoactive endogenous mediators
- Predisposing host factors:
  1. General medical condition
  2. Age
  3. Immunosuppressive therapy
  4. Recent surgery
  5. Granulocytopenia
  6. Hyposplenism
  7. Diabetes
  8. Instrumentation

Dx DIAGNOSIS

DIFFERENTIAL DIAGNOSIS
- Cardiogenic shock
- Acute pancreatitis
- Pulmonary embolism
- Systemic vasculitis
- Toxic ingestion
- Exposure-induced hypothermia
- Fulminant hepatic failure
- Collagen-vascular diseases

WORKUP
- Evaluation should focus on identifying a specific pathogen and localizing the site of primary infection.
- Hemodynamic, metabolic, coagulation disorders should be carefully characterized.
- Intensive monitoring, including the use of central venous or Swan-Ganz catheters, may be necessary.

LABORATORY TESTS
- Cultures of blood and examination and culture of sputum, urine, wound drainage, stool, and CSF
- CBC with differential, coagulation profile
- Routine chemistries, LFTs
- ABGs, lactic acid level; procalcitonin might be useful as a general marker of infection/sepsis
- Urinalysis

IMAGING STUDIES
- Chest x-ray examination
- Other radiographic and radioisotope procedures according to suspected site of primary infection

Rx TREATMENT

NONPHARMACOLOGIC THERAPY
- Tissue oxygenation: mixed venous oxygen saturation maintained >70% if possible; early mechanical ventilation
- Focal infection drained, if possible

ACUTE GENERAL Rx
- Blood pressure support, rapid IV fluid resuscitation and vasopressors, if needed, with the goal of reestablishing a mean arterial blood pressure >65 mm Hg; reduction in blood lactate and mixed venous oxygen saturation >70% within 6 hr of recognition of septic shock is associated with improved survival
  1. IV hydration; crystalloids are as effective as colloids as resuscitation fluids.
  2. Therapy with vasopressors (e.g., dopamine, norepinephrine, vasopressin) if mean blood pressure of 70 to 75 mm Hg cannot be maintained by hydration alone. A recent trial comparing low-dose vasopressin with norepinephrine revealed that low-dose vasopressin did not reduce mortality rates as compared with norepinephrine among patients with septic shock who were treated with catecholamine vasopressors.
- Correction of acidosis by improving the tissue perfusion, not by giving bicarbonate
  1. Mechanical ventilation
- Antibiotics
  1. Directed at the most likely sources of infection. Table 1-162 describes initial antibiotic recommendations for septic patients.
  2. Should generally provide broad coverage of gram-positive and gram-negative bacteria (or fungi if clinically indicated).
  3. Typical regimens:
    a. For hospital-acquired sepsis (pending culture results): vancomycin plus cefepime, imipenem, aztreonam, quinolones, or an aminoglycoside. Monotherapy with appropriate agents appears to be as effective as combination therapy in immunocompetent hosts, but a recent study indicates combination therapy might be better in severely ill patients with a high risk of death.
    b. For community-acquired infection in the absence of granulocytopenia: previously listed or single-drug therapy with third-generation cephalosporin.
    c. For infection in the granulocytopenic host: previously listed or dual gram-negative coverage (e.g., cephalosporin and aminoglycoside).
  4. Biological treatment Drotrecogin alfa (Xigris), a genetically engineered form of activated protein C, is approved for use in patients with severe sepsis with multiorgan dysfunction (or APACHE II score >24); when combined with conventional therapy, there may be a reduction in mortality.

5. The role of corticosteroids in the acute management of septicemia has long been debated. Patients with relative adrenal insufficiency may benefit from low-dose therapy with hydrocortisone (50 mg IV q6h) and fludrocortisone (50 microgram daily PO) given together for 7 days. Recent trials however revealed that hydrocortisone did not improve survival or reversal of shock, either overall or in patients who did not have a response to corticotropin, although hydrocortisone hastened reversal of shock in patients in whom shock was reversed.

CHRONIC Rx
- Adjust antibiotic therapy on the basis of culture results.
- In general, continue therapy for a minimum of 2 wk.

DISPOSITION
All patients with suspected septicemia should be hospitalized and given access to intensive monitoring and nursing care.

REFERRAL
- To infectious diseases expert
- To physician experienced in critical care

PEARLS & CONSIDERATIONS

COMMENTS
Mortality rises quickly if antibiotic therapy is not instituted promptly and metabolic derangements are not treated aggressively.

EVIDENCE
available at www.expertconsult.com

SUGGESTED READINGS
available at www.expertconsult.com

AUTHOR: **STEVEN M. OPAL, M.D.**

TABLE 1-162 Initial Antibiotic Recommendations for Septic Patients*

Empiric coverage	Vancomycin 15 mg/kg q12h plus either piperacillin-tazobactam[†] 3.375 g IV q6h or imipenem 0.5 g IV q6h or meropenem 1.0 g IV q8h with or without an aminoglycoside (e.g., tobramycin 5 mg/kg IV q24).[‡]
Community-acquired pneumonia	Ceftriaxone 1 g IV q24h plus azithromycin 500 mg IV q24h or a fluoroquinolone (e.g., moxifloxacin 400 mg IV q24h or levofloxacin 750 mg IV q24h).[§]
Community-acquired urosepsis	Ciprofloxacin 400 mg IV q24h or ampicillin 2 g IV q6h plus gentamicin 5 mg/kg IV q24h.
Meningitis	Vancomycin 500-750 mg IV q6h plus ceftriaxone 2 g IV q12h plus dexamethasone 0.15 mg/kg IV q6h × 2-4 days preferably before antibiotics; add ampicillin 2 g IV q4h if *Listeria* is suspected.
Nosocomial pneumonia	Vancomycin 15 mg/kg q12h plus either piperacillin-tazobactam 4.5 g IV q6h or imipenem 0.5 g IV q6h or meropenem 1 g IV q8h or cefepime 2 g IV q12h plus either an aminoglycoside (e.g., amikacin 15 mg/kg IV q24h or tobramycin 7 mg/kg IV q24h) or levofloxacin 750 mg IV q24h. Some authorities would substitute linezolid 600 mg IV q12h for vancomycin if MRSA is of significant concern or known to be the cause.
Neutropenia	Cefepime 2 g IV q8h; add vancomycin 15 mg/kg IV q12h if a central line is present and infection is a concern. Add antifungal coverage with liposomal amphotericin B 3-5 mg/kg q24h or caspofungin 70 mg IV × 1 then 50 mg IV q24h if fever persists ≥5 days. If invasive aspergillosis is highly suspected or proven, voriconazole 6 mg/kg IV q12h × 2 then 4 mg/kg IV q12h should be used.
Cellulitis and skin infections	Vancomycin 15 mg/kg IV q12h. Add piperacillin-tazobactam 4.5 g IV q6h in diabetics or immunocompromised patients. If necrotizing fasciitis is suspected, add clindamycin 900 mg IV; surgical débridement is crucial.

Andreoli TE, Benjamin IJ, Griggs RC, Wing EJ: *Andreoli and Carpenter's cecil essentials of medicine,* ed 8, Philadelphia, 2010, Saunders.
*Assumes normal renal function; dose adjustments required with impaired creatinine clearance.
[†]Substitute aztreonam 2 g IV q8h if penicillin allergic.
[‡]Monitor drug levels of aminoglycosides (i.e., peak and trough).
[§]Use ceftriaxone and azithromycin if the patient is admitted to the intensive care unit.
MRSA, Methicillin-resistant *Staphylococcus aureus*.

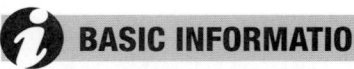 BASIC INFORMATION

DEFINITION

Serotonin syndrome (SS) refers to a group of symptoms resulting from increased activity of serotonin (5-hydroxytryptamine) in the CNS. SS is a drug-induced disorder that is classically characterized by a change in mental status and alteration in neuromuscular activity and autonomic function.

SYNONYMS

SS
Hyperserotonemia
Serotonergic syndrome
Serotonin toxicity

ICD-9CM CODES
333.99 Syndrome serotonin

EPIDEMIOLOGY & DEMOGRAPHICS

- The incidence of SS is not known.
- SS is seen in all age groups, from neonates to elderly.
- SS classically occurs in patients receiving two or more serotonergic drugs, but it can also occur with monotherapy—selective serotonin reuptake inhibitor (SSRI) monotherapy has an incidence of 0.5 to 0.9 cases of SS per 1000 patient-mo. Although there is an FDA alert, it has been argued that there is a lack of sufficient evidence showing that SSRIs and triptans cause serious SS.
- Concomitant use of an SSRI with a monoamine oxidase inhibitor (MAOI) poses the greatest risk of developing SS.
- Combination of SSRIs with other serotonergic drugs (e.g., tryptophan, illicit drugs like cocaine and MDMA, "ecstasy") or drugs with serotonin properties (e.g., lithium, meperidine, triptans) may also lead to SS.

PHYSICAL FINDINGS & CLINICAL PRESENTATION

- Findings of clonus with hyperreflexia in the setting of recent (<5 wk) use of serotonergic agents strongly suggests the diagnosis of SS.
- Symptoms can manifest within minutes to hours after starting a new psychopharmacologic treatment, increasing the dose of a serotonergic drug, or after administering a second serotonergic drug.
- Clonus (inducible, spontaneous, and ocular) is the key finding in establishing a diagnosis of SS.
- Other pertinent findings include:
  - Confusion, agitation, hypomania
  - Fever >38° C (100° F), tachycardia, and tachypnea
  - Nausea, vomiting, abdominal pain, and diaphoresis
  - Diarrhea, tremors, shivering, and seizures
  - Hyperreflexia and muscle rigidity

ETIOLOGY

- Hyperstimulation of the brainstem and spinal cord serotonin receptors leading to the neuromuscular and autonomic symptoms.
- Psychopharmacologic drugs—in particular, fluoxetine and sertraline co-administered with MAOI (e.g., tranylcypromine and phenelzine)—have been cited in the literature as a common cause of SS. Triptans (serotonin-receptor agonists used in the treatment of migraines) may also precipitate the SS when used in combination with SSRIs and serotonin-norepinephrine reuptake inhibitors (SNRIs).

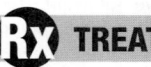 DIAGNOSIS

- The diagnosis of SS is made on clinical grounds. There are no specific laboratory tests for SS. A high index of suspicion along with a detailed medication history is the mainstay of diagnosis.
- Diagnostic criteria: most accurate is Hunter Serotonin Toxicity Criteria (sensitivity 84%, specificity 97%, confirmation by toxicologist).
- To fulfill Hunter criteria a patient must have consumed a serotonergic drug and have one of the following:
  1. Spontaneous clonus
  2. Inducible clonus plus agitation or diaphoresis
  3. Ocular clonus plus agitation or diaphoresis
  4. Tremor and hyperreflexia
  5. Temperature greater than 38° C (100° F) plus hypertonia plus ocular clonus or inducible clonus

DIFFERENTIAL DIAGNOSIS

- Neuroleptic malignant syndrome (NMS), substance abuse (e.g., cocaine, amphetamines), anticholinergic toxicity, thyroid storm, infection (e.g., meningitis, encephalitis), alcohol and opioid withdrawal.
- Classic features in differentiation of NMS from SS are that SS develops over 24 hr, involves neuromuscular hyperactivity, and begins to resolve within 24 hr with appropriate therapy, whereas NMS develops gradually over days to weeks, involves sluggish neuromuscular response, and resolves over an average period of 1 wk to 10 days.

WORKUP

- Because SS is a clinical diagnosis, there is no laboratory test that confirms the diagnosis, and serum serotonin concentration does not correlate with clinical picture. Other causes are described in "Differential Diagnosis." Thus, all patients should have blood tests and diagnostic imaging studies to rule out infectious, toxic, and metabolic causes.
- Additional laboratory tests are performed to exclude complicating features of SS (e.g., renal failure secondary to rhabdomyolysis).

LABORATORY TESTS

- CBC with differential to rule out sepsis
- Electrolytes, BUN, and creatinine to rule out acidosis and renal failure
- Blood and urine toxicology screen
- Thyroid function tests
- Creatine-phosphokinase (CPK) with isoenzymes
- Urine and blood cultures
- ECG because ventricular rhythm disturbance is a potentially fatal complication

IMAGING STUDIES

Imaging studies are not specific in the diagnosis of SS and are only ordered to exclude other causes with similar clinical presentations as SS.

TREATMENT

- Once a diagnosis of SS is established, appropriate consultation with a medical toxicologist, clinical pharmacologist, and/or poison control center should be sought.
- Management includes:
  - Discontinue use of all potential precipitating drugs
  - Provide supportive management
  - Control agitation
  - Administer serotonin antagonists
  - Control autonomic instability
  - Control hyperthermia
  - Reassess the need to resume the use of the serotonergic agent once the symptoms have resolved

NONPHARMACOLOGIC THERAPY

- Discontinuation of the drug is the mainstay of therapy.
- Treatment is supportive: maintaining oxygenation and blood pressure and monitoring respiratory status. Hypotensive patients may require both IV fluids and vasopressor therapy.
- Patients who are severely hyperthermic with temperatures greater than 41° C (106° F) should be given IV sedation, paralyzed, and intubated. Cooling blankets can be used for patients with mild to moderate hyperthermia. There is no role of acetaminophen here.
- Intubation is recommended for patients unable to protect their airways as a result of mental status changes or seizures.

ACUTE GENERAL Rx

- Benzodiazepines for control of agitation is preferred to physical restraints.
  1. Lorazepam 1 to 2 mg IV every 30 min has been used effectively in treating agitation, muscle rigidity, myoclonus, and seizure complications.
  2. Diazepam is an alternative choice.
- Blood pressure management with short-acting agents such as esmolol and nitroprusside.
- Serotonin antagonists should be titrated to clinical effectiveness in patients for whom nonpharmacologic therapy and benzodiazepines are not achieving adequate response, though substantial and rigorous data is lacking.
  1. Cyproheptadine 4-mg tablet or 2 mg/5 ml syrup is given 12 mg initially followed by 2 mg every 2 hr until therapeutic response is achieved in adults (up to 32 mg/day), children ages 7 to 14 should receive 4 mg every 6 hr (up to 16 mg/day), children ages 2 to 6 should receive 2 mg every 6 hr (up to 12 mg/day), and children

younger than 2 yr should receive a maximum of 0.25 mg/kg/day as 0.06 mg/kg every 6 hr.

2. Atypical antipsychotic agents with serotonin antagonist properties (e.g., olanzapine 10 mg SL) have been tried with some success.

3. Chlorpromazine 50 to 100 mg IM may be considered in severe cases.

CHRONIC Rx

For patients not requiring hospital admission, cyproheptadine and lorazepam can be given in an oral dose on a prn basis with close follow-up.

DISPOSITION

• SS is a potentially life-threatening condition if not recognized early, though it does exist on a spectrum.

• Prompt diagnosis and withdrawal of the medication results in improvement of symptoms within 24 hr.

• Seizures, rhabdomyolysis, hyperthermia, ventricular arrhythmia, respiratory arrest, and coma are all complicating features of SS.

REFERRAL

All cases of SS secondary to psychotropic medications should be referred to a psychiatrist.

PREVENTION

Modify prescription practices by avoiding multidrug regimens.

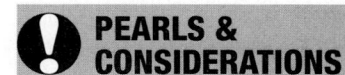

PEARLS & CONSIDERATIONS

The combined use of SSRIs and MAOIs is contraindicated.

COMMENTS

• The use of SSRIs and other serotonergic agents is not an absolute contraindication; however, prompt withdrawal of the medication is recommended if any symptoms suggesting SS occur.

• SS is usually found in patients being treated for depression, bipolar disorders, obsessive-compulsive disorder, attention-deficit disorder, and Parkinson's disease.

SUGGESTED READINGS
available at www.expertconsult.com

AUTHOR: **MARK F. BRADY, M.D., M.P.H., M.M.S.**

S

Diseases
and Disorders

I

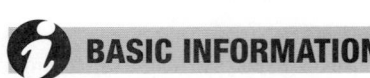

BASIC INFORMATION

DEFINITION

Severe acute respiratory syndrome (SARS) is a respiratory illness caused by a coronavirus called SARS-associated coronavirus (SARS-CoV).

CLINICAL CRITERIA:

A. Asymptomatic or mild respiratory illness
B. Moderate respiratory illness
   1. Temperature of >100.4° F (>38° C)* *and*
   2. One or more clinical findings of respiratory illness (e.g., cough, shortness of breath, difficulty breathing, hypoxia)
C. Severe respiratory illness
   1. Temperature of >100.4° F (>38° C)* *and*
   2. One or more clinical findings of respiratory illness (e.g., cough, shortness of breath, difficulty breathing, hypoxia) *and*
      a. Radiographic evidence of pneumonia, *or*
      b. Respiratory distress syndrome, *or*
      c. Autopsy findings consistent with pneumonia or respiratory distress syndrome without an identifiable cause

EPIDEMIOLOGIC CRITERIA:

- Travel (including transit in an airport) within 10 days of onset of symptoms to an area with current or previously documented or suspected community transmission of SARS, *or*
- Close contact[†] within 10 days of onset of symptoms with a person known or suspected to have SARS.
- The Chinese horseshoe bat, which is a healthy carrier of SARS, has been identified as the reservoir of the virus in nature. The spread of the virus was facilitated by people eating bats or using bat feces in traditional medicine for asthma, kidney ailments, and general malaise.

Laboratory criteria:
- Confirmed:
   1. Detection of antibody to SARS-CoV in a serum sample, *or*

---

*A measured documented temperature of >100.4° F (>38° C) is preferred. However, clinical judgment should be used when evaluating patients for whom a measured temperature of >100.4° F (>38° C) has not been documented. Factors that might be considered include patient self-report of fever, use of antipyretics, presence of immunocompromising conditions or therapies, lack of access to health care, and inability to obtain a measured temperature. Reporting authorities should consider these factors when classifying patients who do not strictly meet the clinical criteria for this case definition.

[†]Close contact is defined as having cared for or lived with a person known to have SARS or having a high likelihood of direct contact with respiratory secretions and/or body fluids of a patient known to have SARS. Examples of close contact include kissing or embracing, sharing eating or drinking utensils, close conversation (<3 ft), physical examination, and any other direct physical contact between persons. Close contact does not include activities such as walking by a person or sitting across a waiting room or office for a brief period.

---

   2. Detection of SARS-CoV RNA by reverse-transcription polymerase chain reaction (PCR) confirmed by a second PCR assay by using a second aliquot of the specimen and a different set of PCR primers, *or*
   3. Isolation of SARS-CoV
- Negative:
   1. Absence of antibody to SARS-CoV in a convalescent-phase serum sample obtained >28 days after symptom onset[‡]
- Undetermined:
   1. Laboratory testing either not performed or incomplete

Case classification[§]:
- Probable case: meets the clinical criteria for severe respiratory illness of unknown etiology and epidemiologic criteria for exposure; laboratory criteria confirmed or undetermined.
- Suspect case: meets the clinical criteria for moderate respiratory illness of unknown etiology and epidemiologic criteria for exposure; laboratory criteria confirmed or undetermined.

Exclusion criteria: a case may be excluded as a suspect or probable SARS case if:
- An alternative diagnosis can fully explain the illness.
- The case has a convalescent-phase serum sample (i.e., obtained >28 days after symptom onset) that is negative for antibody to SARS-CoV.[‡]
- The case was reported on the basis of contact with an index case that was subsequently excluded as a case of SARS, provided other possible epidemiologic exposure criteria are not present.

SYNONYMS

SARS

ICD-9CM CODES
Not available

[‡]The World Health Organization has specified that the surveillance period for China should begin on November 1; the first recognized cases in Hong Kong, Singapore, and Hanoi (Vietnam) had onset in February 2003. The date for Toronto is linked to the occurrence of a laboratory confirmed case of SARS in a U.S. resident who had traveled to Toronto; the date for Taiwan is linked to the Centers for Disease Control and Prevention (CDC) issuing travel recommendations.

[§]The last date for illness onset is 10 days (i.e., one incubation period) after removal of a CDC travel alert. The case patient's travel should have occurred on or before the last date the travel alert was in place.

Assays for the laboratory diagnosis of SARS-CoV infection include enzyme-linked immunosorbent assay, indirect fluorescent-antibody assay, and reverse-transcription PCR assays of appropriately collected clinical specimens (Source: CDC: *Guidelines for collection of specimens from potential cases of SARS.* Available at http://www.cdc.gov/ncidod/sars/specimen_collection_sars2.htm). Absence of SARS-CoV antibody from serum obtained <28 days after illness onset,[‡] a negative PCR test, or a negative viral culture does not exclude SARS-CoV infection and is not considered a definitive laboratory result. In these instances a convalescent serum sample obtained >28 days after illness is needed to determine infection with SARS-CoV.

EPIDEMIOLOGY & DEMOGRAPHICS

- The disease was first recognized in Asia in February 2003 and spread to more than 2 dozen countries in North and South America, Europe, and Asia over the next several months, affecting more than 8000 patients and resulting in more than 750 deaths. In July 2003, cases were no longer being reported, and SARS outbreaks worldwide were considered contained.
- Most reported cases of SARS in the United States were attributed to exposure through foreign travel to countries with community transmission of SARS, with only limited secondary spread to close contacts such as family members and health care workers.
- Incubation period is 2 to 10 days.
- Evidence of airborne transmission of the SARS virus and laboratory-acquired SARS have now been documented.

PHYSICAL FINDINGS & CLINICAL PRESENTATION[¶]

- Early manifestations: fever, myalgias, and headache. Fever is often high and associated with chills or rigors. Fever may be absent in elderly patients.
- Dry, nonproductive cough occurs within 2 to 4 days of onset of fever.
- Diarrhea may occur in up to 25% of cases.
- Dyspnea and hypoxemia follow the cough and may require intubation in nearly 20% of patients.
- A biphasic course of illness may occur with initial improvement followed by subsequent deterioration in some patients.

ETIOLOGY

SARS-associated coronavirus

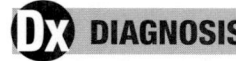 **DIAGNOSIS**

DIFFERENTIAL DIAGNOSIS

- Legionella pneumonia
- Influenza A and B
- Respiratory syncytial virus
- Acute respiratory distress syndrome (ARDS)

WORKUP

Initial diagnostic testing for suspected SARS patients should include chest radiograph, pulse oximetry, blood cultures, sputum Gram stain and culture, and testing for viral respiratory pathogens, notably influenza A and B and respiratory syncytial virus. A specimen for Legionella and pneumococcal urinary antigen testing should also be considered.

LABORATORY TESTS

When to test for SARS:
- In the absence of documented SARS transmission, diagnostic testing for SARS-

---

[¶]Asymptomatic SARS-CoV infection or clinical manifestations other than respiratory illness might be identified as more is learned about SARS-CoV infection.

associated coronavirus (SARS-CoV) should *not* be considered unless the clinician and health department have a high index of suspicion for SARS (e.g., a hospitalized pneumonia patient has a possible SARS exposure during travel and no other explanation for their pneumonia).

- Respiratory specimens should be collected as soon as possible in the course of the illness. The likelihood of recovering most viruses diminishes markedly >72 hours after symptom onset.
- Three types of specimens may be collected for viral or bacterial isolation and PCR. These include (1) nasopharyngeal wash/aspirates, (2) nasopharyngeal swabs, or (3) oropharyngeal swabs. Nasopharyngeal aspirates are the specimen of choice for detection of respiratory viruses and are the preferred collection method among children aged <2 yr.
- Laboratory testing on initial evaluation should also include CBC with differential, platelet count, liver enzymes, LDH, and CPK. Common laboratory abnormalities in SARS include thrombocytopenia, lymphopenia, elevated LDH, and elevated CPK, ALT, AST.

IMAGING STUDIES
- Chest x-ray: patchy focal infiltrates or consolidation with peripheral distribution.
- Chest x-ray may be normal in up to 25% of patients.
- Pleural effusions generally are not present.

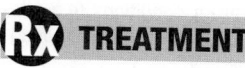 **TREATMENT**

NONPHARMACOLOGIC THERAPY
- Supportive care.
- Nearly 25% of cases will require ventilator assistance.
- Nutritional support.

ACUTE GENERAL Rx
- There is no specific treatment currently available for SARS.
- Broad-spectrum antibiotics (quinolone or macrolide) are generally started pending laboratory testing.

- Use of corticosteroids (methylprednisolone 40 mg bid or doses up to 2 mg/kg/day) is controversial but may be beneficial in patients with significant hypoxemia and progressive pulmonary infiltrates.
- In a preliminary, uncontrolled study of patients with SARS, use of interferon alfacon-1 plus corticosteroids was beneficial.

DISPOSITION
- Case fatality rate is 3% to 12%.
- Mortality rate is higher in elderly and immunocompromised patients and lower in pediatric age group.

REFERRAL
- Infectious disease consultation and pulmonary consultation is recommended in all cases.
- Notification of state Department of Health is mandatory.

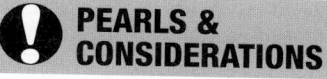 **PEARLS & CONSIDERATIONS**

COMMENTS
- Persons who may have been exposed to SARS should be vigilant for fever (i.e., measure temperature twice daily) and respiratory symptoms over the 10 days after exposure. During this time, in the absence of both fever and respiratory symptoms, persons who may have been exposed to SARS patients need not limit their activities outside the home and should not be excluded from work, school, out-of-home child care, church, or other public areas.
- Exposed persons should notify their health care provider immediately if fever or respiratory symptoms develop.
- Symptomatic persons exposed to SARS should follow the following infection control precautions:
  1. If fever or respiratory symptoms develop, the person should limit interactions outside the home and not go to work, school, out-of-home child care, church, or other public areas. In addition, the person

should use infection control precautions in the home to minimize the risk for transmission, and continue to measure temperature twice daily.
  2. If symptoms improve or resolve within 72 hr after first symptom onset, the person may be allowed, after consultation with local public health authorities, to return to work, school, out-of-home child care, church, or other public areas, and infection control precautions can be discontinued.
  3. For persons who meet or progress to meet the case definition for suspected SARS (e.g., develop fever and respiratory symptoms), infection control precautions should be continued until 10 days after the resolution of fever, provided respiratory symptoms are absent or improving.
  4. If the illness does not progress to meet the case definition, but the individual has persistent fever or unresolving respiratory symptoms, infection control precautions should be continued for an additional 72 hr, at the end of which time a clinical evaluation should be performed. If the illness progresses to meet the case definition, infection control precautions should be continued as described earlier. If case definition criteria are not met, infection control precautions can be discontinued after consultation with local public health authorities and the evaluating clinician.
- Persons who meet or progress to meet the case definition for suspected SARS (e.g., develop fever and respiratory symptoms) or whose illness does not meet the case definition, but who have persistent fever or unresolving respiratory symptoms over the 72 hr after onset of symptoms, should be tested for SARS coronavirus infection.

SUGGESTED READINGS
available at www.expertconsult.com

AUTHOR: **FRED F. FERRI, M.D.**

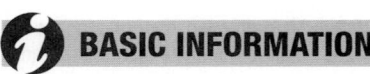

BASIC INFORMATION

DEFINITION

A sexual dysfunction in a woman is any disorder that interferes with female sexuality and that causes marked distress to that person. These disorders are generally categorized into four types:
1. Disorders of desire (most common)
2. Disorders of arousal
3. Orgasmic disorders
4. Sexual pain disorders (including dyspareunia, vaginismus, and vulvodynia)

Female sexual dysfunction is also further categorized as lifelong (primary) or acquired (secondary), situational (e.g., current partner) or generalized (all partners and settings).

SYNONYMS

Female sexual dysfunction

ICD-9CM CODES
302.70 Decreased libido
302.72 Disorders of arousal
302.73 Orgasmic disorders
625.x Sexual pain disorders

EPIDEMIOLOGY & DEMOGRAPHICS

INCIDENCE: According to the National Health and Social Life Survey, in 1999, ~20% to 50% of women reported some form of sexual dysfunction during their lifetimes. One third of women reported a decrease in sexual interest, and one fourth reported an inability to achieve orgasm.
PREVALENCE: A more recent survey of women 18 yr of age and older found an age-adjusted prevalence of any sexual problem to be ~43%.
PREDOMINANT AGE: Sexually related personal distress was more common in middle-aged women (aged 45 to 64) than in younger or older women.
RISK FACTORS: Correlates of distressing sexual problems include poor self-assessed health, low education level, depression, anxiety, thyroid conditions, and urinary incontinence.

PHYSICAL FINDINGS & CLINICAL PRESENTATION

- History:
  - Important to obtain the patient's definition of the dysfunction, including its onset and duration; to determine whether the dysfunction is situational or global; and to determine whether more than one dysfunction exists and the interrelationship among the dysfunctions
  - Related medical and gynecologic conditions (including prior gynecologic surgery)
  - Psychosocial factors, including sexual abuse, sexual orientation, depression, and anxiety, status of current relationships and sexual activity, personal and family beliefs about sexuality

  - Current medications including OTC and herbal preparations, alcohol, tobacco and drug use, and birth control method
- Physical examination:
  - The gynecologic examination can aid in identifying signs of decreased estrogen and androgen levels, infection, endometriosis, pelvic floor dysfunction, and systemic disease
  - Other body systems as indicated (e.g., cardiovascular, thyroid)

ETIOLOGY

- Chronic medical conditions (e.g., diabetes, coronary vascular disease, arthritis, urinary incontinence)
- Medication induced (e.g., antihypertensives, selective serotonin reuptake inhibitors (SSRIs)
- Gynecologic conditions (e.g., cystitis, posthysterectomy, gynecologic cancers, breast cancer [femininity/self-image issues; chemotherapy effects], postpregnancy, postmenopausal)
- Psychosocial (e.g., religion, taboos, identity conflicts, guilt, relationship problems, abuse, rape, life stressors)

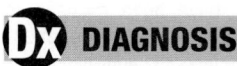

DIAGNOSIS

DIFFERENTIAL DIAGNOSIS

- Depression
- Psychosocial stressors
- Medical disease (e.g., thyroid dysfunction)

LABORATORY TESTS

- Cervical cultures and vaginal swabs for infectious disease
- Pap smear
- Appropriate laboratory tests if comorbid or chronic disease is suspected

IMAGING STUDIES

Appropriate imaging studies if comorbid or chronic disease is suspected

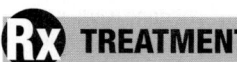

TREATMENT

NONPHARMACOLOGIC THERAPY

- Education including a discussion of normal sexual behavior
- Stress management
- Activities to enhance stimulation and eliminate routine
- Distraction techniques
- Noncoital behavior
- Position changes (e.g., female astride)
- Lubricants (e.g., nonpetroleum based). Zestra is an over-the-counter botanical massage oil applied to female genitalia that, according to manufacturer, increases sensation and facilitates arousal

ACUTE GENERAL Rx

NSAIDs before intercourse for sexual pain disorders

CHRONIC Rx

- Treat underlying medical, gynecologic, or psychologic conditions.
- Reduce comorbidities.
- For medication-induced conditions, decrease dose or change medication.
- For postmenopausal women or those with hypoestrogenism, try estrogen replacement therapy with or without progesterone.
- Testosterone therapy (some RCTs show an increase in satisfying sexual activity and sexual desire with treatment).
- Sildenafil (evidence from RCTs for use in patients with neurodegenerative disease and antidepressant-induced FSD after traditional therapy have failed). Data is conflicting. Phosphodiesterase inhibitors may increase blood flow to the genitalia but generally appear to have little benefit in treating female sexual dysfunction.
- Bupropion 300 to 400 mg/day was shown to increase sexual arousal and orgasm completion in a recent trial.
- Behavioral therapy (e.g., cognitive-behavioral therapy to reduce anxiety).

REFERRAL

- Gynecologic referral for conditions that may be amenable to surgical therapy
- Psychologic referral for conditions (e.g., depression, abuse) that may benefit from counseling or psychotherapy
- Social services referrals for active abuse issues

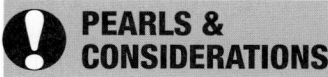

PEARLS & CONSIDERATIONS

COMMENTS

Identify the earliest cause in the chain and treat that first.

PATIENT/FAMILY EDUCATION

When appropriate, involve the patient's partner or significant other in treatment.

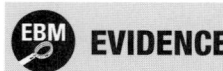

EVIDENCE

available at www.expertconsult.com

SUGGESTED READINGS

available at www.expertconsult.com

AUTHOR: **ANNGENE A. GIUSTOZZI, M.D., M.P.H., F.A.A.F.P.**

BASIC INFORMATION

DEFINITION

Sheehan's syndrome is a state of hypopituitarism resulting from an infarct of the pituitary secondary to postpartum hemorrhage or shock, causing partial or complete loss of the anterior pituitary hormones (adrenocorticotropic hormone [ACTH], follicle-stimulating hormone [FSH], luteinizing hormone [LH], growth hormone [GH], prolactin [PRL], thyroid-stimulating hormone [TSH]) and their target organ functions.

ICD-9CM CODES
253.2 Sheehan's syndrome

EPIDEMIOLOGY & DEMOGRAPHICS

INCIDENCE: One case in 10,000 deliveries (perhaps more rare in the U.S.)
PREDOMINANT SEX: Affects only females
RISK FACTORS:
- Hypovolemic shock
- Type 1 (insulin-dependent) diabetes mellitus (secondary to microvascular disease)
- Sickle cell anemia (secondary to occlusion of the small vessels in the pituitary)

ONSET OF SYMPTOMS: Average delay of 5 to 7 yr between onset of symptoms and diagnosis of disease.

PHYSICAL FINDINGS & CLINICAL PRESENTATION

- Failure of lactation
- Infertility
- Failure to resume menses after delivery
- Failure to regrow shaved pubic or axillary hair
- Skin depigmentation (including areola)
- Rapid breast involution
- Superinvolution of the uterus
- Hypothyroidism
- Adrenal cortical insufficiency
- Diabetes insipidus (rare)

ETIOLOGY

- Compromise of the blood supply to the low-pressure pituitary sinusoidal system may occur with postpartum hemorrhage or shock, resulting in pituitary infarct and/or necrosis.
- It is hypothesized that locally released factors may mediate vascular spasm of the pituitary blood supply.
- Severity of postpartum hemorrhage does not always correlate with the presence of Sheehan's syndrome.

DIAGNOSIS

DIFFERENTIAL DIAGNOSIS

- Chronic infections
- HIV
- Sarcoidosis
- Amyloidosis
- Rheumatoid disease
- Hemochromatosis
- Metastatic carcinoma
- Lymphocytic hypophysitis

WORKUP

- Target gland deficiency should be investigated by measuring levels of ACTH, FSH, LH, TSH (which may be normal or low), and T_4. Cortisol and estradiol (which may be low) should also be measured.
- Provocative testing of pituitary hormone reserves (e.g., metyrapone test, insulin tolerance test, and cosyntropin test): normal, subnormal, or delayed responses may suggest the presence of islands of pituitary cells that no longer have the support of the hypothalamic-portal circulation.
- Measurement of insulin-like growth factor-I to screen for GH deficiency: subnormal levels suggest decreased GH.
- Impaired prolactin response to TRH or dopamine antagonist stimulation is frequently found.
- During pregnancy, adjustments must be made in interpreting both hormone levels and responses to various stimuli because of normal physiologic changes.

IMAGING STUDIES

- Study of choice: MRI of the pituitary
  1. Sella turcica partially or totally empty
  2. Rules out mass lesion
- CT scan of the pituitary when MRI is unavailable or contraindicated

TREATMENT

ACUTE GENERAL Rx

- Acute form can be lethal, presenting with hypotension, tachycardia, failure to lactate, and hypoglycemia.
- A high degree of suspicion is required with any woman who has undergone postpartum hemorrhage and shock.
- IV corticosteroids and fluid replacement should be given initially.
- Diagnosis is confirmed with a full endocrinologic workup, as noted previously.
- Thyroid hormone is replaced as L-thyroxin in doses of 0.1 to 0.2 mg qd.

CHRONIC Rx

- With late-onset disease (symptoms of general hypopituitarism, such as oligomenorrhea or amenorrhea, vaginal atrophic changes, and loss of libido): a full endocrinologic workup and replacement of the appropriate hormones are needed.
- With symptoms of adrenal insufficiency: corticosteroids should be given.
  1. A maintenance dose of cortisone acetate or prednisone may be given.
  2. Because adrenal production of cortisol is not entirely dependent on ACTH, replacement of mineralocorticoids is rarely necessary.
  3. Stress doses of glucocorticoids should be administered during surgery or during labor and delivery.

DISPOSITION

Patients who receive early diagnosis and adequate hormonal replacement may expect favorable outcomes, including subsequent pregnancy.

REFERRAL

Patients should have yearly examinations by an endocrinologist.

SUGGESTED READING
available at www.expertconsult.com

AUTHORS: **BETH J. WUTZ, M.D.,** and **RUBEN ALVERO, M.D.**

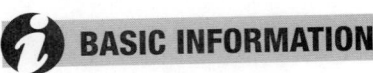

BASIC INFORMATION

DEFINITION
Shigellosis is an inflammatory disease of the bowel caused by one of several species of *Shigella*. It is the most common cause of bacillary dysentery in the U.S.

SYNONYMS
Bacillary dysentery

ICD-9CM CODES
004.9 Shigellosis

EPIDEMIOLOGY & DEMOGRAPHICS
INCIDENCE (IN U.S.): Approximately 15,000 cases/yr
PREDOMINANT SEX: Male homosexuals at increased risk
PREDOMINANT AGE: Young children
PEAK INCIDENCE: Summer
GENETICS: Neonatal infection: rare but severe

PHYSICAL FINDINGS & CLINICAL PRESENTATION
- Possibly asymptomatic, but incubation period can range from 1 to 7 days with an average of 3 days
- Mild illness that is usually self-limited, resolving in a few days
- Fever
- Watery diarrhea
- Bloody diarrhea
- Dysentery (abdominal cramps, tenesmus, and numerous, small-volume stools with blood, mucus, and pus)
- Descending intestinal tract illness, reflecting infection of small bowel first and then the colon
- Severe disease is more common in children and elderly and outside of U.S.
- Complications of severe illness:
  1. Seizures
  2. Megacolon
  3. Intestinal perforation
  4. Death
- Extraintestinal manifestations are rare
- Bacteremia is more common in children; in adults it has been described in patients with AIDS, the elderly, and diabetics
- Hemolytic-uremic syndrome (HUS): usually occurs as the initial illness seems to be resolving
- Reactive arthritis, sometimes as part of Reiter's syndrome

ETIOLOGY
- Shigella
  1. *S. flexneri*
  2. *S. dysenteriae*
  3. *S. sonnei*
  4. *S. boydii*
- *S. sonnei* is the most commonly isolated species in the U.S., and it usually causes a mild watery diarrhea.
- Direct person-to-person transmission is thought to be the most common route. Outbreaks among men who have sex with men have occurred because of direct or indirect oral-anal contact.
- Contaminated food or water may transmit disease.
- A recent outbreak occurred at a community wading pool frequented by toddlers.

DIAGNOSIS

DIFFERENTIAL DIAGNOSIS
- May mimic any bacterial or viral gastroenteritis
- Dysentery also caused by *Entamoeba histolytica*
- Bloody diarrhea may resemble disease caused by enterotoxigenic *E. coli*

LABORATORY TESTS
- Total WBCs may be low, normal, or high. Leukemoid reactions can occur in children.
- Stool should be cultured from fresh samples, because the yield is increased by processing the specimen soon after passage. The best yield is from the mucoid part of the stool.
- Serology is available but rarely useful.
- Polymerase chain reaction may be diagnostic.
- Fecal leukocyte preparation may show WBCs.

IMAGING STUDIES
Abdominal radiographs may suggest megacolon or perforation in rare, severe cases.

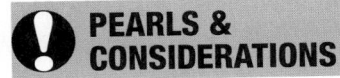 TREATMENT

NONPHARMACOLOGIC THERAPY
- Adequate hydration
- Electrolyte replacement

ACUTE GENERAL Rx
Antibiotics:
- To shorten course of illness.
- To limit transmission of illness.
- For children: IV ceftriaxone (50 mg/kg/day) for severe disease. For oral therapy, can use SMX/TMP or ampicillin for 5 days for susceptible strains. Azithromycin can be used for 5 days when susceptibilities still not known or in areas of high resistance (12 mg/kg for the first day, then 6 mg/kg/day for 4 days).
- For adults: Pending susceptibilities, ciprofloxacin 500 mg PO bid for 5 days should be used. If susceptible, can also use SMX/TMP one DS PO bid for 5 days. Azithromycin is a second alternative.

DISPOSITION
- Most disease is self-limited.
- Severe illness may be fatal.

REFERRAL
For severe illness or complications

PEARLS & CONSIDERATIONS

COMMENTS
- *Shigella* is one cause of "gay bowel syndrome."
- Illness is worsened by agents that decrease intestinal motility.
- Food handlers, child care providers, and health care workers should have a negative stool culture documented following treatment.

SUGGESTED READINGS
available at www.expertconsult.com

AUTHORS: **GLENN G. FORT, M.D., M.P.H.,** and **DENNIS J. MIKOLICH, M.D.**

BASIC INFORMATION

DEFINITION

Short bowel syndrome is a malabsorption syndrome that results from extensive small intestinal resection.

SYNONYMS

Short bowel

ICD-9CM CODES
579.3 (postsurgical malabsorption)

EPIDEMIOLOGY & DEMOGRAPHICS

- Parallels Crohn's disease (see "Crohn's Disease" in Section I), which is the most common cause of the syndrome in adults.
- In children, two thirds of short bowels are related to congenital abnormalities (intestinal atresia, gastroschisis, volvulus, aganglionosis) and one third are related to necrotizing enterocolitis.
- Prevalence: 10,000 to 20,000 cases are estimated to exist in the U.S.

PHYSICAL FINDINGS & CLINICAL PRESENTATION

- Diarrhea and steatorrhea
- Weight loss
- Anemia related to iron or vitamin B_{12} absorption
- Bleeding diathesis related to vitamin K malabsorption
- Osteoporosis/osteomalacia related to vitamin D and calcium malabsorption
- Hyponatremia, hypokalemia
- Hypovolemia
- Other macronutrient or micronutrient deficiency states

ETIOLOGY

- Extensive bowel resection for treatment of the conditions mentioned previously (see "Epidemiology").
- Pathogenesis (Fig. 1-342).

The human intestine is 3 to 8 m in length. Removal of up to half of the small intestine produces no disruption in nutrient absorption, and most patients can maintain nutritional balance on oral feeding if they have more than 100 cm (3 ft) of jejunum. Similarly, 100 cm of intact jejunum can maintain a normal water, sodium, and potassium balance under normal circumstances. The presence of an intact colon can compensate for some small intestine loss.

Site-specific functions:

- Calcium, magnesium, phosphorus, iron, and vitamins are absorbed in the duodenum and proximal jejunum.

- Vitamin B_{12} and bile acids are absorbed in the ileum. The resection of more than 60 cm of ileum results in vitamin B_{12} malabsorption. The loss of more than 100 cm results in fat malabsorption (from the loss of bile acids).
- The loss of gastrointestinal endocrine hormones can affect intestinal motility.
- Intestinal bacterial overgrowth may also occur, especially if the ileocecal valve is lost.

DIAGNOSIS

Presence of macronutrient and/or micronutrient loss in a patient with a known history of bowel resection

DIFFERENTIAL DIAGNOSIS

Because the history of significant bowel resection is typically known, there is no differential diagnosis. If that history is not known, all causes of weight loss, malabsorption, and diarrhea must be considered.

TREATMENT

Extensive small bowel resection with colectomy (<100 cm of jejunum)
- Rx: long-term total parenteral nutrition (TPN). Some patients can switch to oral intake after 1 to 2 yr of TPN. In jejunostomy patients, excessive fluid loss can be reduced with H_2 blockers, proton pump inhibitors, or octreotide. Micronutrients are supplemented.

Extensive small bowel resection with partial colectomy (usually patients with Crohn's disease)
- Rx: oral intake alone is possible in all patients with >100 cm of jejunum. In addition to vitamin B_{12} deficiency, these patients often have diarrhea. Consider lactose malabsorption and bacterial overgrowth treated, respectively, with lactose restriction and antibiotics (tetracycline 250 mg tid or metronidazole 500 mg tid for 2 wk). Nonspecific antidiarrheal agents may also be indicated (e.g., Imodium or codeine). The patient must be monitored for micronutrient losses.

COMPLICATIONS

- Oxalate kidney stones
- Cholesterol gallstones
- D-Lactic acidosis

PROGNOSIS

Directly dependent on the extent of the bowel resection and in the case of Crohn's disease by the underlying illness

AUTHOR: **FRED F. FERRI, M.D.**

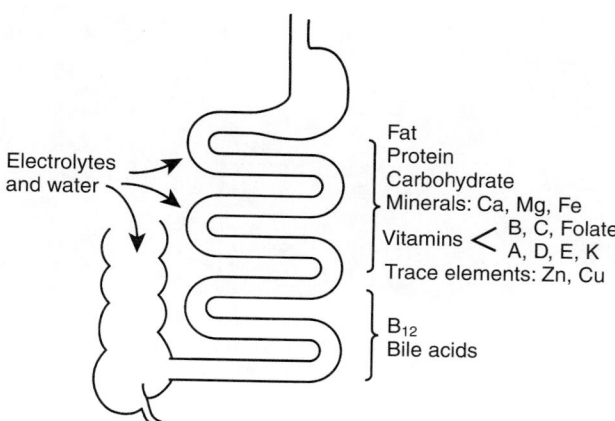

FIGURE 1-342 Specific areas of absorption of constituents of diet and secretions in the gastrointestinal tract. Macronutrients and micronutrients are predominantly absorbed in the proximal jejunum. Bile acids and vitamin B_{12} are only absorbed in the ileum. Electrolytes and water are absorbed in both the small and the large intestine. (From Feldman M et al [eds]: *Sleisenger and Fortran's gastrointestinal and liver disease: pathophysiology, diagnosis, and management,* ed 6, Philadelphia, 1998, WB Saunders.)

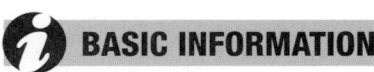
BASIC INFORMATION

DEFINITION
Sialadenitis is an inflammation of the salivary glands.

ICD-9CM CODES
527.2 Sialadenitis

EPIDEMIOLOGY & DEMOGRAPHICS
Parotid or submandibular glands are most frequently affected (Fig. 1-343).

PHYSICAL FINDINGS & CLINICAL PRESENTATION
- Pain and swelling of the affected salivary gland
- Increased pain with meals
- Erythema, tenderness at the duct opening
- Purulent discharge from duct orifice
- Induration and pitting of the skin, with involvement of the masseteric and submandibular spatial planes in severe cases

ETIOLOGY
- Ductal obstruction is generally from a mucus plug caused by stasis of saliva with increased viscosity with subsequent stasis and infection.
- Most frequent infecting organisms are *Staphylococcus aureus, Pseudomonas, Enterobacter, Klebsiella, Enterococcus, Proteus,* and *Candida* spp.
- Sjögren's syndrome, trauma, radiation therapy, chemotherapy, dehydration, and chronic illness are predisposing factors.

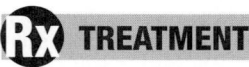
DIAGNOSIS

DIFFERENTIAL DIAGNOSIS
- Salivary gland neoplasm
- Ductal stricture
- Sialolithiasis
- Decreased salivary secretion as a result of medications (e.g., amitriptyline, diphenhydramine, anticholinergics)

WORKUP
- Generally not necessary
- Ultrasound or CT scan in patients not responding to medical treatment

LABORATORY TESTS
- Generally not indicated
- Complete blood count with differential to possibly reveal leukocytosis with left shift

IMAGING STUDIES
- Ultrasound or CT scan may be needed in patients not responding to medical therapy.
- Sialography should not be performed during the acute phase.

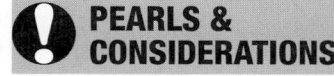
TREATMENT

NONPHARMACOLOGIC THERAPY
- Massage of the gland: may express pus and relieve some of the pressure
- Rehydration
- Warm compresses
- Oral cavity irrigations

ACUTE GENERAL Rx
- Amoxicillin-clavulanate 500 to 875 mg or cefuroxime 250 to 500 mg bid should be given for 10 days. Clindamycin is an alternative choice in patients allergic to penicillin.
- IV antibiotics (e.g., cefoxitin, nafcillin) can be given in severe cases.

DISPOSITION
Complete recovery unless the patient has underlying obstruction (e.g., ductal stricture, tumor, or stone)

REFERRAL
- To ear-nose-throat specialist for nonresolving cases despite appropriate antibiotic therapy
- For salivary gland incision and drainage, which may be necessary in resistant cases

PEARLS & CONSIDERATIONS

COMMENTS
Prevention of dehydration will decrease the risk of sialadenitis.

AUTHOR: **FRED F. FERRI, M.D.**

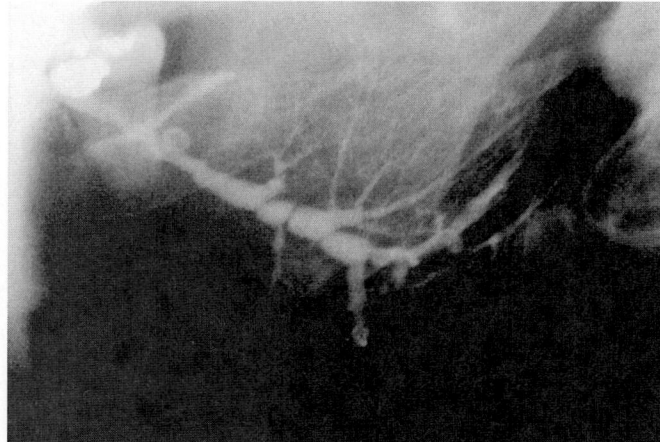

FIGURE 1-343 Sialogram of patient with chronic sialadenitis showing sausage link–like patterns and massive duct dilation. (From Blitzer CE et al: Sialadenitis. In Johnson JT, Yu VL [eds]: *Infectious diseases and antimicrobial therapy of the ears, nose, and throat,* Philadelphia, 1997, WB Saunders.)

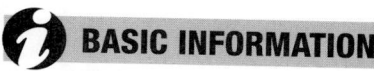

BASIC INFORMATION

DEFINITION

Sialolithiasis is the existence of hardened intra-luminal deposits in the ductal system of a salivary gland.

SYNONYMS

Salivary gland stone
Salivary calculus

ICD-9CM CODES
527.5 Sialolithiasis

EPIDEMIOLOGY & DEMOGRAPHICS

Affects patients mostly in the fifth to eighth decades and occurs most commonly in the submandibular gland (80%); only 14% are located in a parotid gland.

PHYSICAL FINDINGS & CLINICAL PRESENTATION

- Symptoms: colicky postprandial pain and swelling of a salivary gland. Tends to have a remitting/relapsing course.
- Signs: swelling and tenderness of a salivary gland. The stone may be felt by palpation of the floor of the mouth (Fig. 1-344).

ETIOLOGY

- The cause is unknown. Contributing factors include saliva stagnation, sialadenitis (inflammation of a salivary gland), ductal inflammation, or injury.
- Salivary calculus composition is mainly calcium phosphate and carbonate, often combined with small proportions of magnesium, zinc, ammonium salts, and organic materials or debris.

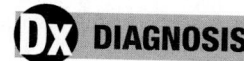

DIAGNOSIS

DIFFERENTIAL DIAGNOSIS

- Lymphadenitis
- Salivary gland tumor
- Salivary gland bacterial (*Staphylococcus* or *Streptococcus*), viral (mumps), or fungal infection (sialadenitis)
- Noninfectious salivary gland inflammation (e.g., Sjögren's syndrome, sarcoidosis, lymphoma)
- Salivary duct stricture
- Dental abscess

IMAGING STUDIES

- Plain radiograph
- Sialography

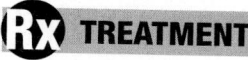

TREATMENT

- Warm soaks to area
- Antibiotics if associated bacterial sialadenitis is present
- Bland diet; avoid citrus fruit and spices
- Manual stone extraction sometimes associated with incisional enlargement of the ductal orifice
- Surgical salivary gland removal for retained hilar calculi

REFERRAL

To otorhinolaryngologist

AUTHOR: **FRED F. FERRI, M.D.**

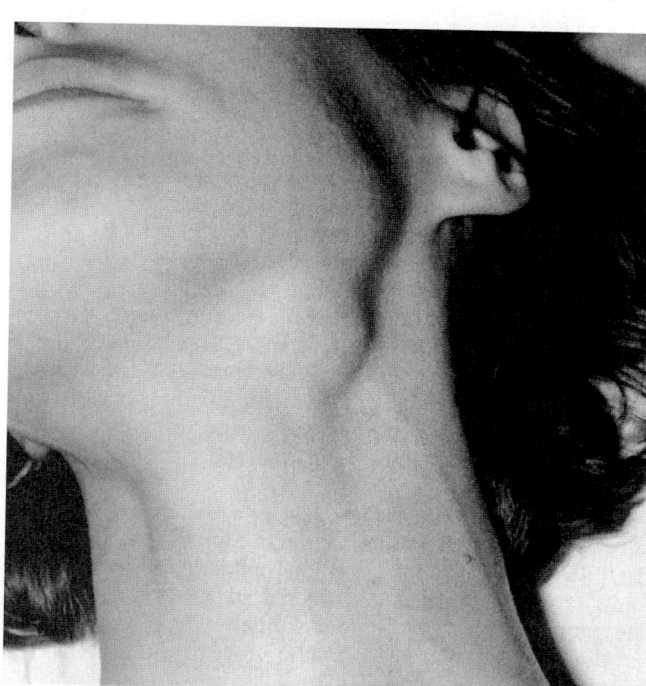

FIGURE 1-344 Patient with large calculus and obstruction of the left submandibular gland. (From Blitzer CE et al: Sialadenitis. In Johnson JT, Yu VL [eds]: *Infectious diseases and antimicrobial therapy of the ears, nose, and throat,* Philadelphia, 1997, WB Saunders.)

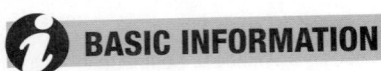 **BASIC INFORMATION**

DEFINITION

Sick sinus syndrome is a group of cardiac rhythm disturbances characterized by abnormalities of the sinus node including: (1) sinus bradycardia, (2) sinus arrest or exit block, (3) combinations of sinoatrial or atrioventricular conduction defects, and (4) alternating with paroxysmal supraventricular tachyarrhythmias (bradycardia-tachycardia syndrome) that result in atrial rates that are inappropriate for physiologic needs.

SYNONYMS

Bradycardia-tachycardia syndrome

ICD-9CM CODES
427.81 Sick sinus syndrome

EPIDEMIOLOGY & DEMOGRAPHICS

- In children: associated with congenital heart disease.
- In adults: primarily a disease of the elderly resulting from degenerative disease of the conduction system. It can also be seen at any age resulting from destruction of the sinus node due to other causes (i.e., ischemia or infarction, infiltrative diseases, endocrinologic abnormalities, etc.).

PHYSICAL FINDINGS & CLINICAL PRESENTATION

- Light-headedness, dizziness, syncope, palpitations.
- Physical examination may be normal or reveal abnormalities (e.g., heart murmurs or gallop sounds) associated with the underlying heart disease.

ETIOLOGY

- Fibrosis or fatty infiltration involving the sinus node, which may also affect the atrioventricular node, the His bundle, or its branches.
- In addition, inflammatory or degenerative changes of the nerves and ganglia surrounding the sinus nodes and other sclerodegenerative changes may be found.

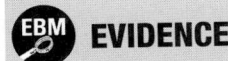 **DIAGNOSIS**

DIFFERENTIAL DIAGNOSIS

- Bradycardia: atrioventricular block
- Tachycardia: atrial fibrillation
- Atrial flutter
- Paroxysmal atrial tachycardia
- Sinus tachycardia

WORKUP

- ECG
- Ambulatory cardiac rhythm monitoring
- 24-hour ambulatory ECG (Holter) (Fig. 1-345)
- Event recorder
- Electrophysiologic testing, including sinus nodal recovery time and sino-atrial conduction time

Rx TREATMENT

- Permanent pacemaker placement. Indications for sinus node dysfunction are described in Table 1-163.
- In bradycardia-tachycardia syndrome, the drug treatment of the tachycardia (e.g., with digitalis or calcium channel blockers) may worsen or bring out the bradycardia and become the reason for pacemaker requirement.

REFERRAL

To cardiologist

EBM EVIDENCE

available at www.expertconsult.com

SUGGESTED READINGS

available at www.expertconsult.com

AUTHORS: **ALEXANDER G. TRUESDELL, M.D., FRED F. FERRI, M.D.,** and **WEN-CHIH WU, M.D.**

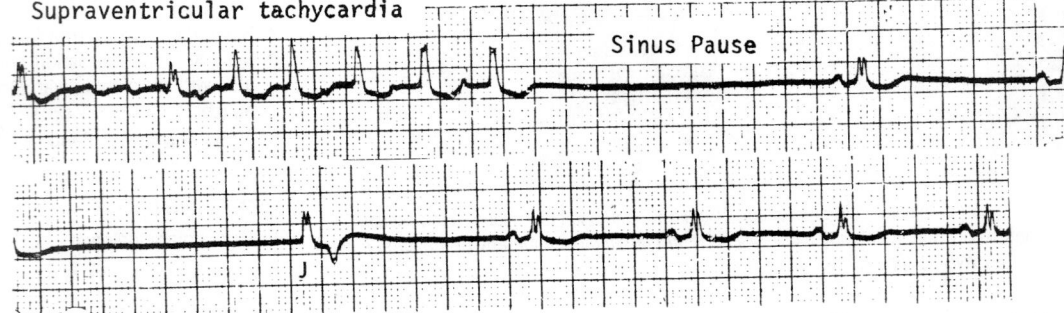

FIGURE 1-345 Brady-tachy (sick sinus) syndrome. This rhythm strip shows a narrow-complex tachycardia (probably atrial flutter) followed by a sinus pause, an AV junctional escape beat *(J)*, and then sinus rhythm. (From Goldberger AL: *Clinical electrocardiography*, ed 5, St Louis, 1994, Mosby.)

TABLE 1-163	Indications for Permanent Pacing in Sinus Node Dysfunction
Class	Indications
I	Sinus node dysfunction with documented symptomatic bradycardia. In some patients the bradycardia is iatrogenic and will occur as a consequence of essential long-term therapy of a type and dose for which there are no acceptable alternatives.
IIa	Sinus node dysfunction, occurring spontaneously or as a result of necessary drug therapy, with a heart rate of less than 40 bpm when a clear association between significant symptoms consistent with bradycardia has not been documented.
IIb	A chronic heart rate of less than 30 bpm, while awake, in the minimally symptomatic patient.
III	Sinus node dysfunction in asymptomatic patients, including those in whom substantial sinus bradycardia (heart rate of less than 40 bpm) is a consequence of long-term drug treatment. Sinus node dysfunction in which symptoms suggestive of bradycardia are clearly documented as not associated with a slow heart rate.

Crawford MH, DiMaxcro JP, Paulus WJ (eds): *Cardiology*, ed 2, St Louis, 2004, Mosby.

BASIC INFORMATION

DEFINITION

Sickle cell disease is a hemoglobinopathy characterized by the production of hemoglobin S caused by substitution of the amino acid valine for glutamic acid in the sixth position of the gamma-globin chain. When exposed to lower oxygen tension, red blood cells (RBCs) assume a sickle shape, resulting in stasis of RBCs in capillaries. Painful crises are caused by ischemic tissue injury resulting from obstruction of blood flow produced by sickled erythrocytes. Vasoocclusive crises are the main reason for hospital admission of children with SCD.

SYNONYMS

Sickle cell anemia
SCA
SCD
Hemoglobin S disease

ICD-9CM CODES
286.60 Sickle cell anemia

EPIDEMIOLOGY & DEMOGRAPHICS

- Sickle cell hemoglobin S is transmitted by an autosomal-recessive gene. It is found mostly in blacks (one in 400 black Americans).
- Sickle cell trait occurs in approximately 300 million people worldwide, with the highest prevalence of approximately 30% to 40% in sub-Saharan Africa. In the United States, it is found in nearly 10% of black Americans.
- It is estimated that 2000 babies are born with sickle cell disease in the U.S. each year.
- There is no predominant sex.

PHYSICAL FINDINGS & CLINICAL PRESENTATION

- Physical examination is variable depending on the degree of anemia and presence of acute vaso-occlusive syndromes or neurologic, cardiovascular, genitourinary, and musculoskeletal complications. Pain in adults with sickle cell disease is the rule rather than the exception and is far more prevalent and severe than reported in older large-scale surveys.
- There is no clinical laboratory finding that is pathognomonic of painful crisis of sickle cell disease. The diagnosis of a painful episode is made solely on the basis of the medical therapy and physical examination.
- Bones are the most common site of pain. Dactylitis, or hand-foot syndrome (acute, painful swelling of the hands and feet), is the first manifestation of sickle cell disease in many infants. Irritability and refusal to walk are other common symptoms. After infancy, musculoskeletal pain can be symmetric, asymmetric, or migratory, and it may or may not be associated with swelling, low-grade fever, redness, or warmth.
- In both children and adults, sickle vaso-occlusive episodes are difficult to distinguish

from osteomyelitis, septic arthritis, synovitis, rheumatic fever, or gout.
- When abdominal or visceral pain is present, care should be taken to exclude sequestration syndromes (spleen, liver) or the possibility of an acute condition such as appendicitis, pancreatitis, cholecystitis, urinary tract infection, pelvic inflammatory disease, or malignancy.
- Pneumonia develops during the course of 20% of painful events and can present as chest and abdominal pain. In adults chest pain may be a result of vaso-occlusion in the ribs and often precedes a pulmonary event. The lower back is also a frequent site of painful crisis in adults.
- The acute chest syndrome manifests with chest pain, fever, wheezing, tachypnea, and cough. Chest radiograph reveals pulmonary infiltrates. Common causes include infection (mycoplasma, chlamydia, viruses), infarction, and fat embolism.
- Musculoskeletal and skin abnormalities seen in sickle cell anemia include leg ulcers (particularly on the malleoli) and limb-girdle deformities caused by avascular necrosis of the femoral and humeral heads.
- Endocrine abnormalities include delayed sexual maturation and late physical maturation, especially evident in boys.
- Neurologic abnormalities on examination may include seizures and altered mental status.
- Infections, particularly involving *Salmonella, Mycoplasma,* and *Streptococcus,* are relatively common.
- Severe splenomegaly as a result of sequestration often occurs in children before splenic atrophy.

DIAGNOSIS

DIFFERENTIAL DIAGNOSIS

- Thalassemia
- Iron-deficiency anemia, leukemia
- The differential diagnosis of patients presenting with a painful crisis is discussed in "Physical Findings"

WORKUP

- Screening of all newborns regardless of racial background is recommended. Screening can be performed with sodium metabisulfite reduction test (Sickledex test).
- Hemoglobin electrophoresis will also confirm the diagnosis and is useful to identify hemoglobin variants such as fetal hemoglobin and hemoglobin A2.

LABORATORY TESTS

- Anemia (resulting from chronic hemolysis), reticulocytosis, leukocytosis, and thrombocytosis are common.
- Elevations of bilirubin and lactate dehydrogenase are also common.
- Peripheral blood smear may reveal sickle cells, target cells, poikilocytosis, and hypochromia (Fig. 1-346).
- Elevated blood urea nitrogen and creatinine may be present in patients with progressive renal insufficiency.
- Urinalysis may reveal hematuria and proteinuria.

IMAGING STUDIES

- Chest radiography is useful in patients presenting with chest syndrome. Cardiomegaly may be present on chest x-ray.
- Bone scan is useful to rule out osteomyelitis (usually the result of *Salmonella*). MRI scan is also effective in diagnosing osteomyelitis.
- CT scan or MRI of brain is often needed in patients with neurologic complications such as transient ischemic attack, cerebrovascular accident, seizures, or altered mental status.
- Transcranial Doppler ultrasonograhy (TCD) is a useful commodity to identify children with sickle cell anemia who are at risk for stroke, in adults magnetic resonance angiography (MRA) can be used instead of TCD.
- Doppler echocardiography can be used to diagnose pulmonary hypertension.

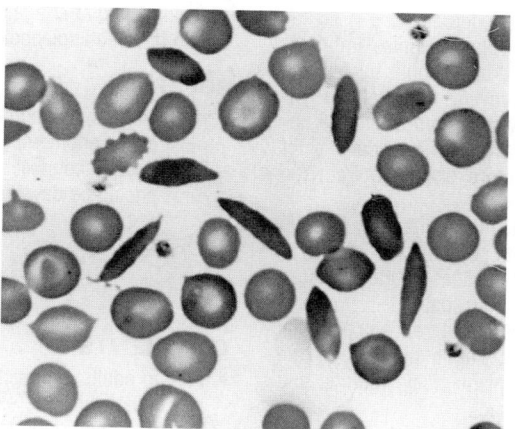

FIGURE 1-346 Photomicrograph of peripheral blood smear with sickle cells, typical of sickle cell anemia. (From Andreoli TE [ed]: *Cecil essentials of medicine,* ed 4, Philadelphia, 1997, WB Saunders.)

TREATMENT

NONPHARMACOLOGIC THERAPY

- Patients should be instructed to avoid conditions that may precipitate sickling crisis, such as hypoxia, infections, acidosis, and dehydration.
- Maintain adequate hydration (PO or IV).
- Correct hypoxia.

ACUTE GENERAL Rx

- Aggressively diagnose and treat suspected infections (*Salmonella* osteomyelitis and pneumococcal infections occur more often in patients with sickle cell anemia because of splenic infarcts and atrophy). Combination therapy with a cephalosporin and erythromycin plus incentive spirometry and bronchodilators is useful in patients with acute chest syndrome.
- Provide pain relief during the vaso-occlusive crisis. The fear of creating or perpetuating addiction or being deceived by patients often causes physicians to prescribe subtherapeutic dosages of opioids. However, available evidence suggests that the prevalence of drug addiction among patients with sickle cell anemia is no higher than in the overall U.S. population. Medications should be administered on a fixed time schedule with a dosing interval that does not extend beyond the duration of the desired pharmacologic effect.
  1. Meperidine is contraindicated in patients with renal dysfunction or central nervous system disease because its metabolite, normeperidine (which is excreted by the kidneys), can cause seizures.
  2. Narcotics (e.g., morphine 0.1 mg/kg IV q3-4h or 0.3 mg/kg PO q4h) should be given on a fixed schedule (not prn for pain), with rescue dosing for breakthrough pain as needed.
  3. Except when contraindications exist, concomitant use of nonsteroidal antiinflammatory drugs should be standard treatment.
  4. Nurses should be instructed not to give narcotics if the patient is heavily sedated or respirations are depressed.
  5. When the patient shows signs of improvement, narcotic drugs should be tapered gradually to prevent withdrawal syndrome. It is advisable to observe the patient on oral pain relief medications for 12 to 24 hr before discharge from the hospital.
  6. Analgesic medications should be used in combination with psychologic, behavioral, and physical modalities in the management of sickle cell disease.
- Aggressively diagnose and treat any potential complications (e.g., septic necrosis of the femoral head, priapism, bony infarcts, and acute chest syndrome).
- Avoid "routine" transfusions but consider early transfusions for patients at high risk for complications. Indications for transfusion include aplastic crises, severe hemolytic crises (particularly during third trimester of pregnancy), acute chest syndrome, and high risk of stroke.
- Hydroxyurea (15 mg/kg body weight per day in patients with normal creatinine clearance) increases hemoglobin F levels and reduces the incidence of vaso-occlusive complications. It is generally well tolerated. Side effects consist primarily of mild, reversible neutropenia. It should be avoided in patients with existing leukopenia, thrombocytopenia, or severe hypoplastic anemia. It is indicated for adults with sickle cell anemia who have moderate to severe disease, typically those with three or more acute painful crises or episodes of the acute chest syndrome in the previous year.
- Replace folic acid (1 mg PO qd) due to loss from increased utilization of folic acid stores due to chronic hemolysis. Sickle cell patients also often have mineral and vitamin deficiencies (calcium, zinc, and vitamins A, C, D, and E) and may need vitamin and nutritional supplementation.

CHRONIC Rx

- Guidelines for prompt management of fever, infections, pain, and specific complications should be reviewed.
- Genetic counseling is recommended in all cases.
- Avoid unnecessary transfusions. Exchange transfusions may be necessary for patients with acute neurologic signs, in aplastic crisis, or undergoing surgery. The target hemoglobin level is 10 to 11 g/dl (hematocrit 30%). Transfusing to a higher Hb/Hct should be avoided due to associated hyperviscosity if there is a substantial portion of HbS in the blood.
- Allogeneic stem cell transplantation can be curative in young patients with symptomatic sickle cell disease; however, the death rate from the procedure is nearly 10%, the marrow recipients are likely to be infertile, and there is an undefined risk of chemotherapy-induced malignancy.
- Penicillin V 125 mg PO bid should be administered by age 2 mo and increased to 250 mg bid by age 3 yr. Penicillin prophylaxis can be discontinued after age 5 yr except in children who have had splenectomy.

REFERRAL

- Hospitalization is generally recommended for most crises and complications.
- Psychosocial counseling and support structures should be developed.

ⓘ PEARLS & CONSIDERATIONS

COMMENTS

- Pain in adults with sickle cell disease is the rule rather than the exception and needs to be treated appropriately.
- Patients and their families should receive genetic counseling and should be made aware of the difference between sickle cell trait and sickle cell disease.
- Regular immunizations and pneumococcal vaccination are recommended. The prophylactic administration of penicillin soon after birth and the timely administration of pneumococcal and *Haemophilus influenzae* type b vaccines have resulted in a significant decline in the incidence of these infections. The heptavalent conjugated pneumococcal vaccine (Prevan) should be administered from 2 mo of age. The 23-valent unconjugated pneumococcal vaccine is given from age 2 yr and can be boosted once 3 yr later. Influenza vaccination can be given after 6 mo of age.
- Patients should be instructed on a well-balanced diet and appropriate folic acid supplementation.
- The presence of dactylitis, Hb 7, or leukocytosis in the absence of infection during the first 2 yr of life indicates a higher risk of severe sickle cell disease later in life.
- Among patients with sickle cell disease, acute chest syndrome is commonly precipitated by fat embolism and infection, especially community-acquired pneumonia. Among older patients and those with neurologic symptoms, the syndrome often progresses to respiratory failure.
- Poloxamer 188, a nonionic surfactant with hemorrheologic and antithrombotic properties, has been reported to produce a significant but relatively small decrease in the duration of painful episodes and an increase in the proportion of patients who achieved resolution of the symptoms. A more significant effect was observed in patients who received concomitant hydroxyurea.
- Pulmonary hypertension is a complication of chronic hemolysis and is associated with a high risk of death. It can be detected by Doppler echocardiography in more than 30% of adult patients with sickle cell disease. Cardiac catheterization will confirm the diagnosis. It is resistant to hydroxyurea therapy.
- Neurocognitive brain dysfunction is common in SCD. Trials have shown that compared with healthy controls, adults with SCD have a poorer cognitive performance, which is associated with anemia and age.
- Among patients with SCD hospitalized with vaso-occlusive pain crisis, the use of inhaled nitric oxide compared with placebo did not improve time to crisis resolution.
- The average lifespan of individuals with sickle cell trait is similar to that of the general population. However, it is associated with a higher incidence of renal medullary cancer.

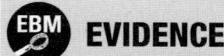 **EVIDENCE**

available at www.expertconsult.com

SUGGESTED READINGS

available at www.expertconsult.com

AUTHOR: **FRED F. FERRI, M.D.**

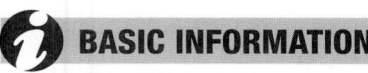

BASIC INFORMATION

DEFINITION

Silicosis is a lung disease attributable to the inhalation of silica (silicon dioxide) in crystalline form (quartz) or in cristobalite or tridymite forms.

SYNONYMS

Pneumoconiosis caused by silica

ICD-9CM CODES
502 Silicosis, occupational
503 Pneumoconiosis caused by other inorganic dust

EPIDEMIOLOGY & DEMOGRAPHICS

- Occupational disease affecting men and women involved in gathering, milling, processing, or using silica-containing rock or sand
- An estimated 1 million Americans are exposed

PHYSICAL FINDINGS & CLINICAL PRESENTATION

- Dyspnea
- Cough
- Wheezing
- Abnormal chest radiograph in an asymptomatic person

ETIOLOGY

- Silica particles are ingested by alveolar macrophages, which in turn release oxidants causing cell injury and cell death, attract fibroblasts, and activate lymphocytes, increasing immunoglobulins in the alveolar space.
- Hyperplasia of alveolar epithelial cells occurs.
- Collagen accumulates in the interstitium.
- Neutrophils also accumulate and secrete proteolytic enzymes, which leads to tissue destruction and emphysema.
- Silica dust may be carcinogenic (not proven).
- Exposure to silicosis predisposes to tuberculosis.
- Some patients develop rheumatoid silicotic pulmonary nodules and may have arthritic symptoms of rheumatoid arthritis (Caplan's syndrome). Scleroderma has also been associated with silicosis.

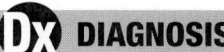

DIAGNOSIS

DIFFERENTIAL DIAGNOSIS

- Other pneumoconiosis, berylliosis, hard metal disease, asbestosis
- Sarcoidosis
- Tuberculosis
- Interstitial lung disease
- Hypersensitivity pneumonitis
- Lung cancer
- Langerhans' cell granulomatosis (histiocytosis X)
- Granulomatous pulmonary vasculitis

WORKUP

- History of occupational exposure
- Chest radiograph (Fig. 1-347)

Chronic silicosis:
- Characteristic finding: small, rounded lung parenchymal opacities
- Hilar lymphadenopathy with "eggshell" calcifications
- Pleural plaques (uncommon)

Accelerated silicosis (progressive massive fibrosis):
- Large parenchymal lesions resulting from coalesced small nodules

Acute silicosis:
- Ground-glass appearance of the lung fields
- Chest CT scan
- Pulmonary function tests
- Combination of obstructive and restrictive changes with or without reduction in diffusing capacity
- Bronchoscopy with lung biopsy in uncertain cases

COURSE

Chronic silicosis:
- May not progress with absence of further exposure
- Accelerated silicosis: progressive respiratory failure and cor pulmonale

Acute silicosis:
- Fatal course from respiratory failure over several months to a few years

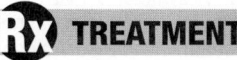

TREATMENT

- Prevention (industrial hygiene)
- Treatment of associated tuberculosis if present
- Supportive measures (oxygen, bronchodilators)
- Lung transplant

AUTHOR: **FRED F. FERRI, M.D.**

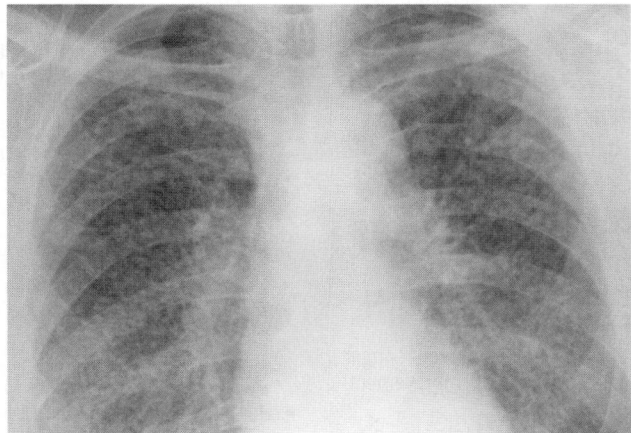

FIGURE 1-347 Simple silicosis. There are multiple small (2- to 4-mm) nodules distributed throughout the lungs, with an upper lobe predominance. (From McLoud TC: *Thoracic radiology: the requisites,* St Louis, 1998, Mosby.)

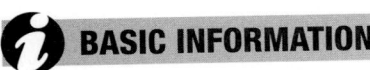

BASIC INFORMATION

DEFINITION

Sinusitis is inflammation of the mucous membranes lining one or more of the paranasal sinuses. The various presentations are:

- Acute sinusitis: infection lasting <4 wk, with complete resolution of symptoms.
- Subacute infection: lasts from 4 to 12 wk, with complete resolution of symptoms.
- Recurrent acute infection: episodes of acute infection lasting <30 days, with resolution of symptoms, which recur at intervals at least 10 days apart.
- Chronic sinusitis: inflammation lasting >12 wk, with persistent upper respiratory symptoms.
- Acute bacterial sinusitis superimposed on chronic sinusitis: new symptoms that occur in patients with residual symptoms from prior infection(s). With treatment, the new symptoms resolve but the residual ones do not.

SYNONYMS

Rhinosinusitis: sinusitis is almost always accompanied by inflammation of the nasal mucosa; thus it is now the preferred term.

ICD-9CM CODES

473.9 Sinusitis (accessory) (nasal) (hyperplastic) (nonpurulent) (purulent) (chronic)
461.9 Acute sinusitis

EPIDEMIOLOGY & DEMOGRAPHICS

INCIDENCE (IN U.S.): Seems to correlate with the incidence of upper respiratory tract infections
PEAK INCIDENCE: Fall, winter, spring: September through March

PHYSICAL FINDINGS & CLINICAL PRESENTATION

- Patients often give a history of a recent upper respiratory illness with some improvement, then a relapse.
- Mucopurulent secretions in the nasal passage:
  1. Purulent nasal and postnasal discharge lasting 7 to 10 days
  2. Facial tightness, pressure, or pain
  3. Nasal obstruction
  4. Headache
  5. Decreased sense of smell
  6. Purulent pharyngeal secretions, brought up with cough, often worse at night
- Erythema, swelling, and tenderness over the infected sinus in a small proportion of patients:
  1. Diagnosis cannot be excluded by the absence of such findings.
  2. These findings are not common, and do not correlate with number of positive sinus aspirates.
- Intermittent low-grade fever in about half of adults with acute bacterial sinusitis.

- Toothache is a common complaint when the maxillary sinus is involved.
- Periorbital cellulitis and excessive tearing with ethmoid sinusitis:
  1. Orbital extension of infection: chemosis, proptosis, impaired extraocular movements
- Characteristics of acute sinusitis in children with upper respiratory tract infections:
  1. Persistence of symptoms
  2. Cough
  3. Bad breath
- Symptoms of chronic sinusitis (may or may not be present):
  1. Nasal or postnasal discharge
  2. Fever
  3. Facial pain or pressure
  4. Headache
- Nosocomial sinusitis is typically seen in patients with nasogastric tubes or nasotracheal intubation.

ETIOLOGY

- Each of the four paranasal sinuses is connected to the nasal cavity by narrow tubes (ostia), 1 to 3 mm in diameter; these drain directly into the nose through the turbinates. The sinuses are lined with a ciliated mucous membrane (mucoperiosteum).
- Acute viral infection:
  1. Infection with the common cold or influenza
  2. Mucosal edema and sinus inflammation
  3. Decreased drainage of thick secretions/obstruction of the sinus ostia
  4. Subsequent entrapment o f bacteria
     a. Multiplication of bacteria
     b. Secondary bacterial infection
- Other predisposing factors:
  1. Tumors
  2. Polyps
  3. Foreign bodies
  4. Congenital choanal atresia
  5. Other entities that cause obstruction of sinus drainage
  6. Allergies
  7. Asthma
- Dental infections lead to maxillary sinusitis.
- Viruses recovered alone or in combination with bacteria (in 16% of cases):
  1. Rhinovirus
  2. Coronavirus
  3. Adenovirus
  4. Parainfluenza virus
  5. Respiratory syncytial virus
- The principal bacterial pathogens in sinusitis are *Streptococcus pneumoniae*, nontypeable *Haemophilus influenzae*, and *Moraxella catarrhalis*.
- In the remainder of cases find *Streptococcus pyogenes*, *Staphylococcus aureus*, beta-hemolytic streptococci, and mixed anaerobic infections (*Peptostreptococcus, Fusobacterium, Bacteroides, Prevotella* spp.).
- Infection is polymicrobial in about one third of cases.
- Anaerobic infections are seen more often in cases of chronic sinusitis and in cases asso-

ciated with dental infection; anaerobes are unlikely pathogens in sinusitis in children.
- Fungal pathogens are isolated with increasing frequency in immunocompromised patients but remain uncommon pathogens in the paranasal sinuses. Fungal pathogens include: *Phaeohyphomycoses, Aspergillus, Pseudallescheria, Sporothrix,* and *Zygomycetes* spp.
- Nosocomial infections: occur in patients with nasogastric tubes, nasotracheal intubation, cystic fibrosis, and patients who are immunocompromised.
  1. *S. aureus* (including MRSA)
  2. *Pseudomonas aeruginosa*
  3. *Klebsiella pneumoniae*
  4. *Enterobacter* spp.
  5. *Proteus mirabilis*
- Organisms typically isolated in chronic sinusitis:
  1. *S. aureus*
  2. *S. pneumoniae*
  3. *H. influenzae*
  4. *P. aeruginosa*
  5. Anaerobes

DIAGNOSIS

DIFFERENTIAL DIAGNOSIS

- Temporomandibular joint disease
- Migraine headache
- Cluster headache
- Dental infection
- Trigeminal neuralgia
- Allergic rhinitis
- Drugs (cocaine, decongestants overuse)
- GERD
- Wegener granulomatosis
- Cystic fibrosis

WORKUP

- The diagnosis is generally based on clinical signs and symptoms (purulent rhinorrhea and facial pain). Radiologic tests and cultures are not recommended initially and should be considered only when treatment is ineffective and sinusitis persists.
- In the normal healthy host, the paranasal sinuses should be sterile. Although the contiguous structures are colonized with bacteria and likely contaminate the sinuses, the mucociliary lining functions to remove these bacteria.
- Gold standard for diagnosis: recovery of bacteria in high density $\geq 10^4$ colony-forming units/ml from a paranasal sinus, in the setting of a patient with history of upper respiratory infection and symptoms persisting for 7 to 10 days. Sinus aspiration is the best method for obtaining cultures; however, it must be performed by an otorhinolaryngologist and is not practical for the primary care practitioner. Therefore, most diagnoses are based on the clinical history and presentation, possibly supported by radiologic evaluations.

1. Standard four-view sinus radiographs
   a. Complete opacification and air-fluid levels are most specific findings (average 85% and 80%, respectively)
   b. Mucosal thickening has low specificity (40% to 50%)
   c. Absence of all three of the previous findings has estimated sensitivity of 90%
   d. Overall, standard radiographs are of limited use in diagnosis, although negative films are strong evidence against the diagnosis
2. CT scans:
   a. Much more sensitive than plain radiographs in detecting acute changes and disease in the sinuses
   b. Recommended for patients requiring surgical intervention, including sinus aspiration; it is a useful adjunct to guide therapy
3. Transillumination:
   a. Used for diagnosis of frontal and maxillary sinusitis
   b. Place transilluminator in the mouth or against cheek to assess maxillary sinuses, under medial aspect of the supraorbital ridge to assess frontal sinuses
   c. Absence of light transmission indicates that sinus is filled with fluid
   d. Dullness (decreased light transmission) is less helpful in diagnosing infection
4. Endoscopy:
   a. Used to visualize secretions coming from the ostia of infected sinuses
   b. Culture collection via endoscopy often contaminated by nasal flora; not nearly as good as sinus puncture
5. Sinus puncture:
   a. Gold standard for collecting sinus cultures
   b. Generally reserved for treatment failures, suspected intracranial extension, and nosocomial sinusitis

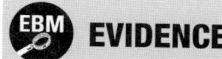 **TREATMENT**

NONPHARMACOLOGIC THERAPY

To help promote sinus drainage:
- Air humidification with vaporizers (for steam) or humidifiers (for a cool mist)
- Application of hot, wet towel over the face
- Sipping hot beverages
- Hydration

ACUTE GENERAL Rx

- Sinus drainage:
  1. Nasal vasoconstrictors, such as phenylephrine nose drops, 0.25% or 0.5%
  2. Topical decongestants should not be used for more than a few days because of the risk of rebound congestion

3. Systemic decongestants
4. Nasal or systemic corticosteroids, such as nasal beclomethasone, short course oral prednisone
5. Nasal irrigation, with hypertonic or normal saline (saline may act as a mild vasoconstrictor of nasal blood flow)
6. Use of antihistamines has no proven benefit, and the drying effect on the mucous membranes may cause crusting, which blocks the ostia, thus interfering with sinus drainage

- Analgesics, antipyretics

Antimicrobial therapy:
- Most cases of acute sinusitis have a viral cause and will resolve within 2 wk without antibiotics.
- Current treatment recommendations favor symptomatic treatment for those with mild symptoms. Physicians grossly overprescribe antibiotics for presumed bacterial sinusitis despite a much higher prevalence of viral infections.
- Antibiotics should be reserved for those with moderate to severe symptoms who meet the criteria for diagnosis of sinusitis.
- Antibiotic therapy is usually empiric, targeting the common pathogens:
  1. First-line antibiotics include amoxicillin, erythromycin, TMP-SMX.
  2. Second-line antibiotics include the newer macrolides: clarithromycin, azithromycin, amoxicillin/clavulanate, cefuroxime axetil, cefprozil, cefaclor, loracarbef, ciprofloxacin, levofloxacin, moxifloxacin, clindamycin, metronidazole, and others.
  3. For patients with uncomplicated acute sinusitis, the less expensive first-line agents appear to be as effective as the costlier second-line agents.
- Hospitalization and IV antibiotics may be required for more severe infection and those with suspected intracranial complications. Broader-spectrum antibiotic coverage may be indicated in severe cases, to cover for MRSA, *Pseudomonas,* and fungal pathogens.
- Duration of therapy generally 10 to 14 days, although some have success with much shorter regimens.

Surgery:
- Surgical drainage indicated
  1. If intracranial or orbital complications suspected
  2. Many cases of frontal and sphenoid sinusitis
  3. Chronic sinusitis recalcitrant to medical therapy
- Surgical debridement imperative in the treatment of fungal sinusitis

Complications:
- Untreated, sinusitis may lead to a number of serious, life-threatening complications.
- Intracranial complications include meningitis, brain abscess, and epidural and subdural empyema.

- Intracranial sequelae are more common with frontal and ethmoid infections.
- Extracranial complications include orbital cellulitis, blindness, orbital abscess, osteomyelitis.
- Extracranial sequelae are more commonly seen with ethmoid sinusitis.

CHRONIC Rx

- Broad-spectrum antibiotics that cover both aerobes and anaerobes
- Duration of therapy not clearly established: range 3 to 6 wk
- Adjunctive therapy: one or more of the various options listed previously
- Surgical intervention may be necessary in nonresponders

DISPOSITION

Appropriate diagnosis and treatment are necessary to avoid the various sequelae that can occur without proper therapy.

REFERRAL

- To infectious disease specialist if failure to respond to initial therapy
- To otorhinolaryngologist for:
  1. Failure to respond to therapy
  2. Suspected fungal infection
  3. Suspected intracranial or orbital complications

❗ PEARLS & CONSIDERATIONS

- Recurrent sinusitis is usually related to anatomic defects, poor drainage, or immunocompromised states; such patients deserve a thorough workup by an ENT specialist and/or an infectious disease specialist.
- Nosocomial sinusitis from obstruction by nasotracheal or nasogastric tubes is not uncommon and can be difficult to recognize in patients in the critical care units.

EBM EVIDENCE

available at www.expertconsult.com

SUGGESTED READINGS

available at www.expertconsult.com

AUTHORS: **GLENN G. FORT, M.D., M.P.H.,** and **DENNIS J. MIKOLICH, M.D.**

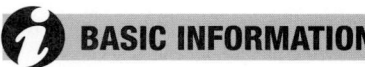

BASIC INFORMATION

DEFINITION

Sjögren's syndrome (SS) is an autoimmune disorder characterized by lymphocytic and plasma cell infiltration and destruction of salivary and lacrimal glands with subsequent diminished lacrimal and salivary gland secretions.
- Primary: dry mouth (xerostomia) and dry eyes (xerophthalmia) develop as isolated entities.
- Secondary: associated with other disorders.

SYNONYMS

SS
Sicca syndrome

ICD-9CM CODES
710.2 Sjögren's syndrome

EPIDEMIOLOGY & DEMOGRAPHICS

INCIDENCE & PREVALENCE: 1-2 million persons in the U.S. are affected. Prevalence is 0.05%-4.8% of population; secondary SS is also common and can affect up to one third of patients with systemic lupus erythematosus (SLE) and nearly 20% of rheumatoid arthritis (RA) patients.

PREDOMINANT SEX: Females are affected much more often than males.

PREDOMINANT AGE: Peak incidence is in the sixth decade.

PHYSICAL FINDINGS & CLINICAL PRESENTATION

- Dry mouth with dry lips (cheilosis), erythema of tongue (Fig. 1-348) and other mucosal surfaces, carious teeth
- Dry eyes (conjunctival injection, decreased luster, and irregularity of the corneal light reflex)
- Possible salivary gland enlargement and dysfunction, with subsequent difficulty in chewing and swallowing food and in speaking without frequent water intake
- Purpura (nonthrombocytopenic, hyperglobulinemic, vasculitic) may be present
- Evidence of associated conditions (e.g., RA or other connective tissue disease, lymphoma, hypothyroidism, chronic obstructive pulmonary disease, trigeminal neuropathy, chronic liver disease, polymyopathy)

ETIOLOGY

Autoimmune disorder

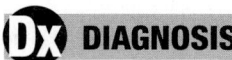

DIAGNOSIS

DIFFERENTIAL DIAGNOSIS

- Medication-related dryness (e.g., anticholinergics)
- Age-related exocrine gland dysfunction
- Mouth breathing
- Anxiety
- Other: sarcoidosis, primary salivary hypofunction, radiation injury, amyloidosis

WORKUP

Workup involves ocular and oral examination and laboratory and radiographic testing to demonstrate the following criteria for diagnosis of primary and secondary SS.

PRIMARY:
- Symptoms and objective signs of ocular dryness:
  1. Schirmer's test: <8 mm wetting per 5 min
  2. Positive rose bengal or fluorescein staining of cornea and conjunctiva to demonstrate keratoconjunctivitis sicca
- Symptoms and objective signs of dry mouth:
  1. Decreased parotid flow using Lashley cups or other methods
  2. Abnormal biopsy result of minor salivary gland (focus score >2 based on average of four assessable lobules)
- Evidence of systemic autoimmune disorder:
  1. Elevated titer of rheumatoid factor >1:320
  2. Elevated titer of antinuclear antibody (ANA) >1:320
  3. Presence of anti-SS A (Ro) or anti-SS B (La) antibodies

SECONDARY:
- Characteristic signs and symptoms of SS
- Clinical features sufficient to allow a diagnosis of RA, SLE, polymyositis, or scleroderma

LABORATORY TESTS

- Positive ANA (>60% of patients) with autoantibodies anti-SS A and anti-SS B may be present.
- Additional laboratory abnormalities may include elevated erythrocyte sedimentation rate, anemia (normochromic, normocytic), abnormal liver function studies, elevated serum $beta_2$ microglobulin levels, rheumatoid factor.
- A definite diagnosis of SS can be made with a salivary gland biopsy.

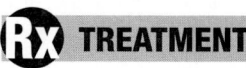

TREATMENT

NONPHARMACOLOGIC THERAPY

- Adequate fluid replacement. Ameliorate skin dryness by gently blotting dry after bathing, leaving a small amount of moisture, and then applying a moisturizer.
- Proper oral hygiene (daily topical fluoride use and antimicrobial mouth rinses) to reduce the incidence of caries. Sugar-free chewing gum and sour lemon lozenges to stimulate salivary secretion.
- Periodic dental and ophthalmology evaluations to screen for complications.

GENERAL Rx

- Use artificial tears frequently.
- Pilocarpine 5 mg PO qid is useful to improve dryness. A cyclosporine 0.05% ophthalmic emulsion (Restasis) may also be useful for dry eyes. Recommended dose is one drop bid in both eyes.
- Cevimeline (Evoxac), a cholinergic agent with muscarinic agonist activity, 30 mg PO tid is effective for the treatment of dry mouth in patients with SS.
- Interferon-alfa, 150 IU tid for 12 wk, has been shown to significantly improve stimulated whole saliva output and decrease reports of xerostomia.
- Hydroxychloroquine may be useful for arthralgias. Antitumor necrosis factor agents have not shown clinical efficacy and larger controlled trials are needed to establish the efficacy of rituximab for severe inflammatory manifestations.

PEARLS & CONSIDERATIONS

COMMENTS

- Unusual presentations of SS may occur in association with polymyalgia rheumatica, chronic fatigue syndrome, fever of unknown origin, and inflammatory myositis.
- The most serious complication of primary SS is the development of non-Hodgkin's lymphoma and other lymphoproliferative disorders.

SUGGESTED READING

available at www.expertconsult.com

AUTHOR: **FRED F. FERRI, M.D.**

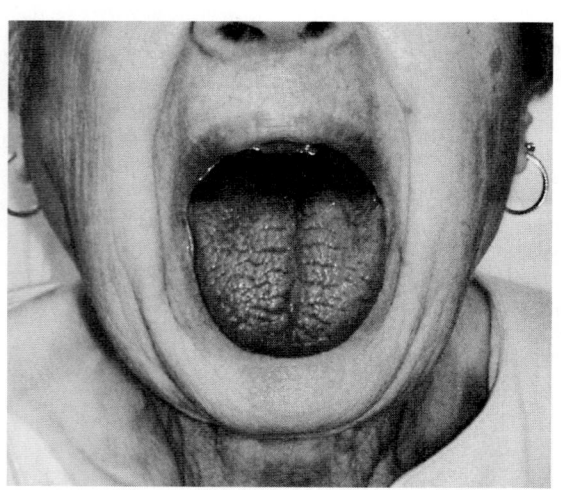

FIGURE 1-348 "Crocodile tongue" in a patient with Sjögren's syndrome. (From Noble J: *Primary care medicine*, ed 3, St Louis, 2001, Mosby.)

BASIC INFORMATION

DEFINITION

The *International Classification of Sleep Disorders, Second Edition*, classifies sleep-disordered breathing disorders into three categories: central sleep apnea syndrome, obstructive sleep apnea (OSA), and sleep-related hypoventilation/hypoxic syndromes. The American Academy of Sleep Disorders defines OSA as repetitive episodes of upper airway obstruction that occur during sleep and that are typically associated with oxyhemoglobin desaturations.

SYNONYMS

Sleep apnea syndrome
Sleep-disordered breathing
Obstructive sleep apnea syndrome
Obstructive sleep apnea–hypopnea syndrome

ICD-9CM CODES
327.2 Organic sleep apnea
327.21 Organic sleep apnea, unspecified
327.23 Obstructive sleep apnea (adult) (pediatric)

EPIDEMIOLOGY & DEMOGRAPHICS

OSA is a common disease in the U.S. Data from the Wisconsin Cohort Study indicated that the prevalence of OSA in people between the ages of 30 and 60 yr is 9% to 24% for men and 4% to 9% for women. The estimated prevalence of OSA is 4% for men and 2% for women. The prevalence is higher in obese and hypertensive patients. ~2% of children have OSA, which develops more commonly between the ages of 2 and 8 yr when adenotonsillar size is largest relative to size of the airway.

PHYSICAL FINDINGS & CLINICAL PRESENTATION

- Nocturnal symptoms.
- Snoring that can be loud, habitual, and bothersome to others.
- Witnessed apneas that often interrupt the snoring and that end with a snort.
- Gasping or choking sensations that arouse the patient from sleep.
- Restless sleep associated with frequent arousals.
- Daytime symptoms:
  - Nonrestorative sleep
  - Not feeling refreshed upon awakening
  - Morning headache
  - Dry mouth or throat upon awakening
  - Excessive daytime sleepiness, typically during quiet activities
  - Daytime fatigue or tiredness
  - Problems with memory, concentration, and cognitive function, especially with executive functioning
  - Easily angered, short tempered, and inattentive
  - Hyperactivity in children
- Systemic hypertension.
- Obesity (body mass index >30 kg/m^2).
- Mood swings, anxiety, depression, and decreased libido.
- A neck circumference of >43 cm (17 in) in men and of >37 cm (15 in) in women has been associated with an increased risk for OSA.
- The oropharynx may be erythematous as a result of snoring.
- Adenotonsillar hypertrophy, excessive soft tissue, high-arched hard palate, pendulous uvula, prominent tongue, large degree of overjet, and retrognathia or micrognathia can be present.
- A narrowing of the lateral airway walls is an independent predictor of OSA in men but not in women.
- Craniofacial skeletal abnormalities can lead to OSA, particularly among children and non-obese adults.
- A positive family history increases an individual's risk with each additional close family member with OSA.

ETIOLOGY

- Narrowing of upper airway as a result of obesity or increased peripharyngeal fat deposition, retrognathia and/or micrognathia, adenotonsillar hypertrophy, macroglossia, or neuromuscular weakness
- Upper airway muscular weakness as a result of neuromuscular disorders, primary central nervous system disorders (e.g., stroke), or metabolic disorders
- Other diseases associated with the development of OSA (e.g., hypothyroidism, acromegaly)

DIAGNOSIS

DIFFERENTIAL DIAGNOSIS

- Anemia
- Anxiety or panic disorder
- Behaviorally induced insufficient sleep syndrome
- Cardiac or heart disease
- Central sleep apnea
- Circadian rhythm disorder
- Depression
- Drug or alcohol abuse
- Hypothyroidism
- Idiopathic hypersomnia with long or short sleep time
- Inadequate sleep hygiene
- Insomnia
- Medication effect
- Narcolepsy
- Nocturnal asthma
- Nocturnal gastroesophageal reflux
- Obesity–hypoventilation syndrome (i.e., Pickwickian syndrome)
- Parasomnias
- Parkinson's disease
- Periodic limb movement disorder
- Primary snoring
- Pulmonary or lung disease
- Restless legs syndrome
- Sleep fragmentation (multiple causes)

WORKUP

- Evaluation should include questions about snoring, witnessed apneas, gasping or choking episodes, restless sleep, and excessive daytime sleepiness.
- Mood swings and personality changes should be addressed.
- Job performance and difficulty driving or previous motor vehicle accidents related to excessive daytime sleepiness should be discussed.
- Additional historic concerns include morning dry mouth or throat, morning headaches, alcohol intake, weight gain, and mood or personality changes.
- A thorough drug history should include muscle relaxants and sedatives.
- A family history should target any family members with OSA.
- The physical examination is frequently normal in patients with OSA except for the presence of obesity, enlarged neck circumference, and hypertension.
- OSA is confirmed by nocturnal polysomnography (PSG), which is the gold standard for diagnosis. The PSG should be performed during the patient's typical sleeping hours; it should all stages of sleep as well as sleep in the supine position.
- The severity of the OSA is determined by the apnea–hypopnea index (AHI), which is derived from the total number of apneas and hypopneas divided by the total sleep time.
- Recommended severity cutoff levels for the AHI are as follows:
  - Mild: 5 to 15 episodes per hour (with symptoms)
  - Moderate: 15 to 30 episodes per hour
  - Severe: >30 episodes per hour
- Criteria for the treatment of mild OSA often require symptoms, including excessive daytime sleepiness, cardiovascular disease, hypertension, and mood swings.
- In-home respiratory monitoring is an effective alternative to PSG for the evaluation of OSA.

LABORATORY TESTS

- Arterial blood gas testing should be performed if a patient has suspected pulmonary hypertension or cor pulmonale to rule out daytime hypoxemia or hypercapnia.
- The thyroid-stimulating hormone level should be obtained if hypothyroidism is suspected.
- A fasting glucose level is recommended since OSA increases the risk of developing diabetes independent of other risk factors.
- A CBC is helpful to look for anemia, and iron studies are indicated if anemia is detected.
- Pulmonary function testing is indicated if a pulmonary disorder is suspected or to assess the severity of neuromuscular disease, if present.
- An ECG or possibly an echocardiogram is indicated if a cardiac disorder (e.g., arrhythmia, pulmonary hypertension) is suspected.

IMAGING STUDIES

- Plain radiography of the neck can be helpful to assess the soft tissues of patients with suspected anatomic abnormalities.
- Chest x-ray is indicated if pulmonary disease is suspected.

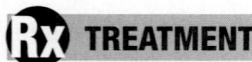 **TREATMENT**

NONPHARMACOLOGIC THERAPY

- Behavioral modifications:
  - Weight loss in overweight and obese patients, with consideration of bariatric surgery. Weight loss is effective for reducing the severity of OSA, and if significant, it may potentially allow some patients to discontinue continuous positive airway pressure (CPAP) therapy.
  - Avoidance of alcohol for 4 to 6 hr before bedtime
  - Avoidance of muscle relaxants and sedating medications
  - Sleep hygiene training
  - Avoidance or elimination of supine sleeping positions
- Medical treatment:
  - Continuous positive airway pressure (CPAP) is the primary therapy for OSA. It provides a pneumatic splint that relieves the upper airway obstruction.
  - An oral appliance constructed by a reputable and qualified dentist may be effective for the treatment of mild OSA in certain patients, especially those with retrognathia.
  - The optimal treatment of allergic rhinitis is needed; nasal corticosteroids are often helpful.
  - Symptoms of excessive daytime sleepiness may linger and require further investigation or medical therapy.

  - Patients should be considered for surgery if multiple attempts at CPAP therapy have failed and if an oral appliance is not an option. If the patient opts for surgery, ensure that the surgery is performed by a reputable and qualified otolaryngologist and that the surgery is based on the location of airway collapse.
- Surgical treatment:
  - Adenotonsillectomy is often curative for children with OSA.
  - Nasal septoplasty should be considered for patients with nasoseptal deformities.
  - Uvulopalatopharyngoplasty, which involves the resection of the uvula and the soft palate, is effective for a small number of patients. However, predicting which patients will benefit from the procedure is difficult.
  - Tracheostomy is typically reserved for patients with very severe OSA who cannot tolerate CPAP or who have cor pulmonale.

DISPOSITION

- The short-term prognosis for excessive daytime sleepiness and snoring is good to excellent with the regular use of nasal CPAP, but no studies have been performed to address the long-term effects in a large population of patients.
- Residual symptoms of excessive daytime sleepiness can occur in some patients with OSA despite regular CPAP use. This has led the U.S. Food and Drug Administration to approve modafinil (Provigil) for the management of residual sleepiness.

REFERRAL

- Highly trained sleep specialists with expertise in caring for patients with OSA are recommended, especially for complex cases.

- Surgical referral to otolaryngology should be considered for children and for adults who are unresponsive to weight loss and CPAP therapy.
- Referral to a qualified dentist for treatment with an oral appliance may be useful for certain patients with mild OSA.

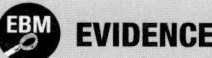 **PEARLS & CONSIDERATIONS**

- OSA is a common disorder that is underrecognized and underdiagnosed, so the identification of risk factors is crucial for making the correct diagnosis.
- The prevalence of OSA increases among women after menopause.
- The degree of tonsillar hypertrophy does not correlate with the presence of OSA in children.
- A 10% weight loss can decrease the AHI of a patient with OSA by as much as 50%.
- The single most effective therapy for OSA is nasal CPAP.
- Patients with OSA are more vulnerable than healthy persons to the effects of alcohol consumption and sleep restriction with regard to various driving performance variables.

EBM **EVIDENCE**

available at www.expertconsult.com

SUGGESTED READINGS
available at www.expertconsult.com

AUTHOR: **DON HAYES, JR., M.D.**

BASIC INFORMATION

DEFINITION

Smallpox infection is caused by the variola virus, a DNA virus member of the genus *Orthopoxvirus*. It is a human virus with no known nonhuman reservoir of disease. Natural infection occurs after implantation of the virus on the oropharyngeal or respiratory mucosa.

ICD-9CM CODES
050.9 Smallpox NOS
V01.3 Smallpox exposure
050.0 Smallpox, hemorrhagic (pustular)
050.1 Variola minor (alastrim)
050.0 Variola major

EPIDEMIOLOGY & DEMOGRAPHICS

- Smallpox infection was eliminated from the world in 1977. The last cases of smallpox, from laboratory exposure, occurred in 1978. The threat of bioterrorism has brought on renewed interest in the smallpox virus.
- Routine vaccination against smallpox ended in 1972.
- Smallpox is spread from person to person by infected saliva droplets in face-to-face contact with the ill person.
- Persons with smallpox are most infectious during the first week of illness, when the largest amount of virus is present in saliva; however, some risk of transmission lasts until all scabs have fallen off.
- The incubation period is approximately 12 days (range, 7 to 17 days) after exposure.
- Contaminated clothing or bed linens can also spread the virus. Special precautions need to be taken to ensure that all bedding and clothing of patients are cleaned appropriately with bleach and hot water. Disinfectants such as bleach and quaternary ammonia can be used for cleaning contaminated surfaces.

PHYSICAL FINDINGS & CLINICAL PRESENTATION

- Initial symptoms include high fever, fatigue, and headaches and backaches. A characteristic rash, most prominent on the face, arms, and legs, follows in 2 to 3 days (Fig. 1-349).
- The rash starts with flat red lesions that evolve at the same rate. The rash follows a centrifugal pattern.
- Lesions are firm to the touch, domed, or umbilicated. They become pus filled and begin to crust early in the second week.
- Scabs develop and then separate and fall off after approximately 3 to 4 wk. Depigmentation persists at the base of the skin lesions for 3 to 6 mo after illness. Scarring is usually most extensive on the face.
- Associated with the rash may be fever, headache, generalized malaise, vomiting, and colicky abdominal pain.
- Variola major may produce a rapidly fatal toxemia in some patients.

- Complications of smallpox include dehydration, pneumonia, blepharitis, conjunctivitis, and corneal ulcerations.

ETIOLOGY

Smallpox is caused by the variola virus. There are at least two strains of the virus, the most virulent known as *variola major* and a less virulent strain known as *variola minor* (alastrim).

DIAGNOSIS

DIFFERENTIAL DIAGNOSIS

- Rash from other viral illnesses (e.g., hemorrhagic chickenpox, measles, Coxsackie virus)
- Abdominal pain may mimic appendicitis
- Meningococcemia
- Insect bites
- Impetigo
- Dermatitis herpetiformis
- Pemphigus
- Papular urticaria

WORKUP & LABORATORY TESTS

- Laboratory examination requires high-containment (BL-4) facilities.
- Electron microscopy of vesicular scrapings can be used to distinguish poxvirus particles from varicella-zoster virus or herpes simplex. To obtain vesicular or pustular fluid it may be necessary to open lesions with the blunt edge of a scalpel. A cotton swab may be used to collect the fluid.
- In the absence of electron microscopy, light microscopy can be used to visualize variola viral particles (Guarnieri bodies) after Giemsa staining.
- Polymerase chain reaction techniques and restriction fragment-length polymorphisms can rapidly identify variola.

IMAGING STUDIES

Chest radiograph in patients with suspected pneumonia

TREATMENT

NONPHARMACOLOGIC THERAPY

- Supportive therapy
- IV hydration in severe cases
- A suspect case of smallpox should be placed in strict respiratory and contact isolation

ACUTE GENERAL Rx

- There is no proven treatment for smallpox. Vaccination administered within 3 to 4 days may prevent or significantly ameliorate subsequent illness. Vaccinia immune globulin can be used for treatment of vaccine complications and for administration with vaccine to those for whom vaccine is otherwise contraindicated.
- Patients can benefit from supportive therapy (e.g., IV fluids, acetaminophen for pain or fever).
- Antibiotics are indicated only if secondary bacterial infections occur. Penicillinase-resistant antimicrobial agents should be used if smallpox lesions are secondarily infected.
- Topical idoxuridine should be considered for corneal lesions.

DISPOSITION

- The mortality rate for variola major is 20% to 50%. Variola minor has a mortality rate of 1%.
- After severe smallpox, pitted lesions (most commonly on the face) are seen in up to 80% of survivors.
- Panophthalmitis and blindness from viral keratitis or secondary eye infection occur in 1% of patients.
- Arthritis caused by viral infection of the metaphysis of growing bones occurs in 2% of children.

REFERRAL

ID consultation and notification of local health authorities is mandatory in all cases of smallpox.

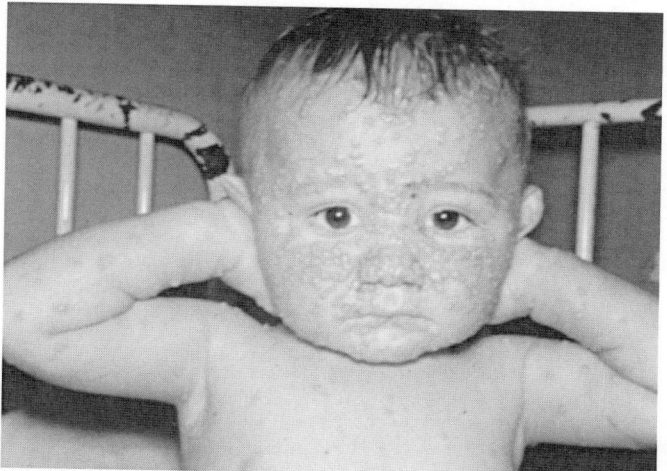

FIGURE 1-349 Appearance of the rash of smallpox on days 6 to 7. All the lesions are in the same stage of development. (From Gorbach SL: *Infectious diseases,* ed 2, Philadelphia, 1998, WB Saunders.)

! PEARLS & CONSIDERATIONS

- The smallpox virus is fragile; in the event of an aerosol release, all viruses will be inactivated or dissipated within 1 to 2 days. Buildings exposed to the initial aerosol release of the virus do not need to be decontaminated. By the time the first cases are identified, typically 2 wk after release, the virus in the building will be gone. Infected patients, however, will be capable of spreading the virus and possibly contaminating surfaces while they are sick. Standard hospital-grade disinfectants such as quaternary ammonias are effective in killing the virus on surfaces and should be used for disinfecting hospitalized patients' rooms or other contaminated surfaces. In the hospital setting, patients' linens should be autoclaved or washed in hot water with bleach added. Infectious waste should be placed in biohazard bags and autoclaved before incineration.
- Symptomatic patients with suspected or confirmed smallpox are capable of spreading the virus. Patients should be placed in medical isolation to avoid spread of the virus. In addition, people who have come into close contact with smallpox patients should be vaccinated immediately and closely watched for symptoms of smallpox.

COMMENTS

- In people exposed to smallpox, the vaccine can lessen the severity of or even prevent illness if given within 4 days of exposure.
- The vaccine against smallpox contains another live virus called *vaccinia*. The vaccine does not contain smallpox virus. Smallpox vaccination produces a skin lesion that is infectious. Vaccine virus in the skin lesion can be transferred to others if the skin lesion is touched directly or if the bandage is handled casually with ungloved hands. The vaccination site is infectious until the scab falls off, approximately 21 days after vaccination.
- Primary vaccination confers full immunity to smallpox in more than 95% of persons for up to 10 yr.

SUGGESTED READINGS

available at www.expertconsult.com

AUTHOR: **FRED F. FERRI, M.D.**

BASIC INFORMATION

DEFINITION

Social anxiety disorder (SAD) is a persistent and significant fear of being embarrassed or humiliated in social and/or performance situations. SAD commonly presents as excessive anxiety or fear in situations involving social interactions (e.g., conversing with one or a group of other individuals, with sexually attractive others, with authority figures) and/or performance situations (e.g., public speaking, acting/performing in front of an audience). The anxiety must persist in these situations for at least 6 mo in individuals younger than age 18. The anxiety often results in avoidance of these situations, thus leading to significant occupational, academic, and/or social impairment as well as marked distress. Currently two subtypes are described: specific (fear of one or only a few situations) and generalized (fear of many social situations).

SYNONYMS

Social phobia
SAD

ICD-9CM CODES
F40.1 (DSM-IV Code 300.23)

EPIDEMIOLOGY & DEMOGRAPHICS

INCIDENCE (IN U.S.): ~8% over a 12-mo period in epidemiologic samples
PEAK INCIDENCE: Highest standardized incidence rates per person-yr between 10 and 19 yr of age
PREVALENCE (IN U.S.): Lifetime prevalence of 12% in epidemiologic samples; point prevalence of up to 30% in outpatient clinical settings
PREDOMINANT SEX: More common in women than in men (ratio of 3:2) in epidemiologic samples; the two genders are equally represented in clinical settings
PREDOMINANT AGE: Mean age of onset ~16 yr of age; onset rarely occurs after age 25
GENETICS:
- Heritability ranges from 20% to 50%.
- 15% to 26% risk of SAD among first-degree relatives of those with SAD.

PHYSICAL FINDINGS & CLINICAL PRESENTATION

- Physical symptoms such as heart palpitations, sweating, shaking, and/or blushing, which may take the form of a panic attack.
- Fear that others will observe these physical symptoms in social situations and negatively judge them; fears that they will "say something stupid," make a mistake, or offend others also are common.
- Report being "shy" most of their lives.

- Comorbid psychiatric disorders (e.g., major depression, other anxiety disorders) and substance abuse (e.g., alcohol/cannabis) are common.
- Few seek treatment specifically for SAD, and instead initially seek treatment for other psychiatric disorders (e.g., major depression, other anxiety disorders).
- The onset of SAD often precedes that of the other comorbid psychiatric conditions.

ETIOLOGY

- There is no clear etiology and likely is a combination of multiple factors.
- Research has examined developmental psychology factors (e.g., lack of modeling of socialization by parents), temperamental factors (e.g., behavioral inhibition), and occurrence of prior traumatic social experiences (e.g., significant teasing by peers, being embarrassed or humiliated in a social or performance situation).
- The risk of SAD also may be increased with family history.

Dx DIAGNOSIS

DIFFERENTIAL DIAGNOSIS

- Other anxiety disorders (e.g., panic disorder with agoraphobia).
- As a consequence of mood disorders (e.g., avoidance of social situations associated with major depression).
- Pervasive developmental disorder (e.g., Asperger's disorder).
- Personality disorders (e.g., schizoid personality disorder); however, in the case of avoidant personality disorder, both may be diagnosed.
- Anxiety associated with medical conditions such as stuttering or Parkinson's disease.

WORKUP

- Psychiatric history is required for a diagnosis.
- Screening measures may improve detection of SAD as it is a chronic, disabling condition for which many individuals do not seek treatment.
- Physical examination may be useful in ruling out other explanations for physical symptoms that are present, and to rule out presence of social anxiety due to a medical condition.

Rx TREATMENT

NONPHARMACOLOGIC THERAPY

- Cognitive-behavior therapy (CBT)
- Exposure therapy
- Social skills training

PHARMACOLOGIC THERAPY

- SSRIs/SNRIs
- Benzodiazepines (less favored)

- MAOIs (less favored)
- Beta blockers (e.g., propanolol, atenolol: for performance-related anxiety)

ACUTE GENERAL Rx

- SAD is a chronic condition; therefore acute treatment is rarely indicated.
- However, benzodiazepines or beta blockers may be prescribed on an as-needed basis for acute performance anxiety; caution should be taken when prescribing benzodiazepines due to the possibility of dependence or misuse and high incidence of relapse following discontinuation.
- Beta blockers may also be prescribed on an as-needed basis, particularly for physical symptoms experienced during performance situations.

CHRONIC Rx

- SSRIs/SNRIs (e.g., paroxetine, sertraline, venlafaxine) are effective in the treatment of SAD and are a first-line pharmacologic treatment.
- MAOIs previously were considered "gold standard" treatment for SAD, but currently are less favorable due to side effects and dietary restrictions.
- CBT also is effective.
- Combination treatment of SSRI/SNRI and CBT is effective for SAD.

DISPOSITION

- SAD is a chronic condition, typically unremitting without treatment.
- Treatment may significantly improve SAD, although symptoms and impairment may continue to be present for some individuals following treatment.

REFERRAL

- If comorbid psychiatric conditions are present.
- If the symptoms do not improve upon treatment or response to treatment is not optimal.

EBM EVIDENCE

available at www.expertconsult.com

SUGGESTED READINGS
available at www.expertconsult.com

AUTHOR: **KRISTY L. DALRYMPLE, PH.D.**

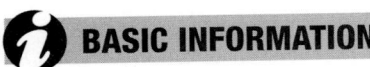

BASIC INFORMATION

DEFINITION

Somatization disorder refers to a pattern of recurring multiple somatic complaints that begin before the age of 30 yr and persist over several years. Patients complain of multiple sites of pain (a minimum of four), gastrointestinal symptoms (a minimum of two), a sexual or reproductive symptom, and a pseudoneurologic symptom. These cannot be explained by a medical condition or are in excess of an expected disability from a coexisting medical condition.

SYNONYMS

Briquet's syndrome
Nonorganic physical symptoms
Medically unexplained symptoms
Functional somatic symptoms

ICD-9CM CODES
300.81 Somatization disorder

EPIDEMIOLOGY & DEMOGRAPHICS

PREVALENCE (IN U.S.): Lifetime rates of 0.25% to 2% in women, ≤0.2% in men
PEAK INCIDENCE: Typically before age 25 yr
PREDOMINANT SEX: Women are more commonly affected in the U.S. (10:1 ratio)
PREDOMINANT AGE: Onset occurs before age 30 yr and usually in adolescence.
GENETICS: In males, there is a high risk of associated substance abuse or antisocial personality disorder.

PHYSICAL FINDINGS & CLINICAL PRESENTATION

- Onset is characteristically in the teens; course is marked by frequent, unexplained, and frequently disabling pain and physical complaints.
- Patient frequently undergoes multiple procedures and seeks treatment from multiple physicians. Symptom focus rotates periodically with new physicians sought for new complaints.
- Patient often has a comorbid psychiatric disorder, most commonly generalized anxiety, panic disorder, or depression.

ETIOLOGY

- Believed to be the physical expression of psychologic distress; there appears to be a biologic predisposition.
- May be more common in individuals without sufficient verbal or intellectual capacity to communicate psychologic distress, individuals with alexithymia (inability to describe emotional states), or individuals from cultural backgrounds that consider emotional distress as an undesirable quality.
- Some aspects of somatization behavior possibly learned from somatizing parents.

DIAGNOSIS

DIFFERENTIAL DIAGNOSIS

- Undifferentiated somatoform disorder (ICD-10 F45.1, DMS-IV 300.81): one or more physical complaints that cannot be explained by a medical condition are present for at least 6 mo (NOTE: Somatization disorder is more severe and less common).
- Conversion disorder: an alteration or loss of voluntary motor or sensory function without demonstrable physical cause and related to a psychologic stress or a conflict (NOTE: With multiple complaints, the diagnosis of conversion is not made).
- Pain disorder: distinguished from somatization disorder by the latter featuring multiple nonpain symptoms.
- Factitious disorder (e.g., Munchausen's syndrome) and malingering: the psychologic basis of the complaints in somatization disorder is not conscious as in factitious disorder, in which the goal is to be in the patient role, and malingering, in which symptoms are also produced consciously but for some secondary gain like a monetary award in litigation or opioids.

WORKUP

- Rule out a general medical condition.
- If somatization is suspected on the basis of a history of repeated, multiple, unexplained complaints, restraint in ordering tests is recommended.

LABORATORY TESTS

No specific laboratory tests are required.

IMAGING STUDIES

No specific imaging studies are required.

TREATMENT

NONPHARMACOLOGIC THERAPY

- Legitimize patient's complaints.
- Minimize diagnostic investigation and symptomatic treatment. Only do invasive testing or procedures when there are clear-cut signs, not just symptom reports.
- Set attainable treatment goals. Patients may benefit from realizing that even though they cannot be cured, that they will be cared for. This may help reassure them that they will continue to have a relationship with the physician.
- Treat coexisting psychiatric conditions such as depression and anxiety.

ACUTE GENERAL Rx

- At each visit do a brief physical examination focusing on the area of complaint.
- Gently praise increased functioning rather than focusing on symptoms.

- Explore recent life events and ask how the patient is handling these.
- Convey empathy with the patient's suffering and psychosocial difficulties.
- No specific pharmacologic therapy has been clearly proven effective, although a number of agents, including gabapentin and St. John's wort, have been useful in some studies.

CHRONIC Rx

- Provide one primary care practitioner to manage care.
- Avoid confronting the patient regarding the psychological origin of symptoms.
- Ensure follow-up visits at regular intervals (e.g., 2- to 4-wk intervals that are not symptom contingent; maintain the regularity even if the symptoms improve so that the patient does not need new symptoms to continue the relationship).
- Avoid invasive or expensive diagnostic procedures unless there are clear signs of new illness, not just symptoms.
- Diagnose and treat mood or anxiety disorders.
- Cognitive behavior therapy groups have been helpful for patients with unexplained somatic symptoms and can dramatically improve functioning.

DISPOSITION

A chronic condition with frequent exacerbations

REFERRAL

If the patient is open to discussing psychological issues, a referral for psychotherapy can be made.

PEARLS & CONSIDERATIONS

Patients with somatization disorder respond best to establishing a regular, working relationship with a primary care provider. Avoiding confrontations about the origins of symptoms, investigating symptoms when related to actual signs of disease, and gently investigating concurrent stressors will help avoid most of the common problems with this population.

Patients with subsyndromal symptoms (i.e., failing to meet the full criteria but having three or more medically unexplained symptoms) may be just as challenging and chronic. They warrant similar approaches as utilized for the full syndrome.

SUGGESTED READINGS
available at www.expertconsult.com

AUTHOR: **STUART J. EISENDRATH, M.D.**

BASIC INFORMATION

DEFINITION

Exaggerated tone, which displays a velocity-dependent increase in resistance of muscles to a passive stretch stimulus

SYNONYMS

Hypertonicity

ICD-9CM CODES

782.85 Spasm of muscle
342.1, 343.0-344.9 Spastic paralysis
781.0 Abnormal involuntary movements/ Spasms NOS
781.2 Abnormality of gait/spastic
342.1 Spastic hemiplegia
344.0-344.9 Spastic paralysis specified as noncongenital or noninfantile
343 Infantile cerebral palsy/spastic infantile paralysis

EPIDEMIOLOGY & DEMOGRAPHICS

INCIDENCE: Spasticity affects between 47% and 70% of people with multiple sclerosis, 32% to 36% of those with spinal cord injury, approximately 20% of those with stroke, more than 90% with cerebral palsy, and approximately 50% of patients with traumatic brain injury.

PREDOMINANT SEX AND AGE: Spasticity is not affected by sex, race, or age group, nor is it more prevalent in any of those groups.

RISK FACTORS: Multiple sclerosis, stroke, spinal cord injury, cerebral palsy, traumatic brain injury

PHYSICAL FINDINGS & CLINICAL PRESENTATION

- Patient may present with impaired gait, impaired limb function, decreased mobility, or discomfort due to increased muscle tone.
- Examine active and passive motion, reflexes, and function:
  - Strength may be normal to decreased. Isometric strength is typically greater than concentric strength.
  - Tone may be slightly to severely (modified Ashworth scale; see Table 1-164) increased to passive range of motion.
  - Reflexes are typically brisk.
  - Patient may have accompanied extensor plantar signs, clonus, or spontaneous flexor spasms.
  - Function may be impaired or enhanced due to increased tone.

ETIOLOGY

Upper motor neuron injury, most commonly due to multiple sclerosis, stroke, spinal cord injury, cerebral palsy, traumatic brain injury

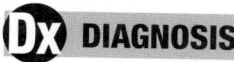

DIAGNOSIS

DIFFERENTIAL DIAGNOSIS

Rigidity, clonus, dystonia, dyskinesia, myotonia, tetanus, muscle contracture, cramps

WORKUP

- The diagnosis of spasticity can be established on a clinical basis alone.
- Investigate for reversible exacerbating causes of spasticity: underlying infection, bladder distention, bowel impaction, fracture, pain.

LABORATORY TESTS

Urinalysis, complete blood count, metabolic panel

IMAGING STUDIES

Chest x-ray, abdominal x-ray series, bladder ultrasound

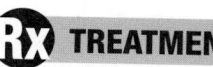

TREATMENT

First treat reversible causes of worsened spasticity (see "Workup"), then proceed to physical and pharmacologic therapeutics. Lastly, consider surgical intervention in severe, refractory cases.

NONPHARMACOLOGIC THERAPY

- Physical therapeutics include range of motion and muscle stretching, serial casting or orthotics, muscle cooling, electrical stimulation.
- Surgical procedures include tenotomy, tendon lengthening, and tendon transfers. More invasive surgical interventions include peripheral neurectomy, myelotomy, and rhizotomy.

ACUTE GENERAL Rx

- Oral medications: baclofen, tizanidine, diazepam, dantrolene (see Table 1-165)
- Other interventions: intrathecal baclofen, botulism toxin intramuscular injections, chemical nerve blocks (with bupivacaine, phenol, or ethyl alcohol)

COMPLEMENTARY & ALTERNATIVE MEDICINE

EMG biofeedback

DISPOSITION

Typically nonprogressive, but medications may lose efficacy after long duration of use. Drug holidays (with use of alternate spasmolytic) may be beneficial.

REFERRAL

- Physicians: neurologist or physiatrist with expertise in botulism toxin injection and/or intrathecal spasmolytic therapy is recommended in cases where oral medication is ineffective or not tolerated.
- Therapists: physical or occupational are recommended.

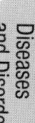

TABLE 1-164 Modified Ashworth Scale

0	No increase in muscle tone
1	Slight increase in muscle tone, manifested by a catch and release or by minimal resistance at the end range of motion when the part is moved in flexion or extension/ abduction or adduction
1+	Slight increase in muscle tone, manifested by a catch, followed by minimal resistance throughout the remainder (less than half) of the range of motion
2	More marked increase in muscle tone through most of the range of motion, but the affected part is easily moved
3	Considerable increase in muscle tone, passive movement is difficult
4	Affected part is rigid in flexion or extension (abduction or adduction)

From Stein J: Spasticity. In Frontera (ed): *Essentials of physical medicine and rehabilitation*, ed 2, Philadelphia, 2008, Saunders.

TABLE 1-165 Commonly Used Oral Spasmolytic Medications

Medication	Mechanism of Action	Starting Dose	Maximum Dose	Common Side Effects	Considerations†
Baclofen	GABA-B agonist	5 mg tid	20 mg qid*	Sedation, rare hepatotoxicity	Cognitive impairment
Diazepam	GABA-A agonist	2 mg bid	10 mg qid	Sedation, dependence or tolerance	History of substance abuse, cognitive impairment
Tizanidine	α-2 agonist	2 mg tid	12 mg tid	Sedation, hypotension, hepatotoxicity	Cognitive impairment
Dantrolene	Blocks Ca^{2+} release from sarcoplasmic reticulum	25 mg daily	100 mg qid	Weakness, hepatotoxicity	Liver disease

*Approved by the U.S. Food and Drug Administration only up to 80 mg/day, but many clinicians exceed this in patients who tolerate this medication well but do not respond to smaller doses.
†Baclofen, diazepam, and tizanidine are centrally acting and may exacerbate cognitive impairment. Dantrolene acts peripherally; however, it has the rare but fatal side effect of hepatotoxicity.
Modified from Stein J: Spasticity. In Frontera (ed): *Essentials of physical medicine and rehabilitation*, ed 2, Philadelphia, 2008, Saunders.

PEARLS & CONSIDERATIONS

- Assess whether the spasms recently increased in severity or intensity (as would occur with reversible exacerbating causes).
- Consider whether patient's tone is beneficial or detrimental to patient's functionality or overall health status.

- Spasticity may contribute to posture and mobility, as well as maintain muscle mass and bone mineralization, reduce dependent edema, and prevent deep venous thromboses.
- Spasticity may impair patient's functionality, interfere with activities of daily living, interfere with sleep, and cause discomfort.
- Monitor liver function with dantrolene and tizanidine, as these drugs may cause hepatotoxicity.

SUGGESTED READINGS
available at www.expertconsult.com

AUTHOR: **KARA A. KENNEDY, D.O.**

BASIC INFORMATION

DEFINITION

Spina bifida is the term for a group of neural tube disorders that involve the spinal column, including spina bifida occulta and spina bifida cystica. Anencephaly and cranium bifidum (i.e., encephalocele) are also classified as neural tube disorders, but these involve the cranium and brain and thus deserve a separate classification.

Spina bifida occulta is a midline defect that involves the closure of the posterior vertebral arches and laminae and that usually involves the L5-S1 area of the spinal cord.

Spina bifida cystica involves both meningocele and myelomeningocele. Meningocele is a midline defect in which meninges herniate through the posterior vertebral arch defect with a normal spinal cord in a normal position in the spinal canal; this condition makes up about 5% of cases of spina bifida cystica. Myelomeningocele is the most severe form of disease in the spectrum of spina bifida. The meninges, fragments of bone and cartilage, and the spinal cord herniate through the vertebral arches or the skin; this condition makes up about 95% of cases. The majority of these defects (~75%) are located in the lumbosacral area (Figs. 1-350 and 1-351).

SYNONYMS

Dysraphism
Meningomyelocele
Neural tube disorders

ICD-9CM CODES

756.17 Spina bifida occulta
741.9   Meningocele/myelomeningocele
        (without mention of hydrocephalus)

EPIDEMIOLOGY & DEMOGRAPHICS

INCIDENCE:
- Spina bifida occulta: 10% of the general pediatric population
- Spina bifida cystica: 0.15% of Caucasians, 0.04% of African Americans
- Highest in Ireland and lowest in Japan
- Influenced by season, economic status, maternal age, heat exposure, and a mother who has had other children with neural tube defects

PREVALENCE: About 12 infants are born daily with spina bifida or anencephaly.

PREDOMINANT SEX: Females are affected more frequently than males.

RISK FACTORS:
- Nutritional deficiency (specifically folate)
- Prior children with neural tube defects (risk increases 1.5% to 2%)
- If two prior children had spinal column defects, the risk increases 6% to 10%

GENETICS: Unknown

PHYSICAL FINDINGS & CLINICAL PRESENTATION

- Spina bifida occulta:
  - Most patients are asymptomatic and have a normal neurological examination.
  - In some cases, patients may have a patch of hair, a lipoma, skin discoloration, or a dermal sinus overlying the defect.
  - The condition is occasionally associated with syringomyelia, diastematomyelia, and a tethered cord.
- Meningocele:
  - Patients typically have a normal neurological examination; however, lesions may be accompanied by tethering, syringomyelia, or diastematomyelia.
  - Constipation or bladder dysfunction can develop as a result of an enlargement of the lesion.
- Myelomeningocele:
  - The lesion can be completely exposed, or it may have a skinlike membrane that covers it.

- The extent of the neurologic deficits depends on the level of the lesion:
  - Thoracolumbar: hypertonic bladder with normal anal tone
  - Below L2: flaccid tone; areflexic paraparesis; sensory loss in L3-L4 dermatomes; bladder and bowel incontinence; and poor anal sphincter tone, which can result in rectal prolapse
  - Below S3: motor deficits are absent; bladder and anal sphincter paralysis with saddle anesthesia
- Joint deformities include contractures, hip dislocations, scoliosis, clubfoot, and rocker-bottom foot.
- Hydrocephalus with Chiari type II malformations occurs in up to 90% of lumbosacral myelomeningoceles, and it is seen in more than half of cases at birth.
- Tethered cord disease manifests with a loss of motor function, spasticity with contractures, a rapid progression of scoliosis with bent posture, back pain, and changes in urodynamics.
- The condition is associated with disorders of cell migration that cause brain malformations, including heterotopia and schizencephaly.
- With this disease, there may also be multiorgan developmental disease (e.g., renal agenesis/anomalies, duodenal atresia, cardiac malformations, tracheoesophageal fistulas).

ETIOLOGY

- The posterior neuropore closes at about 26 to 28 days of gestation, which is typically before

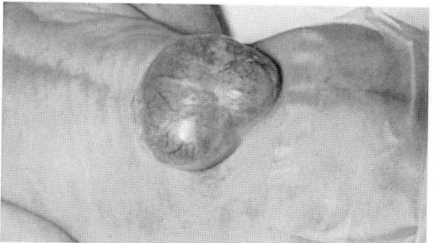

FIGURE 1-350 Lumbosacral myelomeningocele covered by an epithelialized membrane. (From Kliegman RM [ed]: *Nelson textbook of pediatrics*, ed 18, Philadelphia, 2007, Saunders.)

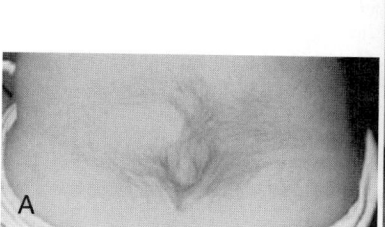
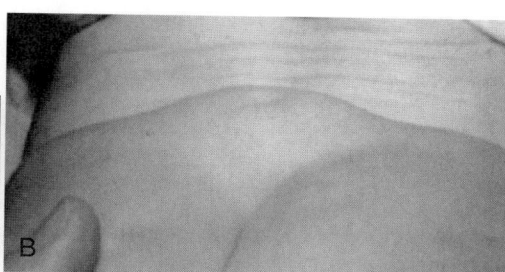
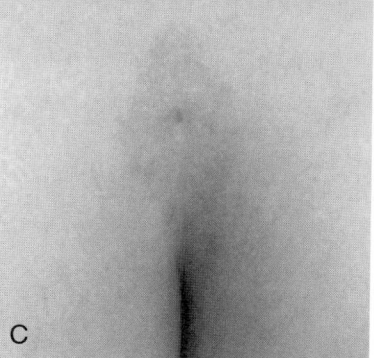

FIGURE 1-351 Examples of cutaneous malformations associated with spina bifida occulta. **A,** Tuft of hair. **B,** Sacral lipoma. **C,** Sinus tract that communicates with a dermoid tumor. (From Zitelli BJ, Davis HW [eds]: *Atlas of pediatric physical diagnosis,* ed 5, Philadelphia, 2007, Saunders.)

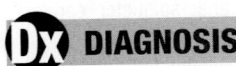

the mother has knowledge of the pregnancy. The failure of the closure results in any of the neural tube disorders, with the severity being dependent on the stage of development at closure (i.e., earlier in development results in spina bifida cystica vs. spina bifida occulta).

- The cause of the failure to close is unknown, but it is thought to be multifactorial and to involve genetic defects, environmental toxins, and folate deficiency.

Dx DIAGNOSIS

DIFFERENTIAL DIAGNOSIS
Isolated to this group of disorders

WORKUP
- Spina bifida occulta: none, unless foot deformities, neurogenic bladder, or neurologic deficits develop, which would be concerning for spinal cord pathology
- Spina bifida cystica: mostly includes imaging studies

LABORATORY TESTS
None

IMAGING STUDIES
- Ultrasound
- MRI of head and spine
- Computed tomography is a quicker study and would not require sedation; however, this method exposes the patient to radiation and therefore should be minimized.

Rx TREATMENT

- Spina bifida occulta: if asymptomatic with normal examination, none
- Meningocele: none
- Myelomeningocele: antiepileptic medications, if warranted

NONPHARMACOLOGIC THERAPY
- Spina bifida occulta: These is no nonpharmacologic therapy used for this condition, unless the patient develops neurological disease that is suggestive of underlying spinal cord disease.
- Meningocele: Most of these defects are covered by skin, so there is minimal risk of infection. If the patient has a normal examination with full-thickness skin, surgery can be delayed. However, if cerebrospinal fluid begins to leak or if the skin is thin, then immediate surgical correction is warranted.
- Myelomeningocele: Initial sac closure with a ventriculoperitoneal shunt is usually performed during the first 48 hr of life.
- The in utero closure of spinal lesions has been successful in a few centers, but there is a lack of evidence to support this procedure. The theory is that early closure possibly results in less severe motor disease, joint deformities, and sensory loss.

CHRONIC RX
- Involves a multidisciplinary approach that includes primary care, neurology, urology, orthopedic surgery, neurosurgery, and intense physical and occupational therapy
- Bladder catheterization to ensure the complete emptying of the bladder and the minimization of renal scarring
- Urodynamic evaluations
- Bowel training with stool softeners and enemas (An appendicostomy may be placed for antegrade enemas, if warranted.)
- The goal is to prevent the further loss of function and to maximize ambulation:
  - Close monitoring via physical examination for further worsening of clubfoot, spasticity, sensory loss as a result of possible shunt malfunction, or tethering of cord, which would warrant neurosurgical intervention
  - Orthotics
  - Physical and occupational therapy

- Frequent skin examinations to monitor for decubitus ulcer formation

DISPOSITION
- 70% of patients have normal intelligence; this is affected by episodes of meningitis and encephalitis
- Higher incidence of learning disorders and seizures as compared with the general population, which is likely related to brain malformations

! PEARLS & CONSIDERATIONS

PREVENTION
All women of childbearing age should take a daily multivitamin for folate supplementation (0.4 mg/day), because more than half of pregnancies are unplanned, and the greatest benefit is seen when supplements are taken for about 1 mo before conception. In addition, women who are taking valproic acid, carbamazepine, methotrexate, sulfamethoxazole/trimethoprim, and other medications that affect folate metabolism probably need a higher dose (e.g., 1 mg/day).

PATIENT/FAMILY EDUCATION
Spina Bifida Family Support and Spina Bifida Central have websites where families can share their experiences and information about their children.

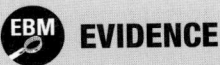 **EVIDENCE**
available at www.expertconsult.com

SUGGESTED READINGS
available at www.expertconsult.com

AUTHOR: **DONITA DILLON LIGHTNER, M.D.**

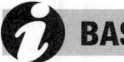 **BASIC INFORMATION**

DEFINITION

Spinal cord compression is the neurologic loss of spine function. Lesions may be complete or incomplete and develop gradually or acutely. Incomplete lesions often present as distinct syndromes, as follows:
- Central cord syndrome
- Anterior cord syndrome
- Brown-Séquard syndrome
- Conus medullaris syndrome
- Cauda equina syndrome

ICD-9CM CODES
344.89 Brown-Séquard syndrome
344.60 Cauda equina syndrome
336.8   Conus medullaris syndrome
Other lesions listed by site

PHYSICAL FINDINGS & CLINICAL PRESENTATION

Clinical features reflect the amount of spinal cord involvement:
- Motor loss and sensory abnormalities
- Babinski testing usually positive
- Clonus
- Gradual compression, often manifested by progressive difficulty walking, clonus with weight bearing, and involuntary spasm; development of sensory symptoms; bladder dysfunction (late)
- Central cord syndrome: results in a variable quadriparesis with the upper extremities more severely involved than the lower extremities; some sensory sparing

- Anterior cord syndrome: results in motor, pain, and temperature loss below the lesion
- Brown-Séquard syndrome:
  1. Spinal cord syndrome caused by injury to either half of the spinal cord and resulting in the loss of motor function, position, vibration, and light touch on the affected side
  2. Pain and temperature sense loss on the opposite side
- Conus medullaris syndrome: results in variable motor loss in the lower extremities with loss of bowel and bladder function
- Cauda equina syndrome: typical low back pain, weakness in both lower extremities, saddle anesthesia, and loss of voluntary bladder and bowel control

ETIOLOGY
- Trauma
- Tumor
- Infection
- Inflammatory processes
- Degenerative disk conditions with spinal stenosis
- Acute disk herniation
- Cystic abnormalities

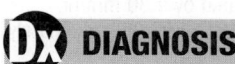 **DIAGNOSIS**

DIFFERENTIAL DIAGNOSIS
- See "Etiology."
- Section II describes the differential diagnosis of paraplegia.

WORKUP
- Spinal cord compression: requires an immediate referral for radiographic and neurologic assessment
- Laboratory results usually unremarkable unless infectious or inflammatory causes suspected

IMAGING STUDIES
- Depend on the suspected etiology
- MRI usually required

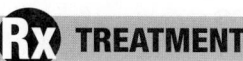 **TREATMENT**

Urgent surgical decompression is usually indicated as soon as the etiology is established.

DISPOSITION
Important indicators regarding prognosis:
- The greater the distal motor and sensory sparing, the greater the expected recovery.
- When a plateau of recovery is reached, no further improvement is expected.
- The quicker the recovery, the greater the recovery.

REFERRAL
Immediate referral for radiographic and neurologic evaluation and treatment in all suspected cases of spinal cord compression

SUGGESTED READINGS
available at www.expertconsult.com

AUTHOR: **LONNIE R. MERCIER, M.D.**

S

Diseases and Disorders

BASIC INFORMATION

DEFINITION

A spinal epidural abscess (SEA) is a focal suppurative infection occurring in the spinal epidural space.

ICD-9CM CODES
324.1 Spinal epidural abscess

EPIDEMIOLOGY & DEMOGRAPHICS

INCIDENCE (IN U.S.):
- 2 to 25 cases/100,000 hospitalized patients/yr
- May be increasing over the past 3 decades

PREDOMINANT AGE:
- Median age of onset approximately 50 yr (35 yr in intravenous drug users)
- Peak incidence in seventh and eighth decades of life

PHYSICAL FINDINGS & CLINICAL PRESENTATION

- The presentation of SEA can be nonspecific.
- Fever, malaise, and back pain are the most consistent early symptoms.
- Pain is often focal. It may initially be mild but can progress to become severe.
- As the disease progresses, root pain can occur, followed by motor weakness, sensory changes, bladder and bowel dysfunction, and paralysis.
- Physical findings may be limited to fever or spinal tenderness.
- The evolution to neurologic deficits can occur as quickly as a few hours, or over weeks to months.
- Once paralysis occurs, it may quickly become irreversible without the appropriate intervention.

ETIOLOGY

- Pyogenic bacteria account for the majority of cases in the U.S. Immigrants from TB-endemic areas may present with tuberculous SEAs. Fungi and parasites can also cause this condition. The most common causative organism is *Staphylococcus aureus*. Most posterior SEAs are thought to

originate from distant focus (e.g., skin and soft tissue infections), while anterior SEAs are commonly associated with diskitis or vertebral osteomyelitis. No source was found in approximately one third of cases.
- Associated predisposing conditions include diabetes mellitus, alcoholism, cancer, AIDS, and chronic renal failure, or following epidural anesthesia, spinal surgery or trauma, or IV drug use. No predisposing condition is found in approximately 20% of patients.
- Damage to the spinal cord can be caused by direct compression of the spinal cord, vascular compromise, bacterial toxins, and inflammation.

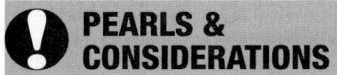 **DIAGNOSIS**

DIFFERENTIAL DIAGNOSIS

- Herniated disc
- Vertebral osteomyelitis and diskitis
- Metastic tumors
- Meningitis

LABORATORY TESTS

- WBC may be normal or elevated.
- ESR is usually elevated over 30 mm/hr.
- Blood cultures are positive in approximately 60% of patients with SEA.
- CSF cultures are positive in 19%, but lumbar puncture is unnecessary, and may be contraindicated.
- Once imaging is done, CT-guided aspiration or open biopsy should be done to determine causative organism. Abscess content culture is positive in 90% of patients.

IMAGING STUDIES

- MRI with gadolinium is the imaging modality of choice; CT scan with contrast may show the abscess but is less sensitive than MRI.
- CT with myelography is more sensitive for cord compression.

TREATMENT

NONPHARMACOLOGIC THERAPY

- Surgical decompression is the mainstay of treatment. Decompression within the first

24 hr has been related to an improved prognosis.
- Nonsurgical treatment is effective in some patients, but failure rate may be excessive. This approach should not be considered and should only be attempted in the absence of signs of compressive myelopathy and with very careful follow-up.

ACUTE GENERAL Rx

- In addition to surgery, antibiotics directed at the most likely organism should be initiated.
- If the organism is unknown, broad coverage against staphylococci, streptococci, and gram-negative bacilli should be initiated. The regimen can be adjusted according to culture results. Therapy should continue for at least 4 to 6 wk.

CHRONIC Rx

Neurologic deficits may remain despite aggressive treatment.

DISPOSITION

Irreversible paralysis and death can occur in up to 25% of patients.

REFERRAL

All cases should be referred to a neurosurgeon and an infectious disease specialist.

PEARLS & CONSIDERATIONS

It is critically important to recognize this process early; the prognosis is generally excellent if treatment is initiated while symptoms are localized and before evidence of myelopathy develops.

SUGGESTED READINGS
available at www.expertconsult.com

AUTHORS: **GLENN G. FORT, M.D., M.P.H.,** and **DENNIS J. MIKOLICH, M.D.**

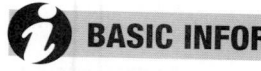 **BASIC INFORMATION**

DEFINITION

Spinal stenosis is the pathologic condition caused by the compressing or narrowing of the spinal canal, nerve root canal, or intervertebral foramina at the lumbar region.

SYNONYMS

Central spinal stenosis
Lateral spinal stenosis
Spondylosis

ICD-9CM CODES
724.02 Spinal stenosis lumbar, lumbosacral

EPIDEMIOLOGY & DEMOGRAPHICS

More common between 50 and 60 yr of age

PHYSICAL FINDINGS & CLINICAL PRESENTATION

- Symptoms caused by direct mechanical compression or indirect vascular compression of the nerve roots or the cauda equina.
- Neurogenic claudication: leg, buttock, or back pain precipitated by walking and relieved by sitting.
- Pain may radiate down to ankles and is associated with numbness, tingling, and weakness.
- Taking a flexed posture reduces symptoms because it increases the available space in the lumbar spinal canal.
- Decreased lumbar extension.
- Normal peripheral pulses.
- Positive Romberg's sign (decreased proprioception).
- Wide-based gait.
- Reduced knee and ankle reflex.
- Urine incontinence.

ETIOLOGY

Spinal stenosis may be primary or secondary
- Primary stenosis (congenital or developmental narrowing)
  1. Idiopathic
  2. Achondroplasia
  3. Morquio-Ullrich syndrome
- Secondary stenosis (acquired)
  1. Degenerative (hypertrophy of the articular processes, disk degeneration, ligamentum flavum hypertrophy, spondylolisthesis)
  2. Fracture/trauma
  3. Postoperative (postlaminectomy)
  4. Paget's disease
  5. Ankylosing spondylitis
  6. Tumors
  7. Acromegaly

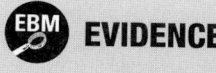 **DIAGNOSIS**

DIFFERENTIAL DIAGNOSIS

- Osteoarthritis of the knee or hip
- Acute cauda equina syndrome, resulting from compression by epidural abscess or tumors
- Pain and weakness caused by multiple myeloma or osteomyelitis
- Intermittent claudication—peripheral vascular disease

- Peripheral neuropathy such as that caused by a herniated nucleus pulposus
- Scoliosis or spondylolisthesis
- Rheumatoid diseases: ankylosing spondylitis, Reiter's syndrome, fibromyalgia
- Table 1-166 compares clinical features of spinal stenosis, peripheral vascular disease, and disc disease.

WORKUP

History, physical examination, and specific imaging studies

IMAGING STUDIES

- Lumbar spine film sensitivity 66%, specificity 93%.
- Ultrasound of the spinal canal has also been used.
- CT scan of the lumbosacral spine: sensitivity (75% to 85%), specificity (80%).
- MRI of the lumbosacral spine: sensitivity (80% to 90%), specificity (95%).
- Myelogram: sensitivity (77%), specificity (72%). Absolute stenosis is defined as the anterior-posterior (AP) diameter of the spinal canal <10 mm. Relative stenosis: 10 to 12 mm AP diameter.
- Electromyography (EMG) and nerve conduction velocity (NCV) are additional studies particularly useful in differentiating peripheral neuropathy from lumbar spinal stenosis.

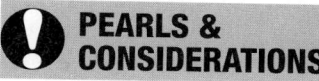 **TREATMENT**

NONPHARMACOLOGIC THERAPY

- Physiotherapy
- Lumbar corsets
- Back exercises
- Abdominal muscle strengthening
- Aquatic exercises

ACUTE GENERAL Rx

- Surgery is indicated in patients with significant compression of nerve roots as determined by MRI or CT and incapacitating symptoms limiting activities of daily living or bladder and bowel incontinence.
- Surgical procedures include decompressive laminectomy, arthrodesis, hemilaminectomy, and medial facetectomy.
- Lumbar interspinous process decompression using X-STOP device: a titanium oval spacer placed between the two adjacent spinous processes of the affected level; provides an unloading distractive force to the stenotic middle column part of the motion segment.

CHRONIC Rx

- Conservative therapy with NSAIDs (ibuprofen 800 mg PO tid, naproxen 500 mg PO bid) may be tried for symptomatic relief in addition to acetaminophen 1 g PO qid.
- Epidural steroid injections may provide temporary relief.

DISPOSITION

- Approximately 20% of patients having surgery require repeat surgery within 10 yr. Nearly one third of these patients continue to experience pain.
- The natural history of spinal stenosis is one of slow progression. Although not very common, cord compression with resultant bowel and bladder incontinence and paresis can occur.
- Operative treatment is more effective in reducing pain and disability than nonoperative treatment.

REFERRAL

- Patients who have spinal stenosis should be referred to an orthopedic surgeon specializing in back surgery or to a neurosurgeon.
- Pain clinic referrals should be made if surgery is contraindicated or if the patient does not want surgery.

PEARLS & CONSIDERATIONS

COMMENTS

- Approximately one third of patients have coexisting peripheral vascular disease.
- The severity of cauda equina constriction is directly related to the walking ability and the pain intensity in the legs and back.
- Spinal stenosis is also a cause of chronic low back pain in the young.

EBM EVIDENCE

available at www.expertconsult.com

SUGGESTED READINGS
available at www.expertconsult.com

AUTHOR: **JORGE A. VILLAFUERTE, M.D.**

TABLE 1-166 Comparative Clinical Features of Spinal Stenosis, Peripheral Vascular Disease, and Disc Disease

Feature	Spinal Stenosis	Disc Prolapse	Peripheral Vascular Disease
Reduced straight leg raise	Rarely	Usually	No
Neurologic deficit	Sometimes	Often	No
Leg pain on walking	Yes	Usually	Yes
Leg pain on sitting	No	Usually	Yes
Pain relief on standing still	No	Yes	No
Pain relief on sitting	No	No	Yes
Numbness/paresthesia	Yes	Yes	Sometimes

(From Carr A, Hamilton W: Orthopedics in primary care, ed 2, Philadelphia, 2005, Elsevier.)

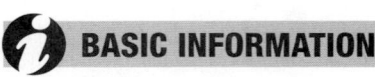

BASIC INFORMATION

DEFINITION

The spinocerebellar ataxias (SCAs) are a heterogeneous group of autosomal dominantly inherited genetic conditions that cause progressive ataxia.

SYNONYMS

Autosomal-dominant cerebellar ataxia (ADCA)
Machado-Joseph disease (eponym for SCA3; this may be the most common SCA)

ICD-9CM CODES

334.2 Primary cerebellar degeneration

EPIDEMIOLOGY & DEMOGRAPHICS

PREVALENCE: The prevalence of the condition is approximately 3 persons per 100,000. The most common SCAs are 1, 2, 3, 6, and 7.
PREDOMINANT SEX: SCA demonstrates no gender preference.
PREDOMINANT AGE: The age of onset is often during the 30s or 40s. However, this can be highly variable, even within family groups; SCAs can occur anytime from childhood to late adulthood.
GENETICS: All SCAs are inherited in an autosomal dominant fashion; however, reduced penetrance can be present.

PHYSICAL FINDINGS & CLINICAL PRESENTATION

- Chronically progressive ataxia is the predominant symptom of all of the SCAs. It typically presents as a combination of balance and gait difficulty, limb incoordination, and dysarthria.
- Previous nomenclature had grouped these conditions into ADCA type I (i.e., ataxia plus other neurologic symptoms, such as pyramidal, extrapyramidal, ophthalmoplegia, dementia, dystonia, or others); ADCA type II (i.e., ataxia with progressive retinopathy); and ADCA type III (i.e., pure cerebellar dysfunction). Current terminology preferentially involves the use of the SCA genetic classification.
- More than 30 different genetic subtypes of SCA have been described to date. Although certain clinical characteristics are common to specific SCA subtypes, there is significant overlap among and variability within these conditions, so making a diagnosis on the basis of the clinical presentation alone can be challenging and sometimes impossible without genetic testing. Some of the more common SCAs and their features include the following:
  - SCA1 can be characterized by ataxia, nystagmus, spasticity, and neuropathy.
  - SCA2 can be characterized by ataxia, slow saccades, gaze palsy, neuropathy, and sometimes parkinsonism or dementia.
  - SCA3, which is also known as *Machado-Joseph disease,* can be characterized by

ataxia, neuropathy, amyotrophy, parkinsonism, and dystonia.
  - SCA6 is generally felt to be a pure cerebellar syndrome with ataxia and nystagmus (gaze evoked and downbeat) as well as a frequently later age of onset.
  - SCA7 is characterized by ataxia, vision loss caused by a pigmentary maculopathy, and sometimes ophthalmoplegia.
  - Knowledge in this area is constantly expanding and being updated. Online sources of information (e.g., Online Mendelian Inheritance in Man [http://www.ncbi.nlm.nih.gov/omim]) can be invaluable for tracking new developments.

ETIOLOGY

Several of the SCAs are the result of polyglutamine CAG repeat expansions; this causes the accumulation of mutant proteins inside neurons, which is thought to cause dysfunction and cell death. Higher numbers of repeats are correlated with an earlier onset of symptoms, and anticipation may be present. Other types of repeat expansions and point mutations have been found with several SCAs; for others, the affected gene has not been identified.

DIAGNOSIS

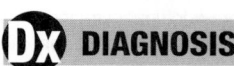

DIFFERENTIAL DIAGNOSIS

- Structural cerebellar abnormality: includes cerebellar tumor, inflammation (e.g., multiple sclerosis), stroke, or hemorrhage; the time course for these causes is typically more acute or subacute than chronic
- Endocrine dysfunction: hypothyroidism or hypoparathyroidism can uncommonly cause ataxia
- Alcoholic cerebellar degeneration: caused by heavy alcohol use; gait ataxia predominates
- Other toxin-induced ataxias: antiepileptic medications, lithium, and chemotherapeutic agents
- Creutzfeldt-Jakob disease: rapidly progressive ataxia, dementia, and myoclonus
- Paraneoplastic cerebellar degeneration: found in association with primary malignancies (e.g., small-cell lung cancer, breast cancer); subacute onset ataxia that progresses rapidly
- Celiac disease: gluten-sensitive enteropathy with malabsorption may be associated with ataxia; autoantibodies such as antigliadin or antiendomysial antibodies are typically present
- Multiple system atrophy: cerebellar variant of this disorder causes ataxia; there is typically associated parkinsonism with some degree of autonomic dysfunction (e.g., orthostatic hypotension, urinary incontinence)
- Friedreich's ataxia: autosomal recessive inheritance, generally younger age of onset (i.e., mean 15 yr of age), lower limb areflexia, and posterior column dysfunction
- Ataxia associated with vitamin E deficiency: can be an autosomal recessive disorder or acquired; clinically resembles Friedreich's

ataxia, with areflexia and loss of position sense
- Ataxia telangiectasia: autosomal recessive inheritance, childhood onset, oculocutaneous telangiectases, and immunodeficiency
- Wilson's disease: can cause hepatic dysfunction and a variety of movement disorders, including ataxia; particularly important to screen for this in patients who are young at onset because it is treatable
- Dentatorubral pallidoluysian atrophy: autosomal dominant like SCA but typically has ataxia with associated choreoathetosis, myoclonus, epilepsy, and dementia
- Fragile X–associated tremor/ataxia syndrome: premutation of the fragile X mutation gene; more common among males than females; late onset of ataxia (i.e., >50 yr), tremor, and sometimes parkinsonism; MRI often shows T2 hyperintensity in the middle cerebellar peduncle
- Box 1-17 shows the classification of the various causes of ataxia.

LABORATORY TESTS

- Rule out acquired causes of ataxia, depending on the clinical scenario, with thyroid studies, toxicology screening, and the determination of the vitamin E level or presence of paraneoplastic antibodies.
- Screen for Wilson's disease with ceruloplasmin and, if indicated, a 24-hour urinary copper determination.
- Genetic testing is commercially available for many but not all of the SCAs.

IMAGING STUDIES

- MRI of the brain should be performed to exclude structural abnormalities.
- Cerebellar or brain stem atrophy can be seen with several of the SCA subtypes.

TREATMENT

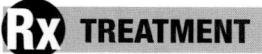

NONPHARMACOLOGIC THERAPY

- Speech therapy for dysarthria and dysphagia
- Physical therapy
- Occupational therapy

CHRONIC Rx

Treatment is symptomatic and supportive. In some cases, parkinsonism can respond to levodopa. Clonazepam can be helpful if tremor is prominent. Spasticity can be treated with baclofen or tizanidine. Dystonia may benefit from botulinum toxin injections.

DISPOSITION

All SCA disorders are progressive, although the speed is variable from subtype to subtype and from patient to patient. On average, patients become wheelchair bound 15 yr after the onset of ataxia, and death can occur after 20 to 25 yr.

REFERRAL

Referral to a general neurologist or to a movement disorders center is appropriate.

BOX 1-17 Classification of Ataxia

Congenital Ataxias

Hereditary Ataxias

Autosomal Recessive Ataxias
- Friedreich's ataxia
- Ataxia–telangiectasia
- Ataxia with oculomotor apraxia type 1
- Ataxia with oculomotor apraxia type 2
- Autosomal recessive spastic ataxia of Charlevoix-Saguenay
- Abetalipoproteinemia
- Ataxia with isolated vitamin E deficiency
- Refsum's disease
- Cerebrotendinous xanthomatosis
- Marinesco-Sjögren syndrome
- Autosomal recessive ataxia with known gene locus
- Early-onset cerebellar ataxia

X-Linked Ataxias
- Fragile X tremor ataxia syndrome

Autosomal Dominant Ataxias
- Spinocerebellar ataxias
- Dentatorubral–pallidoluysian atrophy
- Episodic ataxias

Nonhereditary Degenerative Ataxias
- Multiple system atrophy, cerebellar type
- Sporadic adult-onset ataxia of unknown etiology

Acquired Ataxias
- Alcoholic cerebellar degeneration
- Ataxia as a result of other toxic causes (e.g., antiepileptic medications, lithium, solvents)
- Paraneoplastic cerebellar degeneration
- Other immune-mediated ataxias (e.g., gluten ataxia, ataxia associated with anti-glutamic acid decarboxylase antibodies)
- Acquired vitamin E deficiency
- Hypothyroidism
- Ataxia as a result of physical causes (e.g., heat stroke, hyperthermia)

(From Goetz CG: *Textbook of clinical neurology*, ed 3, Philadelphia, 2007, Saunders.)

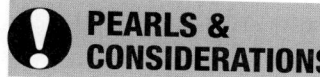

PEARLS & CONSIDERATIONS

COMMENTS
- Genetic testing can have consequences for both the patient and the family. These issues should be discussed during the informed consent process. Patients who desire asymptomatic testing as a result of a relevant family history should undergo genetic counseling before testing.
- In symptomatic patients with a family history of dominantly inherited ataxia, the diagnostic process is relatively straightforward. Genetic testing that is directed toward likely mutations by phenotype and ethnic origin should be the first step.

PATIENT/FAMILY EDUCATION
Patient educational materials as well as contact information for support and advocacy groups are available on the website of the National Ataxia Foundation: http://www.ataxia.org.

SUGGESTED READINGS
available at www.expertconsult.com

AUTHOR: **ANDREW DUKER, M.D.**

Diseases and Disorders

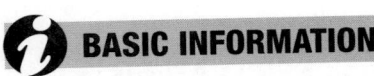 **BASIC INFORMATION**

DEFINITION

Spontaneous miscarriage is fetal loss before week 20 of pregnancy, calculated from the patient's last menstrual period or the delivery of a fetus weighing <500 g. Early loss is before menstrual week 12, whereas late loss refers to losses from weeks 12 to 20.

Miscarriage can also be classified as incomplete (partial passage of fetal tissue through partially dilated cervix), complete (spontaneous passage of all fetal tissue), threatened (uterine bleeding without cervical dilation or passage of tissue), inevitable (bleeding with cervical dilation without passage of fetal tissue), or missed abortion (intrauterine fetal demise without passage of tissue).

Recurrent miscarriage involves three or more spontaneous pregnancy losses before week 20.

SYNONYMS

Abortion

ICD-9CM CODES
634.0 Spontaneous abortion

EPIDEMIOLOGY & DEMOGRAPHICS

INCIDENCE: 5% to 20% of clinically recognized pregnancies, with 80% of miscarriages occurring in the first trimester. Recurrent miscarriage occurs in approximately 1% of couples attempting to have children.

GENETICS:
- Distribution of abnormal karyotypes: autosomal trisomy (50%), monosomy 45,X (20%), triploidy (15%), tetraploidy (10%), structural chromosomal abnormalities (5%).
- With two or more spontaneous miscarriages, a karyotype should be performed to evaluate for balanced translocation, which has 80% risk for abortion, and, if the pregnancy is carried to term, has 3% to 5% risk for unbalanced karyotype.

RISK FACTORS: Prior pregnancy history (risk after live birth, 5%; prior pregnancy aborted, 20% subsequent risk) is the most significant risk factor. Vaginal bleeding, especially >3 days, carries with it a 15% to 20% chance of miscarriage.

PHYSICAL FINDINGS & CLINICAL PRESENTATION

- Profuse bleeding and cramping have a higher association with miscarriage than bleeding without cramping, which is more consistent with a threatened miscarriage.
- Cervical dilation with history or finding of fetal tissue at cervical os may be present.
- In cases of missed abortion, uterine size may be smaller than menstrual dating, in contrast to molar gestation, where size may be greater than dates.

ETIOLOGY

- In a general overview the etiology can be classified in terms of maternal (environmental) and fetal (genetic) factors, with the majority of miscarriages being related to genetic or chromosomal causes.
- Causes: uterine anomalies (unicornuate uterus risk, 50%; bicornuate or septate uterus risk, 25% to 30%); incompetent cervix (iatrogenic or congenital, associated with 20% of mid-trimester losses); diethylstilbestrol exposure in utero (T-shaped uterus); submucous leiomyomas; intrauterine adhesions or synechiae; luteal phase or progesterone deficiency; autoimmune disease such as anticardiolipin antibodies; uncontrolled diabetes mellitus. Rare or controversial causes include: human leukocyte antigen associations between mother and father; infections such as tuberculosis, *Chlamydia*, and *Ureaplasma*; smoking and alcohol use; irradiation; and environmental toxins.

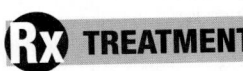 **DIAGNOSIS**

DIFFERENTIAL DIAGNOSIS

- Normal pregnancy
- Hydatidiform molar gestation
- Ectopic pregnancy
- Dysfunctional uterine bleeding
- Pathologic endometrial or cervical lesions

WORKUP

- All patients with bleeding in the first trimester should have an evaluation for possible ectopic pregnancy.
- If there are three early, prior pregnancy losses, a workup and treatment for recurrent miscarriage should begin before next conception. If there is a strong history for second-trimester loss, consideration for cerclage should be given, especially if the history is consistent with incompetent cervix (e.g., painless cervical dilation).

LABORATORY TESTS

- Type and antibody screen are used to evaluate the need for Rh immune globulin.
- During the preconception period, hemoglobin A1C, anticardiolipin antibody, lupus anticoagulant, Factor V Leiden, MTHFR, antithrombin III, prothrombin gene 2210A, karyotyping, endometrial biopsy with progesterone level, and cervical cultures or serum antibodies can be checked for suspected disease processes.

- Progesterone level <5 mg/dl indicates nonviable gestation versus >25 mg/dl, which suggests a good prognosis.

IMAGING STUDIES

Transabdominal or transvaginal sonogram (preferably) can be used in combination with menstrual dating and serum quantitative human chorionic gonadotropin to document pregnancy location, fetal heart presence, gestational sac size, and adnexal pathology.

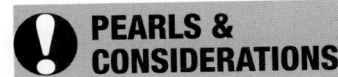 **TREATMENT**

NONPHARMACOLOGIC THERAPY

Depending on the patient's clinical status, desire to continue the pregnancy, and certainty of the diagnosis, expectant management can be considered. In pregnancies <6 wk or >14 wk, complete expulsion of fetal tissue usually occurs and surgical intervention such as dilation and curettage (D&C) can be avoided.

ACUTE GENERAL Rx

- Incomplete miscarriage between 6 and 14 wk can be associated with large amounts of blood loss; thus these patients should undergo D&C.
- In cases of missed abortion, if fetal demise has occurred >6 wk before or gestational age is >14 wk, there is an increased risk of hypofibrinogenemia with disseminated intravascular coagulation. Thus D&C should be performed early in the disease course. Consider use of misoprostol (Cytotec) 200 mg PO q6h.
- Rh-negative patients should be given Rhogam 300 mcg IM to prevent Rh isoimmunization.

REFERRAL

Refer to obstetrician/gynecologist

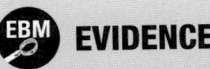 **PEARLS & CONSIDERATIONS**

Spontaneous pregnancy loss is recommended as a replacement for the term *abortion* and to acknowledge the emotional aspects of losing a pregnancy.

EBM **EVIDENCE**

available at www.expertconsult.com

SUGGESTED READINGS
available at www.expertconsult.com

AUTHORS: **SCOTT J. ZUCCALA, D.O.,** and **RUBEN ALVERO, M.D.**

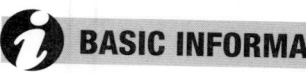

BASIC INFORMATION

DEFINITION

Sporotrichosis is a granulomatous disease caused by the dimorphic fungus *Sporothrix schenckii*.

SYNONYMS

Lymphocutaneous sporotrichosis
Cutaneous sporotrichosis
Pulmonary sporotrichosis

ICD-9CM CODES
117.1 Sporotrichosis

EPIDEMIOLOGY & DEMOGRAPHICS

PREDOMINANT SEX: The most common form, lymphocutaneous sporotrichosis, occurs equally in both sexes. Males predominate in both pulmonary and osteoarticular sporotrichosis.
PREDOMINANT AGE: Generally, lymphocutaneous sporotrichosis occurs in people 35 yr of age or younger, and pulmonary sporotrichosis occurs in people between the ages of 30 and 60 yr, often alcoholic men with COPD.
GENETICS: Neonatal infection: at least one case of transmission from the cheek lesions of the mother to the skin of the infant has been reported.

PHYSICAL FINDINGS & CLINICAL PRESENTATION

- Cutaneous disease
  1. Arises at the site of inoculation, often the site of soil exposure
  2. Initial lesion usually located on the distal part of an extremity (Fig. 1-352), although any area may be affected, including the face
  3. Variable incubation period of approximately 3 wk once introduced into the skin
  4. Granulomatous reaction provoked
  5. Lesion becomes papulonodular, erythematous, elastic, variable in size
  6. Subsequently, nodule becomes fluctuant, undergoes central necrosis, breaks down,

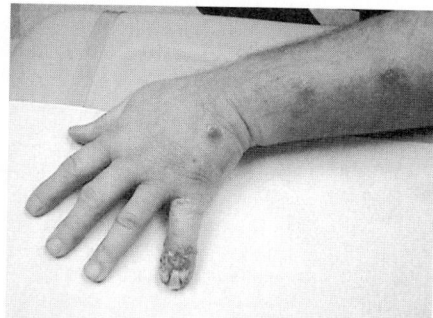

FIGURE 1-352 Sporotrichosis of the fifth finger in a gardener. Three nodular lesions are visible on the hand and arm. (From Mandell GL, Bennett JE, Dolin R: *Principles and practice of infectious diseases,* ed 7, Philadelphia, 2010, Elsevier.)

discharges mucoid pus from which fungus may be isolated
  7. Indolent ulcer with raised erythematous or violaceous borders
  8. Secondary lesions:
     a. Develop along superficial lymphatic channels
     b. Evolve in the same manner as the primary lesion, with subsequent inflammation, induration, and suppuration
- Fixed, or plaque form
  1. Erythematous verrucous, ulcerated, or crusted lesions
  2. Does not spread locally
  3. Does not involve lymphatic vessels
  4. Rarely undergoes spontaneous resolution
  5. More often persists for years without systemic symptoms and within a setting of normal laboratory examinations
- Osteoarticular involvement
  1. Most common extracutaneous form
  2. Usually presents as monoarticular arthritis
  3. Left untreated, may progress to:
     a. Synovitis
     b. Osteitis
     c. Periostitis
     d. All involving elbows, knees, wrists, and ankles
  4. Joint inflamed
     a. Associated with an effusion
     b. Painful on motion
- Early pulmonary disease
  1. Usually associated with a paucity of clinical findings
     a. Low-grade fever
     b. Cough
     c. Fatigue
     d. Malaise
     e. Weight loss
  2. Untreated
     a. Cavitary pulmonary disease
     b. Frank pulmonary dysfunction
  3. Meningitis uncommon
     a. Except perhaps in the immunocompromised patient
     b. Presents with few signs or symptoms of neurologic involvement, usually headache
  4. Few reported cases
     a. Infection of the ocular adnexa
     b. Endophthalmitis without antecedent trauma
     c. Infection of the testes and epididymis

ETIOLOGY

- *Sporothrix schenckii*
  1. Global in distribution
  2. Often isolated from soil, plants, and plant products
  3. Majority of case reports from tropical and subtropical regions of the Americas
- Occupational or recreational exposure
  1. Hay
  2. Straw
  3. Sphagnum moss
  4. Timber
  5. Thorny plants (e.g., roses and barberry bushes)
- Animal contact
  1. Armadillos
  2. Cats
  3. Squirrels
- Human-to-human transmission
- Tattooing

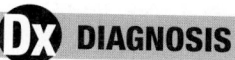

DIAGNOSIS

DIFFERENTIAL DIAGNOSIS

- Fixed, or plaque, sporotrichosis
  1. Bacterial pyoderma
  2. Foreign body granuloma
  3. Tularemia
  4. Anthrax
  5. Other mycoses: blastomycosis, chromoblastomycosis
- Lymphocutaneous sporotrichosis
  1. *Nocardia brasiliensis*
  2. *Leishmania braziliensis*
  3. Atypical mycobacterial disease: *M. marinum, M. kansasii*
- Pulmonary sporotrichosis
  1. Pulmonary TB
  2. Histoplasmosis
  3. Coccidioidomycosis
- Osteoarticular sporotrichosis
  1. Pigmented villonodular synovitis
  2. Gout
  3. Rheumatoid arthritis
  4. Infection with *M. tuberculosis*
  5. Atypical mycobacteria: *M. marinum, M. kansasii, M. avium-intracellulare*
- Meningitis
  1. Histoplasmosis
  2. Cryptococcosis
  3. TB

WORKUP

- The diagnosis should be considered in individuals who are occupationally exposed to soil, decaying plant matter, and thorny plants (gardeners, horticulturists, farmers) who present with chronic nonhealing ulcers or lesions with or without associated arthritis or pulmonary symptoms.
- Diagnosis is made by culture:
  1. Pus
  2. Joint fluid
  3. Sputum
  4. Blood
  5. Skin biopsy
- Isolation of the fungus from any site is considered diagnostic of infection.
- Saprophytic colonization of the respiratory tract has been described.
- A positive blood culture may indicate infection in an immunocompromised host.
- Increasingly sensitive laboratory culturing systems may detect the fungus in the normal host.
- Biopsy specimens are diagnostic if characteristic cigar-shaped, round, oval, or budding yeast forms are seen.

- Despite special staining, the yeast may remain difficult to detect unless multiple sections are examined.
- No standard method of serologic testing is available.
- Previously described techniques have been hampered by the presence of antibody in the absence of infection.

LABORATORY TESTS

- CBCs and serum chemistries are generally normal.
- Elevated ESR is seen with extracutaneous disease.
- CSF analysis in meningeal disease reveals:
  1. Lymphocytic pleocytosis
  2. Elevated protein
  3. Hypoglycorrhachia
- Nested polymerase chain reaction (PCR) assay represents a future clinical modality to rapidly detect *Sporothrix schenckii.*

IMAGING STUDIES

- Chest x-ray examination: unilateral or bilateral upper lobe cavitary or noncavitary lesions
- Radiographic findings of affected joints:
  1. Loss of articular cartilage
  2. Periosteal reaction
  3. Periarticular osteopenia
  4. Cystic changes

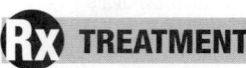 **TREATMENT**

NONPHARMACOLOGIC THERAPY

Local heat and prevention of bacterial superinfection in cutaneous or plaque form

ACUTE GENERAL Rx

CUTANEOUS AND LYMPHOCUTANEOUS SPOROTRICHOSIS:

- Itraconazole at doses of 200 mg/day is the drug of choice and should be given for 2 to 4 wk after the lesions have resolved.
- Alternative treatment: Use saturated solution of potassium iodide (SSKI) 5 to 10 drops PO tid or 1.5 ml PO tid, gradually increasing to 40 to 50 drops PO tid or 3 ml PO tid after meals.
- Maximum tolerated dose should be continued until cutaneous lesions have resolved, approximately 6 to 12 wk.
- Adjunctive therapy with heat is useful and occasionally curative.
- Side effects of SSKI:
  1. Nausea
  2. Anorexia

  3. Diarrhea
  4. Parotid or lacrimal gland hypertrophy
  5. Acneiform rash

DEEP-SEATED MYCOSES (E.G., OSTEOARTICULAR, NONCAVITARY PULMONARY DISEASE):

- Itraconazole
  1. Appropriate initial chemotherapy
  2. Probably as effective as amphotericin B
  3. Less toxic than amphotericin B
  4. Better tolerated than ketoconazole
  5. 100 to 200 mg bid for 1 to 2 yr with continued lifelong suppressive therapy in selected patients
  6. Absence of relapses from 40 to 68 mo has been documented when at least 200 mg/day administered for 24 mo
  7. Insufficient data for use in disseminated disease (e.g., fungemia and meningitis)
  8. Drug levels should be monitored to assess absorption.
- Parenteral amphotericin B, total course of 2 to 2.5 g or more, results in cure in approximately two thirds of cases. Lipid Am B 3 to 5 mg/kg/day is also recommended and less toxic.
  1. Relapses are common.
  2. Amphotericin B-resistant isolates of *Sporothrix schenckii* have been reported.
  3. Remains the drug of choice for severely ill patients with disseminated disease.
  4. In cavitary pulmonary disease, given perioperatively as an adjunct to surgical resection.
- Fluconazole
  1. Less effective than itraconazole
  2. The latest IDSA guidelines recommend fluconazole only as an alternative treatment for lymphocutaneous disease
  3. Requires daily doses of 400 mg/day for lymphocutaneous disease and 800 mg/day for visceral or osteoarticular disease

CHRONIC Rx

For lymphocutaneous and visceral disease, therapy with itraconazole 200 mg/day for periods of 24 mo or greater. Sporothrix is resistant to voriconazole. It is sensitive *in vitro* to posaconazole, but existing data is very limited at present.

DISPOSITION

- Prognosis for cutaneous disease is good.
- Prognosis is less satisfactory for extracutaneous disease, especially if associated with

abnormal immunologic states or other underlying systemic diseases.

REFERRAL

To surgeon; with an established diagnosis of pulmonary sporotrichosis, cavitary lesions require resection of involved tissue
Infectious disease physician

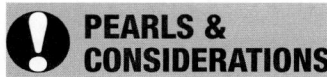 **PEARLS & CONSIDERATIONS**

COMMENTS

- In patients with underlying immunosuppression (e.g., hematologic malignancy or infection with HIV), progression of the initial infection may develop into multifocal extracutaneous sporotrichosis.
- In this subset of patients, dissemination of cutaneous lesions is accompanied by hematogenous spread to lungs, bone, mucous membranes, CNS.
- Osteoarticular and pulmonary manifestations predominate with the development of polyarticular arthritis and osteolytic bone lesions.
- In the absence of therapy, the infection is ultimately fatal.
- Patients with underlying immunosuppressive states should be carefully evaluated even when presenting with single cutaneous lesions.
- Diagnostic modalities should include:
  1. Radiographic examination of chest
  2. Technetium pyrophosphate bone scan
  3. Culture of synovial fluid, blood, skin lesion(s)
- In patients with AIDS, itraconazole appears to be the drug of choice, although meningitis and pulmonary disease may warrant the use of amphotericin B.
- In patients with AIDS, lifetime suppressive therapy with itraconazole should follow initial therapy because of the potential for relapse and dissemination. Treatment may be terminated when CD4 counts exceed 200.

SUGGESTED READINGS

available at www.expertconsult.com

AUTHOR: **PATRICIA CRISTOFARO, M.D.**

BASIC INFORMATION

DEFINITION

- Complex pathophysiological process affecting the brain, induced by traumatic biomechanical forces. It may be caused by a direct blow to the head, face, neck, or elsewhere on the body with an "impulsive" force transmitted to the head.
- Concussion typically results in the rapid onset of short-lived impairment of neurologic function that resolves spontaneously. It may result in neuropathologic changes, but the acute clinical symptoms largely reflect a functional disturbance rather than a structural injury.
- Concussion results in a graded set of clinical syndromes that may or may not involve loss of consciousness. Resolution of the clinical symptoms typically follows a sequential course. It is typically associated with grossly normal structural neuroimaging studies.

SYNONYMS

Sports-related mild traumatic brain injury (mTBI)

TABLE 1-167 Symptoms and Signs of Concussion

Mental Status Changes

Amnesia
Confusion
Disorientation
Easily distracted
Excessive drowsiness
Feeling dinged, stunned, or foggy
Impaired level of consciousness
Inappropriate play behaviors
Poor concentration and attention
Seeing stars or flashing lights
Slow to answer questions or to follow directions

Physical or Somatic

Ataxia or loss of balance
Blurry vision
Decreased performance or playing ability
Dizziness
Double vision
Fatigue
Headache
Lightheadedness
Nausea, vomiting
Poor coordination
Ringing in the ears
Seizures
Slurred, incoherent speech
Vacant stare/glassy-eyed
Vertigo

Behavior or Psychosomatic

Emotional lability
Irritability
Low frustration tolerance
Personality changes
Nervousness, anxiety
Sadness, depressed mood

From Patel DR et al: Sports related concussions in adolescents, *Pediatr Clin N Am* 57:652, 2010.

ICD-9-CM CODES

850.0 Concussion (no loss of consciousness)
850.11 Concussion (loss of consciousness of ≤30 min)
850.9 Concussion unspecified

EPIDEMIOLOGY & DEMOGRAPHICS

INCIDENCE: 1.6 million to 3.8 million sports and recreation related concussions occur each year in the United States.
PREVALENCE: Each year, U.S. emergency departments treat an estimated 135,000 sports- and recreation-related TBIs, including concussions, among children ages 5 to 18.
PREDOMINANT SEX AND AGE: Children and teens are more likely to get a concussion and take longer to recover than adults.
RISK FACTORS: High-impact sports and recreation; six times more likely in organized sports than leisure physical activity.

PHYSICAL FINDINGS & CLINICAL PRESENTATION

See Table 1-167.

ETIOLOGY

- Concussion occurs when rotational or angular acceleration forces are applied to the brain, resulting in shear strain of the underlying neural elements.
- This may be associated with a blow to the skull; however, direct impact to the head is not required.

DIAGNOSIS

DIFFERENTIAL DIAGNOSIS

See "Postconcussive Syndrome"

WORKUP

- Sideline assessment:
  - No athlete with a suspected concussion should return to play that day.

- Neurologic assessment using a standardized tool, such as
  SCAT2 (Sport Concussion Assessment Tool)
  SAC (Standardized Assessment of Concussion)
  - Monitor for deterioration; no athlete should be left alone
- Neurocognitive testing:
  - Computer-based programs, such as ImPACT, ANAM, CogSport
  - Neuropsychiatric testing administered by a neuropsychologist
- Gait/balance testing with a tool such as the Balance Error Scoring System (BESS)
- When used in combination, symptom assessment, balance assessment, and neurocognitive testing provide a sensitivity of >90% for the identification of concussion.

IMAGING STUDIES

- CT imaging is indicated in any athlete with a Glasgow Coma Scale score of ≤15 or a rapidly changing neurologic exam
- Neuroimaging using PECARN guidelines

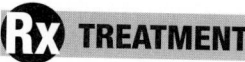 TREATMENT

ACUTE GENERAL Rx

- Removal from game
- Physical rest
  - No return to play until asymptomatic for 24 hr
  - Follow return-to-play guidelines (Table 1-168)
- Cognitive rest to limit symptoms
  - Modifications at school
  - Modifications at home/recreation
  - Encourage sleep

CHRONIC Rx

See "Postconcussive Syndrome"

DISPOSITION

See Table 1-168

REFERRAL

Sports-medicine physician, neuropsychology or concussion center

TABLE 1-168 Graduated Return to Play Protocol

Rehabilitation Stage	Functional Exercise at Each Stage of Rehabilitation	Objective of Each Stage
1. No activity	Complete physical and cognitive rest	Recovery
2. Light aerobic exercise	Walking, swimming, or stationary cycling, keeping intensity <70% maximum predicted heart rate. No resistance training	Increase heart rate
3. Sport-specific exercise	Skating drills in ice hockey, running drills in soccer. No head impact activities	Add movement
4. Noncontact training drills	Progression to more complex training drills, e.g., passing drills in football and ice hockey. May start progressive resistance training	Exercise, coordination, and cognitive load
5. Full contact practice	After medical clearance, participate in normal training activities	Restore confidence and assess functional skills by coaching staff
6. Return to play	Normal game play	

From Putukian M: The acute symptoms of sports-related concussion: diagnosis and on-field management, *Clin Sports Med* 30(58), 2011.

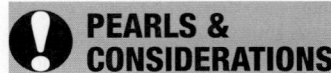

PEARLS & CONSIDERATIONS

PREVENTION
- Preparticipation evaluations for all athletes
- Preparticipation neurocognitive and balance testing to establish a baseline

PATIENT/FAMILY EDUCATION

Centers for Disease Control and Prevention: http://www.cdc.gov/concussion/support.html.

SUGGESTED READINGS

available at www.expertconsult.com

AUTHORS: **PETER J. SELL, D.O.,** and **AMITY RUBEOR, D.O.**

BASIC INFORMATION

DEFINITION

Squamous cell carcinoma (SCC) is a malignant tumor of the skin arising in the epithelium.

SYNONYMS

SCC
Skin cancer

ICD-9CM CODES

173.9 Skin neoplasm, site unspecified

EPIDEMIOLOGY & DEMOGRAPHICS

- SCC is the second most common cutaneous malignancy, comprising 20% of all cases of nonmelanoma skin cancer.
- Incidence is highest in lower latitudes (e.g., southern U.S., Australia).
- Male-to-female ratio is 2:1.
- Incidence increases with age and sun exposure.
- Average age at diagnosis is 66 yr.

PHYSICAL FINDINGS & CLINICAL PRESENTATION

- SCC commonly affects the scalp, neck region, back of hands, superior surface of the pinna, and the lip.
- The lesion may have a scaly, erythematous macule or plaque.
- Telangiectasia, central ulceration may also be present (Fig. 1-353).
- Most SCCs present as exophytic lesions that grow over a period of months.

ETIOLOGY

Risk factors include ultraviolet B radiation and immunosuppression (kidney transplant recipients have a threefold increased risk).

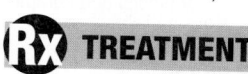

DIAGNOSIS

DIFFERENTIAL DIAGNOSIS

- Keratoacanthomas
- Actinic keratosis
- Amelanotic melanoma
- Basal cell carcinoma
- Benign tumors
- Healing traumatic wounds
- Spindle cell tumors
- Warts

WORKUP

Diagnosis is made by full-thickness skin biopsy (incisional or excisional).

TREATMENT

ACUTE GENERAL Rx

- Electrodesiccation and curettage for small SCCs (<2 cm in diameter), superficial tumors, and lesions located in extremity and trunk.
- Tumors thinner than 4 mm can be managed by simple local removal.
- Lesions between 4 and 8 mm thick or those with deep dermal invasion should be excised.
- Tumors penetrating the dermis can be treated with several modalities, including excision and Mohs' surgery, radiation therapy, and chemotherapy.
- Metastatic SCC can be treated with cryotherapy and combination of chemotherapy using 13-*cis*-retinoic acid and interferon-alpha 2A.

DISPOSITION

- Survival is related to size, location, degree of differentiation, immunologic status of the patient, depth of invasion, and presence of metastases. Risk factors for metastasis include lesions on the lip or ear, increasing lesion depth, and poor cell differentiation.
- Patients whose tumors penetrate through the dermis or exceed 8 mm in thickness are at risk of tumor recurrence.
- The most common metastatic locations are regional lymph nodes, liver, and lung.
- Tumors on the scalp, forehead, ears, nose, and lips also carry a higher risk.
- SCCs originating in the lip and pinna metastasize in 10% to 20% of cases.
- Five-year survival for metastatic squamous cell carcinoma is 34%.

REFERRAL

Oncology referral for metastatic SCC

PEARLS & CONSIDERATIONS

COMMENTS

SCC arising in areas of prior radiation, thermal injury, and areas of chronic ulcers or chronic draining sinuses are more aggressive and have a higher frequency of metastasis than those originating in actinic damaged skin.

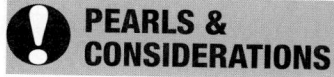

EVIDENCE

available at www.expertconsult.com

SUGGESTED READING

available at www.expertconsult.com

AUTHOR: **FRED F. FERRI, M.D.**

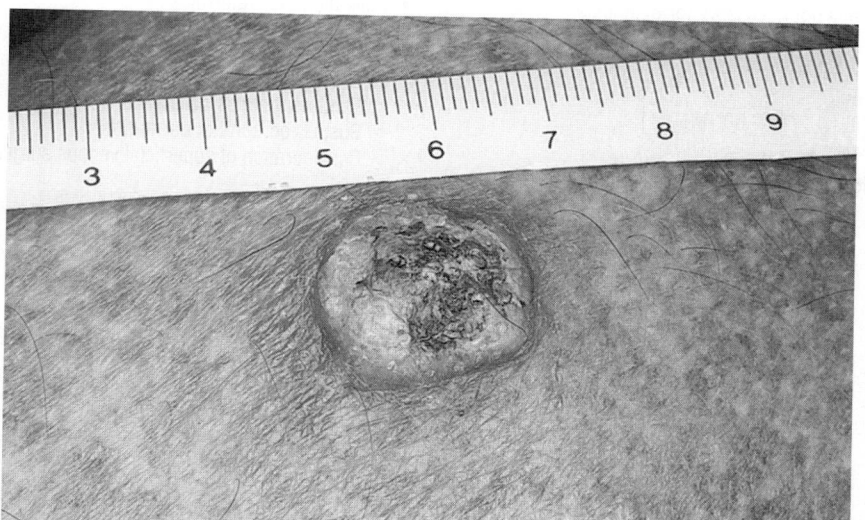

FIGURE 1-353 Squamous cell carcinoma. Nodular hyperkeratotic lesion with central erosion. (From Noble J et al: *Textbook of primary care medicine*, ed 3, St Louis, 2001, Mosby.)

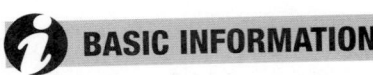

BASIC INFORMATION

DEFINITION

Stasis dermatitis refers to an inflammatory skin disease of the lower extremities, commonly seen in patients with chronic venous insufficiency (Fig. 1-354).

SYNONYMS

Chronic venous insufficiency

ICD-9CM CODES
454.1 Varicose veins of lower extremities with inflammation

EPIDEMIOLOGY & DEMOGRAPHICS

- Prevalence of stasis dermatitis increases with age and obesity
- Rarely seen before age 50 yr
- Twice as common in women than men, although men tend to have more severe disease
- No ethnic predilection for disease

PHYSICAL FINDINGS & CLINICAL PRESENTATION

- Insidious onset
- Pruritus
- Chronic lower extremity edema, sometimes unilateral, often described as "brawny" because of dermal fibrosis
- Ill-defined erythema
- Eczematous patches
- Commonly located over the medial malleolus
- Progressive pigment changes can occur as a result of extravasation of red blood cells and hemosiderin deposition within the cutaneous tissue
- Secondary infections can occur

ETIOLOGY

- Stasis dermatitis is believed to occur as a result of venous incompetence. Common etiologies include:
  1. Deep vein thrombosis
  2. History of lower extremity injury
  3. Pregnancy
  4. Vein stripping or vein harvesting in patients requiring coronary artery bypass grafting

- Venous insufficiency subsequently results in venous hypertension, causing skin inflammation and the aforementioned physical findings and clinical presentation

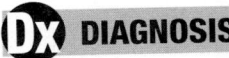

DIAGNOSIS

The diagnosis of stasis dermatitis is primarily made by a detailed history and physical examination

DIFFERENTIAL DIAGNOSIS

- Contact dermatitis
- Atopic dermatitis
- Cellulitis
- Dermatophyte infection
- Pretibial myxedema
- Nummular eczema
- Lichen simplex chronicus
- Xerosis
- Asteatotic eczema
- Deep vein thrombosis

WORKUP

Directed at excluding potential life-threatening causes (e.g., deep vein thrombosis) and complications (e.g., cellulitis and sepsis).

LABORATORY TESTS

Generally not helpful unless a secondary infection is present

IMAGING STUDIES

- Radiograph, CT scans, and MRIs are generally not necessary for diagnosis
- Doppler studies are indicated in any patient suspected of having deep vein thrombosis

TREATMENT

NONPHARMACOLOGIC THERAPY

- Leg elevation above heart level for 30 min three to four times a day (avoid in arterial occlusive diseases)
- Compression stocking with a gradient of at least 30 to 40 mm Hg; in obese patients, intermittent pneumatic compression pump is recommended
- For weeping skin lesions, wet to dry dressing changes are helpful

ACUTE GENERAL Rx

- The mainstay of treatment of stasis dermatitis is to control leg edema and prevent venous stasis ulcers from developing.
- In patients with acute stasis dermatitis, a compression (Unna) boot can be applied.
- Topical corticosteroid creams or ointments (e.g., triamcinolone 0.1% bid) are used frequently to help reduce inflammation and itching. Steroids should not be applied to stasis ulcers.
- Secondary infections should be treated with appropriate antibiotics. Most secondary infections are the result of Staphylococcus or Streptococcus organisms.
- Diuretics for controlling edema.

CHRONIC Rx

- Patients with chronic stasis dermatitis can be treated with topical emollients (e.g., white petrolatum, lanolin, Eucerin)
- Surgical therapy:
  ○ Venous stripping
  ○ Superficial and deep perforator vein ligation
  ○ Endovenous stenting

COMPLEMENTARY & ALTERNATIVE MEDICINE

Oral horse chestnut seed extract

REFERRAL

- Dermatology
- Vascular surgery
- Indications for referral:
  ○ Nonhealing ulcers
  ○ Uncertainty in the diagnosis
  ○ Associated arterial insufficiency
  ○ Persistent stasis dermatitis
  ○ Suspected contact dermatitis
  ○ Consideration of superficial venous surgery

PEARLS & CONSIDERATIONS

COMMENTS

- Inflammatory skin changes from stasis dermatitis are believed to result from poor oxygen perfusion to the lower extremity skin tissue.
- Venous disease is irreversible. Goal of treatment is to alleviate symptoms and prevent progression.
- Stasis ulcers are often associated with stasis dermatitis. Refer to Section I, "Venous Ulcers," for more information.

EVIDENCE

available at www.expertconsult.com

SUGGESTED READINGS

available at www.expertconsult.com

AUTHORS: **KACHIU LEE, B.A.,** and **JESSICA RISSER, M.D., M.P.H.**

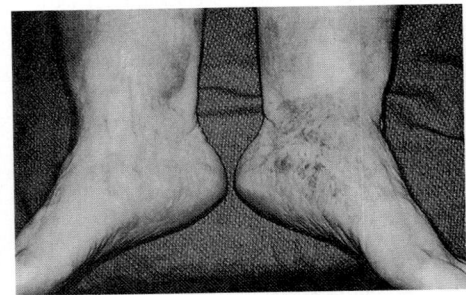

FIGURE 1-354 Moderate stasis dermatitis with hyperpigmentation and bilateral venous insufficiency. (Courtesy Department of Dermatology, University of North Carolina at Chapel Hill. From Goldstein BG, Goldstein AO: *Practical dermatology*, ed 2, St Louis, 1997, Mosby.)

BASIC INFORMATION

DEFINITION

Status epilepticus is a medical neurologic emergency. It is historically defined as 30 min of continuous seizure activity or two or more seizures without full recovery of consciousness between seizures. However, in practice a continuous seizure that last >5 min may be considered and treated as status epilepticus.

SYNONYMS

Convulsive status epilepticus
Nonconvulsive status epilepticus

ICD-9CM CODES
345.3 Grand mal status

EPIDEMIOLOGY & DEMOGRAPHICS

INCIDENCE: 40 to 100 cases per 100,000 persons
PEAK INCIDENCE: It is most common among children younger than 1 yr and adults older than 60 yr.
PREDOMINANT SEX AND AGE: No gender preference.

PHYSICAL FINDINGS & CLINICAL PRESENTATION

- Patients can present with repetitive tonic clonic movements of the body (convulsive status epilepticus); other patients are comatose and nonresponsive (nonconvulsive status epilepticus).
- Lethargy, intermittent confusion, involuntary movements can also present in these patients.

ETIOLOGY

- Status epilepticus can be the result of an acute neurologic injury, such as stroke, meningitis, etc.
- In patients with epilepsy, abrupt discontinuation of antiepileptic drugs can result in status epilepticus.
- See Table 1-169 for causes of status epilepticus.

TABLE 1-169 Causes of Status Epilepticus

- Stroke (ischemic/hemorrhagic)
- CNS infections
- Traumatic head injury
- CNS toxicity: certain medications, drugs, ethanol
- Brain tumors or other mass lesions
- Metabolic disturbances: hypoglycemia, hyponatremia
- Abrupt discontinuation of antiepileptic drugs in patient with epilepsy
- Cryptogenic

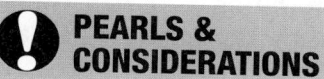 **DIAGNOSIS**

DIFFERENTIAL DIAGNOSIS

- Convulsive syncope
- Nonepileptic spells
- Encephalopathies: Metabolic, infectious, toxic, etc.

WORKUP

- ABCs
- ICU admission
- Emergent electroencephalogram (EEG)
- Continuous video EEG in refractory cases

LABORATORY TESTS

- Routine blood workup (CBC, CMP, glucose, electrolytes)
- Urine drug screen
- Lumbar puncture and CSF analysis in patients with suspected meningitis

IMAGING STUDIES

- Immediate CT scan of the head.
- MRI of the brain should be performed once the patient is in a stable condition.

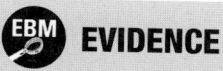 **TREATMENT**

- Patients with continuous seizure activity over 3 min need intravenous lorazepam 0.1 mg/kg at 2 mg/min (or diazepam 0.2 mg/kg at 5 mg/min only when lorazepam is not available).
- Lorazepam is followed by intravenous fosphenytoin 20 mg/kg (PE) at a rate not greater that 150 mg/min.
- An alternate to fosphenytoin is phenytoin 20 mg/kg IV at up to 50 mg/min as tolerated. Vital signs should be monitored during the infusion.
- If seizures continue intravenous phenobarbital, midazolam or propofol is an alternative. Other agents used include intravenous valproic acid and intravenous levetiracetam.

NONPHARMACOLOGIC THERAPY

An EEG is useful emergently for monitoring response to therapy in patients who do not clear clinically. Continuous EEG monitoring is ideal.

GENERAL Rx

It is important to find out the etiology of the status epilepticus (e.g., metabolic disturbance, infection, etc.). The appropriate treatment/understanding of the underlying cause of the status epilepticus will impact the successful treatment.

CHRONIC Rx

- The chronic treatment of patient with status epilepticus depends on the etiology.
- Patient with status epilepticus due to epilepsy will need chronic treatment.

COMPLEMENTARY AND ALTERNATIVE MEDICINE

Not applicable

DISPOSITION

- Response to treatment depends on the etiology of the status epilepticus.
- When there is no CNS injury as a cause or result from the status epilepticus, the prognosis is good.
- No driving until seizure freedom in accordance with local laws and regulations.

REFERRAL

Status epilepticus is a neurologic emergency; therefore immediate neurologic consultation is warranted.

PEARLS & CONSIDERATIONS

COMMENTS

- Status epilepticus is a medical emergency that carries a high risk of mortality.
- Continuous video EEG is crucial in the treatment of these patients because some of them may not be clinically seizing (convulsing) but electrographically they may still have subclinical repetitive seizures or subclinical status epilepticus.

PREVENTION

Medication compliance is crucial in patients with epilepsy.

PATIENT/FAMILY EDUCATION

- Patients with epilepsy have normal lives.
- The goal of treatment is no seizures and no side effects to medications.
- Patient education and information can be obtained at the Epilepsy Foundation: www.epilepsyfoundation.org
- Pregnant women with epilepsy should visit the Antiepileptic Drug Pregnancy Registry website for information and assistance: www2.massgeneral.org/aed
- Patients with ongoing seizures are forbidden from driving; check your State regulations and laws regarding driving and epilepsy.

EBM EVIDENCE

available at www.expertconsult.com

SUGGESTED READINGS
available at www.expertconsult.com

AUTHOR: PATRICIO SEBASTIAN ESPINOSA, M.D., M.P.H.

BASIC INFORMATION

DEFINITION

Stevens-Johnson syndrome (SJS) is a rare, severe vesiculobullous form of erythema multiforme affecting the skin, mouth, eyes, and genitalia.

SYNONYMS

SJS
Herpes iris
Febrile mucocutaneous syndrome

ICD-9CM CODES
695.1 Stevens-Johnson syndrome

EPIDEMIOLOGY & DEMOGRAPHICS

- SJS affects predominantly children and young adults.
- Male/female ratio is 2:1.

PHYSICAL FINDINGS & CLINICAL PRESENTATION

- The cutaneous eruption is generally preceded by vague, nonspecific symptoms of low-grade fever and fatigue occurring 1 to 14 days before the skin lesions. Cough is often present. Fever may be high during the active stages.
- Bullae generally occur on the conjunctiva, mucous membranes of the mouth, nares, and genital regions.
- Corneal ulcerations may result in blindness.
- Ulcerative stomatitis results in hemorrhagic crusting.
- Flat, atypical target lesions or purpuric maculae may be distributed on the trunk or be widespread (Fig. 1-355).
- The pain from oral lesions may compromise fluid intake and result in dehydration.
- Thick, mucopurulent sputum and oral lesions may interfere with breathing.

ETIOLOGY

- Drugs (e.g., phenytoin, sulfonamides, lamotrigine, allopurinol, phenobarbitol) are the most common cause.
- Upper respiratory tract infections (e.g., *Mycoplasma pneumoniae*) and herpes simplex viral infections have also been implicated in SJS.

DIAGNOSIS

DIFFERENTIAL DIAGNOSIS

- Toxic erythema (drugs or infection)
- Pemphigus
- Pemphigoid
- Urticaria
- Hemorrhagic fevers
- Serum sickness
- *Staphylococcus* scalded-skin syndrome
- Behçet's syndrome

WORKUP

- Diagnosis is generally based on clinical presentation and characteristic appearance of the lesions.
- Skin biopsy is generally reserved for when classic lesions are absent and diagnosis is uncertain.

LABORATORY TESTS

Complete blood count with differential, cultures in cases of suspected infection

IMAGING STUDIES

Chest radiographs may show patchy changes in patients with pulmonary involvement.

TREATMENT

NONPHARMACOLOGIC THERAPY

- Withdrawal of any potential drug precipitants
- Careful skin nursing to prevent secondary infection

ACUTE GENERAL Rx

- Treatment of associated conditions (e.g., acyclovir for herpes simplex virus infection, azithromycin for *Mycoplasma* infection)
- Antihistamines for pruritus
- Treatment of the cutaneous blisters with cool, wet Burow's compresses
- Relief of oral symptoms by frequent rinsing with lidocaine (Xylocaine Viscous)
- Liquid or soft diet with plenty of fluids to ensure proper hydration
- Treatment of secondary infections with antibiotics
- Corticosteroids: use remains controversial and should be used only in severe cases early in the disease; when used, prednisone 20 to 30 mg bid until new lesions no longer appear, then rapidly tapered
- Topical steroids: may use to treat papules and plaques; however, should not be applied to eroded areas
- Vitamin A: may be used for lacrimal hyposecretion
- Consider intravenous immunoglobulins in severe cases

DISPOSITION

- Prognosis varies with severity of disease. It is generally good in patients with limited disease; however, mortality rate may approach 10% in patients with extensive involvement.
- Oral lesions may continue for several months.
- Scarring and corneal abnormalities may occur in 20% of patients.

REFERRAL

- Hospital admission in a unit used for burn care is recommended in severe cases.
- Urethral involvement may necessitate catheterization.
- Ocular involvement should be monitored by an ophthalmologist.

EVIDENCE

available at www.expertconsult.com

SUGGESTED READING
available at www.expertconsult.com

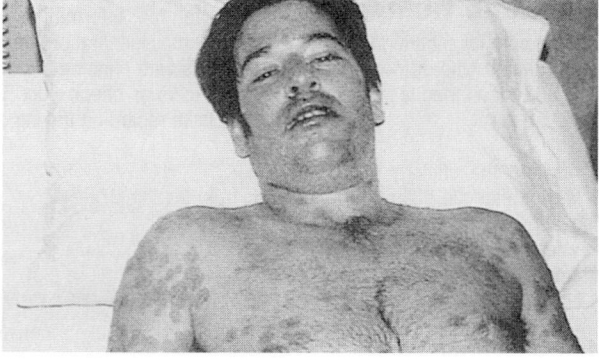

FIGURE 1-355 Stevens-Johnson syndrome. (From Stein JH: *Internal medicine,* ed 5, St Louis, 1998, Mosby.)

AUTHOR: **FRED F. FERRI, M.D.**

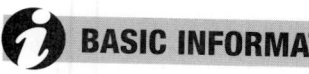

BASIC INFORMATION

DEFINITION

Stomatitis is inflammation involving the oral mucous membranes.

SYNONYMS

Heterogeneous grouping of unrelated illnesses, each with their own designation(s)

ICD-9CM CODES
528.0 Stomatitis
054.2 (herpetic)
528.2 (aphthous)
112.0 (monilial)

PHYSICAL FINDINGS & CLINICAL PRESENTATION

WHITE LESIONS:
- Candidiasis (thrush)
- Caused by yeast infection (*Candida albicans*)
- Examination: white, curdlike material that when wiped off leaves a raw bleeding surface
- Epidemiology: seen in the very young and the very old, those with immunodeficiency (AIDS, cancer), persons with diabetes, and patients treated with antibacterial agents
- Other
  1. Leukoedema: filmy opalescent-appearing mucosa, which can be reverted to normal appearance by stretching. This condition is benign.
  2. White sponge nevus: thick, white corrugated folds involving the buccal mucosa. Appears in childhood as an autosomal dominant trait. Benign condition.
  3. Darier's disease (keratosis follicularis): white papules on the gingivae, alveolar mucosa, and dorsal tongue. Skin lesions also present (erythematous papules). Inherited as an autosomal-dominant trait.
  4. Chemical injury: white sloughing mucosa.
  5. Nicotine stomatitis: whitened palate with red papules.
  6. Lichen planus: linear, reticular, slightly raised striae on buccal mucosa. Skin is involved by pruritic violaceous papules on forearms and inner thighs.
  7. Discoid lupus erythematosus: lesion resembles lichen planus.
  8. Leukoplakia: white lesions that cannot be scraped off; 20% are premalignant epi-

thelial dysplasia or squamous cell carcinoma.
  9. Hairy leukoplakia: shaggy white surface that cannot be wiped off; seen in HIV infection, caused by Epstein-Barr virus.

RED LESIONS:
- Candidiasis may present with red lesions instead of the more frequent white. Median rhomboid glossitis is a chronic variant.
- Benign migratory glossitis (geographic tongue): area of atrophic depapillated mucosa surrounded by a keratotic border. Benign lesion, no treatment required.
- Hemangiomas.
- Histoplasmosis: ill-defined, irregular patch with a granulomatous surface, sometimes ulcerated.
- Allergy.
- Anemia: atrophic reddened glossal mucosa seen with pernicious anemia.
- Erythroplakia: red patch usually caused by epithelial dysplasia or squamous cell carcinoma.
- Burning tongue (glossopyrosis): normal examination; sometimes associated with denture trauma, anemia, diabetes, vitamin B_{12} deficiency, psychogenic problems.

DARK LESIONS (BROWN, BLUE, BLACK):
- Coated tongue: accumulation of keratin; harmless condition that can be treated by scraping
- Melanotic lesions: freckles, lentigines, lentigo, melanoma, Peutz-Jeghers syndrome, Addison's disease
- Varices
- Kaposi's sarcoma: red or purple macules that enlarge to form tumors; seen in patients with AIDS

RAISED LESIONS:
- Papilloma
- Verruca vulgaris
- Condyloma acuminatum
- Fibroma
- Epulis
- Pyogenic granuloma
- Mucocele
- Retention cyst

BLISTERS:
- Primary herpetic gingivostomatitis
- Caused by herpes simplex virus type 1 or, less frequently, type 2
- Course: day 1: malaise, fever, headache, sore throat, cervical lymphadenopathy; days 2 and 3: appearance of vesicles that develop into

painful ulcers of 2 to 4 mm in diameter; duration of up to 2 wk
- Recurrent intraoral herpes: rare; recurrences typically involve only the keratinized epithelium (lips)
- Pemphigus and pemphigoid
- Hand-foot-mouth disease: caused by coxsackievirus group A
- Erythema multiforme
- Herpangina: caused by echovirus
- Traumatic ulcer
- Primary syphilis
- Perlèche (or angular cheilitis)
- Recurrent aphthous stomatitis (canker sores)
- Behçet's syndrome (aphthous ulcers, uveitis, genital ulcerations, arthritis, and aseptic meningitis)
- Reiter's syndrome (conjunctivitis, urethritis, and arthritis with occasional oral ulcerations)
- Unknown cause

Course: solitary or multiple painful ulcers may develop simultaneously and heal over 10 to 14 days. The size of the lesions and the frequency of recurrences are variable.

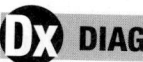 DIAGNOSIS

WORKUP
- White lesions: Candidiasis (thrush) diagnosis: ovoid yeast and hyphae seen in scrapings treated with KOH culture
- Blisters:
  - Exfoliative cytology
  - Viral culture
  - Immunofluorescence for herpes antigen

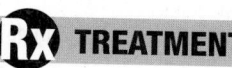 TREATMENT

White lesions: candidiasis (thrush) treatment:
- Topical with nystatin or clotrimazole
- Systemic with ketoconazole or fluconazole

Blisters:
- Supportive
- Consider acyclovir

Recurrent intraoral herpes: topical corticosteroids or systemic steroids for severe cases

SUGGESTED READINGS
available at www.expertconsult.com

AUTHOR: **FRED F. FERRI, M.D.**

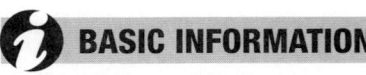
BASIC INFORMATION

DEFINITION
Strabismus is a condition of the eyes in which the visual axes of the eyes are not straight in the primary position or in which the eyes do not follow each other in the different positions of gaze.

SYNONYMS
Esotropia
Exotropia
Restrictive eye movement

ICD-9CM CODES
378.9 Strabismus

EPIDEMIOLOGY & DEMOGRAPHICS
INCIDENCE (IN U.S.): 2% of all children
PEAK INCIDENCE: Childhood
PREDOMINANT SEX: None
PREDOMINANT AGE: Birth to age 5 yr
GENETICS: None known

PHYSICAL FINDINGS & CLINICAL PRESENTATION
- Conjugate gaze loss in both eyes with the eyes focusing independently (Fig. 1-356).
- Amblyopia (a decrease in best-corrected visual acuity in an otherwise structurally healthy eye) may occur with untreated strabismus.

ETIOLOGY
- Many cases are congenital.
- Accommodative cases occur later with focusing.
- Rarely, there is neurologic disease or severe refractive errors.
- Hereditary form is common, with hyperopia (far-sightedness) the most common.

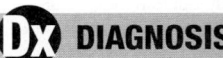
DIAGNOSIS

DIFFERENTIAL DIAGNOSIS
- Measuring eye position and movement
- Vision testing
- Refractive errors
- Central nervous system (CNS) tumors
- Orbital tumors
- Brain and CNS dysfunction

WORKUP
- Eye examination. Strabismus is classified according to the type and magnitude of misalignment. Esotropia refers to an inward deviation of the nonfixing eye and exotropia to the outward deviation of the nonfixing eye. Hypertropia is a vertical deviation in which the nonfixing eye is higher, and hypotropia is a vertical deviation in which the nonfixing eye is lower.
- Visual field
- MRI to rule out tumors that develop later with no apparent cause

LABORATORY TESTS
Generally not needed

IMAGING STUDIES
Necessary only if other neurologic findings are found

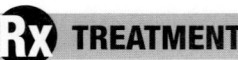
TREATMENT

NONPHARMACOLOGIC THERAPY
- Glasses
- Patching: best between age 3 and 7 yr; vision most improved by 3 to 6 mo
- Prisms
- Atropine: same as patching most of the time, although patching may give better results in resistant cases

CHRONIC Rx
- Glasses
- Alternate eye patching
- Surgery
- Prisms

DISPOSITION
- The earlier the condition is treated, the more likely the child will have normal vision in both eyes.
- After age 7 yr, visual loss is usually permanent from amblyopia.

REFERRAL
- Early for full rehabilitation of eye cosmetically and functionally
- To an ophthalmologist for management (usually)

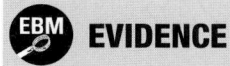
EVIDENCE
available at www.expertconsult.com

SUGGESTED READING
available at www.expertconsult.com

AUTHOR: **MELVYN KOBY, M.D.**

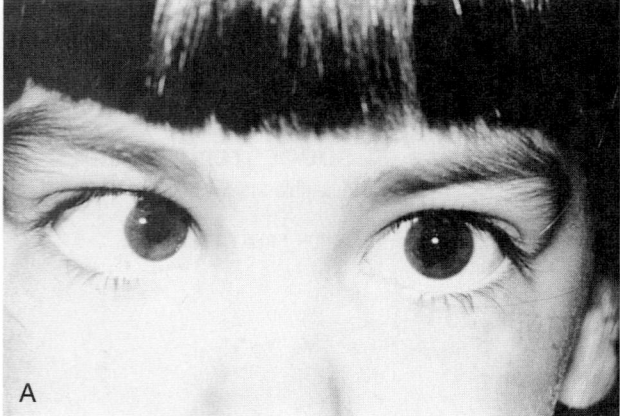
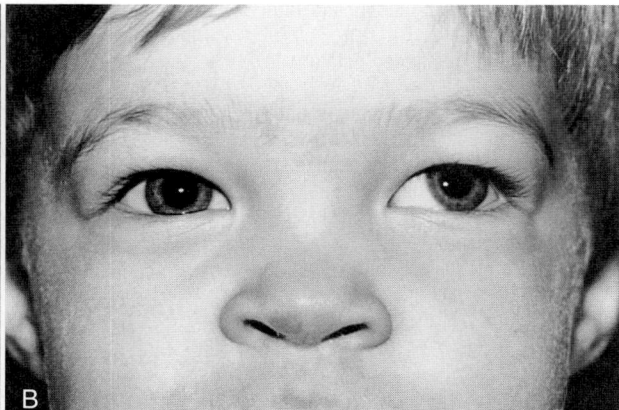

FIGURE 1-356 A, Note the nasal deviation of the right eye with the corneal light reflection temporally displaced on the right eye and centered in the left pupil, indicating an esotropia. **B,** Divergent strabismus of the left eye, defining an exotropia. (From Hodkelman [ed]: *Primary pediatric care*, ed 3, St Louis, 1997, Mosby.)

BASIC INFORMATION

DEFINITION

Ischemic stroke is the sudden onset of a focal neurologic deficit as a result of ischemia. Acute ischemic stroke may be defined as relating to the first few days after onset. However, the purpose of this chapter is to help the provider to make decisions regarding the acute stroke patient within the first several hours of symptoms; this is the crucial time for definitive treatment interventions.

SYNONYMS

Stroke
Brain attack
Cerebrovascular attack (This is a nonspecific term and should not be used.)

ICD-9CM CODES
494.31 Ischemic stroke
436 Acute stroke

EPIDEMIOLOGY & DEMOGRAPHICS

INCIDENCE:
- ~750,000 new or recurrent strokes occur each year in the U.S.
- Stroke is the number three cause of death and the leading cause of long-term disability in the U.S.

PREVALENCE: There are ~4.5 million stroke survivors in the U.S.

RISK FACTORS: Hypertension, dyslipidemia, diabetes mellitus, and smoking are the four major risk factors. Other risk factors include atrial fibrillation, mechanical heart valve, patent foramen ovale, recent myocardial infarction, carotid stenosis, hypercoaguable states, and sickle cell disease.

GENETICS: Multifactorial

PHYSICAL FINDINGS & CLINICAL PRESENTATION

The presentation of ischemic stroke varies with the artery involved and the region of the central nervous system affected. Following are some common syndromic presentations. Please note that this list is not comprehensive and that all findings for a particular syndrome may not be listed here.

- Large- to medium-sized arteries:
  - Left middle cerebral artery: right face, arm, and leg weakness and sensory loss with aphasia (expressive, receptive, or both); possible hemianopia
  - Right middle cerebral artery: right face, arm, and leg weakness and sensory loss with hemineglect; possible hemianopia
  - Basilar artery: typically an acute loss of consciousness preceded by vertigo, nausea, vomiting, and diplopia; quadriparesis or quadriplegia may be seen, including the "locked-in" syndrome
  - Posterior cerebral artery: unilateral hemianopia
  - Anterior cerebral artery: unilateral leg weakness and sensory loss

  - Cerebellum: ataxia (typically of the limbs), often with vertigo, nausea, and vomiting
- Small arteries (common lacunar syndromes)
  - Lateral medullary (Wallenberg's) syndrome
  - Posterior limb internal capsule

ETIOLOGY

Etiologies include atherosclerosis, cardioembolism, artery-to-artery embolism, small-vessel lipohyalinosis, arteritis, arterial dissection, and vasospasm.

DIAGNOSIS

DIFFERENTIAL DIAGNOSIS

The differential diagnosis of acute ischemic stroke includes hemorrhagic stroke (primarily intracerebral hemorrhage), seizure with postictal paralysis, migraine with hemiparesis, syncope, hypoglycemia, hypertensive encephalopathy, and conversion disorder.

LABORATORY TESTS

- Immediate (Box 1-18): CBC, metabolic panel that includes blood glucose and renal function, PT/INR, aPTT, cardiac enzymes, troponin I, and urinalysis
- National Institutes of Health Stroke Scale: a brief, focused neurologic examination aimed at providing a numeric estimate of the severity of stroke; can be performed by any provider trained in its use; may increase the likelihood of the correct assessment of stroke
- ECG and telemetry monitoring

IMAGING STUDIES

- Immediate (Fig. 1-357): computed tomography (CT) of the head without contrast or MRI of the brain with stroke protocol to rule out

---

BOX 1-18 Immediate Diagnostic Studies: Evaluation of a Patient with Suspected Acute Ischemic Stroke

All Patients
Noncontrast brain computed tomographic scan or magnetic resonance image
Blood glucose level
Serum electrolyte and renal function tests
Electrocardiography
Markers of cardiac ischemia
Complete blood count, including platelet count*
Prothrombin time/international normalized ratio*
Activated partial thromboplastin time*
Oxygen saturation

Selected Patients
Hepatic function tests
Toxicology screen
Blood alcohol level
Pregnancy test
Arterial blood gas tests (if hypoxia is suspected)
Chest radiography (if lung disease is suspected)
Lumbar puncture (if subarachnoid hemorrhage is suspected and computed tomography scan is negative for blood)
Electroencephalogram (if seizures are suspected)

*Although it is desirable to know the results of these tests before giving a patient tissue plasminogen activator, thrombolytic therapy should not be delayed while awaiting the results unless (1) there is clinical suspicion of a bleeding abnormality or thrombocytopenia; (2) the patient has received heparin or warfarin; or (3) the patient's use of anticoagulants is not known.

From Christensen H et al: Abnormalities on ECG and telemetry predict stroke outcome at 3 months, *J Neurol Sci* 234:99-103, 2005.

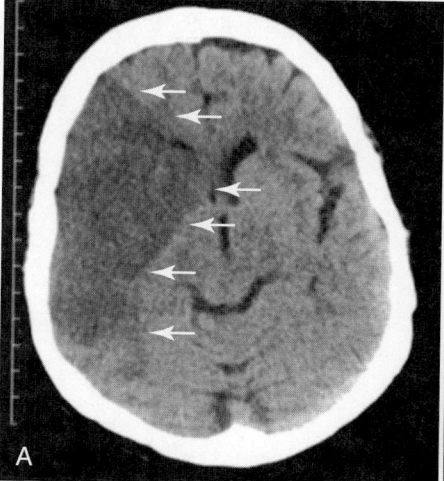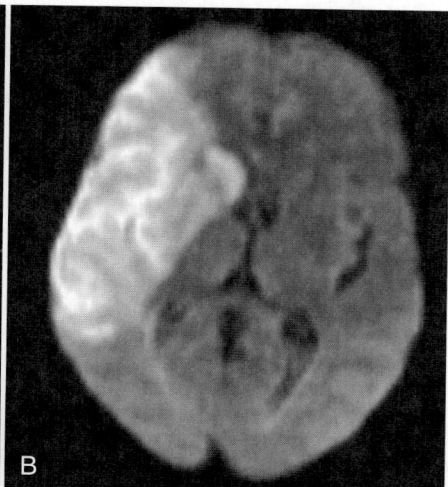

FIGURE 1-357 Large right middle cerebral artery infarct on **A,** an unenhanced computed tomographic scan and **B,** a diffusion-weighted magnetic resonance image. There is a mass effect, and this patient is at risk for cerebral herniation syndromes.

hemorrhage and, if possible, to assess the extent of stroke. (Because CT typically will not show an ischemic stroke for several hours, it may also be useful to estimating how long ischemia has been present for cases in which the time of onset is unclear.)

- Several other neuroimaging studies are useful during the early stages of acute stroke to assess whether there is a thrombus that is amenable to intervention (Table 1-170).

Cross Reference: See "Transient Ischemic Attack" for general workup, which is identical to that for ischemic stroke.

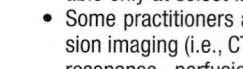

TREATMENT

NONPHARMACOLOGIC THERAPY

GENERAL CONSIDERATIONS:

- Airway and breathing should be maintained.
- Supplemental oxygen should be provided to keep the oxygen saturation at ≥92%.
- Fever is harmful during acute stroke. Ascertaining and addressing the cause while lowering an elevated temperature is strongly advised.
- Pneumatic compression devices or pharmacologic means should be applied to help prevent deep venous thromboses.
- Avoid any and all oral intake until swallowing is clearly unimpaired; this helps to avoid aspiration pneumonia.
- Early mobilization for rehabilitation is desirable.
- Consider neurosurgical intervention for craniectomy in select cases. Typical cases in which craniectomy may be performed include cerebellar ischemia with compression of the brain stem or the fourth ventricle and large right middle cerebral artery ischemia.

IMMEDIATE CATHETER CEREBRAL ANGIOGRAPHY FOR ENDOVASCULAR INTERVENTION

(Figs. 1-358 and 1-359): Methods Available:

1. The Merci® clot retrieval system is approved by the U.S. FDA for use up to 8 hr after the onset of symptoms.
2. The Penumbra System is also available at some centers.
3. Intraarterial tissue plasminogen activator (TPA) is used routinely for up to 6 hr after the onset of symptoms, although it is not approved by the U.S. FDA for this purpose.

Pearls and Caveats:

- Multimodal therapy (i.e., thrombectomy and intraarterial TPA) is sometimes performed.
- Endovascular treatment may be performed for select cases in which intravenous (IV) TPA has failed to recanalize an occluded artery.
- Endovascular intervention may be an option for cases in which there are systemic contraindications to IV TPA.
- Endovascular intervention is useful only for large, accessible thrombi. Therefore, if a stroke patient is a candidate for IV TPA, then he or she should probably receive IV TPA.
- One can reasonably expect a recanalization rate of 60% in appropriate patients.
- Complications can ensue from the angiogram procedure itself, including an intracerebral hemorrhage rate that is similar to that associated with IV TPA.

- Endovascular intervention is typically available only at select large stroke centers.
- Some practitioners are making use of perfusion imaging (i.e., CT perfusion and magnetic resonance perfusion) to assess whether there is salvageable brain tissue before performing the procedure. In some cases, this may lead to a dramatic expansion of traditional time windows; this practice is currently being studied in clinical trials.

ACUTE GENERAL Rx

INTRAVENOUS THROMBOLYSIS:

- IV TPA is the only medical therapy approved by the U.S. FDA for the treatment of ischemic stroke.
- The time window for administration is within 3 hr of symptom onset.
- There are strict criteria for the administration of IV TPA (see Box 1-19).
- The protocol is weight based, with 90 mg being the maximum allowable dose.
- The risk of brain hemorrhage with IV TPA is about 5% in stroke patients.

TABLE 1-170 Imaging Modalities for Stroke

Imaging Modality	Advantage	Disadvantage
Cerebral catheter angiography	• Allows for the definitive assessment of cerebral circulation (gold standard) • Allows for the deployment of intra-arterial thrombolysis and thrombectomy devices if a thrombus is found • Allows for the assessment of collateral circulation	• Invasive (significant risks) • High cost • Not available at all facilities
Doppler studies	• Noninvasive • May be performed at the patient's bedside	• Can be limited by the patient's body habitus • Operator dependent
Magnetic resonance angiography	• Excellent view of the large arteries of the neck and brain • No contrast material needed	• Cannot be performed in patients who are critically ill, who are unable to tolerate supine positioning, who have a pacemaker or other ferromagnetic hardware, or who are claustrophobic
Magnetic resonance perfusion	• Assesses cerebral hemodynamics • May show ischemic penumbra (i.e., the area of the brain that may be saved by timely intervention)	• Not commonly available • Not well standardized
CT angiography	• Excellent view of the large arteries of the neck and brain • Similar to magnetic resonance angiography with regard to resolution	• Requires intravenous contrast
CT perfusion	• Assesses cerebral hemodynamics • May show ischemic penumbra (i.e., the area of the brain that may be saved by timely intervention)	• Challenging to interpret in some cases • Not routinely available at many facilities • Requires intravenous contrast

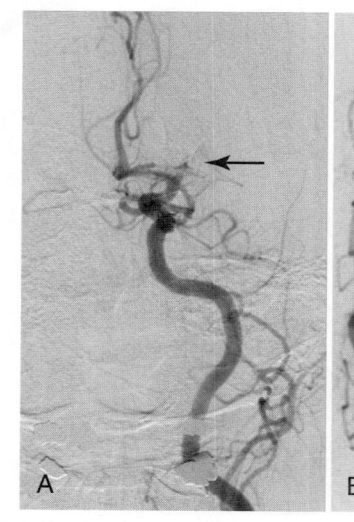 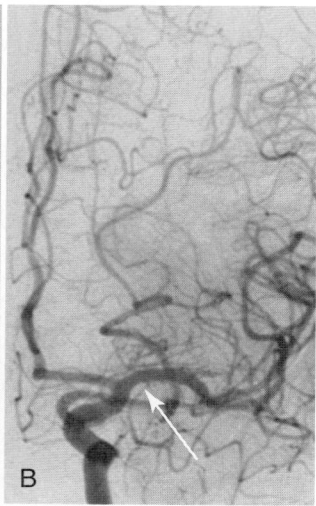

FIGURE 1-358 A, A catheter angiogram showing left middle cerebral artery occlusion, which caused severe stroke symptoms for several hours. **B,** The artery was opened with the Merci® clot retrieval system, and this resulted in normal flow.

- Some new data suggest that IV TPA can be administered safely and with benefit in select patients up to 4.5 hours after symptom onset. As of this writing, this should probably not be routine practice. There are additional exclusion criteria if IV TPA is given beyond the 3-hr window.

HYPERTENSION: Elevated blood pressure is common during acute stroke, and it often subsides without specific therapy. In general, hypertension is not treated acutely unless it is extremely high (e.g., >220 mm Hg systolic blood pressure); unless there is evidence of organ damage caused by the hypertension; or unless thrombolysis is being considered, in which case the blood pressure needs to come down (if it can be safely accomplished) to <185/110 mm Hg. It is risky to severely decrease blood pressure in the presence of acute ischemic stroke. A 15% to 25% decrease over the first 24 hours is recommended.

HYPOGLYCEMIA: Hypoglycemia can mimic stroke. The prompt assessment of the serum glucose level and replacement as necessary are important.

HYPERGLYCEMIA: The presence of hyperglycemia worsens ischemic stroke outcome. Hyperglycemia should be managed aggressively.

HYPOTENSION: The presence of systemic hypotension in acute ischemic stroke portends a poor outcome. The cause should be sought, and volume depletion should be corrected with normal saline. Cardiac arrhythmias should be treated. Induced hypertension with vasopressor agents may be useful for select cases with an ischemic penumbra that is at risk, but caution is strongly advised.

ANTIPLATELET THERAPY: Beginning the oral or feeding tube administration of aspirin (325 mg/day) within 48 hours of stroke onset is advised. This will decrease the likelihood of a repeat ischemic stroke. Another oral antiplatelet regimen approved for secondary stroke prophylaxis (e.g., clopidogrel, aspirin plus extended-release dipyridamole) will also suffice and may be superior in the long term.

DISPOSITION

Patients with acute ischemic stroke should be cared for in a stroke unit or an intensive care unit. Nurses with skills in stroke care and telemetry monitoring should be routine. After the patient is stable and the workup is complete, rehabilitation should be arranged.

REFERRAL

Patients with acute ischemic stroke should be transported to a hospital in which providers are skilled with regard to the treatment of stroke. Depending on the severity and duration of symptoms, the patient may qualify for immediate endovascular intervention at a comprehensive stroke center, even if he or she is not a candidate for IV TPA. If complications from brain edema develop, further evaluation by a neurosurgeon may be helpful during the acute phase.

BOX 1-19 Three-Hour Criteria for Tissue Plasminogen Activator (Alteplase [Activase]) Use in Patients with Thromboembolic Stroke

Criteria for considering TPA as a treatment option:
- Noncontrast CT scan without evidence of hemorrhage
- Time since onset of symptoms clearly <3 hr before TPA administration would begin

Criteria for excluding TPA as a treatment option:
- Historic and clinical findings
- Clinical presentation suggestive of subarachnoid hemorrhage, even if CT scan is normal
- Sudden, severe headache, often with a loss of consciousness at onset
- Vomiting common
- Active internal bleeding, increased risk of bleeding, or known bleeding diathesis, including as a result of the following:
  - Recent use of warfarin with an INR of ≥1.7
  - Use of heparin within 48 hr with a prolonged aPTT
  - Platelet count of <100,000/mm^3
  - History of intracranial hemorrhage
  - Known arteriovenous malformation or aneurysm
- GI or GU bleeding within the past 21 days
- Arterial puncture within the past 7 days
- Recent lumbar puncture
- Stroke, intracranial surgery, or head trauma within the previous 3 mo
- Major surgery or serious trauma within the preceding 14 days
- Systolic blood pressure >185 mm Hg or diastolic blood pressure >110 mm Hg that does not decrease below that range with treatment
- Seizure at stroke onset
- Rapidly improving neurologic signs
- Isolated mild neurologic deficits
- Acute myocardial infarction
- Post–myocardial infarction pericarditis
- Blood glucose <50 mg/dl or >400 mg/dl
- Patient who is pregnant or lactating
- CT findings
- Evidence of intracranial hemorrhage
- Hypodensity or effacement of the sulci in one third of the territory of the middle cerebral artery

(From Rakel RE [ed]: *Principles of family practice,* ed 6, Philadelphia, 2002, WB Saunders.)
TPA, Tissue plasminogen activator; *CT,* computed tomography; *INR,* international normalized ratio; *aPTT,* activated partial thromboplastin time; *GI,* gastrointestinal; *GU,* genitourinary.

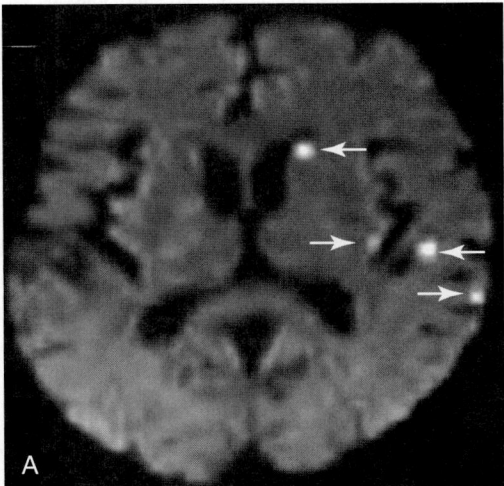
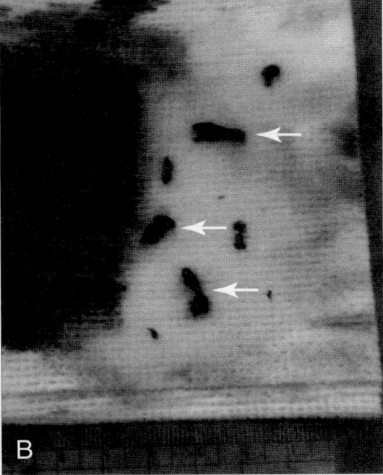

FIGURE 1-359 A, A diffusion-weighted magnetic resonance image of the same patient as shown in previous figure, this time showing only mild left cerebral ischemia after intervention. The patient was clinically normal. **B,** Thrombi removed from the middle cerebral artery with the use of the Merci® clot retrieval system.

PEARLS & CONSIDERATIONS

PREVENTION

The prevention of acute ischemic stroke depends on the aggressive management of risk factors in individual patients.

Cross reference: stroke, secondary prevention

PATIENT/FAMILY EDUCATION

Patients and families need to be taught about ways to reduce the risk for recurrent stroke, including lifestyle modifications. Education about rehabilitation goals, when appropriate, should also be accomplished.

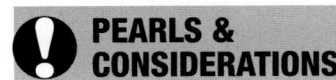 **EVIDENCE**

available at www.expertconsult.com

SUGGESTED READINGS
available at www.expertconsult.com

AUTHOR: **MICHAEL R. DOBBS, M.D.**

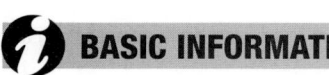

BASIC INFORMATION

DEFINITION
Hemorrhagic stroke is the sudden onset of a focal neurologic deficit caused by hemorrhage into or around the brain.

SYNONYMS
Intracerebral hemorrhage
Intracranial hemorrhage
Cerebrovascular attack (This is a nonspecific term and should not be used.)
The term *subarachnoid hemorrhage* refers to a specific location for hemorrhage, which commonly occurs as a result of a ruptured aneurysm. Please see "Subarachnoid Hemorrhage" for additional information.

ICD-9CM CODES
431 Intracerebral hemorrhage
432.9 Unspecified intracranial hemorrhage

EPIDEMIOLOGY & DEMOGRAPHICS
INCIDENCE: There are ~750,000 new or recurrent strokes per year in the United States, of which ~10% to 15% are hemorrhagic.
RISK FACTORS:
- Hypertension
- Anticoagulant use
- Thrombolysis
- Alcoholism
- Illicit drug use (e.g., cocaine)
- Cerebral amyloid angiopathy
GENETICS: Multifactorial

PHYSICAL FINDINGS & CLINICAL PRESENTATION
The presentation varies with the region of the brain that is affected. The following are common locations for hemorrhage:
- Basal ganglia
- Cerebellum
- Pons
- Lobar (i.e., amyloid angiopathy)

ETIOLOGY
- Rupture of vessels
- Aneurysm
- Arteriovenous malformation
- Brain tumor
- Amyloid angiopathy

DIAGNOSIS

DIFFERENTIAL DIAGNOSIS
- Ischemic stroke
- Seizure with postictal paralysis
- Migraine with hemiparesis
- Syncope
- Conversion disorder

LABORATORY TESTS
- CBC, metabolic panel including blood glucose and renal function, PT/INR, aPTT, urinalysis, and toxicology screens
- ECG and telemetry monitoring

IMAGING STUDIES
- Immediate: CT scanning of the head without contrast is highly sensitive for hemorrhage (Fig. 1-360).
- MRI of the brain with a gradient echo sequence is also highly sensitive for hemorrhage, including intracerebral microhemorrhages that may not be visible with computed tomography scanning.

TREATMENT

NONPHARMACOLOGIC THERAPY
- Surgery should be performed promptly for cases of cerebellar hemorrhage of >3 cm when the patient is deteriorating clinically or showing brain stem edema or hydrocephalus.
- Surgery for lobar or deep brain clots may be considered for select cases, although the level of evidence for efficacy is not high.

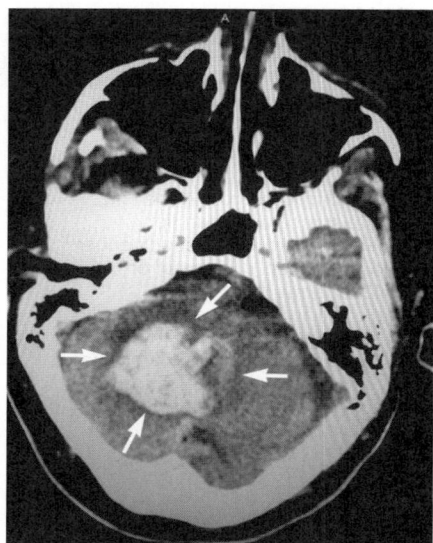

FIGURE 1-360 Nonenhanced computed tomographic scan of a patient with large cerebellar hemorrhage, mass effect, and compression of the fourth ventricle.

- Pneumatic compression devices should be applied to help prevent deep venous thromboses.
- Early mobilization for rehabilitation is desirable.

ACUTE GENERAL Rx
- Hypertension (Box 1-20): Blood pressure should be quickly lowered by 15% and then gradually and safely brought to the individual patient's target range. In theory, this may diminish the expansion of the hematoma.
- Hyperglycemia: A high blood glucose level predicts a worse outcome. Markedly elevated glucose levels should be lowered to <300 mg/dl.
- Seizures: If seizures occur, they should be treated aggressively, including with intravenous medications, if needed.
- Elevated intracranial pressure: This condition should be treated with a graded approach, which may include the elevation of the head of the bed elevation, analgesia/sedation, hyperventilation, and osmotic therapy.
- Antipyretics should be administered for cases that involve fever in addition to searching for a cause of the fever.
- Protamine sulfate is used to treat cases of heparin-induced intracerebral hemorrhage.
- Vitamin K is given for warfarin-associated intracerebral hemorrhage. In addition, recombinant factor VIIa and fresh frozen plasma are sometimes used.
- Recommendations for thrombolytic-associated intracerebral hemorrhage treatment include the consideration of the infusion of platelets and cryoprecipitate.

DISPOSITION
For large hemorrhages or unstable patients, immediate referral to a stroke center

REFERRAL
Patients with hemorrhagic stroke should be transported to a hospital where providers are skilled in the treatment of stroke. Depending on the severity and duration of symptoms, the patient may require neurosurgical intervention.

BOX 1-20 Suggested Recommended Guidelines for the Treatment of Elevated Blood Pressure in Patients with Spontaneous Intracerebral Hemorrhage

1. SBP of >200 mm Hg or MAP of >150 mm Hg: Consider the aggressive reduction of BP with continuous intravenous infusion, with BP monitoring every 5 min.
2. SBP of >180 mm Hg or MAP of >130 mm Hg with evidence or suspicion of elevated ICP: Consider ICP monitor and reducing BP with intermittent or continuous intravenous medications to keep cerebral perfusion pressure >60 to 80 mm Hg.
3. SBP of >180 mm Hg or MAP of >130 mm Hg without evidence or suspicion of elevated ICP: Consider a modest reduction of BP (e.g., MAP of 110 mm Hg or target blood pressure of 160/90 mm Hg) with intermittent or continuous intravenous medications, and clinically reexamine the patient every 15 min.

BP, Blood pressure; *ICP,* intracranial pressure; *MAP,* mean arterial pressure; *SBP,* systolic blood pressure. Modified from Broderick J et al: Guidelines for the management of spontaneous intracerebral hemorrhage in adults: 2007 update, *Stroke* 38:2001-2023, 2007.

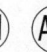
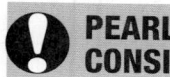

PEARLS & CONSIDERATIONS

- Outcomes are inversely correlated with hemorrhage size.
- Specific reversal agents may be useful for warfarin-, heparin-, or thrombolysis-associated hemorrhage.
- Although they have been investigated in placebo-controlled trials, no procoagulant medications have yet been shown to be safe and effective for the mitigation of spontaneous intracerebral hemorrhage.

PREVENTION

Prevention depends on the aggressive management of risk factors in individual patients, including hypertension, smoking, alcohol use, and cocaine use.

PATIENT/FAMILY EDUCATION

Patients and families need to understand that most patients will not soon achieve functional independence and that rehabilitation will be a long process. Education about avoiding antithrombotic agents should be stressed as appropriate for individual circumstances.

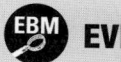 **EVIDENCE**

available at www.expertconsult.com

SUGGESTED READING

available at www.expertconsult.com

AUTHOR: **MICHAEL R. DOBBS, M.D.**

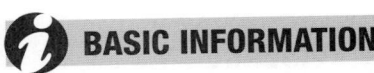

DEFINITION

Secondary prevention of stroke involves preventing the recurrence of a cerebral vascular ischemic or hemorrhagic stroke after a primary event.

SYNONYMS

Brain attack
Stroke
Cerebral thrombosis
Cerebral hemorrhage
Brain infarct

ICD-9CM CODES

433 Precerebral vessel occlusion
434 Cerebral vessel thrombosis or occlusion

EPIDEMIOLOGY

Stroke is the third leading cause of death in the U.S. and the leading cause of morbidity. There are a total of 750,000/yr, of which approximately 200,000 are recurrent strokes. Thus, the secondary prevention of ischemic stroke remains the best treatment. Secondary prevention is specifically targeted toward modifiable risk factors.

RISK FACTORS: Age is the most important non-modifiable risk factor for stroke. Modifiable risk factors include hypertension, hyperlipidemia, cigarette smoking, excessive alcohol consumption, physical inactivity, obesity (i.e., a body mass index of >25 kg/m^2), and diabetes mellitus.

GENETICS: Multifactorial

PHYSICAL FINDINGS & CLINICAL PRESENTATION

- Stroke can present in many ways, and the clinical history and the physical findings can provide the most important clues regarding how to proceed. Typically, the individual has a sudden definable loss of motor, sensory, visual, or cognitive functions that have a clear time of onset and that are noticed by others or by the individual themselves.
- Physical findings such as weakness in one limb or on one side of the body, the sudden loss of a visual field, or the inability to understand or communicate with others raises one's suspicion of a stroke event.
- In addition, there may be eye deviation, facial droop, numbness of the face or extremities, and definable weakness on one side of the body.
- The inability to understand or communicate with others may lead others to classify the person as psychotic or confused; this finding is known as *aphasia*.

ETIOLOGY

- Strokes are broadly divided into ischemic or hemorrhagic (i.e., intraparenchymal or subarachnoid hemorrhage)
- The main causes of ischemic stroke include atherosclerosis; cardioembolic causes (e.g., atrial fibrillation); and lacunar stroke (i.e.,

small-vessel disease). Rare causes that result from drug use (e.g., cocaine abuse); dissection; and hypercoaguable states need to be considered when ischemic stroke occurs among younger individuals.
- The most common cause of intracerebral hemorrhage is uncontrolled hypertension. Spontaneous rupture of a brain aneurysm causes subarachnoid hemorrhage.

DIAGNOSIS

DIFFERENTIAL DIAGNOSIS

- Seizure and postictal states
- Complicated migraine
- Hypoglycemia
- Brain tumor
- Somatization disorder
- Metabolic disorder

WORKUP

- Blood glucose level at the bedside or in the office
- aPTT, PT/INR, CBC, and CMP
- Fasting lipid panel
- Hypercoagulability tests for young stroke patients with no obvious risk factors

IMAGING STUDIES

- Computed tomography scanning of the head without contrast can differentiate between ischemic and hemorrhagic stroke. MRI of the brain is a more specific test.
- Carotid ultrasound and transcranial Doppler are used to detect large-vessel atherosclerosis. Magnetic resonance and computed tomography angiography are good alternatives.
- Echocardiogram and ECG can be used to detect a cardioembolic source.

TREATMENT

The secondary prevention of stroke is targeted toward modifiable risk factors and toward preventing strokes in specific conditions. Lifestyle modifications, including appropriate diet and exercise, need to be emphasized for every stroke patient. It is important to note that, for all patients with noncardioembolic ischemic stroke or transient ischemic attack (TIA), aspirin (50 to 325 mg/day), the combination of aspirin and extended-release dipyridamole, and clopidogrel are all acceptable options for initial therapy. Both the combination of aspirin and extended-release dipyridamole and clopidogrel were found to be superior to aspirin in comparison trials. A consultation with a neurologist should be considered for young stroke patients and for patients with no obvious cause or with stroke from unusual causes (e.g., hypercoaguable states, dissections).

PREVENTING STROKE IN SPECIFIC CONDITIONS:

1. Cardioembolic strokes as a result of atrial fibrillation: Try to maintain an international normalized ratio between 2.0 and 3.0. For patients who are unable to take oral antico-

agulants, aspirin (325 mg/day) is recommended. A recent study suggested that a combination of aspirin and clopidogrel is slightly better than aspirin alone.
2. Cardioembolic strokes as a result of a prosthetic metallic valve: Try to obtain an international normalized ratio between 2.5 and 3.5.
3. Strokes as a result of large-vessel atherosclerois (i.e., symptomatic carotid stenosis): For patients with recent TIA or ischemic stroke within the last 6 months and ipsilateral severe (70% to 99%) carotid artery stenosis, carotid endarterectomy (CEA) performed by a surgeon is recommended and results in a perioperative morbidity and mortality rate of <6%. For patients with recent TIA or ischemic stroke and ipsilateral moderate (50% to 69%) carotid stenosis, CEA is recommended. When the degree of stenosis is <50%, there is no indication for CEA. Carotid stenting is not indicated except for cases in which surgery is high risk.
4. Symptomatic intracranial atherosclerosis: The optimal therapy in these cases is unclear. Warfarin is not superior to aspirin according to the WASID study. Angioplasty/stenting is believed by many to be the treatment of choice, but this remains investigational (Fig. 1-361). Trials are ongoing, but treatment is available at many stroke centers.

RISK FACTOR MODIFICATION:

1. Hypertension: Antihypertensive treatment is recommended for both the prevention of recurrent stroke and the prevention of other vascular events in persons who have had an ischemic stroke or a TIA. An absolute target blood pressure level and reduction are uncertain and should be individualized. Normal blood pressure levels have been defined as <120/80 mm Hg by the JNC-7. Several lifestyle modifications have been associated with blood pressure reduction and should be included as part of a comprehensive antihypertension treatment plan.
2. Diabetes: The goal for the hemoglobin A_{1c} level should be $\leq 7\%$.
3. Hyperlipidemia: For patients with ischemic stroke or TIA with elevated cholesterol levels, statin agents are recommended. The target goals for cholesterol lowering are an LDL-C level of <100 mg/dl and an LDL-C level of <70 mg/dl for very high-risk persons with multiple risk factors (e.g., both coronary artery disease and diabetes).
4. Cigarette smoking: Absolute cessation is required.
5. Obesity: Weight reduction may be considered for all overweight ischemic stroke and TIA patients to maintain the goal of a body mass index of between 18.5 and 24.9 kg/m^2 and a waist circumference of <35 in for women and <40 in for men.
6. Excessive alcohol consumption: Patients with ischemic stroke or TIA who are heavy drinkers should eliminate or reduce their consumption of alcohol. Light to moderate levels of no more than two drinks per day for men and one drink per day for nonpregnant women may be considered.

DISPOSITION

Secondary stroke prevention is a multifaceted approach of lifestyle modification and pharmacological intervention that is aimed at preventing or limiting disability.

REFERRAL

- For complicated recurrent strokes, a referral to a neurologist who specializes in stroke is recommended.

- Obtaining previously suggested radiologic studies and laboratory tests before referral is recommended.

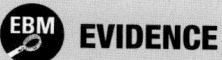

PEARLS & CONSIDERATIONS

The modification of risk factors is the best prevention of stroke. Lifestyle modification is a very important aspect of secondary stroke prevention.

PREVENTION

Prevention is the goal of treatment, and compliance is the most important factor. Review risk factor reduction and pharmacologic therapy as previously discussed.

PATIENT/FAMILY EDUCATION

More information can be obtained from the following sources:

- American Heart Association, National Center, 7272 Greenville Avenue, Dallas, TX 75231
- American Stroke Association, 1-888-4-STROKE or 1-888-478-7653
- H.O.P.E. for Stroke, 250 Duck Pond Drive, Wantagh, NY 11793, 516-804-8495

EBM EVIDENCE

available at www.expertconsult.com

SUGGESTED READINGS

available at www.expertconsult.com

AUTHOR: **NAWAZ HACK, M.D.**

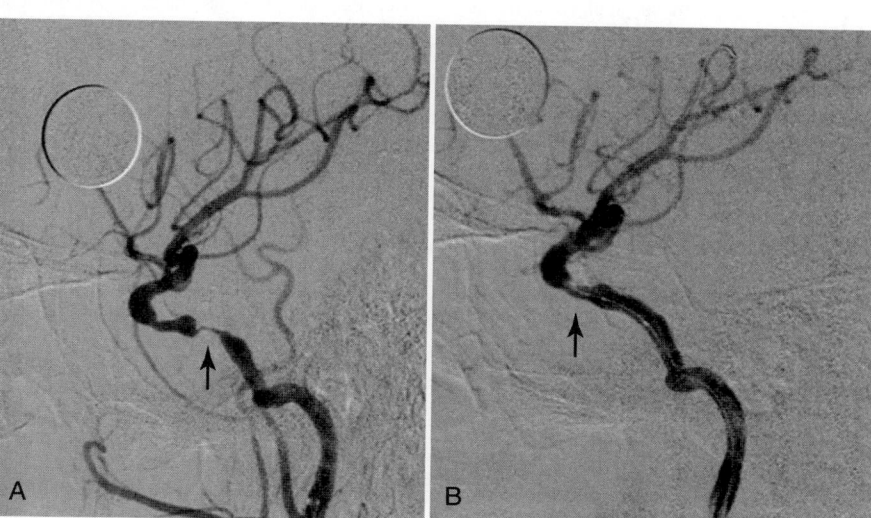

FIGURE 1-361 **A,** Intracranial high-grade symptomatic stenosis. **B,** This patient failed aggressive medical therapy and responded only to angioplasty and stenting.

Diseases and Disorders

S

I

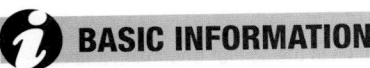

DEFINITION

Sturge-Weber syndrome (SWS) is a sporadic congenital disorder characterized by a dermal capillary malformation (port-wine stain) occurring in association with vascular malformations of the leptomeninges and the eye.

Sturge first described a patient with epilepsy, a facial capillary malformation, and buphthalmos in 1879. Parkes Weber better characterized the pattern and distribution of the characteristic intracranial calcifications. The complete syndrome generally includes the triad of facial dermal capillary malformation (port-wine stain), ipsilateral central nervous system (CNS) vascular malformation (leptomeningeal angiomatosis), and vascular malformation of the choroid of the eye associated with glaucoma. Partial forms have been reported.

SYNONYMS

Sturge (-Weber) (-Dimitri) disease or syndrome
Encephalocutaneous angiomatosis

ICD-9CM CODES
759.6

EPIDEMIOLOGY & DEMOGRAPHICS

SWS is not a heritable disorder; thus recurrence is unlikely.

PHYSICAL FINDINGS & CLINICAL PRESENTATION

SWS is characterized by a facial angioma (port-wine stain) and an associated leptomeningeal angioma. These vascular malformations are associated with specific ocular and neurologic abnormalities.

CUTANEOUS MANIFESTATIONS:

- Cutaneous port-wine stain is the most common type of vascular malformation, occurring in 0.3% of newborns (Fig. 1-362, A). However, only a small number of children with port-wine stains have SWS.
- In SWS, the port-wine stain typically is present on the forehead and upper eyelid, primarily in the distribution of the first or second division of the trigeminal nerve. Extension of the skin lesion to both sides of the face and the trunk and extremities is common.
- The distribution of the cutaneous angioma influences the risk of an associated leptomeningeal angioma. Leptomeningeal angioma occurs in approximately 90% of cases when the port-wine stain involves both the upper and lower eyelids compared with 10% when only one eyelid is affected.
- The skin lesion usually is obvious at birth. However, its appearance changes with age and its size increases as the patient grows. In the newborn, the lesion is flat and usually light pink in color. It typically darkens with age to a deep red, port-wine appearance and vascular ectasias develop (Fig. 1-362, B). The vascular ectasias produce nodularity and superficial blebbing, which lead to overgrowth of the underlying soft tissues and sometimes the bone.
- It may extend to mucosal surfaces with concomitant gingival hypertrophy, which may be even further accentuated in patients being treated with phenytoin for seizures. Some patients exhibit accelerated eruption of teeth.

LEPTOMENINGEAL ANGIOMA:

- Leptomeningeal angioma occurs in 10% to 20% of cases when a typical facial lesion is present. The intracerebral lesion usually occurs on the same side as the port-wine stain. Leptomeningeal angiomatosis seldom occurs without an accompanying facial angioma.
- The parietal and occipital areas are affected most commonly, although any portion of the cerebrum can be involved.
- The pathologic appearance of the leptomeninges includes thickening and discoloration caused by the increased vascularity. The angiomatous tissue typically fills the subarachnoid space in the sulci, and large, tortuous venous structures drain superficially or into the deep venous system. The underlying parenchyma may be atrophic and contain multiple calcific granular deposits. The intraparenchymal calcification may result from chronic tissue hypoxia caused by venous stasis.

OCULAR MANIFESTATIONS:

- Ocular features of SWS include glaucoma and vascular malformations of the conjunctiva, episclera, choroid, and retina.
- The predominant ocular abnormality is glaucoma (increased intraocular pressure), which occurs in 30% to 70% of affected patients. The risk of glaucoma is highest in the first decade. Congenital glaucoma is seen in approximately one half of patients with SWS and presents in newborns with enlargement of the globe (buphthalmos). Patients occasionally develop glaucoma as adults. Thus continued vigilance is needed, even in patients with initially normal intraocular pressure.
- Angioma of the choroid occurs in 30% to 40% of patients with SWS and can lead to increased intraocular pressure. These lesions may be diffuse or localized within the retina.
- Episcleral and conjunctival lesions include anomalous vessels or true angiomata. These may be caused by increased venous pressure in the eye.
- Weber originally noted heterochromia of the iris. The more deeply pigmented iris usually is ipsilateral to the facial angioma. The pigmentation is caused by aggregated melanocytic hamartomata on the anterior surface of the iris.

NEUROLOGIC FEATURES:

- The neurologic features of SWS are progressive and include seizures, focal neurologic deficits, and mental retardation. These disorders occur with variable severity. A small proportion of patients have no neurologic abnormalities.
- The reasons for neurologic progression are uncertain. A possible mechanism is hypoxic-ischemic injury to tissue adjacent to the leptomeningeal angioma. Other proposed mechanisms are venous occlusion and increased venous pressure.

SEIZURES:

1. Seizures occur in 80% of patients with SWS and are more common with bilateral than unilateral port-wine stains. Seizures may develop at any age, although they usually start in early childhood.
2. Seizures are often the first symptom to appear. Initially, seizures are typically focal but often become generalized tonic-clonic. Less often, infantile spasms or myoclonic or atonic seizures are seen. The occurrence of seizures, the age at onset, and the response to treatment affect prognosis. Onset before age 1 yr and poor response to anticonvulsant therapy are associated with a greater likelihood of cognitive impairment.
   - Hemiparesis: often develops acutely in conjunction with the onset of seizures. The deficit occurs contralateral to the facial and intracranial lesions. The affected extremity usually does not grow at a normal rate, resulting in hemiatrophy. Some affected children have progressive loss of motor function or have a series of stroke-like events.
   - Mental retardation: children with SWS typically develop normally for several months after birth, then manifest devel-

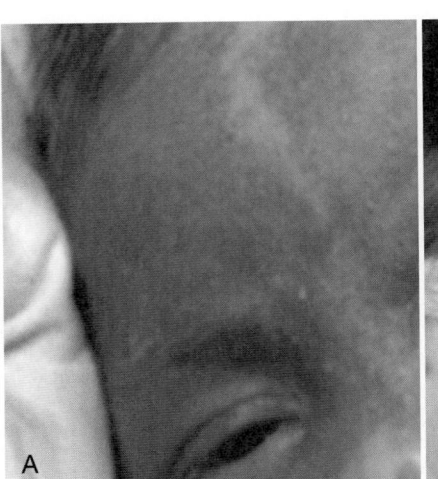
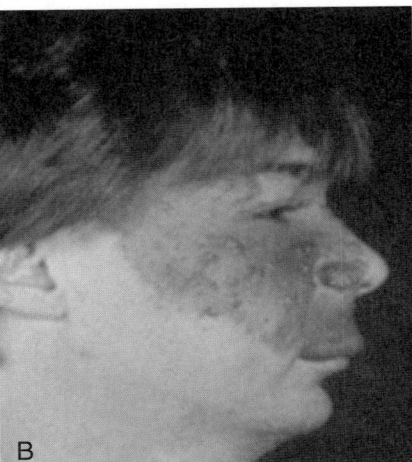

FIGURE 1-362 Port-wine stain at different stages.

opmental delay. However, impairment can be obvious soon after birth, especially in infants with extensive brain involvement. Cognitive function is poorest in patients with bilateral intracerebral lesions. In one report, only 8% of patients with bilateral leptomeningeal angiomata were intellectually normal.

- Behavior problems: are more common in SWS patients than in their unaffected siblings. Higher risk for psychological problems is associated with poorer cognitive function and frequent seizures. However, behavior problems can occur in patients with normal intelligence.
- Other deficits: many patients have visual field defects, typically homonymous hemianopia. This is from the involvement of the leptomeningeal angioma with one or both occipital lobes or optic tracts. Hydrocephalus also may occur. This disorder is believed to result from increased venous pressure caused by thrombosis of the deep venous channels or extensive arteriovenous anastomoses.

ETIOLOGY

The etiology of SWS is unknown. One hypothesis suggests that the capillary angiomata result from somatic mutations in fetal ectodermal tissues that cause inappropriate control or maturation of capillary blood vessel formation.

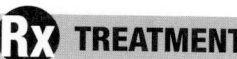 DIAGNOSIS

DIFFERENTIAL DIAGNOSIS

- Klippel-Trenaunay-Weber syndrome (extensive capillary angiomata associated with dysplastic veins involving the limbs and trunk, often with hypertrophy of the affected extremity)
- Von Hippel-Lindau disease (associated with capillary retinal angiomata in contrast to cavernous angiomata seen in SWS)

WORKUP

SWS should be suspected in all patients with facial capillary malformations involving the trigeminal dermatome. At-risk infants should undergo careful physical examination to determine the extent of the malformation.

IMAGING STUDIES

- Most children with facial port-wine stains without an intracranial lesion would be expected to develop normally. Therefore performing neuroimaging studies is helpful to provide prognostic information.
- Plain radiographs of the skull may detect intracranial calcifications, revealing the classic "tram line" appearance, but calcifications are often not present before age 2 yr. Newer radiographic techniques have made plain films obsolete.
- The preferred technique is MRI with gadolinium contrast, which demonstrates the presence of the leptomeningeal angioma and the extent of involvement with brain structures (Fig. 1-363).
- If MRI is not readily available, cranial CT reliably identifies brain calcification and provides some anatomic information.
- In some cases leptomeningeal involvement may not be detected by neuroimaging during infancy and only becomes apparent later. There is no absolute way to exclude intracerebral lesions during the first year after birth.

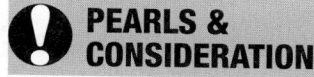 TREATMENT

No specific treatment exists for SWS. The cutaneous, ocular, and neurologic manifestations are treated with mixed success.

ACUTE GENERAL & CHRONIC Rx
Port-wine stain:
- Port-wine stains can be treated by selective photothermolysis with a pulsed-dye laser. Treatment can be further optimized for individual patients so that blanching of the lesion can be accomplished in the fewest possible sessions.
- The response of facial port-wine stains to laser treatment depends on the location and size of the lesion and the patient's age. The greatest decrease in size occurs in the smallest lesions and in the youngest children

(<1 yr). The greater success in the youngest patients may reflect treatment before the development of ectasias.
- Complications of laser therapy include scarring and transient hyperpigmentation. Retinal injury can occur if the eyes are not shielded properly.

Glaucoma:
- The development of new medications has improved the medical management of glaucoma in SWS. However, topical treatment often is ineffective in normalizing intraocular pressure. In these cases, the surgical treatment depends on the etiology of the glaucoma.

Seizures:
- Management of seizures in SWS often is difficult. The success of controlling seizures with anticonvulsant medication is variable and unpredictable. Carbamazepine is the recommended antiepileptic of choice. In refractory cases, hemispherectomy or more limited surgical resection of epileptogenic tissue may be beneficial, although risks often outweigh benefits.

REFERRAL

- Initial ophthalmologic evaluation should be performed in the neonatal period because of the risk of congenital glaucoma.
- If the first complete ophthalmologic evaluation is normal, it should be repeated frequently (some authors have suggested quarterly evaluations) for the first 2 yr of life.
- If the examination results remain normal, the vision should be reevaluated at least annually throughout the patient's lifetime.
- Periodic evaluation by a pediatric neurologist is an essential component of the management of SWS.

⊘ PEARLS & CONSIDERATIONS

COMMENTS

- The prognosis for SWS depends on the extent of the leptomeningeal angioma and its effect on the perfusion of the cerebral cortex as well as the severity of ocular involvement.
- Prognosis also is affected by the age of onset of seizures and whether they can be controlled.
- Neurologic function may deteriorate with age. As a result, approximately half of affected adults are impaired, including those who initially were normal.

PATIENT & FAMILY EDUCATION

- The Sturge-Weber Foundation is an active support group for patients and families (http://www.sturge-weber.com).

SUGGESTED READINGS
available at www.expertconsult.com

AUTHOR: RUBY SATPATHY, M.D.

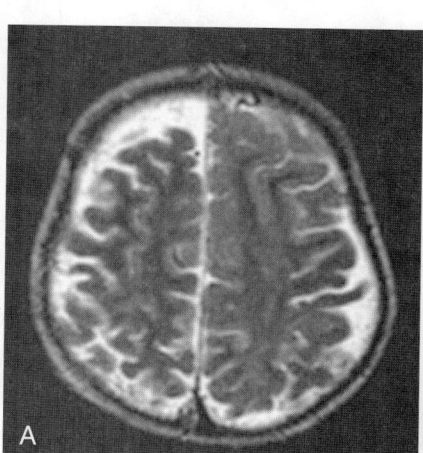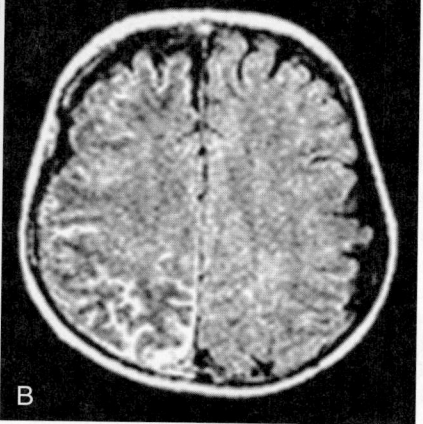

FIGURE 1-363 Axial magnetic resonance image of child with Sturge-Weber syndrome demonstrating atrophy of the left hemisphere and contrast enhancement of the surface of the left hemisphere particularly prominent over the occipital lobe.

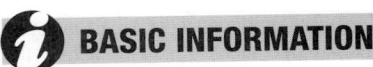

DEFINITION

Subarachnoid hemorrhage (SAH) is defined as hemorrhage into the subarachnoid space. There are several causes of SAH, with the most common being head trauma and the rupture of an intracerebral aneurysm.

SYNONYMS

Subarachnoid bleed

ICD-9CM CODES
430 Subarachnoid hemorrhage

EPIDEMIOLOGY & DEMOGRAPHICS

INCIDENCE: ~6 to 8 cases/100,000 persons per yr
PREDOMINANT SEX: Women aged >55 yr were found to have a 25% greater risk of developing SAH compared with men of the same age.
PREDOMINANT AGE: The mean age at onset is 55 yr.
PEAK INCIDENCE: Most aneurysmal SAH occurs in people who are between the ages of 55 and 60 yr.
GENETICS:
- First-degree relatives have a 5 to 12 times greater risk of developing SAH compared with the general population.
- If someone has two or more first-degree relatives who have experienced aneurysmal SAH, screening may be worthwhile.
- Autosomal dominant polycystic kidney disease is known to be associated with cerebral aneurysms in 8% of cases; screening is recommended in families with this condition in which one family member has experienced a ruptured aneurysm.

RISK FACTORS: Although genetics seem to play a factor in SAH, lifestyle factors are more important for determining overall risk. These risk factors include smoking, hypertension, oral contraception, pregnancy, and cocaine use.

PHYSICAL FINDINGS & CLINICAL PRESENTATION

- The primary symptom is a sudden, severe headache in 97% of cases. This is classically described as the "worst headache of my life" and also called a thunderclap headache.
- 30% to 60% of patients report a history of sentinel bleeds with short last headaches during the weeks before the hemorrhage.
- The onset of the headache may be associated with a brief loss of consciousness, a seizure, nausea or vomiting, and meningismus.
- Altered mental status and coma may result from the direct effect of the SAH causing a mass effect and increased intracranial pressure.
- A posterior communication aneurysm may cause a third cranial nerve palsy.

ETIOLOGY

- Trauma is the most common cause of SAH.
- 75% to 80% of cases of spontaneous SAH are caused by the rupture of a cerebral aneurysm.
- Idiopathic SAH, which is also known as angiogram-negative SAH, is found in 15% to 20% of cases of spontaneous SAH. In these cases, no angiographic cause of the hemorrhage is found.
- Other culprits include arteriovenous malformations, bleeding into preexisting tumors, vasculitis, and cerebral artery dissection.
- Cocaine abuse, sickle cell anemia, coagulopathies, and pituitary apoplexy can also result in SAH.

DIAGNOSIS

DIFFERENTIAL DIAGNOSIS

- Intracerebral hemorrhage as a result of trauma, tumors, and stroke with hemorrhagic conversion
- Other causes of headache, including migraines, tension headaches, and cluster headaches

WORKUP

- Look for a history that is suggestive of SAH (e.g., thunderclap headache, "worst headache of my life").
- Computed tomography (CT) will be positive in more than 95% of cases, especially during the acute phase (i.e., 24 to 48 hr) after the onset of bleeding (Fig. 1-364).
- Lumbar puncture is a very important part of the workup, especially because 3% of patients with normal CT scans show evidence of hemorrhage on lumbar puncture. An RBC count of more than 100,000/m³ is strongly suggestive of SAH. If RBC counts drop between the first and fourth tubes, then the tap is most likely traumatic. The presence of xanthochromia or bilirubin in the cerebrospinal fluid is a sign of SAH.
- A CT angiogram or a cerebral angiogram is imperative for determining the origin of the SAH. Angiography may also be extremely useful, because it may offer a therapeutic benefit via the coiling of the aneurysm.

LABORATORY TESTS

- Basic laboratory values, including CBC, chemistry panel, prothrombin time, partial thromboplastin time, and platelet count
- Troponin and sodium levels also important to guide management

IMAGING STUDIES

- High-resolution CT scanning (Fig. 1-364) correctly identifies more than 95% of SAH cases, with blood appearing hyperdense in the subarachnoid spaces.
- Cerebral angiography is the gold standard for diagnosis and may offer a therapeutic option via coiling.

- MRI is not a good imaging modality during the acute phase; however, its sensitivity increases after 4 to 7 days.

TREATMENT

NONPHARMACOLOGIC THERAPY

- Patients with a depressed level of consciousness may need to be intubated and mechanically ventilated in an intensive care unit setting.
- A lumbar drain or a ventriculostomy is required should the patient develop hydrocephalus and increased intracranial pressure.

ACUTE GENERAL Rx

- Initial management strategies are geared toward stabilizing the patient and preventing rehemorrhage and hydrocephalus.
- Tight blood pressure control is paramount. This can be done with the use of drips (e.g., nipride) or as-needed medications. A systolic blood pressure of 120 to 150 mm Hg is recommended.
- After an aneurysm has been identified, measures to secure it should be undertaken; this can be done by either clipping or coiling the aneurysm. Clipping consists of placing a clip around the neck of the aneurysm and is performed via intra-arterial angiography; it consists of deploying platinum coils inside the aneurysm to cause thrombosis of the aneurysmal sac.
- Pain control is performed with the use of short-acting and less-sedating medications (e.g., codeine, low-dose morphine).
- Seizures occur in about 3% of patients during the acute phase; however, the use of prophylactic antiepileptics is still controversial.
- Vasospasm, which typically begins around day 3 after the hemorrhage and reaches a

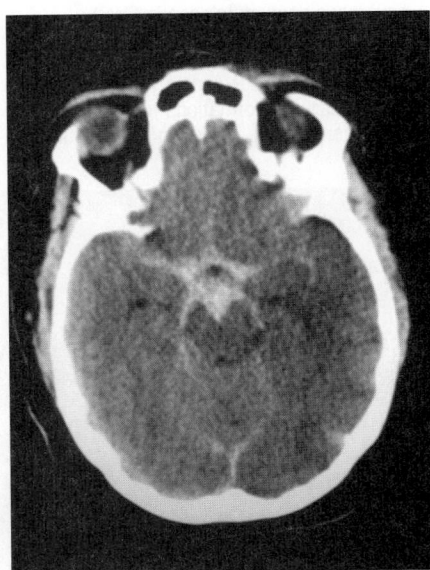

FIGURE 1-364 Noncontrast CT of brain in patient with subarachnoid hemorrhage.

peak on day 6 to 8, is the leading cause of death and disability after aneurysm rupture. Nimodipine has been shown to improve outcomes if it is administered between days 4 and 21 after the hemorrhage, even if it does not significantly reduce the amount of vasospasm detected on angiography. After vasospasm develops, "triple H" therapy—to achieve *H*ypertension, *H*ypervolemia, and *H*emodilution—is used in an attempt to provide adequate cerebral perfusion.

CHRONIC Rx

Chronic treatment usually involves the management of the complications of SAH through means such as intensive physical therapy and rehabilitation.

DISPOSITION

- SAH is often associated with a poor outcome. The death rate associated with SAH is between 40% and 50%, with 10% to 15% of patients dying before they reach the hospital.
- More than 46% of those who survive hospitalization have cognitive impairments that affect their lifestyles.

REFERRAL

Patients should be transferred as soon as possible to a facility with neurosurgical care.

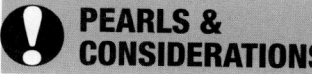

COMMENTS

- After the diagnosis of SAH is made, the patient should be transferred to a facility where neurosurgical care in an intensive care unit setting is available.
- All anticoagulation and antiplatelet therapy should be withheld, and coagulopathy should be corrected.
- Patients should be adequately hydrated, and Nimotop should be started to prevent poor outcomes of vasospasm.
- Measures to prevent rebleeding include adequate control of blood pressure and aneurysm treatment with the use of coiling or clipping.

PREVENTION

Controlling some of the modifiable risk factors, including smoking and blood pressure, may help to decrease the risk of aneurysmal rupture.

PATIENT/FAMILY EDUCATION

- SAH is a devastating condition, with most survivors developing significant cognitive deficits. A good support system and an adequate physical and cognitive rehabilitation program may prove useful to survivors.
- Screening may be useful for patients with two or three relatives with SAH.

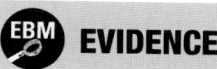

available at www.expertconsult.com

SUGGESTED READINGS
available at www.expertconsult.com

AUTHORS: **WISSAM S. Z. ASFAHANI, M.D.,** and **CHRISTIAN N. RAMSEY, III, M.D.**

S

Diseases and Disorders

BASIC INFORMATION

DEFINITION

Subclavian steal syndrome is an occlusion or severe stenosis of the proximal subclavian artery leading to decreased antegrade flow or retrograde flow in the ipsilateral vertebral artery and neurologic symptoms referable to the posterior circulation.

SYNONYMS

Proximal subclavian (or innominate) artery stenosis or occlusion

ICD-9CM CODES
435.2 Subclavian steal syndrome

EPIDEMIOLOGY & DEMOGRAPHICS

- Similar to that of other manifestations of atherosclerosis (coronary artery disease, cerebrovascular disease, or peripheral vascular disease)
- Affects middle-aged persons (men somewhat younger than women on average) with arteriosclerotic risk factors, including family history, smoking, diabetes mellitus, hyperlipidemia, hypertension, and sedentary lifestyle

PHYSICAL FINDINGS & CLINICAL PRESENTATION

Symptoms:
- Many patients are asymptomatic.
- Upper extremity ischemic symptoms: fatigue, exercise-related aching, coolness, numbness of the involved upper extremity.
- Neurologic symptoms are reported by 25% of patients with known unilateral subclavian steal. These include brief spells of:
  1. Vertigo
  2. Diplopia
  3. Decreased vision
  4. Oscillopsia
  5. Gait unsteadiness

These spells are only occasionally provoked by exercising the ischemic upper extremity (classic subclavian steal). Left subclavian steal is more common than right, but the latter is more serious.
- Posterior circulation stroke related to subclavian steal is rare.
- Innominate artery stenosis can cause decreased right carotid artery flow and cerebrovascular symptoms of the anterior cerebral circulation, but this is uncommon.

Physical findings:
- Delayed and smaller volume pulse (wrist or antecubital) in the affected upper extremity
- Lower blood pressure in the affected upper extremity
- Supraclavicular bruit

NOTE: Inflating a blood pressure cuff will increase the bruit if it originates from a vertebral artery stenosis and decrease the bruit if it originates from a subclavian artery stenosis.

ETIOLOGY & PATHOGENESIS

Etiology:
- Atherosclerosis
- Arteritis (Takayasu's disease and temporal arteritis)
- Embolism to the subclavian or innominate artery
- Cervical rib
- Long-term use of a crutch
- Occupational (baseball pitchers and cricket bowlers)

Pathogenesis: The vertebral artery originates from the subclavian artery. For subclavian steal to occur, the occlusion must be proximal to the takeoff of the vertebral artery. On the right side, only a small distance separates the bifurcation of the innominate artery and the takeoff of the vertebral artery, explaining why the condition occurs less commonly on the right side. Occlusion of the innominate artery must affect right carotid artery flow.

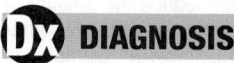

DIAGNOSIS

The carotid arteries should be evaluated at least noninvasively in all cases.

DIFFERENTIAL DIAGNOSIS

- Posterior circulation transient ischemic attack or stroke
- Upper extremity ischemia
  1. Distal subclavian artery stenosis or occlusion
  2. Raynaud's syndrome
  3. Thoracic outlet syndrome

WORKUP

- Noninvasive upper extremity arterial flow studies
- Doppler sonography of the vertebral, subclavian, and innominate arteries
- Arteriography

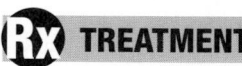

TREATMENT

- In most patients the disease is benign and requires no treatment other than atherosclerosis risk factor modification and aspirin. Symptoms tend to improve over time as collateral circulation develops.
- Vascular surgical reconstruction requires a thoracotomy; it may be indicated in innominate artery stenosis or when upper extremity ischemia is incapacitating.

AUTHOR: **FRED F. FERRI, M.D.**

BASIC INFORMATION

DEFINITION

A subdural hematoma (SDH) is a collection of blood or blood products between the arachnoidal (superficial) layer of the brain and the dura or meningeal layer of the brain.

SYNONYMS

Subdural hemorrhage

ICD-9CM CODES
852.10 Subdural hematoma

EPIDEMIOLOGY & DEMOGRAPHICS

INCIDENCE: SDH is a common finding, especially among trauma patients.
PREVALENCE: Unknown
PEAK INCIDENCE: SDH most commonly occurs in the elderly and alcoholic populations as a result of cerebral atrophy and in the infant population (e.g., shaken baby) as a result of the increasing traction on the bridging veins between the brain parenchyma and the dura mater. SDHs are more common than epidural hematomas.
RISK FACTORS: Any conditions that predispose patients to hemorrhage (e.g., anticoagulants, antiplatelet therapy); atrophy of the brain (e.g., dementia, alcoholism); or falls and trauma (e.g., movement disorders, previous stroke)

PHYSICAL FINDINGS & CLINICAL PRESENTATION

Symptoms vary on the basis of acuity, size, and location. Acute traumatic SDHs are often seen in comatose patients. When they are associated with a midline shift (i.e., >5 mm), they can cause signs of cerebral herniation (e.g., ipsilateral pupil dilation, contralateral weakness). Chronic and subacute SDHs present with variable symptoms of headache, mild weakness, slowness of mentation, aphasia, mobility problems, and abulia.

ETIOLOGY

SDH is usually the result of shear and of the tearing of a bridging vein. It can be caused by any source of bleeding into the subdural space (i.e., contusion, extension of parenchymal hemorrhage, rarely other vascular abnormalities [e.g., arteriovenous malformation, aneurysm]).

DX **DIAGNOSIS**

DIFFERENTIAL DIAGNOSIS

Other causes of subdural collections, such as hygromas, abscesses, and tumor infiltrations.

WORKUP

- Patient history, including medications with anticoagulant properties, alcohol abuse, trauma, cancer, and recent bacterial infections
- Physical examination, including alertness, pupil and facial symmetry, and motor weakness (i.e., pronator drift)

LABORATORY TESTS

- Prothrombin time (international normalized ratio)
- partial thromboplastin time

IMAGING STUDIES

A noncontrast computed tomographic (CT) scan of the head should be obtained (Fig. 1-365). For comatose and trauma patients, include a cervical spine CT scan. Contrast is only needed if there are concerns about tumor or infection.

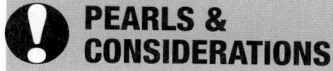 **TREATMENT**

1. Correction of underlying coagulopathy, if present (e.g., Coumadin reversal)
2. The majority of SDH can be managed without surgery in awake patients with normal neurologic examinations.

NONPHARMACOLOGIC THERAPY

1. For acute SDH with mass effect, midline shift, and clinical effects (e.g., coma, weakness), surgical evacuation is required.
2. For chronic SDH with a mass effect, a change in the clinical examination from the baseline evacuation, or enlargement, evacuation via craniotomy or burr hole should be considered.

COMPLEMENTARY AND ALTERNATIVE MEDICINE

Remember that some herbal and alternative medicines can be associated with coagulopathy.

DISPOSITION

Depending on the size and location of the SDH and the examination of the patient, observation can range from the intensive care unit to outpatient management. When observation of the patient is considered, clinical examinations should be serially performed. Patient baseline and follow-up clinical examinations are more important than CT scan findings.

REFERRAL

Neurosurgical and operative consultation should be made available.

! **PEARLS & CONSIDERATIONS**

COMMENTS

- Many elderly patients have small chronic SDHs or hygromas. Unless these are associated with seizures or clinical or radiographic progression, they are usually not emergent. The important thing is to recognize the cause (e.g., medication, fall risk).
- Recurrence after surgical management for chronic SDH is common.
- SDHs in elderly patients can have a mixed hyperdense and hypodense appearance on noncontrast CT scan; this is suggestive of acute and chronic components.

PREVENTION

Fall risk and prevention, especially among the elderly, are very important when considering anticoagulant medications.

PATIENT/FAMILY EDUCATION

Individuals with SDHs are at higher risk for seizure, so surveillance is important.

AUTHOR: **CHRISTIAN N. RAMSEY, M.D.**

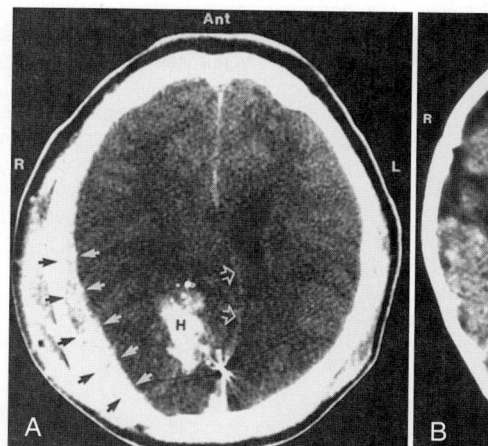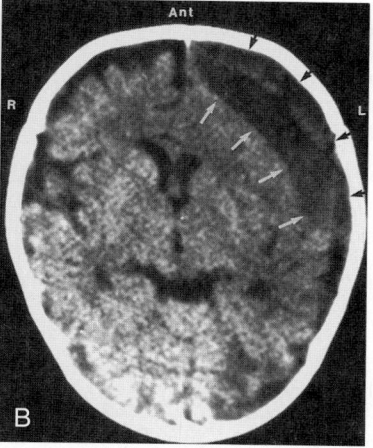

FIGURE 1-365 Subdural hematomas. A, A noncontrast computed tomographic scan of an acute subdural hematoma shows a crescentic area of increased density in the right posterior parietal region between the brain and the skull *(black and white arrows)*. An area of intraparenchymal hemorrhage *(H)* is also seen. **B,** A chronic subdural hematoma for a different patient is shown. There is an area of decreased density in the left frontoparietal region *(arrows)* that effaces the sulci, compresses the anterior horn of the left lateral ventricle, and shifts the midline somewhat to the right. (From Mettler FA [ed]: *Primary care radiology,* Philadelphia, 2000, WB Saunders.)

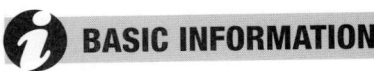

BASIC INFORMATION

DEFINITION

Suicide is the intentional ending of one's own life.

SYNONYMS

Self-murder

ICD-9CM CODES

Categorized by method

EPIDEMIOLOGY & DEMOGRAPHICS

INCIDENCE (IN U.S.): Mortality (CDC)

All suicides
- Number of deaths: 34,598
- Deaths per 100,000 population: 11.5
- Cause of death rank: 11

Firearm suicides
- Number of deaths: 17,352
- Deaths per 100,000 population: 5.8

Suffocation suicides
- Number of deaths: 8161
- Deaths per 100,000 population: 2.7

Poisoning suicides
- Number of deaths: 6358
- Deaths per 100,000 population: 2.1

Suicidal deaths are only part of the problem. More people survive suicide attempts than actually die. They are often seriously injured and need medical care.

AGE-RELATED DATA:
- Incidence of suicide increases with age (13.1 cases/100,000 persons ages 15 to 24 yr, 16.9 cases/100,000 persons ages 65 to 74 yr, and 23.5 cases/100,000 persons ages 75 to 84 yr)
- During 2002 to 2006, the greatest percentage of suicides occurred by firearm among all race/ethnicity groups for persons ages 65 yr and older. Except for Asian/Pacific Islanders, suffocation accounted for the highest percentage of suicides among those 65 yr and older (52.6%).

GENDER DIFFERENCES:
- Women attempt suicide about two to three times as often as men.
- Males succeed at taking their own lives at nearly four times the rate of females and represent 79% of all U.S. suicides.
- Suicide is the seventh leading cause of death for males and sixteenth leading cause for females.

- Firearms are the most common method of suicide among males (56%).
- Poisoning is the most common method in women (40.3%).

ENVIRONMENTAL FACTORS
- Suicide rates traditionally decrease in times of war and increase in times of economic crises.
- After adjusting for age, suicide rates are highest in the western and northwestern regions of the United States.

MARITAL STATUS: Suicide rates are highest among the divorced, separated, and widowed and lowest among the married.

SUBSTANCE USE: CDC data:
- 33.3% of suicides tested positive for alcohol and 16.4% for opiates.

RISK FACTORS:
- Previous suicide attempt(s).
- History of depression or other mental illness (bipolar, psychosis, PTSD, and others).
- Anxiety.
- Alcohol or drug abuse.
- Family history of suicide or violence.
- Physical illness.
- Feeling alone.
- Individuals with a mental or substance use disorder account for >90% of suicides.
- The concurrence of more than one condition (e.g., depression and alcohol abuse) greatly increases the risk.
- Hopelessness is a strong predictor of suicide potential.
- Rates are higher in developing countries.
- Rates vary by occupation, ethnicity, and employment status.

SUICIDAL BEHAVIOR:
- All suicidal behavior should be taken seriously, as a failed attempt may lead to a completed suicide in the future.
- Nearly half of suicides are preceded by an attempt that does not end in death.
- Those with a history of attempts are 23 times more likely to eventually end their own lives than those without.
- A suicidal gesture does not have death as a goal, but can serve as a dramatic way of alerting others to some type of ongoing distress.
- Risky behaviors such as speeding or disregarding traffic laws, or abusing drugs, are considered parasuicide when the person shows total disregard for whether the actions might result in his or her death.

- Unsuccessful suicide attempts may also result from miscalculations in the plan. These people are at high risk for attempting suicide again.

EVALUATION:
- The provider must directly inquire into the presence of suicidal ideation. Approximately one half to two thirds of individuals who commit suicide visit physicians within 1 mo of taking their lives.
- Explicit suicidal intent, hopelessness, and a well-formulated plan indicate high risk. Clinicians can use the mnemonic SAL: Is the method specific? Is it available? Is it lethal?
- The concurrence of multiple psychiatric problems, substance abuse, and multiple physical problems increases the risk.
- Covert suicidal ideation occurs in patients primarily with multiple vague physical complaints, depression, anxiety, or substance abuse.

ACUTE INTERVENTIONS

- Place patient in a safe environment (usually hospitalization in a psychiatric unit or a medical unit with continuous observation).
- Emergency medical stabilization and clearance as required, related to severity and lethality of attempt, age, comorbid medical issues, and overall clinical presentation.

ACUTE PSYCHOPHARMACOLOGICAL INTERVENTIONS

- Benzodiazepines may be useful in reducing extreme anxiety and dysphoria in an acutely suicidal patient; however, these agents should not be prescribed until the means of the suicidal attempt are known (not a benzodiazepine overdose) and patient is medically stable (i.e., respiratory system, vital signs, cognitive functioning are stable).
- Antipsychotics (typicals or atypicals) can be used if psychosis is present (e.g., voices telling patient to hurt self) and to manage acute agitation.
- If indicated, mood stabilizers and antidepressants can be started in the acute setting but may have up to a 2-wk latency period. However, awareness of increased risk of suicidal thoughts/behavior with these medications in some populations is required.

TABLE 1-171 Suicide and Risk Factors: A Summary

Primary Diagnosis	Demographics	Personality Factors	Comorbidities	Social Factors	Other Factors
Bipolar	Male	Borderline	Substance abuse	Divorced	Means available
Schizophrenia	Older Age	Narcissistic	Panic disorder	Widower	History of child abuse
MDD	White race	Antisocial	Anxiety	Lives alone	Few reasons to live
Dysthymia	Homosexuality	Conduct disorder	Axis III dx	Isolated	Lots of adverse events
Adjustment d/o	History of attempt	Impulsive		Money worries	Change grades
Conduct D/O	Family History			Other losses	Change friends
Psychosis	Suicidal ideas			No religion	Giving things away
	Hopeless				Guns in the home
	Helpless				

From Kaplan & Sadock: Comprehesive textbook of psychiatry, ed 9, Wolters Kluwer Health/Lippincott Williams Wilkins, 2009.

THERAPY

- Long-term: psychotherapy aimed at factors that underlie the decision to pursue suicide or at the risk factors contributing to suicidal behavior
- Substance abuse treatment (e.g., Alcoholics Anonymous, Narcotics Anonymous) when substance use disorder is present
- Therapy should be aimed at the underlying condition (e.g., antidepressants for depression, anxiolytics or antidepressants for anxiety, substance abuse treatment, or psychotherapy for chronic low self-esteem, hopelessness).
- In elderly, loneliness and medical disability are major reasons for suicide and therefore major targets for intervention.
- Involvement of family members, spouse, loved one, care givers if possible for therapy and management.

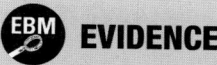

EVIDENCE

available at www.expertconsult.com

SUGGESTED READINGS

available at www.expertconsult.com

AUTHOR: **ALI KAZIM, M.D.**

S

Diseases and Disorders

I

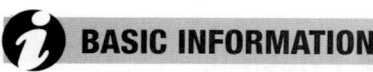

BASIC INFORMATION

DEFINITION

Superior vena cava syndrome is a set of symptoms that results when a mediastinal mass compresses the superior vena cava (SVC) or the veins that drain into it.

ICD-9CM CODES
453.2 Vena cava thrombosis

EPIDEMIOLOGY & DEMOGRAPHICS

- SVC syndrome occurs in 15,000 persons in the U.S. every year.
- Mirrors lung cancer (especially small-cell carcinoma) and lymphoma (see "Lung Neoplasm" and "Lymphoma" in Section I).

PHYSICAL FINDINGS & CLINICAL PRESENTATION

The pathophysiology of the syndrome involves the increased pressure in the venous system draining into the SVC, producing edema of the head, neck, and upper extremities. Symptoms develop over a period of 2 wk in one third of patients and include:
- Shortness of breath
- Chest pain
- Cough
- Dysphagia, hoarseness, stridor
- Headache
- Syncope
- Visual trouble

Signs:
- Chest wall vein distention (Fig. 1-366)
- Neck vein distention

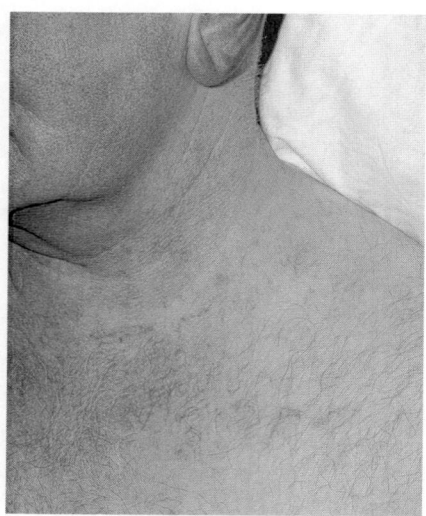

FIGURE 1-366 Superior vena cava obstruction causing dilated veins and plethora of the upper trunk and neck in a patient with bronchial carcinoma. Patients with superior vena cava obstruction are occasionally referred to dermatologists with suspected contact allergy (eyelid swelling) or angioedema (facial or hand swelling). (From White GM, Cox NH [eds]: *Diseases of the skin, a color atlas and text*, ed 2, St Louis, 2006, Mosby.)

- Facial edema
- Upper extremity swelling
- Cyanosis

ETIOLOGY

- Lung cancer (80% of all cases, of which half are small-cell lung cancer)
- Lymphoma (15%)
- Thymoma
- Tuberculosis
- Goiter
- Aortic aneurysm (arteriosclerotic or syphilitic)
- SVC thrombosis
  1. Primary: associated with a central venous catheter
  2. Secondary: as a complication of SVC syndrome associated with one of the above-mentioned causes
- Inflammatory process, fibrosing mediastinitis
- Table 1-172 summarizes common malignancies associaed with SVC syndrome in adults

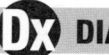

DIAGNOSIS

CT of the chest with contrast is the most useful diagnostic study. MRI is usually adequate to establish the diagnosis of SVC obstruction and to assist in the differential diagnosis of probable cause.

DIFFERENTIAL DIAGNOSIS

The syndrome is characteristic enough to exclude other diagnoses. The differential diagnosis concerns the underlying etiologies listed above.

WORKUP

- Chest radiograph
- Chest CT with contrast or MRI (in patient who cannot tolerate contrast medium)
- Venography: warranted only when an intervention (e.g., stent or surgery) is planned
- Percutaneous needle biopsy (usually the initial diagnostic modality used to establish a histologic diagnosis)
- Bronchoscopy
- Mediastinoscopy
- Thoracotomy

TREATMENT

- Although invasive procedures such as mediastinoscopy or thoracotomy are associated with higher than usual risk of bleeding, a tissue diagnosis is usually needed before commencing therapy.
- Management is guided by the severity of the symptoms and the underlying etiology.
- Emergency empiric radiation is indicated in critical situations such as respiratory failure or central nervous system signs associated with increased intracranial pressure.
- Treatment of the underlying malignancy:
  1. Radiotherapy: the majority of tumors causing SVC syndrome are sensitive to radiotherapy
  2. Systemic chemotherapy
- Anticoagulant or fibrinolytic therapy in patients who do not respond to cancer treatment within a week or if an obstructing thrombus has been documented.
- Loop diuretics are often used, but their effect is limited.
- Upright positioning and fluid restriction until collateral channels develop and allow for clinical regression are useful modalities for SVC syndrome secondary to benign disease.
- Steroids (dexamethasone 4 mg q6h) may be useful in reducing the tumor burden in lymphoma and thymoma.
- Percutaneous self-expandable stents that can be placed under local anesthesia with radiologic manipulation are useful in the treatment of SVC syndrome to bypass the obstruction, especially in cases associated with malignant tumors.
- Surgical bypass grafting is infrequently used to treat SVC syndrome.

REFERRAL

To a thoracic surgeon, pulmonary specialist, or oncologist

AUTHOR: **FRED F. FERRI, M.D.**

TABLE 1-172 Malignancies Associated with Superior Vena Cava (SVC) Syndrome in Adults*

Neoplastic Diagnosis	Percentage of SVC	Percentage of Disease-Associated SVC
Lung cancer, stage 3B or 4:	48-81	
Small cell lung cancer		15-45
Squamous cell cancer		20-25
Adenocarcinoma		5-25
Large cell carcinoma		4-30
Lymphoma:	2-21	
Diffuse large cell lymphoma		64
Lymphoblastic lymphoma		33
Breast cancer	11	

Zipes DP, Libby P, Bonow RO, Braunwald E (eds): *Braunwald's heart disease*, ed 7, Philadelphia, 2005, Elsevier.
*Include lung cancer, lymphomas, and metastases from other solid tumors. 75% to 85% of patients with SVC have neoplastic disease.

BASIC INFORMATION

DEFINITION

Syncope is the transient loss of consciousness that results from an acute global reduction in cerebral blood flow. Syncope should be distinguished from other causes of transient loss of consciousness.

ICD-9CM CODES
720.2 Syncope

EPIDEMIOLOGY & DEMOGRAPHICS

- Syncope accounts for 3% to 5% of emergency department visits.
- 30% of the adult population will experience at least one syncopal episode during their lifetimes.
- Incidence of syncope is highest in elderly men and young women.

PHYSICAL FINDINGS & CLINICAL PRESENTATION

- Blood pressure: if low, consider orthostatic hypotension; if unequal in both arms (difference >20 mm Hg), consider subclavian steal or dissecting aneurysm. (NOTE: Blood pressure [BP] and heart rate should be recorded in the supine and standing positions.) If there is a drop in BP but no change in heart rate (HR), the patient may be taking a beta-blocker or may have an autonomic neuropathy.
- Pulse: if patient has tachycardia, bradycardia, or irregular rhythm, consider arrhythmia.
- Heart: if there are murmurs present, consider syncope attributable to left ventricular outflow obstruction; if there are jugular venous distension and distal heart sounds, consider cardiac tamponade.
- Carotid sinus pressure: can be diagnostic if it reproduces symptoms and other causes are excluded; a pause >3 sec or a systolic BP drop >50 mm Hg without symptoms or <30 mm Hg with symptoms when sinus pressure is applied separately on each side for <5 sec is considered abnormal. This test should be avoided in patients with carotid bruits or cerebrovascular disease. ECG monitoring, IV access, and bedside atropine should be available when carotid sinus pressure is applied.

ETIOLOGY

- Neurally mediated syncope
  1. Psychophysiologic (emotional upset, panic disorders, hysteria, hyperventilation)
  2. Visceral reflex (micturition, defecation, food ingestion, coughing, ventricular contraction; glossopharyngeal neuralgia)
  3. Carotid sinus pressure
  4. Reduction of venous return caused by Valsalva maneuver
- Orthostatic hypotension
  1. Hypovolemia
  2. Vasodilator medications
  3. Autonomic neuropathy (diabetes, amyloid, Parkinson's disease, multisystem atrophy)
  4. Pheochromocytoma
  5. Carcinoid syndrome
- Cardiac
  1. Reduced cardiac output
     a. Left ventricular outflow obstruction (aortic stenosis, hypertrophic cardiomyopathy)
     b. Obstruction to pulmonary flow (pulmonary embolism, pulmonic stenosis, primary pulmonary hypertension)
     c. Myocardial infarct with pump failure
     d. Cardiac tamponade
     e. Mitral stenosis
     f. Reduction of venous return (atrial myxoma, valve thrombus)
     g. Beta-blocker therapy
  2. Arrhythmias or asystole
     a. Extreme tachycardia (>160 to 180 beats/min)
     b. Severe bradycardia (<30 to 40 beats/min)
     c. Sick sinus syndrome
     d. Atrioventricular block (second or third degree)
     e. Ventricular tachycardia or fibrillation
     f. Long QT syndrome
     g. Pacemaker malfunction
     h. Psychotropic medications and beta-blockers

DIAGNOSIS

DIFFERENTIAL DIAGNOSIS

1. Seizure (see "Workup.")
2. Vertebrobasilar transient ischemic attack (TIA) usually manifests as diplopia, vertigo, or ataxia but not loss of consciousness. Isolated episodes of transient loss of consciousness (TLOC) without accompanying neurologic symptoms are unlikely to be TIAs.
3. Recreational drugs or alcohol.
4. Functional causes, such as stress and somatoform disorders.
5. Sleep disorders, such as sleep attacks and narcolepsy, are also in the differential for TLOC.
6. Head trauma.

WORKUP

The history is crucial to diagnosing the cause of syncope and may suggest a diagnosis that can be evaluated with directed testing. History is also important to determine other etiologies for TLOC, such as seizure.

- Sudden LOC: consider cardiac arrhythmias.
- Gradual LOC: consider orthostatic hypotension, vasodepressor syncope, hypoglycemia.
- History of aura before LOC or prolonged confusion (>1 min), amnesia, or lethargy after LOC suggests seizure rather than syncope.
- Patient's activity at the time of syncope:
  1. Micturition, coughing, defecation: consider syncope caused by decreased venous return.
  2. Turning head or while shaving: consider carotid sinus syndrome.
  3. Physical exertion in a patient with murmur: consider aortic stenosis.
  4. Arm exercise: consider subclavian steal syndrome.
  5. Assuming an upright position: consider orthostatic hypotension.
- Associated events:
  1. Chest pain: consider myocardial infarction, pulmonary embolism.
  2. Palpitations: consider arrhythmias.
  3. Incontinence (urine or fecal) and tongue biting are associated with seizure or syncope.
  4. Brief, transient shaking after LOC may represent myoclonus from global cerebral hypoperfusion and not seizures. However, sustained tonic/clonic muscle action is more suggestive of seizure.
  5. Focal neurologic symptoms or signs point to a neurologic event such as a seizure with residual deficits (e.g., Todd's paralysis) or cerebral ischemic injury.
  6. Psychologic stress: syncope may be vasovagal.
- Review current medications, particularly antihypertensive and psychotropic drugs.

LABORATORY TESTS

Routine blood tests rarely yield diagnostically useful information and should be done only if they are specifically suggested by the results of the history and physical examination. The following are commonly ordered tests:

- Pregnancy test in women of childbearing age
- Complete blood count to look for anemia and signs of infection
- Electrolytes, blood urea nitrogen, creatinine, magnesium, and calcium to look for electrolyte abnormalities and evaluate fluid status
- Serum glucose level
- Cardiac isoenzymes, especially if the patient gives a history of chest pain before the syncopal episode
- Drug and alcohol levels with suspected toxicity

IMAGING STUDIES

- Echocardiography.
- If seizure is suspected, CT scan and/or MRI of the head and electroencephalogram may be useful.
- If head trauma or neurologic signs on examination, CT or MRI may be helpful.
- If arrhythmias are suspected, a 24-hr Holter monitor or admission to a telemetry unit is appropriate. In general, Holter monitoring is rarely useful, revealing a cause for syncope in <3% of cases. Loop recorders that can be activated after syncopal episode to retrieve information about the cardiac rhythm during the preceding 4 min add considerable diagnostic yield in patients with unexplained syncope.
- Implantable cardiac monitors that function as permanent loop recorders or implantable cardioverter-defibrillators, which are placed subcutaneously in the pectoral region with the patient under local anesthesia, are useful in patients with cardiac syncope.

- Electrophysiologic studies may be indicated in patients with structural heart disease and/or recurrent syncope.
- ECG to rule out arrhythmias; may be diagnostic in 5% to 10% of patients.

TILT-TABLE TESTING

- Useful to support a diagnosis of neurally mediated syncope. Patients age >50 yr should have stress testing before tilt-table testing. Positive results would preclude tilt-table testing.
- Indicated in patients with recurrent episodes of unexplained syncope as well as patients in high-risk occupations (e.g., pilots, bus drivers) (Fig. 1-367). The test is also useful for identifying patients with prominent bradycardic response who may benefit from implantation of a permanent pacemaker.
- It is performed by keeping the patient in an upright posture on a tilt table with footboard support. The angle of the tilt table varies from 60 to 80 degrees. The duration of upright posture during tilt-table testing varies from 25 to 45 min.
- The hallmark of neurally mediated syncope is severe hypotension associated with a para-doxic bradycardia triggered by a specific stimulus. The diagnosis of neurally mediated syncope is likely if upright tilt testing reproduces these hemodynamic changes in <15 min and causes presyncope or syncope.

PSYCHIATRIC EVALUATION

- May be indicated in young patients without heart disease who have frequently recurring transient loss of consciousness and other somatic symptoms.
- Generalized anxiety disorder, pain disorder, and major depression predispose patients to neurally mediated reactions and may result in syncope.

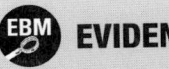 **TREATMENT**

NONPHARMACOLOGIC THERAPY

- Ensure proper hydration; consider thromboembolic stockings and salt tablets in appropriate patients.
- Eliminate medications that may induce hypotension.

ACUTE GENERAL Rx

- Varies with the underlying etiology of syncope (e.g., pacemaker in patients with syncope resulting from complete heart block).
- Syncope caused by orthostatic hypotension is treated with volume replacement in patients with intravascular volume depletion. Also consider midodrine to promote venous return by adrenergic-mediated vasoconstriction and Florinef for its mineralocorticoid effects to increase intravascular volume.

DISPOSITION

Prognosis varies with the age of the patient and the etiology of the syncope. In general:

- Benign prognosis (very low 1-yr morbidity rate) in patients:
  1. Age <30 yr and having noncardiac syncope
  2. Age <70 yr and having vasovagal or psychogenic syncope or syncope of unknown cause
- Poor prognosis (high mortality and morbidity rates) in patients with cardiac syncope.
- Patients with the following risk factors have a higher 1-yr mortality rate: abnormal ECG, history of ventricular arrhythmia, history of congestive heart failure.

REFERRAL

Hospital admission in elderly patients without prior history of syncope or unknown etiology of their syncope and in any patients suspected of having cardiac syncope.

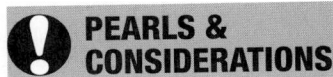 **PEARLS & CONSIDERATIONS**

COMMENTS

- Section III, "Syncope," describes an algorithmic approach to the patient.
- The etiology of syncope is identified in <50% of cases during the initial evaluation.
- A thorough history and physical examination are the most productive means of establishing a diagnosis in patients with syncope.

EVIDENCE

available at www.expertconsult.com

SUGGESTED READINGS

available at www.expertconsult.com

AUTHOR: **SEAN I. SAVITZ, M.D.**

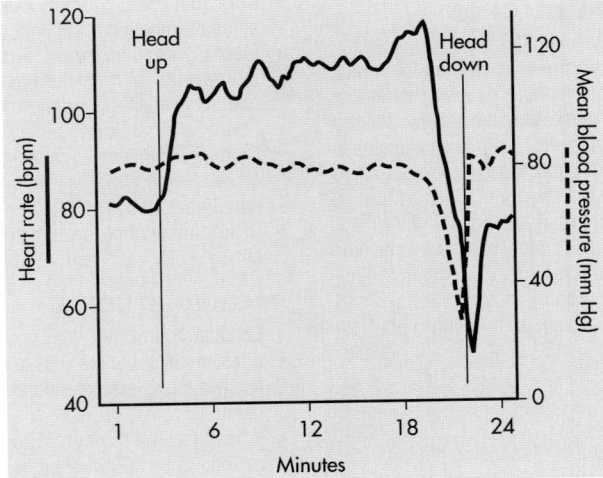

FIGURE 1-367 Head-up tilt test performed on an 18-year-old woman with a history of syncope associated with pain, preceded by a prodrome of dizziness, graying vision, and diaphoresis. A similar prodrome preceded syncope during the test. Note the precipitous and nearly simultaneous decline of heart rate and blood pressure after an initial rise in heart rate. Vital signs returned to normal rapidly after the head was lowered. (Courtesy Robert F. Sprung, University of Utah. In Goldman L, Ausiello D [eds]: *Cecil textbook of medicine,* ed 22, Philadelphia, 2004, WB Saunders.)

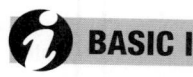

BASIC INFORMATION

DEFINITION

Syndrome of inappropriate antidiuresis (SIAD) is a syndrome characterized by excessive secretion of antidiuretic hormone (ADH) in absence of normal osmotic or physiologic stimuli (increased serum osmolarity, decreased plasma volume, hypotension).

SYNONYMS

SIAD
SIADH
Syndrome of inappropriate antidiuretic hormone secretion
Inappropriate secretion of antidiuretic hormone

ICD-9CM CODES
276.9 Inappropriate secretion of antidiuretic hormone

EPIDEMIOLOGY & DEMOGRAPHICS

The syndrome of inappropriate antidiuresis is the most frequent cause of hyponatremia. Nearly 50% of hyponatremia detected in the hospital setting is caused by SIAD.

PHYSICAL FINDINGS & CLINICAL PRESENTATION

- The patient is generally normovolemic or slightly hypervolemic; edema is absent.
- Delirium, lethargy, and seizures may be present if the hyponatremia is severe or of rapid onset.
- Manifestations of the underlying disease may be evident (e.g., fever from an infectious process or headaches and visual field defects from an intracranial mass).
- Diminished reflexes and extensor plantar responses may occur with severe hyponatremia.

ETIOLOGY

- Neoplasm: lung, oropharynx, stomach, duodenum, pancreas, brain, thymus, bladder, prostate, endometrium, mesothelioma, lymphoma, Ewing's sarcoma
- Pulmonary disorders: pneumonia, aspergillosis, pulmonary abscess, TB, bronchiectasis, emphysema, cystic fibrosis, status asthmaticus, respiratory failure associated with positive-pressure breathing.
- Intracranial pathology: trauma, neoplasms, infections (meningitis, encephalitis, brain abscess), hemorrhage, hydrocephalus, MS, Guillain-Barré syndrome
- Postoperative period: surgical stress, ventilators with positive pressure, anesthetic agents
- Drugs: nicotine, chlorpropamide, thiazide diuretics, vasopressin, desmopressin, oxytocin, chemotherapeutic agents (vincristine, vinblastine, cyclophosphamide), carbamazepine, phenothiazines, MAO inhibitors, tricyclic antidepressants, narcotics, nicotine, clofibrate, haloperidol, SSRIs, NSAIDs

- Other: acute intermittent porphyria, myxedema, psychosis, delirium tremens, ACTH deficiency (hypopituitarism), general anesthesia, endurance exercise

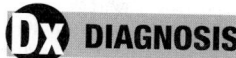

DIAGNOSIS

DIFFERENTIAL DIAGNOSIS

- Hyponatremia associated with hypervolemia (congestive heart failure, cirrhosis, nephrotic syndrome)
- Factitious hyponatremia (hyperglycemia, abnormal proteins, hyperlipidemia)
- Hyponatremia associated with hypovolemia (e.g., burns, GI fluid loss)

WORKUP

- Demonstration through laboratory evaluation (see "Laboratory Tests") of excessive secretion of ADH in absence of appropriate osmotic or physiologic stimuli (abnormal result on test of water load, elevated plasma arginine vasopressin levels despite the presence of hypotonicity and clinical euvolemia)
- Demonstration of normal thyroid, adrenal, and cardiac function
- No recent or concurrent use of diuretics
- Failure to correct hyponatremia after 0.9% saline infusion
- Correction of hyponatremia through fluid restriction

LABORATORY TESTS

- Hyponatremia
- Decreased effective osmolality (<275 mOsm/kg of water)
- Urine osmolality >100 mOsm/kg of water during hypotonicity
- Urinary osmolarity > serum osmolarity
- Urinary sodium usually >40 mEq/L with normal dietary salt intake
- Normal BUN, creatinine (indicative of normal renal function and absence of dehydration), normal TSH
- Decreased uric acid

IMAGING STUDIES

Chest radiograph to rule out neoplasm or infectious process

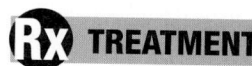

TREATMENT

NONPHARMACOLOGIC THERAPY

Fluid restriction to 500 to 800 ml/day with close monitoring of levels of urinary and plasma electrolytes. Adequate intake of dietary protein and salt should be encouraged.

ACUTE GENERAL Rx

- In emergency situations (seizures, coma) SIAD can be treated with combination of:
  1. Hypertonic saline solution (slow infusion of 250 ml of 3% NaCl). Infuse 3% saline (513 mmol/L) at a rate of 1 to 2 ml/kg of body weight per hour to increase the serum sodium level by 1 to 2 mmol/L/hr.
  2. Furosemide, 20 to 40 mg IV. This combination increases the serum sodium by causing diuresis of urine that is more dilute than plasma and prevents extracellular fluid volume expansion.
- The rapidity of correction varies depending on the degree of hyponatremia and if the hyponatremia is acute or chronic; generally the serum sodium should be corrected only halfway to normal in the initial 24 hr. A prudent approach is to increase serum sodium by <0.5 mEq/L/hr and limit the total increase to 8 to 12 mmol/L during the first 24 hr.
- Close monitoring of the rate of correction (every 2 to 3 hr) is recommended to avoid overcorrection. In patients with hyponatremia of chronic duration, correction of serum sodium level by >12 mmol/L over a period of 24 hr increases the risk of osmotic demyelination.
- Conivaptan (20 to 40 mg/day IV) or tolvaptan (15 mg/day PO initially) are selective arginine-vasopressin (AVP) antagonists useful in selected hospitalized patients with moderate-to-severe hypervolemic and euvolemic hyponatremia. Their direct antagonism of the renal V_2 receptors increases urine water excretion, resulting in an increase in free water clearance (aquaresis). With these agents there is a significant increase in serum sodium concentration in as early as 8 hours and the change is maintained for several days. Potential problems associated with these agents are risk of osmotic demyelination if serum sodium levels are corrected too rapidly and are infusion-site reactions (50% of patients) with conivaptan.

CHRONIC Rx

- Depending on the underlying etiology, fluid restriction may be needed indefinitely. Monthly monitoring of electrolytes is recommended in patients with chronic SIAD.
- Demeclocycline 300 to 600 mg PO bid reduces urinary osmolality and increases serum sodium levels. It may be useful in patients with chronic SIAD (e.g., secondary to neoplasm) but use with caution in patients with hepatic disease; its side effects include nephrogenic diabetes insipidus (DI) and photosensitivity. This medication is also very expensive.
- Successful treatment of chronic nephrogenic SIAD with urea to induce osmotic diuresis has been reported in children and adults. However, oral intake of urea (30 g/day) is generally poorly tolerated.

DISPOSITION

- Prognosis varies depending on the cause. Generally, prognosis is benign when SIAD is caused by an infectious process.

- Morbidity and mortality are high (>40%) when serum sodium concentration is <110 mEq/L.

REFERRAL

Hospital admission depending on severity of symptoms and degree of hyponatremia

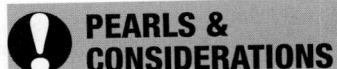

COMMENTS

- Use of hypertonic (3%) saline is contraindicated in patients with CHF, nephrotic syndrome, or cirrhosis.

- Too rapid correction of hyponatremia can cause demyelination and permanent central nervous system damage.

SUGGESTED READING

available at www.expertconsult.com

AUTHOR: **FRED F. FERRI, M.D.**

BASIC INFORMATION

DEFINITION

Syphilis is a systemic sexually transmitted treponemal disease, acute and chronic, characterized by primary skin lesions; secondary eruption involving skin and mucous membranes; long periods of latency; and late lesions of the skin, bone, viscera, central nervous system, and cardiovascular system.

SYNONYMS

Lues

ICD-9CM CODES
097.9 Syphilis, acquired unspecified

EPIDEMIOLOGY & DEMOGRAPHICS

- Widespread, primarily involving ages 20 to 35 yr. Racial differences in incidence are related to social factors. Usually more prevalent in urban areas. Estimated annual incidence of 90,000 cases in the U.S. Increase in incidence in the late 1980s to 1990s, likely related to illicit drug use and prostitution. Increase occurred primarily in lower socioeconomic groups.
- Communicability is indefinite and variable. Communicable during primary, secondary, and latent mucocutaneous lesions in up to first 4 yr of latency. Most probable congenital transmission occurs in early maternal syphilis. Adequate penicillin treatment ends infectivity within 24 to 48 hr.

PHYSICAL FINDINGS & CLINICAL PRESENTATION

PRIMARY SYPHILIS: Characteristic lesion is a painless chancre on genitalia, mouth, or anus; atypical primary lesions may occur. Usually appears 3 wk after exposure and may spontaneously involute.

SECONDARY SYPHILIS:
- Localized or diffuse mucocutaneous lesions and generalized lymphadenopathy. Common to have constitutional symptoms, flulike symptoms. May begin approximately 4 to 6 wk after appearance of primary lesion. Manifestations may resolve in 1 wk to 12 mo.
- 60% to 80% of patients have maculopapular lesions on their palms and soles.
- Condylomata lata intertriginous papules form at areas of friction and moisture, such as the vulva.
- 21% to 58% have mucocutaneous or mucosal lesions (pharyngitis, tonsillitis, "mucous patch" lesion on oral and genital mucosa).

EARLY LATENT (≤1 YR): Generally asymptomatic

LATE LATENT (>1 YR):
- Characterized by gummas (nodular, ulcerative lesions) that can involve the skin, mucous membranes, skeletal system, and viscera.
- Manifestations of cardiovascular syphilis include aortitis, aneurysm, or aortic regurgitation.
- Neurosyphilis may be asymptomatic or symptomatic. Tabes dorsalis, meningovascular syphilis, general paralysis, or insanity may

occur. Iritis, choroidoretinitis, and leukoplakia may also occur.

ETIOLOGY
- *Treponema pallidum,* a spirochete
- Spread by sexual intercourse or by intrauterine transfer

DIAGNOSIS

DIFFERENTIAL DIAGNOSIS
- Other genitoulcerative diseases such as herpes, chancroid (see Section II)
- See Section III for a clinical algorithm for the evaluation of genital ulcer disease

WORKUP
Confirmation is primarily through laboratory diagnosis.

LABORATORY TESTS
- Dark-field microscopy of fluid from lesion to look for treponeme is the definitive method for diagnosis of early syphilis.
- Serologic testing, both nontreponemal (VDRL, RPR) and treponemal (FTA, MHA). The use of only one type of serologic test is insufficient for diagnosis because each type of test has limitations, including the possibility of false-positive test results in persons without syphilis. False-positive nontreponemal test results can be associated with various medical conditions unrelated to syphilis, including autoimmune conditions, older age, and injection-drug use; therefore, persons with a reactive nontreponemal test should receive a treponemal test to confirm the diagnosis of syphilis.
- Lumbar puncture for cerebrospinal fluid VDRL (CSF-VDRL) in patients with evidence of latent syphilis. When reactive in the absence of substantial contamination of CSF with blood, it is considered diagnostic of neurosyphilis.

TREATMENT

ACUTE GENERAL Rx
- Early (primary, secondary, early latent): penicillin G benzathine 2.4 million U IM × 1
- Late (late latent, cardiovascular, gumma): penicillin G benzathine 2.4 million U IM qwk × 3 wk or doxycycline 100 mg PO bid × 4 wk
- Neurosyphilis: aqueous crystalline penicillin G 18 to 24 million U/day, administered as 3 to 4 million U IV q4h × 10 to 14 days or procaine penicillin 2.4 million U IM/day plus probenecid 500 mg PO qid, both for 10 to 14 days
- Congenital syphilis: aqueous crystalline penicillin G 50,000 U/kg/dose IV q12h × first 7 days of life and q8h after that for total of 10 days or procaine penicillin G 50,000 U/kg/dose IM/day × 10 days
- Penicillin-allergic patients with primary or secondary syphilis: doxycycline 100 mg PO bid × 14 days, or tetracycline 500 mg PO qid × 14 days, or ceftriaxone 1 g IM or IV × 8 to 10 days. A recent large study has shown that a single oral dose of azithromycin (2 g admin-

istered as 4 500-mg tablets) can be curative in patients with early syphilis
- Latent syphilis in penicillin-allergic patient: doxycycline 100 mg PO bid or tetracycline 500 mg qid for 28 days
- Tetracyclines are contraindicated in pregnancy. If pregnant and penicillin allergic, must be desensitized prior to treatment

DISPOSITION
- Repeat quantitative nontreponemal tests at 3, 6, and 12 mo. Pregnancy requires monthly tests until delivery.
- If a fourfold increase in titer occurs, if initial high titer fails to drop by fourfold within a year, or signs persist retreatment may be indicated. Use treatment regimen for late syphilis.
- Pregnant women without a fourfold drop in titer in a 3-mo period need to be retreated.
- Cases should be reported to local or state health department for referral, follow-up, and partner notification.

REFERRAL
- Pregnant and possible congenital syphilis
- Pregnant and allergic to penicillin, with need to be desensitized
- Late latent syphilis with serious central nervous system, cardiovascular, or other organ system compromise

PEARLS & CONSIDERATIONS

- Jarisch-Herxheimer reaction (fever, myalgia, tachycardia, hypotension) may occur within 24 hr of treatment.
- One third of untreated patients develop central nervous system and/or cardiovascular sequelae.
- Up to 80% of those treated during late stages remain seropositive indefinitely.
- Treponemal tests remain positive even after adequate therapy.
- Male circumcision does not decrease the incidence of syphilis (unlike HIV, HSV-2, and HPV infection).
- Partner notification and treatment:
  ○ Persons who are exposed within 90 days preceding the diagnosis of primary, secondary, or early latent syphilis in a sex partner might be infected even if seronegative; therefore, such persons should be treated presumptively.
  ○ Persons who were exposed ≥90 days before the diagnosis of syphilis in a sex partner should be treated presumptively if serologic test results are not available immediately and the opportunity for follow-up is uncertain.

EVIDENCE

available at www.expertconsult.com

SUGGESTED READINGS

available at www.expertconsult.com

AUTHORS: **MARIA A. CORIGLIANO, M.D.,** and **RUBEN ALVERO, M.D.**

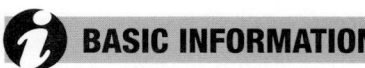

BASIC INFORMATION

DEFINITION

Syringomyelia is a disease of the spine characterized by the formation of fluid-filled cavities within the spinal cord, sometimes extending into the brain stem.

ICD-9CM CODES
336.0 Syringomyelia

PHYSICAL FINDINGS & CLINICAL PRESENTATION

- Onset is usually insidious, with symptoms often not beginning until the third or fourth decade.
- Cervical spine is the most commonly affected area.
  1. Intrinsic hand atrophy, weakness, and anesthetic sensory loss may develop.
  2. The latter may lead to unnoticed burns or other injuries in the hand.
  3. Loss of pain and temperature sensation may occur, but tactile sense in the upper extremity is preserved.
  4. Sharp testing elicits no pain, but patient often perceives the sharpness of the object.
  5. A Charcot joint in the shoulder or elbow may develop.
- Reflexes are absent in the upper extremity.
- Spasticity and hyperreflexia are present in the lower extremity.
- Scoliosis is common.
- Nystagmus and Horner's syndrome may also occur.
- Trophic skin changes eventually develop in many cases.

ETIOLOGY

- Cause is unknown, but condition is believed to result from obstruction of the outlet of the fourth ventricle, often associated with a Chiari I malformation, which causes fluid to be diverted down the central cord.
- A history of birth injury often exists.
- Syringes later in life may be the result of trauma or an intramedullary tumor.

DIAGNOSIS

DIFFERENTIAL DIAGNOSIS

- Amyotrophic lateral sclerosis
- Multiple sclerosis
- Spinal cord tumor
- Tabes dorsalis
- Progressive spinal muscular atrophy

WORKUP

- Plain radiographs usually reveal widening of the bony canal in the region of involvement.
- Bony anomalies are often present at the base of the skull and at the C1-C2 spinal segments.
- Myelography, MRI (Fig. 1-368), and other imaging studies are recommended.

TREATMENT

Drainage and operative repair of any bony anomalies are undertaken, often with decompression laminectomy of C1 and C2.

DISPOSITION

- Condition is slowly progressive in most cases but course may be quite variable, ranging from death in a few months to slow incapacitation over several years; progression may halt at any time.
- Surgical intervention often stops progression but frequently does not lead to improvement in neurologic findings.

REFERRAL

For neurosurgical consultation when diagnosis is suspected

EVIDENCE

available at www.expertconsult.com

SUGGESTED READINGS

available at www.expertconsult.com

AUTHOR: **LONNIE R. MERCIER, M.D.**

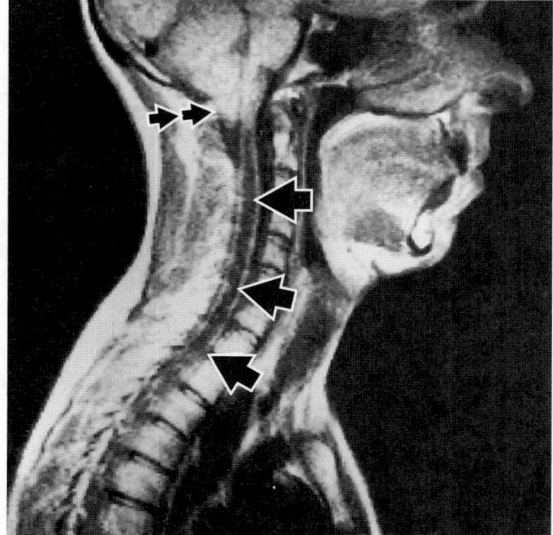

FIGURE 1-368 Midsagittal magnetic resonance image of Arnold-Chiari malformation *(small black arrows)* and syringomyelia *(three large black arrows)* in a 31-yr-old man. Note the cerebellar tonsils extending below the posterior rim of the foramen magnum *(dark structure* immediately above the *black arrow).* The syrinx extends from the medulla well into the thoracic cord. (From Andreoli TE [ed]: *Cecil essentials of medicine,* ed 4, Philadelphia, 1997, WB Saunders.)

ℹ️ BASIC INFORMATION

DEFINITION
Systemic lupus erythematosus (SLE) is a chronic, multisystemic disease characterized by production of autoantibodies and protean clinical manifestations.

SYNONYMS
SLE

ICD-9CM CODES
710.0 Systemic lupus erythematosus

EPIDEMIOLOGY & DEMOGRAPHICS
PREVALENCE: 20 cases per 100,000 persons. Ethnic groups, such as those of African or Asian ancestry, are at greatest risk of developing the disorder.
PREDOMINANT SEX: Female/male ratio of 9:1
PREDOMINANT AGE: 20 to 45 yr (childbearing years)

PHYSICAL FINDINGS & CLINICAL PRESENTATION
- Skin: erythematous rash over the malar eminences (Fig. 1-369), generally with sparing of the nasolabial folds (butterfly rash); alopecia; raised erythematous patches with subsequent edematous plaques and adherent scales (discoid lupus); leg, nasal, or oropharyngeal ulcerations; livedo reticularis; pallor (from anemia); petechiae (from thrombocytopenia)
- Joints: tenderness, swelling, or effusion, generally involving peripheral joints

- Cardiac: pericardial rub (in patients with pericarditis), heart murmurs (if endocarditis or valvular thickening or dysfunction)
- Other: fever, conjunctivitis, dry eyes, dry mouth (sicca syndrome), oral ulcers, abdominal tenderness, decreased breath sounds (pleural effusions)

ETIOLOGY
Unknown. Autoantibodies are typically present many years before the diagnosis of SLE. A haplotype of STAT4 is associated with increased risk for both rheumatoid arthritis and SLE, suggesting a shared pathway for these illnesses. Genetic susceptibility to lupus is inherited as a complex trait. An interval on the long arm of chromosome 1, 1q23-24 has been linked with SLE in many populations.

🅳🆇 DIAGNOSIS

DIFFERENTIAL DIAGNOSIS
- Other connective tissue disorders (e.g., rheumatoid arthritis, mixed connective tissue disease, progressive systemic sclerosis)
- Metastatic neoplasm
- Infection

WORKUP
The diagnosis of SLE can be made by demonstrating the presence of any four or more of the following criteria of the American Rheumatism Association:
1. Butterfly rash
2. Discoid rash
3. Photosensitivity (particularly leg ulcerations)

4. Oral ulcers
5. Arthritis
6. Serositis (pleuritis, pericarditis)
7. Renal disorder (persistent proteinuria >0.5 g/day or 3+ if quantitation not performed, cellular casts)
8. Neurologic disorder (seizures, psychosis [in absence of offending drugs or metabolic derangement])
9. Hematologic disorder:
   a. Hemolytic anemia with reticulocytosis
   b. Leukopenia ($<4000/mm^3$ total on two or more occasions)
   c. Lymphopenia ($<1500/mm^3$ on two or more occasions)
   d. Thrombocytopenia ($<100,000/mm^3$ in the absence of offending drugs)
10. Immunologic disorder:
   a. Positive SLE cell preparation
   b. Anti-DNA (presence of antibody to native DNA in abnormal titer)
   c. Anti-Sm (presence of antibody to Smith nuclear antigen)
   d. False-positive STS known to be positive for at least 6 mo and confirmed by negative TPI or FTA tests
11. Antinuclear antibody (ANA): an abnormal titer of ANA by immunofluorescence or equivalent assay at any time in the absence of drugs known to be associated with "drug-induced lupus" syndrome

LABORATORY TESTS
Suggested initial laboratory evaluation of suspected SLE:
- Immunologic evaluation: ANA, anti-DNA antibody, anti-Sm antibody
- Other laboratory tests: complete blood count with differential, platelet count (Coombs test if anemia detected), urinalysis (24-hr urine collection for protein if proteinuria is detected), partial thromboplastin time and anticardiolipin antibodies in patients with thrombotic events, blood urea nitrogen, creatinine to evaluate renal function

IMAGING STUDIES
- Chest radiograph for evaluation of pulmonary involvement (e.g., pleural effusions, pulmonary infiltrates)
- Echocardiogram to screen for significant valvular heart disease (present in 18% of patients with SLE); echocardiography can identify a subset of lesions (valvular thickening and dysfunction) other than verrucous (Libman-Sacks) endocarditis that are prone to hemodynamic deterioration

🅡🆇 TREATMENT

NONPHARMACOLOGIC THERAPY
Patients with photosensitivity should avoid sunlight and use high-factor sunscreen.

GENERAL Rx
- Joint pain and mild serositis are generally well controlled with nonsteroidal antiinflammatory drugs; antimalarials are also effective (e.g., hydroxychloroquine [Plaquenil]).

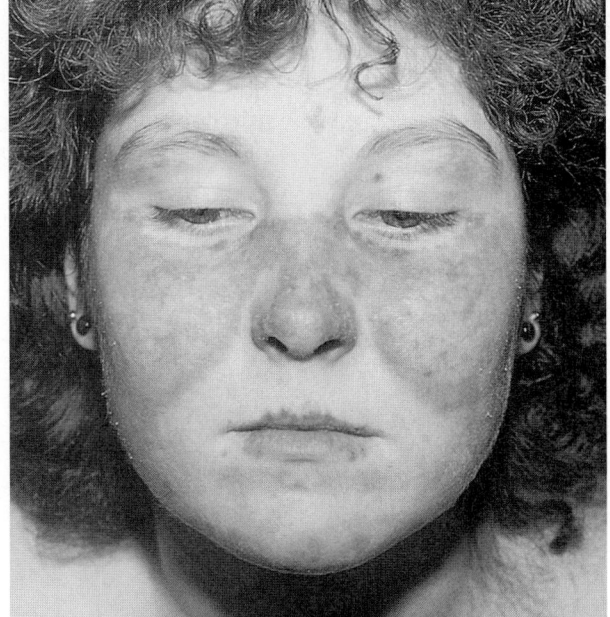

FIGURE 1-369 Acute cutaneous lupus erythematosus (LE) (systemic LE). The classic butterfly rash occurs in 10% to 50% of patients with acute LE. (From Habif TP: *Clinical dermatology: a color guide to diagnosis and therapy,* ed 3, St Louis, 1996, Mosby.)

- Cutaneous manifestations are treated with the following:
  1. Topical corticosteroids; intradermal corticosteroids are helpful for individual discoid lesions, especially in the scalp
  2. Antimalarials (e.g., hydroxychloroquine [Plaquenil] and quinacrine)
  3. Sunscreens that block ultraviolet (UV) A and UVB radiation
  4. Immunosuppressive drugs (methotrexate or azathioprine) are used as steroid-sparing drugs
- Renal disease (lupus nephritis)
  1. The use of high-pulsed doses of cyclophosphamide given at monthly intervals is more effective in preserving renal function than is treatment with glucocorticoids alone. The present standard of care with monthly high-dose IV cyclophosphamide has been challenged on several fronts. Alternative ways of administering cyclophosphamide in much lower doses for shorter periods have emerged. The combination of methylprednisolone and cyclophosphamide is superior to bolus therapy with methylprednisolone or cyclophosphamide alone in patients with lupus nephritis. For patients with proliferative lupus nephritis, short-term therapy with IV cyclophosphamide followed by maintenance therapy with mycophenolate mofetil or azathioprine appears to be more efficacious and safer than long-term therapy with IV cyclophosphamide. In the treatment of severe proliferative lupus nephritis, mycophenolate mofetil represents an excellent alternative to cyclophosphamide.
  2. The use of plasmapheresis in combination with immunosuppressive agents (to prevent the rebound phenomenon of antibody levels after plasmapheresis) is generally reserved for rapidly progressive renal failure or life-threatening systemic vasculitis.
- Central nervous system involvement: treatment generally consists of corticosteroid therapy; however, its efficacy is uncertain, and it is generally reserved for organic brain syndrome. Anticonvulsants and antipsychotics are also indicated in selected cases; headaches are treated symptomatically.

- Hemolytic anemia: treatment of Coombs-positive hemolytic anemia consists of high doses of corticosteroids; nonhemolytic anemia (secondary to chronic disease) does not require specific therapy.
- Thrombocytopenia
  1. Initial treatment consists of corticosteroids.
  2. In patients with poor response to steroids, encouraging results have been reported with the use of danazol, vincristine, and immunoglobulins. Combination chemotherapy with cyclophosphamide and prednisone combined with vincristine, vincristine and procarbazine, or etoposide may be useful in patients with severe refractory idiopathic thrombocytopenic purpura.
  3. Splenectomy generally does not cure the thrombocytopenia of SLE, but it may be necessary as an adjunct in managing selected cases.
- Infections are common because of compromised immune function secondary to SLE and the use of corticosteroid, cytotoxic, and antimetabolite drugs; pneumococcal bacteremia is associated with high mortality rate.
- Close monitoring for exacerbation of the disease and for potential side effects from medications (corticosteroids, cytotoxic agents) with frequent laboratory evaluation and office visits is necessary in all patients with SLE.
- Valvular heart disease is present in 18% of patients with SLE. The prevalence of infective endocarditis is approximately 1% (similar to the prevalence after prosthetic valve surgery, but greater than that after rheumatic valvulitis). Valvular heart disease in patients with SLE frequently changes over time (e.g., vegetations can appear unexpectedly for the first time, resolve, or change in size or appearance). These frequent changes are temporarily unrelated to other clinical features of SLE and can be associated with substantial morbidity and mortality rates.
- Newer treatment modalities include the use of rituximab (a chimeric human-murine monoclonal antibody directed against CD20 on B cells and their precursors) to induce substantial remissions in patients previously unresponsive to conventional agents. Intravenous immunoglobulins are also increasingly

being used in the treatment of patients with resistant lupus.

DISPOSITION
- Most patients with SLE experience remissions and exacerbations.
- The leading cause of death in SLE is infection (one third of all deaths); active nephritis causes approximately 18% of deaths, and central nervous system disease causes 7% of deaths; the survival rate is 75% over the first 10 yr. Blacks and Hispanics generally have a worse prognosis.
- Symptomatic pericarditis occurs in one fourth of patients with SLE at some point during the course of the disease. Asymptomatic involvement is estimated to be more than 60% based on autopsy reports.
- Renal histologic studies and evaluation of renal function are useful in determining disease activity and predicting disease outcome (e.g., serum creatinine levels >3 mg/dl or evidence of diffuse proliferative involvement on renal biopsy are poor prognostic factors).
- Atherosclerosis occurs prematurely in patients with SLE and is independent of traditional risk factors for cardiovascular disease.
- Antiphospholipid syndrome with thrombotic manifestations is a major predictor of irreversible organ damage and death in patients with SLE.

REFERRAL
- Rheumatology consultation in all patients with SLE
- Hematology consultation in patients with significant hematologic abnormalities (e.g., severe hemolytic anemia or thrombocytopenia)
- Nephrology consultation in patients with significant renal involvement

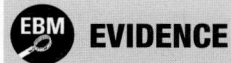

EVIDENCE

available at www.expertconsult.com

SUGGESTED READINGS
available at www.expertconsult.com

AUTHOR: **FRED F. FERRI, M.D.**

BASIC INFORMATION

DEFINITION

Tabes dorsalis is a form of tertiary neurosyphilis affecting the dorsal columns of the spinal cord and peripheral nerves, characterized by paroxysmal pain, particularly in the abdomen and legs; sensory ataxia; normal strength; autonomic dysfunction; and Argyll-Robertson pupils.

SYNONYMS

Posterior spinal sclerosis
Tabetic neurosyphilis
Syphilitic myeloneuropathy

ICD-9CM CODES
094.0 Tabes dorsalis, ataxia, locomotor

EPIDEMIOLOGY & DEMOGRAPHICS

INCIDENCE (IN U.S.): Rare, but increasing with HIV/AIDS
PEAK INCIDENCE: 15 to 20 yr after initial infection
PREVALENCE (IN U.S.): Rare; more common with HIV/AIDS epidemic. Ten percent of untreated patients with syphilis develop neurosyphilis, 2% to 5% of whom may develop tabes dorsalis. Relative prevalence of tabes dorsalis is reduced compared with the preantibiotic era. This may be the only clinical manifestation of neurosyphilis that has been altered during the antibiotic era.
PREDOMINANT SEX: Male

PHYSICAL FINDINGS & CLINICAL PRESENTATION

- Argyll-Robertson pupils are common (pupil reacts poorly to light but well to accommodation)
- Loss of position and vibration at ankles (wide-based gait, inability to walk in the dark, sensory ataxia)
- Loss of deep pain sensation, resulting in deep foot ulcers
- Degenerative joint disease, especially in knees, caused by severe neuropathy (Charcot joints)
- Normal strength with areflexia in the legs
- Lightning pains in the legs
- Severe intermittent visceral pains, such as gastrointestinal and laryngeal (visceral crises)
- Autonomic dysfunction (urinary and fecal incontinence)

ETIOLOGY

Infectious *(Treponema pallidum)*

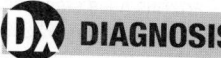

DIAGNOSIS

DIFFERENTIAL DIAGNOSIS

- Vitamin B_{12} deficiency (subacute combined degeneration of the spinal cord)
- Vitamin E deficiency
- Chronic nitrous oxide abuse
- Spinal cord neoplasm (involving conus medullaris)
- Lyme's disease

WORKUP

Thorough neurologic history and examination

LABORATORY TESTS

- Lumbar puncture for elevated Venereal Disease Research Laboratory (VDRL) and Fluorescent Treponemal Antigen-Antibody test (FTA-ABS) titers. False-positive cerebrospinal fluid (CSF) VDRL titers may occur with traumatic tap. CSF mononuclear pleocytosis (>5 white cells/μL) with increased protein support the diagnosis.
- Serum VDRL test. Results may be normal in 25% to 30% of patients. Serum microhemagglutination-*Treponema pallidum* (MHA-TP) or FTA-ABS is necessary if clinical suspicion high.
- False-positive serum VDRL may occur in Lyme disease, nonvenereal treponematoses, genital herpes simplex, pregnancy, systemic lupus erythematosus, alcoholic cirrhosis, scleroderma, and mixed connective tissue disease.

IMAGING STUDIES

Not necessary if diagnosis confirmed

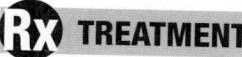

TREATMENT

ACUTE GENERAL Rx

- Procaine penicillin 2 million to 4 million U IM qd, along with probenecid 500 mg PO qid, for 14 days or aqueous penicillin G 3 million to 4 million U IV q4h for 10 to 14 days.
- If patient is penicillin allergic, doxycycline 200 mg PO bid for 4 wk.
- Many of the symptoms—degenerative neuropathic joint disease, lightning pains—persist after treatment.

CHRONIC Rx

- Physical therapy
- Analgesics, carbamazepine, gabapentin, or steroids may help lightning pain
- Supportive care (wheelchair, toileting issues, etc.)

DISPOSITION

- Close follow-up required. Repeat lumbar puncture is recommended every 6 mo until CSF pleocytosis normalizes. If pleocytosis does not normalize in 6 mo or CSF is still abnormal in 2 yr, repeat treatment.
- Further indication for retreatment: if there is a fourfold increase in titers or a failure of titers >1:32 to decrease at least fourfold by 12 to 24 mo.

REFERRAL

Joint replacement in moderate cases

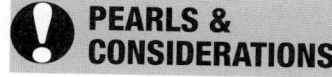

PEARLS & CONSIDERATIONS

COMMENTS

Diagnosis should be considered in all patients with a progressive neuropsychiatric disorder with signs of spinal cord dysfunction and peripheral neuropathy.

SUGGESTED READINGS
available at www.expertconsult.com

AUTHOR: **EROBOGHENE E. UBOGU, M.D.**

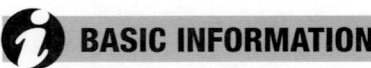

DEFINITION

Takayasu's arteritis is a chronic systemic granulomatous large-vessel vasculitis. It often presents as a pulseless disease caused by widespread arterial stenosis.

SYNONYMS

Pulseless disease
Aortitis syndrome
Aortic arch arteritis
Nonspecific aortoarteritis

ICD-9CM CODES
446.7 Takayasu disease or syndrome

EPIDEMIOLOGY & DEMOGRAPHICS

- Most cases have been reported in Japan, China, India, and Mexico.
- The incidence in the United States is 2.6:1 million persons.
- The female-to-male ratio is 9:1.
- The age of onset is usually between 10 and 40 yr.

PHYSICAL FINDINGS & CLINICAL PRESENTATION

- The early phase of Takayasu's arteritis often manifests as constitutional symptoms, including the following:
  1. Low-grade fever
  2. Malaise
  3. Weight loss
  4. Fatigue
  5. Arthralgia and myalgia
  6. Night sweats
  7. Anemia
  8. Serum blood tests reveal elevated erythrocyte sedimentation rate (ESR)
- Takayasu's arteritis may result in stenosis or aneurysms of the aorta and its primary branches, and may therefore manifest as follows:
  - Arm or leg claudication, weakness, and numbness
  - Amaurosis fugax, diplopia, headache, orthostasis, vertigo, or syncope
  - Angina or myocardial infarction
  - Vascular bruits of the carotid artery, subclavian artery, and aorta
  - Discrepancy of blood pressures between the upper extremities, typically of >10 mm Hg
  - Diminished or absent pulses, ischemic ulcerations, or gangrene in advanced disease
  - Hypertension
  - Retinopathy
  - Aortic insufficiency as a result of aortic root dilatation and aneurysm formation
- In the late stage, weakness of the arterial walls may give rise to localized aneurysms. Raynaud's phenomenon is commonly found in this disease.

ETIOLOGY

- The cause of Takayasu's arteritis is poorly understood. Cell-mediated mechanisms are thought to be important to the pathogenesis.
- The infiltration of inflammatory cells (lymphocytes, macrophages, and multinucleated giant cells) into the vasa vasorum and media of the large elastic arteries leads to fibrosis, thickening and narrowing or obliteration. Patients with Takayasu's arteritis have stenoses in >90% of cases, and aneurysms in ~25% of cases. Release of metalloproteinases and reactive oxygen species may result in local aneurysms.

Dx DIAGNOSIS

Diagnostic criteria for Takayasu's arteritis were established by the American College of Rheumatology in 1990 and include the following:
- Age of disease onset <40 yr
- Claudication of extremities
- Decreased brachial artery pulse
- Systolic blood pressure difference >10 mm Hg between left and right arms
- Bruit over subclavian arteries or abdominal aorta
- Abnormal arteriogram, not related to arteriosclerosis or fibromuscular dysplasia
- Takayasu's arteritis is diagnosed if at least three of the six criteria are present; this results in a sensitivity of 90% and a specificity of 98%

DIFFERENTIAL DIAGNOSIS

Other causes of inflammatory aortitis must be excluded:
- Giant cell arteritis
- Syphilis
- Tuberculosis
- Systemic lupus erythematosus
- Rheumatoid arthritis
- Buerger's disease
- Behçet's disease
- Cogan's syndrome
- Kawasaki disease
- Spondyloarthropathies

WORKUP

Any young patient with findings of absent pulses and loud bruits merits a workup for Takayasu's arteritis. The workup generally includes blood testing to look for signs of inflammation as well as imaging studies, with the angiogram being the diagnostic gold standard.

LABORATORY TESTS

- A CBC may reveal a normal or elevated white blood cell count as well as anemia of chronic disease.

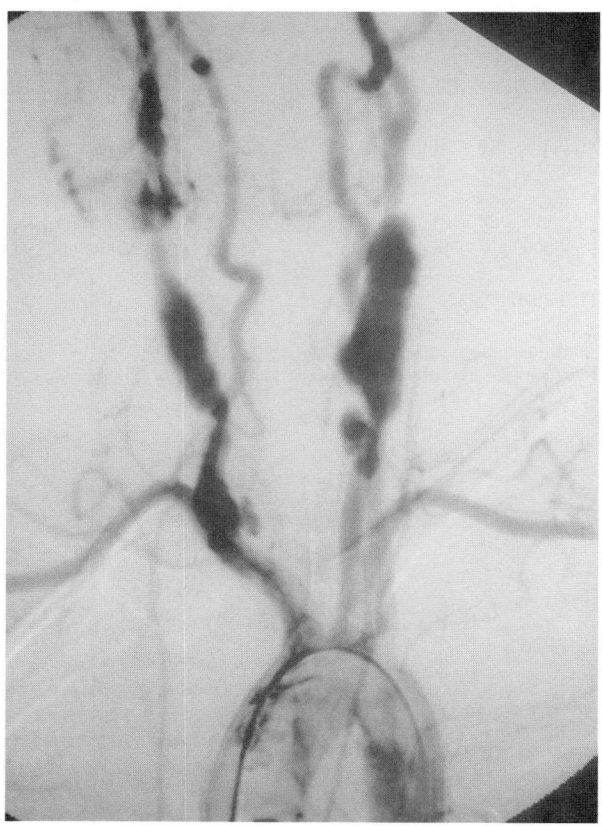

FIGURE 1-370 An angiogram of a child with Takayasu's arteritis that shows massive bilateral carotid dilation, stenosis, and poststenotic dilation. (From Behrman RE: *Nelson textbook of pediatrics,* ed 16, Philadelphia, 2000, WB Saunders.)

- Erythrocyte sedimentation rate (ESR) and serum C-reactive protein levels are usually elevated, but can be normal even in the setting of active vasculitis.

IMAGING STUDIES

- Ultrasound: Carotid, thoracic, and abdominal ultrasound are useful adjunctive imaging studies to diagnose the occlusive disease that results from Takayasu's arteritis (Fig. 1-370).
- Doppler and noninvasive upper and lower extremity studies are helpful to assess blood flow and absent pulses.
- Computed tomographic scanning and MRI may be used to assess the thickness of the large arteries.
- Angiography can show the narrowing of the aorta and its branches, aneurysm formation, and poststenotic dilation. Collateral circulation may also be visualized. Angiographic findings are classified into four types:
  1. Type I: lesions that involve only the aortic arch and its branches
  2. Type II: lesions that involve only the abdominal aorta and its branches
  3. Type III: lesions that involve the aorta above and below the diaphragm
  4. Type IV: lesions that involve the pulmonary artery

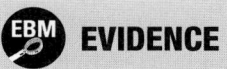

TREATMENT

ACUTE GENERAL Rx

- Glucocorticoids are effective to suppress systemic symptoms and to stop the progression of Takayasu's arteritis. Prednisone (40 to 60 mg PO daily or 1 mg/kg/day) can be used for 3 mo.
- Patients are monitored for symptoms and ESR. Attempts to taper prednisone can be made in accordance with the resolution of constitutional symptoms, ESR and C-reactive protein levels, and imaging studies. Patients often relapse when prednisone is tapered.

CHRONIC Rx

- Long-term low-dose prednisone may be necessary to stop the progression of arterial stenoses.
- Although there have been no randomized controlled trials, use of steroid-sparing immunosuppressants is increasing. Ethotrexate is the most commonly used agent, although there are also data supporting the use of azathioprine or antitumor necrosis factor as adjunctive or alternative therapy with glucocorticoids to patients who are in relapse or resistant to other treatments. There is limited experience with cyclophosphamide.
- Percutaneous angioplasty or bypass grafts should be considered for irreversible arterial stenoses with severe ischemia (cardiac or cerebral), severe hypertension in renal artery stenosis, or aneurysmal enlargement with risk of rupture.
- Aortic regurgitation may require valve replacement or repair by surgery.

DISPOSITION

- Immunosuppressants may achieve clinical remission.
- No studies have proved that treatment results in regression of stenosis, although there are limited case reports describing the return of pulses with treatment.
- With the addition of a second agent for patients with treatment resistance or relapse, 50% remission has been seen.
- Quality of life is comparable to that of patients with rheumatoid arthritis or ankylosing spondylitis.

- Mortality results are mixed, with high rates in reports from Asia and lower rates in studies performed in the United States (2%).
- Death can occur suddenly from a ruptured aneurysm, a myocardial infarction, or a stroke.

REFERRAL

Whenever the diagnosis of vasculitis is suspected, a rheumatology consultation is appropriate. Vascular surgery and cardiology consultations are recommended for any evidence of carotid, peripheral, or coronary artery disease or if a large abdominal aneurysm is found.

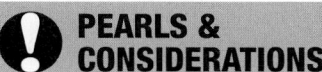

PEARLS & CONSIDERATIONS

With long-term glucocorticoid use, consider measures to protect against bone loss. Bisphosphonates have been studied prospectively with corticosteroid use in this fashion; remember to ensure adequate dietary calcium and vitamin D intake as well.

COMMENTS

The long-term prognosis of patients with treated Takayasu's disease varies by geography, and 10-yr survival ranges from 80% to 96%.

EBM **EVIDENCE**

available at www.expertconsult.com

SUGGESTED READINGS

available at www.expertconsult.com

AUTHORS: **JEANNETTE P. LIN, M.D.,** and **PRANAV M. PATEL, M.D.**

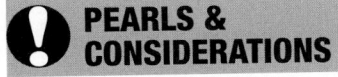

BASIC INFORMATION

DEFINITION

Four species of adult tapeworm may infect humans as the definitive host: *Taenia saginata* (beef tapeworm), *Taenia solium* (pork tapeworm), *Diphyllobothrium latum* (fish tapeworm), and *Hymenolepis nana*. In addition, *T. solium* may infect humans in its larval form (cysticercosis), and several animal tapeworms (see "Echinococcosis" in Section I) may cause infection in an analogous manner.

SYNONYMS

Cysticercosis (larval infection by *T. solium*)

ICD-9CM CODES
123.9 Tapeworm infestation

EPIDEMIOLOGY & DEMOGRAPHICS

INCIDENCE (IN U.S.):
- Diagnosed primarily in immigrants
- Varies widely by country of origin and dietary practices

PREVALENCE (IN U.S.):
- *T. saginata:* <0.1%
- *D. latum:* <0.05%
- *T. solium:* <0.1%
- *H. nana:* sporadic, often in setting of outbreak

PREDOMINANT SEX: Equal sex distribution

PREDOMINANT AGE:
- *T. saginata, T. solium, D. latum:* 20 to 39 yr of age
- *H. nana* in setting of institution outbreaks: children

PHYSICAL FINDINGS & CLINICAL PRESENTATION

Adult worms
1. Attach to bowel mucosa
2. Feed and grow
3. Cause minimal or no symptoms or sequelae

Cysticercosis
1. Mass lesions of brain (neurocysticercosis), soft tissue, viscera
2. Neurocysticercosis may cause seizures, hydrocephalus

Prolonged infection with *D. latum*
1. Vitamin B_{12} deficiency
2. Megaloblastic anemia

ETIOLOGY

TAPEWORM:
- Adult worm resides in small or large bowel; proglottids and eggs are passed in stool.
- Eggs are ingested by the animal intermediate host.
- Eggs hatch into larvae.
- Larvae disseminate largely in skeletal muscle, brain, viscera.
- Humans eat infected beef (*T. saginata*), infected pork (*T. solium*), or infected fish (*D. latum*).
- Larvae mature into adults within the GI lumen.
- *H. nana* infection is acquired by ingesting eggs in human or rodent feces.

CYSTICERCOSIS:
- Humans ingest eggs of *T. solium* in food contaminated with human feces that contain the eggs.
- Eggs hatch into larvae in gut.
- Larvae disseminate widely through tissues (particularly soft tissue and CNS) forming cystic lesions containing either viable or nonviable larvae.

DIAGNOSIS

WORKUP
- Stool examination for eggs or proglottids (tapeworm)
- Cerebral CT scan (neurocysticercosis)
- Serum antibody (neurocysticercosis)

IMAGING STUDIES
- Tapeworm: incidental finding on upper GI series
- Neurocysticercosis:
  1. Cerebral cysts are readily demonstrated by CT scan or MRI.
  2. Calcified lesions are an incidental finding.

TREATMENT

ACUTE GENERAL Rx
- All patients with intestinal tapeworm infections should be treated with a single oral dose of praziquantel.
  1. *T. solium:* 5 mg/kg
  2. *T. saginata:* 20 mg/kg

  3. *D. latum:* 10 mg/kg
  4. *H. nana:* 25 mg/kg
- An alternative therapy to praziquantel for tapeworm infections is niclosamide, 2 g PO once or 500 mg PO daily for 3 days.
- Therapy that may be considered for symptomatic cysticercosis:
  1. May regress spontaneously
  2. Surgery
  3. Albendazole 15 mg/kg PO qid in three doses for 28 days
  4. Praziquantel 50 mg/kg PO qid in three doses for 15 days
- Therapy contraindicated with:
  1. Ocular infections
  2. Cerebral infections in which local inflammation caused by destruction of the parasite may cause significant damage

CHRONIC Rx
- Retreatment if required
- Avoidance of undercooked pork, meat, or fish
- Cysticercosis: proper hand washing, proper disposal of human waste

DISPOSITION
- Neurologic follow-up for patients with neurocysticercosis
- Ophthalmologic follow-up for patients with ocular involvement

REFERRAL

Patients treated for neurocysticercosis should be evaluated by a physician experienced in managing this infection, if possible.

PEARLS & CONSIDERATIONS

COMMENTS

T. solium is the most dangerous of the tapeworms because of the potential for cysticercosis by means of autoinfection.

SUGGESTED READINGS
available at www.expertconsult.com

AUTHORS: **GLENN G. FORT, M.D., M.P.H.,** and **DENNIS J. MIKOLICH, M.D.**

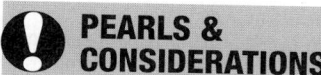BASIC INFORMATION

DEFINITION

Tardive dyskinesia (TD) is a syndrome of involuntary movements associated with the long-term use of antipsychotic medication, particularly first-generation antipsychotics. Patients exhibit rapid, repetitive, stereotypic movements that mostly involve the oral, lingual, trunk, and limb areas.

SYNONYMS

Orofacial dyskinesia
Tardive syndrome

ICD-9CM CODES
333.85 Tardive dyskinesia

EPIDEMIOLOGY & DEMOGRAPHICS

- The disorder is caused by dopamine-blocking antipsychotics (e.g., haloperidol) and antiemetics (e.g., metoclopramide, prochlorperazine, and promethazine).
- With first-generation antipsychotics, at least 20% of patients are affected with TD, and ~5% are expected to develop TD with each year of antipsychotic treatment.
- The incidence of TD is declining with the increased use of second-generation antipsychotics. ~0.5% to 1% of all adults develop TD yearly while taking these medications.
- Risk increases with the duration of antipsychotic treatment, in elderly patients, and in patients with nonschizophrenia diagnoses.

PHYSICAL FINDINGS & CLINICAL PRESENTATION

- TD is classically described as a chronic condition of insidious onset, but symptoms are variable over time and may even improve despite continued antipsychotic therapy.
- The condition typically appears with the reduction or withdrawal of the antipsychotic medications.
- TD primarily involves stereotypic movements of the mouth and tongue, including lip smacking and puckering, tongue twisting and protrusion, and facial grimacing.
- TD may also involve slow, writhing movements of the trunk or choreoathetotic movements of the fingers and toes.
- The involuntary mouth movements associated with TD may be suppressed by voluntary actions (e.g., putting food in the mouth, talking).
- Variants of TD with similar treatment include: tardive dystonia (e.g., torticollis, blepharospasm), tardive myoclonus, tardive akathisia, and tardive tics.

ETIOLOGY

TD is generally thought to result from chronic exposure to dopamine-receptor–blocking agents, which are primarily used to treat psychosis. TD has not been reported with dopamine depleters (e.g., reserpine), and it is less common with second-generation antipsychotic drugs. Some drugs used to treat nausea (e.g., metoclopramide, prochlorperazine) can also cause TD. TD is believed to be caused by the upregulation and increased sensitivity of dopamine receptors in the basal ganglia and by antipsychotic-induced damage to striatal cholinergic neurons.

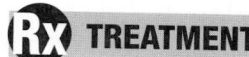DIAGNOSIS

DIFFERENTIAL DIAGNOSIS

- Acute extrapyramidal symptoms (e.g., short-term withdrawal dyskinesias, parkinsonism, akathisia)
- Basal ganglia movement disorders (e.g., Huntington's chorea, Tourette's syndrome, Levodopa-induced dyskinesia in Parkinson's disease, Wilson's disease)
- Autoimmune diseases (Sydenham's chorea, multiple sclerosis)
- Other causes of neurologic damage (e.g., lead or mercury toxicity, HIV, neurosyphilis, head injury, neurodegeneration from illicit substances)
- Mannerisms associated with disorganized type or catatonic type schizophrenia
- Hyperthyroidism-induced choreoathetosis
- Edentulous dyskinesias and improperly fitted dentures
- Rabbit syndrome (a rare variant of extrapyramidal symptoms) with vertical orofacial movements without tongue involvement; may respond to anticholinergic agents

WORKUP

TD is a diagnosis of exclusion, with emphasis on a complete neuropsychiatric and medication history and a thorough physical examination.

IMAGING STUDIES

Brain imaging is normal in patients with TD.

TREATMENT

ACUTE GENERAL Rx

- Treatment is predicated on prevention: limit the indications for antipsychotics; use the lowest effective dose; discontinue the drugs, when feasible; and monitor patients frequently.
- Switch to second-generation antipsychotics, if possible.

CHRONIC Rx

- Clozapine has the best evidence for improving the symptoms of TD, although olanzapine and amisulpride may also be of benefit.
- Tetrabenazine, benzodiazepines, vitamin E, vitamin B_6, donepezil, piracetam, and melatonin may be helpful, although controlled trial evidence is weak.
- For disabling TD, deep brain stimulation of the globus pallidus has been reported to provide significant symptom reduction without exacerbation of psychiatric symptoms.
- TD is potentially irreversible in nearly two-thirds of patients; thus, patients undergoing long-term treatment with dopamine receptor–blocking medications require frequent monitoring and aggressive management at the onset of TD symptoms.

REFERRAL

Movement disorder specialist consultation if symptoms are severe

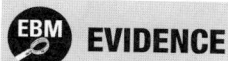PEARLS & CONSIDERATIONS

- First-generation antipsychotics should be resumed to treat TD in the absence of active psychosis only as a last resort for persistent, disabling, and treatment-resistant TD.
- Avoid the use of anticholinergic medications (e.g., benztropine), which may exacerbate TD symptoms.
- A worsening of the overall psychopathology in patients with schizophrenia is longitudinally associated with the emergence of TD and suggestive of a worse prognosis.
- Recent evidence suggests increased overall mortality among patients with TD, which highlights the need for referral for more aggressive specialized interventions.

EVIDENCE

available at www.expertconsult.com

SUGGESTED READINGS

available at www.expertconsult.com

AUTHOR: **JOHN A. GRAY, M.D., PH.D.**

Diseases and Disorders

T

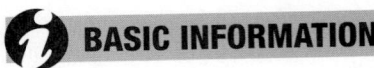

DEFINITION

Tarsal tunnel syndrome is the most common compressive neuropathy in the foot and ankle. The syndrome is secondary to a pathologic, structural, or biomechanical factor that causes compression of the posterior tibial nerve or its branches (medial calcaneal, medial plantar, lateral plantar branches), within or distal to the tarsal canal (Fig. 1-371).

ICD-9CM CODES
355.5 Tarsal tunnel syndrome

EPIDEMIOLOGY & DEMOGRAPHICS

PREVALENCE: Most common entrapment neuropathy in the foot/ankle.
PREDOMINANT SEX: Relatively equal

PHYSICAL FINDINGS & CLINICAL PRESENTATION

- Symptoms can vary between neuritic and localized heel pain.
- Common presentations include medial ankle pain, heel pain, distal numbness/shooting pain and generalized foot/ankle pain that keeps the patient awake at night.
- Percussion over the porta pedis resulting in Tinel's sign (distal radiation of symptoms)
- Valleix phenomenon (producing proximal symptomatology) is consistent with tarsal tunnel syndrome. Holding the foot in a dorsiflexed and everted subtalar joint position may reproduce symptoms.
- Look for: localized edema, varicosities, palpable soft tissue masses, biomechanical abnormalities, and signs of trauma.
- Loss of motor function and loss of sensation are extremely rare.

ETIOLOGY

- Inflammatory (adjacent tendonitis, recent ankle trauma)
- Compressive pathology: (ganglion cyst, lipoma, varicosities)
- Structural (osseous): Exostosis, severe arthritis, fracture of rearfoot/ankle
- Biomechanical: Abnormal calcaneal eversion or inversion, subtalar joint pronation
- Systemic causes of neuropathy: Diabetes, hypothyroidism, Reiter's syndrome, and more

DX DIAGNOSIS

DIFFERENTIAL DIAGNOSIS

- Plantar fasciitis
- Calcaneal fracture/other osseous trauma.
- Ankle sprain/strain or chronic ST injury. Posterior tibial tendonitis often overlooked

- Systemic causes of peripheral neuropathy: diabetes, hypothyroidism, Reiter's syndrome
- Radiculopathy
- Peripheral vascular disease

DIAGNOSTIC STUDIES

- X-rays: Rule out trauma, bone tumor, structural deformity.
- MRI: Look for soft tissue mass, edema, trauma.
- EMG and nerve conduction studies can support the clinical diagnosis. False negatives are common.
- Local diagnostic injections: Evaluate local versus proximal source of neuropathy.

Rx TREATMENT

- First line: rest, ice, limit aggravating activity
- Avoid shoegear that is too small (length, width), overtightened, too loose (allowing increased pathologic motion)
- Nonsteroidal anti-inflammatory drugs
- Custom-molded orthotics for optimal biomechanical function/stabilization
- Heel lifts promote ankle plantar flexion, which can reduce pressure within the tarsal tunnel
- Ankle bracing if ankle instability present/causative factor
- Physical therapy (iontophoresis, other therapeutic modalities, strength/flexibility work)
- Local steroid injection
- If persistent, offloading with cast or cast walker may yield resolution in 3 to 6 wk
- Surgical: Decompress tarsal tunnel or remove aggravating mass/varicosities

DISPOSITION

Can yield lifelong, chronic pain with unknown specific etiology or can follow a limited course once causative factor resolved (mechanical, healed ankle sprain, soft tissue mass resection, etc.)

REFERRAL

- Physical therapy for various treatment modalities.
- Podiatric or foot/ankle orthopedic surgeon for biomechanical evaluation, orthotic treatment, injection expertise and surgery if necessary.

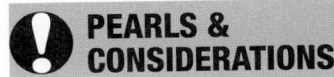 PEARLS & CONSIDERATIONS

- Be sure to rule out etiologies such as calcaneal fracture and bone or soft tissue tumor.
- Differentiation from plantar fasciitis can be difficult, yet the initial therapy can be identical (refer to "Plantar Fasciitis").

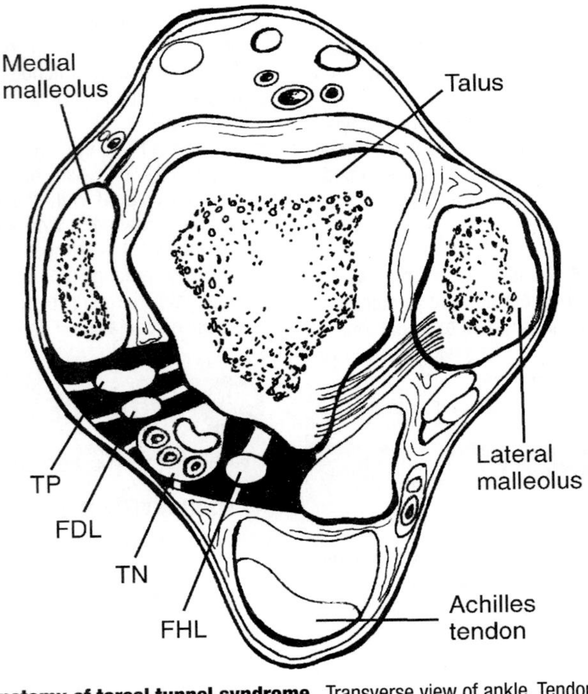

SUGGESTED READINGS
available at www.expertconsult.com

AUTHOR: **BROOKE E. KEELEY, D.P.M.**

FIGURE 1-371 Anatomy of tarsal tunnel syndrome. Transverse view of ankle. Tendons and neurovascular elements are included in individual fibrous septa that connect periosteum with the deep fascia. *FDL,* Flexor digitorum longus; *FHL,* flexor hallucis longus tendon; *TN,* tibial nerve (single contour), posterior tibial artery, veins; *TP,* tibialis posterior tendon. (From Canoso J: *Rheumatology in primary care,* Philadelphia, 1997, WB Saunders.)

BASIC INFORMATION

DEFINITION

Temporomandibular joint (TMJ) syndrome refers to a group of disorders leading to symptoms of the temporomandibular joint.

SYNONYMS

Temporomandibular dysfunction
Painful temporomandibular joint

ICD-9CM CODES
524.60 Temporomandibular joint pain-dysfunction syndrome

EPIDEMIOLOGY & DEMOGRAPHICS

- 15% of the population have TMJ disorders
- Females are affected more often than males (4:1 ratio)
- Occurs between the second and fourth decades of life
- Usually unilateral, affecting either side with equal frequency

PHYSICAL FINDINGS & CLINICAL PRESENTATION

- Often unilateral pain in the muscles of mastication, usually described as a "dull" ache
- Otalgia
- Odontalgia
- Headaches (frontal, temporal, retro-orbital)
- Tinnitus
- Dizziness
- Clicking or popping sounds with movement of the TMJ
- Joint locking
- Tender to palpation
- Limited range of motion of the TMJ
- Symptoms usually appear in association with a stressful life event

ETIOLOGY

- Multifactorial, encompassing local anatomic anomalies to systemic disease processes.
- Myofascial pain-dysfunction syndrome: the most common cause of TMJ syndrome and results from teeth grinding and clenching the jaw (bruxism)
- Internal TMJ derangement: abnormal connection of the articular disk to the mandibular condyle
- Degenerative joint disease
- Rheumatoid arthritis
- Gouty arthritis
- Pseudogout
- Ankylosing spondylitis

- Trauma
- Prior surgery (orthodontic, intraarticular steroid injection)
- Tumors

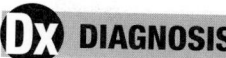 **DIAGNOSIS**

Can be made based on history and physical examination in most cases.

DIFFERENTIAL DIAGNOSIS

Includes the list provided above. Myofascial pain-dysfunction syndrome, internal TMJ derangement, and degenerative joint disease represent >90% of all causes of TMJ syndrome. Others not mentioned include dental problems such as loss of posterior teeth support and Eagle's syndrome (stylohyoid syndrome, carotidynia, and trigeminal neuralgia).

WORKUP

Radiographic imaging evaluation is used to exclude anatomic or systemic causes of disease when conservative management has failed.

LABORATORY TESTS

Laboratory examination is not very helpful.

IMAGING STUDIES

- Plain radiographs: the most common views are the panoramic, transorbital, and transpharyngeal in both opened and closed positions.
- Arthrography is helpful in looking for meniscus involvement but is seldom performed anymore.
- CT scan is highly accurate in diagnosing meniscal and osseous derangements of the TMJ.
- MRI is the procedure of choice and has replaced arthrography in cases of disabling pain or if locking occurs. It is used to determine disc position and morphology along with degenerative bony changes.

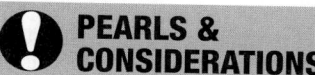 **TREATMENT**

NONPHARMACOLOGIC THERAPY

- Soft diet to rest the muscles of mastication
- Heat 15 to 20 min four to six times per day
- Massage of the masseter and temporalis muscles
- Formed splints or bite appliances
- Range-of-motion exercises

ACUTE GENERAL Rx

- Nonsteroidal antiinflammatory drugs: ibuprofen 800 PO mg tid prn, naproxen 500 PO mg bid prn, titrated to relieve symptoms

- Muscle relaxants at bedtime: diazepam 2.5 to 5 mg PO tid prn or amitriptyline 5 to 100 mg PO qd prn
- In degenerative joint disease of the TMJ, intraarticular steroid injection can be tried
- Botulism toxin injections into the masticatory muscles

CHRONIC Rx

- Most of the above treatments are used for myofascial pain-dysfunction syndrome; however, they can be applied to other causes of TMJ syndrome. Surgery is usually a measure of last resort in patients who do not respond to nonpharmacologic and acute general treatment.
- Surgical procedures include:
  1. Meniscoplasty
  2. Meniscectomy
  3. Subcondylar osteotomy
  4. TMJ reconstruction

DISPOSITION

The course depends on the underlying etiology; however, a lengthy course with exacerbations of symptoms can be expected.

REFERRAL

All patients with TMJ syndrome refractory to conservative nonpharmacologic and acute therapy should be referred to a periodontist, oral maxillofacial surgeon, or ear-nose-throat surgeon.

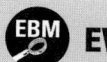 **PEARLS & CONSIDERATIONS**

Patients with rheumatoid arthritis involving the TMJ usually have bilateral involvement.

COMMENTS

Frequently, emotional stress initiates the myofascial pain-dysfunction, which accounts for 85% of all cases of TMJ syndrome.

EBM EVIDENCE

available at www.expertconsult.com

SUGGESTED READINGS

available at www.expertconsult.com

AUTHORS: **RYAN W. ZUZEK, M.D.,** and **DOUGLAS BURTT, M.D.**

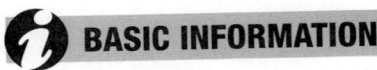

BASIC INFORMATION

DEFINITION

Testicular neoplasms are primary cancers originating in a testis.

SYNONYMS

Testis tumor
Testicular neoplasms

ICD-9CM CODES
186.9   Testicular neoplasm
M906/3   (seminoma)
M9101/3 (embryonal carcinoma or teratoma)
M9100/3 (choriocarcinoma)

EPIDEMIOLOGY & DEMOGRAPHICS

INCIDENCE: 5.4 cases per 100,000 men annually. White men have the highest incidence at 6.3 cases/100,000 men. Testicular cancer is the most common cancer diagnosis in men between the ages of 15 and 35 yr. The incidence has been gradually increasing since 1975.
PREVALENCE: 1% to 2% of all cancers in males
PREDOMINANT AGE: Can occur in any age but most common in young adults; average age for embryonal cell carcinoma: 30 yr; average age for seminoma: 36 yr

PHYSICAL FINDINGS & CLINICAL PRESENTATION

- Testicular cancer typically presents as a painless mass in the testis. Any mass within the testicle should be considered cancer until proven otherwise. It may be found by the patient, who brings it to the attention of a physician, or it may be found by a physician on a routine examination.
- Symptoms other than scrotal or testicular swelling are typically absent unless the cancer has metastasized (5% of patients at diagnosis). Occasionally a patient may report scrotal fullness or heaviness. Gynecomastia from tumors that secrete beta-human chorionic gonadotropin (hCG) is found in 1% of men with testicular cancer.
- Testicular palpation should be performed with two hands. Transillumination may distinguish a solid mass (e.g., cancer) and a fluid-filled lesion (e.g., hydrocele or spermatocele). The mass is nontender; indeed, it is less sensitive than a normal testicle.

ETIOLOGY & PATHOLOGY

- Cryptorchidism (undescended testes) is a major risk factor even if corrected by orchiopexy; however, treatment of undescended testis before puberty decreases the risk of testicular cancer from fivefold to twofold. Other risk factors are family history, infertility, tobacco use, and white race.

- Pathology:

Cell Type	Frequency (%)
Seminoma	42
Embryonal cell carcinoma	26
Teratocarcinoma	26
Teratoma	5
Choriocarcinoma	1

- Other rare types:
  - Yolk sac carcinoma
  - Mixed germ cell tumors
  - Carcinoid tumor
  - Sertoli cell tumors
  - Leydig cell tumors
  - Lymphoma
  - Metastatic cancer to the testes
- TNM staging system for testicular cancer
  - T_0: No apparent primary
  - T_1: Testis only (excludes rete testis)
  - T_2: Beyond the tunica albuginea
  - T_3: Rete testis or epididymal involvement
  - T_4: Spermatic cord
    1. Spermatic cord
    2. Scrotum
  - N_0: No nodal involvement
  - N_1: Ipsilateral regional nodal involvement
  - N_2: Contralateral or bilateral abdominal or groin nodes
  - N_3: Palpable abdominal nodes or fixed groin nodes
  - N_4: Juxtaregional nodes
  - M_0: No distant metastases
  - M_1: Distant metastases present

The clinical stages consist of stage A, with tumor confined to the testis and cord structures; stage B, with tumor confined to the retroperitoneal lymph nodes; and stage C, with tumor involving the abdominal viscera or disease above the diaphragm.

DIAGNOSIS

DIFFERENTIAL DIAGNOSIS

- Spermatocele
- Varicocele
- Hydrocele
- Epididymitis
- Epidermoid cyst of the testicle
- Epididymis tumors

WORKUP

Physical examination, laboratory tests, and imaging studies (see Section III, "Testicular Mass")

LABORATORY TESTS

- Serum hCG
- Serum alpha-fetoprotein (AFP)
One or both of these tumor markers will be elevated in 70% of cases of testicular cancer.
- Serum lactate dehydrogenase (LDH) level
- Testicular biopsy contraindicated

IMAGING STUDIES

- Ultrasound
- CT scan or MRI of pelvis and abdomen
- Chest radiograph
- CT of the chest in patients with suspected mediastinal, hilar, or lung parenchymal disease; MRI of the brain in patients with neurologic symptoms

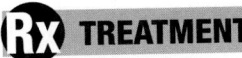

TREATMENT

- Surgical exploration of the testicle through an inguinal incision with a noncrushing clamp placed on the cord before direct testicular examination. If a mass is confined within the body of the testicle, an orchiectomy is performed.
- Retroperitoneal lymph node dissection for clinical stage A and low stage B (lymph nodes <6 cm in greatest diameter) provides cure in 70%.
- Chemotherapy: cisplatin, vinblastine, and bleomycin
  1. Not indicated in clinical stage A
  2. Controversial in low stage B
  3. Cornerstone of treatment in high stage B or stage C
- Radiation therapy for stage A and low stage B seminoma provides cure in 85%
- Posttreatment surveillance for testicular cancer survivors (annually)
  1. General maintenance
  2. Fertility assessment
  3. Sexuality status
  4. Skin examination (increased risk of dysplastic nevi)
  5. Testicular examination (3% to 4% risk of second testicular cancer)
  6. Serum tumor markers (hCG, AFP)
  7. Chest radiograph (for late relapse)
  8. Complications of cisplatin: hypertension, hyperlipidemia, renal failure, hypomagnesemia, hearing loss, tinnitus, peripheral neuropathy, and infertility

DISPOSITION

The overall cure for testicular cancer is >95% (80% for metastatic disease). Because treatment produces favorable outcomes even in advanced stages, the U.S. preventive task force recommends against screening asymptomatic men for testicular cancer.

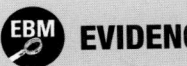 EVIDENCE

available at www.expertconsult.com

SUGGESTED READINGS
available at www.expertconsult.com

AUTHOR: **FRED F. FERRI, M.D.**

BASIC INFORMATION

DEFINITION

Testicular torsion is a twisting of the spermatic cord leading to cessation of testicular blood flow, ischemia, and infarction if left untreated.

SYNONYMS

Spermatic cord torsion

ICD-9CM CODES
608.2 Testicular torsion

EPIDEMIOLOGY & DEMOGRAPHICS

INCIDENCE: Affects one in 4000 males aged <25 yr
PREDOMINANT AGE: Two thirds of all cases occur between the ages of 12 and 18 yr, but may occur at any age, including antenatally.

PHYSICAL FINDINGS & CLINICAL PRESENTATION

- Typical sequence is sudden onset of hemiscrotal pain, then swelling, nausea, and vomiting without fever or urinary symptoms.
- Physical examination may reveal a tender firm testis, high-riding testis, horizontal lie of testis, absent cremasteric reflex, and no pain with elevation of testis. Absence of the cremasteric reflex (stroking or pinching the medial thigh normally causes contraction of the cremaster muscle and elevation of the testis) is the most sensitive physical finding.
- Painless testicular swelling occurs in 10%.
- One out of three patients reports previous episodes of spontaneously remitting scrotal pain.
- In the neonate, testicular torsion should be presumed in patients with a painless, discolored hemiscrotal swelling.
- In rare cases, torsion may involve an undescended testicle. In such situations an empty hemiscrotum is palpated together with a tender lump in the inguinal area.

ETIOLOGY

- There are two types of testicular torsion: extravaginal, caused by nonadherence of the tunica vaginalis to the dartos layer, and intravaginal, caused by malrotation of the spermatic cord with the tunica vaginalis. Intravaginal torsion accounts for 90% of cases.
- Torsion usually occurs in the absence of any precipitating events. Trauma accounts for <10% of cases.

DIAGNOSIS

Diagnosis is made mainly by clinical suspicion. Color Doppler ultrasound evaluation or a nuclear testicular scan (Fig. 1-372) may help with the diagnosis. Ultrasonography will show absent or decreased blood flow; scintigraphy reveals decreased perfusion on symptomatic side.

DIFFERENTIAL DIAGNOSIS

See also Section II.
- Torsion of the testicular appendages (appendix testis)
- Testicular tumor
- Epididymitis
- Incarcerated inguinoscrotal hernia
- Orchitis
- Spermatocele
- Hydrocele, varicocele

WORKUP

The diagnosis is usually based on history and physical examination.

IMAGING STUDIES

- Radionuclide scrotal scanning (technetium-99m): cold testicle
- Doppler ultrasonic stethoscope (Doppler flowmetry)

TREATMENT

Surgical derotation of the spermatic cord followed by bilateral testicular fixation with nonabsorbable sutures. If the affected testis is nonviable, orchiectomy of the affected testis and orchiopexy of the contralateral side are performed. Attempts at manual detorsion should not delay surgical consultation.

PROGNOSIS

- The degree of ischemia depends on the duration of torsion and the degree of rotation of the spermatic cord.
- There is an 80% testicular salvage rate if detorsion occurs within 12 hr of onset.
- After 24 hr, irreversible testicular infarction is expected.
- Because the contralateral testes can be affected (immunologic process), when treatment is delayed and return of blood flow does not occur after detorsion, some recommend orchiectomy of the infarcted testicle.

REFERRAL

To urologist

PEARLS & CONSIDERATIONS

- Manual detorsion by external rotation of the testis toward the thigh can be attempted for adolescent intravaginal torsion if an operating facility is not readily available.
- Extravaginal torsion is diagnosed in the newborn. Intravaginal torsion can occur at any age but is usually diagnosed in males ages 12 to 18 yr.

SUGGESTED READING

available at www.expertconsult.com

AUTHOR: **FRED F. FERRI, M.D.**

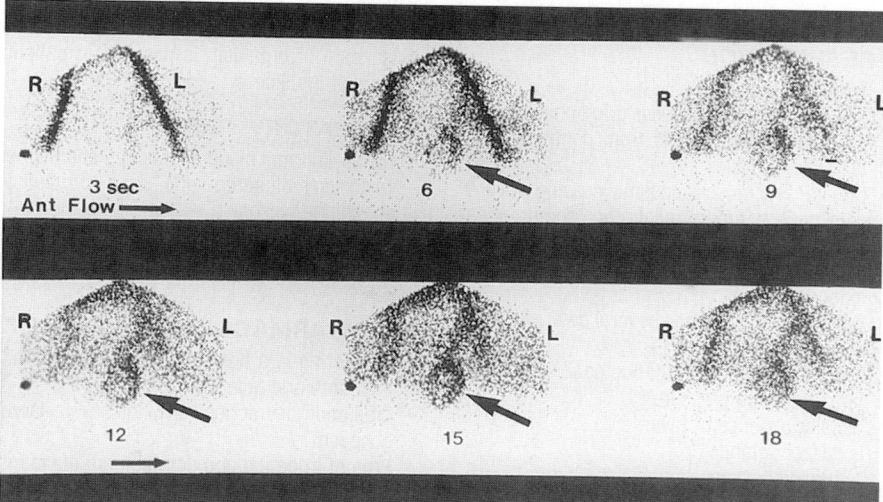

FIGURE 1-372 Testicular torsion. Evaluation of blood flow to the testicle has been done by giving an intravenous bolus of radioactive material. The right and left iliac vessels are clearly identified, and sequential images are obtained every 3 sec. Here, increased flow is seen to the rim of the left testicle *(arrows)*, and there is no blood flow centrally. This is the appearance of a testicular torsion in which the torsion has been present for more than approximately 24 hr. (From Mettler FA [ed]: *Primary care radiology,* Philadelphia, 2000, WB Saunders.)

T

Diseases and Disorders

I

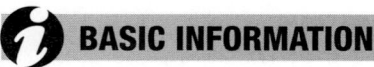

BASIC INFORMATION

DEFINITION

Tetanus is a life-threatening illness manifested by muscle rigidity and spasms; it is caused by a neurotoxin (tetanospasmin) produced by *Clostridium tetani*.

SYNONYMS

Lockjaw
Generalized tetanus
Neonatal tetanus
Cephalic tetanus
Localized tetanus

ICD-9CM CODES
037 Tetanus

EPIDEMIOLOGY & DEMOGRAPHICS

INCIDENCE (IN U.S.): 48 to 64 cases reported annually since 1986
INCIDENCE (WORLDWIDE): About 1 million cases of tetanus are reported worldwide annually, suggesting a global incidence of about 18 per 100,000 persons per year and an estimated 300,000 to 500,000 deaths per year. Tetanus is an expected complication when disasters strike in developing countries where tetanus immunization coverage is low
PREDOMINANT AGE: >60 yr of age
GENETICS:
Neonatal infection:
- Rare in U.S.
- Among the leading causes of neonatal mortality in many parts of the world (caused by infection of the umbilical cord stump)

PHYSICAL FINDINGS & CLINICAL PRESENTATION

- Trismus ("lockjaw")
- Risus sardonicus (peculiar grin), characteristic grimace that results from contraction of the facial muscles
- Generalized muscle spasms causing severe pain and, at times, respiratory compromise and death
- Rigid abdominal muscles, flexed arms, and extended legs
- Autonomic dysfunction several days after onset of illness
- Leading cause of death: fluctuations in heart rate and blood pressure
- Usually, absence of fever
- Localized tetanus
  1. Rigidity of muscles near the injury
  2. Weakness as a result of lower motor neuron injury
  3. May be self-limited and resolve spontaneously

4. More often progresses to generalized tetanus
5. Cephalic tetanus:
   a. May occur with head injuries or chronic otitis with localized ear or mastoid infection with *C. tetani*
   b. Can manifest as cranial nerve dysfunction

ETIOLOGY

- *C. tetani* is a gram-positive, spore-forming bacillus that resides primarily in the soil.
- Majority of cases are caused by punctures and lacerations.
- Toxin is elaborated from organisms in a contaminated wound.
- Local symptoms are caused by inhibition of neurotransmitter at presynaptic sites.
  1. Over the next 2 to 14 days, the toxin travels up the neurons to the CNS, where it acts on inhibitory neurons to prevent neurotransmitter release.
  2. Unopposed motor activity results in tonic contractions of muscles.

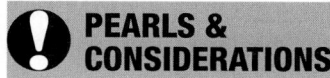

DIAGNOSIS

DIFFERENTIAL DIAGNOSIS

- Strychnine poisoning
- Dystonic reaction caused by neuroleptic agents
- Local infection (dental or masseter muscle) causing trismus
- Severe hypocalcemia
- Hysteria

WORKUP

- Positive wound culture is not helpful in diagnosis.
- Isolation of organism is possible in patients without the illness.

LABORATORY TESTS

- Usually, normal blood counts and chemistries
- Toxicology of serum and urine to rule out strychnine poisoning

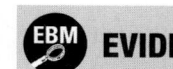

TREATMENT

NONPHARMACOLOGIC THERAPY

- Monitoring in a hospital ICU: keep surroundings dark and quiet
- Intubation or tracheostomy for severe laryngospasm
- Prompt irrigation and debridement of wound

ACUTE GENERAL Rx

- Human tetanus immunoglobulin (HTIg) 500 U via IM injection

- Tetanus toxoid (Td) 0.5 ml by IM injection at a different site
- Metronidazole 500 mg IV q6h, or penicillin G 1 million U IV q4h for 10 days. Metronidazole is the preferred antimicrobial
- IV diazepam to control muscle spasms. Alternative agents are baclofen, magnesium, dantrolene, barbiturates, and chlorpromazine
- Neuromuscular blockade if necessary

CHRONIC Rx

- Supportive care. Beta-blockers, magnesium, and morphine can improve autonomic dysfunction
- Possible mechanical ventilation. If ventilator support is not available, benzodiazepines are the preferred agent to manage respiratory failure
- Minimal external stimuli
- Control of heart rate and blood pressure:
  1. Labetalol for sympathetic hyperactivity
  2. Pacemaker for sustained bradycardia
- Physical therapy once spasms subside

DISPOSITION

Full recovery over weeks to months if complications can be avoided

REFERRAL

- To emergency department
- To infectious disease specialist

PEARLS & CONSIDERATIONS

COMMENTS

- Illness is preventable.
- Boosters of Td should be given every 10 yr to maintain immune status.
- Passive as well as active immunization (HTIg and Td) should be given for patients with tetanus-prone wounds who have not been adequately immunized in the previous 5 yr.
- A recent U.S. study showed that only 72% of people older than 6 yr had protective levels of antibody.

EVIDENCE

available at www.expertconsult.com

SUGGESTED READINGS
available at www.expertconsult.com

AUTHORS: **GLENN G. FORT, M.D., M.P.H.,** and **DENNIS J. MIKOLICH, M.D.**

BASIC INFORMATION

DEFINITION

Tetralogy of Fallot (TOF) is a congenital heart deformity that consists of the following four features (Fig. 1-373):

1. Ventricular septal defect (VSD)
2. Infundibular stenosis that leads to the obstruction of the right ventricular (RV) outflow tract
3. An aorta that overrides the VSD by <50% of its diameter
4. Concentric RV hypertrophy

ICD-9CM CODES
745.2 Tetralogy of Fallot

EPIDEMIOLOGY & DEMOGRAPHICS

- TOF is the most common cyanotic congenital heart malformation that is diagnosed in patients after the age of 1 yr.
- TOF accounts for nearly 10% of all cases of congenital heart disease.
- TOF occurs in approximately 3000 newborns/yr.

PHYSICAL FINDINGS & CLINICAL PRESENTATION

- Of the four major features of TOF, infundibular stenosis that leads to RV outflow tract obstruction and VSD are the primary defects that result in clinical manifestations. The degree of RV outflow obstruction determines the age and symptoms at presentation. RV outflow tract obstruction and the VSD result in the following:
  - Right-to-left shunting and hypoxemia
  - Altered RV hemodynamics
  - Decreased pulmonary blood flow
- The aforementioned pathophysiologic concepts result in common manifestations of TOF, including the following:
  - Cyanosis of the nail beds and lips as a result of the shunting of deoxygenated blood from the RV through the VSD into the left ventricle, thus bypassing the lungs
  - Dyspnea on exertion
  - Digital clubbing
  - The child assuming a squatting position after exercise to increase systemic vascular resistance, thereby decreasing right-to-left shunting
  - Low birth weight and growth rate
  - Palpable RV impulse
  - Systolic thrill along the left sternal border
  - Single second heart sound with an inaudible P2 component
  - A harsh systolic crescendo/decrescendo murmur that results from RV outflow tract obstruction and that is usually heard along the left mid to upper sternal border with posterior radiation
- After repair, patients may have a low-pitched diastolic murmur at the pulmonic area that is consistent with pulmonary regurgitation or a pansystolic murmur that is consistent with a VSD patch leak. If the patient only has a palliative shunt, a continuous murmur may be heard from the site of the shunt.

ETIOLOGY

TOF likely results from the maldevelopment of the embryologic conotruncus, but the exact mechanism is unknown.

DIAGNOSIS

- The diagnosis of TOF is suspected in any neonate, infant, or child who presents with cyanosis and a heart murmur.
- VSD is associated with other cardiac defects:
  - Persistent foramen ovale/atrial septal defect
  - Pulmonary artery anomalies
  - Right aortic arch
  - Left superior vena cava to coronary sinus
  - Additional VSDs
  - Coronary artery anomalies
- Associated syndromes include the following:
  - DeGeorge
  - DeLange
  - Goldenhar
  - Klippel-Feil
  - VACTERL
  - CHARGE

DIFFERENTIAL DIAGNOSIS

- Asthma
- Isolated VSD
- Pulmonary atresia
- Patent ductus arteriosus
- Aortic stenosis
- Pneumothorax

WORKUP

- Detailed history and physical examination, including pulse oximetry
- Echocardiogram, chest radiograph, 12-lead ECG, and routine laboratory tests

LABORATORY TESTS

- The CBC shows polycythemia from long-standing hypoxemia.
- Arterial blood gas levels show hypoxemia, normal pH, and pCO_2 (carbon dioxide levels).
- ECG commonly demonstrates right axis deviation, RV hypertrophy, and right atrial enlargement. The QRS duration may reflect the degree of RV dilation.
- Exercise testing may help to evaluate functional capacity and exertional arrhythmias.

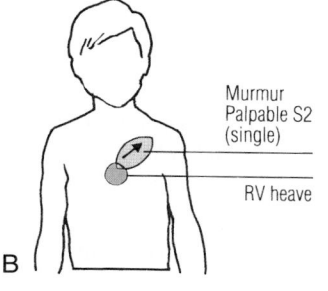

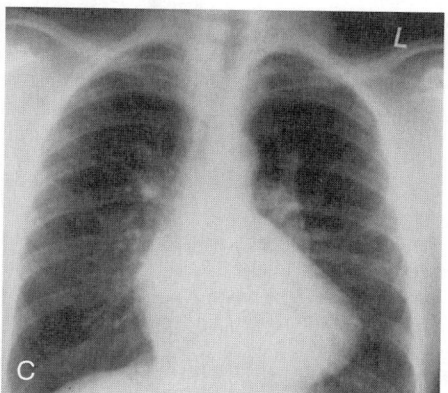

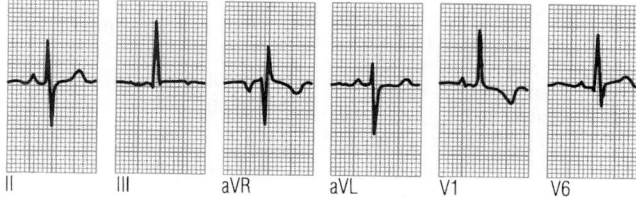

FIGURE 1-373 Features of Fallot tetralogy. A, Diagram of abnormality. VSD = Ventricular septal defect; PA = pulmonary artery; Ao = aorta. B, Physical signs. C, Chest x-ray showing right ventricular hypertrophy, typical 'coeur en sabol.' D, ECG showing right atrial and ventricular hypertrophy and right axis deviation. (Souhami RL, Moxham J: *Textbook of medicine*, ed 4, London, 2002, Churchill Livingstone.)

IMAGING STUDIES

- Chest radiography reveals a boot-shaped heart that is commonly described as *coeur en sabot;* a prominent RV with decreased pulmonary vascularity; and a heart size that is usually normal. Cardiomegaly may reflect important pulmonary or tricuspid regurgitation, and a right-sided aortic arch may be seen.
- Echocardiography demonstrates VSD with a stenotic RV outflow tract and an overriding aorta. After repair, echocardiography can assess the severity of residual RV outflow tract obstruction, pulmonary regurgitation, and any tricuspid regurgitation that may be present. Right ventricular systolic pressures may also be assessed. A residual VSD may be seen, and RV size and function can be determined qualitatively.
- Cardiac catheterization and angiography help to determine hemodynamics, the severity of right-to-left shunting, the localization of the VSD, the flow across a persistent foramen ovale or atrial septal defect, and the severity of the pulmonic regurgitation; it can also be used to anatomically assess the RV outflow tract and the anatomy of the pulmonary artery and the coronary artery. Interventions are also possible, such as the elimination of collateral vessels or systemic–pulmonic artery shunts, dilation or stent implantation for obstructed pulmonary arteries, and possible percutaneous pulmonic valve replacement.
- Cardiac MRI is used for the localization of the VSD, the anatomic assessment of the RV outflow tract, the assessment of RV function, the quantification of pulmonary regurgitation, and the detection of RV myocardial fibrosis. Magnetic resonance angiography can be a noninvasive alternative to cardiac catheterization for the evaluation of pulmonary vascular anatomy and the ascending aorta.
- Multislice spiral computed tomography can be used for diagnosis, and it is extremely important during the planning of the repair procedure. Its use may be limited by the risks associated with radiation exposure in children. It can also be used to make assessments that are similar to those usually made by MRI for patients who are unable to undergo MRI.

(Rx) TREATMENT

NONPHARMACOLOGIC THERAPY

- Oxygen
- Prostaglandins at time of birth to keep a patent ductus and to maintain ductal flow to the lungs
- Knee–chest position during hypoxemic spells to help reduce venous return and to increase systemic vascular resistance, thereby decreasing right-to-left shunting

ACUTE GENERAL Rx

The acute treatment of any infant or child with TOF who is cyanotic with respiratory distress is aimed at increasing systemic vascular resistance and decreasing right-to-left shunting (e.g., phenylephrine 0.1 to 0.5 mcg/kg/min intravenously). Intravenous β-blockers (e.g., pro-

pranolol 0.15 to 0.25 mg/kg via slow intravenous push) are used to decrease RV outflow tract contractility, and subcutaneous morphine can be used to decrease venous return.

CHRONIC Rx

- Palliative repair includes procedures to increase pulmonary blood flow, thus reducing right-to-left shunting and allowing for pulmonary development. Examples of palliative procedures include the Blalock-Taussig shunt, in which a shunt is made between the subclavian artery and the pulmonary artery; the Waterston shunt, which attaches the ascending aorta to the right pulmonary artery; and the Potts shunt, which attaches the descending aorta to the left pulmonary artery. These are generally performed when the patient is still an infant.
- Complete surgical repair has good success and involves closing the VSD with a Dacron patch and relieving the RV outflow tract obstruction by simple resection of the infundibular stenosis, patch augmentation of the RV outflow, or the placement of a transannular patch). Patients who have the repair before the age of 2 yr are usually symptom free and can generally lead a normal life. If the repair is performed during adulthood, pulmonary valve replacement may be required.
- Postoperative issues include the following:
  - Residual pulmonic regurgitation
  - RV dilation and dysfunction from pulmonary regurgitation
  - Residual RV outflow tract obstruction
  - Branch pulmonary artery stenosis or hypoplasia
  - Sustained ventricular tachycardia
  - Sudden cardiac death
  - Atrioventricular block, atrial flutter, and atrial fibrillation
  - Progressive aortic regurgitation
  - Syndromal associations

DISPOSITION

- Almost all patients with TOF have either palliative or complete surgical repair before they reach adulthood.
- <3% of patients with TOF reach the age of 40 yr without surgery.
- Survival after the complete operative repair of TOF is excellent if the RV outflow tract obstruction has been relieved and the VSD has been closed.
- The 35-yr survival rate for patients after TOF repair is 85%.
- The need for pulmonary valve replacement increases after the second decade of life. It is indicated in symptomatic patients with severe pulmonary regurgitation or asymptomatic patients with severe pulmonary stenosis or regurgitation with signs of progressive or severe RV enlargement or dysfunction.
- A prolonged QRS duration on the preoperative ECG predicts an increased risk of postoperative supraventricular or ventricular arrhythmia. Prolongation of the QRS beyond 180 msec identifies patients who are at increased risk of ventricular tachycardia after surgery.
- Ventricular arrhythmia can lead to sudden cardiac death in 8.3% of surgically repaired

patients by the age of 35 yr. Monomorphic ventricular tachycardia is likely the result of a reentry circuit from a scar caused by the surgery.
- Patients with signs or symptoms of arrhythmia should undergo hemodynamic and electrophysiologic testing. Treatment is tailored to the testing results and may include pulmonic valve replacement, residual VSD closure, mapping and ablation of an arrhythmia, antiarrhythmic medication, or the placement of an implantable cardiac defibrillator.
- Reduced exercise capacity is usually the result of chronic pulmonary regurgitation or residual RV outflow tract obstruction.
- Women with repaired TOF should be assessed by a cardiologist before considering pregnancy to determine if pulmonic valve replacement is needed first. The offspring of patients with TOF are more likely to have congenital anomalies than the offspring of the general population.
- Selected patients with normal RV pressures and function without evidence of residual shunt and without atrial or ventricular tachyarrhythmia are eligible to participate in competitive sports.

REFERRAL

- Infants and children with cyanotic heart disease should be referred to a pediatric cardiologist for further diagnostic evaluation. After being diagnosed with TOF, patients should be referred to centers with experience in palliative and complete surgical repair.
- Adult patients with repaired TOF should be comanaged with a cardiologist who specializes in adults with congenital heart disease.

(!) PEARLS & CONSIDERATIONS

- TOF was first described by the French physician Etienne Fallot in 1888.
- The first palliative surgical treatment for TOF was performed by Dr. Alfred Blalock at Johns Hopkins University in 1945 (i.e., the Taussig-Blalock shunt).
- The first surgical repair for TOF was performed by Dr. C. Walton Lillehei at the University of Minnesota in 1954.

COMMENTS

- The severity of RV outflow tract obstruction is the primary determinant of clinical symptoms and outcomes.
- TOF requires subacute bacterial endocarditis prophylaxis before any dental work or nonsterile surgical procedures (e.g., surgery of the bowel or bladder).
- Children with TOF are at risk for neurodevelopmental delay when they reach school age.

SUGGESTED READINGS
available at www.expertconsult.com

AUTHORS: **SCOTT COHEN, M.D.,** and **WEN-CHIH WU, M.D.**

BASIC INFORMATION

DEFINITION

Thalassemias are a heterogeneous group of disorders of hemoglobin synthesis that have in common a deficient synthesis of one or more of the polypeptide chains of the normal human hemoglobin, resulting in a quantitative abnormality of the hemoglobin thus produced. There are no qualitative changes such as those encountered in the hemoglobinopathies (e.g., sickle cell disease).

SYNONYMS

Mediterranean anemia
Cooley's anemia

ICD-9CM CODES
282.4 Thalassemia

EPIDEMIOLOGY & DEMOGRAPHICS

- Thalassemia is among the most common genetic disorders worldwide. Approximately 4.83% of the world's population carry globin variants, including 1.67% of the population that are heterozygous for alpha-thalassemia and beta-thalassemia.
- The highest concentration of alpha-thalassemia is found in Southeast Asia and the African west coast. For example, the prevalence is 5% to 10% in Thailand. It is also common among blacks, with a prevalence of approximately 5%.
- The worldwide prevalence of beta-thalassemia is approximately 3%; in certain regions of Italy and Greece the prevalence reaches 15% to 30%. This high prevalence can be found in Americans of Italian or Greek descent.
- The distribution of thalassemia in Europe and Africa parallels that of malaria, suggesting that thalassemic persons are more resistant to the parasite, thus permitting evolutionary survival advantage.

CLASSIFICATION

Beta-thalassemia:
- Beta (+) thalassemia (suboptimal beta-globin synthesis)
- Beta (o) thalassemia (total absence of beta-globin synthesis)
- Delta-beta-thalassemia (total absence of both delta-globin and beta-globin synthesis)
- Lepore hemoglobin (synthesis of small amounts of fused delta-beta-globin and total absence of delta- and beta-globin)
- Hereditary persistence of fetal hemoglobin (HPHF) (increased hemoglobin F synthesis and reduced or absence of delta- and beta-globin)

Alpha-thalassemia:
- Silent carrier (three alpha-globin genes present)
- Alpha thalassemia trait (two alpha-globin genes present)

- Hemoglobin H disease (one alpha-globin gene present)
- Hydrops fetalis (no alpha-globin gene)
- Hemoglobin constant sprint (elongated alpha-globin chain)

Thalassemic hemoglobinopathies:
- Hb Terre Haute, Hb Quong Sze, HbE, Hb Knossos

PHYSICAL FINDINGS & CLINICAL PRESENTATION

Beta-thalassemia:
- Heterozygous beta-thalassemia (thalassemia minor): no or mild anemia, microcytosis and hypochromia, mild hemolysis manifested by slight reticulocytosis and splenomegaly
- Homozygous beta-thalassemia (thalassemia major): intense hemolytic anemia; transfusion dependency; bone deformities (skull and long bones); hepatomegaly; splenomegaly; iron overload leading to cardiomyopathy, diabetes mellitus, and hypogonadism; growth retardation; pigment gallstones; susceptibility to infection
- Thalassemia intermedia caused by combination of beta- and alpha-thalassemia or beta-thalassemia and Hb Lepore: resembles thalassemia major but is milder

Alpha-thalassemia:
- Silent carrier: no symptoms.
- Alpha-thalassemia trait: microcytosis only.
- Hemoglobin H disease: moderately severe hemolysis with microcytosis and splenomegaly.
- The loss of all four alpha-globin genes is incompatible with life (stillbirth of hydropic fetus). NOTE: Pregnancies with hydrops fetalis are associated with a high incidence of toxemia.

ETIOLOGY

- Beta-thalassemia: it is caused by more than 200 point mutations and, rarely, by deletions. The reduction of beta-globin synthesis results in redundant alpha-globin chains (Heinz bodies), which are cytotoxic and cause intramedullary hemolysis and ineffective erythropoiesis. Fetal hemoglobin may be increased.
- Alpha-thalassemia: several mutations can result in insufficient amounts of alpha-globin available for combination with non–alpha-globins.

DIAGNOSIS

LABORATORY TESTS

Beta-thalassemia:
- Microcytosis (mean cell volume: 55 to 80 FL)
- Normal red blood cell (RBC) distribution width index (RDW)
- Smear: nucleated RBCs, anisocytosis, poikilocytosis, polychromatophilia, Pappenheimer and Howell-Jolly bodies

- Hemoglobin electrophoresis: absent or reduced hemoglobin A, increased fetal hemoglobin, variable increase in the amount of hemoglobin A_2
- Markers of hemolysis: elevated indirect bilirubin and lactate dehydrogenase, decreased haptoglobin

Alpha-thalassemia:
- Microcytosis in the absence of iron deficiency
- Hemoglobin electrophoresis normal except for the presence of hemoglobin H in hemoglobin H disease

 TREATMENT

- Thalassemia minor: no treatment, but avoid iron administration for incorrect diagnosis of iron deficiency.
- Beta-thalassemia major (and hemoglobin H disease):
  1. Transfusion as required together with chelation of iron with desferrioxamine (by IV or subcutaneous administration, 8 to 12 hr nightly, 5 to 6 days a week at a dose of 2 to 6 g/day with a portable infusion pump).
  2. Splenectomy for hypersplenism if present.
  3. Bone marrow transplantation. Although hematopoietic stem cell transplantation is the only curative approach for thalassemia, it has been limited by the high cost and scarcity of human leukocyte antigen–matched donors. Before transplantation, it is necessary to administer myeloablative regimens to eradicate the endogenous thalassemic bone marrow. Commonly used agents are hydroxyurea, azathioprine, fludarabine, busulfan, and cyclophosphamide.
  4. Hydroxyurea may increase the level of hemoglobin F.

PEARLS & CONSIDERATIONS

- Polymerase chain reaction can be used to detect point mutations or deletions in chorionic villous samples, enabling first-trimester, DNA-based testing for thalassemia.
- Preimplantation genetic diagnosis can be extended to human leukocyte antigen typing on embryonic biopsies, allowing the selection of an embryo that is not affected by thalassemia and that may also serve as a stem cell donor for a previously affected child within the same family.

SUGGESTED READING
available at www.expertconsult.com

AUTHOR: **FRED F. FERRI, M.D.**

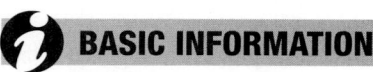

BASIC INFORMATION

DEFINITION

Thoracic outlet syndrome describes a condition producing upper extremity symptoms believed to result from neurovascular compression at the thoracic outlet. Three types are described on the basis of point of compression: (1) cervical rib and scalenus syndrome, in which abnormal scalene muscles or the presence of a cervical rib may cause compression; (2) costoclavicular syndrome, in which compression may occur under the clavicle; and (3) hyperabduction syndrome, in which compression may occur in the subcoracoid area.

ICD-9CM CODES
353.0 Thoracic outlet syndrome

EPIDEMIOLOGY & DEMOGRAPHICS

PREVALENCE: Varies from source to source; presence of cervical ribs in 0.5% to 1% of population (50% bilateral), but most are asymptomatic
PREDOMINANT SEX: Females affected more often than males (ratio of 3.5:1)
PREDOMINANT AGE: Rare in those aged <20 yr

PHYSICAL FINDINGS & CLINICAL PRESENTATION

- Symptoms and signs are related to the degree of involvement of each of the various structures at the level of the first rib.
- True venous or arterial involvement is not common.
- Diagnosis is most often used in the consideration of neural pain affecting the arm, which suggests involvement of the brachial plexus.
  1. Arterial compression: pallor, paresthesias, diminished pulses, coolness, digital gangrene, and a supraclavicular bruit or mass
  2. Venous compression: edema and pain; thrombosis causing superficial venous dilation in the shoulder area
  3. "True" neural compression: lower trunk (C8, T1) findings with intrinsic weakness and diminished sensation to the ring finger and small fingers and ulnar aspect of the forearm
  4. Possible supraclavicular tenderness
  5. Provocative tests (Adson's, Wright's): may reproduce pain but are of disputed usefulness

ETIOLOGY

- Congenital cervical rib or fibrous extension of cervical rib (Fig. 1-374)
- Abnormal scalene muscle insertion
- Drooping of shoulder girdle from generalized hypotonia or trauma
- Narrowed costoclavicular interval as a result of downward and backward pressure on shoulder (sometimes seen in individuals who carry heavy backpacks)
- Acute venous thrombosis with exercise (effort thrombosis)
- Bony abnormalities of first rib
- Abnormal fibromuscular bands
- Malunion of clavicle fracture

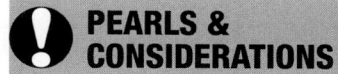

DIAGNOSIS

DIFFERENTIAL DIAGNOSIS

- Carpal tunnel syndrome
- Cervical radiculopathy
- Brachial neuritis
- Ulnar nerve compression
- Reflex sympathetic dystrophy
- Superior sulcus tumor

WORKUP

Except for venous or arterial pathology, no ancillary diagnostic tests are reliable for diagnostic confirmation.

IMAGING STUDIES

- Arteriography or venography when vascular pathology is strongly suspected clinically
- Cervical spine radiographs to rule out cervical disk disease
- Chest radiograph to rule out lung tumor
- Electromyography, nerve conduction velocity studies to rule out carpal tunnel syndrome, cervical radiculopathy

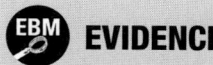

TREATMENT

ACUTE GENERAL Rx

- Sling for pain relief
- Physical therapy modalities plus shoulder girdle–strengthening exercises
- Postural reeducation
- Nonsteroidal anti-inflammatory drugs

DISPOSITION

- Surgery: generally successful for vascular disorders
- Nonsurgical treatment: often successful for patients with pain as the primary symptom

REFERRAL

For vascular surgery consultation when venous or arterial impairment is present

PEARLS & CONSIDERATIONS

COMMENTS

- True thoracic outlet syndrome is probably an uncommon condition.
- Diagnosis is often used to describe a wide variety of clinical symptoms.
- Considerable disagreement exists regarding the frequency of this disorder.

EBM EVIDENCE

available at www.expertconsult.com

SUGGESTED READINGS
available at www.expertconsult.com

AUTHOR: **LONNIE R. MERCIER, M.D.**

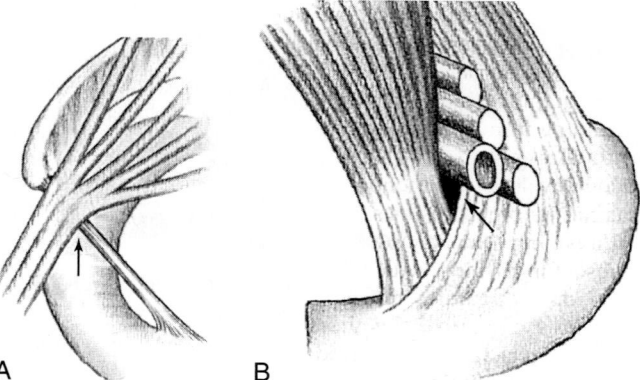

FIGURE 1-374 A, Compression caused by a cervical rib *(arrow).* **B,** Abnormal scalene muscle insertions that may cause compression at the cervicobrachial region *(arrow).* (From Mercier LR: *Practical orthopedics,* ed 5, St Louis, 2000, Mosby.)

BASIC INFORMATION

DEFINITION

Thromboangiitis obliterans (TAO, Buerger's disease) is a relatively rare, segmental, and nonatherosclerotic, inflammatory occlusive disease that commonly affects small- and medium-sized arteries, veins, and nerves of the extremities.

SYNONYMS

Buerger's disease
Presenile gangrene
TAO

ICD-9CM CODES
443.1 Thromboangiitis obliterans (Buerger's disease)

EPIDEMIOLOGY & DEMOGRAPHICS

- TAO occurs with the least frequency in Western Europe (0.5% to 5.6% of patients with peripheral arterial disease, PAD) and the most commonly among Ashkenazi Jews in Israel (80% of cases of PAD).
- A genetic predisposition has been proposed on the basis of the higher incidence in Israel among Jews of Ashkenazi ancestry with peripheral artery disease.
- High morbidity is also observed in India (45% to 63%), Korea and Japan (16% to 66%).
- The prevalence has been estimated at 12.6 per 100,000 in the United States.
- The symptoms almost always begin before the age of 45 yr (mean age 42.9 yr female and 39.8 yr male), and almost all patients affected are smokers.
- TAO predominantly affects young males. However, there has been a recent increase in the prevalence of TAO among females (percentage of female patients 9.8%), which has been attributed to increased smoking in this patient population.
- Amputation is common, and major amputations (limbs rather than fingers or toes) are almost twice as common among patients who continue to smoke.

PHYSICAL FINDINGS & CLINICAL PRESENTATION

- The most common symptoms on presentation include the following: intermittent claudication, superficial thrombophlebitis, parestesias from ischemic neuropathy, Raynaud's phenomenon; and more rarely and typically with more advanced disease, rest pain as the first symptom; and necrosis and ulceration.
- The lower extremities are involved in 100% of cases, while the upper extremities in 40% to 50%. The disease rarely affects the vessels proximal to the popliteal artery.
- Involvement of both the upper and lower extremities and the size and location of affected vessels help distinguish TAO from atherosclerosis. Superficial thrombophlebitis further differentiates TAO from other vasculitides (excluding Behcet's disease).
- Superficial thrombophlebitis may be present before the onset of ischemic symptoms. Patients often describe a migratory pattern of tender nodules that follow a venous distribution.
- Rare atypical clinical manifestations have been reported: abdominal involvement resulting in small and large intestine ischemia; transient ischemic attack (TIA); coronary artery involvement along with internal thoracic arteries; and renal artery involvement.
- Rest pain generally occurs on the forefoot and causes continuous pain; patients may therefore sleep with their legs dangling downward.
- There can be evidence of prolonged capillary refill with dependent rubor.
- Although nonspecific, a positive Allen's test in a young smoker with digital ischemia is suggestive of the disease.

ETIOLOGY

- The etiology of TAO remains unclear; however, a multifactorial mechanism has been proposed that involves a combination of genetic susceptibility, tobacco exposure, and immune and coagulary responses.
- Inflammatory markers such as C-reactive protein (CRP) and erythrocyte sedimentation rate (ESR) and commonly measured autoantibodies are typically normal; however, abnormalities in immunoreactivity are believed to drive the inflammatory process.
- Prothrombotic factors may play a role in the pathophysiology: presence of prothrombin gene mutation 20210 and anticardiolipin antibodies are associated with increased risk.
- Pathologic studies have described three phases of TAO:
  1. The acute phase of the disease is characterized by the formation of an occlusive, highly cellular, inflammatory thrombus composed of polymorphonuclear neutrophils, microabcesses, and multinucleated giant cells;
  2. A subacute phase where progressive organization of the thrombus occurs;
  3. A chronic phase with organized thrombus and vascular fibrosis that may mimic atherosclerosis.
- Although debated, TAO in any stage is distinguished from atherosclerosis and other vasculitides by the preservation of the internal elastic lamina.

DIAGNOSIS

DIFFERENTIAL DIAGNOSIS

- Limb ischemia as a result of emboli or atherosclerotic occlusive disease
- Antiphospholipid antibody syndrome
- Autoimmune disorders
- Acrocyanosis
- Carpal tunnel syndrome
- CREST syndrome (i.e., Calcinosis cutis, Reynaud's phenomenon, Esophageal motility disorder, Sclerodactyly, and Telangiectasia)
- Systemic lupus erythematosus
- Diabetes mellitus
- Repetitive vibratory equipment use
- Hypothenar hammer syndrome
- Raynaud's phenomenon
- Ergotamine intoxication
- Polyarteritis nodosa
- Cannabis arteritis
- Peripheral neuropathy

WORKUP

- TAO is a clinical diagnosis that is supported by a compatible history, physical findings, and diagnostic vascular abnormalities on imaging studies.
- Although a definitive diagnosis is made with histopathologic identification of acute phase lesions in patients with signs of the disease, several common clinical criteria may be helpful, including:
  1. PAD occurring in those aged <45 yr.
  2. Current or recent history of tobacco use.
  3. Presence of distal ischemia affecting both the lower (infrapopliteal) and upper extremities rather than just the lower extremities, as is seen with atherosclerosis.
  4. Presence of migratory thrombophlebitis.
  5. Exclusion of thrombophilia or autoimmune disease.
  6. Absence of atherosclerotic risk factors other than smoking (diabetes, hyperlipidemia, hypertension).
  7. Exclusion of a proximal source of embolization.
  8. Consistent angiographic findings.
- Angiographic criteria (see "Imaging Studies" later in this topic).
- TAO is an inflammatory disease; however, in contrast with all the major forms of arteritis, fibrinoid necrosis of the arterial wall is not observed, and the vascular wall is preserved. This feature distinguishes TAO from other types of systemic vasculitis and from atherosclerosis, in which there is usually disruption of the internal elastic lamina and media.

LABORATORY TESTS

The primary goal of laboratory testing in patients with suspected TAO is to exclude alternative diagnoses. Along with basic laboratory studies, inflammatory markers should be obtained such as CRP and ESR, which are typically normal in patients with TAO. Serological markers of autoimmune disease are typically negative in TAO. Lupus anticoagulant and anticardiolipin antibodies are detected in some patients but may also indicate an isolated thrombophilia.

IMAGING STUDIES

- Computed tomographic angiography (CTA), magnetic resonance angiography (MRA), or invasive catheter-based contrast angiography may be performed to define anatomy and extent of disease.
- Echocardiography may be indicated in certain cases when acute distal arterial occlusion caused by cardiac thromboembolism is suspected.
- Angiography findings of TAO include the following:
  - Involvement of distal small- and medium-sized vessels
  - Occlusions that are segmental, multiple, smooth, and tapered

- Collateral circulation that gives a "tree root" or "spider leg" appearance (Fig. 1-375)
- Involvement of both the upper and lower extremities

Rx TREATMENT

NONPHARMACOLOGIC THERAPY

The goal of medical therapy is to provide relief from ischemic pain and to heal ischemic ulcerations. The prognosis for patients with TAO depends largely on the ability to avoid both active and passive smoking exposure. An increased rate of limb amputation due to progression of disease has been demonstrated in patients who continue tobacco use.

ACUTE GENERAL Rx

- Discontinuation of tobacco use is the definitive therapy for TAO. Pharmacotherapy and smoking cessation groups should be offered to patients. Nicotine replacement therapy should be avoided as it may contribute to disease activity.
- Patients should be treated with antiplatelet agents as well as walking exercises. Patient with critical limb ischemia should be hospitalized.
- Therapeutic options have been limited to vasodilators, intermittent pneumatic compression, spinal cord stimulation, and peripheral periarterial sympathectomy:
  - Treatment of patients in the acute phase of TAO with the prostanoid vasodilator iloprost (intravenous only as oral therapy has no significant clinical effect) has been associated with reduced rest pain, greater healing of ischemic ulcers, and a two thirds reduction in the amputation rate. (Alprostadil alphadex, another prostanoid, is also available for the treatment of TAO).

- Critical limb ischemia can also been treated with prostanoids but with limited effectiveness.
  - Other vasodilators (α-blockers, calcium channel blockers, and sildenafil) may be helpful but have not been studied in prospective clinical trials.
  - Pneumatic compression has been used to augment perfusion to the lower extremities in patients with severe claudication or critical limb ischemia who are not revascularization candidates.
  - Epidural spinal cord stimulation has been shown to improve regional perfusion.
  - Peripheral periarterial sympathectomy may be considered for patients with refractory pain and digital ischemia.

CHRONIC Rx

- As with medical treatment, surgical procedures have limited efficacy in patients given progression of the disease in native vessels and poor patency rates of graft vessels in patients who continue to smoke.
- Surgical revascularization is usually not feasible in patients with TAO due to the distal and diffuse nature of the disease. Surgical bypass grafting below the knee is associated with a high percentage of graft reocclusion.
- Revascularization may be considered in patients with critical limb ischemia and suitable distal target vessels.
- Surgical bypass grafting can be considered in patients with distal disease and ischemic ulcerations given the high rate of healing (upward of 90%) in these patients despite short-term survival of the grafts.
- Short-term results with intramusculary-administered vascular endothelial growth factor to promote angiogenesis have been promising with healing of ischemic ulcers and re-

ducing ischemic rest pain in patients with critical limb ischemia.
- Intramuscular transplantation of autologous bone marrow mononuclear cells and related treatments remain controversial therapeutic options.

DISPOSITION

Periods of exacerbation and remission are characteristic of TAO. The disease typically intensifies at the age of 30 to 40 and then symptoms diminish. Patients aged 60 yr or older rarely have recurrence of symptoms. The diagnosis is associated with a higher risk of limb amputation, which can be modified by tobacco cessation. There is a debated reduction in survival of patients with TAO that cannot be modified by stopping smoking exposure. The prognosis of TAO can be dramatically modified by the cessation of tobacco.

REFERRAL

Smoking cessation counseling, rheumatology consultation, and vascular surgery consultation are recommended for any young smoker with claudication and ischemic ulcers, especially if both the upper and lower extremities are involved.

(!) PEARLS & CONSIDERATIONS

COMMENTS

- TAO is most commonly seen among Ashkenazi Jews in Israel (80% of cases of PAD).
- The pathogenesis of the disease is still poorly understood.
- A multifactorial mechanism has been proposed that involves a combination of genetic susceptibility, tobacco exposure, and immune and coaguable responses.
- No diagnostic criteria are fully accepted by international circles.
- Discontinuation of tobacco use is the definitive therapy for TAO.

PATIENT/FAMILY EDUCATION

Patients with TAO must be warned about tobacco use and secondhand passive smoke. Information for patients can be obtained from the following organizations:
- Vascular Disease Foundation (http://www.vdf.org)
- Mayo Foundation for Medical Education and Research (http://www.mayoclinic.com)

EBM EVIDENCE

available at www.expertconsult.com

SUGGESTED READINGS

available at www.expertconsult.com

AUTHORS: **AHMAD EDRIS, M.D.,** and **PRANAV M. PATEL, M.D.**

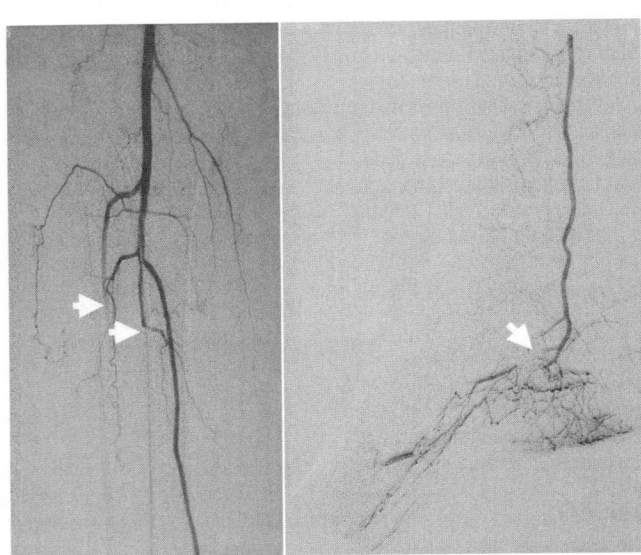

FIGURE 1-375 Angiogram of a young woman with thromboangiitis obliterans. The left panel demonstrates occlusion of the anterior tibial and peroneal arteries *(arrows)*. The right panel demonstration an occlusion of the distal portion of the posterior tibial artery *(arrow)* with bridging collateral vessels. (From Zipes DP et al [eds]: *Braunwauld's heart disease*, ed 7, Philadelphia, 2005, Elsevier.)

BASIC INFORMATION

DEFINITION

Thrombocytosis is defined by an elevated platelet count (>450,000/μl) in peripheral blood. It is caused by overproduction of platelets (reactive thrombocytosis), or it may be caused by clonal expansion of megakaryocytes (autonomous thrombocytosis). Reactive thrombocytosis is driven by excessive cytokines induced by various stimuli, such as trauma or inflammation. The latter is defined as chronic myeloproliferative disorders (CMPD), of which four subgroups are well characterized: chronic myelogenous leukemia (CML), polycythemia vera (PV), primary myelofibrosis (PMF), and essential thrombocythemia (ET). In addition, platelet count can be spuriously elevated in some conditions (see differential diagnosis). Extreme thrombocytosis is defined as platelet count >1 million/μl.

SYNONYMS

Thrombocythemia

ICD-9CM CODES
289.9 Unspecified diseases of blood and blood-forming organs
238.71 Essential thrombocytosis

EPIDEMIOLOGY & DEMOGRAPHICS

Reactive thrombocytosis is much more frequent than autonomous thrombocytosis (70% vs. 22% in one series) for essential thrombocytosis.
INCIDENCE: 2.5 new cases/100,000 population/yr
PREVALENCE: Estimated as 24 cases/100,000 population
PREDOMINANT SEX AND AGE: The median age at diagnosis is 60 yr. Female-to-male ratio of 2:1

PHYSICAL FINDINGS & CLINICAL PRESENTATION

- Regardless of the cause, a high platelet count may be associated with vasomotor symptoms such as headache, visual disturbances, dizziness, atypical chest pain, acral dysesthesia, and erythromelalgia.
- Thrombotic and bleeding complications can occur.
- Symptoms and complications are much more likely to occur in association with autonomous thrombocytosis than reactive thrombocytosis.
- The degree of thrombocytosis cannot predict the likelihood of autonomous thrombocytosis, and does not generally correlate to the risk of thrombosis.
- Splenomegaly is common with CMPD.
- Coexistent leukocytosis and erythrocytosis are common with CML and PV.
- Disease transformation from ET to PV, PMF and acute myeloid leukemia (AML) is uncommon. The incidences have been reported as 2.7%, 4%, and 1.4%, respectively after median follow-up with 9.2 yr.

ETIOLOGY

- *JAK2* mutation is frequent in CMPD (100% in PV, 50% in ET, and 40% to 60% in PMF).
- *MPL* mutation in 1% to 4% of ET patients.

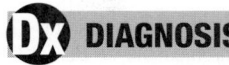

DIAGNOSIS

DIFFERENTIAL DIAGNOSIS

- Spurious thrombocytosis
  - Mixed cryoglobulinemia
  - Circulating cytoplasmic fragments in patients with leukemia, lymphoma, or severe hemolysis or burns can be counted as platelets
- Reactive thrombocytosis
  - Benign hematologic disorders
    Acute hemorrhage, iron deficiency anemia, hemolytic anemia
  - Chronic infection, such as tuberculosis
  - Acute and chronic inflammatory disorders
    Rheumatologic disorders
    Inflammatory bowel disease
    Celiac disease
  - Functional and surgical asplenia
  - Tissue damage
    Trauma, thermal burn
    Myocardial infarction
    Acute pancreatitis
    Recent surgery
  - Renal failure, nephrotic syndrome
  - Exercise
  - Medications, such as vincristine, epinephrine
- Autonomous thrombocytosis
  - Chronic myelogenous leukemia
  - Polycythemia vera
  - Primary myelofibrosis
  - Myelodysplastic syndrome (5q−syndrome)
  - AML with inv(3), t(3;3)
  - Essential thrombocytosis

WORKUP

- Repeat CBC with peripheral blood smear to exclude spurious thrombocytosis.
- Comprehensive history and physical examination to exclude many of the common causes of reactive thrombocytosis: history and physical examination suggestive of acute blood loss, iron deficiency, acute or chronic infection/inflammation, medication use, asplenia, malignancy and trauma should be looked for.

LABORATORY TESTS

- CBC with peripheral blood smear: Howell-Jolly bodies and target cells are present in patients with asplenia; nucleated RBC, teardrop RBC and WBC precursors in patients with PMF
- Serum ferritin level: low ferritin level suggests iron deficiency
- Serum C-reactive protein (CRP), ESR and plasma fibrinogen: nonspecific markers of infection or inflammation
- Philadelphia chromosome or BCR-ABL rearrangement: positive in CML

- Serum erythropoietin assay: low to normal in PV and ET
- *JAK2* mutation analysis: PV and ET
- Bone marrow chromosome analysis: 5q−syndrome and other myelodysplastic syndrome, CML

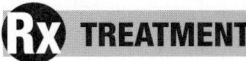

TREATMENT

Treatment for ET will be addressed in this chapter. Reactive thrombocytosis has been rarely associated with thrombosis or bleeding and generally does not require specific therapy.

ACUTE GENERAL Rx

- Vasomotor symptoms easily manageable with low-dose aspirin (40 to 81 mg/day).
- Bleeding
  - Discontinue any platelet antiaggregating agent, such as aspirin or nonsteroidal anti-inflammatory agents.
  - Evaluate for disseminated intravascular coagulopathy and coagulation factor deficiency. Acquired factor V deficiency is occasionally present in association with autonomous thrombocytosis. In that case, treat with fresh frozen plasma infusion.
  - In case of extreme thrombocytosis, acquired von Willebrand disease may occur. Immediate platelet apheresis with definitive therapy with a platelet-lowering agent is essential in this instance.
- Thrombosis
  - If the platelet count is >800,000/μl, platelet apheresis coupled with a platelet-lowering agent (see later) should be started with the goal of platelet count <400,000/ μl.
  - Initial workup should include additional thrombophilic diseases, such as proteins C and S, abnormality, antithrombin, anticardiolipin antibody, mutations of factor V and II, and plasma homocysteine.
  - Anticoagulant therapy for 3 to 9 mo based on the presence or absence of additional thrombophilic defects.

CHRONIC Rx

Treatment strategies for ET are based on the presence or absence of risk factors for thrombosis. The cytoreductive therapy is indicated in high-risk patients aged 60 yr or older and/or with previous history of thrombosis.
- Low-dose aspirin (<81 mg/day) may be safe and possibly effective in preventing vascular events.
- Hydroxyurea (HU) vs. anagrelide: HU plus aspirin is suggested to be safer and more effective than anagrelide plus aspirin in regard to thrombosis, bleeding, and transformation to PMF at 5 yr in a randomized trial.
- The incidence of leukemic conversion in patients with ET treated with HU alone is reported as 0% to 5%.
- Interferon alpha may be effective for controlling platelet count in patients failing treatment with HU.

- In low-risk patients without cardiovascular risk or *JAK2* mutation, observation may be adequate.

DISPOSITION

Most patients with ET have a normal life expectancy without disease-related complications.

REFERRAL

Refer to hematologist/oncologist when platelet count is consistently elevated >450,000/μl without causes for reactive thrombocytosis.

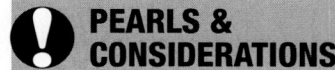

PEARLS & CONSIDERATIONS

COMMENTS

- Some patients with clinically apparent ET have Philadelphia chromosome or *BCR-ABL* rearrangement, even in the absence of other features of CML. It is suggested that it should be tested in all ET patients due to its potential therapeutic implications.

- The risk of bleeding with aspirin use in patients with ET is increased when the platelet count is >1 million/μl.

PATIENT/FAMILY EDUCATION

Smoking cessation is encouraged in both patients with ET and reactive thrombocytosis.

SUGGESTED READINGS

available at www.expertconsult.com

AUTHOR: **ETSUKO AOKI, M.D., PH.D.**

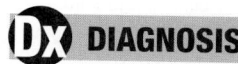

BASIC INFORMATION

DEFINITION

Superficial thrombophlebitis is inflammatory thrombosis in subcutaneous veins. Superficial suppurative thrombophlebitis is an inflammation of the vein wall caused by the presence of microorganisms and occurring as a complication of either dermal infection or use of an indwelling intravenous catheter.

SYNONYMS

Phlebitis
Superficial suppurative thrombophlebitis
Superficial venous thrombosis
SVT

ICD-9CM CODES

451.0 Thrombophlebitis, superficial

EPIDEMIOLOGY & DEMOGRAPHICS

- 10% to 20% of superficial thrombophlebitis cases are associated with occult deep vein thrombosis (DVT).
- Catheter-related thrombophlebitis incidence is 100 in 100,000. The disease occurs more frequently when plastic catheters are inserted in the lower extremities. The mean duration of preceding venous cannulation is 4.8 days, and the latent interval from removal of the catheter to development of symptoms ranges from 2 to 10 days.

PHYSICAL FINDINGS & CLINICAL PRESENTATION

- Subcutaneous vein is palpable, tender; tender cord is present with erythema and edema of the overlying skin and subcutaneous tissue.
- Induration, redness, and tenderness are localized along the course of the vein. This linear appearance rather than circular appearance is useful to distinguish thrombophlebitis from other conditions (cellulitis, erythema nodosum).
- There is no significant swelling of the limb (superficial thrombophlebitis generally does not produce swelling of the limb).
- Low-grade fever may be present. High fever and chills are suggestive of septic phlebitis.
- Superficial suppurative thrombophlebitis may be difficult to identify because local findings of inflammation may be absent. Fever is present in >70% of cases but rigors are rare. Local findings (warmth, erythema, tenderness, swelling, lymphangitis) are present in only one third of patients.

ETIOLOGY

- Trauma to preexisting varices.
- Intravenous cannulation of veins (most common cause).
- Abdominal cancer (e.g., carcinoma of pancreas).

- Infection: *Staphylococcus aureus* was the most common pathogen, found in 65% to 78% of the cases of superficial suppurative thrombophlebitis before 1970; now most cases are caused by Enterobacteriaceae, especially *Klebsiella-Enterobacter* spp. These agents are acquired nosocomially and are often resistant to multiple antibiotics. Infection with fungi or gram-negative aerobic bacilli is often seen in patients who are receiving broad-spectrum antibiotics at the time of the superficial suppurative phlebitis.
- Hypercoagulable state.
- DVT.

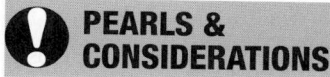

DIAGNOSIS

DIFFERENTIAL DIAGNOSIS

- Lymphangitis
- Cellulitis
- Erythema nodosum
- Panniculitis
- Kaposi's sarcoma

WORKUP

Laboratory evaluation to exclude infectious etiology and imaging studies to rule out DVT in suspected cases

LABORATORY TESTS

- Complete blood count with differential, blood cultures, culture of IV catheter tip (when secondary to intravenous cannulation). Bacteremia occurs in 80% to 90% of the cases of superficial suppurative thrombophlebitis.
- Culture of the catheter may be misleading because even though bacteria are isolated in 60% of the cases, a positive culture does not correlate with inflammation.
- Exploratory venotomy may be necessary in suspected superficial suppurative thrombophlebitis.

IMAGING STUDIES

- Serial compression ultrasound or whole leg compression ultrasound in patients with suspected DVT
- CT scan of abdomen and pelvis in patients with suspected malignancy (Trousseau's syndrome: recurrent migratory thrombophlebitis)

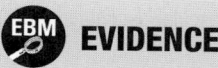

TREATMENT

NONPHARMACOLOGIC THERAPY

- Warm, moist compresses.
- It is not necessary to restrict activity; however, if there is extensive thrombophlebitis, bed rest with the leg elevated will limit the thrombosis and improve symptoms.

ACUTE GENERAL Rx

- Nonsteroidal anti-inflammatory drugs to relieve symptoms.

- Treatment of septic thrombophlebitis with antibiotics with adequate coverage of Enterobacteriaceae and *Staphylococcus*. Initial empirical treatment with a semisynthetic penicillin (IV nafcillin 2 g q4-6h plus either an aminoglycoside [gentamicin 1 mg/kg IV q8h] or a third-generation cephalosporin [cefotaxime] or a quinolone [ciprofloxacin]).
- Oral dicloxacillin or cephalexin may be adequate for outpatient treatment or mild cases of superficial thrombophlebitis.
- Ligation and division of the superficial vein at the junction to avoid propagation of the clot in the deep venous system when the thrombophlebitis progresses toward the junction of the involved superficial vein with deep veins.
- The role of antifungal therapy for superficial suppurative thrombophlebitis caused by *Candida albicans* is controversial. Most of these infections can be cured by vein excision. Because of the propensity of these infections for hematogenous spread, a 10- to 14-day course of amphotericin B or fluconazole is advisable.

DISPOSITION

Clinical improvement within 7 to 10 days

REFERRAL

Surgical referral in selected cases (see "Acute General Rx")

PEARLS & CONSIDERATIONS

COMMENTS

- Patients with positive cultures should be evaluated and treated for endocarditis.
- Suppurative thrombophlebitis is a particular problem in burned patients; it represents a common cause of death from infection.
- Septic thrombophlebitis is more common in IV drug addicts.
- A substantial number of patients with superficial vein thrombosis exibit venous thromboembolism at presentation and some who do not can develop this complication in the subsequent 3 mo. The efficacy and safety of anticoagulant treatment for superficial vein thrombosis in the legs without concomitant DVT or pulmonary embolism (PE) have not been established. Trial with fundaparinux (2.5 mg SC qd for 45 days) found it effective in preventing DVT or PE and without serious side effects.

EBM EVIDENCE

available at www.expertconsult.com

SUGGESTED READINGS

available at www.expertconsult.com

AUTHOR: **FRED F. FERRI, M.D.**

BASIC INFORMATION

DEFINITION

Thrombotic thrombocytopenic purpura (TTP) is a rare disorder characterized by thrombocytopenia (often accompanied by purpura) and micro-angiopathic hemolytic anemia; neurologic impairment, renal dysfunction, and fever may also be present.

SYNONYMS

TTP

ICD-9CM CODES
446.6 Thrombotic thrombocytopenic purpura

EPIDEMIOLOGY & DEMOGRAPHICS

- TTP primarily affects females between ages 10 and 50 yr.
- Frequency is 11 cases annually per 1 million persons.

PHYSICAL FINDINGS & CLINICAL PRESENTATION

- Most patients present with nonspecific constitutional symptoms (weakness, nausea, abdominal pain, vomiting)
- Purpura (secondary to thrombocytopenia)
- Jaundice, pallor (from hemolysis)
- Mucosal bleeding
- Fever
- Fluctuating levels of consciousness (caused by thrombotic occlusion of the cerebral vessels)
- Renal failure and neurologic events are usually end-stage features

ETIOLOGY

- TTP is caused in some patients by an acquired deficiency of a circulating metalloproteinase. It can also be caused, in very rare cases, by a hereditary deficiency of ADAMTS13.
- Many drugs, including clopidogrel, penicillin, antineoplastic agents, oral contraceptives, quinine, and ticlopidine, have been associated with TTP. Other precipitating causes include infectious agents, pregnancy, malignancies, allogenic bone marrow transplantation, and neurologic disorders.

DIAGNOSIS

DIFFERENTIAL DIAGNOSIS

- Disseminated intravascular coagulation (DIC)
- Malignant hypertension
- Vasculitis
- Eclampsia or preeclampsia
- Hemolytic-uremic syndrome (typically encountered in children, often after a viral infection)
- Gastroenteritis as a result of a serotoxin-producing serotype of *Escherichia coli*
- Medications: clopidogrel, ticlopidine, penicillin, antineoplastic chemotherapeutic agents, oral contraceptives

WORKUP

- A comprehensive history, physical examination, and laboratory evaluation usually confirm the diagnosis.
- The disease often begins as a flulike illness ultimately followed by clinical and laboratory abnormalities.
- An algorithm for the diagnosis of TTP is described in Section III.

LABORATORY TESTS

- Severe anemia and thrombocytopenia (platelet count <50,000 or >50% reduction from previous counts
- Elevated blood urea nitrogen and creatinine
- Evidence of hemolysis: elevated reticulocyte count, indirect bilirubin, lactate dehydrogenase, decreased haptoglobin
- Urinalysis: hematuria (red blood cells [RBCs] and RBC casts in urine sediment) and proteinuria
- Peripheral smear: severely fragmented RBCs (schistocytes). More than 4% RBC fragments in the peripheral blood.
- No laboratory evidence of DIC (normal fibrin degradation product, fibrinogen)
- The ADAMTS13 level is not necessary and metalloproteinase deficiency need not be proved for diagnosis of TTP

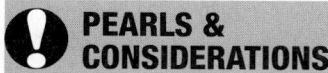

TREATMENT

ACUTE GENERAL Rx

- Discontinue potential offending agents.
- The American Association of Blood Banks, the American Society for Apheresis, and the British Committee for Standards in Haematology recommend daily plasma exchange with replacement of 1.0 to 1.5 times the predicted plasma volume of the patient as standard therapy for TTP. The British guidelines recommend that plasma exchange therapy be continued for a minimum of 2 days after the platelet count returns to normal (>150,000 cells/m³).
- Corticosteroids (prednisone 1 to 2 mg/kg/day) use is controversial. They may be effective alone in patients with mild disease or may be administered concomitantly with plasmapheresis plus plasma exchange with fresh frozen plasma.
- High-dose plasma infusion (25 ml/kg/day) may be useful only if plasma exchange cannot be promptly started and for patients with very severe or refractory disease between plasma exchange sessions. High-dose plasma infusions can cause volume overload in patients with renal insufficiency.
- The monoclonal antibody rituximab has also been used for treatment of TTP.
- Platelet transfusions are contraindicated except in severely thrombocytopenic patients with documented bleeding.
- Use of antiplatelet agents (acetylsalicylic acid, dipyridamole) is controversial.
- Splenectomy is performed in refractory cases.

CHRONIC Rx

- Relapsing TTP may be treated with plasma exchange.
- Remission of chronic TTP that is unresponsive to conventional therapy has been reported after treatment with cyclophosphamide and the monoclonal antibody rituximab.
- Splenectomy done while the patients are in remission has been used in some centers to decrease the frequency of relapse in TTP.

DISPOSITION

- Survival of patients with TTP currently exceeds 80% with plasma exchange therapy.
- Relapse occurs in 20% to 40% of patients who have TTP in remission.

REFERRAL

Surgical referral for splenectomy in selected patients (see "Acute General Rx" and "Chronic Rx.")

PEARLS & CONSIDERATIONS

COMMENTS

- Thrombotic microangiopathy can also be associated with administration of cyclosporine and mitomycin C and with HIV infection.
- The diagnosis of TTP/hemolytic uremic syndrome should be considered in pregnant women with vague neurologic, gastrointestinal, or renal symptoms to either the obstetric triage or emergency department areas.

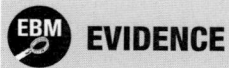

EVIDENCE

available at www.expertconsult.com

SUGGESTED READINGS
available at www.expertconsult.com

AUTHOR: **FRED F. FERRI, M.D.**

BASIC INFORMATION

DEFINITION

Thyroid carcinoma is a primary neoplasm of the thyroid. There are four major types of thyroid carcinoma: papillary, follicular, anaplastic, and medullary.

SYNONYMS

Papillary carcinoma of thyroid
Follicular carcinoma of thyroid
Anaplastic carcinoma of thyroid
Medullary carcinoma of thyroid

ICD-9CM CODES
193 Malignant neoplasm of thyroid

EPIDEMIOLOGY & DEMOGRAPHICS

- Thyroid cancer is the most common endocrine cancer, with an annual incidence of 14,000 new cases in the U.S. and approximately 1100 deaths.
- Female/male ratio is 3:1.
- Most common type (50% to 60%) is papillary carcinoma.
- Median age at diagnosis: 45 to 50 yr.

PHYSICAL FINDINGS & CLINICAL PRESENTATION

- Presence of thyroid nodule
- Hoarseness and cervical lymphadenopathy
- Painless swelling in the region of the thyroid

ETIOLOGY

- Risk factors: prior neck irradiation
- Multiple endocrine neoplasia II (medullary carcinoma)

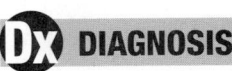

DIAGNOSIS

DIFFERENTIAL DIAGNOSIS

- Multinodular goiter
- Lymphocytic thyroiditis
- Ectopic thyroid

WORKUP

The workup of thyroid carcinoma includes laboratory evaluation and diagnostic imaging. However, diagnosis is confirmed with fine-needle aspiration or surgical biopsy. The characteristics of thyroid carcinoma vary with the type:

- Papillary carcinoma:
  1. Most frequently occurs in women during second or third decades
  2. Histologically, psammoma bodies (calcific bodies present in papillary projections) are pathognomonic; found in 35% to 45% of papillary thyroid carcinomas
  3. Majority are not papillary lesions but mixed papillary follicular carcinomas
  4. Spread is by lymphatics and by local invasion
- Follicular carcinoma:
  1. More aggressive than papillary carcinoma
  2. Incidence increases with age

3. Tends to metastasize hematogenously to bone, producing pathologic fractures
4. Tends to concentrate iodine (useful for radiation therapy)
- Anaplastic carcinoma:
  1. Very aggressive neoplasm
  2. Two major histologic types: small cell (less aggressive, 5-yr survival approximately 20%) and giant cell (death usually within 6 mo of diagnosis)
- Medullary carcinoma:
  1. Unifocal lesion: found sporadically in elderly patients
  2. Bilateral lesions: associated with pheochromocytoma and hyperparathyroidism; this combination is known as MEN-II and is inherited as an autosomal-dominant disorder

LABORATORY TESTS

- Thyroid function studies are generally normal. Thyroid-stimulating hormone (TSH), T_4, and serum thyroglobulin levels should be obtained before thyroidectomy in patients with confirmed thyroid carcinoma.
- Increased plasma calcitonin assay in patients with medullary carcinoma (tumors produce thyrocalcitonin).
- Fine-needle aspiration biopsy is the best method to assess a thyroid nodule (see "Thyroid Nodule" in Section I).

IMAGING STUDIES (Fig. 1-376)

- Thyroid ultrasound can detect solitary solid nodules that have a high risk of malignancy. However, a negative ultrasound does not exclude diagnosis of thyroid carcinoma.
- Thyroid scanning with iodine-123 or technetium-99m can identify hypofunctioning (cold) nodules, which are more likely to be malignant. However, warm nodules can also be malignant.

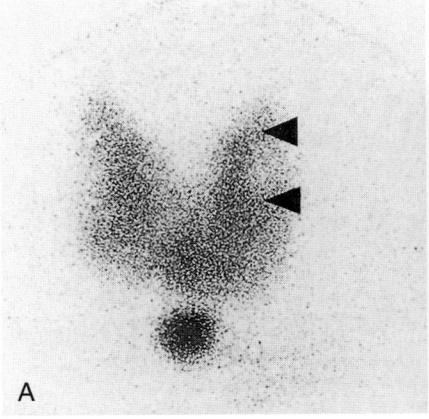
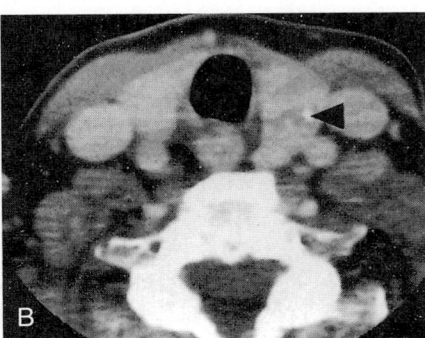

FIGURE 1-376 Papillary adenocarcinoma. A 74-year-old woman presented with a thyroid nodule. **A,** An I123 thyroid scan (anterior view) demonstrates a "cold" nodule *(arrows)* in the upper portion of the left thyroid lobe. The "hot" spot below the thyroid is a suprasternal marker. **B,** An axial CT scan demonstrates an irregular density within the left thyroid lobe at the level of the lesion seen on the radionuclide scan. The lesion contains a single area of calcification *(arrow)* and is not sharply demarcated from normal thyroid tissue. At operation, there proved to be extracapsular extension. (From Skarin AT: *Atlas of diagnostic oncology,* ed 3, St Louis, 2003, Mosby.)

TREATMENT

ACUTE GENERAL Rx

- Papillary carcinoma:
  1. Total thyroidectomy is indicated if the patient has:
     a. Extrapyramidal extension of carcinoma
     b. Papillary carcinoma limited to thyroid but a positive history of irradiation to the neck
     c. Lesion >2 cm
  2. Lobectomy with isthmectomy may be considered in patients with intrathyroid papillary carcinoma <2 cm and no history of neck or head irradiation; most follow surgery with suppressive therapy with thyroid hormone because these tumors are TSH responsive. The accepted practice is to suppress serum TSH concentrations to <0.1 mcU/ml.
  3. Radiotherapy with iodine-131 (after total thyroidectomy), followed by thyroid suppression therapy with triiodothyronine, can be used in metastatic papillary carcinoma.
- Follicular carcinoma:
  1. Total thyroidectomy followed by TSH suppression, as previously noted
  2. Radiotherapy with iodine-131 followed by thyroid suppression therapy with triiodothyronine is useful in patients with metastasis
- Anaplastic carcinoma:
  1. At diagnosis, this neoplasm is rarely operable; palliative surgery is indicated for extremely large tumor compressing the trachea.
  2. Management is usually restricted to radiation therapy or chemotherapy (combination of doxorubicin, cisplatin, and other

antineoplastic agents); these measures rarely provide significant palliation.

- Medullary carcinoma:
  1. Thyroidectomy should be performed.
  2. Patients and their families should be screened for pheochromocytoma and hyperparathyroidism.

DISPOSITION

Prognosis varies with the type of thyroid carcinoma: 5-yr survival approaches 80% for follicular carcinoma and is approximately 5% with anaplastic carcinoma (see Table 1-173).

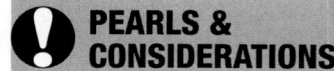

COMMENTS

Family members of patients with medullary carcinoma should be screened; DNA analysis for the detection of mutations in the *RET* gene structure permits the identification of *MEN IIA* gene carriers.

Motesanib, an oral inhibitor of vascular endothelial growth factor (VEGF) receptors, has been reported effective in inducing partial responses in patients with advanced or metastatic differentiated thyroid cancer that is progressive.

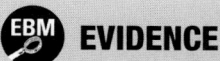

available at www.expertconsult.com

SUGGESTED READINGS

available at www.expertconsult.com

AUTHOR: **FRED F. FERRI, M.D.**

TABLE 1-173 Characteristics of Thyroid Cancers

Type of Cancer	Percentage of Thyroid Cancers	Age of Onset (Yr)	Treatment	Prognosis
Papillary	80	40-80	Thyroidectomy, followed by radioactive iodine ablation	Good
Follicular	15	45-80	Thyroidectomy, followed by radioactive iodine ablation	Fair to good
Medullary	3	20-50	Thyroidectomy and central compartment lymph node dissection	Fair
Anaplastic	1	50-80	Isthmusectomy followed by palliative x-ray treatment	Poor
Lymphoma	1	25-70	X-ray therapy and/or chemotherapy	Fair

Andreoli TE, Benjamin IJ, Griggs RC, Wing EJ: *Andreoli and Carpenter's cecil essentials of medicine,* ed 8, Philadelphia, 2010, Saunders.

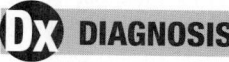

BASIC INFORMATION

DEFINITION

A thyroid nodule is an abnormality found on physical examination of the thyroid gland; nodules can be benign (70%) or malignant.

ICD-9CM CODES
241.0 Nodule, thyroid

EPIDEMIOLOGY & DEMOGRAPHICS

- Palpable thyroid nodules occur in 4% to 7% of the population.
- Thyroid nodules can be found in 50% of autopsies; however, only one in 10 is palpable.
- Malignancy is present in 5% to 30% of palpable nodules.
- Incidence of thyroid nodules increases after age 45 yr. They are found more frequently in women.
- History of prior head and neck irradiation increases the risk of thyroid cancer.
- Increased likelihood that nodule is malignant: nodule increasing in size or >2 cm, regional lymphadenopathy, fixation to adjacent tissues, age <40 yr, symptoms of local invasion (dysphagia, hoarseness, neck pain, male sex, family history of thyroid cancer or polyposis [Gardner syndrome]), rapid growth during levothyroxine therapy.

PHYSICAL FINDINGS & CLINICAL PRESENTATION

- Palpable, firm, and nontender nodule in the thyroid area should prompt suspicion of carcinoma. Signs of metastasis are regional lymphadenopathy and inspiratory stridor.
- Signs and symptoms of thyrotoxicosis can be found in functioning nodules.

ETIOLOGY

- History of prior head and neck irradiation
- Family history of pheochromocytoma, carcinoma of the thyroid, and hyperparathyroidism (medullary carcinoma of the thyroid is a component of MEN-II)

DIAGNOSIS

DIFFERENTIAL DIAGNOSIS

- Thyroid carcinoma
- Multinodular goiter
- Thyroglossal duct cyst
- Epidermoid cyst
- Laryngocele
- Nonthyroid neck neoplasm
- Branchial cleft cyst

WORKUP

- Fine-needle aspiration (FNA) biopsy is the best diagnostic study; the accuracy can be >90%, but it is directly related to the level of experience of the physician and the cytopathologist interpreting the aspirate.
- FNA biopsy is less reliable with thyroid cystic lesions; surgical excision should be considered for most thyroid cysts not abolished by aspiration.
- A diagnostic approach to thyroid nodule is described in Section III.

LABORATORY TESTS

- Thyroid-stimulating hormone (TSH), T_4, and serum thyroglobulin levels should be obtained before thyroidectomy in patients with confirmed thyroid carcinoma on FNA biopsy.
- Serum calcitonin at random or after pentagastrin stimulation is useful when suspecting medullary carcinoma of the thyroid and in anyone with a family history of medullary thyroid carcinoma.
- Serum thyroid autoantibodies (see "Thyroiditis" in Section I) are useful when suspecting thyroiditis.

IMAGING STUDIES

- Thyroid ultrasound is useful to evaluate the size of the thyroid and the number, composition (solid vs. cystic), and dimensions of the thyroid nodule; solid thyroid nodules have a higher incidence of malignancy, but cystic nodules can also be malignant.
- The introduction of high-resolution ultrasonography has made it possible to detect many nonpalpable nodules (incidentalomas) in the thyroid (found at autopsy in 30% to 60% of cadavers). Most of these lesions are benign. For most patients with nonpalpable nodules that are incidentally detected by thyroid imaging, simple follow-up neck palpation is sufficient.
- Thyroid scan can be performed with technetium-99m pertechnetate, iodine-123, or iodine-131. Iodine isotopes are preferred because up to 35% of nodules that appear functioning on pertechnetate scanning may appear nonfunctioning on radioiodine scanning. A thyroid scan:
  1. Classifies nodules as hyperfunctioning (hot), normally functioning (warm), or nonfunctioning (cold); cold nodules have a higher incidence of malignancy.
  2. Scan has difficulty evaluating nodules near the thyroid isthmus or at the periphery of the gland.
  3. Normal tissue over a nonfunctioning nodule might mask the nodule as "warm" or normally functioning.
- Both thyroid scan and ultrasound provide information about the risk of malignant neoplasia based on the characteristics of the thyroid nodule, but their value in the initial evaluation of a thyroid nodule is limited because neither provides a definite tissue diagnosis.

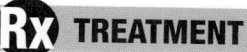

TREATMENT

GENERAL Rx

- Evaluation of results of FNA:
  1. Normal cells: may repeat biopsy during present evaluation or reevaluate patient after 3 to 6 mo of suppressive therapy (I-thyroxine, prescribed in doses to suppress the TSH level to 0.1 to 0.5)
     a. Failure to regress indicates increased likelihood of malignancy.
     b. Reliance on repeat FNA biopsy is preferable to routine surgery for nodules not responding to thyroxine.
  2. Malignant cells: surgery
  3. Hypercellularity: thyroid scan
     a. Hot nodule: ^{131}I therapy if the patient is hyperthyroid
     b. Warm or cold nodule: surgery (rule out follicular adenoma vs. carcinoma)

DISPOSITION

Variable with results of FNA biopsy

REFERRAL

Surgical referral for FNA biopsy

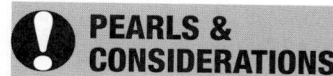

PEARLS & CONSIDERATIONS

COMMENTS

- Most solid, benign nodules grow; therefore an increase in nodule volume alone is not a reliable predictor of malignancy.
- Surgery is indicated in hard or fixed nodule, presence of dysphagia or hoarseness, and rapidly growing solid masses regardless of "benign" results on FNA.
- Suppressive therapy of malignant thyroid nodules postoperatively with thyroxine is indicated. The use of suppressive therapy for benign solitary nodules is controversial.
- The preferred approach when repeated FNA fails to yield an adequate specimen remains a challenge. Immunohistochemical markers (galectin-3, human bone marrow endothelial cell) have shown promise in preliminary studies. Routine calcitonin measurement for early detection of medullary carcinoma remains controversial because of the low frequency of this cancer and the high cost associated with case detection.

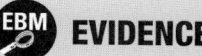

available at www.expertconsult.com

SUGGESTED READINGS
available at www.expertconsult.com

AUTHOR: **FRED F. FERRI, M.D.**

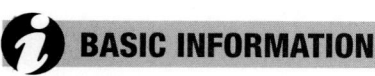 **BASIC INFORMATION**

DEFINITION

Thyroiditis is an inflammatory disease of the thyroid. It is a multifaceted disease with various etiologies, different clinical characteristics (depending on the stage), and distinct histopathology. Thyroiditis can be subdivided into three common types (Hashimoto's, painful, and painless) and two rare forms (suppurative and Riedel's). To add to the confusion, there are various synonyms for each form, and there is no internationally accepted classification of autoimmune thyroid disease.

SYNONYMS

Hashimoto's thyroiditis: chronic lymphocytic thyroiditis, chronic autoimmune thyroiditis, lymphadenoid goiter

Painful subacute thyroiditis: subacute thyroiditis, giant cell thyroiditis, de Quervain's thyroiditis, subacute granulomatous thyroiditis, pseudogranulomatous thyroiditis

Painless postpartum thyroiditis: subacute lymphocytic thyroiditis, postpartum thyroiditis

Painless sporadic thyroiditis: silent sporadic thyroiditis, subacute lymphocytic thyroiditis

Suppurative thyroiditis: acute suppurative thyroiditis, bacterial thyroiditis, microbial inflammatory thyroiditis, pyogenic thyroiditis

Riedel's thyroiditis: fibrous thyroiditis

ICD-9CM CODES
245.2 Hashimoto's thyroiditis
245.1 Subacute thyroiditis
245.9 Silent thyroiditis
245.0 Suppurative thyroiditis
245.3 Riedel's thyroiditis

PHYSICAL FINDINGS & CLINICAL PRESENTATION

- Hashimoto's: patients may have signs of hyperthyroidism (tachycardia, diaphoresis, palpitations, weight loss) or hypothyroidism (fatigue, weight gain, delayed reflexes) depending on the stage of the disease. Usually there is diffuse, firm enlargement of the thyroid gland; the gland may also be of normal size (atrophic form with clinically manifested hypothyroidism).
- Painful subacute: exquisitely tender, enlarged thyroid, fever; signs of hyperthyroidism are initially present; signs of hypothyroidism can subsequently develop.
- Painless thyroiditis: clinical features are similar to subacute thyroiditis except for the absence of tenderness of the thyroid gland.
- Suppurative: patient is febrile with severe neck pain, focal tenderness of the involved portion of the thyroid, erythema of the overlying skin.
- Riedel's: slowly enlarging hard mass in the anterior neck; often mistaken for thyroid cancer; signs of hypothyroidism occur in advanced stages.

ETIOLOGY

- Hashimoto's: autoimmune disorder that begins with the activation of CD4 (helper) T-lymphocytes specific for thyroid antigens. The etiologic factor for the activation of these cells is unknown.
- Painful subacute: possibly postviral; usually follows a respiratory illness not considered to be a form of autoimmune thyroiditis.
- Painless thyroiditis: frequently occurs postpartum.
- Suppurative: infectious etiology, generally bacterial, although fungi and parasites have also been implicated; often occurs in immunocompromised hosts or after a penetrating neck injury.
- Riedel's: fibrous infiltration of the thyroid; etiology unknown.
- Drug induced: lithium, interferon-alfa, amiodarone, interleukin-2.

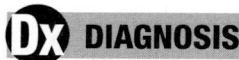 **DIAGNOSIS**

DIFFERENTIAL DIAGNOSIS

- The hyperthyroid phase of Hashimoto's, subacute, and silent thyroiditis can be mistaken for Graves' disease.
- Riedel's thyroiditis can be mistaken for carcinoma of the thyroid.
- Painful subacute thyroiditis can be mistaken for infections of the oropharynx and trachea or for suppurative thyroiditis.
- Factitious hyperthyroidism can mimic silent thyroiditis.

WORKUP

- The diagnostic workup includes laboratory and radiologic evaluation to rule out other conditions that may mimic thyroiditis (see above) and differentiate the various forms of thyroiditis.
- The patient's medical history may be helpful in differentiating the various types of thyroiditis (e.g., presentation after childbirth is suggestive of silent [postpartum, painless] thyroiditis; occurrence after a viral respiratory infection suggests subacute thyroiditis; history of penetrating injury to the neck indicates suppurative thyroiditis).

LABORATORY TESTS

- Thyroid-stimulating hormone, free T_4: may be normal or indicative of hypothyroidism or hyperthyroidism depending on the stage of the thyroiditis.
- White blood cell (WBC) with differential: increased WBC with left shift occurs with subacute and suppurative thyroiditis.
- Antimicrosomal antibodies: detected in >90% of patients with Hashimoto's thyroiditis and 50% to 80% of patients with silent thyroiditis.
- Serum thyroglobulin levels are elevated in patients with subacute and silent thyroiditis; this test is nonspecific but may be useful in monitoring the course of subacute thyroiditis and distinguishing silent thyroiditis from factitious hyperthyroidism (low or absent serum thyroglobulin level).

IMAGING STUDIES

Twenty-four-hour radioactive iodine uptake (RAIU) is useful to distinguish Graves' disease (increased RAIU) from thyroiditis (normal or low RAIU).

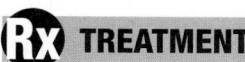 **TREATMENT**

ACUTE GENERAL Rx

- Treat hypothyroid phase with levothyroxine 25 to 50 mcg/day initially and monitor serum thyroid-stimulating hormone initially every 6 to 8 wk.
- Control symptoms of hyperthyroidism with beta-blockers (e.g., propranolol 20 to 40 mg PO q6h).
- Control pain in patients with subacute thyroiditis with nonsteroidal antiinflammatory drugs. Prednisone 20 to 40 mg qd may be used if nonsteroidals are insufficient, but it should be gradually tapered off over several weeks.
- Use IV antibiotics and drain abscess (if present) in patients with suppurative thyroiditis.

DISPOSITION

- Hashimoto's thyroiditis: long-term prognosis is favorable; most patients recover their thyroid function.
- Painful subacute thyroiditis: permanent hypothyroidism occurs in 10% of patients.
- Painless thyroiditis: 6% of patients have permanent hypothyroidism.
- Suppurative thyroiditis: there is usually full recovery after treatment.
- Riedel's thyroiditis: hypothyroidism occurs when fibrous infiltration involves the entire thyroid.

REFERRAL

Surgical referral in patients with compression of adjacent neck structures and in some patients with suppurative thyroiditis

SUGGESTED READINGS
available at www.expertconsult.com

AUTHOR: **FRED F. FERRI, M.D.**

BASIC INFORMATION

DEFINITION

Thyrotoxic storm is the abrupt and severe exacerbation of thyrotoxicosis.

ICD-9CM CODES
242.9 Thyrotoxic storm
242.0 With goiter
242.2 Multinodular
242.3 Adenomatous
242.8 Thyrotoxicosis factitia

PHYSICAL FINDINGS & CLINICAL PRESENTATION

- Goiter
- Tremor, tachycardia, fever
- Warm, moist skin
- Lid lag, lid retraction, proptosis
- Altered mental status (psychosis, coma, seizures)
- Other: evidence of precipitating factors (infection, trauma)

ETIOLOGY

- Major stress (e.g., infection, myocardial infarction [MI], diabetic ketoacidosis) in an undiagnosed hyperthyroid patient
- Inadequate therapy in a hyperthyroid patient

 DIAGNOSIS

The clinical presentation is variable. The patient may present with the following signs and symptoms:
- Fever
- Marked anxiety and agitation, psychosis
- Hyperhidrosis, heat intolerance
- Marked weakness and muscle wasting
- Tachyarrhythmias, palpitations
- Diarrhea, nausea, vomiting
- Elderly patients may have a combination of tachycardia, congestive heart failure (CHF), and mental status changes

DIFFERENTIAL DIAGNOSIS

- Psychiatric disorders
- Alcohol or other drug withdrawal
- Pheochromocytoma
- Metastatic neoplasm

WORKUP

- Laboratory evaluation to confirm hyperthyroidism (elevated free T_4, decreased thyroid-stimulating hormone [TSH])
- Evaluation for precipitating factors (e.g., ECG and cardiac enzymes in suspected MI, blood and urine cultures to rule out sepsis)
- Elimination of disorders noted in the differential diagnosis (e.g., psychiatric history, evidence of drug and alcohol abuse)

LABORATORY TESTS

- Free T_4, TSH
- Complete blood count with differential
- Blood and urine cultures
- Glucose
- Liver enzymes
- Blood urea nitrogen, creatinine
- Serum calcium
- Creatine phosphokinase

IMAGING STUDIES

Chest radiograph to exclude infectious process, neoplasm, CHF in suspected cases

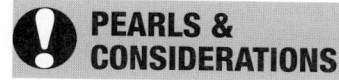 TREATMENT

NONPHARMACOLOGIC THERAPY

- Nutritional care: replace fluid deficit aggressively (daily fluid requirement may reach 6 L); use solutions containing glucose and add multivitamins to the hydrating solution.
- Monitor for fluid overload and CHF in the elderly and in those with underlying cardiovascular or renal disease.
- Treat significant hyperthermia with cooling blankets.

ACUTE GENERAL Rx

- Inhibition of thyroid hormone synthesis:
  1. Administer propylthiouracil (PTU) 300 to 600 mg initially (PO or by nasogastric tube), then 150 to 300 mg q6h.
  2. If the patient is allergic to PTU, use methimazole (Tapazole) 80 to 100 mg PO or rectally followed by 30 mg PR q8h.
- Inhibition of stored thyroid hormone:
  1. Iodide can be administered as sodium iodine 250 mg IV q6h, saturated solution of potassium iodide, 5 gtt PO q8h, or Lugol's solution, 10 gtt q8h. It is important to administer PTU or methimazole 1 hr *before*

the iodide to prevent the oxidation of iodide to iodine and its incorporation in the synthesis of additional thyroid hormone.
  2. Corticosteroids: dexamethasone 2 mg IV q6h or hydrocortisone 100 mg IV q6h for approximately 48 hr is useful to inhibit thyroid hormone release, impair peripheral conversion of T_3 from T_4, and provide additional adrenocortical hormone to correct deficiency (if present).
- Suppression of peripheral effects of thyroid hormone:
  1. Beta-adrenergic blockers: administer propranolol 80 to 120 mg PO q4-6h. Propranolol may also be given IV 1 mg/min for 2 to 10 min under continuous ECG and blood pressure monitoring. Beta-adrenergic blockers must be used with caution in patients with severe CHF or bronchospasm. Cardioselective beta-blockers (e.g., esmolol or metoprolol) may be more appropriate for patients with bronchospasm, but these patients must be closely monitored for exacerbation of bronchospasm because these agents lose their cardioselectivity at high doses.
- Control of fever with acetaminophen 325 to 650 mg q4h; avoidance of aspirin because it displaces thyroid hormone from its binding protein
- Consider digitalization of patients with CHF and atrial fibrillation (these patients may require higher than usual digoxin doses)
- Treatment of any precipitating factors (e.g., antibiotics if infection is strongly suspected)

DISPOSITION

Patients with thyrotoxic crisis should be treated and appropriately monitored in the ICU.

REFERRAL

Endocrinology referral is appropriate in patients with thyrotoxic crisis.

PEARLS & CONSIDERATIONS

COMMENTS

If the diagnosis is strongly suspected, therapy should be started immediately without waiting for laboratory confirmation.

AUTHOR: **FRED F. FERRI, M.D.**

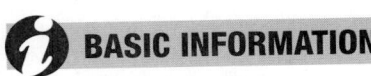

BASIC INFORMATION

DEFINITION

Tinea capitis is a dermatophyte infection of the scalp.

SYNONYMS

Ringworm of the scalp, ringworm of the head, gray patch tinea capitis, black dot tinea capitis, tinea tonsurans, superficial mycosis, dermatophytosis, kerion

ICD-9CM CODES
110.0 Tinea capitis

EPIDEMIOLOGY & DEMOGRAPHICS

Tinea capitis is the most common dermatophytosis of childhood, primarily affecting children between 3 and 9 yr of age. About 3% to 8% of American children are affected, although it is more common among black children, and 34% of household contacts are asymptomatic carriers. Adult and geriatric populations are less frequently affected, possibly because of the fungistatic effect of the sebum found in older persons. In urban populations, large family size, low socioeconomic status, and crowded living conditions may contribute to an increased incidence of tinea capitis. Infection of the scalp with *Trichophyton tonsurans* results from person-to-person transmission. Transmission occurs via infected persons or asymptomatic carriers, fallen infected hairs, animal vectors, and fomites. *Microsporum audouinii* is commonly spread by dogs and cats. Infectious fungal particles may remain viable for many months.

PHYSICAL FINDINGS & CLINICAL PRESENTATION

- Triad of scalp scaling, alopecia, and cervical adenopathy
- Primary lesions including plaques, papules, pustules, or nodules on the scalp (usually occipital region)
- Secondary lesions include scales, alopecia (usually reversible), erythema, exudates, and edema
- Two distinctly different forms:
  - Gray patch: Lesions are scaly and well demarcated. The hairs within the patch break off a few millimeters above the scalp. One or several lesions may be present; sometimes the lesions join to form larger ones.
  - Black dot: Early lesions with erythema and scaling patch are easily overlooked until areas of alopecia develop. Hairs within the patches break at the surface of the scalp, leaving behind a pattern of swollen black dots.
- Scalp pruritus may be present
- Fever, pain, and lymphadenopathy (commonly postcervical) with inflammatory lesions
- Kerion: inflamed, exudative, pustular, boggy, tender nodules exhibiting marked edema,

and hair loss seen in severe tinea capitis. Caused by immune response to the fungus. May lead to some scarring.
- Favus: production of scutula (hair matted together with dermatophyte hyphae and keratin debris), characterized by yellow cup-shaped crusts around hair shafts. A fetid odor may be present.

ETIOLOGY

Although the organism remains viable on combs, hairbrushes, and other fomites for long periods of time, the role of fomites in causative organisms may vary in different geographic areas. *T. tonsurans* is the predominant cause of tinea capitis, present in more than 90% of cases in North and Central America. *Microsporum canis*, *M. audouinii*, and *Trichophyton mentagrophytes* are less common. Most common causative species for black dot tinea capitis is *T. tonsurans* and for gray patch tinea capitis are *M. andouinii* and *M. canis*.

DIAGNOSIS

DIFFERENTIAL DIAGNOSIS

Alopecia areata, impetigo, pediculosis, trichotillomania, traction alopecia, folliculitis, pseudopelade, seborrhea/atopic dermatitis, psoriasis, carbuncles, pyoderma, lichen ruber planus, lupus erythematosus

WORKUP

- KOH testing of hair shaft extracted from the lesion, not the scale, because the *T. tonsurans* spores attach to or reside inside hair shafts and will rarely be found in the scales.
- Wood's ultraviolet light fluoresces blue-green on hair shafts for *Microsporum* infections but will fail to identify *T. tonsurans*.
- Fungal culture of hairs and scales on fungal medium such as Sabouraud's agar may be used to confirm the diagnosis, especially if uncertain.
- Histology of biopsies with fungal staining in cases where mycology tests are negative because of treatment initiation.

TREATMENT

- Griseofulvin is the gold standard FDA-approved treatment, which costs less than other treatments and has an excellent long-term safety profile. Micronized and ultramicronized preparations are absorbed better, and side effects are infrequent, especially when administered with fatty meals. Periodic monitoring of hematologic, liver, and renal function may be indicated, especially in prolonged treatment over 8 wk.
  Children: Griseofulvin is approved for children age >2: microsize griseofulvin 10 to 20 mg/kg per day (maximum, 1 g) or ultramicrosize griseofulvin, 5 to 15 mg/kg per day (maximum, 750 mg), is given orally once daily. Optimally, griseofulvin is given after a meal containing fat (e.g., peanut butter

or ice cream). Treatment for 4 to 6 wk typically is necessary and should be continued 2 wk beyond clinical resolution (until hair regrowth occurs). Some children may require higher doses to achieve clinical cure.
  Adults: 250 mg orally bid or 500 mg qd (or 250 mg tid for a few cases of black dot type) for 4 to 12 weeks.
- New alternative treatments: oral terbinafine, itraconazole, or fluconazole are comparable in efficacy and safety to griseofulvin, with possibly shorter treatment and better patient compliance. Preferred when resistant or when an allergy to griseofulvin is of concern. Monitoring of CBC, liver function tests, and renal function may be indicated.
  - Terbinafine—6-wk course of therapy as effective as with griseofulvin. Dosages are 67.5 mg/day for patients weighing <20 kg; 125 mg/day for patients weighing 20 to 40 kg; and 250 mg for patients weighing >40 kg.
  - Itraconazole—3.5 mg/kg daily for 4 to 6 weeks or pulse therapy of 5 mg/kg daily for 1 wk each month for 2 to 3 mo (not approved for children)
  - Fluconazole—the only oral antifungal agent approved for children <2 yr, 6 mg/kg/day for 6 wk in children (3 to 6 wk in adults) or 8 mg/kg weekly for 8 to 12 wk (cap at 150 mg weekly for adults)
- The adjuvant use of antifungal shampoos may be recommended for all patients and household contacts. Shampoo like selenium sulfide 2.5% used for 5 min or ketoconazole shampoo used 2 to 3 times/week can help prevent infection or eradicate asymptomatic carrier state by inhibiting fungal growth.
- Severe inflammatory kerion can be managed with additional prednisone 40 mg daily (1 mg/kg/day in children) and tapering over 2 wk.

PEARLS & CONSIDERATIONS

- Systemic antifungal therapy is required for tinea capitis because topical antifungal medications are not effective.
- Prompt treatment is indicated, as is examination of siblings and other household contacts for evidence of tinea capitis.
- Shaving of the head, haircuts, or wearing a cap or scarf during treatment are unnecessary.
- Sharing of combs, hair ribbons, and hairbrushes should be discouraged. Children receiving treatment for tinea capitis may attend school once they start therapy with griseofulvin or other effective systemic agent.

COMMENTS

- Confirming the diagnosis of tinea capitis with a laboratory specimen is important because misdiagnosis will result in delay or improper treatment.

- Patients and their families should look for sources of infections and disinfect contaminated objects such as combs, brushes, towels, and headgear. Avoid sharing personal hygiene utensils.
- Culture of hairs and scalp dander facilitates carrier identification and prevention.

- Pets that are infected or asymptomatic carriers should be treated.
- Recommend follow-up visit every 2 to 4 wk with Wood's light, microscopic study, and fungal culture. A mycologically documented cure is the goal of treatment.

SUGGESTED READINGS
available at www.expertconsult.com

AUTHORS: **MARIE ELIZABETH WONG, M.D.,** and **JEFFREY BORKAN, M.D., Ph.D.**

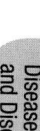

Diseases and Disorders

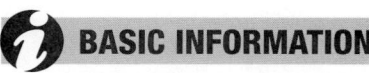

BASIC INFORMATION

DEFINITION

Tinea corporis is a dermatophyte fungal infection caused by the genera *Trichophyton* or *Microsporum*.

SYNONYMS

Ringworm
Body ringworm
Tinea circinata

ICD-9CM CODES
110.5 Tinea corporis

EPIDEMIOLOGY & DEMOGRAPHICS

- The disease is more common in warm climates.
- There is no predominant age or sex.

PHYSICAL FINDINGS & CLINICAL PRESENTATION

- Typically appears as single or multiple annular lesions with an advancing scaly border; the margin is slightly raised, reddened, and may be pustular.
- The central area becomes hypopigmented and less scaly as the active border progresses outward (Fig. 1-377).
- The trunk and legs are primarily involved.
- Pruritus is variable.
- It is important to remember that recent topical corticosteroid use can significantly alter the appearance of the lesions.

ETIOLOGY

Trichophyton rubrum is the most common pathogen.

DIAGNOSIS

DIFFERENTIAL DIAGNOSIS

- Pityriasis rosea
- Erythema multiforme
- Psoriasis
- Cutaneous systemic lupus erythematosus
- Secondary syphilis
- Nummular eczema
- Eczema
- Granuloma annulare
- Lyme disease
- Tinea versicolor
- Contact dermatitis

WORKUP

Diagnosis is usually made on clinical grounds. It can be confirmed by direct visualization under the microscope of a small fragment of the scale using wet mount preparation and potassium hydroxide solution; dermatophytes appear as translucent branching filaments (hyphae) with lines of separation appearing at irregular intervals.

LABORATORY TESTS

- Microscopic examination of hyphae
- Mycotic culture is usually not necessary
- Biopsy is indicated only when the diagnosis is uncertain and the patient has not responded to treatment

TREATMENT

NONPHARMACOLOGIC THERAPY

Affected areas should be kept clean and dry.

ACUTE GENERAL Rx

- Various creams are effective; the application area should include normal skin approximately 2 cm beyond the affected area:
  1. Butenafine cream applied qd for 14 days
  2. Terbinafine cream applied bid for 14 days
- Systemic therapy is reserved for severe cases and is usually given up to 4 wk; commonly used agents:
  1. Fluconazole, 200 mg qd
  2. Terbinafine, 250 mg qd

DISPOSITION

Majority of cases resolve without sequelae within 3 to 4 wk of therapy.

REFERRAL

Dermatology referral in patients with persistent or recurrent infections

SUGGESTED READINGS
available at www.expertconsult.com

AUTHOR: **FRED F. FERRI, M.D.**

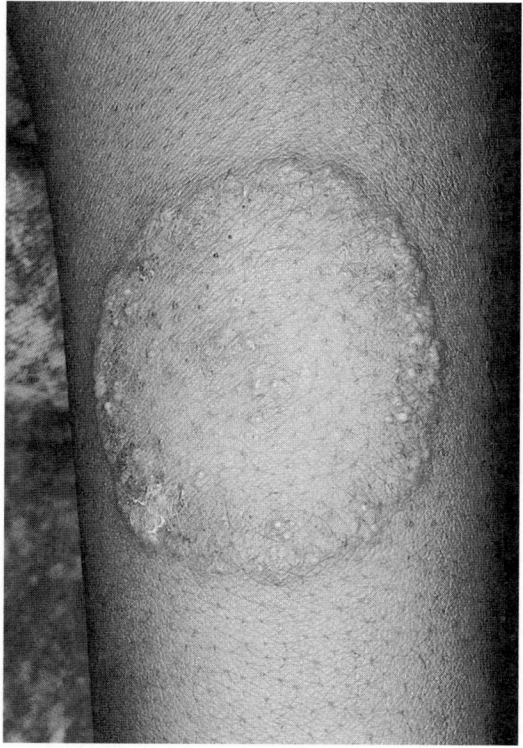

FIGURE 1-377 Annular lesion (tinea corporis). Note raised erythematous, scaling border and central clearing. (From Noble J et al: *Textbook of primary care medicine,* ed 3, St Louis, 2001, Mosby.)

BASIC INFORMATION

DEFINITION

Tinea cruris is a dermatophyte infection of the groin.

SYNONYMS

Jock itch
Ringworm

ICD-9CM CODES

110.3 Tinea cruris

EPIDEMIOLOGY & DEMOGRAPHICS

- Most common during the summer in adolescent and young adult males.
- Males are affected more frequently than females; however, it has become more common in postpubertal females who are overweight or who often wear tight jeans or pantyhose.
- The infection often coexists with tinea pedis.

PHYSICAL FINDINGS & CLINICAL PRESENTATION

- Erythematous plaques have a half-moon shape and a scaling border.
- The acute inflammation tends to move down the inner thigh and usually spares the scrotum; in severe cases the fungus may spread onto the buttocks.
- Itching may be severe.
- Red papules and pustules may be present.
- An important diagnostic sign is the advancing well-defined border with a tendency toward central clearing (Fig. 1-378).

ETIOLOGY

- Dermatophytes of the genera *Trichophyton*, *Epidermophyton*, and *Microsporum*. *T. rubrum* and *E. floccosum* are the most common infecting agents.
- Transmission from direct contact (e.g., infected persons, animals). The patient's feet should be evaluated as a source of infection because tinea cruris is often associated with tinea pedis.

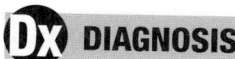

DIAGNOSIS

DIFFERENTIAL DIAGNOSIS

- Candidal intertrigo
- Psoriasis
- Seborrheic dermatitis
- Erythrasma
- Contact dermatitis
- Tinea versicolor

WORKUP

Diagnosis is based on clinical presentation and demonstration of hyphae microscopically using potassium hydroxide.

LABORATORY TESTS

- Microscopic examination
- Cultures are generally not necessary

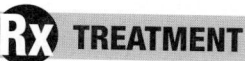

TREATMENT

NONPHARMACOLOGIC THERAPY

- Keep infected area clean and dry.
- Boxer shorts are preferred to regular underwear.

ACUTE GENERAL Rx

- Various topical antifungal agents are available:
  1. Butenafine cream, applied qd × 14 days
  2. Terbinafine cream, applied bid × 14 days
- Drying powders (e.g., Miconazole nitrate) may be useful in patients with excessive perspiration.
- Oral antifungal therapy is generally reserved for cases unresponsive to topical agents or can be used along with topical agents in severe cases. Effective medications are fluconazole 200 mg qd × 10 days and terbinafine 250 mg qd × 30 days.

DISPOSITION

Most cases respond promptly to therapy with complete resolution within 2 to 3 wk.

SUGGESTED READINGS

available at www.expertconsult.com

AUTHOR: **FRED F. FERRI, M.D.**

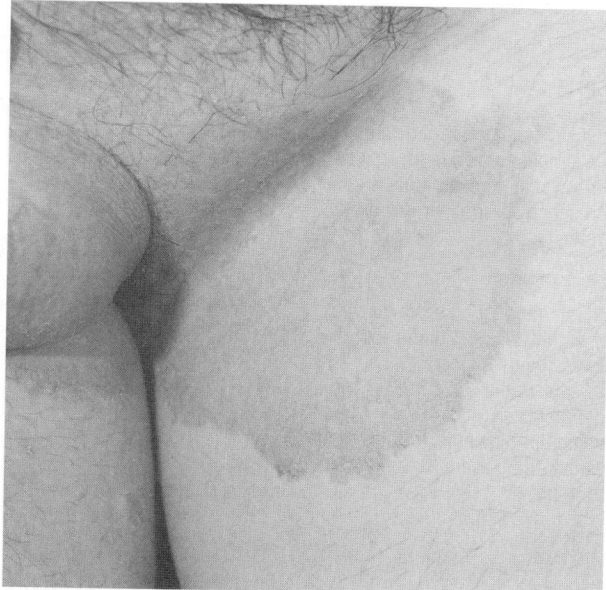

FIGURE 1-378 Tinea cruris. A half-moon–shaped plaque has a well-defined, scaling border. (From Habif TB: *Clinical dermatology: a color guide to diagnosis and therapy*, ed 3, St Louis, 1996, Mosby.)

Diseases and Disorders

T

I

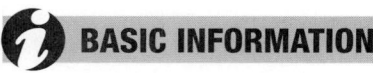

BASIC INFORMATION

DEFINITION
Tinea pedis is a dermatophyte infection of the feet.

SYNONYMS
Athlete's foot

ICD-9CM CODES
110.4 Tinea pedis

EPIDEMIOLOGY & DEMOGRAPHICS
- Most common dermatophyte infection
- Increased incidence in hot humid weather; occlusive footwear is a contributing factor
- Occurrence is rare before adolescence
- More common in adult males

PHYSICAL FINDINGS & CLINICAL PRESENTATION
- Typical presentation is variable and ranges from erythematous scaling plaques (Fig. 1-379) and isolated blisters to interdigital maceration.

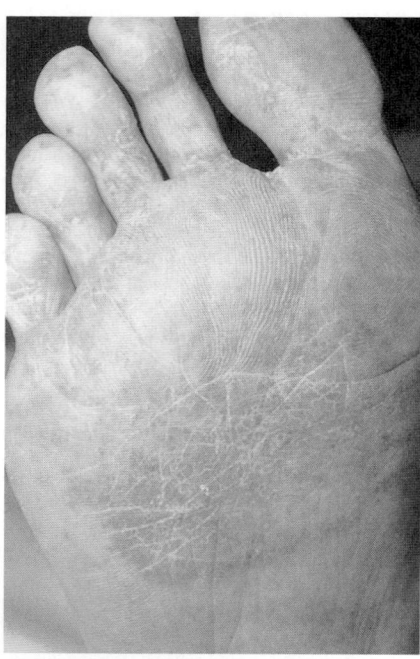

FIGURE 1-379 Tinea pedis. (From Goldstein BG, Goldstein AO: *Practical dermatology,* ed 2, St Louis, 1997, Mosby.)

- The infection usually starts in the interdigital spaces of the foot. Most infections are found in the toe webs or on the soles.
- Fourth or fifth toes are most commonly involved.
- Pruritus is common and is most intense after removal of shoes and socks.
- Infection with *tinea rubrum* often manifests with a "moccasin" distribution affecting the soles and lateral feet.

ETIOLOGY
Dermatophyte infection caused by *T. rubrum, T. mentagrophytes,* or less commonly *E. floccosum*

DIAGNOSIS
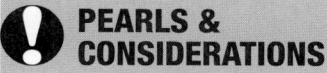

DIFFERENTIAL DIAGNOSIS
- Contact dermatitis
- Toe web infection (bacterial or candidal infection)
- Eczema
- Psoriasis
- Keratolysis exfoliativa
- Juvenile plantar dermatosis

WORKUP
- Diagnosis is usually made by clinical observation.
- Laboratory testing, when performed, generally consists of a simple potassium hydroxide preparation with mycologic examination under a light microscope to confirm the presence of dermatophytes.

LABORATORY TESTS
- Microscopic examination of a scale or the roof of a blister with 10% KOH under low or medium power will reveal hyphae.
- Mycologic culture is rarely indicated in the diagnosis of tinea pedis.
- Biopsy is reserved for when the diagnosis remains in question after testing or failure to respond to treatment.

TREATMENT
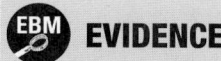

NONPHARMACOLOGIC THERAPY
- Keep infected area clean and dry. Aerate feet by using sandals when possible.

- Use 100% cotton socks rather than nylon socks to reduce moisture.
- Areas likely to become infected should be dried completely before being covered with clothes.

ACUTE GENERAL Rx
- Benzylamines: Butenafine HCL 1% cream applied bid for 1 wk or qd for 4 wk is effective in interdigital tinea pedis.
- Allylamines: Terbinafine cream applied bid × 14 days, or naftifine 1% cream applied qd or naftifine gel applied bid for 4 wk produce a significantly high cure rate.
- Imidazoles: Econazole, ketoconazole, miconazole, or clotrimazole cream are also effective agents. Clotrimazole 1% cream is an over-the-counter treatment. It should be applied to affected and surrounding area bid for up to 4 wk.
- Ciclopirox and tolnaftate are other antifungal agents available in cream, suspension, or gel. Tolnaftate is also available as a lotion, spray, or powder.
- When using topical preparations, the application area should include normal skin approximately 2 cm beyond the affected area.
- Areas of maceration can be treated with Burow's solution soaks for 10 to 20 min bid followed by foot elevation.
- Oral agents (fluconazole 150 mg once per week for 4 wk) can be used in combination with topical agents in resistant cases.

PEARLS & CONSIDERATIONS

Combination therapy of antifungal and corticosteroid (clotrimazole/betamethasone [Lotrisone]) should only be used when the diagnosis of fungal infection is confirmed and inflammation is a significant issue.

EBM EVIDENCE

available at www.expertconsult.com

SUGGESTED READING
available at www.expertconsult.com

AUTHOR: **FRED F. FERRI, M.D.**

BASIC INFORMATION

DEFINITION

Tinea versicolor is a fungal infection of the skin caused by the yeast *Pityrosporum orbiculare* (*Malassezia furfur*).

SYNONYMS

Pityriasis versicolor

ICD-9CM CODES
111.0 Tinea versicolor

EPIDEMIOLOGY & DEMOGRAPHICS

- Increased incidence in adolescence and young adulthood
- More common during the summer (hypopigmented lesions are more evident when the skin is tanned)

PHYSICAL FINDINGS & CLINICAL PRESENTATION

- Most lesions begin as multiple small, circular macules of various colors.
- The macules may be darker or lighter than the surrounding normal skin and will scale with scraping.
- Most frequent site of distribution is trunk.
- Facial lesions are more common in children (forehead is most common facial site).
- Eruption is generally of insidious onset and asymptomatic.
- Lesions may be hyperpigmented in blacks.
- Lesions may be inconspicuous in fair-complexioned individuals, especially during the winter.
- Most patients become aware of the eruption when the involved areas do not tan (Fig. 1-380).

ETIOLOGY

The infection is caused by the lipophilic yeast *P. orbiculare* (round form) and *P. ovale* (oval form), which are normal inhabitants of the skin flora. Factors that favor proliferation are pregnancy, malnutrition, immunosuppression, oral contraceptives, and excess heat and humidity.

DIAGNOSIS

DIFFERENTIAL DIAGNOSIS

- Vitiligo
- Pityriasis alba
- Secondary syphilis
- Pityriasis rosea
- Seborrheic dermatitis

WORKUP

Diagnosis is based on clinical appearance; identification of hyphae and budding spores ("spaghetti and meatballs" appearance) with microscopy confirms diagnosis.

LABORATORY TESTS

Microscopic examination with potassium hydroxide confirms diagnosis.

TREATMENT

NONPHARMACOLOGIC THERAPY

Sunlight accelerates repigmentation of hypopigmented areas.

ACUTE GENERAL Rx

- Topical treatment: selenium sulfide 2.5% suspension (Selsun or Exsel) applied daily for 10 min for 7 consecutive days results in a cure rate of 80% to 90%.
- Antifungal topical agents (e.g., miconazole, ciclopirox, clotrimazole) are also effective.

- Oral treatment can be given along with topical agents but is generally reserved for resistant cases. Effective agents are ketoconazole 200 mg qd for 5 days, or single 400-mg dose (cure rate >80%), fluconazole 400 mg given as a single dose (cure rate >70% at 3 wk after treatment), or itraconazole 200 mg/day for 5 days.

DISPOSITION

The prognosis is good, with death of the fungus usually occurring within 3 to 4 wk of treatment; however, recurrence is common.

PEARLS & CONSIDERATIONS

COMMENTS

Patients should be informed that the hypopigmented areas will not disappear immediately after treatment and that several months may be necessary for the hypopigmented areas to regain their pigmentation.

AUTHOR: **FRED F. FERRI, M.D.**

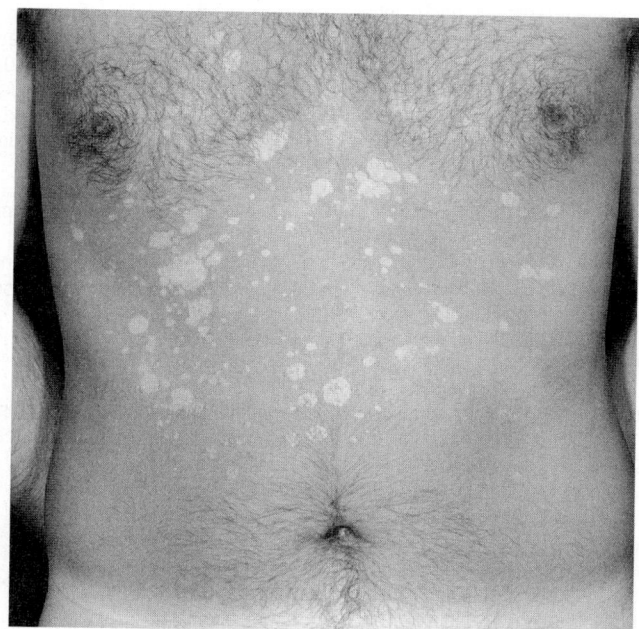

FIGURE 1-380 The classic presentation of tinea versicolor with white, oval, or circular patches on tan skin. (From Habif TB: *Clinical dermatology: a color guide to diagnosis and therapy*, ed 3, St Louis, 1996, Mosby.)

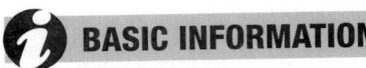

BASIC INFORMATION

DEFINITION

Tinnitus is a perception of sound in the absence of external sounds; an unwanted auditory perception of internal origin. The name is derived from the Latin word *tinnitus,* meaning "ringing."

SYNONYMS   Ringing in the ear(s)

ICD-9CM CODES
388.30 Tinnitus

EPIDEMIOLOGY & DEMOGRAPHICS

Tinnitus increases with age. The most recent prevalence statistics from the National Center for Health Statistics (1999) indicate that tinnitus affects ~18% of the population. The American Tinnitus Association reports that 50 million Americans have tinnitus. It is slightly more common in men, frequently associated with hearing impairment, and more common in whites than African Americans. The prevalence is double in the southern states compared to the northern states. It is most prevalent at ages 40 to 70 yr.

PHYSICAL FINDINGS & CLINICAL PRESENTATION

- Patient complaints are of sounds in ears. Determine onset, localization, pitch, loudness, duration, and nature—can be pulsatile, or described as ringing, buzzing, cricketlike, hissing, humming, or whistling.
- Objective tinnitus is pulsatile, with bursts of sound energy coinciding with the pulse.

ETIOLOGY

- Tinnitus has multiple causes and is often a secondary symptom to hearing loss caused by abnormalities in the brain or at any point along the auditory pathway. Although the exact etiology is unclear, possibilities include injured cochlear hair cells, spontaneous activity in auditory nerve fibers, hyperactivity in the auditory nuclei in the brain stem, or a reduction in suppressive activity of the central auditory cortex. Current theory posits that tinnitus may arise when normal auditory signals are no longer received by the brain.
- Medications implicated in tinnitus are aspirin, NSAIDs, aminoglycosides, chloramphenicol, erythromycin, tetracycline, vancomycin, bleomycin, cisplatin, mechlorethamine, vincristine, bumetanide, ethacrynic acid, furosemide, chloroquine, heavy metals, heterocyclic antidepressants, and quinine.
- Generally classified as objective vs. subjective tinnitus:
  - Objective tinnitus is provoked by sound generated in the body that reaches the ear through conduction in body tissues, while subjective tinnitus is composed of sounds without any associated meanings or physical source and can be heard only by the suffering person.
  - Objective causes: (1) vascular: arterial bruit, venous hum, AV malformation, vascular tumors, acoustic neuromas; (2) neurologic: palatomyoclonus, idiopathic stapedial muscle spasm; (3) patulous (lax) eustachian tube.
  - Subjective causes: (1) otologic: hearing loss, Meniere's disease, acoustic neuroma, cerumen impaction; (2) ototoxic medications; (3) neurologic: multiple sclerosis, head injury; (4) metabolic: thyroid disorder, hyperlipidemia, vitamin B_{12} deficiency; (5) psychogenic: depression, anxiety, fibromyalgia; and (6) Infectious: otitis media, Lyme disease, meningitis, syphilis.

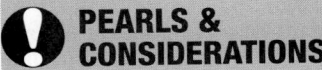

DIAGNOSIS

DIFFERENTIAL DIAGNOSIS

Subjective or objective tinnitus

WORKUP

- History including the onset, associated symptoms (such as hearing loss), and possible exposure to ototoxic substances or disease processes that predispose to tinnitus
- Association with depression: screen for depression
- Focused physical exam: Blood pressure, examination of eyes for nystagmus, and a full examination of the ears. This should include inspection of the external canal and tympanic membrane for signs of cerumen impaction, perforation, or infection. The cranial nerves should be examined for evidence of brain stem damage or hearing loss, including specific testing for conductive or sensorineural hearing loss (performing the Weber-Rinne tests using a 512-Hz or 1,024-Hz tuning fork). Also recommended is auscultation over the neck, periauricular area, orbits, and mastoid and compression of the jugular veins.

LABORATORY TESTS

- Audiometry, tympanometry, pitch masking generally performed
- Consider evaluating for metabolic abnormalities: thyroid disease, hyperlipidemia, anemia, B_{12} deficiency, zinc deficiency, CBC, complete blood chemistry

IMAGING STUDIES

- MRI/CT: Consider brain imaging to rule out multiple sclerosis, acoustic neuroma, brain stem tumor
- MRI/MRA for pulsatile tinnitus

TREATMENT

NONPHARMACOLOGIC THERAPY

Unknown effectiveness: psychotherapy, biofeedback, acupuncture, tinnitus-masking devices

ACUTE GENERAL Rx

A number of psychopharmacologic drugs may be useful in the clinical management of tinnitus, both as candidate triggers and as potential therapies. However, at present, there are no FDA-approved medications for this disorder and there are strong methodologic issues that limit the reliability of research on the topic. Although not FDA approved, antidepressants (tricyclics), some SSRIs and SNRIs (e.g., sertraline and venlafaxine), anxiolytics (e.g., benzodiazepines), and $GABA_B$ agonists, antiepileptics, mood stabilizers, and other pharmacologic agents may be effective—however, they should be used with caution.

CHRONIC Rx

- Long-term behavioral therapies and emerging therapies exist, although there are insufficient RCTs to determine their relative value
  - Tinnitus retraining therapy (TRT): a form of habituation therapy composed of education, support, counseling, feedback device, multidisciplinary team, and long duration of therapy
  - Tinnitus masking (TM)
  - Neuromonics
  - Transcranial magnetic stimulation

COMPLEMENTARY & ALTERNATIVE MEDICINE

- Possibly effective: acupuncture, relaxation therapy, hypnosis (based on systemic reviews)
- *Ginkgo biloba* unlikely to be effective, but study results are conflicting

DISPOSITION

Evaluate for all treatable causes, careful history to raise awareness of pulsatile tinnitus: subjective or objective

REFERRAL

- Consider referring in cases where tinnitus comes on rapidly, is pulsatile, or is associated with sudden hearing loss or with other significant symptoms such as loss of balance, psychiatric changes, movement or speech disorders, etc.
- ENT, neurology

PEARLS & CONSIDERATIONS

COMMENTS

- Up to 18% of population may have tinnitus, with 0.5% severely effected; be aware of high prevalence.
- Treatments may be effective in reducing symptoms and suffering, whether or not there are treatable underlying causes
- Be aware of concurrent depression; screen and treat for it. Treat all treatable underlying causes.

PREVENTION

Avoid ototoxic drugs and loud, chronic noise exposure.

PATIENT & FAMILY EDUCATION

Counsel families and patients that tinnitus may be irreversible but that there are approaches that can help, and be aware of the effect on their lives.

- American Tinnitus Association: 800-634-8978, http://www.ata.org
- American Academy of Audiology: 800-AAA-2336, http://www.audiology.org
- Hear USA: http://www.hearusa.org

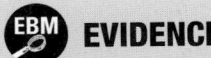 **EVIDENCE**

available at www.expertconsult.com

SUGGESTED READINGS

available at www.expertconsult.com

AUTHOR: **JEFFREY BORKAN, M.D., Ph.D.**

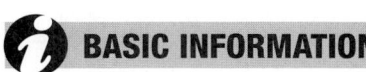

BASIC INFORMATION

DEFINITION

Torticollis is a contraction or contracture of the muscles of the neck that causes the head to be tilted to one side. It is usually accompanied by rotation of the chin to the opposite side with flexion (Fig. 1-381). Usually it is a symptom of some underlying disorder. This term is often used incorrectly in cases when the torticollis may simply be positional.

SYNONYMS

Twisted neck
"Wry neck"

ICD-9CM CODES
723.5   Spastic (intermittent) torticollis
754.1   Congenital muscular
         (sternocleidomastoid)
300.11   Hysterical
714.0   Rheumatoid
333.83   Spasmodic

PHYSICAL FINDINGS & CLINICAL PRESENTATION

- Congenital muscular torticollis:
  1. Palpable soft tissue "mass" in the sternocleidomastoid shortly after birth
  2. Mass gradually subsides, leaving a shortened, contracted sternocleidomastoid muscle
  3. Head characteristically tilted toward the side of the mass and rotated in the opposite direction
  4. Facial asymmetry and other secondary changes persisting into adulthood
- Spasmodic torticollis:
  1. "Spasms" in the cervical musculature; may be bilateral and uncontrollable
  2. Head often tilted toward the affected side
- Findings in other cases depend on etiology

ETIOLOGY

Torticollis has been found to have more than 50 different causes:
- Localized fibrous shortening of unknown cause involving the sternocleidomastoid, leading to the condition termed *congenital muscular torticollis*
- Spasmodic torticollis: of uncertain etiology, possibly a variant of dystonia musculorum deformans
- Infection, specifically pharyngitis, tonsillitis, retropharyngeal abscess
- Miscellaneous rare causes: congenital musculoskeletal deformities, trauma, inflammation from rheumatoid arthritis, vestibular disturbances, posterior fossa tumor, syringomyelia, neuritis of spinal accessory nerve, and drug reactions

DIAGNOSIS

DIFFERENTIAL DIAGNOSIS

- Usually involves separating each disorder from the others
- Acquired positional disorders (e.g., ocular disturbances, acute disk herniation)

WORKUP

- Workup depends on the clinical situation.
- Laboratory studies are usually not helpful unless infection or rheumatoid disease is suspected.
- Section II describes a differential diagnosis for the evaluation and therapy of neck pain.
- Any child with a gradually increasing torticollis should have a complete eye examination.

IMAGING STUDIES

- Plain radiographs in cases of trauma or to rule out congenital abnormalities
- MRI in appropriate cases
- Electrodiagnostic studies: only rarely indicated to rule out neurologic causes

TREATMENT

- Congenital muscular torticollis: gentle stretching exercises carried out by the parent
- Spasmodic torticollis: physical therapy, psychotherapy, cervical braces, biofeedback, and pain control
- Other forms: treated according to etiology

DISPOSITION

- Most patients with congenital muscular torticollis respond well to conservative treatment.
- Spasmodic torticollis is often resistant to normal conservative treatment.
- Prognosis of other forms of torticollis depends on etiology.

REFERRAL

- Torticollis often requires a multidisciplinary approach unless the etiology is obvious.
- Children usually do not require any specific studies; however, an orthopedic consultation is recommended.
- Fixed deformity in the child; may need orthopedic referral for surgical release.

SUGGESTED READINGS
available at www.expertconsult.com

AUTHOR: **LONNIE R. MERCIER, M.D.**

Diseases and Disorders

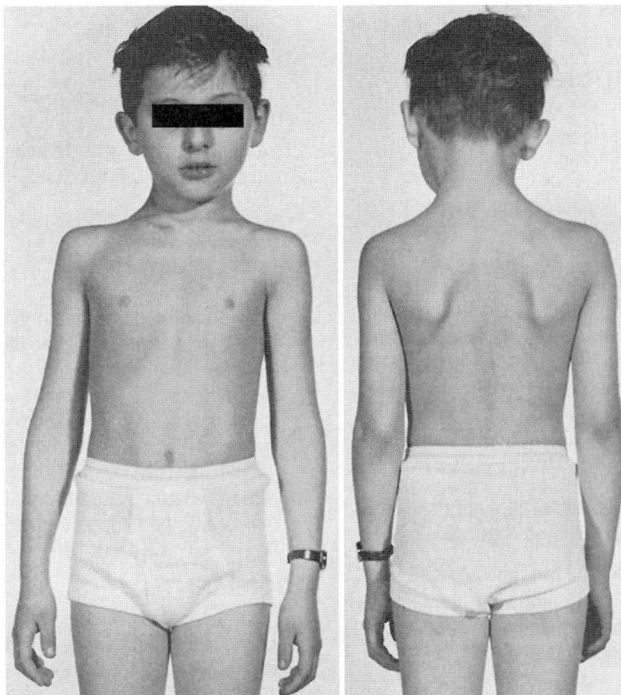

FIGURE 1-381 Torticollis. In this child, the right sternocleidomastoid muscle is contracted. (From Brinker MR, Miller MD: *Fundamentals of orthopaedics,* Philadelphia, 1999, WB Saunders.)

BASIC INFORMATION

DEFINITION

Tics are sudden, brief, intermittent involuntary or semivoluntary movements (motor tics) or sounds (phonic or vocal tics) that mimic fragments of normal behavior.

Tourette's syndrome (TS) is an inherited neuropsychiatric disorder characterized by multiple motor and vocal tics that change during the course of the illness. Onset is typically before age 18 (new-onset tics can occasionally occur after age 18 yr, but for DSM-IV criteria of TS, they must begin before this age).

SYNONYMS

Gilles de la Tourette syndrome
TS
Tourette's disorder

ICD-9CM CODES
307.23 Gilles de la Tourette disorder

EPIDEMIOLOGY & DEMOGRAPHICS

PREVALENCE (IN U.S.): Unknown; estimates range from 0.7% to 5%
PREDOMINANT SEX: Approximate male/female ratio of 3:1
PREDOMINANT AGE: Typical age of onset is between 2 and 15 yr (mean 5 to 7 yr)

PHYSICAL FINDINGS & CLINICAL PRESENTATION

- Neurologic examination is normal.
- Vocal tics (clearing of throat, repetitive short phrases, e.g., "you bet," swearing [coprolalia]).
- Motor tics can be simple (e.g., blinking, grimacing, head jerking) or complex (e.g., gesturing). Tics wax, wane, and change over time. Often they can be suppressed for short periods. Commonly they are preceded by an urge to perform the tic.
- TS is often associated with a variety of behavioral symptoms, most commonly attention deficit hyperactivity disorder (ADHD) and obsessive-compulsive disorder (OCD).

TS can be diagnosed using the DSM-IV-TR criteria as follows:
1. Both multiple motor and one or more vocal tics must be present at some time during the illness.
2. Tics occur many times a day (usually in bouts over >1 year, during which time there must be no tic-free period of >3 consecutive mo.
3. Age at onset is <18 yr.
4. Disturbance is not attributable to the direct physiologic effects of a substance (e.g., stimulants) or a general medical condition (e.g., Huntington's disease or postviral encephalitis).

ETIOLOGY

There is a large genetic contribution to TS. There is a strong family history of OCD or TS in patients with tics, and twin studies provide evidence for the importance of genetic factors. Recent analysis of linkage in a two-generation pedigree has led to the identification of a mutation in the HDC gene encoding L-histidine decarboxylase, the rate-limiting enzyme in histamine biosynthesis, pointing to a role for histaminergic neurotransmission in the mechanism and modulation of Tourette's syndrome and tics.

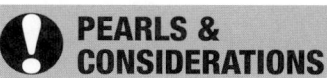 **DIAGNOSIS**

DIFFERENTIAL DIAGNOSIS

- Sydenham's chorea: occurs after infection with group A *Streptococcus.*
- PANDAS: pediatric autoimmune neuropsychiatric disorder associated with streptococcal infection.
- Sporadic tic disorders: tend to be motor or vocal but not both.
- Head trauma.
- Drug intoxication: many drugs are known to induce or exacerbate tic disorder, including methylphenidate, amphetamines, pemoline, anticholinergics, and antihistamines.
- Postinfectious encephalitis.
- Inherited disorders: Huntington's disease, Hallervorden Spatz, and neuroacanthocytosis. All these conditions should have other observed abnormalities on neurologic examination.

WORKUP

Clinical observation and history to confirm diagnosis

LABORATORY TESTS

No definitive laboratory tests

IMAGING STUDIES

CT scan and MRI of brain are normal and unnecessary in the absence of abnormal neurologic examination.

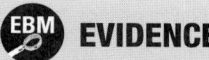 **TREATMENT**

NONPHARMACOLOGIC THERAPY

Multidisciplinary: parents, teachers, psychologists, school nurses. Cognitive behavioral therapy termed habit-reversal treatment is efficacious in suppressing tics

ACUTE GENERAL Rx

Dopamine-blocking agents may be used to reduce severity of tics acutely (e.g., haloperidol 0.25 mg PO qhs initially). There are risks of side effects, such as acute dystonic reactions.

CHRONIC Rx

Tics only require treatment when they interfere with psychosocial, educational, and occupational functioning of a person.
TICS:
- Clonidine: many choose this as a first-line agent because of fewer long-term side effects. Start at 0.05 mg and slowly titrate to approximately 0.45 mg daily (needs tid/qid dosing). May also help with symptoms of ADHD.
- Guanfacine is another alpha-agonist similar to clonidine but can be administered once daily. Typical starting dose is 0.5 mg titrating to 1 to 3 mg qd.
- Tetrabenazine: dopamine-depleting agent that recently became available in the U.S. Avoids many of the typical side effects of the neuroleptics; most notably does not cause tardive dyskinesias.
- Atypical antipsychotics such as ziprasidone, risperidone, and olanzapine. These may have fewer side effects than typical neuroleptics.
- Dopamine-blocking agents: neuroleptics (pimozide, haloperidol, fluphenazine). These should be avoided until other options have been exhausted.
- Dopamine agonists: the dopamine depleter tetrabenazine may also be effective in reducing tics. A few small, open-label studies have found that ropinirole and pramipexole in low doses may be effective in reducing tic severity.
- Botulinum toxin local injection is effective for eye blinking and neck and shoulder tics. The benefits are temporary, lasting 3 to 6 mo.
- Surgical treatment with deep-brain stimulation has also been reported effective in some patients with disabling tics that are refractory to medication.

ADHD: Stimulants (dextroamphetamine, methylphenidate) are useful for symptoms of ADHD but may exacerbate tics.
OCD: Selective serotonin reuptake inhibitors, such as fluoxetine, are the most effective.

DISPOSITION

- In the later teen years, intensity and frequency of tics typically diminish.
- One third of patients will achieve significant remission, although complete, lifelong remission is rare.
- One third will have mild, persistent, but "non-impairing" tics.

REFERRAL

To a neurologist to confirm initial diagnosis and for treatment in difficult cases

! **PEARLS & CONSIDERATIONS**

- Tics do not need treatment unless they interfere with an individual's ability to function.
- Greater improvement in symptom severity among children with Tourette and chronic tic disorder has been reported with a comprehensive behavioral intervention compared with supportive therapy and education.
- An important part of treatment is appropriate evaluation and therapy of coexisting conditions (e.g., ADHD, OCD).

COMMENTS

Patient education may be obtained from the Tourette's Syndrome Association, 4240 Bell Blvd., Bayside, NY 11361-2864; 800-237-0717 or 718-224-2999; http://www.tsa-usa.org.

EBM **EVIDENCE**

available at www.expertconsult.com

SUGGESTED READINGS

available at www.expertconsult.com

AUTHOR: **CINDY ZADIKOFF, M.D.**

BASIC INFORMATION

DEFINITION

Toxic shock syndrome (TSS) is an acute febrile illness resulting in multiple organ system dysfunction caused most commonly by a bacterial exotoxin. Disease characteristics also include hypotension, vomiting, myalgia, watery diarrhea, vascular collapse, and an erythematous sunburnlike cutaneous rash that desquamates during recovery.

ICD-9CM CODES
040.89 Toxic shock syndrome

EPIDEMIOLOGY & DEMOGRAPHICS

- Case reported incidence peak: 14 cases per 100,000 menstruating women annually in 1980; has since fallen to one case per 100,000 persons
- Occurs most commonly between ages 10 and 30 yr in healthy, young, menstruating white females
- Case fatality ratio of 3%

PHYSICAL FINDINGS & CLINICAL PRESENTATION

- Fever (>38.0° C).
- Diffuse macular erythrodermatous rash that involves both skin and mucous membranes that resembles sunburn and also involves the palms and soles. The rash then desquamates 1 to 2 wk after disease onset in survivors.
- Orthostatic hypotension.
- Gastrointestinal symptoms: vomiting, diarrhea, abdominal tenderness.
- Constitutional symptoms: myalgia, headache, photophobia, rigors, altered sensorium, conjunctivitis, arthralgia.
- Respiratory symptoms: dysphagia, pharyngeal hyperemia, strawberry tongue.
- Genitourinary symptoms: vaginal discharge, vaginal hyperemia, adnexal tenderness.
- End-organ failure.
- Severe hypotension and acute renal failure.
- Hepatic failure.
- Cardiovascular symptoms: disseminated intravascular coagulation, pulmonary edema, acute respiratory distress syndrome (ARDS), endomyocarditis, heart block.

ETIOLOGY

- Menstruation-associated TSS: 45% of cases associated with tampons, diaphragm, or vaginal sponge use.
- Non–menstruation-associated TSS: 55% of cases associated with puerperal sepsis, post–cesarean section endometritis, mastitis, sinusitis, wound or skin infection, septohinoplasty, pelvic inflammatory disease, respiratory infections following influenza, enterocolitis, and burns.
- Causative agent: *Staphylococcus aureus* infection of a susceptible individual (10% of population lacking sufficient levels of antitoxin antibodies), which liberates the disease mediator TSST-1 (exotoxin). While most

cases are caused by methicillin-susceptible *S. aureus* (MSSA), cases of TSS from methicillin-resistant *S. aureus* (MRSA) have occurred, particularly those due to the more virulent community-associated MRSA strains.
- *S. aureus* exotoxins are superantigens that can activate large numbers of T cells (up to 20% at one time) resulting in a massive cytokine production: interleukin(Il-1), Il-2, TNF, and interferon gamma that then mediate the signs and symptoms of the disease.
- Other causative agents: coagulase-negative streptococci producing enterotoxins B or C, and exotoxin-A—producing group A beta-hemolytic streptococci.

DIAGNOSIS

DIFFERENTIAL DIAGNOSIS

- Staphylococcal food poisoning
- Septic shock
- Mucocutaneous lymph node syndrome
- Scarlet fever
- Rocky Mountain spotted fever
- Meningococcemia
- Toxic epidermal necrolysis
- Kawasaki's syndrome
- Leptospirosis
- Legionnaires' disease
- Hemolytic-uremic syndrome
- Stevens-Johnson syndrome
- Scalded skin syndrome
- Erythema multiforme
- Acute rheumatic fever

WORKUP

Broad-spectrum syndrome with multiorgan system involvement and variable but acute clinical presentation, including the following:
- Fever (>38.0° C)
- Classic desquamating rash (1 to 2 wk)
- Hypotension/orthostatic systolic blood pressure ≤90 mm Hg
- Syncope
- Negative throat and cerebrospinal fluid cultures
- Negative serologic test for Rocky Mountain spotted fever, rubeola, and leptospirosis

- Clinical involvement of three or more of the following:
  - Cardiopulmonary: ARDS, pulmonary edema, endomyocarditis, second- or third-degree atrioventricular block
  - Central nervous system: altered sensorium without focal neurologic findings
  - Hematologic: thrombocytopenia (platelets <100,000)
  - Liver: elevated liver function test results
  - Renal: >5 cells/high-powered field, negative urine cultures, azotemia, and increased creatinine (double normal)
  - Mucous membrane involvement: vagina, oropharynx, conjunctiva
  - Musculoskeletal: myalgia, creatine phosphokinase twice normal
  - Gastrointestinal: vomiting, diarrhea

LABORATORY TESTS

- Pan culture (cervix and vagina, throat, nasal passages, urine, blood, cerebrospinal fluid, wound) for *Staphylococcus, Streptococcus,* and other pathogenic organisms (Table 1-174)
- Electrolytes to detect hypokalemia, hyponatremia
- Complete blood count with differential and clotting profile for anemia (normocytic or normochromic), thrombocytopenia, leukocytosis, coagulopathy, and bacteremia
- Chemistry profile to detect decreased protein, increased aspartate aminotransferase, increased alanine aminotransferase, hypocalcemia, elevated blood urea nitrogen and creatinine, hypophosphatemia, increased lactate dehydrogenase, increased creatine phosphokinase
- Urinalysis to detect white blood cells (>5 cells/high-powered field), proteinemia, microhematuria
- Arterial blood gases to assess respiratory function and acid–base status
- Serologic tests considered for Rocky Mountain spotted fever, rubeola, and leptospirosis

IMAGING STUDIES

- Chest x-ray examination to evaluate pulmonary edema
- ECG to evaluate arrhythmia

TABLE 1-174 Staphylococcal versus Streptococcal Toxic Shock Syndrome

Feature	Staphylococcal	Streptococcal
Age	Primarily 15-35 yr	Primarily 20-50 yr
Gender	Higher frequency in women	Men and women equally affected
Severe pain	Rare	Common
Hypotension	100%	100%
Erythroderma rash	Very common	Less common
Renal failure	Common	Common
Bacteremia	Low frequency	60%
Tissue necrosis	Rare	Common
Predisposing factors	Tampons, surgery	Cuts, burns, varicella
Thrombocytopenia	Common	Common
Mortality rare	<3%	30-70%

Mandell GL et al: *Principles and practice in infections diseases,* ed 7, Philadelphia, 2008, Elsevier.

- Sonography, CT scan, or MRI considered if pelvic abscess or tubo-ovarian abscess suspected

Rx TREATMENT

NONPHARMACOLOGIC THERAPY

- For optimal outcome: high index of suspicion and early and aggressive supportive management in an ICU setting
- Aggressive fluid resuscitation (maintenance of circulating volume, cardiac output, systolic blood pressure)
- Thorough search for a localized infection or nidus: incision and drainage, debridement, removal of tampon or vaginal sponge
- Central hemodynamic monitoring, Swan-Ganz catheter and arterial line for surveillance of hemodynamic status and response to therapy
- Foley catheter to monitor hourly urine output
- Possible military antishock trousers as temporary measure
- Acute ventilator management if severe respiratory compromise
- Renal dialysis for severe renal impairment
- Surgical intervention for indicated conditions (i.e., ruptured tubo-ovarian abscess, wound abscess, mastitis)

ACUTE GENERAL Rx

- Isotonic crystalloid (normal saline solution) for volume replacement following "7–3" rule (refers to the response in millimeters of mercury [mm Hg] of the pulmonary artery wedge pressure to volume replacement).
- Electrolyte replacement (K+, Ca+)
- Packed red blood cells, coagulation factor replacement, fresh frozen plasma to treat anemia or dilation and curettage.
- Vasopressor therapy for hypotension refractory to fluid volume replacement (e.g., dopamine beginning at 2 to 5 μg/kg/min)
- Steroids have been used but are not generally recommended due to lack of evidence of benefit.
- It is not clear whether antibiotics alter the course of acute TSS. Most authors recommend that patients receive 10 to 14 days of combination antibiotic therapy. Clindamycin (600 mg IV every 8 hr in adults or 25 to 40 mg/kg per day in children) plus vancomycin (adults: 30 mg/kg per day IV in two divided doses; children: 40 mg/kg per day IV in four divided doses). Oxacillin or nafcillin sodium (2 g IV every 4 hr in adults; children: 100 to 150 mg/kg per 24 hr divided in four doses) can be used instead of Vancomycin if TSS due to MSSA. An alternative to vancomycin is linezolid.

- Broad-spectrum antibiotic including gram-negative coverage added if concurrent sepsis suspected.
- Intravenous immune globulin (IVIG): while no controlled trials exist, most authors recommend IVIG (400 mg/kg in a single dose administered over several hours) in severe cases of TSS that are not responding to fluids or vasopressors. It may neutralize superantigen and decrease tissue damage.
- Tetracycline added if considering Rocky Mountain spotted fever.

CHRONIC Rx

- Severely ill patient: may require prolonged hospitalization and supportive management with gradual recovery and/or sequelae from severe end-organ involvement (ARDS or renal failure requiring dialysis)
- Majority of patients: complete recovery
- Early late-onset complications (within 2 wk):
  - Skin desquamation
  - Impaired digit sensation
  - Denuded tongue
  - Vocal cord paralysis
  - Acute tubular necrosis
  - ARDS
- Late-onset complications (after 8 wk):
  - Nail splitting and loss
  - Alopecia
  - Central nervous system sequelae
  - Renal impairment
  - Cardiac dysfunction
- Recurrent TSS:
  - More common in menstruation-related cases.
  - Less common in patients treated with beta-lactamase–resistant antistaphylococcal antibiotics.

- Patients with history of TSS: if suspect signs and symptoms occur, have high index of suspicion and low threshold for evaluation and treatment.
- Screen for nasal carriage of *S. aureus* in patients with *S. aureus* TSS and treat with mupirocin in those with positive cultures.

PREVENTION

- Avoidance of tampons or use of low-absorbency tampons only (<4 hr in situ) and alternate with napkins
- Education for patients concerning signs and symptoms of TSS
- Avoidance of tampons for patients with history of TSS

DISPOSITION

- Complete recovery for most patients
- Long-term management of early- and late-onset complications for minority of patients

REFERRAL

- For multidisciplinary management, involving primary physician, gynecologist, internist, infectious disease specialist, and other supportive care specialists
- To tertiary-level hospital

⚠ PEARLS & CONSIDERATIONS

COMMENTS

Patient information is available from American College of Gynecologists and Obstetricians.

EBM EVIDENCE

available at www.expertconsult.com

SUGGESTED READINGS

available at www.expertconsult.com

AUTHORS: **GLENN G. FORT, M.D., M.P.H.,** and **DENNIS J. MIKOLICH, M.D.**

BASIC INFORMATION

DEFINITION

Toxoplasmosis is an infection caused by the protozoal parasite *Toxoplasma gondii.*

ICD-9CM CODES
130.9 Toxoplasmosis

EPIDEMIOLOGY & DEMOGRAPHICS

INCIDENCE (IN U.S.):
- 3% to 70% of healthy adults
- Increases with age
- Increases with certain activities
  1. Slaughterhouse workers
  2. Cat owners
- Increases with certain geographic locations: high prevalence of cats

PREDOMINANT SEX: Equal gender distribution
PREDOMINANT AGE:
- Infancy (congenital infection)
- Prevalence increases with age

PEAK INCIDENCE: Temperate climates
GENETICS: Congenital infection:
- Incidence and severity vary with the trimester of gestation during which the mother acquired infection.
  1. 10% to 25% (first trimester)
  2. 30% to 54% (second trimester)
  3. 60% to 65% (third trimester)
- Congenital infection occurring in the first trimester is the most severe.
- 89% to 100% of infections in the third trimester are asymptomatic.
- Risk to the fetus is not correlated with symptoms in the mother.

PHYSICAL FINDINGS & CLINICAL PRESENTATION

- Acquired (immunocompetent host)
  1. 80% to 90% asymptomatic
  2. Adenopathy (usually cervical)
  3. Fever
  4. Myalgias
  5. Malaise
  6. Sore throat
  7. Maculopapular rash
  8. Hepatosplenomegaly
  9. Chorioretinitis rare
- Acquired (in patients with AIDS)
  1. 89% of symptomatic cases
     a. Encephalitis
     b. Intracerebral mass lesions
  2. Pneumonitis
  3. Chorioretinitis
  4. Other end organ
- Acquired (immunocompromised patients)
  1. Encephalitis
  2. Myocarditis (especially in heart transplant patients)
  3. Pneumonitis
- Ocular infection in the immunocompetent host
  1. Congenital infection
  2. Blurred vision
  3. Photophobia
  4. Pain

5. Loss of central vision if macula involved
6. Focal necrotizing retinitis
7. Typically presents in second or third decade
- Congenital
  1. Results from acute infection acquired by the mother within 6 to 8 wk before conception or during gestation
  2. Usually, asymptomatic mother
  3. No sign of disease
  4. Chorioretinitis
  5. Blindness
  6. Epilepsy
  7. Psychomotor or mental retardation
  8. Intracranial calcifications
  9. Hydrocephalus
  10. Microcephaly
  11. Encephalitis
  12. Anemia
  13. Thrombocytopenia
  14. Hepatosplenomegaly
  15. Lymphadenopathy
  16. Jaundice
  17. Rash
  18. Pneumonitis
  19. Most infected infants are asymptomatic at birth

ETIOLOGY

- *Toxoplasma gondii*
  1. Ubiquitous intracellular protozoan
  2. Present worldwide
  3. Cat is definitive host
- Human infection
  1. Ingestion of oocysts shed by cats
  2. Ingestion of meat containing tissue cysts
  3. Vertical transmission

Dx DIAGNOSIS

DIFFERENTIAL DIAGNOSIS

- Lymphadenopathy
  1. Infectious mononucleosis
  2. CMV mononucleosis
  3. Cat-scratch disease
  4. Sarcoidosis
  5. Tuberculosis
  6. Lymphoma
  7. Metastatic cancer
- Cerebral mass lesions in immunocompromised host
  1. Lymphoma
  2. Tuberculosis
  3. Bacterial abscess
- Pneumonitis in immunocompromised host
  1. *Pneumocystis jirovecii (carinii)* pneumonia
  2. Tuberculosis
  3. Fungal infection
- Chorioretinitis
  1. Syphilis
  2. Tuberculosis
  3. Histoplasmosis (competent host)
  4. CMV
  5. Syphilis
  6. Herpes simplex
  7. Fungal infection
  8. Tuberculosis (AIDS patient)

- Myocarditis
  1. Organ rejection in heart transplant recipients
- Congenital infection
  1. Rubella
  2. CMV
  3. Herpes simplex
  4. Syphilis
  5. Listeriosis
  6. Erythroblastosis fetalis
  7. Sepsis

WORKUP

- Acute infection, immunocompetent host
  1. CBC
  2. *Toxoplasma* serology (IgG, IgM) in serial blood specimens 3 wk apart
  3. Lymph node biopsy if diagnosis uncertain
- Immunocompromised host
  1. CNS symptoms
     a. Cerebral CT scan or MRI if CNS symptoms present
     b. Spinal tap, if safe
     c. Brain biopsy if no response to empiric therapy
  2. Ocular symptoms
     a. Funduscopic examination
     b. Serologic studies
     c. Rarely, vitreous tap
  3. Pulmonary symptoms
     a. Chest x-ray examination
     b. Bronchoalveolar lavage
     c. Transbronchial or open-lung biopsy
  4. Myocarditis
     a. Cardiac enzymes
     b. Electrocardiogram
     c. Endomyocardial biopsy for definitive diagnosis
- Toxoplasmosis in pregnancy
  1. Initial maternal screening with IgM and IgG
     a. If negative, mother at risk of acute infection and should be retested monthly
     b. If both IgG and IgM positive, obtain IgA and IgE ELISA, AC/HS test
     c. IgA and IgE ELISA, AC/HS test elevated in acute infection
     d. Ig high for 1 yr or more
     e. IgG repeated 3 to 4 wk later to determine if titer is stable
  2. Acute maternal infection not excluded or documented
     a. Fetal blood sampling (for culture, Ig, IgA, IgE)
     b. Amniotic fluid polymerase chain reaction (PCR)
  3. Fetal ultrasound every other wk if maternal infection documented
- Congenital toxoplasmosis
  1. Placental histology
  2. Specific IgM or IgA in infant's blood

LABORATORY TESTS

- Antibody studies
  1. More than one test necessary to establish diagnosis of acute toxoplasmosis

2. IgM antibody
   a. Appears 5 days into infection
   b. Peaks at 2 wk
   c. Falls to low level or disappears within 2 mo
   d. May persist at low levels for 1 yr or more
3. Antibody not measurable
   a. Ocular toxoplasmosis
   b. Reactivation
   c. Immunocompromised hosts
4. IgA ELISA, IgE ELISA, and IgE ASAGA
   a. More sensitive tests
   b. Disappear more rapidly than Ig, establishing diagnosis of acute infection
5. IgG antibody
   a. Appears 1 to 2 wk after infection
   b. Peaks at 6 to 8 wk
   c. Gradually declines over months to years

IMAGING STUDIES

- Chest x-ray if pulmonary involvement suspected
- Cerebral CT scan (Fig. 1-382) or MRI if encephalitis suspected

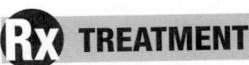

TREATMENT

NONPHARMACOLOGIC THERAPY

- Selected cases of ocular infection
  1. Photocoagulation
  2. Vitrectomy
  3. Lentectomy
- Selected cases of congenital cerebral infection
  1. Ventricular shunting

ACUTE GENERAL Rx

- Acute infection, immunocompetent host
  1. No treatment, unless severe and persistent symptoms or vital organ damage

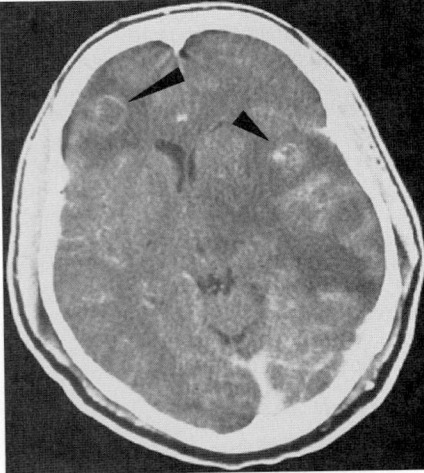

FIGURE 1-382 Toxoplasmic encephalitis in person who has AIDS. A cranial CT scan shows bilateral contrast-enhanced ring lesions with peripheral edema and mass effect. (From Cohen J, Powderly WG: *Infectious diseases,* ed 2, St Louis, 2004, Mosby.)

- Acute infection, immunocompromised host, non-AIDS
  1. Treat even if asymptomatic
  2. Duration
     a. Until 4 to 6 wk after resolution of all signs and symptoms
     b. Usually 6 mo or longer
- Reactivated infection, immunocompromised host, non-AIDS
  1. Treat if symptomatic
- Acute or reactivated infection, AIDS
  1. Treat in all cases
  2. Induction course
     a. 3 to 6 wk.
     b. Maintenance therapy continued for life; consider discontinuation of suppressive therapy if the patient has a good response to highly active antiretroviral therapy and if the CD4 count remains >200 cell/mm^3 for more than 3 mo.
  3. Empiric therapy
     a. AIDS with positive IgG
     b. Multiple ring-enhancing lesions on cerebral CT scan or MRI
     c. Response seen by day 7 in 71% and day 14 in 91%
- Ocular infection
  1. Treat in all cases
  2. Therapy continued for 1 mo or longer if needed
  3. Response seen in 70% within 10 days
  4. Retreat as needed
  5. Steroids may be indicated
  6. Surgical treatment in selected cases
- Treatment regimens
  1. Pyrimethamine 100 to 200 mg loading dose once PO, then 25 mg PO qid (50 to 75 mg in AIDS), plus
  2. Leucovorin 10 to 20 mg PO qid, plus
  3. Sulfadiazine 1 to 1.5 g PO q6h

Other treatment options (if sulfa-hypersensitivity or allergy is present): pyrimethamine 50 to 75 mg/day PO with leucovorin 10 to 20 mg/day PO and either (1) clindamycin 600 mg IV or PO q6h, or (2) clarithromycin 1 gm PO bid, or (3) dapsone 100 mg/day PO, or (4) atovaquone 750 mg PO q6h.

- Acute infection in pregnancy
  1. Treat immediately
  2. Risk of fetal infection reduced by 60% with treatment
     a. First trimester
        i. Spiramycin 3 g PO qid in two to four divided doses
        ii. Sulfadiazine 4 g PO qid in four divided doses
     b. Second and third trimester
        i. Sulfadiazine as previously described, *plus*
        ii. Pyrimethamine 25 mg PO qid, *plus*
        iii. Leucovorin 5 to 15 mg PO qid
        iv. Spiramycin as previously described
- Congenital infection
  1. Sulfadiazine 50 mg/kg PO bid, plus
  2. Pyrimethamine 2 mg/kg PO for 2 days, then 1 mg/kg PO, three times weekly, plus
  3. Leucovorin 5 to 20 mg PO three times weekly
  4. Minimum duration of treatment: 12 mo

CHRONIC Rx

- Maintenance therapy in AIDS patients because of the high risk (80%) of relapse
  1. Pyrimethamine 25 mg PO qid
  2. Sulfadiazine 500 mg PO qid
  3. Leucovorin 10 to 20 mg PO qid

DISPOSITION

- Prognosis
  1. Excellent in the immunocompetent host
  2. Good in ocular infection (although relapses are common)
- Treatment of acute infection in pregnancy
  1. Reduces incidence and severity of congenital toxoplasmosis
- Treatment of congenital infection
  1. Improvement in intellectual function
  2. Regression of retinal lesions
- AIDS
  1. 70% to 95% response to therapy

REFERRAL

- To infectious disease expert:
  1. Immunocompromised hosts
  2. Pregnant women
  3. Difficulty in making a diagnosis or deciding on treatment
- To pediatric infectious disease expert:
  1. Congenital infection
- To obstetrician:
  1. Pregnant seronegative mother
  2. Acute seroconversion
- To ophthalmologist:
  1. Congenital infection
  2. Any case of ocular infection

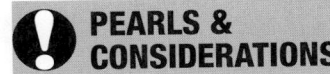

PEARLS & CONSIDERATIONS

COMMENTS

- Prevention of toxoplasmosis is most important in seronegative pregnant women and immunocompromised hosts.
- Patient instructions:
  1. Cook meat to 66° C.
  2. Cook eggs.
  3. Do not drink unpasteurized milk.
  4. Wash hands thoroughly after handling raw meat.
  5. Wash kitchen surfaces that come in contact with raw meat.
  6. Wash fruits and vegetables.
  7. Avoid contact with materials potentially contaminated with cat feces.

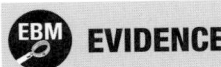 **EVIDENCE**

available at www.expertconsult.com

SUGGESTED READINGS

available at www.expertconsult.com

AUTHORS: **GLENN G. FORT, M.D., M.P.H.,** and **DENNIS J. MIKOLICH, M.D.**

BASIC INFORMATION

DEFINITION

Bacterial tracheitis is an acute infectious disease affecting the trachea and large conducting airways. Tracheal inflammation may be caused by a large number of inhaled stimuli, but bacterial infection is a life-threatening illness associated with purulent secretions and subglottic edema.

SYNONYMS

Bacterial tracheobronchitis
Pseudomembranous croup
Membranous laryngotracheobronchitis

ICD-9CM CODES
464.10 Tracheitis

EPIDEMIOLOGY & DEMOGRAPHICS

INCIDENCE (IN U.S.):
- Uncommon
- May be the most common cause of acute upper airway obstruction requiring admission to pediatric ICUs

PEAK INCIDENCE: Three fourths of cases reported in winter
PREDOMINANT SEX: Boys > girls in one series
PREDOMINANT AGE:
- 1 mo to 8 yr
- Almost all <13 yr (most <3 yr)

GENETICS:
- Down syndrome is a possible predisposing factor.
- Congenital infection: Some cases have been found in those with anatomic abnormalities of the upper airways.

PHYSICAL FINDINGS & CLINICAL PRESENTATION

- Croupy or "brassy" cough
- Inspiratory stridor (frequent)
- Wheezing (unusual)
- Fever (often >102° F)
- Thick, purulent secretions expectorated
  1. Minority of patients expectorate "ricelike" pellets.
  2. Most patients are unable to mobilize secretions.
     a. Become inspissated
     b. Form pseudomembranes

ETIOLOGY

- *Staphylococcus aureus*
- *Haemophilus influenzae*
- β-Hemolytic streptococcal infection

- Secondary to viral infections of the respiratory tract
  1. Primary influenza
  2. RSV
  3. Parainfluenza
- Many cases follow measles
  1. Especially when accompanied by chest radiographic infiltrates
  2. Sometimes fatal outcome
  3. Associated with prolonged endotracheal intubation

DIAGNOSIS

DIFFERENTIAL DIAGNOSIS

- Viral croup
- Epiglottitis
- Diphtheria
- Necrotizing herpes simplex infection in the elderly
- CMV in immunocompromised patients
- Invasive aspergillosis in immunocompromised patients

WORKUP

Direct laryngoscopy
1. Typical secretions
   a. May form pseudomembranes
   b. Airway obstruction
2. Normal epiglottis rules out epiglottitis
3. Possible subglottic edema

LABORATORY TESTS

- WBC is sometimes elevated.
- On differential, left shift is almost universal.
- Gram stain and culture of tracheal secretions confirm diagnosis.
- Blood cultures are positive in a minority.

IMAGING STUDIES

- Lateral x-ray examination of neck
  1. Normal epiglottis
  2. Vague density or a "dripping candle" appearance of tracheal mucosa
     a. Secretions
     b. Pseudomembranes
- Chest radiograms
  1. Not diagnostic
  2. Should not be performed on patients in acute respiratory distress, because severe or fatal upper airway obstruction can develop suddenly
- Pneumonic infiltrates frequent
- Atelectasis: unusual but can lead to lobar collapse

TREATMENT

NONPHARMACOLOGIC THERAPY

- Aggressive maintenance of a patent airway
  1. Laryngoscopy or bronchoscopy used diagnostically and therapeutically to strip away pseudomembranes
  2. Voluminous and tenacious secretions suctioned from the underlying friable mucosa
     a. May extend from between the vocal cords to the main carina
     b. Larger channels of rigid instruments for more effective suctioning
- Prevention of complete large airway obstruction
  1. Nasotracheal intubation
  2. Humidification of inspired gas
  3. Frequent saline instillation and suctioning
  4. Intubation with general anesthesia, performed in the operating room, is preferred by some
- Ventilatory support necessary with initial management in ICU

ACUTE GENERAL Rx

- Antibiotic therapy: start immediately, generally continued for 1 to 2 wk
- Initial therapy directed against *H. influenzae* and *S. aureus* (e.g., cefotaxime and vancomycin)
- Oral therapy is usually sufficient after 5 or 6 days of IV administration

DISPOSITION

- Most patients are extubated in 5 to 6 days after initiating antibiotic therapy.
- Anoxic encephalopathy is reported in 7% of survivors.

REFERRAL

Suspected diagnosis

PEARLS & CONSIDERATIONS

COMMENTS

- Infants are at increased risk of airway obstruction because of the small airway dimension.
- Presence of pneumonia and a staphylococcal cause are thought to worsen prognosis.
- Reported complications: toxic shock syndrome, persistent postextubation stridor, pneumothorax, and volutrauma

SUGGESTED READINGS
available at www.expertconsult.com

AUTHORS: **GLENN G. FORT, M.D., M.P.H.,** and **DENNIS J. MIKOLICH, M.D.**

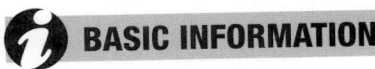 **BASIC INFORMATION**

DEFINITION

Hemolytic transfusion reaction is acute intravascular hemolysis caused by mismatches in the ABO system. It is caused by complement-fixing immunoglobulin (Ig) and IgG antibodies to group A and B red blood cells. Hemolytic transfusion reactions can also be caused by minor antigen systems; however, they are usually less severe. In delayed serologic transfusion reactions, hemolysis with hemoglobinemia is unusual; in delayed reactions the only manifestations may be the development of a newly positive Coombs test and fever. The clinical severity of an ABO-incompatible blood transfusion is significantly influenced by the degree of complement activation and cytokine stimulation.

ICD-9CM CODES
999.8 Other transfusion reaction

EPIDEMIOLOGY & DEMOGRAPHICS

- Acute intravascular hemolysis occurs in one to five per 50,000 transfusions.
- From 1996 to 2007, there were 213 ABO-incompatible RBC transfusions with 24 deaths.

PHYSICAL FINDINGS & CLINICAL PRESENTATION

- Hypotension.
- Pain at the infusion site.
- Fever, tachycardia, chest pain, dyspnea, dizziness, bronchospasm.
- Lower back pain due to ischemic muscle pain or vasospasm rather than kidney pain from developing renal failure.
- Severe reactions often occur in surgical patients under anesthesia who are unable to give any warning signs.

See Table 1-175.

ETIOLOGY

Most fatal hemolytic reactions are caused by clerical errors and mislabeled specimens.

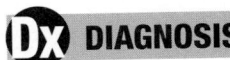 **DIAGNOSIS**

DIFFERENTIAL DIAGNOSIS

- Bacterial contamination of blood
- Hemoglobinopathies

WORKUP

The transfusion must be stopped immediately. The blood bank must be notified, and the donor transfusion bag must be returned to the blood bank along with a freshly drawn posttransfusion specimen.

LABORATORY TESTS

- Positive Coombs test, elevated BUN, creatinine, LDH bilirubin (especially indirect bilirubin).
- Analyze urine for hemoglobinuria (wine-colored urine), observe plasma for hemoglobinemia (pink plasma).
- Decreased hematocrit and serum haptoglobin (haptoglobin low to 0 mg/dl).
- The direct antiglobulin test (DAT) usually becomes positive in an immune hemolytic reaction (if tested before all the incompatible RBCs are destroyed). Preparation of an antibody eluate is necessary to identify the offending antibody.
- Monitor coagulation status (PT, aPTT, fibrinogen).

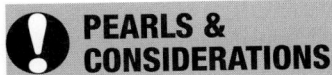 **TREATMENT**

NONPHARMACOLOGIC THERAPY

- Stop transfusion immediately. Test anticoagulated blood from the recipient for the presence of free hemoglobin in the plasma.
- Monitor vital signs closely, and maintain IV access and adequate airway.

ACUTE GENERAL Rx

- Vigorous IV hydration (0.9% NaCl or some other suitable crystalloid solution) to maintain urine flow at >100 ml/hr until hypotension is corrected and hemoglobinuria clears. IV furosemide may be necessary to maintain adequate renal flow.
- The addition of mannitol may prevent renal damage (controversial). Mannitol, if chosen, must be used with caution, if acute tubular necrosis occurs before mannitol infusion, pulmonary edema may occur as a result of the acute increase in intravascular volume secondary to fluid expansion.
- Monitor for the presence of disseminated intravascular coagulation. PT, aPTT, and fibrinogen levels should be closely monitored.
- If sepsis is suspected, culture as appropriate.

DISPOSITION

Mortality rate exceeds 50% in severe transfusion reactions.

PEARLS & CONSIDERATIONS

COMMENTS

Hemolysis caused by minor antigen systems is generally less severe and may be delayed 5 to 10 days after transfusion.

SUGGESTED READING
available at www.expertconsult.com

AUTHOR: **FRED F. FERRI, M.D.**

TABLE 1-175 Signs and Symptoms of Acute Adverse Reactions to Blood Transfusion

Reaction	Fever	Chills/ Rigors	Nausea/ Vomiting	Chest Discomfort/ Pain	Facial Flushing	Wheezing/ Dyspnea	Back/ Lumbar Pain	Discomfort at Infusion Site	Hypotension
Acute hemolytic	X	X	X	X	X	X	X	X	X
Febrile nonhemolytic	X	X		X	X				
Nonimmune hemolysis									
Acute lung injury	X			X		X			X
Allergic									
Massive transfusion complications									
Anaphylaxis	X	X	X	X	X	X	X	X	X
Passive cytokine infusion	X	X	X			X			
Hypervolemia						X			
Bacterial sepsis	X	X	X				X	X	X
Air embolus				X		X			

From Goldman L, Bennett JC (eds): *Cecil textbook of medicine*, ed 22, Philadelphia, 2004, WB Saunders.

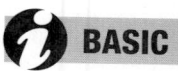 **BASIC INFORMATION**

DEFINITION

Transient ischemic attack (TIA) is a transient episode of neurologic dysfunction caused by focal brain, spinal cord, or retinal ischemia without permanent tissue damage. TIA symptoms typically resolve within 60 min and almost always within 24 hr.

SYNONYMS

TIA
Amaurosis fugax
"Mini-stroke"
Pre-stroke

ICD-9CM CODES
435.9 Unspecified transient cerebral ischemia

EPIDEMIOLOGY & DEMOGRAPHICS

INCIDENCE: 49 to 83 cases per 100,000 persons annually
PEAK INCIDENCE: After age 60 yr
PREVALENCE: 200,000 to 500,000 persons in the United States
PREDOMINANT SEX AND RACE: Males > females; African American > Caucasian
RISK FACTORS: Same as for ischemic stroke

PHYSICAL FINDINGS & CLINICAL PRESENTATION

Transient ischemic attacks often present with ipsilateral transient monocular blindness (amaurosis fugax), contralateral numbness or weakness, contralateral homonymous hemianopsia, and/or aphasia.

ETIOLOGY

Embolic (cardioembolism in 10% to 15%), large vessel atherothrombotic disease (20% to 25%), lacunar disease, hypoperfusion, hypercoagulable state, arteritis

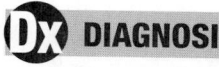 **DIAGNOSIS**

DIFFERENTIAL DIAGNOSIS

Seizures, hypoglycemia, complicated migraine, intracranial hemorrhage, mass lesion, vestibular disease, Bell's palsy, meningitis, multiple sclerosis, conversion disorder, subdural hematoma, brain abscess, cervical or lumbar spine disease

WORKUP

Given the high risk of stroke within the first 48 hr following TIA (up to 10%), hospital admission for workup is advised.

LABORATORY TESTS

Complete blood count, basic metabolic panel, prothrombin time, activated partial thromboplastin time, sedimentation rate, fasting lipid panel, serum glucose and hemoglobin A_{1c} (to detect latent diabetes mellitus)

IMAGING STUDIES

- CT scan should be obtained to exclude hemorrhage unless MRI with diffusion weighting is immediately available.
- Imaging of the vessels should be obtained via magnetic resonance angiography (MRA), computed tomography angiography (CTA), or carotid Dopplers/transcranial Dopplers (CD/TCD).
  - If symptoms are referable to the posterior circulation, MRA or CTA should be obtained in lieu of CD/TCD.
  - Transthoracic echocardiogram should be obtained.
    An echocardiogram with bubble should be obtained in all patients younger than 50 yr with TIA symptoms.
- Electrocardiogram should be obtained to exclude the presence of arrhythmias, namely atrial fibrillation.
- At least 24 hr of heart rhythm monitoring should be accomplished to screen for arrhythmia.

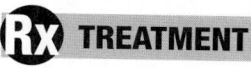 **TREATMENT**

NONPHARMACOLOGIC THERAPY

- Carotid endarterectomy or carotid stenting should be considered for patients found to have carotid stenosis as the cause for TIA. Please refer to "Carotid Stenosis" chapter for more information.
- Intracranial angioplasty and stenting may be considered in cases of symptomatic intracranial atherosclerosis. Clinical trials are ongoing.

ACUTE GENERAL Rx

- In the absence of contraindications, patients who are identified to have atrial fibrillation should be considered for anticoagulation with intravenous heparin (or therapeutic lovenox) along with warfarin until the prothrombin time is between 2.0 and 3.0.
- Although no compelling evidence exist for the use of heparin in the acute treatment of TIAs, patients who develop recurrent symptoms within the same vascular territory that increase in duration, severity, and/or frequency (crescendo TIA/stuttering TIA) may benefit from its use.

CHRONIC Rx

- Chronic therapy should be aimed at modifying the four major risk factors: blood pressure control, control of dyslipidemia, control of blood sugars, and smoking cessation.
- Antiplatelet therapy should be used to reduce the risk of recurrent TIAs or subsequent stroke. Three antiplatelet agents are commonly used in stroke prevention: aspirin, aspirin/dipyridimole, and clopidigrel. All are reasonable choices but practitioners should consider their individual patient's comorbidities when selecting an antiplatelet agent.
- Dose-adjusted warfarin (INR 2.0 to 3.0) is indicated for prevention of future strokes in atrial fibrillation patients. Dabigatran, a direct thrombin inhibitor, is an emerging alternative treatment to warfarin for stroke prevention in atrial fibrillation.

DISPOSITION

Disposition and prognosis depend on the duration of symptoms and underlying etiology.

REFERRAL

All patients that have symptoms of TIA should be referred to a neurologist for further evaluation.

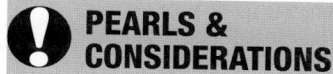 **PEARLS & CONSIDERATIONS**

Despite complete symptom resolution, 20% to 50% of patients with TIA have evidence of acute tissue infarction on MRI.

PREVENTION

Prevention of carotid stenosis should be guided at pursuing a healthy lifestyle and management of risk factors.

PATIENT/FAMILY EDUCATION

Patients should be counseled on the early signs of stroke symptoms and instructed to promptly seek medical attention if they develop symptoms concerning for stroke. Patients should be encouraged to pursue a healthy lifestyle to include exercise and smoking cessation. In addition, patients should take an active role in controlling blood pressure and blood glucose. Further educational materials can be found online at http//www.strokecenter.org/education.

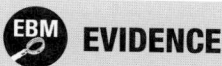 **EVIDENCE**

available at www.expertconsult.com

SUGGESTED READINGS

available at www.expertconsult.com

AUTHOR: **JOSEPH R. OWENS, M.D.**

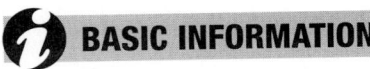

BASIC INFORMATION

DEFINITION

Trichinosis is an infection by one of various species of *Trichinella*.

SYNONYMS

Trichinella spiralis muscle infection

ICD-9CM CODES
124 Trichinosis

EPIDEMIOLOGY & DEMOGRAPHICS

INCIDENCE (IN U.S.): <100 cases/yr
GENETICS: Congenital infection:
- Abrupt delivery of stillbirths in infected pregnant women
- Vertical infection of the fetus

PHYSICAL FINDINGS & CLINICAL PRESENTATION

- Symptoms:
  1. May vary widely depending on the time from ingestion of contaminated meat and on worm burden
  2. Most people asymptomatic
- Enteral phase:
  1. Correlates with penetration of ingested larvae into the intestinal mucosa
  2. May last from 2 to 6 wk
  3. Mild, transient diarrhea and nausea
  4. Abdominal pain
  5. Diarrhea or constipation
  6. Vomiting
  7. Malaise
  8. Low-grade fevers
- Migratory or parenteral phase:
  1. In the intestine, maturation and mating
  2. Newborn larvae
     a. Penetrate into lymphatic and blood vessels
     b. Migrate to muscles, where they penetrate into muscle cells, enlarge, coil, and develop a cyst wall
  3. Patients may present with:
     a. Fever
     b. Myalgias
     c. Periorbital or facial edema
     d. Headache
     e. Skin rash
     f. Other symptoms caused by the penetration of tissues by the newborn migrating larvae
  4. Peak in symptoms 2 to 3 wk after infection, then slowly subside
- Severe complications:
  1. Brain damage by granulomatous inflammation or occlusion of arteries
  2. Cardiac involvement
  3. Can lead to death

ETIOLOGY

- The nematode responsible for this illness is an obligate intracellular parasite belonging to the genus *Trichinella*.
- It is one of the most ubiquitous parasites in the world and may be found in virtually all warm-blooded animals.
- Infection in humans occurs by the ingestion of contaminated animal meat that is raw or partially cooked and contains viable cysts.
- Most cases are now related to the consumption of poorly processed pork or wild game (bear, wild boar, cougar, and walrus).

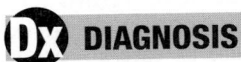

DIAGNOSIS

DIFFERENTIAL DIAGNOSIS

- Different presentations have different differential diagnoses.
- Early illness may resemble gastroenteritis.

- Later symptoms may be confused with:
  1. Measles
  2. Dermatomyositis
  3. Glomerulonephritis

WORKUP

- Antibody assay of serum is usually positive by approximately 2 wk after infection.
- Muscle biopsy is used to detect the larva in muscle tissue if diagnosis unclear; best done by placing the tissue between two slides.

LABORATORY TESTS

- CBC: leukocytosis with prominent eosinophilia
- ESR: usually normal
- Elevation of muscle enzymes common (i.e., CPK, aldolase)

IMAGING STUDIES

Soft-tissue radiographs may show calcified cyst walls.

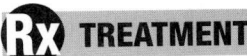

TREATMENT

NONPHARMACOLOGIC THERAPY

Bed rest for myalgias

ACUTE GENERAL Rx

- Albendazole 400 mg PO for 1 to 2 wk.
- Salicylates to decrease muscle discomfort.
- Steroids in critically ill patients.
- Mebendazole 200 mg PO tid for 3 days, followed by mebendazole 400 mg PO tid, is an alternative to albendazole.

DISPOSITION

- Most symptoms subside over time.
- Reports of long-term sequelae:
  1. Myalgias
  2. Headaches
- Occasionally, death occurs.

REFERRAL

Diagnosis uncertain

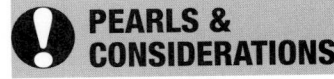

COMMENTS

- Prevention by thorough cooking of meats.
- Inadequate to smoke, cure, or dry meats.
- Freezing at specified temperatures kills *T. spiralis* larvae in pork.
- *T. nativa* is a freeze-resistant species that remains viable after freezing, even for months or years; it has been associated with infection from ingestion of bear meat.

SUGGESTED READINGS

available at www.expertconsult.com

AUTHORS: **GLENN G. FORT, M.D., M.P.H.,** and **DENNIS J. MIKOLICH, M.D.**

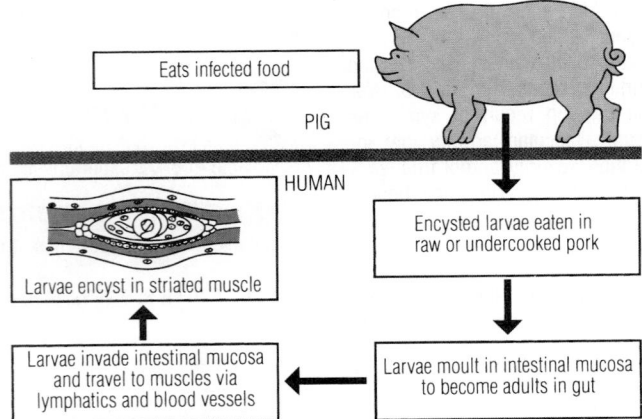

FIGURE 1-383 Lifecycle of *Trichinella spiralis*. (Souhami RL, Moxham J: *Textbook of medicine*, ed 4, London, 2002, Churchill Livingstone.)

Eats infected food

PIG

HUMAN

Encysted larvae eaten in raw or undercooked pork

Larvae encyst in striated muscle

Larvae invade intestinal mucosa and travel to muscles via lymphatics and blood vessels

Larvae moult in intestinal mucosa to become adults in gut

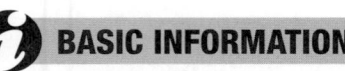

BASIC INFORMATION

DEFINITION

Tricuspid regurgitation (TR) refers to an abnormal flow of blood from the right ventricle to the right atrium (Fig. 1-384).

SYNONYMS

Tricuspid insufficiency
Tricuspid incompetence

ICD-9CM CODES
397.0 Diseases of the tricuspid valve
424.2 Tricuspid valve disorders, specified as non-rheumatic

EPIDEMIOLOGY & DEMOGRAPHICS

- In the adult population, TR is usually functional rather than structural.
- In adolescents and young adults, most cases of TR are the result of congenital cardiac abnormalities.
- In patients with rheumatic heart disease, TR rarely occurs alone; it is usually associated with mitral or aortic valve disease.
- A small degree (i.e., trace to mild) of TR is present in approximately 70% of normal adults. On echocardiography, this "normal" degree of regurgitation is localized to a small region adjacent to valve closure, it often does not extend throughout systole, and it has a low signal strength.

PHYSICAL FINDINGS & CLINICAL PRESENTATION

- Isolated TR can cause nonspecific symptoms (e.g., exercise intolerance).
- Signs and symptoms in the presence of TR are usually the result of an underlying cause.
- Signs and symptoms may be caused by accompanying right-sided heart failure (e.g., jugular venous distension, peripheral edema, ascites, hepatomegaly, right-sided S3).
- A lower-left parasternal holosystolic murmur may be found; the murmur becomes louder during inspiration (Carvallo's sign) and during maneuvers that increase venous return.
- Prominent V waves in the jugular venous waveform can occur (see Fig. 1-384).
- Severe TR may produce systolic propulsion of the eyeballs, pulsatile varicose veins, a venous systolic thrill and murmur in the neck, a mid-diastolic murmur in severe regurgitation, and systolic hepatic pulsation.
- Atrial fibrillation or flutter is common as a result of right atrial enlargement.

ETIOLOGY

- Tricuspid valve dysfunction can occur with structurally normal (functional TR) or abnormal valves (structural TR).
- Functional TR involves conditions that lead to the dilation of the tricuspid annulus or right ventricular enlargement, including the following:
  - Any cause of pulmonary hypertension (e.g., chronic obstructive pulmonary disease, pulmonary embolism, restrictive lung disease, collagen vascular disease, primary pulmonary hypertension)
  - Left-sided heart failure that leads to right-sided heart failure
  - Dilated cardiomyopathy
  - Right ventricular infarction
- Structural TR involves conditions directly affect the tricuspid valve apparatus, including the following:
  - Rheumatic valvulitis
  - Congenital conditions (e.g., Ebstein's anomaly, tricuspid atresia)
  - Endocarditis, either bacterial (particularly related to intravenous drug use) or marantic (e.g., systemic lupus erythematosus, rheumatoid arthritis)
  - Tricuspid valve prolapse or chordae rupture
  - Carcinoid syndrome
  - Marfan's syndrome
  - Iatrogenic damage to the valve (e.g., pacemaker, implantable cardioverter defibrillator, myocardial biopsy, anorectic drugs)
  - External trauma (e.g., deceleration injury)
  - Right atrial myxoma
  - Collagen vascular diseases
  - Radiation injury

DIAGNOSIS

The diagnosis of TR is made noninvasively by physical examination and imaging techniques (e.g., echocardiography) and invasively by right-sided heart catheterization in selected cases.

DIFFERENTIAL DIAGNOSIS

On the basis of heart auscultation, the diagnosis of TR may be confused with other causes of systolic murmurs, such as mitral regurgitation, aortic stenosis, pulmonary stenosis, ventricular septal defect, and hypertrophic cardiomyopathy.

WORKUP

Any patient suspected of having significant TR should undergo the following:
- Chest x-ray
- ECG
- Echocardiogram (confirmatory)
- Right-sided cardiac heart catheterization (in selected cases)

LABORATORY TESTS

ECG may show evidence of the following:
- Right atrial enlargement (e.g., P-wave amplitude in leads II or III or aVF of >2.5 mV)
- Right ventricular enlargement or hypertrophy (e.g., R wave > S wave in lead V_1)
- Right axis deviation of >100 degrees
- Atrial fibrillation

IMAGING STUDIES

- A chest x-ray may show the following:
  - Evidence of chronic obstructive pulmonary disease (e.g., flattened diaphragms, barrel chest, dilated pulmonary arteries, increased retrosternal air space) or restrictive lung disease
  - Enlarged right atrium
  - Enlarged right ventricle
- An echocardiogram (either transthoracic or transesophageal) will do the following:
  - Assess tricuspid valve structure and motion, measure annular size, and identify other cardiac abnormalities
  - Estimate the severity of TR
  - Estimate the pulmonary artery pressure
  - Exclude vegetation, mass, or prolapse
  - Assess left and right ventricular function
- Right-sided cardiac heart catheterization shows the following:
  - Elevated right atrial and right ventricular systolic and end-diastolic pressures
  - Large V waves

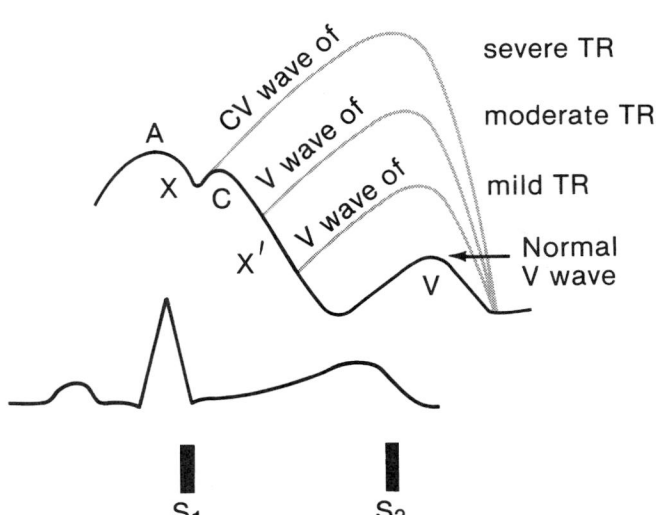

FIGURE 1-384 The jugular venous pulse in tricuspid regurgitation. The jugular venous pulse wave normally drops during ventricular systole. As tricuspid regurgitation becomes more severe, the CV wave becomes more obvious during ventricular systole. (From Conn R: *Current diagnosis,* ed 9, Philadelphia, 1997, WB Saunders.)

Diseases and Disorders

Rx TREATMENT

The treatment of TR is usually directed at the underlying cause.

NONPHARMACOLOGIC THERAPY

Oxygen therapy is beneficial for patients with functional TR caused by underlying pulmonary hypertension provoked by alveolar hypoxia.

ACUTE GENERAL Rx

- Functional TR caused by left-sided heart failure is treated in the standard way with preload reduction, afterload reduction, or inotropic therapy (see "Congestive Heart Failure").
- The reversal of pulmonary hypertension with vasodilators or pulmonary thromboendarterectomy has been shown to reverse functional TR.
- Structural TR treatment depends on the underlying cause of heart disease.

CHRONIC Rx

- The 2006 American College of Cardiology/American Heart Association Guidelines Pertaining to the Surgical Management of Tricuspid Valve Disease/Regurgitation include the following:
  - Class I: Tricuspid valve repair is beneficial for severe TR in patients with mitral valve (MV) disease that requires MV surgery. **B**
  - Class IIa: Tricuspid valve replacement or annuloplasty is reasonable for a symptomatic patient with severe primary TR and for severe TR as a result of diseased or abnormal tricuspid valve leaflets that are not amenable to annuloplasty or repair. **C**
  - Class IIb: Tricuspid annuloplasty may be considered for less-than-severe TR in patients who are undergoing MV surgery when there is pulmonary hypertension or tricuspid annular dilatation (usually >21 mm/m² body surface area [BSA]). **C**
  - Class III: Tricuspid valve replacement or annuloplasty is not indicated for asymptomatic patients with TR whose pulmonary artery pressure is <60 mm Hg in the presence of a normal MV or for those with mild TR. **C**
- Patients with severe TR of any cause have poor long-term outcomes as a result of right ventricular dysfunction or systemic venous congestion.
- During recent years, annuloplasty has become an established surgical approach to significant TR. A recent study showed that tricuspid valve (TV) repair with an annuloplasty ring results in improved long-term outcomes.
- When the valve leaflets themselves are diseased, abnormal, or destroyed, valve replacement with a low-profile mechanical valve or bioprosthesis is often necessary.
- A biologic prosthesis is preferred because of the high rate of thromboembolic complications that occur with mechanical prostheses in the tricuspid position.

DISPOSITION

- Regardless of the cause, a greater-than-mild degree of TR is associated with decreased survival.
- Clinically insignificant TR can be detected by color Doppler imaging in many normal people. This is not an indication for either routine follow-up or prophylaxis against bacterial endocarditis.
- Isolated TR should not pose a significant problem during pregnancy, although greater care may be necessary for protection from diuretic-induced hypoperfusion.
- Isolated TR with normal right ventricular function does not preclude an individual's involvement in competitive sports.

REFERRAL

For patients with significant symptomatic TR, a cardiology consultation is recommended.

! PEARLS & CONSIDERATIONS

- TR that results from tricuspid valve prolapse is often associated with concurrent MV prolapse.
- Secondary TR commonly occurs in combination with left-sided valvular heart disease. It often does not improve, despite correction of the left-sided valve dysfunction.
- Functional tricuspid insufficiency, if left uncorrected, carries serious long-term consequences.

COMMENTS

- Antibiotic prophylaxis for dental, gastrointestinal, or genitourinary procedures is no longer recommended for patients with only structural tricuspid valve abnormalities.
- Tricuspid annuloplasty at the time of MV surgery results in improved functional capacity without any increase in perioperative morbidity or mortality.
- During TR of the donor heart after cardiac transplantation, tricuspid valve replacement with a biologic prosthesis is a safe, durable, and effective method of treating TR after transplantation. This allows for future endomyocardial biopsies to be performed. Mechanical valves should be avoided.

EBM EVIDENCE

available at www.expertconsult.com

SUGGESTED READINGS
available at www.expertconsult.com

AUTHORS: **VIKRAM BEHERA, M.D.,** and **GAURAV CHOUDHARY, M.D.**

BASIC INFORMATION

DEFINITION

Tricuspid stenosis (TS) is an uncommon valvular pathology that is caused by the narrowing of the tricuspid valve orifice, which results in the restriction of right atrial emptying. TS is most often rheumatic in origin, and it often presents with a combination of regurgitation and stenosis.

SYNONYMS

Tricuspid valve stenosis
TS

ICD-9CM CODES
397.0 Disease of the tricuspid valve

EPIDEMIOLOGY & DEMOGRAPHICS

- TS is most commonly caused by rheumatic heart disease, and it almost always occurs with associated mitral or aortic valve disease.
- Antibiotic therapy has made rheumatic heart disease and TS in the U.S. very rare.
- TS is present at autopsy in 15% of patients with rheumatic heart disease, but it is clinically significant in only 5%.

PHYSICAL FINDINGS & CLINICAL PRESENTATION

- Obstruction to tricuspid flow limits cardiac output.
- Symptoms and physical examination findings usually depend on the presence and severity of concomitant mitral or aortic valve disease.
- Symptoms of right heart failure include fatigue, right upper quadrant abdominal pain (from hepatic congestion), ascites, hepatomegaly, and peripheral edema.
- Jugular venous distention, a prominent a wave, and a palpable hepatic pulsation are noted during the sinus rhythm.
- A right atrial pulsation may be palpated to the right of the sternum, and a diastolic thrill that increases with inspiration may be felt over the left sternal edge.
- An opening snap and a low-frequency diastolic murmur are best heard along the left sternal border of the fourth intercostal space. These are augmented by inspiration (i.e., Carvallo's sign), leg raises, isotonic exercise, and squatting.

ETIOLOGY

- Rheumatic heart disease results in the scarring of the valve leaflets, the shortening of the chordae tendineae, and the fusion of the commissures, thereby leading to the immobility of the valve leaflets and the narrowing of the tricuspid valve orifice.
- Other causes are congenital, infectious (e.g., endocarditis), metabolic, and enzymatic abnormalities (e.g., carcinoid syndrome, Whipple's disease, Fabry's disease); right atrial or metastatic tumors; and, rarely, scarring and adhesions as a result of complications of pacemaker placement.

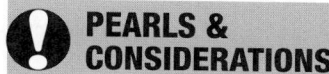

DIAGNOSIS

DIFFERENTIAL DIAGNOSIS

- Congenital tricuspid atresia
- Right heart diastolic dysfunction: endomyocardial fibrosis or constrictive pericarditis
- Extrinsic compression of the right ventricle: severe pectum excavatum, massive ascites, pleural effusion, pericardial effusion, or tumor
- Obstruction of right atrial emptying: right atrial myxoma, metastatic tumor, right atrial thrombi, or tricuspid valve vegetation (particularly in association with a permanent pacemaker lead)

WORKUP

- Echocardiography is the diagnostic test of choice to evaluate the tricuspid valve.
- ECG is recommended to look for atrial arrhythmias, atrial fibrillation, or atrial flutter as a result of an enlarged right atrium.
- Chest x-ray.
- Right heart catheterization is an option when echocardiography cannot be used to make a definitive diagnosis.

IMAGING STUDIES

- Echocardiography reveals the thickening and shortening of the tricuspid valve leaflets, the restriction of the movement of the leaflets and the leaflet tips, a reduction in the diameter of the annulus, and diastolic doming of the valve. Evidence of right atrial enlargement is present in most cases.
- Doppler echocardiography or cardiac catheterization demonstrates a reduced tricuspid valve area (severe when <1 cm^2) and a diastolic pressure gradient across the tricuspid valve (normal gradient, <1 mm Hg).
- Chest radiography may reveal an enlarged right atrium and a reduced pulmonary blood volume.

TREATMENT

NONPHARMACOLOGIC THERAPY

Salt and fluid restriction are essential to decrease peripheral edema.

ACUTE GENERAL Rx

- Assess and treat the underlying cause of the valvular pathology.
- Treat bacterial endocarditis with antibiotics.
- Manage right atrium volume overload with diuretics.
- Prescribe rate-controlling atrioventricular nodal blockers and anticoagulants, especially for patients with atrial arrhythmia.

CHRONIC Rx

- Symptoms of systemic venous hypertension and congestion can be controlled with diuretics and angiotensin-converting inhibitors or angiotensin receptor antagonists.
- Balloon valvuloplasty or dilation of the stenosed tricuspid valve has been shows to be effective. Tricuspid regurgitation that is more than mild is generally considered a contraindication to valvotomy. Tumor masses, vegetations, and thrombi are also contraindications to valvotomy.
- Surgery for TS is usually recommended when the valve is not treatable by balloon valvuloplasty and the valve area is <2 cm^2 with a mean diastolic gradient across the tricuspid valve of >5 mm Hg.
- Isolated tricuspid valve replacement surgery almost never occurs. It is typically performed in the setting of concomitant mitral or aortic valve surgery.
- Surgical procedures for TS include commissurotomy and tricuspid valve replacement.

DISPOSITION

The natural course of severe TS is not well known.

REFERRAL

TS may be difficult to diagnose, so consultation with a cardiologist is recommended.

PEARLS & CONSIDERATIONS

- Rheumatic heart disease accounts for $>90\%$ of stenotic tricuspid valves.
- Rheumatic TS almost always occurs in association with mitral valve disease and sometimes with aortic valve disease.
- The majority of cases present with tricuspid regurgitation or a combination of regurgitation and stenosis.

COMMENTS

Tricuspid valve replacement carries a 30-day operative morbidity and mortality rate of 5% to 7% in addition to a high risk of right heart thrombus formation. Therefore, surgical procedures are reserved for patients who are not candidates for balloon dilation techniques. Unlike patients with mitral stenosis, patients with TS typically do not report dyspnea, orthopnea, or paroxysmal nocturnal dyspnea.

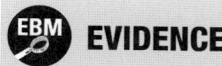 EVIDENCE

available at www.expertconsult.com

SUGGESTED READINGS
available at www.expertconsult.com

AUTHORS: **VIKRAM BEHERA, M.D.,** and **GAURAV CHOUDHARY, M.D.**

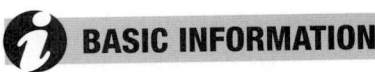

BASIC INFORMATION

DEFINITION

Tricyclic antidepressants (TCAs) are secondary or tertiary amines that have variable abilities to inhibit reuptake of neurotransmitters (norepinephrine, dopamine, and serotonin) and to be anticholinergic, antihistaminic, and sedating. These properties are important to consider when prescribing these agents and when managing an intentional or accidental overdose.

SYNONYMS

Tricyclic antidepressant intoxication or poisoning
TCA OD

ICD-9CM CODES
969.0

EPIDEMIOLOGY & DEMOGRAPHICS

- TCAs are one of the most common cause of death from prescription drug overdose in the U.S.
- Available TCAs: amitriptyline, imipramine, desipramine, nortriptyline, doxepin, amoxapine, clomipramine, protriptyline, and others.

PHYSICAL FINDINGS & CLINICAL PRESENTATION

Cardiovascular:
- Intraventricular conduction delay (QRS prolongation)
- Sinus tachycardia
- Atrioventricular block
- Prolongation of the QT interval
- Ventricular tachycardia
- Wide complex tachycardia without P waves
- Refractory hypotension (the most common cause of death from TCA overdose)
- Late arrhythmias or sudden death (in addition to the arrhythmias, which occur during the first 24 to 48 hr; late problems can occur up to 5 days after the overdose)
- Fig. 1-385 illustrates a common ECG rhythm abnormality in tricyclic overdose

Central nervous system:
- Coma
- Delirium
- Myoclonus
- Seizures

Other:
- Hyperthermia
- Ileus
- Urinary retention

- Pulmonary complications (e.g., aspiration pneumonitis)
- Life-threatening overdose exists with the ingestion of more than 1 g of a TCA. Among patients who reach a hospital, most deaths occur within the first 24 hr; lack of initial symptoms can be deceptive.

ETIOLOGY & PATHOGENESIS

- Mechanisms of tricyclic antidepressant cardiovascular toxicity (Table 1-176)
- CNS toxicity:
  1. Cholinergic blockade is believed to cause hyperthermia, ileus, urinary retention, pupillary dilation, delirium, and coma.
  2. The mechanism of myoclonus and seizures is not fully understood.

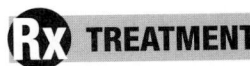

DIAGNOSIS

DIFFERENTIAL DIAGNOSIS

Cardiotoxicity from TCA can be confused with intoxication by drugs that cause QRS prolongation. These include class Ia antiarrhythmic agents (disopyramide, procainamide, quinidine), class Ic antiarrhythmic agents (encainide, flecainide, propafenone), cocaine, propranolol, quinine, chloroquine, neuroleptics, propoxyphene, and digoxin. Other causes of QRS prolongation include hyperkalemia, ischemic heart disease, cardiomyopathy, and cardiac conduction system dysfunction.

WORKUP

- Clinical presentation
- Knowledge of the overdose
- Serum drug levels (TCA concentration >1 mcg/ml is life threatening; TCA concentration >3 mcg/ml is often fatal)
- Baseline complete blood count, prothrombin time, blood urea nitrogen, creatinine, and electrolytes

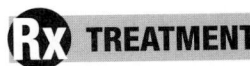

TREATMENT

ACUTE GENERAL Rx

1. Initial measures:
   - Hospitalization with cardiac monitoring as well as monitoring of vital signs and temperature

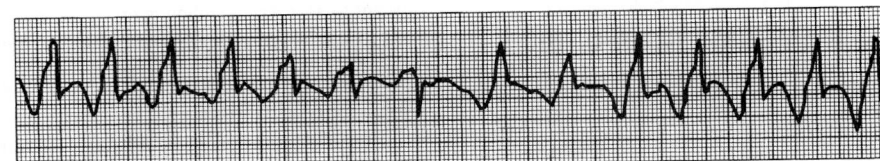

FIGURE 1-385 Rhythm ECG in tricyclic overdose. (Souhami RL, Moxham J: *Textbook of medicine,* ed 4, London, 2002, Churchill Livingstone.)

TABLE 1-176 Mechanism of Tricyclic Antidepressant Cardiovascular Toxicity

Toxic Effect	Mechanism
Conduction Delays, Arrhythmias	
QRS prolongation atrioventricular block	Cardiac sodium channel → slowed depolarization in atrioventricular node, His-Purkinje fibers, and ventricular myocardium
Sinus tachycardia	Cholinergic blockade, inhibition of norepinephrine reuptake
Ventricular tachycardia	
Monomorphic	Cardiac sodium channel inhibition → reentry
Torsades de pointes	Cardiac potassium channel inhibition → prolonged repolarization
Ventricular bradycardia	Impaired cardiac automaticity
Hypotension	
Vasodilation	Vascular alpha-adrenergic receptor blockade
Decreased cardiac contractility	Cardiac sodium channel inhibition → impaired excitation-contraction coupling

- Initiate IV access
- Administer activated charcoal with sorbitol
- Large-bore tube gastric lavage is of unproven benefit
- Ipecac is contraindicated
- 12-Lead ECG
- If no evidence of cardiotoxicity has been noted during the first 6 hr of observation, further monitoring is not necessary; if there is evidence of cardiotoxicity, monitoring should continue for 24 hr after all signs of toxicity have resolved
2. See Table 1-177 for treatment of specific complications of TCA toxicity.
3. When the patient is medically stable, psychiatric evaluation should be obtained.

SUGGESTED READING
available at www.expertconsult.com

AUTHOR: **FRED F. FERRI, M.D.**

TABLE 1-177 Treatment of Complications of Tricyclic Antidepressant Toxicity

Toxic Effect	Treatment
Cardiovascular	
QRS prolongation	Hypertonic NaHCO$_3$ if QRS prolongation is marked or progressing; not clear if treatment is needed in the absence of hypotension or arrhythmias
Hypotension	Intravascular volume expansion, NaHCO$_3$ Vasopressors (norepinephrine) or inotropic agents (dopamine) Correct hyperthermia, acidosis, seizures Consider mechanical support
Ventricular tachycardia	NaHCO$_3$, lidocaine, overdrive, pacing Correct hypotension, hypothermia, acidosis, seizures
Torsades de pointes	Overdrive, pacing
Ventricular bradycardia	Chronotropic agent (epinephrine), pacemaker
Sinus tachycardia	Treatment rarely needed
Atrioventricular block type II second or third degree	Pacemaker
Hypertension	Rapidly titratable antihypertensive agent (nitroprusside)
Central Nervous System	
Delirium	Restraints, benzodiazepine Neuromuscular blockade for hyperthermia, acidosis
Seizures	Benzodiazepine Neuromuscular blockade for hyperthermia, acidosis
Coma	Intubation, ventilation if needed
Other	
Hyperthermia	Control seizures, agitation Cooling measures
Acidosis	NaHCO$_3$ Correct hypotension, hypoventilation

Diseases and Disorders

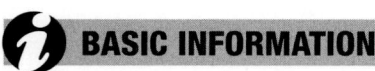

DEFINITION

Intense, usually unilateral, paroxysmal, stabbing pain in the distribution of the fifth cranial nerve

SYNONYMS

Tic douloureux ("painful tics/spasms")

ICD-9CM CODES
350.1 Trigeminal neuralgia

EPIDEMIOLOGY & DEMOGRAPHICS

INCIDENCE: 4 per 100,000
PEAK INCIDENCE: Incidence increases with age, peaks at 67 yr
PREVALENCE: 155 in 1 million
PREDOMINANT SEX AND AGE: Male to female ratio is 1:1.5
RISK FACTORS: Most cases are idiopathic; age and multiple sclerosis are risk factors

PHYSICAL FINDINGS & CLINICAL PRESENTATION

- Patients present with unilateral facial pain that is usually described as shock-like, stabbing, or electric (Fig. 1-386).
- In severe cases, facial spasms can accompany the pain.
- The pain seldom lasts more than a few seconds to a minute.
- There is usually no sensory or motor loss.

ETIOLOGY

- Idiopathic or "classic": cause usually unknown, likely an aberrant artery or vein compressing cranial nerve V at or near the pons
- Secondary: compression by lesions that are not vessels (multiple sclerosis, meningioma, cysts, etc.)

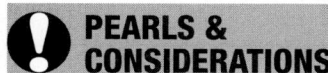 **DIAGNOSIS**

DIFFERENTIAL DIAGNOSIS

- Glossopharyngeal neuralgia
- Temporomandibular joint pain
- Unilateral, neuralgiform headache
- Dental pain

WORKUP

Trigeminal neuralgia is a clinical diagnosis (see above)

IMAGING STUDIES

Neuroimaging (MRI/magnetic resonance angiogram [MRA]) should be considered in young patient with atypical symptoms (sensory loss, bilateral symptoms)

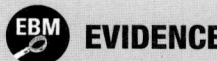 **TREATMENT**

NONPHARMACOLOGIC THERAPY

Patients with refractory pain eventually need secondary intervention, such as nerve root de-

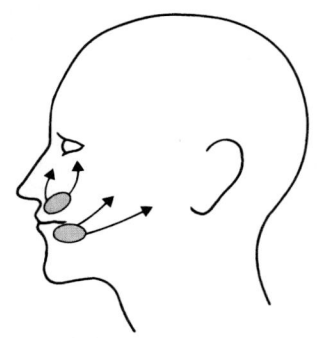

FIGURE 1-386 Trigeminal neuralgia. The two most common sites of origin and radiation of pain are shown: mouth-ear and nose-orbit. Pain usually starts in the region of the encircled area and radiates in the directions shown. (From Souhami RL, Moxham J: *Textbook of medicine,* ed 4, London, 2002, Churchill Livingstone.)

compression, chemical ablation, or gamma knife radiosurgery.

CHRONIC Rx

- Carbamazepine 100 to 200 mg bid is the recommended initial treatment. This can be titrated to pain relief by 200 mg daily to a maximum of 1200 mg divided bid.
- Oxcarbazepine can be used if carbamazepine is not tolerated due to side effects. Others medications include baclofen, lamotrigine, and phenytoin.

DISPOSITION

Most patients are very responsive to pharmacologic treatment. Spontaneous remission is possible.

REFERRAL

Referral to a neurologist is appropriate if uncertain about diagnosis or refractory to conservative management.

PEARLS & CONSIDERATIONS

In secondary disease, no medications have been established for treatment. Initial therapy should address underlying secondary causes.

EVIDENCE

available at www.expertconsult.com

SUGGESTED READINGS
available at www.expertconsult.com

AUTHOR: **WILLIAM F. DOTSON II, M.D.**

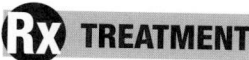

BASIC INFORMATION

DEFINITION

Trigger finger, or digital stenosing tenosynovitis, refers to an inflammatory process of the digital flexor tendon sheath.

SYNONYMS   Digital stenosing tenosynovitis

ICD-9CM CODES
727.03 Trigger finger (acquired)

EPIDEMIOLOGY & DEMOGRAPHICS

- Trigger finger can be found in all age groups but is commonly found in patients >45 yr
- More frequently affects females (4:1)
- Repetitive use occupational risk groups: meat cutters, seamstress, tailors, and dentists
- In adults, the middle finger is most often affected (Fig. 1-387)
- In children, the thumb is most often affected

PHYSICAL FINDINGS & CLINICAL PRESENTATION

- Tenosynovitis of the flexor tendon always precedes the mechanical symptoms of triggering
- Painful triggering or snapping with flexion of the affected digit
- Locking or loss of active digital extension is the most common symptom
- The digit is usually fixed in flexion (trapped or incarcerated)
- Usually affects one digit
- If more digits are involved, a systemic cause is most likely present (e.g., diabetes, rheumatoid arthritis)

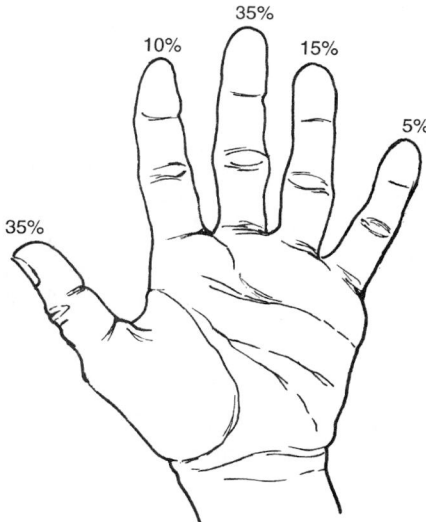

FIGURE 1-387 Trigger finger. Frequency of trigger finger according to digit in adults. In children, virtually all cases occur in the thumb. (From Canoso J: *Rheumatology in primary care,* Philadelphia, 1997, WB Saunders.)

- A palpable tender nodule is noted at the metacarpophalangeal (MCP) joint of the affected digit
- Pain over the flexor tendon with resisting flexion isometrically
- Pain with passive stretching

ETIOLOGY

Trigger finger is described as being primary or secondary:
- Primary (idiopathic)
- Secondary
  1. Diabetes
  2. Rheumatoid arthritis
  3. Hypothyroidism
  4. Histiocytosis
  5. Amyloidosis
  6. Gout

DIAGNOSIS

Clinical history and physical examination

DIFFERENTIAL DIAGNOSIS

- Dupuytren's contracture
- De Quervain's tenosynovitis
- Acute digital tenosynovitis
- Proliferative tenosynovitis
- Ulnar collateral ligament injury (gamekeeper's thumb)
- Carpal tunnel syndrome
- Flexion tendon rupture
- Posttraumatic MCP osteoarthritis

WORKUP

Pursued if a secondary cause is suspected.

LABORATORY TESTS

- Complete blood count with differential
- Electrolytes, blood urea nitrogen, creatinine
- Blood glucose
- Thyroid function tests
- Uric acid
- Rheumatoid factor

IMAGING STUDIES

Radiograph studies are not helpful unless a secondary cause has affected other organs (e.g., rheumatoid lung).

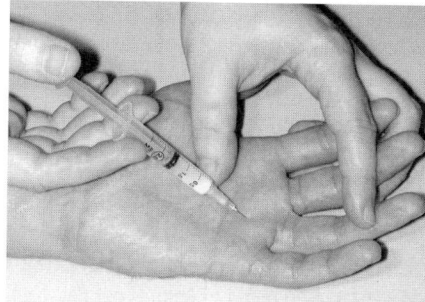

FIGURE 1-388 Injection into the palm for trigger finger. (From Carr A, Hamilton W: *Orthopedics in primary care,* ed 2, Philadelphia, 2005, Elsevier.)

TREATMENT

The goals of treatment are to reduce swelling and inflammation in the flexor tendon sheath and allow smooth movement of the tendon under the A-1 pulley of the MCP joint.

NONPHARMACOLOGIC THERAPY

Splinting or buddy taping to the adjacent finger for 4 to 6 wk

ACUTE GENERAL Rx

- In idiopathic trigger finger, steroid injection with 15 to 20 mg depot methylprenisolone acetate in 1 ml 1% Xylocaine (Fig. 1-388) has been used with success if conservative immobilization has failed.
- Triamcinolone 10 mg with 1 ml 1% Xylocaine is an alternative steroid for patients who do not respond to the first injection.
- If symptoms do not resolve in 6 wk, a repeat injection can be tried.

CHRONIC Rx

- Surgical release is indicated in patients with refractory symptoms (e.g., locked digits) despite nonpharmacologic and acute treatment.
- Surgery is also indicated in patients with recurrent symptoms despite two steroid injections.

DISPOSITION

- After steroid injection, symptoms usually resolve in 3 to 5 days, and locking resolves in 60% of the cases in 2 to 3 wk.
- If symptoms recur, a repeat steroid injection improves the symptoms in ≥80% of patients.
- Diabetic patients do not have the same success rate with steroid injections as the idiopathic group.

REFERRAL

If steroid injection therapy is considered, a rheumatology consult is requested.

PEARLS & CONSIDERATIONS

COMMENTS

If more than one digit is involved, a workup for a secondary systemic cause is in order.

EVIDENCE

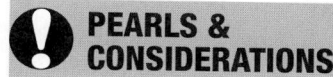

available at www.expertconsult.com

SUGGESTED READINGS
available at www.expertconsult.com

AUTHORS: **RYAN W. ZUZEK, M.D.,** and **PAUL GORDON, M.D.**

BASIC INFORMATION

DEFINITION

Trochanteric bursitis is a presumed inflammation or irritation of the gluteus maximus bursa or the bursa separating the greater trochanter from the gluteus medius and gluteus minimus (Fig. 1-389).

SYNONYMS

Greater trochanteric pain syndrome

ICD-9CM CODES
726.5 Bursitis trochanteric area

EPIDEMIOLOGY & DEMOGRAPHICS

- Trochanteric bursitis is commonly associated with other conditions:
  1. Osteoarthritis of the hip
  2. Lumbar spinal degenerative joint disease
  3. Rheumatoid arthritis
- Incidence peaks between the fourth and sixth decades of life but can occur at any age group
- Occurs in females more often than males (ratio of 4:1)

PHYSICAL FINDINGS & CLINICAL PRESENTATION

- Hip pain is the most common symptom. The pain is chronic, intermittent, and located over the lateral thigh.
- Numbness can be present.
- Pain is precipitated with prolonged lying or standing on the affected side.
- Walking, climbing, and running exacerbate the pain.
- Point tenderness over the greater trochanter is noted.
- Pain is reproduced with resisted hip abduction.

ETIOLOGY

- The specific cause of trochanteric bursitis is not known, although repetitive high-intensity use of the hip joint, trauma, infection (tuberculosis and bacterial), and crystal deposition can precipitate the disease.
- Trochanteric bursitis can occur when other conditions such as osteoarthritis of the knee and hip and bunions of the feet cause changes in the patient's gait, placing varus stress on the hip joint.

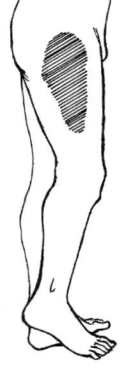

FIGURE 1-389 Typical location of pain in trochanteric bursitis syndrome. This is also a frequent pain radiation site for lumbar spine lesion, various nerve compression syndromes, and hip disease, particularly in osteonecrosis of the femoral head. (From Canoso JJ: *Rheumatology in primary care*, Philadelphia, 1997, WB Saunders.)

DIAGNOSIS

A detailed physical examination and clinical presentation usually make the diagnosis of trochanteric bursitis. Laboratory tests and x-ray images are helpful adjunctive studies used to exclude other conditions either associated with or mimicking trochanteric bursitis.

DIFFERENTIAL DIAGNOSIS

- Osteoarthritis of the hip
- Osteonecrosis of the hip
- Stress fracture of the hip
- Osteoarthritis of the lumbar spine
- Fibromyalgia
- Iliopsoas bursitis
- Trochanteric tendonitis
- Gout
- Pseudogout
- Trauma
- Neuropathy
- Tuberculosis of the greater trochanter
- Metastatic bone disease

WORKUP

A workup is indicated if suspected associated conditions exist; otherwise treatment can be started on clinical grounds alone.

LABORATORY TESTS

- Complete blood count with differential may show elevated white blood cell count if infection is present.
- Erythrocyte sedimentation rate is elevated in an inflammatory process.

IMAGING STUDIES

- Plain radiographs of the hip generally are not helpful in diagnosing trochanteric bursitis. Sometimes calcifications may be seen around the greater trochanter.
- Bone scan can be done but is usually not necessary.
- CT and MRI may show bursitis but are usually not warranted because they will not alter treatment.

TREATMENT

NONPHARMACOLOGIC THERAPY

- Heat 15 to 20 min 4 to 6 times per day
- Ultrasound therapy
- Rest

- Partial weight bearing
- Physical therapy to strengthen back, hip, and knee muscles

ACUTE GENERAL Rx

- Nonsteroidal anti-inflammatory drugs (NSAIDs) for pain relief: ibuprofen 800 mg PO tid or naproxen 500 mg PO bid
- Acetaminophen 500-mg tablet, 1 to 2 tablets PO q6h prn, can be used with NSAIDs or alternating with NSAIDs.
- Corticosteroid injection (30 to 40 mg depot methylprednisolone acetate mixed with 3 ml 1% Xylocaine).

CHRONIC Rx

Although rarely done, surgical removal of the bursa is possible for patients with refractory symptoms or infection.

DISPOSITION

- Most patients respond to NSAIDs and/or nonpharmacologic therapy.
- If steroid injection is used, approximately 70% of patients respond after the first injection and more than 90% respond to two injections.
- 25% of patients receiving steroid injection may develop a relapse.

REFERRAL

A rheumatology or orthopedics referral is made if steroid injection therapy is needed or if the etiology is believed to be infectious.

PEARLS & CONSIDERATIONS

Patients with trochanteric bursitis will commonly report "hip" pain. The physical examination readily distinguishes true hip pain from trochanteric bursitis.

COMMENTS

- The absence of pain with flexion and extension differentiates trochanteric bursitis from degenerative joint disease of the hip.
- Localization of pain over the lateral thigh differentiates trochanteric bursitis from pain caused by meralgia paresthetica located over the anterolateral thigh and pain from osteoarthritis located over the inner thigh groin area.

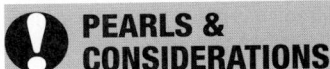
SUGGESTED READINGS
available at www.expertconsult.com

AUTHOR: **MEL L. ANDERSON, M.D.**

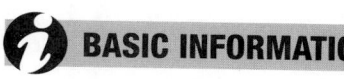 **BASIC INFORMATION**

DEFINITION

Tropical sprue is a malabsorption syndrome occurring primarily in tropical regions, including Puerto Rico, India, and Southeast Asia.

SYNONYMS

Postinfectious tropical malabsorption
"Tropical enteropathy," referring to a subclinical form of tropical sprue

ICD-9CM CODES
579.1 Tropical sprue

EPIDEMIOLOGY & DEMOGRAPHICS

- Tropical sprue is endemic in tropical regions of Venezuela, Colombia, the Middle East, the Far East, the Caribbean (Puerto Rico, Haiti, Dominican Republic, Cuba), and India.
- The disease affects mainly adults, although it has been reported in all age groups.

PHYSICAL FINDINGS & CLINICAL PRESENTATION

- The classic clinical features of tropical sprue are nonspecific and simply reflect the symptom of malabsorption. Onset is generally not insidious, and most patients can pinpoint when their disorder began.
- Diffuse, nonspecific abdominal tenderness and distention. Abdominal pain is crampy in nature.
- Low-grade fever.
- Glossitis, cheilosis, hyperkeratosis, hyperpigmentation.
- Diarrhea, often with mucus and foul-smelling stools from fat malabsorption.
- Nausea, which leads to decreased appetite and decreased oral intake.
- Lactose intolerance often develops early in the course of tropical sprue.

ETIOLOGY

- Unknown. There is a strong presumption that it is caused by an enteric infection, perhaps in individuals predisposed by some nutritional deficiency.
- Associated with overgrowth of predominantly coliform bacteria in the small intestine.

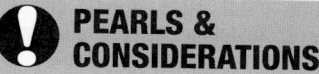 **DIAGNOSIS**

The clinical features of tropical sprue include anorexia, diarrhea, weight loss, abdominal pain, and steatorrhea; these symptoms can develop in expatriates even several months after returning to temperate regions.

DIFFERENTIAL DIAGNOSIS

- Celiac disease
- Parasitic infestation
- Inflammatory bowel disease
- Other causes of malabsorption (e.g., Whipple's disease)
- Lymphoma
- Pancreatic tumor
- Intestinal tuberculosis
- Microsporidia-associated HIV enteropathy

WORKUP

Diagnostic workup includes a comprehensive history (especially travel history), physical examination, laboratory evidence of malabsorption (see below), and jejunal biopsy; the biopsy results are nonspecific, with blunting, atrophy, and even disappearance of the villi and subepithelial lymphocytic infiltration. Partial villus atrophy distinguishes tropical sprue histologically from celiac sprue, which reveals flattened mucosa.

LABORATORY TESTS

- Megaloblastic anemia (>50% of cases)
- Vitamin B_{12} deficiency, folate deficiency
- Abnormal D-xylose absorption (72-hr fecal fat determination or serum carotene concentration)
- Stool examination to exclude *Giardia* spp.

IMAGING STUDIES

Gastrointestinal series with small-bowel follow-through may reveal coarsening of the jejunal folds.

TREATMENT

NONPHARMACOLOGIC THERAPY

Monitoring of weight and calorie intake

ACUTE GENERAL Rx

- Folic acid therapy (5 mg bid for 2 wk followed by a maintenance dose of 1 mg tid) will im-

prove anemia and malabsorption in more than two thirds of patients.
- Tetracycline 250 mg qid for 4 to 6 wk in individuals who have returned to temperate zones, up to 6 mo in patients in endemic areas; ampicillin 500 mg bid for at least 4 wk in patients intolerant to tetracycline.
- Correction of vitamin B_{12} deficiency: vitamin B_{12} 1000 mcg IM weekly for 4 wk, then monthly for 3 to 6 mo.
- Correction of other nutritional deficiencies (e.g., calcium, iron).

DISPOSITION

Complete recovery with appropriate therapy

REFERRAL

Gastrointestinal referral for jejunal biopsy

PEARLS & CONSIDERATIONS

COMMENTS

- Tropical sprue should be considered in any patient who presents with chronic diarrhea, weight loss, and malabsorption, especially if there is significant travel and exposure history.
- Important factors in the medical history in addition to travel history are use of medications that may predispose to a small-bowel overgrowth, HIV exposure (increased risk of chronic diarrhea), and any surgical procedure that may predispose to blind loop syndrome.
- Most of the functional changes in tropical sprue may be related to small-bowel mucosal damage; however, there is also dysfunctional hormonal regulation of the gut (increased enteroglucagon, motilin levels, decreased postprandial insulin and gastric inhibitory peptide) and decreased ability of the colon to absorb water.
- Even with prolonged therapy relapses can occur; however, some may be attributable to reexposure to an infecting organism rather than relapsing disease.

AUTHOR: **FRED F. FERRI, M.D.**

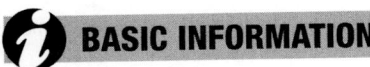

BASIC INFORMATION

DEFINITION
Miliary tuberculosis (TB) is an infection of disseminated hematogenous disease, caused by the bacterium *Mycobacterium tuberculosis* (Mtb), and is often characterized as resembling millet seeds on examination. Extrapulmonary disease may occur in virtually every organ site.

SYNONYMS
Disseminated TB

ICD-9CM CODES
018.94 Miliary tuberculosis

EPIDEMIOLOGY & DEMOGRAPHICS
INCIDENCE (IN U.S.): >38% of AIDS patients with TB have disseminated disease, often with concurrent pulmonary and extrapulmonary active sites. (See "Pulmonary Tuberculosis" in Section I.)
PREVALENCE (IN U.S.):
- Undetermined
- Highest prevalence
  1. AIDS patients
  2. Minorities
  3. Children
  4. Foreign-born persons
  5. Elderly

PREDOMINANT SEX:
- No specific predilection
- Male predominance in AIDS, shelters, and prisons reflected in disproportionate male TB incidence

PREDOMINANT AGE: Predominantly among 24- to 45-yr-olds
PEAK INCIDENCE: HIV-positive patients, regardless of age

PHYSICAL FINDINGS & CLINICAL PRESENTATION
- See also "Etiology"
- Common symptoms
  1. High intermittent fever (93%)
  2. Night sweats (79%)
  3. Weight loss (85%)
  4. Dyspnea (64%)
  5. Cough (82%)
- Symptoms referable to individual organ systems may predominate
  1. Meninges
  2. Pericardium
  3. Liver
  4. Kidney
  5. Bone
  6. GI tract
  7. Lymph nodes
  8. Serous spaces
     a. Pleural
     b. Pericardial
     c. Peritoneal
     d. Joint
  9. Skin
  10. Lung: cough, shortness of breath
- Adrenal insufficiency possible, caused by infection of adrenal gland

- Pancytopenia
  1. With fever and weight loss *or*
  2. Without other localizing symptoms or signs *or*
  3. With only splenomegaly
- TB hepatitis
  1. Tender liver
  2. Obstructive enzymes (alkaline phosphatase) elevated out of proportion to minimal hepatocellular enzymes (SGOT, SGPT) and bilirubin
- TB meningitis
  1. Gradual-onset headache
  2. Minimal meningeal signs
  3. Malaise
  4. Low-grade fever (may be absent)
  5. Sudden stupor or coma
  6. Cranial nerve VI palsy
- TB pericarditis
  1. Effusions resembling TB pleurisy
  2. Cardiac tamponade
- Skeletal TB
  1. Large joint arthritis (with effusions resembling TB pericarditis)
  2. Bone lesions (especially ribs)
  3. Pott's disease
     a. TB spondylitis, especially of lower thoracic spine
     b. Paraspinous TB abscess
     c. Possible psoas abscess
     d. Frequent cord compression (often relieved by steroids)
- Genitourinary TB
  1. Renal TB
     a. Papillary necrosis
     b. Destruction of renal pelvis
     c. Strictures of upper third of ureters
     d. Hematuria
     e. Pyuria with misleading bacterial cultures
     f. Preserved renal function
  2. TB orchitis or epididymitis
     a. Scrotal mass
     b. Draining abscess
  3. Chronic prostatic TB
- GI TB
  1. Diarrhea
  2. Pain
  3. Obstruction
  4. Bleeding
  5. Especially common with AIDS
  6. Bowel lesions
     a. Circumferential ulcers
     b. Short strictures
     c. Calcified granulomas
     d. TB mesenteric caseous adenitis
     e. Abscess, but rare fistula formation
     f. Often difficult to distinguish from granulomatous bowel disease (Crohn's disease)
- TB peritonitis
  1. Fluid resembles TB pleurisy
  2. PPD often negative
  3. Tender abdomen
  4. Doughy peritoneal consistency, often with ascites
  5. Peritoneal biopsy indicated for diagnosis

- TB lymphadenitis (scrofula)
  1. May involve all node groups
  2. Common adenopathies
     a. Cervical
     b. Supraclavicular
     c. Axillary
     d. Retroperitoneal
  3. Biopsy generally needed for diagnosis
  4. Surgical resection of nodes may be necessary
  5. Especially common with AIDS
- Cutaneous TB
  1. Skin infection from autoinoculation or dissemination
  2. Nodules or abscesses
  3. Tuberculids (possibly allergic reactions)
  4. Erythema nodosum
- Miscellaneous presentations
  1. TB laryngitis
  2. TB otitis
  3. Ocular TB
     a. Choroidal tubercles
     b. Iritis
     c. Uveitis
     d. Episcleritis
  4. Adrenal TB
  5. Breast TB

ETIOLOGY
- See also "Pulmonary Tuberculosis" in Section I
- Mtb, a slow-growing, aerobic, non–spore forming, nonmotile bacillus
- Humans are the only reservoir for Mtb
- Pathogenesis:
  1. Acid fast bacilli (AFB) (Mtb) are ingested by macrophages in alveoli, then transported to regional lymph nodes where spread is contained.
  2. Some AFB reach the bloodstream and disseminate widely.
  3. Immediate active disseminated disease may ensue or a latent period may develop.
  4. During latent period, T-cell immune mechanisms contain infection in granulomas until later reactivation occurs as a result of immunosuppression or other undefined factors in conjunction with reactivated pulmonary TB or alone.
- Miliary TB may occur as a consequence of the following:
  1. Primary infection: inability to contain primary infection leads to a hematogenous spread and progressive disseminated disease.
  2. In late chronic TB and in those with advanced age or poor immunity, a continuous seeding of the blood may develop and lead to disseminated disease.

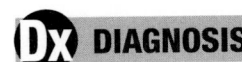

DIAGNOSIS

DIFFERENTIAL DIAGNOSIS
Widespread sites of possible dissemination associated with myriad differential diagnostic possibilities:
- Lymphoma
- Typhoid fever

- Brucellosis
- Other tumors
- Collagen-vascular disease

WORKUP

- Prompt evaluation is essential
- Sputum for AFB stain and culture
- Chest x-ray examination
- PPD
- Fluid analysis and culture wherever available
  1. Sputum
  2. Blood: particularly helpful in patients with AIDS
  3. Urine
  4. CSF
  5. Pleural
  6. Pericardial
  7. Peritoneal
  8. Gastric aspirates
- Biopsy of any involved tissue is advisable to make immediate diagnosis
  1. Transbronchial biopsy preferred and easily accessible
  2. Bone marrow
  3. Lymph node
  4. Scrotal mass if present
  5. Any other involved site
  6. Positive granuloma or AFB on biopsy specimen is diagnostic
- Imaging studies as needed

LABORATORY TESTS

- Culture and fluid analysis as described previously
- Smear-negative sputum often is positive weeks later on culture
- CBC is usually normal
- ESR is usually elevated

IMAGING STUDIES

- Chest x-ray examination (may or may not be positive) (see "Pulmonary Tuberculosis" in Section I)
- CT scan or MRI of brain and spinal cord (Fig. 1-390)
  1. Tuberculoma
  2. Basilar arachnoiditis
- Barium studies of bowel

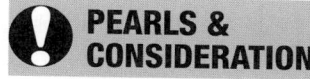 **TREATMENT**

NONPHARMACOLOGIC THERAPY

- Bed rest during acute phase of treatment
- High-calorie, high-protein diet to reverse malnutrition and enhance immune response to TB
- Isolation in negative-pressure rooms with high-volume air replacement and circulation (with health care provider wearing proper protective 0.5- to 1-micron filter respirators)
  1. Until three consecutive sputum AFB smears are negative, if pulmonary disease coexists
  2. Isolation not required for closed-space TB infections

ACUTE GENERAL Rx

- See "Pulmonary Tuberculosis" in Section I.
- Therapy should be initiated immediately. Do not wait for definitive diagnosis.
- More rapid response to chemotherapy by disseminated TB foci than cavitary pulmonary TB.
- Treatment for 6 mo with INH plus rifampin plus PZA.
  1. Treatment for 12 mo often required for bone and renal TB.

2. Prolonged treatment often required for CNS and pericardial.
3. Prolonged treatment often required for all disseminated TB in infants.
- Compliance (rigid adherence to treatment regimen) is the chief determinant of success.
  1. Supervised directly observed therapy (DOT) is recommended for all patients.
  2. Supervised DOT is mandatory for unreliable patients.
- Steroids are often helpful additions in fulminant miliary disease with the hypoxemia and DIC.

CHRONIC Rx

- Generally not indicated beyond treatment described previously
- Prolonged treatment supervised by infectious disease expert required in a few complicated infections caused by resistant organisms

DISPOSITION

- Monthly follow-up by physician experienced in TB treatment
- Confirm sensitivity testing, and alter treatment appropriately (see "Pulmonary Tuberculosis" in Section I)

REFERRAL

- To infectious disease expert for:
  1. HIV-positive patient
  2. Patient with suspected drug-resistant TB
  3. Patient previously treated for TB
  4. Patient whose fever has not decreased and sputum (if positive) has not converted to negative in 2 to 4 wk
  5. Patients with overwhelming pulmonary or extrapulmonary TB
- To pulmonary, orthopedic, or GI physicians for examinations or biopsy

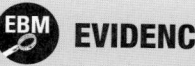 **PEARLS & CONSIDERATIONS**

COMMENTS

- Consider acute TB in critically ill patients with enigmatic acute respiratory distress syndrome, shock, or DIC.
- All contacts (especially close household contacts and infants) should be properly tested for PPD conversions >3 mo following exposure.
- Those with positive PPD should be evaluated for active TB and properly treated or given prophylaxis.

EBM **EVIDENCE**

available at www.expertconsult.com

SUGGESTED READINGS

available at www.expertconsult.com

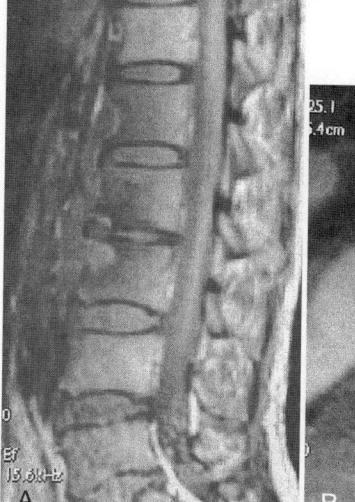

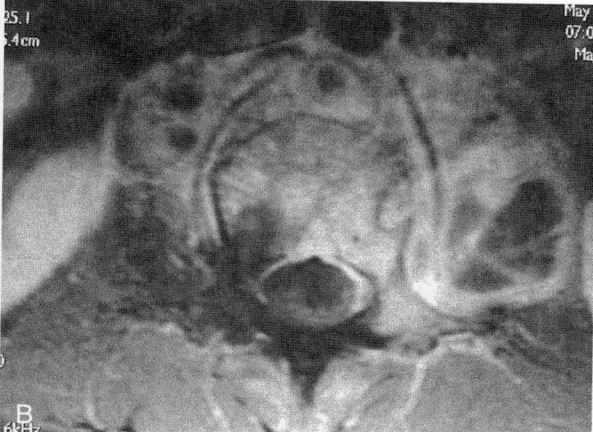

FIGURE 1-390 A, B, MR images of tuberculous spinal osteomyelitis with scalloping of the vertebrae (tuberculous caries) and paraspinal "cold" abscesses. (From Grainger RG, Allison D: *Grainger & Allison's diagnostic radiology, a textbook of medical imaging,* ed 4, 2001, Churchill Livingstone.)

AUTHORS: **GLENN G. FORT, M.D., M.P.H.,** and **DENNIS J. MIKOLICH, M.D.**

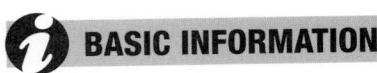

BASIC INFORMATION

DEFINITION

Pulmonary tuberculosis (TB) is an infection of the lung and, occasionally, surrounding structures, caused by the bacterium *Mycobacterium tuberculosis* (Mtb). Multidrug resistant (MDR) TB is defined as disease caused by strains of Mtb that are at least resistant to treatment with isoniazid and rifampin; extensively drug-resistant (XDR) TB refers to disease caused by multidrug-resistant strains that are also resistant to treatment with any fluoroquinolone and any of the injectable drugs used in the treatment of second line antituberculosis drugs.

SYNONYMS

TB

ICD-9CM CODES
011.9 Pulmonary tuberculosis

EPIDEMIOLOGY & DEMOGRAPHICS

INCIDENCE (IN U.S.):
- Approximately 7 cases/100,000 persons—lowest in reported history
- >90% of new cases each yr from reactivated prior infections
- 9% newly infected
- Only 10% of patients with purified protein derivative (PPD) conversions (higher [8%/yr] in HIV-positive patients) will develop TB, most within 1 to 2 yr
- Two thirds of all new cases in racial and ethnic minorities
- 80% of new cases in children in racial and ethnic minorities
- Occurs most frequently in geographic areas and among populations with highest AIDS prevalence
  1. Urban blacks and Hispanics between 25 and 45 yr old
  2. Poor, crowded urban communities
- Nearly 36% of new cases from new immigrants
- In 2008, 440,000 cases of MDR TB emerged globally with India and China accounting for nearly 50% of the world's total cases

PREVALENCE (IN U.S.):
- Estimated 10 million people infected
- Varies widely among population groups

PREDOMINANT SEX:
- No specific predilection
- Male predominance in AIDS, shelters, and prisons reflected in disproportionate male incidence

PREDOMINANT AGE:
- 24 to 45 yr old
- Childhood cases common among minorities
- Nursing home outbreaks among elderly

PEAK INCIDENCE:
- Infancy
- Teenage years
- Pregnancy
- Elderly
- HIV-positive patients, regardless of age, at highest risk

GENETICS:
- Populations with widespread low native resistance have been intensely infected when initially exposed to TB.
- Following elimination of those with least native resistance, incidence and prevalence of TB tend to decline.

PHYSICAL FINDINGS & CLINICAL PRESENTATION
- See "Etiology"
- Primary pulmonary TB infection generally asymptomatic
- Reactivation pulmonary TB
  1. Fever
  2. Night sweats
  3. Cough
  4. Hemoptysis
  5. Scanty nonpurulent sputum
  6. Weight loss
- Progressive primary pulmonary TB disease: same as reactivation pulmonary TB
- TB pleurisy
  1. Pleuritic chest pain
  2. Fever
  3. Shortness of breath
- Rare massive, suffocating, fatal hemoptysis secondary to erosion of pulmonary artery within a cavity (Rasmussen's aneurysm)
- Chest examination
  1. Not specific
  2. Usually underestimates extent of disease
  3. Rales accentuated following a cough (posttussive rales)

ETIOLOGY
- Mtb, a slow-growing, aerobic, non-spore-forming, nonmotile bacillus, with a lipid-rich cell wall:
  1. Lacks pigment
  2. Produces niacin
  3. Reduces nitrate
  4. Produces heat-labile catalase
  5. Mtb staining, acid-fast and acid-alcohol fast by Ziehl-Neelsen method, appearing as red, slightly bent, beaded rods 2 to 4 microns long (acid-fast bacilli [AFB]), against a blue background
  6. Polymerase chain reaction (PCR) to detect <10 organisms/ml in sputum (compared with the requisite 10,000 organisms/ml for AFB smear detection)
  7. Culture
     a. Growth on solid media (Löwenstein-Jensen; Middlebrook 7H11) in 2 to 6 wk
     b. Growth in liquid media (BACTEC, using a radioactive carbon source for early growth detection) often in 9 to 16 days
     c. Enhanced in a 5% to 10% carbon dioxide atmosphere
  8. DNA fingerprinting (based on restriction fragment length polymorphism [RFLP])
     a. Facilitates immediate identification of Mtb strains in early growing cultures
     b. False negatives possible if growth suboptimal

9. Humans are the only reservoir for Mtb
10. Transmission
    a. Facilitated by close exposure to high-velocity cough (unprotected by proper mask or respirators) from patient with AFB-positive sputum and cavitary lesions, producing aerosolized droplets containing AFB, which are inhaled directly into alveoli
    b. Occurs within prisons, nursing homes, and hospitals
- Pathogenesis
  1. AFB (Mtb) ingested by macrophages in alveoli, then transported to regional lymph nodes, where spread is contained
  2. Some AFB may reach bloodstream and disseminate widely
  3. Primary TB (asymptomatic, minimal pneumonitis in lower or midlung fields, with hilar lymphadenopathy) essentially an intracellular infection, with multiplication of organisms continuing for 2 to 12 wk after primary exposure, until cell-mediated hypersensitivity (detected by positive skin test reaction to tuberculin PPD) matures, with subsequent containment of infection
  4. Local and disseminated AFB thus contained by T-cell-mediated immune responses
     a. Recruitment of monocytes
     b. Transformation of lymphocytes with secretion of lymphokines
     c. Activation of macrophages and histiocytes
     d. Organization into granulomas, where organisms may survive within macrophages (Langhans' giant cells), but within which multiplication essentially ceases (95%) and from which spread is prohibited
  5. Progressive primary pulmonary disease
     a. May immediately follow the asymptomatic phase
     b. Necrotizing pulmonary infiltrates
     c. Tuberculous bronchopneumonia
     d. Endobronchial TB
     e. Interstitial TB
     f. Widespread miliary lung lesions
  6. Postprimary TB pleurisy with pleural effusion
     a. Develops after early primary infection, although often before conversion to positive PPD
     b. Results from pleural seeding from a peripheral lung lesion or rupture of lymph node into pleural space
     c. May produce a large (sometimes hemorrhagic) exudative effusion (with polymorphonuclear cells early, rapidly replaced by lymphocytes), frequently without pulmonary infiltrates
     d. Generally resolves without treatment
     e. Portends a high risk of subsequent clinical disease, and therefore must be diagnosed and treated early (pleural biopsy and culture) to prevent future catastrophic TB illness

f. May result in disseminated extrapulmonary infection

7. Reactivation pulmonary TB
   a. Occurs months to years following primary TB
   b. Preferentially involves the apical posterior segments of the upper lobes and superior segments of the lower lobes
   c. Associated with necrosis and cavitation of involved lung, hemoptysis, chronic fever, night sweats, weight loss
   d. Spread within lung occurs via cough and inhalation

8. Reinfection TB
   a. May mimic reactivation TB
   b. Ruptured caseous foci and cavities, which may produce endobronchial spread

9. Mtb in both progressive primary and reactivation pulmonary TB
   a. Intracellular (macrophage) lesions (undergoing slow multiplication)
   b. Closed caseous lesions (undergoing slow multiplication)
   c. Extracellular, open cavities (undergoing rapid multiplication)
   d. INH and rifampin are cidal in all three sites
   e. Pyrazinamide (PZA) especially active within acidic macrophage environment
   f. Extrapulmonary reactivation disease also possible

10. Rapid local progression and dissemination in infants with devastating illness before PPD conversion occurs

11. Most symptoms (fever, weight loss, anorexia) and tissue destruction (caseous necrosis) from cytokines and cell-mediated immune responses

12. Mtb has no important endotoxins or exotoxins

13. Granuloma formation related to tumor necrosis factor (TNF) secreted by activated macrophages

(Dx) DIAGNOSIS

DIFFERENTIAL DIAGNOSIS
- Necrotizing pneumonia (anaerobic, gram-negative)
- Histoplasmosis
- Coccidioidomycosis
- Melioidosis
- Interstitial lung diseases (rarely)
- Cancer
- Sarcoidosis
- Silicosis
- Rare pneumonias
  1. *Rhodococcus equi* (cavitation)
  2. *Bacillus cereus* (50% hemoptysis)
  3. *Eikenella corrodens* (cavitation)

WORKUP
- Sputum for AFB stains
- Chest x-ray (Fig. 1-391)

- PPD (tuberculin skin test [TST])
  1. Recent conversion from negative to positive within 3 mo of exposure is highly suggestive of recent infection.
  2. Single positive PPD is not helpful diagnostically.
  3. Negative PPD never rules out acute TB.
  4. Be certain that positive PPD does not reflect "booster phenomenon" (prior positive PPD may become negative after several yr and return to positive only after second repeated PPD; repeat second PPD within 1 wk), which thus may mimic skin test conversion.
  5. Positive PPD reaction is determined as follows:
     a. Induration after 72 hr of intradermal injection of 0.1 ml of 5 TU-PPD
     b. 5-mm induration if HIV-positive (or other severe immunosuppressed state affecting cellular immune function), close contact of active TB, fibrotic chest lesions
     c. 10-mm induration if in high–medical risk groups (immunosuppressive disease or therapy, renal failure, gastrectomy, silicosis, diabetes), foreign-born high-risk group (Southeast Asia, Latin America, Africa, India), low socioeconomic groups, IV drug addict, prisoner, health care worker
     d. 15-mm induration if low risk
  6. Anergy antigen testing (using mumps, *Candida,* tetanus toxoid) may identify patients who are truly anergic to PPD and these antigens, but results are often confusing. Not recommended.

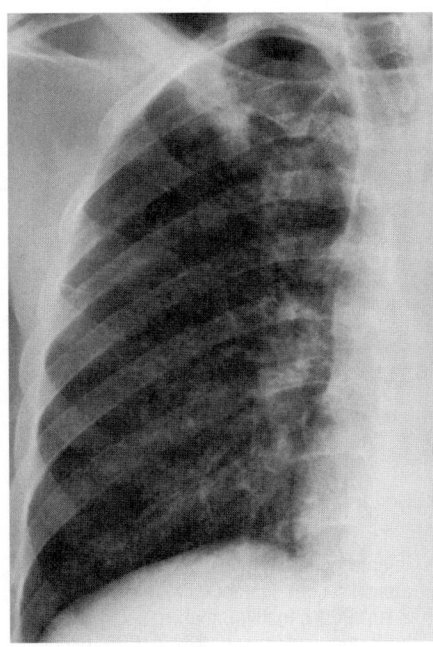

FIGURE 1-391 Miliary pattern in tuberculosis consists of numerous nodules of uniform size. (From Grainger RG et al [eds]: *Grainger & Allison's diagnostic radiology,* ed 4, Philadelphia, 2001, Churchill Livingstone.)

  7. Patients with TB may be selectively anergic only to PPD.
  8. Positive PPD indicates prior infection but does not itself confirm active disease.
- Interferon gamma release assays (IGRAs): diagnostic test for latent TB infection, known is the quantaferon test (QFT-G). This is a blood test that measures interferon response to specific Mtb antigens. The test is FDA approved and is available in some large TB centers and state health departments. It may assist in distinguishing true positive reactions, from individuals with latent TB, from PPD reactions related to: nontuberculous mycobacteria; prior BCG vaccination; or difficult-to-interpret skin test results from people with dermatologic conditions or immediate allergic reactions to PPD. The diagnostic utility of the test as a replacement or supplement to the standard PPD is not yet fully determined. The enzyme-linked immunospot assay (Elispot plus) incorporating a novel antigen, RV3879c, when used in combination with tuberculin testing, has been reported to enable rapid exclusion of active infection in patients with moderate to high pretest probability of TB. Other IGRAs now available for detection of TB using blood include QFT-GIT and T-spot.
- The Xpert MTB/RIF is an automated molecular test for mycobacterium tuberculosis (MTB) and resistance to rifampin (RIF) that provides sensitive detection of tuberculosis and rifampin resistance directly from untreated sputum in less than 2 hr with minimal hands-on time.

LABORATORY TESTS
- Sputum for AFB stains and culture
  1. Induced sputum if patient not coughing productively
- Sputum from bronchoscopy if high suspicion of TB with negative expectorated induced sputum for AFB
  1. Positive AFB smear is essential before or shortly after treatment to ensure subsequent growth for definitive diagnosis and sensitivity testing
  2. Consider lung biopsy if sputum negative, especially if infiltrates are predominantly interstitial
- AFB stain-negative sputum may grow Mtb subsequently
- Gastric aspirates reliable, especially in HIV-negative patients
- CBC
  1. Variable values
     a. WBCs: low, normal, or elevated (including leukemoid reaction: >50,000)
     b. Normocytic, normochromic anemia often
  2. Rarely helpful diagnostically
- ESR usually elevated
- Thoracentesis
  1. Exudative effusion
     a. Elevated protein
     b. Decreased glucose

c. Elevated WBCs (polymorphonuclear leukocytes early, replaced later by lymphocytes)
d. May be hemorrhagic
2. Pleural fluid usually AFB-negative
3. Pleural biopsy often diagnostic—may need to be repeated for diagnosis
4. Culture pleural biopsy tissue for AFB
- Bone marrow biopsy is often diagnostic in difficult-to-diagnose cases, especially miliary TB

IMAGING STUDIES

- Chest radiograph
1. Primary infection reflected by calcified peripheral lung nodule with calcified hilar lymph node
2. Reactivation pulmonary TB
   a. Necrosis
   b. Cavitation (especially on apical lordotic views)
   c. Fibrosis and hilar retraction
   d. Bronchopneumonia
   e. Interstitial infiltrates
   f. Miliary pattern
   g. Many of previous findings may also accompany progressive primary TB
3. TB pleurisy
   a. Pleural effusion, often rapidly accumulating and massive
4. TB activity not established by single chest x-ray examination
5. Serial chest x-ray examinations are excellent indicators of progression or regression

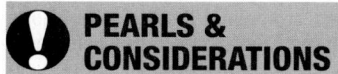 **TREATMENT**

NONPHARMACOLOGIC THERAPY

- Increased rest during acute phase of treatment
- High-calorie, high-protein diet to reverse malnutrition and enhance immune response to TB
- Isolation in negative-pressure rooms with high-volume air replacement and circulation, with health care provider wearing proper protective 0.5- to 1-micron filter respirators, until three consecutive sputum AFB smears are negative

ACUTE GENERAL Rx

- Compliance (rigid adherence to treatment regimen) chief determinant of success.
1. Supervised directly observed therapy (DOT) recommended for all patients and mandatory for unreliable patients
- Preferred adult regimen: DOT.
1. Isoniazid (INH) 15 mg/kg (max 900 mg), rifampin 600 mg, ethambutol (EMB) 30 mg/kg (max 2500 mg), and pyrazinamide (PZA) (2 g [<50 kg]; 2.5 g [51 to 74 kg]; 3 g [>75 kg]) thrice weekly for 6 mo
2. Alternative, more complicated DOT regimens

- Rifapentine, a rifampin derivative with a much longer serum half-life, was shown to be as effective when administered weekly (with weekly isoniazid) as conventional regimens for drug-sensitive pulmonary TB in non–HIV-infected patients.
- Short-course daily therapy: adult.
1. HIV-negative patient: 6 mo total therapy (2 mo INH 300 mg, rifampin 600 mg, and EMB 15 mg/kg [max 2500 mg]) and PZA (1.5 g [<50 kg]; 2 g [51 to 74 kg]; 2.5 g [>75 kg]) daily and until smear negative and sensitivity confirmed; then INH and rifampin daily for 4 mo
2. HIV-positive patient: 9 mo total therapy (2 mo INH, rifampin, EMB, and PZA daily until smear negative and sensitivity confirmed; then INH and rifampin qid for 7 mo)
3. Continue treatment at least 3 mo following conversion to negative cultures
- Drug resistance (often multiple drug resistance TB [MDRTB]) increased by:
1. Prior treatment
2. Acquisition of TB in developing countries
3. Homelessness
4. AIDS
5. Prisoners
6. IV drug addicts
7. Known contact with MDRTB
- Never add single drug to failing regimen.
- Never treat TB with fewer than two to three drugs or two to three new additional drugs.
- Monitor for clinical toxicity (especially hepatitis).
1. Patient and physician awareness that anorexia, nausea, right upper quadrant pain, and unexplained malaise require immediate cessation of treatment
2. Evaluation of liver function testing
   a. Minimal SGOT/SGPT elevations without symptoms generally transient and not clinically significant
- Preventive treatment for PPD conversion only (infection without disease).
1. Must be certain that chest x-ray examination is negative and patient has no symptoms of TB
2. INH 300 mg daily for 9 to 12 mo; at least 12 mo if HIV-positive patient
3. Most important groups:
   a. HIV-positive and other severely immunocompromised patients
   b. Close contact with active TB
   c. Recent converter
   d. Old TB on chest x-ray examination
   e. IV drug addict
   f. Medical risk factor
   g. High-risk foreign country
   h. Homeless
- Infants generally given prophylaxis immediately if recent contact with active TB (even if infant PPD negative), then retested with PPD in 3 mo (continuing INH if PPD becomes positive and stopping INH if PPD remains negative).

- Chronic, stable PPD (several yr) given INH prophylaxis generally only if patient is <35 yr old.
1. INH toxicity may outweigh benefit
2. Individualize decision
- Preventive therapy for suspected INH-resistant organisms is unclear.

CHRONIC Rx

- Generally not indicated beyond treatment described previously
- Prolonged treatment, supervised by infectious disease expert, in a few very complicated infections caused by resistant organisms

DISPOSITION

- Monthly follow up by physician experienced in TB treatment
- Confirm sensitivity testing and alter treatment appropriately
- Frequent sputum samples until culture is negative
- Confirm chest x-ray regression at 2 to 3 mo

REFERRAL

- To infectious disease expert for:
1. HIV-positive patient
2. Patient with suspected drug-resistant TB
3. Patients previously treated for TB
4. Patients whose fever has not decreased and sputum has not converted to negative in 2 to 4 wk
5. Patients with overwhelming pulmonary or extrapulmonary TB
- To pulmonologist for bronchoscopy or pleural biopsy

ⓘ PEARLS & CONSIDERATIONS

COMMENTS

- All contacts (especially close household contacts and infants) should be properly tested for PPD conversions during 3 mo following exposure.
- Those with positive PPD should be evaluated for active TB and properly treated or given prophylaxis.
- Previous treatment is a common risk factor for extensively drug-resistant and multidrug-resistant TB.

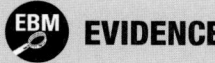 **EVIDENCE**

available at www.expertconsult.com

SUGGESTED READINGS

available at www.expertconsult.com

AUTHORS: **GLENN G. FORT, M.D., M.P.H.,** and **DENNIS J. MIKOLICH, M.D.**

BASIC INFORMATION

DEFINITION

Tuberous sclerosis (TS) is an inherited neurocutaneous disorder that is characterized by pleomorphic features involving many organ systems, including multiple benign neoplasms (hamartomas) of the brain, kidney, and skin.

ICD-9CM CODES
759.5 Tuberous sclerosis

EPIDEMIOLOGY & DEMOGRAPHICS

INCIDENCE: TS has an estimated incidence of 1 case per 6000 live births. Thus, it is the second most common neurocutaneous syndrome after neurofibromatosis.

PREVALENCE: The disorder affects about 1 in 10,000 persons in the general population.

PREDOMINANT SEX: TS has no predilection for gender or race.

GENETICS:

- TS is an autosomal dominant disorder with almost complete penetrance but a wide range of clinical severity. However, only one third of cases are familial. The apparently nonfamilial cases can represent either spontaneous mutations or mosaicism.
- Genetic research has identified two TS genes. One is located on chromosome 9 (*TSC1* gene) and the other on chromosome 16 (*TSC2* gene). About 68% of cases occur as a result of new gene mutations. Because of the genetic transmission and new mutations, antenatal diagnosis is difficult.

PHYSICAL FINDINGS & CLINICAL PRESENTATION

- Dermatologic manifestations may be the only clues the family physician has to the diagnosis of the disorder, which is also marked by childhood seizures and mental retardation (Figs. 1-392 through 1-394).
- The diagnostic criteria for TS were recently revised at a consensus conference. Major and minor features are listed in Table 1-178.
- The classic diagnostic triad of seizures, mental retardation, and facial angiofibromas (Vogt's triad) occurs in fewer than 50% of patients with TS.

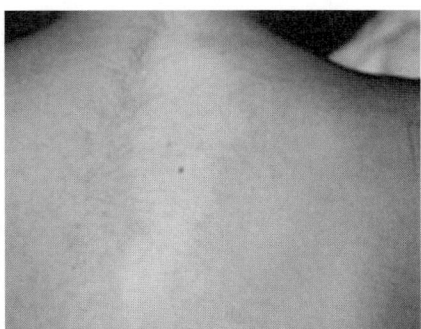

FIGURE 1-392 Hypomelanotic macules ("ash left" spots).

- All of the clinical features of TS may not be apparent in the first yr of life. Thus, a child is often initially diagnosed with possible or probable TS and the diagnosis of definite TS is made after additional features are identified.
- Dermatologic manifestations: A careful skin examination of patients at risk for TS continues to be the easiest and most accessible method of establishing the diagnosis (Table 1-179).
- Neurologic manifestations: These are the leading cause of morbidity and mortality in patients with TS. Brain hamartomas in the form of cortical tubers, subependymal nodules, and subependymal giant cell astrocytomas are often responsible for intractable seizures, most commonly as infantile spasms. Approximately 90% to 96% of TS patients suffer from seizures. Approximately 85% of patients have their first epileptic episode in the first 2 yr of life. Behavioral and cognitive dysfunction, including autism and mental retardation, can be seen in 40% to 50% of patients.
- Renal and pulmonary manifestations are strongly associated with TS.
- Angiomyolipoma is the most common renal lesion found in TS patients. Clinically evident pulmonary involvement in TS patients is relatively rare, with an estimated incidence of 1% to 6%. The most common lesion is lymphangiomyomatosis (LAM), a progressive cystic lung disease with progressive dyspnea and spontaneous pneumothorax in a childbearing woman.

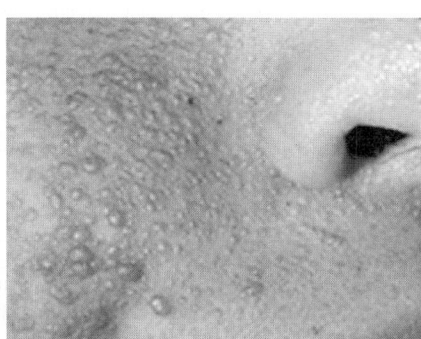

FIGURE 1-393 Facial angiofibromas.

- Cardiovascular manifestations: These are often the earliest diagnostic findings in patients with TS. Rhabdomyoma is the most common primary cardiac tumor in infants and children. Its incidence in TS patients ranges between 47% and 60%. In fact, 80% to 95% of patients with cardiac rhabdomyomas have TS.
- The most common ocular findings in TS are retinal hamartomas, appearing in 40% to 50% of patients.

ETIOLOGY

TS is an autosomal dominant disorder.

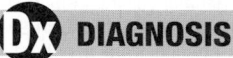

DIAGNOSIS

DIFFERENTIAL DIAGNOSIS

Cutaneous manifestations:
- Nevus anemicus
- Nevus depigmentosus (nevus achromicus)
- Vitiligo

WORKUP

- The dermatologic manifestations of TS are helpful in diagnosing this disorder. When TS has been inherited in the autosomal dominant form, dermatologic signs are almost universally present in one of the patient's parents.

TABLE 1-178 Revised Diagnostic Criteria for Tuberous Sclerosis Complex (TSC)

Major features

1. Facial angiofibromas or forehead plaque
2. Nontraumatic ungual or periungual fibroma
3. Hypomelanotic macule (3 or more)
4. Shagreen patch (connective tissue nevus)
5. Multiple retinal nodular hamartomas
6. Cortical tuber
7. Subependymal nodule
8. Subependymal giant cell astrocytoma
9. Cardiac rhabdomyoma, single or multiple
10. Lymphangiomyomatosis
11. Renal angiomyolipoma

Minor features

1. Multiple, randomly distributed pits in dental enamel
2. Hamartomatous rectal polyps
3. Bone cysts
4. Cerebral white matter radial migration lines
5. Gingival fibromas
6. Nonrenal hamartomas
7. Retinal achromic patch
8. "Confetti" skin lesions
9. Multiple renal cysts

Definite TSC: Either two major features or one major feature plus two minor features. Probable TSC: One major plus one minor feature. Possible TSC: Either one major feature or two or more minor features.

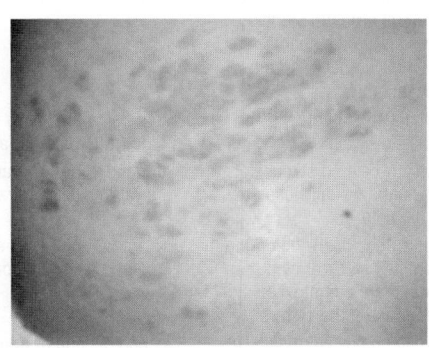

FIGURE 1-394 Shagreen patches.

- No specific prenatal laboratory test is available.
- Early recognition of TS is vital because prompt implementation of the recommended diagnostic evaluation (neuroimaging studies, EEG, ECG, renal ultrasonography, and chest CT) may prevent serious clinical consequences.

LABORATORY TESTS

- Molecular genetic testing: In recent years, molecular genetic testing for TS has become clinically available. Such testing identifies mutations in the *TSC1* and *TSC2* genes by one of several methods, most commonly polymerase chain reaction (PCR) amplification of individual exons, followed by DNA sequencing on DNA obtained from a patient's blood sample.
- DNA testing for TS is potentially useful in several settings:
  - First, it can be helpful in confirming a clinical diagnosis of TS, especially in young patients in whom many clinical signs and symptoms have yet to develop.
  - Second, in many families with a history of TS in which there is a sporadic case of TS in a new child, genetic testing can provide reassurance to parents, children, and other family members that they do not carry the TS gene mutation.
  - Third, DNA testing is useful for prenatal diagnosis.

Rx TREATMENT

The management of TS complex (TSC) is presently symptomatic.

NONPHARMACOLOGIC THERAPY

Genetic counseling should be offered to families with affected members, even though accurate counseling remains difficult because of the variability of gene expression.

ACUTE GENERAL Rx & CHRONIC Rx

- Treatment methods currently available for patients with disfiguring facial angiofibromas include cryosurgery, curettage, dermabrasion, chemical peeling, excision, and laser therapy.
- Some patients have been treated successfully with antiepileptic medications; unfortunately, there are multiple cases of intractable seizure in which medical treatment is ineffective. In some cases of intractable epilepsy, neurosurgical intervention becomes a life-saving option.
- In such drug-resistant cases of TS, the early administration of vigabatrin (a-vinyl-gamma aminobutyric acid), a selective irreversible inhibitor of GABA-transaminase, has been proven to result in 80% to 100% cessation rates of infantile spasms. Vigabatrin is marketed in many European countries, but remains unavailable in the U.S. and has not been approved by the FDA.
- Embolization and/or renal sparing surgery are treatment options for renal angiomyolipomas.
- Oopherectomy, medroxyprogesterone, and tamoxifen use have been advocated in patients with LAM, but therapeutic benefit is unclear. Lung transplantation is reserved for patients with end-stage LAM.
- Most rhabdomyomas tend to regress with increasing age, although tumor growth has been documented in some at puberty. Surgery

is recommended only for life-threatening situations, such as hemodynamic compromise.
- Oral rapamycin or sirolimus therapy can induce regression of brain astrocytomas associated with TS. Ongoing therapeutic trials with rapamycin in lymphangioleiomyomatosis appear promising.
- Neurosurgical resection is the standard treatment for subependymal giant-cell astrocytomas in patients with the tuberous sclerosis complex. Trials with everolimus, which inhibits the mammalian target of rapamycin, a protein regulated by gene products involved in the tuberous sclerosis complex, have shown marked reduction in volume of subependymal giant-cell astrocytomas and seizure frequency.

REFERRAL

A multidisciplinary team including genetics, neurology, ophthalmology, nephrology, dermatology, neurosurgery, and plastic surgery should evaluate children suspected of having TS.

! PEARLS & CONSIDERATIONS

PREVENTION

It is speculated that if one could establish the prenatal diagnosis of TS and begin using rapamycin early, one might prevent the development of TS manifestations.

SUGGESTED READINGS
available at www.expertconsult.com

AUTHOR: **RUBY SATPATHY, M.D.**

TABLE 1-179 Cutaneous Manifestations Associated with Tuberous Sclerosis Complex (TSC)

Cutaneous Lesions	Descriptions	Age of Onset	Prevalence	Diagnostic Classification
Hypomelanotic macules ("ash leaf" spots) or Fitzpatrick patches	Leaf-shaped or polygonal white spots enhanced by Wood's lamp examination	Earliest cutaneous lesion; usually present at birth or infancy on buttocks	97.2%	Major
Facial angiofibromas	Red to pink papules with a smooth surface, symmetrically distributed over the centrofacial areas, sparing the upper lips	Second to fifth yr of life; become more prominent with age	74.5%	Major
Shagreen patches	Slightly elevated patch or plaque, usually found on the dorsal body surfaces, especially the lumbosacral area; its rough surface resembles an orange peel; represents a connective tissue nevus, sometimes called collagenoma	Rare during infancy; tend to increase in size and number with age	48.1%	Major
Molluscum pendulum	Multiple soft pedunculated skin growths on neck; rarely in axilla or groin	More common during first decade of life; rare during infancy	22.6%	Minor
Forehead fibrous plaque	Yellowish-brown or skin-colored plaques of variable size and shape, usually located on the forehead or scalp	Common at any age and can be seen at birth or early infancy	18.9%	Major
Periungual fibromas	Skin-colored or reddish nodules seen on the lateral nail groove, nail plate, or along the proximal nail folds; more commonly found on the toes than on the fingers	Present at puberty or soon after; become more common with age	15.1%	Major
"Confetti-like" macules	Multiple 1-2 mm white spots symmetrically distributed over extremities	Second decade or adulthood	2.8%	Minor

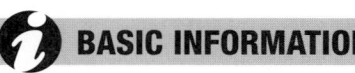

BASIC INFORMATION

DEFINITION

Acute tubular necrosis (ATN) refers to intrinsic tubular damage induced by hypoperfusion or direct toxic injury to renal parenchymal cells, particularly tubular epithelium, that results in an acute decrease in renal function.

SYNONYMS

Acute kidney injury (AKI)
Acute tubular injury
Ischemic or nephrotoxic acute renal failure (ARF)

ICD-9CM CODES
586   Renal failure, unspecified
584.5 Acute renal failure with lesion of
      tubular necrosis
997.5 Urinary complications

EPIDEMIOLOGY & DEMOGRAPHICS

- Most common cause of intrinsic renal failure among hospitalized patients, especially in critical care units and on surgical services in patients undergoing major cardiovascular surgery or in intensive care units in patients suffering severe trauma, hemorrhage, sepsis, or volume depletion.
- Hospital-acquired ARF is often caused by more than one insult.
- Early identification is important because causes are often reversible.

PHYSICAL FINDINGS & CLINICAL PRESENTATION

No apparent physical findings. Clinical features include recent hemorrhage, hypotension, or surgery, thereby suggesting ischemic ARF. Recent radiocontrast study, nephrotoxic drugs, history suggestive of rhabdomyolysis, hemolysis, or myeloma may suggest toxin-mediated ARF.
- The classic progression of ATN includes three phases, but can be highly variable:
  1. Initiation phase (hours to days)—renal hypoperfusion, evolving ischemia. Acute decrease in GFR (glomerular filtration rate), sudden rise in BUN and serum creatinine, and decrease in urine output.
  2. Maintenance phase (1 to 2 wk)—renal cell injury established, GFR stabilizes at its nadir (5 to 10 ml/min), urine output at its lowest (usually 40 to 400 cc/day), and complications arise such as hyperkalemia, metabolic acidosis, uremia, and salt and water overload. Some patients have nonoliguric ATN, where urine output does not decrease, which usually signifies a more benign course.
  3. Recovery phase (>2 wk)—renal parenchymal cell repair and regeneration, gradual return of GFR to premorbid levels; may be complicated by a marked diuretic phase due to excretion of retained salt

and water and other solutes, continued use of diuretics, or delayed recovery of epithelial cell function (solute and water reabsorption) relative to glomerular filtration.

PATHOLOGIC FINDINGS

- Ischemic ARF—patchy and focal necrosis of tubule epithelium with detachment from its basement membrane and occlusion of tubule lumens with casts composed of epithelial cells, cellular debris, Tamm-Horsfall mucoprotein (represents the matrix of all urinary casts), and pigments. Also present is leukocyte accumulation in vasa recta (capillaries that return the NaCl and water reabsorbed in the loop of Henle and medullary collecting tubule to the systemic circulation). Morphology of glomeruli and renal vasculature remain normal. Necrosis most severe in pars recta (straight portion of proximal tubule and thick ascending limb of loop of Henle).
- Nephrotoxic ARF-morphologic changes in convoluted and straight portion of proximal tubule. Tubule cell necrosis less pronounced than in ischemic ARF.

ETIOLOGY

- Ischemia from any cause, including hypotension or shock, prolonged pre renal azotemia, and postoperative sepsis syndrome. Hypoperfusion may occur without clinically apparent hypotension, so ischemic acute renal failure should be considered even in patients who have had normal blood pressures.
- Medications: NSAIDs, antimicrobial drugs (acyclovir, foscarnet, aminoglycosides, amphotericin B, pentamidine, cephalosporins), calcineurin inhibitors, cisplatin, ifosfamide, thiazides, anesthetics.
- Radiocontrast (contrast nephropathy).
- Hemoglobin and myoglobin (rhabdomyolysis, transfusion reactions).
- Heavy metals.
- Crystals (urate, oxalate, acute phosphate nephropathy).
- Hypercalcemia.
- Immunoglobulin light chain disease (amyloidosis, multiple myeloma, MGUS).

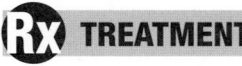

DIAGNOSIS

DIFFERENTIAL DIAGNOSIS

Allergic interstitial nephritis, acute bilateral pyelonephritis

LABORATORY TESTS

- Urinalysis for specific gravity (SG), U_{Na}, P_{Cr}, P_{Na}, U_{Cr}.
- Urine microscopic analysis.
- Calculate fractional excretion of sodium $(FE_{Na}) = [(U_{Na} \times P_{Cr}) / (P_{Na} \times U_{Cr})] \times 100$.
- Trial of fluid repletion can distinguish prerenal azotemia from ATN. Improvement in urine

output and renal function with intravenous fluids suggests prerenal disease.
- Potential biomarkers for early diagnosis of ATN are currently under investigation.

LABORATORY FINDINGS

$FE_{Na} > 1\%$
$U_{Na} > 20$ mmol/L
"Muddy brown" granular and epithelial cell casts
$SG < 1.015$

IMAGING STUDIES

Not necessary

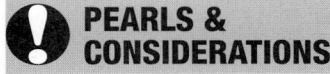

TREATMENT

ACUTE GENERAL Rx

Should focus on providing etiology-specific supportive care or correction of primary hemodynamic abnormality. No specific therapies for established ATN. Peritoneal or hemodialysis for replacement of renal function may be necessary until regeneration and repair restore renal function. Diuretic use is not recommended.

DISPOSITION

Recovery typically takes 1 to 2 wk after normalization of renal perfusion as it requires repair and regeneration of renal cells. Prognosis depends heavily on clinical context, but patients who do not have complications or underlying illness can have a 95% chance of recovery. However, with sepsis or multiorgan failure mortality can be more than 50%.

REFERRAL

Renal consultation for severe cases of ATN requiring dialysis.

PEARLS & CONSIDERATIONS

COMMENTS

Prevention is paramount.

PREVENTION

- Aggressive restoration of intravascular volume in surgical/trauma patients to prevent ischemic ARF.
- Tailoring dosage of potential nephrotoxins to body size and GFR to limit renal injury.
- Low volume contrast, pre-study intravenous fluids, and acetylcysteine (600 mg PO BID × 2 days or 600 to 1200 mg IV BID) may help prevent contrast-induced nephropathy.

SUGGESTED READINGS
available at www.expertconsult.com

AUTHOR: **ELIZABETH BROWN, M.D.**

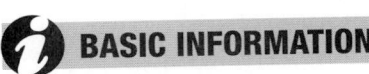

DEFINITION

Tularemia is a zoonosis caused by small, facultative gram-negative intracellular coccobacillus *Francisella tularensis*. Clinical manifestations range from asymptomatic illness to septic shock and death.

SYNONYMS

Rabbit fever
Deerfly fever
O'Hara's disease

ICD-9CM CODES
021.9 Tularemia

EPIDEMIOLOGY & DEMOGRAPHICS

INCIDENCE (IN U.S.): Highest overall incidence in Arkansas, Missouri, and Oklahoma. It is also found in Canada, Mexico, European countries, Turkey, Israel, China, and Japan.
PREDOMINANT SEX: Male
PREDOMINANT AGE: Occurs at any age
PEAK INCIDENCE: June through August and in December

PHYSICAL FINDINGS & CLINICAL PRESENTATION

Physical findings:
- Incubation period is 3 to 5 days but may range from 1 to 21 days.
- Most common initial signs and symptoms:
  1. Fever
  2. Chills
  3. Headache
  4. Malaise
  5. Anorexia
  6. Fatigue
  7. Cough
  8. Myalgias
  9. Chest discomfort
  10. Vomiting
  11. Abdominal pain
  12. Diarrhea
  13. Conjunctivitis
  14. Lymphadenitis

Clinical presentation:
- Ulceroglandular and glandular: account for 75% to 80% of cases. Fever and a single erythematous papuloulcerative lesion with a central eschar accompanied by tender lymphadenopathy (Fig. 1-395).
- Oculoglandular: accounts for 1% to 2% of cases. Painful inflamed conjunctiva with numerous yellowish nodules and pinpoint ulcers. Purulent conjunctivitis with regional lymphadenopathy. Corneal perforation may occur.
- Oropharyngeal and gastrointestinal: account for 1% to 4% of cases. Acute exudative membranes pharyngitis associated with cervical lymphadenopathy. Ulcerative intestinal lesion associated with mesenteric lymphadenopathy, diarrhea, abdominal pain, nausea, vomiting, and GI bleeding.

- Pulmonary: occurs often in the elderly and has a higher mortality. Symptoms include nonproductive cough, dyspnea, or pleuritic chest pain.
- Typhoidal: 10% of all cases of tularemia. Rare in U.S. Symptoms include high continuous fever, signs of endotoxemia, and severe headache. Mortality can approach 30%.

COMPLICATIONS

1. Intravascular coagulation
2. Renal failure
3. Rhabdomyolysis
4. Jaundice
5. Hepatitis
6. Meningitis
7. Encephalitis
8. Pericarditis
9. Peritonitis
10. Osteomyelitis
11. Splenic rupture
12. Thrombophlebitis
13. Myositis and septicemia

ETIOLOGY

- Caused by infection with *F. tularensis*.
- Two main biovars of *F. tularensis*: Type A and Type B. Type A produces severe disease in humans. Type B produces milder subclinical infection.
- Transmitted by ticks, tabanid flies, and mosquitoes. Also acquired by inhalation and ingestion.
- Cases also occur after exposure to animals (wild rabbit, squirrels, birds, sheep, beavers, muskrats, and domestic dogs and cats) or animal products.
- Laboratory acquisition is possible.
- Pathogenesis: after inoculation into the skin the organism multiplies locally within 2 to 5 days, then it produces erythematous tender or pruritic papule. The papule rapidly enlarges and forms an ulcer with a black base. The bacteria spread to the regional lymph nodes producing lymphadenopathy, and with bacteremia may spread to distant organs.

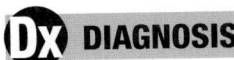

DIFFERENTIAL DIAGNOSIS

- Rickettsial infections
- Meningococcal infections
- Cat-scratch disease
- Infectious mononucleosis
- Atypical pneumonia
- Group A strep pharyngitis
- Typhoid fever
- Fungal infection—sporotrichosis
- Anthrax
- Plague
- Bacterial skin infections

WORKUP

- CBC
- Chest x-ray examination
- Cultures of blood, lymph node, pleural fluid, wounds, sputum, and gastric aspirate
- Antigen detection in urine
- Polymerase chain reaction (PCR)
- Serology

LABORATORY TESTS

- WBC count and ESR normal or elevated.
- Rarely seen on gram-stained smears or tissue biopsies.
- Antibodies to *F. tularensis* demonstrated by tube agglutination, microagglutination, hemagglutination, and ELISA; definitive serologic diagnosis requires a fourfold or greater rise in titer between acute and convalescent specimens.
- PCR to facilitate early diagnosis.

IMAGING STUDIES

Chest x-ray examination to show bilateral patchy infiltrate, lobar parenchymal infiltrate, cavitary lesion, pleural effusion, or emphysema

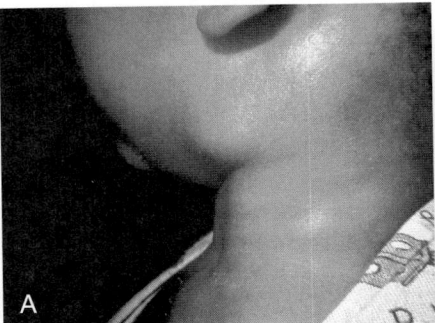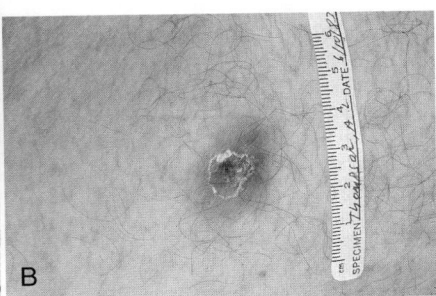

FIGURE 1-395 Examples of primary lesions seen in ulceroglandular tularemia. A, Large cervical and submandibular lymph nodes in a young child; an ulcer was found under the hairline on her forehead at the site of a tick bite. **B,** Papule undergoing central necrosis with desquamation on the thigh of a middle-aged man. (**A** Courtesy of Dr. Joseph A. Bocchini, Louisiana State University Health Sciences Center, Shreveport, LA. **B** From Mandell GL, Bennett JE, Dolin R: *Principles and practice of infectious diseases,* ed 6, Philadelphia, 2005, Elsevier.)

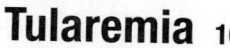 **Tularemia** 1053

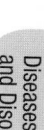 T

Diseases and Disorders

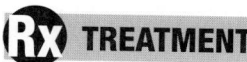 **TREATMENT**

ACUTE GENERAL Rx

- Immediate therapy to limit extent of acute illness and complication.
- Streptomycin 10 mg/kg IM q12h (daily dose should not exceed 2 g) or gentamicin 3 to 5 mg/kg/day in 2 or 3 divided doses.
- Tetracycline 500 mg PO qid or doxycycline 100 mg PO bid or chloramphenicol 25 to 50 mg/kg q6h (do not exceed 6 g).
- Quinolones offer new options for the treatment of tularemia.
- Combination antibiotics required for tularemic meningitis—chloramphenicol plus streptomycin.
- Surgical therapies are limited to drainage of abscessed lymph nodes and chest tube drainage of empyemas.

PROGNOSIS

The mortality rate of severe untreated infection (tularemic pneumonia and typhoidal tularemia) can be as high as 30%. Overall mortality associated with tularemia is 2% to 4% with appropriate treatment. Lifelong immunity usually follows tularemia.

DISPOSITION

Follow-up as outpatient

PREVENTION

- Educate the public to prevent sick or dead animals.
- Use insect repellants.
- Remove ticks promptly.
- Drink only potable water.
- Adequately cook wild meats.
- Tularemia vaccine has been developed but is not commercially available in the U.S.; however, it is available from the Centers for Disease Control and Prevention (CDC). Vaccination of high-risk individuals working with large quantities of cultured organism is recommended.
- Avoid skinning wild animals, especially rabbits; wear gloves while handling animal carcasses.
- Do not use wells or other water that is contaminated by dead animals.
- Hospitalized patients with tularemia do not need special isolation (no person to person transmission). Standard universal precautions for contaminated secretion are adequate when handling drainage from wounds.
- Laboratory personnel should be notified of potential danger of growing this organism in the laboratory and generation of an infectious aerosol from dried culture media.

REFERRAL

- For consultation with infectious diseases specialist in suspected cases.
- A cluster of tularemia cases, particularly in an urban area or nonendemic regions, should prompt concern over the possibility of bioterrorism; the local public health authorities should be contacted immediately to investigate the possibility of deliberate release of tularemia as a weapon of terror.

PEARLS & CONSIDERATIONS

- Alert the microbiology laboratory to the possibility of tularemia; this is a major biohazard in the laboratory.
- Do not use doxycycline or tetracycline in children or pregnant women.
- Because of its highly contagious nature with low inoculums, tularemia is considered an agent that could be used by terrorists. It is classified as a category A critical biologic agent by the CDC.

SUGGESTED READINGS

available at www.expertconsult.com

AUTHOR: **STEVEN M. OPAL, M.D.**

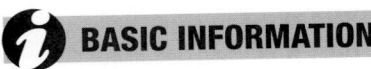

BASIC INFORMATION

DEFINITION

Turner's syndrome is a pattern of malformation characterized by short stature, ovarian hypofunction, loose nuchal skin, and cubitus valgus, as described by Turner in 1938. An associated 45,X chromosome constitution was recognized by Ford et al in 1959.

ICD-9CM CODES
758.6 Syndrome, Turner's

EPIDEMIOLOGY & DEMOGRAPHICS

One case in every 2500 to 5000 live female births

PHYSICAL FINDINGS & CLINICAL PRESENTATION

- Turner's phenotype is recognizable at any point on the developmental spectrum.
- In spontaneous abortions it is the most common sex chromosome abnormality detected (45,X chromosome constitution) and accounts for 20% of such cases.
- In fetuses, it is suspected with ultrasonographic manifestations such as thickening of the nuchal folds, frank nuchal cystic hygromas, or mild shortness of the femur at midtrimester.
- In infants:
  1. At birth may display loose nuchal skin (pterygium colli) and edema on the dorsa of hands and feet
  2. Canthal folds reflecting midface hypoplasia and redundant skin in the periorbital region
  3. Nipples appearing widely spaced
  4. Heart and cardiovascular system: murmur of aortic stenosis or bicuspid aortic valve or diminished femoral pulses suggestive of aortic coarctation
  5. Renal ultrasonography: renal ectopia such as pelvic kidney or horseshoe kidneys
- In older children:
  1. Slow linear growth
  2. Short stature: may be improved with growth hormone therapy
  3. Delayed or absent menses: secondary sex characteristics possibly normalized with estrogen replacement therapy
  4. Intelligence is often normal, but delays in spatial perception or visual-motor integration are commonly observed; frank mental retardation is rare

ETIOLOGY

- Phenotype caused by absence of the second sex chromosome, whether X or Y
- 45,X chromosome constitution in approximately 50% of affected individuals
- Other chromosome aberrations (40% of cases): isochromosome Xq (46,X,i[Xq]) or mosaicism (XX/X)
- With deletions involving the short (or "p") arm of the X chromosome: short stature but little ovarian hypofunction
- Deletions involving Xq13-q27: ovarian failure
- Usually a deficiency of paternal contribution of sex chromosome, reflecting paternal nondisjunction

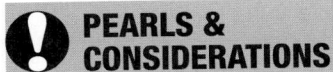

DIAGNOSIS

DIFFERENTIAL DIAGNOSIS

- Noonan syndrome, an autosomally dominant inherited disorder also characterized by loose nuchal skin, midface hypoplasia, canthal folds, and stenotic cardiac valvular defects and affecting males and females equally; also have normal chromosome constitutions
- Other conditions in the differential diagnosis of loose skin, whether or not associated with edema:
  1. Fetal hydantoin syndrome (loose nuchal skin, midface hypoplasia, distal digital hypoplasia)
  2. Disorders of chromosome constitution (trisomy 21, tetrasomy 12p mosaicism)
  3. Congenital lymphedema (Milroy edema)

WORKUP

- Giemsa banded karyotype to confirm clinical diagnosis
- Once diagnosis is established: cardiologic consultation for evaluation for cardiac valvular abnormalities or aortic coarctation
- Renal ultrasonography
- Endocrine evaluations in older patients with short stature or amenorrhea
- Psychometrics to document known or suspected learning disabilities

LABORATORY TESTS

- As noted, routine Giemsa banded karyotype on peripheral lymphocytes to confirm the clinical impression in all suspected cases of Turner's syndrome
- Important to exclude the presence of Y chromosome in mosaics
- Recognition of associated medical problems, such as hypergonadotropic hypogonadism or autoimmune thyroiditis, prompting periodic evaluation of these potential areas

IMAGING STUDIES

- Echocardiogram
- Renal ultrasonography
- Abdominal ultrasonography for evaluation of ovarian and uterine size and morphology
- MRI of brain (especially in cases with known or suspected neurologic impairment)
- Radiographs (for evaluation of carpal/metacarpal abnormalities, radioulnar synostosis)
- Bone age (for evaluation of short stature)

TREATMENT

Recognition of the multisystem involvement of Turner's syndrome necessitates multiple medical specialists working in concert with the primary care provider to maximize and improve outcome while minimizing unnecessary or redundant testing.

NONPHARMACOLOGIC THERAPY

General medical care guided by normal medical standards with special attention paid to identifying such age-related problems as developmental delays, learning disabilities, slow growth, or amenorrhea.

ACUTE GENERAL Rx

Specific treatment geared to the specific medical problem (e.g., cardiac or renal dysfunction)

CHRONIC Rx

- Estrogen-replacement therapy in early adolescence
- Some benefit from recombinant human growth hormone therapy

REFERRAL

- To geneticist: clinical diagnosis, differential diagnosis, recurrence risk counseling, cytogenetic tests
- To endocrinologist (pediatric): evaluation of short stature, estrogen or growth hormone replacement therapy
- To cardiologist: for cardiac valvular abnormalities or aortic coarctation

PEARLS & CONSIDERATIONS

COMMENTS

- Although newer studies are optimistic regarding outcomes, previous reports suffered from retrospective observations, case reports, and ascertainment bias, contributing to a generally poor interaction between physician and patient.
- Affected individuals and families often benefit from the contemporary experiences and expertise of members of genetic support groups. The Turner Syndrome Society of the United States (800-365-9944; http://www.turnersyndrome.org) and the Alliance of Genetic Support Groups (800-336-4363 or 202-966-5557; http://geneticalliance.org) are valuable resources.
- A Turner syndrome diagnosis should be considered in all girls with short stature or primary amenorrhea.
- Almost all women with Turner syndrome are infertile, although some conceive with assisted reproduction.

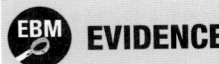

EVIDENCE

available at www.expertconsult.com

SUGGESTED READINGS
available at www.expertconsult.com

AUTHORS: **LUTHER K. ROBINSON, M.D.,** and **RUBEN ALVERO, M.D.**

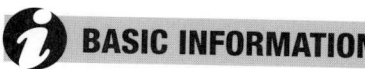

BASIC INFORMATION

DEFINITION

Typhoid fever is a systemic infection caused by *Salmonella typhi.*

SYNONYMS

Typhoid
Enteric fever

ICD-9CM CODES
002.0 Typhoid fever

EPIDEMIOLOGY & DEMOGRAPHICS

INCIDENCE (IN U.S.): Approximately 250 cases of *S. typhi* infections are reported annually in recent surveys. Over three quarters of the cases reported in the U.S. are now associated with foreign travel (most from Asia, Africa, and Central America).

PHYSICAL FINDINGS & CLINICAL PRESENTATION

- Incubation period of a few days to several wk.
- Usual manifestations:
  1. Prolonged fever
  2. Myalgias
  3. Headache
  4. Cough
  5. Sore throat
  6. Malaise
  7. Anorexia, at times with abdominal pain and hepatosplenomegaly
  8. Diarrhea or constipation may occur early in the course of illness
  9. Rose spots, which are faint, maculopapular, blanching lesions, may sometimes be seen on the chest or abdomen
- In the untreated patient, fever may last 1 to 2 mo. The main complication of untreated disease is GI bleeding as a result of perforation from ulceration of Peyer's patches in the ileum. Mental status changes and shock are rare complications. The relapse rate is approximately 10%.

ETIOLOGY

- *Salmonella typhi.*
- *S. paratyphi.*
- *S. typhi* or *S. paratyphi* found only in humans.
- Acquisition of disease by ingestion of food or water contaminated by other humans.
- In the U.S. most cases are acquired either during foreign travel or by ingestion of food

prepared by chronic carriers, many of whom acquired the organism outside of the U.S.

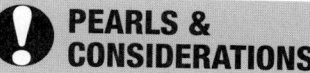

DIAGNOSIS

DIFFERENTIAL DIAGNOSIS

- Malaria
- Tuberculosis
- Brucellosis
- Amebic liver abscess

WORKUP

- Blood, stool, and urine cultures are helpful.
- Cultures should be repeated if initially negative.
- Blood cultures are more likely to be positive early in the course of illness.
- Stool and urine cultures are more commonly positive in the second and third wk of illness.
- Bone marrow biopsy cultures are 90% positive, although this procedure is usually not necessary.
- Serology using Widal test is helpful in retrospect, showing a fourfold increase in convalescent titers.

LABORATORY TESTS

- Neutropenia is common.
- Transaminitis is possible.
- Culture:
  1. Blood
  2. Body fluids
  3. Biopsy specimens

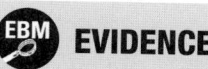

TREATMENT

ACUTE GENERAL Rx

- Ciprofloxacin 500 mg PO bid or 400 mg IV bid for 14 days
- Ceftriaxone 2 g IV qd for 14 days
- If organism sensitive
  1. SMX/TMP, 1 to 2 DS tabs PO bid *or*
  2. Amoxicillin, 2 g PO q8h to complete 14 days
- Dexamethasone, 3 mg/kg IV initially, followed by 1 mg/kg IV q6h for 8 doses for patients with septic shock or mental status changes

CHRONIC Rx

- Carrier states possible
- More common in age >60 yr and in people with gallstones
- Usual site of colonization: gallbladder
- Treatment in those with persistently positive stool cultures and in food handlers

- Suggested regimens for eradication of carrier state
  1. Ciprofloxacin 500 mg PO bid for 4 wk
  2. SMX/TMP 1 to 2 tabs PO bid for 6 wk (if susceptible)
  3. Amoxicillin, 2 g PO q8h for 6 wk (if susceptible)
- Cholecystectomy possibly required in carriers with gallstones who fail medical therapy

DISPOSITION

- Treated patients usually respond to therapy, with a small percentage becoming chronic carriers.
- The relapse rate is approximately 10%.
- Untreated patients may have serious complications.

REFERRAL

- Failure of therapy
- Chronic carrier

PEARLS & CONSIDERATIONS

COMMENTS

- Oral and parenteral vaccines are available for travelers to areas of high risk.
- Vaccines are about 70% effective and well tolerated but are infrequently used.
- Immunity wanes after several yr.
- Parenteral preparations are accompanied by frequent side effects:
  1. Pain at injection site
  2. Fever
  3. Malaise
  4. Headaches
- Infection with antimicrobial-resistant *S. typhi* strains among U.S. patients with typhoid fever is associated with travel to the Indian subcontinent, and an increasing proportion of these infections are due to *S. typhi* strains with decreased susceptibility to fluoroquinolones.

EVIDENCE

available at www.expertconsult.com

SUGGESTED READINGS
available at www.expertconsult.com

AUTHOR: **STEVEN M. OPAL, M.D.**

BASIC INFORMATION

DEFINITION Ulcerative colitis is a chronic inflammatory bowel disease of undetermined etiology. Accumulating evidence suggests that it may result from an inappropriate inflammatory response to intestinal microbes in the genetically susceptible host.

SYNONYMS Inflammatory bowel disease (IBD); idiopathic proctocolitis; IBD

ICD-9CM CODES 556.9 Ulcerative colitis

EPIDEMIOLOGY & DEMOGRAPHICS
INCIDENCE:
- 50 to 150 cases per 100,000 persons; most common between ages 15 and 40 yr, with a second peak between 50 and 80 yr. The disease affects men and women at similar rates.
- Appendectomy for an inflammatory condition (appendicitis or lymphadenitis) but not for nonspecific abdominal pain is associated with a low risk of subsequent ulcerative colitis. This inverse relation is limited to patients who undergo surgery before age 20 yr.

PHYSICAL FINDINGS & CLINICAL PRESENTATION
- Patients with ulcerative colitis often present with bloody diarrhea accompanied by tenesmus, fever, dehydration, weight loss, anorexia, nausea, and abdominal pain.
- Abdominal distention and tenderness.
- Bloody diarrhea.
- Fever, evidence of dehydration.
- Evidence of extraintestinal manifestations may be present in nearly 25% of patients: liver disease, sclerosing cholangitis, iritis, uveitis, episcleritis, arthritis, erythema nodosum, pyoderma gangrenosum, aphthous stomatitis.

DIAGNOSIS

DIFFERENTIAL DIAGNOSIS
- Crohn's disease
- Bacterial infections
  1. Acute: *Campylobacter, Yersinia, Salmonella, Shigella, Chlamydia, Escherichia coli, Clostridium difficile,* gonococcal proctitis
  2. Chronic: Whipple's disease, tuberculosis, enterocolitis
- Irritable bowel syndrome
- Protozoal and parasitic infections (amebiasis, giardiasis, cryptosporidiosis)
- Neoplasm (intestinal lymphoma, carcinoma of colon)
- Ischemic bowel disease
- Diverticulitis
- Celiac sprue, collagenous colitis, radiation enteritis, endometriosis, gay bowel syndrome

WORKUP
Diagnostic workup includes:
- Comprehensive history, physical examination
- Laboratory tests (see "Laboratory Tests")
- Colonoscopy to establish the presence of mucosal inflammation; typical endoscopic findings in ulcerative colitis are friable mucosa; diffuse, uniform erythema replacing the usual mucosal vascular pattern; and pseudopolyps. Rectal involvement is invariably present if the disease is active.

LABORATORY TESTS
- Anemia and high erythrocyte sedimentation rate (in severe colitis) are common.
- Potassium, magnesium, calcium, and albumin may be decreased.
- Stool examinations for ova and parasites, stool culture, and testing for *Clostridium difficile* toxin may be useful to eliminate other causes of chronic diarrhea.
- Antineutrophil cytoplasmic antibodies (ANCA) with a perinuclear staining pattern (pANCA) can be found in >45% of patients; there is an increased frequency in treatment-resistant left-sided colitis, suggesting a possible association between these antibodies and a relative resistance to medical therapy in patients with ulcerative colitis.
- Calprotectin is a protein that is measured in feces as a marker of intestinal mucosa leukocyte activity that may be useful for screening of patients with suspected IBD. Trials have shown that based on a pretest probability of IBD of 32% in adults, an abnormal fecal calprotectin test would increase the posttest probability to 91% and a normal result would reduce the probability to 3%.

IMAGING STUDIES Image studies are generally not indicated. A double-contrast barium enema and small-bowel follow-through, when used (in cases in which colonic strictures prevent a thorough evaluation), may reveal continuous involvement (including the rectum), pseudopolyps, decreased mucosal pattern, and fine superficial ulcerations.

TREATMENT

NONPHARMACOLOGIC THERAPY
- Correct nutritional deficiencies; total parenteral nutrition with bowel rest may be necessary in severe cases. Folate supplementation may reduce the incidence of dysplasia and cancer in chronic ulcerative colitis.
- Avoid oral feedings during acute exacerbation to decrease colonic activity; a low-roughage diet may be helpful in early relapse.
- Psychotherapy is useful in most patients. Referral to self-help groups is also important because of the chronicity of the disease and the young age of the patients.

ACUTE GENERAL Rx
The therapeutic options vary with the degree of disease (mild, severe, fulminant) and areas of involvement (distal, extensive).
- Mild or moderate disease can be treated with mesalamine. It can be administered as an enema (40 mg once daily at bedtime for 3 to 6 wk) or suppository (500 mg bid) for patients with distal colonic disease. Oral forms in which the 5-acetyl salicylic acid is in a slow-release or pH-dependent matrix (Pentasa 1 g qid, Asacol 800 mg PO tid) can deliver therapeutic concentrations to the more proximal small bowel or distal ileum.
- Olsalazine can be useful for maintenance of remission of ulcerative colitis in patients intolerant to sulfasalazine. Usual dose is 500 mg bid taken with food.
- Balsalazide is indicated for mild to moderately active ulcerative colitis. Usual dose is three 750-mg capsules tid.
- Severe disease usually responds to oral corticosteroids (e.g., prednisone 40 to 60 mg/day); corticosteroid suppositories or enemas are also useful for distal colitis. The immunosuppressant azathioprine also provides effective long-term treatment for Crohn's disease.
- Infliximab, a chimeric monoclonal antibody, has been shown to be effective in patients who have not responded to corticosteroid therapy.
- Fulminant disease generally requires hospital admission and parenteral corticosteroids (e.g., IV hydrocortisone 100 mg q6h). When bowel movements have returned to normal and the patient is able to eat normally, oral prednisone is resumed. IV cyclosporine can also be used in severe refractory cases; renal toxicity is a potential complication.
- Surgery is indicated in patients who do not respond to intensive medical therapy. Colectomy is usually curative in these patients and also eliminates the high risk of developing adenocarcinoma of the colon (10% to 20% of patients develop it after 10 yr with the disease); newer surgical techniques allow preservation of the sphincter.

CHRONIC Rx
- Colonoscopic surveillance and multiple biopsies should be instituted approximately 10 yr after diagnosis because of the increased risk of colon carcinoma.
- Erythropoietin is useful in patients with anemia refractory to treatment with iron and vitamins.
- In patients on long-term steroid therapy, periodic bone density scans are recommended to screen for glucocorticoid-induced osteoporosis.

DISPOSITION The clinical course is variable. ~66% of patients will achieve clinical remission with medical therapy, and nearly 80% of treatment compliant patients maintain remission. 15% to 20% of patients eventually require colectomy; >75% of patients treated medically will experience relapse.

REFERRAL
- Gastrointestinal consultation for initial diagnostic sigmoidoscopy/colonoscopy in suspected cases
- Surgical referral for patients with severe disease unresponsive to medical therapy

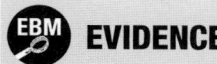

EVIDENCE

available at www.expertconsult.com

SUGGESTED READINGS
available at www.expertconsult.com

AUTHOR: **FRED F. FERRI, M.D.**

BASIC INFORMATION

DEFINITION

Urethritis is a well-defined clinical syndrome manifested by dysuria, a urethral discharge, or both.

ICD-9CM CODES
597.80 Urethritis, unspecified
098.20 Gonococcal

EPIDEMIOLOGY & DEMOGRAPHICS

- The major single specific etiology of acute urethritis is *Neisseria gonorrhoeae,* producing gonococcal urethritis (GCU). Urethritis of all other etiologies is called *nongonococcal urethritis* (NGU).
- NGU is twice as common as GCU in the U.S. NGU is the most common sexually transmitted disease (STD) syndrome occurring in men, accounting for 6 million office visits annually. NGU is more frequently encountered in higher socioeconomic groups. GCU is more common in homosexual males than heterosexual males with acute urethritis.
- *N. gonorrhoeae* is a gram-negative, kidney-shaped diplococcus with flattened opposed margins. The urethra is the most common site of infection in all men. In the United States, the rates of gonorrhea are 40 times higher in black adolescent males than in white adolescent males. In heterosexual men, the pharynx is infected in 7%, and in homosexual men the pharynx is infected in 40% and the rectum in 25%. A single episode of intercourse with an infected partner carries a transmission risk of 20% for males; female partners of an infected male will contract the disease 80% of the time.

PHYSICAL FINDINGS & CLINICAL PRESENTATION

- Symptoms of gonococcal urethritis: urethral discharge and dysuria are the most common symptoms. There is complaint of urethral itching. Prostatic involvement can cause frequency, urgency, and nocturia. It can involve the epididymis through spreading down the vas deferens, causing acute epididymitis.
- Incubation period: 3 to 10 days. Without treatment urethritis persists for 3 to 7 wk, with 95% of men becoming asymptomatic after 3 mo. GCU is asymptomatic in up to 60% of contacts.
- Signs of gonococcal urethritis: yellow-brown discharge, meatal edema, urethral tenderness to palpation. Rectal bleeding with pus is seen with gonococcal proctitis. Periurethritis leading to urethral stenosis can occur. Disseminated infection can occur. Tenosynovitis and

arthritis can occur. Rarely, hepatitis, myocarditis, endocarditis, and meningitis can occur.

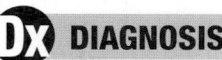

DIAGNOSIS

DIFFERENTIAL DIAGNOSIS

- NGU
- Herpes simplex virus

LABORATORY TESTS

- Nucleic acid amplification tests (NAATs): these tests have largely replaced culture in many settings where persons are screened for asymptomatic genital infection. They are not more sensitive than culture for detecting *N. gonorrhoeae* in cervical or urethral specimen; however, they have specificities of >99% and retain sensitivity when used to test voided urine or self-collected vaginal swabs.
- Calcium alginate or rayon swab on a metal shaft (not cotton-tipped swabs, which are bactericidal) of the urethra should be performed anywhere from 2 to 4 hr after voiding to prevent bacterial washout with voiding. Gram staining with modified Thayer-Martin media is indicated. Cultures of the pharynx and rectum when indicated.
- Concomitant serologic testing for syphilis on all patients.
- Concomitant *Chlamydia* testing on all patients.
- Offer of HIV counseling and testing to all patients.

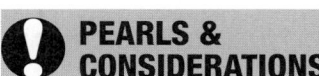

TREATMENT

NONPHARMACOLOGIC THERAPY

Behavioral management: avoid intercourse until cure has been attained and sexual partners have been evaluated and treated.

ACUTE GENERAL Rx

Uncomplicated infections of the urethra:
- Ceftriaxone 250 mg IM in a single dose or, if not an option
- Cefixime 400 mg orally in a single dose or
- Single dose injectable cephalosporin regimens
  PLUS
azithromycin 1 g orally in a single dose
  or
doxycycline 100 mg a day for 7 days
- Resistance to penicillins, fluoroquinolones, sulfonamides, and tetracyclines is now widespread.
- The proportion of gonorrhea cases in heterosexual men that are fluoroquinolone resistant (QRNG) has reached 6.7%, an elevenfold increase from 0.6% in 2001. Fluoroquinolone

antibiotics are no longer recommended to treat gonorrhea in the U.S.
- Dual treatment for gonococcal and chlamydial infections is based on theory and expert opinion rather than evidence from clinical trials.

CHRONIC Rx

Postgonococcal urethritis (PGU): reinfection is the most common cause of recurrence. Repeat swab and culture of the urethra, pharynx, and rectum (where applicable) are mandatory. Persistence of polymorphonuclear cells (PMNs) with the absence of gram-negative intracellular diplococci suggests a diagnosis of postgonococcal urethritis. This occurs when GCU is treated with a regimen that is ineffective against coincident chlamydial infection; it represents NGU after GCU. The syndrome should be treated as NGU. Persistence of *N. gonorrhoeae* by smear or culture requires treatment for *N. gonorrhoeae*.

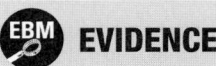

PEARLS & CONSIDERATIONS

COMMENTS

- Partner notification: the names and contact information of sexual partners should be gathered at the time of the visit and referred to the health department or the patient notifies the contact directly. Expedited partner treatment is recommended by the Centers for Disease Control and Prevention (CDC) and approved in several states. This consists of giving prescriptions to the infected patient for their partner(s) who has not been evaluated by a physician and is unlikely to seek medical care.
- On examination of the urethral smear, the presence of small numbers of PMNs provides objective evidence of urethritis. The complete absence of PMNs on a urethral smear argues against urethritis. If in addition to the PMNs there are gram-negative, intracellular diplococci, the diagnosis of gonorrhea is established.

EVIDENCE

available at www.expertconsult.com

SUGGESTED READINGS

available at www.expertconsult.com

AUTHORS: **PHILIP J. ALIOTTA, M.D., M.S.H.A.,** and **RUBEN ALVERO, M.D.**

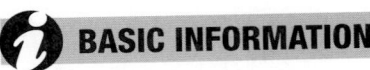

DEFINITION

Nongonococcal urethritis (NGU) is urethral inflammation caused by any of several organisms.

SYNONYMS

NGU

ICD-9CM CODES
099.40 Nongonococcal
099.41 Chlamydial

EPIDEMIOLOGY & DEMOGRAPHICS

- Occurrence is 50% in sexually transmitted disease clinics.
- NGU most commonly affects men in a higher socioeconomic class, affecting heterosexual men more frequently than homosexual men.
- NGU carries a greater morbidity rate than gonococcal urethritis (GCU).

PHYSICAL FINDINGS & CLINICAL PRESENTATION

- Incubation period: 2 to 35 days.
- Symptoms: dysuria, whitish-clear urethral discharge (see Fig. 1-396), and urethral itching. The onset of symptoms in NGU is less acute than GCU.

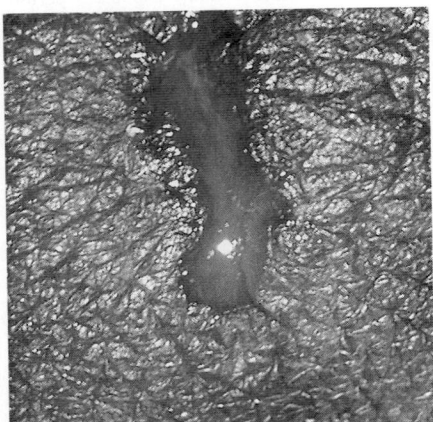

FIGURE 1-396 Urethral discharge from a man with nongonococcal urethritis. (From Mandell GL et al: *Principles and practice of infectious diseases*, ed 7, Philadelphia, 2009, Elsevier.)

- Signs: whitish-clear urethral discharge, meatal edema, and erythema. Infected women manifest pyuria, and the disease can present as acute urethral syndrome.

COMPLICATIONS

Epididymitis in heterosexual men may be linked to nonbacterial prostatitis, proctitis in homosexual men, or Reiter's syndrome.

ETIOLOGY

- Most common agent is *Chlamydia* spp., an obligate intracellular parasite possessing both DNA and RNA, which replicates by binary fission. It causes 20% to 50% of NGU cases. Two species exist:
  - *Chlamydia psittaci*
  - *Chlamydia trachomatis* with its 15 serotypes
    Serotypes A through C cause hyperendemic-blinding trachoma.
    Serotypes D through K cause genital tract infection.
    Serotypes L1 through L3 cause lymphogranuloma venereum.
- Other causes of NGU: *Ureaplasma urealyticum,* causing 15% to 30% of the cases of NGU; *Trichomonas vaginalis;* and herpes simplex virus. The cause of 20% of the cases of NGU has not been identified.
- Asymptomatic infection occurs in 28% of the contacts of women with chlamydial cervical infection.

 DIAGNOSIS

DIFFERENTIAL DIAGNOSIS

- GCU
- Herpes simplex virus
- Trichomoniasis

LABORATORY TESTS

- Requires demonstration of urethritis and exclusion of infection with *N. gonorrhoeae.*
- Nucleic acid amplification tests (NAATs): these tests have largely replaced culture in many settings where persons are screened for asymptomatic genital infection.
- The appearance of PMNs on urethral smear confirms the diagnosis of urethritis. Because *Chlamydia* is an intracellular parasite of the columnar epithelium, the best specimen for

culture is an endourethral swab taken from an area 2 to 4 cm inside the urethra. For culture, a Dacron-tipped swab is used; avoid calcium alginate or cotton swabs. The organism can only be grown in tissue culture, which is expensive.

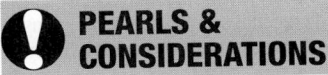 **TREATMENT**

Because it is impossible to differentiate among the common etiologies of NGU, the condition is treated syndromically, including in the initial treatment regimen those drugs effective against the common causative agents. In patients with isolated uncomplicated nongonococcal urethritis, recommended regimens are azithromycin 1 g orally single dose or doxycline 100 mg bid × 7 days. In patients with confirmed urethritis and unclear etiology, concurrent treatment for gonorrhea and *Chlamydia* is recommended. In these patients, uncomplicated infections of the urethra can be treated with combination of a single 1-g dose of oral azithromycin or 100 mg doxycycline bid × 7 days *plus*
- Cefixime 400 mg PO × 1 dose or
- Ceftriaxone 125 mg IM × 1 dose

PEARLS & CONSIDERATIONS

COMMENTS

Partner notification: The names and contact information of sexual partners should be gathered at the time of the visit and referred to the health department or the patient notifies the contact directly. Expedited partner treatment is recommended by the CDC and approved in several states. This consists of giving prescriptions to the infected patient for their partner(s) who has not been evaluated by a physician and is unlikely to seek medical care.

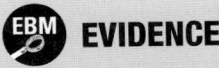 **EVIDENCE**

available at www.expertconsult.com

SUGGESTED READINGS

available at www.expertconsult.com

AUTHORS: **PHILIP J. ALIOTTA, M.D., M.S.H.A.,** and **RUBEN ALVERO, M.D.**

BASIC INFORMATION

DEFINITION

Urinary tract infection (UTI) is a term that encompasses a broad range of clinical entities that have in common a positive urine culture. A conventional threshold is growth of >100,000 colony-forming units per milliliter from a midstream-catch urine sample. In symptomatic patients, a smaller number of bacteria (between 100 and 10,000 colony-forming units per milliliter of midstream urine) is recognized as an infection.

SYNONYMS

UTI

ICD-9CM CODES
595.0 Acute cystitis
595.3 Trigonitis
595.2 Chronic cystitis
590.1 Acute pyelonephritis
590.0 Chronic pyelonephritis
590.8 Nonspecific pyelonephritis

CLASSIFICATION

- First infection: the first documented UTI; tends to be uncomplicated and is easily treated.
- Unresolved bacteriuria: UTI in which the urinary tract is not sterilized during therapy. Main causes are bacterial resistance, patient noncompliance with medication, resistance, mixed bacterial infection, rapid reinfection, azotemia, infected stones, Münchhausen syndrome, and papillary necrosis.
- Bacterial persistence: UTI in which the urine cultures become sterile during therapy, but a persistent source of infection from a site within the urinary tract that was excluded from the high urinary concentrations gives rise to reinfection by the same organism. Causes include infected stone, chronic bacterial prostatitis, atrophic infected kidney, vesicovaginal or enterovesical fistulas, obstructive uropathy, infected pyelocaliceal diverticula, infected ureteral stump after nephrectomy, infected necrotic papillae from papillary necrosis, infected urachal cysts, infected medullary sponge kidney, urethral diverticula, and foreign bodies.
- Reinfection: UTI in which a new infection occurs with new pathogens at variable intervals after a previous infection has been eradicated.
- Relapse: the less common form of recurrent infection; occurs within 2 wk of treatment when the same organism reappears in the same site as the previous infection. Relapsing infections of the urinary tract most commonly occur in pyelonephritis, kidney obstruction from a stone, and prostatitis.

EPIDEMIOLOGY & DEMOGRAPHICS

INCIDENCE:

- In neonates: more common in boys as a result of anatomic abnormalities.
- In preschool children: more common in girls (4.5% vs. 0.5% for boys).

- In adulthood: more common in women, with a 1% to 3% prevalence in nonpregnant women. In pregnancy at 12 wk, the incidence of asymptomatic bacteriuria is similar to non-pregnant women, at 2% to 10%. However, 70% to 80% of women with asymptomatic bacteriuria develop acute pyelonephritis, especially in the second and third trimesters, and have a pyelonephritic recurrence rate of 10%. In adults aged ≥65 yr, at least 10% of men and 20% of women have bacteriuria.

PHYSICAL FINDINGS & CLINICAL PRESENTATION

- UTI presentation is inconsistent and cannot be relied on to diagnose UTI accurately or to localize the site of infection. Patients report:
  - Urinary frequency, urgency
  - Dysuria
  - Urge incontinence
  - Suprapubic pain
  - Gross or microscopic hematuria
- When negative cultures are associated with significant pyuria, vaginal discharge, or hematuria, infections with *Chlamydia trachomatis*, *Neisseria gonorrhoeae*, and *Trichomonas vaginalis* should be considered.
- Acute pyelonephritis presents with fever, flank or abdominal pain, chills, malaise, vomiting, and diarrhea. It is these systemic symptoms that distinguish pyelonephritis from cystitis. Complications of acute pyelonephritis are renal abscess, perinephric abscess, emphysematous pyelonephritis, and pyonephrosis.

ETIOLOGY & PATHOGENESIS

- Four major pathways:
  - Ascending from the urethra
  - Lymphatic
  - Hematogenous
  - Direct extension from another organ system
- Other risk factors: neurologic diseases, renal failure, diabetes; anatomic abnormalities: bladder outlet obstruction, urethral stricture,

vesicoureteral reflux, fistula, urinary diversion, megacystis, infected stones, age, pregnancy, instrumentation, poor patient compliance, poor hygiene, infrequent voiding, diaphragm contraceptives, tampon use, douches, and catheters.

- Catheters: all patients who require a long-term Foley catheter eventually develop significant levels of bacteriuria. Treatment is reserved for individuals who become symptomatic (leukocytosis, fever, chills, malaise, loss of appetite, etc.) Using prophylactic antibiotics to treat patients who have chronic catheters is to be discouraged because of the risk of acquiring bacteria resistant to antibiotic therapy.
- Once bacteria reach the urinary tract, three factors determine whether the infection occurs (Box 1-21). These factors also determine the anatomic level of the UTI:
  - Virulence of the microorganism
  - Inoculum size
  - Adequacy of the host defense mechanisms
- Urinary pathogens: in 95% of UTIs the infecting organism is a member of the Enterobacteriaceae, enterococci, or, in young women, *Staphylococcus saprophyticus*. In contrast, the organisms that commonly colonize the distal urethra and skin of both men and women and the vagina of women are *Staphylococcus epidermidis*, diphtheroides, lactobacilli, *Gardnerella vaginalis*, and a variety of anaerobes that rarely cause UTIs. In general, the isolation of two or more bacterial species from a urine culture signifies a contaminated specimen unless the patient is being managed with an indwelling catheter or urinary diversion or has a chronic complicated infection.
- Defense mechanisms against cystitis: low pH and high osmolarity, mucopolysaccharide glycosaminoglycan protective layer, normal bladder that empties completely and has no incontinence, and the presence of estrogen.

BOX 1-21 Bacterial Factors

- The size of the inoculum
  - The virulence of the infecting organism:
  - Virulence factors:
    P-fimbriae facilitate the adherence of bacteria to biologic surfaces.
    K-antigens facilitate adherence and protect the organisms from the host-immune response.
    O-antigens are an important source of the systemic reactions, such as fever and shock, that occur with bacterial infections.
    H-antigens are associated with flagella and are related to bacterial locomotion.
    Hemolysin may potentiate tissue damage and facilitate local bacterial growth.
    Urease alkalinizes the urine and facilitates stone formation, thus potentiating infection.
  - Biofilms harbor bacteria on prosthetic devices and may be a source of recurrent infections.
  - The presence of sialosyl galactosyl globoside on the surface of kidney cells. This compound is a highly powerful receptor for *Escherichia coli* bacteria.
  - Women with a deficiency in human beta-defensin-1 are at greater risk for urinary tract infection.
- Adequacy of host defense mechanisms

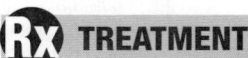

DIAGNOSIS

DIFFERENTIAL DIAGNOSIS

- Interstitial cystitis
- Vaginitis
- Urethritis (gonococcal, nongonococcal, *Trichomonas*)
- Frequency-urgency syndrome, prostatitis (acute and chronic)
- Obstructive uropathy
- Infected stones
- Fistulas
- Papillary necrosis
- Vesicoureteral reflux

LABORATORY TESTS

- Urinalysis with microscopic evaluation of clean-catch urine for bacteria and pyuria
- Urine culture and sensitivity
- Complete blood count with differential (shows leukocytosis)
- Antibody-coated bacteria are seen with pyelonephritis

IMAGING STUDIES

- Warranted only if renal infection or genitourinary abnormality is suspected
- KUB (kidneys, ureter, and bladder); voiding cystourethrogram; renal sonogram; intravenous pyelogram; CT scan; nuclear scan
- Specialty examination: cystoscopy with occasional retrograde pyelography to rule out obstructive uropathy; stenting the obstruction possibly required

TREATMENT

NONPHARMACOLOGIC THERAPY

- Hot sitz baths, anticholinergics, urinary analgesics
- For pyelonephritis: bed rest, analgesics, antipyretics, and IV hydration

ACUTE GENERAL Rx

- Conventional therapy of 7 days; short-term therapy of 1, 3, or 5 days.

- Agents of choice: amoxicillin/clavulanate, cephalosporins, fluoroquinolones, nitrofurantoin, and trimethoprim plus sulfonamide.
- For pyelonephritis: hospitalization until afebrile and stable, then at home by home care agency with IV antibiotic composed of aminoglycoside plus cephalosporin for 1 wk followed by oral agents (based on sensitivity) for 2 wk. Moderate forms of pyelonephritis have been successfully treated with fluoroquinolone therapy for 21 days without requiring hospitalization. Most important, complicating factors such as obstructive uropathy or infected stones must be identified and treated.
- "Urinary Tract Infection" in Section III describes an approach to the management of UTI.

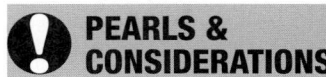

PEARLS & CONSIDERATIONS

COMMENTS

- Asymptomatic bacteriuria: occurs in both anatomically normal and abnormal urinary tracts. This can clear spontaneously, persist, or lead to symptomatic kidney infection. Treatment is recommended in patients with vesicoureteral reflux, stones, obstructive uropathy, parenchymal renal disease, or diabetes mellitus and in pregnant or immunocompromised patients.
- Pregnancy: 20% to 40% of pregnant women with untreated bacteriuria develop pyelonephritis. This is associated with prematurity and low-birth-weight infants. Confirmed significant bacteriuria should be treated with an aminopenicillin and cephalosporin.
- Recurrent UTI: caused by an unresolved infection, vaginal colonization of the originally infecting organism, or reinfection with a new strain. Management of recurrent UTI includes continuous antibiotic prophylaxis, intermittent self-treatment, and postcoital prophylaxis. Prophylaxis is recommended for women who have two or more symptomatic UTIs over a 6-mo period or three or more episodes over a 12-mo period.

- Changes after menopause: lower levels of lactobacilli, decreased estrogen, senile atrophy of the genitalia, and loss of bladder elasticity (compliance).
- Biologic factors altering defense systems: the presence of sialosyl galactosyl globoside on the surface of the kidney acts as a powerful receptor for *Escherichia coli* and increases the risk for UTI; the presence of the blood group P1 causes increased binding of *E. coli* that is resistant to normal infection-fighting mechanisms in the body. It is believed that some individuals are deficient in a compound called human beta-defensin-1, a naturally occurring antibiotic that fights *E. coli* within the urinary tract.

RESISTANCE:

- Because of the overuse of antibiotics, organisms once sensitive to a number of antimicrobial agents are now increasingly more resistant, making effective management of UTI and pyelonephritis more difficult and potentially more dangerous. Most important has been the increasing resistance to trimethoprim plus sulfamethoxazole (TMP-SMX), the current primary care provider drug of choice for acute uncomplicated UTI in women.
- When choosing a treatment regimen, physicians should consider such factors as:
  - In vitro susceptibility
  - Adverse effects
  - Cost effectiveness
  - Resistance rates in their respective communities

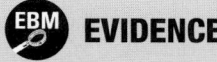

EVIDENCE

available at www.expertconsult.com

SUGGESTED READING

available at www.expertconsult.com

AUTHORS: **PHILIP J. ALIOTTA, M.D., M.S.H.A.,** and **RUBEN ALVERO, M.D.**

BASIC INFORMATION

DEFINITION

Urolithiasis is the presence of calculi within the urinary tract. The five major types of urinary stones are calcium oxalate (>50%), calcium phosphate (10% to 20%), uric acid (7%), struvite (7%), and cystine (3%) (see Table 1-180).

SYNONYMS

Kidney stones
Renal colic
Nephrolithiasis

ICD-9CM CODES
592.9 Urinary calculus

EPIDEMIOLOGY & DEMOGRAPHICS

- Urinary stone disease afflicts 250,000 to 750,000 persons in the U.S. annually.
- The male/female ratio is 4:1; after the sixth decade, it is 1.5:1.
- The incidence of symptomatic nephrolithiasis is greatest during the summer as a result of increased humidity and temperatures with a concomitant increased risk of dehydration and concentrated urine.
- Calcium oxalate or mixed calcium oxalate/calcium phosphate stones account for 70% of uroliths. Supersaturation, often expressed as the ratio of urinary calcium oxalate or calcium phosphate concentration to its solubility, is the driving force in stone formation. At levels above 1, crystals can nucleate and grow, promoting stone formation.

PHYSICAL FINDINGS & CLINICAL PRESENTATION

Stones may be asymptomatic, or they may cause the following signs and symptoms as a result of obstruction:
- Sudden onset of flank tenderness
- Nausea and vomiting

- The patient being in constant movement in an attempt to lessen the pain (Patients with an acute abdomen are usually still because movement exacerbates the pain.)
- Pain that is referred to the testes or labium by the progression of stone down the urinary ureter
- Fever and chills that accompany the acute colic if there is superimposed infection
- Pain that may radiate anteriorly over to the abdomen and result in intestinal ileus

ETIOLOGY

- Supersaturation, often expressed as the ratio of urinary calcium oxalate or calcium phosphate concentration to its solubility, is the driving force in calcium kidney stone formation
- Increased absorption of calcium in the small bowel: type I absorptive hypercalciuria (i.e., independent of calcium intake)
- Idiopathic hypercalciuria nephrolithiasis (This is the most common diagnosis for patients with calcium stones; the diagnosis is made only if there is no hypercalcemia and no known cause of the hypercalciuria.)
- Increased vitamin D synthesis (e.g., as a result of renal phosphate loss: type III absorptive hypercalciuria)
- Renal tubular malfunction with inadequate reabsorption of calcium and resulting hypercalciuria
- Heterozygous mutations in the NPT2a gene that result in hypophosphatemia and urinary phosphate loss
- Hyperparathyroidism with resulting hypercalcemia
- Elevated uric acid level (e.g., metabolic defects, dietary excess)
- Chronic diarrhea (e.g., inflammatory bowel disease) with increased oxalate absorption
- Type I (distal tubule) renal tubular acidosis (<1% of calcium stones)
- Long-term hydrochlorothiazide treatment

- Chronic infections with urease-producing organisms (e.g., *Proteus, Providencia, Pseudomonas, Klebsiella*) (Struvite, or magnesium ammonium phosphate crystals, are produced when the urinary tract is colonized by bacteria, thus producing elevated concentrations of ammonia.)
- Abnormal excretion of cystine
- Chemotherapy for malignancies
- Estrogen supplements

DIAGNOSIS

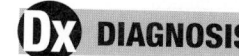

DIFFERENTIAL DIAGNOSIS

- Urinary tract infection
- Pyelonephritis
- Diverticulitis
- Pelvic inflammatory disease
- Ovarian pathology
- Factitious (i.e., in drug addicts)
- Appendicitis
- Small-bowel obstruction
- Ectopic pregnancy

The differential diagnosis of obstructive uropathy is described in Section II.

WORKUP

- Laboratory and imaging studies: Stone analysis should be performed on recovered stones.
- A clinical algorithm for the evaluation of nephrolithiasis is described in Section III.
- Box 1-22 describes events in the medical history that may be significant with regard to urolithiasis.

LABORATORY TESTS

- Urinalysis: Hematuria may be present; however, its absence does not exclude urinary stones. The evaluation of the urinary pH is of value for the identification of the type of stone: a pH of >7.5 is associated with struvite stones, whereas a pH of <5 generally is seen with uric acid or cystine stones. A low

TABLE 1-180 Stone Composition and Relative Occurrence

Stone Composition	Occurrence (%)
Calcium-Containing Stones	
Ca oxalate	60
Mixed Ca oxalate/hydroxyapatite	20
Brushite	2
Non-Calcium-Containing Stones	
Uric Acid	7
Magnesium Ammonium Phosphate (Struvite)	7
Cystine	1-3 (10% of stones in children)
Xanthine	<1
Medication-Related Stones	<1

Lipshultz LI, Khera M, Atwal DT: *Urology and the primary care practitioner,* ed 3, Philadelphia, 2008, Elsevier.

BOX 1-22 Components of the Medical History That Are Significant for Urolithiasis

- Diseases associated with disturbances of calcium metabolism: primary hyperparathyroidism, Wilson's disease, medullary sponge kidney, osteoporosis, immobilization, sarcoidosis, osteolytic metastases, plasmacytoma, neuroendocrine tumors, Paget's disease
- Dietary history: purine gluttony, calcium excess, milk alkali, oxalate excess, sodium excess, low citrus fruit intake
- Medications: uricosurics, diuretics, analgesics, vitamins C and D, antacids (especially phosphorus-binding agents), acetazolamide, calcium channel blockers, triamterene, estrogens, theophylline, protease inhibitors (indinavir), sulfonamides
- Diseases associated with disturbances of oxalate metabolism: primary hyperoxaluria types I and II, Crohn's disease, ulcerative colitis, intestinal bypass surgery (especially jejunoileal bypass), ileal resection
- Diseases associated with disturbances of purine metabolism
- Intrinsic metabolic disorders: anemia, neoplastic disorders (especially leukemias), intoxication, myocardial infarction, irradiation, cytotoxic chemotherapy
- Enzyme deficiency: primary gout, Lesch-Nyhan syndrome
- Altered excretion: renal insufficiency, metabolic acidosis
- Infectious history: organisms (particularly *Proteus* and *Klebsiella*), febrile, upper tract involvement, and dates (if hospitalized)

Modified from Nseyo UO (ed): *Urology for primary care physicians,* Philadelphia, 1999, WB Saunders.

serum bicarbonate concentration with a urine pH of ≥6 is suggestive of renal tubular acidosis.
- Urine culture and sensitivity results should be obtained for all patients.
- Serum chemistries should include calcium, electrolytes, phosphate, and uric acid.
- Additional tests: 24-hr urine collection for calcium, uric acid, phosphate, oxalate, and citrate excretion is generally reserved for patients with recurrent stones.

IMAGING STUDIES

- Plain films of the abdomen can identify radiopaque stones (e.g., calcium, uric acid) of ≥5mm in diameter.
- Renal sonogram is generally not sensitive for small stones, but it may be helpful for identifying associated hydronephrosis.
- Unenhanced (noncontrast) helical computed tomography scanning can be used to visualize the calculus, which is identified by the "rim sign" or "halo" that represents the edematous ureteral wall around the stone. The test is fast and accurate (sensitivity, 15% to 100%; specificity, 94% to 96%), and it can be used to readily identify all stone types in all locations. This modality is being used increasingly during the initial assessment of renal colic.
- Intravenous pyelography demonstrates the size and location of the stone as well as the degree of obstruction. However, this modality has largely been replaced by computed tomography.

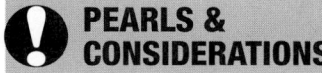

NONPHARMACOLOGIC THERAPY

- An increase in water or other fluid intake is recommended; in fact, a doubling of previous fluid intake should occur unless the patient has a history of congestive heart failure or fluid overload. Generally, patients at increased risk for the development of stones should increase their fluid intake to >2 L/day (68 oz/day) to maintain a urine volume of >2 L/day.
- Normal dietary calcium intake is recommended. If one does not consume enough calcium, less is available to bind to dietary oxalate; as a result, more oxalate reaches the colon, is absorbed into the bloodstream, and excreted as calcium oxalate, thus setting the stage for calcium urolithiasis.
- Sodium restriction to decrease calcium excretion and decreased protein intake to 1 g/kg/day to decrease uric acid, calcium, and oxalate excretion should be considered.
- Increasing the amount of bran in the diet may decrease bowel transit time with an increased binding of calcium and a subsequent decrease in urinary calcium.

ACUTE GENERAL Rx

- Pain control: Ketorolac (60 mg intramuscularly) can be used for moderate pain. However, the use of narcotics is generally indicated because of the severity of pain.
- Specific therapy is tailored to the stone type:
  - Uric acid calculi: control of hyperuricosuria with allopurinol 100 to 300 mg/day; increase urinary pH with potassium citrate 10-mEq tablets tid. Alkalinization of the urine may help prevent uric acid stones and cystine stones.
  - Calcium stones:
    1. Hydrochlorothiazide 25 to 50 mg qd in patients with type I absorptive hypercalciuria
    2. Decrease bowel absorption of calcium with cellulose phosphate 10 g/day in patients with type I absorptive hypercalciuria
    3. Orthophosphates to inhibit vitamin B synthesis in patients with type III absorptive hypercalciuria
    4. Potassium citrate supplementation for patients with hypocitraturic calcium nephrolithiasis
    5. Purine dietary restrictions or allopurinol for patients with hyperuricosuric calcium nephrolithiasis
    6. Paradoxically, calcium restriction is not warranted for patients who have had calcium stones and may even be harmful
  - Struvite stones:
    1. Most of these stones are large and cause obstruction and bleeding.
    2. Extracorporeal shockwave lithotripsy (ESWL) and percutaneous nephrolithotomy are generally necessary. Percutaneous nephrolithotomy is very effective for large stones in the kidney and is especially indicated for struvite stones.
    3. The prolonged use of antibiotics directed against the predominant urinary tract organism may be beneficial to prevent recurrence.
  - Cystine stones: hydration and alkalization of the urine to pH >6.5; penicillamine and tiopronin can be used to reduce the formation of cystine; captopril is also beneficial and causes fewer side effects.
- Possibly useful medications to help with the passage of distal ureteral stones of <10 mm in diameter are tamsulosin (alpha-adrenergic antagonist) and nifedipine (calcium channel blocker used for ureteral dilatation and relaxation). Side effects may include dizziness with tamsulosin and hypotension with nifedipine.
- Administer antibiotics if fever or pyuria (>5 to 20 leukocytes/high-power field) are present.
- Surgical treatment for patients with severe pain that is unresponsive to medication and patients with persistent fever or nausea or significant impediment of urine flow:
  - Ureteroscopic stone extraction
  - ESWL for most renal stones
- In 1997, the American Urological Association issued the following guidelines for the treatment of ureteral stones:
  - Proximal ureteral stones <1 cm in diameter: The options are ESWL, percutaneous nephroureterolithotomy, and ureteroscopy.
  - Proximal ureteral stones >1 cm in diameter: The options are ESWL, percutaneous nephroureterolithotomy, and ureteroscopy. The placement of a ureteral stent should be considered if the stone is causing high-grade obstruction.
  - Distal ureteral stones <1 cm in diameter: Most of these stones pass spontaneously. ESWL and ureteroscopy are two accepted modes of therapy.
  - Distal ureteral stones >1 cm in diameter: The options are watchful waiting, ESWL, and ureteroscopy (after stone fragmentation).

Section III describes an approach to the management of ureteral calculi.

CHRONIC Rx

The maintenance of proper hydration and dietary restrictions (see "Acute General Rx")

DISPOSITION

- >50% of patients will pass the stone within 48 hr.
- Stones will recur in approximately 50% of patients within 5 yr if no medical treatment is provided.

REFERRAL

A urology referral should be undertaken for patients with complicated or recurrent urolithiasis. Most patients with small uncomplicated ureteral or renal calculi can be followed up as outpatients, whereas patients with persistent vomiting, suspected urinary tract infection, pain that is unresponsive to oral analgesics, or obstructing calculus associated with a solitary kidney should be admitted.

PEARLS & CONSIDERATIONS

COMMENTS

- The early identification and aggressive treatment of urinary tract infections is indicated for all patients with struvite stones.
- The alkalinization of urine (i.e., getting to a pH of >7.5 with the use of penicillamine) is useful for patients with recurrent cystine stones.
- Stones <5 mm in diameter often pass spontaneously whereas stones >10 mm generally do not.
- An algorithmic approach to the management of ureteral calculi is described in Section III.

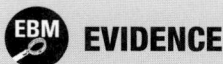 **EVIDENCE**

available at www.expertconsult.com

SUGGESTED READINGS

available at www.expertconsult.com

AUTHORS: **PHILIP J. ALIOTTA, M.D., M.S.H.A.,** and **RUBEN ALVERO, M.D.**

BASIC INFORMATION

DEFINITION

Urticaria is a pruritic rash involving the epidermis and the upper portions of the dermis caused by localized capillary vasodilation and followed by transudation of protein-rich fluid in the surrounding tissue and manifesting clinically with the presence of hives. Urticaria is classified according to its chronicity into acute (<6-wk duration) and chronic (>6-wk duration).

SYNONYMS

Hives
Wheals

ICD-9CM CODES
708.8 Other unspecified urticaria

EPIDEMIOLOGY & DEMOGRAPHICS

- 12% to 24% of the population will have one episode of hives during their lifetime.
- Incidence is increased in atopic patients.
- The etiology of chronic urticaria (hives lasting >6 wk) is determined in only 5% to 20% of cases.

PHYSICAL FINDINGS & CLINICAL PRESENTATION

- Presence of elevated, erythematous, or white nonpitting plaques that change in size and shape over time; they generally last a few hours and disappear without a trace.
- Annular configuration with central pallor (Fig. 1-397).
- Angioedema occurs in approximately 40% of cases of urticaria and is caused by mast cell mediator release in the subcutaneous tissue and deep dermis.

ETIOLOGY

- Foods (e.g., shellfish, eggs, strawberries, nuts)
- Drugs (e.g., penicillin, aspirin, sulfonamides)
- Systemic diseases (e.g., systemic lupus erythematosus, serum sickness, autoimmune thyroid disease, polycythemia vera)

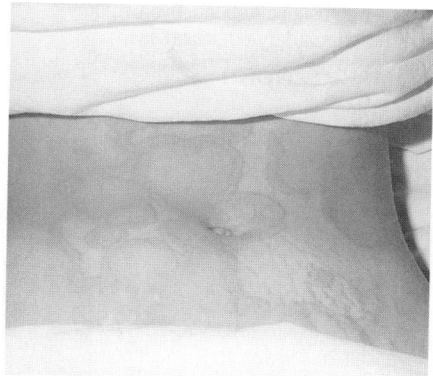

FIGURE 1-397 Wheal (urticaria). Note central cleaning, giving annular configuration. (From Noble J et al: *Textbook of primary care medicine,* ed 3, St Louis, 2001, Mosby.)

- Food additives (e.g., salicylates, benzoates, sulfites)
- Infections (viral infections, fungal infections, chronic bacterial infections)
- Physical stimuli (e.g., pressure urticaria, exercise-induced, solar urticaria, cold urticaria)
- Inhalants (e.g., mold spores, animal dander, pollens)
- Contact (nonimmunologic) urticaria (e.g., caterpillars, plants)
- Other: hereditary angioedema, urticaria pigmentosa, pregnancy, cryoglobulinemia, hair bleaches, chemicals, saliva, cosmetics, perfumes, pemphigoid, emotional stress, malignancy (lymphomas, endocrine tumors)

DIAGNOSIS

DIFFERENTIAL DIAGNOSIS

- Erythema multiforme
- Erythema marginatum
- Erythema infectiosum
- Urticarial vasculitis
- Herpes gestationis
- Drug eruption
- Multiple insect bites
- Bullous pemphigoid

WORKUP

- It is useful to determine whether hives are acute or chronic; a medical history focused on various etiologic factors is necessary before embarking on extensive laboratory testing.
- Most cases of acute urticaria resolve spontaneously and diagnostic testing is not required.
- A diagnostic approach to chronic urticaria is described in Section III.

LABORATORY TESTS

- Complete blood count with differential.
- Stool for ova and parasites in patients with suspected parasitic infestations.
- Skin testing with allergic extracts and screening for dermatographism by attempting to elicit a wheal after application of linear skin pressure should be performed only after withholding antihistamines for 36 to 72 hr to prevent false-negative results.
- Antinuclear antibody, erythrocyte sedimentation rate, thyroid-stimulating hormone, antithyroid antibodies, *Helicobacter pylori* serology, liver function tests, and eosinophil count are indicated only in patients with chronic urticaria.
- Measurement of C_4 may be helpful in patients who present with angioedema alone.
- Skin biopsy is helpful in patients with fever, arthralgias, and elevated erythrocyte sedimentation rate. Histologic evidence of leukocytoclasia (neutrophilic infiltration with fragmentation of nuclei) is indicative of urticarial vasculitis.
- When suspecting food allergy in acute urticaria, testing can be performed using skin prick, immunoCAP, and radioallergosorbent testing.

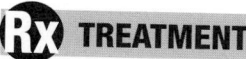

TREATMENT

NONPHARMACOLOGIC THERAPY

- Remove suspected etiologic agents (e.g., stop aspirin and all nonessential drugs), and restrict diet (e.g., elimination of tomatoes, nuts, eggs, shellfish).
- Elimination of yeast should be attempted in patients with chronic urticaria (*Candida albicans* sensitivity may be a factor in patients with chronic urticaria).

ACUTE GENERAL Rx

- Oral antihistamines: use of nonsedating antihistamines (e.g., loratadine 10 mg qd, cetirizine 10 mg qd, fexofenadine 180 mg qd, levocetirizine 5 mg qd) is preferred over first-generation antihistamines (e.g., hydroxyzine, diphenhydramine).
- Doxepin (a tricyclic antidepressant) that blocks both H_1 and H_2 receptors 25 to 75 mg qhs may be effective in patients with chronic urticaria.
- Oral corticosteroids should be reserved for refractory cases (e.g., prednisone 20 mg qd or 20 mg bid).
- H_2 receptor antagonists (cimetidine, ranitidine, famotidine) can be added to H_1 antagonists in refractory cases.

CHRONIC Rx

- Use of nonsedating antihistamines, doxepin, and/or oral corticosteroids (see "Acute General Rx").
- Low dose of the immunosuppressant cyclosporine (2.5 to 3 mg/kg body weight/day) has been shown to be effective and corticosteroid sparing in chronic urticaria.
- There are insufficient data to support use of leukotriene antagonists (zafirlukast, montelukast) in patients with chronic urticaria.

DISPOSITION

- Most cases of urticaria resolve within 6 wk.
- Only 25% of patients with a history of chronic urticaria are completely cured after 5 yr.

PEARLS & CONSIDERATIONS

COMMENTS

Local treatment (e.g., starch baths or oatmeal baths) may be helpful in selected patients; however, local treatment is generally not rewarding.

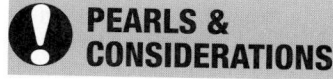 EVIDENCE

available at www.expertconsult.com

SUGGESTED READING
available at www.expertconsult.com

AUTHOR: **FRED F. FERRI, M.D.**

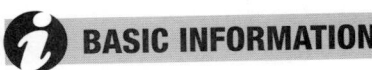 **BASIC INFORMATION**

DEFINITION

Uterine fibroids are benign tumors of muscle cell origin. They are discrete nodular tumors that vary in size and number and that may be found as subserosal, intramural, or submucosal masses. They can also be located in the cervix, broad ligament, or on a stalk (pedunculated).

SYNONYMS

Uterine leiomyomas
Uterine myomas

ICD-9CM CODES
218.9 Leiomyomas, fibroids

EPIDEMIOLOGY & DEMOGRAPHICS

- Estimated prevalence of 20% of reproductive age women
- The most common benign uterine tumor
- More common in black women than white women
- Asymptomatic fibroids may be present in 40% to 50% of women aged >40 yr
- May occur singly but are often multiple
- Fewer than half of all fibroids are estimated to produce symptoms
- Frequently diagnosed incidentally on pelvic examination
- There is increased familial incidence
- Potential to enlarge during pregnancy as well as regress after menopause
- Infrequent primary cause of infertility in <3% of infertile patients
- Symptomatic fibromas are the primary indication for approximately 30% of all hysterectomies

PHYSICAL FINDINGS & CLINICAL PRESENTATION

- Enlarged, irregular uterus on pelvic examination.
- Presenting symptoms:
  1. Menorrhagia (most common)
  2. Chronic pelvic pain (dysmenorrhea, dyspareunia, pelvic pressure)
  3. Acute pain (torsion of pedunculated fibroma, infarction, and degeneration)
  4. Urinary symptoms (frequency from bladder pressure, partial ureteral obstruction, complete ureteral obstruction)
  5. Rectosigmoid compression with constipation or intestinal obstruction
  6. Prolapse through cervix of pedunculated submucosal tumor
  7. Venous stasis of lower extremities
  8. Polycythemia
  9. Ascites

ETIOLOGY

Incompletely understood. It is suggested that fibromas arise from an original single smooth muscle cell in the myometrium. Each individual fibroma is monoclonal (all the cells are derived from one progenitor myocyte). Malignant degeneration of preexisting leiomyoma is extremely uncommon (<0.5%).

 DIAGNOSIS

DIFFERENTIAL DIAGNOSIS

Leiomyosarcoma, ovarian mass (neoplastic, non-neoplastic, endometrioma), inflammatory mass, pregnancy

WORKUP

- Complete pelvic examination, rectovaginal examination, Pap test
- Estimation of size of mass in centimeters
- Endometrial sampling may be indicated (biopsy or dilation and curettage) when abnormal bleeding and pelvic mass are present
- If urinary symptoms are prominent, cystometry, cystoscopy to rule out bladder lesions, intravenous pyelogram to rule out impingement on urinary system

LABORATORY TESTS

- Pregnancy test
- Pap smear
- Complete blood count, erythrocyte sedimentation rate
- Fecal occult blood

IMAGING STUDIES

- Pelvic ultrasound (transvaginal may have higher diagnostic accuracy) is useful.
- CT scan is helpful in planning treatment if malignancy is strongly suspected.
- Hysteroscopy may provide direct evidence of intrauterine pathology or submucosal leiomyoma that distorts uterine cavity.

 **TREATMENT**

Management should be based on primary symptoms and may include observation with close follow-up, temporizing surgical therapies, medical management, or definitive surgical procedures. Treatment is generally indicated only when symptoms are present and are severe enough to be unacceptable to the patient.

NONSURGICAL Rx

- Patient observation and follow-up with periodic repeat pelvic examinations to ensure that tumors are not growing rapidly.
- Gonadotropin-releasing hormone (GnRH) agonist use results in 40% to 60% reduction in uterine volume. Hypoestrogenism, reversible bone loss, and hot flushes are associated with use. Limit to short-term use and consider low-dose hormonal replacement to minimize hypoestrogenic effects.
- Regrowth occurs in approximately 50% of women treated a few months after cessation.
- Indications for GnRH:
  1. Fertility preservation in women with large myomas before attempting conception or preoperative myectomy treatment
  2. Anemia treatment to normalize hemoglobin before surgery
  3. Women approaching menopause to avoid surgery
  4. Preoperative for large myomas to make vaginal hysterectomy, hysteroscopic resection/ablation, or laparoscopic destruction more feasible
  5. Women with medical contraindications for surgery
  6. Personal or medical indications for delaying surgery
- Progestational agents may also result in decrease in uterine size and amenorrhea, allowing iron therapy to treat anemia with limited success.
- Other drugs used and under investigation:
  1. Danazol: androgen and multienzyme inhibitor of steroidogenesis
  2. Mifepristone: antiprogestogen shown to reduce the fibroid volume by 40% to 50% with amenorrhea
  3. Raloxifene: selective estrogen receptor modulator, either alone or with a GnRHa, shown to reduce the fibroid volume 70% up to 1 yr but only in postmenopausal women
  4. Fadrozole: aromatase inhibitor reported to have produced a 71% reduction in volume

SURGICAL Rx

- Indications
  1. Abnormal uterine bleeding with anemia refractory to hormonal therapy
  2. Chronic pain with severe dysmenorrhea, dyspareunia, or lower abdominal pressure/pain
  3. Acute pain, torsion, or prolapsing submucosal fibroid
  4. Urinary symptoms or signs such as hydronephrosis
  5. Rapid uterine enlargement premenopausal or any growth after menopause
  6. Infertility or recurrent pregnancy loss with submucous leiomyoma as only finding
  7. Enlarged uterus with compression symptoms or discomfort
- Procedures
  1. Hysterectomy (definitive procedure): Nearly 15% of women with uterine fibroids and a mean age of 45 yr require hysterectomy.
  2. Abdominal myomectomy (to preserve fertility)
  3. Vaginal myomectomy for prolapsed pedunculated submucous fibroid
  4. Hysteroscopic resection
  5. Laparoscopic/robotic myomectomy
  6. Uterine artery embolization

COMPLICATIONS

- Red degeneration
- Leiomyosarcoma (<0.1%)

REFERRAL

Consultation with gynecologic oncologist if suspicion of malignancy

EBM EVIDENCE

available at www.expertconsult.com

SUGGESTED READINGS

available at www.expertconsult.com

AUTHORS: **ARUNDATHI G. PRASAD, M.D.,** and **RUBEN ALVERO, M.D.**

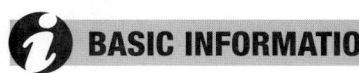 **BASIC INFORMATION**

DEFINITION

Uterine malignancy includes tumors from the endometrium and sarcomas. Uterine sarcoma is an abnormal proliferation of cells originating from the mesenchymal, or connective tissue, elements of the uterine wall.

SYNONYMS

Leiomyosarcomas
Endometrial stromal sarcoma
Malignant mixed Müllerian tumors
Adenosarcomas

ICD-9CM CODES

182.0 Malignant neoplasm of body of uterus (corpus uteri), except isthmus
182.1 Malignant neoplasm of body of uterus, isthmus
182.8 Malignant neoplasm of body of uterus, other specified sites of body of uterus

EPIDEMIOLOGY & DEMOGRAPHICS

INCIDENCE: 17.1 cases per 1 million females. Endometrial cancer remains the most common gynecologic malignancy in the U.S.
PREVALENCE: Uterine sarcoma accounts for 4.3% of all cancers of the uterine corpus and is the most lethal gynecologic malignancy.
MEAN AGE AT DIAGNOSIS: 52 yr
RISK FACTORS: Similar to endometrial carcinoma

PHYSICAL FINDINGS & CLINICAL PRESENTATION

- Abnormal vaginal bleeding is the most common symptom
- May also present as pelvic pain or pressure and pelvic mass on examination
- May appear as tumor protruding through the cervix
- Vaginal discharge may also be a presenting symptom
- Rapidly enlarging uterus

ETIOLOGY

- The exact etiology is unknown.
- Prior pelvic radiation is a risk factor for sarcoma.
- Black women may be at higher risk.

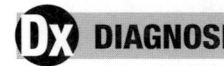 **DIAGNOSIS**

DIFFERENTIAL DIAGNOSIS

Leiomyoma

WORKUP

Diagnosis is made histologically by biopsy for abnormal bleeding.

LABORATORY TESTS

Chest radiography, CT scans, and MRI are used to evaluate spread.

BOX 1-23   Uterine Sarcoma: Key Points

The disease mainly affects postmenopausal women.
Most patients present early with postmenopausal bleeding.
The primary treatment is hysterectomy.
Adjuvant radiotherapy to the pelvis is used if poor prognosis features in Stage 1 or if spread has occurred beyond the corpus.

Greer IA, Cameron IT, Kitchner HC, Prentice A: *Mosby's color atlas and text of obstetrics and gynecology,* London, 2001, Harcourt.

IMAGING STUDIES

- Chest radiography is usually done as routine preoperative testing.
- CT scans and MRI are good for assessing tumor spread once diagnosis is made.

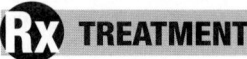 **TREATMENT**

NONPHARMACOLOGIC THERAPY

- Surgical excision is the mainstay of treatment.
- Grade and stage of tumor affect prognosis.
- The benefit of adjuvant radiotherapy in stage I endometrial adenocarcinoma to improve pelvic disease control and improve survival remains controversial despite several phase 3 trials.
- Chemotherapeutic agents have produced only partial and short-term responses.

DISPOSITION

- Survival varies with each type of sarcoma but is generally very poor.
- Five-year survival for leiomyosarcoma ranges from 48% for stage I to 0% for stage IV.
- Five-year survival for malignant mixed mesodermal tumor ranges from 36% for stage I to 6% for stage IV.

REFERRAL

Uterine sarcoma should be managed by a gynecologic oncologist and radiation oncologist. Key points in the management of uterine sarcoma are described in Box 1-23.

SUGGESTED READINGS
available at www.expertconsult.com

AUTHORS: **GIL M. FARKASH, M.D.,** and **RUBEN ALVERO, M.D.**

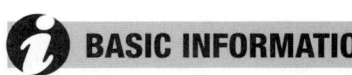

BASIC INFORMATION

DEFINITION

Uveitis is inflammation of the uveal tract, including the iris, ciliary body, and choroid. It may also involve other closed structures such as the sclera, retina, and vitreous humor.

SYNONYMS

Anterior uveitis
Posterior uveitis
Acute or chronic uveitis
Granulomatous or nongranulomatous uveitis
Iritis
Chroroiditis
Pars planitis
Iridocyclitis

ICD-9CM CODES
364.3 Unspecified iridocyclitis, uveitis

EPIDEMIOLOGY & DEMOGRAPHICS

INCIDENCE (IN U.S.): Common; busy ophthalmologist will see two or more cases per week.
PEAK INCIDENCE: Middle age or older; uveitis in childhood rare; equal in boys and girls; 25% idiopathic and 75% related to toxoplasmosis, juvenile rheumatoid arthritis, pars planitis, toxicaris canis, or Behçet's disease
PREVALENCE (IN U.S.): 17 cases per 100,000 persons
PREDOMINANT SEX: None
PREDOMINANT AGE: 38 yr. Although uveitis is less common in children than adults, it is believed to be more severe with an increased risk for vision-threatening complications.

PHYSICAL FINDINGS & CLINICAL PRESENTATION

- Symptoms of uveitis depend on the site of involvement and whether process is acute or insidious:
  - Acute anterior uveitis: pain and photophobia. Vision may not be affected initially.
  - Posterior uveitis: floaters, hazy vision. Involvement of the retina may produce blind spots or flashing lights.
  - Insidious anterior uveitis: symptoms may not be present until scarring cataracts and loss of vision occur.
- Photophobia
- Blurred visual acuity
- Irregular pupil
- Hazy cornea
- Abnormal cells and flare in anterior chamber or vitreous humor
- Retinal hemorrhage, vascular sheathing
- Conjunctival injection
- Ciliary flush
- Keratitic precipitates (precipitates on the cornea)
- Hazy vitreous
- Retinal inflammation
- Iris nodules
- Glaucoma
- Rheumatoid arthritis
- Scleritis
- Systemic symptoms related to etiology

ETIOLOGY

- Infections: herpes simplex virus, cytomegalovirus, toxoplasmosis, tuberculosis, syphilis, HIV
- Systemic disorders: sarcoidosis, Behçet's syndrome, HLA-B27–associated diseases (e.g., ankylosing spondylitis, reactive arthritis), inflammatory bowel disease, juvenile idiopathic arthritis
- Idiopathic

DIAGNOSIS

DIFFERENTIAL DIAGNOSIS

- Glaucoma
- Conjunctivitis
- Retinal detachment
- Retinopathy
- Keratitis
- Scleritis
- Episcleritis
- Masquerading syndromes: lymphoma, uveal melanoma, metastases (breast, lung, renal), leukemia, retinitis pigmentosa, retinoblastoma

WORKUP

- Associated with arthritis, syphilis, tuberculosis, granulomatous disease, collagen-vascular disease, allergies, AIDS, sarcoid, Behçet's disease, histoplasmosis, toxoplasmosis, and toxicaris canis
- Slit lamp examination, indirect ophthalmoscopy

LABORATORY TESTS

- Complete blood count
- Laboratory tests for specific inflammatory causes cited previously in "Workup" (e.g., antinuclear antibody, erythrocyte sedimentation rate, syphilis (VDRL), HLA-B27, purified protein derivative, Lyme titer)
- Visual field testing

IMAGING STUDIES

- Chest radiograph in suspected sarcoidosis, tuberculosis, histoplasmosis
- Sacroiliac radiograph in suspected ankylosing spondylitis

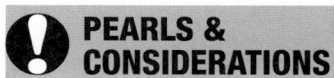

TREATMENT

NONPHARMACOLOGIC THERAPY

- Treat the underlying disease. Treatment is often multidisciplinary (ophthalmologist, internist, rheumatologist, internal disease specialist).
- Treat photophobia and local pain.

ACUTE GENERAL Rx

- Corticosteroids are the mainstay of therapy for noninfectious causes. The route of administration depends on the location of inflammation, the severity, and the presence of systemic disease. Cycloplegic drops (cyclopentolate) or cycloplegic agents (homatropine hydrobromide 1gtt q3 to 4h while awake) and topical steroids (prednisone acetate 1% 1 gtt qh during day, prn at night until favorable response,

then q4 to 6h); avoid topical corticosteroids in infectious uveitis. Periocular corticosteroid injections can be used for posterior disease; they have the advantage of achieving high intraocular levels of steroids without the systemic side effects of oral corticosteroids.
- Antibiotics for bacterial infections and antiviral agents, when infection is suspected, should be started to prevent retinal damage.
- Systemic steroids if appropriate for the underlying disease. Systemic corticosteroid therapy is generally reserved for patients with systemic disorders and those with bilateral disease that is refractory to local medication or those with major ocular disability or retinitis.
- Antimetabolites when indicated. Immunosuppressive medications used in steroid-dependent or refractory uveitis include methotrexate, sulfasalazine, azathioprine, cyclosporine, and tacrolimus. These medications can have significant toxicity and should be prescribed only by physicians experienced with their use.
- High-dose IV daclizumab has been reported as effective in reducing active inflammation in active JIA-associated anterior uveitis. Additional trials are needed to better assess efficacy and safety.

CHRONIC Rx

- Topical steroids and cycloplegics
- Treat underlying cause

DISPOSITION

Urgent referral to ophthalmologist for diagnosis and treatment

REFERRAL

- Eye problem should be monitored early on by an ophthalmologist.
- Underlying medical disease should be treated by the primary care physician.

PEARLS & CONSIDERATIONS

COMMENTS

- In 90% of cases the condition is idiopathic.
- Associated causes are found approximately 10% of the time, usually chronic and recurrent.
- Chronic glaucoma, cataracts, retinal degeneration, and other severe eye problems occur with the disease and the treatment.
- Chronic anterior uveitis is the most common form of intraocular inflammation in children. Juvenile idiopathic arthritis (JIA) is the most common cause.

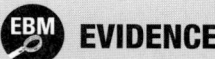 EVIDENCE

available at www.expertconsult.com

SUGGESTED READINGS
available at www.expertconsult.com

AUTHOR: **MELVYN KOBY, M.D.**

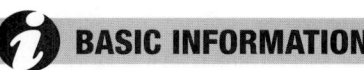 **BASIC INFORMATION**

DEFINITION

Bleeding per vagina at any time during pregnancy must be regarded as abnormal and is associated with an increased likelihood of pregnancy complications.

SYNONYMS

Hemorrhage

ICD-9CM CODES

634.9	Spontaneous abortion
633.9	Ectopic pregnancy
630/631	Molar pregnancy
622.7	Cervical polyps
180.9/180.0/180.8	Cervical dysplasia/cancer
616.0	Cervicitis
616.10	Vulvovaginitis
184.0	Vaginal cancer
644.2	Premature labor term labor
641.1	Placenta previa
641.2	Placental abruption

EPIDEMIOLOGY & DEMOGRAPHICS

- Common in U.S.; 20% to 25% of patients have vaginal spotting/bleeding in first trimester; of those, miscarriage occurs in 50%.
- Occurs in women of childbearing age.
- Between 1% and 2% of all pregnancies in the U.S. are ectopic.
- After one ectopic pregnancy, the chance of another is 7% to 15%.
- Ectopic pregnancy is the leading cause of maternal mortality in the first trimester.
- Average reported frequency for placental abruption is about 1 in 150 deliveries (0.3%).
- Incidence of placenta previa is <1 in 200 deliveries (0.5%).

PHYSICAL FINDINGS & CLINICAL PRESENTATION

- Bleeding: ranges from scant to life-threatening with hemodynamic instability
- Color: brown to bright red
- Can be painless or painful (cramps, back pain, severe abdominal pain)
- Fetal compromise: ranges from none to fetal demise

ETIOLOGY

- Influenced by gestational age
- Vaginal
- Cervical
- Uterine

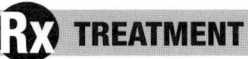 **DIAGNOSIS**

DIFFERENTIAL DIAGNOSIS

- Any gestational age:
  1. Cervical lesions: polyps, decidual reaction, neoplasia
  2. Vaginal trauma
  3. Cervicitis/vulvovaginitis
  4. Postcoital trauma
  5. Bleeding dyscrasias
- Gestation <20 wk:
  1. Spontaneous abortion
  2. Presence of intrauterine device
  3. Ectopic pregnancy
  4. Molar pregnancy
  5. Implantation bleeding
  6. Low-lying placenta
- Gestation >20 wk:
  1. Molar pregnancy
  2. Placenta previa
  3. Placental abruption
  4. Vasa previa
  5. Marginal separation of the placenta
  6. Bloody show at term
  7. Preterm labor
- Section II describes the differential diagnosis of vaginal bleeding in pregnancy.

WORKUP

- Gestation <20 wk (Section III, "Bleeding, Early Pregnancy")
  1. Pelvic examination
  2. Culdocentesis
  3. Laparoscopy
  4. Laparotomy
  5. Ultrasound to verify viable intrauterine pregnancy
- Gestation >20 wk:
  1. Ultrasound to locate placenta before pelvic examination
  2. If placenta previa, no speculum or bimanual examination
  3. If preterm labor, appropriate evaluation done

LABORATORY TESTS

- Urine pregnancy test: if positive, get quantitative β human chorionic gonadotropin (hCG). The following are typical although not entirely exclusive patterns:
  1. Early pregnancy: follow serially every 48 hr
  2. Normal pregnancy: hCG doubles approximately every 48 hr
  3. Spontaneous abortion: hCG level will fall
  4. Ectopic pregnancy: hCG level will rise inappropriately
  5. Molar pregnancy: hCG level is extremely high

- CBC
- Blood type and screen (Rh-negative patients need RhoGAM)
- Coagulation profile (useful in missed abortion and abruption)
- Cervical cultures/wet mount
- Pap smear for cervical malignancy; caution with biopsy, because cervix can bleed extensively

IMAGING STUDIES

Ultrasound:
- 5 to 6 wk: gestational sac (transvaginally); hCG >2500 mIU/ml (third IS) or >1000 mIU/ml (second IS)
- 8 to 9 wk: fetal cardiac activity
- Molar pregnancy: characteristic cluster of cysts
- Location of placenta
- Degree of placental separation: difficult to assess

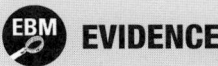 **TREATMENT**

NONPHARMACOLOGIC THERAPY

- Pelvic rest: no coitus, douching, or tampons
- Bed rest, if >20 wk
- Counseling: genetic, bereavement

ACUTE GENERAL Rx

- Hemodynamic stabilization
- Emergency D&C, laparotomy, or cesarean section as necessary

CHRONIC Rx

Depends on diagnosis

DISPOSITION

Depends on diagnosis

REFERRAL

- If patient is unstable and needs emergency ob/gyn management and/or surgery
- If patient has diagnosis of ectopic or molar pregnancy, because immediate surgical treatment is indicated
- Perinatal consultation for high-risk pregnancy

EBM **EVIDENCE**

available at www.expertconsult.com

SUGGESTED READING
available at www.expertconsult.com

AUTHORS: **GEORGE T. DANAKAS, M.D.,** and **RUBEN ALVERO, M.D.**

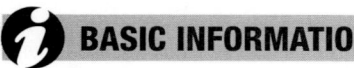

BASIC INFORMATION

DEFINITION

Vaginal malignancy is an abnormal proliferation of vaginal epithelium demonstrating malignant cells below the basement membrane.

SYNONYMS

Squamous cell carcinoma of the vagina
Adenocarcinoma of the vagina
Melanoma of the vagina
Sarcoma of the vagina
Endodermal sinus tumor

ICD-9CM CODES

184.0 Vagina, vaginal neoplasm

EPIDEMIOLOGY & DEMOGRAPHICS

INCIDENCE: 0.42 cases per 100,000 persons
PREVALENCE: Vaginal cancer is the second rarest gynecologic cancer. It comprises 2% of malignancies of the female genital tract.
MEAN AGE AT DIAGNOSIS: Predominantly a disease of menopause. Mean age at diagnosis is 60 yr.

PHYSICAL FINDINGS & CLINICAL PRESENTATION

- Majority of cases are asymptomatic
- Postmenopausal vaginal bleeding and/or vaginal discharge are the most common symptoms
- May also present as pelvic pain or pressure, dyspareunia, dysuria, malodor, or postcoital bleeding
- May present as a vaginal lesion or abnormal Pap smear

ETIOLOGY

- The exact etiology is unknown.
- Vaginal intraepithelial neoplasia is believed to be a precursor for squamous cell carcinoma of the vagina.
- Long-term pessary use has been associated with vaginal malignancy.
- Prior pelvic radiation may be a risk factor.
- Clear-cell adenocarcinoma is related to in utero diethylstilbestrol exposure.

DIAGNOSIS

DIFFERENTIAL DIAGNOSIS

- Extension from other primary carcinoma more common than primary vaginal cancer
- Vaginitis

WORKUP

- Diagnosis is made histologically by biopsy.
- Colposcopy and biopsy should follow suspicious Pap smear.
- Cystoscopy, proctosigmoidoscopy, chest radiography, IV urography, and barium enema may be used for clinical staging.
- CT scan (Fig. 1-399), FDG, PET scan, and MRI are used to evaluate spread.
- Staging I to IV (Fig. 1-398).

IMAGING STUDIES

- Chest radiography, IV urography, and barium enema are used for staging.
- CT scan and MRI are good for assessing tumor spread.

TREATMENT

NONPHARMACOLOGIC THERAPY

- Radiation therapy is the mainstay of treatment.
- Stage I tumors that are small and confined to the posterior, upper third of the vagina may be treated with radical surgery.
- Other stages require a whole-pelvis, interstitial, and/or intracavitary radiation therapy.
- Chemotherapy is used in conjunction with radiotherapy in rare select cases.

DISPOSITION

Five-year survival ranges from 80% for stage I to 17% for stage IV.

REFERRAL

Vaginal cancer should be managed by a gynecologic oncologist and radiation oncologist.

EVIDENCE

available at www.expertconsult.com

SUGGESTED READING

available at www.expertconsult.com

AUTHORS: **GIL M. FARKASH, M.D.,** and **RUBEN ALVERO, M.D.**

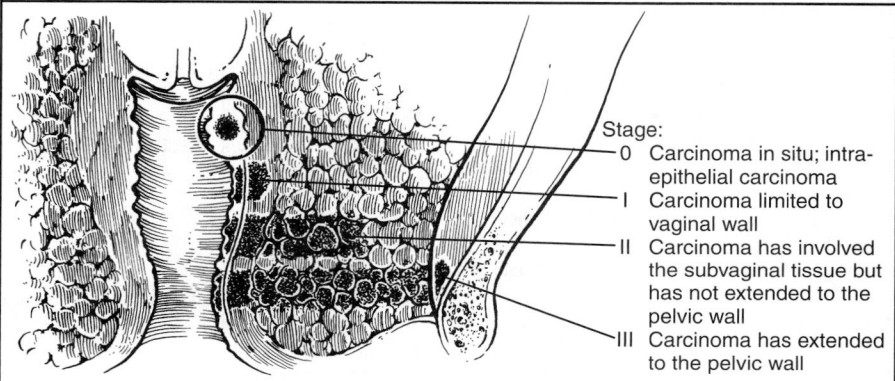

Stage:
- 0 Carcinoma in situ; intraepithelial carcinoma
- I Carcinoma limited to vaginal wall
- II Carcinoma has involved the subvaginal tissue but has not extended to the pelvic wall
- III Carcinoma has extended to the pelvic wall

FIGURE 1-398 Staging system for vaginal cancer. Metastatic disease that involves the bladder or rectum is stage IV-a. Metastatic disease beyond the pelvis is stage IV-b. (From Copeland LJ: *Textbook of gynecology,* ed 2, Philadelphia, 2000, WB Saunders.)

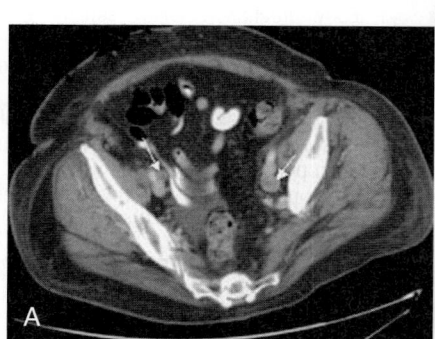 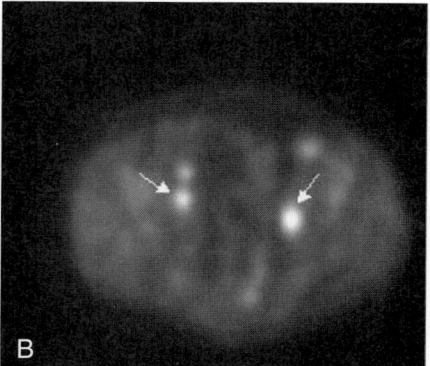

FIGURE 1-399 Vaginal cancer with lymphadenopathy. A, CT of pelvis showing mildly enlarged external iliac nodes suggestive of metastases (arrows). **B,** Axial FDG PET scan showing hypermetabolic nodes as hyperintense spots confirming metastases. Abeloff MD: *Clinical oncology,* ed 3, Philadelphia, 2004, Elsevier.

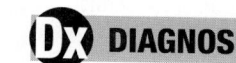

BASIC INFORMATION

DEFINITION

Vaginismus refers to the involuntary spasm of the vaginal, introital, and/or levator ani muscles, preventing penetration or causing painful intercourse.

ICD-9CM CODES
300.11 Hysterical vaginismus
306.51 Psychogenic or functional vaginismus
625.1 Reflex vaginismus

EPIDEMIOLOGY & DEMOGRAPHICS

INCIDENCE: Estimated at 11.7% to 42% of women presenting to sexual dysfunction clinics
PREVALENCE: Affects approximately 1 in 200 women
PREDOMINANT SEX: Affects only females
RISK FACTORS: Any previous sexual trauma, including incest or rape

PHYSICAL FINDINGS & CLINICAL PRESENTATION

- Fear of pain with coitus
- Dyspareunia
- Orgasmic dysfunction

ETIOLOGY

- Learned conditioned response to real or imagined painful vaginal experience (e.g., traumatic speculum examination, incest, rape)
- Vaginitis
- Pelvic inflammatory disease
- Endometriosis
- Anatomic anomalies
- Atrophic vaginitis
- Mucosal tears
- Inadequate lubrication
- Focal vulvitis
- Painful hymenal tags
- Scarring secondary to episiotomy
- Skin disorders
- Topical allergies
- Postherpetic neuralgia

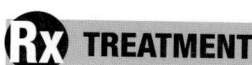

DIAGNOSIS

WORKUP

- Thorough history (including sexual history)
- Careful pelvic examination
- Behavioral therapy

TREATMENT

NONPHARMACOLOGIC THERAPY

- Deconditioning the response by systematic self-administered progressive dilation techniques using fingers or dilators
- Behavioral and/or psychosexual therapy

ACUTE GENERAL Rx

- Botulinum toxin therapy given locally has been shown to relieve the perineal muscle spasms associated with vaginismus, allowing resumption of intercourse.
  1. Acts by preventing neuromuscular transmission, causing muscle weakness
  2. Considered experimental treatment for vaginismus at this time
- Cause should be determined by history and explained to the patient so that she understands the mechanics of the muscle spasms.
- Patient must be motivated to desire painless vaginal insertion for such reasons as pleasurable coitus, tampon insertion, or gynecologic examination.
- Patient (and her partner) must be willing to patiently undergo the process of systematic desensitization and counseling.

DISPOSITION

A high percentage of successfully treated patients

REFERRAL

To a gynecologist or sex therapist

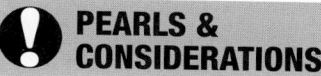

PEARLS & CONSIDERATIONS

COMMENTS

- May uncover early sexual abuse or an aversion to sexuality in general
- American Association of Sex Educators, Counselors and Therapists, 11 Dupont Circle, NW, Washington, DC, 20036.
- Sex Information and Education Council of the U.S. (SIECUS), 85th Avenue, New York, NY 10022.

SUGGESTED READINGS

available at www.expertconsult.com

AUTHORS: **BETH J. WUTZ, M.D.,** and **RUBEN ALVERO, M.D.**

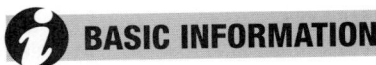

DEFINITION

Bacterial vaginosis (BV) is a thin, gray, homogenous, malodorous vaginal discharge that results from a shift in the vaginal flora from a predominance of lactobacilli to high concentrations of anaerobic bacteria.

SYNONYMS

Before 1955: nonspecific vaginitis
1955: *Haemophilus vaginalis* vaginitis
1963: *Corynebacterium vaginalis* vaginitis
1980: *Gardnerella vaginalis* vaginitis
1990: Bacterial vaginosis

ICD-9CM CODES
616.10 Vaginitis, bacterial

EPIDEMIOLOGY & DEMOGRAPHICS

- Most common vaginal infection
- *Gardnerella, Mycoplasma,* and *Mobiluncus* are harbored in the urethra of male partners; however:
  1. Male partners are asymptomatic.
  2. There is no improved cure rate or lower reinfection rate if the infected patient's male partner is treated.
  3. Abstinence from intercourse or condom use while the patient completes her treatment regimen may improve cure rates and lessen recurrences.

PHYSICAL FINDINGS & CLINICAL PRESENTATION

- 50% of patients are asymptomatic
- A thin, dark, or dull gray homogenous discharge that adheres to the vaginal walls
- An offensive, "fishy" odor that is accentuated after intercourse or menses
- Pruritus (only in 13%)

ETIOLOGY

- *Gardnerella vaginalis* is detected in 40% to 50% of vaginal secretions.
  1. Increase in vaginal pH caused by decrease in hydrogen peroxide–producing lactobacilli

2. Anaerobes predominate and produce amines
- Amines, when alkalinized by semen, menstrual blood, the use of alkaline douches, or the addition of 10% potassium hydroxide, volatilize and cause the unpleasant "fishy" odor.
- In BV:
  1. *Bacteroides* (anaerobes) species are increased 1000× the usual concentration.
  2. *G. vaginalis* are 100× normal.
  3. *Peptostreptococcus* are 10× normal.
  4. *Mycoplasma hominis* and Enterobacteriaceae members are present in increased concentrations.

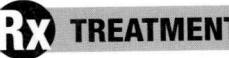

DIAGNOSIS

WORKUP

Seattle Group criteria:
- The presence of three of the four following signs will diagnose 90% correctly, with <10% false-positive results:
  1. Thin, gray, homogenous, malodorous discharge that adheres to the vaginal walls
  2. Elevated pH >4.5
  3. Positive potassium hydroxide whiff test
  4. Clue cells present on wet mount
- Cultures are unnecessary.
- Pap smear will not identify *G. vaginalis*.
- Gram stain of vaginal secretions will reveal clue cells and abnormal mixed bacteria (Fig. 1-400).

TREATMENT

ACUTE GENERAL Rx

- Recommended regimens (equal efficacy):
  1. Metronidazole 500 mg PO bid for 7 days
  2. 0.75% metronidazole gel in vagina bid for 5 days
  3. 2% clindamycin cream qd for 7 days
- Alternate regimens (lower efficacy for BV):
  1. Clindamycin ovules 100 g intravaginally qhs for 3 days
  2. Clindamycin 300 mg PO bid for 7 days (increased incidence of diarrhea)

3. Metronidazole ER 750 mg PO qd for 7 days
4. Metronidazole 2 g PO single dose (higher relapse rate)
- Patients should be advised to avoid alcohol while taking metronidazole and for 24 hr thereafter.
- Treatment in pregnancy:
  ○ All pregnant patients proven to have BV should be treated because of its association with preterm labor, chorioamnionitis, and premature rupture of membranes (PROM).
- Recommended regimens:
  1. Metronidazole 250 mg PO tid for 7 days
  2. Clindamycin 300 mg PO bid for 7 days
- Existing data do not support the use of topical agents during pregnancy.
- Multiple studies and meta-analyses have not demonstrated associations between metronidazole use during pregnancy and teratogenic effects in newborns.
  3. Tinidazole, an oral antiprotozoal drug, is now FDA approved for treatment of bacterial vaginosis. Dosage is 2 gm once/day for 2 days or 1 gm qd x 5 days
- Recurrent BV:
  1. Condom use may help reduce the risk of recurrence.
  2. Concurrent treatment of male partner is controversial. Consider treating the male partner if there is recurrent vaginitis or any suspicion of associated upper genital tract infection.

PEARLS & CONSIDERATIONS

- Bacterial vaginosis has been associated with pelvic inflammatory disease, cystitis, posthysterectomy vaginal cuff cellulitis, postabortal infection, preterm delivery, PROM, amnionitis, chorioamnionitis, and postpartum endometritis. New evidence also shows BV increases women's risk of acquiring HIV.
- Higher cumulative cure rates have been found at 3 to 4 wk for a 7-day regimen of metronidazole (500 mg twice daily) than with a single dose (2 g).
- Persistent bacterial vaginosis is associated with several bacteria in the *Clostridiales* order, *Megasphaera* phylotype 2, and *P. lacrimalis*.

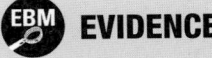 **EVIDENCE**

available at www.expertconsult.com

SUGGESTED READINGS
available at www.expertconsult.com

AUTHORS: **ARUNDATHI G. PRASAD, M.D.,** and **RUBEN ALVERO, M.D.**

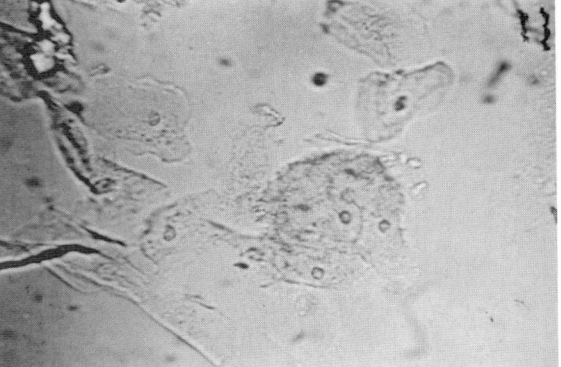

FIGURE 1-400 Clue cells characteristic of bacterial vaginosis, squamous epithelial cells whose borders are obscured by bacteria. (From Carlson K [ed]: *Primary care of women,* St Louis, 1995, Mosby.)

BASIC INFORMATION

DEFINITION

Varicella is a common viral illness that is characterized by the acute onset of a generalized vesicular rash and fever.

SYNONYMS

Chickenpox

ICD-9CM CODES
052.9 Varicella

EPIDEMIOLOGY & DEMOGRAPHICS

- Varicella is extremely contagious. More than 90% of unvaccinated contacts become infected.
- The incubation period of chickenpox ranges from 9 to 21 days.
- The peak incidence is during the springtime.
- The predominant age is 5 to 10 yr.
- The infectious period begins 2 days before the onset of clinical symptoms and lasts until all of the lesions have crusted.
- Most patients will have lifelong immunity after an attack of chickenpox; protection from the virus after a varicella vaccine is approximately 6 yr.

PHYSICAL FINDINGS & CLINICAL PRESENTATION

- Findings vary with the clinical course. Initial symptoms consist of fever, chills, backache, generalized malaise, and headache.
- Symptoms are generally more severe in adults.
- Initial lesions generally occur on the trunk (centripetal distribution) and occasionally on the face; these lesions consist primarily of 3- to 4-mm red papules with an irregular outline and a clear vesicle on the surface (i.e., the appearance of dewdrops on a rose petal).
- Intense pruritus generally accompanies the initial stage.
- New lesion development generally ceases by the fourth day, with subsequent crusting by the sixth day.
- Lesions generally spread to the face and the extremities (i.e., centrifugal spread).
- Patients generally present with lesions that are in different stages at the same time.
- Crusts generally fall off within 5 to 14 days.
- The fever is usually highest during the eruption of the vesicles; the patient's temperature generally returns to normal after the disappearance of vesicles.
- Signs of potential complications (e.g., bacterial skin infections, neurologic complications, pneumonia, hepatitis) may be present on physical examination.
- Mild constitutional symptoms (e.g., anorexia, myalgias, headaches, restlessness) may be present; these are most common among adults.
- Excoriations may be present if scratching is prominent.

ETIOLOGY

Varicella-zoster virus is a human herpes virus III that can manifest with either varicella or herpes zoster (i.e., shingles, which is a reactivation of varicella).

DIAGNOSIS

DIFFERENTIAL DIAGNOSIS

- Other viral infection
- Impetigo
- Scabies
- Drug rash
- Urticaria
- Dermatitis herpetiformis
- Smallpox

WORKUP

The diagnosis is usually made on the basis of the patient's history and clinical presentation.

LABORATORY TESTS

- Laboratory evaluation is generally not necessary.
- The CBC may reveal leukopenia and thrombocytopenia.
- Serum varicella titers (i.e., a significant rise in the serum varicella immunoglobulin G antibody level), skin biopsies, or Tzanck smears are used only when diagnosis is in question.

TREATMENT

NONPHARMACOLOGIC THERAPY

- Use antipruritic lotions for symptomatic relief.
- Avoid scratching to prevent excoriations and superficial skin infections.
- Use a mild soap for bathing.
- Hands should be washed often.

ACUTE GENERAL Rx

- Use acetaminophen for fever and myalgias; aspirin should be avoided because of the associated increased risk for Reye's syndrome.
- Oral acyclovir (20 mg/kg qid for 5 days) initiated at the earliest sign (i.e., within 24 hr of illness) is useful for healthy, nonpregnant individuals 13 yr old or older to decrease the duration and severity of signs and symptoms. Immunocompromised hosts should be treated with intravenous acyclovir 500 mg/m^2 or 10 mg/kg q8h for 7 to 10 days.
- Varicella is most contagious from 2 days before to a few days after the onset of the rash. Varicella vaccine is available for children and adults; protection lasts at least 6 yr. Healthy, nonimmune adults and children exposed to varicella-zoster virus should receive prophylaxis with live attenuated varicella vaccine (Varivax). Patients with HIV or other immunocompromised patients should not receive the live attenuated vaccine.
- Exposed patients with contraindications to varicella vaccine can be treated with varicella-zoster immunoglobulin (VariZIG), which effectively prevents varicella in susceptible individuals. The dose is 12.5 U/kg IM up to a maximum of 625 U. VariZIG must be administered as early as possible after presumed exposure (i.e., within 4 days). If VariZIG cannot be obtained and administered within 4 days, providers should consider the use of intravenous immunoglobulin within 4 days of exposure.
- Pruritus from chickenpox can be controlled with antihistamines (e.g., hydroxyzine 25 mg q6h) and oral antipruritic lotions (e.g., calamine).
- Oral antibiotics are not routinely indicated and should be used only in patients with secondary infection and infected lesions; the most common infective organisms are *Streptococcus* sp. and *Staphylococcus* sp.

DISPOSITION

- The course is generally benign in immunocompetent adults and children.
- Infants who develop chickenpox are incapable of controlling the infection and should be given varicella-zoster immunoglobulin or gamma globulin if VariZIG is not available.

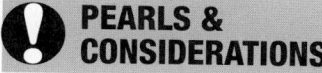

PEARLS & CONSIDERATIONS

COMMENTS

- VariZIG can be obtained from the nearest regional Red Cross Blood Center or the Centers for Disease Control and Prevention in Atlanta.
- Varicella immunization is recommended for all who have not had chickenpox; the dosage for adults and adolescents (>13 yr old) is two 0.5-ml doses 4 to 8 wk apart.

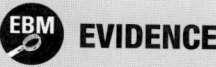

EVIDENCE

available at www.expertconsult.com

AUTHOR: **FRED F. FERRI, M.D.**

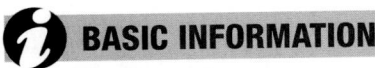
BASIC INFORMATION

DEFINITION
A varicocele is a collection of dilated and tortuous veins in the pampiniform plexus surrounding the spermatic cord in the scrotum.

SYNONYMS
Sometimes referred to as "bag of worms" (Fig. 1-401)

ICD-9CM CODES
456.4

EPIDEMIOLOGY & DEMOGRAPHICS
PREVALENCE: A varicocele is present in up to 20% of all males. It occurs in approximately 30% of infertile men. However, only 10% to 15% of males with varicoceles have fertility problems.
RISK FACTORS: There are no reliable data on epidemiologic risk factors for varicocele, such as a family history or environmental exposures.

PHYSICAL FINDINGS & CLINICAL PRESENTATION
- Patients may report a mass lying posterior to and above the testis. When the patient is supine, dilation of the veins is generally decreased. Dilation and tortuosity of the veins are increased when the patient is upright and when the patient performs a Valsalva maneuver.
- The majority of cases occur more commonly on the left side because the left spermatic vein enters the left renal vein at a 90-degree angle, whereas the right testicular vein drains directly into the vena cava.

ETIOLOGY
Varicoceles are caused by dysfunction of the valves in the spermatic vein, which allows pooling of blood in the pampiniform plexus.

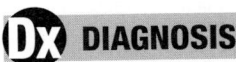
DIAGNOSIS

DIFFERENTIAL DIAGNOSIS
- Hydrocele
- Spermatocele
- Epididymal orchitis
- Testicular tumor

WORKUP
Patient should be examined in an upright position and supine position.

LABORATORY TESTS
Semen analysis if a varicocele is detected and the patient is infertile

IMAGING
High-resolution color-flow Doppler ultrasound or Doppler ultrasound are the most common and least invasive technique to confirm a varicocele and differentiate from other scrotal abnormalities.

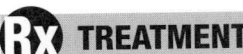
TREATMENT

Once a varicocele is identified, providers must document bilateral testicular size at regular intervals. If the testicle on the affected side is small, spermatogenesis may have been adversely affected.

SURGERY
- Varicocelectomy is performed by ligation of the veins of the pampiniform plexus through an inguinal incision or by ligating the internal spermatic vein in the retroperitoneum. This is generally performed as an ambulatory surgery.
- The goal of varicocelectomy is to maximize chances for fertility.
- Surgical treatment is indicated when there is significant disparity in testicular size or pain. Also, surgery should be performed if the contralateral testis is diseased or absent. Surgery may be considered if the varicocele is large, even without a disparity in testicular size.
- Postoperatively the involved testis typically enlarges and catches up to the uninvolved side in 1 to 2 yr. Semen parameters also improve significantly in 65%.
- The success rate of surgical repair is close to 98%; that of percutaneous repair is significantly lower.

PEARLS & CONSIDERATIONS

- A varicocele in a boy <10 yr or on the right side may be indicative of an abdominal or retroperitoneal mass. Ultrasound should be performed.
- The sudden occurrence of a left-sided varicocele in an older man indicates occlusion of the spermatic vein and should prompt evaluation for a renal tumor.

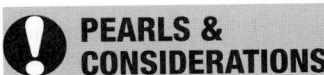
EVIDENCE

available at www.expertconsult.com

SUGGESTED READINGS
available at www.expertconsult.com

AUTHORS: **BETH NOWAK, M.D.,** and
JANICE PATACSIL-TRULL, M.D.

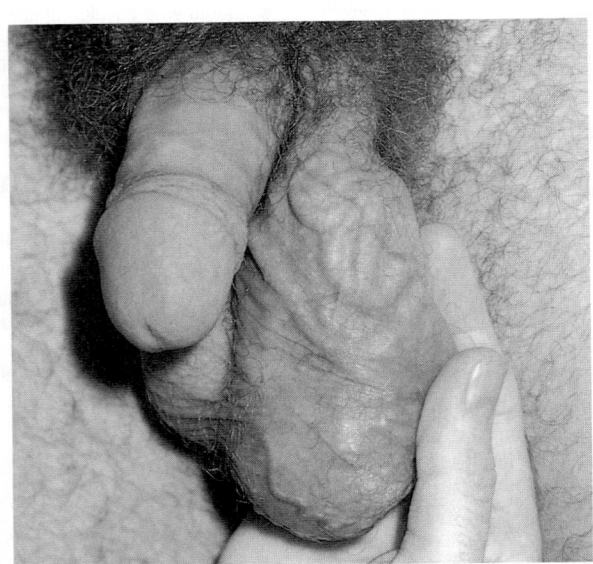
FIGURE 1-401 Varicocele. (From Swartz MH: *Textbook of physical diagnosis*, ed 5, Philadelphia, 2006, Saunders.)

BASIC INFORMATION

DEFINITION

Veins in the leg are soft, thin-walled tubes that return blood back to the heart. This is accomplished by the presence of one-way valves and the action of the calf pump. Superficial venous insufficiency develops when venous return is impaired by valvular incompetence, obstruction, or calf muscle pump failure.

Varicose veins, the most common clinical manifestation of chronic venous disease are bulging (>3 mm in diameter), tortuous conduits. Reticular veins often called "feeder veins" are bluish subdermal veins about 1 to 3 mm in diameter that give rise to telangiectasisa. Spider veins or telangiectasias are very small (≤1 mm in diameter) thread veins found commonly in cluster on the surface of the skin.

SYNONYMS

Chronic venous disorder

ICD-9CM CODES
448.1 Spider veins/telangiectasias
454.9 Varicose veins
454.8 Varicose veins with symptoms

EPIDEMIOLOGY

PREVALENCE: One large U.S. cohort study found the biannual incidence of varicose veins was 3% in women and 2% in men.

The prevalence of varicose veins in Western populations was estimated in one study to be about 25% to 30% in women and 10% to 20% in men.
RISK FACTORS:
Gender: female
Genetics: family history of varicose veins
Increasing age
Multiple pregnancies

SYMPTOMS AND PHYSICAL FINDINGS

Leg complaints consistent with chronic venous disease include aching, heaviness, subjective swelling, cramps, itching, tingling, and pain. These symptoms can be exacerbated by menses, heat, and prolonged standing.

CLINICAL PRESENTATION

- Chronic vein disease is the result of the introduction of high pressures into a normal low-pressure superficial venous system.
- This increased pressure or venous hypertension causes superficial veins to distend to such a degree that vein valves fail to close causing reflux and pooling of blood in surface veins.
- Manifested clinically by two syndromes:
  - Junctional: failure of the terminal valve at the intersection between the saphenous vein trunks and the deep system. If the great saphenous vein is involved large varicose veins are found mainly above medial knee or calf. When the small saphenous vein is involved large varicose veins are found in posterior knee or calf

area. If the anterior accessory of great saphenous vein is involved large varicose veins are found mainly in anterior or lateral thigh.
  - Perforator: failure of valves located in perforating vein. Large varicose veins are found most commonly in medial calf and proximal thigh region.

CLASSIFICATION

Chronic venous disease can now be classified using the CEAP criteria to allow for a precise description of the type of venous disease being discussed and provides an orderly framework for decision making (Table 1-181).

ETIOLOGY

- The underlying etiology of varicose veins remains uncertain.
- Important structural changes that occur: failure of vein valve function and vein wall dilatation from fragmentation of the muscle layer.

COMPLICATIONS

- Superficial venous thrombophlebitis (SVT): a very common disorder with an incidence of 125,000 new cases per year in the U.S. The most frequent predisposing risk factors are varicose veins. The clinical findings include the presence of erythema, tenderness and a palpable cord. Pain, increased warmth, and swelling are also present. Diagnosis is made by ultrasonography, which is useful to identify associated deep vein thrombosis that can occur in approximately 15% of patients. The location of the SVT determines the course of

---

TABLE 1-181   CEAP Classification of Chronic Venous Disease

C: Clinical

C_0: no visible or palpable signs of venous disease
C_1: telangiectasias or reticular veins
C_2: varicose veins
C_3: edema
C_4: pigmentation or eczema
C_5: healed venous ulcer
C_6: active venous ulcer

E: Etiological

c: congenital
p: primary
s: secondary or post thrombotic
n: no venous cause identified

A: Anatomic

s: superficial veins
p: perforator veins
d: deep veins
n: no venous location identified

P: Pathophysiological

r: reflux
o: obstruction
r,o: reflux and obstruction
n: no venous pathophysiology identified

---

treatment, if the proximal great saphenous vein (GSV) is involved then a 1-mo course of LMWH plus compression stockings has been found to be more effective than vein ligation. If SVT involves branch varicosities, treatment is usually symptomatic (control of pain).
- Bleeding: is a more common complication than traditionally suspected. It is associated with thin-walled ectatic veins known as "blue blebs" that are found predominantly in the medial lower calf and ankle region. The best emergency treatment consists of pressure wrapping and not suture ligation which results in delayed healing of the bleeding site. Sclerotherapy of these veins is the definitive treatment to prevent further bleeding.
- Varicose eczema: see "Veus Ulcers" section.
- Atrophe blanche: see "Venous Ulcers" section.
- Lipodermosclerosis: see "Venous Ulcers" section.
- Venous stasis ulcer: see "Venous Ulcers" section.

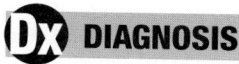

DIAGNOSIS

DIFFERENTIAL DIAGNOSIS

Other conditions that cause leg pain:
- Stress fracture
- Arthritis hip/knee joint
- Gout
- Degenerative disc disease of lower back
- Intermittent claudication secondary to peripheral arterial disease (PAD)
- Medications such as allopurinol and statins
Other conditions that cause leg swelling:
- Cellulitis
- Soft tissue injury to leg/ankle/foot
- Obesity
- Diabetes
- Advancing age
- Medications such as calcium channel blockers, steroids, MAO inhibitors, and tricyclics

WORKUP

The diagnosis of chronic venous disorders is predominantly clinical. Initial evaluation consists of a thorough history and physical exam with classification of disease according to the Clinical-Etiology-Anatomy-Pathophysiology (CEAP) criteria.

LABORATORY TESTS

Laboratory tests are not useful in patients with varicose veins.

IMAGING STUDIES

Duplex ultrasonography:
- Gold-standard imaging modality for the diagnosis, prognostic evaluation, pretreatment mapping, and posttreatment assessment of therapeutic intervention.
- Duplex ultrasound is used to identify and quantify points of valvular reflux within the superficial venous system.
- Assessment of valvular reflux is done with patient in the upright position which physio-

logically approximates the condition in which valvular reflux occurs.

- Reverse flow of greater than 0.5 sec after distal compression is considered abnormal.

Other tests:

- Air plethysmography: may be useful in patients who have reflux in both superficial and deep venous systems or in patients with an unusual presentation of leg pain.
- Venography: has been largely replaced by duplex ultrasonagraphy still retains a critical role in the evaluation of chronic venous insufficiency prior to venous reconstruction.

Rx TREATMENT

CONSERVATIVE THERAPY:

- Aerobic exercise regularly for 30 min a day.
- Elevate legs above heart level to reduce swelling.
- Flex ankles frequently at work, during air travel or long car travel.
- Maintain proper weight.
- Graduated compression stockings (below knee) to alleviate symptoms in patients who are not candidates or do not desire to undergo treatment of their varicose veins.

SCLEROTHERAPY:

- Small- to medium-sized varicose veins such as spider veins and reticular varices in the absence of reflux in sahenous trunks are best treated with liquid sclerotherapy.
- The three principal sclerosants used in the U.S. are hypertonic saline, sodium tetradecyl-

sulfate, and the newly FDA-approved solution, polidoconol.

- These agents are injected into vessels using 27-gauge or 30-gauge needles at concentrations of 23.4%, 0.1%, or 0.5%, respectively causing injury to the endothelium with the resultant disappearance of the vein over period of time (usually 8 to 12 wk).

AMBULATORY PHLEBECTOMY:

- A procedure in which large varicose vein branches are removed with special hook instruments through a small puncture—incisions are made with an #18-gauge needle or #11 blade
- Performed safely under local anesthesia in an office setting and offers excellent cosmetic results and relief of symptoms
- Most commonly performed in conjunction with endovenous ablation procedures

ENDOVENOUS ABLATION:

- Ablation of diseased saphenous vein trunks, large incompetent tributaries or perforating veins can be achieved by using:
  ○ Radiofrequency energy
  ○ Laser energy
  ○ Ultrasound-guided foam sclerotherapy.
- The first two accomplish thermal injury to the vein in situ via an intraluminal catheter or bare-tipped laser wire. Chemical ablation uses a solution (polidoconol or sodium tetradecylsulfate) that is injected directly into the vein in the form of foam.

- Endovenous ablation can be performed in an office setting using local anesthesia. Patients can return to their normal daily activities immediately.
- The efficacy of these endovenous ablation procedures have been borne out by numerous published reports with occlusion rates over 95% and reflux free rates over 5-yr follow-up of 86%.

DISPOSITION

- It is important that the physician educate the patient to understand that varicose veins are a chronic and progressive disease.
- Any treatment is at best palliative, as patients in time will develop varicose veins in other areas.

REFERRAL

To either a phlebologist, preferably board certified by the newly created American Board of Phlebology or a residency-trained vascular surgeon

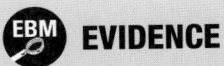 **EVIDENCE**

available at www.expertconsult.com

SUGGESTED READINGS

available at www.expertconsult.com

AUTHOR: **FRANK G. FORT, M.D., F.A.C.S.**

BASIC INFORMATION

DEFINITION

Venous ulcers account for more than 80% of all lower extremity ulcerations and are typically irregular and shallow, with granulation tissue and fibrin present in the ulcer base. They are usually located above the medial malleolus and below the knee ("gaiter" region) and may be accompanied by varicose veins, edema, hyperpigmentation, and lipodermatosclerosis. These ulcerations develop in patients with chronic venous insufficiency as a result of incompetent valves, obstructed veins, or immobility.

SYNONYMS

Stasis ulcers
Peripheral venous insufficiency
Venous leg ulcers

ICD-9CM CODES

459.3   Chronic venous hypertension, including stasis edema
459.81 Peripheral venous insufficiency
707.1   Ulcer of the lower limb (calf: 2, ankle: 3)

EPIDEMIOLOGY & DEMOGRAPHICS

In industrialized nations up to 1.5% of the population will suffer from venous ulcers. In patients ≥65 yr, the incidence is 4%. In the United States, more than 500,000 people suffer from stasis ulcers and 10% to 35% of the U.S. adult population has some form of chronic venous insufficiency (CVI). The lack of effective therapies and high recurrence of ulcers places a heavy burden on the health-care system that has been estimated at more than $1 billion a year.

RISK FACTORS:

- Obesity
- Women are more likely to develop ulcers than men
- Sedentary lifestyle
- Increasing age
- Family history of chronic venous insufficiency
- History of venous thromboembolism

PHYSICAL FINDINGS & CLINICAL PRESENTATION

- Elevated venous pressure is the cause for many of the skin manifestations of chronic venous insufficiency. The spectrum of cutaneous changes in the affected leg include:
  - Varicose eczema: the most common and earliest sign and involves skin above the medial ankle and consists of pruritic, red, and scaly eczematous patches and plaques (Fig. 1-402).
  - Hyperpigmentation: caused by the breakdown of red blood cells leads to hemosiderin deposition and dark staining of the skin (Fig. 1-403).
  - Atrophie blanche: usually presents as hypopigmented white patches with focal red punctuate dots or telangiectasias surrounded by hyperpigmentation. Skin in this

condition is avascular and prone to ulceration (Fig. 1-404).
  - Lipodermatosclerosis: a slow, chronic induration of the skin and underlying fat that usually involves the skin from medial malleolus up to the lower border of the calf. Progression of the disease leads to an "inverted champagne bottle" appearance. The induration and lack of perfusion of the skin in this area makes it susceptible to ulcer formation (Fig. 1-405).

ETIOLOGY

The exact mechanism of the role of venous hypertension in the etiology of venous ulcers is not certain. Recent histologic and immunocytochemical analyses of venous leg ulcers suggest

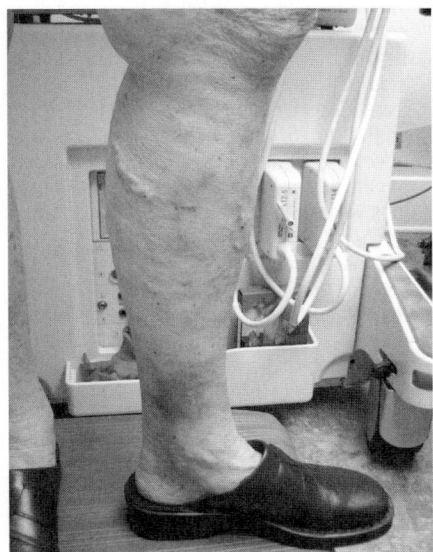

FIGURE 1-402 Varicose eczema.

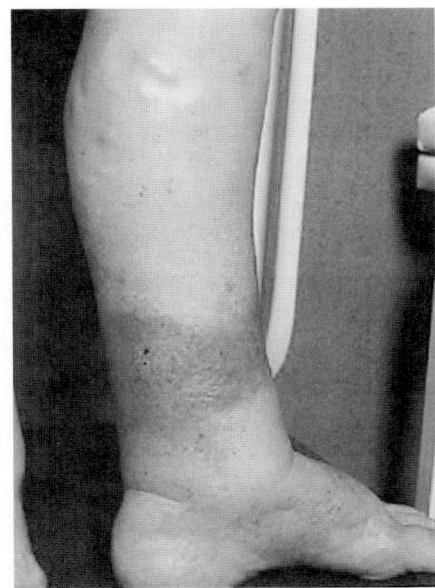

FIGURE 1-403 Hyperpigmentation.

that lesions observed in the different stages of chronic venous insufficiency (CVI) may be related to an inflammatory process that leads to fibrosclerotic remodeling of the skin and then to ulceration. The vascular network of the most superficial layers of the skin appears to be the target of the inflammatory reaction. Hemodynamic forces such as venous hypertension, circulatory stasis, and modified conditions of shear stress appear to play an important role in an inflammatory reaction accompanied by leukocyte activation which clinically leads to venous dermatitis and venous ulceration.

DIAGNOSIS

DIFFERENTIAL DIAGNOSIS

- Arterial ulcer
- Neurotrophic ulcers (located predominantly in the foot)
- Traumatic and self inflicted ulcers
- Vasculitis
- Pyoderma gangrenosum
- Ulcerated skin tumors like basal cell or squamous cell carcinoma (Marjolin's ulcer)
- Rheumatoid arthritis

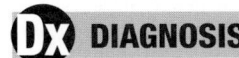
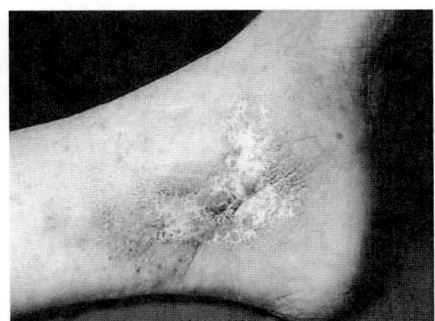

FIGURE 1-404 Atrophe blanche.

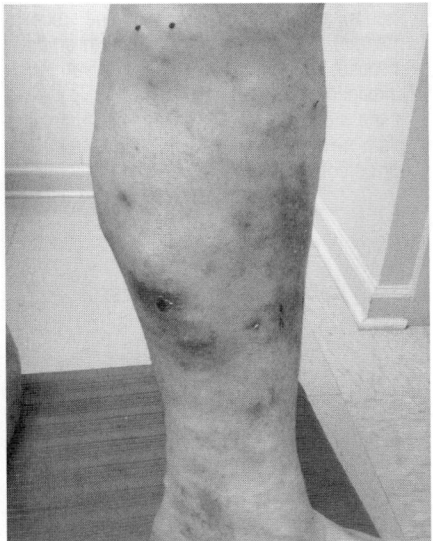

FIGURE 1-405 Lipodermosclerosis.

WORKUP

- The history and clinical signs and symptoms of leg ulcers are often misleading and may not differentiate venous ulcers from other leg ulcers; about 20% of leg ulcers are not of venous origin.
- Measurement of the ankle-brachial index (ABI) is essential in excluding peripheral arterial disease (PAD), which can be present in 20% of patients and is required before starting compression therapy. Arterial insufficiency is suggested by an ankle-brachial index of <1.0.
- Patients with lower-extremity ulcers should also be evaluated for diabetes.
- Coagulation defects have been found in 40% of patients with leg ulcers. This finding suggests that many patients with leg ulcers have a known or suspected history of deep venous thrombosis and a thrombophilia workup is indicated.
- If vasculitis is suspected, a biopsy of the edge of the ulcer can confirm the diagnosis.
- Any wound that has failed to improve after therapy of 4 wk should be biopsied to rule out malignancy.

IMAGING STUDIES

- Evaluation of patients with venous leg ulcer should include duplex sonography to identify reflux in the superficial, deep, and perforating veins as well as possible obstruction of the deep veins.
- Any detected pathology should be classified according to the CEAP classification (Clinical, Etiological, Anatomical, Pathophysiological). The clinical portion consists of categories C_0 to C_6. The etiological portion is based on the congenital and primary and secondary causes of venous dysfunction. The anatomic portion describes whether the superficial, deep, or perforating venous systems may be involved. The pathophysiological portion describes the underlying mechanism resulting in CVI, including reflux, obstruction, or both.
- Plethysmography, venous pressure measurements, and venography may be recommended for patients with postthrombotic disease, especially if surgical intervention is considered.
- If the ulcer appears to be infected, consider plain x-ray films and bone scan to evaluate for osteomyelitis.

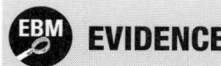 TREATMENT

NONPHARMACOLOGIC THERAPY

- The goal of therapy is to improve venous return to the heart, thereby decreasing edema, inflammation, and tissue ischemia.
- Surgical debridement in order to remove all nonviable material can be accomplished in the office setting with the use of a topical xylocaine gel (1% to 4%). Debridement produces the release of growth factors that allow the development of healthy granulation tissue and the initiation of the healing process.
- The first-line treatment of ulcers includes compression stockings, which can be safely used only if the ankle brachial index is at least 0.8 because compression can cause limb ischemia.
- There is level-A evidence that graduated compression stockings alone can lead to healing of a venous ulcer. Below knee stockings with graded pressure that provide at least 35 to 40 mm Hg of pressure at the ankle and 20 to 25 mm Hg at the knee are most effective. The stockings should be worn during the day and removed at night. The stockings wear out and need to be replaced every 6 mo.
- Patients should maintain a normal weight and quit smoking.
- Regular, brisk walking 30 min a day, 5 times a week is recommended.
- Elevate leg above heart level and raise the foot of bed with 3-in blocks to reduce edema.
- Role of surgery: in a randomized controlled trial, endovenous catheter ablation of superficial reflux showed no improvement in the healing rate of ulcers but did demonstrate a reduction of ulcer recurrence from 28% to 12% at 12 mo.

ACUTE GENERAL Rx

- Dressings are used under compression stockings to provide a clean, moist environment to promote healing.
- Modern more complex dressings have been developed and include occlusive, and semiocclusive dressings, classified according to their physical composition and ability to control wound drainage.
- Semiocclusive dressings have varying ability to absorb wound drainage. Some examples of this type are hydrocolloids (DuoDerm), hy-drogels (Duoderm hydrogel), foam dressings (Allevyn), and alginates.
- Biological wound dressings (Apligraf) and tissue engineered products (Oasis) have been developed, and these products can either directly provide growth factors or indirectly stimulate growth factors in the ulcer bed.
- Underlying systemic hypertension and diabetes should be aggressively treated.
- Pentoxifylline (800 mg tid) has been shown to be an effective adjuvant to compression therapy as reported in a meta-analysis of nine clinical trials.
- Skin grafting should be considered for large or refractory ulcers as long as the wound is clean and there is healthy granulation tissue.
- Systemic antibiotics are not indicated unless there are obvious clinical signs of infection.
- Published randomized clinical trials on the value of the different types of dressings in the management of leg ulcers have not shown effects on ulcer healing. Despite the lack of evidence to support their use, modern dressings remain a part of the standard of care. Decisions regarding their use should be based on local cost of the dressings and the physician's clinical experience.

DISPOSITION

The overall prognosis for this condition is poor; the healing rate depends on the initial size of the ulcer. Although 65% to 70% of venous ulcers are healed within 6 mo, the 5-yr recurrence rate of healed venous ulcers can be as high as 40%. Maintenance of lifelong compression therapy is recommended.

REFERRAL

- Referral to a wound clinic should be considered for patients with large (>5 × 5 cm) or longstanding wounds.
- All patients should be evaluated weekly during the first month of therapy. Nonhealing ulcers with little to no improvement should also be referred to a wound care clinic.

EBM EVIDENCE

available at www.expertconsult.com

SUGGESTED READINGS
available at www.expertconsult.com

AUTHOR: **FRANK G. FORT, M.D., F.A.C.S.**

BASIC INFORMATION

DEFINITION

- Ventricular septal defect (VSD) refers to an abnormal communication through the septum that separates the right and left ventricles of the heart.
- VSDs may be large or small and single or multiple.
- VSDs are located at various anatomic regions of the septum and classified as follows:
  - Membranous (75% to 80%): This is the most common type of defect, and it extends into the membranous portion of the interventricular septum. The septal leaflet of the tricuspid valve may become adherent and form a "pouch" of the septum that can limit the left-to-right shunting.
  - Muscular or trabecular (5% to 20%): This defect is entirely surrounded by muscular tissue.
  - Canal or inlet (8%): This defect commonly lies beneath the septal leaflet of the tricuspid valve; it is often seen in patients with Down's syndrome.
  - Subarterial, outlet, infundibular, or supracristal (5% to 7%): This is the least common type of defect. It is usually found beneath the aortic valve, and it may lead to aortic regurgitation.

SYNONYMS

VSD

ICD-9CM CODES

745.4 Ventricular septal defect

EPIDEMIOLOGY & DEMOGRAPHICS

- VSD was first described by Dalrymple in 1847.
- VSDs are one of the most common congenital heart abnormalities, accounting for 30% of all congenital cardiac defects.
- VSD accounts for ~25% of all congenital heart defects in children and for approximately 10% of defects in adults (the decrease is a result of spontaneous closure that occurs by adulthood).
- The prevalence of VSD is 3 to 3.5 infants per 1000 live births and 0.5/1000 adults.
- VSD is found with equal frequency among both males and females.
- VSD may be associated with the following conditions:
  - Atrial septal defect (35%)
  - Patent ductus arteriosus (22%)
  - Coarctation of the aorta (17%)
  - Subvalvular aortic stenosis (4%)
  - Subpulmonic stenosis, usually associated with progressive aortic regurgitations caused by prolapsed of the aortic cusp through the defect
- Multiple VSDs are more prevalent among patients with tetralogy of Fallot and double-outlet right ventricular defects.

PHYSICAL FINDINGS & CLINICAL PRESENTATION

- Clinical presentation depends on the direction and volume of the VSD shunt, which is dictated by the size of the defect and the ratio of the pulmonary vascular resistance.
  - Defects of ≤25% of the aortic annulus diameter are small defects that typically involve small left-to-right shunts, no left ventricular volume overload, and no pulmonary artery hypertension.
  - Defects that are 25% to 75% of aortic annulus diameter are considered to be moderate in size, with small to moderate left-to-right shunting, mild to moderate left ventricular volume overload, and mild or no pulmonary artery hypertension. Patients may have symptoms of congestive heart failure that may improve with medical therapy or with age as the defect decreases in size relative to increasing body size.
  - Defects of ≥75% of the aortic annulus diameter usually have moderate to large left-to-right shunting, left ventricular volume overload, and pulmonary artery hypertension. These patients usually have a history of congestive heart failure, or they may possibly develop right-to-left shunting in the setting of Eisenmenger's syndrome during late childhood, adolescence, or young adulthood.
- Infants may be asymptomatic at birth because of elevated pulmonary artery resistance. During the first few weeks of life, pulmonary arterial resistance decreases, thereby allowing for more left-to-right shunting through the VSD. This results in a subsequent increase in flow into the lungs, the left atrium, and the left ventricle, which can potentially cause left ventricular volume overload. Tachypnea, failure to thrive, and congestive heart failure may then ensue.
- In adults with VSD, the shunt is left to right in the absence of pulmonary stenosis and pulmonary hypertension. Patients typically manifest symptoms of left-sided heart failure (e.g., shortness of breath, orthopnea, dyspnea on exertion).
- A spectrum of physical findings may be seen, including the following:
  - Machinelike holosystolic murmur that is heard best along the left sternal border (i.e., shorter duration of the murmur as right ventricular pressure increases)
  - Systolic thrill
  - Mid-diastolic rumble heard at the apex
  - S_3 heart sound
  - Rales
- With the development of pulmonary hypertension, the following occur:
  - An augmented pulmonic component of the S_2 heart sound
  - Cyanosis, clubbing, right ventricular heave, and signs of right heart failure (i.e., as seen with Eisenmenger's complex, with a reversal of the shunt in a right-to-left direction)

ETIOLOGY

- VSD is usually congenital (which is the focus of this review), but it may occur after myocardial infarction.
- After acute myocardial infarction, the rupture of the intraventricular septum typically occurs 1 to 5 days after the event in 0.2% of patients in the current fibrinolytic, primary angioplasty era.

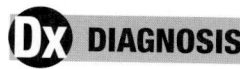 DIAGNOSIS

The diagnosis of VSD can be suspected during a physical examination. Imaging studies—particularly transthoracic echocardiography with color Doppler—establish the diagnosis.

DIFFERENTIAL DIAGNOSIS

On the basis of the physical examination alone, the diagnosis of VSD may be confused with other causes of systolic murmurs, such as mitral regurgitation, tricuspid regurgitation, aortic stenosis, pulmonary stenosis, and hypertrophic cardiomyopathy.

WORKUP

Any person who is suspected of having a VSD should undergo an ECG, a chest radiograph, and an echocardiogram.

LABORATORY TESTS

- Laboratory tests are not specific but may offer insight into the severity of the disease.
- The CBC may show polycythemia, especially in patients with Eisenmenger's complex.
- Arterial blood gas results may demonstrate hypoxemia.

IMAGING STUDIES

- ECG findings vary in accordance with the size of the VSD and depending on whether pulmonary hypertension is present. With large VSDs with pulmonary hypertension, right-axis deviation is seen, along with evidence of right ventricular hypertrophy.
- Chest x-ray findings in patients with VSD include the following:
  - Cardiomegaly that results from left ventricular volume overload that directly relates to the magnitude of the shunt
  - The enlargement of the proximal pulmonary arteries along with the redistribution and pruning of the distal pulmonary vessels as a result of sustained pulmonary hypertension (Fig. 1-406, A)
- Echocardiography is the imaging modality of choice for the diagnosis of VSD:
  - Two-dimensional echocardiography and color Doppler display the size and location of the VSD (Fig. 1-406, B), the chamber sizes, ventricular function, the presence of aortic valve prolapse or regurgitation, outflow tract obstruction, and the presence of tricuspid regurgitation.
  - Continuous-wave Doppler approximates the gradient between the left and right ventricle and estimates the pulmonary artery pressure.

- The magnitude of the shunt can be determined by the calculation of the pulmonary-to-systemic flow ratio with the use of echocardiography.
- Heart catheterization is primarily indicated to assess operability of VSD patients with PAH, and in patients whom the noninvasive testing was inconclusive, and further information, such as quantification of shunting and assessment of pulmonary pressures, is required.
- Ventriculography may help to locate the VSD:
  - MRI and computed tomography scanning can be useful to assess the pulmonary artery, the pulmonary vein, and the aortic anatomy and to confirm the anatomy of unusual VSDs (e.g., inlet or apical defects) that are not seen well with echocardiography.

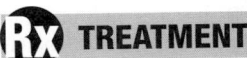 **TREATMENT**

The decision to close a VSD depends on the type, size, and shunt severity as well as the patient's pulmonary vascular resistance, functional capacity, and associated valvular abnormalities.

NONPHARMACOLOGIC THERAPY

- In young children and adults, a small, asymptomatic VSD with a large left-to-right ventricular pressure gradient, a pulmonary-to-systemic blood flow ratio of less than 1.5:1, and no evidence of pulmonary hypertension can be observed (i.e., restrictive defect).

- Oxygen for hypoxemia and a low-salt diet are recommended for patients with congestive heart failure.

ACUTE GENERAL & CHRONIC RX

Closure is indicated for the following patients:
- Infants with congestive heart failure
- Children between the ages of 1 and 6 yr with persistent VSD and a pulmonary-to-systemic blood flow ratio (Qp/Qs) of >2:1
- Adults with a Qp/Qs of ≥2 and clinical evidence of left ventricular volume overload (class I):
  - Positive history of infective endocarditis (class I)
  - Adults with a Qp/Qs of >1.5 with pulmonary artery pressure that is less than two thirds of the systemic pressure and pulmonary vascular resistance that is less than two thirds of the systemic vascular resistance (class IIa)
  - Adults with a Qp/Qs of >1.5 in the presence of left ventricular systolic or diastolic failure (class IIa)
  - Surgical closure is not indicated for VSD with severe irreversible PAH.

Surgical closure with Dacron or Gore-Tex patches or primary surgical closure has long been the gold standard of therapy. However, with improvements in cardiac imaging and catheter devices, percutaneous transcatheter closure has risen in popularity.

Catheter-based closure in muscular VSD may be considered, especially if the VSD is remote from the tricuspid valve and the aorta, if the VSD is associated with severe left-sided heart chamber enlargement, or if there is PAH (class2b). Device closure is indicated in residual defects after prior attempts at surgical closure, restrictive VSDs with either a significant left-to-right shunt (Qp/Qs >1.5/1 or hx of IE, trauma, or iatrogenic artifacts after surgical replacement of the aortic valve.

Some studies have shown similar success rates for both surgical and percutaneous closures, and there are significantly fewer complications, days in the hospital, and blood transfusions after percutaneous closures. Postinfarct VSDs usually carry a high mortality rate, and surgical closure is still the preferred method of treatment for this type.

DISPOSITION

- The natural history of an isolated VSD depends on the type of defect, its size, and any associated abnormalities.
- ~75% to 80% of small VSDs close spontaneously by the time the patient reaches the age of 10 yr.
- Only 10% to 15% of large VSDs will close spontaneously.
- Large VSDs that are left untreated may lead to arrhythmias, congestive heart failure, pulmonary hypertension, and Eisenmenger's complex.
- Eisenmenger's complex carries a poor prognosis, with most patients dying before the age of 40 yr.

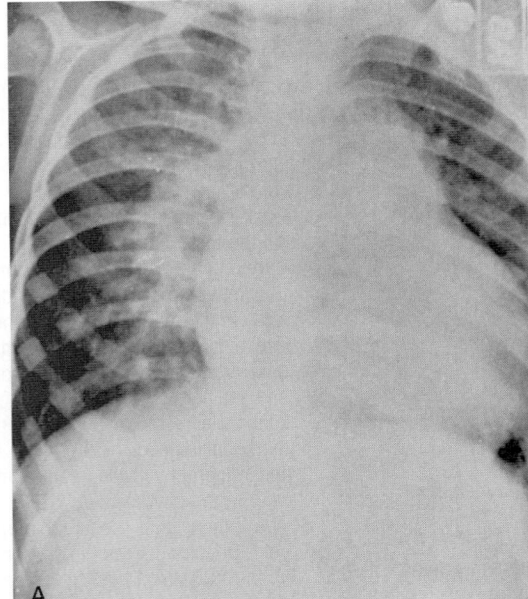
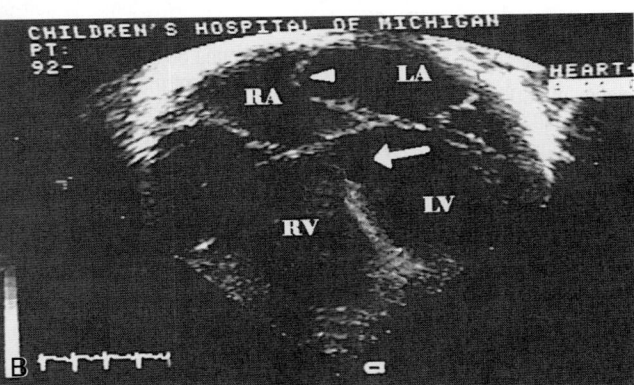

FIGURE 1-406 A, Chest roentgenogram of a child with a large ventricular septal defect, large pulmonary blood flow, and pulmonary hypertension but only mild elevation of peripheral vascular resistance. This is reflected in the evidence of left and right ventricular enlargement, the enlargement of the main pulmonary artery, and a marked increase in pulmonary blood flow. **B,** Apical four-chamber echocardiographic view of ventricular septal defect *(large arrow).* The small arrow points to the interatrial septum. *LA,* Left atrium; *LV,* left ventricle; *RA,* right atrium; *RV,* right ventricle. (**A,** From Pacifico AD et al: Surgical treatment of ventricular septal defect. In Sabiston DC Jr, Spencer FC [eds]: *Surgery of the chest,* ed 5, Philadelphia, 1990, WB Saunders. **B,** Courtesy of Richard Humes, MD, Children's Hospital of Michigan, Detroit.)

- Issues to monitor in adults with unrepaired or repaired and catheter-closed VSDs include the following:
  - Development of aortic regurgitation
  - Assessment of associated coronary artery disease
  - Development of tricuspid regurgitation
  - Assessment of the degree of left-to-right shunting (in unrepaired or residual VSD after repair)
  - Ventricular dysfunction
  - Assessment of pulmonary pressure
  - Development of subpulmonary stenosis (usually as a result of a double-chambered right ventricle)
  - Development of discrete subaortic stenosis
  - Development of arrhythmia or heart block
  - Thromboembolic complications
  - Infective endocarditis
- After closure, late survival is excellent when ventricular function is normal. Pulmonary artery hypertension may improve, progress, or remain the same. Late operations may be required for tricuspid or aortic regurgitation.

REFERRAL

All infants and children diagnosed with VSD should be referred to a pediatric cardiologist. Adults with VSD should be referred to an adult cardiologist. Cardiothoracic surgeons who have experience with congenital heart disease surgery should be consulted if surgery is indicated.

FOLLOW-UP

- Adults with no residual VSD, no associated lesions, and normal pulmonary artery pressure do not require continued follow-up at a regional ACHD center except on referral from the patient's cardiologist or physician.
- Adults with VSD with residual heart failure, shunts, PAH, AR, or RV outflow tract (RVOT) or LV outflow tract (LVOT) obstruction should be seen at least annually at an ACHD regional center (level of evidence: C).
- Adults with a small residual VSD and no other lesions should be seen every 3 to 5 yr at an ACHD regional center (level of evidence: C).
- Adults with device closure of a VSD should be followed up every 1 to 2 yr at an ACHD center depending on the location of the VSD and other factors.
- Patients who develop bifascicular block or transient trifascicular block after VSD closure are at risk in later years for the development of complete heart block and should be followed up yearly by history and ECG and have periodic ambulatory monitoring and/or exercise testing.

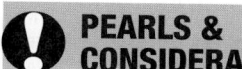

PEARLS & CONSIDERATIONS

COMMENTS

- A loud murmur does not imply a large VSD. Small, hemodynamically insignificant VSDs can cause loud murmurs.
- In patients with Eisenmenger's complex, the right-to-left shunting across the VSD is usually not associated with an audible murmur.
- The risk of patients with unrepaired VSD developing infective endocarditis is 4%. The risk is higher if aortic insufficiency is present.
- For patients with endocarditis, routine antibiotic prophylaxis for dental or surgical procedures is no longer indicated for isolated VSDs, except in the following circumstances:
  - In the presence of complex congenital heart disease with cyanosis
  - In the presence of a residual VSD after surgical closure
  - During the first 6 mo after surgical patch or percutaneous transcatheter closure
- Any patient with a newly diagnosed murmur or hemodynamic compromise after a myocardial infarction should undergo evaluation for possible VSD.
- Pregnancy with a VSD is generally well tolerated in women with small VSDs, no pulmonary artery hypertension, and no associated lesions. Women with large shunts may experience arrhythmias, ventricular dysfunction, and the progression of pulmonary hypertension.
- Women with VSDs and severe pulmonary artery hypertension or Eisenmenger's physiology should be counseled against pregnancy because of associated excessive maternal and fetal mortality.
- Minimally invasive periventricular device closure of ventricular septal defect without cardiopulmonary bypass under guidance of transesophageal echocardiography is a promising technique, but it needs long-term follow-up.

SUGGESTED READINGS

available at www.expertconsult.com

AUTHORS: **SCOTT COHEN, M.D., WEN-CHIH WU, M.D.,** and **ABDULRAHMAN ABDULBAKI, M.D.**

Diseases and Disorders

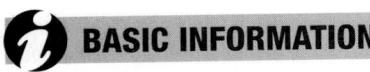

BASIC INFORMATION

DEFINITION

Vertebral compression fractures (VCFs) are defined as fractures of spinal vertebrae in which a bony surface is driven toward another bony surface. These fractures are classified as radiographic reductions in vertebral body height of more than 15% to 20%.

SYNONYMS

Thoracolumbar vertebral compression fractures
Osteoporotic fractures

ICD-9CM CODES
805.8 Compression fracture, spine
805.4 Compression fracture, lumbar vertebra
805.2 Compression fracture, thoracic vertebra
733.13 Compression fracture, L2 vertebra

EPIDEMIOLOGY & DEMOGRAPHICS

~750,000 VCFs occur in the United States each year, and they affect up to 25% of postmenopausal women. The prevalence increases with age, reaching a peak of 40% to 50% among women aged >80 yr. Compression fractures are also a major concern among men, although their rates of VCF are lower.

RISK FACTORS:
- Modifiable: tobacco or alcohol use, osteoporosis, estrogen deficiency (i.e., early menopause, bilateral ovariectomy, premenopausal amenorrhea for >1 yr), frailty, impaired vision, abusive situations, inadequate physical activity, low body mass index, and dietary deficiency of vitamin D or calcium
- Nonmodifiable: advanced age, female gender, dementia, Caucasian, history of fractures in adulthood and among first-degree relatives, and falls

PHYSICAL FINDINGS & CLINICAL PRESENTATION

- Asymptomatic: Most VCFs are asymptomatic, except for height loss or kyphosis (i.e., dowager hump), which is often a sign of multiple VCFs.
- Symptomatic: Many VCFs often present as acute back pain after activity (e.g., bending, lifting) or coughing; neck strain and rib pain may also be present.

ETIOLOGY

- VCFs take place when the combination of bending and the axial load on the spine exceed the strength of the vertebral body.
- The primary etiology of VCF is osteoporosis.

DIAGNOSIS

DIFFERENTIAL DIAGNOSIS
- Hyperparathyroidism
- Osteomalacia
- Granulomatous diseases (e.g., tuberculosis)
- Hematologic/oncologic diseases (e.g., multiple myeloma, malignancy)

WORKUP
- Only one third of VCFs are diagnosed.
- VCF can be clinically suspected from the history and physical alone.
- There may or may not be a specific injury or a remembered event that led to the VCF.

LABORATORY TESTS

Tests to rule out infection or cancer may be helpful, such as a CBC, an erythrocyte sedimentation rate, an alkaline phosphatase level, and a C-reactive protein level; these tests can be reserved for individuals for whom there is clinical suspicion.

IMAGING STUDIES

- Plain frontal and lateral radiographs (x-rays) are the initial imaging method (Fig. 1-407) and may be sufficient, particularly when no neurologic abnormalities are present. MRI and computed tomography (CT) scans may be uncomfortable or painful for the patient, especially during the acute phase.
- Although CT scans are not routinely necessary, they can be helpful for visualizing fractures that are not seen on plain films, for evaluating the integrity of the posterior vertebral wall, for ruling out other causes of back pain, for detecting spinal canal narrowing, and for assessing instability.
- MRI may be useful when spinal cord compression is suspected, if neurologic symptoms are present, or to distinguish malignancy from osteoporosis (e.g., in patients <55 yr with VCR after minimum or no trauma).
- Bone density studies may be helpful to determine the severity of osteoporosis, which is a key risk factor for future fractures.

TREATMENT

NONPHARMACOLOGIC THERAPY

- Physical therapy
- External back braces
- Exercise programs: Getting the person active as soon as possible is extremely important for both the short and long term.

ACUTE GENERAL Rx

- Analgesics for pain control, including acetaminophen and opioids (oral or parenteral). The prevention of constipation is important with opioids.
- Nonsteroidal anti-inflammatory drugs are helpful but must be used with caution among elderly patients or when contraindicated.
- Muscle relaxants should be used judiciously.
- The efficacy of vertebroplasty and kyphoplasty is controversial: percutaneous vertebroplasty involves the injection of acrylic bone cement into the affected vertebral body in an effort to stabilize the fracture and reduce pain, while in kyphoplasty a high-pressure inflatable bone tamp or balloon is expanded before the injection of bone cement into the cavity in the fractured vertebral body.

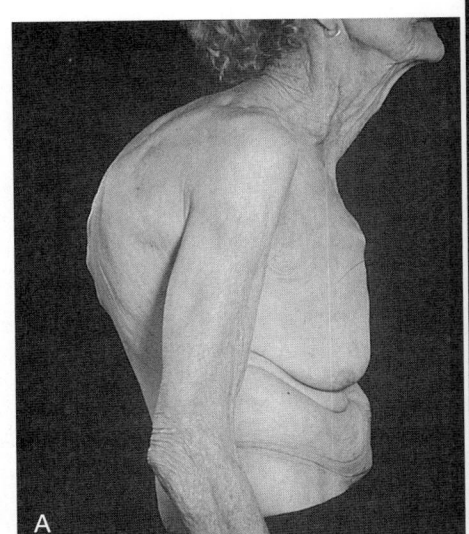
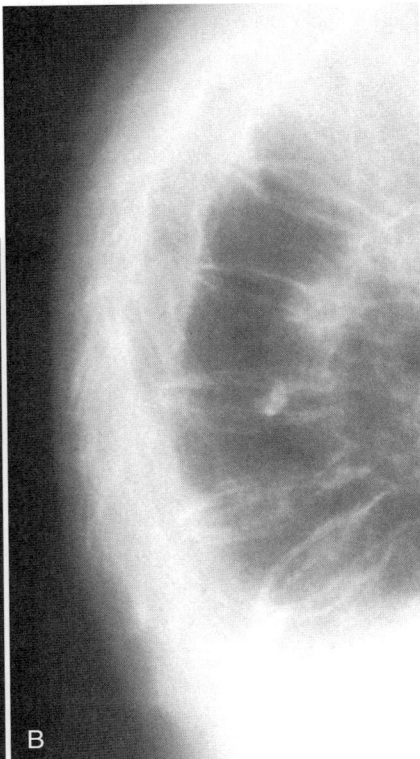

FIGURE 1-407 Dowager's hump. A, Marked thoracic kyphosis due to multiple osteoporotic fractures in an elderly woman with **B,** corresponding radiograph. (From Hochberg MC et al [eds]: *Rheumatology,* ed 3, St Louis, 2003, Mosby.)

These two procedures were thought to be helpful in patients who did not respond to conservative therapy; however, more recently studies have shown them to be no more effective than sham procedures (Buchbinder et al., 2009; Kallmes et al., 2009). Nonetheless, Klazen et al. (2010) demonstrated that for the subgroup of patients with acute osteoporotic vertebral compression fractures and persistent pain, percutaneous vertebroplasty may provide immediate pain relief, sustained for at least a year, which may be significantly greater than that achieved with conservative treatment. Further questions exist regarding the amount of time that conservative therapy alone should be pursued and which procedure, if any, should be advised.

CHRONIC Rx

Osteoporosis should be treated with the reduction of risk factors (e.g., smoking, alcohol), diet exercise, calcium and vitamin D supplements, and potentially the use of medications that are more commonly used to treat osteoporosis (e.g., bisphosphonates).

REFERRAL

Referral is indicated for neurologic abnormalities, unremitting pain, instability, continued disability, or when the investigation of the cause of the fracture reveals serious underlying pathology.

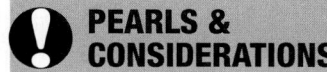
PEARLS & CONSIDERATIONS

Prevention of osteoporosis and conservative therapy remain the mainstay.

COMMENTS

- VCFs should be suspected in anyone aged >50 yr with the acute onset of low back pain. There are many opportunities for diagnosis and treatment that are easy to miss, especially for males.
- Solitary vertebral fractures higher than T7 are unusual and may be suspicious for other pathologic causes.

- Diagnosing and treating osteoporosis reduces the incidence of VCFs.
- Getting people with VCF physically active as soon as possible will be efficacious both acutely and in the long term.
- In general, VCF can perhaps be best managed through a partnership of the patient, the primary care physician, an orthopedist, a physical therapist, a dietician, and a social worker.

PREVENTION

Reducing the effects of modifiable risk factors is key.

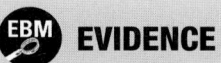
EVIDENCE

available at www.expertconsult.com

SUGGESTED READINGS

available at www.expertconsult.com

AUTHOR: **JEFFREY BORKAN, M.D., PH.D**

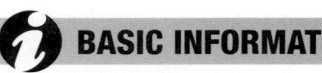 **BASIC INFORMATION**

DEFINITION

Vestibular neuronitis is a syndrome of sudden-onset, often severe, prolonged vertigo of peripheral origin.

SYNONYMS

Labyrinthitis, vestibular neuritis, acute neuritis, neurolabyrinthitis

ICD-9CM CODES
078.81 Vestibular neuronitis
386.12 Neuronitis, vestibular

EPIDEMIOLOGY & DEMOGRAPHICS

Viral origin supported by the fact that it occurs in epidemics, may affect several family members, and occurs more commonly in spring and early summer. Male-to-female ratio is similar. Thought to result from selective inflammation of the vestibular nerve; etiology presumed to be viral. There is selective damage to the superior part of the vestibular labyrinth, supplied by the superior division of the vestibular nerve.

PHYSICAL FINDINGS & CLINICAL PRESENTATION

- Course: develops over period of hours, resolves over periods of days, although with frequent long-term sequelae; may have viral prodrome.
- Symptoms of vertigo, spontaneous peripheral nystagmus, positive head-thrust test, imbalance. Patient reports intense sensation of rotation, difficulty standing and walking, tends to veer toward affected side, autonomic symptoms with pallor, sweating, nausea, and vomiting.

ETIOLOGY

Thought to be viral in origin, possibly thought to be due to herpes zoster, but trial of valacyclovir with and without methylprednisolone showed no efficacy for valacyclovir, but efficacy for the steroid.

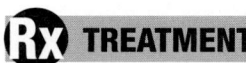 **DIAGNOSIS**

DIFFERENTIAL DIAGNOSIS

- Labyrinthitis: similar etiology, but includes hearing loss
- Labyrinthine infarction
- Perilymph fistula
- Brain stem and cerebellar infarction
- Migraine-associated vertigo
- Multiple sclerosis

WORKUP

- Patient may fall toward affected side when attempting ambulation or during Romberg tests.
- Head-thrust test: grasp patient's head, apply brief small-amplitude rapid head turn, first to one side and then the other; patient fixates on examiner's nose: positive test is lack of corrective eye movements "saccades" on affected side.

LABORATORY TESTS

- Electronystagmography (ENG): testing of the vestibular apparatus with physical challenges, unilateral lack of caloric response
- Audiogram: normal

IMAGING STUDIES

Brain imaging: CT or MRI—normal

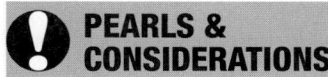 **TREATMENT**

NONPHARMACOLOGIC THERAPY

Vestibular exercises, when tolerated, will accelerate recovery.

ACUTE GENERAL Rx

- Corticosteroids: clinical recovery—especially long-term recovery—may not be better in patients receiving corticosteroids, although they may improve the caloric extent and recovery of canal paresis. Nonetheless, corticosteroids are often prescribed.
- Antihistamines: meclizine, dimenhydrinate, promethazine.
- Anticholinergics: scopolamine.

- Anti-emetics: droperidol, prochlorperazine.
- Benzodiazepines: diazepam, valium.

CHRONIC Rx

- Vestibular rehabilitation exercises
- Anti-GABA agents
- Antihistamines

DISPOSITION

Most patients can be treated as outpatients, but if dehydrated because of severe vomiting, they may require brief parenteral therapy.

REFERRAL

- ENT: if diagnosis uncertain, and if these patients are at risk for BPPV subsequently; also symptoms may linger.
- Neurology: if question of central origin or migraine.

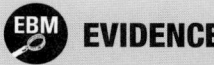 **PEARLS & CONSIDERATIONS**

COMMENTS

- Diagnosis unlikely to be vestibular neuronitis if hearing is impaired or other neurologic signs and symptoms present.
- Although patients may recover from dramatic acute symptoms, subtle vestibular deficits may linger for prolonged period, if not indefinitely.
- Program of vestibular habituation head movement exercises can reduce imbalance symptoms.

PATIENT/FAMILY EDUCATION

Vestibular Disorders Association: http://www.vestibular.org

EBM **EVIDENCE**

available at www.expertconsult.com

SUGGESTED READINGS
available at www.expertconsult.com

AUTHORS: **JEFFREY M. BORKAN, M.D., Ph.D.,** and **JUDITH NUDELMAN, M.D.**

BASIC INFORMATION

DEFINITION Vitiligo is the acquired loss of epidermal pigmentation that is characterized histologically by the absence of epidermal melanocytes. There are two major forms: nonsegmental (generalized) vitiligo, which accounts for >80% of cases, and segmental vitiligo, which accounts for 30% of childhood cases.

ICD-9CM CODES
709.1 Vitiligo

EPIDEMIOLOGY & DEMOGRAPHICS

PREVALENCE: Vitiligo affects 0.5% to 1% of the population; it is the most common depigmenting disorder.

PREDOMINANT AGE: Vitiligo can begin at any age, but the age at onset is <20 yr for half of patients.

GENETICS: A positive family history is present in 25% to 30% of patients, and both sexes are equally affected. There are no differences in the rates of occurrence with regard to skin type or race.

PHYSICAL FINDINGS & CLINICAL PRESENTATION

- Hypopigmented and depigmented lesions (Figure 1-408) favor sun-exposed regions, intertriginous areas, genitalia, and sites over bony prominences (i.e., nonsegmental or type A vitiligo).
- Areas around the body orifices are also frequently involved.
- The lesions tend to be symmetric.
- Occasionally the lesions are linear or pseudo-dermatomal (i.e., segmental or type B vitiligo).
- Vitiligo lesions may occur at trauma sites (i.e., Koebner's phenomenon).
- The hair in affected areas may be white.
- The margins of the lesions are usually well demarcated; when a ring of hyperpigmentation is seen, the term *trichrome vitiligo* is used.
- The term *marginal inflammatory vitiligo* is used to describe lesions with raised borders.
- Initially the disease is limited, but the lesions tend to become more extensive over time.

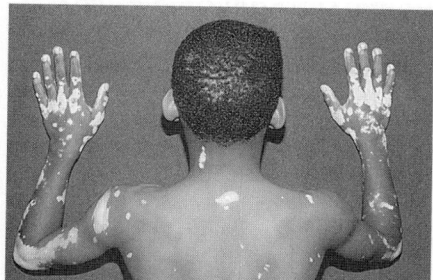

FIGURE 1-408 Multiple, sharply demarcated, symmetric, depigmented areas of vitiligo. (From Behrman RE: *Nelson textbook of pediatrics,* Philadelphia, 2006, WB Saunders.)

- Type B vitiligo is more common among children.
- Vitiligo may begin around pigmented nevi and produce a halo (i.e., Sutton's nevus); in such cases, the central nevus often regresses and disappears over time.

ETIOLOGY & PATHOGENESIS

- Three pathophysiologic theories:
  1. Autoimmune theory (i.e., autoantibodies against melanocytes)
  2. Neural theory (i.e., neurochemical mediators selectively destroy melanocytes)
  3. Self-destructive process in which melanocytes fail to protect themselves against cytotoxic melanin precursors
- Although vitiligo is considered to be an acquired disease, 25% to 30% of cases are familial. The mode of transmission is unknown; the condition seems to be polygenic or autosomal dominant with incomplete penetrance and variable expression.
- Associated disorders:
  - Alopecia areata
  - Type 1 diabetes mellitus
  - Adrenal insufficiency
  - Hyperthyroidism and hypothyroidism
  - Mucocutaneous candidiasis
  - Pernicious anemia
  - Polyglandular autoimmune syndromes
  - Melanoma

DIAGNOSIS

DIFFERENTIAL DIAGNOSIS

- Acquired hypopigmentation disorders:
  - Chemical-induced (e.g., chloroquine, imatinib, phenolic-catecholic derivatives [e.g., adhesives, deodorants, latex gloves, lacquer resins, varnish, soap antioxidants, insecticides, printing ink, paints, motor oil additives, disinfectants])
  - Halo nevus
  - Idiopathic guttate hypomelanosis
  - Leprosy
  - Leukoderma associated with melanoma
  - Pityriasis alba
  - Postinflammatory hypopigmentation
  - Tinea versicolor
  - Vogt-Koyanagi syndrome (i.e., vitiligo, uveitis, and deafness)
  - Melasma
  - Mycosis fungoides
- Congenital hypopigmentation disorders:
  - Albinism, partial (piebaldism)
  - Albinism, total
  - Nevus anemicus
  - Nevus depigmentosus
  - Tuberous sclerosis
  - Ito's hypomelanosis

WORKUP

- Inquire about a personal and family history of autoimmune disease.
- Perform a physical examination.

- A Wood's light examination may enhance the lesions of light-skinned individuals.

TREATMENT

Treatment is indicated primarily for cosmetic purposes when depigmentation causes emotional or social distress. Depigmentation is more noticeable among patients with darker complexions.

- Cosmetic masking agents (e.g., Dermablend, Covermark) or stains (e.g., DY-O-Derm, Vitadye)
- Sunless tanning lotions (e.g., dihydroxyacetone)
- Repigmentation (This is achieved by the activation and migration of melanocytes from hair follicles; therefore, skin with little or no hair responds poorly to treatment.)
- Narrow-band ultraviolet B radiation (This is the preferred treatment for nonsegmental vitiligo. It is given twice weekly [not on successive days] during sessions that last from 5 to 10 min. The best results are achieved on the face, trunk, and limbs.)
- Psoralens and sunlight (e.g., PUVAsol)
- Topical mid-potency steroids (e.g., triamcinolone 0.1% or desonide 0.05% cream qd for 3 to 4 mo)
- Topical calcineurin inhibitors for face and neck lesions
- Intralesional steroid injection
- Systemic steroids (e.g., betamethasone 5 mg qd on two consecutive days per week for 2 to 4 mo)
- Total depigmentation in cases of extensive vitiligo with 20% monobenzyl ether or hydroquinone (This is a permanent procedure, and patients will require lifelong protection from sun exposure.)
- Topical immunomodulators (e.g., tacrolimus, pimecrolimus) (These substances can also induce the repigmentation of vitiliginous skin lesions. However, their potential for systemic immunosuppression or for increasing the risk of skin or other malignancies remains to be defined.)
- Calcipotriol, which is a synthetic analog of vitamin D_3 (This has also been used in combination with ultraviolet light or clobetasol, with limited results.)
- Surgical techniques

EVIDENCE

available at www.expertconsult.com

SUGGESTED READING
available at www.expertconsult.com

AUTHOR: **FRED F. FERRI, M.D.**

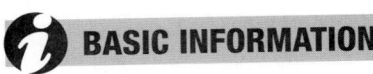
DEFINITION

Von Hippel-Lindau disease (VHL) is a rare, autosomal-dominant, inherited disorder that is characterized by the formation of hemangioblastomas, cysts, and malignancies that involve multiple organ systems.

SYNONYMS

Hippel-Lindau syndrome
Cerebelloretinal hemangioblastomatosis
Retinocerebellar angiomatosis

ICD-9CM CODES
759.6 von Hippel-Lindau disease

EPIDEMIOLOGY & DEMOGRAPHICS

- The incidence of VHL is 1 case/36,000 live births.
- The mean age at the onset of clinical manifestations is 26 yr, but the disease can present from infancy until the seventh decade of life.
- In the U.S., approximately 6000 to 7000 people have VHL.
- Affected individuals are at risk for the development of renal cell carcinoma, pheochromocytoma, pancreatic islet cell tumor, endolymphatic sac tumor, and hemangioblastomas of the cerebellum and the retina.

PHYSICAL FINDINGS & CLINICAL PRESENTATION

- There are two clinical types of VHL:
  - Type 1 has no pheochromocytoma
  - Type 2 has pheochromocytoma:
    1. Type 2A: hemangioblastoma in the central nervous system (CNS) with no renal cell carcinoma
    2. Type 2B: renal cell carcinoma and other tumors
    3. Type 2C: only pheochromocytoma; associated with Chuvash polycythemia
- Retinal angiomas (60% prevalence):
  1. Usually occurs by age 25 yr with both VHL type 1 and VHL type 2
  2. Often multifocal and bilateral
  3. Detached retina
  4. Glaucoma
  5. Blindness
- CNS hemangioblastomas (70% prevalence):
  1. Cerebellum and spinal cord are the most common sites, followed by the medulla
  2. Usually multiple; mean age at diagnosis is 25 yr; found with VHL types 1, 2A, and 2B
  3. Headache, ataxia, slurred speech, nystagmus, vertigo, nausea, and vomiting
- Renal cysts (approximately 60% prevalence) and clear cell renal cell carcinoma (RCC; approximately 25% to 45% prevalence):
  1. Usually occur by the age of 40 yr
  2. May be asymptomatic or cause abdominal and flank pain
  3. RCC is bilateral in 75% of patients

- Pancreatic cysts:
  1. Usually asymptomatic
  2. Large cysts can cause biliary obstructive symptoms
  3. Diarrhea and diabetes may develop if enough of the pancreas is replaced by cysts
- Pheochromocytoma (7% to 18% prevalence):
  1. Found with VHL types 2A, 2B, and 2C
  2. Bilateral in 50% to 80% of cases
  3. Hypertension, palpitations, sweating, and headache
  4. Commonly occurs with pancreatic islet cell tumors
- Papillary cystadenoma of the epididymis (25% to 60% of men with VHL):
  1. Palpable scrotal mass
  2. May be unilateral or bilateral
- Papillary cystadenoma of the broad ligaments (unknown prevalence):
  1. Usually asymptomatic
  2. Reported symptoms include pain, dyspareunia, and menorrhagia
- Endolymphatic sac tumors of the middle ear (approximately 15% prevalence):
  1. Vertigo
  2. Hearing loss
  3. Facial paralysis

ETIOLOGY

VHL is primarily caused by a mutation of the von Hippel-Lindau gene, which is located on the short arm of chromosome 3. The VHL gene codes for a cytoplasmic protein that functions in tumor suppression.

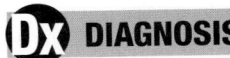 **DIAGNOSIS**

DIFFERENTIAL DIAGNOSIS

Table 1-182 compares genetic diseases associated with the development of pancreatic or gut endocrine tumors.

WORKUP

- A clinical diagnosis is established in the presence of a positive family history plus a single CNS hemangioblastoma or a visceral lesion (e.g., RCC, pheochromocytoma, pancreatic cysts or tumors).
- If no clear family history is present, two or more hemangioblastomas or one hemangioblastoma with a visceral lesion are required to make the diagnosis.

- Genetic screening is up to 100% sensitive and specific, although, in the 20% of patients with de novo VHL mutations, the test may be falsely negative as a result of somatic mosaicism.
- Screening family members is essential for the early detection of VHL disease.

WORKUP

Screening laboratory values and ophthalmoscopic, genetic, and imaging studies to look for sites of involvement

LABORATORY TESTS

- CBC may reveal erythrocytosis that requires periodic phlebotomies
- Electrolytes and renal function tests
- Urine for norepinephrine, epinephrine, and vanillylmandelic acid to look for pheochromocytoma
- Genetic studies: complete sequencing of coding region, Southern blot, and fluorescent in situ hybridization

IMAGING STUDIES

- Indirect and direct ophthalmoscopy, fluorescein angiography, and tonometry are used to screen for retinal angiomas and glaucoma.
- Computed tomographic scanning of the abdomen is used for the screening, detection, and monitoring of patients with renal cysts or tumors, pheochromocytomas, and pancreatic cysts or tumors:
  1. Renal cysts grow an average of 0.5 cm/yr.
  2. Renal tumors grow an average of 1.5 cm/yr.
  3. Computed tomography scans are performed every 6 mo for the first 2 yr and every year for life in patients who have had surgery for RCC.
- MRI with gadolinium is used for the screening and evaluation of CNS and spinal cord hemangioblastomas, endolymphatic sac tumors, and pheochromocytomas.
- Angiography may be performed before CNS surgery.

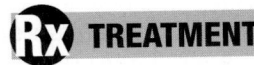 **TREATMENT**

NONPHARMACOLOGIC THERAPY

Genetic counseling

TABLE 1-182   Genetic Diseases Associated with the Development of Pancreatic or Gut Endocrine Tumors

Gene	Disease	Phenotype
Menin	Multiple endocrine neoplasia type 1	Parathyroid, pituitary, and pancreatic endocrine tumors
VHL	von Hippel-Lindau disease	Pancreatic endocrine tumors, hemangiomas, and multiple neoplasms
NF-1	Neurofibromatosis	Neurofibromas and pheochromocytomas
TSC1/2	Tuberous sclerosis	Pancreatic endocrine tumors and hamartomas

From Larsen PR et al: *Williams textbook of endocrinology*, ed 10, Philadelphia, 2003, WB Saunders.

ACUTE GENERAL RX

- Laser photocoagulation and cryotherapy are used for patients with retinal angiomas to prevent blindness (Table 1-183).
- For cerebellar hemangioblastomas, treatment is surgical. External-beam radiation and stereotactic radiosurgery can also be performed.
- For renal tumors, surgery is delayed until one of the renal tumors reaches 3 cm in diameter.

Nephron-sparing surgery is the preferred approach.
- Pancreatic islet cell tumors usually require surgical removal.
- Adrenalectomy is performed for pheochromocytoma.
- Antiangiogenic therapy has been shown to improve the survival of patients with RCC, with studies ongoing to assess combination therapy.

CHRONIC RX

- Dialysis has been delayed for many patients with the use of nephron-sparing surgery.
- Renal transplantation is usually delayed for 1 yr after bilateral nephrectomy for renal tumors to ensure that no metastases have occurred.

DISPOSITION

The median life expectancy of patients with this condition is 49 yr.

REFERRAL

Geneticist, neurosurgeon, urologist, nephrologist, ophthalmologist, otolaryngologist, neurologist, endocrinologist, and radiation oncologist referrals should be considered.

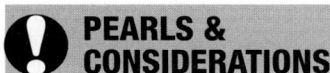

PEARLS & CONSIDERATIONS

- The most common cause of death in patients with VHL is RCC.
- More information for patients can be obtained at from the von Hippel-Lindau Family Alliance (http://vhl.org).

SUGGESTED READINGS
available at www.expertconsult.com

AUTHORS: **MARK F. BRADY, M.D., M.P.H.,** and **WEN-Y. WU-CHEN, M.D.**

TABLE 1-183 The Management of Different Manifestations of von Hippel-Lindau Disease

Tumor	Treatment	Screening
Retinal angiomas	If small, laser photocoagulation/cryotherapy; in severe cases, the removal of the affected eye	Retinal examinations once per year soon after birth
Central nervous system hemangioblastomas	Surgical resection for symptomatic patients or large tumors; gamma knife if difficult to remove from primary site	MRI for patients >10 yr once per year
Renal cysts/carcinomas	For tumors <3 cm in diameter, observation; for one tumor >3 cm in diameter, remove all tumors by enucleation or partial nephrectomy; percutaneous radiofrequency ablation and cryosurgery are also performed; surgical resection is not recommended for any cyst without a tumor inside of it; nephrectomy is indicated for patients with end-stage renal disease who require dialysis because of the malignancy potential	CT/MRI scan once yearly; if the patient has relatives with the condition, he or she is checked once per year with CT before the age of 20 yr
Pancreatic cysts	Partial resection of the pancreas, depending on the site of the cyst	
Pheochromocytomas	Preferable to remove only the tumor itself and thus to conserve adrenal function	CT scan once per year for patients <10 yr old

CT, Computed tomography; *MRI,* magnetic resonance imaging.

BASIC INFORMATION

DEFINITION

Von Willebrand's disease is a congenital disorder of hemostasis characterized by defective or deficient von Willebrand factor (vWF). There are several subtypes of von Willebrand's disease. The most common type (80% of cases) is type I, which is caused by a quantitative decrease in vWF; type IIA and type IIB are results of qualitative protein abnormalities; and type III is a rare, autosomal recessive disorder characterized by a near-complete quantitative deficiency of vWF. Acquired von Willebrand's disease (AvWD) is a rare disorder that usually occurs in elderly patients and usually presents with mucocutaneous bleeding abnormalities and no clinically meaningful family history. It is often accompanied by a hematoproliferative or autoimmune disorder. Successful treatment of the associated illness can reverse the clinical and laboratory manifestations.

SYNONYMS

Pseudohemophilia
vWD

ICD-9CM CODES
286.4 von Willebrand's disease

EPIDEMIOLOGY & DEMOGRAPHICS

- Autosomal-dominant disorder
- Most common inherited bleeding disorder
- Prevalence is 1% to 2% in general population, according to screening studies; estimates based on referral for symptoms of bleeding suggest a prevalence of 30 to 100 cases per million

PHYSICAL FINDINGS & CLINICAL PRESENTATION

- Generally normal physical examination
- Mucosal bleeding (gingival bleeding, epistaxis) and gastrointestinal bleeding may occur
- Easy bruising
- Postpartum bleeding, bleeding after surgery or dental extraction, menorrhagia

ETIOLOGY

Quantitative or qualitative deficiency of vWF (see "Definition")

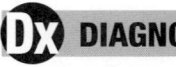 **DIAGNOSIS**

The diagnosis of vWD generally requires two criteria: (1) a personal history, family history, or physical evidence of mucocutaneous bleeding and (2) a qualitative or quantitative decrease in functional activity of vWF. The American Society of Hematology states that a definitive diagnosis of vWD may be made if vWF antigen levels are less than 30 IU/dL. It also describes a gray zone of 30 to 50 IU/dL, designated as "low vWF."

DIFFERENTIAL DIAGNOSIS

Platelet function disorders, clotting factor deficiencies

WORKUP

- Laboratory evaluation (see "Laboratory Tests")
- Initial testing includes partial thromboplastin time (increased), platelet count (normal), and bleeding time (prolonged)
- Subsequent tests include vWF level (decreased), factor VIII:C (decreased), and ristocetin agglutination (increased in type II B) (Table 1-184)

LABORATORY TESTS

- Normal platelet number and morphology
- Prolonged bleeding time
- Decreased factor VIII coagulant activity
- Decreased vWF antigen or ristocetin cofactor
- Normal platelet aggregation studies
- Type II A von Willebrand disease can be distinguished from type I by absence of ristocetin cofactor activity and abnormal multimer
- Type IIB von Willebrand disease is distinguished from type I by abnormal multimer

TREATMENT

NONPHARMACOLOGIC THERAPY

- Avoidance of aspirin and other nonsteroidal antiinflammatory drugs.
- Evaluation for likelihood of bleeding (with measurement of bleeding time) before surgical procedures. When a patient undergoes surgery or receives repeated therapeutic doses of concentrates, factor VIII activity should be assayed every 12 hr on the day a dose is administered and every 24 hr thereafter.

GENERAL Rx

- The mainstay of treatment in von Willebrand's disease is the replacement of the deficient protein at the time of spontaneous bleeding or before invasive procedures are performed.
- Desmopressin acetate (DDAVP) is useful to release stored vWF from endothelial cells. It is used to cover minor procedures and traumatic bleeding in mild type I von Willebrand's disease. Dose is 0.3 mcg/kg in 100 ml of normal saline solution IV infused >20 min. DDAVP is also available as a nasal spray (dose of 150 mcg spray administered to each nostril) as a preparation for minor surgery and management of minor bleeding episodes. DDAVP is not effective in type IIA von Willebrand's disease and is potentially dangerous in type IIB (increased risk of bleeding and thrombocytopenia).
- In patients with severe disease, replacement therapy in the form of cryoprecipitate is the method of choice. The standard dose is 1 bag of cryoprecipitate per 10 kg of body weight.
- Factor VIII concentrate rich in vWF (Humate-P) is useful to correct bleeding abnormalities in type IIA, IIB, and type III von Willebrand's disease without alloantibodies. Alloantibodies that inactivate vWF and form circulating immune complexes develop in 15% of patients with type III von Willebrand's disease who have received multiple transfusions. In these patients, recombinant factor VIII is preferred because autoantibodies can elicit life-threatening anaphylactic reactions because of complement activation by immune complexes.
- Life-threatening hemorrhage unresponsive to therapy with cryoprecipitate or factor VIII concentrate may require transfusion of normal platelets.

SUGGESTED READINGS
available at www.expertconsult.com

AUTHOR: **FRED F. FERRI, M.D.**

TABLE 1-184   Genetic and Laboratory Findings in von Willebrand's Disease

Parameter Type	BT	VIII-c	vw-Ag	R-cof	Ripa	Multimer Structure	Mode of Inheritance
I (classic)	P	R	R	R	R	Normal	AD
II							
A	P	N/R	N/R	R	R	Abnormal	AD
B	P	N/R	N/R	N/R	I	Abnormal	AD
III	P	R	R	R	R	Variable	AR

From Behrman RE: *Nelson textbook of pediatrics*, ed 17, Philadelphia, 2004, WB Saunders.

AD, Autosomal dominant; *AR,* autosomal recessive; *BT,* bleeding time; *I,* increased; *N/R,* normal or reduced; *P,* prolonged; *R,* reduced; *R-Cof,* ristocetin cofactor; *RIPA,* ristocetin-induced platelet aggregation (agglutination); *vW-Ag,* von Willebrand antigen (protein); *VIII-C,* factor VIII coagulant activity.

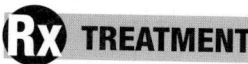

BASIC INFORMATION

DEFINITION

Vulvar cancer is an abnormal cell proliferation arising on the vulva and exhibiting malignant potential. The majority are of squamous cell origin; however, other types include adenocarcinoma, basal cell carcinoma, sarcoma, and melanoma.

SYNONYMS

Squamous cell carcinoma of the vulva (90%)
Basal cell carcinoma of the vulva
Adenocarcinoma of the vulva
Melanoma of the vulva
Bartholin gland carcinoma
Verrucous carcinoma of the vulva
Vulvar sarcoma

ICD-9CM CODES
184.4 Vulvar neoplasm

EPIDEMIOLOGY & DEMOGRAPHICS

INCIDENCE: 2.2 cases per 100,000 persons
PREVALENCE: Vulvar cancer is uncommon. It comprises 4% of malignancies of the female genital tract. It is the fourth most common gynecologic malignancy.
MEAN AGE AT DIAGNOSIS: Predominantly a disease of menopause. Mean age at diagnosis is 65 yr.

PHYSICAL FINDINGS & CLINICAL PRESENTATION

- Vulvar pruritus or pain is present.
- May produce a malodorous discharge or present as bleeding.
- Raised lesion that may have fleshy, ulcerated, leukoplakic, or warty appearance; may have multifocal lesions.
- Lesions are usually located on labia majora but may be seen on labia minora, clitoris, and perineum.
- The lymph nodes of groin may be palpable.

ETIOLOGY

- The exact etiology is unknown.
- Vulvar intraepithelial neoplasia has been reported in 20% to 30% of invasive squamous cell carcinoma of the vulva, but the malignant potential is unknown.
- Human papillomavirus is found in 30% to 50% of vulvar carcinoma, but its exact role is unclear.
- Chronic pruritus, wetness, industrial wastes, arsenicals, hygienic agents, and vulvar dystrophies have been implicated as causative agents.
- Vulvar cancer in younger women is more directly dependent on HPV infection, vulvar dysplasia, and tobacco use.

DIAGNOSIS

DIFFERENTIAL DIAGNOSIS

- Lymphogranuloma inguinale
- Tuberculosis
- Vulvar dystrophies
- Vulvar atrophy
- Paget's disease

WORKUP

- Diagnosis is made histologically by biopsy
- Thorough examination of the lesion and assessment of spread. Table 1-185 describes FIGO staging of vulvar cancer
- Possible colposcopy of adjacent areas
- Cytologic smear of vagina and cervix
- Cystoscopy and proctosigmoidoscopy may be necessary

IMAGING STUDIES

- Chest radiography
- CT scan and MRI for assessing local tumor spread

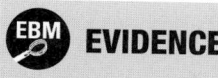

TREATMENT

NONPHARMACOLOGIC THERAPY

- Treatment is individualized depending on the stage of the tumor.
- Stage I tumors with <1 mm stromal invasion are treated with complete local excision without groin node dissection. Imiquimod 5% cream, a topical immune response modulator, is also effective in the treatment of vulvar intraepithelial neoplasia.
- Stage I tumors with >1 mm stromal invasion are treated with complete local excision with groin node dissection.
- Stage II tumors require radical vulvectomy with bilateral groin node dissection.
- Advanced-stage disease may require the addition of radiation and chemotherapy to the surgical regimen.
- Section III describes a treatment algorithm for management of vulvar cancer.

DISPOSITION

Five-year survival ranges from 90% for stage I to 15% for stage IV.

REFERRAL

Vulvar cancer should be managed by a gynecologic oncologist and radiation oncologist.

EVIDENCE

available at www.expertconsult.com

SUGGESTED READINGS
available at www.expertconsult.com

AUTHORS: **GIL M. FARKASH, M.D.,** and **RUBEN ALVERO, M.D.**

TABLE 1-185   FIGO Staging of Vulval Cancer

Stage I	Tumor confined to the vulva—2 cm or less in diameter. Nodes are not involved. A. Lesions less than 1 mm depth invasion B. Other lesions less than 2 cm in diameter
Stage II	Tumor confined to the vulva—more than 2 cm in diameter. Nodes are not involved.
Stage III	Tumor of any size with: Adjacent spread to the lower urethra and/or the vagina, the perineum and the anus, and/or unilateral lymph node involvement.
Stage IV	Tumor of any size with bilateral groin lymph node involvement: A. Infiltrating the bladder mucosa or the rectal mucosa, or both, including the upper part of the urethral mucosa B. Fixed to the bone or other distant metastases. Fixed or ulcerated nodes in either one or both groins.

Symonds EM, Symonds IM: *Essential obstetrics and gynecology*, ed 4, London, 2004, Churchill Livingstone.

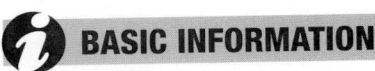

BASIC INFORMATION

DEFINITION

Bacterial vulvovaginitis is inflammation affecting the vagina, only rarely affecting the vulva, caused by anaerobic and aerobic bacteria.

SYNONYMS

Bacterial vaginosis
Gardnerella vaginalis
Haemophilus vaginalis
Corynebacterium vaginalis

ICD-9CM CODES
616.10 Vulvovaginitis

EPIDEMIOLOGY & DEMOGRAPHICS

- Most prevalent form of vaginal infection of reproductive age women in the U.S.
- 32% to 64% in patients visiting STD clinics
- 12% to 25% in other clinic populations
- 10% to 26% in patients visiting obstetric clinics
- May be associated with adverse pregnancy outcomes: premature rupture of membranes, preterm labor, preterm birth
- Organisms frequently found in postpartum or postcesarean endometritis

PHYSICAL FINDINGS & CLINICAL PRESENTATION

- >50% of all women may be without symptoms.
- Unpleasant, fishy, or musty vaginal odor in about 50% to 70% of all patients. Odor exacerbated immediately after intercourse or during menstruation.
- Vaginal discharge is increased.
- Vaginal itching and irritation occur.

ETIOLOGY

- Synergistic polymicrobial infection characterized by an overgrowth of bacteria normally found in the vagina
- Anaerobics: *Bacteroides* spp., *Peptostreptococcus* spp., *Mobiluncus* spp.
- Facultative anaerobes: *G. vaginalis, Mycoplasma hominis*
- Concentration of anaerobic bacteria increased to 100 to 1000 times normal
- Lactobacilli are absent or greatly reduced

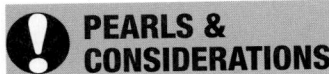

DIAGNOSIS

DIFFERENTIAL DIAGNOSIS

- Fungal vaginitis
- *Trichomonas* vaginitis
- Atrophic vaginitis
- Cervicitis

WORKUP

- Pelvic examination
- Speculum examination
- Normal saline and 10% KOH slide of discharge
- Amsel criteria for diagnosis (three of four should be present):
  1. pH >4.5
  2. Clue cells (epithelial cells covered with bacteria) on saline solution slide
  3. Positive whiff test on 10% KOH
  4. Homogeneous, white, adherent discharge
- Section III, "Vaginal Discharge," describes the evaluation of discharge

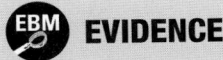

TREATMENT

ACUTE GENERAL Rx

- Metronidazole 500 mg PO bid × 7 days, >90% cure rate
- Metronidazole 2 g PO × 1 day, 67% to 92% cure rate
- Metronidazole gel 5 g, intravaginal bid × 5 days
- Clindamycin 2% cream 5 g, intravaginal qd × 7 days
- Clindamycin 300 mg PO bid × 7 days in pregnancy

CHRONIC Rx

Clindamycin 300 mg PO bid × 7 days; cure rate similar to those achieved with metronidazole
Related to adverse pregnancy outcomes
- Metronidazole 250 mg PO bid × 7 days
- Metronidazole zympoxidase
- Clindamycin 300 mg PO bid × 7 days
- Good hygiene: avoidance of douching, harsh shower gels, bubble baths; cotton underwear

DISPOSITION

- Reevaluate if not cured with treatment
- Recurrence fairly common

REFERRAL

Refer to obstetrician/gynecologist for recurrence or pregnant patient with bacterial vaginosis

PEARLS & CONSIDERATIONS

COMMENTS

Treating sexual partners has failed to demonstrate a benefit.

EVIDENCE

available at www.expertconsult.com

SUGGESTED READINGS

available at www.expertconsult.com

AUTHORS: **JULIE ANNE SZUMIGALA, M.D.,** and **RUBEN ALVERO, M.D.**

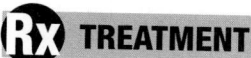

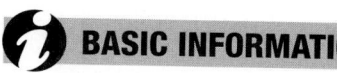 **BASIC INFORMATION**

DEFINITION

Estrogen-deficient vulvovaginitis is the irritation and/or inflammation of the vulva and vagina because of progressive thinning and atrophic changes secondary to estrogen deficiency (Fig. 1-409).

SYNONYMS

Atrophic vaginitis

ICD-9CM CODES
616.10 Vulvovaginitis

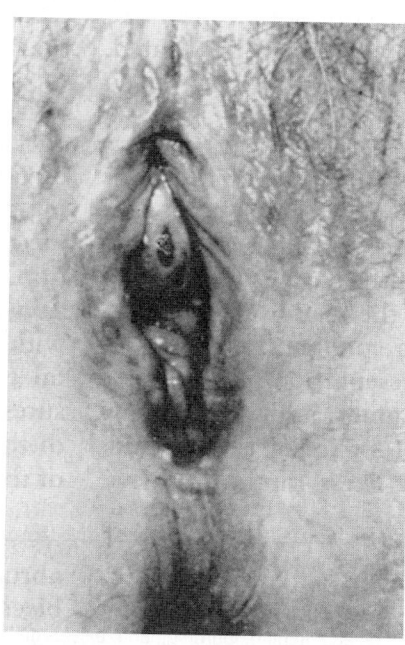

FIGURE 1-409 Advanced postmenopausal atrophy of the vulva in a 72-year-old woman. (From Symonds EM, Macpherson MBA: Color atlas of obstetrics and gynecology, St Louis, 1994, Mosby.)

EPIDEMIOLOGY & DEMOGRAPHICS
- Seen most often in postmenopausal women
- Average age of menopause is 52 yr
- In 1990, there were 36 million women 50 yr of age or older

PHYSICAL FINDINGS & CLINICAL PRESENTATION
- Thinning of pubic hair, labia minora and majora
- Decreased secretions from the vestibular glands, with vaginal dryness
- Regression of subcutaneous fat
- Vulvar and vaginal itching
- Dyspaereunia
- Dysuria and urinary frequency
- Vaginal spotting

ETIOLOGY
Estrogen deficiency

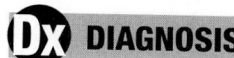 **DIAGNOSIS**

DIFFERENTIAL DIAGNOSIS
- Infectious vulvovaginitis
- Squamous cell hyperplasia
- Lichen sclerosus
- Vulvar malignancy
- Vaginal malignancy
- Cervical and endometrial malignancy

WORKUP
- Pelvic examination
- Speculum examination
- Pap smear
- Possible endometrial biopsy if bleeding

LABORATORY TESTS
FSH and estradiol: generally after menopause, estradiol <15 pg and FSH >40 mIU/ml (diagnosis of menopause usually made on a clinical basis and does not usually require FSH and/or estradiol testing)

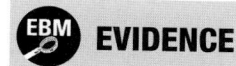 **TREATMENT**

ACUTE GENERAL Rx
- Premarin 0.625 mg PO qd.
- Estraderm patch 0.05 mg × 2 per week.
- If uterus present:
  1. Estrogen + 2.5 mg PO Provera qd *or*
  2. Estrogen + 10 mg PO Provera × 10 days each mo
- Conjugated estrogen vaginal cream intravaginally. Estradiol vaginal cream 0.01%. 2 to 4 g/day × 2 wk then 1 to 2 g/day × 2 wk then 1 to 2 g × 3 days/wk
- Vagifem (estradiol vaginal tablets) 25 mg inserted intravaginally daily for 2 wk then twice weekly. May take up to 12 wk to feel the full benefits of the medication.
- Conjugated estrogen vaginal cream: 2 to 4 g qd (3 wk on, 1 wk off) for 3 to 5 mo.

CHRONIC Rx
See "Acute General Rx." May discontinue vaginal estrogen cream once symptoms alleviate.

DISPOSITION
The symptoms should be improved with the therapy. Caution for vaginal bleeding if uterus present.

REFERRAL
To obstetrician/gynecologist if vaginal bleeding

EBM EVIDENCE

available at www.expertconsult.com

AUTHORS: **JULIE ANNE SZUMIGALA, M.D.,** and **RUBEN ALVERO, M.D.**

V

Diseases and Disorders

I

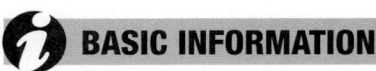

BASIC INFORMATION

DEFINITION

Fungal vulvovaginitis is the inflammation of vulva and vagina caused by *Candida* spp.

SYNONYMS

Monilial vulvovaginitis
Vulvovaginal candidiasis
VVC

ICD-9CM CODES

112.1 Vulvovaginitis, monilial

EPIDEMIOLOGY & DEMOGRAPHICS

- Second most common cause of vaginal infection.
- Approximately 13 million people were affected in 1990.
- 75% of women will have at least one episode during their childbearing years, and ~40% to 50% of these will have a second attack.
- No symptoms in 20% to 40% of women who have positive cultures.

PHYSICAL FINDINGS & CLINICAL PRESENTATION

- Intense vulvar and vaginal pruritus
- Edema and erythema of vulva
- Thick, curd-like vaginal discharge
- Adherent, dry, white, curdy patches attached to vaginal mucosa

ETIOLOGY

- *Candida albicans* is responsible for 80% to 95% of vaginal fungal infections.
- *Candida tropicalis* and *Torulopsis glabrata* (*Candida glabrata*) are the most common nonalbicans *Candida* species that can induce vaginitis.

PREDISPOSING HOST FACTORS

- Pregnancy
- Oral contraceptives (high-estrogen)
- Diabetes mellitus
- Antibiotics
- Immunosuppression (e.g., HIV)
- Tight, poorly ventilated, nylon underclothing, with increased local perineal moisture and temperature

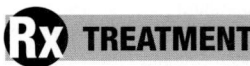 DIAGNOSIS

DIFFERENTIAL DIAGNOSIS

- Bacterial vaginosis
- *Trichomonas* vaginitis
- Atrophic vaginitis

Section II describes the differential diagnosis of vaginal discharges and infections.

WORKUP

- Pelvic examination
- Speculum examination
- Hyphae or budding spores on 10% KOH preparation (positive in 50% to 70% of individuals with yeast infection)

Section III, "Vaginal Discharge," describes the evaluation of discharge.

LABORATORY TESTS

Culture, especially recurrence for identification

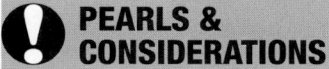 TREATMENT

ACUTE GENERAL Rx

- Cure rate of the various azole derivatives 85% to 90%; little evidence of superiority of one azole agent over another
- No significant differences in persistent symptoms with oral or vaginal treatment
- Fluconazole 150 mg PO × 1 is preferred treatment
- Cure rate of polyene cream and suppositories: 75% to 80%
- Miconazole 200-mg suppository, one suppository × 3 days or 2% vaginal cream, one applicator full intravaginally qhs × 7
- Clotrimazole 200-mg vaginal tablet, one tablet intravaginally qhs × 3 or 100-mg vaginal tablet one tablet intravaginally qhs × 7, or 1% vaginal cream intravaginally qhs × 7
- Butoconazole 2% cream one applicator intravaginally qhs × 3
- Terconazole 80-mg suppository or 0.8% vaginal cream, one suppository or one applicator intravaginally qhs × 3 or 0.4% vaginal cream, one applicator intravaginally qhs × 7
- Gynecazole-1 vaginal cream one applicator intravaginally × 1
- Tioconazole 6.5% ointment (Vagi-stat), one applicator intravaginally × 1

CHRONIC Rx (FOUR OR MORE SYMPTOMATIC EPISODES ANNUALLY)

- Resistance or recurrence
  - 14- to 21-day course of 7-day regimens mentioned in "Acute General Rx" above
  - Fluconazole 150 mg PO × 2

  - Ketoconazole 200 mg PO bid × 5 to 14 days
  - Itraconazole 200 mg PO qd × 3 days
  - Boric acid 600-mg capsule intravaginally bid × 14 days
- Prophylactic regimens
  - Clotrimazole one 500-mg vaginal tablet each month
  - Ketoconazole 200 mg PO bid × 5 days each month
  - Fluconazole 150 mg PO × 1 each month
  - Miconazole 100-mg vaginal tablet × 2 weekly

DISPOSITION

- If symptoms do not resolve completely with treatment, or if they recur within a 2- to 3-mo period, further evaluation is indicated.
- Reexamination and possibly culture are necessary.
- Positive culture in absence of symptoms should not lead to treatment. Approximately 30% of women harbor *Candida* spp. and other species in the vagina.

REFERRAL

To obstetrician/gynecologist for recurrence

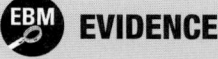 PEARLS & CONSIDERATIONS

COMMENTS

- No evidence that treating a woman's male sexual partner significantly improves woman's infection or reduces their rate of relapse.
- Many *Candida albicans* strains produce hyaluronidase, which is an enzyme that degrades hyaluronan. Elevated hyaluronan levels in vaginal secretions are associated with increased itching, burning, and discharge in women with recurrent vulvovaginal candidiasis.

EBM EVIDENCE

available at www.expertconsult.com

SUGGESTED READING

available at www.expertconsult.com

AUTHORS: **JULIE ANNE SZUMIGALA, M.D.,** and **RUBEN ALVERO, M.D.**

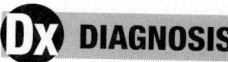

BASIC INFORMATION

DEFINITION

Prepubescent vulvovaginitis is an inflammatory condition of the vulva and vagina.

ICD-9CM CODES
616.10 Vulvovaginitis

EPIDEMIOLOGY & DEMOGRAPHICS

- Most common gynecologic problem of the premenarcheal female.
- Prepubertal girl is susceptible to irritation and trauma because of the absence of protective hair and labial fat pads and the lack of estrogenization with atrophic vaginal mucosa.
- Symptoms of vulvovaginitis and introital irritation and discharge account for 80% to 90% of gynecologic visits.
- Nonspecific etiology in approximately 75% of children with vulvovaginitis.
- Majority of vulvovaginitis in children involves a primary irritation of the vulva with secondary involvement of the lower third of the vagina.

PHYSICAL FINDINGS & CLINICAL PRESENTATION

- Vulvar pain, dysuria, pruritus
  1. Discharge is not a primary symptom.
  2. If present, vaginal discharge may be foul smelling or bloody.

ETIOLOGY

- Infections
  1. Bacterial
  2. Protozoal
  3. Mycotic
  4. Viral
- Endocrine disorders
- Labial adhesions
- Poor hygiene
- Sexual abuse
- Allergic substance
- Trauma
- Foreign body
- Masturbation
- Constipation

Section II describes the differential diagnosis of vaginal discharge in prepubertal girls.

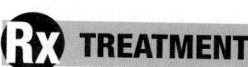

DIAGNOSIS

DIFFERENTIAL DIAGNOSIS

- Physiologic leukorrhea
- Foreign body
- Bacterial vaginosis
- Gonorrhea
- Fungal vulvovaginitis
- *Trichomonas* vulvovaginitis
- Sexual abuse
- Pinworms

WORKUP

- Pelvic, genital examination
- Speculum examination
- Rectal examination
- KOH and normal saline preparation of discharge

Section III, "Vaginal Discharge," describes the evaluation of discharge.

LABORATORY TESTS

- Urinalysis to rule out urinary tract infection and diabetes
- Cultures including sexually transmitted diseases

TREATMENT

NONPHARMACOLOGIC THERAPY

- Avoid tight clothing
- Perineal hygiene
- Avoid irritant chemicals
- Reassurance

ACUTE GENERAL Rx

- Group A beta *Streptococcus* and *Streptococcus pneumoniae:* penicillin V potassium 125 to 250 mg PO qid × 10 days
- *Chlamydia trachomatis:* erythromycin 50 mg/kg/day PO × 10 days
  ○ Children >8 yr, doxycycline 100 mg bid PO × 7 days
- *Neisseria gonorrhoeae:* ceftriaxone 125 mg IM × 1 day
  ○ Children >8 yr should also be given doxycycline 100 mg bid PO × 7 days
- *Staphylococcus aureus:* amoxicillin-clavulanate 20 to 40 mg/kg/day PO × 7 to 10 days
- *Haemophilus influenzae:* amoxicillin 20 to 40 mg/kg/day PO × 7 days
- *Trichomonas:* metronidazole 125 mg (15 mg/kg/day) tid PO × 7 to 10 days
- Pinworms: mebendazole 100-mg tablet chewable, repeat in 2 wk
- Labial agglutination: spontaneous resolution or topical estrogen cream for 7 to 10 days

CHRONIC Rx

See "Referral."

DISPOSITION

Further education:
- Young child: hygiene
- Adolescent: pregnancy prevention and safe sexual practices

REFERRAL

- To obstetrician/gynecologist
- To pediatrician

SUGGESTED READING
available at www.expertconsult.com

AUTHORS: **JULIE ANNE SZUMIGALA, M.D.,** and **RUBEN ALVERO, M.D.**

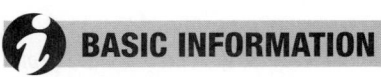

BASIC INFORMATION

DEFINITION
Trichomonas vulvovaginitis is the inflammation of vulva and vagina caused by *Trichomonas* spp.

SYNONYMS
Trichomonas vaginalis
Trichomoniasis
TV

ICD-9CM CODES
131.01 Vulvovaginitis, trichomonal

EPIDEMIOLOGY & DEMOGRAPHICS
- Acquired through sexual contact
- Diagnosed in
  - 50% to 75% of prostitutes
  - 5% to 15% of women visiting gynecology clinics
  - 7% to 32% of women in sexually transmitted disease (STD) clinics
  - 5% of women in family planning clinics

PHYSICAL FINDINGS & CLINICAL PRESENTATION
- Profuse, yellow, malodorous vaginal discharge and severe vaginal itching
- Vulvar itching
- Dysuria
- Dyspareunia
- Intense erythema of the vaginal mucosa
- Cervical petechiae ("strawberry cervix")
- Asymptomatic in ~50% of women and 90% of men

ETIOLOGY
Single-cell protozoan *Trichomonas vaginalis*

RISK FACTORS
- Multiple sexual partners
- History of previous STDs

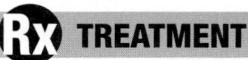

DIAGNOSIS

DIFFERENTIAL DIAGNOSIS
(Table 1-186)
- Bacterial vaginosis
- Fungal vulvovaginitis
- Cervicitis
- Atrophic vulvovaginitis

WORKUP
- Pelvic examination.
- Speculum examination.

- Mobile trichomonads seen on normal saline preparation: 70% sensitivity.
- Elevated pH (>5) of vaginal discharge.
- Culture is considered the traditional gold standard laboratory test for diagnosis of TV.
- Nucleic acid amplification tests (NAATs) have been developed that combine excellent performance characteristics with a more rapid turnaround time compared with culture; however, they are not commercially readily available.
- APTIMA assays utilize target capture and transcription-mediated amplification (TMA) to selectively purify, amplify, and detect species-specific 16 S ribosomal RNA. APTIMA *Trichomonas vaginalis* transcription-mediated amplification may be a better laboratory test than culture based on sensitivity and time frame for results.

LABORATORY TESTS
- Culture (modified Diamond media): 90% sensitivity
- Direct enzyme immunoassay
- Fluorescein-conjugated monoclonal antibody test
- Pap test 40% detected

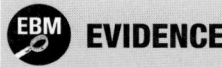

TREATMENT

NONPHARMACOLOGIC THERAPY
Condom use

ACUTE GENERAL Rx
Metronidazole 2 g PO × 1 or 500 mg PO bid × 7 days *or* Tindamax (tinidazole) single 2 g oral dose in both sexes

CHRONIC Rx
- Metronidazole gel: less likely to achieve therapeutic levels; therefore not recommended.
- Metronidazole (retreat): 500 mg PO bid × 7 days.
- Treatment of future recurrences: metronidazole 2 g PO qd × 3 to 5 days.
- Allergy, intolerance, or adverse reactions: alternatives to metronidazole are not available. Patients who are allergic to metronidazole can be managed by desensitization.
- Pregnancy:
  - Associated with adverse outcomes (i.e., premature rupture of membranes)
  - Metronidazole 2 g PO × 1 day

DISPOSITION
Trichomonas infection is considered an STD; therefore treatment of the sexual partner is necessary.

REFERRAL
To obstetrician/gynecologist for recurrence and pregnancy

EBM EVIDENCE

available at www.expertconsult.com

SUGGESTED READINGS
available at www.expertconsult.com

AUTHORS: **JULIE ANNE SZUMIGALA, M.D.,** and **RUBEN ALVERO, M.D.**

Characteristics of Vaginal Discharge	*C. Albicans* Vaginitis	*T. Vaginalis* Vaginitis	Bacterial Vaginosis
pH	4.5	>5.0	>5.0
White curd	Usually	No	No
Odor with KOH	No	Yes	Yes
Clue cells	No	No	Usually
Motile trichomonads	No	Usually	No
Yeast cells	Yes	No	No

TABLE 1-186 Differential Diagnosis of Vaginitis

From Goldman L, Ausiello D (eds): *Cecil textbook of medicine,* ed 22, Philadelphia, 2004, WB Saunders.

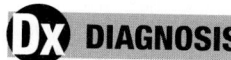

BASIC INFORMATION

DEFINITION

Waldenström's macroglobulinemia (WM) is a plasma cell dyscrasia (B-cell malignancy) characterized by lymphoplasmacytic infiltration in the bone marrow or lymphatic tissue and a monoclonal immunoglobulin M protein (IgM) in the serum.

SYNONYMS

WM
Monoclonal macroglobulinemia
Lymphoplasmacytic lymphoma

ICD-9CM CODES
273.3 Waldenström's macroglobulinemia

EPIDEMIOLOGY & DEMOGRAPHICS

- Accounts for 2% of all hematologic cancers
- 1500 people diagnosed every year in the United States
- Overall incidence: 3.4 per million person-yr in men, 1.7 per million person-yr in women
- Median age approximately 63 yr
- More common among men than women and among whites than blacks

PHYSICAL FINDINGS & CLINICAL PRESENTATION

- Weakness
- Fatigue
- Weight loss
- Pallor
- Headache, dizziness, vertigo, deafness, and seizures (hyperviscosity syndrome)
- Easy bleeding (e.g., epistaxis)
- Retinal vein link-sausage shaped
- Lymphadenopathy (15%)
- Hepatomegaly (20%)
- Most commonly encountered neurological presentation is symmetric polyneuropathy (5%)
- Splenomegaly (15%)
- Purpura
- Fever and night sweats

ETIOLOGY

- The exact cause of WM is not known.
- Multiple reports suggest familial clustering, which indicates a genetic predisposition. In one study, chromosomal deletions in 6q21–22.1 were confirmed in 42% of WM patients, regardless of family history. In another study, the strongest evidence of linkage was found on chromosomes 1q and 4q.
- The main risk factor for development of WM is having IgM monoclonal gammopathy of unknown significance (MGUS).
- Radiation exposure, occupational chemicals, viral infection, and chronic inflammatory stimulation have been suggested, but there is insufficient evidence to substantiate these hypotheses.
- There is a twofold to threefold increased risk of WM in people with a personal history of autoimmune diseases with autoantibodies, there is also increased risk with HIV, hepatitis, and rickettsiosis.

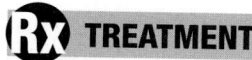

DIAGNOSIS

The diagnosis of WM is usually established by laboratory blood tests and by bone marrow biopsy.

DIFFERENTIAL DIAGNOSIS

- MGUS
- Multiple myeloma
- Chronic lymphocytic leukemia
- Hairy-cell leukemia
- Lymphoma
- Smoldering macroglobulinemia

WORKUP

In any patient suspected of having WM, specific blood tests (CBC, erythrocyte sedimentation rate [ESR], serum or urine protein electrophoresis [SPEP or UPEP, respectively], IgM level, beta 2-microglobulin, serum viscosity) should be ordered. Bone marrow biopsy confirms the diagnosis.

LABORATORY TESTS

- CBC with differential:
  - Anemia is a common finding, with a median hemoglobin value of approximately 10 g/dl. WBC count is usually normal; thrombocytopenia can occur.
  - Peripheral smear may reveal "stacked coin" rouleaux formations and malignant lymphoid cells in terminal patients.
- Elevated ESR.
- SPEP: homogeneous M spike (monoclonal gammopathy)
- Immunoelectrophoresis: confirms IgM responsible for the M spike. Table 1-187 describes physiochemical and immunological properties of the monoclonal IgM protein in Waldenström macroglobulinemia.
- Urine immunoelectrophoresis: monoclonal light chains are usually kappa chains. Bence Jones protein can be seen, but is not the typical finding in WM.
- IgM levels are high, generally >3 g/dl.
- Beta 2-microglobulin: elevated in 55%, high levels are associated with poor prognosis.
- Serum viscosity: symptoms usually occur when the serum viscosity is four times the viscosity of normal serum; classical feature although present in only 15% of cases.
- Cryoglobulins, rheumatoid factor, or cold agglutinins may be present.
- Bone marrow biopsy: lymphoplasmacytoid cells are characteristic.

IMAGING STUDIES

Chest radiograph can be obtained to rule out pulmonary involvement.

TREATMENT

- Because of the incurable nature of WM, the aim of treatment is to relieve symptoms and reduce the risk of organ damage. Patients with smoldering or asymptomatic WM and preserved hematologic function should be

TABLE 1-187 Physicochemical and Immunologic Properties of Monoclonal Immunoglobulin Protein in Waldenström's Macroglobulinemia

Properties of Monoclonal Immunoglobulin Protein	Diagnostic Condition	Clinical Manifestations
Pentameric structure	Hyperviscosity	Headaches, blurred vision, epistaxis, retinal hemorrhages, leg cramps, impaired mentation, and intracranial hemorrhage
Prescription on cooling	Cryoglobulinemia (type I)	Raynaud's phenomenon, acrocyanosis, ulcers, purpura, and cold urticaria
Autoantibody activity to myelin-associated glycoprotein, ganglioside M1, and sulfatide moieties on peripheral nerve sheaths	Peripheral neuropathies	Sensorimotor neuropathies, painful neuropathies, ataxic gait, and bilateral foot drop
Autoantibody activity to immunoglobulin G	Cryoglobulinemia (type II)	Purpura, arthralgias, renal failure, and sensorimotor neuropathies
Autoantibody activity to red blood cell antigens	Cold agglutinins	Hemolytic anemia, Raynaud's phenomenon, acrocyanosis, and livedo reticularis
Tissue deposition as amorphous aggregates	Organ dysfunction	Skin: bullous skin disease, papules, and Schnitzler syndrome Gastrointestinal: diarrhea, malabsorption, and bleeding Kidney: proteinuria and renal failure (light-chain component)
Tissue deposition as amyloid fibrils (light-chain fibrils commonly the largest component)	Organ dysfunction	Fatigue, weight loss, edema, periorbital purpura, hepatomegaly, macroglossia, and organ dysfunction of the involved organs: heart, kidney, liver, and peripheral sensory and autonomic nerves

From Hoffmann R et al: *Hematology, basic principles and practice*, ed 5, Philadelphia, 2009, Churchill Livingstone.

observed without therapy. Considerations for the initiation of treatment include the following: hemoglobin concentration less than 100 $\times$ 10^9/L, significant adenopathy or organomegaly, symptomatic hyperviscosity, severe neuropathy, amyloidosis, cryoglobulinemia, cold-agglutinin disease, or evidence of disease transformation.
- Treatment is directed at both hyperviscocity and the lymphoproliferative disorder itself.

NONPHARMACOLOGIC THERAPY

Asymptomatic patients do not require treatment, and these patients should be monitored periodically for the onset of symptoms or changes in blood tests (e.g., worsening anemia, thrombocytopenia, rising IgM, and serum viscosity).

ACUTE GENERAL Rx

- Plasmapheresis is the treatment used to alleviate symptoms of hyperviscosity.
- Treatment of the lymphoproliferative disorder includes single or combination therapy; although guidance has been suggested in the Mayo Stratification of Macroglobulinemia and Risk-Adapted Therapy (mSMART) Guidelines, there is no universally agreed upon standard of care:
  - Rituximab, a monoclonal anti-CD 20 antibody, can be used in symptomatic patients with modest hematologic compromise, IgM-related neuropathy, or hemolytic anemia unresponsive to corticosteroids.
  - Plasmapheresis should be initial treatment in patients with symptoms of hyperviscosity.
  - DRC regimen (dexamethasone, rituximab, cyclophosphamide) in patients with severe constitutional symptoms, symptomatic bulky disease, hyperviscosity, or profound hematologic compromise.

CHRONIC Rx

- Refractory patients can be retried on original therapy if length of response from initial therapy is >2 yr. If the response from the initial therapy was <2 yr, alternative first-line agents such as fludarabine or cladribine can be used.
- Other treatment options: interferon alpha, thalidomide, and autologous stem cell transplantation.

DISPOSITION

- The onset of WM is slow and insidious. Most patients die from progression of the disease with hyperviscosity, hemorrhage, and infection, or from congestive heart failure.
- Some patients develop acute myelogenous leukemia, immunoblastic sarcoma, or chronic myelogenous leukemia as a preterminal event.
- Median survival in patients with WM is about 4 to 5 yr.
- ~10% of patients will achieve complete remission, with prognosis being more favorable (median survival 11 yr).

- A staging system using serum beta 2-microglobulin concentration, hemoglobin concentration, and serum IgM concentration before treatment provides insight into prognosis and survival.
- Other factors can negatively affect the survival: age >65, male gender, the presence of organomegaly and the presence of cytopenias.

REFERRAL

If WM is suspected, a hematology consultation is helpful in guiding future workup, treatment, and monitoring. Autologous stem cell transplant should be considered in all eligible patients with relapsed disease

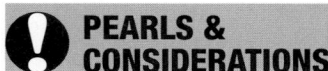

PEARLS & CONSIDERATIONS

COMMENTS

- WM was first described in 1944 by the Swedish physician Jan Gosta Waldenström.
- Amyloidosis is rare, occurring in 5% of patients with WM.

SUGGESTED READINGS

available at www.expertconsult.com

AUTHOR: **MARK F. BRADY, M.D., M.P.H., M.M.S.**

BASIC INFORMATION

DEFINITION

Warts are benign epidermal lesions caused by human papillomavirus (HPV).

SYNONYMS

Verruca vulgaris (common warts)
Verruca plana (flat warts)
Condyloma acuminatum (venereal warts)
Verruca plantaris (plantar warts)
Mosaic warts (cluster of many warts)

ICD-9CM CODES
078.10 Viral warts
078.19 Venereal wart (external genital organs)

EPIDEMIOLOGY & DEMOGRAPHICS

- Risk factors include use of communal showers, occupational handling of meat, and immunosuppression. Common warts occur most frequently in children and young adults.
- Anogenital warts are most common in young, sexually active patients. Genital warts are the most common viral sexually transmitted disease in the United States, with up to 24 million Americans carrying the causative virus.
- Common warts are longer lasting and more frequent in immunocompromised patients (e.g., lymphoma, AIDS, immunosuppressive drugs).
- Plantar warts occur most frequently at points of maximal pressure (over the heads of the metatarsal bones or on the heels).

PHYSICAL FINDINGS & CLINICAL PRESENTATION

- Common warts (Fig. 1-410) have an initial appearance of a flesh-colored papule with a rough surface; they subsequently develop a hyperkeratotic appearance with black dots on the surface (thrombosed capillaries). They may be single or multiple and are most common on the hands.
- Warts obscure normal skin lines (important diagnostic feature). Cylindrical projections from the wart may become fused, forming a mosaic pattern.
- Flat warts generally are pink or light yellow, slightly elevated, and often found on the forehead, back of hands, mouth, and beard area. They often occur in lines corresponding to trauma (e.g., a scratch), are often misdiagnosed (particularly when present on the face), and inappropriately treated with topical corticosteroids.
- Filiform warts have a fingerlike appearance with various projections; they are generally found near the mouth, beard, or periorbital and paranasal regions.
- Plantar warts are slightly raised and have a roughened surface; they may cause pain when walking; as they involute, small hemorrhages (caused by thrombosed capillaries) may be noted.
- Genital warts are generally pale pink with several projections and a broad base. They may coalesce in the perineal area to form masses with a cauliflower-like appearance.
- Genital warts on the cervical epithelium can produce subclinical changes that may be noted on Pap smear or colposcopy.

ETIOLOGY

- HPV infection; >60 types of viral DNA have been identified. Transmission of warts is by direct contact.
- Genital warts 90% are caused by HPV types 6 or 11. HPV types 16, 18, 31, 33, and 35 are found occasionally in visible genital warts (usually as coinfections with HPV 6 or 11) and can be associated with foci of high-grade, intraepithelial neoplasia, particularly in persons who are infected with HIV infection. In addition to warts on genital areas, HPV types 6 and 11 have been associated with conjunctival, nasal, oral, and laryngeal warts.

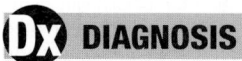

DIAGNOSIS

DIFFERENTIAL DIAGNOSIS

- *Molluscum contagiosum*
- *Condyloma latum*
- Acrochordon (skin tags) or seborrheic keratosis
- Epidermal nevi
- Hypertrophic actinic keratosis
- Squamous cell carcinomas
- Acquired digital fibrokeratoma
- Varicella zoster virus in patients with AIDS
- Recurrent infantile digital fibroma
- Plantar corns (may be mistaken for plantar warts)

WORKUP

- Diagnosis is generally based on clinical findings.
- Suspect lesions should be biopsied.
- The application of 3% to 5% acetic acid, which causes skin color to turn white, has been used by some providers to detect HPV-infected genital mucosa. However, acetic acid application is not a specific test for HPV infection. Therefore, the routine use of this procedure for screening to detect mucosal changes attributed to HPV infection is not recommended.

LABORATORY TESTS

Colposcopy with biopsy of patients with cervical squamous cell changes

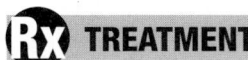

TREATMENT

NONPHARMACOLOGIC THERAPY

- Importance of use of condoms to reduce transmission of genital warts should be emphasized.
- Watchful waiting is an acceptable option in the treatment of warts because many warts will disappear without intervention over time.
- Plantar warts that are not painful do not need treatment.
- Factors that influence selection of treatment include wart size, wart number, anatomic site of the wart, wart morphology, patient preference, cost of treatment, convenience, adverse effects, and provider experience. Factors that might affect response to therapy include the presence of immunosuppression and compliance with therapy.

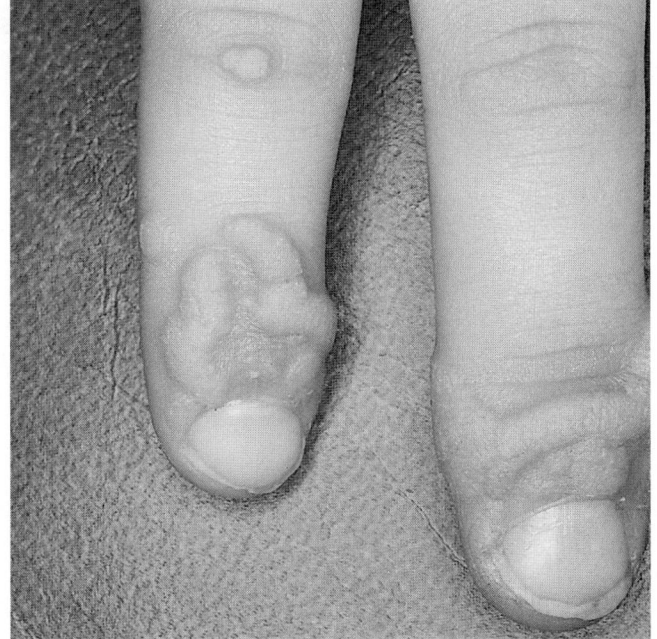

FIGURE 1-410 Verruca vulgaris, or common viral warts. These papules often have verrucous surface changes. (From Callen JP: *Color atlas of dermatology,* ed 2, Philadelphia, 2000, WB Saunders.)

GENERAL Rx

- Common warts:
  - Application of topical salicylic acid 17%. Soak area for 5 min in warm water and dry. Apply thin layer once or twice daily for up to 12 wk, avoiding normal skin. Bandage.
  - Liquid nitrogen and electrocautery are also common methods of removal.
  - Blunt dissection can be used in large lesions or resistant lesions.
  - Duct tape occlusion is also effective for treating common warts. It is cut to cover warts and left in place for 6 days. It is removed after 6 days and the warts are soaked in water and then filed with pumice stones. New tape is applied 12 hr later. This treatment can be repeated until warts resolve.
- Filiform warts: surgical removal is necessary.
- Flat warts: generally more difficult to treat.
  - Tretinoin cream applied at bedtime over the involved area for several weeks may be effective.
  - Application of liquid nitrogen.
  - Electrocautery.
  - 5-Fluorouracil cream applied once or twice a day for 3 to 5 wk is also effective. Persistent hyperpigmentation may occur after Efudex use.
- Plantar warts:
  - Salicylic acid therapy (e.g., Occlusal-HP). Soak wart in warm water for 5 min, remove loose tissue, dry. Apply to area, allow to dry, reapply. Use once or twice daily; maximum 12 wk. Use of 40% salicylic acid plasters (Mediplast) is also a safe, nonscarring treatment; it is particularly useful in treating mosaic warts covering a large area.
  - Blunt dissection is also a fast and effective treatment modality.
  - Laser therapy can be used for plantar warts and recurrent warts; however, it leaves open wounds that require 4 to 6 wk to fill with granulation tissue.

- Interlesional bleomycin is also effective but generally used when all other treatments fail.
- Genital warts:
  - Can be effectively treated with 20% podophyllin resin in compound tincture of benzoin applied with a cotton tip applicator by the treating physician and allowed to air dry. The treatment can be repeated weekly if necessary.
  - Podofilox (Condylox 0.5% gel) is available for application by the patient. Local adverse effects include pain, burning, and inflammation at the site.
  - Cryosurgery with liquid nitrogen delivered with a probe or as a spray is effective for treating smaller genital warts.
  - Carbon dioxide laser can also be used for treating primary or recurrent genital warts (cure rate >90%).
  - Imiquimod cream, 5%, is a patient-applied immune response modifier effective in the treatment of external genital and perianal warts (complete clearing of genital warts in >70% of females and >30% of males in 4 to 16 wk). Sexual contact should be avoided while the cream is on the skin. It is applied 3 times per week before normal sleeping hours and is left on the skin for 6 to 10 hr.
  - Sinecatechins (Veregen), a botanical drug product, is also effective for treatment of external genital and perianal warts. Formulation is a 15% ointment applied to affected area tid for up to 16 wk.
- Application of trichloroacetic acid or bichloroacetic acid 80% to 90% is also effective for external genital warts. A small amount should be applied only to warts and allowed to dry, at which time a white "frosting" develops. This treatment can be repeated weekly if necessary.

DISPOSITION

- Warts can be effectively treated with the previous modalities with complete resolution in the majority of patients; however, the recurrence rate is high.
- Cervical carcinomas and precancerous lesions in women are associated with genital papillomavirus infection.
- Squamous cell anal cancer is also associated with a history of genital warts.

REFERRAL

- Dermatology referral for warts resistant to conservative therapy
- Surgical referral in selected cases
- Sexually transmitted disease counseling for patients with anogenital warts

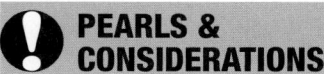

PEARLS & CONSIDERATIONS

COMMENTS

- Subungual and periungual warts are generally more resistant to treatment. Dermatology referral for cryosurgery is recommended in resistant cases.
- Examination of sex partners is not necessary for the management of genital warts because no data indicate that reinfection plays a role.
- Sexually transmitted HPV infections contribute to nearly 20,000 cases of invasive cancer in the U.S. affecting cervix, anus, vagina, penis, and oral cavity. HPV vaccination is available for females aged 11 to 26 and males aged 9 to 26.

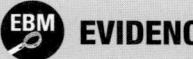 **EVIDENCE**

available at www.expertconsult.com

SUGGESTED READINGS
available at www.expertconsult.com

AUTHOR: **FRED F. FERRI, M.D.**

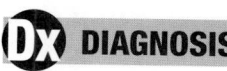

BASIC INFORMATION

DEFINITION

Wegener granulomatosis is a multisystem disease generally consisting of the classic triad of:
1. Necrotizing granulomatous lesions in the upper or lower respiratory tract
2. Generalized focal necrotizing vasculitis involving both arteries and veins
3. Focal glomerulonephritis of the kidneys
   "Limited forms" of the disease can also occur and may evolve into the classic triad; Wegener granulomatosis can be classified using the "ELK" classification, which identifies the three major sites of involvement: *E*, ears, nose, and throat or respiratory tract; *L*, lungs; *K*, kidneys.

ICD-9CM CODES
446.4 Wegener's granulomatosis

EPIDEMIOLOGY & DEMOGRAPHICS

INCIDENCE: 3/100,000 persons, equal in men and women
MEAN AGE AT ONSET: 41 yr

PHYSICAL FINDINGS & CLINICAL PRESENTATION

- Clinical manifestations often vary with the stage of the disease and degree of organ involvement. 90% of patients present with symptoms involving the upper or lower airways or both.
- Frequent manifestations are:
  1. Upper respiratory tract: chronic sinusitis, chronic otitis media, mastoiditis, nasal crusting, obstruction and epistaxis, nasal septal perforation, nasal lacrimal duct stenosis, saddle nose deformities (resulting from cartilage destruction)
  2. Lung: hemoptysis, multiple nodules, diffuse alveolar pattern
  3. Kidney: renal insufficiency, glomerulonephritis
  4. Skin: necrotizing skin lesions
  5. Nervous system: mononeuritis multiplex, cranial nerve involvement
  6. Joints: monarthritis or polyarthritis (nondeforming), usually affecting large joints
  7. Mouth: chronic ulcerative lesions of the oral mucosa, "mulberry" gingivitis
  8. Eye: proptosis, uveitis, episcleritis, retinal and optic nerve vasculitis

ETIOLOGY
Unknown

DIAGNOSIS

DIFFERENTIAL DIAGNOSIS

- Other granulomatous lung diseases (e.g., sarcoidosis, lymphomatoid granulomatosis, Churg-Strauss syndrome, necrotizing sarcoid granulomatosis, bronchocentric granulomatosis, sarcoidosis); the differential diagnosis of granulomatous lung disease is described in Section II
- Neoplasms (especially lymphoproliferative disease)
- Goodpasture's syndrome
- Bacterial or fungal sinusitis
- Midline granuloma
- Viral infections
- Other causes of glomerulonephritis (e.g., poststreptococcal nephritis)

WORKUP

- Wegener granulomatosis should be suspected in anyone presenting with sinus disease that does not respond to conventional treatment, pulmonary hemorrhage, glomerulonephritis, mononeuritis multiplex resulting in wrist or foot drop, progressive migratory arthralgias or arthritis, and unexplained multisystem disease.
- Chest x-ray, laboratory evaluation, PFTs, and tissue biopsy.

LABORATORY TESTS

- Positive test for cytoplasmic pattern of ANCA (c-ANCA).
- Anemia, leukocytosis.
- Urinalysis: may reveal hematuria, RBC casts, and proteinuria.
- Elevated serum creatinine, decreased creatinine clearance.
- Increased ESR, positive rheumatoid factor, and elevated C-reactive protein may be found.

IMAGING STUDIES

- Chest x-ray: may reveal bilateral multiple nodules, cavitated mass lesions, pleural effusion (20%). Up to one third of patients without pulmonary signs or symptoms have an abnormal chest x-ray (Fig. 1-411).
- PFTs: useful in detecting stenosis of the airways.
- Biopsy of one or more affected organs should be attempted; the most reliable source for tissue diagnosis is the lung. Lesions in the nasopharynx (if present) can be easily biopsied but biopsy is positive in only 20%. Biopsy of radiographically abnormal pulmonary parenchyma provides the highest yield (>90%).

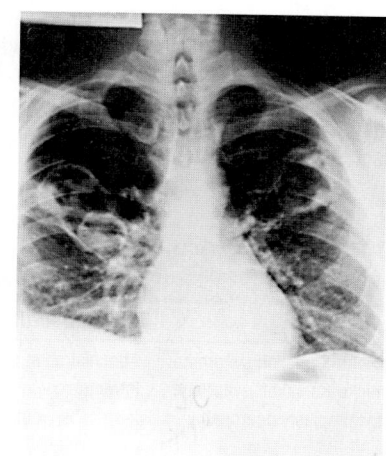

FIGURE 1-411 Chest radiograph shows multiple cavitary pulmonary nodules in patient with Wegener granulomatosis. (From Weinberg SE et al: *Principles of pulmonary medicine*, ed 5, Philadelphia, 2008, Saunders.)

TREATMENT

NONPHARMACOLOGIC THERAPY

- Ensure proper airway drainage.
- Give nutritional counseling.

ACUTE GENERAL Rx

- Prednisone 60 to 80 mg/day and cyclophosphamide 2 mg/kg are generally effective and are used to control clinical manifestations; once the disease comes under control, prednisone is tapered and cyclophosphamide is continued. Other potentially useful agents in patients intolerant to cyclophosphamide are rituximab, methotrexate, azathioprine, and mycophenolate mofetil. Recent trials involving rituximab show that it is not inferior to daily cyclophosphamide treatment for induction of remission in severe ANCA-associated vasculitis and may be superior in relapsing disease.
- TMP-SMX therapy may represent a useful alternative in patients with lesions limited to the upper or lower respiratory tracts in absence of vasculitis or nephritis. Treatment with TMP-SMX (160 mg/800 mg bid) also reduces the incidence of relapses in patients with Wegener granulomatosis in remission. It is also useful in preventing *Pneumocystis jirovecii* pneumonia, which occurs in 10% of patients receiving induction therapy. When used for prophylaxis, dose of TMP-SMX (160 mg/800 mg) is 1 tablet three times/wk.

DISPOSITION

Five-year survival with aggressive treatment is approximately 80%; without treatment 2-yr survival is <20%.

REFERRAL

Surgical referral for biopsy

PEARLS & CONSIDERATIONS

COMMENTS

- Methotrexate (20 mg/wk) represents an alternative to cyclophosphamide in patients who do not have immediately life-threatening disease.
- C-ANCA levels should not dictate changes in therapy, because they correlate erratically with disease activity.
- The incidence of venous thrombotic events in Wegener granulomatosis is significantly higher than the general population. Clinicians should maintain a heightened awareness of the risks of venous thrombosis and a lower threshold for evaluating patients for possible DVT or pulmonary embolism.

EVIDENCE

available at www.expertconsult.com

SUGGESTED READINGS
available at www.expertconsult.com

AUTHOR: **FRED F. FERRI, M.D.**

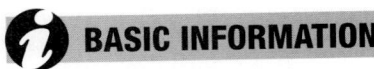

BASIC INFORMATION

DEFINITION

An acute neuropsychiatric disorder characterized by the classic triad of ophthalmoplegia, ataxia, and disturbances of mental activity or consciousness due to a deficiency of thiamine often associated with chronic alcoholism.

SYNONYMS

Wernicke encephalopathy (WE)
Gayet-Wernicke encephalopathy
Cerebral beriberi
Wernicke's superior hemorrhagic polioencephalitis

ICD-9CM CODES

265.1 Wernicke's encephalopathy, disease, or syndrome (superior hemorrhagic polioencephalitis)
294.0 Wernicke-Korsakoff's syndrome or psychosis, non-alcoholic
291.1 Wernicke-Korsakoff's syndrome or psychosis, alcoholic

EPIDEMIOLOGY & DEMOGRAPHICS

PREVALENCE:
- Higher prevalence of WE based on lesions from autopsy (0.8% to 2.8%) than predicted by clinical studies (0.04% to 0.13%) in the general population
- WE lesions on autopsy of alcoholic abusers: 12.5%
- Alcohol-related deaths with WE lesions on autopsy estimated to 29% to 59%
- WE lesions confirmed on autopsy of alcoholics and AIDS patients missed by clinical examination: 75% to 80%
- WE lesions confirmed on autopsy of children missed by clinical examination: 58%

PREDOMINANT SEX AND AGE:
- Male-to-female ratio of 1.7 to 1
- Estimated mortality: 17%

GENETICS:
- Thiamine-dependent enzyme, transketolase, has been shown by biochemical studies with fibroblasts from patients with WE to have a decrease affinity for thiamine pyrophosphate.
- Wet (cardiovascular) beriberi is more commonly seen in the Asian population compared to Dry beriberi with polyneuropathy and WE seen in the European population.

RISK FACTORS:
- Alcohol abuse/misuse
- Diet
  - Malnutrition/unbalanced nutrition/infant formulas
  - Intravenous hyperalimentation without thiamine supplementation
  - Magnesium depletion—cofactor required by enzymes: transketolase and thiamine pyrophospokinase
- Gastrointestinal disorders including recurrent vomiting or chronic diarrhea
  - Hyperemesis gravidarum

- Gastrointestinal surgical procedures (excluding portions of the gastrointestinal tract)
  - Bariatric surgery in young woman with vomiting: 4 to 12 wk postoperatively
  - Poor digestion with consequent malabsorption secondary to reduced surface area of gastric and duodenal mucosa
- Systemic cancers
  - Most common underlying disorder onset for WE in children
  - Consumption of thiamine by fast-growing neoplastic cells
- Chemical compounds/drugs or chemotherapeutic treatments
- Systemic diseases
  - Peritoneal or hemodialysis
  - HIV/AIDS
  - Prolonged infectious febrile disease
  - Hypermetabolic states
  - Thyrotoxicosis

PHYSICAL FINDINGS & CLINICAL PRESENTATION

- WE remains a clinical diagnosis in the setting of the classic triad of ophthalmoplegia, ataxia, and disturbances of mental activity or consciousness – although this triad is only seen in 16% of all patients.
- Eye movement abnormalities: nystagmus, external rectus palsies, and reduced conjugate gaze.
- Fundoscopic findings: swelling of the optic disks and retinal hemorrhages.
- Clinical suspicion must remain high in patients with those risk factors listed above, especially in the setting of poor nutrition.
- Confirmed by response of neurologic signs after the administration of parenteral thiamine.
- Aided by labs and other paraclinical studies, although labs should not postpone a trial of parenteral administration of thiamine.

ETIOLOGY

- The biologically active form of vitamin B_1 or thiamine, thiamine pyrophosphate (TP), a coenzyme for several important biochemical pathways, such as energy production, lipid metabolism, and production of amino acids and glucose-derived neurotransmitters.

- Body's reserve for thiamine is sufficient for 18 days.
- Malnutrition for 2 to 3 wk or a diet disproportionately high in carbohydrates and low in thiamine intake can lead to an impaired function of enzymes requiring TP.

DIAGNOSIS

DIFFERENTIAL DIAGNOSIS

- Other acute encephalopathies (see Table 1-188)
- Paramedian thalamic infarction
- Ventriculoencephalitis, paraneoplastic encephalitis, herpes simplex encephalitis
- Miller-Fisher syndrome
- Primary cerebral lymphoma
- Multiple sclerosis, Behcet's disease, Leigh's disease
- Variant Creutzfeldt-Jakob disease

WORKUP

- Lumbar puncture: cerebrospinal fluid (CSF) may have elevated protein.
- Electroencephalogram: may show only nonspecific diffuse slowing in the late stages of WE.

LABORATORY TEST(S)

- Blood thiamine concentration.
- Functional measurement of erythrocyte thiamine transketolase (ETKA) before and after administration of parenteral thiamine. A diagnosis may be confirmed if ETKA is low followed by a 25% increase after thiamine supplementation.
- High-performance liquid chromatography method for assessment of thiamine, thiamine mono- and di-phosphate in human erythrocytes.
- Serum magnesium (depletion).

IMAGING STUDIES

- MRI is most valuable tool in diagnosis.
- Bilaterally, symmetrical increase in T2 signal at the paraventricular regions of the thalamus and mammillary bodies. Other areas include hypothalamus, periaqueductal region, floor of the fourth ventricle, and midline cerebellum.

TABLE 1-188 Acute and Subacute Presentation of Nutritional Deficiency Syndromes

Syndrome	Clinical Setting
Wernicke-Korsakoff syndrome	Administration of intravenous glucose to a thiamine-deficient alcoholic patient
Wernicke-Korsakoff syndrome	Intractable vomiting due to hyperemesis gravidarum or gastroplasty
Postgastroplasty neuropathy	Intractable vomiting and severe weight loss in patients following weight reduction surgical procedures
Vitamin B_{12} myeloneuropathy	Nitrous oxide administration in cobalamin-deficient patients
Central pontine myelinolysis	Sudden change in tissue osmolarity in critically ill patients or alcoholics

From Goetz CG, Pappert EJ: *Textbook of clinical neurology*, Philadelphia, 1999, Saunders.

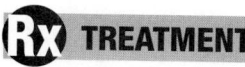

TREATMENT

ACUTE GENERAL Rx

- Alcoholics with WE: treat with 500 mg of thiamine hydrochloride (dissolved in 100 ml of normal saline) infused intravenously over 30 min, 3 times daily for 2 to 3 days.
- If a response is observed, continue with 250 mg of thiamine hydrochloride intravenously or intramuscular daily until clinical improvement ceases.
- Nonalcoholics with WE: treat with 200 mg of thiamine hydrochloride (dissolved in 100 ml of normal saline) infused intravenously over 30 min, 3 times daily for 2 to 3 days.
- Parenteral side effects may include generalized pruritis, transient local irritation, or rarely, anaphylactic or anaphylactoid reactions.
- Parenteral magnesium: infused concurrently with thiamine.

CHRONIC Rx

Recommended oral dose after treatment for WE: thiamine 30 to 100 mg twice daily

DISPOSITION

- If prompt treatment with thiamine is not administered during the potential reversible stages of WE, Korsakoff's syndrome may develop consisting of a typical pattern of memory loss emerging after the acute global confusional state of WE resolves.
- Approximately 80% who survive with WE develop Korsakoff's syndrome.

REFERRAL

In cases of altered mental status, ophthalmoplegia or ataxia or gait, consider neurology consultation. However, if WE is even suspected, do not delay treatment for consultation.

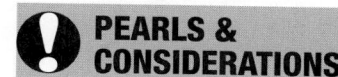

PEARLS & CONSIDERATIONS

COMMENTS

Pathologic features include periventricular petechial hemorrhages and neuropil breakdown in the diencephalon and brainstem.

PREVENTION

- Prophylactic treatment for patient with severe alcohol withdrawal, poorly nourished, or signs of malnutrition: thiamine 250 mg intramuscular daily for 3 to 5 days.
- In individuals susceptible to WE, 100 mg of intravenous thiamine should precede any glucose infusion.
- Recommended daily dose of thiamine for an average, healthy adult: 1.4 mg or 0.5 mg per 1000 kcal of carbohydrates consumed.
- Higher dose recommended for children, critically ill conditions, and during pregnancy and lactation.

PATIENT/FAMILY EDUCATION

In cases of known alcohol abuse or severe illness, the patient and family should be counseled on the importance of proper nutrition including vitamin supplementation.

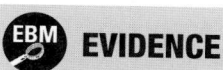

EVIDENCE

available at www.expertconsult.com

SUGGESTED READINGS

available at www.expertconsult.com

AUTHOR: **D. BRANDON BURTIS, D.O.**

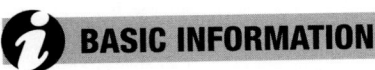

BASIC INFORMATION

DEFINITION
West Nile virus (WNV) infection is an illness affecting the CNS, caused by the mosquito-borne WNV.

SYNONYMS
West Nile virus fever
West Nile virus encephalitis
Neuroinvasive West Nile virus infection
Nonneuroinvasive West Nile virus infection

ICD-9CM CODES
066.4 West Nile virus infection

EPIDEMIOLOGY & DEMOGRAPHICS
- Before 1999, WNV infection was confined to areas in the Middle East, with occasional outbreaks in Europe. The infection began being diagnosed in the Western hemisphere in 1999. First seen in the northeast and mid-Atlantic states, WNV virus infection has spread steadily each year to new regions of the U.S., with a general westward migration pattern. In 2003, a record number of cases were reported from the U.S., with over 7000 cases reported, resulting in several hundred deaths. Most deaths occur in elderly patients with WNV encephalitis. In 2003, Illinois, Ohio, Michigan, and Louisiana were hardest hit. Since 2004 the incidence of WNV infection diminished gradually as it spread to the western states. Human cases of WNV infection have now been reported across all the contiguous continental U.S. (sparing only Hawaii and Alaska). A total of 720 neuroinvasive and non-neuroinvasive cases, with 33 deaths from WNV, were reported in the U.S. in 2009.
- The virus is carried by a number of species of birds, as well as horses and several other animals. It is transmitted to humans through the bite of an infected mosquito. For this reason, WNV infection is seen primarily from mid-summer to mid-autumn, the period of maximum mosquito intensity.
- The majority of severe cases have been reported among individuals >50 yr of age. There is no gender predilection.
- Person-to-person transmission is fortunately rare but has been reported to occur by blood transfusion, organ transplantation, breast-feeding, and perhaps by perinatal transmission; the blood supply is now routinely tested by nucleic acid testing methods to reduce the risk of transmission-acquired WNV in the U.S.

PHYSICAL FINDINGS & CLINICAL PRESENTATION
- Less than 20% of infected individuals develop symptomatic disease. The initial phase of illness is nonspecific, with abrupt onset of fever accompanied by malaise, eye pain, anorexia, headache, and, occasionally, rash and lymphadenopathy. Less commonly, myocarditis, hepatitis, or pancreatitis may occur.
- In approximately 1 in 150 cases, especially among elderly patients, severe neurologic sequelae will occur. Most common among these are ataxia, cranial nerve palsies, optic neuritis, seizures, myelitis, and polyradiculitis.

ETIOLOGY
The WNV is a member of the flavivirus group, along with the yellow fever, dengue, St Louis, and Japanese encephalitis viruses. It has a large reservoir in nature, infecting many species of birds, as well as certain mammals, and is thought to be spread to humans exclusively by various species of mosquito. Neurologic disease is caused by direct invasion of the CNS.

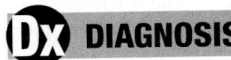

DIAGNOSIS

DIFFERENTIAL DIAGNOSIS
- Meningitis or encephalitis caused by more common viruses (e.g., enteroviruses, herpes simplex)
- Bacterial meningitis
- Vasculitis
- Fungal meningitis (e.g., cryptococcal infection)
- Tuberculous meningitis

LABORATORY TESTS
- CBC, electrolytes (hyponatremia common)
- Spinal tap and CSF examination: typically demonstrates lymphocytic pleocytosis with normal level of glucose and elevated level of protein
- CSF WNV IgM antibody level: rare false-positive results in people recently vaccinated against Japanese encephalitis or yellow fever viruses

IMAGING STUDIES
CT or MRI studies of the brain to exclude mass lesions and cerebral edema

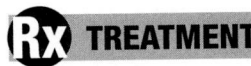

TREATMENT

NONPHARMACOLOGIC THERAPY
Hospitalization, IV hydration, ventilator support may be necessary.

ACUTE GENERAL Rx
No specific therapy has been established in clinical trials. Ribavirin and interferon alfa-2b have been shown to have in vitro activity against the virus. IV immunoglobulin (IVIG) from convalescent patient plasma is under study but no controlled trials have been reported as yet.

CHRONIC Rx
Chronic rehabilitation therapy usually necessary for patients with severe neurologic impairment. Mental status defects following WNV neuroinvasive disease appear to be more common and severe than initially recognized.

DISPOSITION
Chronic rehabilitation as needed following recovery from acute infection. Physical and mental outcome measures seem to normalize within approximately 1 yr in patients with WNV. The presence of preexisting comorbid conditions is associated with longer recovery.

REFERRAL
- Infectious disease consultant
- Public health authorities

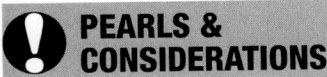

PEARLS & CONSIDERATIONS

COMMENTS
- Diagnosis requires a high index of suspicion, because disease course may be nonspecific and may mimic other, more common disorders.
- Specific laboratory diagnostic studies are available only through public-health laboratories.
- Best means of prevention is reduction in mosquito population by draining of stagnant water deposits and, if necessary, insecticide spraying.
- Individuals may reduce risk by covering arms and legs in areas where mosquitoes are likely to be found and using insect repellent containing DEET.

SUGGESTED READINGS
available at www.expertconsult.com

AUTHOR: **STEVEN M. OPAL, M.D.**

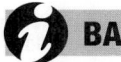 **BASIC INFORMATION**

DEFINITION

Whiplash refers to a hyperextension injury to the neck, often the result of being struck from behind by a fast-moving vehicle.

SYNONYMS

Acceleration flexion-extension neck injury

ICD-9CM CODES
847.0 Whiplash injury or syndrome

EPIDEMIOLOGY & DEMOGRAPHICS

- Whiplash occurs in more than 1 million people each year.
- Most injuries (40%) are the result of rear-end motor vehicle accidents.
- Whiplash occurs at all ages, in both sexes, and at all socioeconomic levels.
- Incidence is 4 per 1000 persons and is higher in women than men.
- Nearly 50% of patients with whiplash seek legal advice.
- Whiplash is also seen in shaken baby syndrome.

PHYSICAL FINDINGS & CLINICAL PRESENTATION

- Most present with a history of being involved in a motor vehicle accident and being rear-ended by another vehicle
- Pain not present initially but usually develops hr to a few days later
- Neck tightness and stiffness
- Occipital headache
- Shoulder, arm, and back pain
- Numbness in the arms
- Tinnitus
- Temporomandibular jaw (TMJ) pain
- Dysphagia (retropharyngeal hematoma)
- Decreased range of motion of the neck
- Depressive symptoms

ETIOLOGY

- The mechanism of injury is the result of the sudden acceleration of the body forward, forcing the neck to hyperextend backward, causing injury to ligaments, muscles, bone, and/or intervertebral disk. At the end of the accident the head is thrust forward in a flexion position, sometimes causing injury to the cervical spine: C5-C6-C7.
- Motor vehicle accidents, trauma from falls, contact sports, physical abuse, and altercations are all possible causes of whiplash.
- The incidence of whiplash injury following polytrauma is low.
- Low-velocity crashes constitute a major cause of whiplash injury.

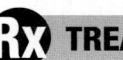 **DIAGNOSIS**

DIFFERENTIAL DIAGNOSIS

- Osteoarthritis
- Cervical disk disease
- Fibrositis
- Neuritis
- Torticollis
- Spinal cord tumor
- TMJ syndrome
- Tension headache
- Migraine headache

WORKUP

Any patient who presents with symptoms of whiplash and musculoskeletal or neurologic signs merits a workup to exclude cervical spine fractures or herniated disk disease.

LABORATORY TESTS

Laboratory studies are not helpful.

IMAGING STUDIES

- Plain C-spine films (antero-posterior, lateral, and odontoid views)
- Flexion/extension x-rays
- CT scan to exclude fracture
- MRI as alternative or in addition to CT in selected cases

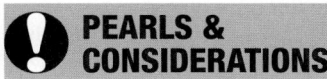 **TREATMENT**

NONPHARMACOLOGIC THERAPY

- Soft cervical collar for no longer than 72 hr
- Moist heat 15 to 20 min four to six times per day.
- Continue with usual activities.

TABLE 1-189 Factors Associated with Persistent and Severe Whiplash Injuries
Severe Whiplash Injury
High-speed injury
Intense and rapid onset of pain
Severe restriction of movement at presentation
Abnormal neurology
Bony injuries
Persistent Whiplash Injury
High-speed injury
Intense and rapid onset of pain
Severe restriction of movement at presentation
Abnormal neurology
Bony injuries
Increasing age
Upper limb paraesthesiae
Cervical spondylosis

Carr A, Hamilton W: *Orthopedics in primary care,* ed 2, Philadelphia, 2005, Elsevier.

ACUTE GENERAL Rx

- Analgesics
  1. Ibuprofen 800 mg PO tid
  2. Naproxen 500 mg PO bid
  3. Acetaminophen 1 g PO qid
- Muscle relaxants (short-term use)
  1. Cyclobenzaprine 10 mg PO tid
  2. Methocarbamol 1 g PO qid
  3. Carisoprodol 350 mg PO qid

CHRONIC Rx

NSAIDs can be used long term.

DISPOSITION

- Most patients recover from the acute whiplash injury within weeks.
- Factors associated with persistent and severe whiplash injuries are described in Table 1-189.
- 20% to 40% may develop chronic whiplash syndrome (symptoms of headache, neck pain, and psychiatric complaints that persist for 6 mo).
- Older age, female gender, lawyer involvement, and at work at entry to the clinic were found to be prognostic factors associated with a negative outcome.

REFERRAL

Orthopedic

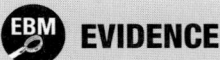 **PEARLS & CONSIDERATIONS**

- Nearly one third of all personal injury cases involve cervical injuries.
- There is no dose-response relationship between trauma severity and incidence of whiplash injury.

COMMENTS

The entity of chronic whiplash syndrome remains elusive. Some authorities argue that financial motivation is a factor leading to persistent neck symptoms. Other studies do not substantiate this, showing a true chronic injury to the soft tissues of the neck.

EBM **EVIDENCE**

available at www.expertconsult.com

SUGGESTED READINGS
available at www.expertconsult.com

AUTHOR: **JORGE A. VILLAFUERTE, M.D.**

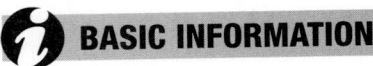

BASIC INFORMATION

DEFINITION

Whipple's disease is a multisystem illness characterized by malabsorption and its consequences, lymphadenopathy, arthritis, cardiac involvement, ocular symptoms, and neurologic problems; it is caused by the gram-positive bacillus *Tropheryma whippelii.*

SYNONYMS

Intestinal lipodystrophy (name used by Whipple in 1907)

ICD-9CM CODES
040.2 Whipple's disease

EPIDEMIOLOGY & DEMOGRAPHICS

- Uncommon illness (only about 1000 cases have been reported to date)
- Peak age: 30 to 60 yr; mean age at diagnosis 50 yr
- More frequent in men than women and in Caucasians
- Specific environmental factors have not been associated with Whipple's disease

PHYSICAL FINDINGS & CLINICAL PRESENTATION

PHYSICAL FINDINGS:
- Abdominal distention, sometimes with tenderness and less commonly fullness or mass, which represents enlarged mesenteric lymph nodes
- Signs of weight loss, cachexia
- Clubbing
- Lymphadenopathy
- Inflamed joints
- Heart murmur or rub
- Sensory loss or motor weakness related to peripheral neuropathy
- Abnormal mental status examination
- Pallor

CLINICAL PRESENTATION: Whipple's disease is characterized by two stages: a prodromal stage and a much later steady-state stage. The prodromal stage is marked by protean symptoms and chronic arthralgias and arthritis. The steady-state stage, which follows the prodromal stage by an average time of 6 yr, is manifested by weight loss, diarrhea, or both. When the disease presents with extraintestinal symptoms (e.g., arthralgia), few clinicians will suspect the diagnosis unless or until gastrointestinal (GI) symptoms are present. Weight loss, diarrhea, and arthropathies are found together in 75% of patients at time of diagnosis. The GI manifestations are those seen in malabsorption of any cause:
- Diarrhea: five to 10 semiformed, malodorous steatorrheic stools per day
- Abdominal bloating and cramps
- Anorexia

Extraintestinal manifestations of malabsorption:
- Weight loss, fatigue
- Anemia
- Bleeding diathesis
- Edema and ascites
- Osteomalacia

Extraintestinal involvement:
- Arthritis (intermittent, migratory; affecting small, large, and axial joints)
- Pleuritic chest pain and cough
- Pericarditis, endocarditis
- Dementia, ophthalmoplegia, myoclonus, and many other symptoms because any portion of the central nervous system may be a disease site
- Fever

ETIOLOGY & PATHOGENESIS

- Infectious disease caused by *Tropheryma whippelii,* an actinobacter.
- The bacillus has never been cultured, nor has direct transmission from patient to patient ever been documented; however, the agent can be seen in tissue samples by electron microscopy and identified by polymerase chain reaction (PCR).
- Predictable response to appropriate antibiotic therapy confirms the pathogenic role of the infection.
- Tissue infiltration by macrophages is believed to be the mechanism of specific organ dysfunction and symptoms.
- Subtle defects of the cell-mediated immunity exist in active and inactive Whipple's disease that may predispose certain individuals to clinical manifestations. HLA-B27 positivity is found in 26% of patients (four times higher than expected).

DIAGNOSIS

DIFFERENTIAL DIAGNOSIS

Malabsorption/maldigestion:
- Celiac disease
- *Mycobacterium avium-intracellulare* intestinal infection in patients with AIDS
- Intestinal lymphoma
- Abetalipoproteinemia
- Amyloidosis
- Systemic mastocytosis
- Radiation enteritis
- Crohn's disease
- Short bowel syndrome
- Pancreatic insufficiency
- Intestinal bacterial overgrowth
- Lactose deficiency
- Postgastrectomy syndrome
- Other cause of diarrhea (see Section III, "Diarrhea, Acute" and "Diarrhea, Chronic")
- Seronegative inflammatory arthritis
- Pericarditis and pleuritis
- Lymphadenitis
- Neurologic disorders

WORKUP

Laboratory tests and imaging studies are useful; however, the diagnosis of Whipple's disease is usually made by upper endoscopy and biopsy. Endoscopic findings reveal a pale yellow, shaggy mucosa alternating with an erythematous, erosive, or friable mucosa in the duodenum or jejunum.

LABORATORY TESTS

- Anemia (iron, folate, or vitamin B_{12} deficiency)
- Hypokalemia
- Hypocalcemia
- Hypomagnesemia
- Hypoalbuminemia
- Prolonged prothrombin time
- Low serum carotene
- Low cholesterol
- Leukocytosis
- Steatorrhea demonstrated by a Sudan fecal fat stain
- 72-hr stool collection demonstrating more than 7 g/24 hr of fat in the stool is impractical to perform, especially in ambulatory patients
- Defective d-xylose absorption

IMAGING STUDIES

Small bowel radiographs after barium ingestion often show thickening of mucosal folds.

BIOPSY

Infiltration of the intestinal lamina propria by PAS-positive macrophages containing gram-positive, acid-fast negative bacilli, associated with lymphatic dilation (diagnostic); PCR of the involved tissue in uncertain cases. If PAS staining of the small-bowel biopsy specimen is positive and the PCR assay is negative, the diagnosis of Whipple's disease must be confirmed; this can be done by immunohistochemical testing with an antibody to *T. whippelii.* If this test is positive, Whipple's disease is confirmed.

TREATMENT

- Antibiotics: TMP/SMX DS bid for 12 to 24 mo, usually preceded by parenteral administration of streptomycin (1 g/day) together with penicillin G (1.2 million U/day) or ceftriaxone (2 g/day) for 2 wk.
- Alternative regimen consists of doxycycline (200 mg/day) plus hydroxychloroquine (200 mg tid).
- Treat specific vitamin, mineral, and nutrient deficiencies.
- Patients with a neurologic recurrence of Whipple's disease have a poor prognosis. Interferon gamma has been proposed for treatment of recurrent central nervous system disease.

SUGGESTED READING
available at www.expertconsult.com

AUTHOR: **FRED F. FERRI, M.D.**

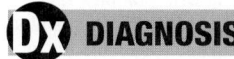 **BASIC INFORMATION**

DEFINITION

Wilson's disease is a disorder of copper transport with inadequate biliary copper excretion, leading to an accumulation of the metal in liver, brain, kidneys, and corneas.

SYNONYMS

Progressive hepatolenticular degeneration

ICD-9CM CODES
275.1 Wilson's disease

EPIDEMIOLOGY & DEMOGRAPHICS

PREVALENCE: One case in 30,000
PREDOMINANT SEX: Affects men and women equally (autosomal recessive gene)
ONSET OF SYMPTOMS: Ages 3 to 40 yr

PHYSICAL FINDINGS & CLINICAL PRESENTATION

Hepatic presentation:
- Acute hepatitis with malaise, anorexia, nausea, jaundice, elevated transaminase, prolonged prothrombin time; rarely fulminant hepatic failure
- Chronic active (or autoimmune) hepatitis with fatigue, malaise, rashes, arthralgia, elevated transaminase, elevated serum immunoglobulin G, positive antinuclear antibody and anti-smooth muscle antibody
- Chronic liver disease/cirrhosis with hepatosplenomegaly, ascites, low serum albumin, prolonged prothrombin time, portal hypertension

Neurologic presentation:
- Movement disorder: tremors, ataxia
- Spastic dystonia: masklike facies, rigidity, gait disturbance, dysarthria, drooling, dysphagia

Ophthalmic:
- Kaiser-Fleisher ring
- Sunflower cataracts

Psychiatric presentation:
- Depression, obsessive-compulsive disorder, psychopathic behaviors, neuroses

Other organs:
- Hemolytic anemia
- Renal disease (i.e., Fanconi's syndrome with hematuria, phosphaturia, renal tubular acidosis, vitamin D–resistant rickets)
- Cardiomyopathy
- Arthritis
- Hypoparathyroidism
- Hypogonadism

PHYSICAL FINDINGS:
- Ocular: the Kayser-Fleischer ring is a gold-yellow ring seen at the periphery of the iris (Fig. 1-412); these should be sought with slit-lamp examination by a skilled examiner.
- Stigmata of acute or chronic liver disease.
- Neurologic abnormalities: see previous.

ETIOLOGY & PATHOGENESIS
- Dietary copper is transported from the intestine to the liver, where normally it is metabolized into ceruloplasmin. In Wilson's disease, defective incorporation of copper into ceruloplasmin and a decrease of biliary copper excretion lead to accumulation of this mineral.
- The gene for Wilson's disease is located in chromosome 13.

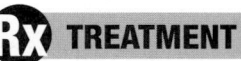 **DIAGNOSIS**

DIFFERENTIAL DIAGNOSIS
- Hereditary hypoceruloplasminemia.
- Menkes' disease.
- Consider the diagnosis of Wilson's disease in all cases of acute or chronic liver disease for which another cause has not been established.
- Consider Wilson's disease in patients with movement disorders or dystonia even without symptomatic liver disease.

LABORATORY TESTS
- Abnormal liver function tests (note that aspartate aminotransferase may be higher than alanine aminotransferase)
- Low serum ceruloplasmin level (<200 mg/L)
- Low serum copper (<65 mcg/L)
- 24-hr urinary copper excretion greater than 100 mcg (normal <30 mcg); increases to greater than 1200 mcg/24 hr after 500 mg of d-penicillamine (normal <500 mcg/24 hr)
- Low serum uric acid and phosphorus
- Abnormal urinalysis (hematuria)

BIOPSY
- Early:
  - Steatosis, focal necrosis, glycogenated hepatocyte nuclei
  - May reveal inflammation and piecemeal necrosis
- Late: cirrhosis
- Hepatic copper content (>250 mcg/g of dry weight) (normal is 20 to 50 mcg)
- Histochemical confirmation of excess copper can be helpful in diagnosis, but if absent, does not exclude Wilson's disease. The lack of immunoreactivity to copper-binding protein can occur because of the diffuse presence of copper in the cytoplasm and because of the assay's low sensitivity. Rhodamine and rubeanic acid stains can show dense granular lysosomal copper deposition in hepatocytes at the stage of cirrhotic nodular regeneration.

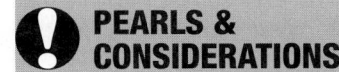 **TREATMENT**

- Penicillamine: (chelator therapy)
  - 0.75 to 1.5 g/day divided bid (with pyridoxine 25 mg/day)
  - Monitor complete blood count (CBC) and urinalysis weekly
- Trientine: (triethylene tetramine) (chelator therapy)
  - 1 to 2 g/day divided tid
  - Monitor CBC
- Zinc: (inhibits intestinal copper absorption)
  - 50 mg tid
  - Monitor zinc level
- Ammonium tetrathiomolybdate for neurologic symptoms
- Antioxidants
- Liver transplantation (for severe hepatic failure unresponsive to chelation); liver transplantation corrects the underlying pathophysiology and can be lifesaving

PROGNOSIS
Good with early chelation treatment

REFERRAL
To gastroenterologist, neurologist

 PEARLS & CONSIDERATIONS

COMMENTS
Family screening of first-degree relatives must be undertaken. Genetic diagnosis is also useful in patients with indeterminate clinical and biochemical features.

EBM **EVIDENCE**

available at www.expertconsult.com

SUGGESTED READING
available at www.expertconsult.com

AUTHOR: **FRED F. FERRI, M.D.**

Diseases and Disorders

I

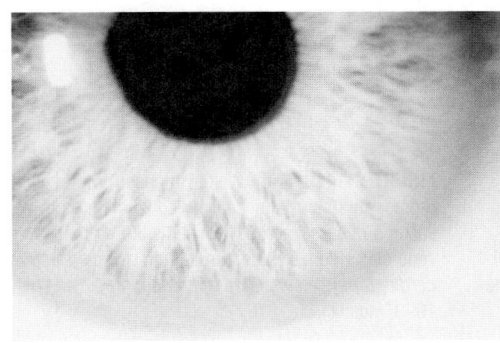

FIGURE 1-412 **Wilson's disease.** A Kayser-Fleisher ring, which is a gold-yellow ring, extends to the limbus without a clear interval. (From Palay D [ed]: *Ophthalmology for the primary care physician*, St Louis, 1997, Mosby.)

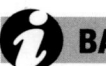

BASIC INFORMATION

DEFINITION

Wolff-Parkinson-White (WPW) syndrome is defined as the presence of preexcitation of the ventricles of the heart due to an abnormal electrical communication from the atria to the ventricles through an accessory pathway. It is typically manifested by a short PR interval (i.e., <120 msec) and the presence of a delta wave in the ECG (WPW pattern).

SYNONYMS

Preexcitation syndrome
WPW

ICD-9CM CODES	
426.7	Wolff-Parkinson-White syndrome
426.81	Lown-Ganong-Levine syndrome

EPIDEMIOLOGY & DEMOGRAPHICS

- The prevalence of a WPW pattern on the surface ECG is 0.15% to 0.25% in the general population. The prevalence is increased to 0.55% in first-degree relatives of affected patients.
- In a study of a presumed healthy population of more than 20,000 patients, the WPW pattern was recognized in 0.25%. Of these patients, only 1.8% had documented arrhythmias that were consistent with the WPW syndrome.
- The prevalence of WPW is higher among males and decreases with age.
- Most patients with WPW syndrome have structurally normal hearts, but associations with mitral valve prolapse, cardiomyopathies, and Ebstein's anomaly have been reported.

PHYSICAL FINDINGS & CLINICAL PRESENTATION

- The physical examination may be entirely normal.
- Symptoms are typically related to tachyarrhythmias, including the following:
  - Palpitations
  - Syncope or near syncope
  - Sudden cardiac death (rarely)
- The type of tachycardia can be any of the following:
  - Supraventricular tachycardia: atrioventricular (AV) reentrant tachycardia (either through the orthodromal pathway [narrow complex] or the antidromal pathway [wide complex]; 80%)
  - Atrial fibrillation (~10% to 30%)
  - Atrial flutter (~5%)
  - Ventricular tachycardia or ventricular fibrillation: rare. Potentially fatal consequence if atrial fibrillation is conducted down the accessory pathway.

ETIOLOGY & PATHOGENESIS

- The existence of an accessory pathway allows for conduction from the atria to the ventricles while bypassing the AV node.

- If the accessory pathway is capable of anterograde conduction, two parallel routes of AV conduction are possible: one is subject to delay through the AV node, and the other occurs without delay through the accessory pathway. The resulting QRS complex is a fusion beat, with the delta wave representing rapid ventricular activation through the accessory pathway and the later ventricular activation occurring via conduction through the AV node (Figure 1-413).
- Tachycardias occur when conduction is anterograde in one pathway (usually the normal AV pathway) and retrograde in the other (usually the accessory pathway) as a result of different refractory periods. Some patients (~5% to 10%) with WPW syndrome have multiple accessory pathways.
- In patients with WPW syndrome, the development of atrial fibrillation may be associated with very rapid ventricular rates from AV conduction over the accessory AV pathway.
- In patients with atrial fibrillation with rapid ventricular response, rapid conduction to the ventricles by way of the accessory pathway may result in degeneration into ventricular fibrillation.

DIAGNOSIS

- Three basic features characterize the ECG abnormalities associated with WPW syndrome (Figure 1-414):
  1. PR interval <120 msec
  2. QRS complex >120 msec with a slurred, slowly rising onset of QRS in some leads (i.e., delta wave)
  3. Secondary ST-T wave changes

- Variants:
  - Lown-Ganong-Levine syndrome: atriohisian pathway with a short PR interval and a normal QRS complex on ECG (i.e., no delta wave)
  - Atriofascicular accessory pathways: duplication of the AV node with normal baseline ECG

TREATMENT

- There is no definitive recommendation for treatment in the absence of tachyarrhythmias. However, there is an American Heart Association/American College of Cardiology class IIa recommendation for radiofrequency ablation for asymptomatic patients whose lifestyles may be adversely affected by a tachyarrhythmia.
- For the acute termination of narrow complex regular tachyarrhythmias, carotid sinus massage or the Valsalva maneuver may be successful. First-line pharmacologic therapy includes adenosine or verapamil for patients WITHOUT atrial fibrillation or flutter.
- For patients with a rapid ventricular response with hemodynamic compromise, urgent electrical cardioversion is warranted.
- Digitalis should not be used, because it can reduce refractoriness in the accessory pathway and accelerate the tachycardia.
- Drug therapy for the chronic prevention of narrow complex regular tachyarrhythmias includes class IC antiarrhythmics, β-blockers, calcium channel blockers, amiodarone, or sotalol. The choice of drug therapy is dictated by the underlying mechanism of the tachyarrhythmia.

WPW: Sinus Rhythm

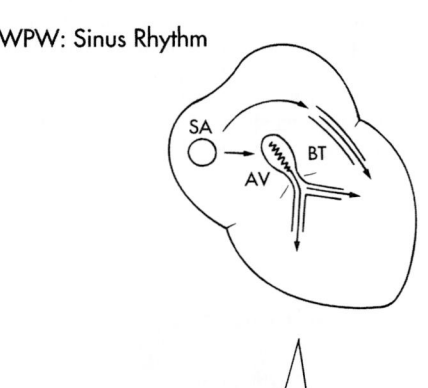

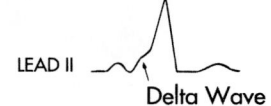

FIGURE 1-413 With Wolff-Parkinson-White syndrome, an abnormal accessory conduction pathway called a *bypass tract (BT)* connects the atria and the ventricles. (From Goldberger AL [ed]: *Clinical electrocardiography: a simplified approach,* ed 6, St Louis, 1999, Mosby.)

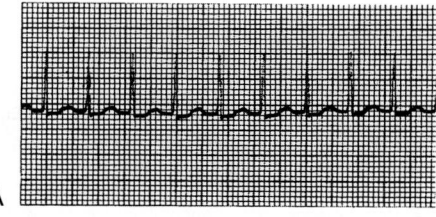

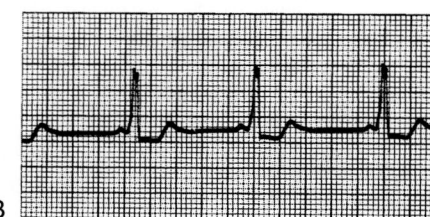

FIGURE 1-414 A, Supraventricular tachycardia in a child with Wolff-Parkinson-White syndrome. Note the normal QRS complexes during the tachycardia. **B,** Later, the typical features of Wolff-Parkinson-White syndrome are apparent: a short P-R interval, a delta wave, and a wide QRS. (From Behrman RE: *Nelson textbook of pediatrics,* ed 18, Philadelphia, 2007, WB Saunders.)

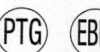
- For the treatment of atrial fibrillation in patients with WPW, the administration of AV nodal-blocking agents may not slow the ventricular rate, because the accessory pathways capable of rapid conduction do not respond to AV-blocking agents. Procainamide is the drug of choice for controlling the ventricular rate and restoring the sinus rhythm in patients with WPW who have atrial fibrillation.
- When medical therapy fails or the patient cannot tolerate the tachyarrythmias, radiofrequency ablation should be performed (class I indication).

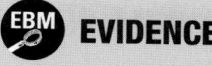 **EVIDENCE**

available at www.expertconsult.com

SUGGESTED READINGS

available at www.expertconsult.com

AUTHORS: **JOSHUA R. SILVERSTEIN, M.D., FRED F. FERRI, M.D., and WEN-CHIH WU, M.D.**

W

Diseases
and Disorders

I

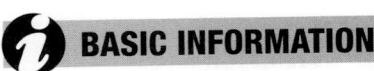

BASIC INFORMATION

DEFINITION

Yellow fever is a mosquito-borne infection, primarily of the liver, with systemic manifestations caused by the yellow fever virus (YFV). The clinical spectrum ranges from asymptomatic infection to life-threatening disease with severity and mortality highest in the elderly.

SYNONYMS

Tropical hemorrhagic fever from YFV

ICD-9CM CODES
060.9 Yellow fever

EPIDEMIOLOGY & DEMOGRAPHICS
GEOGRAPHIC DISTRIBUTION:
- South America and Africa, in countries between +15 and −15 degrees latitude.
- The World Health Organization estimates there are more than 200,000 cases a yr with 30,000 deaths per yr. More than 90% of cases occur in Africa.

INCIDENCE: Approximate attack rates of 3% in Africa and Amazon

PREVALENCE: Endemic areas: 20% of population

PREDOMINANT SEX: In Africa and the Amazon, male agricultural workers.

PHYSICAL FINDINGS & CLINICAL PRESENTATION
- Most subclinical.
- The onset of illness appears suddenly 3 to 6 days after the bite of an infected mosquito.
- Viremic (early) phase:
  1. Fever, chills
  2. Severe headache
  3. Lumbosacral pain
  4. Myalgias, nausea, malaise
  5. Conjunctivitis
  6. Relative bradycardia (Faget's sign)
- After brief recovery, toxic phase:
  1. Jaundice
  2. Oliguria
  3. Albuminuria
  4. Hemorrhage
  5. Encephalopathy
  6. Shock
  7. Acidosis
- Case fatality rate 25% to 50%.

ETIOLOGY
- YFV (L. flavus)
  1. Flavivirus infects hepatic cells.
  2. Late in infection, cytopathic effects (antibody- and cell-mediated) produce pathology.
- Vector
  1. Aedes aegypti (urban).
  2. Aedes spp., Haemagogus (especially in Amazon) mosquitos (sylvan).
  3. Primary hosts: humans and simian species.
  4. Exists in two transmission cycles:
     a. Sylvatic or jungle cycle involving mosquitos and nonhuman primates.
     b. Urban cycle involving mosquitos and humans.

PATHOGENESIS & PATHOLOGY
- Virus replication begins at site of mosquito bite, spreading to lymphatic channels and regional lymph nodes. Viremic spread to other organs, especially liver, spleen, and bone marrow.
- Shock and fatal illness result from direct damage to organs and vasoactive cytokines.
- Viral antigen found in hepatocytes, kidneys, and myocardium.
- Midzone of liver lobules primarily affected.
- Hemorrhages of mucosal surfaces of GI tract.

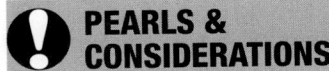

DIAGNOSIS

DIFFERENTIAL DIAGNOSIS
- Viral hepatitis
- Leptospirosis
- Malaria
- Typhoid fever
  1. Typhus
  2. Relapsing fever
- Other hemorrhagic fevers such as Dengue

LABORATORY TESTS
- CBC
  1. Mild leukopenia
  2. Thrombocytopenia
  3. Anemia
- LFTs
  1. AST levels exceed ALT levels.
  2. Alkaline phosphatase normal or slightly elevated.
  3. Elevated bilirubin levels.
- Elevated BUN and creatinine
- Proteinuria
- Coagulation studies
  1. Demonstrate abnormal prothrombin time *or*
  2. Reveal DIC
- Terminal hypoglycemia
- CSF
  1. Pleocytosis
  2. Elevated protein count
- Specific diagnosis confirmed by:
  1. Viral isolation from blood
  2. Viral antigen in serum (ELISA)
  3. Viral RNA by polymerase chain reaction (PCR)
  4. IgM-capture ELISA
     a. Preferred serologic test.
     b. Appears within 5 to 7 days.
     c. Rising Ab confirmed by paired sera.
     d. Cross-reactivity with other flavivirus infections.
  5. Immunohistochemical staining of post-mortem liver biopsy specimens

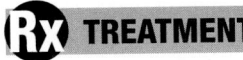

TREATMENT

ACUTE GENERAL Rx
- Acetaminophen (for headache and fever) and H_2 blockers (GI bleeding); avoid aspirin because of bleeding risk
- Blood transfusion, volume replacement for hemorrhage and shock
- Dialysis for renal failure
- Avoidance of sedatives and drugs dependent on hepatic metabolism

DISPOSITION

Follow up until hepatic, renal, CNS disease resolved. Infection in humans is capable of producing hemorrhagic fever and is fatal in 20% to 50% of persons with severe disease

REFERRAL

To infectious diseases expert for accurate diagnosis and management

PEARLS & CONSIDERATIONS

PREVENTION
- Yellow fever is preventable.
- Recovery from yellow fever confers lasting immunity.
- Live, attenuated yellow fever vaccine (YF-Vax) provides protective immunity in 95% of vaccinated patients within 10 days of vaccination. Reimmunization at 10-yr intervals for travelers. Vaccine certificate to verify immunization status is required before travel in many tropical countries in South America and Africa.
- Vaccine contraindicated in:
  1. Infants <6 mo (postvaccinal encephalitis)
  2. Immunosuppressed patients
  3. Pregnant women and nursing mothers
  4. Patients with egg hypersensitivity
- Adverse effects of vaccine:
  1. General
     a. Mild headaches, myalgias, low-grade fevers (25% vaccinees in clinical trials).
     b. Immediate hypersensitivity reaction (history of egg allergy).
  2. Vaccine-associated neurotropic disease (postvaccine encephalitis) (1.8 cases per million)
     a. Primarily among infants.
     b. Adult cases only in first-time vaccine recipients.
  3. Vaccine-associated viscerotropic disease (2.2 cases per million)
     a. Disease syndrome resembling wild-type yellow fever, often fatal.
     b. All cases in first-time vaccinees; age >60 yr are at particular risk.

SUGGESTED READINGS
available at www.expertconsult.com

AUTHOR: **STEVEN M. OPAL, M.D.**

BASIC INFORMATION

DEFINITION
Zenker's diverticulum (ZD) refers to the acquired physiologic obstruction of the esophageal introitus that results from mucosal herniation posteriorly between the cricopharyngeus muscle and the inferior pharyngeal constrictor muscle (Fig. 1-415).

SYNONYMS
Pharyngoesophageal diverticulum
Pulsion diverticulum

ICD-9CM CODES
530.6 Zenker's diverticulum (esophagus)

EPIDEMIOLOGY & DEMOGRAPHICS
- The most common type of diverticulum of the upper gastrointestinal tract
- Rare disease with annual incidence estimated 1/50,000 per year
- Most commonly presents after the age of 60 yr, more commonly seen in males
- Peak incidence is seventh to ninth decades
- Associated with gastroesophageal reflux disease (GERD) and hiatal hernia

PHYSICAL FINDINGS & CLINICAL PRESENTATION
A small ZD may be asymptomatic. As it becomes larger, symptoms may include:
- Dysphagia to solids and liquids (most common)
- Regurgitation of undigested food
- Sensation of globus or fullness in the neck
- Cough
- Halitosis
- Aspiration pneumonia
- Weight loss
- Voice changes
- Sialorrhea (excessive drooling)

ETIOLOGY
- The specific cause is not known. The leading hypothesis suggests a discoordination of the swallowing muscles (specifically, incomplete relaxation of the cricopharyngeus muscle) that leads to an increased pressure on the mucosa of the hypopharynx, resulting in a progressive distention of that mucosa in its weakest area (posterior wall in "Killian's triangle," the point between the oblique fibers of the inferior pharyngeal muscle and the horizontal fibers of the cricopharyngeus muscle). The end result is the formation of a false diverticulum where food elements and secretions may be lodged, causing the symptoms listed previously.
- ZD may also occur after anterior spinal surgery or cervical spine injury.

DIAGNOSIS
- Clinical presentation and barium swallow typically make the diagnosis of ZD.
- Neck ultrasound can also be used.
- Esophageal manometry can help elucidate the pathogenesis but not required for diagnosis

DIFFERENTIAL DIAGNOSIS
The differential diagnosis is similar to anyone presenting with dysphagia:
- Achalasia
- Esophageal spasm
- Esophageal carcinoma
- Esophageal webs
- Peptic stricture
- Lower esophageal (Schatzki) ring
- Foreign bodies
- Central nervous system disorders (stroke, Parkinson's disease, amyotrophic lateral sclerosis, multiple sclerosis, myasthenia gravis, muscular dystrophies)

- Dermatomyositis
- Infection

WORKUP
Barium swallow is the test of choice. Upper endoscopy runs the risk of perforation.

LABORATORY TESTS
Not specific

IMAGING STUDIES
- Barium swallow: demonstrates a herniated sac with a narrow diverticular neck that typically originates proximal to the cricopharyngeus at the level of C5–C6 (Fig. 1-416).
- Endoscopy is only indicated if barium studies show mucosal irregularities to rule out neoplasia.
- Oropharyngeal-esophageal scintigraphy has recently been shown to be an effective, sensitive, and simple diagnostic study for both qualitative and quantitative analyses.
- A chest x-ray is performed in cases of suspected aspiration pneumonia.

TREATMENT

NONPHARMACOLOGIC THERAPY
- Soft mechanical diet can be tried in patients with symptoms of dysphagia.
- Avoid seeds, skins, and nuts.

ACUTE GENERAL Rx
- Surgical repair is the conventional treatment for symptomatic patients (dysphagia, cough, aspiration) with excellent relief of symptoms in nearly all patients and low procedural mortality (<1.5%). Procedures include:
  1. Cervical diverticulectomy with cricopharyngeal myotomy (most common approach)
  2. Diverticulopexy or diverticular inversion with cricopharyngeal myotomy
  3. Diverticulectomy alone
  4. Cricopharyngeal myotomy alone
- Endoscopic techniques (esophagodiverticulostomy) have largely replaced conventional surgery and include:
  1. Endoscopic stapler diverticulotomy (may be the initial treatment of choice)
  2. Microendoscopic carbon dioxide laser surgical diverticulotomy
  3. Diverticula <3 cm is a contraindication to endosurgical approach
  4. Head-to-head comparison with surgical repairs showed endoscopic techniques to be similar in results, relief of symptoms, and patient satisfaction

CHRONIC Rx
In patients not having surgery, treatment is directed toward any complications that may occur:
- Antibiotics for aspiration pneumonia
- H_2 antagonists for ulcerations that can develop within the diverticulum
- Botulinum toxin for temporary relief of dysphagia

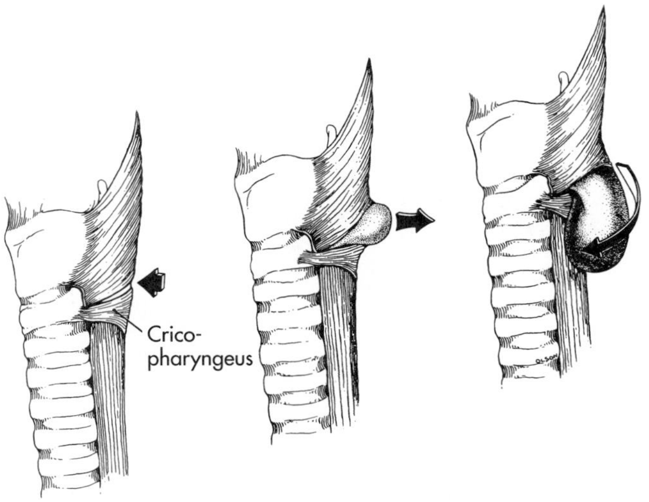

FIGURE 1-415 Formation of pharyngoesophageal (Zenker's) diverticulum. *Left,* Herniation of the pharyngeal mucosa and submucosa occurs at the point of transition *(arrow)* between the oblique fibers of the thyropharyngeus muscle and the more horizontal fibers of the cricopharyngeus muscle. *Center and right,* As the diverticulum enlarges, it dissects toward the left side and downward into the superior mediastinum in the prevertebral space. (From Sabiston D: *Textbook of surgery,* ed 15, Philadelphia, 1997, WB Saunders.)

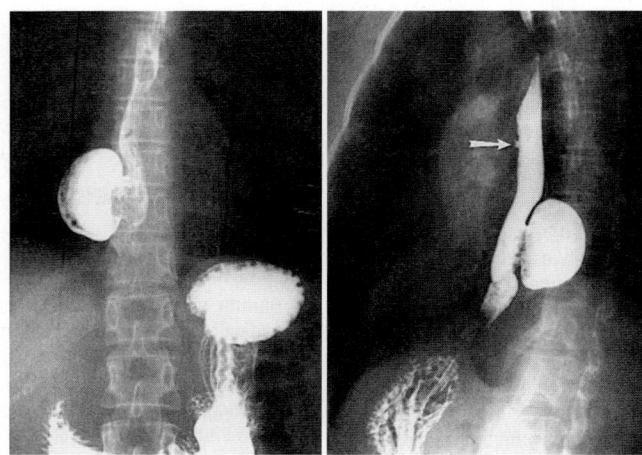

FIGURE 1-416 Posteroanterior *(left)* and oblique *(right)* views from barium esophagogram showing both a typical diverticulum of the junction of the mid-esophagus and distal esophagus and a small traction diverticulum *(arrow)* of the mid-esophagus. (From Sabiston D: *Textbook of surgery,* ed 15, Philadelphia, 1997, Saunders.)

DISPOSITION

- If left untreated, progressive enlargement of the diverticulum occurs.
- The risk of complications (e.g., aspiration pneumonia) increases with the size of the diverticulum.
- Postsurgical recurrence can occur (4%); however, these are usually asymptomatic.

REFERRAL

Any patient with dysphagia requires a gastroenterology consultation. A thoracic surgical, ENT, or head and neck surgeon may be consulted if surgery is considered.

COMMENTS

The association with cancer is rare (0.4%).

SUGGESTED READINGS

available at www.expertconsult.com

AUTHORS: **ROBERT M. KIRCHNER, M.D.,** and **PAUL GORDON, M.D.**

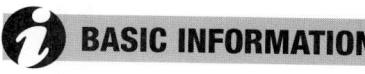
BASIC INFORMATION

DEFINITION

Zollinger-Ellison (ZE) syndrome is a hypergastrinemic state caused by a pancreatic or extrapancreatic non–beta islet cell tumor (gastrinoma) resulting in peptic acid disease.

SYNONYMS

Gastrinoma

ICD-9CM CODES
251.5 Zollinger-Ellison syndrome

EPIDEMIOLOGY & DEMOGRAPHICS

- Incidence is unknown, but 0.1% of all duodenal ulcers are believed to be caused by ZE.
- Occurs in both genders and at any age (most common in ages 30 to 50 yr).
- Two thirds of gastrinomas are sporadic, and one third are associated with multiple endocrine neoplasia type 1 (MEN-1), an autosomal-dominant genetic disorder that also includes hyperparathyroidism and pituitary tumors.
- Approximately 60% of gastrinomas are malignant.
- The incidence and prevalence of pancreatic neuroendocrine tumors are increasing. They represent 1.3% of all cases of pancreatic cancer.

PHYSICAL FINDINGS & CLINICAL PRESENTATION

- The majority of patients (95%) present with symptoms of peptic ulcer (see Section I, "Peptic Ulcer Disease").
- 60% of patients have symptoms related to gastroesophageal reflux disease (see Section I, "Gastroesophageal Reflux Disease").
- One third of patients with ZE have diarrhea and, less commonly, steatorrhea.

The following circumstances warrant suspicion of ZE syndrome:
- Ulcers distal to the first portion of the duodenum
- Multiple peptic ulcers
- Ineffective treatment for peptic ulcer disease with the usual drug doses and schedules
- Peptic ulcer and diarrhea
- Familial history of peptic ulcer
- Patients with a personal or family history suggesting parathyroid or pituitary tumors of dysfunction
- Peptic ulcer and urinary tract calculi
- Patients with peptic ulcer who are negative for *Helicobacter pylori* and do not have a history of nonsteroidal antiinflammatory drug use

ETIOLOGY

- The pathophysiologic manifestations of ZE syndrome are related to the effects of hypergastrinemia. Gastrin stimulates gastric acid secretion, which in turn is responsible for the development of duodenal ulcers and diarrhea. Gastrin also promotes gastric mucosal epithelial cell growth and resulting parietal cell hyperplasia.
- Gastrinomas are usually small (0.1 to 2 cm) but sometimes large (>20 cm) tumors.
- 60% of gastrinomas are malignant, with liver and regional lymph nodes the most common site of metastases. Histology is not a good predictor of the biology of gastrinomas.
- 60% of patients with MEN-1 have gastrinomas.
- 10% of patients with ZE syndrome have islet cell hyperplasia rather than gastrinomas; in 10% to 20% of patients with gastrinoma the tumors cannot be located because of small size.

DIAGNOSIS

DIFFERENTIAL DIAGNOSIS

- Peptic ulcer disease (see Section I, "Peptic Ulcer Disease")
- Gastroesophageal reflux disease (see Section I, "Gastroesophageal Reflux Disease")
- Diarrhea (see Section III, "Diarrhea, Acute" and "Diarrhea, Chronic")

WORKUP

- Diagnosis of peptic ulcer:
  - Upper gastrointestinal series (may also show prominent gastric rugal folds)
  - Endoscopy
- Gastric acid secretion:
  - Serum gastrin level (fasting) >150 pg/ml (causes of false-positive results: pernicious anemia, renal failure, retained gastric antrum syndrome, diabetes mellitus, rheumatoid arthritis)
- Provocative gastrin level tests:
  - Secretin stimulation
  - Calcium stimulation
  - Standard test meal stimulation
- Gastrinoma localization:
  - Arteriography
  - Abdominal sonography
  - Abdominal CT scan
  - Abdominal MRI
  - Selective portal vein branch gastrin level
  - Octreotide scan

TREATMENT

- Surgical resection of the gastrinoma (NOTE: 90% of gastrinomas can be located, resulting in a 40% overall cure rate)
- Total gastrectomy or vagotomy (palliative in some patients)
- Medical treatment
  - Proton pump inhibitors (e.g., omeprazole, lansoprazole)
  - Somatostatin or octreotide
  - Chemotherapy for metastatic gastrinoma with streptozotocin, 5-fluorouracil, and doxorubicin
  - Early trials with everolimus, an oral inhibitor of mammalian target of rapamycin (mTOR) have shown antitumor activity in patients with advanced pancreatic neuroendocrine tumors with significant prolongation of progression-free survival and low rates of severe adverse events
  - Preliminary trials with the tyrosine kinase inhibitor sunitinib have shown encouraging results on prolongation of survival

PROGNOSIS

Five-yr survival:
- Two thirds of all patients
- 20% with liver metastases
- 90% without liver metastases

REFERRAL

To gastroenterologist and surgeon

SUGGESTED READINGS
available at www.expertconsult.com

AUTHOR: **FRED F. FERRI, M.D.**

Differential Diagnosis

ABDOMINAL DISTENTION
ICD-9CM # 787.3

NONMECHANICAL OBSTRUCTION
Excessive intraluminal gas.
Intraabdominal infection.
Trauma.
Retroperitoneal irritation (renal colic, neoplasms, infections, hemorrhage).
Vascular insufficiency (thrombosis, embolism).
Mechanical ventilation.
Extraabdominal infection (sepsis, pneumonia, empyema, osteomyelitis of spine).
Metabolic/toxic abnormalities (hypokalemia, uremia, lead poisoning).
Chemical irritation (perforated ulcer, bile, pancreatitis).
Peritoneal inflammation.
Severe pain, pain medications.

MECHANICAL OBSTRUCTION
Neoplasm (intraluminal, extraluminal).
Adhesions, endometriosis.
Infection (intraabdominal abscess, diverticulitis).
Gallstones.
Foreign body, bezoars.
Pregnancy.
Hernias.
Volvulus.
Stenosis at surgical anastomosis, radiation stenosis.
Fecaliths.
Inflammatory bowel disease.
Gastric outlet obstruction.
Hematoma.
Other: parasites, superior mesenteric artery (SMA) syndrome, pneumatosis intestinalis, annular pancreas, Hirschsprung's disease, intussusception, meconium.

ABDOMINAL PAIN, ADOLESCENCE[26]
ICD-9CM # 789.67

Acute gastroenteritis.
Appendicitis.
Inflammatory bowel disease.
Peptic ulcer disease (PUD).
Cholecystitis.
Neoplasm.
Diabetic ketoacidosis.
Functional abdominal pain.
Pelvic inflammatory disease (PID).
Pregnancy.
Pyelonephritis.
Renal stone.
Trauma.

ABDOMINAL PAIN, CHILDHOOD[26]
ICD-9CM # 789.67

Acute gastroenteritis.
Appendicitis.
Constipation.
Cholecystitis, acute.

Intestinal obstruction.
Pancreatitis.
Neoplasm.
Inflammatory bowel disease.
Other:
    Functional abdominal pain.
    Pyelonephritis.
    Pneumonia.
    Diabetic ketoacidosis.
    Heavy metal poisoning.
    Sickle cell crisis.
    Trauma.

ABDOMINAL PAIN, CHRONIC LOWER[38]
ICD-9CM # 789.64 Abdominal Pain Left Lower Quadrant
789.63 Abdominal Pain Right Lower Quadrant
789.85 Abdominal Pain Suprapubic

ORGANIC DISORDERS
Common
Gynecological disease.
Lactase deficiency.
Diverticulitis.
Crohn's disease.
Intestinal obstruction.
Uncommon
Chronic intestinal pseudoobstruction.
Mesenteric ischemia.
Malignancy (e.g., ovarian carcinoma).
Abdominal wall pain.
Spinal disease.
Testicular disease.
Metabolic diseases (e.g., diabetes mellitus, familial Mediterranean fever, C1 esterase deficiency [angioneurotic edema], porphyria, lead poisoning, tabes dorsalis, renal failure).

FUNCTIONAL DISORDERS
Common
Irritable bowel syndrome.
Functional abdominal bloating.
Uncommon
Functional abdominal pain.

ABDOMINAL PAIN, DIFFUSE
ICD-9CM # 789.67

Early appendicitis.
Aortic aneurysm.
Gastroenteritis.
Intestinal obstruction.
Diverticulitis.
Peritonitis.
Mesenteric insufficiency or infarction.
Pancreatitis.
Inflammatory bowel disease.
Irritable bowel.
Mesenteric adenitis.
Metabolic: toxins, lead poisoning, uremia, drug overdose, diabetic ketoacidosis (DKA), heavy metal poisoning.
Sickle cell crisis.
Pneumonia (rare).

Trauma.
Urinary tract infection, PID.
Other: acute intermittent porphyria, tabes dorsalis, periarteritis nodosa, Henoch-Schönlein purpura, adrenal insufficiency.

ABDOMINAL PAIN, EPIGASTRIC
ICD-9CM # 789.66

Gastric: PUD, gastric outlet obstruction, gastric ulcer.
Duodenal: PUD, duodenitis.
Biliary: cholecystitis, cholangitis.
Hepatic: hepatitis.
Pancreatic: pancreatitis.
Intestinal: high small bowel obstruction, early appendicitis.
Cardiac: angina, MI, pericarditis.
Pulmonary: pneumonia, pleurisy, pneumothorax.
Subphrenic abscess.
Vascular: dissecting aneurysm, mesenteric ischemia.

ABDOMINAL PAIN, INFANCY[26]
ICD-9CM # 789.67

Acute gastroenteritis.
Appendicitis.
Intussusception.
Volvulus.
Meckel diverticulum.
Other: colic, trauma.

ABDOMINAL PAIN, LEFT LOWER QUADRANT
ICD-9CM # 789.64

Intestinal: diverticulitis, intestinal obstruction, perforated ulcer, inflammatory bowel disease, perforated descending colon, inguinal hernia, neoplasm, appendicitis.
Reproductive: ectopic pregnancy, ovarian cyst, torsion of ovarian cyst, tuboovarian abscess, mittelschmerz, endometriosis, seminal vesiculitis.
Renal: renal or ureteral calculi, pyelonephritis, neoplasm.
Vascular: leaking aortic aneurysm.
Psoas abscess.
Trauma.

ABDOMINAL PAIN, LEFT UPPER QUADRANT
ICD-9CM # 789.32

Gastric: PUD, gastritis, pyloric stenosis, hiatal hernia.
Pancreatic: pancreatitis, neoplasm, stone in pancreatic duct or ampulla.
Cardiac: MI, angina pectoris.
Splenic: splenomegaly, ruptured spleen, splenic abscess, splenic infarction.

Renal: calculi, pyelonephritis, neoplasm.
Pulmonary: pneumonia, empyema, pulmonary infarction.
Vascular: ruptured aortic aneurysm.
Cutaneous: herpes zoster.
Trauma.
Intestinal: high fecal impaction, perforated colon, diverticulitis.

ABDOMINAL PAIN, NONSURGICAL CAUSES
ICD-9CM # 789.9

Irritable bowel syndrome.
Urinary tract infection, pyelonephritis, salpingitis, PID.
Gastroenteritis, gastritis, peptic ulcer.
Diverticular spasm.
Hepatitis, mononucleosis.
Pancreatitis.
Inferior wall myocardial infarction.
Basilar pneumonia, pulmonary embolism.
Diabetic ketoacidosis.
Strain or hematoma of rectus muscle.
Ruptured Graafian follicle.
Herpes zoster.
Nerve root compression.
Sickle cell crisis.
Acute adrenal insufficiency.
Other: acute porphyria, familial Mediterranean fever, tabes dorsalis.

ABDOMINAL PAIN, PERIUMBILICAL
ICD-9CM # 789.65

Intestinal: small bowel obstruction or gangrene, early appendicitis.
Vascular: mesenteric thrombosis, dissecting aortic aneurysm.
Pancreatic: pancreatitis.
Metabolic: uremia, DKA.
Trauma.

ABDOMINAL PAIN, POORLY LOCALIZED[26]
ICD-9CM # 789.60

EXTRAABDOMINAL
Metabolic
DKA, acute intermittent porphyria, hyperthyroidism, hypothyroidism, hypercalcemia, hypokalemia, uremia, hyperlipidemia, hyperparathyroidism.
Hematologic
Sickle cell crisis, leukemia or lymphoma, Henoch-Schönlein purpura.
Infectious
Infectious mononucleosis, Rocky Mountain spotted fever, acquired immunodeficiency syndrome (AIDS), streptococcal pharyngitis (in children), herpes zoster.
Drugs and Toxins
Heavy metal poisoning, black widow spider bites, withdrawal syndromes, mushroom ingestion.

Referred Pain
Pulmonary: pneumonia, pulmonary embolism, pneumothorax.
Cardiac: angina, MI, pericarditis, myocarditis.
Genitourinary: prostatitis, epididymitis, orchitis, testicular torsion.
Musculoskeletal: rectus sheath hematoma.
Functional
Somatization disorder, malingering, hypochondriasis, Munchausen syndrome.

INTRAABDOMINAL
Early appendicitis, gastroenteritis, peritonitis, pancreatitis, abdominal aortic aneurysm, mesenteric insufficiency or infarction, intestinal obstruction, volvulus, ulcerative colitis.

ABDOMINAL PAIN, PREGNANCY[26]
ICD-9CM # 789.67

GYNECOLOGIC (GESTATIONAL AGE IN PARENTHESES)
Miscarriage	(<20 wk; 80% <12 wk)
Septic abortion	(<20 wk)
Ectopic pregnancy	(<14 wk)
Corpus luteum cyst rupture	(<12 wk)
Ovarian torsion	(especially <24 wk)
Pelvic inflammatory disease	(<12 wk)
Chorioamnionitis	(>16 wk)
Abruptio placentae	(>16 wk)

NONGYNECOLOGIC
Appendicitis	(Throughout)
Cholecystitis	(Throughout)
Hepatitis	(Throughout)
Pyelonephritis	(Throughout)
Preeclampsia	(>20 wk)

ABDOMINAL PAIN, RIGHT LOWER QUADRANT
ICD-9CM # 789.63

Intestinal: acute appendicitis, regional enteritis, incarcerated hernia, cecal diverticulitis, intestinal obstruction, perforated ulcer, perforated cecum, Meckel diverticulitis.
Reproductive: ectopic pregnancy, ovarian cyst, torsion of ovarian cyst, salpingitis, tuboovarian abscess, mittelschmerz, endometriosis, seminal vesiculitis.
Renal: renal and ureteral calculi, neoplasms, pyelonephritis.
Vascular: leaking aortic aneurysm.
Psoas abscess.
Trauma.
Cholecystitis.

ABDOMINAL PAIN, RIGHT UPPER QUADRANT
ICD-9CM # 789.61

Biliary: calculi, infection, inflammation, neoplasm.
Hepatic: hepatitis, abscess, hepatic congestion, neoplasm, trauma.
Gastric: PUD, pyloric stenosis, neoplasm, alcoholic gastritis, hiatal hernia.
Pancreatic: pancreatitis, neoplasm, stone in pancreatic duct or ampulla.
Renal: calculi, infection, inflammation, neoplasm, rupture of kidney.
Pulmonary: pneumonia, pulmonary infarction, right-sided pleurisy.
Intestinal: retrocecal appendicitis, intestinal obstruction, high fecal impaction, diverticulitis.
Cardiac: myocardial ischemia (particularly involving the inferior wall), pericarditis.
Cutaneous: herpes zoster.
Trauma.
Fitz-Hugh-Curtis syndrome (perihepatitis).

ABDOMINAL PAIN, SUPRAPUBIC
ICD-9CM # 789.85

Intestinal: colon obstruction or gangrene, diverticulitis, appendicitis.
Reproductive system: ectopic pregnancy, mittelschmerz, torsion of ovarian cyst, PID, salpingitis, endometriosis, rupture of endometrioma.
Cystitis, rupture of urinary bladder.

ABDOMINAL WALL MASSES[38]
ICD-9CM # varies with specific diagnosis

LUMPS ARISING IN THE SKIN AND SUBCUTANEOUS FAT (THAT COULD OCCUR ANYWHERE ON THE BODY)
Lipoma.
Sebaceous cyst.

LUMPS ARISING IN THE SKIN AND SUBCUTANEOUS FAT (SPECIFIC TO THE ANTERIOR ABDOMINAL WALL)
Tumor nodule of the umbilicus (secondary to the intraperitoneal malignancy, also called Sister Mary Joseph nodule).

LUMPS ARISING IN THE FASCIA AND MUSCLE
Rectus sheath hematoma (usually painful).
Desmoid tumor (associated with Gardner's syndrome).

HERNIA

Incisional	It has an overlying scar. The sac may be very much larger than the neck of the hernia.
Umbilical	The hernia is through the umbilical scar. Those presenting at birth commonly resolve in the first years of life.
Paraumbilical	The neck is just lateral to the umbilical scar. Patients usually present later in life.
Epigastric	It occurs in the midline between the xiphoid process and the umbilicus. They are usually small (<2 cm). They result when a knuckle of extraperitoneal fat extrudes through a small defect in the linea alba. Commonly irreducible and without an expansile cough impulse.
Spigelian	A rare hernia found along the linea semilunaris at the lateral edge of the rectus sheath, most commonly a third of the way between the umbilicus and the pubis.

DIVARICATION OF THE RECTI

Supraumbilical elliptical swelling of the attenuated linea alba (no cough impulse).

ABORTION, RECURRENT
ICD-9CM # 761.8

Congenital anatomic abnormalities.
Adhesions (uterine synechiae).
Uterine fibroids.
Endometriosis.
Endocrine abnormalities (luteal phase insufficiency, hypothyroidism, uncontrolled diabetes mellitus [DM]).
Parenteral chromosome abnormalities.
Maternal infections (cervical mycoplasma, ureaplasma, chlamydia).
DES exposure, heavy metal exposure.
Thrombocytosis.
Allogenic immunity, autoimmunity, lupus anticoagulant.

ACHES AND PAINS, DIFFUSE[24]
ICD-9CM # 719.49

Postviral arthralgias/myalgias.
Bilateral soft tissue rheumatism.
Overuse syndromes.
Fibrositis.
Hypothyroidism.
Metabolic bone disease.
Paraneoplastic syndrome.
Myopathy (polymyositis, dermatomyositis).
Rheumatoid arthritis (RA).
Sjögren's syndrome.
Polymyalgia rheumatica.
Hypermobility.

Benign arthralgias/myalgias.
Chronic fatigue syndrome.
Hypophosphatemia.

ACIDOSIS, LACTIC
ICD-9CM # 276.2

TISSUE HYPOXIA
Shock (hypovolemic, cardiogenic, endotoxic).
Respiratory failure (asphyxia).
Severe CHF.
Severe anemia.
Carbon monoxide or cyanide poisoning.

ASSOCIATED WITH SYSTEMIC DISORDERS
Neoplastic diseases (e.g., leukemia, lymphoma).
Liver or renal failure.
Sepsis.
DM.
Seizure activity.
Abnormal intestinal flora.
Alkalosis.
HIV.

SECONDARY TO DRUGS OR TOXINS
Salicylates.
Ethanol, methanol, ethylene glycol.
Fructose or sorbitol.
Biguanides (phenformin, metformin [usually occurring in patients with renal insufficiency]).
Isoniazid.
Streptozocin.
Nucleoside reverse transcriptase inhibitors (zidovudine, didanosine, stavudine).

HEREDITARY DISORDERS
G6PD deficiency and others.

ACIDOSIS, METABOLIC
ICD-9CM # 276.2

METABOLIC ACIDOSIS WITH INCREASED AG (AG ACIDOSIS)
Lactic acidosis.
Ketoacidosis (DM, alcoholic ketoacidosis).
Uremia (chronic renal failure).
Ingestion of toxins (paraldehyde, methanol, salicylate, ethylene glycol).
High-fat diet (mild acidosis).

METABOLIC ACIDOSIS WITH NORMAL AG (HYPERCHLOREMIC ACIDOSIS)
Renal tubular acidosis (including acidosis of aldosterone deficiency).
Intestinal loss of HCO_3^- (diarrhea, pancreatic fistula).
Carbonic anhydrase inhibitors (e.g., acetazolamide).
Dilutional acidosis (as a result of rapid infusion of bicarbonate-free isotonic saline).
Ingestion of exogenous acids (ammonium chloride, methionine, cystine, calcium chloride).
Ileostomy.
Ureterosigmoidostomy.

Drugs: amiloride, triamterene, spironolactone, β-blockers.

ACIDOSIS, RESPIRATORY
ICD-9CM # 276.2

Pulmonary disease (COPD, severe pneumonia, pulmonary edema, interstitial fibrosis).
Airway obstruction (foreign body, severe bronchospasm, laryngospasm).
Thoracic cage disorders (pneumothorax, flail chest, kyphoscoliosis).
Defects in muscles of respiration (myasthenia gravis, hypokalemia, muscular dystrophy).
Defects in peripheral nervous system (amyotrophic lateral sclerosis, poliomyelitis, Guillain-Barré syndrome, botulism, tetanus, organophosphate poisoning, spinal cord injury).
Depression of respiratory center (anesthesia, narcotics, sedatives, vertebral artery embolism or thrombosis, increased intracranial pressure).
Failure of mechanical ventilator.

ACUTE SCROTUM
ICD-9CM # 608.9

Testicular torsion.
Epididymitis.
Testicular neoplasm.
Orchitis.

ADNEXAL MASS[26]
ICD-9CM # varies with specific disorder

Ovary (neoplasm, endometriosis, functional cyst).
Fallopian tube (ectopic pregnancy, neoplasm, tuboovarian abscess, hydrosalpinx, paratubal cyst).
Uterus (fibroid, neoplasm).
Retroperitoneum (neoplasm, abdominal wall hematoma or abscess).
Urinary tract (pelvic kidney, distended bladder, urachal cyst).
Inflammatory bowel disease.
GI tract neoplasm.
Diverticular disease.
Appendicitis.
Bowel loop with feces.

ADRENAL MASSES[36]
ICD-9CM # 194.0 Adrenocortical Carcinoma
255.8 Adrenal Hyperplasia

UNILATERAL ADRENAL MASSES
Functional Lesions
Adrenal adenoma.
Adrenal carcinoma.
Pheochromocytoma.
Primary aldosteronism, adenomatous type.
Nonfunctional Lesions
Incidentaloma of adrenal.
Ganglioneuroma.
Myelolipoma.
Hematoma.
Adenolipoma.
Metastasis.

BILATERAL ADRENAL MASSES
Functional Lesions
ACTH-dependent Cushing's syndrome.
Congenital adrenal hyperplasia.
Pheochromocytoma.
Conn's syndrome, hyperplastic variety.
Micronodular adrenal disease.
Idiopathic bilateral adrenal hypertrophy.
Nonfunctional Lesions
Infection (tuberculosis, fungi).
Infiltration (leukemia, lymphoma).
Replacement (amyloidosis).
Hemorrhage.
Bilateral metastases.

ADRENOCORTICAL HYPERFUNCTION[1]
ICD-9CM # 255.1

SYNDROMES OF ADRENOCORTICAL HYPERFUNCTION
States of Glucocorticoid Excess
Physiologic states
Stress.
Strenuous exercise.
Last trimester of pregnancy.
Pathologic states
Psychiatric conditions (pseudo-Cushing's disorders).
 Depression.
 Alcoholism.
 Anorexia nervosa.
 Panic disorders.
 Alcohol and drug withdrawal.
ACTH-dependent states.
 Pituitary adenoma (Cushing's disease).
 Ectopic ACTH syndrome.
 • Bronchial carcinoid.
 • Thymic carcinoid.
 • Islet cell tumor.
 • Small cell lung carcinoma.
 Ectopic CRH secretion.
ACTH-independent states.
 Adrenal adenoma.
 Adrenal carcinoma.
 Micronodular adrenal disease.
Exogenous sources
Glucocorticoid intake.
ACTH intake.
States of Mineralocorticoid Excess
Primary aldosteronism
Aldosterone-secreting adenoma.
Bilateral adrenal hyperplasia.
Aldosterone-secreting carcinoma.
Glucocorticoid-suppressible hyperaldosteronism.
Adrenal Enzyme Deficiencies
11β-hydroxylase deficiency.
17α-hydroxylase deficiency.
11β-hydroxysteroid dehydrogenase, type II.
Exogenous Mineralocorticoids
Licorice.
Carbenoxolone.
Fludrocortisone.

Secondary hyperaldosteronism
Associated with hypertension.
 Accelerated hypertension.
 Renovascular hypertension.
 Estrogen administration.
 Renin-secreting tumors.
Without hypertension.
 Bartter syndrome.
 Sodium-wasting nephropathy.
 Renal tubular acidosis.
 Diuretic and laxative abuse.
 Edematous states (cirrhosis, nephrosis, congestive heart failure).

ACTH, Adrenocorticotropin hormone; *CRH,* corticotropin-releasing hormone.

ADRENOCORTICAL HYPOFUNCTION
ICD-9CM # 255.4

SYNDROMES OF ADRENOCORTICAL HYPOFUNCTION
Primary Adrenal Disorders
Combined glucocorticoid and mineralocorticoid deficiency
Autoimmune:
 Isolated autoimmune disease (Addison disease).
 Polyglandular autoimmune syndrome, type I.
 Polyglandular autoimmune syndrome, type II.
Infectious:
 Tuberculosis.
 Fungal.
 Cytomegalovirus.
 Human immunodeficiency virus.
Vascular:
 Bilateral adrenal hemorrhage.
 Sepsis.
 Coagulopathy.
 Thrombosis; embolism.
 Adrenal infarction.
Infiltration:
 Metastatic carcinoma and lymphoma.
 Sarcoidosis.
 Amyloidosis.
 Hemochromatosis.
Congenital:
 Congenital adrenal hyperplasia.
 • 21-hydroxylase deficiency.
 • 3β-ol dehydrogenase deficiency.
 • 20,22-desmolase deficiency.
 Adrenal unresponsiveness to ACTH.
 Congenital adrenal hypoplasia.
 Adrenoleukodystrophy.
 Adrenomyeloneuropathy.
Iatrogenic
Bilateral adrenalectomy.
Drugs: metyrapone, aminoglutethimide, trilostane, ketoconazole, o,p′-DDD, mifepristone.
Mineralocorticoid deficiency without glucocorticoid deficiency:
Corticosterone methyl oxidase deficiency.
Isolated zona glomerulosa defect.
Heparin therapy.
Critical illness.
Converting-enzyme inhibitors.

Secondary Adrenal Disorders
Secondary adrenal insufficiency
Hypothalamic-pituitary dysfunction.
Exogenous glucocorticoids.
After removal of an ACTH-secreting tumor.
Hyporeninemic Hypoaldosteronism
Diabetic nephropathy.
Tubulointerstitial diseases.
Obstructive uropathy.
Autonomic neuropathy.
Nonsteroidal anti-inflammatory drugs.
β-Adrenergic drugs.

ACTH, Adrenocorticotropic hormone.

ADYNAMIC ILEUS[26]
ICD-9CM # 560.1

Abdominal trauma.
Infection (retroperitoneal, pelvic, intrathoracic).
Laparotomy.
Metabolic disease (hypokalemia).
Renal colic.
Skeletal injury (rib fracture, vertebral fracture).
Medications (e.g., narcotics).

AEROPHAGIA (BELCHING, ERUCTATION)
ICD-9CM # 787.3

Anxiety disorders.
Rapid food ingestion.
Carbonated beverages.
Nursing infants (especially when nursing in horizontal position).
Eating or drinking in supine position.
Gum chewing.
Poorly fitting dentures, orthodontic appliances.
Hiatal hernia, gastritis, nonulcer dyspepsia.
Cholelithiasis, cholecystitis.
Ingestion of legumes, onions, peppers.

AIR-SPACE OPACIFICATION ON X-RAY[16a]
ICD-9CM # varies with specific diagnosis

CAUSES OF AIR-SPACE OPACIFICATION
Edema
Cardiogenic.
Non-cardiogenic.
Inflammation/Infection
Wegener's granulomatosis.
Cryptogenic organizing pneumonia.
Blood
Idiopathic pulmonary haemosiderosis.
Antibasement membrane antibody disease.
Systemic lupus erythematosus.
Miscellaneous Causes
Eosinophilic pneumonia.
Alveolar proteinosis.
Alveolar cell carcinoma.
Alveolar microlithiasis.
Lymphoma (MALToma).
Sarcoidosis.

AIRWAY OBSTRUCTION, PEDIATRIC AGE[19]

ICD-9CM # 496	Obstruction Due to Bronchospasm
934.9	Obstruction Due to Foreign Body
478.75	Obstruction Due to Laryngospasm
506.9	Obstruction Due to Inhalation of Fumes or Vapors

CONGENITAL CAUSES

Craniofacial dysmorphism.
Hemangioma.
Laryngeal cleft/web.
Laryngoceles, cysts.
Laryngomalacia.
Macroglossia.
Tracheal stenosis.
Vascular ring.
Vocal cord paralysis.

ACQUIRED INFECTIOUS CAUSES

Acute laryngotracheobronchitis.
Epiglottitis.
Laryngeal papillomatosis.
Membranous croup (bacterial tracheitis).
Mononucleosis.
Retropharyngeal abscess.
Spasmodic croup.
Diphtheria.

ACQUIRED NONINFECTIOUS CAUSES

Anaphylaxis.
Foreign body aspiration.
Supraglottic hypotonia.
Thermal/chemical burn.
Trauma.
Vocal cord paralysis.
Angioneurotic edema.

AKINETIC/RIGID SYNDROME[1]

ICD-9CM # code not available

Parkinsonism (idiopathic, drug-induced).
Catatonia (psychosis).
Progressive supranuclear palsy.
Multisystem atrophy (Shy-Drager syndrome, olivopontocerebellar atrophy).
Diffuse Lewy-body disease.
Toxins (MPTP, manganese, carbon monoxide).
Huntington's disease and other hereditary neurodegenerative disorders.

ALKALOSIS, METABOLIC

ICD-9CM # 276.3

CHLORIDE-RESPONSIVE

Vomiting.
Nasogastric (NG) suction.
Diuretics.
Posthypercapnic alkalosis.
Stool losses (laxative abuse, cystic fibrosis, villous adenoma).

Massive blood transfusion.
Exogenous alkali administration.

CHLORIDE-RESISTANT

Hyperadrenocorticoid states (Cushing's syndrome, primary hyperaldosteronism, secondary mineralocorticoidism [licorice, chewing tobacco]).
Hypomagnesemia.
Hypokalemia.
Bartter's syndrome.

ALKALOSIS, RESPIRATORY

ICD-9CM # 276.3

Hypoxemia (pneumonia, pulmonary embolism, atelectasis, high-altitude living).
Drugs (salicylates, xanthenes, progesterone, epinephrine, thyroxine, nicotine).
Central nervous system (CNS) disorders (tumor, cerebrovascular accident [CVA], trauma, infections).
Psychogenic hyperventilation (anxiety, hysteria).
Hepatic encephalopathy.
Gram-negative sepsis.
Hyponatremia.
Sudden recovery from metabolic acidosis.
Assisted ventilation.

ALOPECIA[14,28]

ICD-9CM # 704.00	Alopecia NOS
704.01	Alopecia, Androgenic
704.01	Alopecia Areata
757.4	Alopecia, Congenital
316	Alopecia, Psychogenic

SCARRING ALOPECIA

Congenital (aplasia cutis).
Tinea capitis with inflammation (kerion).
Bacterial folliculitis.
Discoid lupus erythematosus.
Lichen planopilaris.
Folliculitis decalvans.
Neoplasm.
Trauma.

NONSCARRING ALOPECIA

Cosmetic treatment.
Tinea capitis.
Structural hair shaft disease.
Trichotillomania (hair pulling).
Anagen arrest.
Telogen arrest.
Alopecia areata.
Androgenetic alopecia.

ALVEOLAR CONSOLIDATION

ICD-9CM # 514

Infection.
Neoplasm (bronchoalveolar carcinoma, lymphoma).
Aspiration.
Trauma.
Hemorrhage (Wegener's Goodpasture, bleeding diathesis).
ARDS.
CHF.

Renal failure.
Eosinophilic pneumonia.
Bronchiolitis obliterans.
Pulmonary alveolar proteinosis.

ALVEOLAR HEMORRHAGE[28]

ICD-9CM # 770.3

Hematologic disorders (coagulopathies, thrombocytopenia).
Goodpasture syndrome (anti–basement-membrane antibody disease).
Wegener's vasculitis.
Immune complex–mediated vasculitis.
Idiopathic pulmonary hemosiderosis.
Drugs (penicillamine).
Lymphangiogram contrast.
Mitral stenosis.

AMENORRHEA

ICD-9CM # 626.0

PREGNANCY

EARLY MENOPAUSE

HYPOTHALAMIC DYSFUNCTION: defective synthesis or release of LHRH, anorexia nervosa, stress, exercise.
PITUITARY DYSFUNCTION: neoplasm, postpartum hemorrhage, surgery, radiotherapy.
OVARIAN DYSFUNCTION: gonadal dysgenesis, 17-α-hydroxylase deficiency, premature ovarian failure, polycystic ovarian disease, gonadal stromal tumors.

UTEROVAGINAL ABNORMALITIES

Congenital: imperforate hymen, imperforate cervix, imperforate or absent vagina, Müllerian agenesis.
Acquired: destruction of endometrium with curettage (Asherman's syndrome), closure of cervix or vagina caused by traumatic injury, hysterectomy.

OTHER

Metabolic diseases (liver, kidney), malnutrition, rapid weight loss, exogenous obesity, endocrine abnormalities (Cushing's syndrome, Graves' disease, hypothyroidism).

AMNESIA

ICD-9CM # 292.83	Drug Induced
300.12	Hysterical
780.9	Retrograde
437.7	Transient Global

Degenerative diseases (e.g., Alzheimer's, Huntington's disease).
CVA (especially when involving thalamus, basal forebrain, and hippocampus).
Head trauma.
Postsurgical (e.g., mammillary body surgery, bilateral temporal lobectomy).
Infections (herpes simplex encephalitis, meningitis).
Wernicke-Korsakoff syndrome.
Cerebral hypoxia.
Hypoglycemia.

Differential Diagnosis

II

CNS neoplasms.
Creutzfeldt-Jakob disease.
Medications (e.g., midazolam and other benzo-diazepines).
Psychosis.
Malingering.

AMNIONIC FLUID ALPHA-FETOPROTEIN ELEVATION[16a]

ICD-9CM # V28.1

CAUSES OF ELEVATED AMNIOTIC FLUID α-FETOPROTEIN

Craniospinal defect (open neural tube defect).
Omphalocele.
Gastroschisis.
Duodenal atresia.
Congenital nephrosis.
Cystic hygroma.
Unbalanced D/G dislocation.
Down, Tay–Sachs, Klinefelter's, Turner's syndromes.
Fetal tumors.
Epidermolysis bullosa.
Pilonidal sinus.
Rhesus disease.
Fetal demise.
Incorrect dates.
Multiple pregnancy.

ANAL ABSCESS AND FISTULA[38]

ICD-9CM # 566

Primary anal gland infection.
Secondary abscess:
    Inflammatory bowel disease:
      • Crohn's disease.
      • Ulcerative colitis.
    Infection:
      • Tuberculosis.
      • Actinomycosis.
      • Threadworm.
    Trauma.
    Leucopenia.
    Immunosuppression:
      • HIV.
      • Drugs.
    Rectal cancer.
    Diabetes mellitus.

ANAL INCONTINENCE[26]

ICD-9CM # 787.6

TRAUMATIC

Nerve injured in surgery.
Spinal cord injury.
Obstetric trauma.
Sphincter injury.

NEUROLOGIC

Spinal cord lesions.
Dementia.
Autonomic neuropathy (e.g., DM).
Obstetrics: pudendal nerve stretched during surgery.
Hirschsprung's disease.

MASS EFFECT

Carcinoma of anal canal.
Carcinoma of rectum.
Foreign body.
Fecal impaction.
Hemorrhoids.

MEDICAL

Procidentia.
Inflammatory disease.
Diarrhea.
Laxative abuse.

PEDIATRIC

Congenital.
Meningocele.
Myelomeningocele.
Spina bifida.
After corrective surgery for imperforate anus.
Sexual abuse.
Encopresis.

ANAPHYLAXIS[21]

ICD-9CM # 995.0

PULMONARY

Laryngeal edema.
Epiglottitis.
Foreign body aspiration.
Pulmonary embolus.
Asphyxiation.
Hyperventilation.

CARDIOVASCULAR

Myocardial infarction.
Arrhythmia.
Hypovolemic shock.
Cardiac arrest.

CNS

Vasovagal reaction.
CVA.
Seizure disorder.
Drug overdose.

ENDOCRINE

Hypoglycemia.
Pheochromocytoma.
Carcinoid syndrome.
Catamenial (progesterone-induced anaphylaxis).

PSYCHIATRIC

Vocal cord dysfunction syndrome.
Munchausen syndrome.
Panic attack/globus hystericus.

OTHER

Hereditary angioedema.
Cord urticaria.
Idiopathic urticaria.
Mastocytosis.
Serum sickness.
Idiopathic capillary leak syndrome.
Sulfite exposure.
Scombroid poisoning (tuna, blue fish, mackerel).

ANDROGEN EXCESS, REPRODUCTIVE-AGE WOMAN

ICD-9CM # varies with specific disorder

Polycystic ovary syndrome.
Idiopathic.
Medications (e.g., anabolizing agents, testosterone, danazol).
Pregnancy (luteoma, hyperreactio luteinalis).
Sertoli-Leydig ovarian neoplasm.
Adrenal adenoma or hyperplasia.
Cushing's syndrome.
Glucocorticoid resistance.
Hypothyroidism.
Hyperprolactinemia.

ANEMIA, APLASTIC[20]

ICD-9CM # 284

ACQUIRED APLASTIC ANEMIA

Secondary aplastic anemia.
Irradiation.
Drugs and chemicals.
Regular effects.
Cytotoxic agents.
Benzene.
Idiosyncratic reactions.
Chloramphenicol.
Nonsteroidal anti-inflammatory drugs.
Antiepileptics.
Gold.
Other drugs and chemicals.
Viruses.
Epstein-Barr virus (infectious mononucleosis).
Hepatitis virus (non-A, non-B, non-C, non-G hepatitis).
Parvovirus (transient aplastic crisis, some pure red cell aplasia).
Human immunodeficiency virus (acquired immunodeficiency syndrome).
Immune diseases.
Eosinophilic fasciitis.
Hyperimmunoglobulinemia.
Thymoma and thymic carcinoma.
Graft-versus-host disease in immunodeficiency.
Paroxysmal nocturnal hemoglobinuria.
Pregnancy.
Idiopathic aplastic anemia.

INHERITED APLASTIC ANEMIA

Fanconi anemia.
Dyskeratosis congenita.
Shwachman-Diamond syndrome.
Reticular dysgenesis.
Amegakaryocytic thrombocytopenia.
Familial aplastic anemias.
Preleukemia (e.g., monosomy 7).
Nonhematologic syndromes (e.g., Down, Dubowitz, Seckel).

ANEMIA, APLASTIC, DUE TO DRUGS AND CHEMICALS[1]

ICD-9CM # 284.89

Agents that regularly produce marrow depression as a major toxic effect when used in commonly employed doses or normal exposures:

Cytotoxic drugs used in cancer chemotherapy.
Alkylating agents (busulfan, melphalan, cyclophosphamide).
Antimetabolites (antifolic compounds, nucleotide analogs), antimitotics (vincristine, vinblastine, colchicine).
Some antibiotics (daunorubicin, doxorubicin [Adriamycin]).
Benzene (and less often benzene-containing chemicals; kerosene, carbon tetrachloride, Stoddard solvent, chlorophenols).

Agents probably associated with aplastic anemia but with a relatively low probability relative to their use:

Chloramphenicol.
Insecticides.
Antiprotozoals (quinacrine and chloroquine).
Nonsteroidal anti-inflammatory drugs (including phenylbutazone, indomethacin, ibuprofen, sulindac, diclofenac, naproxen, piroxicam, fenoprofen, fenbufen, aspirin).
Anticonvulsants (hydantoins, carbamazepine, phenacemide, ethosuximide).
Gold, arsenic, and other heavy metals such as bismuth and mercury.
Sulfonamides as a class.
Antithyroid medications (methimazole, methylthiouracil, propylthiouracil).
Antidiabetes drugs (tolbutamide, carbutamide, chlorpropamide).
Carbonic anhydrase inhibitors (acetazolamide, methazolamide, mesalazine).
D-Penicillamine.
2-Chlorodeoxyadenosine.

Agents more rarely associated with aplastic anemia:

Antibiotics (streptomycin, tetracycline, methicillin, ampicillin, mebendazole and albendazole, sulfonamides, flucytosine, mefloquine, dapsone).
Antihistamines (cimetidine, ranitidine, chlorpheniramine).
Sedatives and tranquilizers (chlorpromazine, prochlorperazine, piperacetazine, chlordiazepoxide, meprobamate, methyprylon, remoxipride).
Antiarrhythmics (tocainide, amiodarone).
Allopurinol (can potentiate marrow suppression by cytotoxic drugs).
Ticlopidine.
Methyldopa.
Quinidine.
Lithium.
Guanidine.
Canthaxanthin.
Thiocyanate.
Carbimazole.
Cyanamide.
Deferoxamine.
Amphetamines.

ANEMIA, DRUG-INDUCED[17]

ICD-9CM # 283.0

DRUGS THAT MAY INTERFERE WITH RED CELL PRODUCTION BY INDUCING MARROW SUPPRESSION OR APLASIA

Alcohol.
Antineoplastic drugs.
Antithyroid drugs.
Antibiotics.
Oral hypoglycemic agents.
Phenylbutazone.
Azidothymidine (AZT).

DRUGS THAT INTERFERE WITH VITAMIN B_{12}, FOLATE, OR IRON ABSORPTION OR UTILIZATION

Nitrous oxide.
Anticonvulsant drugs.
Antineoplastic drugs.
Isoniazid, cycloserine A.

DRUGS CAPABLE OF PROMOTING HEMOLYSIS

Immune Mediated
Penicillins.
Quinine.
Alpha-methyldopa.
Procainamide.
Mitomycin C.
Oxidative Stress
Antimalarials.
Sulfonamide drugs.
Nalidixic acid.

DRUGS THAT MAY PRODUCE OR PROMOTE BLOOD LOSS

Aspirin.
Alcohol.
Nonsteroidal anti-inflammatory agents.
Corticosteroids.
Anticoagulants.

ANEMIA, HYPOCHROMIC[20]

ICD-9CM # varies with specific diagnosis
280.9 Iron deficiency
285.0 Sideroblastic

DECREASED BODY IRON STORES

Iron-deficiency anemia.

NORMAL OR INCREASED BODY IRON STORES

Impaired iron metabolism.
Anemia of chronic disease.
Defective absorption, transport, or use of iron.
Disorders of globin synthesis:
• Thalassemia.
• Other microcytic hemoglobinopathies.
Disorders of heme synthesis: sideroblastic anemias:
• Hereditary.
• Acquired.

ANEMIA, LOW RETICULOCYTE COUNT[1]

ICD-9CM # 285.9

MICROCYTIC ANEMIA (MCV <80)

Iron deficiency.
Thalassemia minor.
Sideroblastic anemia.
Lead poisoning.

MACROCYTIC ANEMIA (MCV >100)

Megaloblastic anemias.
Folate deficiency.
Vitamin B_{12} deficiency.
Drug-induced megaloblastic anemia.
Nonmegaloblastic macrocytosis.
Liver disease.
Hypothyroidism.

NORMOCYTIC ANEMIA (MCV 80-100)

Early iron deficiency.
Aplastic anemia.
Myelophthisic disorders.
Endocrinopathies.
Anemia of chronic disease.
Uremia.
Mixed nutritional deficiency.

ANEMIA, MEGALOBLASTIC[36]

ICD-9CM # 281.0 Pernicious Anemia
281.1 B_{12} Deficiency
281.2 Folate Deficiency
281.3 B_{12} with Folate Deficiency
281.4 Protein or Amino Acid Deficiency
281.8 Nutritional
281.9 NOS

COBALAMIN (CBL) DEFICIENCY

NUTRITIONAL CBL DEFICIENCY (INSUFFICIENT CBL INTAKE): vegetarians, vegans, breastfed infants of mothers with pernicious anemia.
ABNORMAL INTRAGASTRIC EVENTS (INADEQUATE PROTEOLYSIS OF FOOD CBL): atrophic gastritis, partial gastrectomy with hypochlorhydria.
LOSS/ATROPHY OF GASTRIC OXYNTIC MUCOSA (DEFICIENT IF MOLECULES): total or partial gastrectomy, pernicious anemia (PA), caustic destruction (lye).
ABNORMAL EVENTS IN SMALL BOWEL LUMEN:
Inadequate pancreatic protease (R-CBL not degraded, CBL not transferred to IF).
• Insufficiency of pancreatic protease—pancreatic insufficiency.
• Inactivation of pancreatic protease—Zollinger-Ellison syndrome.
Usurping of luminal CBL (inadequate CBL binding to IF).
• By bacteria—stasis syndromes (blind loops, pouches of diverticulosis, strictures, fistulas, anastomoses); impaired bowel

motility (scleroderma, pseudoobstruction), hypogammaglobulinemia.
- By *Diphyllobothrium latum.*

DISORDERS OF ILEAL MUCOSA/IF RECEPTORS (IF-CBL NOT BOUND TO IF RECEPTORS):

Diminished or absent IF receptors—ileal bypass/resection/fistula.

Abnormal mucosal architecture/function—tropical/nontropical sprue, Crohn's disease, TB ileitis, infiltration by lymphomas, amyloidosis.

IF-/post IF-receptor defects—Imerslund-Graesbeck syndrome, TC II deficiency.

Drug-induced effects (slow K, biguanides, cholestyramine, colchicine, neomycin, PAS).

DISORDERS OF PLASMA CBL TRANSPORT (TC II-CBL NOT DELIVERED TO TC II RECEPTORS)

Congenital TC II deficiency, defective binding of TC II-CBL to TC II receptors (rare).

METABOLIC DISORDERS (CBL NOT UTILIZED BY CELL)

Inborn enzyme errors (rare).

Acquired disorders: (CBL oxidized to cob[III]alamin)—N_2O inhalation.

FOLATE DEFICIENCY

Nutritional Causes

Decreased dietary intake—poverty and famine (associated with kwashiorkor, marasmus), institutionalized individuals (psychiatric/nursing homes), chronic debilitating disease/goats' milk (low in folate), special diets (slimming), cultural/ethnic cooking techniques (food folate destroyed) or habits (folate-rich foods not consumed).

Decreased diet and increased requirements:
- Physiologic: pregnancy and lactation, prematurity, infancy.
- Pathologic: intrinsic hematologic disease (autoimmune hemolytic disease), drugs, malaria; hemoglobinopathies (SS, thalassemia), RBC membrane defects (hereditary spherocytosis, paroxysmal nocturnal hemoglobinopathy); abnormal hematopoiesis (leukemia/lymphoma, myelodysplastic syndrome, agnogenic myeloid metaplasia with myelofibrosis); infiltration with malignant disease; dermatologic (psoriasis).

Folate Malabsorption

With normal intestinal mucosa:
- Some drugs (controversial).
- Congenital folate malabsorption (rare).

With mucosal abnormalities—tropical and nontropical sprue, regional enteritis.

Defective Cellular Folate Uptake—Familial Aplastic Anemia (Rare) Inadequate Cellular Utilization

Folate antagonists (methotrexate).

Hereditary enzyme deficiencies involving folate.

Drugs (Multiple Effects on Folate Metabolism)

Alcohol, sulfasalazine, triamterene, pyrimethamine, trimethoprim-sulfamethoxazole, diphenylhydantoin, barbiturates.

MISCELLANEOUS MEGALOBLASTIC ANEMIAS (NOT CAUSED BY CBL OR FOLATE DEFICIENCY)

Congenital Disorders of DNA Synthesis (Rare)

Orotic aciduria, Lesch-Nyhan syndrome, congenital dyserythropoietic anemia.

Acquired Disorders of DNA Synthesis

Thiamine-responsive megaloblastosis (rare).

Malignancy—erythroleukemia—refractory sideroblastic anemias—all antineoplastic drugs that inhibit DNA synthesis.

Toxic—alcohol.

ANERGY, CUTANEOUS[36]
ICD-9CM # 279.9

IMMUNOLOGIC

Acquired (AIDS, acute leukemia, carcinoma, CLL, Hodgkin's lymphoma, NHL).

Congenital (ataxia-telangiectasia, Di George's syndrome, severe combined immunodeficiency, Wiskott-Aldrich syndrome).

INFECTIONS

Bacterial (bacterial pneumonia, brucellosis).

Disseminated mycotic infections.

Mycobacterial (lepromatous leprosy, TB).

Viral (varicella, hepatitis, influenza, mononucleosis, measles, mumps).

IMMUNOSUPPRESSIVE MEDICATIONS

Systemic corticosteroids.

Methotrexate, cyclophosphamide.

Rifampin.

OTHER

Alcoholic cirrhosis, biliary cirrhosis, sarcoidosis, rheumatic disease.

Diabetes, Crohn's disease, uremia.

Anemia, pyridoxine deficiency, sickle cell anemia.

Burns, malnutrition, pregnancy, old age, surgery.

ANEURYSMS, THORACIC AORTA
ICD-9CM # 441.2

Trauma.

Infection.

Inflammatory (syphilis, Takayasu's disease).

Collagen vascular disease (RA, ankylosing spondylitis).

Annuloaortic ectasia (Marfan's syndrome, Ehlers-Danlos syndrome).

Congenital.

Coarctation.

Cystic medial necrosis.

ANHYDROSIS
ICD-9CM # 705.1

Drugs (anticholinergics).

Dehydration.

Hysteria.

Obstruction of sweat ducts (e.g., inflammation, miliaria).

Local radiant heat or pressure.

CNS lesions (medulla, hypothalamus, pons).

Spinal cord lesions.

Lesions of sympathetic nerves.

Congenital sweat gland disturbances.

ANION GAP INCREASE
ICD-9CM # 276.9

Uremia.

Ketoacidosis (diabetic, starvation, alcoholic).

Lactic acidosis.

Ethylene glycol poisoning.

Salicylate overdose.

Methanol poisoning.

ANISOCORIA
ICD-9CM # 379.41

Mydriatic or miotic drugs.

Prosthetic eye.

Inflammation (keratitis, iridocyclitis).

Infections (herpes zoster, syphilis, meningitis, encephalitis, TB, diphtheria, botulism).

Subdural hemorrhage.

Cavernous sinus thrombosis.

Intracranial neoplasm.

Cerebral aneurysm.

Glaucoma.

CNS degenerative diseases.

Internal carotid ischemia.

Toxic polyneuritis (alcohol, lead).

Adie's syndrome.

Horner's syndrome.

DM.

Trauma.

Congenital.

ANOREXIA[38]
ICD-9CM # 783.0

SELECTED CAUSES OF ANOREXIA

Gastrointestinal Tract/Liver

Gastric outlet obstruction or small bowel obstruction.

Gastric cancer.

Hepatic metastases.

Acute viral hepatitis.

Metabolic

Addison's disease.

Hypopituitarism.

Hyperparathyroidism.

Functional

Extremely unpleasant sight/smell.

Systemic

Chronic pain.

Renal failure.

Severe congestive heart failure.

Respiratory failure.

Psychiatric

Depression.

Anorexia nervosa.

Medications
Digoxin.
Narcotic analgesics.
Diuretics.
Antihypertensives.
Chemotherapeutic agents.
Amphetamines.

Miscellaneous
Excessive smoking.
Excessive alcohol intake.
Oral cavity disease.
Thiamine deficiency.
Early pregnancy.
Hypogeusia or dysgeusia.

ANOVULATION
ICD-9CM # 628.0

Anorexia and bulimia.
Strenuous exercise.
Weight loss/malnutrition.
Empty sella syndrome.
Pituitary disorders (infarction, infection, trauma, irradiation, surgery, microadenomas, macroadenomas).
Idiopathic hypopituitarism.
Drug induced.
Thyroid dysfunction (hypothyroidism, hyperthyroidism).
Systemic diseases (e.g., liver disease).
Adrenal hyperfunction (Cushing's syndrome, congenital adrenal hyperplasia).
Polycystic ovarian syndrome.
Isolated gonadotropin deficiency.

APPETITE LOSS IN INFANTS AND CHILDREN[19]
ICD-9CM # 783.0   Appetite Loss
            307.59 Appetite Loss,
                   Psychogenic Origin

ORGANIC DISEASE

Infection (Acute or Chronic)
Neurologic
Congenital degenerative disease.
Hypothalamic lesion.
Increased intracranial pressure (including a brain tumor).
Swallowing disorders (neuromuscular).

Gastrointestinal
Oral lesions (e.g., thrush or herpes simplex).
Gastroesophageal reflux.
Obstruction (especially with gastric or intestinal distention).
Inflammatory bowel disease.
Celiac disease.
Constipation.

Cardiac
Congestive heart failure (especially associated with cyanotic lesions).

Metabolic
Renal failure and/or renal tubule acidosis.
Liver failure.
Congenital metabolic disease.
Lead poisoning.

Nutritional
Marasmus.
Iron deficiency.
Zinc deficiency.

Fever
RA.
Rheumatic fever.

Drugs
Morphine.
Digitalis.
Antimetabolites.
Methylphenidate.
Amphetamines.

Miscellaneous
Prolonged restriction of oral feedings, beginning in the neonatal period.
Systemic lupus erythematosus (SLE).
Tumor.

PSYCHOLOGIC FACTORS

Anxiety, fear, depression, mania (limbic influence on the hypothalamus).
Avoidance of symptoms associated with meals (abdominal pain, diarrhea, bloating, urgency, dumping syndrome).
Anorexia nervosa.
Excessive weight loss and food aversion in athletes, simulating anorexia nervosa.

ARTERIAL OCCLUSION[15]
ICD-9CM # 444.22 Arterial Occlusion, Lower
                    Extremities
            444.21 Arterial Occlusion, Upper
                    Extremities

Thromboembolism (post-MI, mitral stenosis, rheumatic valve disease, atrial fibrillation, atrial myxoma, marantic endocarditis, bacterial endocarditis, Libman-Sacks endocarditis).
Atheroembolism (microemboli composed of cholesterol, calcium, and platelets from proximal atherosclerotic plaques).
Arterial thrombosis (endothelial injury, altered arterial blood flow, trauma, severe atherosclerosis, acute vasculitis).
Vasospasm.
Trauma.
Hypercoagulable states.
Miscellaneous (irradiation, drugs, infections, necrotizing).

ARTHRITIS AND ABDOMINAL PAIN
ICD-9CM # varies with specific disorder

Viral syndrome.
Inflammatory bowel disease.
Celiac disease.
Vasculitis.
SLE.
RA.
Scleroderma.
Amyloidosis.
Chronic hepatitis C.
Whipple's disease.
Polyarteritis nodosa.
Behçet's disease.
Familial Mediterranean fever.
Blind loop syndrome.

ARTHRITIS AND DIARRHEA
ICD-9CM # varies with specific disorder

Viral syndrome.
Inflammatory bowel disease.
Celiac disease.
Whipple's disease.
Enterogenic (bacterial) reactive arthritis.
Collagenous colitis.
Behçet's disease.
Hyperthyroidism.
Spondyloarthropathy.
Blind loop syndrome.

ARTHRITIS AND EYE LESIONS[6]
ICD-9CM # varies with specific diagnosis

SLE.
Sjögren's syndrome.
Behçet's syndrome.
Sarcoidosis.
Subacute bacterial endocarditis (SBE).
Lyme disease.
Wegener's granulomatosis.
Giant cell arteritis.
Takayasu's arteritis.
RA, JRA.
Scleroderma.
Inflammatory bowel disease.
Whipple's disease.
Ankylosing spondylitis.
Reactive arthritis.
Psoriatic arthritis.

ARTHRITIS AND HEART MURMUR[6]
ICD-9CM # varies with specific diagnosis

SBE.
Cardiac myxoma.
Ankylosing spondylitis.
Reactive arthritis.
Acute rheumatic fever.
RA.
SLE with Libman-Sacks endocarditis.
Relapsing polychondritis.

ARTHRITIS AND MUSCLE WEAKNESS[8]
ICD-9CM # varies with specific diagnosis

RA.
Ankylosing spondylitis.
Polymyositis.
Dermatomyositis.
SLE, scleroderma, mixed connective tissue disease.
Sarcoidosis.
HIV-associated arthritis.
Whipple's disease.

Differential Diagnosis

ARTHRITIS AND RASH[6]

ICD-9CM # varies with specific diagnosis

Chronic urticaria.
Vasculitic urticaria.
SLE.
Dermatomyositis.
Polymyositis.
Psoriatic arthritis.
Reactive arthritis.
Chronic sarcoidosis.
Serum sickness.
Sweet's syndrome.
Leprosy.

ARTHRITIS AND SUBCUTANEOUS NODULES[6]

ICD-9CM # varies with specific diagnosis

RA.
Gout.
Pseudogout (rare).
Sarcoidosis.
Light chain (LA) amyloidosis (primary, multiple myeloma).
Acute rheumatic fever (ARF).
Hemochromatosis.
Whipple's disease.
Multicentric reticulohistiocytosis.

ARTHRITIS AND WEIGHT LOSS[6]

ICD-9CM # varies with specific diagnosis

Severe RA.
RA with vasculitis.
Reactive arthritis.
RA or psoriatic arthritis or ankylosing spondylitis with amyloidosis.
Cancer.
Enteropathic arthritis (Crohn's, ulcerative colitis).
HIV infection.
Whipple's disease.
Blind loop syndrome.
Scleroderma with intestinal bacterial overgrowth.

ARTHRITIS, AXIAL SKELETON

ICD-9CM # 720.0 Arthritis, Rheumatoid, Spine
696.0 Arthritis, Psoriatic
715.9 Arthritis, Degenerative, NOS
720.0 Ankylosing Spondylitis

RA.
Psoriatic arthritis.
Reiter's syndrome.
Ankylosing spondylitis.
Juvenile RA.
Degenerative disease of the nucleus pulposus.
Spondylosis deformans.
Diffuse idiopathic skeletal hyperostosis (DISH).
Alkaptonuria.
Infection.

ARTHRITIS, FEVER, AND RASH[6]

ICD-9CM # varies with specific diagnosis

Rubella, parvovirus B-19.
Gonococcemia, meningococcemia.
Secondary syphilis, Lyme borreliosis.
Adult acute rheumatic fever, adult Still's disease, adult Kawasaki disease.
Vasculitic urticaria.
Acute sarcoidosis.
Familial Mediterranean fever.
Hyperimmunoglobulinemia D and periodic fever syndrome.

ARTHRITIS, MONOARTICULAR AND OLIGOARTICULAR[2]

ICD-9CM # 715.3 Osteoarthritis, Localized
711.9 Infectious Arthritis
716.6 Monoarticular Arthritis; 5th digit to be added to the above depending on site of arthritis
0. Site Unspecified
1. Shoulder Region
2. Upper Arm
3. Forearm
4. Hand
5. Pelvic Region and Thigh
6. Lower Leg
7. Ankle and/or Foot
8. Other Specified Except Spine

Septic arthritis (*S. aureus, Neisseria gonorrhea, Meningococci, Streptococci, S. pneumoniae*, enteric gram-negative bacilli).
Crystalline-induced arthritis (gout, pseudogout, calcium oxalate, hydroxyapatite and other basic calcium/phosphate crystals).
Traumatic joint injury.
Hemarthrosis.
Monoarticular or oligoarticular flare of an inflammatory polyarticular rheumatic disease (RA, psoriatic arthritis, Reiter's syndrome, SLE).

ARTHRITIS, PEDIATRIC AGE[19]

ICD-9CM # 711.9 Infectious Arthritis
714.30 Juvenile Chronic or Unspecified
714.31 Juvenile Rheumatoid Polyarticular Acute
714.32 Juvenile Rheumatoid Pauciarticular
714.33 Juvenile Rheumatoid Monoarticular

RHEUMATIC DISEASES OF CHILDHOOD

Acute rheumatic fever.
SLE.
Juvenile ankylosing spondylitis.
Polymyositis and dermatomyositis.
Vasculitis.

Scleroderma.
Psoriatic arthritis.
Mixed connective tissue disease and overlap syndromes.
Kawasaki disease.
Behçet's syndrome.
Familial Mediterranean fever.
Reiter's syndrome.
Reflex sympathetic dystrophy.
Fibromyalgia (fibrositis).

INFECTIOUS DISEASES

Bacterial arthritis.
Viral or postviral arthritis.
Fungal arthritis.
Osteomyelitis.
Reactive arthritis.

NEOPLASTIC DISEASES

Leukemia.
Lymphoma.
Neuroblastoma.
Primary bone tumors.

NONINFLAMMATORY DISORDERS

Trauma.
Avascular necrosis syndromes.
Osteochondroses.
Slipped capital femoral epiphysis.
Diskitis.
Patellofemoral dysfunction (chondromalacia patellae).
Toxic synovitis of the hip.
Overuse syndromes.

GENETIC OR CONGENITAL SYNDROMES

Hematologic Disorders
Sickle cell disease.
Hemophilia.

INFLAMMATORY BOWEL DISEASE

Miscellaneous
Growing pains.
Psychogenic arthralgias (conversion reactions).
Hypermobility syndrome.
Villonodular synovitis.
Foreign body arthritis.

ARTHRITIS, POLYARTICULAR

ICD-9CM # 715.09 Generalized Osteoarthritis, Multiple Sites
716.89 Arthritis, Multiple Sites
714.31 Juvenile Rheumatoid, Polyarticular, Acute

RA, juvenile (rheumatoid) polyarthritis.
SLE, other connective tissue diseases, erythema nodosum, palindromic rheumatism, relapsing polychondritis.
Psoriatic arthritis, ankylosing spondylitis.
Sarcoidosis.
Lyme arthritis, bacterial endocarditis, *Neisseria gonorrhoeae* infection, rheumatic fever, Reiter's disease.
Crystal deposition disease.
Hypersensitivity to serum or drugs.

Hepatitis B, HIV, rubella, mumps.
Other: serum sickness, leukemias, lymphomas, enteropathic arthropathy, Whipple's disease, Behçet's syndrome, Henoch-Schönlein purpura, familial Mediterranean fever, hypertrophic pulmonary osteoarthropathy.

ASCITES

ICD-9CM # 789.5 Ascites NOS
197.6 Ascites, Cancerous (Malignant)
457.8 Ascites, Chylous

Hypoalbuminemia: nephrotic syndrome, protein-losing gastroenteropathy, starvation.
Cirrhosis.
Hepatic congestion: CHF, constrictive pericarditis, tricuspid insufficiency, hepatic vein obstruction (Budd-Chiari syndrome), inferior vena cava or portal vein obstruction.
Peritoneal infections: TB and other bacterial infections, fungal diseases, parasites.
Neoplasms: primary hepatic neoplasms, metastases to liver or peritoneum, lymphomas, leukemias, myeloid metaplasia.
Lymphatic obstruction: mediastinal tumors, trauma to the thoracic duct, filariasis.
Ovarian disease: Meigs' syndrome, struma ovarii.
Chronic pancreatitis or pseudocyst: pancreatic ascites.
Leakage of bile: bile ascites.
Urinary obstruction or trauma: urine ascites.
Myxedema.
Chylous ascites.

ASTHENIA

ICD-9CM # 780.79

Depression.
Chronic fatigue syndrome.
Sleep disorders.
Anemia.
Hypothyroidism.
Sedentary lifestyle.
Medications (e.g., narcotics, sedatives).
Infections.
Dehydration/electrolyte disorders.
COPD and other pulmonary disorders.
Renal failure.
CHF.
Diabetes.
Addison's disease.
Paraneoplastic syndrome.

ASTHMA, CHILDHOOD[4]

ICD-9CM # 493.0 use 5th digit
0. Without Mention of Status Asthmaticus
1. With Status Asthmaticus

INFECTIONS

Bronchiolitis (RSV).
Pneumonia.
Croup.
Tuberculosis, histoplasmosis.
Bronchiectasis.
Bronchiolitis obliterans.

Bronchitis.
Sinusitis.

ANATOMIC, CONGENITAL

Cystic fibrosis.
Vascular rings.
Ciliary dyskinesia.
B-lymphocyte immune defect.
Congestive heart failure.
Laryngotracheomalacia.
Tumor, lymphoma.
H-type tracheoesophageal fistula.
Repaired tracheoesophageal fistula.
Gastroesophageal reflux.

VASCULITIS, HYPERSENSITIVITY

Allergic bronchopulmonary aspergillosis.
Allergic alveolitis, hypersensitivity pneumonitis.
Churg-Strauss syndrome.
Periarteritis nodosa.

OTHER

Foreign body aspiration.
Pulmonary thromboembolism.
Psychogenic cough.
Sarcoidosis.
Bronchopulmonary dysplasia.
Vocal cord dysfunction.

ATAXIA

ICD-9CM # 781.3 Ataxia NOS
303.0 Alcoholic, Acute
303.9 Alcoholic, Chronic
334.3 Cerebellar
331.89 Cerebral
334.0 Friedreich's
300.11 Hysterical

Vertebral-basilar artery ischemia.
Diabetic neuropathy.
Tabes dorsalis.
Vitamin B_{12} deficiency.
Multiple sclerosis and other demyelinating diseases.
Meningomyelopathy.
Cerebellar neoplasms, hemorrhage, abscess, infarct.
Nutritional (Wernicke's encephalopathy).
Paraneoplastic syndromes.
Parainfectious: Guillain-Barré syndrome, acute ataxia of childhood and young adults.
Toxins: phenytoin, alcohol, sedatives, organophosphates.
Wilson's disease (hepatolenticular degeneration).
Hypothyroidism.
Myopathy.
Cerebellar and spinocerebellar degeneration: ataxia/telangiectasia, Friedreich's ataxia.
Frontal lobe lesions: tumors, thrombosis of anterior cerebral artery, hydrocephalus.
Labyrinthine destruction: neoplasm, injury, inflammation, compression.
Hysteria.
AIDS.

ATAXIA, ACUTE OR RECURRENT[11]

ICD-9CM # varies with specific diagnosis
781.3 Ataxia NOS
0.94 Locomotor ataxia
334.0 Friedreich's ataxia
334.2 Cerebellar ataxia, primary
334.3 Other cerebellar ataxia
334.8 Ataxia-telangiectasia

Drug ingestion (e.g., phenytoin, carbamazepine, sedatives, hypnotics, and phencyclidine) or intoxication (e.g., alcohol, ethylene glycol, hydrocarbon fumes, lead, mercury, or thallium).
Postinfectious (cerebellitis [e.g., varicella], acute disseminated encephalomyelitis).
Head trauma.
Basilar migraine.
Benign paroxysmal vertigo (migraine equivalent).
Brain tumor or neuroblastoma (if accompanied by opsoclonus or myoclonus [i.e., "dancing eyes, dancing feet"]).
Hydrocephalus.
Infection (e.g., labyrinthitis, abscess).
Seizure (ictal or postictal).
Vascular events (e.g., cerebellar hemorrhage or stroke).
Miller-Fisher variant of Guillain-Barré syndrome (ataxia, ophthalmoplegia, and areflexia). Warning: If bulbar signs present, disease is likely progressive; patient may lose ability to protect airway and/or ability to breathe.
Inherited ataxias.
Inborn errors of metabolism (e.g., mitochondrial disorders, amino-acidopathies, urea cycle defects).
Conversion reaction.
Multiple sclerosis.

ATAXIA, CEREBELLAR, ADULT ONSET[34a]

ICD-9CM # 334.2

CAUSES OF ADULT ONSET CEREBELLAR ATAXIA

Inherited
Later onset SCA syndromes.
Rarely Friedreich's ataxia.
Congenital
Arnold–Chiari malformation (cerebellar ectopia).
Inflammatory
Multiple sclerosis.
Sarcoidosis.
Infections (TB, viral).
Neoplastic
Often metastatic in adults.
Meningioma, neurofibroma.
Haemangioblastoma.
Paraneoplastic
Usually with small-cell bronchial carcinoma.
Vascular
Infarction, hemorrhage.
Arteriovenous malformations.

Trauma
Head injury.
Postsurgical.
Toxic
Alcohol, phenytoin, solvent abuse.
Endocrine
Hypothyroidism (very rare).
Degenerative
Multiple system atrophy (MSA).

ATAXIA, CEREBELLAR, CHILDREN[34a]

ICD-9CM # 334.2

CAUSES OF CEREBELLAR ATAXIA IN CHILDREN

Congenital Malformations
Cerebellar agenesis/hypoplasia.
Dandy–Walker syndrome.*
Arnold–Chiari malformation.**
Hereditary Ataxias
Friedreich's ataxia.
Trauma
Birth trauma.*
Head injury in childhood.*
Infectious
Secondary to bacterial meningitis.
Secondary to encephalitis.
Hydrocephalus*
Tumors
Medulloblastoma.
Astrocytoma.
Haemangioblastoma.

*May persist into adult life.
**May present in adult life.

ATAXIA, CHRONIC OR PROGRESSIVE[11]

ICD-9CM # varies with specific diagnosis
781.3   Ataxia NOS
0.94   Locomotor ataxia
334.0   Friedreich's ataxia
334.2   Cerebellar ataxia, primary
334.3   Other cerebellar ataxia
334.8   Ataxia-telangiectasia

Hydrocephalus.
Hypothyroidism.
Tumor or paraneoplastic syndrome.
Low vitamin E levels (e.g., cystic fibrosis).
Wilson disease.
Inborn errors of metabolism.
Inherited ataxias (e.g., ataxia-telangiectasia, Friedreich's ataxia).

ATELECTASIS

ICD-9CM # 518.0

Lung neoplasm (primary or metastatic).
Infection (pneumonia, TB, fungal, histoplasmosis).
Postoperative (lower lobes).
Sarcoidosis.
Mucoid impaction.
Foreign body.
Postinflammatory (middle lobe syndrome).

Pneumothorax.
Pleural effusion.
Pneumoconiosis.
Interstitial fibrosis.
Bulla.
Mediastinal or adjacent mass.

ATRIAL ENLARGEMENT, LEFT ATRIUM[16a]

ICD-9CM # varies with specific diagnosis

CAUSES OF LARGE LEFT ATRIUM

Causes Due to Volume Overload
Mitral regurgitation (often with left ventricular failure).
Ventricular septal defect.
Patent ductus arteriosus.
Atrial septal defect with shunt reversal (i.e., pulmonary hypertension).
ASD with tricuspid atresia (obligatory shunt reversal).
Aortopulmonary window.
Causes Due to Pressure Overload
Mitral stenosis.
Noncompliant left ventricle: hypertension, hypertrophic cardiomyopathy, aortic stenosis.
Left ventricular failure (often with secondary mitral regurgitation).
Left atrial myxoma.
Other Causes (Both Rare)
Atrial fibrillation.
Isolated/idiopathic.

ATRIUM ENLARGEMENT, RIGHT ATRIUM

ICD-9CM # varies with specific disorder

Right ventricular failure.
Atrial septal defect.
Tricuspid regurgitation.
Tricuspid stenosis.
Pulmonary hypertension.
Restrictive cardiomyopathy.
Right atrial myxoma.
Ebstein's anomaly.
Anomalous pulmonary venous drainage to the right atrium.
Endomyocardial fibrosis.
Sinus of Valsalva fistula.
Arrhythmogenic right ventricular dysplasia.

ATYPICAL LYMPHOCYTOSIS, HETEROPHIL NEGATIVE, INFECTIOUS CAUSES[1]

ICD-9CM # 288.61

MOST COMMON INFECTIOUS CAUSES OF HETEROPHIL-NEGATIVE ATYPICAL LYMPHOCYTOSIS

Babesiosis.
Chickenpox.
Cytomegalovirus.
Epstein-Barr virus (particularly in children).
Human herpesvirus 6.

Human immunodeficiency virus (especially during acute seroconversion).
Infectious mononucleosis.
Malaria.
Measles.
Toxoplasmosis.
Varicella.
Infectious hepatitis.

AV NODAL BLOCK[15]

ICD-9CM # 426.10 AV Block (Incomplete, Partial)
426.0   AV Block, Complete

Idiopathic fibrosis (Lenègre's disease).
Sclerodegenerative processes (e.g., Lev's disease with calcification of the mitral and aortic annuli).
AV node radiofrequency ablation procedure.
Medications (e.g., digoxin, beta-blockers, calcium channel blockers, class III antiarrhythmics).
Acute inferior wall MI.
Myocarditis.
Infections (endocarditis, Lyme disease).
Infiltrative diseases (e.g., hemochromatosis, sarcoidosis, amyloidosis).
Trauma (including cardiac surgical procedures).
Collagen vascular diseases.
Aortic root diseases (e.g., spondylitis).
Electrolyte abnormalities (e.g., hyperkalemia).

BACK PAIN

ICD-9CM # 724.5   Back Pain (Postural)
724.2   Low Back Pain
307.89 Back Pain Psychogenic
724.8   Stiff Back
847.9   Back Strain
724.6   Backache, Sacroiliac

Trauma: injury to bone, joint, or ligament.
Mechanical: pregnancy, obesity, fatigue, scoliosis.
Degenerative: osteoarthritis.
Infections: osteomyelitis, subarachnoid or spinal abscess, TB, meningitis, basilar pneumonia.
Metabolic: osteoporosis, osteomalacia.
Vascular: leaking aortic aneurysm, subarachnoid or spinal hemorrhage/infarction.
Neoplastic: myeloma, Hodgkin's disease, carcinoma of pancreas, metastatic neoplasm from breast, prostate, lung.
GI: penetrating ulcer, pancreatitis, cholelithiasis, inflammatory bowel disease.
Renal: hydronephrosis, calculus, neoplasm, renal infarction, pyelonephritis.
Hematologic: sickle cell crisis, acute hemolysis.
Gynecologic: neoplasm of uterus or ovary, dysmenorrhea, salpingitis, uterine prolapse.
Inflammatory: ankylosing spondylitis, psoriatic arthritis, Reiter's syndrome.
Lumbosacral strain.
Psychogenic: malingering, hysteria, anxiety.
Endocrine: adrenal hemorrhage or infarction.

BACK PAIN, CHILDREN AND ADOLESCENTS
ICD-9CM # 724.2

Trauma (muscle strain, vertebral fracture).
Idiopathic scoliosis, kyphosis.
Psychological problem.
Infection (pyelonephritis, osteomyelitis).
Inflammatory spondyloarthropathy.
Tumor.
Herniated disc.
Spondylolysis, spondylolisthesis.
Sickle cell crisis.
Syrinx.

BACK PAIN, LOW, ACUTE[2]
ICD-9CM # 724.2

DIFFERENTIAL CONSIDERATIONS IN ACUTE LOW BACK PAIN
Emergent
Aortic dissection.
Cauda equina syndrome.
Epidural abscess or hematoma.
Meningitis.
Ruptured/expanding aortic aneurysm.
Spinal fracture or subluxation with cord or root impingement.
Urgent
Back pain with neurologic deficits.
Disk herniation causing neurologic compromise.
Malignancy.
Sciatica with motor nerve root compression.
Spinal fractures without cord impingement.
Spinal stenosis.
Transverse myelitis.
Vertebral osteomyelitis.
Common or Stable
Acute ligamentous injury.
Acute muscle strain.
Ankylosing spondylitis.
Degenerative joint disease.
Intervertebral disk disease without impingement.
Pathologic fracture without impingement.
Seropositive arthritis.
Spondylolisthesis.
Referred or Visceral
Cholecystitis.
Esophageal disease.
Nephrolithiasis.
Ovarian torsion, mass, or tumor.
Pancreatitis.
Peptic ulcer disease.
Pleural effusion.
Pneumonia.
Pulmonary embolism.
Pyelonephritis.
Retroperitoneal hemorrhage or mass.

BACK PAIN, VISCEROGENIC ORIGIN
ICD-9CM # varies with specific disorder

Urolithiasis.
Aortic aneurysm.
Colorectal carcinoma.

Endometriosis.
Tubal pregnancy.
Prostatitis.
Peptic ulcer.
Pancreatitis.
Diverticular spasm.
Metastatic neoplasm (e.g., bladder, uterus, ovary, kidney).

BACTERIAL OVERGROWTH, SMALL INTESTINE[38]
ICD-9CM # varies with specific diagnosis

Gastric surgery—Billroth II.
Small bowel diverticula.
Small bowel stricture:
- Crohn's disease.
- Radiation enteritis.

Impaired small intestinal motility:
- Scleroderma.
- Diabetes mellitus.
- Chronic intestinal pseudoobstruction.

Miscellaneous/multifactorial
- Elderly.
- Immune deficiency syndrome.
- Chronic pancreatitis.
- Cirrhosis.

BALLISM*
ICD-9CM # 333.5

Cerebral infarction or hemorrhage.
Medications (e.g., dopamine agonists, phenytoin).
CNS neoplasm (primary or metastatic).
Nonketotic hyperosmolar state.

*Violent, flinging, nonpatterned rapid movements

BILE DUCT, DILATED[38]
ICD-9CM # varies with specific diagnosis

Normal variant.
Post-cholecystectomy.
Unsuspected bile duct stone.
Sphincter of Oddi stenosis.
Occult bile duct stricture.
Previous bile duct injury.
Early carcinoma of the pancreas, carcinoma of the bile duct or carcinoma of the ampulla.
Extrinsic compression of the bile duct by a primary or secondary neoplasm.

BLEEDING, LOWER GI
ICD-9CM # 578.9

(ORIGINATING BELOW THE LIGAMENT OF TREITZ)
Small Intestine
Ischemic bowel disease (mesenteric thrombosis, embolism, vasculitis, trauma).
Small bowel neoplasm: leiomyomas, carcinoids.
Hereditary hemorrhagic telangiectasia (Rendu-Osler-Weber syndrome).
Meckel diverticulum and other small intestine diverticula.
Aortoenteric fistula.

Intestinal hemangiomas: blue rubber-bleb nevi, intestinal hemangiomas, cutaneous vascular nevi.
Hamartomatous polyps: Peutz-Jeghers syndrome (intestinal polyps, mucocutaneous pigmentation).
Infections of small bowel: tuberculous enteritis, enteritis necroticans.
Volvulus.
Intussusception.
Lymphoma of small bowel, sarcoma, Kaposi's sarcoma.
Irradiation ileitis.
AV malformation of small intestine.
Inflammatory bowel disease.
Polyarteritis nodosa.
Other: pancreatoenteric fistulas, Henoch-Schönlein purpura, Ehlers-Danlos syndrome, SLE, amyloidosis, metastatic melanoma.
Colon
Carcinoma (particularly left colon).
Diverticular disease.
Inflammatory bowel disease.
Ischemic colitis.
Colonic polyps.
Vascular abnormalities: angiodysplasia, vascular ectasia.
Radiation colitis.
Infectious colitis.
Uremic colitis.
Aortoenteric fistula.
Lymphoma of large bowel.
Hemorrhoids.
Anal fissure.
Trauma, foreign body.
Solitary rectal/cecal ulcers.
Long-distance running.

BLEEDING, LOWER GI, PEDIATRIC[2]
ICD-9CM # 578.9

<3 MO
Swallowed maternal blood.
Infectious colitis.
Milk allergy.
Bleeding diathesis.
Intussusception.
Midgut volvulus.
Meckel diverticulum.
Necrotizing enterocolitis.

<2 YR
Anal fissure.
Infectious colitis.
Milk allergy.
Colitis.
Intussusception.
Meckel diverticulum.
Polyp.
Duplication.
Hemolytic uremic syndrome.
Inflammatory bowel disease.
Pseudomembranous enterocolitis.

<5 YR

Differential Diagnosis

II

Infectious colitis.
Anal fissure.
Polyp.
Intussusception.
Meckel diverticulum.
Henoch-Schönlein purpura.
Hemolytic-uremic syndrome.
Inflammatory bowel disease.
Pseudomembranous enterocolitis.

5 TO 18 YR

Infectious colitis.
Inflammatory bowel disease.
Pseudomembranous enterocolitis.
Polyp.
Hemolytic-uremic syndrome.
Hemorrhoid.

BLEEDING, RECTAL[38]

ICD-9CM # 578.9

IN PATIENTS <40 YR

Very Common:
Hemorrhoids.
Anal fissure.
Inflammatory bowel disease (mainly proctitis).
Less Common:
Polyps (hamartomatous or adenomatous).
Infective colitis.
Meckel's diverticulum.
Intussusception.
Rare:
Colorectal cancer.

IN PATIENTS >40 YR

Hemorrhoids.
Anal fissure.
Colorectal cancer.
Colorectal polyps (mostly adenomas).
Angiodysplasia.
Diverticular disease.
Inflammatory bowel disease.
Ischemic colitis.
Infective colitis.

BLEEDING, UPPER GI

ICD-9CM # 578.9

(ORIGINATING ABOVE THE LIGAMENT OF TREITZ)

Oral or pharyngeal lesions: swallowed blood from nose or oropharynx.
Swallowed Hemoptysis
Esophageal: varices, ulceration, esophagitis, Mallory-Weiss tear, carcinoma, trauma.
Gastric: peptic ulcer (including Cushing and Curling's ulcers), gastritis, angiodysplasia, gastric neoplasms, hiatal hernia, gastric diverticulum, pseudoxanthoma elasticum, Rendu-Osler-Weber syndrome.
Duodenal: peptic ulcer, duodenitis, angiodysplasia, aortoduodenal fistula, duodenal diverticulum, duodenal tumors, carcinoma of ampulla of Vater, parasites (e.g., hookworm), Crohn's disease.

Biliary: hematobilia (e.g., penetrating injury to liver, hepatobiliary malignancy, endoscopic papillotomy).

BLEEDING, UPPER GI, PEDIATRIC[2]

ICD-9CM # 578.9

<3 MO

Swallowed maternal blood.
Gastritis.
Ulcer, stress.
Bleeding diathesis.
Foreign body (NG tube).
Vascular malformation.
Duplication.

<2 YR

Esophagitis.
Gastritis.
Ulcer.
Pyloric stenosis.
Mallory-Weiss syndrome.
Vascular malformation.
Duplication.

<5 YR

Esophagitis.
Gastritis.
Ulcer.
Esophageal varices.
Foreign body.
Mallory-Weiss syndrome.
Hemophilia.
Vascular malformations.

5 TO 18 YR

Esophagitis.
Gastritis.
Ulcer.
Esophageal varices.
Mallory-Weiss syndrome.
Inflammatory bowel disease.
Hemophilia.
Vascular malformation.

BLINDNESS, GERIATRIC AGE

ICD-9CM # 369.4

Cataracts.
Glaucoma.
Diabetic retinopathy.
Macular degeneration.
Trauma.
CVA.
Corneal scarring.
Giant cell arteritis.
Ocular herpes zoster.

BLINDNESS, MONOCULAR, TRANSIENT

ICD-9CM # 369.67

Migraine (vasospasm).
Embolic cerebrovascular disease.
Intermittent angle-closure glaucoma.
Partial retinal vein occlusion.

Hyphema.
Optic disc edema.
Giant cell arteritis.
Psychogenic.
Hypotension.
Hypercoagulopathy disorders.
Multiple sclerosis.

BLINDNESS, PEDIATRIC AGE[23]

ICD-9CM # varies with specific disorder

CONGENITAL

Optic nerve hypoplasia or aplasia.
Optic coloboma.
Congenital hydrocephalus.
Hydranencephaly.
Porencephaly.
Microencephaly.
Encephalocele, particularly occipital type.
Morning glory disc.
Aniridia.
Anterior microphthalmia.
Peter's anomaly.
Persistent pupillary membrane.
Glaucoma.
Cataracts.
Persistent hyperplastic primary vitreous.

PHAKOMATOSES

Tuberous sclerosis.
Neurofibromatosis (special association with optic glioma).
Sturge-Weber syndrome.
von Hippel–Lindau disease.

TUMORS

Retinoblastoma.
Optic glioma.
Perioptic meningioma.
Craniopharyngioma.
Cerebral glioma.
Posterior and intraventricular tumors when complicated by hydrocephalus.
Pseudotumor cerebri.

NEURODEGENERATIVE DISEASES

Cerebral storage disease.
Gangliosidoses, particularly Tay-Sachs disease (infantile amaurotic familial idiocy), Sandhoff's variant, generalized gangliosidosis.
Other lipidoses and ceroid lipofuscinoses, particularly the late-onset amaurotic familial idiocies such as those of Jansky-Bielschowsky and of Batten-Mayou-Spielmeyer-Vogt.
Mucopolysaccharidoses, particularly Hurler's syndrome and Hunter's syndrome.
Leukodystrophies (dysmyelination disorders), particularly metachromatic leukodystrophy and Canavan's disease.
Demyelinating sclerosis (myelinoclastic diseases), especially Schilder's disease and Devic's neuromyelitis optica.
Special types: Dawson's disease, Leigh's disease, Bassen-Kornzweig syndrome, Refsum's disease.
Retinal degenerations: retinitis pigmentosa and its variants, Leber's congenital type.

Optic atrophies: congenital autosomal recessive type, infantile and congenital autosomal dominant types, Leber's disease, and atrophies associated with hereditary ataxias—the types of Behr, of Marie, and of Sanger-Brown.

INFECTIOUS PROCESSES

Encephalitis, especially in the prenatal infection syndromes caused by *Toxoplasma gondii*, cytomegalovirus, rubella virus, *Treponema pallidum*, herpes simplex.
Meningitis, arachnoiditis.
Chorioretinitis.
Endophthalmitis.
Keratitis.

HEMATOLOGIC DISORDERS

Leukemia with central nervous system involvement.

VASCULAR AND CIRCULATORY DISORDERS

Collagen vascular diseases.
Arteriovenous malformations—intracerebral hemorrhage, subarachnoid hemorrhage.
Central retinal occlusion.

TRAUMA

Contusion or avulsion of optic nerves, chiasm, globe, cornea.
Cerebral contusion or laceration.
Intracerebral, subarachnoid, or subdural hemorrhage.

DRUGS AND TOXINS

Other
Retinopathy of prematurity.
Sclerocornea.
Conversion reaction.
Optic neuritis.
Osteopetrosis.

BLISTERS, SUBEPIDERMAL
ICD-9CM # 919.2

Burns.
Porphyria cutanea tarda.
Bullous pemphigoid.
Bullous drug reaction.
Arthropod bite reaction.
Toxic epidermal necrosis.
Dermatitis herpetiformis.
Polymorphous light eruption.
Variegate porphyria.
SLE.
Epidermolysis bullosa.
Pseudoporphyria.
Acute graft-versus-host reaction.
Linear IgA disease.
Leukocytoclastic vasculitis.
Pressure necrosis.
Urticaria pigmentosa.
Amyloidosis.

BONE DENSITY, DECREASED, GENERALIZED[16a]
ICD-9CM # 733.00

DISORDERS ASSOCIATED WITH GENERALIZED LOSS OF BONE DENSITY

Disorders of Multiple or Uncertain Cause
Senile osteoporosis.*
Juvenile osteoporosis.
Osteogenesis imperfecta.†
Secondary Bone Disorders
Endocrine
Adrenal cortex.†
    Cushing's disease.
    Addison's disease.
Gonadal disorders.
    Postmenopausal osteoporosis.*
    Hypogonadism.†
Pituitary.
    Acromegaly.
    Hypopituitarism.
Pancreas.
    Diabetes mellitus.*
Thyroid.
    Hyperthyroidism.
    Hypothyroidism.
Parathyroid.
    Hyperparathyroidism.*
Marrow replacement and expansion
Myeloma.
Leukemia.
Lymphoma.
Metastatic disease.*
Gaucher's disease.
Anemias (sickle cell, thalassaemia, hemophilia).†
Drugs and other substances
Steroids.*†
Heparin (osteoporosis).
Anticonvulsants (osteomalacia).
Immunosuppressants.
Alcohol.*
Chronic disease
Chronic renal disease.†
Hepatic insufficiency.†
GI malabsorption syndromes.
Chronic inflammatory polyarthropathies.
Chronic debility or immobilization.

---

*Common cause of decrease in bone density in adults.
†Common cause of decrease in bone density in children.

BONE DENSITY, DECREASED, LOCALIZED[16a]
ICD-9CM # V17.81

DISORDERS ASSOCIATED WITH LOCALIZED LOSS OF BONE DENSITY

Disuse osteoporosis.*
Reflex sympathetic dystrophy (Sudeck's).*

Osteolytic syndromes.
    Acro-osteolysis, primary and secondary.
    Massive osteolytic of Gorham.
    Carpotarsal osteolysis.
Transient regional osteoporosis.
Neuromuscular disorders.
Infection.*
Arthropathies.*
Tumors, primary and secondary, myelomatosis.

*Common causes.

BONE LESIONS, PREFERENTIAL SITE OF ORIGIN[35]

ICD-9CM # 170.0 Skull and Face
        170.1 Mandible
        170.2 Vertebral Column
        170.3 Ribs, Sternum, Clavicle
        170.4 Scapula, Long Bones Upper Limb
        170.5 Short Bones and Upper Limb
        170.6 Pelvic Bones, Sacrum Coccyx
        170.7 Long Bones Lower Limb
        170.8 Short Bones Lower Limb
        170.9 Bone Cancer NOS
        198.5 Bone Cancer, Metastatic

EPIPHYSIS

Chondroblastoma.
Giant-cell tumor—after fusion of growth plate.
Langerhans' cell histiocytosis.
Clear cell chondrosarcoma.
Osteosarcoma.

METAPHYSIS

Parosteal sarcoma.
Chondrosarcoma.
Fibrosarcoma.
Nonossifying fibroma.
Giant-cell tumor—before fusion of growth plate.
Unicameral bone cyst.
Aneurysmal bone cyst.

DIAPHYSIS

Myeloma.
Ewing's tumor.
Reticulum cell sarcoma.

METADIAPHYSEAL

Fibrosarcoma.
Fibrous dysplasia.
Enchondroma.
Osteoid osteoma.
Chondromyofibroma.

BONE MARROW FAILURE SYNDROMES, INHERITED[20]
ICD-9CM # 284

BI-LINEAGE AND TRI-LINEAGE CYTOPENIAS

Fanconi anemia.
Shwachman-Diamond syndrome.

Dyskeratosis congenita.
Amegakaryocytic thrombocytopenia:
- Other inherited thrombocytopenia disorders.

Other genetic syndromes:
- Down syndrome.
- Dubowitz syndrome.
- Seckel syndrome.
- Reticular dysgenesis.
- Schimke immunoosseous dysplasia.
- Noonan syndrome.
- Cartilage-hair hypoplasia.
- Familial marrow failure (non-Fanconi).

UNI-LINEAGE CYTOPENIA

Diamond-Blackfan anemia.
Kostmann syndrome/Congenital neutropenia:
- *ELA2* mutations.
- *HAX1* mutations.
- *GFI1* mutations.
- *WASP* mutations.
- Constitutive cell surface G-CSF-R mutations.

Other inherited neutropenia syndromes:
- Barth syndrome.
- Glycogen storage disease 1b.
- Miscellaneous.

Thrombocytopenia with absent radii.
Congenital dyserythropoietic anemias (CDAs):
- Types I, II, III, IV.
- Variants.
- Nonclassifiable CDAs.
- Groups IV, V, VI, VII.

BONE MARROW FIBROSIS[14]

ICD-9CM # 289.9

MYELOID DISORDERS

Myelofibrosis with myeloid metaplasia.
Metastatic cancer.
Chronic myeloid leukemia.
Myelodysplastic syndrome.
Atypical myeloid disorder.
Acute megakaryocytic leukemia.
Other acute myeloid leukemias.
Gray platelet syndrome.

LYMPHOID DISORDERS

Hairy cell leukemia.
Multiple myeloma.
Lymphoma.

NONHEMATOLOGIC DISORDERS

Connective tissue disorder.
Infections (tuberculosis, kala-azar).
Vitamin D–deficiency rickets.
Renal osteodystrophy.

BONE MASS, LOW[1]

ICD-9CM # varies 733.0

SECONDARY CAUSES OF LOW BONE MASS

Endocrine Diseases
Female hypogonadism.
Hyperprolactinemia.
Hypothalamic amenorrhea.

Anorexia nervosa.
Premature and primary ovarian failure.
Female athlete triad.
Male hypogonadism.
Primary gonadal failure (e.g., Klinefelter's syndrome).
Secondary gonadal failure (e.g., idiopathic hypogonadotropic hypogonadism, androgen deprivation therapy for prostate cancer).
Hyperthyroidism.
Hyperparathyroidism.
Hypercortisolism.
Vitamin D insufficiency or deficiency.

Gastrointestinal Diseases
Subtotal gastrectomy.
Gastric bypass surgery.
Malabsorption syndromes.
Chronic obstructive jaundice.
Primary biliary cirrhosis and other cirrhoses.

Bone Marrow Disorders
Multiple myeloma.
Monoclonal gammopathy of unknown significance (MGUS).
Lymphoma.
Leukemia.
Hemolytic anemias.
Systemic mastocytosis.
Disseminated carcinoma.

Connective Tissue Diseases
Osteogenesis imperfecta.
Ehlers-Danlos syndrome.
Marfan syndrome.
Homocystinuria.

Drugs
Alcohol.
Antiseizure medications.
Aromatase inhibitors.
Chemotherapy.
Cyclosporine.
Depo-medroxyprogesterone.
Excess thyroid hormone.
Glucocorticoids.
Gonadotropin-releasing hormone agonists.
Heparin.

Miscellaneous Causes
Immobilization.
Rheumatoid arthritis.
Chronic obstructive pulmonary disease.
Weight loss.

BONE MINERAL DENSITY, INCREASED

ICD-9CM # 733.99

Paget's disease of bone.
Skeletal metastases.
DISH.
Osteonecrosis.
Sarcoidosis.
Hypoparathyroidism, pseudohypoparathyroidism.
Milk-alkali syndrome.
Osteopetrosis.
Hypervitaminosis A or D.
Dysplasias (craniodiaphyseal, craniometaphyseal, frontometaphyseal).
Endosteal hyperostosis.
Fluorosis.

Heavy metal poisoning.
Ionizing radiation.
Other: lymphoma, leukemia, mastocytosis, multiple myeloma, polycythemia vera.

BONE PAIN

ICD-9CM # code not available

Trauma.
Neoplasm (primary or metastatic).
Osteoporosis with compression fracture.
Paget's disease of bone.
Infection (osteomyelitis, septic arthritis).
Osteomalacia.
Viral syndrome.
Sickle cell disease.
Anxiety.

BONE RESORPTION[35]

ICD-9CM # 733.90 Bone Disorder

DISTAL CLAVICLE

Hyperparathyroidism.
RA.
Scleroderma.
Posttraumatic osteolysis.
Progeria.
Pycnodysostosis.
Cleidocranial dysplasia.

INFERIOR ASPECT OF RIBS

Vascular impression, associated with but not limited to coarctation of the aorta.
Hyperparathyroidism.
Neurofibromatosis.

TERMINAL PHALANGEAL TUFTS

Scleroderma.
Raynaud's phenomenon.
Vascular disease.
Frostbite, electrical burns.
Psoriasis.
Tabes dorsalis.
Hyperparathyroidism.

GENERALIZED RESORPTION

Paraplegia.
Myositis ossificans.
Osteoporosis.

BRADYCARDIA, SINUS[15]

ICD-9CM # 427.89

Idiopathic.
Degenerative processes (e.g., Lev's disease, Lenègre's disease).

Medications
Beta-blockers.
Some calcium channel blockers (diltiazem, verapamil).
Digoxin (when vagal tone is high).
Class I antiarrhythmic agents (e.g., procainamide).
Class III antiarrhythmic agents (amiodarone, sotalol).
Clonidine.
Lithium carbonate.

Acute Myocardial Ischemia and Infarction
Right or left circumflex coronary artery occlusion or spasm.
High vagal tone (e.g., athletes).

BREAST INFLAMMATORY LESION[12]

ICD-9CM # 611.0 Acute Mastitis
611.72 610.1 Chronic Cystic Mastitis
771.5 Neonatal Infective Mastitis
778.7 Neonatal Noninfective Mastitis

Mastitis (*S. aureus*, beta-hemolytic *Streptococcus*).
Trauma.
Foreign body (sutures, breast implants).
Granuloma (TB, fungal).
Fat necrosis post biopsy.
Necrosis or infarction (anticoagulant therapy, pregnancy).
Breast malignancy.

BREAST MASS

ICD-9CM # 611.72

Fibrocystic breasts.
Benign tumors (fibroadenoma, papilloma).
Mastitis (acute bacterial mastitis, chronic mastitis).
Malignant neoplasm.
Fat necrosis.
Hematoma.
Duct ectasia.
Mammary adenosis.

BREATH ODOR[34]

ICD-9CM # 784.9 Halitosis

Sweet, fruity: DKA, starvation ketosis.
Fishy, stale: uremia (trimethylamines).
Ammonia-like: uremia (ammonia).
Musty fish, clover: fetor hepaticus (hepatic failure).
Foul, feculent: intestinal obstruction/diverticulum.
Foul, putrid: nasal/sinus pathology (infection, foreign body, cancer), respiratory infections (empyema, lung abscess, bronchiectasis).
Halitosis: tonsillitis, gingivitis, respiratory infections, Vincent's angina, gastroesophageal reflux, achalasia, certain foods (garlic, onions, protein drinks, etc.)
Cinnamon: pulmonary TB.

BREATHING, NOISY[34]

ICD-9CM # 786.09 Breathing, Labored
789.09 Snoring, Wheezing
786.1 Stridor

Infection: upper respiratory infection, peritonsillar abscess, retropharyngeal abscess, epiglottitis, laryngitis, tracheitis, bronchitis, bronchiolitis.
Irritants and allergens: hyperactive airway, asthma (reactive airway disease), rhinitis, angioneurotic edema.
Compression from outside of the airway: esophageal cysts or foreign body, neoplasms, lymphadenopathy.

Congenital malformation and abnormality: vascular rings, laryngeal webs, laryngomalacia, tracheomalacia, hemangiomas within the upper airway, stenoses within the upper airway, cystic fibrosis.
Acquired abnormality (at every level of the airway): nasal polyps, hypertrophied adenoids and/or tonsils, foreign body, intraluminal tumors, bronchiectasis.
Neurogenic disorder: vocal cord paralysis.

BRONCHIAL OBSTRUCTION[16a]

ICD-9CM # varies with specific diagnosis

CAUSES OF BRONCHIAL OBSTRUCTION

Outside the Bronchus
Lymph nodes and other masses.
In the Wall of the Bronchus
Tumors
Lung carcinoma (commonly squamous cell).
Bronchial carcinoid.
Metastasis.
Hamartoma.
Inflammation
Tuberculosis.
Sarcoidosis.
Wegener's granulomatosis.
Inflammatory bowel disease.
Bronchomalacia
Broncholith.
Inside the Bronchus
Mucus plug.
Inhaled foreign body.

BRONCHOPLEURAL FISTULA[16a]

ICD-9CM # 510.0

CAUSES OF BRONCHOPLEURAL FISTULA

Trauma
Penetrating.
Iatrogenic (especially post-pneumonectomy, post-lobectomy, post-biopsy).
Infection
Necrotizing pneumonia.
Empyema.
Tuberculosis.
Septic embolus.
Infected pulmonary infarct.

BROWN URINE

ICD-9CM # 788.69

Bile pigments.
Myoglobin.
Concentrated urine.
Use of multivitamin supplements.
Medications (antimalarials, metronidazole, nitrofurantoin, levodopa, methyldopa, Phenazopyridine).
Diet rich in fava beans.
Urinary tract infection.

BRUISING

ICD-9CM # 459.89

Medication-induced (warfarin, aspirin, NSAIDs, prednisone).
Alcohol abuse.
Senile purpura.
Purpura simplex.
Physical abuse.
Vasculitis.
Platelet disorders.
Coagulation factor deficiencies.
Cushing's disease.
Vitamin C deficiency.
Marfan's syndrome.
Ehlers-Danlos syndrome.
Disseminated intravascular coagulation.
Leukemia.
Hereditary hemorrhagic telangiectasia.

BULLOUS DISEASES

ICD-9CM # 694.9 Bullous Dermatoses
694.5 Bullous Pemphigoid
694.4 Pemphigus Vulgaris
694.4 Pemphigus Foliaceus

Bullous pemphigoid.
Pemphigus vulgaris.
Pemphigus foliaceus.
Paraneoplastic pemphigus.
Cicatricial pemphigoid.
Erythema multiforme.
Dermatitis herpetiformis.
Herpes gestationis.
Impetigo.
Erosive lichen planus.
Linear IgA bullous dermatosis.
Epidermolysis bullosa acquisita.

CALCIFICATION ON CHEST X-RAY

ICD-9CM # 722.92

Lung neoplasm (primary or metastatic).
Silicosis.
Idiopathic pulmonary fibrosis.
Tuberculosis.
Histoplasmosis.
Disseminated varicella infection.
Mitral stenosis (end-stage).
Secondary hyperparathyroidism.

CALCIFICATIONS, ABDOMINAL, NON-VISCERAL ON X-RAY[16a]

ICD-9CM # 728.10

NONVISCERAL ABDOMINAL CALCIFICATION

Common
Atherosclerosis.
Mesenteric lymph nodes.
Phleboliths.
Aneurysm.
Dermoid cyst.

Differentiate:
  Rib cartilage.
  Injections in the buttocks.
Uncommon
Infestations.
  Armillifer armillatus.
  Cysticercosis.
  Guinea worm.
  Hydatid.
Tumors.
  Lipoma.
  Hemangioma.
  Neuroblastoma.
  Osteo/chondrosarcoma of soft tissues.
  Retroperitoneal sarcoma of soft tissues.
  Peritoneal metastases.
  Pheochromocytoma.
Tuberculosis.
  Peritonitis.
  Psoas abscess.
Meconium peritonitis.
Pseudomyxoma Peritonei
Mesenteric cyst.
Pancreatitis with saponification.
Lithopedion.
Appendices Epiploicae
Ligaments.
Foreign bodies.
Posttraumatic buttock cysts.

CALCIFICATIONS, ADRENAL GLAND ON X-RAY[16a]
ICD-9CM # 275.49

ADRENAL GLAND CALCIFICATION

Common
Idiopathic.
Hemorrhage.
Tuberculosis.
Neuroblastoma/ganglioneuroma.
Pheochromocytoma.
Uncommon
Other tumors:
  Adenoma.
  Carcinoma.
  Dermoid.
Addison's disease.
Cyst.
Histoplasmosis.

CALCIFICATIONS, CARDIAC ON X-RAY[16a]
ICD-9CM # 275.49

CAUSES OF VISIBLE CALCIFICATION WITHIN THE HEART

Coronary Artery
Atherosclerosis.
Aortic Root
Atherosclerotic aorta.
Thrombus.
Syphilis.
Ankylosing spondylitis.
Homograft calcification.
Pericardium
Chronic pericarditis, tuberculosis, hemopericardium, pyogenic or viral pericarditis.

Posttraumatic.
Postoperative.
Uremic pericarditis.
Asbestosis (may be pleural calcification applied to pericardium).
Myocardium
Ventricular aneurysm (may mimic pericardial calcification).
Calcified myocardial infarction.
Postmyocarditis.
Endocardium
Endomyocardial fibrosis.
Thrombus.
Valve Cusps
Calcified valves (particularly mitral and aortic valves).
Mitral annulus calcification.
Homograft calcification.
Old vegetation.
Valve Annulus
Submitral.
Mitral.
Aortic.
Left Atrium
Wall.
Thrombus.
Atrial myxoma.
Pulmonary Artery
Pulmonary hypertension.
Postoperative.
Postoperative Serumoma
Calcified Hydatid Cyst

CALCIFICATIONS, CUTANEOUS
ICD-9CM # 709.3

Calcification, Raynaud's phenomenon, esophageal dysmotility, sclerodactyly, and telangiectasia (CREST) syndrome.
Trauma.
Pancreatitis or pancreatic cancer.
Chronic renal failure.
Sarcoidosis.
Hyperparathyroidism.
Milk-alkali syndrome.
Hypervitaminosis D.
Panniculitis.
Idiopathic.
Iatrogenic (e.g., application of calcium alginate dressing to skin).
Multiple myeloma.
Dermatomyositis.
Parasitic infections.
Leukemia.
Lymphoma.

CALCIFICATIONS, GENITAL TRACT, FEMALE ON X-RAY[16a]
ICD-9CM # 275.49

FEMALE GENITAL TRACT CALCIFICATION

Uterus
Leiomyomas.
Squamous cell carcinoma.
Adenocarcinoma of endometrium.

Leiomyosarcoma.
Lithopedion.
Fallopian Tubes
Ovary.
Dermoid cyst.
Serous cystadenoma/carcinoma.
Tuberculosis.
Cysts.
Autoamputation.

CALCIFICATIONS, LIVER ON X-RAY[16a]
ICD-9CM # 573

LIVER CALCIFICATION

Common
Granuloma (tuberculosis, histoplasmosis, brucellosis).
  • Multiple scattered round densities.
Hydatid cyst.
  • Fine curvilinear in wall, or dense and irregular if contracted.
Primary liver tumor (hemangioma, hepatoblastoma, hepatoma, cholangiocarcinoma).
  • Irregular patterns or multiple nodules.
Metastases (mucinous primary of colon or breast, cystadenocarcinoma of ovary).
  • Finely stippled, may be extensive.
Uncommon
Hepatic artery aneurysm.
Armillifer armillatus infestation.
Chronic granulomatous disease of childhood.
Cyst (congenital or acquired).
Hematoma.
Intrahepatic gallstones.
Old liver abscess.
Portal vein thrombosis.
Differentiate
Hemochromatosis.
Thorotrast, thallium, iron.

CALCIFICATIONS, PANCREAS ON X-RAY[16a]
ICD-9CM # 275.49

PANCREATIC CALCIFICATION

Common
Chronic pancreatitis.
Uncommon
Acute pancreatitis (saponification).
Tumors.
  Cystadenoma.
  Cystadenocarcinoma.
  Islet-cell tumor.
  Metastases.
Hereditary pancreatitis (large clumps).
Hemorrhage.
Hyperparathyroidism.
Pseudocyst.
Cavernous lymphangioma.
Mucoviscidosis.
Kwashiorkor.

CALCIFICATION, SPLEEN ON X-RAY[16a]

ICD-9CM # 275.49

SPLENIC CALCIFICATION

Larger than 10 mm
Splenic artery aneurysm.
Splenic artery atheroma.
Cyst.
   Posttraumatic.
   Dermoid.
   Epidermoid.
   Hydatid.
Hematoma.
Infarct.
Abscess.
Tuberculosis.
Smaller than 10 mm
Histoplasmosis.
Tuberculosis.
Phleboliths.
Armillifer armillatus infestation.
Brucellosis.
Infarcts.

CALCIFICATIONS, VALVULAR ON X-RAY[16a]

ICD-9CM # 275.49

CAUSES OF RADIOGRAPHICALLY VISIBLE VALVE CALCIFICATION

Aortic Valve
Rheumatic aortic valve disease.
Bicuspid aortic valve.
Age/degenerate aortic valve.
Syphilis.
Ankylosing spondylitis.
Homograft calcification.
Mitral Valve
Rheumatic mitral valve disease.
Mitral annulus calcification.
Old vegetation (may only be visible on CT).
Homograft calcification.
Pulmonary Valve
Congenital pulmonary valve stenosis.
Rheumatic pulmonary valve disease (rare).
Fallot's tetralogy (usually after repair).
Pulmonary hypertension.
Homograft calcification.
Tricuspid Valve
Rheumatic tricuspid valve disease.
Old vegetation (may only be visible on ultrafast CT).

CALCIUM STONES

ICD-9CM # 592.9

Medications (e.g., antacids, loop diuretics, vitamin D, acetazolamide, glucocorticoids).
Primary hyperparathyroidism.
Hypercalcemia from malignancy.
Sarcoidosis.
Prolonged immobilization.
Hyperoxaluria (e.g., Crohn's disease, celiac disease, chronic pancreatitis).
Hyperuricosuria (e.g., hyperuricemia, excessive dietary purine, allopurinol, probenecid).
Renal tubular acidosis.
Milk-alkali syndrome.
Thyrotoxicosis.
Hypocitraturia (e.g., metabolic acidosis, hypomagnesemia, hypokalemia).

CARDIAC ARREST, NONTRAUMATIC[26]

ICD-9CM # 427.5 Cardiac Arrest NOS

Cardiac (coronary artery disease, cardiomyopathies, structural abnormalities, valve dysfunction, arrhythmias).
Respiratory (upper airway obstruction, hypoventilation, pulmonary embolism, asthma, COPD exacerbation, pulmonary edema).
Circulatory (tension pneumothorax, pericardial tamponade, PE, hemorrhage, sepsis).
Electrolyte abnormalities (hypokalemia or hyperkalemia, hypomagnesemia or hypermagnesemia, hypocalcemia).
Medications (tricyclic antidepressants, digoxin, theophylline, calcium channel blockers).
Drug abuse (cocaine, heroin, amphetamines).
Toxins (carbon monoxide, cyanide).
Environmental (drowning/near-drowning, electrocution, lightning, hypothermia or hyperthermia, venomous snakes).

CARDIAC DEATH, SUDDEN[1]

ICD-9CM # varies with specific disorder

Ventricular tachycardia.
Bradyarrhythmia, sick sinus syndrome.
Aortic stenosis.
Tetralogy of Fallot.
Pericardial tamponade.
Cardiac tumors.
Complications of infective endocarditis.
Hypertrophic cardiomyopathy (arrhythmia or obstruction).
Myocardial ischemia.
Atherosclerosis.
Prinzmetal's angina.
Kawasaki's arteritis.

CARDIAC ENLARGEMENT[15]

ICD-9CM # 429.3 Cardiomegaly, Idiopathic
       746.89 Cardiomegaly, Congenital
       402.0   Cardiomegaly, Malignant
       402.1   Cardiomegaly, Benign

CARDIAC CHAMBER ENLARGEMENT

Chronic Volume Overload
Mitral or aortic regurgitation.
Left-to-right shunt (PDA, VSD, AV fistula).
Cardiomyopathy
Ischemic.
Nonischemic.

Decompensated Pressure Overload
Aortic stenosis.
Hypertension.
High-Output States
Severe anemia.
Thyrotoxicosis.
Bradycardia
Severe sinus bradycardia.
Complete heart block.

LEFT ATRIUM

LV failure of any cause.
Mitral valve disease.
Myxoma.

RIGHT VENTRICLE

Chronic volume overload.
Tricuspid or pulmonic regurgitation.
Left-to-right shunt (ASD).
Decompensated pressure overload:
   Pulmonic stenosis.
   Pulmonary artery hypertension:
   • Primary.
   • Secondary (PE, COPD).
   Pulmonary venoocclusive disease.

RIGHT ATRIUM

RV failure of any cause.
Tricuspid valve disease.
Myxoma.
Ebstein's anomaly.

MULTICHAMBER ENLARGEMENT

Hypertrophic cardiomyopathy.
Acromegaly.
Severe obesity.

PERICARDIAL DISEASE

Pericardial effusion with or without tamponade.
Effusive constrictive disease.
Pericardial cyst, loculated effusion.

PSEUDOCARDIOMEGALY

Epicardial fat.
Chest wall deformity (pectus excavatum, straight back syndrome).
Low lung volumes.
AP chest x-ray.
Mediastinal tumor, cyst.

CARDIAC MURMURS

ICD-9CM # varies with specific disorder

SYSTOLIC

Mitral regurgitation (MR).
Tricuspid regurgitation (TR).
Ventricular septal defect (VSD).
Aortic stenosis (AS).
Idiopathic hypertrophic subaortic stenosis (IHSS).
Pulmonic stenosis (PS).
Innocent murmur of childhood.
Coarctation of aorta.
Mitral valve prolapse (MVP).

Differential Diagnosis

II

DIASTOLIC

Aortic regurgitation (AR).
Atrial myxoma.
Mitral stenosis (MS).
Pulmonary artery branch stenosis.
Tricuspid stenosis (TS).
Graham Steell murmur (diastolic decrescendo murmur heard in severe pulmonary hypertension).
Pulmonic regurgitation (PR).
Severe mitral regurgitation (MR).
Austin Flint murmur (diastolic rumble heard in severe AR).
Severe VSD and patent ductus arteriosus.

CONTINUOUS

Patent ductus arteriosus.
Pulmonary AV fistula.

CARDIOEMBOLISM
ICD-9CM # 410.9

Acute MI.
Atrial fibrillation.
Left ventricular aneurysm.
Valvular heart disease (e.g., rheumatic mitral valve disease, mitral valve prolapse).
Dilated cardiomyopathy.
Atrial septal defect.
Patent foramen ovale.
Cardioversion for atrial fibrillation.
Infective endocarditis.
Atrial septal aneurysm.
Sick sinus syndrome and cardiac arrhythmias.
Nonbacterial thrombotic endocarditis.
Prosthetic heart valves.
Atrial myxoma and other intracardiac tumors.
Cyanotic heart disease.
Balloon angioplasty.
Coronary artery bypass grafting.
Aneurysms of sinus of Valsalva.
Other: VVI pacing, ventricular support devices, heart transplantation, intracardiac defects with paradoxical embolism.

CARDIOGENIC SHOCK
ICD-9CM # 785.51

Myocardial infarction.
Arrhythmias.
Pericardial effusion/tamponade.
Chest trauma.
Valvular heart disease.
Myocarditis.
Cardiomyopathy.
CHF, end-stage.

CAVITARY LESION ON CHEST X-RAY[16]
ICD-9CM # 793.1 Chest X-Ray Lung Shadow

NECROTIZING INFECTIONS

Bacteria: anaerobes, *Staphylococcus aureus,* enteric gram-negative bacteria, *Pseudomonas aeruginosa, Legionella* species, *Haemophilus influenzae, Streptococcus pyogenes,* Strepto-coccus pneumoniae (?), *Rhodococcus, Actinomyces.*
Mycobacteria: *Mycobacterium tuberculosis, Mycobacterium kansasii,* MAI.
Bacteria-like: *Nocardia* species.
Fungi: *Coccidioides immitis, Histoplasma capsulatum, Blastomyces hominis, Aspergillus* species, *Mucor* species.
Parasitic: *Entamoeba histolytica, Echinococcus, Paragonimus westermani.*

CAVITARY INFARCTION

Bland infarction (with or without superimposed infection).
Lung contusion.

SEPTIC EMBOLISM

S. aureus, anaerobes, others.

VASCULITIS

Wegener's granulomatosis, periarteritis.

NEOPLASMS

Bronchogenic carcinoma, metastatic carcinoma, lymphoma.

MISCELLANEOUS LESIONS

Cysts, blebs, bullae, or pneumatocele with or without fluid collections.
Sequestration.
Empyema with air-fluid level.
Bronchiectasis.

CEREBRAL INFARCTION SECONDARY TO INHERITED DISORDERS
ICD-9CM # 434.91

Homocystinuria.
Marfan's syndrome.
Ehlers-Danlos syndrome.
Rendu-Osler-Weber syndrome.
Pseudoxanthoma elasticum.
Fabry's disease.

CEREBROVASCULAR DISEASE, ISCHEMIC[40]
ICD-9CM # 437.9

VASCULAR DISORDERS

Large-vessel atherothrombotic disease.
Lacunar disease.
Arterial-to-arterial embolization.
Carotid or vertebral artery dissection.
Fibromuscular dysplasia.
Migraine.
Venous thrombosis.
Radiation.
Complications of arteriography.
Multiple, progressive intracranial arterial occlusions.

INFLAMMATORY DISORDERS

Giant cell arteritis.
Polyarteritis nodosa.
SLE.
Granulomatous angiitis.
Takayasu's disease.
Arteritis associated with amphetamine, cocaine, or phenylpropanolamine.
Syphilis, mucormycosis.
Sjögren's syndrome.
Behçet's syndrome.

CARDIAC DISORDERS

Rheumatic heart disease.
Mural thrombus.
Arrhythmias.
Mitral valve prolapse.
Prosthetic heart valve.
Endocarditis.
Myxoma.
Paradoxical embolus.

HEMATOLOGIC DISORDERS

Thrombotic thrombocytopenic purpura.
Sickle cell disease.
Hypercoagulable states.
Polycythemia.
Thrombocytosis.
Leukocytosis.
Lupus anticoagulant.

CHEST PAIN, CHILDREN[4]
ICD-9CM # 786.50 Chest Pain NOS
786.59 Chest Pressure
786.52 Chest Pain, Pleuritic

MUSCULOSKELETAL (COMMON)

Trauma (accidental, abuse).
Exercise, overuse injury (strain, bursitis).
Costochondritis (Tietze's syndrome).
Herpes zoster (cutaneous).
Pleurodynia.
Fibrositis.
Slipping rib.
Sickle cell anemia vasoocclusive crisis.
Osteomyelitis (rare).
Primary or metastatic tumor (rare).

PULMONARY (COMMON)

Pneumonia.
Pleurisy.
Asthma.
Chronic cough.
Pneumothorax.
Infarction (sickle cell anemia).
Foreign body.
Embolism (rare).
Pulmonary hypertension (rare).
Tumor (rare).

GASTROINTESTINAL (LESS COMMON)

Esophagitis (gastroesophageal reflux).
Esophageal foreign body.
Esophageal spasm.
Cholecystitis.
Subdiaphragmatic abscess.
Perihepatitis (Fitz-Hugh-Curtis syndrome).
Peptic ulcer disease.

CARDIAC (LESS COMMON)

Pericarditis.
Postpericardiotomy syndrome.
Endocarditis.
Mitral valve prolapse.
Aortic or subaortic stenosis.
Arrhythmias.
Marfan's syndrome (dissecting aortic aneurysm).
Anomalous coronary artery.
Kawasaki disease.
Cocaine, sympathomimetic ingestion.
Angina (familial hypercholesterolemia).

IDIOPATHIC (COMMON)

Anxiety, hyperventilation.
Panic disorder.

OTHER (LESS COMMON)

Spinal cord or nerve root compression.
Breast-related pathologic condition.
Castleman's disease (lymph node neoplasm).

CHEST PAIN (NONPLEURITIC)[9]

ICD-9CM # 786.50 Chest Pain NOS
786.59 Chest Discomfort

Cardiac: myocardial ischemia/infarction, myocarditis.
Esophageal: spasm, esophagitis, ulceration, neoplasm, achalasia, diverticula, foreign body.
Referred pain from subdiaphragmatic GI structures.
Gastric and duodenal: hiatal hernia, neoplasm, PUD.
Gallbladder and biliary: cholecystitis, cholelithiasis, impacted stone, neoplasm.
Pancreatic: pancreatitis, neoplasm.
Dissecting aortic aneurysm.
Pain originating from skin, breasts, and musculoskeletal structures: herpes zoster, mastitis, cervical spondylosis.
Mediastinal tumors: lymphoma, thymoma.
Pulmonary: neoplasm, pneumonia, pulmonary embolism/infarction.
Psychoneurosis.
Chest pain associated with mitral valve prolapse.

CHEST PAIN (PLEURITIC)

ICD-9CM # 786.52 Chest Pain, Pleuritic

Cardiac: pericarditis, postpericardiotomy/Dressler's syndrome.
Pulmonary: pneumothorax, hemothorax, embolism/infarction, pneumonia, empyema, neoplasm, bronchiectasis, pneumomediastinum, TB, carcinomatous effusion.
GI: liver abscess, pancreatitis, esophageal rupture, Whipple's disease with associated pericarditis or pleuritis.
Subdiaphragmatic abscess.
Pain originating from skin and musculoskeletal tissues: costochondritis, chest wall trauma, fractured rib, interstitial fibrositis, myositis, strain of pectoralis muscle, herpes zoster, soft tissue and bone tumors.

Collagen vascular diseases with pleuritis.
Psychoneurosis.
Familial Mediterranean fever.

CHOLESTASIS[14]

ICD-9CM # 574.71

EXTRAHEPATIC

Choledocholithiasis.
Bile duct stricture.
Cholangiocarcinoma.
Pancreatic carcinoma.
Chronic pancreatitis.
Papillary stenosis.
Ampullary cancer.
Primary sclerosing cholangitis.
Choledochal cysts.
Parasites (e.g., ascaris, clonorchis).
AIDS.
Cholangiography.
Biliary atresia.
Portal lymphadenopathy.
Mirizzi's syndrome.

INTRAHEPATIC

Viral hepatitis.
Alcoholic hepatitis.
Drug induced.
Ductopenia syndromes.
Primary biliary cirrhosis.
Benign recurrent intrahepatic cholestasis.
Byler's disease.
Primary sclerosing cholangitis.
Alagille's syndrome.
Sarcoid.
Lymphoma.
Postoperative.
Total parenteral nutrition.
Alpha-1-antitrypsin deficiency.

CHOREA

ICD-9CM # 333.5

Medications (e.g., neuroleptics, tricyclics, antiparkinsonian drugs).
Cerebral palsy.
Huntington's disease.
Benign hereditary chorea.
Thyroid disorder (hyperthyroidism, hypothyroidism).
Friedreich's ataxia.
Ataxia-telangiectasia.
Hypoglycemia, hyperglycemia.
Electrolyte abnormalities (hyponatremia, hypocalcemia, hypomagnesemia, hypernatremia).
Vitamin B_{12} deficiency.
SLE.
Wilson's disease.
Alcohol.
Cocaine.
Carbon monoxide poisoning.
Mercury poisoning.

CHOREOATHETOSIS[28]

ICD-9CM # 275.1 Choreoathetosis-Agitans
Syndrome
33.5 Choreoathetosis
Paroxysmal

SYSTEMIC DISEASES

SLE.
Polycythemia.
Thyrotoxicosis.
Rheumatic fever.
Cirrhosis of the liver (acquired hepatocerebral degeneration).
DM.
Wilson's disease.

PRIMARY DEGENERATIVE BRAIN DISEASES

Huntington's chorea.
Olivopontocerebellar atrophies.
Neuroacanthocytosis.

FOCAL BRAIN DISEASES

Hemichorea.
Stroke.
Tumor.
Arteriovenous malformation.

DRUG-INDUCED CHOREOATHETOSIS

Parkinson's Disease Drugs
Levodopa.
Epilepsy Drugs
Phenytoin.
Carbamazepine.
Phenobarbital.
Gabapentin.
Valproate.
Psychostimulant Drugs
Cocaine.
Amphetamine.
Methamphetamine.
Dextroamphetamine.
Methylphenidate.
Pemoline.
Psychotropic Drugs
Lithium.
Tricyclic antidepressant drugs.
Oral Contraceptive Drugs
Cimetidine.

CHYLOTHORAX

ICD-9CM # 457.8

Post lymph node dissection of neck or chest.
Subclavian venous catheterization.
Thoracic aneurysm repair.
Trauma to chest and neck.
Mediastinal tumor resection.
Esophagectomy, pneumonectomy.
Lymphangitis, mediastinitis.
Neoplasms (lymphoma, carcinoma of esophagus, lung, mediastinal malignancies).
Sympathectomy.
Venous thrombosis.
Congenital.

Differential Diagnosis

II

CLOUDY URINE
ICD-9CM # 788.69

Concentrated urine.
Use of multivitamin supplements.
Diet high in purine-rich foods.
Pyuria.
Phosphaturia.
Urinary tract infection.
Lipiduria.
Chyluria.
Hyperoxaluria.

CLUBBING
ICD-9CM # 781.5 Clubbing Finger

Pulmonary neoplasm (lung, pleura).
Other neoplasm (GI, liver, Hodgkin's, thymus, osteogenic sarcoma).
Pulmonary infectious process (empyema, abscess, bronchiectasis, TB, chronic pneumonitis).
Extrapulmonary infectious process (subacute bacterial endocarditis, intestinal TB, bacterial or amebic dysentery, arterial graft sepsis).
Pneumoconiosis.
Cystic fibrosis.
Sarcoidosis.
Cyanotic congenital heart disease.
Endocrine (Graves' disease, hyperparathyroidism).
Inflammatory bowel disease.
Celiac disease.
Chronic liver disease, cirrhosis (particularly biliary and juvenile).
Pulmonary AV malformations.
Idiopathic.
Thyroid acropachy.
Hereditary (pachydermoperiostosis).
Chronic trauma (jackhammer operators, machine workers).

COBALAMIN DEFICIENCY[20]
ICD-9CM # 266.2

ETIOPATHOPHYSIOLOGIC CLASSIFICATION OF COBALAMIN DEFICIENCY

Nutritional cobalamin deficiency (i.e., insufficient cobalamin intake):
Vegetarians, poverty-imposed near-vegetarians, breastfed infants of mothers with pernicious anemia.
Abnormal intragastric events (i.e., inadequate proteolysis of food cobalamin):
Atrophic gastritis, partial gastritis with hypochlorhydria, proton-pump inhibitors, H_2 blockers.
Loss or atrophy of gastric oxyntic mucosa (i.e., deficient intrinsic factor [IF] molecules):
Total or partial gastrectomy, pernicious anemia, caustic destruction (lye).
Abnormal events in small bowel lumen:
Inadequate pancreatic protease (e.g., R-cobalamin not degraded, cobalamin not transferred to IF):
• Insufficient pancreatic protease (i.e., pancreatic insufficiency).

• Inactivation of pancreatic protease (i.e., Zollinger–Ellison syndrome).
Usurping of luminal cobalamin (i.e., inadequate cobalamin binding to IF):
• By bacteria, during stasis syndromes (e.g., blind loops, pouches of diverticulosis, strictures, fistulas, anastomosis), impaired bowel motility (e.g., scleroderma), hypogammaglobulinemia.
• By *Diphyllobothrium latum* (fish tapeworm).
Disorders of ileal mucosa/IF–cobalamin receptors (i.e., IF–cobalamin not bound to IF–cobalamin receptors):
Diminished or absent IF–cobalamin receptors (e.g., ileal bypass, resection, fistula).
Abnormal mucosal architecture/function (e.g., tropical or nontropical sprue, Crohn's disease, tuberculosis ileitis, infiltration by lymphomas, amyloidosis).
IF-/post-IF–cobalamin receptor defects (e.g., Imerslund–Gräsbeck syndrome, transcobalamin II [TC II] deficiency).
Drug effects (e.g., slow K, metformin, cholestyramine, colchicine, neomycin).
Disorders of plasma cobalamin transport (i.e., TC II–cobalamin not delivered to TC II receptors):
Congenital TC II deficiency, defective binding of TC II–cobalamin to TC II receptors (rare).
Metabolic disorders (i.e., cobalamin not used by cells):
Inborn enzyme errors (rare).
Acquired disorders (e.g., cobalamin functionally inactivated by irreversible oxidation, N_2O inhalation).

COLIC, ACUTE ABDOMINAL[38]
ICD-9CM # 789.0

Acute gastroenteritis.
Food poisoning.
Nonspecific causes.
Constipation.
Gastric outlet obstruction:
• Chronic peptic ulceration.
• Gastric cancer.
Small bowel obstruction:
Adhesions:
• Postsurgical.
• Inflammatory (e.g., diverticular).
• Radiation.
• Meckel's diverticulum.
• Metastatic.
Stricture:
• Ischemic.
• Radiation.
• Inflammatory (e.g., Crohn's disease).
Volvulus Intussusception:
• Tumor (e.g., Peutz-Jegher's syndrome).
• Superior mesenteric artery syndrome.
Intraluminal bolus:
• Gallstone.
• Bezoar.
Hernia:
• Abdominal wall.
• Internal.

Neoplasm:
• Benign (e.g., leiomyoma).
• Malignant (e.g., carcinoid tumor, adenocarcinoma).
Large bowel obstruction:
• Colon cancer.
• Diverticular disease.
• Volvulus.
Uterine:
• Missed abortion.
• Parturition.
• Period pain.

COLOR CHANGES, CUTANEOUS[34]
ICD-9CM # 709.00 Pigmentation Anomaly

BROWN
Generalized: pituitary, adrenal, liver disease, ACTH-producing tumor (e.g., oat cell lung carcinoma).
Localized: nevi, neurofibromatosis.

WHITE
Generalized: albinism.
Localized: vitiligo, Raynaud's syndrome.

RED (ERYTHEMA)
Generalized: fever, polycythemia, urticaria, viral exanthems.
Localized: inflammation, infection, Raynaud's syndrome.

YELLOW
Generalized: liver disease, chronic renal disease, anemia.
Generalized (except sclera): hypothyroidism, increased intake of vegetables containing carotene.
Localized: resolving hematoma, infection, peripheral vascular insufficiency.

BLUE
Lips, mouth, nail beds: cardiovascular and pulmonary diseases, Raynaud's.

COMA
ICD-9CM # 780.01

Vascular: hemorrhage, thrombosis, embolism.
CNS infections: meningitis, encephalitis, cerebral abscess.
Cerebral neoplasms with herniation.
Head injury: subdural hematoma, cerebral concussion, cerebral contusion.
Drugs: narcotics, sedatives, hypnotics.
Ingestion or inhalation of toxins: CO, alcohol, lead.
Metabolic disturbances.
Hypoxia.
Acid-base disorders.
Hypoglycemia, hyperglycemia.
Hepatic failure.
Electrolyte disorders.
Uremia.
Hypothyroidism.

Hypothermia, hyperthermia.
Hypotension, malignant hypertension.
Postictal.

COMA, NORMAL COMPUTED TOMOGRAPHY[1]
ICD-9CM # 780.01

MENINGEAL DISORDERS
Subarachnoid hemorrhage (uncommon).
Bacterial meningitis.
Encephalitis.
Subdural empyema.

EXOGENOUS TOXINS
Sedative drugs and barbiturates.
Anesthetics and γ-hydroxybutyrate.*
Alcohols.
Stimulants:
  Phencyclidines.[†]
  Cocaine and amphetamines.[‡]
Psychotropic drugs:
  Cyclic antidepressants.
  Phenothiazines.
  Lithium.
Anticonvulsants.
Opioids.
Clonidine.[§]
Penicillins.
Salicylates.
Anticholinergics.
Carbon monoxide, cyanide, and methemoglobinemia.

ENDOGENOUS TOXINS/ DEFICIENCIES/DERANGEMENTS
Hypoxia and ischemia.
Hypoglycemia.
Hypercalcemia.
Osmolar:
  Hyperglycemia.
  Hyponatremia.
  Hypernatremia.
Organ system failure:
  Hepatic encephalopathy.
  Uremic encephalopathy.
  Pulmonary insufficiency (carbon dioxide narcosis).

SEIZURES
Prolonged postical state.
Spike-wave stupor.

HYPOTHERMIA OR HYPERTHERMIA
Brain stem ischemia.
Basilar artery stroke.
Brain stem or cerebellar hemorrhage.
Conversion or malingering.

*General anesthetic, similar to γ-aminobutyric acid; recreational drug and body building aid. Rapid onset, rapid recovery often with myoclonic jerking and confusion. Deep coma (2-3 hr; Glasgow Coma Scale = 3) with maintenance of vital signs.
[†]Coma associated with cholinergic signs: lacrimation, salivation, bronchorrhea, and hyperthermia.

[‡]Coma after seizures or status (i.e., a prolonged postictal state).
[§]An antihypertensive agent active through the opiate receptor system; frequent overdose when used to treat narcotic withdrawal.

COMA, PEDIATRIC POPULATION[31]
ICD-9CM # 780.01

ANOXIA
Birth asphyxia.
Carbon monoxide poisoning.
Croup/epiglottitis.
Meconium aspiration.

INFECTION
Hemolysis.
Blood loss.
Hydrops fetalis.
Infection.
Meningoencephalitis.
Sepsis.
Postimmunization encephalitis.

INCREASED INTRACRANIAL PRESSURE
Anoxia.
Inborn metabolic errors.
Toxic encephalopathy.
Reye's syndrome.
Head trauma/intracranial bleed.
Hydrocephalus.
Posterior fossa tumors.

HYPERTENSIVE ENCEPHALOPATHY
Coarctation of aorta.
Nephritis.
Vasculitis.
Pheochromocytoma.

ISCHEMIA
Hypoplastic left heart.
Shunting lesions.
Aortic stenosis.
Cardiovascular collapse (any cause).

PURPURIC CAUSES
Disseminated intravascular coagulation.
Hemolytic-uremic syndrome.
Leukemia.
Thrombotic purpura.

HYPERCAPNIA
Cystic fibrosis.
Bronchopulmonary dysplasia.
Congenital lung anomalies.

NEOPLASM
Medulloblastoma.
Glioma of brain stem.
Posterior fossa tumors.

DRUGS/TOXINS
Maternal sedation.
Alcohol.
Any drug.
Lead.
Salicylism.
Arsenic.
Pesticides.

ELECTROLYTE ABNORMALITIES
Hypernatremia (diarrhea, dehydration, salt poisoning).
Hyponatremia (SIADH, androgenital syndrome, gastroenteritis).
Hyperkalemia (renal failure, salicylism, androgenitalism).
Hypokalemia (diarrhea, hyperaldosteronism, salicylism, DKA).
Hypocalcemia (vitamin D deficiency, hyperparathyroidism).
Severe acidosis (sepsis, cold injury, salicylism, DKA).

HYPOGLYCEMIA
Birth injury or stress.
Diabetes.
Alcohol.
Salicylism.
Hyperinsulinemia.
Iatrogenic.

POSTSEIZURE
Renal Causes
Nephritis.
Hypoplastic kidneys.
Hepatic Causes
Acute hepatitis.
Fulminant hepatic failure.
Inborn metabolic errors.
Bile duct atresia.

CONGESTIVE HEART FAILURE AND CARDIOMYOPATHY[1]
ICD-9CM # 428.0 Congestive heart failure
425.9 Cardiomyopathy, secondary, unspecified

CAUSES OF CONGESTIVE HEART FAILURE AND CARDIOMYOPATHY
Coronary Artery Disease
Acute ischemia.
Myocardial infarction.
Ischemic cardiomyopathy with hibernating myocardium.
Idiopathic
Idiopathic dilated cardiomyopathy.*
Idiopathic restrictive cardiomyopathy.
Peripartum.
Pressure Overload
Hypertension.
Aortic stenosis.
Volume Overload
Mitral regurgitation.
Aortic insufficiency.
Anemia.
Atrioventricular fistula.
Toxins
Ethanol.
Cocaine.
Doxorubicin (Adriamycin).
Methamphetamine.

Differential Diagnosis

Metabolic-Endocrine
Thiamine deficiency.
Diabetes.
Hemochromatosis.
Thyrotoxicosis.
Obesity.
Hemochromatosis.
Infiltrative
Amyloidosis.
Inflammatory
Viral myocarditis.
Hereditary
Hypertrophic.
Dilated.

---

*Genetic bases for these cardiomyopathies have been identified in a large number of individual patients and families. Most of the mutations have been found in cardiac contractile or structural proteins.

CONJUNCTIVAL NEOPLASM

ICD-9CM # varies with specific disorder

MALIGNANT

Squamous cell carcinoma.
Melanoma.
Sebaceous carcinoma.
Kaposi's sarcoma.
Metastatic neoplasms.

BENIGN

Melanocytic nevus.
Squamous papilloma.
Hemangioma.
Lymphangioma.
Myxoma.

CONSTIPATION

ICD-9CM # 564.0

Intestinal obstruction.
Fecal impaction.
Diverticular disease.
GI neoplasm.
Strangulated femoral hernia.
Gallstone ileus.
Tuberculous stricture.
Adhesions.
Ameboma.
Volvulus.
Intussusception.
Inflammatory bowel disease.
Hematoma of bowel wall, secondary to trauma or anticoagulants.
Poor dietary habits: insufficient bulk in diet, inadequate fluid intake.
Change from daily routine: travel, hospital admission, physical inactivity.
Acute abdominal conditions: renal colic, salpingitis, biliary colic, appendicitis, ischemia.
Hypercalcemia or hypokalemia, uremia.
Irritable bowel syndrome, pregnancy, anorexia nervosa, depression.
Painful anal conditions: hemorrhoids, fissure, stricture.
Decreased intestinal peristalsis: old age, spinal cord injuries, myxedema, diabetes, multiple sclerosis, Parkinsonism and other neurologic diseases.

Drugs: codeine, morphine, antacids with aluminum, verapamil, anticonvulsants, anticholinergics, disopyramide, cholestyramine, alosetron, iron supplements.
Hirschsprung's disease, meconium ileus, congenital atresia in infants.

CONSTIPATION, ADULT PATIENT[38]

ICD-9CM # 564

NO GROSS STRUCTURAL ABNORMALITY

Inadequate fiber intake.
Irritable bowel syndrome (associated with abdominal pain) or functional constipation.
Idiopathic slow-transit constipation.
"Obstructed defecation"—pelvic floor dysfunction (or dyssynergia).

STRUCTURAL DISORDERS

Anal fissure, infection or stenosis.
Colon cancer or stricture.
Aganglionosis and/or abnormal myenteric plexus:
- Hirschsprung's disease.
- Chagas' disease.
- Neuropathic pseudoobstruction.
Abnormal colonic muscle:
- Myopathy.
- Dystrophia myotonica.
- Systemic sclerosis.
Idiopathic megarectum and/or megacolon.
Proximal megacolon.

NEUROLOGIC CAUSES

Diabetic autonomic neuropathy.
Damage to the sacral parasympathetic outflow.
Spinal cord damage or disease (e.g., multiple sclerosis).
Parkinson's disease.
Blunting of consciousness, mental retardation, psychosis.
Pain induced by straining (e.g., sciatic nerve compression).

ENDOCRINE OR METABOLIC CAUSES

Hypothyroidism.
Hypercalcemia.
Porphyria.
Pregnancy.

PSYCHOLOGIC DISORDERS

Depression.
Anorexia nervosa.
Denied bowel habit.

DRUG SIDE EFFECTS

CORNEAL SENSATION, DECREASED

ICD-9CM # 371.89

Herpes (simplex, zoster).
Contact lens wear.
Topical agents (NSAIDs, anesthetics, beta-blockers).

Diabetes.
Eye trauma.
Postsurgery.

COUGH

ICD-9CM # 786.2

Infectious process (viral, bacterial).
Postinfectious.
"Smoker's cough."
Rhinitis (allergic, vasomotor, postinfectious).
Asthma.
Exposure to irritants (noxious fumes, smoke, cold air).
Drug-induced (especially ACE inhibitors, beta-blockers).
GERD.
Interstitial lung disease.
Lung neoplasms.
Lymphomas, mediastinal neoplasms.
Bronchiectasis.
Cardiac (CHF, pulmonary edema, mitral stenosis, pericardial inflammation).
Recurrent aspiration.
Inflammation of larynx, pleura, diaphragm, mediastinum.
Cystic fibrosis.
Anxiety.
Other: pulmonary embolism, foreign body inhalation, aortic aneurysm, Zenker's diverticulum, osteophytes, substernal thyroid, thyroiditis, PMR.

CUTANEOUS INFECTIONS, ATHLETES

ICD-9CM # 686.9

Tinea pedis.
Tinea cruris.
Molluscum contagiosum.
Herpes simplex.
Verruca vulgaris.
Folliculitis.
Impetigo.
Furuncles.
Otitis externa.
Erythrasma.

CYANOSIS[2]

ICD-9CM # 782.5

DIFFERENTIAL DIAGNOSIS OF CYANOSIS

Peripheral Cyanosis
Low cardiac output states
Shock.
Left ventricular failure.
Hypovolemia.
Environmental exposure (cold)
Air or water.
Arterial occlusion
Thrombosis.
Embolism.
Vasospasm (Raynaud's phenomenon).
Peripheral vascular disease.
Venous obstruction
Redistribution of blood flow from extremities

Central Cyanosis

Decreased arterial oxygen saturation
High altitude (>8000 ft).
Impaired pulmonary function.
  Hypoventilation.
  Impaired oxygen diffusion.
  Ventilation-perfusion mismatching.
- Pulmonary embolism.
- Acture respiratory distress syndrome.
- Pulmonary hypertension.

  Respiratory compromise.
- Upper airway obstruction.
- Pneumonia.
- Diaphragmatic hernia.
- Tension pneumothorax.
- Polycythemia.

Anatomic Shunts
Pulmonary arteriovenous fistulae and intrapulmonary shunts.
Cerebral, hepatic, peripheral arteriovenous fistulae.
Cyanotic congenital heart disease.
  Endocardial cushion defects.
  Ventricular septal defects.
  Coarctation of aorta.
  Tetralogy of Fallot.
  Total anomalous pulmonary venous drainage.
  Hypoplastic left ventricle.
  Pulmonary vein stenosis.
  Tricuspid atresia and anomalies.
  Premature closure of foramen ovale.
  Dextrocardia.
  Pulmonary stenosis of atrial septal defect.
  Patent ductus arteriosis with reversed shunt.

Abnormal Hemoglobin
Methemoglobinemia.
  Hereditary.
  Acquired.
Sulfhemoglobinemia.
Mutant hemoglobin with low oxygen affinity (e.g., hemoglobin Kansas).

DAYTIME SLEEPINESS

ICD-9CM # varies with specific disorder

Sleep deprivation.
Medication induced (e.g., benzodiazepines, beta-blockers, narcotics, sedative antidepressants, gabapentin).
Depression.
Obstructive sleep apnea.
Medical illness (e.g., severe anemia, hypothyroidism, COPD, hepatic failure, renal insufficiency, CHF, electrolyte disturbances).
Circadian rhythm abnormalities (e.g., jet lag, shift work sleep disorder).
Restless legs syndrome.
Posttrauma.
Narcolepsy.
Neurologic disorders (e.g., neurodegenerative disorders; parkinsonism; multiple sclerosis; lesions affecting thalamus, hypothalamus, or brain stem).

DELAYED PASSAGE OF MECONIUM[16a]

ICD-9CM # 777.1

Ileal atresia.
Meconium ileus.
Functional immaturity of the colon.
Colon atresia.
Anorectal malformations.
Hirschsprung's disease.
Megacystis-microcolon-intestinal hypoperistalsis syndrome.
Extrinsic compression of the distal bowel by a mass lesion.
  Mesenteric cyst.
  Enteric duplication cyst.
Paralytic ileus, sepsis, drugs, and metabolic upset.

DELIRIUM[26]

ICD-9CM # 780.09 Delirium NOS
        293.0 Acute Delirium

PHARMACOLOGIC AGENTS
Anxiolytics (benzodiazepines).
Antidepressants (e.g., amitriptyline, doxepin, imipramine).
Cardiovascular agents (e.g., methyldopa, digitalis, reserpine, propranolol, procainamide, captopril, disopyramide).
Antihistamine.
Cimetidine.
Corticosteroids.
Antineoplastics.
Drugs of abuse (alcohol, cannabis, amphetamines, cocaine, hallucinogens, opioids, sedative-hypnotics, phencyclidine).

METABOLIC DISORDERS
Hypercalcemia.
Hypercarbia.
Hypoglycemia.
Hyponatremia.
Hypoxia.

INFLAMMATORY DISORDERS
Sarcoidosis.
SLE.
Giant cell arteritis.

ORGAN FAILURE
Hepatic encephalopathy.
Uremia.

NEUROLOGIC DISORDERS
Alzheimer's disease.
CVA.
Encephalitis (including HIV).
Encephalopathies.
Epilepsy.
Huntington's disease.
Multiple sclerosis.
Neoplasms.
Normal pressure hydrocephalus.
Parkinson's disease.
Pick's disease.
Wilson's disease.

ENDOCRINE DISORDERS
Addison's disease.
Cushing's disease.
Panhypopituitarism.
Parathyroid disease.
Postpartum psychosis.
Recurrent menstrual psychosis.
Sydenham's chorea.
Thyroid disease.

DEFICIENCY STATES
Niacin.
Thiamine, vitamin B_{12}, and folate.

DELIRIUM, AGITATED[2]

ICD-9CM # 293.1

Metabolic causes:
  Electrolyte abnormalities.
  Hypoglycemia.
  Hypoxia.
  Uremia/hyperammonemia.
Structural lesions of the CNS:
  Trauma.
  Stroke.
  Hemorrhage.
  Mass.
Endocrine disease:
  Thyrotoxicosis.
Infections:
  Bacterial/viral meningitis/encephalitis.
Toxicologic causes:
  Sympathomimetic/stimulants.
- Cocaine.
- Amphetamines and derivatives.
- Caffeine.
- Phencyclidine/ketamine.

  Anticholinergics.
  Serotonin syndrome.
  Sedative-hypnotic withdrawal.
Heatstroke
Postictal state

CNS, Central nervous system.

DELIRIUM, DIALYSIS PATIENT[26]

ICD-9CM # 293.0 Acute Delirium
        293.9 Encephalopathy from Dialysis

STRUCTURAL
Cerebrovascular accident (particularly hemorrhage).
Subdural hematoma.
Intracerebral abscess.
Brain tumor.

METABOLIC
Disequilibrium syndrome.
Uremia.
Drug effects.
Meningitis.
Hypertensive encephalopathy.
Hypotension.
Postictal state.
Hypernatremia or hyponatremia.

Hypercalcemia.
Hypermagnesemia.
Hypoglycemia.
Severe hyperglycemia.
Hypoxemia.
Dialysis dementia.

DEMYELINATING DISEASES[40]
ICD-9CM # 341.9

MULTIPLE SCLEROSIS
Relapsing and chronic progressive forms.
Acute multiple sclerosis.
Neuromyelitis optica (Devic's disease).

DIFFUSE CEREBRAL SCLEROSIS
Schilder's encephalitis periaxialis diffusa.
Baló's concentric sclerosis.

ACUTE DISSEMINATED ENCEPHALOMYELITIS
After measles, chickenpox, rubella, influenza, mumps.
After rabies or smallpox vaccination.

NECROTIZING HEMORRHAGIC ENCEPHALITIS
Hemorrhagic leukoencephalitis.

LEUKODYSTROPHIES
Krabbe's globoid leukodystrophy.
Metachromatic leukodystrophy.
Adrenoleukodystrophy.
Adrenomyeloneuropathy.
Pelizaeus-Merzbacher leukodystrophy.
Canavan's disease.
Alexander's disease.

DIAPHRAGM ELEVATION, BILATERAL, SYMMETRICAL[16a]
ICD-9CM # 519.4

CAUSES OF BILATERAL SYMMETRICAL ELEVATION OF THE DIAPHRAGM
Supine position.
Poor inspiration.
Obesity.
Pregnancy.
Abdominal distention (ascites, intestinal obstruction, abdominal mass).
Diffuse pulmonary fibrosis.
Lymphangitis carcinomatosa.
Disseminated lupus erythematosus.
Bilateral basal pulmonary emboli.
Painful conditions (after abdominal surgery).
Bilateral diaphragmatic paralysis.

DIAPHRAGM ELEVATION, UNILATERAL[16a]
ICD-9CM # 519.4

CAUSES OF UNILATERAL ELEVATION OF THE DIAPHRAGM
Posture—lateral decubitus position (dependent side).

Gaseous distention of stomach or colon.
Dorsal scoliosis.
Pulmonary hypoplasia.
Pulmonary collapse.
Phrenic nerve palsy.
Eventration.
Pneumonia or pleurisy.
Pulmonary thromboembolism.
Rib fracture and other painful conditions.
Subphrenic infection.
Subphrenic mass.

DIARRHEA, ACUTE WATERY AND BLOODY[38]
ICD-9CM # varies with specific diagnosis
    009.3 Infectious diarrhea
    558.9 Non-infectious diarrhea
    564.5 Functional diarrhea
    787.91 Diarrhea

ACUTE WATERY DIARRHEA
Gastrointestinal infections:
- Protozoal (e.g., *Giardia*).
- Bacterial (e.g., enterotoxigenic *Escherichia coli*, cholera).
- Viral (e.g., rotavirus, Norwalk virus).

Drugs.
Toxins.
Dietary constituents (e.g., lactose intolerance).
Onset of chronic diarrheal illness.

ACUTE BLOODY DIARRHEA
Infectious colitis:
- Confluent proctocolitis (e.g., *Shigella*, *Campylobacter*, *Salmonella*, *Entamoeba histolytica*).
- Segmental colitis (e.g., *Campylobacter*, *Salmonella*, enteroinvasive *E. coli*, *Aeromonas*, *E. histolytica*).

Drug-induced colitis (e.g., nonsteroidal anti-inflammatory drugs [NSAIDs]).
Inflammatory bowel disease.
Ischemic colitis (usually elderly patient with underlying heart disease or arrhythmias).
Antibiotic-associated colitis.

DIARRHEA, INFECTIOUS[2]
ICD-9CM # 009.2

ETIOLOGIC AGENTS OF INFECTIOUS DIARRHEA
Viral (60% of Cases)
Astrovirus.
Calicivirus.
Coronavirus.
Cytomegalovirus.*
Enteric adenovirus.
Hepatitis A through G.
Herpes simplex virus.
HIV enteropathy.
Norwalk-like agents.
Pararotavirus.
Norwalk virus.
Picornavirus.
Rotavirus.
Small round viruses.

Bacterial (20% of Cases)
Invasive*
Aeromonas spp.
Campylobacter spp.
Clostridium difficile.
Enteroinvasive *E. coli*.
Mycobacterium spp.
Plesiomonas shigelloides.
Salmonella spp.
Shigella spp.
Vibrio fluvialis.
Vibrio parahaemolyticus.
Vibrio vulnificus.
Yersinia enterocolitica.
Yersinia pseudotuberculosis.
Toxigenic
Food poisoning with preformed toxins.
  Bacillus cereus.
  Clostridium botulinum.
  Staphylococcus aureus.
Toxin formation after colonization.
  Aeromonas hydrophila.
  Clostridium perfringens.
  Enterohemorrhagic *E. coli* O157:H7.*
  Enterotoxigenic *E. coli*.
  Klebsiella pneumoniae.
  Shigella spp.
  Vibrio cholerae.
Other bacteria
Parasitic (5% of Cases)
Protozoa
Balantidium coli.*
Blastocystis hominis.
Cryptosporidium.
Cyclospora.
Dientamoeba fragilis.
Entamoeba histolytica.*
Entamoeba polecki.
Enteromonas hominis.
Giardia lamblia.
Isospora belli.
Microsporidia.
Sarcocystis hominis.
Helminths
Angiostrongylus costaricense.
Anisakiasis.
Ascaris lumbricoides.
Diphyllobothrium latum.
Enterobius vermicularis.
Hookworms.
Schistosoma spp.
Strongyloides stercoralis.
Taenia spp.
Trichinella spiralis.
Trichuris trichiura.

---

*Associated with fever, abdominal pain, and fecal red blood cells or white blood cells. % indicates the estimated contribution to total cases.

DIARRHEA, NONINFECTIOUS[2]
ICD-9CM # 564.5

CAUSES OF NONINFECTIOUS DIARRHEA
Toxins
Drugs
ACE inhibitors.
Alprazolam.

Antacids (Mg).
Antibiotics.
Antidepressants.
Antiepileptic drugs.
Antihypertensives.
Antiparkinson drugs.
Beta-blockers.
Caffeine.
Cardiac antiarrhythmics.
Chemotherapy agents.
Cholesterol-lowering drugs.
Cholinergic agents.
Cholinesterase inhibitors.
Colchicine.
Digitalis.
Diuretics.
Flurouracil.
Fluoxetine.
Histamine H_2-receptor antagonists.
Hydralazine.
Lactulose.
Laxatives/cathartics.
Levodopa.
Lithium.
NSAIDs.
Neomycin.
Podophyllin.
Procainamide.
Prostaglandins.
Quinidine.
Ricinoleic acid.
Theophylline.
Thyroid hormone.
Valproic acid.
Dietetic foods
Mannitol.
Sorbitol.
Xylitol.
Fish-associated toxins
Amnestic shellfish poisoning.
Ciguatera.
Echinoderms.
Neurotoxic shellfish poisoning.
Paralytic shellfish poisoning.
Scombroid.
Tetroton.
Plant-associated toxins
Herbal preparations.
Horse chestnut.
Mushrooms—*Amanita* spp.
Nicotine.
Other plant toxins:
  Pesticides—organophosphates.
  Pokeweed.
  Rhubarb.
Miscellaneous:
  Allergic reactions.
  Carbon monoxide poisoning.
  Ethanol.
  Heavy metals.
  Monosodium glutamate (MSG).
  Opiate withdrawal.
Gastrointestinal Pathology
Appendicitis.
Autonomic dysfunction.
Bile acid malabsorption.
Blind loop.
Bowel obstruction.

Celiac disease.
Cirrhosis.
Defects in amino acid transport.
Diverticular disease.
Familial dysautonomia.
Fecal impaction.
Fecal incontinence.
GI bleed.
GI cancer.
Hirschsprung's disease.
Inflammatory bowel disease (ulcerative colitis, Crohn's disease).
Intussusception.
Irritable bowel syndrome.
Ischemic bowel.
Lactose/fructose intolerance.
Malabsorption syndromes.
Malrotation.
Postsurgical.
Postvagotomy.
Radiation therapy.
Short gut syndrome.
Small bowel resection.
Strictures.
Toxic megacolon.
Tropical sprue.
Volvulus.
Whipple's disease.
Endocrine-related
Carcinoid syndrome (serotonin).
Hormonal hypersecretion.
Hyperthyroidism (thyroid hormone).
Medullary carcinoma of the thyroid (calcitonin).
Pancreatic cholera (VIP).
Somatostatinoma (somatostatin).
Systemic mastocytosis (histamine).
Zollinger-Ellison syndrome (gastrin).
Endocrine pathology
Adrenal insufficiency.
Diabetes enteropathy.
Hypoparathyroidism.
Pancreatic insufficiency.
Systemic Illness/Other
Alcoholism.
Amyloidosis.
Connective tissue disease.
Cystic fibrosis.
Ectopic pregnancy.
Hemolytic-uremic syndrome.
Henoch-Schönlein purpura.
Lymphoma.
Otitis media—infants.
Pelvic inflammatory disease.
Pneumonia/sepsis.
Pyelonephritis.
Scleroderma/SLE.
Severe malnutrition.
Stevens-Johnson syndrome.
Toxic shock syndrome.
Wilson's disease.
Miscellaneous:
  Factitious diarrhea.
  Runner's diarrhea.

ACE, Angiotensin-converting enzyme; *GI*, gastrointestinal; *NSAIDs*, nonsteroidal anti-inflammatory drugs; *SLE*, systemic lupus erythematosus; *VIP*, vasoactive intestinal polypeptide.

DIARRHEA, TUBE-FED PATIENT[14]
ICD-9CM # 564.4

COMMON CAUSES UNRELATED TO TUBE FEEDING
Elixir medications containing sorbitol.
Magnesium-containing antacids.
Antibiotic-induced sterile gut.
Pseudomembranous colitis.

POSSIBLE CAUSES RELATED TO TUBE FEEDING
Inadequate fiber to form stool bulk.
High fat content of formula (in the presence of fat malabsorption syndrome).
Bacterial contamination of enteral products and delivery systems (causal association with diarrhea not documented).
Rapid advancement in rate (after the GI tract is unused for prolonged periods).

UNLIKELY CAUSES RELATED TO TUBE FEEDING
Formula hyperosmolality (proven not to be the cause of diarrhea).
Lactose (absent from nearly all enteral feeding formulas).

DIPLOPIA, BINOCULAR
ICD-9CM # 368.2

Cranial nerve palsy (3rd, 4th, 6th).
Thyroid eye disease.
Myasthenia gravis.
Decompensated strabismus.
Orbital trauma with blowout fracture.
Orbital pseudotumor.
Cavernous sinus thrombosis.

DIPLOPIA, MONOCULAR
ICD-9CM # 368.2

Postoperative corrected longstanding tropia.
Defective contact lenses.
Poorly fitting bifocals.
Trauma to iris.
Corneal disorder (e.g., dry eye, astigmatism).
Cataracts.
Lens subluxation.
Nystagmus.
Eyelid twitching.
Foreign body in aqueous or vitreous media.
Migraine.
Lesions of occipital cortex.
Psychogenic.

DIPLOPIA, VERTICAL
ICD-9CM # 368.2

Myasthenia.
Superior oblique palsy.
Myositis or pseudotumor with orbital involvement.
Lymphoma or metastases affecting the orbits.
Brain stem or cerebellar lesions.
Hydrocephalus.

Differential Diagnosis
II

Third nerve palsy.
Botulism.
Wernicke's encephalopathy.
Dysthyroid orbitopathy (muscle infiltration).

DIZZINESS
ICD-9CM # 780.4

Viral syndrome.
Anxiety, hyperventilation.
Benign positional paroxysmal vertigo.
Medications (e.g., sedatives, antihypertensives, analgesics).
Withdrawal from medications (e.g., benzodiazepines, SSRIs).
Alcohol or drug abuse.
Postural hypotension.
Hypoglycemia, hyperglycemia.
Hematologic disorders (e.g., anemia, polycythemia, leukemia).
Head trauma.
Menière's disease.
Vertebrobasilar ischemia.
Cervical osteoarthritis.
Cardiac abnormalities (arrhythmias, cardiomyopathy, CHF, pericarditis).
Multiple sclerosis.
Peripheral vestibulopathy.
Air or sea travel.
Electrolyte abnormalities.
Eye problems (cornea, lens, retina).
Migraine.
Brain stem infarct.
Autonomic neuropathy.
Chronic otomastoiditis.
Complex partial seizures.
Ramsey Hunt syndrome.
Arteritis.
Syncope and presyncope.
Perilymph fistula.
Cerebellopontine tumor.
Hepatic or renal disease.

DRY EYE
ICD-9CM # 375.15

Contacts.
Medications (antihistamines, clonidine, beta-blockers, ibuprofen, scopolamine).
Keratoconjunctivitis sicca.
Trauma.
Environmental causes (air conditioning in patient with contacts).

DYSPAREUNIA[12]
ICD-9CM # 625.0 Dyspareunia
        608.89 Dyspareunia, Male
        302.76 Dyspareunia, Psychogenic

INTROITAL
Vaginismus.
Intact or rigid hymen.
Clitoral problems.
Vulvovaginitis.
Vaginal atrophy: hypoestrogen.
Vulvar dystrophy.
Bartholin or Skene gland infection.

Inadequate lubrication.
Operative scarring.

MIDVAGINAL
Urethritis.
Trigonitis.
Cystitis.
Short vagina.
Operative scarring.
Inadequate lubrication.

DEEP
Endometriosis.
Pelvic infection.
Uterine retroversion.
Ovarian pathology.
GI.
Orthopedic.
Abnormal penile size or shape.

DYSPHAGIA
ICD-9CM # 787.2

Esophageal obstruction: neoplasm, foreign body, achalasia, stricture, spasm, esophageal web, diverticulum, Schatzki's ring.
Peptic esophagitis with stricture, Barrett's stricture.
External esophageal compression: neoplasms (thyroid neoplasm, lymphoma, mediastinal tumors), thyroid enlargement, aortic aneurysm, vertebral spurs, aberrant right subclavian artery (dysphagia lusoria).
Hiatal hernia, GERD.
Oropharyngeal lesions: pharyngitis, glossitis, stomatitis, neoplasms.
Hysteria: globus hystericus.
Neurologic and/or neuromuscular disturbances: bulbar paralysis, myasthenia gravis, ALS, multiple sclerosis, Parkinsonism, CVA, diabetic neuropathy.
Toxins: poisoning, botulism, tetanus, postdiphtheritic dysphagia.
Systemic diseases: scleroderma, amyloidosis, dermatomyositis.
Candida and herpes esophagitis.
Presbyesophagus.

DYSPHAGIA, OROPHARYNGEAL[38]
ICD-9CM # 787.22

FUNCTIONAL DISORDERS
Central Nervous System
Stroke.
Head injury.
Parkinson's disease.
Motor neuron disease.
Multiple sclerosis.
Tumor.
Drugs (e.g., phenothiazines).
Malformations (e.g., syrinx, Arnold–Chiari).
Neural
Motor neuron disease.
Myasthenia gravis.
Radiotherapy.
Poliomyelitis.
Familial dysautonomia.

Muscle
Autoimmune myopathy (polymyositis, dermatomyositis, systemic lupus erythematosus).
Thyrotoxic myopathy.
Guillain-Barré motor neuropathy.
Muscular dystrophies.

STRUCTURAL DISORDERS
Head/neck surgery.
Stricture.
Radiotherapy.
Tumor.
Pharyngeal pouch.
Web.
Extrinsic (e.g., osteophytes).

MISCELLANEOUS
Xerostomia.

DYSPNEA
ICD-9CM # 786.00

Upper airway obstruction: trauma, neoplasm, epiglottitis, laryngeal edema, tongue retraction, laryngospasm, abductor paralysis of vocal cords, aspiration of foreign body.
Lower airway obstruction: neoplasm, COPD, asthma, aspiration of foreign body.
Pulmonary infection: pneumonia, abscess, empyema, TB, bronchiectasis.
Pulmonary hypertension.
Pulmonary embolism/infarction.
Parenchymal lung disease.
Pulmonary vascular congestion.
Cardiac disease: ASHD, valvular lesions, cardiac dysrhythmias, cardiomyopathy, pericardial effusion, cardiac shunts.
Space-occupying lesions: neoplasm, large hiatal hernia, pleural effusions.
Disease of chest wall: severe kyphoscoliosis, fractured ribs, sternal compression, morbid obesity.
Neurologic dysfunction: Guillain-Barré syndrome, botulism, polio, spinal cord injury.
Interstitial pulmonary disease: sarcoidosis, collagen vascular diseases, DIP, Hamman-Rich pneumonitis, etc.
Pneumoconioses: silicosis, berylliosis, etc.
Mesothelioma.
Pneumothorax, hemothorax, pleural effusion.
Inhalation of toxins.
Cholinergic drug intoxication.
Carcinoid syndrome.
Hematologic: anemia, polycythemia, hemoglobinopathies.
Thyrotoxicosis, myxedema.
Diaphragmatic compression caused by abdominal distention, subphrenic abscess, ascites.
Lung resection.
Metabolic abnormalities: uremia, hepatic coma, DKA.
Sepsis.
Atelectasis.
Psychoneurosis.
Diaphragmatic paralysis.
Pregnancy.

DYSURIA

ICD-9CM # 788.1 Dysuria
306.53 Dysuria, Psychogenic

Urinary tract infection.
Estrogen deficiency (in postmenopausal female).
Vaginitis.
Genital infection (e.g., herpes, condyloma).
Interstitial cystitis.
Chemical irritation (e.g., deodorant aerosols, douches).
Meatal stenosis or stricture.
Reiter's syndrome.
Bladder neoplasm.
GI etiology (diverticulitis, Crohn's disease).
Impaired bladder or sphincter action.
Urethral carbuncle.
Chronic fibrosis posttrauma.
Radiation therapy.
Prostatitis.
Urethritis (gonococcal, *Chlamydiae*).
Behçet's syndrome.
Stevens-Johnson syndrome.

EARACHE[33]

ICD-9CM # 388.70 Earache
388.72 Ear Pain, Referred

Otitis media.
Serous otitis media.
Eustachitis.
Otitis externa.
Otitic barotrauma.
Mastoiditis.
Foreign body.
Impacted cerumen.
Referred otalgia, as with TMJ dysfunction, dental problems, and tumors.

ECTOPIC ACTH SECRETION[14]

ICD-9CM # 255.0

Small cell carcinoma of lung.
Endocrine tumors of foregut origin.
  Thymic carcinoid.
  Islet cell tumor.
  Medullary carcinoid, thyroid.
  Bronchial carcinoid.
Pheochromocytoma.
Ovarian tumors.

EDEMA, CHILDREN[19]

ICD-9CM # 782.3 Edema NOS

CARDIOVASCULAR

Congestive heart failure.
Acute thrombi or emboli.
Vasculitis of many types.

RENAL

Nephrotic syndrome.
Glomerulonephritis of many types.
End-stage renal failure.

ENDOCRINE OR METABOLIC

Thyroid disease.
Starvation.
Hereditary angioedema.

IATROGENIC

Drugs (diuretics and steroids).
Water or salt overload.

HEMATOLOGIC

Hemolytic disease of the newborn.

GASTROINTESTINAL

Hepatic cirrhosis.
Protein-losing enteritis.
Lymphangiectasis.
Cystic fibrosis.
Celiac disease.
Enteritis of many types.

LYMPHATIC ABNORMALITIES

Congenital (gonadal dysgenesis).
Acquired.

EDEMA, GENERALIZED

ICD-9CM # 782.3 Edema NOS

Congestive heart failure (CHF).
Cirrhosis.
Nephrotic syndrome.
Pregnancy.
Idiopathic.
Acute nephritic syndrome.
Myxedema.
Medications (NSAIDs, estrogens, vasodilators).

EDEMA, LEG, UNILATERAL[26]

ICD-9CM # 782.3

WITH PAIN

DVT.
Postphlebitic syndrome.
Popliteal cyst rupture.
Gastrocnemius rupture.
Cellulitis.
Psoas or other abscess.

WITHOUT PAIN

DVT.
Postphlebitic syndrome.
Other venous insufficiency (after saphenous vein harvest, varicosities).
Lymphatic obstruction/lymphedema (carcinoma, lymphoma, sarcoidosis, filariasis, retroperitoneal fibrosis).

EDEMA OF LOWER EXTREMITIES

ICD-9CM # 782.3

CHF (right-sided).
Hepatic cirrhosis.
Nephrosis.
Myxedema.
Lymphedema.
Pregnancy.
Abdominal mass: neoplasm, cyst.
Venous compression from abdominal aneurysm.
Varicose veins.
Bilateral cellulitis.
Bilateral thrombophlebitis.
Vena cava thrombosis, venous thrombosis.
Retroperitoneal fibrosis.

EJECTION SOUND OR CLICK

ICD-9CM # 785.3

Aortic regurgitation.
Aortic root dilatation.
Systemic hypertension.
Chronic pulmonary hypertension.
Tetralogy of Fallot.
Atrial septal defect.
Pulmonary valve stenosis.
Aortic aneurysm.

ELBOW PAIN

ICD-9CM # 719.42

Trauma.
Infection.
Inflammatory arthritis.
Lateral or medial epicondylitis.
Entrapment neuropathy.
Olecranon bursitis.
Osteoarthritis.
Gout.
Cervical disease (referred pain).
Shoulder disease (referred pain).
Partial subluxation.
Synovial osteochondromatosis.
Loose body.

ELEVATED HEMIDIAPHRAGM

ICD-9CM # 519.4 Diaphragm Disorder
519.4 Diaphragm Paralysis
756.6 Diaphragm Eventration, Congenital

Neoplasm (bronchogenic carcinoma, mediastinal neoplasm, intrahepatic lesion).
Substernal thyroid.
Infectious process (pneumonia, empyema, TB, subphrenic abscess, hepatic abscess).
Atelectasis.
Idiopathic.
Eventration.
Phrenic nerve dysfunction (myelitis, myotonia, herpes zoster).
Trauma to phrenic nerve or diaphragm (e.g., surgery).
Aortic aneurysm.
Intraabdominal mass.
Pulmonary infarction.
Pleurisy.
Radiation therapy.
Rib fracture.

EMBOLI, ARTERIAL[26]

ICD-9CM # 444.22 Embolism, Artery, Lower Extremity
444.21 Embolism, Artery, Upper Extremity

Myocardial infarction with mural thrombi.
Atrial fibrillation.
Cardiomyopathies.
Prosthetic heart valves.
CHF.
Endocarditis.
Left ventricular aneurysm.
Left atrial myxoma.

Sick sinus syndrome.
Paradoxical embolus from venous thrombosis.
Aneurysms of large blood vessels.
Atheromatous ulcers of large blood vessels.

EMESIS, PEDIATRIC AGE[19]
ICD-9CM # 787.03

INFANCY
Gastrointestinal Tract
Congenital:
Regurgitation—chalasia, gastroesophageal reflux.
Atresia—stenosis (tracheoesophageal fistula, prepyloric diaphragm, intestinal atresia).
Duplication.
Volvulus (errors in rotation and fixation, Meckel diverticulum).
Congenital bands.
Hirschsprung's disease.
Meconium ileus (cystic fibrosis), meconium plug.
Acquired:
Acute infectious gastroenteritis, food poisoning (staphylococcal, clostridial).
Pyloric stenosis.
Gastritis, duodenitis.
Intussusception.
Incarcerated hernia—inguinal, internal secondary to old adhesions.
Cow's milk protein intolerance, food allergy, eosinophilic gastroenteritis.
Disaccharidase deficiency.
Celiac disease—presents after introduction of gluten in diet; inherited risk.
Adynamic ileus—the mediator for many nongastrointestinal causes.
Neonatal necrotizing enterocolitis.
Chronic granulomatous disease with gastric outlet obstruction.
Nongastrointestinal Tract
Infectious—otitis, urinary tract infection, pneumonia, upper respiratory tract infection, sepsis, meningitis.
Metabolic—aminoaciduria and organic aciduria, galactosemia, fructosemia, adrenogenital syndrome, renal tubular acidosis, diabetic ketoacidosis, Reye's syndrome.
Central nervous system—trauma, tumor, infection, diencephalic syndrome, rumination, autonomic responses (pain, shock).
Medications—anticholinergics, aspirin, alcohol, idiosyncratic reaction (e.g., codeine).

CHILDHOOD
Gastrointestinal Tract
Peptic ulcer—vomiting is a common presentation in children younger than 6 yr old.
Trauma—duodenal hematoma, traumatic pancreatitis, perforated bowel.
Pancreatitis—mumps, trauma, cystic fibrosis, hyperparathyroidism, hyperlipidemia, organic acidemias.
Crohn's disease.
Idiopathic intestinal pseudoobstruction.
Superior mesenteric artery syndrome.

Nongastrointestinal Tract
Central nervous system—cyclic vomiting, migraine, anorexia nervosa, bulimia.

ENCEPHALOMYELITIS, NONVIRAL CAUSES[25]
ICD-9CM # varies with specific disorder

Subacute bacterial endocarditis.
Rocky Mountain spotted fever.
Typhus.
Ehrlichia.
Q fever.
Chlamydia.
Mycoplasma.
Legionella.
Brucellosis.
Listeria.
Whipple's disease.
Cat-scratch disease.
Syphilis (meningovascular).
Relapsing fever.
Lyme disease.
Leptospirosis.
Nocardia.
Actinomycosis.
Tuberculosis.
Cryptococcus.
Histoplasma.
Toxoplasma.
Plasmodium falciparum.
Trypanosomiasis.
Behçet's disease.
Vasculitis.
Carcinoma.
Drug reactions.

ENCEPHALOPATHY, METABOLIC[36]

ICD-9CM #	
291.2	Alcoholic Encephalopathy
572.2	Hepatic Encephalopathy
251.2	Hypoglycemic Encephalopathy
349.82	Toxic Encephalopathy
984.9	Lead Encephalopathy
293.9	Encephalopathy

Substrate deficiency: hypoxia/ischemia, carbon monoxide poisoning, hypoglycemia.
Cofactor deficiency: thiamine, vitamin B_{12}, pyridoxine (INH administration).
Electrolyte disorders: hyponatremia, hypercalcemia, carbon dioxide narcosis, dialysis, hypermagnesemia, disequilibrium syndrome.
Endocrinopathies: DKA, hyperosmolar coma, hypothyroidism, hyperadrenocorticism, hyperparathyroidism.
Endogenous toxins: liver disease, uremia, porphyria.
Exogenous toxins: drug overdose (sedative/hypnotics, ethanol, narcotics, salicylates, tricyclic antidepressants), drug withdrawal, toxicity of therapeutic medications, industrial toxins (e.g., organophosphates, heavy metals), sepsis.
Heat stroke.
Epilepsy (postictal).

ENTHESOPATHY
ICD-9CM # code not available

Viremia or bacteremia.
Ankylosing spondylitis.
Psoriatic arthritis.
Drug-induced (quinolones, etretinate).
Reactive arthritis.
DISH.
Reiter's syndrome.

EOSINOPHILIC LUNG DISEASE[16a]
ICD-9CM # 495.8

IDIOPATHIC
Simple pulmonary eosinophilia (Löffler's syndrome).
Acute eosinophilic pneumonia.
Chronic eosinophilic pneumonia.
Hypereosinophilic syndrome.

DRUG-INDUCED
Aminosalicylic acid.
Para-arminosalicylic acid.
NSAIDs.
Captopril.
Cocaine.
Minocycline.
Nitrofurantoin.
Phenytoin.

INFECTION
Parasitic (ascariasis, paragonomiasis, tropical eosinophilia).
Fungal (aspergillus).
Bacterial (TB, atypical mycobacterial infection, brucella).
Viral (respiratory syncytial virus).

IMMUNOLOGICAL DISEASES
Wegener's granulomatosis.
Churg–Strauss syndrome.
Rheumatoid disease.
Sarcoidosis.

NEOPLASMS
Brochogenic carcinoma.
Bronchial carcinoid.
Lymphoma (Hodgkin's, non-Hodgkin's).

EPIGASTRIC PAIN[38]
ICD-9CM # 789.66

No specific cause found.
Peptic ulceration (uncomplicated).*
Peptic ulceration (perforated).*
Biliary colic.*
Acute pancreatitis.*
Abdominal aortic aneurysm.

*Conditions that also cause right upper quadrant pain.

EPILEPSY

ICD-9CM # 345.9 Epilepsy NOS

Psychogenic spells.
Transient ischemic attack.
Hypoglycemia.
Syncope.
Narcolepsy.
Migraine.
Paroxysmal vertigo.
Arrhythmias.
Drug reaction.

EPISTAXIS

ICD-9CM # 784.7

Trauma.
Medications (nasal sprays, NSAIDs, anticoagulants, antiplatelets).
Nasal polyps.
Cocaine use.
Coagulopathy (hemophilia, liver disease, DIC, thrombocytopenia).
Systemic disorders (hypertension, uremia).
Infections.
Anatomic malformations.
Rhinitis.
Nasal polyps.
Local neoplasms (benign and malignant).
Desiccation.
Foreign body.

ERECTILE DYSFUNCTION, ORGANIC[31]

ICD-9CM # 607.84

Neurogenic abnormalities: Somatic nerve neuropathy, central nervous system abnormalities.
Psychogenic causes: Depression, performance anxiety, marital conflict.
Endocrine causes: Hyperprolactinemia, hypogonadotropic hypogonadism, testicular failure, estrogen excess.
Trauma: Pelvic fracture, prostate surgery, penile fracture.
Systemic disease: DM, renal failure, hepatic cirrhosis.
Medications: Diuretics, antidepressants, H_2 blockers, exogenous hormones, alcohol, antihypertensives, nicotine abuse, finasteride, etc.
Structural abnormalities: Peyronie's disease.

EROSIONS, GENITALIA

ICD-9CM # 599.84

Candidiasis.
Intraepithelial neoplasia.
Squamous cell carcinoma.
Lichen planus.
Pemphigus vulgaris.
Erythema multiforme.
Lichen sclerosus.
Bullous pemphigoid.
Extramammary Paget's disease.
Impetigo.

ERYTHEMATOUS ANNULAR SKIN LESIONS

ICD-9CM # varies with diagnosis

Tinea corporis.
Warfarin plaques.
Erythema multiforme.
Erythema annulare.
Cutaneous lupus.
Cutaneous sarcoidosis.
Trauma.
Acute febrile neutrophilic dermatosis (Sweet's syndrome).

ERYTHROCYTOSIS[20]

ICD-9CM # 289.6

CAUSES OF ERYTHROCYTOSIS

Relative or Spurious Erythrocytosis (Normal Red Cell Mass)
Hemoconcentration secondary to dehydration (diarrhea, diaphoresis, diuretics, water deprivation, emesis, ethanol, hypertension, preeclampsia, pheochromocytoma, carbon monoxide intoxication).
True or Absolute Erythrocytosis
Polycythemia vera.
Primary congenital polycythemia.
Secondary erythrocytosis caused by:
Congenital causes (e.g., activating mutation of erythropoietin receptor).
Hypoxia caused by carbon monoxide poisoning, high oxygen affinity hemoglobin, high-altitude residence, chronic pulmonary disease, hypoventilation syndromes such as sleep apnea, right to left cardiac shunt, neurologic defects involving the respiratory center.
Nonhypoxic causes with pathologic erythropoietin production.
- Renal disease (cysts, hydronephrosis, renal artery stenosis, focal glomerulonephritis, renal transplantation).
- Tumors (renal cell cancer, hepatocellular carcinoma, cerebellar hemangioblastoma, uterine fibromyoma, adrenal tumors, meningioma, pheochromocytoma).
Drug-associated causes:
- Androgen therapy.
- Exogenous erythropoietin growth factor therapy.

ERYTHRODERMA

ICD-9CM # 695.9   Secondary
            696.2   Maculopapular
            696.1   Psoriaticum
            695.89 Exfoliative
            778.8   Neonatorum

Drug reaction (e.g., allopurinol, ampicillin, phenytoin, vancomycin, dapsone, omeprazole, carbamazepine).
Atopic dermatitis.
Psoriasis.
Contact dermatitis.
Idiopathic.
Pityriasis rubra.

Chronic actinic dermatitis.
Bullous pemphigoid.
Paraneoplastic.
Cutaneous T-cell lymphoma.
Connective tissue disease.
Hypereosinophilia syndrome.

ESOPHAGEAL PERFORATION[26]

ICD-9CM # 530.4   Perforation, Nontraumatic
             862.22 Injury, Traumatic

Trauma.
Caustic burns.
Iatrogenic.
Foreign bodies.
Spontaneous rupture (Boerhaave's syndrome).
Postoperative breakdown of anastomosis.

ESOPHAGITIS[25]

ICD-9CM # 530.12

INFECTIOUS

Candidiasis.
Cytomegalovirus.
Herpes simplex virus.
HIV infection, acute.

NONINFECTIOUS

Gastroesophageal reflux.
Mucositis from cancer chemotherapy.
Mucositis from radiation therapy.
Aphthous ulcers.

ESOTROPIA

ICD-9CM # Nonaccommodative 378.00
            Accommodative 378.35
            Alternating 378.05

Congenital.
Accommodative esotropia.
Myasthenia gravis.
Abducens palsy.
Pseudo-sixth nerve palsy.
Medial rectus entrapment (e.g., blowout fracture).
Posterior internuclear ophthalmoplegia.
Wernicke's encephalopathy.
Thyroid myopathy.
Chiari malformation.

EXANTHEMS[28]

ICD-9CM # 782.1

Measles.
Rubella.
Erythema infectiosum (fifth disease).
Roseola exanthema.
Varicella.
Enterovirus.
Adenovirus.
Epstein-Barr virus.
Kawasaki disease.
Staphylococcal scalded skin.
Scarlet fever.
Meningococcemia.
Rocky Mountain spotted fever.

Differential Diagnosis

II

EYELID NEOPLASM

ICD-9CM # varies with specific disorder

MALIGNANT

Melanoma.
Basal cell carcinoma.
Squamous cell carcinoma.
Bowen's disease.
Sebaceous cell carcinoma.
Metastatic lymphoma/leukemia.

BENIGN

Melanocytic nevus.
Pilar, eccrine, or apocrine tumor.
Neurofibroma.
Keratosis.
Squamous papilloma.
Keratoacanthoma.

EYELID RETRACTION

ICD-9CM # 374.89

Congenital.
Graves' ophthalmopathy.
Myasthenia gravis.
Postsurgical.
Guillain-Barré syndrome.
Cerebellar disease.
Horizontal gaze palsy.
Partial palsy of superior rectus muscle.
Encephalitis.
Closed head injury.
Disseminated sclerosis.
Eye trauma.
Contact lens wear.
Proptosis.
Eyelid neoplasm.
Atopic dermatitis.
Herpes zoster ophthalmicus.
Botulinum toxin injection.
Cyclic oculomotor paralysis.
Spheroid wing meningioma.
Hepatic cirrhosis.
Down syndrome.
Essential hypertension.
Meningitis.
Paget's disease of bone.

EYE PAIN

ICD-9CM # 379.91

Foreign body.
Herpes zoster.
Trauma.
Conjunctivitis.
Iritis.
Iridocyclitis.
Uveitis.
Blepharitis.
Ingrown lashes.
Orbital or periorbital cellulitis/abscess.
Sinusitis.
Headache.
Glaucoma.
Inflammation of lacrimal gland.
Tic douloureux.
Cerebral aneurysm.

Cerebral neoplasm.
Entropion.
Retrobulbar neuritis.
UV light.
Dry eyes.
Irritation or inflammation from eye drops, dust, cosmetics, etc.

FACIAL PAIN

ICD-9CM # 784.0

Infection, abscess.
Postherpetic neuralgia.
Trauma, posttraumatic neuralgia.
Tic douloureux.
Cluster headache, "lower-half headache."
Geniculate neuralgia.
Anxiety, somatization syndrome.
Glossopharyngeal neuralgia.
Carotidynia.

FACIAL PARALYSIS[28]

ICD-9CM # 351.0 Facial (7th Nerve) Palsy

INFECTION

Bacterial: otitis media, mastoiditis, meningitis, Lyme disease.
Viral: herpes zoster, mononucleosis, varicella, rubella, mumps, Bell's palsy.
Mycobacterial: TB, meningitis, leprosy.
Miscellaneous: syphilis, malaria.

TRAUMA

Temporal bone fracture, facial laceration.
Surgery.

NEOPLASM

Malignant: squamous cell carcinoma, basal cell and adenocystic tumors, leukemia, parotid neoplasms, metastatic tumors.
Benign: facial nerve neuroma, vestibular schwannoma, congenital cholesteatoma.

IMMUNOLOGIC

Guillain-Barré syndrome, periarteritis nodosa.
Reaction to tetanus antiserum.

METABOLIC

Pregnancy.
Hypothyroidism.
DM.

FAILURE TO THRIVE

ICD-9CM # 783.4

MALABSORPTION

Cow's milk protein allergy.
Cystic fibrosis.
Celiac disease.
Biliary atresia.

INSUFFICIENT CALORIC INTAKE

Parental neglect.
Feeding difficulties (CNS lesion, severe reflux, oromotor abnormalities).
Use of diluted formula preparation.
Food shortage (poverty).

INCREASED NEEDS

Hyperthyroidism.
Congenital heart defects.
Malignancy.
Renal or hepatic disease.
HIV.

IMPROPER UTILIZATION

Storage disorders.
Amino acid disorders.
Trisomy 13, 21, 18.

FATIGUE

ICD-9CM # 780.7 Fatigue NOS
300.5 Fatigue Psychogenic
780.7 Chronic Fatigue Syndrome

Depression.
Anxiety, emotional stress.
Inadequate sleep.
Chronic fatigue syndrome.
Prolonged physical activity.
Pregnancy and postpartum period.
Anemia.
Hypothyroidism.
Medications (beta-blockers, anxiolytics, antidepressants, sedating antihistamines, clonidine, methyldopa).
Viral or bacterial infections.
Sleep apnea syndrome.
Dieting.
Renal failure, CHF, COPD, liver disease.

FATTY LIVER

ICD-9CM # 571.8

Obesity.
Alcohol abuse.
DM.
Acute fatty liver of pregnancy.
Medications (tetracycline, valproic acid, glucocorticoids, amiodarone, estrogen, methotrexate).
Reye's syndrome.
Wilson's disease.
Nonalcoholic steatosis.

FEVER AND JAUNDICE

ICD-9CM # 789.6 Fever
782.4 Jaundice

Cholecystitis.
Hepatic abscess (pyogenic, amebic).
Ascending cholangitis.
Pancreatitis.
Malaria.
Neoplasm (hepatic pancreatic, biliary tract, metastatic).
Mononucleosis.
Viral hepatitis.
Sepsis.
Babesiosis.
HIV (cryptosporidium).
Biliary ascariasis.
Toxic shock syndrome.
Yersinia infection, leptospirosis, yellow fever, Dengue fever, relapsing fever.

FEVER AND RASH

ICD-9CM # 782.1 Exanthem
57.9 Exanthem Viral
789.6 Fever

Drug hypersensitivity: penicillin, sulfonamides, thiazides, anticonvulsants, allopurinol.
Viral infection: measles, rubella, varicella, erythema infectiosum, roseola, enterovirus infection, viral hepatitis, infectious mononucleosis, acute HIV.
Other infections: meningococcemia, staphylococcemia, scarlet fever, typhoid fever, *Pseudomonas* bacteremia, Rocky Mountain spotted fever, Lyme disease, secondary syphilis, bacterial endocarditis, babesiosis, brucellosis, listeriosis.
Serum sickness.
Erythema multiforme.
Erythema marginatum.
Erythema nodosum.
SLE.
Dermatomyositis.
Allergic vasculitis.
Pityriasis rosea.
Herpes zoster.

FEVER IN RETURNING TRAVELERS AND IMMIGRANTS[28]

ICD-9CM # varies with specific disorder

Differential diagnosis of some selected systemic febrile illnesses to consider in returned travelers and immigrants.*

COMMON

Acute respiratory tract infection (worldwide).
Gastroenteritis (worldwide) [foodborne, waterborne, fecal-oral].
Enteric fever, including typhoid (worldwide) [food, water].
Urinary tract infection (worldwide) [sexual contact].
Drug reactions [antibiotics, prophylactic agents, other] {rash frequent}.
Malaria (tropics, limited areas of temperate zones) [mosquitoes].
Arboviruses (Africa; tropics) [mosquitoes, ticks, mites].
Dengue (Asia, Caribbean, Africa) [mosquitoes].
Viral hepatitis (worldwide).
Hepatitis A (worldwide) [food, fecal-oral].
Hepatitis B (worldwide, especially Asia, sub-Saharan Africa) [sexual contact] {long incubation period}.
Hepatitis C (worldwide) [blood or sexual contact].
Hepatitis E (Asia, North Africa, Mexico, others) [food, water].
Tuberculosis (worldwide) [airborne, milk] {long period to symptomatic infection}.
Sexually transmitted diseases (worldwide) [sexual contact].

LESS COMMON

Filariasis (Asia, Africa, South America) [biting insects] {long incubation period, eosinophilia}.
Measles (developing world) [airborne] {in susceptible individual}.
Amebic abscess (worldwide) [food].
Brucellosis (worldwide) [milk, cheese, food, animal contact].
Listeriosis (worldwide) [foodborne] {meningitis}.
Leptospirosis (worldwide) [animal contact, open fresh water] {jaundice, meningitis}.
Strongyloidiasis (warm and tropical areas) [soil contact] {eosinophilia}.
Toxoplasmosis (worldwide) [undercooked meat].

RARE

Relapsing fever (western Americas, Asia, northern Africa) [ticks, lice].
Hemorrhagic fevers (worldwide) [arthropod and nonarthropod transmitted].
Yellow fever (tropics) [mosquitoes] {hepatitis}.
Hemorrhagic fever with renal syndrome (Europe, Asia, North America) [rodent urine] {renal impairment}.
Hantavirus pulmonary syndrome (western North America, other) [rodent urine] {respiratory distress syndrome}.
Lassa fever (Africa) [rodent excreta, person to person] {high mortality rate}
Other—chikungunya, Rift Valley, Ebola-Marburg, etc. (various) [insect bites, rodent excreta, aerosols, person to person] {often severe}.
Rickettsial infections {rashes and eschars}.
Leishmaniasis, visceral (Middle East, Mediterranean, Africa, Asia, South America) [biting flies] {long incubation period}.
Acute schistosomiasis (Africa, Asia, South America, Caribbean) [fresh water].
Chagas' disease (South and Central America) [reduviid bug bites] {often asymptomatic}.
African trypanosomiasis (Africa) [tsetse fly bite] {neurologic syndromes, sleeping sickness}.
Bartonellosis (South America) [sandfly bite; cb] {skin nodules}.
HIV infection/AIDS (worldwide) [sexual and blood contact].
Trichinosis (worldwide) [undercooked meat] {eosinophilia}.
Plague (temperate and tropical plains) [animal exposures and fleas].
Tularemia (worldwide) [animal contact, fleas, aerosols] {ulcers, lymph nodes}.
Anthrax (worldwide) [animal, animal product contact] {ulcers}.
Lyme disease (North America, Europe) [tick bites] {arthritis, meningitis, cardiac abnormalities}.

---

*Diagnoses for which particular symptoms are indicative are in *italics*. Exposure to regions of the world that are most likely to be significant to the diagnosis are presented in (parentheses). Vectors, risk behaviors, and sources associated with acquisition are presented in [brackets]. Special clinical characteristics are listed within {braces}.

FEVER, NONINFECTIOUS CAUSES[2]

ICD-9CM # 780.60

DIFFERENTIAL DIAGNOSIS— NONINFECTIOUS CAUSES OF FEVER

Critical Diagnoses
Acute myocardial infarction.
Pulmonary embolism/infarction.
Intracranial hemorrhage.
Cerebrovascular accident.
Neuroleptic-malignant syndrome.
Thyroid storm.
Acute adrenal insufficiency.
Transfusion reaction.
Pulmonary edema.
Emergent Diagnoses
Congestive heart failure.
Dehydration.
Recent seizure.
Sickle cell disease.
Transplant rejection.
Pancreatitis.
Deep vein thrombosis.
Nonemergent Diagnoses
Drug fever.
Malignancy.
Gout.
Sarcoidosis.
Crohn's disease.
Postmyocardiotomy syndrome.

FINGER LESIONS, INFLAMMATORY

ICD-9CM # varies with specific disorder

Paronychia.
Herpes simplex type 1 (herpetic whitlow).
Dyshidrotic eczema (pompholyx).
Herpes zoster.
Bacterial endocarditis (Osler's nodes).
Psoriatic arthritis.

FLATULENCE AND BLOATING[33]

ICD-9CM # 787.3

Ingestion of nonabsorbable carbohydrates.
Ingestion of carbonated beverages.
Malabsorption: pancreatic insufficiency, biliary disease, celiac disease, bacterial overgrowth in small intestine.
Lactase deficiency.
Irritable bowel syndrome.
Anxiety disorders.
Food poisoning, giardiasis.

FLUSHING[27]

ICD-9CM # 782.62

Physiologic flushing: menopause, ingestion of monosodium glutamate (Chinese restaurant syndrome), ingestion of hot drinks.

Drugs: alcohol (with or without disulfiram, metronidazole, or chlorpropamide), nicotinic acid, diltiazem, nifedipine, levodopa, bromocriptine, vancomycin, amyl nitrate.
Neoplastic disorders: carcinoid syndrome, VIPoma syndrome, medullary carcinoma of thyroid, systemic mastocytosis, basophilic chronic myelocytic leukemia, renal cell carcinoma.
Anxiety.
Agnogenic flushing.

FOLATE DEFICIENCY[20]
ICD-9CM # 281.2

ETIOPATHOPHYSIOLOGIC CLASSIFICATION OF FOLATE DEFICIENCY
Nutritional causes:
Decreased dietary intake:
- Poverty and famine.
- Institutionalized individuals (e.g., psychiatric, nursing homes), chronic debilitating disease.
- Prolonged feeding of infants with goat's milk, special slimming diets or food fads (i.e., folate-rich foods not consumed), cultural or ethnic cooking techniques (i.e., food folate destroyed).
Decreased diet and increased requirements:
- Physiologic (e.g., pregnancy and lactation, prematurity, hyperemesis gravidarum, infancy).
- Pathologic (e.g., intrinsic hematologic diseases involving hemolysis with compensatory erythropoiesis, abnormal hematopoiesis, or bone marrow infiltration with malignant disease and dermatologic disease such as psoriasis).
Folate malabsorption:
With normal intestinal mucosa:
- Some drugs (controversial).
- Congenital folate malabsorption (rare).
With mucosal abnormalities (e.g., tropical and nontropical sprue, regional enteritis).
Defective cellular folate uptake:
Familial aplastic anemia (rare).
Acute cerebral folate deficiency.
Inadequate cellular use:
Folate antagonists (e.g., methotrexate).
Hereditary enzyme deficiencies involving folate.
Drugs:
Multiple effects on folate metabolism (e.g., alcohol, sulfasalazine, triamterene, pyrimethamine, trimethoprim-sulfamethoxazole, diphenylhydantoin, barbiturates).
Acute folate deficiency:
Intensive care unit setting.
Uncertain origin.

FOOT AND ANKLE PAIN, IN DIFFERENT AGE GROUPS[8]
ICD-9CM # varies with specific diagnosis

COMMON CAUSES OF FOOT AND ANKLE PAIN IN DIFFERENT AGE GROUPS
Childhood (2-10 yr)
Intraarticular:
Club foot.
Congenital midfoot and forefoot deformities.
Septic arthritis.
Periarticular:
Osteomyelitis.
Adolescence (10-18 yr)
Intraarticular:
Arch disorders (pes cavus, pes planus).
Periarticular:
Osteomyelitis.
Tumors.
Early Adulthood (18-30 yr)
Intraarticular:
Metatarsalgia.
Hallux valgus.
Hallux rigidus.
Osteochondritis.
Accessory ossicles.
Periarticular:
Achilles tendonitis.
Achilles tendon rupture.
Fasciitis.
Referred:
Lumbar spine.
Knee.
Adulthood (30-50 yr)
Intraarticular:
Osteoarthritis.
Inflammatory arthritis.
Gout.
Metatarsalgia.
Hallux valgus.
Hallux rigidus.
Osteochondritis.
Accessory ossicles.
Periarticular:
Ischemic foot pain.
Diabetes.
Bursitis.
Tendonitis.
Plantar fasciitis.
Corns.
Referred:
Lumbar spine.
Knee.
Old Age (>50 yr)
Intraarticular:
Osteoarthritis.
Inflammatory arthritis.
Gout.
Metatarsalgia.
Hallux valgus.
Hallux rigidus.
Periarticular:
Ischemic foot pain.
Diabetes.

Bursitis.
Tendonitis.
Plantar fasciitis.
Corns.
Referred:
Lumbar spine.
Knee.

FOOT DERMATITIS
ICD-9CM # varies with specific disorder

Tinea pedis.
Dyshidrotic eczema.
Tylosis (mechanically induced hyperkeratosis, fissuring, and dryness).
Allergic contact dermatitis.
Psoriasis.
Peripheral vascular insufficiency.
Neuropathic foot ulcers (DM, poorly fitting shoes).
Acquired plantar keratoderma.
Sézary's syndrome.

FOOTDROP
ICD-9CM # varies with specific disorder

Peripheral neuropathy.
L5 radiculopathy.
Peroneal nerve compression.
Sciatic nerve palsy.
Scapuloperoneal syndromes.
Spasticity.
Peroneal nerve compression.
Myopathy.
Dystonia.

FOOT LESION, ULCERATING
ICD-9CM # 917.9

Cellulitis.
Plantar wart.
Squamous cell carcinoma.
Actinomycosis (Madura foot).
Plantar fibromatosis.
Pseudoepitheliomatous hyperplasia.

FOOT PAIN
ICD-9CM # varies with specific diagnosis

Trauma (fractures, musculoskeletal and ligamentous strain).
Inflammation (plantar fasciitis, Achilles tendonitis or bursitis, calcaneal apophysitis).
Arterial insufficiency, Raynaud's phenomenon, thromboangiitis obliterans.
Gout, pseudogout.
Calcaneal spur.
Infection (cellulitis, abscess, lymphangitis, gangrene).
Decubitus ulcer.
Paronychia, ingrown toenail.
Thrombophlebitis, postphlebitic syndrome.

FOREARM AND HAND PAIN

ICD-9CM # 959.3 Forearm Injury
959.4 Hand Injury

Epicondylitis.
Tenosynovitis.
Osteoarthritis.
Cubital tunnel syndrome.
Carpal tunnel syndrome.
Trauma.
Herpes zoster.
Peripheral vascular insufficiency.
Infection (cellulitis, abscess).

GAIT ABNORMALITY

ICD-9CM # 781.2 Gait Abnormality

Parkinsonism.
Degenerative joint disease (hips, back, knees).
Multiple sclerosis.
Trauma, foot pain.
CVA.
Cerebellar lesions.
Infections (tabes, encephalitis, meningitis).
Sensory ataxia.
Dystonia, cerebral palsy, neuromuscular disorders.
Metabolic abnormalities.

GALACTORRHEA[28]

ICD-9CM # 611.6

Prolonged suckling.
Drugs (INH, phenothiazines, reserpine derivatives, amphetamines, spironolactone and tricyclic antidepressants).
Major stressors (surgery, trauma).
Hypothyroidism.
Pituitary tumors.

GASTRIC DILATATION[16a]

ICD-9CM # 536.1

CAUSES OF A MASSIVELY DILATED STOMACH

Mechanical Gastric Outlet Obstruction
Duodenal or pyloric canal ulceration.
Carcinoma of pyloric antrum.
Extrinsic compression.
Paralytic Ileus
Surgery.
Trauma.
Peritonitis.
Pancreatitis.
Cholecystitis.
Diabetes.
Hepatic coma.
Drugs.
Gastric Volvulus
Intubation.
Air swallowing.

GASTRIC EMPTYING, DELAYED[1]

ICD-9CM # 578.89

CAUSES OF DELAYED GASTRIC EMPTYING

Mechanical Causes
Peptic ulcer disease, scarred pylorus.
Malignancy: gastric cancer, gastric lymphoma, pancreatic cancer.
Gastric surgery: vagotomy, gastric resection, roux-en-Y anastomosis.
Crohn's disease.
Endocrine and Metabolic Causes
Diabetes mellitus.
Hypothyroidism.
Hypoadrenal states.
Electrolyte abnormalities.
Chronic renal failure.
Medications.
Anticholinergics.
Opiates.
Dopamine agonists.
Tricyclic antidepressants.
Abnormalities of Gastric Smooth Muscle
Scleroderma.
Polymyositis, dermatomyositis.
Amyloidosis.
Pseudo-obstruction.
Myotonic dystrophy.
Neuropathy.
Scleroderma.
Amyloidosis.
Autonomic neuropathy.
Central Nervous System or Psychiatric Disorders
Brain stem tumors.
Spinal cord injury.
Anorexia nervosa.
Stress.
Miscellaneous
Idiopathic gastroparesis.
Gastroesophageal reflux disease.
Nonulcer (functional) dyspepsia.
Cancer cachexia or anorexia.

GASTRIC EMPTYING, RAPID

ICD-9CM # 536.8 Gastric Motility Disorder

Pancreatic insufficiency.
Dumping syndrome.
Peptic ulcer.
Celiac disease.
Promotility agents.
Zollinger-Ellison disease.

GENITAL DISCHARGE, FEMALE[12]

ICD-9CM # 629.9

Physiologic discharge: cervical mucus, vaginal transudation, bacteria, squamous epithelial cells.
Individual variation.
Pregnancy.
Sexual response.
Menstrual cycle variation.
Infection.
Foreign body: tampon, cervical cap, other.
Neoplasm.
Fistula.
IUD.
Cervical ectropion.
Spermicide.
Nongenital causes: urinary incontinence, urinary tract fistula, Crohn's disease, rectovaginal fistula.

GENITAL SORES[1]

ICD-9CM # 054.10 Genital Herpes
91.0 Genital Syphilis
078.11 Condyloma Acuminatum
099.0 Chancroid
099.2 Granuloma Inguinale
099.1 Lymphogranuloma Venereum
629.8 Ulcer, Genital Site, Female
608.89 Ulcer, Genital Site, Male

Herpes genitalis.
Syphilis.
Chancroid.
Lymphogranuloma venereum.
Granuloma inguinale.
Condyloma acuminatum.
Neoplastic lesion.
Trauma.

GLOMERULONEPHRITIS, RAPIDLY PROGRESSIVE[1]

ICD-9CM # 583.4

DIFFERENTIAL DIAGNOSIS OF RAPIDLY PROGRESSIVE GLOMERULONEPHRITIS

Linear Immune Staining
Anti-GBM disease.
Goodpasture's syndrome.
Rarely membranous glomerulonephritis.
Granular Immune Staining
Subacute bacterial endocarditis (past infectious).
Lupus nephritis.
Cryoglobulinemia.
Membranoproliferative glomerulonephritis (type II more than type I).
Immunoglobulin A nephropathy, Henoch-Schönlein purpura.
Idiopathic.
No Immune Staining (Pauci-immune)
Antineutrophil cytoplasmic antibody-associated vasculitis (Wegener granulomatosis, microscopic polyangiitis, Churg-Strauss syndrome).
Idiopathic.

GLOMERULOPATHIES, THROMBOTIC, MICROANGIOPATHIC[1]

ICD-9CM # 446.6

THROMBOTIC MICROANGIOPATHIC GLOMERULOPATHIES

Thrombotic thrombocytopenic purpura.
Hemolytic-uremic syndrome.
Malignant hypertension.
Scleroderma renal crisis.
Preeclampsia, eclampsia.
HELLP syndrome (hemolysis, elevated liver enzymes, low platelets).
Antiphospholipid antibody syndrome.
Drugs: oral contraceptives, quinine, cyclosporine, tacrolimus, ticlopidine, clopidogrel.

GLOMERULOSCLEROSIS, FOCAL SEGMENTAL[1]

ICD-9CM # 582.1

ETIOLOGY OF FOCAL SEGMENTAL GLOMERULOSCLEROSIS (FSGS)

Primary idiopathic FSGS.
Secondary FSGS.
HIV (usually collapsing variant).
Reflux nephropathy.
Heroin abuse.
Sickle cell disease.
Oligomenganephronia.
Renal dysgenesis or agenesis (low nephron mass).
Radiation nephritis.
Familial podocytopathies.
NPHS1 (nephrin) mutation.
NPHS2 (podocin) mutation.
TRPC6 (cation channel) mutation.
ACTN4 (α-actinin 4 mutation).

GLOSSODYNIA[38]

ICD-9CM # 529.6

DENTURE-RELATED

Dentures (ill-fitting, monomer from denture base).
Dental plaque.
Oral parafunction.

INFECTIVE/DERMATOLOGICAL

Candidiasis.
Lichen planus.

DEFICIENCY STATES

Iron, B_{12}, folate, B_2 (riboflavin), B_6 (pyridoxine), zinc.

ENDOCRINE

Diabetes.
Myxedema.*
Hormonal changes occurring during menopause.*

NEUROLOGICALLY MEDIATED

Referred from tonsils, teeth.
Lingual nerve neuropathy.
Glossopharyngeal neuralgia.
Esophageal reflux.*

IATROGENIC

Mouthwash.

XEROSTOMIA

PSYCHOGENIC

IDIOPATHIC

*Unproven associations

GLUCOCORTICOID DEFICIENCY[14]

ICD-9CM # 255.4

ACTH-independent causes.
TB.
Autoimmune (idiopathic).
Other rare causes:
  Fungal infection.
  Adrenal hemorrhage.
  Metastases.
  Sarcoidosis.
  Amyloidosis.
  Adrenoleukodystrophy.
  Adrenomyeloneuropathy.
  HIV infection.
  Congenital adrenal hyperplasia.
  Medications (e.g., ketoconazole).
ACTH-dependent causes:
Hypothalamic-pituitary-adrenal suppression.
  Exogenous.
  Glucocorticoid.
  ACTH.
  Endogenous—cure of Cushing's syndrome.
Hypothalamic-pituitary lesions.
  Neoplasm:
   • Primary pituitary tumor.
   • Metastatic tumor.
   • Craniopharyngioma.
  Infection:
   • Tuberculosis.
   • Actinomycosis.
   • Nocardiosis.
  Sarcoid.
  Head trauma.
  Isolated ACTH deficiency.

GOITER

ICD-9CM # 240.9 Goiter, Unspecified
        241.9 Goiter, Adenomatous
        246.1 Goiter, Congenital
        240.9 Goiter, Nontoxic Diffuse
        241.1 Goiter, Nontoxic Multinodular
        240.0 Simple Goiter
        242.1 Thyrotoxic Goiter

Thyroiditis.
Toxic multinodular goiter.
Graves' disease.
Medications (PTU, methimazole, sulfonamides, sulfonylureas, ethionamide, amiodarone, lithium, etc.).
Iodine deficiency.
Sarcoidosis, amyloidosis.
Defective thyroid hormone synthesis.
Resistance to thyroid hormone.

GRANULOMATOUS DERMATITIDES

ICD-9CM # varies with specific disorder

Granuloma annulare.
Sarcoidosis.
Necrobiosis lipoidica diabeticorum.
Cutaneous Crohn's disease.
Rheumatoid nodules.
Annular elastolytic giant cell granuloma (actinic granuloma).
Foreign body granuloma.

GRANULOMATOUS DISORDERS[32]

ICD-9CM # 446.4 Granulomatosis
        288.1 Granulomatous Disease

INFECTIONS

Fungi
Histoplasma.
Coccidioides.
Blastomyces.
Sporothrix.
Aspergillus.
Cryptococcus.
Protozoa
Toxoplasma.
Leishmania.
Metazoa
Toxocara.
Schistosoma.
Spirochetes
Treponema pallidum.
T. pertenue.
T. carateum.
Mycobacteria
M. tuberculosis.
M. leprae.
M. kansasii.
M. marinum.
M. avian.
Bacille Calmette-Guérin (BCG) vaccine.
Bacteria
Brucella.
Yersinia.
Other Infections
Cat scratch.
Lymphogranuloma.

NEOPLASIA

Carcinoma.
Reticulosis.
Pinealoma.
Dysgerminoma.
Seminoma.
Reticulum cell sarcoma.
Malignant nasal granuloma.

CHEMICALS

Beryllium.
Zirconium.
Silica.
Starch.

IMMUNOLOGIC ABERRATIONS

Sarcoidosis.
Crohn's disease.
Primary biliary cirrhosis.
Wegener's granulomatosis.
Giant-cell arteritis.
Peyronie's disease.
Hypogammaglobulinemia.
SLE.
Lymphomatoid granulomatosis.
Histiocytosis X.
Hepatic granulomatous disease.
Immune complex disease.
Rosenthal-Melkersson syndrome.
Churg-Strauss allergic granulomatosis.

LEUKOCYTE OXIDASE DEFECT

Chronic granulomatous disease of childhood.

EXTRINSIC ALLERGIC ALVEOLITIS

Farmer's lung.
Bird fancier's.
Mushroom worker's.
Suberosis (cork dust).
Bagassosis.
Maple bark stripper's.
Paprika splitter's.
Coffee bean.
Spatlese lung.

OTHER DISORDERS

Whipple's disease.
Pyrexia of unknown origin.
Radiotherapy.
Cancer chemotherapy.
Panniculitis.
Chalazion.
Sebaceous cyst.
Dermoid.
Sea urchin spine injury.

GRANULOMATOUS LIVER DISEASE
ICD-9CM # 572.8

Sarcoidosis.
Wegener's granulomatosis.
Vasculitis.
Inflammatory bowel disease.
Allergic granulomatosis.
Erythema nodosum.
Infections (fungal, viral, parasitic).
Primary biliary cirrhosis.
Lymphoma.
Hodgkin's disease.
Drugs (e.g., allopurinol, hydralazine, sulfonamides, penicillins).
Toxins (copper sulfate, beryllium).

GREEN OR BLUE URINE
ICD-9CM # 788.69

Pseudomonal urinary tract infection
Medications: triamterene, amitriptyline, IV cimetidine, IV promethazine.
Biliverdin.
Dyes (methylene blue, indigo carmine).

GROIN LUMP[38]
ICD-9CM # varies with specific diagnosis

COMMON CAUSES

Inguinal hernia.
Femoral hernia.
Lymph node.

OTHER CAUSES

Saphena varix.
Femoral artery aneurysm/pseudoaneurysm.
Psoas abscess.
Lipoma of the cord.
Encysted hydrocele of the cord (male).
Testicular maldescent (male).
Hydrocele of canal of Nuck (female).

GROIN MASSES
ICD-9CM # 959.1

Hernia (inguinal, femoral).
Hydrocele.
Varicocele.
Sebaceous cyst.
Hydradenitis of inguinal apocrine glands.
Neoplasm: lymphoma, metastases.
Lipoma.
Hematoma.
Reactive inguinal adenopathy, femoral adenitis.
Folliculitis, psoas abscess.
Epididymitis, testicular torsion, ectopic testes.
Aneurysm or pseudoaneurysm of femoral artery.

GROIN PAIN, ACTIVE PATIENT[37]
ICD-9CM # 959.1 Groin Injury
848.8 Groin Pain

MUSCULOSKELETAL

Avascular necrosis of the femoral head.
Avulsion fracture (lesser trochanter, anterior superior iliac spine, anterior inferior iliac spine).
Bursitis (iliopectineal, trochanteric).
Entrapment of the ilioinguinal or iliofemoral nerve.
Gracilis syndrome.
Muscle tear (adductors, iliopsoas, rectus abdominis, gracilis, sartorius, rectus femoris).
Myositis ossificans of the hip muscles.
Osteitis pubis.
Osteoarthritis of the femoral head.
Slipped capital femoral epiphysis.
Stress fracture of the femoral head or neck and pubis.
Synovitis.

HERNIA-RELATED

Avulsion of the internal oblique muscle in the conjoined tendon.
Defect at the insertion of the rectus abdominis muscle.
Direct inguinal hernia.
Femoral ring hernia.
Indirect inguinal hernia.
Inguinal canal weakness.

UROLOGIC

Epididymitis.
Fracture of the testis.
Hydrocele.
Kidney stone.
Posterior urethritis.
Prostatitis.
Testicular cancer.
Torsion of the testis.
Urinary tract infection.
Varicocele.

GYNECOLOGIC

Ectopic pregnancy.
Ovarian cyst.
Pelvic inflammatory disease.
Torsion of the ovary.
Vaginitis.

LYMPHATIC ENLARGEMENT IN GROIN

GYNECOMASTIA
ICD-9CM # 611.1 Gynecomastia, Nonpuerperal

Physiologic (puberty, newborns, aging).
Drugs (estrogen and estrogen precursors, digitalis, testosterone and exogenous androgens, clomiphene, cimetidine, spironolactone, ketoconazole, amiodarone, ACE inhibitors, isoniazid, phenytoin, methyldopa, metoclopramide, phenothiazine).
Increased prolactin level (prolactinoma).
Liver disease.
Adrenal disease.
Thyrotoxicosis.
Increased estrogen production (hCG-producing tumor, testicular tumor, bronchogenic carcinoma).
Secondary hypogonadism.
Primary gonadal failure (trauma, castration, viral orchitis, granulomatous disease).
Defects in androgen synthesis.
Testosterone deficiency.
Klinefelter's syndrome.

HALITOSIS
ICD-9CM # 784.9

Tobacco use.
Alcohol use.
Dry mouth (mouth breathing, inadequate fluid intake).
Foods (onion, garlic, meats, nuts, protein drinks).

Disease of mouth or nose (infections, cancer, inflammation).
Medications (antihistamines, antidepressants).
Systemic disorders (diabetes, uremia).
GI disorders (esophageal diverticula, hiatal hernia, GERD, achalasia).
Sinusitis.
Pulmonary disorders (bronchiectasis, pneumonia, neoplasms, TB).

HAND PAIN AND SWELLING[6]

ICD-9CM # varies with specific diagnosis

Trauma.
Gout.
Pseudogout.
Cellulitis.
Lymphangitis.
DVT of upper extremity.
Thrombophlebitis.
RA.
Remitting seronegative symmetrical synovitis with pitting edema (RS3PE).
Polymyalgia rheumatica.
Mixed connective tissue disease.
Scleroderma.
Rupture of the olecranon bursa.
Metzger's syndrome (neoplasia).
The puffy hand of drug addiction.
Reflex sympathetic dystrophy.
Eosinophilic fasciitis.
Sickle cell (hand-foot syndrome).
Leprosy.
Factitial (the rubber band syndrome).

HEADACHE[13]

ICD-9CM # 784.0	Headache NOS
307.81	Headache, Tension
346.2	Headache, Cluster
346.9	Headache, Migraine
784.0	Headache, Vascular

Vascular: migraine, cluster headaches, temporal arteritis, hypertension, cavernous sinus thrombosis.
Musculoskeletal: neck and shoulder muscle contraction, strain of extraocular and/or intraocular muscles, cervical spondylosis, temporomandibular arthritis.
Infections: meningitis, encephalitis, brain abscess, sepsis, sinusitis, osteomyelitis, parotitis, mastoiditis.
Cerebral neoplasm.
Subdural hematoma.
Cerebral hemorrhage/infarct.
Pseudotumor cerebri.
Normal pressure hydrocephalus (NPH).
Postlumbar puncture.
Cerebral aneurysm, arteriovenous malformations.
Posttrauma.
Dental problems: abscess, periodontitis, poorly fitting dentures.
Trigeminal neuralgia, glossopharyngeal neuralgia.
Otitis and other ear diseases.
Glaucoma and other eye diseases.
Metabolic: uremia, carbon monoxide inhalation, hypoxia.

Pheochromocytoma, hypoglycemia, hypothyroidism.
Effort induced: benign exertional headache, cough, headache, coital cephalalgia.
Drugs: alcohol, nitrates, histamine antagonists.
Paget's disease of the skull.
Emotional, psychiatric.

HEADACHE, ACUTE[11]

ICD-9CM # 784.0

DIFFERENTIAL DIAGNOSIS OF ACUTE HEADACHE

Evaluation of the first acute headache should exclude pathologic causes listed here before consideration of more common etiologies..
Increased intracranial pressure (ICP): Trauma, hemorrhage, tumor, hydrocephalus, pseudotumor cerebri, abscess, arachnoid cyst, cerebral edema.
Decreased ICP: After ventriculoperitoneal shunt, lumbar puncture, cerebrospinal fluid leak from basilar skull fracture.
Meningeal inflammation: Meningitis, leukemia, subarachnoid or subdural hemorrhage.
Vascular: Vasculitis, arteriovenous malformation, hypertension, cerebrovascular accident.
Bone, soft tissue: Referred pain from scalp, eyes, ears, sinuses, nose, teeth, pharynx, cervical spine, temporomandibular joint.
Infection: Systemic infection, encephalitis, sinusitis, etc.
First migraine.

HEADACHE AND FACIAL PAIN[36]

ICD-9CM # 784.0 Headache NOS
784.0 Facial Pain

VASCULAR HEADACHES

Migraine
Migraine with headaches and inconspicuous neurologic features:
- Migraine without aura ("common migraine").
Migraine with headaches and conspicuous neurologic features:
- With transient neurologic symptoms: Migraine with typical aura ("classic migraine").
  Sensory, basilar, and hemiplegic migraine.
- With prolonged or permanent neurologic features ("complicated migraine"): Ophthalmoplegic migraine.
  Migrainous infarction.
Migraine without headaches but with conspicuous neurologic features ("migraine equivalents"):
- Abdominal migraine.
- Benign paroxysmal vertigo of childhood.
- Migraine aura without headache ("isolated auras," transient migrainous accompaniments).

Cluster Headaches
Episodic cluster headache ("cyclic cluster headaches").

Chronic cluster headaches.
Chronic paroxysmal hemicrania.
Other Vascular Headaches
Headaches of reactive vasodilation (fever, drug-induced, postictal, hypoglycemia, hypoxia, hypercarbia, hyperthyroidism).
Headaches associated with arterial hypertension:
- Chronic severe hypertension (diastolic 120 mm Hg).
- Paroxysmal severe hypertension (pheochromocytoma, some coital headaches).
Headaches caused by cranial arteritis:
- Giant cell arteritis ("temporal arteritis").
- Other vasculitides.

HEADACHES ASSOCIATED WITH DEMONSTRABLE MUSCLE SPASM

Headache caused by posturally induced or perilesional muscle spasm:
- Headaches of sustained or impaired posture (e.g., prolonged close work, driving).
- Headaches associated with cervical spondylosis and other diseases of cervical spine.
- Myofascial pain dysfunction syndrome (headache or facial pain associated with disorders of teeth, jaws, and related structures, or "TMJ syndrome").
Headaches caused by psychophysiologic muscular contraction ("muscle contraction headaches," or tension-type headache associated with disorder of pericranial muscles).

HEADACHES AND FACIAL PAIN WITHOUT DEMONSTRABLE PHYSICAL SUBSTRATE

Headaches of uncertain etiology:
- "Tension headaches" (tension-type headache unassociated with disorder of pericranial muscles).
- Some forms of posttraumatic headache.
Psychogenic headaches (e.g., hypochondriacal, conversional, delusional, malingered).
Facial pain of uncertain etiology ("atypical facial pain").

COMBINED TENSION-MIGRAINE HEADACHES

Episodic migraine superimposed on chronic tension headaches.
Chronic daily headaches:
- Associated with analgesic and/or ergotamine overuse ("rebound headaches").
- Not associated with drug overuse.

HEADACHES AND HEAD PAINS CAUSED BY DISEASES OF EYES, EARS, NOSE, SINUSES, TEETH, OR SKULL

HEADACHES CAUSED BY MENINGEAL INFLAMMATION

Subarachnoid hemorrhage.
Meningitis and meningoencephalitis.
Others (e.g., meningeal carcinomatosis).

HEADACHES ASSOCIATED WITH ALTERED INTRACRANIAL PRESSURE ("TRACTION HEADACHES")

Increased Intracranial Pressure
Intracranial mass lesions (neoplasm, hematoma, abscess, etc.).
Hydrocephalus.
Benign intracranial hypertension.
Venous sinus thrombosis.

Decreased Intracranial Pressure
Post–lumbar puncture headaches.
Spontaneous hypoliquorrheic headaches.

HEADACHES AND HEAD PAINS CAUSED BY CRANIAL NEURALGIAS

Presumed Irritation of Superficial Nerves
Occipital neuralgia.
Supraorbital neuralgia.

Presumed Irritation of Intracranial Nerves
Trigeminal neuralgia ("tic douloureux").
Glossopharyngeal neuralgia.

HEADACHE, CHRONIC[11]
ICD-9CM # 784.0

DIFFERENTIAL DIAGNOSIS OF RECURRENT OR CHRONIC HEADACHES
Migraine (with or without aura).
Tension.
Analgesic rebound.
Caffeine withdrawal.
Sleep deprivation (e.g., in children with sleep apnea) or chronic hypoxia.
Tumor.
Psychogenic: Conversion disorder, malingering.
Cluster headache.

HEAD AND NECK, SOFT TISSUE MASSES
ICD-9CM # varies with specific diagnosis

Lipoma.
Pilar cyst.
Epidermal inclusion cyst.
Dermoid cyst.
Bone cyst.
Hemangioma.
Eosinophilic granuloma.
Other: facial nerve neuroma, teratoma, rhabdomyoma, rhabdomyosarcoma, branchial cleft cyst.

HEARING LOSS, ACUTE[26]
ICD-9CM # 388.2

Infectious: mumps, measles, influenza, herpes simplex, herpes zoster, CMV, mononucleosis, syphilis.
Vascular: macroglobulinemia, sickle cell disease, Berger's disease, leukemia, polycythemia, fat emboli, hypercoagulable states.
Metabolic: diabetes, pregnancy, hyperlipoproteinemia.

Conductive: cerumen impaction, foreign bodies, otitis media, otitis externa, barotrauma, trauma.
Medications: aminoglycosides, loop diuretics, antineoplastics, salicylates, vancomycin.
Neoplasm: acoustic neuroma, metastatic neoplasm.

HEARTBURN AND INDIGESTION[33]
ICD-9CM # 787.1 Heartburn
536.8 Indigestion

Reflux esophagitis.
Gastritis.
Nonulcer dyspepsia.
Functional GI disorder (anxiety disorder, social/environmental stresses).
Excessive intestinal gas (ingestion of flatulogenic foods, GI stasis, constipation).
Gas entrapment (hepatitis or splenic flexure syndrome).
Neoplasm (adenocarcinoma of stomach or esophagus, lymphoma).
Gallbladder disease.

HEART FAILURE, ACUTE[2]
ICD-9CM # 428.9

COMMON PRECIPITATING CAUSES OF ACUTE HF
Systemic hypertension.
Myocardial infarction or ischemia.
Dysrhythmia.
Systemic infection.
Anemia.
Dietary, physical, environmental, and emotional excesses.
Pregnancy.
Thyrotoxicosis or hypothyroidism.
Acute myocarditis.
Acute valvular dysfunction.
Pulmonary embolus.
Pharmacologic complications.

HEART FAILURE, PREGNANCY
ICD-9CM # 428.90

Congenital valvular heart disease exacerbated by pregnancy.
Peripartum cardiomyopathy.
Untreated thyrotoxicosis.
Hypothyroidism.
Pulmonary hypertension.
Myocardial infarction.

HEEL PAIN
ICD-9CM # varies with specific diagnosis

Achilles tendonitis/tendinopathy (insertional, noninsertional).
Retrocalcaneal bursitis (superficial, deep).
Plantar fasciopathy.
Neuropathy (tarsal tunnel, posterior tibial nerve [medial calcaneal branch], abductor digiti quinti).

Calcaneal stress fracture.
Puncture wound, foreign body.
Cellulitis.
Spondyloarthropathy.
Fat pad atrophy.
Soft tissue tumor.
S1 radiculopathy.
Paget's disease of bone.
Haglund deformity.
Primary or metastatic bone tumor.

HEEL PAIN, PLANTAR[24]
ICD-9CM # 729.5

SKIN
Keratoses.
Verruca.
Ulcer.
Fissure.

CONNECTIVE TISSUE
Fat
Atrophy.
Panniculitis.
Dense Connective Tissue
Inflammatory fasciitis.
Fibromatosis.
Enthesopathy.
Bursitis.
Bone (Calcaneus)
Stress fracture.
Paget's disease.
Benign bone cyst/tumor.
Malignant bone tumor.
Metabolic bone disease (osteopenia).
Nerve
Tarsal tunnel.
Plantar nerve entrapment.
S1 nerve root radiculopathy.
Painful peripheral neuropathy.

INFECTION
Dermatomycoses.
Acute osteomyelitis.
Plantar abscess.

MISCELLANEOUS
Foreign body.
Nonunion calcaneus fracture.
Psychogenic.
Idiopathic.

HEMARTHROSIS
ICD-9CM # 848.9 Hemarthrosis (Sprain) NOS

Trauma.
Anticoagulant therapy.
Thrombocytopenia, thrombocytosis.
Bleeding disorders (e.g., von Willebrand's disease).
Charcot's joint.
Idiopathic.
Other: pigmented villonodular synovitis, hemangioma, synovioma, AV fistula, ruptured aneurysm.

HEMATEMESIS[38]
ICD-9CM # 578.0

CAUSES OF HEMATEMESIS
Very common
Gastric or duodenal ulcer or erosions.
Common
Mallory-Weiss tear (a laceration at the gastro-esophageal junction).
Ulcerative esophagitis.
Esophageal varices.
Uncommon
Vascular malformations.
Ulcerated gastrointestinal stromal tumor.
Carcinoma of esophagus or stomach.
Aortoenteric fistula.

HEMATURIA
ICD-9CM # 599.7 Hematuria, Benign
(Essential)

Use the mnemonic TICS:
  T (trauma): blow to kidney, insertion of Foley catheter or foreign body in urethra, prolonged and severe exercise, very rapid emptying of overdistended bladder.
  (tumor): hypernephroma, Wilms' tumor, papillary carcinoma of the bladder, prostatic and urethral neoplasms.
  (toxins): turpentine, phenols, sulfonamides and other antibiotics, cyclophosphamide, NSAIDs.
  I (infections): glomerulonephritis, TB, cystitis, prostatitis, urethritis, *Schistosoma haematobium,* yellow fever, blackwater fever.
  (inflammatory processes): Goodpasture's syndrome, periarteritis, postirradiation.
  C (calculi): renal, ureteral, bladder, urethra.
  (cysts): simple cysts, polycystic disease.
  (congenital anomalies): hemangiomas, aneurysms, AVM.
  S (surgery): invasive procedures, prostatic resection, cystoscopy.
  (sickle cell disease and other hematologic disturbances): hemophilia, thrombocytopenia, anticoagulants.
  (somewhere else): bleeding genitals, factitious (drug addicts).

HEMATURIA, DIFFERENTIAL BASED ON AGE AND SEX
ICD-9CM # 599.7 Hematuria Benign
(Essential)
other codes vary with cause

0 TO 20 YR
Acute urinary tract infections.
Acute glomerulonephritis.
Congenital urinary tract anomalies with obstruction.
Trauma to genitals.

20 TO 40 YR
Acute urinary tract infection.
Trauma to genitals.
Urolithiasis.
Bladder cancer.

40 TO 60 YR (WOMEN)
Acute urinary tract infection.
Bladder cancer.
Urolithiasis.

40 TO 60 YR (MEN)
Acute urinary tract infection.
Bladder cancer.
Urolithiasis.

60 YR AND OLDER (WOMEN)
Acute urinary tract infection.
Bladder cancer.
Vaginal trauma or irritation.
Urolithiasis.

60 YR AND OLDER (MEN)
Acute urinary tract infection.
Benign prostatic hyperplasia.
Bladder cancer.
Urolithiasis.
Trauma.

HEMATURIA, IN CHILDREN[2]
ICD-9CM # 599.7

EXTRARENAL
Trauma.
Meatal stenosis or posterior urethral valves.
Exercise.
Menstruation or rectal bleeding.
Foreign bodies.
Cystitis, urethritis, or epididymitis.

INTRARENAL
Pyelonephritis.
Renal or bladder stones or tumors.
Poststreptococcal or idiopathic glomerulonephritis.
Acute interstitial nephritis.
Acute tubular necrosis.
Basement membrane glomerular disease.
Renal vein or arterial thrombosis.
Recurrent familial hematuria.
Polycystic kidney disease.

SYSTEMIC
Henoch-Schönlein purpura.
Systemic lupus erythematosus.
Hemolytic-uremic syndrome.
Infectious mononucleosis.
Sickle cell disease or other hemoglobinopathies.
Bacterial endocarditis or artificial cardiac valves.
Bleeding disorders, warfarin, or aspirin.
Medications such as amitriptyline or chlorpromazine, radiocontrast dyes.
Munchausen syndrome or factitious.

HEMIPARESIS/HEMIPLEGIA
ICD-9CM # 436.0 Acquired Due to Acute
CVA, Flaccid
436.1 Acquired Due to CVA,
Acute, Spastic

CVA.
Transient ischemic attack.
Cerebral neoplasm.

Multiple sclerosis or other demyelinating disorder.
CNS infection.
Migraine.
Hypoglycemia
Subdural hematoma.
Vasculitis.
Todd's paralysis.
Epidural hematoma.
Metabolic (hyperosmolar state, electrolyte imbalance).
Psychiatric disorders.
Congenital disorders.
Leukodystrophies.

HEMOLYSIS AND HEMOGLOBINURIA
ICD-9CM # 773.2 Hemolysis
791.2 Hemoglobinuria

Erythrocyte trauma (prosthetic cardiac valves, marching and severe trauma, extensive burns).
Infections (malaria, *Bartonella, Clostridium Welchii*).
Brown recluse spider bite.
Incompatible blood transfusions.
Hemolytic uremic syndrome.
Thrombotic thrombocytopenic purpura (TTP).
Paroxysmal nocturnal hemoglobinuria (PNH).
Drugs (penicillins, quinidine, methyldopa, sulfonamides, nitrofurantoin).
Erythrocyte enzyme deficiencies (e.g., exposure to fava beans in patients with glucose-6-phosphate dehydrogenase deficiency).

HEMOLYSIS, INTRAVASCULAR
ICD-9CM # 283.2

Infections.
Exertional hemolysis (e.g., prolonged march).
Valve hemolysis.
Microangiopathic hemolytic anemia.
Osmotic and chemical agents.
Thermal injury.
Cold agglutinins.
Venoms (snakes, spiders).
Paroxysmal nocturnal hemoglobinuria (PNH).

HEMOLYSIS, MECHANICAL
ICD-9CM # 283.19

Prosthetic heart valves.
Aortic stenosis.
Malignant hypertension.
Metastatic adenocarcinoma.
Traumatic exercise.
Renal transplants.
Renal cortical necrosis.
Glomerulonephritis.
Thrombotic thrombocytopenic purpura (TTP), hemolytic-uremic syndrome (HUS).
Renal vasculitis.
Scleroderma.
Diabetes.

HEMOPERITONEUM

ICD-9CM # 568.81

Ruptured Graafian follicle.
Ruptured spleen.
Ectopic pregnancy.
Traumatic laceration of liver.
Ruptured aneurysm.
Ruptured bladder.
Traumatic laceration of bowel, pancreas, uterus.

HEMOPTYSIS

ICD-9CM # 786.3

CARDIOVASCULAR

Pulmonary embolism/infarction.
Left ventricular failure.
Mitral stenosis.
AV fistula.
Severe hypertension.
Erosion of aortic aneurysm.

PULMONARY

Neoplasm (primary or metastatic).
Infection.
Pneumonia: *Streptococcus pneumoniae, Klebsiella pneumoniae, Staphylococcus aureus, Legionella pneumophila.*
Bronchiectasis.
Abscess.
TB.
Bronchitis.
Fungal infections (aspergillosis, coccidioidomycosis).
Parasitic infections (amebiasis, ascariasis, paragonimiasis).
Vasculitis: Wegener's granulomatosis, Churg-Strauss syndrome, Henoch-Schönlein purpura.
Goodpasture's syndrome.
Trauma (needle biopsy, foreign body, right-sided heart catheterization, prolonged and severe cough).
Cystic fibrosis, bullous emphysema.
Pulmonary sequestration.
Pulmonary AV fistula.
SLE.
Idiopathic pulmonary hemosiderosis.
Drugs: aspirin, anticoagulants, penicillamine.
Pulmonary hypertension.
Mediastinal fibrosis.

OTHER

Epistaxis, trauma.
Laryngeal bleeding (laryngitis, laryngeal neoplasm).
Hematologic disorders (clotting abnormalities, DIC, thrombocytopenia).

HEPATIC CYSTS[36]

ICD-9CM # 751.62 Hepatic Cyst, Congenital
122.8 Echinococcus Infection, Liver

CONGENITAL HEPATIC CYSTS

Parenchymal: solitary cyst, polycystic disease.
Ductal: localized dilatation, multiple cystic dilatations of intrahepatic ducts (Caroli's disease).

ACQUIRED HEPATIC CYSTS

Inflammatory cysts: retention cysts, echinococcal cyst, amebic cyst.
Neoplastic cyst.
Peliosis hepatis.

HEPATIC GRANULOMAS[1]

ICD-9CM # 572.8

INFECTIONS

Bacterial, spirochetal: TB and atypical mycobacterial infections, tularemia, brucellosis, leprosy, syphilis, Whipple's disease, listeriosis.
Viral: mononucleosis, CMV.
Rickettsial: Q fever.
Fungal: coccidioidomycosis, histoplasmosis, cryptococcal infections, actinomycosis, aspergillosis, nocardiosis.
Parasitic: schistosomiasis, clonorchiasis, toxocariasis, ascariasis, toxoplasmosis, amebiasis.

HEPATOBILIARY DISORDERS

Primary biliary cirrhosis, granulomatous hepatitis, jejunoileal bypass.

SYSTEMIC DISORDERS

Sarcoidosis, Wegener's granulomatosis, inflammatory bowel disease, Hodgkin's disease, lymphoma.

DRUGS/TOXINS

Beryllium, parenteral foreign material (starch, talc, silicone, etc.), phenylbutazone, α-methyldopa, procainamide, allopurinol, phenytoin, nitrofurantoin, hydralazine.

HEPATITIS, ACUTE[25]

ICD-9CM # varies with specific disorder

Infectious:
    Hepatitis A, B, C, D, G.
    Epstein-Barr virus.
    Cytomegalovirus.
    Herpes simplex virus.
    Yellow fever.
    Leptospirosis.
    Q fever.
    HIV.
    Brucellosis.
    Lyme disease.
    Syphilis.
Noninfectious:
    Drug induced.
    Autoimmune.
    Ischemic.
    Acute fatty liver of pregnancy.
    Acute Budd-Chiari syndrome.
    Wilson's disease.

HEPATITIS, CHRONIC[25]

ICD-9CM # 571.40 Hepatitis, Noninfectious, Chronic
072.22 Hepatitis B, Chronic
070.44 Hepatitis C, Chronic

Chronic viral hepatitis:
    Hepatitis B.
    Hepatitis C.
    Hepatitis D.

Autoimmune hepatitis and variant syndromes.
Hereditary hemochromatosis.
Wilson's disease.
α-Antitrypsin deficiency.
Fatty liver and nonalcoholic steatohepatitis.
Alcoholic liver disease.
Drug-induced liver disease.
Hepatic granulomas:
    Infectious.
    Drug induced.
    Neoplastic.
    Idiopathic.

HEPATOMEGALY

ICD-9CM # 789.1

FREQUENT JAUNDICE

Infectious hepatitis.
Toxic hepatitis.
Carcinoma: liver, pancreas, bile ducts, metastatic neoplasm to liver.
Cirrhosis.
Obstruction of common bile duct.
Alcoholic hepatitis.
Biliary cirrhosis.
Cholangitis.
Hemochromatosis with cirrhosis.

INFREQUENT JAUNDICE

CHF.
Amyloidosis.
Liver abscess.
Sarcoidosis.
Infectious mononucleosis.
Alcoholic fatty infiltration.
Nonalcoholic steatohepatitis.
Lymphoma.
Leukemia.
Budd-Chiari syndrome.
Myelofibrosis with myeloid metaplasia.
Familial hyperlipoproteinemia type 1.
Other: amebiasis, hydatid disease of liver, schistosomiasis, kala-azar *(Leishmania donovani)*, Hurler's syndrome, Gaucher's disease, kwashiorkor.

HEPATOMEGALY, BY SHAPE OF LIVER[38]

ICD-9CM # 789.1

DIFFUSELY ENLARGED AND SMOOTH

Massive
Metastatic disease.
Alcoholic liver disease with fatty infiltration.
Myeloproliferative diseases (e.g., polycythemia rubra vera, myelofibrosis).
Moderate
The above causes.
Hemochromatosis.
Hematological disease (e.g., chronic myeloid leukemia, lymphoma).
Fatty liver (e.g., diabetes mellitus, obesity).
Infiltrative disorders (e.g., amyloid).
Mild
The above causes.
Hepatitis (viral, drugs).
Cirrhosis.

Biliary obstruction.
Granulomatous disorders (e.g., sarcoid).
HIV infection.

DIFFUSELY ENLARGED AND IRREGULAR

Metastatic disease.
Cirrhosis.
Hydatid disease.
Polycystic liver disease.

LOCALIZED SWELLINGS

Riedel's lobe (a normal variant—the lobe may be palpable in the right lumbar region).
Metastasis.
Large simple hepatic cyst.
Hydatid cyst.
Hepatoma.
Liver abscess (e.g., amoebic abscess).

HERMAPHRODITISM[4]

ICD-9CM # 752.7 Hermaphroditism, Congenital

FEMALE PSEUDOHERMAPHRODITISM

Androgen exposure:
Fetal source:
- 21-Hydroxylase (P450 c21) deficiency.
- 11β-Hydroxylase (P450 c11) deficiency.
- 3β-Hydroxysteroid dehydrogenase II (3β-HSD II) deficiency.
- Aromatase (P450arom) deficiency.
Maternal source.
Virilizing ovarian tumor.
Virilizing adrenal tumor.
Androgenic drugs.
Undetermined origin:
Associated with genitourinary and GI tract defects.

MALE PSEUDOHERMAPHRODITISM

Defects in testicular differentiation:
Denys-Drash syndrome (mutation in WT1 gene).
WAGR syndrome (Wilms tumor, aniridia, genitourinary malformation, retardation).
Deletion of 11p13.
Camptomelic syndrome (autosomal gene at 17q24.3-q25.1) and SOX 9 mutation.
XY pure gonadal dysgenesis (Swyer syndrome).
- Mutation in SRY gene.
- Unknown cause.
XY gonadal agenesis.
Deficiency of testicular hormones:
Leydig cell aplasia.
Mutation in LH receptor.
Lipoid adrenal hyperplasia (P450 scc) deficiency; mutation in StAR (steroidogenic acute regulatory protein).
3b-HSDII deficiency.
17-Hydroxylase/17, 20-lyase (P450 c17) deficiency.

Persistent Müllerian duct syndrome.
- Gene mutations, Müllerian-inhibiting substance (MIS).
- Receptor defects for MIS.
Defect in androgen action:
5α-Reductase II mutations.
Androgen receptor defects:
- Complete androgen insensitivity syndrome.
- Partial androgen insensitivity syndrome.
- Reifenstein and other syndromes.
- Smith-Lemli-Opitz syndrome.
Defect in conversion of 7-dehydrocholesterol to cholesterol.

TRUE HERMAPHRODITISM

XX.
XY.
XX/XY chimeras.

HICCUPS[21]

ICD-9CM # 786.8

TRANSIENT HICCUPS

Sudden excitement, emotion.
Gastric distention.
Esophageal obstruction.
Alcohol ingestion.
Sudden change in temperature.

PERSISTENT OR CHRONIC HICCUPS

Toxic/metabolic: uremia, DM, hyperventilation, hypocalcemia, hypokalemia, hyponatremia, gout, fever.
Drugs: benzodiazepines, steroids, α-methyldopa, barbiturates.
Surgery/general anesthesia.
Thoracic/diaphragmatic disorders: pneumonia, lung cancer, asthma, pleuritis, pericarditis, myocardial infarction, aortic aneurysm, esophagitis, esophageal obstruction, diaphragmatic hernia or irritation.
Abdominal disorders: gastric ulcer or cancer, hepatobiliary or pancreatic disease, IBD, bowel obstruction, intraabdominal or subphrenic abscess, prostatic infection or cancer.
Central nervous system disorders: traumatic, infectious, vascular, structural.
Ear, nose, and throat disorders: pharyngitis, laryngitis, tumor, irritation of auditory canal.
Psychogenic disorders.
Idiopathic disorders.

HIP PAIN WITHOUT OBVIOUS FRACTURE[2]

ICD-9CM # 338

DIFFERENTIAL DIAGNOSIS OF A PAINFUL HIP WITHOUT OBVIOUS FRACTURE

Referred pain (lumbar spine, hip, or knee).
Avascular necrosis of the femoral head.
Degenerative joint disease or osteoarthritis.
Herniation of a lumbar disk.
Diskitis.

Toxic synovitis of the hip.
Septic arthritis.
Bursitis.
Tendonitis.
Ligamentous injuries of the knee or hip.
Occult fracture.
Slipped capital femoral epiphysis.
Perthes' disease.
Tumor (lymphoma).
Deep venous thrombosis.
Arterial insufficiency.
Osteomyelitis.
Iliopsoas abscess.
Retroperitoneal hematoma.
Inguinal hernia.
Inguinal lymphadenopathy.
Genitourinary complaints.
Sports-related hernia.

HIP PAIN, CHILDREN[26]

ICD-9CM # 959.6 Hip Injury
719.95 Hip Joint Disorder
843.9 Hip Strain

TRAUMA

Hip or pelvis fractures.
Overuse injuries.

INFECTION

Septic arthritis.
Osteomyelitis.

INFLAMMATION

Transient synovitis.
Juvenile RA.
Rheumatic fever.

NEOPLASM

Leukemia.
Osteogenic or Ewing's sarcoma.
Metastatic disease.

HEMATOLOGIC DISORDERS

Hemophilia.
Sickle cell anemia.

MISCELLANEOUS

Legg-Calvé-Perthes disease.
Slipped capital femoral epiphysis.

HIP PAIN, IN DIFFERENT AGE GROUPS[8]

ICD-9CM # 719.45

COMMON CAUSES OF HIP PAIN IN DIFFERENT AGE GROUPS

Childhood (2-10 yr)
Intraarticular:
Developmental dislocation of the hip.
Perthes' disease.
Irritable hip.
Rickets.
Periarticular:
Osteomyelitis.
Referred:
Abdominal.

Adolescence (10-18 yr)
Intraarticular:
Slipped upper femoral epiphysis.
Torn labrum.
Periarticular:
Trochanteric bursitis.
Snapping hip.
Osteomyelitis.
Tumors.
Referred:
Abdominal.
Lumbar spine.
Early Adulthood (18-30 yr)
Intraarticular:
Inflammatory arthritis.
Torn labrum.
Periarticular:
Bursitis.
Referred:
Abdominal.
Lumbar spine.
Adulthood (30-50 yr)
Intraarticular:
Osteoarthritis.
Inflammatory arthritis.
Osteonecrosis.
Transient osteoporosis.
Periarticular:
Bursitis.
Referred:
Abdominal.
Lumbar spine.
Old Age (>50 yr)
Intraarticular:
Osteoarthritis.
Inflammatory arthritis.
Referred:
Abdominal.
Lumbar spine.

HIRSUTISM

ICD-9CM # 704.1

Idiopathic: familial, possibly increased sensitivity to androgens.
Menopause.
Polycystic ovarian syndrome.
Drugs: androgens, anabolic steroids, methyltestosterone, minoxidil, diazoxide, phenytoin, glucocorticoids, cyclosporine.
Congenital adrenal hyperplasia.
Adrenal virilizing tumor.
Ovarian virilizing tumor: arrhenoblastoma, hilus cell tumor.
Pituitary adenoma.
Cushing's syndrome.
Hypothyroidism (congenital and juvenile).
Acromegaly.
Testicular feminization.

HIV INFECTION, ANORECTAL LESIONS[26]

ICD-9CM # 042 HIV infection, symptomatic
V08 HIV infection, asymptomatic

COMMON CONDITIONS

Anal fissure.
Abscess and fistula.
Hemorrhoids.
Pruritus ani.
Pilonidal disease.

COMMON STDs

Gonorrhea.
Chlamydia.
Herpes.
Chancroid.
Syphilis.
Condylomata acuminata.

ATYPICAL CONDITIONS

Infectious: TB, CMV, actinomycosis, cryptococcus.
Neoplastic: lymphoma, Kaposi's sarcoma, squamous cell carcinoma.
Other: idiopathic and ulcer.

HIV INFECTION, CHEST RADIOGRAPHIC ABNORMALITIES[26]

ICD-9CM # 042 HIV infection, symptomatic
V08 HIV infection, asymptomatic

DIFFUSE INTERSTITIAL INFILTRATION

Pneumocystis carinii.
Cytomegalovirus.
Mycobacterium tuberculosis.
Mycobacterium avium complex.
Histoplasmosis.
Coccidioidomycosis.
Lymphoid interstitial pneumonitis.

FOCAL CONSOLIDATION

Bacterial pneumonia.
Mycoplasma pneumoniae.
Pneumocystis carinii.
Mycobacterium tuberculosis.
Mycobacterium avium complex.

NODULAR LESIONS

Kaposi's sarcoma.
Mycobacterium tuberculosis.
Mycobacterium avium complex.
Fungal lesions.
Toxoplasmosis.

CAVITARY LESIONS

Pneumocystis carinii.
Mycobacterium tuberculosis.
Bacterial infection.

PLEURAL EFFUSION

Kaposi's sarcoma.
(Small effusion may be associated with any infection).

ADENOPATHY

Kaposi's sarcoma.
Lymphoma.
Mycobacterium tuberculosis.
Cryptococcus.

PNEUMOTHORAX

Kaposi's sarcoma.

HIV INFECTION, COGNITIVE IMPAIRMENT[25]

ICD-9CM # 042 HIV Infection, Symptomatic

EARLY TO MID-STAGE HIV DISEASE

Depression.
Alcohol and substance abuse.
Medication-induced cognitive impairment.
Metabolic encephalopathies.
HIV-related cognitive impairment.

ADVANCED HIV DISEASE (CD4+ <100/mm^3)

Opportunistic infection of CNS.
Neurosyphilis.
CNS lymphoma.
Progressive multifocal leukoencephalopathy.
Depression.
Metabolic encephalopathies.
Medication-induced cognitive impairment.
Stroke.
HIV dementia.

HIV INFECTION, CUTANEOUS MANIFESTATIONS[21]

ICD-9CM # 042 HIV Infection, Symptomatic
V08 HIV Infection, Asymptomatic

BACTERIAL INFECTION

Bacillary angiomatosis: Numerous angiomatous nodules associated with fever, chills, weight loss.
Staphylococcus aureus: Folliculitis, ecthyma, impetigo, bullous impetigo, furuncles, carbuncles.
Syphilis: May occur in different forms (primary, secondary, tertiary); chancre may become painful because of secondary infection.

FUNGAL INFECTION

Candidiasis: Mucous membranes (oral, vulvovaginal), less commonly candida intertrigo or paronychia.
Cryptococcoses: Papules or nodules that strongly resemble molluscum contagiosum; other forms include pustules, purpuric papules, and vegetating plaques.
Seborrheic dermatitis: Scaling and erythema in the hair-bearing areas (eyebrows, scalp, chest, and pubic area).

ARTHROPOD INFESTATIONS

Scabies: Pruritus with or without rash, usually generalized but can be limited to a single digit.

VIRAL INFECTION

Herpes simplex: Vesicular lesion in clusters; perianal, genital, orofacial, or digital; can be disseminated.
Herpes zoster: Painful dermatomal vesicles that may ulcerate or disseminate.
HIV: Discrete erythematous macules and papules on the upper trunk, palms, and soles are the most characteristic cutaneous finding of acute HIV infection.

Differential Diagnosis

II

Human papillomavirus: Genital warts (may become unusually extensive).

Kaposi's sarcoma (herpesvirus): Erythematous macules or papules; enlarge at varying rates; violaceous nodules or plaques; occasionally painful.

Molluscum contagiosum: Discrete umbilicated papules commonly on the face, neck, and intertriginous sites (axilla, groin, or buttocks).

NONINFECTIOUS

Drug reactions: More frequent and severe in HIV patients.

Nutritional deficiencies: Mainly seen in children and patients with chronic diarrhea; diffuse skin manifestations, depending upon the deficiency.

Psoriasis: Scaly lesions; diffuse or localized; can be associated with arthritis.

Vasculitis: Palpable purpuric eruption (can resemble septic emboli).

HIV INFECTION, ESOPHAGEAL DISEASE

ICD-9CM # varies with specific diagnosis

Candida infection.
Cytomegalovirus infection.
Aphthous ulcer.
Herpes simplex.

HIV INFECTION, HEPATIC DISEASE[25]

ICD-9CM # 042 HIV Infection, Symptomatic

VIRUSES

Hepatitis A.
Hepatitis B.
Hepatitis C.
Hepatitis D (with HBV).
Epstein-Barr virus.
Cytomegalovirus.
Herpes simplex virus.
Adenovirus.
Varicella-zoster virus.

MYCOBACTERIA

Mycobacterium avium complex.
Mycobacterium tuberculosis.

FUNGI

Histoplasma capsulatum.
Cryptococcus neoformans.
Coccidioides immitis.
Candida albicans.
Pneumocystis carinii.
Penicillium marneffei.

PROTOZOA

Toxoplasma gondii.
Cryptosporidium parvum.
Microsporida spp.
Schistosoma.

BACTERIA

Bartonella henselae (peliosis hepatis).

MALIGNANCY

Kaposi's sarcoma (HHV-8).
Non-Hodgkin's lymphoma.
Hepatocellular carcinoma.

MEDICATIONS

Zidovudine.
Didanosine.
Ritonavir.
Other HIV-1 protease inhibitors.
Fluconazole.
Macrolide antibiotics.
Isoniazid.
Rifampin.
Trimethoprim-sulfamethoxazole.

HIV INFECTION, LOWER GI TRACT DISEASE[25]

ICD-9CM # 042 HIV Infection, Symptomatic

CAUSES OF ENTEROCOLITIS

Bacteria
Campylobacter jejuni and other spp.
Salmonella spp.
Shigella flexneri.
Aeromonas hydrophila.
Plesiomonas shigelloides.
Yersinia enterocolitica.
Vibrio spp.
Mycobacterium avium complex.
Mycobacterium tuberculosis.
Escherichia coli (enterotoxigenic, enteroadherent).
Bacterial overgrowth.
Clostridium difficile (toxin).
Parasites
Cryptosporidium parvum.
Microsporida (*Enterocytozoon bieneusi, Septata intestinalis*).
Isospora belli.
Entamoeba histolytica.
Giardia lamblia.
Cyclospora cayetanensis.
Viruses
Cytomegalovirus.
Adenovirus.
Calicivirus.
Astrovirus.
Picobirnavirus.
Human immunodeficiency virus.
Fungi
Histoplasma capsulatum.

CAUSES OF PROCTITIS

Bacteria
Chlamydia trachomatis.
Neisseria gonorrhoeae.
Treponema pallidum.
Viruses
Herpes simplex.
Cytomegalovirus.

HIV INFECTION, OCULAR MANIFESTATIONS[36]

ICD-9CM # 042 HIV Infection, Symptomatic
V08 HIV Infection, Asymptomatic

EYELIDS

Molluscum contagiosum.
Kaposi's sarcoma.

CORNEA/CONJUNCTIVA

Keratoconjunctivitis sicca.
Bacterial/fungal ulcerative keratitis.
Herpes simplex.
Herpes zoster ophthalmicus.
Conjunctival microvasculopathy.
Kaposi's sarcoma.

RETINA, CHOROID, AND VITREOUS

Microvasculopathy.
Endophthalmitis.
Cytomegalovirus retinitis.
Acute retinal necrosis.
Syphilis.
Toxoplasmosis.
Pneumocystis choroidopathy.
Cryptococcosis.
Mycobacterial infection.
Intraocular lymphoma.
Candidiasis.
Histoplasmosis.

DRUGS ASSOCIATED WITH OCULAR TOXICITY

Rifabutin.
Didanosine.

NEUROOPHTHALMIC

Disc edema.
Primary or secondary optic neuropathy.
Cranial nerve palsies.

ORBITAL

Lymphoma.
Infection.
Pseudotumor.

HIV INFECTION, PULMONARY DISEASE[25]

ICD-9CM # 042 HIV Infection, Symptomatic

MYCOBACTERIAL

M. tuberculosis.
M. kansasii.
M. avium complex.
Other nontuberculous mycobacteria.

OTHER BACTERIAL

Streptococcus pneumoniae.
Staphylococcus aureus.
Haemophilus influenzae.
Enterobacteriaceae.
Pseudomonas aeruginosa.
Moraxella catarrhalis.

Group A *Streptococcus*.
Nocardia spp.
Rhodococcus equi.
Chlamydia pneumoniae.

FUNGAL

Pneumocystis carinii.
Cryptococcus neoformans.
Histoplasma capsulatum.
Coccidioides immitis.
Aspergillus spp.
Blastomyces dermatitidis.
Penicillium marneffei.

VIRAL

Cytomegalovirus.
Herpes simplex virus.
Adenovirus.
Respiratory syncytial virus.
Influenza viruses.
Parainfluenza virus.

OTHER

Toxoplasma gondii.
Strongyloides stercoralis.
Kaposi's sarcoma.
Lymphoma.
Lung cancer.
Lymphocytic interstitial pneumonitis.
Nonspecific interstitial pneumonitis.
Bronchiolitis obliterans with organizing pneumonia.
Pulmonary hypertension.
Emphysema-like or bullous disease.
Pneumothorax.
Congestive heart failure.
Diffuse alveolar damage.
Pulmonary embolus.

HOARSENESS

ICD-9CM # 784.49

Allergic rhinitis.
Infections (laryngitis, epiglottitis, tracheitis, croup).
Vocal cord polyps.
Voice strain.
Irritants (tobacco smoke).
Vocal cord trauma (intubation, surgery).
Neoplastic involvement of vocal cord (primary or metastatic).
Neurologic abnormalities (multiple sclerosis, ALS, parkinsonism).
Endocrine abnormalities (puberty, menopause, hypothyroidism).
Other (laryngeal webs or cysts, psychogenic, muscle tension abnormalities).

HYDROCEPHALUS

ICD-9CM # 331.4

Head trauma.
Brain neoplasm (primary or metastatic).
Spinal cord tumor.
Cerebellar infarction.
Exudative or granulomatous meningitis.
Cerebellar hemorrhage.

Subarachnoid hemorrhage.
Aqueductal stenosis.
Third ventricle colloid cyst.
Hindbrain malformation.
Viral encephalitis.
Metastases to leptomeninges.

HYPERCALCEMIA

ICD-9CM # 275.42 Hypercalcemia Disorder

Malignancy: increased bone resorption via osteoclast-activating factors, secretion of PTH-like substances, prostaglandin E2, direct erosion by tumor cells, transforming growth factors, colony-stimulating activity. Hypercalcemia is common in the following neoplasms:
  Solid tumors: breast, lung, pancreas, kidneys, ovary.
  Hematologic cancers: myeloma, lymphosarcoma, adult T-cell lymphoma, Burkitt's lymphoma.
Hyperparathyroidism: increased bone resorption, GI absorption, and renal absorption; etiology:
  Parathyroid hyperplasia, adenoma.
  Hyperparathyroidism or renal failure with secondary hyperparathyroidism.
Granulomatous disorders: increased GI absorption (e.g., sarcoidosis).
Paget's disease: increased bone resorption, seen only during periods of immobilization.
Vitamin D intoxication, milk-alkali syndrome; increased GI absorption.
Thiazides: increased renal absorption.
Other causes: familial hypocalciuric hypercalcemia, thyrotoxicosis, adrenal insufficiency, prolonged immobilization, vitamin A intoxication, recovery from acute renal failure, lithium administration, pheochromocytoma, disseminated SLE.

HYPERCALCEMIA, MALIGNANCY-INDUCED

ICD-9CM # 275.42

Lung carcinoma	(6% frequency, 35% of hypercalcemic cases)
Breast carcinoma	(10% frequency, 25% of hypercalcemic cases)
Multiple myeloma	(33% frequency, 10% of hypercalcemic cases)
Lymphoma	(4% of hypercalcemic cases)
Genitourinary cancer	(6% of hypercalcemic cases)

HYPERCAPNIA, PERSISTENT[36]

ICD-9CM # 786.09

Hypercapnia with normal lungs: CNS disturbances (CVA, parkinsonism, encephalitis), metabolic alkalosis, myxedema, primary alveolar hypoventilation, spinal cord lesions.
Diseases of the chest wall (e.g., kyphoscoliosis, ankylosing spondylitis).

Neuromuscular disorders (e.g., myasthenia gravis, Guillain-Barré syndrome, amyotrophic lateral sclerosis, muscular dystrophy, poliomyelitis).
COPD.

HYPERCOAGULABLE STATE, ASSOCIATED DISORDERS[20]

ICD-9CM # 289.82

Systemic lupus erythematosus in association with the presence of a lupus anticoagulant or antiphospholipid antibodies.
Malignancy:
  Disease-related: includes migratory superficial thrombophlebitis (Trousseau syndrome), nonbacterial thrombotic endocarditis, thrombosis associated with chronic DIC, thrombotic microangiopathy.
  Treatment-related: associated with the administration of various chemotherapeutic agents (L-asparaginase, mitomycin, some adjuvant chemotherapeutic agents for treatment of breast cancer, thalidomide or lenalidomide in conjunction with high doses of dexamethasone).
Infusion of prothrombin complex concentrates.
Nephrotic syndrome.
Heparin-induced thrombocytopenia.
Myeloproliferative disorders.
Paroxysmal nocturnal hemoglobinuria.

DIC, Disseminated intravascular coagulopathy.

HYPERGASTRINEMIA

ICD-9CM # varies with specific disorder

Decreased gastrin release inhibition from medications (proton pump inhibitors [PPIs], H_2 receptor antagonists), vagotomy.
Chronic renal failure.
Hypochlorhydria due to atrophic gastritis, gastric carcinoma, pernicious anemia.
Gastrinoma (Zollinger-Ellison syndrome).
Pyloric obstruction.
Hyperplasia of antral G cells.
RA.

HYPERHIDROSIS[4]

ICD-9CM # 780.8 hyperhidrosis

CORTICAL

Emotional.
Familial dysautonomia.
Congenital ichthyosiform erythroderma.
Epidermolysis bullosa.
Nail-patella syndrome.
Jadassohn-Lewandowsky syndrome.
Pachyonychia congenita.
Palmoplantar keratoderma.

HYPOTHALAMIC

Drugs
Antipyretics.
Emetics.
Insulin.
Meperidine.

Exercise Infection
Defervescence.
Chronic illness.
Metabolic
Debility.
DM.
Hyperpituitarism.
Hyperthyroidism.
Hypoglycemia.
Obesity.
Porphyria.
Pregnancy.
Rickets.
Infantile scurvy.
Cardiovascular
Heart failure.
Shock.
Vasomotor
Cold injury.
Raynaud phenomenon.
RA.
Neurologic
Abscess.
Familial dysautonomia.
Postencephalitic.
Tumor.
Miscellaneous
Chédiak-Higashi syndrome.
Compensatory.
Phenylketonuria.
Pheochromocytoma.
Vitiligo.
Medullary
Physiologic gustatory sweating.
Encephalitis.
Granulosis rubra nasi.
Syringomyelia.
Thoracic sympathetic trunk injury.
Spinal
Cord transection.
Syringomyelia.
Changes in Blood Flow
Mallucci syndrome.
Arteriovenous fistula.
Klippel-Trenaunay syndrome.
Glomus tumor.
Blue rubber bleb nevus syndrome.

HYPERKALEMIA

ICD-9CM # 276.7

Pseudohyperkalemia.
  Hemolyzed specimen.
    Severe thrombocytosis (platelet count 0.106 ml).
    Severe leukocytosis (white blood cell count 0.105 ml).
  Fist clenching during phlebotomy.
Excessive potassium intake (often in setting of impaired excretion).
  Potassium replacement therapy.
  High-potassium diet.
  Salt substitutes with potassium.
  Potassium salts of antibiotics.
Decreased renal excretion.
  Potassium-sparing diuretics (e.g., spironolactone, triamterene, amiloride).

Renal insufficiency.
Mineralocorticoid deficiency.
Hyporeninemic hypoaldosteronism (DM).
Tubular unresponsiveness to aldosterone (e.g., SLE, multiple myeloma, sickle cell disease).
Type 4 RTA.
ACE inhibitors.
Heparin administration.
NSAIDs.
Trimethoprim-sulfamethoxazole.
Beta-blockers.
Pentamidine.
Redistribution (excessive cellular release).
  Acidemia (each 0.1 decrease in pH increases the serum potassium by 0.4 to 0.6 mEq/L). Lactic acidosis and ketoacidosis cause minimal redistribution.
  Insulin deficiency.
  Drugs (e.g., succinylcholine, markedly increased digitalis level, arginine, beta-adrenergic blockers).
  Hypertonicity.
  Hemolysis.
  Tissue necrosis, rhabdomyolysis, burns.
  Hyperkalemic periodic paralysis.

HYPERKINETIC MOVEMENT DISORDERS[30]

ICD-9CM # 314.8 Hyperkinetic Syndrome
    275.1 Choreoathetosis
    335.5 Hemiballism
    333.7 Dystonia Due to Drugs
    333.6 Dystonia, Idiopathic

Chorea, choreoathetosis: drug-induced, Huntington's chorea, Sydenham's chorea.
Tardive dyskinesia (e.g., phenothiazines).
Hemiballismus (lacunar CVA near subthalamic nuclei in basal ganglia, metastatic lesions, toxoplasmosis [in AIDS]).
Dystonia (idiopathic, familial, drug-induced [prochlorperazine, metoclopramide]), Wilson's disease.
Liver failure.
Thyrotoxicosis.
SLE, polycythemia.

HYPERMAGNESEMIA

ICD-9CM # 275.2

Renal failure (decreased GFR).
Decreased renal excretion secondary to salt depletion.
Abuse of antacids and laxatives containing magnesium in patients with renal insufficiency.
Endocrinopathies (deficiency of mineralocorticoid or thyroid hormone).
Increased tissue breakdown (rhabdomyolysis).
Redistribution: acute DKA, pheochromocytoma.
Other: lithium, volume depletion, familial hypocalciuric hypercalcemia.

HYPEROSTOSIS, CORTICAL BONE[16a]

ICD-9CM # varies with specific diagnosis

DISORDERS ASSOCIATED WITH HYPEROSTOSIS OF CORTICAL BONE

Progressive diaphyseal dysplasia.
Endosteal hyperostosis.
Pachydermoperiostosis.
Hypertrophic oseoarthropathy.
Thyroid acropachy.
Hypervitaminosis A.
Paget's disease.
Infantile cortical hyperostosis.

HYPERPHOSPHATEMIA

ICD-9CM # 275.3

Excessive phosphate administration.
Excessive oral intake or IV administration.
Laxatives containing phosphate (phosphate tablets, phosphate enemas).
Decreased renal phosphate excretion.
Acute or chronic renal failure.
Hypoparathyroidism or pseudohypoparathyroidism.
Acromegaly, thyrotoxicosis.
Bisphosphonate therapy.
Tumor calcinosis.
Sickle cell anemia.
Transcellular shift out of cells.
Chemotherapy of lymphoma or leukemia, tumor lysis syndrome, hemolysis.
Acidosis.
Rhabdomyolysis, malignant hyperthermia.
Artifact: in vitro hemolysis.
Pseudohyperphosphatemia: hyperlipidemia, paraproteinemia, hyperbilirubinemia.

HYPERPIGMENTATION[5]

ICD-9CM # 709.00

Addison's disease.*
Arsenic ingestion.
ACTH- or MSH-producing tumors (e.g., oat cell carcinoma of the lung).*
Drug induced (i.e., antimalarials, some cytotoxic agents).
Hemochromatosis ("bronze" diabetes).
Malabsorption syndrome (Whipple's disease and celiac sprue).
Melanoma.
Melanotropic hormone injection.*
Pheochromocytoma.
Porphyrias (porphyria cutanea tarda and variegate porphyria).
Pregnancy.
Progressive systemic sclerosis and related conditions.
PUVA therapy (psoralen administration) for psoriasis and vitiligo.*

ACTH, Adrenocorticotropic hormone; *MSH,* melanocyte-stimulating hormone; *PUVA,* psoralen plus ultraviolet A.
*Accentuation on sun-exposed surfaces.

HYPERSPLENISM, ASSOCIATED CONDITIONS

ICD-9CM # 289.4

Cirrhosis.
Portal vein thrombosis.
Myeloproliferative diseases.
Lymphomas.
Leukemias.
Splenic vein thrombosis.
Autoimmune disease.
Sickle cell disease.
Thalassemias.
Gaucher's disease.
Niemann-Pick disease.

HYPERTENSION, IN CHILDREN[2]

ICD-9CM # 401

PRIMARY

Essential hypertension.

SECONDARY

Renal
Glomerulonephritis.
Henoch-Schönlein purpura.
Pyelonephritis.
Obstruction of reflux.
Polycystic kidney disease.
Diabetic nephropathy.
Trauma.
Renal transplant or hemodialysis.
Tuberous sclerosis.
Systemic lupus nephritis.
Endocrine
Pheochromocytoma.
Cushing's syndrome.
Congenital adrenal hyperplasia.
Corticosteroid treatment.
Hyperthyroidism.
Neuroblastoma.
Ovarian tumor.
Cardiac
Congestive heart failure.
Coarctation of the aorta.
Vascular
Hemolytic-uremic syndrome.
Kawasaki syndrome.
Renal artery thrombosis or stenosis.
Neurologic
Central nervous system tumor or infection.
Central nervous system trauma or abuse.
Increased intracranial pressure.
Guillain-Barré syndrome.
Neoplastic
Neuroblastoma.
Wilms' tumor.
Pheochromocytoma.
Adrenal carcinoma.
Drugs
Corticosteroids.
Cocaine.
Sympathomimetics.
Oral contraceptives.

Phencyclidine.
Beta-blocker or clonidine withdrawal.
Lead, mercury.
Others
Iatrogenic fluid overload.
Volume overload from end-stage renal disease.

HYPERTRICHOSIS[7]

ICD-9CM # 704.1 Hypertrichosis NOS
　　　　　　 757.4 Hypertrichosis, Congenital

DRUGS

Dilantin.
Streptomycin.
Hexachlorobenzene.
Penicillamine.
Diazoxide.
Minoxidil.
Cyclosporine.

SYSTEMIC ILLNESS

Hypothyroidism.
Anorexia nervosa.
Malnutrition.
Porphyria.
Dermatomyositis.

IDIOPATHIC

HYPERTROPHIC OSTEOARTHROPATHY

ICD-9CM # 731.2

Idiopathic.
Pulmonary disease (e.g., pulmonary fibrosis, cystic fibrosis, sarcoidosis).
Bronchogenic carcinoma.
AIDS.
GI neoplasm (e.g., esophagus, colon).
Hepatic neoplasm, cirrhosis.
Cardiovascular diseases, aortic aneurysm, aortic prosthesis.
Congenital cyanotic heart disease, patent ductus arteriosus.
Pulmonary infections, bacterial endocarditis, amebic dysentery.
Inflammatory bowel disease.
Connective tissue diseases.
Lymphomas.
Thyroid acropachy.

HYPERVENTILATION, PERSISTENT[36]

ICD-9CM # 786.01

Fibrotic lung disease.
Metabolic acidosis (e.g., diabetes, uremia).
CNS disorders (midbrain and pontine lesions).
Hepatic coma.
Salicylate intoxication.
Fever.
Sepsis.
Psychogenic (e.g., anxiety).

HYPOCALCEMIA

ICD-9CM # 275.41

Renal insufficiency: hypocalcemia caused by:
　Increased calcium deposits in bone and soft tissue secondary to increased serum PO423 level.
　Decreased production of 1,25-dihydroxyvitamin D.
　Excessive loss of 25-OHD (nephrotic syndrome).
Hypoalbuminemia: each decrease in serum albumin (g/L) will decrease serum calcium by 0.8 mg/dl but will not change free (ionized) calcium.
Vitamin D deficiency:
　Malabsorption (most common cause).
　Inadequate intake.
　Decreased production of 1,25-dihydroxyvitamin D (vitamin D–dependent rickets, renal failure).
　Decreased production of 25-OHD (parenchymal liver disease).
　Accelerated 25-OHD catabolism (phenytoin, phenobarbital).
　End-organ resistance to 1,25-dihydroxyvitamin D.
Hypomagnesemia: hypocalcemia caused by:
　Decreased PTH secretion.
　Inhibition of PTH effect on bone.
Pancreatitis, hyperphosphatemia, osteoblastic metastases: hypocalcemia is secondary to increased calcium deposits (bone, abdomen).
Pseudohypoparathyroidism (PHP): autosomal recessive disorder characterized by short stature, shortening of metacarpal bones, obesity, and mental retardation; the hypocalcemia is secondary to congenital end-organ resistance to PTH.
Idiopathic hypoparathyroidism, surgical removal of parathyroids (e.g., neck surgery).
"Hungry bones syndrome": rapid transfer of calcium from plasma into bones after removal of a parathyroid tumor.
Sepsis.
Massive blood transfusion (as a result of EDTA in blood).

HYPOCAPNIA

ICD-9CM # 786.01

Hyperventilation.
Pneumonia, pneumonitis.
Fever, sepsis.
Medications (salicylates, beta-adrenergic agonists, progesterone, methylxanthines).
Pulmonary disease (asthma, interstitial fibrosis).
Pulmonary embolism.
Hepatic failure.
Metabolic acidosis.
High altitude.
CHF.
Pregnancy.
Pain.
CNS lesions.

Differential Diagnosis

II

HYPOGLYCEMIA

ICD-9CM # 251.2 Spontaneous
250.3 Diabetic
251.0 Due to Insulin
579.3 Postoperative
251.2 Reactive

Oral hypoglycemics (therapeutic, factitious).
Exogenous insulin (therapeutic, factitious).
Postoperative gastric emptying (alimentary hyperinsulinism).
Severe malnutrition.
Liver disease.
Hypermetabolic state (sepsis).
Ketotic hypoglycemia.
Insulinoma.
Antibodies to endogenous insulin.
Hormone deficiencies (glucagon, growth hormone, hypoadrenalism).
Enzyme disorders in metabolism of glycogen, hexose, glycolysis, and Krebs cycle.
Idiopathic.

HYPOGONADISM

ICD-9CM # 256.3 Female
257.2 Male
256.3 Ovarian
253.4 Pituitary
257.2 Testicular

HYPERGONADOTROPIC HYPOGONADISM

Hormone resistance (androgen, LH insensitivity).
Gonadal defects (e.g., Klinefelter's syndrome, myotonic dystrophy).
Drug-induced (e.g., spironolactone, cytotoxins).
Alcoholism, radiation-induced.
Mumps orchitis.
Anatomic defects, castration.

HYPOGONADOTROPIC HYPOGONADISM

Pituitary lesions (neoplasms, granulomas, infarction, hemochromatosis, vasculitis).
Drug-induced (e.g., glucocorticoids).
Hyperprolactinemia.
Genetic disorders (Laurence-Moon-Biedl syndrome, Prader-Willi).
Delayed puberty.
Other: chronic disease, nutritional deficiency, Kallmann's syndrome, idiopathic isolated LH or FSH deficiency.

HYPOKALEMIA

ICD-9CM # 276.8

Cellular shift (redistribution) and undetermined mechanisms.
Alkalosis (each 0.1 increase in pH decreases serum potassium by 0.4 to 0.6 mEq/L).
Insulin administration.
Vitamin B_{12} therapy for megaloblastic anemias, acute leukemias.
Hypokalemic periodic paralysis: rare familial disorder manifested by recurrent attacks of flaccid paralysis and hypokalemia.

Beta-adrenergic agonists (e.g., terbutaline), decongestants, bronchodilators, theophylline, caffeine.
Barium poisoning, toluene intoxication, verapamil intoxication, chloroquine intoxication.
Correction of digoxin intoxication with digoxin antibody fragments (Digibind).
Increased renal excretion.
Drugs:
Diuretics, including carbonic anhydrase inhibitors (e.g., acetazolamide).
Amphotericin B.
High-dose sodium penicillin, nafcillin, ampicillin, or carbenicillin.
Cisplatin.
Aminoglycosides.
Corticosteroids, mineralocorticoids.
Foscarnet sodium.
RTA: distal (type 1) or proximal (type 2).
Diabetic ketoacidosis (DKA), ureteroenterostomy.
Magnesium deficiency.
Postobstruction diuresis, diuretic phase of ATN.
Osmotic diuresis (e.g., mannitol).
Bartter's syndrome: hyperplasia of juxtaglomerular cells leading to increased renin and aldosterone, metabolic alkalosis, hypokalemia, muscle weakness, and tetany (seen in young adults).
Increased mineralocorticoid activity (primary or secondary aldosteronism), Cushing's syndrome.
Chronic metabolic alkalosis from loss of gastric fluid (increased renal potassium secretion).
GI loss:
Vomiting, nasogastric suction.
Diarrhea.
Laxative abuse.
Villous adenoma.
Fistulas.
Inadequate dietary intake (e.g., anorexia nervosa).
Cutaneous loss (excessive sweating).
High dietary sodium intake, excessive use of licorice.

HYPOMAGNESEMIA

ICD-9CM # 275.2

GASTROINTESTINAL AND NUTRITIONAL

Defective GI absorption (malabsorption).
Inadequate dietary intake (e.g., alcoholics).
Parenteral therapy without magnesium.
Chronic diarrhea, villous adenoma, prolonged nasogastric suction, fistulas (small bowel, biliary).

EXCESSIVE RENAL LOSSES

Diuretics.
RTA.
Diuretic phase of ATN.
Endocrine disturbances (DKA, hyperaldosteronism, hyperthyroidism, hyperparathyroidism), SIADH, Bartter's syndrome, hypercalciuria, hypokalemia.

Cisplatin, alcohol, cyclosporine, digoxin, pentamidine, mannitol, amphotericin B, foscarnet, methotrexate.
Antibiotics (gentamicin, ticarcillin, carbenicillin).
Redistribution: hypoalbuminemia, cirrhosis, administration of insulin and glucose, theophylline, epinephrine, acute pancreatitis, cardiopulmonary bypass.
Miscellaneous: sweating, burns, prolonged exercise, lactation, "hungry-bones" syndrome.

HYPONATREMIA

ICD-9CM # 276.1

Renal loss from renal disease, diuretics.
GI loss (diarrhea, vomiting, suction).
Hypertonic hyponatremia (e.g., increased serum osmolality from hyperglycemia).
Transcutaneous loss (extensive burns, excessive sweating).
Fluid sequestration (e.g., ascites).
Osmotic diuresis (e.g., mannitol, glucose).
Dilutional (psychogenic polydipsia, iatrogenic).
Syndrome of inappropriate antidiuretic hormone secretion.
Edema with water and sodium retention.
Artifact (e.g., severe hyperlipidemia).
Laboratory error.
Adrenal insufficiency.

HYPOPHOSPHATEMIA

ICD-9CM # 275.3

Decreased intake (prolonged starvation [alcoholics], hyperalimentation, or IV infusion without phosphate).
Malabsorption.
Phosphate-binding antacids.
Renal loss:
RTA.
Fanconi syndrome, vitamin D–resistant rickets.
ATN (diuretic phase).
Hyperparathyroidism (primary or secondary).
Familial hypophosphatemia.
Hypokalemia, hypomagnesemia.
Acute volume expansion.
Glycosuria, idiopathic hypercalciuria.
Acetazolamide.
Transcellular shift into cells:
Alcohol withdrawal.
DKA (recovery phase).
Glucose-insulin or catecholamine infusion.
Anabolic steroids.
Total parenteral nutrition.
Theophylline overdose.
Severe hyperthermia; recovery from hypothermia.
"Hungry bones" syndrome.

HYPOPIGMENTATION

ICD-9CM # 709.00

Vitiligo.
Tinea versicolor.
Atopic dermatitis.
Chemical leukoderma.
Idiopathic hypomelanosis.

Sarcoidosis.
SLE.
Scleroderma.
Oculocutaneous albinism.
Phenylketonuria.
Nevoid hypopigmentation.

HYPOTENSION, POSTURAL

ICD-9CM # 458.0

Antihypertensive medications (especially α-blockers, diuretics, ACE inhibitors).
Volume depletion (hemorrhage, dehydration).
Impaired cardiac output (constrictive pericarditis, aortic stenosis).
Peripheral autonomic dysfunction (DM, Guillain-Barré).
Idiopathic orthostatic hypotension.
Central autonomic dysfunction (Shy-Drager syndrome).
Peripheral venous disease.
Adrenal insufficiency.

ILIAC FOSSA PAIN, LEFT SIDED[38]

ICD-9CM # varies with specific diagnosis

GASTROINTESTINAL CAUSES OF ACUTE LEFT ILIAC FOSSA PAIN

Nonspecific left iliac fossa pain including constipation.
Acute gastroenteritis.
Acute diverticulitis.
Colonic carcinoma.
Colonic ischemia.
Localized small bowel perforation.

ILIAC FOSSA PAIN, RIGHT SIDED[38]

ICD-9CM # varies with specific diagnosis

DIFFERENTIAL DIAGNOSIS OF RIGHT ILIAC FOSSA PAIN

Gastrointestinal Causes
Nonspecific right iliac fossa pain.
Acute appendicitis.
Mesenteric adenitis.
Terminal ileitis.
Acute inflammation of Meckel's diverticulum.
Crohn's disease of the terminal ileum.
Cecal carcinoma.
Inflammatory cecal lesion (e.g., diverticulitis in a solitary cecal diverticulum).
Inflammatory lesion of the terminal ileum (e.g., foreign body perforation).
Non-Gastrointestinal Causes
Ruptured ovarian follicle (mittelschmerz).
Acute salpingitis (pelvic inflammatory disease).
Rupture/torsion or hemorrhage of an ovarian cyst.
Endometriosis.
Ectopic pregnancy.
Urinary tract infection.

IMPOTENCE[27]

ICD-9CM # 302.72 Psychosexual
607.84 Organic
997.99 Organic Postprostatectomy

Psych`ogenic.
Endocrine: hyperprolactinemia, DM, Cushing's syndrome, hypothyroidism or hyperthyroidism, abnormality of hypothalamic-pituitary-testicular axis.
Vascular: arterial insufficiency, venous leakage, AV malformation, local trauma.
Medications.
Neurogenic: autonomic or sensory neuropathy, spinal cord trauma or tumor, CVA, multiple sclerosis, temporal lobe epilepsy.
Systemic illness: renal failure, COPD, cirrhosis of liver, myotonic dystrophy.
Peyronie's disease.
Prostatectomy.

INCONTINENCE, FECAL[38]

ICD-9CM # 787.6

NORMAL SPHINCTER

Diarrhea.
Anorectal conditions:
- Rectal carcinoma.
- Inflammatory bowel disease.
- Hemorrhoids.
- Mucosal prolapse.
- Fissure-in-ano.
- Abnormal rectal sensation.

ABNORMAL SPHINCTER

Congenital abnormalities.
Anal sepsis.
Neurological conditions.
Rectal prolapse.
Sphincter trauma.
Neurogenic (idiopathic) incontinence.

INFERTILITY, FEMALE[14]

ICD-9CM # 628.9

FALLOPIAN TUBE PATHOLOGY

PID or puerperal infection.
Congenital anomalies.
Endometriosis.
Secondary to past peritonitis of nongenital origin.
Amenorrhea and anovulation.
Minor anovulatory disturbances.

CERVICAL AND UTERINE FACTORS

Leiomyomas and polyps.
Uterine anomalies.
Intrauterine synechiae (Asherman's syndrome).
Destroyed endocervical glands (postsurgery or postinfection).

VAGINAL FACTORS

Congenital absence of vagina.
Imperforate hymen.

Vaginismus.
Vaginitis.

IMMUNOLOGIC FACTORS

Sperm-immobilizing antibodies.
Sperm-agglutinating antibodies.

NUTRITIONAL AND METABOLIC FACTORS

Thyroid disorders.
DM.
Severe nutritional disturbances.

INFERTILITY, MALE[14]

ICD-9CM # 606.9

DECREASED PRODUCTION OF SPERMATOZOA

Varicocele.
Testicular failure.
Endocrine disorders.
Cryptorchidism.
Stress, smoking, caffeine, nicotine, recreational drugs.

DUCTAL OBSTRUCTION

Epididymal (postinfection).
Congenital absence of vas deferens.
Ejaculatory duct (postinfection).
Postvasectomy.

INABILITY TO DELIVER SPERM INTO VAGINA

Ejaculatory disturbances.
Hypospadias.
Sexual problems (i.e., impotence), medical or psychological.

ABNORMAL SEMEN

Infection.
Abnormal volume.
Abnormal viscosity.
Abnormal sperm motion.

IMMUNOLOGIC FACTORS

Sperm-immobilizing antibodies.
Sperm-agglutinating antibodies.

INSOMNIA[33]

ICD-9CM # 780.52 Insomnia NOS
307.42 Insomnia, Chronic Associated with Anxiety or Depression
780.51 Insomnia with Sleep Apnea

Anxiety disorder, psychophysiologic insomnia.
Depression.
Drugs (e.g., caffeine, amphetamines, cocaine), hypnotic-dependent sleep disorder.
Pain, fibromyalgia.
Inadequate sleep hygiene.
Restless leg syndrome.
Obstructive sleep apnea.
Sleep bruxism.
Medical illness (e.g., GERD, sleep-related asthma, parkinsonism and movement disorders).

Differential Diagnosis

II

Narcolepsy.
Other: periodic leg movement of sleep, central sleep apnea, REM behavioral disorder.

INTESTINAL PSEUDOOBSTRUCTION[36]

ICD-9CM # 560.1 Adynamic Intestinal Obstruction
564.9 Intestinal Disorder, Functional

"PRIMARY" (IDIOPATHIC INTESTINAL PSEUDOOBSTRUCTION)

Hollow visceral myopathy:
  Familial.
  Sporadic.
Neuropathic:
  Abnormal myenteric plexus.
  Normal myenteric plexus.

SECONDARY

Scleroderma.
Myxedema.
Amyloidosis.
Muscular dystrophy.
Hypokalemia.
Chronic renal failure.
DM.
Drug toxicity caused by:
  Anticholinergics.
  Opiate narcotics.
Ogilvie's syndrome.

INTRA-ABDOMINAL MASS LESION, NEONATAL[16a]

ICD-9CM # 789.3

CAUSES OF A NEONATAL INTRA-ABDOMINAL MASS LESION

Complicated meconium ileus.
Dilated bowel proximal to an obstruction.
Mesenteric or duplication cyst.
Abscess.
GU Causes:
  Hydronephrosis.
  Renal cystic disease.
  Mesoblastic nephroma.
  Wilms' tumor.
  Adrenal hemorrhage.
  Neuroblastoma.
  Retroperitoneal teratoma.
  Ovarian cyst.
  Hydrometrocolpos.
Hemangioendothelioma.
Hepatoblastoma.
Choledochal, hepatic, or splenic cysts.

INTRACEREBRAL HEMORRHAGE, NONHYPERTENSIVE CAUSES

ICD-9CM # 431

Trauma.
Anticoagulation.
Intracranial tumors.

Vascular malformations.
Bleeding disorders.
Vasculitides (e.g., polyarteritis nodosa, granulomatous angiitis).
Cocaine and other sympathomimetic agents.
Cerebral amyloid angiopathy.

INTRACRANIAL LESION

ICD-9CM # 348.8

Tumor (primary or metastatic).
Abscess.
Stroke.
Intracranial hemorrhage.
Angioma.
Multiple sclerosis (initial single lesion).
Granuloma.
Herpes encephalitis.
Artifact.

INTRAOCULAR NEOPLASM

ICD-9CM # varies with specific disorder

MALIGNANT

Retinoblastoma.
Melanoma.
Reticulum cell sarcoma.
Metastatic tumor.

BENIGN

Melanocytic nevus.
Hemangioma.
Reactive lymphoid hyperplasia.

IRON OVERLOAD[20]

ICD-9CM # 275.0

HEREDITARY IRON OVERLOAD

Hereditary hemochromatosis:
  HFE-associated (type 1).
  Non–HFE-associated:
    • Transferrin receptor 2–associated (type 3).
Juvenile hemochromatosis (type 2):
  Hemojuvelin-associated (type 2A).
  Hepcidin-associated (type 2B).
Autosomal dominant hemochromatosis:
  Ferroportin-associated (type 4).
DMT1-associated hemochromatosis.
Atransferrinemia.
Aceruloplasminemia.

ACQUIRED IRON OVERLOAD

Iron-loading anemias (refractory anemias with hypercellular erythroid marrow).
Chronic liver disease.
Porphyria cutanea tarda.
Insulin resistance–associated hepatic iron overload.
African dietary iron overload.[a]
Medical iron ingestion.[a]
Parenteral iron overload:
  Transfusional iron overload.
  Inadvertent iron overload from therapeutic injections.

PERINATAL IRON OVERLOAD

Neonatal hemochromatosis.
Trichohepatoenteric syndrome.

Cerebrohepatorenal syndrome.
GRACILE[b] (Fellman) syndrome.

FOCAL SEQUESTRATION OF IRON

Idiopathic pulmonary hemosiderosis.
Renal hemosiderosis.
Associated with neurologic abnormalities:
  Pantothenate kinase–associated neurodegeneration (formerly called Hallervorden-Spatz syndrome).
  Neuroferritinopathy.
  Friedreich's ataxia.

---

[a]May have a genetic component.
[b]GRACILE, growth retardation, aminoaciduria, cholestasis, iron overload, lactic acidosis, and early death.

ISCHEMIC COLITIS, NONOCCLUSIVE[21]

ICD-9CM # 557.1

ACUTE DIMINUTION OF COLONIC INTRAMURAL BLOOD FLOW

Small Vessel Obstruction
Collagen-vascular disease.
Vasculitis, diabetes.
Oral contraceptives.
Nonocclusive Hypoperfusion
Hemorrhage.
CHF, MI, arrhythmias.
Sepsis.
Vasoconstricting agents: vasopressin, ergot.
Increased viscosity: polycythemia, sickle cell disease, thrombocytosis.

INCREASED DEMAND ON MARGINAL BLOOD FLOW

Increased Motility
Mass lesion, stricture.
Constipation.
Increased Intraluminal Pressure
Bowel obstruction.
Colonoscopy.
Barium enema.

ISCHEMIC NECROSIS OF CARTILAGE AND BONE[14]

ICD-9CM # 733.90

ENDOCRINE/METABOLIC

Ethanol abuse.
Glucocorticoid therapy.
Cushing's disease.
DM.
Hyperuricemia.
Osteomalacia.
Hyperlipidemia.

STORAGE DISEASES (E.G., GAUCHER'S DISEASE)

Hemoglobinopathies (e.g., sickle cell disease).
Trauma (e.g., dislocation, fracture).
HIV infection.
Dysbaric conditions (e.g., caisson disease).
Collagen-vascular disorders.
Irradiation.

Pancreatitis
Organ transplantation.
Hemodialysis.
Burns.
Intravascular coagulation.
Idiopathic, familial.

JAUNDICE

ICD-9CM # 782.4 Jaundice NOS
576.8 Jaundice, Obstructive
277.4 Bilirubin Excretion
Disorders

PREDOMINANCE OF DIRECT (CONJUGATED) BILIRUBIN

Extrahepatic obstruction.
Common duct abnormalities: calculi, neoplasm, stricture, cyst, sclerosing cholangitis.
Metastatic carcinoma.
Pancreatic carcinoma, pseudocyst.
Ampullary carcinoma.
Hepatocellular disease: hepatitis, cirrhosis.
Drugs: estrogens, phenothiazines, captopril, methyltestosterone, labetalol.
Cholestatic jaundice of pregnancy.
Hereditary disorders: Dubin-Johnson syndrome, Rotor's syndrome.
Recurrent benign intrahepatic cholestasis.

PREDOMINANCE OF INDIRECT (UNCONJUGATED) BILIRUBIN

Hemolysis: hereditary and acquired hemolytic anemias.
Inefficient marrow production.
Impaired hepatic conjugation: chloramphenicol.
Neonatal jaundice.
Hereditary disorders: Gilbert's syndrome, Crigler-Najjar syndrome.

JAUNDICE, CLASSIFICATION[1]

ICD-9CM # 782.4

PREHEPATIC (PREDOMINANTLY UNCONJUGATED HYPERBILIRUBINEMIA)

Overproduction

Hemolysis (e.g., spherocytosis, sickle cell disease, hemolysis of the newborn, autoimmune disorders).
Ineffective erythropoiesis (e.g., megaloblastic anemias).
Hematomas.
Pulmonary emboli.

HEPATIC (UNCONJUGATED HYPERBILIRUBINEMIA)

Decreased Hepatic Uptake

Gilbert syndrome.
Drugs (e.g., rifampin, radiographic contrast agents)
Neonatal jaundice
Posthepatitis
Decreased cystolic binding proteins (e.g., newborn or premature infants)
Portocaval shunt
Prolonged fasting

Decreased Conjugation Due to Limited Glucuronyl Transferase Activity

Gilbert's disease.
Crigler-Najjar syndrome, types I and II.
Neonatal jaundice.
Breast-milk jaundice.
Chronic persistent hepatitis.
Wilson's disease.
Noncirrhotic portal fibrosis.
Drug inhibition (e.g., chloramphenicol).

PREDOMINANTLY CONJUGATED HYPERBILIRUBINEMIA

Impaired Hepatic Excretion

Familial disorders (Dubin-Johnson syndrome, Rotor syndrome, benign recurrent cholestasis, cholestasis of pregnancy).
Hepatocellular infiltrative disorders.
Liver metastasis.
Liver cirrhosis.
Hepatitis (viral, bacterial, parasitic, autoimmune, ethanol, and drug-induced).
Drug-induced cholestasis (especially chlorpromazine, erythromycin estolate, isoniazid, halothane).
Primary biliary cirrhosis.
Primary sclerosing cholangitis.
Pericholangitis.
Congestive heart failure.
Shock.
Toxemia of pregnancy.
Sarcoidosis.
Hepatic trauma.
Amyloidosis.
Autoimmune cholangiopathy.
Vanishing bile duct syndrome.
Sepsis.
Postoperative complications.

EXTRAHEPATIC

Extrahepatic Biliary Obstruction

Gallstones, choledocholithiasis.
Cholecystitis.
Tumors of the head of the pancreas (adenocarcinoma, mucinous duct ectasia, neuroendocrine tumors, metastasis).
Tumors of bile ducts (cholangiocarcinoma, Klatskin tumor: cholangiocarcinoma at the bifurcation).
Gallbladder cancer.
Tumors of the ampulla of Vater (adenoma, adenocarcinoma).
Tumors of the duodenum (adenocarcinoma, lymphoma).
Hemobilia (blood in the biliary tree).
Biliary strictures (postcholecystectomy, post-liver transplantation, primary sclerosing cholangitis).
Congential disorders (biliary atresia, idiopathic dilation of common bile duct, cystic fibrosis).
Metastasis to the hepatic hilum.
Primary bile duct lymphoma.
Cholangiopathy of acquired immunodeficiency syndrome.
Choledochal cysts.
Infectious cholangiopathy (Clonorchis sinensis, Ascaris lumbricoides, Fasciola hepatica).
Chronic pancreatitis (fibrosis of the head of the pancreas).

JAUNDICE, NEONATAL[1]

ICD-9CM # 774.6

PREHEPATIC

Hereditary spherocytosis.
Nonspherocytic hemolytic anemia (glucose-6-phosphate dehydrogenase deficiency, α-thalassemia, vitamin K_3–induced hemolysis, pyruvate kinase deficiency).

HEPATIC

Crigler-Najjar syndrome, types I and II.
α_1-antitrypsin deficiency.
Sepsis.
Drug-induced.
Hypothyroidism.
Breast-milk jaundice.
Fetomaternal blood group incompatibility (Rhesus, Landsteiner groups ABO).

POSTHEPATIC

Extrahepatic biliary obstruction.
Biliary atresia.
Bile duct paucity.
Alagille syndrome.

JOINT PAIN, ANTERIOR HIP, MEDIAL THIGH, KNEE[28]

ICD-9CM # 719.4 add 5th digit
0 Site NOS
1 Shoulder Region
2 Upper Arm (Elbow, Humerus)
3 Forearm (Radius, Wrist, Ulna)
4 Hand
5 Pelvic Region and Thigh
6 Lower Leg (Fibula, Patella, Tibia)
7 Ankle and/or Foot

ACUTE

Acute rheumatic fever.
Adductor muscle strain.
Avascular necrosis.
Crystal arthritis.
Femoral artery (pseudo) aneurysm.
Fracture (femoral neck or intertrochanteric).
Hemarthrosis.
Hernia.
Herpes zoster.
Iliopectineal bursitis.
Iliopsoas tendinitis.
Inguinal lymphadenitis.
Osteomalacia.
Painful transient osteoporosis of hip.
Septic arthritis.

SUBACUTE AND CHRONIC

Adductory muscle strain.
Amyloidosis.
Acute rheumatic fever.
Femoral artery aneurysm.
Hernia (inguinal or femoral).
Iliopectineal bursitis.
Iliopsoas tendinitis.
Inguinal lymphadenopathy.
Osteochondromatosis.
Osteomyelitis.

Osteitis deformans (Paget's disease).
Osteomalacia (pseudofracture).
Postherpetic neuralgia.
Sterile synovitis (e.g., RA, psoriatic, SLE).

JOINT PAIN, HIP, LATERAL THIGH[28]

ICD-9CM # 959.6 Hip Injury
719.95 Hip Joint Disorder
843.9 Hip Strain

ACUTE

Herpes zoster.
Iliotibial tendinitis.
Impacted fracture of femoral neck.
Lateral femoral cutaneous neuropathy (meralgia paresthetica).
Radiculopathy: L4-5.
Trochanteric avulsion fracture (greater trochanter).
Trochanteric bursitis.
Trochanteric fracture.

SUBACUTE AND CHRONIC

Lateral femoral cutaneous neuropathy (meralgia paresthetica).
Osteomyelitis.
Postherpetic neuralgia.
Radiculopathy: L4-5.
Tumors.

JOINT PAIN, POLYARTICULAR

ICD-9CM # 719.40

Osteoarthritis.
RA.
Fibromyalgia.
Viral syndrome (e.g., human parvovirus B19 infection).
SLE.
Psoriatic arthritis.
Ankylosing spondylitis.

JOINT PAIN, POSTERIOR HIPS, THIGH, BUTTOCKS[28]

ICD-9CM # 719.4 add 5th digit
0 Site NOS
1 Shoulder Region
2 Upper Arm (Elbow, Humerus)
3 Forearm (Radius, Wrist, Ulna)
4 Hand
5 Pelvic Region and Thigh
6 Lower Leg (Fibula, Patella, Tibia)
7 Ankle and/or Foot

ACUTE

Gluteal muscle strain.
Herpes zoster.
Ischial bursitis.
Ischial or sacral fracture.
Osteomalacia (pseudofracture).
Sciatic neuropathy.
Radiculopathy: L5-S1.

SUBACUTE AND CHRONIC

Gluteal muscle strain.
Ischial bursitis.
Lumbar spinal stenosis.
Osteoarthritis of hip.
Osteitis deformans (Paget's disease).
Osteomyelitis.
Osteochondromatosis.
Osteomalacia (pseudofracture).
Postherpetic neuralgia.
Radiculopathy: L5-S1.
Tumors.

JOINT SWELLING

ICD-9CM # 719.0 add 5th digit
0 Site NOS
1 Shoulder Region
2 Upper Arm (Elbow, Humerus)
3 Forearm (Radius, Wrist, Ulna)
4 Hand
5 Pelvic Region and Thigh
6 Lower Leg (Fibula, Patella, Tibia)
7 Ankle and/or Foot

Trauma.
Osteoarthritis.
Gout.
Pyogenic arthritis.
Pseudogout.
RA.
Viral syndrome.

JUGULAR VENOUS DISTENTION

ICD-9CM # 459.89 Increased Venous Pressure

Right-sided heart failure.
Cardiac tamponade.
Constrictive pericarditis.
Goiter.
Tension pneumothorax.
Pulmonary hypertension.
Cardiomyopathy (restrictive).
Superior vena cava syndrome.
Valsalva maneuver.
Right atrial myxoma.
COPD.

KERATITIS, NONINFECTIOUS

ICD-9CM # 370.9

Collagen vascular disease.
Atopic keratoconjunctivitis.
Chemical injury.
Thermal injury.
Ectropion/entropion.
Lid defects.
Exophthalmos.
Keratoconjunctivitis sicca.
Erythema multiforme.
Mucous membrane pemphigoid.
DM (delayed epithelial healing).
Neuroparalytic (cranial nerve VII).
Neurotrophic (diabetes, cranial nerve V).

KIDNEY ENLARGEMENT, UNILATERAL[38]

ICD-9CM # 591

Hydronephrosis (may be bilateral).
Polycystic kidney (may be bilateral).
Simple cyst of kidney.
Renal cell carcinoma.
Pyonephrosis (may be bilateral).
Acute renal vein thrombosis.

KNEE PAIN[28]

ICD-9CM # 844.1 Collateral Ligament Sprain, Medial
844.2 Cruciate Ligament Sprain
716.96 Knee Inflammation
959.7 Knee Injury
718.86 Knee Instability
836.1 Lateral Meniscus Tear
836.0 Medial Meniscus Tear
844.8 Patellar Sprain
719.56 Knee Stiffness
719.06 Knee Swelling

DIFFUSE

Articular.
Anterior.
Prepatellar bursitis.
Patellar tendon enthesopathy.
Chondromalacia patellae.
Patellofemoral osteoarthritis.
Cruciate ligament injury.
Medial plica syndrome.

MEDIAL

Anserine bursitis.
Spontaneous osteonecrosis.
Osteoarthritis.
Medial meniscal tear.
Medial collateral ligament bursitis.
Referred pain from hip and L3.
Fibromyalgia.

LATERAL

Iliotibial band syndrome.
Meniscal cyst.
Lateral meniscal tear.
Collateral ligament.
Peroneal tenosynovitis.

POSTERIOR

Popliteal cyst (Baker's cyst).
Tendinitis.
Aneurysms, ganglions, sarcoma.

KNEE PAIN, IN DIFFERENT AGE GROUPS[8]

ICD-9CM # 719.46

COMMON CAUSES OF KNEE PAIN IN DIFFERENT AGE GROUPS

Childhood (2-10 yr)
Intraarticular:
Juvenile arthritis.
Osteochondritis dissecans.

Infection.
Torn discoid meniscus.
Periarticular:
Osteomyelitis.
Referred:
Perthes' disease.
Irritable hip.
Adolescence (10-18 yr)
Intraarticular:
Osteochondritis dissecans.
Torn meniscus.
Anterior knee pain syndrome.
Patellar instability.
Periarticular:
Osgood–Schlatter disease.
Sinding–Larsen–Johansson syndrome.
Osteomyelitis.
Bone tumors.
Referred:
Slipped upper femoral epiphysis.
Early Adulthood (18-30 yr)
Intraarticular:
Torn meniscus.
Patellar instability.
Anterior knee pain syndrome.
Inflammatory arthritis.
Periarticular:
Ligament injuries.
Bursitis.
Adulthood (30-50 yr)
Intraarticular:
Degenerate meniscal tears.
Osteoarthritis.
Inflammatory arthritis.
Periarticular:
Bursitis.
Referred:
Osteoarthritis of hip.
Spinal disorders.
Old Age (>50 yr)
Intraarticular:
Osteoarthritis.
Inflammatory arthritis.
Periarticular:
Bursitis.
Referred:
Osteoarthritis of hip.
Spinal disorders.

LARGE BOWEL STRICTURE[16a]

ICD-9CM # 751.2

CAUSES OF LARGE-BOWEL STRICTURES

Physiological:
 Spasm.
 Distended bladder.
Maligant:
 Annular carcinoma.
 Scirrhous carcinoma.
 Lymphoma.
Diverticular disease:
 Muscle thickening.
 Pericolic abscess.
 Superimposed malignancy.
Ischemia.

Radiation colitis.
Inflammatory bowel disease:
 Ulcerative colitis.
 Crohn's disease.
 Tuberculosis.
 Lymphogranuloma venereum.
 Amebiasis.
Extrinsic disease:
 Intraabdominal masses.
 Melastatic carcinoma.
 Endometriosis.
 Pelvic lipomatosis.
 Cholecystitis.
 Pancreatitis.
Miscellaneous:
 Postoperative anastomosis.
 Trauma.
 Hirschsprung's disease.

LEFT AXIS DEVIATION[22]

ICD-9CM # 426.3 Left Bundle Branch Block
 426.2 Left Bundle Branch Hemiblock
 429.3 Left Ventricular Hypertrophy

Normal variation.
Left anterior fascicular block (hemiblock).
Left bundle branch block.
Left ventricular hypertrophy.
Mechanical shifts causing a horizontal heart, high diaphragm, pregnancy, ascites.
Some forms of ventricular tachycardia.
Endocardial cushion defects and other congenital heart disease.

LEFT BUNDLE BRANCH BLOCK

ICD-9CM # 426.3

Ischemic heart disease.
Electrolyte abnormalities (e.g., hyperkalemia).
Cardiomyopathy.
Idiopathic.
LVH.
Pulmonary embolism.
Cardiac trauma.
Bacterial endocarditis.

LEG CRAMPS, NOCTURNAL

ICD-9CM # 729.82 Muscle Cramps

Diabetic neuropathy.
Medications.
Electrolyte abnormalities (hypokalemia, hyponatremia, hypocalcemia, hyperkalemia, hypophosphatemia).
Respiratory alkalosis.
Uremia.
Hemodialysis.
Peripheral nerve injury.
ALS.
Alcohol use.
Heat cramps.
Vitamin B_{12} deficiency.
Hyperthyroidism.

Contractures.
DVT.
Hypoglycemia.
Peripheral vascular insufficiency.
Baker's cyst.

LEG LENGTH DISCREPANCIES[23]

ICD-9CM # 736.81 Leg Length Discrepancy, Acquired
 755.30 Leg Length Discrepancy, Congenital

CONGENITAL

Proximal femoral local deficiency.
Coxa vara.
Hemiatrophy-hemihypertrophy (anisomelia).
Development dysplasia of the hip.

DEVELOPMENTAL

Legg-Calvé-Perthes disease.

NEUROMUSCULAR

Polio.
Cerebral palsy (hemiplegia).

INFECTIOUS

Pyogenic osteomyelitis with physeal damage.

TRAUMA

Physeal injury with premature closure.
Overgrowth.
Malunion (shortening).

TUMOR

Physeal destruction.
Radiation-induced physeal injury.
Overgrowth.

LEG MOVEMENT WHEN STANDING, INVOLUNTARY

ICD-9CM # varies with specific disorder

Benign essential tremor.
Orthostatic tremor.
Spastic ataxia.
Cerebellar truncal tremor.
Postanoxic myoclonus.

LEG PAIN WITH EXERCISE

ICD-9CM # 729.82 Muscle Cramps

Shin splints.
Arteriosclerosis obliterans.
Neurogenic (spinal cord compression or ischemia).
Venous claudication.
Popliteal cyst.
DVT.
Thromboangiitis obliterans.
Adventitial cysts.
Popliteal artery entrapment syndrome.
McArdle syndrome.

Differential Diagnosis

II

LEG ULCERS[28]

ICD-9CM #	440.23	Lower Limb, Arteriosclerotic
	707.1	Lower Limb, Chronic
	707.1	Lower Limb, Neurogenic
	250.70	Lower Limb, Chronic DM Type 2
	250.71	Lower Limb, Chronic, DM Type 1

VASCULAR

Arterial: arteriosclerosis, thromboangiitis obliterans, AV malformation, cholesterol emboli.
Venous: superficial varicosities, incompetent perforators, DVT, lymphatic abnormalities.

VASCULITIS HEMATOLOGIC

Sickle cell anemia, thalassemia, polycythemia vera, leukemia, cold agglutinin disease.
Macroglobulinemia, protein C and protein S deficiency, cryoglobulinemia, lupus anticoagulant, antiphospholipid syndrome.

INFECTIOUS

Fungus: Blastomycosis, coccidioidomycosis, histoplasmosis, sporotrichosis.
Bacterial: Furuncle, ecthyma, septic emboli.
Protozoal: leishmaniasis.

METABOLIC

Necrobiosis lipoidica diabeticorum.
Localized bullous pemphigoid.
Gout, calcinosis cutis, Gaucher's disease.

TUMORS

Basal cell carcinoma, squamous cell carcinoma, melanoma.
Mycosis fungoides, Kaposi's sarcoma, metastatic neoplasms.

TRAUMA

Burns, cold injury, radiation dermatitis.
Insect bites.
Factitial, excessive pressure.

NEUROPATHIC

Diabetic trophic ulcers.
Tabes dorsalis, syringomyelia.

DRUGS

Warfarin, IV colchicine extravasation, methotrexate, halogens, ergotism, hydroxyurea.

PANNICULITIS

Weber-Christian disease.
Pancreatic fat necrosis, alpha-antitrypsinase deficiency.

LEPTOMENINGEAL LESIONS

ICD-9CM # varies with specific disorder

Metastases.
Multiple sclerosis.
Bacterial or viral meningitis.
Vasculitis.
Lyme disease.
Tuberculosis.

Fungal infections (e.g., *Cryptococcus*).
Sarcoidosis.
Wegener's granulomatosis.
Neurocysticercosis.
Rheumatoid nodules.
Histiocytosis.

LEUKOCORIA

ICD-9CM # 379.90

Cataract.
Retinal detachment.
Retinoblastoma.
Retinal telangiectasia.
Retrolenticular vascularized membrane.
Familial exudative vitreoretinopathy.

LIMP

ICD-9CM #	781.2	Gait Abnormality
	719.75	Gait Disorder Due to Joint Abnormality in Hip, Buttock, or Femur
	719.76	Gait Disorder Due to Joint Abnormality in Lower Leg
	719.77	Gait Disorder Due to Joint Abnormality in Ankle and/ or Foot
	300.11	Hysterical Gait Disorder

Degenerative joint disease, osteochondritis dissecans, chondromalacia patellae.
Trauma to extremities, vertebral disc, hips.
Poorly fitting shoes, foreign body in shoe, unequal leg length.
Splinter in foot.
Joint infection (septic arthritis, osteomyelitis), viral arthritis.
Abdominal pain (e.g., appendicitis, incarcerated hernia), testicular torsion.
Polio, neuromuscular disorders, Guillain-Barré syndrome, multiple sclerosis.
Osgood-Schlatter disease.
Legg-Calvé-Perthes disease.
Factitious, somatization syndrome.
Neoplasm (local or metastatic).
Other: diskitis, periostitis, sickle cell disease, hemophilia.

LIMPING, PEDIATRIC AGE[23]

ICD-9CM # 781.2 Gait Abnormality

TODDLER (1-3 YR)

Infection:
 Septic arthritis:
 • Hip.
 • Knee.
 Osteomyelitis.
 Diskitis.
Occult trauma:
 Toddler's fracture.
Neoplasia.

CHILDHOOD (4-10 YR)

Infection:
 Septic arthritis:
 • Hip.
 • Knee.

 Osteomyelitis.
 Diskitis.
 Transient synovitis, hip.
LCPD.
Tarsal coalition.
Rheumatologic disorder:
 JRA.
Trauma.
Neoplasia.

ADOLESCENCE (11+ YR)

SCFE.
Rheumatologic disorder:
 JRA.
Trauma.
Tarsal coalition.
Hip dislocation (DDH).
Neoplasia.

DDH, Developmental dysplasia of the hip; *JRA*, juvenile RA; *LCPD*, Legg-Calvé-Perthes disease; *SCFE*, slipped capital femoral epiphysis.

LIVEDO RETICULITIS

ICD-9CM # code not available

Emboli (SBE, left atrial myxoma, cholesterol emboli).
Thrombocythemia or polycythemia.
Antiphospholipid antibody syndrome.
Cryoglobulinemia, cryofibrinogenemia.
Leukocytoclastic vasculitis.
SLE, RA, dermatomyositis.
Pancreatitis.
Drugs (quinine, quinidine, amantadine, catecholamines).
Physiologic (cutis marmorata).
Congenital.

LIVER DISEASE, PREGNANCY[38]

ICD-9CM # varies with specific diagnosis

INCIDENTAL TO PREGNANCY

Viral hepatitis.
Alcohol related.
Autoimmune chronic active hepatitis.

RELATED TO PREGNANCY (possibly influenced by hormones present in pregnancy)

Complicated gallstone disease.
Hepatic adenoma.
Focal nodular hyperplasia.
Budd-Chiari syndrome.

SPECIFIC TO PREGNANCY

Severe hyperemesis gravidarum.
Benign intrahepatic cholestasis.
Acute fatty liver of pregnancy.
Pre-eclampsia (HELLP).

LIVER LESIONS, BENIGN, OFTEN CONFUSED WITH MALIGNANCY
ICD-9CM # 573.8

Fatty infiltration.
Adenoma.
Hemangioma.
Cysts.
Flow artifacts.
Focal nodular hyperplasia.
Nonenhanced vessels.

LOW-VOLTAGE ECG
ICD-9CM # 794.31

Hypothyroidism.
Obesity.
Pericardial effusion.
Anasarca.
Pleural effusion.
Pneumothorax.
Amyloidosis.
Aortic stenosis.

LUNG CANCER, OCCUPATIONAL CAUSES[16a]
ICD-9CM # 162.9

CAUSES OF OCCUPATIONAL LUNG CANCER

Asbestos	Lagging, insulation
Arsenic	Metal smelting, pesticide manufacture
Beryllium	Electronics, dental prosthetic manufacture
Chromium	Coloring pigment production, electroplating
Nickel	Electroplating
Silica	Grinding, quarrying, sandblasting
Radon	Mining
Uranium	Mining

LYMPHADENOPATHY[14]
ICD-9CM # 785.6

GENERALIZED
AIDS.
Lymphoma: Hodgkin's disease, non-Hodgkin's lymphoma.
Leukemias, reticuloendotheliosis.
Infectious mononucleosis, CMV, and other viral infections.
Diffuse skin infection: generalized furunculosis, multiple tick bites.
Parasitic infections: toxoplasmosis, filariasis, leishmaniasis, Chagas' disease.
Serum sickness.
Collagen vascular diseases (RA, SLE).
Dengue (arbovirus infection).
Sarcoidosis and other granulomatous diseases.
Drugs: INH, hydantoin derivatives, antithyroid and antileprosy drugs.
Secondary syphilis.
Hyperthyroidism, lipid-storage diseases.

LOCALIZED
Cervical Nodes
Infections of the head, neck, ears, sinuses, scalp, pharynx.
Mononucleosis.
Lymphoma.
TB.
Malignancy of head and neck.
Rubella.
Scalene/Supraclavicular Nodes
Lymphoma.
Lung neoplasm.
Bacterial or fungal infection of thorax or retroperitoneum.
GI malignancy.
Axillary Nodes
Infections of hands and arms.
Cat-scratch disease.
Neoplasm (lymphoma, melanoma, breast carcinoma).
Brucellosis.
Epitrochlear Nodes
Infections of the hand.
Lymphoma.
Tularemia.
Sarcoidosis, secondary syphilis (usually bilateral).
Inguinal Nodes
Infections of leg or foot, folliculitis (pubic hair).
LGV, syphilis.
Lymphoma.
Pelvic malignancy.
Pasteurella pestis.
Hilar Nodes
Sarcoidosis.
TB.
Lung carcinoma.
Fungal infections, systemic.
Mediastinal Nodes
Sarcoidosis.
Lymphoma.
Lung neoplasm.
TB.
Mononucleosis.
Histoplasmosis.
Abdominal/Retroperitoneal Nodes
Lymphoma.
TB.
Neoplasm (ovary, testes, prostate, and other malignancies).

LYMPHANGITIS[25]
ICD-9CM # 457.2

Acute:
  Group A streptococci.
  Staphylococcus aureus.
  Pasteurella multocida.
Chronic:
  Sporothrix schenckii (sporotrichosis).
  Mycobacterium marinum (swimming pool granuloma).
  Mycobacterium kansasii.
  Nocardia brasiliensis.
  W. bancrofti.

LYMPHOCYTOSIS, ATYPICAL[25]
ICD-9CM # 288.8

Epstein-Barr virus primary infection (infectious mononucleosis).
Cytomegalovirus primary infection (heterophile-negative mono).
Human herpesvirus 6 primary infection (roseola).
Primary HIV infection.
Toxoplasmosis.
Acute viral hepatitis.
Rubella, mumps.
Drug reactions (e.g., phenytoin, sulfa).

MACROTHROMBOCYTOPENIA, INHERITED[20]
ICD-9CM # varies with specific diagnosis

Bernard-Soulier syndrome.
MHY9-related disorders:
- May-Hegglin anomaly.
- Sebastian syndrome.
- Fechtner syndrome.
- Epstein syndrome.
Gray platelet syndrome.
Montreal platelet syndrome.
Mediterranean macrothrombocytopenia.
Mediterranean stomatocytosis/macrothrombocytenia.
GATA1 mutations.
Sialyl-Lewis-S antigen deficiency.
Paris-Trousseau syndrome.
Platelet-type von Willebrand's disease.

MALABSORPTION[38]
ICD-9CM # 579

CAUSES OF MALABSORPTION
More Common
Celiac disease.
Chronic pancreatitis.
Post gastrectomy.
Crohn's disease.
Small bowel resection.
Small intestinal bacterial overgrowth.
Lactase deficiency.
Less Common
AIDS (*Myobacterium avium* intracellulare, AIDS enteropathy).
Whipple's disease.
Intestinal lymphoma.
Immunoproliferative small intestinal disease (alpha heavy chain disease).
Radiation enteritis.
Collagenous sprue.
Tropical sprue.
Non-granulomatous ulcerative jejunoileitis.
Eosinophilic gastroenteritis.
Amyloidosis.
Zollinger-Ellison syndrome.
Intestinal lymphangiectasia.
Systemic mastocytosis.
Chronic mesenteric ischemia.
Abetalipoproteinemia (autosomal recessive).

Differential Diagnosis

MEDIASTINAL COMPARTMENTS, ANATOMY AND PATHOLOGY[39]

ICD-9CM # varies with specific diagnosis

ANTERIOR
Normal Structures
Lymph nodes.
Connective tissue.
Thymus (remnant in adults).
Masses
Thymoma.
Germ cell neoplasm.
Lymphoma.
Thyroid enlargement (intrathoracic goiter).
Other tumors.

MIDDLE
Normal Structures
Pericardium.
Heart.
Vessels: Ascending aorta, venae cavae, main pulmonary arteries.
Trachea.
Lymph nodes.
Nerves: Phrenic, upper vagus.
Masses
Carcinoma.
Lymphoma.
Pericardial cyst.
Bronchogenic cyst.
Benign lymph node enlargement (granulomatous disease).

POSTERIOR
Normal Structures
Vessels: Descending aorta.
Esophagus.
Vertebral column.
Nerves: Sympathetic chain, lower vagus.
Lymph nodes.
Connective tissue.
Masses
Neurogenic tumor.
Diaphragmatic hernia.

MEDIASTINAL MASSES OR WIDENING ON CHEST X-RAY

ICD-9CM # 785.6 Adenopathy
          519.3 Disease NEC
          793.2 Shift (CXR)

Lymphoma: Hodgkin's disease and non-Hodgkin's lymphoma.
Sarcoidosis.
Vascular: aortic aneurysm, ectasia or tortuosity of aorta or bronchocephalic vessels.
Carcinoma: lungs, esophagus.
Esophageal diverticula.
Hiatal hernia.
Achalasia.
Prominent pulmonary outflow tract: pulmonary hypertension, pulmonary embolism, right-to-left shunts.
Trauma: mediastinal hemorrhage.
Pneumomediastinum.

Lymphadenopathy caused by silicosis and other pneumoconioses.
Leukemias.
Infections: TB, viral (rare), *Mycoplasma* (rare), fungal, tularemia.
Substernal thyroid.
Thymoma.
Teratoma.
Bronchogenic cyst.
Pericardial cyst.
Neurofibroma, neurosarcoma, ganglioneuroma.

MEDIASTINITIS, ACUTE[25]

ICD-9CM # 519.2

Esophageal perforation.
Iatrogenic.
EGD, esophageal dilation, esophageal variceal sclerotherapy, nasogastric tube, Sengstaken-Blackmore tube, endotracheal intubation, esophageal surgery, paraesophageal surgery, transesophageal echocardiography, anterior stabilization of cervical vertebral bodies.
Swallowed foreign bodies.
Trauma.
Spontaneous perforation (e.g., emesis, carcinoma).
Head and neck infections (e.g., tonsillitis, pharyngitis, parotitis, epiglottitis, odontogenic).
Infections originating at another site (e.g., TB, pneumonia, pancreatitis, osteomyelitis of sternum, clavicle, ribs).
Cardiothoracic surgery (median sternotomy) (e.g., CABG, valve replacement, other types of cardiothoracic surgery).

MELANONYCHIA

ICD-9CM # varies with specific disorder

Pregnancy.
Trauma.
Medications (e.g., AZT, 5-fluorouracil, doxorubicin, psoralens).
Nail matrix nevus.
HIV infection.
Onychomycosis.
Melanocyte hyperplasia.
Verrucae.
Pustular psoriasis.
Lichen planus.
Basal cell carcinoma.
Nail matrix melanoma.
Subungual keratosis.
Addison's disease.
Bowen's disease.

MEMORY LOSS SYMPTOMS, ELDERLY PATIENTS

ICD-9CM # varies with specific disorder

Age-related mild cognitive impairment.
Depression (pseudodementia).
Medications (e.g., anticholinergics, sedatives).
Hypothyroidism.
Chronic hypoxia.
Cerebrovascular infarcts.
Alzheimer's disease.
Hepatic disease.

Chronic renal failure.
Hyperthyroidism.
Frontotemporal dementia.
Lewy body dementia.

MENINGITIS, CHRONIC[26]

ICD-9CM # 322.2

TB.
Fungal CNS infection.
Tertiary syphilis.
CNS neoplasm.
Metabolic encephalopathies.
Multiple sclerosis.
Chronic subdural hematoma.
SLE cerebritis.
Encephalitides.
Sarcoidosis.
NSAIDs.
Behçet's syndrome.
Anatomic defects (traumatic, congenital, postoperative).
Granulomatous angiitis.

MENINGITIS, RECURRENT[25]

ICD-9CM # varies with specific disorder

Drug induced (with rechallenge).
Parameningeal focus.
Infection (sinusitis, mastoiditis, osteomyelitis, brain abscess).
Tumor (epidermoid cyst, craniopharyngioma).
Posttraumatic (bacterial).
Mollaret's meningitis.
SLE.
Herpes simplex virus.

MENTAL STATUS CHANGES AND COMA[2]

ICD-9CM # 780.97

METABOLIC/SYSTEMIC ETIOLOGY OF ALTERED MENTAL STATUS AND COMA

Hypoxia
Severe pulmonary disease (hypoventilation).
Severe anemia.
Environmental/toxin:
Methemoglobinemia.
Cyanide.
Carbon monoxide.
Decreased atmospheric oxygen (high altitude).
Near-drowning.
Disorders of Glucose
Hypoglycemia:
Chronic alcohol abuse and liver disease.
Excessive use of insulin or other hypoglycemic agents.
Insulinoma.
Hyperglycemia:
Diabetic ketoacidosis.
Nonketotic hyperosmolar coma.
Decreased Cerebral Blood Flow
Hypovolemic shock.
Cardiac:
Vasovagal syncope.
Arrhythmias.

Myocardial infarction.
Valvular disorders.
Congestive heart failure.
Pericardial effusion/tamponade.
Myocarditis.
Infectious:
Septic shock.
Bacterial meningitis.
Vascular/hematologic:
Hypertensive encephalopathy.
Pseudotumor cerebri.
Hyperviscosity (sickle cell, polycythemia).
Hyperventilation.
Cerebral lupus vasculitis.
Thrombotic thrombocytopenic purpura.
Disseminated intravascular coagulation.

Metabolic Cofactor Deficiency
Thiamine (Wernicke-Korsakoff syndrome).
Pyridoxine (isoniazid overdose).
Folic acid (chronic alcohol abuse).
Cyanocobalamine.
Niacin.

Electrolye/pH Disturbances
Acidosis/alkalosis.
Hypernatremia/hyponatremia.*
Hypercalcemia/hypocalcemia.
Hypophosphatemia.
Hypermagnesemia/hypomagnesemia.

Endocrine Disorders
Myxedema coma, thyrotoxicosis.
Hypopituitarism.
Addison's disease (primary or secondary).
Cushing's disease.
Pheochromocytoma.
Hyperparathyroidism/hypoparathyroidism.

Endogenous Toxins
Hyperammonemia (liver failure).
Uremia (renal disease).
Carbon dioxide narcosis (pulmonary disease).
Porphyria.

Exogenous Toxins
Alcohols:
Ethanol, isopropyl alcohol, methanol, ethylene glycol.
Acid poisons:
Salicylates.
Paraldehyde.
Ammonium chloride.
Antidepressant medications:
Lithium.
Tricyclic antidepressants (TCAs).
Selective serotonin reuptake inhibitors (SSRIs).
Monamine oxidase inhibitors (MAOIs).
Stimulants:
Amphetamines/methamphetamines.
Cocaine.
Over-the-counter sympathomimetics.
Narcotics/opiates:
Morphine.
Heroin.
Codeine, oxycodone, meperidine, hydrocodone.
Methadone.
Fentanyl.
Propoxyphene.
Sedative-hypnotics:
Benzodiazepines.
Barbiturates.

Rohypnol.
Bromide.
Hallucinogens:
Lysergic acid diethylamide (LSD).
Marijuana.
Mescaline, peyote.
Mushrooms.
Phencyclidine (PCP).
Herbs/plants:
Aconite.
Jimson weed.
Morning glory.
Volatile substances:
Hydrocarbons (gasoline, butane, toluene, benzene, chloroform).
Nitrites.
Anesthetic agents (nitrous oxide, ether).
Other:
γ-Hydroxybutyrate (GHB).
Ketamine.
Penicillin.
Cardiac glycosides.
Anticonvulsants.
Steroids.
Heavy metals.
Cimetidine.
Organophosphates.

Disorders of Temperature Regulation/Environmental
Hypothermia.
Heat stroke.
Malignant hyperthermia.
Neuroleptic malignant syndrome.
High-altitude cerebral edema (HACE).
Dysbarism.

Primary Glial or Neuronal Disorders
Adrenoleukodystrophy.
Creutzfeldt-Jakob disease.
Progressive multifocal leukoencephalopathy.
Marchiava-Bignami disease.
Gliomatosis cerebri.
Central pontine myelinolysis.

Other Disorders of Unknown Etiology
Seizures.
Postictal states.
Reye's syndrome.†
Intussuception.†

---

*Can be associated with dilution of formula in infant feeding.
†Prominent in the pediatric population.

MESENTERIC ARTERIAL EMBOLISM, ASSOCIATED FACTORS[2]

ICD-9CM # 557.0

FACTORS ASSOCIATED WITH MESENTERIC ARTERIAL EMBOLISM

Coronary artery disease.
Post-myocardial infarction mural thrombi.
Congestive heart failure.
Valvular heart disease.
Rheumatic mitral valve disease.
Nonbacterial endocarditis.

Arrhythmias.
Chronic atrial fibrillation.
Aortic aneurysms or dissections.
Coronary angiography.

MESENTERIC ISCHEMIA, NONOCCLUSIVE[26]

ICD-9CM # 557.0	Mesenteric Artery Embolism or Infarction
557.1	Mesenteric Artery Insufficiency, Chronic
902.39	Mesenteric Vein Injury

Cardiovascular disease resulting in low-flow states (CHF, cardiogenic shock, post cardiopulmonary bypass, dysrhythmias).
Septic shock.
Drug induced (cocaine, vasopressors, ergot alkaloid poisoning).

MESENTERIC VENOUS THROMBOSIS[26]

ICD-9CM # 557.0

Hypercoagulable states (protein C or S deficiency, antithrombin III deficiency, Factor V Leyden, malignancy, polycythemia vera, sickle cell disease, homocystinemia, lupus anticoagulant, cardiolipin antibody).
Trauma (operative venous injury, abdominal trauma, postsplenectomy).
Inflammatory conditions (pancreatitis, diverticulitis, appendicitis, cholangitis).
Other: CHF, renal failure, portal hypertension, decompression sickness.

METASTATIC NEOPLASMS

ICD-9CM # 198.5	Bone and Bone Marrow
198.3	Brain and Spinal Cord
197.7	Liver
197.0	Lung

To: Bone	To: Brain
Breast	Lung
Lung	Breast
Prostate	Melanoma
Thyroid	GU tract
Kidney	Colon
Bladder	Sinuses
Endometrium	Sarcoma
Cervix	Skin
Melanoma	Thyroid
To: Liver	**To: Lung**
Colon	Breast
Stomach	Colon
Pancreas	Kidney
Breast	Testis
Lymphomas	Stomach
Bronchus	Thyroid
Lung	Melanoma
Sarcoma	
Choriocarcinoma	
Kidney	

MICROCEPHALY[4]

ICD-9CM # 742.1 Microcephalus

PRIMARY (GENETIC)

Familial (autosomal recessive).
Autosomal dominant.
Syndromes:
    Down (21-trisomy).
    Edward (18-trisomy).
    Cri-du-chat (5 p-).
    Cornelia de Lange.
    Rubinstein-Taybi.
    Smith-Lemli-Opitz.

SECONDARY (NONGENETIC)

Radiation.
Congenital infections:
    Cytomegalovirus.
    Rubella.
    Toxoplasmosis.
Drugs:
    Fetal alcohol.
    Fetal hydantoin.
Meningitis/encephalitis.
Malnutrition.
Metabolic.
Hyperthermia.
Hypoxic-ischemic encephalopathy.

MICROPENIS[27]

ICD-9CM # 752.69 Penile Agenesis or Atresia
              607.89 Penile Atrophy
              752.64 Micropenis (Congenital)

HYPOGONADOTROPIC HYPOGONADISM (HYPOTHALAMIC OR PITUITARY DEFICIENCIES)

Kallmann's syndrome: autosomal dominant; associated with hyposmia.
Prader-Willi syndrome: hypotonia, mental retardation, obesity, small hands and feet.
Rud syndrome: hyposomia, ichthyosis, mental retardation.
De Morsier's syndrome (septooptic dysplasia): hypopituitarism, hypoplastic optic discs, absent septum pellucidum.

HYPERGONADOTROPIC HYPOGONADISM

Primary testicular defect: disorders of testicular differentiation or inborn errors of testosterone synthesis.
Klinefelter's syndrome.
Other X polysomies (i.e., XXXXY, XXXY).
Robinow's syndrome: brachymesomelic dwarfism, dysmorphic facies.

PARTIAL ANDROGEN INSENSITIVITY

Idiopathic
Defective morphogenesis of the penis.

MIOSIS

ICD-9CM # 379.42 Miosis, Persistent not
              Due to Miotics

Medications (e.g., morphine, pilocarpine).
Neurosyphilis.
Congenital.
Iritis.
CNS pontine lesion.
CNS infections.
Cavernous sinus thrombosis.
Inflammation/irritation of cornea or conjunctiva.

MONOARTHRITIS, ACUTE

ICD-9CM # 716.60

Overuse.
Trauma.
Gout.
Pseudogout.
Osteoarthritis.
Infectious arthritis (e.g., gonococcal, Lyme disease, viral, mycobacteria, fungi).
Osteomyelitis.
Avascular necrosis of bone.
Hemarthrosis.
Bowel disease–associated arthritis.
Bone malignancy.
Psoriatic arthritis.
Juvenile RA.
Sarcoidosis.
Hemoglobinopathies.
Vasculitic syndromes.
Behçet's syndrome.
Foreign body synovitis.
Hypertrophic pulmonary osteoarthropathy.
Amyloidosis, familial Mediterranean fever.

MONOCYTOSIS[20]

ICD-9CM # 288.63

Inflammatory diseases:
    Infectious diseases:
    • Tuberculosis.
    • Syphilis.
    • Subacute bacterial endocarditis.
    • Fever of unknown origin.
    Autoimmune/granulomatous.
    Systemic lupus erythematosus.
    Rheumatoid arthritis.
    Temporal arteritis.
    Myositis.
    Polyarteritis.
    Ulcerative colitis.
    Regional enteritis.
    Sarcoidosis.
Malignant disorders:
    Preleukemia.
    Nonlymphocytic leukemia.
    Histiocytoses.
    Hodgkin's disease.
    Non-Hodgkin's lymphoma.
    Carcinomas.
Miscellaneous:
    Chronic neutropenia.
    Post splenectomy.

MONONEUROPATHY

ICD-9CM # 355.9

Herpes zoster.
Herpes simplex.
Vasculitis.
Trauma, compression.
Diabetes.
Postinfectious or inflammatory.

MONONEUROPATHY, ISOLATED[2]

ICD-9CM # varies with specific diagnosis

UPPER EXTREMITY

Radial nerve.
    Axilla.
    Humerus.
    Elbow (posterior interosseous neuropathy).
    Wrist (superficial cutaneous radial neuropathy).
Ulnar nerve.
    Axilla.
    Humerus.
    Elbow.
    Condylar groove.
    Cubital tunnel.
Wrist (Guyon's canal).
Hand.
    Superficial terminal ulnar neuropathy.
    Deep terminal ulnar neuropathy.
    • Proximal hypothenar.
    • Distal hypothenar.
Median nerve.
Axilla.
Humerus (musculocutaneous mononeuropathy).
Forearm.
    Anterior interosseus.
    Pronator syndrome (?).
Wrist (carpal tunnel).
Hand (recurrent motor branch).
Suprascapular mononeuropathy.
    Axillary mononeuropathy.

LOWER EXTREMITY

Sciatic nerve.
Femoral nerve.
    Iliacus compartment (proximal).
    Saphenous mononeuropathy (distal).
Lateral femoral cutaneous (meralgia paresthetica).
Peroneal nerve.
    Common peroneal mononeuropathy (fibular head, popliteal fossa).
    Deep peroneal mononeuropathy (anterior compartment).
Tibial nerve.
    Popliteal fossa (proximal).
    Tarsal tunnel (distal).
Sural nerve.
    Popliteal fossa, calf (proximal).
    Fifth metatarsal base (distal).
Plantar nerve.
    Distal to tarsal tunnel.
    Interdigital neuropathies (Morton's neuroma).
Obturator mononeuropathy.

MONONUCLEOSIS, MONOSPOT NEGATIVE[1]

ICD-9CM # 075

DIFFERENTIAL DIAGNOSIS OF MONOSPOT-NEGATIVE MONONUCLEOSIS

Acute HIV infection.
EBV mononucleosis (particularly in children).
Cytomegalovirus.
Acute toxoplasmosis.
Streptococcal pharyngitis.
Acute hepatitis B infection.

EBV, Epstein-Barr virus; *HIV,* human immunodeficiency virus.

MUSCLE DISEASE[34a]

ICD-9CM # 728

CLASSIFICATION OF MUSCLE DISEASE

Muscular Dystrophies
Duchenne.
Becker.
Limb girdle.
Childhood.
Facioscapulohumeral.
Myotonic Disorders
Dystrophia myotonica.
Myotonica congenita.
Inflammatory
Infective: bacterial, viral, parasitic.
Unknown cause: polymyositis, dermatomyositis, sarcoidosis.
Endocrine
Thyroid disease—hyper- and hypothyroidism.
Cushing's disease.
Addison's disease.
Hyperparathyroidism.
Metabolic
Glycogen storage diseases.
Periodic paralyses.
Mitochondrial diseases.
Drug-induced
Corticosteroids.
Chloroquine.
Amiodarone.
Penicillamine.
Alcohol.
Zidovudine.
Clofibrate.
Other
Inclusion body myositis.

MUSCLE WEAKNESS

ICD-9CM # 728.9

Physical deconditioning.
Impaired cardiac output (e.g., mitral stenosis, mitral regurgitation).
Uremia, liver failure.
Electrolyte abnormalities (hypokalemia, hyperkalemia, hypophosphatemia, hypercalcemia), hypoglycemia.
Drug induced (e.g., statin myopathy).

Muscular dystrophies.
Steroid myopathy.
Alcoholic myopathy.
Myasthenia gravis, Lambert-Eaton syndrome.
Infections (polio, botulism, HIV, hepatitis, diphtheria, tick paralysis, neurosyphilis, brucellosis, TB, trichinosis).
Pernicious anemia, other anemias, beriberi.
Psychiatric illness (depression, somatization syndrome).
Organophosphate or arsenic poisoning.
Inflammatory myopathies (e.g., collagen vascular disease, RA, sarcoidosis).
Endocrinopathies (e.g., adrenal insufficiency, hypothyroidism), diabetic neuropathy.
Other: motor neuron disease, mitochondrial myopathy, L-tryptophan (eosinophilia-myalgia), rhabdomyolysis, glycogen storage disease, lipid storage disease.

MUSCLE WEAKNESS, LOWER MOTOR NEURON VERSUS UPPER MOTOR NEURON[40]

ICD-9CM # 728.9

LOWER MOTOR NEURON

Weakness, usually severe.
Marked muscle atrophy.
Fasciculations.
Decreased muscle stretch reflexes.
Clonus not present.
Flaccidity.
No Babinski sign.
Asymmetric and may involve one limb only in the beginning to become generalized as the disease progresses.

UPPER MOTOR NEURON

Weakness, usually less severe.
Minimal disuse muscle atrophy.
No fasciculations.
Increased muscle stretch reflexes.
Clonus may be present.
Spasticity.
Babinski sign.
Often initial impairment of only skilled movements.
In the limbs the following muscles may be the only ones weak or weaker than the others: triceps; wrist and finger extensors; interossei; iliopsoas; hamstrings; and foot dorsiflexors, inverters, and extroverters.

MYDRIASIS

ICD-9CM # 379.43 Mydriasis, Persistent not Due to Mydriatics

Coma.
Medications (cocaine, atropine, epinephrine, etc.).
Glaucoma.
Cerebral aneurysm.
Ocular trauma.
Head trauma.
Optic atrophy.
Cerebral neoplasm.
Iridocyclitis.

MYELIN DISORDERS

ICD-9CM # varies with specific disorder

Multiple sclerosis.
Vitamin B_{12} deficiency.
Radiation.
Hypoxia.
Toxicity from carbon monoxide, alcohol, mercury.
Progressive multifocal encephalopathy.
Acute disseminated encephalomyelitis.
Acute hemorrhagic leukoencephalopathy.
Phenylketonuria.
Adrenoleukodystrophy.
Krabbe's disease.

MYELOPATHY AND MYELITIS[36]

ICD-9CM # 722.70 Myelopathy, Discogenic Intervertebral NOS
336.9 Myelopathy, Nondiscogenic Unspecified

INFLAMMATORY

Infectious: spirochetal TB, zoster, rabies, HIV, polio, rickettsial, fungal, parasitic.
Noninfectious: idiopathic transverse myelitis, multiple sclerosis.

TOXIC/METABOLIC

DM, pernicious anemia, chronic liver disease, pellagra, arsenic.

TRAUMA COMPRESSION

Spinal neoplasm, cervical spondylosis, epidural abscess, epidural hematoma.

VASCULAR

AV malformation, SLE, periarteritis nodosa, dissecting aortic aneurysm.

PHYSICAL AGENTS

Electrical injury, irradiation.

NEOPLASTIC

Spinal cord tumors, paraneoplastic myelopathy.

MYOCARDIAL ISCHEMIA[36]

ICD-9CM # 414.8 Ischemia (Chronic)
411.89 Ischemia, Acute without MI

Atherosclerotic obstructive coronary artery disease.
Nonatherosclerotic coronary artery disease:
Coronary artery spasm.
Congenital coronary artery anomalies:
Anomalous origin of coronary artery from pulmonary artery.
Aberrant origin of coronary artery from aorta or another coronary artery.
Coronary arteriovenous fistula.
Coronary artery aneurysm.

Acquired disorders of coronary arteries:
Coronary artery embolism.
Dissection:
- Surgical.
- During percutaneous coronary angioplasty.
- Aortic dissection.
- Spontaneous (e.g., during pregnancy).
Extrinsic compression:
- Tumors.
- Granulomas.
- Amyloidosis.
Collagen-vascular disease:
- Polyarteritis nodosa.
- Temporal arteritis.
- RA.
- SLE.
- Scleroderma.
Miscellaneous disorders:
- Irradiation.
- Trauma.
- Kawasaki disease.
Syphilis.
Hereditary disorders:
Pseudoxanthoma elasticum.
Gargoylism.
Progeria.
Homocystinuria.
Primary oxaluria.
"Functional" causes of myocardial ischemia in absence of anatomic coronary artery disease:
Syndrome X.
Hypertrophic cardiomyopathy.
Dilated cardiomyopathy.
Muscle bridge.
Hypertensive heart disease.
Pulmonary hypertension.
Valvular heart disease; aortic stenosis, aortic regurgitation.

MYOCLONUS
ICD-9CM # 333.2

Physiologic (e.g., exercise or anxiety induced).
Renal failure.
Hepatic failure.
Hyponatremia.
Hypoglycemia or severe hyperglycemia.
Postdialysis.
Epileptic myoclonus.
Postencephalitis.
CNS lesion (stroke, neoplasm).
CNS trauma.
Parkinson's disease.
Medications (e.g., tricyclics, L-dopa).
Friedreich's ataxia.
Ataxia telangiectasia.
Wilson's disease.
Huntington's disease.
Progressive supranuclear palsy.
Heavy metal poisoning.
Benign familial.

MYOPATHIES, INFECTIOUS
ICD-9CM # 359.8

HIV.
Viral myositis.
Trichinosis.
Toxoplasmosis.
Cysticercosis.

MYOPATHIES, INFLAMMATORY
ICD-9CM # 359.9

SLE, RA.
Sarcoidosis.
Paraneoplastic syndrome.
Polymyositis, dermatomyositis.
Polyarteritis nodosa.
Mixed connective tissue disease.
Scleroderma.
Inclusion body myositis.
Sjögren's syndrome.
Cimetidine, D-penicillamine.

MYOPATHIES, TOXIC[1]
ICD-9CM # 359.4

Inflammatory: cimetidine, D-penicillamine.
Noninflammatory necrotizing or vacuolar: cholesterol-lowering agents, chloroquine, colchicine.
Acute muscle necrosis and myoglobinuria: cholesterol-lowering drugs, alcohol, cocaine.
Malignant hyperthermia: halothane, ethylene, others; succinylcholine.
Mitochondrial: zidovudine.
Myosin loss: nondepolarizing neuromuscular blocking agents; glucocorticoids.

MYOSITIS, INFLAMMATORY[1]
ICD-9CM # 729.1

INFECTIOUS
Viral myositis:
Retroviruses (HIV, HTLV-I).
Enteroviruses (echovirus, Coxsackievirus).
Other viruses (influenza, hepatitis A and B, Epstein-Barr virus).
Bacterial: pyomyositis.
Parasites: trichinosis, cysticercosis.
Fungi: candidiasis.

IDIOPATHIC
Granulomatous myositis (sarcoid, giant cell).
Eosinophilic myositis.
Eosinophilia-myalgia syndrome.

ENDOCRINE/METABOLIC DISORDERS
Hypothyroidism.
Hyperthyroidism.
Hypercortisolism.
Hyperparathyroidism.
Hypoparathyroidism.
Hypocalcemia.
Hypokalemia.

METABOLIC MYOPATHIES
Myophosphorylase deficiency (McArdle's disease).
Phosphofructokinase deficiency.
Myoadenylate deaminase deficiency.
Acid maltase deficiency.
Lipid storage diseases.
Acute rhabdomyolysis.

DRUG-INDUCED MYOPATHIES
Alcohol.
D-Penicillamine.
Zidovudine.
Colchicine.
Chloroquine, hydroxychloroquine.
Lipid-lowering agents.
Cyclosporine.
Cocaine, heroin, barbiturates.
Corticosteroids.

NEUROLOGIC DISORDERS
Muscular dystrophies.
Congenital myopathies.
Motor neuron disease.
Guillain-Barré syndrome.
Myasthenia gravis.

NAIL CLUBBING
ICD-9CM # 703.9

COPD.
Pulmonary malignancy.
Cirrhosis.
Inflammatory bowel disease.
Chronic bronchitis.
Congenital heart disease.
Endocarditis.
AV malformations.
Asbestosis.
Trauma.
Idiopathic.

NAIL, HORIZONTAL WHITE LINES (BEAU'S LINES)
ICD-9CM # 703.8

Malnutrition.
Idiopathic.
Trauma.
Prolonged systemic illnesses.
Pemphigus.
Raynaud's disease.

NAIL KOILONYCHIA
ICD-9CM # 703.8

Trauma.
Iron deficiency.
SLE.
Hemochromatosis.
Raynaud's disease.
Nail-patella syndrome.
Idiopathic.

NAIL ONYCHOLYSIS
ICD-9CM # 703.8

Infection.
Trauma.
Psoriasis.
Connective tissue disorders.
Sarcoidosis.
Hyperthyroidism.
Amyloidosis.
Nutritional deficiencies.

NAIL PITTING
ICD-9CM # 703.8

Psoriasis.
Alopecia areata.
Reiter's syndrome.
Trauma.
Idiopathic.

NAIL SPLINTER HEMORRHAGE
ICD-9CM # 703.8

SBE.
Trauma.
Malignancies.
Oral contraceptives.
Pregnancy.
SLE.
Antiphospholipid syndrome.
Psoriasis.
RA.
Peptic ulcer disease.

NAIL STRIATIONS
ICD-9CM # 703.8

Psoriasis.
Alopecia areata.
Trauma.
Atopic dermatitis.
Vitiligo.

NAIL TELANGIECTASIA
ICD-9CM # 703.8

RA.
Scleroderma.
Trauma.
SLE.
Dermatomyositis.

NAIL WHITENING (TERRY'S NAILS)
ICD-9CM # 703.8

Malnutrition.
Trauma.
Liver disease (cirrhosis, hepatic failure).
DM.
Hyperthyroidism.
Idiopathic.

NAIL YELLOWING
ICD-9CM # 703.8

Tobacco abuse.
Nephrotic syndrome.
Chronic infections (TB, sinusitis).
Bronchiectasis.
Lymphedema.
Raynaud's disease.
RA.
Pleural effusions.
Thyroiditis.
Immunodeficiency.

NASAL AND PARANASAL SINUS TUMORS[16a]
ICD-9CM # 873.23

BENIGN AND MALIGNANT NASAL AND PARANASAL SINUS TUMORS
Epithelial Tumors
Benign
Papilloma.
Adenoma.
Inverting papilloma.
Malignant
Squamous carcinoma.
Adenocarcinoma.
Melanoma.
Adenoid cystic carcinoma.
Malignant salivary tumors.
Mesenchymal Tumors
Benign
Osteoma.
Ossifying fibroma complex.
Angiofibroma.
Chondroma.
Malignant
Osteogenic sarcoma.
Fibrosarcoma.
Angiosarcoma.
Chondrosarcoma.
Lymphoma.
Rhabdomyosarcoma.

NASAL MASSES, CONGENITAL[16a]
ICD-9CM # 478.19

Dermoid.
Nasal cerebral heterotopia (glioma).
Frontal meningoencephalocele.
Nasolacrimal duct mucocele.
Nasal hamartoma.
Nasal hemangioma.

NAUSEA AND VOMITING
ICD-9CM # 787.01

Infections (viral, bacterial).
Intestinal obstruction.
Metabolic (uremia, electrolyte abnormalities, DKA, acidosis, etc.).
Severe pain.
Anxiety, fear.
Psychiatric disorders (bulimia, anorexia nervosa).
Pregnancy.
Medications (NSAIDs, erythromycin, morphine, codeine, aminophylline, chemotherapeutic agents, etc.).
Withdrawal from substance abuse (drugs, alcohol).
Head trauma.
Vestibular or middle ear disease.
Migraine headache.
CNS neoplasms.
Radiation sickness.
PUD.
Carcinoma of GI tract.
Reye's syndrome.
Eye disorders.
Abdominal trauma.

NECK AND ARM PAIN
ICD-9CM # 723.1   Neck Pain
            847.0   Neck Strain
            959.09 Neck Injury
            959.2   Arm Injury
            840.9   Arm Strain

Cervical disc syndrome.
Trauma, musculoskeletal strain.
Rotator cuff syndrome.
Bicipital tendonitis.
Glenohumeral arthritis.
Acromioclavicular arthritis.
Thoracic outlet syndrome.
Pancoast tumor.
Infection (cellulitis, abscess).
Angina pectoris.

NECK MASS[28]
ICD-9CM # 784.2

CONGENITAL ANOMALIES
Thyroglossal duct cyst.
Bronchial apparatus anomalies.
Teratomas.
Ranula.
Dermoid cysts.
Hemangioma.
Laryngoceles.
Cystic hygroma.

NONNEOPLASTIC INFLAMMATORY ETIOLOGIES
Folliculitis.
Adenopathy secondary to peritonsillar abscess.
Retropharyngeal or parapharyngeal abscess.
Salivary gland infections.
Viral infections (mononucleosis, HIV, CMV).
TB.
Cat-scratch disease.
Toxoplasmosis.
Actinomyces.
Atypical mycobacterium.
Jugular vein thrombus.

NEOPLASM (PRIMARY OR METASTATIC)
Lipoma.

NECK PAIN[28]

ICD-9CM # 723.1 Neck Pain
                 (Nondiscogenic)
       959.09 Neck Injury

INFLAMMATORY DISEASES
RA.
Spondyloarthropathies.
Juvenile RA.

NONINFLAMMATORY DISEASE
Cervical osteoarthritis.
Diskogenic neck pain.
Diffuse idiopathic skeletal hyperostosis.
Fibromyalgia or myofascial pain.

INFECTIOUS CAUSES
Meningitis.
Osteomyelitis.
Infectious diskitis.

NEOPLASMS
Primary.
Metastatic.

REFERRED PAIN
Temporomandibular joint pain.
Cardiac pain.
Diaphragmatic irritation.
GI sources (gastric ulcer, gallbladder, pancreas).

NECROTIZING PNEUMONIAS[1]

ICD-9CM # 482.8

COMMON
Tuberculosis.
Staphylococcus.
Gram-negative bacilli.
Anaerobes.
Fungi.
Pneumocystis jirovecii.

RARE
Streptococcus pneumoniae.
Legionella.
Viruses.
Mycoplasma pneumoniae.

NEPHRITIC SYNDROME, ACUTE[1]

ICD-9CM # 580.89

LOW SERUM COMPLEMENT LEVEL
Acute postinfectious glomerulonephritis.
Membranoproliferative glomerulonephritis.
SLE.
Subacute bacterial endocarditis.
Visceral abscess "shunt" nephritis.
Cryoglobulinemia.

NORMAL SERUM COMPLEMENT LEVEL
IgA nephropathy.
Idiopathic rapidly progressive glomerulonephritis.
Antiglomerular basement membrane disease.

Polyarteritis nodosa.
Wegener's glomerulonephritis.
Henoch-Schönlein purpura.
Goodpasture's syndrome.

NEPHROCALCINOSIS

ICD-9CM # 275.49

Sarcoidosis.
Hyperparathyroidism.
Chronic glomerulonephritis.
Milk-alkali syndrome.
Distal renal tubular acidosis.
Medullary sponge kidney.
Bartter's syndrome.
Hypervitaminosis D.
Idiopathic hypercalciuria.
Hyperoxaluria.
Cortical necrosis.
Tuberculosis.
Idiopathic hypercalciuria.
Rapidly progressive osteoporosis.

NEUROGENIC BLADDER[29]

ICD-9CM # 396.54

SUPRATENTORIAL
CVA.
Parkinson's disease.
Alzheimer's disease.
Cerebral palsy.

SPINAL CORD
Spinal cord injury.
Spinal stenosis.
Central cord syndrome.
ALS.
Multiple sclerosis.
Myelodysplasia.

PERIPHERAL NEUROPATHY
Diabetes.
Alcohol.
Shingles.
Syphilis.

NEUROLOGIC DEFICIT, FOCAL[26]

ICD-9CM # 436 CVA
       435.9 TIA

TRAUMATIC: INTRACRANIAL, INTRASPINAL
Subdural hematoma.
Intraparenchymal hemorrhage.
Epidural hematoma.
Traumatic hemorrhagic necrosis.

INFECTIOUS
Brain abscess.
Epidural and subdural abscesses.
Meningitis.

NEOPLASTIC
Primary central nervous system tumors.
Metastatic tumors.
Syringomyelia.

Vascular.
Thrombosis.
Embolism.
Spontaneous hemorrhage: arteriovenous mal-
    formation, aneurysm, hypertensive.

METABOLIC
Hypoglycemia.
B_{12} deficiency.
Postseizure.
Hyperosmolar nonketotic.

OTHER
Migraine.
Bell's palsy.
Psychogenic.

NEUROLOGIC DEFICIT, MULTIFOCAL[26]

ICD-9CM # 436 CVA
       435.9 TIA

Acute disseminated encephalomyelitis: postviral
    or postimmunization.
Infectious encephalomyelitis: poliovirus, entero-
    viruses, arbovirus, herpes zoster, Epstein-
    Barr virus.
Granulomatous encephalomyelitis: sarcoid.
Autoimmune: SLE.
Other: Familial spinocerebellar degenerations.

NEUROMUSCULAR JUNCTION DYSFUNCTION[1]

ICD-9CM # varies with specific diagnosis

DISORDERS OF THE NEUROMUSCULAR JUNCTION
Autoimmune
Myasthenia gravis.
Lambert-Eaton myasthenic syndrome.
Congenital
Presynaptic defects in ACh resynthesis, packag-
    ing, or release.
Synaptic defect: congenital end plate AChE defi-
    ciency.
Postsynaptic defects: slow-channel syndromes.
Postsynaptic defects: decreased response to
    ACh.
    Fast-channel syndromes.
    AChR deficiency without kinetic abnormality.
Familial limb-girdle myasthenia.
Toxic
Botulism.
Drug-induced disorders.
Organophosphate intoxication.

Ach, Acetylcholine; *AChE,* acetylcholinesterase;
AChR, acetylcholine receptor.

NEURONOPATHIES, SENSORY (GANGLIONOPATHIES)[2]

ICD-9CM # varies with specific diagnosis

Herpes:
    Herpes simplex I and II.
    Varicella zoster (shingles).
Inflammatory sensory polyganglionopathy (ISP).

Paraneoplastic.
Primary biliary cirrhosis.
Sjögren's syndrome (keratoconjunctivitis sicca).
Toxin-induced:
  Pyridoxine (vitamin B$_6$) overdose.
  Metals:
    • Platinum (cisplatin).
    • Methyl mercury.
Vitamin E deficiency.

NEUROPATHIC BLADDER

ICD-9CM # 596.59

Diabetes.
Stroke.
Multiple sclerosis.
Parkinson's disease.
Dementia.
Encephalopathy.
Brain trauma.
Spinal cord trauma.
Pelvic surgery.
Spina bifida.

NEUROPATHIES WITH FACIAL NERVE INVOLVEMENT

ICD-9CM # varies with specific disorder

Sarcoidosis.
HIV.
Lyme disease.
Guillain-Barré.
Others: chronic inflammatory polyneuropathy, Tangier disease, amyloidosis.

NEUROPATHIES, PAINFUL[40]

ICD-9CM #	
355.9	Neuropathy NOS
357.5	Alcoholic
357.8	Chronic Progressive or Relapsing
356.2	Congenital Sensory
356.0	Dejerine-Sottas
356.60	Diabetic Polyneuropathy, type II
356.61	Diabetic Polyneuropathy type I

MONONEUROPATHIES

Compressive neuropathy (carpal tunnel, meralgia paresthetica).
Trigeminal neuralgia.
Ischemic neuropathy.
Polyarteritis nodosa.
Diabetic mononeuropathy.
Herpes zoster.
Idiopathic and familial brachial plexopathy.

POLYNEUROPATHIES

DM.
Paraneoplastic sensory neuropathy.
Nutritional neuropathy.
Multiple myeloma.
Amyloid.
Dominantly inherited sensory neuropathy.
Toxic (arsenic, thallium, metronidazole).
AIDS-associated neuropathy.
Tangier disease.
Fabry's disease.

NEUROPATHIES, PERIPHERAL, ASYMMETRICAL PROXIMAL/DISTAL[2]

ICD-9CM # varies with specific diagnosis

BRACHIAL PLEXOPATHY

Open
Direct plexus injury (knife or gunshot wound).
Neurovascular (plexus ischemia).
Iatrogenic (central line insertion).
Closed
Traction injuries:
  "Stingers."
  Traction neurapraxia.
  Partial or complete nerve root avulsion.
Radiation.
Neoplastic.
Idiopathic brachial plexitis.
Throracic outlet.

LUMBOSACRAL PLEXOPATHIES

Open
Closed
Traction injuries:
  Pelvic double vertical shearing fracture.
  Posterior hip dislocation.
  Retroperitoneal hemorrhage.
Vasospastic (deep buttock injection).
Neoplastic.
Radiation.
Idiopathic lumbosacral plexitis.
Infectious:
  Herpesvirus (sacrococcygeal).
  Herpes simplex II.
  Herpes zoster.
Cytomegalovirus (CMV) polyradiculopathy (HIV).

NEUTROPENIA WITH DECREASED MARROW RESERVE[20]

ICD-9CM # 288.09

PRIMARY

Severe congenital neutropenia.
Shwachman–Diamond syndrome.
Cyclic neutropenia.

SECONDARY

Lymphoproliferative disorder of granular lymphocytes.
Chemotherapy.
Drug induced (nonimmune).
Nutritional.
Viral infection (varicella, EBV, measles, CMV, hepatitis, HIV).

NEUTROPENIA WITH NORMAL MARROW RESERVE[20]

ICD-9CM # 288.0

Chronic benign neutropenia of infancy and childhood.
Ethnic or benign familial neutropenia.

Autoimmune neutropenia.
Alloimmune neutropenia.
Drug induced neutropenia.
Infection-related neutropenia.
Hypersplenism.

NEUTROPHILIA[20]

ICD-9CM # 288.60

CLASSIFICATION OF NEUTROPHILIA

Primary (No Other Evident Associated Disease)
Hereditary neutrophilia.
Chronic idiopathic neutrophilia.
Chronic myelogenous leukemia (CML) and other myeloproliferative diseases.
Familial myeloproliferative disease.
Congenital anomalies and leukemoid reaction.
Leukocyte adhesion factor deficiency (LAD).
Familial cold urticaria and leukocytosis.
Secondary
Infection.
Stress neutrophilia.
Chronic inflammation.
Drug induced.
Nonhematologic malignancy.
Generalized marrow stimulation as in hemolysis.
Asplenia and hyposplenism.

NIPPLE LESIONS

ICD-9CM # varies with specific disorder

Contact dermatitis.
Trauma.
Paget's disease.
Sebaceous hyperplasia.
Neurofibroma.
Accessory nipple.
Papillary adenoma.
Nevoid hyperkeratosis.
Cellulitis.

NODULAR LESIONS, SKIN

ICD-9CM # 782.2

Lipoma.
Cherry angioma.
Angiokeratoma.
Hemangioma.
Classic Kaposi's sarcoma.
Nodular melanoma.
Pyogenic granuloma.
Angiosarcoma.
Eccrine poroma.

NODULES, PAINFUL

ICD-9CM # varies with specific disorder

Arthropod bite or sting.
Erythema nodosum.
Glomus tumor.
Neuroma.
Leiomyoma.
Angiolipoma.
Dermatofibroma.
Osler's node.

Blue rubber bleb nevus.
Vasculitis.
Sweet's syndrome.

NYSTAGMUS

ICD-9CM # 379.50 Nystagmus NOS
          386.11 Benign Positional
          386.2 Central Positional
          379.59 Congenital

Medications (meperidine, barbiturates, pheny-
  toin, phenothiazines, etc.).
Multiple sclerosis.
Congenital.
Neoplasm (cerebellar, brain stem, cerebral).
Labyrinthine or vestibular lesions.
CNS infections.
Optic atrophy.
Other: Arnold–Chiari malformation, syringobul-
  bia, chorioretinitis, meningeal cysts.

NYSTAGMUS, MONOCULAR

ICD-9CM # 379.50

Amblyopia.
Strabismus.
Multiple sclerosis.
Monocular blindness.
Internuclear ophthalmoplegia.
Lid fasciculations.
Brain stem infarct.

ODYNOPHAGIA[38]

ICD-9CM # varies with specific diagnosis

CAUSES OF ODYNOPHAGIA
Infections
Herpes simplex virus.
Cytomegalovirus.
Candidiasis.
Chemical, Inflammatory
Gastroesophageal reflux.
Drug induced (Slow-K, tetracyclines, quinidine).
Radiation.
Graft-versus-host disease.
Crohn's disease.
Dermatological diseases (pemphigus and pem-
  phigoid).

OPACIFICATION OF HEMIDIAPHRAGM ON X-RAY[16a]

ICD-9CM # 419.4

CAUSES OF OPACIFICATION OF A HEMITHORAX
Pleural effusion.
Consolidation.
Collapse.
Massive tumor.
Fibrothorax.
Combination of above lesions.
Pneumonectomy.
Lung agenesis.

OPHTHALMOPLEGIA[1]

ICD-9CM # 378.9 Ophthalmoplegia NOS
          378.52 Cerebellar Ataxia
                 Syndrome
          376.22 Exophthalmic

BILATERAL
Botulism.
Myasthenia gravis.
Wernicke's encephalopathy.
Acute cranial polyneuropathy.
Brain stem stroke.

UNILATERAL
Carotid-posterior (3rd cranial nerve, pupil in-
  volved communicating aneurysm).
Diabetic-idiopathic (3rd or 6th cranial nerve,
  pupil spared).
Myasthenia gravis.
Brain stem stroke.

OPSOCLONUS*

ICD-9CM # 379.59

Multiple sclerosis.
Encephalitis.
CNS lymphoma.
Hydrocephalus.
Pontine hemorrhage.
Thalamic disorder (glioma, hemorrhage).
Hyperosmolar coma.
Carcinoma, paraneoplastic.
Cocaine.
Medications (e.g., phenytoin, haloperidol, ami-
  triptyline, diazepam, vidarabine).

*Spontaneous, multivector, chaotic eye movement

OPTIC ATROPHY[34a]

ICD-9CM # 377.1

CAUSES OF OPTIC ATROPHY
Optic nerve compression
Pituitary tumor.
Carotid aneurysm.
Glaucoma.
Optic nerve tumor.
Sphenoid meningioma.
Olfactory groove meningioma.
Optic neuritis
Following longstanding papilloedema
Central retinal artery occlusion
Toxic/metabolic
Diabetes.
Methyl alcohol.
Tobacco.
Quinine.
Ethambutol.
Lead and arsenic.
Anemia.
Secondary to retinal disease
Senile macular degeneration.
Retinitis pigmentosa.
Severe chorioretinitis.
Secondary to trauma
Orbital fracture.

Hereditary
Leber's optic atrophy.
Hereditary ataxias.
Spinocerebellar degeneration.

ORAL MUCOSA, ERYTHEMATOUS LESIONS[9]

ICD-9CM # 528.3 Oral Abscess
          528.9 Oral Disease (Soft Tissue)
          528.8 Hyperplasia (Tongue)

Allergy.
Erythroplakia.
Candidiasis.
Geographic tongue.
Stomatitis areata migrans.
Plasma cell gingivitis.
Pemphigus vulgaris.

ORAL MUCOSA, PIGMENTED LESIONS[9]

ICD-9CM # 528.3 Oral Abscess
          528.9 Oral Disease (Soft Tissue)
          528.8 Hyperplasia (Tongue)

Racial pigmentation.
Oral melanotic macule.
Peutz-Jeghers syndrome.
Neurofibromatosis.
Albright's syndrome.
Addison's disease.
Chloasma.
Drug reaction: quinacrine, Minocin, chlorproma-
  zine, Myleran.
Amalgam tattoo.
Lead line.
Smoker's melanosis.
Nevi.
Melanoma.

ORAL MUCOSA, PUNCTATE EROSIVE LESIONS[9]

ICD-9CM # 528.3 Oral Abscess
          528.9 Oral Disease (Soft Tissue)
          528.8 Hyperplasia (Tongue)

Viral lesion: Herpes simplex, coxsackievirus (A,
  B, A16), herpes zoster.
Aphthous stomatitis.
Sutton's disease (giant aphthae).
Behçet's syndrome.
Reiter's syndrome.
Neutropenia.
Acute necrotizing ulcerative gingivostomatitis
  (ANUG).
Drug reaction.
Inflammatory bowel disease.
Contact allergy.

ORAL MUCOSA, WHITE LESIONS[9]

ICD-9CM # 528.3 Oral Abscess
          528.9 Oral Disease (Soft Tissue)
          528.8 Hyperplasia (Tongue)

Leukoplakia.
White, hairy leukoplakia.

Squamous cell carcinoma.
Lichen planus.
Stomatitis nicotinica.
Benign intraepithelial dyskeratosis.
White spongy nevus.
Leukoedema.
Darier-White disease.
Pachyonychia congenita.
Candidiasis.
Allergy.
SLE.

ORAL ULCERS, ACUTE

ICD-9CM # varies with diagnosis
528.9 Traumatic Ulcer of Oral Mucosa

Trauma (including thermal trauma).
Aphthous stomatitis.
Syphilis.
Herpes simplex infection.
Herpes zoster.

ORAL VESICLES AND ULCERS[1]

ICD-9CM # 528.9

Aphthous stomatitis.
Primary herpes simplex infection.
Vincent's stomatitis.
Syphilis.
Coxsackievirus A (herpangina).
Fungi (histoplasmosis).
Behçet's syndrome.
SLE.
Reiter's syndrome.
Crohn's disease.
Erythema multiforme.
Pemphigus.
Pemphigoid.

ORBITAL LESIONS, CALCIFIED

ICD-9CM # 376.89

Chronic inflammation.
Phlebolith.
Dermoid cyst.
Mucocele walls.
Tumors (lacrimal gland, fibro-osseous).
Meningioma (optic sheath).
Lymphangioma.
Orbital varix.

ORBITAL LESIONS, CYSTIC

ICD-9CM # 376.9

Sweat gland cyst.
Dermoid cyst.
Lacrimal gland cyst.
Abscess.
Conjunctival cyst.
Lymphangioma.
Schwannoma.

ORGASM DYSFUNCTION[12]

ICD-9CM # 302.73 Orgasm Inhibited, Female Psychosexual
302.74 Orgasm Inhibited, Male Psychosexual

Anorgasmia: inadequate stimulation or learning.
Spinal cord lesion or injury.
Multiple sclerosis.
Alcoholic neuropathy.
Amyotrophic lateral sclerosis.
Spinal cord accident.
Spinal cord trauma.
Peripheral nerve damage.
Radical pelvic surgery.
Herniated lumbar disk.
Hypothyroidism.
Addison's disease.
Cushing's disease.
Acromegaly.
Hypopituitarism.
Pharmacologic agents (e.g., SSRIs, beta-blockers).
Psychogenic.

OROFACIAL PAIN

ICD-9CM # 784.0

Dental abscess.
Sinusitis.
Otitis media.
Otitis externa.
Wisdom tooth eruption.
Sialoadenitis.
Herpes zoster.
Trigeminal neuralgia.
Parotitis.
Anxiety disorder.
Malingering.

OSTEOPOROSIS, SECONDARY CAUSES

ICD-9CM # 733.00

Medication induced (e.g., glucocorticoids, anticonvulsants, heparin, LHRH agonists or antagonists).
Hyperparathyroidism.
Hyperthyroidism.
Prolonged immobilization.
Chronic renal failure.
Sickle cell disease.
Multiple myeloma.
Myeloproliferative diseases.
Leukemias and lymphomas.
Acromegaly.
Prolactinoma.
DM.
Total parenteral nutrition.
Malabsorption.
Chronic hypophosphatemia.
Connective tissue disorders (e.g., osteogenesis imperfecta, Marfan's syndrome, Ehlers-Danlos).
Hepatobiliary disease.
Postgastrectomy.
Aluminum containing antacids.

Systemic mastocytosis.
Homocystinuria.

OSTEOSCLEROSIS, DIFFUSE[16a]

ICD-9CM # varies with specific diagnosis

DISORDERS ASSOCIATED WITH DIFFUSE OSTEOSCLEROSIS

Neoplastic Causes*
Prostate carcinoma, breast carcinoma, gastrointestinal adenocarcinoma, carcinoid tumors, transitional cell carcinoma of the bladder, myeloma, lymphoma, leukemia.
Haematological Causes*
Sickle cell disorders, mastocytosis, myelofibrosis, polycythaemia vera.
Metabolic Causes*
Renal osteodystrophy, primary hyperparathyoidism, familial hypophosphataemic osteomalacia, hypervitaminosis D, fluorosis, hypoparathyroidism, pseudohypoparathyroidism.
Primary Osseous Disorders†
Osteoporosis.
Pyknodysostosis.
Paget's disease.

*Involvement principally of cancellous bone
†Involvement of cancellous and cortical bone

OVULATORY DYSFUNCTION[21]

ICD-9CM # 628.0 Anovulatory Cycle
626.5 Ovulation Pain

HYPERANDROGENIC ANOVULATION

Polycystic ovarian syndrome.
Late-onset congenital adrenal hyperplasias.
Ovarian hyperthecosis.
Androgen-producing ovarian tumors.
Androgen-producing adrenal tumors.
Cushing's syndrome.

HYPOESTROGENIC ANOVULATION (HYPOTHALAMIC OR PITUITARY ETIOLOGY)

Hypogonadotropic Hypoestrogenic States
Reversible:
Functional hypothalamic amenorrheas:
- Eating disorders (anorexia nervosa, excessive weight loss).
- Excessive athletic training.
Neoplastic:
Craniopharyngioma.
Pituitary stalk compression.
Infiltrative diseases:
Histiocytosis-X.
Sarcoidosis.
Hypophysitis.
Pituitary adenomas:
Hyperprolactinemia.
Euprolactinemic galactorrhea.
Endocrinopathies:
Hypothyroidism/hyperthyroidism.
Cushing's disease.
Irreversible:

Irreversible:
    Kallmann's syndrome.
    Isolated gonadotropin deficiency (hypotha-
        lamic or pituitary origin).
    Panhypopituitarism/pituitary insufficiency:
    • Sheehan's syndrome, pituitary apoplexy.
    • Pituitary irradiation or ablation.

Hypergonadotropic Hypoestrogenic States
Physiologic states:
    Menopause.
    Perimenopause.
Premature ovarian failure.
Immune-related:
    Radiation/chemotherapy-induced.
Ovarian dysgenesis.
Turner's syndrome.
46XX with mutations of X.
Androgen insensitivity syndrome.

MISCELLANEOUS

Endometriosis.
Luteal phase defect.

PAIN, MIDFOOT
ICD-9CM # 719.47

MEDIAL ASPECT

Tendonitis of posterior tibialis.
Tendonitis of flexor digitorum longus.
Tendonitis of flexor hallucis longus.
Infection (osteomyelitis, septic arthritis, celluli-
    tis) of foot.
Peripheral vascular insufficiency.
Fracture.
Osteoarthritis.
Gout, pseudogout.
Neuropathy.
Tumor.

LATERAL ASPECT

Peroneus longus tendonitis.
Peroneus brevis tendonitis.
Infection (osteomyelitis, septic arthritis, celluli-
    tis) of foot.
Peripheral vascular insufficiency.
Fracture.
Osteoarthritis.
Gout, pseudogout.
Neuropathy.
Tumor.

PAIN, PLANTAR ASPECT, HEEL
ICD-9CM # 719.47

Plantar fasciitis.
Tarsal tunnel syndrome.
Neuroma.
Infection (osteomyelitis, septic arthritis, celluli-
    tis) of foot.
Peripheral vascular insufficiency.
Fracture.
Bone cyst.
Osteoarthritis.
Gout, pseudogout.
Neuropathy.
Tumor.

Heel pad atrophy.
Plantar fascia rupture.

PAIN, POSTERIOR HEEL
ICD-9CM # 729.5

Achilles tendonitis.
Retrocalcaneal bursitis.
Retroachilles bursitis.
Infection (osteomyelitis, septic arthritis, celluli-
    tis) of foot.
Peripheral vascular insufficiency.
Fracture.
Osteoarthritis.
Gout, pseudogout.
Neuropathy.
Tumor.

PALINDROMIC RHEUMATISM[6]
ICD-9CM # 719.3 use 5th digit
        0. Site Unspecified
        1. Shoulder Region
        2. Upper Arm (Elbow, Humerus)
        3. Forearm (Radius, Wrist, Ulna)
        4. Hand (Carpal, Metacarpal,
            Fingers)
        5. Pelvic Region and Thigh
        6. Lower Leg
        7. Ankle and Foot
        8. Other
        9. Multiple

Palindromic RA.
Essential palindromic rheumatism.
Crystal synovitis (gout, CPPD, pseudogout, cal-
    cific periarthritis).
Lyme borreliosis, stages 2 and 3.
Sarcoidosis.
Whipple's disease.
Acute rheumatic fever.
Reactive arthritis (rare).

PALMOPLANTAR HYPERKERATOSIS
ICD-9CM # 701.1

Superficial skin infection.
Chronic eczema.
Repeated trauma.
Psoriasis.
Reiter's syndrome.
Paraneoplastic acrokeratosis.

PALPITATIONS[33]
ICD-9CM # 785.1 Palpitations

Anxiety.
Electrolyte abnormalities (hypokalemia, hypo-
    magnesemia).
Exercise.
Hyperthyroidism.
Ischemic heart disease.
Ingestion of stimulant drugs (cocaine, amphet-
    amines, caffeine).
Medications (digoxin beta-blockers, calcium
    channel antagonists, hydralazines, diuretics,
    minoxidil).

Hypoglycemia in type 1 DM.
Mitral valve prolapse.
Wolff-Parkinson-White (WPW) syndrome.
Sick sinus syndrome.

PANCREATIC CALCIFICATIONS
ICD-9CM # 577.8

Chronic pancreatitis.
Hyperparathyroidism.
Metastatic neoplasm.
Pseudocyst.
Hereditary pancreatitis.
Cystoadenoma.
Cystoadenocarcinoma.
Cavernous lymphangioma.
Hemorrhage.
Acute pancreatitis (saponification).

PANCREATITIS, DRUG-INDUCED[2]
ICD-9CM # 577.0

DEFINITE

Acetaminophen.
Azathioprine.
Cimetidine.
Cisplatin.
Corticosteroids.
Didanosine.
Erythromycin.
Estrogens.
Ethyl alcohol.
Furosemide.
L-Asparaginase.
Mercaptopurine.
Metronidazole.
Methyldopa.
Nitrofurantoin.
Octreotide.
Organophosphates.
Pentamidine.
Ranitidine.
Tetracycline.
Salicylates.
Sulfonamides, trimethoprim-sulfamethoxazole,
    sulfasalazine.
Sulindac.
Valproic acid.

POSSIBLE

Bumetanide.
Carbamazepine.
Chlorthalidone.
Clonidine.
Colchicine.
Cyclosporine.
Cytarabine.
Diazoxide.
Enalapril.
Ergotamine.
Ethacrynic acid.
Indomethacin.
Isoniazid.
Isotretinoin.
Mefenamic acid.
Opiates.
Phenformin.

Piroxicam.
Procainamide.
Rifampin.
Thiazides.

PANCYTOPENIA[20]
ICD-9CM # 284.1

PANCYTOPENIA WITH HYPOCELLULAR BONE MARROW

Acquired aplastic anemia.
Inherited aplastic anemia (Fanconi anemia and others).
Some myelodysplasia syndromes.
Rare aleukemic leukemia (acute myelogenous leukemia).
Some acute lymphoblastic leukemias.
Some lymphomas of bone marrow.

PANCYTOPENIA WITH CELLULAR BONE MARROW

Primary bone marrow diseases.
Myelodysplasia syndromes.
Paroxysmal nocturnal hemoglobinuria.
Myelofibrosis.
Some aleukemic leukemias.
Myelophthisis.
Bone marrow lymphoma.
Hairy cell leukemia.
Secondary to systemic diseases.
Systemic lupus erythematosus, Sjögren syndrome.
Hypersplenism.
Vitamin B_{12}, folate deficiency (familial defect).
Overwhelming infection.
Alcohol.
Brucellosis.
Ehrlichiosis.
Sarcoidosis.
Tuberculosis and atypical mycobacteria.

HYPOCELLULAR BONE MARROW ± CYTOPENIA

Q fever.
Legionnaires disease.
Mycobacteria.
Tuberculosis.*
Anorexia nervosa, starvation.
Hypothyroidism.

---

*Pancytopenia in tuberculosis only rarely is associated with a hypocellular bone marrow at biopsy or autopsy. Marrow failure in the setting of tuberculosis is almost always fatal; exceptional patients probably had underlying myelodysplasia or acute leukemia.

PAPILLEDEMA
ICD-9CM # 377.00 Papilledema NOS
        377.02 With Decreased Ocular Pressure
        377.01 With Increased Intracranial Pressure
        377.03 With Retinal Disorder

CNS infections (viral, bacterial, fungal).
Medications (lithium, cisplatin, corticosteroids, tetracycline, etc.).

Head trauma.
CNS neoplasm (primary or metastatic).
Pseudotumor cerebri.
Cavernous sinus thrombosis.
SLE.
Sarcoidosis.
Subarachnoid hemorrhage.
Carbon dioxide retention.
Arnold–Chiari malformation and other developmental or congenital malformations.
Orbital lesions.
Central retinal vein occlusion.
Hypertensive encephalopathy.
Metabolic abnormalities.

PAPULOSQUAMOUS DISEASES[14]
ICD-9CM # 709.8

Psoriasis.
Pityriasis rubra pilaris.
Pityriasis rosea.
Lichen planus.
Lichen nitidus.
Secondary syphilis.
Pityriasis lichenoides.
Parapsoriasis.
Mycosis fungoides.
Dermatophytosis.
Tinea versicolor.

PARANEOPLASTIC NEUROLOGIC SYNDROMES
ICD-9CM # varies with specific disorder

Lambert-Eaton myasthenic syndrome.
Myasthenia gravis.
Guillain-Barré syndrome.
Amyotrophic lateral sclerosis.
Dermatomyositis.
Carcinoid myopathy.
Cerebellar degeneration.
Encephalomyelitis.
Optic neuritis, uveitis, retinopathy.
Stiff-man syndrome.
Autonomic neuropathy.
Brachial neuritis.
Sensory neuropathy.
Progressive multifocal leukoencephalopathy.

PARANEOPLASTIC SYNDROMES, ENDOCRINE[36]
ICD-9CM # varies with specific disorder

Hypercalcemia.
Syndrome of inappropriate secretion of antidiuretic hormone.
Hypoglycemia.
Zollinger-Ellison syndrome.
Ectopic secretion of human chorionic gonadotropin.
Cushing's syndrome.

PARANEOPLASTIC SYNDROMES, NONENDOCRINE[36]
ICD-9CM # varies with specific disorder

CUTANEOUS

Dermatomyositis.
Acanthosis nigricans.
Sweet's syndrome.
Erythema gyratum repens.
Systemic nodular panniculitis (Weber-Christian disease).

RENAL

Nephrotic syndrome.
Nephrogenic diabetes insipidus.

NEUROLOGIC

Subacute cerebellar degeneration.
Progressive multifocal leukoencephalopathy.
Subacute motor neuropathy.
Sensory neuropathy.
Ascending acute polyneuropathy (Guillain-Barré syndrome).
Myasthenic syndrome (Eaton-Lambert syndrome).

HEMATOLOGIC

Microangiopathic hemolytic anemia.
Migratory thrombophlebitis (Trousseau's syndrome).
Anemia of chronic disease.

RHEUMATOLOGIC

Polymyalgia rheumatica.
Hypertrophic pulmonary osteoarthropathy.

PARAPARESIS, ACUTE OR SUBACUTE[34a]
ICD-9CM # varies with specific diagnosis

CAUSES OF ACUTE OR SUBACUTE PARAPARESIS

Trauma to a Previously Normal Spine
Vertebral disease
Metastatic carcinoma.
Cervical spondylosis.
Dorsal disc prolapse.
Paget's disease.
Rheumatoid arthritis.
Pott's disease of spine.
Tumors
Extradural or intradural carcinoma, lymphoma, myeloma, leukemia.
Dorsal meningioma.
Neurofibroma.
Hematological disease
Any cause of thrombocytopenia.
Other clotting disorders.
Leukemia.
Anticoagulant treatment.
Epidural or intramedullary hemorrhage.
Infection
Epidural abscess.
TB abscess.

Syphilitic myelitis.
HIV infection.
Vascular myelopathy.
Vascular
Anterior spinal artery occlusion.
Infarction secondary to hypotension.
Embolic infarction.
Infarction secondary to aortic dissection.
Arteriovenous malformation: infarction or hemorrhage.
Primary intramedullary hemorrhage.
Vasculitis—polyarteritis nodosa (PAN).
Inflammatory
Myelitis of unknown cause.
Multiple sclerosis.
Systemic lupus erythematosus.
Sarcoidosis.
Metabolic
Subacute degeneration of the cord.

PARAPARESIS, CHRONIC PROGRESSIVE[34a]

ICD-9CM # varies with specific diagnosis

CAUSES OF CHRONIC PROGRESSIVE PARAPARESIS

Vertebral Disease
Cervical spondylosis.
Dorsal disc prolapse.
Rheumatoid arthritis.
Pott's disease of spine.
Ankylosing spondylitis.
Tumors
Meningioma.
Neurofibroma.
Glioma.
Ependymoma.
Chordoma.
Lipoma.
Syringomyelia
With Arnold–Chiari malformation.
With tumor.
Posttraumatic.
Infection
Tropical spastic paraparesis (HTLV 1 infection).
Syphilitic myelitis.
Vascular
Arteriovenous malformation.
Inflammatory
Multiple sclerosis.
Sarcoidosis.
Radiation myelopathy.
Arachnoiditis.
Metabolic
Subacute combine degeneration of the cord.
Paget's disease.
Degenerative
Motor neuron disease.
Hereditary
Hereditary spastic paraplegia.

PARAPLEGIA

ICD-9CM # 344.1 Paraplegia, Acquired
343.0 Paraplegia, Congenital
438.50 Paraplegia, Late Effect of CVA

Trauma: penetrating wounds to motor cortex, fracture-dislocation of vertebral column with compression of spinal cord or cauda equina, prolapsed disk, electrical injuries.
Neoplasm: parasagittal region, vertebrae, meninges, spinal cord, cauda equina, Hodgkin's disease, NHL, leukemic deposits, pelvic neoplasms.
Multiple sclerosis and other demyelinating disorders.
Mechanical compression of spinal cord, cauda equina, or lumbosacral plexus: Paget's disease, kyphoscoliosis, herniation of intervertebral disk, spondylosis, ankylosing spondylitis, RA, aortic aneurysm.
Infections: spinal abscess, syphilis, TB, poliomyelitis, leprosy.
Thrombosis of superior sagittal sinus.
Polyneuritis: Guillain-Barré syndrome, diabetes, alcohol, beriberi, heavy metals.
Heredofamilial muscular dystrophies.
ALS.
Congenital and familial conditions: syringomyelia, myelomeningocele, myelodysplasia.
Hysteria.

PARESTHESIAS

ICD-9CM # 782.0

Multiple sclerosis.
Nutritional deficiencies (thiamin, vitamin B_{12}, folic acid).
Compression of spinal cord or peripheral nerves.
Medications (e.g., INH, lithium, nitrofurantoin, gold, cisplatin, hydralazine, amitriptyline, sulfonamides, amiodarone, metronidazole, dapsone, disulfiram, chloramphenicol).
Toxic chemicals (e.g., lead, arsenic, cyanide, mercury, organophosphates).
DM.
Myxedema.
Alcohol.
Sarcoidosis.
Neoplasms.
Infections (HIV, Lyme disease, herpes zoster, leprosy, diphtheria).
Charcot-Marie-Tooth syndrome and other hereditary neuropathies.
Guillain-Barré neuropathy.

PARKINSONISM-PLUS SYNDROMES

ICD-9CM # varies with specific disorder

Parkinson's disease.
Shy-Drager syndrome.
Corticobasal degeneration.
Olivo-ponto-cerebellar atrophy.
Dementia with Lewy bodies.
Progressive supranuclear palsy.
Striatonigral degeneration.

PAROTID SWELLING[3]

ICD-9CM # 527.2 Allergic Parotitis
72.9 Infectious Parotitis
527.8 Salivary Gland Obstruction
527.5 Salivary Gland Obstruction with Calculus
527.8 Salivary Gland Stricture
527.3 Salivary Gland Abscess
235.1 Salivary Gland Neoplasm

INFECTIOUS

Mumps.
Parainfluenza.
Influenza.
Cytomegalovirus infection.
Coxsackievirus infection.
Lymphocytic choriomeningitis.
Echovirus infection.
Suppuration (bacterial).
Actinomyces infection.
Mycobacterial infection.
Cat-scratch disease.

NONINFECTIOUS

Drug hypersensitivity (thiouracil, phenothiazines, thiocyanate, iodides, copper, isoprenaline, lead, mercury, phenylbutazone).
Sarcoidosis.
Tumors, mixed.
Hemangioma, lymphangioma.
Sialectasis.
Sjögren's syndrome.
Mikulicz's syndrome (scleroderma, mixed connective tissue disease, SLE).
Recurrent idiopathic parotitis.
Pneumoparotitis.
Trauma.
Sialolithiasis.
Foreign body.
Cystic fibrosis.
Malnutrition (marasmus, alcohol cirrhosis).
Dehydration.
DM.
Waldenström's macroglobulinemia.
Reiter's syndrome.
Amyloidosis.

NONPAROTID SWELLING

Hypertrophy of masseter muscle.
Lymphadenopathy.
Rheumatoid mandibular joint swelling.
Tumors of jaw.
Infantile cortical hyperostosis.

PELVIC MASS

ICD-9CM # 789.39

Hemorrhagic ovarian cyst.
Simple ovarian cyst (follicle or corpus luteum).
Ovarian carcinoma, carcinoma of fallopian tube, colorectal carcinoma, metastatic carcinoma, prostate carcinoma, bladder carcinoma, lymphoma, Hodgkin's disease.
Cystadenoma, teratoma, endometrioma.
Leiomyoma.
Leiomyosarcoma.
Diverticulitis, diverticular abscess.

Appendiceal abscess, tuboovarian abscess.
Ectopic pregnancy, intrauterine pregnancy.
Paraovarian cyst.
Hydrosalpinx.

PELVIC PAIN, CAUSES IN WOMEN[2]

ICD-9CM # 338.4

POTENTIAL CAUSES OF PELVIC PAIN IN WOMEN

Reproductive Tract
Ovarian torsion.
Ovarian cyst.
Salpingitis/tubo-ovarian abscess.
Septic pelvic thrombophlebitis.
Endometritis.
Endometriosis.
Uterine perforation.
Uterine fibroids.
Dysmenorrhea.
Pregnancy-related
First trimester
Ectopic pregnancy.
Threatened abortion.
Nonviable pregnancy.
Ovarian hyperstimulation syndrome.
Second and third trimesters
Placenta previa.
Placental abruption.
Round ligament pain.
Intestinal Tract
Appendicitis.
Diverticulitis.
Ischemic bowel.
Perforated viscus.
Bowel obstruction.
Incarcerated/strangulated hernia.
Inflammatory bowel disease.
Gastroenteritis.
Urinary Tract
Pyelonephritis.
Cystitis.
Ureteral stone.

PELVIC PAIN, CHRONIC[7]

ICD-9CM # 625.9 Pelvic Pain, Female
            789.09 Pelvic Pain, Male

GYNECOLOGIC DISORDERS

Primary dysmenorrhea.
Endometriosis.
Adenomyosis.
Adhesions.
Fibroids.
Retained ovary syndrome after hysterectomy.
Previous tubal ligation.
Chronic pelvic infection.

MUSCULOSKELETAL DISORDERS

Myofascial pain syndrome.

GASTROINTESTINAL DISORDERS

Irritable bowel syndrome.
Inflammatory bowel disease.

URINARY TRACT DISORDERS

Interstitial cystitis.
Nonbacterial urethritis.

PELVIC PAIN, GENITAL ORIGIN[26]

ICD-9CM # 625.9 Pelvic Pain, Female
            789.09 Pelvic Pain, Male

PERITONEAL IRRITATION

Ruptured ectopic pregnancy.
Ovarian cyst rupture.
Ruptured tuboovarian abscess.
Uterine perforation.

TORSION

Ovarian cyst or tumor.
Pedunculated fibroid.

INTRATUMOR HEMORRHAGE OR INFARCTION

Ovarian cyst.
Solid ovarian tumor.
Uterine leiomyoma.

INFECTION

Endometritis.
Pelvic inflammatory disease.
Trichomonas cervicitis or vaginitis.
Tuboovarian abscess.

PREGNANCY-RELATED

First Trimester
Ectopic pregnancy.
Abortion.
Corpus luteum hematoma.
Late Pregnancy
Placental problems.
Preeclampsia.
Premature labor.

MISCELLANEOUS

Endometriosis.
Foreign objects.
Pelvic adhesions.
Pelvic neoplasm.
Primary dysmenorrhea.

PENILE RASH

ICD-9CM # 782.1

Herpes simplex 2.
Balanitis (candida).
Condyloma acuminata.
Molluscum contagiosum.
Scabies.
Pediculosis pubis.
Pearly penile papules.
Lichen nitidus.
Fox-Forcyte disease (follicular papules).

PERIANAL PAIN[38]

ICD-9CM # 569.42

Fissure-in-ano
Anal sepsis
• Anal abscess
• Anal fistula

Hemorrhoids
• Internal hemorrhoids
• External hemorrhoids
Pruritus ani
Proctalgia fugax
Chronic perianal pain syndromes
• Coccygodynia
• Descending perineum syndrome
• Levator ani syndrome
• Idiopathic perineal pain

PERICARDIAL EFFUSION

ICD-9CM # 420.90

Pericarditis.
Uremia.
Myxedema.
Neoplasm (leukemia, lymphoma, metastatic).
Hemorrhage (trauma, leakage of thoracic aneurysm).
SLE, rheumatoid disease.
Myocardial infarction.

PERIODIC PARALYSIS, HYPERKALEMIC

ICD-9CM # 344.9

Chronic renal failure.
Renal insufficiency with excessive potassium supplementation.
Potassium-sparing diuretics.
Endocrinopathies (hypoaldosteronism, adrenal insufficiency).

PERIODIC PARALYSIS, HYPOKALEMIC

ICD-9CM # 344.9

Chronic diarrhea (laxative abuse, sprue, villous adenoma).
Potassium depleting diuretics.
Medications (amphotericin B, corticosteroids).
Chronic licorice ingestion.
Thyrotoxicosis.
Renal tubular acidosis.
Conn's syndrome.
Barter's syndrome.
Barium intoxication.

PERITONEAL CARCINOMATOSIS[14]

ICD-9CM # 197.6

PRIMARY DISORDERS OF THE PERITONEUM: MESOTHELIOMA

Metastatic spread from:
Stomach.
Colon.
Pancreas.
Carcinoid.
Other Intraabdominal Organs
Ovary.
Pseudomyxoma peritonei.
Extraabdominal Primary Tumors
Breast.
Lung.
Hematologic Malignancy
Lymphoma.

PERITONEAL EFFUSION[18]

ICD-9CM # 792.9

TRANSUDATES

Increased hydrostatic pressure or decreased plasma oncotic pressure.
Congestive heart failure.
Hepatic cirrhosis.
Hypoproteinemia.

EXUDATES

Increased capillary permeability or decreased lymphatic resorption.
Infections (TB, spontaneous bacterial peritonitis, secondary bacterial peritonitis).
Neoplasms (hepatoma, metastatic carcinoma, lymphoma, mesothelioma).
Trauma.
Pancreatitis.
Bile peritonitis (e.g., ruptured gallbladder).

CHYLOUS EFFUSION

Damage or obstruction to thoracic duct.
Trauma.
Lymphoma.
Carcinoma.
Tuberculosis.
Parasitic infection.

PERIUMBILICAL SWELLING

ICD-9CM # 789.3

Umbilical hernia.
Lipoma.
Epigastric hernia.
Umbilical granuloma.
Omphalocele.
Gastroschisis.
Caput medusae.

PHOTODERMATOSES[14]

ICD-9CM # 692.72

Polymorphous light eruption.
Chronic actinic dermatitis.
Solar urticaria.
Phototoxicity and photoallergy.
Porphyrias.

PHOTOSENSITIVITY

ICD-9CM # 692.72

Solar urticaria.
Photoallergic reaction.
Phototoxic reaction.
Polymorphous light eruption.
Porphyria cutanea tarda.
SLE.
Drug induced (e.g., tetracyclines).

PIGMENTURIA[2]

ICD-9CM # varies with specific diagnosis

HEMOGLOBINURIA

Hemolysis.

HEMATURIA

Renal causes.
Trauma.

ACUTE INTERMITTENT PORPHYRIA

Bilirubinuria
Food
Beets.
Drugs
Vitamin B_{12}.
Rifampin.
Phenytoin.
Laxatives.

PITUITARY REGION TUMORS[16a]

ICD-9CM # varies with specific diagnosis

PRIMARY TUMORS IN THE SELLAR AND PARASELLAR REGION

Tumor
Pituitary macroadenoma.
Meningioma.
Schwannoma (e.g., of fifth nerve).
Chordoma.
Chondrosarcoma.
Crangiopharyngioma.
Rathke's cleft cyst.
Dermoid.
Epidermoid.
Tuber cinerum hamartoma.
Optic glioma.
Germ cell tumors.

PLEURAL EFFUSIONS

ICD-9CM # 511.9 Pleural Effusion, Unspecified

EXUDATIVE

Neoplasm: bronchogenic carcinoma, breast carcinoma, mesothelioma, lymphoma, ovarian carcinoma, multiple myeloma, leukemia, Meigs' syndrome.
Infections: viral pneumonia, bacterial pneumonia, *Mycoplasma*, TB, fungal and parasitic diseases, extension from subphrenic abscess.
Trauma.
Collagen vascular diseases: SLE, RA, scleroderma, polyarteritis, Wegener's granulomatosis.
Pulmonary infarction.
Pancreatitis.
Postcardiotomy/Dressler's syndrome.
Drug-induced SLE (hydralazine, procainamide).
Postabdominal surgery.
Ruptured esophagus.
Chronic effusion secondary to congestive failure.

TRANSUDATIVE

CHF.
Hepatic cirrhosis.
Nephrotic syndrome.
Hypoproteinemia from any cause.
Meigs' syndrome.

PLEURAL EFFUSIONS, MALIGNANCY-ASSOCIATED

ICD-9CM # 197.2

Lung cancer	(30% to 40%)
Breast cancer	(20% to 25%)
Lymphoma	(10% to 15%)
Leukemia	(5% to 10%)
GI tract	(5%)
GU tract	(5%)
Reproductive	(3%)

PNEUMATOSIS INTESTINALIS IN NEONATE AND OLDER CHILD[16a]

ICD-9CM # varies with specific diagnosis

CAUSES OF PNEUMATOSIS INTESTINALIS IN THE NEONATE AND THE OLDER CHILD

Necrotizing enterocolitis.
Bowel ischemia, inflammation, and obstruction.
Cyanotic congenital heart disease.
Hirschsprung's disease.
Gastroschisis.
Anorectal atresia.
Inflammatory bowel disease.
Lymphoma.
Leukemia.
CMV and rotavirus gastroenteritis.
Colonoscopy.
Caustic ingestion.
Short bowel syndrome.
Congenital immune deficiency states.
Clostridium infection.
Chronic steroid use.
Posthepatic, renal, or bone marrow transplant.
Collagen vascular disease.
Graft-versus-host disease.
AIDS.

PNEUMONIA, RECURRENT

ICD-9CM # 482.9 Bacterial Pneumonia
480.9 Viral Pneumonia
484.1 Fungal Pneumonia
485 Segmental Pneumonia

Mechanical obstruction from neoplasm.
Chronic aspiration (tube feeding, alcoholism, CVA, neuromuscular disorders, seizure disorder, inability to cough).
Bronchiectasis.
Kyphoscoliosis.
COPD, CHF, asthma, silicosis, pulmonary fibrosis, cystic fibrosis.
Pulmonary TB, chronic sinusitis.
Immunosuppression (HIV, corticosteroids, leukemia, chemotherapy, splenectomy).

PNEUMOPERITONEUM, NEONATAL[16a]

ICD-9CM # varies with specific diagnosis

CAUSES OF NEONATAL PNEUMOPERITONEUM

Necrotizing enterocolitis.
Spontaneous perforation of a hollow viscus.
  Stomach.
  Duodenum.
  Ileum.
  Colon.
Malrotation and volvulus.
Distal obstruction.
Perforation of Meckel's diverticulum.
Anterior abdominal wall defects.
  Pentalogy of Cantrell.
  Omphalocele.
  Gastroschisis.
  Cloacal exstrophy.
Stress and peptic ulcers.
Mechanical ventilation (air leak) or resuscitation ("bagging").
Post-laparotomy.
Iatrogenic gastric perforation with an orogastric tube.
Iatrogenic colon perforation.
  Thermometer.
  During an enema.
Indomethacin.
Dexamethasone treatment.

POLYCYTHEMIA

ICD-9CM # 790.0

Tobacco abuse.
Chronic lung disease.
High altitude.
Sleep apnea.
Right-to-left cardiac shunts.
Erythropoietin administration.
Androgens/anabolic steroids.
Polycystic kidney disease.
Renal cell carcinoma.
Hepatocellular carcinoma.
Polycythemia vera.
Carbon monoxide exposure.
Primary familial and congenital polycythemia.
High-oxygen–affinity hemoglobins.
Uterine leiomyoma, meningioma, pheochromocytoma, parathyroid carcinoma.
Cobalt exposure.

POLYCYTHEMIA, RELATIVE VERSUS ABSOLUTE[20]

ICD-9CM # 790.0

RELATIVE OR SPURIOUS POLYCYTHEMIA

Decreased plasma volume—reduced fluid intake, marked loss of body fluids (diaphoresis, vomiting, diarrhea, "third-spacing").
Gaisböck syndrome.
Overfilling of blood in collection vacuum tubes.

ABSOLUTE POLYCYTHEMIA
Primary Congenital and Familial Polycythemia
Secondary Polycythemia:
Acquired:
  Hypoxia:
   • Pulmonary disease.
   • Cyanotic congenital heart disease.
   • Hypoventilation syndromes—sleep apnea, Pickwickian syndrome.
  High altitude.
  Smokers' polycythemia, carbon monoxide intoxication due to industrial exposure.
  Postrenal transplantation erythrocytosis.
  Aberrant erythropoietin production:
   • Tumors—renal cell carcinoma, Wilms' tumor, hepatic carcinoma, uterine leiomyomata, virilizing ovarian tumors, vascular cerebellar tumors.
   • Miscellaneous renal and hepatic disorders—solitary renal cysts, polycystic kidney disease, renal artery stenosis hydronephrosis, viral hepatitis.
  Endocrine disorders—Cushing's syndrome, primary aldosteronism.
  Androgen use.
  Erythropoietin use.
Congenital:
  Abnormal high-affinity hemoglobin variants.
  Bisphosphoglycerate deficiency.
  Congenital methemoglobinemia.
  Chuvash polycythemia (von Hippel–Lindau mutations).
  Prolyl hydroxylase mutations.
Polycythemia Vera

POLYNEUROPATHY[40]

ICD-9CM # 357.9

PREDOMINANTLY MOTOR

Guillain-Barré syndrome.
Porphyria.
Diphtheria.
Lead.
Hereditary sensorimotor neuropathy, types I and II.
Paraneoplastic neuropathy.

PREDOMINANTLY SENSORY

Diabetes.
Amyloidosis.
Leprosy.
Lyme disease.
Paraneoplastic neuropathy.
Vitamin B_{12} deficiency.
Hereditary sensory neuropathy, types I-IV.

PREDOMINANTLY AUTONOMIC

Diabetes.
Amyloidosis.
Alcoholic neuropathy.
Familial dysautonomias.

MIXED SENSORIMOTOR

Systemic diseases: renal failure, hypothyroidism, acromegaly, RA, periarteritis nodosa, SLE, multiple myeloma, macroglobulinemia, remote effect of malignancy.

Medications: isoniazid, nitrofurantoin, ethambutol, chloramphenicol, chloroquine, vincristine, vinblastine, dapsone, disulfiram, diphenylhydantoin, cisplatin, 1-tryptophan.
Environmental toxins: N-hexane, methyl N-butyl ketone, acrylamide, carbon disulfide, carbon monoxide, hexachlorophene, organophosphates.
Deficiency disorders: malabsorption, alcoholism, vitamin B_1 deficiency, Refsum's disease, metachromatic leukodystrophy.

POLYNEUROPATHY, DEMYELINATING[2]

ICD-9CM # varies with specific diagnosis

Guillain-Barré syndrome.
  Acute inflammatory demyelinating polyradiculoneuropathy (AIDP).
  Acute motor axonal neuropathy (AMAN).
  Acute motor and sensory axonal neuropathy (AMSAN).
  Miller Fisher syndrome.
Chronic inflammatory demyelinating polyradiculoplexo-neuropathy.
Malignancy.
HIV.
Hepatitis B.
Buckthorn.
Diphtheria.

POLYNEUROPATHY, DISTAL SENSORIMOTOR[2]

ICD-9CM # •••

Diabetes mellitus.
Alcoholism.
Neoplastic or paraneoplastic.
Hereditary motor and sensory neuropathies (Charcot-Marie-Tooth).
Cryptogenic sensorimotor polyneuropathies (CSPN).
HIV.
Toxins:
  Organic or industrial agents:
  • Acrylamide.
  • Allyl chloride.
  • Carbon disulfide.
  • Ethylene oxide.
  • Hexacarbons.
  • Methyl bromide.
  • Organophosphate-induced delayed polyneuropathy (OPIDP).
  • Polychlorinated biphenyls (PCBs).
  • Trichloroethylene.
  • Vacor.
  Metals:
  • Arsenic.
  • Gold.
  • Mercury (inorganic).
  • Thallium.
  Therapeutic agents:
  • Amiodarone.
  • Antiretrovirals.
  • Dapsone.
  • Disulfiram.
  • Isoniazid.

Differential Diagnosis

II

- Metronidazole.
- Nitrofurantoin.
- Paclitaxel (Taxol).
- Phenytoin.
- Statins (HMG-CoA reductase inhibitors).
- Thalidomide.
- Vinca alkaloids (vincristine, vinblastin).

Nutritional:
- Beriberi (thiamine or vitamin B_1).
- Pellagra (niacin, B vitamins).
- Pernicious anemia (vitamin B_{12}).
- Pyridoxine deficiency (vitamin B_6).

End-organ dysfunction:
- Acromegaly.
- Chronic pulmonary disease.
- Hypothyroidism.
- Renal failure (uremic neuropathy).

Paraproteinemias:
- Amyloidosis.
- Monoclonal gammopathy of unknown significance (MGUS).
- Multiple myeloma.
- Waldenström's macroglobulinemia.

Porphyria.

HMG-CoA, Hydroxymethylglutaryl coenzyme A.

POLYNEUROPATHY, DRUG-INDUCED[40]

ICD-9CM # 357.6

DRUGS IN ONCOLOGY

Vincristine.
Procarbazine.
Cisplatin.
Misonidazole.
Metronidazole (Flagyl).
Taxol.

DRUGS IN INFECTIOUS DISEASES

Isoniazid.
Nitrofurantoin.
Dapsone.
ddC (dideoxycytidine).
ddl (dideoxyinosine).

DRUGS IN CARDIOLOGY

Hydralazine.
Perhexiline maleate.
Procainamide.
Disopyramide.

DRUGS IN RHEUMATOLOGY

Gold salts.
Chloroquine.

DRUGS IN NEUROLOGY AND PSYCHIATRY

Diphenylhydantoin.
Glutethimide.
Methaqualone.

MISCELLANEOUS

Disulfiram (Antabuse).
Vitamin: pyridoxine (megadoses).

POLYNEUROPATHY, SYMMETRIC[40]

ICD-9CM # 357.9

ACQUIRED NEUROPATHIES

Toxic:
  Drugs.
  Industrial toxins.
  Heavy metals.
  Abused substances.
Metabolic/endocrine:
  Diabetes.
  Chronic renal failure.
  Hypothyroidism.
  Polyneuropathy of critical illness.
Nutritional deficiency:
  Vitamin B_{12} deficiency.
  Alcoholism.
  Vitamin E deficiency.
Paraneoplastic:
  Carcinoma.
  Lymphoma.
Plasma cell dyscrasia:
  Myeloma, typical, atypical, and solitary forms.
  Primary systemic amyloidosis.
Idiopathic chronic inflammatory demyelinating polyneuropathies.
Polyneuropathies associated with peripheral nerve autoantibodies.
Acquired immunodeficiency syndrome.

INHERITED NEUROPATHIES

Neuropathies with Biochemical Markers
Refsum's disease.
Bassen-Kornzweig disease.
Tangier disease.
Metachromatic leukodystrophy.
Krabbe's disease.
Adrenomyeloneuropathy.
Fabry's disease.
Neuropathies without Biochemical Markers or Systemic Involvement
Hereditary motor neuropathy.
Hereditary sensory neuropathy.
Hereditary sensorimotor neuropathy.

POLYURIA

ICD-9CM # 788.42

DM.
Diabetes insipidus.
Primary polydipsia (compulsive water drinking).
Hypercalcemia.
Hypokalemia.
Postobstructive uropathy.
Diuretic phase of renal failure.
Drugs: diuretics, caffeine, alcohol, lithium.
Sickle cell trait or disease, chronic pyelonephritis (failure to concentrate urine).
Anxiety, cold weather.

POPLITEAL SWELLING

ICD-9CM #	
459.2	Venous Obstruction
747.4	Vein Anomaly, Lower Limb Vessel
442.3	Artery Aneurysm
904.41	Artery Injury
447.8	Entrapment Syndrome
727.51	Baker's Cyst
451.2	Phlebitis, Lower Extremity
727.67	Rupture of Achilles Tendon

Phlebitis (superficial).
Lymphadenitis.
Trauma: fractured tibia or fibula, contusion, traumatic neuroma.
DVT.
Ruptured varicose vein.
Baker's cyst.
Popliteal abscess.
Osteomyelitis.
Ruptured tendon.
Aneurysm of popliteal artery.
Neoplasm: lipoma, osteogenic sarcoma, neurofibroma, fibrosarcoma.

PORTAL HYPERTENSION[1]

ICD-9CM # 572.3

INCREASED RESISTANCE TO FLOW

Presinusoidal
Portal or splenic vein occlusion (thrombosis, tumor).
Schistosomiasis.
Congenital hepatic fibrosis.
Sarcoidosis.
Sinusoidal
Cirrhosis (all causes).
Alcoholic hepatitis.
Postsinusoidal
Venoocclusive disease.
Budd-Chiari syndrome.
Constrictive pericarditis.

INCREASED PORTAL BLOOD FLOW

Splenomegaly not caused by liver disease.
Arterioportal fistula.

POSTMENOPAUSAL BLEEDING

ICD-9CM # 627.1

Hormone replacement therapy.
Neoplasm (uterine, ovarian, cervical, vaginal, vulvar).
Atrophic vaginitis.
Vaginal infection.
Polyp.
Extragenital (GI, urinary).
Tamoxifen.
Trauma.

POSTURAL HYPOTENSION, NONNEUROLOGIC CAUSES

ICD-9CM # 458.0

Diuretics and hypertensive agents.
GI hemorrhage.
Alcohol.
Excessive heat.
Rapid volume loss from diarrhea, vomiting.
Hemodialysis.
Extensive burns.
Pyrexia.
Aortic stenosis (impaired output).
Constrictive pericarditis, atrial myxoma (impaired cardiac filling).
Adrenal insufficiency.
Diabetes insipidus.
Vasodilatory agents (e.g., nitrates).

PREMATURE GRAYING, SCALP HAIR

ICD-9CM # varies with specific disorder

Chemical exposure (e.g., phenol/catechol derivatives, sulfhydryls, arsenic).
Physical agents (e.g., ionizing radiation, lasers).
Hyperthyroidism.
Vitamin B_{12} deficiency.
Down's syndrome.
Chronic and severe protein deficiency.
Vitiligo.
Idiopathic.
Myotonic dystrophy.
Ataxia telangiectasia.
Progeria.
Werner's syndrome.

PREMATURE VENTRICULAR CONTRACTIONS AND VENTRICULAR TACHYCARDIA[2]

ICD-9CM # 427.6

CAUSES OF PREMATURE VENTRICULAR CONTRACTIONS AND VENTRICULAR TACHYCARDIA

Acute or previous myocardial infarction/ischemia.
Hypokalemia.
Hypoxemia.
Ischemic heart disease.
Valvular disease.
Catecholamine excess.*
Other drug intoxications (especially cyclic antidepressants).
Idiopathic causes.[†]
Digitalis toxicity.
Hypomagnesemia.
Hypercapnia.
Class I/antidysrhythmic agents.
Ethanol.
Myocardial contusion.
Cardiomyopathy.
Acidosis.

Alkalosis.
Methylxanthine toxicity.

*Relative increase in sympathetic tone from drugs (direct or indirect) or conditions that augment catecholamine release or decrease parasympathetic tone.
[†]Isolated premature ventricular contractions (PVCs) can occur in up to 50% of young subjects without obvious cardiac or noncardiac disease; however, multiform and repetitive PVCs and ventricular tachycardia are rarely seen in this population.

PROPTOSIS[30]

ICD-9CM # 376.30

Thyrotoxicosis.
Orbital pseudotumor.
Optic nerve tumor.
Cavernous sinus AV fistula, cavernous sinus thrombosis.
Cellulitis.
Metastatic tumor to orbit.

PROPTOSIS AND PALATAL NECROTIC ULCERS

ICD-9CM # 528.9   Ulcer of Palate
            376.30 Proptosis

Cavernous sinus thrombosis.
Bacterial orbital cellulitis.
Metastatic neoplasm.
Rhinocerebral mucormycosis.
Ecthyma gangrenosum.
CNS aspergillosis.

PROTEINURIA

ICD-9CM # 791.0

Nephrotic syndrome as a result of primary renal diseases.
Malignant hypertension.
Malignancies: multiple myeloma, leukemias, Hodgkin's disease.
CHF.
DM.
SLE, RA.
Sickle cell disease.
Goodpasture's syndrome.
Malaria.
Amyloidosis, sarcoidosis.
Tubular lesions: cystinosis.
Functional (after heavy exercise).
Pyelonephritis.
Pregnancy.
Constrictive pericarditis.
Renal vein thrombosis.
Toxic nephropathies: heavy metals, drugs.
Radiation nephritis.
Orthostatic (postural) proteinuria.
Benign proteinuria: fever, heat, or cold exposure.

PRURITUS

ICD-9CM # 698.9 Pruritus NOS
            697.0 Pruritus Ani
            698.1 Pruritus, Genital Organs

Dry skin.
Drug-induced eruption, fiberglass exposure.
Scabies.

Skin diseases.
Myeloproliferative disorders: mycosis fungoides, Hodgkin's lymphoma, multiple myeloma, polycythemia vera.
Cholestatic liver disease.
Endocrine disorders: DM, thyroid disease, carcinoid, pregnancy.
Carcinoma: breast, lung, gastric.
Chronic renal failure.
Iron deficiency.
AIDS.
Neurosis.
Sjögren's syndrome.

PRURITUS ANI[26]

ICD-9CM # 697.0

FECAL IRRITATION

Poor hygiene.
Anorectal conditions (fissure, fistula, hemorrhoids, skin tags, perianal clefts).
Spicy foods, citrus foods, caffeine, colchicine, quinidine.

CONTACT DERMATITIS

Anesthetic agents, topical corticosteroids, perfumed soap.

DERMATOLOGIC DISORDERS

Psoriasis, seborrhea, lichen simplex or sclerosus.

SYSTEMIC DISORDERS

Chronic renal failure, myxedema, DM, thyrotoxicosis, polycythemia vera, Hodgkin's disease.

SEXUALLY TRANSMITTED DISEASES

Syphilis, herpes simplex virus, human papillomavirus.

OTHER INFECTIOUS AGENTS

Pinworms.
Scabies.
Bacterial infection, viral infection.

PRURITUS VULVAE[34a]

ICD-9CM # 698.1

CAUSES OF PRURITUS VULVAE

Diseases special to vulval skin
Lichen sclerosus et atrophicus.
Leukoplakia.
Carcinoma.
Skin disease
Psoriasis.
Atopic dermatitis.
Irritant and allergic contact dermatitis (especially medicaments).
Infection
Candidiasis.
Trichomonas.
Infestation
Pediculosis.
Psychogenic
Anxiety.
Depression.
Unknown

PSEUDOCYANOSIS, ETIOLOGY

ICD-9CM # varies with etiology

Medications: amiodarone, minocycline, chlor-promazine.
Heavy metals:
Gold (systemic absorption).
Silver (systemic absorption).
Local contact with color dyes, gold, silver.

PSEUDOHERMAPHRODITISM, FEMALE

ICD-9CM # 255.2 Adrenal
752.7 Without Adrenocortical Disorder

Congenital adrenal hyperplasia.
Maternal use of testosterone or related steroids.
Virilizing ovarian or adrenal tumor.
Virilizing luteoma of pregnancy.
Disturbances in differentiation of urogenital structures, non-androgen related.
Maternal virilizing adrenal hyperplasia.
Fetal P450 aromatase deficiency.

PSEUDOHERMAPHRODITISM, MALE

ICD-9CM # 255.2 Adrenal
752.7 Without Adrenocortical Disorder

Maternal ingestion of progestogens.
End-organ resistance to androgenic hormones.
5-Alpha-reductase-2 deficiency.
XY gonadal dysgenesis.
Testicular regression syndrome.
Defects in testosterone metabolism by peripheral tissues.
Testosterone biosynthesis defects.

PSEUDOINFARCTION[22]

ICD-9CM # code not available

Cardiac tumors, primary and secondary.
Cardiomyopathy (particularly hypertrophic and dilated).
Chagas' disease.
Chest deformity.
COPD (particularly emphysema).
HIV infection.
Hyperkalemia.
Left anterior fascicular block.
Left bundle branch block.
Left ventricular hypertrophy.
Myocarditis and pericarditis.
Normal variant.
Pneumothorax.
Poor R wave progression, rotational changes, and lead placement.
Pulmonary embolism.
Trauma to chest (nonpenetrating).
Wolff-Parkinson-White syndrome.
Rare causes: pancreatitis, amyloidosis, sarcoidosis, scleroderma.

PSYCHOSIS[28]

ICD-9CM # 298.9 Psychosis NOS
298.90 Psychosis, Affective
291.0 Psychosis, Alcoholic
290.41 Psychosis, Acute Arteriosclerotic

PRIMARY

Schizophrenia related.*
Major depression.
Dementia.
Bipolar disorder.

SECONDARY

Drug use.[†]
Drug withdrawal.[‡]
Drug toxicity.[§]
Charles Bonnet syndrome.
Infections (pneumonia).
Electrolyte imbalance.
Syphilis.
Congestive heart failure.
Parkinson's disease.
Trauma to temporal lobe.
Postpartum psychosis.
Hypothyroidism/hyperthyroidism.
Hypomagnesemia.
Epilepsy.
Meningitis.
Encephalitis.
Brain abscess.
Herpes encephalopathy.
Hypoxia.
Hypercarbia.
Hypoglycemia.
Thiamine deficiency.
Postoperative states.

---

*Includes schizophrenia, schizophreniform disorder, brief reactive psychosis.
[†]Includes hypnotics, glucocorticoids, marijuana, phencyclidine, atropine, dopaminergic agents (e.g., amantadine, bromocriptine, L-dopa), immunosuppressants.
[‡]Includes alcohol, barbiturates, benzodiazepines.
[§]Includes digitalis, theophylline, cimetidine, anticholinergics, glucocorticoids, catecholaminergic agents.

PTOSIS

ICD-9CM # 374.30 Ptosis NOS
743.61 Congenital
374.33 Mechanical
374.32 Myogenic
374.31 Paralytic

Third nerve palsy.
Myasthenia gravis.
Horner's syndrome.
Senile ptosis.

PUBERTY, DELAYED[27]

ICD-9CM # 259.0

NORMAL OR LOW SERUM GONADOTROPIN LEVELS

Constitutional delay in growth and development.
Hypothalamic and/or pituitary disorders:
Isolated deficiency of growth hormone.
Isolated deficiency on Gn-RH.
Isolated deficiency of LH and/or FSH.
Multiple anterior pituitary hormone deficiencies.
Associated with congenital anomalies: Kallmann's syndrome; Prader-Willi syndrome; Laurence-Moon-Biedl syndrome; Friedreich's ataxia.
Trauma.
Postinfection.
Hyperprolactinemia.
Postirradiation.
Infiltrative disease (histiocytosis).
Tumor.
Autoimmune hypophysitis.
Idiopathic.
Functional:
Chronic endocrinologic or systemic disorders.
Emotional disorders.
Drugs: cannabis.

INCREASED SERUM GONADOTROPIN LEVELS

Gonadal abnormalities:
Congenital:
- Gonadal dysgenesis.
- Klinefelter's syndrome.
- Bilateral anorchism.
- Resistant ovary syndrome.
- Myotonic dystrophy in males.
- 17-Hydroxylase deficiency in females.
- Galactosemia.
Acquired:
- Bilateral gonadal failure resulting from trauma or infection or after surgery, irradiation, or chemotherapy.
- Oophoritis: isolated or with other autoimmune disorders.
Uterine or vaginal disorders:
Absence of uterus and/or vagina.
Testicular feminization: complete or incomplete androgen insensitivity.

PUBERTY, PRECOCIOUS

ICD-9CM # 255.2

Idiopathic.
Congenital virilizing adrenal hyperplasia.
Hypothalamic tumors.
Head trauma.
Hydrocephalus.
Degenerative CNS disease.
Arachnoid cyst.
Sex chromosome abnormalities (e.g., 47, XXY, 48, XXXY).
Perinatal asphyxia.
CNS infection (e.g., meningitis, encephalitis).

PULMONARY CRACKLES

ICD-9CM # code not available

Pneumonia.
Left ventricular failure.
Asbestosis, silicosis, interstitial lung disease.
Chronic bronchitis.
Alveolitis (allergic, fibrosing).
Neoplasm.

PULMONARY CYSTS ON X-RAY[16a]
ICD-9CM # 793.1

CAUSES OF CYSTS IN THE LUNG ON CHEST RADIOGRAPH
Cystic fibrosis.
Cystic bronchiectasis.
Bronchopulmonary dysplasia (neonate and older).
Tuberculosis (apical thick walled).
Pulmonary abscess (thick wall, fluid level).
Empyema.
Streptococcal pneumatocele (thin wall, postinfective).
Cavitating pneumonia.
Mycetoma (apical cyst with contents).
Cystic congenital adenomatoid malformation (basal cysts of varying size).
Diaphragmatic hernia (cysts of similar size).
Hiatal hernia (posterior).
Morgagni hernia (midline anterior).
Bronchopulmonary sequestration (basal).
Congenital lobar emphysema.
Hydatid disease (in endemic areas).
Kerosene inhalation (pneumatocele).
Histiocytosis and other causes of interstitial disease.

PULMONARY EDEMA, NON-CARDIOGENIC[16a]
ICD-9CM # 518.4

CAUSES OF NONCARDIOGENIC PULMONARY EDEMA
Adult respiratory distress syndrome.
Drowning.
Asphyxia.
Upper airway obstruction (usually with cardiomegaly).
High altitude.
Increased intracranial pressure.
Postical.
Noxious gases:
  Smoke.
  Nitrous dioxide (silo filler's disease).
  Sulphur dioxide.
  Nitrogen mustard.
Drugs:
  Asprin.
  Diazepam, chlordiazepoxide, barbiturates.
  Narcotics (heroin, methadone, morphine).
  Beta adrenergic drugs (terbutaline).
  Contrast media.
  Colchicine.
  Fluorescein.
  Hydrochlorothiazide.
  Nitrofurantoin.
  Propoxyphene.
Poisons:
  Parathion.
Transfusion reactions.
Renal failure: transplantation.
Bone marrow transplantation.
Fat embolism.
Pancreatitis.

PULMONARY HEMORRHAGIC SYNDROMES, DIFFUSE[16a]
ICD-9CM # 770.3

CLASSIFICATION OF DIFFUSE PULMONARY HEMORRHAGE SYNDROMES

Non-immunocompromised patients
Antibasement membrane antibody disease/Goodpasture's syndrome.
Diseases of presumed immune aetiology, with or without nephropathy:
  Systemic lupus erythematosus.
  Rheumatoid arthritis.
  Systemic sclerosis.
  Systemic necrotizing vasculitis.
  Wegener's granulomatosis.
  Microscopic polyarteritis.
Diseases with no known immune etiology:
  Idiopathic pulmonary hemosiderosis.
  Rapidly progressive glomerulonephritis without immune complexes.
  Fibrillary glomerulonephritis.
  Drug-induced (anticoagulants, trimellitic anhydride, cocaine, lymphangiography).
  Valvular heart disease.
  Disseminated intravascular coagulation.
  Acute lung injury.
  Tumors.
Immunocompromised patients
Blood dyscrasias.
Infection.
Tumors.

PULMONARY INFILTRATES, IMMUNOCOMPROMISED HOST[39]
ICD-9CM # 518.3

CAUSES OF PULMONARY INFILTRATES IN THE IMMUNOCOMPROMISED HOST
Infections:
  Bacteria:
  • Gram-positive cocci, especially *Staphylococcus.*
  • Gram-negative bacilli.
  • *Mycobacterium tuberculosis.*
  • Nontuberculous mycobacteria.
  • *Nocardia.*
  Viruses:
  • Cytomegalovirus.
  • Herpesvirus.
  Fungi:
  • *Aspergillus.*
  • *Cryptococcus.*
  • *Candida.*
  • *Mucor.*
  • *Pneumocystis jiroveci.*
  Protozoa:
  • *Toxoplasma gondii* (rare).
Pulmonary effects of therapy:
  Chemotherapeutic agents.
  Radiation therapy.
Pulmonary hemorrhage.
Congestive heart failure.

Disseminated malignancy.
Nonspecified interstitial pneumonitis (no defined etiology).

PULMONARY LESIONS
ICD-9CM # 518.3 Pulmonary Infiltrate
          518.89 Pulmonary Nodule
          508.9 Pulmonary Disorder Due to Unspecified External Agent
          861.20 Pulmonary Injury NOS

TB.
Legionella pneumonia.
Mycoplasma pneumonia.
Viral pneumonia.
Pneumocystis carinii.
Hypersensitivity pneumonitis.
Aspiration pneumonia.
Fungal disease (aspergillosis, histoplasmosis).
ARDS associated with pneumonia.
Psittacosis.
Sarcoidosis.
Septic emboli.
Metastatic cancer.
Multiple pulmonary emboli.
Rheumatoid nodules.

PULMONARY MASS, SOLITARY, CAUSES[16a]
ICD-9CM # 793.1

CAUSES OF A SOLITARY PULMONARY MASS
Bronchial carcinoma.
Bronchial carcinoid.
Granuloma.
Hamartoma.
Metastasis.
Chronic pneumonia or abscess.
Hydatid cyst.
Pulmonary hematoma.
Bronchocele.
Fungus ball.
Massive fibrosis in coal workers.
Bronchogenic cyst.
Sequestration.
Atriovenous malformation.
Pulmonary infarct.
Round atelectasis.

PULMONARY MASS, SOLITARY, MIMICS[16a]
ICD-9CM # varies with specific diagnosis

SIMULANTS OF A SOLITARY PULMONARY MASS
Extrathoracic artifacts.
Cutaneous masses.
Bony lesions.
Pleural tumors or plaques.
Encysted pleural fluid.
Pulmonary vessels.

Differential Diagnosis

PULMONARY NODULE, SOLITARY

ICD-9CM # 518.89

Bronchogenic carcinoma.
Granuloma from histoplasmosis.
TB granuloma.
Granuloma from coccidioidomycosis.
Metastatic carcinoma.
Bronchial adenoma.
Bronchogenic cyst.
Hamartoma.
AV malformation.
Other: fibroma, intrapulmonary lymph node, sclerosing hemangioma, bronchopulmonary sequestration.

PULSELESS ELECTRICAL ACTIVITY

ICD-9CM # code not available

Hypovolemia.
Hypoxia.
Hyperkalemia.
Acidosis.
Cardiac tamponade.
Tension pneumothorax.
Pulmonary embolus.
Drug overdose.
Hypothermia.

PUPILLARY DILATATION, POOR RESPONSE TO DARKNESS

ICD-9CM # varies with specific disorder

Drugs (narcotics, general anesthetics, cholinergics).
Acute trauma (spasm from prostaglandin release).
Inflammation, infection (interruption of inhibitory fibers to the Edinger-Westphal nucleus).
Old age (loss of inhibition at midbrain from reticular activating formation).
Horner's syndrome (sympathetic neuron interruption).
Adie's syndrome tonic pupil.
Lymphoma.
Congenital miosis.

PURPURA

ICD-9CM # 287.2 Purpura NOS
  287.0 Autoimmune
  287.0 Henoch-Schönlein
  287.3 Idiopathic thrombocytopenic
  446.6 Thrombocytopenic

THROMBOTIC

Trauma.
Septic emboli, atheromatous emboli.
DIC.
Thrombocytopenia.
Meningococcemia.
Rocky Mountain spotted fever.
Hemolytic-uremic syndrome.

Viral infection: echo, coxsackie.
Scurvy.
Other: left atrial myxoma, cryoglobulinemia, vasculitis, hyperglobulinemic purpura.

PURPURA, NONPALPABLE[20]

ICD-9CM # 287.2

INCREASED TRANSMURAL PRESSURE GRADIENT

Acute (Valsalva, coughing, vomiting, high altitude, weight lifting).
Chronic—Venous stasis.

DECREASED MECHANICAL INTEGRITY OF MICROCIRCULATION AND SUPPORTING TISSUES

Age related (infancy and actinic purpura).
Glucocorticoid excess—Cushing syndrome and glucocorticoid therapy.
Vitamin C deficiency (scurvy).
Abnormal connective tissue—Ehlers-Danlos syndrome.
Amyloid infiltration of blood vessels.
Colloid milium.
Hormonal—Female easy bruising syndrome (purpura simplex).
Lorenzo's oil.
MELAS syndrome.

TRAUMA TO BLOOD VESSELS

Physical:
  • Injuries.
  • Child abuse.
  • Factitial purpura.
Ultraviolet purpura:
  • Purpuric sunburn.
  • Solar purpura.
Infectious:
  • Bacterial.
  • Rickettsial.
  • Fungal.
  • Viral.
  • Parasitic.
Embolic:
  • Infectious organisms.
  • Atheroemboli (cholesterol crystal emboli).
  • Fat emboli.
Allergic and/or inflammatory:
  • Serum sickness.
  • Pigmented purpuric eruptions.
  • Pyoderma gangrenosum.
  • Contact dermatitis.
  • Familial Mediterranean fever.
Neoplastic.
Metabolic:
  • Erythropoietic porphyria.
  • Calciphylaxis.
Immunoglobulin related (hyperglobulinemic purpura of Waldenström and light-chain vasculitis).
Drug related.
Thrombotic:
  • Disseminated intravascular coagulation.
  • Warfarin (coumadin)-induced skin necrosis.

  • Protein C or protein S deficiency, factor V Leiden, prothrombin G20201A.
  • Purpura fulminans.
  • Paroxysmal nocturnal hemoglobinuria.
  • Antiphospholipid antibody syndrome.
  • Hemangioma with thrombocytopenia and consumptive coagulopathy (Kasabach-Merritt syndrome).

UNKNOWN CAUSE— PSYCHOGENIC PURPURA

PURPURA, NONPURPURIC DISORDERS SIMULATING PURPURA[1]

ICD-9CM # varies with specific diagnosis

Disorders with telangiectasias:
  Cherry angiomas.
  Hereditary hemorrhagic telangiectasia.
  Chronic actinic telangiectasia.
  Scleroderma.
  CREST syndrome.
  Ataxia-telangiectasia.
  Chronic liver disease.
  Pregnancy-related telangiectasia.
Kaposi sarcoma and other vascular sarcomas.
Fabry disease.
Neonatal extramedullary hematopoiesis.
Angioma serpiginosum.

PURPURA, PALPABLE[20]

ICD-9CM # 287.2

Cutaneous vasculitis:
  Systemic vasculitides.
  Paraneoplastic vasculitis.
  Henoch-Schönlein purpura.
  Acute hemorrhagic edema of infancy.
  Livedoid vasculitis.
  Idiopathic.
  Urticarial.
Cryoglobulinemia.
Cryofibrinogenemia.
Primary cutaneous diseases.

QT INTERVAL PROLONGATION[22]

ICD-9CM # 794.31

Drugs:
  Class I antiarrhythmics (e.g., disopyramide, procainamide, quinidine).
  Class III antiarrhythmics.
  Tricyclic antidepressants.
  Phenothiazines.
  Astemizole.
  Terfenadine.
  Adenosine.
  Antibiotics (e.g., erythromycin and other macrolides).
  Antifungal agents.
  Pentamidine, chloroquine.
Ischemic heart disease.
Cerebrovascular disease.

Rheumatic fever.
Myocarditis.
Mitral valve prolapse.
Electrolyte abnormalities.
Hypocalcemia.
Hypothyroidism.
Liquid protein diets.
Organophosphate insecticides.
Congenital prolonged QT syndrome.

RECTAL MASS, PALPABLE[38]

ICD-9CM # varies with specific diagnosis

Rectal carcinoma.
Rectal polyp.
Hypertrophied anal papilla.
Diverticular phlegmon (prolapsing into the pouch of Douglas).
Sigmoid colon carcinoma (prolapsing into the pouch of Douglas).
Metastatic deposits at the pelvic reflection (Blumer's shelf).
Primary pelvic malignancy (uterine, ovarian, prostatic or cervical).
Mesorectal lymph nodes.
Endometriosis.
Solitary rectal ulcer syndrome.
Foreign body.
Feces (indent).
Presacral cyst.
Amoebic granuloma.
Vaginal tampon and even the pubic bone may be mistaken for a rectal mass.

RECTAL PAIN

ICD-9CM # 569.42

Anal fissure.
Thrombosed hemorrhoid.
Anorectal abscess.
Foreign bodies.
Fecal impaction.
Endometriosis.
Neoplasms (primary or metastatic).
Pelvic inflammatory disease.
Inflammation of sacral nerves.
Compression of sacral nerves.
Prostatitis.
Other: proctalgia fugax, uterine abnormalities, myopathies, coccygodynia.

RED BLOOD CELL APLASIA, ACQUIRED, ETIOLOGY

ICD-9CM # 284.0

Idiopathic (>50% of cases).
Medications (most frequent with phenytoin).
Non-Hodgkin's lymphoma.
Viral infections (parvovirus B-19, EB virus, mumps, hepatitis).
Myelodysplastic syndromes.
Thymoma.
Autoimmune diseases.
Allogenic bone marrow transplant from ABO incompatible donor.
Pregnancy.

RED EYE

ICD-9CM # 379.93

Infectious conjunctivitis (bacterial, viral).
Allergic conjunctivitis.
Acute glaucoma.
Keratitis (bacterial, viral).
Iritis.
Trauma.

RED HOT JOINT

ICD-9CM # varies with specific disorder

Trauma.
Gout.
Infection (septic joint).
Pseudogout (calcium pyrophosphate dehydrate crystal deposition).
Psoriatic arthropathy.
Reactive arthritis.
Palindromic rheumatism.

RED URINE

ICD-9CM # 788.69

Hematuria.
Porphyrins.
Hemoglobinuria.
Myoglobinuria.
Medications (phenazopyridine, aminosalicylic acid, deferoxamine, phenazopyridine, phenolphthalein, NSAIDs, rifampin, phenytoin, methyldopa, doxorubicin, phenacetin).
Foods (beets, berries, maize).
Urate crystalluria.

RENAL ARTERY OCCLUSION, CAUSES

ICD-9CM # 593.81

Atrial fibrillation.
Angiography or stent placement.
Abdominal aortic surgery.
Trauma.
Renal artery aneurysm/dissection.
Vasculitis.
Thrombosis in patient with fibromuscular dysplasia.
Atherosclerosis.
Septic embolism.
Mural thrombus thromboembolism.
Atrial myxoma thromboembolism.
Mitral stenosis thromboembolism.
Prosthetic valve thromboembolism.
Renal cell carcinoma.

RENAL CYSTIC DISORDERS

ICD-9CM # varies with specific disorder

Simple cysts.
Acquired cystic kidney disease.
Autosomal dominant polycystic kidney disease.
Autosomal recessive polycystic kidney disease.
Medullary cystic disease.
Medullary sponge kidney.

RENAL FAILURE, ACUTE, PIGMENT-INDUCED[2]

ICD-9CM # 586

CAUSES OF PIGMENT-INDUCED ACUTE RENAL FAILURE

Rhabdomyolysis and myoglobinuria.
Vigorous exercise.
Arterial embolization.
Status epilepticus.
Status asthmaticus.
Coma-induced and pressure-induced myonecrosis.
Heat stress.
Diabetic ketoacidosis.
Myopathy.
Alcoholism.
Hypokalemia.
Hypophosphatemia.
Hemoglobinuria.
Transfusion reactions.
Snake envenomation.
Malaria.
Mechanical destruction of RCBs by prosthetic valves.
G6PD deficiency.

G6PD, Glucose-6-phosphate dehydrogenase; *RBCs*, red blood cells.

RENAL FAILURE, INTRINSIC OR PARENCHYMAL CAUSES[36]

ICD-9CM # 584. Acute, use 4th digit
    5. With Acute Tubular Necrosis
    6. With Cortical Necrosis
    7. With Medullary Necrosis
    8. With Other Unspecified Pathologic Condition in Kidney
    9. Renal Failure Unspecified
    585 Renal Failure, Chronic

ABNORMALITIES OF THE VASCULATURE

Renal arteries: atherosclerosis, thromboembolism, arteritis.
Renal veins: thrombosis.
Microvasculature: vasculitis, thrombotic microangiopathy.

ABNORMALITIES OF GLOMERULI (ACUTE GLOMERULONEPHRITIS)

Antiglomerular membrane disease (Goodpasture's syndrome).
Immune complex glomerulonephritis: SLE, post-infectious, idiopathic, membranoproliferative.

ABNORMALITIES OF INTERSTITIUM (ACUTE INTERSTITIAL NEPHRITIS)

Drugs (e.g., antibiotics, NSAIDs, diuretics, anticonvulsants, allopurinol).
Infectious pyelonephritis.
Infiltrative: lymphoma, leukemia, sarcoidosis.

Differential Diagnosis

II

ABNORMALITIES OF TUBULES

Physical obstruction (uric acid, oxalate, light chains).

Acute tubular necrosis:
Ischemic.
Toxic (antibiotics, chemotherapy, immuno-suppressives, radiocontrast dyes, heavy metals, myoglobin, hemolysed RBCs).

RENAL FAILURE, POSTRENAL CAUSES[36]

ICD-9CM # 584. Acute, use 4th digit
5. With Acute Tubular Necrosis
6. With Cortical Necrosis
7. With Medullary Necrosis
8. With Other Unspecified Pathologic Condition in Kidney
9. Renal Failure Unspecified
585 Renal Failure, Chronic

URETER AND RENAL PELVIS

Intrinsic obstruction:
Blood clots.
Stones.
Sloughed papillae: diabetes, sickle cell disease, analgesic nephropathy.
Inflammatory: fungus ball.
Extrinsic obstruction:
Malignancy.
Retroperitoneal fibrosis.
Iatrogenic: inadvertent ligation of ureters.

BLADDER

Prostatic hypertrophy or malignancy.
Neuropathic bladder.
Blood clots.
Bladder cancer.
Stones.

URETHRAL

Strictures.
Congenital valves.

RENAL FAILURE, PRERENAL CAUSES[36]

ICD-9CM # 584. Acute, use 4th digit
5. With Acute Tubular Necrosis
6. With Cortical Necrosis
7. With medullary necrosis
8. With Other Unspecified Pathologic Condition in Kidney
9. Renal Failure Unspecified
585 Renal Failure, Chronic

DECREASED CARDIAC OUTPUT

CHF.
Arrhythmias.
Pericardial constriction or tamponade.
Pulmonary embolism.

HYPOVOLEMIA

GI tract loss (vomiting, diarrhea, nasogastric suction).
Blood losses (trauma, GI tract surgery).
Renal losses (diuretics, mineralocorticoid deficiency, postobstructive diuresis).
Skin losses (burns).

VOLUME REDISTRIBUTION (DECREASE IN EFFECTIVE BLOOD VOLUME)

Hypoalbuminemic states (cirrhosis, nephrosis).
Sequestration of fluid in "third" space (ischemic bowel, peritonitis, pancreatitis).
Peripheral vasodilation (sepsis, vasodilators, anaphylaxis).

ALTERED RENAL VASCULAR RESISTANCE

Increase in afferent vascular resistance (NSAIDs, liver disease, sepsis, hypercalcemia, cyclosporine).
Decrease in efferent arteriolar tone (ACE inhibitors).

RENAL PARENCHYMAL DISEASE, CHRONIC[16a]

ICD-9CM # 593.9

DIFFERENTIAL DIAGNOSIS OF CHRONIC RENAL PARENCHYMAL DISEASE

No Papillary/Caliceal Abnormality
Diffuse parenchymal loss
Bilateral:
Chronic glomerulonephritis.
Diffuse small-vessel disease.
Hereditary nephropathies.
Unilateral:
Renal artery stenosis.
Postirradiation.
Rare:
• Hypoplastic kidney.
• Postobstructive atrophy.
Focal parenchymal loss
Infarct.
Previous trauma.
Papillary/Caliceal Abnormality
Diffuse parenchymal loss
Obstructive nephropathy.
Generalized reflux nephropathy.
No Parenchymal Loss
Papillary necrosis.
TB.
Medullary sponge kidney.
Megacalices.
Pelvicaliceal cyst.
Focal Parenchymal Loss
Focal reflux nephropathy (chronic atrophic pyelonephritis).
TB.
Calculus disease.

RENAL VEIN THROMBOSIS, CAUSES

ICD-9CM # 453.3

Nephrotic syndrome.
Renal cell carcinoma.
Aortic aneurysm causing compression.
Lymphadenopathy.
Retroperitoneal fibrosis.
Estrogen therapy.
Pregnancy.
Renal cell carcinoma with vein invasion.
Severe dehydration.

RESPIRATORY FAILURE, HYPOVENTILATORY[28]

ICD-9CM # 518.81 Respiratory Failure

ABNORMAL RESPIRATORY CAPACITY (NORMAL RESPIRATORY WORKLOADS)

Acute depression of central nervous system:
Various causes.
Chronic central hypoventilation syndromes:
Obesity-hypoventilation syndrome.
Sleep apnea syndrome.
Hypothyroidism.
Shy-Drager syndrome (multisystem atrophy syndrome).
Acute toxic paralysis syndromes:
Botulism.
Tetanus.
Toxic ingestion or bites.
Organophosphate poisoning.
Neuromuscular disorders (acute and chronic):
Myasthenia gravis.
Guillain-Barré syndrome.
Drugs.
Amyotrophic lateral sclerosis.
Muscular dystrophies.
Polymyositis.
Spinal cord injury.
Traumatic phrenic nerve paralysis.

ABNORMAL PULMONARY WORKLOADS

Chronic obstructive pulmonary disease:
Chronic bronchitis.
Asthmatic bronchitis.
Emphysema.
Asthma and acute bronchial hyperreactivity syndromes.
Upper airway obstruction.
Interstitial lung diseases.

ABNORMAL EXTRAPULMONARY WORKLOADS

Chronic thoracic cage disorders:
Severe kyphoscoliosis.
After thoracoplasty.
After thoracic cage injury.
Acute thoracic cage trauma and burns.
Pneumothorax.
Pleural fibrosis and effusions.
Abdominal processes.

RETINOPATHY, HYPERTENSIVE

ICD-9CM # 362.11

Retinal venous obstruction.
Diabetic retinopathy.
Ocular ischemic syndrome.
Hyperviscosity.
Tortuosity of retinal artery.

RHINITIS

ICD-9CM # 472.0

Allergic rhinitis.
Infectious rhinitis.
Vasomotor rhinitis.
Exercise-induced rhinitis.
Emotional rhinitis.
Rhinitis medicamentosa.
Hormone-mediated rhinitis (menses, pregnancy, oral contraceptives, hypothyroidism).
GERD.
Chemical- or irritant-induced rhinitis.
Rhinitis mimics:
  Deviated septum.
  Enlarged adenoids.
  Nasal polyps/tumors.
  Foreign bodies.
  CSF rhinorrhea.
  Sarcoidosis.
  Midline granuloma.
  Wegener's granulomatosis.
  SLE.
  Sjögren's syndrome.

RIB DEFECTS ON X-RAY[16a]

ICD-9CM # varies with specific diagnosis

CAUSES OF SUPERIOR MARGINAL RIB DEFECTS

Normal
Isolated defects.
Projectional artifacts (due to lordosis).
Neurological
Paralytic poliomyelitis.
Quadriparesis.
Collagen Vascular Disease
Rheumatoid arthritis.
SLE.
Systemic sclerosis.
Local Pressure
Chest drainage tube.
Osteochondroma.
Neural tumor.
Coarctation of aorta.
Hyperparathyroidism
Miscellaneous
Osteogenesis imperfecta.
Marfan's syndrome.

RIB NOTCHING ON X-RAY[16a]

ICD-9CM # varies with specific diagnosis

CAUSES OF INFERIOR RIB NOTCHING

Arterial
Aortic obstruction
Aortic coarctation.
Aortic thrombosis.
Aortitis.
Subclavian artery obstruction
Blalock-Taussig operation.
Arteritis.
Atherosclerotic occlusion.

Pulmonary oligaemia
Pulmonary atresia.
Tetralogy of Fallot.
Multiple pulmonary arterial stenoses.
Venous
Chronic superior vena caval obstruction
Arteriovenous
Arteriovenous malformation
Pulmonary.
Chest wall.
Neural
Neurofibromas

RIGHT AXIS DEVIATION[22]

ICD-9CM # varies with specific diagnosis

Normal variation.
Right ventricular hypertrophy.
Left posterior fascicular block.
Lateral myocardial infarction.
Pulmonary embolism.
Dextrocardia.
Mechanical shifts or emphysema causing a vertical heart.

SALIVARY GLAND ENLARGEMENT

ICD-9CM # 527.1

Neoplasm.
Sialolithiasis.
Infection (mumps, bacterial infection, HIV, TB).
Sarcoidosis.
Idiopathic.
Acromegaly.
Anorexia/bulimia.
Chronic pancreatitis.
Medications (e.g., phenylbutazone).
Cirrhosis.
DM.

SALIVARY GLAND SECRETION, DECREASED

ICD-9CM # 527.7

Medications (antihistamines, antidepressants, neuroleptics, antihypertensives).
Dehydration.
Anxiety.
Sjögren's syndrome.
Sarcoidosis.
Mumps.
Amyloidosis.
CNS disorders.
Head and neck radiation.

SCLERODERMA-LIKE SYNDROMES[1]

ICD-9CM # varies with specific diagnosis

OTHER DISEASES

Morphea.
Eosinophilic fasciitis.
Scleredema (of Buschke).
Scleromyxedema.
Graft-versus-host disease.
Nephrogenic-fibrosing dermopathy.

Environmental Agents and Drugs
Bleomycin.
L-tryptophan.
Organic solvents.
Pentazocine.
Toxic oil syndrome.
Vinyl chloride disease.
Gadolinium.

SCROTAL PAIN[28]

ICD-9CM # 878.2 Scrotal Injury, Traumatic
608.9 Scrotal Disorder NOS
608.4 Scrotal Cellulitis
608.83 Scrotal Hemorrhage, Nontraumatic
608.4 Scrotal Nodule, Inflammatory

Torsion:
  Appendages.
  Spermatic cord.
Infection:
  Orchitis.
  Abscess.
  Epididymitis.
Neoplasia:
  Benign.
  Malignant.
Incarcerated hernia.
Trauma.
Hydrocele.
Spermatocele.
Varicocele.

SCROTAL SWELLING

ICD-9CM # 608.86

Hydrocele.
Varicocele.
Neoplasm.
Acute epididymitis.
Orchitis.
Trauma.
Hernia.
Torsion of spermatic cord.
Torsion of epididymis.
Torsion of testis.
Insect bite.
Folliculitis.
Sebaceous cyst.
Thrombosis of spermatic vein.
Other: lymphedema, dermatitis, fat necrosis, Henoch-Schönlein purpura, idiopathic scrotal edema.

SEIZURE

ICD-9CM # 780.39

Syncope.
Alcohol abuse/withdrawal.
TIA.
Hemiparetic migraine.
Psychiatric disorders.
Carotid sinus hypersensitivity.
Hyperventilation, prolonged breath holding.
Hypoglycemia.
Narcolepsy.
Movement disorders (tics, hemiballismus).

Differential Diagnosis

II

Hyponatremia.
Brain tumor (primary or metastatic).
Tetanus.
Strychnine, phencyclidine poisoning.

SEIZURE, PEDIATRIC[2]

ICD-9CM # 780.39 Infantile Seizures
729.0 Seizures, Newborn

FIRST MONTH OF LIFE

First Day
Hypoxia.
Drugs.
Trauma.
Infection.
Hyperglycemia.
Hypoglycemia.
Pyridoxine deficiency.
Day 2-3
Infection.
Drug withdrawal.
Hypoglycemia.
Hypocalcemia.
Developmental malformation.
Intracranial hemorrhage.
Inborn error of metabolism.
Hyponatremia or hypernatremia.
Day >4
Infection.
Hypocalcemia.
Hyperphosphatemia.
Hyponatremia.
Developmental malformation.
Drug withdrawal.
Inborn error of metabolism.

1 TO 6 MO

As above.

6 MO TO 3 YR

Febrile seizures.
Birth injury.
Infection.
Toxin.
Trauma.
Metabolic disorder.
Cerebral degenerative disease.

>3 YR

Idiopathic.
Infection.
Trauma.
Cerebral degenerative disease.

SEIZURES MIMICS[1]

ICD-9CM # varies with specific diagnosis

NON-EPILEPTIC EPISODIC DISORDERS THAT MAY RESEMBLE SEIZURES

Movement disorders: myoclonus, paroxysmal choreoathetosis, episodic ataxias, hyperexplexia (startle disease).
Migraine: confusional, vertebrobasilar, visual auras.
Syncope.

Behavioral and psychiatric: psychogenic non-epileptic attacks (pseudoseizures), hyperventilation syndrome, panic or anxiety disorder, dissociative states.
Cataplexy (usually associated with narcolepsy).
Transient ischemic attack.
Alchoholic blackouts.
Hypoglycemia.

SEXUAL DYSFUNCTION, FEMALE[1]

ICD-9CM # 302.7

FACTORS THAT MAY INFLUENCE SEXUAL FUNCTIONING IN WOMEN

Biological
Medications (e.g., antidepressants, antihypertensives).
Vaginal atrophy, pain with intercourse.
Low testosterone levels (e.g., bilateral oophorectomy).
Illness (e.g., diabetes, hypothyroidism, cerebrovascular accident).
Sleep disturbances, fatigue.
Disability or pain from illness (e.g., arthritis).
Incontinence.
Psychological
Depression.
Body image.
Interpersonal
Marital issues.
Poor communication.
Partner's sexual problems (e.g., erectile dysfunction).
Partner's health problems (e.g., myocardial infarction).
Sociocultural
Ageism ("too old" to want sex).
Multiple other obligations and commitments.
Lack of partner.

SEXUALLY TRANSMITTED DISEASES, ANORECTAL REGION[26]

ICD-9CM # 569.49 Infection and Region

ULCERATIVE

Lymphogranuloma venereum.
Herpes simplex virus.
Early (primary) syphilis.
Chancroid *(Haemophilus ducreyi).*
Cytomegalovirus.
Idiopathic (usually HIV positive).

NONULCERATIVE

Condyloma acuminatum.
Gonorrhea.
Chlamydia *(Chlamydia trachomatis).*
Syphilis.

SEXUAL PRECOCITY[41]

ICD-9CM # 259.1

TRUE PRECOCIOUS PUBERTY

Premature reactivation of LHRH pulse generator.

INCOMPLETE SEXUAL PRECOCITY

(Pituitary gonadotropin independent).
Males
Chorionic gonadotropin-secreting tumor.
Leydig cell tumor.
Familial testotoxicosis.
Virilizing congenital adrenal hyperplasia.
Virilizing adrenal tumor.
Premature adrenarche.
Females
Granulosa cell tumor (follicular cysts may be manifested similarly).
Follicular cyst.
Feminizing adrenal tumor.
Premature thelarche.
Premature adrenarche.
Late-onset virilizing congenital adrenal hyperplasia.
In both sexes
McCune-Albright syndrome.
Primary hypothyroidism.

SHOULDER PAIN

ICD-9CM # 952.2 Shoulder Injury
718.81 Shoulder Instability
726.19 Shoulder Ligament or Muscle Instability
840.9 Shoulder Strain, Site Unspecified

WITH LOCAL FINDINGS IN SHOULDER

Trauma: contusion, fracture, muscle strain, trauma to spinal cord.
Arthrosis, arthritis, RA, ankylosing spondylitis.
Bursitis, synovitis, tendinitis, tenosynovitis.
Aseptic (avascular) necrosis.
Local infection: septic arthritis, osteomyelitis, abscess, herpes zoster, TB.

WITHOUT LOCAL FINDINGS IN SHOULDER

Cardiovascular disorders: ischemic heart disease, pericarditis, aortic aneurysm.
Subdiaphragmatic abscess, liver abscess.
Cholelithiasis, cholecystitis.
Pulmonary lesions: apical bronchial carcinoma, pleurisy, pneumothorax, pneumonia.
GI lesions: PUD, gastric neoplasm, peptic esophagitis.
Pancreatic lesions: carcinoma, calculi, pancreatitis.
CNS abnormalities: neoplasm, vascular abnormalities.
Multiple sclerosis.
Syringomyelia.
Polymyositis/dermatomyositis.
Psychogenic.
Polymyalgia rheumatica.
Ectopic pregnancy.

SHOULDER PAIN BY LOCATION

ICD-9CM # 952.2   Shoulder Injury
             726.19   Shoulder Ligament or
                        Muscle Instability
             840.8   Shoulder Separation

TOP OF SHOULDER (C4)

Cervical source.
Acromioclavicular.
Sternoclavicular.
Diaphragmatic.

SUPEROLATERAL (C5)

Rotator cuff tendinitis.
Impingement.
Adhesive capsulitis.
Glenohumeral arthritis.

ANTERIOR

Bicipital tendinitis and rupture.
Glenoid labral tear.
Adhesive capsulitis.
Glenohumeral arthritis.
Osteonecrosis.

AXILLARY

Neoplasm (Pancoast's, mediastinal).
Herpes zoster.

SHOULDER PAIN, IN DIFFERENT AGE GROUPS[8]

ICD-9CM # 719.41

COMMON CAUSES OF SHOULDER PAIN IN DIFFERENT AGE GROUPS

Childhood (2-10 yr)
Intraarticular:
Instability.
Periarticular:
Osteochondromas.
Adolescence (10-18 yr)
Intraarticular:
Instability.
Early Adulthood (18-30 yr)
Intraarticular:
Instability.
Acromioclavicular joint sprain.
Periarticular:
Calcific tendonitis.
Impingement.
Referred:
Cervical.
Adulthood (30-60 yr)
Intraarticular:
Osteochondritis.
Osteoarthritis.
Frozen shoulder.
Inflammatory arthritis.
Periarticular:
Calcific tendonitis.
Impingement.
Rotator cuff tear.
Bicipital tendinitis.
Referred:
Cervical.

Old Age (>60 yr)
Intraarticular:
Osteochondritis.
Osteoarthritis.
Frozen shoulder.
Inflammatory arthritis.
Periarticular:
Impingement.
Rotator cuff tear.
Referred:
Cervical.

SMALL BOWEL MASSES[38]

ICD-9CM # varies with specific diagnosis

Cyst:
     Mesenteric cyst.
Tumor:
     Benign.
     Malignant.
Intussusception.
Inflammation:
     Crohn's disease.

SMALL BOWEL OBSTRUCTION[26]

ICD-9CM # 751.1   Small Intestine
                    Obstruction, Congenital
           560.81   Small Intestine
                    Obstruction Due
                    to Adhesion

INTRINSIC

Congenital (atresia, stenosis).
Inflammatory (Crohn's, radiation enteritis).
Neoplasms (metastatic or primary).
Intussusception.
Traumatic (hematoma).

EXTRINSIC

Hernias (internal and external).
Adhesions.
Volvulus.
Compressing masses (tumors, abscesses, hematomas).

INTRALUMINAL

Foreign body.
Gallstones.
Bezoars.
Barium.
Ascaris infestation.

SMALL INTESTINE ULCERATION

ICD-9CM # 569.82

Inflammatory bowel disease.
Celiac disease.
Vasculitis, SLE, Behçet's syndrome.
Uremia.
Infections (*Campylobacter*, TB, *Yersinia*, parasites, typhoid, cytomegalovirus [CMV], *Clostridium*).
Mesenteric insufficiency.
Neoplasms.
Radiation.

Drugs (salicylates, potassium, indomethacin, antimetabolites).
Meckel diverticulum.
Zollinger-Ellison syndrome.
Lymphocytic enterocolitis.
Stomal ulceration.

SMELL DISTURBANCE

ICD-9CM # varies with specific disorder

Upper respiratory tract infection.
Nasal or paranasal sinus disease.
Exposure to noxious vapors.
Head trauma.
Idiopathic.
Dental caries, periodontal disease.
Medications.

SORE THROAT[2]

ICD-9CM # 484.1

DIFFERENTIAL DIAGNOSIS FOR SORE THROAT

Infectious Causes
Aerobes
Common:
     Streptococcus pyogenes (GABHS).
     GABHS.
     Peptostreptococcus sp.
     Non–group A streptococcus.
     Neisseria gonorrhoeae.
     Neisseria meningitides.
     Mycoplasma pneumoniae.
     Arcanobacterium hemolyticum.
     Chlamydia trachomatis.
     Staphylococcus aureus.
Uncommon:
     Haemophilus influenzae.
     Haemophilus parainfluenzae.
     Coccidioides sp.
     Corynebacterium diphtheriae.
     Streptococcus pneumoniae.
     Yersinia enterocolitica.
     Treponema pallidum.
     Francisella tularensis.
     Legionella pneumophila.
     Mycobacterium sp.
Anaerobes
Bacteroides sp.
Peptococcus sp.
Clostridium sp.
Fusobacterium sp.
Prevotella sp.
Other
Candida sp.
Viral
Rhinovirus.
Adenovirus.
Coronavirus.
Herpes simplex 1,2.
Influenza A, B.
Parainfluenza.
Cytomegalovirus.
Epstein-Barr.
Varicella-zoster.
Hepatitis virus.

Differential Diagnosis

II

Noninfectious causes
Systemic
Kawasaki disease.
Stevens-Johnson syndrome.
Cyclic neutropenia.
Thyroiditis.
Connective tissue disease
Trauma, miscellaneous
Penetrating injury.
Angioneurotic edema.
Retained foreign body.
Anomalous aortic arch.
Laryngeal fracture.
Calcific retropharyngeal tendinitis.
Retropharyngeal hematoma.
Caustic exposure.
Tumor
Tongue.
Larynx.
Thyroid.
Leukemia.

SPASTIC PARAPLEGIAS

ICD-9CM # 344.1

Cervical spondylosis.
Friedreich's ataxia.
Multiple sclerosis.
Spinal cord tumor.
HIV.
Tertiary syphilis.
Vitamin B_{12} deficiency.
Spinocerebellar ataxias.
Syringomyelia.
Spinal cord AV malformations.
Adrenoleukodystrophy.

SPINAL CORD COMPRESSION, EPIDURAL

ICD-9CM # varies with specific disorder

Osteoarthritis.
Meningioma.
Spinal epidural abscess.
Spinal epidural hematoma.
Spinal epidural vascular malformations.
RA.
Metastatic cancer (vertebral, intramedullary, leptomeninges).
Radiation myelopathy.
Neurofibroma.
Sarcoidosis.
Paraneoplastic myelopathy.
Histiocytosis.

SPINAL CORD DYSFUNCTION

ICD-9CM #		
	336.9	Spinal Cord Compression
	336.9	Spinal Cord Disease NOS
	742.9	Spinal Cord Disease, Congenital
	281.1	Spinal Cord Degeneration, B_{12} Deficiency Anemia
	336.8	Spinal Cord Atrophy, Acute
	336.10	Spinal Cord Atrophy, Adult

Trauma.
Multiple sclerosis.

Transverse myelitis.
Neoplasm (primary, metastatic).
Syringomyelia.
Spinal epidural abscess.
HIV myelopathy.
Diskitis.
Spinal epidural hematoma.
Spinal cord infarction.
Spinal AV malformation.
Subarachnoid hemorrhage.

SPINAL CORD DYSFUNCTION, NON-TRAUMATIC[2]

ICD-9CM # 742.9

NONTRAUMATIC ETIOLOGIES OF SPINAL CORD DYSFUNCTION
Processes Affecting the Spinal Cord or Blood Supply Directly
Multiple sclerosis.
Transverse myelitis.
Spinal arteriovenous malformation/subarachnoid hemorrhage.
Syringomyelia.
HIV myelopathy.
Other myelopathies.
Spinal cord infarction.
Compressive Lesions Affecting the Spinal Cord
Spinal epidural abscess.
Spinal epidural hematoma.
Diskitis.
Neoplasm.
Metastatic.
Primary CNS.

HIV, Human immunodeficiency virus; *CNS*, central nervous system.

SPINAL CORD ISCHEMIC SYNDROMES

ICD-9CM # varies with specific disorder

Systemic hypotension.
Venous or arterial occlusion.
Arterial dissection.
Thromboembolism.
Endovascular procedures.
Vasculitis.
Fibrocartilaginous embolism.
Regional hemodynamic compromise.

SPINAL TUMORS[14]

ICD-9CM # 299.7

EXTRADURAL
Metastases.
Primary bone tumors arising in spine.

INTRADURAL EXTRAMEDULLARY
Meningiomas.
Neurofibromas.
Schwannomas.
Lipomas.
Arachnoid cysts.
Epidermoid cysts.
Metastasis.

INTRAMEDULLARY
Ependymoma.
Glioma.
Hemangioblastoma.
Lipoma.
Metastases.

SPLENOMEGALY

ICD-9CM #		
	789.2	Splenomegaly Unspecified
	289.51	Chronic Congestive
	759.0	Congenital
	789.2	Unknown Origin

Hepatic cirrhosis.
Neoplastic involvement: CML, CLL, lymphoma, multiple myeloma.
Bacterial infections: TB, infectious endocarditis, typhoid fever, splenic abscess.
Viral infections: infectious mononucleosis, viral hepatitis, HIV.
Gaucher's disease and other lipid storage diseases.
Sarcoidosis.
Parasitic infections (malaria, kala-azar, histoplasmosis).
Hereditary and acquired hemolytic anemias.
Idiopathic thrombocytopenic purpura (ITP).
Collagen vascular disorders: SLE, RA (Felty's syndrome), polyarteritis nodosa.
Serum sickness, drug hypersensitivity reaction.
Splenic cysts and benign tumors: hemangioma, lymphangioma.
Thrombosis of splenic or portal vein.
Polycythemia vera, myeloid metaplasia.

SPLENOMEGALY AND HEPATOMEGALY[38]

ICD-9CM #		
	789.2	Splenomegaly
	789.1	Hepatomegaly

CAUSES OF SPLENOMEGALY AND HEPATOSPLENOMEGALY
Massive Splenomegaly
Hematological disease (e.g., chronic myeloid leukemia, myelofibrosis).
Moderate Splenomegaly
The above causes.
Portal hypertension.
Hematological disease (e.g., lymphoma, leukemia, thalassemia).
Storage disease (e.g., Gaucher's disease).
Small Splenomegaly
The above causes.
Infective (hepatitis, leptospirosis, malaria, bacterial endocarditis).
Hematological disease (e.g., hemolytic anemias, essential thrombocythemia, polycythemia rubra vera).
Connective tissue diseases or vasculitis (e.g., rheumatoid arthritis, systemic lupus erythematosus, polyarteritis nodosa).
Solitary cyst, polycystic syndrome, hydatid cyst.
Infiltration (amyloid, sarcoid).
Hepatosplenomegaly
Chronic liver disease with portal hypertension.
Hematological disease (e.g., myeloproliferative disease, lymphoma).

Infection (e.g., amyloid, sarcoid).
Connective tissue disease (e.g., systemic lupus erythematosus).

SPLENOMEGALY, CHILDREN[20]
ICD-9CM # 782.2

DISORDERS OF THE BLOOD
Hemolytic anemia: congenital/acquired.
Thalassemia.
Sickle cell disease.
Leukemia.
Osteopetrosis.
Myelofibrosis/myeloid metaplasia/thrombocythemia.

INFECTIONS: ACUTE AND CHRONIC
Viral:
    Congenital (e.g., TORCH association).
    Mononucleosis (e.g., EBV, CMV infection).
    Virus-associated hemophagocytic syndrome.
    Human immunodeficiency virus.
Bacterial:
    Sepsis/abscess.
    Brucellosis.
    Salmonellosis.
    Tularemia.
    Tuberculosis.
    Subacute bacterial endocarditis.
    Syphilis.
    Lyme disease.
Fungal:
    Histoplasmosis (disseminated).
Rickettsial:
    Rocky Mountain spotted fever.
    Cat scratch disease.
Parasitic:
    Toxoplasmosis.
    Malaria.
    Leishmaniasis (kala-azar).
    Schistosomiasis.
    Echinococcosis.

HEPATIC/PORTAL SYSTEM DISORDERS
Acute/chronic active hepatitis.
Cirrhosis/hepatic fibrosis/biliary atresia.
Portal or splenic venous obstruction (Banti syndrome).

AUTOIMMUNE DISEASE
Juvenile rheumatoid arthritis.
Systemic lupus erythematosus.
Autoimmune lymphoproliferative syndrome (Canale–Smith syndrome).

NEOPLASMS/CYSTS
Lymphomas (Hodgkin and non-Hodgkin).
Hemangiomas/lymphangiomas.
Hamartomas.
Congenital or acquired (posttraumatic) cysts.

STORAGE DISEASES/INBORN ERRORS OF METABOLISM
Lipidoses: Gaucher disease, Niemann–Pick disease, others.
Mucopolysaccharidoses.

Defects in carbohydrate metabolism: galactosemia, fructose intolerance.
Sea-blue histiocyte syndrome.

MISCELLANEOUS DISORDERS
Histiocytoses:
    Reactive.
    Langerhans cell.
    Malignant.
Sarcoidosis.
Congestive heart failure.
Familial Mediterranean fever.

CMV, Cytomegalovirus; *EBV,* Epstein-Barr virus; *TORCH,* toxoplasmosis, other infections, rubella, cytomegalovirus infection, herpes simplex.

STEATOHEPATITIS
ICD-9CM # 571.8

Alcohol abuse.
Obesity.
DM.
Parenteral nutrition.
Medications (high-dose estrogen, amiodarone, corticosteroids, methotrexate, nifedipine).
Jejunoileal bypass.
Abetalipoproteinemia.
Wilson's disease, Weber-Christian disease.

STOMATITIS, BULLOUS
ICD-9CM # 528.0

Erythema multiforme.
Erosive lichen planus.
Bullous pemphigoid.
SLE.
Pemphigus vulgaris.
Mucous membrane pemphigoid.

STRIDOR, PEDIATRIC AGE[4]
ICD-9CM # 786.1 Stridor
           748.3 Stridor Laryngeal
                 Congenital

RECURRENT
Allergic (spasmodic) croup.
Respiratory infections in a child with otherwise asymptomatic anatomic narrowing of the large airways.
Laryngomalacia.

PERSISTENT
Laryngeal obstruction:
    Laryngomalacia.
    Papillomas, other tumors.
    Cysts and laryngoceles.
    Laryngeal webs.
    Bilateral abductor paralysis of the cords.
    Foreign body.
Tracheobronchial disease:
    Tracheomalacia.
    Subglottic tracheal webs.
Endotracheal, endobronchial tumors.
Subglottic tracheal stenosis.
Congenital.
Acquired.
Extrinsic masses.
Mediastinal masses.

Vascular ring.
Lobar emphysema.
Bronchogenic cysts.
Thyroid enlargement.
Esophageal foreign body.
Tracheoesophageal fistulas.
Other.
Gastroesophageal reflux.
Macroglossia, Pierre Robin syndrome.
Cri-du-chat syndrome.
Hysterical stridor.
Hypocalcemia.

STROKE[36]
ICD-9CM # 436 Acute Stroke

Hypoglycemia.
Drug overdose or intoxication.
Hysterical conversion reaction.
Hyperventilation.
Metabolic encephalopathy.
Migraine.
Syncope.
Transient global amnesia.
Seizures.
Vestibular vertigo.

STROKE, PEDIATRIC AGE[23]
ICD-9CM # 436 Stroke, Acute

CARDIAC DISEASE
Congenital:
    Aortic stenosis.
    Mitral stenosis; mitral prolapse.
    Ventricular septal defects.
    Patent ductus arteriosus.
    Cyanotic congenital heart disease involving right-to-left shunt.
Acquired:
    Endocarditis (bacterial, SLE).
    Kawasaki disease.
    Cardiomyopathy.
    Atrial myxoma.
    Arrhythmia.
    Paradoxical emboli through patent foramen ovale.
    Rheumatic fever.
    Prosthetic heart valve.

HEMATOLOGIC ABNORMALITIES
Hemoglobinopathies:
    Sickle cell (SS) disease.
    Sickle (SC) disease.
Polycythemia.
Leukemia/lymphoma.
Thrombocytopenia.
Thrombocytosis.
Disorders of coagulation:
    Protein C deficiency.
    Protein S deficiency.
    Factor V Leiden.
    Antithrombin III deficiency.
    Lupus anticoagulant.
Oral contraceptive pill use.
Pregnancy and the postpartum state.
Disseminated intravascular coagulation.
Paroxysmal nocturnal hemoglobinuria.
Inflammatory bowel disease (thrombosis).

INFLAMMATORY DISORDERS

Meningitis:
  Viral.
  Bacterial.
  Tuberculosis.
Systemic infection:
  Viremia.
  Bacteremia.
  Local head and neck infections.
Drug-induced inflammation:
  Amphetamine.
  Cocaine.
Autoimmune disease:
  SLE.
  Juvenile RA.
  Takayasu's arteritis.
  Mixed connective tissue disease.
  Polyarteritis nodosum.
  Primary CNS vasculitis.
  Sarcoidosis.
  Behçet's syndrome.
  Wegener's granulomatosis.

METABOLIC DISEASE ASSOCIATED WITH STROKE

Homocystinuria.
Pseudoxanthoma elasticum.
Fabry's disease.
Sulfite oxidase deficiency.
Mitochondrial disorders:
  MELAS.
  Leigh syndrome.
Ornithine transcarbamylase deficiency.

INTRACEREBRAL VASCULAR PROCESSES

Ruptured aneurysm.
Arteriovenous malformation.
Fibromuscular dysplasia.
Moyamoya disease.
Migraine headache.
Postsubarachnoid hemorrhage vasospasm.
Hereditary hemorrhagic telangiectasia.
Sturge-Weber syndrome.
Carotid artery dissection.
Postvaricella.

TRAUMA AND OTHER EXTERNAL CAUSES

Child abuse.
Head trauma/neck trauma.
Oral trauma.
Placental embolism.
ECMO therapy.

CNS, Central nervous system; *ECMO,* extracorporeal membrane oxygenation; *MELAS,* mitochondrial encephalomyopathy, lactic acidosis, and stroke.

STROKE, YOUNG ADULT, CAUSES[1]

ICD-9CM # 436

Cardiac factors (ASD, MVP, patent foramen ovale).
Inflammatory factors (SLE, polyarteritis nodosa).
Infections (endocarditis, neurosyphilis).
Drugs (cocaine, heroin, oral contraceptives, decongestants).

Arterial dissection.
Hematolic factors (DIC, TTP, deficiency of protein S, protein C, antithrombin III).
Migraine.
Postpartum angiopathy.
Other: premature atherosclerosis, fibromuscular dysplasia.

ST SEGMENT ELEVATIONS, NONISCHEMIC

ICD-9CM # 794.31

Early repolarization.
Acute pericarditis.
LVH.
Normal pattern variant.
LBBB.
Pulmonary embolism.
Hyperkalemia.
Postcardioversion.

SUDDEN DEATH, PEDIATRIC AGE[4]

ICD-9CM # varies with specific disorder

SIDS AND SIDS "MIMICS"

SIDS.
Long QT syndromes.
Inborn errors of metabolism.
Child abuse.
Myocarditis.
Duct-dependent congenital heart disease.

CORRECTED OR UNOPERATED CONGENITAL HEART DISEASE

Aortic stenosis.
Tetralogy of Fallot.
Transposition of great vessels (postoperative atrial switch).
Mitral valve prolapse.
Hypoplastic left heart syndrome.
Eisenmenger's syndrome.

CORONARY ARTERIAL DISEASE

Anomalous origin.
Anomalous tract.
Kawasaki disease.
Periarteritis.
Arterial dissection.
Marfan's syndrome.
Myocardial infarction.

MYOCARDIAL DISEASE

Myocarditis.
Hypertrophic cardiomyopathy.
Dilated cardiomyopathy.
Arrhythmogenic right ventricular dysplasia.

CONDUCTION SYSTEM ABNORMALITY/ARRHYTHMIA

Long Q-T syndromes.
Proarrhythmic drugs.
Preexcitation syndromes.
Heart block.
Commotio cordis.
Idiopathic ventricular fibrillation.
Heart tumor.

MISCELLANEOUS

Pulmonary hypertension.
Pulmonary embolism.
Heat stroke.
Cocaine.
Anorexia nervosa.
Electrolyte disturbances.

SIDS, Sudden infant death syndrome.

SUDDEN DEATH, YOUNG ATHLETE

ICD-9CM # varies with specific diagnosis

Hypertrophic cardiomyopathy.
Coronary artery anomalies.
Myocarditis.
Ruptured aortic aneurysm (Marfan's syndrome).
Arrhythmias.
Aortic valve stenosis.
Asthma.
Trauma (cerebral, cardiac).
Drug and alcohol abuse.
Heat stroke.
Cardiac sarcoidosis.
Atherosclerotic coronary artery disease.
Dilated cardiomyopathy.

SWOLLEN LIMB

ICD-9CM # 729.81 Swollen Arm or Hand
            729.81 Swollen Leg or Foot

Trauma.
Insect bite.
Abscess.
Lymphedema.
Thrombophlebitis.
Lipoma.
Neurofibroma.
Postphlebitic syndrome.
Myositis ossificans.
Nephrosis, cirrhosis, CHF.
Hypoalbuminemia.
Varicose veins.

TALL STATURE[27]

ICD-9CM # 253.0 Growth Hormone
            Overproduction, Gigantism

Constitutional (familial or genetic)—most common cause

ENDOCRINE CAUSES

Growth hormone excess—gigantism.
Sexual precocity (tall as children, short as adults):
  True sexual precocity.
  Pseudosexual precocity.
Androgen deficiency:
  Klinefelter's syndrome.
  Bilateral anorchism.

GENETIC CAUSES

Klinefelter's syndrome.
Syndromes of XYY, XXYY.

MISCELLANEOUS SYNDROMES AND DISORDERS

Cerebral gigantism or Sotos' syndrome: prominent forehead, hypertelorism, high arched palate, dolichocephaly, mental retardation, large hands and feet, and premature eruption of teeth. Large at birth, with most rapid growth in first 4 yr of life.

Marfan's syndrome: disorder of mesodermal tissues, subluxation of the lenses, arachnodactyly, and aortic aneurysm.

Homocystinuria: same phenotype as Marfan's syndrome.

Obesity: tall as infants, children, and adolescents.

Total lipodystrophy: large hands and feet, generalized loss of subcutaneous fat, insulin-resistant DM, and hepatomegaly.

Beckwith-Wiedemann syndrome: neonatal tallness, omphalocele, macroglossia, and neonatal hypoglycemia.

Weaver-Smith syndrome: excessive intrauterine growth, mental retardation, megalocephaly, widened bifrontal diameter, hypertelorism, large ears, micrognathia, camptodactyly, broad thumbs, and limited extension of elbows and knees.

Marshall-Smith syndrome: excessive intrauterine growth, mental retardation, blue sclerae, failure to thrive, and early death.

TARDIVE DYSKINESIA[13]

ICD-9CM # 781.3   Dyskinesia
            300.11 Hysterical Dyskinesia
            333.82 Orofacial Dyskinesia
            307.9 Psychogenic Dyskinesia

DIFFERENTIAL DIAGNOSIS:

Medications (antidepressants, anticholinergics, amphetamines, lithium, L-dopa, phenytoin).

Brain neoplasms.

Ill-fitting dentures.

Huntington's disease.

Idiopathic dystonias (tics, blepharospasm, aging).

Wilson's disease.

Extrapyramidal syndrome (postanoxic or postencephalitic).

Torsion dystonia.

TASTE AND SMELL LOSS[1]

ICD-9CM # 781.1 Smell and Taste Disturbance of Sensation

TASTE

Local: radiation therapy.

Systemic: cancer, renal failure, hepatic failure, nutritional deficiency (vitamin B_{12}, zinc), Cushing's syndrome, hypothyroidism, DM, infection (influenza), drugs (antirheumatic and antiproliferative).

Neurologic: Bell's palsy, familial dysautonomia, multiple sclerosis.

SMELL

Local: allergic rhinitis, sinusitis, nasal polyposis, bronchial asthma.

Systemic: renal failure, hepatic failure, nutritional deficiency (vitamin B_{12}), Cushing's syndrome, hypothyroidism, DM, infection (viral hepatitis, influenza), drugs (nasal sprays, antibiotics).

Neurologic: head trauma, multiple sclerosis, Parkinson's disease, frontal brain tumor.

TELANGIECTASIA

ICD-9CM # 448.9

Oral contraceptive agents.

Pregnancy.

Rosacea.

Varicose veins.

Trauma.

Drug induced (corticosteroids, systemic or topical).

Spider telangiectases.

Hepatic cirrhosis.

Mastocytosis.

SLE, dermatomyositis, systemic sclerosis.

TENDINOPATHY[26]

ICD-9CM # 727.9

INTRINSIC FACTORS

Anatomic Factors

Malalignment.

Muscle weakness or imbalance.

Muscle inflexibility.

Decreased vascularity.

Systemic Factors

Inflammatory conditions (e.g., SLE).

Pregnancy.

Quinolone-induced tendinopathy.

Age-Related Factors

Tendon degeneration.

Increased tendon stiffness.

Tendon calcification.

Decreased vascularity.

EXTRINSIC FACTORS

Repetitive Mechanical Load

Excessive duration.

Excessive frequency.

Excessive intensity.

Poor technique.

Workplace factors.

Equipment Problems

Footwear.

Athletic field surface.

Equipment factors (e.g., racquet size).

Protective gear.

TESTICULAR FAILURE[10]

ICD-9CM # 257.1 Testicular Failure

PRIMARY

Klinefelter's syndrome (XXY).

XYY.

Vanishing testes syndrome (in utero or early postnatal torsion).

Noonan's syndrome.

Varicocele.

Myotonic dystrophy.

Orchitis (mumps, gonorrhea).

Cryptorchidism.

Chemical exposure.

Irradiation to testes.

Spinal cord injury.

Polyglandular failure.

Idiopathic oligospermia or azoospermia.

Germinal cell aplasia (Sertoli cell–only syndrome).

Idiopathic testicular failure.

Testicular torsion.

Testicular trauma.

Diethylstilbestrol (maternal use during pregnancy leading to in utero estrogen exposure).

Testicular tumor with subsequent irradiation therapy, chemotherapy, or surgery (retroperitoneal lymph node dissection or orchiectomy).

SECONDARY

Delayed puberty.

Kallmann's syndrome.

Isolated gonadotropin deficiency.

Prader-Labhart-Willi syndrome.

Lawrence-Moon-Biedl syndrome.

Central nervous system irradiation.

Prepubertal panhypopituitarism.

Postpubertal panhypopituitarism.

Hypogonadism secondary to hyperprolactinemia.

Adrenogenital syndrome.

Chronic liver disease.

Chronic renal failure/uremia.

Hemochromatosis.

Cushing's syndrome.

Malnutrition.

Massive obesity.

Sickle cell anemia.

Hyper/hypothyroidism.

Anabolic steroid use.

TESTICULAR PAIN

ICD-9CM # 608.9

Testicular torsion.

Trauma.

Epididymitis.

Orchitis.

Neoplasm.

Urolithiasis.

Inguinal hernia.

Infection (cellulitis, abscess, folliculitis).

Anxiety.

TESTICULAR SIZE VARIATIONS[10]

ICD-9CM # 608.3 Testicular Atrophy
            608.89 Testicular Mass
            257.2 Hypogonadism

SMALL TESTES

Hypothalamic-pituitary dysfunction.

Gonadotropin deficiency.

Growth hormone deficiency.

Normal variant.

Primary hypogonadism.

Autoimmune destruction, chemotherapy, cryptorchidism, irradiation, Klinefelter's syndrome, orchiditis, testicular regression syndrome, torsion, trauma.

LARGE TESTES

Adrenal rest tissue.
Compensatory.
Fragile X syndrome.
Idiopathic.
Tumor.

TETANUS[26]

ICD-9CM # 037

Acute abdomen.
Black widow spider bite.
Dental abscess.
Dislocated mandible.
Dystonic reaction.
Encephalitis.
Head trauma.
Hyperventilation syndrome.
Hypocalcemia.
Meningitis.
Peritonsillar abscess.
Progressive fluctuating muscular rigidity (stiff-man syndrome).
Psychogenic.
Rabies.
Sepsis.
Subarachnoid hemorrhage.
Status epilepticus.
Strychnine poisoning.
Temporomandibular joint syndrome.

THROMBOCYTOPENIA

ICD-9CM # 287.3 Congenital or Primary
287.4 Secondary
287.5 Thrombocytopenia NOS

INCREASED DESTRUCTION

Immunologic

Drugs: quinine, quinidine, digitalis, procainamide, thiazide diuretics, sulfonamides, phenytoin, aspirin, penicillin, heparin, gold, meprobamate, sulfa drugs, phenylbutazone, nonsteroidal anti-inflammatory drugs (NSAIDs), methyldopa, cimetidine, furosemide, INH, cephalosporins, chlorpropamide, organic arsenicals, chloroquine, platelet glycoprotein IIb/IIIa receptor inhibitors, ranitidine, indomethacin, carboplatin, ticlopidine, clopidogrel.
Idiopathic thrombocytopenic purpura (ITP).
Transfusion reaction: transfusion of platelets with plasminogen activator (PLA) in recipients without PLA-1.
Fetal/maternal incompatibility.
Collagen vascular diseases (e.g., SLE).
Autoimmune hemolytic anemia.
Lymphoreticular disorders (e.g., CLL).

Nonimmunologic

Prosthetic heart valves.
Thrombotic thrombocytopenic purpura (TTP).
Sepsis.
DIC.
Hemolytic-uremic syndrome (HUS).
Giant cavernous hemangioma.

DECREASED PRODUCTION

Abnormal marrow.
Marrow infiltration (e.g., leukemia, lymphoma, fibrosis).
Marrow suppression (e.g., chemotherapy, alcohol, radiation).
Hereditary disorders.
Wiskott-Aldrich syndrome: X-linked disorder characterized by thrombocytopenia, eczema, and repeated infections.
May-Hegglin anomaly: increased megakaryocytes but ineffective thrombopoiesis.
Vitamin deficiencies (e.g., vitamin B_{12}, folic acid).

SPLENIC SEQUESTRATION, HYPERSPLENISM

DILUTIONAL, AS A RESULT OF MASSIVE TRANSFUSION

THROMBOCYTOPENIA, IN PREGNANCY[20]

ICD-9CM # 287.4

Incidental thrombocytopenia of pregnancy (gestational thrombocytopenia).
Preeclampsia/eclampsia.*
Disseminated intravascular coagulation (DIC) secondary to:
    Abruptio placentae.
    Endometritis.
    Amniotic fluid embolism.
    Retained fetus.
Preeclampsia/eclampsia:*
    Peripartum/postpartum thrombotic microangiopathy.
    Thrombotic thrombocytopenic purpura.
    Hemolytic uremic syndrome.

---

*Preeclampsia/eclampsia usually is not associated with overt DIC.

THROMBOCYTOPENIA, INHERITED DISORDERS[1]

ICD-9CM # 287.3

Amegakaryocytic thrombocytopenia.
Thrombocytopenia absent radii.
MYH9-related thrombocytopenia:
    May-Hegglin anomaly.
    Fechtner syndrome.
    Epstein syndrome.
    Sebastian syndrome.
X-linked macrothrombocytopenia.
Wiskott-Aldrich syndrome.
X-linked thrombocytopenia.
Thrombocytopenia and radioulnar synostosis.
Familial platelet disorder—AML.
Familial dominant thrombocytopenia.
Paris-Trousseau thrombocytopenia.
Bernard-Soulier syndrome.
Bernard-Soulier carrier/Mediterranean macrothrombocytopenia.

THROMBOCYTOSIS

ICD-9CM # 289.9 Thrombocytosis, Essential

Iron deficiency.
Posthemorrhage.
Neoplasms (GI tract).
CML.
Polycythemia vera.

Myelofibrosis with myeloid metaplasia.
Infections.
After splenectomy.
Postpartum.
Hemophilia.
Pancreatitis.
Cirrhosis.
Idiopathic.

THROMBOSIS OR THROMBOTIC DIATHESIS[1]

ICD-9CM # 444

DIFFERENTIAL DIAGNOSIS OF THE PATIENT PRESENTING WITH THROMBOSIS OR THROMBOTIC DIATHESIS

Inherited (Primary) Hypercoagulable States

Activated protein C resistance caused by factor V Leiden mutation.
Prothrombin gene mutation (G to A transition at position 20210 in the 3 -untranslated region).
Antithrombin III deficiency.
Protein C deficiency.
Protein S deficiency.
Dysfibrinogenemias (rare).

Acquired (Secondary) Hypercoagulable States

In association with physiologic or thrombogenic stimuli:
    Pregnancy (especially the postpartum period).
    Estrogen use (oral contraceptives, hormone replacement therapy).
    Immobilization.
    Trauma.
    Postoperative state.
Advancing age.
Obesity.
Prolonged air travel.
Lupus anticoagulant or antiphospholipid antibody syndrome.
In association with other clinical disorders .

Mixed/Unknown

Activated protein C resistance in the absence of factor V Leiden.
Elevated factor VIII level.
Elevated factor XI level.
Elevated factor IX level.
Elevated thrombin activatable fibrinolysis inhibitor (TAFI) level.
Decreased free tissue factor pathway inhibitor (TFPI) level.
Decreased plasma fibrinolytic activity.

THYROMEGALY

ICD-9CM # varies with specific diagnosis

Goiter.
Graves' disease.
Thyroiditis (lymphocytic, granulomatous, suppurative).
Toxic adenoma.
Neoplasm (primary, metastatic).

TICK-RELATED INFECTIONS

ICD-9CM # 082.0 Rocky Mountain Spotted Fever
          066.1 Colorado Tick Fever
          088.82 Babesiosis
          082.8 Ehrlichiosis
          088.81 Lyme Disease

Lyme disease.
Rocky Mountain spotted fever.
Babesiosis.
Tularemia.
Q fever.
Colorado tick fever.
Ehrlichiosis.
Relapsing fever.

TICS

ICD-9CM # 307.20

Tourette's syndrome.
Physiologic tic.
Anxiety disorder.
Huntington's disease.
Medications (e.g., antipsychotics, carbamazepine, phenytoin, phenobarbital).
Encephalitis.
Head trauma.
Schizophrenia.
Carbon monoxide poisoning.
Stroke.
Sydenham's chorea.
Creutzfeldt-Jakob disease.

TORSADES DE POINTES[22]

ICD-9CM # code not available

Antiarrhythmics known to increase the QT interval (e.g., quinidine, procainamide, amiodarone, disopyramide, sotalol).
Tricyclic antidepressants and phenothiazines.
Histamine (H1) antagonists (e.g., astemizole, terfenadine).
Antiviral and antifungal agents and antibiotics.
Hypokinemia.
Hypomagnesemia.
Insecticide poisoning.
Bradyarrhythmias.
Congenital long QT syndrome.
Subarachnoid hemorrhage.
Chloroquinine, pentamidine.
Cocaine abuse.

TRACHEOBRONCHIAL NARROWING ON X-RAY[16a]

ICD-9CM # varies with specific diagnosis

CAUSES OF TRACHEOBRONCHIAL NARROWING

Long-segment/Diffuse Narrowing
Sarcoidosis.
Amyloidosis.
Wegener's granulomatosis.
Relapsing polychondritis.
Tracheobronchopathia osteochondroplastica.
Pemphigoid.

Short-segment Narrowing
Previous intubation or tracheostomy.
Congenital stenosis or web.
Extrinsic compression (from thyroid).
Adenoid cystic carcinoma.
Squamous carcinoma.

TREMOR

ICD-9CM # 781.0 Tremor NOS
          333.1 Benign Essential Tremor
          333.1 Familial Tremor

REST TREMORS

Parkinson's disease.
Other parkinsonian syndromes (less commonly).
Midbrain (rubral) tremor: rest < postural < kinetic.
Wilson's disease (also acquired hepatocerebral degeneration).
Essential tremor—only if severe: rest < postural and action.

POSTURAL AND ACTION (TERMINAL) TREMORS

Physiological tremor.
Exaggerated physiological tremor (these factors can also aggravate other forms of tremor).
  Stress, fatigue, anxiety, emotion.
  Endocrine: hypoglycemia, thyrotoxicosis, pheochromocytoma, adrenocorticosteroids.
  Drugs and toxins: β-agonists, dopamine agonists, amphetamines, lithium, tricyclic antidepressants, neuroleptics, theophylline, caffeine, valproic acid, alcohol withdrawal, mercury (Hatter's shakes), lead, arsenic, others.
Essential tremor (familial or sporadic) ?subtypes.
Primary writing tremor.
With other CNS disorders.
  Parkinson's disease.
  Other akinetic-rigid syndromes.
  Idiopathic dystonia, including focal dystonias.
With peripheral neuropathy.
  Charcot-Marie-Tooth syndrome (controversial whether to call this the Roussy-Levy syndrome).
  Variety of other peripheral neuropathies (especially dysgammaglobulinemia).
Cerebellar tremor.

KINETIC (INTENTION) TREMOR

Disease of cerebellar outflow (dentate nucleus and superior cerebellar peduncle): multiple sclerosis, trauma, tumor, vascular disease, Wilson's acquired hepatocerebral degeneration, drugs, toxins (e.g., mercury), others.

MISCELLANEOUS RHYTHMICAL MOVEMENT DISORDERS

Psychogenic tremor.
Orthostatic tremor.
Rhythmical movements in dystonia (dystonic tremor).
Rhythmical myoclonus (segmental myoclonus—e.g., palatal or branchial myoclonus, spinal myoclonus, limb myorhythmia).
Oscillatory myoclonus.
Asterixis.

Clonus.
Epilepsia partialis continua.
Hereditary chin quivering.
Spasmus nutans.
Head bobbing with third ventricular cysts.
Nystagmus.

TUBULOINTERSTITIAL DISEASE, ACUTE[14]

ICD-9CM # 584.5

DRUGS

Antibiotics, penicillins, cephalosporins, rifampin.
Sulfonamides: cotrimoxazole, sulfamethoxazole.
NSAIDs: propionic acid derivatives.
Miscellaneous: phenytoin, thiazides, allopurinol, cimetidine, ifosfamide.

INFECTIONS

Invasion of renal parenchyma.
Reaction to systemic infections: streptococcal, diphtheria, hantavirus.

SYSTEMIC DISEASES

Immune mediated: SLE, transplanted kidney, cryoglobulinemias.
Metabolic: Urate, oxalate.
Neoplastic: Lymphoproliferative diseases.

IDIOPATHIC

TUBULOINTERSTITIAL KIDNEY DISEASE[14]

ICD-9CM # 584.5

Ischemic and toxic acute tubular necrosis.
Allergic interstitial nephritis.
Interstitial nephritis secondary to immune complex-related collagen vascular disease (e.g., SLE, Sjögren's).
Granulomatous diseases (sarcoidosis, uveitis).
Pigment-related tubular injury (myoglobinuria, hemoglobinuria).
Hypercalcemia with nephrocalcinosis.
Tubular obstruction (drugs such as indinavir, uric acid in tumor lysis syndrome).
Myeloma kidney or cast nephropathy.
Infection-related interstitial nephritis: *Legionella, Leptospira*.
Infiltrative diseases (e.g., lymphoma).

TUMOR MARKERS ELEVATION[38]

ICD-9CM # 795.8

CAUSES OF ELEVATED LEVELS OF TUMOR MARKERS

Carcinoembryonic Antigen (CEA)
Colonic cancer (higher levels if the tumor is more differentiated or is extensive or has spread to the liver).
Lung or breast cancer; seminoma.
Cigarette smokers.
Cirrhosis, inflammatory bowel disease, rectal polyps, pancreatitis.
Advanced age.

Alpha Fetoprotein

Hepatocellular cancer: very high titers or a rising titer is strongly suggestive, but >10% of patients do not have an elevated level.

Hepatic regeneration (e.g., cirrhosis, alcoholic or viral hepatitis).

Cancer of the stomach, colon, pancreas, or lung.

Teratocarcinoma or embryonal cell carcinoma (testis, ovary, extragonadal).

Pregnancy.

Ataxia telangiectasia.

Normal variant.

Prostate-Specific Antigen

Prostate carcinoma (localized disease).

Prostatic hyperplasia.

Prostatitis.

Prostatic infarction.

Cancer-Associated Antigen (CA-19-9)*

Pancreatic carcinoma (80% with advanced, well-differentiated cancer have an elevated level).

Other gastrointestinal cancers: colon, stomach, bile duct.

Acute or chronic pancreatitis.

Chronic liver disease.

Biliary tract disease.

---

*Patients who cannot synthesize Lewis blood group antigens (~5% of the population) do not produce CA-19-9 antigen.

URETERAL COLIC[24a]
ICD-9CM # 788.0

DIAGNOSTIC DIFFERENTIALS OF RENAL OR URETERAL COLIC

Acute cholecystitis, acute cholelithiasis.

Acute appendicitis.

Pelvic inflammatory disease.

Diverticulosis and/or diverticulitis.

Intestinal obstruction.

Leaking abdominal aortic aneurysm.

Musculoskeletal sprains.

Herniated disc.

Hepes zoster (shingles).

Gastrointestinal dysfunction with ileus and/or toxic colonic dilatation.

URETERIC OBSTRUCTION, CONGENITAL[16a]
ICD-9CM # 593.4

CONGENITAL CAUSES OF URETERIC OBSTRUCTION

Primary megaureter.

Ureterocele (ectopic and orthotopic).

Ureteric valve.

Distal ureteric stenosis.

Ureteric atresia.

Circumcaval ureter and variants.

Bladder diverticulum.

URETHRAL DISCHARGE AND DYSURIA
ICD-9CM # 788.7 Urethral Discharge
            599.9 Urethral Discharge Bloody
            788.1 Dysuria

Urethritis (gonococcal, chlamydial, trichomonal).

Cystitis.

Prostatitis.

Vaginitis (candidiasis, chemical).

Meatal stenosis.

Interstitial cystitis.

Trauma (foreign body, masturbation, horseback or bike riding).

URETHRAL OBSTRUCTION, CHILDREN[16a]
ICD-9CM # 593.4

CAUSES OF URETHRAL OBSTRUCTION IN CHILDREN

Intrinsic lesions

Valve (posterior, anterior, saccular diverticulum).

Stenosis, atresia.

Inflammatory stricture.

Traumatic stricture:

External trauma (saddle injury, and so on).

Iatrogenic trauma (catheter, cystoscopy, surgery).

Urethral "tumors":

Girls: leiomyoma.

Boys: polyp, rhabdomyosarcoma.

Miscellaneous (epidemolysis bullosa).

Extrinsic lesions

Presacral mass dissecting inferiorly (tumor, cyst).

Fecal impaction (Hirschsprung's, postrepair anal atresia, habitual constipation, neuropathy).

Mass originating in genital organs:

Boys: utricle cyst, prostate rhabdomyosarcoma, seminal vesicle cyst, Cowper's duct cyst.

Girls: hydrometrocolpos, hydrocolpos, fused labia.

URIC ACID STONES
ICD-9CM # 792.9

Hyperuricemia.

Excessive dietary purine.

Medications (salicylates, allopurinol, probenecid).

Urine pH <5.5 (e.g., diarrhea, high animal protein diet).

Decreased urine output (dehydration, malabsorption, diarrhea, inadequate fluid intake).

Tumor lysis.

Hemolytic anemia.

Myeloproliferative disorders.

URINARY RETENTION[24a]
ICD-9CM # 788.20

COMMON CAUSES OF URINARY RETENTION

Obstructive Cause

Urethral stricture.

Enlarged prostate.

Lower genitourinary tract malignancy.

Pelvic malignancy.

Bladder stones.

Foreign body.

Blood clot.

Posterior urethral valves.

Ureterocele.

Primary Detrusor Insufficiency

Detrusor areflexia.

Multiple sclerosis.

Iatrogenic injury during abdominal or back surgery.

Spinal cord injury.

Myelomeningocele.

URINARY RETENTION, ACUTE
ICD-9CM # 788.20

Mechanical obstruction: urethral stone, foreign body, urethral stricture, BPH, prostate carcinoma, prostatitis, trauma with hematoma formation.

Neurogenic bladder.

Neurologic disease (MS, parkinsonism, tabes dorsalis, CVA).

Spinal cord injury.

CNS neoplasm (primary or metastatic).

Spinal anesthesia.

Lower urinary tract instrumentation.

Medications (antihistamines, antidepressants, narcotics, anticholinergics).

Abdominal or pelvic surgery.

Alcohol toxicity.

Pregnancy.

Anxiety.

Encephalitis.

Postoperative pain.

Spina bifida occulta.

URINE CASTS
ICD-9CM # 791.7

Normal finding.

Pyelonephritis.

Chronic renal disease.

Nephrotic syndrome.

Acute tubular necrosis.

Interstitial nephritis.

Nephritic syndrome.

Glomerulonephritis.

Eclampsia.

Heavy metal ingestion.

Allograft rejection.

Hypothyroidism.

URINE COLOR ABNORMALITIES[24a]
ICD-9CM # 791.9

COMMON CAUSES OF ABNORMAL URINE COLOR

Colorless

Disease

Diabetes mellitus.

Diabetes insipidus.

Drug

Ethyl alcohol.

Diuretics.

Miscellaneous
Overhydration.
Yellow-orange
Drug
Tetracycline.
Flutamide.
Pyridium.
Azo Gantrisin (Roche Labs, Nutley, NJ).
Sulfasalazine.
Vitamin B.
Miscellaneous
Dehydration.
Milky white
Disease
Urinary tract infection/pyuria.
Blue-green
Disease
Pseudomonas urinary tract infection.
Drug
Methylene blue.
Urised (Polymedica Pharmaceuticals, Woburn, MA).
Indigo carmine.
Doan's pills (Novartis Consumer Health, Parsippany, NJ).
Clorets (Cadbury Adams, Parsippany, NJ).
Amitriptyline.
Red-brown
Disease
Hematuria.
Hemolytic anemia.
Hemoglobinuria.
Lead poisoning.
Mercury poisoning.
Porphyria.
Drug
Rifampin.
Ex-Lax (Novartis Consumer Health, Parsippany, NJ).
Phenolphthalein.
Phenothiazines.
Nitrofurantoin.
Doxorubicin.
Miscellaneous
Beets.
Blackberries.
Rhubarb.
Brown-black
Disease
Fecaluria.
Methemoglobinuria.
Melaninuria.
Drug
Metronidazole.
Methyldopa.
Methocarbamol.
Miscellaneous
Fava beans.
Aloe.

URINE, RED[29]

ICD-9CM # varies with specific diagnosis

WITH A POSITIVE DIPSTICK
Hematuria.
Hemoglobinuria: negative urinalysis.
Myoglobinuria: negative urinalysis.

WITH A NEGATIVE DIPSTICK
Drugs
Aminosalicylic acid.
Deferoxamine mesylate.
Ibuprofen.
Phenacetin.
Phenolphthalein.
Phensuximide.
Rifampin.
Anthraquinone laxatives.
Doxorubicin.
Methyldopa.
Phenazopyridine.
Phenothiazine.
Phenytoin.
Dyes
Azo dyes.
Eosin.
Foods
Beets, berries, maize.
Rhodamine B.
Metabolic
Porphyrins.
Serratia marcescens (red diaper syndrome).
Urate crystalluria.

UROPATHY, OBSTRUCTIVE[36]

ICD-9CM # 599.6

INTRINSIC CAUSES
Intraluminal
Intratubular deposition of crystals (uric acid, sulfas).
Stones.
Papillary tissue.
Blood clots.
Intramural
Functional.
Ureter (ureteropelvic or ureterovesical dysfunction).
Bladder (neurogenic): spinal cord defect or trauma, diabetes, multiple sclerosis, Parkinson's disease, cerebrovascular accidents.
Bladder neck dysfunction.
Anatomic
Tumors.
Infection, granuloma.
Strictures.

EXTRINSIC CAUSES
Originating in the Reproductive System
Prostate: benign hypertrophy or cancer.
Uterus: pregnancy, tumors, prolapse, endometriosis.
Ovary: abscess, tumor, cysts.
Originating in the Vascular System
Aneurysms (aorta, iliac vessels).
Aberrant arteries (ureteropelvic junction).
Venous (ovarian veins, retrocaval ureter).
Originating in the Gastrointestinal Tract
Crohn's disease.
Pancreatitis.
Appendicitis.
Tumors.
Originating in the Retroperitoneal Space
Inflammations.
Fibrosis.
Tumor, hematomas.

UROSEPSIS[24a]

ICD-9CM # 995.91

COMMON CAUSES OF UROSEPSIS
Obstructing ureteral stone with pyonephrosis.
Staghorn calculus with urinary tract infection.
Ureteral obstruction with proximal urinary tract infection.
Urinary retention with urinary tract infection.
Acute prostatitis with prostatic abscess.
Perinephric abscess or renal carbuncle.
Urethral stricture with periurethral abscess.
Fournier gangrene.
Foreign body within urinary tract (e.g., Foley catheter).

UTERINE BLEEDING, ABNORMAL[12]

ICD-9CM # 626.9

PREGNANCY
Threatened abortion.
Incomplete abortion.
Complete abortion.
Molar pregnancy.
Ectopic pregnancy.
Retained products of conception.

OVULATORY
Vulva: infection, laceration, tumor.
Vagina: infection, laceration, tumor, foreign body.
Cervix: polyps, cervical erosion, cervicitis, carcinoma.
Uterus: fibroids (submucous fibroids most likely to cause abnormal bleeding), polyps, adenomyosis, endometritis, intrauterine device, atrophic endometrium.
Pregnancy complications: ectopic pregnancy; threatened, incomplete, complete abortion; retained products of conception.
Abnormality of clotting system.
Midcycle bleeding.
Halban's disease (persistent corpus luteum).
Menorrhagia.
Pelvic inflammatory disease.

ANOVULATORY
Physiologic causes:
  Puberty.
  Perimenopausal.
Pathologic causes:
  Ovarian failure (FSH over 40 IU/ml).
  Hyperandrogenism.
  Hyperprolactinemia.
  Obesity.
  Hypothalamic dysfunction (polycystic ovaries); LH/FSH ratio greater than 2:1.
  Hyperplasia.
  Endometrial carcinoma.
  Estrogen-producing tumors.
  Hypothyroidism.

Differential Diagnosis

II

VAGINAL BLEEDING, PREGNANCY[7]

ICD-9CM # 626.6 Irregular Vaginal Bleeding

FIRST TRIMESTER

Implantation bleeding.
Abortion.
   Threatened.
   Complete.
   Incomplete.
   Missed.
Ectopic pregnancy.
Neoplasia.
Hydatidiform mole.
Cervix.

THIRD TRIMESTER

Placenta previa.
Placental abruption.
Premature labor.
Choriocarcinoma.

VAGINAL DISCHARGE, PREPUBERTAL GIRLS[19]

ICD-9CM # 623.5 Vaginal Discharge

Irritative (bubble baths, sand).
Poor perineal hygiene.
Foreign body.
Associated systemic illness (group A streptococci, chickenpox).
Infections.
Escherichia coli with foreign body.
Shigella organisms.
Yersinia organisms.
Infections (consider sexual abuse).
   Chlamydia trachomatis.
   Neisseria gonorrhoeae.
   Trichomonas vaginalis.
Tumor (rare).

VALVULAR HEART DISEASE[1]

ICD-9CM # varies with specific diagnosis

MAJOR CAUSES OF VALVULAR HEART DISEASE IN ADULTS

Aortic Stenosis
Bicuspid aortic valve.
Rheumatic fever.
Degenerative stenosis.
Aortic Regurgitation
Bicuspid aortic valve.
Aortic dissection.
Endocarditis.
Rheumatic fever.
Aortic root dilation.
Mitral Stenosis
Rheumatic fever.
Mitral Regurgitation
Chronic
Mitral valve prolapse.
Left ventricular dilation.
Posterior wall myocardial infarction.
Rheumatic fever.
Endocarditis.

Acute
Posterior wall or papillary muscle ischemia.
Papillary muscle or chordal rupture.
Endocarditis.
Prosthetic valve dysfunction.
Systolic anterior motion of mitral valve.
Tricuspid Regurgitation
Functional (annular) dilation.
Tricuspid valve prolapse.
Endocarditis.
Carcinoid heart disease.

VASCULITIS, CLASSIFICATION[26]

ICD-9CM # 447.6

LARGE VESSEL DISEASE

Arteritis
Giant cell arteritis.
Takayasu's arteritis.
Arteritis associated with Reiter's syndrome, ankylosing spondylitis.

MEDIUM AND SMALL VESSEL DISEASE

Polyarteritis Nodosa
Primary (idiopathic).
Associated with viruses (Hepatitis B or C, CMV, HIV, herpes zoster).
Associated with malignancy (hairy cell leukemia).
Familial Mediterranean fever.
Granulomatous Vasculitis
Wegener's granulomatosis.
Lymphomatoid granulomatosis.
Behçet's Disease
Kawasaki Disease (Mucocutaneous Lymph Node Syndrome)

PREDOMINANTLY SMALL VESSEL DISEASE

Hypersensitivity Vasculitis (Leukocytoclastic Vasculitis)
Henoch-Schönlein purpura.
Mixed cryoglobulinemia.
Serum sickness.
Vasculitis associated with connective tissue diseases (SLE, Sjögren's syndrome).
Vasculitis associated with specific syndromes:
   Primary biliary cirrhosis.
   Lyme disease.
   Chronic active hepatitis.
   Drug-induced vasculitis.
Churg-Strauss Syndrome
Goodpasture's Syndrome
Erythema Nodosum
Panniculitis
Buerger's Disease (Thrombophlebitis Obliterans)

VASCULITIS (DISEASES THAT MIMIC VASCULITIS)[28]

ICD-9CM # varies with specific disease

EMBOLIC DISEASE

Infectious or marantic endocarditis.
Cardiac mural thrombus.

Atrial myxoma.
Cholesterol embolization syndrome.

NONINFLAMMATORY VESSEL WALL DISRUPTION

Atherosclerosis.
Arterial fibromuscular dysplasia.
Drug effects (vasoconstrictors, anticoagulants).
Radiation.
Genetic disease (neurofibromatosis, Ehlers-Danlos syndrome).
Amyloidosis.
Intravascular malignant lymphoma.

DIFFUSE COAGULATION

Disseminated intravascular coagulation.
Thrombotic thrombocytopenic purpura.
Hemolytic-uremic syndrome.
Protein C and S deficiencies, factor V/Leiden mutation.
Antiphospholipid syndrome.

VEGETATIVE STATE, PERSISTENT[1]

ICD-9CM # 780.03

PERSISTENT VEGETATIVE STATE: COMMON CAUSES*

Trauma (diffuse axonal injury).
Cardiac arrest and hypoperfusion (laminar necrosis of cortical mantle and/or thalamic necrosis).
Bihemispheric infarctions.
Purulent meningitis or encephalitis (cortical injury).
Carbon monoxide.
Prolonged hypoglycemic coma.

---

*A vegetative state may not necessarily begin with coma but can also develop as the end stage of neurodegenerative diseases (e.g., Alzheimer's disease) of adults or children and can accompany severe congenital developmental abnormalities of the brain such as anencephaly.

VENTILATION–PERFUSION MISMATCH ON LUNG SCAN

ICD-9CM # varies with specific disorder

Pulmonary embolism.
Emphysema.
Irradiation.
Pulmonary hypertension.
AV malformations.
Pulmonary thrombosis.
External compression of pulmonary artery (neoplasm, cysts, fibrosing mediastinitis).
Vasculitis.
Tuberculosis.
Pulmonary thrombosis.
Congenital (pulmonary artery hypoplasia, congenital heart disease with upper lobe diversion).
Sequestered segment.
Parasitic lung disease.
Intraluminal obstruction from catheter fragments.

VENTRICULAR FAILURE
ICD-9CM # 429.9 Ventricular Dysfunction

LEFT VENTRICULAR FAILURE
Systemic hypertension.
Valvular heart disease (AS, AR, MR).
Cardiomyopathy, myocarditis.
Bacterial endocarditis.
Myocardial infarction.
Idiopathic hypertrophic subaortic stenosis.

RIGHT VENTRICULAR FAILURE
Valvular heart disease (mitral stenosis).
Pulmonary hypertension.
Bacterial endocarditis (right-sided).
Right ventricular infarction.

BIVENTRICULAR FAILURE
Left ventricular failure.
Cardiomyopathy.
Myocarditis
Arrhythmias.
Anemia.
Thyrotoxicosis.
Arteriovenous fistula.
Paget's disease.
Beriberi.

VERRUCOUS LESIONS
ICD-9CM # varies with specific disorder

Warts.
Seborrheic keratosis.
Lichen simplex.
Acanthosis nigricans.
Scabies (Norwegian, crusted).
Verrucous carcinoma.
Nevus sebaceous.
Deep fungal infection.

VERTIGO
ICD-9CM # 780.4 Vertigo NOS
386.11 Benign Paroxysmal Positional
386.2 Central Origin
386.10 Peripheral
386.12 Vestibular (Neuronitis)

PERIPHERAL
Otitis media.
Acute labyrinthitis.
Vestibular neuronitis.
Benign positional vertigo.
Ménière's disease.
Ototoxic drugs: streptomycin, gentamicin.
Lesions of the eighth nerve: acoustic neuroma, meningioma, mononeuropathy, metastatic carcinoma.
Mastoiditis.

CNS OR SYSTEMIC
Vertebrobasilar artery insufficiency.
Posterior fossa tumor or other brain tumors.
Infarction/hemorrhage of cerebral cortex, cerebellum, or brainstem.
Basilar migraine.
Metabolic: drugs, hypoxia, anemia, fever.

Hypotension/severe hypertension.
Multiple sclerosis.
CNS infections: viral, bacterial.
Temporal lobe epilepsy.
Arnold–Chiari malformation, syringobulbia.
Psychogenic: ventilation, hysteria.

VESICULOBULLOUS DISEASES[14]
ICD-9CM # 709.8

IMMUNOLOGICALLY MEDIATED DISEASES
Bullous pemphigoid.
Herpes gestationis.
Mucous membrane pemphigoid.
Epidermolysis bullosa acquisita.
Dermatitis herpetiformis.
Pemphigus (vulgaris, foliaceus, paraneoplastic).

HYPERSENSITIVITY DISEASES
Erythema multiforme minor.
Erythema multiforme major (Stevens-Johnson syndrome).
Toxic epidermal necrolysis.

METABOLIC DISEASES
Porphyria cutanea tarda.
Pseudoporphyria.
Diabetic blisters.

INHERITED GENETIC DISORDERS
Epidermolysis bullosa.
Simplex.
Junctional.
Dystrophic.

INFECTIOUS DISEASES
Impetigo.
Staphylococcal scalded skin syndrome.
Herpes simplex.
Varicella.
Herpes zoster.

VISION LOSS, ACUTE, PAINFUL
ICD-9CM # 368.11 Vision Loss, Sudden

Acute angle-closure glaucoma.
Corneal ulcer.
Uveitis.
Endophthalmitis.
Factitious.
Somatization syndrome.
Trauma.

VISION LOSS, ACUTE, PAINLESS
ICD-9CM # 368.11 Vision Loss, Sudden

Retinal artery occlusion.
Optic neuritis.
Retinal vein occlusion.
Vitreous hemorrhage.
Retinal detachment.
Exudative macular degeneration.
CVA.

Ischemic optic neuropathy.
Factitious.
Somatization syndrome, anxiety reaction.

VISION LOSS, CHILDREN
ICD-9CM # 368.9

Craniopharyngioma.
Hereditary optic atrophy.
Optic nerve glioma.
Glioma of chiasm.
Albinism.
Optic nerve hypoplasia.

VISION LOSS, CHRONIC, PROGRESSIVE
ICD-9CM # 369.9 Vision Loss NOS

Cataract.
Macular degeneration.
Cerebral neoplasm.
Refractive error.
Open-angle glaucoma.

VISION LOSS, MONOCULAR, TRANSIENT
ICD-9CM # 369.9

Thromboembolism.
Vasculitis.
Migraine (vasospasm).
Anxiety reaction.
CNS tumor.
Temporal arteritis.
Multiple sclerosis.

VOCAL CORD PARALYSIS
ICD-9CM # 478.30 Unspecified
478.31 Unilateral Partial
478.32 Unilateral Complete
478.33 Bilateral Partial
478.34 Bilateral Complete

Neoplasm: primary or metastatic (e.g., lung, thyroid, parathyroid, mediastinum).
Neck surgery (parathyroid, thyroid, carotid endarterectomy, cervical spine).
Idiopathic.
Viral, bacterial, or fungal infection.
Trauma (intubation, penetrating neck injury).
Cardiac surgery.
RA.
Multiple sclerosis.
Parkinsonism.
Toxic neuropathy.
CVA.
CNS abnormalities: hydrocephalus, Arnold–Chiari malformation, meningomyelocele.

VOLUME DEPLETION[1]
ICD-9CM # 276.5

GI losses:
Upper: bleeding, nasogastric suction, vomiting.
Lower: bleeding, diarrhea, enteric or pancreatic fistula, tube drainage.

Renal losses:
  Salt and water: diuretics, osmotic diuresis, postobstructive diuresis, acute tubular necrosis (recovery phase), salt-losing nephropathy, adrenal insufficiency, renal tubular acidosis.
Water loss: diabetes insipidus.
Skin and respiratory losses:
  Sweat, burns, insensible losses.
Sequestration without external fluid loss:
  Intestinal obstruction, peritonitis, pancreatitis, rhabdomyolysis, internal bleeding.

VOLUME EXCESS[1]

ICD-9CM # varies with specific diagnosis

PRIMARY RENAL SODIUM RETENTION (INCREASED EFFECTIVE CIRCULATING VOLUME)

Renal failure, nephritic syndrome, acute glomerulonephritis.
Primary hyperaldosteronism.
Cushing's syndrome.
Liver disease.

SECONDARY RENAL SODIUM RETENTION (DECREASED EFFECTIVE CIRCULATING VOLUME)

Heart failure.
Liver disease.
Nephrotic syndrome (minimal change disease).
Pregnancy.

VOMITING

ICD-9CM # 787.03

GI disturbances:
  Obstruction: esophageal, pyloric, intestinal.
  Infections: viral or bacterial enteritis, viral hepatitis, food poisoning, gastroenteritis.
  Pancreatitis.
  Appendicitis.
  Biliary colic.
  Peritonitis.
  Perforated bowel.
  Diabetic gastroparesis.
Other: gastritis, PUD, IBD, GI tract neoplasms.
Drugs: morphine, digitalis, cytotoxic agents, bromocriptine.
Severe pain: MI, renal colic.
Metabolic disorders: uremia, acidosis/alkalosis, hyperglycemia, DKA, thyrotoxicosis.
Trauma: blows to the testicles, epigastrium.
Vertigo.
Reye's syndrome.
Increased intracranial pressure.
CNS disturbances: trauma, hemorrhage, infarction, neoplasm, infection, hypertensive encephalopathy, migraine.
Radiation sickness.
Nausea and vomiting of pregnancy, hyperemesis gravidarum.
Motion sickness.
Bulimia, anorexia nervosa.
Psychogenic: emotional disturbances, offensive sights or smells.

Severe coughing.
Pyelonephritis.
Boerhaave's syndrome.
Carbon monoxide poisoning.

VULVAR LESIONS[12]

ICD-9CM #		
	625.8	Vulvar Mass
	098.0	Vulvar Ulcer, Gonococcal
	091.0	Vulvar Ulcer, Syphilitic
	616.51	Behçet's
	624.0	Leukoplakia
	624.8	Dysplasia
	233.3	Carcinoma
	616.9	Inflammatory Lesion
	624.4	Vulvar Scar (Old)
	624.1	Vulvar Atrophy

RED LESION

Infection/Infestation
Fung I infection:
  Candida.
  Tinea cruris.
  Intertrigo.
  Pityriasis versicolor.
Sarcoptes scabiei.
Erythrasma: *Corynebacterium minutissimum.*
Granuloma inguinale: *Calymmatobacterium granulomatis.*
Folliculitis: *Staphylococcus aureus.*
Hidradenitis suppurativa.
Behçet's syndrome.

Inflammation
Reactive vulvitis.
Chemical irritation:
  Detergent.
  Dyes.
  Perfume.
  Spermicide.
  Lubricants.
  Hygiene sprays.
  Podophyllum.
  Topical 5-FU.
  Saliva.
  Gentian violet.
  Semen.
Mechanical trauma: scratching.
Vestibular adenitis.
Essential vulvodynia.
Psoriasis.
Seborrheic dermatitis.

Neoplasm
Vulvar intraepithelial neoplasia (VIN):
  Mild dysplasia.
  Moderate dysplasia.
  Severe dysplasia.
  Carcinoma-in-situ.
Vulvar dystrophy.
Bowen's disease.
Invasive cancer:
  Squamous cell carcinoma.
  Malignant melanoma.
  Sarcoma.
  Basal cell carcinoma.
  Adenocarcinoma.
  Paget's disease.
  Undifferentiated.

WHITE LESION

Vulvar dystrophy:
  Lichen sclerosus.
  Vulvar dystrophy.
  Vulvar hyperplasia.
  Mixed dystrophy.
VIN.
Vitiligo.
Partial albinism.
Intertrigo.
Radiation treatment.

DARK LESION

Lentigo.
Nevi (mole).
Neoplasm (see Neoplasm, Vulvar, below).
Reactive hyperpigmentation.
Seborrheic keratosis.
Pubic lice.

ULCERATIVE LESION

Infection
Herpes simplex.
Vaccinia.
Treponema pallidum.
Granuloma inguinale.
Pyoderma.
Tuberculosis.

Noninfection
Behçet's disease.
Crohn's disease.
Pemphigus.
Pemphigoid.
Hidradenitis suppurativa (see Neoplasm, Vulvar, below).

Neoplasm
Basal cell carcinoma.
Squamous cell carcinoma.
Vulvar tumor <1 cm:
  Condyloma acuminatum.
  Molluscum contagiosum.
  Epidermal inclusion.
  Vestibular cyst.
  Mesonephric duct.
  VIN.
  Hemangioma.
  Hidradenoma.
  Neurofibroma.
  Syringoma.
  Accessory breast tissue.
  Acrochordon.
  Endometriosis.
  Fox-Fordyce disease.
  Pilonidal sinus.
Vulvar tumor >1 cm:
  Bartholin cyst or abscess.
  Lymphogranuloma venereum.
  Fibroma.
  Lipoma.
  Verrucous carcinoma.
  Squamous cell carcinoma.
  Hernia.
  Edema.
  Hematoma.
  Acrochordon.
  Epidermal cysts.
  Neurofibromatosis.
  Accessory breast tissue.

WEAKNESS, ACUTE, EMERGENT[26]

ICD-9CM # 780.7

Demyelinating disorders (Guillain-Barré, chronic inflammatory demyelinating polyneuropathy [CIDP]).
Myasthenia gravis.
Infectious (poliomyelitis, diphtheria).
Toxic (botulism, tick paralysis, paralytic shellfish toxin, puffer fish, newts).
Metabolic (acquired or familial hypokalemia, hypophosphatemia, hypermagnesemia).
Metal poisoning (arsenic, thallium).
Porphyria.

WEAKNESS, GRADUAL ONSET

ICD-9CM # 780.7

Depression.
Malingering.
Anemia.
Hypothyroidism.
Medications (e.g., sedatives, antidepressants, narcotics).
CHF.
Renal failure.
Liver failure.
Respiratory insufficiency.
Alcoholism.
Nutritional deficiencies.
Disorders of motor unit.
Basal ganglia disorders.
Upper motor neuron lesions.

WEAKNESS, NONNEUROMUSCULAR CAUSES

ICD-9CM # 780.79

Anxiety disorder.
Infectious process.
Anemia.
Renal insufficiency.
Hyperventilation.
Malignancy.
Hypothyroidism.
Hypotension.
Hypercapnia.
Hypoglycemia.
Cardiac arrhythmias.
Hepatic insufficiency.
Electrolyte imbalance.
Malnutrition.
Cerebrovascular insufficiency.

WEIGHT GAIN

ICD-9CM # 783.1   Abnormal Weight Gain
             278.00 Obesity

Sedentary lifestyle.
Fluid overload.
Discontinuation of tobacco abuse.

Endocrine disorders (hypothyroidism, hyperinsulinism associated with maturity-onset DM, Cushing's syndrome, hypogonadism, insulinoma, hyperprolactinemia, acromegaly).
Medications (nutritional supplements, oral contraceptives, glucocorticoids, etc.).
Anxiety disorders with compulsive eating.
Laurence-Moon-Biedl syndrome, Prader-Willi syndrome, other congenital diseases.
Hypothalamic injury (rare; <100 cases reported in medical literature).

WEIGHT LOSS

ICD-9CM # 783.2 Abnormal Weight Loss

Malignancy.
Psychiatric disorders (depression, anorexia nervosa).
New-onset DM.
Malabsorption.
COPD.
AIDS.
Uremia, liver disease.
Thyrotoxicosis, pheochromocytoma, carcinoid syndrome.
Addison's disease.
Intestinal parasites.
Peptic ulcer disease.
Inflammatory bowel disease.
Food faddism.
Postgastrectomy syndrome.

WHEEZING

ICD-9CM # 786.09

Asthma.
COPD.
Interstitial lung disease.
Infections (pneumonia, bronchitis, bronchiolitis, epiglottitis).
Cardiac asthma.
GERD with aspiration.
Foreign body aspiration.
Pulmonary embolism.
Anaphylaxis.
Obstruction of airway (neoplasm, goiter, edema or hemorrhage from trauma, aneurysm, congenital abnormalities, strictures, spasm).
Carcinoid syndrome.

WHEEZING, PEDIATRIC AGE[4]

ICD-9CM # 786.09 Wheezing

Reactive airways disease.
Atopic asthma.
Infection-associated airway reactivity.
Exercise-induced asthma.
Salicylate-induced asthma and nasal polyposis.
Asthmatic bronchitis.
Other hypersensitivity reactions:
    Hypersensitivity pneumonitis.
    Tropical eosinophilia.
    Visceral larva migrans.
    Allergic bronchopulmonary aspergillosis.
Aspiration:
    Foreign body.
    Food, saliva, gastric contents.
    Laryngotracheoesophageal cleft.

Tracheoesophageal fistula, H-type.
Pharyngeal incoordination or neuromuscular weakness.
Cystic fibrosis.
Primary ciliary dyskinesia.
Cardiac failure.
Bronchiolitis obliterans.
Extrinsic compression of airways:
    Vascular ring.
    Enlarged lymph node.
    Mediastinal tumor.
    Lung cysts.
Tracheobronchomalacia.
Endobronchial masses.
Gastroesophageal reflux.
Pulmonary hemosiderosis.
Sequelae of bronchopulmonary dysplasia.
"Hysterical" glottic closure.
Cigarette smoke, other environmental insults.

WRIST AND HAND PAIN, IN DIFFERENT AGE GROUPS[8]

ICD-9CM # 959.3

COMMON CAUSES OF WRIST AND HAND PAIN IN DIFFERENT AGE GROUPS

Childhood (2-10 yr)
Intraarticular:
Infection.
Periarticular:
Fracture.
Osteomyelitis.
Adolescence (10-18 yr)
Intraarticular:
Infection.
Periarticular:
Trauma.
Osteomyelitis.
Tumors.
Ganglion.
Idiopathic wrist pain.
Early adulthood (18-30 yr)
Intraarticular:
Inflammatory arthritis.
Infection.
Osteoarthritis.
Periarticular:
Peripheral nerve entrapment.
Tendonitis.
Referred:
Cervical.
Adulthood (30-50 yr)
Intraarticular:
Inflammatory arthritis.
Infection.
Osteoarthritis.
Periarticular:
Peripheral nerve entrapment.
Tendonitis.
Referred:
Cervical.
Chest.
Cardiac.
Old age (>50 yr)
Intraarticular:
Inflammatory arthritis.
Osteoarthritis.

Differential Diagnosis

II

Periarticular:
Peripheral nerve entrapment.
Tendonitis.
Referred:
Cervical.
Chest.
Cardiac.

WRIST PAIN
ICD-9CM # 959.3

MECHANICAL
Osteoarthritis.
Ligament tear.
Fracture.
Ganglion.
De Quervain's tenosynovitis.
Avascular necrosis (scaphoid, lunate).
Nonunion of scaphoid or lunate.
Neoplasm.

METABOLIC
Pregnancy.
Diabetes.
Gout.
Pseudogout.
Paget's disease.
Acromegaly.
Hypothyroidism.
Hyperparathyroidism.

INFECTIOUS
Osteomyelitis.
Septic arthritis.
Cat-scratch disease.
Tick bite (Lyme disease, babesiosis).
Tuberculosis.

NEUROLOGIC
Peripheral neuropathy.
Nerve injury (median, ulnar, radial nerve).
Thoracic outlet compression syndrome.
Distal posterior interosseous nerve syndrome.

RHEUMATOLOGIC
Psoriasis.
RA.
SLE, mixed connective tissue disorder (MCTD).
Scleroderma.

MISCELLANEOUS
Granulomatous (sarcoidosis).
Amyloidosis.
Multiple myeloma.
Leukemia.

XEROPHTHALMIA[28]
ICD-9CM # 372.53 Xerophthalmia

MEDICATIONS
Tricyclic antidepressants: amitriptyline (Elavil), doxepin (Sinequan).
Antihistamines: diphenhydramine (Benadryl), chlorpheniramine (Chlor-Trimeton), promethazine (Phenergan), and many cold and decongestant preparations.
Anticholinergic agents: antiemetics such as scopolamine, antispasmodic agents such as oxybutynin chloride (Ditropan).

ABNORMALITIES OF EYELID FUNCTION
Neuromuscular disorders.
Aging.
Thyrotoxicosis.

ABNORMALITIES OF TEAR PRODUCTION
Hypovitaminosis A.
Stevens-Johnson syndrome.
Familial diseases affecting sebaceous secretions.

ABNORMALITIES OF CORNEAL SURFACES
Scarring from past injuries and herpes simplex infection.

XEROSTOMIA[28]
ICD-9CM # 527.7

MEDICATIONS
Tricyclic antidepressants: amitriptyline (Elavil), doxepin (Sinequan).
Antihistamines: diphenhydramine (Benadryl), chlorpheniramine (Chlor-Trimeton), promethazine (Phenergan), and many cold and decongestant preparations.
Anticholinergic agents: antiemetics such as scopolamine, antispasmodic agents such as oxybutynin chloride (Ditropan).

DEHYDRATION
Debility.
Fever.

POLYURIA
Alcohol intake.
Arrhythmia.
Diabetes.

PREVIOUS HEAD AND NECK IRRADIATION SYSTEMIC DISEASES
Sjögren's syndrome.
Sarcoidosis.
Amyloidosis.
Human immunodeficiency virus (HIV) infection.
Graft-versus-host disease.

YELLOW URINE
ICD-9CM # 788.69

Normal coloration.
Concentrated urine.
Use of multivitamin supplements.
Diet rich in carrots.
Use of Cascara.
Urinary tract infection.

REFERENCES

1. Andreoli TE (ed): *Cecil essentials of medicine,* ed 5, Philadelphia, 2001, WB Saunders.
2. Barkin RM, Rosen P: *Emergency pediatrics: a guide to ambulatory care,* ed 5, St Louis, 1998, Mosby.
3. Baude AI: *Infectious diseases and medical microbiology,* ed 2, Philadelphia, 1986, WB Saunders.
4. Behrman RE: *Nelson textbook of pediatrics,* ed 16, Philadelphia, 2000, WB Saunders.
5. Callen JP: *Color atlas of dermatology,* ed 2, Philadelphia, 2000, WB Saunders.
6. Canoso J: *Rheumatology in primary care,* Philadelphia, 1997, WB Saunders.
7. Carlson KJ: *Primary care of women,* ed 2, St Louis, 2000, Mosby.
8. Carr A, Hamilton W: *Orthopedics in primary care,* ed 2, Philadelphia, 2005, Elsevier.
9. Conn R: *Current diagnosis,* ed 9, Philadelphia, 1997, WB Saunders.
10. Copeland LJ: *Textbook of gynecology,* ed 2, Philadelphia, 2000, WB Saunders.
11. Custer JW, Rau RE: *The Harriet Lane handbook,* ed 18, St Louis, Mosby, 2009.
12. Danakas G (ed): *Practical guide to the care of the gynecologic/obstetric patient,* St Louis, 1997, Mosby.
13. Goldberg RJ: *The care of the psychiatric patient,* ed 3, St Louis, 2006, Mosby.
14. Goldman L, Ausiello D: *Cecil textbook of medicine,* ed 21, Philadelphia, 2004, WB Saunders.
15. Goldman L, Braunwauld E (eds): *Primary cardiology,* Philadelphia, 1998, WB Saunders.
16. Gorbach SL: *Infectious diseases,* ed 2, Philadelphia, 1998, WB Saunders.

16a. Grainger RG, Allison D: *Grainger & Allison's diagnostic radiology, a textbook of medical imaging,* ed 4, London, 2001, Churchill Livingstone.

17. Harrington J: *Consultation in internal medicine,* ed 2, St Louis, 1997, Mosby.

18. Henry JB: *Clinical diagnosis and management by laboratory methods,* ed 20, Philadelphia, 2001, WB Saunders.

19. Hoekelman R: *Primary pediatric care,* ed 3, St Louis, 1997, Mosby.

20. Hoffmann R et al: *Hematology, Basic principles and practice,* ed 5, Philadelphia, 2009, Churchill Livingstone.

21. Kassirer J (ed): *Current therapy in adult medicine,* ed 4, St Louis, 1998, Mosby.

22. Khan MG: *Rapid ECG interpretation,* Philadelphia, 2003, WB Saunders.

23. Kliegman R: *Practical strategies in pediatric diagnosis and therapy,* Philadelphia, 1996, WB Saunders.

24. Klippel J (ed): *Practical rheumatology,* London, 1995, Mosby.

24a. Lipshultz LI, Khera M, Atwal DT: *Urology and the primary care practitioner,* ed 3, Philadelphia, 2008, Elsevier.

25. Mandell GL: *Mandell, Douglas, and Bennett's principles and practice of infectious diseases,* ed 6, New York, 2005, Churchill Livingstone.

26. Marx J (ed): *Rosen's emergency medicine: concepts and clinical practice,* ed 5, St Louis, 2002, Mosby.

27. Moore WT, Eastman RC: *Diagnostic endocrinology,* ed 2, St Louis, 1996, Mosby.

28. Noble J (ed): *Primary care medicine,* ed 3, St Louis, 2001, Mosby.

29. Nseyo UO: *Urology for primary care physicians,* Philadelphia, 1999, WB Saunders.

30. Palay D (ed): *Ophthalmology for the primary care physician,* St Louis, 1997, Mosby.

31. Rakel RE: *Principles of family practice,* ed 6, Philadelphia, 2002, WB Saunders.

32. Schwarz MI: *Interstitial lung disease,* ed 2, St Louis, 1993, Mosby.

33. Seller RH: *Differential diagnosis of common complaints,* ed 4, Philadelphia, 2000, WB Saunders.

34. Siedel HM (ed): *Mosby's guide to physical examination,* ed 4, St Louis, 1999, Mosby.

34a. Souhami RL, Moxham J: *Textbook of medicine,* ed 4, London, 2002, Churchill Livingstone.

35. Specht N: *Practical guide to diagnostic imaging,* St Louis, 1998, Mosby.

36. Stein JH (ed): *Internal medicine,* ed 5, St Louis, 1998, Mosby.

37. Swain R, Snodgrass: *Phys Sportmed* 23:56, 1995.

38. Talley NJ, Martin CJ: *Clinical gastroenterology,* ed 2, Sydney, 2006, Churchill Livingstone.

39. Weinberg SE et al: *Principles of pulmonary medicine,* ed 5, Philadelphia, 2008, Saunders.

40. Wiederholt WC: *Neurology for non-neurologists,* ed 4, Philadelphia, 2000, WB Saunders.

41. Wilson JD: *Williams textbook of endocrinology,* ed 9, Philadelphia, 1998, WB Saunders.

Differential
Diagnosis

II

Clinical Algorithms

PLEASE NOTE: These algorithms are designed to assist clinicians in the evaluation and treatment of patients. They may not apply to all patients with a particular disorder and are not intended to replace the clinician's individual judgment.

Additional algorithms available at www.expertconsult.com:

Clinical Algorithms

III

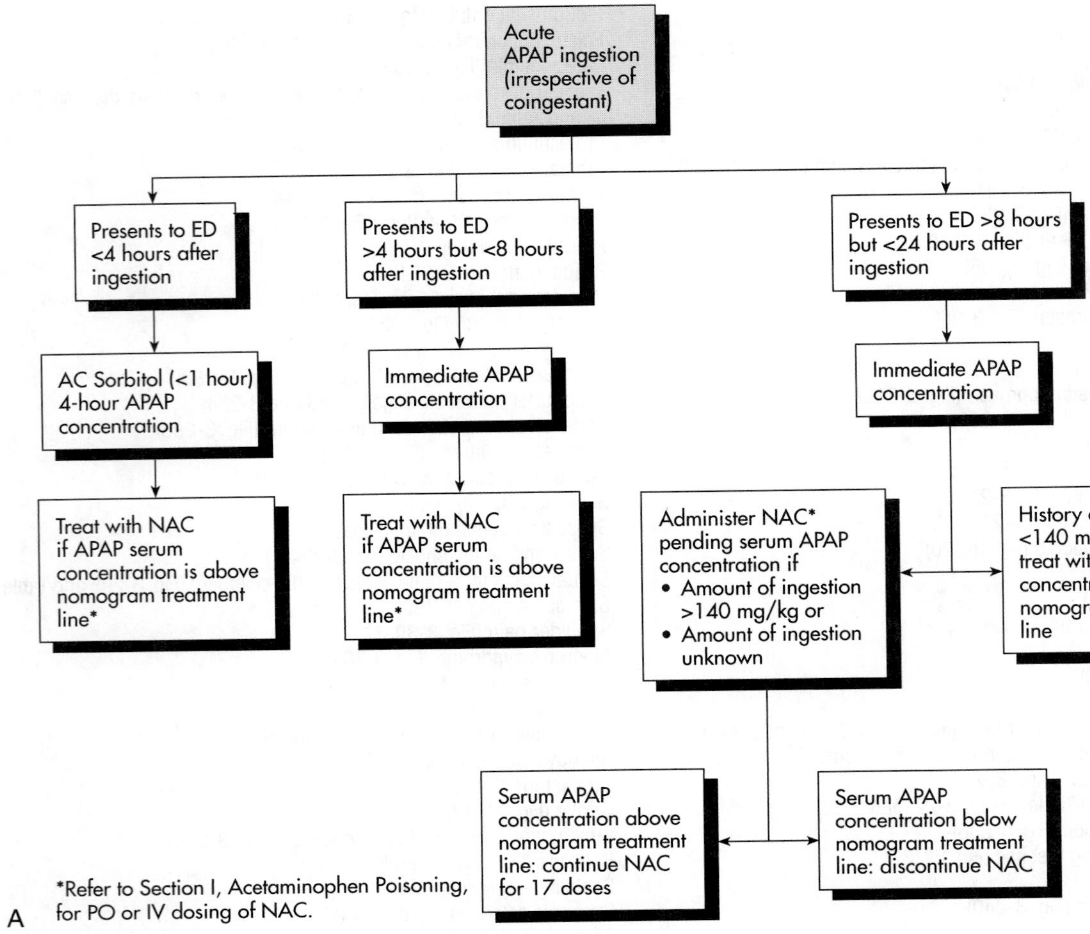

Acute
APAP ingestion
(irrespective of
coingestant)
Presents to ED <4 hours after ingestion
Presents to ED >4 hours but <8 hours after ingestion
Presents to ED >8 hours but <24 hours after ingestion
AC Sorbitol (<1 hour) 4-hour APAP concentration
Immediate APAP concentration
Immediate APAP concentration
Treat with NAC if APAP serum concentration is above nomogram treatment line*
Treat with NAC if APAP serum concentration is above nomogram treatment line*
Administer NAC* pending serum APAP concentration if
• Amount of ingestion >140 mg/kg or
• Amount of ingestion unknown
History of ingestion <140 mg/kg treat with NAC if serum concentration is above nomogram treatment line
Serum APAP concentration above nomogram treatment line: continue NAC for 17 doses
Serum APAP concentration below nomogram treatment line: discontinue NAC
*Refer to Section I, Acetaminophen Poisoning, for PO or IV dosing of NAC.
A

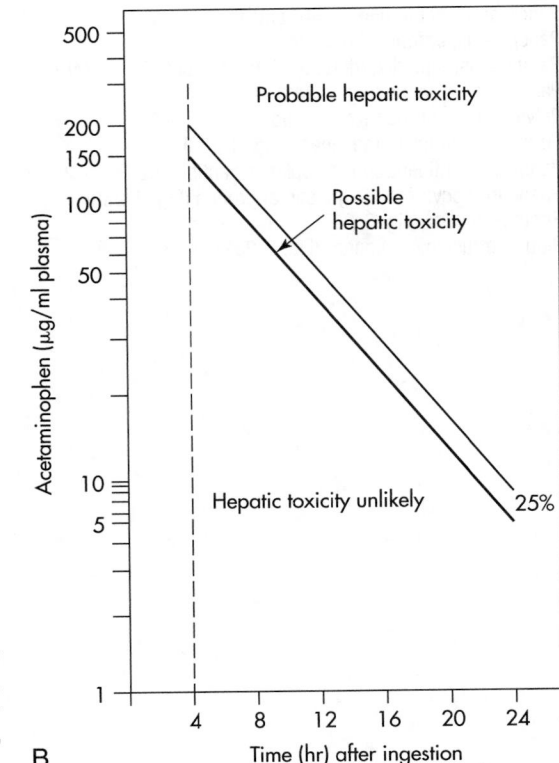

500
200
150
100
50
10
5
1
Acetaminophen (μg/ml plasma)
Probable hepatic toxicity
Possible hepatic toxicity
Hepatic toxicity unlikely
25%
4
8
12
16
20
24
Time (hr) after ingestion
B

FIGURE 3-3 A, Treatment of acetaminophen ingestion. *APAP,* Acetaminophen; *ED,* emergency department; *NAC, N*-acetylcysteine. (From Marx J [ed]: *Rosen's emergency medicine,* ed 5, St Louis, 2002, Mosby.) **B,** Rumack-Matthew nomogram for acetaminophen poisoning. (Modified from Rumack BH, Matthew H: *Pediatrics* 55:871, 1975. In Marx J [ed]: *Rosen's emergency medicine,* ed 6, St Louis, 2006, Mosby.)

ACID-BASE HOMEOSTASIS

ICD-9CM # 276.2 Lactic acidosis
276.2 Metabolic acidosis
276.2 Respiratory acidosis
276.3 Respiratory alkalosis
276.3 Metabolic alkalosis

1213

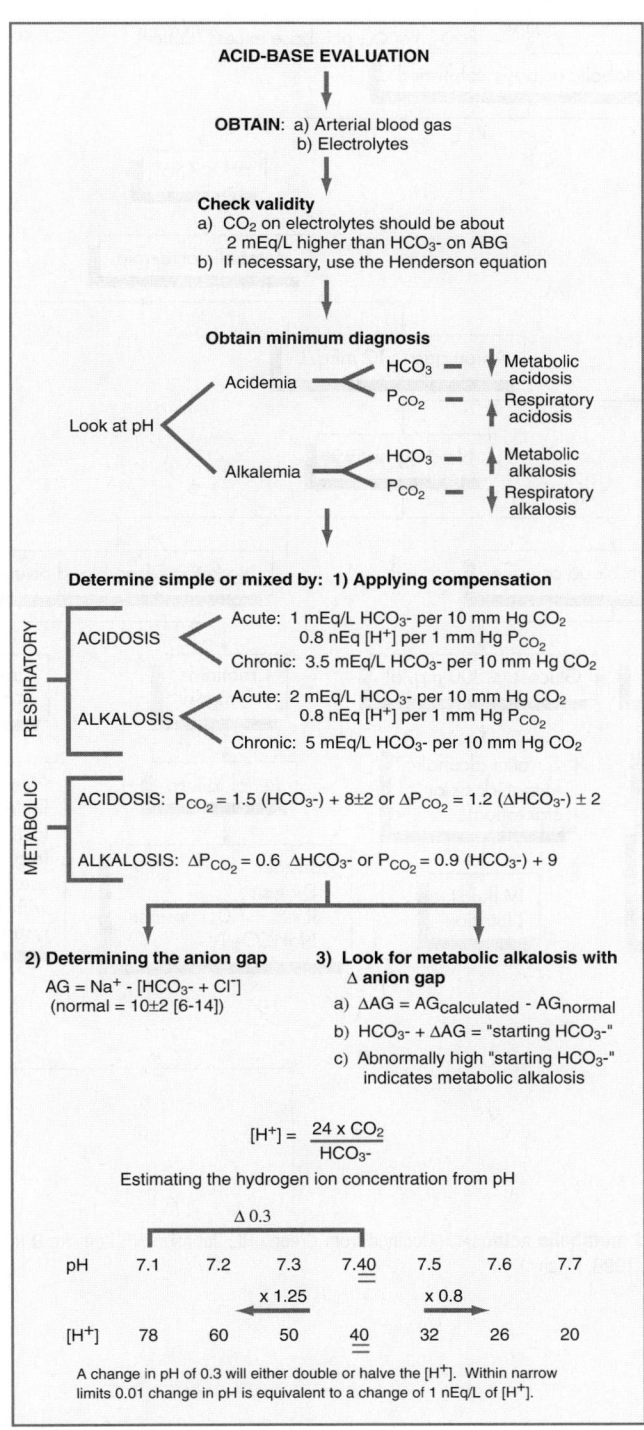

FIGURE 3-4 Scheme for assessing acid-base homeostasis. (From Andreoli TE [ed]: *Cecil essentials of medicine,* ed 7, Philadelphia, 2008, WB Saunders.)

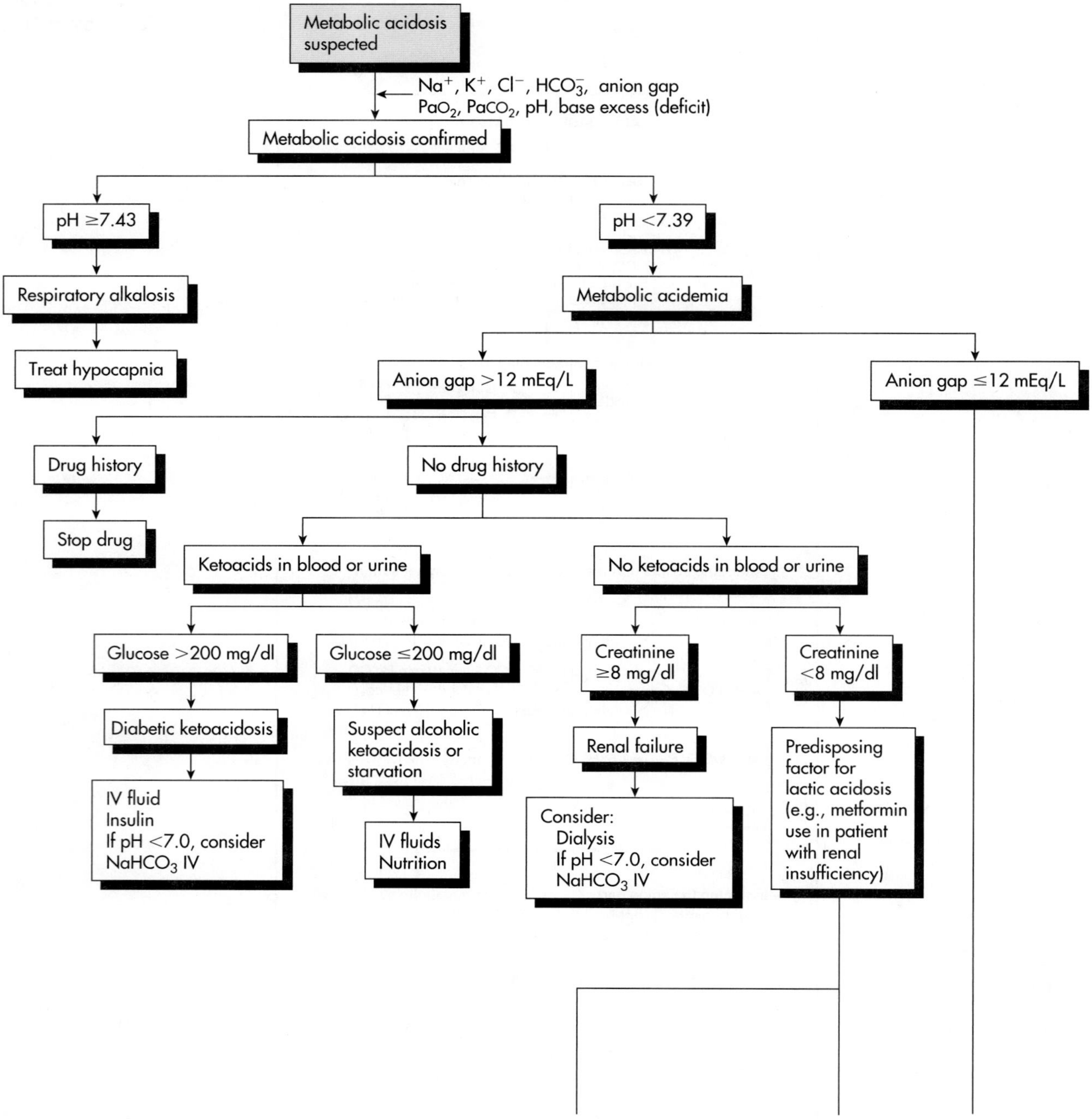

FIGURE 3-5 **Suspected metabolic acidosis.** (Modified from Greene HL, Johnson WP, Lemcke D [eds]: *Decision making in medicine,* ed 2, St Louis, 1998, Mosby.)

(Continued on next page)

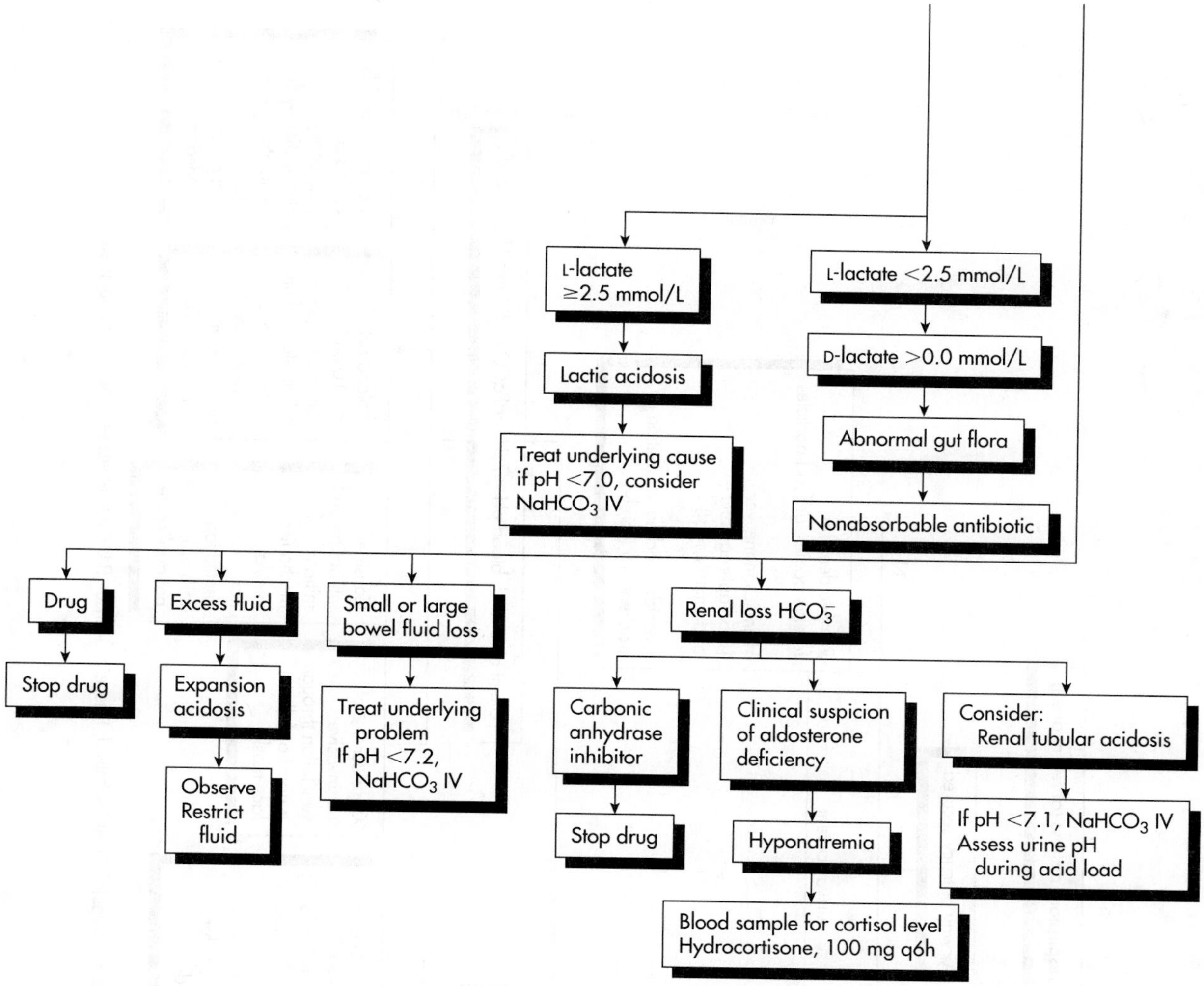

L-lactate
≥2.5 mmol/L

L-lactate <2.5 mmol/L

Lactic acidosis

D-lactate >0.0 mmol/L

Treat underlying cause
if pH <7.0, consider
$NaHCO_3$ IV

Abnormal gut flora

Nonabsorbable antibiotic

Drug

Excess fluid

Small or large
bowel fluid loss

Renal loss HCO_3^-

Stop drug

Expansion
acidosis

Treat underlying
problem
If pH <7.2,
$NaHCO_3$ IV

Carbonic
anhydrase
inhibitor

Clinical suspicion
of aldosterone
deficiency

Consider:
Renal tubular acidosis

Observe
Restrict
fluid

Stop drug

Hyponatremia

If pH <7.1, $NaHCO_3$ IV
Assess urine pH
during acid load

Blood sample for cortisol level
Hydrocortisone, 100 mg q6h

FIGURE 3-5 (Continued)

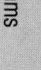

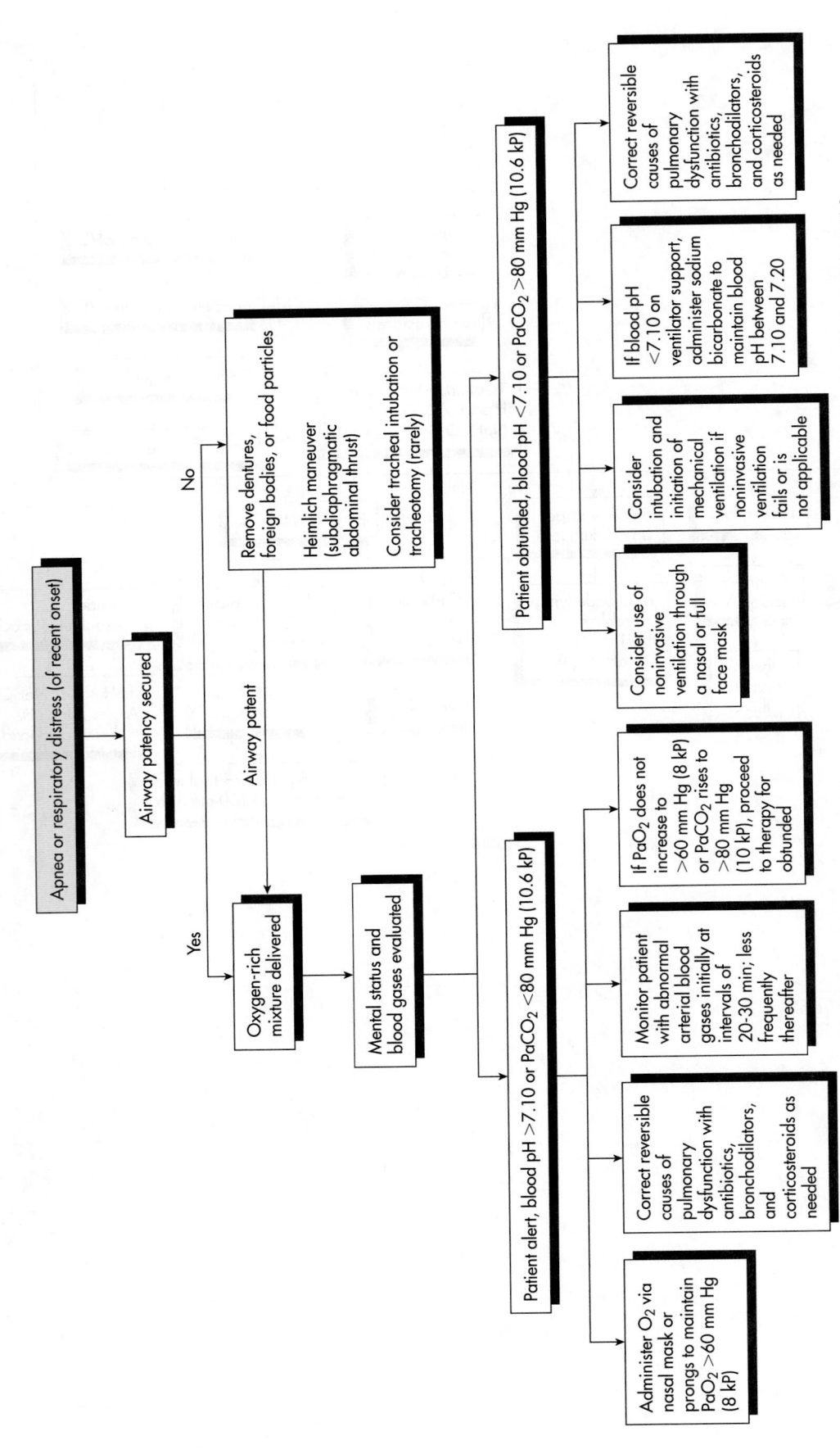

FIGURE 3-6 Algorithm for management of acute respiratory acidosis. (From Feehally J, Floege J, Johnson RJ: *Comprehensive clinical nephrology*, ed 3, St Louis, 2007, Mosby.)

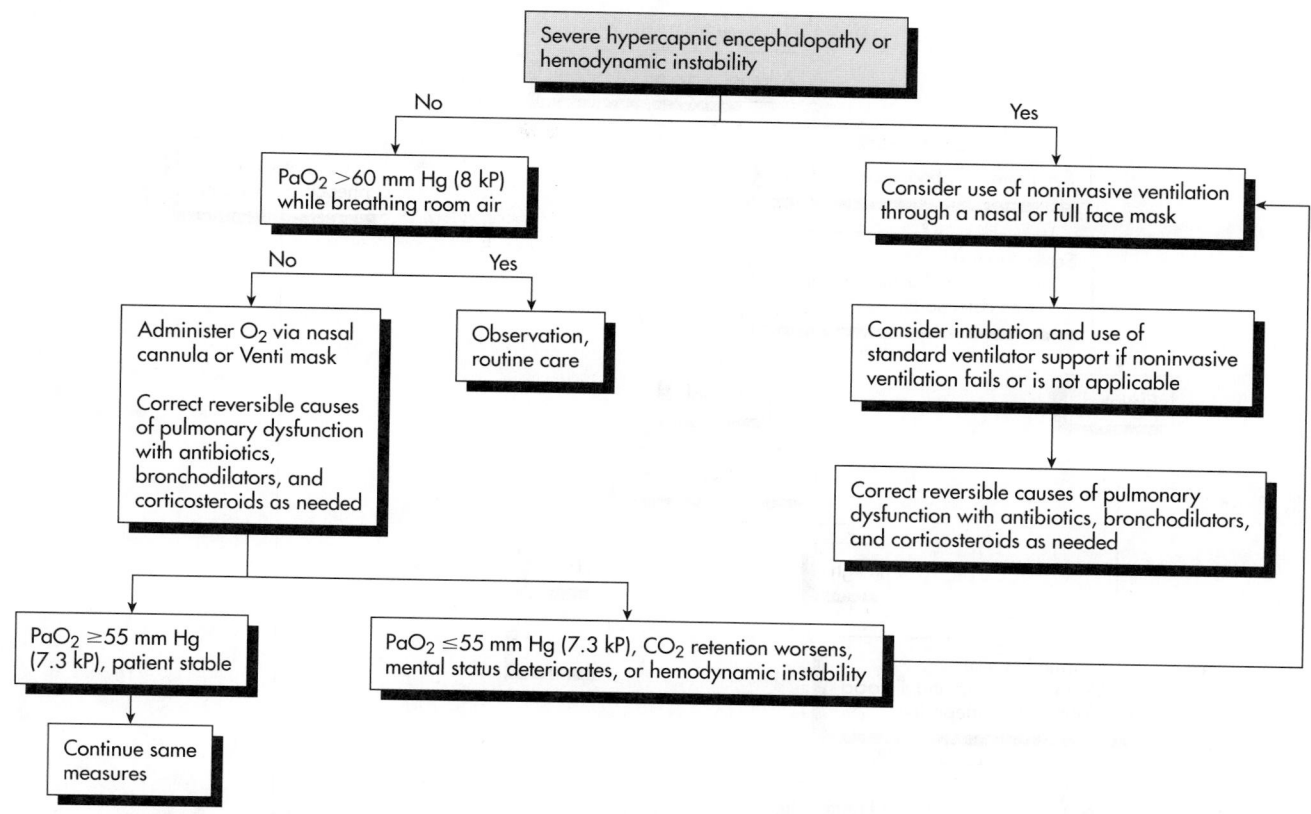

FIGURE 3-7 Algorithm for management of chronic respiratory acidosis. (From Feehally J, Floege J, Johnson RJ: *Comprehensive clinical nephrology,* ed 3, St Louis, 2007, Mosby.)

ICD-9CM # 194.0 Adrenal cortical carcinoma
site NOS M8370/3
255.8 Adrenal hyperplasia

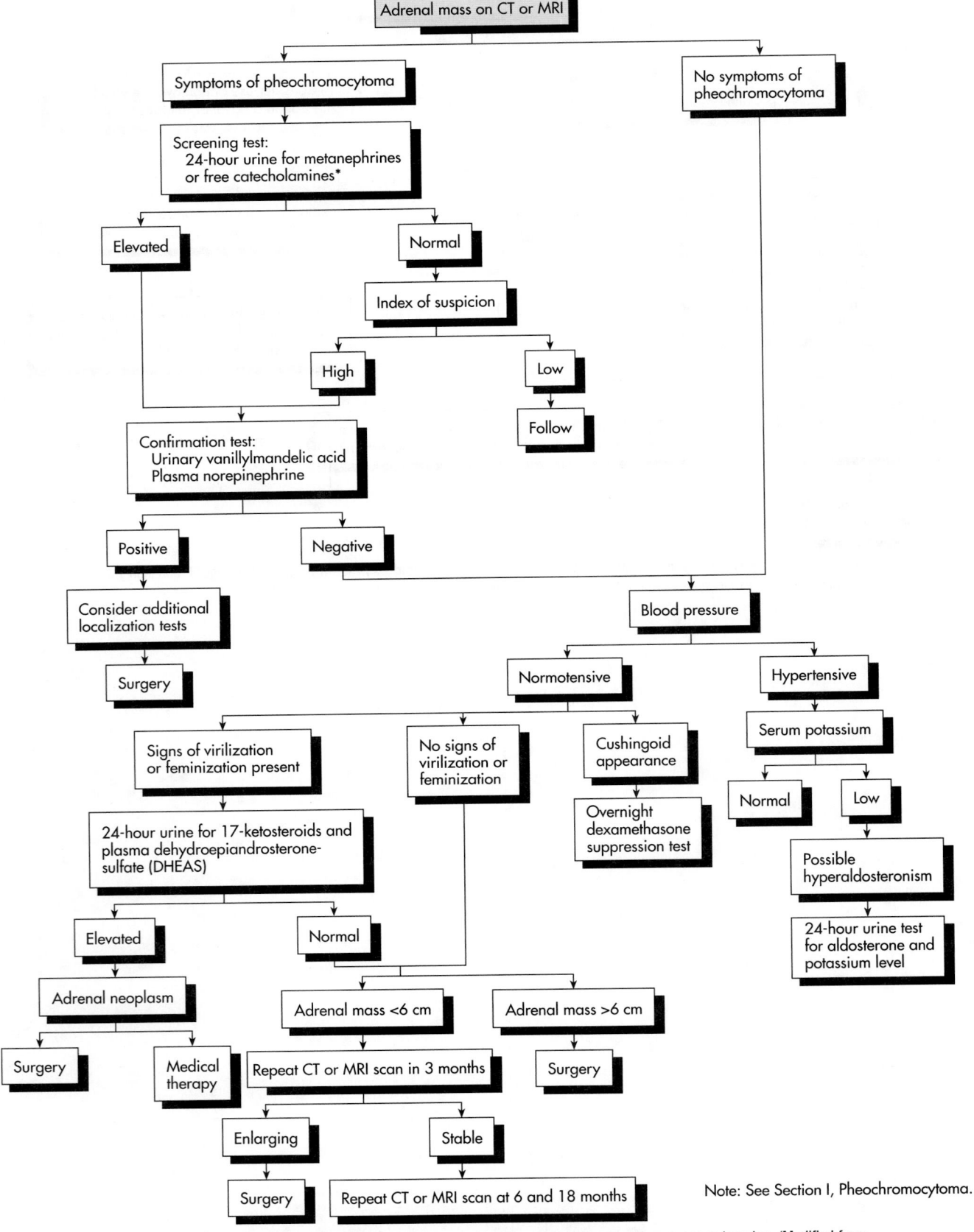

FIGURE 3-11 Evaluation of adrenal mass. *CT,* Computed tomography; *MRI,* magnetic resonance imaging. (Modified from Greene HL, Johnson WP, Lemcke D [eds]: *Decision making in medicine,* ed 2, St Louis, 1998, Mosby.)

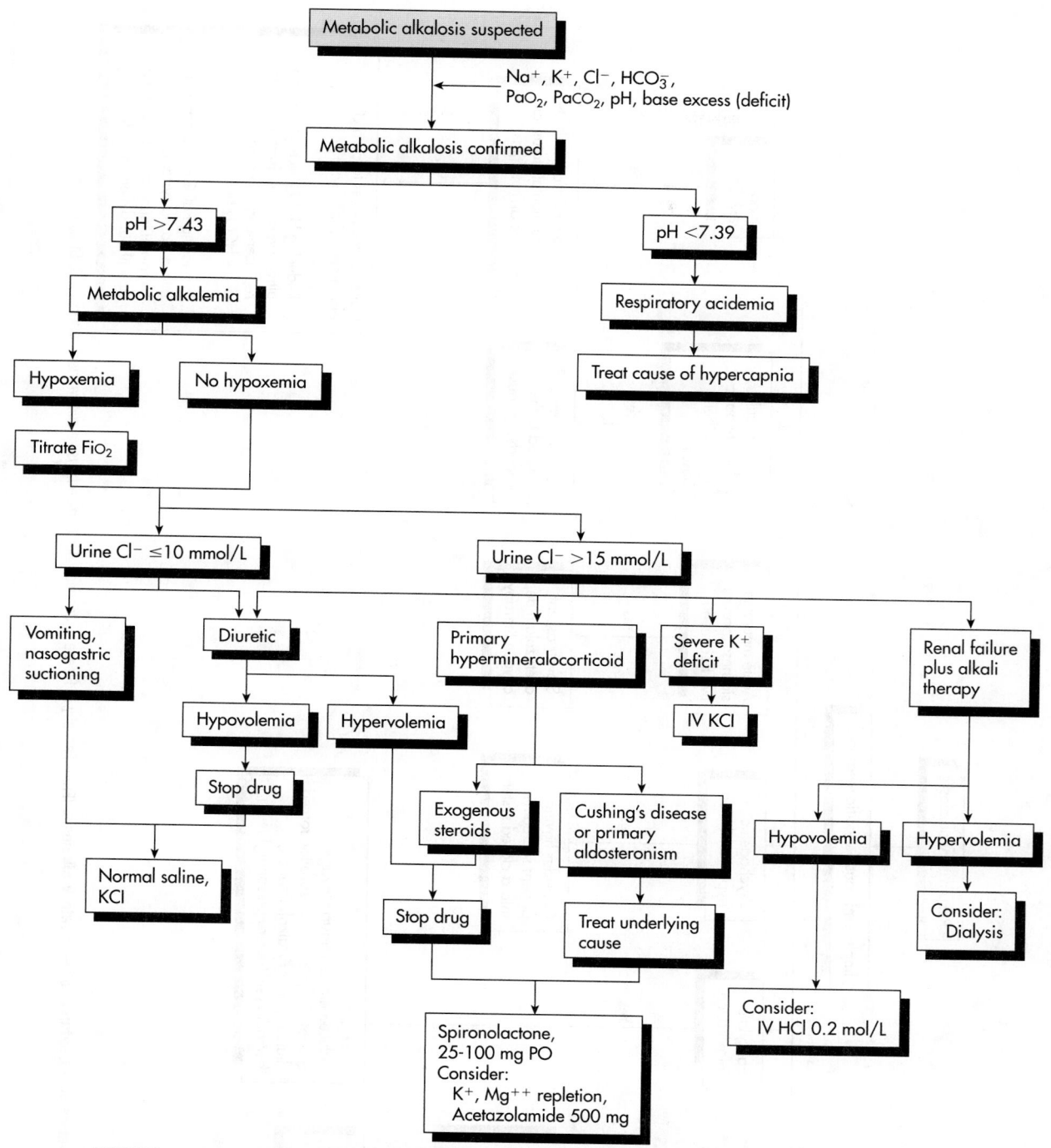

FIGURE 3-15 Suspected metabolic alkalosis. (From Greene HL, Johnson WP, Lemcke D [eds]: *Decision making in medicine,* ed 2, St Louis, 1998, Mosby.)

ALKALOSIS, RESPIRATORY TREATMENT

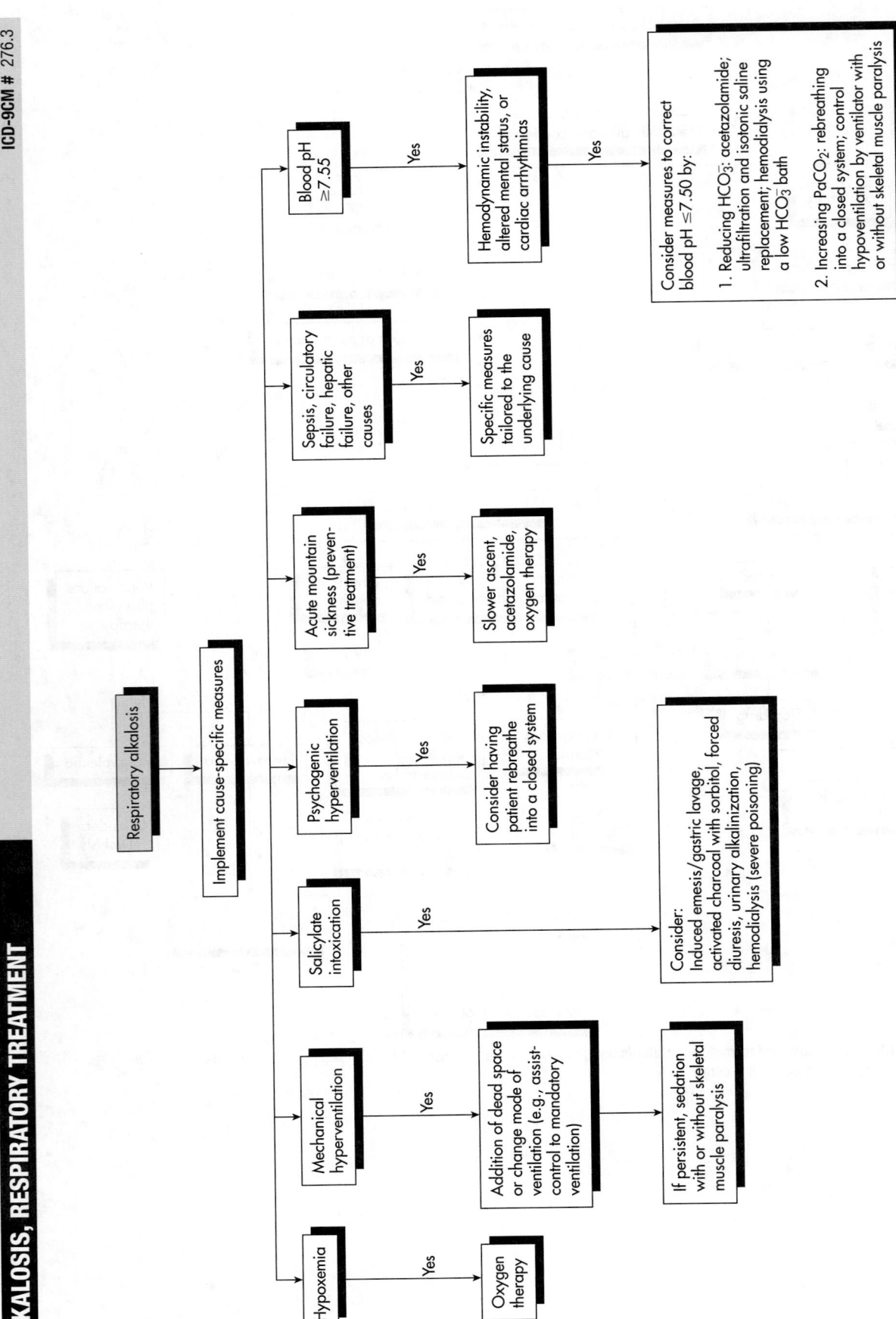

FIGURE 3-16 Recommended treatment of respiratory alkalosis. (From Feehally J, Floege J, Johnson RJ: *Comprehensive clinical nephrology*, ed 3, St Louis, 2007, Mosby.)

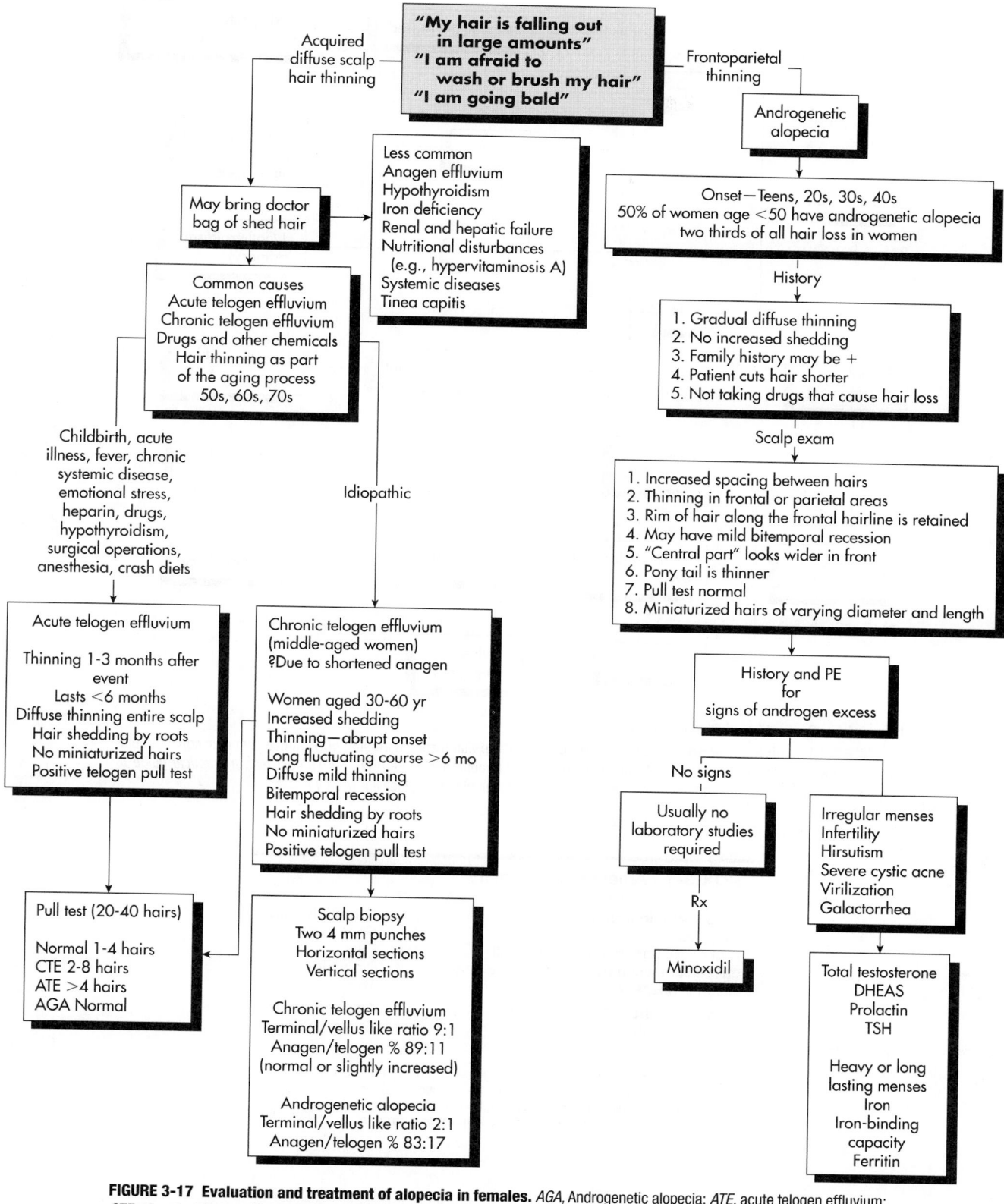

FIGURE 3-17 Evaluation and treatment of alopecia in females. *AGA,* Androgenetic alopecia; *ATE,* acute telogen effluvium; *CTE,* chronic telogen effluvium; *DHEAS,* dehydroepiandrosterone-sulfate; *PE,* physical examination; *TSH,* thyroid-stimulating hormone. (Modified from Habif TA: *Clinical dermatology,* ed 4, St Louis, 2004, Mosby.)

Clinical Algorithms

III

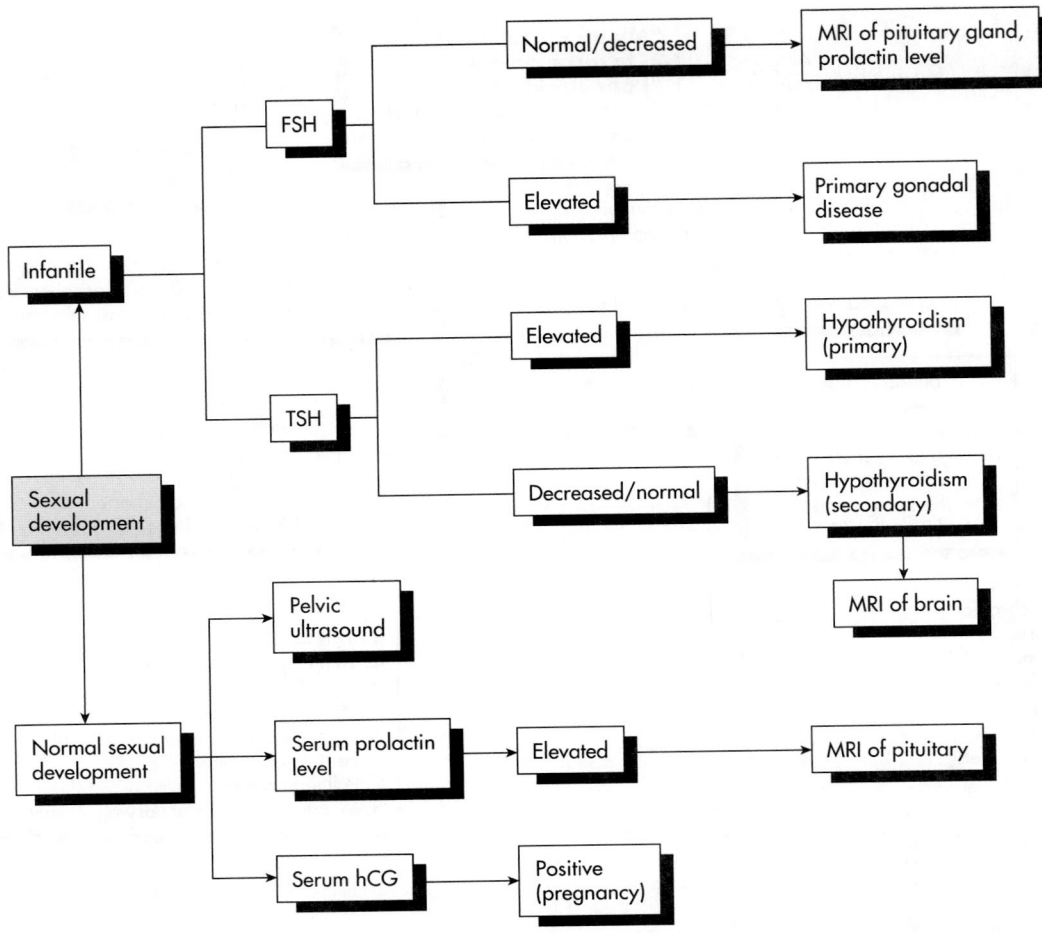

Note: Refer to Section I for additional information on this topic.

FIGURE 3-19 Evaluation of primary amenorrhea. *FSH,* Follicle-stimulating hormone; *hCG,* human chorionic gonadotropin; *MRI,* magnetic resonance imaging; *TSH,* thyroid-stimulating hormone. (From Ferri FF: *Ferri's best test: a practical guide to clinical laboratory medicine and diagnostic imaging,* ed 2, Philadelphia, 2009, Elsevier Mosby.)

BOX 3-1 Amenorrhea, Primary

Diagnostic imaging	**Lab evaluation**
Best test	***Best tests***
MRI of pituitary/hypothalamus with gadolinium when hypothalamic/pituitary lesion is suspected	FSH
	Prolactin
	TSH
Ancillary tests	***Ancillary tests***
Pelvic ultrasound	Serum hCG

From Ferri FF: *Ferri's best test: a practical guide to clinical laboratory medicine and diagnostic imaging,* ed 2, Philadelphia, 2009, Elsevier Mosby.
FSH, Follicle-stimulating hormone; *hCG,* human chorionic gonadotropin; *MRI,* magnetic resonance imaging; *TSH,* thyroid-stimulating hormone.

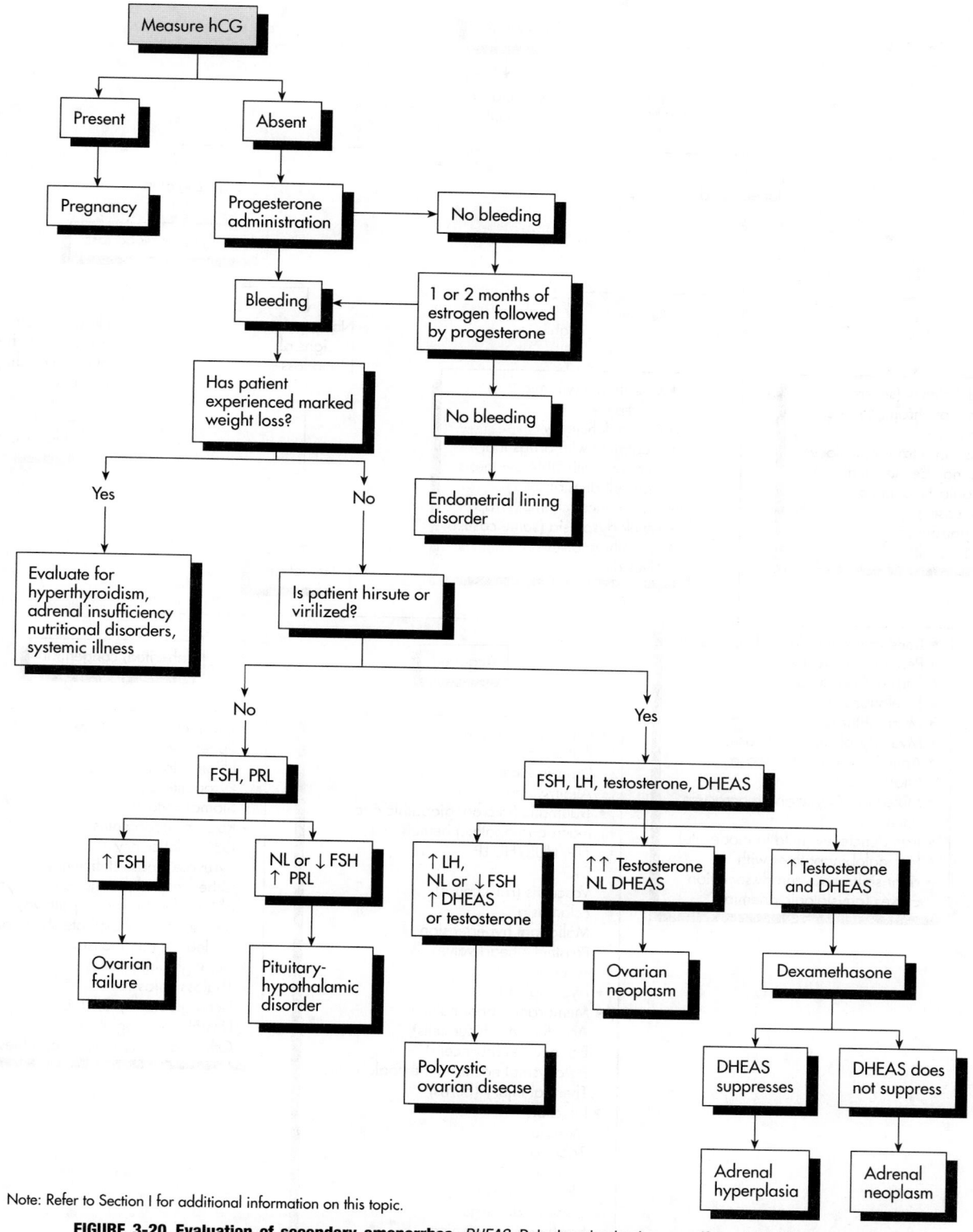

FIGURE 3-20 Evaluation of secondary amenorrhea. *DHEAS,* Dehydroepiandrosterone-sulfate; *FSH,* follicle-stimulating hormone; *hCG,* human chorionic gonadotropin; *LH,* luteinizing hormone; *NL,* normal; *PRL,* prolactin; ↑, increased; ↑↑, markedly increased; ↓, decreased. (From Andreoli TE [ed]: *Cecil essentials of medicine,* ed 7, Philadelphia, 2008, WB Saunders.)

Note: Refer to Section I for additional information on this topic.

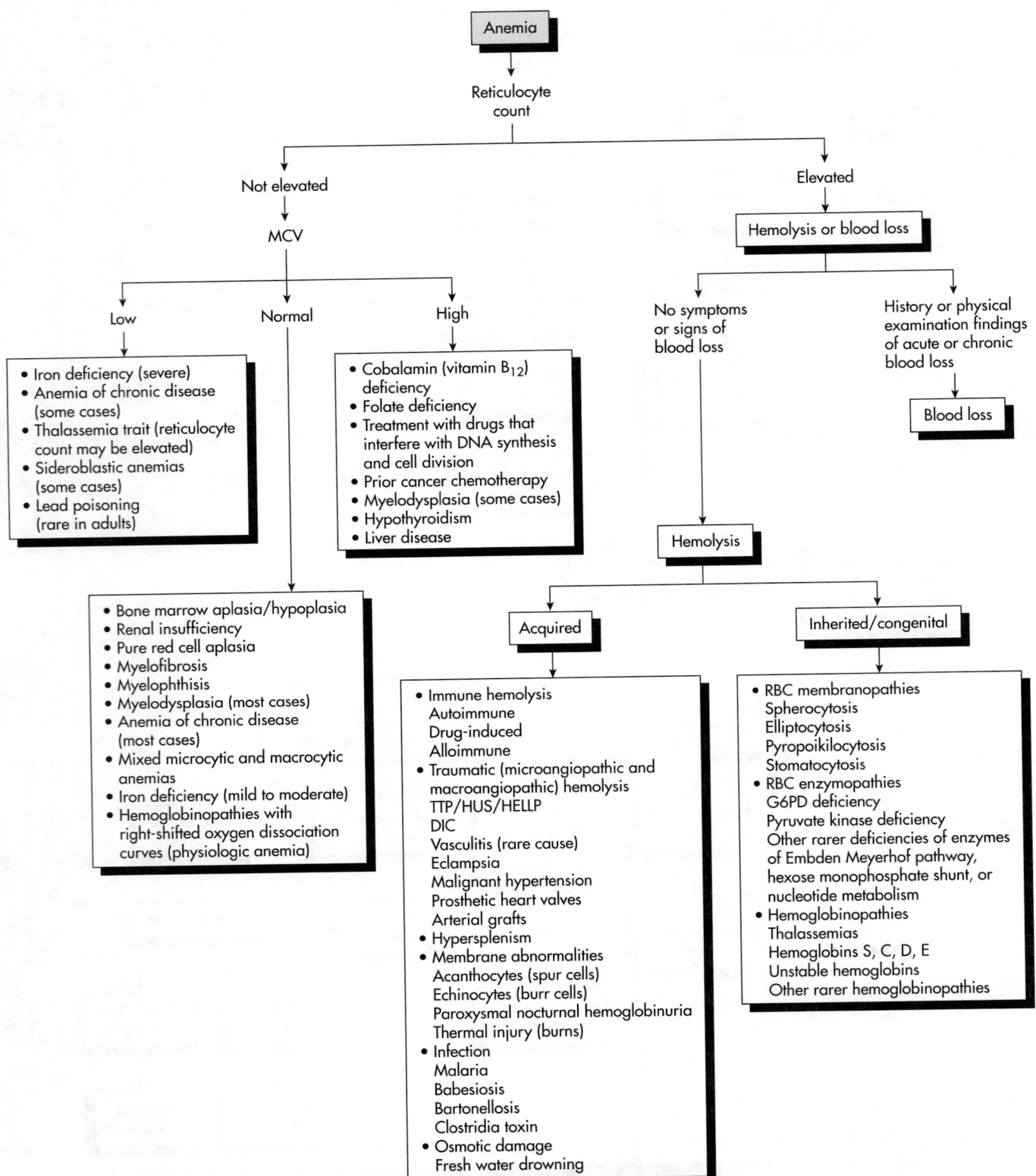

FIGURE 3-22 Algorithm for diagnosis of anemias. *DIC,* Disseminated intravascular coagulation; *G6PD,* glucose-6-phosphate-dehydrogenase; *HELLP,* hepatomegaly-elevated *l*iver (function tests)-*l*ow *p*latelets; *HUS,* hemolytic-uremic syndrome; *MCV,* mean corpuscular volume; *RBC,* red blood cell; *TTP,* thrombotic thrombocytopenic purpura. (From Goldman L, Ausiello D [eds]: *Cecil textbook of medicine,* ed 23, Philadelphia, 2008, WB Saunders.)

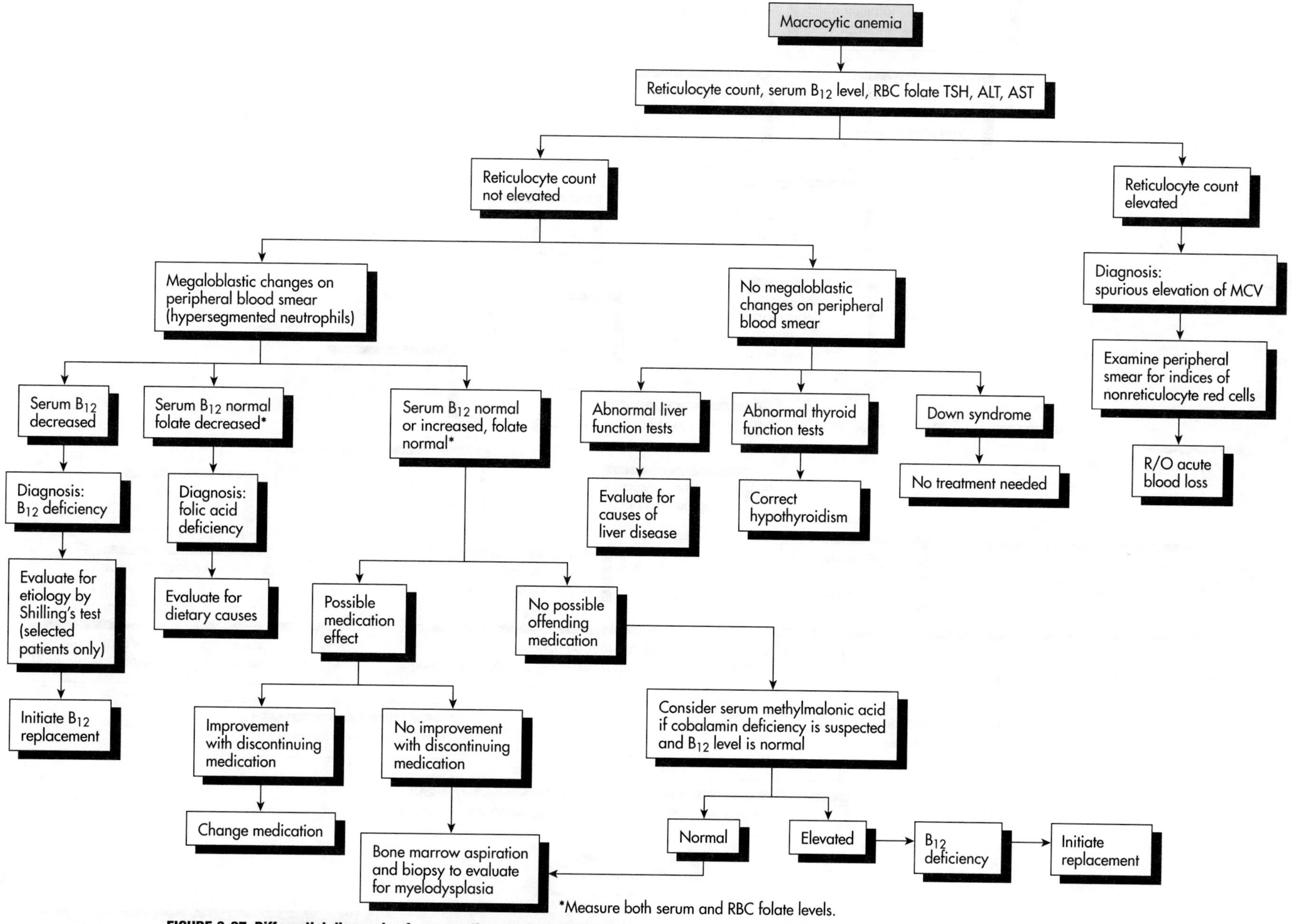

ICD-9CM # 282.4

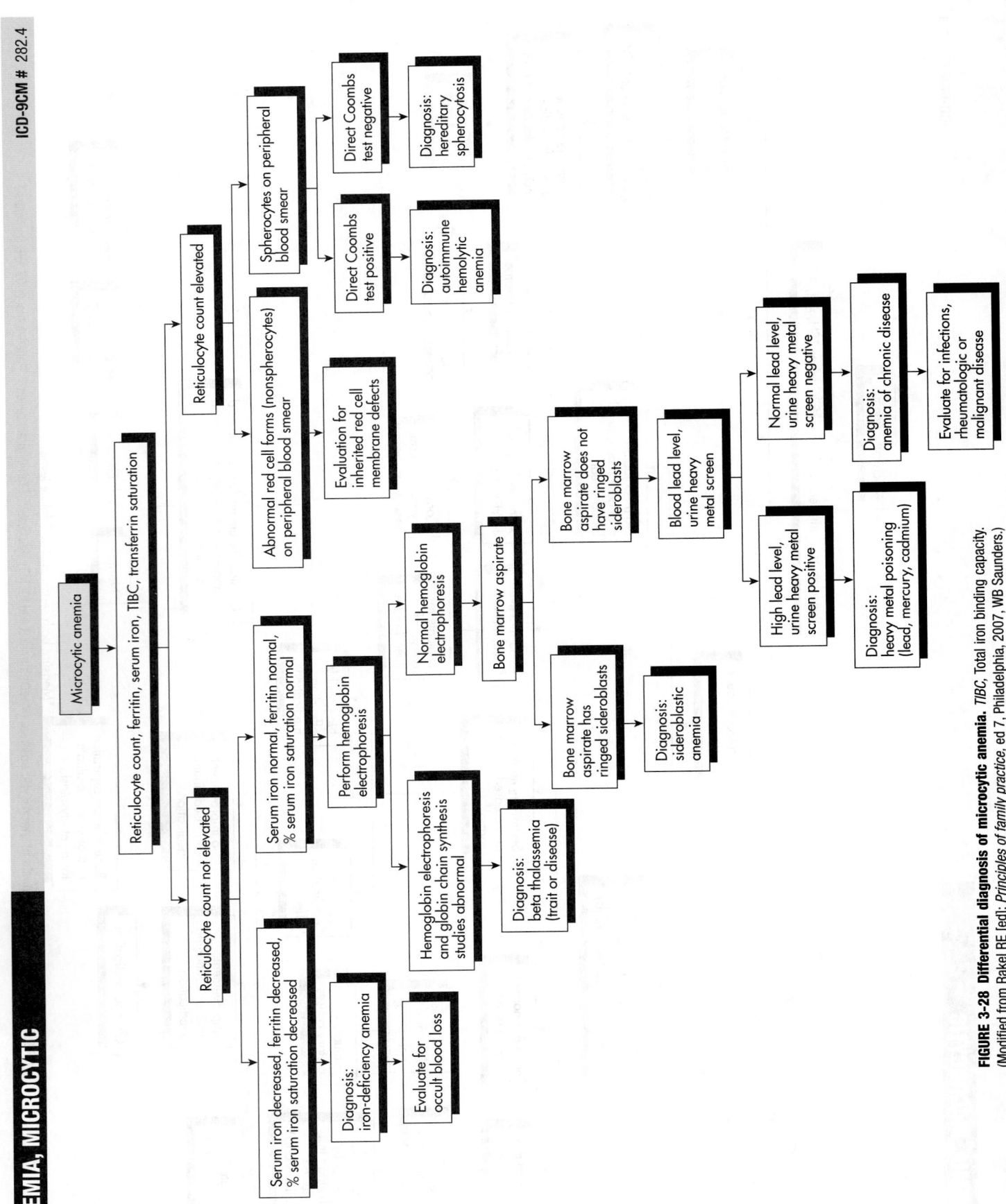

FIGURE 3-28 Differential diagnosis of microcytic anemia. *TIBC,* Total iron binding capacity. (Modified from Rakel RE [ed]: *Principles of family practice,* ed 7, Philadelphia, 2007, WB Saunders.)

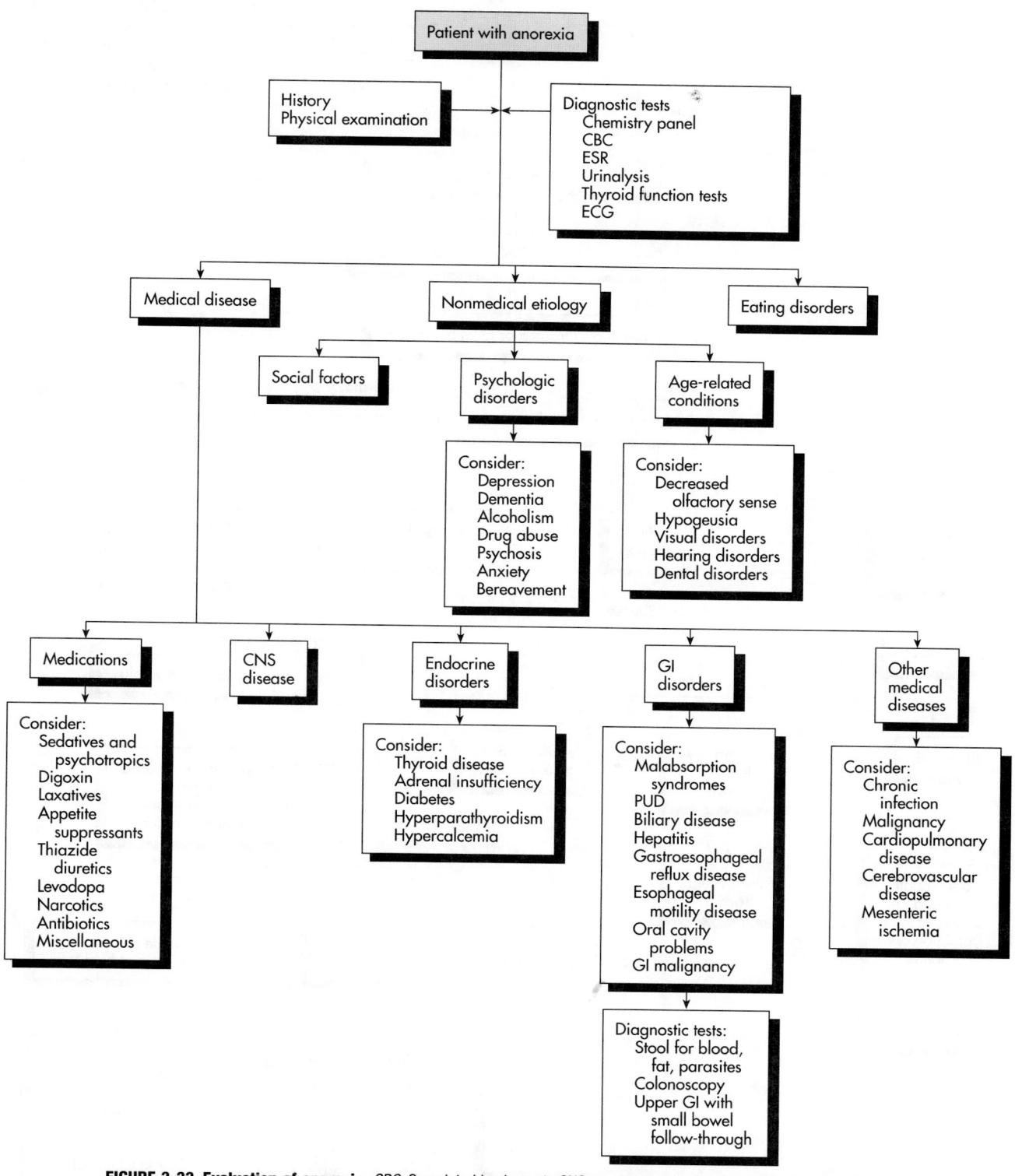

FIGURE 3-33 Evaluation of anorexia. *CBC,* Complete blood count; *CNS,* central nervous system; *ECG,* electrocardiogram; *ESR,* erythrocyte sedimentation rate; *GI,* gastrointestinal; *PUD,* peptic ulcer disease. (Modified from Greene HL, Johnson WP, Lemcke D [eds]: *Decision making in medicine,* ed 2, St Louis, 1998, Mosby.)

Clinical Algorithms

ICD-9CM # 719.40 Arthralgia site NOS
719.41 Arthralgia, shoulder region
719.42 Arthralgia, upper arm
719.43 Arthralgia, forearm
719.44 Arthralgia, hand
719.45 Arthralgia, pelvic region and thigh
719.46 Arthralgia, lower leg
719.47 Arthralgia, ankle and/or foot

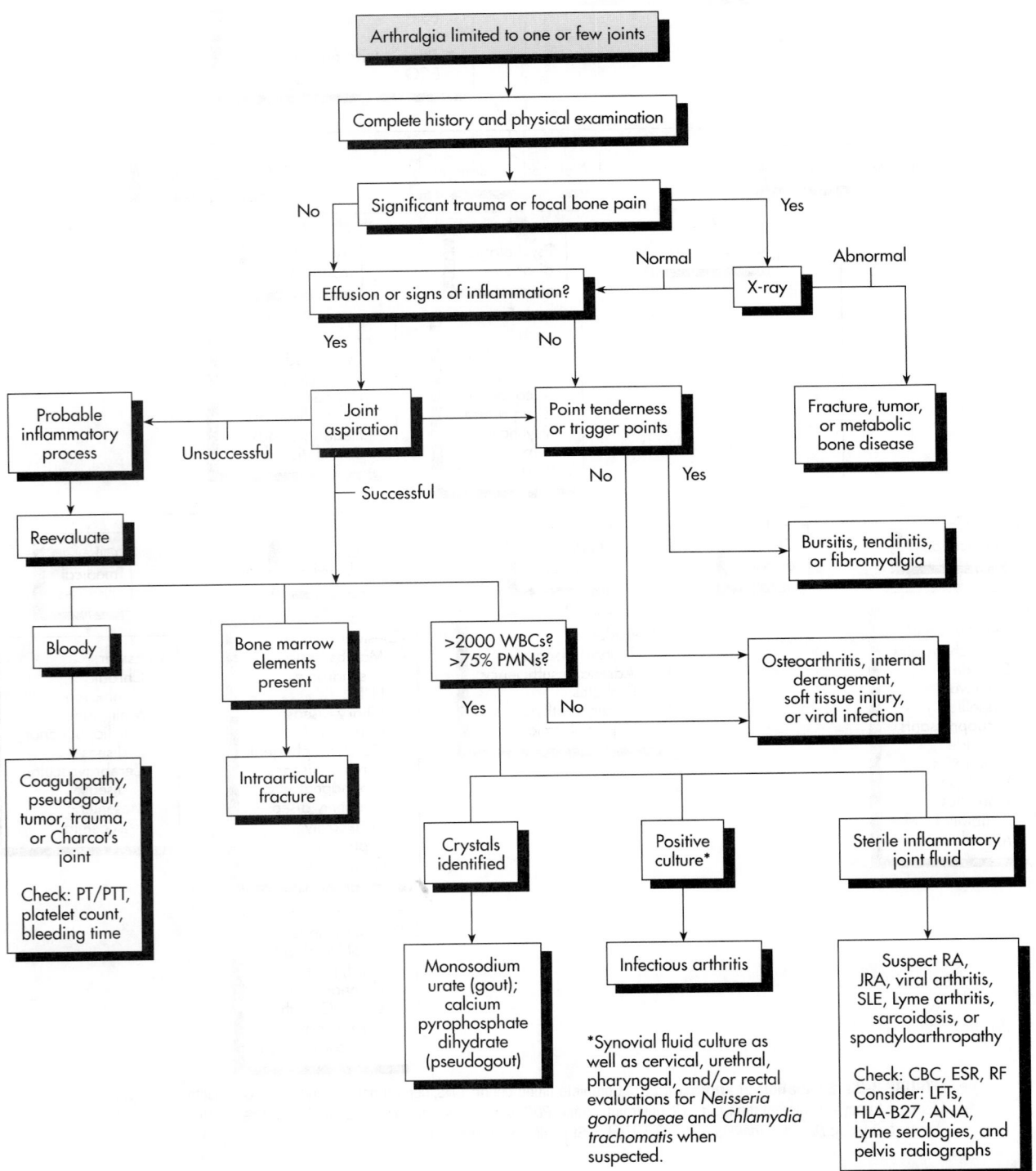

FIGURE 3-39 A diagnostic approach to arthralgia in a few joints. *ANA,* Antinuclear antibodies; *CBC,* complete blood count; *ESR,* erythrocyte sedimentation rate; *JRA,* juvenile rheumatoid arthritis; *LFTs,* liver function tests; *PMNs,* polymorpho-nuclear neutrophils; *PT,* prothrombin time; *PTT,* partial thromboplastin time; *RA,* rheumatoid arthritis; *RF,* rheumatoid factor; *SLE,* systemic lupus erythematosus; *WBCs,* white blood cells. (Modified from American College of Rheumatology Ad Hoc Committee on Clinical Guidelines: *Arthritis Rheum* 39:1, 1996.)

ICD-9CM # 789.5 Ascites NOS
197.6 Ascites, cancerous
(malignant) M8000/6
457.8 Chylous
014.0 Tuberculous

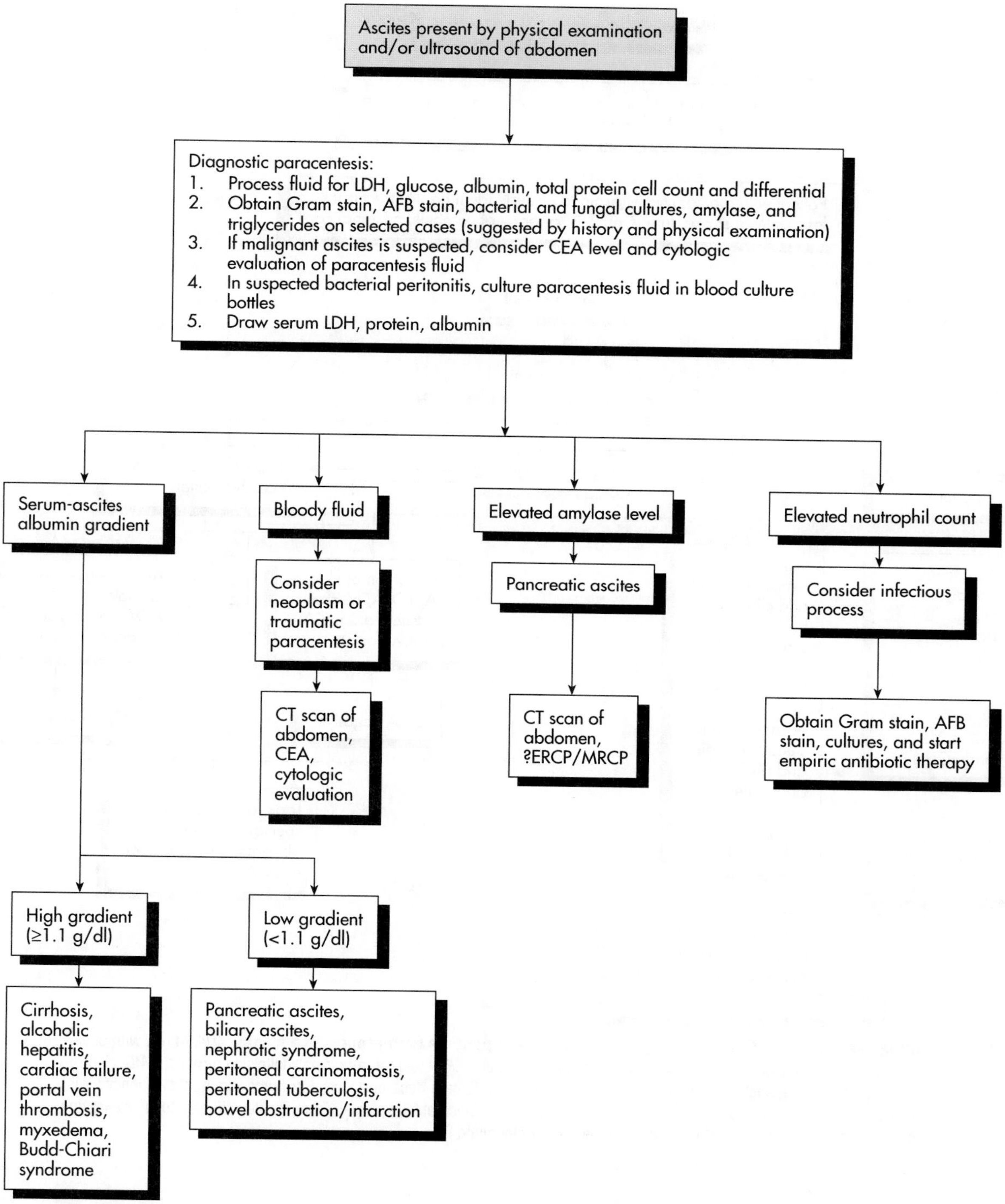

1229

Ascites present by physical examination and/or ultrasound of abdomen

Diagnostic paracentesis:
1. Process fluid for LDH, glucose, albumin, total protein cell count and differential
2. Obtain Gram stain, AFB stain, bacterial and fungal cultures, amylase, and triglycerides on selected cases (suggested by history and physical examination)
3. If malignant ascites is suspected, consider CEA level and cytologic evaluation of paracentesis fluid
4. In suspected bacterial peritonitis, culture paracentesis fluid in blood culture bottles
5. Draw serum LDH, protein, albumin

| Serum-ascites albumin gradient | Bloody fluid | Elevated amylase level | Elevated neutrophil count |

Bloody fluid → Consider neoplasm or traumatic paracentesis → CT scan of abdomen, CEA, cytologic evaluation

Elevated amylase level → Pancreatic ascites → CT scan of abdomen, ?ERCP/MRCP

Elevated neutrophil count → Consider infectious process → Obtain Gram stain, AFB stain, cultures, and start empiric antibiotic therapy

High gradient (≥1.1 g/dl) → Cirrhosis, alcoholic hepatitis, cardiac failure, portal vein thrombosis, myxedema, Budd-Chiari syndrome

Low gradient (<1.1 g/dl) → Pancreatic ascites, biliary ascites, nephrotic syndrome, peritoneal carcinomatosis, peritoneal tuberculosis, bowel obstruction/infarction

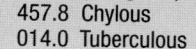

Clinical Algorithms

III

FIGURE 3-40 Evaluation of ascites. *AFB*, Acid-fast bacillus; *CEA*, carcinoembryonic antigen; *CT*, computed tomography; *ERCP*, endoscopic retrograde cholangiopancreatography; *LDH*, lactate dehydrogenase; *MRCP*, magnetic resonance cholangio-pancreatography.

ICD-9CM # 781.3 Ataxia NOS
303.9 Alcoholic, chronic
334.3 Cerebellar
331.89 Cerebral
334.0 Friedreich's

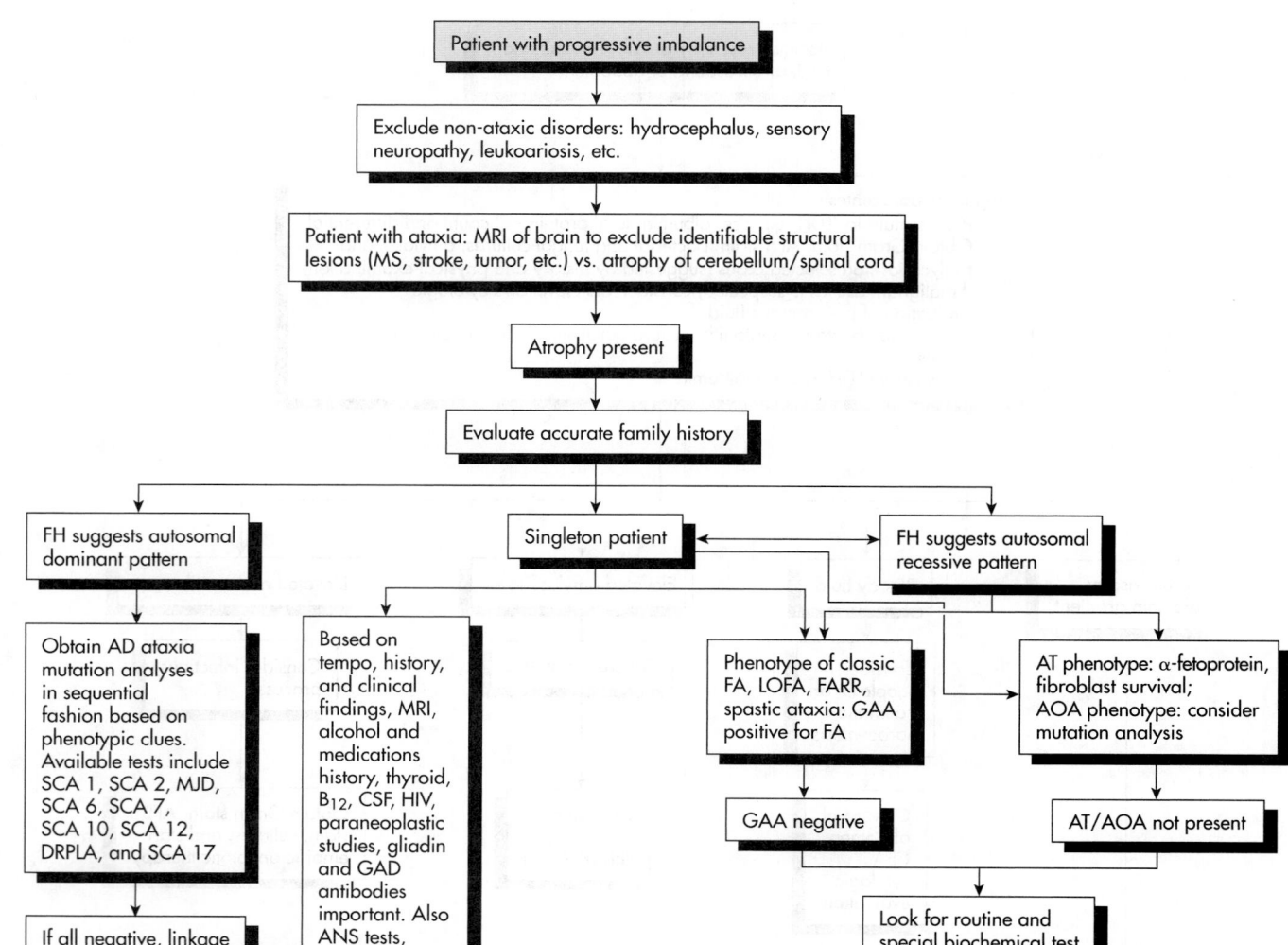

FIGURE 3-47 An algorithm for a diagnostic approach to patients with progressive ataxia. *AOA,* Ataxia with oculomotor apraxia; *AT,* ataxia-telengiectasia; *CSF,* cerebrospinal fluid; *DRPLA,* dentatorubral-pallidoluysian atrophy; *EMG,* electromyelography; *FA,* Friedreich's ataxia; *FH,* family history; *GAD,* glutamate decarboxylase; *HIV,* human immunodeficiency virus; *MRI,* magnetic resonance imaging; *MS,* multiple sclerosis; *SCA,* spinocerebellar ataxia. (From Bradley WG et al [eds]: *Neurology in clinical practice,* ed 4, Philadelphia, 2004, Butterworth Heinemann.)

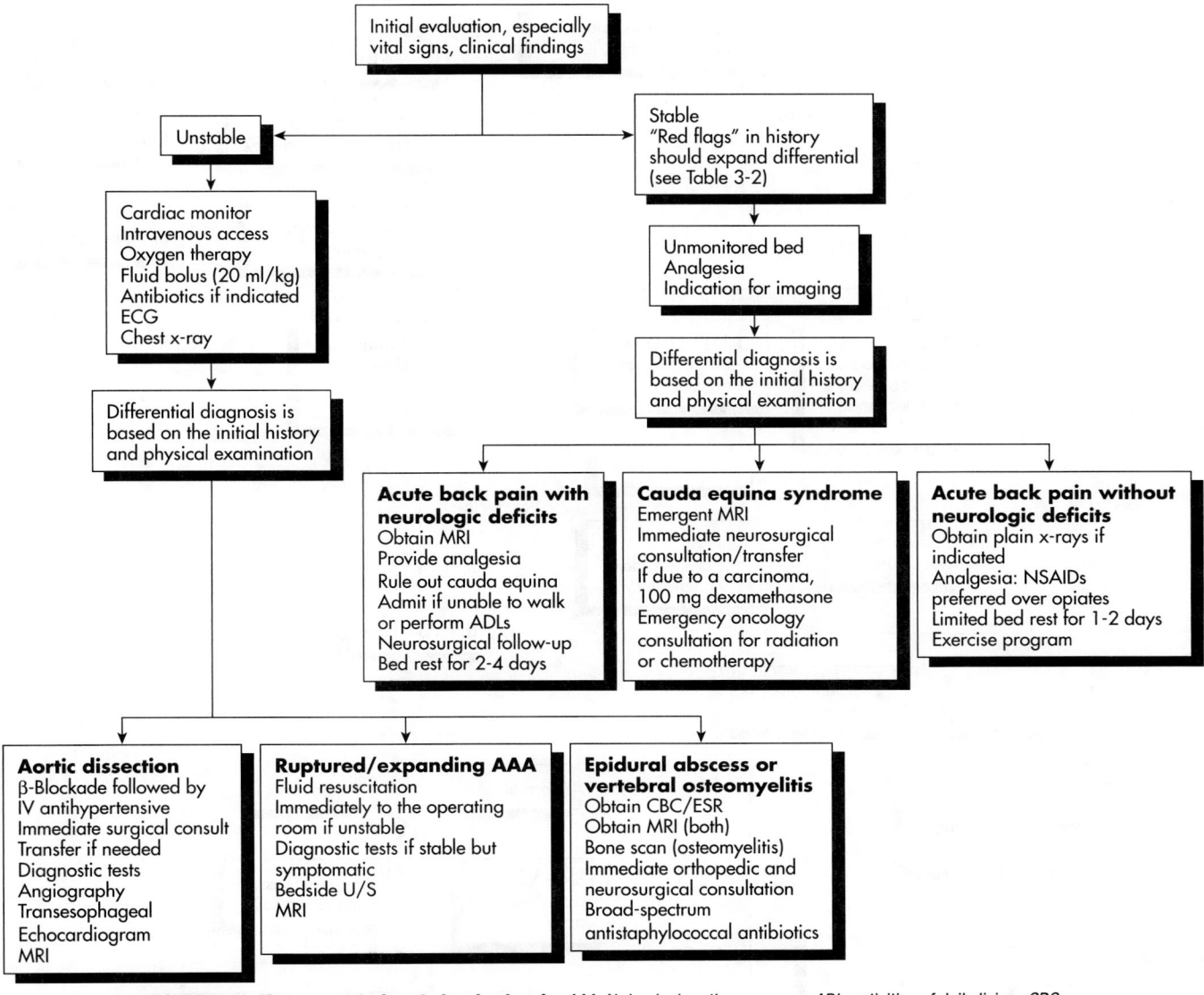

FIGURE 3-51 **Management of acute low back pain.** *AAA,* Abdominal aortic aneurysm; *ADL,* activities of daily living; *CBC,* complete blood count; *ECG,* electrocardiogram; *ESR,* erythrocyte sedimentation rate; *IV,* intravenous; *MRI,* magnetic resonance imaging; *NSAIDs,* nonsteroidal anti-inflammatory drugs; *U/S,* ultrasound. (From Marx JA [ed]: *Rosen's emergency medicine,* ed 6, St Louis, 2006, Mosby.)

TABLE 3-2 Red Flags for Potentially Serious Conditions

Possible Fracture	Possible Tumor or Infection	Possible Cauda Equina Syndrome
From Medical History		
Major trauma, such as vehicle accident or fall from height	Age over 50 or under 20 yr	Saddle anesthesia
Minor trauma or even strenuous lifting (in older or potentially osteoporotic patient)	History of cancer	Recent onset of bladder dysfunction, such as urinary retention, increased frequency, or overflow incontinence
	Constitutional symptoms, such as recent fever or chills or unexplained weight loss	Severe or progressive neurologic deficit in the lower extremity
	Risk factors for spinal infection: recent bacterial infection (e.g., urinary tract infection), intravenous drug abuse, or immune suppression (from steroids, transplant, or human immunodeficiency virus)	
	Pain that worsens when supine; severe nighttime pain	

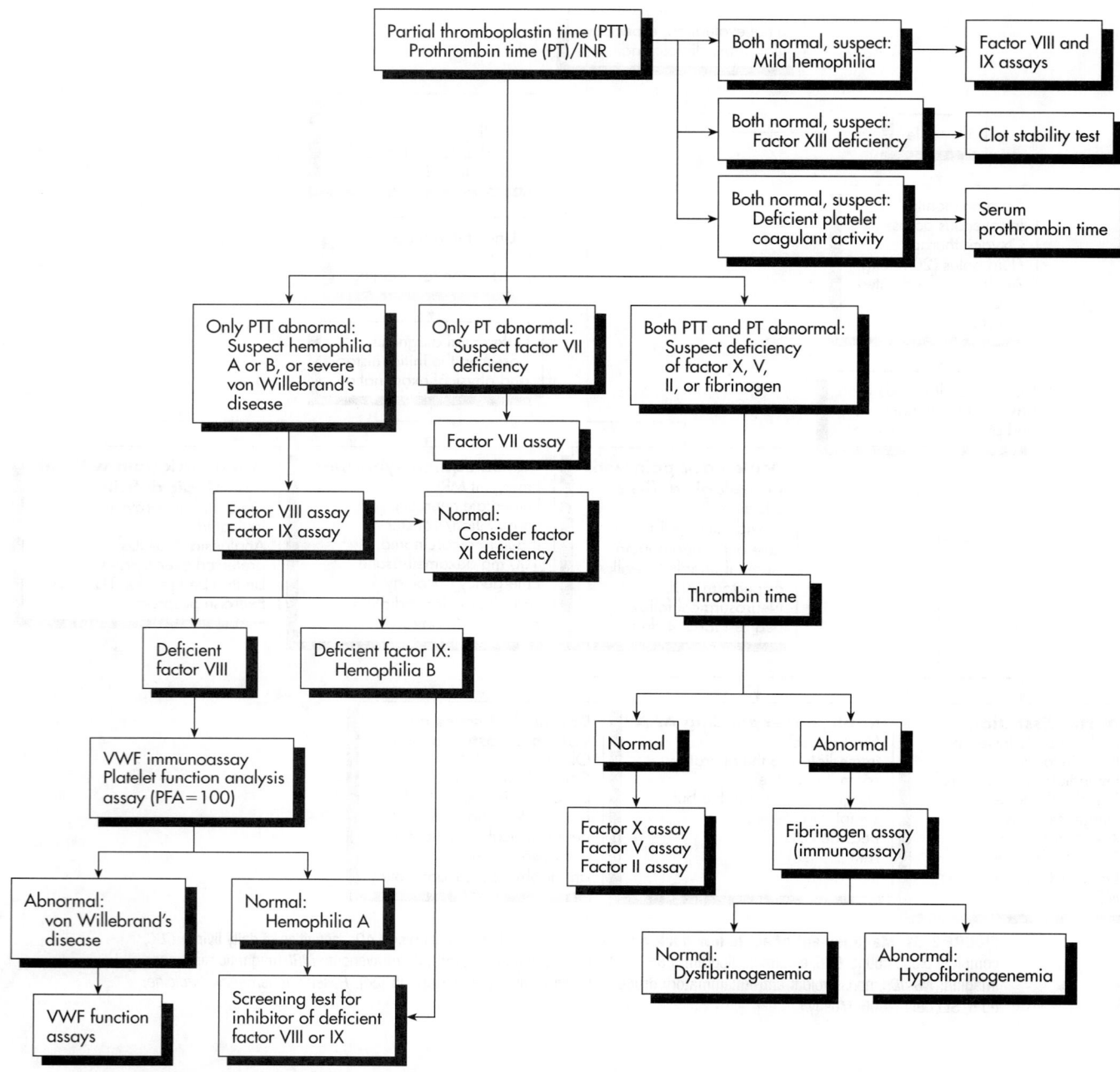

FIGURE 3-53 Laboratory evaluation of a patient with a bleeding disorder in whom the history and physical examination suggest a congenital coagulation disorder. *INR,* International normalized ratio; *VWF,* von Willebrand factor. (Modified from Stein JH [ed]: *Internal medicine,* ed 5, St Louis, 1998, Mosby.)

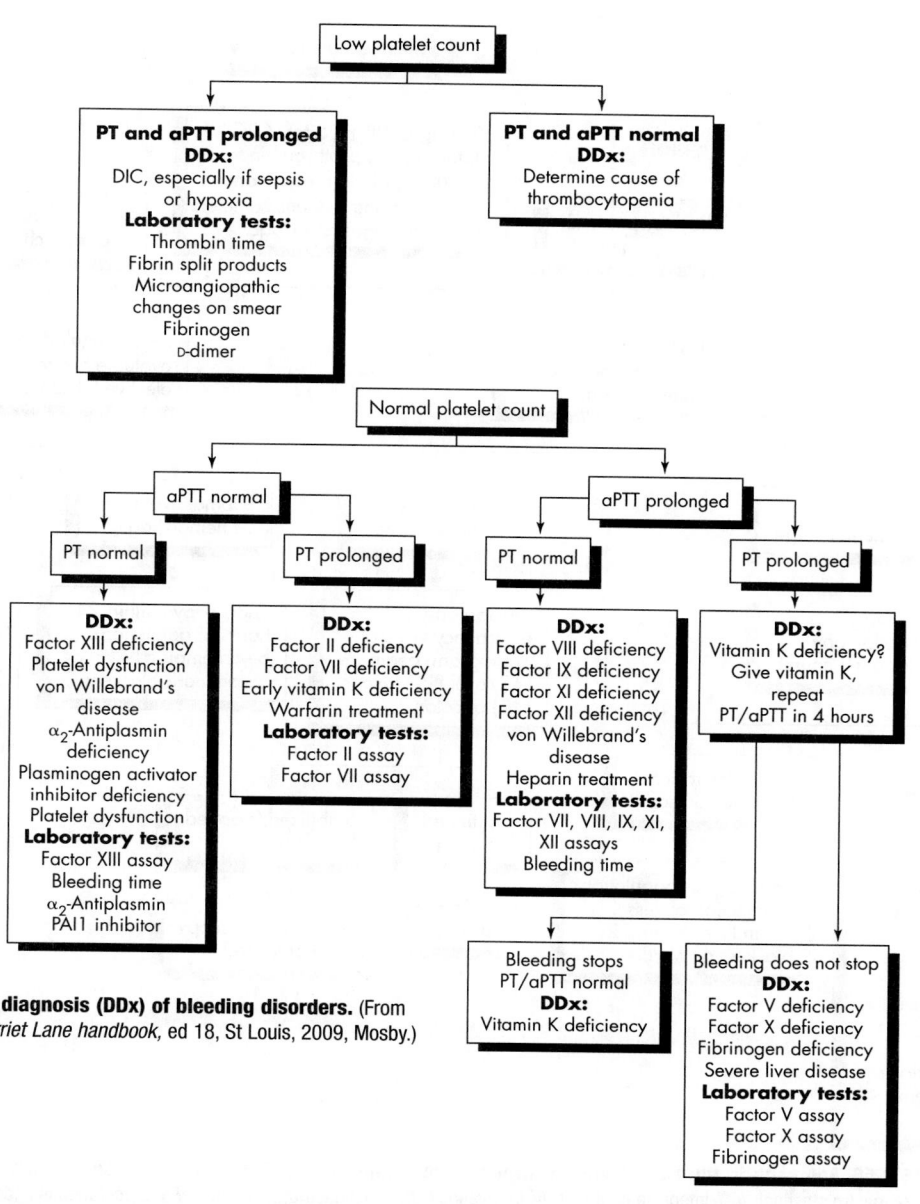

FIGURE 3-54 Differential diagnosis (DDx) of bleeding disorders. (From Cluster JW, Rau RE: *The Harriet Lane handbook,* ed 18, St Louis, 2009, Mosby.)

Clinical
Algorithms

BOX 3-3   Bleeding Disorders

Congenital

Disorder of platelet number or function

Thrombocytopenia: Secondary to bone marrow disease or defective megakaryocyte maturation

Disorders of platelet function: Bernard-Soulier syndrome, Glanzmann thrombasthenia, storage pool diseases

Factor VIII deficiency: See text (Section I)
Factor IX deficiency: See text (Section I)
von Willebrand's disease: See text (Section I)

Acquired

Disseminated intravascular coagulation: Characterized by prolonged PT and aPTT, decreased fibrinogen and platelets, increased fibrin degradation products, and elevated D-dimers. Treatment includes identifying and treating underlying disorder. Replacement of depleted coagulation factors with FFP may be necessary in severe cases, especially when bleeding is present; 10-15 ml/kg will raise clotting factors 20%. Fibrinogen, if depleted, can be given as cryoprecipitate. Platelet transfusions may also be necessary.

Liver disease: The liver is the major site of synthesis of factors V, VII, IX, X, XI, XII, XIII, prothrombin, plasminogen, fibrinogen, protein C and S, and ATIII. Treatment with FFP and platelets may be needed, but this will increase hepatic protein load. Vitamin K should be given to patients with liver disease and clotting abnormalities.

Vitamin K deficiency: Factors II, VII, IX, X, protein C, and protein S are vitamin K dependent. Early vitamin K deficiency may present with isolated prolonged PT because factor VII has the shortest half-life. Fibrinogen should be normal.

Hemolytic-uremic syndrome/thrombotic thrombocytopenic purpura (HUS/TTP): Characterized by the triad of microangiopathic hemolytic anemia, uremia, and thrombocytopenia. HUS/TTP is often triggered by bacterial enteritis, especially caused by *Escherichia coli* O157:H7, although there are a variety of causes. HUS does not typically include coagulation abnormalities, such as those seen in DIC. Avoid blood products in patients with HUS thought to be secondary to pneumococcal infection. TTP includes the triad of HUS in addition to fever and CNS changes and is more common in older adolescents and adults.

(From Custer JW, Rau RE: *The Harriet Lane handbook*, ed 18, St Louis, 2009, Mosby.)

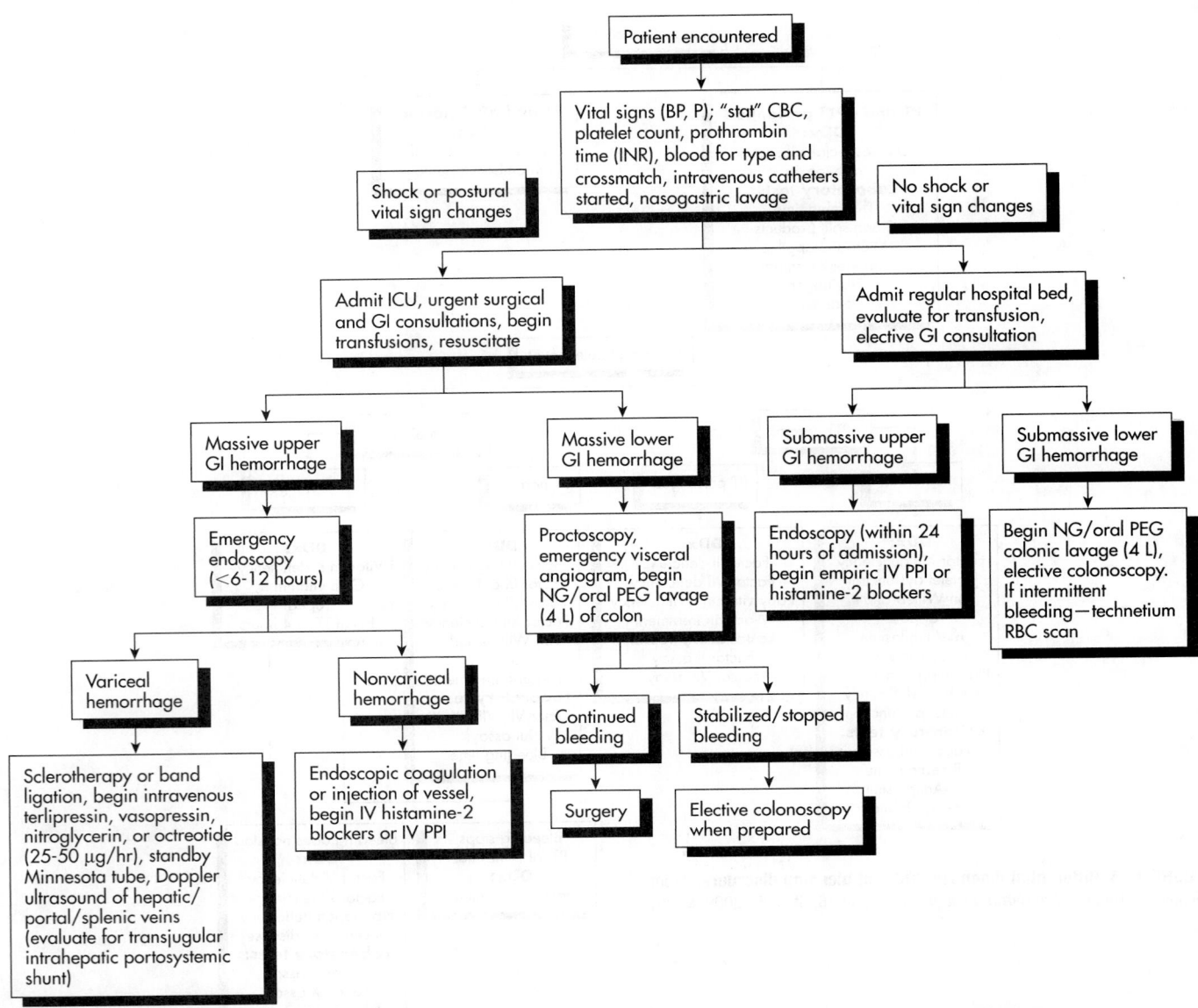

FIGURE 3-56 Approach to the patient with gastrointestinal hemorrhage. *BP*, Blood pressure; *CBC*, complete blood count; *GI*, gastrointestinal; *ICU*, intensive care unit; *IV*, intravenous; *NG*, nasogastric; *P*, weight; *PEG*, percutaneous endoscopic gastrostomy; *PPI*, proton pump inhibitor; *RBC*, red blood cell. (Modified from Goldman L, Ausiello D [eds]: *Cecil textbook of medicine*, ed 23, Philadelphia, 2008, WB Saunders.)

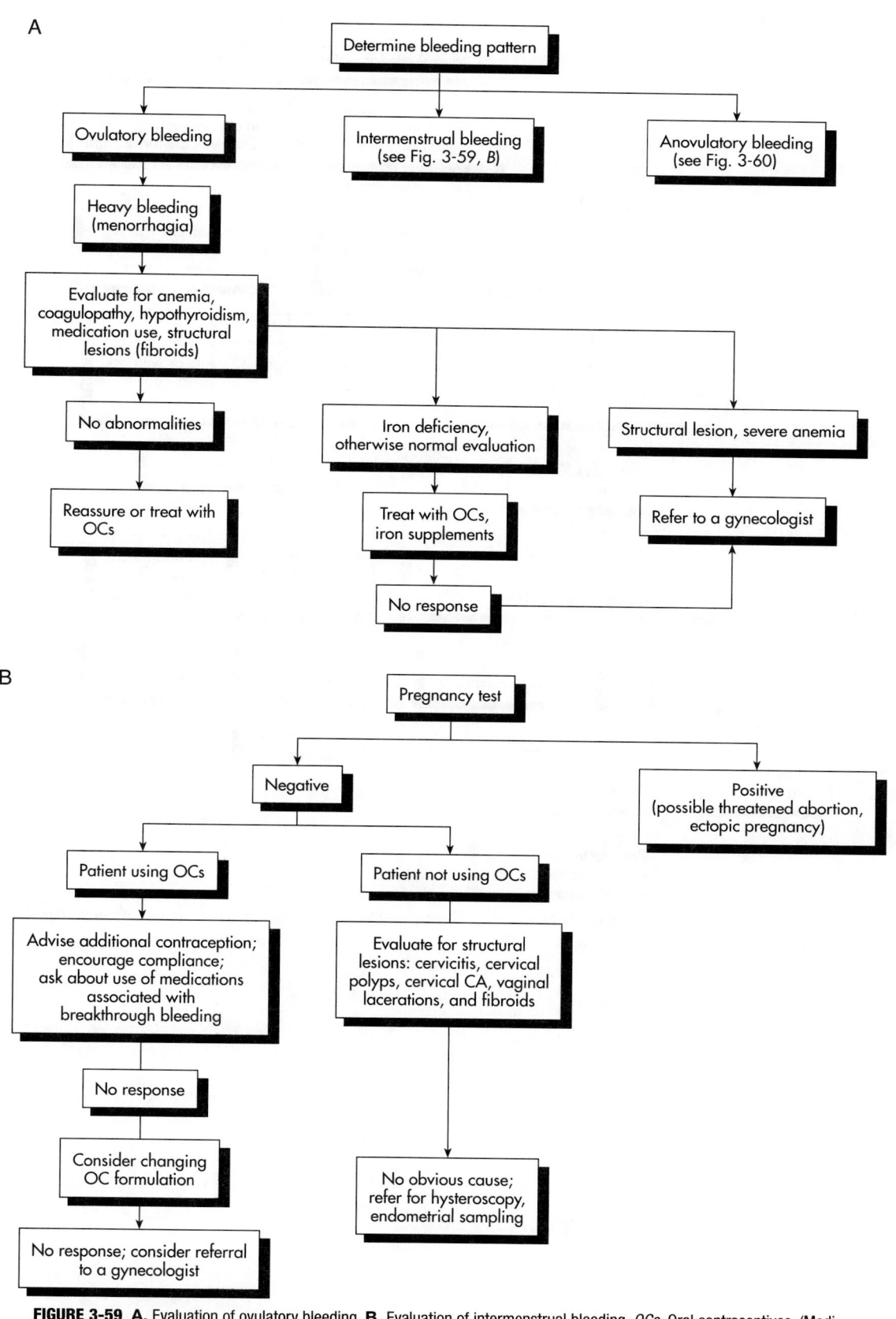

FIGURE 3-59 A, Evaluation of ovulatory bleeding. **B,** Evaluation of intermenstrual bleeding. *OCs,* Oral contraceptives. (Modified from Appleby J, Henderson M, Wathen PI: *Intern Med* Sept:17, 1996.)

Clinical
Algorithms

III

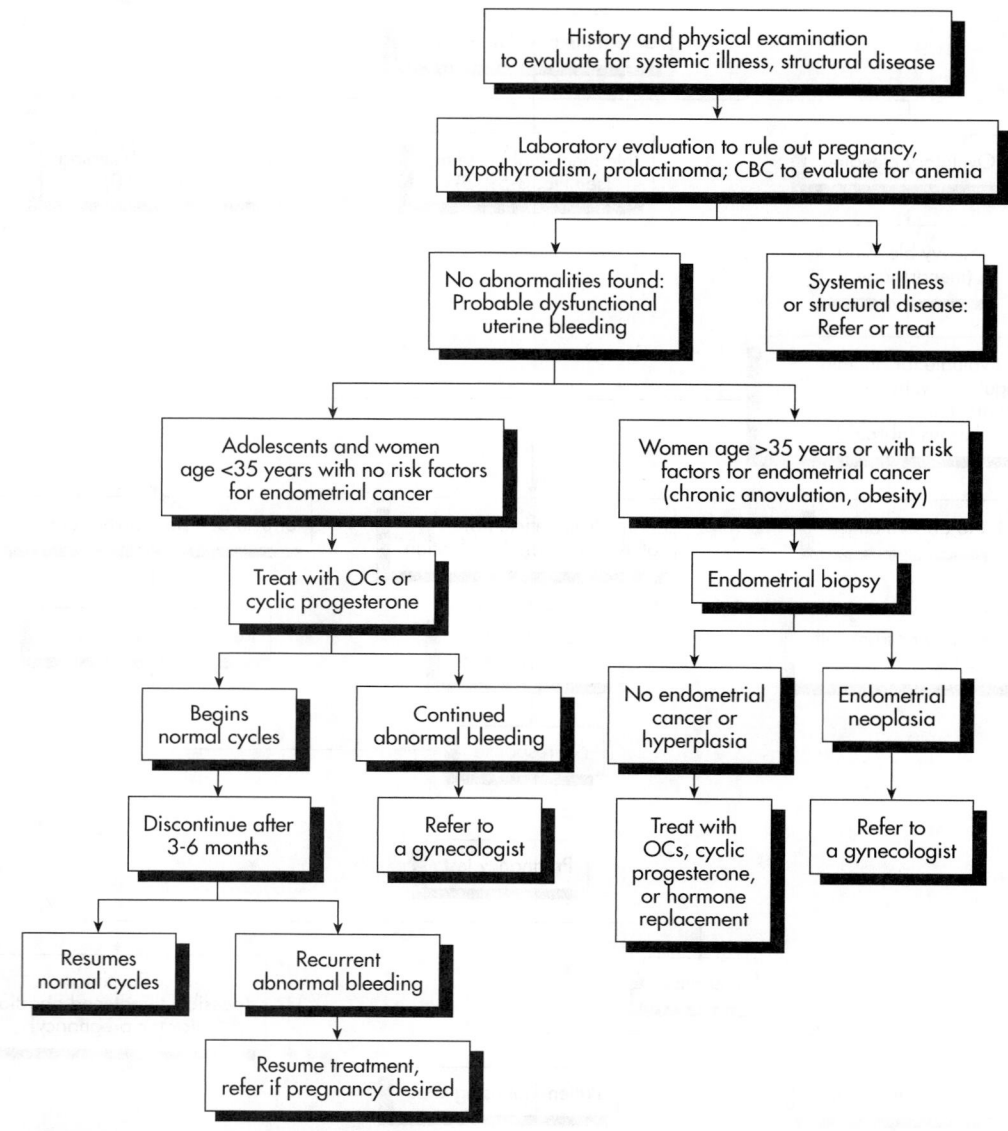

FIGURE 3-60 Evaluation of anovulatory bleeding. *CBC*, Complete blood count; *OCs*, oral contraceptives. (From Appleby J, Henderson M, Wathen PI: *Intern Med*, Sept:17, 1996.)

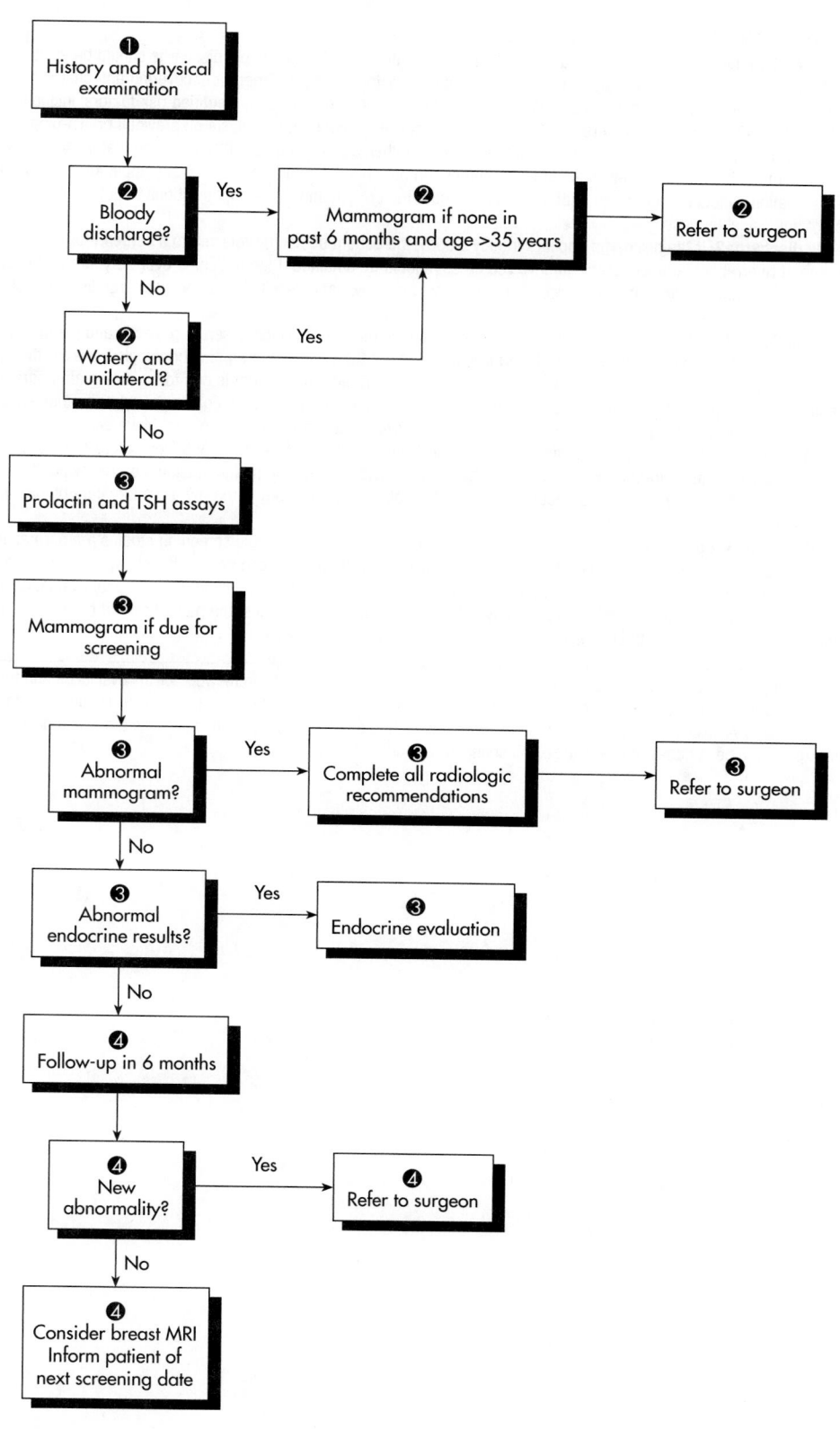

*Without palpable mass.

FIGURE 3-63 Breast cancer screening and evaluation. (Modified from Institute for Clinical Systems Integration, Minneapolis: *Postgrad Med* 100:182, 1996.)

Continued on following page

Clinical
Algorithms

FIGURE 3-63 (Continued)

1. **History and physical examination.*** Patients who present with a complaint of nipple discharge should be evaluated with breast-related history taking and a physical examination. History taking is aimed at uncovering and characterizing any other breast-related symptom. A risk assessment should also be undertaken for identified risk factors, including patient age over 50 years, any past personal history of breast cancer, history of hyperplasia on previous breast biopsies, and family history of breast cancer in first-degree relatives (mother, sister, daughter). Physical examination should include inspection of the breast for any evidence of ulceration or contour changes and inspection of the nipple for Paget's disease. Palpation should be performed with the patient in both the upright and the supine positions to determine the presence of any palpable mass.

2. **Bloody discharge?** If the discharge appears frankly bloody, the patient should be referred to a surgeon for evaluation. At the time of referral, a mammogram of the involved breast should be obtained if the patient is over 35 years of age and has not had a mammogram within the preceding 6 months. Similarly, patients with a watery, unilateral discharge should be referred to a surgeon for evaluation and possible biopsy.

3. **Endocrine tests. Mammogram.** If the discharge appears frankly milky or is bilateral, serum prolactin and serum thyroid-stimulating hormone *(TSH)* assays should be performed to rule out the presence of an endocrinologic basis for the symptoms. At the time of that visit, a mammogram should also be performed if the patient is due for routine mammographic screening according to the recommended intervals. A patient with an abnormal mammogram should be further evaluated radiologically to better characterize the lesion and then be referred to a surgeon if appropriate. Make certain that all recommended additional views, ultrasound examinations, and follow-up studies have been obtained before referral to a surgeon. Should the mammogram appear normal, results of the assays for TSH and prolactin should be reviewed. If the results are abnormal, the patient should undergo appropriate evaluation for etiology, either by a primary care physician or by an endocrinologist.

4. **Six-month follow-up results.** If results of the mammogram and the endocrinologic screening studies are normal, the patient should return for a follow-up visit in 6 months to ensure that there has been no specific change in the character of the discharge, such as development of frank bleeding or Paget's disease, that would warrant surgical evaluation. If the evaluation at that follow-up visit fails to reveal any palpable or visible abnormalities, the patient should be returned to the routine screening process with studies performed at the recommended intervals.

---

*ICSI health care guidelines are designed to assist clinicians by providing an analytic framework for the evaluation and treatment of patients. They are not intended either to replace a clinician's judgment or to establish a protocol for all patients with a particular condition. A guideline will rarely establish the only approach to a problem. In addition, guidelines are "living documents" that are expected to be imperfect and are subject to annual review and revision.

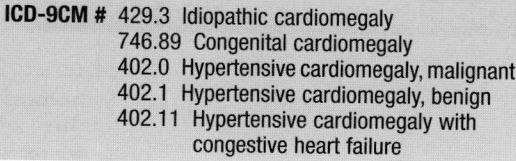

ICD-9CM # 429.3 Idiopathic cardiomegaly
746.89 Congenital cardiomegaly
402.0 Hypertensive cardiomegaly, malignant
402.1 Hypertensive cardiomegaly, benign
402.11 Hypertensive cardiomegaly with
congenital heart failure

Evaluation of cardiomegaly on chest x-ray

↓

Review history
Examination
ECG

↓

Echocardiogram

Left ventricular dilation

Evaluate for:
Valvular heart disease
Coronary artery disease
Cardiomyopathy

Biventricular dilation

Consider right heart failure secondary to left heart failure from various causes of left ventricular dilation

Right ventricular dilation

Pulmonary hypertension?

Yes → Evaluate for:
Pulmonary emboli
Mitral stenosis
Primary pulmonary hypertension
Eisenmenger's syndrome

No → Evaluate for:
Atrial septal defect
Tricuspid regurgitation

Pericardial effusion/thickening/mass

R/O tamponade → ? Pericardiocentesis

? Cause → Consider:
CT
MRI
Surgery/biopsy

No abnormalities

No further workup

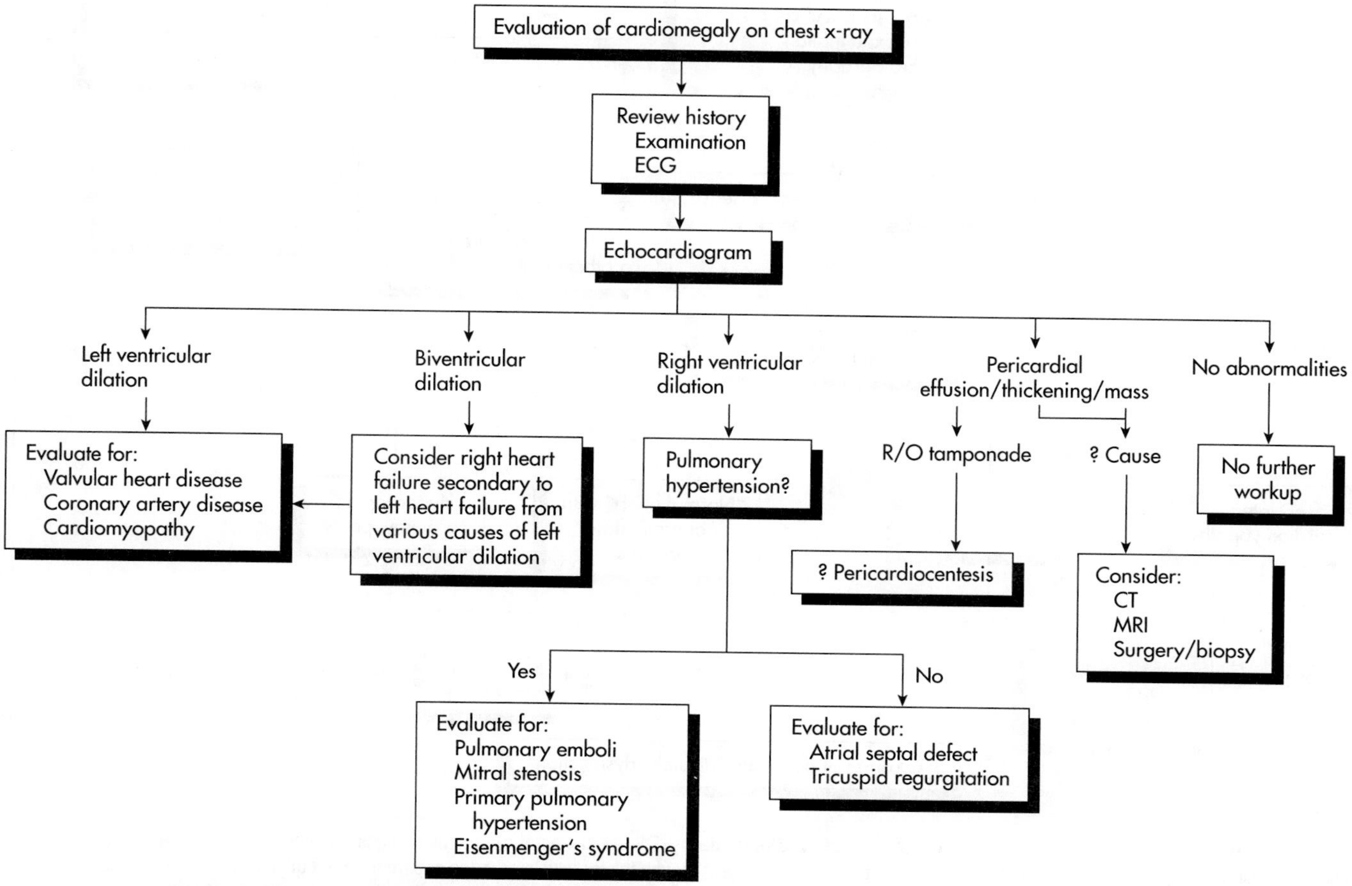

FIGURE 3-69 Approach to the patient with cardiomegaly. When cardiomegaly is found on the chest radiograph, the history and physical examination should be reviewed and an electrocardiogram *(ECG)* performed before obtaining a two-dimensional Doppler echocardiographic study. Cardiomegaly may be explained by left ventricular dilation, biventricular dilation, right ventricular dilation, or pericardial abnormalities, or it may be found to be spurious on the echocardiogram. Rarely, isolated abnormalities of the atrium, particularly the left atrium, may cause abnormalities on the chest radiograph but will not cause true cardiomegaly. Depending on the echocardiographic findings, further tests can help elucidate the cause of echocardiographically confirmed cardiomegaly. *CT,* Computed tomography; *MRI,* magnetic resonance imaging; *R/O,* rule out. (From Goldman L, Braunwald E [eds]: *Primary cardiology,* ed 2, Philadelphia, 2003, WB Saunders.)

Clinical
Algorithms

III

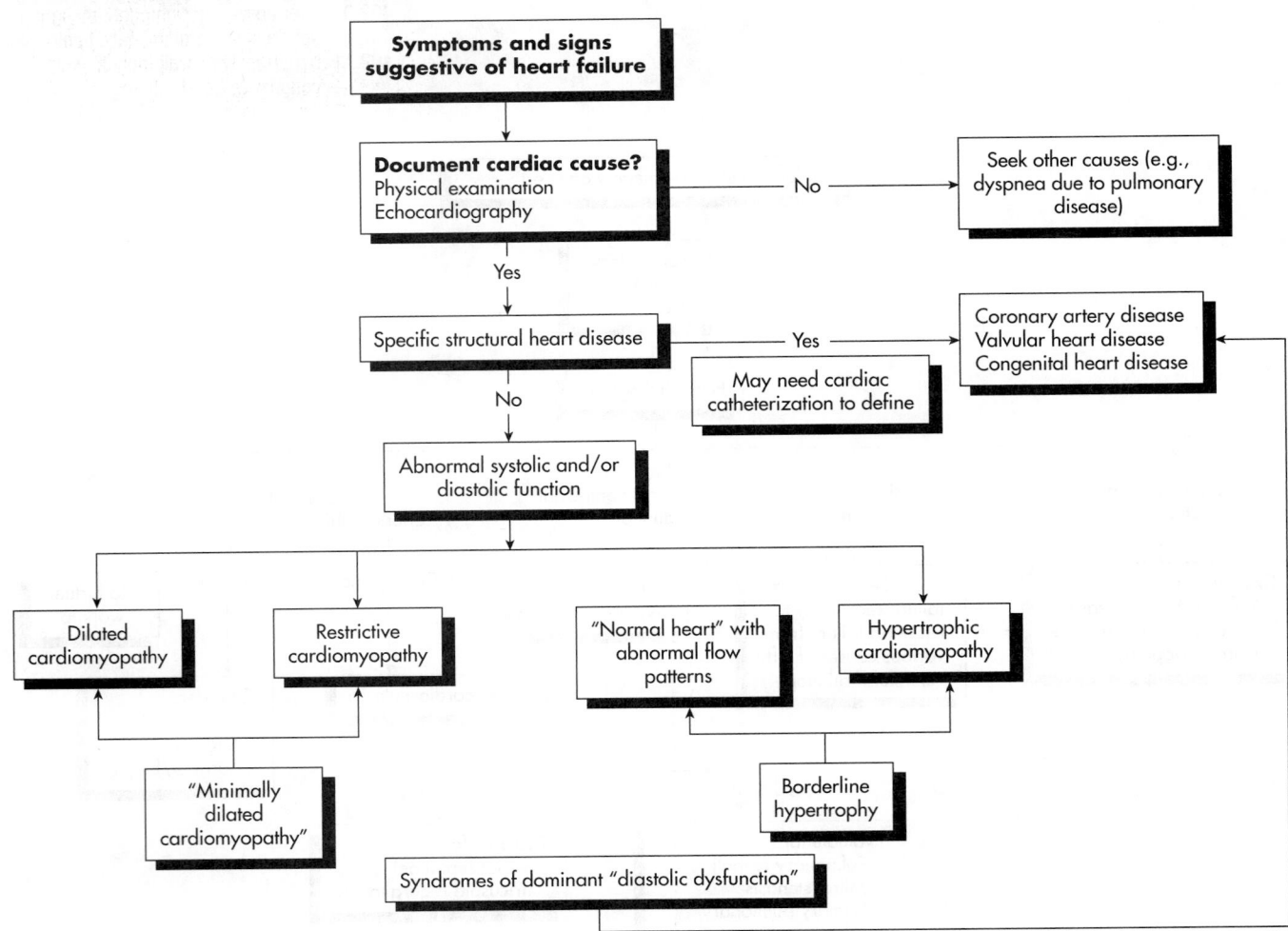

FIGURE 3-70 Initial approach to classification of cardiomyopathy. The evaluation of symptoms or signs consistent with heart failure first includes confirmation that they can be attributed to a cardiac cause. Although this conclusion is often apparent from routine physical examination, echocardiography serves to confirm cardiac disease and provides clues to the presence of other cardiac disease, such as focal abnormalities, suggesting primary valve disease or congenital heart disease. Having excluded these conditions, cardiomyopathy is generally considered to be dilated, restrictive, or hypertrophic. Patients with apparently normal cardiac structure and contraction are occasionally found to demonstrate abnormal intracardiac flow patterns consistent with diastolic dysfunction but should also be evaluated carefully for other causes of their symptoms. Most patients with so-called diastolic dysfunction also demonstrate at least borderline criteria for left ventricular hypertrophy, frequently in the setting of chronic hypertension and diabetes. A moderately decreased ejection fraction without marked dilation or a pattern of restrictive cardiomyopathy is sometimes referred to as "minimally dilated cardiomyopathy," which may represent either a distinct entity or a transition between acute and chronic disease. (From Goldman L, Ausiello D [eds]: *Cecil textbook of medicine,* ed 23, Philadelphia, 2008, WB Saunders.)

TABLE 3-4   Profiles of Symptomatic Cardiomyopathy

	Dilated	**Restrictive**	**Hypertrophic**
Ejection fraction (normal >55%)	<30%	25%-50%	>60%
Left ventricular diastolic dimension (normal <55 mm)	≥60 mm	<60 mm	Often decreased
Left ventricular wall thickness	Decreased	Normal or increased	Markedly increased
Atrial size	Increased	Increased; may be massive	Increased
Valvular regurgitation	Mitral first during decompensation; tricuspid regurgitation in late stages	Frequent mitral and tricuspid regurgitation, rarely severe	Mitral regurgitation
Common first symptoms*	Exertional intolerance	Exertional intolerance, fluid retention	Exertional intolerance; may have chest pain
Congestive symptoms*	Left before right, except right prominent in young adults	Right often exceeds left	Primary exertional dyspnea
Risk for arrhythmia	Ventricular tachyarrhythmias; conduction block in Chagas' disease, giant cell myocarditis, and some families; atrial fibrillation	Ventricular tachyarrhythmias uncommon except in sarcoidosis; conduction block in sarcoidosis and amyloidosis, atrial fibrillation	Ventricular tachyarrhythmias, atrial fibrillation

From Goldman L, Ausiello D [eds]: *Cecil textbook of medicine,* ed 23, Philadelphia, 2008, WB Saunders.
*Left-sided symptoms of pulmonary congestion: dyspnea on exertion, orthopnea, paroxysmal nocturnal dyspnea. Right-sided symptoms of systemic venous congestion: discomfort on bending, hepatic and abdominal distention, peripheral edema.

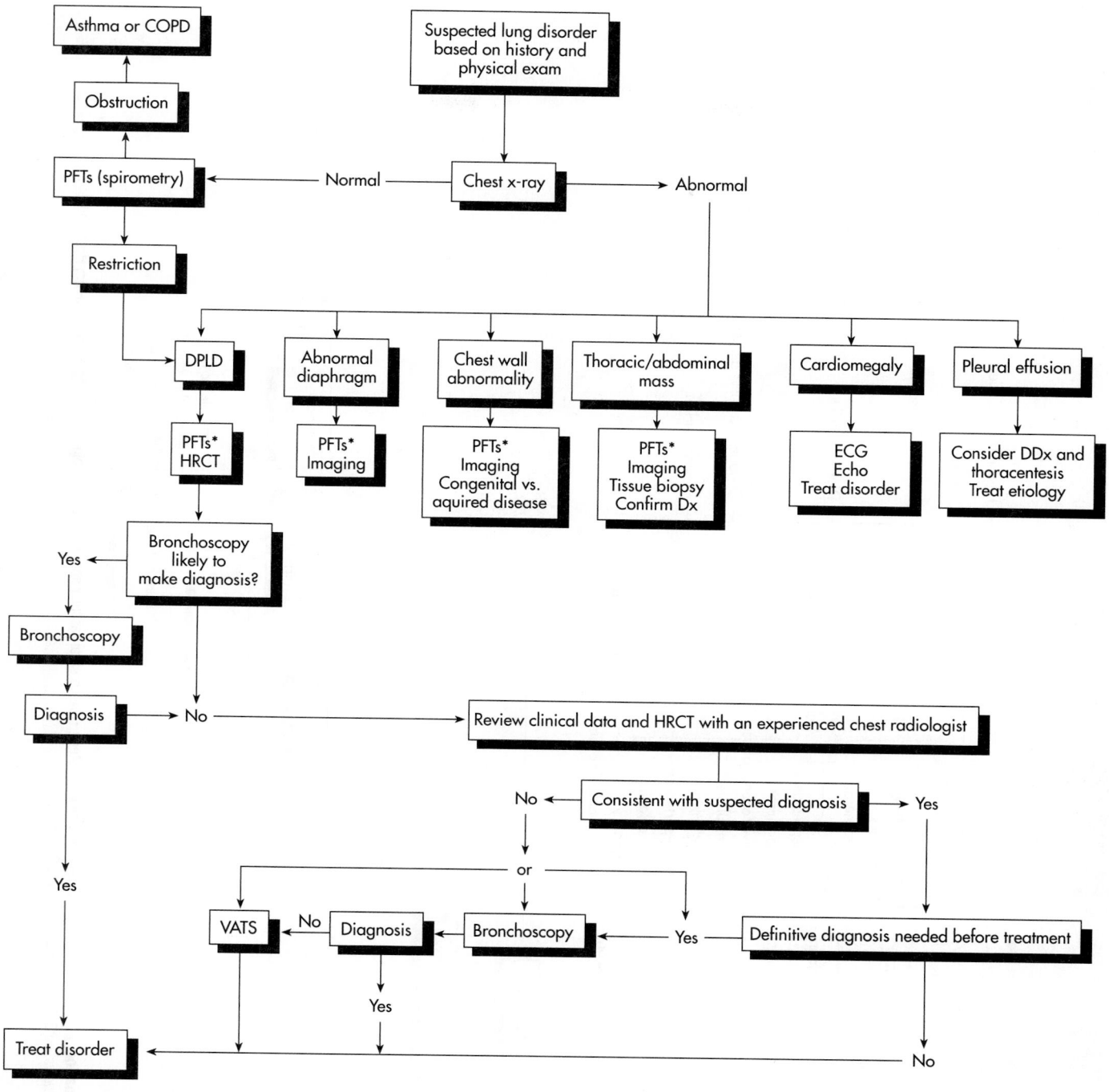

PFTs* = Full set including lung volumes and DLCO

FIGURE 3-75 Diagnostic algorithm. *COPD,* Chronic obstructive pulmonary disease; *DDx,* differential diagnosis; *DLCO,* diffusion capacity; *DPLD,* diffuse parenchymal lung disease; *ECG,* electrocardiogram; *HRCT,* high-resolution computed tomography; *PFTs,* pulmonary function tests; *VATS,* video-assisted thoracoscopic surgery. (Modified from Runge MS, Greganti MA: *Netter's internal medicine,* Philadelphia, 2008, WB Saunders.)

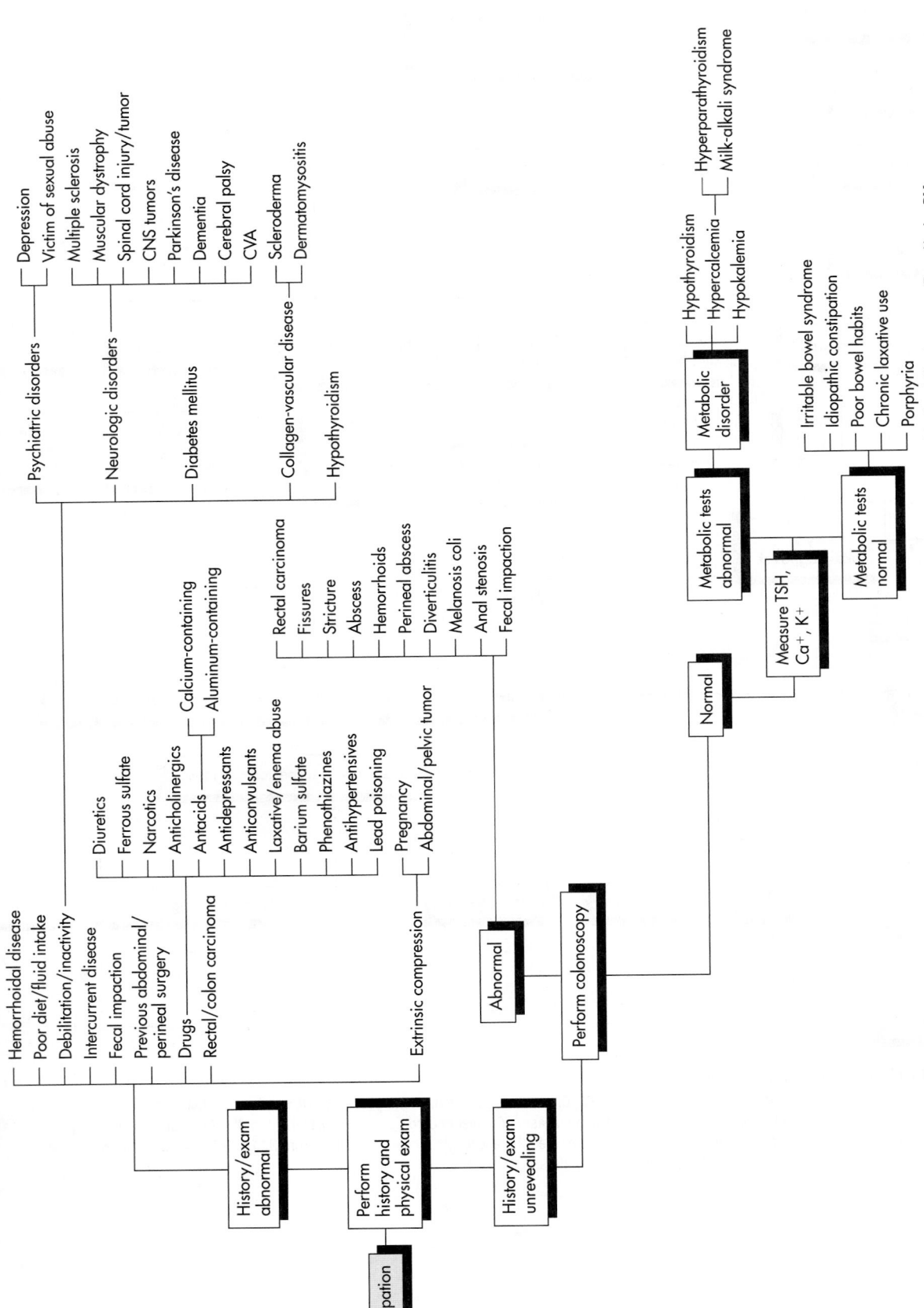

FIGURE 3-77 Constipation. *BE,* Barium enema; *CNS,* central nervous system; *CVA,* cerebral vascular accident; *TSH,* thyroid-stimulating hormone. (From Healey PM: *Common medical diagnosis,* ed 3, Philadelphia, 2000, WB Saunders.)

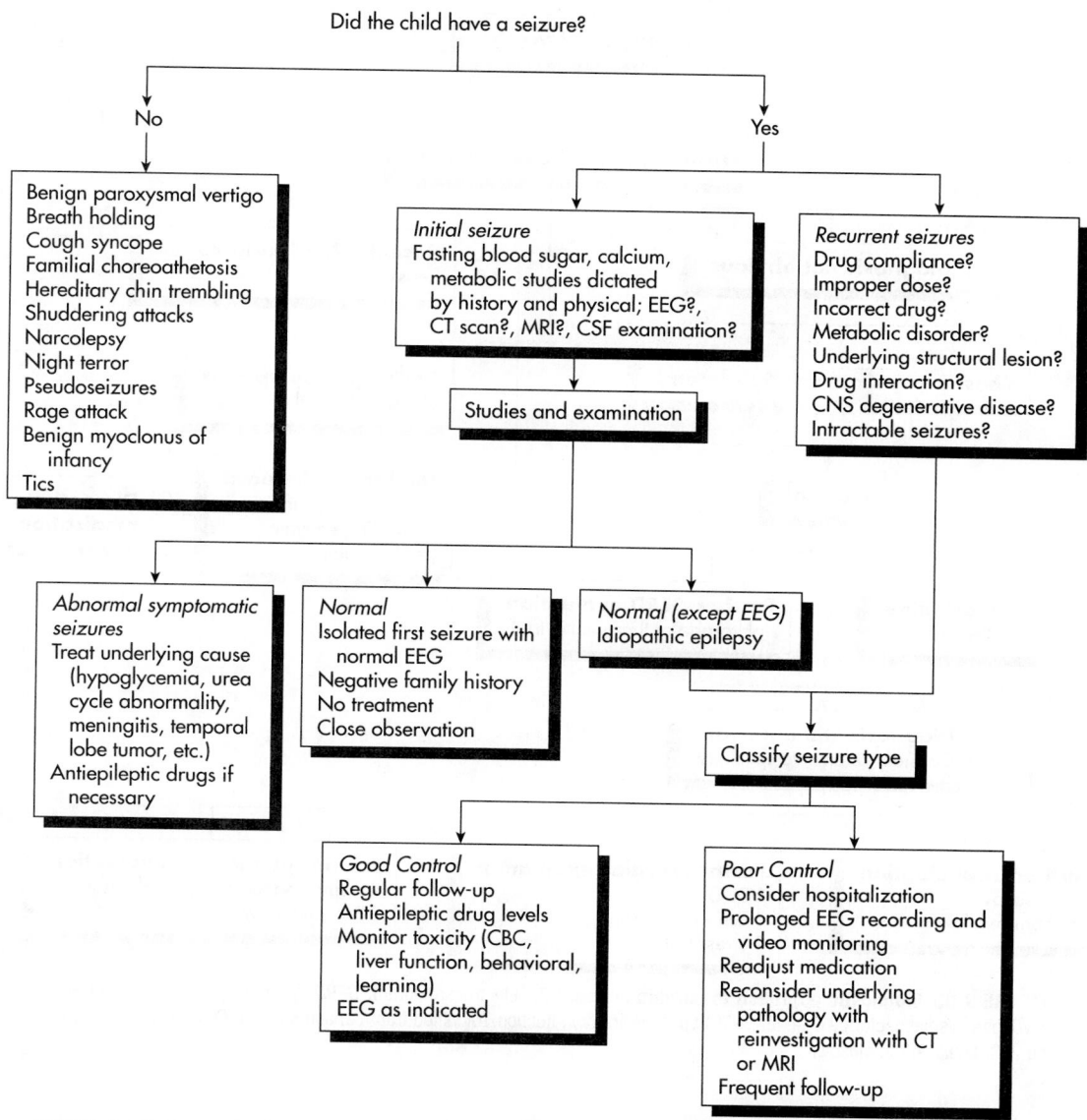

FIGURE 3-80 An approach to the child with a suspected convulsive disorder. *CBC,* Complete blood count; *CNS,* central nervous system; *CSF,* cerebrospinal fluid; *CT,* computed tomography; *EEG,* electroencephalogram; *MRI,* magnetic resonance imaging. (From Behrman RE: *Nelson textbook of pediatrics,* ed 18, Philadelphia, 2007, WB Saunders.)

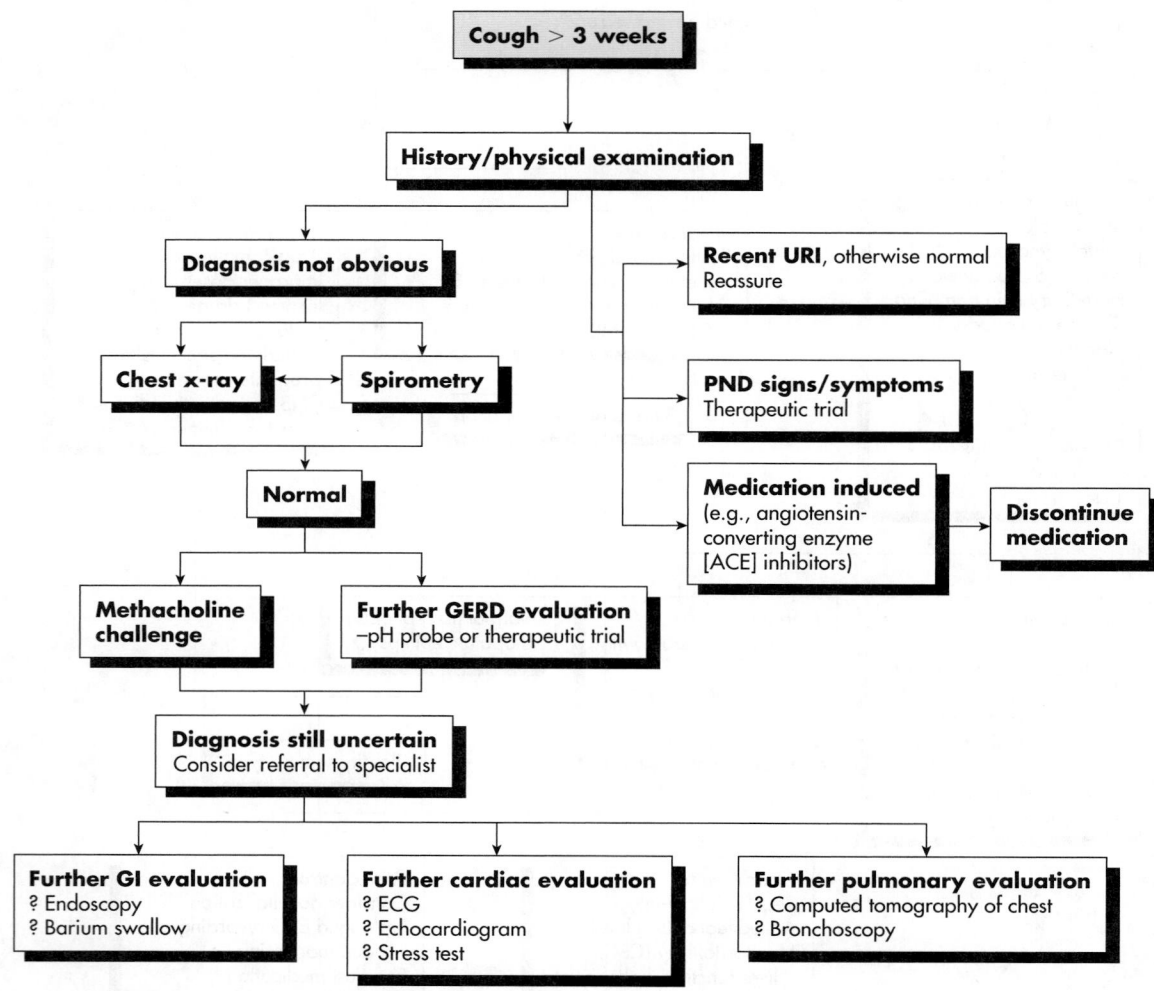

FIGURE 3-83 Diagnostic approach to chronic cough. *ECG,* Electrocardiogram; *GERD,* gastroesophageal reflux disease; *PND,* paroxysmal nocturnal dyspnea; *URI,* upper respiratory infection. (Modified from Carlson KJ et al: *Primary care of women,* ed 2, St Louis, 2002, Mosby.)

CREATINE KINASE ELEVATION

```
Laboratory evaluation

Patient with elevated creatine kinase level
    │
    └──> Determine origin
         MB Fractionation
              │
    ┌─────────┼──────────────────────┐
    │         │                      │
Cardiac    Brain (BB)            Muscle (MM)
 (MB)         │                      │
    │      CT or MRI            History
    │      of brain           Physical examination
    │                               │
Cardiac troponin levels,     ┌──────┼──────────┬────────────────┐
cardiac evaluation           │      │          │                │
    │                    Normal  Muscle    Drugs,          
    │                            weakness/ medications      
┌───┴────────┐                   tenderness    │
│            │                    │        Discontinue
History of  Positive          Screening    offending
trauma      family            tests:       agent
    │       history             CBC
Repeat CK       │             Electrolytes
analysis    Consider:         Serum aldolase
after        Inherited        Thyroid
several       myopathies      function
weeks         Familial        tests
              idiopathic
              elevated CK
```

Screening
tests:
  CBC
  Serum aldolase
  Electrolytes
  Thyroid
  function
  tests
    │
    ├── Negative ──> Follow patient
    │
    └── Positive ──> Consider:
                      Infection
                      Severe hypokalemia
                      Hypothyroidism

(from muscle weakness/tenderness screening)
    ├── Positive ──> Consider: Infection, Severe hypokalemia, Hypothyroidism
    └── Negative ──> EMG ──>

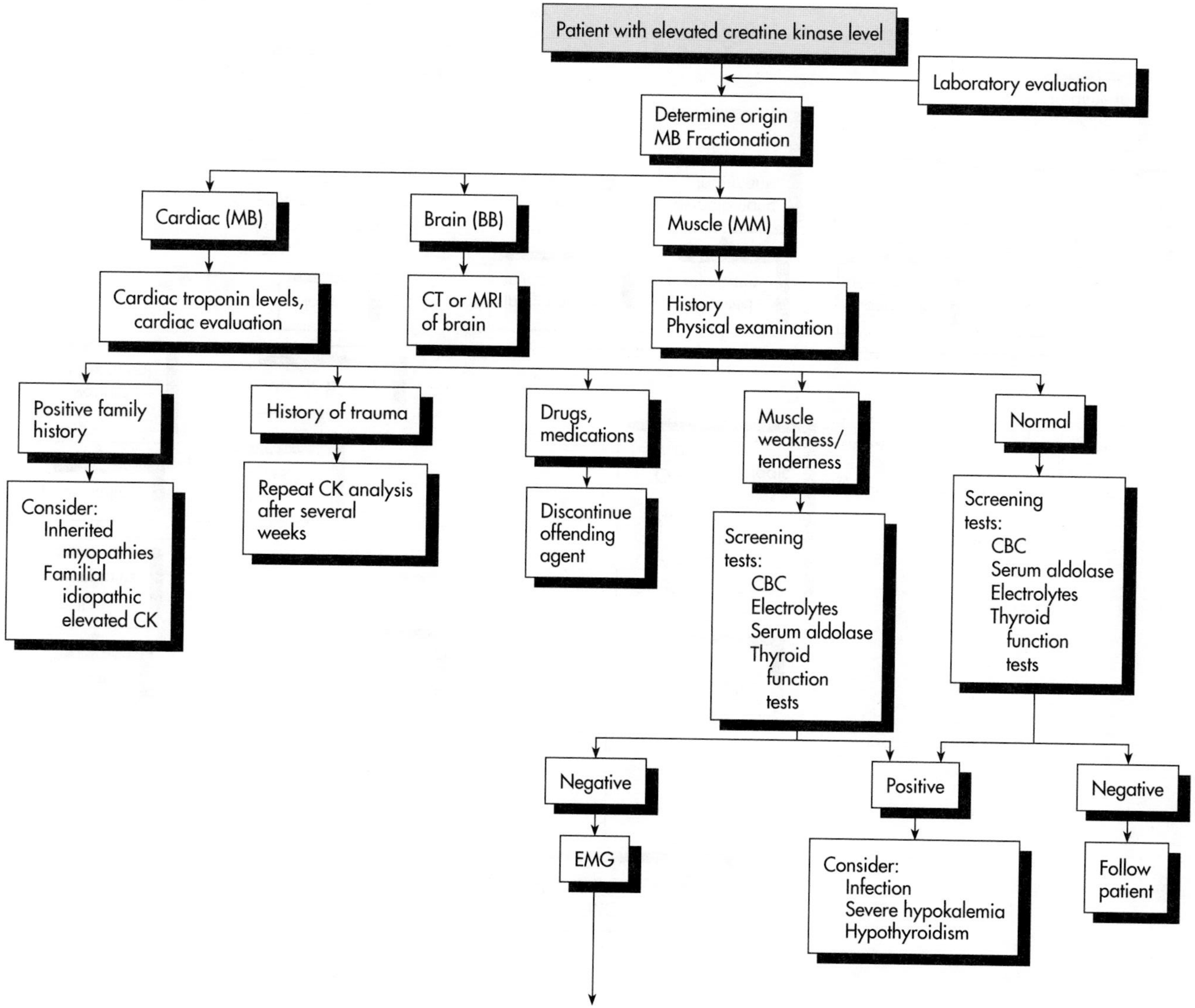

FIGURE 3-84 Evaluation of creatine kinase elevation. *CBC,* Complete blood count; *CK,* creatine kinase; *CT,* computed tomography; *EMG,* electromyography; *MRI,* magnetic resonance imaging. (Modified from Greene HL, Johnson WP, Lemcke D [eds]: *Decision making in medicine,* ed 2, St Louis, 1998, Mosby.)

(Continued on next page)

Clinical
Algorithms

III

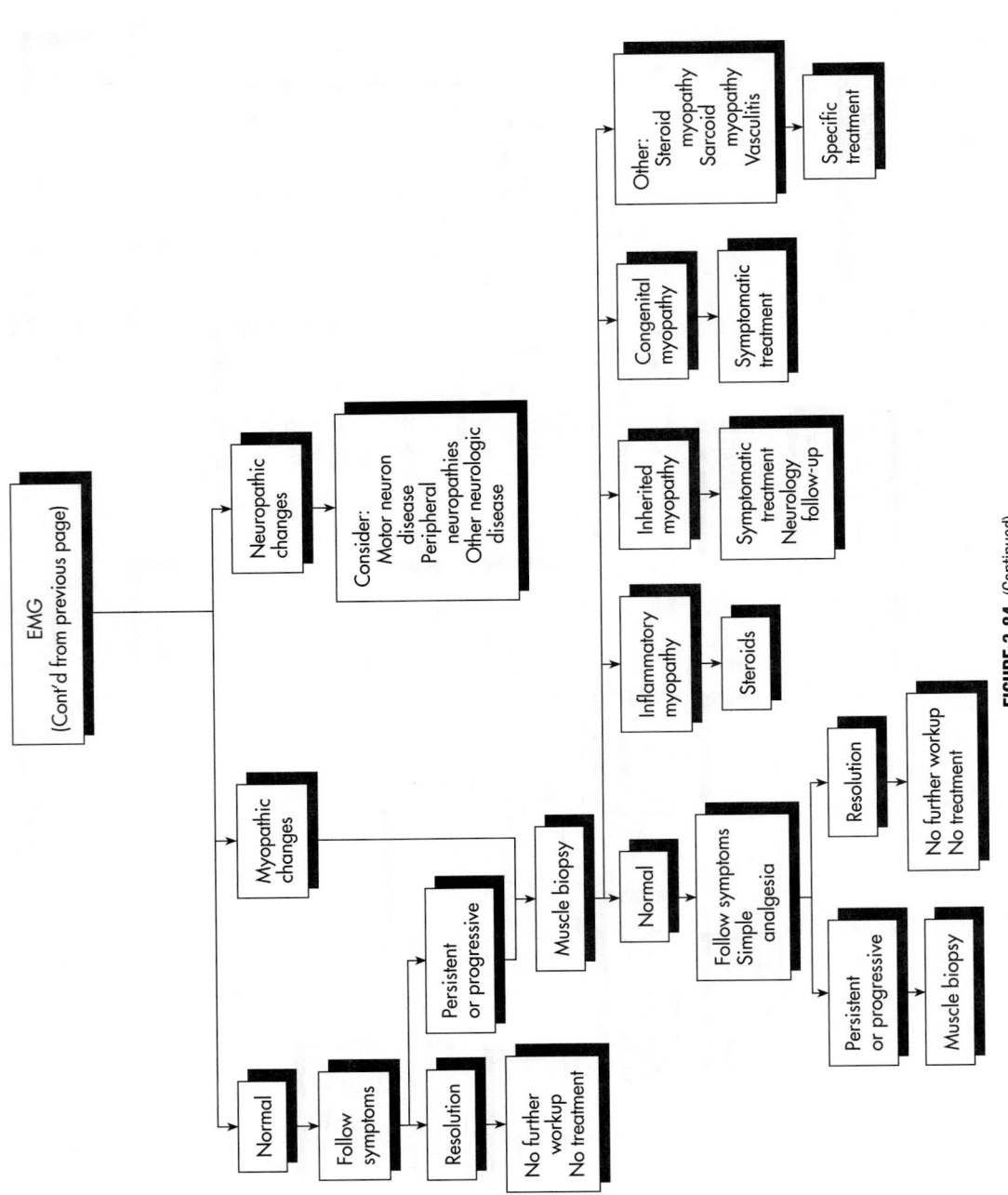

FIGURE 3-84 (Continued)

CYANOSIS

ICD-9CM # 782.5 Cyanosis NOS

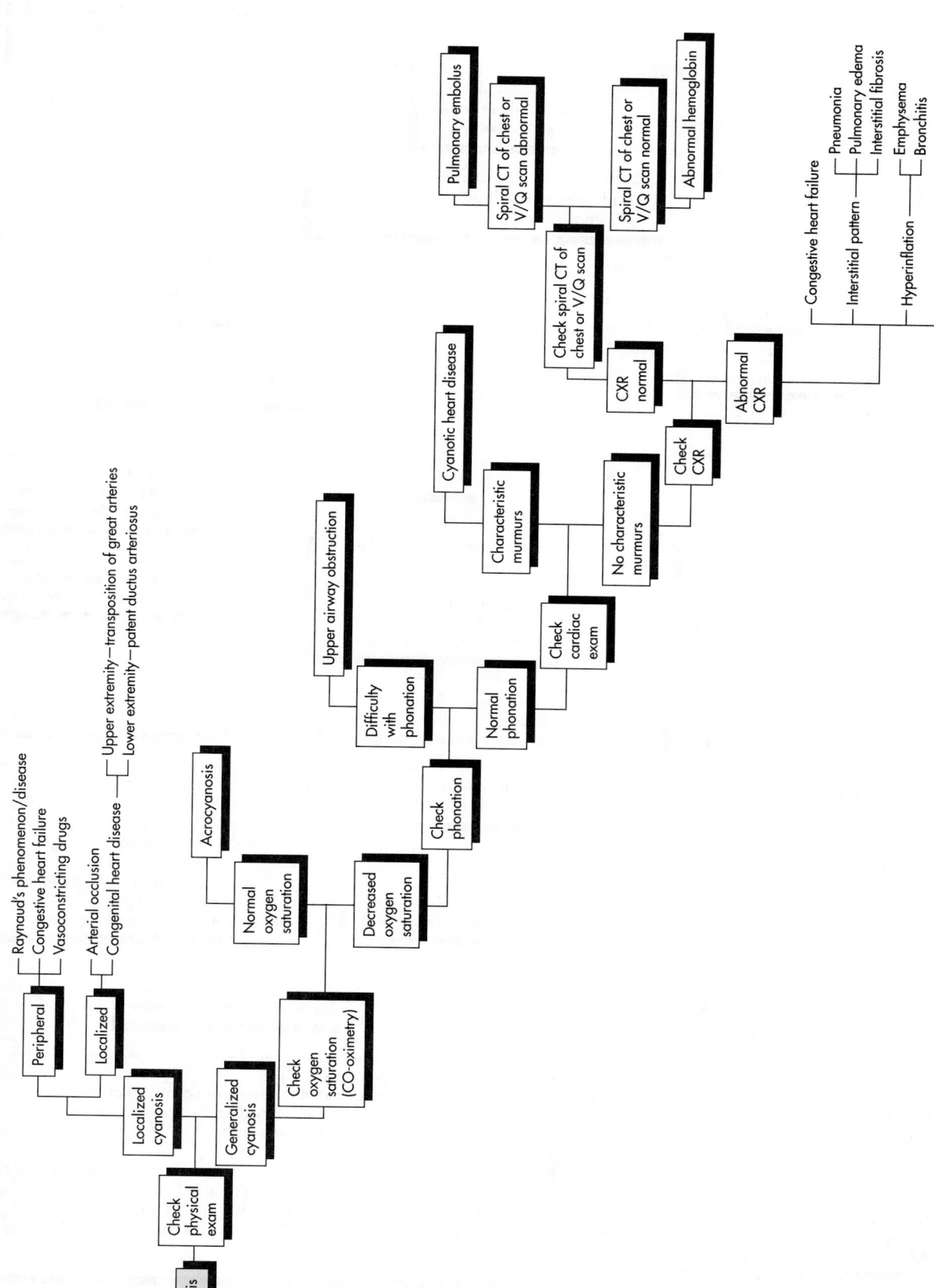

FIGURE 3-87 Cyanosis. *A-V,* Arteriovenous; *CXR,* chest x-ray; *V/Q,* ventilation-perfusion. (From Healey PM: *Common medical diagnosis: an algorithmic approach,* ed 3, Philadelphia, 2000, WB Saunders.)

ICD-9CM #   293.0 Delirium, acute
            292.81 Delirium, drug induced
            293.1 Delirium, subacute
            293.81 Delirium, transient organic with
                   delusions
            293.82 Delirium, transient organic with
                   hallucinations

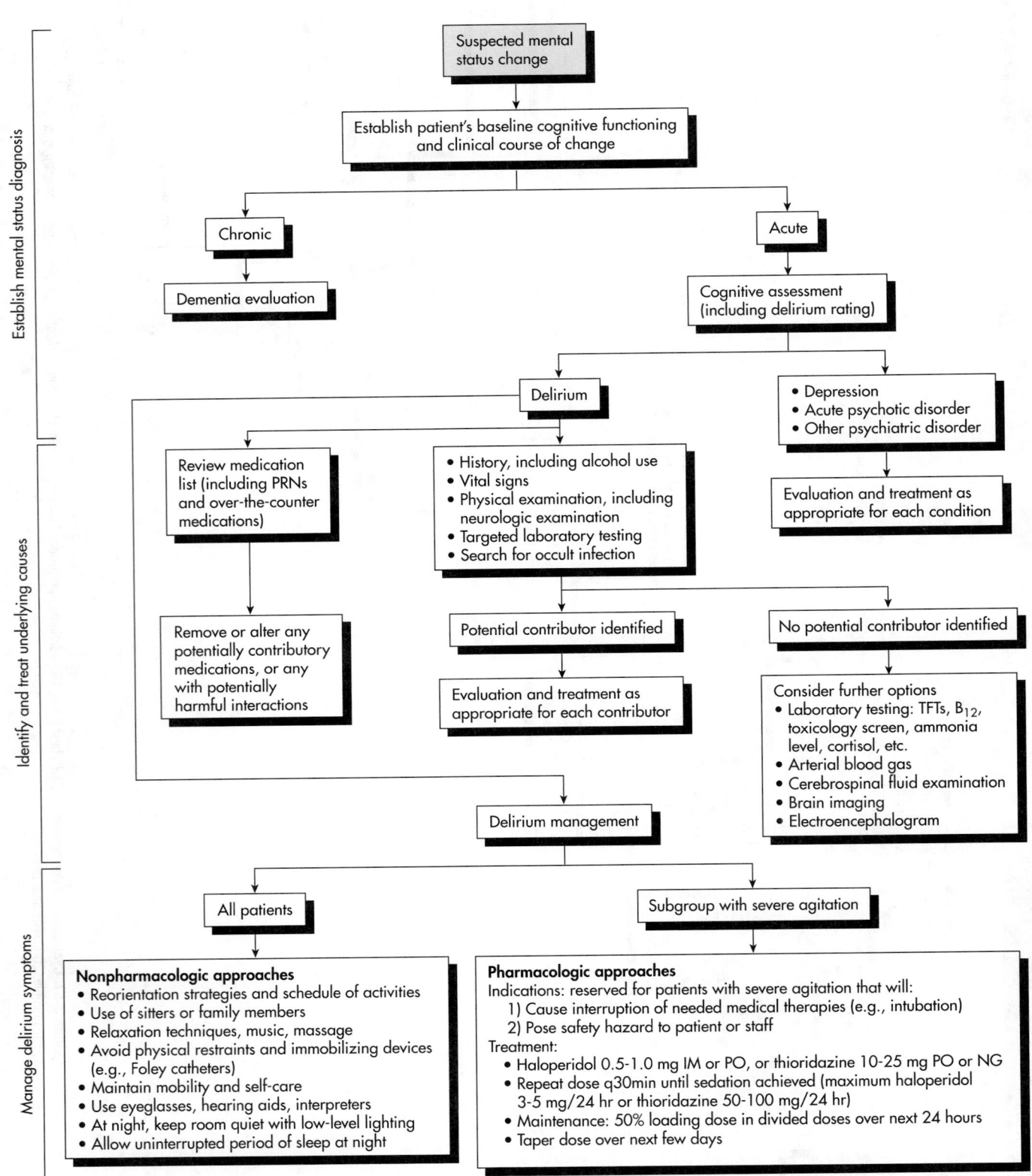

FIGURE 3-94 Algorithm for evaluation of suspected mental status change in an older patient. *IM,* Intramuscular; *NG,* nasogastric; *PO,* by mouth; *PRN,* as needed; *TFTs,* thyroid function tests. (From Goldman L, Ausiello D [eds]: *Cecil textbook of medicine,* ed 23, Philadelphia, 2008, WB Saunders.)

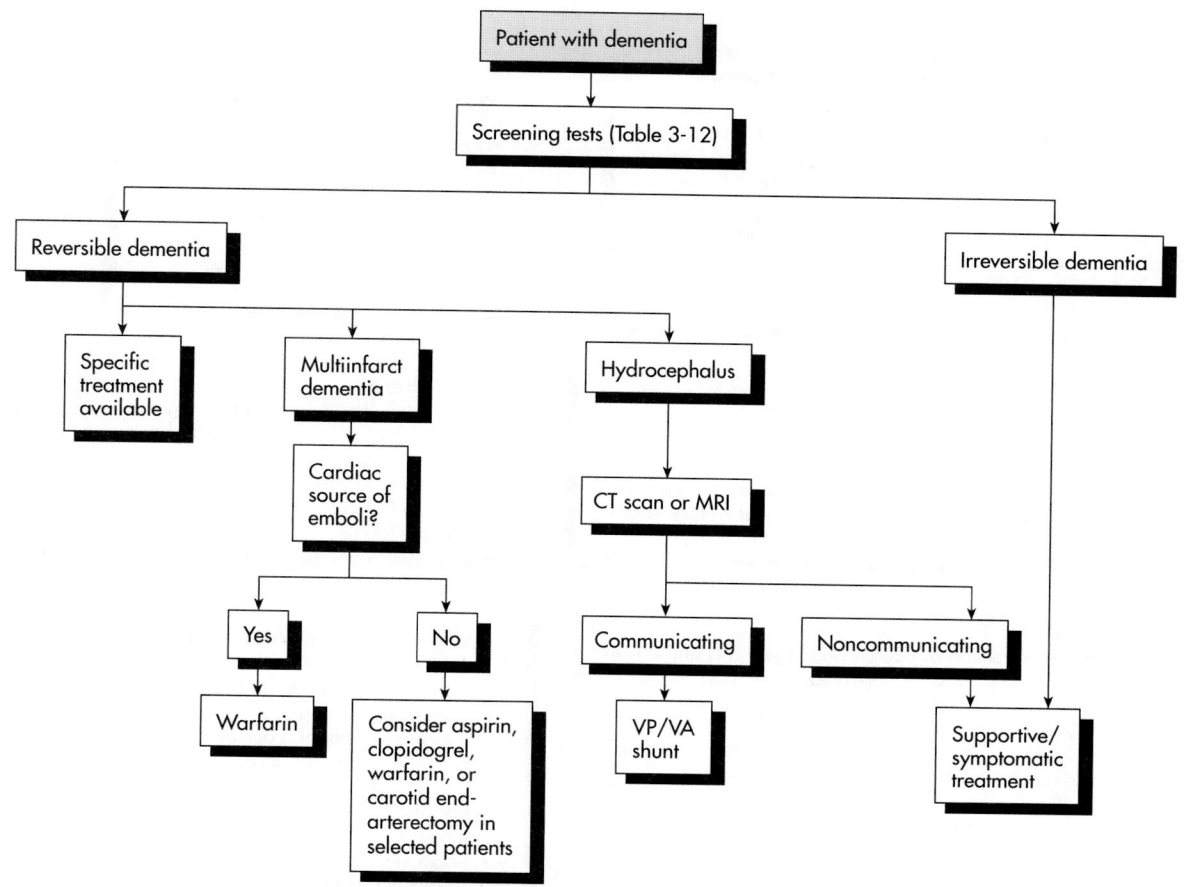

FIGURE 3-95 Management of dementia. *VA,* Ventriculoatrial; *VP,* ventriculoperitoneal.

TABLE 3-12 Screening Tests for Diagnosis of Dementia

Test	Rationale	Remarks
Blood Test		
Complete blood count	Assess general nutritional status	
Serum B_{12} level	Exclude vitamin B_{12} deficiency	Consider Schilling's test if B_{12} level is low
TSH + free T_4 *or* TSH + FTI	Exclude primary and secondary hypothyroidism	
HIV serology	Exclude HIV infection	Perform only if indicated; consent from patient required
Cerebrospinal Fluid		
Cell count/protein level	Exclude chronic meningitis	Perform only if indicated
Cytology	Exclude carcinomatous meningitis	Perform only if indicated
VDRL	Exclude neurosyphilis	Perform only if indicated; check serum TPHA and HIV serology if CSF VDRL is positive
CT Scan/MRI/PET Scan of the Brain		
	Identify infarcts and white matter changes; exclude presence of neoplasm, demyelinating disease, and hydrocephalus; location of atrophy may suggest the diagnosis (e.g., para-hippocampal atrophy in Alzheimer's disease, frontotemporal atrophy in Pick's disease)	
Electroencephalogram		
	Exclude metabolic encephalopathies; useful if Creutzfeldt-Jakob disease or status epilepticus is suspected	Perform only if indicated
Neuropsychologic Evaluation		
	Help to characterize pattern of cognitive impairment, which may aid in the classification of dementia; rule out pseudo-dementia from depression	

Modified from Johnson RT, Griffin JW: *Current therapy in neurologic disease,* ed 5, St Louis, 1997, Mosby.

CSF, Cerebrospinal fluid; *CT,* computed tomography; *FTI,* free thyroxine index; *HIV,* human immunodeficiency virus; *MRI,* magnetic resonance imaging; *PET,* positron emission tomography; *T₄,* thyroxine; *TPHA,* treponema pallidum hemagglutination assay; *TSH,* thyroid-stimulating hormone; *VDRL,* Venereal Disease Research Laboratory.

Clinical Algorithms

III

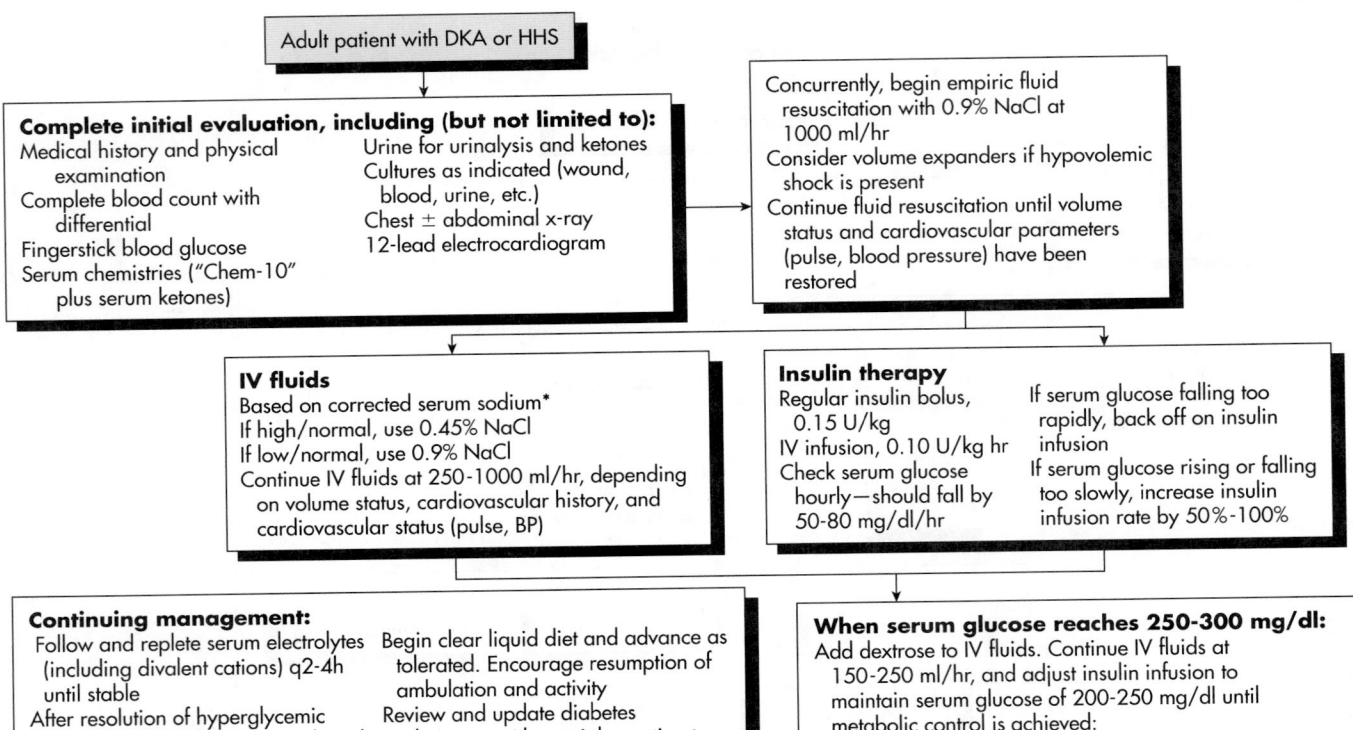

Adult patient with DKA or HHS

Complete initial evaluation, including (but not limited to):
Medical history and physical examination
Complete blood count with differential
Fingerstick blood glucose
Serum chemistries ("Chem-10" plus serum ketones)
Urine for urinalysis and ketones
Cultures as indicated (wound, blood, urine, etc.)
Chest ± abdominal x-ray
12-lead electrocardiogram

Concurrently, begin empiric fluid resuscitation with 0.9% NaCl at 1000 ml/hr
Consider volume expanders if hypovolemic shock is present
Continue fluid resuscitation until volume status and cardiovascular parameters (pulse, blood pressure) have been restored

IV fluids
Based on corrected serum sodium*
If high/normal, use 0.45% NaCl
If low/normal, use 0.9% NaCl
Continue IV fluids at 250-1000 ml/hr, depending on volume status, cardiovascular history, and cardiovascular status (pulse, BP)

Insulin therapy
Regular insulin bolus, 0.15 U/kg
IV infusion, 0.10 U/kg hr
Check serum glucose hourly—should fall by 50-80 mg/dl/hr
If serum glucose falling too rapidly, back off on insulin infusion
If serum glucose rising or falling too slowly, increase insulin infusion rate by 50%-100%

Continuing management:
Follow and replete serum electrolytes (including divalent cations) q2-4h until stable
After resolution of hyperglycemic state, follow blood glucose q4h and initiate sliding scale regular insulin coverage
Convert IV insulin to subcutaneous injections (or resumption of prior therapy), ensuring adequate overlap if treating patients without endogenous insulin secretion
Begin clear liquid diet and advance as tolerated. Encourage resumption of ambulation and activity
Review and update diabetes education, with special attention to prevention of further hyperglycemic crises

When serum glucose reaches 250-300 mg/dl:
Add dextrose to IV fluids. Continue IV fluids at 150-250 ml/hr, and adjust insulin infusion to maintain serum glucose of 200-250 mg/dl until metabolic control is achieved:
For DKA, continue until anion gap has closed and acidosis has resolved
For HHS, continue until plasma osmolality drops below 310 mOsm/kg
Begin more exhaustive search for precipitant of metabolic decompensation

Potassium (K+) repletion
Obtain baseline serum potassium
Obtain 12-lead ECG

$[K^+] \geq 5.5$ mEq/L

Hold K+ therapy

Treat hyperkalemia if ECG changes present

Recheck [K+] in 2 hr

$[K^+] < 5.5$ mEq/L and adequate urine output

Add K+ to IV fluids (Use KCl and/or KPhos)

[K+] = 4.5-5.4: add 20 mEq/L IVF
[K+] = 3.5-4.4: add 30 mEq/L IVF
[K+] < 3.5: add 40 mEq/L IVF

Follow serum [K+] every 2-4 hours until stable: anticipate rapid drop of serum [K+] during therapy, due to dilution and intracellular shifting
Ensure adequate urine output to avoid over-repletion and hyperkalemia
Continue K+ repletion until serum [K+] is stable at between 4-5 mEq/L
If refractory hypokalemia, ensure concurrent magnesium repletion
Repletion may need to be continued for several days, as total body losses may reach up to 500 mEq

Bicarbonate therapy
Obtain ABG
Obtain baseline serum bicarbonate

pH < 6.9

88 mEq/L (2 amps) NaHCO₃ over 2 hr

6.9 ≤ pH < 7.0

44 mEq/L (1 amp) NaHCO₃ over 1 hr

pH ≥ 7.0

Assess need for bicarbonate

Repeat ABG after bicarbonate administration
Repeat NaHCO₃ therapy until pH ≥7.0, then discontinue therapy
Follow serum bicarbonate q4h until stable

*Sodium correction: Serum sodium should be corrected for hyperglycemia. For every 100 mg/dl of glucose elevation above 100 mg/dl, add 1.6 mEq/L to the measured sodium value; this will yield the correction serum sodium concentration.

Note: Refer to Section I for additional information on these topics.

FIGURE 3-100 Management of diabetic ketoacidosis *(DKA)* and hyperosmolar hyperglycemic state *(HHS)*. *ABG,* Arterial blood gas; *DKA,* diabetic ketoacidosis; *ECG,* electrocardiograph. (From Goldman L, Ausiello D [eds]: *Cecil textbook of medicine,* ed 23, Philadelphia, 2008, WB Saunders.)

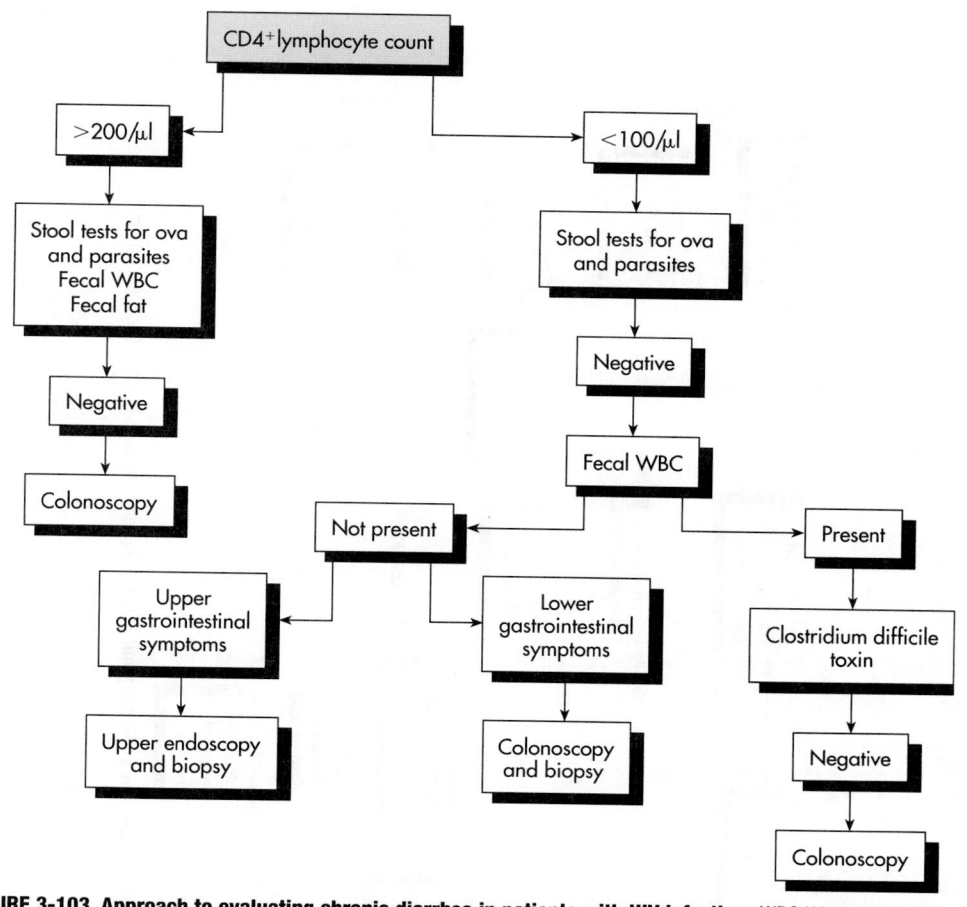

FIGURE 3-103 Approach to evaluating chronic diarrhea in patients with HIV infection. *WBC,* White blood cell count. (Modified from Wilcox CM: *Gastrointest Dis Today* 5:9, 1996.)

TABLE 3-13   Common Gastrointestinal Pathogens Associated with HIV Infection

Pathogen	CD4+ Cells/μL	Stool Volume and Frequency	Abdominal Pain	Weight Loss	Fever	Fecal Leukocytes
Cytomegalovirus*	<100	Mild to moderate	++	++	++	+
Cryptosporidiosis	<100	Moderate to severe	−	++	−	−
Microsporidiosis	<100	Mild to moderate	−	+	−	−
Mycobacterium avium complex†	<100	Mild to moderate	+	+++	+++	−

From Wilcox CM: *Gastrointest Dis Today* 5:9, 1996.
*Can have proctitis symptoms when involving the distal colon.
†Typical presentation is fever and wasting; diarrhea is usually secondary.
+++, Very common; ++, frequent; +, can occur; −, absent.

Clinical Algorithms

III

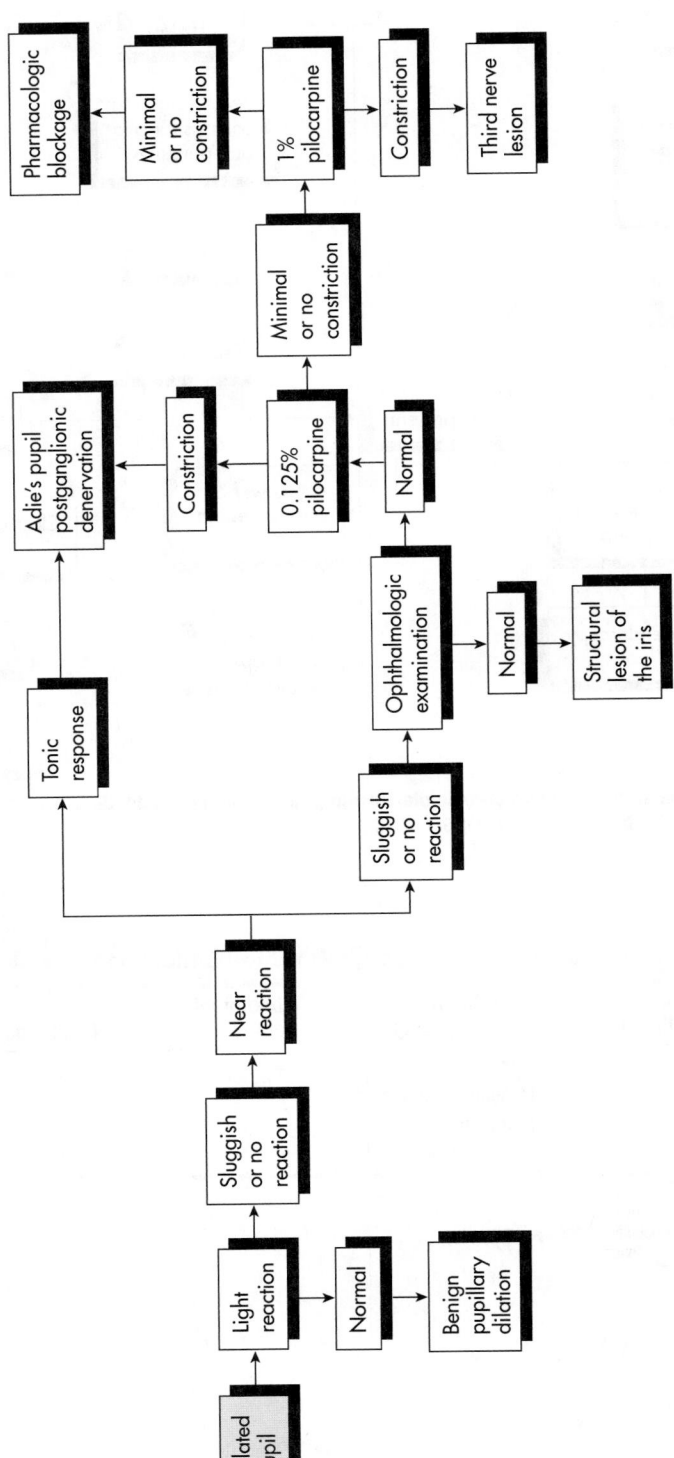

FIGURE 3-104 Use of pilocarpine to help differentiate between different causes of a dilated pupil. (From Goldman L, Ausiello D [eds]: *Cecil textbook of medicine*, ed 23, Philadephia, 2008, WB Saunders.)

CD-9CM #   563.3 Dyspepsia atonic
           536.8 Dyspepsia disorders other unspecified
                  function of stomach
           306.4 Dyspepsia, psychogenic

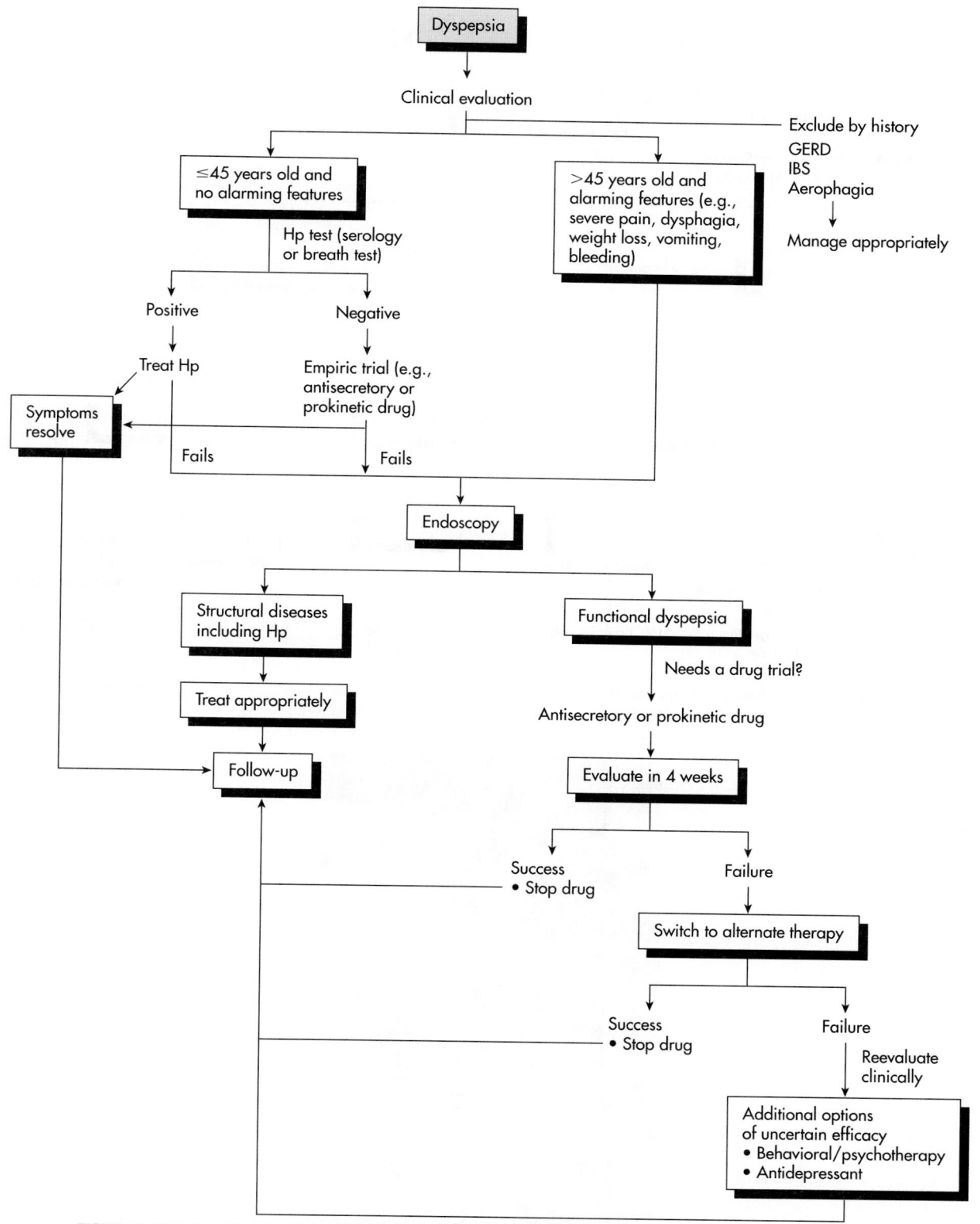

FIGURE 3-107 Algorithm for the evaluation of dyspepsia. *GERD,* Symptomatic gastroesophageal reflux disease; *Hp, Helicobacter pylori; IBS,* irritable bowel syndrome. (From Goldman L, Ausiello D [eds]: *Cecil textbook of medicine,* ed 23, Philadelphia, 2008, WB Saunders.)

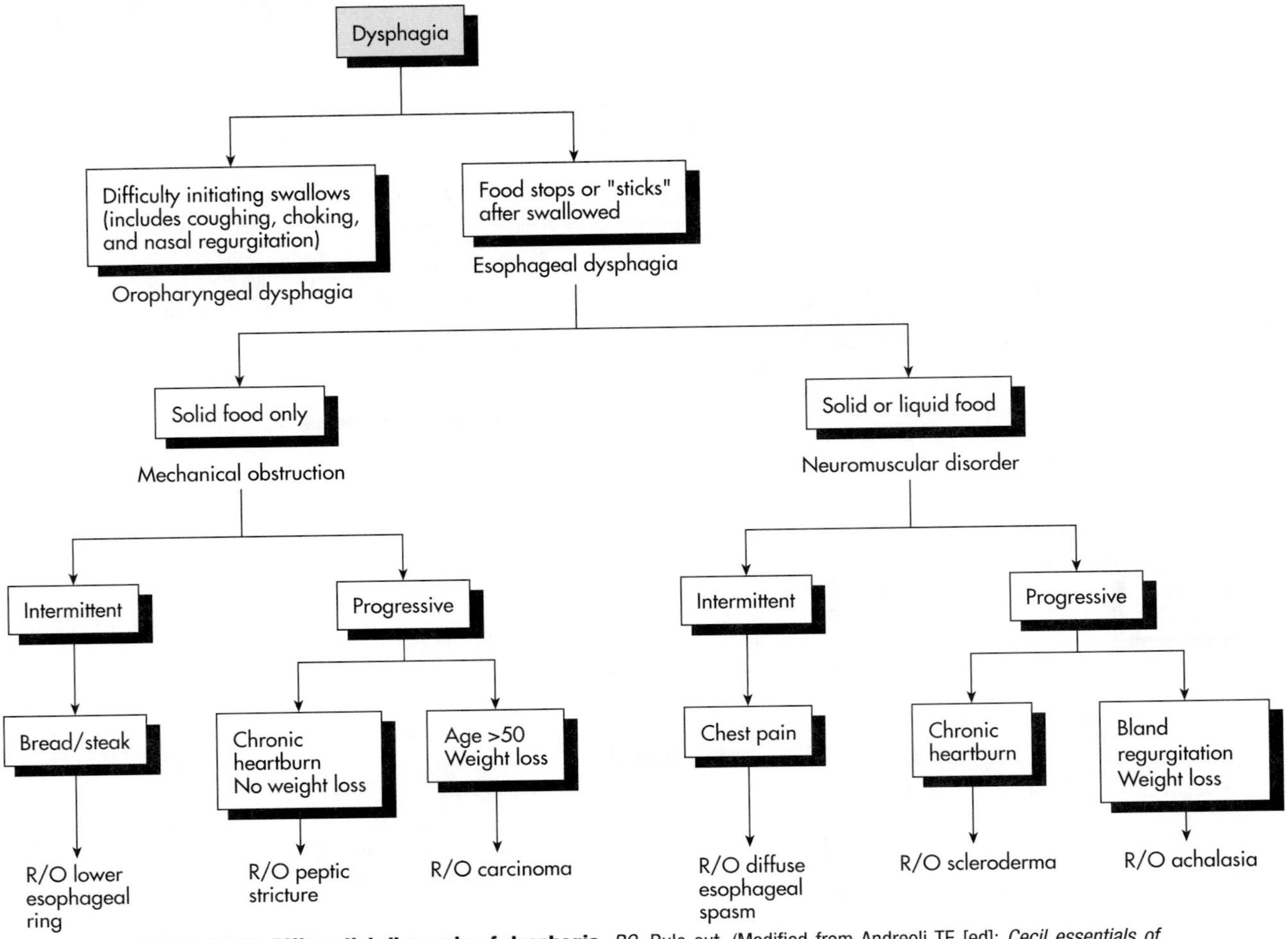

Dysphagia

Difficulty initiating swallows (includes coughing, choking, and nasal regurgitation)

Oropharyngeal dysphagia

Food stops or "sticks" after swallowed

Esophageal dysphagia

Solid food only

Mechanical obstruction

Solid or liquid food

Neuromuscular disorder

Intermittent

Progressive

Intermittent

Progressive

Bread/steak

Chronic heartburn No weight loss

Age >50 Weight loss

Chest pain

Chronic heartburn

Bland regurgitation Weight loss

R/O lower esophageal ring

R/O peptic stricture

R/O carcinoma

R/O diffuse esophageal spasm

R/O scleroderma

R/O achalasia

FIGURE 3-108 Differential diagnosis of dysphagia. *RO,* Rule out. (Modified from Andreoli TE [ed]: *Cecil essentials of medicine,* ed 7, Philadelphia, 2008, WB Saunders.)

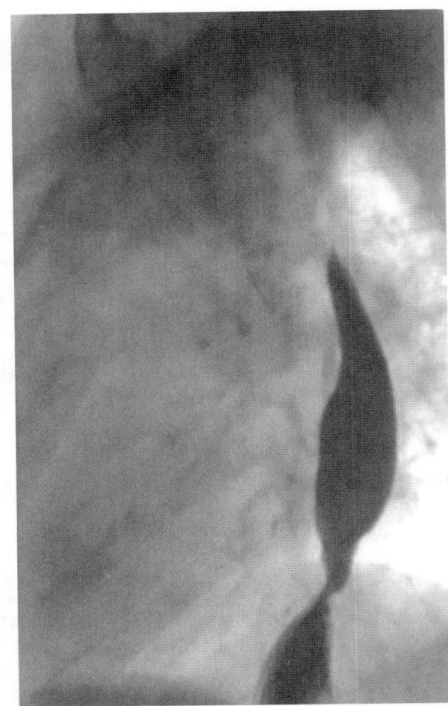

FIGURE 3-109 Barium swallow demonstrating a benign peptic stricture in a patient with gastroesophageal reflux disease and dysphagia. (From Talley NJ, Martin C: *Clinical gastroenterology: a practical problem-based approach,* ed 2, Sydney, 2006, Elsevier.)

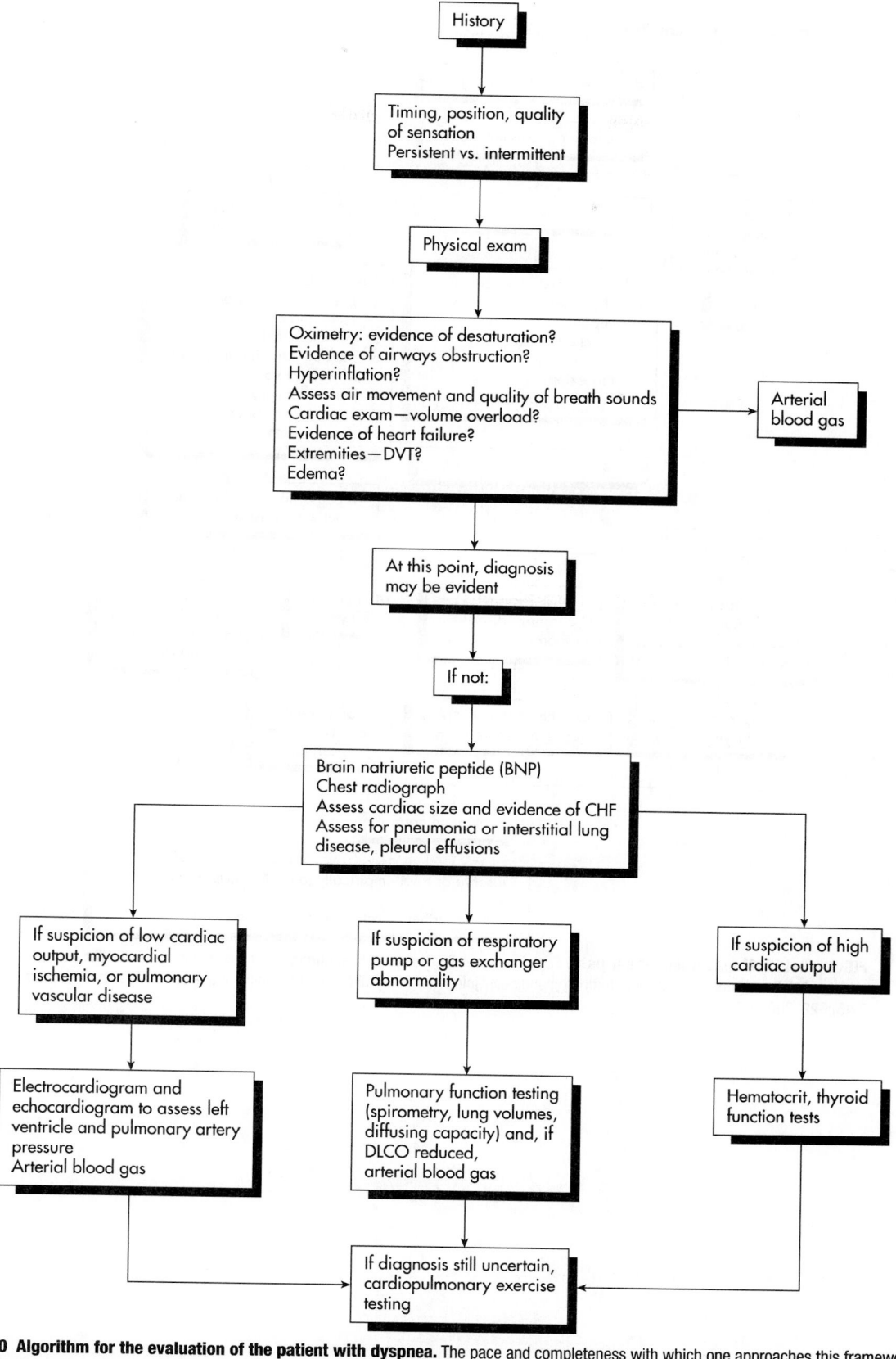

FIGURE 3-110 Algorithm for the evaluation of the patient with dyspnea. The pace and completeness with which one approaches this framework depends on the intensity and acuity of the patient's symptoms. In a patient with severe, acute dyspnea, for example, an arterial blood gas measurement may be one of the first laboratory evaluations, whereas this measurement might not be obtained until much later in the workup in a patient with chronic breathlessness of unclear cause. A therapeutic trial of a medication, for example, a bronchodilator, may be instituted at any point if one is fairly confident of the diagnosis based on the data available at that time. *CHF,* Congestive heart failure; *DLCO,* diffusing capacity of the lung for carbon monoxide; *DVT,* deep venous thrombosis. (Modified from Schwartzstein RM, Feller-Kopman D: Approach to the patient with dyspnea. In Braunwald E, Goldman L [eds]: *Primary cardiology,* ed 2, Philadelphia, 2003, WB Saunders.)

Clinical Algorithms

III

Management of Ear Pain

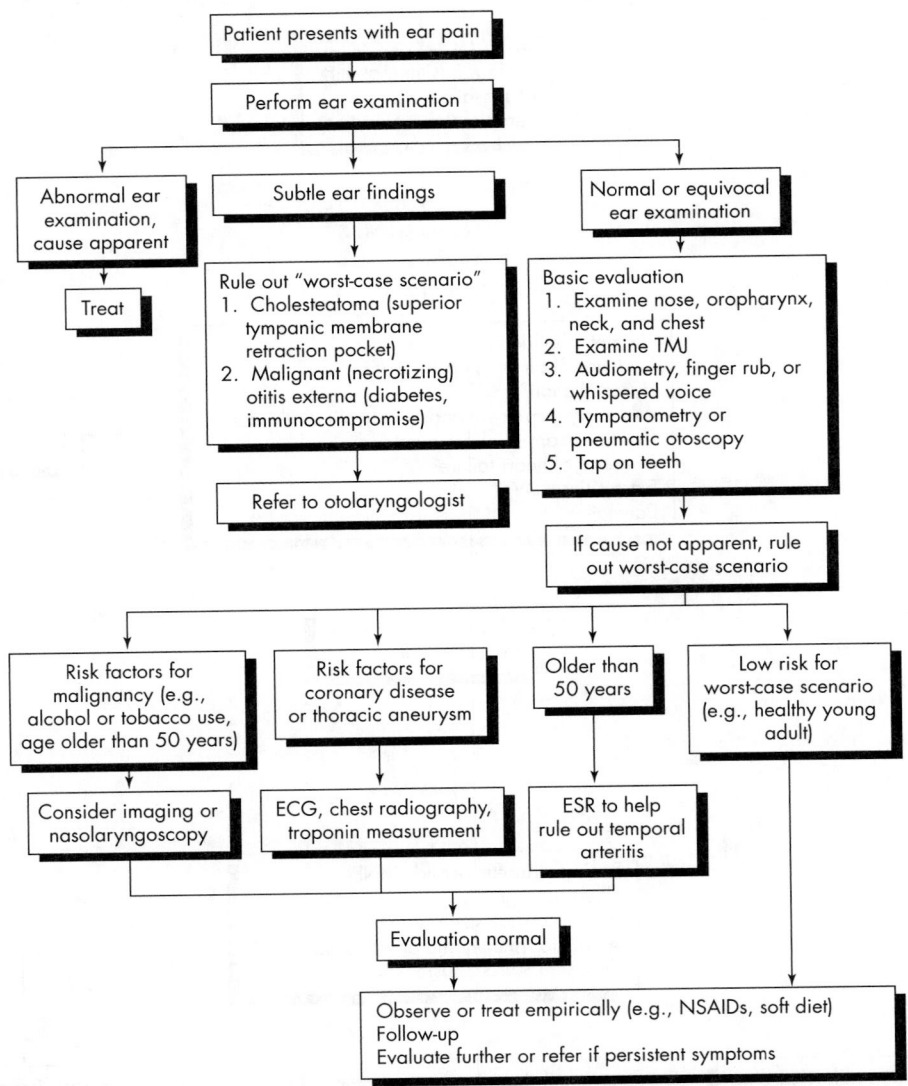

FIGURE 3-112 Management of ear pain. *ECG,* Electrocardiography; *ESR,* erythrocyte sedimentation rate; *NSAIDs,* nonsteroidal anti-inflammatory drugs; *TMJ,* temporomandibular joint. (From Ely JW et al: Diagnosis of ear pain, *Am Fam Physician* 77(5):622, 2008.)

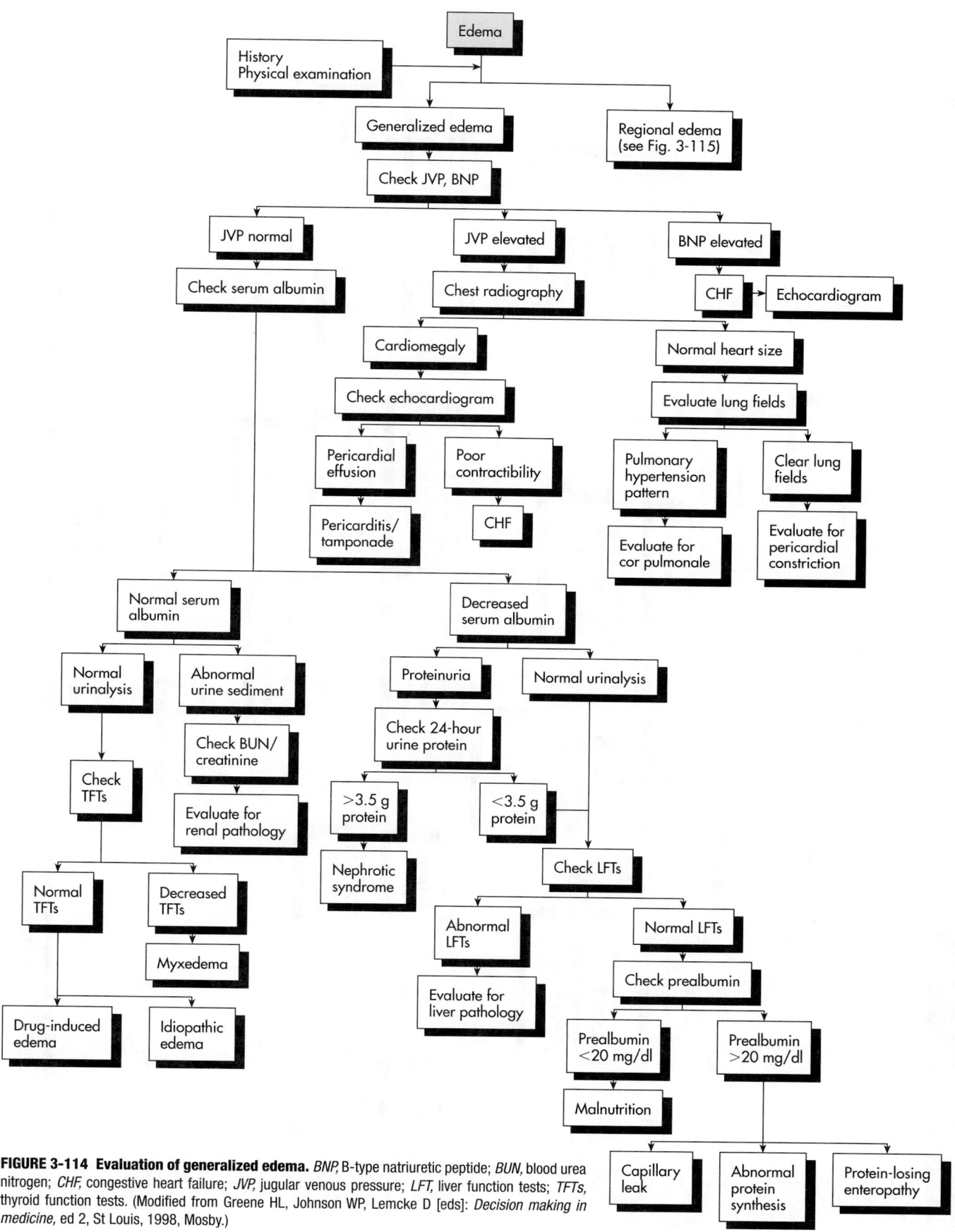

FIGURE 3-114 Evaluation of generalized edema. *BNP,* B-type natriuretic peptide; *BUN,* blood urea nitrogen; *CHF,* congestive heart failure; *JVP,* jugular venous pressure; *LFT,* liver function tests; *TFTs,* thyroid function tests. (Modified from Greene HL, Johnson WP, Lemcke D [eds]: *Decision making in medicine,* ed 2, St Louis, 1998, Mosby.)

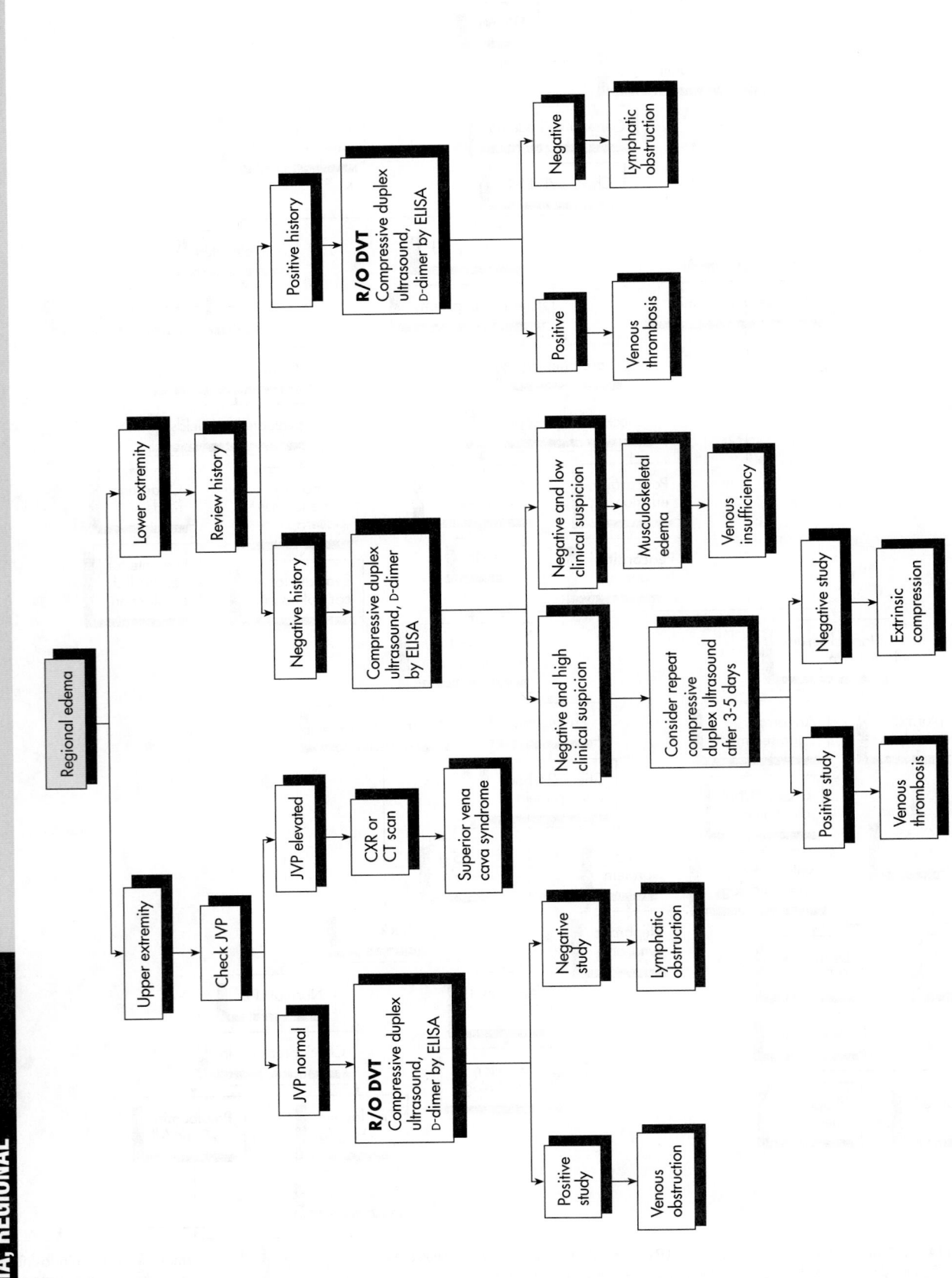

FIGURE 3-115 Evaluation of regional edema. *CT,* Computed tomography; *CXR,* chest x-ray examination; *JVP,* jugular venous pressure. (Modified from Greene HL, Johnson WP, Lemcke D [eds]: *Decision making in medicine,* ed 2, St Louis, 1998, Mosby.)

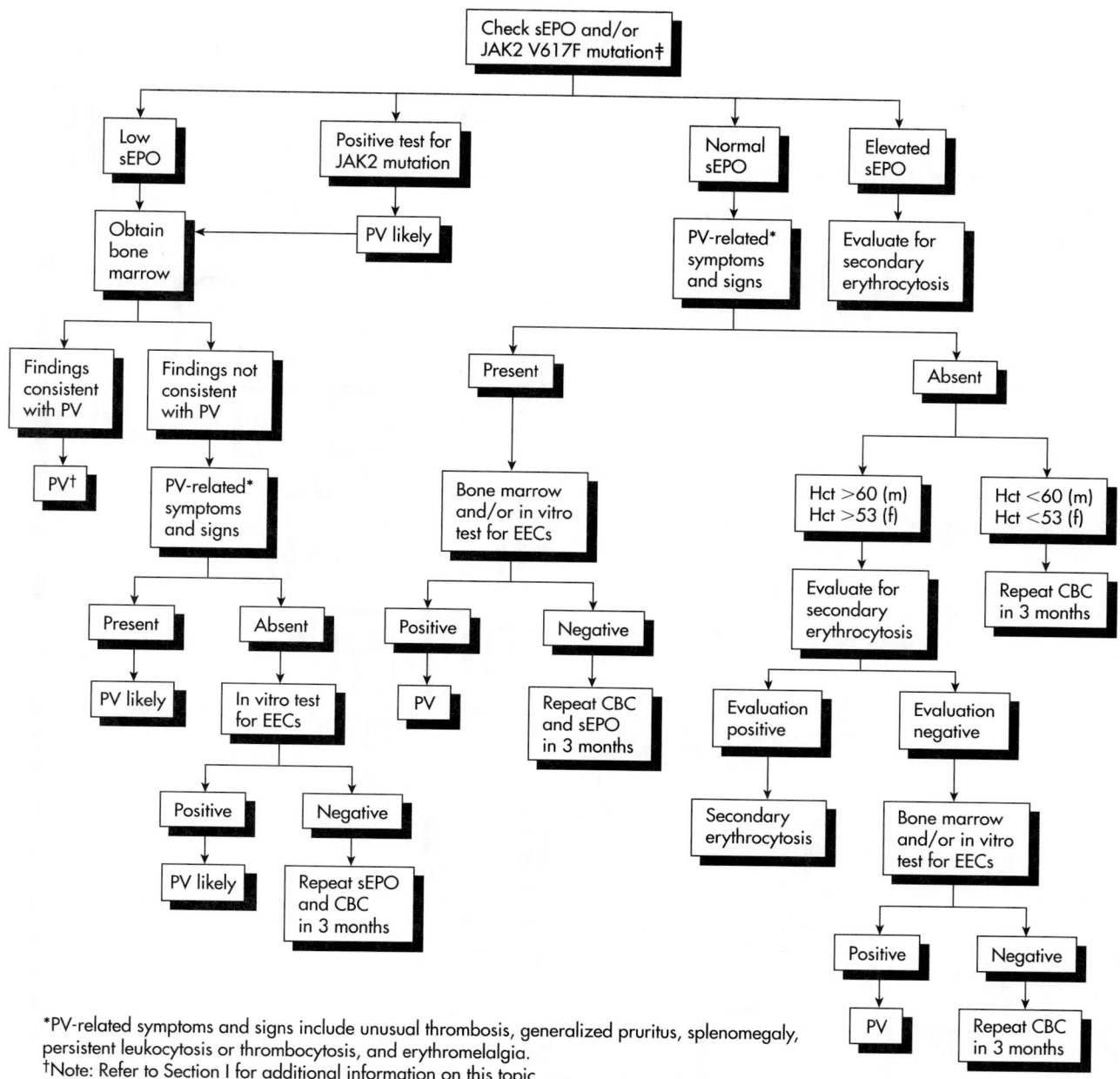

*PV-related symptoms and signs include unusual thrombosis, generalized pruritus, splenomegaly, persistent leukocytosis or thrombocytosis, and erythromelalgia.
†Note: Refer to Section I for additional information on this topic.
‡The JAK2 mutation is found in >95% of patients with PV and can be used for diagnostic purposes.

FIGURE 3-121 A diagnostic approach to acquired erythrocytosis. *CBC,* Complete blood cell count; *EEC,* endogenous (spontaneous) erythroid colonies; *f,* female; *Hct,* hematocrit; *m,* male; *PV,* polycythemia vera; *sEPO,* serum erythropoietin level. (Modified from Goldman L, Ausiello D [eds]: *Cecil textbook of medicine,* ed 23, Philadelphia, 2008, WB Saunders.)

Clinical Algorithms

III

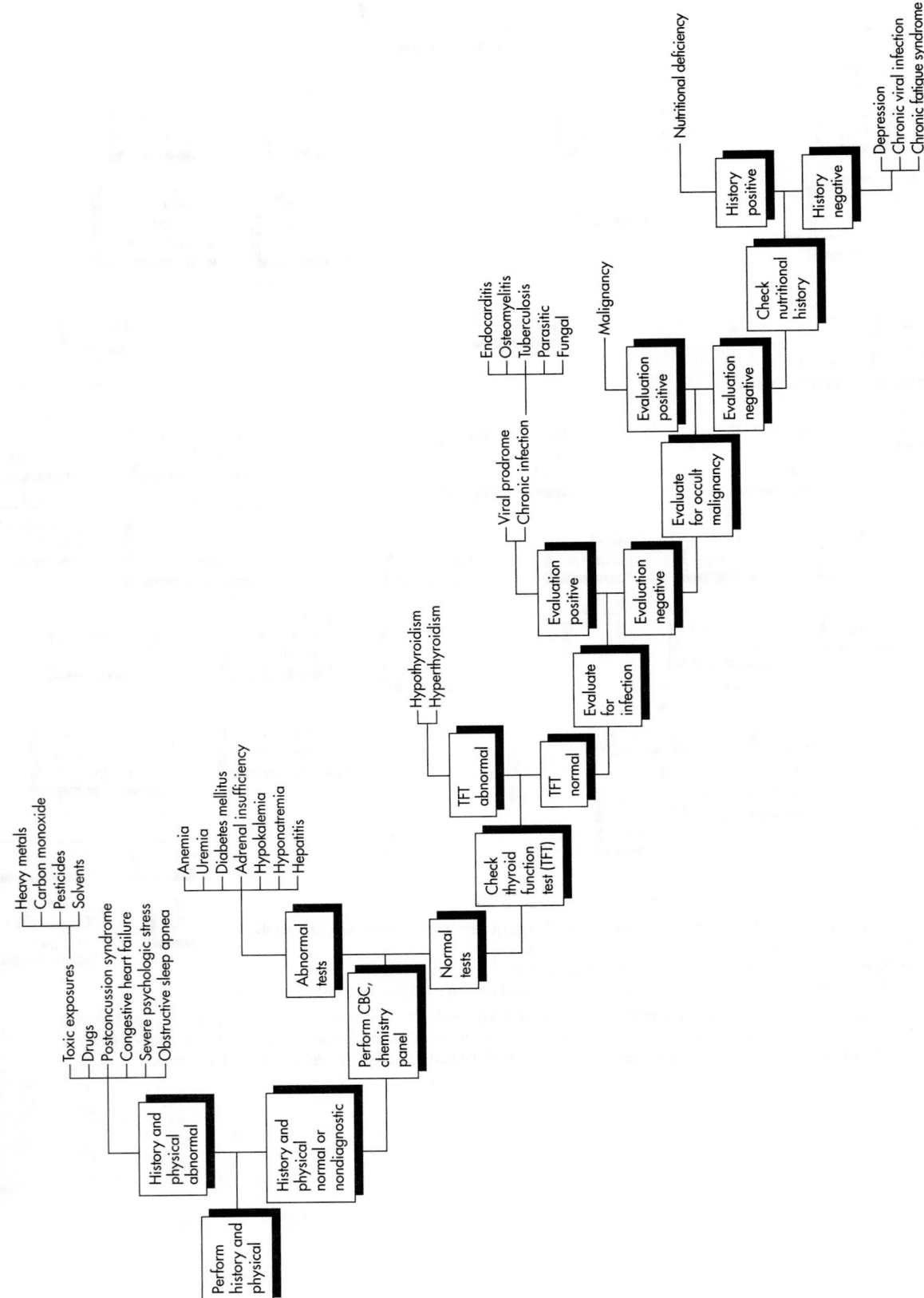

FIGURE 3-123 Evaluation of fatigue. *CBC,* Complete blood count. (Modified from Healey PM: *Common medical diagnosis: an algorithmic approach,* ed 3, Philadelphia, 2000, WB Saunders.)

ICD-9CM # 780.7 Fatigue, general

FATIGUE

Fatigue

Perform history and physical

History and physical abnormal

History and physical normal or nondiagnostic

Toxic exposures
— Heavy metals
— Carbon monoxide
— Pesticides
— Solvents
Drugs
Postconcussion syndrome
Congestive heart failure
Severe psychologic stress
Obstructive sleep apnea

Perform CBC, chemistry panel

Abnormal tests
— Anemia
— Uremia
— Diabetes mellitus
— Adrenal insufficiency
— Hypokalemia
— Hyponatremia
— Hepatitis

Normal tests

Check thyroid function test (TFT)

TFT abnormal
— Hypothyroidism
— Hyperthyroidism

TFT normal

Evaluate for infection

Evaluation positive
— Viral prodrome
— Chronic infection
— Endocarditis
— Osteomyelitis
— Tuberculosis
— Parasitic
— Fungal

Evaluation negative

Evaluate for occult malignancy

Evaluation positive
— Malignancy

Evaluation negative

Check nutritional history

History positive
— Nutritional deficiency

History negative
— Depression
— Chronic viral infection
— Chronic fatigue syndrome

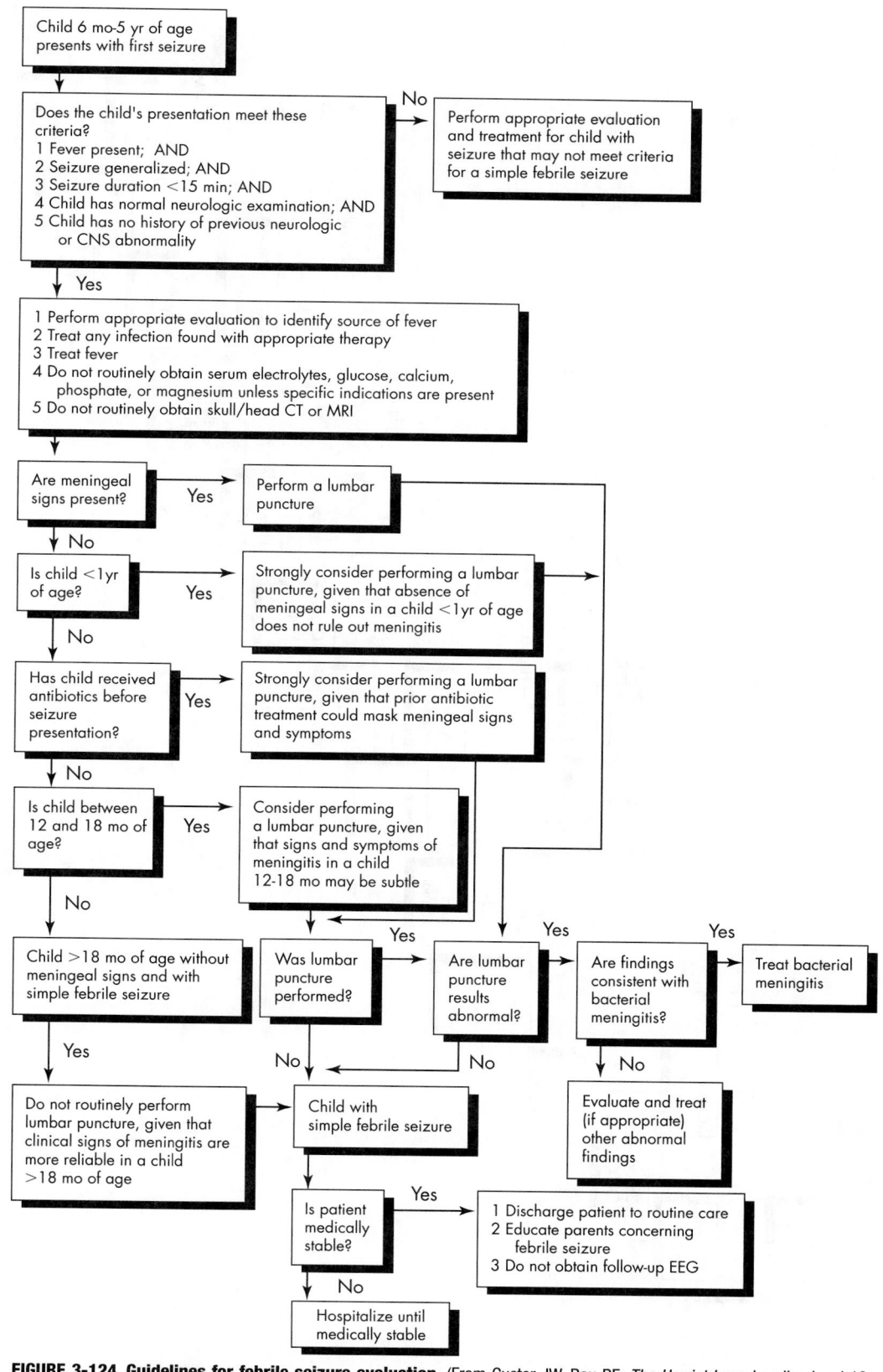

FIGURE 3-124 Guidelines for febrile seizure evaluation. (From Custer JW, Rau RE: *The Harriet Lane handbook,* ed 18, St Louis, 2009, Mosby.)

Clinical Algorithms

FEVER OF UNDETERMINED ORIGIN

ICD-9CM # 780.6 Pyrexia of undetermined origin

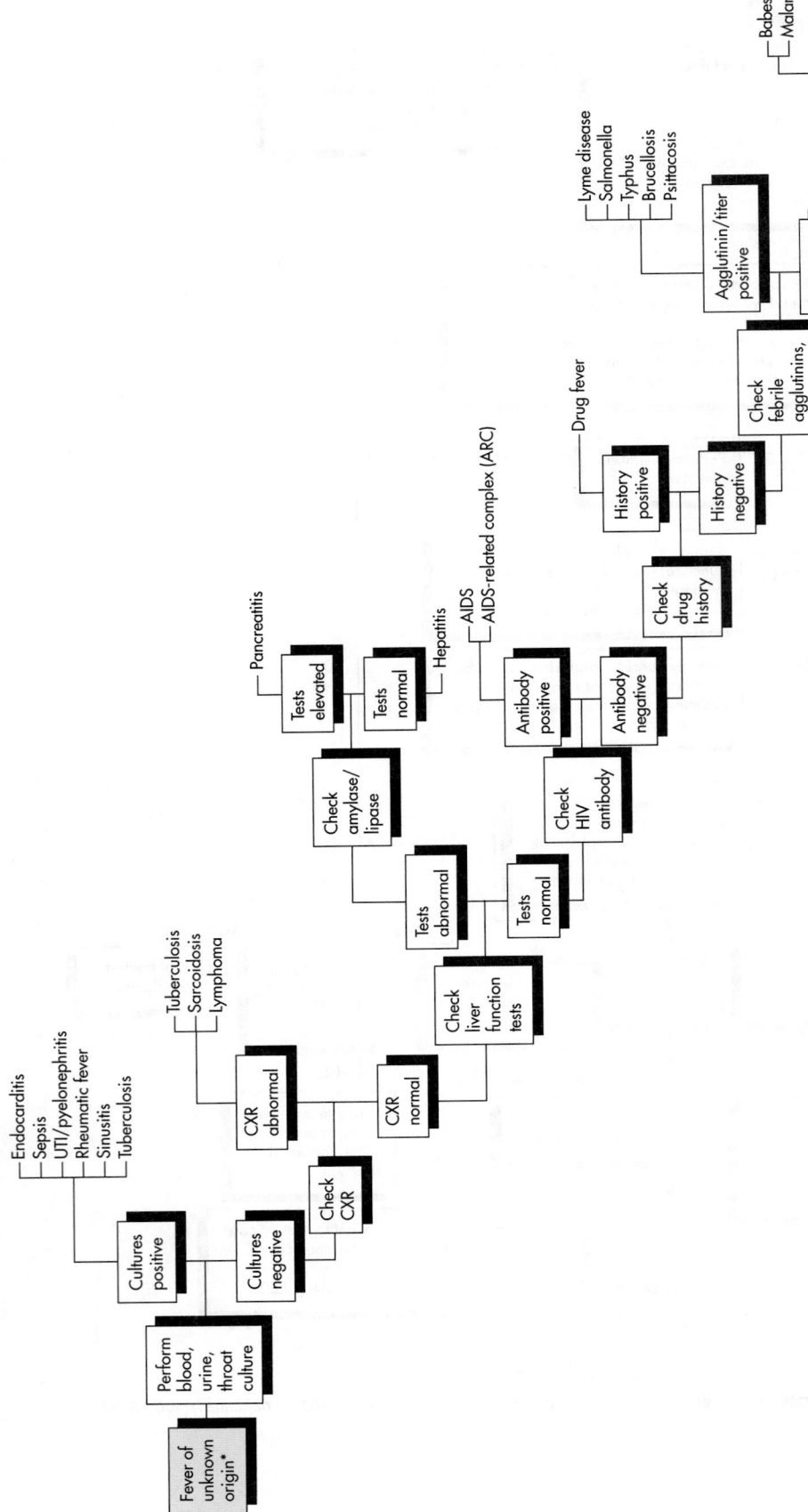

*Note: Refer to Section I for additional information on this topic.

FIGURE 3-128 Approach to the patient with fever of undetermined origin. *AIDS,* Acquired immunodeficiency syndrome; *ANA,* antinuclear antibody; *CT,* computed tomography; *CXR,* chest x-ray; *ESR,* erythrocyte sedimentation rate; *GI,* gastrointestinal; *HIV,* human immunodeficiency virus; *RBC,* red blood cell; *UTI,* urinary tract infection. (Modified from Healey PM: *Common medical diagnosis: an algorithmic approach,* ed 3, Philadelphia, 2000, WB Saunders.)   *(Continued on next page)*

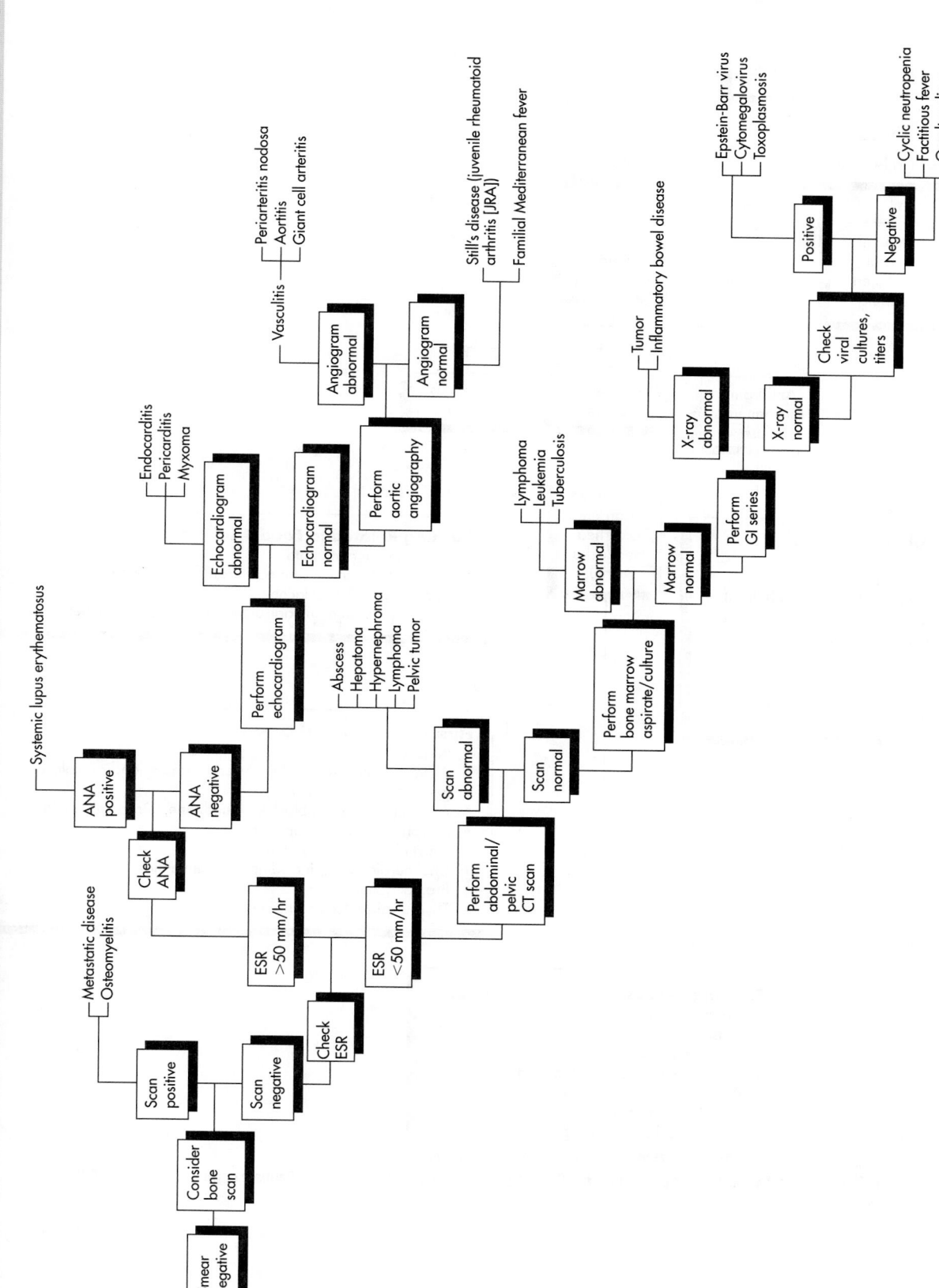

FIGURE 3-128 (Continued)

Flushing

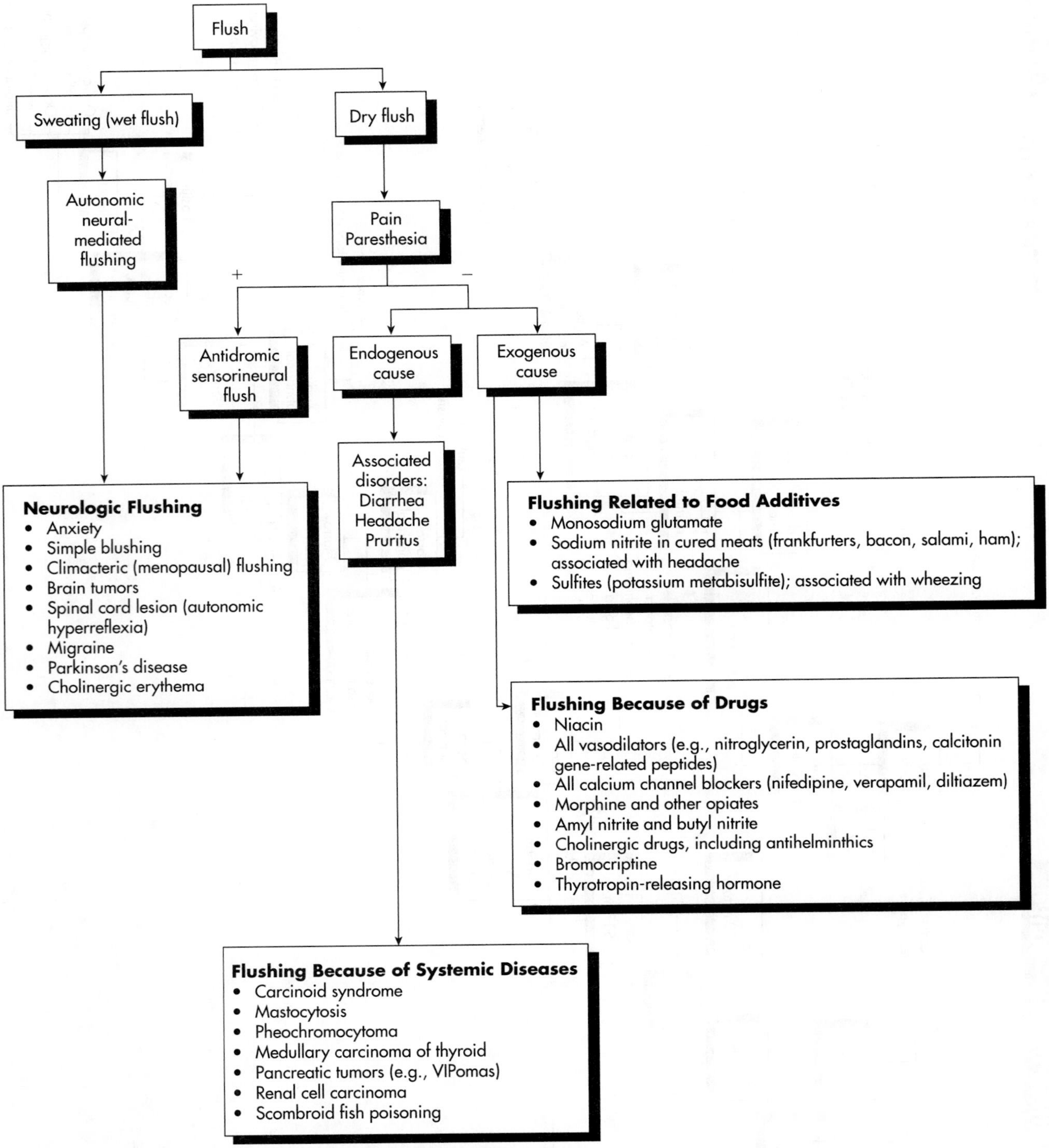

FIGURE 3-130 Evaluation of patients with flushing. (From Bolognia JL et al [eds]: *Dermatology*, ed 2, St Louis, 2008, Mosby.)

ICD-9CM # 054.10 Genital herpes
91.0 Genital syphilis
078.11 Condyloma acuminatum
099.0 Chancroid
099.2 Granuloma inguinale
099.1 Lymphogranuloma venereum
629.8 Ulcer, genital site, female
608.89 Ulcer, genital site, male

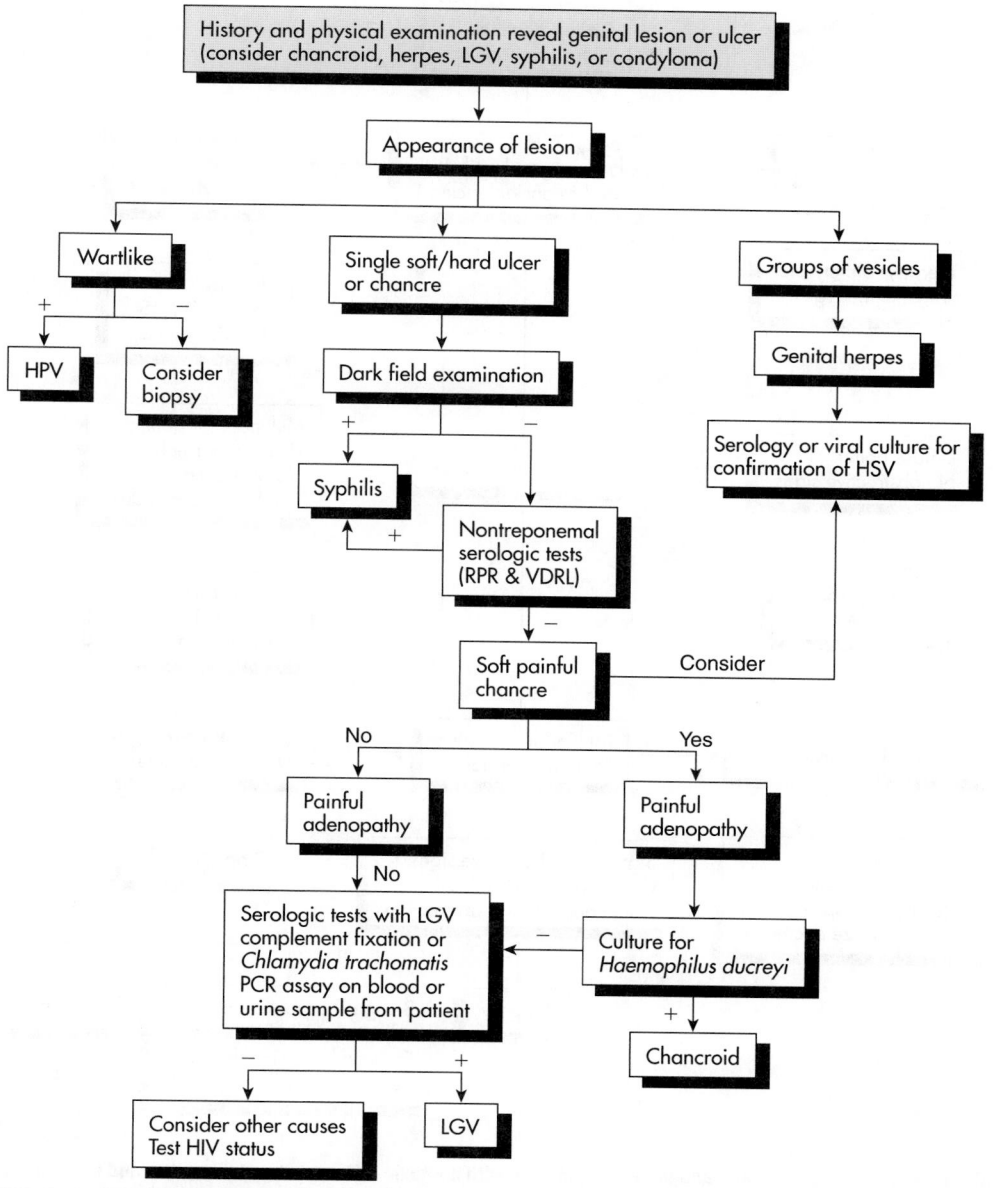

FIGURE 3-132 Evaluation of patients with genital lesions or ulcers. *HIV,* Human immunodeficiency virus; *HPV,* human papillomavirus; *HSV,* herpes simplex virus; *LGV,* lymphogranuloma venereum; *RPR,* rapid plasma reagin; *VDRL,* Venereal Disease Research Laboratory. (Modified from Nseyo UO [ed]: *Urology for primary care physicians,* Philadelphia, 1999, WB Saunders.)

Clinical
Algorithms

III

ICD-9CM # 240.9 Goiter, unspecified
240.0 Goiter, simple
241.9 Goiter, adenomatous
246.1 Goiter, congenital
242.1 Goiter, uninodular with thyrotoxicosos
242.2 Goiter, multinodular with thyrotoxicosos

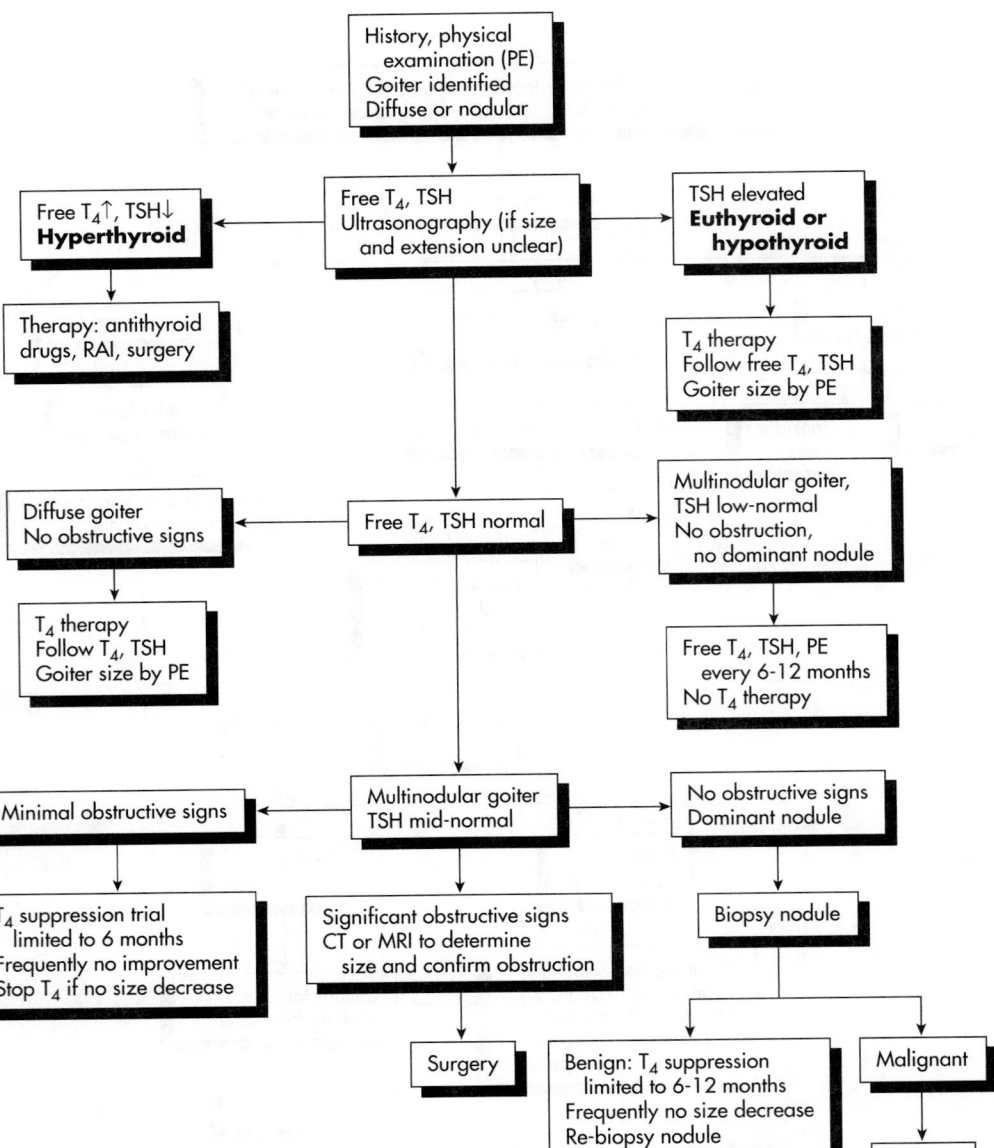

FIGURE 3-135 Evaluation and management of patients with nontoxic diffuse and nodular goiter and undetermined thyroid status. *CT,* Computed tomography; *MRI,* magnetic resonance imaging; *RAI,* radioactive iodine; *TSH,* thyroid-stimulating hormone. (From Goldman L, Ausiello D [eds]: *Cecil textbook of medicine,* ed 23, Philadelphia, 2008, WB Saunders.)

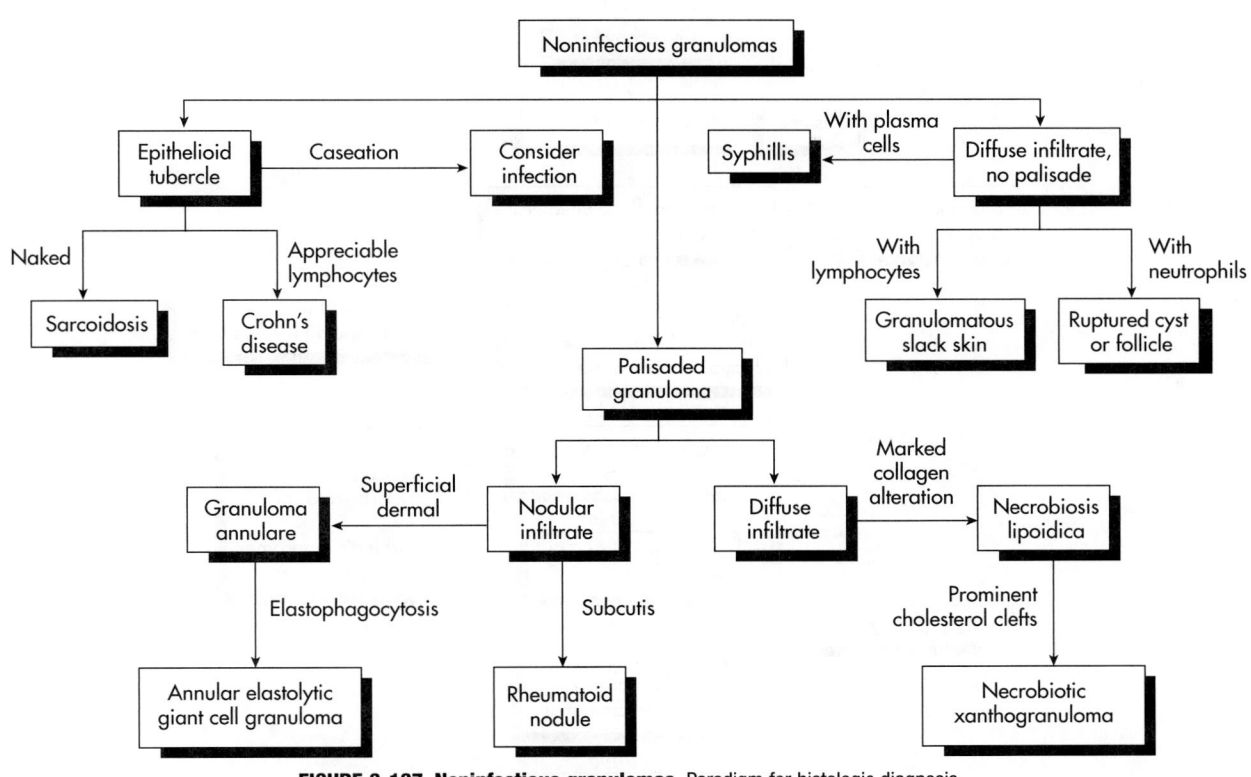

FIGURE 3-137 Noninfectious granulomas. Paradigm for histologic diagnosis.

TABLE 3-15   Clinical Features of the Major Granulomatous Dermatitides

	Sarcoidosis	Classic GA*	NLD	AEGCG	Crohn's Disease	Rheumatoid Nodule
Average age (years)	25-35, 45-65	<30		40	35	30-40
Sex	Female	Female	Female	Female	Female	Female
Racial predilection in United States	African American	None	None	Caucasian	None	None
Site	Symmetric on face, neck, upper trunk, extremities	Hands, feet, extremities	Anterior and lateral distal lower extremities	Face, neck, forearms	Genital areas, lower > upper extremities	Juxtaarticular areas, elbows, hands, ankles, feet
Appearance	Red to red-brown papules and plaques	Papules coalescing into annular plaques	Plaques with elevated borders, telangiec- tasias centrally	Annular plaques	Dusky erythema and swelling, ulceration	Skin-colored, firm, mobile subcuta- neous nodules
Size of lesions	1-5 cm	1-2 mm papules, <5 cm annular plaques	>10 cm	1-6 cm	Variable	1-3 cm
Number of lesions	Variable	1-10	1-10	1-10	1-5	1-10
Associations	Systemic manifesta- tions of sarcoidosis	Rare diabetes mel- litus, malignancy	Diabetes mellitus	Actinic damage	Intestinal Crohn's disease	Rheumatoid arthritis
Special clinical characteristics	Occasional central at- rophy and hypopig- mentation	Central hyperpig- mentation	Yellow-brown atro- phic centers, ulceration	Central atrophy and hypopigmentation	Draining sinuses and fistulae	Occasional ulcer- ation, especially at site of trauma

From Bolognia JL et al: *Dermatology,* ed 2, St Louis, 2008, Mosby.
AEGCG, Annular elastolytic giant cell granuloma; *GA,* granuloma annulare; *NLD,* necrobiosis lipoidica diabeticorum.
*Clinical variants include generalized, micropapular, nodular, perforating, subcutaneous, and patch GA.

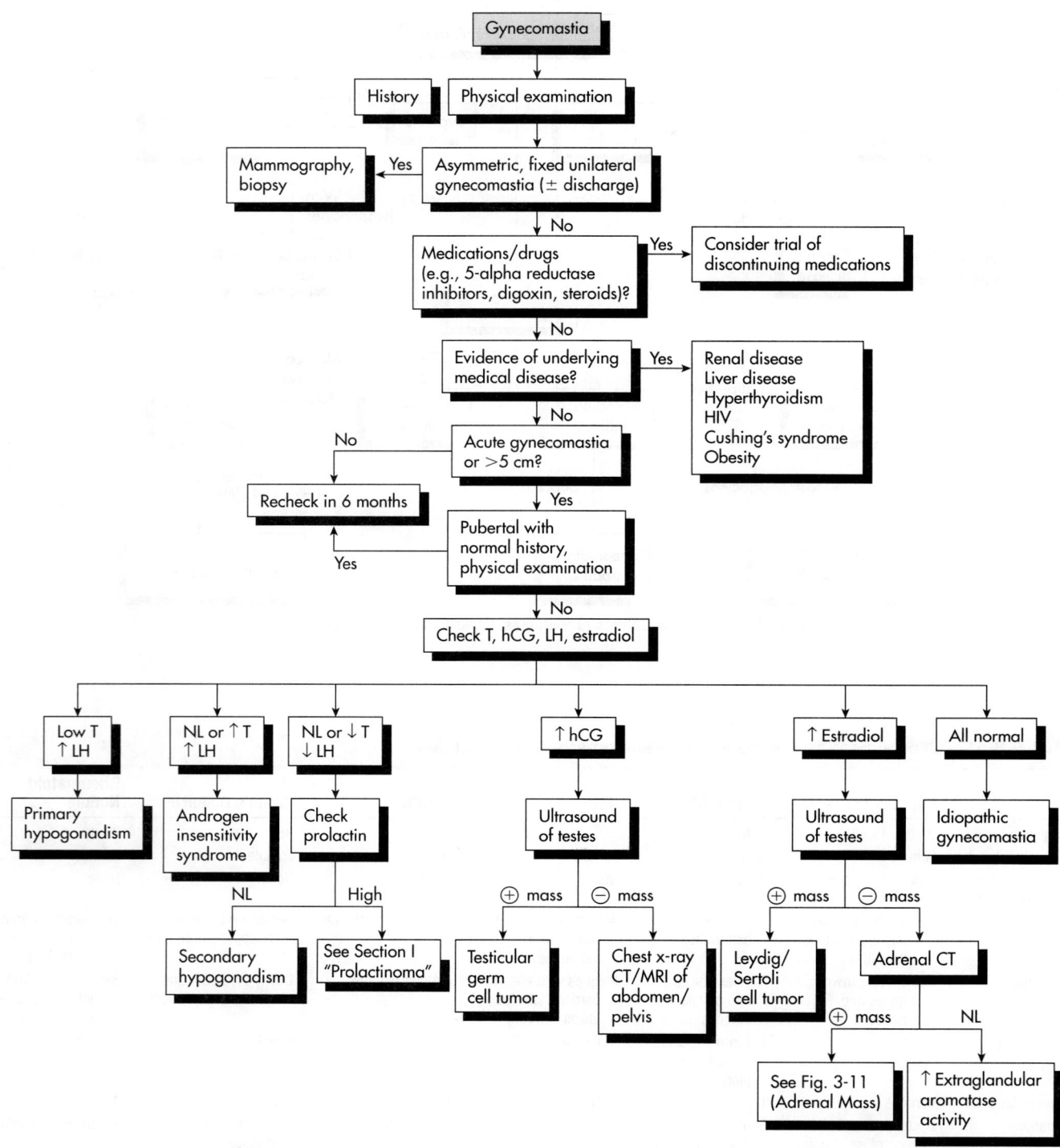

FIGURE 3-138 Evaluation of gynecomastia. *CT,* Computed tomography; *hCG,* human chorionic gonadotropin; *HIV,* human immunodeficiency syndrome; *LH,* luteinizing hormone; *MRI,* magnetic resonance imaging; *NL,* normal limits; *T,* testosterone. (Modified from Noble J: *Primary care medicine,* ed 3, St Louis, 2001, Mosby.)

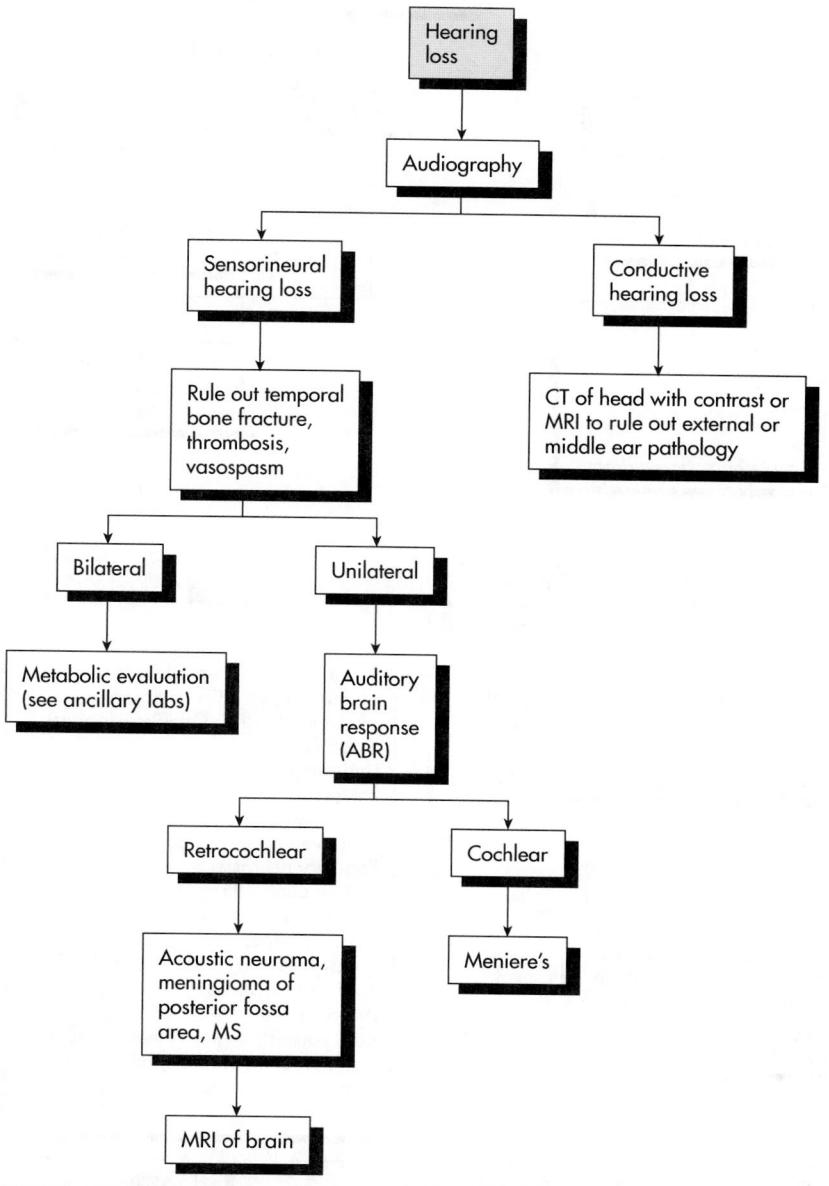

FIGURE 3-139 Evaluation of hearing loss. *CT,* Computed tomography; *MRI,* magnetic resonance imaging; *MS,* multiple sclerosis. (From Ferri FF: *Ferri's best test: a practical guide to clinical laboratory medicine and diagnostic imaging,* ed 2, Philadelphia, 2009, Elsevier Mosby.)

BOX 3-7   Hearing Loss

Diagnostic imaging	Lab evaluation
Best test	**Best test**
None	None
Ancillary tests	**Ancillary tests**
CT of head with contrast or MRI with contrast	CBC
CT of temporal bone without contrast	ALT, AST
	ANA, VDRL
	TSH

From Ferri FF: *Ferri's best test: a practical guide to clinical laboratory medicine and diagnostic imaging,* ed 2, Philadelphia, 2009, Elsevier Mosby.
    ALT, Alanine aminotransferase; *ANA,* antibody to nuclear antigens; *AST,* angiotensin sensitivity test; *CBC,* complete blood count; *CT,* computed tomography; *TSH,* thyroid-stimulating hormone; *VDRL,* Venereal Disease Research Laboratory.

Clinical Algorithms

III

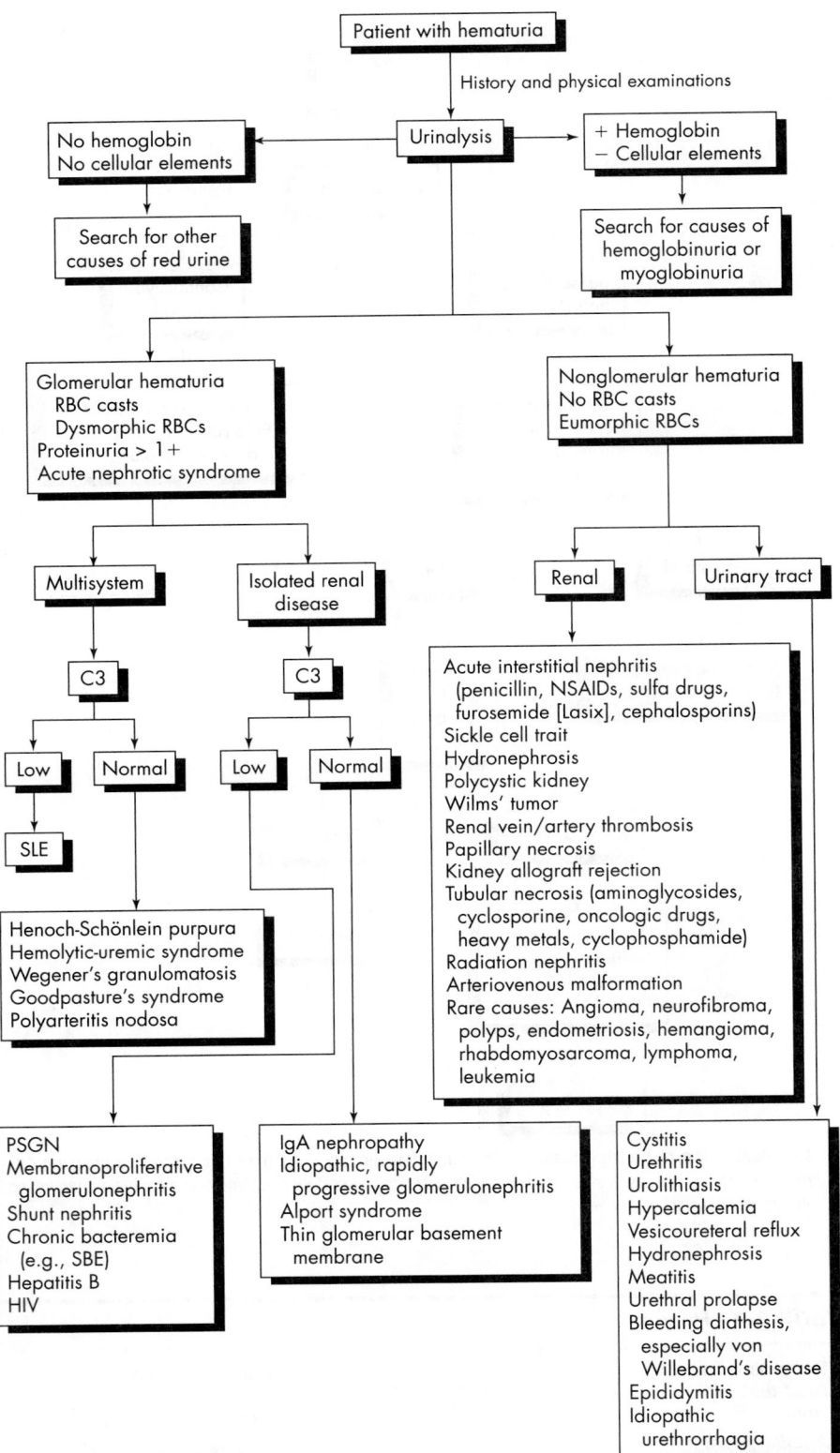

FIGURE 3-142 A diagnostic strategy for hematuria. *HIV,* Human immunodeficiency virus; *NSAIDs,* nonsteroidal anti-inflammatory drugs; *PSGN,* poststreptococcal glomerulonephritis; *RBC,* red blood cell; *SBE,* subacute bacterial endocarditis; *SLE,* systemic lupus erythematosus. (From Custer JW, Rau RE: *The Harriet Lane handbook,* ed 18, St Louis, 2009, Mosby.)

HEMOPTYSIS

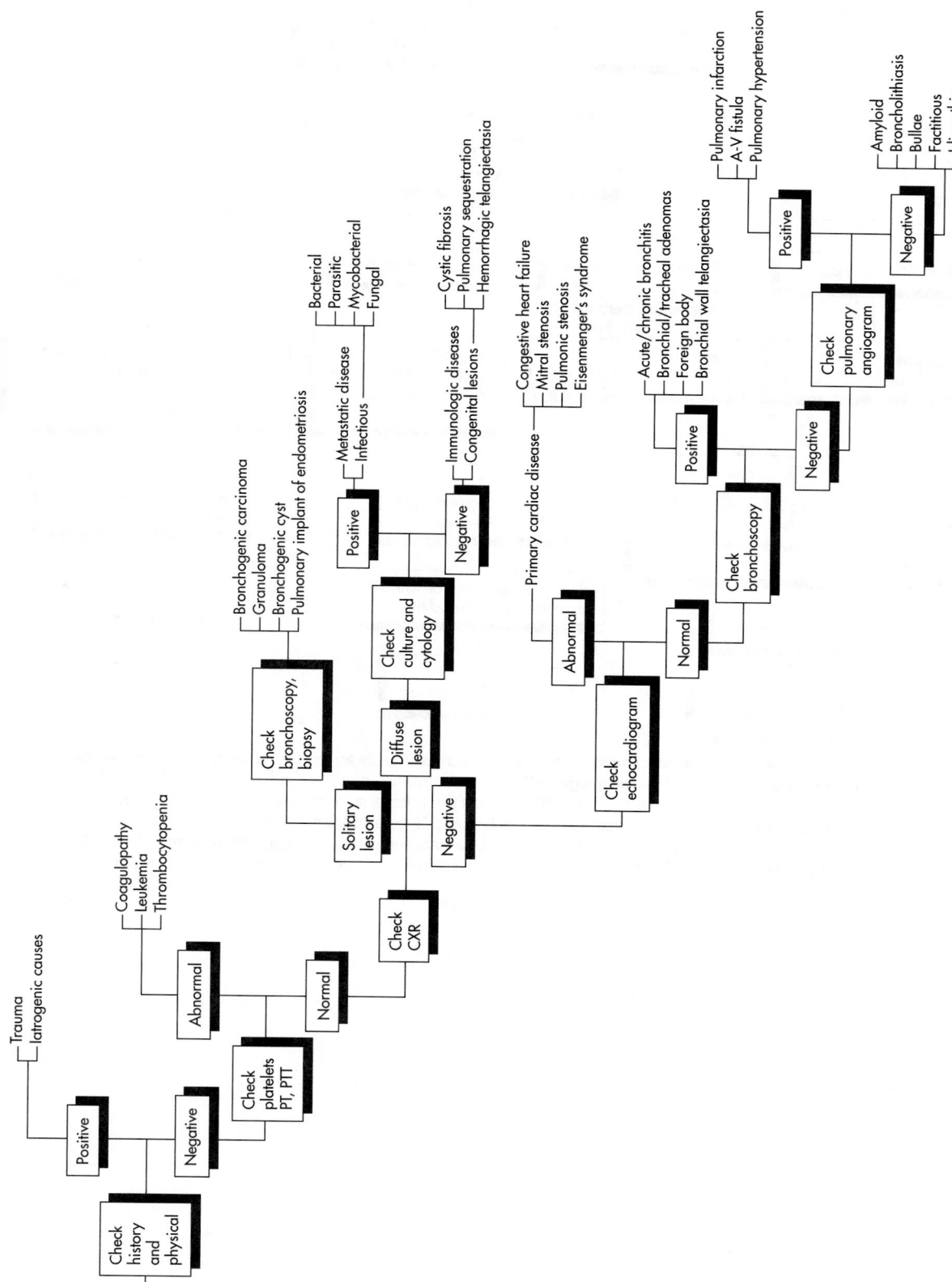

FIGURE 3-144 Evaluation of hemoptysis. *A-V,* Arteriovenous; *CXR,* chest x-ray; *PT,* prothrombin time; *PTT,* partial thromboplastin time. (From Healey PM: *Common medical diagnosis: an algorithmic approach,* ed 3, Philadelphia, 2000, WB Saunders.)

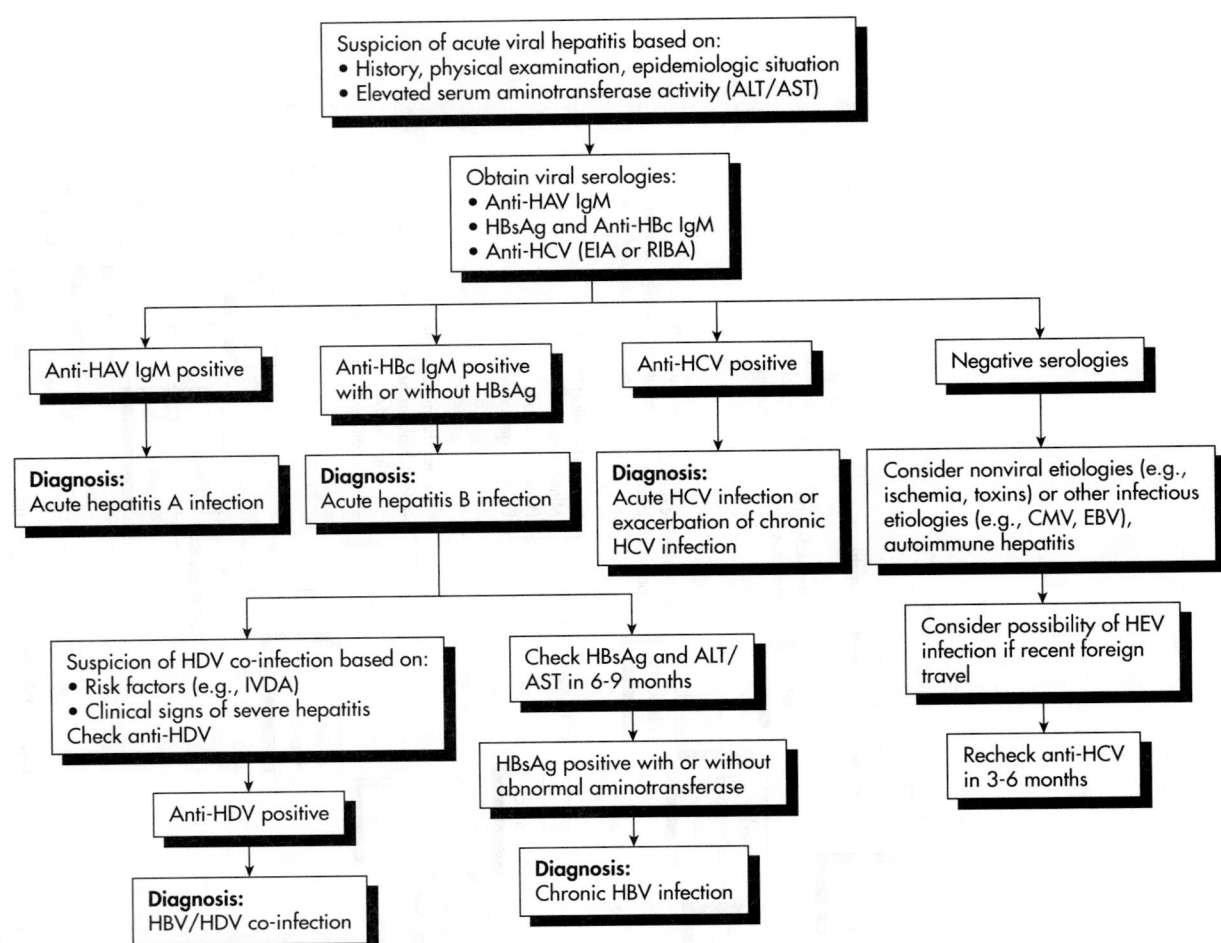

FIGURE 3-146 A flow diagram showing the use of specific serologic tests for the diagnosis of acute viral hepatitis in relation to the clinical and epidemiologic setting. Co-infections and superinfections of chronic hepatitis B or C patients should always be considered in cases that do not fit well with the clinical or serologic picture. *CMV,* Cytomegalovirus; *EBV,* Epstein-Barr virus; *EIA,* enzyme immunoassay; *HBV,* hepatitis B virus; *HCV,* hepatitis C virus; *HDV,* hepatitis D virus; *HEV,* hepatoencephalomyelitis virus; *IVDA,* intravenous drug abuse; *RIBA,* recombinant immunoblot assay. (Modified from Mandell GL: *Mandell, Douglas, and Bennett's principles and practice of infectious diseases,* ed 7, New York, 2008, Churchill Livingstone.)

HEPATOMEGALY

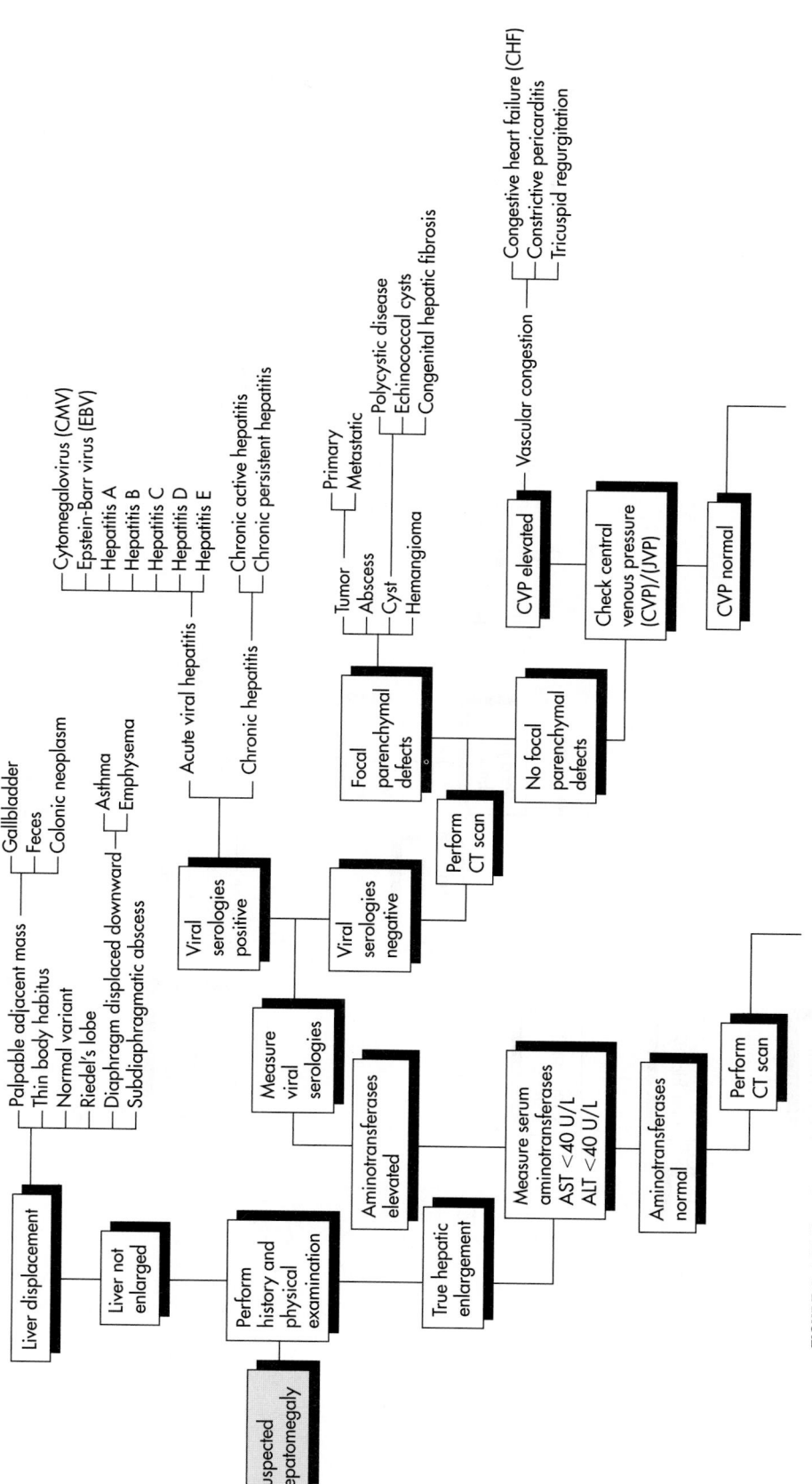

FIGURE 3-147 Hepatomegaly. *ALT*, Alanine aminotransferase; *AST*, aspartate aminotransferase; *CT*, computed tomography; *JVP*, jugular venous pressure. (Modified from Healey PM: *Common medical diagnosis: an algorithmic approach*, ed 3, Philadelphia, 2000, WB Saunders.)

(Continued on next page)

(Continued on next page)

Clinical
Algorithms

III

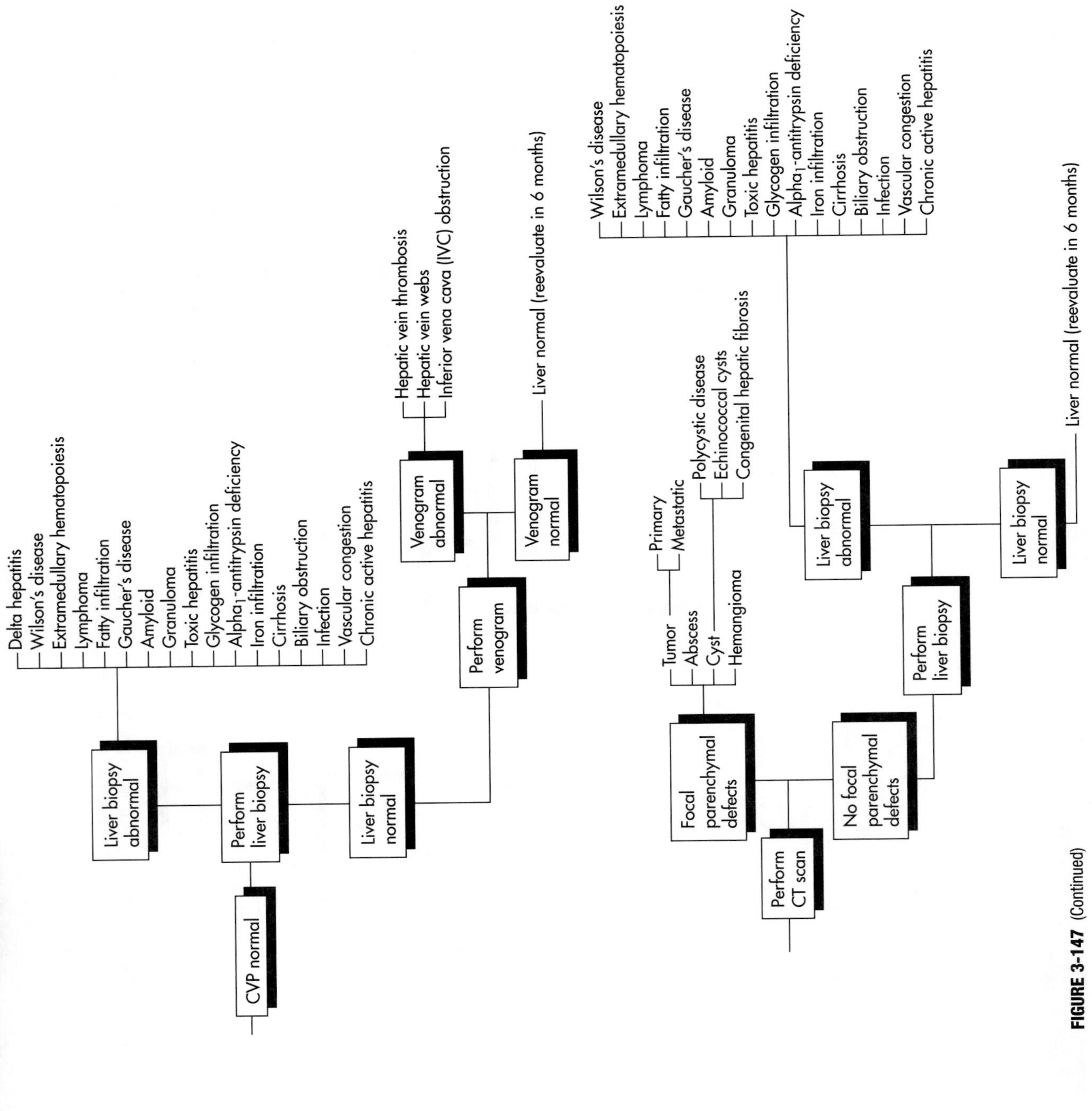

HEPATOMEGALY—cont'd

Delta hepatitis
Wilson's disease
Extramedullary hematopoiesis
Lymphoma
Fatty infiltration
Gaucher's disease
Amyloid
Granuloma
Toxic hepatitis
Glycogen infiltration
Alpha₁-antitrypsin deficiency
Iron infiltration
Cirrhosis
Biliary obstruction
Infection
Vascular congestion
Chronic active hepatitis

Liver biopsy abnormal

Perform liver biopsy

Liver biopsy normal

CVP normal

Hepatic vein thrombosis
Hepatic vein webs
Inferior vena cava (IVC) obstruction

Venogram abnormal

Perform venogram

Venogram normal

Liver normal (reevaluate in 6 months)

Tumor — Primary / Metastatic
Abscess
Cyst
Hemangioma

Polycystic disease
Echinococcal cysts
Congenital hepatic fibrosis

Focal parenchymal defects

Perform CT scan

No focal parenchymal defects

Perform liver biopsy

Wilson's disease
Extramedullary hematopoiesis
Lymphoma
Fatty infiltration
Gaucher's disease
Amyloid
Granuloma
Toxic hepatitis
Glycogen infiltration
Alpha₁-antitrypsin deficiency
Iron infiltration
Cirrhosis
Biliary obstruction
Infection
Vascular congestion
Chronic active hepatitis

Liver biopsy abnormal

Liver biopsy normal

Liver normal (reevaluate in 6 months)

FIGURE 3-147 (Continued)

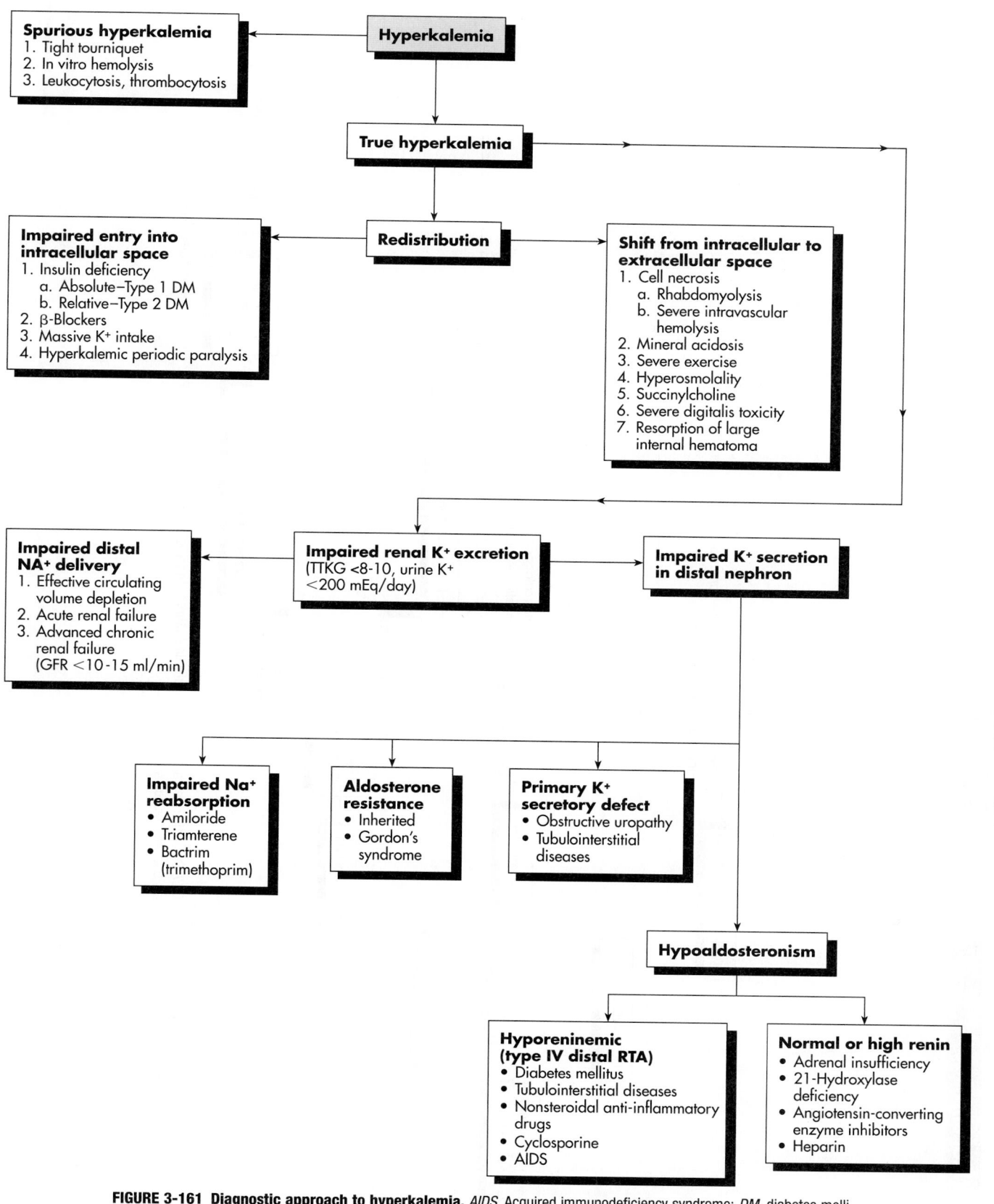

FIGURE 3-161 Diagnostic approach to hyperkalemia. *AIDS,* Acquired immunodeficiency syndrome; *DM,* diabetes mellitus; *GFR,* glomerular filtration rate; *RTA,* renal tubular acidosis; *TTKG,* transtubular potassium gradient. (From Andreoli TE [ed]: *Cecil essentials of medicine,* ed 7, Philadelphia, 2008, WB Saunders.)

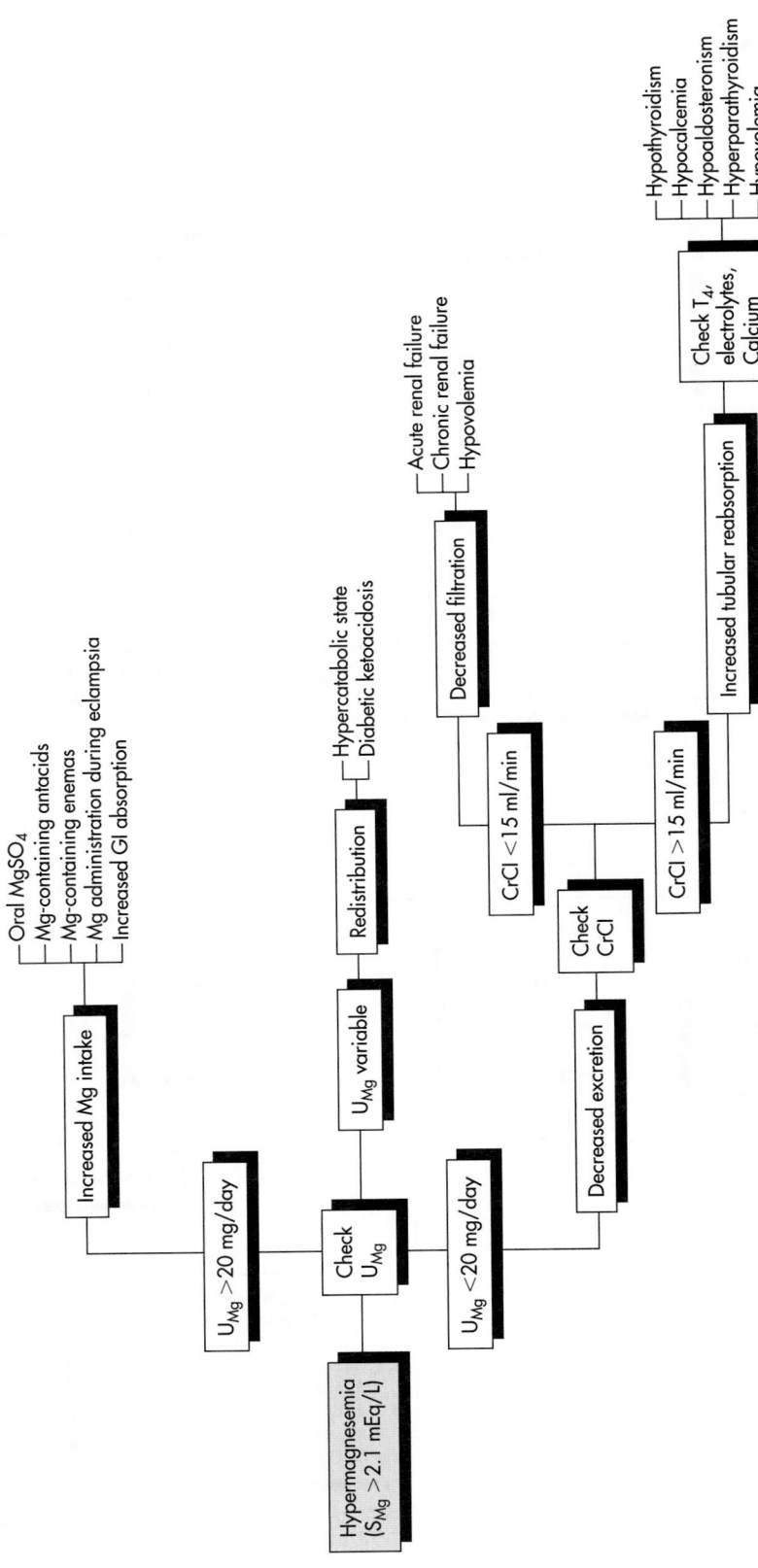

FIGURE 3-164 Hypermagnesemia. *CrCl,* Creatinine clearance; *GI,* gastrointestinal; *MgSO₄,* magnesium sulfate. (From Healey PM: *Common medical diagnosis: an algorithmic approach,* ed 3, Philadelphia, 2000, WB Saunders.)

HYPERNATREMIA

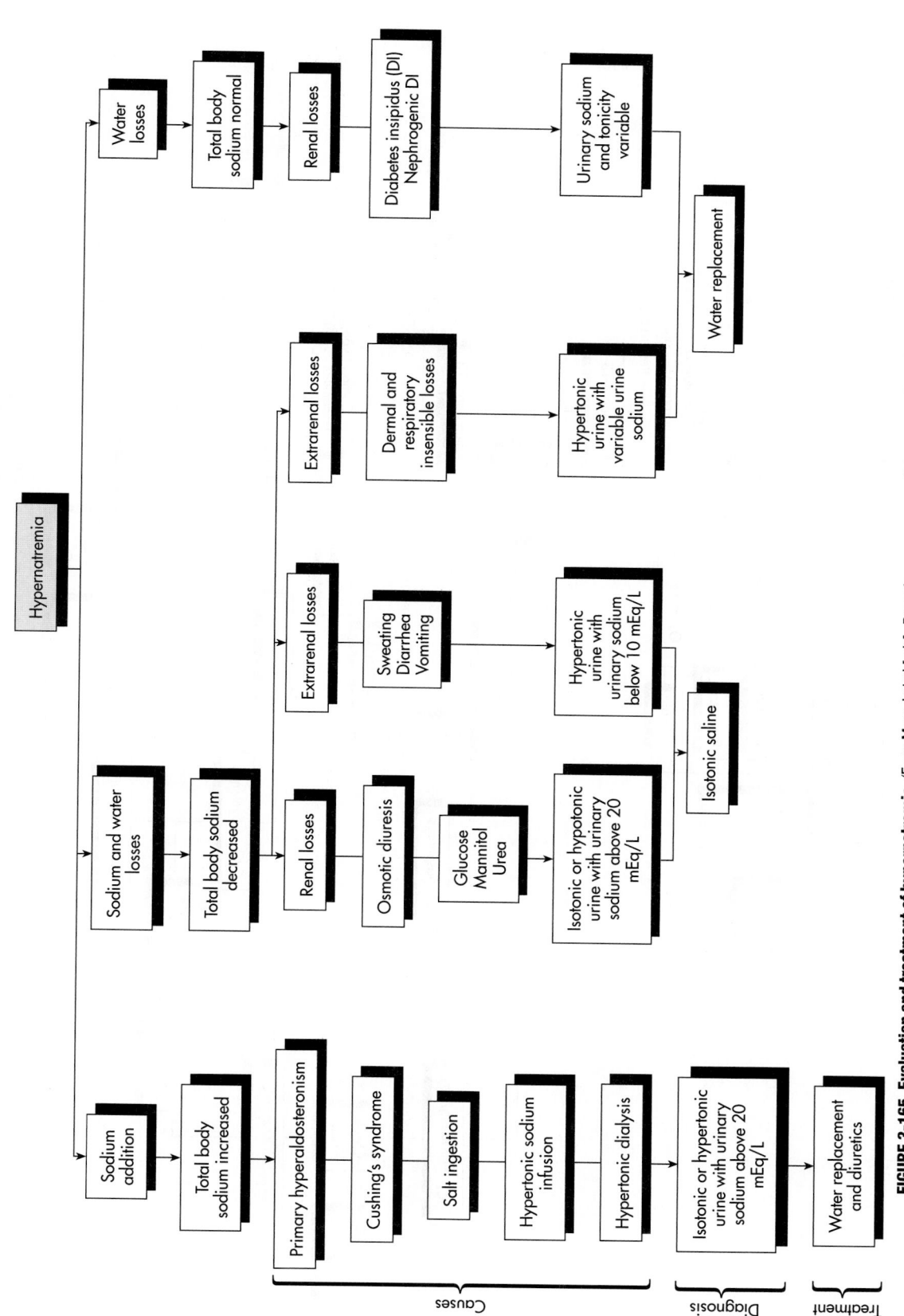

FIGURE 3-165 Evaluation and treatment of hypernatremia. (From Marx J et al [eds]: *Rosen's emergency medicine: concepts and clinical practice*, ed 6, St Louis, 2006, Mosby.)

Clinical
Algorithms

III

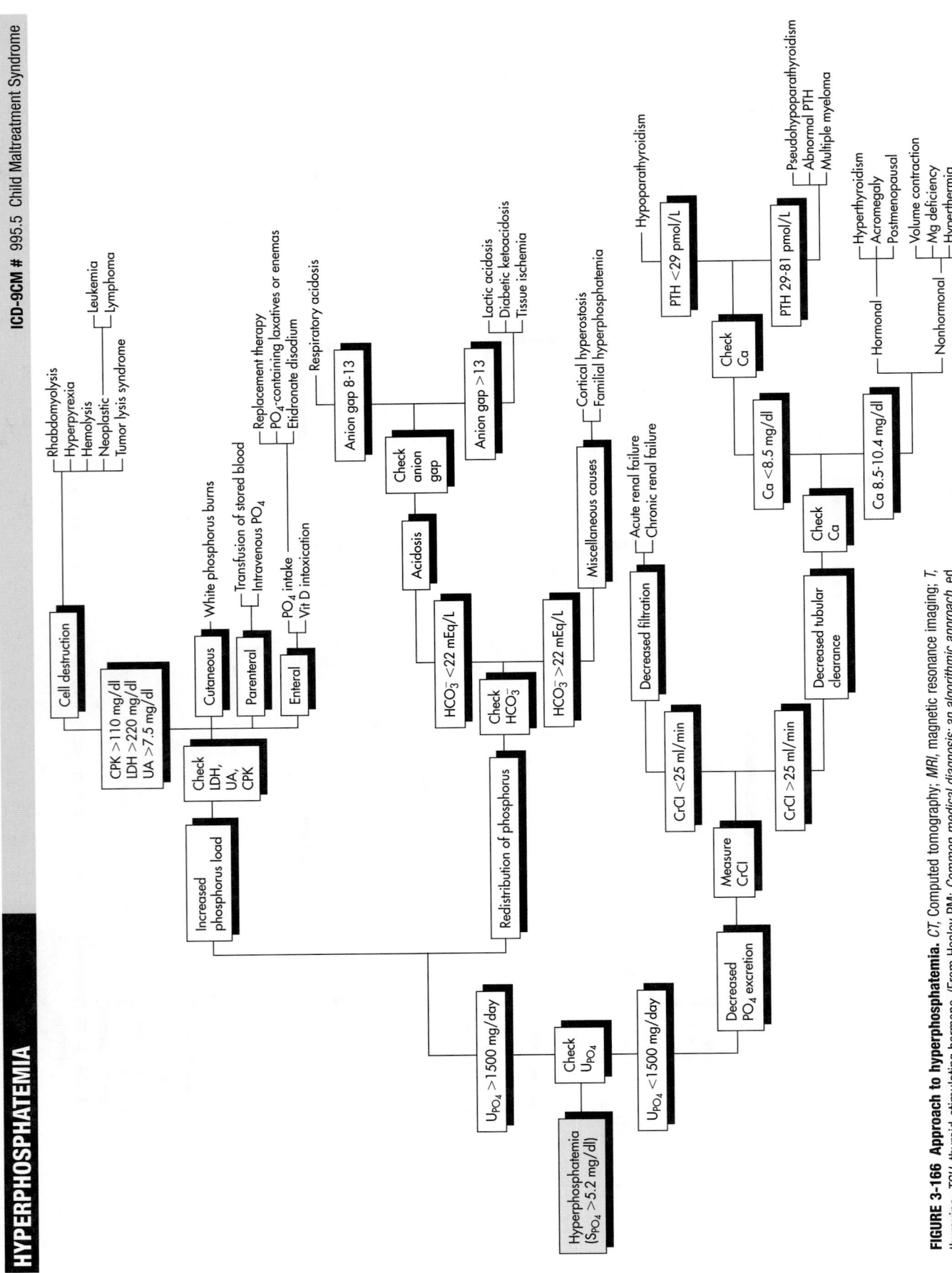

FIGURE 3-166 Approach to hyperphosphatemia. *CT,* Computed tomography; *MRI,* magnetic resonance imaging; *T,* thyroxine; *TSH,* thyroid-stimulating hormone. (From Healey PM: *Common medical diagnosis: an algorithmic approach,* ed 3, Philadelphia, 2000, WB Saunders.)

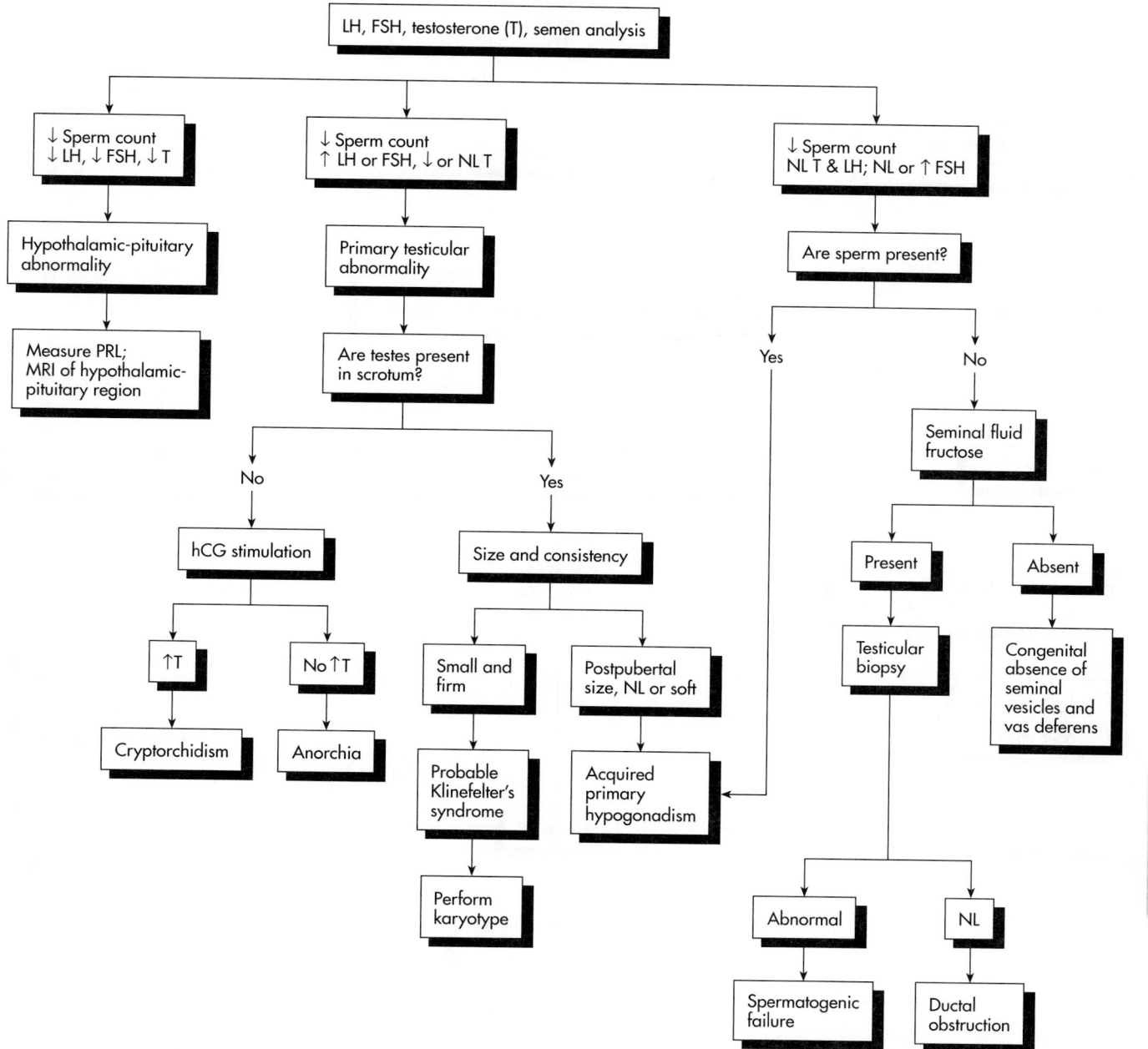

FIGURE 3-177 Laboratory evaluation of hypogonadism. *FSH*, Follicle-stimulating hormone; *hCG*, human chorionic gonadotropin; *LH*, luteinizing hormone; *MRI*, magnetic resonance imaging; *NL*, normal; *PRL*, prolactin; ↑, elevated; ↓, decreased or low. (From Andreoli TE [ed]: *Cecil essentials of medicine*, ed 7, Philadelphia, 2008, WB Saunders.)

Clinical
Algorithms

III

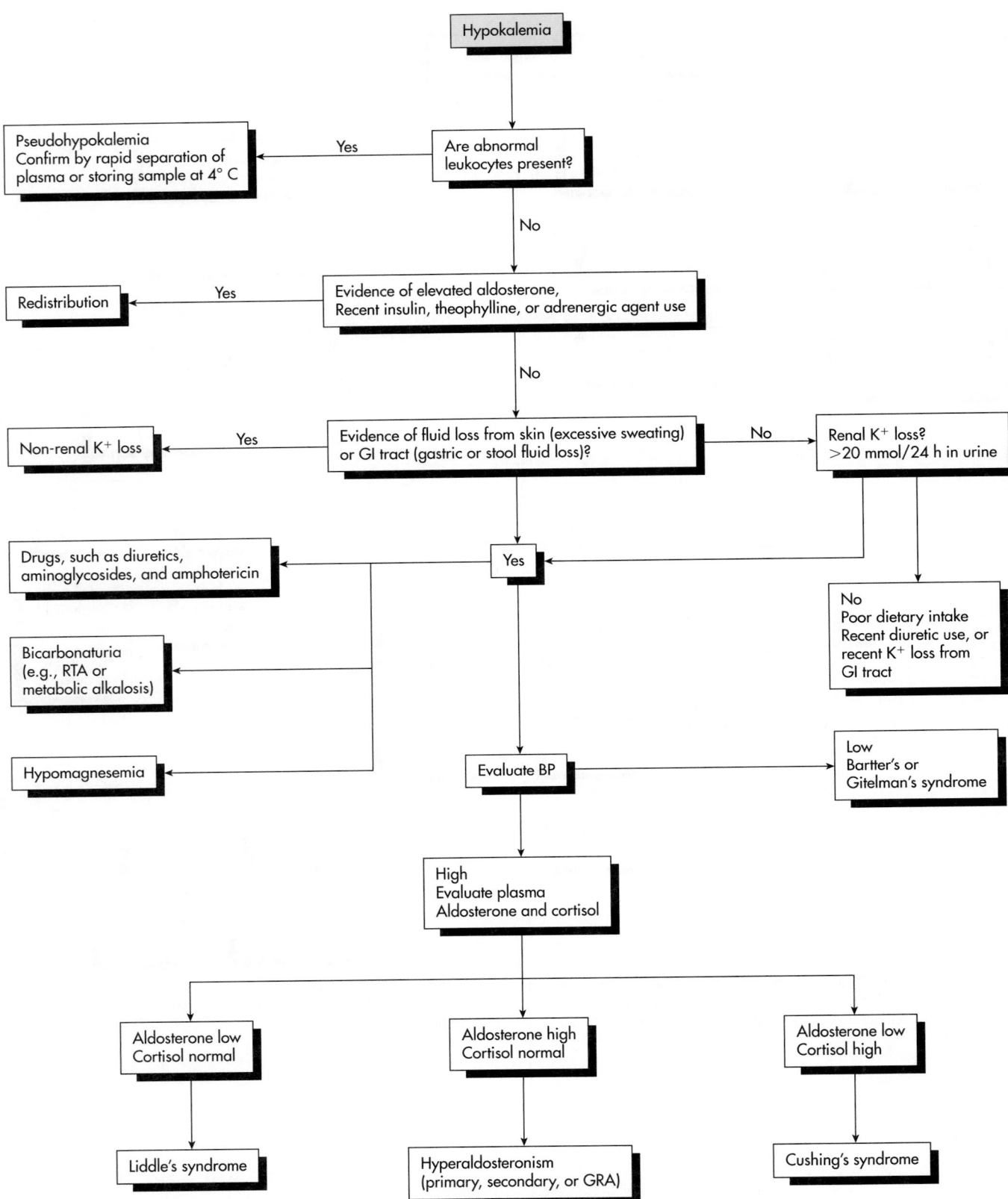

FIGURE 3-178 Diagnostic evaluation of hypokalemia. *BP,* Blood pressure; *GI,* gastrointestinal; *GRA,* glucose remediable aldosteronism; *RTA,* renal tubular acidosis. (From Feehally J, Floege J, Johnson RJ: *Comprehensive clinical nephrology,* ed 3, St Louis, 2007, Mosby.)

HYPOMAGNESEMIA

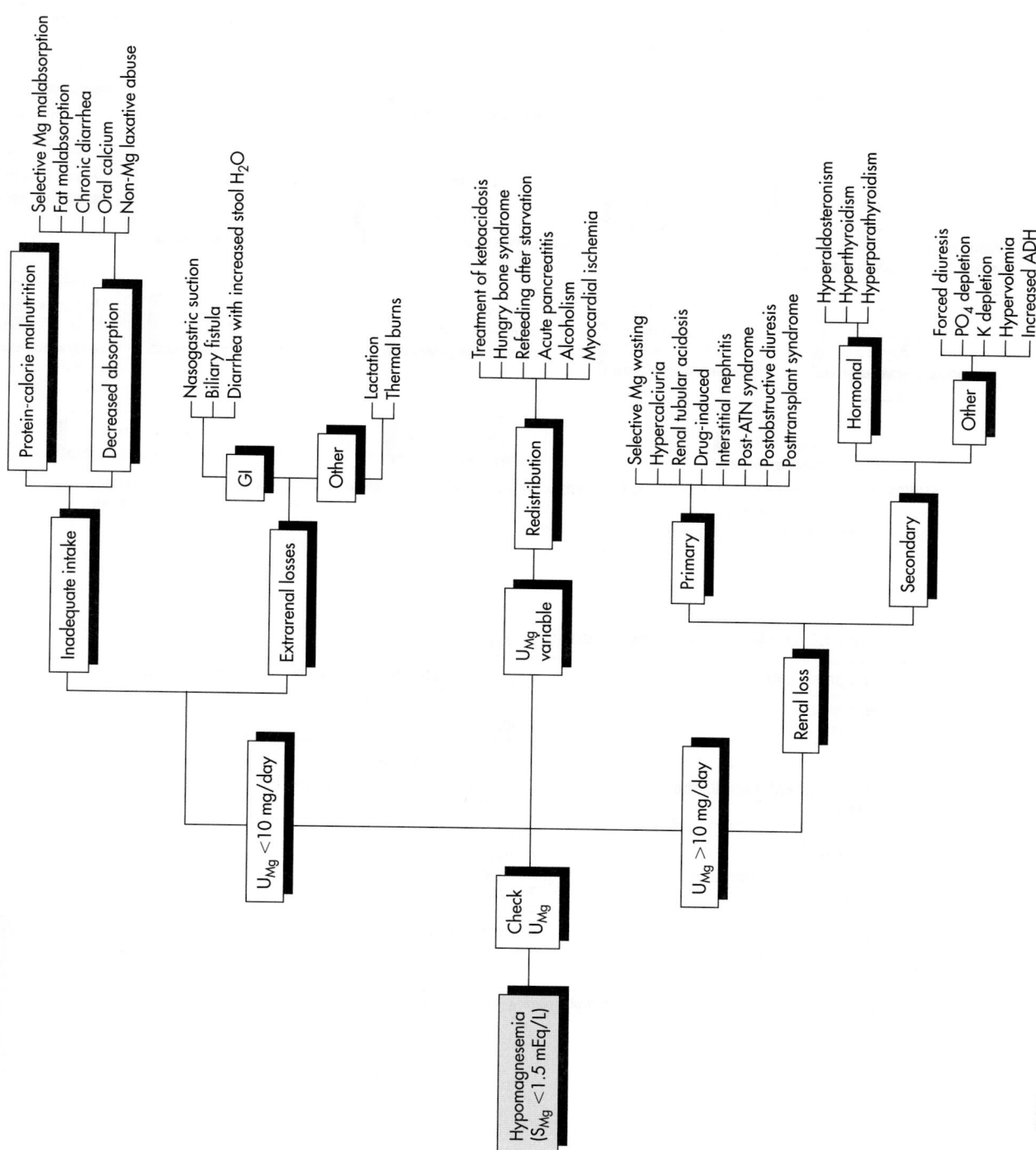

FIGURE 3-179 Hypomagnesemia. *ADH,* Antidiuretic hormone; *GI,* gastrointestinal; *post-ATN,* post acute tubular necrosis. (From Healy PM: *Common medical diagnosis: an algorithmic approach,* ed 3, Philadelphia, 2000, WB Saunders.)

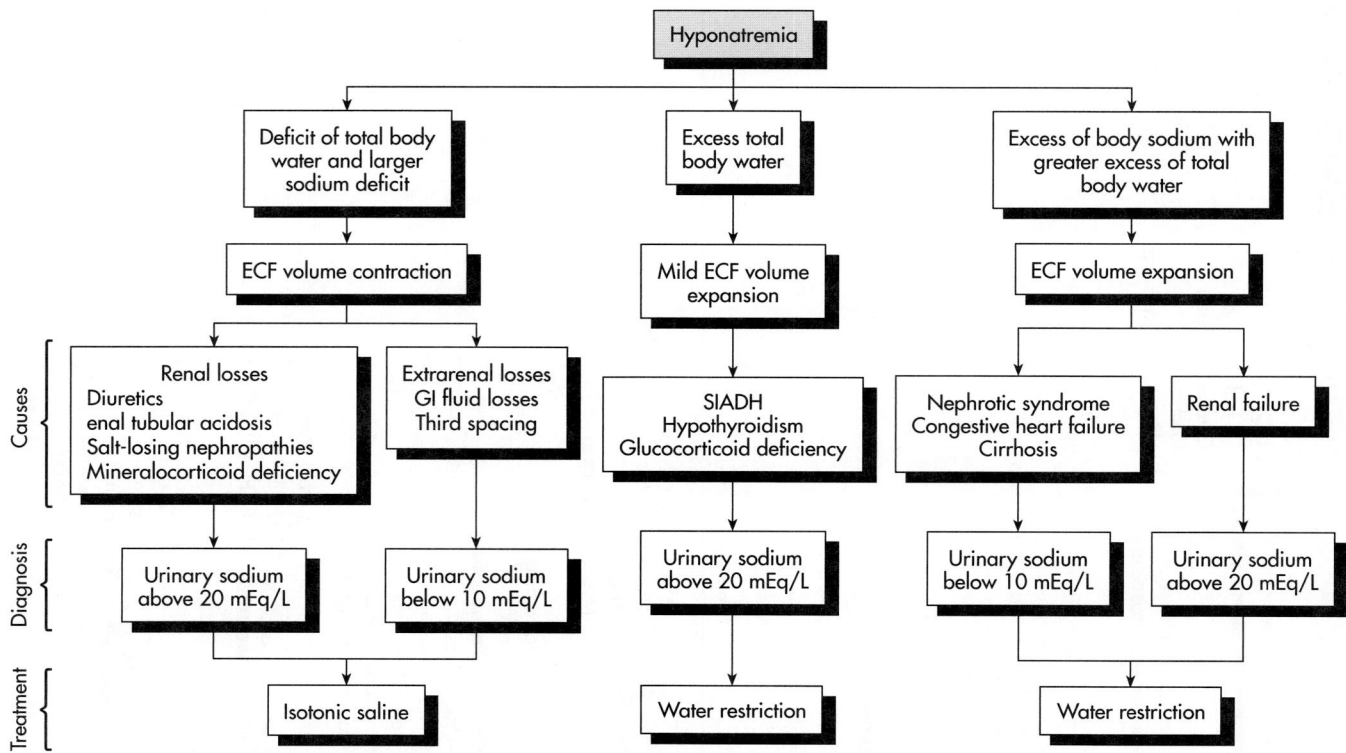

FIGURE 3-180 Evaluation and treatment of asymptomatic, mild hyponatremia. *ECF,* Extracellular fluid; *GI,* gastrointestinal; *SIADH,* syndrome of inappropriate secretion of antidiuretic hormone. (From Marx J et al [eds]: *Rosen's emergency medicine: concepts and clinical practice,* ed 6, St Louis, 2006, Mosby.)

TABLE 3-19 Drugs Associated with Hyponatremia*

Vasopressin Analogs	Drugs that Potentiate Renal Action of Vasopressin
Desmopressin (DDAVP)	Chlorpropamide
Oxytocin	Cyclophosphamide
	Nonsteroidal anti-inflammatory agents
	Acetaminophen (paracetamol)
Drugs that Enhance Vasopressin Release	**Drugs that Cause Hyponatremia by Unknown Mechanisms**
Chlorpropamide	*Haloperidol*
Clofibrate	Fluphenazine
Carbamazepine–oxycarbazepine	Amitriptyline
Vincristine	Thioradazine
Nicotine	Fluoxetine
Narcotics	*Methamphetamine (MDMA or Ecstacy)*
Antipsychotics/antidepressants	Sertraline
Ifosfamide	

(From Johnson RJ, Feehally J: *Comprehensive clinical nephrology,* ed 2, St Louis, 2000, Mosby.)
Italics: The common causes
*Not including diuretics

HYPOTENSION

ICD-9CM # 458.9 Hypotension, NOS
458.1 Hypotension, chronic
458.2 Hypotension, iatrogenic
458.0 Hypotension, orthostatic or postural

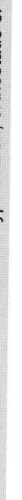

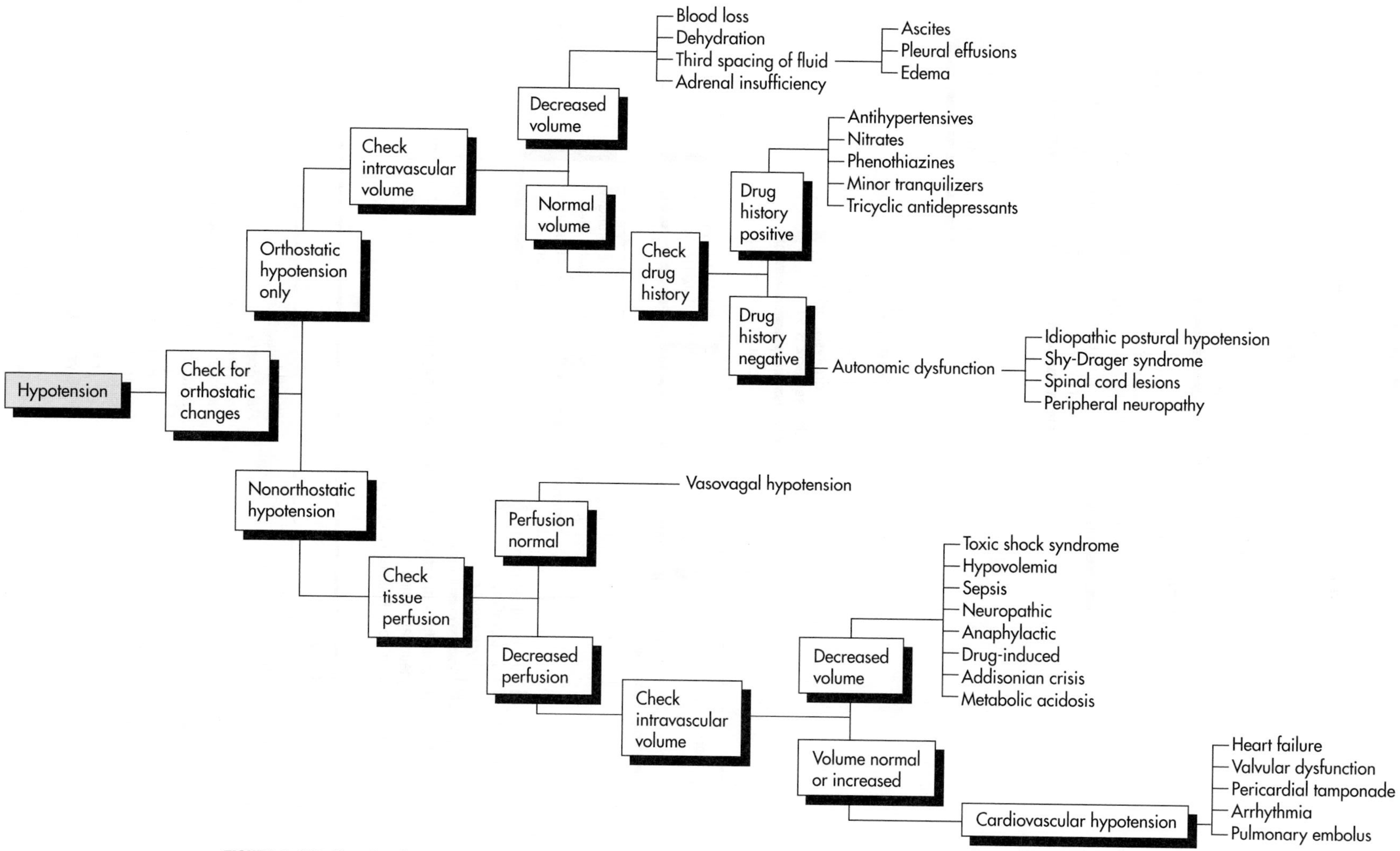

Blood loss
Dehydration
Third spacing of fluid — Ascites / Pleural effusions / Edema
Adrenal insufficiency

Antihypertensives
Nitrates
Phenothiazines
Minor tranquilizers
Tricyclic antidepressants

Idiopathic postural hypotension
Shy-Drager syndrome
Spinal cord lesions
Peripheral neuropathy

Autonomic dysfunction

Drug history positive
Drug history negative
Check drug history
Decreased volume
Normal volume
Check intravascular volume
Orthostatic hypotension only
Check for orthostatic changes
Hypotension
Nonorthostatic hypotension
Vasovagal hypotension
Check tissue perfusion
Perfusion normal
Decreased perfusion
Check intravascular volume
Decreased volume
Volume normal or increased

Toxic shock syndrome
Hypovolemia
Sepsis
Neuropathic
Anaphylactic
Drug-induced
Addisonian crisis
Metabolic acidosis

Cardiovascular hypotension

Heart failure
Valvular dysfunction
Pericardial tamponade
Arrhythmia
Pulmonary embolus

FIGURE 3-182 Hypotension. (From Healey PM: *Common medical diagnosis: an algorithmic approach*, ed 3, Philadelphia, 2000, WB Saunders.)

Clinical Algorithms

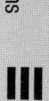

III

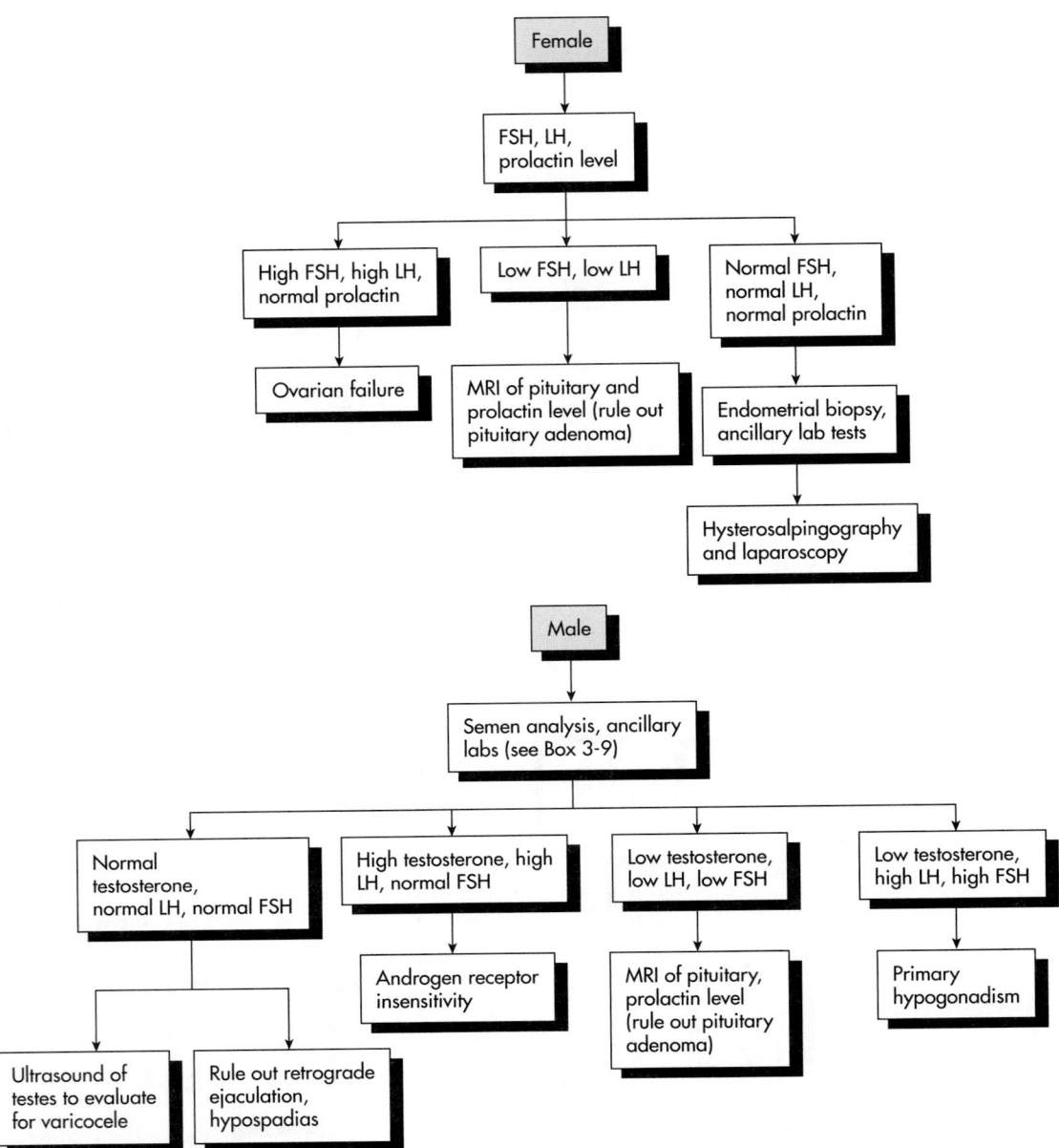

FIGURE 3-186 Approach to infertility diagnosis and management. *FSH,* Follicle-stimulating hormone; *LH,* luteinizing hormone; *MRI,* magnetic resonance imaging. (From Ferri FF: *Ferri's best test: a practical guide to clinical laboratory medicine and diagnostic imaging,* ed 2, Philadelphia, 2009, Elsevier Mosby.)

BOX 3-9   Infertility

Diagnostic imaging
Best test
None

Ancillary tests
MRI of pituitary with contrast
Hysterosalpingography
Testicular ultrasound

Lab evaluation
Best tests
Male: semen analysis
Female: endometrial biopsy

Ancillary tests
FSH, LH
Prolactin
Serum testosterone (male)
TSH
CBC, ESR, FBS
Urinalysis, VDRL, *Mycoplasma* culture, chlamidiae serology

Ferri FF: *Ferri's best test: a practical guide to clinical laboratory medicine and diagnostic imaging,* ed 2, Philadelphia, 2009, Elsevier Mosby.
   CBC, Complete blood count; *ESR,* erythrocyte sedimentation rate; *FBS,* fasting blood sugar; *FSH,* follicle-stimulating hormone; *LH,* luteinizing hormone; *MRI,* magnetic resonance imaging; *VDRL,* Venereal Disease Research Laboratory (test).

LEG ULCER

ICD-9CM # 440.23 Ulcer, lower limb, arteriosclerotic
707.1   Ulcer, lower limb, chronic
707.1   Ulcer, lower limb, neurogenic
707.9   Ulcer, non-healing
707.0   Pressure ulcer

1285

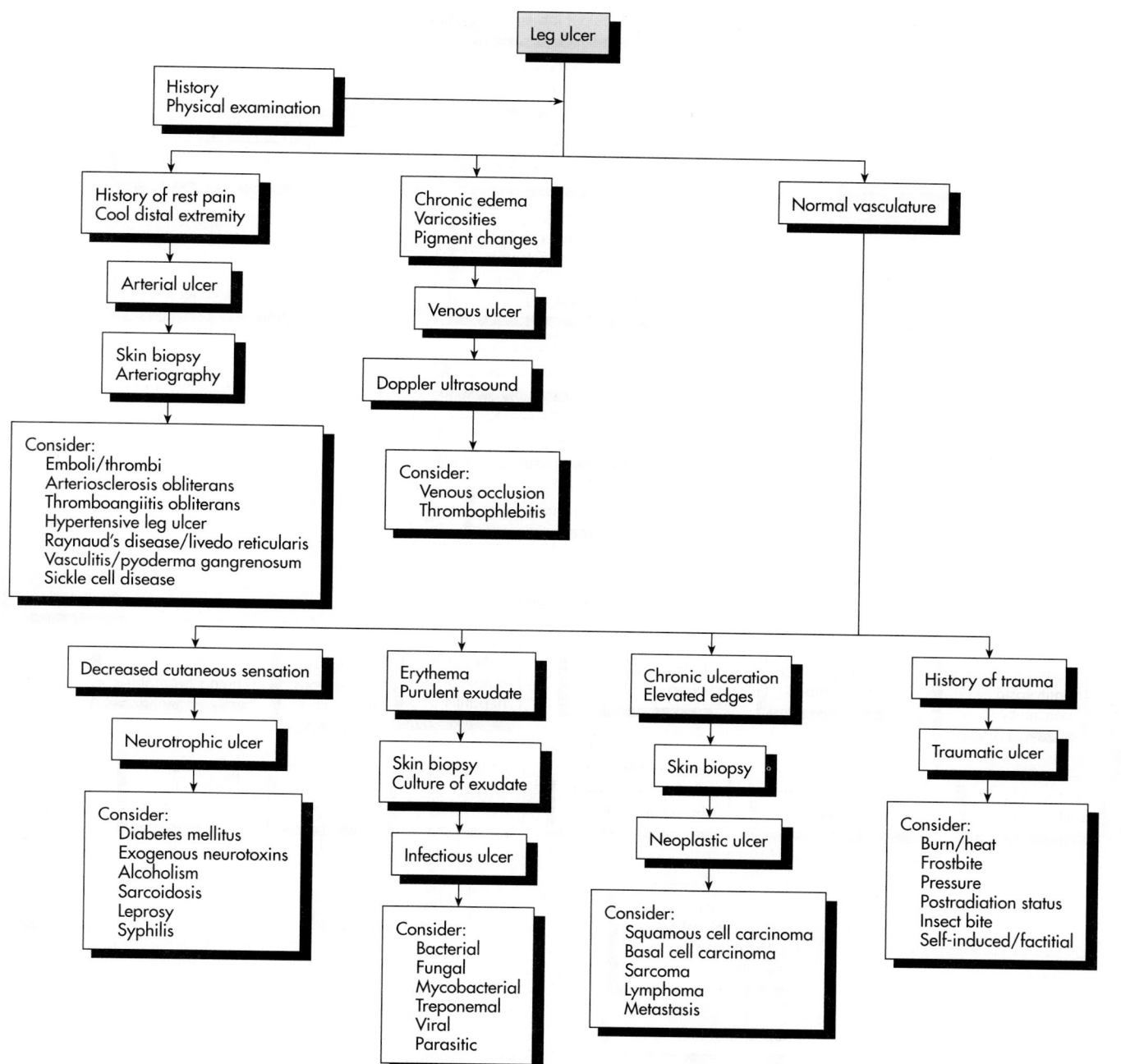

FIGURE 3-197 Leg ulcer. (From Greene HL, Johnson WP, Lemcke D [eds]: *Decision making in medicine*, ed 2, St Louis, 1998, Mosby.)

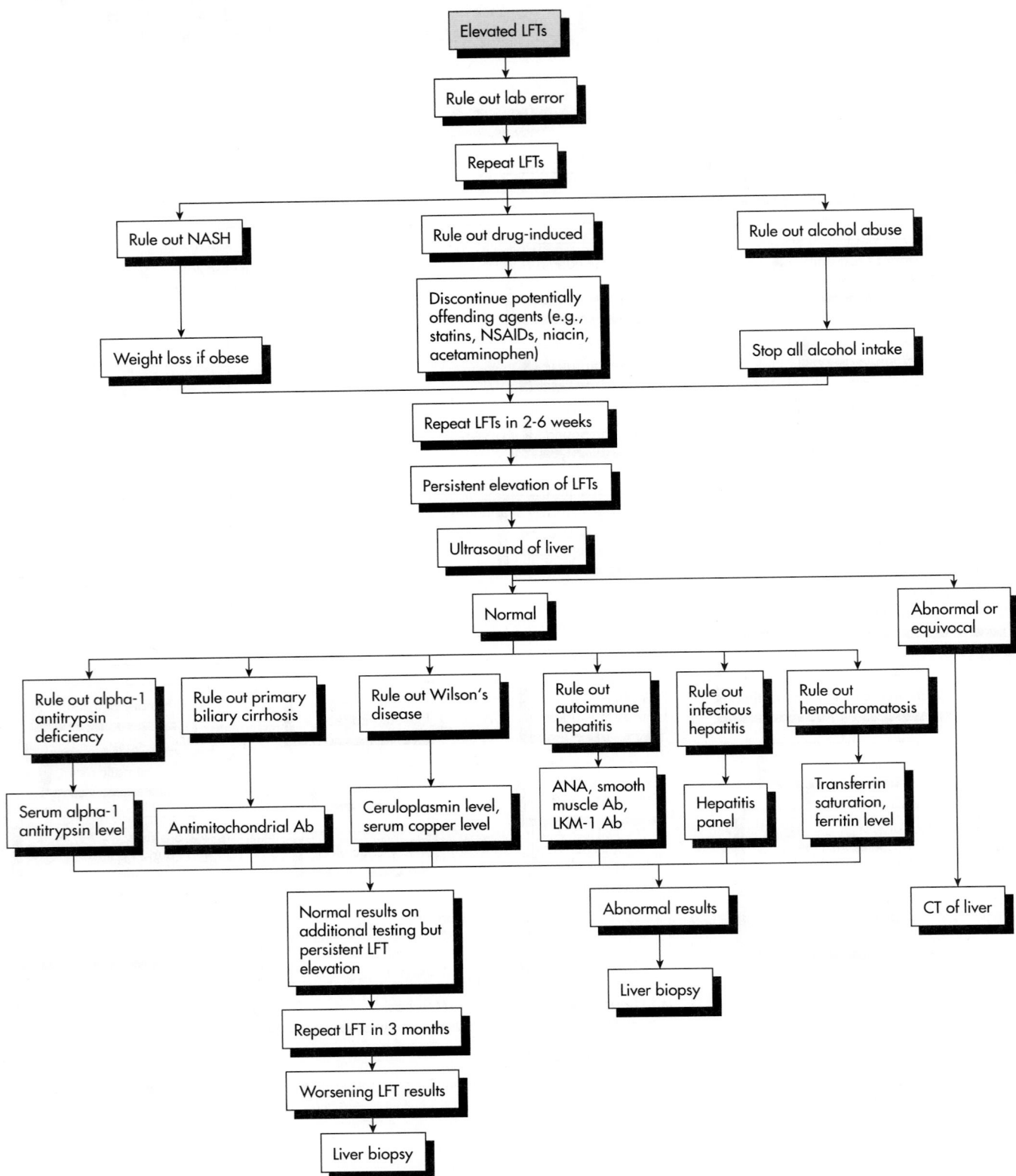

FIGURE 3-199 Liver function test elevations. *Ab,* Antibody; *ANA,* antibody to nuclear antigens; *CT,* computed tomography; *IEP,* immuno-electrophoresis; *LFTs,* liver function test; *LKM,* liver-kidney microsome; *NASH,* nonalcoholic steatohepatitis; *NSAIDs,* nonsteroidal anti-inflammatory drugs.

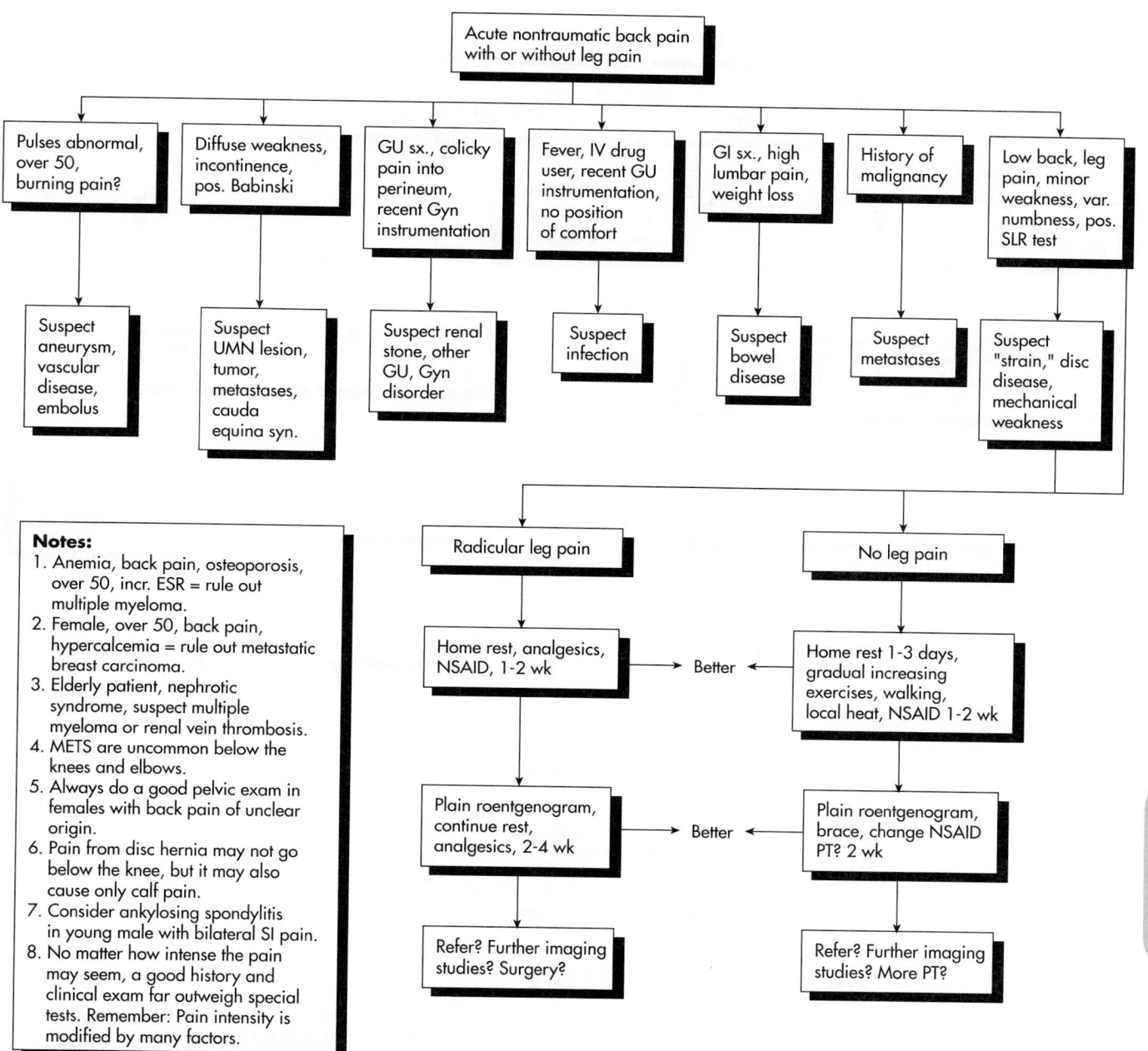

FIGURE 3-200 Algorithm for low back and/or leg pain. *GI*, Gastrointestinal; *GU*, genitourinary; *IV*, intravenous; *METS*, metabolic equivalents; *NSAID*, nonsteroidal anti-inflammatory drug; *PT*, physical therapy; *SLR*, straight-leg raising; *UMN*, upper motor neuron. (From Mercier LR: *Practical orthopedics*, ed 2, St Louis, 2000, Mosby.)

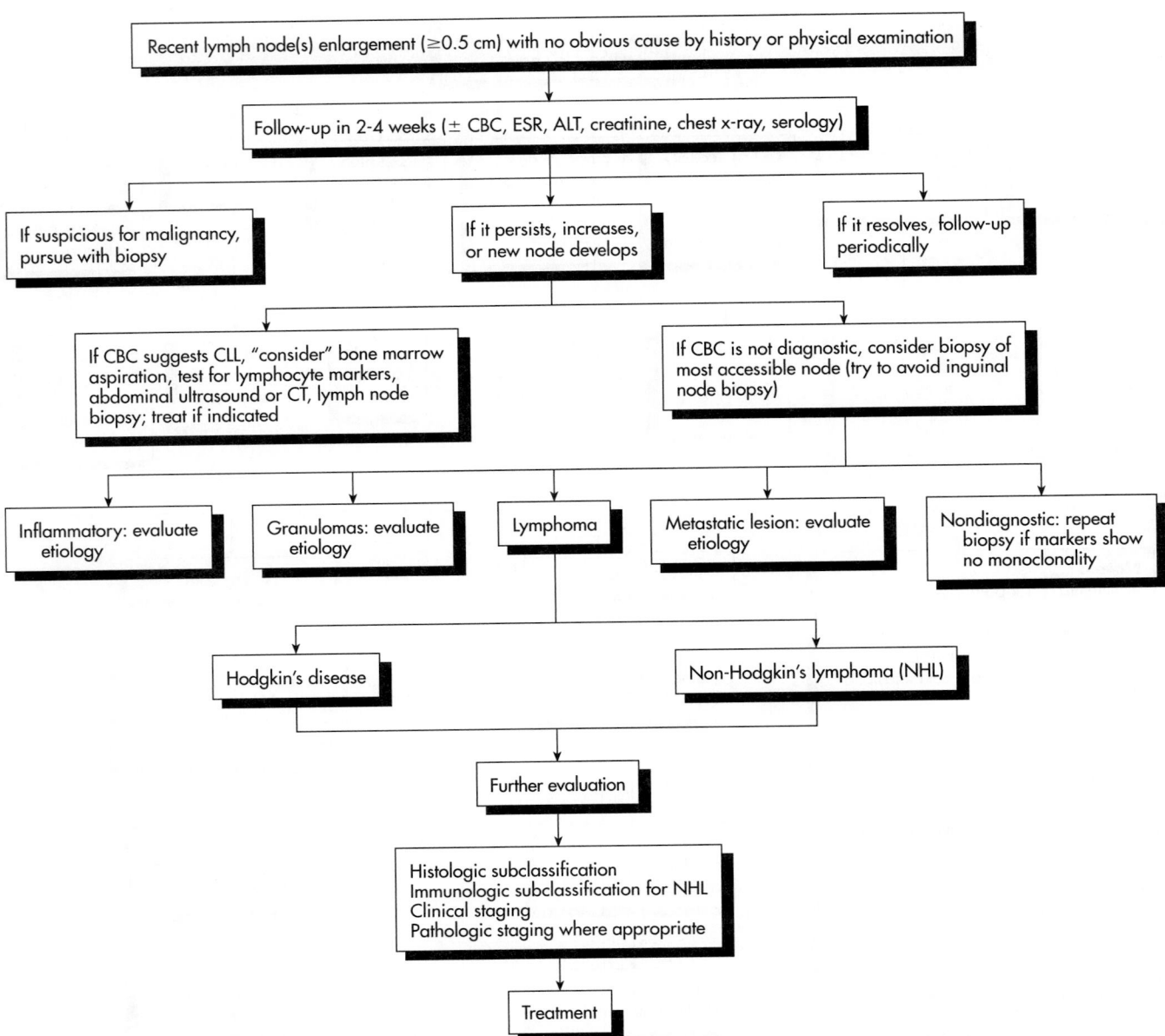

FIGURE 3-204 Workup of lymphadenopathy. *ALT,* Alanine aminotransferase; *CBC,* complete blood count; *CLL,* chronic lymphocytic leukemia; *CT,* computed tomography; *ESR,* erythrocyte sedimentation rate. (Modified from Noble J [ed]: *Primary care medicine*, ed 3, St Louis, 2001, Mosby.)

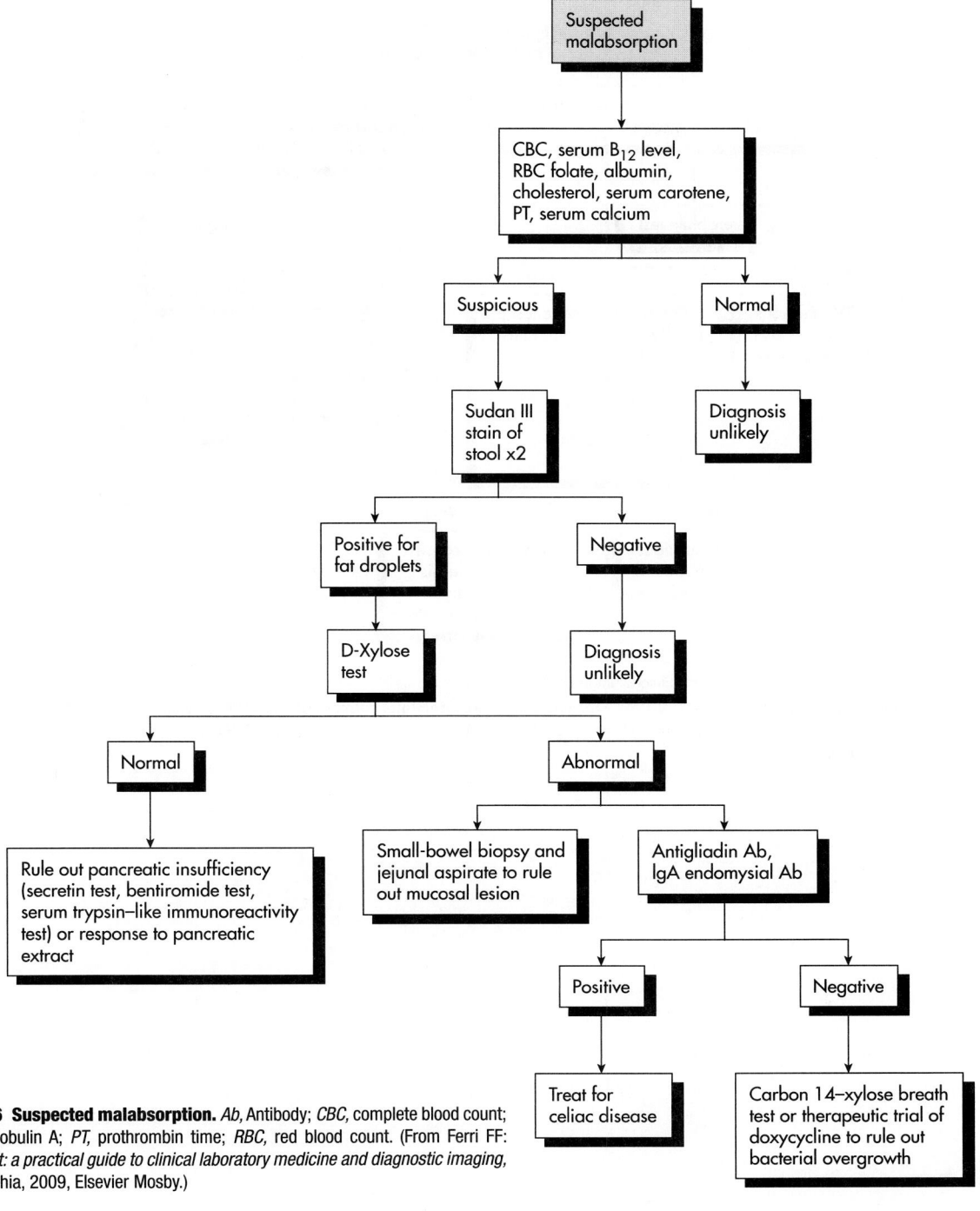

FIGURE 3-206 Suspected malabsorption. *Ab,* Antibody; *CBC,* complete blood count; *IgA,* immunoglobulin A; *PT,* prothrombin time; *RBC,* red blood count. (From Ferri FF: *Ferri's best test: a practical guide to clinical laboratory medicine and diagnostic imaging,* ed 2, Philadelphia, 2009, Elsevier Mosby.)

BOX 3-10   Malabsorption, Suspected

Diagnostic imaging
Best test
Small-bowel series

Ancillary test
CT of pancreas with IV contrast

Lab evaluation
Best test
Biopsy of small bowel

Ancillary tests
Albumin, total protein
ALT, AST, PT
Serum lytes, BUN, creatinine
Sudan III stain of stool for fecal leukocytes
CBC, RBC folate, serum iron, serum carotene, cholesterol, serum calcium
Hydrogen 14-C xylose breath test
D-Xylose test, secretin test
Quantitative fecal test
Antigliadin antibody, IgA endomysial antibody

From Ferri FF: *Ferri's best test: a practical guide to clinical laboratory medicine and diagnostic imaging,* ed 2, Philadelphia, 2009, Elsevier Mosby.
   ALT, Alanine aminotransferase; AST, aspartate aminotransferase; BUN, blood urea nitrogen; CBC, complete blood count; CT, computed tomography; IgA, immunoglobulin A; IV, intravenous; PT, prothrombin time; RBC, red blood count.

Diagnostic Algorithm for EBV Infection and Infectious Mononucleosis*

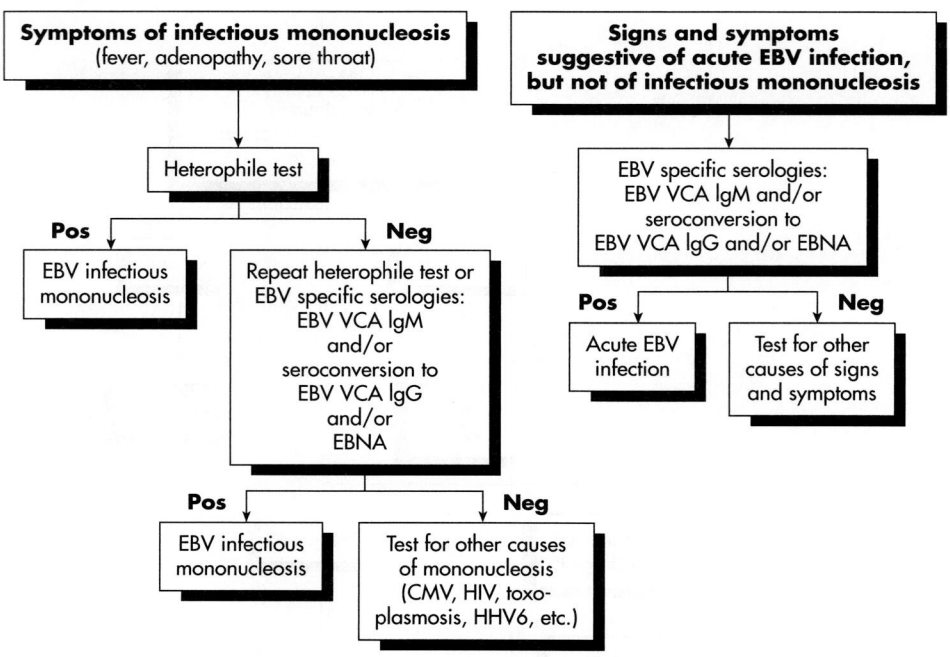

*Note: Refer to Section I for additional information on this topic.

FIGURE 3-210 Diagnostic algorithm for EBV infection and infectious mononucleosis. *CMV,* Cytomegalovirus; *EBV,* Epstein-Barr virus; *HIV,* human immunodeficiency virus. (From Young NS, Gerson SL, High KA [eds]: *Clinical hematology,* St Louis, 2006, Mosby.)

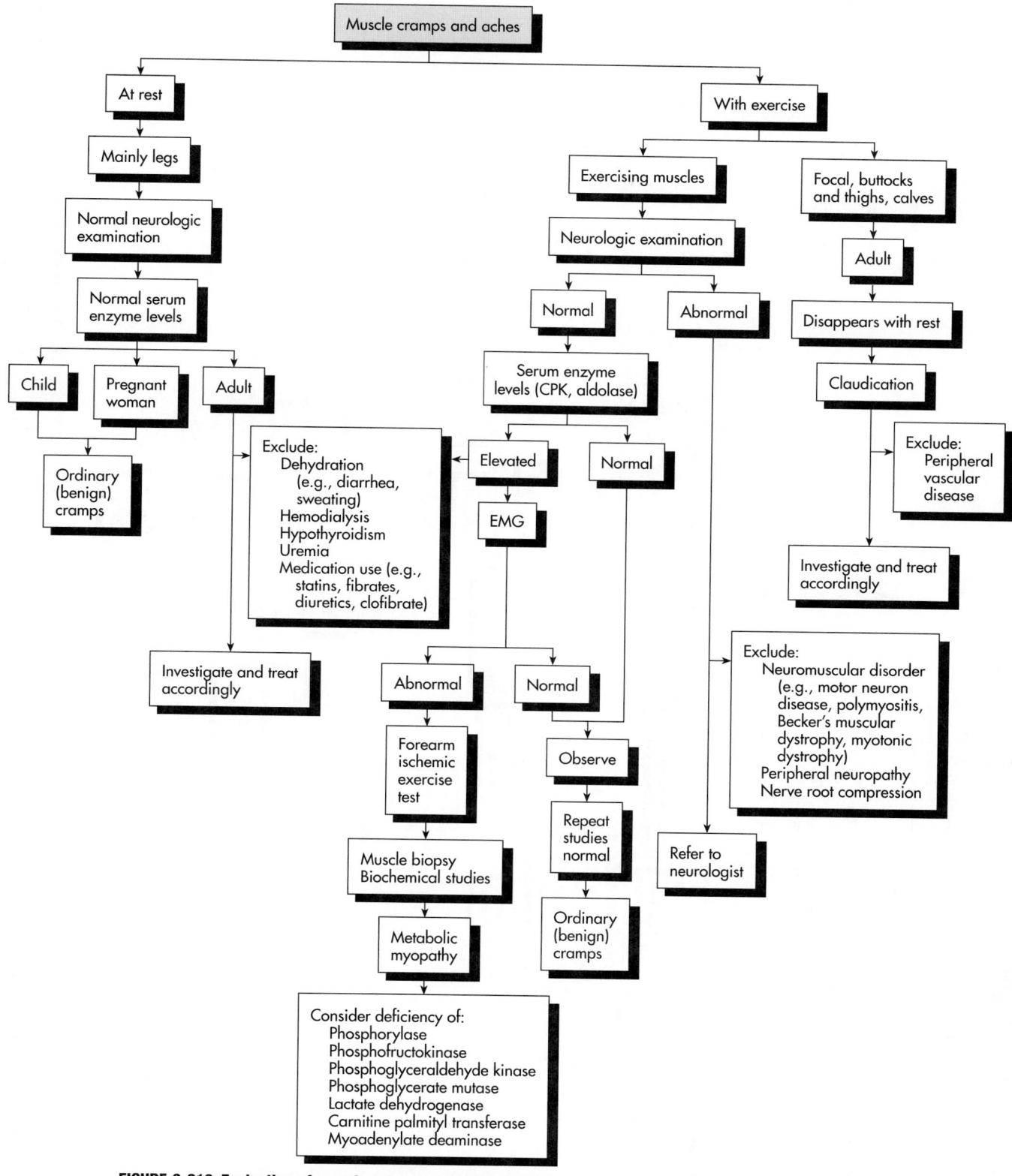

FIGURE 3-216 Evaluation of muscle cramps and aches. *CPK,* Creatine phosphokinase; *EMG,* electromyography. (From Greene HL, Johnson WP, Lemcke D [eds]: *Decision making in medicine,* ed 2, St Louis, 1998, Mosby.)

Clinical Algorithms

III

MUSCLE WEAKNESS

ICD-9CM # 782.9

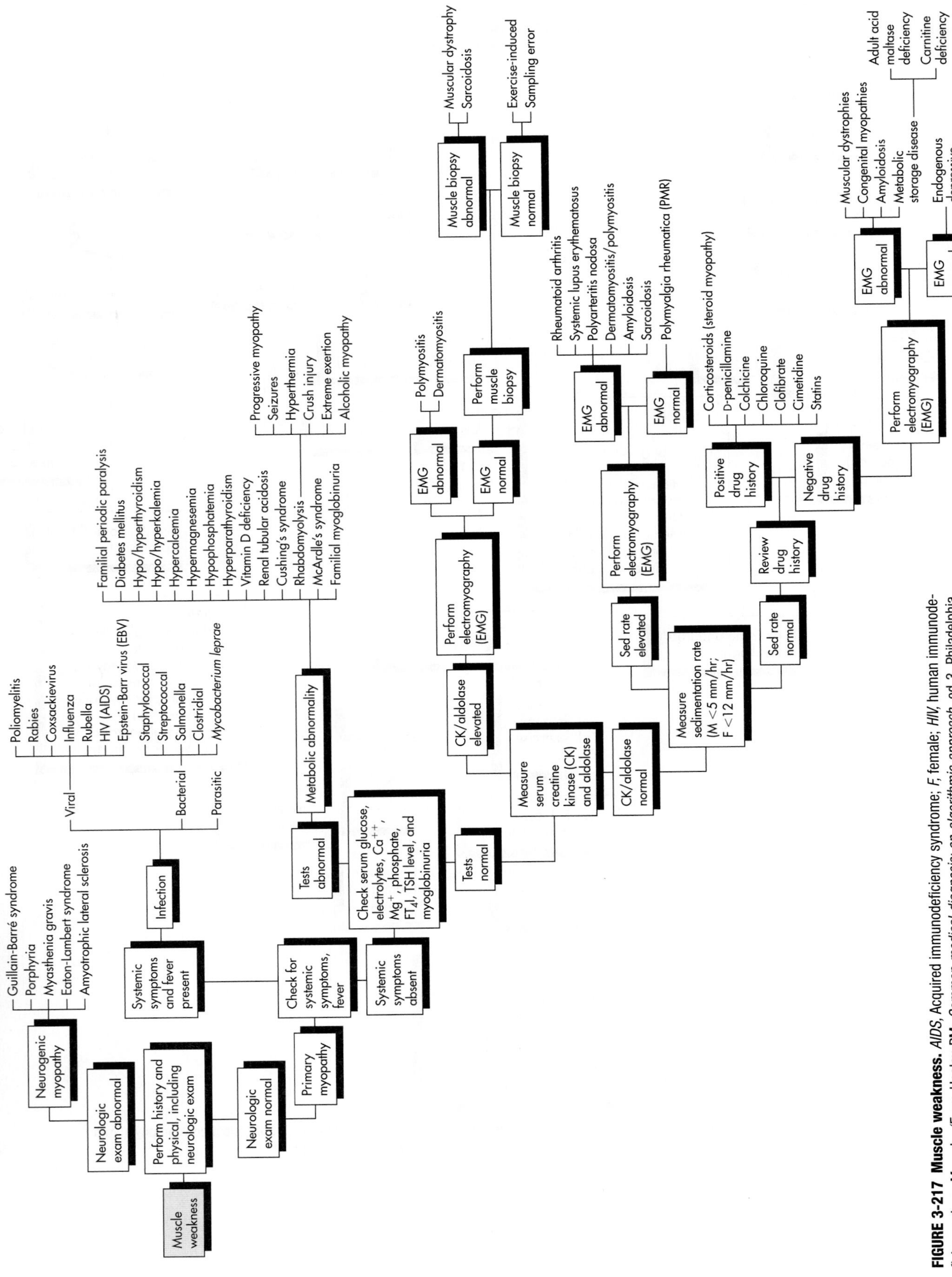

FIGURE 3-217 Muscle weakness. *AIDS*, Acquired immunodeficiency syndrome; *F*, female; *HIV*, human immunodeficiency virus; *M*, male. (From Healey PM: *Common medical diagnosis: an algorithmic approach*, ed 3, Philadelphia, 2000, WB Saunders.)

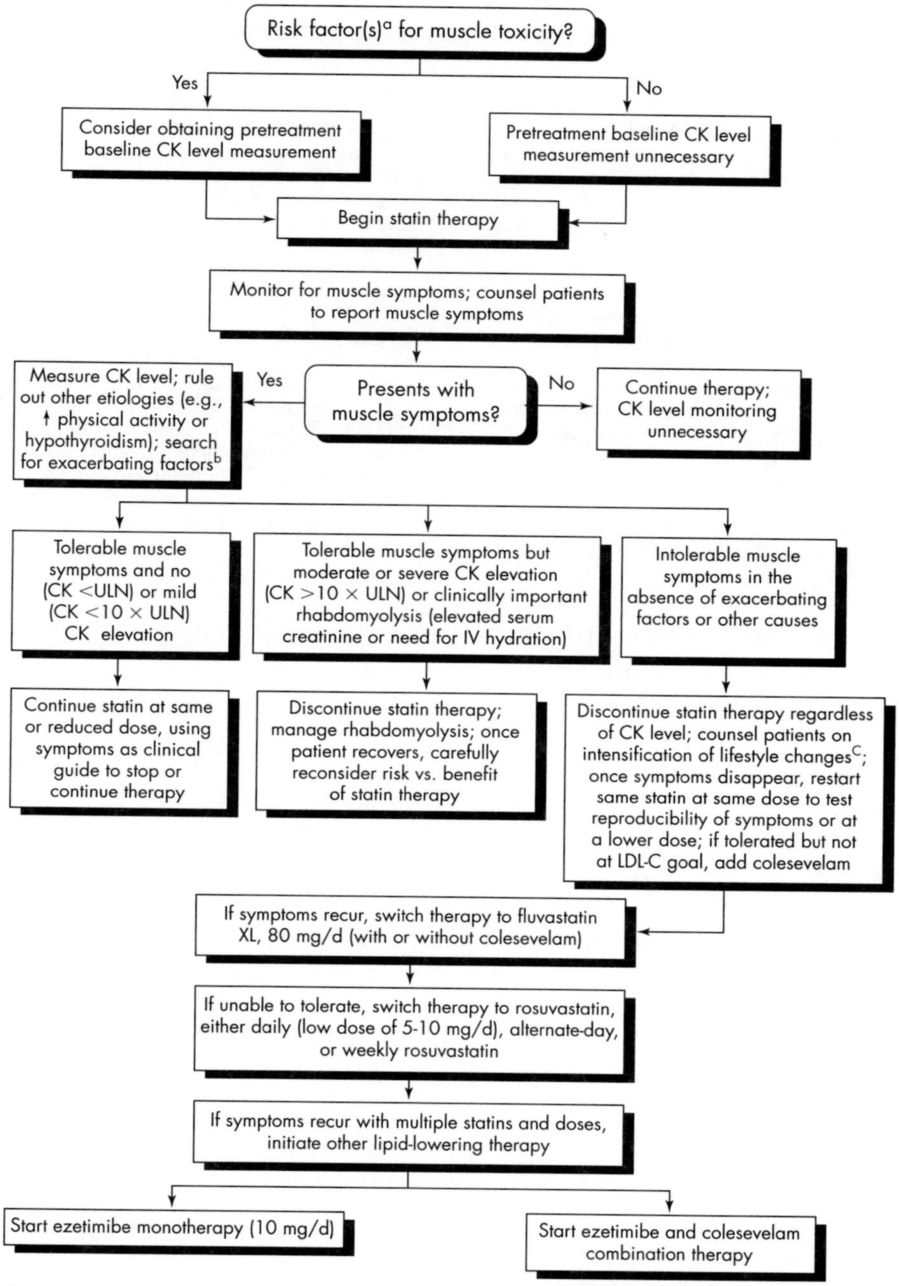

Clinical Algorithms

FIGURE 3-221 Algorithm for monitoring and management of suspected statin-associated myopathy. a, Risk factors for muscle toxicity include advanced age and frailty, small body frame, deteriorating renal function, infection, untreated hypothyroidism, interacting drugs, perioperative periods, and alcohol abuse. **b,** Causes for elevated CK levels/muscle toxicity are increased physical activity, trauma, falls, accidents, seizure, shaking chills, hypothyroidism, infections, carbon monoxide poisoning, polymyositis, dermatomyositis, alcohol abuse, and drug abuse (cocaine, amphetamines, heroin, or PCP). **c,** Patient counseling regarding intensification of therapeutic lifestyle changes (reduced intake of saturated fats and cholesterol, increased physical activity, and weight control) should be an integral part of management in all patients with statin-associated intolerable muscle symptoms. *CK,* Creatine kinase; *IV,* intravenous; *LDL-C,* low-density lipoprotein cholesterol; *PCP,* phencyclidine; *ULN,* upper limit of normal; *XL,* extended release. (Modified from Jacobson TA: Toward "pain-free" statin prescribing, *Mayo Clin Proc* 83[60]: 696, 2008.)

BOX 3-11   Recommendations to Health Care Professionals Regarding Statin and Muscle Safety

Whenever muscle symptoms or an increased CK level are encountered in patients receiving statin therapy, health professionals should attempt to rule out other causes, because these are most likely to explain the findings. Other comon causes include increased physical activity, trauma, falls, accidents, seizure, shaking chills, hypothyroidism, infections, carbon monoxide poisoning, polymyositis, dermatomyositis, alcohol abuse, and drug abuse (cocaine, amphetamines, heroin, or PCP).

Obtaining a pretreatment, baseline CK level can be considered in patients who are at high risk of experiencing muscle toxicity (e.g., older patients or those combining a statin with an agent known to increase myotoxicity), but this is not routinely necessary in other patients.

It is unnecessary to measure CK levels in asymptomatic patients during the course of statin therapy, because marked, clinically important CK elevations are rare and are usually related to physical exertion or other causes.

Patients receiving statin therapy should be counseled about the increased risk of muscle symptoms, particularly if initiation of vigorous, sustained endurance exercise or a surgical operation is being contemplated; they should be advised to report such muscle symptoms to a health professional.

Creatine kinase measurements should be obtained in symptomatic patients to help gauge the severity of muscle damage and facilitate decision of whether to continue therapy or alter doses.

In patients who develop intolerable muscle symptoms with or without CK elevation and for whom other etiologies have been ruled out, the statin should be discontinued. Once symptoms disappear, the same or different statin at the same or a lower dose can be restarted to test the reproducibility of symptoms. Recurrence of symptoms with multiple statins and doses requires initiation of other lipid-altering therapy.

In patients who develop tolerable muscle symptoms or have no symptoms but have a CK level $<10 \times$ ULN, statin therapy may be continued at the same or reduced doses and symptoms may be used as the clinical guide to stop or continue therapy.

In patients who develop rhabdomyolysis (CK $>10,000$ IU/L or $>10 \times$ ULN with an elevation in serum creatinine or need for intravenous hydration therapy), statin therapy should be stopped. Intravenous hydration therapy in a hospital should be instituted if indicated for patients experiencing rhabdomyolysis. Once patients recover, risk vs benefit of statin therapy should be carefully reconsidered.

From McKenney JM et al: Final conclusions and recommendations of the National Lipid Association Statin Safety Assessment Task Force, *Am J Cardiol,* 97 (suppl 8A):89C-94C, 2006.

CK, Creatine kinase; *PCP,* phencyclidine; *ULN,* upper limit of normal.

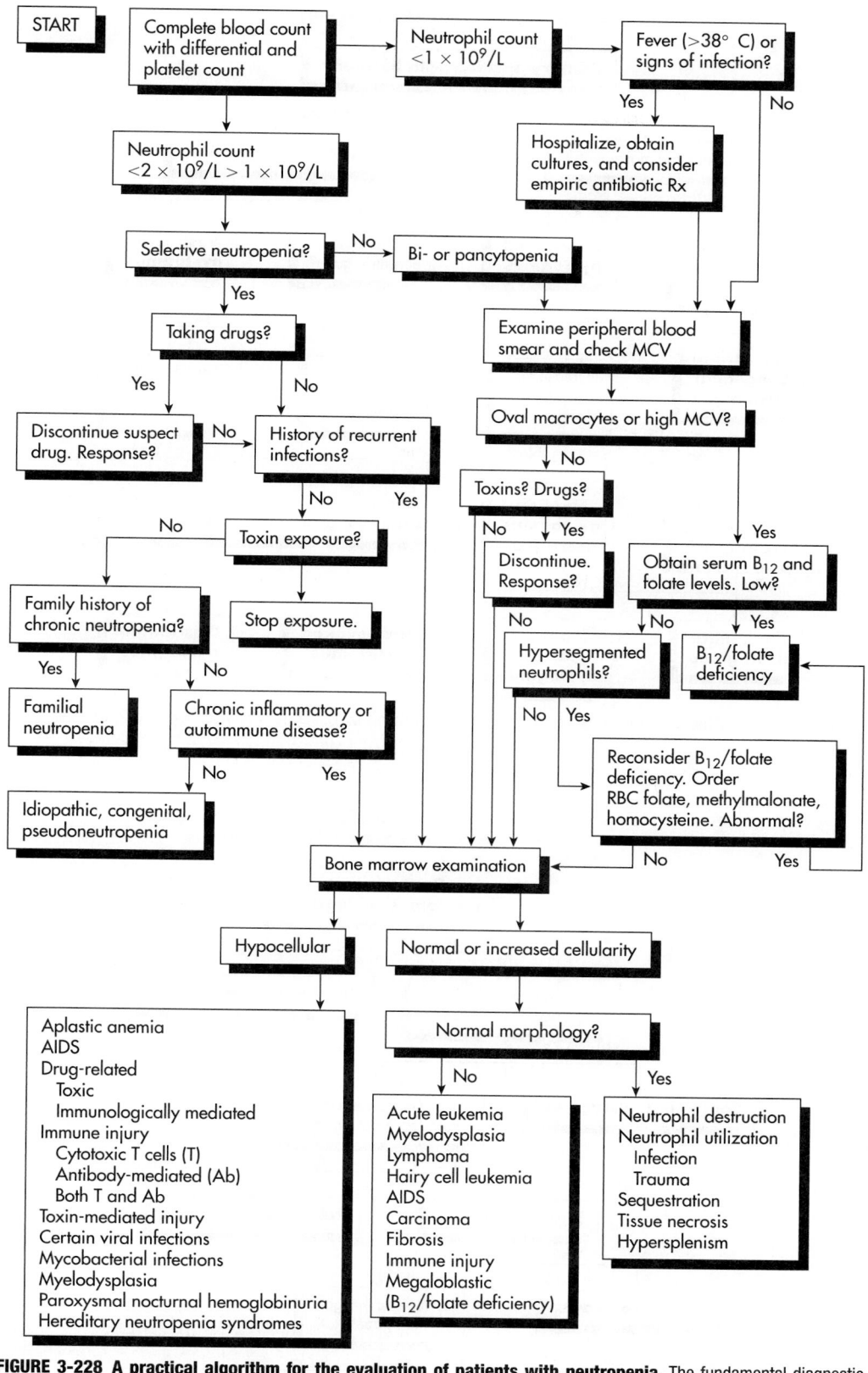

FIGURE 3-228 A practical algorithm for the evaluation of patients with neutropenia. The fundamental diagnostic principle is that for patients with severe neutropenia or for those with bicytopenia or pancytopenia, bone marrow examination will likely be necessary unless the following diagnoses are made: (1) a nutritional (folate or vitamin B_{12}) deficiency or (2) drug- or toxin-induced neutropenia in a patient whose neutropenia resolves after discontinuation of the offending agent. *AIDS*, Acquired immunodeficiency syndrome; *MCV*, mean corpuscular volume; *RBC*, red blood cell. (From Goldman L, Ausiello D [eds]: *Cecil textbook of medicine*, ed 23, Philadelphia, 2008, WB Saunders.)

Clinical Algorithms

Identification of Types of Nystagmus

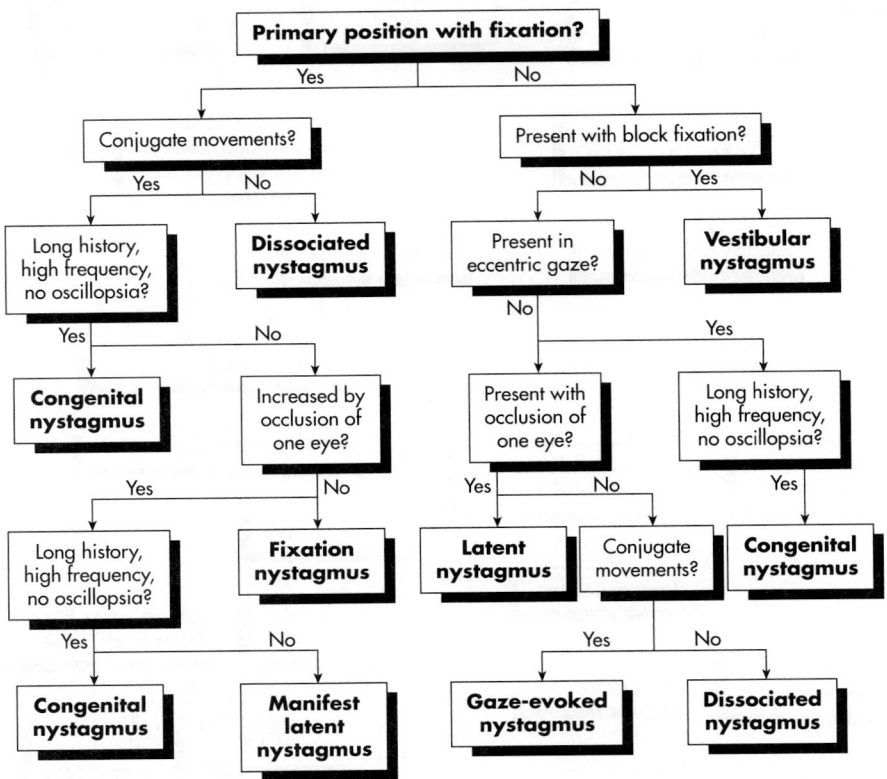

FIGURE 3-232 **Identification of types of nystagmus.** (From Yanoff M, Duker JS: *Ophthalmology,* ed 2, St Louis, 2004, Mosby.)

Identification of Types of Gaze-Evoked Nystagmus

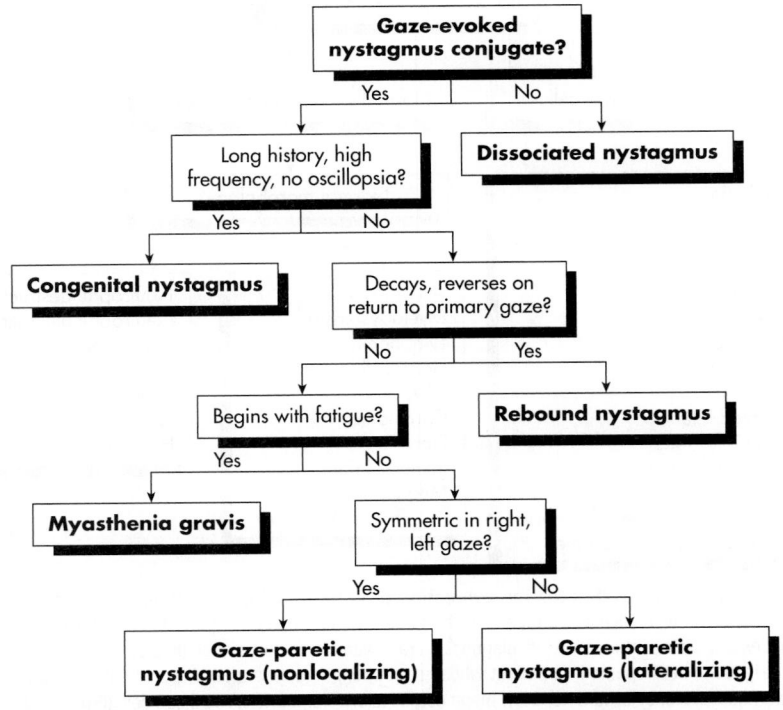

FIGURE 3-234 **Identification of types of gaze-evoked nystagmus.** (From Yanoff M, Duker JS: *Ophthalmology,* ed 2, St Louis, 2004, Mosby.)

(Continued on next page)

Identification
of Types of Dissociated Nystagmus

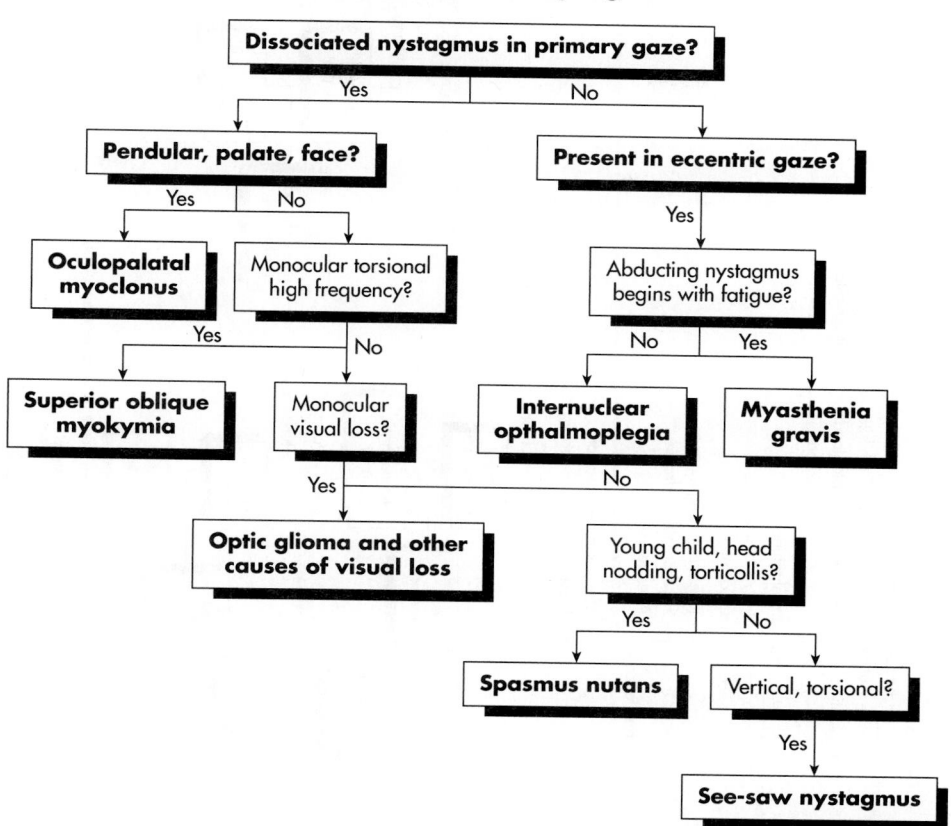

FIGURE 3-235 Identification of types of dissociated nystagmus. (From Yanoff M, Duker JS: *Ophthalmology,* ed 2, St Louis, 2004, Mosby.)

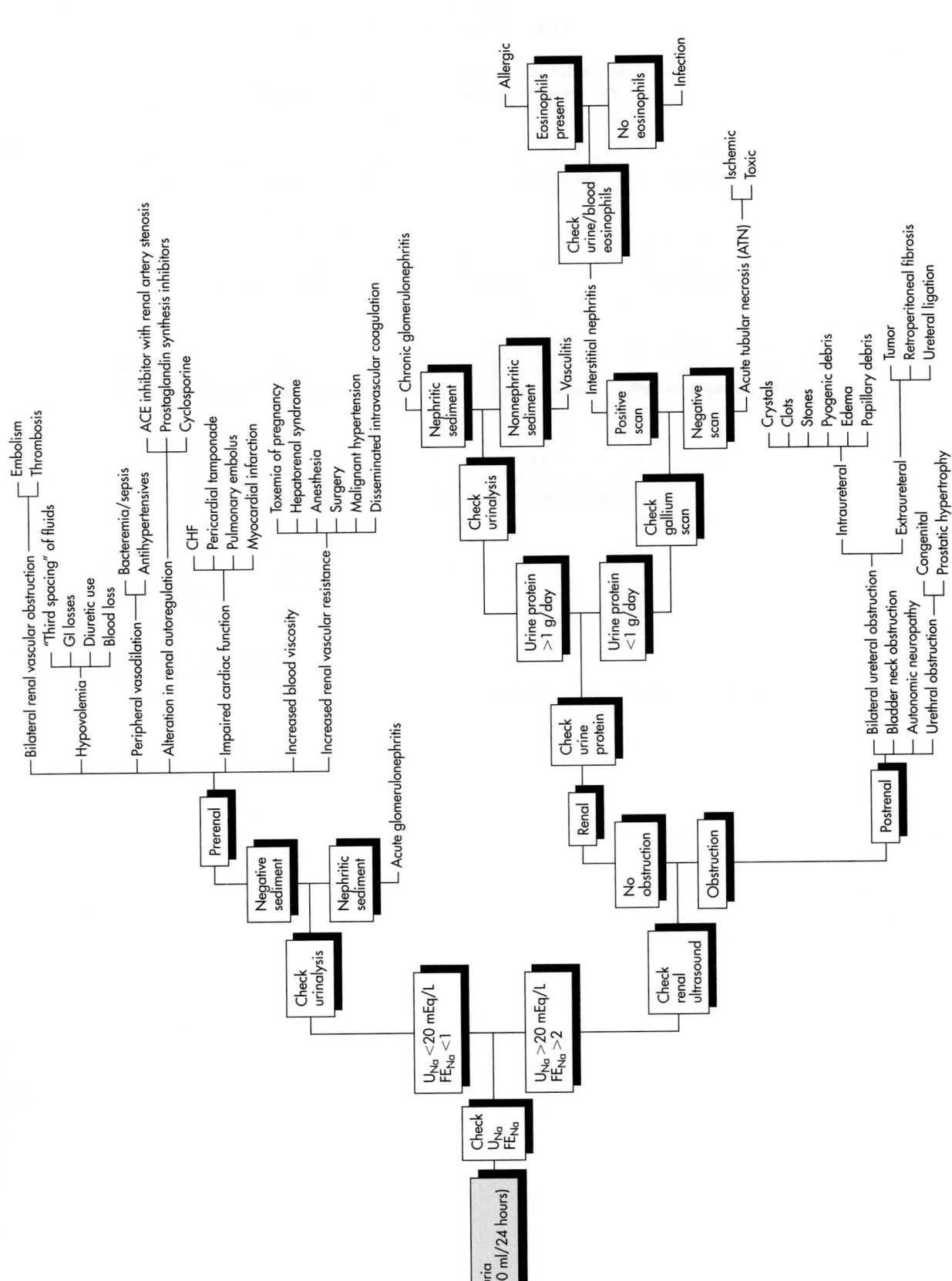

FIGURE 3-238 Evaluation of oliguria. *ACE,* Angiotensin-converting enzyme; *CHF,* congestive heart failure; *GI,* gastrointestinal. (From Healey PM: *Common medical diagnosis: an algorithmic approach,* ed 3, Philadelphia, 2000, WB Saunders.)

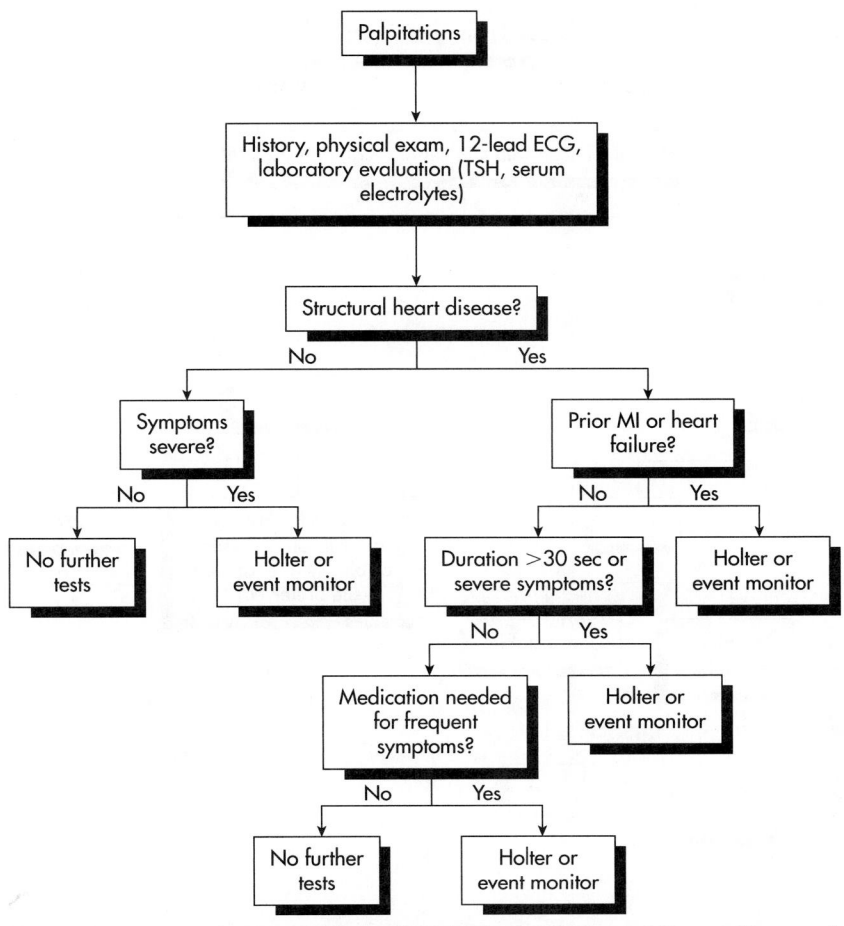

FIGURE 3-243 Diagnostic approach to the patient with palpitations. *ECG,* Electrocardiogram; *MI,* myocardial infarction; *TSH,* thyroid-stimulating hormone. (From Hiatky MA: Approach to the patient with palpitations. In Braunwald E, Goldman L [eds]: *Primary cardiology,* ed 2, Philadelphia, 2003, WB Saunders.)

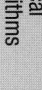

TABLE 3-24   Items to be Covered in History of Patient with Palpitation

Does the Palpitation Occur:	If So, Suspect:
As isolated "jumps" or "skips"?	Extrasystoles
In attacks known to be of abrupt beginning, with a heart rate of 120 beats/min or over, with regular or irregular rhythm?	Paroxysmal rapid heart action
Independent of exercise or excitement adequate to account for the symptom?	Atrial fibrillation, atrial flutter, thyrotoxicosis, anemia, febrile states, hypoglycemia, anxiety state
In attacks developing rapidly though not absolutely abruptly, unrelated to exertion or excitement?	Hemorrhage, hypoglycemia, tumor of the adrenal medulla
In conjunction with the taking of drugs?	Tobacco, coffee, tea, alcohol, epinephrine, ephedrine, aminophylline, atropine, thyroid extract, monoamine oxidase inhibitors
On standing?	Postural hypotension
In middle-aged women, in conjunction with flushes and sweats?	Menopausal syndrome
When the rate is known to be normal and the rhythm regular?	Anxiety state

(From Goldman L, Braunwald E: Chest discomfort and palpitation. In Isselbacher KJ, Braunwald E et al [eds]: *Harrison's principles of internal medicine,* ed 13, New York, 1994, McGraw-Hill.)

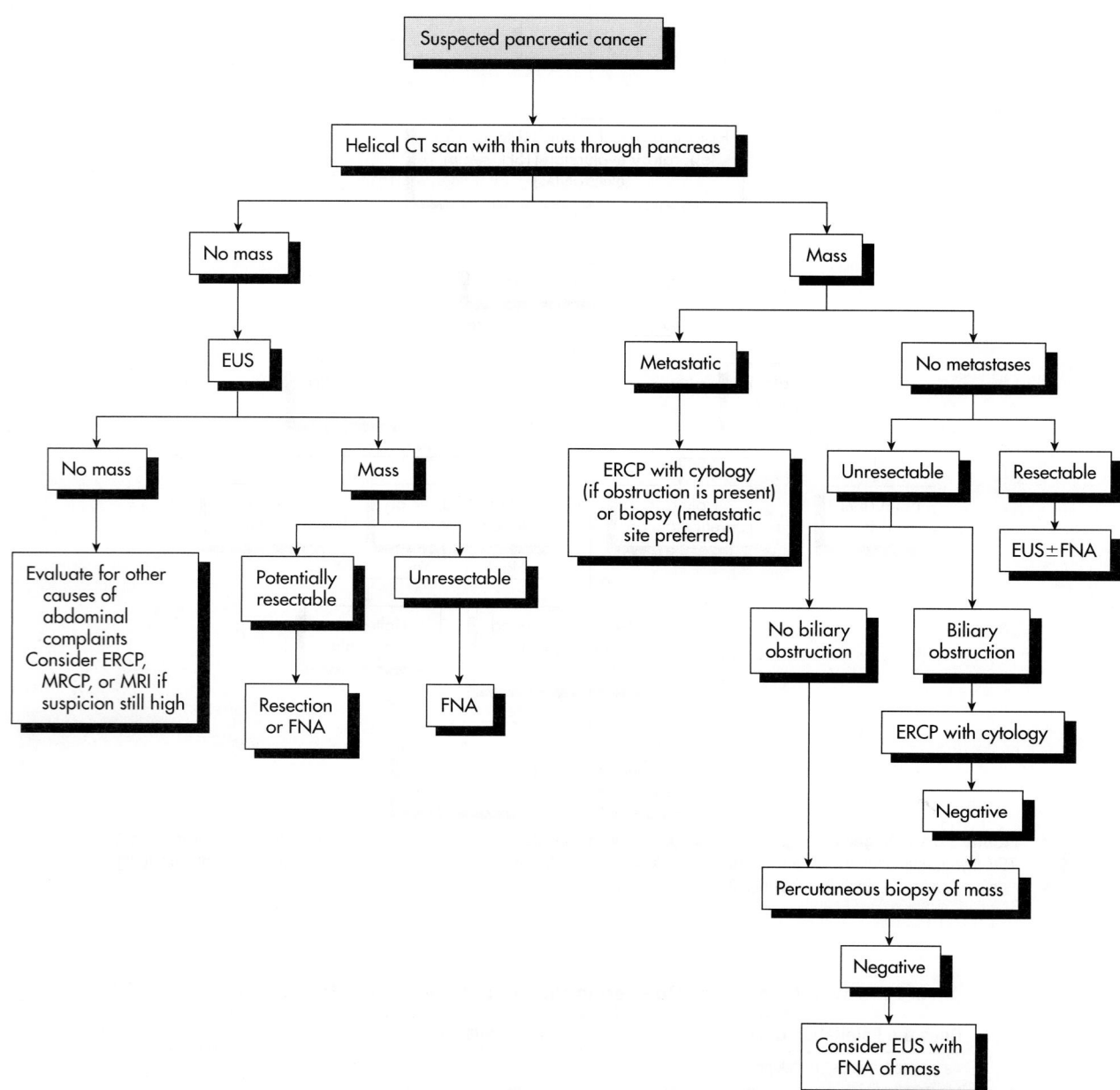

FIGURE 3-245 Diagnostic algorithm for pancreatic cancer. Intraoperative fine-needle aspiration (FNA) if found inoperable during surgery. *CT,* Computed tomography; *ERCP,* endoscopic retrograde cholangiopancreatography; *EUS,* endoscopic ultrasonography; *MRI,* magnetic resonance imaging. (From Goldman L, Ausiello D [eds]: *Cecil textbook of medicine,* ed 23, Philadelphia, 2008, WB Saunders.)

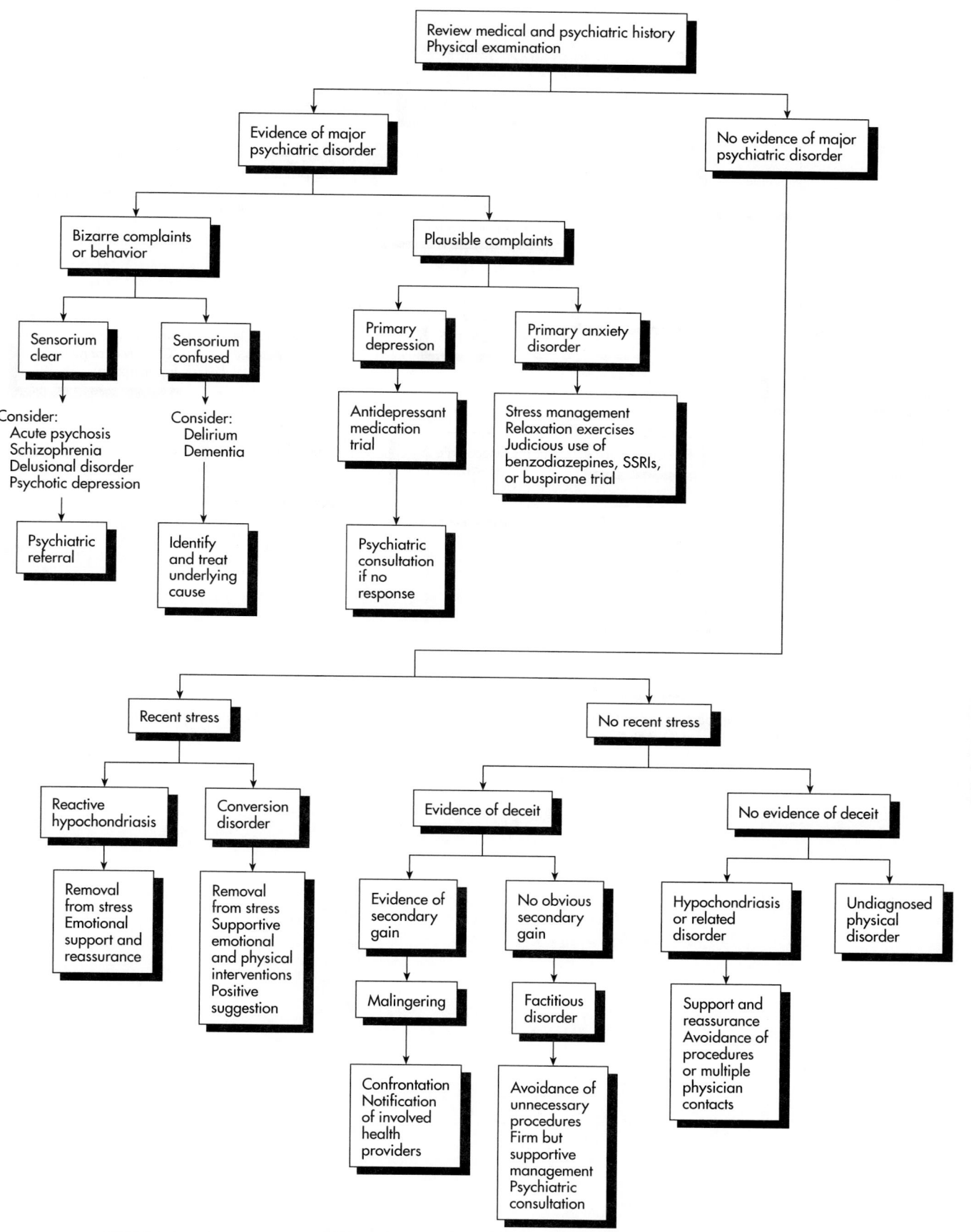

FIGURE 3-250 Patient with ill-defined physical complaints. Previous or recent evaluations are noncontributory. *SSRIs,* Selective serotonin reuptake inhibitors. (From Greene H, Johnson WP, Lemcke D [eds]: *Decision making in medicine,* ed 2, St Louis, 1998, Mosby.)

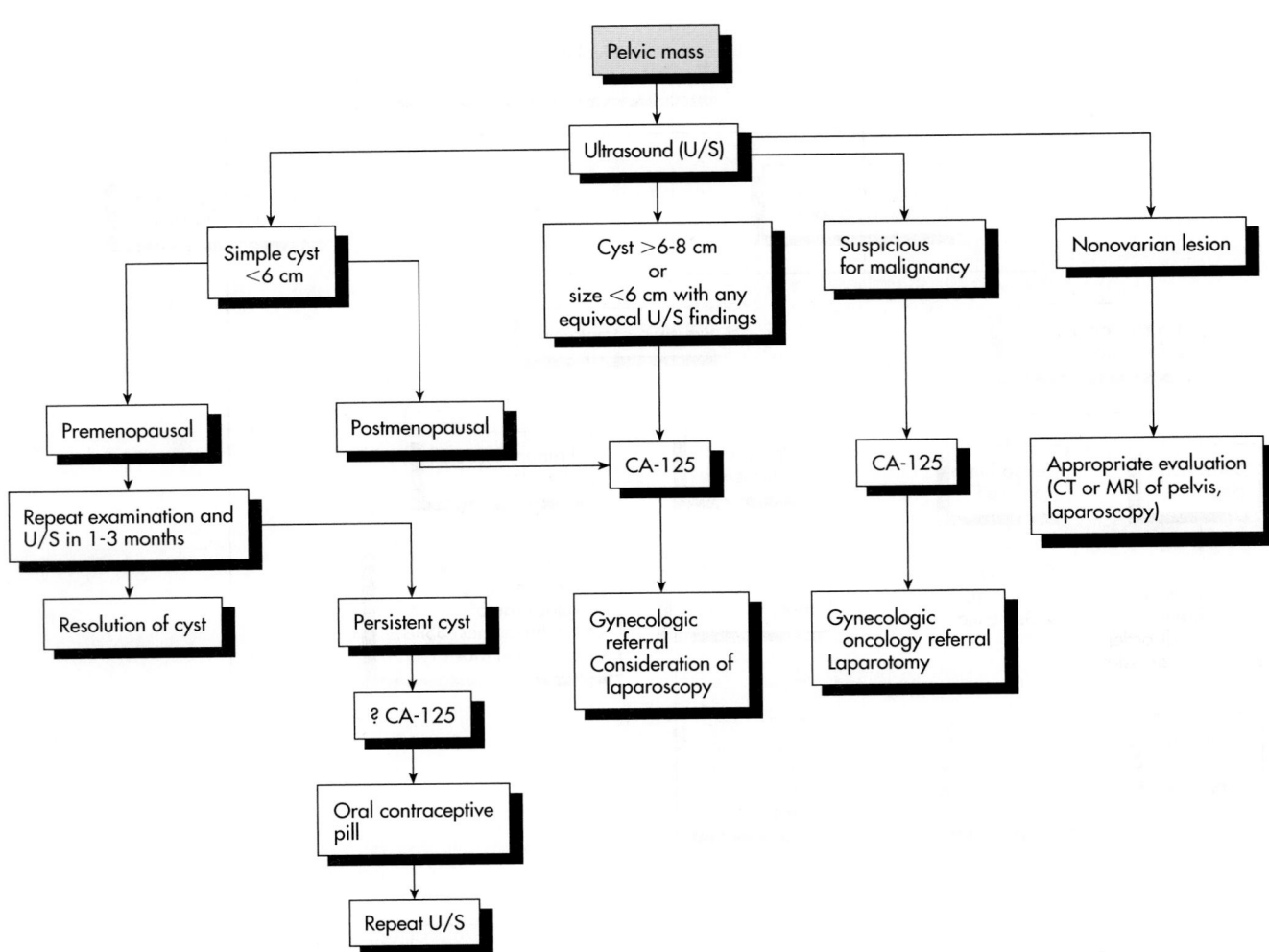

FIGURE 3-251 Approach to the patient with a pelvic mass. *CT,* Computed tomography; *MRI,* magnetic resonance imaging. (Modified from Carlson KJ et al: *Primary care of women,* ed 2, St Louis, 2002, Mosby.)

PERIPHERAL NEUROPATHY

ICD-9CM # 356.9 Peripheral nerve neuropathy
355.10 Lower extremity neuropathy
354.11 Upper extremity neuropathy

1303

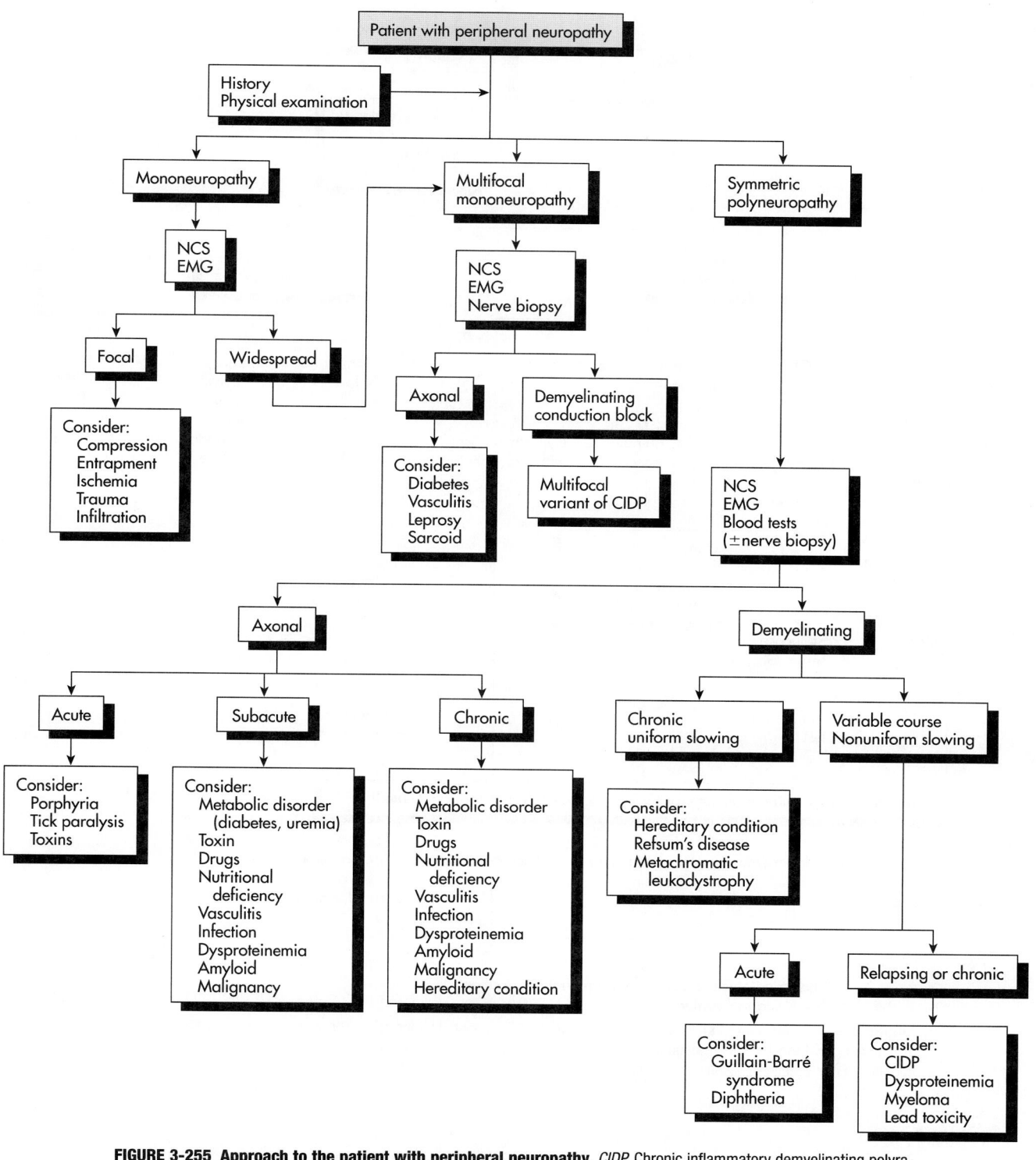

FIGURE 3-255 Approach to the patient with peripheral neuropathy. *CIDP*, Chronic inflammatory demyelinating polyra-dioneuropathy; *EMG*, electromyogram; *NCS*, nerve conduction studies. (From Greene HL, Johnson WP, Lemcke DL: *Decision making in medicine*, ed 2, St Louis, 1988, Mosby.)

ICD-9CM # 253 Pituitary adenoma
253.0 Acromegaly
253.1 Prolactinoma

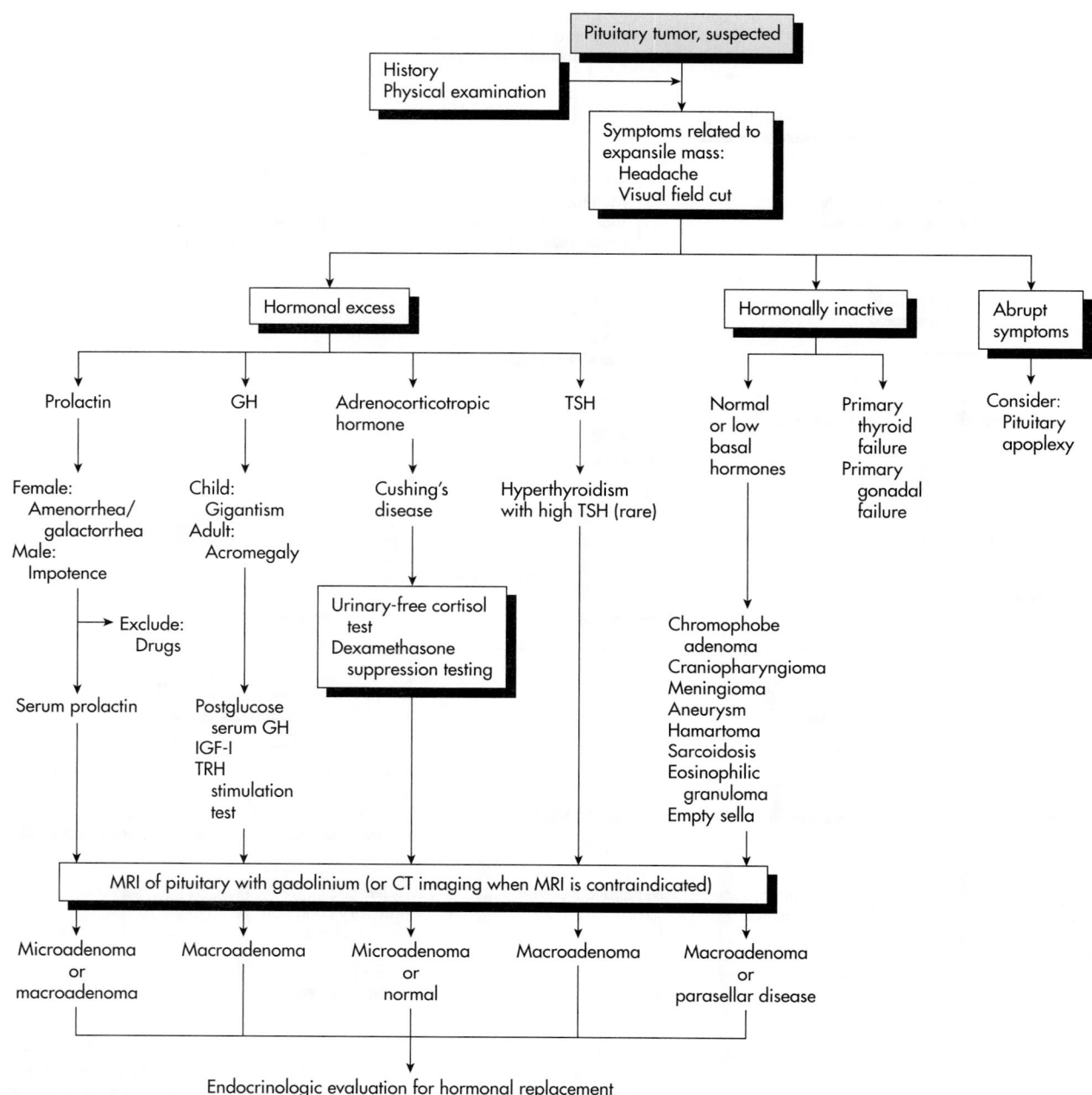

FIGURE 3-258 Evaluation of suspected pituitary tumor. *CT,* Computed tomography; *GH,* growth hormone; *IGF-I,* one of the insulin-like growth factors; *MRI,* magnetic resonance imaging; *TRH,* thyrotropin-releasing hormone; *TSH,* thyroid-stimulating hormone. (From Greene HL, Johnson WP, Lemcke DL: *Decision making in medicine,* ed 2, St Louis, 1998, Mosby.)

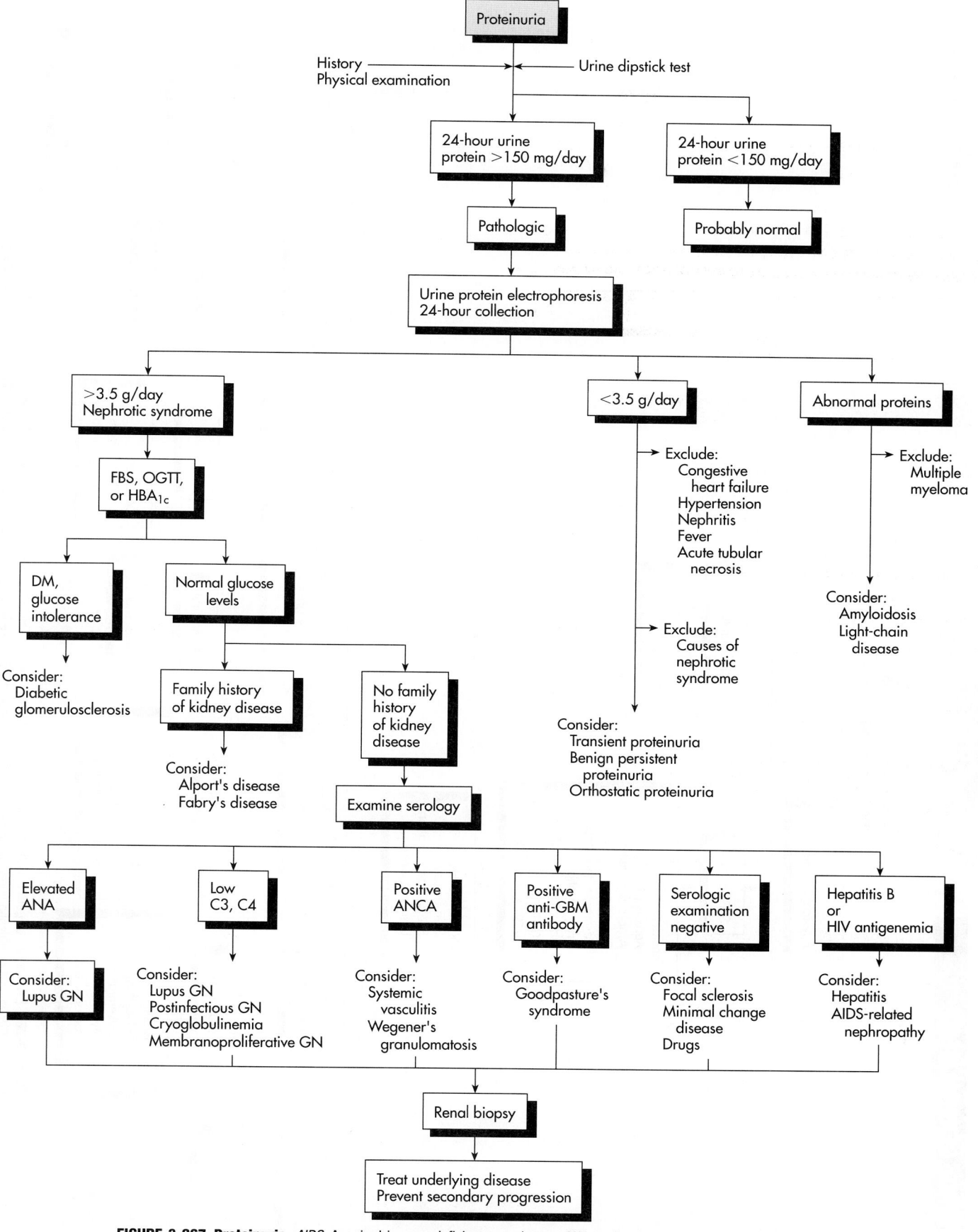

FIGURE 3-267 Proteinuria. *AIDS,* Acquired immunodeficiency syndrome; *ANA,* antinuclear antibody; *ANCA,* antineutrophil cytoplasmic autoantibody; *anti-GBM,* anti–glomerular basement membrane; *FBS,* fasting blood sugar; *GN,* glomerulonephritis; *OGTT,* oral glucose tolerance test. (Modified from Greene HL, Johnson WP, Lemcke DL [eds]: *Decision making in medicine,* ed 2, St Louis, 1998, Mosby.)

PRURITUS, GENERALIZED

ICD-9CM # 698.9 Pruritus NOS

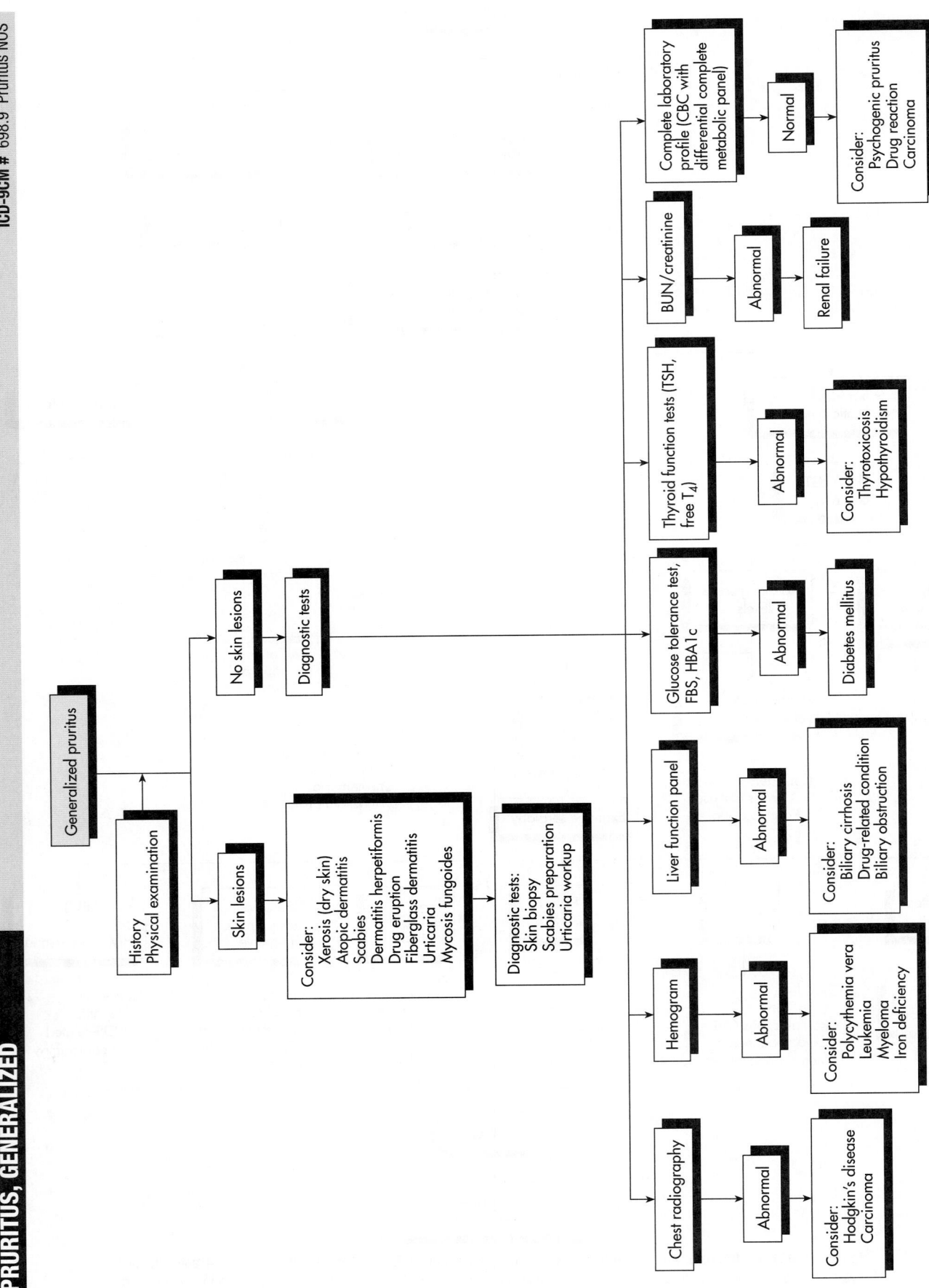

FIGURE 3-268 Evaluation of generalized pruritus. *BUN,* Blood urea nitrogen; *CBC,* complete blood count; *FBS,* fasting blood sugar; *HBA1c,* hemoglobin A1c; *T₄,* thyroxine; *TSH,* thyroid-stimulating hormone. (From Greene HL, Johnson WP, Lemcke DL [eds]: *Decision making in medicine,* ed 2, St Louis, 1998, Mosby.)

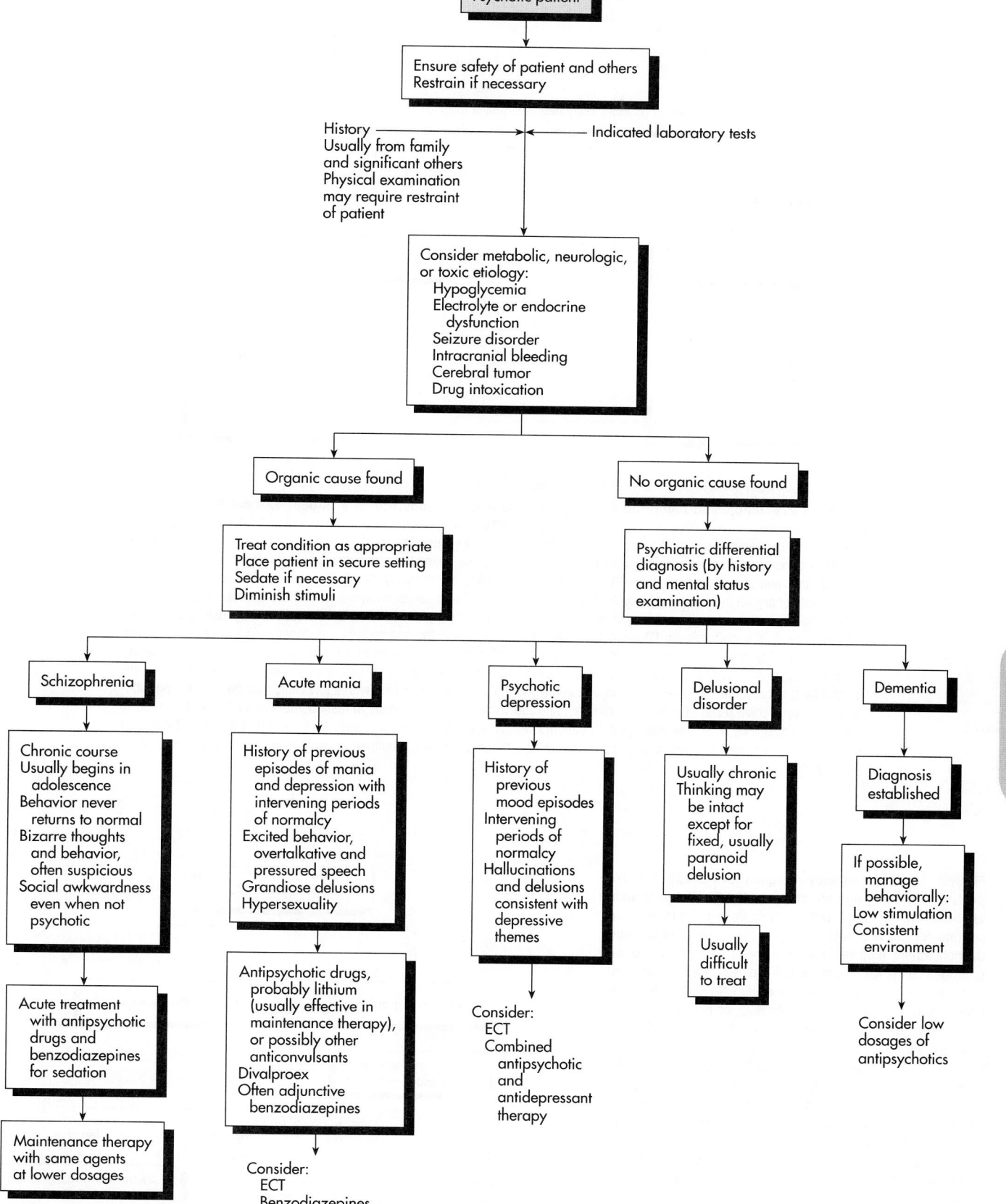

FIGURE 3-273 Evaluation of psychotic patient. *ECT,* Electroconvulsive therapy. (Modified from Greene HL, Johnson WP, Lemcke DL [eds]: *Decision making in medicine,* ed 2, St Louis, 1998, Mosby.)

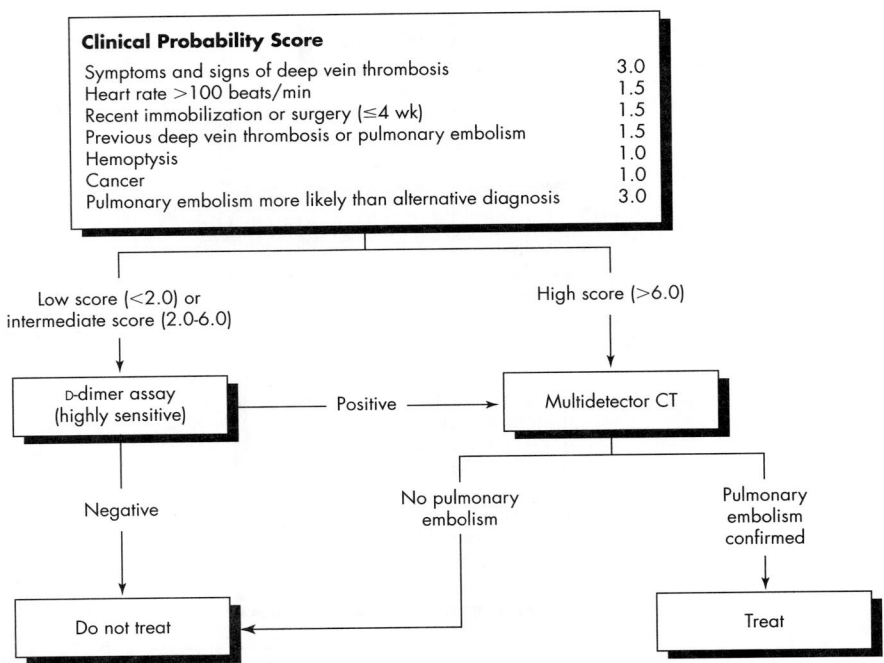

Note: Refer to Section I for additional information on this topic.

FIGURE 3-276 Diagnostic algorithm for suspected pulmonary embolism in a patient without hypotension or shock. This assessment of clinical probability is based on the Wells score (which has a range of 0 to 12.5, with higher scores indicating higher clinical probability). The revised Geneva score may be used as an alternative. If a moderately sensitive latex-derived D-dimer assay is used instead of the highly sensitive enzyme-linked immunosorbent D-dimer assay, pulmonary embolism can be ruled out only in patients with a low clinical probability. Alternatively, the Wells score can be dichotomized, classifying pulmonary embolism as unlikely (≤4.0) or likely (>4.0). For patients in whom pulmonary embolism is considered unlikely, either a highly sensitive or a moderately sensitive D-dimer assay can be used to rule out the diagnosis without need for further testing. If multidetector CT pulmonary angiography, with or without venography, is negative in a patient with a high clinical probability, the possibility of a false negative result should be considered and further testing performed to rule out pulmonary embolism. Options include serial venous ultrasonography, ventilation-perfusion lung scanning, and pulmonary angiography. If a multidetector CT scan shows only subsegmental defects in a patient with a low clinical probability, the possibility of a false positive result should be considered, and further testing (e.g., venous ultrasonography) should be performed to confirm the diagnosis. This may also apply to patients with an intermediate clinical probability, although the need for further tests is less well established for these patients. (From Konstantinides S: Acute pulmonary embolism, *N Engl J Med* 359:2804, 2806, 2008.)

FIGURE 3-277 Emergency diagnostic workup for suspected pulmonary embolism in a patient with hypotension or shock. A direct sign of pulmonary embolism on a transthoracic or transesophageal echocardiogram is the presence of thrombi in the right atrium, right ventricle, or pulmonary artery. Thrombi may protrude into the left atrium through a patent foramen ovale. Indirect signs include right ventricular dysfunction (identified by the finding of dilation, free-wall hypokinesia, or paradoxical septal-wall motion); a systolic pressure gradient between the right ventricle and the right atrium of more than 30 mm Hg; and a pulmonary arterial flow acceleration time of less than 80 msec. When direct or indirect signs of pulmonary embolism are present, immediate treatment (without further diagnostic tests) is justified, particularly if CT angiography is still not available and arterial hypotension or shock persists. Adapted from the 2008 Guidelines on the Diagnosis and Management of Acute Pulmonary Embolism of the European Society of Cardiology. Since validation of diagnostic algorithms in prospective trials excluded hemodynamically unstable patients, these recommendations reflect expert opinion. (From Konstantinides S: Acute pulmonary embolism, *N Engl J Med* 359:2804, 2807, 2008.)

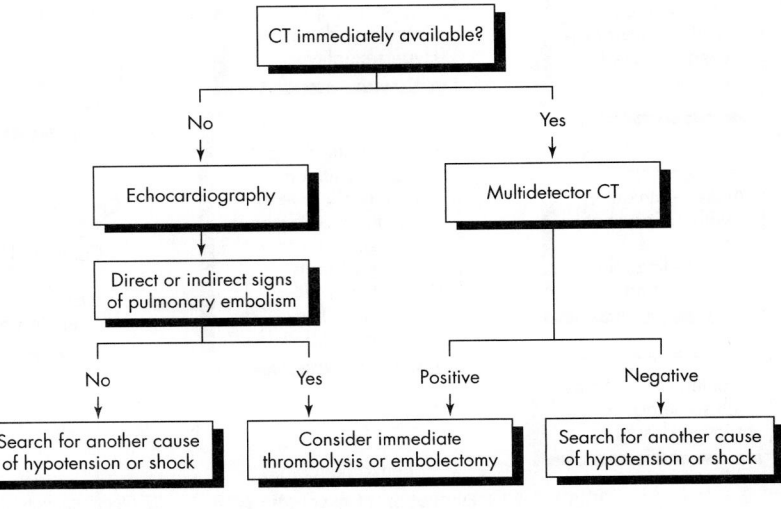

TABLE 3-29 Anticoagulant Drugs for Initial Treatment of Pulmonary Embolism*

Drug	Dose	Remarks
Unfractionated heparin (intravenous infusion)[†]	80 IU/kg of body weight as an intravenous bolus, followed by continuous infusion at the rate of 18 IU/kg/hr	Adjust infusion rate to maintain aPTT between 1.5 and 2.5 times control, corresponding to therapeutic heparin levels (0.3 to 0.7 IU/ml by factor Xa inhibition)[††]; monitor platelet count at baseline and every other day from day 4 to day 14 or until heparin is stopped; investigate for heparin-induced thrombocytopenia if platelet count falls by ≥50% or a thrombotic event occurs.
Low-molecular-weight heparins (subcutaneous injection)[§]		Low-molecular-weight heparins have not been tested in patients with arterial hypotension or shock and thus are not recommended for such patients; monitoring of anti–factor Xa levels may be helpful in patients at increased risk for bleeding, particularly those with moderate or severe renal impairment; the need for monitoring anti–factor Xa levels in pregnant women remains controversial; monitor platelet count at baseline and every 2 to 4 days from day 4 to day 14 or until heparin is stopped.[¶]
Enoxaparin	1.0 mg/kg every 12 hr or 1.5 mg/kg once daily[‖]	If creatinine clearance is <30 ml/min, reduce enoxaparin dose to 1 mg/kg once daily; consider unfractionated heparin infusion as an alternative.
Tinzaparin	175 U/kg once daily	
Fondaparinux[§]	5 mg (body weight, <50 kg); 7.5 mg (body weight, 50-100 kg); or 10 mg (body weight, >100 kg), administered once daily	This drug is contraindicated in patients with severe renal impairment (creatinine clearance, <30 ml/min); no routine platelet monitoring is necessary.

(From Konstantinides S: Acute pulmonary embolism, *N Engl J Med* 359:2804, 2808, 2008.)
*The abbreviation aPTT denotes activated partial thromboplastin time.
[†]Unfractionated heparin is the preferred treatment in patients with severe renal dysfunction (creatinine clearance, <30 ml per minute), since it is not eliminated by the kidneys, and in patients with an increased risk of bleeding (i.e., those with congenital or acquired bleeding diathesis, active ulcerative or angiodysplastic gastrointestinal disease, recent hemorrhagic stroke, recent brain, spinal, or ophthalmologic surgery diabetic retinopathy, or bacterial endocarditis), owing to its short half-life and reversible anticoagulant effects.
[††]It is recommended that the treatment dose be adjusted on the basis of standardized nomograms such as that proposed by Raschke et al.
[§]Tinzaparin and fondaparinux are explicitly approved for the treatment of acute pulmonary embolism. Enoxaparin is approved for the treatment of deep vein thrombosis with or without pulmonary embolism.
[¶]This recommendation applies to postoperative patients and to medical or obstetrical patients who have received unfractionated heparin within the past 100 days. For medical or obstetrical patients who have received only low-molecular-weight heparin, some authorities recommend no routine monitoring of platelet counts.
[‖]Once-daily injection of enoxaparin at a dose of 1.5 mg per kilogram is approved for inpatient treatment of pulmonary embolism in the United States and in some, but not all, European countries.

TABLE 3-30 Stratification of Risk of Death Associated with Pulmonary Embolism and Severity-Adjusted Treatment*

Early Risk of Death	Risk Factor			Recommended Treatment
	Shock or Hypotension (on Clinical Examination)	Right Ventricular Dysfunction (on Echocardiography or Multidetector CT)	Myocardial Injury (on Cardiac Troponin Testing)	
High	Present	Present[†]	NA[††]	Unfractionated heparin plus thrombolysis or embolectomy
Non-high				
Intermediate[§]	Absent	Present	Present	Low-molecular-weight heparin or fondaparinux; as a rule, no early thrombolysis; monitor clinical status and right ventricular function
	Absent	Present	Absent	
	Absent	Absent	Present	
Low	Absent	Absent	Absent	Low-molecular-weight heparin or fondaparinux; consider outpatient treatment

(From Konstantinides S: Acute pulmonary embolism, *N Engl J Med* 359:2804, 2810, 2008.)
*Adapted with modifications from the 2008 Guidelines on the Diagnosis and Management of Acute Pulmonary Embolism of the European Society of Cardiology. NA denotes not applicable.
[†]If RV function is normal on echocardiography, or if a CT scan shows no RV dilatation in a patient with hemodynamic compromise and clinically suspected pulmonary embolism, an alternative diagnosis should be sought.
[††]Troponin test results do not influence risk assessment or treatment in hemodynamically compromised patients with acute pulmonary embolism.
[§]Although it has been suggested that normotensive patients with both RV dysfunction and myocardial injury have a higher risk of death than those with only one of these risk factors, there is currently no definitive proof that they should receive more aggressive treatment.

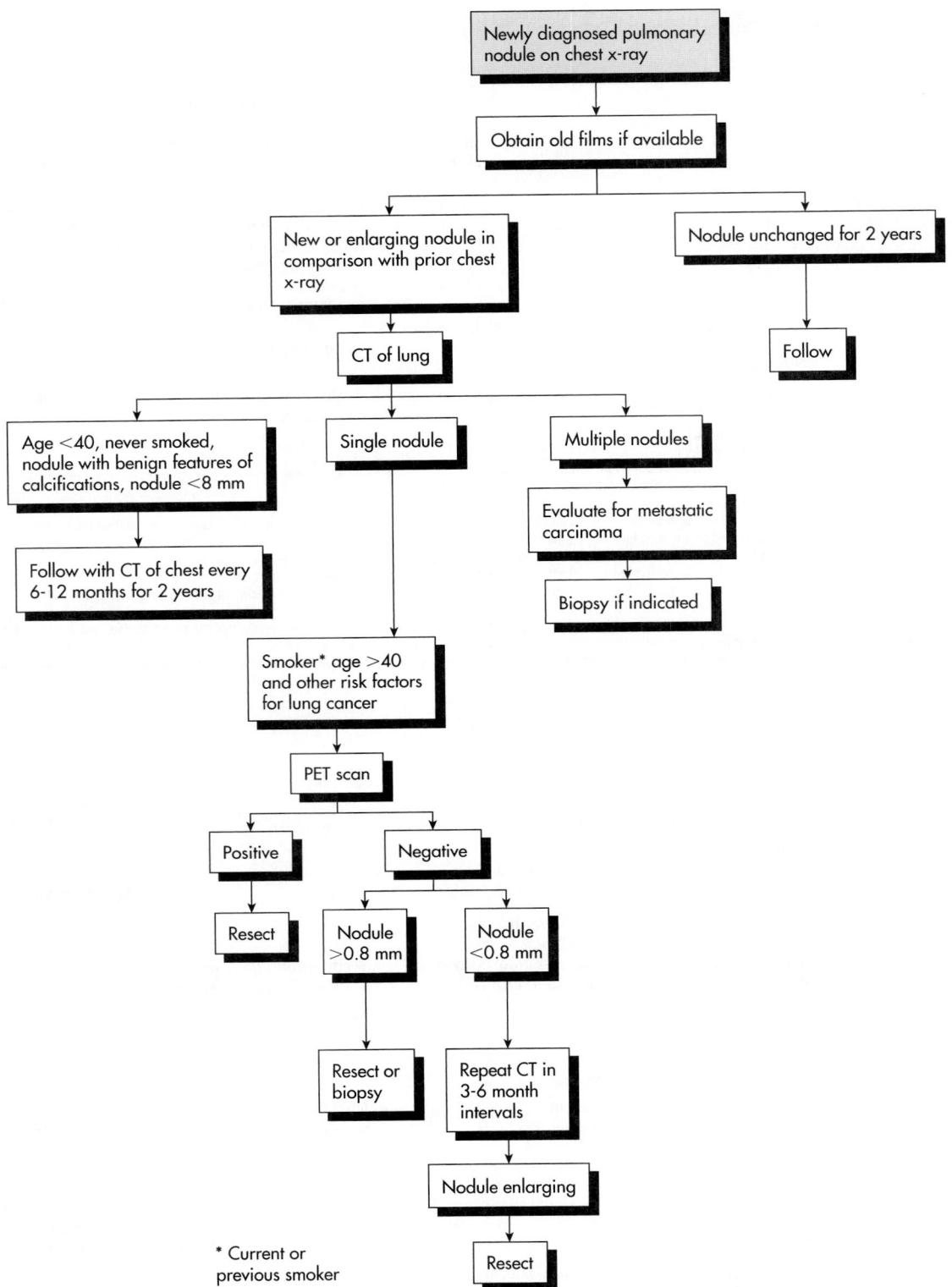

FIGURE 3-278 Pulmonary nodule. *CT*, Computed tomography; *PET*, positron emission tomography.

FIGURE 3-279 Differential diagnosis of purpura. (From Bolognia JL, Jorizzo JL, Rapini RP: *Dermatology,* St Louis, 2003, Mosby.)

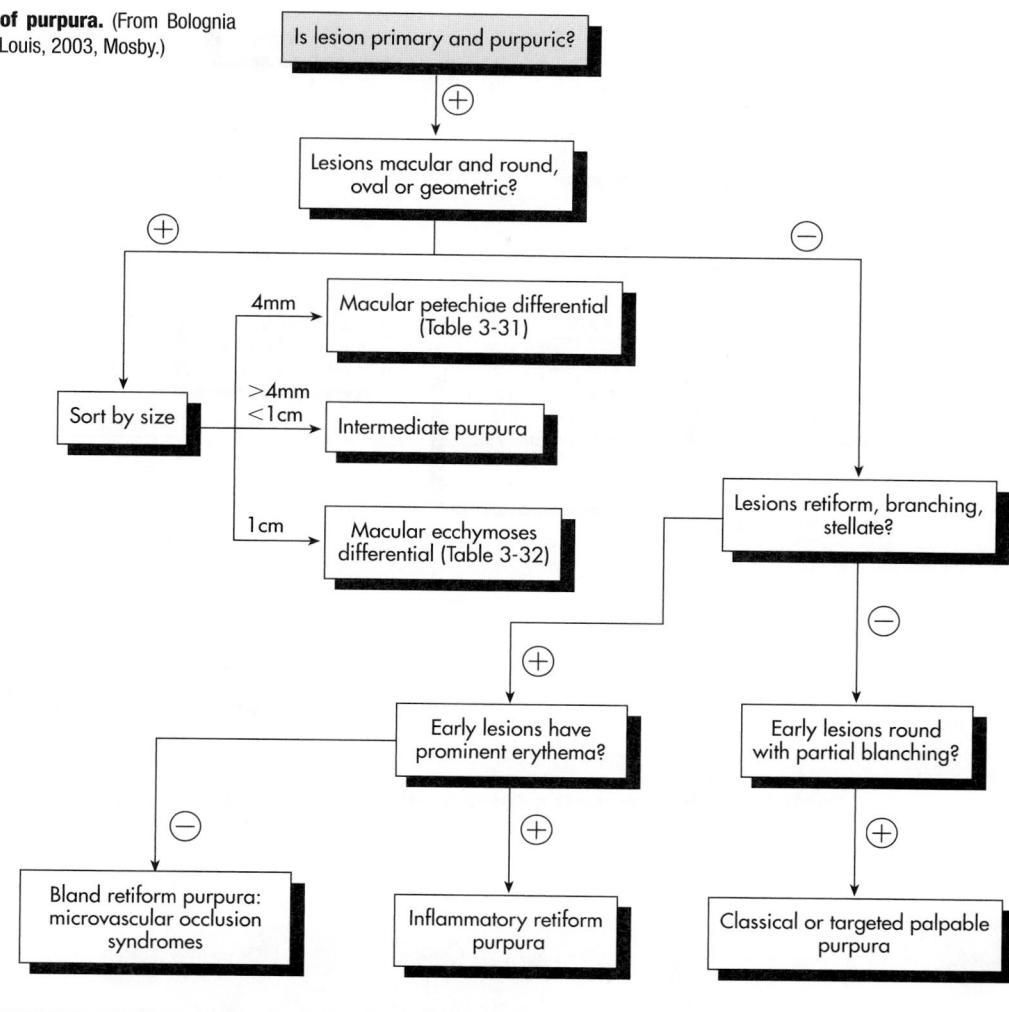

TABLE 3-31 Differential Diagnosis of Petechial Hemorrhage—Non-Palpable, Non-Retiform and ≤4 mm in Diameter

Pathophysiology: hemostatically relevant thrombocytopenia ($<50,000/mm^3$) **

Major etiologies*
1. Idiopathic thrombocytopenic purpura
2. Thrombotic thrombocytopenic purpura
3. Disseminated intravascular coagulation
4. Other acquired thrombocytopenias, including drug-related
   a. Peripheral destruction (e.g., quinine, quinidine)
   b. Decreased production, idiosyncratic or dose-related (e.g., chemotherapy)
   c. Bone marrow infiltration, fibrosis or failure

Pathophysiology: abnormal platelet function

Major etiologies*
1. Congenital or hereditary platelet function defects
2. Acquired platelet function defects
   a. Aspirin, NSAIDs
   b. Renal insufficiency
   c. Monoclonal gammopathy
3. Thrombocytosis in myeloproliferative disease (often $>1,000,000/mm^3$)

Pathophysiology: non-platelet etiologies

Major etiologies*
1. Spiking elevations of intravascular venous pressure (Valsalva maneuver-like, e.g., repetitive vomiting, childbirth, paroxysmal coughing, seizure)
2. Fixed increased pressure (e.g., stasis, ligatures)
3. Trauma (often linear)
4. Perifollicular (vitamin C deficiency)
5. Mildly inflammatory conditions
   a. Chronic pigmented purpura
   b. Hypergammaglobulinemic purpura of Waldenström

TABLE 3-32 Differential Diagnosis for Macular Purpura and Ecchymoses—Non-Palpable and Non-Retiform

Intermediate macular purpura (>4 mm, <1 cm in diameter)

Major etiologies*
1. Hypergammaglobulinemic purpura of Waldenström
2. Infection/inflammation in patients with thrombocytopenia
3. Rarely, minimally inflamed immune complex vasculitis (usually dependent distribution)

Ecchymoses (≥1 cm in diameter)

A. Pathophysiology: procoagulant defect plus minor trauma*
   1. Anticoagulant use
   2. Hepatic insufficiency with poor procoagulant synthesis
   3. Vitamin K deficiency
   4. Disseminated intravascular coagulation (some)
B. Pathophysiology: poor dermal support of vessels plus minor trauma*
   1. Actinic (solar, senile) purpura
   2. Corticosteroid therapy, topical or systemic
   3. Vitamin C deficiency (scurvy)
   4. Systemic amyloidosis (light chain-related, some familial types)
   5. Ehlers-Danlos syndrome (primarily type IV)
C. Pathophysiology: other causes plus minor trauma*
   1. Hypergammaglobulinemic purpura of Waldenström
   2. Platelet function defects, including von Willebrand disease, medications, metabolic diseases
   3. Acquired or congenital thrombocytopenia

*Partial list.
**Most patients do not have petechiae until platelets $≤20,000/mm^3$.

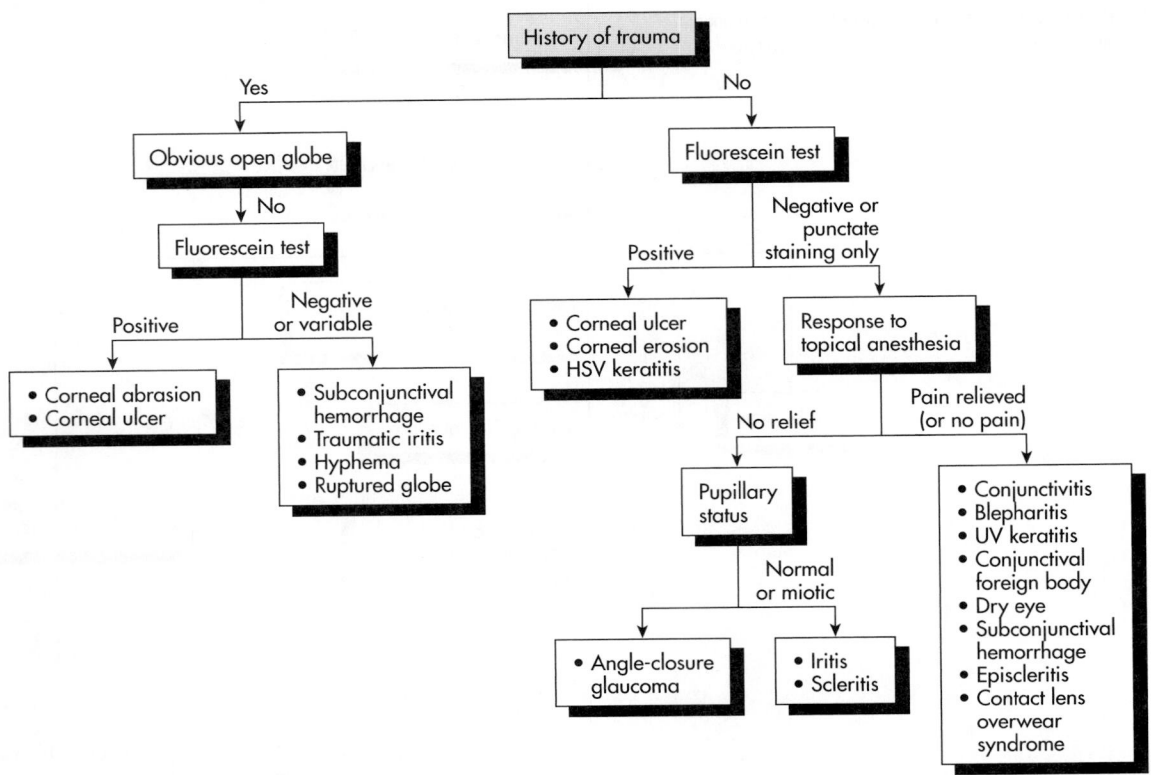

FIGURE 3-281 Algorithm showing diagnostic procedure for the acute red eye. *HSV,* Herpes simplex virus; *UV,* ultra-violet. (From Auerbach PS: *Wilderness medicine,* ed 5, St Louis, 2007, Mosby.)

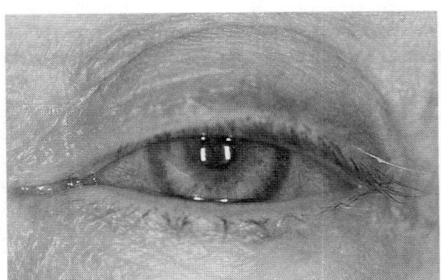

FIGURE 3-282 Contact lens acute red eye. This is often accompanied by pain and photophobia. (From Yanoff M, Duker JS: *Ophthalmology,* ed 2, St Louis, 2004, Mosby.)

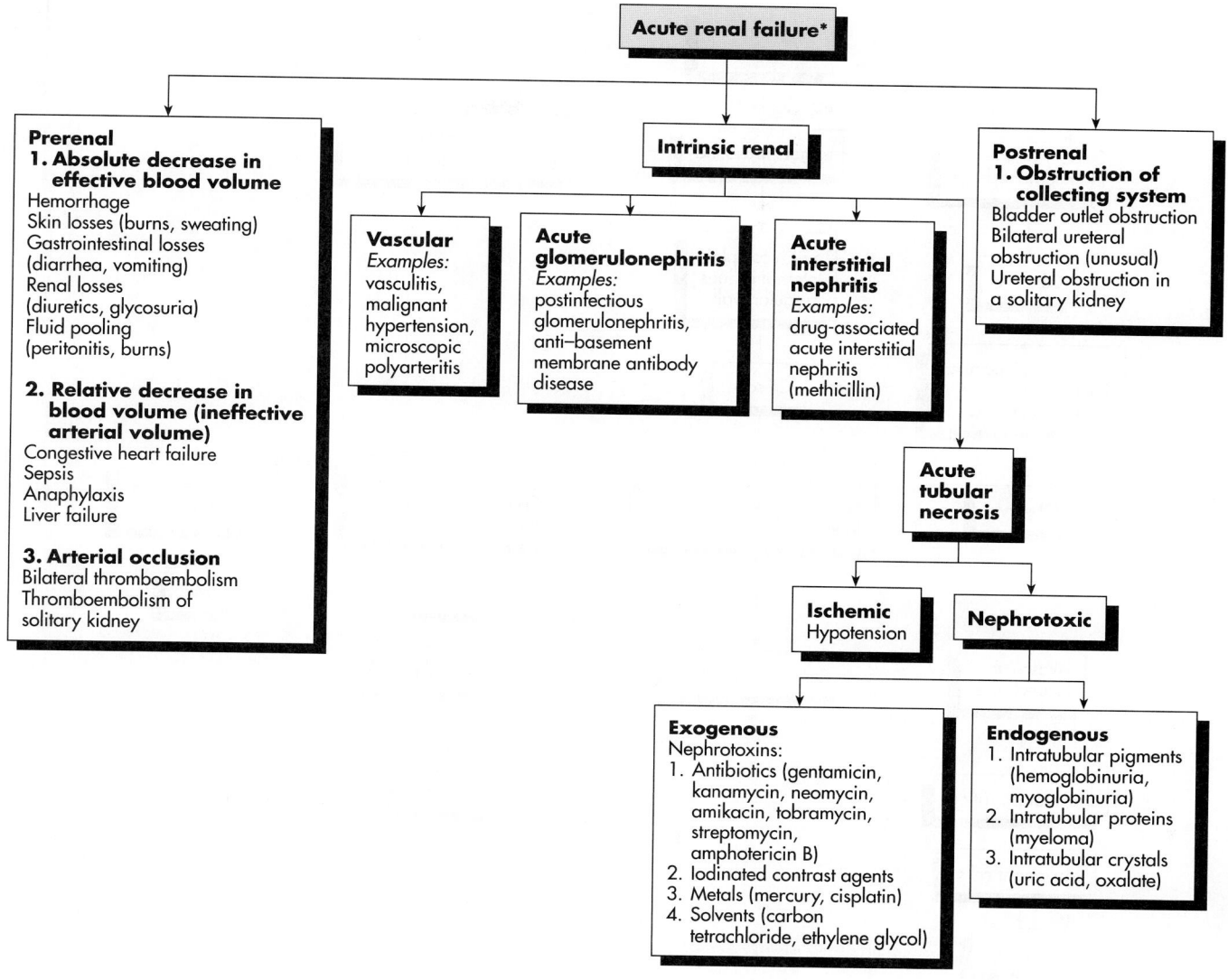

FIGURE 3-286 Causes of acute renal failure. (From Andreoli TE [ed]: *Cecil essentials of medicine*, ed 7, Philadelphia, 2008, WB Saunders.)

*Note: Refer to Section I for additional information on this topic.

Clinical Algorithms

III

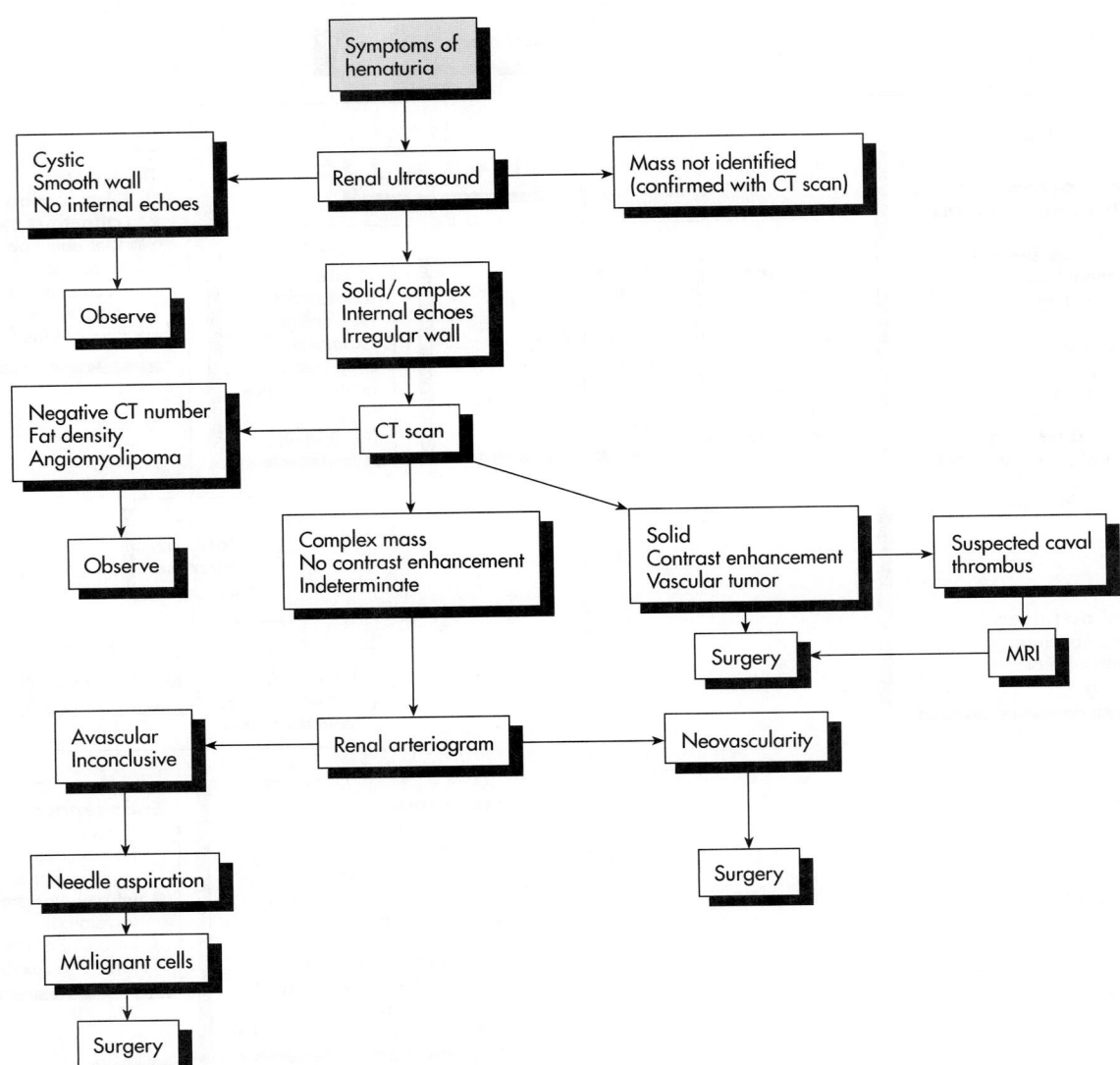

FIGURE 3-287 Evaluation of a patient with a renal mass. *CT,* Computed tomography; *MRI,* magnetic resonance imaging. (Modified from Williams RD: Tumors of the kidney, ureter, and bladder. In Goldman L, Ausiello D [eds]: *Cecil textbook of medicine,* ed 23, Philadelphia, 2008, WB Saunders.)

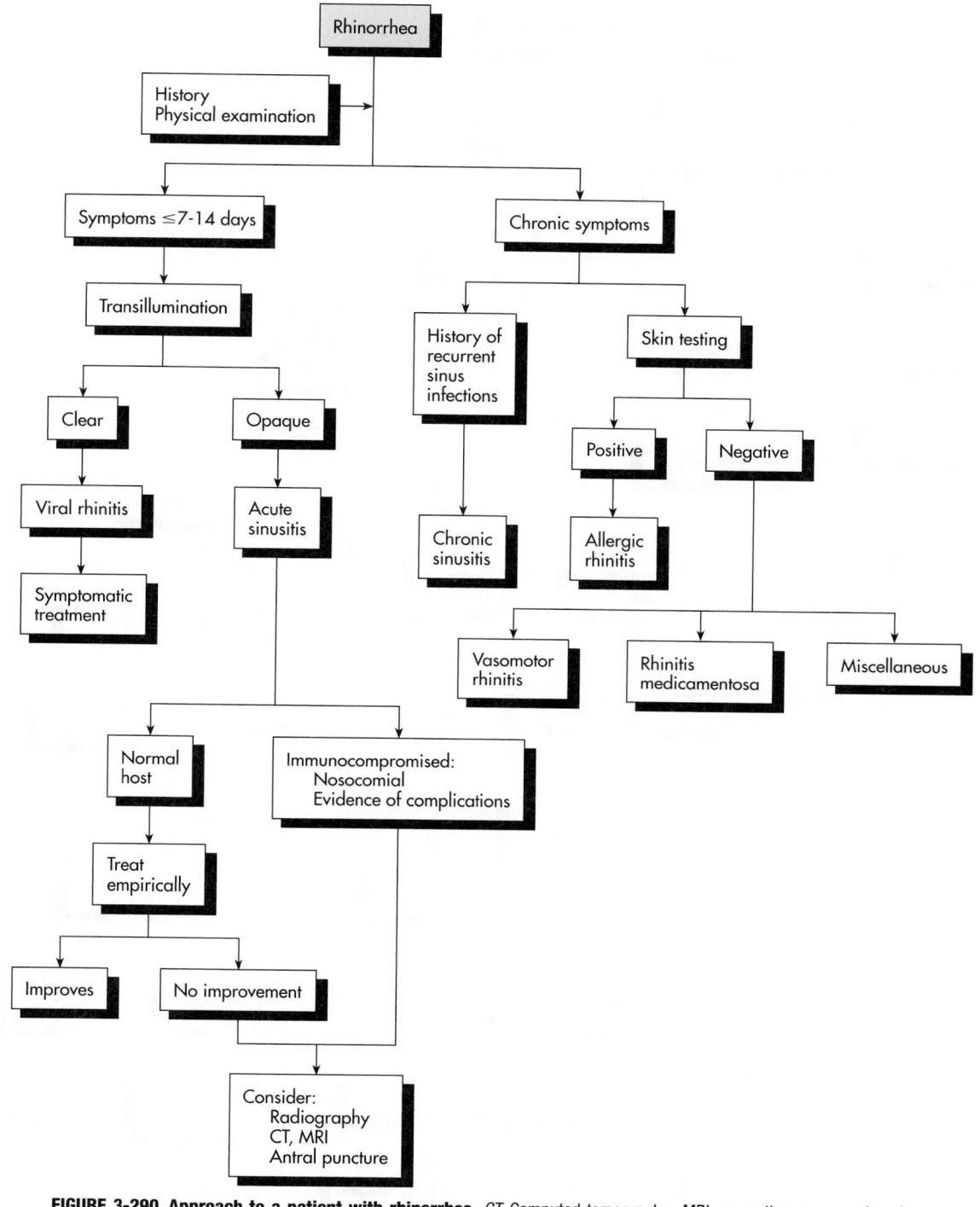

FIGURE 3-290 Approach to a patient with rhinorrhea. *CT,* Computed tomography; *MRI,* magnetic resonance imaging.
(From Noble J [ed]: *Primary care medicine,* ed 3, St Louis, 2001, Mosby.)

Clinical
Algorithms

III

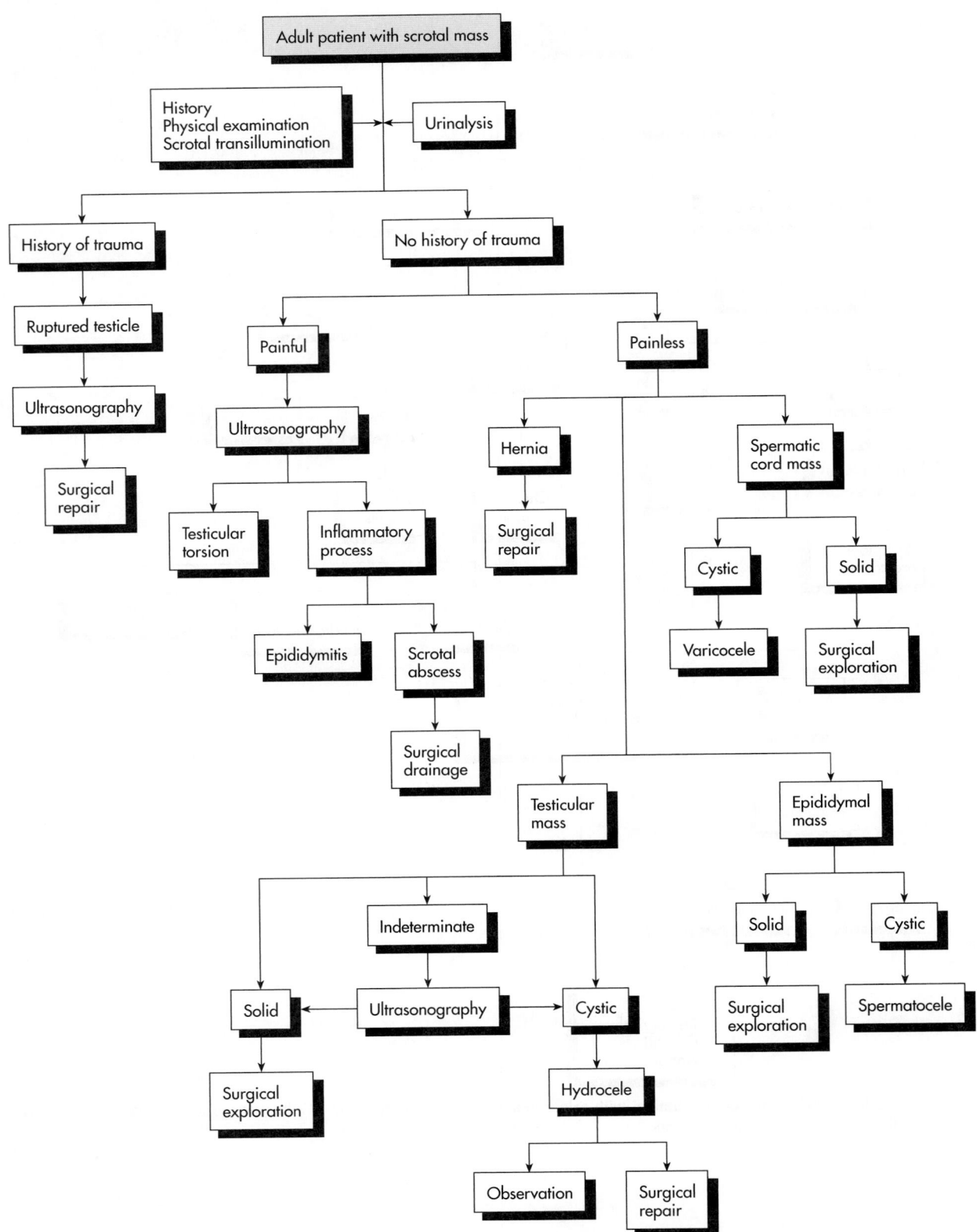

FIGURE 3-293 Evaluation of scrotal mass. (From Greene HL, Johnson WP, Lemcke DL [eds]: *Decision making in medicine,* ed 2, St Louis, 1998, Mosby.)

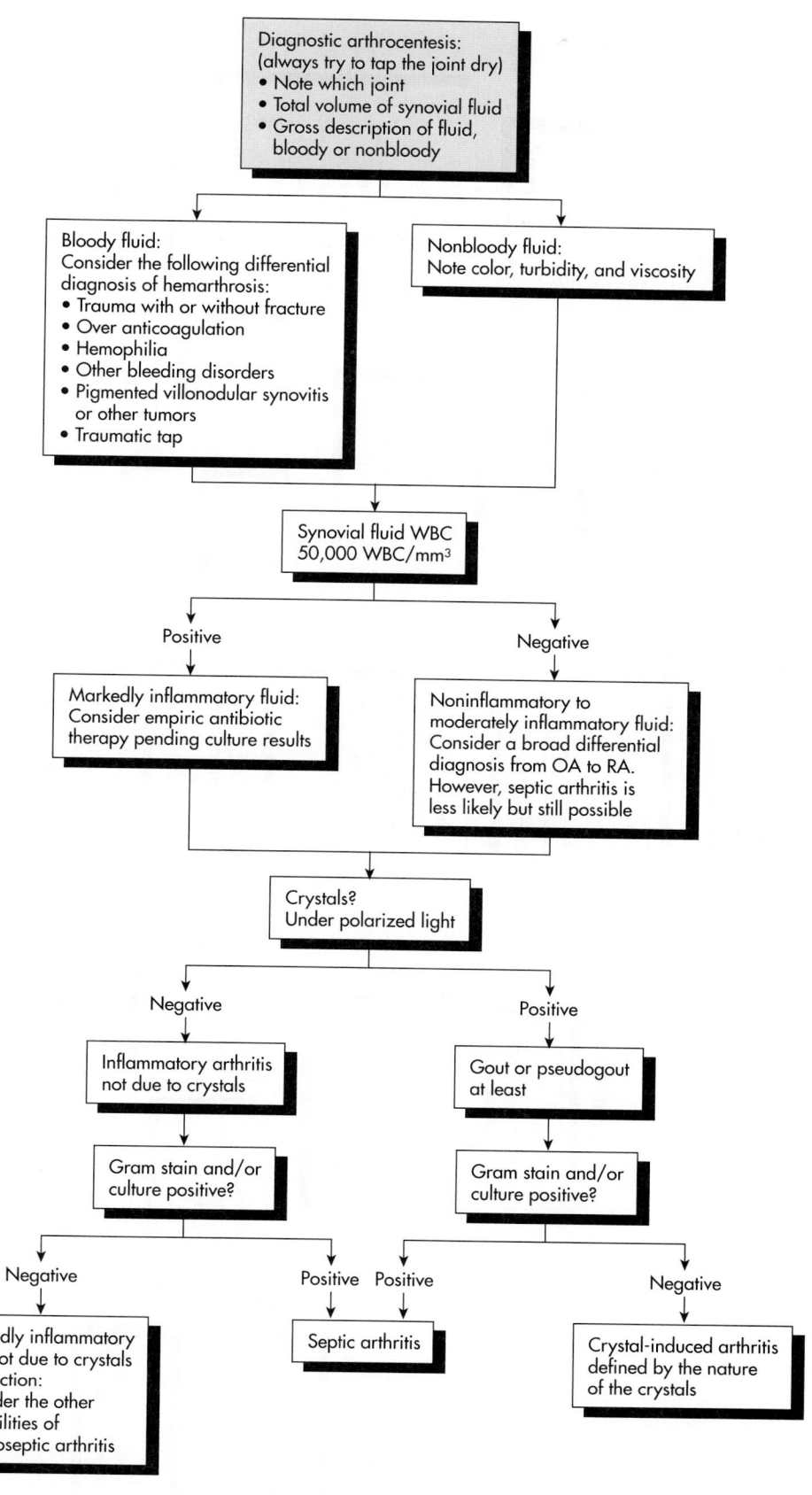

Note: Refer to Section I, Infectious Arthritis, for additional information.

FIGURE 3-295 Algorithm for synovial fluid analysis in septic arthritis. *OA*, Osteoarthritis; *RA*, rheumatoid arthritis; *WBC*, white blood cell count. (From Harris ED et al [eds]: *Kelley's textbook of rheumatology*, ed 7, Philadelphia, 2005, Saunders.)

ICD-9CM # 309.2 Sexual disorder (psychosexual)
V41.7 Sexual function problem

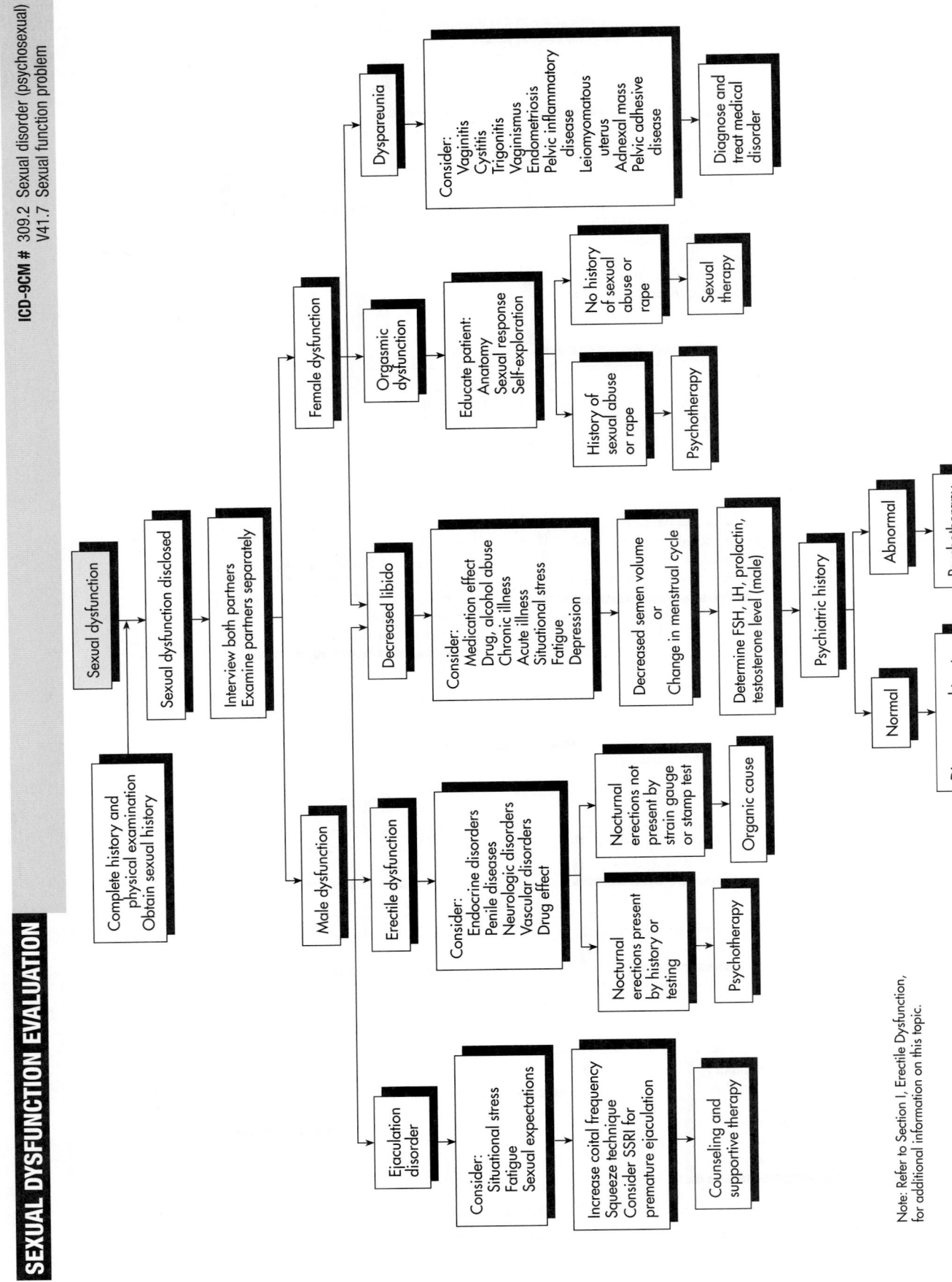

FIGURE 3-296 Evaluation of sexual dysfunction. *FSH*, Follicle-stimulating hormone; *LH*, luteinizing hormone; *SSRI*, selective serotonin reuptake inhibitor. (Modified from Greene HL, Johnson WP, Lemcke DL [eds]: *Decision making in medicine*, ed 2, St Louis, 1998, Mosby.)

Note: Refer to Section I, Erectile Dysfunction, for additional information on this topic.

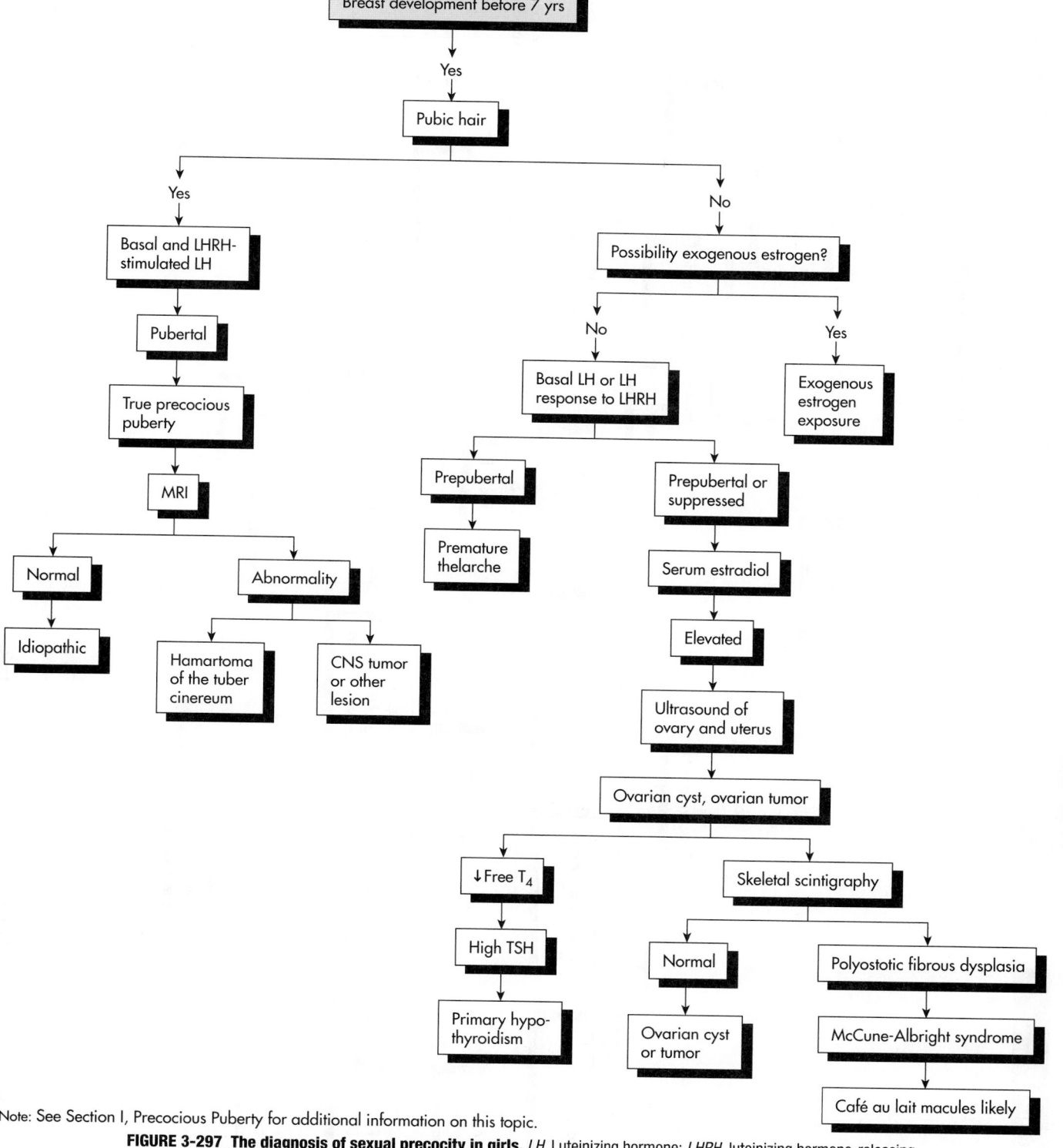

FIGURE 3-297 The diagnosis of sexual precocity in girls. *LH,* Luteinizing hormone; *LHRH,* luteinizing hormone-releasing hormone; *MRI,* magnetic resonance imaging; *T₄,* thyroxine; *TSH,* thyroid-stimulating hormone; *yrs,* years. (From Larsen PR, Kronenberg HM, Memlmed S, Polansky, KS [eds]: *Williams textbook of endocrinology,* ed 11, Philadelphia, 2008, Saunders.)

Note: See Section I, Precocious Puberty for additional information on this topic.

ICD-9CM # 259.1

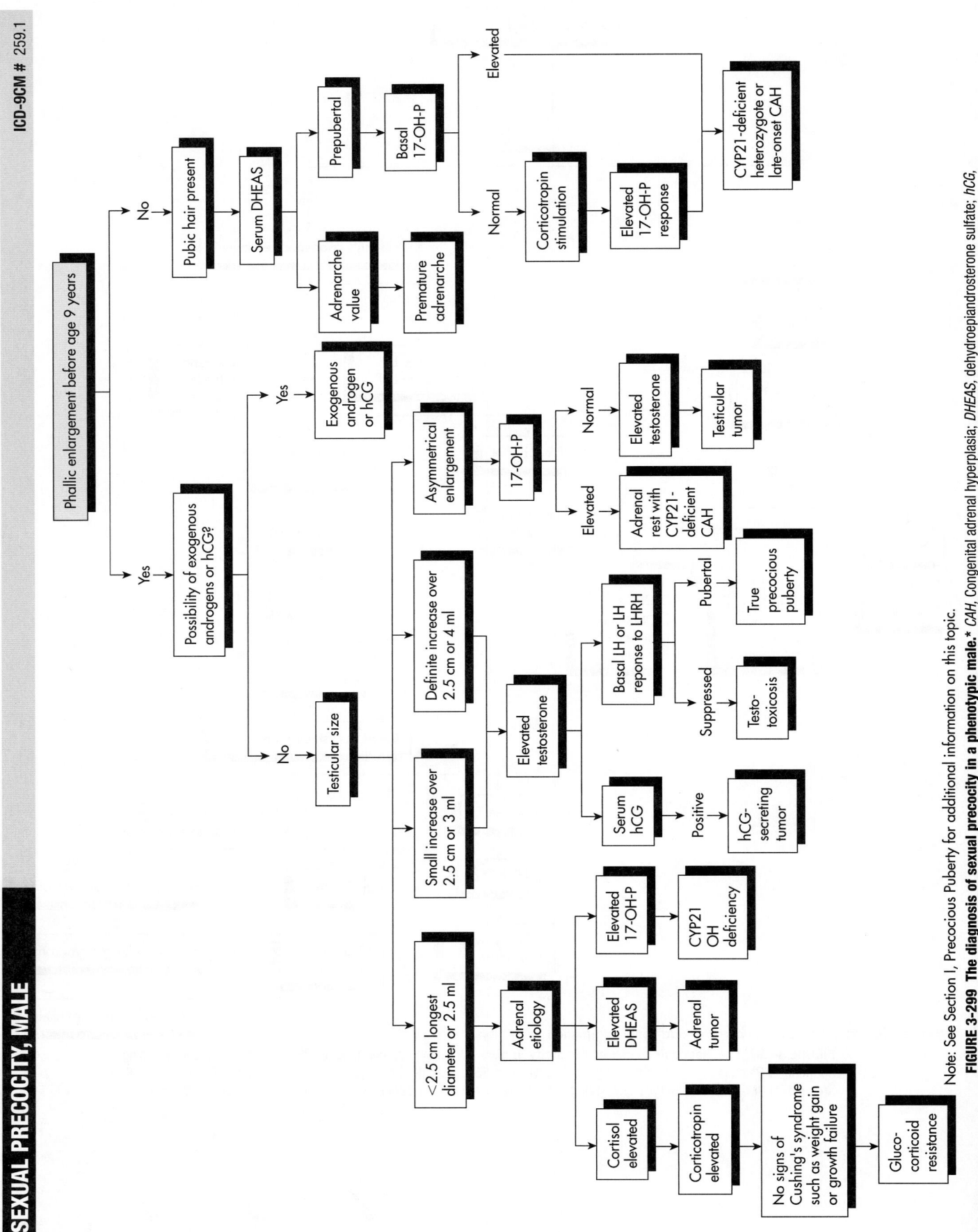

Note: See Section I, Precocious Puberty for additional information on this topic.

FIGURE 3-299 The diagnosis of sexual precocity in a phenotypic male.* *CAH,* Congenital adrenal hyperplasia; *DHEAS,* dehydroepiandrosterone sulfate; *hCG,*

SEXUAL PRECOCITY, MALE—cont'd

ICD-9CM # 259.1

TABLE 3-34 Differential Diagnosis of Sexual Precocity

	Plasma Gonadotropins	LH Response to LHRH	Serum Sex Steroid Concentration	Gonadal Size	Miscellaneous
True Precocious Puberty (premature reactivation of LHRH pulse generator)	Prominent LH pulses, initially during sleep	Pubertal LH response	Pubertal values of testosterone or estradiol	Normal pubertal testicular enlargement or ovarian and uterine enlargement (by ultrasonography)	MRI of brain to rule out CNS tumor or other abnormality; skeletal survey for McCune-Albright syndrome
Incomplete Sexual Precocity (pituitary gonadotropin-independent)					
Males					
Chorionic gonadotropin-secreting tumor in males	High hCG, low LH	Prepubertal LH response	Pubertal value of testosterone	Slight to moderate uniform enlargement of testes	Hepatomegaly suggests hepatoblastoma; CT scan of brain if chorionic gonadotropin-secreting CNS tumor suspected
Leydig cell tumor in males	Suppressed	No LH response	Very high testosterone	Irregular asymmetrical enlargement of testes	
Familial testotoxicosis	Suppressed	No LH response	Pubertal values of testosterone	Testes symmetrical and larger than 2.5 cm but smaller than expected for pubertal development; spermatogenesis occurs	Familial; probably sex-limited, autosomal dominant trait
Virilizing congenital adrenal hyperplasia	Prepubertal	Prepubertal LH response	Elevated 17-OHP in CYP21 deficiency or elevated 11-deoxycortisol in CYP11B1 deficiency	Testes prepubertal	Autosomal recessive, may be congenital or late-onset form, may have salt loss in CYP21 deficiency or hypertension in CYP11B1 deficiency
Virilizing adrenal tumor	Prepubertal	Prepubertal LH response	High DHEAS and androstenedione values	Testes prepubertal	CT, MRI, or ultrasonography of abdomen
Premature adrenarche	Prepubertal	Prepubertal LH response	Prepubertal testosterone, DHEAS, or urinary 17-ketosteroid values appropriate for pubic hair stage 2	Testes prepubertal	Onset usually after 6 years of age; more frequent in CNS-injured children
In Both Sexes					
McCune-Albright syndrome	Suppressed	Suppressed	Sex steroids pubertal or higher	Ovarian (on ultrasound); slight testicular enlargement	Skeletal survey for polyostotic fibrous dysplasia and skin examination for café au lait spots
Primary hypothyroidism	LH prepubertal; FSH may be slightly elevated	Prepubertal FSH may be increased	Estradiol may be pubertal	Testicular enlargement; ovaries cystic	TSH and prolactin elevated; T_4 low

From Larson PR, Kronenberg HM, Memlmed S, Polansky, KS [eds]: *Williams textbook of endocrinology*, ed 11, Philadelphia, 2008, Saunders.

CNS, Central nervous system; *CT*, computed tomography; *DHEAS*, dehydroepiandrosterone sulfate; *hCG*, human chorionic gonadotropin; *LH*, luteinizing hormone; *MRI*, magnetic resonance imaging; *17-OHP*, 17-hydroxy progesterone; T_4, thyroxine; *TSH*, thyrotropin.

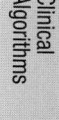
Clinical Algorithms

III

ICD-9CM # 785.50 Shock NOS
995.0 Shock anaphylactic
785.51 Shock cardiogenic
785.59 Shock septic
958.4 Shock traumatic
977.9 Shock due to drug, medicine incorrectly administered

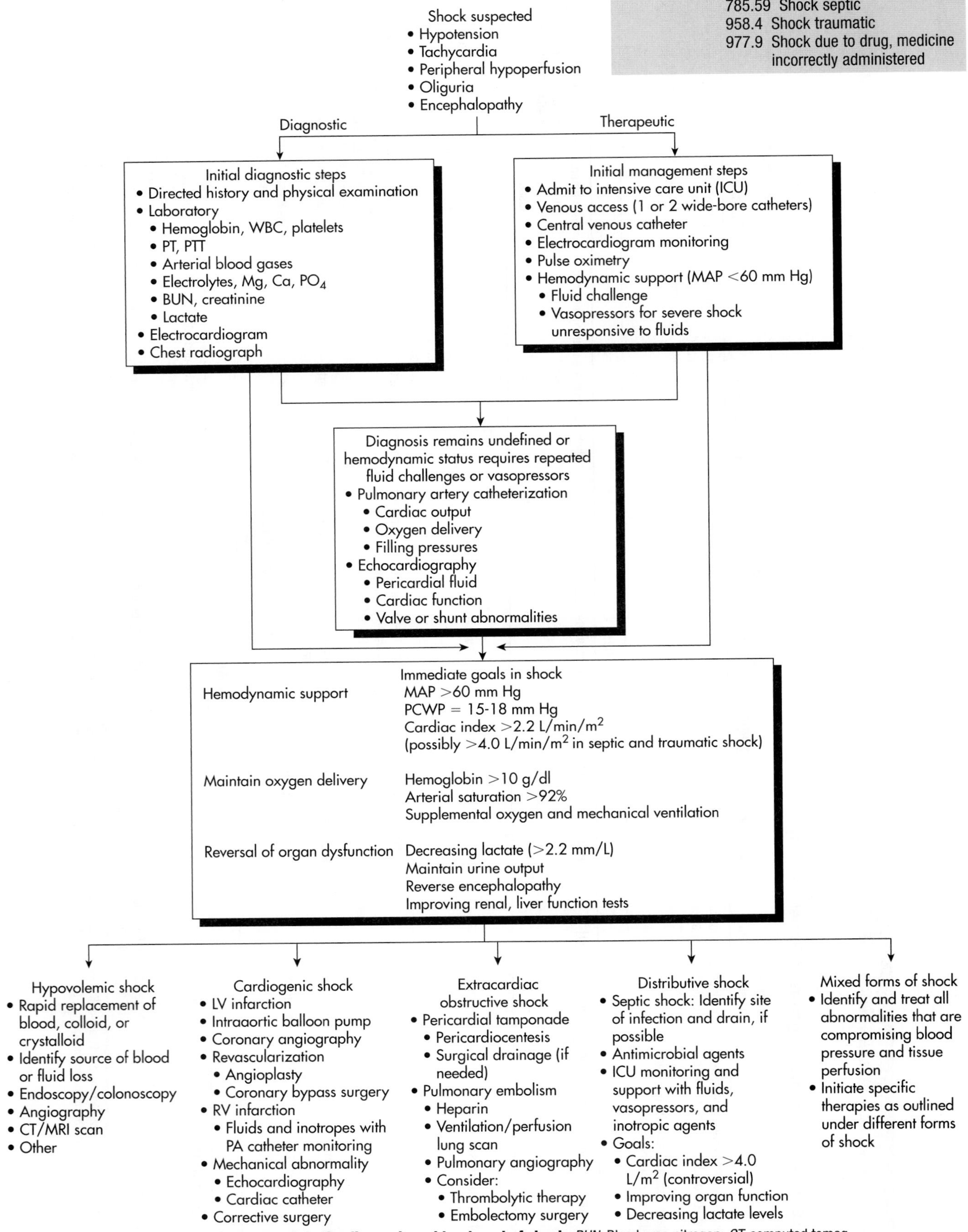

FIGURE 3-301 An approach to the diagnosis and treatment of shock. *BUN,* Blood urea nitrogen; *CT,* computed tomography; *LV,* left ventricular; *MAP,* mean arterial pressure; *MRI,* magnetic resonance imaging; *PA,* pulmonary arterial; *PCWP,* pulmonary capillary wedge pressure; *PT,* prothrombin time; *PTT,* partial thromboplastin time; *RV,* right ventricular; *WBC,* white blood cell count. (From Goldman L, Ausiello D [eds]: *Cecil textbook of medicine,* ed 23, Philadelphia, 2008, WB Saunders.)

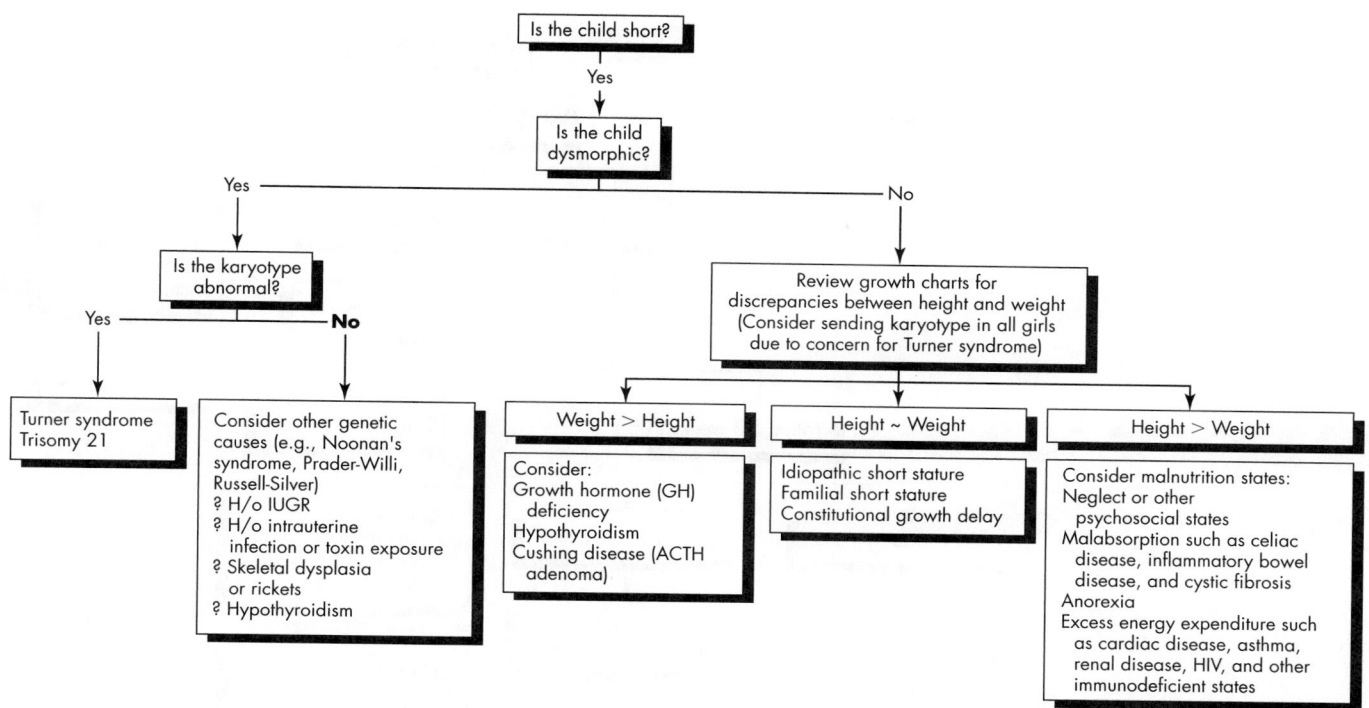

FIGURE 3-302 Differential diagnosis of short stature. (From Custer JW, Rau RE: *The Harriet Lane handbook,* ed 18, St Louis, 2009, Mosby.)

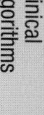

A

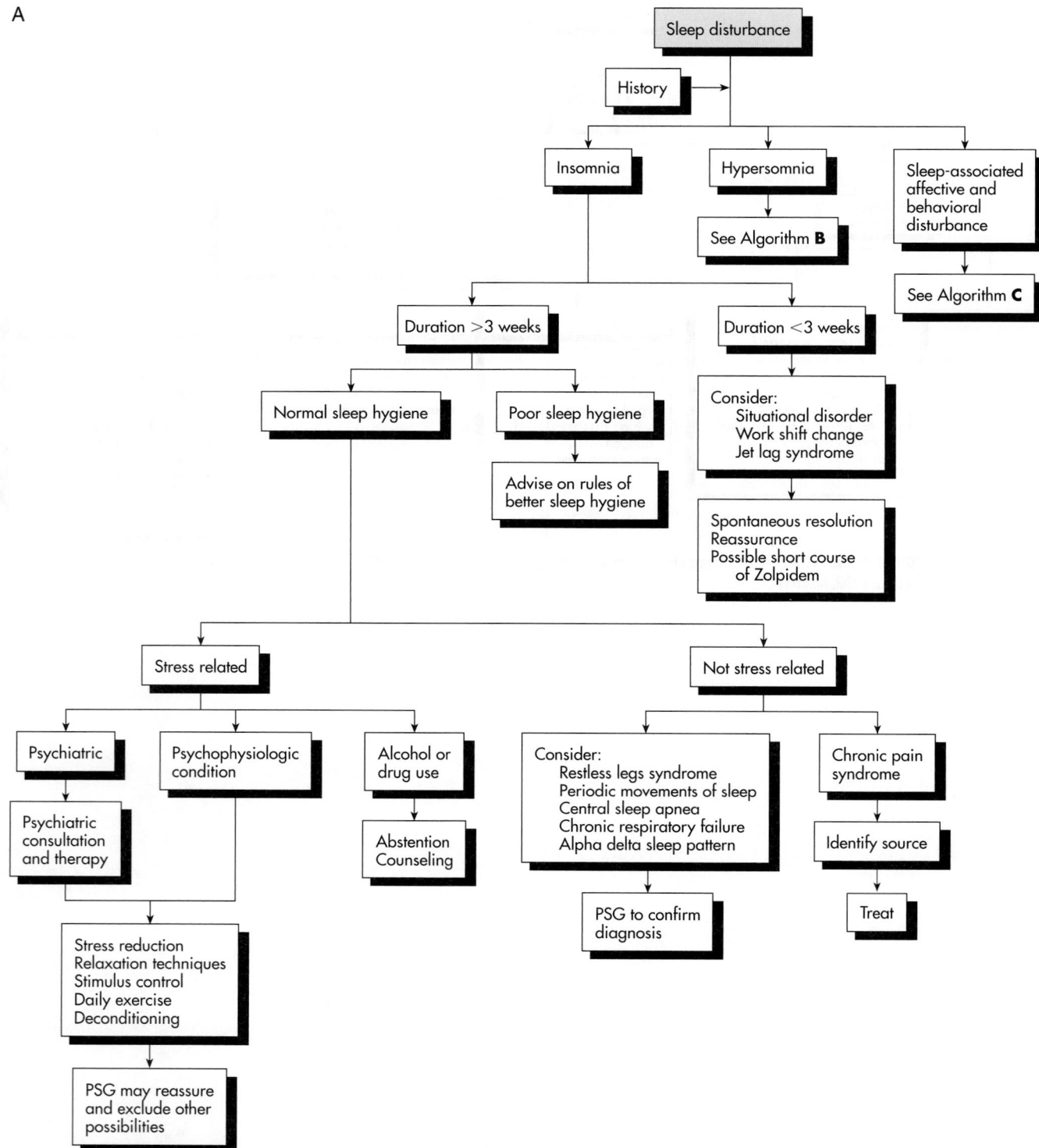

FIGURE 3-306 A, Patient with sleep disturbance. *MSLT,* Multiple sleep latency tests; *PSG,* polysomnography. (Modified from Greene HL, Johnson WP, Lemcke DL [eds]: *Decision making in medicine,* ed 2, St Louis, 1998, Mosby.)

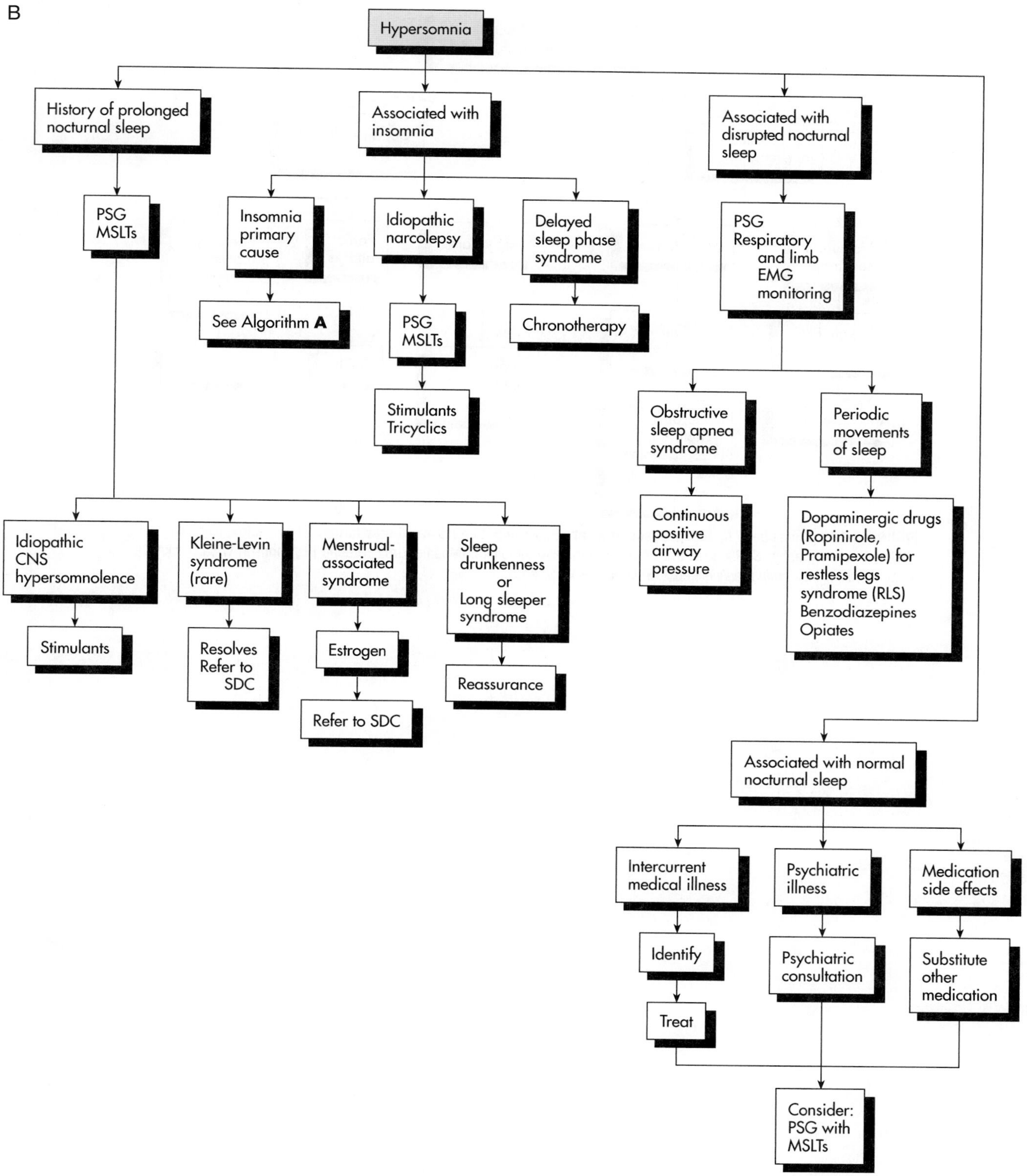

B

Hypersomnia

History of prolonged nocturnal sleep

PSG
MSLTs

Associated with insomnia

Insomnia primary cause

See Algorithm **A**

Idiopathic narcolepsy

PSG
MSLTs

Stimulants
Tricyclics

Delayed sleep phase syndrome

Chronotherapy

Associated with disrupted nocturnal sleep

PSG
Respiratory and limb EMG monitoring

Obstructive sleep apnea syndrome

Continuous positive airway pressure

Periodic movements of sleep

Dopaminergic drugs (Ropinirole, Pramipexole) for restless legs syndrome (RLS) Benzodiazepines Opiates

Idiopathic CNS hypersomnolence

Stimulants

Kleine-Levin syndrome (rare)

Resolves
Refer to SDC

Menstrual-associated syndrome

Estrogen

Refer to SDC

Sleep drunkenness or Long sleeper syndrome

Reassurance

Associated with normal nocturnal sleep

Intercurrent medical illness

Identify

Treat

Psychiatric illness

Psychiatric consultation

Medication side effects

Substitute other medication

Consider:
PSG with MSLTs

Clinical Algorithms

III

FIGURE 3-306 (Continued) **B, Hypersomnia.** *CNS,* Central nervous system; *EMG,* electromyelogram; *MSLTs,* multiple sleep latency tests; *PSG,* polysomnography; *SDC,* sleep disorders clinic. (Modified from Greene HL, Johnson WP, Lemcke DL [eds]: *Decision making in medicine,* ed 2, St Louis, 1998, Mosby.)

Continued on following page

C

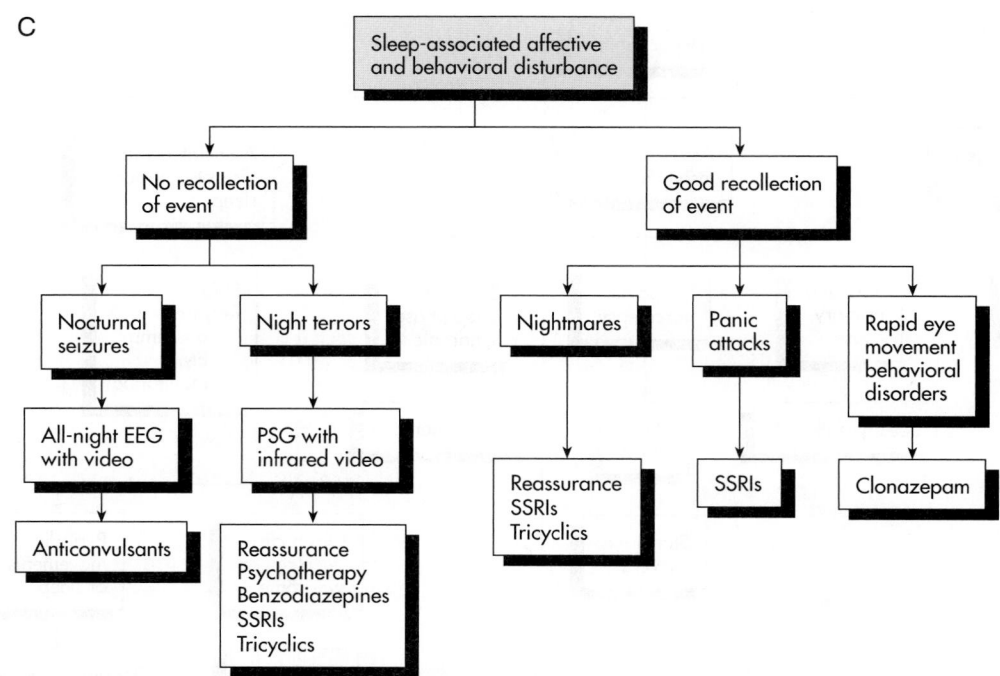

FIGURE 3-306 (Continued) **C, Sleep-associated affective and behavioral disturbance.** *EEG,* Electroencephalogram; *PSG,* polysomnography; *SSRIs,* selective serotonin reuptake inhibitors. (Modified from Greene HL, Johnson WP, Lemcke DL [eds]: *Decision making in medicine,* ed 2, St Louis, 1998, Mosby.)

SPLENOMEGALY

ICD-9CM # 789.2 Splenomegaly, unspecified
289.51 Splenomegaly, chronic congestive
759.0 Splenomegaly, congenital
789.2 Splenomegaly, unknown etiology

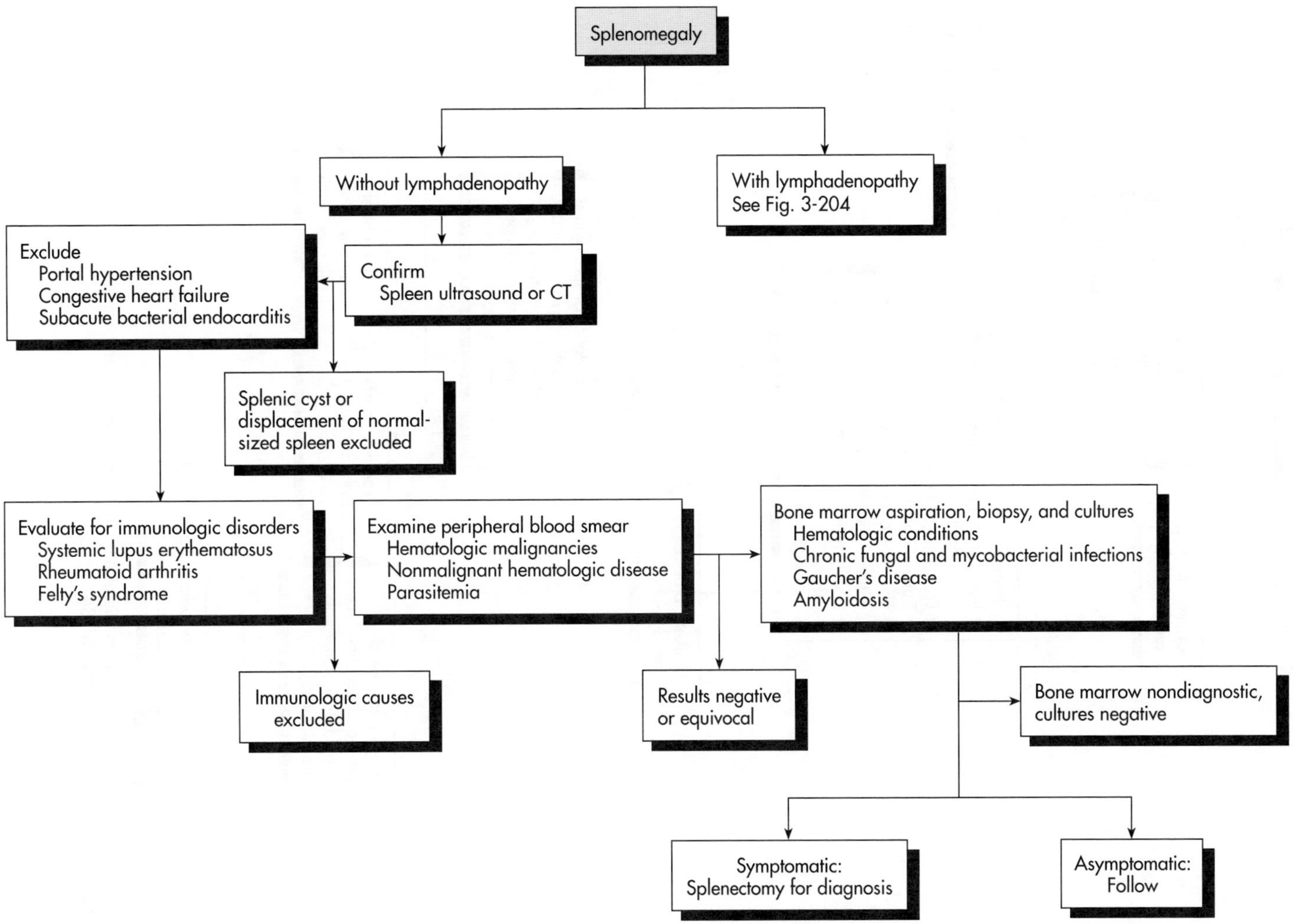

Splenomegaly

With lymphadenopathy
See Fig. 3-204

Without lymphadenopathy

Exclude
Portal hypertension
Congestive heart failure
Subacute bacterial endocarditis

Confirm
Spleen ultrasound or CT

Splenic cyst or
displacement of normal-
sized spleen excluded

Evaluate for immunologic disorders
Systemic lupus erythematosus
Rheumatoid arthritis
Felty's syndrome

Immunologic causes
excluded

Examine peripheral blood smear
Hematologic malignancies
Nonmalignant hematologic disease
Parasitemia

Results negative
or equivocal

Bone marrow aspiration, biopsy, and cultures
Hematologic conditions
Chronic fungal and mycobacterial infections
Gaucher's disease
Amyloidosis

Bone marrow nondiagnostic,
cultures negative

Asymptomatic:
Follow

Symptomatic:
Splenectomy for diagnosis

FIGURE 3-308 Clinical approach to patient with splenomegaly. *CT,* Computed tomography. (Modified from Stein JH [ed]: *Internal medicine,* ed 5, St Louis, 1998, Mosby.)

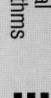

Clinical
Algorithms

III

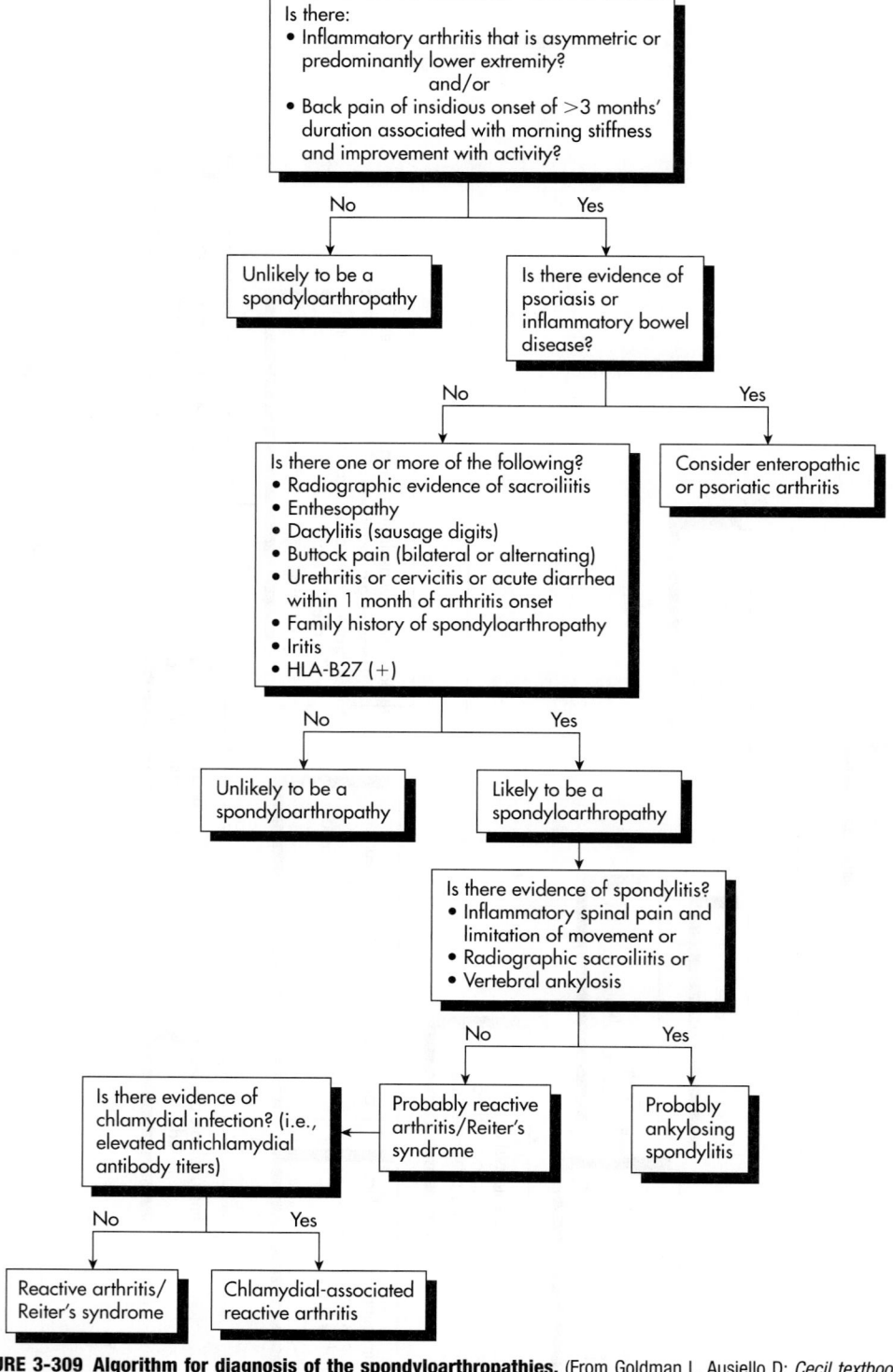

FIGURE 3-309 Algorithm for diagnosis of the spondyloarthropathies. (From Goldman L, Ausiello D: *Cecil textbook of medicine,* ed 23, Philadelphia, 2008, WB Saunders.)

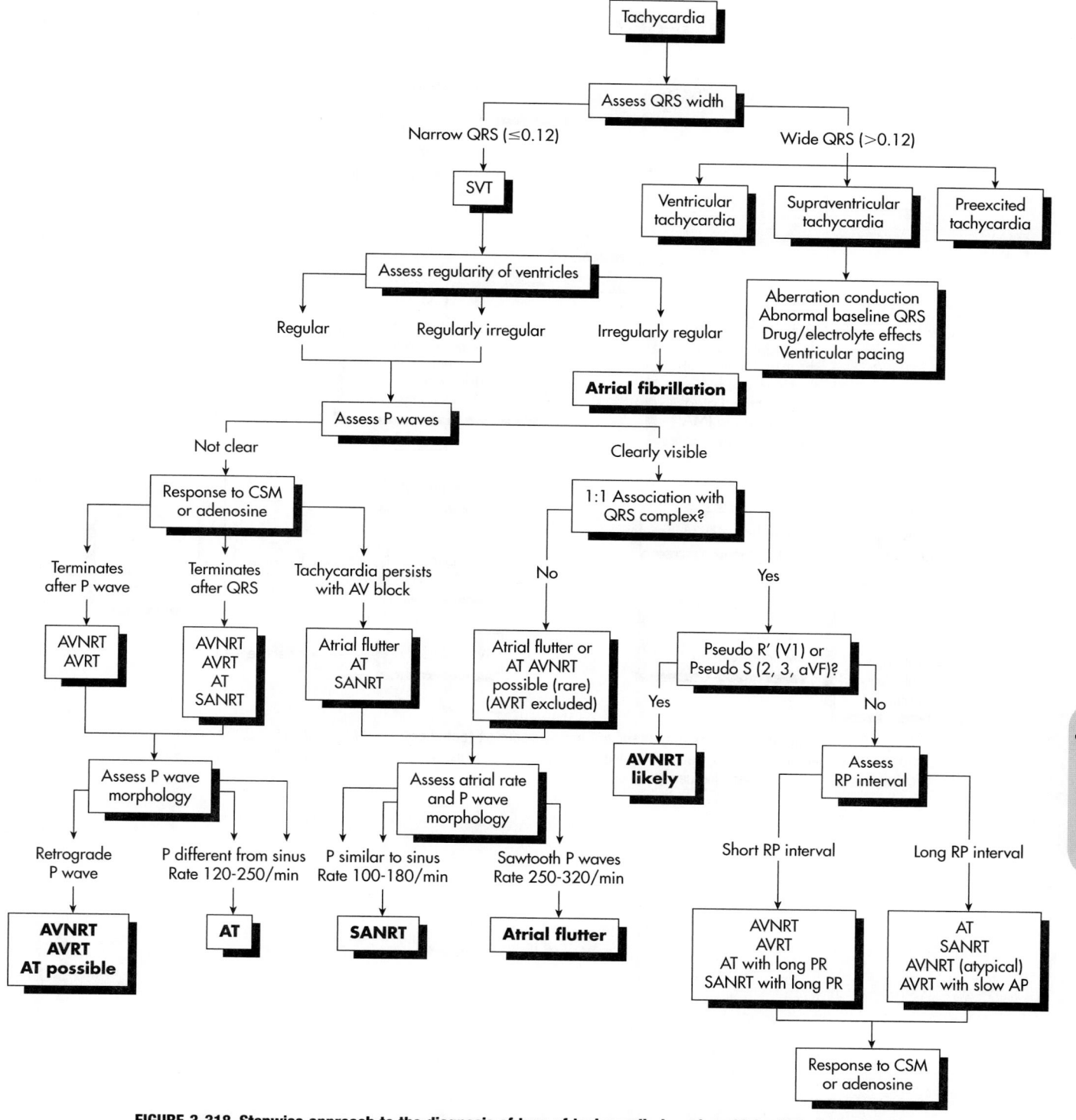

FIGURE 3-318 Stepwise approach to the diagnosis of type of tachycardia based on 12-lead electrocardiogram during the episode. The initial step is to determine whether the tachycardia has a wide or narrow QRS complex (Fig. 3-319). For wide-complex tachycardia, see Figure 3-320; the remainder of the algorithm is helpful in diagnosing the type of narrow-complex tachycardia. *AP,* Accessory pathway; *AT,* atrial tachycardia; *AV,* atrioventricular; *AVNRT,* AV nodal reentrant tachycardia; *AVRT,* AV reciprocating tachycardia; *CSM,* carotid sinus massage; *SANRT,* sinoatrial nodal reentry tachycardia; *SVT,* supraventricular tachycardia. (From Zipes DP, Libby P, Bonow RO, Braunwald E [eds]: *Braunwald's heart disease,* ed 7, Philadelphia, 2005, Elsevier.)

Clinical
Algorithms

III

ICD-9CM # 427.2 Paroxysmal tachycardia
427.0 Supraventricular paroxysmal tachycardia
427.42 Ventricular flutter
427.1 Ventricular paroxysmal tachycardia
427.89 Atrial tachycardia

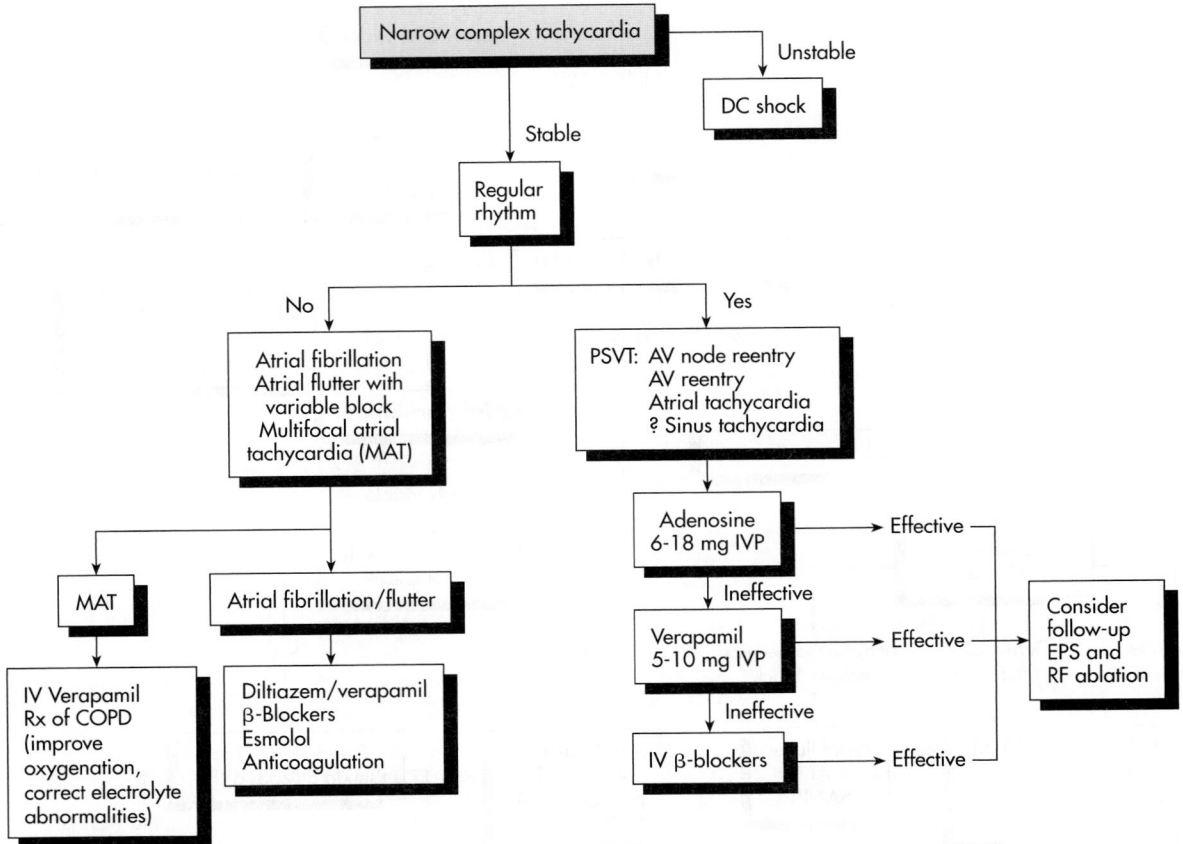

FIGURE 3-319 Evaluation and management of narrow complex tachycardia. *AV,* Atrioventricular; *COPD,* chronic obstructive pulmonary disease; *EPS,* electrophysiologic studies; *IV,* intravenous; *IVP,* intravenous push; *PSVT,* paroxysmal supraventricular tachycardia; *RF,* radiofrequency.

ICD-9CM # 427.2 Paroxysmal tachycardia
427.0 Supraventricular paroxysmal tachycardia
427.42 Ventricular flutter
427.1 Ventricular paroxysmal tachycardia
427.89 Atrial tachycardia

1331

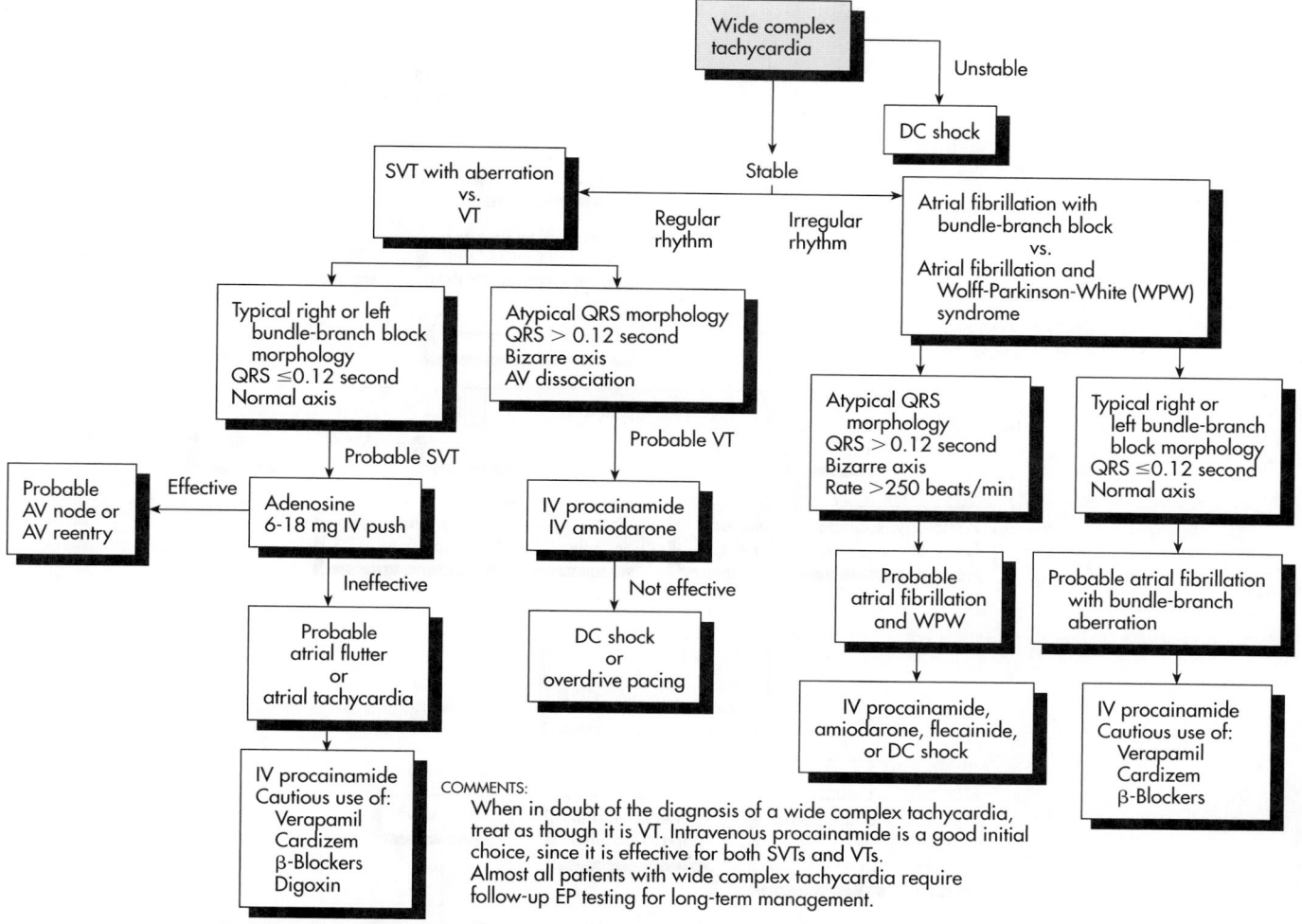

FIGURE 3-320 Evaluation and management of wide complex tachycardia. *AV,* Atrioventricular; *EP,* electrophysiologic; *IV,* intravenous; *SVT,* supraventricular tachycardia; *VT,* ventricular tachycardia. (From Driscoll CE et al: *The family practice desk reference,* ed 3, St Louis, 1996, Mosby.)

COMMENTS:
When in doubt of the diagnosis of a wide complex tachycardia, treat as though it is VT. Intravenous procainamide is a good initial choice, since it is effective for both SVTs and VTs.
Almost all patients with wide complex tachycardia require follow-up EP testing for long-term management.

TABLE 3-36 Major Features in the Differential Diagnosis of Wide QRS Beats Versus Tachycardia

Supports SVT	Supports VT
Slowing or termination by vagal tone	Fusion beats
Onset with premature P wave	Capture beats
RP interval ≤100 msec	AV dissociation
P and QRS rate and rhythm linked to suggest that ventricular activation depends on atrial discharge, e.g., 2:1 AV block rSR′ V1	P and QRS rate and rhythm linked to suggest that atrial activation depends on ventricular discharge, e.g., 2:1 VA block
Long-short cycle sequence	"Compensatory" pause
	Left axis deviation; QRS duration >140 msec
	Specific QRS contours (see text)

(From Zipes DP et al [eds]: *Braunwauld's heart disease,* ed 7, Philadelphia, 2005, Elsevier.)
SVT, Supraventricular tachycardia; *VT,* ventricular tachycardia.

ICD-9CM # 186.9 Testicular neoplasm
M906/3 (seminoma)
M9101/3 (embryonal carcinoma or teratoma)
M9100/3 (choriocarcinoma)

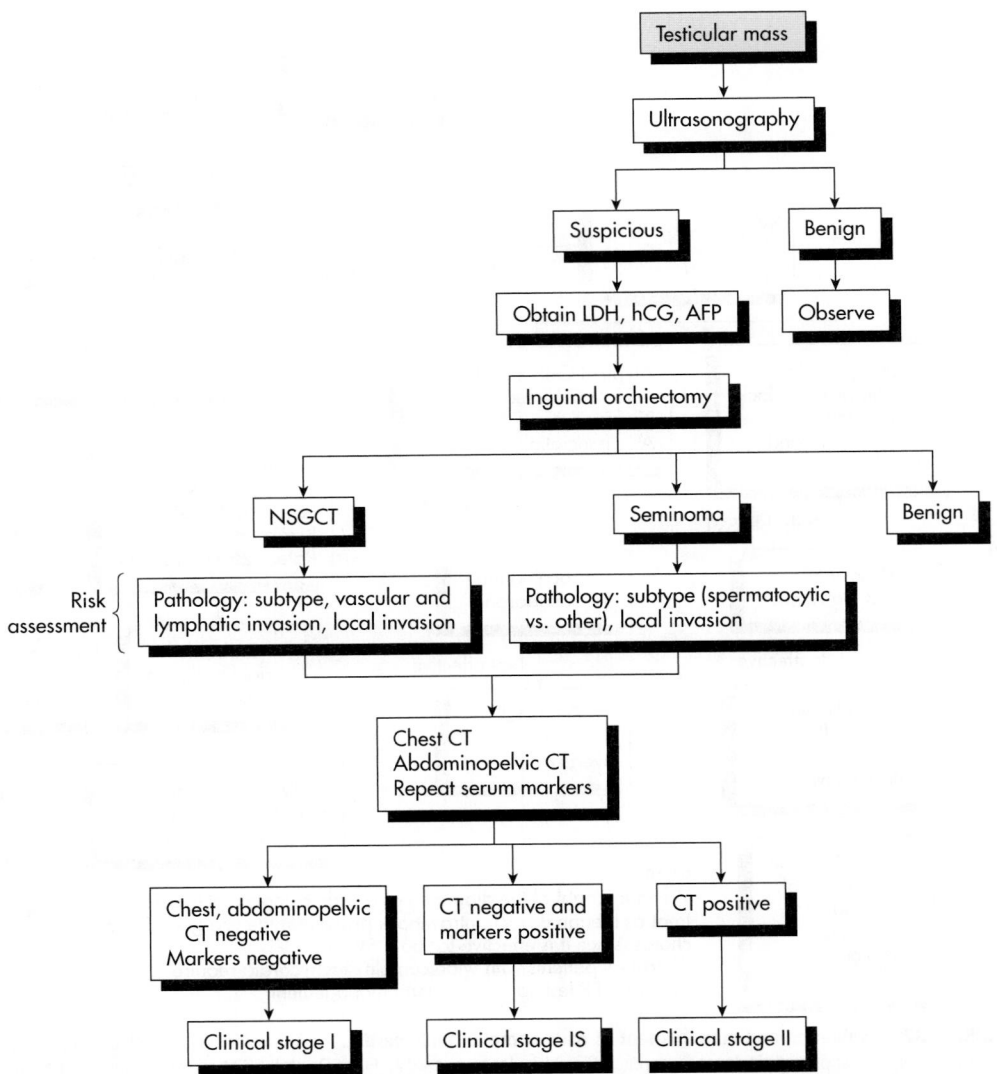

FIGURE 3-321 Diagnosis, staging, and risk assessment of patients with testicular germ cell tumor. *AFP,* α-fetoprotein; *CT,* computed tomography; *hCG,* human chorionic gonadotropin; *LDH,* lactic dehydrogenase; *NSGCT,* nonseminoma germ cell tumor. (From Abeloff MD: *Clinical oncology,* ed 4, New York, 2007, Churchill Livingstone.)

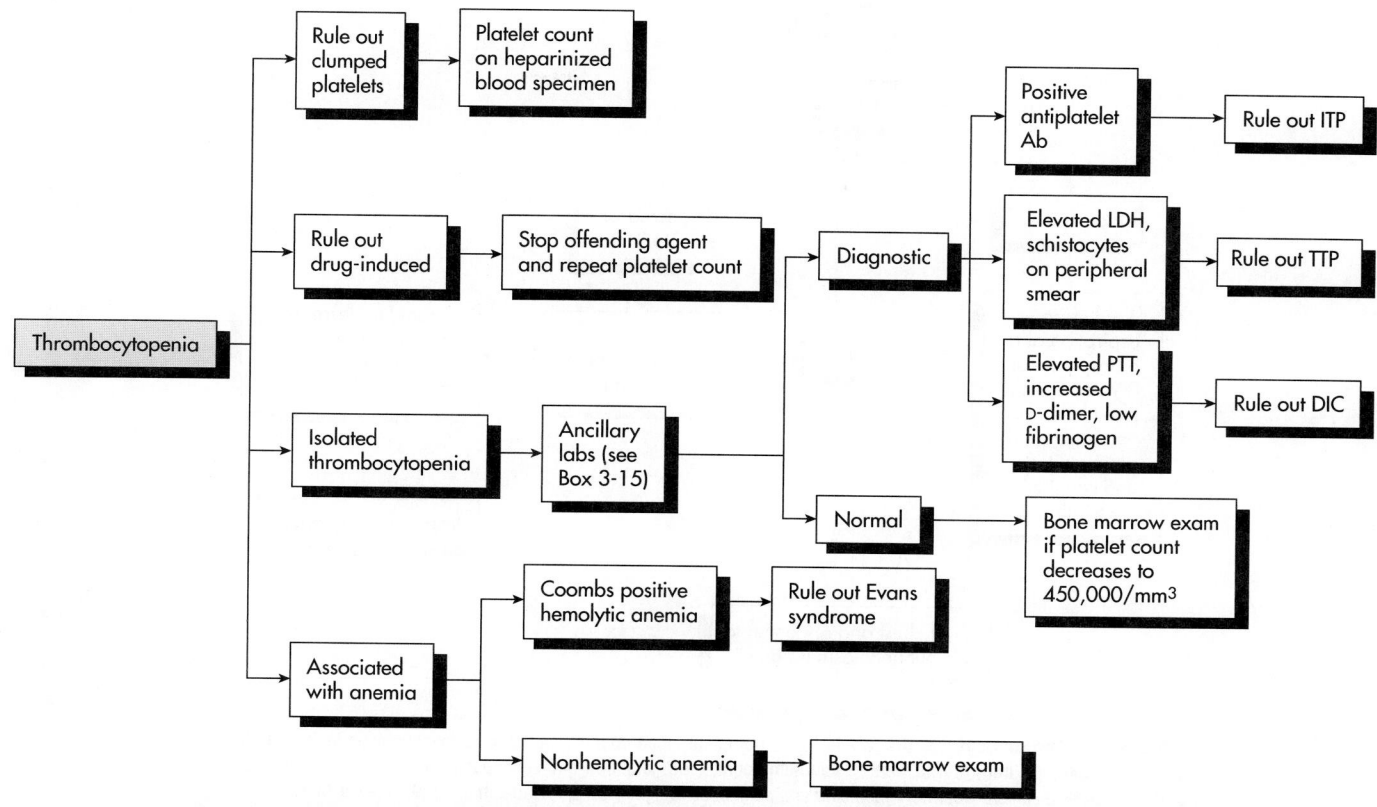

FIGURE 3-323 Evaluation of thrombocytopenia. *DIC,* Disseminated intravascular coagulation; *ITP,* idiopathic thrombocytopenic purpura; *LDH,* lactic dehydrogenase; *PPT,* partial thromboplastin time; *TTP,* thrombotic thrombocytopenic purpura. (From Ferri FF: *Ferri's best test: a practical guide to clinical laboratory medicine and diagnostic imaging,* ed 2, Philadelphia, 2009, Elsevier Mosby.)

Clinical
Algorithms

BOX 3-15 Thrombocytopenia	
Diagnostic imaging **Best Test** None	**Lab evaluation** **Best Test** Bone marrow exam
Ancillary test CT of abdomen if splenomegaly is present	**Ancillary tests** CBC, PT, PTT LDH HIV, ANA Antiplatelet Ab D-dimer Coombs tests

From Ferri FF: *Ferri's best test: a practical guide to clinical laboratory medicine and diagnostic imaging,* ed 2, Philadelphia, 2009, Elsevier Mosby.
ANA, Antibody to nuclear antigens; *CBC,* complete blood count; *CT,* computed tomography; *HIV,* human immunodeficiency virus; *LDH,* lactic dehydrogenase; *PT,* prothrombin time; *PTT,* partial thromboplastin time.

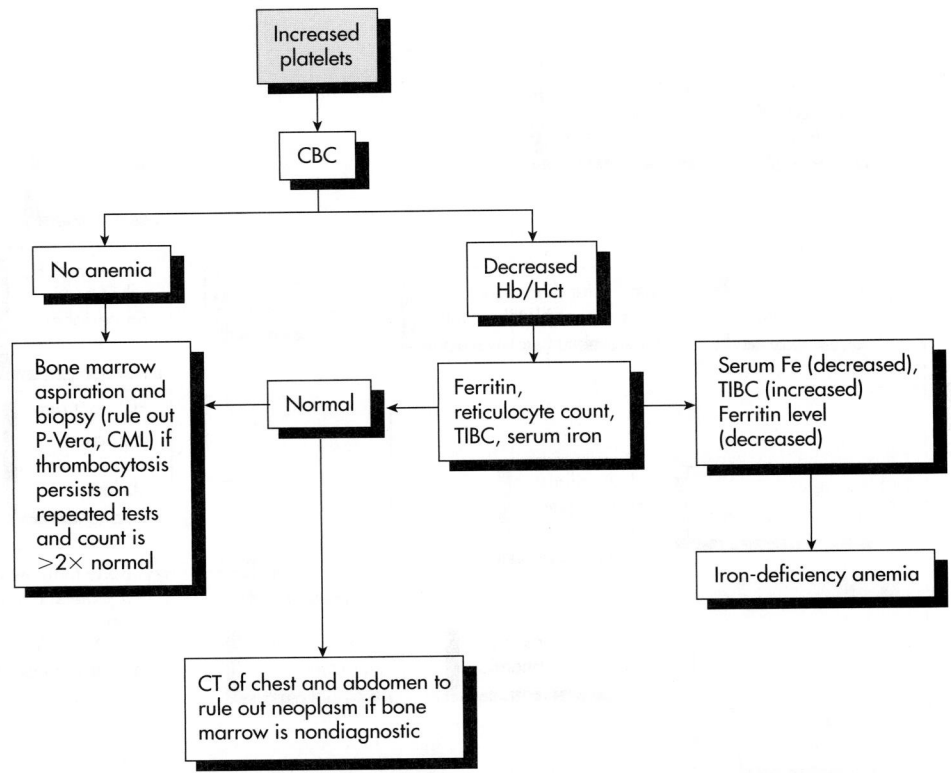

FIGURE 3-324 Thrombocytosis diagnosis. *CBC,* Complete blood count; *CML,* chronic myelogenous leukemia; *CT,* computed tomography; *Fe,* iron; *Hb/Hct,* hemoglobin/hematocrit; *TIBC,* total iron-binding capacity. (From Ferri FF: *Ferri's best test: a practical guide to clinical laboratory medicine and diagnostic imaging,* ed 2, Philadelphia, 2009, Elsevier Mosby.)

BOX 3-16 Thrombocytosis

Diagnostic imaging
Best Test
None

Ancillary test
CT of chest and abdomen

Lab evaluation
Best Test
Bone marrow exam

Ancillary tests
CBC
Reticulocyte count
Stool for OB ×3
Serum ferritin, TIBC, iron

From Ferri FF: *Ferri's best test: a practical guide to clinical laboratory medicine and diagnostic imaging,* ed 2, Philadelphia, 2009, Elsevier Mosby.
　CBC, Complete blood count; *CT,* computed tomography; *OB,* occult blood; *TIBC,* total iron-binding capacity.

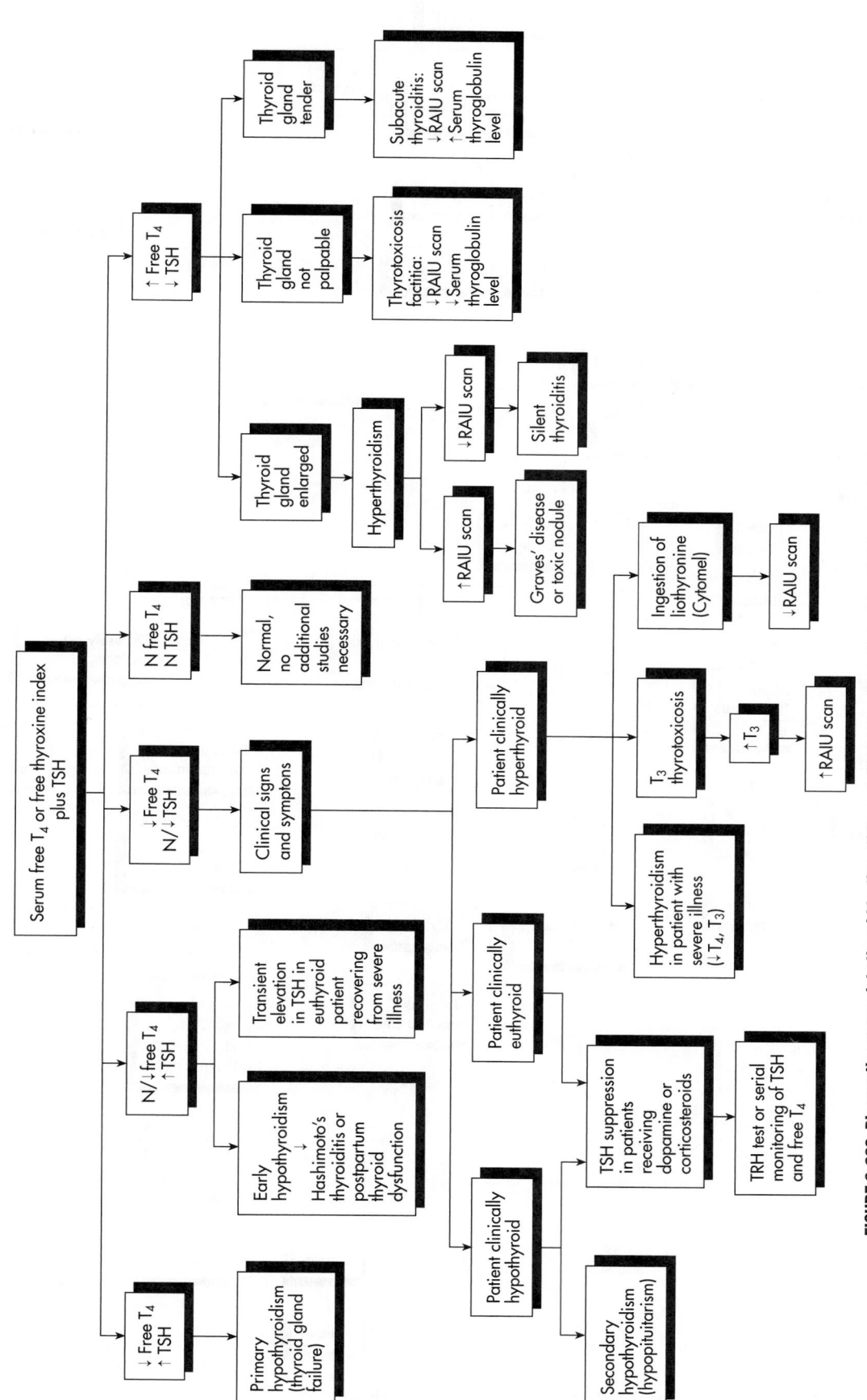

FIGURE 3-328 Diagnostic approach to thyroid testing. *N,* Normal; *RAIU,* radioactive iodine uptake; *TRH,* thyrotropin-releasing hormone; *TSH,* thyroid-stimulating hormone. (From Ferri FF: *Practical guide to the care of the medical patient,* ed 8, St Louis, 2011, Mosby.)

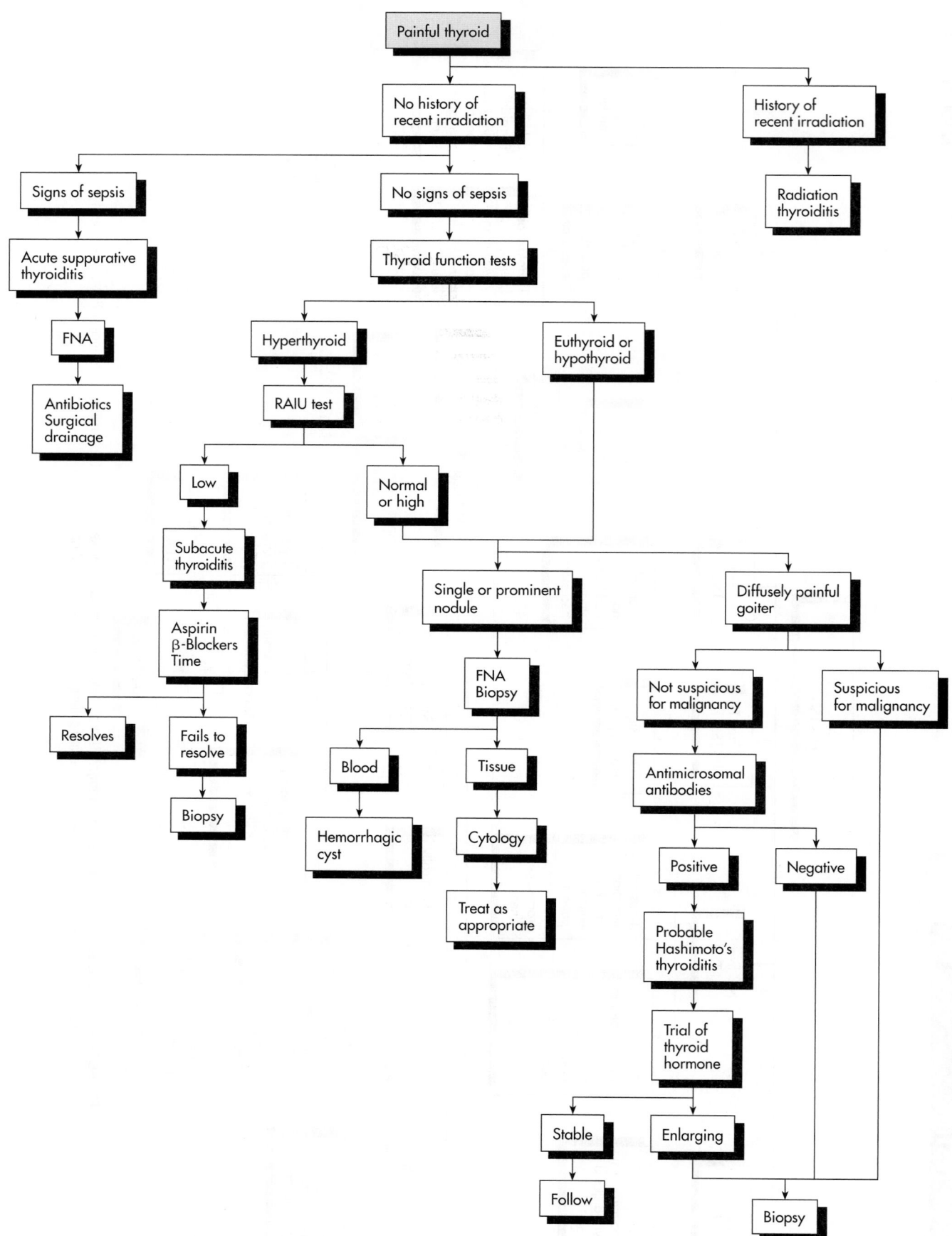

FIGURE 3-329 Painful thyroid. *FNA,* Fine-needle aspiration; *RAIU,* radioactive iodine uptake. (From Greene HL, Johnson WP, Lemcke DL [eds]: *Decision making in medicine,* ed 2, St Louis, 1998, Mosby.)

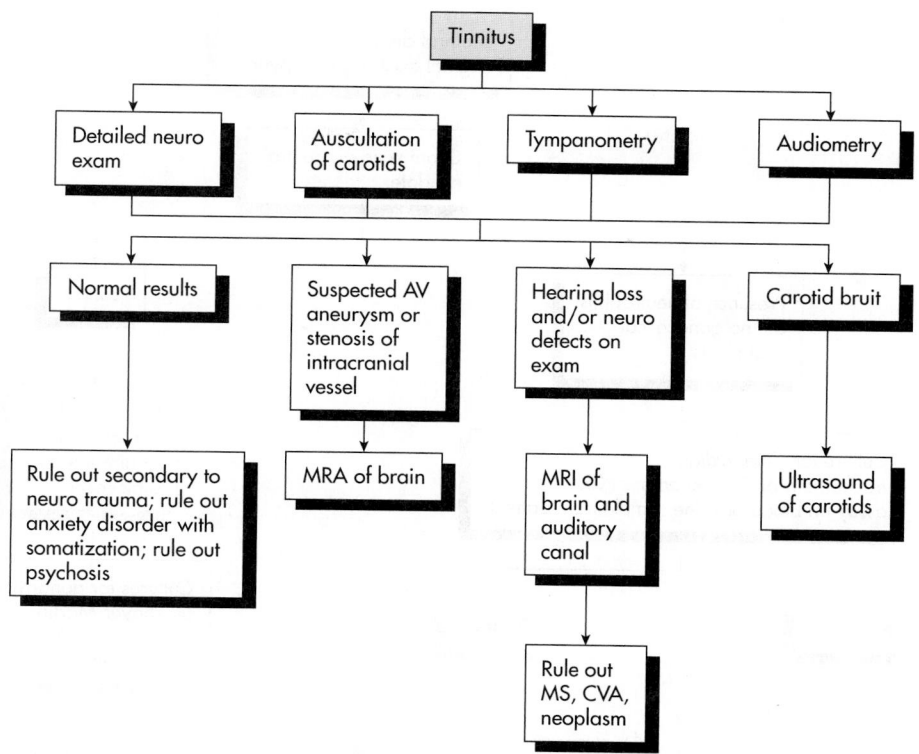

FIGURE 3-330 Tinnitus evaluation. *AV,* Atrioventricular; *CVA,* cerebrovascular accident; *MRA,* magnetic resonance angiography; *MRI,* magnetic resonance imaging; *MS,* multiple sclerosis. (From Ferri FF: *Ferri's best test: a practical guide to clinical laboratory medicine and diagnostic imaging,* ed 2, Philadelphia, 2009, Elsevier Mosby.)

BOX 3-17   Tinnitus

Diagnostic imaging	**Lab evaluation**
Best Test	***Best Test***
None	None
Ancillary tests	***Ancillary tests***
Carotid Doppler ultrasound	CBC
MRI of brain and auditory canals	Lipid panel
Brain MRA	

From Ferri FF: *Ferri's best test: a practical guide to clinical laboratory medicine and diagnostic imaging,* ed 2, Philadelphia, 2009, Elsevier Mosby.
   CBC, Complete blood count; *MRA,* magnetic resonance angiography; *MRI,* magnetic resonance imaging.

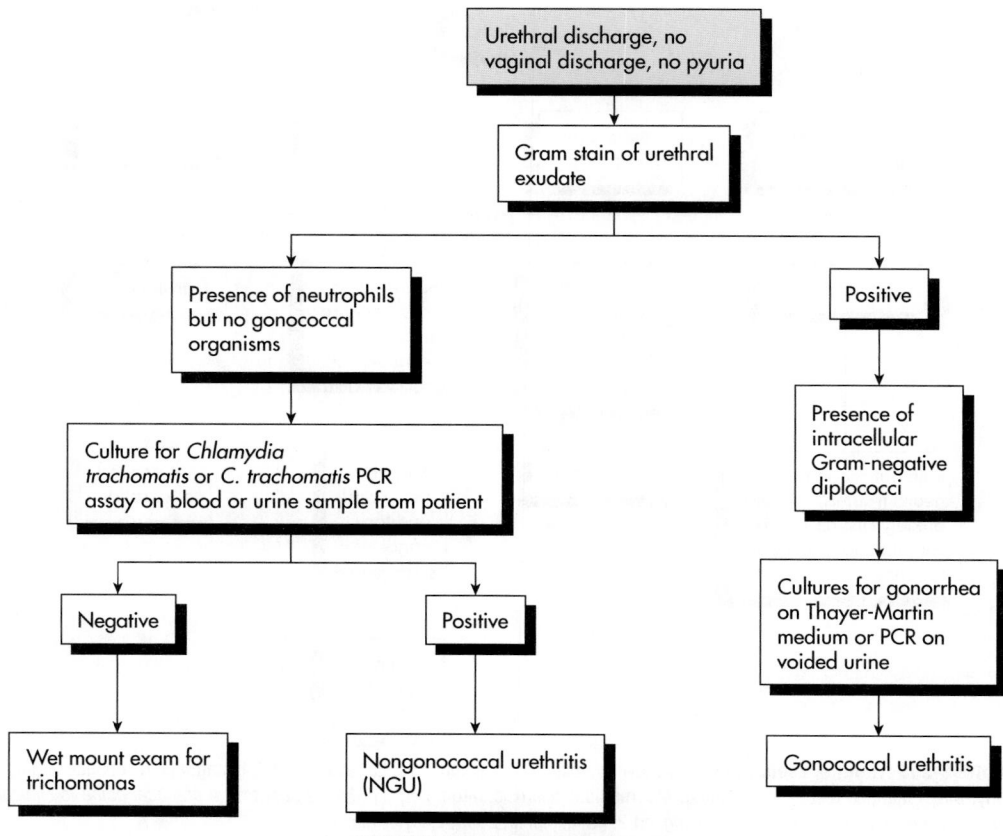

FIGURE 3-334 Urethral discharge.

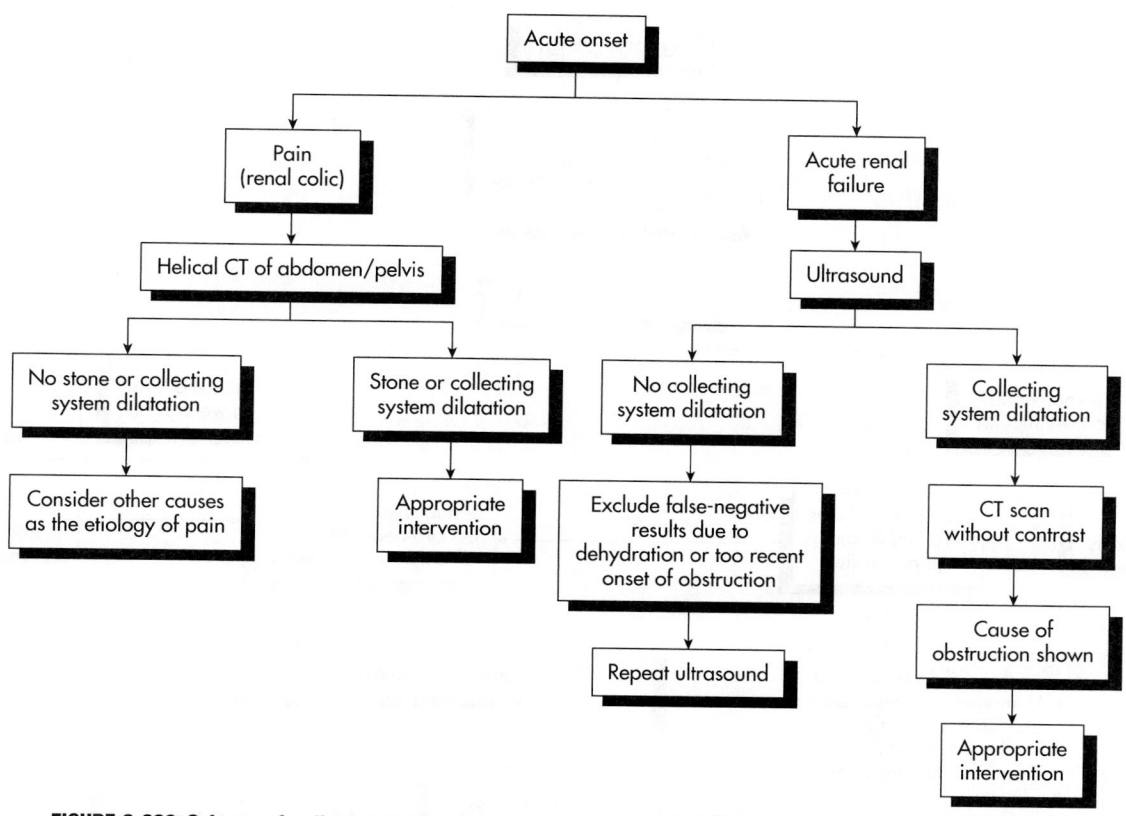

FIGURE 3-336 Scheme of a diagnostic approach to urinary tract obstruction. *CT,* Computed tomography; *IVP,* intravenous pyelography; *KUB,* kidneys, ureter, bladder (a flat film of the abdomen without contrast medium). (Modified from Goldman L, Ausiello D [eds]: *Cecil textbook of medicine,* ed 23, Philadelphia, 2008, WB Saunders.)

BOX 3-18   Diagnostic Tests Used in Obstructive Uropathy

Upper Urinary Tract Obstruction
Sonography (ultrasound)
Plain films of the abdomen (KUB)
Excretory or intravenous pyelography (very rarely needed)
Retrograde pyelography
Isotopic renography
Computed tomography (helical CT)
Magnetic resonance imaging
Pressure flow studies (the Whitaker test)

Lower Urinary Tract Obstruction
Some of the tests listed above
Cystoscopy
Voiding cystourethrogram
Retrograde urethrography
Urodynamic tests
Debimetry
Cystometrography
Electromyography
Urethral pressure profile

KUB, Kidneys, ureter, bladder.

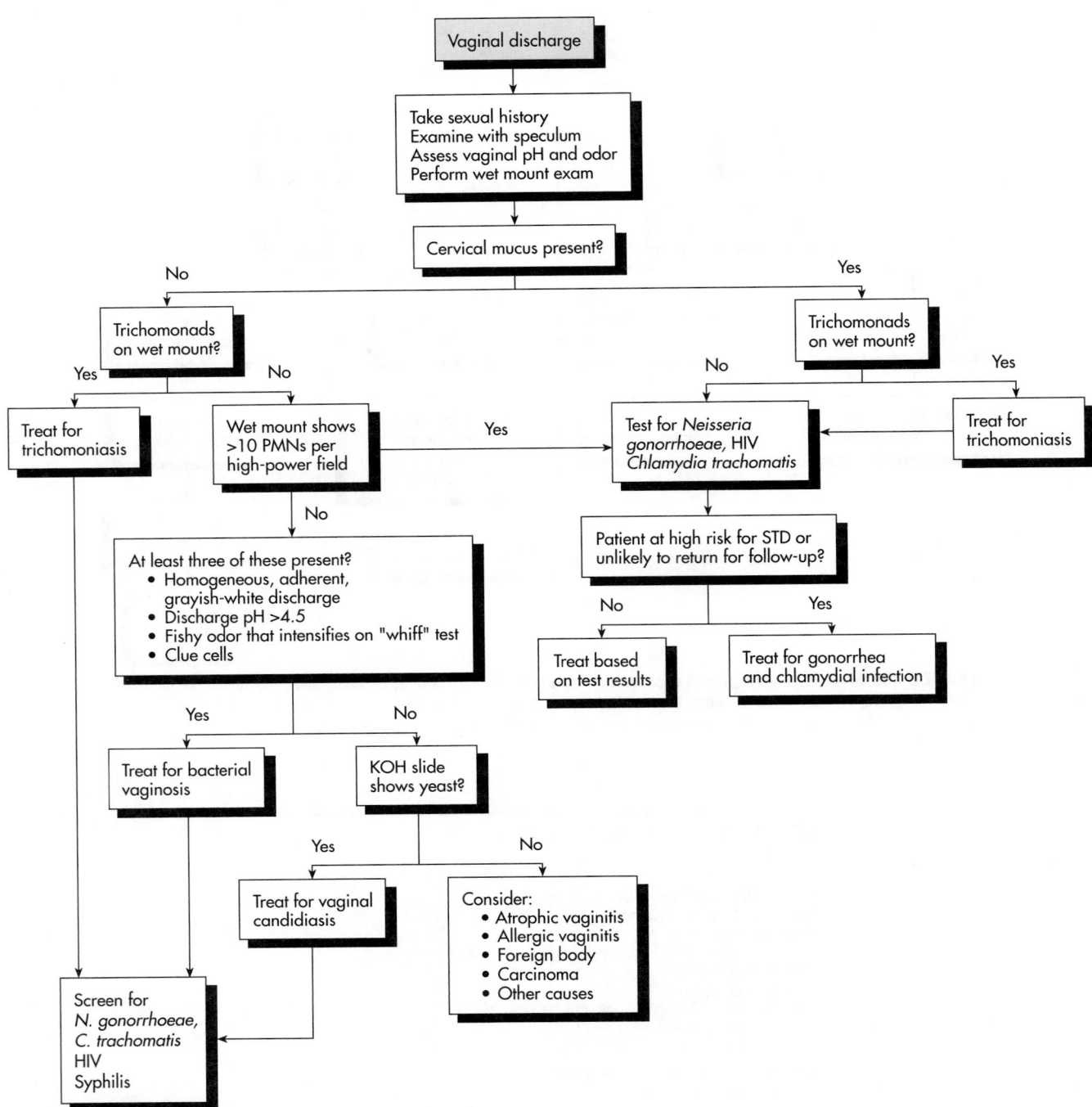

FIGURE 3-340 Evaluation of vaginal discharge. *HIV,* Human immunodeficiency virus; *KOH,* potassium hydroxide; *PMN,* polymorphonuclear leukocyte; *STD,* sexually transmitted disease. (Modified from Fox KK, Behets FMT: *Postgrad Med* 98:87, 1995.)

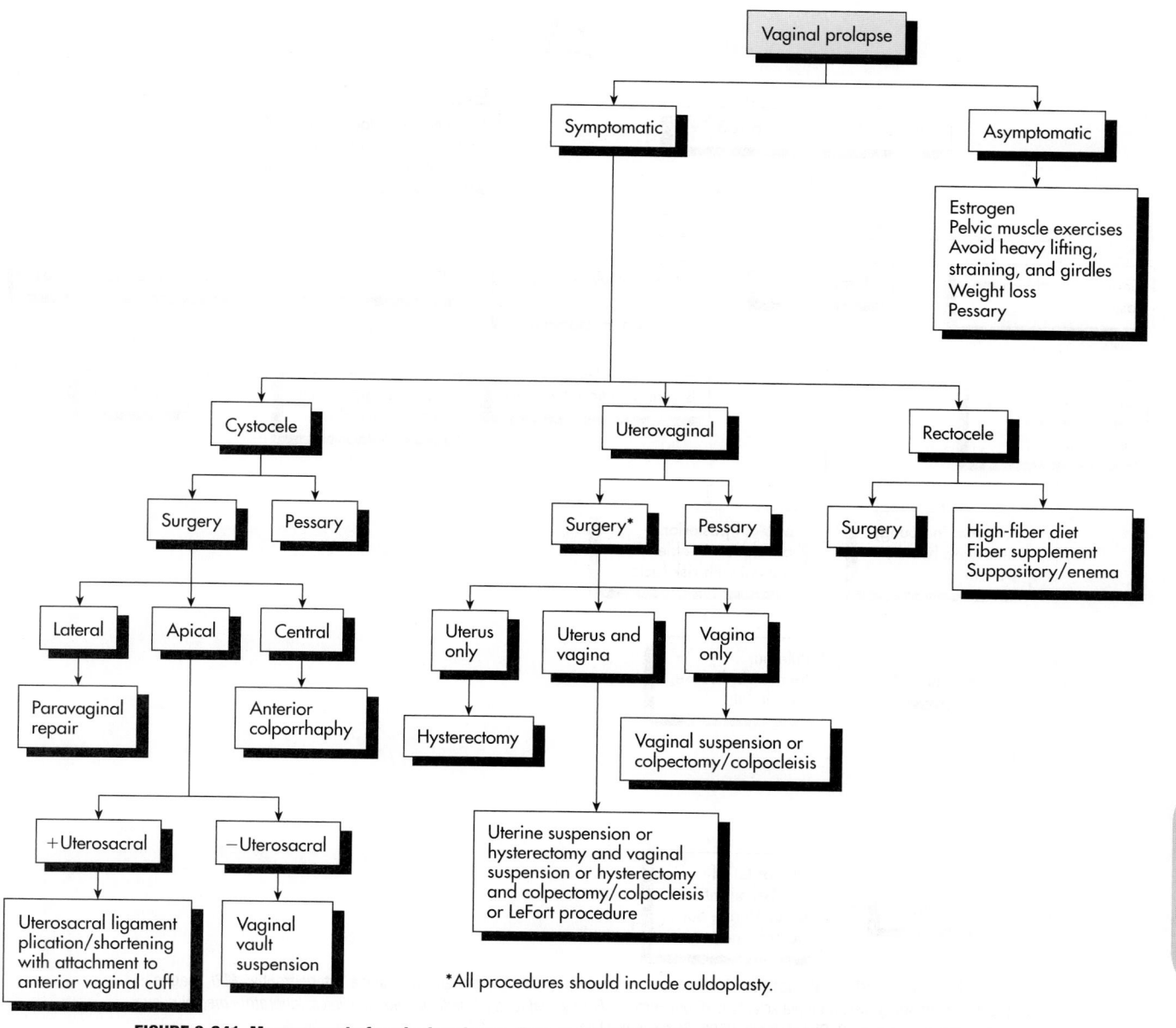

FIGURE 3-341 Management of vaginal prolapse. (From Zuspan FP [ed]: *Handbook of obstetrics, gynecology, and primary care,* St Louis, 1998, Mosby.)

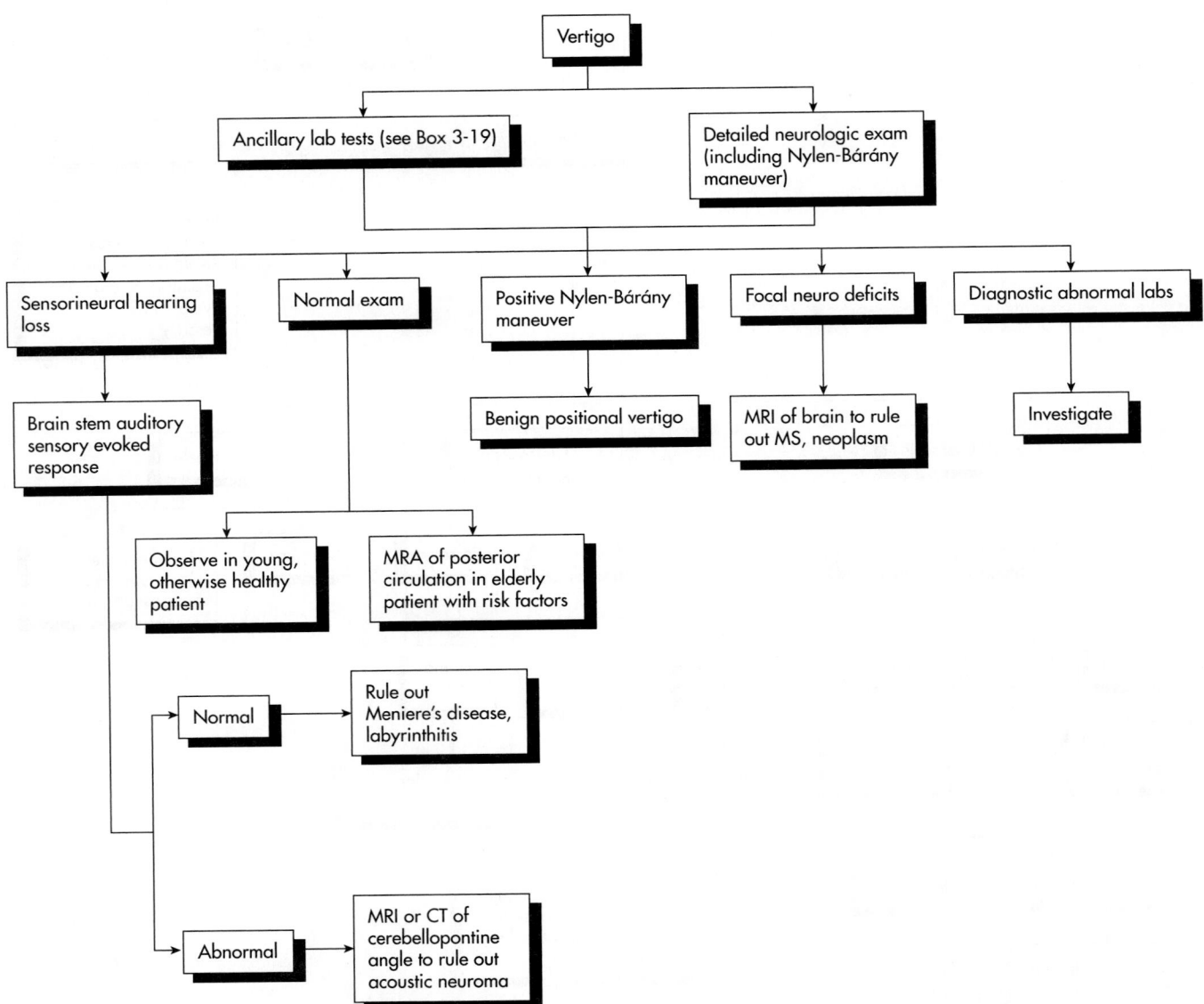

FIGURE 3-342 Vertigo evaluation. *CT,* Computed tomography; *MRA,* magnetic resonance arteriography; *MRI,* magnetic resonance imaging; *MS,* multiple sclerosis. (From Ferri FF: *Ferri's best test: a practical guide to clinical laboratory medicine and diagnostic imaging,* ed 2, Philadelphia, 2009, Elsevier Mosby.)

BOX 3-19 Vertigo

Diagnostic imaging
Best test
MRI of brain

Ancillary tests
MRA of posterior circulation
CT of cerebellopontine region if MRI is contraindicated

Lab evaluation
Best test
None

Ancillary tests
CBC with differential
Serum glucose, creatinine, ALT, electrolytes

From Ferri FF: *Ferri's best test: a practical guide to clinical laboratory medicine and diagnostic imaging,* ed 2, Philadelphia, 2009, Elsevier Mosby.
  ALT, Alanine aminotransferase; *CBC,* complete blood count; *CT,* computed tomography; *MRA,* magnetic resonance angiography; *MRI,* magnetic resonance imaging.

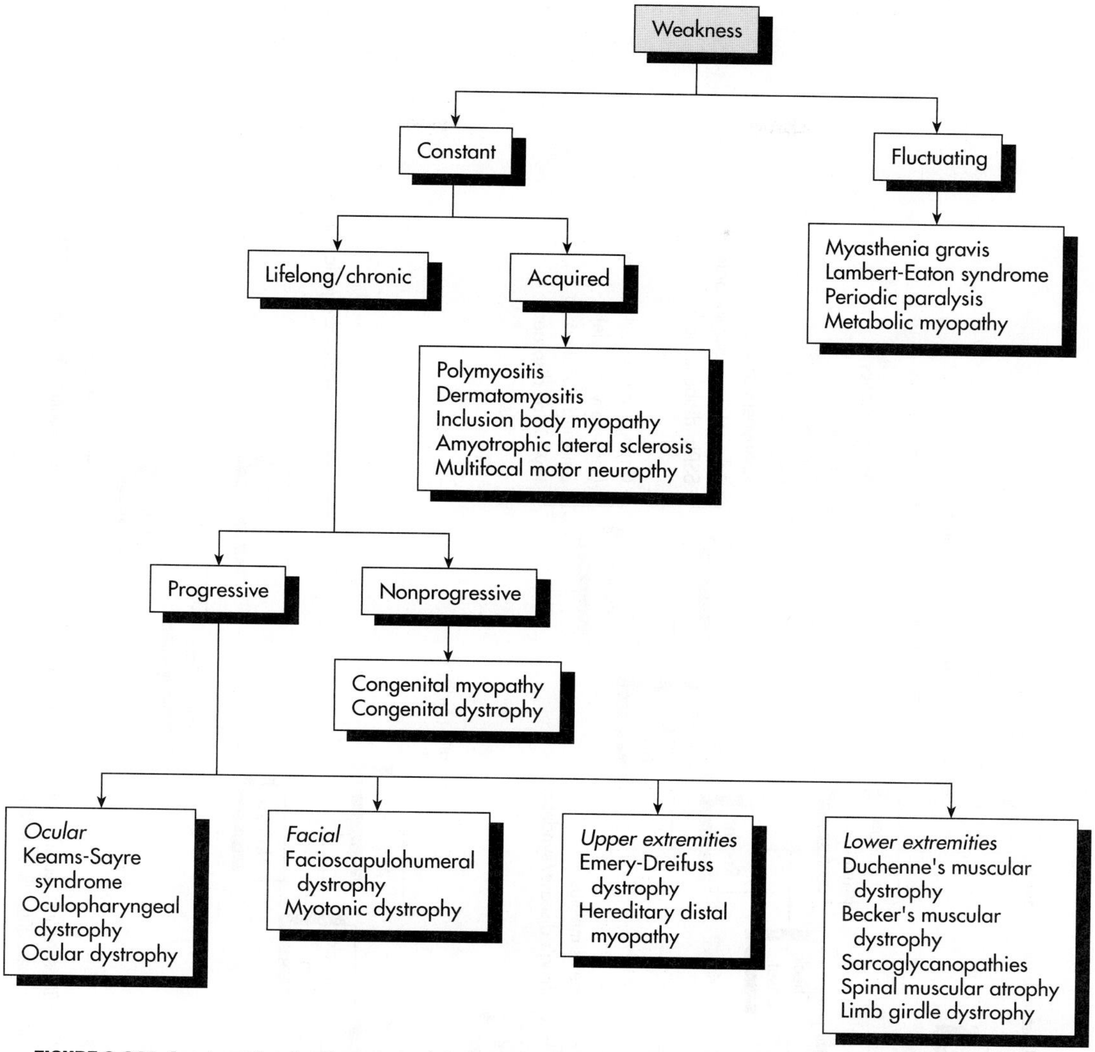

Weakness

Constant

Fluctuating
- Myasthenia gravis
- Lambert-Eaton syndrome
- Periodic paralysis
- Metabolic myopathy

Lifelong/chronic

Acquired
- Polymyositis
- Dermatomyositis
- Inclusion body myopathy
- Amyotrophic lateral sclerosis
- Multifocal motor neuropthy

Progressive

Nonprogressive
- Congenital myopathy
- Congenital dystrophy

Ocular
- Keams-Sayre syndrome
- Oculopharyngeal dystrophy
- Ocular dystrophy

Facial
- Facioscapulohumeral dystrophy
- Myotonic dystrophy

Upper extremities
- Emery-Dreifuss dystrophy
- Hereditary distal myopathy

Lower extremities
- Duchenne's muscular dystrophy
- Becker's muscular dystrophy
- Sarcoglycanopathies
- Spinal muscular atrophy
- Limb girdle dystrophy

FIGURE 3-344 An algorithm for the approach to the patient with weakness. (From Bradley WG, Daroff RB, Fenichel GM, Jankovic J [eds]: *Neurology in clinical practice,* ed 4, Philadelphia, 2004, Butterworth Heinemann.)

Clinical Algorithms

ICD-9CM # 783.1 Abnormal weight gain
278.00 Obesity

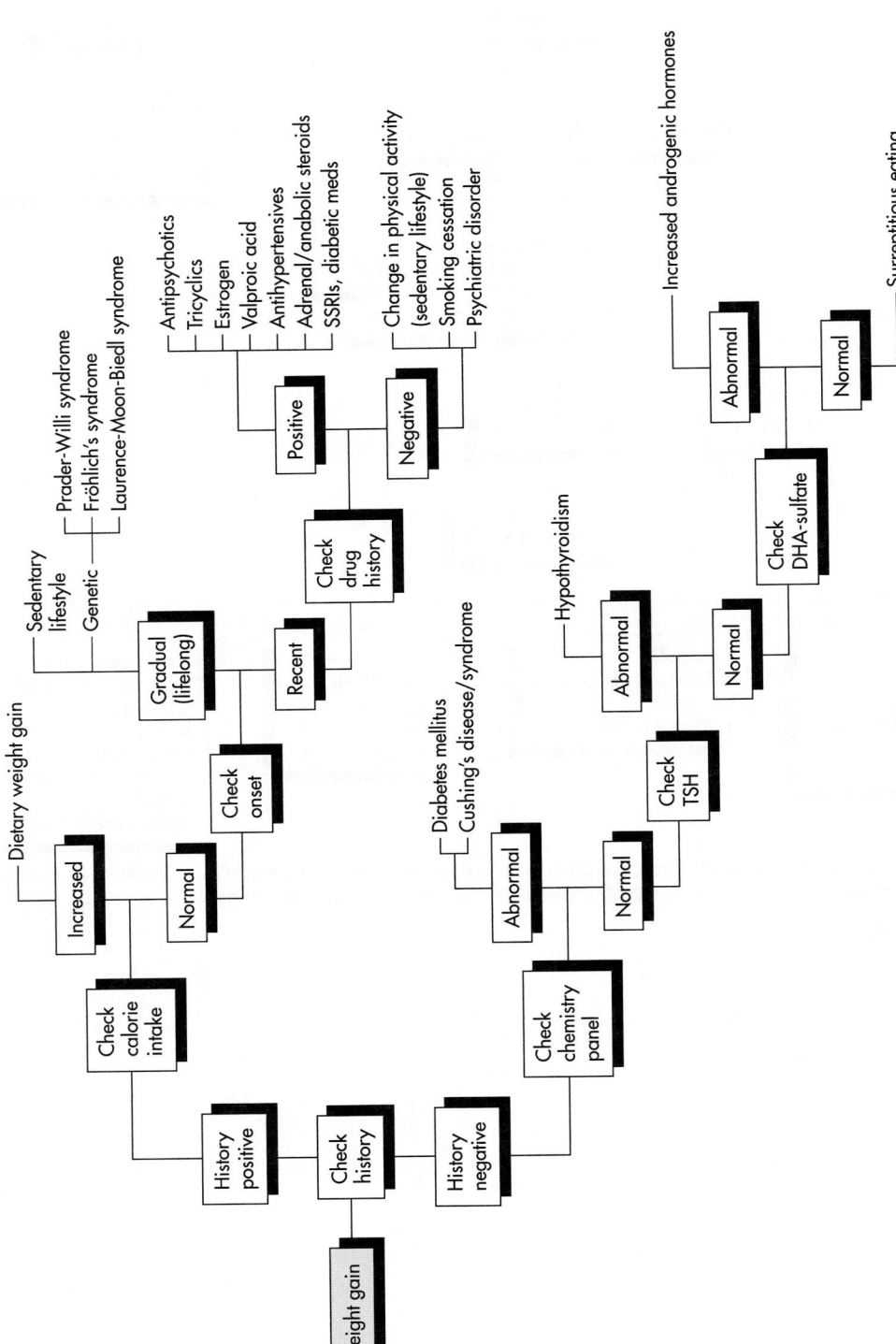

FIGURE 3-345 Weight gain. *DHA,* Dehydroepiandrosterone; *SSRIs,* serotonin reuptake inhibitors; *TSH,* thyroid-stimulating hormone. (Modified from Healey PM: *Common medical diagnosis: an algorithmic approach,* ed 3, Philadelphia, 2000, WB Saunders.)

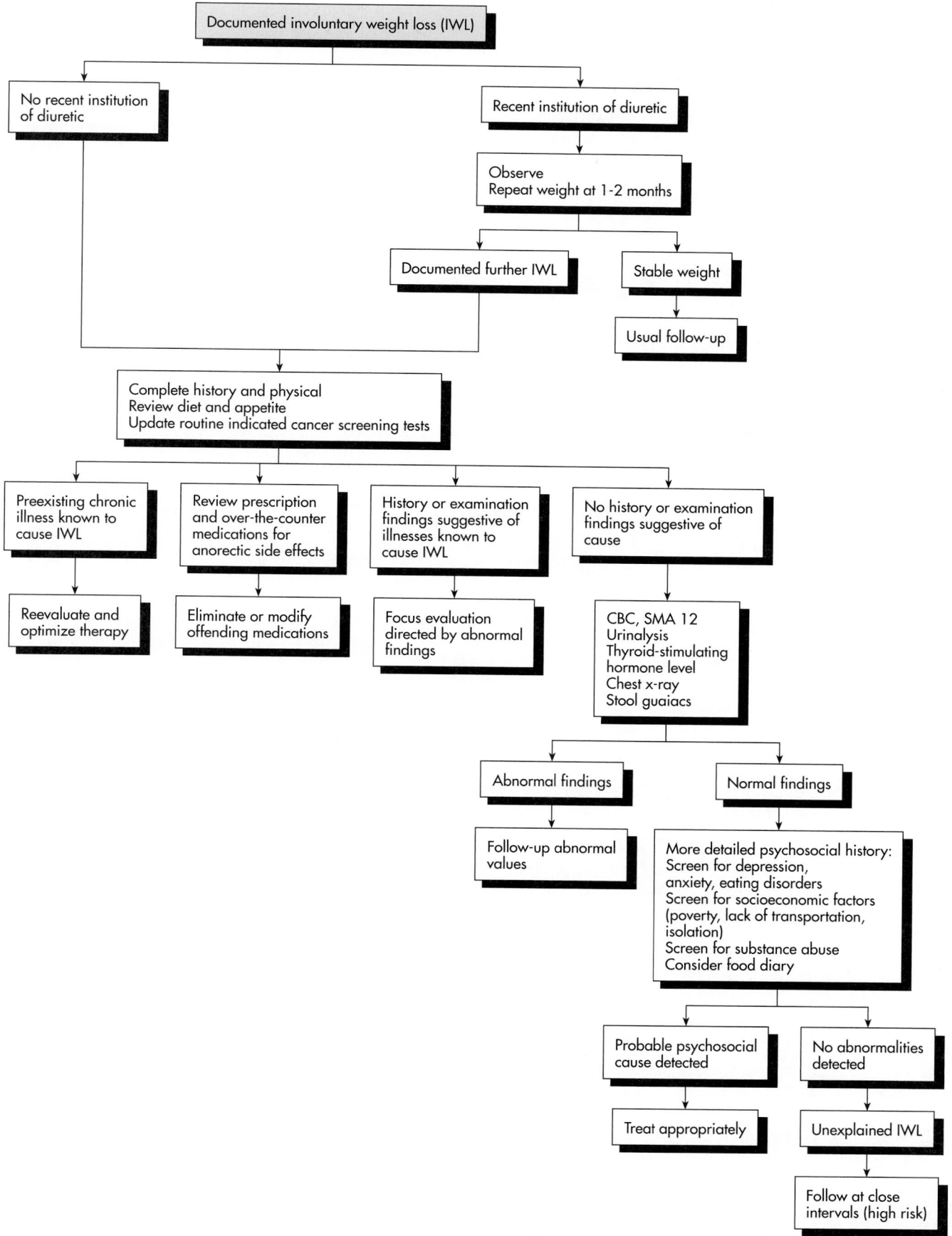

FIGURE 3-346 Involuntary weight loss. *CBC,* Complete blood count. (From Greene HL, Johnson WP, Lemcke DL [eds]: *Decision making in medicine,* ed 2, St Louis, 1998, Mosby.)

Clinical Algorithms

III

Laboratory Tests and Interpretation of Results

This section contains more than 300 commonly performed laboratory tests. In general, the tests are discussed in the following format:

1. Laboratory test.
2. Normal range in adult patients. Normal values are given using the present (traditional) reference interval, followed by the Système Internationale (SI) reference interval, the conversion factor (CF), and the suggested minimum increment (SMI).
3. Common abnormalities, such as positive test, increased or decreased value.
4. Causes of abnormal result.

The normal ranges may differ slightly, depending on the laboratory. The reader should be aware of the "normal range" of the particular laboratory performing the test. Every attempt has been made to present current laboratory test data, with emphasis on practical considerations.

ACE LEVEL
See ANGIOTENSIN-CONVERTING ENZYME

ACETONE (serum or plasma)
Normal: Negative
Elevated in: DKA, starvation, isopropanol ingestion

ACETYLCHOLINE RECEPTOR (AChR) ANTIBODY
Normal: <0.03 nmol/L
Elevated in: Myasthenia gravis. Changes in AChR concentration correlate with the clinical severity of myasthenia gravis following therapy and during therapy with prednisone and immunosuppressants. False-positive AChR antibody results may be found in patients with Eaton-Lambert syndrome.

ACID-BASE REFERENCE VALUES
See Tables 4-1 and 4-2.

ACID PHOSPHATASE (serum)
Normal range: 0-5.5 U/L (0-90 nkat/L [CF: 16.67; SMI: 2 nkat/L])
Elevated in: Carcinoma of prostate, other neoplasms (breast, bone), Paget's disease, osteogenesis imperfecta, malignant invasion of bone, Gaucher's disease, multiple myeloma, myeloproliferative disorders, benign prostatic hypertrophy, prostatic palpation or surgery, hyperparathyroidism, liver disease, chronic renal failure, idiopathic thrombocytopenic purpura, bronchitis

ACID SERUM TEST
See HAM TEST

ACTIVATED CLOTTING TIME (ACT)
Normal: This test is used to determine the dose of protamine sulfate to reverse the effect of heparin as an anticoagulant during angioplasty, cardiac surgery, and hemodialysis. The accepted goal during cardiopulmonary bypass surgery is usually 400-500 sec.

ACTIVATED PARTIAL THROMBOPLASTIN TIME (APTT, aPTT)
See PARTIAL THROMBOPLASTIN TIME

ADRENOCORTICOTROPIC HORMONE
Normal: 9-52 pg/ml
Elevated in: Addison's disease, ectopic ACTH-producing tumors, congenital adrenal hyperplasia, Nelson's syndrome, pituitary-dependent Cushing's disease
Decreased in: Secondary adrenocortical insufficiency, hypopituitarism, adrenal adenoma or adrenal carcinoma

ALANINE AMINOPEPTIDASE
Normal:
Male: 1.11-1.71 mcd/ml
Female: 0.96-1.52 mcg/ml
Elevated in: Liver or pancreatic disease, ethanol use, oral contraceptives use, malignancy, tobacco use, pregnancy
Decreased in: Abortion

ALANINE AMINOTRANSFERASE (ALT, SGPT)
Normal range: 0-35 U/L (0.058 μkat/L [CF: 0.02 μkat/L])
Elevated in: Liver disease (hepatitis, cirrhosis, Reye's syndrome), hepatic congestion, infectious mononucleosis, myocardial infarction, myocarditis,

TABLE 4-1 Commonly Used Acid-Base Reference Values for Arterial and Venous Plasma or Serum (Averaged from Various Sources)

	ARTERIAL		VENOUS	
	Conventional Units	SI Units*	Conventional Units	SI Units*
pH	7.40 (7.35-7.45)	7.40 (7.35-7.45)	7.37 (7.32-7.42)	7.37 (7.32-7.42)
Pco_2	40 mm Hg (35-45)	5.33 kPa (4.67-6.10)	45 mm Hg (45-50)	6.10 kPa (5.33-6.67)
Po_2	80-100 mm Hg	10.66-13.33 kPa	40 mm Hg (37-43)	5.33 kPa (4.93-5.73)
HCO_3 (CO_2 combining power)	24 mEq/L (20-28)	24 mmol/L (20-28)	26 mEq/L (22-30)	26 mmol/L (22-30)
CO_2 content	25 mEq/L (22-28)	25 mmol/L (22-28)	27 mEq/L (24-30)	27 mmol/L (24-30)

Reprinted from Ravel R: *Clinical laboratory medicine,* ed 6, St Louis, 1995, Mosby.
*International system.

TABLE 4-2 Summary of Laboratory Findings in Primary Uncomplicated Respiratory and Metabolic Acid-Base Disorders*

Disorder	Pco_2	pH	Base Excess
Acute primary respiratory hypoactivity (respiratory acidosis)	Increase	Decrease	Normal/positive
Acute primary respiratory hyperactivity (respiratory alkalosis)	Decrease	Increase	Normal/negative
Uncompensated metabolic acidosis	Normal	Decrease	Negative
Uncompensated metabolic alkalosis	Normal	Increase	Positive
Partially compensated metabolic acidosis	Decrease	Decrease	Negative
Partially compensated metabolic alkalosis	Increase	Increase	Positive
Chronic primary respiratory hypoactivity (compensated respiratory acidosis)	Increase	Normal	Positive
Fully compensated metabolic alkalosis	Increase	Normal	Positive
Chronic primary respiratory hyperactivity (compensated respiratory alkalosis)	Decrease	Normal	Negative
Fully compensated metabolic acidosis	Decrease	Normal	Negative

Reprinted from Ravel R: *Clinical laboratory medicine,* ed 6, St Louis, 1995, Mosby.
*Base excess results refer to negative (−) values more than 22 and positive (+) values more than 12.

severe muscle trauma, dermatomyositis/polymyositis, muscular dystrophy, drugs (antibiotics, narcotics, antihypertensive agents, heparin, labetalol, statins, NSAIDs, amiodarone, chlorpromazine, phenytoin), malignancy, renal and pulmonary infarction, convulsions, eclampsia, shock liver

ALBUMIN (serum)
Normal range: 4-6 g/dl (40-60 g/L [CF: 10; SMI: 1 g/L])
Elevated in: Dehydration (relative increase)
Decreased in: Liver disease, nephrotic syndrome, poor nutritional status, rapid IV hydration, protein-losing enteropathies (e.g., inflammatory bowel disease), severe burns, neoplasia, chronic inflammatory diseases, pregnancy, oral contraceptives, prolonged immobilization, lymphomas, hypervitaminosis A, chronic glomerulonephritis

ALCOHOL DEHYDROGENASE
Normal: 0-7 U/L
Elevated in: Drug-induced hepatocellular damage, obstructive jaundice, malignancy, inflammation, infection

ALDOLASE (serum)
Normal range: 0-6 U/L (0-100 nkat/L [CF: 16.67; SMI: 20 nkat/L])
Elevated in: Muscular dystrophy, rhabdomyolysis, dermatomyositis/polymyositis, trichinosis, acute hepatitis and other liver diseases, myocardial infarction, prostatic carcinoma, hemorrhagic pancreatitis, gangrene, delirium tremens, burns
Decreased in: Loss of muscle mass, late stages of muscular dystrophy

ALDOSTERONE
Normal range:
Recumbent: 50-150 ng/L
Upright: 150-300 ng/L
(Highest levels in neonates, decreasing over time to adult levels)
Elevated in: Primary aldosteronism, secondary aldosteronism, pseudoprimary aldosteronism
Decreased in:
Patient with hypertension: diabetes mellitus, Turner's syndrome, acute alcohol intoxication, excess secretion of deoxycorticosterone, corticosterone, and 18-hydroxycorticosterone
Patient without hypertension: Addison's disease, hypoaldosteronism resulting from renin deficiency, isolated aldosterone deficiency

ALKALINE PHOSPHATASE (serum)
Normal range: 30-120 U/L (0.5-2 μkat/L [CF: 0.01667; SMI: 0.1 μkat/L])
Elevated in:
LIVER AND BILIARY TRACT ORIGIN
Extrahepatic bile duct obstruction
Intrahepatic biliary obstruction
Liver cell acute injury
Liver passive congestion
Drug-induced liver cell dysfunction
Space-occupying lesions
Primary biliary cirrhosis
Sepsis
BONE ORIGIN (OSTEOBLAST HYPERACTIVITY)
Physiologic (rapid) bone growth (childhood and adolescence)
Metastatic tumor with osteoblastic reaction
Fracture healing
Paget's disease of bone
CAPILLARY ENDOTHELIAL ORIGIN
Granulation tissue formation (active)
PLACENTAL ORIGIN
Pregnancy
Some parenteral albumin preparations
OTHER
Thyrotoxicosis
Benign transient hyperphosphatasemia
Primary hyperparathyroidism
Decreased in: Hypothyroidism, pernicious anemia, hypophosphatemia, hypervitaminosis D, malnutrition

ALPHA-1-ANTITRYPSIN (serum)
Normal range: 110-140 mg/dl
Decreased in: Homozygous or heterozygous deficiency

ALPHA-1-FETOPROTEIN (serum)
See α-1 FETOPROTEIN

ALT
See ALANINE AMINOTRANSFERASE

ALUMINUM (serum)
Normal range: 0-6 ng/ml
Elevated in: Chronic renal failure on dialysis, parenteral nutrition, industrial exposure

AMEBIASIS SEROLOGIC TEST
Test description: Test is used to support diagnosis of amebiasis caused by *Entamoeba histolytica*. Serum acute and convalescent titers are drawn 1-3 weeks apart. A fourfold increase in titer is the most indicative result.

AMINOLEVULIC ACID (d-ALA) (24-h urine collection)
Normal: 1.5-7.5 mg/day
Elevated in: Acute porphyries, lead poisoning, DKA, pregnancy, anticonvulsant drugs, hereditary tyrosinemia
Decreased in: Alcoholic liver disease

AMMONIA (serum)
Normal range: 10-80 μg/dl (5-50 μmol/L [CF: 0.5872; SMI: 5 μmol/L])
Elevated in: Hepatic failure, hepatic encephalopathy, Reye's syndrome, portacaval shunt, drugs (diuretics, polymyxin B, methicillin)
Decreased in: Drugs (neomycin, lactulose, tetracycline), renal failure

AMYLASE (serum)
Normal range: 0-130 U/L (0-2.17 μkat/L [CF: 0.01667; SMI: 0.01 μkat/L])
Elevated in: Acute pancreatitis, pancreatic neoplasm, abscess, pseudocyst, ascites, macroamylasemia, perforated peptic ulcer, intestinal obstruction, intestinal infarction, acute cholecystitis, appendicitis, ruptured ectopic pregnancy, salivary gland inflammation, peritonitis, burns, diabetic ketoacidosis, renal insufficiency, drugs (morphine), carcinomatosis (of lung, esophagus, ovary), acute ethanol ingestion, mumps, prostate tumors, post–endoscopic retrograde cholangiopancreatography, bulimia, anorexia nervosa
Decreased in: Advanced chronic pancreatitis, hepatic necrosis, cystic fibrosis

AMYLASE, URINE
See URINE AMYLASE

AMYLOID A PROTEIN (serum)
Normal: <10 mcg/ml
Elevated in: Inflammatory disorders (acute phase–reacting protein), infections, acute coronary syndrome, malignancies

ANA
See ANTINUCLEAR ANTIBODY

ANCA
See ANTINEUTROPHIL CYTOPLASMIC ANTIBODY

ANDROSTENEDIONE (serum)
Normal:
Male: 75-205 ng/dl
Female: 85-275 ng/dl
Elevated in: Congenital adrenal hyperplasia, polycystic ovary syndrome, ectopic ACTH-producing tumor, Cushing's syndrome, hirsutism, hyperplasia of ovarian stroma, ovarian neoplasm
Decreased in: Ovarian failure, adrenal failure, sickle cell anemia

ANGIOTENSIN II

Normal: 10-60 pg/ml
Elevated in: Hypertension, CHF, cirrhosis, renin-secreting renal tumor, volume depletion
Decreased in: ACE inhibitor drugs, ARB drugs, primary aldosteronism, Cushing's syndrome

ANGIOTENSIN-CONVERTING ENZYME (ACE level)

Normal range: <40 nmol/ml/min (<670 nkat/L [CF: 16.67; SMI: 10 nkat/L])
Elevated in: Sarcoidosis, primary biliary cirrhosis, alcoholic liver disease, hyperthyroidism, hyperparathyroidism, diabetes mellitus, amyloidosis, multiple myeloma, lung disease (asbestosis, silicosis, berylliosis, allergic alveolitis, coccidioidomycosis), Gaucher's disease, leprosy

ANION GAP

Normal range: 9-14 mEq/L
Elevated in: Lactic acidosis, ketoacidosis (diabetes, alcoholic starvation), uremia (chronic renal failure), ingestion of toxins (paraldehyde, methanol, salicylates, ethylene glycol), hyperosmolar nonketotic coma, antibiotics (carbenicillin)
Decreased in: Hypoalbuminemia, severe hypermagnesemia, IgG myeloma, lithium toxicity, laboratory error (falsely decreased sodium or overestimation of bicarbonate or chloride), hypercalcemia of parathyroid origin, antibiotics (e.g., polymyxin)

ANTICARDIOLIPIN ANTIBODY (ACA)

Normal range: Negative. Test includes detection of IgG, IgM, and IgA antibodies to phospholipid, cardiolipin
Present in: Antiphospholipid antibody syndrome, chronic hepatitis C

ANTICOAGULANT

See CIRCULATING ANTICOAGULANT

ANTIDIURETIC HORMONE

Normal range: mOsm/kg 295-300 4-12 pg/ml[EN4]
Elevated in: SIADH, antipsychotic medications, ectopic ADH from systemic neoplasm, Guillain-Barré syndrome, CNS infections, brain tumors, nephrogenic diabetes insipidus
Decreased in: Central diabetes insipidus, nephritic syndrome, psychogenic polydipsias, demeclocycline, lithium, phenytoin, alcohol

ANTI-DNA

Normal range: Absent
Present in: Systemic lupus erythematosus, chronic active hepatitis, infectious mononucleosis, biliary cirrhosis

ANTI-ds DNA

Normal: <25 U
Elevated in: Systemic lupus erythematosus

ANTIGLOMERULAR BASEMENT ANTIBODY

See GLOMERULAR BASEMENT MEMBRANE ANTIBODY

ANTIHISTONE

Normal: <1 U
Elevated in: Drug-induced lupus erythematosus

ANTIMITOCHONDRIAL ANTIBODY

Normal range: <1:20 titer
Elevated in: Primary biliary cirrhosis (85%-95%), chronic active hepatitis (25%-30%), cryptogenic cirrhosis (25%-30%)

ANTINEUTROPHIL CYTOPLASMIC ANTIBODY (ANCA)

Positive test: Cytoplasmic pattern (cANCA): positive in Wegener's granulomatosis
Perinuclear pattern (pANCA): positive in inflammatory bowel disease, primary biliary cirrhosis, primary sclerosing cholangitis, autoimmune chronic active hepatitis, crescenteric glomerulonephritis

ANTINUCLEAR ANTIBODY (ANA)

Normal range: <1:20 titer
Positive test: Systemic lupus erythematosus (more significant if titer >1:160), drugs (phenytoin, ethosuximide, primidone, methyldopa, hydralazine, carbamazepine, penicillin, procainamide, chlorpromazine, griseofulvin, thiazides), chronic active hepatitis, age over 60 years (particularly age over 80 years), rheumatoid arthritis, scleroderma, mixed connective tissue disease, necrotizing vasculitis, Sjögren's syndrome, tuberculosis, pulmonary interstitial fibrosis. Table 4-3 describes diseases associated with ANA subtypes. Fig. 4-1 illustrates various fluorescent ANA test patterns.

TABLE 4-3 Disease-Associated ANA Subtypes

Nuclear Location	Disease(s)
"Native" DNA (dsDNA, or dsDNA/ssDNA complex)	SLE (60%-70%; range, 35%-75%) Also PSS (5%-55%), MCTD (11%-25%), RA (5%-40%), DM (5%-25%), SS (5%)
sNP	SLE (50%) Also other collagen diseases
DNP (DNA-histone complex)	SLE (52%) Also MCTD (8%), RA (3%)
Histones	Drug-induced SLE (95%) Also SLE (30%), RA (15%-24%)
ENA Sm	SLE (30%-40%; range, 28%-40%) Also MCTD (0%-8%); RNP (U1-RNP) MCTD (in high titer without any other ANA subtype present: 95%-100%) Also SLE (26%-50%), PSS (11%-22%), RA (10%), SS (3%)
SS-A (Ro)*	SS without RA (60%-70%) Also SLE (26%-50%), neonatal SLE (over 95%), PSS (30%), MCTD (50%), SS with RA (9%), PBC (15%-19%)
SS-B (La)	SS without RA (40%-60%) Also SLE (5%-15%), SS with RA (5%)
Scl-70*	PSS (15%-43%)
Centromere*	CREST syndrome (70%-90%; range 57%-96%) Also PSS (4%-20%), PBC (12%)
Nucleolar	PSS (scleroderma) (54%-90%) Also SLE (25%-26%), RA (9%)
RAP (RANA)	SS with RA (60%-76%) Also SS without RA (5%)
Jo-1	Polymyositis (30%)
PM-1	Polymyositis or PMS/PSS overlap syndrome (60%-90%) Also DM (17%)
ssDNA	SLE (60%-70%) Also CAH, infectious mononucleosis, RA, chronic GN, chronic infections, PBC

Cytoplasmic Location	Disease(s)
Mitochondrial	Primary biliary cirrhosis (90%-100%) Also CAH (7%-30%), cryptogenic cirrhosis (30%), acute hepatitis, viral hepatitis (3%), other liver diseases (0%-20%), SLE (5%), SS and PSS (8%)
Microsomal†	Chronic active hepatitis (60%-80%), Hashimoto's thyroiditis (97%)
Ribosomal	SLE (5%-12%)
Smooth muscle‡	Chronic active hepatitis (60%-91%) Also cryptogenic cirrhosis (28%), acute hepatitis, viral hepatitis (5%-87%), infectious mononucleosis (81%), MS (40%-50%), malignancy (67%), PBC (10%-50%)

Reprinted from Ravel R: *Clinical laboratory medicine,* ed 6, St Louis, 1995, Mosby.
CAH, Chronic active hepatitis; *DM,* dermatomyositis; *GN,* glomerulonephritis; *MS,* multiple sclerosis; *PBC,* primary biliary cirrhosis; *SS,* Sjögren's syndrome.
*Not detected using rat or mouse liver or kidney tissue method.
†Not detected by cultured cell method.
‡Detected by cultured cells but better with rat or mouse tissue.

Laboratory Tests

IV

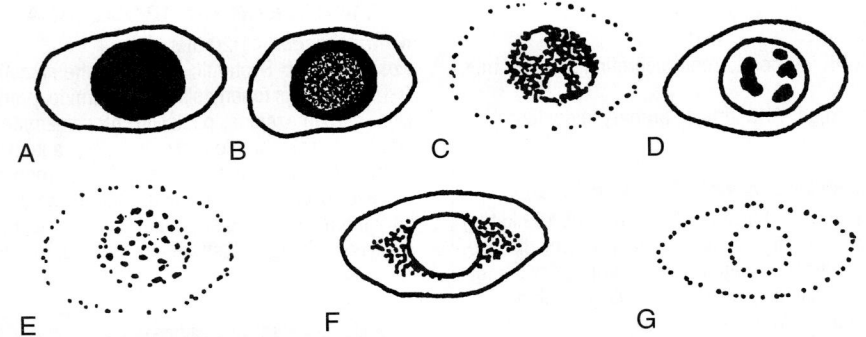

FIGURE 4-1 Fluorescent antinuclear antibody test patterns (HEP-2 cells). A, Solid (homogeneous). **B,** Peripheral (rim). **C,** Speckled. **D,** Nucleolar. **E,** Anticentromere. **F,** Antimitochondrial. **G,** Normal (nonreactive). (Reprinted from Ravel R [ed]: *Clinical laboratory medicine,* ed 6, St Louis, 1995, Mosby.)

ANTI-RNP ANTIBODY

See EXTRACTABLE NUCLEAR ANTIGEN

ANTI-Scl-70

Normal: Absent
Elevated in: Scleroderma

ANTI-Sm (anti-Smith) ANTIBODY

See EXTRACTABLE NUCLEAR ANTIGEN

ANTI-SMOOTH MUSCLE ANTIBODY

See SMOOTH MUSCLE ANTIBODY

ANTISTREPTOLYSIN O TITER (Streptozyme, ASLO titer)

Normal range for adults: <160 Todd units
Elevated in: Streptococcal upper airway infection, acute rheumatic fever, acute glomerulonephritis, increased levels of β-lipoprotein
  NOTE: A fourfold increase in titer between acute and convalescent specimens is diagnostic of streptococcal upper airway infection regardless of the initial titer.

ANTITHROMBIN III

Normal range: 81%-120% of normal activity; 17-30 mg/dl
Decreased in: Hereditary deficiency of antithrombin III, disseminated intravascular coagulation, pulmonary embolism, cirrhosis, thrombolytic therapy, chronic liver failure, postsurgery, third trimester of pregnancy, oral contraceptives, nephrotic syndrome, IV heparin >3 days, sepsis, acute leukemia, carcinoma, thrombophlebitis
Elevated in: Warfarin drugs, post–myocardial infarction

APOLIPOPROTEIN A-1 (Apo A-1)

Normal: Recommended >120 mg/dl
Elevated in: Familial hyperalphalipoproteinemia, statins, niacin, estrogens, weight loss, familial cholesteryl ester transfer protein (CETP) deficiency
Decreased in: Familial hypoalphalipoproteinemia, Tangier disease, diuretics, androgens, cigarette smoking, hepatocellular disorders, chronic renal failure, nephritic syndrome, coronary heart disease, cholestasis

APOLIPOPROTEIN B (Apo B)

Normal: Desirable <100 mg/dl; high risk >120 mg/dl
Elevated in: High saturated fat diet, high-cholesterol diet, hyperapobetalipoproteinemia, familial combined hyperlipidemia, anabolic steroids, diuretics, beta-blockers, corticosteroids, progestins, diabetes, hypothyroidism, chronic renal failure, liver disease, Cushing's syndrome, coronary heart disease
Decreased in: Statins, niacin, low-cholesterol diet, malnutrition, abetalipoproteinemia, hypobetalipoproteinemia, hyperthyroidism

ARTERIAL BLOOD GASES

Normal range:
Po_2: 75-100 mm Hg
Pco_2: 35-45 mm Hg
HCO_3: 24-28 mEq/L
pH: 7.35-7.45
Abnormal values: Acid-base disturbances (see the following)
METABOLIC ACIDOSIS
Metabolic acidosis with increased AG (AG acidosis)
Lactic acidosis
Ketoacidosis (diabetes mellitus, alcoholic ketoacidosis)
Uremia (chronic renal failure)
Ingestion of toxins (paraldehyde, methanol, salicylate, ethylene glycol)
High-fat diet (mild acidosis)
Metabolic acidosis with normal AG (hyperchloremic acidosis)
Renal tubular acidosis (including acidosis of aldosterone deficiency)
Intestinal loss of HCO_3^- (diarrhea, pancreatic fistula)
Carbonic anhydrase inhibitors (e.g., acetazolamide)
Dilutional acidosis (as a result of rapid infusion of bicarbonate-free isotonic saline)
Ingestion of exogenous acids (ammonium chloride, methionine, cystine, calcium chloride)
Ileostomy
Ureterosigmoidostomy
Drugs: amiloride, triamterene, spironolactone, β-blockers
RESPIRATORY ACIDOSIS
Pulmonary disease (COPD, severe pneumonia, pulmonary edema, interstitial fibrosis)
Airway obstruction (foreign body, severe bronchospasm, laryngospasm)
Thoracic cage disorders (pneumothorax, flail chest, kyphoscoliosis)
Defects in muscles of respiration (myasthenia gravis, hypokalemia, muscular dystrophy)
Defects in peripheral nervous system (amyotrophic lateral sclerosis, poliomyelitis, Guillain-Barré syndrome, botulism, tetanus, organophosphate poisoning, spinal cord injury)
Depression of respiratory center (anesthesia, narcotics, sedatives, vertebral artery embolism or thrombosis, increased intracranial pressure)
Failure of mechanical ventilator
METABOLIC ALKALOSIS
Divided into chloride-responsive (urinary chloride <15 mEq/L) and chloride-resistant forms (urinary chloride level >15 mEq/L)
Chloride-responsive
Vomiting
Nasogastric (NG) suction
Diuretics
Posthypercapnic alkalosis
Stool losses (laxative abuse, cystic fibrosis, villous adenoma)
Massive blood transfusion
Exogenous alkali administration

Chloride-resistant
Hyperadrenocorticoid states (Cushing's syndrome, primary hyperaldosteronism, secondary mineralocorticoidism [licorice, chewing tobacco])
Hypomagnesemia
Hypokalemia
Bartter's syndrome
RESPIRATORY ALKALOSIS
Hypoxemia (pneumonia, pulmonary embolism, atelectasis, high-altitude living)
Drugs (salicylates, xanthines, progesterone, epinephrine, thyroxine, nicotine)
Central nervous system (CNS) disorders (tumor, cerebrovascular accident [CVA], trauma, infections)
Psychogenic hyperventilation (anxiety, hysteria)
Hepatic encephalopathy
Gram-negative sepsis
Hyponatremia
Sudden recovery from metabolic acidosis
Assisted ventilation

ARTHROCENTESIS FLUID
Interpretation of results:
1. **Color:** Normally it is clear or pale yellow; cloudiness indicates inflammatory process or presence of crystals, cell debris, fibrin, or triglycerides.
2. **Viscosity:** Normally it has a high viscosity because of hyaluronate; when fluid is placed on a slide, it can be stretched to a string >2 cm in length before separating (low viscosity indicates breakdown of hyaluronate [lysosomal enzymes from leukocytes] or the presence of edema fluid).
3. **Mucin clot:** Add 1 ml of fluid to 5 ml of a 5% acetic acid solution and allow 1 minute for the clot to form; a firm clot (does not fragment on shaking) is normal and indicates the presence of large molecules of hyaluronic acid (this test is nonspecific and infrequently done).
4. **Glucose:** Normally it approximately equals serum glucose level; a difference of more than 40 mg/dl is suggestive of infection.
5. **Protein:** Total protein concentration is <2.5 g/dl in the normal synovial fluid; it is elevated in inflammatory and septic arthritis.
6. **Microscopic examination for crystals**
   a. **Gout:** Monosodium urate crystals
   b. **Pseudogout:** Calcium pyrophosphate dihydrate crystals

ASLO TITER
See ANTISTREPTOLYSIN O TITER

ASPARTATE AMINOTRANSFERASE (AST, SGOT)
Normal range: 0-35 U/L (0-0.58 μkat/L [CF: 0.01667, SMI: 0.01μkat/L])
Elevated in:
HEART
Acute myocardial infarction
Pericarditis (active: some cases)
LIVER
Hepatitis virus, Epstein-Barr, or cytomegalovirus infection
Active cirrhosis
Liver passive congestion or hypoxia
Alcohol- or drug-induced liver dysfunction
Space-occupying lesions (active)
Fatty liver (severe)
Extrahepatic biliary obstruction (early)
Drug-induced
SKELETAL MUSCLE
Acute skeletal muscle injury
Muscle inflammation (infectious or noninfectious)
Muscular dystrophy (active)
Recent surgery
Delirium tremens
KIDNEY
Acute injury or damage
Renal infarct
OTHER
Intestinal infarction
Shock

Cholecystitis
Acute pancreatitis
Hypothyroidism
Heparin therapy (60%-80% of cases)

ATRIAL NATRIURETIC HORMONE (ANH)
Normal: 20-77 pg/ml
Elevated in: CHF, volume overload, cardiovascular disease with high filling pressure
Decreased with: Prazosin and other alpha blockers

B-type NATRIURETIC PEPTIDE
Normal range: up to 100 mcg/L. Natriuretic peptides are secreted to regulate fluid volume, blood pressure, and electrolyte balance. They have activity in both the central and peripheral nervous systems. In humans the main source of circulatory BNP is the heart ventricles.
Elevated in: Heart failure. This test is useful in the emergency department setting to differentiate heart failure patients from those with chronic obstructive pulmonary disease presenting with dyspnea. Levels are also increased in asymptomatic left ventricular dysfunction, arterial and pulmonary hypertension, cardiac hypertrophy, valvular heart disease, arrhythmia, and acute coronary syndrome.

BASOPHIL COUNT
Normal range: 0.4%-1% of total WBC; 40-100/mm^3
Elevated in: Leukemia, inflammatory processes, polycythemia vera, Hodgkin's lymphoma, hemolytic anemia, after splenectomy, myeloid metaplasia, myxedema
Decreased in: Stress, hypersensitivity reaction, steroids, pregnancy, hyperthyroidism, postirradiation

BICARBONATE
Normal: Arterial: 21-28 mEq/L
Venous: 22-29 mEq/L
Elevated in: Metabolic alkalosis, compensated respiratory acidosis, diuretics, corticosteroids, laxative abuse
Decreased in: Metabolic acidosis, compensated respiratory alkalosis, acetazolamide, cyclosporine, cholestyramine, methanol or ethylene glycol poisoning

BILE ACID BREATH TEST (breath test, hydrogen breath test)
Normal: The test determines the radioactivity of $_{14}CO_2$ in breath samples at 2 and 4 hr.
  2 hr after dose: 0.11 ± 0.14
  4 hr after dose: 0.52 ± 0.09
Elevated in: GI bacterial overgrowth, disease or resection of terminal ileum and other H$_2$ blocker USF cimetidine

BILE, URINE
See URINE BILE

BILIRUBIN, DIRECT (conjugated bilirubin)
Normal range: 0-0.2 mg/dl (0-4 μmol/L [CF: 17.10; SMI: 2 μmol/L])
Elevated in: Hepatocellular disease, biliary obstruction, drug-induced cholestasis, hereditary disorders (Dubin-Johnson syndrome, Rotor's syndrome)

BILIRUBIN, INDIRECT (unconjugated bilirubin)
Normal range: 0-1.0 mg/dl (2-18 μmol/L [CF: 17.10; SMI: 2 μmol/L])
Elevated in:
A. Increased bilirubin production (if normal liver, serum unconjugated bilirubin is usually less than 4 mg/100 ml)
  1. Hemolytic anemia
    a. Acquired
    b. Congenital
  2. Resorption from extravascular sources
    a. Hematomas
    b. Pulmonary infarcts

3. Excessive ineffective erythropoiesis
   a. Congenital (congenital dyserythropoietic anemias)
   b. Acquired (pernicious anemia, severe lead poisoning; if present, bilirubinemia is usually mild)
B. Defective hepatic unconjugated bilirubin clearance (defective uptake or conjugation)
   1. Severe liver disease
   2. Gilbert's syndrome
   3. Crigler-Najjar type I or II
   4. Drug-induced inhibition
   5. Portacaval shunt
   6. Congestive heart failure
   7. Hyperthyroidism (uncommon)

BILIRUBIN, TOTAL

Normal range: 0-1.0 mg/dl (2-18 μmol/L [CF: 17.10, SMI: 2 μmol/L])
Elevated in: Liver disease (hepatitis, cirrhosis, cholangitis, neoplasm, biliary obstruction, infectious mononucleosis), hereditary disorders (Gilbert's disease, Dubin-Johnson syndrome), drugs (steroids, statins, niacin, acetaminophen, diphenylhydantoin, phenothiazines, penicillin, erythromycin, clindamycin, captopril, amphotericin B, sulfonamides, azathioprine, isoniazid, 5-aminosalicylic acid, allopurinol, methyldopa, indomethacin, halothane, oral contraceptives, procainamide, tolbutamide, labetalol), hemolysis, pulmonary embolism or infarct, hepatic congestion secondary to congestive heart failure

BILIRUBIN, URINE

See URINE BILE

BLADDER TUMOR ASSOCIATED ANTIGEN

Normal: ≤14 U/ml. Test is used to detect bladder cancer recurrence. Sensitivity 57%-83% and specificity 68%-72%.
Elevated in: Bladder cancer, renal stones, nephritis, UTI, hematuria, renal cancer, cystitis, recent bladder or urinary tract trauma

BLEEDING TIME (modified Ivy method)

Normal range: 2 to 9.5 min
Elevated in: Thrombocytopenia, capillary wall abnormalities, platelet abnormalities (Bernard-Soulier disease, Glanzmann's disease), drugs (aspirin, warfarin, anti-inflammatory medications, streptokinase, urokinase, dextran, β-lactam antibiotics, moxalactam), disseminated intravascular coagulation, cirrhosis, uremia, myeloproliferative disorders, von Willebrand's disease

BLOOD VOLUME, TOTAL

Normal: 60-80 ml/kg
Elevated in: Polycythemia vera, pulmonary disease, CHF, renal insufficiency, pregnancy, acidosis, thyrotoxicosis
Decreased in: Anemia, hemorrhage, vomiting, diarrhea, dehydration, burns, starvation

BORDETELLA PERTUSSIS SEROLOGY

Test description: PCR of nasopharyngeal aspirates or secretions is used to identify *Bordetella pertussis*, the organism responsible for whooping cough.

BRCA ANALYSIS

DESCRIPTION OF ANALYSIS

Comprehensive BRCA analysis:
BRCA1: Full sequence determination in both forward and reverse directions of approximately 5500 base pairs comprising 22 coding exons and one noncoding exon (exon 4) and approximately 800 adjacent base pairs in the noncoding intervening sequence (intron). Exon 1, which is noncoding, is not analyzed. The wild-type *BRCA1* gene encodes a protein comprising 1863 amino acids.
BRCA2: Full sequence determination in both forward and reverse directions of approximately 10,200 base pairs comprising 26 coding exons and approximately 900 adjacent base pairs in the noncoding intervening sequence (intron). Exon 1, which is noncoding, is not analyzed. The wild-type *BRCA2* gene encodes a protein comprising 3418 amino acids.
The noncoding intronic regions of *BRCA1* and *BRCA2* that are analyzed do not extend more than 20 base pairs proximal to the 5′ end and 10 base pairs distal to the 3′ end of each exon.

Single-site bracanalysis: DNA sequence analysis for a specified mutation in *BRCA1* and/or *BRCA2*.
Multisite 3 bracanalysis: DNA sequence analysis of specific portions of *BRCA1* exon 2, *BRCA1* exon 20, and *BRCA2* exon 11 designed to detect only mutations 187delAG and 5385insC in *BRCA1* and 6174delT in *BRCA2*.

Interpretive Criteria:
"Positive for a deleterious mutation": Includes all mutations (nonsense, insertions, deletions) that prematurely terminate ("truncate") the protein product of *BRCA1* at least 10 amino acids from the C-terminus, or the protein product of *BRCA2* at least 110 amino acids from the C-terminus (based on documentation of deleterious mutations in *BRCA1* and *BRCA2*).
In addition, specific missense mutations and noncoding intervening sequence (IVS) mutations are recognized as deleterious on the basis of data derived from linkage analysis of high-risk families, functional assays, biochemical evidence, and/or demonstration of abnormal mRNA transcript processing.
"Genetic variant, suspected deleterious": Includes genetic variants for which the available evidence indicates a likelihood, but not proof, that the mutation is deleterious. The specific evidence supporting such an interpretation will be summarized for individual variants on each such report.
"Genetic variant, favor polymorphism": Includes genetic variants for which available evidence indicates that the variant is highly unlikely to contribute substantially to cancer risk. The specific evidence supporting such an interpretation will be summarized for individual variants on each such report.
"Genetic variant of uncertain significance": Includes missense mutations and mutations that occur in analyzed intronic regions whose clinical significance has not yet been determined, as well as chain-terminating mutations that truncate *BRCA1* and *BRCA2* distal to amino acid positions 1853 and 3308, respectively.
"No deleterious mutation detected": Includes nontruncating genetic variants observed at an allele frequency of approximately 1% of a suitable control population (providing that no data suggest clinical significance), as well as all genetic variants for which published data demonstrate absence of substantial clinical significance. Also includes mutations in the protein-coding region that neither alter the amino acid sequence nor are predicted to significantly affect exon splicing, and base pair alterations in noncoding portions of the gene that have been demonstrated to have no deleterious effect on the length or stability of the mRNA transcript.
There may be uncommon genetic abnormalities in *BRCA1* and *BRCA2* that will not be detected by *BRCA* analysis. This analysis, however, is believed to rule out the majority of abnormalities in these genes, which are believed responsible for most hereditary susceptibility to breast and ovarian cancer.
"Specific variant/mutation not identified": Specific and designated deleterious mutations or variants of uncertain clinical significance are not present in the individual being tested. If one (or rarely two) specific deleterious mutations have been identified in a family member, a negative analysis for the specific mutation(s) indicates that the tested individual is at the general population risk of developing breast or ovarian cancer.

BREATH HYDROGEN TEST (hydrogen breath test)

Normal: This test is for bacterial overgrowth. H_2 excretion fasting: 4.6 ± 5.1, after lactulose, early increase <12. Lactulose usually results in a colonic response >30 min after ingestion.
Elevated in: A high fasting breath H_2 level and an increase of at least 12 ppm within 30 min after lactulose challenge are indicative of bacterial overgrowth in the small intestine. The increase must precede the colonic response.
Fast positives in: Accelerated gastric emptying, laxative use
Fast negatives in: Use of antibiotics and patients who are nonhydrogen producers

BUN

See UREA NITROGEN, BLOOD

C282Y AND H63D MUTATION ANALYSIS

Procedure: Detection of the C282Y and H63D mutations is accomplished by amplification of exons 2 and 4 of the *HFE* gene on chromosome 6 by polymerase chain reaction (PCR) followed by allele-specific hybridization and chemiluminescent detection of hybridized probes. H63D is viewed by some as a polymorphism rather than a mutation because of its prevalence in the population, because 15% of the individuals affected with hereditary hemochromatosis (HH) are compound heterozygotes for C282Y and H63D and about 1% of patients are H63D homozygotes, which suggests that H63D may be causative in the development of the disorder at reduced penetrance.

Interpretation: Homozygosity for the C282Y mutation has been associated with an increased risk of being affected with HH compared with the general population. The genotype is observed in 60%-90% of individuals affected with HH and occurs in less than 1% of the general population. However, approximately 25% of asymptomatic individuals with this genotype do not develop the disorder.

C3

See COMPLEMENT

C4

See COMPLEMENT

CALCITONIN (serum)

Normal range: <100 pg/ml (<100 ng/L [CF: 1; SMI: 10 ng/L])
Elevated in: Medullary carcinoma of the thyroid (particularly if level >1500 pg/ml), carcinoma of the breast, apudomas, carcinoids, renal failure, thyroiditis

CALCIUM (serum)

Normal range: 8.8-10.3 mg/dl (2.2-2.58 μmol/L [CF: 0.2495; SMI: 0.02 μmol/L])

ELEVATED

Relatively common:
Neoplasia
Bone primary
Myeloma
Acute leukemia
Nonbone solid tumors
Breast
Lung
Squamous nonpulmonary
Kidney
Neoplasm secretion of parathyroid hormone-related protein (PTHrP, "ectopic PTH")
Primary hyperparathyroidism
Thiazide diuretics
Tertiary (renal) hyperparathyroidism
Idiopathic
Spurious (artifactual) hypercalcemia
Dehydration
Serum protein elevation
Laboratory technical problem (lab error)

Relatively uncommon:
Sarcoidosis
Hyperthyroidism
Immobilization (mostly seen in children and adolescents)
Diuretic phase of acute renal tubular necrosis
Vitamin D intoxication
Milk-alkali syndrome
Addison's disease
Lithium therapy
Idiopathic hypercalcemia of infancy
Acromegaly
Theophylline toxicity

Table 4-4 describes the laboratory differential diagnosis of hypercalcemia.

DECREASED
Artifactual
Hypoalbuminemia
Hemodilution
Primary hypoparathyroidism
Pseudohypoparathyroidism
Vitamin D–related
Vitamin D deficiency
Malabsorption
Renal failure

TABLE 4-4 Laboratory Differential Diagnosis of Hypercalcemia

Diagnosis	PLASMA TESTS					URINE TESTS			Comments
	Ca	PO$_4$	PTH	25(OH)D	1,25(OH)$_2$D	cAMP	TmP/GFR	Ca	
Primary hyperparathyroidism	↑	N/↓	↑	N	N/↑	↑	↓	↑	Parathyroid adenoma most common
MEN I									Parathyroid hyperplasia; also includes pituitary and pancreatic neoplasms
MEN IIa									Parathyroid hyperplasia; also includes medullary thyroid carcinoma and heochromocytoma
MEN IIb									Parathyroid disease uncommon, primarily medullary thyroid carcinoma and pheochromocytoma
FHH	↑	N	N/↑	N	N	N/↑	N/↓	↓↓	Autosomal dominant inheritance; hypercalcemia present within first decade; benign
Malignancy									
Solid tumor, humoral	↑	N/↓	↓	N	N	↑	↓	↑↑	Primarily epidermoid tumors; PTH-related protein(s) is mediator
Solid tumor, osteolytic	↑	N/↑	↓	N	N	↓	↑	↑↑	
Lymphoma	↑	N/↑	↓	N/↓	↑	↓	↑	↑↑	
Granulomatous disease	↑	N/↑	↓	N/↓	↑↑	↓	↑	↑↑	Sarcoid most common etiology
Vitamin D intoxication	↑	N/↑	↓	↑↑	N	↓	↑	↑↑	
Hyperthyroidism	↑	N	↓	N	N	N	N	↑↑	Plasma concentrations of T$_4$ and/or T$_3$ are elevated

Reprinted from Moore WT, Eastman RC: *Diagnostic endocrinology,* ed 2, St Louis, 1996, Mosby.
Ca, Calcium; *cAMP,* cyclic adenosine monophosphate; *FHH,* familial hypocalciuric hypercalcemia; *GFR,* glomerular filtration rate; *MEN,* multiple endocrine neoplasia; *25(OH)D,* 25 hydroxyvitamin D; *PO$_4$,* phosphate; *PTH,* parathyroid hormone; *T$_3$,* triiodothyronine; *T$_4$,* thyroxine; *TmP,* renal threshold for phosphorus.

Laboratory Tests

IV

TABLE 4-5 Laboratory Differential Diagnosis of Hypocalcemia

Diagnosis	Ca	PO$_4$	PTH	25(OH)D	1,25(OH)$_2$D	cAMP	cAMP after PTH	TmP/GFR	TmP/GFR after PTH	Ca	Comments
				PLASMA TESTS				URINE TESTS			
Hypopara-thyroidism	↓	↑	N/↓	N	↓	↓	↑↑	↑	↓↓	N/↓	Deficiency of PTH
Pseudohypoparathyroidism											
Type I	↓	↑	↑↑	N	↓	↓	NC	↑	↑	N/↓	Resistance to PTH; patients may have Albright's hereditary osteodystrophy and resistance to multiple hormones
Type II	↓	N	↑↑	N	↓	↓	↑	↑	↑	N/↓	Renal resistance to cAMP
Vitamin D deficiency	↓	N/↓	↑↑	↓↓	N/↓	↑	↑	↓	↓	↓↓	Deficient supply (e.g., nutrition) or absorption (e.g., pancreatic insufficiency) of vitamin D
Vitamin D–dependent rickets											
Type I	↓	N/↓	↑↑	N	↓	↑		↓		↓↓	Deficient activity of renal 25(OH)D-1a-hydroxylase
Type II	↓	N/↓	↑↑	N	↑↑	↑		↓		↓↓	Resistance to 1,25(OH)$_2$D

Reprinted from Moore WT, Eastman RC: *Diagnostic endocrinology*, ed 2, St Louis, 1996, Mosby.
Ca, Calcium; *cAMP,* cyclic adenosine monophosphate; *FHH,* familial hypocalciuric hypercalcemia; *GFR,* glomerular filtration rate; *MEN,* multiple endocrine neoplasia; *NC,* no change or small increase; *(OH)D,* hydroxycalciferol D; *PO$_4$,* phosphate; *PTH,* parathyroid hormone; *T$_3$,* triiodothyronine; *T$_4$,* thyroxine; *TmP,* renal threshold for phosphorus.

Magnesium deficiency
Sepsis
Chronic alcoholism
Tumor lysis syndrome
Rhabdomyolysis
Alkalosis (respiratory or metabolic)
Acute pancreatitis
Drug-induced hypocalcemia
Large doses of magnesium sulfate
Anticonvulsants
Mithramycin
Gentamicin
Cimetidine
Table 4-5 describes the laboratory differential diagnosis of hypocalcemia.

CALCIUM, URINE
See URINE CALCIUM

CANCER ANTIGEN 15-3 (CA 15-3)
Normal: <30 U/ml
Elevated in: Approximately 80% of women with metastatic breast cancer. Clinical sensitivity is 0.60, specificity 0.87, positive predictive value 0.91. This test is generally used to predict recurrence of breast cancer and evaluate response to therapy. May also be elevated in liver cancer, pancreatic cancer, ovarian cancer, colorectal cancer. Elevations can also occur with benign breast and liver disease.

CANCER ANTIGEN 27-29 (CA 27-29)
Normal: <38 U/ml
Elevated in: Approximately 75% of women with metastatic breast cancer. Clinical sensitivity is 0.57, specificity 0.97, positive predictive value 0.83, negative predictive value 0.92. This test is generally used to predict recurrence of breast cancer and evaluate response to therapy. May also be elevated in liver cancer, pancreatic cancer, ovarian cancer, colorectal cancer. Elevations can also occur with benign breast and liver disease.

CANCER ANTIGEN 72-4 (CA 72-4)
Normal: <4.0 ng/ml
Elevated in: Gastric cancer (elevated in >50% of patients). Often used in combination with CA 72-4, CA 19.9, and CEA to monitor gastric cancer after treatment.

CANCER ANTIGEN 125 (CA 125)
Normal range: <1.4%
This test uses an antibody against antigen from tissue culture of an ovarian tumor cell line. Various published evaluations report sensitivity of about 75%-80% in patients with ovarian carcinoma. There is also an appreciable incidence of elevated values in nonovarian malignancies and in certain benign conditions (see below). Test values may transiently increase during chemotherapy.
MALIGNANT
Epithelial ovarian carcinoma, 75%-80% (range, 25%-92%; better in serous than mucinous cystadenocarcinoma)
Endometrial carcinoma, 25%-48% (2%-90%)
Pancreatic carcinoma, 59%
Colorectal carcinoma, 20% (15%-56%)
Endocervical adenocarcinoma, 83%
Squamous cervical or vaginal carcinoma, 7%-14%
Lung carcinoma, 32%
Breast carcinoma, 12%-40%
Lymphoma, 35%
BENIGN
Cirrhosis, 40%-80%
Acute pancreatitis, 38%
Acute peritonitis, 75%
Endometriosis, 88%
Acute pelvic inflammatory disease, 33%
Pregnancy first trimester, 2%-24%
During menstruation (occasionally)
Renal failure (?frequency)
Normal persons, 0.6%-1.4%

CAPTOPRIL STIMULATION TEST
Normal: Test performed by giving 25 mg captopril orally after overnight fast. Patient should be seated during test. After captopril, aldosterone <15 ng/dl, renin >2 ng, angiotensin I/ml/hr
Interpretation: In patients with primary aldosteronism, plasma aldosterone remains high and plasma renin activity remains low after captopril.

CARBAMAZEPINE (Tegretol)
Normal therapeutic range: 4-12 mcg/ml

CARBOHYDRATE ANTIGEN 19-9

Normal: <37.0 U/ml
Elevated in: GI cancer, most frequently pancreatic cancer. Amount of elevation has no relation to tumor mass. Elevations can also occur with cirrhosis, cholangitis, and chronic or acute pancreatitis.

CARBON DIOXIDE, PARTIAL PRESSURE

Normal:
Male: 35-48 mm Hg
Female: 32-45 mm Hg
Elevated in: Respiratory acidosis
Decreased in: Respiratory alkalosis

CARBON MONOXIDE

See CARBOXYHEMOGLOBIN

CARBOXYHEMOGLOBIN

Normal range: Saturation of hemoglobin <2%; smokers <9%
Elevated in: Smoking, exposure to smoking, exposure to automobile exhaust fumes, malfunctioning gas-burning appliances

CARCINOEMBRYONIC ANTIGEN (CEA)

Normal range:
Nonsmokers: 0-2.5 ng/ml (0-2.5 μg/L [CF: 1; SMI: 0.1 μg/L])
Smokers: 0-5 ng/ml (0-5 μg/L [CF: 1; SMI: 0.1 μg/L])
Elevated in:
Colorectal carcinomas, pancreatic carcinomas, and metastatic disease (usually produce higher elevations: >20 ng/ml)
Carcinomas of the esophagus, stomach, small intestine, liver, breast, ovary, lung, and thyroid (usually produce lesser elevations)
Benign conditions (smoking, inflammatory bowel disease, hypothyroidism, cirrhosis, pancreatitis, infections) (usually produce levels <10 ng/ml)

CAROTENE (serum)

Normal range: 50-250 μg/dl (0.9-4.6 μmol/L [CF: 0.01863; SMI: 0.1 μmol/L])
Elevated in: Carotenemia, chronic nephritis, diabetes mellitus, hypothyroidism, nephrotic syndrome, hyperlipidemia
Decreased in: Fat malabsorption, steatorrhea, pancreatic insufficiency, lack of carotenoids in diet, high fever, liver disease

CATECHOLAMINES, URINE

See URINE CATECHOLAMINES

CBC

See COMPLETE BLOOD COUNT

CD40 LIGAND

Normal: <5 mcg/L. CD40 ligand is a soluble protein that is shed from activated leukocytes and platelets and used in risk stratification for acute coronary syndrome.
Elevated in: Acute coronary syndrome. Increased CD40 ligand is associated with higher incidence of death or nonfatal MI.

CD4+ T-LYMPHOCYTE COUNT (CD4+ T-cells)

Calculated as total WBC × % lymphocytes × % lymphocytes stained with CD4.

This test is used primarily to evaluate immune dysfunction in HIV infection. It is useful as a prognostic indicator and as a criterion for initiating prophylaxis for several opportunistic infections that are sequelae of HIV infection. Progressive depletion of CD4+ T-lymphocytes is associated with an increased likelihood of clinical complications (Table 4-6). Adolescents and adults with HIV are classified as having AIDS if their CD4+ lymphocyte count is under 200/μL and/or if their CD4+ T-lymphocyte percentage is less than 14%. HIV-infected patients whose CD4+ count is less than 200/μL and who acquire certain infectious diseases or malignancies are also classified as having AIDS. Corticosteroids decrease CD4+ T-cell percentage and absolute number.

TABLE 4-6 Relation of CD4 Lymphocyte Counts to the Onset of Certain HIV-Associated Infections and Neoplasms in North America

CD4 Count (Cells/mm³)*	Opportunistic Infection or Neoplasm	Frequency (%)†
>500	Herpes zoster, polydermatomal	5-10
200-500	*Mycobacterium tuberculosis* infection, pulmonary and extrapulmonary	2-20
	Oral hairy leukoplakia	40-70
	Candida pharyngitis (thrush)	40-70
	Recurrent *Candida* vaginitis	15-30 (F)
	Kaposi's sarcoma, mucocutaneous	15-30 (M)
	Bacterial pneumonia, recurrent	15-20
	Cervical neoplasia	1-2 (F)
100-200	*Pneumocystis carinii* pneumonia	15-60
	Herpes simplex, chronic, ulcerative	5-10
	Histoplasma capsulatum infection, disseminated	0-20
	Kaposi's sarcoma, visceral	3-8 (M)
	Progressive multifocal leukoencephalopathy	2-3
	Lymphoma, non-Hodgkin's	2-5
<100	*Candida* esophagitis	15-20
	Mycobacterium avium-intracellulare, disseminated	25-40
	Toxoplasma gondii encephalitis	5-25
	Cryptosporidium enteritis	2-10
	CMV retinitis	20-35
	Cryptococcus neoformans encephalitis	2-5
	CMV esophagitis or colitis	6-12
	Lymphoma, central nervous system	4-8

Reprinted from Andreoli TE (ed): *Cecil essentials of medicine,* ed 5, Philadelphia, 2000, WB Saunders.
CMV, Cytomegalovirus; *F,* exclusively in women; *HIV,* human immunodeficiency virus; *M,* almost exclusively in men.
*Table indicates CD4 count at which specific infections or neoplasms generally begin to appear. Each infection may recur or progress during the subsequent course of HIV disease.
†Even within the United States, great regional differences in the incidence of specific opportunistic infections are apparent. For example, disseminated histoplasmosis is common in the Mississippi River drainage area but very rare in individuals who have lived exclusively on the East or West Coast.

CEA

See CARCINOEMBRYONIC ANTIGEN

CEREBROSPINAL FLUID (CSF)

Interpretation of results:
1. Appearance of the fluid
   a. Clear: normal.
   b. Yellow color (xanthochromia) in the supernatant of centrifuged CSF within 1 hour or less after collection is usually the result of previous bleeding (subarachnoid hemorrhage); it may also be caused by increased CSF protein, melanin from meningeal melanosarcomas, or carotenoids.
   c. Pinkish color is usually the result of a bloody tap; the color generally clears progressively from tubes 1 to 4 (the supernatant is usually crystal clear in traumatic taps).
   d. Turbidity usually indicates the presence of leukocytes (bleeding introduces approximately 1 WBC/500 RBCs into the CSF).
2. CSF pressure: elevated pressure can be seen with meningitis, meningoencephalitis, pseudotumor cerebri, mass lesions, and intracerebral bleeding.
3. Cell count: in the adult the CSF is normally free of cells (although up to 5 mononuclear cells/mm³ is considered normal); the presence of granulocytes is never normal.
   a. Neutrophils: seen in bacterial meningitis, early viral meningoencephalitis, and early tuberculosis (TB) meningitis.

TABLE 4-7 Cerebrospinal Fluid Findings in Central Nervous System Disorders

Condition	Pressure (mm H$_2$O)	Leukocytes (mm^3)	Protein (mg/dl)	Glucose (mg/dl)	Comments
Normal	50-80	<5, ≥75% lymphocytes	20-45	>50 (or 75% serum glucose)	
Common Forms of Meningitis					
Acute bacterial meningitis	Usually elevated (100-300)	100-10,000 or more; usually 300-2000; PMNs predominate	Usually 100-500	Decreased, usually <40 (or <66% serum glucose)	Organisms usually seen on Gram stain and recovered by culture; latex agglutination of CSF usually positive
Partially treated bacterial meningitis	Normal or elevated	5-10,000; PMNs usual but mononuclear cells may predominate if pretreated for extended period	Usually 100-500	Normal or decreased	Organisms may be seen on Gram stain; latex agglutination CSF may be positive; pretreatment may render CSF sterile
Viral meningitis or meningoencephalitis	Normal or slightly elevated (80-150)	Rarely >1000 cells; eastern equine encephalitis and lymphocytic choriomeningitis may have cell counts of several thousand; PMNs early but mononuclear cells predominate through most of the course	Usually 50-200	Generally normal; may be decreased to <40 in some viral diseases, particularly mumps (15%-20% of cases)	HSV encephalitis is suggested by focal seizures or by focal findings on CT or MRI scans or EEG. Enteroviruses and HSV infrequently recovered from CSF. HSV and enteroviruses may be detected by PCR of CSF.
Uncommon Forms of Meningitis					
Tuberculous meningitis	Usually elevated	10-500; PMNs early but lymphocytes predominate through most of the course	100-3000; may be higher in presence of block	<50 in most cases; decreases with time if treatment is not provided	Acid-fast organisms almost never seen on smear; organisms may be recovered in culture of large volumes of CSF; *Mycobacterium tuberculosis* may be detected by PCR of CSF
Fungal meningitis	Usually elevated	5-500; PMNs early but mononuclear cells predominate through most of the course; cryptococcal meningitis may have no cellular inflammatory response	25-500	<50; decreases with time if treatment is not provided	Budding yeast may be seen; organisms may be recovered in culture; cryptococcal antigen (CSF and serum) may be positive in cryptococcal infection
Syphilis (acute) and leptospirosis	Usually elevated	50-500; lymphocytes predominate	50-200	Usually normal	Positive CSF serology; spirochetes not demonstrable by usual techniques of smear or culture; darkfield examination may be positive
Amoebic (Naegleria) meningoencephalitis	Elevated	1000-10,000 or more; PMNs predominate	50-500	Normal or slightly decreased	Mobile amebae may be seen by hanging-drop examination of CSF at room temperature

Reprinted from Behrman RE: *Nelson textbook of pediatrics*, ed 17, Philadelphia, 2004, WB Saunders.
CNS, Central nervous system; *CSF*, cerebrospinal fluid; *CT*, computed tomography; *EEG*, electroencephalogram; *HSV*, herpes simplex virus; *MRI*, magnetic resonance imaging; *PCR*, polymerase chain reaction; *PMN*, polymorphonuclear neutrophils.

(Table continued on next page)

   b. Increased lymphocytes: TB meningitis, viral meningoencephalitis, syphilitic meningoencephalitis, fungal meningitis.
4. Protein: serum proteins are generally too large to cross the normal blood–CSF barrier; however, increased CSF protein is seen with meningeal inflammation, traumatic tap, increased CNS synthesis, tissue degeneration, obstruction to CSF circulation, and Guillain-Barré syndrome.
5. Glucose
   a. Decreased glucose is seen with bacterial meningitis, TB meningitis, fungal meningitis, subarachnoid hemorrhage, and some cases of viral meningitis.
   b. A mild increase in CSF glucose can be seen in patients with very elevated serum glucose levels.
Table 4-7 describes CSF findings in central nervous system disorders.

CERULOPLASMIN (serum)

Normal range: 20-35 mg/dl (200-350 mg/L [CF: 10; SMI: 10 mg/L])
Elevated in: Pregnancy, estrogens, oral contraceptives, neoplastic diseases (leukemias, Hodgkin's lymphoma, carcinomas), inflammatory states, systemic lupus erythematosus, primary biliary cirrhosis, rheumatoid arthritis
Decreased in: Wilson's disease (values often <10 mg/dl), nephrotic syndrome, advanced liver disease, malabsorption, total parenteral nutrition, Menkes' syndrome

CHLAMYDIA GROUP ANTIBODY SEROLOGIC TEST

Test description: Acute and convalescent sera is drawn 2-4 weeks apart. A fourfold increase in titer between acute and convalescent sera is necessary for confirmation. A single titer ≥1:64 is considered indicative of psittacosis or LGV.

TABLE 4-7   Cerebrospinal Fluid Findings in Central Nervous System Disorders—cont'd

Condition	Pressure (mm H$_2$O)	Leukocytes (mm^3)	Protein (mg/dl)	Glucose (mg/dl)	Comments
Brain and Parameningeal Abscesses					
Brain abscess	Usually elevated (100-300)	5-200; CSF rarely acellular; lymphocytes predominate; if abscess ruptures into ventricle, PMNs predominate and cell count may reach >100,000	75-500	Normal unless abscess ruptures into ventricular system	No organisms on smear or culture unless abscess ruptures into ventricular system
Subdural empyema	Usually elevated (100-300)	100-5000; PMNs predominate	100-500	Normal	No organisms on smear or culture of CSF unless meningitis also present; organisms found on tap of subdural fluid
Cerebral epidural abscess	Normal to slightly elevated	10-500; lymphocytes predominate	50-200	Normal	No organisms on smear or culture of CSF
Spinal epidural abscess	Usually low, with spinal block	10-100; lymphocytes predominate	50-400	Normal	No organisms on smear or culture of CSF
Chemical (drugs, dermoid cysts, myelography dye)	Usually elevated	100-1000 or more; PMNs predominate	50-100	Normal or slightly decreased	Epithelial cells may be seen within CSF by use of polarized light in some children with dermoids
Noninfectious Causes					
Sarcoidosis	Normal or elevated slightly	0-100; mononuclear	40-100	Normal	No specific findings
Systemic lupus erythematosus with CNS involvement	Slightly elevated	0-500; PMNs usually predominate; lymphocytes may be present	100	Normal or slightly decreased	No organisms on smear or culture; LE preparation may be positive; positive neuronal and ribosomal P protein antibodies in CSF
Tumor, leukemia	Slightly elevated to very high	0-100 or more; mononuclear or blast cells	50-1000	Normal to decreased (20-40)	Cytology may be positive

CHLAMYDIA TRACHOMATIS PCR

Test description: Test is performed on endocervical swab, urine, and intraurethral swab
Normal: Negative

CHLORIDE (serum)

Normal range: 95-105 mEq/L (95-105 mmol/L [CF: 1; SMI: 1 mmol/L])
Elevated in: Dehydration, excessive infusion of normal saline solution, cystic fibrosis (sweat test), hyperparathyroidism, renal tubular disease, metabolic acidosis, prolonged diarrhea, drugs (ammonium chloride administration, acetazolamide, boric acid, triamterene)
Decreased in: Congestive heart failure, syndrome of inappropriate antidiuretic hormone secretion, Addison's disease, vomiting, gastric suction, salt-losing nephritis, continuous infusion of D$_5$W, thiazide diuretic administration, diaphoresis, diarrhea, burns, diabetic ketoacidosis

CHLORIDE (sweat)

Normal: 0-40 mmol/L
Borderline/indeterminate: 41-60 mmol/L
Consistent with cystic fibrosis: >60 mmol/L
False low results can occur with edema, excessive sweating, and hypoproteinemia.

CHLORIDE, URINE

See URINE CHLORIDE

CHOLECYSTOKININ-PANCREOZYMIN (CCK, CCK-PZ)

Normal: <80 pg/ml
Elevated in: Pancreatic disease, celiac disease, gastric ulcer, postgastrectomy, IBS, fatty food intolerance

CHOLESTEROL, HIGH-DENSITY LIPOPROTEIN

See HIGH-DENSITY LIPOPROTEIN CHOLESTEROL

CHOLESTEROL, LOW-DENSITY LIPOPROTEIN

See LOW-DENSITY LIPOPROTEIN CHOLESTEROL

CHOLESTEROL, TOTAL

Normal range: Varies with age
Generally <200 mg/dl (<5.20 mmol/L [CF: 0.02586; SMI: 0.05 mmol/L])
Elevated in: Primary hypercholesterolemia, biliary obstruction, diabetes mellitus, nephrotic syndrome, hypothyroidism, primary biliary cirrhosis, high-cholesterol diet, pregnancy third trimester, myocardial infarction, drugs (steroids, phenothiazines, oral contraceptives)
Decreased in: Medications (statins, niacin), starvation, malabsorption, sideroblastic anemia, thalassemia, abetalipoproteinemia, hyperthyroidism, Cushing's syndrome, hepatic failure, multiple myeloma, polycythemia vera, chronic myelocytic leukemia, myeloid metaplasia, Waldenström's macroglobulinemia, myelofibrosis

CHORIONIC GONADOTROPINS, HUMAN (serum)

Normal range, serum: Female, premenopausal: <0.8 IU/L; postmenopausal <3.3 IU/L
Male: <0.7 IU/L
Elevated in:
Pregnancy, choriocarcinoma, gestational trophoblastic neoplasia (including molar gestations), placental site trophoblastic tumors; human antimouse antibodies (HAMA) can produce false serum assay for hCG.
The principal use of this test is to diagnose pregnancy. The concentration of hCG increases significantly during the initial 6 weeks of pregnancy. Peak values approaching 100,000 IU/L occur 60-70 days following implantation.
hCG levels generally double every 1-3 days. In patients with concentration <2000 IU/L, an increase of serum hCG <66% after 2 days is suggestive of spontaneous abortion or ruptured ectopic gestation.

Laboratory Tests

IV

TABLE 4-8 Characteristics of Coagulation Factors

Factor	Descriptive Name	Source	Approximate Half-Life (hr)	Function
I	Fibrinogen	Liver	120	Substrate for fibrin clot (CP)
II	Prothrombin	Liver (VKD)	60	Serine protease (CP)
V	Proaccelerin, labile factor	Liver	12-36	Cofactor (CP)
VII	Serum prothrombin conversion accelerator, proconvertin	Liver (VKD)	6	(?) Serine protease (EP)
VIII	Antihemophilic factor or globulin	Endothelial cells and (?) elsewhere	12	Cofactor (IP)
IX	Plasma thromboplastin component, Christmas factor	Liver (VKD)	24	Serine protease (IP)
X	Stuart-Prower factor	Liver (VKD)	36	Serine protease (CP)
XI	Plasma thromboplastin antecedent	(?) Liver	40-84	Serine protease (IP)
XII	Hageman factor	(?) Liver	50	Serine protease contact activation (IP)
XIII	Fibrin-stabilizing factor	(?) Liver	96-180	Transglutaminase (CP)
Prekallikrein	Fletcher factor	(?) Liver	?	Serine protease contact activation (IP)
High-molecular-weight kininogen	Fitzgerald factor, Flaujeac or Williams factor	(?) Liver	?	Cofactor, contact activation (IP)

Reprinted from Noble J (ed): *Primary care medicine,* ed 3, St Louis, 2001, Mosby.
CP, Common pathway; *EP,* extrinsic pathway; *IP,* intrinsic pathway; *VKD,* vitamin K dependent.

CHYMOTRYPSIN

Normal: <10 mcg/L
Elevated in: Acute pancreatitis, chronic renal failure, oral enzyme preparations, gastric cancer, pancreatic cancer
Decreased in: Chronic pancreatitis, late cystic fibrosis

CIRCULATING ANTICOAGULANT (lupus anticoagulant)

Normal: Negative
Detected in: Systemic lupus erythematosus, drug-induced lupus, long-term phenothiazine therapy, multiple myeloma, ulcerative colitis, rheumatoid arthritis, postpartum, hemophilia, neoplasms, chronic inflammatory states, AIDS, nephrotic syndrome
   NOTE: The name is a misnomer because these patients are prone to hypercoagulability and thrombosis.

CK

See CREATINE KINASE

CLONIDINE SUPPRESSION TEST

Interpretation: Clonidine inhibits neurogenic catecholamine release and will cause a decrease in plasma norepinephrine into the reference interval in hypertensive subjects without pheochromocytoma. Test is performed by giving 4.3 mcg clonidine/kg orally after overnight fast. Norepinephrine is measured at 3 hr. Result should be within established reference range and decrease to <50% of baseline concentration. Lack of decrease in norepinephrine is suggestive of pheochromocytoma.

CLOSTRIDIUM DIFFICILE TOXIN ASSAY (stool)

Normal: Negative
Detected in: Antibiotic-associated diarrhea and pseudomembranous colitis

CO

See CARBOXYHEMOGLOBIN

COAGULATION FACTORS

See Table 4-8 for characteristics of coagulation factors.
Factor reference ranges:
V: >10%
VII: >10%
VIII: 50%-170%
IX: 60%-136%

X: >10%
XI: 50%-150%
XII: >30%
   Table 4-9 describes screening laboratory results in coagulation factor deficiencies.

COLD AGGLUTININS TITER

Normal range: <1:32
Elevated in:
Primary atypical pneumonia (mycoplasma pneumonia), infectious mononucleosis, CMV infection
Others: hepatic cirrhosis, acquired hemolytic anemia, frostbite, multiple myeloma, lymphoma, malaria

COMPLEMENT

Normal range:
C3: 70-160 mg/dl (0.7-1.6 g/L [CF: 0.01; SMI: 0.1 g/L])
C4: 20-40 mg/dl (0.2-0.4 g/L [CF: 0.01; SMI: 0.1 g/L])

TABLE 4-9 Screening Laboratory Results in Coagulation Factor Deficiencies

Deficient Factor	Frequency	PT	PTT	TT
I (fibrinogen)	Rare	↑	↑	↑
II (prothrombin)	Very rare	↑	↑	↑
V 1:1,000,000	↑		↑	NL
VII	1:500,000	↑	NL	NL
VIII	1:5000 (male)	NL	↑	NL
IX	1:30,000 (male)	NL	↑	NL
X 1:500,000	↑		↑	NL
XI	Rare*	NL	↑	NL
XII or HMWK or PK†	Rare	NL	↑	NL
XIII	Rare	NL	NL	NL

Reprinted from Andreoli TE (ed): *Cecil essentials of medicine,* ed 5, Philadelphia, 2001, WB Saunders.
↑ Increased over normal range; *HMWK,* high-molecular-weight kininogen; *NL,* normal; *PK,* prekallikrein; *PT,* prothrombin time; *PTT,* partial thromboplastin time; *TT,* thrombin time.
*Except in those of Ashkenazi Jewish descent (approximately 4% are heterozygous for factor XI deficiency).
†Not associated with clinical bleeding.

Abnormal values:

Decreased C3: Active SLE, immune complex disease, acute glomerulone-phritis, inborn C3 deficiency, membranoproliferative glomerulonephritis, infective endocarditis, serum sickness, autoimmune/chronic active hepatitis

Decreased C4: Immune complex disease, active SLE, infective endocarditis, inborn C4 deficiency, hereditary angioedema, hypergammaglobulin-emic states, cryobulinemic vasculitis

Table 4-10 describes complement deficiency states.

COMPLETE BLOOD COUNT (CBC)

White blood cells 3200-9800 mm^3 (3.2-9.8 × 10^9/L [CF: 0.001; SMI: 0.1 × 10^9/L])

Red blood cells
   Male: 4.3-5.9 × 10^6/mm^3 (4.3-5.9 × 10^{12}/L [CF: 0.001; SMI: 0.1 × 10^{12}/L])
   Female: 3.5-5 × 10^6/mm^3 (3.5-5 × 10^{12}/L [CF: 0.001; SMI: 0.1 × 10^{12}/L])
Hemoglobin
   Male: 13.6-17.7 g/dl (136-172 g/L [CF: 10; SMI: 1 g/L])
   Female: 12-15 g/dl (120-150 g/L [CF: 10; SMI: 1 g/L])
Hematocrit
   Male: 39%-49% (0.39-0.49 [CF: 0.01; SMI: 0.01])
   Female: 33%-43% (0.33-0.43 [CF: 0.01; SMI: 0.01])
Mean corpuscular volume (MCV): 76-100 μm^3 (76-100 fL [CF: 1; SMI: 1 fL])

TABLE 4-10 Complement Deficiency States

Component	No. of Reported Patients	Mode of Inheritance	Functional Defects	Disease Associations
Classic Pathway				
C1qrs	31	ACD	Impaired IC handling, delayed C' activation, impaired immune response	CVD, 48%; infection (encapsulated bacteria), 22%; both, 18%; healthy, 12%
C4	21	ACD	Impaired C' activation in absence of specific antibody	Infection (meningococcal), 74%; healthy, 26%
C2	109	ACD		
Alternative pathway				
D	3	ACD	Impaired IC handling, opson/phag; granulocytosis, CTX, immune response and absent SBA	CVD, 79%; recurrent infection (encapsulated bacteria), 71%
P	70	XL		
Junction of classic and alternative pathways				
C3	19	ACD	Impaired CTX; absent SBA	Infection (*Neisseria*, primarily meningococcal), 58%; CVD, 4%
Terminal components				
C5	27	ACD	Absent SBA	Both, 1%
C6	77	ACD		Healthy, 25%
C7	73	ACD		
C8	73	ACD		
C9	165	ACD	Impaired SBA	Healthy, 91%; infection, 9%
Plasma proteins regulating C' activation				
C1-INH	Many	AD	Uncontrolled generation of an inflammatory mediator on C' activation	Hereditary angioedema
H	13	Acq	Uncontrolled AP activation → low C3	CVD, 40%; CVD plus infection (encapsulated bacteria), 40%; healthy, 20%
I	14	ACD	Uncontrolled AP activation → low C3	Infection (encapsulated bacteria), 100%
Membrane proteins regulating C' activation	Many	Acq	Impaired regulation of C3b and C8 deposited on host RBCs; PMN, platelets → cell lysis	Paroxysmal nocturnal hemoglobinuria
Decay-accelerating factor				
Homologous restriction factor				
CD59	>20	ACD	Impaired PMN adhesive functions (i.e., margination), CTX, C3bi-mediated opson/phag	Infection (*Staphylococcus aureus, Pseudomonas* spp.), 100%
CR3 autoantibodies				
C3 nephritic factors	>59	Acq	Stabilize AP, convertase → low C3	MPGN, 41%; PLD, 25%; infection (encapsulated bacteria), 16%; MPGN plus PLD, 10%; PLD plus infection, 5%; MPGN plus PLD plus infection, 3%; MPGN plus infection, 2%
C4 nephritic factor		Acq	Stabilize CP, C3 convertase → low C3	Glomerulonephritis, 50%; CVD, 50%

Reprinted from Mandell GL: *Mandell, Douglas, and Bennett's principles and practice of infectious diseases*, ed 6, New York, 2005, Churchill Livingstone.
ACD, Autosomal codominant; *Acq,* acquired; *AD,* autosomal dominant; *AP,* alternative pathway; *C',* complement; *CP,* classic pathway; *CTX,* chemotaxis; *CVD,* collagen-vascular disease; *IC,* immune complex, *MPGN,* membranoproliferative glomerulonephritis; *PLD,* partial lipodystrophy; *PMN,* polymorphonuclear neutrophil; *RBCs,* red blood cells; *SBA,* serum bactericidal activity; *XL,* X-linked.

Laboratory Tests

IV

Mean corpuscular hemoglobin (MCH): 27-33 pg (27-33 pg [CF: 1; SMI: 1 pg])

Mean corpuscular hemoglobin concentration (MCHC): 33-37 g/dl (330-370 g/L [CF: 10; SMI: 10 g/L])

Red blood cell distribution width index (RDW): 11.5%-14.5%

Platelet count: 130-400 × 10³/mm³ (130-400 × 10⁹/L [CF: 1; SMI: 5 × 10⁹/L])

Differential:
- 2-6 stabs (bands, early mature neutrophils)
- 60-70 segs (mature neutrophils)
- 1-4 eosinophils
- 0-1 basophils
- 2-8 monocytes
- 25-40 lymphocytes

CONJUGATED BILIRUBIN

See BILIRUBIN, DIRECT

COOMBS, DIRECT

Normal: Negative

Positive: Autoimmune hemolytic anemia, erythroblastosis fetalis, transfusion reactions, drugs (α-methyldopa, penicillins, tetracycline, sulfonamides, levodopa, cephalosporins, quinidine, insulin)

False-positive: May be seen with cold agglutinins

COOMBS, INDIRECT

Normal: Negative

Positive: Acquired hemolytic anemia, incompatible cross-matched blood, anti-Rh antibodies, drugs (methyldopa, mefenamic acid, levodopa)

COPPER (serum)

Normal range: 70-140 μg/dl (11-22 μmol/L [CF: 0.1574, SMI: 0.2 μmol/L])

Decreased in: Wilson's disease, Menkes' syndrome, malabsorption, malnutrition, nephrosis, total parenteral nutrition, acute leukemia in remission

Elevated in: Aplastic anemia, biliary cirrhosis, systemic lupus erythematosus, hemochromatosis, hyperthyroidism, hypothyroidism, infection, iron deficiency anemia, leukemia, lymphoma, oral contraceptives, pernicious anemia, rheumatoid arthritis

COPPER, URINE

See URINE COPPER

CORTICOTROPIN RELEASING HORMONE (CRH) STIMULATION TEST

Normal: A dose of 0.5 mg of dexamethasone is given every 6 hours for 2 days; 2 hours after last dose 1 mcg/kg CRH is given IV. Samples are drawn after 15 min. Normally there is a twofold to fourfold increase in mean baseline concentration of ACTH or cortisol. Cortisol >1.4 mcg/L is virtually 100% specific and 100% diagnostic.

Interpretation:

Normal or exaggerated response: Pituitary Cushing's disease

No response: Ectopic ACTH-secreting tumor

A positive response to CRH or a suppressed response to high-dose dexamethasone has a 97% positive predictive value for Cushing's disease. However, a lack of response to either test excludes Cushing's disease in only 64%-78% of patients. When the tests are considered together, negative responses from both have a 100% predictive value for ectopic ACTH secretion.

CORTISOL, PLASMA

Normal range: Varies with time of collection (circadian variation):

8 AM: 4-19 μg/dl (110-520 nmol/L [CF: 27.59; SMI: 10 nmol/L])

4 PM: 2-15 μg/dl (50-410 nmol/L [CF: 27.59; SMI: 10 nmol/L])

Elevated in: Ectopic adrenocorticotropic hormone production (i.e., oat cell carcinoma of lung), loss of normal diurnal variation, pregnancy, chronic renal failure, iatrogenic, stress, adrenal or pituitary hyperplasia, or adenomas

Decreased in: Primary adrenocortical insufficiency, anterior pituitary hypofunction, secondary adrenocortical insufficiency, adrenogenital syndromes

C-PEPTIDE

Elevated in: Insulinoma, sulfonylurea administration

Decreased in: Insulin-dependent diabetes mellitus, factitious insulin administration

CPK

See CREATINE KINASE

C-REACTIVE PROTEIN

Normal range: 6.8-820 μg/dl (68-8200 μg/L [CF: 10; SMI: 10 μg/L])

Elevated in: Rheumatoid arthritis, rheumatic fever, inflammatory bowel disease, bacterial infections, myocardial infarction, oral contraceptives, third trimester of pregnancy (acute phase reactant), inflammatory and neoplastic diseases

C-REACTIVE PROTEIN, HIGH SENSITIVITY (hs-CRP, cardio-CRP)

This is a cardiac risk marker. It is increased in patients with silent atherosclerosis years before a cardiovascular event and is independent of cholesterol level and other lipoproteins. It can be used to help stratify cardiac risk.

INTERPRETATION OF RESULTS:

Cardio-CRP result (mg/L)	Risk
0.6	Lowest risk
0.7-1.1	Low risk
1.2-1.9	Moderate risk
2.0-3.8	High risk
3.9-4.9	Highest risk
≥5.0	Results may be confounded by acute inflammatory disease. If clinically indicated, a repeat test should be performed in 2 or more weeks.

CREATINE KINASE (CK, CPK)

Normal range: 0-130 U/L (0-2.16 μkat/L [CF: 0.01667; SMI: 0.01 μkat/L])

Elevated in: Myocardial infarction, myocarditis, rhabdomyolysis, myositis, crush injury/trauma, polymyositis, dermatomyositis, vigorous exercise, muscular dystrophy, myxedema, seizures, malignant hyperthermia syndrome, IM injections, cerebrovascular accident, pulmonary embolism and infarction, acute dissection of aorta

Decreased in: Steroids, decreased muscle mass, connective tissue disorders, alcoholic liver disease, metastatic neoplasms

CREATINE KINASE ISOENZYMES

CK-BB:

Elevated in: Cerebrovascular accident, subarachnoid hemorrhage, neoplasms (prostate, gastrointestinal tract, brain, ovary, breast, lung), severe shock, bowel infarction, hypothermia, meningitis

CK-MB:

Elevated in: Myocardial infarction (MI), myocarditis, pericarditis, muscular dystrophy, cardiac defibrillation, cardiac surgery, extensive rhabdomyolysis, strenuous exercise (marathon runners), mixed connective tissue disease, cardiomyopathy, hypothermia

NOTE: CK-MB exists in the blood in two subforms. MB₂ is released from cardiac cells and converted in the blood to MB₁. Rapid assay of CK-MB subforms can detect MI (CK-MB₂ ≥1.0 U/L, with a ratio of CK-MB₂/CK-MB₁ ≥1.5) within 6 hours of onset of symptoms.

Fig. 4-2 illustrates the time course of CK, AST, troponins, and LDH activity after acute MI.

CK-MM:

Elevated in: Crush injury, seizures, malignant hyperthermia syndrome, rhabdomyolysis, myositis, polymyositis, dermatomyositis, vigorous exercise, muscular dystrophy, IM injections, acute dissection of aorta

CREATININE (serum)

Normal range: 0.6-1.2 mg/dl (50-110 μmol/L [CF: 88.4; SMI: 10 μmol/L])

Elevated in: Renal insufficiency (acute and chronic), decreased renal perfusion (hypotension, dehydration, congestive heart failure), urinary tract infection, rhabdomyolysis, ketonemia

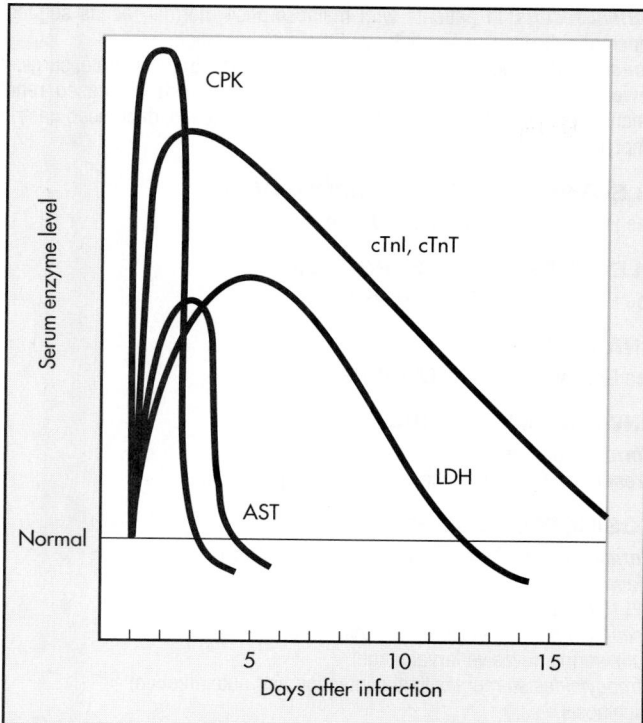

FIGURE 4-2 Evaluation of creatine kinase elevation. *CBC*, Complete blood count; *CK*, creatine kinase; *EMG*, electromyography. (Reprinted from Greene HL, Johnson WP, Lemcke D [eds]: *Decision making in medicine*, ed 2, St Louis, 1998, Mosby.)

Drugs (antibiotics [aminoglycosides, cephalosporins], hydantoin, diuretics, methyldopa)

Falsely elevated in: Diabetic ketoacidosis, administration of some cephalosporins (e.g., cefoxitin, cephalothin)

Decreased in: Decreased muscle mass (including amputees and older persons), pregnancy, prolonged debilitation

CREATININE CLEARANCE

Normal range: 75-124 ml/min (1.24-2.08 ml/sec [CF: 0.01667; SMI: 0.02 ml/sec])

Box 4-1 describes a formula for calculation of creatinine clearance.

The Cockcroft-Gault formula to calculate creatinine clearance is described in Box 4-2.

BOX 4-1   Calculation of the Creatinine Clearance

$C_{cr} = U_{cr} \times V/P_{cr}$
where C_{cr} = clearance of creatinine (ml/min)
  U_{cr} = urine creatinine (mg/dl)
  V = volume of urine (ml/min) (for 24-hr volume: divide by 1440)
  P_{cr} = plasma creatinine (mg/dl)
Normal range: 95 to 105 ml/min/1.75m²

BOX 4-2   Cockcroft-Gault Formula to Calculate Creatinine Clearance (C_{cr})

$$C_{cr} = \frac{(140 - \text{age in year}) \times (\text{lean body weight in kg})}{S_{cr} \text{ in mg/dl} - 72}$$

Elevated in: Pregnancy, exercise
Decreased in: Renal insufficiency, drugs (cimetidine, procainamide, antibiotics, quinidine)

CREATININE, URINE
See URINE CREATININE

CRYOGLOBULINS (serum)
Normal range: Not detectable
Present in: Collagen vascular diseases, chronic lymphocytic leukemia, hemolytic anemias, multiple myeloma, Waldenström's macroglobulinemia, chronic active hepatitis, Hodgkin's disease

CRYPTOSPORIDIUM ANTIGEN BY EIA (stool)
Normal range: Not detected
Present in: Cryptosporidiosis

CSF
See CEREBROSPINAL FLUID

CYSTATIN C
Normal: Cystatin C is a cysteine protease inhibitor that is produced at a constant rate by all nucleated cells. It is freely filtered by the glomerulus and reabsorbed (but not secreted) by the renal tubules with no extrarenal excretion. Its concentration is not affected by diet, muscle mass, or acute inflammation. Normal range when measured by particle-enhanced nephelometric immunoassay (PENIA) is <0.28 mg/L.
Elevated in: Renal disorders. Good predictor of the severity of acute tubular necrosis. Cystatin C increases more rapidly than creatinine in the early stages of GFR impairment. The cystatin C concentration is an independent risk factor for heart failure in older adults and appears to provide a better measure of risk assessment than the serum creatinine concentration.

CYSTIC FIBROSIS PCR
Test description: Test can be performed on whole blood or tissue. Common mutations in the cystic fibrosis transmembrane regulator (CFTR) gene can be used to detect 75%-80% of mutant alleles.

CYTOMEGALOVIRUS BY PCR
Test description: Test can be performed on whole blood, plasma, or tissue. Qualitative PCR is highly sensitive but may not be able to differentiate between latent and active infection.

D-DIMER
Normal range: <0.5 mcg/ml
Elevated in:
DVT, pulmonary embolism, high levels of rheumatoid factor, activation of coagulation and fibrolytic system from any cause
D-dimer assay by ELISA assists in the diagnosis of DVT and pulmonary embolism. This test has significant limitations because it can be elevated whenever the coagulation and fibrinolytic systems are activated and can also be falsely elevated with high rheumatoid factor levels.

DEHYDROEPIANDROSTERONE SULFATE
Normal:
Males:

Ages 19-30:	125-619 mcg/dl
31-50:	59-452 mcg/dl
51-60:	20-413 mcg/dl
61-83:	10-285 mcg/dl

Females:

Ages 19-30:	29-781 mcg/dl
31-50:	12-379 mcg/dl
Postmenopausal:	30-260 mcg/dl

Elevated in: Hirsutism, congenital adrenal hyperplasia, adrenal carcinomas, adrenal adenomas, polycystic ovary syndrome, ectopic ACTH-producing tumors, Cushing's disease, spironolactone

DEHYDROTESTOSTERONE (serum, urine)

Normal:
Serum: Males: 30-85 ng/dl; females: 4-22 ng/dl
Urine, 24 h: Males: 20-50 mcg/day; females: <8 mcg/day
Elevated in: Hirsutism
Decreased in: 5-α-reductase deficiency, hypogonadism

DEOXYCORTICOSTERONE (11-deoxycorticosterone, DOC) (serum)

Normal: 2-19 ng/dl. Normal secretion depends on ACTH and is suppressible by dexamethasone.
Elevated in: Adrogenital syndromes due to 17- and 11-hydroxylase deficiencies, pregnancy
Decreased in: Preeclampsia

DEXAMETHASONE SUPPRESSION TEST, OVERNIGHT

Normal: Test is performed by giving 1 mg dexamethasone orally at 11 PM and measuring serum cortisol at 8 AM the following morning. Normal response is cortisol suppression to <3 mcg/dl; If dose of 4 mg dexamethasone is given, cortisol suppression will be to <50% of baseline.
Interpretation: Cushing's syndrome (>10 mcg/dl), endogenous depression (half of patients suppress test values >5 mcg/dl). Most patients with pituitary Cushing's disease demonstrate suppression, whereas patients with adrenal adenoma, carcinoma, and ectopic ACTH-producing tumors do not.

DIGOXIN

Normal therapeutic range: 0.5-2 ng/ml
Elevated in: Impaired renal function, excessive dosing, concomitant use of quinidine, amiodarone, verapamil, fluoxetine, nifedipine. Toxicity may occur at a lower blood concentration in the presence of hypokalemia, hypomagnesemia, and hypercalcemia.

DILANTIN

See PHENYTOIN

DISACCHARIDE ABSORPTION TESTS

Normal: Test is used to diagnose malabsorption due to disaccharide deficiency. It is performed by giving disaccharide orally 1 g/kg body weight to a total of 25 g. Blood is drawn at 0, 30, 60, 90, and 120 min. Normal response is a change in glucose from fasting value >30 mg/dl, inconclusive when increase is 20-30 mg/dl, abnormal when increase is <20 mg/dl. Test can also be performed by measuring air at 0, 30, 60, 90, and 120 min. Normal is H_2 >20 ppm above baseline level before a colonic response.
Decreased in: Disaccharide deficiency (lactose, fructose, sorbitol), celiac disease, sprue, acute gastroenetetitis

DOC

See DEOXYCORTICOSTERONE

DONATH-LANDSTEINER (D-L) TEST FOR PAROXYSMAL COLD HEMOGLOBINURIA

Normal: No hemolysis
Interpretation: Hemolysis indicates presence of bithermic cold hemolysins or Donath-Landsteiner antibodies (D-L Ab)

DOPAMINE

Normal range: 175 pg/ml
Elevated in: Pheochromocytomas, neuroblastomas, stress, vigorous exercise, certain foods (bananas, chocolate, coffee, tea, vanilla)

d-XYLOSE ABSORPTION

Normal range: 21%-31% excreted in 5 hours
Decreased in: Malabsorption syndrome

d-XYLOSE ABSORPTION TEST

Normal range:
URINE: ≥4 g/5 hours (5-hour urine collection in adults >12 years [25-g dose])
SERUM: ≥25 mg/dl (adult, 1 h, 25-g dose, normal renal function)

Normal results: In patients with malabsorption, normal results suggest pancreatic disease as an etiology of the malabsorption.
Abnormal results: Celiac disease, Crohn's disease, tropical sprue, surgical bowel resection, AIDS. False-positives can occur with decreased renal function, dehydration/hypovolemia, surgical blind loops, decreased gastric emptying, vomiting.

ELECTROPHORESIS, HEMOGLOBIN

See HEMOGLOBIN ELECTROPHORESIS

ELECTROPHORESIS, PROTEIN

See PROTEIN ELECTROPHORESIS

ENA COMPLEX

See EXTRACTABLE NUCLEAR ANTIGEN

ENDOMYSIAL ANTIBODIES

Normal: Not detected
Present in: Celiac disease, dermatitis herpetiformis

EOSINOPHIL COUNT

Normal range: 1%-4% eosinophils (0-440/mm³)
Elevated in:
HELMINTHIC PARASITES
Ascaris lumbricoides (invasive larval stage)
Hookworms (invasive larval stage)
Strongyloides stercoralis (initial infection and autoinfection)
Trichinosis
Filariasis
Echinococcus granulosus and *E. multilocularis*
Toxocara species
Animal hookworms
Angiostrongylus cantonensis and *A. costaricensis*
Schistosomiasis
Liver flukes
Fasciolopsis buski
Anisakiasis
Capillaria philippinensis
Paragonimus westermani
"Tropical eosinophilia" (unidentified microfilariae)
OTHER INFECTIONS/INFESTATIONS
Pulmonary aspergillosis
Severe scabies
ALLERGIES
Asthma
Hay fever
Drug reactions
Atopic dermatitis
AUTOIMMUNE AND RELATED DISORDERS
Polyarteritis nodosa
Necrotizing vasculitis
Eosinophilic fasciitis
Pemphigus
NEOPLASTIC DISEASES
Hodgkin's disease
Mycosis fungoides
Chronic myelocytic leukemia
Eosinophilic leukemia
Polycythemia vera
Mucin-secreting adenocarcinomas
IMMUNODEFICIENCY STATES
Hyperimmunoglobulin E with recurrent infection
Wiskott-Aldrich syndrome
OTHER
Addison's disease
Inflammatory bowel disease
Dermatitis herpetiformis
Toxic/chemical syndrome

Eosinophilic myalgia syndrome, tryptophan, toxic oil syndrome
Hypereosinophilic syndrome (unknown etiology)

EPINEPHRINE, PLASMA

Normal range: 0-90 pg/ml
Elevated in: Pheochromocytomas, neuroblastomas, stress, vigorous exercise, certain foods (bananas, chocolate, coffee, tea, vanilla), hypoglycemia

EPSTEIN-BARR VIRUS SEROLOGY

Normal range: IgG anti-VCA <1:10 or negative
Abnormal:
IgG anti-VCA >1:10 or positive indicates either current or previous infection
IgM anti-VCA >1:10 or positive indicates current or recent infection
Anti-EBNA ≥1.5 or positive indicates previous infection
Table 4-11 and Fig. 4-3 describe test interpretation.

ERYTHROCYTE SEDIMENTATION RATE (ESR, sed rate, sedimentation rate)

Normal range:
Male: 0-15 mm/hr
Female: 0-20 mm/hr
Elevated in: Collagen vascular diseases, infections, myocardial infarction, neoplasms, inflammatory states (acute phase reactant), hyperthyroidism, hypothyroidism, rouleaux formation

Decreased in: Sickle cell disease, polycythemia, corticosteroids, spherocytosis, anisocytosis, hypofibrinogenemia, increased serum viscosity

ERYTHROPOIETIN (EP)

Normal: 3.7-16.0 IU/L by radioimmunoassay
Erythropoietin is a glycoprotein secreted by the kidneys that stimulates RBC production by acting on erythroid-committed stem cells.
Increased in:
Extremely high: Generally seen in patients with severe anemia (Hct <25, <7) such as in cases of aplastic anemia, severe hemolytic anemia, hematologic cancers
Very high: Patients with mild to moderate anemia (Hct, 25-35; Hb, 7-10)
High: Patients with mild anemia (e.g., AIDS, myelodysplasia)
Erythropoietin can be inappropriately elevated in patients with malignant neoplasms, renal cysts, postrenal transplant, meningioma, hemangioblastoma, and leiomyoma.
Decreased in: Renal failure, polycythemia vera, autonomic neuropathy

ESTRADIOL (serum)

Normal range:
Female, premenopausal: 30-400 pg/ml, depending on phase of menstrual cycle
Female, postmenopausal: 0-30 pg/ml
Male, adult: 10-50 pg/ml
Decreased in: Ovarian failure
Elevated in: Tumors of ovary, testis, adrenal, or nonendocrine sites (rare)

TABLE 4-11 Antibody Tests in Epstein-Barr Viral Infection

	Appearance	Peak	Disappears
Heterophil Ab	3-5 days after onset of Sx (range, 0-21 days)	During second wk after onset of Sx (1-4 wk)	2-3 mo after onset of Sx (still found at 1 yr in 20% of cases)
VCA-IgM	Beginning of Sx (1 wk before to 1 wk after Sx begin)	During first wk after onset of Sx (0-21 days)	2-3 mo after onset of Sx (1-6 mo)
VCA-IgG	3 days after onset of Sx (0-2 wk)	During second wk after onset of Sx (1-3 wk)	Decline to lower level, then persists for life
EBNA-IgG	3 wk after onset of Sx (1-4 wk)	8 mo after appearance (3-12 mo)	Lifelong
EA-D	5 days after onset of Sx (during first 1-2 wk after onset of Sx)	14-21 days after onset of Sx (1-4 wk)	9 wk after appearance (2-6 mo)
EBNA-IgM	Same as VCA-IgM	Same as VCA-IgM	Same as VCA-IgM

Reprinted from Ravel R: *Clinical laboratory medicine,* ed 6, St Louis, 1995, Mosby.
Ab, Antibody; *EA,* early antigen; *EBNA,* Epstein-Barr virus nuclear antigen; *Sx,* symptoms; *VCA,* viral capsid antigen.

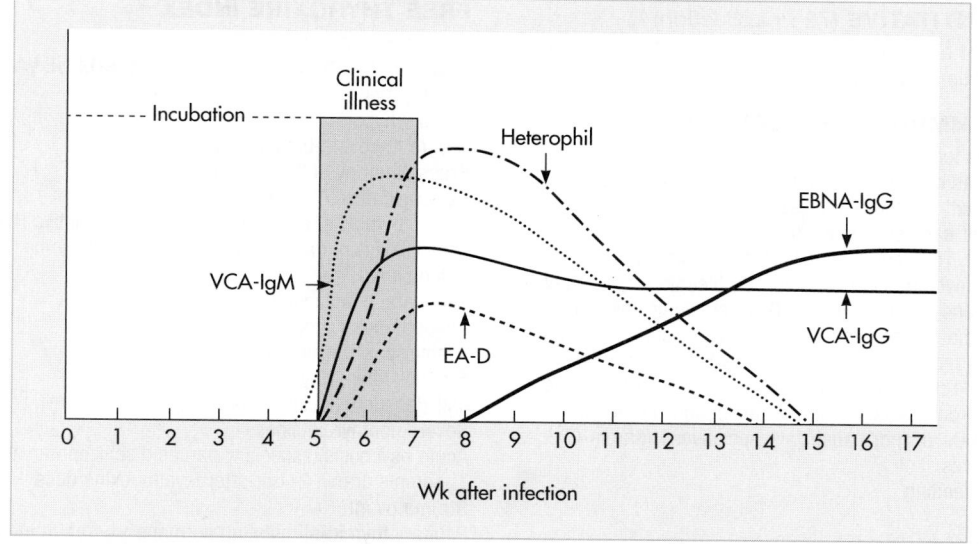

FIGURE 4-3 Tests in Epstein-Barr viral infection. See Table 4-11 for abbreviations. (Reprinted from Ravel R [ed]: *Clinical laboratory medicine,* ed 6, St Louis, 1995, Mosby.)

Laboratory Tests

IV

ESTROGEN

Normal range (serum):
Males: 20-80 pg/ml
Females:
Follicular: 60-200 pg/ml
Luteal: 160-400 pg/ml
Postmenopausal: <130 pg/ml
Normal range (urine):
Males: 4-23 μg/g creatinine
Females:
Follicular: 7-65 μg/g creatinine
Midcycle: 32-104 μg/g creatinine
Luteal: 8-135 μg/g creatinine

Elevated in: Hyperplasia of adrenal cortex, ovarian tumors producing estrogen, granulosa and thecal cell tumors, testicular tumors

Decreased in: Menopause, hypopituitarism, primary ovarian malfunction, anorexia nervosa, hypofunction of adrenal cortex, ovarian agenesis, psychogenic stress, gonadotropin-releasing hormone deficiency

ETHANOL (blood)

Normal range:
Negative (values <10 mg/dl are considered negative)
Ethanol is metabolized at 10-25 mg/dl/hour. Levels ≥80 mg/dl are considered evidence of impairment for driving. Fatal blood concentration is considered to be >400 mg/dl.

EXTRACTABLE NUCLEAR ANTIGEN (ENA complex, anti-RNP antibody, anti-SM, anti-Smith)

Normal: Negative
Present in: Systemic lupus erythematosus, rheumatoid arthritis, Sjögren's syndrome, mixed connective tissue disease

FACTOR V LEIDEN

Test description: PCR test performed on whole blood or tissue. This single mutation, found in 2%-8% of the general Caucasian population, is the single most common cause of hereditary thrombophilia.

FASTING BLOOD SUGAR

See GLUCOSE, FASTING

FBS

See GLUCOSE, FASTING

FDP

See FIBRIN DEGRADATION PRODUCT

FECAL FAT, QUANTITATIVE (72-hr collection)

Normal range: 2-6 g/24 hr (7-21 mmol/dl [CF: 3.515; SMI: 1 mmol/dl])
Elevated in: Malabsorption syndrome

FECAL GLOBIN IMMUNOCHEMICAL TEST

Normal: Negative. This test is performed by immunochromatography on a cellulose strip that has been impregnated with various antibodies. The test uses a small amount of toilet water as the specimen and is placed onto absorbent pads of card similar to traditional OB card. There is no direct handling of stool. This test is specific for the globin portion of the hemoglobin molecule, which confers lower GI bleeding specificity. It specifically detects blood from the lower GI tract; guaic tests are not lower GI specific. It is more sensitive than typical Hemoccult test (detection limit 50 mcg Hb/g feces versus >500 mcg Hb/g feces for Hemoccult). It has no dietary restrictions and gives no false-positives due to plant peroxidases and red meats. It has no medication restrictions. Iron supplements and NSAIDs do not cause false-positives. Vitamin C does not cause false-negatives.
Positive in: Lower GI bleeding

FERRITIN (serum)

Normal range: 18-300 ng/ml (18-300 μg/L [CF: 1; SMI: 10 μg/L])
Elevated in: Hyperthyroidism, inflammatory states, liver disease (ferritin elevated from necrotic hepatocytes), neoplasms (neuroblastomas, lymphomas, leukemia, breast carcinoma), iron replacement therapy, hemochromatosis, hemosiderosis
Decreased in: Iron deficiency anemia

α-1 FETOPROTEIN

Normal range: 0-20 ng/ml (0-20 μg/L [CF: 1; SMI: 1 μg/L])
Elevated in: Hepatocellular carcinoma (usually values >1000 ng/ml), germinal neoplasms (testis, ovary, mediastinum, retroperitoneum), liver disease (alcoholic cirrhosis, acute hepatitis, chronic active hepatitis), fetal anencephaly, spina bifida, basal cell carcinoma, breast carcinoma, pancreatic carcinoma, gastric carcinoma, retinoblastoma, esophageal atresia

FIBRIN DEGRADATION PRODUCT (FDP)

Normal range: <10 μg/ml
Elevated in: Disseminated intravascular coagulation, primary fibrinolysis, pulmonary embolism, severe liver disease
NOTE: The presence of rheumatoid factor may cause falsely elevated FDP.

FIBRINOGEN

Normal range: 200-400 mg/dl (2-4 g/L [CF: 0.01; SMI: 0.1 g/L])
Elevated in: Tissue inflammation or damage (acute phase protein reactant), oral contraceptives, pregnancy, acute infection, myocardial infarction
Decreased in: Disseminated intravascular coagulation, hereditary afibrinogenemia, liver disease, primary or secondary fibrinolysis, cachexia

FOLATE (folic acid)

Normal range:
Plasma: 2-10 ng/ml (4-22 nmol/L [CF: 2.266; SMI: 2 nmol/L])
Red blood cells: 140-960 ng/ml (550-2200 nmol/L [CF: 2.266; SMI: 10 nmol/L])
Decreased in: Folic acid deficiency (inadequate intake, malabsorption), alcoholism, drugs (methotrexate, trimethoprim, phenytoin, oral contraceptives, Azulfidine), vitamin B_{12} deficiency (defective red cell folate absorption), hemolytic anemia
Elevated in: Folic acid therapy

FOLLICLE-STIMULATING HORMONE (FSH)

Normal range: 5-20 mIU/ml
Elevated in: Menopause, primary gonadal failure, alcoholism, castration, Klinefelter's syndrome, gonadotropin-secreting pituitary hormones
Decreased in: Pregnancy, polycystic ovary disease, anorexia nervosa, anterior pituitary hypofunction

FREE T_4

See T_4, FREE

FREE THYROXINE INDEX

Normal range: 1.1-4.3
INCREASED THYROXINE OR FREE THYROXINE VALUES
Laboratory error
Primary hyperthyroidism (T_4/T_3 type)
Severe thyroxine-binding globulin elevation
Excess therapy of hypothyroidism
Excessive dose of levothyroxine
Active thyroiditis (subacute, painless, early active Hashimoto's disease)
Familial dysalbuminemic hyperthyroxinemia (some FT_4 kits, especially analog types)
Peripheral resistance to T_4 syndrome
Amiodarone or propranolol
Postpartum transient toxicosis
Factitious hyperthyroidism
Jod-Basedow (iodine-induced) hyperthyroidism
Severe nonthyroid illness
Acute psychosis (especially paranoid schizophrenia)
T_4 sample drawn 2-4 hr after levothyroxine dose
Struma ovarii
Pituitary thyroid-stimulating hormone–secreting tumor
Certain x-ray contrast media (Telepaque and Oragrafin)
Acute porphyria
Heparin effect (some T_4 and FT_4 kits)

Amphetamine, heroin, methadone, and phencyclidine abuse
Perphenazine or 5-fluorouracil
Antithyroid or anti-IgG heterophil (HAMA) autoantibodies
"T_4" hyperthyroidism
Hyperemesis gravidarum; about 50% of patients
High altitudes

DECREASED THYROXINE OR FREE THYROXINE VALUES
Laboratory error
Primary hypothyroidism
Severe nonthyroid illness*
Lithium therapy
Severe thyroxine-binding globulin decrease (congenital, disease, or drug-induced) or severe albumin decrease*
Dilantin, Depakene, or high-dose salicylate drugs*
Pituitary insufficiency
Large doses of inorganic iodide (e.g., saturated solution of potassium iodide)
Moderate or severe iodine deficiency
Cushing's syndrome
High-dose glucocorticoid drugs
Pregnancy, third trimester (low normal or small decrease)
Addison's disease; some patients (30%)
Heparin effect (a few FT_4 kits)
Desipramine or amiodarone drugs
Acute psychiatric illness

FTA-ABS (serum)
Normal: Nonreactive
Reactive in: Syphilis, other treponemal diseases (yaws, pinta, bejel), SLE, pregnancy

FUROSEMIDE STIMULATION TEST
Normal: Test is performed by giving 60 mg furosemide orally after overnight fast. Patient should be on a normal diet without medications the week before the test. Normal results: renin 1-6 ng angiotensin L/ml/hr.
Elevated in: Renovascular hypertension, Barrter's syndrome, high-renin essential hypertension, pheochromocytoma
No response in: Primary aldosteronism, low-renin essential hypertension, hyporeninemic hypoaldosteronism

GAMMA-GLUTAMYL TRANSFERASE (gGt)
See γ-GLUTAMYL TRANSFERASE

GASTRIN (serum)
Normal range: 0-180 pg/ml (0-180 ng/L [CF: 1; SMI: 10 ng/L])
Elevated in: Zollinger-Ellison syndrome (gastrinoma), pernicious anemia, hyperparathyroidism, retained gastric antrum, chronic renal failure, gastric ulcer, chronic atrophic gastritis, pyloric obstruction, malignant neoplasms of the stomach, H_2-blockers, omeprazole, calcium therapy, ulcerative colitis, rheumatoid arthritis

GASTRIN STIMULATION TEST
Normal: Gastrin stimulation test after calcium infusion is performed by giving a calcium infusion (15 mg Ca/Kg in 500 ml normal saline over 4 hours). Serum is drawn in fasting state before infusion and at 1, 2, 3, and 4 hr. Normal response is little or no increase over baseline gastrin level.
Elevated in: Gastrinoma (gastrin >400 pg/ml), duodenal ulcer (gastrin level increase <400 ng/L)
Decreased in: Pernicious anemia, atrophic gastritis

GLIADIN ANTIBODIES, IgA AND IgG
Normal: <25 U, equivocal 20-25 U, positive >25 U. Test is useful to monitor compliance with gluten-free diet in patients with celiac disease.
Elevated in: Celiac disease with dietary noncompliance

GLOMERULAR BASEMENT MEMBRANE (gBm) ANTIBODY
Normal: Negative
Present in: Goodpasture's syndrome

GLOMERULAR FILTRATION RATE
Normal:
Ages 20-29   116 ml/min/1.73 m²
Ages 30-39   107 ml/min/1.73 m²
Ages 40-49   99 ml/min/1.73 m²
Ages 50-59   93 ml/min/1.73 m²
Ages 60-69   85 ml/min/1.73 m²
Ages >75   75 ml/min/1.73 m²
Decreased in: Renal insufficiency, decreased renal blood flow

GLUCAGON
Normal: 20-100 pg/ml
Elevated in: Glucagonoma (900-7800 pg/ml), chronic renal failure, diabetes mellitus, glucocorticoids, insulin, nifedipine, danazol, sympathomimetic amines
Decreased in: Hyperlipoproteinemia (types III, IV), beta-blockers, secretin

GLUCOSE, FASTING (FBS, Fasting Blood Sugar)
Normal range: 60-99 mg/dl (3.8-6.0 mmol/L [CF: 0.05551; SMI: 0.1 mmol/L])
Elevated in: Diabetes mellitus, stress, infections, myocardial infarction, cerebrovascular accident, Cushing's syndrome, acromegaly, acute pancreatitis, glucagonoma, hemochromatosis, drugs (glucocorticoids, diuretics [thiazides, loop diuretics]), glucose intolerance, impaired fasting glucose
Decreased in: Sulfonylurea therapy, insulin therapy, reactive hypoglycemia (e.g., s/b subtotal gastrectomy), starvation, insulinoma, glycogen storage disorders, severe liver disease or renal disease, ethanol-induced hypoglycemia, mesenchymal tumors that secrete insulin-like hormones

GLUCOSE, POSTPRANDIAL
Normal range: <140 mg/dl (<7.8 mmol/L [CF: 0.05551; SMI: 0.1 mmol/L])
Elevated in: Diabetes mellitus, glucose intolerance
Decreased in: Post-gastrointestinal resection, reactive hypoglycemia, hereditary fructose intolerance, galactosemia, leucine sensitivity

GLUCOSE TOLERANCE TEST
Normal values above fasting:
30 min: 30-60 mg/dl (1.65-3.3 mmol/L [CF: 0.05551; SMI: 0.1 mmol/L])
60 min: 20-50 mg/dl (1.1-2.75 mmol/L [CF: 0.05551; SMI: 0.1 mmol/L])
120 min: 5-15 mg/dl (0.28-0.83 mmol/L [CF: 0.05551; SMI: 0.1 mmol/L])
180 min: fasting level or below
Abnormal in: Glucose intolerance, diabetes mellitus, Cushing's syndrome, acromegaly, pheochromocytoma, gestational diabetes

GLUCOSE-6-PHOSPHATE DEHYDROGENASE (G6PD) SCREEN (blood)
Normal: G6PD enzyme activity detected
Abnormal: If a deficiency is detected, quantitation of G6PD is necessary; a G6PD screen may be falsely interpreted as "normal" after an episode of hemolysis because most G6PD-deficient cells have been destroyed.

γ-GLUTAMYL TRANSFERASE (GGT)
Normal range: 0-30 U/L (0.050 μkat/L [CF: 0.01667; SMI: 0.01 μkat/L])
Elevated in: Chronic alcoholic liver disease, neoplasms (hepatoma, metastatic disease to the liver, carcinoma of the pancreas), systemic lupus erythematosus, congestive heart failure, trauma, nephrotic syndrome, sepsis, cholestasis, drugs (phenytoin, barbiturates)

GLYCATED (glycosylated) HEMOGLOBIN (HbA₁c) (glycohemoglobin)
Normal range: 4.0%-5.9%
Elevated in: Uncontrolled diabetes mellitus (glycated hemoglobin levels reflect the level of glucose control over the preceding 120 days), lead toxicity, alcoholism, iron deficiency anemia, hypertriglyceridemia
Decreased in: Hemolytic anemias, decreased red blood cell survival, pregnancy, acute or chronic blood loss, chronic renal failure, insulinoma, congenital spherocytosis, hemoglobin S, C, and D diseases

Laboratory Tests

IV

GROWTH HORMONE

Normal: Male: 1-9 ng/ml; female: 1-16 ng/ml
Elevated in: Pituitary gigantism, acromegaly, ectopic GH secretion, cirrhosis, renal failure, anorexia nervosa, stress, exercise, prolonged fasting, amphetamines, beta-blockers, insulin, levodopa, metoclopramide, clonidine, vasopressin, human growth hormone (HGH) supplementation
Decreased in: Hypopituitarism, pituitary dwarfism, adrenocortical hyperfunction, bromocriptine, corticosteroids, glucose

GROWTH HORMONE RELEASING HORMONE (GHRH)

Normal: <50 pg/ml
Elevated in: Acromegaly caused by GHRH secretion by neoplasms

GROWTH HORMONE SUPPRESSION TEST
(after glucose)

Normal: Test is done by giving 1.75 g glucose/kg orally after overnight fast. Blood is drawn at baseline, after 60 min, and after 120 min of glucose load. Normal response is growth hormone suppression to <2 ng/ml or undetectable levels.
Abnormal: There is no or incomplete suppression from the high basal level in gigantism or acromegaly.

HAM TEST (acid serum test)

Normal: Negative
Positive in: Paroxysmal nocturnal hemoglobinuria
False-positive in: Hereditary or acquired spherocytosis, recent transfusion with aged red blood cells, aplastic anemia, myeloproliferative syndromes, leukemia, hereditary dyserythropoietic anemia type II

HAPTOGLOBIN (serum)

Normal range: 50-220 mg/dl (0.50-2.2 g/L [CF: 0.01; SMI: 0.01 g/L])
Elevated in: Inflammation (acute phase reactant), collagen vascular diseases, infections (acute phase reactant), drugs (androgens), obstructive liver disease
Decreased in: Hemolysis (intravascular more than extravascular), megaloblastic anemia, severe liver disease, large tissue hematomas, infectious mononucleosis, drugs (oral contraceptives)

HBA$_{1c}$

See GLYCATED HEMOGLOBIN

HDL

See HIGH-DENSITY LIPOPROTEIN CHOLESTEROL

HELICOBACTER PYLORI (serology, stool antigen)

Normal range: Not detected
Detected in: H. pylori infection. Positive serology can indicate current or past infection. Positive stool antigen test indicates acute infection (sensitivity and specificity >90%). Stool testing should be delayed at least 4 weeks after eradication therapy.

HEMATOCRIT

Normal range:
Male: 39%-49% (0.39-0.49 [CF: 0.01; SMI: 0.01])
Female: 33%-43% (0.33-0.43 [CF: 0.01; SMI: 0.01])
Elevated in: Polycythemia vera, smoking, chronic obstructive pulmonary disease, high altitudes, dehydration, hypovolemia
Decreased in: Blood loss (gastrointestinal, genitourinary) anemia

HEMOGLOBIN

Normal range:
Male: 13.6-17.7 g/dl (136-172 g/L [CF: 10; SMI: 1 g/L])
Female: 12.0-15.0 g/dl (120-150 g/L [CF: 10; SMI: 1 g/L])
Elevated in: Hemoconcentration, dehydration, polycythemia vera, chronic obstructive pulmonary disease, high altitudes, false elevations (hyperlipemic plasma, white blood cells >50,000/mm^3), stress
Decreased in: Hemorrhagic (gastrointestinal, genitourinary) anemia

HEMOGLOBIN A$_{1c}$

See GLYCATED HEMOGLOBIN

HEMOGLOBIN ELECTROPHORESIS

Normal range:
HbA$_1$: 95%-98%
HbA$_2$: 1.5%-3.5%
HbF: <2%
HbC: absent
HbS: absent

HEMOGLOBIN, GLYCATED

See GLYCATED HEMOGLOBIN

HEMOGLOBIN, GLYCOSYLATED

See GLYCATED HEMOGLOBIN

HEMOGLOBIN H

Normal: Negative
Present in: Hemoglobin H disease, alpha-thalassemia trait, unstable hemoglobin disorders

HEMOGLOBIN, URINE

See URINE HEMOGLOBIN

HEMOSIDERIN, URINE

See URINE HEMOGLOBIN

HEPARIN-INDUCED THROMBOCYTOPENIA ANTIBODIES

Normal: Antigen assay: Negative, <0.45; weak, 0.45-1.0; strong, >1.0
Elevated in: Heparin-induced thrombocytopenia

HEPATITIS A ANTIBODY

Normal: Negative
Present in: Viral hepatitis A; can be IgM or IgG (if IgM, acute hepatitis A; if IgG, previous infection with hepatitis A)
    See Fig. 4-4 for serologic tests in HAV infection.
HAV-IgM ANTIBODY
Appearance: About the same time as clinical symptoms (3-4 weeks after exposure, range 14-60 days), or just before beginning of AST/ALT elevation (range 10 days before to 7 days after)
Peak: About 3-4 weeks after onset of symptoms (1-6 weeks)
Becomes nondetectable: 3-4 months after onset of symptoms (1-6 months). In a few cases HAV-IgM antibody can persist as long as 12-14 months.
HAV TOTAL ANTIBODY
Appearance: About 3 weeks after IgM becomes detectable (therefore about the middle of clinical symptom period to early convalescence)
Peak: About 1-2 months after onset
Becomes nondetectable: Remains elevated for life but can somewhat slowly fall

HEPATITIS A VIRAL INFECTION

Best all-purpose test(s) to diagnose acute HAV infection = HAV-Ab (IgM)
Best all-purpose test(s) to demonstrate past HAV infection/immunity = HAV-Ab (total)

HEPATITIS B SURFACE ANTIGEN (HBsAg)

Normal: Not detected
Detected in: Acute viral hepatitis type B, chronic hepatitis B
Appearance: 2-6 weeks after exposure (range, 6 days to 6 months); 5%-15% of patients are negative at onset of jaundice
Peak: 1-2 weeks before to 1-2 weeks after onset of symptoms
Becomes nondetectable: 1-3 months after peak (range, 1 week to 5 months)

HEPATITIS B VIRAL INFECTION

Figs. 4-5, 4-6, and 4-7 illustrate antigens and antibodies in hepatitis B infection.

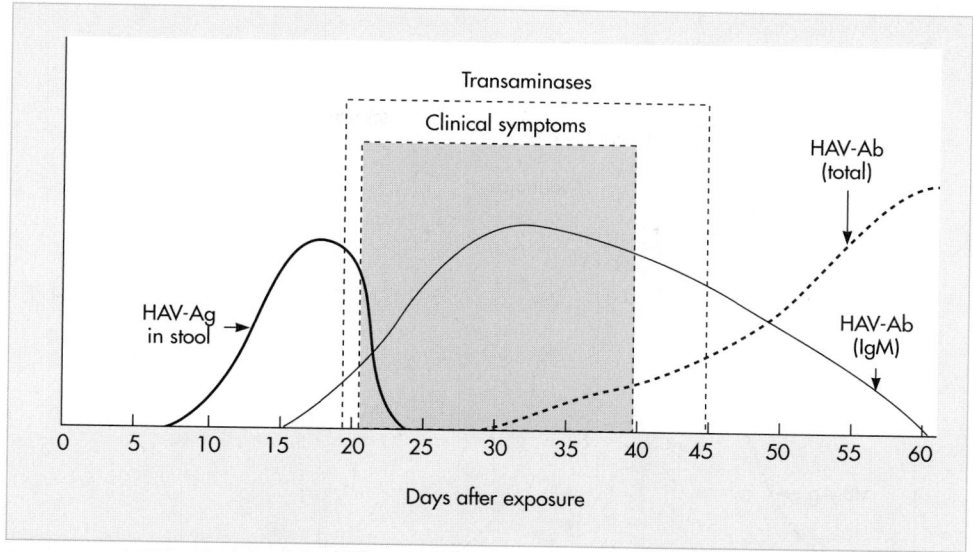

FIGURE 4-4 Serologic tests in HAV infection. (Reprinted from Ravel R [ed]: *Clinical laboratory medicine,* ed 6, St Louis, 1995, Mosby.)

HB$_S$
-Ag
HB$_S$Ag: shows current active HBV infection.
Persistence over 6 months indicates carrier/chronic HBV infection.
HBV nucleic acid probe: present before and longer than HB$_S$Ag.
More reliable marker for increased infectivity than HB$_S$Ag and/or HB$_e$Ag.
-Ab
HB$_S$Ab-total: shows previous healed HBV infection and evidence of immunity.

HB$_C$
-Ab
HB$_C$Ab-IgM: shows either acute or very recent infection by HBV.
In convalescent phase of acute HBV, may be elevated when HB$_S$Ag has disappeared (core window).
Negative HB$_C$Ab-IgM with positive HB$_S$Ag suggests either very early acute HBV or carrier/chronic HBV.
HB$_C$Ab-total: only useful to show past HBV infection if HB$_S$Ag and HB$_C$Ab-IgM are both negative.

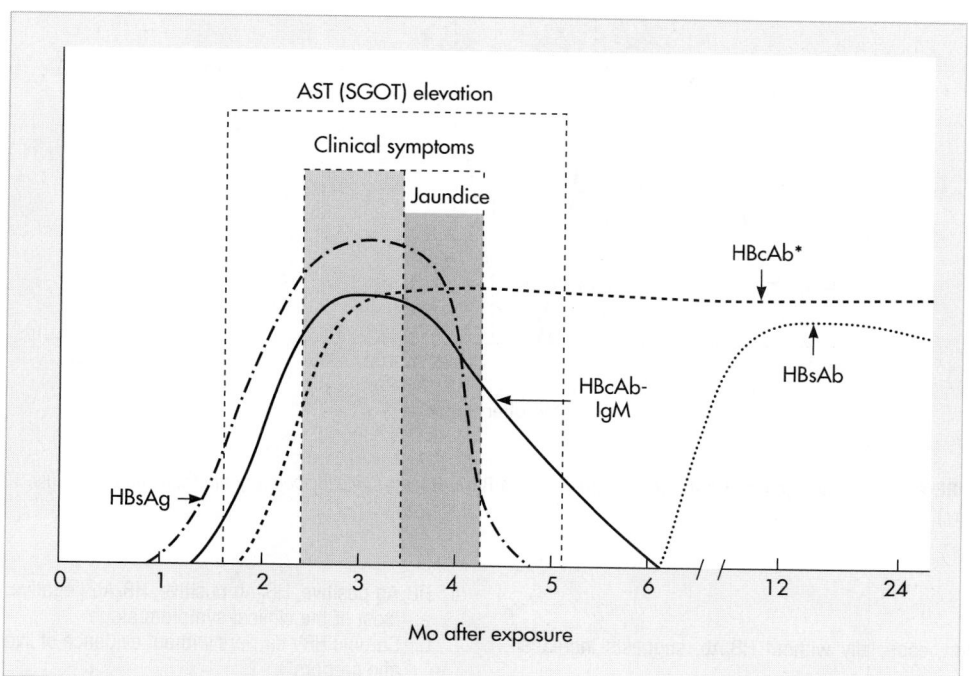

FIGURE 4-5 HBV surface antigen-antibody and core antibodies. Note "core window." *HB$_C$Ab = HB$_C$Ab-IgM + HBCAb-IgG (combined). (Reprinted from Ravel R [ed]: *Clinical laboratory medicine,* ed 6, St Louis, 1995, Mosby.)

Laboratory Tests

IV

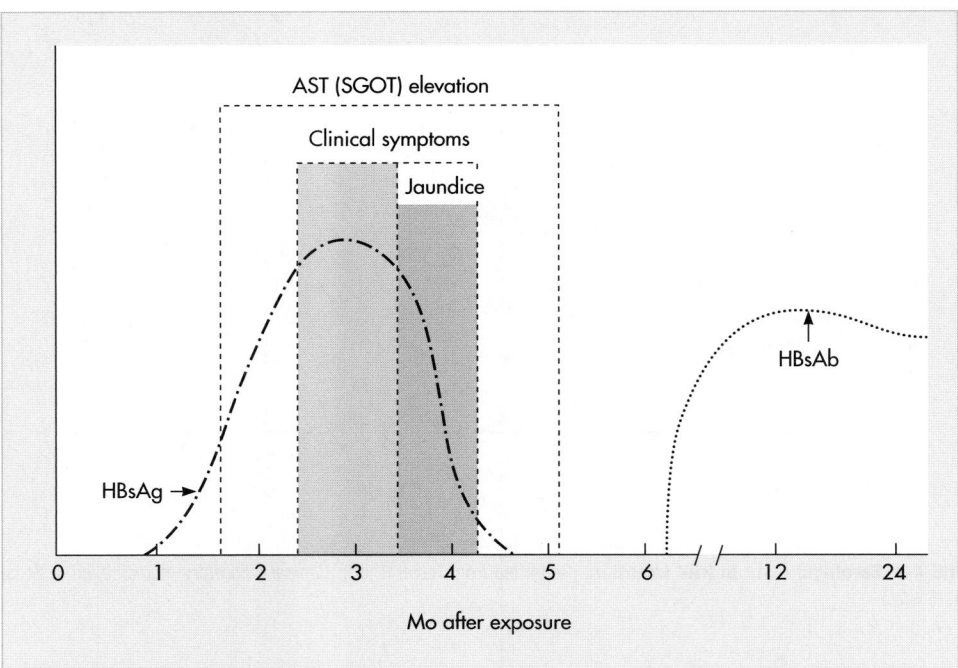

FIGURE 4-6 HBV surface antigen and antibody (HB$_S$Ag and HB$_S$Ab-total). (Reprinted from Ravel R [ed]: *Clinical laboratory medicine,* ed 6, St Louis, 1995, Mosby.)

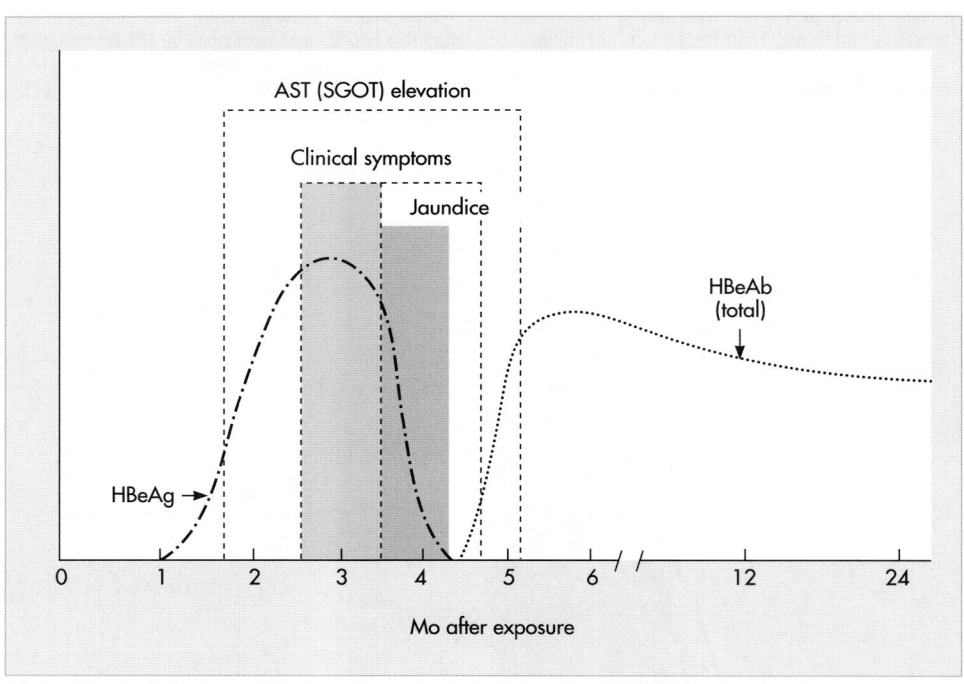

FIGURE 4-7 HBVe antigen and antibody. (Reprinted from Ravel R [ed]: *Clinical laboratory medicine,* ed 6, St Louis, 1995, Mosby.)

HB$_e$
-Ag

HB$_e$-AbAg: when present, especially without HB$_e$Ab, suggests increased patient infectivity.

HB$_e$Ab-total: when present, suggests less patient infectivity.

I. HB$_S$Ag positive, HB$_C$Ab negative*

About 5% (range, 0%-17%) of patients with early-stage HBV acute infection (HB$_C$Ab rises later)

II. HB$_S$Ag positive, HB$_C$Ab positive, HB$_S$Ab negative
   a. Most of the clinical symptom stage
   b. Chronic HBV carriers without evidence of liver disease ("asymptomatic carriers")
   c. Chronic HBV hepatitis (chronic persistent type or chronic active type)

III. HB$_S$Ag negative, HB$_C$Ab positive,* HB$_S$Ab negative
   a. Late clinical symptom stage or early convalescence stage (core window)

b. Chronic HBV infection with HB$_S$Ag below detection levels with current tests
c. Old previous HBV infection
IV. HB$_S$Ag negative, HB$_C$Ab positive, HB$_S$Ab positive
   a. Late convalescence to complete recovery
   b. Old infection

HEPATITIS C VIRAL INFECTION

Fig. 4-8 illustrates antigens and antibodies in hepatitis C infection.

HEPATITIS C RNA

Normal: Negative
Elevated in: Hepatitis C. Detection of hepatitis C-RNA is used to confirm current infection and to monitor treatment. Quantitative assays (viral load) are needed before treatment to assess response (<2 log decrease after 12-week treatment indicates lack of response).

HCV

-Ag
HCV nucleic acid probe: shows current infection by HCV (especially with PCR amplification).
-Ab
HCV-Ab (IgG): current, convalescent, or old HCV infection.

HAV

-Ag
HAV-Ag by EM: shows presence of virus in stool early in infection.
-Ab
HAV-Ab (IgM): current or recent HAV infection.
HAV-Ab (total): convalescent or old HAV infection.

HEPATITIS D VIRAL INFECTION

Fig. 4-9 illustrates antigens and antibodies in hepatitis D infection.
Best current all-purpose screening test = ADV-Ab (total)
Best test to differentiate acute from chronic infection = HDV-Ab (IgM)

DELTA HEPATITIS COINFECTION (acute HDV1 acute HBV) OR SUPERINFECTION (acute HDV1 chronic HBV)

HDV

-Ag
HDV-Ag: shows current infection (acute or chronic) by HDV.
HDV nucleic acid probe: detects antigen before and longer than HDV-Ag by EIA.
-Ab
HDV-Ab (IgM): high elevation in acute HDV; does not persist.
Low or moderate elevation in convalescent HDV; does not persist.
Low to high persistent elevation in chronic HDV (depends on degree of cell injury and sensitivity of the assay).
HDV-Ab (total): high elevation in acute HDV; does not persist.
High persistent elevation in chronic HDV.

HDV-AG

Detected by DNA probe, less often by immunoassay
Appearance: Prodromal stage (before symptoms); just at or after initial rise in ALT (about a week after appearance of HB$_S$Ag and about the time HB$_C$Ab-IgM level begins to rise)
Peak: 2-3 days after onset
Becomes nondetectable: 1-4 days (may persist until shortly after symptoms appear)

HDV-AB (IgM)

Appearance: About 10 days after symptoms begin (range, 1-28 days)
Peak: About 2 weeks after first detection
Becomes nondetectable: About 35 days (range, 10-80 days) after first detection (most other IgM antibodies take 3-6 months to become nondetectable)

HDV-AB (total)

Appearance: About 50 days after symptoms begin (range, 14-80 days); about 5 weeks after HDV-Ag (range, 3-11 weeks)
Peak: About 2 weeks after first detection
Becomes nondetectable: About 7 months after first detection (range, 4-14 months)

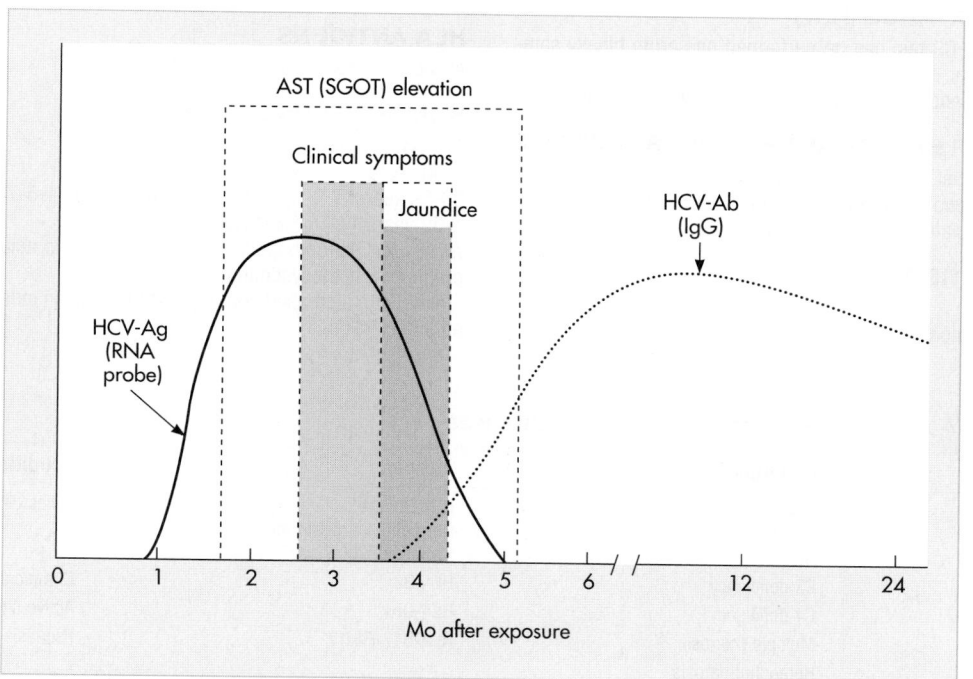

FIGURE 4-8 HCV antigen and antibody. (Reprinted from Ravel R [ed]: *Clinical laboratory medicine,* ed 6, St Louis, 1995, Mosby.)

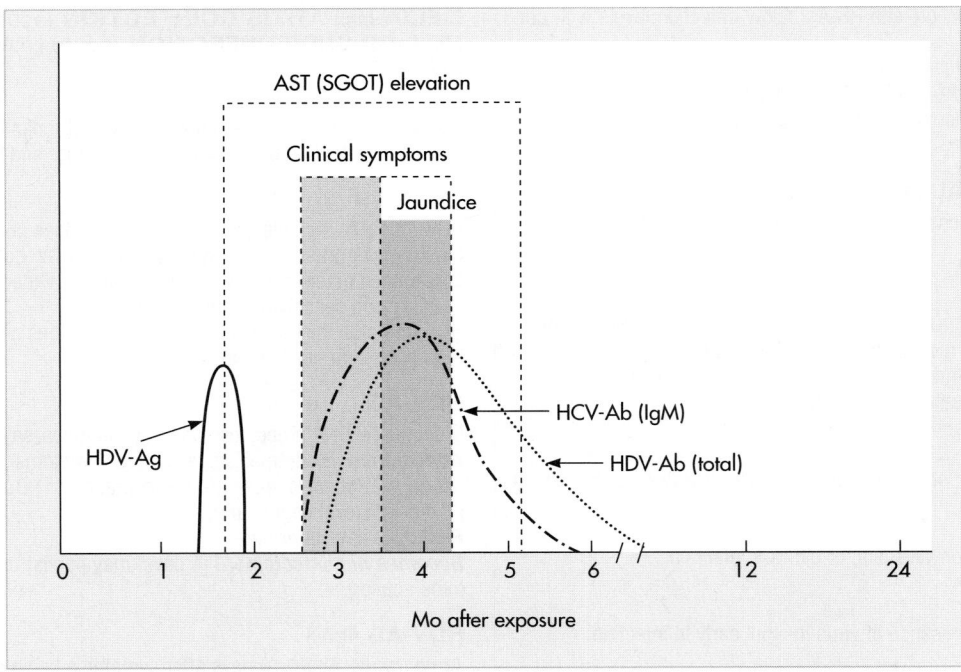

FIGURE 4-9 HDV antigen and antibodies. (Reprinted from Ravel R [ed]: *Clinical laboratory medicine,* ed 6, St Louis, 1995, Mosby.)

HER-2/*NEU*

Normal: Negative

Present in: Present in 25%-30% of primary breast cancers. It can also be found in other epithelial tumors, including lung, hepatocellular, pancreatic, colon, stomach, ovarian, cervical, and bladder cancer. Trastuzumab (Herceptin) is a humanized monoclonal antibody against Her-2/*neu*. This test is useful to identify patients with metastatic; recurrent; and/or treatment refractory, unresectable, locally advanced breast cancer for trastuzumab treatment.

HERPES SIMPLEX VIRUS (HSV)

Test description: The PCR test can be performed on serum biopsy samples, CSF, vitreous humor.

Table 2-3 describes laboratory diagnosis of herpes virus infections.

HFE SCREEN FOR HEREDITARY HEMOCHROMATOSIS

Test description: PCR test can be performed on whole blood or tissue. One mutation (C282Y) and two polymorphisms (H63D, S65C) account for the majority of alleles associated with this disease.

HETEROPHIL ANTIBODY

Normal: Negative

Positive in: Infectious mononucleosis

HIGH-DENSITY LIPOPROTEIN (HDL) CHOLESTEROL

Normal range:

Male: 40-70 mg/dl (0.8-1.8 mmol/L [CF: 0.02586; SMI: 0.05 mmol/L])
Female: 50-90 mg/dl (1.1-2.35 mmol/L [CF: 0.02586; SMI: 0.05 mmol/L])

Increased in: Use of gemfibrozil, statins, fenofibrate, nicotinic acid, estrogens, regular aerobic exercise, small (1 oz) daily alcohol intake

Decreased in: Deficiency of apoproteins, liver disease, probucol ingestion, Tangier disease

NOTE: A cholesterol/HDL ratio >4.0 is associated with increased risk of coronary artery disease.

HLA ANTIGENS

Associated disorders: see Table 4-12.

HOMOCYSTEINE (plasma)

Normal range:

0-30 years: 4.6-8.1 mcmol/L
30-59 years: 6.3-11.2 mcmol/L (males), 4-5-7.9 mcmol/L (females)
>59 years: 5.8-11.9 mcmol/L

Increased: Thrombophilic states, B$_6$, B$_{12}$, folic acid, riboflavin deficiency, pregnancy, homocystinuria

NOTE: An increased homocysteine level is an independent risk factor for atherosclerosis.

TABLE 4-12   HLA Antigens Associated with Specific Diseases

Antigen	Condition	Antigen	Condition
HLA-B27	Ankylosing spondylitis	HLA-B8, Dw3	Celiac disease
Reiter's syndrome	HLA-B8, Dw3	Dermatitis herpetiformis	
Psoriatic arthritis	HLA-B8	Myasthenia gravis	
HLA-A10, B18, Dw2	C2 deficiency	HLA-B8	Chronic active hepatitis in children
HLA-A2, B40, Cw3	C4 deficiency	HLA-Drw4	Active chronic hepatitis in adults
HLA-B7, Dw2	Multiple sclerosis	HLA-B13, Bw17	Psoriasis
HLA-A3	Hemochromatosis		

Reprinted from Cerra FB: *Manual of critical care,* St Louis, 1987, Mosby.
HLA, Human leukocyte antigen.

HUMAN HERPES VIRUS 8 (HHV8)

Test description: PCR test can be performed on whole blood, tissue, bone marrow, and urine. HHV8 is found in all forms of Kaposi's sarcoma.

HUMAN CHORIONIC GONADOTROPIN (hCG)

Normal range: Varies with gestational stage:

1 wk:	5-50 mU/ml
1-2 wk:	50-550 mU/ml
2-3 wk:	up to 5000 mU/ml
3-4 wk:	up to 10,000 mU/ml
4-5 wk:	up to 50,000 mU/ml
2-3 mo:	10,000-100,000 mU/ml

Elevated in: Normal pregnancy, hydatidiform mole, choriocarcinoma, germ cell tumors of testicle, some nontrophoblastic neoplasms (e.g., neoplasms of cervix, gastrointestinal tract, ovary, lung, breast)

HUMAN IMMUNODEFICIENCY VIRUS ANTIBODY, TYPE 1 (HIV-1)

Normal range: Not detected

Abnormal result: HIV antibodies usually appear in the blood 1-4 months after infection.

Testing sequence:

1. ELISA is the recommended initial screening test. Sensitivity and specificity are >99%. False-positive ELISA may occur with autoimmune disorders, administration of immune globulin manufactured before 1985, within 6 weeks of testing, in the presence of rheumatoid factor, in the presence of DLA-DR antibodies in multigravida female, with administration of influenza vaccine within 3 months of testing, with hemodialysis, with positive plasma reagin test, and with certain medical disorders (hemophilia, hypergammaglobulinemia, alcoholic hepatitis).

2. A positive ELISA is confirmed with Western blot. False-positive Western blot may result from connective tissue disorders, human leukocyte antigen antibodies, polyclonal gammopathies, hyperbilirubinemia, presence of antibody to another human retrovirus, or cross-reaction with other non-virus-derived proteins in healthy persons. Undetermined Western blot may occur in AIDS patients with advanced immunodeficiency (caused by loss of antibodies) and in recent HIV infections.

3. PCR is used to confirm indeterminate Western blot results or negative results in persons with suspected HIV infection.

Fig. 4-10 describes tests in HIV infection; indications for plasma HIV RNA testing are described in Table 4-13.

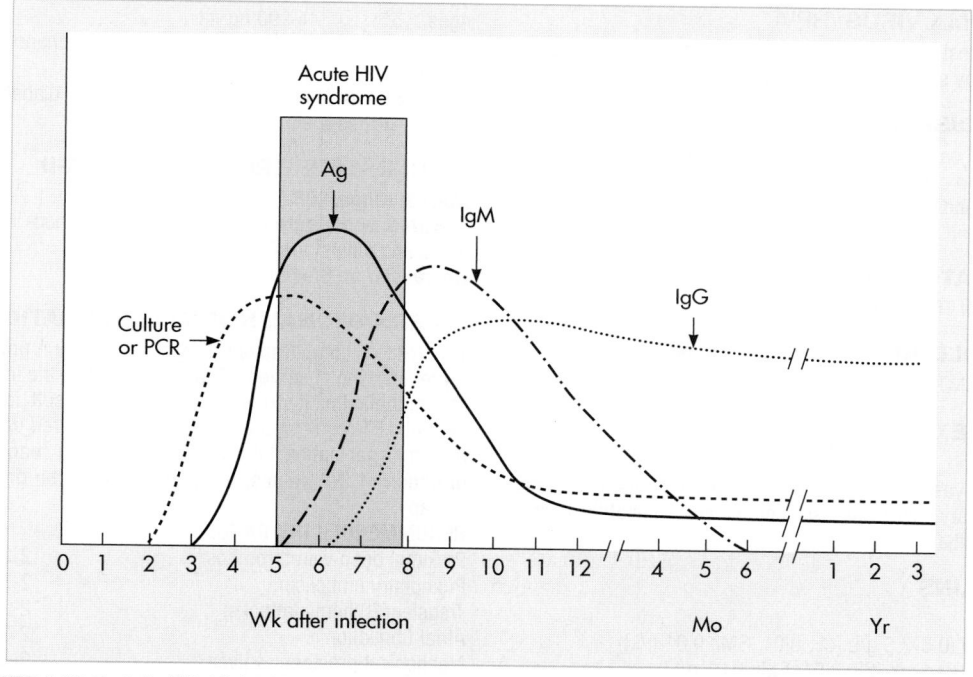

FIGURE 4-10 Tests in HIV-1 infection. (Reprinted from Ravel R [ed]: *Clinical laboratory medicine,* ed 6, St Louis, 1995, Mosby.)

TABLE 4-13   Indications for Plasma HIV RNA Testing*

Clinical Indication	Information	Use
Syndrome consistent with acute HIV infection	Establishes diagnosis when HIV antibody test is negative or indeterminate	Diagnosis[†]
Initial evaluation of newly diagnosed HIV infection	Baseline viral load set point	Decision to start or defer therapy
Every 3-4 mo in patients not on therapy	Changes in viral load	Decision to start therapy
4-8 wk after initiation of antiretroviral therapy	Initial assessment of drug efficacy	Decision to continue or change therapy
3-4 mo after start of therapy	Maximal effect of therapy	Decision to continue or change therapy
Every 3-4 mo in patients on therapy	Durability of antiretroviral effect	Decision to continue or change therapy
Clinical event or significant decline in CD4+ T cells	Association with changing or stable	Decision to continue, initiate, or change

Reprinted from *MMWR,* 47:RR-5, 1998.

*Acute illness (e.g., bacterial pneumonia, tuberculosis, HSV, PCP) and immunizations can cause increase in plasma HIV RNA for 2-4 wk; viral load testing should not be performed during this time. Plasma HIV RNA results should usually be verified with a repeat determination before starting or making changes in therapy. HIV RNA should be measured using the same laboratory and the same assay.

†Diagnosis of HIV infection determined by HIV RNA testing should be confirmed by standard methods (e.g., Western blot serology) performed 2-4 mo after the initial indeterminate or negative test.

HUMAN IMMUNODEFICIENCY VIRUS TYPE 1 (HIV-1) ANTIGEN (p24), QUALITATIVE (p24 antigen)

Normal range: Negative. This test detects uncomplexed HIV-1 p24 antigen. The core protein p24 is the first detectable protein encoded by the group-specific antigen *(gag)* gene. This protein is a marker for viremia. This test should not be used in place of HIV-1 antibody testing as a screen for HIV-1 infection. HIV-1 p24 may be detectable in the first month of acute HIV-1 infection and generally falls to undetectable levels during the asymptomatic stage of HIV-1 infection. A negative result does not exclude the possibility of infection or exposure to HIV-1. It is recommended that a negative result be followed with repeat testing at least 8 weeks after the original test. This test is used primarily for screening of donated blood and plasma and as an aid for the prognosis of HIV-1 infection.

HUMAN IMMUNODEFICIENCY VIRUS TYPE 1 (HIV-1) VIRAL LOAD

Normal range: HIV-1 RNA, quant. bDNA 3: less than 50 copies/ml or less than 1.7 log copies/ml

This test should be used only in individuals with documented HIV-1 infection for monitoring the progression of infection, response to antiretroviral therapy, and disease prognosis. It is not indicated for diagnosis of HIV infection.

HUMAN PAPILLOMA VIRUS (HPV)

Test description: PCR test can be performed on cervical smears, biopsies, scrapings, liquid cytology specimen, and anogenital tissues.

HUNTINGTON'S DISEASE PCR

Test description: PCR can be performed on whole blood. Huntington's disease is caused by the expansion of the trinucleotide repeat CAG within IT 15 (huntingtin). Pre- and post-test counseling should be performed when ordering this test.

HYDROGEN BREATH TEST

See BREATH HYDROGEN TEST

5-HYDROXYINDOLE-ACETIC ACID, URINE

See URINE 5-HYDROXYINDOLE-ACETIC ACID

IMMUNE COMPLEX ASSAY

Normal: Negative
Detected in: Collagen vascular disorders, glomerulonephritis, neoplastic diseases, malaria, primary biliary cirrhosis, chronic acute hepatitis, bacterial endocarditis, vasculitis

IMMUNOGLOBULINS

Normal range:

IgA:	50-350 mg/dl (0.5-3.5 g/L [CF: 0.01; SMI: 0.01 g/L])
IgD:	<6 mg/dl (<60 mg/L [CF: 0.01; SMI: 0.01 g/L])
IgE:	<25 μg/dl (<0.00025 g/L [CF: 0.01; SMI: 0.01 g/L])
IgG:	800-1500 mg/dl (8-15 g/L [CF: 0.01; SMI: 0.01 g/L])
IgM:	45-150 mg/dl (0.45-1.5 g/L [CF: 0.01; SMI: 0.01 g/L])

Elevated in:
IgA: Lymphoproliferative disorders, Berger's nephropathy, chronic infections, autoimmune disorders, liver disease
IgE: Allergic disorders, parasitic infections, immunologic disorders, IgE myeloma
IgG: Chronic granulomatous infections, infectious diseases, inflammation, myeloma, liver disease
IgM: Primary biliary cirrhosis, infectious diseases (brucellosis, malaria), Waldenström's macroglobulinemia, liver disease
Decreased in:
IgA: Nephrotic syndrome, protein-losing enteropathy, congenital deficiency, lymphocytic leukemia, ataxia-telangiectasia, chronic sinopulmonary disease
IgE: Hypogammaglobulinemia, neoplasma (breast, bronchial, cervical), ataxia-telangiectasia
IgG: Congenital or acquired deficiency, lymphocytic leukemia, phenytoin, methylprednisolone, nephrotic syndrome, protein-losing enteropathy
IgM: Congenital deficiency, lymphocytic leukemia, nephrotic syndrome

INFLUENZA A AND B TESTS

Test description: PCR can be performed on nasopharyngeal swab, wash, or aspirate
Normal: Negative

INSULIN AUTOANTIBODIES

Normal: Negative
Present in: Exogenous insulin from insulin therapy. The presence of islet cell antibodies indicates ongoing beta cell destruction. This test is useful in the early diagnosis of type 1a diabetes mellitus and in the identification of patients at high risk for type 1a diabetes.

INSULIN, FREE

Normal: <17 mcU/ml
Elevated in: Insulin overdose, insulin resistance syndromes, endogenous hyperinsulinemia
Decreased in: Inadequately treated type 1 DM

INSULIN-LIKE GROWTH FACTOR-1 (IGF-1) (serum)

Normal range:

Ages 16-24:	182-780 ng/ml
Ages 25-39:	114-492 ng/ml
Ages 40-54:	90-360 ng/ml
Ages >55:	71-290 ng/ml

Elevated in: Adolescence, acromegaly, pregnancy, precocious puberty, obesity
Decreased in: Malnutrition, delayed puberty, diabetes mellitus, hypopituitarism, cirrhosis, old age

INSULIN-LIKE GROWTH FACTOR-II

Normal range: 288-736 ng/ml
Elevated in: Hypoglycemia associated with non–islet cell tumors, hepatoma, and Wilms' tumor
Decreased in: Growth hormone deficiency

INTERNATIONAL NORMALIZED RATIO (INR)

The INR is a comparative rating of prothrombin time (PT) ratios. The INR represents the observed PT ratio adjusted by the International Reference Thromboplastin. It provides a universal result indicative of what the patient's PT result would have been if measured using the primary World Health Organization International Reference reagent. For proper interpretation of INR values, the patient should be on stable anticoagulant therapy.

RECOMMENDED INR RANGES:

Proximal deep vein thrombosis:	2-3
Pulmonary embolism:	2-3
Transient ischemic attacks:	2-3
Atrial fibrillation:	2-3
Mechanical prosthetic valves:	3-4.5
Recurrent venous thromboembolic disease:	3-4.5

INTRINSIC FACTOR ANTIBODIES

Normal: Negative
Present in: Pernicious anemia (>50% of patients). Cyanocobalamin may give false-positive results.

IRON (serum)

Normal: Male: 65-175 mcg/dl; female: 50-1170 mcg/dl
Elevated in: Hemochromatosis, excessive iron therapy, repeated transfusions, lead poisoning, hemolytic anemia, aplastic anemia, pernicious anemia
Decreased in: Iron deficiency anemia, hypothyroidism, chronic infection

IRON-BINDING CAPACITY, TOTAL (TIBC)

Normal range: 250-460 μg/dl (45-82 μmol/L [CF: 0.1791; SMI: 1 μmol/L])
Elevated in: Iron deficiency anemia, pregnancy, polycythemia, hepatitis, weight loss

TABLE 4-14 Serum Iron and Total Iron-Binding Capacity Patterns

SI↓	TIBC↓	Chronic diseases Uremia
SI↓	TIBC↑	Chronic iron deficiency anemia Pregnancy in third trimester
SI↑	TIBC↓	Hemachromatosis Iron therapy overload (TIBC may be normal) Hemolytic anemia; thalassemia; lead poisoning; megaloblastic anemia; aplastic, pyridoxine deficiency, or other sideroblastic anemias
SI↑	TIBC↑	Oral contraceptives Acute hepatitis (some report TIBC is low normal) Chronic hepatitis (some patients)
SI↑	TIBC NL	B_{12} or folate deficiency
SI↓	TIBC NL	Chronic iron deficiency (some patients) Acute infection, surgery, tissue damage
SI NL	TIBC↑	B_{12}/folate deficiency plus iron deficiency

Reprinted from Ravel R: *Clinical laboratory medicine,* ed 6, St Louis, 1995, Mosby.
NL, Normal; *SI,* serum iron; *TIBC,* total iron-binding capacity.

Decreased in: Anemia of chronic disease, hemochromatosis, chronic liver disease, hemolytic anemias, malnutrition (protein depletion)
   Table 4-14 describes TIBC and serum iron abnormalities.

IRON SATURATION (% TRANSFERRIN SATURATION)
Normal:
Male: 20%-50%
Female: 15%-50%
Elevated in: Hemochromatosis, excessive iron intake, aplastic anemia, thalassemia, vitamin B_6 deficiency
Decreased in: hypochromic anemias, GI malignancy

LACTATE (blood)
Normal range: 0.5-2.0 mEq/L
Elevated in: Tissue hypoxia (shock, respiratory failure, severe CHF, severe anemia, carbon monoxide or cyanide poisoning), systemic disorders (liver or renal failure, seizures), abnormal intestinal flora (D-lactic acidosis), drugs or toxins (salicylates, ethanol, methanol, ethylene glycol), G6PD deficiency

LACTATE DEHYDROGENASE (LDH)
Normal range: 50-150 U/L (0.82-2.66 μkat/L [CF: 0.01667; SMI: 0.02 μkat/L])
Elevated in:
Infarction of myocardium, lung, kidney
Diseases of cardiopulmonary system, liver, collagen, central nervous system
Hemolytic anemias, megaloblastic anemias, transfusions, seizures, muscle trauma, muscular dystrophy, acute pancreatitis, hypotension, shock, infectious mononucleosis, inflammation, neoplasia, intestinal obstruction, hypothyroidism

LACTATE DEHYDROGENASE ISOENZYMES
Normal range:
LDH$_1$: 22%-36% (cardiac, red blood cell) (0.22-0.36 [CF: 0.01, SMI: 0.01])
LDH$_2$: 35%-46% (cardiac, red blood cell) (0.35-0.46)
LDH$_3$: 13%-26% (pulmonary) (0.15-0.26)
LDH$_4$: 3%-10% (striated muscle, liver) (0.03-0.1)
LDH$_5$: 2%-9% (striated muscle, liver) (0.02-0.09)
Normal ratios:
LDH$_1$<LDH$_2$
LDH$_5$<LDH$_4$
Abnormal values:
LDH$_1$>LDH$_2$: Myocardial infarction (can also be seen with hemolytic anemias, pernicious anemia, folate deficiency, renal infarct)
LDH$_5$>LDH$_4$: Liver disease (cirrhosis, hepatitis, hepatic congestion)

LACTOSE TOLERANCE TEST (serum)
Normal: Test is performed by giving 2 g/kg body weight lactose orally and drawing glucose level at 0, 30, 45, 60, and 90 min. Normal response is change in glucose from fasting value to >30 mg/dl. Inconclusive response is increase of 20-30 mg/dl, abnormal response is increase <20 mg/dl.
Abnormal in: Lactase deficiency

LAP SCORE
See LEUKOCYTE ALKALINE PHOSPHATASE

LEAD
Normal: Child, <10 mcg/dl; adult, <25 mcg/dl; acceptable for industrial exposure, <50 mcg/dl
Elevated in: Lead exposure, lead poisoning

LDH
See LACTATE DEHYDROGENASE

LDL
See LOW-DENSITY LIPOPROTEIN CHOLESTEROL

LEGIONELLA TITER
Normal: Negative
Positive in: Legionnaire's disease (presumptive: ≥1:256 titer; definitive: fourfold titer increase to ≥1:128)

LEGIONELLA PNEUMOPHILA PCR
Test description: PCR can be performed on lung tissue, water sputum, bronchoalveolar lavage, and other respiratory fluids.

LEUKOCYTE ALKALINE PHOSPHATASE (LAP)
Normal range: 13-100 (33-188 U)
Elevated in: Leukemoid reactions, neutrophilia secondary to infections (except in sickle cell crisis—no significant increase in LAP score), Hodgkin's disease, polycythemia vera, hairy cell leukemia, aplastic anemia, Down's syndrome, myelofibrosis
Decreased in: Acute and chronic granulocytic leukemia, thrombocytopenic purpura, paroxysmal nocturnal hemoglobinuria, hypophosphatemia, collagen disorders

LEUKOCYTE COUNT
See COMPLETE BLOOD COUNT

LIPASE
Normal range: 0-160 U/L (0-2.66 μkat/L [CF: 0.01667; SMI: 0.02 μkat/L])
Elevated in: Acute pancreatitis, perforated peptic ulcer, carcinoma of pancreas (early stage), pancreatic duct obstruction, bowel infarction, intestinal obstruction

LIPOPROTEIN(a)
Normal: Male: 1.35-19.6 mg/dl; female: 1.24-20.1 mg/dl
Elevated in: Coronary artery disease, uncontrolled diabetes, hypothyroidism, chronic renal failure, pregnancy, tobacco use, infections, nephritic syndrome
Decreased in: Niacin, omega-3 fatty acids, estrogens, tamoxifen, statins

LIPOPROTEIN CHOLESTEROL, HIGH-DENSITY
See HIGH-DENSITY LIPOPROTEIN CHOLESTEROL

LIPOPROTEIN CHOLESTEROL, LOW-DENSITY
See LOW-DENSITY LIPOPROTEIN CHOLESTEROL

LIVER KIDNEY MICROSOME TYPE 1 ANTIBODIES (LKM1)
Normal: <20 U
Elevated in: Autoimmune hepatitis type 2

LKM1
See LIVER KIDNEY MICROSOME TYPE 1 ANTIBODIES

Laboratory
Tests

IV

LOW-DENSITY LIPOPROTEIN (LDL) CHOLESTEROL

Normal range: 50-130 mg/dl (1.30-1.68 mmol/L [CF: 0.02586; SMI: 0.05 mmol/L])

<70	Optimal in diabetics, prior MI, and patients with cardiac risk factors
100-129	Near or above optimal
130-159	Borderline high
160-189	High
≥190	Very high

LUPUS ANTICOAGULANT

See CIRCULATING ANTICOAGULANT

LUTEINIZING HORMONE

Normal range: 5-25 mIU/ml

Elevated in: Postmenopause, pituitary adenoma, primary gonadal dysfunction, polycystic ovary syndrome

Decreased in: Severe illness, anorexia nervosa, malnutrition, pituitary or hypothalamic impairment, severe stress

LYME DISEASE ANTIBODY TITER

Normal range: Negative

Positive result: Fig. 4-11 illustrates the usual serologic response in Lyme disease.

A serologic test is not necessary or helpful for several days after a tick bite because it is only 40%-50% sensitive in this stage, and a negative test does not rule out the diagnosis.

LYMPHOCYTES

Normal range: 15%-40%

Total lymphocyte count = 800-2600/mm^3
Total T lymphocyte: = 800-2200/mm^3
CD4 lymphocytes = ≥400/mm^3
CD8 lymphocytes = 200-800/mm^3
   Normal CD4/CD8 ratio is 2.0.

Elevated in: Chronic infections, infectious mononucleosis and other viral infections, chronic lymphocytic leukemia, Hodgkin's disease, ulcerative colitis, hypoadrenalism, idiopathic thrombocytopenia

Decreased in:

AIDS, bone marrow suppression from chemotherapeutic agents or chemotherapy, aplastic anemia, neoplasms, steroids, adrenocortical hyperfunction, neurologic disorders (multiple sclerosis, myasthenia gravis, Guillain-Barré syndrome)

CD4 lymphocytes are calculated as total white blood cells × % lymphocytes × % lymphocytes stained with CD4. They are decreased in AIDS and other immune dysfunction.

Table 4-15 describes various lymphocyte abnormalities in peripheral blood.

MAGNESIUM (serum)

Normal range: 1.8-3.0 mg/dl (0.80-1.20 mmol/L [CF: 0.4114; SMI: 0.02 mmol/L])

CAUSES OF HYPERMAGNESEMIA

I. Decreased renal excretion
   A. Renal failure—glomerular filtration rate less than 30 ml/min
   B. Hyperparathyroidism
   C. Hypothyroidism
   D. Addison's disease
   E. Lithium intoxication
   F. Familial hypocalciuric hypercalcemia
II. Other causes: usually in association with decrease in glomerular filtration rate
   A. Endogenous loads
      1. Diabetic ketoacidosis
      2. Severe tissue injury—burns
   B. Exogenous loads
      1. Gastrointestinal
         a. Magnesium-containing laxatives and antacids
         b. High-dose vitamin D analogs
      2. Parenteral: management of toxemia of pregnancy

CAUSES OF HYPOMAGNESEMIA

Alcoholic abuse
Diuretic use
Renal losses
Acute and chronic renal failure
Postobstructive diuresis
Acute tubular necrosis
Chronic glomerulonephritis
Chronic pyelonephritis
Interstitial nephropathy
Renal transplantation
Gastrointestinal losses
Chronic diarrhea
Nasogastric suctioning
Short bowel syndrome
Protein calorie malnutrition
Bowel fistula
Total parenteral nutrition
Acute pancreatitis
Endocrine
Diabetes mellitus
Hyperaldosteronism
Hyperthyroidism
Hyperparathyroidism
Acute intermittent porphyria
Pregnancy
Drugs

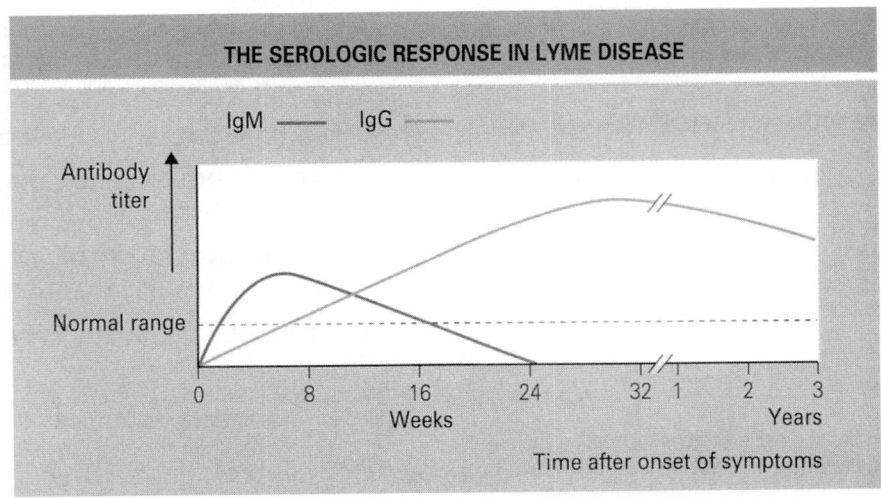

FIGURE 4-11 IgM and IgG responses in Lyme disease.

TABLE 4-15 Differential Diagnosis of Abnormal Lymphocytes in Peripheral Blood

Lymphocyte Type	Usual Disease Association	Cytologic Features	Laboratory Features	Clinical Features
Small lymphocyte	Chronic lymphocytic leukemia	B-cell surface markers with low concentration of surface immunoglobulin, CD5 antigen	Hypogammaglobulinemia in 50%; positive direct Coombs test in 15%; on node biopsy, diffuse, well-differentiated lymphocytic infiltrate	Elderly adults; presentation runs gamut from asymptomatic with lymphocytosis only to bulky disease with adenopathy, splenomegaly, and "packed" bone marrow
Atypical lymphocyte	Infectious mononucleosis, other viral illnesses	Suppressor T-cell markers	Heterophil agglutinin; positive serology for Epstein-Barr virus, cytomegalovirus, toxoplasma, HBsAg	Pharyngitis, fever, adenopathy, rash, splenomegaly, palatal petechiae, jaundice
Plasmacytoid lymphocyte	Waldenström's macroglobulin anemia	Cytoplasmic IgM, periodic acid-Schiff positivity	IgM paraprotein, rouleaux, cryoglobulins	Adenopathy, splenomegaly, absence of bone lesions, hyperviscosity syndrome, cryopathic phenomena
Lymphoblast	ALL	Terminal transferase positivity, common ALL antigen, B- or T-precursor markers	Anemia, granulocytopenia, thrombocytopenia, hyperuricemia, diffuse bone marrow infiltration	Peak incidence in childhood, acute onset, bone pain frequent
Lymphosarcoma cell	Lymphocytic lymphoma	B-cell surface markers with high concentration of monoclonal surface immunoglobulin	Nodular or diffuse, poorly differentiated lymphocytic lymphoma on node biopsy, patchy, peritrabecular bone marrow involvement	Middle-aged to older adults, generalized adenopathy, constitutional symptoms
Sézary cell	Cutaneous lymphomas	T-lymphocyte surface markers	Skin biopsy is diagnostic	Exfoliative erythroderma, cutaneous plaques or tumors
Hairy cell	Hairy cell leukemia	B-lymphocyte markers, cytoplasmic projections, tartrate-resistant acid phosphatase, interleukin-2 receptors, CD11 antigen	Pancytopenia	Middle-aged males, moderate to marked splenomegaly without adenopathy
Prolymphocyte	Prolymphocytic leukemia	B-cell surface markers with high concentration of surface immunoglobulin, CD5 negative	Marked lymphocytosis (frequently >100 × 10^9/L)	Elderly adults, massive splenomegaly, minimum adenopathy, poor response to therapy

Reprinted from Stein JH (ed): *Internal medicine*, ed 5, St Louis, 1998, Mosby.
ALL, Acute lymphoblastic leukemia.

Aminoglycosides
Amphotericin
β-agonists
Cisplatin
Cyclosporine
Diuretics
Foscarnet
Pentamidine
Theophylline
Congenital disorders
Familial hypomagnesemia
Maternal diabetes
Maternal hypothyroidism
Maternal hyperparathyroidism

MEAN CORPUSCULAR VOLUME (MCV)

Normal range: 76-100 μm^3 (76-100 fL) (76-100 fL [CF: 1; SMI: 1 fL])
See Tables 4-16 and 4-17 for descriptions of MCV abnormalities.

METANEPHRINES, URINE

See URINE METANEPHRINES

METHYLMALONIC ACID, SERUM

Normal: <0.2 mcmol/L
Elevated in: Vitamin B$_{12}$ deficiency, pregnancy, methylmalonic acidemia

MITOCHONDRIAL ANTIBODY (AMA)

Normal: Negative
Present in: Primary biliary cirrhosis (>90% of patients)

MONOCYTE COUNT

Normal range: 2%-8%
Elevated in: Viral diseases, parasites, infections, neoplasms, inflammatory bowel disease, monocytic leukemia, lymphomas, myeloma, sarcoidosis
Decreased in: Aplastic anemia, lymphocytic leukemia, glucocorticoid administration

MYCOPLASMA PNEUMONIAE PCR

Test description: PCR can be performed on sputum, bronchoalveolar lavage, nasopharyngeal and throat swabs, other respiratory fluids, and lung tissue

MYELIN BASIC PROTEIN, CEREBROSPINAL FLUID

Normal: <2.5 ng/ml
Elevated in: Multiple sclerosis, CNS trauma, stroke, encephalitis

MYOGLOBIN, URINE

See URINE MYOGLOBIN

NEISSERIA GONORRHOEA PCR

Test description: Test can be performed on endocervical swab, urine, and intraurethral swab
Normal: Negative

NEUTROPHIL COUNT

Normal range: 50%-70%
Subsets:
Stabs (bands, early mature neutrophils): 2%-6%
Segs (mature neutrophils): 60%-70%
Elevated in: Acute bacterial infections, acute myocardial infarction, stress, neoplasms, myelocytic leukemia
Decreased in: Viral infections, aplastic anemias, immunosuppressive drugs, radiation therapy to bone marrow, agranulocytosis, drugs (antibiotics, antithyroidals, clopidogrel), lymphocytic and monocytic leukemias
Table 4-18 describes various drugs that can cause neutropenia.

NOREPINEPHRINE

Normal range: 0-600 pg/ml
Elevated in: Pheochromocytomas, neuroblastomas, stress, vigorous exercise, certain foods (bananas, chocolate, coffee, tea, vanilla)

Laboratory Tests

IV

TABLE 4-16 Some Causes of Increased Mean Corpuscular Volume (Macrocytosis)

Causes	% of all Macrocytosis Patients*	% of Macrocytosis in Each Disease†
Common		
Folate or B_{12} deficiency	20-30 (5-50)‡	80-90 (4-100)
Chronic liver disease	15-20 (6-28)	25-30 (8-65)
Chronic alcoholism	10-12 (3-15)	60 (26-90)
Cytotoxic chemotherapy	10-15 (2-20)	30-40 (13-82)
Cardiorespiratory abnormality	8 (7-9.5)	?
Reticulocytosis	6-7 (0-15)	Depends on severity
Myelodysplastic syndromes	Frequent over age 40 yr	>60 in RAEB and RARS
Unexplained	25 (22.5-27)	—
Normal newborn		
Less Common	**<4%**	
Noncytotoxic drugs		
Zidovudine		
Phenytoin		30 (14-50)
Azathioprine		
Hypothyroidism		20-30 (8-55)
Chronic leukemia/myelofibrosis		
Radiotherapy for malignancy		
Chronic renal disease (occasional patients)		
Distance-runner macrocytosis (some persons)		
Down syndrome		
Artifactual (e.g., cold agglutinins)		

Reprinted from Ravel R: *Clinical laboratory medicine,* ed 6, St Louis, 1995, Mosby.
RAEB, Refractory anemia with excessive blasts; RARS, refractory anemia with ring sideroblasts (formerly called "IASA," or idiopathic acquired sideroblastic anemia).
*Percentage of all patients with macrocytosis.
†Percentage of patients with each condition listed who have macrocytosis.
‡Numbers in parentheses are literature range.

TABLE 4-17 Some Causes of Decreased Mean Corpuscular Volume (Microcytosis)

Common	Less Common
Chronic iron deficiency	Some cases of polycythemia
α- or β-thalassemia (minor)	Some cases of lead poisoning
Anemia of chronic disease	Some cases of congenital spherocytosis
	Some cases of sideroblastic anemia
	Certain abnormal hemoglobins (HbE, Hb Lepore)

Reprinted from Ravel R: *Clinical laboratory medicine,* ed 6, St Louis, 1995, Mosby.

5'-NUCLEOTIDASE

Normal range: 2-16 IU/L (3-27 × 10⁸ kat/L [CF: 1.67 × 10⁸; SMI: 1 × 10⁸ kat/L])
Elevated in: Biliary obstruction, metastatic neoplasms to liver, primary biliary cirrhosis, renal failure, pancreatic carcinoma, chronic active hepatitis

OSMOLALITY (serum)

Normal range: 280-300 mOsm/kg (280-300 mmol/kg [CF: 1; SMI: 1 mmol/kg])
It can also be estimated by the following formula:

$$2([Na] + [K]) + glucose/18 + BuN/2.8$$

Elevated in: Dehydration, hypernatremia, diabetes insipidus, uremia, hyperglycemia, mannitol therapy, ingestion of toxins (ethylene glycol, methanol, ethanol), hypercalcemia, diuretics
Decreased in: Syndrome of inappropriate diuretic hormone secretion, hyponatremia, overhydration, Addison's disease, hypothyroidism

OSMOLALITY, URINE
See URINE OSMOLALITY

TABLE 4-18 Drugs That Cause Neutropenia

Antiarrhythmics
  Tocainide, procainamide, propranolol, quinidine
Antibiotics
  Chloramphenicol, penicillins, sulfonamides, p-aminosalicylic acid (PAS), rifampin, vancomycin, isoniazid, nitrofurantoin
Antimalarials
  Dapsone, quinine, pyrimethamine
Anticonvulsants
  Phenytoin, mephenytoin, trimethadione, ethosuximide, carbamazepine
Hypoglycemic agents
  Tolbutamide, chlorpropamide
Antihistamines
  Cimetidine, brompheniramine, tripelennamine
Antihypertensives
  Methyldopa, captopril
Anti-inflammatory agents
  Aminopyrine, phenylbutazone, gold salts, ibuprofen, indomethacin
Antithyroid agents
  Propylthiouracil, methimazole, thiouracil
Diuretics
  Acetazolamide, hydrochlorothiazide, chlorthalidone
Phenothiazines
  Chlorpromazine, promazine, prochlorperazine
Immunosuppressive agents
  Antimetabolites
Cytotoxic agents
  Alkylating agents, antimetabolites, anthracyclines, Vinca alkaloids, cisplatin, hydroxyurea, dactinomycin
Other agents
  Recombinant interferons, allopurinol, ethanol, levamisole, penicillamine, zidovudine, streptokinase, carbamazepine, clopidogrel, ticlopidine

Modified from Goldman L, Ausiello D (eds): *Cecil textbook of medicine,* ed 22, Philadelphia, 2004, WB Saunders.

OSMOTIC FRAGILITY TEST

Normal: Hemolysis begins at 0.50, w/v [5.0 g/L] and is complete at 0.30, w/v [3.0 g/L] NaCl.

Elevated in: Hereditary spherocytosis, hereditary stomatocytosis, spherocytosis associated with acquired immune hemolytic anemia

Decreased in: Iron deficiency anemia, thalassemias, liver disease, leptocytosis associated with asplenia

PARACENTESIS FLUID

Testing and evaluation of results:

1. Process the fluid as follows:
   a. Tube 1: LDH, glucose, albumin
   b. Tube 2: protein, specific gravity
   c. Tube 3: cell count and differential
   d. Tube 4: save until further notice
2. Draw serum LDH, protein, albumin.
3. Gram stain, AFB stain, bacterial and fungal cultures, amylase, and triglycerides should be ordered only when clearly indicated; bedside inoculation of blood-culture bottles with ascitic fluid improves sensitivity in detecting bacterial growth.
4. If malignant ascites is suspected, consider a carcinoembryonic antigen level on the paracentesis fluid and cytologic evaluation.
5. In suspected spontaneous bacterial peritonitis (SBP) the incidence of positive cultures can be increased by injecting 10 to 20 ml of ascitic fluid into blood culture bottles.
6. Peritoneal effusion can be subdivided as exudative or transudative based on its characteristics (see Section II).
7. The serum-ascites albumin gradient (serum albumin level–ascitic fluid albumin level) correlates directly with portal pressure and can also be used to classify ascite. Patients with gradients ≥1.1 g/dl have portal hypertension, and those with gradients ≤1.1 g/dl do not; the accuracy of this method is >95%.
8. For the differential diagnosis of ascites, refer to Section II.
9. An ascitic fluid polymorphonuclear leukocyte count >500/μl is suggestive of SBP.
10. A blood-ascitic fluid albumin gradient.

PARATHYROID HORMONE (PTH)

Normal:
Serum, intact molecule 10-65 pg/ml
Plasma 1.0-5.0 pmol/L

Elevated in: hyperparathyroidism (primary or secondary), pseudohypoparathyroidism, anticonvulsants, corticosteroids, lithium, INH, rifampin, phosphates, ZE syndrome, hereditary vitamin D deficiency

Decreased in: hypoparathyroidism, sarcoidosis, cimetidine, beta-blockers, hyperthyroidism, hypomagnesemia

PARIETAL CELL ANTIBODIES

Normal: Negative

Present in: Pernicious anemia (>90%), atrophic gastritis (up to 50%), thyroiditis (30%), Addison's disease, myasthenia gravis, Sjögren's syndrome, type 1 DM

PARTIAL THROMBOPLASTIN TIME (PTT), ACTIVATED PARTIAL THROMBOPLASTIN TIME (APTT)

Normal range: 25-41 sec

Elevated in: Heparin therapy, coagulation factor deficiency (I, II, V, VIII, IX, X, XI, XII), liver disease, vitamin K deficiency, disseminated intravascular coagulation, circulating anticoagulant, warfarin therapy, specific factor inhibition (PCN reaction, rheumatoid arthritis), thrombolytic therapy, nephrotic syndrome

NOTE: Useful to evaluate the intrinsic coagulation system.

PEPSINOGEN I

Normal: 124-142 ng/ml

Elevated in: ZE syndrome, duodenal ulcer, acute gastritis

Decreased in: Atrophic gastritis, gastric carcinoma, myxedema, pernicious anemia, Addison's disease

pH, BLOOD

Normal values:
Arterial: 7.35-7.45
Venous: 7.32-7.42
  For abnormal values, refer to ARTERIAL BLOOD GASES.

pH, URINE

See URINE pH

PHENOBARBITAL

Normal therapeutic range: 15-30 mcg/ml for epilepsy control

PHENYTOIN (Dilantin)

Normal therapeutic range: 10-20 mcg/ml

PHOSPHATASE, ACID

See ACID PHOSPHATASE

PHOSPHATASE, ALKALINE

See ALKALINE PHOSPHATASE

PHOSPHATE (serum)

Normal range: 2.5-5 mg/dl (0.8-1.6 mmol/L [CF: 0.3229; SMI: 0.05 mmol/L])

DECREASED
Parenteral hyperalimentation
Diabetic acidosis
Alcohol withdrawal
Severe metabolic or respiratory alkalosis
Antacids that bind phosphorus
Malnutrition with refeeding using low-phosphorus nutrients
Renal tubule failure to reabsorb phosphate (Fanconi's syndrome; congenital disorder; vitamin D deficiency)
Glucose administration
Nasogastric suction
Malabsorption
Gram-negative sepsis
Primary hyperthyroidism
Chlorothiazide diuretics
Therapy of acute severe asthma
Acute respiratory failure with mechanical ventilation

INCREASED
Renal failure
Severe muscle injury
Phosphate-containing antacids
Hypoparathyroidism
Tumor lysis syndrome

PLASMINOGEN

Normal: Immunoassay (antigen): <20 mg/dl

Elevated in: infection, trauma, neoplasm, myocardial infarction (acute phase reactant), pregnancy, bilirubinemia

Decreased in: DIC, severe liver disease, thrombolytic therapy with streptokinase or urokinase, alteplase

PLATELET AGGREGATION

Normal: Full aggregation (generally >60%) in response to epinephrine, thrombin, ristocetin, ADP, collagen

Elevated in: Heparin, hemolysis, lipemia, nicotine, hereditary and acquired disorders of platelet adhesion, activation, and aggregation

Decreased in: Aspirin, some penicillins, chloroquine, chlorpromazine, clofibrate, captopril, Glanzmann's thrombasthenia, Bernard-Soulier syndrome, Wiskott-Aldrich syndrome, cyclooxygenase deficiency. In von Willebrand's disease there is normal aggregation with ADP, collagen, and epinephrine but abnormal agglutination with ristocetin.

PLATELET ANTIBODIES
Normal: Absent
Present in: ITP (>90% of patients with chronic ITP). Patients with nonimmune thrombocytopenias may have false-positive results.

PLATELET COUNT
Normal range: 130-400 × 10^3/mm^3 (130-400 × 10^9/L [CF: 1; SMI: 5 × 10^9/L])
Elevated in:
REACTIVE THROMBOCYTOSIS
Infections or inflammatory states—vasculitis, allergic reactions, etc.
Surgery and tissue damage—myocardial infarction, pancreatitis, etc.
Postsplenectomy state
Malignancy—solid tumors, lymphoma
Iron deficiency anemia, hemolytic anemia, acute blood loss
Uncertain etiology
Rebound effect after chemotherapy or immune thrombocytopenia
Renal disorders—renal failure, nephrotic syndrome
MYELOPROLIFERATIVE DISORDERS
Chronic myeloid leukemia
Primary thrombocythemia
Polycythemia vera
Idiopathic myelofibrosis
Decreased:
A. Increased destruction
  1. Immunologic
    a. Drugs: quinine, quinidine, digitalis, procainamide, thiazide diuretics, sulfonamides, phenytoin, aspirin, penicillin, heparin, gold, meprobamate, sulfa drugs, phenylbutazone, NSAIDs, methyldopa, cimetidine, furosemide, INH, cephalosporins, chlorpropamide, organic arsenicals, chloroquine
    b. Idiopathic thrombocytopenic purpura
    c. Transfusion reaction: transfusion of platelets with platelet antigen HPA-1a (PL^{A1}) in recipients without PL^{A1}
    d. Fetal/maternal incompatibility
    e. Vasculitis (e.g., systemic lupus erythematosus)
    f. Autoimmune hemolytic anemia
    g. Lymphoreticular disorders (e.g., chronic lymphocytic leukemia)
  2. Nonimmunologic
    a. Prosthetic heart valves
    b. Thrombotic thrombocytopenic purpura
    c. Sepsis
    d. Disseminated intravascular coagulation
    e. Hemolytic-uremic syndrome
    f. Giant cavernous hemangioma
B. Decreased production
  1. Abnormal marrow
    a. Marrow infiltration (e.g., leukemia, lymphoma, fibrosis)
    b. Marrow suppression (e.g., chemotherapy, alcohol, radiation)
  2. Hereditary disorders
    a. Wiskott-Aldrich syndrome: X-linked disorder characterized by thrombocytopenia, eczema, and repeated infections
    b. May-Hegglin anomaly: increased megakaryocytes but ineffective thrombopoiesis
  3. Vitamin deficiencies (e.g., vitamin B$_{12}$, folic acid)
C. Splenic sequestration, hypersplenism
D. Dilutional, secondary to massive transfusion

PLATELET FUNCTION ANALYSIS 100 ASSAY (PFA)
Normal: This test is a two-component assay where blood is aspirated through two capillary tubes, one of which is coated with collagen and ADP (COL/ADP) and the other with collagen and epinephrine (COL/EPI). The test measures the ability of platelets to occlude an aperture in a biologically active membrane treated with COL/ADP and COL/EPI. During the test, the platelets adhere to the surface of the tube and cause blood flow to cease. The closing time refers to the cessation of blood flow and is reported in conjunction with the hematocrit and platelet count. Hematocrit count must be >25% and platelet count >50 K/microliter for the test to be performed
  COL/ADP: 70-120 sec
  COL/EPI: 75-120 sec

Elevated in: acquired platelet dysfunction, von Willebrand's disease, anemia, thrombocytopenia, use of aspirin and NSAIDs

POTASSIUM (serum)
Normal range: 3.5-5 mEq/L (3.5-5 mmol/L [CF: 1; SMI: 0.1 mmol/L])
CAUSES OF HYPERKALEMIA
I. Pseudohyperkalemia
  A. Hemolysis of sample
  B. Thrombocytosis
  C. Leukocytosis
  D. Laboratory error
II. Increased potassium intake and absorption
  A. Potassium supplements (oral and parenteral)
  B. Dietary—salt substitutes
  C. Stored blood
  D. Potassium-containing medications
III. Impaired renal excretion
  A. Acute renal failure
  B. Chronic renal failure
  C. Tubular defect in potassium secretion
    1. Renal allograft
    2. Analgesic nephropathy
    3. Sickle cell disease
    4. Obstructive uropathy
    5. Interstitial nephritis
    6. Chronic pyelonephritis
    7. Potassium-sparing diuretics
    8. Miscellaneous (lead, systemic lupus erythematosus, pseudohypoaldosteronism)
  D. Hypoaldosteronism
    1. Primary (Addison's disease)
    2. Secondary
      a. Hyporeninemic hypoaldosteronism (type IV RTA)
      b. Congenital adrenal hyperplasia
      c. Drug-induced
        (1) NSAIDs
        (2) ACE inhibitors
        (3) Heparin
        (4) Cyclosporine
IV. Transcellular shifts
  A. Acidosis
  B. Hypertonicity
  C. Insulin deficiency
  D. Drugs
    1. β-blockers
    2. Digitalis toxicity
    3. Succinylcholine
  E. Exercise
  F. Hyperkalemic periodic paralysis
V. Cellular injury
  A. Rhabdomyolysis
  B. Severe intravascular hemolysis
  C. Acute tumor lysis syndrome
  D. Burns and crush injuries
CAUSES OF HYPOKALEMIA
I. Decreased intake
  A. Decreased dietary potassium
  B. Impaired absorption of potassium
  C. Clay ingestion
  D. Kayexalate
II. Increased loss
  A. Renal
    1. Hyperaldosteronism
      a. Primary
        (1) Conn's syndrome
        (2) Adrenal hyperplasia
      b. Secondary
        (1) Congestive heart failure
        (2) Cirrhosis

(3) Nephrotic syndrome
(4) Dehydration
  c. Bartter's syndrome
2. Glycyrrhizic acid (licorice, chewing tobacco)
3. Excessive adrenal corticosteroids
  a. Cushing's syndrome
  b. Steroid therapy
  c. Adrenogenital syndrome
4. Renal tubular defects
  a. Renal tubular acidosis
  b. Obstructive uropathy
  c. Salt-wasting nephropathy
5. Drugs
  a. Diuretics
  b. Aminoglycosides
  c. Mannitol
  d. Amphotericin
  e. Cisplatin
  f. Carbenicillin
B. Gastrointestinal
1. Vomiting
2. Nasogastric suction
3. Diarrhea
4. Malabsorption
5. Ileostomy
6. Villous adenoma
7. Laxative abuse
C. Increased losses from the skin
1. Excessive sweating
2. Burns
III. Transcellular shifts
A. Alkalosis
1. Vomiting
2. Diuretics
3. Hyperventilation
4. Bicarbonate therapy
B. Insulin
1. Exogenous
2. Endogenous response to glucose
C. β₂-Agonists (albuterol, terbutaline, epinephrine)
D. Hypokalemia periodic paralysis
1. Familial
2. Thyrotoxic
IV. Miscellaneous
A. Anabolic state
B. Intravenous hyperalimentation
C. Treatment of megaloblastic anemia
D. Acute mountain sickness

POTASSIUM, URINE

See URINE POTASSIUM

PROCAINAMIDE

Normal therapeutic range: 4-10 mcg/ml

PROGESTERONE (serum)

Normal:
Female: Follicular phase: 15-70 ng/dl
Luteal phase: 200-2500 ng/dl
Male: 15-70 ng/dl
Elevated in: Congenital adrenal hyperplasia, clomiphene, corticosterone, 11-deoxycortisol, dihydroprogesterone, molar pregnancy, lipoid ovarian tumor
Decreased in: Primary or secondary hypogonadism, oral contraceptives, ampicillin, threatened abortion

PROLACTIN

Normal range: <20 ng/ml (<20 μg/L [CF: 1; SMI: 1 μg/L])
Elevated in: Prolactinomas (level >200 highly suggestive), drugs (phenothiazines, cimetidine, tricyclic antidepressants, metoclopramide, estrogens,

antihypertensives [methyldopa], verapamil, haloperidol), postpartum, stress, hypoglycemia, hypothyroidism

PROSTATE-SPECIFIC ANTIGEN (PSA)

Normal range: 0-4 ng/ml
  Table 4-19 describes age-specific reference ranges for PSA.
Elevated in: Benign prostatic hypertrophy, carcinoma of prostate, prostatitis, postrectal examination, prostate trauma.
  Factors affecting serum PSA are described in Table 4-20.
  NOTE: Measurement of free PSA is useful to assess the probability of prostate cancer in patients with normal digital rectal examination and total PSA between 4 and 10 ng/ml. In these patients, the global risk of prostate cancer is 25%; however, if the free PSA is >25%, the risk of prostate cancer decreases to 8%, whereas if the free PSA is <10%, the risk of cancer increases to 56%. Free PSA is also useful to evaluate the aggressiveness of prostate cancer. A low free PSA percentage generally indicates a high-grade cancer, whereas a high free PSA percentage is generally associated with a slower growing tumor.
Decreased in: 5 alpha-reductase inhibitors (finasteride, dutasteride), saw palmetto use, antiandrogens

PROSTATIC ACID PHOSPHATASE

Normal: 0-0.8 U/L
Elevated in: Prostate cancer (especially in metastatic prostate cancer), BPH, prostatitis, post–prostate surgery or manipulation, hemolysis, androgens, clofibrate
Decreased in: Ketoconazole

PROTEIN (SERUM)

Normal range: 6-8 g/dl (60-80 g/L [CF: 10; SMI: 1 g/L])
Elevated in: Dehydration, multiple myeloma, Waldenström's macroglobulinemia, sarcoidosis, collagen vascular diseases

TABLE 4-19 Age-Specific Reference Ranges for PSA

Age (yr)	Serum PSA (ng/ml)		
	Whites	Japanese	African Americans
40-49	0-2.5	0-2.0	0-2.0
50-59	0-3.5	0-3.0	0-4.0
60-69	0-4.5	0-4.0	0-4.5
70-79	0-6.5	0-5.0	0-5.5

Reprinted from Nseyo UO (ed): *Urology for primary care physicians*, Philadelphia, 1999, WB Saunders.
PSA, Prostate-specific antigen.

TABLE 4-20 Factors Affecting Serum PSA

Factors Affecting Serum PSA	Duration of Effect
Prostate cell number	NA
Prostate size	NA
Recent ejaculation	6-48 hours
Prostate manipulation	
Vigorous massage	1 week
Cystoscopy	1 week
Prostate biopsy	4-6 weeks
Prostatitis	
Acute	3-6 months
Chronic	Unknown
Prostate cancer	NA
Drugs: finasteride (Proscar)*	3-6 months

Reprinted from Nseyo UO (ed): *Urology for primary care physicians*, Philadelphia, 1999, WB Saunders.
NA, Not applicable; *PSA*, prostate-specific antigen.
*Lowers PSA for as long as patient is on the medication.

Laboratory Tests

IV

Decreased in: Malnutrition, low-protein diet, overhydration, malabsorption, pregnancy, severe burns, neoplasms, chronic diseases, cirrhosis, nephrosis

PROTEIN C ASSAY

Normal: 70%-140%
Elevated in: Oral contraceptives, stanozol
Decreased in: Congenital protein C deficiency, warfarin therapy, Vitamin K deficiency, renal insufficiency, consumptive coagulopathies

PROTEIN ELECTROPHORESIS (serum)

Normal range:
Albumin: 60%-75% (0.6-0.75 [CF: 0.01; SMI: 0.01])
  α-1: 1.7%-5% (0.02-0.05)
  α-2: 6.7%-12.5% (0.07-0.13)
  β: 8.3%-16.3% (0.08-0.16)
  γ: 10.7%-20% (0.11-0.2)
Albumin: 3.6-5.2 g/dl (36-52 g/L [CF: 0.01; SMI: 1 g/L])
  α-1: 0.1-0.4 g/dl (1-4 g/L)
  α-2: 0.4-1 g/dl (4-10 g/L)

  β: 0.5-1.2 g/dl (5-12 g/L)
  γ: 0.6-1.6 g/dl (6-16 g/L)
Elevated in:
Albumin: dehydration
α-1: neoplastic diseases, inflammation
α-2: neoplasms, inflammation, infection, nephrotic syndrome
β: hypothyroidism, biliary cirrhosis, diabetes mellitus
γ: See IMMUNOGLOBULINS
Decreased in:
Albumin: malnutrition, chronic liver disease, malabsorption, nephrotic syndrome, burns, systemic lupus erythematosus
α-1: emphysema (α-1 antitrypsin deficiency), nephrosis
α-2: hemolytic anemias (decreased haptoglobin), severe hepatocellular damage
β: hypocholesterolemia, nephrosis
γ: See IMMUNOGLOBULINS
  Fig. 4-12 describes serum protein electrophoretic patterns.

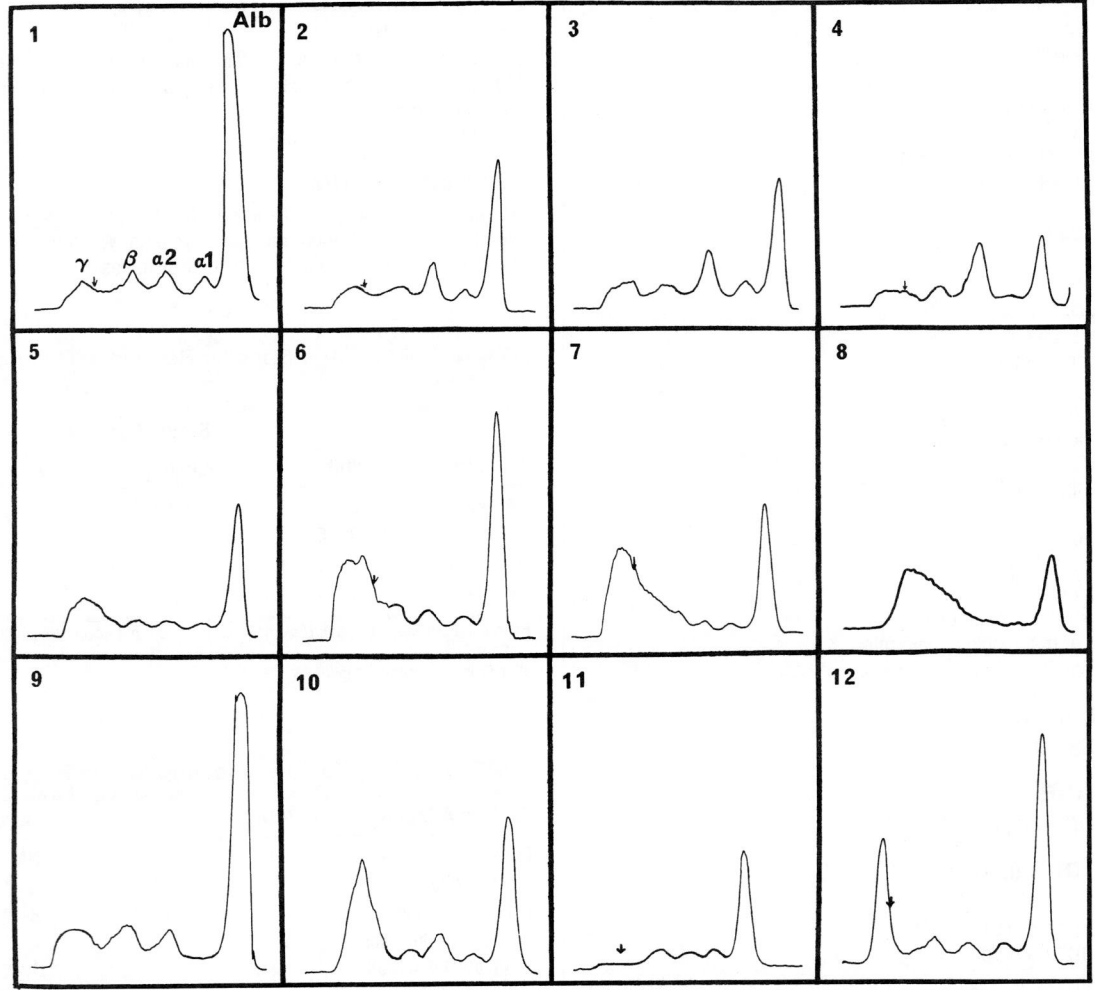

FIGURE 4-12 Typical serum protein electrophoretic patterns. *1,* Normal (*arrow* near γ region indicates serum application point). *2,* Acute reaction pattern. *3,* Acute reaction or nephrotic syndrome. *4,* Nephrotic syndrome. *5,* Chronic inflammation, cirrhosis, granulomatous diseases, rheumatoid-collagen group. *6,* Same as 5, but γ elevation is more pronounced. There is also partial (but not complete) β-γ fusion. *7,* Suggestive of cirrhosis but could be found in the granulomatous diseases or the rheumatoid-collagen group. *8,* Characteristic pattern of cirrhosis. *9,* α-1 Antitrypsin deficiency with mild γ elevation suggesting concurrent chronic disease. *10,* Same as 5, but the γ elevation is marked. The configuration of the γ peak superficially mimics that of myeloma, but is more broad-based. There are superimposed acute reaction changes. *11,* Hypogammaglobulinemia or light-chain myeloma. *12,* Myeloma, Waldenström's macroglobulinemia, idiopathic or secondary monoclonal gammopathy. (Reprinted from Ravel R [ed]: *Clinical laboratory medicine,* ed 6, St Louis, 1995, Mosby.)

PROTEIN S ASSAY

Normal: 65%-140%
Elevated in: Presence of lupus anticoagulant
Decreased in: Hereditary deficiency, acute thrombotic events, DIC, surgery, oral contraceptives, pregnancy, hormone replacement therapy, L-asparaginase treatment

PROTHROMBIN TIME (PT)

Normal range: 10-12 sec
Elevated in: Liver disease, oral anticoagulants (warfarin), heparin, factor deficiency (I, II, V, VII, X), disseminated intravascular coagulation, vitamin K deficiency, afibrinogenemia, dysfibrinogenemia, drugs (salicylate, chloral hydrate, diphenylhydantoin, estrogens, antacids, phenylbutazone, quinidine, antibiotics, allopurinol, anabolic steroids)
Decreased in: Vitamin K supplementation, thrombophlebitis, drugs (glutethimide, estrogens, griseofulvin, diphenhydramine)

PROTOPORPHYRIN (free erythrocyte)

Normal range: 16-36 μg/dl of red blood cells (0.28-0.64 μmol/L [CF: 0.0177; SMI: 0.02 μmol/L])
Elevated in: Iron deficiency, lead poisoning, sideroblastic anemias, anemia of chronic disease, hemolytic anemias, erythropoietic protoporphyria

PSA

See PROSTATE-SPECIFIC ANTIGEN

PT

See PROTHROMBIN TIME

PTH

See PARATHYROID HORMONE

PTT

See PARTIAL THROMBOPLASTIN TIME

RDW

See RED BLOOD CELL DISTRIBUTION WIDTH

RED BLOOD CELL (RBC) COUNT

Normal range:
Male: $4.3-5.9 \times 10^6/mm^3$ ($4.3-5.9 \times 10^{12}/L$ [CF: 1; SMI: $0.1 \times 10^{12}/L$])
Female: $3.5-5 \times 10^6/mm^3$ ($3.5-5 \times 10^{12}/L$ [CF: 1; SMI: $0.1 \times 10^{12}/L$])

Elevated in: Polycythemia vera, smokers, high altitude, cardiovascular disease, renal cell carcinoma and other erythropoietin-producing neoplasms, stress, hemoconcentration/dehydration
Decreased in: Anemias, hemolysis, chronic renal failure, hemorrhage, failure of marrow production

RED BLOOD CELL DISTRIBUTION WIDTH (RDW)

Measures variability of red cell size (anisocytosis)
Normal range: 11.5-14.5
Normal RDW and elevated mean corpuscular volume (MCV): Aplastic anemia, preleukemia
Normal MCV: Normal, anemia of chronic disease, acute blood loss or hemolysis, chronic lymphocytic leukemia (CLL), chronic myelocytic leukemia, nonanemic enzymopathy or hemoglobinopathy
Decreased MCV: Anemia of chronic disease, heterozygous thalassemia
Elevated RDW and elevated MCV: Vitamin B_{12} deficiency, folate deficiency, immune hemolytic anemia, cold agglutinins, CLL with high count, liver disease
Normal MCV: Early iron deficiency, early vitamin B_{12} deficiency, early folate deficiency, anemic globinopathy
Decreased MCV: Iron deficiency, red blood cell fragmentation, HbH disease, thalassemia intermedia

RED BLOOD CELL FOLATE

See FOLATE

RED BLOOD CELL MASS (volume)

Normal range:
Male: 20-36 ml/kg body weight ($1.15-1.21$ L/m^2 body surface area)
Female: 19-31 ml/kg body weight ($0.95-1.00$ L/m^2 body surface area)
Elevated in: Polycythemia vera, hypoxia (smokers, high altitude, cardiovascular disease), hemoglobinopathies with high oxygen affinity, erythropoietin-producing tumors (renal cell carcinoma)
Decreased in: Hemorrhage, chronic disease, failure of marrow production, anemias, hemolysis

RED BLOOD CELL MORPHOLOGY

See Fig. 4-13.

RENIN (serum)

Elevated in: Drugs (thiazides, estrogen, minoxidil), chronic renal failure, Bartter's syndrome, pregnancy (normal), pheochromocytoma, renal hypertension, reduced plasma volume, secondary aldosteronism

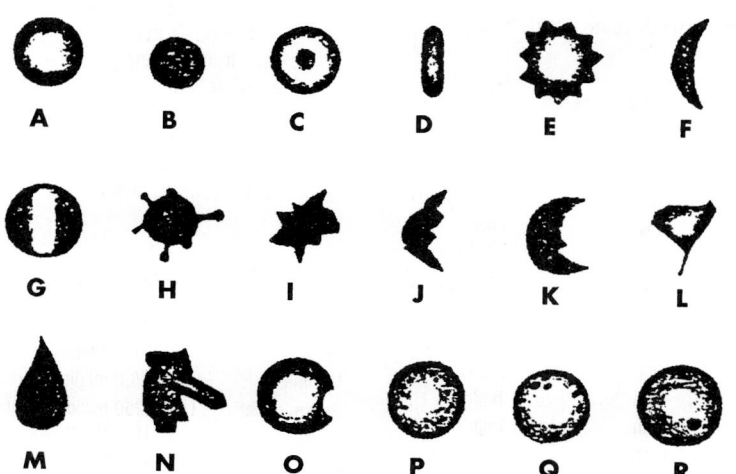

FIGURE 4-13 Abnormal red blood cells (RBCs). A, Normal RBC. **B,** Spherocyte. **C,** Target cell. **D,** Elliptocyte. **E,** Echinocyte. **F,** Sickle cell. **G,** Stomatocyte. **H,** Acanthocyte. **I** to **L,** Schistocytes. **M,** Teardrop RBC. **N,** Distorted RBC with Hb C crystal protruding. **O,** Degmacyte. **P,** Basophilic stippling. **Q,** Pappenheimer bodies. **R,** Howell-Jolly body. (Reprinted from Ravel R [ed]: *Clinical laboratory medicine,* ed 6, St Louis, 1995, Mosby.)

Decreased in: Adrenocortical hypertension, increased plasma volume, primary aldosteronism, drugs (propranolol, reserpine, clonidine)

Table 4-21 describes typical renin-aldosterone patterns in various conditions.

RESPIRATORY SYNCYTIAL VIRUS (RSV) SCREEN

Test description: PCR test can be performed on nasopharyngeal swab, wash, or aspirate

RETICULOCYTE COUNT

Normal range: 0.5%-1.5%

Elevated in: Hemolytic anemia (sickle cell crisis, thalassemia major, autoimmune hemolysis), hemorrhage, postanemia therapy (folic acid, ferrous sulfate, vitamin B_{12}), chronic renal failure

Decreased in: Aplastic anemia, marrow suppression (sepsis, chemotherapeutic agents, radiation), hepatic cirrhosis, blood transfusion, anemias of disordered maturation (iron deficiency anemia, megaloblastic anemia, sideroblastic anemia, anemia of chronic disease)

RHEUMATOID FACTOR

Normal: Negative. Present in titer >1:20

RHEUMATIC DISEASES

Rheumatoid arthritis
Sjögren's syndrome
Systemic lupus erythematosus
Polymyositis/dermatomyositis
Mixed connective tissue disease
Scleroderma

INFECTIOUS DISEASES

Subacute bacterial endocarditis
Tuberculosis
Infectious mononucleosis
Hepatitis
Syphilis
Leprosy
Influenza

MALIGNANCIES

Lymphoma
Multiple myeloma
Waldenström's macroglobulinemia
Postradiation or postchemotherapy

MISCELLANEOUS

Normal adults, especially the elderly
Sarcoidosis
Chronic pulmonary disease (interstitial fibrosis)

Chronic liver disease (chronic active hepatitis, cirrhosis)
Mixed essential cryoglobulinemia
Hypergammaglobulinemic purpura

RNP

See EXTRACTABLE NUCLEAR ANTIGEN

ROTAVIRUS SEROLOGY

Test description: PCR test is performed on stool specimen
Normal: Negative

SED RATE

See ERYTHROCYTE SEDIMENTATION RATE

SEDIMENTATION RATE

See ERYTHROCYTE SEDIMENTATION RATE

SEMEN ANALYSIS

Table 4-22 describes semen analysis reference ranges.

SGOT

See ASPARTATE AMINOTRANSFERASE

SGPT

See ALANINE AMINOTRANSFERASE

SICKLE CELL TEST

Normal: Negative
Positive in: Sickle cell anemia, sickle cell trait, combination of *Hb S* gene with other disorders such as alpha-thalassemia, beta-thalassemia.

SMOOTH MUSCLE ANTIBODY

Normal: Negative
Present in: Chronic acute hepatitis ($\geq$1:80), primary biliary cirrhosis ($\leq$1:80), infectious mononucleosis

SODIUM (serum)

Normal range: 135-147 mEq/L (135-147 mmol/L [CF: 1; SMI: 1 mmol/L])

HYPONATREMIA

A. Sodium and water depletion (deficit hyponatremia)
   1. Loss of gastrointestinal secretions with replacement of fluid but not electrolytes
      a. Vomiting
      b. Diarrhea
      c. Tube drainage
   2. Loss from skin with replacement of fluids but not electrolytes
      a. Excessive sweating
      b. Extensive burns
   3. Loss from kidney
      a. Diuretics
      b. Chronic renal insufficiency (uremia) with acidosis
   4. Metabolic loss
      a. Starvation with acidosis
      b. Diabetic acidosis

TABLE 4-21 Typical Renin-Aldosterone Patterns in Various Conditions

	Plasma Renin	Aldosterone
Primary aldosteronism	Low	High
"Low-renin" essential hypertension	Low	Normal
Cushing's syndrome	Low	Low-normal
Licorice ingestion syndrome	Low	Low
High-salt diet	Low	Low
Oral contraceptives	High	Normal
Cirrhosis	High	High
Malignant hypertension	High	High
Unilateral renal disease	High	High
"High-renin" essential hypertension	High	High
Pregnancy	High	High
Diuretic overuse	High	High
Juxtaglomerular tumor (Bartter's syndrome)	High	High
Low-salt diet	High	High
Addison's disease	High	Low
Hypokalemia	High	Low

Reprinted from Ravel R: *Clinical laboratory medicine*, ed 6, St Louis, 1995, Mosby.

TABLE 4-22 Semen Analysis Reference Ranges

Color	Grayish white
pH	7.3-7.8 (literature range, 7.0-7.8)
Volume	2.0-5.0 ml (literature range, 1.5-6.0 ml)
Sperm count	20-250 million/ml (literature range for upper limit varies from 100-250 million/ml)
Motility	>60% motile <3 hours after specimen is obtained (literature range, >40% to >70%)
% Normal sperm	>60% (literature range, >60% to >70%)
Viscosity	Can be poured from a pipet in droplets rather than a thick strand

From Ravel R (ed): *Clinical laboratory medicine*, ed 6, St Louis, 1995, Mosby.

5. Endocrine loss
   a. Addison's disease
   b. Sudden withdrawal of long-term steroid therapy
6. Iatrogenic loss from serous cavities
   a. Paracentesis or thoracentesis

B. Excessive water (dilution hyponatremia)
   1. Excessive water administration
   2. Congestive heart failure
   3. Cirrhosis
   4. Nephrotic syndrome
   5. Hypoalbuminemia (severe)
   6. Acute renal failure with oliguria

C. Inappropriate antidiuretic hormone (IADH) syndrome
D. Intracellular loss (reset osmostat syndrome)
E. False hyponatremia (actually a dilutional effect)
   1. Marked hypertriglyceridemia
   2. Marked hyperproteinemia
   3. Severe hyperglycemia

HYPERNATREMIA

Dehydration is the most frequent overall clinical finding in hypernatremia.

1. Deficient water intake (either orally or intravenously)
2. Excess kidney water output (diabetes insipidus, osmotic diuresis)
3. Excess skin water output (excess sweating, loss from burns)
4. Excess gastrointestinal tract output (severe protracted vomiting or diarrhea without fluid therapy)
5. Accidental sodium overdose
6. High-protein tube feedings

STREPTOZYME

See ANTISTREPTOLYSIN O TITER

SUCROSE HEMOLYSIS TEST (sugar water test)

Normal: Absence of hemolysis
Positive in:
Paroxysmal nocturnal hemoglobinuria
False-positive: autoimmune hemolytic anemia, megaloblastic anemias
False-negative: may occur with use of heparin or EDTA

SUDAN III STAIN (qualitative screening for fecal fat)

Normal: Negative. Test should be preceded by diet containing 100-150 g of dietary fat/day for 1 week, avoidance of high-fiber diet, and avoidance of suppositories or oily material before specimen collection.
Positive in: Steatorrhea, use of castor oil or mineral oil droplets

SYNOVIAL FLUID ANALYSIS

Table 4-23 describes the classification and interpretation of synovial fluid analysis.

T_3 (triiodothyronine)

See Table 4-24 for T_3 abnormalities.
Normal range: 75-220 ng/dl (1.2-3.4 nmol/L [CF: 0.01536; SMI: 0.1 nmol/L])
Abnormal values:

A. Elevated in hyperthyroidism (usually earlier and to a greater extent than serum T_4).

TABLE 4-23 Classification and Interpretation of Synovial Fluid Analysis

Group	Diseases	Appearance	Viscosity	Mucin Clot	WBC/mm³	% PMN	Glucose (mg/dl) (Blood-Synovial Fluid)	Protein (g/dl)
Normal	—	Clear	↑	Firm	<200	<25	<10	<2.5
I (noninflammatory)	Osteoarthritis, aseptic necrosis, traumatic arthritis, erythema nodosum, osteochondritis dissecans	Clear, yellow (may be xanthochromic if traumatic arthritis)	↑	Firm	↑ Up to 10,000	<25	<10	<2.5
II (inflammatory)	Crystal-induced arthritis, rheumatoid arthritis, Reiter's syndrome, collagen vascular disease, psoriatic arthritis, serum sickness, rheumatic fever	Clear, yellow, turbid	↓	Friable	↑↑ Up to 100,000	40-90	<40	>2.5
III (septic)	Bacterial (staphylococcal, gonococcal, tuberculosis)	Turbid	↓/↑	Friable	↑↑↑ Up to 5 million	40-100	20-100	>2.5

↑, Elevated; ↑↑, markedly high; ↓, decreased; *PMN*, polymorphonuclear leukocytes. Note that there is considerable overlap in the numbers listed above.

TABLE 4-24 Findings in Thyroid Function Tests in Various Clinical Conditions

TRH Condition	T_4	FT_4I	T_3	FT_3I	TSH	TSI	Stimulation
Hyperthyroidism							
Graves' disease	↑	↑	↑	↑	↓	+	↓
Toxic nodular goiter	↑	↑	↑	↑	↓	−	↓
Pituitary TSH-secreting tumors	↑	↑	↑	↑	↑	−	↓
T_3 thyrotoxicosis	N	N	↑	↑	↓	+, −	↓
T_4 thyrotoxicosis	↑	↑	N	N	↓	+, −	↓
Hypothyroidism							
Primary	↓	↓	↓	↓	↑	+, −	↑
Secondary	↓	↓	↓	↓	↓ N	−	↓
Tertiary	↓	↓	↓	↓	↓, N	−	N
Peripheral unresponsiveness	↑, N	↑, N	↑, N	↑	↑, N	−	N, ↑

Reprinted from Tilton RC, Barrows A: *Clinical laboratory medicine*, St Louis, 1992, Mosby.
↑, Increased; ↓, decreased; +, − variable; *N*, normal.

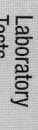
Laboratory Tests

IV

B. Useful in diagnosing:
1. T₃ hyperthyroidism (thyrotoxicosis): increased T₃, normal FTI.
2. Toxic nodular goiter: increased T₃, normal or increased T₄.
3. Iodine deficiency: normal T₃, possibly decreased T₄.
4. Thyroid replacement therapy with liothyronine (Cytomel): normal T₄, increased T₃ if patient is symptomatically hyperthyroid.

Not ordered routinely but indicated when hyperthyroidism is suspected and serum-free T₄ or FTI inconclusive.

T₃ RESIN UPTAKE (T₃RU)

Normal range: 25%-35%
Abnormal values: Increased in hyperthyroidism. T₃ resin uptake (T₃RU or RT₃U) measures the percentage of free T₄ (not bound to protein); it does not measure serum T₃ concentration; T₃RU and other tests that reflect thyroid hormone binding to plasma protein are also known as *thyroid hormone-binding ratios* (THBR).

T₄, FREE (free thyroxine)

Normal range: 0.8-2.8 ng/dl
Elevated in:
Graves' disease, toxic multinodular goiter, toxic adenoma, iatrogenic and factitious causes, transient hyperthyroidism
Serum-free T₄ directly measures unbound thyroxine. Free T₄ can be measured by equilibrium dialysis (gold standard of free T₄ assays) or by immunometric techniques (influenced by serum levels of lipids, proteins, and certain drugs). The free thyroxine index (FTI) can also be easily calculated by multiplying T₄ times T₃RU and dividing the result by 100; the FTI corrects for any abnormal T₄ values secondary to protein binding: $FTI = T_4 \times T_3RU/100$.
Normal values equal 1.1 to 4.3.

T₄, SERUM T₄

Normal range: 0.8-2.8 ng/dl (10-36 pmol/L [CF: 12.87; SMI: 1 pmol/L])
Abnormal values: Serum thyroxine (T₄)
Elevated in:
1. Graves' disease
2. Toxic multinodular goiter
3. Toxic adenoma
4. Iatrogenic and factitious
5. Transient hyperthyroidism
   a. Subacute thyroiditis
   b. Hashimoto's thyroiditis
   c. Silent thyroiditis
6. Rare causes: hypersecretion of TSH (e.g., pituitary neoplasms), struma ovarii, ingestion of large amounts of iodine in a patient with preexisting thyroid hyperplasia or adenoma (Jod-Basedow phenomenon), hydatidiform mole, carcinoma of thyroid, amiodarone therapy of arrhythmias.
Serum thyroxine test measures both circulating thyroxine bound to protein (represents >99% of circulating T₄) and unbound (free) thyroxine. Values vary with protein binding; changes in the concentration of T₄ secondary to changes in thyroxine-binding globulin (TBG) can be caused by the following:

Increased TBG (↑T₄)	Decreased TBG (↓T₄)
Pregnancy	Androgens, glucocorticoids
Estrogens	Nephrotic syndrome, cirrhosis
Acute infectious	Acromegaly
hepatitis	Hypoproteinemia
Oral contraceptives	Familial
Familial	Phenytoin, ASA and other heroin, methadone,
Fluorouracil, clofibrate	NSAIDs, high-dose penicillin, asparaginase
	Chronic debilitating illness

To eliminate the suspected influence of protein binding on thyroxine values, two additional tests are available: T₃ resin uptake and serum free thyroxine.

TEGRETOL

See CARBAMAZEPINE and Table 4-24, under T₃ (Triiodothyronine).

TESTOSTERONE (total testosterone)

Normal range: Variable with age and sex
Serum/plasma
Males: 280-1100 ng/dl   Females: 15-70 ng/dl
Urine
Males: 50-135 μg/day   Females: 2-12 μg/day
Elevated in: Testicular tumors, ovarian masculinizing tumors, testosterone replacement therapy
Decreased in: Hypogonadism, sleep apnea

THEOPHYLLINE

Normal therapeutic range: 10-20 mcg/ml

THORACENTESIS FLUID

Testing and evaluation of results:
1. Pleural effusion fluid should be differentiated in exudate or transudate. The initial laboratory studies should be aimed only at distinguishing an exudate from a transudate.
   a. Tube 1: protein, LDH, albumin.
   b. Tubes 2, 3, 4: save the fluid until further notice. In selected patients with suspected empyema, a pH level may be useful (generally ≤7.0). See following for proper procedure to obtain a pH level from pleural fluid.
      NOTE: Do not order further tests until the presence of an exudate is confirmed on the basis of protein and LDH determinations (see Section III); however, if the results of protein and LDH determinations cannot be obtained within a reasonable time (resulting in unnecessary delay), additional laboratory tests should be ordered at the time of thoracentesis.
2. A serum/effusion albumin gradient of ≤1.2 g/dl is indicative of exudative effusions, especially in patients with congestive heart failure (CHF) treated with diuretics.
3. Note the appearance of the fluid:
   a. A grossly hemorrhagic effusion can be a result of a traumatic tap, neoplasm, or an embolus with infarction.
   b. A milky appearance indicates either of the following:
      (1) Chylous effusion: caused by trauma or tumor invasion of the thoracic duct; lipoprotein electrophoresis of the effusion reveals chylomicrons and triglyceride levels >115 mg/dl.
      (2) Pseudochylous effusion: often seen with chronic inflammation of the pleural space (e.g., TB, connective tissue diseases).
4. If transudate, consider CHF, cirrhosis, chronic renal failure, and other hypoproteinemic states and perform subsequent workup accordingly.
5. If exudate, consider ordering these tests on the pleural fluid:
   a. Cytologic examination for malignant cells (for suspected neoplasm).
   b. Gram stain, cultures (aerobic and anaerobic), and sensitivities (for suspected infectious process).
   c. AFB stain and cultures (for suspected TB).
   d. pH: a value <7.0 suggests parapneumonic effusion or empyema; a pleural fluid pH must be drawn anaerobically and iced immediately; the syringe should be prerinsed with 0.2 ml of 1:1000 heparin.
   e. Glucose: a low glucose level suggests parapneumonic effusions and rheumatoid arthritis.
   f. Amylase: a high amylase level suggests pancreatitis or ruptured esophagus.
   g. Perplexing pleural effusions are often a result of malignancy (e.g., lymphoma, malignant mesothelioma, ovarian carcinoma), TB, subdiaphragmatic processes, prior asbestos exposure, and postcardiac injury syndrome.

THROMBIN TIME (TT)

Normal range: 11.3-18.5 sec
Elevated in: Thrombolytic and heparin therapy, disseminated intravascular coagulation, hypofibrinogenemia, dysfibrinogenemia

THYROGLOBULIN
Normal: 3-40 ng/ml. Thyroglobulin is a tumor marker for monitoring the status of patients with papillary or follicular thyroid cancer following resection.
Elevated in: Papillary or follicular thyroid cancer, Hashimoto's thyroiditis, Graves' disease, subacute thyroiditis

THYROID MICROSOMAL ANTIBODIES
Normal: Undetectable. Low titers may be present in 5%-10% of normal individuals
Elevated in: Hashimoto's disease, thyroid carcinoma, early hypothyroidism, pernicious anemia

THYROID-STIMULATING HORMONE (TSH)
Normal range: 2-11 μU/ml (2-11 mU/L [CF: 1; SMI: 1 mU/L])
CONDITIONS THAT INCREASE SERUM THYROID-STIMULATING HORMONE VALUES
Laboratory error
Primary hypothyroidism
Synthroid therapy with insufficient dose
Lithium or amiodarone; some patients
Hashimoto's thyroiditis in later stage
Large doses of inorganic iodide (e.g., SSKI)
Severe nonthyroid illness in recovery phase
Iodine deficiency (moderate or severe)
Addison's disease
TSH specimen drawn in evening (peak of diurnal variation)
Pituitary TSH-secreting tumor
Therapy of hypothyroidism (3-6 wk after beginning therapy [range, 1-8 wk]; sometimes longer when pretherapy TSH is over 100 μU/ml)
Acute psychiatric illness
Peripheral resistance to T_4 syndrome
Antibodies (e.g., HAMA) interfering with monoclonal sandwich method of TSH assay
Telepaque (iopanoic acid) and Oragrafin (ipodate) x-ray contrast media
Amphetamines
High altitudes
CONDITIONS THAT DECREASE SERUM THYROID-STIMULATING HORMONE VALUES
Laboratory error
T_4/T_3 toxicosis (diffuse or nodular etiology)
Excessive therapy for hypothyroidism
Active thyroiditis (subacute, painless, or early active Hashimoto's disease)
Multinodular goiter containing areas of autonomy
Severe nonthyroid illness (especially acute trauma, dopamine, or glucocorticoid)
T_3 toxicosis
Pituitary insufficiency
Cushing's syndrome (and some patients on high-dose glucocorticoid)
Jod-Basedow (iodine-induced) hyperthyroidism
Thyroid-stimulating hormone drawn 2-4 hr after levothyroxine dose
Postpartum transient toxicosis
Factitious hyperthyroidism
Struma ovarii
Radioimmunoassay, surgery, or antithyroid drug therapy for hyperthyroidism 4-6 weeks (range, 2 wk to 2 yr) after the treatment
Interleukin-2 drugs (3%-6% of cases) or α-interferon therapy (1% of cases)
Hyperemesis gravidarum
Amiodarone therapy

THYROTROPIN (TSH) RECEPTOR ANTIBODIES
Normal: <130% of basal activity
Elevated in: Values between 1.3 and 2.0 are found in 10% of patients with thyroid disease other than Graves' disease. Values >2.8 have been found only in patients with Graves' disease.

THYROTROPIN RELEASING HORMONE (TRH) STIMULATION TEST
Elevated in: Celiac disease (specificity, 94%-97%; sensitivity, 90%-98%), dermatitis herpetiformis

THYROXINE (T_4)
Normal range: 4-11 μg/dl (51-142 nmol/L [CF: 12.87; SMI: 1 nmol/L])

TIBC
See IRON-BINDING CAPACITY

TISSUE TRANSGLUTAMINASE ANTIBODY
Normal: Negative
Present in: Celiac disease (specificity, 94%-97%, sensitivity, 90%-98%), dermatitis herpetiformis

TRANSFERRIN
Normal range: 170-370 mg/dl (1.7-3.7 g/L [CF: 0.01; SMI: 0.01 g/L])
Elevated in: Iron deficiency anemia, oral contraceptive administration, viral hepatitis, late pregnancy
Decreased in: Nephrotic syndrome, liver disease, hereditary deficiency, protein malnutrition, neoplasms, chronic inflammatory states, chronic illness, thalassemia, hemochromatosis, hemolytic anemia

TRIGLYCERIDES
Normal range: <150 mg/dl (<1.80 mmol/L [CF: 0.01129; SMI: 0.02 mmol/L])
Elevated in: Hyperlipoproteinemias (types I, IIb, III, IV, V), hypothyroidism, pregnancy, estrogens, acute myocardial infarction, pancreatitis, alcohol intake, nephrotic syndrome, diabetes mellitus, glycogen storage disease
Decreased in: Malnutrition, congenital abetalipoproteinemias, drugs (e.g., gemfibrozil, fenofibrate, nicotinic acid, clofibrate)

TRIIODOTHYRONINE
See T_3

TROPONINS, SERUM
Normal range: 0-0.4 ng/ml (negative). If there is clinical suspicion of evolving acute MI or ischemic episode, repeat testing in 5-6 hours is recommended.
Indeterminate: 0.05-0.49 ng/ml. Suggest further tests. In a patient with unstable angina and this troponin I level, there is an increased risk of a cardiac event in the near future.
Strong probability of acute MI:
≥0.05 ng/ml
Cardiac troponin T (CTNT) is a highly sensitive marker for myocardial injury for the first 48 hours after MI and for up to 5-7 days (see Fig. 4-2, under "Creatine Kinase Isoenzymes"). It may also be elevated in renal failure, chronic muscle disease, and trauma.
Cardiac troponin I (CTNI) is highly sensitive and specific for myocardial injury (≥CK-MB) in the initial 8 hours, peaks within 24 hours and lasts up to 7 days. With progressively higher levels of cTnI, the risk of mortality increases because the amount of necrosis increases.

TSH
See THYROID-STIMULATING HORMONE

TT
See THROMBIN TIME

TUBERCULIN TEST (PPD)
Abnormal results: see Boxes 4-3 and 4-4 for interpretation.

IV

BOX 4-3 PPD Reaction Size Considered "Positive" (Intracutaneous 5 TU Mantoux Test at 48 hr)

5 mm or More
- HIV infection or risk factors for HIV
- Close recent contact with active TB case
- Persons with chest x-ray consistent with healed TB

10 mm or More
- Foreign-born persons from countries with high TB prevalence in Asia, Africa, and Latin America
- IV drug users
- Medically underserved low-income population groups (including Native Americans, Hispanics, and blacks)
- Residents of long-term care facilities (nursing homes, mental institutions)
- Medical conditions that increase risk for TB (silicosis, gastrectomy, undernourishment, diabetes mellitus, high-dose corticosteroids or immunosuppression Rx, leukemia or lymphoma, other malignancies)
- Employees of long-term care facilities, schools, child-care facilities, health care facilities

15 mm or More
- All others not already listed

TB, Tuberculosis; *TU,* tuberculin units.

BOX 4-4 Factors Associated with False-Negative Tuberculin Tests

Technical Errors
- Improper administration
- Inaccurate reading
- Loss of potency of antigen

Patient-Related Factors (Anergy)
- Age (elderly)
- Nutritional status
- Medications: corticosteroids, immunosuppressive agents
- Severe tuberculosis
- Coexisting diseases
  - HIV infection
  - Viral illness or vaccination
  - Lymphoreticular malignancies
  - Sarcoidosis
  - Solid tumors
  - Lepromatous leprosy
  - Sjögren's syndrome
  - Ataxia telangiectasia
  - Uremia
  - Primary biliary cirrhosis
  - Systemic lupus erythematosus
- Severe systemic disease of any etiology

Reprinted from Stein JH (ed): *Internal medicine,* ed 4, St Louis, 1994, Mosby.

UNCONJUGATED BILIRUBIN

See BILIRUBIN, DIRECT

UREA NITROGEN, BLOOD (BUN)

Normal range: 8-18 mg/dl (3-6.5 mmol/L [CF: 0.357; SMI: 0.5 mmol/L])
Box 4-5 describes factors affecting BUN level independent of renal function.

Elevated in: Drugs (aminoglycosides and other antibiotics, diuretics, lithium, corticosteroids), dehydration, gastrointestinal bleeding, decreased renal blood flow (shock, congestive heart failure, myocardial infarction), renal disease (glomerulonephritis, pyelonephritis, diabetic nephropathy), urinary tract obstruction (prostatic hypertrophy)

Decreased in: Liver disease, malnutrition, third trimester of pregnancy, overhydration, acromegaly, celiac disease

BOX 4-5 Factors Affecting Blood Urea Nitrogen Level Independent of Renal Function

Disproportionate Increase in Blood Urea Nitrogen
- Volume depletion ("prerenal azotemia")
- Gastrointestinal hemorrhage
- Corticosteroid or cytotoxic agents
- High-protein diet
- Obstructive uropathy
- Sepsis
- Catabolic states tissue breakdown

Disproportionate Decrease in Blood Urea Nitrogen
- Low-protein diet
- Liver disease

Reprinted from Andreoli TE (ed): *Cecil essentials of medicine,* ed 5, Philadelphia, 2001, WB Saunders.

URIC ACID (serum)

Normal range: 2-7 mg/dl
Elevated in: Renal failure, gout, excessive cell lysis (chemotherapeutic agents, radiation therapy, leukemia, lymphoma, hemolytic anemia), hereditary enzyme deficiency (hypoxanthine-guanine-phosphoribosyl transferase), acidosis, myeloproliferative disorders, diet high in purines or protein, drugs (diuretics, low doses of ASA, ethambutol, nicotinic acid), lead poisoning, hypothyroidism, Addison's disease, nephrogenic diabetes insipidus, active psoriasis, polycystic kidneys
Decreased in: Drugs (allopurinol, febuxostat, high doses of ASA, probenecid, warfarin, corticosteroid), deficiency of xanthine oxidase, syndrome of inappropriate antidiuretic hormone secretion, renal tubular deficits (Fanconi's syndrome), alcoholism, liver disease, diet deficient in protein or purines, Wilson's disease, hemochromatosis

URINALYSIS

Normal range:
Color: light straw
Appearance: clear
Ketones: absent
pH: 4.5-8 (average, 6)
Protein: absent
Glucose: absent
Specific gravity: 1.005-1.030
Occult blood absent
Microscopic examination:
  Red blood cells: 0-5 (high-power field)
  White blood cells: 0-5 (high-power field)
  Bacteria (spun specimen): absent
  Casts: 0-4 hyaline (low-power field)
  Abnormalities in the microscopic examination of urine are described in Table 4-25.

URINE AMYLASE

Normal range: 35-260 U Somogyi/hr (6.5-48.1 U/hr [CF: 0.185; SMI: 1 U/hr])
Elevated in: Pancreatitis, carcinoma of the pancreas

URINE BILE

Normal: Absent
Abnormal:
Urine bilirubin: hepatitis (viral, toxic, drug-induced), biliary obstruction
Urine urobilinogen: hepatitis (viral, toxic, drug-induced), hemolytic jaundice, liver cell dysfunction (cirrhosis, infection, metastases)

TABLE 4-25 Microscopic Examination of the Urine

Finding	Associations
Casts	
Red blood cell	Glomerulonephritis, vasculitis
White blood cell	Interstitial nephritis, pyelonephritis
Epithelial cell	Acute tubular necrosis, interstitial nephritis, glomerulonephritis
Granular	Renal parenchymal disease (nonspecific)
Waxy, broad	Advanced renal failure
Hyaline	Normal finding in concentrated urine
Fatty	Heavy proteinuria
Cells	
Red blood cell	Urinary tract infection, urinary tract inflammation
White blood cell	Urinary tract infection, urinary tract inflammation
Eosinophil	Acute interstitial nephritis
(Squamous) epithelial cell	Contaminants
Crystals	
Uric acid	Acid urine, acute uric acid nephropathy, hyperuricosuria
Calcium phosphate	Alkaline urine
Calcium oxalate	Acid urine, hyperoxaluria, ethylene glycol poisoning
Cystine	Cystinuria
Sulfur	Sulfa-containing antibiotics

From Andreoli TE (ed): *Cecil essentials of medicine,* ed 5, Philadelphia, 2001, WB Saunders.

URINE CALCIUM

Normal range: <250 mg/24 hr (<6.2 mmol/dl [CF: 0.02495; SMI: 0.1 mmol/dl])
Elevated in: Primary hyperparathyroidism, hypervitaminosis D, bone metastases, multiple myeloma, increased calcium intake, steroids, prolonged immobilization, sarcoidosis, Paget's disease, idiopathic hypercalciuria, renal tubular acidosis
Decreased in: Hypoparathyroidism, pseudohypoparathyroidism, vitamin D deficiency, vitamin D–resistant rickets, diet low in calcium, drugs (thiazide diuretics, oral contraceptives), familial hypocalciuric hypercalcemia, renal osteodystrophy, potassium citrate therapy

URINE cAMP

Elevated in: Hypercalciuria, familial hypocalciuric hypercalcemia, primary hyperparathyroidism, pseudohypoparathyroidism, rickets
Decreased in: Vitamin D intoxication, sarcoidosis

URINE CATECHOLAMINES

Normal range:
Norepinephrine: <100 μg/24 hr (<590 nmol/day [CF: 5.911; SMI: 10 nmol/day])
Epinephrine: <10 μg/24 hr (55 nmol/day [CF: 5.458; SMI: 5 nmol/day])
Elevated in: Pheochromocytoma, neuroblastoma, severe stress

URINE CHLORIDE

Normal range: 110-250 mEq/day (110-250 mmol/day [CF: 1; SMI: 1 mmol/day])
Elevated in: Corticosteroids, Bartter's syndrome, diuretics, metabolic acidosis, severe hypokalemia
Decreased in: Chloride depletion (vomiting), colonic villous adenoma, chronic renal failure, renal tubular acidosis

URINE COPPER

Normal range: <40 μg/24 hr (<0.6 μmol/day [CF: 0.01574; SMI: 0.2 μmol/day])

URINE CORTISOL, FREE

Normal range: 10-110 μg/24 hr (30-300 nmol/day [CF: 2.759; SMI: 10 nmol/day])
Elevated: See CORTISOL, PLASMA

URINE CREATININE (24 hr)

Normal range:
Male: 0.8-1.8 g/day (7-16 mmol/day [CF: 8.840; SMI: 0.1 mmol/day])
Female: 0.6-1.6 g/day (5.3-14 mmol/day)
  NOTE: Useful test as an indicator of completeness of 24-hr urine collection.

URINE CRYSTALS

Uric acid: acid urine, hyperuricosuria, uric acid nephropathy
Sulfur: antibiotics containing sulfa
Calcium oxalate: ethylene glycol poisoning, acid urine, hyperoxaluria
Calcium phosphate: alkaline urine
Cystine: cystinuria

URINE EOSINOPHILS

Normal: Absent
Present in: Interstitial nephritis, acute tubular necrosis, urinary tract infection, kidney transplant rejection, hepatorenal syndrome

URINE GLUCOSE (QUALITATIVE)

Normal: Absent
Present in: Diabetes mellitus, renal glycosuria (decreased renal threshold for glucose), glucose intolerance

URINE HEMOGLOBIN, FREE

Normal: Absent
Present in: Hemolysis (with saturation of serum haptoglobin binding capacity and renal threshold for tubular absorption of hemoglobin)

URINE HEMOSIDERIN

Normal: Absent
Present in: Paroxysmal nocturnal hemoglobinuria, chronic hemolytic anemia, hemochromatosis, blood transfusion, thalassemias

URINE 5-HYDROXYINDOLE-ACETIC ACID (URINE 5-HIAA)

Normal range: 2-8 mg/24 hr (10-40 μmol/day [CF: 5.23; SMI: 5 μmol/day])
Elevated in: Carcinoid tumors, after ingestion of certain foods (bananas, plums, tomatoes, avocados, pineapples, eggplant, walnuts), drugs (monoamine oxidase inhibitors, phenacetin, methyldopa, glycerol guaiacolate, acetaminophen, salicylates, phenothiazines, imipramine, methocarbamol, reserpine, methamphetamine)

URINE INDICAN

Normal: Absent
Present in: Malabsorption secondary to intestinal bacterial overgrowth

URINE KETONES (semiquantitative)

Normal: Absent
Present in: Diabetic ketoacidosis, alcoholic ketoacidosis, starvation, isopropanol ingestion

URINE METANEPHRINES

Normal range: 0-2.0 mg/24 hr (0-11.0 μmol/day [CF: 5.458; SMI: 0.5 μmol/day])
Elevated in: Pheochromocytoma, neuroblastoma, drugs (caffeine, phenothiazines, monoamine oxidase inhibitors), stress

URINE MYOGLOBIN

Normal: Absent
Present in: Severe trauma, hyperthermia, polymyositis/dermatomyositis, carbon monoxide poisoning, drugs (narcotic and amphetamine toxicity), hypothyroidism, muscle ischemia

Laboratory Tests

IV

URINE NITRITE
Normal: Absent
Present in: Urinary tract infections

URINE OCCULT BLOOD
Normal: Negative
Positive in: Trauma to urinary tract, renal disease (glomerulonephritis, pyelonephritis), renal or ureteral calculi, bladder lesions (carcinoma, cystitis), prostatitis, prostatic carcinoma, menstrual contamination, hematopoietic disorders (hemophilia, thrombocytopenia), anticoagulants, ASA

URINE OSMOLALITY
Normal range: 50-1200 mOsm/kg (50-1200 mmol/kg [CF: 1; SMI: 1 mmol/kg])
Elevated in: Syndrome of inappropriate antidiuretic hormone secretion, dehydration, glycosuria, adrenal insufficiency, high-protein diet
Decreased in: Diabetes insipidus, excessive water intake, IV hydration with D_5W, acute renal insufficiency, glomerulonephritis

URINE pH
Normal range: 4.6-8 (average, 6)
Elevated in: Bacteriuria, vegetarian diet, renal failure with inability to form ammonia, drugs (antibiotics, sodium bicarbonate, acetazolamide)
Decreased in: Acidosis (metabolic, respiratory), drugs (ammonium chloride, methenamine mandelate), diabetes mellitus, starvation, diarrhea

URINE PHOSPHATE
Normal range: 0.8-2.0 g/24 hr
Elevated in: Acute tubular necrosis (diuretic phase), chronic renal disease, uncontrolled diabetes mellitus, hyperparathyroidism, hypomagnesemia, metabolic acidosis, metabolic alkalosis, neurofibromatosis, adult-onset vitamin D–resistant hypophosphatemic osteomalacia
Decreased in: Acromegaly, acute renal failure, decreased dietary intake, hypoparathyroidism, respiratory acidosis

URINE POTASSIUM
Normal range: 25-100 mEq/24 hr (25-100 mmol/day [CF: 1; SMI: 1 mmol/day])
Elevated in: Aldosteronism (primary, secondary), glucocorticoids, alkalosis, renal tubular acidosis, excessive dietary potassium intake
Decreased in: Acute renal failure, potassium-sparing diuretics, diarrhea, hypokalemia

URINE PROTEIN (quantitative)
Normal range: <150 mg/24 hr (<0.15 g/day [CF: 0.001; SMI: 0.01 g/day])
Elevated in:
Nephrotic syndrome as a result of primary renal diseases
Malignant hypertension
Malignancies: multiple myeloma, leukemias, Hodgkin's disease
Congestive heart failure
Diabetes mellitus
Systemic lupus erythematosus, rheumatoid arthritis
Sickle cell disease
Goodpasture's syndrome
Malaria
Amyloidosis, sarcoidosis
Tubular lesions: cystinosis
Functional (after heavy exercise)
Pyelonephritis
Pregnancy
Constrictive pericarditis
Renal vein thrombosis
Toxic nephropathies: heavy metals, drugs
Radiation nephritis
Orthostatic (postural) proteinuria
Benign proteinuria: fever, heat or cold exposure

URINE SEDIMENT
See Fig. 4-14 for evaluation of common abnormalities.

URINE SODIUM (quantitative)
Normal range: 40-220 mEq/day (40-220 mmol/day [CF: 1; SMI: 1 mmol/day])
Elevated in: Diuretic administration, high sodium intake, salt-losing nephritis, acute tubular necrosis, vomiting, Addison's disease, syndrome of inappropriate antidiuretic hormone secretion, hypothyroidism, congestive heart failure, hepatic failure, chronic renal failure, Bartter's syndrome, glucocorticoid deficiency, interstitial nephritis caused by analgesic abuse, mannitol, dextran, or glycerol therapy, milk-alkali syndrome, decreased renin secretion, postobstructive diuresis
Decreased in: Increased aldosterone, glucocorticoid excess, hyponatremia, prerenal azotemia, decreased salt intake

URINE SPECIFIC GRAVITY
Normal range: 1.005-1.03
Elevated in: Dehydration, excessive fluid losses (vomiting, diarrhea, fever), x-ray contrast media, diabetes mellitus, congestive heart failure, syndrome of inappropriate antidiuretic hormone secretion, adrenal insufficiency, decreased fluid intake
Decreased in: Diabetes insipidus, renal disease (glomerulonephritis, pyelonephritis), excessive fluid intake or IV hydration

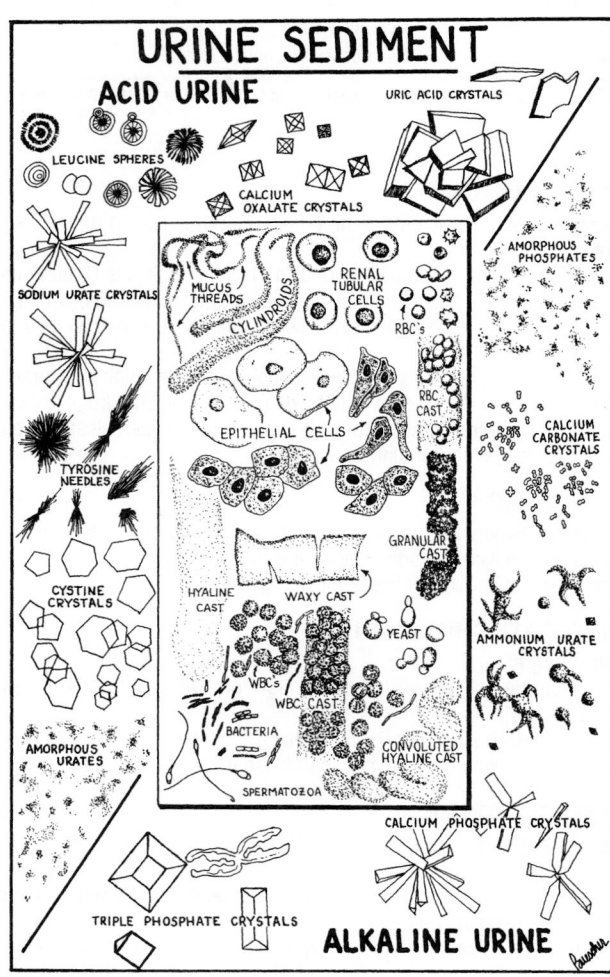

FIGURE 4-14 Microscopic examination of urinary sediment. (Reprinted from Grigorian Greene M: *The Harriet Lane handbook: a manual for pediatric house officers,* ed 17, St Louis, 2007, Mosby.)

URINE VANILLYIMANDELIC ACID (VMA)

Normal range: <6.8 mg/24 hr (<35 μmol/day [CF: 5.046; SMI: 1 μmol/day])

Elevated in: Pheochromocytoma, neuroblastoma, ganglioblastoma, drugs (isoproterenol, methocarbamol, levodopa, sulfonamides, chlorpromazine), severe stress, after ingestion of bananas, chocolate, vanilla, tea, coffee

Decreased in: Drugs (monoamine oxidase inhibitors, reserpine, guanethidine, methyldopa)

VARICELLA-ZOSTER VIRUS (VZV) SEROLOGY

Test description: Test can be performed on whole blood, tissue, skin lesions, and CSF

VASOACTIVE INTESTINAL PEPTIDE (VIP)

Normal: <50 pg/ml

Elevated in: Pancreatic VIP-omas, neuroblastoma, pancreatic islet call hyperplasia, liver disease, MEN I, ganglioneuroma, ganglioneuroblastoma

VDRL

Normal range: Negative

Positive test: Syphilis, other treponemal diseases (yaws, pinta, bejel)

  NOTE: A false-positive test may be seen in patients with systemic lupus erythematosus and other autoimmune diseases, infectious mononucleosis, HIV, atypical pneumonia, malaria, leprosy, typhus fever, rat-bite fever, relapsing fever.

  NOTE: See Table 4-26 for interpretation of serologic tests for syphilis.

VISCOSITY (serum)

Normal range: 1.4-1.8 relative to water (1.10-1.22 centipoise)

Elevated in: Monoclonal gammopathies (Waldenström's macroglobulinemia, multiple myeloma), hyperfibrinogenemia, systemic lupus erythematosus, rheumatoid arthritis, polycythemia, leukemia

VITAMIN B$_{12}$

Normal:

190-900 ng/ml

Causes of vitamin B$_{12}$ deficiency:

1. Pernicious anemia (antibodies against intrinsic factor and gastric parietal cells)
2. Dietary (strict lacto-ovovegetarians, food faddists)
3. Malabsorption (achlorhydria, gastrectomy, ileal resection, pancreatic insufficiency, drugs [omeprazole, cholestyramine])

Falsely low levels occur in patients with severe folate deficiency, in patients using high doses of ascorbic acid, and when cobalamin levels are measured after nuclear medicine studies (radioactivity interferes with cobalamin radioimmunoassay).

Falsely high or normal levels in patients with cobalamin deficiency can occur in severe liver disease and chronic granulocytic leukemia.

The absence of anemia or macrocytosis does not exclude the diagnosis of cobalamin deficiency.

VITAMIN D, 1,25 DIHYDROXY CALCIFEROL

Normal: 16-65 pg/ml

Elevated in: Tumor calcinosis, primary hyperparathyroidism, sarcoidosis, tuberculosis, idiopathic hypercalciuria

Decreased in: Postmenopausal osteoporosis, chronic renal failure, hypoparathyroidism, tumor-induced osteomalacia, rickets, tumor-induced osteomalacia, elevated blood lead levels

VITAMIN K

Normal: 0.10-2.20 ng/ml

Decreased in: Primary biliary cirrhosis, anticoagulants, antibiotics, choelstyramine, GI disease, pancreatic disease, cystic fibrosis, obstructive jaundice, hypoprothrombinemia, hemorrhagic disease of the newborn

---

TABLE 4-26   Interpretation of Serologic Tests for Syphilis*

Nontreponemal Tests	Treponemal Tests	Interpretation of Finding: Is Syphilis Present?*
Nonreactive	Nonreactive	Early primary syphilis is not ruled out by negative serologic tests. Early syphilis is present in 13%-30% of patients who have a negative microhemagglutination *Treponema pallidum* test; in about 30% of patients who present with chancre but have a nonreactive reagin test; and in about 10% of patients who have a negative FTA-ABS test. Late syphilis is present in a very small fraction of patients. Adequately treated syphilis in remote past may produce these results, but treponemal tests usually remain reactive.
	Reactive	Observed in about 10% of patients with chancre. The treponemal tests may turn positive shortly before the reagin tests. Reagin tests repeated after several days are generally positive. In adequately treated early syphilis, the reagin test may return to nonreactive within 1-2 yr, whereas the treponemal tests generally do not. Late syphilis is not ruled out by a negative reagin test. The sensitivity of the reagin tests is lower than that of treponemal tests in untreated late syphilis. In secondary syphilis, rarely, a highly reactive serum appears negative when tested undiluted with a reagain test because flocculation is inhibited by relative antibody excess. Not reported to occur with treponemal tests. Quantitative reagin tests are positive. False-positive treponemal tests occur in 40% of patients with Lyme disease.
Reactive	Nonreactive borderline (FTA-ABS)	Finding is not diagnostic of syphilis but constitutes a classic biologic false-positive reaction. Not diagnostic of syphilis; most patients (90%) with this pattern do not develop clinical or serologic evidence of syphilis. Repeat test is indicated. Chronic borderline results are associated with a variety of conditions other than syphilis.
	Beaded (FTA-ABS)	Not diagnostic of syphilis. Seen with collagen vascular disease.
	Reactive	Findings diagnostic of syphilis or other treponemal disease. In adequately treated syphilis, one would expect (1) a sustained fourfold drop in titer of reagin test, although reagin test may remain positive after adequate therapy; (2) treponemal tests remain positive after adequate therapy. Concurrent false-positive results on both nontreponemal and treponemal tests could occur in rare instances. It may be impossible to rule out syphilis in an individual with this test profile.

Reprinted from Stein JH (ed): *Internal medicine,* ed 4, St Louis, 1994, Mosby.
FTA-ABS, Fluorescent treponemal antibody, absorbed.

*Serologic data must always be interpreted in the light of a total clinical evaluation. Diagnosis based on serologic criteria alone is fraught with error. Serologic tests apparently in conflict with clinical diagnosis should be confirmed by repetition or possibly referral to a reference laboratory.

Laboratory Tests

IV

VON WILLEBRAND FACTOR

Normal: Levels vary according to blood type; blood type O: 50-150 U/dl; blood type non-O: 90-200 U/dl

Decreased in: von Willebrand's disease (however, in type II von Willebrand's disease the antigen may be normal but the function is impaired)

WWBC

See COMPLETE BLOOD COUNT

WESTERGREN

See ERYTHROCYTE SEDIMENTATION RATE

WHITE BLOOD COUNT

See COMPLETE BLOOD COUNT

Clinical Practice Guidelines

PART A
THE PERIODIC HEALTH EXAMINATION*

Age-Specific Charts, 1396

PART B
IMMUNIZATIONS AND CHEMOPROPHYLAXIS

Childhood and Adolescent Immunizations, 1405

*Data modified from U.S. Preventive Services Task Force: *Guide to clinical preventive services: report of the U.S. Preventive Services Task Force,* ed 2, Washington, DC, 1996 (revised 2001), U.S. Department of Health and Human Services. Text downloaded from http://text.nlm.nih.gov

General Recommendations on Immunization, 1410

Immunizations for Adults, 1422

PART C
GUIDE TO CLINICAL PREVENTIVE SERVICES

PART A • THE PERIODIC HEALTH EXAMINATION

Age-Specific Charts

TABLE 5-1 Birth to 10 Years

Interventions considered and recommended for the Periodic Health Examination	Leading causes of death
	Conditions originating in perinatal period
	Congenital anomalies
	Sudden infant death syndrome
	Unintentional injuries (non–motor vehicle)
	Motor vehicle injuries

INTERVENTIONS FOR THE GENERAL POPULATION

Screening

Height and weight

Blood pressure

Vision screen (ages 3-4 yr)

Hemoglobinopathy screen (birth)[1]

Phenylalanine level (birth)[2]

Thyroxine and/or thyroid-stimulating hormone (birth)[3]

Counseling

Injury prevention

Child safety car seats (age <5 yr)

Lap/shoulder belts (age ≥5 yr)

Bicycle helmet; avoid bicycling near traffic

Smoke detector, flame-retardant sleepwear

Hot water heater temperature <120°-130° F

Window/stair guards, pool fence

Safe storage of drugs, toxic substances, firearms, and matches

Syrup of ipecac, poison control phone number

CPR training for parents/caretakers

Diet and exercise

Breastfeeding, iron-enriched formula and foods (infants and toddlers)

Limit fat and cholesterol; maintain caloric balance; emphasize grains, fruits, vegetables (age ≥2 yr)

Regular physical activity*

Substance use

Effects of passive smoking*

Antitobacco message*

Dental health

Regular visits to dental care provider*

Floss, brush with fluoride toothpaste daily*

Advice about baby bottle tooth decay*

Immunizations

Diphtheria-tetanus-pertussis (DTaP)[4]

Inactivated poliovirus vaccine (IPV)[5]

Measles-mumps-rubella (MMR)[6]

H. influenzae type b (Hib) conjugate[7]

Hepatitis A vaccine (HR4)

Hepatitis B[8]

Varicella[9]

Pneumococcal vaccine[10]

Influenza[11]

Meningococcal conjugate vaccine (MCV)[12]

Rotavirus (RV)[13]

Human papillomavirus vaccine (HPV)[14]

Chemoprophylaxis

Ocular prophylaxis (birth)

INTERVENTIONS FOR HIGH-RISK POPULATIONS

Population	*Potential Interventions (see detailed high-risk definitions)*
Preterm or low birth weight	Hemoglobin/hematocrit (HR1)
Infants of mothers at risk for HIV	HIV testing (HR2)
Low income; immigrants	Hemoglobin/hematocrit (HR1); PPD (HR3)
TB contacts	PPD (HR3)
Native American/Alaska Native	Hemoglobin/hematocrit (HR1); PPD (HR3); pneumococcal vaccine (HR5)
Residents of long-term care facilities	PPD (HR3); hepatitis A vaccine (HR4); influenza vaccine (HR6)
Certain chronic medical conditions	PPD (HR3); pneumococcal vaccine (HR5); influenza vaccine (HR6)
Increased individual or community lead exposure	Blood lead level (HR7)
Inadequate water fluoridation	Daily fluoride supplement (HR8)
Family history of skin cancer; nevi; fair skin, eyes, hair	Avoid excess/midday sun, use protective clothing* (HR9)

HR, High risk; *PPD,* purified protein derivative; *TB,* tuberculosis.

[1]Whether screening should be universal or targeted to high-risk groups depends on the proportion of high-risk individuals in the screening area and other considerations. [2]If done during first 24 hr of life, repeat by age 2 wk. [3]Optimally between day 2 and 6, but in all cases before newborn nursery discharge. [4]2, 4, 6, and 12-18 mo; once between age 4-6 yr. [5]2, 4, 6-18 mo; once between age 4-6 yr. [6]12-15 mo and 4-6 yr. [7]2, 4, 6 and 12-15 mo; no dose needed at 6 mo if PRP-OMP vaccine is used for first 2 doses. [8]Birth, 1 mo, 6 mo; or, 0-2 mo, 1-2 mo later, and 6-18 mo. If not done in infancy: current visit, and 1 and 6 mo later. [9]12-18 mo; or any child without history of chickenpox or previous immunization. Include information on risk in adulthood, duration of immunity, and potential need for booster doses. Administer a second dose of varicella vaccine at age 4-6 yr. [10]Pneumococcal polysaccharide vaccine (PPSV) can be administered at the same time as the other childhood vaccines at a separate site. [11]Influenza vaccine is recommended in children 6 mo-18 yr of age. [12]Administer meningococcal conjugate vaccine (MCV) to children aged 2 through 10 yr with terminal complement component deficiency, anatomic or functional asplenia, and certain other high risk groups (see *MMWR* 54[RR-7], 2005). Persons who received MPSV 3 or more years previously and who remain at increased risk for meningococcal disease should be revaccinated with MCV. [13]Administer first dose at 2 mo. If Rotarix® is administered at ages 2 and 4 mo, a dose at 6 mo is not indicated. [14]HPV4 may be administered in a 3-dose series to males aged 9 through 26 yr and females aged 11 to 26 yr to reduce the likelihood of acquiring genital warts.

*The ability of clinician counseling to influence this behavior is unproven.

HR1: Infants aged 6-12 mo who are living in poverty, black, Native American or Alaska Native, immigrants from developing countries, preterm and low-birth-weight infants, infants whose principal dietary intake is unfortified cow's milk.

HR2: Infants born to high-risk mothers whose HIV status is unknown. Women at high risk include past or present injection drug users; persons who exchange sex for money or drugs and their sex partners; injection drug–using, bisexual, or HIV-positive sex partners currently or in past; persons seeking treatment for STDs; persons who received a blood transfusion between 1978 and 1985.

HR3: Persons infected with HIV, close contacts of persons with known or suspected TB, persons with medical risk factors associated with TB, immigrants from countries with high TB prevalence, medically underserved low-income populations (including homeless), residents of long-term care facilities.

HR4: Hepatitis A vaccine (Hep A) is recommended for all children at 1 yr of age (i.e., 12-23 mo). The two doses in the series should be administered at least 6 mo apart. Children who are not vaccinated by 2 yr of age can be vaccinated at subsequent visits.

HR5: Immunocompetent persons ≥ 2 yr with certain medical conditions, including chronic cardiac or pulmonary disease, diabetes mellitus, and anatomic asplenia, as well as cochlear implant candidates and recipients. Immunocompetent persons ≥ 2 yr living in high-risk environments or social settings (e.g., certain Native American and Alaska Native populations).

HR6: Annual vaccinations of children ≥ 6 mo who are residents of chronic care facilities or who have chronic cardiopulmonary disorders, metabolic diseases (including diabetes mellitus), hemoglobinopathies, immunosuppression, or renal dysfunction.

HR7: Children approximately age 12 mo who (1) live in communities in which the prevalence of lead levels requiring individual intervention, including residential lead hazard control or chelation, is high or undefined; (2) live in or frequently visit a home built before 1950 with dilapidated paint or with recent or ongoing renovation or remodeling; (3) have close contact with a person who has an elevated lead level; (4) live near lead industry or heavy traffic; (5) live with someone whose job or hobby involves lead exposure; (6) use lead-based pottery; or (7) take traditional ethnic remedies that contain lead.

HR8: Children living in areas with inadequate water fluoridation (<0.6 ppm).

HR9: Persons with a family history of skin cancer; a large number of moles; atypical moles; poor tanning ability; or light skin, hair, and eye color.

TABLE 5-2 Ages 11 to 24 Years

Interventions considered and recommended for the Periodic Health Examination	Leading causes of death
	Motor vehicle accidents/other unintentional injuries
	Homicide
	Suicide
	Malignant neoplasms
	Heart diseases

INTERVENTIONS FOR THE GENERAL POPULATION

Screening

Height and weight

Blood pressure[1]

Papanicolaou (Pap) test[2] (females)

Chlamydia screen[3] (females <25 yr)

HIV screening

Lipid panel (in high-risk young adults only)

Rubella serology or vaccination history[4] (females >12 yr)

Assess for problem drinking

Counseling

Injury prevention

Lap/shoulder belts

Bicycle/motorcycle/ATV helmets*

Smoke detector*

Safe storage/removal of firearms*

Substance use

Avoid tobacco use

Avoid underage drinking and illicit drug use*

Avoid alcohol/drug use while driving, swimming, boating, etc.*

Sexual behavior

STD prevention: abstinence*; avoid high-risk behavior*; condoms/female barrier with spermicide*

Unintended pregnancy: contraception

Diet and exercise

Limit fat and cholesterol; maintain caloric balance; emphasize grains, fruits, vegetables

Adequate calcium intake (females)

Regular physical activity*

Dental health

Regular visits to dental care provider*

Floss, brush with fluoride toothpaste daily

Immunizations

Tetanus, diphtheria, pertussis[†]

Hepatitis B[5]

Measles-mumps-rubella (MMR) (11-12 yr)[6]

Varicella (11-12 yr)[7]

Rubella (females >12 yr)[4]

Meningococcal[8]

Human papilloma virus (females 11-26 yr, males 9-26 yr)[9]

Influenza[10]

Pneumococcal polysaccharide vaccine (PPSV)[11]

Chemoprophylaxis

Multivitamin with folic acid (females)

INTERVENTIONS FOR HIGH-RISK POPULATIONS

Population	Potential Interventions (see detailed high-risk definitions)
High-risk sexual behavior	RPR/VDRL (HR1); screen for gonorrhea (female) (HR2), HIV (HR3), chlamydia (female) (HR4); hepatitis A vaccine (HR5)
Injection or street drug use	RPR/VDRL (HR1); HIV screen (HR3); hepatitis A vaccine (HR5); PPD (HR6); advice to reduce infection risk (HR7)
TB contacts; immigrants; low income	PPD (HR6)
Native Americans/Alaska Natives	Hepatitis A vaccine (HR5); PPD (HR6); pneumococcal vaccine (HR8)
Travelers to developing countries	Hepatitis A vaccine (HR5)
Certain chronic medical conditions	PPD (HR6); pneumococcal vaccine (HR8); influenza vaccine (HR9)
Settings where adolescents and young adults congregate	Second MMR (HR10)
Susceptible to varicella, measles, mumps	Varicella vaccine (HR11); MMR (HR12)
Blood transfusion between 1975 and 1985	HIV screen (HR3)
Institutionalized persons; health care/lab workers	Hepatitis A vaccine (HR5); PPD (HR6); influenza vaccine (HR9)
Family history of skin cancer; nevi; fair skin, eyes, hair	Avoid excess/midday sun, use protective clothing* (HR13)
Prior pregnancy with neural tube defect	Folic acid 4.0 mg (HR14)
Inadequate water fluoridation	Daily fluoride supplement (HR15)
Pregnancy	HIV screen

ATV, All-terrain vehicle; *HR,* high risk; *PPD,* purified protein derivative; *RPR,* rapid plasmin reagin; *STD,* sexually transmitted disease; *TB,* tuberculosis; *VDRL,* Venereal Disease Research Laboratory.
[1]Periodic blood pressure for persons aged ≥21 yr. [2]If sexually active at present or in the past: q ≤3 yr. If sexual history is unreliable, begin Pap tests at age 21 yr. [3]If sexually active. [4]Serologic testing, documented vaccination history, and routine vaccination against rubella (preferably with MMR) are equally acceptable alternatives. [5]If not previously immunized: current visit and 1 and 6 mo later. [6]If no previous second dose of MMR. [7]If susceptible to chickenpox. [8]Meningococcal conjugate vaccine (MCV) can be administered at 11-12 yr visit, at high school entry, or at beginning of college (especially indicated in students living in college dormitories). [9]Quadrivalent human papillomavirus (types 6, 11, 16, 18) recombinant vaccine (Gardasil) should be given to all females aged 11-26 yr who have not been previously vaccinated. The vaccine is indicated for the prevention of cervical cancer and genital warts caused by the human papilloma virus (HPV) 6, 11, 16, or 18. Gardasil is an intramuscular injection for administration to the thigh or upper arm. The schedule consists of three 0.5-ml doses, with the second dose given 2 mo after the first, and the final dose administered 6 mo after the initial dose. HPV4 may also be administered in a 3-dose series to males aged 9 through 26 years to reduce their likelihood of acquiring genital warts. [10]Influenza vaccine is recommended for children 6 mo to 18 yr of age. [11]Administer to children with certain underlying medical conditions (see *MMWR* 46[RR-8], 1997), including a cochlear implant. A single revaccination should be administered to children with functional or anatomic asplenia or other immunocompromising condition after 5 yr.
*The ability of clinician counseling to influence this behavior is unproven.
[†]Tdap vaccine is recommended for adolescents aged 11-12 yr who have completed the recommended childhood DTP/DTaP vaccination series and have not received a Td booster dose. Adolescents aged 13-18 yr who missed the 11- 12-yr Td/Tdap booster dose should also receive a single dose of Tdap if they have completed the recommended childhood DTP/DTaP vaccination series. A 5-yr interval from the last Td dose is encouraged when Tdap is used as a booster drug; however, a shorter interval may be used if pertussis immunity is needed.

HR1: Persons who exchange sex for money or drugs and their sex partners, persons with other STDs (including HIV), and sexual contacts of persons with active syphilis. Clinicians should also consider local epidemiology.

HR2: Females who have had two or more sex partners in the last year or a sex partner with multiple sexual contacts; exchanged sex for money or drugs; or have a history of repeated episodes of gonorrhea. Clinicians should also consider local epidemiology.

HR3: Males who had sex with males after 1975; past or present injection drug users; persons who exchange sex for money or drugs and their sex partners; injection drug–using, bisexual, or HIV-positive sex partner currently or in the past; recipients of a blood transfusion between 1978 and 1985; persons seeking treatment for STDs. Clinicians should also consider local epidemiology and screening for HIV in general population.

HR4: Sexually active females with multiple risk factors, including history of prior STD, new or multiple sex partners, age <25 yr, nonuse or inconsistent use of barrier contraceptives, or cervical ectopy. Clinicians should consider local epidemiology of the disease in identifying other high-risk groups.

HR5: Persons living in, traveling to, or working in areas where the disease is endemic and where periodic outbreaks occur (e.g., countries with high or intermediate endemicity; certain Alaska Native, Pacific Island, Native American, and religious communities); men who have sex with men; injection or street drug users; persons with clotting factor disorders or chronic liver disease. Vaccine may be considered for institutionalized persons and workers in these institutions; military personnel; and day-care, hospital, and laboratory workers. Clinicians should also consider local epidemiology.

HR6: HIV-positive, close contacts of persons with known or suspected TB, health care workers, persons with medical risk factors associated with TB, immigrants from countries with high TB prevalence, medically underserved low-income populations (including homeless), alcoholics, injection drug users, and residents of long-term care facilities.

HR7: Persons who continue to inject drugs.

HR8: Immunocompetent persons with certain medical conditions, including chronic cardiac or pulmonary disease, diabetes mellitus, cochlear implants candidates and recipients, and anatomic asplenia. Immunocompetent persons who live in high-risk environments or social settings (e.g., certain Native American and Alaska Native populations).

HR9: Annual vaccination of residents of chronic care facilities; persons with chronic cardiopulmonary disorders, metabolic diseases (including diabetes mellitus), hemoglobinopathies, immunosuppression, or renal dysfunction; and health care providers for high-risk patients.

HR10: Adolescents and young adults in settings where such individuals congregate (e.g., high schools and colleges) if they have not previously received a second dose.

HR11: Healthy persons aged ≥13 yr without a history of chickenpox or previous immunization. Consider serologic testing for presumed susceptible persons aged ≥13 yr.

HR12: Persons born after 1956 who lack evidence of immunity to measles or mumps (e.g., documented receipt of live vaccine on or after the first birthday, laboratory evidence of immunity, or a history of physician-diagnosed measles or mumps).

HR13: Persons with a family or personal history of skin cancer; a large number of moles; atypical moles; poor tanning ability; or light skin, hair, and eye color.

HR14: Women with prior pregnancy affected by neural tube defect who are planning pregnancy.

HR15: Persons aged <17 yr living in areas with inadequate water fluoridation (<0.6 ppm).

TABLE 5-3 Ages 25 to 64 Years

Interventions considered and recommended
  for the Periodic Health Examination

Leading causes of death
  Malignant neoplasms
  Heart diseases
  Motor vehicle and other unintentional injuries
  HIV infection
  Suicide and homicide

INTERVENTIONS FOR THE GENERAL POPULATION

Screening

Blood pressure

Height and weight

Lipid panel (men aged 35-64 yr, women aged 45-64 yr)

HIV screening

Papanicolaou (Pap) test (women)[1]

Fecal occult blood test[2] and/or colonoscopy (≥50 yr)

Mammogram ± clinical breast examination[3] (women 40-69 yr)

Bone density scan in postmenopausal women

Assess for problem drinking

Rubella serology or vaccination history[4] (women of childbearing age)

Counseling

Substance use

Tobacco cessation

Avoid alcohol/drug use while driving, swimming, boating, etc.*

Diet and exercise

Limit fat and cholesterol; maintain caloric balance; emphasize grains, fruits,
  vegetables

Adequate calcium intake (women)

Regular physical activity*

Injury prevention

Lap/shoulder belts

Motorcycle/bicycle/ATV helmets*

Smoke detector*

Safe storage/removal of firearms*

Sexual behavior

STD prevention: avoid high-risk behavior*; condoms/female barrier with spermicide*

Unintended pregnancy: contraception

Dental health

Regular visits to dental care provider*

Floss, brush with fluoride toothpaste daily*

Immunizations

Tetanus-diphtheria (Td) boosters

Rubella[4] (women of childbearing age)

Influenza vaccine†

Human papilloma virus[5]

Herpes zoster (≥60 yr)[6]

Chemoprophylaxis

Multivitamin with folic acid (women planning or capable of pregnancy)

INTERVENTIONS FOR HIGH-RISK POPULATIONS

Population	*Potential Interventions (see detailed high-risk definitions)*
High-risk sexual behavior	RPR/VDRL (HR1); screen for gonorrhea (female) (HR2), HIV (HR3), Chlamydia (female) (HR4); hepatitis B vaccine (HR5); hepatitis A vaccine (HR6)
Injection or street drug use	RPR/VDRL (HR1); HIV screen (HR3); hepatitis B vaccine (HR5); hepatitis A vaccine (HR6); PPD (HR7); advice to reduce infection risk (HR8)
Low income; TB contacts; immigrants; alcoholics	PPD (HR7)
Native Americans/Alaska Natives	Hepatitis A vaccine (HR6); PPD (HR7); pneumococcal vaccine (HR9)
Travelers to developing countries	Hepatitis B vaccine (HR5); hepatitis A vaccine (HR6)
Certain chronic medical conditions	PPD (HR7); pneumococcal vaccine (HR9); influenza vaccine (HR10)
Blood product recipients	HIV screen (HR3); hepatitis B vaccine (HR5); hepatitis C screen
Susceptible to measles, mumps, or varicella	MMR (HR11); varicella vaccine (HR12)
Institutionalized persons	Hepatitis A vaccine (HR6); PPD (HR7); pneumococcal vaccine (HR9); influenza vaccine (HR10)
Health care/lab workers	Hepatitis B vaccine (HR5); hepatitis A vaccine (HR6); PPD (HR7); influenza vaccine (HR10)
Family history of skin cancer; fair skin, eyes, hair	Avoid excess/midday sun, use protective clothing* (HR13)
Previous pregnancy with neural tube defect	Folic acid 4.0 mg (HR14)
Cardiovascular risk factors	Lipid panel (HR 15)
Pregnancy	HIV screen

ATV, All-terrain vehicle; *HR*, high risk; *MMR*, measles-mumps-rubella; *PPD*, purified protein derivative; *RPR*, rapid plasma reagin; *STD*, sexually transmitted disease; *TB*, tuberculosis; *VDRL*, Venereal Disease Research Laboratory.

[1]Women who are or have been sexually active and who have a cervix: q ≤3 yr. Routine pap smear screening is unnecessary for women who have undergone a complete hysterectomy for benign disease. The American College of Obstetricians and Gynecologists (ACOG) recommends routine paps should start at age 21. Women 30 and older should wait 3 yrs between paps once they have had three consecutive clear tests. [2]Annually. [3]Mammogram q1-2 yr, or mammogram q1-2 yr with annual clinical breast examination. [4]Serologic testing, documented vaccination history, and routine vaccination (preferably with MMR) are equally acceptable. [5]Quadrivalent human papillomavirus (types 6, 11, 16, 18) recombinant vaccine (Gardasil) should be given to all females aged 9-26 yr who have not been previously vaccinated. The vaccine is indicated for the prevention of cervical cancer and genital warts caused by the human papilloma virus (HPV) 6, 11, 16, or 18. Gardasil is an intramuscular injection for administration to the thigh or upper arm. The schedule consists of three 0.5-ml doses, with the second dose given 2 mo after the first, and the final dose administered 6 mo after the initial dose. Gardasil is also indicated in males aged 9 to 26 yr for prevention of genital warts. [6]Herpes zoster vaccine (Zostavax) is indicated for prevention of herpes zoster (shingles) in individuals 60 yr or older. Zostavax is administered as a single dose subcutaneously. It is a lyophilic preparation of the Oka/Merck strain of live, attenuated varicella zoster virus (VZV). It should not be administered to individuals with a history of primary or acquired immunodeficiency states, persons on immunosuppressive therapy (including high-dose corticosteroids), those with active untreated tuberculosis, and those who may be pregnant.

*The ability of clinician counseling to influence this behavior is unproven.
†A live attenuated influenza vaccine (LAIV, Flumist) administered intranasally is available for healthy persons aged 2 to 49 yr.

HR1: Persons who exchange sex for money or drugs and their sex partners, persons with other STDs (including HIV), and sexual contacts of persons with active syphilis. Clinicians should also consider local epidemiology.

HR2: Women who exchange sex for money or drugs or who have had repeated episodes of gonorrhea. Clinicians should also consider local epidemiology.

HR3: Men who had sex with men after 1975; past or present injection drug users; persons who exchange sex for money or drugs and their sex partners; persons with current or past injection drug–using, bisexual, or HIV-positive sex partners; recipients of a blood transfusion between 1978 and 1985; persons seeking treatment for STDs. Clinicians should also consider local epidemiology and HIV screening in the general population.

HR4: Sexually active women with multiple risk factors, including history of STD, new or multiple sex partners, nonuse or inconsistent use of barrier contraceptives, or cervical ectopy. Clinicians should also consider local epidemiology.

HR5: Blood product recipients (including hemodialysis patients), persons with frequent occupational exposure to blood or blood products, men who have sex with men, injection drug users and their sex partners, persons with multiple recent sex partners, persons with other STDs (including HIV), travelers to countries with endemic hepatitis B.

HR6: Persons living in, traveling to, or working in areas where the disease is endemic and where periodic outbreaks occur (e.g., countries with high or intermediate endemicity; certain Alaska Native, Pacific Island, Native American, and religious communities); men who have sex with men; injection or street drug users; patients with clotting factor disorders or chronic liver disease. Consider for institutionalized persons and workers in these institutions; military personnel; and day-care, hospital, and laboratory workers. Clinicians should also consider local epidemiology.

HR7: HIV-positive, close contacts of persons with known or suspected TB, health care workers, persons with medical risk factors associated with TB, immigrants from countries with high TB prevalence, medically underserved low-income populations (including homeless), alcoholics, injection drug users, and residents of long-term care facilities.

HR8: Persons who continue to inject drugs.

HR9: Immunocompetent institutionalized persons aged ≥50 yr and immunocompetent persons with certain medical conditions, including chronic cardiac or pulmonary disease, anatomic asplenia, or diabetes mellitus; cochlear implant candidates and recipients. Immunocompetent persons who live in high-risk environments or social settings (e.g., certain Native American and Alaska Native populations).

HR10: Annual vaccination of residents of long-term care facilities; persons with chronic cardiopulmonary disorders, metabolic diseases (including diabetes mellitus), hemoglobinopathies, immunosuppression, or renal dysfunction; and health care providers of high-risk patients.

HR11: Persons born after 1956 who lack evidence of immunity to measles or mumps (e.g., documented receipt of live vaccine on or after the first birthday, laboratory evidence of immunity, or a history of physician-diagnosed measles or mumps).

HR12: Healthy adults without a history of chickenpox or previous immunization. Consider serologic testing for presumed susceptible adults.

HR13: Persons with a family or personal history of skin cancer; a large number of moles; atypical moles; poor tanning ability; or light skin, hair, and eye color.

HR14: Women with previous pregnancy affected by neural tube disorder who are planning pregnancy.

HR15: Clinicians should consider a fasting serum lipid panel on a case-by-case basis.

TABLE 5-4 Ages 65 and Older

Interventions considered and recommended for the Periodic Health Examination	Leading causes of death
	Heart diseases
	Malignant neoplasms (lung, colorectal, breast)
	Cerebrovascular disease
	Chronic obstructive pulmonary disease
	Pneumonia and influenza

INTERVENTIONS FOR THE GENERAL POPULATION

Screening

Blood pressure

Height and weight

Fecal occult blood test[1] and/or colonoscopy

Mammogram $\pm$ clinical breast examination[2] (women $\leq$69 yr)

Papanicolaou (Pap) test (women)[3]

Bone density scan in postmenopausal patients

Vision screening

Assess for hearing impairment

Assess for problem drinking

Offer HIV screen

Counseling

Substance use

Tobacco cessation

Avoid alcohol/drug use while driving, swimming, boating, etc.*

Diet and exercise

Limit fat and cholesterol; maintain caloric balance; emphasize grains, fruits, vegetables

Adequate calcium intake (women)

Regular physical activity*

Injury prevention

Lap/shoulder belts

Motorcycle and bicycle helmets*

Fall prevention*

Safe storage/removal of firearms*

Smoke detector*

Set hot water heater to <120°-130° F

CPR training for household members

Dental health

Regular visits to dental care provider*

Floss, brush with fluoride toothpaste daily*

Sexual behavior

STD prevention: avoid high-risk sexual behavior*; use condoms

Immunizations

Pneumococcal vaccine

Influenza[1]

Tetanus-diphtheria (Td) boosters

Herpes zoster[4]

INTERVENTIONS FOR HIGH-RISK POPULATIONS

Population	Potential Interventions (see detailed high-risk definitions)
Institutionalized persons	PPD (HR1); hepatitis A vaccine (HR2); amantadine/rimantadine (HR4)
Chronic medical conditions; TB contacts; low income; immigrants; alcoholics	PPD (HR1)
Persons $\geq$75 yr or $\geq$70 yr with risk factors for falls	Fall prevention intervention (HR5)
Cardiovascular disease risk factors	Consider lipid screening (HR6)
Family history of skin cancer; nevi; fair skin, eyes, hair	Avoid excess/midday sun, use protective clothing* (HR7)
Native Americans/Alaska Natives	PPD (HR1); hepatitis A vaccine (HR2)
Travelers to developing countries	Hepatitis A vaccine (HR2); hepatitis B vaccine (HR8)
Blood product recipients	HIV screen (HR3); hepatitis B vaccine (HR8)
High-risk sexual behavior	Hepatitis A vaccine (HR2); HIV screen (HR3); hepatitis B vaccine (HR8); RPR/VDRL (HR9)
Injection or street drug use	PPD (HR1); hepatitis A vaccine (HR2); HIV screen (HR3); hepatitis B vaccine (HR8); RPR/VDRL (HR9); advice to reduce infection risk (HR10)
Health care/lab workers	PPD (HR1); hepatitis A vaccine (HR2); amantadine/rimantadine (HR4); hepatitis B vaccine (HR8)
Persons susceptible to varicella	Varicella vaccine (HR11)
Men aged 65 to 75 who have ever smoked	Ultrasound of abdominal aorta (HR12)

HR, High risk; *PPD*, purified protein derivative; *RPR*, rapid plasma reagin; *STD*, sexually transmitted disease; *TB*, tuberculosis; *VDRL*, Venereal Disease Research Laboratory.

[1]Annually. [2]Mammogram q1-2 yr, or mammogram q1-2 yr with annual clinical breast exam. [3]All women who are or have been sexually active and who have a cervix. Consider discontinuation of testing after age 65 yr if previous regular screening with consistently normal results. [4]Herpes zoster vaccine (Zostavax) is indicated for prevention of herpes zoster (shingles) in individuals age $\geq$60 yr. Zostavax is administered as a single dose subcutaneously. It is a lyophilic preparation of the Oka/Merck strain of live, attenuated varicella zoster virus (VZV). It should not be administered to individuals with a history of primary or acquired immunodeficiency states, persons on immunosuppressive therapy (including high-dose corticosteroids), those with active untreated tuberculosis, and those who may be pregnant.

*The ability of clinician counseling to influence this behavior is unproven.

HR1: HIV-positive, close contacts of persons with known or suspected TB, health care workers, persons with medical risk factors associated with TB, immigrants from countries with high TB prevalence, medically underserved low-income populations (including homeless), alcoholics, injection drug users, and residents of long-term care facilities.

HR2: Persons living in, traveling to, or working in areas where the disease is endemic and where periodic outbreaks occur (e.g., countries with high or intermediate endemicity; certain Alaska Native, Pacific Island, Native American, and religious communities); men who have sex with men; injection or street drug users; persons with clotting factor disorders or chronic liver disease. Consider for institutionalized persons and workers in these institutions and day-care, hospital, and laboratory workers. Clinicians should also consider local epidemiology and HIV screening in the general population.

HR3: Men who had sex with men after 1975; past or present injection drug users; persons who exchange sex for money or drugs and their sex partners; persons with current or past injection drug–using, bisexual, or HIV-positive sex partners; recipients of a blood transfusion between 1978 and 1985; persons seeking treatment for STDs. Clinicians should also consider local epidemiology.

HR4: Consider for persons who have not received influenza vaccine or are vaccinated late, when the vaccine may be ineffective because of major antigenic changes in the virus; for unvaccinated persons who provide home care for high-risk persons; as supplemental protection in persons who are expected to have a poor antibody response; and for high-risk persons in whom the vaccine is contraindicated.

HR5: Persons aged ≥75 yr or 70-74 yr with one or more additional risk factors, including use of certain psychoactive and cardiac medications (e.g., benzodiazepines, antihypertensives); use of four or more prescription medications; impaired cognition, strength, balance, or gait. Intensive individualized, home-based multifactorial fall prevention intervention is recommended in settings where adequate resources are available to deliver such services.

HR6: Clinicians should consider fasting lipid panel screening on a case-by-case basis for persons aged 65 to 75 yr, especially in those with additional risk factors (e.g., smoking, diabetes, or hypertension).

HR7: Persons with a family or personal history of skin cancer; a large number of moles; atypical moles; poor tanning ability; or light skin, hair, and eye color.

HR8: Blood product recipients (including hemodialysis patients), persons with frequent occupational exposure to blood or blood products, men who have sex with men, injection drug users and their sex partners, persons with multiple recent sex partners, persons with other STDs (including HIV), travelers to countries with endemic hepatitis B.

HR9: Persons who exchange sex for money or drugs and their sex partners, persons with other STDs (including HIV), and sexual contacts of persons with active syphilis. Clinicians should also consider local epidemiology.

HR10: Persons who continue to inject drugs.

HR11: Healthy adults without a history of chickenpox or previous immunization. Consider serologic testing for presumed susceptible adults.

HR12: Consider ultrasound of abdominal aorta to screen for abdominal aortic aneurysm in all men aged 65 to 75 yr who have ever smoked.

TABLE 5-5 Pregnant Women*

Interventions considered and recommended for the Periodic Health Examination

---

INTERVENTIONS FOR THE GENERAL POPULATION

Screening

First visit

Blood pressure

Hemoglobin/hematocrit

Hepatitis B surface antigen (HBsAg)

RPR/VDRL

Chlamydia screen (<25 yr)

Rubella serology or vaccination history

D(Rh) typing, antibody screen

Offer CVS (<13 wk)[1] or amniocentesis (15-18 wk)[1] (age ≥35 yr)

Offer hemoglobinopathy screening

Assess for problem or risk drinking

Offer HIV screening[2]

Follow-up visits

Blood pressure

Urine culture (12-16 wk)

Offer amniocentesis (15-18 wk)[1] (age ≥35 yr)

Offer multiple marker testing[1] (15-18 wk)

Offer serum α-fetoprotein[1] (16-18 wk)

Counseling

Tobacco cessation; effects of passive smoking

Alcohol/other drug use

Nutrition, including adequate calcium intake

Encourage breastfeeding

Lap/shoulder belts

Infant safety car seats

STD prevention: avoid high-risk sexual behavior[†]; use condoms[†]

Chemoprophylaxis

Multivitamin with folic acid[3]

INTERVENTIONS FOR HIGH-RISK POPULATIONS

Population	*Potential Interventions (see detailed high-risk definitions)*
High-risk sexual behavior	Screen for chlamydia (first visit) (HR1), gonorrhea (first visit) (HR2), HIV (first visit) (HR3); HBsAg (third trimester) (HR4); RPR/VDRL (third trimester) (HR5)
Blood transfusion between 1978 and 1985	HIV screen (first visit) (HR3)
Injection drug use	HIV screen (HR3); HBsAg (third trimester) (HR4); advice to reduce infection risk (HR6)
Unsensitized D-negative women	D(Rh) antibody testing (24-28 wk) (HR7)
Risk factors for Down syndrome	Offer CVS (first trimester), amniocentesis (15-18 wk)[1] (HR8)
Prior pregnancy with neural tube defect	Offer amniocentesis (15-18 wk),[1] folic acid 4.0 mg[3] (HR9)

CVS, Chorionic villus sampling; *HR*, high risk; *RPR*, rapid plasma reagin; *VDRL*, Venereal Disease Research Laboratory.
[1]Women with access to counseling and follow-up services, reliable standardized laboratories, skilled high-resolution ultrasound and, for those receiving serum marker testing, amniocentesis capabilities. [2]Universal screening is recommended. [3]Beginning at least 1 mo before conception and continuing through the first trimester.
*See Tables 5-2 and 5-3 for other preventive services recommended for women of this age group.
[†]The ability of clinician counseling to influence this behavior is unproven.

HR1: Women with history of STD or new or multiple sex partners. Clinicians should also consider local epidemiology. Chlamydia screen should be repeated in third trimester if at continued risk.

HR2: Women younger than 25 yr with two or more sex partners in the last year or whose sex partner has multiple sexual contacts, women who exchange sex for money or drugs, and women with a history of repeated episodes of gonorrhea. Clinicians should also consider local epidemiology. Gonorrhea screen should be repeated in the third trimester if at continued risk.

HR3: Universal screening for HIV infection is recommended for all pregnant women. It is especially important in women with the following individual risk factors: past or present injection drug use; history of exchanging sex for money or drugs; injection drug–using, bisexual, or HIV-positive sex partner currently or in the past; recipients of a blood transfusion between 1978 and 1985; persons seeking treatment for STDs.

HR4: Women who are initially HBsAg negative who are at high risk because of injection drug use, who have suspected exposure to hepatitis B during pregnancy, and who have had multiple sex partners.

HR5: Women who exchange sex for money or drugs, women with other STDs (including HIV), and sexual contacts of persons with active syphilis. Clinicians should also consider local epidemiology.

HR6: Women who continue to inject drugs.

HR7: Unsensitized D-negative women.

HR8: Prior pregnancy affected by Down syndrome, advanced maternal age (≥35 yr), known carriage of chromosome rearrangement.

HR9: Women with previous pregnancy affected by neural tube defect.

PART B • IMMUNIZATIONS AND CHEMOPROPHYLAXIS

Childhood and Adolescent Immunizations

TABLE 5-6 Recommended Immunization Schedule for Persons Aged 0-6 Years—United States
(For those who fall behind or start late, see the catch-up schedule)

Vaccine ▼ Age ▶	Birth	1 Month	2 Months	4 Months	6 Months	12 Months	15 Months	18 Months	19-23 Months	2-3 Years	4-6 Years	
Hepatitis B[1]	HepB	HepB		See footnote 1		HepB						Range of recommended ages
Rotavirus[2]			RV	RV	RV[2]							
Diphtheria, tetanus, pertussis[3]			DTaP	DTaP	DTaP	See footnote 3	DTaP				DTaP	
Haemophilus influenzae type b[4]			Hib	Hib	Hib[4]	Hib						
Pneumococcal[5]			PCV	PCV	PCV	PCV				PPSV		Certain high-risk groups
Inactivated poliovirus			IPV	IPV		IPV					IPV	
Influenza[6]						Influenza (yearly)						
Measles, mumps, rubella[7]						MMR		See footnote 7			MMR	
Varicella[8]						Varicella		See footnote 8			Varicella	
Hepatitis A[9]						HepA (2 doses)				HepA Series		
Meningococcal[10]										MCV		

This schedule indicates the recommended ages for routine administration of currently licensed vaccines for children aged 0-6 years. Any dose not administered at the recommended age should be administered at any subsequent visit, when indicated and feasible. Licensed combination vaccines may be used whenever any components of the combination are indicated and other components of the vaccine are not contraindicated and if approved by the Food and Drug Administration for that dose of the series. Providers should consult the relevant Advisory Committee on Immunization Practices statement for detailed recommendations, including high-risk conditions: http://www.cdc.gov/vaccines/pubs/acip-list.htm. Clinically significant adverse events that follow immunization should be reported to the Vaccine Adverse Event Reporting System (VAERS). Guidance about how to obtain and complete a VAERS form is available at http://www.vaers.hhs.gov or by telephone, 800-822-7967.

1. **Hepatitis B vaccine (HepB).** *(Minimum age: birth)*
   At birth:
   - Administer monovalent HepB to all newborns before hospital discharge.
   - If mother is hepatitis B surface antigen (HBsAg)-positive, administer HepB and 0.5 ml of hepatitis B immune globulin (HBIG) within 12 hours of birth.
   - If mother's HBsAg status is unknown, administer HepB within 12 hours of birth. Determine mother's HBsAg status as soon as possible and, if HBsAg-positive, administer HBIG (no later than age 1 week).
   After the birth dose:
   - The HepB series should be completed with either monovalent HepB or a combination vaccine containing HepB. The second dose should be administered at age 1 or 2 months. Monovalent HepB vaccine should be used for doses administered before age 6 weeks. The final dose should be administered no earlier than age 24 weeks.
   - Infants born to HBsAg-positive mothers should be tested for HBsAg and antibody to HBsAg (anti-HBs) after completion of at least 3 doses of the HepB series, at age 9 through 18 months (generally at the next well-child visit).
   4-month dose:
   - Administration of 4 doses of HepB to infants is permissible when combination vaccines containing HepB are administered after the birth dose. The fourth dose should be administered no earlier than age 24 weeks.
2. **Rotavirus vaccine (RV).** *(Minimum age: 6 weeks)*
   - Administer the first dose at age 6 through 14 weeks *(maximum age: 14 weeks 6 days).* Vaccination should not be initiated for infants aged 15 weeks or older (i.e., 15 weeks, 0 days or older).
   - Administer the final dose in the series by age 8 months 0 days.
   - If Rotarix® is administered at ages 2 and 4 months, a dose at 6 months is not indicated.
3. **Diphtheria and tetanus toxoids and acellular pertussis vaccine (DTaP).** *(Minimum age: 6 weeks)*
   - The fourth dose may be administered as early as age 12 months, provided at least 6 months have elapsed since the third dose.
   - Administer the final dose in the series at age 4 through 6 years.
4. **Haemophilus influenzae type b conjugate vaccine (Hib).** *(Minimum age: 6 weeks)*
   - If PRP-OMP (PedvaxHIB® or Comvax® [HepB-Hib]) is administered at ages 2 and 4 months, a dose at age 6 months is not indicated.
   - TriHiBit® (DTaP/Hib) should not be used for doses at ages 2, 4, or 6 months but can be used as the final dose in children aged 12 months or older.
5. **Pneumococcal vaccine.** *(Minimum age: 6 weeks for pneumococcal conjugate vaccine [PCV]; 2 years for pneumococcal polysaccharide vaccine [PPSV])*
   - PCV is recommended for all children aged younger than 5 years. Administer 1 dose of PCV to all healthy children aged 24 through 59 months who are not completely vaccinated for their age.
   A 13-valent pneumococcal conjugate vaccine (PCV13; Prevnar 13) has replaced PCV7. A single supplemental dose of PCV13 is recommended for healthy children 14 through 59 mo

of age who have been completely vaccinated with PCV7. An interval of at least 8 wk is recommended between the final dose of PCV7 and the supplemental dose of PCV13. A supplemental dose is also recommended for children 14 through 71 mo of age who are at high risk of pneumococcal disease (e.g., those with chronic heart and lung disease, diabetes mellitus, sickle cell anemia, asplenia, HIV, cochlear implant, CSF leak or other immunocompromising conditions) and have been completely immunized with PCV7.

6. **Influenza vaccine.** *(Minimum age: 6 months for trivalent inactivated influenza vaccine [TIV]; 2 years for live, attenuated influenza vaccine [LAIV])*
   - Administer annually to children aged 6 months through 18 years
   - For healthy nonpregnant persons (i.e., those who do not have underlying medical conditions that predispose them to influenza complications) aged 2 through 49 years, either LAIV or TIV may be used.
   - Children receiving TIV should receive 0.25 ml if aged 6 through 35 months or 0.5 ml if aged 3 years or older.
   - Administer 2 doses (separated by at least 4 weeks) to children aged younger than 9 years who are receiving influenza vaccine for the first time or who were vaccinated for the first time during the previous influenza season but only received 1 dose.
7. **Measles, mumps, and rubella vaccine (MMR).** *(Minimum age: 12 months)*
   - Administer the second dose at age 4-6 years. However, the second dose may be administered before age 4, provided at least 28 days have elapsed since the first dose.
8. **Varicella vaccine.** *(Minimum age: 12 months)*
   - Administer the second dose at age 4 through 6 years. However, the second dose may be administered before age 4, provided at least 3 months have elapsed since the first dose.
   - For children aged 12 months through 12 years the minimum interval between doses is 3 months. However, if the second dose was administered at least 28 days after the first dose, it can be accepted as valid.
9. **Hepatitis A vaccine (HepA).** *(Minimum age: 12 months)*
   - Administer to all children aged 1 year (i.e., aged 12 through 23 months). Administer 2 doses at least 6 months apart.
   - Children not fully vaccinated by age 2 years can be vaccinated at subsequent visits.
   - HepA also is recommended for children older than 1 year who live in areas where vaccination programs target older children or who are at increased risk of infection. See *MMWR* 2006;55(No. RR-7).
10. **Meningococcal vaccine.** *(Minimum age: 2 years for meningococcal conjugate vaccine [MCV] and for meningococcal polysaccharide vaccine [MPSV])*
    - Administer MCV to children aged 2 through 10 years with terminal complement component deficiency, anatomic or functional asplenia, and certain other high-risk groups. See *MMWR* 2005;54(No. RR-7).
    - Persons who received MPSV 3 or more years previously and who remain at increased risk for meningococcal disease should be revaccinated with MCV.

Note: The National Childhood Vaccine Injury Act requires that health care providers provide dparents or patients with copies of vaccine information statements before administering each dose of the vaccines listed in the schedules.

Clinical Practice Guidelines

V

The recommended immunization schedules for persons aged 0 to 18 yr are approved by the Advisory Committee on Immunization Practices (http://www.cdc.gov/vaccines/recs/acip), the American Academy of Pediatrics (http://www.aap.org), and the American Academy of Family Physicians (http://www.aafp.org).

TABLE 5-7 Recommended Immunization Schedule for Persons Aged 7-18 Years—United States
(For those who fall behind or start late, see the schedule below and the catch-up schedule)

Vaccine ▼ Age ▶	7-10 years	11-12 years	13-18 years	
Tetanus, diphtheria, pertussis[1]	See footnote 1	Tdap	Tdap	Range of recommended ages
Human papillomavirus[2]	See footnote 2	HPV (3 doses)	HPV Series	
Meningococcal[3]	MCV	MCV	MCV	
Influenza[4]	Influenza (yearly)			Catch-up immunization
Pneumococcal[5]	PPSV			
Hepatitis A[6]	HepA Series			
Hepatitis B[7]	HepB Series			Certain high-risk groups
Inactivated poliovirus[8]	IPV Series			
Measles, mumps, rubella[9]	MMR Series			
Varicella[10]	Varicella Series			

This schedule indicates the recommended ages for routine administration of currently licensed vaccines for children aged 7-18 years. Any dose not administered at the recommended age should be administered at any subsequent visit, when indicated and feasible. Licensed combination vaccines may be used whenever any components of the combination are indicated and other components of the vaccine are not contraindicated and if approved by the Food and Drug Administration for that dose of the series. Providers should consult the respective Advisory Committee on Immunization Practices statement for detailed recommendations, including high-risk conditions: http://www.cdc.gov/vaccines/pubs/acip-list.htm. Clinically significant adverse events that follow immunization should be reported to the Vaccine Adverse Event Reporting System (VAERS). Guidance about how to obtain and complete a VAERS form is available at http://www.vaers.hhs.gov or by telephone, 800-822-7967.

1. **Tetanus and diphtheria toxoids and acellular pertussis vaccine (Tdap).** *(Minimum age: 10 years for BOOSTRIX® and 11 years for ADACEL®)*
   - Administer at age 11 or 12 years for those who have completed the recommended childhood DTP/DTaP vaccination series and have not received a tetanus and diphtheria toxoid (Td) booster dose.
   - Persons aged 13 to 18 years who have not received Tdap should receive a dose.
   - A 5-year interval from the last Td dose is encouraged when Tdap is used as a booster dose; however, a shorter interval may be used if pertussis immunity is needed.
2. **Human papillomavirus vaccine (HPV).** *(Minimum age: 9 years)*
   - Two HPV vaccines are licensed: A quadrivalent vaccine (HPV4) for the prevention of cervical, vaginal, and vulvar cancer (in females) and genital warts (in females and males) and a bivalent vaccine (HPV2) for the prevention of cervical cancers in females.
   - HPV4 is recommended for the prevention of cervical, vaginal, and vulvar precancers and cancers and genital warts in females and genital warts in males.
   - Administer the first dose to females at age 11 or 12 years.
   - Administer the second dose 2 months after the first dose and the third dose 6 months after the first dose (at least 24 weeks after the first dose).
   - Administer the series to females at age 13 to 18 years if not previously vaccinated.
   - HPV4 may be administered in a 3-dose series to males aged 9 through 18 years to reduce the likelihood of acquiring genital warts.
3. **Meningococcal conjugate vaccine (MCV).**
   - Administer at age 11 or 12 years, or at age 13 to 18 years if not previously vaccinated.
   - Administer to previously unvaccinated college freshmen living in a dormitory.
   - Administer MCV4 to children aged 2 through 10 years with complement component deficiency, anatomic or functional asplenia, or certain other conditions placing them at high risk.
   - Administer to children previously vaccinated with MCV4 or MPSV4 who remain at increased risk after 3 years (if first dose administered at age 7 years or older). Persons whose only risk factor is living in on-campus housing are not recommended to receive an additional dose. See *MMWR* 2009;58:1042-1043.
4. **Influenza vaccine.**
   - Administer annually to children aged 6 months to 18 years.
   - For healthy, nonpregnant persons (i.e., those who do not have underlying medical conditions that predispose them to influenza complications) aged 2 to 49 years, either LAIV or TIV may be used.

   - Administer 2 doses (separated by at least 4 weeks) to children aged younger than 9 years who are receiving influenza vaccine for the first time or who were vaccinated for the first time during the previous influenza season but only received 1 dose.
5. **Pneumococcal polysaccharide vaccine (PPSV).**
   - Administer to children with certain underlying medical conditions (see *MMWR* 1997;46[No. RR-8]), including a cochlear implant. A single revaccination should be administered to children with functional or anatomic asplenia or other immunocompromising condition after 5 years. (See previous page, pneumococcal vaccine.)
6. **Hepatitis A vaccine (HepA).**
   - Administer 2 doses at least 6 months apart.
   - HepA is recommended for children older than 23 months who live in areas where vaccination programs target older children, who are at increased risk for infection, or for whom immunity against hepatitis A is desired.
7. **Hepatitis B vaccine (HepB).**
   - Administer the 3-dose series to those not previously vaccinated.
   - A 2-dose series (separated by at least 4 months) of adult formulation Recombivax HB® is licensed for children aged 11 to 15 years.
8. **Inactivated poliovirus vaccine (IPV).**
   - For children who received an all-IPV or all-oral poliovirus (OPV) series, a fourth dose is not necessary if the third dose was administered at age 4 years or older.
   - If both OPV and IPV were administered as part of a series, a total of 4 doses should be administered, regardless of the child's current age.
9. **Measles, mumps, and rubella vaccine (MMR).**
   - If not previously vaccinated, administer 2 doses or the second dose for those who have received only 1 dose, with at least 28 days between doses.
10. **Varicella vaccine.**
    - For persons aged 7 to 18 years without evidence of immunity (see *MMWR* 2007;56[No. RR-4]), administer 2 doses if not previously vaccinated or the second dose if they have received only 1 dose.
    - For persons aged 7 to 12 years, the minimum interval between doses is 3 months. However, if the second dose was administered at least 28 days after the first dose, it can be accepted as valid.
    - For persons aged 13 years and older, the minimum interval between doses is 28 days.

The recommended immunization schedules for persons aged 0 to 18 yr are approved by the Advisory Committee on Immunization Practices (http://www.cdc.gov.vaccines.recs.acip), the American Academy of Pediatrics (http://www.aap.org), and the American Academy of Family Physicians (http://www.aafp.org).

This table provides catch-up schedules and minimum intervals between doses for children whose vaccinations have been delayed. A vaccine series does not need to be restarted regardless of the time that has elapsed between doses. Use the section appropriate for the child's age.

CATCH-UP SCHEDULE FOR PERSONS AGED 4 MONTHS TO 6 YEARS

Vaccine	Minimum Age for Dose 1	Minimum Interval Between Doses			
		Dose 1 to Dose 2	Dose 2 to Dose 3	Dose 3 to Dose 4	Dose 4 to Dose 5
Hepatitis B[1]	Birth	4 weeks	8 weeks (and at least 16 weeks after first dose)		
Rotavirus[2]	6 weeks	4 weeks	4 weeks[2]		
Diphtheria,tetanus, pertussis[3]	6 weeks	4 weeks	4 weeks	6 months	6 months[3]
Haemophilus influenzae type b[4]	6 weeks	4 weeks if first dose administered at younger than 12 months of age / 8 weeks (as final dose) if first dose administered at age 12-14 months / No further doses needed if first dose administered at age 15 months or older	4 weeks[4] if current age is younger than 12 months / 8 weeks (as final dose)[4] if current age is 12 months or older and second dose administered at younger than 15 months / No further doses needed if previous dose administered at age 15 months or older	8 weeks (as final dose) This dose only necessary for children aged 12 months through 59 months who received 3 doses before age 12 months	
Pneumococcal[5]	6 weeks	4 weeks if first dose administered at younger than 12 months of age / 8 weeks (as final dose for healthy children) if first dose administered at age 12 months or older or current age 24 to 59 months / No further doses needed for healthy children if first dose administered at age 24 months or older	4 weeks if current age is younger than 12 months / 8 weeks (as final dose for healthy children) if current age is 12 months or older / No further doses needed for healthy children if previous dose administered at age 24 months or older	8 weeks (as final dose) This dose only necessary for children aged 12 months to 59 months who received 3 doses before age 12 months or for high-risk children who received 3 doses at any age	
Inactivated poliovirus[6]	6 weeks	4 weeks	4 weeks	4 weeks[6]	
Measles, mumps, rubella[7]	12 months	4 weeks			
Varicella[8]	12 months	3 months			
Hepatitis A[9]	12 months	6 months			

CATCH-UP SCHEDULE FOR PERSONS AGED 7 TO 18 YEARS

Vaccine	Minimum Age for Dose 1	Dose 1 to Dose 2	Dose 2 to Dose 3	Dose 3 to Dose 4	Dose 4 to Dose 5
Tetanus, diphtheria/tetanus, diphtheria, pertussis[10]	7 years[10]	4 weeks	4 weeks if first dose administered at younger than 12 months of age / 6 months if first dose administered at age 12 months or older	6 months if first dose administered at younger than 12 months of age	
Human papillomavirus[11]	9 years	Routine dosing intervals are recommended[11]			
Hepatitis A[9]	12 months	6 months			
Hepatitis B[1]	Birth	4 weeks	8 weeks (and at least 16 weeks after first dose)		
Inactivated poliovirus[6]	6 weeks	4 weeks	4 weeks	6 months	
Measles, mumps, rubella[7]	12 months	4 weeks			
Varicella[8]	12 months	3 months if the person is younger than age 13 years of age / 4 weeks if the person is aged 13 years or older			

1. **Hepatitis B vaccine (HepB).**
   - Administer the 3-dose series to those not previously vaccinated.
   - A 2-dose series (separated by at least 4 mo) of adult formulation Recombivax HB is licensed for children aged 11 to 15 yr.
2. **Rotavirus vaccine (RV).**
   - The maximum age for the first dose is 14 wk 6 days. Vaccination should not be initiated for infants aged 15 wk or older (i.e., 15 wk 0 days or older).
   - Administer the final dose in the series by age 8 mo 0 days.
   - If Rotarix was administered for the first and second doses, a third dose is not indicated.
3. **Diphtheria and tetanus toxoids and acellular pertussis vaccine (DTaP).**
   - The fifth dose is not necessary if the fourth dose was administered at age 4 yr or older.
4. **Haemophilus influenzae type b conjugate vaccine (Hib).**
   - Hib vaccine is not generally recommended for persons aged 5 yr or older. No efficacy data are available on which to base a recommendation concerning use of Hib vaccine for older children and adults. However, studies suggest good immunogenicity in persons who have sickle cell disease, leukemia, or HIV infection, or who have had a splenectomy; administering 1 dose of Hib vaccine to these persons is not contraindicated.
   - If the first 2 doses were PRP-OMP (PedvaxHIB or Comvax), and administered at age 11 mo or younger, the third (and final) dose should be administered at age 12 to 15 mo and at least 8 wk after the second dose.
   - If the first dose was administered at age 7 to 11 mo, administer 2 doses separated by 4 wk and a final dose at age 12 to 15 mo.
5. **Pneumococcal vaccine.**
   - Administer 1 dose of pneumococcal conjugate vaccine (PCV) to all healthy children aged 24 to 59 mo who have not received at least 1 dose of PCV on or after age 12 mo.
   - For children aged 24 to 59 mo with underlying medical conditions, administer 1 dose of PCV if 3 doses were received previously or administer 2 doses of PCV at least 8 wk apart if fewer than 3 doses were received previously.
   - Administer pneumococcal polysaccharide vaccine (PPSV) to children aged 2 yr or older with certain underlying medical conditions (see *MMWR* 49(RR-9), 2000), including a cochlear implant, at least 8 wk after the last dose of PCV. (See Table 5-6, pneumococcal vaccine.)

6. **Inactivated poliovirus vaccine (IPV).**
   - The final dose in the series should be administered on or after the fourth birthday and at least 6 months following the previous dose.
   - A fourth dose is not necessary if the third dose was administered at age 4 or older and at least 6 months following the previous dose.
   - In the first 6 months of life, minimum age and minimum intervals are only recommended if the person is at risk for imminent exposure to circulating poliovirus (i.e., travel to a polio-endemic region or during an outbreak).
7. **Measles, mumps, and rubella vaccine (MMR).**
   - Administer the second dose at age 4 to 6 yr. However, the second dose may be administered before age 4, provided at least 28 days have elapsed since the first dose.
   - If not previously vaccinated, administer 2 doses with at least 28 days between doses.
8. **Varicella vaccine.**
   - Administer the second dose at age 4 to 6 yr. However, the second dose may be administered before age 4, provided at least 3 mo have elapsed since the first dose.
   - For persons aged 12 mo to 12 yr, the minimum interval between doses is 3 mo. However, if the second dose was administered at least 28 days after the first dose, it can be accepted as valid.
   - For persons aged 13 yr and older, the minimum interval between doses is 28 days.
9. **Hepatitis A vaccine (HepA).**
   - HepA is recommended for children older than 1 yr who live in areas where vaccination programs target older children or who are at increased risk of infection. See *MMWR* 55(RR-7), 2006.
10. **Tetanus and diphtheria toxoids vaccine (Td) and tetanus and diphtheria toxoids and acellular pertussis vaccine (Tdap).**
   - Doses of DTaP are counted as part of the Td/Tdap series.
   - dap should be substituted for a single dose of Td in the catch-up series or as a booster for children aged 10 to 18 yr; use Td for other doses.
11. **Human papillomavirus vaccine (HPV).**
   - Administer the series to females at age 13 to 18 yr if not previously vaccinated and to males aged 9 to 26.
   - Use recommended routine dosing intervals for series catch-up (i.e., the second and third doses should be administered at 2 and 6 mo after the first dose). However, the minimum interval between the first and second doses is 4 wk. The minimum interval between the second and third doses is 12 wk, and the third dose should be given at least 24 wk after the first dose.

Information about reporting reactions after immunization is available online at http://www.vaers.hhs.gov or by telephone, 800-822-7967. Suspected cases of vaccine-preventable diseases should be reported to the state or local health department. Additional information, including precautions and contraindications for immunization, is available from the National Center for Immunization and Respiratory Diseases at http://www.cdc.gov/vaccines or by telephone at 800-CDC-INFO (800-232-4636).

QUADRIVALENT HUMAN PAPILLOMAVIRUS (HPV) VACCINE*

SUMMARY OF RATIONALE FOR QUADRIVALENT HPV VACCINE RECOMMENDATIONS*

The availability of a quadrivalent HPV vaccine offers an opportunity to decrease the burden of HPV infection and its sequelae, including cervical cancer precursors, cervical cancer, other anogenital cancers, and genital warts, in the United States. Quadrivalent HPV vaccine is licensed for use among females and males aged 9 to 26 years. HPV4 may also be administered in a 3-dose series to males aged 9 through 18 years to reduce their likelihood of acquiring genital warts. In this age group, clinical trials indicate that the vaccine is safe and immunogenic. Trials among females aged 16 to 26 years indicated the vaccine (Gardasil) to be effective against HPV types 6-, 11-, 16-, and 18-related cervical, vaginal, and vulvar cancer precursors and dysplastic lesions and genital warts. HPV 16 and 18 cause approximately 70% of cervical cancers; HPV 6 and 11 cause approximately 90% of genital warts. A new HPV vaccine (Cervarix) has been approved. Cervarix is bivalent and targets two oncogenic types, HPV 16 and 18. Because HPV is sexually transmitted and often acquired soon after onset of sexual activity, vaccination should ideally occur before first sexual activity. The recommended age for vaccination is 11 to 12 years; vaccine can be administered to girls as young as age 9 years. At the beginning of a vaccination program, females older than 12 years will exist who did not have the opportunity to receive vaccine at age 11 to 12 years. Catch-up vaccination is recommended for females aged 13 to 26 years who have not yet been vaccinated.

The recommendation for routine vaccination of girls aged 11 to 12 years is based on several considerations, including studies suggesting that quadrivalent HPV vaccine among adolescents will be safe and effective, high antibody titers achieved after vaccination at age 11 to 12 years, data on HPV epidemiology and age of sexual debut in the United States, and the high probability of HPV acquisition within several years of first sexual activity. Ideally, HPV vaccine should be administered before first sexual activity, and duration of protection should extend for many years, providing protection when exposure through sexual activity might occur. The vaccine has been demonstrated to provide protection for at least 5 years without evidence of waning. Long-term follow-up studies are under way to determine duration of protection. The recommendation also considered cost-effectiveness evaluations and the established young adolescent health care visit at age 11 to 12 years recommended by several professional organizations, when other vaccines are also recommended.

Although routine vaccination is recommended at age 11 to 12 years, the majority of females aged 13 to 26 years also can benefit from vaccination. Females not yet sexually active can be expected to receive the full benefit of vaccination. Although sexually active females in this age group might have been infected with one or more vaccine HPV types, type-specific prevalence studies in the United States suggest that a small percentage of sexually active females have been infected with all four of the HPV vaccine types. These data, available from North American females aged 16 to 24 years who participated in the quadrivalent vaccine trials, are from women who were more likely to have ever had sex than similarly aged females in the general U.S. population. Among those sexually active females, the median number of lifetime sex partners (two) was similar in trial participants and females in the general U.S. population. The vaccine does not appear to protect against persistent infection, cervical cancer precursor lesions, or genital warts caused by an HPV type that females are infected with at the time of vaccination. However, females already infected with one or more vaccine HPV types before vaccination would be protected against disease caused by the other vaccine HPV types. Therefore although overall vaccine effectiveness would be lower when administered to a population of females who are sexually active and would decrease with older age and likelihood of HPV exposure with increasing number of sex partners, the majority of females in this age group will derive at least partial benefit from vaccination.

*From CDC: Quadrivalent human papillomavirus vaccine: recommendations of the Advisory Committee on Immunization Practices (ACIP), *MMWR* 56(RR-2):16-18, 2007.

RECOMMENDATIONS FOR USE OF HPV VACCINE
RECOMMENDATIONS FOR ROUTINE USE AND CATCH-UP
Routine Vaccination of Females Aged 11 to 12 Years
The Advisory Committee on Immunization Practices (ACIP) recommends routine vaccination of females aged 11 to 12 years with 3 doses of quadrivalent HPV vaccine. The vaccination series can be started as young as age 9 years.

Catch-Up Vaccination of Females Aged 13-26 Years
Vaccination also is recommended for females aged 13 to 26 years who have not been previously vaccinated or who have not completed the full series. Ideally, vaccine should be administered before potential exposure to HPV through sexual contact; however, females who might have already been exposed to HPV should be vaccinated. Sexually active females who have not been infected with any of the HPV vaccine types would receive full benefit from vaccination. Vaccination would provide less benefit to females if they have already been infected with one or more of the four vaccine HPV types. However, clinicians cannot assess the extent to which sexually active persons would benefit from vaccination, and the risk for HPV infection might continue as long as persons are sexually active. Pap testing and screening for HPV DNA or HPV antibody are not needed before vaccination at any age.

Dosage and Administration
The vaccine should be shaken well before administration. The dose of quadrivalent HPV vaccine is 0.5 ml, administered intramuscularly (IM), preferably in the deltoid muscle.

Recommended Schedule
Quadrivalent HPV vaccine is administered in a 3-dose schedule. The second and third doses should be administered 2 and 6 months after the first dose.

Minimum Dosing Intervals and Management of Persons Who Were Incorrectly Vaccinated
The minimum interval between the first and second doses of vaccine is 4 weeks. The minimum recommended interval between the second and third doses of vaccine is 12 weeks. Inadequate doses of quadrivalent HPV vaccine or vaccine doses received after a shorter-than-recommended dosing interval should be readministered.

Interrupted Vaccine Schedules
If the quadrivalent HPV vaccine schedule is interrupted, the vaccine series does not need to be restarted. If the series is interrupted after the first dose, the second dose should be administered as soon as possible and separated from the third dose by an interval of at least 12 weeks. If only the third dose is delayed, it should be administered as soon as possible.

Simultaneous Administration with Other Vaccines
Although no data exist on administration of quadrivalent HPV vaccine with vaccines other than hepatitis B vaccine, quadrivalent HPV vaccine is not a live vaccine and has no components that adversely affect safety or efficacy of other vaccinations. Quadrivalent HPV vaccine can be administered at the same visit as other age-appropriate vaccines, such as the diphtheria, tetanus, pertussis (DTP), and quadrivalent meningococcal conjugate (MCV4) vaccines. Administering all indicated vaccines together at a single visit increases the likelihood that adolescents and young adults will receive each of the vaccines on schedule. Each vaccine should be administered by a separate syringe at a different anatomic site.

Cervical Cancer Screening among Vaccinated Females
Cervical cancer screening recommendations have not changed for females who receive HPV vaccine. HPV types in the vaccine are responsible for approximately 70% of cervical cancers; females who are vaccinated could subsequently be infected with a carcinogenic HPV type for which the quadrivalent vaccine does not provide protection. Furthermore, those who were sexually active before vaccination could have been infected with a vaccine-type HPV before vaccination. Health care providers administering quadrivalent HPV vaccine should educate women about the importance of cervical cancer screening.

Vaccination of Males

Quadrivalent HPV vaccine is now licensed for use in males ages 9 to 26 for the prevention of genital warts.

GROUPS FOR WHICH VACCINE IS NOT LICENSED
Vaccination of Females Aged <9 Years and >26 Years

Quadrivalent HPV vaccine is not licensed for use in girls younger than 9 years or women older than 26 years. Studies are ongoing among women older than 26 years. No studies are underway among girls younger than 9 years.

SPECIAL SITUATIONS AMONG FEMALES AGED 9 TO 26 YEARS
Equivocal or Abnormal Pap Test or Known HPV Infection

Females who have an equivocal or abnormal Pap test could be infected with any of approximately 40 high-risk or low-risk genital HPV types. Such females are unlikely to be infected with all four HPV vaccine types, and they might not be infected with any HPV vaccine type. Vaccination would provide protection against infection with HPV vaccine types not already acquired. With increasing severity of Pap test findings, the likelihood of infection with HPV 16 or 18 increases and the benefit of vaccination would decrease. Women should be advised that results from clinical trials do not indicate the vaccine will have any therapeutic effect on existing HPV infection or cervical lesions.

Females who have a positive HC2 high-risk test result conducted in conjunction with a Pap test could have infection with any of 13 high-risk types. This assay does not identify specific HPV types, and testing for specific HPV types is not conducted routinely in clinical practice. Women with a positive HC2 high-risk test result might not have been infected with any of the four HPV vaccine types. Vaccination would provide protection against infection with HPV vaccine types not already acquired. However, women should be advised that results from clinical trials do not indicate the vaccine will have any therapeutic effect on existing HPV infection or cervical lesions.

Genital Warts

A history of genital warts or clinically evident genital warts indicates infection with HPV, most often types 6 or 11. However, these females might not have infection with both HPV 6 and 11 or infection with HPV 16 or 18. Vaccination would provide protection against infection with HPV vaccine types not already acquired. However, females should be advised that results from clinical trials do not indicate the vaccine will have any therapeutic effect on existing HPV infection or genital warts.

Lactating Women

Lactating women can receive the HPV vaccine.

Immunocompromised Persons

Because quadrivalent HPV vaccine is a noninfectious vaccine, it can be administered to females who are immunosuppressed as a result of disease or medications. However, the immune response and vaccine efficacy might be less than that in persons who are immunocompetent.

Vaccination during Pregnancy

Quadrivalent HPV vaccine is not recommended for use in pregnancy. The vaccine has not been causally associated with adverse outcomes of pregnancy or adverse events in the developing fetus. However, data on vaccination during pregnancy are limited. Until additional information is available, initiation of the vaccine series should be delayed until after completion of the pregnancy. If a woman is found to be pregnant after initiating the vaccination series, the remainder of the 3-dose regimen should be delayed until after completion of the pregnancy. If a vaccine dose has been administered during pregnancy, no intervention is needed. A vaccine-in-pregnancy registry has been established; patients and health care providers should report any exposure to quadrivalent HPV vaccine during pregnancy by calling 800-986-8999.

PRECAUTIONS AND CONTRAINDICATIONS
Acute Illnesses

Quadrivalent HPV vaccine can be administered to persons with minor acute illnesses (e.g., diarrhea or mild upper respiratory tract infections with or without fever). Vaccination of persons with moderate or severe acute illnesses should be deferred until after the patient improves.

Hypersensitivity or Allergy to Vaccine Components

Quadrivalent HPV vaccine is contraindicated for persons with a history of immediate hypersensitivity to yeast or to any vaccine component. Data from passive surveillance in the Vaccine Adverse Event Reporting System (VAERS) indicate that recombinant yeast-derived vaccines pose a minimal risk for anaphylactic reactions in persons with a history of allergic reactions to Saccharomyces cerevisiae (baker's yeast).

Preventing Syncope after Vaccination

Syncope (i.e., vasovagal or vasodepressor reaction) can occur after vaccination, most commonly among adolescents and young adults. Among reports to VAERS for any vaccine that was coded as triggering syncope from 1990 to 2004, 35% of these episodes were reported among persons aged 10 to 18 years. Through January 2007, the second most common report to VAERS after receipt of HPV vaccine was syncope (Centers for Disease Control and Prevention, unpublished data, 2007). Vaccine providers should consider observing patients for 15 minutes after they receive HPV vaccine.

General Recommendations on Immunization

TABLE 5-9 Recommended and Minimum Ages and Intervals between Vaccine Doses of Routinely Recommended Vaccines[a]

Vaccine and Dose Number	Recommended Age for this Dose	Minimum Age for this Dose	Recommended Interval to Next Dose	Minimum Interval to Next Dose
Hepatitis B (HepB)-1[b]	Birth	Birth	1-4 mo	4 wk
HepB-2	1-2 mo	4 wk	2-17 mo	8 wk
HepB-3[c]	6-18 mo	24 wk	—	—
Diphtheria-tetanus-acellular pertussis (DTaP)-1[b]	2 mo	6 wk	2 mo	4 wk
DTaP-2	4 mo	10 wk	2 mo	4 wk
DTaP-3	6 mo	14 wk	6-12 mo[d]	6 mo[d,e]
DTaP-4	15-18 mo	12 mo	3 yr	6 mo[d]
DTaP-5	4-6 yr	4 yr	—	—
Haemophilus influenzae type b (Hib)-1[b,f]	2 mo	6 wk	2 mo	4 wk
Hib-2	4 mo	10 wk	2 mo	4 wk
Hib-3[g]	6 mo	14 wk	6-9 mo[d]	8 wk
Hib-4	12-15 mo	12 mo	—	—
Inactivated poliovirus (IPV)-1[b]	2 mo	6 wk	2 mo	4 wk
IPV-2	4 mo	10 wk	2-14 mo	4 wk
IPV-3	6-18 mo	14 wk	3-5 yr	4 wk
IPV-4	4-6 yr	18 wk	—	—
Pneumococcal conjugate (PCV)-1[f]	2 mo	6 wk	2 mo	4 wk
PCV-2	4 mo	10 wk	2 mo	4 wk
PCV-3	6 mo	14 wk	6 mo	8 wk
PCV-4	12-15 mo	12 mo	—	—
Measles-mumps-rubella (MMR)-1[h]	12-15 mo	12 mo	3-5 yr	4 wk
MMR-2[h]	4-6 yr	13 mo	—	—
Varicella (Var)-1[h]	12-15 mo	12 mo	3-5 yr	12 wk[i]
Var-2[h]	4-6 yr	15 mo	—	—
Hepatitis A (HepA)-1[b]	12-23 mo	12 mo	6-18 mo[d]	6 mo[d]
HepA-2	18-41 mo	18 mo	—	—
Influenza inactivated[j]	6-59 mo	6 mo[k]	1 mo	4 wk
Influenza live attenuated[j]	—	5 yr	6-10 wk	6 wk
Meningococcal conjugate[b]	11-12 yr	11 yr	—	—
Meningococcal polysaccharide (MPSV)-1	—	2 yr	5 yr[k]	5 yr[l]
MPSV-2[m]	—	7 yr	—	—
Tetanus-diphtheria	11-12 yr	7 yr	10 yr	5 yr
Tetanus-diphtheria acellular pertussis (Tdap)[n]	≥11 yr	10 yr	—	—
Pneumococcal polysaccharide (PPV)-1	—	2 yr	5 yr	5 yr
PPV-2[o]	—	7 yr	—	—
Human papillomavirus (HPV)-1[p]	11-12 yr	9 yr	2 mo	4 wk
HPV-2	11-12 yr (+2 mo)	109 mo	4 mo	12 wk
HPV-3	11-12 yr (+6 mo)	112 mo	—	—
Rotavirus (RV)-1[q]	2 mo	6 wk	2 mo	4 wk
RV-2	4 mo	10 wk	2 mo	4 wk
RV-3	6 mo	14 wk	—	—
Zoster[r]	60 yr	60 yr	—	—

TABLE 5-9 Recommended and Minimum Ages and Intervals between Vaccine Doses of Routinely Recommended Vaccines—cont'd

From CDC: General recommendations on immunization: recommendations of the Advisory Committee on Immunization Practices (ACIP), *MMWR* 55:(RR-15), 2006.

[a]Combination vaccines are available. Use of licensed combination vaccines is preferred over separate injections of their equivalent component vaccines. (Source: CDC: Combination vaccines for childhood immunization: recommendations of the Advisory Committee on Immunization Practices [ACIP], the American Academy of Pediatrics [AAP], and the American Academy of Family Physicians [AAFP], *MMWR* 48:[RR-5], 1999.) When administering combination vaccines, the minimum age for administration is the oldest age for any of the individual components; the minimum interval between doses is equal to the greatest interval of any of the individual components.

[b]Combination vaccines containing the hepatitis B component are available (HepB-Hib, DTaP-HepB-IPV, and HepA-HepB). These vaccines should not be administered to infants aged <6 wk because of the other components (i.e., Hib, DTaP, HepA, and IPV).

[c]HepB-3 should be administered at least 8 wk after HepB-2 and at least 16 wk after HepB-1 and should not be administered before age 24 wk.

[d]Calendar months.

[e]The minimum recommended interval between DTaP-3 and DTaP-4 is 6 mo. However, DTaP-4 need not be repeated if administered at least 4 mo after DTaP-3.

[f]For Hib and PCV, children receiving the first dose of vaccine at age ≥7 mo require fewer doses to complete the series. (Source: Centers for Disease Control and Prevention: Recommended childhood and adolescent immunization schedule—United States, 2006, *MMWR* 54[51 & 52]:Q1-Q4, 2005.)

[g]If PRP-OMP (Pedvax-Hib, Merck) was administered at age 2 and 4 mo, a dose at age 6 mo is not required.

[h]Combination measles-mumps-rubella-varicella (MMRV) vaccine can be used for children aged 12 mo to 12 yr.

[i]The minimum interval from VAR-1 to VAR-2 for persons beginning the series at age ≥13 yr is 4 wk.

[j]Two doses of influenza vaccine are recommended for children aged <9 yr who are receiving the vaccine for the first time. Children aged <9 yr who have previously received influenza vaccine and persons aged ≥9 yr require only 1 dose per influenza season.

[k]The minimum age for inactivated influenza vaccine varies by vaccine manufacturer. Only Fluzone (Sanofi Pasteur) is approved for children aged 6-35 mo. The minimum age for Fluvirin (Novartis) is 4 yr. For Fluarix and FluLeval (GlaxoSmithKline), the minimum age is 18 yr.

[l]Certain experts recommend a second dose of MPSV 3 yr after the first dose for persons at increased risk for meningococcal disease.

[m]A second dose of meningococcal vaccine is recommended for persons previously vaccinated with MPSV who remain at high risk for meningococcal disease. MCV4 is preferred when revaccinating persons aged 11-55 yr, but a second dose of MPSV is acceptable. (Source: Centers for Disease Control and Prevention: Prevention and control of meningococcal disease: recommendations of the Advisory Committee on Immunization Practices [ACIP], *MMWR* 54:[RR-7], 2005.)

[n]Only 1 dose of Tdap is recommended. Subsequent doses should be administered as Td. If vaccination to prevent tetanus and/or diphtheria disease is required for children aged 7-9 yr, Td should be administered (minimum age for Td is 7 yr). For one brand of Tdap, the minimum age is 11 yr. The preferred interval between Tdap and a previous dose of Td is 5 yr. In persons who have received a primary series of tetanus-toxoid-containing vaccine, for management of a tetanus-prone wound, the minimum interval after a previous dose of any tetanus-containing vaccine is 5 yr.

[o]A second dose of PPV is recommended for persons at highest risk for serious pneumococcal infection and those who are likely to have a rapid decline in pneumococcal antibody concentration. Revaccination 3 yr after the previous dose can be considered for children at highest risk for severe pneumococcal infection who would be aged <10 yr at the time of revaccination. (Source: Centers for Disease Control and Prevention: Prevention of pneumococcal disease: recommendations of the Advisory Committee on Immunization Practices [ACIP], *MMWR* 46:[RR-8], 1997.)

[p]HPV is approved for both males and females aged 9-26 yr.

[q]The first dose of RV must be administered at age 6-12 wk. The vaccine series should not be started at age ≥13 wk. RV should not be administered to children aged ≥33 wk regardless of the number of doses received at age 6-32 wk.

[r]Herpes zoster vaccine is approved as a single dose for persons who are aged ≥60 yr with a history of varicella.

TABLE 5-10   Guidelines for Spacing of Live and Inactivated Antigens

Antigen Combination	Recommended Minimum Interval between Doses
Two or more inactivated*	Can be administered simultaneously or at any interval between doses
Inactivated and live	Can be administered simultaneously or at any interval between doses
Two or more live intranasal or injectable†	4-wk minimum interval if not administered simultaneously

From Centers for Disease Control and Prevention: General recommendations on immunization: recommendations of the Advisory Committee on Immunization Practices (ACIP), *MMWR* 55:(RR-15), 2006.

*Certain experts suggest a 1-mo interval between tetanus toxoid, reduced diphtheria toxoid, and reduced acellular pertussis vaccine and quadrivalent meningococcal conjugate vaccine if they are not administered simultaneously.

†Live oral vaccines (e.g., Ty21a typhoid vaccine and rotavirus vaccine) can be administered simultaneously or at any interval before or after inactivated or live injectable vaccines.

TABLE 5-11   Guidelines for Administering Antibody-Containing Products* and Vaccines

SIMULTANEOUS ADMINISTRATION

Combination	Recommended Minimum Interval between Doses
Antibody-containing products and inactivated antigen	Can be administered simultaneously at different sites or at any time interval between doses.
Antibody-containing products and live antigen	Should not be administered simultaneously.† If simultaneous administration of measles-containing vaccine or varicella vaccine is unavoidable, administer at different sites and revaccinate or test for seroconversion after the recommended interval.

NONSIMULTANEOUS ADMINISTRATION

PRODUCT ADMINISTERED		
First	Second	Recommended Minimum Interval between Doses
Antibody-containing products	Inactivated antigen	Not applicable
Inactivated antigen	Antibody-containing products	Not applicable
Antibody-containing products	Live antigen	Dose-related†‡§
Live antigen	Antibody-containing products	2 weeks†

From Centers for Disease Control and Prevention: General recommendations on immunization: recommendations of the Advisory Committee on Immunization Practices (ACIP), *MMWR* 55(RR-15), 2006.

*Blood products containing substantial amounts of immunoglobulin include intramuscular and intravenous immune globulin, specific hyperimmune globulin (e.g., hepatitis B immune globulin, tetanus immune globulin, varicella zoster immune globulin, and rabies immune globulin), whole blood, packed red cells, plasma, and platelet products.

†Yellow fever, oral Ty21a typhoid vaccine, and live-attenuated influenza vaccine are exceptions to these recommendations. These live-attenuated vaccines can be administered at any time before, after, or simultaneously with an antibody-containing product without substantially decreasing the antibody response.

‡Rotavirus vaccine (RV) should be deferred for 6 wk after receipt of an antibody-containing product if possible. However, if the 6-wk deferral would cause the first dose of RV to be scheduled for age >13 wk, a shorter deferral interval should be used to ensure the first dose of RV is administered no later than age 13 wk.

§The duration of interference of antibody-containing products with the immune response to the measles component of measles-containing vaccine, and possibly varicella vaccine, is dose related.

TABLE 5-12 Suggested Intervals between Administration of Antibody-Containing Products for Different Indications and Measles-Containing Vaccine and Varicella-Containing Vaccine*

Product/Indication	Dose, Including mg Immunoglobulin G (IgG)/kg Body Weight*	Recommended Interval before Measles or Varicella-Containing Vaccine Administration (mo)
Respiratory syncytial virus immune globulin (IG) monoclonal antibody (Synagis)[†]	15 mg/kg intramuscularly (IM)	None
Tetanus IG	250 units (10 mg IgG/kg) IM	3
Hepatitis A IG		
Contact prophylaxis	0.02 ml/kg (3.3 mg IgG/kg) IM	3
International travel	0.06 ml/kg (10 mg IgG/kg) IM	3
Hepatitis B IG	0.06 ml/kg (10 mg IgG/kg) IM	3
Rabies IG	20 international units/kg (22 mg IgG/kg) IM	4
Measles prophylaxis IG		
Standard (i.e., nonimmunocompromised) contact	0.25 ml/kg (40 mg IgG/kg) IM	5
Immunocompromised contact	0.50 ml/kg (80 mg IgG/kg) IM	6
Blood transfusion		
Red blood cells (RBCs), washed	10 ml/kg negligible IgG/kg intravenously (IV)	None
RBCs, adenine-saline added	10 ml/kg (10 mg IgG/kg) IV	3
Packed RBCs (hematocrit 65%)[‡]	10 ml/kg (60 mg IgG/kg) IV	6
Whole blood (hematocrit 35%-50%)[‡]	10 ml/kg (80-100 mg IgG/kg) IV	6
Plasma/platelet products	10 ml/kg (160 mg IgG/kg) IV	7
Cytomegalovirus intravenous immune globulin (IGIV)	150 mg/kg maximum	6
IGIV		
Replacement therapy for immune deficiencies[§]	300-400 mg/kg IV[§]	8
Immune thrombocytopenic purpura	400 mg/kg IV	8
Postexposure varicella prophylaxis[¶]	400 mg/kg IV	8
Immune thrombocytopenic purpura	1000 mg/kg IV	10
Kawasaki disease	2 g/kg IV	11

From Centers for Disease Control and Prevention: General recommendations on immunization: recommendations of the Advisory Committee on Immunization Practices (ACIP), *MMWR* 55:(RR-15), 2006.

*This table is not intended to provide the correct indications and dosages for using antibody-containing products. Unvaccinated persons might not be fully protected against measles during the entire recommended interval, and additional doses of immune globulin or measles vaccine might be indicated after measles exposure. Concentrations of measles antibody in an immune globulin preparation can vary by manufacturer's lot. Rates of antibody clearance after receipt of an immune globulin preparation also may vary. Recommended intervals are extrapolated from an estimated half-life of 30 days for passively acquired antibody and an observed interference with the immune response to measles vaccine for 5 mo after a dose of 80 mg IgG/kg.

[†]Contains antibody only to respiratory syncytial virus.

[‡]Assumes a serum IgG concentration of 16 mg/ml.

[§]Measles and varicella vaccinations are recommended for children with asymptomatic or mildly symptomatic human immunodeficiency virus (HIV) infection but are contraindicated for persons with severe immunosuppression from HIV or any other immunosuppressive disorder.

[¶]The investigational product VariZIG, similar to licensed VZIG, is a purified human immune globulin preparation made from plasma containing high levels of antivaricella antibodies (immunoglobulin class G [IgG]). When indicated, health care providers should make every effort to obtain and administer VariZIG. In situations in which administration of VariZIG does not appear possible within 96 hours of exposure, administration of immune globulin intravenous (IGIV) should be considered as an alternative. IGIV also should be administered within 96 hours of exposure. Although licensed IGIV preparations are known to contain antivaricella antibody titers, the titer of any specific lot of IGIV that might be available is uncertain because IGIV is not routinely tested for antivaricella antibodies. The recommended IGIV dose for postexposure prophylaxis of varicella is 400 mg/kg administered once. For pregnant women who cannot receive VariZIG within 96 hours of exposure, clinicians can choose either to administer IGIV or closely monitor the women for signs and symptoms of varicella and institute treatment with acyclovir if illness occurs. (Source: Centers for Disease Control and Prevention: A new product for postexposure prophylaxis available under an investigational new drug application expanded access protocol, *MMWR* 55 [RR-8]:209-210, 2006.)

TABLE 5-13 Contraindications to and Precautions for Commonly Used Vaccines[a]

Vaccine	True Contraindications and Precautions[a]	Untrue (Vaccines Can Be Administered)
General for all routine vaccines, including diphtheria and tetanus toxoids and acellular pertussis vaccine (DTaP); pediatric diphtheria-tetanus toxoid (DT); adult tetanus-diphtheria toxoid (Td); tetanus-reduced-diphtheria toxoid and acellular pertussis vaccine (Tdap), inactivated poliovirus vaccine (IPV); measles, mumps, and rubella vaccine (MMR); *Haemophilus influenzae* type b vaccine (Hib); hepatitis A vaccine; hepatitis B vaccine; varicella vaccine; Rotavirus vaccine; pneumococcal conjugate vaccine (PCV); inactivated influenza vaccine (TIV); live-attenuated influenza vaccine (LAIV); pneumococcal polysaccharide vaccine (PPV); meningococcal conjugate vaccine (MCV4); meningococcal polysaccharide vaccine (MPSV); human papillomavirus vaccine (HPV); and herpes zoster vaccine (HZ)	*Contraindication* Severe allergic reaction (e.g., anaphylaxis) after a previous vaccine dose or to a vaccine component *Precaution* Moderate or severe acute illness with or without fever	Mild acute illness with or without fever Mild-to-moderate local reaction (e.g., swelling, redness, and soreness), low-grade or moderate fever Lack of previous physical examination in well-appearing person after current antimicrobial therapy[b] Previous convalescent preterm birth (hepatitis B vaccine is an exception in certain circumstances)[c] phase of illness dose Recent exposure to an infectious disease History of penicillin allergy, other nonvaccine allergies, relatives with allergies, receiving allergen extract immunotherapy Breastfeeding
DTaP	*Contraindications* Severe allergic reaction (e.g., anaphylaxis) after a previous vaccine dose or to a vaccine component Encephalopathy (e.g., coma, decreased level of consciousness, prolonged seizures) not attributable to another identifiable cause within 7 days of administration of previous dose of DTP or DTaP Progressive neurologic disorder, including infantile spasms, uncontrolled epilepsy, progressive encephalopathy: defer DTaP until neurologic status clarified and stabilized *Precautions* Temperature of ≥105° F (≥40.5° C) ≤48 hours after vaccination with a previous dose of DTP or DTaP Collapse or shocklike state (i.e., hypotonic hyporesponsive episode) ≤48 hours after receiving a previous dose of DTP/DTaP Seizure ≤3 days after receiving a previous dose of DTP/DTaP[d] Persistent, inconsolable crying lasting ≥3 hours within 48 hr after receiving a previous dose of DTP/DTaP Guillain-Barré syndrome (GBS) <6 wk after previous dose of tetanus toxoid–containing vaccine Moderate or severe acute illness with or without fever	Temperature of ≤104° F (≤40.5° C), fussiness, or mild drowsiness after a previous dose of diphtheria toxoid-tetanus toxoid-pertussis vaccine (DTP/DTaP) Family history of seizures[d] Family history of sudden infant death syndrome Family history of an adverse event after DTP or DTaP administration Stable neurologic conditions (e.g., cerebral palsy, well-controlled seizure disorder, developmental delay)
DT, Td	*Contraindication* Severe allergic reaction (e.g., anaphylaxis) after a previous vaccine dose or to a vaccine component *Precautions* GBS <6 wk after previous dose of tetanus toxoid–containing vaccine Moderate or severe acute illness with or without fever	
Tdap	*Contraindications* Severe allergic reaction (e.g., anaphylaxis) after a previous vaccine dose or to a vaccine component Encephalopathy (e.g., coma, decreased level of consciousness, and prolonged seizures) not attributable to another identifiable cause within 7 days of administration of previous dose of DTP, DTaP, or Tdap *Precautions* Moderate or severe acute illness with or without fever GBS ≤6 wk after a previous dose of tetanus-toxoid-containing vaccine Progressive or unstable neurologic disorder, uncontrolled seizures or progressive encephalopathy until a treatment regimen has been established and the condition has stabilized History of arthus-type hypersensitivity reactions following a previous dose of tetanus toxoid–containing vaccine: defer vaccination until at least 10 yr have elapsed since the last tetanus toxoid–containing vaccine	Temperature of >104° F (>40.5° C) ≤48 hours after vaccination with a previous dose of DTP or DTaP Collapse or shocklike state (i.e., hypotonic hyporesponsive episode) ≤48 hours after receiving a previous dose of DTP/DTaP Seizure ≤3 days after receiving a previous dose of DTP/DTaP[d] Persistent, inconsolable crying lasting ≥3 hours within 48 hours after receiving a previous dose of DTP/DTaP History of extensive limb swelling after DTP/DTaP/Td that is not an arthus-type reaction Stable neurologic disorder Brachial neuritis Latex allergy that is not anaphylactic Breastfeeding Immunosuppression

TABLE 5-13 Contraindications to and Precautions for Commonly Used Vaccines—cont'd

Vaccine	True Contraindications and Precautions[a]	Untrue (Vaccines Can Be Administered)
IPV	**Contraindication** Severe allergic reaction (e.g., anaphylaxis) after a previous vaccine dose or to a vaccine component **Precautions** Pregnancy Moderate or severe acute illness with or without fever	Previous receipt of one or more doses of oral polio vaccine
MMR[e]	**Contraindications** Severe allergic reaction (e.g., anaphylaxis) after a previous vaccine dose or to a vaccine component Pregnancy Known severe immunodeficiency (e.g., hematologic and solid tumors, receiving chemotherapy, congenital immunodeficiency, long-term immunosuppressive therapy,[f] or patients with HIV infection who are severely immunocompromised) **Precautions** Recent ($\leq$11 mo) receipt of antibody-containing blood product (specific interval depends on product)[h] History of thrombocytopenia or thrombocytopenic purpura Moderate or severe acute illness with or without fever	Positive tuberculin skin test Simultaneous tuberculosis skin testing[g] Breastfeeding Pregnancy of recipient's mother or other close or household contact Recipient is female of childbearing age Immunodeficient family member or household contact Asymptomatic or mildly symptomatic HIV infection Allergy to eggs
Hib	**Contraindications** Severe allergic reaction (e.g., anaphylaxis) after a previous vaccine dose or to a vaccine component Age <6 wk **Precaution** Moderate or severe acute illness with or without fever	
Hepatitis B	**Contraindication** Severe allergic reaction (e.g., anaphylaxis) after a previous vaccine dose or to a vaccine component **Precautions** Infant weighing <2000 g[c] Moderate or severe acute illness with or without fever	Pregnancy Autoimmune disease (e.g., systemic lupus erythematosus or rheumatoid arthritis)
Hepatitis A	**Contraindication** Severe allergic reaction (e.g., anaphylaxis) after a previous vaccine dose or to a vaccine component **Precautions** Pregnancy Moderate or severe acute illness with or without fever	
Varicella	**Contraindications** Severe allergic reaction (e.g., anaphylaxis) after a previous vaccine dose or to a vaccine component Substantial suppression of cellular immunity Pregnancy **Precautions** Recent ($\leq$11 mo) receipt of antibody-containing blood product (specific interval depends on product)[h] Moderate or severe acute illness with or without fever	Pregnancy of recipient's mother or other close or household contact Immunodeficient family member or household contact[i] Asymptomatic or mildly symptomatic HIV infection Humoral immunodeficiency (e.g., a gamma-globulinemia)[j]
PCV	**Contraindication** Severe allergic reaction (e.g., anaphylaxis) after a previous vaccine dose or to a vaccine component **Precaution** Moderate or severe acute illness with or without fever	
TIV	**Contraindication** Severe allergic reaction (e.g., anaphylaxis) after a previous vaccine dose or to a vaccine component **Precaution** Moderate or severe acute illness with or without fever	Nonsevere (e.g., contact) allergy to latex or thimerosal Concurrent administration of warfarin or aminophylline

Continued on following page

TABLE 5-13 Contraindications to and Precautions for Commonly Used Vaccines—cont'd

Vaccine	True Contraindications and Precautions[a]	Untrue (Vaccines Can Be Administered)
LAIV	***Contraindications*** Severe allergic reaction (e.g., anaphylaxis) after a previous vaccine dose or to a vaccine component Pregnancy Known severe immunodeficiency (e.g., hematologic and solid tumors, receiving chemotherapy, congenital immunodeficiency, long-term immunosuppressive therapy,[f] or patients with HIV infection who are severely immunocompromised) Previous history of GBS Certain chronic medical conditions[k] ***Precaution*** Moderate or severe acute illness with or without fever	
PPV	***Contraindication*** Severe allergic reaction (e.g., anaphylaxis) after a previous vaccine dose or to a vaccine component ***Precaution*** Moderate or severe acute illness with or without fever	History of invasive pneumococcal disease or pneumonia
MCV4	***Contraindication*** Severe allergic reaction (e.g., anaphylaxis) after a previous vaccine dose or to a vaccine component ***Precautions*** Moderate or severe acute illness with or without fever History of GBS (if not at high risk for meningococcal disease)	
MPSV	***Contraindication*** Severe allergic reaction after a previous dose or to a vaccine component ***Precaution*** Moderate or severe acute illness with or without fever	
HPV	***Contraindication*** Severe allergic reaction after a previous dose or to a vaccine component ***Precautions*** Moderate or severe acute illness with or without fever Pregnancy	
Rotavirus	***Contraindication*** Severe allergic reaction after a previous dose or to a vaccine component ***Precautions*** Moderate or severe acute illness with or without fever Immunosuppression Receipt of an antibody-containing blood product within 6 wk[l] Preexisting gastrointestinal disease Previous history of intussusception	Preterm births Immunosuppression in household contacts Pregnant household contacts

From Centers for Disease Control and Prevention: General recommendations on immunization: recommendations of the Advisory Committee on Immunization Practices (ACIP), *MMWR* 55:(RR-15), 2006.

[a]Events or conditions listed as precautions should be reviewed carefully. Benefits of and risks for administering a specific vaccine to a person under these circumstances should be considered. If the risk from the vaccine is believed to outweigh the benefit, the vaccine should not be administered. If the benefit of vaccination is believed to outweigh the risk, the vaccine should be administered. Whether and when to administer DTaP to children with proven or suspected underlying neurologic disorders should be decided on a case-by-case basis.

[b]Antibacterial drugs and mefloquine might interfere with Ty21a oral typhoid vaccine, and certain antiviral drugs might interfere with varicella-containing and live-attenuated influenza virus vaccine.

[c]Hepatitis B vaccination should be deferred for infants weighing <2000 g if the mother is documented to be hepatitis B surface antigen (HBsAg) negative at the time of the infant's birth. Vaccination can begin at chronologic age 1 mo. For infants born to women who are HBsAg positive, hepatitis B immunoglobulin and hepatitis B vaccine should be administered at or soon after birth regardless of weight.

[d]Acetaminophen or other appropriate antipyretic can be administered to infants and children with a history of previous seizures at the time of DTaP vaccination and every 4 hours for 24 hours thereafter to reduce the possibility of postvaccination fever. (Source: American Academy of Pediatrics: Active immunization. In Pickering LK, Baker CJ, Long SS, et al (eds): *2006 red book: report of the Committee on Infectious Diseases*, ed 27, Elk Grove Village, IL, 2006, American Academy of Pediatrics.)

[e]MMR and varicella vaccines can be administered on the same day. If not administered on the same day, these vaccines should be separated by at least 28 days.

[f]Substantially immunosuppressive steroid dose is considered to be ≥2 wk of daily receipt of ≥20 mg or ≥2 mg/kg body weight of prednisone or equivalent.

[g]Measles vaccination might suppress tuberculin reactivity temporarily. Measles-containing vaccine can be administered on the same day as tuberculin skin testing. If testing cannot be performed until after the day of MMR vaccination, the test should be postponed for ≥4 wk after the vaccination. If an urgent need exists to skin test, do so with the understanding that reactivity might be reduced by the vaccine.

[h]See text for details.

[i]If a patient experiences a presumed vaccine-related rash 7-25 days after vaccination, he or she should avoid direct contact with immunocompromised persons for the duration of the rash if possible.

[j]Vaccine should be deferred for the appropriate interval if replacement immune globulin products are being administered.

[k]For details see Centers for Disease Control and Prevention: Prevention and control of influenza: recommendations of the Advisory Committee on Immunization Practices (ACIP), *MMWR* 55:(RR-10), 2006.

[l]Rotavirus vaccine (RV) should be deferred for 6 wk after receipt of an antibody-containing product if possible. However, if the 6-wk deferral would cause the first dose of RV to be scheduled for age ≥13 wk, a shorter deferral interval should be used to ensure the first dose of RV is administered no later than age 13 wk.

TABLE 5-14 Dose and Route of Administration for Selected Vaccines

Vaccines	Dose	Route
Diphtheria, tetanus, pertussis (DTaP, DT, Td, Tdap)	0.5 ml	IM
Diphtheria, tetanus, acellular pertussis, inactivated polio, hepatitis B vaccine (DTaP-IPV-HepB)	0.5 ml	IM
Diphtheria, tetanus, acellular pertussis, *Haemophilus influenzae* type b vaccine (DTaP-Hib)	0.5 ml	IM
Haemophilus influenzae type b (Hib)	0.5 ml	IM
Haemophilus influenzae type b–Hepatitis B (Hib-HepB)	0.5 ml	IM
Hepatitis A (HepA)	≤18 yr: 0.5 ml ≥19 yr: 1.0 ml	IM
HepB	≤19 yr: 0.5 ml* ≥20 yr: 1.0 ml	IM
HepA/HepB	≥18 yr: 1.0 ml	IM
Influenza, live attenuated	0.5 ml	Intranasal spray
Influenza, trivalent inactivated	6-35 mo: 0.25 ml ≥3 yr: 0.5 ml	IM
Measles, mumps, rubella	0.5 ml	SC
Measles, mumps, rubella, varicella	0.5 ml	SC
Meningococcal conjugate	0.5 ml	IM
Meningococcal polysaccharide	0.5 ml	SC
Pneumococcal conjugate	0.5 ml	IM
Pneumococcal polysaccharide	0.5 ml	IM or SC
Human papillomavirus	0.5 ml	IM
Polio, inactivated	0.5 ml	IM or SC
Rotavirus	2.0 ml	Oral
Varicella	0.5 ml	SC
Zoster	0.7 ml	SC

From CDC: General recommendations on immunization: recommendations of the Advisory Committee on Immunization Practices (ACIP), *MMWR* 55:(RR-15), 2006. Adapted from Immunization Action Coalition (http://www.immunize.org).

IM, Intramuscularly; *SC,* subcutaneously.

*Persons aged 11-15 yr can be administered Recombivax HB (Merck) 1.0 ml (adult formulation) on a 2-dose schedule.

VACCINE ADMINISTRATION*

INFECTION CONTROL AND STERILE TECHNIQUE

Persons administering vaccines should follow appropriate precautions to minimize risk for spread of disease. Hands should be cleansed with an alcohol-based, waterless antiseptic hand rub or washed with soap and water between each patient contact. Occupational Safety and Health Administration (OSHA) regulations do not require that gloves be worn when administering vaccinations unless persons administering vaccinations are likely to come into contact with potentially infectious body fluids or have open lesions on their hands. Needles used for injections must be sterile and disposable to minimize the risk for contamination. A separate needle and syringe should be used for each injection. Changing needles between drawing vaccine from a vial and injecting it into a recipient is not necessary. Different vaccines should never be mixed in the same syringe unless specifically licensed for such use, and no attempt should be made to transfer between syringes.

For all intramuscular injections, the needle should be long enough to reach the muscle mass and prevent vaccine from seeping into subcutaneous tissue but not so long as to involve underlying nerves, blood vessels, or bone. Vaccinators should be familiar with the anatomy of the area where they are injecting vaccine. Intramuscular injections are administered at a 90-degree angle to the skin, preferably into the anterolateral aspect of the thigh or the deltoid muscle of the upper arm depending on the age of the patient.

Decision on needle size and site of injection must be made for each person on the basis of the size of the muscle, the thickness of adipose tissue at the injection site, the volume of the material to be administered, injection technique, and the depth below the muscle surface into which the material is to be injected (Fig. 5-1). Aspiration before injection of vaccines or toxoids (i.e., pulling back on the syringe plunger after needle insertion before injection) is not required because no large blood vessel exists at the recommended injection sites.

INFANTS (AGED <12 MONTHS)

For the majority of infants, the anterolateral aspect of the thigh is the recommended site for injection because it provides a large muscle mass (Fig. 5-2). The muscles of the buttock have not been used for administration of vaccines in infants and children because of concern about potential injury to the sciatic nerve, which is well documented after injection of antimicrobial agents into the buttock. If the gluteal muscle must be used, care

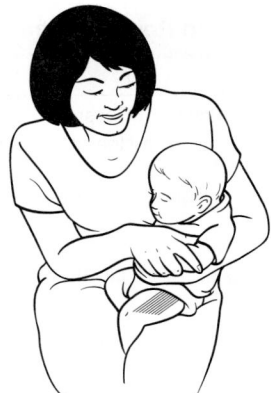

FIGURE 5-2 Intramuscular/subcutaneous site of administration: anterolateral thigh. (Adapted from Minnesota Department of Health. In Centers for Disease Control and Prevention: General recommendations on immunization: recommendations of the Advisory Committee on Immunization Practices [ACIP], *MMWR* 55[RR-15]:6, 2006.)

should be taken to define the anatomic landmarks.[†] Injection technique is the most important parameter to ensure efficient intramuscular vaccine delivery. If the subcutaneous and muscle tissue are bunched to minimize the chance of striking bone, a 1-inch needle is required to ensure intramuscular administration in infants. For the majority of infants, a 1-inch, 22- to 25-gauge needle is sufficient to penetrate muscle in an infant's thigh. For newborn (first 28 days of life) and premature infants, a ⅝-inch-long needle usually is adequate if the skin is stretched flat between thumb and forefinger and the needle inserted at a 90-degree angle to the skin.

TODDLERS AND OLDER CHILDREN (AGED 12 MONTHS TO 10 YEARS)

The deltoid muscle should be used if the muscle mass is adequate. The needle size for deltoid site injections can range from 22 to 25 gauge and from ⅝ to 1 inch on the basis of the size of the muscle and the thickness of adipose tissue at the injection site (Fig. 5-3). A ⅝-inch needle is adequate only for the deltoid muscle and only if the skin is stretched flat between the thumb and forefinger and the needle inserted at a 90-degree

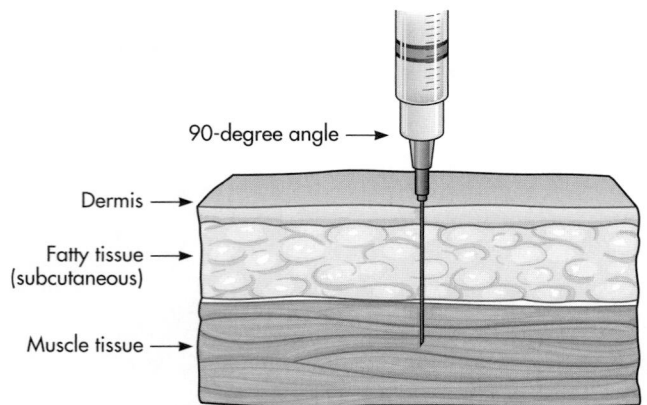

FIGURE 5-1 Intramuscular needle insertion.

90-degree angle

Dermis

Fatty tissue (subcutaneous)

Muscle tissue

FIGURE 5-1 Intramuscular needle insertion. (Adapted from California Immunization Branch. In Centers for Disease Control and Prevention: General recommendations on immunization: recommendations of the Advisory Committee on Immunization Practices [ACIP], *MMWR* 55[RR-15]:16, 2006.)

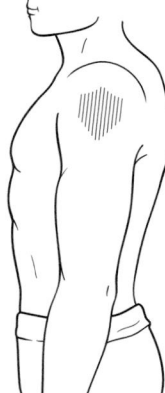

FIGURE 5-3 Intramuscular site of administration: deltoid. (Adapted from Minnesota Department of Health. In Centers for Disease Control and Prevention: General recommendations on immunization: recommendations of the Advisory Committee on Immunization Practices [ACIP], *MMWR* 55[RR-15]:17, 2006.)

---

*From Centers for Disease Control and Prevention: General recommendations on immunization: recommendations of the Advisory Committee on Immunization Practices (ACIP), *MMWR* 55(RR-15):14-16, 2006.

†If the gluteal muscle is chosen, injection should be administered lateral and superior to a line between the posterior superior iliac spine and the greater trochanter or in the ventrogluteal site, the center of a triangle bounded by the anterior superior iliac spine, the tubercle of the iliac crest, and the upper border of the greater trochanter.

angle to the skin. For toddlers, the anterolateral thigh can be used, but the needle should be at least 1 inch in length.

ADOLESCENTS AND ADULTS (AGED >11 YEARS)

For adults and adolescents, the deltoid muscle is recommended for routine intramuscular vaccinations. The anterolateral thigh also can be used. For men and women weighing <130 lb (<60 kg) a ⅝- to 1-inch needle is sufficient to ensure intramuscular injection. For women weighing 130 to 200 lb (60 to 90 kg) and men 130 to 260 lb (60 to 118 kg), a 1- to 1½-inch needle is needed. For women weighing >200 lb (>90 kg) or men weighing >260 lb (>118 kg), a 1½-inch needle is required.

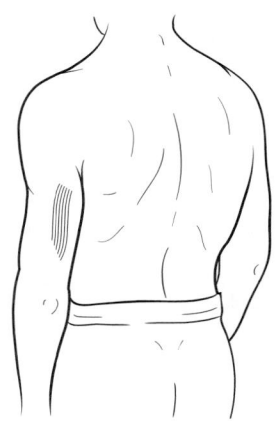

FIGURE 5-4 Subcutaneous site of administration: triceps. (Adapted from Minnesota Department of Health. In Centers for Disease Control and Prevention: General recommendations on immunization: recommendations of the Advisory Committee on Immunization Practices [ACIP], *MMWR* 55[RR-15]:17, 2006.)

SUBCUTANEOUS INJECTIONS

Subcutaneous injections are administered at a 45-degree angle, usually into the thigh for infants younger than 12 months and in the upper-outer triceps area of persons aged 12 months and older. Subcutaneous injections can be administered into the upper-outer triceps area of an infant if necessary. A ⅝-inch, 23- to 25-gauge needle should be inserted into the subcutaneous tissue (Figs. 5-4 and 5-5).

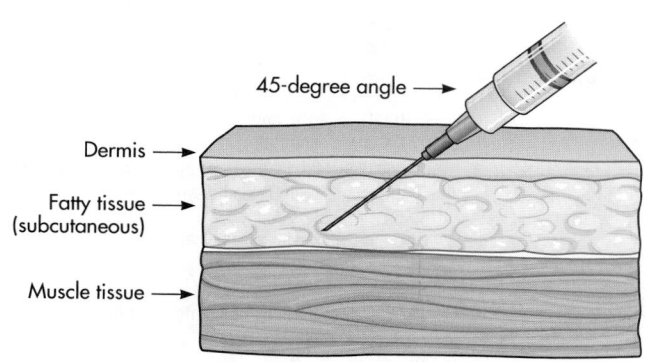

FIGURE 5-5 Subcutaneous needle insertion. (Adapted from California Administration Branch. In Centers for Disease Control and Prevention: General recommendations on immunization: recommendations of the Advisory Committee on Immunization Practices [ACIP], *MMWR* 55[RR-15]:17, 2006.)

TABLE 5-15 Treatment of Anaphylaxis with Intramuscular or Oral Pharmaceuticals

Drug	Dosage
Child	
Primary regimen	
Epinephrine 1:1000 (aqueous) (1 mg/ml)*	0.01 mg/kg up to 0.5 mg (administer 0.01 ml/kg/dose up to 0.5 ml) IM repeated every 10-20 min up to 3 doses
Secondary regimen	
Diphenhydramine	1-2 mg/kg oral, IM or IV, every 4-6 hr (maximum single dose: 100 mg)
Hydroxyzine	0.5-1 mg/kg oral, IM, every 4-6 hr (maximum single dose: 100 mg)
Prednisone	1.5-2 mg/kg oral (maximum single dose: 60 mg); use corticosteroids as long as needed
Adult	
Primary regimen	
Epinephrine 1:1000 (aqueous)*	0.01 mg/kg up to 0.5 mg (give 0.01 ml/kg/dose up to 0.5 ml) IM repeated every 10-20 min up to 3 doses
Secondary regimen	
Diphenhydramine	1-2 mg/kg up to 100 mg IM or oral every 4-6 hr

From Centers for Disease Control and Prevention: General recommendations on immunization: recommendations of the Advisory Committee on Immunization Practices (ACIP), *MMWR* 55:(RR-15), 2006. Adapted from American Academy of Pediatrics: Passive immunization. In Pickering LK, Baker CJ, Long SS, et al (eds): *Red book: 2006 report of the Committee on Infectious Diseases,* ed 27, Elk Grove, IL, 2006, American Academy of Pediatrics; and Immunization Action Coalition: Medical management of anaphylaxis in adult patients. Available at http://www.immunize.org/catg.d/p3082.pdf, and Mosby's Drug Consult 2005.
IM, Intramuscularly; *IV,* intravenously.
*If agent causing anaphylactic reaction was administered by injection, epinephrine can be injected into the same site to slow absorption.

TABLE 5-16 Vaccination of Persons with Primary and Secondary Immune Deficiencies

Category	Specific Immunodeficiency	Vaccines Contraindicated*	Risk-Specific Vaccines Recommended*	Effectiveness and Comments
PRIMARY				
B-lymphocyte (humoral)	Severe antibody deficiencies (e.g., X-linked agammaglobulinemia and common variable immunodeficiency)	Oral poliovirus (OPV)[†] Smallpox Live-attenuated influenza vaccine (LAIV) BCG Live oral typhoid (Ty21a)	Pneumococcal Influenza (TIV) Consider measles and varicella vaccination	The effectiveness of any vaccine will be uncertain if it depends only on the humoral response; IV immune globulin interferes with the immune response to measles vaccine and possibly varicella vaccine
	Less severe antibody deficiencies (e.g., selective IgA deficiency and IgG subclass deficiency)	OPV[†] Other live vaccines appear to be safe	Pneumococcal influenza (TIV)	All vaccines probably effective; immune response may be attenuated
T-lymphocyte (cell mediated and humoral)	Complete defects (e.g., severe combined immunodeficiency [SCID] disease, complete DiGeorge syndrome)	All live vaccines[‡§]	Pneumococcal influenza (TIV)	Vaccines may be ineffective
	Partial defects (e.g., the majority of patients with DiGeorge syndrome, Wiskott-Aldrich syndrome, ataxia-telangiectasia)	All live vaccines[‡§]	Pneumococcal Meningococcal *Haemophilus influenza* type b (Hib) (if not administered in infancy) Influenza (TIV)	Effectiveness of any vaccine depends on degree of immune suppression
Complement	Deficiency of early components (C1, C2, C3, and C4)	None	Pneumococcal Meningococcal Influenza (TIV)	All routine vaccines probably effective
	Deficiency of late components (C5-C9) and C3, properdin, factor B	None	Pneumococcal Meningococcal Influenza (TIV)	All routine vaccines probably effective
Phagocytic function	Chronic granulomatous disease, leukocyte adhesion defect, and myeloperoxidase deficiency	Live bacterial vaccines[‡]	Pneumococcal[‖] Influenza (TIV) (to decrease secondary bacterial infection)	All inactivated vaccines safe and probably effective Live viral vaccines probably safe and effective
SECONDARY				
	HIV/AIDS	OPV Smallpox BCG LAIV Withhold MMR and varicella in severely immunocompromised persons	Influenza (TIV) Pneumococcal Consider Hib (if not administered in infancy) and meningococcal vaccination	Measles, mumps, rubella (MMR); varicella; and all inactivated vaccines, including inactivated influenza, might be effective[¶]
	Malignant neoplasm, transplantation, immunosuppressive or radiation therapy	Live viral and bacterial, depending on immune status	Influenza (TIV) Pneumococcal	Effectiveness of any vaccine depends on degree of immune suppression
	Asplenia	None	Pneumococcal Meningococcal Hib (if not administered in infancy)	All routine vaccines probably effective
	Chronic renal disease	LAIV	Pneumococcal Influenza (TIV) Hepatitis B	All routine vaccines probably effective

From Centers for Disease Control and Prevention (CDC): General recommendations on immunization: recommendations of the Advisory Committee on Immunization Practices (ACIP), *MMWR* 55(RR-15), 2006. Modified from American Academy of Pediatrics: Passive immunization. In Pickering LK, Baker CJ, Long SS, et al (eds): *Red book: 2006 report of the Committee on Infectious Diseases,* ed 27, Elk Grove, IL, 2006, American Academy of Pediatrics; and CDC: Use of vaccines and immune globulins in persons with altered immunocompetence: recommendations of the Advisory Committee on Immunization Practices (ACIP), *MMWR* 42(RR-4):42, 1993.

BCG, Bacille Calmette-Guérin; *Ig,* immunoglobulin; *IV,* intravenous.

*Other vaccines that are universally or routinely recommended should be administered if not contraindicated.

[†]OPV is no longer available for routine use in the United States.

[‡]Live bacterial vaccines: BCG and Ty21a *Salmonella typhi* vaccine.

[§]Live viral vaccines: MMR, OPV, LAIV, yellow fever, and varicella, including measles-mumps-rubella-varicella (MMRV) and herpes zoster (HZ) vaccine, and vaccinia (smallpox). Smallpox vaccine is not recommended for children or the general public.

[‖]Pneumococcal vaccine is not indicated for children with chronic granulomatous disease.

[¶]Children infected with HIV should receive IG after exposure to measles and can receive varicella and measles vaccine if CD4+ lymphocyte count is >15%.

TABLE 5-17 Approaches to the Evaluation and Vaccination of Internationally Adopted Children with No or Questionable Vaccination Records

Vaccine	Recommended Approach	Alternative Approach
Measles, mumps, and rubella (MMR)	Revaccinate with MMR	Serologic testing for immunoglobulin G (IgG) antibody to measles, mumps, and rubella
Haemophilus influenzae type b (Hib)	Age-appropriate revaccination	—
Hepatitis A	Age-appropriate revaccination	Serologic testing for IgG antibody to hepatitis A virus
Hepatitis B (Hep B)	Age-appropriate revaccination and serologic testing for HBsAg*	—
Poliovirus	Revaccinate with inactivated poliovirus vaccine (IPV)	Serologic testing for neutralizing antibody to poliovirus types 1, 2, and 3 (limited availability)
Diphtheria and tetanus toxoids and acellular pertussis (DTaP)	Revaccination with DTaP, with serologic testing for specific IgG antibody to tetanus and diphtheria toxins in the event of a severe local reaction	Children whose records indicate receipt of ≥3 doses: serologic testing for specific IgG antibody to diphtheria and tetanus toxins before administering additional doses or administer a single booster dose of DTaP, followed by serologic testing after 1 mo for specific IgG antibody to diphtheria and tetanus toxins with revaccination as appropriate
Varicella	Age-appropriate vaccination of children who lack evidence of varicella immunity	—
Pneumococcal conjugate	Age-appropriate vaccination	—

From Centers for Disease Control and Prevention (CDC): General recommendations on immunization: recommendations of the Advisory Committee on Immunization Practices (ACIP), *MMWR* 55:(RR-15), 2006.

*Very rarely, Hep B vaccine can give a false-positive hepatitis B surface antigen (HBsAg) result up to 18 days after vaccination; therefore blood should be drawn to test for HBsAg before vaccinating. (Source: CDC: A comprehensive immunization strategy to eliminate transmission of hepatitis B virus infection in the United States: recommendations of the Advisory Committee on Immunization Practices [ACIP]; Part I: immunization in infants, children, and adolescents, *MMWR* 54[RR-16], 2005.)

Immunizations for Adults

TABLE 5-18   Recommended Adult Immunization Schedule, by Vaccine and Age Group—United States

Note: These recommendations *must* be read with the footnotes that follow containing number of doses, intervals between doses, and other important information.

VACCINE ▼ AGE GROUP ▶	19-26 years	27-49 years	50-59 years	60-64 years	≥65 years
Tetanus, diphtheria, pertussis (Td/Tdap)[1],*	Substitute 1-time dose of Tdap for Td booster; then boost with Td every 10 yr				Td booster every 10 yrs
Human papillomavirus (HPV)[2],*	3 doses				
Varicella[3],*	2 doses				
Zoster[4]				1 dose	
Measles, mumps, rubella (MMR)[5],*	1 or 2 doses		1 dose		
Influenza[6],*			1 dose annually		
Pneumococcal (polysaccharide)[7,8]	1 or 2 doses				1 dose
Hepatitis A[9],*	2 doses				
Hepatitis B[10],*	3 doses				
Meningococcal[11],*	1 or more doses				

*Covered by the Vaccine Injury Compensation Program.

☐ For all persons in this category who meet the age requirements and who lack evidence of immunity (e.g., lack documentation of vaccination or have no evidence of prior infection)

■ Recommended if some other risk factor is present (e.g., on the basis of medical, occupational, lifestyle, or other indications)

☐ No recommendation

*These schedules indicate the recommended age groups and medical indications for which administration of currently licensed vaccines is commonly indicated for adults ages 19 years and older, as of January 1, 2010. Licensed combination vaccines may be used whenever any components of the combination are indicated and when the vaccine's other components are not contraindicated. For detailed recommendations on all vaccines, including those used primarily for travelers or that are issued during the year, consult the manufacturers' package inserts and the complete statements from the Advisory Committee on Immunization Practices (http://www.cdc.gov/vaccines/pubs/acip-list.htm).

Report all clinically significant postvaccination reactions to the Vaccine Adverse Event Reporting System (VAERS). Reporting forms and instructions on filing a VAERS report are available at www.vaers.hhs.gov or by telephone, 800-822-7967.

Information on how to file a Vaccine Injury Compensation Program claim is available at www.hrsa.gov/vaccinecompensation or by telephone, 800-338-2382. To file a claim for vaccine injury, contact the U.S. Court of Federal Claims, 717 Madison Place, N.W., Washington, D.C. 20005; telephone, 202-357-6400.

Additional information about the vaccines in this schedule, extent of available data, and contraindications for vaccination is also available at www.cdc.gov/vaccines or from the CDC-INFO Contact Center at 800-CDC-INFO (800-232-4636) in English and Spanish, 24 hours a day, 7 days a week.

Use of trade names and commercial sources is for identification only and does not imply endorsement by the U.S. Department of Health and Human Services.

[1]**Tetanus, diphtheria, and acellular pertussis (Td/Tdap) vaccination**

Tdap should replace a single dose of Td for adults aged 19 through 64 yr who have not received a dose of Tdap previously.

Adults with uncertain or incomplete history of primary vaccination series with tetanus and diphtheria toxoid–containing vaccines should begin or complete a primary vaccination series. A primary series for adults is 3 doses of tetanus and diphtheria toxoid–containing vaccines; administer the first 2 doses at least 4 wk apart and the third dose 6-12 mo after the second. However, Tdap can substitute for any one of the doses of Td in the 3-dose primary series. The booster dose of tetanus and diphtheria toxoid–containing vaccine should be administered to adults who have completed a primary series and if the last vaccination was received 10 or more yr previously. Tdap or Td vaccine may be used, as indicated.

If a woman is pregnant and received the last Td vaccination 10 or more yr previously, administer Td during the second or third trimester. If the woman received the last Td vaccination less than 10 yr previously, administer Tdap during the immediate postpartum period. A dose of Tdap is recommended for postpartum women, close contacts of infants age less than 12 mo, and all health care personnel with direct patient contact if they have not previously received Tdap. An interval as short as 2 yr from the last Td is suggested; shorter intervals can be used. Td may be deferred during pregnancy and Tdap substituted in the immediate postpartum period, or Tdap may be administered instead of Td to a pregnant woman after an informed discussion with the woman.

Consult the ACIP statement for recommendations for administering Td as prophylaxis in wound management.

[2]**Human papillomavirus (HPV) vaccination**

HPV vaccination is recommended for all females and males aged 11 through 26 yr (and may begin at age 9 yr) who have not completed the vaccine series. History of genital warts, abnormal Papanicolaou test result, or positive HPV DNA test result is not evidence of prior infection with all vaccine HPV types; HPV vaccination is recommended for persons with such histories.

Ideally, vaccine should be administered before potential exposure to HPV through sexual activity; however, persons who are sexually active should still be vaccinated consistent with age-based recommendations. Sexually active persons who have not been infected with any of the 4 HPV vaccine types receive the full benefit of the vaccination. Vaccination is less beneficial for persons who have already been infected with 1 or more of the HPV vaccine types.

A complete series consists of 3 doses. The second dose should be administered 2 mo after the first dose; the third dose should be administered 6 mo after the first dose.

HPV vaccination is not specifically recommended for persons with the medical indications described in Table 5-19. Because it is not a live-virus vaccine, it can be administered to persons with the medical indications noted. However, the immune response and vaccine efficacy might be less for persons with the noted medical indications than in persons who do not have the medical indications described or who are immunocompetent. Health care personnel are not at increased risk because of occupational exposure and should be vaccinated consistent with age-based recommendations.

HPV4 may be given to males aged 9 through 26 years to reduce the likelihood of acquiring genital warts.

HPV4 would be most effective when given before exposure to HPV through sexual contact.

[3]**Varicella vaccination**

All adults without evidence of immunity to varicella should receive 2 doses of single-antigen varicella vaccine if not previously vaccinated or the second dose if they have received only 1 dose, unless they have a medical contraindication. Special consideration should be given to those who 1) have close contact with persons at high risk for severe disease (e.g., health care personnel and family contacts of persons with immunocompromising conditions) or 2) are at high risk for exposure or transmission (e.g., teachers; child care employees; residents and staff members of institutional settings, including correctional institutions; college students; military personnel; adolescents and adults living in households with children; nonpregnant women of childbearing age; and international travelers).

Evidence of immunity to varicella in adults includes any of the following: 1) documentation of 2 doses of varicella vaccine at least 4 wk apart; 2) U.S.-born before 1980 (although for health care personnel and pregnant women, birth before 1980 should not be considered evidence of immunity); 3) history of varicella based on diagnosis or verification of varicella by a health care provider (for a patient reporting a history of or presenting with an atypical case, a mild case, or both, health care providers should seek either an epidemiologic link to a typical varicella case or to a laboratory-confirmed case or evidence of laboratory confirmation, if it was performed at the time of acute disease); 4) history of herpes zoster based on health care provider diagnosis or verification of herpes zoster by a health care provider; or 5) laboratory evidence of immunity or laboratory confirmation of disease.

TABLE 5-18 Recommended Adult Immunization Schedule, by Vaccine and Age Group—United States—cont'd

Pregnant women should be assessed for evidence of varicella immunity. Women who do not have evidence of immunity should receive the first dose of varicella vaccine upon completion or termination of pregnancy and before discharge from the health care facility. The second dose should be administered 4-8 wk after the first dose.

⁴Herpes zoster vaccination
A single dose of zoster vaccine is recommended for adults aged 60 yr and older regardless of whether they report a prior episode of herpes zoster. Persons with chronic medical conditions may be vaccinated unless their condition constitutes a contraindication.

⁵Measles, mumps, rubella (MMR) vaccination
Measles component: Adults born before 1957 generally are considered immune to measles. Adults born during or after 1957 should receive 1 or more doses of MMR unless they have a medical contraindication, documentation of 1 or more doses, history of measles based on health care provider diagnosis, or laboratory evidence of immunity.
A second dose of MMR is recommended for adults who 1) have been recently exposed to measles or are in an outbreak setting; 2) have been vaccinated previously with killed measles vaccine; 3) have been vaccinated with an unknown type of measles vaccine during 1963-1967; 4) are students in postsecondary educational institutions; 5) work in a health care facility; or 6) plan to travel internationally.
Mumps component: Adults born before 1957 generally are considered immune to mumps. Adults born during or after 1957 should receive 1 dose of MMR unless they have a medical contraindication, history of mumps based on health care provider diagnosis, or laboratory evidence of immunity.
A second dose of MMR is recommended for adults who 1) live in a community experiencing a mumps outbreak and are in an affected age group; 2) are students in postsecondary educational institutions; 3) work in a health care facility; or 4) plan to travel internationally. For unvaccinated health care personnel born before 1957 who do not have other evidence of mumps immunity, administering 1 dose on a routine basis should be considered and administering a second dose during an outbreak should also be strongly considered.
Rubella component: 1 dose of MMR vaccine is recommended for women whose rubella vaccination history is unreliable or who lack laboratory evidence of immunity. For women of childbearing age, regardless of birth yr, rubella immunity should be determined and women should be counseled regarding congenital rubella syndrome. Women who do not have evidence of immunity should receive MMR vaccine upon completion or termination of pregnancy and before discharge from the health care facility.

⁶Influenza vaccination
Medical indications: Chronic disorders of the cardiovascular or pulmonary systems, including asthma; chronic metabolic diseases, including diabetes mellitus, renal or hepatic dysfunction, hemoglobinopathies, or immunocompromising conditions (including immunocompromising conditions caused by medications or HIV); any condition that compromises respiratory function or the handling of respiratory secretions or that can increase the risk of aspiration (e.g., cognitive dysfunction, spinal cord injury, or seizure disorder or other neuromuscular disorder); and pregnancy during the influenza season. No data exist on the risk for severe or complicated influenza disease among persons with asplenia; however, influenza is a risk factor for secondary bacterial infections that can cause severe disease among persons with asplenia.
Occupational indications: All health care personnel, including those employed by long-term care and assisted-living facilities, and caregivers of children younger than 5 yr.
Other indications: Residents of nursing homes and other long-term care and assisted-living facilities; persons likely to transmit influenza to persons at high risk (e.g., in-home household contacts and caregivers of children younger than 5 yr, persons 65 yr and older, and persons of all ages with high-risk condition[s]); and anyone who would like to decrease their risk of getting influenza. Healthy, nonpregnant adults younger than 50 yr without high-risk medical conditions who are not contacts of severely immunocompromised persons in special care units can receive either intranasally administered live, attenuated influenza vaccine (FluMist) or inactivated vaccine. Other persons should receive the inactivated vaccine.

⁷Pneumococcal polysaccharide (PPSV) vaccination
Medical indications: Chronic lung disease (including asthma); chronic cardiovascular diseases; diabetes mellitus; chronic liver diseases, cirrhosis; chronic alcoholism, chronic renal failure, or nephrotic syndrome; functional or anatomic asplenia (e.g., sickle cell disease or splenectomy [if elective splenectomy is planned, vaccinate at least 2 wk before surgery]); immunocompromising conditions; and cochlear implants and cerebrospinal fluid leaks. Vaccinate as close to HIV diagnosis as possible.
Other indications: Residents of nursing homes or other long-term care facilities and persons who smoke cigarettes. Routine use of PPSV is not recommended for Alaska Native or American Indian persons younger than 65 yr unless they have underlying medical conditions that are PPSV indications. However, public health authorities may consider recommending PPSV for Alaska Natives and American Indians 50 through 64 yr of age who are living in areas in which the risk of invasive pneumococcal disease is increased.

⁸Revaccination with PPSV
One-time revaccination after 5 yr for persons with chronic renal failure or nephrotic syndrome, functional or anatomic asplenia (e.g., sickle cell disease or splenectomy), and persons with immunocompromising conditions. For persons aged 65 yr or older, 1-time revaccination if they were vaccinated 5 or more yr previously and were younger than 65 yr at the time of primary vaccination.

⁹Hepatitis A vaccination
Medical indications: Persons with chronic liver disease and persons who receive clotting factor concentrates.
Behavioral indications: Men who have sex with men and persons who use illegal drugs.
Occupational indications: Persons working with hepatitis A virus (HAV)–infected primates or with HAV in a research laboratory setting.
Other indications: Persons traveling to or working in countries that have high or intermediate endemicity of hepatitis A (a list of countries is available at wwwn.cdc.gov/travel/contentdiseases.aspx) and any person seeking protection from HAV infection. Unvaccinated persons who anticipate close personal contact (e.g., household contact or regular babysitting) with an international adoptee from a country of high or intermediate endemicity during the first 60 days following arrival of the adoptee in the United States should consider vaccination. The first dose of the 2-dose HepA series should be administered as soon as adoption is planned, ideally 2 or more weeks before the arrival of the adoptee.
Single-antigen vaccine formulations should be administered in a 2-dose schedule at either 0 and 6-12 mo (Havrix) or 0 and 6-18 mo (Vaqta). If the combined hepatitis A and hepatitis B vaccine (Twinrix) is used, administer 3 doses at 0, 1, and 6 mo; alternatively, a 4-dose schedule, administered on days 0, 7, and 21 to 30 followed by a booster dose at mo 12 may be used.

¹⁰Hepatitis B vaccination
Medical indications: Persons with end-stage renal disease, including patients receiving hemodialysis; persons with HIV infection; and persons with chronic liver disease.
Occupational indications: Health care personnel and public-safety workers who are exposed to blood or other potentially infectious body fluids.
Behavioral indications: Sexually active persons who are not in a long-term, mutually monogamous relationship (e.g., persons with more than 1 sex partner during the previous 6 mo); persons seeking evaluation or treatment for a sexually transmitted disease (STD); current or recent injection-drug users; and men who have sex with men.
Other indications: Household contacts and sex partners of persons with chronic hepatitis B virus (HBV) infection; clients and staff members of institutions for persons with developmental disabilities; international travelers to countries with high or intermediate prevalence of chronic HBV infection (a list of countries is available at wwwn.cdc.gov/travel/contentdiseases.aspx); and any adult seeking protection from HBV infection.
Hepatitis B vaccination is recommended for all adults in the following settings: STD treatment facilities, HIV testing and treatment facilities, facilities providing drug-abuse treatment and prevention services, health care settings targeting services to injection-drug users or men who have sex with men, correctional facilities, end-stage renal disease programs and facilities for chronic hemodialysis patients, and institutions and nonresidential day care facilities for persons with developmental disabilities.
If the combined hepatitis A and hepatitis B vaccine (Twinrix) is used, administer 3 doses at 0, 1, and 6 mo; alternatively, a 4-dose schedule, administered on days 0, 7, and 21 to 30 followed by a booster dose at mo 12 may be used.
Special formulation indications: For adult patients receiving hemodialysis or with other immunocompromising conditions, 1 dose of 40 μg/ml (Recombivax HB) administered on a 3-dose schedule or 2 doses of 20 μg/mL (Engerix-B) administered simultaneously on a 4-dose schedule at 0, 1, 2, and 6 mo.

¹¹Meningococcal vaccination
Medical indications: Adults with anatomic or functional asplenia or terminal complement component deficiencies.
Other indications: First-yr college students living in dormitories; microbiologists who are routinely exposed to isolates of *Neisseria* meningitidis; military recruits; and persons who travel to or live in countries in which meningococcal disease is hyperendemic or epidemic (e.g., the "meningitis belt" of sub-Saharan Africa during the dry season [December-June]), particularly if their contact with local populations will be prolonged. Vaccination is required by the government of Saudi Arabia for all travelers to Mecca during the annual Hajj.
Meningococcal conjugate vaccine (MCV4) is preferred for adults aged 56 years and older. Revaccination with MCV4 after 5 years is recommended for adults previously vaccinated with MCV4 or MPSV4 who remain at increased risk for infection (e.g., adults with anatomic or functional asplenia). Persons whose only risk factor is living in on-campus housing are not recommended to receive an additional dose.

¹²Selected conditions for which Haemophilus influenzae type b (Hib) vaccine may be used
Hib vaccine generally is not recommended for persons aged 5 years and older. No efficacy data are available on which to base a recommendation concerning use of Hib vaccine for older children and adults. However, studies suggest good immunogenicity in patients who have sickle cell disease, leukemia, or HIV infection or who have had a splenectomy; administering 1 dose of vaccine to these patients is not contraindicated.

¹³Immunocompromising conditions
Inactivated vaccines generally are acceptable (e.g., pneumococcal, meningococcal, and influenza [trivalent inactive influenza vaccine]) and live vaccines generally are avoided in persons with immune deficiencies or immuno-compromising conditions. Information on specific conditions is available at http://www.cdc.gov/vaccines/pubs/acip-list.htm.

Clinical Practice Guidelines

V

TABLE 5-19 Vaccines That Might Be Indicated for Adults Based on Medical and Other Indications—United States

Note: These recommendations *must* be read with the footnotes that follow containing number of doses, intervals between doses, and other important information.

INDICATION ▶ / VACCINE ▼	Pregnancy	Immuno-compromising conditions (excluding human immunodeficiency virus [HIV])[13]	HIV infection[3,12,13] CD4+ T lymphocyte count <200 cells/µL	HIV infection[3,12,13] CD4+ T lymphocyte count ≥200 cells/µL	Diabetes, heart disease, chronic lung disease, chronic alcoholism	Asplenia[12] (including elective splenectomy and terminal complement component deficiencies)	Chronic liver disease	Kidney failure, end-stage renal disease, receipt of hemodialysis	Health care personnel
Tetanus, diphtheria, pertussis (Td/Tdap)[1,*]	Td	Substitute 1-time dose of Tdap for Td booster; then boost with Td every 10 yrs							
Human papillomavirus (HPV)[2,*]		3 doses for females and males through age 26 yrs							
Varicella[3,*]	Contraindicated			2 doses					
Zoster[4]	Contraindicated			1 dose					
Measles, mumps, rubella (MMR)[5,*]	Contraindicated			1 or 2 doses					
Influenza[6,*]	1 dose TIV annually								1 dose TIV or LAIV annually
Pneumococcal (polysaccharide)[7,8]	1 or 2 doses								
Hepatitis A[9,*]	2 doses								
Hepatitis B[10,*]	3 doses								
Meningococcal[11,*]	1 or more doses								

*Covered by the Vaccine Injury Compensation Program.

For all persons in this category who meet the age requirements and who lack evidence of immunity (e.g., lack documentation of vaccination or have no evidence of prior infection)

Recommended if some other risk factor is present (e.g., on the basis of medical, occupational, lifestyle, or other indications)

No recommendation

These schedules indicate the recommended age groups and medical indications for which administration of currently licensed vaccines is commonly indicated for adults ages 19 years and older. Licensed combination vaccines may be used whenever any components of the combination are indicated and when the vaccine's other components are not contraindicated. For detailed recommendations on all vaccines, including those used primarily for travelers or that are issued during the year, consult the manufacturers' package inserts and the complete statements from the Advisory Committee on Immunization Practices (http://www.cdc.gov/vaccines/pubs/acip-list.htm).

[1]Tetanus, diphtheria, and acellular pertussis (Td/Tdap) vaccination

Tdap should replace a single dose of Td for adults aged 19 through 64 yr who have not received a dose of Tdap previously.

Adults with uncertain or incomplete history of primary vaccination series with tetanus and diphtheria toxoid–containing vaccines should begin or complete a primary vaccination series. A primary series for adults is 3 doses of tetanus and diphtheria toxoid–containing vaccines; administer the first 2 doses at least 4 wk apart and the third dose 6-12 mo after the second. However, Tdap can substitute for any one of the doses of Td in the 3-dose primary series. The booster dose of tetanus and diphtheria toxoid–containing vaccine should be administered to adults who have completed a primary series and if the last vaccination was received 10 or more yr previously. Tdap or Td vaccine may be used, as indicated.

If a woman is pregnant and received the last Td vaccination 10 or more yr previously, administer Td during the second or third trimester. If the woman received the last Td vaccination less than 10 yr previously, administer Tdap during the immediate postpartum period. A dose of Tdap is recommended for postpartum women, close contacts of infants age less than 12 mo, and all health care personnel with direct patient contact if they have not previously received Tdap. An interval as short as 2 yr from the last Td is suggested; shorter intervals can be used. Td may be deferred during pregnancy and Tdap substituted in the immediate postpartum period, or Tdap may be administered instead of Td to a pregnant woman after an informed discussion with the woman. Consult the ACIP statement for recommendations for administering Td as prophylaxis in wound management.

[2]Human papillomavirus (HPV) vaccination

HPV vaccination is recommended for all females and males aged 11 through 26 yr (and may begin at age 9 yr) who have not completed the vaccine series. History of genital warts, abnormal Papanicolaou test result, or positive HPV DNA test result is not evidence of prior infection with all vaccine HPV types; HPV vaccination is recommended for persons with such histories.

Ideally, vaccine should be administered before potential exposure to HPV through sexual activity; however, persons who are sexually active should still be vaccinated consistent with age-based recommendations. Sexually active persons who have not been infected with any of the 4 HPV vaccine types receive the full benefit of the vaccination. Vaccination is less beneficial for persons who have already been infected with 1 or more of the HPV vaccine types.

A complete series consists of 3 doses. The second dose should be administered 2 mo after the first dose; the third dose should be administered 6 mo after the first dose.

HPV vaccination is not specifically recommended for persons with the medical indications described in Table 5-19. Because it is not a live-virus vaccine, it can be administered to persons with the medical indications noted. However, the immune response and vaccine efficacy might be less for persons with the noted medical indications than in persons who do not have the medical indications described or who are immunocompetent. Health care personnel are not at increased risk because of occupational exposure and should be vaccinated consistent with age-based recommendations.

[3]Varicella vaccination

All adults without evidence of immunity to varicella should receive 2 doses of single-antigen varicella vaccine if not previously vaccinated or the second dose if they have received only 1 dose, unless they have a medical contraindication. Special consideration should be given to those who 1) have close contact with persons at high risk for severe disease (e.g., health care personnel and family contacts of persons with immunocompromising conditions) or 2) are at high risk for exposure or transmission (e.g., teachers; child care employees; residents and staff members of institutional settings, including correctional institutions; college students; military personnel; adolescents and adults living in households with children; nonpregnant women of childbearing age; and international travelers).

Evidence of immunity to varicella in adults includes any of the following: 1) documentation of 2 doses of varicella vaccine at least 4 wk apart; 2) U.S.-born before 1980 (although for health care personnel and pregnant women, birth before 1980 should not be considered evidence of immunity); 3) history of varicella based on diagnosis or verification of varicella by a health care provider (for a patient reporting a history of or presenting with an atypical case, a mild case, or both, health care providers should seek either an epidemiologic link to a typical varicella case or to a laboratory-confirmed case or evidence of laboratory confirmation, if it was performed at the time of acute disease); 4) history of herpes zoster based on health care provider diagnosis or verification of herpes zoster by a health care provider; or 5) laboratory evidence of immunity or laboratory confirmation of disease.

Pregnant women should be assessed for evidence of varicella immunity. Women who do not have evidence of immunity should receive the first dose of varicella vaccine upon completion or termination of pregnancy and before discharge from the health care facility. The second dose should be administered 4-8 wk after the first dose.

TABLE 5-19 Vaccines That Might Be Indicated for Adults Based on Medical and Other Indications—United States—cont'd

[4]**Herpes zoster vaccination**

A single dose of zoster vaccine is recommended for adults aged 60 yr and older regardless of whether they report a prior episode of herpes zoster. Persons with chronic medical conditions may be vaccinated unless their condition constitutes a contraindication.

[5]**Measles, mumps, rubella (MMR) vaccination**

Measles component: Adults born before 1957 generally are considered immune to measles. Adults born during or after 1957 should receive 1 or more doses of MMR unless they have a medical contraindication, documentation of 1 or more doses, history of measles based on health care provider diagnosis, or laboratory evidence of immunity.

A second dose of MMR is recommended for adults who 1) have been recently exposed to measles or are in an outbreak setting; 2) have been vaccinated previously with killed measles vaccine; 3) have been vaccinated with an unknown type of measles vaccine during 1963-1967; 4) are students in postsecondary educational institutions; 5) work in a health care facility; or 6) plan to travel internationally.

Mumps component: Adults born before 1957 generally are considered immune to mumps. Adults born during or after 1957 should receive 1 dose of MMR unless they have a medical contraindication, history of mumps based on health care provider diagnosis, or laboratory evidence of immunity.

A second dose of MMR is recommended for adults who 1) live in a community experiencing a mumps outbreak and are in an affected age group; 2) are students in postsecondary educational institutions; 3) work in a health care facility; or 4) plan to travel internationally. For unvaccinated health care personnel born before 1957 who do not have other evidence of mumps immunity, administering 1 dose on a routine basis should be considered and administering a second dose during an outbreak should also be strongly considered.

Rubella component: 1 dose of MMR vaccine is recommended for women whose rubella vaccination history is unreliable or who lack laboratory evidence of immunity. For women of childbearing age, regardless of birth yr, rubella immunity should be determined and women should be counseled regarding congenital rubella syndrome. Women who do not have evidence of immunity should receive MMR vaccine upon completion or termination of pregnancy and before discharge from the health care facility.

[6]**Influenza vaccination**

Medical indications: Chronic disorders of the cardiovascular or pulmonary systems, including asthma; chronic metabolic diseases, including diabetes mellitus, renal or hepatic dysfunction, hemoglobinopathies, or immunocompromising conditions (including immunocompromising conditions caused by medications or HIV); any condition that compromises respiratory function or the handling of respiratory secretions or that can increase the risk of aspiration (e.g., cognitive dysfunction, spinal cord injury, or seizure disorder or other neuromuscular disorder); and pregnancy during the influenza season. No data exist on the risk for severe or complicated influenza disease among persons with asplenia; however, influenza is a risk factor for secondary bacterial infections that can cause severe disease among persons with asplenia.

Occupational indications: All health care personnel, including those employed by long-term care and assisted-living facilities, and caregivers of children younger than 5 yr.

Other indications: Residents of nursing homes and other long-term care and assisted-living facilities; persons likely to transmit influenza to persons at high risk (e.g., in-home household contacts and caregivers of children younger than 5 yr, persons 65 yr and older, and persons of all ages with high-risk condition[s]); and anyone who would like to decrease their risk of getting influenza. Healthy, nonpregnant adults younger than 50 yr without high-risk medical conditions who are not contacts of severely immunocompromised persons in special care units can receive either intranasally administered live, attenuated influenza vaccine (FluMist) or inactivated vaccine. Other persons should receive the inactivated vaccine.

[7]**Pneumococcal polysaccharide (PPSV) vaccination**

Medical indications: Chronic lung disease (including asthma); chronic cardiovascular diseases; diabetes mellitus; chronic liver diseases, cirrhosis; chronic alcoholism, chronic renal failure, or nephrotic syndrome; functional or anatomic asplenia (e.g., sickle cell disease or splenectomy [if elective splenectomy is planned, vaccinate at least 2 wk before surgery]); immunocompromising conditions; and cochlear implants and cerebrospinal fluid leaks. Vaccinate as close to HIV diagnosis as possible.

Other indications: Residents of nursing homes or other long-term care facilities and persons who smoke cigarettes. Routine use of PPSV is not recommended for Alaska Native or American Indian persons younger than 65 yr unless they have underlying medical conditions that are PPSV indications. However, public health authorities may consider recommending PPSV for Alaska Natives and American Indians 50 through 64 yr of age who are living in areas in which the risk of invasive pneumococcal disease is increased.

[8]**Revaccination with PPSV**

One-time revaccination after 5 yr for persons with chronic renal failure or nephrotic syndrome, functional or anatomic asplenia (e.g., sickle cell disease or splenectomy), and persons with immunocompromising conditions. For persons age 65 yr or older, 1-time revaccination if they were vaccinated 5 or more yr previously and were younger than 65 yr at the time of primary vaccination.

[9]**Hepatitis A vaccination**

Medical indications: Persons with chronic liver disease and persons who receive clotting factor concentrates.

Behavioral indications: Men who have sex with men and persons who use illegal drugs.

Occupational indications: Persons working with hepatitis A virus (HAV)–infected primates or with HAV in a research laboratory setting.

Other indications: Persons traveling to or working in countries that have high or intermediate endemicity of hepatitis A (a list of countries is available at wwwn.cdc.gov/travel/contentdiseases.aspx) and any person seeking protection from HAV infection.

Single-antigen vaccine formulations should be administered in a 2-dose schedule at either 0 and 6-12 mo (Havrix) or 0 and 6-18 mo (Vaqta). If the combined hepatitis A and hepatitis B vaccine (Twinrix) is used, administer 3 doses at 0, 1, and 6 mo; alternatively, a 4-dose schedule, administered on days 0, 7, and 21 to 30 followed by a booster dose at mo 12 may be used.

[10]**Hepatitis B vaccination**

Medical indications: Persons with end-stage renal disease, including patients receiving hemodialysis; persons with HIV infection; and persons with chronic liver disease.

Occupational indications: Health care personnel and public-safety workers who are exposed to blood or other potentially infectious body fluids.

Behavioral indications: Sexually active persons who are not in a long-term, mutually monogamous relationship (e.g., persons with more than 1 sex partner during the previous 6 mo); persons seeking evaluation or treatment for a sexually transmitted disease (STD); current or recent injection-drug users; and men who have sex with men.

Other indications: Household contacts and sex partners of persons with chronic hepatitis B virus (HBV) infection; clients and staff members of institutions for persons with developmental disabilities; international travelers to countries with high or intermediate prevalence of chronic HBV infection (a list of countries is available at wwwn.cdc.gov/travel/contentdiseases.aspx); and any adult seeking protection from HBV infection.

Hepatitis B vaccination is recommended for all adults in the following settings: STD treatment facilities, HIV testing and treatment facilities, facilities providing drug-abuse treatment and prevention services, health care settings targeting services to injection-drug users or men who have sex with men, correctional facilities, end-stage renal disease programs and facilities for chronic hemodialysis patients, and institutions and nonresidential day care facilities for persons with developmental disabilities.

If the combined hepatitis A and hepatitis B vaccine (Twinrix) is used, administer 3 doses at 0, 1, and 6 mo; alternatively, a 4-dose schedule, administered on days 0, 7, and 21 to 30 followed by a booster dose at mo 12 may be used.

Special formulation indications: For adult patients receiving hemodialysis or with other immunocompromising conditions, 1 dose of 40 μg/ml (Recombivax HB) administered on a 3-dose schedule or 2 doses of 20 μg/mL (Engerix-B) administered simultaneously on a 4-dose schedule at 0, 1, 2, and 6 mo.

[11]**Meningococcal vaccination**

Medical indications: Adults with anatomic or functional asplenia or terminal complement component deficiencies.

Other indications: First-yr college students living in dormitories; microbiologists who are routinely exposed to isolates of Neisseria meningitidis; military recruits; and persons who travel to or live in countries in which meningococcal disease is hyperendemic or epidemic (e.g., the "meningitis belt" of sub-Saharan Africa during the dry season [December-June]), particularly if their contact with local populations will be prolonged. Vaccination is required by the government of Saudi Arabia for all travelers to Mecca during the annual Hajj.

Meningococcal conjugate vaccine (MCV) is preferred for adults with any of the preceding indications who are aged 55 years or younger, although meningococcal polysaccharide vaccine (MPSV) is an acceptable alternative. Revaccination with MCV after 5 years might be indicated for adults previously vaccinated with MPSV who remain at increased risk for infection (e.g., persons residing in areas in which disease is epidemic).

[12]**Selected conditions for which Haemophilus influenzae type b (Hib) vaccine may be used**

Hib vaccine generally is not recommended for persons aged 5 years and older. No efficacy data are available on which to base a recommendation concerning use of Hib vaccine for older children and adults. However, studies suggest good immunogenicity in patients who have sickle cell disease, leukemia, or HIV infection or who have had a splenectomy; administering 1 dose of vaccine to these patients is not contraindicated.

[13]**Immunocompromising conditions**

Inactivated vaccines generally are acceptable (e.g., pneumococcal, meningococcal, and influenza [trivalent inactive influenza vaccine]) and live vaccines generally are avoided in persons with immune deficiencies or immuno-compromising conditions. Information on specific conditions is available at http://www.cdc.gov/vaccines/pubs/acip-list.htm.

TABLE 5-20   Immunization and Pregnancy

Vaccine	Before Pregnancy	During Pregnancy	After Pregnancy	Type of Vaccine	Route
Hepatitis A	If at high risk for disease	If at high risk for disease	If at high risk for disease	Inactivated	IM
Hepatitis B	Yes, if at risk	Yes, if at risk	Yes, if at risk	Inactivated	IM
Human papillomavirus (HPV)	Yes, if 9 to 26 years of age	No, under study	Yes, if 9 to 26 years of age	Inactivated	IM
Influenza TIV	Yes	Yes	Yes	Inactivated	IM
Influenza LAIV	Yes, if <50 years and healthy; avoid conception for 4 weeks	No	Yes, if <50 years and healthy; avoid conception for 4 weeks	Live	Nasal spray
MMR	Yes, avoid conception for 4 weeks	No	Yes, give immediately postpartum if susceptible to rubella	Live	SC
Meningococcal:	If indicated	If indicated	If indicated		
• Polysaccharide				Inactivated	SC
• Conjugate				Inactivated	IM
Pneumococcal polysaccharide	If indicated	If indicated	If indicated	Inactivated	IM or SC
Tetanus/diphtheria Td	Yes, Tdap preferred	If indicated	Yes, Tdap preferred	Toxoid	IM
Tdap, one dose only	Yes, preferred	If high risk of pertussis; otherwise, Td preferred	Yes, preferred	Toxoid/inactivated	IM
Varicella	Yes, avoid conception for 4 weeks	No	Yes, give immediately postpartum if susceptible	Live	SC

TABLE 5-21 Immunizing Agents and Immunization Schedules for Health Care Workers (HCWs)*

Generic Name	Primary Schedule and Booster(s)	Indications	Major Precautions and Contraindications	Special Considerations
Immunizing Agents Strongly Recommended for Health Care Workers				
Hepatitis B (HB) recombinant vaccine	Two doses IM 4 wk apart; third dose 5 mo after second; booster doses not necessary	**Preexposure:** HCWs at risk for exposure to blood or body fluids	Based on limited data no risk of adverse effects to developing fetuses is apparent. Pregnancy should *not* be considered a contraindication to vaccination of women. Previous anaphylactic reaction to common baker's yeast is a contraindication to vaccination.	The vaccine produces neither therapeutic nor adverse effects on HB-infected persons. Prevaccination serologic screening is not indicated for persons being vaccinated because of occupational risk. HCWs who have contact with patients or blood should be tested 1-2 mo after vaccination to determine serologic response.
Hepatitis B immune globulin (HBIG)	0.06 ml/kg IM as soon as possible after exposure. A second dose of HBIG should be administered 1 mo later if the HB vaccine series has not been started.	**Postexposure prophylaxis:** For persons exposed to blood or body fluids containing HBsAg and who are not immune to HBV infection—0.06 ml/kg IM as soon as possible (but no later than 7 days after exposure)		
Influenza vaccine (inactivated whole-virus and split-virus vaccines)	Annual vaccination with current vaccine Administered IM	HCWs who have contact with patients at high risk for influenza or its complications; HCWs who work in long-term care facilities; HCWs with high-risk medical conditions or who are aged ≥65 yr	History of anaphylactic hypersensitivity to egg ingestion	No evidence exists of risk to mother or fetus when the vaccine is administered to a pregnant woman with an underlying high-risk condition. Influenza vaccination is recommended during second and third trimesters of pregnancy because of increased risk for hospitalization.
Measles live-virus vaccine	One dose SC; second dose at least 1 mo later	HCWs[†] born during or after 1957 who do not have documentation of having received two doses of live vaccine on or after the first birthday **or** a history of physician-diagnosed measles or serologic evidence of immunity. Vaccination should be considered for all HCWs who lack proof of immunity, including those born before 1957.	Pregnancy; immunocompromised persons,[‡] including HIV-infected persons who have evidence of severe immunosuppression; anaphylaxis after gelatin ingestion or administration of neomycin; recent administration of immune globulin.	MMR is the vaccine of choice if recipients are likely to be susceptible to rubella and/or mumps as well as measles. Persons vaccinated between 1963 and 1967 with a killed measles vaccine alone, killed vaccine followed by live vaccine, or with a vaccine of unknown type should be revaccinated with two doses of live measles virus vaccine.
Mumps live-virus vaccine	One dose SC; second dose at least 1 mo later	HCWs[†] believed to be susceptible can be vaccinated. Adults born before 1957 can be considered immune.	Pregnancy; immunocompromised persons,[‡] history of anaphylactic reaction after gelatin ingestion or administration of neomycin	MMR is the vaccine of choice if recipients are likely to be susceptible to measles and rubella, as well as mumps.
Hepatitis A virus (HAV) vaccine	Two doses of vaccine either 6-12 mo apart (HAVRIX), or 6 mo apart (VAQTA)	Not routinely indicated for HCWs in the United States. Persons who work with HAV-infected primates or with HAV in a research laboratory setting should be vaccinated.	History of anaphylactic hypersensitivity to alum or, for HAVRIX, the preservative 2-phenoxyethanol. The safety of the vaccine in pregnant women has not been determined; the risk associated with vaccination should be weighed against the risk for hepatitis A in women who may be at high risk for exposure to HAV.	
Meningococcal polysaccharide vaccine (tetravalent A, C, W135, and Y)	One dose in volume and by route specified by manufacturer; need for boosters unknown	Not routinely indicated for HCWs in the United States.	The safety of the vaccine in pregnant women has not been evaluated; it should not be administered during pregnancy unless the risk for infection is high.	

Modified from *MMWR* 46(RR-18), 1998.

HBsAg, Hepatitis B surface antigen; *HBV,* hepatitis B virus; *HIV,* human immunodeficiency virus; *IM,* intramuscularly; *MMR,* measles, mumps, rubella vaccine; *SC,* subcutaneously; *TB,* tuberculosis.

*Persons who provide health care to patients or work in institutions that provide patient care (e.g., physicians, nurses, emergency medical personnel, dental professionals and students, medical and nursing students, laboratory technicians, hospital volunteers, and administrative and support staff in health care institutions).

[†]All HCWs (i.e., medical or nonmedical, paid or volunteer, full time or part time, student or nonstudent, with or without patient-care responsibilities) who work in health care institutions (e.g., inpatient and outpatient, public and private) should be immune to measles, rubella, and varicella.

[‡]Persons immunocompromised because of immune deficiency diseases, HIV infection, leukemia, lymphoma or generalized malignancy, or immunosuppressed as a result of therapy with corticosteroids, alkylating drugs, antimetabolites, or radiation.

Continued on following page

TABLE 5-21 Immunizing Agents and Immunization Schedules for Health Care Workers (HCWs)—cont'd

Generic Name	Primary Schedule and Booster(s)	Indications	Major Precautions and Contraindications	Special Considerations
Typhoid vaccine, IM, SC, and oral	IM vaccine: One 0.5-ml/dose, booster 0.5 ml every 2 yr SC vaccine: Two 0.5-ml doses, ≥4 wk apart, booster 0.5 ml SC or 0.1 ID every 3 yr if exposure continues Oral vaccine: Four doses on alternate days. The manufacturer recommends revaccination with the entire 4-dose series every 5 yr	Workers in microbiology laboratories who frequently work with *Salmonella typhi*	Severe local or systemic reaction to a previous dose. Ty21a (oral) vaccine should not be administered to immunocompromised persons[†] or to persons receiving antimicrobial agents.	Vaccination should not be considered an alternative to the use of proper procedures when handling specimens and cultures in the laboratory.
Vaccinia vaccine (smallpox)	One dose administered with a bifurcated needle; boosters administered every 10 yr	Laboratory workers who directly handle cultures with vaccinia, recombinant vaccinia viruses, or orthopox viruses that infect human beings	The vaccine is contraindicated in pregnancy, in persons with eczema or a history of eczema, and in immunocompromised persons[†] and their household contacts.	Vaccination may be considered for HCWs who have direct contact with contaminated dressings or other infectious material from volunteers in clinical studies involving recombinant vaccinia virus.

Other Vaccine-Preventable Diseases

Generic Name	Primary Schedule and Booster(s)	Indications	Major Precautions and Contraindications	Special Considerations
Tetanus and diphtheria (toxoids [Td])	Two IM doses 4 wk apart; third dose 6-12 mo after second dose; booster every 10 yr	All adults	Except in the first trimester, pregnancy is not a precaution. History of a neurologic reaction or immediate hypersensitivity reaction after a previous dose. History of severe local (arthus-type) reaction after a previous dose. Such persons should not receive further routine or emergency doses of Td for 10 yr.	Tetanus prophylaxis in wound management[‡]
Pneumococcal polysaccharide vaccine (23 valent)	One dose, 0.5 ml, IM or SC; revaccination recommended for those at highest risk ≥5 yr after the first dose	Adults who are at increased risk of pneumococcal disease and its complications because of underlying health conditions; older adults, especially those age ≥65 who are healthy	The safety of vaccine in pregnant women has not been evaluated; it should not be administered during pregnancy unless the risk for infection is high. Previous recipients of any type of pneumococcal polysaccharide vaccine who are at highest risk for fatal infection or antibody loss may be revaccinated ≥5 yr after the first dose.	
Rubella live-virus vaccine	One dose SC; second dose at least 1 mo later	Indicated for HCWs,[†] both men and women, who do not have documentation of having received live vaccine on or after their first birthday **or** laboratory evidence of immunity. Adults born before 1957, **except women who can become pregnant,** can be considered immune.	Pregnancy; immunocompromised persons[†]; history of anaphylactic reaction after administration of neomycin	The risk for rubella vaccine–associated malformations in the offspring of women pregnant when vaccinated or who become pregnant within 3 mo after vaccination is negligible. Such women should be counseled regarding the theoretic basis of concern for the fetus. MMR is the vaccine of choice if recipients are likely to be susceptible to measles or mumps as well as rubella.
Varicella zoster live-virus vaccine	Two 0.5-ml doses SC 4-8 wk apart if ≥13 yr	Indicated for HCWs[†] who do not have either a reliable history of varicella or serologic evidence of immunity	Pregnancy, immunocompromised persons,[‡] history of anaphylactic reaction after receipt of neomycin or gelatin. Avoid salicylate use for 6 wk after vaccination.	Vaccine is available from the manufacturer for certain patients with acute lymphocytic leukemia in remission. Because 71%-93% of persons without a history of varicella are immune, serologic testing before vaccination is likely to be cost effective.

TABLE 5-21 Immunizing Agents and Immunization Schedules for Health Care Workers (HCWs)—cont'd

Generic Name	Primary Schedule and Booster(s)	Indications	Major Precautions and Contraindications	Special Considerations
Varicella-zoster immune globulin (VZIG)	Persons <50 kg: 125 μ/10 kg IM; persons ≥50 kg: 625 μ[§]	Persons known or likely to be susceptible (particularly those at high risk for complications, e.g., pregnant women) who have close and prolonged exposure to a contact case or to an infectious hospital staff worker or patient		Serologic testing may help in assessing whether to administer VZIG. If use of VZIG prevents varicella disease, patient should be vaccinated subsequently.
BCG Vaccination				
Bacille Calmette-Guérin (BCG) vaccine (TB)	One percutaneous dose of 0.3 ml; no booster dose recommended	Should be considered only for HCWs in areas where multidrug TB is prevalent, a strong likelihood of infection exists, and where comprehensive infection control precautions have failed to prevent TB transmission to HCWs	Should not be administered to immunocompromised persons,[‡] pregnant women	In the United States TB-control efforts are directed toward early identification, treatment of cases, and preventive therapy with isoniazid.
Other Immunobiologics that Are or May Be Indicated for HCWs				
Immune globulin (hepatitis A)	**Postexposure**—One IM dose of 0.02 ml/kg administered ≤2 wk after exposure	Indicated for HCWs exposed to feces of infectious patients	Contraindicated in persons with IgA deficiency; do not administer within 2 wk after MMR vaccine or 3 wk after varicella vaccine. Delay administration of MMR vaccine for ≥3 mo and varicella vaccine ≥5 mo after administration of immune globulin	Administer in large muscle mass (deltoid, gluteal).

Modified from *MMWR* 46(RR-18), 1998.

HBsAg, Hepatitis B surface antigen; *HBV,* hepatitis B virus; *HIV,* human immunodeficiency virus; *IM,* intramuscular; *MMR,* measles, mumps, rubella vaccine; *SC,* subcutaneous; *TB,* tuberculosis.

*Persons who provide health care to patients or work in institutions that provide patient care (e.g., physicians, nurses, emergency medical personnel, dental professionals and students, medical and nursing students, laboratory technicians, hospital volunteers, and administrative and support staff in health care institutions).

[†]All HCWs (i.e., medical or nonmedical, paid or volunteer, full time or part time, student or nonstudent, with or without patient-care responsibilities) who work in health care institutions (e.g., inpatient and outpatient, public and private) should be immune to measles, rubella, and varicella.

[‡]Persons immunocompromised because of immune deficiency diseases, HIV infection, leukemia, lymphoma or generalized malignancy, or immunosuppressed as a result of therapy with corticosteroids, alkylating drugs, antimetabolites, or radiation.

[§]Some experts recommend 125 μ/10 kg regardless of total body weight.

TABLE 5-22 Recommendations for Persons with Medical Conditions Requiring Special Vaccination Considerations

Condition	Td	MMR	Varicella	HBV	HAV	Pneumovax[a]	Influenza[b]	HbCV	Meningococcal	IPV	Other Live Vaccines[c]	Other Killed Vaccines[d]
HIV infection	Rou	Rou/Contr[e]	Contr[f]	Rou[g]	Rou	Rec	Rec	Cons	Rou	Rou	Contr	Rou
Severe immunocompromise[h]	Rou	Contr	Contr[f]	Rou[g]	Rou	Rec	Rec	Rou[i]	Rou	Rou	Contr	Rou
Renal failure	Rou	Rou	Rou	Rec[g]	Rou	Rec	Rec	Rou	Rou	Rou	Rou	Rou
Diabetes	Rou	Rou	Rou	Rou	Rou	Rec	Rec	Rou	Rou	Rou	Rou	Rou
Chronic liver disease	Rou	Rou	Rou	Rou	Rec	Rec	Rec	Rou	Rou	Rou	Rou	Rou
Cardiac disease	Rou	Rou	Rou	Rou	Rou	Rec	Rec	Rou	Rou	Rou	Rou	Rou
Pulmonary disease	Rou	Rou	Rou	Rou	Rou	Rec	Rec	Rou	Rou	Rou	Rou	Rou
Alcoholism	Rou	Rou	Rou	Rou	Rou	Rec	Rec	Rou	Rou	Rou	Rou	Rou
Functional/anatomic asplenia	Rou	Rou	Rou	Rou	Rou	Rec[j]	Rec	Rec[j]	Rec[j]	Rou	Rou	Rou
Terminal complement deficiency	Rou	Rou	Rou	Rou	Rou	Rou	Rou	Rou	Rec	Rou	Rou	
Clotting factor disorders	Rou	Rou	Rou	Rec	Rec	Rou	Rou	Rou	Rou	Rou	Rou	Rou

Modified and updated from *MMWR* 42(RR-4):16, 1993.

Cons, Consider vaccination; *Contr,* contraindicated; *HbCV, Haemophilus influenzae* conjugate vaccine; *HBV,* hepatitis B virus; *IPV,* inactivated poliomyelitis vaccine; *MMR,* measles-mumps-rubella; *Rec,* recommended; *Rou,* routine as outlined for all adults.

a Pneumovax should be repeated in 5 yr for patients in whom vaccine is recommended. Asthma without chronic obstructive pulmonary disease is not an indication for the vaccine.

b Influenza vaccine should also be given to caregivers and household members.

c Includes bacille Calmette-Guérin, vaccinia, oral typhoid, yellow fever (if exposure cannot be avoided, persons with HIV can be given yellow fever vaccine; see text).

d Includes rabies (check postvaccination titers in HIV or severely immunocompromised persons), Lyme disease, inactivated typhoid, cholera, plague, and anthrax.

e For asymptomatic, nonseverely immunocompromised persons with HIV, MMR can be used; it is contraindicated in severely immunocompromised persons. MMR can be considered in symptomatic HIV patients without severe immunocompromise.

f Varicella can be given to household members and caregivers, but if varicella-like rash develops after vaccination, contact should be avoided.

g Recommended for persons with severe chronic renal failure approaching or already receiving dialysis, and higher doses should be given. Antibody titers should be measured after vaccination in these patients and in those with HIV or severe immunocompromise (who may require higher doses) to ensure adequate response. Yearly titers should be measured in dialysis patients.

h Severe immunocompromise can result from congenital immunodeficiency, leukemia, lymphoma, malignancy, organ transplant, chemotherapy, radiation therapy, or high-dose corticosteroids.

i Only for persons with Hodgkin's disease.

j Give at least 2 wk in advance of elective splenectomy.

TABLE 5-23 Vaccinations for International Travel

Disease*	Areas Affected†	Prophylaxis Recommended	Ideal Time between Last Vaccine Dose and Travel
Tetanus	All	All travelers; vaccine series/booster	Probably 30 days for series Anamnestic response to booster
Measles	All	If born after 1956; ensure immunity by antibody titer, diagnosed measles, or two doses of vaccine	As MMR, 7-14 days
Rubella	All	If born after 1956 and any female of childbearing age; rubella titer or one dose of vaccine	As MMR, 7-14 days
Mumps	All	If born after 1956; ensure immunity by antibody titer, diagnosed mumps, or one dose of vaccine	As MMR, 7-14 days
Varicella	All	All travelers; antibody titer, reported illness, or vaccine series	7-14 days
Hepatitis B	5%-20% of population are carriers in Africa, Middle East except Israel, all Southeast Asia, Amazon basin, Haiti, and Dominican Republic; 1%-5% of population are carriers in south-central and southwest Asia, Israel, Japan, Americas, Russia, and eastern and southern Europe	Travelers for more than 6 mo in close contact with population or for less time but with high-risk activities (close household contact, seeking dental or medical care, sex); vaccine series	Probably 30 days
Hepatitis A	Developing countries	Travelers to rural areas; eating and drinking in settings of poor sanitation; vaccine or pooled immune globulin	Vaccine, 30 days Pooled IG, 2 days
Influenza	Tropics throughout the year; southern hemisphere from April to September	Travelers for whom vaccine is otherwise indicated; give current vaccine and revaccinate in fall as usual	7-14 days
Meningococcus*	Sub-Saharan Africa "belt" (Senegal to Ethiopia) from December to June; required for pilgrims to Saudi Arabia during Hajj; epidemics reported in other African nations, India, Nepal, and Mongolia	All travelers; vaccine	7-10 days
Rabies	Endemic dog rabies exists in Mexico, El Salvador, Guatemala, Peru, Colombia, Ecuador, India, Nepal, Philippines, Sri Lanka, Thailand, and Vietnam	Travelers staying for more than 30 days or at high risk of exposure to domestic or wild animals; vaccine series/booster	7-14 days
Poliomyelitis	Developing countries not in western hemisphere; at risk all year in tropics; in temperate zones, incidence increases in summer and fall	All travelers; vaccine series/booster	Parenteral vaccine series, 28 day (see text)
Typhoid fever	Many countries in Asia, Africa, Central America, and South America	Travelers with prolonged stay in rural areas with poor sanitation; vaccine series/booster	Oral vaccine, 7 days Parenteral vaccine, probably 14 days
Yellow fever*	North and central South America, forest-savannah zones of Africa; some countries in Africa, Asia, and Middle East require travelers from endemic areas to be vaccinated	All travelers; vaccine/booster at approved yellow fever vaccination center.	10 days
Japanese encephalitis	Seasonally in most areas of Asia, Indian subcontinent, and western Pacific islands; in temperate zones, incidence increases in summer and early fall; in tropics, year-round incidence	Travelers staying for more than 30 days in high-risk rural areas; staying outdoors during transmission season; vaccine series	10 days
Cholera*	Certain undeveloped countries	If required by local authorities, one dose usually suffices; primary series only for those living in high-risk areas under poor sanitary conditions or those with compromised gastric defense mechanisms (achlorhydria, antacid therapy, previous ulcer surgery); booster every 6 mo	Probably 30 days
Plague	Africa, Asia, and Americas in rural mountainous or upland areas	Travelers whose research or field activities bring them in contact with rodents; vaccine series/booster; consider taking tetracycline (500 mg four times a day) for chemoprophylaxis (inferred from clinical experience in treating plague)	Probably 30 days

From Noble J: *Primary care medicine*, ed 3, St Louis, 2001, Mosby.

MMR, Measles-mumps-rubella.

*Only yellow fever vaccine is required for entry by any country; cholera vaccine may be required by some local authorities. Meningococcus vaccine is required for pilgrims to Mecca, in Saudia Arabia, during Hajj. However, it is important to follow Centers for Disease Control and Prevention (CDC) recommendations for all vaccines to prevent disease. If a required vaccine is contraindicated or withheld for any reason, attempts should be made to obtain a waiver from the country's consulate or embassy.

†Because areas affected can change, and for more specific details, consult the CDC's traveler's hotline.

Recommendations and Implementation Strategies for Hepatitis B Vaccination of Adults

BOX 5-1   Adults Recommended to Receive Hepatitis B Vaccination

Persons at Risk for Infection by Sexual Exposure
- Sex partners of persons who are HBsAg positive
- Sexually active persons who are not in a long-term, mutually monogamous relationship (e.g., persons who have had more than one sex partner during the previous 6 months)
- Persons seeking evaluation or treatment for a sexually transmitted disease
- Men who have sex with men

Persons at Risk for Infection by Percutaneous or Mucosal Exposure to Blood
- Current or recent users of injection drugs
- Household contacts of persons who are HBsAg positive
- Residents and staff of facilities for developmentally disabled persons

- Health care and public safety workers with reasonably anticipated risk for exposure to blood or blood-contaminated body fluids
- Persons with end-stage renal disease, including predialysis, hemodialysis, peritoneal dialysis, and home dialysis patients

Others
- International travelers to regions with high or intermediate levels (HBsAg prevalence of $\geq 2\%$) of endemic HBV infection
- Persons with chronic liver disease
- Persons with HIV infection
- All other persons seeking protection from HBV infection

From CDC: A comprehensive immunization strategy to eliminate transmission of hepatitis B virus infection in the United States: recommendations of the Advisory Committee on Immunization Practices (ACIP), *MMWR* 55(RR-16):15, 2006.
HbsAg, Hepatitis B surface antigen.

BOX 5-2   Hepatitis B Vaccine Schedules for Adults (Aged ≥ 20 yr)*

0, 1, and 6 months
0, 1, and 4 months
0, 2, and 4 months
0, 1, 2, and 12 months[†]

From CDC: A comprehensive immunization strategy to eliminate transmission of hepatitis B virus infection in the United States: recommendations of the Advisory Committee on Immunization Practices (ACIP), *MMWR* 55(RR-16):15, 2006.
*All schedules are applicable to single-antigen hepatitis B vaccines; Twinrix (combined hepatitis A and hepatitis B vaccine) may be administered at 0, 1, and 6 months.
[†]A 4-dose schedule of Engerix-B is licensed for all age groups.

TABLE 5-24 Recommended Doses of Currently Licensed Formulations of Adult Hepatitis B Vaccine by Group and Vaccine Type

| | SINGLE-ANTIGEN VACCINE | | | | COMBINATION VACCINE | |
| | Recombivax HB[a] | | Engerix-B[b] | | Twinrix[b,c] | |
Group	Dose (μg)[d]	Vol. (ml)	Dose (μg)[d]	Vol. (ml)	Dose (μg)[d]	Vol. (ml)
Adults (aged ≥20 yr)	10	1.0	20	1.0	20	1.0
Hemodialysis patients and other immunocompromised persons aged ≥20 yr	40[e]	1.0	40[f]	2.0	—[g]	—

From Centers for Disease Control and Prevention: A comprehensive immunization strategy to eliminate transmission of hepatitis B virus infection in the United States: recommendations of the Advisory Committee on Immunization Practices (ACIP), *MMWR* 55(RR-16):10, 2006.
HB, Hepatitis B.
[a]Merck & Co., Inc., Whitehouse Station, New Jersey.
[b]GlaxoSmithKline Biologicals, Rixensart, Belgium.
[c]Combined hepatitis A and hepatitis B vaccine, recommended for persons aged >18 yr who are at increased risk for both hepatitis B virus and hepatitis A virus infections.
[d]Recombinant hepatitis B surface antigen protein dose.
[e]Dialysis formulation administered on a 3-dose schedule at 0, 1, and 6 mo.
[f]Two 1.0-ml doses administered in 1 or 2 injections on a 4-dose schedule at 0, 1, 2, and 6 mo.
[g]Not applicable.

TABLE 5-25 Recommended HIV/AIDS, Sexually Transmitted Disease (STD), and Viral Hepatitis Prevention Services by Risk Population

Risk Population[a]	Recommended Services
High-Risk Heterosexuals	
Persons seeking sexually transmitted disease evaluation or treatment	Hepatitis B vaccination Testing for HIV infection[b] Testing for syphilis, gonorrhea, and chlamydia, as clinically indicated[c]
Sexually active men not in a long-term, mutually monogamous relationship	Hepatitis B vaccination Annual testing for HIV infection[b,d]
Sexually active women not in a long-term, mutually monogamous relationship	Hepatitis B vaccination[e] Annual testing for HIV infection[b,d] Annual testing for chlamydia (NOTE: Also recommended for all sexually active females aged <25 yr)[c]
Men Who Have Sex with Men (MSM)	
All MSM	Hepatitis A vaccination Hepatitis B vaccination[e]
Sexually active MSM not in a long-term, mutually monogamous relationship	Hepatitis A vaccination Hepatitis B vaccination[e] Annual testing for HIV infection[b] Annual testing for syphilis, gonorrhea, and chlamydia[c]
Injection-Drug Users	
	Hepatitis A vaccination[f] Hepatitis B vaccination Testing for hepatitis C virus infection[g] Annual testing for HIV infection[b] Substance-abuse treatment[h]

From Centers for Disease Control and Prevention (CDC): A comprehensive immunization strategy to eliminate transmission of hepatitis B virus infection in the United States: recommendations of the Advisory Committee on Immunization Practices (ACIP), *MMWR* 55(RR-16):17, 2006.
[a]Testing for HIV infection, chlamydia, gonorrhea, syphilis, and hepatitis B surface antigen also is recommended for pregnant women. (CDC: Revised recommendations for HIV testing of adults, adolescents, and pregnant women in health care settings, *MMWR* 55[RR-14], 2006; CDC: Sexually transmitted diseases treatment guidelines, *MMWR* 55[RR-11], 2006; CDC: A comprehensive immunization strategy to eliminate transmission of hepatitis B virus infection in the United States: recommendations of the Advisory Committee on Immunization Practices [ACIP]. Part 1: immunization of infants, children, and adolescents, *MMWR* 54[RR-16], 2005.)
[b]CDC: Revised recommendations for HIV testing of adults, adolescents, and pregnant women in health care settings, *MMWR* 55(RR-14), 2006.
[c]CDC: Sexually transmitted diseases treatment guidelines 2006, *MMWR* 55(RR-11), 2006.
[d]HIV screening is recommended for all persons aged 13-64 yr. Repeat screening is recommended at least annually for persons likely to be at high risk for HIV infection, including MSM or heterosexuals who themselves or whose sex partners have had more than one partner since their most recent HIV test.
[e]Hepatitis B vaccination is recommended for persons who have had more than one sex partner during the previous 6 mo.
[f]CDC: Prevention of hepatitis A through active or passive immunization: recommendations of the Advisory Committee on Immunization Practices (ACIP), *MMWR* 55(RR-7), 2006.
[g]CDC: Recommendations for prevention and control of hepatitis C virus (HCV) infection and HCV-related chronic disease, *MMWR* 47(RR-19), 1998. Recommended frequency of testing for hepatitis C virus infection has not been determined.
[h]CDC: *Substance abuse treatment for injection drug users: a strategy with many benefits,* Atlanta, 2002, U.S. Department of Health and Human Services, CDC. Available at http://www.cdc.gov/idu/facts/treatment.htm.

TABLE 5-26 Guidelines for Postexposure Prophylaxis* of Persons with Nonoccupational Exposures† to Blood or Body Fluids That Contain Blood by Exposure Type and Vaccination Status

	TREATMENT	
Exposure	Unvaccinated Person‡	Previously Vaccinated Person§
HBsAg-Positive Source		
Percutaneous (e.g., bite or needlestick) or mucosal exposure to HBsAg-positive blood or body fluids	Administer hepatitis B vaccine series and hepatitis B immune globulin (HBIG)	Administer hepatitis B vaccine booster dose
Sex or needle-sharing contact with a person who is HBsAg positive	Administer hepatitis B vaccine series and HBIG	Administer hepatitis B vaccine booster dose
Victim of sexual assault/abuse by a perpetrator who is HBsAg positive	Administer hepatitis B vaccine series and HBIG	Administer hepatitis B vaccine booster dose
Source with Unknown HBsAg Status		
Victim of sexual assault/abuse by a perpetrator with unknown HBsAg status	Administer hepatitis B vaccine series	No treatment
Percutaneous (e.g., bite or needlestick) or mucosal exposure to potentially infectious blood or body fluids from a source with unknown HBsAg status	Administer hepatitis B vaccine series	No treatment
Sexual or needle-sharing contact with person with unknown HBsAg status	Administer hepatitis B vaccine series	No treatment

From Centers for Disease Control and Prevention: A comprehensive immunization strategy to eliminate transmission of hepatitis B virus infection in the United States: recommendations of the Advisory Committee on Immunization Practices (ACIP), *MMWR* 55(RR-16):30, 2006.
HBsAg, Hepatitis B surface antigen.
*When indicated, immunoprophylaxis should be initiated as soon as possible, preferably within 24 hours. Studies are limited on the maximum interval after exposure during which postexposure prophylaxis is effective, but the interval is unlikely to exceed 7 days for percutaneous exposures or 14 days for sexual exposures. The hepatitis B vaccine series should be completed.
†These guidelines apply to nonoccupational exposures. Guidelines for management of occupational exposures have been published separately and also can be used for management of nonoccupational exposures if feasible.
‡A person who is in the process of being vaccinated but has not completed the vaccine series should complete the series and receive treatment as indicated.
§A person who has written documentation of a complete hepatitis B vaccine series and did not receive postvaccination testing.

TABLE 5-27 Typical Interpretation of Serologic Test Results for Hepatitis B Virus Infection

SEROLOGIC MARKER				
HBsAg	Total Anti-HBc	IgM Anti-HBc	Anti-HBs	Interpretation
−*	−	−	−	Never infected
+†‡	−	−	−	Early acute infection; transient (up to 18 days) after vaccination
+	+	+	−	Acute infection
−	+	+	+ or −	Acute resolving infection
−	+	−	+	Recovered from past infection and immune
+	+	−	−	Chronic infection
−	+	−	−	False-positive (i.e., susceptible), past infection, "low-level" chronic infection,§ or passive transfer of anti-HBc to infant born to mother who is HBsAg positive
−	−	−	+	Immune if concentration is >10 mIU/ml after vaccine series completion‖; passive transfer after hepatitis B immune globulin administration

From Centers for Disease Control and Prevention: A comprehensive immunization strategy to eliminate transmission of hepatitis B virus infection in the United States: recommendations of the Advisory Committee on Immunization Practices (ACIP), *MMWR* 55(RR-16):4, 2006.
HBc, Antibody to hepatitis B core antigen; *HBs,* antibody to HBsAg; *HBsAg,* hepatitis B surface antigen; *Ig,* immunoglobulin.
*Negative test result.
†Positive test result.
‡To ensure that an HBsAg-positive test result is not a false-positive, samples with reactive HBsAg results should be tested with a licensed neutralizing confirmatory test if recommended in the manufacturer's package insert.
§Persons positive only for anti-HBc are unlikely to be infectious except under unusual circumstances in which they are the source for direct percutaneous exposure of susceptible recipients to large quantities of virus (e.g., blood transfusion or organ transplant).
‖Milliinternational units per milliliter.

Hepatitis A Prophylaxis

TABLE 5-28 Recommended Dosages of Hepatitis A Immune Globulin

Setting	Duration of Coverage	Dose
Preexposure prophylaxis	Short term (<3 mo)	0.02 ml/kg
	Long term (3-5 mo)*	0.06 ml/kg
Postexposure prophylaxis	—	0.02 ml/kg

Modified from Centers for Disease Control and Prevention: Prevention of hepatitis A through active or passive immunization: recommendations of the Advisory Committee on Immunization Practices (ACIP), *MMWR* 55(RR-07):9, 2006.

NOTE: Immune globulin should be administered intramuscularly into the deltoid or gluteal muscle in children younger than 24 mo; it may be administered in the anterolateral thigh muscle.

*Repeat every 5 mo if continued exposure to hepatitis A virus occurs.

TABLE 5-29 Licensed Dosages of Hepatitis A Vaccines

Vaccine	Patient's Age	Dose	Volume (ml)	Number of Doses	Schedule (mo)*
Hepatitis A vaccine, inactivated (Havrix)	12 mo to 18 yr	720 EL.U.	0.5	2	0, 6-12
	≥19 yr	1440 EL.U.	1.0	2	0, 6-12
Hepatitis A vaccine, inactivated (Vaqta)	12 mo to 18 yr	25 U	0.5	2	0, 6-18
	≥19 yr	50 U	1.0	2	0, 6-18
Combined hepatitis A and hepatitis B vaccine (Twinrix)	≥18 yr	720 EL.U. of hepatitis A antigen and 20 mcg of hepatitis B surface antigen protein	1.0	3	0, 1, and 6

Modified from Centers for Disease Control and Prevention: Prevention of hepatitis A through active or passive immunization: recommendations of the Advisory Committee on Immunization Practices (ACIP), *MMWR* 55(RR-07):10, 2006.

*Zero represents the timing of the initial dose; subsequent numbers represent months after the initial dose.

Influenza Treatment and Prophylaxis

BOX 5-3 Summary of Seasonal Influenza Vaccination Recommendations

Children

All children aged 6 months-18 years should be vaccinated annually.

Children and adolescents at higher risk for influenza complications should continue to be a focus for vaccination efforts as providers and programs transition to routinely vaccinating all children and adolescents, including those who:

- are aged 6 months-4 years (59 months)
- have chronic pulmonary (including asthma), cardiovascular (except hypertension), renal, hepatic, cognitive, neurologic/neuromuscular, hematologic, or metabolic disorders (including diabetes mellitus)
- are immunosuppressed (including immunosuppression caused by medications or by human immunodeficiency virus)
- are receiving long-term aspirin therapy and therefore might be at risk for experiencing Reye's syndrome after influenza virus infection
- are residents of long-term care facilities
- will be pregnant during the influenza season

Note: Children aged <6 months cannot receive influenza vaccination. Household and other close contacts (e.g., day-care providers) of children aged <6 months, including older children and adolescents, should be vaccinated.

Adults

Annual vaccination against influenza is recommended for any adult who wants to reduce the risk of becoming ill with influenza or of transmitting it to others. Vaccination is recommended for all adults without contraindications in the following groups, because these persons either are at higher risk for influenza complications, or are close contacts of the persons at higher risk:

- persons aged ≥50 years
- women who will be pregnant during the influenza season
- persons who have chronic pulmonary (including asthma), cardiovascular (except hypertension), renal, hepatic, cognitive, neurologic/neuromuscular, hematologic, or metabolic disorders (including diabetes mellitus)
- persons who have immunosuppression (including immunosuppression caused by medications or by human immunodeficiency virus)
- residents of nursing homes and other long-term care facilities
- health-care personnel
- household contacts and caregivers of children aged <5 years and adults aged ≥50 years, with particular emphasis on vaccinating contacts of children aged <6 months
- household contacts and caregivers of persons with medical conditions that put them at higher risk for severe complications from influenza

Modified from *MMWR* 58:(RR-8), 2009.

RECOMMENDED VACCINES FOR DIFFERENT AGE GROUPS

When vaccinating children aged 6 to 35 months with TIV, health care providers should use TIV that has been licensed by the FDA for this age group (i.e., TIV manufactured by Sanofi Pasteur [FluZone]). TIV from Novartis (Fluvirin) is FDA approved in the United States for use among persons aged 4 years and older. TIV from GlaxoSmithKline (Fluarix and FluLaval) or CSL Biotherapies (Afluria) is labeled for use in persons aged 18 years and older because data to demonstrate efficacy among younger persons have not been provided to the FDA. LAIV from MedImmune (FluMist) is licensed for use by healthy, nonpregnant persons aged 2 to 49 years. A vaccine dose does not need to be repeated if inadvertently administered to a person who does not have an age indication for the vaccine formulation given. Expanded age and risk group indications for licensed vaccines are likely over the next several years, and vaccination providers should be alert to these changes. In addition, several new vaccine formulations are being evaluated in immunogenicity and efficacy trials; when licensed, these new products will increase the influenza vaccine supply and provide additional vaccine choices for practitioners and their patients.

INFLUENZA VACCINES AND USE OF INFLUENZA ANTIVIRAL MEDICATIONS

Administration of TIV and influenza antivirals during the same medical visit is acceptable. The effect on safety and effectiveness of LAIV coadministration with influenza antiviral medications has not been studied. However, because influenza antivirals reduce replication of influenza viruses, LAIV should not be administered until 48 hours after cessation of influenza antiviral therapy, and influenza antiviral medications should not be administered for 2 weeks after receipt of LAIV. Persons receiving antivirals within the period 2 days before to 14 days after vaccination with LAIV should be revaccinated at a later date.

PERSONS WHO SHOULD NOT BE VACCINATED WITH TIV

TIV should not be administered to persons known to have anaphylactic hypersensitivity to eggs or other components of the influenza vaccine. Prophylactic use of antiviral agents is an option for preventing influenza among such persons. Information about vaccine components is located in package inserts from each manufacturer. Persons with moderate to severe acute febrile illness usually should not be vaccinated until their symptoms have abated. However, minor illnesses with or without fever do not contraindicate use of influenza vaccine. Guillaine-Barré syndrome within 6 weeks after a previous dose of TIV is considered a precaution for use of TIV.

CONSIDERATIONS WHEN USING LAIV

LAIV is an option for vaccination of healthy, nonpregnant persons aged 2 to 49 years, including health care providers and other close contacts of high-risk persons (except severely immunocompromised persons who require care in a protected environment). No preference is indicated for LAIV or TIV when considering vaccination of healthy, nonpregnant persons aged 2 to 49 years. Use of the term *healthy* in this recommendation refers to persons who do not have any of the underlying medical conditions that confer high risk for severe complications (see "Persons Who Should Not Be Vaccinated with LAIV"). However, during periods when inactivated vaccine is in short supply, use of LAIV is encouraged when feasible for eligible persons (including health care providers) because use of LAIV by these persons might increase availability of TIV for persons in groups targeted for vaccination but who cannot receive LAIV. Possible advantages of LAIV include its potential to induce a broad mucosal and systemic immune response in children, its ease of administration, and possibly increased acceptability of an intranasal rather than intramuscular route of administration.

If the vaccine recipient sneezes after administration, the dose should not be repeated. However, if nasal congestion is present that might impede delivery of the vaccine to the nasopharyngeal mucosa, deferral of administration should be considered until resolution of the illness, or TIV should be administered instead. No data exist about concomitant use of nasal corticosteroids or other intranasal medications.

Although FDA licensure of LAIV excludes children aged 2 to 4 years with a history of asthma or recurrent wheezing, the precise risk, if any, of wheezing caused by LAIV among these children is unknown because experience with LAIV among these young children is limited. Young children might not have a history of recurrent wheezing if their exposure to respiratory viruses has been limited because of their age. Certain children might have a history of wheezing with respiratory illnesses but have not had asthma diagnosed. The following screening recommendations should be used to assist persons who administer influenza vaccines in providing the appropriate vaccine for children aged 2 to 4 years.

Clinicians and vaccination programs should screen for possible reactive airways diseases when considering use of LAIV for children aged 2 to 4 years and should avoid use of this vaccine in children with asthma or a recent wheezing episode. Health care providers should consult the medical record, when available, to identify children aged 2 to 4 years with asthma or recurrent wheezing that might indicate asthma. In addition, to identify children who might be at greater risk for asthma and possibly at increased risk for wheezing after receiving LAIV, parents or caregivers of children aged 2 to 4 years should be asked, "In the past 12 months, has a health care provider ever told you that your child had wheezing or asthma?" Children whose parents or caregivers answer "yes" to this question and children who have asthma or who had a wheezing episode noted in the medical record during the preceding 12 months should not receive LAIV. TIV is available for use in children with asthma or possible reactive airways diseases.

LAIV can be administered to persons with minor acute illnesses (e.g., diarrhea or mild upper respiratory tract infection with or without fever). However, if nasal congestion is present that might impede delivery of the vaccine to the nasopharyngeal mucosa, deferral of administration should be considered until resolution of the illness.

PERSONS WHO SHOULD NOT BE VACCINATED WITH LAIV

The effectiveness or safety of LAIV is not known for the following groups, who should not be vaccinated with LAIV:

- Persons with a history of hypersensitivity, including anaphylaxis, to any of the components of LAIV or eggs
- Persons younger than 2 years or aged 50 years or older
- Persons with any of the underlying medical conditions that serve as an indication for routine influenza vaccination, including asthma, reactive airways disease, or other chronic disorders of the pulmonary or cardiovascular systems; other underlying medical conditions, including metabolic diseases such as diabetes, renal dysfunction, and hemoglobinopathies; or known or suspected immunodeficiency diseases or immunosuppressed states
- Children aged 2 to 4 years whose parents or caregivers report that a health care provider has told them during the preceding 12 months that their child had wheezing or asthma, or whose medical record indicates a wheezing episode has occurred during the preceding 12 months
- Children or adolescents receiving aspirin or other salicylates (because of the association of Reye syndrome with wild-type influenza virus infection)
- Persons with a history of Guillaine-Barré syndrome after influenza vaccination
- Pregnant women

Concurrent Administration of Influenza Vaccine with Other Vaccines

Use of LAIV concurrently with measles, mumps, rubella (MMR) alone, and MMR and varicella vaccine among children aged 12 to 15 months has been studied, and no interference with immunogenicity to antigens in any of the vaccines was observed. Among adults aged 50 years or older, the safety and immunogenicity of zoster vaccine and TIV were similar whether administered simultaneously or spaced 4 weeks apart. In the absence of specific data indicating interference, following ACIP's general recommendations for vaccination is prudent. Inactivated vaccines do not interfere with the immune response to other inactivated vaccines or to live vaccines. Inactivated or live vaccines can be administered simultaneously with LAIV. However, after administration of a live vaccine, at least 4 weeks should pass before another live vaccine is administered.

TABLE 5-30 Live Attenuated Influenza Vaccine (LAIV) Compared with Inactivated Influenza Vaccine (TIV) for Seasonal Influenza, United States Formulations

Factor	LAIV	TIV
Route of administration	Intranasal spray	Intramuscular injection
Type of vaccine	Live virus	Noninfectious virus (i.e.,inactivated)
Number of included virus strains	3 (2 influenza A, 1 influenza B)	3 (2 influenza A, 1 influenza B)
Vaccine virus strains updated	Annually	Annually
Frequency of administration	Annually*	Annually*
Approved age	Persons aged 2-49 yr	Persons aged ≥6 mo
Interval between 2 doses recommended for children aged ≥6 mo to 8 yr who are receiving influenza vaccine for the first time	4 wk	4 wk
Can be administered to persons with medical risk factors for influenza-related complications[†]	No	Yes
Can be administered to children with asthma or children aged 2-4 yr with wheezing during the preceding year[§]	No	Yes
Can be administered to family members or close contacts of immunosuppressed persons not requiring a protected environment	Yes	Yes
Can be administered to family members or close contacts of immunosuppressed persons requiring a protected environment (e.g., hematopoietic stem cell transplant recipient)	No	Yes
Can be administered to family members or close contacts of persons at high risk but not severely immunosuppressed	Yes	Yes
Can be simultaneously administered with other vaccines	Yes[¶]	Yes**
If not simultaneously administered, can be administered within 4 wk of another live vaccine	Prudent to space 4 wk apart	Yes
If not simultaneously administered, can be administered within 4 wk of an inactivated vaccine	Yes	Yes

Modified from *MMWR* 56(RR-6), 2007.
LAIV, Live attenuated influenza vaccine; *TIV,* inactivated influenza vaccine.
*Children aged 6 months-8 years who have never received influenza vaccine before should receive 2 doses. Those who only receive 1 dose in their first year of vaccination should receive 2 doses in the following year, spaced 4 weeks apart.
[†]Persons at higher risk for complications of influenza infection because of underlying medical conditions should not receive LAIV. Persons at higher risk for complications of influenza infection because of underlying medical conditions include adults and children with chronic disorders of the pulmonary or cardiovascular systems; adults and children with chronic metabolic diseases (including diabetes mellitus), renal dysfunction, hemoglobinopathies, or immunosuppression; children and adolescents receiving long-term aspirin therapy (at risk for developing Reye's syndrome after wild-type influenza infection); persons who have any condition (e.g., cognitive dysfunction, spinal cord injuries, seizure disorders, or other neuromuscular disorders) that can compromise respiratory function or the handling of respiratory secretions or that can increase the risk for aspiration; pregnant women; and residents of nursing homes and other chronic-care facilities that house persons with chronic medical conditions.
[§]Clinicians and immunization programs should screen for possible reactive airways diseases when considering use of LAIV for children aged 2-4 years and should avoid use of this vaccine in children with asthma or a recent wheezing episode. Health care providers should consult the medical record, when available, to identify children aged 2-4 years with asthma or recurrent wheezing that might indicate asthma. In addition, to identify children who might be at greater risk for asthma and possibly at increased risk for wheezing after receiving LAIV, parents or caregivers of children aged 2-4 years should be asked: "In the past 12 months, has a health care provider ever told you that your child had wheezing or asthma?" Children whose parents or caregivers answer "yes" to this question and children who have asthma or who had a wheezing episode noted in the medical record during the preceding 12 months should not receive LAIV.
[¶]LAIV coadministration has been evaluated systematically only among children aged 12–15 months who received measles, mumps, and rubella vaccine or varicella vaccine.
**TIV coadministration has been evaluated systematically only among adults who received pneumococcal polysaccharide or zoster vaccine.

INDICATIONS FOR USE OF ANTIVIRALS

PERSONS FOR WHOM ANTIVIRAL TREATMENT SHOULD BE CONSIDERED

If possible, antiviral treatment should be started within 48 hours of influenza illness onset. The effectiveness of initiating antiviral treatment more than 48 hours after illness onset has not been established. Persons for whom antiviral treatment should be considered include:

- Persons hospitalized with laboratory-confirmed influenza (limited data suggest benefit even for persons whose antiviral treatment is initiated more than 48 hours after illness onset)
- Persons with laboratory-confirmed influenza pneumonia
- Persons with laboratory-confirmed influenza and bacterial coinfection
- Persons with laboratory-confirmed influenza infection who are at higher risk for influenza complications
- Persons presenting to medical care with laboratory-confirmed influenza within 48 hours of influenza illness onset who want to decrease the duration or severity of their symptoms and transmission of influenza to others at higher risk for complications

PERSONS FOR WHOM ANTIVIRAL CHEMOPROPHYLAXIS SHOULD BE CONSIDERED DURING PERIODS OF INCREASED INFLUENZA ACTIVITY IN THE COMMUNITY

- Persons at high risk during the 2 weeks after influenza vaccination (after the second dose for children younger than 9 years who have not previously been vaccinated) if influenza viruses are circulating in the community
- Persons at high risk for whom influenza vaccine is contraindicated
- Family members or health care providers who are unvaccinated and are likely to have ongoing, close exposure to persons at high risk or unvaccinated persons or infants younger than 6 months
- Persons and their family members and close contacts and health care workers when circulating strains of influenza virus in the community are not matched with vaccine strains
- Persons with immune deficiencies or those who might not respond to vaccination (e.g., persons infected with HIV or other immunosuppressed conditions or who are receiving immunosuppressive medications)
- Unvaccinated staff and persons during response to an outbreak in a closed institutional setting with residents at high risk (e.g., extended-care facilities)

Modified from *MMWR* 57(RR-7), 2008.

Note: Recommended antiviral medications (neuraminidase inhibitors) are not licensed for chemoprophylaxis of children younger than 1 year (oseltamivir) or younger than 5 years (zanamivir). Updates or supplements to these recommendations (e.g., expanded age or risk group indications for licensed vaccines) might be required. Health care providers should be alert to announcements of recommendation updates and should check the CDC influenza website periodically for additional information (http://www.cdc.gov/flu).

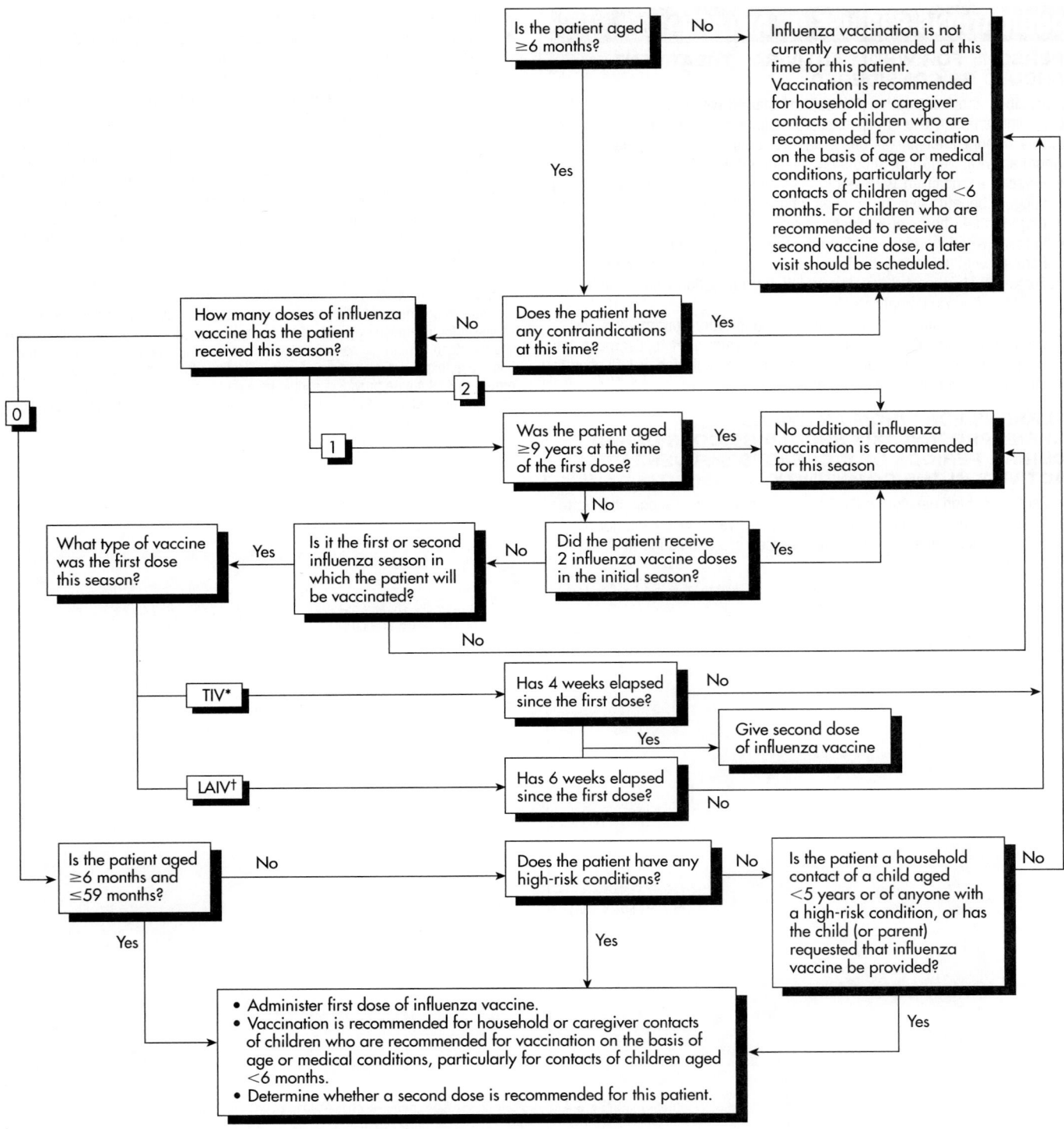

*Trivalent inactivated influenza vaccine.
†Live, attenuated influenza vaccine.

FIGURE 5-6 Algorithm for determining recommended influenza immunization actions for children. (Modified with permission from the American Academy of Pediatrics' Committee on Infectious Diseases: Prevention of influenza: recommendations for influenza immunization of children, 2006-2007, *Pediatrics* 119:846-51.315, 2007.)

HIV Testing and Postexposure Prophylaxis

RECOMMENDATIONS FOR HIV TESTING OF ADULTS, ADOLESCENTS, AND PREGNANT WOMEN

RECOMMENDATIONS FOR ADULTS AND ADOLESCENTS*

The CDC recommends that diagnostic human immunodeficiency virus (HIV) testing and opt-out HIV screening be a part of routine clinical care in all health care settings while also preserving the patient's option to decline HIV testing and ensuring a provider-patient relationship conducive to optimal clinical and preventive care. The recommendations are intended for providers in all health care settings, including hospital emergency departments, urgent-care clinics, inpatient services, sexually transmitted disease (STD) clinics or other venues offering clinical STD services, tuberculosis (TB) clinics, substance abuse treatment clinics, other public health clinics, community clinics, correctional health care facilities, and primary care settings. The guidelines address HIV testing in health care settings only; they do not modify existing guidelines concerning HIV counseling, testing, and referral for persons at high risk for HIV who seek or receive HIV testing in nonclinical settings (e.g., community-based organizations, outreach settings, or mobile vans).

SCREENING FOR HIV INFECTION

- In all health care settings, screening for HIV infection should be performed routinely for all patients aged 13 to 64 years. Health care providers should initiate screening unless prevalence of undiagnosed HIV infection in their patients has been documented to be less than 0.1%. In the absence of existing data for HIV prevalence, health care providers should initiate voluntary HIV screening until they establish that the diagnostic yield is less than 1 per 1000 patients screened, at which point such screening is no longer warranted.
- All patients initiating treatment for TB should be screened routinely for HIV infection.
- All patients seeking treatment for STDs, including all patients visiting STD clinics, should be screened routinely for HIV during each visit for a new complaint, regardless of whether the patient is known or suspected to have specific behavior risks for HIV infection.

REPEAT SCREENING

- Health care providers should subsequently test all persons likely to be at high risk for HIV at least annually. Persons likely to be at high risk include users of injection drugs and their sex partners, persons who exchange sex for money or drugs, sex partners of persons who are HIV infected, and men who have sex with men (MSM) or heterosexual persons who themselves or whose sex partners have had more than one sex partner since their most recent HIV test.
- Health care providers should encourage patients and their prospective sex partners to be tested before initiating a new sexual relationship.
- Repeat screening of persons not likely to be at high risk for HIV should be performed on the basis of clinical judgment.
- Unless recent HIV test results are immediately available, any person whose blood or body fluid is the source of an occupational exposure for a health care provider should be informed of the incident and tested for HIV infection at the time the exposure occurs.

CONSENT AND PRETEST INFORMATION

- Screening should be voluntary and undertaken only with the patient's knowledge and understanding that HIV testing is planned.
- Patients should be informed orally or in writing that HIV testing will be performed unless they decline (opt-out screening). Oral or written information should include an explanation of HIV infection and the meanings of positive and negative test results, and the patient should be offered an opportunity to ask questions and decline testing. With such notification, consent for HIV screening should be incorporated into the patient's

general informed consent for medical care on the same basis as are other screening or diagnostic tests; a separate consent form for HIV testing is not recommended.
- Easily understood informational materials should be made available in the languages of the commonly encountered populations within the service area. The competence of interpreters and bilingual staff to provide language assistance to patients with limited English proficiency must be ensured.
- If a patient declines an HIV test, this decision should be documented in the medical record.

DIAGNOSTIC TESTING FOR HIV INFECTION

- All patients with signs or symptoms consistent with HIV infection or an opportunistic illness characteristic of acquired immunodeficiency syndrome (AIDS) should be tested for HIV.
- Clinicians should maintain a high level of suspicion for acute HIV infection in all patients who have a compatible clinical syndrome and who report recent high-risk behavior. When acute retroviral syndrome is a possibility, a plasma RNA test should be used in conjunction with an HIV antibody test to diagnose acute HIV infection.
- Patients or persons responsible for the patient's care should be notified orally that testing is planned, advised of the indication for testing and the implications of positive and negative test results, and offered an opportunity to ask questions and decline testing. With such notification, the patient's general consent for medical care is considered sufficient for diagnostic HIV testing.

HIV SCREENING FOR PREGNANT WOMEN AND THEIR INFANTS*

UNIVERSAL OPT-OUT SCREENING

- All pregnant women in the United States should be screened for HIV infection.
- Screening should occur after a woman is notified that HIV screening is recommended for all pregnant patients and that she will receive an HIV test as part of the routine panel of prenatal tests unless she declines (opt-out screening).
- HIV testing must be voluntary and free from coercion. No woman should be tested without her knowledge.
- Pregnant women should receive oral or written information that includes an explanation of HIV infection, a description of interventions that can reduce HIV transmission from mother to infant, and the meanings of positive and negative test results. They should be offered an opportunity to ask questions and decline testing.
- No additional process or written documentation of informed consent beyond what is required for other routine prenatal tests should be required for HIV testing.
- If a patient declines an HIV test, this decision should be documented in the medical record.

ADDRESSING REASONS FOR DECLINING TESTING

- Providers should discuss and address reasons for declining an HIV test (e.g., lack of perceived risk, fear of the disease, and concerns regarding partner violence or potential stigma or discrimination).
- Women who decline an HIV test because they have had a previous negative test result should be informed of the importance of retesting during each pregnancy.
- Logistical reasons for not testing (e.g., scheduling) should be resolved.
- Certain women who initially decline an HIV test might accept at a later date, especially if their concerns are discussed. Certain women will continue to decline testing, and their decisions should be respected and documented in the medical record.

TIMING OF HIV TESTING

- To promote informed and timely therapeutic decisions, health care providers should test women for HIV as early as possible during each pregnancy. Women who decline the test early in prenatal care should be encouraged to be tested at a subsequent visit.

*MMWR 57(RR-10), 2008.

- A second HIV test during the third trimester, preferably less than 36 weeks of gestation, is cost effective even in areas of low HIV prevalence and may be considered for all pregnant women. A second HIV test during the third trimester is recommended for women who meet one or more of the following criteria:
  - Women who receive health care in jurisdictions with elevated incidence of HIV or AIDS among women aged 15 to 45 years. In 2004, these jurisdictions included Alabama, Connecticut, Delaware, the District of Columbia, Florida, Georgia, Illinois, Louisiana, Maryland, Massachusetts, Mississippi, Nevada, New Jersey, New York, North Carolina, Pennsylvania, Puerto Rico, Rhode Island, South Carolina, Tennessee, Texas, and Virginia.[†]
  - Women who receive health care in facilities in which prenatal screening identifies at least one pregnant woman who is infected with HIV per 1000 women screened.
  - Women who are known to be at high risk for acquiring HIV (e.g., users of injection drugs and their sex partners, women who exchange sex for money or drugs, women who are sex partners of persons who are infected with HIV, and women who have had a new or more than one sex partner during this pregnancy).
  - Women who have signs or symptoms consistent with acute HIV infection. When acute retroviral syndrome is a possibility, a plasma RNA test should be used in conjunction with an HIV antibody test to diagnose acute HIV infection.

[†]A second HIV test in the third trimester is as cost effective as other common health interventions when HIV incidence among women of childbearing age is ≥17 HIV cases per 100,000 person-years. In 2004, in jurisdictions with available data on HIV case rates, a rate of 17 new HIV diagnoses per year per 100,000 women aged 15 to 45 years was associated with an AIDS case rate of at least nine AIDS diagnoses per year per 100,000 women aged 15 to 45 years (CDC, unpublished data, 2005). As of 2004, the jurisdictions listed above exceeded these thresholds. The list of specific jurisdictions where a second test in the third trimester is recommended will be updated periodically based on surveillance data.

RAPID TESTING DURING LABOR
- Any woman with undocumented HIV status at the time of labor should be screened with a rapid HIV test unless she declines (opt-out screening).
- Reasons for declining a rapid test should be explored (see "Addressing Reasons for Declining Testing").
- Immediate initiation of appropriate antiretroviral prophylaxis should be recommended to women on the basis of a reactive rapid test result without waiting for the result of a confirmatory test.

POSTPARTUM/NEWBORN TESTING
- When a woman's HIV status is still unknown at the time of delivery, she should be screened immediately postpartum with a rapid HIV test unless she declines (opt-out screening).
- When the mother's HIV status is unknown postpartum, rapid testing of the newborn as soon as possible after birth is recommended so that antiretroviral prophylaxis can be offered to infants exposed to HIV. Women should be informed that identifying HIV antibodies in the newborn indicates that the mother is infected.
- For infants whose HIV exposure status is unknown and who are in foster care, the person legally authorized to provide consent should be informed that rapid HIV testing is recommended for infants whose biologic mothers have not been tested.
- The benefits of neonatal antiretroviral prophylaxis are best realized when it is initiated within 12 hours after birth.

CONFIRMATORY TESTING
- Whenever possible, uncertainties regarding laboratory test results indicating HIV infection status should be resolved before final decisions are made regarding reproductive options, antiretroviral therapy, cesarean delivery, or other interventions.
- If the confirmatory test result is not available before delivery, immediate initiation of appropriate antiretroviral prophylaxis should be recommended to any pregnant patient whose HIV screening test result is reactive to reduce the risk for perinatal transmission.

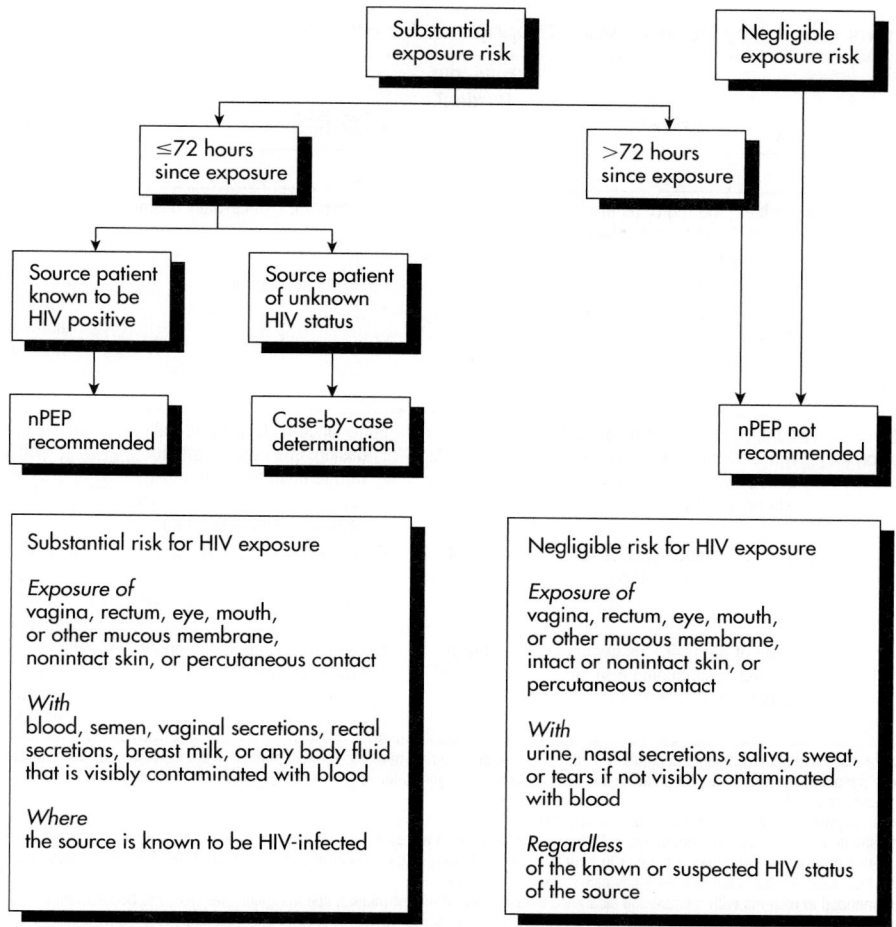

FIGURE 5-7 Algorithm for evaluation and treatment of possible nonoccupational HIV exposure. *nPEP,* Nonoccupational postexposure prophylaxis. (Modified from *MMWR* 54[RR-2], 2005.)

TABLE 5-31   HIV Exposure, Estimated Per-Act Risk

Exposure Route	Risk per 10,000 Exposures to an Infected Source
Blood transfusion	9000
Needle-sharing injection drug use	67
Receptive anal intercourse	50
Percutaneous needle stick	30
Receptive penile-vaginal intercourse	10
Insertive anal intercourse	6.5
Insertive penile-vaginal intercourse	5
Receptive oral intercourse	1
Insertive oral intercourse	0.5

Modified from *MMWR* 54(RR-2), 2005.
Estimates of risk for transmission from sexual exposures assume no condom use.
Source refers to oral intercourse performed on a man.

TABLE 5-32 Regimens for 28-Day Postexposure Prophylaxis for HIV Infection*

Regimen	Dose	Daily Pill Burden[†] no.	Advantages	Disadvantages
Two-Drug Regimens				
Tenofovir–emtricitabine (Truvada)[‡]	One tablet (300 mg of tenofovir with 200 mg of emtricitabine) once daily	1	Well-tolerated; once-daily dosing	Potential nephrotoxicity
Zidovudine–lamivudine (Combivir)[§]	One tablet (300 mg of zidovudine with 150 mg of lamivudine) twice daily	2	Preferred in pregnancy	Twice-daily dosing; less well-tolerated than tenofovir–emtricitabine (nausea, asthenia, neutropenia, anemia, abnormal liver-enzyme levels)
Three-Drug Regimens[¶]				
Ritonavir–lopinavir (Kaletra) (plus either tenofovir–emtricitabine or zidovudine–lamivudine)	Two tablets (50 mg of ritonavir with 200 mg of lopinavir per tablet) twice daily, or four tablets once daily	5 or 6	Either once-daily or twice-daily dosing; one copayment; no refrigeration required; most experience in pregnancy; high genetic barrier to resistance	Gastrointestinal side effects such as diarrhea; may cause elevated liver-enzyme levels or hepatitis
Ritonavir plus atazanavir (plus either tenofovir–emtricitabine or zidovudine–lamivudine)	100 mg of ritonavir plus 300 mg of atazanavir once daily	3 or 4	Once-daily dosing; well tolerated	Ritonavir must be refrigerated; potential for asymptomatic jaundice, renal stones; may cause elevated liver-enzyme levels or hepatitis
Ritonavir plus darunavir (plus either tenofovir–emtricitabine or zidovudine–lamivudine)	100 mg of ritonavir plus two tablets, each containing 400 mg of darunavir, once daily	4 or 5	Once-daily dosing; high genetic barrier to resistance	Ritonavir must be refrigerated; gastrointestinal side effects; may cause elevated liver-enzyme levels or hepatitis

*Tenofovir, emtricitabine, and lamivudine all have activity against hepatitis B. Patients with chronic active hepatitis B (i.e., patients who are positive for hepatitis B surface antigen) may have flares of hepatitis on withdrawal of these agents at the completion of postexposure prophylaxis treatment. Referral to a hepatitis specialist or serial monthly monitoring of liver-enzyme levels for up to 6 months after treatment should be considered.

[†]The daily pill burden in the three-drug regimens depends on which two-drug regimen is chosen.

[‡]The dose of tenofovir–emtricitabine should be reduced to one tablet every 48 hours in patients with a creatinine clearance of 30 to 49 ml per minute. Tenofovir–emtricitabine is not recommended in patients with a creatinine clearance of less than 30 ml per minute or in patients who are undergoing hemodialysis; see the guidelines from the Department of Health and Human Services for considerations regarding doses of individual agents in patients with advanced renal dysfunction.

[§]Zidovudine–lamivudine is not recommended in patients with a creatinine clearance of less than 50 ml per minute; see the guidelines from the Department of Health and Human Services for considerations regarding doses of individual agents in patients with renal dysfunction.

[¶]The boosting agent ritonavir is not considered to be an active drug in tabulating the number of agents in the three-drug regimen.

From Landovitz RJ, Currier JS: Postexposure prophylaxis for HIV infection, *N Engl J Med* 361:1768-75, 2009.

TABLE 5-33 Highly Active Antiretroviral Therapy Medications, Adult Dosage, and Side Effects

Medication	Adult Dosage*	Side Effects and Toxicities
Combination Tablets		
Lopinavir/ritonavir (Kaletra)‡	3 tablets twice daily 400 mg lopinavir/100 mg ritonavir	Diarrhea, nausea, vomiting; asthenia; elevated transaminases; hyperglycemia; fat redistribution; lipid abnormalities; possible increased bleeding in persons with hemophilia; pancreatitis
Zidovudine/lamivudine (Combivir)	1 tablet twice daily 300 mg zidovudine/150 mg lamivudine	See following individual medications
Zidovudine/lamivudine/abacavir (Trizivir)	1 tablet twice daily 300 mg zidovudine/150 mg lamivudine/ 300 mg abacavir	See following individual medications
Lamivudine/abacavir (Epzicom)	1 tablet once daily 300 mg lamivudine/600 mg abacavir	See following individual medications
Emtricitabine/tenofovir (Truvada)	1 tablet once daily 200 mg emtricitabine/300 mg tenofovir	See following individual medications
Single Agents		
Nucleoside and nucleotide reverse transcriptase inhibitors (side effects as a class: lactic acidosis, severe hepatomegaly with steatosis, including some fatal cases)		
Abacavir (Ziagen, ABC)‡	300 mg twice daily or 600 mg once daily	Severe hypersensitivity reaction (can be fatal); nausea; vomiting
Didanosine (Videx, ddl)‡	>60 kg (132 lb) body weight: 200 mg twice daily or 400 mg daily; if with tenofovir, 250 mg/daily <60 kg (132 lb): 125 mg twice daily or 250 mg daily; if with tenofovir, dose not established Do not use with stavudine (d4T, Zerit) during pregnancy; avoid ddl/d4T combination in general because of increased risk for adverse events (e.g., neuropathy, pancreatitis, and hyperlactatemia)	Pancreatitis; nausea, diarrhea; peripheral neuropathy
Emtricitabine (Emtriva, FTC)	200 mg once daily	Minimal toxicity; lactic acidosis and hepatic steatosis a rare but possibly life-threatening event
Lamivudine (Epivir, 3TC)‡	150 mg twice daily or 300 mg once daily	Minimal toxicity; lactic acidosis and hepatic steatosis a rare but possibly life-threatening event
Stavudine (Zerit, d4T)‡	>60 kg (132 lb) body weight: 40 mg twice daily <60 kg (132 lb) body weight: 30 mg twice daily Do not use with didanosine (ddl, Videx) during pregnancy; avoid ddl/d4T combination in general because of increased risk of adverse events (e.g., neuropathy, pancreatitis, and hyperlactatemia)	Pancreatitis; peripheral neuropathy; rapidly progressive ascending neuromuscular weakness (rare)
Tenofovir (Viread)	300 mg daily	Nausea, vomiting, diarrhea; headache; asthenia; flatulence; renal impairment
Zidovudine (Retrovir, AZT)‡	200 mg three times daily or 300 mg twice daily	Bone marrow suppression (anemia, neutropenia); gastrointestinal intolerance; headache; insomnia; asthenia; and myopathy
Nonnucleoside reverse transcriptase inhibitors (side effects as a class: Stevens-Johnson syndrome)		
Efavirenz (Sustiva)	600 mg daily at bedtime	Rash; central nervous system symptoms (e.g., dizziness, impaired concentration, insomnia, and abnormal dreams); transaminase elevation; false-positive cannabinoid test
Protease inhibitors (side effects as a class: gastrointestinal intolerance, hyperlipidemia, hyperglycemia, diabetes, fat redistribution, and possible increased bleeding in hemophiliacs; do not use during known or possible pregnancy)		
Atazanavir (Reyataz)	400 mg once daily; if administered with tenofovir plus ritonavir, 300 mg once daily	Indirect hyperbilirubinemia; prolonged PR interval (use caution in patients with underlying cardiac conduction defects or on concomitant medications that can cause PR prolongation)
Fosamprenavir (Lexiva)‡	1400 mg twice daily	Gastrointestinal intolerance, nausea, vomiting, diarrhea; rash; elevated transaminases; headache
Indinavir (Crixivan)	800 mg q8h With ritonavir (might increase risk for renal adverse events): 800 mg indinavir and 100 mg ritonavir q12h or 800 mg indinavir and 200 mg ritonavir every q12h	Gastrointestinal intolerance, nausea; nephrolithiasis; headache; asthenia; blurred vision; metallic taste; thrombocytopenia; hemolytic anemia; indirect hyperbilirubinemia (inconsequential)
Nelfinavir (Viracept)‡	750 mg three times daily or one 250 mg twice daily	Diarrhea; elevated transaminases
Ritonavir (Norvir)‡	See doses used in combination with other specific protease inhibitors	Gastrointestinal intolerance; nausea, vomiting, diarrhea; paresthesias; hepatitis; pancreatitis; asthenia; taste perversion; many drug interactions
Saquinavir (hard-gel capsule) (Invirase)	With ritonavir: 400 mg saquinavir and 400 mg ritonavir twice daily or 1000 mg saquinavir and 100 mg ritonavir twice daily	Gastrointestinal intolerance; nausea, diarrhea; headache; elevated transaminases
Saquinavir (soft-gel capsule) (Fortavase)	With ritonavir: 400 mg saquinavir and 400 mg ritonavir twice daily or 1000 mg saquinavir and 100 mg ritonavir twice daily	Gastrointestinal intolerance; nausea, diarrhea; abdominal pain; dyspepsia; headache; elevated transaminases

*For pediatric dosing information, see *Guidelines for Use of Antiretroviral Agents in Pediatric HIV Infection*, available at http://www.aidsinfo.nih.gov/guidelines/default_db2.asp?id=51.
‡Pediatric formulation available.

Sources: Modified from U.S. Department of Health and Human Services and the Henry J. Kaiser Family Foundation. Guidelines for the use of antiretroviral agents in HIV-infected adults and adolescents. Available at http://www.aidsinfo.nih.gov/guidelines/default_db2.asp?id=50 (refer to website for updated versions). Bartlett JG, Finkbeiner AK: HIV drugs: the guide to living with HIV infection, 2001. Available at http://www.thebody.com/jh/bartlett/drugs.html.

TABLE 5-34 Laboratory Tests Generally Recommended for Persons after Exposure to HIV*

TEST	RECOMMENDED DURING TREATMENT		RECOMMENDED AT FOLLOW-UP		
	Baseline	Symptom-Directed†	4-6 wk	12 wk	24 wk
ELISA for HIV antibodies	Yes	Yes	Yes	Yes	Yes
Creatinine, liver function, and complete blood count with differential count	Yes	Yes	No	No	No
HIV viral load	No	Yes	No	No	No
Anti-HBs antibodies	Yes‡	No	No	No	No
HBsAg	Yes‡§	No	No	No	No
HCV antibodies	Yes	No	Yes	Yes	Yes
HCV RNA¶	No	Yes	Yes	Yes	Yes
Screening, including rapid plasma reagin test, for other sexually transmitted infections‖	Yes	Yes	No	Yes	No

*Patients who receive zidovudine plus lamivudine–based regimens should have a complete blood count and measurement of liver-enzyme levels at 2 weeks of treatment, irrespective of the presence or absence of clinical symptoms. Tenofovir plus emtricitabine–based regimens generally involve few side effects, and symptom-directed assessment of serum creatinine or liver-enzyme levels should be considered. The addition of a ritonavir-boosted protease inhibitor should be followed by symptom-directed assessment of liver-enzyme levels, serum glucose levels, or both. Anti-HBs antibodies denotes hepatitis B virus surface antibodies, ELISA enzyme-linked immunosorbent assay, HBsAg hepatitis B surface antigen, and HCV hepatitis C virus.
†Symptom-directed tests are for signs or symptoms of toxic effects (rash, nausea, vomiting, or abdominal pain) or HIV seroconversion (fever, fatigue, lymphadenopathy, rash, or oral or genital ulcers).
‡If tests for anti-HBs antibodies and HBsAg are both negative, a vaccination series against HBV infection should be initiated and completed.
§If the patient is HBsAg-positive, he or she should have monthly follow-up of liver-function tests after discontinuation of postexposure prophylactic regimens containing tenofovir, lamivudine, or emtricitabine; referral to a specialist in viral hepatitis should be considered.
¶HCV RNA testing may identify early HCV seroconversion; early detection and treatment during acute HCV infection may avert or ameliorate chronic disease. Data are from Dienstag and McHutchison.
‖Rapid plasma reagin testing and testing of urethral-swab and rectal-swab specimens for gonorrhea and chlamydia and of pharyngeal-swab specimens for gonorrhea should be performed as appropriate, according to the patient's sexual risk-taking behaviors and the type of exposure to HIV.
From Landovitz RJ, Currier JS: *Postexposure Prophylaxis for HIV infection,* N Engl J Med 361:1768-75, 2009

BOX 5-4 Situations for Which Expert Consultation for HIV Postexposure Prophylaxis Is Advised*

- Delayed (i.e., later than 24-36 hours) exposure report
  - The interval after which there is no benefit from postexposure prophylaxis (PEP) is undefined
- Unknown source (e.g., needle in sharps disposal container or laundry)
  - Decide use of PEP on a case-by-case basis
  - Consider the severity of the exposure and the epidemiologic likelihood of HIV exposure
  - Do not test needles or other sharp instruments for HIV
- Known or suspected pregnancy in the exposed person
  - Does not preclude the use of optimal PEP regimens
  - Do not deny PEP solely on the basis of pregnancy
- Resistance of the source virus to antiretroviral agents
  - Influence of drug resistance on transmission risk is unknown
  - Selection of drugs to which the source person's virus is unlikely to be resistant is recommended if the source person's virus is known or suspected to be resistant to one or more of the drugs considered for the PEP regimen
  - Resistance testing of the source person's virus at the time of the exposure is not recommended
- Toxicity of the initial PEP regimen
  - Adverse symptoms such as nausea and diarrhea are common with PEP
  - Symptoms often can be managed without changing the PEP regimen by prescribing antimotility and/or antiemetic agents
  - Modification of dose intervals (i.e., administering a lower dose of drug more frequently throughout the day, as recommended by the manufacturer) in other situations might help alleviate symptoms

*Local experts and/or the National Clinicians' Postexposure Prophylaxis Hotline (PEPline [888-448-4911]).

BOX 5-5 Occupational Exposure Management Resources

National Clinicians' Postexposure Prophylaxis Hotline (PEPline)
Run by University of California–San Francisco/San Francisco General Hospital staff; supported by the Health Resources and Services Administration, Ryan White CARE Act, HIV/AIDS Bureau, AIDS Education and Training Centers, and CDC

Phone: 888-448-4911
Internet: http://www.ucsf.edu/hivcntr

Needlestick!
A website to help clinicians manage and document occupational blood and body fluid exposures. Developed and maintained by the University of California, Los Angeles (UCLA), Emergency Medicine Center, UCLA School of Medicine, and funded in part by CDC and the Agency for Healthcare Research and Quality

Internet: http://www.needlestick.mednet.ucla.edu

Hepatitis Hotline

Phone: 888-443-7232
Internet: http://www.cdc.gov/ncidod/diseases/hepatitis/index.htm

Reporting to CDC: Occupationally acquired HIV infections and failures of PEP

Phone: 800-893-0485

HIV Antiretroviral Pregnancy Registry

Phone: 800-258-4263
Fax: 800-800-1052
Address: 1410 Commonwealth Dr., Suite 215, Wilmington, NC 28405
Internet: http://www.glaxowellcome.com/preg_reg/antiretroviral

Food and Drug Administration
Report unusual or severe toxicity to antiretroviral agents

Phone: 800-332-1088
Address: MedWatch, HF-2, FDA, 5600 Fishers Lane, Rockville, MD 20857
Internet: http://www.fda.gov/medwatch

HIV/AIDS Treatment Information Service

Internet: http://www.hivatis.org

BOX 5-6 Management of Occupational Blood Exposures

Provide immediate care to the exposure site:
- Wash wounds and skin with soap and water
- Flush mucous membranes with water

Determine risk associated with exposure:
- Type of fluid (e.g., blood, visibly bloody fluid, other potentially infectious fluid or tissue, and concentrated virus)
- Type of exposure (e.g., percutaneous injury, mucous membrane or nonintact skin exposure, and bites resulting in blood exposure)

Evaluate exposure source:
- Assess the risk of infection using available information
- Test known sources for HBsAg, anti-HCV, and HIV antibodies (consider using rapid testing)
- For unknown sources, assess risk of exposure to HBV, HCV, or HIV infection
- Do not test discarded needles or syringes for virus contamination

Evaluate the exposed person:
- Assess immune status for HBV infection (i.e., by history of hepatitis B vaccination and vaccine response)

Give PEP for exposures posing risk of infection transmission:
- HBV: See Table 5-26
- HCV: PEP not recommended
- HIV: See Tables 5-34, 5-35, and 5-36 and Figure 5-7
  - Initiate PEP as soon as possible, preferably within hours of exposure
  - Offer pregnancy testing to all women of childbearing age not known to be pregnant
  - Seek expert consultation if viral resistance is suspected
  - Administer PEP for 4 weeks if tolerated

Perform follow-up testing and provide counseling:
- Advise exposed persons to seek medical evaluation for any acute illness occurring during follow-up

HBV exposures
- Perform follow-up anti-HBs testing in persons who receive hepatitis B vaccine
  - Test for anti-HBs 1 to 2 months after last dose of vaccine
  - Anti-HBs response to vaccine cannot be ascertained if HBIG was received in the previous 3 to 4 months

HCV exposures
- Perform baseline and follow-up testing for anti-HCV and alanine aminotransferase 4 to 6 months after exposures
- Perform HCV RNA at 4 to 6 weeks if earlier diagnosis of HCV infection desired
- Confirm repeatedly reactive anti-HCV enzyme immunoassays with supplemental tests

HIV exposures
- Perform HIV-antibody testing for at least 6 months after exposure (e.g., at baseline, 6 weeks, 3 months, and 6 months)
- Perform HIV-antibody testing if illness compatible with an acute retroviral syndrome occurs
- Advise exposed persons to use precautions to prevent secondary transmission during the follow-up period
- Evaluate exposed persons taking PEP within 72 hr after exposure and monitor for drug toxicity for at least 2 weeks

HBIG, Hepatitis B immune globulin; *HBsAg,* hepatitis B surface antigen; *HBV,* hepatitis B virus; *HCV,* hepatitis C virus; *HIV,* human immunodeficiency virus; *PEP,* post-exposure prophylaxis; *RNA,* ribonucleic acid.

Endocarditis Prophylaxis*

TABLE 5-35 Cardiac Conditions Associated with the Highest Risk of Adverse Outcome from Endocarditis for Which Prophylaxis with Dental Procedures Is Recommended

Prosthetic cardiac valve

Previous infective endocarditis

CHD*

Unrepaired cyanotic CHD, including palliative shunts and conduits

Completely repaired congenital heart defect with prosthetic material or device, whether placed by surgery or by catheter intervention, during the first 6 mo after the procedure†

Repaired CHD with residual defects at the site or adjacent to the site of a prosthetic patch or prosthetic device (that inhibit endothelialization)

Cardiac transplant recipients who develop cardiac valvulopathy

CHD, Congenital heart disease.

*Except for the conditions listed above, antibiotic prophylaxis is no longer recommended for any other form of CHD.

†Prophylaxis is recommended because endothelialization of prosthetic material occurs within 6 mo after the procedure.

TABLE 5-36 Dental Procedures for Which Endocarditis Prophylaxis Is Recommended for Patients in Table 5-35

All dental procedures that involve manipulation of gingival tissue or the periapical region of teeth or perforation of the oral mucosa*

*The following procedures and events do not need prophylaxis: routine anesthetic injections through noninfected tissue, taking dental radiographs, placement of removable prosthodontic or orthodontic appliances, adjustment of orthodontic appliances, placement of orthodontic brackets, shedding of deciduous teeth, and bleeding from trauma to the lips or oral mucosa.

TABLE 5-37 Regimens for a Dental Procedure

Situation	REGIMEN: SINGLE DOSE 30-60 MIN BEFORE PROCEDURE		
	Agent	Adults	Children
Oral	Amoxicillin	2 g	50 mg/kg
Unable to take oral medication	Ampicillin OR	2 g IM or IV	50 mg/kg IM or IV
	Cefazolin or ceftriaxone*	1 g IM or IV	50 mg/kg IM or IV
Allergic to penicillins or ampicillin, oral	Cephalexin*† OR	2 g	50 mg/kg
	Clindamycin OR	600 mg	20 mg/kg
	Azithromycin or clarithromycin	500 mg	15 mg/kg
Allergic to penicillins or ampicillin and unable to take oral medicine	Cefazolin or ceftriaxone† OR	1 g IM or IV	50 mg/kg IM or IV
	Clindamycin	600 mg IM or IV	20 mg/kg IM or IV

IM, Intramuscular; *IV*, intravenous.

*Or other first-generation or second-generation oral cephalosporin in equivalent adult or pediatric dosage.

†Cephalosporins should not be used in an individual with a history of anaphylaxis, angioedema, or urticaria with penicillins or ampicillin.

*From Prevention of infective endocarditis. A guideline from the American Heart Association Rheumatic Fever, Endocarditis, and Kawasaki Disease Committee, Council on Cardiovascular Disease in the Young, and the Council on Clinical Cardiology, Council on Cardiovascular Surgery and Anesthesia, and the Quality of Care and Outcomes Research Interdisciplinary Working Group. *Circulation* published online Apr 19, 2007, DOI: 10.1161/CIRCULATIONAHA.106.183095. Copyright © 2007 American Heart Association. All rights reserved. Print ISSN: 0009-7322. Online ISSN: 1524-4539.

TABLE 5-38 Summary of Major Changes in Updated Recommendations

We concluded that bacteremia resulting from daily activities is much more likely to cause IE than bacteremia associated with a dental procedure.

We concluded that only an extremely small number of cases of IE might be prevented by antibiotic prophylaxis even if prophylaxis is 100% effective.

Antibiotic prophylaxis is not recommended based solely on an increased lifetime risk of acquisition of IE.

Limit recommendations for IE prophylaxis only to those conditions listed in Table 5-37.

Antibiotic prophylaxis is no longer recommended for any other form of CHD, except for the conditions listed in Table 5-37.

Antibiotic prophylaxis is recommended for all dental procedures that involve manipulation of gingival tissues or periapical region of teeth or perforation of oral mucosa only for patients with underlying cardiac conditions associated with the highest risk of adverse outcome from IE (see Table 5-37).

Antibiotic prophylaxis is recommended for procedures on respiratory tract or infected skin, skin structures, or musculoskeletal tissue only for patients with underlying cardiac conditions associated with the highest risk of adverse outcome from IE (see Table 5-37).

Antibiotic prophylaxis solely to prevent IE is not recommended for GU or GI tract procedures.

The writing group reaffirms the procedures noted in the 1997 prophylaxis guidelines for which endocarditis prophylaxis is not recommended and extends this to other common procedures, including ear and body piercing, tattooing, and vaginal delivery and hysterectomy.

A guide to the clinical preventive services described is available online at http://www.ahrq.gov/clinic/pocketgd07/.

CHD, Congenital heart disease; *GI*, gastrointestinal; *GU*, genitourinary; *IE*, infective endocarditis.

PART C • GUIDE TO CLINICAL PREVENTIVE SERVICES*

1. Cancer
   a. Screening for bladder cancer in adults
   b. Genetic risk assessment and BRCA mutation testing for breast and ovarian cancer susceptibility
   c. Screening for breast cancer
   d. Screening for cervical cancer
   e. Screening for colorectal cancer
   f. Lung cancer screening
   g. Screening for ovarian cancer
   h. Screening for pancreatic cancer
   i. Screening for prostate cancer
   j. Counseling to prevent skin cancer
   k. Screening for testicular cancer
2. Heart and vascular diseases
   a. Screening for abdominal aortic aneurysm
   b. Aspirin for the primary prevention of cardiovascular events
   c. Screening for coronary heart disease
   d. Screening for lipid disorders in adults
   e. Screening for peripheral arterial disease
3. Infectious diseases
   a. Screening for asymptomatic bacteriuria
   b. Screening for chlamydial infection
   c. Screening for genital herpes
   d. Screening for gonorrhea
   e. Screening for hepatitis B virus infection
   f. Screening for hepatitis C in adults
   g. Screening for syphilis infection
4. Injury and violence
   a. Screening for family and intimate partner violence
5. Mental health conditions and substance abuse
   a. Screening and behavioral counseling interventions in primary care to reduce alcohol misuse
   b. Screening for dementia
   c. Screening for depression
   d. Screening for suicide risk
6. Counseling to prevent tobacco use and tobacco-caused disease
7. Metabolic, nutritional, and endocrine conditions
   a. Behavioral counseling in primary care to promote a healthy diet
   b. Hormone therapy for the prevention of chronic conditions in post-menopausal women
   c. Screening for obesity in adults
   d. Behavioral counseling in primary care to promote physical activity
   e. Screening for thyroid disease
   f. Screening for type 2 diabetes mellitus in adults
8. Musculoskeletal conditions
   a. Primary care interventions to prevent low back pain in adults
   b. Screening for osteoporosis in postmenopausal women
9. Vision disorders
   a. Screening for glaucoma

*Available online.

I. Complementary and Alternative Medicine

II. Primary Care Procedures
(available online)

APPENDIX

I. Complementary and Alternative Medicine

II. Primary Care Procedures
(available online)

Dietary Supplements: What Every Primary Care Provider Should Know

Primary care providers must be knowledgeable regarding the safety, efficacy, and drug interactions associated with common dietary supplements because of the following:

- An estimated 38% of adults ages 18 years and older reported the use of at least one form of complementary and alternative medicine (CAM) according to the National Health Interview Survey in 2007.
- Almost 17.8% of adults specifically reported the use of dietary supplements, with fish oil, glucosamine, echinacea, flaxseed, and ginseng most frequently used.
- Although the use of dietary supplements has plateaued as a result of consumer concerns about effectiveness and potential adverse effects, usage remains common and potentially dangerous.

COMMON TERMINOLOGY

- A *dietary supplement* is defined as an oral product containing vitamins, minerals, herbs, or other botanicals; amino acids; dietary substances used to supplement the diet by increasing the total dietary intake; or a concentrate, metabolite, constituent, extract, or combination.
- *CAM* refers to the broad domain of healing practices that include diverse health systems, modalities, and practices and their accompanying theories and beliefs (see glossary of terms in Appendix Id).
- *Complementary therapies* are those that are used *in addition to* conventional therapies, whereas *alternative therapies* are those that are used *instead of* conventional therapies. Most consumers in the United States use dietary supplements as a complementary therapy.
- *Standardization* refers to the practice of producing dietary supplements with a specific amount of a given compound that may or may not include the actual active ingredient. For example, feverfew has been standardized to its parthenolide content.

LEGISLATION

The U.S. Food and Drug Administration (FDA) is frequently criticized for not closely regulating dietary supplements and monitoring their safety. However, although the agency regulates prescription drugs and over-the-counter (OTC) products, the FDA has limited regulatory authority over dietary supplements. This is because the Dietary Supplement and Health Education Act (DSHEA) of 1994 and its resulting regulations limit the FDA's authority. As a result of DSHEA, the FDA is able to act only when a dietary supplement has been documented to contain a prescription drug, as was the case with glyburide in a natural treatment for diabetes and diazepam in an osteoarthritis preparation. In addition, the FDA can act when safety issues related to a product have been clearly documented, although these cases are frequently challenged in the courts.

HEALTH CLAIMS

Dietary supplements generally are marketed under three types of health claims. The first category is the "nutrient content" claim, in which the product is identified as an excellent source of, typically, a mineral such as calcium, based on recommended daily values. The second type is the "significant scientific agreement" claim; these claims are used when some evidence of the product's efficacy exists (e.g., fish oil supplements). The third and most common type of health claim is called a "structure/function" claim; these claims state that the product has some effect on health—for example, "helps to maintain a healthy heart." However, dietary supplements are not permitted to carry claims stating that they are effective in preventing, treating, or curing diseases.

INFORMATION RESOURCES

Appendix 1b provides a brief overview of common dietary supplements. Until recently, few evidence-based resources on dietary supplements were available. Clinical studies and systematic reviews on dietary supplements are now widely available through PubMed, EMBASE, and the Cochrane Database of Systematic Reviews. Although more information is available, references on specific products vary in their interpretation of the available evidence and may exhibit an unintentional bias, either pro or con, regarding the safety and efficacy of dietary supplements.

"Gold standard" evidence-based databases on dietary supplements (subscription required) include the following:

- Natural Medicines Comprehensive Database (http://www.naturaldatabase.com): This database includes listings for many dietary supplements and is organized in a clinician-friendly manner. Monographs include the different common and scientific names; uses and likely effectiveness for different uses; chemical constituents; interactions with drugs, diseases, foods, and laboratory tests; adverse effects; and cautions. The information is extensively referenced and is updated on a daily basis. The primary limitation is that the evaluation of data on clinical effectiveness could be more rigorous.
- Natural Standard (http://www.naturalstandard.com): This database includes listings for dietary supplements and other forms of complementary and alternative medicine. The evidence supporting the assessments in this database is critically evaluated and rigorous in nature. The primary limitation is that many fewer dietary supplements are included in this database.

Evidence-based free websites on dietary supplements include the following:

- National Center for Complementary and Alternative Medicine (NCCAM) (http://nccam.nih.gov)
- Office of Dietary Supplements International Bibliographic Information on Dietary Supplements (http://dietary-supplements.info.nih.gov/Health_Information/IBIDS.aspx)
- Memorial Sloan-Kettering Cancer Center (http://www.mskcc.org/mskcc/html/11570.cfm)

DRUG INTERACTIONS

Clinically significant interactions have been documented between dietary supplements and prescription or OTC drugs. The challenge for primary care providers is to identify real, clinically relevant interactions versus potential or theoretical interactions. Data on interactions with dietary supplements are usually based on isolated case reports or on studies enrolling healthy volunteers. As with drug-drug interactions, the likelihood of an interaction and its severity are influenced especially by concomitant medical conditions, such as heart failure and presence or absence of impaired kidney and liver function.

Appendix Ic lists interactions between selected natural products and prescription and nonprescription drugs. The following two broad interactions are particularly important in primary care practice:

- St. John's wort, commonly used for depression, is a potent inducer of cytochrome P450 3A4 isoenzymes and has been documented to increase the clearance of many drugs that are metabolized through this (and other) pathways. (For a list of common drugs cleared in this manner, readers should consult http://medicine.iupui.edu/flockhart/clinlist.htm.) In addition, St. John's wort may also induce p-glycoprotein transporter systems that are important for digoxin and some chemotherapeutic agents. St. John's wort has also been associated with the development of serotonin syndrome when used with drugs that have significant serotonergic activity.
- Dietary supplements such as garlic, ginkgo, and feverfew, as well as many others, have been purported to either have antiplatelet activity or have effects on the clotting cascade. This may be important for adults also taking aspirin (and other platelet-active agents) or warfarin.

COUNSELING POINTS

The single most important counseling point related to dietary supplements is always to ask patients about their use of these products and to do so in an open, nonjudgmental manner. The approach should emphasize that many consumers have been interested in vitamins, minerals, herbs, teas, and so on, to maintain their health or to treat illness. If the clinician is unaware of the safety, efficacy, and interactions of a specific product, several websites are available to quickly scan for information. Also, access to drug information centers at colleges of pharmacy is almost always available, and some hospitals now offer programs in integrative medicine.

Patients should be asked about their goals in using the product, as well as how long they have taken it and in what dosage. Allergies to plants should be documented because cross-allergies are common. Clinicians should appreciate that an individual who uses dietary supplements may be interested in making lifestyle changes and potentially decreasing their use of prescription drugs. In addition, if an individual is also consulting an alternative medicine practitioner, clinicians should recognize that some alternative health systems discourage the use of established therapies such as vaccines.

Although problems with safety and efficacy have been identified, many dietary supplements are benign except for their cost. Some patients are at higher risk for adverse outcomes from the use of dietary supplements (e.g., those with chronic kidney and liver disease). Patients should be counseled specifically to avoid purchasing dietary supplements over the Internet.

RESEARCH ISSUES

Many clinical and observational studies of dietary supplements have been published. In the past, clinicians frequently stated that published studies of dietary supplements either did not exist or only a few were available. The reason for this finding was that until recently the National Library of Medicine did not abstract from the peer-reviewed alternative medicine literature. Fortunately, much more research is now readily available. As with all research, the more rigorous the study methodology, the less likely the dietary supplement is to demonstrate clinical benefit.

In evaluating published studies of dietary supplements, the following should be considered:

- Has the correct plant and part of the plant (root, stem, leaf) been used? This critical information may not be known to many clinicians. Consulting a resource such as the National Medicines Comprehensive Database can usually provide the needed information to judge this component of the study.
- Has the content of active ingredients been verified throughout the study? In a recent review of 81 major randomized controlled trials of herbal products, only 12 (15%) reported performing tests to quantify actual contents, and 3 (4%) provided adequate data to compare actual with expected content values of at least one chemical constituent.
- Is the severity of the disease appropriate for study? Negative studies with dietary supplements sometimes inappropriately enroll participants who have moderate-to-severe disease (e.g., those with depression or benign prostatic hyperplasia) when only mild disease would be appropriate.
- Is the duration of the study appropriate? Early studies comparing glucosamine and nonsteroidal anti-inflammatory agents (NSAIA) demonstrated greater efficacy with the NSAIA because of an inadequate study duration for glucosamine to show any benefit.
- Is a placebo group included? Recent studies with dietary supplements for menopausal symptoms and osteoarthritis have demonstrated placebo responses over 40% to 50%.
- Was the blinding maintained throughout the study? Some dietary supplements, such as saw palmetto, have distinctive odors and tastes that are not easily masked.
- Is the preparation commercially available? Most importantly, when a study with dietary supplements does show benefit, it frequently is difficult to use the product in practice because the specific formulation studied is not commercially available.

AUTHOR: **ANNE L. HUME, PHARM.D.**

Overview of Selected Natural Products

This table includes a few of the common uses and side effects of selected natural products. The evidence supporting the uses and side effects of these products varies considerably and may be based on anecdotal information or theoretical concerns with the natural products.

Natural Products	Common Use(s)	Adverse Effects/Potential Concerns
African plum (Pygeum)	Benign prostatic hyperplasia	Nausea and abdominal pain have been reported, but pygeum is generally well tolerated. Pygeum does not decrease prostate size or influence PSA concentrations.
Andrographis	Prevention and treatment of viral respiratory infections	Headache, fatigue, rash, diarrhea, and vomiting. Products are standardized to 4%-6% andrographolide; this botanical is commonly used in combination products.
Black cohosh	Menopausal symptoms (hot flashes), induction of labor in pregnant women, premenstrual syndrome	Dyspepsia, rash, weight gain, headache, and cramping have been reported. Concern exists that black cohosh causes liver toxicity. The potential development of mild estrogen-like adverse effects, especially endometrial hyperplasia, is of concern.
Butterbur	Prevention of migraine headaches; allergic rhinitis; urinary tract spasms; pain	Diarrhea, stomach upset, fatigue, belching, headache, and drowsiness may occur. Due to concern about hepatotoxicity, butterbur products should be free of pyrrolizidine alkaloids. Products should be standardized to 15% petasin and isopetasin.
Chamomile (German)	Motion sickness, anxiety, insomnia; gastrointestinal spasms; mucositis	Allergic reactions occur on rare occasion. Patients with a ragweed allergy should use chamomile with caution.
Chasteberry	Premenstrual dysphoric disorder, premenstrual syndrome, menopausal symptoms, female infertility, mastalgia	Gastrointestinal upset, headache, rash, acne, weight gain, and menstrual bleeding have been reported.
Chitosan	Weight loss, Crohn's disease, hypercholesterolemia, anemia	Gastrointestinal upset, nausea, flatulence, and constipation have been reported. Patients with a shellfish allergy should avoid the use of chitosan.
Chondroitin sulfate	Osteoarthritis, osteoporosis, hyperlipidemia	Gastrointestinal upset, nausea, diarrhea, constipation, and alopecia. Concern exists that chondroitin may have anticoagulant activity due to its structural similarity to part of heparin.
Cinnamon	Type 2 diabetes mellitus, flatulence, gastrointestinal spasms, anorexia, menopausal symptoms, impotence	Cassia cinnamon is one of three types of cinnamon in commercial food products; this is the only type that may have minor effects to improve blood glucose concentrations.
Coenzyme Q10	Congestive heart failure, angina, dilated cardiomyopathy, statin-induced myopathy, Parkinson's disease, chronic fatigue syndrome, HIV/AIDS	Nausea, vomiting, diarrhea, anorexia, heartburn, and rash have been reported. Coenzyme Q10 is structurally similar to vitamin K; concern exists about potential interaction with warfarin.
Cranberry	Prevention and treatment of urinary tract infections; type 2 diabetes mellitus; chronic fatigue syndrome; pleurisy	Gastrointestinal upset and diarrhea have been reported with large doses of cranberry. Uric acid kidney stone formation is also possible with large doses of cranberry over prolonged periods of time.
Dehydroepiandrosterone (DHEA)	Slow or reverse aging, weight loss, metabolic syndrome, erectile dysfunction, immune stimulant, osteoporosis, systemic lupus erythematosus, multiple sclerosis, depression, schizophrenia	Acne and other androgenic effects commonly occur in women. Alopecia, insulin resistance, hepatic dysfunction, and hypertension have been reported. Ingested wild yam and soy cannot be converted into DHEA by humans.
Devil's claw	Osteoarthritis, atherosclerosis, gout, myalgias, fever, migraines	Diarrhea, nausea, and vomiting, as well as allergic reactions, have been reported.

AIDS, Acquired immune deficiency syndrome; *HIV,* human immunodeficiency virus.

Continued on following page **1457**

Natural Products	Common Use(s)	Adverse Effects/Potential Concerns
Echinacea	Prevention and treatment of viral respiratory infections; urinary tract infections; chronic fatigue syndrome; attention deficit hyperactivity disorder	Nausea, vomiting, diarrhea, heartburn, headaches, dizziness, arthralgias, and allergic reactions have been reported with echinacea. Patients with a ragweed allergy should use echinacea with caution because the risk of allergic reactions may be increased.
Eleuthero (Siberian ginseng)	Maintenance of a normal blood pressure; atherosclerosis; Alzheimer's disease; chronic fatigue syndrome; diabetes; herpes simplex infections	Drowsiness, anxiety, and irritability have been reported.
Evening primrose oil (EPO)	Premenstrual syndrome, mastalgia, osteoporosis, asthma, menopausal symptoms, eczema, chronic fatigue syndrome	EPO is well tolerated.
Fenugreek	Type 2 diabetes mellitus, anorexia, atherosclerosis; also used as galactogogue	Gastrointestinal upset, flatulence, and hypoglycemia are possible side effects. Patients with a peanut allergy (and an allergy to related plants) should use fenugreek with caution. Nursing mothers who use fenugreek may notice a "maple syrup" smell in their sweat and in the urine of their infants. This may be mistaken to be "Maple Syrup Urine Disease" in the infant.
Feverfew	Prevention of migraines; fever; menstrual-related problems; arthritis; infertility; asthma	Gastrointestinal side effects are the most common with feverfew. A "post-feverfew syndrome" has been reported in individuals who have taken feverfew for prolonged periods of time and then have abruptly stopped the herbal.
Fish oil	Hypertriglyceridemia, coronary heart disease, hypertension, asthma, depression, rheumatoid arthritis, osteoporosis, psoriasis	Heartburn, nausea, rash, and a "fishy" aftertaste can occur. Contamination with pesticides (as well as with mercury and other heavy metals) is a potential concern, although this is unlikely.
Garlic	Hyperlipidemia, hypertension, peripheral arterial disease, type 2 diabetes mellitus	Nausea, vomiting, heartburn, and body odor are most common. "Deodorized" garlic products may lack the active ingredient, allicin.
Ginger	Nausea and vomiting secondary to pregnancy, chemotherapy, motion sickness, surgery	Heartburn, belching, and dermatitis have been reported. In overdoses, ginger has been associated with central nervous system depression and arrhythmias. Efficacy for hyperemesis gravidarum is unknown, and use is not recommended.
Ginkgo	Alzheimer's disease, vascular dementias, tinnitus, acute mountain sickness, intermittent claudication	Gastrointestinal side effects, headaches, dizziness, and allergic skin reactions. Seizures have been reported in several case reports. Products should contain 24% ginkgo flavone glycosides and 6% terpenoids.
Ginseng (Panax)	Increased resistance to stress and improved well-being; increased physical stamina; depression; diabetes; erectile dysfunction	Insomnia has been reported with ginseng. Vaginal bleeding, mastalgia, and amenorrhea have also been reported.
Glucosamine sulfate	Osteoarthritis	Nausea, heartburn, skin reactions, and headache have been reported. Increased glucose concentrations have been a concern but have not been well documented. Patients with a shellfish allergy should use glucosamine with caution.
Green tea	Improve cognitive performance; prevention of breast, prostate, and colon cancer; hyperlipidemia; Parkinson's disease; obesity; diabetes; cardiovascular disease	Nausea, vomiting, dyspepsia, dizziness, insomnia, and nervousness have been reported. Side effects may be a result of the large amount of caffeine in green tea products. Hepatotoxicity has been a potential concern with green tea.
Hawthorn	Mild heart failure, angina, arrhythmias, hypertension	Mild gastrointestinal effects, dizziness, rash, palpitations, and nervousness have been reported.
Hoodia	Obesity	Side effects have not been reported. Many products lack the actual ingredient.
Horse chestnut	Chronic venous insufficiency, including varicose veins; benign prostate hyperplasia; diarrhea	Mild nausea, vomiting, dizziness, headache, and itching. Products are standardized to 16%-20% aescin.
Huperzine	Alzheimer's disease, increased alertness and energy, myasthenia gravis, memory enhancement	Nausea, vomiting, diarrhea, sweating, and blurred vision as a result of the cholinergic effects of huperzine have been reported.
Kava	Anxiety, insomnia, restlessness, seizure disorders, depression, chronic fatigue syndrome	Gastrointestinal upset, headache, dizziness, "kava" dermopathy, and allergic skin reactions. Hepatotoxicity is the primary concern with kava; some countries have banned the use of kava.
Melatonin	Jet lag, insomnia, migraine, chronic fatigue syndrome, breast cancer, osteoporosis; also used for insomnia in children with ADHD	Daytime drowsiness, headache, and dizziness have been reported. Vaginal bleeding has occurred in perimenopausal women. Melatonin from animal sources should be avoided.
Melissa	Cold sores (topically), anxiety, insomnia, Alzheimer's disease, hypertension, dyspepsia	Nausea, vomiting, dizziness, and wheezing have occurred with oral melissa.
Methylsulfonylmethane (MSM)	Chronic pain, arthritis, diabetes, osteoporosis, allergies, obesity, premenstrual syndrome	Nausea, bloating, diarrhea, fatigue, and insomnia have been associated with MSM. This substance is used frequently in combination with glucosamine and chondroitin.
Milk thistle	Protective agent against liver damage due to alcohol, acetaminophen, and carbon tetrachloride; hepatitis C	Nausea, abdominal fullness, diarrhea, and allergic reactions. Patients with a ragweed allergy should use milk thistle with caution.
Peppermint	Irritable bowel syndrome, sinusitis, morning sickness, dysmenorrhea	Heartburn has been reported, as well as laryngeal and bronchial spasm in infants and children.

Natural Products	Common Use(s)	Adverse Effects/Potential Concerns
Policosanol	Hyperlipidemia, intermittent claudication, atherosclerosis	Migraines, insomnia, dizziness, skin rash, and bleeding have been reported with policosanol. The product has antiplatelet effects.
Probiotics	Treatment and prevention of diarrhea including antibiotic-associated diarrhea; irritable bowel syndrome; atopic dermatitis; Crohn's disease	Theoretically, probiotic products may increase risk of infections in immunocompromised individuals.
Red clover phytoestrogens	Menopausal symptoms, premenstrual syndrome, asthma	Rash, myalgias, headaches, and vaginal bleeding have been reported. Theoretically, endometrial hyperplasia is an adverse effect from the use of these compounds.
Red yeast rice	Hyperlipidemia, indigestion, diarrhea, circulatory conditions, HIV/AIDS	Gastrointestinal upset and dizziness may occur. Red yeast rice may contain lovastatin-like compounds and potentially cause rhabdomyolysis.
S-adenosylmethionine (SAM-e)	Depression, anxiety, dementia, osteoarthritis, heart disease	Nausea, vomiting, diarrhea, headache, and nervousness have been reported. Concern exists that SAM-e raises homocysteine levels.
St. John's wort	Depression, anxiety, chronic fatigue syndrome, HIV/AIDS	Anxiety, gastrointestinal upset, vaginal bleeding, neuropathy, and rash can occur. Hypomania has been induced by St. John's wort.
Tea tree oil	Topical use for acne, fungal infections, lice, scabies	Local inflammation and contact dermatitis may occur.
Valerian	Insomnia, depression, chronic fatigue syndrome, menstrual cramps	Headaches, gastrointestinal upset, and drowsiness can occur. Hepatotoxicity is a potential concern with valerian.

AUTHOR: **ANNE L. HUME, PHARM.D.**

Natural Products and Drug Interactions

This table lists interactions between selected natural products and prescription and nonprescription drugs. Although many of the listed interactions are theoretical in nature and have not been documented to occur in humans, those involving St. John's wort are potentially life threatening in nature, depending on the individual drug. Other interactions are based on small studies of healthy volunteers and use pharmaceutical-quality natural products that may or may not be commercially available.

Natural Products	Drugs	Interactions
Andrographis	Immune suppressants	Andrographis may stimulate immune function, potentially decreasing the effectiveness of drugs such as cyclosporine, tacrolimus, and prednisone.
	Antihypertensive agents	Andrographis may lower blood pressure, potentiating the hypotensive effects of antihypertensive agents.
	Antiplatelet and anticoagulant agents	Andrographis may have antiplatelet activity, potentially increasing the risk of bleeding.
Black cohosh	Hepatotoxic drugs	Concern exists that the risk of hepatotoxicity with black cohosh is increased in the presence of hepatotoxic drugs such as acetaminophen.
	Cisplatin	Animal studies suggest that the efficacy of cisplatin against breast cancer cells may be decreased by black cohosh.
	CYP2D6 substrates	Black cohosh may modestly inhibit CYP2D6 enzyme activity to result in higher drug concentrations.
Butterbur	CYP3A4 inducers (Rifampin, carbamazepine, etc.)	Drugs that induce the activity of CYP3A4 increase the risk of the formation of hepatotoxic metabolites from pyrrolizidine alkaloids from some butterbur products.
Chamomile	CNS depressants (benzodiazepines, opiates, barbiturates, etc.)	Chamomile may have additive CNS depressant effects.
	CYP1A2 substrates	Chamomile may inhibit CYP1A2 enzyme activity to result in higher drug concentrations.
	CYP3A4 substrates	Chamomile may inhibit CYP3A4 enzyme activity to result in higher drug concentrations.
	Estrogens	Chamomile may compete for estrogen receptors.
	Tamoxifen	Chamomile may interfere with the effects of tamoxifen because of its estrogenic effects.
Chaste tree berry	Antipsychotic agents	Chaste tree berry may antagonize the effects of antipsychotic agents through its dopaminergic activity.
	Metoclopramide	Chaste tree berry may antagonize the effects of metoclopramide through its dopaminergic activity.
	Dopamine agonists	Chaste tree berry may possess additive effects to drugs such as levodopa and ropinirole through its dopaminergic activity.
	Oral contraceptives/estrogens	Chaste tree berry may possess additive hormonal effects.
Chondroitin	Warfarin	High-dose chondroitin has structural similarity to a heparinoid and may possess weak anticoagulant effects.
Cinnamon	Hypoglycemic agents	Cinnamon may possess additive effects on blood glucose to those of hypoglycemic agents.
Coenzyme Q10	Antihypertensive agents	Coenzyme Q10 may possess additive effects on blood pressure to those of antihypertensive agents.
	Warfarin	Coenzyme Q10 may lessen the anticoagulant effects of warfarin because of its structural similarity to vitamin K.
	Chemotherapy	The antioxidant effects of coenzyme Q10 may blunt the efficacy of certain chemotherapeutic agents that depend on the formation of free radicals.
Cranberry	CYP2C9 substrates (warfarin)	Cranberry may inhibit CYP2C9 enzyme activity to result in higher drug concentrations; evidence with warfarin is contradictory.
Dehydroepiandrosterone (DHEA)	Tamoxifen and aromatase inhibitors such as anastrozole and exemestane	DHEA may interfere with the antiestrogenic effects of these drugs.
	CYP3A4 substrates	DHEA may slightly inhibit CYP3A4 enzyme activity to result in higher drug concentrations.

AChE, Acetylcholinesterase; CCB, calcium channel blockers; CNS, central nervous system; MAOI, monoamine oxidase inhibitor; PPI, proton pump inhibitors; SSRI, selective serotonin reuptake inhibitors.

Continued on following page

Natural Products	Drugs	Interactions
Devil's claw	Antihypertensive agents	Devil's claw may possess additive effects on blood pressure to those of antihypertensive agents.
	Hypoglycemic agents	Devil's claw may possess additive effects on blood glucose to those of hypoglycemic agents.
	H$_2$ antagonists and PPI	Devil's claw may raise gastric pH and blunt the efficacy of H$_2$ antagonists and PPI.
	CYP3A4 substrates	Devil's claw may inhibit CYP3A4 enzyme activity to result in higher drug concentrations.
	CYP2C9 substrates	Devil's claw may inhibit CYP2C9 enzyme activity to result in higher drug concentrations.
	CYP2C19 substrates	Devil's claw may inhibit CYP2C19 enzyme activity to result in higher drug concentrations.
	Warfarin	Devil's claw may inhibit CYP2C9 enzyme activity to result in higher concentrations of warfarin; purpura has been reported.
Echinacea	Immune suppressants	Echinacea may stimulate immune function, potentially decreasing the effectiveness of drugs such as cyclosporine, tacrolimus, and prednisone.
	CYP3A4 substrates	Echinacea may modestly induce hepatic CYP3A4 enzyme activity to result in lower drug concentrations.
	CYP1A2 substrates	Echinacea may inhibit CYP1A2 enzyme activity to result in higher drug concentrations.
Eleuthero (Siberian ginseng)	CNS depressants (benzodiazepines, opiates, barbiturates, etc.)	Eleuthero may have additive CNS depressant effects.
	Antiplatelet and anticoagulant agents	Eleuthero may have antiplatelet activity, potentially increasing the risk of bleeding.
	CYP3A4 substrates	Eleuthero may inhibit CYP3A4 enzyme activity to result in higher drug concentrations.
	CYP1A2 substrates	Eleuthero may modestly inhibit CYP1A2 enzyme activity to result in higher drug concentrations.
	CYP2C9 substrates	Eleuthero may modestly inhibit CYP2C9 enzyme activity to result in higher drug concentrations.
	CYP2D6 substrates	Eleuthero may inhibit CYP2D6 enzyme activity to result in higher drug concentrations.
	Digoxin	Concentration of digoxin has been reported to increase but without evidence of toxicity.
Evening primrose oil (EPO)	Antiplatelet and anticoagulant agents	EPO may have anticoagulant activity, potentially increasing the risk of bleeding.
Fenugreek	Antiplatelet and anticoagulant agents	Fenugreek may have antiplatelet activity, potentially increasing the risk of bleeding.
	Hypoglycemic agents	Fenugreek may potentially lower blood glucose concentrations and have additive effects with hypoglycemic agents.
Feverfew	Antiplatelet and anticoagulant agents	Feverfew may have antiplatelet activity, potentially increasing the risk of bleeding.
	CYP3A4 substrates	Feverfew may inhibit CYP3A4 enzyme activity to result in higher drug concentrations.
	CYP1A2 substrates	Feverfew may inhibit CYP1A2 enzyme activity to result in higher drug concentrations.
	CYP2C9 substrates	Feverfew may inhibit CYP2C9 enzyme activity to result in higher drug concentrations.
	CYP2C19 substrates	Feverfew may inhibit CYP2C19 enzyme activity to result in higher drug concentrations.
Fish oils (omega-3 fatty acids)	Antiplatelet and anticoagulant agents	Fish oils may have antiplatelet activity, potentially increasing the risk of bleeding, although this has not been documented in humans.
	Antihypertensive agents	Fish oils may possess additive effects on blood pressure to those of antihypertensive agents.
	Oral contraceptives	Oral contraceptives may potentially interfere with the triglyceride-lowering effects of fish oil.
Garlic	Antiplatelet and anticoagulant agents	Garlic may have antiplatelet activity, potentially increasing the risk of bleeding.
	CYP3A4 substrates	Garlic may potentially induce CYP3A4 enzyme activity to result in lower drug concentrations; evidence is contradictory.
	CYP2E1 substrates	Garlic may modestly inhibit CYP2E1 enzyme activity to result in higher drug concentrations.
Ginger	Antiplatelet and anticoagulant agents	Ginger may have antiplatelet activity, potentially increasing the risk of bleeding.
	Hypoglycemic agents	Ginger may potentially lower blood glucose concentrations and have additive effects with hypoglycemic agents.
Ginkgo	Antiplatelet and anticoagulant agents	Ginkgo may have antiplatelet activity, potentially increasing the risk of bleeding.
	CYP2C19 substrates	Ginkgo may induce CYP2C19 enzyme activity to result in lower drug concentrations.
	CYP1A2 substrates	Ginkgo may modestly inhibit CYP1A2 enzyme activity to result in higher drug levels.
	CYP2C9 substrates	Ginkgo may modestly inhibit CYP2C9 enzyme activity to result in higher drug concentrations.
	CYP2D6 substrates	Ginkgo may inhibit CYP2D6 enzyme activity to result in higher drug concentrations.
Ginseng (Panax)	Antiplatelet and anticoagulant agents	Panax ginseng may have antiplatelet properties; American ginseng may decrease the effectiveness (international normalized ration [INR]) of warfarin.
	CYP2D6 substrates	Panax ginseng may modestly inhibit CYP2D6 enzyme activity to result in higher drug concentrations.
	Immune suppressants	Panax ginseng may stimulate immune function, potentially decreasing the effectiveness of drugs such as cyclosporine, tacrolimus, and prednisone.
	Hypoglycemic agents	Panax ginseng may potentially lower blood glucose levels and have additive effects with hypoglycemic agents.
Glucosamine	Warfarin	High-dose glucosamine (along with high-dose chondroitin) may have additive effects to those of warfarin because of structural similarity to heparin.

AChE, Acetylcholinesterase; *CCB*, calcium channel blockers; *CNS*, central nervous system; *MAOI*, monoamine oxidase inhibitor; *PPI*, proton pump inhibitors; *SSRI*, selective serotonin reuptake inhibitors.

Natural Products	Drugs	Interactions
Green tea extract	Antiplatelet agents	Green tea possesses compounds that may have antiplatelet activity, potentially increasing the risk of bleeding.
	Amphetamines	Caffeine in green tea may increase the risk of CNS toxicity.
	Cocaine	Caffeine in green tea may increase the risk of CNS toxicity.
	Oral contraceptives	Oral contraceptives may decrease the clearance of caffeine in green tea.
	Warfarin	Small amounts of vitamin K have been reported to be present in green tea, potentially decreasing the effectiveness of warfarin.
	Theophylline	Caffeine potentially decreases theophylline clearance.
	Verapamil	Verapamil decreases caffeine clearance, resulting in increased concentrations.
	Quinolone antibiotics	Some quinolone antibiotics decrease the clearance of caffeine.
	Hepatotoxic drugs	Concern exists that the risk of hepatotoxicity with green tea is increased in the presence of hepatotoxic drugs such as acetaminophen.
Hawthorn	β-blockers	Hawthorn and β-blockers may have additive effects on blood pressure and heart rate.
	CCB, nitrates	Hawthorn and CCB (or nitrates) may have additive effects due to coronary vasodilation.
	Digoxin	Hawthorn may have additive effects to those of digoxin.
	Phosphodiesterase inhibitors	Hawthorn may have additive vasodilatory and hypotensive effects with sildenafil, tadalafil, and vardenafil.
Horse chestnut seed extract (HCSE)	Antiplatelet and anticoagulant agents	HCSE may have antiplatelet activity, potentially increasing the risk of bleeding.
	Hypoglycemic agents	HCSE may potentially lower blood glucose concentrations and have additive effects with hypoglycemic agents.
Huperzine	AChE inhibitors (donepezil, etc.)	Huperzine may have additive effects when combined with AChE inhibitors.
	Anticholinergic drugs	The effectiveness of huperzine and/or the anticholinergic drug may be decreased by their concomitant administration.
	Cholinergic drugs (bethanechol, neostigmine, etc.)	Huperzine may have additive effects when combined with cholinergic drugs.
Kava	CYP3A4 substrates	Kava may inhibit CYP3A4 enzyme activity to result in higher drug concentrations.
	CYP1A2 substrates	Kava may inhibit CYP1A2 enzyme activity to result in higher drug concentrations.
	CYP2C9 substrates, CYP2C19 substrates	Kava may inhibit CYP2C9 and CYP2C19 enzyme activity to result in higher drug concentrations.
	CYP2D6 substrates	Kava may inhibit CYP2D6 enzyme activity to result in higher drug concentrations.
	P-glycoprotein substrates (digoxin; etoposide, paclitaxel, vinblastine, vincristine; itraconazole; diltiazem, verapamil; and many other drugs)	Kava may inhibit P-glycoprotein transporter systems.
	Hepatotoxic drugs	Concern exists that the risk of hepatotoxicity from kava is increased in the presence of hepatotoxic drugs such as acetaminophen.
Melatonin	Antiplatelet and anticoagulant agents	Melatonin may potentiate the effects of antiplatelets and anticoagulants, although the mechanism is unknown.
	CNS depressants	Melatonin may have additive CNS depressant effects.
	Fluvoxamine	Fluvoxamine may increase levels of melatonin.
	Immune suppressants	Melatonin may stimulate immune function, potentially decreasing the effectiveness of drugs such as cyclosporine, tacrolimus, and prednisone.
	Hypoglycemic agents	Melatonin may impair glucose utilization and may decrease the efficacy of hypoglycemic agents.
Milk thistle	Estrogens (and other drugs that undergo glucuronidation)	Silymarin may increase the clearance of estrogens.
	CYP2C9 substrates	Milk thistle may modestly inhibit CYP2C9 enzyme activity to result in higher drug concentrations.
Peppermint oil	H_2 antagonists and proton pump inhibitors	Peppermint oil may raise gastric pH and blunt efficacy of H_2 antagonists and PPI.
	CYP3A4 substrates	Peppermint oil may modestly inhibit CYP3A4 enzyme activity to result in higher drug concentrations.
	CYP1A2 substrates	Peppermint oil may modestly inhibit CYP1A2 enzyme activity to result in higher drug concentrations.
	CYP2C9 substrates, CYP2C19 substrates	Peppermint oil may modestly inhibit CYP2C9 and CYP2C19 enzyme activity to result in higher drug concentrations.
Policosanol	Antiplatelet and anticoagulant agents	Policosanol may have antiplatelet activity, potentially increasing the risk of bleeding.
Probiotics	Antibiotics	Antibiotics may kill the live organisms in different probiotic preparations.
	Immune suppressants	Theoretically, probiotics may cause bacterial or fungal infections in patients who are taking immune suppressants chronically.

Continued on following page

Natural Products	Drugs	Interactions
Red clover phytoestrogens	Antiplatelet and anticoagulant agents	Theoretically, red clover may possess coumarins, which increase the risk of bleeding with antiplatelet and anticoagulants.
	Tamoxifen/aromatase inhibitors	
	CYP3A4 substrates	Red clover may inhibit CYP3A4 enzyme activity to result in higher drug concentrations.
	CYP2C9 substrates, CYP2C19 substrates	Red clover may inhibit CYP2C9 and CYP2C19 enzyme activity to result in higher drug concentrations.
	CYP1A2 substrates	Red clover may inhibit CYP1A2 enzyme activity to result in higher drug concentrations.
Red yeast rice	CYP3A4 inhibitors	Drugs that inhibit CYP3A4 may decrease the metabolism of lovastatin in red yeast rice.
	Statins	Red yeast rice contains lovastatin and increases the risk of myopathy (and hepatotoxicity).
	Fibrates and niacin	Fibrates and niacin may increase concentrations of lovastatin in red yeast rice.
S-adenosylmethionine (SAM-e)	Antidepressants (including MAOIs)	Additive effects are possible, and there is potential for toxicity.
	Serotonergic drugs (triptans, SSRIs, tramadol, meperidine, dextromethorphan, etc.)	SAM-e may increase the risk of development of serotonin syndrome when used concomitantly.
Soy phytoestrogens	Antibiotics	Antibiotics may decrease the efficacy of soy because intestinal bacteria convert isoflavones into more active forms.
	Estrogens	Soy potentially may inhibit the effects of estrogen.
	Tamoxifen/aromatase inhibitors	Soy's estrogenic effects may antagonize the antitumor effects of tamoxifen/aromatase inhibitors.
	MAOIs	Fermented soy products may contain tyramine.
St. John's wort	CYP3A4 substrates	St. John's wort strongly induces CYP3A4 enzyme activity to result in lower drug concentrations.
	CYP1A2 substrates	St. John's wort modestly induces CYP1A2 enzyme activity to result in lower drug levels.
	CYP2C9 substrates	St. John's wort induces CYP2C9 enzyme activity to result in lower drug concentrations.
	P-glycoprotein substrates (digoxin; etoposide, paclitaxel, vinblastine, vincristine; itraconazole; diltiazem, verapamil; and other drugs)	St. John's wort induces P-glycoprotein transporter systems.
	Serotonergic drugs (triptans, SSRIs, tramadol, meperidine, dextromethorphan, etc.)	St. John's wort may increase the risk of development of serotonin syndrome when used concomitantly.
Valerian	CNS depressants (benzodiazepines, opiates, barbiturates, alcohol, etc.)	Valerian may increase the sedative effects of CNS depressants.
	CYP3A4 substrates	Valerian may modestly inhibit the CYP3A4 enzyme activity.

AChE, Acetylcholinesterase; *CCB,* calcium channel blockers; *CNS,* central nervous system; *MAOI,* monoamine oxidase inhibitor; *PPI,* proton pump inhibitors; *SSRI,* selective serotonin reuptake inhibitors.

EXAMPLES OF DRUGS METABOLIZED BY CYP ENZYMES

The following are example drugs that are metabolized through the different cytochrome P450 isoenzymes:

CYP1A2 substrates: theophylline, imipramine, clozapine, naproxen
CYP2C9 substrates: warfarin, tamoxifen, irbesartan, ibuprofen, glipizide
CYP2C19 substrates: omeprazole and other proton pump inhibitors, phenytoin, phenobarbital, cyclophosphamide

CYP2D6 substrates: S-metoprolol, propafenone, paroxetine, risperidone, tramadol
CYP2E1 substrates: acetaminophen, alcohol
CYP3A4 substrates: most statins, indinavir, amlodipine, verapamil, alprazolam, buspirone
(For a complete list of drugs and their respective metabolic pathways through the cytochrome P450 isoenzyme systems go to http://medicine.iupui.edu/flockhart.)

AUTHOR: **ANNE L. HUME, PHARM.D.**

Definitions of Complementary and Alternative Medicine Terms

Acupuncture Thin needles are inserted superficially on the skin at locations throughout the body. These points are located along "channels" of energy. Heat can be applied by burning (moxibustion), electric current (electroacupuncture), or pressure (acupressure). Healing is proposed by the restoration of a balance of energy flow called *Qi.* Another explanation suggests that, possibly, the stimulation activates endorphin receptors.

Alexander Technique A bodywork technique in which rebalancing of "postural sets" (i.e., physical alignment) is taught by mentally focusing on the way correct alignments should look and feel and through verbal and tactile guidance by the practitioner.

Applied Kinesiology A form of treatment that uses nutrition, physical manipulation, vitamins, diets, and exercise to restore and energize the body. Weak muscles are proposed as a source of dysfunctional health.

Aromatherapy A form of herbal medicine that uses various oils from plants. Route of administration can be through absorption in the skin or inhalation. The aromatic biochemical structures of certain herbs are thought to act in areas of the brain related to past experiences and emotions (e.g., limbic system).

Ayurveda A major health system that originated in India and incorporates the body, mind, and spirit to prevent and treat disease. Includes special types of diets, herbs, and minerals.

Biofeedback A mind-body therapy procedure in which sensors are placed on the body to measure muscle tension, heart rate, and sweat responses or neural activity. Information is provided by visual, auditory, or body-muscle cell activation so as to teach either to increase or decrease physiologic activity, which, when reconstituted, is proposed to improve health problems (e.g., pain, anxiety, or high blood pressure). In some cases, relaxation exercises complement this procedure.

Chelation Therapy Involves the removal—through intravenous infusion of a chelating agent (synthetic amino acid ethylenediamine tetraacetic acid [EDTA])—of heavy metals, including lead, nickel, and cadmium, as a way to treat certain diseases. Ancillary treatments include the use of vitamins, changes in diet, and exercise.

Cognitive Therapy Psychologic therapy in which the major focus is altering and changing irrational beliefs through a type of Socratic dialogue and self-evaluation of certain illogical thoughts. Conditioning and learning are important components of this therapy.

Craniosacral Therapy A form of gentle manual manipulation used for diagnosis and for making corrections in a system made up of cerebrospinal fluid, cranial and dural membranes, cranial bones, and sacrum. This system is proposed to be dynamic, with its own physiologic frequency. Through touch and pressure, tension is proposed to be reduced and cranial rhythms normalized, leading to improvement in health and disease.

Diathermy The use of high-frequency electrical currents as a form of physical therapy and in surgical procedures. The term *diathermy,* derived from the Greek words *dia* and *therma,* literally means "heating through." The three forms of diathermy used by physical therapists are short wave, ultrasound, and microwave.

Eye Movement Desensitization and Reprocessing (EMDR) A technique that proposes to remove painful memories by behavioral techniques. Rhythmic, multisaccadic eye movements are produced by allowing the patient to track and follow a moving object while imagining a stressful memory or event. By using deconditioning, including verbal interaction with the therapist, the painful memory is extinguished and health improved.

Feldenkrais Method A bodywork technique that integrates physics, judo, and yoga. The practitioner directs sequences of movement using verbal or hands-on techniques or teaches a system of self-directed exercise to treat physical impairments through the learning of new movement patterns.

Hatha Yoga The branch of yoga practice that involves physical exercise, breathing practices, and movement. These exercises are designed to have a salutary effect on posture, flexibility, and strength and are intended ultimately to prepare the body to remain still for long periods of meditation.

Hellerwork A bodywork technique that treats and improves proper body alignment through the development of a more complete awareness of the physical body. The goal is to realign fascia for improvement of standing, sitting, and breathing using "body energy," verbal feedback, and changing emotions and attitudes.

Homeopathy A form of treatment in which substances (minerals, plant extracts, chemicals, or disease-producing germs), which in sufficient doses would produce a set of illness symptoms in healthy individuals, are given in microdoses to produce a "cure" of those same symptoms. The *symptom* is not thought to be part of the illness but part of a curative process.

Hyperbaric Oxygen A therapy in which 100% oxygen is given at or above atmospheric pressure. An increase in oxygen in the tissue is proposed to increase blood circulation and improve healing and health and influence the course of disease.

Jin Shin Jyutsu An ancient bodywork technique to harmonize body, mind, and spirit by gentle touch that uses specific "healing points" at the body surface. The points are proposed to overlie flowing energy (Qi). The therapist's fingers are used to "redirect, balance, and provide a more efficient energy flow" to and throughout the body.

Light Therapy Natural light or light of specified wavelengths is used to treat disease. This may include ultraviolet light, colored light, or low-intensity laser light. Generally, the eye is the initial entry point for the light because of its direct connection to the brain.

Magnetic Therapy Magnets are placed directly on the skin, theoretically stimulating living cells and increasing blood flow by ionic currents that are created from polarities on the magnets.

Modified from Spencer JW: *Complementary/alternative medicine: an evidence-based approach*, St Louis, 1999, Mosby.

Mediterranean Diet   A diet that is thought to provide optimal distribution of daily caloric intake of different nutrients and includes 50% to 60% carbohydrates, 30% fats, and 10% proteins. The diet is derived from the eating habits of people in the Mediterranean area, who were shown to have reduced rates of cardiovascular disease.

Mind-Body Therapies   A group of therapies that emphasize using the mind or brain in conjunction with the body to assist healing. Mind-body therapies can involve varying degrees of levels of consciousness, including *hypnosis,* in which selective attention is used to induce a specific altered state (trance) for memory retrieval, relaxation, or suggestion; *visual imagery,* in which the focus is on a target visual stimulus; *yoga,* which involves integration of posture and controlled breathing, relaxation, and/or meditation; *relaxation,* which includes lighter levels of altered states of consciousness through indirect or direct focus; and *meditation,* in which there is an intentional use of posture, concentration, contemplation, and visualization.

Muscle Energy Technique   A manual therapy in osteopathic medicine that includes both passive mobilization and muscle reeducation. Diagnosis of somatic dysfunction is performed by the practitioner, after which the patient is guided to provide corrective muscle contraction.

Music Therapy   The use of music in an either active or passive mode. Used mainly to reduce stress, anxiety, and pain.

Naturopathy   A major health system that includes practices that emphasize diet, nutrition, homeopathy, acupuncture, herbal medicine, manipulation, and various mind-body therapies. Focal points include self-healing and treatment through changes in lifestyle and emphasis on health prevention.

Ornish Diet   A life-choice program based on eating a vegetarian diet containing less than 10% fat. The diet is high in complex carbohydrates and fiber. Meat and fish are generally avoided.

Oslo Diet   An eating plan that emphasizes increased intake of fish and reduced total fat intake. Diet is combined with regular endurance exercise.

Pilates   An educational and exercise approach using the proper body mechanics, movements, truncal and pelvic stabilization, coordinated breathing, and muscle contractions to promote strengthening. Attention is paid to the entire musculoskeletal system.

Prayer   The use of prayer(s) that are offered to "some higher being" or authority to heal and/or arrest disease. May be practiced by the individual patient, by groups, or by other(s) with or without the patient's knowledge (e.g., intercessory).

Pritikin Diet   A weight management plan that is based on a vegetarian framework. Meals are low in fat, high in fiber, and high in complex carbohydrates.

Qi Gong   A form of Chinese exercise-stimulation therapy that proposes to improve health by redirecting mental focus, breathing, coordination, and relaxation. The goal is to "rebalance" the body's own healing capacities by activating proposed electrical or energetic currents that flow along meridians located throughout the body. These meridians, however, do not follow conventional nerve or muscle pathways. In Chinese medical training and practice this therapy includes "external Qi," which is energy transmitted from one person to another so as to heal.

Raja Yoga   Yoga practice that includes all of the other forms of yoga. The practitioner is instructed to follow moral directives, physical exercises, breathing exercises, meditation, devotion, and service to others to facilitate religious awakening.

Reflexology   A bodywork technique that uses reflex points on the hands and feet. Pressure is applied at points that correspond to various body parts, to eliminate blockages thought to produce pain or disease.

Reiki   Comes from the Japanese word meaning "universal life force energy." The practitioner serves as a conduit for healing energy directed into the body or energy field of the recipient without physical contact with the body.

Rolfing   A bodywork technique that involves the myofascia. The body is realigned by using the hands to apply deep pressure and friction that allows more sufficient posture, movement, and the "release" of emotions from the body.

Shiatsu   A Japanese bodywork technique involving finger pressure at specific points on the body mainly to balance "energy" in the body. The major focus is on prevention by keeping the body healthy. The therapy uses more than 600 points on the skin that are proposed to be connected to pathways through which energy flows.

T'ai Chi   A technique that uses slow, purposeful motor-physical movements of the body to control and achieve a more balanced physiologic and psychologic state.

Therapeutic Touch   A body energy field technique in which hands are passed over the body without actually touching to recreate and change proposed "energy imbalances" for restoring innate healing forces. Verbal interaction between patient and therapist helps maximize effects.

Traditional Chinese Medicine   An ancient form of medicine that focuses on prevention and secondarily treats disease with an emphasis on maintaining balance through the body by stimulating a constant, smooth-flowing Qi energy. Herbs, acupuncture, massage, diet, and exercise are also used.

Trager Psychophysical Integration   A bodywork technique in which the practitioner enters a meditative state and guides the client through gentle, light, rhythmic, nonintrusive movements. "Mentastics" exercises using self-healing movements are taught to the clients.

AUTHOR: **ANNE L. HUME, PHARM.D.**

Relaxation Techniques

Relaxation Techniques

Relaxation Technique	Summary	Further Resources
Breathing exercise	This is the foundation of most relaxation techniques. Have patients place one hand on the chest and the other on the abdomen. Instruct them to take a slow, deep breath, as if they were sucking in all the air in the room. While doing this, the hand on the abdomen should rise higher than the hand on the chest. This promotes diaphragmatic breathing that increases alveolar expansion in the bases of the lungs. Have them hold the breath for a count of 7 and then exhale. Exhalation should take twice as long as inhalation. Repeat this for a total of five breaths, and encourage patients to do this three times a day.	*Conscious Breathing* by Gay Hendricks is one of many good resources on using breathing for relaxation and health.
Meditation		
Transcendental/The relaxation response	To prevent distracting thoughts, the subject repeats a mantra (a word or sound) over and over again while sitting in a comfortable position. If a distracting thought comes to mind, it is accepted and let go, with the mind focusing again on the mantra.	www.mindbody.harvard.edu or *The Relaxation Response* by Herbert Benson; www.tm.org for information on transcendental meditation.
Mindful meditation	This represents the philosophy of living in the present or in the moment. The *body scan* is one technique where the subject uses breathing to obtain a relaxed state while lying or sitting. The mind progressively focuses on different parts of the body, where it feels any and all sensations intentionally but nonjudgmentally before moving on to another part of the body. A patient with back pain may focus on the quality and characteristics of the pain as if to better understand it and bring it under control.	*Full Catastrophe Living* by Jon Kabat-Zinn describes this technique in full and the program for stress reduction at the University of Massachusetts Medical Center.
Centering prayer	This is a form similar to transcendental meditation that has a more religious foundation. The subject repeats a "sacred word" similar to a mantra. As thoughts come to mind, they are accepted and let go, clearing the mind to become more centered on the spirit within, as if the mind's preoccupied thoughts are the layers of an onion that are peeled away, allowing better understanding of the spirit at the core.	www.Centeringprayer.com; look under "method of centering prayer" for a nondenominational discussion.
Progressive muscle relaxation (PMR)	A form of relaxation in which the subject is attuned to the difference in feeling when the muscles are tensed and then relaxed. In a comfortable position, start by tensing the whole body from head to toe. While doing this, notice the feelings of tightness. Take a deep breath in and as you let it out, let the tension release and the muscles relax. This is then followed by progressive tension and relaxation throughout the body. One may start by clenching the fists and then tensing the arms, shoulders, chest, abdomen, hips, legs, and so on, with each step followed by relaxation.	www.uaex.edu/publications/pub/fshei28.htm is a good review of PMR as well as other relaxation exercises. It is sponsored by the University of Arkansas. *You Must Relax* is a book by the founder of this technique, Edmund Jacobson.
Visualization/Self-hypnosis	The subject uses visualization to recruit images that create a relaxed state. For example, if a person is anxious, visualizing images of a place and a time that were peaceful and comforting would help induce relaxation. This is best used in conjunction with a breathing exercise.	There are many audiocassettes that can guide people through a visualization "script" that can result in relaxation. Emmett Miller is one well-known author.
Autogenic training	This induces a physiologic response by using simple phrases. For example, "My legs are heavy and warm" is meant to increase the blood flow to this area, resulting in relaxation. This is done progressively from head to toe with the use of deep breathing and repetition of the phrase. After completing this, focus attention on any body part that may still be tense, and then focus the breath and phrase to that area until the whole body is relaxed.	The British Autogenic Society at www.autogenictherapy.org.uk is a good resource for more information.

From Rakel RE (ed): *Principles of family practice,* ed 6, Philadelphia, 2002, WB Saunders.

Continued on following page

Relaxation Techniques—cont'd		
Relaxation Technique	**Summary**	**Further Resources**
Exercise/Movement Aerobic	While performing an aerobic exercise, focus attention on a phrase, sound, word, or prayer and passively disregard other thoughts that may enter the mind. Some may focus on their breathing, saying to themselves, "In" with inhalation and "Out" with exhalation, or repeating "one-two, one-two" with each step they take with jogging. Doing this will help the mind focus, preventing other thoughts that may cause tension.	*Beyond the Relaxation Response* by Herbert Benson includes discussion of his research on inducing the relaxation response while exercising.
Yoga	This has been practiced for thousands of years in India. In America, it has been divided into three aspects: breathing (pranayama yoga), bodily postures or asanas (hatha yoga), and meditation to maintain balance and health. Regular practice induces relaxation.	For the following therapies, it is best to encourage patients to take a class at a local community center or gym and to pick up an introductory book at a library or bookstore.
T'ai chi	An ancient Chinese martial art that uses slow, graceful movements combined with inner mindfulness and breathing techniques to help bring balance between the mind and body.	See above.
Qi gong	A traditional Chinese practice that uses movement, meditation, and controlled breathing to balance the body's vital energy force, Qi.	See above.

A

AA, **68-69**
AAA, **68-69**
AAT, **43**
Abacavir, for AIDS/HIV, 27, 493
Abciximab
  for Kawasaki disease, 565
  for myocardial infarction, 677
Abdominal aorta aneurysm, **68-69**, 69f
Abdominal calcifications, non-visceral on x-ray, 1129-1130
Abdominal distention, 1113
Abdominal ovarian malignancy, 626
Abdominal pain
  adolescence, 1113
  arthritis and, 1121
  childhood, 1113
  chronic lower, 1113
  differential diagnosis of, 1113-1114
  diffuse, 1113
  epigastric, 1113
  infancy, 1113
  left lower quadrant, 1113
  left upper quadrant, 1113-1114
  by location, 1113
  nonsurgical causes of, 1114
  periumbilical, 1114
  poorly localized, 1114
  in pregnancy, 1114
  right lower quadrant, 1114
  right upper quadrant, 1114
  suprapubic, 1114
Abdominal pregnancy. *See* Ectopic pregnancy.
Abdominal wall masses, 1114-1115
Abortion
  missed, 958
  recurrent, differential diagnosis of, 1115
  spontaneous miscarriage, **958**
  threatened, 958
ABPA. *See* Allergic bronchopulmonary aspergillosis.
Abrasion, corneal, **264**
Abruptio placentae, **3-130**
Abscess
  brain, **4-5**, 1358-1359t
  breast, **6**
  liver, **7-8**
  lung, **9-10**
  pancreatic, 740
  parameningeal, 1358-1359t
  parapharyngeal, 1173
  pelvic, **11**
  perirectal, **12**
  peritonsillar, **776,** 1173
  pilonidal
    acne, 783
    chronic, 783
  retropharyngeal, **889-890**, 889f, 890f, 1173
  spinal epidural, **954**
  tuboovarian, **11**
  vaginal cuff, **11**
Absence epilepsy
  childhood, 920
  juvenile, 920
Absence seizures, **920**

Abstinence, 259
Abuse
  alcohol. *See* Alcohol abuse.
  child, **13-15**
    clinical algorithm, 1212f
    sexual, 758-759
  drug, **16-17,** 16t
  elder, **18**
    clinical algorithm, 1213f
ACA, 1351
Acamprosate
  for alcohol withdrawal, 17, 40
  for alcoholism, 40
Acarbose
  for diabetes mellitus, 305
  for dumping syndrome, 319
Acceleration flexion-extension neck injury, **1101**
Accutane. *See* Isotretinoin (Accutane).
ACE. *See* Angiotensin-converting enzyme.
Acetaminophen
  for chickenpox, 1071
  for Colorado Tick Fever, 248
  for lumbar spinal stenosis, 955
  for mastitis, 619
  for mucormycosis, 659
  overdose, **19**
  for Paget's disease of bone, 735
  for pharyngitis/tonsillitis, 780
  poisoning, **19,** 1212f
  for rheumatoid arthritis, 895
  for roseola, 901
  for thyrotoxic storm, 1017
  for trochanteric bursitis, 1042
  for Varicella, 1071
  for whiplash injury, 1101
  for Yellow fever, 1106
Acetazolamide
  for altitude sickness, 45
  for hypertension, idiopathic intracranial, 534
  for myotonia, 683
Acetic acid, 728
Acetone, serum or plasma, 1349
Acetylcholine receptor (AChR) antibody, 1349
Acetylcysteine (Mucomyst). *See* N-acetylcysteine (Mucomyst).
Acetylsalicylic acid. *See* Aspirin.
Achalasia, **20-21**
Aches and pains. *See also* Pain.
  diffuse, differential diagnosis, 1115
  muscle cramps and aches, 1291f
Achilles tendinitis, 1146
Achilles tendon rupture, **22**
Acid phosphatase, serum, 1349
Acid serum test, 1368
Acid–base disorders, 1349t
Acid–base homeostasis, 1213f
Acid–base reference values, 1349t
Acidosis
  correction of, 924
  diabetic ketoacidosis, **307-308**
    clinical algorithm, 1250f
  with heat exhaustion and heat stroke, 442
  lactic, 1115
  metabolic
    arterial blood gases, 1352
    clinical algorithm for, 1214f
    differential diagnosis, 1115
    laboratory findings in, 1349t
  renal tubular, **880**

Acidosis *(Continued)*
  respiratory
    acute, clinical algorithm for, 1216f
    arterial blood gases, 1352
    chronic, clinical algorithm for, 1217f
    differential diagnosis, 1115
    laboratory findings in, 1349t
    tricyclic antidepressant, 1039t
Acitretin, 593
Acne, **23-24**
Acne inversa, **475-476,** 475f
Acne rosacea, **900**
Acne vulgaris, **23-24**
Acoustic neurofibromatosis, bilateral, 694
Acoustic neuroma, **25**
Acquired hydronephrosis, **498-499,** 498f
Acquired idiopathic sideroblastic anemia, **67**
Acquired immunodeficiency syndrome, **26-27.** *See also* Human immunodeficiency virus.
  chest radiographic, abnormalities in, 1155
  conditions in, 26
  esophageal disease in, 1156
  histoplasmosis in, 481
  neck mass in, 1173
  nonnucleoside reverse transcriptase inhibitors, 27
  ocular manifestations of, 1156
  protease inhibitors, 27
  toxoplasmosis in, 1029-1030, 1030f
Acquired red cell aplasia, **858-859**
Acrodermatitis chronica atrophicans. *See* Lyme disease.
Acromegaly, **28**
  diagnostic workup for, 785-786
  differential diagnosis of, 785
  pharmacologic therapy for, 786
  typical appearances of, 28f
Actigall, 226
Actinomyces infection. *See* Actinomycosis.
Actinomycosis, **29-30**
  neck mass with, 1173
  thoracic, 29
Activated clotting time (ACT), 1349
Activated partial thromboplastin time, 1379
Acupuncture
  for chronic pain management, 234
  for dysmenorrhea, 323
  for dyspareunia, 325
  for posttraumatic stress disorder, 817
  for tinnitus, 1024
Acute back pain, low, 1125
Acute brain syndrome, **288**
Acute chest syndrome, 937
Acute confusional state, **344.** *See also* Delirium.
Acute conjunctivitis. *See* Conjunctivitis.
Acute cor pulmonale, **262-263,** 262f
Acute coronary syndrome, **32-34,** 32t
  right coronary artery
    after successful percutaneous stenting during STEMI, 33f
    totally occluded proximally, 33f
    timing of release of cardiac biomarkers in, 32f
Acute cranial polyneuropathy, 1175
Acute fatty metamorphosis, **377**
Acute hepatitis, 1153
Acute ischemic stroke, **969-971**
  diagnostic studies, immediate, 969b
  imaging studies, 969-970, 969f, 970f, 970t
  intravenous TPA, 969b, 970-971
Acute labyrinthitis, **571**

Respiratory syncytial virus *(Continued)*
  physical findings and clinical presentation of, 797
  predominant age of, 797
  prophylaxis, 1413t
Respiratory syncytial virus (RSV) screen, 1384
Respiratory tract infection, acute, 1145
Restless legs syndrome, **883**
  diagnostic criteria, 883t
Restlessness, 669t
Restrictive cardiomyopathy, **195-196**
  caused by amyloidosis, 195, 195f
  constrictive pericarditis, differentiated from, 196t
Restrictive eye movement. *See* Strabismus.
Resveratrol, for blepharitis, 159
Reticulocyte count, 1384
Reticuloendotheliosis, leukemic, **591,** 591f
Retinal angioma, 1085
Retinal artery occlusion, 1203
Retinal detachment, **884,** 884f
  differential diagnosis, 1203
Retinal hemorrhage, **885,** 885f
Retinal pigment epithelium, congenital hypertrophy
  of, 398
Retinal trauma, **885,** 885f
Retinal vein occlusion, 1203
Retinitis, CMV, 282
Retinitis pigmentosa, **886,** 886f
Retinoblastoma, **887**
Retinocerebellar angiomatosis, **1084-1085**
Retinoic acid, 593
Retinoids, topical
  for oral hairy leukoplakia, 592
  for oral lichen planus, 593
Retinopathy
  diabetic, 301, **888,** 888f
  high-altitude, **885,** 885f
  hypertensive, 1190
Retrobulbar neuritis. *See* Optic neuritis.
Retrograde ejaculation, 335
Retropatellar pain syndrome, **752**
Retropharyngeal abscess, **889-890,** 889f, 890f
Revascularization
  for angina pectoris, 72
  for renal artery stenosis, 873
Reversible sideroblastic anemias, **67**
Rewarming
  active core, 531
  active external, 531
Reye's syndrome, **891**
  clinical staging of, 891t
Rh immune globulin, for spontaneous miscarriage, 958
Rh incompatibility, **892**
Rh isoimmunization, **892**
Rhabdomyolysis, **893,** 893f
Rheumatic carditis, **894**
Rheumatic diseases, of childhood, 1122
Rheumatic fever, **894**
Rheumatism
  nonarticular. *See* Fibromyalgia.
  palindromic, 1178
  psychogenic. *See* Fibromyalgia.
Rheumatoid arthritis, **895-896,** 895f
  eye lesions, 1121
  Felty's syndrome, **378**
  juvenile, eye lesions, 1121
  selective disease-modifying antirheumatic drugs,
    896t
  seropositive, 895, 895f
Rheumatoid factor, 1384
Rhinitis, 1191
Rhinitis, allergic, **897**
Rhinorrhea, 1315f
Rhizopus infection, 659
Rhizotomy, selective dorsal, for cerebral palsy, 208
Rhythm method (natural family planning), 259
Rib defects on x-ray, 1191
Rib notching on x-ray, 1191

Ribavirin
  for hepatitis C, 462
  for respiratory syncytial virus, 882
  for viral pneumonia, 798
  for West Nile virus infection, 1100
Ribavirin aerosol, for RSV pneumonia, 798
Ribs, bone resorption at inferior aspect of, 1128
RICE (rest, ice, compression, elevation), 77
Rickets, **898**
  vitamin D-resistant, 898
  X-linked hypophosphatemic, 898, 898f
Rickettsia rickettsii infection, **899**
  differential diagnosis of, 1145
Rickettsial infections, in returning travelers and im-
    migrants, 1145
Riedel's thyroiditis, 1016
Rifampin
  for bacterial meningitis, 633t
  for brucellosis, 175
  for cirrhosis, primary biliary, 240
  for endocarditis, 347
  for human granulocytic ehrlichiosis, 491
  for leprosy, 581
  for miliary tuberculosis, 1045
  for pulmonary tuberculosis, 1048
  for Q fever, 863
Rifamycin, for hepatic encephalopathy, 455
RIG. *See* Rabies immunoglobulin.
Right arm, focal dystonia of, 329, 329f
Right axis deviation, 1191
Right subclavian steal, 980
Right ventricular failure, 1203
Right ventricular hypertrophy, 1003-1004
Rigidity, 746
Rimantadine
  for avian influenza, 549
  for influenza, 549
    avian influenza, 549
  for viral pneumonia, 798
Ringworm, **1021,** 1021f. *See also* Tinea corporis.
  of nails. *See* Onychomycosis.
  of the scalp, **1018-1019**
Ringworm of the nails, **710-711,** 710f
Risedronate, for osteoporosis, 726
Risk reduction in patients undergoing invasive proce-
    dures, **825-826**
Risperidone
  for autistic disorder, 129
  for autistic spectrum disorders, 129
  for bipolar disorder, 146-147
  for delirium, 288
  for schizophrenia, 912
  for Tourette's syndrome, 1026
Ritalin. *See* Methylphenidate (Ritalin).
Rituximab
  for antiphospholipid antibody syndrome, 88
  for immune thrombocytopenic purpura, 538
  for leukemia, chronic lymphocytic, 589
  for pemphigus vulgaris, 765
  for Waldenström's macroglobulinemia, 1094
Rivastigmine (Exelon)
  for Alzheimer's disease, 47t
  for cognitive impairment, mild, 646t
  for dementia with Lewy bodies, 290
Rizatriptan, for migraine headaches, 430t
Rocky Mountain spotted fever, **899**
  common history, signs, or symptoms of, 899t
  differential diagnosis of, 1144, 1199
  fatality rate, 899
  fulminant, 899
  rash associated with, 1145
Rocky Mountain wood tick, 1199
Romano-Ward syndrome, 596
Romiplostim, for immune thrombocytopenic purpura,
    538
Ropinirole (Requip), 747
  for restless legs syndrome, 883

Rosacea, **900**
Roseola, **901**
Roseola exanthem, 1143
Roseola infantum, **901**
Rosiglitazone, for diabetes mellitus, 303
Rotator cuff syndrome, **902,** 902f
Rotavirus serology, 1384
Rotavirus vaccine
  contraindications and precautions, 1414-1416t
  dose and route of administration, 1417t
  recommended ages and intervals between doses,
    1410t
  recommended childhood/adolescent immunization
    schedule, 1405t, 1406t
Round worms, **102**
RSD, **252**
RSV, **882**
RTA, **880,** 880t
Rubella (German measles), **903**
  acquired, 903
  congenital, 903, 1170
  differential diagnosis of, 1145
  immunization, 903. *See also* Measles, mumps, ru-
    bella vaccine.
Rubeola, **624,** 624f. *See also* Measles (Rubeola).
Rubinstein-Taybi syndrome, 1170
"Rule of nines," 184f
Runner's knee, **752**
Russula intoxication, 669
RVA, for rabies, 864
RVH. *See* Renovascular hypertension.

S

S. haematobium, 911
S. intercalatum, 911
S. japonicum, 911
S. mansoni, 911
S. mekongi, 911
Sacral cervicopexy, 763
SAD, **947**
Salicylate
  for hypertrophic osteoarthropathy, 521
  for trichinosis muscle-related discomfort,
    1034
Salicylic acid (Duofilm, Mediplast, Occlusal-HP)
  for molluscum contagiosum, 655
  for psoriasis, 845
  for warts, 1095
Saline, for electromechanical dissociation, 857
Salivary calculus, **935,** 935f
Salivary gland stone, **935,** 935f
Salivary glands, 934
  enlargement, 1191
  infections, 1173
  neoplasms, **904**
  secretion, decreased, 1191
Salmon calcitonin, synthetic, 726
Salmonella
  food poisoning, 391
  gastroenteritis, 391
Salmonella typhi, 905, 905f
  invasion, 1055
Salmonellosis, **905-906**
Salpingectomy, 332
Salpingitis, 760-761
Salpingostomy, 332
Salt. *See also* Sodium.
  high-salt diet, 1384t
  low-salt diet, 1384t
San Joaquin Valley fever. *See* Coccidioidomycosis.
Sand worm eruption. *See* Cutaneous larva migrans.
Sandimmune. *See* Cyclosporin.
Saquinavir-ritonavir, for AIDS/HIV, 494
Sarcoidosis, **907-908**
  cardiomyopathy, restrictive, 195
  corticosteroids for, 907, 908t

Meningioma I
Meningomyelocele I
Mental status changes and coma II
Mild cognitive impairment I
Mononeuropathies, isolated II
Motion sickness I
Multiple sclerosis I
Muscle disease II
Muscle weakness, algorithm III
Muscular dystrophy I
Myasthenia gravis I
Myelin disorders II
Myoclonus I
Myopathies, idiopathic inflammatory I
Myotonia I
Narcolepsy I
Neuroblastoma I
Neuromuscular junction dysfunction II
Neuronopathies, sensory (ganglionopathies) II
Neuropathic bladder II
Neuropathic pain I
Neuropathies, peripheral, asymmetrical
 proximal/distal II
Neuropathies with facial nerve involvement II
Neuropathy, hereditary I
Nystagmus, monocular II
Opsoclonus II
Optic atrophy II
Optic neuritis I
Osteosclerosis, diffuse II
Otosclerosis (otospongiosis) I
Paraneoplastic neurologic syndromes II
Paraparesis, acute or subacute II
Paraparesis, chronic progressive II
Parkinsonism-plus syndromes II
Parkinson's disease I
Poliomyelitis I
Polyneuropathies, demyelinating II
Polyneuropathies, distal, sensorimotor II
Postconcussive syndrome I
Postpoliomyelitis syndrome I
Progressive supranuclear palsy I
Ramsay Hunt syndrome I
Reflex sympathetic dystrophy I
Restless legs syndrome I
Seizures, absence I
Seizures, febrile I
Seizures, generalized onset I
Seizures, mimics II
Seizures, partial onset I
Smell disturbance II
Spacticity I
Spina bifida I
Spinal cord compression I
Spinal cord compression, epidural II
Spinal cord dysfunction, non-traumatic II
Spinal cord ischemic syndromes II
Spinal stenosis I
Spinocerebellar ataxia I
Sports-related concussion I
Status epilepticus I
Stroke, acute ischemic I
Stroke, hemorrhagic I
Stroke, secondary prevention I
Subarachnoid hemorrhage I
Subclavian steal syndrome I
Subdural hematoma I
Syncope I
Syringomyelia I
Tabes dorsalis I
Tardive dyskinesia I
Tics II
Tinnitus I
Transient ischemic attack I
Tremors II
Trigeminal neuralgia I
Tuberous sclerosis I
Unconscious patient III
Vegetative state, persistent II
Vertigo, algorithm III
Vestibular neuronitis I
Weakness, neuromuscular III
Wernicke's encephalopathy I
Whiplash I
Wilson's disease I

OPHTHALMOLOGY
Amaurosis fugax I
Amblyopia I
Anisocoria III
Blepharitis I
Blindness, monocular, transient II
Cataracts I
Conjunctival neoplasm II
Conjunctivitis I
Corneal abrasion I
Corneal disorders III

Corneal sensation, decreased II
Corneal ulceration I
Cytomegalovirus infection I
Dilated pupil III
Diplopia, monocular II
Diplopia, vertical II
Episcleritis I
Esotropia II
Eyelid neoplasm II
Eyelid retraction II
Glaucoma, primary angle-closure I
Hordeolum (stye) I
Horner's syndrome I
Intraocular neoplasm II
Keratitis, noninfectious II
Macular degeneration I
Nystagmus, diagnosis III
Nystagmus, monocular II
Ocular foreign body I
Opsoclonus II
Optic atrophy I, II
Optic neuritis I
Orbital lesions, calcified II
Orbital lesions, cystic II
Primary open-angle glaucoma I
Pupillary dilatation, poor response to darkness II
Ramsay Hunt syndrome I
Red eye, acute III
Reiter's syndrome (reactive arthritis) I
Retinal detachment I
Retinal hemorrhage I
Retinitis pigmentosa I
Retinoblastoma I
Retinopathy, diabetic I
Retinopathy, hypertensive II
Scleritis I
Sjögren's syndrome I
Strabismus I
Tuberous sclerosis I
Uveitis I
Von Hippel-Lindau disease I
Wilson's disease I

ORTHOPEDICS
Achilles tendon rupture I
Ankle fracture I
Ankle sprain I
Ankylosing spondylitis I
Arthralgia limited to one or few joints III
Arthritis, granulomatous I
Arthritis, infectious I
Arthritis, psoriatic I
Aseptic necrosis I
Back pain, algorithm III
Back pain, low, acute II
Back pain, viscerogenic origin II
Baker's cyst I
Biceps tendonitis I
Bone tumor, primary malignant I
Bursitis I
Carpal tunnel syndrome I
Cervical disk syndromes I
Charcot's joint I
Costochondritis I
Cubital tunnel syndrome I
De Quervain's tenosynovitis I
Dupuytren's contracture I
Elbow pain II
Epicondylitis I
Femoral neck fracture (hip fracture) I
Fibromyalgia I
Foot and ankle pain, in different age groups II
Footdrop II
Foot lesion, ulcerating II
Fracture, bone III
Frozen shoulder I
Ganglia I
Glenohumeral dislocation I
Gout I
Heel pain II
Hip pain, in different age groups II
Hip pain without obvious fracture II
Hypertrophic osteoarthropathy I
Inflammatory arthritis III
Juvenile idiopathic arthritis I
Knee pain, anterior III
Knee pain, in different age groups II
Legg-Calvé-Perthes disease I
Lumbar disk syndrome I
Metatarsalgia I
Morton's neuroma I
Muscle cramps and aches III
Muscle weakness, algorithm III
Osgood-Schlatter disease I
Osteoarthritis I
Osteochondritis dissecans I
Osteomyelitis I

Osteoporosis I
Osteoporosis, secondary causes II
Paget's disease of the bone I
Patellofemoral pain syndrome I
Plantar fasciitis I
Pronator syndrome I
Pseudogout I
Reflex sympathetic dystrophy I
Rheumatoid arthritis I
Rib defects on x-ray II
Rib notching on x-ray II
Rotator cuff syndrome I
Scoliosis I
Shin splints III
Shoulder pain III
Shoulder pain, in different age groups II
Spinal cord compression I
Spinal cord compression, epidural II
Spinal stenosis, lumbar I
Spine tumor III
Spondyloarthropathy, diagnosis III
Spondyloarthropathy, treatment III
Spondylosis, cervical III
Sports-related concussion I
Tarsal tunnel syndrome I
Temporomandibular joint syndrome I
Thoracic outlet syndrome I
Torticollis I
Trigger finger I
Trochanteric bursitis I
Vertebral compression fractures I
Whiplash I
Wrist and hand pain, in different age groups II
Wrist pain II

OTORHINOLARYNGOLOGY (ENT)
Acoustic neuroma I
Allergic rhinitis I
Behçet's disease I
Bruxism I
Burning mouth syndrome I
Dysphagia III
Epiglottitis I
Epistaxis I
Gingivitis I
Glossitis I
Goiter evaluation and management III
Head and neck, soft tissue masses II
Hearing loss III
Hemoptysis, algorithm III
Herpangina I
Labyrinthitis I
Laryngeal carcinoma I
Laryngitis I
Mastoiditis I
Meniere's disease I
Mononucleosis I
Motion sickness I
Mucormycosis I
Mumps I
Otitis externa I
Otitis media I
Otosclerosis (otospongiosis) I
Peritonsillar abscess I
Pharyngitis/tonsillitis I
Rhinorrhea III
Salivary gland neoplasms I
Sialadenitis I
Sialolithiasis I
Sinusitis I
Sleep apnea, obstructive I
Smell disturbance I
Stomatitis I
Temporomandibular joint syndrome I
Thyroid carcinoma I
Thyroid nodule I
Thyroid, painful III
Thyroiditis I
Tinnitus I
Torticollis I
Tracheitis I
Vertigo, algorithm III

PEDIATRICS
Abuse, child I
Anemia in newborn III
Appendicitis, acute I
Asthma I
Ataxia, cerebellar, children II
Attention deficit hyperactivity disorder I
Autistic spectrum disorders I
Bleeding neonate III
Bone marrow failure syndromes, inherited II
Breastfeeding difficulties III
Bruxism I
Childhood and adolescent immunizations V
Colic, acute abdominal II